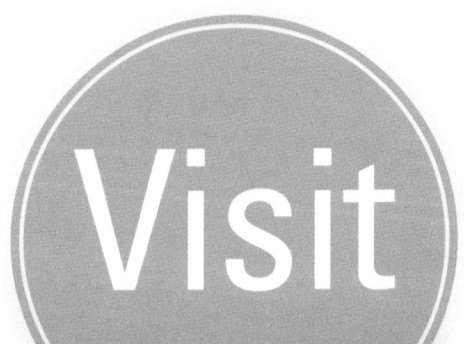
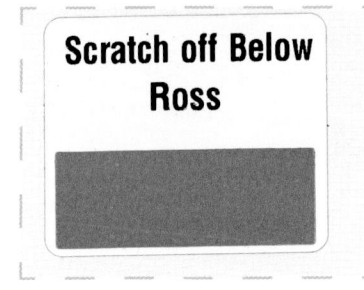
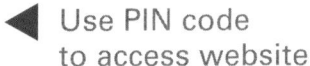
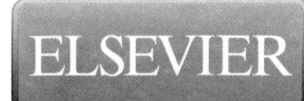

DIAGNOSIS AND MANAGEMENT OF

Lameness
IN THE Horse

DIAGNOSIS AND MANAGEMENT OF
Lameness
IN THE Horse

SECOND EDITION

Mike W. Ross, DVM, Dipl ACVS
Professor of Surgery
Department of Clinical Studies
University of Pennsylvania School of Veterinary Medicine
New Bolton Center
Kennett Square, Pennsylvania, United States

Sue J. Dyson, MA, VetMB, PhD, DEO, FRCVS
Head of Clinical Orthopaedics
Centre for Equine Studies
Animal Health Trust
Newmarket
Suffolk, England

ELSEVIER
SAUNDERS

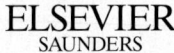

3251 Riverport Lane
St. Louis, Missouri 63043

Notices

Knowledge and best practice in this field are constantly changing. As new research and experience broaden our understanding, changes in research methods, professional practices, or medical treatment may become necessary.

Practitioners and researchers must always rely on their own experience and knowledge in evaluating and using any information, methods, compounds, or experiments described herein. In using such information or methods they should be mindful of their own safety and the safety of others, including parties for whom they have a professional responsibility.

With respect to any drug or pharmaceutical products identified, readers are advised to check the most current information provided (i) on procedures featured or (ii) by the manufacturer of each product to be administered, to verify the recommended dose or formula, the method and duration of administration, and contraindications. It is the responsibility of practitioners, relying on their own experience and knowledge of their patients, to make diagnoses, to determine dosages and the best treatment for each individual patient, and to take all appropriate safety precautions.

To the fullest extent of the law, neither the Publisher nor the authors, contributors, or editors, assume any liability for any injury and/or damage to persons or property as a matter of products liability, negligence or otherwise, or from any use or operation of any methods, products, instructions, or ideas contained in the material herein.

Library of Congress Cataloging-in-Publication Data

Diagnosis and management of lameness in the horse / [edited by] Mike W. Ross, Sue J. Dyson. – 2nd ed.
     p. ; cm.
  Includes bibliographical references and index.
  ISBN 978-1-4160-6069-7 (hardcover : alk. paper) 1. Lameness in horses. I. Ross, Mike W. II. Dyson, Sue J.
  [DNLM: 1. Horse Diseases. 2. Lameness, Animal. 3. Horses–injuries. SF 959.L25]
  SF959.L25R67 2011
  636.1'089758–dc22

                                               2010035776

Publishing Director: Linda Duncan
Acquisitions Editor: Penny Rudolph
Associate Developmental Editor: Lauren Harms
Publishing Services Manager: Catherine Jackson
Senior Project Manager: David Stein
Design Direction: Karen Pauls
Cover Art: Fabio Torre

Working together to grow
libraries in developing countries

www.elsevier.com | www.bookaid.org | www.sabre.org

ELSEVIER   BOOK AID International   Sabre Foundation

Printed in the United States

Last digit is the print number: 9 8 7 6 5 4 3 2 1

Contributors

Rick M. Arthur, DVM
Equine Medical Director
School of Veterinary Medicine
University of California, Davis
Davis, California

Greg Baldwin, BSc, BVSc
Australian Equine Laminitis Research Unit
School of Veterinary Science
The University of Queensland
Queensland, Australia

Lance H. Bassage II, VMD, DACVS
Staff Surgeon
Rhinebeck Equine, LLP
Rhinebeck, New York

Andrew P. Bathe, MA, VetMB, DEO, DECVS, MRCVS
Partner, Head of Equine Sports Injuries Clinic
Rossdale Diagnostic Centre
Rossdale and Partners
Newmarket, Suffolk, United Kingdom

Jill Beech, VMD, DACVIM
Georgia E. and Philip B. Hofmann Professor of Medicine and
    Reproduction
Department of Clinical Studies
University of Pennsylvania
New Bolton Center
Kennett Square, Pennsylvania

Scott D. Bennett, DVM
Equine Services Clinic
Simpsonville, Kentucky

Philippe H. Benoit, DVM, MS
Clinique Equine
Les Breviaires, France

William V. Bernard, DVM, DACVIM
Owner/Manager
Lexington Equine Surgery
Lexington, Kentucky

Alicia L. Bertone, DVM, PhD, DACVS
Trueman Family Endowed Chair and Professor
Veterinary Clinical Sciences
The Ohio State University
Columbus, Ohio

Jerry B. Black, DVM
Director of Undergraduate Programs
Equine Sciences
Colorado State University
Fort Collins, Colorado

James T. Blackford, DVM, MS, DACVS
Professor of Large Animal Surgery
Large Animal Clinical Sciences
University of Tennessee
College of Veterinary Medicine
Knoxville, Tennessee

Jeff A. Blea, DVM
President
Southern California Equine Foundation
Arcadia, California
Partner
Von bluecher, Blea, Hunkin, Inc.
Sierra Madre, California

Jane C. Boswell, MA, VetMB, Cert VA, Cert ES(Orth), DECVS, MRCVS
Partner
The Liphook Equine Hospital
Liphook, Hampshire
United Kingdom

Robert P. Boswell, DVM
Equine Sports Medicine and Diagnostic Imaging
Wellington, Florida

Robert M. Bowker, VMD, PhD
Professor
College of Veterinary Medicine
Michigan State University
East Lansing, Michigan

Julia Brooks, DO, MSc
Haywards Heath and Burgess Hill Osteopathic Practices
West Sussex, United Kingdom

Herbert J. Burns, VMD
Pine Bush Equine
Pine Bush, New York

John P. Caron, DVM
Professor, Equine Surgery
Large Animal Clinical Sciences
Michigan State University
East Lansing, Michigan

G. Kent Carter, DVM, DACVIM
Professor
College of Veterinary Medicine
Texas A & M University
College Station, Texas

Eddy R.J. Cauvin, DVM, MVM, PhD, HDR, CertVetRad, DECVS
Azurvet
Hippodrome de la Côte d'Azur
Cagnes-Sur-Mer, France

Mark W. Cheney, DVM
Veterinary Practice
Lexington, Kentucky

Jennifer M. Cohen, VMD, DACVS
Associate Veterinarian
Manor Equine Hospital
Monkton, Maryland

Chris Colles, BVetMed, PhD, HonFWCF, MRCVS
Director
Avonvale Veterinary Practice
Banbury, United Kingdom

Simon N. Collins, PhD, BSc (Hons)
Australian Equine Laminitis Research Unit (AELRU)
School of Veterinary Science
The University of Queensland
Gatton, Queensland
Australia
Orthopaedic Research Consultant
Centre for Equine Studies
Animal Health Trust
Newmarket, United Kingdom

Robin M. Dabareiner, DVM, PhD, DACVS
Associate Professor of Lameness
Texas A & M University
Large Animal Clinical Sciences
College Station, Texas

Robert Andrew Dalglish, BVM&S, MRCVS
Senior Veterinarian
Veterinary Department
Al Wathba Stables
Abu Dhabi, United Arab Emirates

Elizabeth J. Davidson, DVM, DACVS
Assistant Professor of Sports Medicine
Department of Clinical Studies
University of Pennsylvania
Kennett Square, Pennsylvania

Jean-Marie Denoix, DVM, PhD, Agrégé
Professor
Director CIRALE–Ecole Vétérinaire d'Alfort
Goustranville, France

Stephen P. Dey III, VMD
Dey Equine Veterinarians
Allentown, New Jersey

Janet Douglas, MA, Vet MB, MSc, PhD, MRCVS
Special Lecturer in Equine Orthopaedics
School of Veterinary Medicine and Science
University of Nottingham
Sutton Bonington, Nottinghamshire, England

Matthew Durham, DVM
Associate Veterinarian
Steinbeck Country Equine Clinic
Salinas, California

David R. Ellis, BvetMed, DEO, FRCVS
Newmarket Equine Hospital
Newmarket
Suffolk, United Kingdom

Kristiina Ertola
Tempereen Hevosklinikka
Tampere Equine Clinic
Ravirata
Tampere, Finland

Franco Ferrero, Med. Vet. Specialista in Patologia Equina
Pontirolo Nuovo, Italy

Lisa Fortier, DVM, PhD
Associate Professor of Surgery
Clinical Sciences
Cornell University
Ithaca, New York

David D. Frisbie, DVM, PhD, DACVS
Associate Professor
Department of Clinical Sciences
Colorado State University
Equine Orthopaedic Research Center
Fort Collins, Colorado

José M. García-López, VMD, DACVS
Assistant Professor of Surgery
Large Animal Surgery
Department of Clinical Sciences
Tufts University
Cummings School of Veterinary Medicine
North Grafton, Massachusetts

Ronald L. Genovese, VMD
Cleveland Equine Clinic, LLC
Ravenna, Ohio

Howard E. Gill, DVM
Pine Bush, New York

Dallas O. Goble, DVM
Strawberry Plains, Tennessee

Nancy L. Goodman, DVM
Loveland, Colorado

Barrie D. Grant, DVM
San Luis Rey Equine Hospital
Bonsall, California

Kevin K. Haussler, DVM, DC, PhD, DACVSMR
Assistant Professor
Department of Clinical Sciences
Colorado State University
Fort Collins, Colorado

Dan L. Hawkins, DVM, MS, DACVS
Gainesville, Florida

W. Theodore Hill, VMD
Racing Steward
The Jockey Club
New York Racing Association
Jamaica, New York

Jukka Houttu, DVM
Tempereen Hevosklinikka
Tampere Equine Clinic
Ravirata
Tampere, Finland

Robert J. Hunt, DVM, MS, DACVS
Surgeon
Davidson Surgery Center
Hagyard Equine Medical Institute
Lexington, Kentucky

Kjerstin M. Jacobs, DVM
Private Practice
Chicago, Illinois

Joan S. Jorgensen, DVM, PhD, DACVIM
Assistant Professor
Department of Comparative Biosciences
University of Wisconsin
Madison, Wisconsin

Chris E. Kawcak, DVM, PhD, DACVS
Associate Professor
Equine Orthopaedic Research Center
Department of Clinical Sciences
Colorado State University
Fort Collins, Colorado

Kevin P. Keane, DVM
Member
Sports Medicine Associates of Chester County
Kennett Square, Pennsylvania

Kevin G. Keegan, DVM, MS, DACVS
Professor and Director
E. Paige Laurie Endowed Program in Equine Lameness
Department of Veterinary Medicine and Surgery
University of Missouri
College of Veterinary Medicine
Columbia, Missouri

John C. Kimmel, VMD
Tequesta, Florida

Simon Knapp, BVetMed, MRCVS
Straight Mile Farm
Billingbear
Wokingham
Berkshire, United Kingdom

Svend E. Kold, DrMedVet, CUEW, RFP, MRCVS
RCVS Specialist in Equine Surgery (Orthopaedics)
Senior Consultant to B&W Equine Group
Willesley Equine Clinic
Tetbury, Gloucestershire, England

John Maas, DVM, MS, DACVIM
Veterinarian/Specialist in Cooperative Extension
Veterinary Medicine Extension
School of Veterinary Medicine
University of California, Davis
Davis, California

Benson B. Martin Jr., VMD, DACVS
Associate Professor of Sports Medicine
Dept. of Clinical Studies
University of Pennsylvania
New Bolton Center
Kennett Square, Pennsylvania

Scott R. McClure, DVM, PhD, DACVS
Associate Professor
Veterinary Clinical Sciences
Iowa State University
Ames, Iowa

William H. McCormick, VMD, FAAVA
President, CEO
Middleburg Equine Clinic, Inc.
Middleburg, Virginia

Andrew M. McDiarmid, BVM&S, Cert ES(Orth), MRCVS
Partner
Clyde Vet Group Equine Hospital
Lanark, Scotland, United Kingdom

Sue M. McDonnell, PhD
University of Pennsylvania School of Veterinary Medicine
New Bolton Center
Kennett Square, Pennsylvania

C. Wayne McIlwraith, BVSc, PhD, DSc, Dr. med. vet. (hc), DSc (hc) FRCVS, DACVS
University Distinguished Professor
Barbara Cox Anthony University Chair in Orthopedics
Director of Orthopaedic Research Center
Colorado State University
Fort Collins, Colorado

P.J. McMahon, MVB, MRCVS
Kings Park
Plaistow
Billingshurst
West Sussex, United Kingdom

Rose M. McMurphy, DVM, DACVA, ACVECC
Professor
Department of Clinical Sciences
Kansas State University
College of Veterinary Medicine
Manhattan, Kansas

Christopher (Kit) B. Miller
Miller & Associates
North Salem, New York

Martha M. Misheff, DVM
Associate Veterinarian
Dubai Equine Hospital
Dubai, United Arab Emirates

James B. Mitchell, DVM
John R. Steele & Associates Inc.
Vernon, New York

John S. Mitchell, DVM
Pompano Beach, Florida

Richard D. Mitchell, DVM
President
Fairfield Equine Associates, P.C.
Newtown, Connecticut

Patrick J. Moloney, DVM
Stuart, Florida

William A. Moyer, DVM
Texas A & M University
College of Veterinary Medicine
Large Animal Medicine & Surgery
College Station, Texas

Graham Munroe, BVSc, PhD, DECVS, CertEO, DESM, FRCVS
Flanders Veterinary Services
Greenlaw
Duns
Berwickshire, United Kingdom

Rachel C. Murray, MA, VetMB, MS, PhD, DACVS, MRCVS
Senior Orthopaedic Advisor
Centre for Equine Studies
Animal Health Trust
Newmarket
Suffolk, United Kingdom

Alastair Nelson, MA VetMB CertVR CertESM MRCVS[†]
Rainbow Equine Clinic
Rainbow Farm
Old Malton
Malton
North Yorkshire, United Kingdom

Frank A. Nickels, DVM, MS, DACVS
Professor
Large Animal Clinical Sciences
College of Veterinary Medicine
Michigan State University
East Lansing, Michigan

Paul M. Nolan, DVM
Equine Sports Medicine
Boca Raton, Florida

David M. Nunamaker, VMD
Jacques Jenny Professor Emeritus of Orthopedic Surgery
Department of Clinical Studies
University of Pennsylvania School of Veterinary Medicine
New Bolton Center
Kennett Square, Pennsylvania

Timothy R. Ober, DVM
Associate Veterinarian
John R. Steele & Associates
Vernon, New York

[†]Deceased.

Thomas P.S. Oliver, DVM
Equine Sports Medicine
Lahaska, Pennsylvania

Gene Ovnicek, RMF
President, Chief Technician
Equine Digit Support System, Inc.
Penrose, Colorado

Joe D. Pagan, PhD
President
Kentucky Equine Research, Inc.
Versailles, Kentucky

Eric J. Parente, DVM, DACVS
Associate Professor of Surgery
University of Pennsylvania
New Bolton Center
Kennett Square, Pennsylvania

**Tim D.H. Parkin, BSc, BVSc, PhD, DECVPH
(Population Medicine), MRCVS**
Boyd Orr Centre for Population and Ecosystem Health
Institute of Comparative Medicine
Faculty of Veterinary Medicine
University of Glasgow
Glasgow, United Kingdom

Andrew H. Parks, VetMB, MRCVS, DACVS
Professor of Large Animal Surgery
Department of Large Animal Medicine
College of Veterinary Medicine
University of Georgia
Athens, Georgia

**Richard J. Piercy, MA, VetMB, MS, PhD, DACVIM,
MRCVS**
Senior Lecturer in Equine Medicine and Neurology
Veterinary Clinical Sciences
Royal Veterinary College
London, United Kingdom

Robert C. Pilsworth, MA, VetMB, BSc, CertVR, MRCVS
Associate
Newmarket Equine Hospital
Newmarket
Suffolk, United Kingdom
Associate Lecturer
Equine Hospital
The Queen's School of Veterinary Medicine
Cambridge
Cambridgeshire, United Kingdom

Christopher C. Pollitt, BVSc, PhD
Honorary Professor of Equine Medicine
School of Veterinary Science
The University of Queensland
Gatton Campus, Australia

Joanna Price, BSc, BVSc, PhD, MRCVS
School of Veterinary Science
University of Bristol
Langford
Bristol, United Kingdom

Sarah M. Puchalski, DVM, DACVR
Assistant Professor of Diagnostic Imaging
Department of Surgical and Radiological Sciences
University of California, Davis
Davis, California

Norman W. Rantanen, DVM, MS, DACVR
Fallbrook, California

Virginia B. Reef, DVM, ACVIM (LAIM)
Mark Whittier & Lila Griswold Allam Professor of Medicine
Chief Section of Sports Medicine and Imaging
Department of Clinical Studies
New Bolton Center
University of Pennsylvania
Kennett Square, Pennsylvania

Patrick T. Reilly
Chief of Farrier Service
Applied Polymer Research Laboratory
University of Pennsylvania School of Veterinary Medicine
New Bolton Center
Kennett Square, Pennsylvania

Dean W. Richardson, DVM, DACVS
Charles W. Raker Professor of Surgery
University of Pennsylvania School of Veterinary Medicine
New Bolton Center
Kennett Square, Pennsylvania

Mark C. Rick, DVM
Alamo Pintado Equine Medical Center, Inc.
Los Olivos, California

Bradley S. Root, DVM
Albuquerque Equine Clinic
Albuquerque, New Mexico

Alan J. Ruggles, DVM, DACVS
Partner, Staff Surgeon
Department of Surgery
Rood and Riddle Equine Hospital
Lexington, Kentucky

Allen M. Schoen, MS, DVM
Allen M. Schoen, DVM & Associates, LLC
Sherman, Connecticut
Director/Founder
Veterinary Institute for Therapeutic Alternatives (VITA)
Sherman, Connecticut

Michael C. Schramme, DVM, CertEO, DECVS, PhD
Associate Professor, Equine Surgery
Department of Clinical Sciences
North Carolina State University
Raleigh, North Carolina

**Robert Sigafoos, CJF/Farrier Program/Planning
Committee**
Kennett Square, Pennsylvania

**Roger K.W. Smith, MA, VetMB, PhD, DEO, DECVS,
MRCVS**
Professor of Equine Orthopaedics
Veterinary Clinical Sciences
The Royal Veterinary College
London, United Kingdom

Van E. Snow, DVM†
Santa Ynez, California

Sharon J. Spier, DVM, PhD, Dipl ACVIM
Professor
Department of Medicine and Epidemiology
School of Veterinary Medicine
University of California
Davis, California

Vivian S. Stacy, CNMT
Widener Hospital
School of Veterinary Medicine
University of Pennsylvania
Kennett Square, Pennsylvania

James C. Sternberg, DVM
Powell Animal Hospital
Powell, Tennessee

Anthony Stirk
Stirk & Associates Ltd.
North Yorkshire, United Kingdom

Amanda Sutton, MSc Vet Phys.
Chartered Physiotherapist
Clinical Director
Suttons Animal Physiotherapy
Winchester
Hampshire, United Kingdom

Alain P. Théon, DVM, MS, DACVR-RO
Professor
Department of Surgery and Radiology
Oncology Service Chief
Veterinary Medical Teaching Hospital
School of Veterinary Medicine
University of California, Davis
Davis, California

Fabio Torre, DVM, DECVS, DAMS
Director
Clinica Equina Bagnarola
Bagnarola, Bologna, Italy

Stephanie J. Valberg, DVM, PhD, DACVIM
Professor
Veterinary Population Medicine
University of Minnesota
College of Veterinary Medicine
St. Paul, Minnesota

Robert Joseph Van Pelt, BVSc, BSc, CertEP, MRCVS
Partner
The Arundel Equine Hospital
Arundel
West Sussex, England

John P. Walmsley, MA, VetMB, Cert EO, DECVS, HonFRCVS
The Liphook Equine Hospital
Forest Mere, Liphook
Hants, United Kingdom

Tim Watson, PhD, BSc, MCSP
Professor of Physiotherapy
School of Health and Emergency Professions
University of Hertfordshire
Hertfordshire, United Kingdom

Renate Weller DMV, PhD, MRCVS, FHEA
Senior Lecturer in Veterinary Diagnostic Imaging
Veterinary Clinical Sciences
The Royal Veterinary College
Hatfield, Hertfordshire, United Kingdom

R. Chris Whitton, BVSc, FACVSc, PhD
Associate Professor
Equine Centre
University of Melbourne
Werribee, Victoria, Australia

Jeffrey A. Williams, DVM
Rhinebeck Equine LLP
Rhinebeck, New York

Alan Wilson, BVSc, BVMS, PhD, MRCVS
Professor
Structure and Motion Laboratory
Royal Veterinary College
North Mymms, United Kingdom

Paul Wollenman, DVM
Palm Beach Equine Clinic, LLC
Wellington, Florida

James Wood, BSc, BVetMed, MSc, MA, PhD, DipECVPH, DLSHTM
Professor of Equine and Farm Animal Science
Department of Veterinary Medicine
University of Cambridge
Cambridge, United Kingdom

Foreword

My first employer, the late Gordon Carter, and a man of real wisdom, once said to me: "You won't know the meaning of 'experience' as a clinician until you have been in practice for 20 years, and then you will realise you don't have any." At the time I had no idea what he was talking about. I know now.

The longer one is in practice, the less dogmatic and certain one often becomes. Horses accumulate, which just will not fit neatly into their diagnostic buckets. Prognoses, which were once certain fact, become turned on their heads by the horse that defies the clinician's worst predictions, and comes back from injury against all the odds. Nerve blocks seem increasingly to eliminate pain from regions that were not their target, or do not abolish pain from areas that were. Radiography repeatedly shows no abnormalities in bones when magnetic resonance imaging (MRI) demonstrates gross and marked pathology.

When meeting this plethora of square circles for the first time, the previously available textbooks just made one feel even more hopeless. Nerve blocks were either not needed at all for a diagnosis because a clinician of experience did not NEED to block a horse to know where the problem was. When it WAS employed, diagnostic analgesia eliminated pain in a totally predictable and specific way. All was black and white, clear cut, and specific. This was not the world of equine lameness that I was picking my way through as a novice clinician. Was I simply doing it wrong? Or was it perhaps that there are reasons why biological systems refuse to be pigeon-holed in the neat manner we would like them to be pigeon-holed?

The first edition of *Diagnosis and Management of Lameness in the Horse* was a revelation in that respect. Here were clinicians determined to use a scientific and methodical approach to their horses, but at the same time describing all the many and varied ways that diagnostic tests could mislead. Moreover, here were clinicians who were even admitting to sometimes not making a diagnosis at all.

The feeling of excitement one experienced in realising, as one read succeeding chapters, that other people were groping slowly forward in the same dark tunnel, with the same dim candles as one was oneself, was invigorating. Mike Ross and Sue Dyson redefined the equine lameness textbook in a way that was truly new, breathtaking in its breadth and depth of coverage, and for the first time addressing the fact that horses who perform in the many different disciplines we serve have many different clinical problems. Even horses with the same problems may be managed differently. For the first time each of our specialities was addressed in a clinically relevant manner, often by people at the height of their clinical powers. Although no substitute for experience itself, this massive accumulation of wisdom was put into the public domain, available to novice and expert alike. The very title uses the word "management," acknowledging that although we cannot always expect a total cure with treatment, the horse may be useful or may compete with careful management nonetheless.

Isaac Newton once said "If I have seen a little further than others, it is only because I have stood upon the shoulders of giants." We are in a golden age of equine diagnostic imaging, with ultrasonography, radiography, scintigraphy, computed tomography, and MRI all in frequent clinical use, allowing us to define with greater clarity the damage that produces the pain and therefore lameness in our patients. So who were those giants to whom we collectively owe so much? Many were mentioned in the Foreword to the first edition of this book, and some are omitted here solely through lack of space rather than respect. Ron Genovese and Norman Rantanen set up the field of ultrasonographic examination in the horse for us all to enjoy. In radiography, almost every useful paper in my formative years seemed to have the name Tim O'Brien on it somewhere. He, along with Bill Hornof and other colleagues at the University of Davis, California, United States described the oblique images of the third carpal bone, the flexed image of the distal aspect of the third metacarpal bone, and the "skyline" flexor surface image of the navicular bone, so valuable and yet now taken for granted.

A single issue of *Veterinary Clinics of North America* devoted to Racetrack Practice published in 1990 advanced our knowledge vastly in the field of lameness in this field thanks to all of the authors, but from my own perspective, especially from the work of Roy Pool and Greg Ferraro, masters of their craft. Roy Pool was able to highlight the dramatic role that chronic, daily, repetitive microdamage played in the development of many "spontaneous" fractures. The days of the single misstep as the cause of the majority of fractures were becoming numbered, and even the acute carpal "chip" was shown to be anything but acute in most horses, certainly in terms of aetiology. I was fortunate in my early career to share a month "seeing practice" with Greg Ferraro, Tim O'Brien, and that pantheon of orthopaedics, Larry Bramlage, and that month altered the way I worked for the remainder of my career. There cannot be three people of greater wisdom, clinical skill, and willingness to share that expertise with others on the planet. As an equine orthopaedic surgeon also of great tact and humility (something of an oxymoron), Bramlage has also been a wonderful ambassador to our profession. He, along with Wayne McIlwraith, Dean Richardson, Ian Wright, and David Nunamaker, have added greatly to our knowledge of lameness from a surgical perspective.

Scintigraphy was perhaps the biggest diagnostic leap forward for the racehorse, and has been useful in most other disciplines. This was only because of the dedication and willingness to share openly their knowledge with others by its founding fathers, and their able technicians. These include Gottlieb Ueltschi, Bob Twardock, Mike O' Callaghan, and one of the editors of this book, Mike Ross, all giants indeed, to whom we should be grateful.

In the field of MRI and diagnostic analgesia, the other editor of this book has made an enormous contribution. The name Sue Dyson has become a by-word for elegant, meticulous, probing studies by her and her team at the Animal Health Trust, Newmarket, England, carried out with great scientific integrity, documented in detail and published for all to share. She has made a unique and lasting contribution to studies of equine lameness, and the interlocking problems of the atypical consequences of the use of diagnostic analgesia, without in any way diminishing their importance as the foundation stone of lameness work—in fact, just the reverse. In MRI studies she joins other giants such as Russ Tucker and Rachel Murray who have opened up and explained this fascinating technique to the equine practitioner, and whose insights into the structural damage that leads to pain and consequently lameness have added so much to the various sections of this new edition.

We must not forget the value of thorough clinical examination. The previous generation of lameness clinicians had no recourse to the advanced imaging modalities listed above, but they nevertheless diagnosed and treated horses, many of which returned to a useful life. We can argue that their presumptive diagnoses may have been incorrect in the light of what we know now, but they accumulated experience of which factors worked in restoring a horse with a specific set of clinical signs to soundness. Lameness practice, as pointed out in the first edition, is both an art and a science. The science is often dogma, a "best fit" for the current facts, but the art is a more continuous and constant tradition that many of the contributors to this second edition uphold and in turn pass on. An example of this would be pain which is abolished by both proximal palmar metacarpal (subcarpal) nerve blocks and later also by intraarticular analgesia of the middle carpal joint in a Thoroughbred racehorse. Many of these horses have slight thickening, possibly mild tenderness to palpation of the proximal suspensory ligament, and increased severity of lameness after carpal flexion, but no clinically significant lesion on ultrasonographic examination or radiography. For my generation, MRI is an available option, and in these circumstances one often finds a combination of injuries to the most proximal part of the suspensory ligament or its bone origin, the origin of the accessory ligament of the deep digital flexor tendon, the palmar carpal ligament, the interosseous ligaments between the third

and second and fourth metacarpal bones, or in areas of the third and radial carpal bones simply not visible radiologically. Ray Hopes, my mentor, previous employer, and now good friend, who founded the racing division of the Rossdale practice in Newmarket, England could not have recognised these injuries. Did he diagnose the condition of horses with the blocking history we have outlined? Yes he did. Did he treat these horses and successfully manage their return to training and competition? Very much so. He could not have known the true nature of the lesions. No-one in that era could have done so, but he accumulated enough wisdom and experience to know what one had to do, in terms of rest, therapy, and rehabilitation, to get those horses back to work, a legacy we still employ to the same end point today, possibly for different reasons and with more knowledge now of why it works.

This second edition is not simply a reprint with minor changes to some sections. Every single chapter has been updated, some such as "The Tarsus" and "Navicular Disease" virtually rewritten; such is the avalanche of new knowledge that has come our way in the intervening 8 years. Almost all of the figures have been replaced with better quality digital images that significantly enhance the text. In addition some subjects not previously covered have now been included. Alan Wilson and Renate Weller contribute a new Chapter, "The Biomechanics of the Equine Limb and Its Effect on Lameness." Whilst it may sometimes seem to us that all horses are lame, the majority of course are not. Careful study of biomechanics, particularly in the context of conformation and shoeing, may help us understand why one horse goes lame when its cohort group remains sound under the same exercise regimen.

There are certain seminal textbooks that become so widely known, used, and respected in their field that the title of the book becomes subsumed by the name of the author in the public mind, as succeeding editions are updated and published. Sisson (anatomy), Lehninger (biochemistry), and Roitt (immunology) are books of this type. With this second edition, "Ross and Dyson" is about to join that list. It has become THE textbook on equine lameness. Clinicians certainly do not write textbooks with financial rewards in mind, or if they do, they have been wickedly deceived by their publishers! One has to hope that the knowledge that entire generations of equine practitioners will be enthralled, educated, and engaged by this masterly work will serve as just reward.

Rob Pilsworth
Newmarket, England
January 2010

Second Foreword

The production of veterinary texts addressing lameness in the horse has been very enlightening and, needless to say, a valuable tool to the equine practitioner. It is remarkable that the majority of the veterinary texts have been formulated within the past 50 years. Naturally, this incentive to produce texts has come from the resurgence of the number of horses in the United States. In the late 1920s, the number of horses in the United States was reported to be approximately 27 million. *Dollar's Veterinary Surgery* was a text of note during this period, first being published in 1912; the second edition appeared in 1920, the third in 1937, and the fourth in 1950. In the Preface to the Fourth Edition, JJ O'Connor, MRCVS, who edited the third and fourth editions, made note of the nine additions of new material it contained. The last of the additions was "the examination of horses as to soundness" (approximately 200 pages). This time period is significant because the number of horses in the United States had dramatically dropped to approximately 750,000 by 1957. This precipitous drop in the number of horses prompted a general prediction that if the practice of equine veterinary medicine was not going to completely disappear, it would be a very limited part of veterinary medicine. Consequently, research into equine issues of note was very limited, if at all, and publications of scientific articles relevant to horses were also very limited. Basically no texts were produced after Dollar's fourth edition until the early 1960s; however, in the 1950s a small number of devoted veterinarians, both practitioners and college professors, were diligent in pursuing the cause for the diagnosis and treatment of the lame horse. At the same time, there was a reversal in the decline of the number of horses in the United States. This stimulated more interest in equine veterinary medicine and spawned the resurgence of written material relevant to the lame horse. A reference point to this increase is the fact that the number of horses was reported to be 9.2 million (American Horse Council's DeLoitte Report, June 5, 2005). Concurrently, the American Association of Equine Practitioners (AAEP) was born; this association has served since its inception as a medium to accumulate and disseminate information relevant to the lame horse. It was through the AAEP that I became familiar with the contribution by Dr. Mike Ross and Dr. Sue Dyson.

In the first edition of *Diagnosis and Management of Lameness in the Horse,* in 2003, "Part I: Diagnosis of Lameness," "Section 1: The Lameness Examination," "Chapter 1, Lameness Examination: Historical Perspective," Dr. Mike Ross states "in the mid to late 1900s Adams had the most profound influence by his teachings and writings." He further references O.R. Adams' 1957 "Veterinary Notes on Lameness and Shoeing of Horses" becoming the classic textbook, *Lameness in Horses.* As a graduate of Colorado State University in 1957, I consider it to be one of the privileges of my veterinary career to have been a student of Adams, a part of his notes in 1957, and then a very close friend. Until Adams' first edition of *Lameness in Horses* was published, his notes were invaluable to me. The historical perspective by Dr. Mike Ross echoes my thoughts regarding the assessment of the texts and information relevant to the study of the lame horse, including his reference to those that have influenced the molding of modern lameness detectives. An insight into the history of the printed material directed toward the diagnostic and therapeutic management of the lame horse allows a better insight into the appreciation of the modern printed texts relevant to this subject. Specifically the editors, in the first edition, presented the contents throughout the text in a very logical manner, providing excellent approaches to the resolution of the lame horse's problems. The contents reflect the objective thinking of both editors and their contributors. The first nine chapters are vital to the lameness examination; the CD-ROM component enhances this segment in an extremely useful manner. When those principles are applied, then the logical application of the material in Chapters 10, 11, 12, 13, and 14 will follow as necessary.

Paramount to lameness management is the identification of the pain site causing the lameness. When that has been accomplished, the direction to be taken to resolve the issue will be set. Certainly the material provided in Section 2 of Part I will be utilized as the next step in arriving at the specific site of the infirmity; however, when the factors described in Section 1 of Part I are carefully followed, resolution of the problem may not require the employment of diagnostic imaging. The approach outlined by Section 1 Part I serves as a reminder that the modern "lameness detectives" are provided with the faculties of observation, palpation, and a brain. When used properly, these will facilitate a diagnosis without the necessity of further diagnostic modalities; however, when necessary, diagnostic imaging is vital to the identification of the pain-producing lesions. Certainly the advancements in the diagnostic imaging modalities have enhanced our ability to arrive at a more precise diagnosis with the obvious benefit of arriving at a more complete treatment and prognosis. The second edition contains the revelation of more diagnostic detail than was available in the first edition.

The editors have clearly provided a logical progression by structuring the contents of the text with the foot (Part II) following the general remarks regarding the diagnosis of lameness (Part I). Incorporation of recent discoveries of Robert Bowker, Christopher Pollitt, the editors, and others involved in studies of the foot will be useful information. The assessment of the information and input by the editors with their clinical experience should prove to make the understanding of the foot even more applicable to management of the information encountered in arguably the most common site of lameness in the horse.

The flow of the text continues in a manner in which the diagnostician should proceed to arrive at an informed solution to the lameness problem. The incorporation of the axial skeleton (Part V) in the first edition continues to remind the equine practitioner that its evaluation is very much a part of the assessment of the lame horse. Certainly in my career the axial skeleton has gone from being of very little consideration to its importance today. The inclusion of recent approaches to the diagnosis of axial skeleton issues is going to be another welcomed event.

The contributions to lameness other than those involving the skeleton and articulations as outlined in Parts VI, VII, and VIII of the first edition are updated as well. Certainly, there have been several new therapeutic modalities available for the management of lameness since the first edition. Again, the experience of the contributors and the editors will provide welcome information. Since publication of the first edition, the value of complementary therapy in equine practice continues to evolve, to demonstrate where it fits in Western medicine and the management of the lame horse.

Part V, "Lameness in the Sport Horse" in the first edition provided valuable information into not only the differences between the types of lameness encountered in various athletic endeavors of horses, but also those differences encountered throughout varying geographic locations. There is a difference in the degree of lameness from navicular disease and other soft tissue causes of palmar foot pain at 1609 meters compared with those at sea level.

The CD-ROM component of the first edition has evolved into the website feature of the second edition. The 47 narrated videos of equine lameness provide not only insight into evaluating the more common types of lameness, but also provides examples of unusual cases that escape accurate description by the written word.

I am confident that this second edition of *Diagnosis and Management of Lameness in the Horse* will be a major addition to the libraries of equine practitioners around the world. As a recipient of the contents of the texts that have been produced over the past years, I am extremely grateful and appreciative of the time and effort the editors, Mike W. Ross and Sue J. Dyson, and the contributors have put into this text. Not only does this information and the information provided by other similar literature aid the practitioner, but it has materially improved the health and welfare of the horses we care for.

Marvin Beeman
Littleton, Colorado, United States
January 2010

Preface

The second edition of *Diagnosis and Management of Lameness in the Horse* has been substantially revised. The knowledge that has been accrued through the clinical application of magnetic resonance imaging (MRI) and, to a lesser extent, computed tomography has revolutionized our understanding of many conditions, most especially those of foot pain. This is reflected by the greatly expanded section on the foot. In each chapter we have tried to reflect both our own advances in knowledge and those of our authors, as well as what has been published in the literature. Relevant new references are cited. We have introduced many new images, most acquired digitally and therefore of superior quality, but space constraints restrict what can be included. Some original illustrations reflecting unique conditions have been preserved.

Some chapters have been written by different authors. This did not necessarily reflect that we were unhappy with the original authors, but rather that we wanted a different approach in some instances. We have again added editorial comments to some chapters when our personal experiences differed greatly from those of an author.

As we work daily with lame horses our own knowledge and experience continue to grow. It is also inevitable that between submission of the material for the second edition to the publishers and the book's publication, new literature has been published. Therefore although this new edition reflects as far as possible state-of-the-art information, there are inevitably a few minor omissions.

A major criticism of the first edition of the book was the quality of the binding. We were delighted to learn that the book was being used to such an extent that the bindings failed. We suspect that the second edition, being bigger, unfortunately may also suffer in the same way.

We continue to learn by looking and seeing and encourage readers to watch the videos on the companion web site and listen to the commentaries, which we believe provide a fundamental background to the art of assessing a lame horse. We continue to hold the philosophy that a comprehensive clinical examination, combined with a logical approach to investigation, usually results in an accurate diagnosis, while acknowledging that a minority of horses elude diagnosis. There is a danger that with advances in imaging technology there is a temptation to utilize these tools excessively. We must remember that in many horses a correct diagnosis can be achieved by accurate palpation, observation, and use of diagnostic analgesia, combined with radiography and ultrasonography.

Sue J. Dyson and Mike W. Ross
Suffolk, United Kingdom and Pennsylvania,
United States, December 2009

PREFACE—COMPANION WEB SITE

WWW.ROSSANDDYSON.COM

When approached with the idea of developing the first edition of *Diagnosis and Management of Lameness in the Horse* we immediately determined that having video segments to accompany the text was a necessity, a way of providing moving figures to teach the fundamentals of the lameness examination during movement. At that time there were few textbooks with accompanying digital media and it was necessary to convert to digital format existing analog video footage. We then added newly acquired digital video segments to create the 47 individual files used in the CD-ROM that accompanied the first edition. It was not our intent to capture on video each and every nuance of the lame horse. We did, however, feel strongly in presenting the fundamentals of the lameness examination and the gaits and movement of the normal horse, and to contrast movement with the horses that have pain causing lameness, neurological abnormalities, mechanical deficits, and in brief esoteric gait disturbances. The art of the lameness examination during movement was captured.

Although our views are similar in determining the end result of our examination during movement, we differ in our visual appraisal of the lame horse; for instance, Sue sees more vividly the downward movement of the pelvis when a horse with hindlimb pain causing lameness is in motion, whereas Mike sees the upward movement during a different portion of the stride. These differences and the different venues at which we complete our lameness examination are thoroughly explained in the narration.

Examples are given of horses with unilateral and bilateral forelimb lameness, some with pain originating from common locations such as the foot or lower forelimb, while in others we contrast movement of these horses with those with pain emanating from the upper forelimb. Unilateral and bilateral hindlimb lameness is demonstrated and the concept of hindlimb lameness causing a head and neck nod—a situation during which a lameness diagnostician can confuse hindlimb with forelimb pain—is demonstrated in several video clips. The effect and use of circling a horse during lameness examination, a useful maneuver used to exacerbate lameness, is shown in horses with forelimb and hindlimb pain causing lameness. Concurrent forelimb and hindlimb lameness, the effect of a rider, and gait restriction as a result of thoracolumbar and sacroiliac region pain are demonstrated. Four horses with neurological gait abnormalities ranging from obvious to subtle, six horses with classic mechanical gait deficits causing lameness, and, finally, esoteric causes of gait abnormalities are shown.

Listed below is the table of contents of the narrated video segments included in the web site accompanying the second edition of Ross and Dyson's *Diagnosis and Management of Lameness in the Horse.* Using technological advances developed in the 8 years since the first edition was published we have changed the appearance of the media and improved its efficiency and utility. We have chosen to retain the original video segments and narration, feeling strongly that we have captured the essence of the lameness examination during movement and demonstrated the numerous principles of the lame horse. We debated endlessly whether to expand and include many more examples, to discuss flexion tests, to describe responses to local analgesic techniques and all the associated nuances, and to describe the many different clinical manifestations of pain arising from specific areas. Ultimately we decided not to, but we encourage readers to think about their own experiences and to share these with others.

The video segments, moving figures, have been numbered from 1 to 47, and in the right margin of the text, when appropriate, we have printed an icon ⓥ referring the reader to one or more of the video segments included in the accompanying web site we feel will be helpful to visually evaluate a horse during movement.

TABLE OF CONTENTS OF COMPANION WEBSITE

Normal Gait
1. Gait of a normal horse when evaluated in-hand and while lunged
2. Gait of a normal horse while ridden

Unilateral Forelimb Lameness
3. Left forelimb lameness
4. Right forelimb lameness
5. Unilateral forelimb lameness resulting from upper limb pain
6. Unilateral forelimb lameness resulting from upper limb pain

Bilateral Forelimb Lameness
7. Bilateral forelimb lameness worse in the right forelimb

Effect of Circling on Forelimb Lameness
8. Right forelimb lameness
9. Bilateral forelimb lameness
10. Characteristics of carpal region pain

Hindlimb Lameness without a Head and Neck Nod
11. Left hindlimb lameness in a horse with stifle pain
12. Left hindlimb lameness in a horse with bilateral suspensory desmitis
13. Right hindlimb lameness in a horse with peritarsal soft-tissue injury
14. Right hindlimb lameness
15. Left hindlimb lameness, effect of the pace and trot during lameness examination

Hindlimb Lameness with an Associated Head and Neck Nod
16. Severe right hindlimb lameness from pain associated with fracture of the central tarsal bone
17. Severe left hindlimb lameness
18. Right hindlimb lameness as a result of severe osteoarthritis of the medial femorotibial joint
19. Severe left hindlimb lameness

Bilateral Hindlimb Lameness
20. Bilateral hindlimb lameness and plaiting while trotting
21. Bilateral hindlimb lameness exhibited as a reluctance to work

Effect of Circling on Hindlimb Lameness
22. Right hindlimb lameness and toe drag
23. Toe dragging while circling
24. Right hindlimb lameness worse going to the right

Concurrent Forelimb and Hindlimb Lameness
25. Left forelimb and left hindlimb lameness
26. Left forelimb and left hindlimb lameness in a Standardbred racehorse
27. Left hindlimb and right forelimb lameness causing a "rocking-type" gait
28. Left hindlimb and right forelimb lameness in a trotter before and after low plantar diagnostic analgesia
29. Bilateral hindlimb and mild forelimb lameness in a Thoroughbred racehorse with mal- or nonadaptive subchondral bone remodeling

Other Aspects of Hindlimb Lameness
30. Hindlimb lameness while ridden
31. Gait restriction from thoracolumbar pain
32. Gait restriction from sacroiliac region pain

Neurological Gait Deficits
33. Gait deficit in a horse with a cervical spinal cord lesion
34. Hindlimb ataxia and right shoulder instability
35. Hindlimb weakness
36. Gait deficit in a horse with cervical stenotic myelopathy

Mechanical Gait Deficits
37. Fibrotic myopathy
38. Stringhalt
39. Shivers
40. Upward fixation of the patella
41. Fibularis (peroneus) tertius injury in a mature horse
42. Fibularis tertius avulsion injury in a foal

Esoteric Gait Abnormalities
43. Right hindlimb gait abnormality
44. Running type of hindlimb gait
45. Aortoiliac thrombosis
46. Left hindlimb lameness and gait deficit in a horse with gastrocnemius origin injury
47. Idiopathic shortening of the cranial phase of the stride in a right hindlimb

Mike W. Ross
Sue J. Dyson
December 18, 2009

Acknowledgments

Just as when we wrote the first edition of *Diagnosis and Management of Lameness in the Horse,* we owe tremendous gratitude to our co-authors, many of whom have updated their original chapters, updated and changed figures, and continued to provide us with their unique lameness experiences. In most instances we have returned to the original authors for this second edition, but found it necessary to change authors and to proceed in a new direction with some of the chapters. We give wholehearted thanks to previous authors not included in this edition and welcome our new contributors. Writing textbook chapters is often a thankless job, with little remuneration, and we appreciate the efforts of all who have contributed. In many ways the project to complete the second edition was an easier task than our previous mission, because the skeleton of the textbook, including the major subsections of the written text, remained largely the same. We are grateful to all who inspired the development of the first edition and remain indebted to their initial and continued support.

We are honored by the continued support of our friend, colleague, and co-author, Fabio Torre, who once again has provided us with inspirational cover art. Fabio's original paintings for the first edition hang with pride in each of our homes, reminding us daily of Fabio's unique contribution to the success of this book. The artwork on the cover of the second edition continues a theme dedicated to the movement of the horse, in the form of images of racing Thoroughbred and Standardbred horses in motion. Movement is an integral part of the lameness examination and is captured in still form in Fabio's artwork.

We have both continued to be blessed to work with true professionals, our co-workers, at the Animal Health Trust and New Bolton Center, University of Pennsylvania and are thankful for their continued help and support as we revised this textbook and continue our interest and work in the area of equine lameness. The constant support and professionalism of the staff at Elsevier Health Science, including Lauren Harms and Penny Rudolph, was felt throughout. We also thank Alex Baker whose high standard of artwork we admire, and who has produced a number of new drawings for this edition.

Both of us have learned the art and science of the lame horse by dedicated and experienced lameness diagnosticians who preceded us and then taught us through their own experiences and in their own unique way. Sue continues to acknowledge the timeless support of Bill Moyer, Charlie Reid, Ron Genovese, and Midge Leitch. Sue also acknowledges the knowledge about riding, feeling, and horse management taught by David Arthur and Sheila Willcox. Mike believes strongly his career path was hugely influenced and supported by many high-quality lameness detectives, but singles out Jack Lowe, Loren Evans, and Gene Gill as particularly influential in practice, and in life.

While working on the first edition and now in the years subsequent to its publication we have had a special opportunity to learn from each other, often sharing our own unique experiences and perspectives, questioning each other, keeping each other "on their toes," occasionally with timely and critical questions, and sometimes with answers. We have often shared a podium with each other, listening to and learning first hand from each other's work. Sue has made an indelible contribution to Mike's professional life, and has become a much loved, close friend.

We both greatly appreciate the love and support given us by our families. The time commitment necessary to complete this project and the countless hours we have both invested in refining our skills and interest in the lame horse invariably took time away from our loved ones. John and Beth, our partners, we thank you for your love and willingness to provide us time to complete this edition, and for your countless suggestions and enthusiasm. Mike gives special thanks to Stone, Kennedy, and Allie for their unwavering love, and his parents. Neither one of us will ever forget the horse.

Sue J. Dyson
Mike W. Ross
December 17, 2009

Contents

PART I: DIAGNOSIS OF LAMENESS

Section 1: The Lameness Examination

1 Lameness Examination: Historical Perspective, 1
Mike W. Ross

2 Lameness in Horses: Basic Facts Before Starting, 3
Mike W. Ross

3 Anamnesis (History), 8
Mike W. Ross

4 Conformation and Lameness, 15
Mike W. Ross, C. Wayne McIlwraith

5 Observation: Symmetry and Posture, 32
Mike W. Ross

6 Palpation, 43
Mike W. Ross

The Churchill Hock Test, 60
Dan L. Hawkins

Saphenous Filling Time, 61
Mike W. Ross

7 Movement, 64
Mike W. Ross

8 Manipulation, 80
Mike W. Ross

9 Applied Anatomy of the Musculoskeletal System, 88
Matthew Durham, Sue J. Dyson

10 Diagnostic Analgesia, 100
Lance H. Bassage II, Mike W. Ross

11 Neurological Examination and Neurological Conditions Causing Gait Deficits, 135
William V. Bernard, Jill Beech

12 Unexplained Lameness, 145
Sue J. Dyson

13 Assessment of Acute-Onset, Severe Lameness, 159
Sue J. Dyson

14 The Swollen Limb, 164
Sue J. Dyson

Section 2: Diagnostic Imaging

15 Radiography and Radiology, 168
Sue J. Dyson

16 Ultrasonographic Evaluation of the Equine Limb: Technique, 182
Norman W. Rantanen, Joan S. Jorgensen, Ronald L. Genovese

17 Ultrasonographic Examination of Joints, 206
Jean-Marie Denoix

18 Ultrasonography and Orthopedic (Nonarticular) Disease, 212
Virginia B. Reef

19 Nuclear Medicine, 215
Mike W. Ross, Vivian S. Stacy

20 Computed Tomography, 234
Sarah M. Puchalski

21 Magnetic Resonance Imaging, 239
Rachel C. Murray, Sue J. Dyson

22 Gait Analysis for the Quantification of Lameness, 245
Kevin G. Keegan

23 Arthroscopic Examination, 251
Mike W. Ross

24 Tenoscopy and Bursoscopy, 260
Eddy R.J. Cauvin

25 Thermography: Use in Equine Lameness, 266
Andrew P. Bathe

PART II: THE FOOT

26 The Biomechanics of the Equine Limb and Its Effect on Lameness, 270
Alan Wilson, Renate Weller

27 The Foot and Shoeing, 282
Foot Balance, Conformation, and Lameness, 282
Andrew H. Parks

Horseshoes and Shoeing, 293
Andrew H. Parks

Natural Balance Trimming and Shoeing, 303
Gene Ovnicek

Hoof Reconstruction Materials and Glue-On Shoes, 306
Robert Sigafoos, Patrick T. Reilly

28 Trauma to the Sole and Wall, 309
Robin M. Dabareiner, William A. Moyer, G. Kent Carter

Penetrating Wounds to the Navicular Bursa (Bursa Podotrochlearis), Infectious (Septic) Navicular Bursitis, "Streetnail," 316
Mike W. Ross, Sue J. Dyson
Canker, 319
Mike W. Ross, Sue J. Dyson

29 Functional Anatomy of the Palmar Aspect of the Foot, 320
Robert M. Bowker

30 Navicular Disease, 324
Sue J. Dyson

31 Fracture of the Navicular Bone and Congenital Bipartite Navicular Bone, 343
Sue J. Dyson

32 Primary Lesions of the Deep Digital Flexor Tendon within the Hoof Capsule, 344
Sue J. Dyson

33 The Distal Phalanx and Distal Interphalangeal Joint, 349
Sue J. Dyson

34 Laminitis, 366
  Pathophysiology of Laminitis, 366
    Christopher C. Pollitt
  Diagnosis of Laminitis, 371
    Sue J. Dyson
  Medical Therapy of Laminitis, 372
    Christopher C. Pollitt
  Chronic Laminitis, 374
    Christopher C. Pollitt, Simon N. Collins
  Venography, 377
    Christopher C. Pollitt, Simon N. Collins, Greg Baldwin
  Hoof Care of a Laminitic Horse, 379
    Frank A. Nickels
  Deep Digital Flexor Tenotomy for Managing Laminitis, 382
    Robert J. Hunt
  Other Management Aspects of Laminitis, 384
    Sue J. Dyson, Mike W. Ross

PART III: THE FORELIMB
35 The Proximal and Middle Phalanges and Proximal Interphalangeal Joint, 387
    Alan J. Ruggles
36 The Metacarpophalangeal Joint, 394
    Dean W. Richardson, Sue J. Dyson
37 The Metacarpal Region, 411
    Sue J. Dyson
38 The Carpus, 426
    Mike W. Ross
39 The Antebrachium, 449
    Lance H. Bassage II, Mike W. Ross
40 The Elbow, Brachium, and Shoulder, 456
    Sue J. Dyson

PART IV: THE HINDLIMB
41 The Hind Foot and Pastern, 475
    Mike W. Ross
42 The Metatarsophalangeal Joint, 480
    Mike W. Ross
43 The Metatarsal Region, 499
    Mike W. Ross
44 The Tarsus, 508
    Sue J. Dyson, Mike W. Ross
45 The Crus, 526
    Mike W. Ross
46 The Stifle, 532
    John P. Walmsley
47 The Thigh, 550
    Dan L. Hawkins, Mike W. Ross
  The Gluteal Syndrome, 550
    Dan L. Hawkins
  Trochanteric Bursitis, 552
    Dan L. Hawkins
48 Mechanical and Neurological Lameness in the Forelimbs and Hindlimbs, 555
    Sue J. Dyson, Mike W. Ross

PART V: THE AXIAL SKELETON
49 Diagnosis and Management of Pelvic Fractures in the Thoroughbred Racehorse, 564
    Robert C. Pilsworth
50 Lumbosacral and Pelvic Injuries in Sports and Pleasure Horses, 571
    Sue J. Dyson
51 Diagnosis and Management of Sacroiliac Joint Injuries, 583
    Kevin K. Haussler
52 Thoracolumbar Spine, 592
    Jean-Marie Denoix, Sue J. Dyson
53 The Cervical Spine and Soft Tissues of the Neck, 606
    Sue J. Dyson

PART VI: DEVELOPMENTAL ORTHOPEDIC DISEASE AND LAMENESS
54 Pathogenesis of Osteochondrosis, 617
    Janet Douglas
55 The Role of Nutrition in Developmental Orthopedic Disease: Nutritional Management, 625
    Joe D. Pagan
56 Diagnosis and Management of Osteochondrosis and Osseous Cystlike Lesions, 631
    Dean W. Richardson
57 Physitis, 638
    David R. Ellis
58 Angular Limb Deformities, 640
    José M. García-López, Eric J. Parente
  Surgical Management, 642
    José M. García-López
59 Flexural Limb Deformities in Foals, 645
    Robert J. Hunt
60 Cervical Stenotic Myelopathy, 649
    Richard J. Piercy

PART VII: ARTHRITIS
61 Osteoarthritis, 655
    John P. Caron
62 Markers of Osteoarthritis: Implications for Early Diagnosis and Monitoring of the Pathological Course and Effects of Therapy, 668
    David D. Frisbie
63 Gene Therapy, 671
    C. Wayne McIlwraith, David D. Frisbie
64 Models of Equine Joint Disease, 673
    Chris E. Kawcak
65 Infectious Arthritis and Fungal Infectious Arthritis, 677
    Alicia L. Bertone, Jennifer M. Cohen
  Infectious Arthritis, 677
    Alicia L. Bertone
  Fungal Infectious Arthritis, 684
    Jennifer M. Cohen

66 Noninfectious Arthritis, 687
Alicia L. Bertone

67 Other Joint Conditions, 691
Chris E. Kawcak

PART VIII: THE SOFT TISSUES

68 Pathophysiology of Tendon Injury, 694
Roger K.W. Smith

69 Superficial Digital Flexor Tendonitis, 706
Mike W. Ross, Ronald L. Genovese, Sue J. Dyson, Joan S. Jorgensen

Superficial Digital Flexor Tendonitis in Racehorses, 706
Joan S. Jorgensen, Ronald L. Genovese, Mike W. Ross

Surgical Management of Superficial Digital Flexor
Tendonitis, 715
Mike W. Ross

Superficial Digital Flexor Tendonitis in Event Horses, Show Jumpers,
Dressage Horses, and Pleasure Horses, 721
Sue J. Dyson

70 The Deep Digital Flexor Tendon, 726
Sue J. Dyson

71 Injuries of the Accessory Ligament of the Deep
Digital Flexor Tendon, 734
Sue J. Dyson

72 The Suspensory Apparatus, 738
Sue J. Dyson, Ronald L. Genovese

73 Clinical Use of Stem Cells, Marrow
Components, and Other Growth
Factors, 761
Lisa Fortier

74 Diseases of the Digital Flexor Tendon Sheath,
Palmar Annular Ligament, and Digital Annular
Ligaments, 764
Michael C. Schramme, Roger K.W. Smith

75 The Carpal Canal and Carpal Synovial
Sheath, 777
Sue J. Dyson

76 The Tarsal Sheath, 780
Eddy R.J. Cauvin

77 Extensor Tendon Injury, 785
Jane C. Boswell, Michael C. Schramme

78 Curb, 792
Mike W. Ross, Ronald L. Genovese

79 Bursae and Other Soft Tissue Swellings, 799
Sue J. Dyson

80 Other Soft Tissue Injuries, 802
Sue J. Dyson

81 Tendon Lacerations, 806
Sue J. Dyson, Alicia L. Bertone

82 Soft Tissue Injuries of the Pastern, 810
Virginia B. Reef, Ronald L. Genovese

83 Skeletal Muscle and Lameness, 818
Stephanie J. Valberg, Sue J. Dyson

Nutritional Myopathies, 834
John Maas, Stephanie J. Valberg

Hyperkalemic Periodic Paralysis, 838
Sharon J. Spier

PART IX: THERAPEUTICS

Section 1: Traditional Therapy

84 Principles and Practices of Joint Disease
Treatment, 840
C. Wayne McIlwraith

85 Analgesia and Hindlimb Lameness, 852
Rose M. McMurphy

86 Bandaging, Splinting, and Casting, 858
Alan J. Ruggles, Sue J. Dyson

87 External Skeletal Fixation, 863
David M. Nunamaker

88 Counterirritation, 867
David R. Ellis, Stephen P. Dey III

89 Cryotherapy, 869
Kjerstin M. Jacobs, Thomas P.S. Oliver

90 Radiation Therapy, 872
Alain P. Théon

91 Rest and Rehabilitation, 877
Barrie D. Grant

Section 2: Complementary (Nontraditional) Therapy

92 Acupuncture, 881
Equine Acupuncture for Lameness Diagnosis and Treatment, 881
Allen M. Schoen

Acupuncture Channel Palpation and Equine Musculoskeletal
Pain, 887
William H. McCormick

93 Chiropractic Evaluation and Management of
Musculoskeletal Disorders, 892
Kevin K. Haussler

94 Electrophysical Agents in Physiotherapy, 901
Amanda Sutton, Tim Watson

95 Osteopathic Treatment of the Axial Skeleton of
the Horse, 907
Chris Colles, Julia Brooks

96 Shock Wave Therapy, 914
Scott R. McClure

PART X: LAMENESS IN THE SPORTS HORSE

Section 1: Poor Performance

97 Poor Performance and Lameness, 920
Sue J. Dyson

98 Experiences Using a High-Speed Treadmill to
Evaluate Lameness, 925
Benson B. Martin Jr., Sue J. Dyson, Mike W. Ross

Section 2: The Racehorse

99 The Sales Yearling, 928
Purchase Examination of a Thoroughbred Sales Yearling in North
America, 928
Benson B. Martin Jr., John C. Kimmel, Mark W. Cheney

Purchase Examination of a Thoroughbred Sales Yearling
in Europe, 930
David R. Ellis

North American Standardbred Sales Yearling, 932
Mike W. Ross

100 Pathophysiology and Clinical Diagnosis of
         Cortical and Subchondral Bone Injury, 935
         Elizabeth J. Davidson

101 Bone Biomarkers, 947
         Joanna Price

102 The Bucked-Shin Complex, 953
         Etiology, Pathogenesis, and Conservative Management, 953
         David M. Nunamaker

         Stress Fractures of the Third Metacarpal Bone: Surgical
         Management, 959
         Alan J. Ruggles

103 On-the-Track Catastrophes in the Thoroughbred
         Racehorse, 960
         W. Theodore Hill

104 Catastrophic Injuries, 968
         Dean W. Richardson

105 Track Surfaces and Lameness: Epidemiological
         Aspects of Racehorse Injury, 972
         Tim D.H. Parkin

106 The North American Thoroughbred, 977
         *Rick M. Arthur, Jeff A. Blea, Mike W. Ross,
         Patrick J. Moloney, Mark W. Cheney*

107 The European Thoroughbred, 994
         Robert C. Pilsworth

108 The North American Standardbred, 1014
         James B. Mitchell, John S. Mitchell, Paul M. Nolan, Mike W. Ross

109 The European and Australasian
         Standardbreds, 1036
         The European Standardbred, 1036
         Fabio Torre

         The Australasian Standardbred, 1047
         R. Chris Whitton

110 The Racing Quarter Horse, 1051
         Nancy L. Goodman

111 Lameness in the Arabian Racehorse: Middle East
         and North America, 1057
         Robert Andrew Dalglish, Mark C. Rick

112 National Hunt Racehorse, Point to Point Horse,
         and Timber Racing Horse, 1062
         *Sue J. Dyson, Robert Joseph Van Pelt, Kevin P. Keane, James Wood,
         Anthony Stirk*

113 The Finnish Horse and Other Scandinavian
         Cold-Blooded Trotters, 1076
         Kristiina Ertola, Jukka Houttu

Section 3: Nonracing Sports Horses

114 Prepurchase Examination of the Performance
         Horse, 1081
         Richard D. Mitchell, Sue J.Dyson

115 Lameness in the Show Hunter and Show
         Jumper, 1096
         *Robert P. Boswell, Richard D. Mitchell, Timothy R. Ober, Philippe H. Benoit,
         Christopher (Kit) B. Miller, Sue J. Dyson*

116 Lameness in the Dressage Horse, 1112
         Svend E. Kold, Sue J. Dyson

117 Lameness in the Three Day Event Horse, 1123
         Andrew P. Bathe

118 Lameness in Endurance Horses, 1137
         Martha M. Misheff

119 Lameness in the Polo Pony, 1149
         Paul Wollenman, P.J. McMahon, Simon Knapp, Mike W. Ross

120 The Western Performance Horse, 1165
         The Cutting Horse, 1165
         Jerry B. Black, Robin M. Dabareiner

         The Roping Horse, 1170
         Robin M. Dabareiner

         The Reined Cow Horse, 1176
         Van E. Snow

         Barrel-Racing Horses, 1180
         Robin M. Dabareiner

         The European Western Performance Horse, 1183
         Franco Ferrero

121 Walking Horses, 1186
         James T. Blackford, James C. Sternberg

122 Lameness in the American Saddlebred
         and Other Trotting Breeds with
         Collection, 1188
         Scott D. Bennett

123 Lameness in the Arabian and Half-Arabian
         Show Horse, 1195
         Jeffrey A. Williams, Bradley S. Root

124 Lameness in the Driving Horse, 1205
         Kevin P. Keane, Graham Munroe

125 Lameness in Draft Horses, 1216
         Dallas O. Goble

126 Lameness in the Pony, 1228
         Andrew M. McDiarmid

127 Lameness in Breeding Stallions and
         Broodmares, 1235
         Benson B. Martin Jr., Sue M. McDonnell

128 Lameness in Foals, 1242
         Robert J. Hunt

129 Pleasure Riding Horse, 1252
         Herbert J. Burns

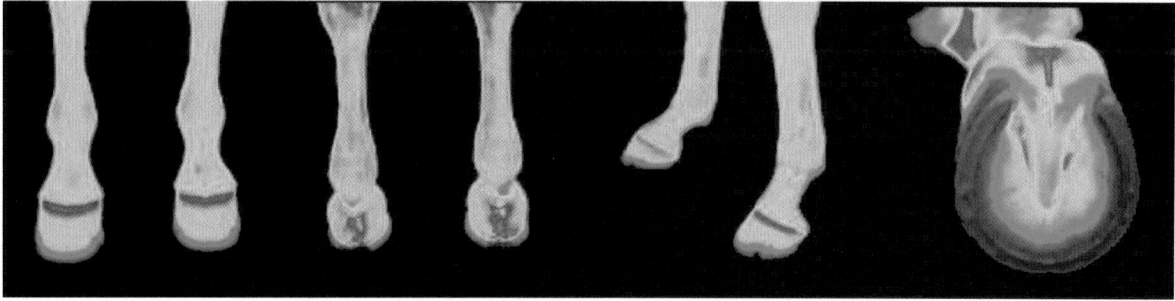

Color Plate 1 • Normal dorsal, palmar, left lateral, and solar thermographic images of the distal aspect of the forelimbs of a horse. There is good symmetry between the limbs. The coronary band is the warmest area, and the rest of the hoof becomes colder in a regular pattern closer to the ground surface. The palmar image shows a normal increase in temperature between the heel bulbs. On the solar image there is a V-shaped pattern of increased temperature representing the sulci of the frog.

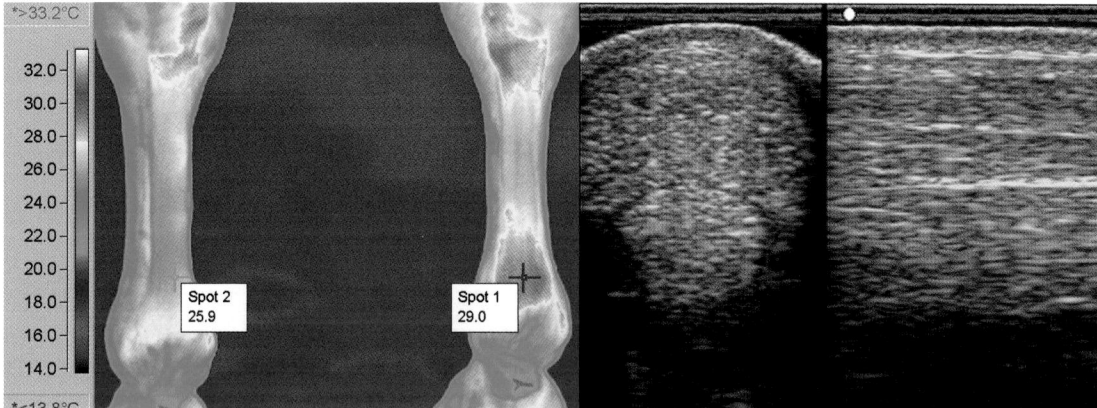

Color Plate 2 • An advanced event horse with previous history of midbody superficial digital flexor tendonitis of the right forelimb. More recently peritendonous edema had developed distally in the right forelimb. Ultrasonographic images show increased cross-sectional area of the superficial digital flexor tendon, and areas of hyperechogenicity and hypoechogenicity. It was not possible to determine if there was active pathology or if this was the level of healing that had been reached from the previous injury. The palmar thermographic image shows rectangular clip artifacts on both limbs. There is a clinically significant increase in temperature of the distal palmar aspect of the right forelimb compared with the left, indicating inflammation, and thus the image suggests recurrent tendon injury.

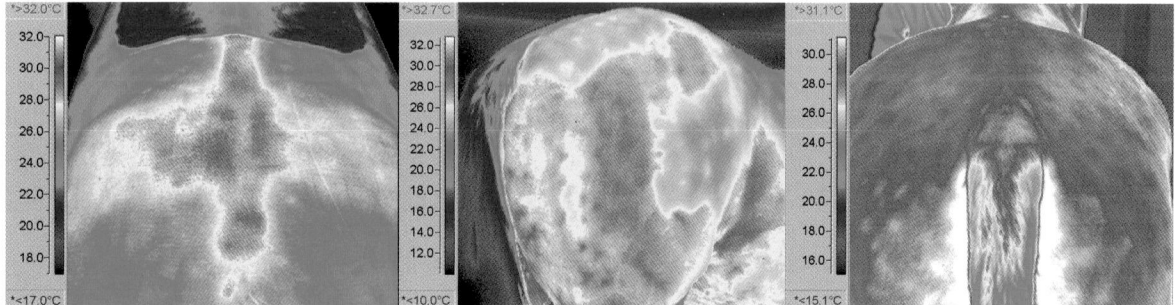

Color Plate 3 • Three examples of muscle injury. The left thermographic image shows a left gluteal injury with increased heat signature. The middle image shows an increase in temperature over the biceps femoris muscle. The right image is of a chronic gluteal injury with fibrosis, which has a cooler thermal pattern.

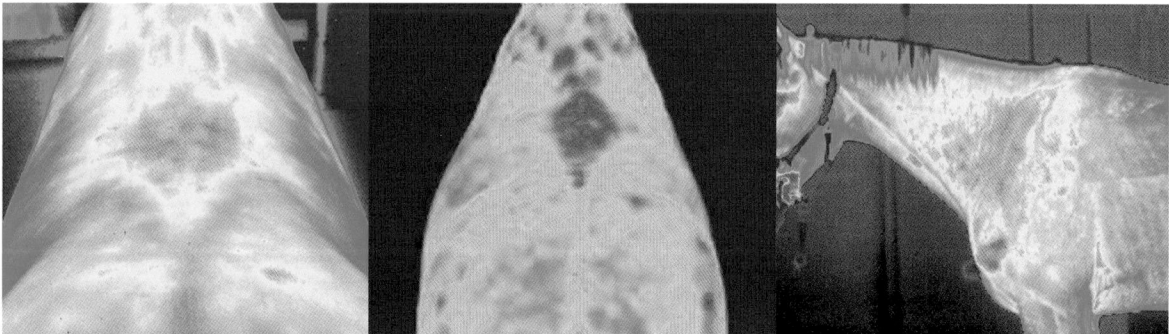

Color Plate 4 • The left and middle thermographic images are caudodorsal views of the back, showing areas of increased temperature associated with clinical signs of back pain and impinging dorsal spinous processes evident radiologically. The lateral view of the neck is from a horse with marked caudal cervical facet joint osteoarthritis. There is an increase in superficial blood flow in this region.

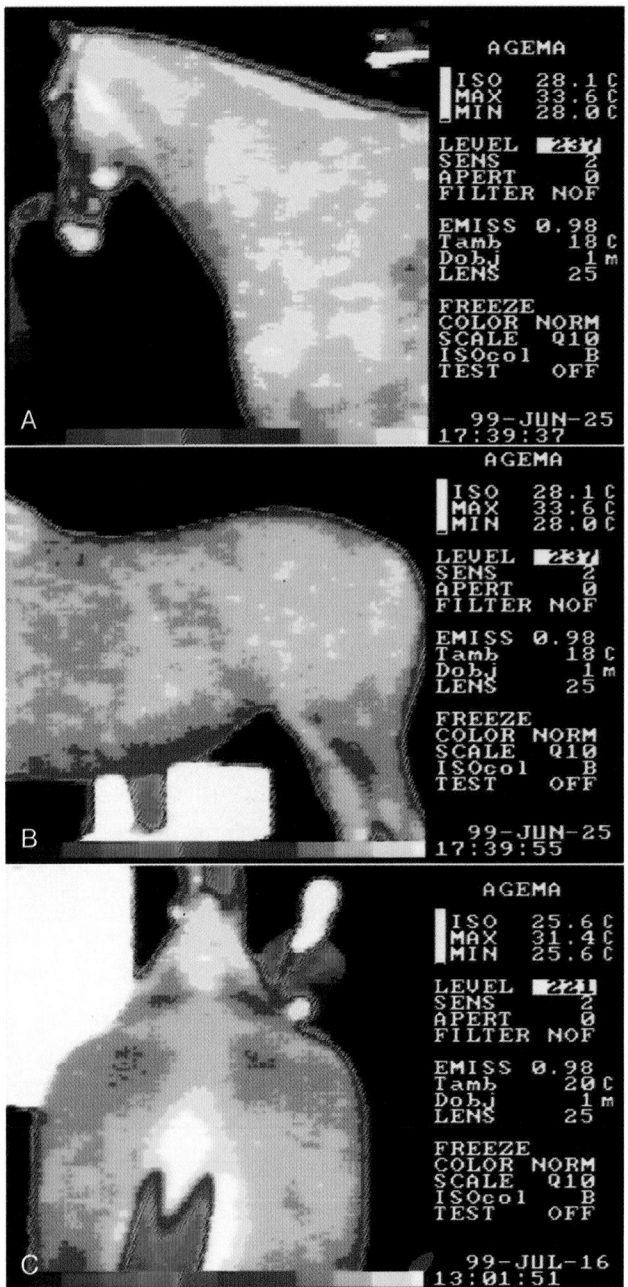

Color Plate 5 • Thermographs show the appearance of normal horses. The color scale represents 5.6° C, using 10 colors; that is, each color represents about a 0.5° C change in temperature. The color bar under the image shows the colors used; those to the right side are the hottest, and those to the left are the coldest. White is above the top of the scale, and black below the scale. **A,** Lateral image of the head, neck, and shoulder. **B,** Lateral image of the thorax, abdomen, and hindquarters. **C,** Oblique dorsal image from behind the horse looking toward its head and neck. Temperature variation is 1° C over the neck, trunk, and hindquarters. A warm midline dorsal stripe along the back extends from the withers to the base of the tail, with symmetrical muscle temperature on either side.

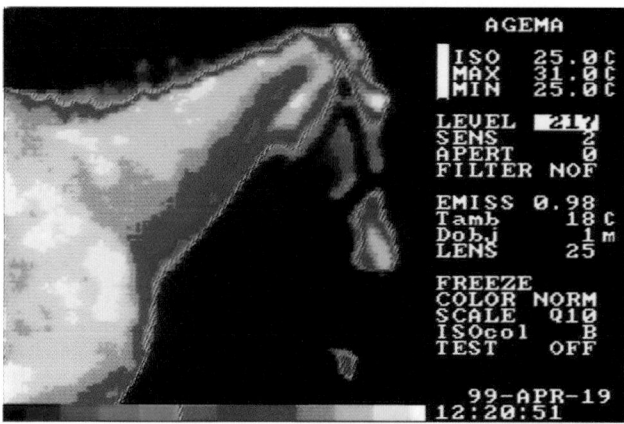

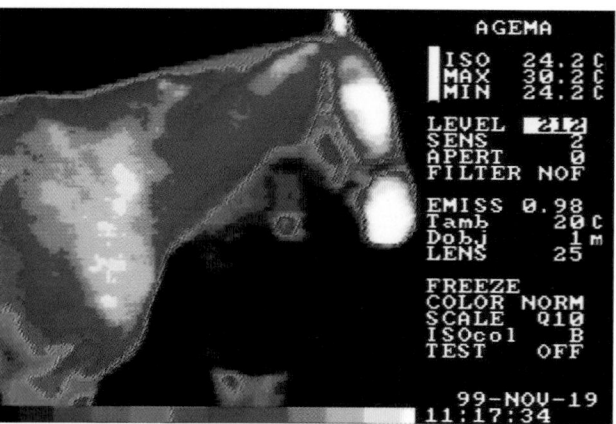

Color Plate 6 • Lateral image of the neck of a horse with reduced mobility in the occipitoatlantal and atlantoaxial joints. A cool line *(red)* runs obliquely from the region of the atlantoaxial joint caudally to the base of the neck and is 1.5° C cooler than the surrounding muscle, indicating an area of sympathetic dystonia.

Color Plate 7 • Lateral image of the neck of horse with reduced mobility in the neck. Note the cooling *(red area)* from the occiput back to the level of the sixth and seventh cervical vertebrae, indicating a problem involving all joints in the neck.

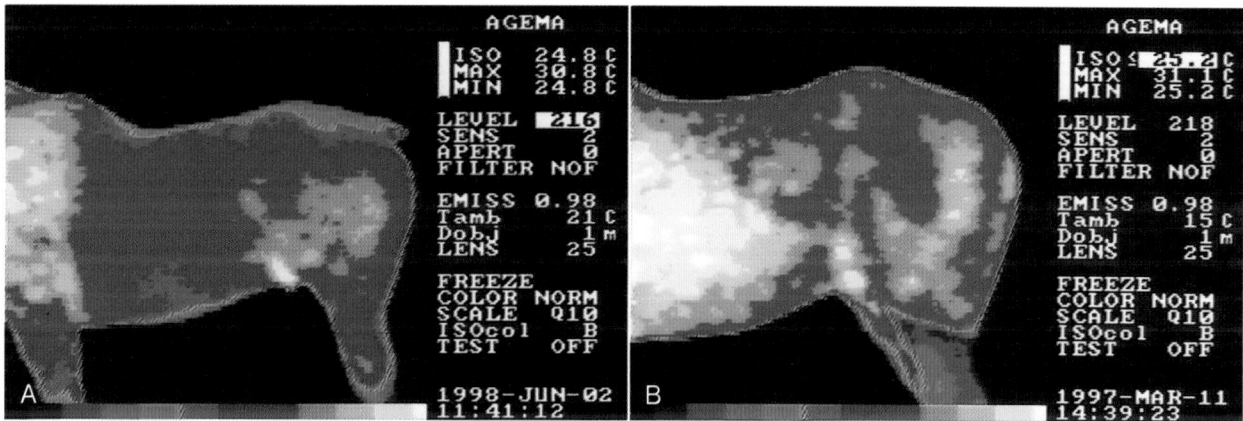

Color Plate 8 • Lateral images of the thoracolumbar area of two horses, both showing clinically significant cooling *(red area)* in the musculature of the dorsal spine from the saddle region caudally. **A,** The vertical cranial boundary to the zone of cooling indicates that the injured area is in the region of the cervicothoracic junction, but the shoulder muscles overlying this area receive innervation from the lower neck, partly masking the muscles supplied by the upper thoracic area. **B,** The typical appearance of cooling in the muscle resulting from an injury to the region of the twelfth thoracic vertebra, with the cranial border of the region running obliquely down and back. This horse has been clipped, but long hair left on the hindlimb shows as an area 5° C cooler than the surface temperature of the thorax of the horse.

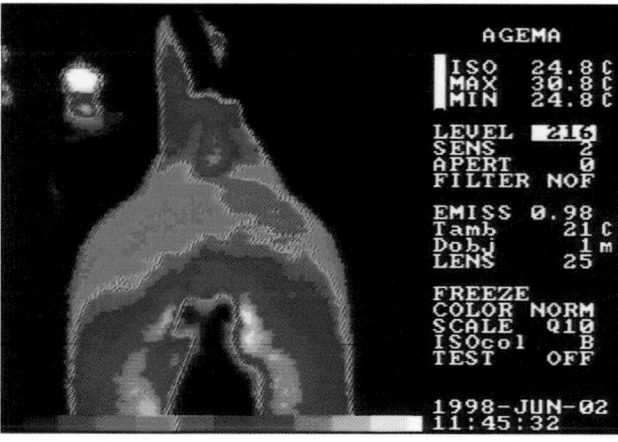

Color Plate 9 • Dorsal image of a horse with abnormal temperature patterns of the thoracolumbar spine. Note the complete loss of the normal central stripe (compare with Color Plate 5, *C*), with cooling indicating the presence of reduced mobility of the entire thoracolumbar spine and pelvis. The asymmetrical nature of the temperature pattern indicates the horse is likely to move with an asymmetrical gait, resulting from increased muscle tone on the left side of the body.

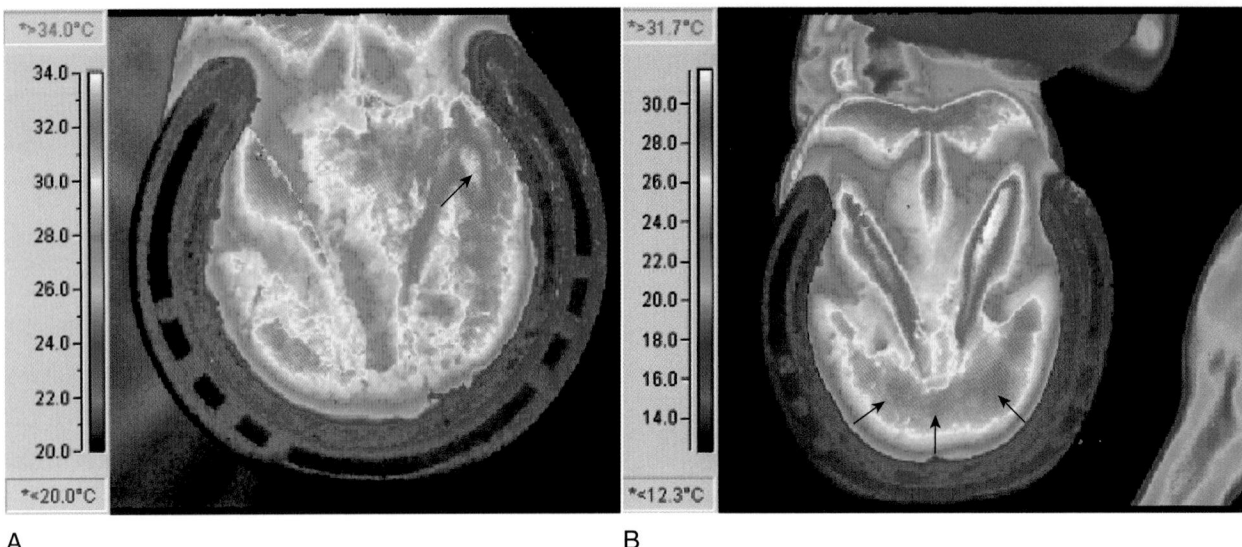

Color Plate 10 • Examples of different thermographic foot patterns (solar images). **A,** This hoof has a medial corn *(arrow)*, manifested as a focal hot spot *(white)* within an area of increased temperature. **B,** This hoof has subacute laminitis, with a pattern of increased temperature in the region of the tip of the distal phalanx *(arrows)*.

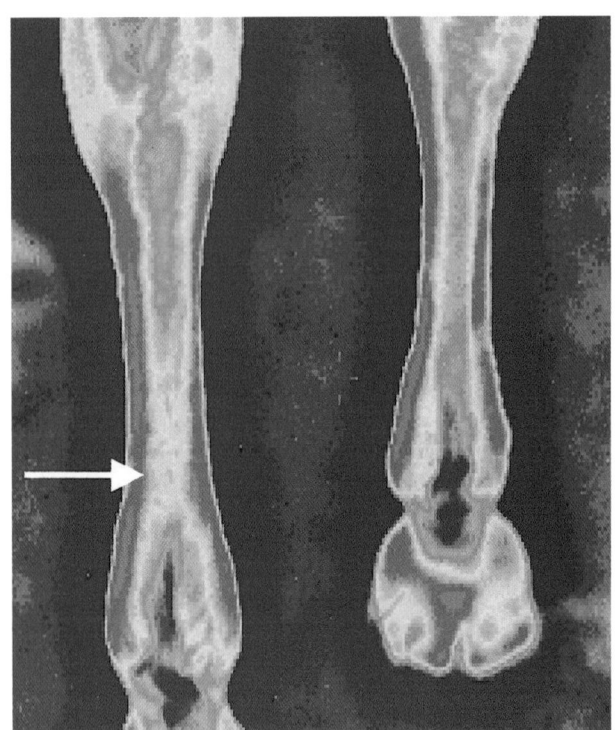

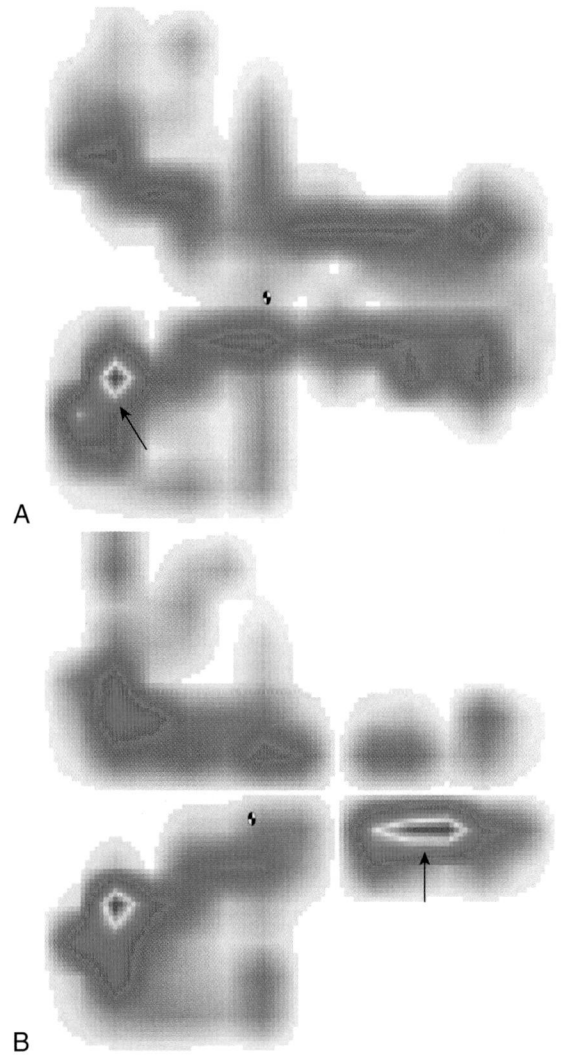

Color Plate 11 • Palmar thermographic image and subsequent transverse *(left)* and longitudinal ultrasonographic images (see Figure 117-5) of an advanced event horse 10 days after successfully completing a Three Day Event. The horse was having a routine examination, and no clinical localizing signs were evident in the tendon. The thermogram demonstrates a focal hot spot over the left distal superficial digital flexor tendon *(arrow)*, and the ultrasonographic images reveal a hypoechoic core lesion in the same region.

Color Plate 12 • Computerized saddle pressure analysis images. Cranial is to the left, and left is to the bottom. **A,** This image shows a poorly fitting saddle, with a focal pressure point in the left withers region *(arrow)*. **B,** This image demonstrates failure of a gel pad to alleviate the pressure point and the development of an additional pressure point caudally *(arrow)*.

PART I

Diagnosis of Lameness

SECTION 1
The Lameness Examination

| Chapter | 1 |

Lameness Examination: Historical Perspective

Mike W. Ross

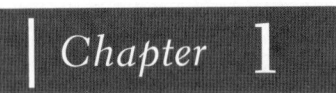
References
on page
1255

If your horse is lame in his shoulder, take off his shoes.... Young and inexperienced practitioners are quite too apt to commit the error of overlooking the examination of the foot, looking upon it as a matter of secondary importance, and attending to it as a routine and formal affair only.

A. Liautard, 1888[1]

As the twenty-first century continues, the extent of change in the diagnosis of lameness in the horse depends on the individual's clinical and ideological perspective. A veritable explosion of new imaging methods such as digital radiography, computed tomography, and magnetic resonance imaging has advanced the current understanding of many musculoskeletal abnormalities. Yet to accurately assess clinical relevance, the clinician must possess a feel for the horse, developed only by careful clinical examination, a procedure that has changed little in hundreds of years. Successful detection of equine lameness does not so much require knowledge of science as it does art. Inasmuch as *art* is defined as "skilled workmanship, craft, or studied action,"[2] the lameness examination demands artistic experience acquired by years of clinical practice and working and learning from experienced practitioners. From Liautard's advice more than 100 years ago to that of modern lameness diagnosticians, the change in the basic skills of lameness diagnosis may be small.

Development of the artistic skills needed to become a true lameness diagnostician requires a thorough, somewhat methodical approach, much like that of a crime scene detective. I often refer to the lameness diagnostician as a *lameness detective*, and although this statement may lack sophistication, in reality, how boring would the task be if the horse could talk? To make a horse talk to you through careful palpation and observation is the essence of the

lameness examination, yet most difficult to teach. Great lameness diagnosticians likely possess this ability to read or feel the horse and skilled, workmanship-like qualities to appreciate the art in lameness diagnosis. Some, with the added ability to share this knowledge effectively, have influenced clinicians more than others simply by writing about those experiences. In the early twenty-first century, Ross and Dyson's *Diagnosis and Management of Lameness in the Horse* chronicled the exhaustive clinical experience of over 100 authors worldwide to capture the essence of the subject at that time.[3] Moving figures captured as video segments on an accompanying CD and individual chapters detailing lameness distribution among different sporting activities complemented basic and advanced material.[3] The book quickly became a staple of every lameness diagnostician's library. In the mid-to-late 1900s, Adams had the most profound influence with his teachings and writings. His former students and friends acknowledge his artistic talent, gained primarily from a ground-up approach to the lame horse, and his profound interest in corrective shoeing. More important, Adams' original lameness notes became his classic textbook.[4] For most clinicians, *Lameness in Horses* represented the "lameness Bible," an excellent resource of information on equine lameness. Adams himself revised the textbook several times; most recently, his respected colleague, Ted S. Stashak, has continued in Adams' footsteps. This important work served as the foundation for learning the fundamentals of equine lameness for many during this period.

Adams was influenced greatly by the work of Dollar and Lacroix. Adams' original notes contain many drawings similar to those originally published in Dollar's *A Handbook of Horseshoeing*,[5] a wonderful collection of drawings and excellent descriptions of shoeing, conformation, and lameness of the equine foot. Adams references the work of Lacroix[6] in the late 1800s. In fact, until Adams' treatise on lameness, scant information about equine lameness existed. The information available in the American literature during most of the 1900s consisted of only sporadic case reports or case series in the *Journal of the American Veterinary Medical Association*. A potential explanation may lie in the importance of the World Wars or other important social events in the early-to-mid 1900s. Experience in the cavalry also may have influenced later writings in the 1900s.

Peters'[7] work detailing lameness in the Thoroughbred racehorse emphasized the importance of lameness in the racetrack practice and the most common cause of poor performance. Many problems he observed in 1939 still exist, although treatment options have expanded considerably. Early important writings included manuscripts by Churchill[8] and Wheat and Rhode[9] on surgical removal of proximal sesamoid bone fractures (the Churchill approach), Forssell[10] on surgical management of navicular bursitis and tendonitis, and Lundvall[11] and later Delahanty[12] debating the subject of the existence or nonexistence of fibular fractures. An early reference of note was the surgical textbook by Frank.[13] Originally written in 1939, with several subsequent editions, this influential and often quoted textbook contained information about numerous musculoskeletal problems and often sensational examples of common and rare abnormalities.

In the late 1800s, several informative, interesting, and entertaining textbooks about equine lameness were written, primarily by European authors. Most publications contained wonderful descriptions of lame horses, and many emphasized shoeing techniques, a mainstay in management of the lame horse both then and now. The writings of Percivall[14] and Gamgee[15] are particularly informative. Although a definitive reason was not provided, Gamgee observed that 42% of horses in the United Kingdom were lame, whereas only 9% of horses in Paris were lame. Disorders of the foot, many of which increased in frequency with age, were most common, and marked remodeling of the distal phalanx was seen in horses undergoing postmortem examination.[15] In addition to the time-honored management technique of shoeing the lame horse, conformation and its relationship to lameness also were emphasized. In *How to Judge a Horse*, Bach[16] emphasized balance, body part length and angulation, and distal extremity conformational faults. In modern day lameness examinations, conformation and its role in the development of lameness are often given cursory emphasis but remain an important part in the art of the examinations. In a chapter entitled "Horse-Docturing [sic] in the Nineteenth Century," Dunlop and Williams[17] emphasized the contribution of Mayhew, described as artist, activist, and veterinary surgeon. Mayhew described and illustrated many common abnormalities of the locomotor system recognized at that time, including splints, spavin, curb, tendon sprains, and thoroughpin, most of which are still recognized today.[17] Of interest, Mayhew was credited for trying "experimental" injections into inflamed areas, an obviously important treatment modality practiced today.[17] Detailed descriptions of laminitis, navicular disease, and other common conditions of the equine foot were provided.[17] Dunlop and Williams,[17] in their treatise on the history of veterinary medicine, also detailed the transition from farriery to veterinary medicine that occurred in the 1700s, although the close association and harmonious working relationships between blacksmiths and equine diagnosticians remain integral parts of a successful lameness management team today. In fact, "the term *veterinarian* came into use when colleges were established in different parts of Europe for improving, or rather for creating the art of treating disease in the lower animals."[17] The first veterinary school was founded in France in 1761, and soon veterinary schools were formed in the United Kingdom.[18]

Although an exhaustive historical review might be interesting, this brief review highlights critical issues central to modern lameness diagnosis. First, the basics have not changed for hundreds of years and will likely not change in the foreseeable future. Second, with the exception of Adams' work, and more recently that of Ross and Dyson, few comprehensive reports on lameness diagnosis were written before the twenty-first century. The modern lameness detective likely has learned most from experience working with accomplished lameness diagnosticians and by word of mouth. Third, many of our most knowledgeable colleagues have not published writings but have made their contributions in day-to-day teachings in academic settings, private practice, and small gatherings at national meetings.

Since 1955 the annual convention of the American Association of Equine Practitioners has played a special role in the dissemination of information and ideas about lameness. Early meetings included a handful of practitioners, gathering and discussing equine medicine and surgery, sometimes late into the night. Much current lameness experience can be traced to these early meetings and practitioners such as Adams, Peters, Frank, Farquharson, Churchill, Goddall, Gabel, and Delahanty. Loren Evans and Howard "Gene" Gill influenced the molding of many modern lameness detectives, including me. Emphasizing the value of acquiring horse sense and spending time palpating and "learning" the horse, Gill often quotes Will Rogers, "… the outside of a horse is good for the inside of a man."

In the United Kingdom the British Equine Veterinary Association was established in 1961, providing a similar formula for dissemination of information through its annual congress and regular day meetings. The establishment of the *Equine Veterinary Journal* in 1968 provided a high-quality, refereed journal. The standard for the journal was set by the first editor, John Hickman, an astute observer of lame horses and an influence on many practitioners.

No substitute exists for careful clinical examination and observation, experience gained over many years of treating and developing a feel for the lame horse. The second edition of this textbook on lameness is once again a collection of the best and most knowledgeable lameness diagnosticians worldwide. Some are "household lameness names," whereas others are less renowned. All have one thing in common: they practice the art of lameness diagnosis and management in the horse.

Chapter 2

Lameness in Horses: Basic Facts Before Starting

Mike W. Ross

References
on page
1255

Lameness is therefore not so much an original evil, a disease per se, as it is a symptom and manifestation of some antecedent vital physical lesion, either isolated or complicated, affecting one or several parts of the locomotive apparatus.

A. Liautard, 1888[1]

DEFINITION

The clinical manifestations of lameness in the horse are well known, but an exact definition is difficult. The word *lame* is an adjective, meaning "crippled or physically disabled, as a person or animal … in the foot or leg so as to limp or walk with difficulty."[2] A medical dictionary defines *lameness* as "incapable of normal locomotion, deviation from the normal gait."[3] The noun *lameness* can be, but infrequently is, used interchangeably with *claudication,* described as "limping or lameness."[3]

Lameness is simply a clinical sign—a manifestation of the signs of inflammation, including pain, or a mechanical defect—that results in a gait abnormality characterized by limping. The definition is simple, but recognition, localization, characterization, and management are complex.

LOCALIZATION OF PAIN

In certain conditions, characteristic gait abnormalities allow immediate and straightforward recognition and localization of the problem. Sweeny, fibrotic myopathy, upward fixation of the patella, stringhalt, shivers, and radial nerve paresis are examples. However, similar gait deficits exist for a variety of lameness problems, complicating recognition and localization. A fundamental concept in lameness diagnosis is the application of diagnostic analgesic techniques to localize the source of pain causing lameness. The sequence of properly determining the lame leg (recognition) and then abolishing the clinical sign of lameness by use of diagnostic analgesia (localization), only to have lameness return when the local anesthetic effects abate, is essential for accurate diagnosis. In essence diagnostic analgesia establishes *clinical relevance,* a most important concept to the lameness diagnostician. With experience and under certain circumstances, this step in lameness diagnosis can be omitted. The degree of lameness, certain gait characteristics, and palpation findings allow the clinician to strongly suspect a certain diagnosis. The next step may be diagnostic imaging. For example, a racehorse with prominent lameness after training may be suspected of having a stress or incomplete fracture. Performing radiographic and scintigraphic examinations before proceeding

with diagnostic analgesia is a prudent choice. Trial and error also occasionally work and in some instances may be the preferred approach. Intraarticular analgesia can be performed in selected joints without disrupting distal-to-proximal perineural techniques later during the same examination. However, because pathognomonic signs are rare, proficiency in diagnostic analgesic techniques is mandatory for the lameness diagnostician.

BASELINE AND INDUCED LAMENESS

Baseline, or primary, lameness is the gait abnormality recognized when the horse is examined at a walk or trot in hand before flexion or manipulative tests are used. The clinician usually recognizes this abnormality by watching the horse on a firm or hard surface, while it is being trotted in a straight line. Diagnostic analgesia is used to abolish this lameness. Changing the surface or nature of the exercise by lunging, or circling the horse at a trot in hand, potentially changes the baseline lameness. The surface and exercise (gait and speed) must be consistent. In some horses no observable lameness is present at a walk or trot in hand. Lameness may be evident when the horse is ridden, and this lameness becomes the baseline lameness.

Flexion tests and other forms of manipulation are used to exacerbate baseline lameness or to induce lameness. An induced lameness is one that is observed after flexion or manipulative tests, but induced lameness may not be the same as the baseline lameness. Manipulative tests are expected to, and often do, exacerbate the primary lameness. However, flexion and manipulative tests can cause development of additional lameness, unrelated to the primary or baseline lameness, and test results must be interpreted carefully.

COEXISTENT LAMENESS

Horses often have several sites of pain, although one usually is most obvious and the cause of baseline lameness. In many horses, secondary or compensatory (sometimes referred to as *complementary*) lameness develops in predictable sites or limbs. Concomitant bilateral forelimb or hindlimb lameness is common, but horses often demonstrate more prominent clinical signs in one limb. In horses with palmar foot pain, initially pronounced single forelimb lameness that is abolished by palmar digital analgesia may be present, with subsequent recognition of contralateral forelimb lameness. In racehorses, bilateral lameness, such as in the carpi or metacarpophalangeal or metatarsophalangeal joints, is common. The clinician should carefully examine the contralateral limb. Predictable compensatory or secondary lameness often exists in the ipsilateral or contralateral forelimb when primary lameness is present in the hindlimb, or vice versa. In a Thoroughbred (TB) racehorse with left forelimb lameness, compensatory problems in the right forelimb and left hindlimb are not uncommon, because these limbs presumably are succumbing to excessive loads while protecting the primary source of pain. In a trotter, diagonal lameness often occurs (primary lameness in the left hindlimb and compensatory lameness in the right forelimb), whereas in pacers, ipsilateral lameness is most common (primary right forelimb and compensatory right hindlimb). When several limbs are involved, identification of the primary or major source of pain is important. If forelimb and hindlimb lameness exist simultaneously, diagnostic analgesic techniques should begin in the hindlimb (see Chapter 10). A common secondary lameness abnormality, proximal suspensory desmitis, can develop in the compensating forelimb or hindlimb.

Coexistent lameness can make assigning primary or baseline lameness to a particular limb during lameness examination difficult (see Chapter 7). Bilaterally symmetrical pain may cause a short, choppy gait, but primary or baseline lameness often cannot be seen when the horse is examined in a straight line in hand. Often, horses with coexistent lameness must be circled, lunged, or ridden for primary or baseline lameness to be observed. The lameness diagnostician may have to arbitrarily assign lameness to a limb and begin diagnostic analgesia in this manner. Often, once the primary source of pain has been identified, horses show pronounced lameness of much greater magnitude than expected in another limb, vivid clinical evidence that coexistent lameness exists.

LAMENESS DISTRIBUTION

Among all types of horses, forelimb lameness is more common than hindlimb lameness. A horse's center of gravity or balance, while dictated to a certain extent by conformation (see Chapter 4), is not located in the center of the horse but is closer to the forelimbs than the hindlimbs. Thus the forelimb/hindlimb (F/H) weight (load) distribution ratio is approximately 60%:40% (Figure 2-1). Higher loads are expected on the individual forelimbs (30% each), predisposing the horse to greater injury.

At certain times during the stride cycle of gaits such as the canter (three-beat gait) and gallop (four-beat gait), a single forelimb is weight bearing, which predisposes the limb to injury. The weight of a rider may shift F/H load distribution to 70%:30% (Figure 2-2). Two-beat gaits, such as the pace and trot, allow more equal load sharing between forelimbs and hindlimbs because a forelimb and hindlimb (ideally, if the gait is balanced perfectly) hit the ground simultaneously. In pacers and trotters the proportion of forelimb lameness is less than in the TB racehorse. The added load of pulling a sulky, cart, or any heavy load increases the likelihood of hindlimb lameness in Standardbreds (STBs), other harness breeds, and draft horses (Figure 2-3). The F/H distribution of lameness in STB racehorses is 55%:45%. Sporting activities such as dressage and jumping also may shift lameness distribution to the hindlimbs because collection (working off the hindlimbs) and propulsion needed by horses to perform these activities may predispose to hindlimb lameness. The tendency of good moving dressage horses to show advanced diagonal placement in trot results in a single hindlimb bearing weight.

In the forelimb, up to 95% of lameness problems occur at the level of or distal to the carpus.[4] The distal parts of the limb always should be excluded as a potential source

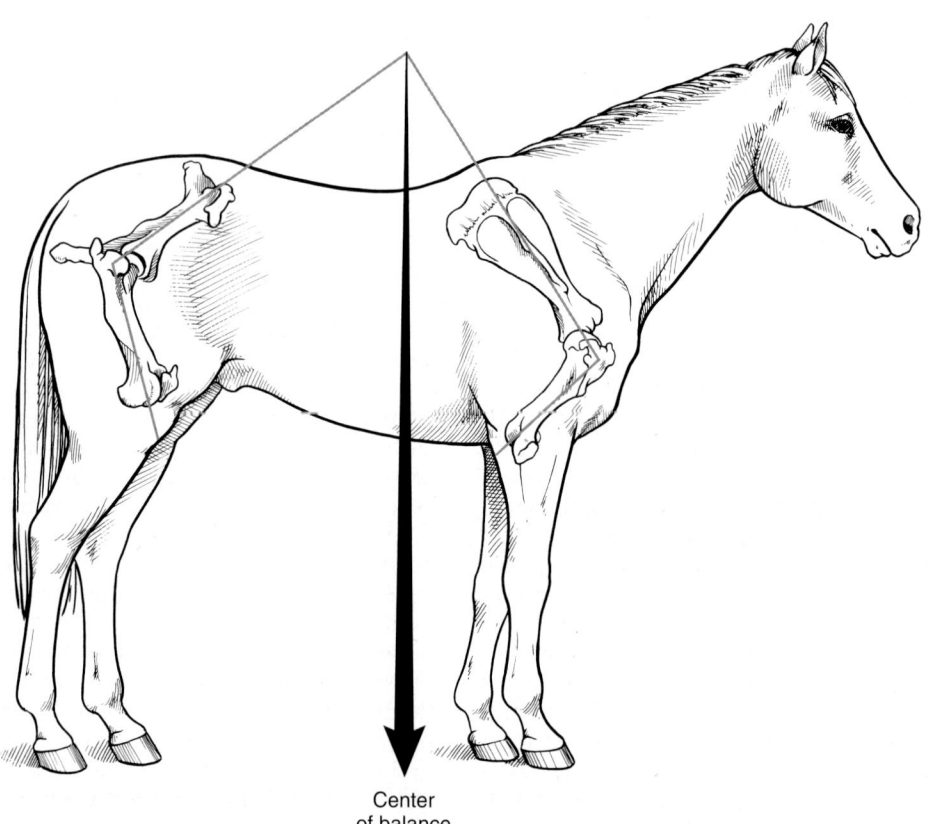

Center
of balance

Fig. 2-1 • The center of balance (gravity) of the horse is located closer to the forelimbs, which accounts for the load distribution difference between the forelimbs and hindlimbs. Conformation, namely the angles of the shoulder and rump, and weight of the head and neck and gait can change this load distribution.

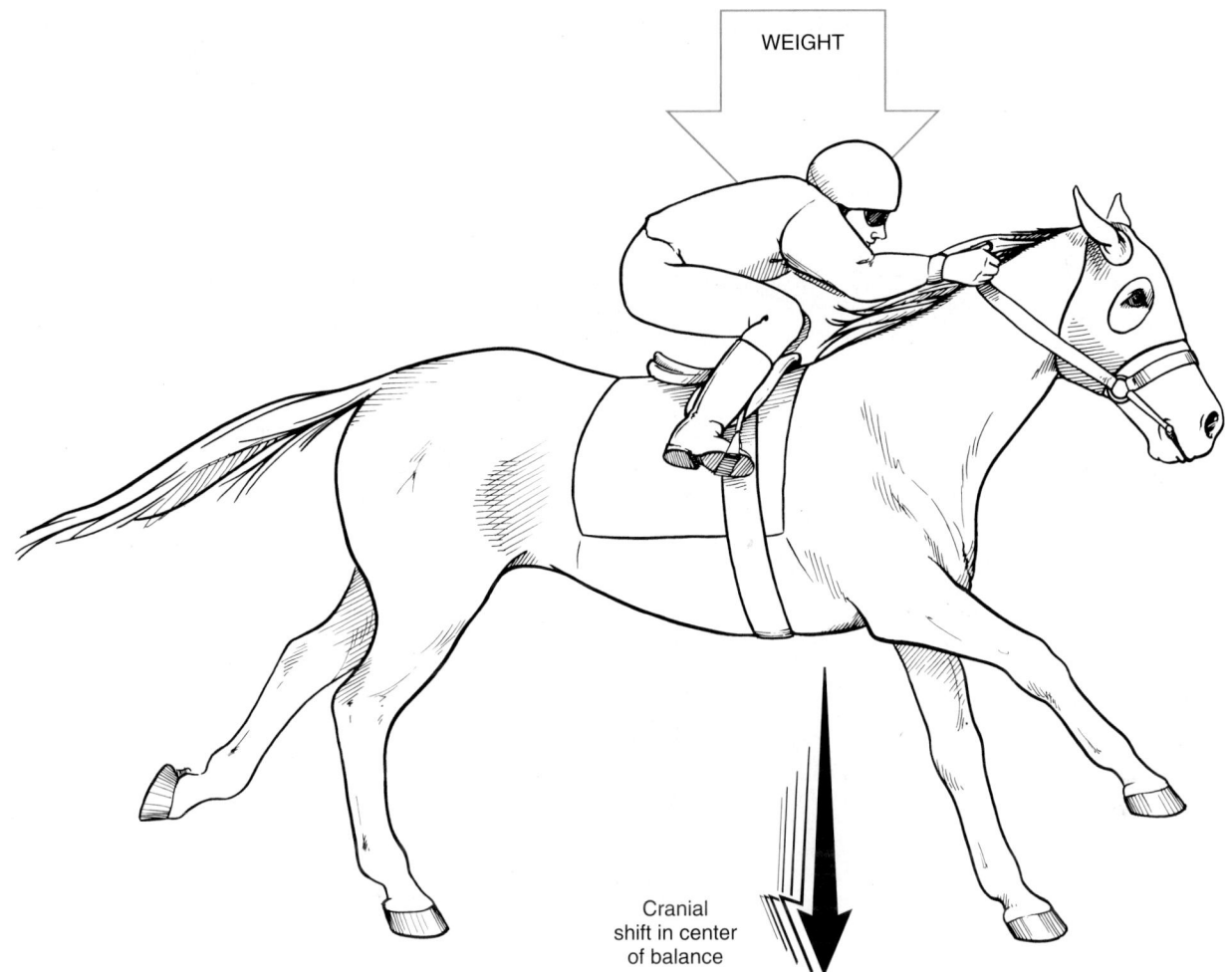

Fig. 2-2 • Gaits such as the canter and gallop (depicted) and the added weight of a rider, as shown here in a Thoroughbred racehorse, increase load on the forelimbs by shifting the center of balance, thus increasing the likelihood of forelimb lameness.

of lameness before the upper limb is addressed, although many owners believe otherwise and may try to mislead an inexperienced practitioner. The foot should be suspected first. Pain in the foot is one of the most common causes of forelimb lameness in all types of horses, and in draft breed horses, the foot is also the most common site of pain in the hindlimb.

Hindlimb Lameness

Hindlimb lameness should not be underplayed, although its recognition is more difficult. In the forelimb lameness–prone TB racehorse, many hindlimb lameness problems are overlooked. However, a rider or jockey often may suspect a hindlimb problem when the lameness actually exists in the forelimb.

A practitioner should consider carefully the distribution of sites of hindlimb lameness. Historically, the hock has been regarded as the major source of problems, and although it is an important source of hindlimb lameness, other sites also are important. For instance, in both the TB and STB racehorse the metatarsophalangeal joint is a major source of lameness that historically has been overlooked.[5,6] Maladaptive or nonadaptive bone remodeling of the distal aspect of the third metatarsal bone cannot be seen

radiologically in early stages and requires careful diagnostic analgesic techniques to achieve localization. Scintigraphic examination is mandatory for definitive diagnosis.[7] Lameness of the metatarsophalangeal joint in STBs is almost as common as that of the hock, but without careful examination and the use of diagnostic analgesia, hock lameness is suspected in many such horses and they are treated for it. In sports horses proximal suspensory desmitis is now recognized as a more important cause of lameness than hock pain. The combined use of diagnostic analgesia, ultrasonography, and scintigraphy has increased clinical knowledge of the broad spectrum of lameness conditions in the hindlimbs.

In the draft horse, lameness in the hindlimb most commonly develops in the foot. Lameness in this area reflects the work performed by these horses, and innate characteristics of the draft horse foot, which predispose the foot to conditions such as laminitis. In jumping and dressage horses, problems in the fetlock region such as osteoarthritis and tenosynovitis are common and reflect the stress imposed by these disciplines. Although owners, trainers, and veterinarians often suspect an upper hindlimb lameness, gait characteristics of lower limb lameness problems often are similar. Only use of diagnostic analgesia allows an accurate diagnosis.

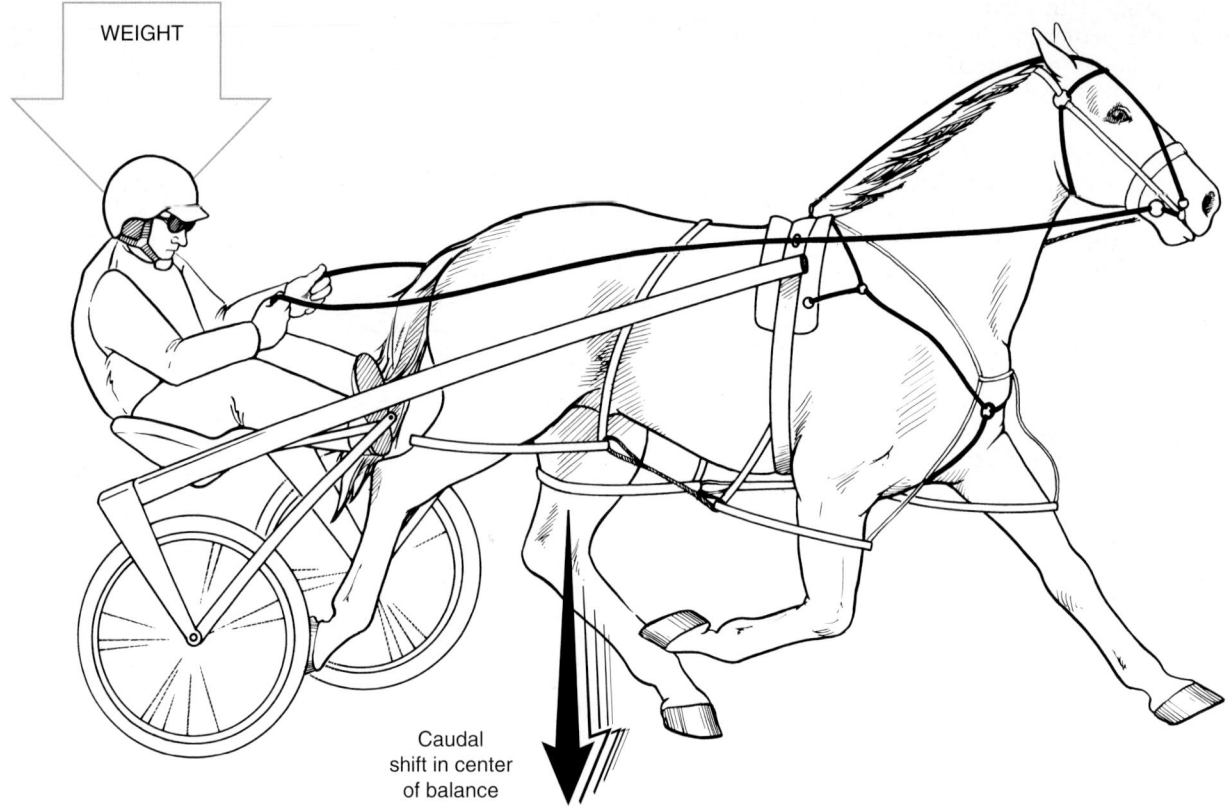

WEIGHT

Caudal
shift in center
of balance

Fig. 2-3 • In a Standardbred racehorse (pacer depicted), the hindlimbs share added load compared with a Thoroughbred racehorse because of a caudal shift in the center of balance. The type of harness with the overcheck bit, the added weight of the sulky and driver, and the necessity of pulling a load increase the likelihood of hindlimb lameness in this breed.

RELATIONSHIP OF LAMENESS AND CONFORMATION

Conformation of the distal extremities, and to a lesser extent the overall body, plays a major role in the development of forelimb and hindlimb lameness (see Chapter 4). When a practitioner examines a weanling or yearling with poor conformation, predicting the time and the exact way the lameness will occur may be difficult, but many well-recognized conformational faults can lead directly to lameness problems. Conformational faults of the carpus, such as carpus varus or valgus, back-at-the-knee, and offset knees, can be important factors in carpal and lower forelimb lameness. In the hindlimbs, excessively straight hindlimbs ("straight behind") and sickle-hocked and in-at-the-hock conformation can lead directly to predictable lameness conditions. Although exceptions do exist, in the case of poor conformation, predictable lameness conditions consistently develop in poorly conformed horses. Evaluation of conformation is therefore an essential part of a lameness examination.

POOR PERFORMANCE

Convincing trainers and owners may be difficult, but the leading cause of poor performance in racehorses is lameness, and lameness is the most prevalent health problem among all horses.[8-11] In one study, 50% of North American

operations with three or more horses had one or more lame horses, and 5% of the horses could be expected to be lame.[10] In another study, 74% of racehorses evaluated for poor racing performance had substantial musculoskeletal abnormalities contributing to poor performance. Lameness examination was emphasized as a most important aspect of comprehensive performance evaluation.[12,13] Others have emphasized the importance of lameness in epidemiological studies evaluating wastage in TB racehorses.[14,15] Recently, lameness was once again found to be the most important condition causing missed training days in TB racehorses training in the United Kingdom.[16] Two-year-olds missed training days significantly more than 3-year-olds, and stress fractures were the most important cause of lameness.[16] Disappointingly, there has been little change in the importance of lameness and missed training days in the United Kingdom over a 20-year period.[16] The same is likely true among all sports horses, particularly those competing at upper levels, although comprehensive studies have not been performed. Obvious lameness need not be demonstrated for performance to be compromised in horses, especially those competing at high speeds or upper levels. The possibility of achieving maximal performance in horses with substantial lameness is a common misconception. I have examined numerous top-level STB and TB racehorses in which easily recognized lameness is seen when the horses are trotted in hand on a hard surface. Notwithstanding the ignorance of many in the horse industry, the ability of many horses with obvious lameness to compete is a tribute to their mental and physical toughness. For example, bilateral forelimb or hindlimb lameness is common in race-horses but in some instances goes unrecognized if the condition is of similar severity in both limbs. Unilateral lameness of this magnitude would be recognized easily, but because the lameness is bilateral, horses still race, albeit at a lower level. Bilateral third carpal slab fractures and sagittal fractures of the proximal phalanx have been diagnosed in horses examined for poor racing performance but, if seen unilaterally, would have caused pronounced lameness. Part of the art of the lameness examination is separating those horses capable of performing with moderate pain at a high level from those that cannot do so.

GAIT DEFICITS NOT CAUSED BY LAMENESS

Gait abnormalities can exist with or without the presence of clinically apparent lameness. Deficits such as stringhalt, mild intermittent upward fixation of the patella, and shivers (see Chapter 48) can be present without obvious lameness and may complicate diagnosis of a completely different primary source of pain causing lameness. Horses with neurological disease may have gait deficits that are considered the result of painful lameness conditions (see Chapter 11). Horses with lower motor neuron diseases, such as equine protozoal myelitis, may have lameness associated with muscle atrophy or unexplained low-grade lameness associated with the disease. Concomitant lameness conditions can and do occur in these horses. Recurrent exertional rhabdomyolysis can cause stiffness and in some instances lameness, or it can cause poor racing performance, all of which can be misinterpreted as lameness (see Chapter 83).

UNEXPLAINED LAMENESS

A diagnosis is made for most, but not all, lame horses through careful clinical examination and ancillary imaging modalities. Even with advanced imaging techniques, a solution is not always found (see Chapter 12), but it is hoped that future innovations in clinical examination and imaging will result in the continued expansion of the science of lameness diagnosis.

COMPONENTS OF THE LAMENESS EXAMINATION AND LAMENESS STRATEGY

Lameness Examination

Lameness examinations should be performed in an orderly, step-by-step way, but many factors may change or abbreviate the examination (Box 2-1). Owner financial constraints may not allow performance of certain diagnostic tests and may curtail the time necessary to complete the entire examination. Drug testing of competing racehorses or show horses may limit a practitioner's ability to perform diagnostic analgesic techniques and restrict management options. Clients do not always understand the need for diagnostic analgesia. Education about the value of this technique, and the difficulties of interpretation of the results of diagnostic imaging without it, is vital.

Abbreviated lameness examinations often are performed in horses that exhibit severe lameness compatible with a

---

> **BOX 2-1**
> ### Components of the Lameness Examination
>
> History—anamnesis
> Examination from a distance—conformation, symmetry, posture
> Palpation
>   Hoof tester examination
> Physical examination—other ancillary testing
> Movement
>   Baseline
>   Additional movement
> Selected examinations—manipulation, flexion, direct pressure, wedge
> Diagnostic analgesia
> Imaging
> Diagnosis
>   Certain, presumptive, open
> Management
> Follow-up examination

fracture. Typical or obvious clinical signs may accompany severe lameness, and in many instances prolonged or extensive lameness examination is contraindicated. If incomplete fractures are suspected, diagnostic analgesic techniques may be dangerous and should be performed only in certain situations. A clinician may proceed directly to conventional or advanced imaging techniques before completing the initial steps of a conventional lameness examination.

Many other factors affect the ability to complete a comprehensive evaluation. Time constraints (usually of the veterinarian) often are cited, although shortcuts, if taken, usually create future problems. Omission of a diagnostic block or failure to perform detailed palpation often leads to misdiagnosis. Omission of a brief physical examination, including assessment of the horse's temperature, can lead to embarrassing situations.

The footing available on which to complete the lameness examination can be problematic. A dry, flat, hard surface or space for lunging or riding may be unavailable. The horse's temperament may preclude adequate movement and often limits the practitioner's ability to perform diagnostic analgesia. Many ill-tempered horses are referred for advanced imaging techniques, such as scintigraphic examination, because diagnostic analgesic techniques are dangerous to the veterinarian and handler.

Lameness Etiquette

Owners frequently request an opinion from more than one veterinarian. Therefore professional, ethical conduct is important, with practitioner acknowledgment that horses can appear very different every day and that response to diagnostic analgesia is not always consistent. For example, differences of opinion concerning radiological interpretation can exist. A good working relationship with the client or agent is essential but should extend also to the farrier and any paraprofessionals involved in the management of the horse, even when opinions differ.

Prognosis Assessment

Assessment of prognosis for performance is important, but because few published data relating to many sports disciplines are available, clinicians often must rely on personal experience based on an understanding of the sport. Owners and trainers should consider prognosis carefully when making decisions to pursue therapeutic options, particularly when a long layoff period is required. I prefer to define prognosis as the "chance the horse will return to its previous level of competition." However, this may not be a fair or reasonable definition.

Retrospective studies can be used to evaluate prognosis after surgical or conservative management for various conditions in racehorses. Objective data such as numbers of race starts, race times, earnings per start, and time from treatment to first race start can be assessed. Earnings per start is an important criterion because it establishes racing class or level of competition. However, in most retrospective studies, earnings per start decrease after treatment. The question is whether practitioners can accurately state that the horse will drop in class after treatment and whether this drop in class is the result of the injury, treatment, or aging of the horse an additional year before returning to racing. Use of this information is not easy.

Most owners and trainers have a different view of prognosis than the veterinarian. In considering the prognosis for a horse undergoing arthroscopic surgical removal of a small osteochondral fracture of the carpus, most owners emphasize the surgery rather than the original injury. Clinicians must explain thoroughly the magnitude of the injury and related damage and discuss prognosis, using terminology that clearly indicates that the extent of injury is the factor that determines prognosis.

Expecting a racehorse to return to its previous racing class may be an unrealistic expectation or at least a very strict definition for success. In a retrospective study of postoperative racing performance of STBs treated for carpal chip fractures, 74% of horses made at least one race start after surgery.[17] Median earnings per start significantly decreased, but the median race mark (best winning time) also significantly decreased, indicating that horses made less money but raced faster after surgery.[17] These results must be compared with a normal population of STBs as the horses age, without considering injury, because STB racing performance is not standard over time.[18] Average earnings per start is highest in 2-year-old horses and decreases exponentially until retirement.[18] A population of horses undergoing any long-term layoff that requires recommencement of racing the following year can be expected naturally (unrelated to the original injury) to have lower earnings per start, regardless of whether an injury occurred or treatment was given. Therefore retrospective studies may underestimate prognosis associated with injuries and management choices.

Success criteria and outcome assessment must be standardized to compare treatment results and to define prognosis. The current standard for racehorses is comparison of performance for five starts before and after injury and treatment. This criterion is strict; a practitioner first may prefer to predict the chance of the horse returning to racing and then assess the chance that the horse will perform at or near its previous level.

Other statistical methods have been used to evaluate racing performance in TBs using a regression model accounting for variables such as track surface, race distance, and age.[19-21] To date, this performance analysis has been restricted to evaluation of horses after upper respiratory tract surgery but probably will be applied to horses with musculoskeletal injuries.

When comparing published information regarding management of various types of lameness, the clinician should be clear about criteria for inclusion of cases and be sure to compare "apples to apples." For instance, comparing results of management of horses with chronic, recurrent hindlimb suspensory desmitis to those with acute forelimb suspensory desmitis is unfair.

Chapter 3

Anamnesis (History)

Mike W. Ross

The importance of a detailed clinical history, the anamnesis, cannot be overemphasized. Information is divided into two categories: basic facts necessary for every horse, and additional information from questions tailored to the specific horse. The veterinarian must understand the breed, use, and level of competition of each horse, because prognosis varies greatly among different types of sports horses. Firsthand experience of the particular type of sports horse being examined is useful but is not essential. Clinicians must understand the language associated with the particular sporting event, and this may be a challenge. For some sporting events, understanding the clinical history and having the ability to ask the right questions are like speaking a different language. A veterinarian unfamiliar with the sporting activity should briefly review the type of activities performed and the array of potential lameness problems encountered with them (see Chapters 106 to 129). In some instances the veterinarian may lose credibility when talking to trainers or riders, particularly those involved in upper-level competition, if they perceive unfamiliarity.

The veterinarian must understand the difference between subjective and objective information in the clinical history. Objective information is gained from the horse, and subjective information is perceived by the rider or owner. Knowledge about a horse's performance such as "the horse is bearing out," "the horse is on the right line," "the horse is lugging in," "the horse has just started to refuse fences," or "the horse no longer takes the right lead" is valuable objective information. Common examples of information perceived by the owner or rider include "the horse feels off behind," "the horse is stiff behind," or "the horse is lame behind" and it "feels up high." Such information generally is useful and indicates a change in the horse's gait, but only an experienced rider or trainer can discriminate accurately between forelimb and hindlimb lameness at any gait. Erroneous information obtained from the rider can complicate communication during lameness examination, particularly if the individual is strong-willed and seemingly authoritative; this situation occurs if riders or trainers insist they are correct and the veterinarian disagrees. In my experience, many horses considered to have hindlimb lameness by a rider actually are lame in front, but convincing a disbelieving trainer is difficult. Similarly, lameness perceived as "up high" (in the upper hindlimb, pelvis, or back) in most horses originates from the lower part of the hindlimb. The veterinarian must understand that everyone is trying to resolve the problem, but sometimes diplomacy is needed for successful communication. The veterinarian must be forthright and objective to determine the current source of lameness, even if the determination contradicts well-intentioned but strong-willed trainers.

Clinical history is important but should not override clinical findings. In racehorses that perform at high speed, physical examination generally supports the finding that a horse bears away from the source of pain. During counterclockwise racing or training and with left forelimb lameness, a Thoroughbred (TB) will lug out (away from the inside of the track) and a Standardbred (STB) will be on the "left line" (bearing out; the driver must pull harder on the left line). Some horses, however, especially STBs with medial right forelimb pain, bear out particularly in the turns, presumably because the source of pain is medial or on the compression side of the limb.

The veterinarian must seek out as much information as possible, particularly if the problem is complex or not readily apparent. Videotapes are useful, particularly if the gait deficit, behavioral problem, or any other circumstances necessary to elicit the suspected lameness cannot be duplicated during the examination. Paraprofessionals working with the horse provide useful information, but not everyone may agree about the source of the problem, and in some instances diplomacy is key to negotiating among concerned individuals.

CLINICAL HISTORY: BASIC INFORMATION
Signalment

Age
The age, sex, breed, and use of the horse are basic vital facts (Box 3-1). Flexural deformities, physitis, other manifestations of osteochondrosis, and angular limb deformities are age-related problems. Infectious arthritis (hematological origin), lateral luxation of the patella, and rupture of the common digital extensor tendon are conditions usually unique to foals. Emphasis on training skeletally immature, 2- and 3-year-old racehorses causes predictable soft tissue and bone changes, often resulting in stress-related cortical or subchondral bone injury. Liautard observed more than 100 years ago: "When an undeveloped colt, whose stamina is not yet established and constitution not yet confirmed, with tendons and ligaments relatively tender and weak, and bones scarcely out of the gristle, is unwisely condemned to hard labor, it is irrational to expect any other results than lesions of one or another portion of the abused apparatus of locomotion. They will be fortunate if they

---

BOX 3-1

Anamnesis: Basic and Specific Information

Basic Information

Signalment: age, sex, breed, use
Current lameness: what is the problem?
  History of trauma
  Duration of lameness
  Deterioration or improvement of lameness
  Circumstances when lameness worsens or improves
  Effects of exercise: worsening or improvement in lameness
  Management changes
    Changes in shoeing and related issues
    Changes in training or performance intensity
    Changes in surface
    Changes in diet and health
    Changes in housing
  Current medication and response; response to rest
Past lameness problems

Specific Information

Type of sporting activity
  Level of competition: current and future
Additional sources
  Videotapes
  Images
  Records
  Discussions with others

BOX 3-2

Summary of Lameness Conditions of the Geriatric Horse

Chronic, progressive osteoarthritis
  Proximal and distal interphalangeal joints
  Metacarpophalangeal joint
  Carpometacarpal joint*
  Coxofemoral joint*
  Femorotibial joints
  Tarsus
  Progressive osteoarthritis—previous injury (usually retired racehorses)
Navicular disease
Unexplained, severe soft tissue injuries*
  Superficial digital flexor tendonitis
  Flexural deformity
  Suspensory desmitis
Fractures during recovery from general anesthesia

*Some of these conditions are unique to the older horse and often are unexplainable.

---

escape a fate still worse, and become sufferers from nothing worse than mere lameness."[1] This statement aptly summarizes the situation then and now. The high value of races for 2- and 3-year-olds results in high-intensity training for early 2-year-olds, which may result in injury such as maladaptive or nonadaptive remodeling of the third carpal bone (C3), precluding racing at a young age.

Some problems are unique to older horses (Box 3-2). Overall, osteoarthritis (OA) and other degenerative

References on page 1255

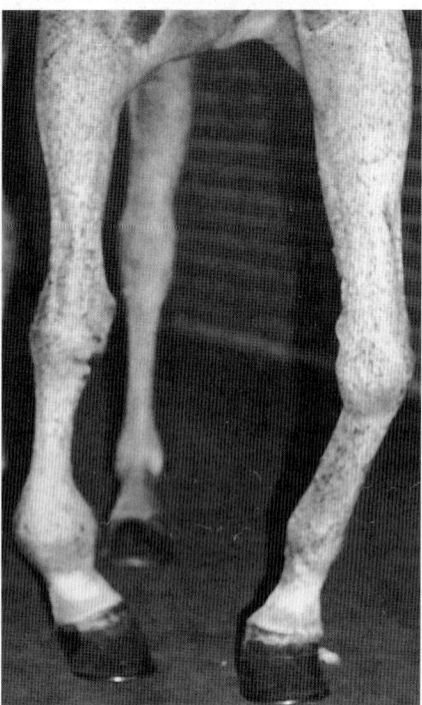

Fig. 3-1 • An aged Thoroughbred broodmare with severe forelimb deformity caused by primary severe osteoarthritis of the right metacarpophalangeal joint and secondary or compensatory (chronic overload) carpus varus in the left forelimb.

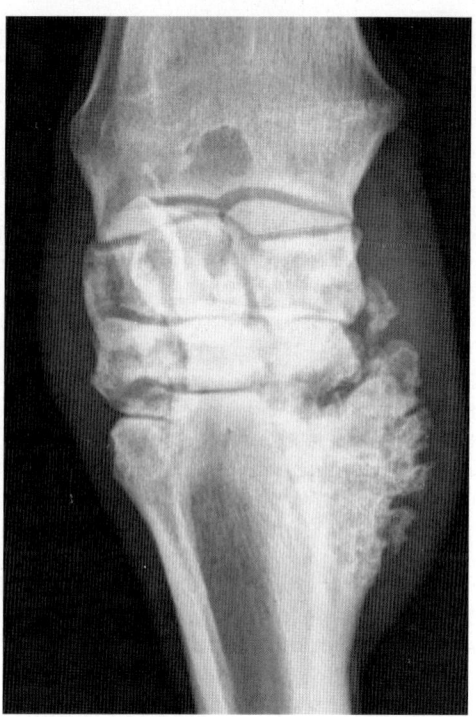

Fig. 3-2 • Dorsopalmar digital radiographic image of the right carpus in a 13-year-old Arabian mare with pronounced lameness as a result of severe, progressive osteoarthritis of the carpometacarpal and middle carpal joints (medial is to the right). There is substantial varus limb deformity present. Comfort improved after partial carpal arthrodesis. (Courtesy Dr. Dean Richardson.)

conditions such as navicular disease are most common but certainly are not unique to the geriatric horse. Some horses have a remarkably early onset of navicular disease or OA despite little physical work, suggesting a genetic predisposition to the condition. These problems worsen with advancing age, particularly if several limbs are involved. In former racehorses, progressive OA is of particular concern; this condition most commonly affects the carpal and metacarpophalangeal joints (Figure 3-1). Occasionally in older horses, severe, progressive OA of the carpometacarpal joint occurs without any history of carpal lameness (Figure 3-2). In some horses, angular deformities (the most common is carpus varus) develop at the carpometacarpal joint. Inexplicably severe OA of the carpometacarpal and middle carpal joints is most commonly seen in Arabian horses (see Chapter 38). Primary OA of this joint is rare in young horses, even in racehorses with middle carpal joint abnormalities, unless C3 slab fracture or infectious arthritis occurs. OA of the coxofemoral joint is rare in horses with the exception of young horses with osteochondrosis, but it does occur in older horses.

An unusual group of soft tissue injuries of unknown origin occurs in older horses. Superficial digital flexor tendonitis and suspensory desmitis generally are considered overuse injuries and usually occur in upper-level performance horses or racehorses. However, severe tendonitis and desmitis do occur, often suddenly and without provocation, in older (teenage) horses. Horses usually are turned out at pasture when initial lameness is observed. In some horses, superficial digital flexor tendonitis is severe and progressive, later leading to flexural deformity because of adhesions. Suspensory desmitis may be unilateral or bilateral, may involve the forelimbs or hindlimbs but is more common in the hindlimbs, and is most common in the older broodmares. The name *degenerative suspensory (ligament) desmitis* (DSD) was given to a syndrome, often seen in older horses and most common in Peruvian Pasos, in which severe, often bilateral suspensory desmitis occurred[2-4] (see Chapter 72). In a recent study horses other than Peruvian Pasos were affected, and an alternative name—*equine systemic proteoglycan accumulation*—was proposed, because abnormal accumulation of proteoglycans in many connective tissues was found.[4] However this has recently been disputed[5]; the suspensory ligaments (SLs) and other tissues from affected Peruvian Pasos and unaffected STB and Quarter Horses were examined using Safranin-O staining for detection of proteoglycan. Proteoglycan deposition was not unique to the affected Peruvian Pasos, being present in the nuchal ligament, heart, muscle, and other tissues, with similar or greater amounts in the control horses. However greater amounts were detected in the SLs of affected horses compared with control horses. It was concluded that cartilage metaplasia and associated proteoglycan deposition in affected SLs was the response to injury rather than the cause. Further work is needed to define this important disease.

Older horses, particularly older broodmares, are at greater risk than younger horses to fracture long bones during recovery from general anesthesia.[6] From 1988 to 1994, 9 of 14 horses with catastrophic fractures or dislocations that developed during recovery from general anesthesia were older than 10 years of age.

Age prominently affects prognosis. A common premise in considering lameness in foals is that young horses have time to outgrow the problem. Maturation will aid in angular limb deformities, some forms of osteochondrosis, and distal phalanx and diaphyseal fractures. However, fractures of important physes such as the proximal tibia may result in progressive angular deformities or disparity in limb length, limiting future prognosis. Early surgical management of flexural deformity of the distal interphalangeal (DIP) joint before 6 to 8 months of age optimizes future soundness and the possibilities for normal hoof conformation. In one study the reported success rate was 80%.[7] If surgical management is undertaken later in life or when deformity is severe, the prognosis decreases substantially. The prognosis for survival of foals treated for infectious arthritis is reasonable, but only 31% of TB foals and 36% of STB foals started one or more races, indicating that the prognosis for future racing performance is poor, because articular healing even in young foals is not possible.[8]

In middle-aged (12 to 18 years of age), upper-level performance horses, prognosis is difficult to assess, particularly in horses with several problems. Level of competition rather than age may be the most important factor, and often performance level declines.

Sex

Most lameness conditions affect stallions, geldings, and mares with similar frequency. Sex-specific conditions are unusual but do exist. The most important consideration, however, regarding the horse's sex is future breeding potential or lack thereof in the case of geldings. In many types of horses, and specifically in racehorses, decisions about future performance or racing potential often are important when management options and financial aspects are considered. This factor is particularly important when life-or-death decisions must be made after catastrophic injury (see Chapters 13 and 104). Frank discussions about the prognosis for return to the current sporting activity or level of performance often are necessary, and the clinician should consider reproductive capability of the horse. Owners are more likely to refrain from racing females and elect treatment for geldings and, in some instances, stallions. Future stallion prospects usually must prove race or performance success, thereby putting pressure on trainers to continue horses in training or racing.

Behavioral abnormalities associated with the estrous cycle in fillies or mares are well recognized and may cause performance problems confused or misinterpreted as lameness (refusing fences, going off stride, striking) (see Chapter 12). An ill-defined behavioral problem in middle-aged nonracehorse mares could explain sudden performance problems often associated with or misinterpreted as lameness.[9] Recurrent exertional rhabdomyolysis (RER) is more common in female TB racehorses[10] and event horses.[11] An association between sex and RER in STBs may exist and RER may be more common in fillies administered anabolic steroids.

Obscure or unexplained hindlimb lameness has been attributed, rightly or wrongly, to retained testicles. The origin of lameness in these horses is difficult to prove without removing the retained testicle, and anecdotal reports suggest that hindlimb lameness has resolved after castration in some horses. The origin of pain in an abdominal cryptorchid is difficult to explain and questionable. The source of pain may be easier to understand in a horse with a testicle located within the inguinal canal. Activity of the external and internal abdominal oblique muscles and tension on the spermatic cord are possible explanations.

Breed and Use

Most lameness conditions affect all breeds of horses. Although breed has considerable influence on sporting activity, sporting activity or use primarily has the greatest impact on lameness distribution (see Chapters 106 through 129).

Current Lameness

Determination of the Problem

Accurate information is necessary to determine precisely the horse's current problem. Obtaining reliable information may be difficult if the horse has been purchased recently, if the horse has been claimed or changed trainers, or if you are giving a second opinion and have no past history with the horse. Additional objective information may be necessary to assess the effect of lameness on the horse's performance. Evaluation of the horse's race record may indicate when the problem began and if it is ongoing or new. The groom, rider (if not the owner), assistant trainer, blacksmith, and other paraprofessionals may have other pertinent information. Horses with poor performance usually are lame, although respiratory problems, rhabdomyolysis, shoeing, tack or equipment, and other medical problems can contribute.

The horse's past history is important in determining the cause of the current problem, particularly in racehorses training or racing with existing low-grade OA that develop new overload injury to supporting limbs (secondary or compensatory lameness). Existing problems such as OA worsen insidiously but may reach critical levels, causing sudden, severe unexpected lameness. OA of the metacarpophalangeal joint may exist for months in racehorses without causing obvious lameness, although in many horses joint effusion ultimately leads to treatment ("maintenance injections"). The horse suddenly may be much lamer after racing or training, and the trainer may assume the cause is different. Because intraarticular analgesia may only partially relieve lameness, persuading the trainer that the problem is still the fetlock may be difficult. Horses can endure extensive cartilage damage in any joint for many months, but at some point they reach a threshold level beyond which they cannot tolerate the pain.

History of Trauma

Many lameness problems develop during or shortly after a traumatic incident, but unfortunately many owners presume trauma played a role even when no one witnessed an alleged incident. A common but often erroneous assumption when examining a lame foal is that the dam stepped on it, but usually infection is the cause. Clinical signs of osteochondritis dissecans of the shoulder or stifle often are expressed after a traumatic incident, and yet most lame weanlings or yearlings are assumed to be lame because of trauma, not a developmental problem. Some lameness problems appear after specific forms of trauma. Palmar carpal fractures occur most commonly in jumpers, but horses recovering from general anesthesia are at risk for this injury. Horses may be only mildly lame immediately after recovery, and the extent of injury is often not discovered until nonsteroidal antiinflammatory medication is discontinued, sometimes 7 to 10 days after the surgical procedure. A common history of horses with subluxation of the scapulohumeral joint (often called *Sweeny* or *suprascapular nerve injury*) is sudden profound lameness after being outside in a thunderstorm. Injury likely occurs when a horse runs into a solid object such as a tree, fence post, or building.

Duration

The veterinarian must understand the duration of the current lameness problem and determine whether a preexisting chronic, low-grade lameness exists and a sudden exacerbation of this problem has occurred, or a completely unrelated new problem has developed.

Worsening of Condition

The veterinarian must establish if the horse's current problem is worsening or improving, under which conditions or circumstances the lameness deteriorates or improves, and if the horse responds to treatment such as shoeing or management changes. Most lameness problems worsen with time, particularly if training or performance continues despite owner or trainer recognition. Racehorses with stress-related bone injury often are noticeably lame after work but become sound relatively quickly, within 1 to 3 days. A minimal number of other clinical signs are present, particularly because the most commonly affected bones (tibia, humerus) are difficult to palpate and buried by soft tissue. This cycle of lame-sound-work-lame is an important part of the history.

Improvement of lameness with rest is important from historical and therapeutic perspectives. Lameness in most horses with severe articular damage, usually from severe OA, does not improve substantially with rest. Severe OA most commonly appears in the fetlock, femorotibial, and tarsocrural joints. Horses with fractures or mild to moderate soft tissue injuries generally improve with rest.

Warming into Lameness

Warming into lameness means the horse's lameness worsens during the exercise period. *Warming out of lameness* means the lameness improves. This concept is important. Lameness associated with stress or incomplete fractures, soft tissue injuries (tendonitis and suspensory desmitis), splints, curb, and foot soreness worsens with exercise. In racehorses a worsening lameness appears as progressive bearing in or out during training or racing. In riding horses, this may be progressive stumbling, problems taking leads, progressive asymmetry in diagonals, or refusing to jump later fences. Horses with OA may be stiff and obviously lame at a walk, but lameness may improve with work. In western performance horses, OA of the proximal and distal interphalangeal joints and in some horses navicular syndrome cause lameness with this characteristic. The most dramatic example is distal hock joint pain, particularly in racehorses. Horses may be noticeably lame at a walk and trot, warm out of the lameness to the point of racing

successfully, and then show pronounced lameness after a race.

One frequent statement at the racetrack is that the horse throws the lameness away at speed. This decrease occurs with some lameness conditions, such as distal hock joint pain, but two other factors are important. A horse may be able to race with lameness but not be able to perform at peak, particularly if lameness is bilateral. Horses often can race with bilateral conditions and show minimal signs of lameness, but performance is reduced. Lameness at the gallop may be impossible to perceive, and even at the fast trot or pace, most persons have difficulty seeing lameness. The same limitation occurs in observing a dressage or jumping horse at the canter. The veterinarian may gain some information by observing that a horse is reluctant to take either the left or right lead, but lameness is difficult if not impossible to detect at the canter. Unless slow-motion video analysis is available, the horse appears to be able to "throw lameness away," but lameness *is* present but difficult to see. In this situation, horses do not warm out of lameness but simply cope with the pain while racing. Horses in this situation are at risk for developing compensatory problems.

Older horses with OA may have difficulty in getting up and later may warm out of the lameness. Horses of any age with pelvic fractures or severe lameness may have difficulty in rising.

Recent Management Changes

Many lameness conditions start after a change in management. Changes in shoeing, training or performance intensity, surface, housing, and diet or other medical issues can have a profound effect on the musculoskeletal system. Changes in ownership often dictate changes in exercise intensity and certainly in owner expectations. The veterinarian must be careful in questioning and responding to questions if a horse has been purchased recently, especially if a colleague performed a prepurchase examination. Clinicians should avoid implying that a condition may have been preexisting or missed.

Shoeing

The veterinarian should determine when the horse was last shod and whether the shoeing strategy was changed. Nail bind often causes acute progressive lameness related temporally to shoe application. Abscesses that result from a "close nail" may take several days to cause lameness.

Foot balance is critical and, in some horses, changing foot angles results in lameness. A substantial increase or decrease in heel angle in a horse with chronic laminitis may exacerbate lameness. In horses with palmar foot pain, raising the heel angle may produce an obvious improvement in clinical signs briefly, whereas in horses with subchondral pain of the distal phalanx, raising the heel may worsen clinical signs. In racehorses with "sore feet" resulting from soft tissue and bone pain, changing shoes may result in improvement, related in part to temporary reduction in weight bearing in the painful area of the foot.

Temporary lameness often occurs in horses with recently trimmed but unshod hooves, particularly if the horses' hooves are trimmed aggressively or the ground is unusually hard for that time of year. The veterinarian must remember that a horse with recently trimmed hooves often shows bilateral forelimb lameness when trotted on flat or uneven hard surfaces, regardless of the primary cause of the current lameness. The horse should be reassessed on a soft surface.

Attempts to make both front feet symmetrical may create substantial lameness immediately after trimming. Horses may cope well with different size and shaped front feet, but when radical trimming is performed, they may develop severe lameness.

The veterinarian must determine whether any recent or past changes in shoeing either improved or worsened lameness. Lameness in a STB trotter with foot pain may be improved by changing from conventional shoes, such as half-round or flat steel shoes in the front to a "flip-flop" shoe.

The farrier often first notices a common problem that a horse is reluctant to pick up the hindlimbs. In some horses this problem is purely behavioral, whereas in others it is a real sign of pain. This history most often is associated with conditions such as OA of one or more joints but also may be a sign of pelvic or sacroiliac pain. In Warmbloods, draft breeds, and draft-cross horses, reluctance to pick up a hindlimb may be an early sign of shivers.

Training or Performance Intensity

Lameness that worsens in response to recent increase in training intensity may be related to stress-related subchondral or cortical bone injury. Stress fractures, bucked shins, or maladaptive or nonadaptive stress-related injuries of subchondral bone occur typically during defined periods of training and often after brief periods of rest. When horses in active race training are given time off, even brief periods such as 7 to 21 days, bone undergoes detraining, leaving it subject to stress-related injury. If training resumes at the prerest level or is accelerated, stress fractures or bucked shins often develop. In 3-year-old TBs, stress fractures of the humerus often occur within 4 to 8 weeks after returning to training. Bucked shins often develop in 2-year-old TB racehorses after a brief rest period for an unrelated medical condition.

Surface

Most lameness conditions worsen if the horse performs on a harder surface. In show horses such as the Arabian or half-Arabian breeds, foot lameness often results when horses are warmed up or shown on harder surfaces. An association exists between fracture development and hard racing surfaces. A dramatic change in any racing surface may lead to unexpected episodic lameness in racehorses. On breeding farms, anecdotal evidence suggests drought conditions causing harder than normal pastures lead to a higher prevalence of osteochondrosis or distal phalanx fractures.

Lameness that is most pronounced on hard surfaces is often seen with conditions of the foot. Lameness that worsens on softer surfaces, however, may be associated with soft tissue injuries such as proximal suspensory desmitis. Uneven surfaces may exacerbate lameness and other gait abnormalities. Horses prone to stumbling on uneven surfaces may have palmar foot pain, proximal suspensory desmitis, or neurological disease. Horses with bilateral lameness may be lame in one leg going in a particular direction on a banked surface (such as a racetrack) and lame in the opposite leg going the other way. Bilateral lameness may be confused with other causes of poor performance because of inconsistencies in gait. Lameness may worsen or improve when a horse goes uphill or downhill.

Diet and Health

Changes in diet or dietary factors may lead to or exacerbate existing lameness conditions. Dietary factors, especially dietary excesses or deficiencies, are important in the many manifestations of developmental orthopedic disease (see Chapter 55). Sudden changes in diet, such as those associated with turning horses out on lush pastures or consumption of large quantities of grain (grain overload), may cause laminitis or exacerbate existing chronic laminitis. Overweight horses normally consuming a high-grain diet may be prone to laminitis or gastrointestinal tract disturbances that lead to laminitis.

Lameness may be associated with, or result from, other medical conditions. Obvious associations exist in foals; for example, conditions such as infectious arthritis and physitis are associated with umbilical, gastrointestinal, or respiratory tract infections. Immune-mediated synovitis also occurs in older foals with chronic infections (see Chapter 66). In adult horses, infectious arthritis generally develops after intraarticular injections or penetrating wounds, but may result from hematological spread of bacteria. Occasionally, horses develop distal extremity edema and lameness after vaccination, presumably caused by vasculitis or other immune-related mechanisms. Similar signs appear in horses with purpura hemorrhagica or viral illnesses such as equine viral arteritis.

Housing

Many lameness conditions develop while a horse is turned out, or as the result of turnout, often as the result of trauma such as kick wounds or fence-related injuries. Sudden changes in weather may excite horses, particularly those turned out at pasture. Minimizing problems with turnout requires the use of well-groomed and well-maintained pastures or paddocks with individual paddocks to reduce horse-to-horse interactions.

Dramatic housing changes have a substantial impact on the development of lameness. Shipping to and from sales, foaling, and weaning are associated with soft tissue injuries, puncture or kick wounds, and other injuries.

Current Medication Changes and Response

The veterinarian must establish if the horse currently is receiving medication or was administered medication recently and the response to treatment. Response to medication or a management change is important information in formulating a treatment plan. For example, recent improvement with rest and the administration of nonsteroidal antiinflammatory drugs indicates more of the same treatment may be reasonable. The veterinarian must establish dosages of medication because a horse may not respond to phenylbutazone because of underdosage.

Many owners and trainers do not understand that although intraarticular analgesia relieves lameness, intraarticular medication may not, thus causing doubt about the diagnosis. This characteristic commonly appears in horses with subchondral bone pain and is useful in diagnosis. Horses with early OA and negative or equivocal radiological signs, or those with short, incomplete fractures, often do not respond to intraarticular medication. Negative radiological findings are a good sign because dramatic radiological evidence of subchondral lucency or fracture reduces the prognosis considerably. However, convincing the trainer of the validity of the diagnosis may be difficult.

The amount of rest is important. Many acquired conditions, such as OA, or degenerative conditions, such as navicular syndrome, take many months and usually years to develop. Therefore expectation that a horse will show marked improvement with a brief rest period is unreasonable. Lameness in many horses with severe OA may not improve substantially, even with prolonged rest. In horses with early OA in which pain occurs primarily in subchondral bone and for which radiological findings are negative or equivocal, rest or controlled exercise for 3 to 6 months may be necessary. The same regimen applies for horses with navicular syndrome, fractures, and many soft tissue injuries.

Quality of rest is equally important. Did the horse receive absolute box stall rest with handwalking, or was it lunged or turned out in a paddock or field with other horses? Was a brief rest period followed by an attempt to ride or train the horse? Those associated with the horse often consider this type of intermittent rest *complete* rest, but many conditions remain chronically active. Without adequate rest, reinjury follows temporary improvement and early healing, highlighting that, in my opinion, *turnout is the antithesis of healing!*

Past Lameness History

Obtaining the horse's entire lameness history may not be necessary or possible, but the veterinarian should gather as much information as is practically available. Prognosis for many injuries is affected adversely by recurrence, and often management options differ in these situations. Recurrence may prompt more aggressive therapy, considerations for referral, or perhaps surgical evaluation if the problem involves a joint. If a reliable diagnosis was made previously, retreatment for the past problem may be a reasonable or preferred management approach, particularly between races or competitions. If a horse responded previously to intraarticular medication, reinjection may be reasonable. However, in many horses with progressive OA, results of

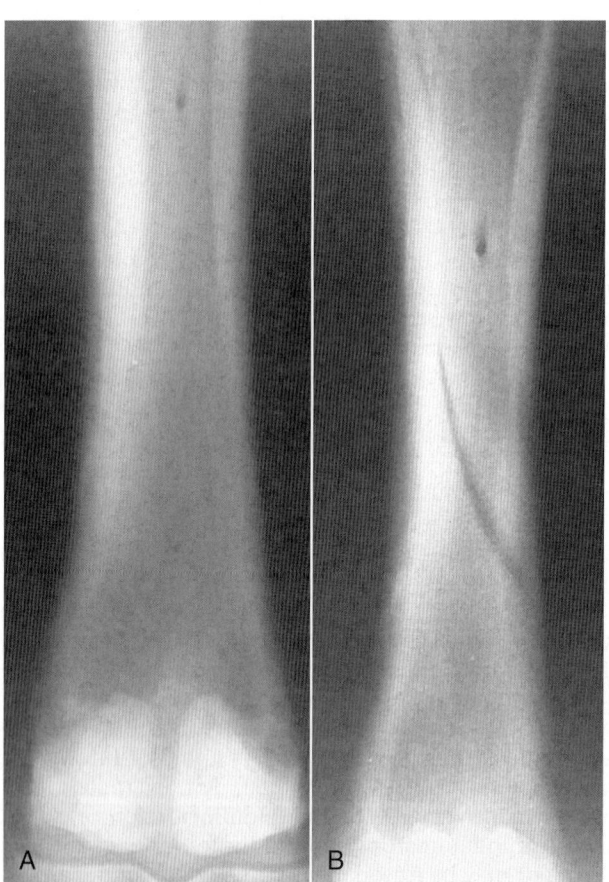

Fig. 3-3 • Initial **(A)** and 2-week follow-up **(B)** dorsopalmar radiographic image of the left third metacarpal bone in an 18-year-old Thoroughbred gelding. The initial image was obtained after the horse was found to have a small skin wound in the region but was sound. Acute, severe lameness developed 9 days after initial injury, and the follow-up radiograph shows a long oblique fracture of the third metacarpal bone. (Courtesy Dr. Janet Durso, 2001.)

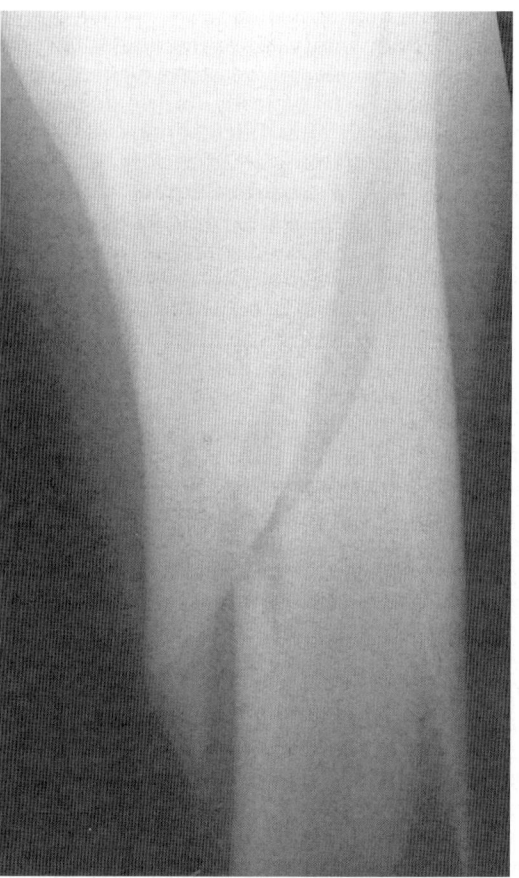

Fig. 3-4 • Craniocaudal radiographic image of the left antebrachium of a 5-year-old Thoroughbred mare showing a displaced, long oblique fracture of the radius. This filly had sustained a small puncture wound to the lateral aspect of the antebrachium 5 days earlier but was sound. The mare was turned out and developed acute, severe lameness and was later euthanized.

additional therapy often are diminished. The veterinarian should not assume that the failed response to intraarticular medication means the problem lies elsewhere because medication does not affect subchondral bone pain in early or late OA.

Recent history is important. Small, innocuous-looking wounds over the third metacarpal bone or third metatarsal bone, radius, or tibia may be associated with bone trauma with delayed-onset severe lameness. Incomplete or spiral fractures may develop from small cortical defects (Figure 3-3). Catastrophic failure of long bones occurs even when initial radiographs show no or minimal cortical trauma. The radius appears to be at greatest risk (Figure 3-4).

New problems may and often do arise despite a long history of recurrent lameness. Comprehensive reevaluation is the best and safest approach to avoid delays in proper diagnosis and treatment.

FURTHER INFORMATION

Full understanding of a horse's use, type and level of sporting activity, and value, all of which help the veterinarian assess prognosis, requires specific information. If a horse previously was under the veterinary care of another individual in the same or a different practice, it is important to obtain accurate case records and view previous radiographs and other images.

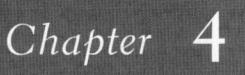

Conformation and Lameness

Mike W. Ross and C. Wayne McIlwraith

References on page 1255

The idea of a good horse with poor legs is a misnomer; the legs are the essence of the horse, and every other part of the equine machine is of only subservient and tributary importance.

A. Liautard[1]

The thought that the way a horse is conformed determines the way it moves is well accepted. The relationship of conformation, especially of the distal extremities, and lameness also is well recognized. "Conformation determines the shape, wear, flight of the foot, and distribution of weight."[2] Veterinarians often are asked to comment on conformation during lameness and prepurchase examinations, especially with regard to the suitability of the horse to perform the intended task. In some instances, as in the case of presale yearling evaluations, the veterinarian's opinion is paramount, and purchase is contingent on judgment of the yearling's potential to perform as a racehorse, given its conformation, or in some instances its conformational faults (see Chapter 99). "It is by a study of conformation that we assign to a horse the particular place and purpose to which he is best adapted as a living machine and estimate his capacity for work, and the highest success in this connection will be best attained by the judicious blending of practice with science."[3] Evaluation of conformation and its influence on lameness is based largely on observation, experience, and pattern recognition. Recognizing desirable conformational traits in horses suited for a particular sporting activity and learning when to overlook a minor fault that has little clinical relevance are important.

RELEVANCE OF EVALUATION OF CONFORMATION

Conformation is one piece of the complex puzzle of a lame horse, although poor conformation does not necessarily condemn a horse to lameness: "faulty conformation is not an unsoundness ... it is a warning sign."[2] All lameness diagnosticians should evaluate conformation briefly at the beginning of each examination. The association of lameness and faulty conformation will be obvious. The clinician must evaluate the horse from afar, assessing the whole horse for balance, angles and lengths, and posture and symmetry. The clinician must remember that horses come in all shapes, sizes, and types, and therefore conformation varies accordingly, but certain conformational faults produce predictable lameness conditions and are undesirable. However, good conformation is not synonymous with success, and although horses of certain body types tend to have longer strides and are more athletic than others, intelligence, aggression, "will to win," and other intangible factors are important. It is our opinion that a well-bred horse from a successful family can endure faulty conformation much better than one with poor or mediocre breeding.

HEREDITARY ASPECTS OF CONFORMATION

Certain conformational faults appear to be highly heritable traits. Evaluation of broodmares and foals often reveals that the early conformational defects seen in a foal are present in the dam. The dam seems to contribute more to faulty conformation than does the sire, although the stallion also is important. This difference may be explained in part by the fact that fillies with faulty conformation may develop problems or be retired early and subsequently bred, whereas most stallions usually are proven performers with exceptional conformation. Conformational faults such as toed in and toed out commonly are passed down from generation to generation. Back-at-the-knee (calf-knee), offset (bench) knee, tied-in below the knee, sickle-hocked, and straight-behind conditions appear to be highly heritable. In a recent study abnormal sire phenotype (offset carpi and outward rotation) was associated with faulty yearling carpal conformation.[4] Heavier foals and yearlings were more likely to have faulty carpal conformation and inward rotation of the fetlock joints.[4]

Certain lameness conditions are common in horses with faulty conformation, but similar lameness conditions develop inexplicably in some breeding lines year after year in offspring with apparently acceptable conformation. Lameness of the carpus or tarsus appears to be most important. For example, in Standardbreds (STBs), siblings commonly develop similar lameness conditions, such as proximal suspensory avulsion injury, carpal osteochondral fragments, distal hock joint pain, or curb.

OBJECTIVE EVALUATION OF CONFORMATION: IS IT POSSIBLE?

An attempt to quantify conformation using a linear assessment trait evaluation system that allows the observer to assess where, given a particular trait, a single horse falls within a population of horses, was described in 1996.[5] A population of 101 Irish Thoroughbred (TB) flat racehorses and 19 top stallions was used and 27 common conformational traits were evaluated, including various heights, lengths and angles, and distal extremity conformation. Of the 27 traits, six were significantly linked to age (withers' height and conformation, back length, neck size, carpal conformation, and hind pastern conformation), and five were linked to sex (head and neck shape; neck size at the poll, the larynx the withers, and the manubrium of the sternum; and forelimb hoof pastern axis). Most traits exhibited large phenotypic variation within the population, but 21 of 27 non–age-linked traits were judged suitable for possible inclusion in a linear assessment protocol.[4] Researchers judged a high percentage of horses to be toed out, suggesting this trait may even be desirable.

More recent studies have used video-image analysis, but direct physical measurements may be more accurate than those obtained by analyzing videotapes or photographs.[6] Potential errors in image analysis occur because of movement of skin markers over selected bony protuberances, a phenomenon more common in the upper limb and in motion studies.[6,7] Skin marker location is critical for evaluation of joint angulation and movement during locomotion or conformation analysis. Instantaneous center (or axis) of rotation (ICR) is defined as the point with zero velocity during movement of that joint; accurate measurements of joint angulation require positioning markers at the ICR.[8] Conventional positions of skin markers and ICR in most joints agree well, but use of traditional marker sites on the scapulohumeral and femorotibial joints results in overestimation and underestimation, respectively, of caudal joint angles.[9] Although video-image analysis may be fraught with potential or in some instances real error, objectivity is a major advantage. Other advantages include the ability to replay images, reduction of observer fatigue, elimination of observations and measurements in real time, and permanent recording of the observation. Ideally, objective measurements would withstand statistical evaluation, distinguish between desirable and undesirable traits, and account for differences among different types of horses.[6]

A combination of direct measurement and photography was used to evaluate conformation of Swedish Warmblood (WBL) and elite sports horses.[10,11] Whereas most of the conformational defects were mild or moderate, 80% of WBL horses were toed out behind, suggesting this may be a normal finding in this breed as in the STB trotter. More than 50% of horses had bench knees and 5% were toed out in front, contrary to findings in STB trotters.[10,12] Many of the elite horses were bucked kneed, whereas the riding school horses tended to have calf-knees. It was speculated that this occurred because elite horses were evaluated after competition, and muscle fatigue may have contributed to the tendency to be over at the knee. Sex had a significant influence on conformation; females were smaller and had longer bodies and smaller forearms and metacarpal regions. There were interesting findings regarding hock angle. A sickle hock is defined as a hock angle of 53 degrees or less; a large hock angle is referred to as *straight behind*. Sickle-hocked conformation was nearly absent in elite horses, and it was hypothesized that sickle-hocked conformation either predisposed a horse to lameness or impaired a horse's ability to achieve upper levels of competition.[10] A positive relationship between larger hock angles and soundness in STB trotters also exists.[13] All results must be viewed in moderation, because it is our clinical impression that horses with excessively large hock angles (straight behind) are substantially predisposed to suspensory desmitis. In forelimbs of WBL show jumpers and the forelimbs and hindlimbs of STB trotters, smaller fetlock joint angles (less upright) were desirable.[10,13]

Radiology was used to assess the degree of hyperextension of the carpus to study the potential effect of back-at-the-knee (calf-knee) conformation on the subsequent development of carpal chip fractures.[14] Lateromedial radiographic images of 21 horses with carpal chip fractures and of 10 normal horses were obtained, with and without the contralateral limb raised. No relationship between measured carpal angle and carpal chip fracture formation existed, suggesting that this group of TB racehorses did not develop carpal chip fractures as a result of calf-kneed conformation. The sample size was small, however, and a larger study may produce different results. Horses with severe calf-kneed conformation may develop other problems and not advance enough in training to develop carpal chip fractures. They may be judged poor surgical candidates, are not referred, or are slow.

Two recent studies evaluated TBs and Quarter Horses (QHs) using skin markers, photography (three views: front, side, back), and computer-image analysis.[15,16] Of the two studies done in TBs, one evaluated longitudinal development of conformation from weaning to 3 years of age. A strong relationship between long bone lengths and withers heights for all ages supported the theory that horses are proportional. Longitudinal bone growth in the distal limb increased only 5% to 7% and was presumably completed before the yearling year. Withers height, croup height, and length of neck topline, neck bottom line, scapula, humerus, radius, and femur increased significantly from age 0 to 1 year and age 1 to 2 years. Hoof lengths (medial and lateral, right and left) grew significantly from the ages of 0 to 1 and 1 to 2 years but decreased in length from age 2 to 3 years (presumably associated with trimming).[15] Changes in growth measures indicated that growth rate either slowed or reached a plateau at 2 to 3 years of age. Horses also became more offset in the right forelimb between weaning and age 3, but the offset ratios did not change with age in the left forelimb. Shoulder angle increased in all age groups (becoming more upright), and this contributed to the increase in measured height at the withers. Dorsal hoof angle (both front and hind) decreased significantly from ages 0 to 1 and 1 to 2 years but did not change in the 2- and 3-year-old groups. This study provided objective information regarding conformation and skeletal growth in the TB, which could potentially be used for selection and recognition of important conformational abnormalities.[15] Measurements of length and angle were obtained from photographs in which a tape measure was used for objective criteria and an objective method was developed for measuring offset knees (Figures 4-1 to 4-4).[15]

In another study the role of conformation in the development of musculoskeletal problems in the racing TB was evaluated.[16] Conformation measurements were obtained

from photographs of horses with markers at specific reference points and digitally analyzed as previously described.[15] Clinical observations were recorded regularly for each horse, and stepwise (forward) logistic regression analysis was performed to investigate the relationship between binary response of clinical outcomes probability and conformation variables by the method of maximum likelihood. Clinical outcomes significantly ($P < .05$) associated with conformational variables included effusion of the front fetlock joints, effusion of the right carpal joint, effusion of the carpal joints, effusion of the hind fetlock joints, fractures of the left or right carpus, and right front fetlock and left hind fetlock lameness. Offset knees contributed to fetlock lameness (for every 10% increase in the right offset ratio, the risk of effusion in the right front fetlock increased 1.8 times and the odds of right front fetlock lameness increased by a factor of 1.26). Long pasterns increased the odds of forelimb fracture. Surprisingly, an increase in the carpal angle as viewed from the front (carpus valgus) appeared to act as a protective mechanism, because odds for the development of carpal fracture and carpal effusion decreased with increase in carpal angle (for every 1 degree increase in right carpal angle as viewed from the front, the odds of effusion in the right carpus decreased by a factor of 0.68 and the odds of a right carpal fracture decreased by a factor of 0.24).[16] Horses with long shoulders had decreased odds of developing forelimb fracture (odds ratio [OR] = 0.50), but horses with long pasterns had increased odds for forelimb fracture (OR = 4.55). Long sloping pasterns were suggested as a potential cause of carpal chip fractures.[14]

In the second TB study described previously, ORs were created for increase in bone length of 2.54 cm (1 inch) or

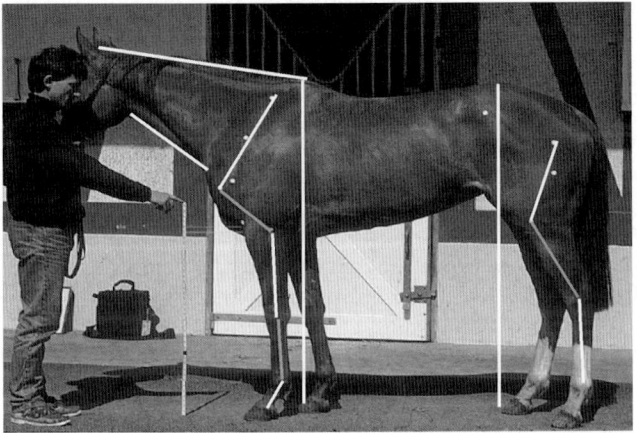

Fig. 4-1 • Length measurements (centimeters) recorded from the left lateral view in a Thoroughbred conformational study.[15] (Reproduced with permission from Anderson TM, McIlwraith CW: Longitudinal development of equine conformation from weanling to age 3 years in the Thoroughbred, *Equine Vet J* 36:563, 2004.)

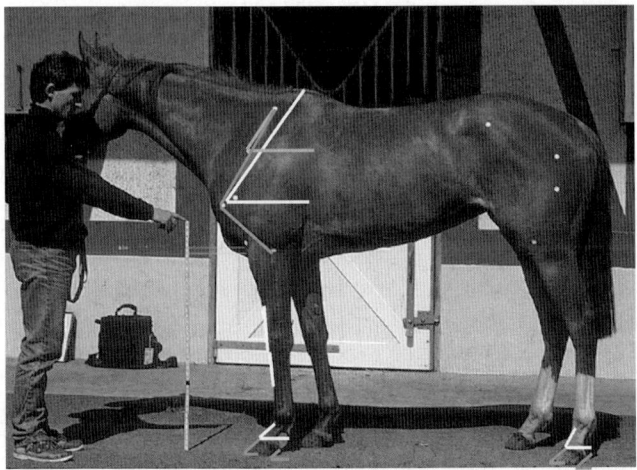

Fig. 4-2 • Angle measurements (degrees) recorded from the left lateral view in a Thoroughbred study.[15] (Reproduced with permission from Anderson TM, McIlwraith CW: Longitudinal development of equine conformation from weanling to age 3 years in the Thoroughbred, *Equine Vet J* 36:563, 2004.)

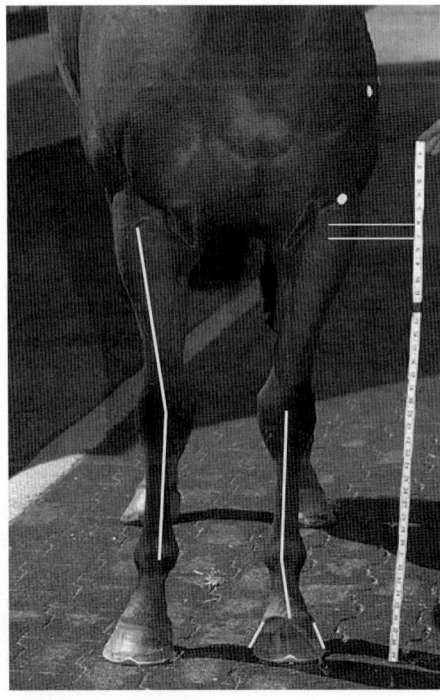

Fig. 4-3 • Length (centimeters) and angle measurements (degrees) recorded from the front view in a Thoroughbred study.[15] (Reproduced with permission from Anderson TM, McIlwraith CW: Longitudinal development of equine conformation from weanling to age 3 years in the Thoroughbred, *Equine Vet J* 36:563, 2004.)

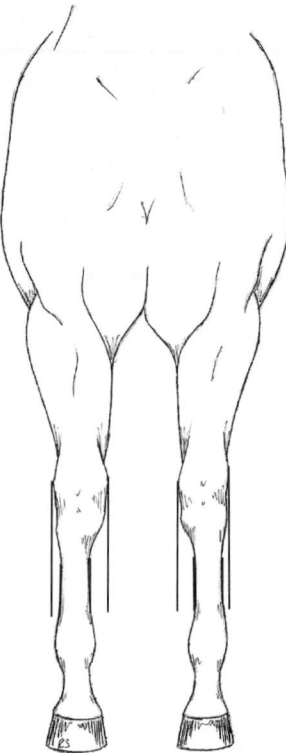

Fig. 4-4 • Lines drawn to determine offset ratios. A bench-knee measurement, called an offset ratio, of the medial width/lateral width determines the amount of third metacarpal bone that is offset laterally. The medial/lateral width is the distance (centimeters) from a line drawn along the medial or lateral aspect of the third metacarpal bone to a line from the medial or lateral distal lateral radial physis parallel with the third metacarpal bone. A ratio of greater than 1.0 represents bench-kneed conformation. (Reproduced with permission from Anderson TM, McIlwraith CW: Longitudinal development of equine conformation from weanling to age 3 years in the Thoroughbred, *Equine Vet J* 36:563, 2004.)

joint angle of 1 degree and development of lameness.[16] For every 2.5 cm increase in humeral length, odds for fracture of the proximal phalanx or carpal synovitis or capsulitis increased. Increased length from elbow to ground and increased toe length increased chances for carpal fracture, and in horses with offset knees greater than 10% the potential for carpal or fetlock synovitis or capsulitis increased. The potential for fracture of the proximal phalanx increased with an increase in shoulder angle.[16]

A study examining conformation in 160 racing QHs in training at Los Alamitos Race Course found humeral length had a significant association with several clinical entities.[17] For every 10-cm increase in humeral length the odds of an osteochondral fracture fragment of the dorsoproximal aspect of the left front proximal phalanx increased by a factor of 9.06. Similarly, ORs for carpal synovitis and capsulitis and for sustaining carpal chip fracture (8.12 in the left forelimb and 10.17 in the right forelimb) rose significantly with each 10-cm incremental increase in humeral length. The length of the left front toe was important.[17] For each 1-cm increase in toe length, the odds of sustaining carpal chip fractures increased by a factor of 58.90.[17] Horses with upright shoulders were at increased risk for development of osteochondral fragmentation of the

proximal phalanx and those with offset carpi were at increased risk for development of synovitis and capsulitis in both forelimbs (OR = 2.26).[17]

The relationship of many lower limb lameness conditions with limb length is interesting and somewhat unexpected because longer limb length generally is considered desirable. In addition, a relationship between longer toes and carpal fracture is interesting. Longer toes may delay breakover of the foot, altering forelimb biomechanics, but an effect on a distant joint such as the carpus cannot be easily explained. The relationship between offset knees and lower limb lameness was expected, but unexpected were fewer carpal fractures in TBs with this conformational fault. Because development of lameness, termed *clinical outcomes* in these studies, is complex, confounding variables such as track conditions, training regimen, breeding, individual horse ability, and experimental error could have contributed to outcome.

Little doubt exists that acquiring objective information is useful, not only to determine what is abnormal but also to define what is normal in a population. In both WBLs and STB trotters in Europe, toed-out conformation in the hindlimbs should likely be considered normal because a majority of both breeds have this conformational trait.[10,12] These populations differed, however, in forelimb conformation. Few STB trotters had bench-kneed conformation, a finding supported by one of our (MWR) clinical observations that this conformational fault is highly undesirable in this breed (see Chapter 108). Recently, variation in conformation of National Hunt racehorses established guidelines with which individual horses could be compared and highlighted significant variations in horses with different origins (Irish and French horses differed significantly in girth and intermandibular width measurements).[18] Circumference and length measurements were significantly associated with withers height. No underlying pattern of combinations of conformational parameters was found, but variations were identified between left and right measurements and in hoof, stifle angle, and coxofemoral angle measurements.[18]

EVALUATION OF CONFORMATION

Conformation determines the way a horse moves, and it is intuitive that a relationship exists between faulty conformation and the development of lameness. Therefore assessment of conformation should be an integral part of lameness examination. Conformation evaluation has four basic components: assessment of (1) balance, (2) lengths, angles, and heights, (3) muscling, and (4) conformation of the limbs. All are intertwined but should be evaluated separately, considering the whole horse not just the limbs, and then consolidated. The clinician should evaluate the horse on firm, level ground, preferably a smooth, nonslip surface that does not obscure the view of the feet. The horse should stand squarely with equal weight on all four limbs. Dynamic assessment of limb conformation while the horse is walking also is essential.

Balance

Balance is the way all parts of the horse fit together and is linked directly with assessment of lengths, angles, and heights. The horse should be proportional and thus well

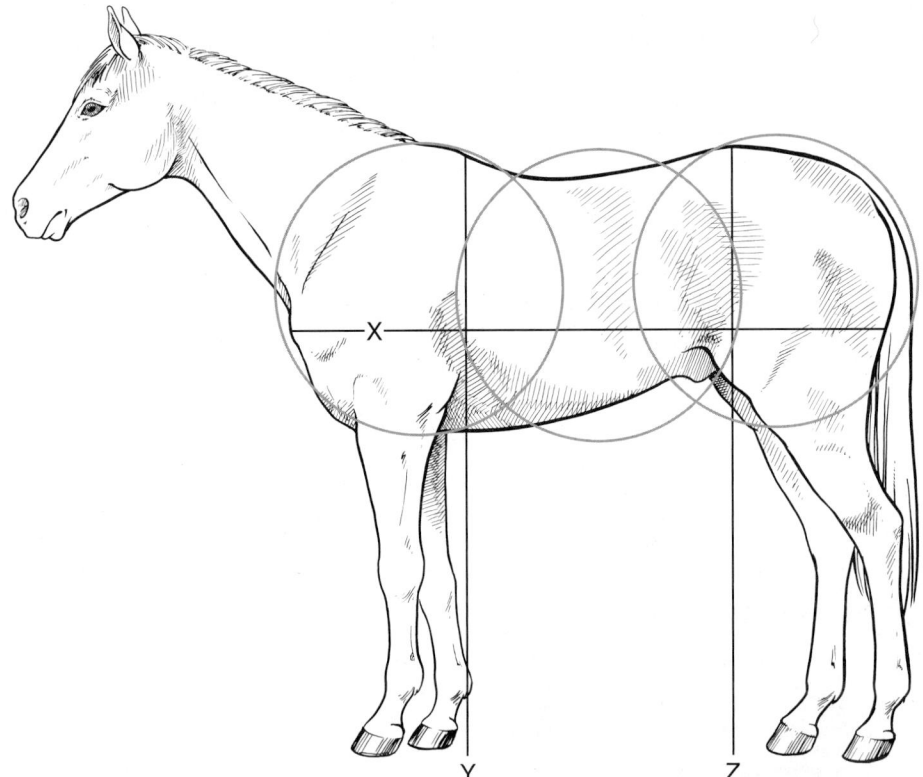

Fig. 4-5 • Diagrammatic depiction of assessing balance during conformation evaluation. Three circles (from left to right: forehand, midbody, hindquarters) are visualized and should overlap by approximately one third. Excessive overlapping of circles (short coupled) or scant overlapping of circles (long, weak in the back) are common conformational abnormalities. Body length *(X)* should be equal to or slightly longer than withers height *(Y)*, and withers height and rump height *(Z)* should be the same.

balanced. A horse may be visualized in thirds—the forehand, the midbody, and the hindquarters—by drawing three circles incorporating these areas (Figure 4-5). The circles should overlap but not excessively. Horses in good balance are likely to be superior athletes. Horses with a short, thick (throatlatch and shoulder regions) neck are often heavy and straight in the shoulders (Figure 4-6). A horse with a short back has naturally closer dorsal spinous processes which may be predisposed to impingement or overriding, whereas a horse with a long back (Figure 4-7) may have difficulty engaging the hindlimbs properly. The clinician must assess the relative heights of the withers and hindquarters. A horse that is taller behind than in front (rump height is greater than height at the withers) is predisposed to forelimb lameness. A horse that also is underdeveloped in the shoulders and upper forelimbs (weak up front) and heavy behind is more at risk. Limb lengths should be proportional to body size and height. In general, the body length (point of shoulder to point of rump) should be equal or slightly longer than withers height (see Figure 4-5).

Head conformation is not relevant to lameness, but the size of the head relative to the body and the angulation between the head and neck influence the ease with which the horse can work "on the bit" (see Chapters 97 and 116). A horse's ability to see is important. A horse with ocular abnormalities may exhibit bizarre behavioral abnormalities or unusual head and neck carriages, possibly misinterpreted as the result of pain. A rare cause of "being on a line" occurs in driving horses, such as a STB with unilateral

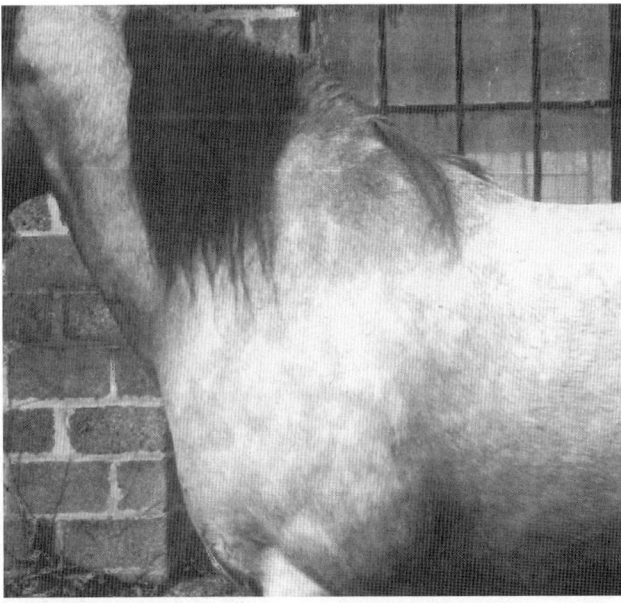

Fig. 4-6 • Horse with short, heavy neck; heavy, short, and straight shoulder; and withers set forward. This horse is prone to forelimb lameness and likely to have a short stride.

blindness. The horse turns the head toward the blind side to see with the opposite eye and thus is on the contralateral line (to straighten the head, the driver must pull on the contralateral line). This mimics a contralateral (to the blind eye) lameness.

Lengths, Angles, and Heights

Body length is important in determining stride length (see Figure 4-5). Short-coupled conformation predisposes horses to short strides and problems with interference, especially racehorses. If horses are too long, they can be weak in the back. The length of the neck is important in assessing balance and should be proportional to the overall body length. Some horses have long, weak necks. The neck may be "set on low" relative to the shoulder, with a depression (ventral deviation) of the dorsal topline cranial to the withers (ewe necked), giving the appearance of prominent

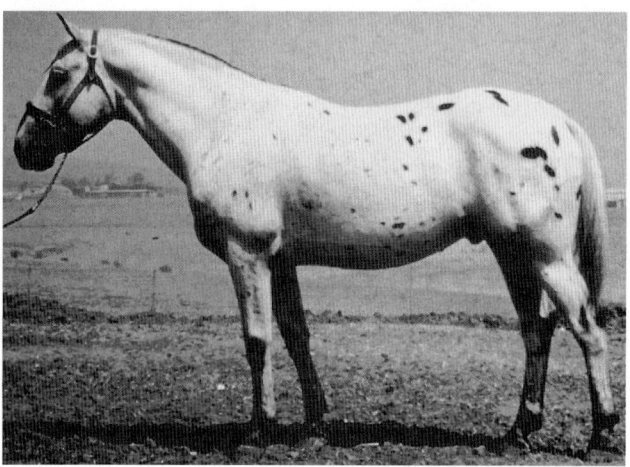

Fig. 4-7 • Unbalanced Appaloosa gelding that is long and weak in the barrel (back). Rump height is slightly higher than withers height.

withers laid too far caudally. Horses should have adequate depth in the girth region (depth of girth).

Shoulder length (top of the withers to the point of the shoulder) may be related directly to stride length, and horses with longer shoulders usually have longer strides (Figure 4-8). Those with short shoulders usually have shorter strides (see Figure 4-8). Shoulder length and shoulder angle often are related; long shoulders often are more sloping (smaller shoulder angle), and short shoulders often are straight. Good shoulder length appears to be important and desirable, but recent objective data from TB and QH racehorses suggest that horses with long limbs may be at increased risk for lower limb lameness.[16,17]

In TBs particularly a long radius (forearm) and short, strong third metacarpal bone (McIII) have been considered desirable for adequate strength and maximum stride length. However, more recent work[16] suggests that a long forearm would lead to a long metacarpal bone, and because horses are proportional we must question this long-held impression. Chest width should be commensurate with overall body size. A wide chest with a base-narrow forelimb stance (the front feet are close when the horse is evaluated from the front) or a narrow chest with a base-wide stance are undesirable. In STB pacers a good chest width is desirable, but in trotters a narrow chest is preferred (see Chapter 108).

Rump length also is important in determining stride length, and a longer length of the rump is desirable. Many horses with long rumps have larger rump angles (flat croup), and those with short rumps have smaller rump angles (steep croup). Long, flat croup regions are desirable. The ideal

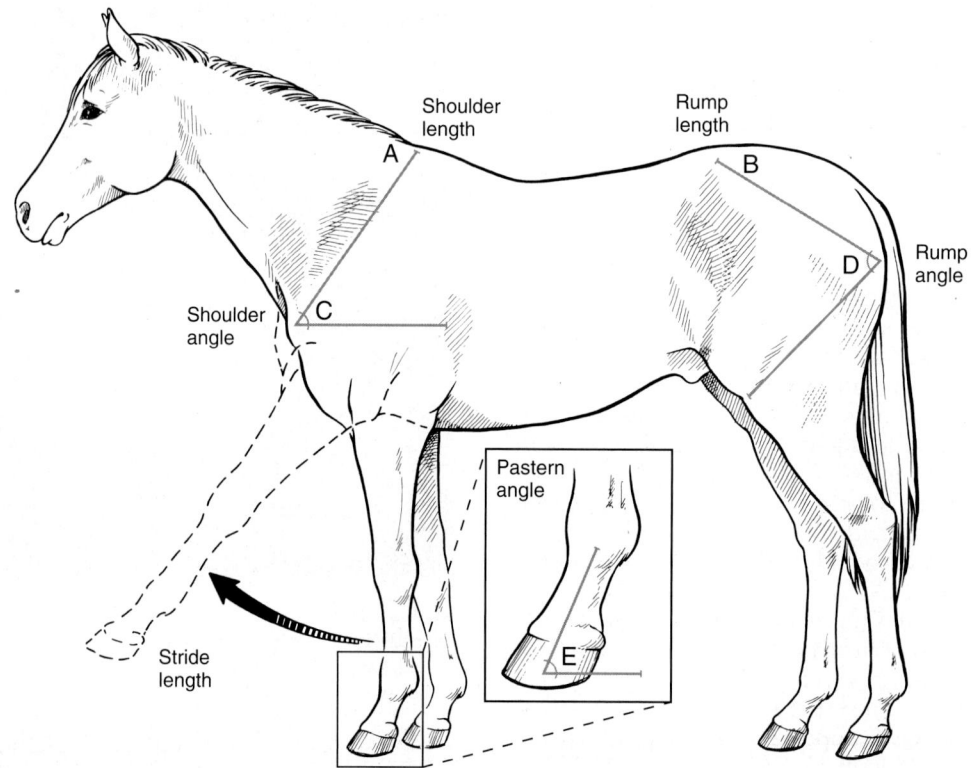

Fig. 4-8 • Measurement of shoulder length *(A)*, rump length *(B)*, shoulder angle *(C)*, and rump angle *(D)*. The pastern angle *(E)* should be equal to the shoulder angle. Shoulder angle and length are important in determining stride length.

horse should have a long gaskin (crus) and a short, strong metatarsal region (the hocks close to the ground) to maximize stride length.

The angles of the shoulder and rump are important factors in determining stride length and balance. Undesirable shoulder and rump angles often accompany other conformational faults and may predispose to lameness. The ideal angle of the shoulder (relative to the ground) has classically been determined to be 45 degrees (see Figure 4-8). Horses with steep shoulder angles (>50 to 55 degrees) usually have short shoulders and short, upright pasterns, which predispose to lower limb lameness. The forelimb pastern angle should be equal to the shoulder angle. A steep shoulder angle shifts the center of gravity forward, predisposing to forelimb lameness. Horses with a flat rump or croup generally have longer rump lengths and longer strides (Figure 4-9). Horses with short, steep rumps (goose rump) often have short, choppy gaits, and many have hindlimb lameness (Figure 4-10). A steep rump angle shifts the center of gravity caudally, predisposing to hindlimb lameness.

Limbs

It is critical to evaluate limb conformation with the horse standing squarely on a firm, flat surface and with an experienced handler who can make the horse cooperate. If the clinician observes a fault that may result from how the horse is standing, he or she should reevaluate the horse after repositioning. Horses often stand camped out, both behind and in front, simply as the result of improper positioning.

The plumb line concept allows evaluation of each limb from the front or back and the side (Figure 4-11). For example, a vertical line from the point of the shoulder should bisect the limb. The clinician also should evaluate the horse while it is walking because some defects are dynamic. Horses that toe in or toe out, or those with fetlock or carpus varus deformities, may stand reasonably well, particularly with corrective trimming and shoeing,

but the defect may be readily apparent while the horse is walking.

FORELIMB CONFORMATION

Front Perspective

Several forelimb conformational abnormalities are apparent when a horse is evaluated from the front. *Base-wide* conformation may occur alone or in combination with toed-in or toed-out conditions (Figure 4-12). Horses that are base wide stand with the forelimbs lateral to the plumb line and generally are narrow in the chest, resulting in overload of the medial aspect of the lower limb, predisposing to lameness. Horses that are *base wide, toed in* tend to wing out or paddle during protraction (Figures 4-12, *B* and 4-13, *A*). Winging out predisposes trotters to interference with the ipsilateral hindlimb. *Base-wide, toed-out* conformation appears most often in horses with uncorrected carpus valgus deformities (Figures 4-12, *C* and 4-13, *B*) and results in excessive loading on the medial aspect of the foot and misshapen feet. Interference with the contralateral forelimb may occur in severely affected horses.

Base-narrow conformation may occur alone or in combination with toed-in or toed-out conformation (Figure 4-14). Horses that are base narrow stand with the forelimbs inside each plumb line and overload the outside of the lower limb and foot. Horses that are *base narrow, toed in* tend to wing out, and those that are *base narrow, toed out* tend to wing in during protraction (see Figures 4-13 and 4-14).

With *in-at-the-knee*, knock-kneed, or carpus valgus conformation (Figure 4-15) the carpi are medial to the plumb

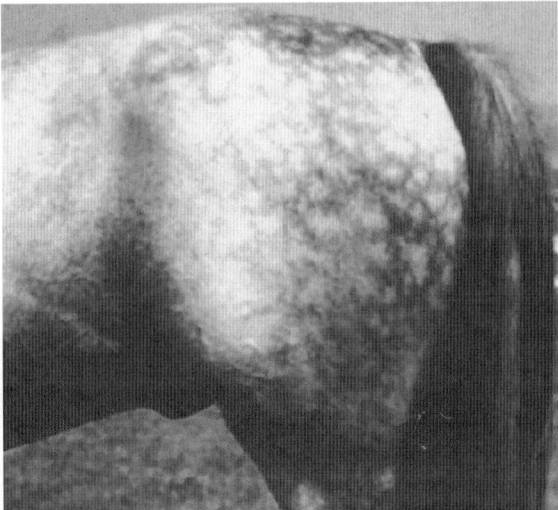

Fig. 4-9 • Desirable hindlimb conformation. The flat rump angle and good rump length would likely increase stride length and allow good support and strength of the hindlimbs.

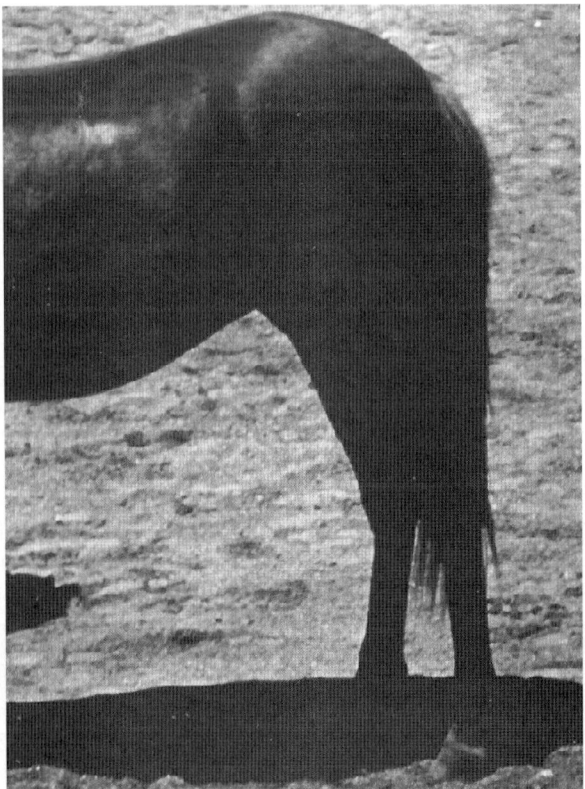

Fig. 4-10 • Undesirable hindlimb conformation characterized by a short, steep rump (goose rump), predisposing to hindlimb lameness.

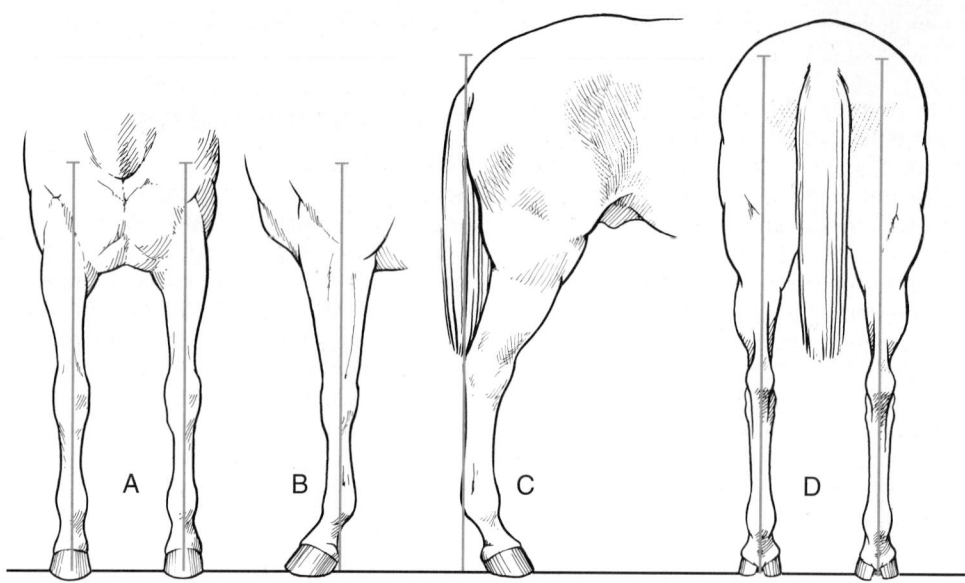

Fig. 4-11 • Diagram demonstrating use of plumb lines to evaluate limb conformation from three perspectives. Vertical lines are visualized from **A,** the front forelimb (line runs from point of the shoulder, bisecting the limb), **B,** the side forelimb (line bisects elbow joint, carpus, and fetlock joint and intersects the ground approximately 5 cm behind the solar surface of the heel), and **C,** the side hindlimb (line runs from point of rump to the ground, touching the point of the hock and plantar aspect of the metatarsal region and intersecting the ground approximately 7.5 to 10 cm behind the heel) and from **D,** the back hindlimb (line drawn from point of rump, bisecting the hindlimb).

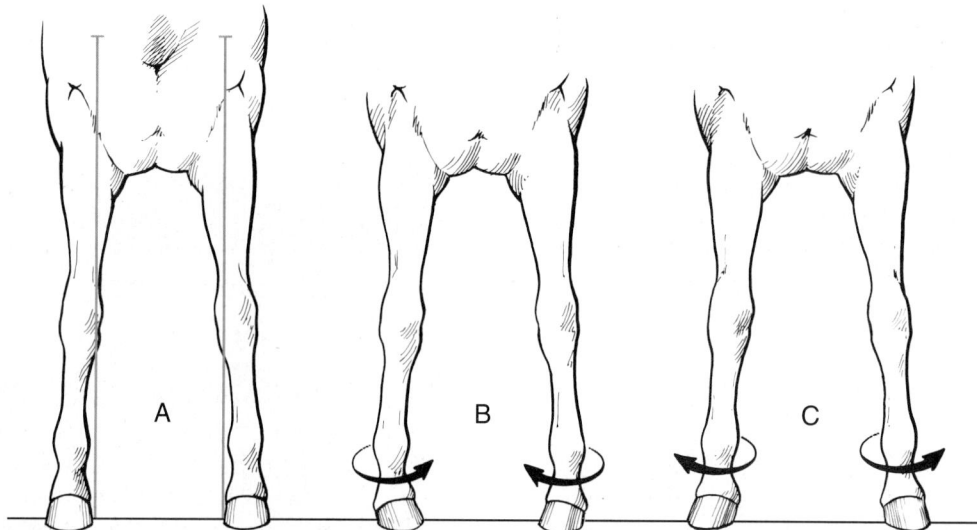

Fig. 4-12 • Three variations of base-wide forelimb conformation, including **(A)** simple base wide, **(B)** base wide, toed in, and **(C)** base wide, toed out.

line, creating an angular deformity and concentrating the weight of the horse on the medial aspect of the carpus and proximal metacarpal region. This condition, if severe, may predispose the horse to carpal lameness and splints. However, recent objective data have suggested that a certain degree of carpal valgus is protective for synovitis and capsulitis, as well as chip fractures in the carpus.[16] Predisposition to carpal lameness and splints with carpal valgus conformation probably applies only to horses with severe abnormalities. In some horses, particularly foals, carpus valgus may be accompanied by external rotation of the entire limb or just the distal aspect (toed out). Severely

affected horses wear the inside aspect of the hoof or shoe abnormally.

Out-at-the-knee (bowlegged, bandy-legged) conformation usually is a consequence of early carpus varus and usually is career-limiting (Figure 4-16). The carpus is bowed outward, lateral to the plumb line. Many horses are also toed in, accentuating abnormal forces on the lateral aspect of the entire distal forelimb, predisposing to osteoarthritis (OA) of the carpus or fetlock or lateral suspensory branch desmitis and sesamoiditis. In most foals with carpus varus, there is coexistent lateral deviation of the elbow, giving the appearance that the angular deformity might be arising

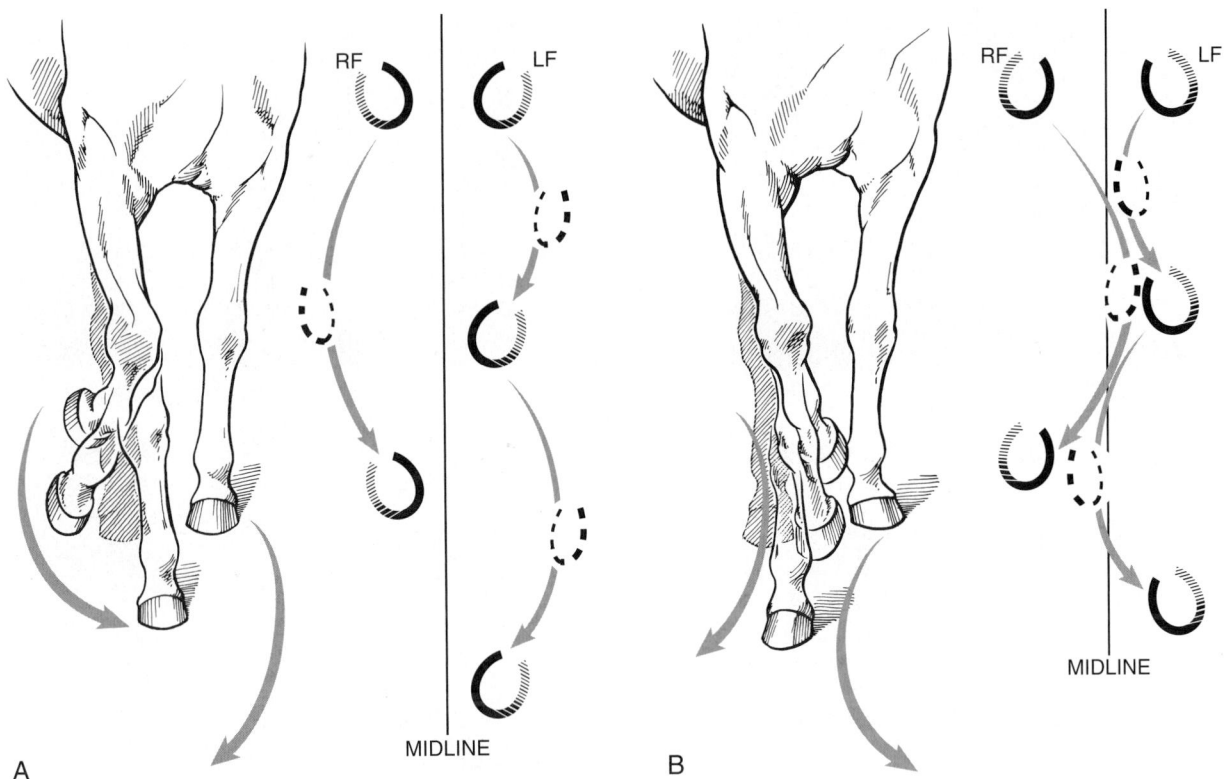

Fig. 4-13 • **A,** Toed-in conformation often causes horses to wing out or paddle during advancement of the forelimb. **B,** Toed-out conformation causes horses to wing in, predisposing to interference with the contralateral forelimb.

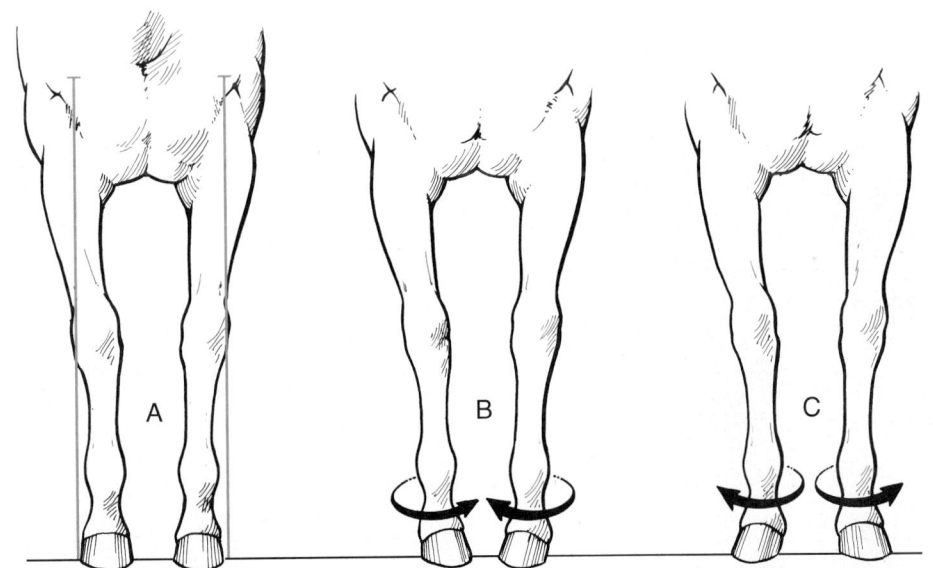

Fig. 4-14 • Three variations of base-narrow forelimb conformation including **(A)** simple base narrow, **(B)** base narrow, toed in, and **(C)** base narrow, toed out.

from asymmetrical growth in the physes associated with the elbow joint. Correction is difficult but usually involves transphyseal retardation of the distal lateral radial physis.

Offset or *bench-knee* conformation is classically defined as lateral positioning of the metacarpal region relative to the central axis of the radius (Figure 4-17). However, radiographs demonstrate that the actual displacement usually is at the antebrachiocarpal joint. Displacement may be

unilateral or bilateral with differing degrees of severity on each side. This conformation has been often associated with carpal or metacarpal lameness (Figure 4-18). Many 2-year-old STBs with offset knees are precocious during early training but often develop carpal lameness at 3 or 4 years of age. TBs with offset knees are believed to perform better on the soft turf tracks in Europe, as opposed to the firm turf or dirt tracks in the United States. In recent

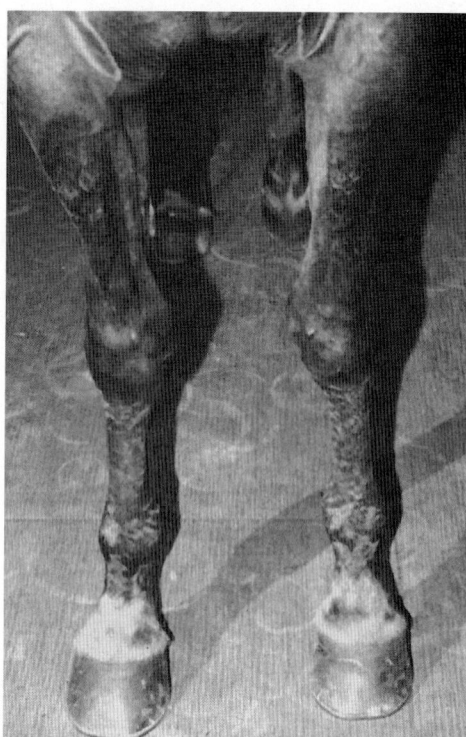

Fig. 4-15 • A horse with in-at-the-knee conformation that is worse in the right forelimb.

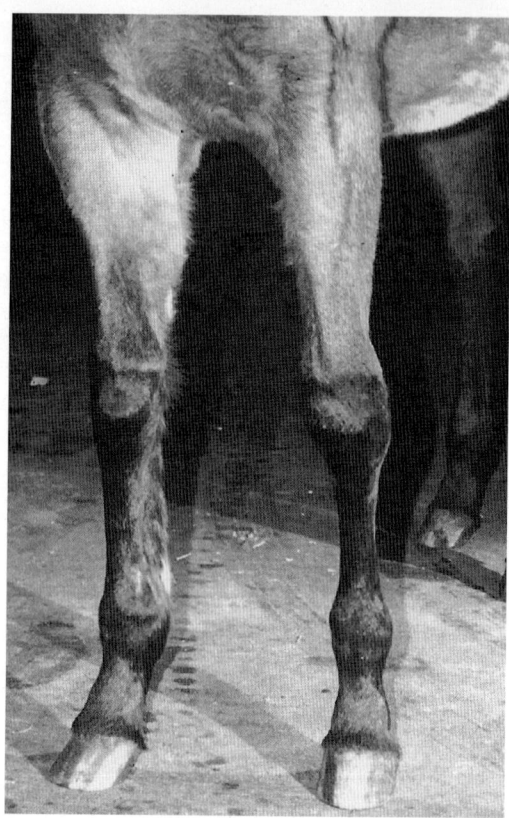

Fig. 4-17 • Standardbred with a prominently offset (bench) knee in the left forelimb. An apparent lateral deviation or shifting (offset) of the cannon bone and distal extremity occurs relative to the plumb line dropped through the left radius.

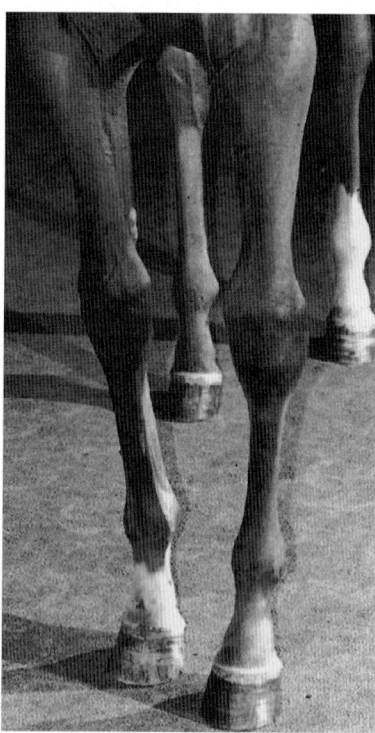

Fig. 4-16 • Two-year-old Thoroughbred filly with moderate-to-severe carpus varus (out-at-the-knee) conformation in the left forelimb and mild deformity in the right forelimb. The filly also is toed in, a common finding in horses with this type of conformation. Another common finding is lateral deviation or bowing of the elbow, prompting clinical suspicion that a deformity also exists at this joint.

studies, a relationship between offset knees and carpal lameness was not found, but horses with this conformational abnormality were at risk for fetlock lameness.[16,17]

Toed-in conformation, or internal rotation of the distal extremity, exists alone or in combination with abnormalities of stance (base narrow or base wide), other conformational faults such as carpus varus and offset knees, and being wide in the chest (see Figure 4-16). Horses that are toed in usually wing out (paddle) (see Figure 4-13). Toed-in conformation is particularly undesirable in a trotter because of potential interference at speed. Toed-in conformation predisposes horses to lateral splints, lameness of the lateral aspect of the fetlock joint region (e.g., lateral branch suspensory desmitis), and OA of the interphalangeal joints. Horses that are toed in wear the outside aspect of the foot.

Toed-out conformation, or external rotation of the distal extremity, is common and if mild may be considered normal or inconsequential (Figure 4-19). Mild toed-out conformation appears in 50% of STBs and is common behind in STBs and WBLs.[10,12] It first develops in foals and, if pronounced, persists in the mature horse. In foals, toed-out conformation often accompanies carpus valgus deformities but may result from external rotation primarily from the fetlock joint distally or, in more severe deformities, from further proximally (Figure 4-20). Mild toed-out conformation usually resolves as a foal matures and with corrective trimming. Toed-out conformation results in abnormal wear on the inside aspect of the foot. Horses tend

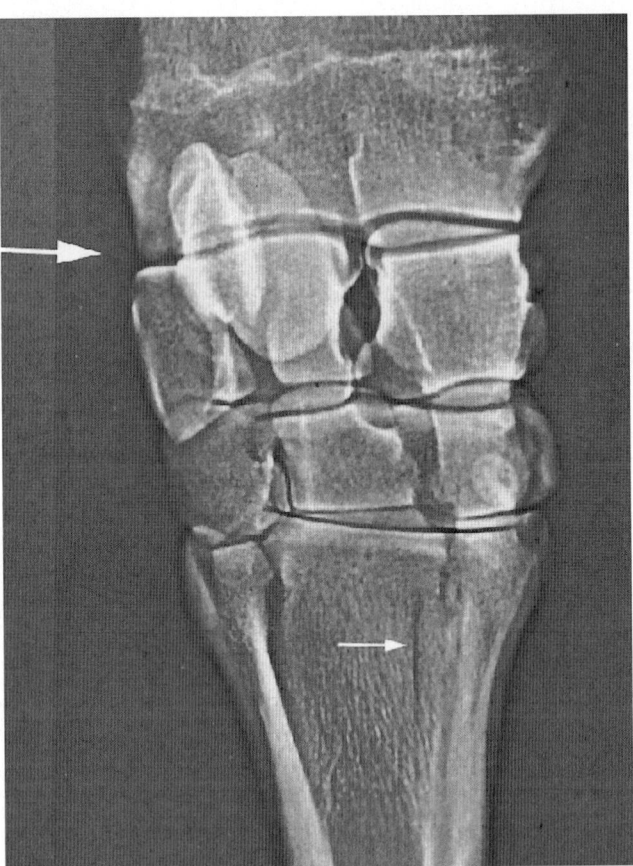

Fig. 4-18 • Dorsopalmar xeroradiograph of 3-year-old Standardbred colt with longitudinal fracture of the third metacarpal bone *(small arrow)*. Medial is to the right. The lateral displacement ("step") at the antebrachio-carpal joint *(large arrow)* gives the clinical appearance of an offset (bench) knee.

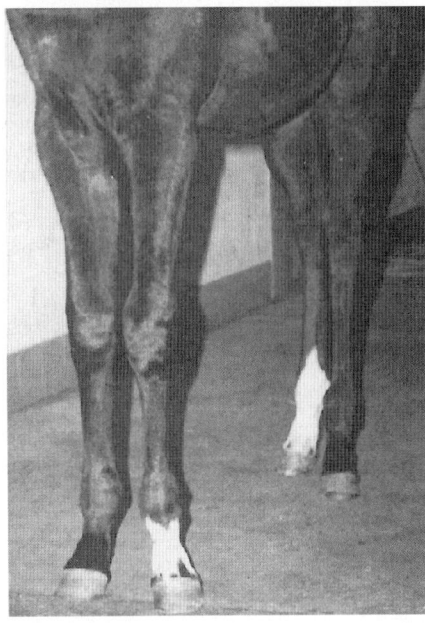

Fig. 4-20 • Thoroughbred foal with pronounced external rotation or toed-out left forelimb limb conformation. The deformity involves the entire limb, beginning well above the carpus.

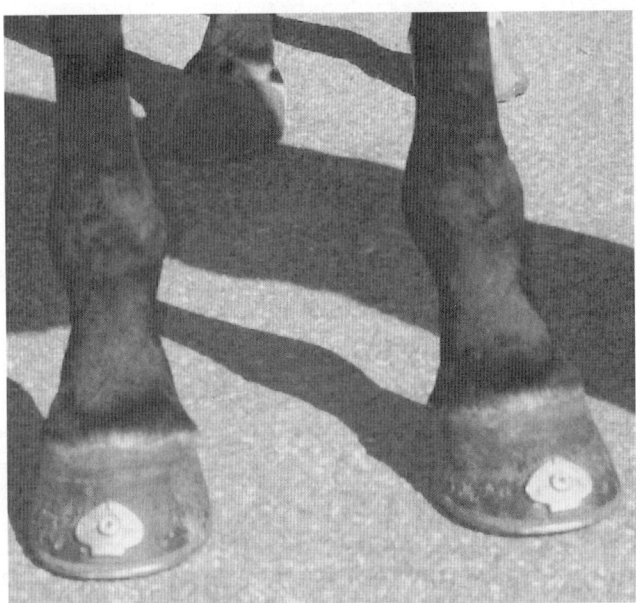

Fig. 4-19 • Trotter showing inconsequential mild toed-out conformation. Toe weights often are used in trotters to balance gait and correct interference.

to wing in; if winging in is severe, particularly if accompanied by base-narrow conformation, it may interfere with the opposite forelimb (see Figure 4-13). Exostoses (splints) on the second metacarpal bone (McII) or McIII may develop, requiring protective boots to be worn during exercise. In STB pacers, interference injury occurs as high as the distal aspect of the radius.

Lateral Perspective

Horses camped out in front stand consistently with an entire forelimb ahead of the plumb line, but this conformation usually is a temporary problem with the horse's stance and can be corrected by repositioning the horse, or it reflects pain caused by laminitis, for example. *Camped under in front* is unusual and usually also results from temporary malpositioning of the horse (Figure 4-21). If a horse prefers to stand camped under and is otherwise sound, however, this trait may be a sign of "extreme speed."[19]

Back-at-the-knee or *calf-knee* (sheep-knee) conformation describes a concave dorsal aspect of the limb, with the carpus behind the plumb line (Figures 4-22 to 4-24). On radiographs of a normal carpus the proximal and distal rows of carpal bones are aligned in a proximal-to-distal direction, and the dorsal faces of these bones are parallel to the radius and the McIII (Figure 4-23, *A*). With back-at-the-knee conformation the proximal row of carpal bones is set back (Figure 4-23, *B*). Horses that stand back at the knee are considered predisposed to carpal injuries because of the natural tendency of the carpus to hyperextend (larger carpal angle) during fatigue. In our experience, TB racehorses are particularly at risk, despite limited contrary evidence (see page 16).[14] While no associations were made between horses with back-at-the-knee conformation and lameness in recent studies in TBs and QHs, horses

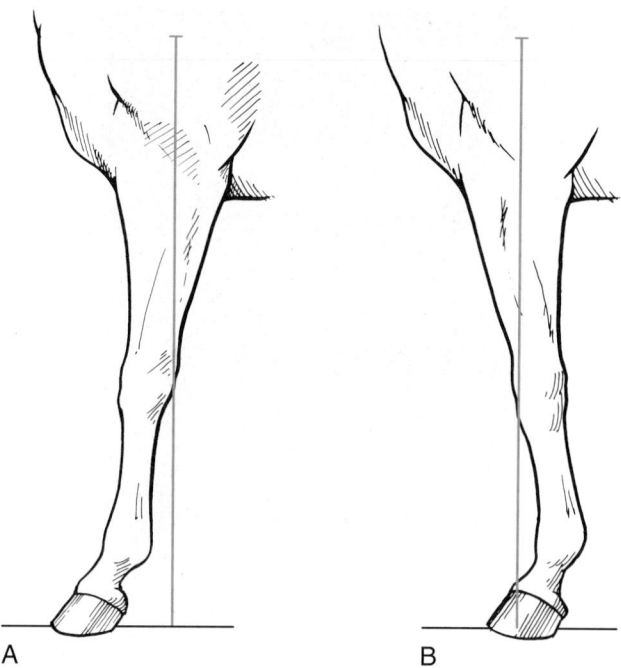

Fig. 4-21 • Diagram showing **(A)** camped-out in front and **(B)** camped-under in front conformation, both in relation to plumb lines.

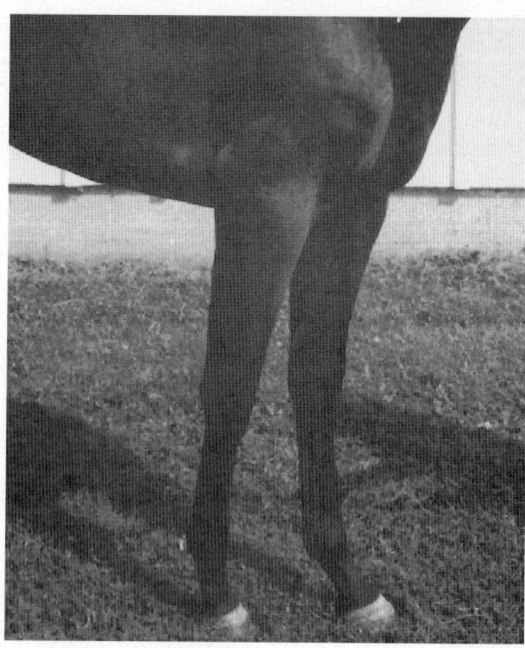

Fig. 4-22 • Thoroughbred yearling with back-at-the-knee (calf-knee) conformation most noticeable in the left forelimb. This conformational fault is undesirable, particularly in racing breeds.

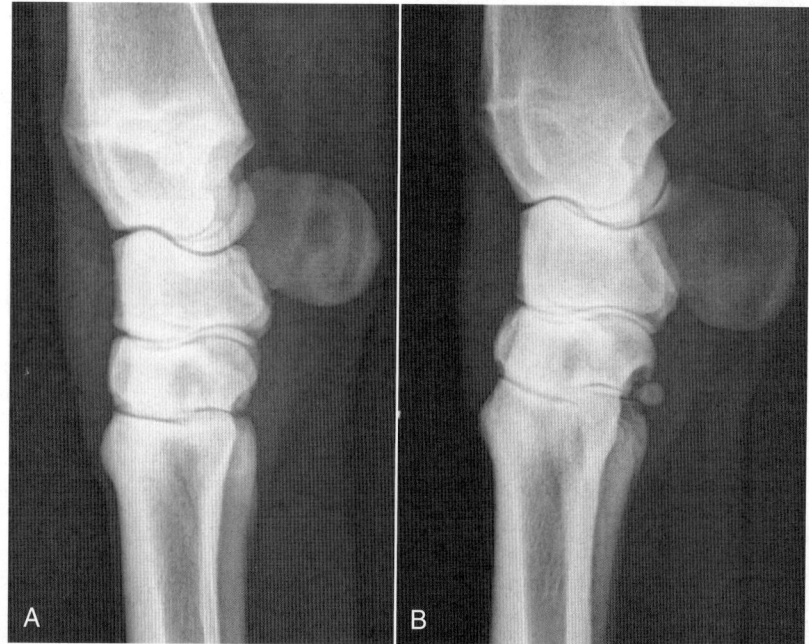

Fig. 4-23 • Lateromedial radiographs of the left carpi of two 2-year-old Thoroughbred racehorses. **A,** There is normal carpal conformation, and the proximal and distal rows of carpal bones are aligned and parallel to the radius and third metacarpal bone. **B,** In a horse with carpal lameness there is palmar deviation of the proximal row of carpal bones. This radiological appearance is typical of back-at-the-knee conformation.

included in those studies were elite, and any foals with obvious back-at-the-knee conformation may have been eliminated from the case population before the studies commenced.[16,17] In a different study TB foals that were back-at-the-knee improved as they matured from 1, 2, and 3 years of age.[15]

In the STB, mild calf-knee conformation is common in pacers and acceptable, whereas in the trotter this defect is undesirable. In other breeds, mild calf-knee conformation may not directly lead to lameness. In young horses with lameness from unrelated sources such as osteochondrosis or fracture of the distal phalanx, back-at-the-knee

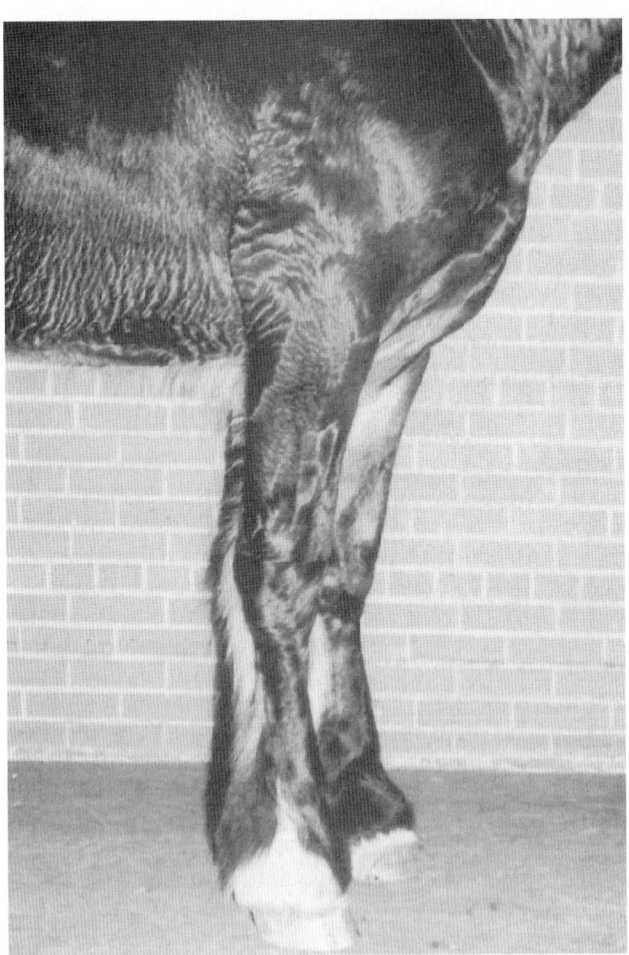

Fig. 4-24 • Clydesdale yearling with calf-knee conformation and clubfoot secondary to osteochondrosis of the shoulder joint. This conformation is primarily the result of chronic lameness, decreased weight bearing, and the development of a flexural deformity.

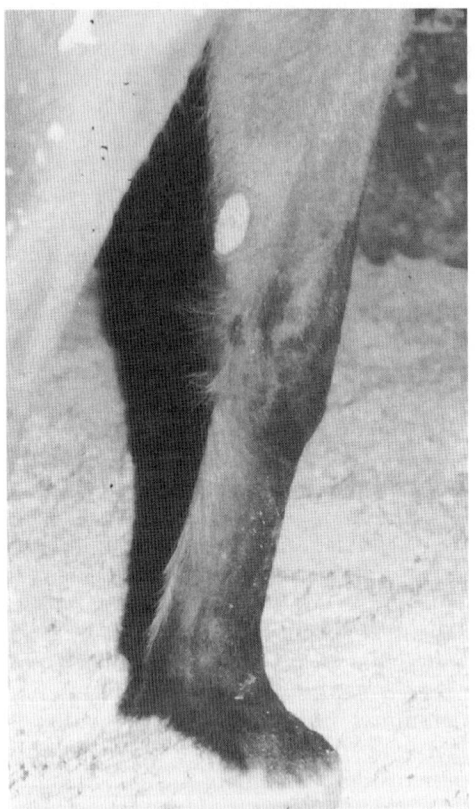

Fig. 4-25 • Older horse without obvious lameness with over-at-the-knee (bucked-knee) conformation.

conformation and clubfoot (a small, upright foot) may accompany flexural deformity of the limb (see Figure 4-24). This deformity is a combination of contraction (clubfoot) and laxity (calf-knee) caused by chronic lameness and partial weight bearing and warrants a guarded prognosis.

Over-at-the-knee, bucked-knee (knee-sprung), or hanging-knee conformation describes a convex dorsal surface of the carpus, with the carpus in front of the plumb line (Figure 4-25). In young, untrained horses, bucked-knee conformation may be a predictor of lameness, but in mature horses it appears to be an acquired characteristic and occurs primarily in horses that jump. Older cross-country horses, steeplechasers, jumpers, or field hunters are prone to bucked-knee conformation and often stand over at the knee with no obvious lameness. These horses may exhibit a tendency to buck forward to such an extent that they appear on the verge of collapse or prone to stumbling yet show good stability. Lame horses that stand over at the knee are often found to have pain in the proximal palmar metacarpal area or carpal sheath. *Tied in below the knee* (Figure 4-26) describes a distinct notch just distal to the accessory carpal bone on the palmar aspect of the limb. Normally, the McIII and the digital flexor tendons are in parallel alignment from the

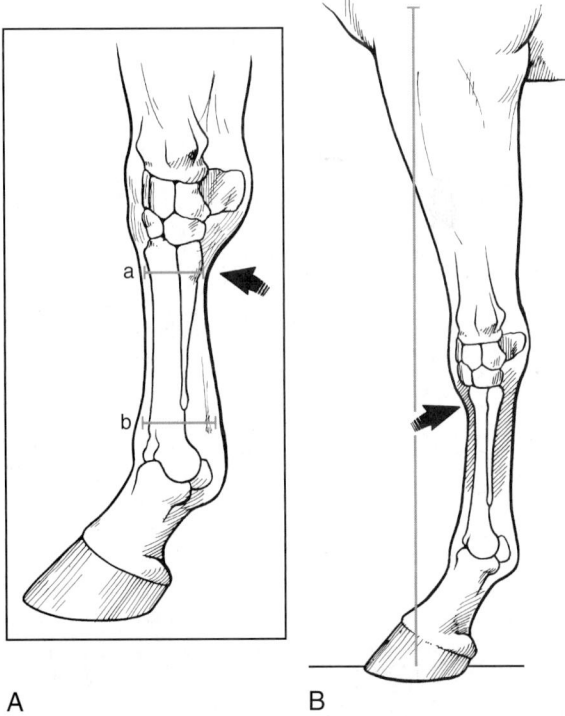

Fig. 4-26 • **A,** Diagrammatic representation of tied in below the knee. The dorsal-palmar length of *a* is less than *b*, giving the appearance that the digital flexor tendons run obliquely, proximally to enter the distal carpal region more dorsally than expected. **B,** A horse that is cut-out under the knee has a concave appearance of the dorsal aspect of the distal carpus and proximal metacarpal region (*arrow*).

accessory carpal bone to the proximal sesamoid bones. With tied-in conformation the digital flexor tendons appear to enter the carpus in a dorsoproximal direction. If the horse also is bucked kneed, the tied-in appearance is accentuated. Young horses are prone to superficial digital flexor tendonitis. In STBs this defect is worse for a pacer than a trotter.

The junction of the carpus and McIII should be flat. *Cut out under knee* describes a notch under the dorsal surface of the carpus (see Figure 4-26). In horses with this defect, the McIII appears thin (dorsopalmar direction) and weak. Horses with this conformational abnormality also are often back at the knee, predisposing them to carpal and metacarpal problems. Some young racehorses, typically late yearlings or early 2-year-olds in training, appear to have distention of the middle carpal joint capsule or an unusually prominent distal radial epiphysis. These findings give the impression of an unusually large gap between these structures, described as "open at the knee." The first author has not seen a correlation between this clinical observation and obvious radiological changes, although in young horses with this conformation the distal radial physis remains visible. Whether this conformation is relevant to lameness in young racehorses is debatable.

Over at the fetlock usually is seen in young horses with flexural deformity of this joint (see Chapter 59). This conformational fault may persist in a mature horse, causing upright pasterns or knuckling of the fetlock joint. In some horses this condition causes a progressive, permanent deformity and severe lameness, whereas in others a dynamic, intermittent knuckling occurs and some of these horses remain surprisingly sound. Knuckling also may be a sequel to desmitis of the accessory ligament of the deep digital flexor tendon.

HINDLIMB CONFORMATION
Lateral Perspective
Hindlimb conformational faults generally are less numerous and problematic than those in the forelimb because of differences in weight distribution and center of gravity. Plumb lines also are useful in evaluating conformation of the hindlimbs with the horse standing squarely, loading all limbs (see Figure 4-11). Camped-out conformation is unusual and generally results from faulty positioning of the horse during the examination. Horses that are truly camped out usually have short strides and poor athletic ability. Camped under behind often is associated with sickle-hocked conformation but also appears in horses that are straight behind (Figures 4-27 and 4-28). Horses with this type of conformation often have short, choppy strides (Figure 4-29).

A particularly severe conformational fault that leads directly to lameness is *straight behind,* otherwise called *straight hocks* or *post* (posty) leg. Horses that are straight behind have larger stifle and hock angles but smaller fetlock joint angles compared with ideal hindlimb conformation (see Figures 4-27 and 4-28). Straight-behind, sickle-hocked, and in-at-the-hock conformation are the three most important hindlimb conformational faults, and all may lead directly to lameness. Horses that are straight behind often develop upward fixation of the patella, a condition seen most often in WBLs. Suspensory desmitis and fetlock OA also occur frequently. Horses with normal initial hindlimb conformation may become straight behind if they develop severe suspensory desmitis and lose support of the fetlock joint (see Chapter 72).

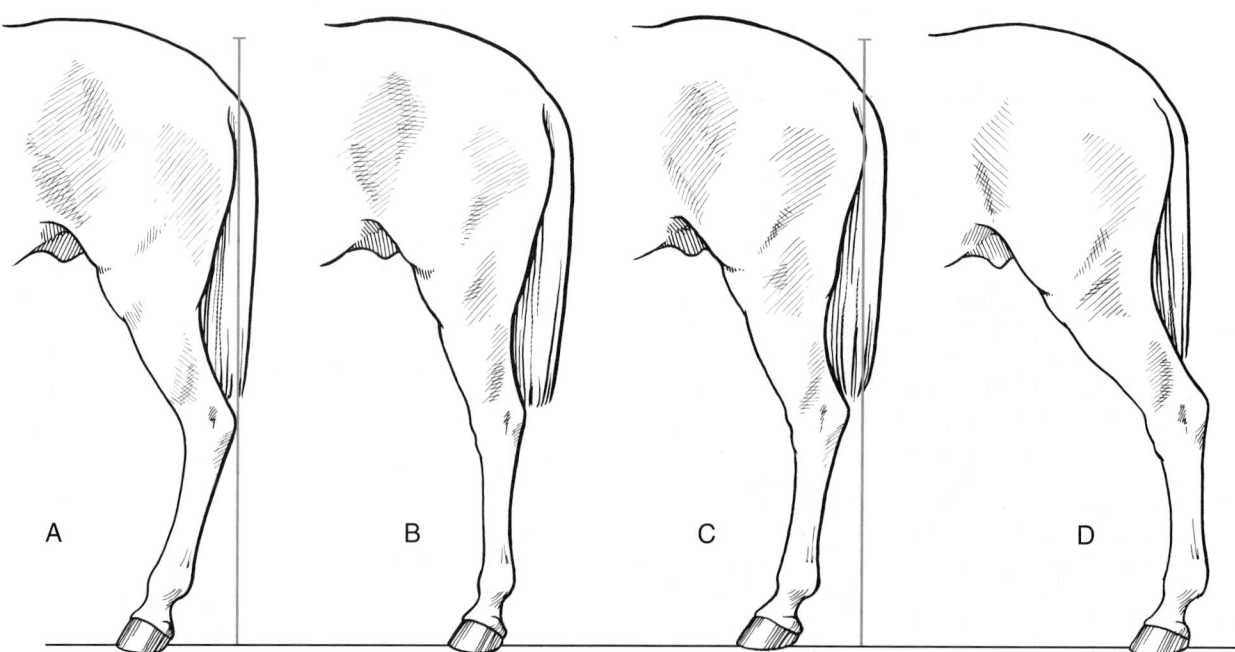

Fig. 4-27 • Diagrammatic representation of conformational faults of the hindlimb from the lateral perspective. Compared with ideal conformation, horses with sickle-hocked conformation (**A**) have a concave dorsal surface of the limb with the distal extremity dorsal to the plumb line, but those that are straight behind (**B**) have large stifle and hock joint angles but smaller fetlock joint angles. Horses that are camped under (**C**) often are sickle hocked as well. Camped-out conformation (**D**) is unusual and most often results from faulty positioning of the horse.

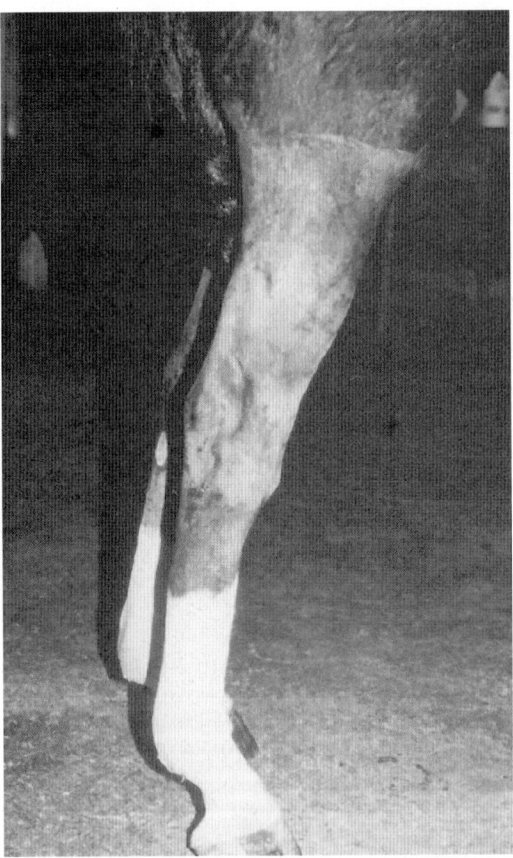

Fig. 4-28 • Standardbred filly with straight hindlimb conformation and suspensory desmitis.

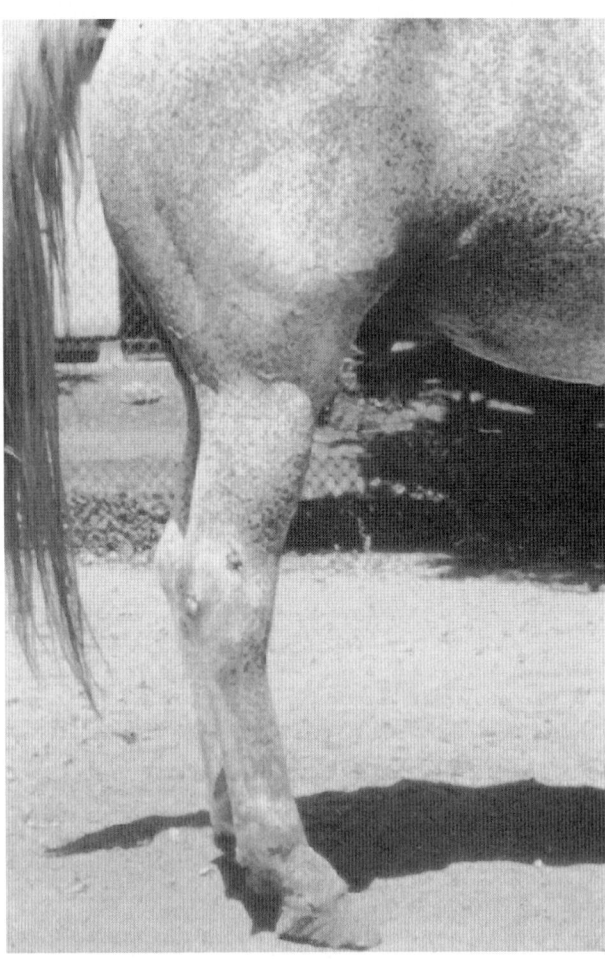

Fig. 4-29 • Horse with camped-under and mild sickle-hocked conformation, a combination leading to a short, choppy gait.

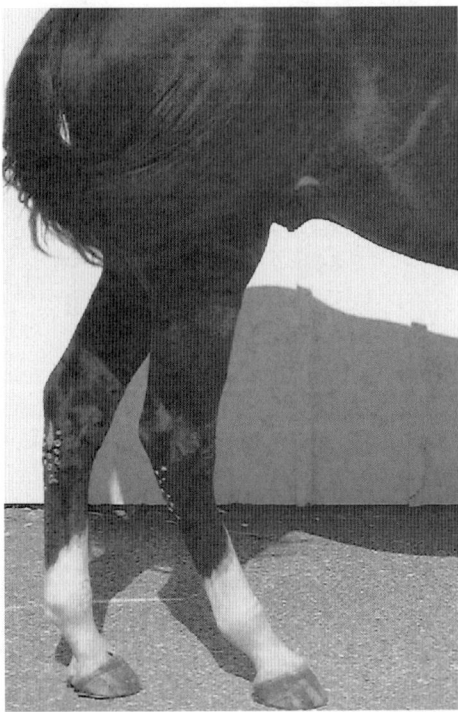

Fig. 4-30 • This 4-year-old Standardbred has sickle-hocked conformation and has developed curb, which has been treated by freeze-firing, resulting in white marks on the plantar aspect of the hocks.

Sickle-hocked conformation is one of the most common conformational faults, and it leads directly to lameness of the tarsus and plantar soft tissues. Horses that are sickle hocked stand with the lower hindlimb well ahead of the plumb line, with an exaggerated concave dorsal surface of the hindlimb (resembling a sickle), creating a smaller than normal hock angle (see Figures 4-27, 4-29, 4-30, and 4-31). This type of conformation is often called *curby* conformation because horses frequently develop curb (see Chapter 78). Sickle-hocked conformation concentrates load in the distal, plantar aspect of the hock, predisposing to curb and to distal hock joint pain. In a recent study evaluating tarsal angles and joint kinematics and kinetics, horses with large hock angles (straighter behind) had less absorbed concussion during impact, smaller vertical impulse, and less extensor movement, characteristics thought to predispose these horses to OA.[20] One of us (MWR) feels results of this study could be interpreted differently, since clinical experience contradicts this finding; horses with larger hock angles are at less risk of the development of OA of the distal hock joints and less absorbed concussion by the tarsus may make other structures such as the suspensory ligament at risk of injury. However, smaller net movement in horses with larger hock angles may be protective for the development of plantar tarsal

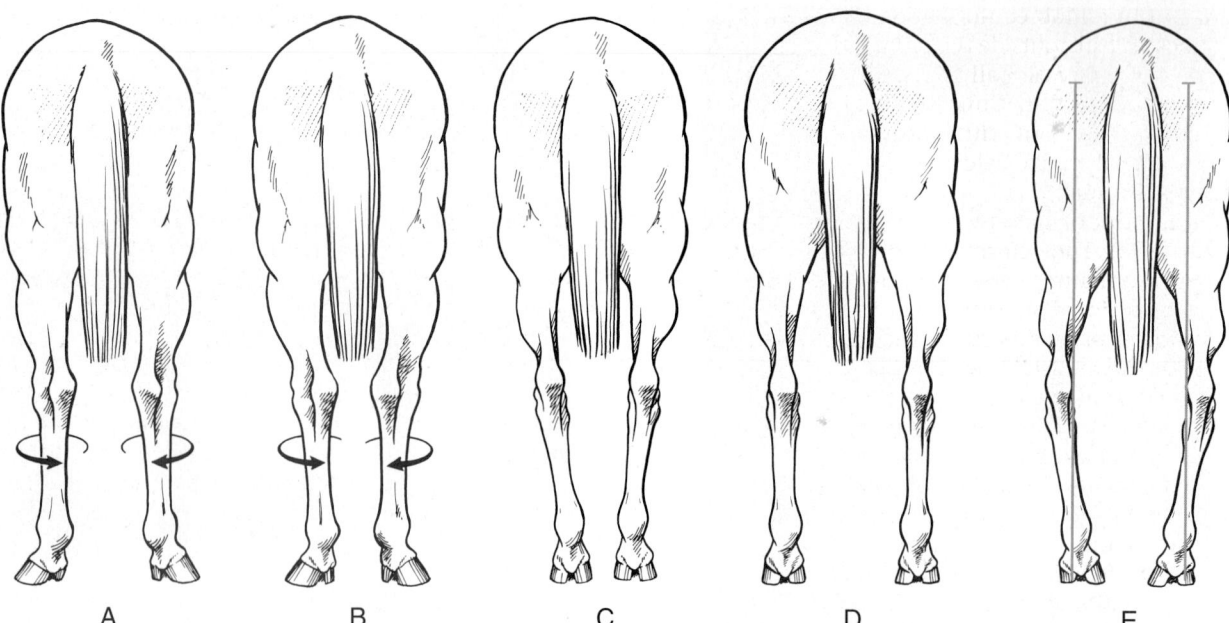

Fig. 4-31 • Hindlimb conformational abnormalities viewed from the rear. **A,** Cow-hocked conformation is a common fault characterized by external rotation of the limb, usually without angular deformity, causing the hocks to be too close together. Mild external rotation of the hindlimbs is common and does not appear to cause lameness. **B,** Cow-hocked, base-narrow conformation. **C,** Base-narrow conformation. **D,** Base-wide conformation is uncommon. **E,** Bowlegged conformation is uncommon and undesirable.

conditions such as curb, a finding that correlates well with my clinical impressions.[20] In foals with incomplete or delayed ossification of the tarsal bones, marked sickle-hocked conformation may occur (see Chapters 44 and 128). Sickle-hocked conformation is undesirable, particularly in racing breeds, but if mild is not detrimental. In STB pacers, some prefer a mild degree of sickle-hocked conformation because horses can extend the hindlimbs farther forward without risk of interference. In STB trotters the condition often predisposes to distal hock joint pain and curb, but these horses tend to be fast, although unsound. In Western reining horses, sickle-hocked horses may be better able to perform sliding stops.

Rear Perspective

A majority of STB and WBL horses toe out behind, which should be considered normal. Horses with mild external rotation of the distal extremity are said to be toed out and usually also have external rotation of hocks, causing the points of the hocks to be closer than normal. This fault is called *cow-hocked* conformation and is a *rotational* change of the hindlimb (Figure 4-31). Cow-hocked conformation occurs in combination with base-wide or base-narrow deformities or independently. Cow-hocked and base-narrow conformation is most common. Base-wide and base-narrow conformation may occur without cow-hocked conformation. These conformational faults seldom lead to lameness but have a substantial effect on gait in some horses. Horses that are base narrow travel closely behind, particularly at a walk. Some travel closely at a trot, pace, or gallop, whereas others seem to widen out when going faster, thus avoiding interference. Those that travel closely at speed often interfere, causing injury to the medial aspect of the contralateral hindlimb.

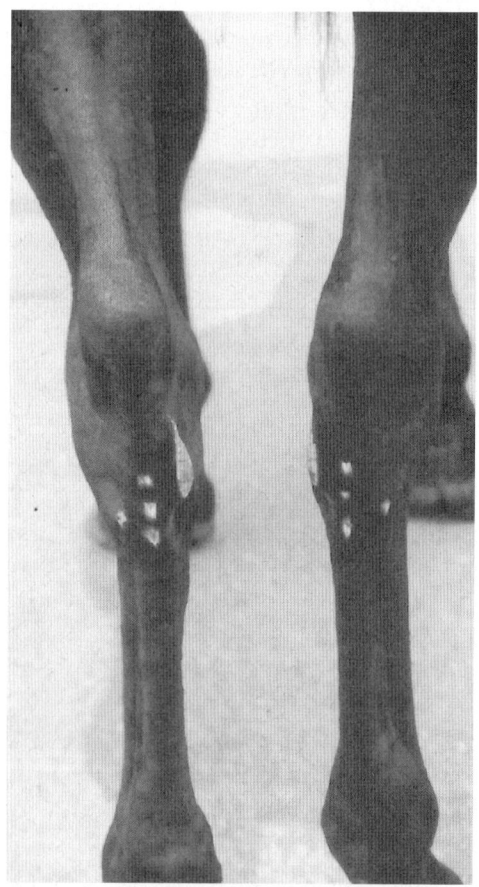

Fig. 4-32 • Mature Standardbred racehorse with in-at-the-hock (tarsus valgus) conformation. This conformational abnormality is characterized by an angular deformity as opposed to the rotational deformity seen in cow-hocked conformation. The characteristic white marks were produced by cryotherapy for treatment of bilateral curb.

Bowlegged hindlimb conformation, in which the point of both hocks is truly outside the plumb line, is uncommon (see Figure 4-31). Occasionally horses that are base narrow appear to be bowlegged. Unilateral bowlegged conformation occurs in foals born with windswept deformity or in those with tarsal varus deformity. Bilateral tarsal varus deformity is unusual.

In at the hock or tarsus valgus is an *angular* deformity (see Figure 4-32). The deformity can be corrected in foals. If it persists in a mature horse, particularly a racehorse with other conformational abnormalities, such as sickle hocks, abnormal forces or load occur in the tarsal region, predisposing the horse to distal hock joint pain, curb, and proximal metatarsal lameness.

Horses can be toed in or toed out behind, but in general the conformational abnormality starts above the fetlock joint, causing the lower limb abnormality to be linked with the upper limb. Thus a horse that is toed in generally is bowlegged, and one that is toed out is cow hocked. In some foals, however, fetlock varus occurs independent of upper limb conformational abnormalities. This abnormality usually appears in windswept foals in which upper limb deformities have resolved, leaving a fetlock varus. This is an angular deformity, but with abnormal hoof wear, toed-in conformation can develop. Fetlock varus and the resulting toed-in conformational defect may cause OA of the fetlock and interphalangeal joints and can be career-limiting.

CONFORMATION OF THE DIGIT

More detailed aspects of conformation of the foot and limb flight characteristics are discussed in Chapters 5, 7, and 27. Many of the changes in hoof growth or conformational changes in the hoof are the result of wear, shoeing, and exercise demands of training and performance and often are not present in a young horse.

The pastern angle has traditionally been thought to be similar to the angle of the shoulder (see Figure 4-8). However, in the recent TB study front pastern angle was only mildly correlated to the scapular spine angle, and there was variability.[15] Variability was likely from shoeing and lowering of the heel. There was a good correlation between pastern and hoof angles.[15] The foot-pastern axis should be straight. The pastern should be neither excessively sloped (low angle) nor upright (high angle). The angle of the pastern is important in determining the amount of load on the lower limb structures. In general, the more upright the pastern (steeper pastern angle), the shorter the stride and vice versa. Horses with upright pasterns appear to be prone to foot lameness and perhaps superficial digital flexor tendonitis. Those with long, sloping pasterns may be at risk to develop OA of the fetlock joint and proximal phalangeal fractures. Horses with short, upright pasterns but relatively normal hoof angles have a broken foot-pastern axis—the foot axis is lower than the pastern axis—and are at risk for developing foot lameness (Figure 4-33). Horses with broken back foot–pastern axis often have underrun heels and other hoof abnormalities and should be evaluated for corrective trimming if lame. If the pastern axis is lower than the foot axis (broken forward foot–pastern axis), called *coon-footed,* it causes undue strain on the soft tissue structures supporting the fetlock joint. This type of conformation may result from severe suspensory desmitis and loss of support of the fetlock joint.

Pastern length is important and usually is related to pastern angle. Horses with long pasterns commonly have more slope or lower pastern angles. The plumb line should drop approximately 5 cm behind the heel in a well-conformed horse. In horses with long, sloping, and weak pasterns, the line drops more than 5 cm behind the heel. Those with short pasterns usually have more upright pasterns, and the plumb line drops through the foot. A variety of pastern lengths and angles occur, but the pastern length should be in proportion to the overall length of the limb.

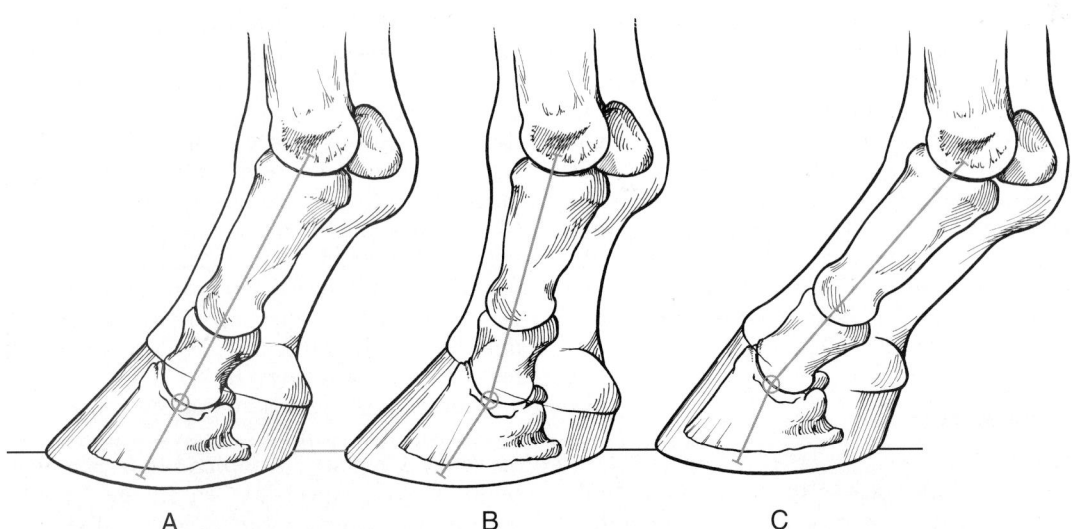

A   B   C

Fig. 4-33 • Diagrammatic representation of ideal pastern and foot conformation and the concept of a broken pastern-foot axis. Ideally the foot and pastern angles **(A)** should be identical to allow full and even weight bearing on all aspects of the foot. A broken foot axis **(B)** occurs when pastern angle is more upright than that of the foot or vice versa **(C).** In both latter situations, uneven load distribution on the foot or soft tissue structures may cause lameness.

Viewed from the front, the plumb line may divide the pastern and foot asymmetrically with more pastern and foot laterally, which often is associated with some degree of distortion of the hoof capsule, with a steeper medial wall and some flaring laterally. This results in asymmetrical loading of the distal limb joints and may predispose to lameness.

Buttress foot is an acquired firm bulge or swelling at and proximal to the dorsal aspect of the coronary band and usually reflects OA of the distal interphalangeal joint (sometimes called *pyramidal disease*). *Bull-nose foot* conformation, an abnormal convex dorsal hoof wall, is uncommon but is occasionally seen in a hind foot (Figure 4-34). It is possible to cause this abnormal hoof conformation by incorrect trimming of the dorsal hoof wall, but in most horses it is caused by faulty hoof growth. One of us (MWR) has seen this type of abnormal hind foot conformation most commonly in the TB racehorse, and it is possible there may be a relationship between bull-nose hoof conformation and lameness of the digit or other areas of the distal aspect of the hindlimb. There may be a relationship between bull-nose foot conformation and long, weak pasterns (see Figure 4-34).

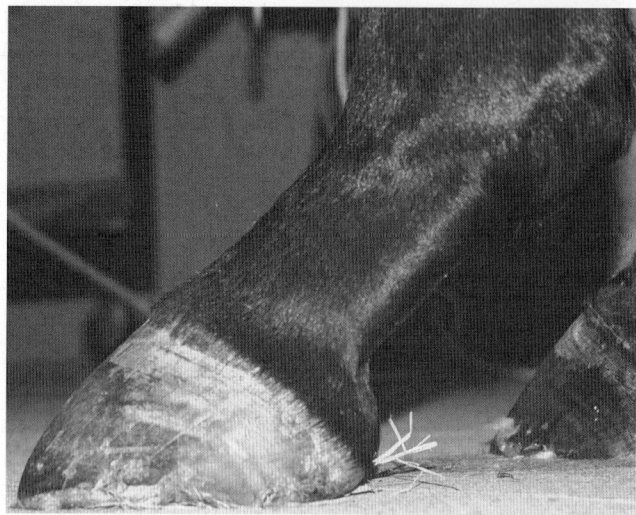

Fig. 4-34 • Bull-nose foot conformation in a 3-year-old Thoroughbred racehorse that developed a medial condylar fracture of the distal aspect of the third metatarsal bone requiring surgical repair. The relationship between poor hoof conformation and lameness is unknown, but in this horse long, weak pasterns are seen and the combination of conformational faults may predispose horses to injury.

Chapter 5

Observation: Symmetry and Posture

Mike W. Ross

Assessments of symmetry and posture are important aspects of a lameness examination. Comparison between the normal and abnormal sides facilitates identification of abnormalities, unless the condition is bilateral so that no recognizable differences exist between the left and right limbs. The horse should be standing squarely on a flat surface in a quiet, insect-free environment. Horses with severe lameness often are reluctant to stand correctly, but information gained about symmetry and posture of severely lame horses is valuable. The veterinarian should look carefully at size, shape, contour, heights, and widths and compare with the opposite side.

FORELIMB SYMMETRY

Muscle Atrophy

The symmetry of skeletal muscle in the forearm, pectoral, and cervical areas should be assessed. Muscle atrophy that occurs in horses with chronic lameness conditions is called *disuse atrophy* and in those with neurological disease is called *neurogenic atrophy*. Horses with muscle atrophy and lower motor neuron disease (see Chapter 11) may be lame, sometimes as a result of muscle pain or nerve root pain,

complicating differentiation between these causes of muscle atrophy. In most but not all horses with neurogenic atrophy, other clinical signs suggestive of neurological disease may be present. Horses with disuse atrophy resulting from chronic lameness usually have generalized atrophy of the ipsilateral forelimb. Muscle loss usually is not pronounced but involves the forearm (extensors are most commonly affected), triceps, and shoulder muscles. Shoulder muscle atrophy involving the infraspinatus and supraspinatus muscles generally is not pronounced, and lateral subluxation of the shoulder joint during weight bearing is not present (see Chapter 40).

Development of disuse atrophy resulting from chronic lameness generally takes weeks to months unless severe lameness exists. In horses with severe or non–weight-bearing lameness, atrophy may develop within 10 to 14 days. In horses with severe forelimb lameness, carpal contraction (flexural deformity of the carpus) may occur simultaneously with muscle atrophy. The most common causes of carpal contraction because of ipsilateral forelimb lameness are olecranon fracture and other elbow lameness, but carpal contraction may occur in horses with severe shoulder or even lower limb lameness. Atrophy of the triceps muscles usually is recognized before other muscle atrophy in severely lame horses.

Horses with neurogenic atrophy may have profound atrophy of one or more muscles in the forearm, pectoral, or cervical regions. Atrophy often is much more pronounced than expected based on the degree of lameness, prompting suspicion of neurological disease. Pronounced, unilateral pectoral or triceps atrophy with mild atrophy of the forearm muscles suggests neurological disease. Severe atrophy localized to the infraspinatus or supraspinatus muscles without subluxation of the shoulder joint usually results from injury of the suprascapular nerve caused by external trauma. Atrophy and subluxation of the shoulder joint is associated with injury of the brachial plexus or nerve roots. Other muscles may also show atrophy.

Localized muscle atrophy or fibrosis occurs in horses with previous injury and subsequent scar tissue formation within muscle bellies. This condition is more common in the hindlimb but occasionally occurs in the forelimb.

Swelling

Swelling, a common sign of inflammation, often causes asymmetry. The presence of swelling and heat should alert the lameness diagnostician to the possibility of an infectious process and may lead to additional examinations such as assessment of body temperature and the acquisition of laboratory data. Swelling within a joint capsule caused by excess joint fluid, *effusion,* is a general reaction of the joint to several traumatic or degenerative processes. Edema, cellulitis (lymphangitis), bleeding, and fibrosis can cause soft tissue swelling. Underlying bony enlargement can mimic soft tissue swelling, particularly in older horses with advanced osteoarthritis. Some swellings are clinically innocuous, such as mild distention of a digital flexor tendon sheath (so-called "windgalls" or "wind puffs"), but a recent change in size, local heat, or marked left-right asymmetry should alert the clinician to a possible problem. Occasionally a well-circumscribed tense spherical swelling is seen palmar to the neurovascular bundle on the side of the fetlock. These synovium-filled masses are usually incidental findings of no clinical significance. *Edema* usually signals acute inflammation, and pits (a distinct impression is visible) when compressed by digital palpation (pitting edema). Horses develop edema around and often distal to the site of inflammation. In some horses, especially racehorses left unbandaged when accustomed to being bandaged, benign mild-to-moderate edema of the distal extremities develops. This process is called "stocking-up" and should not be misinterpreted as a pathological process. In these horses the edematous area is not painful and usually does not pit, and the horse is not lame. Edema in these horses can complicate lameness examination because it is sometimes difficult to palpate underlying structures and to perform diagnostic analgesia.

Cellulitis describes infection within the tissue planes of the distal extremities (see Chapter 14) and is sometimes called *lymphangitis*. Lymphangitis, by definition, is inflammation of the lymphatic circulation of the limb, but the conditions are similar and the terms are used interchangeably. Swelling is firm, warm, and painful, and lameness is often pronounced. "Stovepipe" swelling describes this condition ("the horse is all stoved-up"). Horses generally show systemic signs such as fever and elevated white blood cell count. Cellulitis usually results from small puncture wounds that may be difficult to discover or occurs after articular, periarticular, or subcutaneous injections. Infection develops in subcutaneous tissues or deeper in the dense fascial planes and can be difficult to eradicate.

Blunt trauma or fractures may cause bleeding within tissue planes. Severe lameness and swelling accompany fractures of the scapula and humerus, because large vessels are nearby. Bleeding may be severe and cause a decrease in plasma protein and packed blood cell volume values. In horses with fractures located more distally in the limb, swelling is less pronounced but still prominent. The most

likely location of injury is the swollen area, but swelling may occur distal to the site of injury because of venous and lymphatic congestion.

Fibrosis or scar tissue formation as the result of previous cellulitis or trauma causes asymmetry of the distal extremities but may not be the source of the current lameness. The veterinarian should avoid overinterpreting areas of scar tissue formation unless evidence of recrudescent inflammation exists. Horses may have scars caused by previous application of counterirritants or from healed wounds, leaving large, painless, and thus benign blemishes. Scars from previous surgical procedures, sometimes recognized by small areas of white hair accumulation, should be noted but may have no bearing on the current problem. Previous scars may have more relevance during prepurchase examinations.

Bony swelling is a common cause of asymmetry. Proliferative change results in periosteal or periarticular new bone formation and accompanies myriad problems in the distal extremities. Bony changes may be active, causing the current lameness problem, or old and inactive, causing few or no clinical signs. For example, old inactive bony swelling of the shin or osselets (bony and fibrous swelling of the fetlock joint) may be prominent in ex-racehorses but may have little to no relevance to current lameness.

Angular Deformity

Angular limb deformities in young horses are common, are sometimes associated with lameness or other developmental orthopedic disease, and are discussed elsewhere (see Chapter 58). Abnormalities of conformation should be noted but may have little relevance to the current lameness problem (see Chapter 4). Horses younger than 2 years of age with severe forelimb lameness of several months' duration may develop contralateral varus deformity originating from the carpus or elbow joints.

Horses with severe lameness usually caused by trauma may have luxation or subluxation of joints as a result of collateral ligament injury or fractures and may have an acute change in limb angulation. Angular deviations of limbs are unusual in older horses and generally signal severe injury. Visual examination should be followed by careful palpation during which varus and valgus stress is applied to joints. Stress radiographs can be useful to determine collateral ligament integrity.

Foot Size

Ideally both front feet should be identical in size and shape, or nearly so, and any asymmetry should be noted. Horses with chronic lameness may have disparity in foot size, usually with the smaller foot being ipsilateral to lameness. The small foot often is contracted and more upright (Figure 5-1). Chronic reduction in weight bearing results in foot size disparity in some, but not all, horses. Mild disparity in foot size is a normal finding in some horses. Mild clubfoot conformation, acquired from previous flexural deformity, may be present incidentally in adult horses. Previous lameness may have caused contraction of the foot but has since resolved, resulting in disparity in foot size and shape but no residual lameness. In these horses it would be a mistake to assume current lameness is originating from the foot without confirmation using diagnostic analgesia. Clubfoot conformation appears to be better

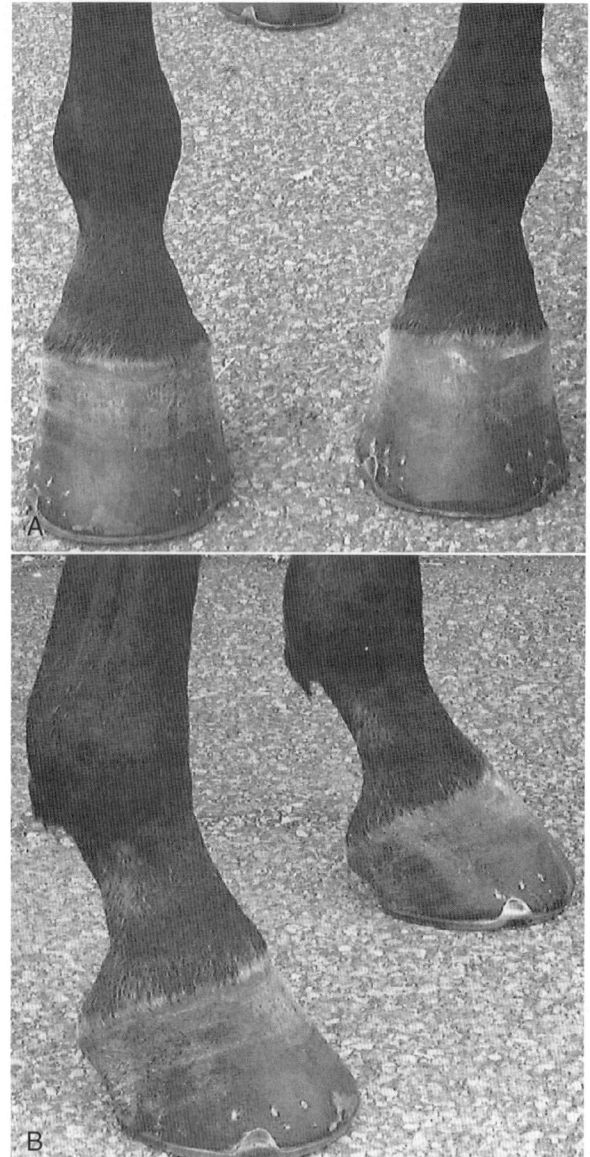

Fig. 5-1 • A horse with disparity in front foot size caused by chronic lameness. The right forelimb foot is smaller compared with the normal left forelimb foot when viewed from the front **(A)** and more upright when viewed from the side **(B).**

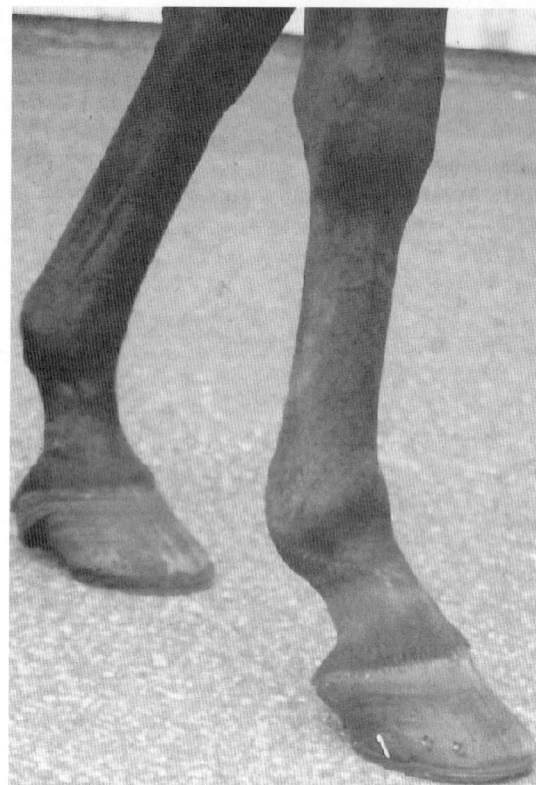

Fig. 5-2 • Standardbred racehorse with severe suspensory desmitis and a "dropped fetlock." The level of the right front fetlock joint is lower than that of the left front, caused by chronic, severe desmitis. Similar clinical signs and severe lameness appear in horses with acute traumatic disruption of the suspensory apparatus.

tolerated in Thoroughbred (TB) than in Standardbred (STB) racehorses.

Fetlock Height

Fetlock position should be assessed in the standing horse and during movement. In a standing horse, fetlock height should be symmetrical, assuming the horse is loading the limbs equally. Horses with severe lameness commonly "point" or hold the limb in front of the opposite forelimb, thus taking weight off the limb. This standing posture obviously causes disparity in fetlock height but should be carefully interpreted. Loss of support of a fetlock in the standing horse causes the affected fetlock to drop and occurs most commonly with acute, traumatic disruption of the suspensory apparatus in racehorses but also appears with chronic, active desmitis (Figure 5-2). Severe superficial digital flexor tendonitis or lacerations resulting in fiber

damage of the deep or superficial digital flexor tendons can cause similar clinical signs.

In horses with mild flexural deformity of the metacarpophalangeal joint, dynamic knuckling (buckling forward, flexion) of the fetlock joint may occur in the standing position (Figure 5-3). Joint position usually returns to normal during movement. In horses with severe flexural deformity, normal fetlock position is never achieved. Knuckling of the fetlock also may result from desmitis of the accessory ligament of the deep digital flexor tendon.

Scapular Height

Disparity in scapular height is a rare clinical sign in a lame horse. The veterinarian must stand behind and above the horse to observe scapular height. The horse's mane may obscure observation from a distance, requiring closer examination by palpation. Traumatic or neurological conditions affect scapular height, causing either injury or dysfunction of the serratus ventralis muscle, respectively. With both conditions the dorsal aspect of the scapula is *higher* on the affected side. The veterinarian may place pieces of white tape or other suitable markers on both sides of the horse and stand back to compare height or may use two assistants to point to the locations. Horses may have disparity in scapular height unrelated to the current lameness condition if there has been resolution of the original injury or neurological problem. Care must be taken to differentiate between genuine differences in the height of each scapula and asymmetrical musculature,

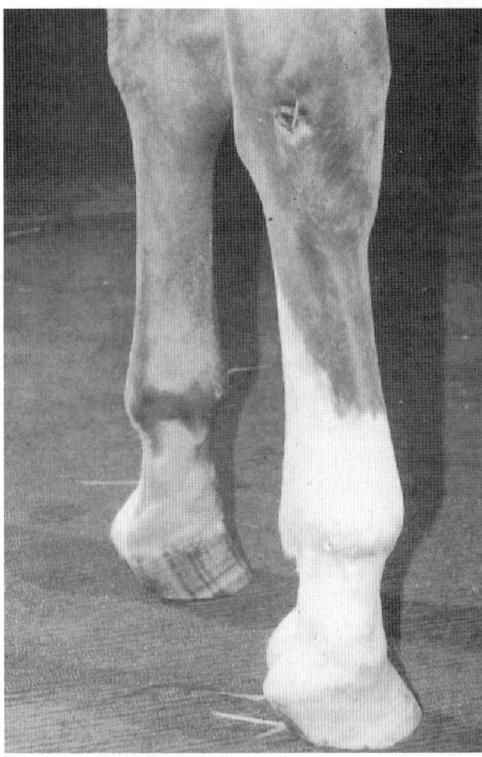

Fig. 5-3 • Knuckling forward of the right front fetlock joint occurs in a standing position in this horse with mild flexural deformity of the metacarpophalangeal joint. This dynamic instability abates somewhat when the horse moves, but the left front fetlock also is straight, indicating the presence of bilateral flexural deformity.

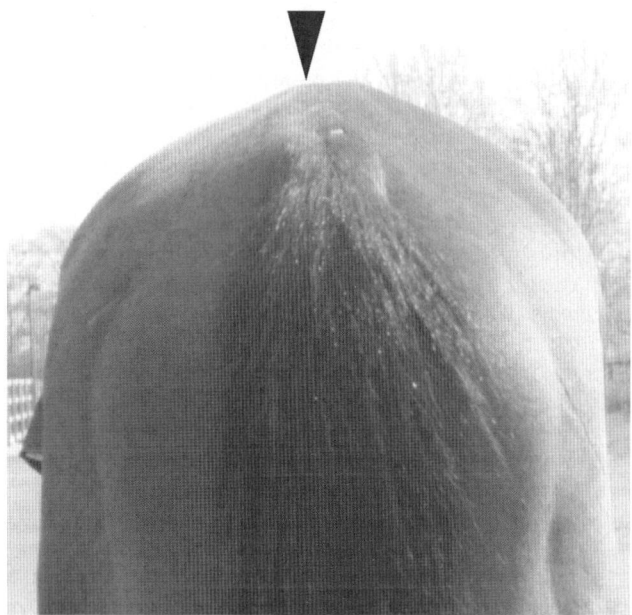

Fig. 5-4 • Three-year-old Thoroughbred filly with subtle disparity in tubera sacrale height. The left tuber sacrale is slightly lower *(arrow)* than the right, caused by a fracture at the base of the tuber sacrale. This clinical finding can easily be missed or confused with mild muscle atrophy.

which occurs much more commonly and may be an incidental observation. Horses with disparity in scapular height or asymmetrical muscle development may have problems with saddle fit.

HINDLIMB SYMMETRY
Muscle Atrophy
Asymmetry of bone and muscle mass in the hindlimbs and pelvis is a common clinical sign but must be differentiated carefully. The horse should stand squarely on a flat, even surface. The clinician must determine whether asymmetry exists, and if so, if the problem involves muscle, bone, or a combination of the tissues. Muscle atrophy is most common and, if unilateral muscle atrophy exists, easily can be confused with bony asymmetry caused by pelvic fractures or asymmetry of the tubera sacrale.

Disuse and neurogenic muscle atrophy occur in the hindlimb. Horses with chronic hindlimb lameness develop ipsilateral gluteal muscle atrophy, but asymmetry may be subtle. Mild muscle atrophy usually first appears just lateral to a tuber sacrale. The veterinarian should differentiate muscle atrophy from disparity in height of the tubera sacrale (Figure 5-4). Recognition of muscle atrophy helps determine the lame leg and provides some information about the duration of the problem. Severe muscle atrophy develops in horses with long-standing, severe lameness or in those with neurological disease (Figure 5-5).

In horses with neurogenic atrophy of the gluteal muscles the degree of muscle loss is inappropriately severe compared

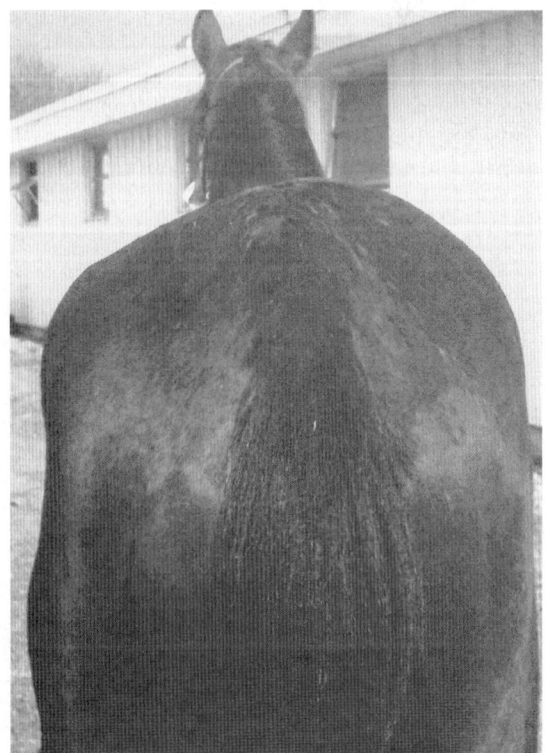

Fig. 5-5 • A 4-year-old Standardbred with severe left gluteal atrophy caused by neurological disease. The presumptive clinical diagnosis was equine protozoal myelitis.

with observed lameness. Neurological signs such as weakness and proprioceptive deficits usually appear in horses with neurogenic atrophy, but early in the course of diseases such as equine protozoal myelitis (EPM) the only observable signs may be muscle atrophy and mild lameness.

Selective atrophy of individual muscles or muscle groups occurs in horses with neurological disease or injuries causing focal muscle loss and scarring. Horses with trauma involving fracture of the tubera ischii may develop focal muscle loss of the semitendinosus or semimembranosus muscles. A depression, sometimes subtle, resulting from localized muscle atrophy replaces initial swelling of the point of the rump. Horses with *fibrotic myopathy,* which in most horses is believed to result from injury and scarring of the semitendinosus muscle, usually have palpable scars or defects of the caudal thigh muscles. Degenerative neuropathy of the nerves supplying the distal aspect of the semitendinosus muscle also may cause fibrotic myopathy[1] (see Chapter 48).

References on page 1256

Swelling

Swelling is especially important in horses with acute, severe lameness when the clinician must differentiate between catastrophic injury, such as pelvic or long bone fracture, and more common conditions, such as cellulitis. Horses with pelvic fractures may develop mild swelling in the thigh, but swelling is not prominent in most horses. In horses with fracture of a tuber coxae or ilial wing or shaft, mild swelling may develop distally but usually is not prominent. Inappropriate lameness and lack of swelling should prompt the clinician to perform a rectal examination, checking for internal asymmetry or crepitus. Horses with femoral fractures develop acute, severe swelling of the thigh, accompanied by severe lameness, instability, and often crepitus (Figure 5-6). Horses may develop severe swelling of the stifle and thigh resulting from trauma and secondary bleeding. Large stifle hematomas resemble the swelling in horses with femoral fractures, and in some

horses hematomas can be confused with severe femoropatellar effusion (Figure 5-7). Excessive bleeding from subcutaneous vessels also may involve the ventral, lateral abdominal region. In horses with stifle hematoma, lameness may not be as prominent as expected, and swelling

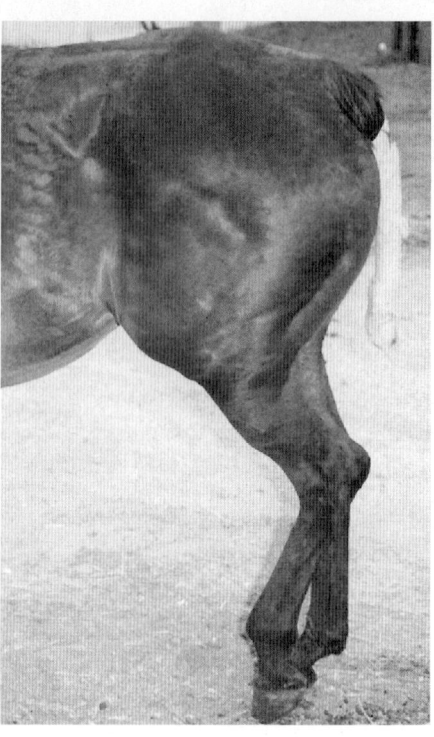

Fig. 5-6 • A Thoroughbred broodmare with severe lameness and swelling of the left thigh caused by a comminuted femoral fracture.

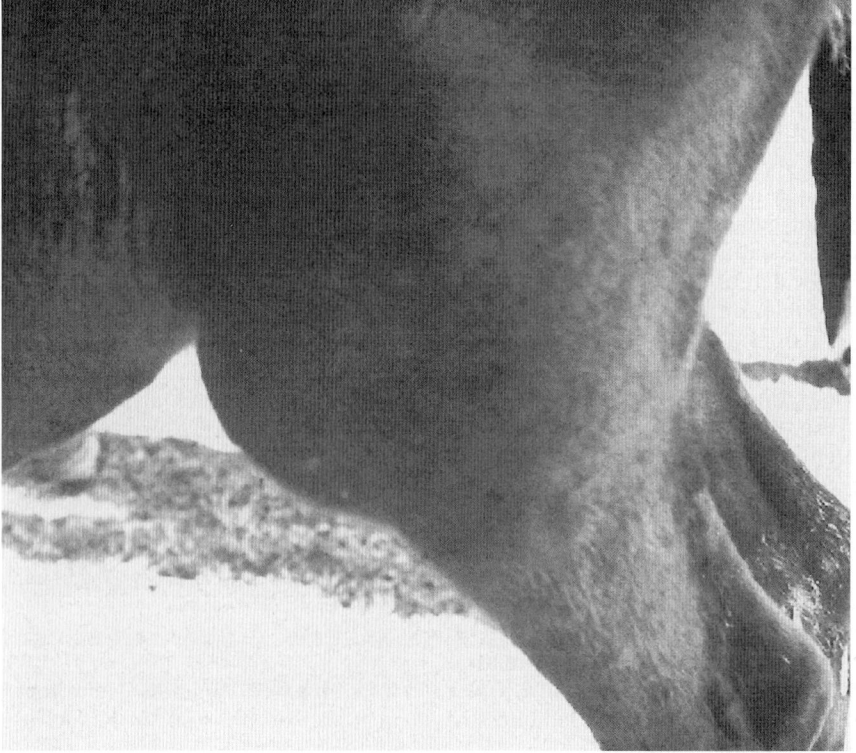

Fig. 5-7 • Moderate, fluctuant soft tissue swelling over the stifle caused by subcutaneous bleeding (hematoma). In this situation, swelling is much more pronounced than expected for the observed degree of lameness.

fluctuates, which is useful in differentiating this cause of lameness from femoral fractures. Generalized, diffuse soft tissue swelling appears in horses with cellulitis or lymphangitis in the hindlimb (Figure 5-8). Horses that negotiate fences such as event and timber horses are at risk for stifle-region trauma and swelling.

Bony Asymmetry

Comparison of the height of the tubera coxae is important to determine the nature and extent of pelvic bony injury (Figure 5-9). Two assistants, one on each side of the horse, may point to the dorsal aspect of the tubera coxae, or the veterinarian may use temporary markers to compare the height. Determining the height of the tubera sacrale may be difficult and requires careful palpation to differentiate bone, ligament, and muscle asymmetry. Accurate determination may be possible only by ultrasonography. Estimating the midline-to-lateral pelvic width also aids in diagnosing acute or chronic pelvic fractures.

Tubera Coxae

Asymmetry in height of the tubera coxae accompanies many different pelvic fractures. The most common fracture involves the tuber coxae itself, often called *knocked-down hip*. Marked ventral and medial displacement of the fracture fragment occurs because of muscle attachment to the bony prominence. The veterinarian also must palpate the actual shape of the tuber coxae, because ventral displacement occurs with other pelvic injuries. Displacement and

rotation occur in horses with fracture of the wing of the ilium caudal to the tuber coxae without an obvious change in size or shape of the tuber coxae. However, with a partial fracture of the ventral aspect of the tuber coxae, there is a change in its shape without displacement of the dorsal aspect of the bone.

Tubera Sacrale

The term *hunter's bump* describes the prominence of the tubera sacrale. This finding may reflect the horse's conformation, poorly developed surrounding musculature, or a change in position of one or both tubera sacrale. Increase or decrease in size of the overlying dorsal sacroiliac ligament also results in apparent asymmetry. Many clinically normal horses have slight apparent asymmetry of the tubera sacrale. Asymmetry in height of the tubera sacrale occurs in horses with acute or chronic sacroiliac joint disruption (Figure 5-10). In horses with acute fractures of the base of the tubera sacrale, the affected side is lower[2] (see Chapters 49 and 50). Ultrasonography and nuclear scintigraphy may help identify the cause of asymmetry.

Midline-to-Lateral Pelvic Width

A change in the relative width of each hemipelvis is a subtle but important clinical sign of pelvic injury. In most horses with pelvic fractures, the injured side is narrower than the normal side. Overriding and displacement of fracture fragments result in compression on the injured side.

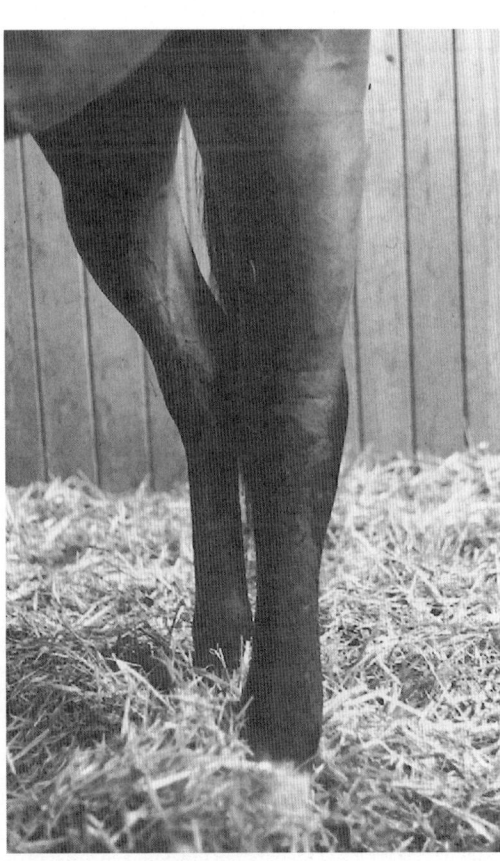

Fig. 5-8 • Soft tissue swelling caused by cellulitis. Firm, painful swelling appears in the entire limb.

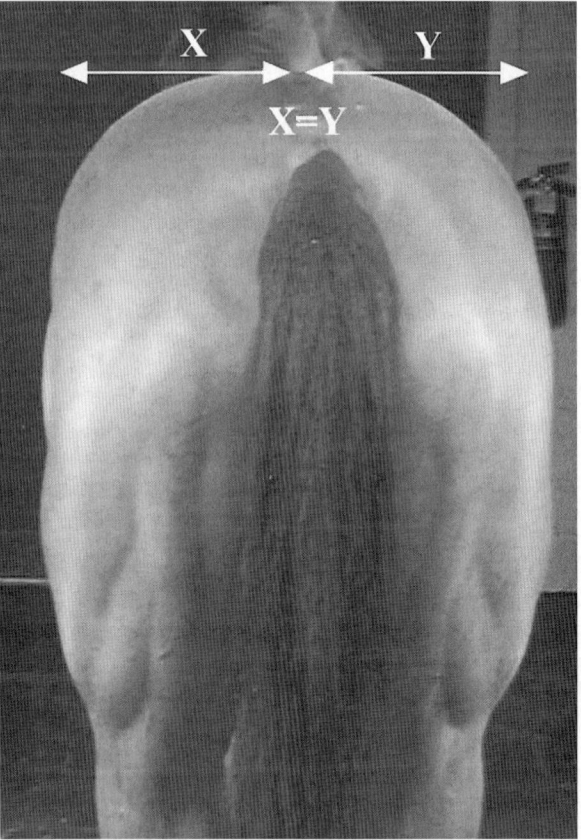

Fig. 5-9 • A horse that is well positioned for determination of tubera coxae height and the midline-to-lateral pelvic width *(X, Y)*. In a normal horse, *X = Y*.

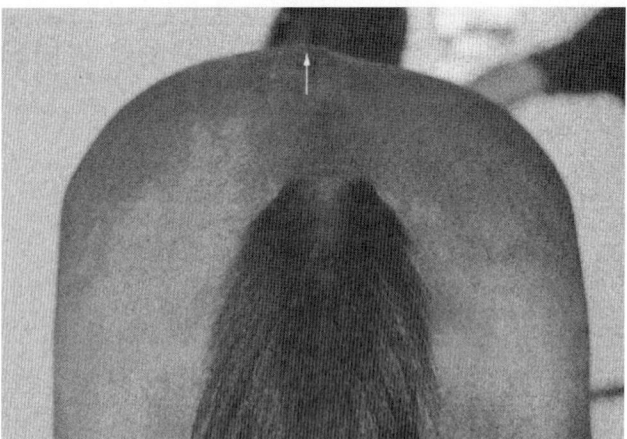

Fig. 5-10 • Asymmetry of the tubera sacrale. The left tuber sacrale *(arrow)* is higher than the right. This horse has chronic left sacroiliac subluxation.

Swelling over the Greater Trochanter

Mild swelling over the lateral aspect of the coxofemoral joint may be a subtle clinical sign of acetabular or proximal femoral fractures. When standing behind the horse, the veterinarian should carefully observe for enlargement over the affected hip joint. This clinical sign usually is not noticeable initially, but soft tissue enlargement is visible within 2 to 3 weeks after intraarticular fracture. The groove between the greater trochanter and the biceps femoris muscle should be compared carefully; usually a slight bulge or subtle enlargement on the affected side is visible.

Crepitus

Bone-on-bone grating is a valuable clinical sign, particularly in horses with pelvic injury. Crepitus can be heard (with or without a stethoscope) or felt (external or rectal palpation) and most often is caused by movement of bone fragments in horses with displaced fractures (see Chapter 6). In horses with pelvic fractures, crepitus usually is not observed for several days to weeks after injury because muscle tone and fracture hematoma apparently stabilize fracture fragments and delay onset. Crepitus also can be felt or heard in horses with end-stage osteoarthritis.

Calcaneus

The points of the hock should be of equal height when observed from the side or from behind. There is dramatic lowering of the point of the hock with complete disruption of the common calcaneal tendon or gastrocnemius tendon alone. Partial injury of the gastrocnemius muscle origin, the musculotendonous junction, or the tendon itself causes varying degrees of asymmetry in height of the point of the hock, both in a standing horse and during movement.[3] Other gait abnormalities such as unusual rotation or instability of the limb usually are present (Figure 5-11).

The point of the hock is elevated in horses with severe pelvic fractures involving the acetabulum, luxation of the coxofemoral joint, and some femoral fractures (Figure 5-12). Evaluating elevation is difficult because horses with severe lameness usually cannot bear weight, causing a dramatic alteration in limb position. However, in horses with true elevation in the point of the hock, the hock is extended,

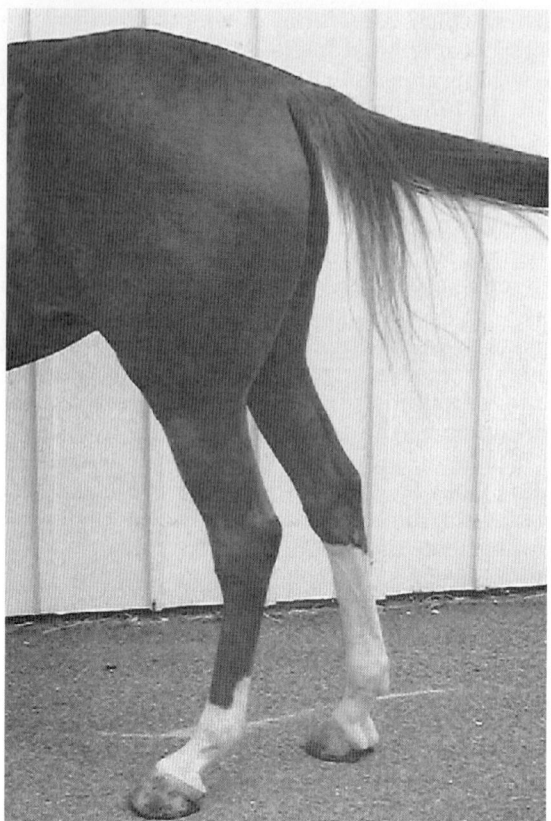

Fig. 5-11 • A horse with partial disruption of the left gastrocnemius. An injury to the origin of the lateral head of the gastrocnemius muscle in this horse caused an unusual gait deficit, lameness, and mild distal displacement (drop) of the hock and fetlock.

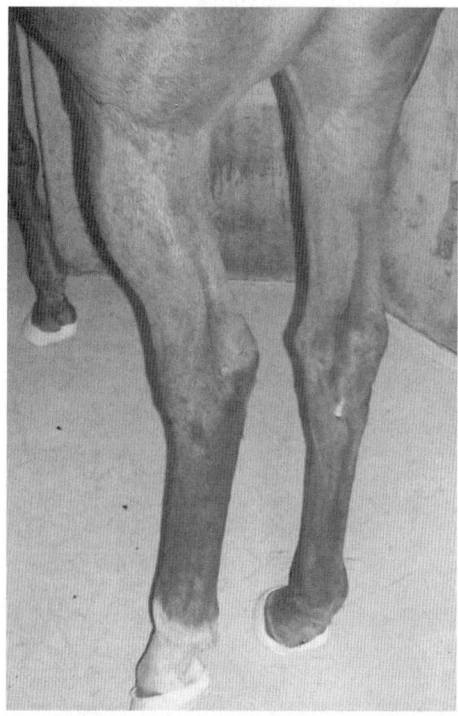

Fig. 5-12 • A horse with a comminuted fracture of the left femur. The point of the left hock is higher than that of the right as a result of overriding of fracture fragments and muscle contraction, effectively shortening the limb.

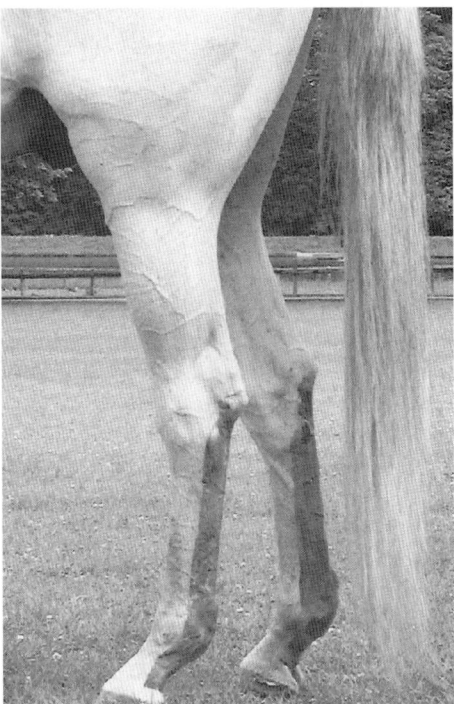

Fig. 5-13 • Warmblood gelding with chronic, severe, bilateral hindlimb suspensory desmitis causing noticeable fetlock drop in the left hindlimb.

whereas with most non–weight-bearing conditions, the hock is flexed.

Fetlock Height

Assessment of fetlock position is as important in the hindlimb as in the forelimb. Horses with excessively straight hindlimb conformation (straight hocks) may have more obvious excursion of the fetlock (fetlock drop) while moving or shifting position during standing. Pathological fetlock drop generally accompanies suspensory desmitis (Figure 5-13) but also occurs with partial disruption of the gastrocnemius and other ligamentous and tendonous injuries.

POSTURE

Body posture provides important clues to the source of lameness, but some abnormalities may be missed unless the horse is observed over long periods. Normal horses tend to rest one hindlimb and may alternate between limbs. Resting a forelimb is uncommon but does occur. Distractions in the environment may make a horse stand normally despite pain. However, abnormal posture because of mechanical or neurological dysfunction usually is evident.

The horse has a well-developed stay apparatus in both the forelimbs and hindlimbs.[4] It is assumed that the main purpose of the stay apparatus is to allow the horse to remain standing for long periods. The stay apparatus in the hindlimbs is better developed than in the forelimbs and includes ligamentous and tendonous structures dictating predictable movement of joints in the limb. If intact, the hindlimb stay apparatus demands reciprocal movement of the hock and stifle and often is called the *reciprocal*

apparatus. A change in posture usually means a part of the reciprocal apparatus is broken.

FORELIMB POSTURE

Pointing

Horses that are severely lame often point or hold the affected forelimb ahead of the unaffected forelimb, or the least affected forelimb in horses with bilateral pain. These horses usually are severely lame at a walk. Horses with severe, bilateral forelimb lameness caused by laminitis may stand camped out in front, attempting to point with both forelimbs simultaneously. However, pointing is not synonymous with the presence of pain or lameness or its degree. Some horses prefer to point one forelimb or another and walk and trot normally. In general, pointing is unusual and often signals resting pain or subtle pain relieved by adopting this posture. Some horses stack bedding under the heel of one or both front feet to stand in a toe-down position, indicating a degree of unilateral or bilateral foot pain. These horses often are not as lame as expected based on the degree of postural change seen at rest. Alternatively a horse may stand with its hindquarters "sitting" on a manger partially to unload the front feet.

Treading

Constant shifting of weight from one forelimb to the other may indicate bilateral forelimb lameness. Laminitis, severe soft tissue injuries such as tendonitis or suspensory desmitis, or severe osteoarthritis may cause treading. Horses with chronic, severe unilateral forelimb lameness often stand with little weight on the affected limb, overload the unaffected limb, and seldom tread. The development of treading in such circumstances is an ominous sign because the horse now is trying to shift weight from the previously unaffected limb, probably because of laminitis.

Buckling Forward at the Knee

Horses with bucked-knee or over-at-the-knee conformation may buckle forward at the knee while standing. In clinically normal older field hunters or other heavily used riding horses with bilateral over-at-the-knee conformation, this may be particularly obvious. The carpus is locked in extension primarily by the action of the extensor muscles. Neurological disease (e.g., EPM) affecting forelimb extensor muscles is a rare cause of buckling forward at the knee, both at rest and during movement. Specific injury of the distal aspect of the radial nerve causes similar clinical signs. In foals, rupture of the common digital extensor tendon or other extensor tendons may cause this posture (see Chapters 77 and 128).

Dropped Elbow

A dropped elbow results from failure of the triceps apparatus to maintain elbow extension (Figure 5-14) and usually results from fracture of the olecranon process. It also may result from injury to the radial nerve or brachial plexus. Similar clinical signs appear in horses with lesions of the nerve roots (neuritis, radiculopathy) or nerve cell bodies in the cervical intumescence, usually the result of lower motor neuron disease. A most unusual cause of this posture appears in horses with root signature (see the section on neck pain).

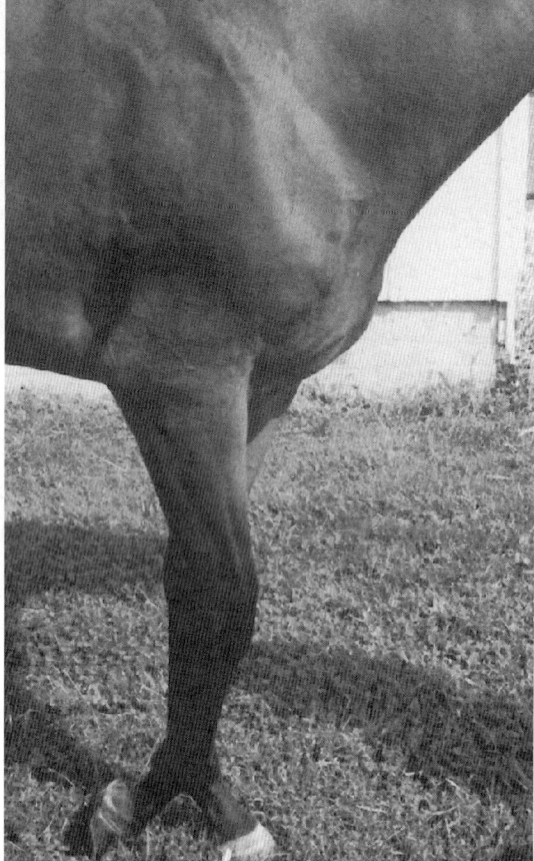

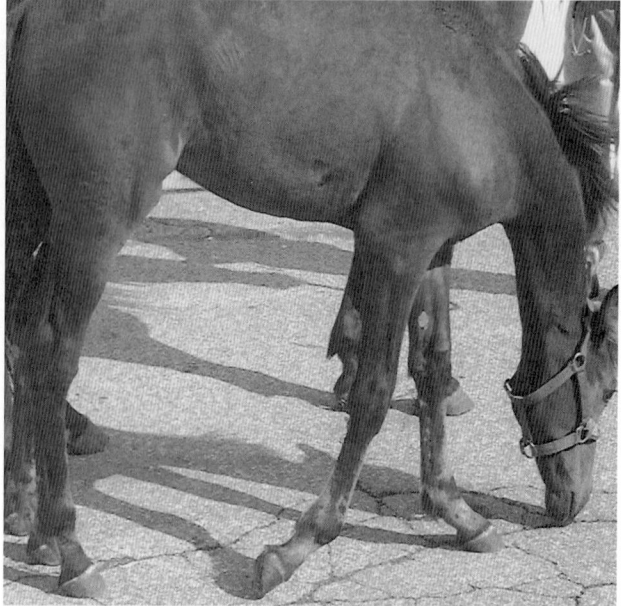

Fig. 5-15 • Forelimb posture in a foal with osteomyelitis (scapula) and infectious arthritis (shoulder joint). With severe lameness of the shoulder or bicipital bursa, horses are reluctant to stand or move normally and often hold the limb caudally. This posture may be difficult to differentiate from that seen with loss of the triceps apparatus (see Figure 5-14).

Fig. 5-14 • Classic forelimb posture most often called *radial nerve paresis* or *paralysis*. The horse cannot extend or fix the elbow, causing the appearance of dropped elbow. The inability to fix the elbow (loss of triceps apparatus) commonly occurs in horses with olecranon fractures.

Severe Lameness of the Shoulder Region

Horses with severe shoulder pain may stand with the affected limb more caudal than usual (Figure 5-15) and often drag the limb with even the slightest movement. This posture is similar to dropped-elbow posture, but in horses with a dropped elbow the limb is held at, or even slightly cranial to, the expected position.

Neck Pain

Horses with neck pain often hold the head and neck lower than expected, at a level equal to or slightly lower than the withers (Figure 5-16). Historically some horses may be observed to get caught in this position. In horses with severe pain, muscle tremors or spasms are visible, especially when one approaches the horse or the horse moves; the horse may stand in a guarded position. The horse may be reluctant to turn or move and may be unable or unwilling to eat food from either the ground or an elevated position. An unusual but characteristic sign of neck pain is posturing of a single forelimb, usually on the side of the lesion. The limb is held extended or pointed in front of the other forelimb; rarely the limb is held in slight flexion (see Figure 53-10, *A*). This sign appears in dogs with cervical pain, most commonly from intervertebral disk disease, and is termed *root signature*.[5,6] Pain associated with the nerve roots supplying the brachial plexus may be the cause. Such a

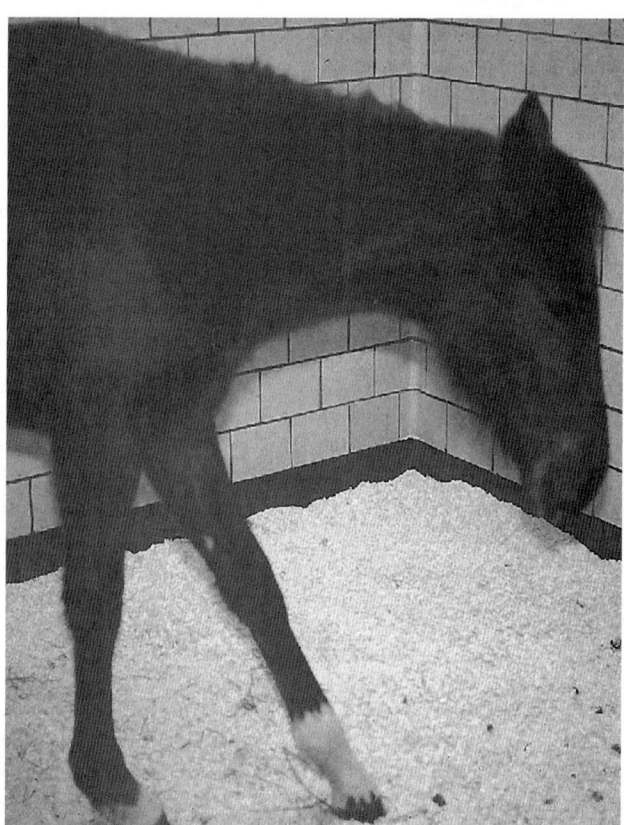

Fig. 5-16 • Yearling Standardbred with neck pain on the left side showing typical stance and head and neck posture.

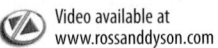

posture has also been seen in a horse with a mediastinal abscess. Some horses with cervical pain also have unilateral forelimb lameness.[7]

HINDLIMB POSTURE

Resting a Hindlimb
Normally a horse rests one hindlimb or another, but immediate resting of a hindlimb after work, or a combination of resting of the hindlimb and trembling in the flank or stifle region, may indicate lameness. Resting of the hindlimb, particularly with trembling of the quadriceps muscles, often prompts handlers to erroneously assume the horse has stifle region pain. Horses with hindlimb pain from other locations will often assume this posture.

Abnormal Tail Position
Horses may carry the tail in an abnormal position during movement, often alerting an observer to possible hindlimb pain. The tail usually is carried away from the lame limb, but this finding is inconsistent. Horses seldom have an abnormal tail posture at rest unless the tail has been traumatized or set or there is severe hindlimb lameness.

External Rotation of the Hindlimb
Cow-hocked conformation is common, but unilateral external rotation may reflect pelvic injury (Figure 5-17). The veterinarian should verify this change in posture by moving and reevaluating the horse. Horses with pronounced unilateral external rotation usually have fractures of the acetabulum or the proximal aspect of the femur but may have nonarticular ilial shaft or wing fractures.

Hindlimb Varus Posture
Horses with chronic, severe unilateral hindlimb lameness may develop varus conformation of the contralateral limb (see Figure 5-17). This posture most often appears in foals and may develop 7 to 10 days after onset of lameness.

Treading
Constant shifting of weight between the hindlimbs, or treading, is an unusual clinical sign and usually indicates pronounced bilateral lameness. Horses with bilateral hindlimb laminitis or severe osteoarthritis of any joint may tread. Horses with chronic, severe unilateral hindlimb lameness can endure 4 to 6 weeks or more of weight bearing on the contralateral limb, but treading may be the earliest sign of traumatic laminitis in the supporting limb.

Camped Under
Camped under appears only in horses with bilateral hindlimb laminitis and is rare. Horses often tread and exhibit an unusual hindlimb gait (shortened caudal phase of the stride) when moved at a walk in hand. Pain arising from the thoracolumbar region may also result in a camped under posture.

Soft Tissue Injuries Altering Hindlimb Posture
Upward fixation of the patella causes rigid extension of all hindlimb joints in a standing horse (Figure 5-18). Patellar dysfunction resulting in fixed extension of the stifle also causes extension of the tarsus and lower limb joints because of the hindlimb reciprocal apparatus. The horse may

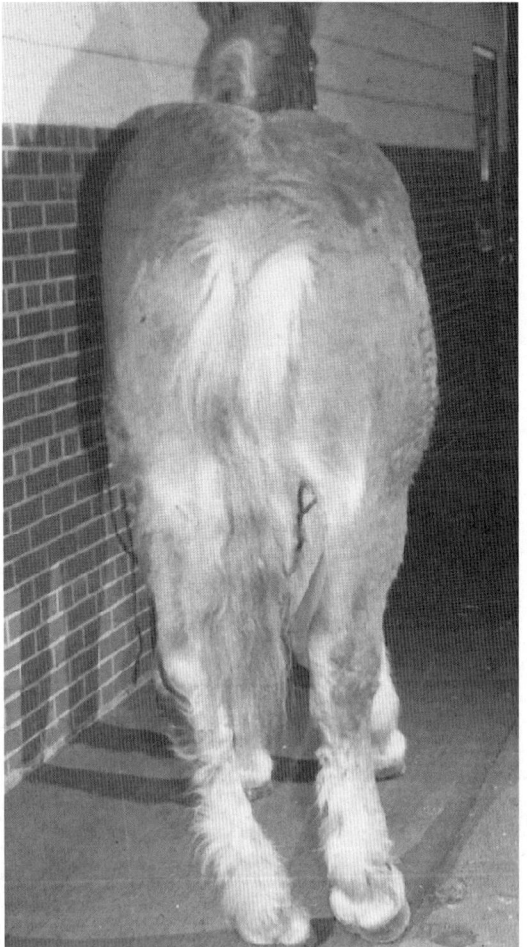

Fig. 5-17 • A 2-year-old Belgian gelding with a fracture of the right femoral head and neck exhibits external rotation of the right hindlimb. Varus deformity of the left hindlimb also is visible.

maintain this posture during movement, or the posture may be intermittent and resolve when the horse is moved. Occasionally a horse with severe hindlimb lameness assumes a similar posture, apparently hanging the limb, but the limb is not locked in extension (Figure 5-19). Normal horses simply resting a hindlimb, or those with severe lameness, usually keep the sole facing the ground.

Foals with unilateral or bilateral lateral patellar luxation have an unusual crouched hindlimb posture similar to femoral nerve paresis. The foal may have difficulty in rising if the condition is bilateral and severe or long-standing.

Disruption of fibularis (peroneus) tertius allows the hock to extend abnormally during weight bearing. Foals occasionally stand excessively straight in the hock (extended) in the affected hindlimb. In foals the injury usually causes tearing at the origin of fibularis tertius from the distal aspect of the femur, but in adults injury may occur in the crus or at the distal aspect of the ligament as it courses over the hock. Swelling and excessive hock extension may occur with the latter injury (Figure 5-20). The diagnosis is confirmed by manipulation: the hock can be extended while the stifle is flexed.

Rupture of the gastrocnemius tendon, or severe injury at any level of the muscle-tendon unit, causes mild or severe hindlimb postural change. During weight bearing,

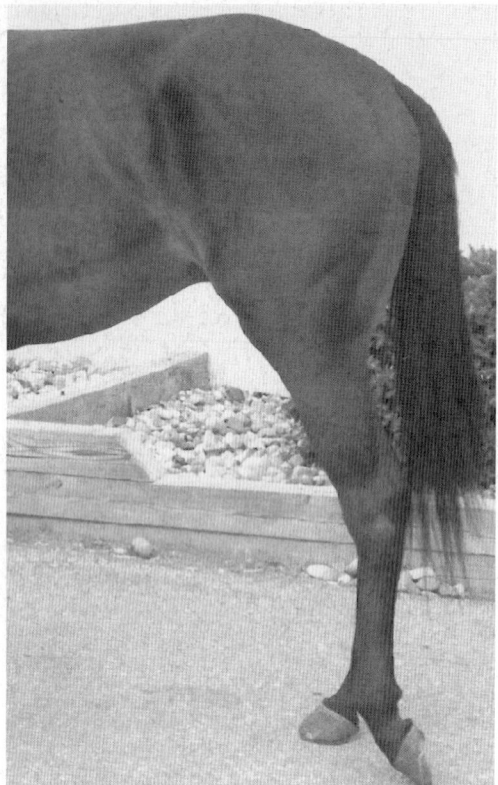

Fig. 5-18 • A horse with the classic posture seen with upward fixation of the patella. All joints are held in rigid extension, and the horse is forced to rest or bear weight on the dorsal aspect of the hoof wall.

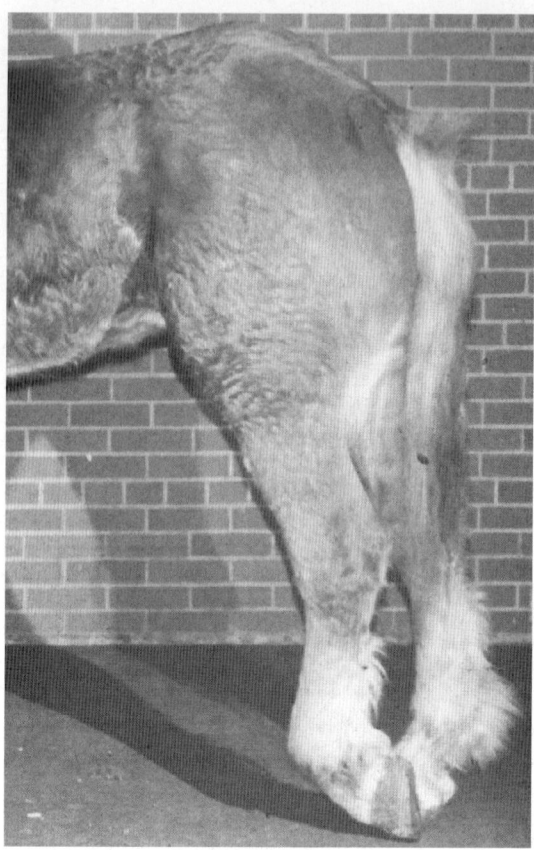

Fig. 5-19 • Belgian gelding shown in Figure 5-17. This horse occasionally rested the left hindlimb in this extended position, similar to that of upward fixation of the patella. Most normal horses, or those with severe lameness, prefer to rest the limb with the sole facing the ground.

the hock flexes excessively as the stifle is held in extension, so the point of the hock drops. This injury is called *disruption of the caudal component of the reciprocal apparatus.*[8,9]

Peripheral Nerve Deficits (see Chapter 11)

Sciatic nerve damage is rare. It occurs in foals as a result of injections into the thigh or rump or may occur transiently after injection of local anesthetic solution caudal to the coxofemoral joint. Horses with sciatic nerve damage support weight but appear to be crouched behind, because innervation to the gastrocnemius, flexor, and extensor muscles causes the hock to drop and fetlock to knuckle forward. Careful observation of stifle action and the ability to support weight are useful for attempting to differentiate this deficit from femoral nerve paresis.

Horses with femoral nerve paresis also assume a crouched hindlimb posture but are unable to bear weight, and the stifle drops substantially (Figure 5-21). Because the reciprocal apparatus is intact, the inability to fix the stifle leads to hock flexion and knuckling (flexion) of the fetlock joint. If the condition is bilateral, the horse is unable to rise for more than a few seconds. Femoral nerve paresis may occur unilaterally or bilaterally after general anesthesia or may result from lower motor neuron disease or injury.

Solitary tibial nerve injury is rare. Fibular (peroneal) nerve injury usually is recognized after general anesthesia and causes characteristic knuckling of the fetlock joint. Tibial nerve injury is differentiated from sciatic injury by lack of involvement of the fibular nerve, and thus normal

positioning of the hock, and from femoral nerve injury, because horses are able to support weight and fix the stifle.

A rare polyneuropathy in Norwegian horses caused unilateral or bilateral knuckling of the hindlimbs, and in some horses paraplegia occurred as a result of peripheral injury of the sciatic nerves.[10] A common epidemiological factor in all horses was the feeding of big bale silage or hay of poor quality.[10] I have seen similar clinical signs in a Warmblood gelding, which developed acute, severe, bilateral hindlimb knuckling (at the fetlock) that resolved completely several days after onset. The cause in this horse was not determined.

Other Unusual Leg Positions

Horses with severe lameness occasionally rest a hindlimb back, forward, or abducted. Often these positions also are maintained during movement. Horses with caudal thigh or pelvic pain prefer to keep the affected hindlimb back, behind the unaffected limb. Horses with shivers may stand with the limb slightly abducted and more caudal than expected, with elevation of the tail head (see Chapter 48).

Stance in Horses with Pelvic Fractures and Conditions Affecting the Coxofemoral Region

Horses with pelvic fractures, in particular those involving the acetabulum, or other severe conditions involving the coxofemoral joint often stand with the limb slightly

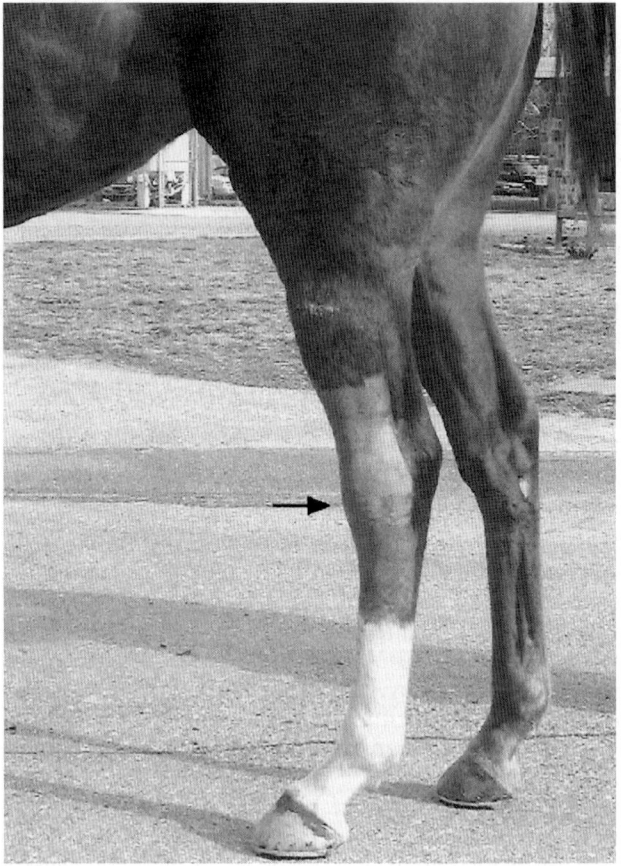

Fig. 5-20 • This Thoroughbred racehorse with fibularis tertius injury has swelling over the dorsal aspect of the hock *(arrow)* and straight-in-the-hock conformation.

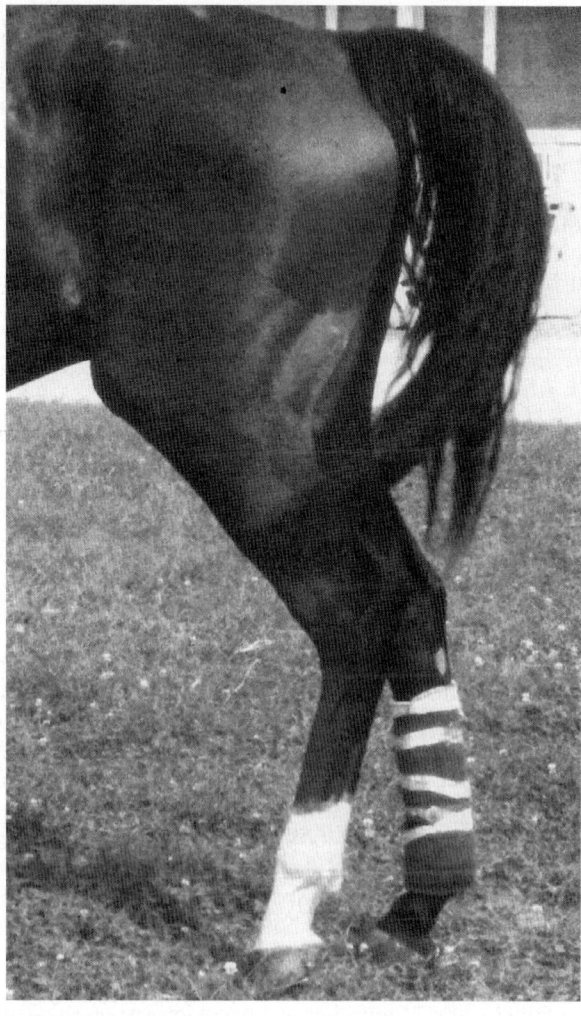

Fig. 5-21 • Thoroughbred with transient, postanesthesia, unilateral (left hindlimb) femoral nerve paresis. The crouched posture of the left hindlimb includes flexion (knuckling) of the fetlock joint.

forward and often are reluctant to place the limb behind the unaffected limb, thus reducing the caudal phase of the stride at the walk. In addition, horses will often stand with the limb externally rotated, and in the rare instance there is coxofemoral luxation, the point of the hock of the affected limb will be slightly proximal to the contralateral point of the hock (see Figure 5-17). I find it interesting that children with infectious arthritis of the coxofemoral joint will often hold the affected hip in flexion, abduction, and external rotation,[11,12] remarkably similar to those clinical

signs seen in the horse. Horses with pain in the medial thigh and groin area stand with the limb abducted and may travel in this manner. Adductor muscle damage, medial thigh abscessation, and scirrhous cord or other inguinal problems also cause this posture.

Chapter 6

Palpation

Mike W. Ross

Palpation is an important part of a lameness examination. In some sports horses, it becomes more important because, for example, suspensory desmitis often is not associated with overt lameness but may compromise performance.

The veterinarian must develop a system to evaluate comprehensively all parts of the musculoskeletal system. I palpate in order each forelimb, the neck, the back, the pelvic regions, and then the hindlimbs. Each limb should be assessed when bearing weight and then again with the limb elevated from the ground. Deep palpation is used to describe direct, digital palpation, with the limb in an elevated position.

If time permits, palpation should be completed *before* the horse is moved, because if the lame limb is identified first, the other limbs may be overlooked and compensatory problems may be missed. For example, in a Thoroughbred (TB) racehorse, superficial digital flexor (SDF) tendonitis is a common compensatory problem caused by contralateral forelimb lameness resulting in overload. If a lame horse with left forelimb lameness is first examined while the horse is moving, and subsequent palpation of the limb reveals signs of possible fetlock osteoarthritis, mild swelling of the right forelimb SDF tendon (SDFT) may be missed. Comprehensive palpation may allow the clinician to make predictions about lameness, to "read" the horse. Palpation before exercise also facilitates identification of localized heat or swelling, because limb temperature increases with exercise, and swelling often decreases.

THE ART OF PALPATION

The veterinarian should palpate and manipulate every possible anatomical structure, using the fingers and hands to push, prod, and feel. Interpretation of an abnormal response requires appreciation of the normal response. There are nerves beneath or adjacent to many structures, and direct pressure may elicit an apparently positive response. Such false-positive responses often occur during palpation of the origin of the suspensory ligament (SL) or the proximal sesamoid bones (PSBs). Care should be taken to apply pressure only in the desired location. During palpation of the PSBs, distal aspect of the SL, and digital flexor tendons, it is easy to apply pressure over the dorsal aspect of the third metacarpal bone (McIII), and a painful response may actually reflect sore shins.

The clinician should look for signs of inflammation: heat, pain, redness, swelling, and loss of function. One side of the horse should be compared with the other, but it should be remembered that both sides may be abnormal. Heat is one of the earliest clinical signs to develop with articular or nonarticular problems and may be the only sign. Subchondral remodeling and sclerosis of the third carpal bone often cause lameness in young racehorses, but effusion of the middle carpal joint and a positive response to flexion are found inconsistently. Usually prominent heat is detectable on the dorsal aspect of the carpus. It is important to recognize normality. A normal horse may have disparity in foot temperature. Horses often have two or three cold feet, but the other foot or feet feel warm. A few hours later, feet that previously were cool may feel warm. Foot temperature often reflects variations in ambient temperature, and care must be taken not to overinterpret this normal finding. In general, palpation is done with the palm side of the hand, although the back of the hand may be more sensitive to detection of warmth.

The veterinarian should assess the quality or strength of the digital pulse. In a normal horse, reliable detection of a digital pulse may be difficult, especially in cold weather or in horses with a thick hair coat. *Increased* or *elevated digital pulse* refers to the detection of increased strength (amplitude) or the bounding nature of the digital pulse. Inflammatory conditions in the foot or pastern region, such as abscesses, laminitis, hoof avulsions, or cracks, are the most common causes of increased digital pulse amplitude. Complete absence of hindlimb digital pulse may occur with aortoiliac thromboembolism or other vascular problems, but care should be taken when interpreting weak or near absent hindlimb digital pulses, because hindlimb digital pulses can be difficult to feel in normal horses.

Redness is difficult to perceive in the horse because of skin pigmentation, but in the foot, solar bruising or redness at the coronary band can be observed, especially in horses with nonpigmented feet. *Swelling* is often detected by observation, but subtle enlargement of structures such as the SL, or presence of effusion may be determined only by careful palpation.

Loss of function of tissues and regions can be assessed during palpation. Manipulation, flexion, and extension of the joints or soft tissues provide a better idea of function or loss of function. Static flexion and extension determine the range of motion of a joint and the horse's response to the procedure. Chronic osteoarthritis of the fetlock or carpal joints often results in reduced range of flexion. However, many horses in work but without lameness resent hard flexion of the lower limbs. Good correlation between a reduction in fetlock flexion range, lameness, and severity of osteoarthritis was found in TB racehorses.[1] A reduction in fetlock flexibility in young Warmbloods may be a predictor of future lameness.[2] The response to rotation of joints also should be assessed.

Crepitus, the grating or crackling sound made by bone rubbing on bone, is an unusual and ominous clinical sign usually determined by palpation, although in horses with prominent osteoarthritis or fractures a grating sound may be heard. A stethoscope may be useful for detection of subtle crepitus.

Other factors may confound the results of palpation. Clipped areas usually are warmer than an adjacent area with normal hair length. Blistering or freeze firing can cause localized pain for weeks after application, even if lameness has resolved. Any type of skin lesion, such as those found in horses with scratches or boot rubs, can cause extreme soreness to palpation but no signs of lameness. Some individual horses are more sensitive to palpation than others, and interpretation of apparent pain can be frustrating.

PALPATION OF THE FORELIMB
Foot

The importance of the foot cannot be overemphasized, and it is for this reason that palpation of the forelimb begins here. The feet are included in evaluation of conformation, symmetry, and posture. Detailed static examination (examination at rest) of the foot must always be supplemented with, and correlated to, dynamic observations of foot flight and foot striking patterns. Some horses continually attempt to pick up the limb as the clinician tries to evaluate it with the horse in the standing position; it may be necessary to stroke the contralateral limb to divert attention. A hoof pick, wire brush, hoof knife, shoe-removing equipment, and hoof testers are required (Figure 6-1). The sole and frog and wall of the foot should be cleaned thoroughly. Removal of the shoe at this stage in the examination usually is indicated only if a subsolar abscess is suspected. The veterinarian should take care to preserve the hoof wall, and if it is cracked, protect it with tape.

Foot and hoof balance are assessed by evaluating toe and heel length, hoof capsule conformation, condition and integrity, type of shoe and shoe position relative to the hoof capsule, hoof and pastern angle (axis), medial-to-lateral hoof balance, coronary band conformation, and

Reference on page 1256

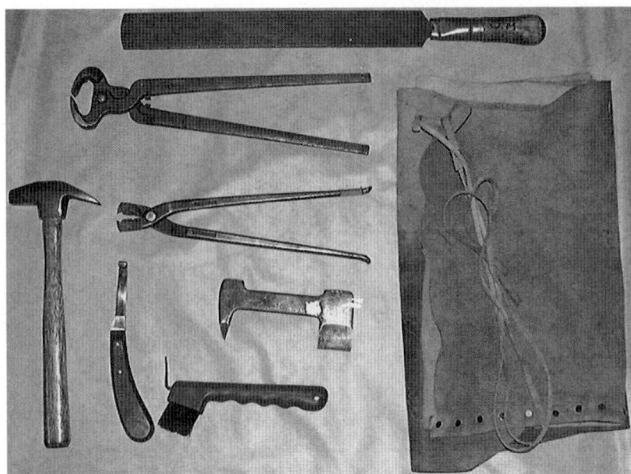

Fig. 6-1 • Instruments needed to examine the hoof, remove a shoe without tearing the hoof wall, and prepare the hoof for radiographic examination. Shown are apron, rasp, shoe pullers, nail pullers, clinch tool, hoof knife, hammer and hoof pick, and wire brush.

distal interphalangeal (coffin) joint capsule distention and response to hoof testers. The coronary band should normally be parallel to the ground surface. Deviation from parallel often indicates mediolateral foot imbalance (Figure 6-2). Medial and lateral wall lengths should be assessed while the horse is standing and again with the limb off the ground, with the foot viewed from palmar to dorsal along the solar aspect. The limb is lifted and held in neutral position so the solar surface is perpendicular to the ground. Sheared and underrun heels are commonly associated with lameness (Figure 6-3). Deformation of the hoof capsule is not necessarily a cause of lameness. Many horses with proximal displacement of the medial heel bulb have level foot strikes and otherwise balanced feet. Toe and heel length should be assessed, and the hoof-pastern axis should be determined. The angle of the hoof and pastern should be equal to allow equal loading of all portions of the foot. Forelimb hoof-pastern angles normally range from 48 to 55 degrees, but the absolute angle should not be overemphasized. A straight (parallel) pastern-foot axis is more important. A long-toe, underrun-heel foot conformation causes a broken foot axis and predisposes to palmar foot pain (Figure 6-4).

The conformation, condition, and integrity of the hoof capsule should be assessed. It is easy to miss hoof wall defects on the medial aspect. Small quarter or heel cracks and defects at the coronary band should not be overlooked. The clinician should evaluate the solar surface, bars, and frog. Thrush, although a reflection of poor management, rarely causes lameness.

The shoe type, shoe wear patterns, and the shoe size relative to the foot need to be assessed. The clinician should note the presence of pads or additions to the shoe, such as toe grabs, borium, and heel caulks. There is an association between toe grabs and suspensory apparatus failure in TB racehorses.[3] Low heel angle also has been associated with injury.[4] Shoe wear is important, because it reflects how the horse has been moving over the last several weeks. The clinician should note the breakover point and whether one branch of the shoe is worn more than the other. Shoe size should be assessed relative to foot size and the fit of the

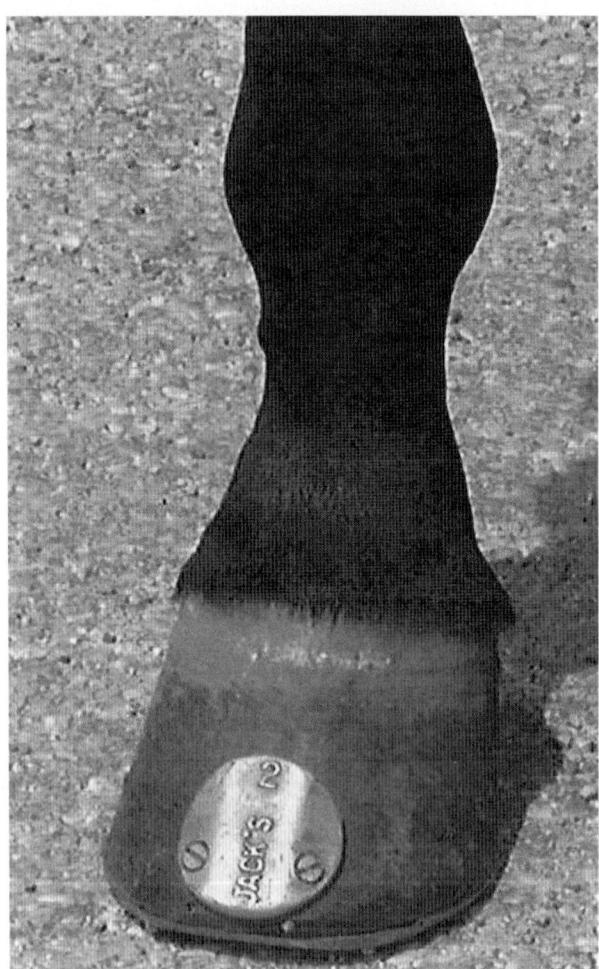

Fig. 6-2 • The coronary band is uneven compared with the ground in this trotter's unbalanced left forelimb hoof. The medial wall *(right)* appears to be shorter than the lateral wall. A toe weight and barium point are also shown.

shoe. A shoe that is too small or set too close to the frog may predispose to lameness.

Careful palpation of the coronary band in the standing and non–weight-bearing position is critical in detecting foot soreness (Figure 6-5). In horses with sore feet, heat and pain often are detected on the sore side of the foot, and a prominent digital pulse usually is present. Effusion of the distal interphalangeal joint capsule accompanies many abnormalities of the foot, from early synovitis to chronic osteoarthritis of the distal interphalangeal joint, and those with non-specific foot soreness. The clinician places one finger lateral to, and another medial to, the common digital extensor tendon and gently pushes in on the joint capsule, first laterally and then medially. *Ballottement* is a useful technique to detect effusion in many synovial structures: with effusion, pushing in on the capsule on one side of the tendon causes elevation of the capsule on the other side. The region of the collateral ligaments of the distal interphalangeal joint should be assessed carefully; focal heat or mild swelling may signify acute injury.

The clinician should palpate the cartilages of the foot, either with the horse standing or with the limb elevated. *Sidebone,* mineralization of the cartilages of the foot, rarely causes lameness. The cartilages of the foot normally are pliable and readily compressed axially. Fracture at the

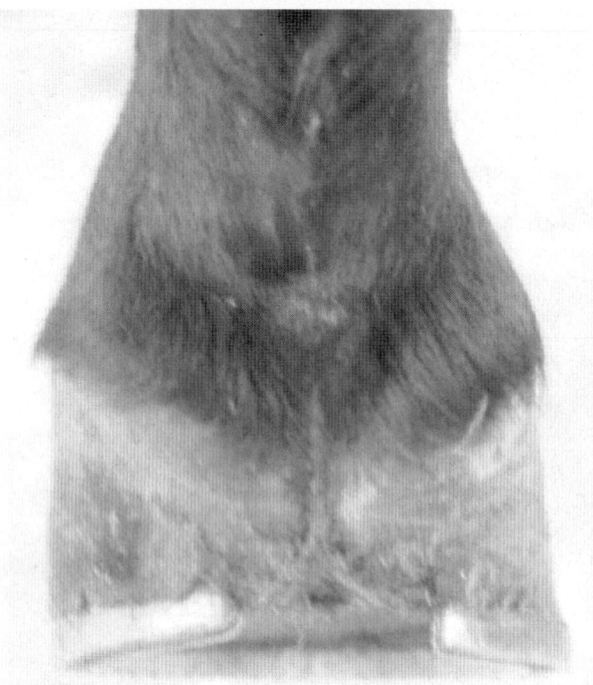

Fig. 6-3 • Elevated foot viewed from the palmar aspects shows that the hairline at the medial bulb of heel (on the right) is displaced proximally compared with the lateral heel bulb. The medial wall is longer. Note also the prominent cleft between the heel bulbs. These features are typical of a sheared heel.

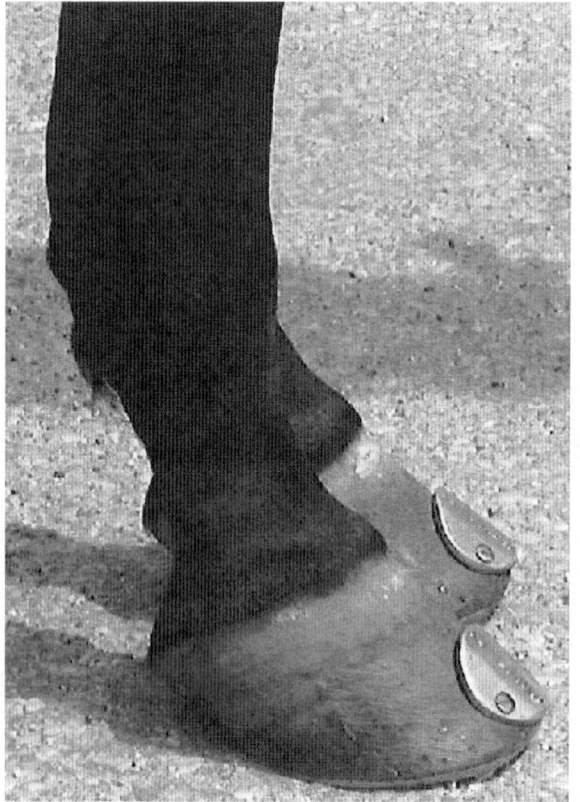

Fig. 6-4 • This trotter has long toe, underrun heel hoof conformation, and broken hoof-pastern axis.

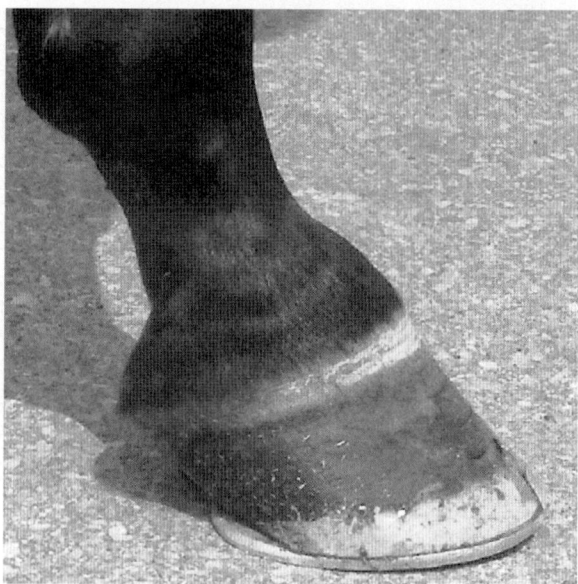

Fig. 6-5 • Palpation of the coronary band should include assessing the dorsal joint pouch of the distal interphalangeal joint. In this horse, distal interphalangeal effusion and fibrosis appear as a bulge just proximal to the coronary band, dorsally.

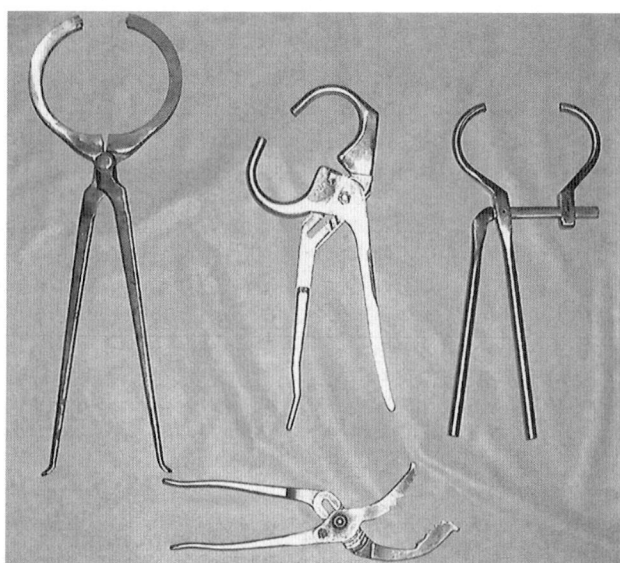

Fig. 6-6 • A variety of hoof testers are available for lameness examinations. I prefer hoof testers that are easily adjusted and used in one hand (two pairs on the right). Large hoof testers *(left)* can be applied only with two hands, and small hoof testers *(bottom)* are inappropriate for medium to large hooves.

attachment of the cartilage of the foot to the distal phalanx is an occasional cause of lameness, and compression of the heel with hoof testers may elicit pain in some horses. Horses with sidebone often have medial-to-lateral hoof imbalance.

Hoof Tester Examination

"… I feel naked going into a stall without my hoof testers!"[5] Hoof testers are essential for evaluation of the foot and are a basic requirement for all lameness examinations. Many types of hoof testers are available (Figure 6-6), but I favor

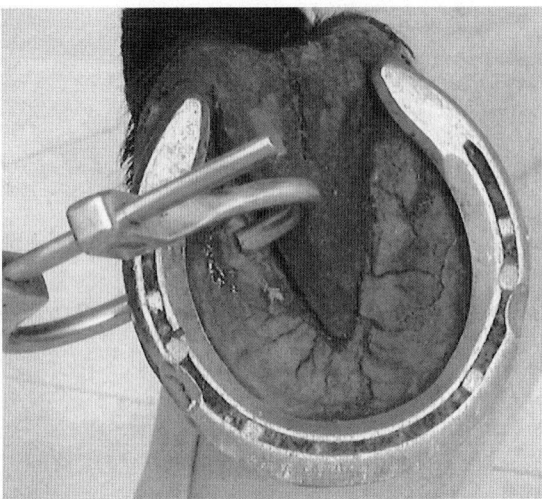

Fig. 6-7 • Hoof testers should be applied from the sole to the wall, from heel to toe, and to both sides of the hoof.

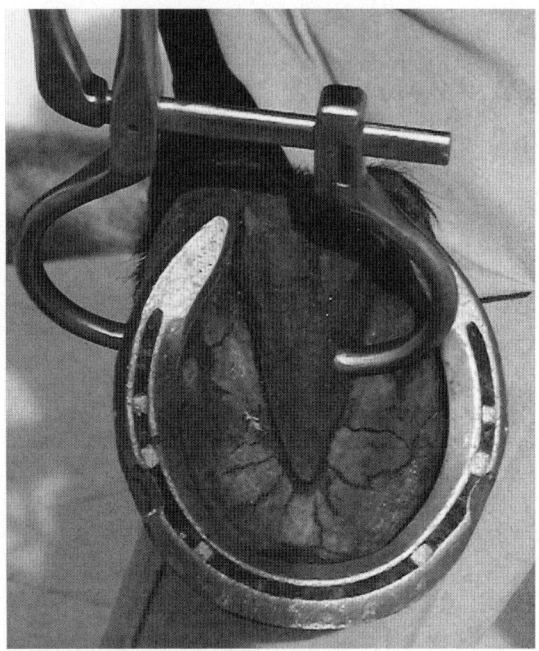

Fig. 6-8 • Hoof testers applied from the middle of the frog to the contralateral hoof wall put pressure on the navicular region. Horses with many abnormal conditions of the hoof may manifest a positive response.

one that is adjustable and can be applied with one hand. A proper evaluation of the foot with hoof testers cannot be done with a pad in place, although useful information can be acquired. The instrument can be applied with or without a shoe in place. The amount of force to apply varies from horse to horse and by region of the hoof, and both false-positive and false-negative responses occur. More force is required when the instrument is used across the heel than when used from sole to quarter. The foot should be held between the clinician's legs in a relaxed manner. The clinician must be able to feel the horse react to subtle pressure, and if the limb is held too tightly or the horse is not calm during the examination, it is difficult to feel a response. The veterinarian should be careful not to place the outside jaw of the instrument too close to the coronary band, because this may cause a false-positive result. Sole sensitivity is assessed by applying the instrument to three to five sites from heel to toe, on both the medial and lateral aspects of the foot, starting from the angle of the sole (seat of the corn) and proceeding dorsally (Figure 6-7). The responses should be compared. If the sole is readily compressible, pain from bruising, a subsolar abscess, laminitis, fracture of the distal phalanx, and other injuries may be elicited, but in horses with hard horn the response may be negative. To evaluate sensitivity of the frog and underlying deeper structures, the hoof testers should be applied from the lateral aspect of the frog to the medial wall, and from the medial aspect of the frog to the lateral wall, each in the palmar, midportion, and dorsal aspects of the frog (Figure 6-8). Pain over the middle third of the frog has been attributed to navicular disease or navicular syndrome, but the specificity of this association is questionable and there are many false-negative responses. Horses with generalized foot soreness or any other cause of palmar foot pain may respond positively or not at all. Only 19 of 42 horses with navicular region pain responded positively to hoof tester examination in the middle third of the frog, with 50% specificity, 50% positive predictive value, and 48% accuracy.[6] Horses with palmar foot pain caused by other conditions were as likely to respond to the test, a finding that obviously prompts questioning of the value of hoof tester examination.[6] It is difficult if not impossible to create adequate pressure to cause pain in large breed horses or if the horn is hard. Application of a poultice or soaking the foot may be necessary to soften a hard foot, and reexamination after several days may be rewarding. Hoof tester application to the small feet of foals or ponies may elicit a false-positive response, and hoof tester size or amount of compression may require adjustment.

Application of hoof testers across the heel may cause pain in horses with palmar foot pain but is not specific (Figure 6-9). Application of the hoof tester to the area of the sole adjacent to each nail, nail hole, or defect in the sole or white line is useful to detect a subsolar abscess or a close nail (Figure 6-10). Areas of pain can be gently explored with a hoof knife, but unless clearly indicated, the veterinarian should refrain from digging too deeply. The hoof tester can then be used as a hammer to percuss each nail in the shoe and the frog and toe regions.

After completing the hoof tester examination, the clinician should reassess the digital pulses. In horses with foot pain the digital pulse may now be bounding. Horses that have recently been shod or trimmed or have raced or performed recently, especially on hard surfaces, may have mild elevations in digital pulse amplitude and may show hoof tester sensitivity normally. Pain causing lameness may not be in the foot.

Wedge Test and Other Forms of Static Manipulation
The wedge test is used most commonly as a dynamic procedure to induce lameness during the movement phase of the examination, but can be used to assess the static response of a horse to dramatic changes in dorsal-to-palmar or medial-to-lateral hoof angles (see Chapter 8, Figure 8-12). A digital extension device, with which the author gauged static painful responses to changes in hoof

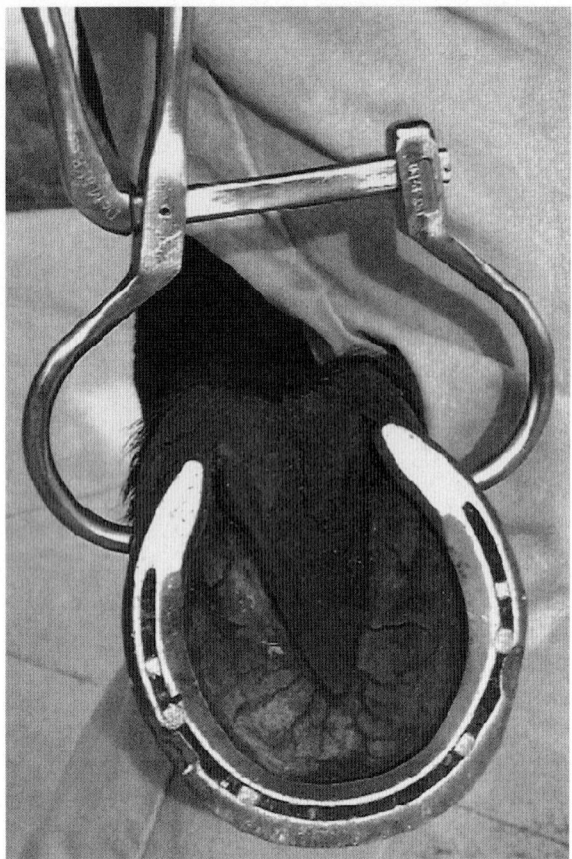

Fig. 6-9 • Adjustable hoof testers are easily placed across the heel. I prefer to apply hoof testers in this manner to assess horses for palmar foot pain during static examination and as a provocative test for lameness.

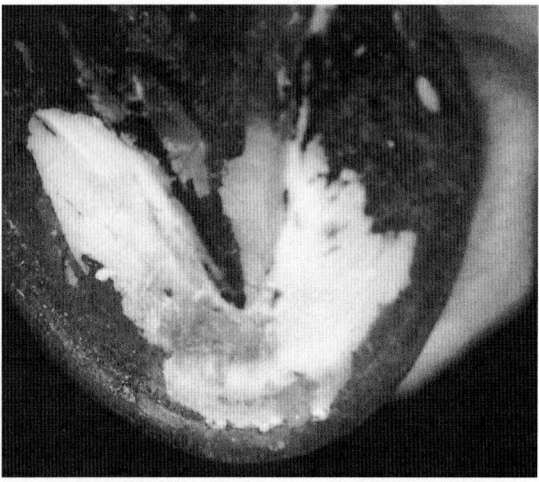

Fig. 6-10 • Acute, severe lameness causing increase in digital pulse and profound hoof tester sensitivity in the toe region resulted from this hoof abscess. Exudate drains from the pared region at the toe. (Courtesy Greg Staller, Pottersville, New Jersey.)

angle to make shoeing recommendations, was recently described.[7]

Pastern

The proximal interphalangeal (pastern) joint capsule is assessed by ballottement, although severe effusion must be

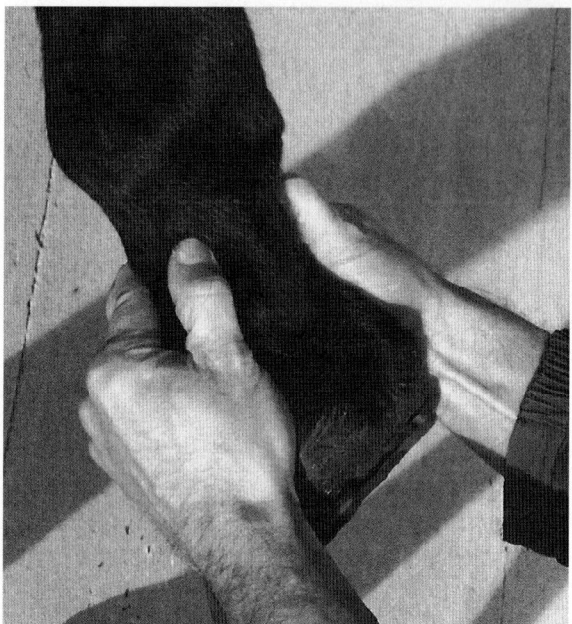

Fig. 6-11 • Palpation of oblique distal sesamoidean ligaments.

present for fluid distention to be perceived. Bony swelling associated with this joint, proximal or high ringbone, is a classic cause of lameness yet an unusual clinical finding. Osteoarthritis of the proximal interphalangeal joint is a common diagnosis, but one made by a combination of clinical findings, diagnostic analgesia, radiography, and sometimes scintigraphy. The distal extent of the digital flexor tendon sheath (DFTS), deep digital flexor tendon (DDFT), and distal sesamoidean ligaments are palpated. Deep pain associated with the origin and insertion of the distal sesamoidean ligaments is assessed by palpation with the limb in flexion (Figure 6-11). In some horses with lesions of the DDFT within the hoof capsule a positive response to compression of the palmar pastern region is present, but this finding is inconsistent and many false-negative responses occur. The oblique sesamoidean ligaments are difficult to differentiate from the branches of the SDFT, but injury of the SDFT is more common. Distal sesamoidean desmitis or chronic suspensory desmitis may result in subluxation of the proximal interphalangeal joint (Figure 6-12). Swelling should prompt ultrasonographic examination if relevance has been confirmed using diagnostic analgesia. The proximal interphalangeal joint is manipulated in a medial-to-lateral direction to assess pain and collateral ligament integrity and is flexed independently of the fetlock joint. The proximal, dorsal aspect of the proximal phalanx is palpated (Figure 6-13). Horses with short, midsagittal fractures or dorsal frontal fractures of the proximal phalanx or proliferation at the attachment of the common digital extensor tendon may show pain. Enthesophyte formation at the common digital extensor tendon attachment, seen most commonly in older ex-racehorses with chronic osteoarthritis of the fetlock joint, results in prominent bony and soft tissue swelling and pain on palpation.

Fetlock

The clinician palpates the joint capsule of the metacarpophalangeal (fetlock) joint with the limb bearing weight,

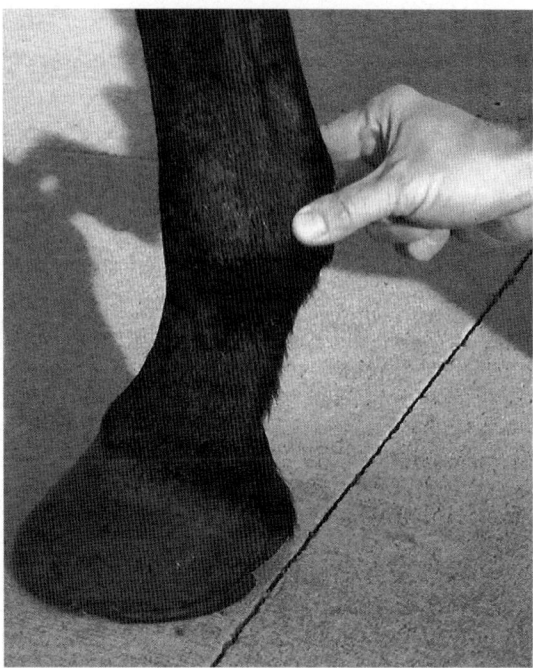

Fig. 6-14 • Digital pulse quality can be assessed easily at the level of the proximal sesamoid bones.

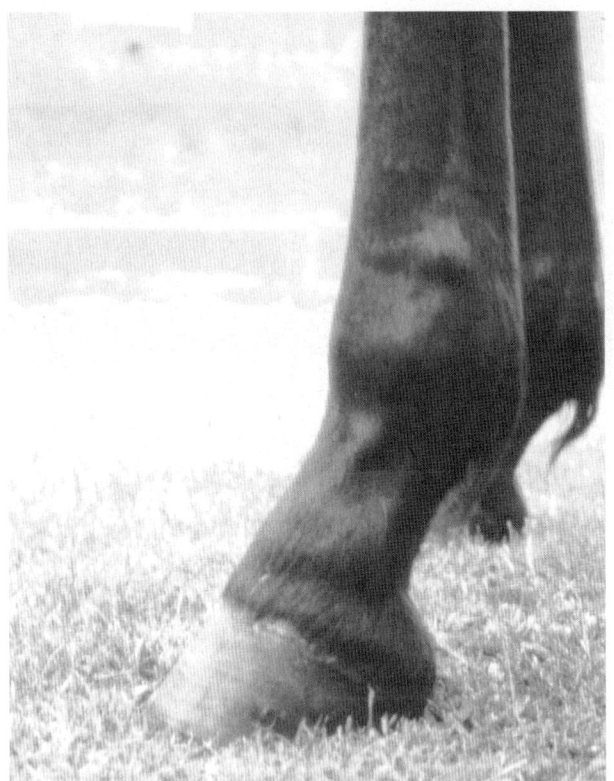

Fig. 6-12 • Subluxation and osteoarthritis of the left front proximal interphalangeal joint resulted from primary suspensory desmitis.

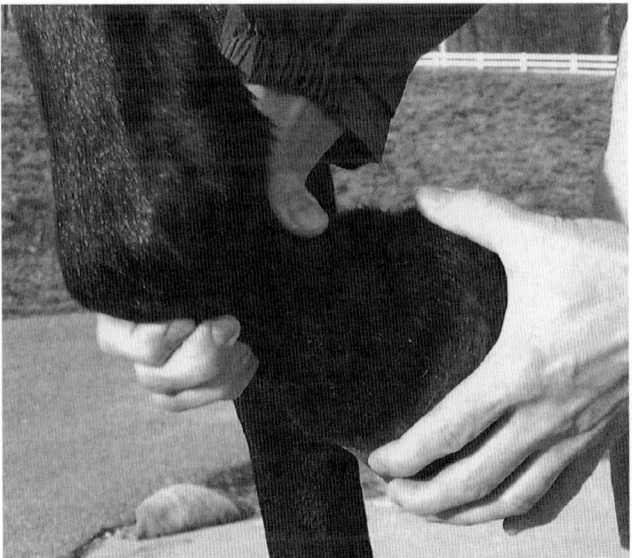

Fig. 6-13 • Proliferative changes at the common digital extensor attachment or pain from midsagittal fracture of the proximal phalanx should be palpated along the dorsal, proximal aspect of the proximal phalanx.

keeping in mind that pain associated with the joint can be present without localizing clinical signs. The dorsal aspect is palpated using ballottement on either side of the common digital extensor tendon. The clinician should determine whether localized heat is present. *Osselets* is a North American term used to describe early osteoarthritis of the metacarpophalangeal joint in young racehorses, with firm bony

and soft tissue swelling on the dorsal, medial aspect of the proximal phalanx, and the distal aspect of the McIII, caused by traumatic capsulitis and early enthesophyte formation. Occasionally in horses with prominent effusion of the metacarpophalangeal joint, a soft tissue swelling can be palpated in the proximal, dorsal aspect of the joint from excessive proliferation of the dorsal synovial pads, called *proliferative* or *villonodular synovitis*. The palmar pouch of the metacarpophalangeal joint is palpated dorsal to the SL branches, both medially and laterally. Mild effusion may be present without associated lameness, especially in older performance horses. The PSBs are palpated and assessed for mild swelling and heat, clinical signs of sesamoiditis, or SL avulsion injury. The digital pulse amplitude is reassessed by placing fingers both medially and laterally, abaxial to both PSBs (Figure 6-14).

The DFTS extends from the distal metacarpal region to the distal palmar aspect of the pastern. Usually no palpable fluid is found. Effusion of the DFTS (tenosynovitis) causes swelling in the palmar fetlock region that must be differentiated from effusion of the metacarpophalangeal joint. Tenosynovitis causes swelling *palmar* to the branches of the SL, medially and laterally. Fluid can be compressed from medial to lateral. With severe effusion, distention is found in the palmar aspect of the pastern, but there may be distention proximal to the palmar annular ligament without obvious distention distally. *Wind puffs* or *windgalls* describe incidental fluid distention of the DFTS, commonly seen in older performance horses unassociated with lameness. Tenosynovitis can cause lameness, but additional diagnostic techniques are required to confirm the diagnosis.

The limb is elevated to assess range of joint motion and the horse's response to flexion. Normally the fetlock can be flexed to 90 degrees (the angle between the proximal phalanx and the McIII) or slightly more. A reduction in fetlock flexion range is indicative of chronic fibrosis but is not necessarily a cause for concern. A pronounced response to static flexion is noteworthy, although many horses resent static flexion but do not show a positive response to dynamic flexion (lower limb or fetlock flexion tests; see Chapter 8). Horses with clinically relevant tenosynovitis usually strongly resent fetlock flexion. With the limb in flexion, the clinician palpates the PSBs and the branches of the SL, avoiding compression of the palmar digital nerves.

Metacarpal Region

The clinician should assess the dorsal aspect of the McIII for heat and swelling. This is a common area for traumatic injury (barked shins) or stress-related bone injury (bucked shin syndrome). Many ex-racehorses have incidental, prominent, chronic, and nonpainful swelling of the McIII caused by extensive modeling and remodeling of the dorsal cortex while in race training. Racehorses currently in training may have heat and pain on deep palpation (performed with the limb elevated), but prominent swelling may be lacking. Any combination of palpation findings is possible in horses with stress-related bone injury of the McIII. It is difficult to apply deep pressure to the dorsal aspect of the McIII without concomitant pressure to the palmar soft tissue structures or PSBs, so the responses should be assessed carefully.

The entire length (abaxial surface) of the second and fourth metacarpal bones (McII/IV) should be palpated with the horse in the standing position to detect exostoses, callus, or fractures. Swelling of the SL branches or body may make this difficult. Palpation of the McII and the McIV should be repeated with the limb elevated, because the axial aspect of these bones is impossible to assess in the weight-bearing position. Splint exostoses are common, particularly in young horses. Therefore the presence of even large bony swellings is not unusual. Exostoses detected axially, possibly impinging on the SL or causing adhesions to the SL (or so-called "blind splints") should be carefully noted. Both false-positive and false-negative results can occur when palpating a splint exostosis and results of palpation and compression should be confirmed using perineural analgesia. Pain from even small exostoses of the McII and the McIV usually is more accurately assessed immediately after training or racing, because pain and lameness resulting from these swellings can be subtle and transient. The clinician should carefully palpate the SL branches. Differentiation of branch or SL body injuries is important: the latter injuries usually are more serious and have a worse prognosis.

The medial and lateral palmar digital vein, artery, and nerve, in dorsal-to-palmar orientation, respectively, are located between the SL and DDFT. The accessory ligament (distal or inferior check ligament) of the DDFT (ALDDFT) normally is difficult to palpate and even when enlarged cannot easily be differentiated from the DDFT, but injuries of the ALDDFT are more common. All soft tissue structures should be palpated carefully, using digital compression, with the limb elevated (Figure 6-15). Acute or chronic swelling should be assessed, as should the horse's response to deep palpation. Obvious swelling and pain indicate the presence of tendonitis or desmitis. In some horses with acute severe tendonitis or desmitis the structure feels "mushy" or soft in the area of fiber damage. This finding, especially in horses with fetlock drop, indicates near rupture of the structure. There are many false-positive and

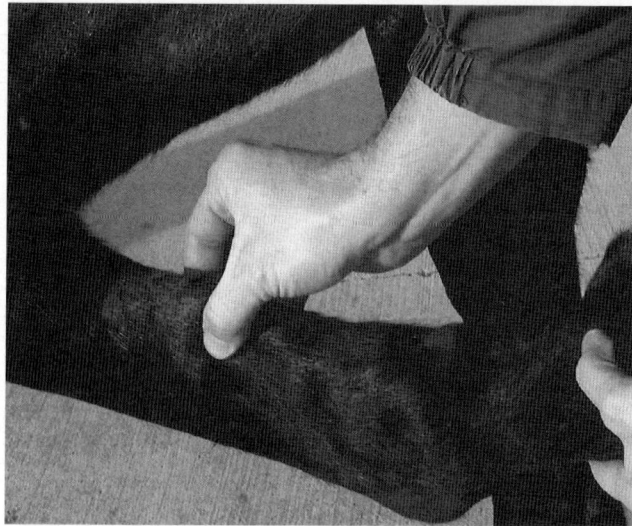

Fig. 6-15 • The soft tissue structures in the palmar metacarpal region should be carefully palpated with the horse in standing and flexed (shown) positions for heat, pain on compression, and swelling. Most ridden horses have mild pain, but in racehorses a painful response is an early sign of tendonitis or desmitis.

even false-negative responses to palpation of the digital flexor tendons and SL. In most ridden performance horses a mild painful response (false-positive) to deep palpation of the SL is normal. However, in racehorses, false-positive responses are less common, and a painful response to deep palpation may indicate the presence of early desmitis or tendonitis. In many horses with foot lameness, secondary, mild suspensory desmitis is common. There is a painful response to palpation of the body and origin of the SL. It may be difficult to decide whether this is a true or false-positive response, a determination that often is made in hindsight after the lameness examination is finished. False-positive and false-negative responses to palpation of the proximal palmar metacarpal region also occur. This is a common site of lameness and should be examined carefully. Palpation must be done with the limb in flexion, and the presence of swelling and pain must be carefully interpreted (Figure 6-16). Horses with acute injuries, such as proximal suspensory desmitis (PSD), avulsion or longitudinal fracture of the McIII, and stress reaction of the McIII at the origin of the SL, may have swelling and pain. Deep palpation may create pressure on the palmar metacarpal nerves resulting in a false-positive pain response, and many horses with PSD have no localizing signs. The most proximal aspect of the SDFT is difficult to palpate with the limb in a flexed position, and mild swelling from tendonitis can easily be missed. When the limb is weight bearing, the expected convex profile associated with SDF tendonitis in the mid-to-distal regions of the metacarpal region is usually not seen because of pressure from the overlying metacarpal fascia. Careful palpation of the proximal aspect of the SDFT, particularly in horses that negotiate fences or in ponies, is necessary to avoid missing subtle lesions. This injury is particularly hard to recognize in horses or ponies with long hair coats.

The proximal dorsal aspect of the McIII should be palpated in a flexed position (Figure 6-17). Occasionally, dorsomedial articular fracture of the McIII results in a subtle

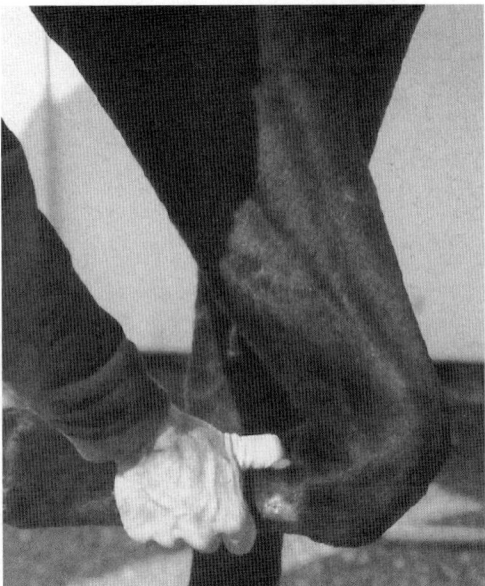

Fig. 6-16 • Palpation of the proximopalmar metacarpal region is essential in diagnosing proximal suspensory desmitis and other conditions of the suspensory origin and differentiating lameness in the region from carpal lameness. (Courtesy Ross Rich, Cave Creek, Arizona.)

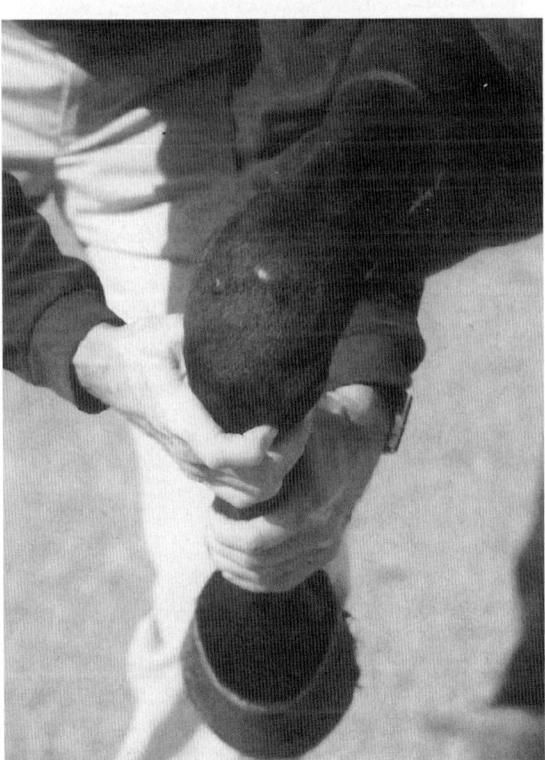

Fig. 6-17 • Careful palpation of the proximal, dorsal metacarpal region identifies pain associated with dorsomedial articular fracture or other fractures of the proximal aspect of the third metacarpal bone. (Courtesy Ross Rich, Cave Creek, Arizona.)

painful swelling. Swelling (effusion) of the carpal sheath may be detected in the proximal medial metacarpal region, but large veins (medial palmar, accessory cephalic, and cephalic veins) may interfere with accurate palpation. With mild tenosynovitis, effusion may be difficult to discern.

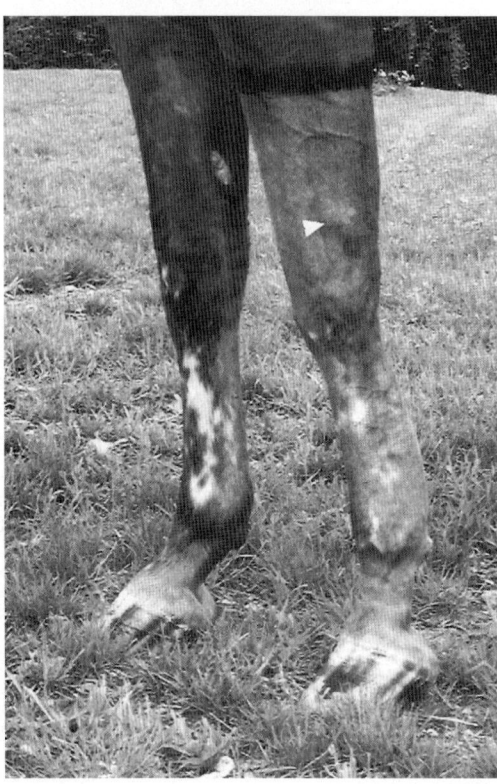

Fig. 6-18 • Carpal tenosynovitis must be differentiated from effusion of the antebrachiocarpal joint. This horse with severe superficial digital flexor tendonitis has moderate distention of the carpal sheath *(arrow)* in the caudal, distal aspect of the antebrachium and medially in the proximal metacarpal region (not shown).

Carpus

Detection of warmth on the dorsal aspect of the carpus is a reliable indicator of underlying inflammation. Obviously, one side should be compared with the other, but bilateral conditions exist commonly. Previous application of counterirritants interferes with the reliable detection of warmth. Carpal joint lameness without obvious signs of synovitis is common, but if present, effusion is easily palpated using ballottement. With the horse in the standing position, a finger is placed dorsolaterally between the extensor carpi radialis and common digital extensor tendons, and another finger is placed just medial to the extensor carpi radialis tendon. These openings are used for palpation and arthrocentesis of both the middle carpal and the antebrachiocarpal joints. The middle carpal and the carpometacarpal joints always communicate, but a small synovial compartment and dense overlying soft tissue structures limit palpation of the carpometacarpal joint. Both the middle carpal and the antebrachiocarpal joints have a palmarolateral pouch that may be distended if effusion is severe. If swelling is detected just caudal to the radius, it is necessary to differentiate distention of the palmarolateral pouch of the antebrachiocarpal joint from the carpal sheath (Figure 6-18). In horses with antebrachiocarpal joint effusion the dorsal outpouchings also should be prominent, whereas in those with carpal sheath effusion, fluid distention is restricted to the palmar aspect and also detected medially, both proximal and distal to the accessory carpal bone.

Tenosynovitis of the extensor carpi radialis, common digital extensor, or lateral digital extensor sheaths results in vertically oriented swellings that traverse the carpal joints, may extend proximal or distal to the carpus, and usually are multilobed, being divided by bands of extensor retinaculum located dorsally and laterally.

Normally the carpus can easily be flexed completely, so that the palmar metacarpal region and bulbs of the heel touch the caudal aspect of the antebrachium. Reduced flexion may be caused by pain, with or without chronic fibrosis, associated with osteoarthritis. Pain during carpal flexion is a reliable indicator of carpal region pain but does not indicate the cause. The carpal sheath is compressed and the extensor tendons are stretched during this maneuver, and conditions involving these structures and the accessory carpal bone can cause pain during flexion. The elbow joint is flexed simultaneously; therefore a positive response to carpal flexion can rarely result from elbow pain. The examiner should palpate the dorsal surfaces of the carpal bones with the limb in partial flexion (Figure 6-19). Many pathological conditions associated with the carpus are manifested dorsally, and pain associated with osteochondral fragmentation, slab fractures or other severe injuries, or osteoarthritis can be assessed with the limb in this position. Focal pain can be identified, and loose fragments associated with the third carpal bone or distal lateral radius occasionally can be identified.

Antebrachium (Forearm)

Digital palpation of the forearm usually is performed with the limb bearing weight. The examiner should look primarily for muscle atrophy, wounds, or mild swelling associated with the radius. Small wounds in the antebrachium may look innocuous, but inappropriately severe lameness and pain on palpation may reflect a spiral radial fracture. The examiner should pay particular attention to the medial aspect of the limb; this area is easily overlooked when palpating from the lateral side. Distally, fluid distention of the carpal sheath or acute swelling associated with injury of the accessory ligament (proximal or superior check ligament) of the SDFT, or the flexor muscles and tendons can occur. The amount of muscle in the extensors and flexors should be compared with that in the contralateral limb, because subtle atrophy may be missed during observation.

Elbow

Frank swelling and prominent lameness accompany many injuries of the elbow region, but other problems of the elbow joint are discovered only after diagnostic analgesia has localized pain to this area or by use of advanced imaging modalities. It is nearly impossible to use diagnostic analgesic techniques to abolish pain in the distal aspect of the humerus and proximal aspects of the radius and ulna; therefore advanced imaging techniques are often required to identify problems in these structures. The clinician should palpate the olecranon process and the lateral and medial collateral ligaments with the limb bearing weight. Effusion is difficult to detect, but excess fluid occasionally can be found using ballottement, by placing fingers both cranial and caudal to the lateral collateral ligament. The elbow is flexed by pulling the distal limb in a cranial and proximal direction and then extended by

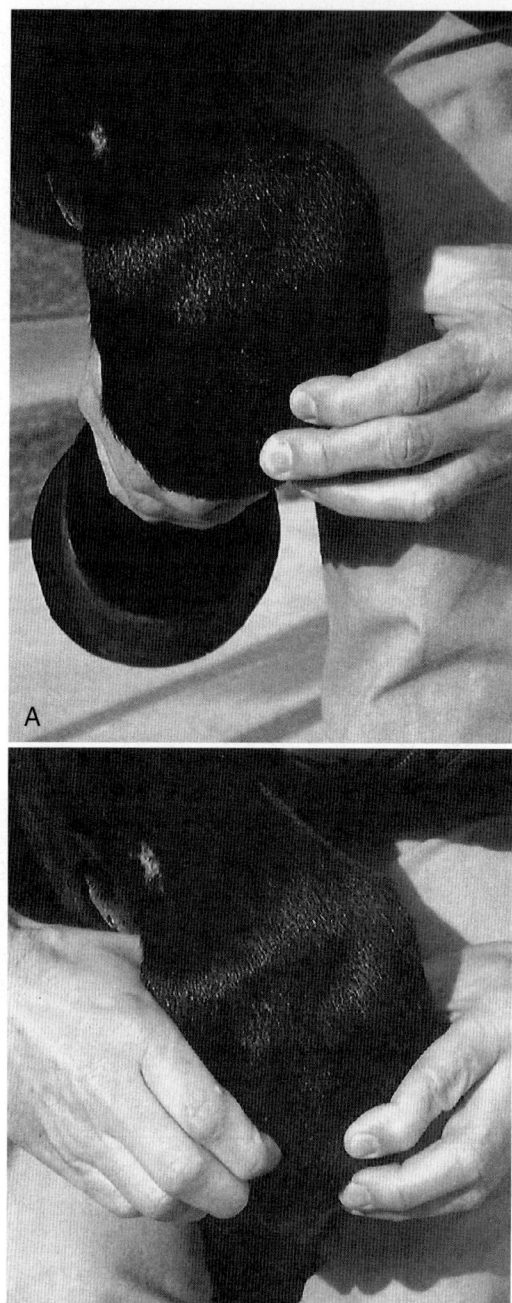

Fig. 6-19 • Careful palpation of the dorsal aspect of each carpal bone can be done with one hand **(A)** or by placing the distal limb between the clinician's legs and using both hands **(B).** A pain response indicates an osteochondral fragment or an osteophyte. Occasionally a loose osteochondral fragment can be palpated.

pulling the lower limb in a caudal direction. The shoulder joint is undergoing the opposite reaction during this manipulation, and pain associated with that joint or the bicipital bursa can cause a positive response during elbow manipulation.

Brachium (Arm) and Shoulder

The shoulder and intertubercular (bicipital) bursa are regularly blamed as the cause of lameness yet are seldom involved. Normal horses may resent palpation of this area. Pain in the muscles surrounding the shoulder joint may develop *secondary* to primary lower limb lameness. In Standardbred (STB) racehorses with carpal lameness, secondary pain often is detected when the bicipital bursa is palpated. A rare cause of lameness is infection as a result of a previous deep injection of the "shoulder bursae," and horses may have only subtle pain on palpation and manipulation of the shoulder region. Infectious bicipital bursitis generally causes severe lameness, a marked shortened cranial phase of the stride, and a marked painful response to shoulder joint flexion.

Palpation of the arm is limited because overlying muscles obscure much of the humerus. Horses with displaced humeral fractures usually are unwilling to bear weight and have severe soft tissue swelling. Those with humeral stress fractures usually have no localizing signs except a positive response to upper limb manipulation. A normal intertubercular bursa is not palpable. Horses with bicipital bursitis usually resent direct compression of the greater tubercle of the humerus, and fluid distention may be palpable, but ballottement is usually limited. Effusion of the scapulohumeral (shoulder) joint is palpable only if severe and even then is easily overlooked.

Upper limb manipulation, including static flexion and extension to assess the range of motion of the shoulder and elbow joints and the presence of a painful response, should always be performed. This can be done during palpation of the elbow or later when the clinician finishes the shoulder region. Most horses with shoulder joint lameness or bicipital bursitis show a painful response when the limb is pulled backward (shoulder flexion, elbow extension), whereas those with elbow lameness may show a painful response when the limb is pulled forward (shoulder extension, elbow flexion).

The examiner should palpate the scapular area and move the mane if necessary. Atrophy of the infraspinatus and supraspinatus muscles may indicate suprascapular nerve or brachial plexus injury (Figure 6-20). Muscle atrophy of these and other forelimb muscles can be caused by other neurogenic causes or by disuse. Upper limb palpation often is used to confirm those findings recognized during observation of the horse. Scapular height is compared manually. Although rare, damage to the innervation of the serratus ventralis muscle or direct trauma to the muscle itself allows abnormal elevation of the injured side when the horse is standing or during movement. Pectoral muscle atrophy can easily be missed during observation, and the pectoral region should be palpated to assess pectoral muscle mass and identify swellings or wounds that may cause lameness.

PALPATION OF THE CERVICAL AND THORACOLUMBAR SPINE

Cervical Spine (Neck)

Palpation of the neck is limited. I usually palpate the brachiocephalicus muscle after shoulder palpation and manipulation, a procedure thought to have predictive but

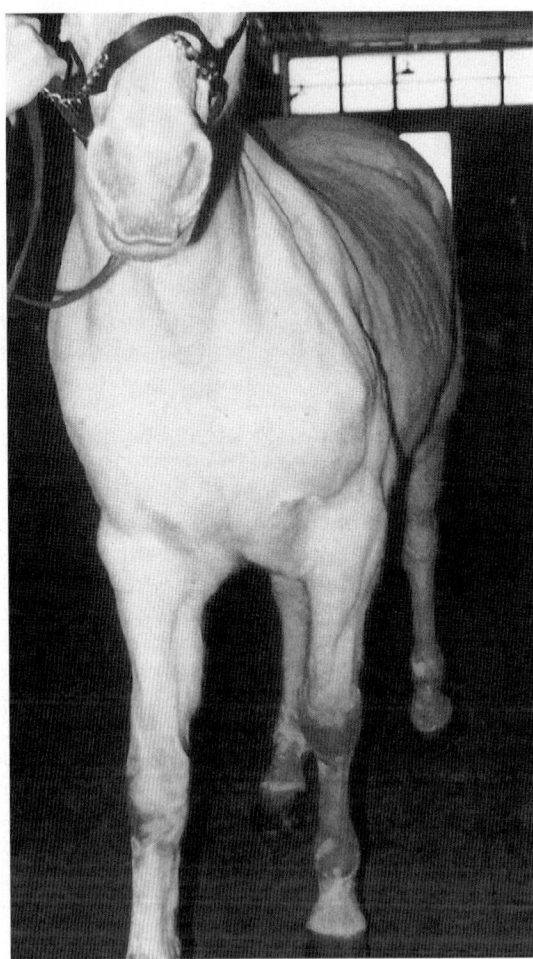

Fig. 6-20 • This horse shows atrophy of the supraspinatus and infraspinatus muscles with concomitant lateral subluxation of the left shoulder joint.

nonspecific value in horses with forelimb lameness.[8] The muscle is squeezed just cranial to the shoulder joint; most horses flinch, but some horses with ipsilateral forelimb lameness show a marked pain response. The examiner should palpate both sides of the neck, noting any swelling or muscle atrophy. Cervical abscessation can cause signs of neck pain and forelimb lameness. Muscle atrophy may indicate long-standing cervical pain or ipsilateral forelimb lameness. Muscle development of the neck may be asymmetrical, especially if viewed from above (the perspective of a rider).[2] Palpation of the poll region is important because undue soreness cranial to the wings of the atlas may be associated with poor performance.[2] The head should be moved from side to side to evaluate the horse's willingness to move the neck. One hand is placed on the midcervical region to use as a fulcrum, and the other hand is used to bend the head and neck toward the examiner. Food also can be used to entice the horse to move the head and neck from side to side. Normally a horse can reach around to the girth region on either side to ingest food, and reluctance to do so may indicate neck pain. This procedure may more closely mimic the horse's natural head and neck movement than using a hand in the midcervical area as a fulcrum. A more comprehensive examination, including neurological or chiropractic evaluations, may be necessary after completion of the lameness examination.

Up-and-down movement of the head also should be assessed. Although usually not a part of a routine lameness examination, evaluation of the temporomandibular joints and the mouth may be necessary in horses with poor performance.[2]

Thoracolumbar Spine (Back)

Additional detailed palpation of the back and pelvis may be necessary once the lameness examination has been completed. Chiropractic manipulation and assessment of acupuncture points may be useful but usually are reserved for specific horses or when history and clinical signs warrant such an examination and if the clinician is qualified to complete it. The cranial thoracic spine has already been briefly evaluated during examination of the shoulder for scapular symmetry. The withers should be examined closely for conformational abnormalities, such as those seen with fracture of the dorsal spinous processes or fistulous withers. The presence of sores may indicate an ill-fitting saddle and can cause performance-related problems. Using a hand on each side of the spine, the examiner should apply digital pressure to assess vertebral height, presence of pain, and muscle atrophy and to confirm symmetry (Figure 6-21). Many horses resent deep and aggressive palpation of the epaxial muscles, and the response of normal horses should be learned before a pathological response is presumed. Most horses readily become mildly lordotic ("scootch") during deep digital palpation or when a blunt object, such as a pen, is used. Some clinicians prefer to use the ends of the fingers to "run" (apply digital pressure while moving the fingers caudally) the muscles from cranial to caudal, parallel to the spinal column. When this is continued along the gluteal muscles and rump, most normal horses become somewhat kyphotic and move forward slightly. Aggressive use of blunt or sharp objects to assess pain should be avoided. Some horses are stoic during palpation, and it may be impossible to stimulate them to extend and flex the thoracolumbar region without the use of a blunt instrument.[2] In these horses, firmly stroking the ventral abdomen may stimulate movement.[2] With one hand on the horse's back during movement of the

thoracolumbar spine, the clinician may be able to feel muscle "cracking" during the release of tension in the epaxial muscles.[2] The observation of muscle fasciculations during or after palpation usually indicates a degree of muscle pain. Failure to exhibit the normal lordotic or kyphotic responses, assumption of a guarded posture, and vocalization during the examination are further signs of back pain.

In many horses, back pain, and more specifically muscle pain, is secondary to hindlimb lameness, resulting from altered gait and posture. Any site of pain in the hindlimb may alter the gait to cause secondary upper limb or back muscle pain. The use of diagnostic analgesia to confirm the primary source of pain (in the hindlimb, or locally in the back) may be required to make the true diagnosis. Back pain often is complex and may be caused by many factors including ill-fitting saddles, poor riding, and other primary problems, such as overriding of dorsal spinous processes or other bony causes. The clinician should palpate carefully to detect localized swelling in the area of the saddle. Even small areas of hair loss without swelling may indicate a loose or ill-fitting saddle, abnormal movement of the saddle associated with hindlimb lameness, or a rider sitting crookedly.[2]

It is doubtful that muscular pain alone can cause unilateral hindlimb lameness. Back pain was induced in STB horses by injection of lactic acid into the left longissimus dorsi muscle and subsequently exercised and observed with high-speed cinematography.[9] Frank lameness was not observed, but there was slight modification of left hindlimb stride and reduced performance. This supports the clinical observation that back pain usually is the result, not the cause, of obvious hindlimb lameness, although it may result in slight alterations in gait. Severe vertebral abnormalities or an abscess in the epaxial muscles may result in lameness or neurological dysfunction.

PALPATION OF THE LATERAL AND VENTRAL THORAX AND ABDOMEN

History or observation of lameness, performance, or behavioral abnormalities seen only when a horse is ridden or wearing tack should prompt examination of the thoracic region. Irritation from an ill-fitting girth or other sores or wounds can contribute to poor performance, and injury of the sternum or ribs can cause pain associated with saddling or being ridden. Traumatically induced hernias of the ventral abdomen can cause gait deficits or guarding of the abdomen.

PALPATION OF THE EXTERNAL GENITALIA

Testicular or inguinal pain should be considered as a cause of gait modification. Swelling, infection from previous castration, scirrhous cord, and mastitis can cause a change in gait. The veterinarian should determine the sex of the horse and the presence of one or both testicles.

PALPATION OF THE PELVIS

Palpation of the pelvis is performed to confirm previous observations. The horse should stand as squarely as possible. The clinician should palpate all bony protuberances,

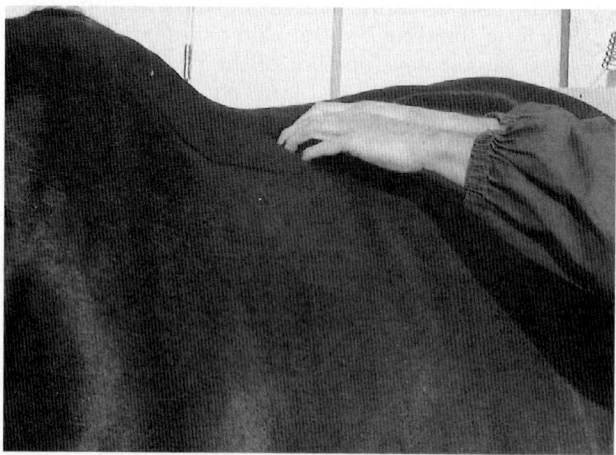

Fig. 6-21 • Palpation of the thoracolumbar region should be performed in a quiet, careful manner. Many horses object to sudden or sharp stimuli applied to this region. Direct, even pressure is applied to the epaxial muscles (shown) and the summits of the dorsal spinous processes.

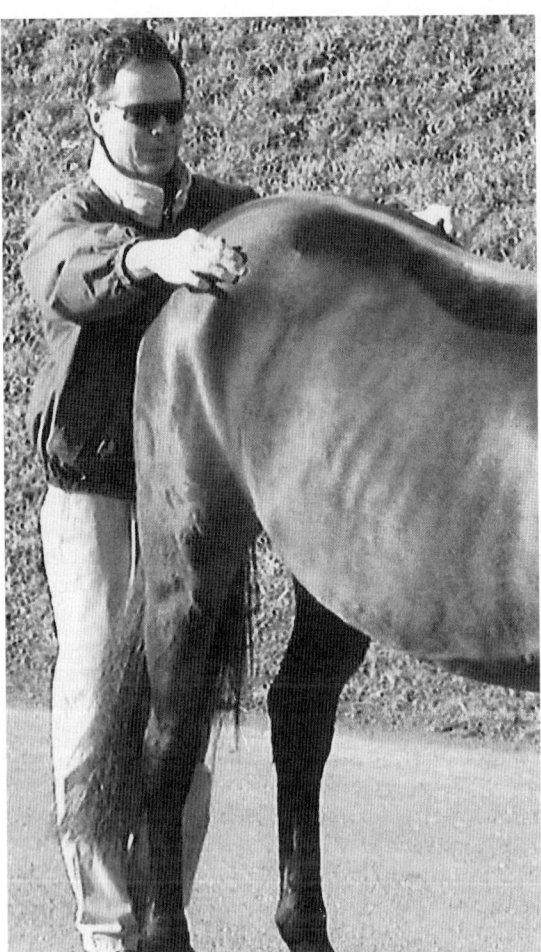

Fig. 6-22 • Although the veterinarian must take care when standing behind any horse, this perspective is crucial in determining pelvic heights and widths. The height of each tuber coxae is compared in this photograph. Alternatively, an assistant on each side can be asked to point to a comparable location, or tape can be applied.

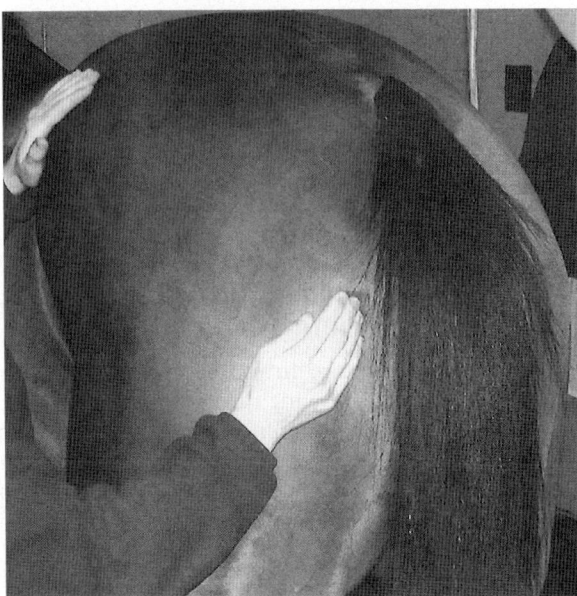

Fig. 6-23 • The tubera ischii (shown) and third trochanters are palpated carefully. Enthesopathy or fracture causes lameness that is difficult to locate without careful palpation or scintigraphic examination. Occasionally, horses with small muscle defects located distal to the tubera ischii have chronic lameness from previous fracture. (Courtesy Carolyn Arnold, College Station, TX.)

Muscle pain and muscle atrophy should be assessed. The clinician carefully examines the gluteal musculature, the origin of the caudal thigh muscles, and the tensor fasciae latae (see Chapter 47 for further discussion of muscle assessment and palpation of the greater trochanter of the femur). Pain or soreness noted during palpation of the semimembranosus and semitendinosus muscles may be associated with injury of the ipsilateral tuber ischium.[2]

PALPATION OF THE PELVIS PER RECTUM

Rectal examination is not part of the routine lameness examination and should be reserved as a special examination procedure if pelvic fracture or aortoiliac thrombosis is suspected. With the wrist just inside the anus the veterinarian should palpate the medial and dorsal aspects of the acetabulum, comparing sides. In young horses, there is a membranous junction between pelvic bones in the center of the acetabulum; a defect and a small amount of motion normally can be felt. Just cranial to the acetabulum is the cranial aspect of the pubis (brim of the pelvis). With the arm at elbow depth the examiner should sweep the arm dorsally on each side to palpate the medial aspect of each ilium. The ventral aspect of the sacrum and sacroiliac region are compared. The clinician should compare the pulse quality between the right and left external iliac arteries and evaluate conformation and pulse quality of the terminal aorta and branches. Horses with aortoiliac thromboembolism have abnormal conformation and altered pulse quality. Crepitus may be felt more easily by gently rocking the horse from side to side, picking up one hindlimb, or walking the horse a short distance with the veterinarian's arm still within the rectum.

Asymmetry, swelling, actual fracture lines, fragments or callus, and crepitus are assessed. In horses with acute pelvic

including the tubera coxae, tubera sacrale, and tubera ischii. The examiner stands behind the horse and palpates these paired protuberances simultaneously if it is safe to do so (Figure 6-22). Fracture of a tuber coxae or an ilial shaft may result in asymmetry, but if the ventral aspect of the tuber coxae is fractured, the height of the dorsal aspect may be equal to that of the contralateral side. The anatomy of the ventral aspect of the tuber coxae is distorted. Small muscle defects may be associated with fracture or enthesopathy of the tubera ischii, but even with a displaced fracture, palpation of this area may be unrewarding (Figure 6-23). If a pelvic injury or fracture is suspected, the clinician should gently rock (move) the horse from side to side. Subtle crepitus may be detected, but in many horses with pelvic fractures this is not apparent until days to weeks after injury and only during the initial portions of the examination before muscle guarding supervenes. The veterinarian should grasp the tail and elevate it. Many horses resist this, but in those with fractures of the base of the tail (most commonly from sitting in the starting gate or trailer), a true pain response is elicited. Subtle swelling also may be present. Lack of tail tone may indicate neurological disease.

fractures, crepitus, fracture fragments or lines, and callus usually are not detectable, but hematoma and soft tissue swelling usually can be felt. In horses with iliac wing or shaft fractures, large fracture hematomas often are present, but the absence of swelling does not preclude presence of iliac fractures. These horses are at risk to develop fatal hemorrhage. Edges of fracture fragments may be evident with comminuted or grossly displaced fractures. With chronic pelvic fractures, crepitus and callus may be more obvious.

PALPATION OF THE HINDLIMB

For safety reasons, I prefer to start proximally and work distally in a hindlimb, allowing the horse to become accustomed to palpation. Horses often object to palpation of the flank and stifle regions, and this should not be misinterpreted as a sign of pain. The clinician should grasp the tail and pull it gently toward himself or herself to keep the ipsilateral hindlimb bearing weight and reduce the chance of the horse kicking. It may be useful to pick up the ipsilateral forelimb. In the large majority of horses the entire limb can be safely examined while bearing weight, but pain in the lame limb or contralateral limb or the horse's behavior may make it difficult or impossible to pick up the limb. Reluctance to pick up the hindlimbs has been attributed to unilateral or bilateral sacroiliac pain.[2] Horses with shivers often are reluctant or anxious to pick up one or both hindlimbs. It may be necessary to spend a small amount of time coaxing the horse to elevate the hindlimb, at first just high enough to examine or pick out the hind foot and then progressing to full flexion. Although historically the hock and stifle joints have been regarded as the principal sources of pain causing hindlimb lameness, there are many other potential sites, and the metatarsal and fetlock regions in particular should be examined with care.

Thigh

The clinician should assess the thigh for swelling, muscle atrophy, or scarring. Horses with femoral fractures usually have obvious severe swelling, crepitus, and instability of the limb. The third trochanter of the femur is difficult to feel, and clinical abnormalities associated with enthesopathy of the insertion of the superficial gluteal muscle or a fracture usually are impossible to detect. Scarring associated with the semitendinosus, the semimembranosus, and rarely the biceps femoris can lead to mechanical gait deficits, known as *fibrotic myopathy*. The gastrocnemius muscle arises from the distal caudal aspect of the femur, and acute tearing of this muscle may cause swelling in the caudal stifle area. This is difficult to perceive, but severe muscle injury results in a marked postural change, which should provoke more careful assessment of this region.

Stifle

Palpation of the stifle is limited to the cranial, lateral, and medial aspects; unfortunately, the caudal and proximal aspects of the joint are inaccessible. Many horses, especially fillies, object to palpation of the stifle, a normal response often misinterpreted as a painful reaction.

The veterinarian should palpate the stifle with the limb bearing weight. The foot should be flat on the ground. This may be impossible if the horse has severe pain prohibiting complete assessment of the stifle. The limb should be in a neutral and not in an abducted position and should be perpendicular to the spine or slightly ahead of the other hindlimb. If the limb is retracted, it is more difficult to palpate the patellar ligaments and joint outpouchings. The middle patellar ligament is identified and followed proximally to the distal aspect of the patella. The clinician should feel the femoropatellar joint capsule between either the middle and medial or the middle and lateral patellar ligaments and should determine the presence of effusion. In horses with osteochondritis dissecans (OCD), fluid distention can be pronounced. However, normal young horses (weanlings to early 2-year-olds) often have prominent bilateral fluid distention of the femoropatellar joint capsules.

The clinician should find the medial patellar ligament and follow it proximally and distally. At the proximal extent, the medial fibrocartilage of the patella can be felt medial to the medial trochlear ridge of the femur. It is this normal arrangement of the medial aspect of the patella and the medial trochlear ridge that allows the veterinarian to determine whether a horse has patellar luxation. The position of the patella is difficult to confirm if the horse is standing with the stifle flexed. True patellar luxation is rare. The examiner should determine if the medial patellar ligament is enlarged, which usually reflects previous desmotomy or dermoplasty. Usually a distinct depression is present between the medial patellar ligament and the medial collateral ligament, but effusion of the medial femorotibial (MFT) joint may result in a substantial "bulge" (Figure 6-24). This may be the only clinical sign indicative of MFT joint injury.

The lateral and middle patellar ligaments are palpated from their origin to insertion. Patellar desmitis is unusual but does occur; it usually involves the middle patellar ligament and may cause mild swelling. Previous injection with counterirritants causes firm, fibrous areas over the patellar ligaments, a common finding in racehorses. Gently rocking the horse from side to side to assess motion of the patella may give some indication of the potential for intermittent upward fixation of the patella (IUFP). In horses prone to IUFP, jerky rather than the normal smooth motion of the patella sometimes is detected.[2] The lateral femorotibial (LFT) joint capsule is accessed between the lateral patellar and lateral collateral ligaments, but even with severe effusion it may be difficult to palpate. Overlying and adjacent soft tissue structures obscure palpation. Effusion of the LFT joint, although rare, is an important palpation finding that should be investigated carefully.

Deep palpation of the medial collateral ligament and the medial patellar ligament with the limb in flexion may elicit a pain response in horses with stifle lameness, but it probably is not specific for the source of pain in the stifle. The medial collateral stress test is perhaps the most reliable manipulative test of the stifle, although horses with lower limb lameness also may respond. With the leg in partial flexion, the shoulder or one hand is used as a fulcrum on the lateral aspect of the stifle, and the distal extremity is pulled laterally, thus placing valgus stress on the stifle (Figure 6-25). Care should be taken because horses may resent this manipulative test. If possible, the valgus motion should be applied by using the shoulder as a fulcrum and both hands on the crus, thus eliminating possible false-positive results from the lower limb. Patellar manipulation may cause a pain response, particularly in horses with

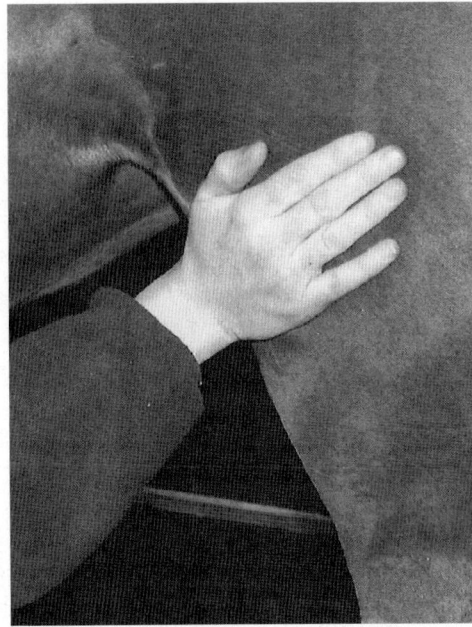

Fig. 6-26 • Used as a static or provocative test, patellar manipulation is performed by placing the palm of the hand over the cranial aspect of the patella and manually forcing the patella proximally several times in succession. This maneuver can exacerbate pain from conditions of the patella and femoropatellar joint and forces the distal femur in a caudal direction. Pain from soft tissue injuries such as patellar, cruciate, or collateral ligament tears and osteoarthritis of the femorotibial joints can be exacerbated, but false-negative and false-positive results are common. (Courtesy Carolyn Arnold, College Station, TX.)

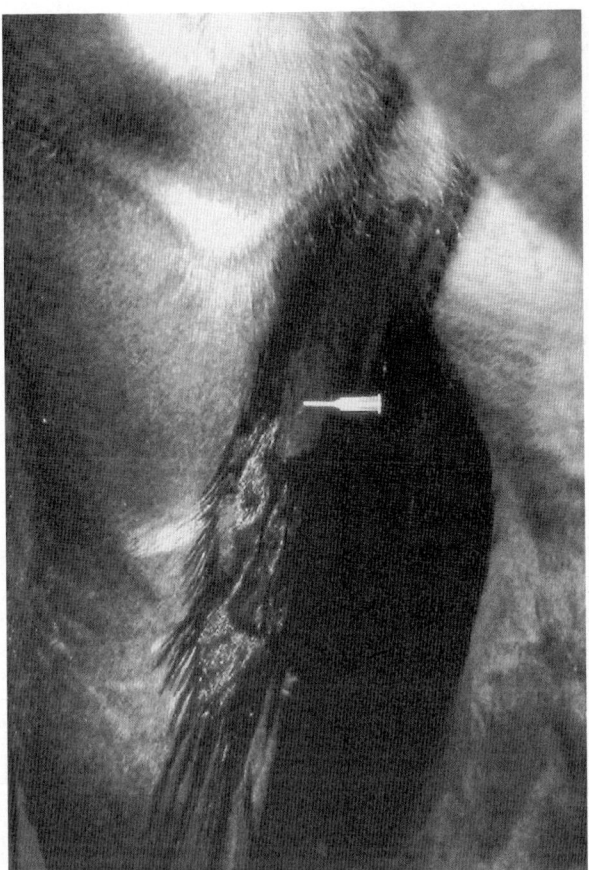

Fig. 6-24 • The medial femorotibial joint (right stifle, cranial view) is the most common location for osteoarthritis of the stifle joint and is palpated medially (needle in joint) between the medial patellar ligament and the medial collateral ligament. Normally a depression is present at this location, but a bulge from effusion can be palpated in this horse.

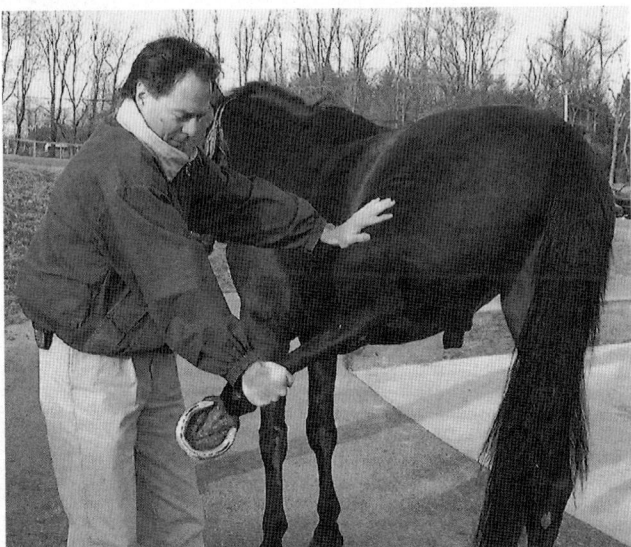

Fig. 6-25 • The valgus stress test of the stifle is difficult to perform and is accomplished by using a hand (shown) or shoulder as a fulcrum. This test can be done during static examination or a provocative test followed by trotting (see Chapter 8).

femorotibial joint disease. During this procedure, caudal movement of the femur also may exacerbate cruciate injuries. With the limb on the ground in a weight-bearing position, the clinician's hand is placed on the distal aspect of the patella, and the patella is forced upward (Figure 6-26). Theoretically during this test, numerous movements of the stifle are induced. The patellar ligaments are stretched, the patella is forced proximally, and on release the patella rapidly moves distally against the trochlear ridges, and the femur is forced caudally. Tests to assess cruciate ligament damage have been described but are dangerous to perform, and I have not found them particularly useful.[10] Complete tearing of the cruciate or collateral ligaments is rare, and partial tearing does not cause clinically detectable instability. In horses with severe lameness and gross stifle instability, it is obvious that the stifle is the source of lameness, and pain usually prohibits manipulation.

Crus

The examiner should palpate the crus using both hands with the limb bearing weight. Subtle swelling of the medial aspect of the tibia can be palpated, but palpation of the caudolateral aspect of the tibia, the area in which stress fractures are diagnosed most frequently, is limited. Often no palpable abnormality is associated with a stress fracture. Any small wound or any form of swelling should be thoroughly investigated for the possibility of underlying bone damage, such as an occult tibial fracture. The veterinarian should palpate the caudal soft tissues.

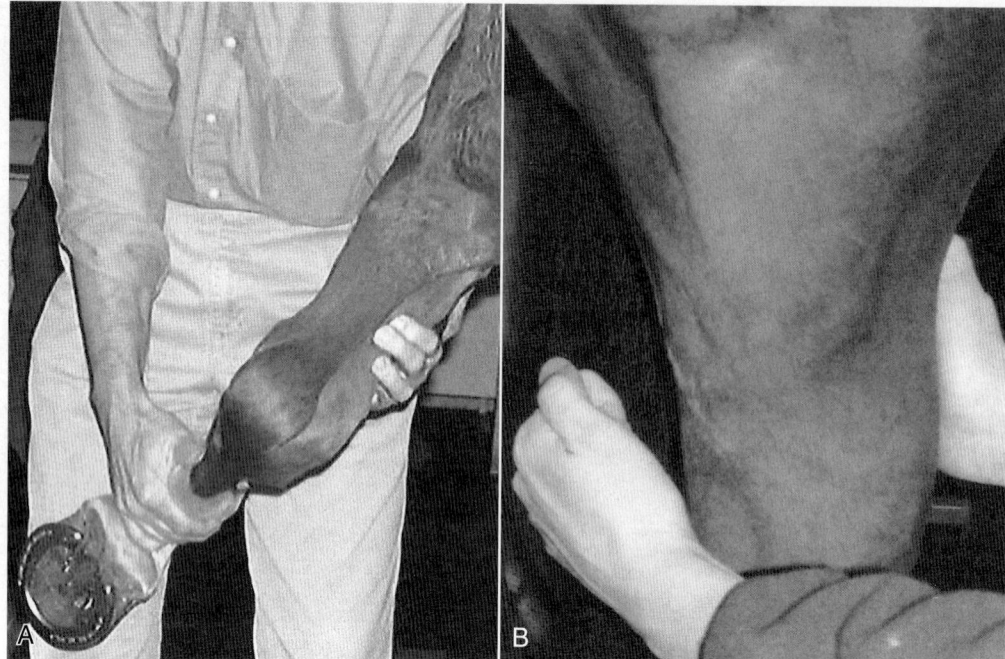

Fig. 6-27 • **A,** Palpation of the medial aspect of the tibia in a flexed position or **B,** tibial percussion in the standing position sometimes elicits pain in horses with tibial stress fractures, but false-positive results are common.

Proximally, the musculotendonous junction of the gastrocnemius muscle is a rare site of pain. The common calcaneal tendon is assessed. Swelling may indicate damage to any one of the contributing tendons. Effusion of the tarsal sheath causes swelling just proximal to the tarsus, at the caudal aspect of the crus, and should be differentiated from bog spavin. Deep palpation of the medial and caudal aspects of the crus is performed with the limb elevated (Figure 6-27). Horses with tibial stress fractures or those with spiral fracture or other tibial trauma may show a pain response, but false-positive responses are frequent. Tibial percussion, performed medially by using a clenched fist (knuckles) as a hammer, may elicit a pain response in horses with stress fractures, but many normal horses resent this test.

Tarsus

Five common swellings of the hock are important to differentiate, but hock swelling is not synonymous with hock pain. *Capped hock* is swelling located at the point of the hock (the proximal aspect of the calcaneus) and usually is an incidental finding, but in some horses the condition does cause lameness (Figure 6-28). The most common form involves the development of firm, fibrous subcutaneous tissue in the false bursa that lies over the point of the hock. This is a common area for abrasions and excoriation, and fibrous tissue formation results in a blemish but usually no lameness. Horses may be sensitive to palpation if the area has been traumatized recently. Infection or trauma leading to osteitis of the calcaneus can cause a clinically important capped hock and severe lameness. In these horses the problem involves the calcaneal bursa, located between the common calcaneal tendon and the calcaneus. If surrounding soft tissue swelling is minimal, fluid distention of the calcaneal bursa may be felt by

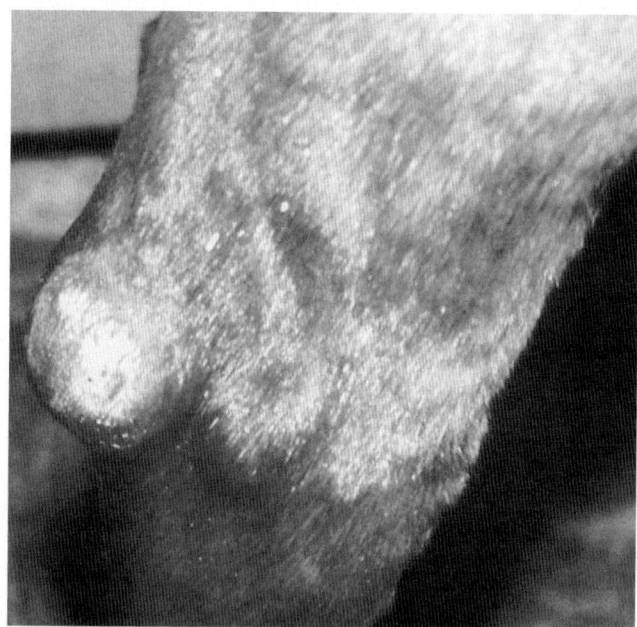

Fig. 6-28 • Capped hock, a firm fibrous swelling of the proximal aspect of the calcaneus (point of the hock), is considered a blemish, but with effusion of the calcaneal bursa (not shown), lameness is substantial.

ballottement. The bursa can be felt both medially and laterally at the proximal aspect of the calcaneus. Lateral, or less commonly, medial dislocation (luxation) of the SDFT results in similar swelling, but in an acute situation, lameness is present. Careful palpation may reveal the SDFT coursing laterally (Figure 6-29), unless excessive soft tissue swelling is present.

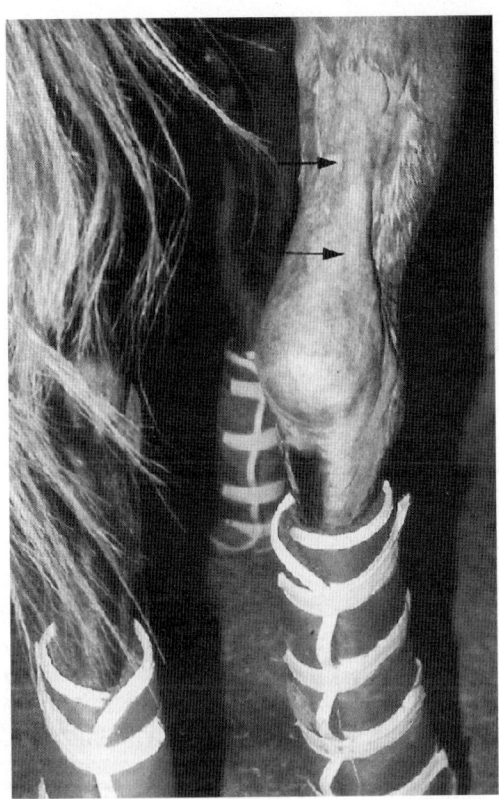

Fig. 6-29 • Lateral dislocation (luxation) of the superficial digital flexor tendon. Instead of attaching to the tuber calcanei, the superficial digital flexor tendon *(arrows)* is now located lateral to the point of the hock. Initial swelling makes this diagnosis difficult.

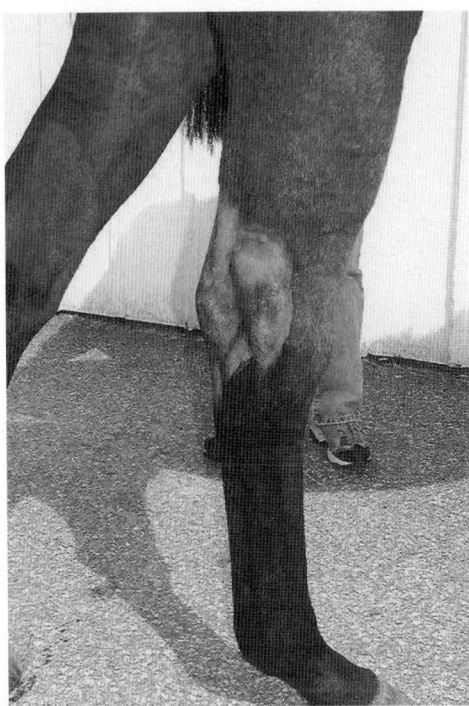

Fig. 6-30 • Thoroughpin, swelling located in the distal, caudal aspect of the crus, usually is caused by distention of the tarsal sheath and must be differentiated from effusion of the plantarolateral pouch of the tarsocrural joint (bog spavin).

Effusion of the tarsal sheath, *thoroughpin,* must be differentiated from bog spavin (see following text). Tarsal tenosynovitis causes swelling both medially and laterally in the depression between the calcaneal tendon and the caudal aspect of the tibia (Figure 6-30). With severe effusion of the tarsal sheath, fluid distention can be palpated distal to the hock on the medial aspect. Thoroughpin usually is an incidental finding, seen most commonly in Western performance horses, but acute lameness accompanied by tarsal tenosynovitis can indicate strain or injury of the sheath, often associated with adjacent bony injury. Unusually, swelling in the distal, caudal aspect of the crus identical to that seen with classic thoroughpin is seen, but communication with and concomitant swelling of the tarsal sheath are absent.

The term *spavin* refers to "any disease of the hock joint of horses in which enlargements occur, often causing lameness ... the enlargement may be due to collection of fluids or to bony growth."[11] *Bog spavin* is fluid distention of the tarsocrural joint capsule. The tarsocrural joint has four outpouchings: dorsolateral, dorsomedial, plantarolateral, and plantaromedial. All joint pouches may be distended, although the dorsomedial and plantarolateral pouches are large and most prominent (Figure 6-31). With ballottement, fluid can be pushed between pouches on the dorsal or plantar aspects, thus differentiating this condition from thoroughpin.

Bone spavin refers to fibrous and bony swelling that results from chronic osteoarthritis of the proximal intertarsal, centrodistal, and tarsometatarsal joints. This swelling

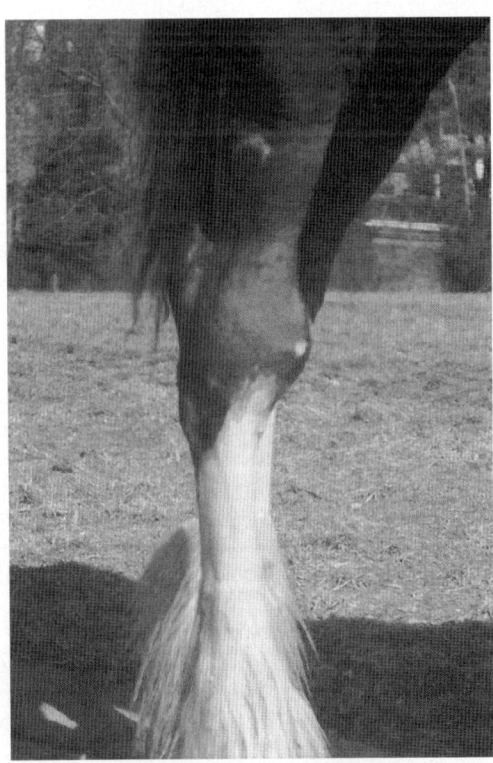

Fig. 6-31 • Moderate-to-severe tarsocrural effusion, bog spavin, in this draft filly was caused by osteochondritis dissecans of the cranial intermediate ridge of the distal aspect of the tibia. Distention of the large dorsomedial pouch and swelling of the dorsolateral, plantarolateral, and plantaromedial pouches was present.

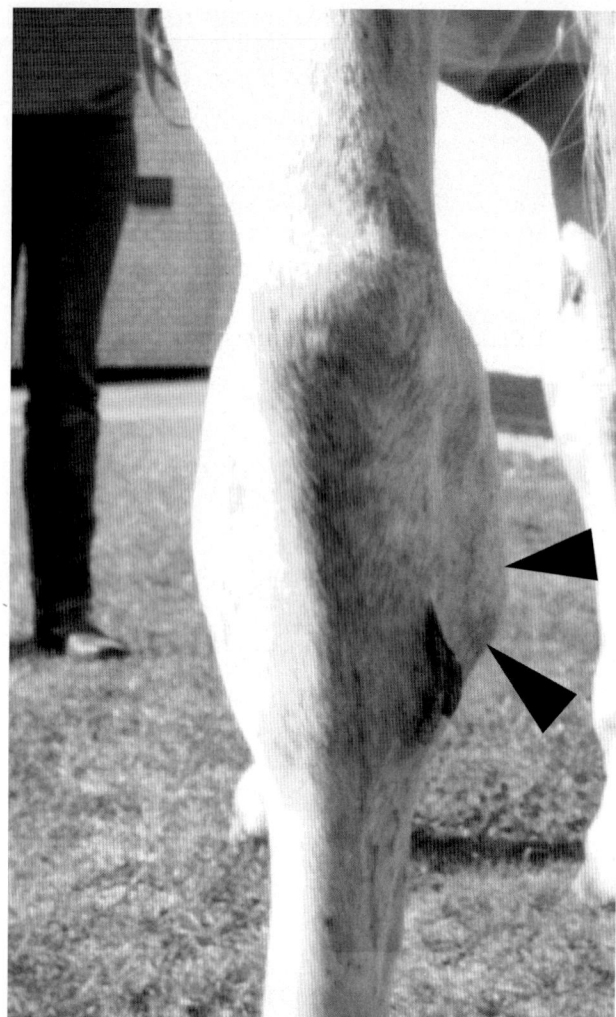

Fig. 6-32 • Bone spavin *(arrows)*, fibrous and bony swelling on the medial aspect of the distal hock joint (left hindlimb) caused by chronic osteoarthritis of the distal hock joints, sometimes appears in older sports horses but is rare in young racehorses. The presence of bone spavin should be noted, and this area should be palpated carefully, but horses can have distal hock pain without bone spavin, and horses with bone spavin can have lameness elsewhere in the limb. Previous cunean tenectomy causes chronic fibrosis in this region.

usually is seen in older horses and can be palpated and observed on the medial side of the hock (Figure 6-32). Although the bony enlargement is the result of proliferation, it does not necessarily mean that the horse is lame as the result of the condition. Most horses with distal hock joint pain do not have palpable enlargement medially, and based on radiological evaluation, the most common area of proliferation and bony change is the dorsolateral aspect of the joints. *Blood spavin* is an old term usually meaning enlargement of the saphenous vein,[3] but it also may have been used to describe a prominent saphenous vein in horses with bog spavin. Saphenous distention is rare, and the term is not used today. *Occult* or *blind spavin* is an obsolete term used to describe horses with clinical signs of hock lameness but no observable bony swelling.[3] *High spavin* is also an obsolete term used to describe bone spavin located close to the tarsocrural joint.[3]

Curb describes swelling along the distal, plantar aspect of the hock and has often erroneously been blamed on long plantar desmitis. In most horses the swelling is actually enlargement of the SDFT or subcutaneous tissues. The swelling is often firm, but in some horses subcutaneous fluid can be present (see Figure 78-1). In horses with acute severe injury the swelling may feel soft and mushy. In some normal horses the proximal aspect of the MtIV is prominent and should not be confused with curb.

Swelling restricted to the medial or lateral aspect of the hock may reflect collateral ligament injury. Localized heat on the medial aspect of the hock or on the proximal aspect of the metatarsal region may be an important finding.

THE CHURCHILL HOCK TEST

Dan L. Hawkins

The Churchill hock test was developed by Dr. E.A. Churchill in the 1950s as a rapid, noninvasive, specific method to screen and identify distal tarsal pain in athletic horses. Although the test has been used by Dr. Churchill and me primarily in STBs, TBs, endurance horses, and Three Day Event horses, it is equally reliable when applied to other equine athletes.

Digital pressure is applied on the plantar aspect of the head of the second metatarsal bone (MtII) and fused first and second tarsal bones with the limb in a non–weight-bearing position. Abduction of the limb is a positive response. To examine the left tarsus, the clinician approaches the horse facing caudally. The left hindlimb is picked up and brought forward, supported by the clinician's right hand cupped under the fetlock or hoof. Holding the limb so that the hoof is approximately 25 to 30 cm above the ground is most comfortable for the horse. The heel of the left hand is positioned on the proximodorsal surface of the third metatarsal bone (MtIII) while the third phalanges of the index and middle or middle and ring fingers are placed around the medial side of the tarsus to engage the bony ridge formed by the head of the MtII and the first and second tarsal bones (the area of insertion of the cunean tendon) (Figure 6-33). The thumb is rested on the dorsal lateral aspect of the tarsus and the proximal aspect of the MtIII. Gentle, firm pressure is applied to the bony ridge by flexing the phalanges of *only the index and middle fingers* (Figure 6-34). The hand does not squeeze the hock. Pressure is applied three times approximately 1 second apart, each time with increasing intensity to a maximum effort on the third time.

Proficiency requires patience and routine practice. Consistent diagnostic information can be obtained safely from more than 90% of fit racehorses. If the limb cannot be picked up, the test cannot be performed. Fussing and repeatedly flexing the hock and limb in an agitated manner while the procedure is performed should not be misinterpreted as a positive response.

The Churchill hock test is useful for horses that are not visibly lame but for which the trainer or rider has a complaint that the horse is doing something uncharacteristic during work or competition associated with decreased performance. The horse may have a changed attitude toward work, lugs in or out, is rough in the turns, refuses to change

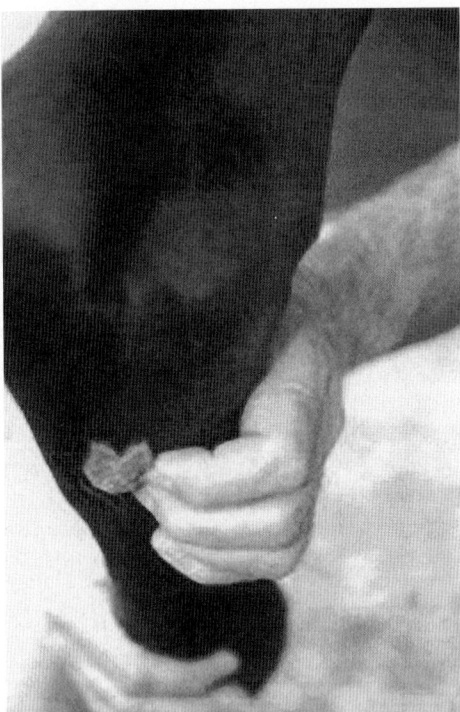

Fig. 6-33 • Correct left hand placement in the left proximal metatarsal region to perform the Churchill hock test. (Courtesy Dan L. Hawkins, Gainesville, FL.)

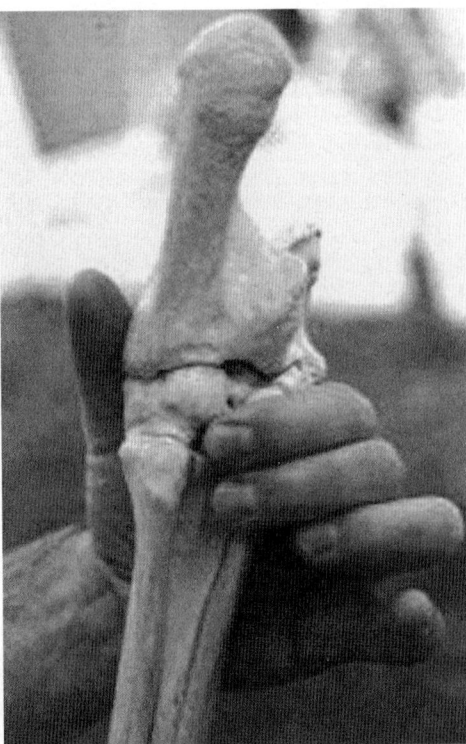

Fig. 6-34 • The Churchill test is demonstrated on an anatomy specimen. The index and middle fingers are flexed and positioned on the bony ridge formed by the third metatarsal bone and the fused first and second tarsal bones, and the heel of the hand rests on the proximodorsal aspect of the third metatarsal bone. The thumb rests against the dorsolateral aspect of the tarsus. (Courtesy Dan L. Hawkins, Gainesville, FL.)

leads, stops at jumps, jumps to one side, or is stiff going in one direction. Although these horses cannot be blocked out at a slow gait, the Churchill hock test may suggest the presence of distal hock joint pain.

SAPHENOUS FILLING TIME

Mike W. Ross

The veterinarian should assess the saphenous vein filling time. Blood flow in the saphenous vein is prevented using digital compression in the proximal metatarsal region, and the blood accumulated in the vein over the tarsocrural joint is pushed proximally to completely collapse the vein. The finger compressing the vein distal to the hock is then removed, and the time it takes for the saphenous vein to fill is observed. Normally, it takes less than 1 second for the vein to fill, but in horses with reduced circulation, prolonged filling time is seen. Pulse quality of the dorsal metatarsal artery, located on the dorsolateral aspect of the MtIII just dorsal to the fourth metatarsal bone (MtIV), can be useful, especially if the history suggests lameness is caused by vascular compromise. The arterial pulse quality is compared with that in the contralateral limb.

Metatarsal Region

The veterinarian should palpate the digital flexor tendons and SL. Tendonitis is unusual in the hindlimb, but occasionally SDF tendonitis occurs in the proximal metatarsal region. This is most common in horses with curb, and tendonitis progresses distally to involve the metatarsal area. The hock angle is evaluated carefully. Occasionally horses with severe curb or those with SDF tendonitis of the metatarsal region have a reduced hock angle (obvious unilateral sickle-hocked conformation), indicating loss of support in the SDFT. Once a general palpation for the presence of heat, swelling, and exostoses associated with the MtIII, the MtII, the MtIV, and the proximal aspect of the DFTS has been completed, the limb is lifted and deep palpation is performed. The clinician should carefully palpate the origin and body of the SL, keeping in mind that both false-positive and false-negative responses can occur (Figure 6-35). Much of the palpation of the SL laterally is indirect, because the MtIV hides the origin and proximal aspect of the body. Because the presence of the splint bones and dense metatarsal fascia prevents substantial swelling, or at least the clinical recognition of swelling of the SL, even mild swelling in the proximal, medial metatarsal region should be carefully interpreted. With the limb in flexion, the axial borders of splint bones are palpated. The dorsal aspect of the MtIII should also be assessed with the limb in flexion, because bony injury of the MtIII does occur and includes dorsal cortical trauma from external injury or interference, dorsal cortical and spiral fractures, and proximal dorsolateral fractures.

Metatarsophalangeal Joint

Many of the common problems of the metatarsophalangeal (MTP) joint, such as short, midsagittal fractures of the proximal phalanx, sesamoiditis, maladaptive or nonadaptive remodeling of the MtIII, and osteochondrosis, cause very few clinical signs, and although palpation is quite important, diagnostic analgesia is often needed to localize pain to

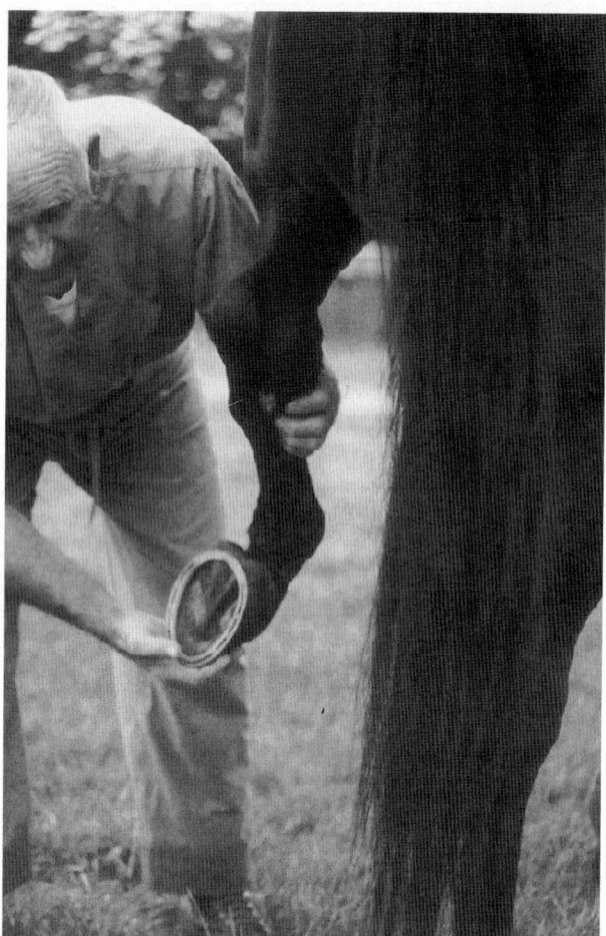

Fig. 6-35 • Deep palpation of the proximal aspect of the suspensory ligament can be performed only with the limb in flexion. The close association of the suspensory origin to the Churchill site explains the need to differentiate proximal plantar metatarsal pain from distal hock joint pain using diagnostic analgesia. (Courtesy Howard "Gene" Gill, Pine Bush, New York.)

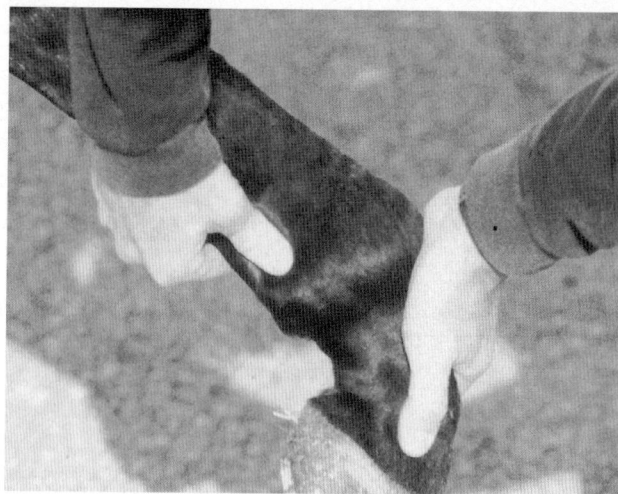

Fig. 6-36 • The metatarsophalangeal joint region often is overlooked during lameness examination. This joint should be palpated carefully with the limb in the standing and flexed *(shown)* positions. (Courtesy Ross Rich, Cave Creek, Arizona.)

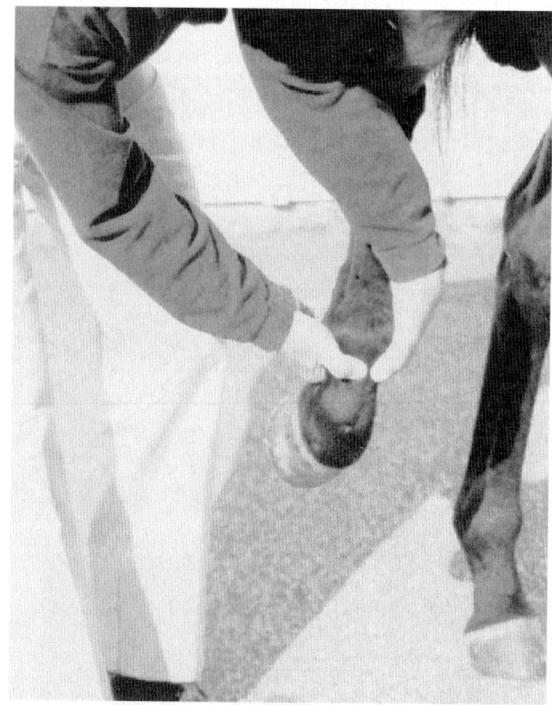

Fig. 6-37 • Palpation of the proximal, dorsal aspect of the proximal phalanx can elicit pain in horses with incomplete mid-sagittal fracture of the proximal phalanx. In trotters, interference injury from the ipsilateral front foot causes pain and swelling in this region. (Courtesy Ross Rich, Cave Creek, Arizona.)

this area. Nonetheless, careful palpation of the fetlock region is mandatory. Some horses have concurrent MTP joint and stifle pain, and when suspicious findings exist in one site, the veterinarian should look carefully at the other for additional, secondary, or complementary problems.

The MTP or hind fetlock joint is evaluated with the limb bearing weight and in flexion. The clinician should assess the MTP joint capsule and the DFTS for the presence of effusion or fibrosis (Figure 6-36). Incidental effusion of both the MTP joint and the DFTS is common in the hindlimb of older performance horses; therefore this finding should not be overinterpreted. In younger horses, particularly racehorses, the presence of effusion can be an important clinical sign associated with osteoarthritis or other problems and should be interpreted accordingly. The clinician should carefully palpate for the presence of heat and mild swelling over the surface of both PSBs, subtle but important signs of sesamoiditis. Sesamoiditis is more prevalent in the hindlimb but can be difficult to detect, and advanced imaging often is necessary for diagnosis. The digital pulse amplitude should be assessed.

With the fetlock joint in flexion, the veterinarian should palpate the proximal, dorsal aspect of the proximal phalanx for the presence of pain or exostoses (Figure 6-37) and should apply pressure to the PSBs, avoiding aggressive compression, which may cause false-positive results. The range of motion of the MTP joint is noted.

Pastern

When the limb is elevated, the reciprocal apparatus causes constant flexion of the digit, which makes palpation of the plantar aspect of the pastern exceedingly difficult. Subtle swelling in the plantar aspect of the pastern is easy to miss. Bony and soft tissue structures should be palpated with the horse in the standing position, and the veterinarian should note the same clinically important areas that were pointed out for the forelimb. High and low ringbone (osteoarthritis of the proximal interphalangeal and distal interphalangeal joints, respectively), osteochondrosis of the pastern joint, and soft tissue problems such as SDF branch tendonitis, distal sesamoidean desmitis, and plantar injury of the pastern joint occur, but with reduced frequency when compared with the forelimb.

Foot

A similar approach to the evaluation of the hind foot as that described for the front foot is used. I spend considerably less time evaluating the hind foot than the front foot, unless the history or horse type dictates otherwise, because this area is relatively infrequently the source of pain. In the draft horse, hind foot pain is as common as in the forelimb, and therefore the hind feet merit considerable attention. Unless specifically indicated by the lameness history, or the horse is severely lame without an obvious cause in the upper limb, I do not routinely perform a hoof tester examination of the hind feet. Pressure with hoof testers over the frog and across the heel in a hind foot often causes a false-positive response in normal horses. The position needed to perform an unassisted hoof tester examination in the hindlimb can be dangerous. The presence of an assistant to elevate the limb may obviate some of the risk.

The examiner should assess the shape, balance, and contour of the foot and observe the shoe (or lack of one) carefully. Hoof angle in the hindlimb ranges from 48 to 58 degrees, and the hoof and pastern axis should be straight. A common finding is a low or underrun heel. An interesting relationship between a low heel and the presence of PSD has been noted.[2] In these horses a lateral radiographic image of the foot shows that the plantar aspect of the distal phalanx is lower than the dorsal aspect.[2] Shoe wear is extremely important in the hindlimb and can give clues to the source of lameness. For instance, horses with distal hock joint pain tend to stab the lower hindlimb during advancement, causing excessive wear of the lateral branch of the shoe (Figure 6-38). Other causes of lower hindlimb lameness, such as osteoarthritis of the MTP joint, can cause a similar gait, but usually abnormal shoe wear is less pronounced. Horses with stifle lameness often wear the medial branch of the shoe. The presence of heel and toe caulks or borium causes additional shear stress on many of the lower limb joints and can exacerbate lameness.

THE ROLE OF PHYSICAL EXAMINATION IN THE LAMENESS EXAMINATION

Body temperature may assist with a clinical diagnosis. The normal temperature range is 37.5° to 38.6° C (99.5° to

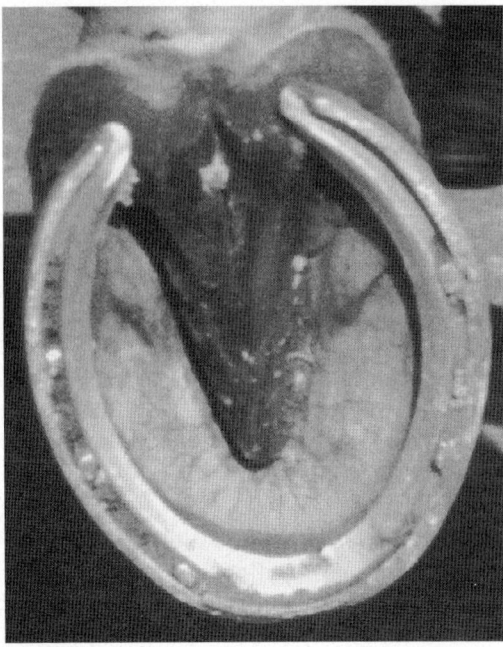

Fig. 6-38 • It is imperative to observe the hind shoes for wear during lameness examination. This right hind shoe (lateral is to the right) has wear along the dorsal and lateral aspects (lateral aspect of toe grab and fullering are worn) consistent with a lower hindlimb lameness, such as distal hock joint or proximal metatarsal region pain.

101.3° F), although in a foal the upper limit may normally be slightly higher. Body temperature in foals rises more abruptly than in adult horses in response to stress, infection, and inflammation. Thus transport of a foal may cause transient low-grade pyrexia, but fever in an adult horse after transport is abnormal. Localized infection in a foal usually causes pyrexia but rarely does so in an adult. The examiner should not *exclude* infectious arthritis in an adult horse simply because fever is *not* present. However, adult horses usually are pyrexic during the early stages of cellulitis or lymphangitis.

Elevation in the pulse and respiratory rates often accompanies severe lameness because of pain. Systemic diseases such as endotoxemia may cause abnormal vital parameter findings in any horse and can lead to conditions such as laminitis.

It is important to remember that diseases of other body systems can cause clinical signs that mimic lameness or cause true gait deficits. For instance, abnormal or stiff gaits can be seen in horses with pleuritis and peritonitis, abdominal, sublumbar, inguinal, thoracic inlet, and pectoral abscesses or tumors. Proliferative new bone associated with hypertrophic osteopathy may be associated with a thoracic or abdominal mass. If an unusual situation arises, the veterinarian should step back and think of the exception rather than the rule, because the "red herring" may be just around the corner.

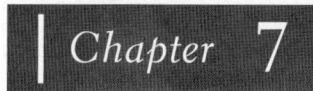

Movement

Mike W. Ross

References
on page
1256

> *"The best time for examining a lame horse is while he is in action. An attendant should lead him on a trot, preferably on hard ground, in a straight line, allowing him freedom of his head, so that his movements may all be natural and unconstrained."*
>
> A. Liautard, 1888[1]

It would be difficult to improve on Liautard's insistence that the lame horse be examined during movement or his description for how it is best accomplished. Although all parts of the lameness examination are important, the key is the determination of the limb or limbs involved. Not all horses with musculoskeletal problems exhibit lameness that is perceptible under normal conditions, or even by use of high-speed or slow-motion cinematography, gait analysis, or other sophisticated imaging devices. Under most circumstances, however, lameness from pain or a mechanical defect in gait is discernible, and the essence of the lameness examination is to determine the source of the pain. This discussion includes relevant experimental findings to support clinical observations, but sometimes experimental findings are confusing rather than informative.

GAIT

Gait, defined as the "manner or style of walking"[2] or "the manner of walking or stepping,"[3] is used to describe the speed and characteristics of a horse in motion. The *natural gaits,* those exhibited when a horse is free in a field, are the walk, trot, and gallop.[4] The canter is a collected gallop. Other gaits including the pace, running walk, rack (a singlefoot or broken amble), fox trot, and amble are *artificial gaits,* although some pacers pace "free-legged" (without the use of hobbles) while on the track, either at a slow speed or racing speed, and occasionally a Standardbred (STB) paces free-legged in a field. In some instances a trotter switches from a trot to the pace, but this change usually is exhibited while the horse is performing at speed and may be associated with lameness or interference. Lame trotters usually "make breaks," going off stride, by switching (breaking) from the trot to the gallop.

The term *beat* describes the number of foot strikes in a single stride cycle regardless of whether one or more feet strike the ground simultaneously. The following abbreviations are used for limbs: left forelimb (LF), right forelimb (RF), left hindlimb (LH), and right hindlimb (RH). The walk is a four-beat gait in which all four feet strike the ground independently without a period of suspension (in which no feet are on the ground). Depending on the part of the stride during which observations begin, the walk can appear to be lateral or diagonal. In general, in a lateral gait, both feet on one side strike the ground before the feet on the contralateral side. In a diagonal gait, one foot strike is followed by a strike of the foot located diagonal and contralateral to the initial foot (e.g., LF followed by the RH).

Lame horses should always be evaluated at the walk. Stride length should be evaluated and compared with observations at the trot. Stride length and sequence of footfalls are easier to see while horses are walking than while they are trotting. Horses with hindlimb lameness may be examined for failure to track up.[5] Horses normally track up, or overtrack. The hind foot is placed in or in front of the imprint of the ipsilateral front foot. Failure to track up usually is caused by hindlimb lameness or poor impulsion, and the hind foot imprint is seen behind that of the ipsilateral front foot.[5] Although unusual, occasionally a horse will be observed to pace while walking, a finding that may indicate the presence of neurological disease. In breeds unassociated with the pace or similar gaits, young horses that pace should undergo careful neurological evaluation. Pacing while walking may be completely normal, and in older, "made" horses (horses that have already achieved an upper level of performance) the finding should not be overinterpreted.

Backing is a diagonal, two-beat gait. Horses seldom back naturally, but backing commonly is required of horses during performance events, while exiting from a trailer, or while driving. Backing is useful during lameness examination to evaluate certain gait deficits, such as those associated with shivers, stringhalt, and neurological disease.

The trot is a diagonal, theoretically two-beat gait, and diagonal pairs of limbs move simultaneously. The trot is theoretically a symmetrical gait, meaning both "halves" (beats) of the stride are identical, and at low speed in a sound horse, symmetry is likely achieved. However, at speed, perfect balance and fine management of weight (of the shoes) are necessary for a trotter to be perfectly symmetrical. There is a moment of suspension between impact of each diagonal pair of limbs. Some elite dressage horses do not have a two-beat gait but show advanced diagonal placement. This means that the hindlimb of a diagonal pair of limbs lands first and therefore is the only limb bearing weight. Hindlimb lameness is present in a higher percentage of horses that perform at speed at the trot compared with galloping horses because of differences in weight distribution in the trot and gallop. Compensatory lameness develops in the diagonal paired limb. LF lameness predisposes to RH lameness. Interference between limbs is more common in horses that trot at speed when compared with those that gallop. Likewise, hindlimb lameness is relatively common in dressage horses.

The pace is a symmetrical, lateral, two-beat gait predominantly in STB racehorses and is characterized by movement of lateral pairs of limbs simultaneously (LH and LF; RH and RF), with a moment of suspension between lateral pairs. Pacers also have a high percentage of hindlimb lameness, but compensatory lameness usually develops in the lateral paired limb. RH lameness predisposes to RF lameness.

The gallop or run is a four-beat gait. In the gallop and the canter the horse leads with the LF or RF, the forelimb that strikes the ground last in the stride sequence. An unrestrained horse usually leads with the LF while turning

Video available at
www.rossanddyson.com
Chapter 7 **Movement** 65

to the left, or the RF while turning to the right. Fatigue also plays a role. A Thoroughbred (TB) racehorse racing counterclockwise leads with the LF on the turns but immediately after entering the stretch switches to the right lead. Failure to switch leads or constantly switching leads in the gallop or canter may reflect fatigue or lameness.

In a *left* lead gallop, the RH strikes the ground first, followed in sequence by the LH, RF, and LF, followed by a period of suspension. When a horse is on the right lead, the RF strikes the ground last, propelling the horse into the suspension phase of the stride. It is often assumed that a horse with RF lameness is reluctant to take the right lead. However, bone stress measured in the radius and the third metacarpal bone (McIII) is greater on the nonlead (trailing) forelimb, and thus a lame horse may change leads to protect the nonlead forelimb.[6] Ground reaction forces (GRFs) are greater in the trailing (nonlead) forelimb, a fact that supports the clinical observation that horses with forelimb lameness may select leads to protect the lame forelimb. A horse with RF lameness may prefer the right lead, allowing the LF to assume the greater forces and bone stress.[5]

The canter (lope) is a three-beat gait. In left lead canter the RH strikes the ground first, then the LH and RF land simultaneously, followed by the LF and then a period of suspension. A horse reluctant to take a lead may be trying to compensate for hindlimb lameness. In the right lead the LH must absorb a considerable amount of concussion and then generate propulsive forces. Proneness of this limb to fatigue seems logical, but a consistent change in stride characteristics of fatigued horses to protect the LH was not seen.[7] Although the LH strikes the ground first, stance time, flexion of the upper limb joints, and GRF are greater in the RH.[5] It could be assumed that a horse lame in the RH would be reluctant to take the right lead and may prefer the left lead.[5] Lead and stride characteristics of fatigued and lame horses are complex because of asymmetry of the gait, and forelimb and hindlimb problems could account for failure or reluctance to take a particular lead and inappropriate lead switching.

Young horses early in training or trained horses that are lame may exhibit a disunited canter. The horse may spontaneously change legs behind, but not in front. In changing from left to right lead canter, or vice versa, the forelimbs and hindlimbs should change simultaneously. Horses with back pain or hindlimb lameness may be reluctant to change leads, or may change in front but not behind.

The Lameness Examination: Which Gait Is Best?
The trot is the most useful gait to determine the location of the lame limb or limbs. Forelimb lameness in particular is difficult to observe at the pace, especially in horses that are led in hand. Lame trotters may pace, supporting the supposition that the pace is an easier gait in a lame STB. I have seen horses with severe forelimb lameness at the trot that looked barely lame when pacing.

Comparing Lameness Seen at the Walk and Trot
Although lameness score should be determined when trotting a horse (see later), it is useful to compare gait deficits at the walk and trot. In horses with forelimb lameness, an exaggerated head and neck nod may be observed while walking horses with upper limb lameness (genuine shoulder region pain, for instance), and, in fact, head and neck excursion may be more pronounced than that seen while the horse is trotting. Some horses may exhibit odd gait deficits while walking, but deficits may abate at the trot. Horses with rare upper forelimb pain from rib fractures or anomalies may manifest abduction of the forelimb during protraction at the walk but not the trot. The stance phase of the stride is relatively longer at the walk than at the trot. The deep digital flexor tendon and the collateral ligaments of the distal interphalangeal joint are stressed maximally with extension of the distal interphalangeal joint. Thus with severe injuries of either structure lameness may be more severe at the walk than at the trot because of greater extension of the distal interphalangeal joint associated with the relatively long stance duration.[5] Horses with hindlimb lameness characterized by a shortened caudal phase of the stride at the walk but shortened cranial phase at the trot often have upper limb lameness, such as that caused by pelvic fractures or osteoarthritis of the coxofemoral joint or from severe pain originating from the foot. In general, horses that have limb flight characteristics that differ between walk and trot should be evaluated carefully because in my experience they often have bona fide pain originating from the upper limb or are affected with an unusual mechanical or neuromuscular deficit.

Relevance of Lameness at a Trot in Hand
Is lameness seen at a trot in hand the same lameness that compromises performance at speed? Is the lameness seen at a trot in hand in a jumping horse the same problem that causes the horse to refuse fences? The answer is usually, but not invariably, yes. For instance, I have seen many STBs show subtle unilateral hindlimb lameness at a trot in hand, but when the horse was later examined at the track and hooked to a cart, pronounced contralateral hindlimb lameness was noted. Differences include the track surface, the act of pulling a cart, the additional weight of the driver, and a faster gait. Lameness often is evaluated on a smooth hard surface useful in exacerbating even subtle problems, but most horses perform on softer surfaces, when other problems may be apparent. More than one lameness problem may exist—one evident at a trot in hand and another while the horse is ridden or driven. Horses can show lameness from one problem when trotted in a straight line but lameness from an entirely different problem while being trotted in a circle. The answer to the first question is complex because performance itself entails the inextricably intertwined relationship between horse and rider or driver and the possible presence of compensatory and coexistent pain. Ideally, to evaluate the role of lameness on poor performance, horses would be evaluated at the speed, at the gait, and in the manner in which they perform, conditions that usually are not always possible to reproduce.

Horse Temperament and Lameness Examination
Safety of the handler, observers, and the horse must always be considered throughout a lameness examination, and with a difficult horse the examination may need to be modified, especially on cold, windy days. In some female horses and geldings, judicious use of the tranquilizer acetylpromazine (0.02 to 0.04 mg/kg intravenously [IV]) permits continuation of the examination. I avoid use of

this tranquilizer in stallions, although the possibility of paraphimosis is remote. Low doses of sedatives such as xylazine can be used (0.15 to 0.30 mg/kg IV) in stallions or other horses but can produce mild ataxia. Detomidine may be a better choice than xylazine because the drug lasts longer, thus allowing diagnostic analgesic procedures to be performed.[5]

I try to avoid using tranquilization and sedation, although some clinicians use them frequently and report that lameness in most horses may be more pronounced and easier to observe. Mild muscle relaxation may reduce the tendency of the horse to guard the lame leg. Mild analgesic effects of sedatives may mask mild pain, and in racehorses care must be taken to avoid use of drugs that may cause a positive result in a drug screen. In big moving, exuberant Warmblood horses, especially dressage horses (particularly stallions), sedation may be essential to accurately assess lameness.[5]

Leading the Horse during Lameness Examination

The horse must be led with a loose lead shank so that it can move the head and neck freely. It is impossible to see a head nod in a fractious or excited horse that is held tightly. Use of a chain lead shank over the nose facilitates control but is resented by some horses, and use of a bridle with a lunge line attached may be preferable.[5]

Horses should move at a consistent speed, not too fast and not too slow. A lazy horse may need encouragement with a whip. Constantly changing speed can make assessment of lameness difficult, but occasionally, assessing a horse during deceleration may reveal useful information about the existence of subtle lameness.[5] A horse may have to be trotted up and down many times. It is sometimes useful for the examiner to lead the horse to assess subtle forelimb lameness, because gait abnormalities may become more obvious.

Surface Characteristics and Lameness Examination

The horse should be examined on a smooth, flat surface. I prefer a hard surface, such as pavement or concrete that creates maximal concussion and may exacerbate subtle lameness. However, the clinical relevance of mild lameness seen on hard surfaces, especially on turns, should not be overinterpreted. Many horses that are actively competing successfully show mild lameness on hard surfaces; it is important to understand that the horse does not perform on a surface of pavement, and foot strike patterns and gait could be much improved if the horse performs on firm but forgiving surfaces. Crushed rock, cobblestone, deep sand, or undulating grassy areas and potentially dangerous slippery surfaces should be avoided.

It is important that the surface be nonslip because some horses appear to lack confidence while moving on hard surfaces and alter the gait. In these situations, horses may shorten the stride for protection rather than from lameness.[5] Horses with studs or caulks on the shoes may develop induced lameness unrelated to the baseline lameness when trotting on hard surfaces.[5]

Ideally the gait on hard and soft surfaces should be compared, to help differentiate soft tissue from bony problems. Horses with foot pain usually perform worse on a hard surface. Lameness from soft tissue injuries, such as suspensory desmitis or tendonitis, tends to be worse on soft

or deep ground. To evaluate lameness during transition from a hard to a soft surface and vice versa, a horse can be examined while circling on a lunge line in an area where both surfaces coexist side by side.[5] Care must be taken to prevent the horse from slipping during this examination.

DETERMINATION, GRADING, AND CHARACTERIZATION OF LAMENESS

Six basic steps are necessary to determine, grade, and characterize lameness. The clinician should determine the following:
1. Primary or baseline lameness or lamenesses
2. Possibility of involvement of more than one limb and presence of compensatory (coexistent) lameness
3. Classification of lameness as supporting, swinging, or mixed
4. Grading of lameness or lamenesses
5. Alteration of the cranial or caudal phase of the stride
6. Presence of abnormal limb flight

The *primary* or *baseline lameness* is the gait abnormality before flexion or manipulative tests are used. The practitioner attempts to abolish baseline lameness using analgesic techniques. Lameness in more than one limb may complicate determination of the worst affected limb. It is important to trot a horse even if it is quite lame at a walk, unless an incomplete or stress fracture is suspected. A horse may take a short step with a limb at walk, or can appear very lame, but trot reasonably soundly. Horses with scratches (palmar or plantar pastern dermatitis) or superficial wounds in the palmar or plantar pastern may appear quite lame at walk but trot relatively well. A STB pacer may walk extremely shortly both in front and behind but pace or trot without lameness. However, only the degree of lameness usually differs between a walk and trot. A horse may appear sound at walk and trot in hand, but lameness may be apparent trotting in a circle, in hand or on the lunge, or while being ridden. *This lameness now becomes the baseline lameness*, and it is under these conditions that the results of diagnostic analgesia should be evaluated. The clinician should try to recognize if the horse has bilateral forelimb or hindlimb lameness that manifests as shortness of stride or poor hindlimb impulsion, or if concurrent forelimb and hindlimb lameness are present. Moderate-to-severe hindlimb lameness can mimic ipsilateral forelimb lameness, although ipsilateral forelimb and hindlimb lameness also occurs. In these horses the veterinarian should perform diagnostic analgesia in the hindlimb first.

Compensatory Lameness

Compensatory (secondary or *complementary) lameness* results from overloading of the other limbs as a result of a primary lameness. It must be differentiated from the stride-to-stride compensation by a horse to avoid interference injury because of a gait deficit, or lameness, or to shift weight (load) during examination. A compensatory problem develops as the result of predictable compensation a horse may make *over time* for a primary lameness in a single limb. However, a horse may compensate for lameness in one limb by shortening the stride in another, a stride-to-stride change in gait that is not the result of lameness. For instance, in some trotters with severe LF lameness, reluctance to extend the LF may induce a compensatory shortening of the cranial phase of the stride in the LH limb, creating what appears to be a hike in the LH. If the veterinarian looks only at the hindlimbs, LH lameness may be diagnosed. A trotter performing at speed with LF lameness is likely to develop compensatory lameness in the RF or RH but not in the LH. However, the horse may appear to be hiking (lame) in the LH to avoid interfering with the LF. Elimination of obvious unilateral forelimb lameness usually resolves an ipsilateral pelvic hike. Most horses with pronounced forelimb lameness examined at a trot in hand will have a concomitant shortening of the cranial phase of the stride in the contralateral hindlimb, giving the false impression of coexistent lameness in this limb and vice versa. Experimental results appear to support this clinical impression. In 6 of 10 horses with stance phase forelimb lameness, compensatory movements of horses created a false lameness in the *contralateral* hindlimb (see following text).[8] Once forelimb lameness is abolished using diagnostic analgesia, the shortened cranial phase of the stride in the contralateral hindlimb will abate.

It is often difficult to know which lameness came first, but it is important to understand how horses compensate for lameness and which limbs are at risk to develop compensatory problems. Compensatory problems range from obvious lameness to only mild palpable abnormalities that may still compromise performance. Several predictable patterns of compensatory lameness are possible; the most common is bilateral forelimb or hindlimb lameness. Horses with a specific lameness in one forelimb are at risk to develop the same condition in the opposite forelimb. This tendency may not always be compensation for the primary lameness but may reflect simultaneous injury or degeneration of bone or soft tissue of both limbs. Abnormal loading of forelimbs or hindlimbs, faulty bilateral conformation, and the same shoeing or foot conditions all likely contribute to bilateral, simultaneous lameness. In horses with bilateral lameness, eliminating lameness in one limb usually results in pronounced contralateral limb lameness. Bilateral lameness may affect both limbs equally, resulting in a short, choppy gait. The horse may be lame in one limb while being circled in one direction and lame in the contralateral limb in the opposite direction.

Racehorses that gallop are most likely to develop compensatory lameness on the contralateral limb or the ipsilateral forelimb or hindlimb. A TB racehorse with a left metatarsophalangeal joint lameness is most likely to develop a similar problem in the RH but may also develop LF lameness. In a trotter the contralateral limb is most at risk, followed by the diagonal forelimb or hindlimb. If a trotter has a right carpal lameness, the left carpus should be examined carefully; compensatory lameness also may occur in the diagonal LH limb. In a pacer the ipsilateral forelimb or hindlimb should be considered after the contralateral limb. In a pacer with LH lameness the RH and LF are at risk.

The most common compensatory lameness is the same problem in the contralateral limb. However, suspensory desmitis is a common compensatory problem in both the contralateral and other limbs. In a TB racehorse or a jumper with LF lameness, RF suspensory desmitis is common. Primary RH lameness may result in suspensory desmitis in

the RF. It is logical that soft tissue structures are particularly vulnerable to the effects of overload. Superficial digital flexor tendonitis may develop secondary to a primary problem in the contralateral limb. In trotters a common pattern is primary carpal lameness and compensatory osteoarthritis of the medial femorotibial joint in the diagonal hindlimb, or vice versa.

Compensatory lameness also can develop in the same limb. In horses with front foot lameness the suspensory ligament (SL) often is sore, and some horses have suspensory desmitis. In horses with lameness abolished by palmar digital analgesia, most with navicular syndrome, scintigraphic examination revealed increased radiopharmaceutical uptake (IRU) in the proximal palmar aspect of the McIII in 30% of horses, indicating possible abnormal loading of the proximal aspect of the SL (Figure 7-1).[9] Complete resolution of lameness may not be achieved until high palmar analgesia is performed.

Horses with primary metatarsophalangeal joint lameness often have associated ipsilateral stifle pain, or vice versa.[10] Determination of the primary site of lameness may be difficult without use of diagnostic analgesia and observing that blocking one site abolishes the majority of lameness. This phenomenon may be most common in STBs, but I have recognized it in all types of sport horses and in TB racehorses.

Supporting, Swinging, and Mixed Lameness

Lameness has classically been divided into three categories in an attempt to characterize the motion associated with the lame leg and to assign a cause to the lameness condition. These categories are described and discussed, but I firmly believe that adequate characterization of most lameness conditions is impossible and may be unnecessary.

Supporting limb lameness describes a lameness that results in pain during the weight-bearing phase of the stride. Most lameness conditions are of this type. Supporting limb lameness also has been referred to as *stance phase lameness,* but this term is inappropriate because the swing phase of the stride is also altered.

Swinging limb lameness describes lameness that primarily affects the way the horse carries the lame limb. However, most horses with painful lameness conditions alter the swing phase of the stride in a typical and repeatable fashion, and it is difficult to make a clear separation between supporting and swinging limb lameness. *Swinging limb lameness* should be a term reserved for mechanical defects of gait, such as fibrotic myopathy, upward fixation of the patella, stringhalt, or other lameness conditions causing a mechanical restriction of gait. In these horses, lameness is manifested in the swing phase of the stride with no apparent pain. Unfortunately, the term *swinging limb lameness* often is used inappropriately to describe the gait deficit in horses with painful, supporting limb lameness. Lameness associated with osteochondrosis of the scapulohumeral joint is often described as a swinging limb lameness because of a markedly shortened cranial phase of the stride. Dramatic improvement in the shortened cranial phase of the stride can be achieved by diagnostic analgesia, eliminating pain associated with lameness. Thus the gait deficit is the direct result of pain, and no clear differentiation between supporting and swinging limb lameness can be made. Horses with painful forelimb lameness almost always

Video available at
www.rossanddyson.com

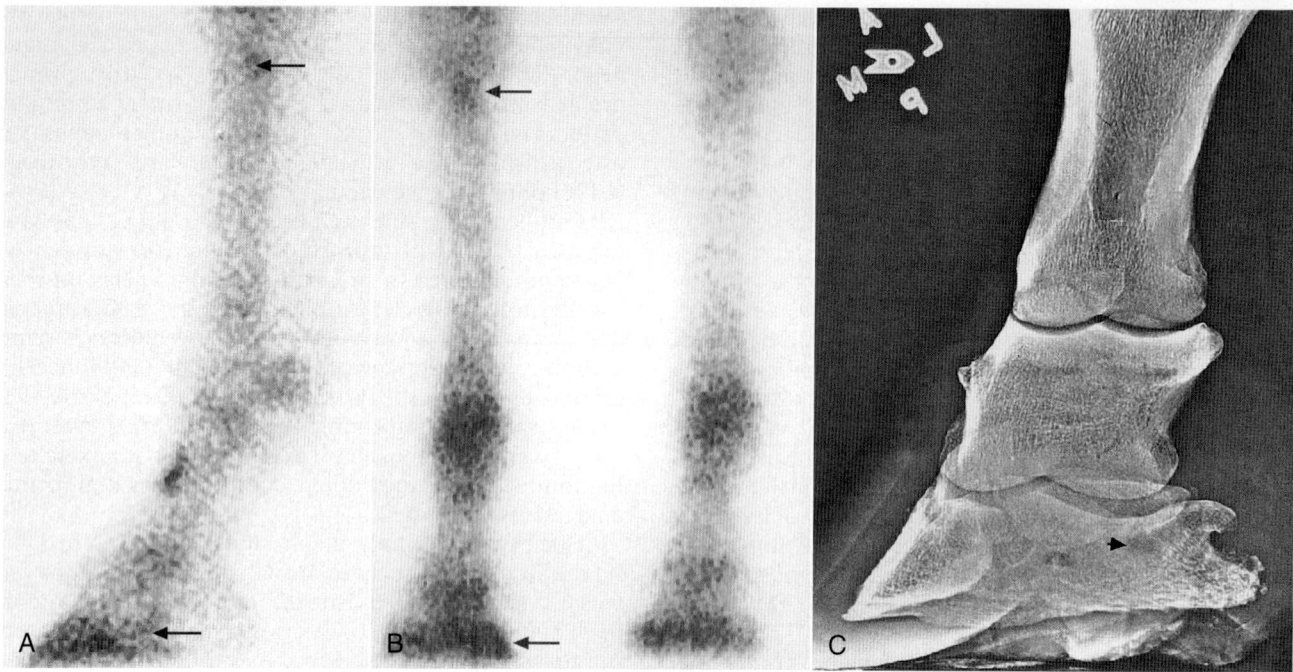

Fig. 7-1 • A, Lateral delayed-phase scintigraphic view showing focal, mild increased radiopharmaceutical uptake (IRU) of the navicular bone *(bottom arrow)* and proximal aspect of the third metacarpal bone (McIII; *top arrow*). Normal modeling is seen in the dorsal aspect of the proximal phalanx. **B,** Dorsal delayed-phase scintigraphic image, and **C,** dorsomedial-palmarolateral oblique xeroradiographic image of a dressage horse with lameness abolished by palmar digital analgesia. IRU of the medial aspect of the distal phalanx *(bottom arrow)* corresponds to the area of subchondral radiolucency seen in the xeroradiographic image (**C,** *arrowhead*). Note the focal area of mild IRU involving the proximal aspect of the McIII (*top arrow,* **A** and **B**). Abnormal loading of the suspensory ligament may occur as a compensatory problem in some horses with navicular syndrome or other sources of palmar foot pain.

shorten the cranial phase of the stride, although perhaps not to the extreme as in a horse with authentic scapulohumeral joint lameness. Horses with any painful hindlimb lameness consistently shorten the cranial phase of the stride, a reliable clinical indicator of which limb is affected, and when pain is abolished, the cranial phase (swing phase) of the stride improves (lengthens). Because the terminology is confusing and often erroneous, I prefer to avoid use of these terms and simply describe lameness as accurately as possible. For instance, describing a horse as grade 2 of 5 LF lame, with a marked shortening of the cranial phase of the stride reminiscent of other horses I have seen with shoulder region lameness, gives the most accurate and useful information.

There is an erroneous tendency to equate a swinging limb lameness with one that is more evident when the lame limb is on the outside of a circle. Upper limb lameness is often presumed yet not confirmed by diagnostic analgesia. It is logical that if a horse is reluctant to swing a limb forward, the lameness may be most prominent when the lame limb is on the outside of a circle. However, many horses with painful weight-bearing lameness show more pronounced lameness with the limb on the outside of a circle, a finding that neither suggests that lameness originates from the upper limb nor indicates the presence of swinging limb lameness (see following text). The outer limbs must stretch further and cover a larger circumference circle than the inside limbs. Slight temporal differences in the stance and swing phases of the inside and outside limbs are necessary to maintain gait symmetry.[5] Therefore the

stance phase of the stride may be relatively longer for the inside hindlimb, resulting in extension of the fetlock for a longer time and stress on the suspensory apparatus, whereas for the outside hindlimb covering a longer distance in the same time, there may be greater extension of the fetlock for a relatively short time, but still with stress on the suspensory apparatus. Thus pain associated with hindlimb proximal suspensory desmitis is worse in some horses with the lame or lamer limb on the inside of the circle, whereas with others lameness is accentuated with the lame limb on the outside of a circle.

The results of cinematographic analysis of gait in lame horses seem to support reservation of the term *swinging limb lameness* for horses with authentic mechanical gait deficits, rather than those induced by painful lameness. In a horse with a supraglenoid tubercle fracture examined at a trot in hand, a marked decrease in the cranial phase of the stride (protraction) was observed, along with a marked head and neck nod. A markedly shortened stride could be equated with swinging leg lameness, but high-speed cinematography showed that the cranial and stance phases of the stride were shorter than in the sound limb.[11] A horse with unilateral semitendinosus fibrotic myopathy had a shortened stride length and a shortened cranial phase of the stride, but the stance phase did not differ from that of the unaffected contralateral limb.[12]

In my experience, most lameness conditions can be considered *mixed lameness,* with changes in gait during weight bearing or the stance phase and during the swing phase of the stride. With the exception of mechanical defects in gait, I have not been able to categorize the clinical characteristics of most lameness conditions into swinging or supporting limb types. However, it has been suggested that swinging limb lameness is caused by muscle injury; supporting limb lameness is caused by bone, tendon, and ligament injury; and mixed lameness is caused by joint, tendon sheath, and periosteal injury.[13] A shortened cranial phase of the stride is a common characteristic in forelimb and hindlimb lameness and should not be considered pathognomonic for the location or type of lameness.

DETERMINING THE LOCATION OF LAMENESS

The horse should be observed at both the walk and the trot from the front, behind, and side. I spend most of my time watching the horse move away and then back toward me. Medial-to-lateral limb flight and foot strike can be evaluated only from this perspective, although cranial and caudal aspects of the stride and fetlock drop (see following discussion) can be evaluated only from the side. Most important, evaluation of lameness from this perspective allows the veterinarian to use the horse as a frame of reference. I find it quite useful to evaluate forelimb lameness when the horse is traveling away from me and hindlimb lameness when the horse is traveling toward me. This perspective allows use of the horse's top line to see a subtle head and neck nod or pelvic hike. Only by observing the horse from the side can the cranial and caudal phases of the stride be determined. When first learning to assess lameness from the side, a linear frame of reference, such as a fence or wall in the background, may be helpful to notice head nod and pelvic hike against an immovable background. Application of pieces of tape or other markers to the horse's head or a fixed point on the pelvis can assist recognition of upward and downward movement of that body part.

Independent observation of the forelimbs and hindlimbs is needed to understand whether a horse has forelimb or hindlimb lameness or a combination. These observations then are amalgamated to form a final clinical impression.

Recognition of Forelimb Lameness

Forelimb lameness often is easier to recognize than hindlimb lameness. *Understanding the concept of the head nod is vital to the correct interpretation of equine lameness.* The head and neck elevate or rise when the lame forelimb is bearing weight or hits the ground and nod down or fall when the sound forelimb hits the ground. "When the [forelimb] is the lame one, the movements of the foot and head occur somewhat in unison. When the lame foot is raised, the head is elevated, but only to fall when the sound leg is brought to a rest."[1] Some clinicians find it easier to appreciate the head nod down, whereas others find it easier to recognize elevation of the head.

When slow-motion videotape of lame horses is evaluated, it is immediately obvious that the elevation of the head and neck is much easier to see than the head nod down. In slow motion the horse appears to be elevating the head and neck just before the lame limb hits the ground, and then, during the later portion of the support or stance phase, the head and neck nod down. In fact, in slow motion it is head and neck elevation from a baseline level and later settling of the head and neck (nod downward) that are seen. The head returns or settles to baseline, giving the distinct impression that the horse is unloading the lame limb rather than loading the sound limb. The head and neck nod occurs as the contralateral limb begins the support or stance phase. Both head elevation and falling are present, but head elevation is much easier to detect when it occurs in unison with the lame limb hitting the ground. It is likely that a combination of visual clues allows the clinician to decide the primary forelimb lameness. Quantification of lameness and description of the actions of the lame and compensatory limbs have been attempted using gait analysis systems. In horses with amphotericin-induced carpal lameness, head movements were the most consistent indicator of lameness, followed by sinusoidal motion, or a rising and falling action, of the head and withers.[14] The motion of the lame limb was assessed, and a falling of the head and withers during the support phase of the lame limb was noted, contrary to clinical perception and evaluation of slow-motion videotape of lame horses. It was suggested that an uncoupling of the weight from the lame forelimb and a "free fall–like" phenomenon occurred during weight bearing.[14] The problem with this description is that it considers only the lame limb and is confusing. When evaluating a lame horse, the observer sees both forelimbs. During the later portion of the support phase of the lame limb, the sound limb is in the later portion of the swing phase and beginning the support or stance phase. Thus the head and withers drop described experimentally appears to occur concomitantly with the sound limb hitting the ground. The observer perceives the early portion of the stance or support phase.

In general, a good correlation between clinical evaluation of forelimb lameness and that described using motion analysis has been observed. There was complete agreement between clinical determination of location of forelimb lameness and that detected by motion analysis using a computerized three-dimensional motion measurement system. However, the degree of lameness differed in 6 of 29 horses.[15] In a more recent study subjective forelimb lameness grades were significantly associated with kinetic parameters, and vertical force peak and impulse had the lowest coefficients of variations and highest correlations with subjective lameness score.[16] In fact, kinetic parameters using GRFs measured by force plate analysis detected subclinical lameness not seen by a trained observer, a finding that may indicate that quantitative lameness analysis may be useful in horses with subtle lameness.[16] The maximal vertical acceleration of the head was the best indicator of forelimb lameness.[17] Although horses with forelimb lameness shifted weight in a caudal direction to the diagonal hindlimb, the amount of withers motion was minimal. The authors reasoned that the tremendous mobility of the head and neck, allowing the horse to asymmetrically elevate the neck and thus load the nonlame forelimb, accounted for the lack of withers movement and the horse's adaptation to forelimb lameness.[17] A similar compensatory ability is not present in the hindlimb. Vertical displacement of the tuber coxae and forward motion or translation of the pelvis occur in horses with hindlimb lameness, because a mechanism such as head and neck movement does not exist.[17] In a computer-generated model of a trotting horse the dynamic effects of head and neck movement accounted for the majority of load shift to the contralateral forelimb and diagonal hindlimb in horses with unilateral forelimb lameness.[18] Load shift and compensation by the diagonal hindlimb in horses with unilateral forelimb lameness lend support to the clinical findings of compensatory lameness in the diagonal limbs in trotters.

Instrumented shoes have been used experimentally to study motion in horses by quantifying GRF but have had limited clinical use.[19,20] Lack of correlation between an in-shoe system and force plate analysis was disappointing, and neither research nor clinical application of the system was recommended.[21] Although these systems are not currently widely available, in the future these or similar systems may be useful to objectively assess lameness and the response to diagnostic analgesic techniques in clinical patients. A remote monitored sensor-based accelerometer-gyroscopic (A-G) system showed good correlation in horses with either forelimb or hindlimb lameness when compared with a video-based motion analysis system used in horses moving on a treadmill.[22] Hindlimb lameness was consistently higher (in grade) using the A-G system, but the system yielded false-positive results in horses with concurrent forelimb lameness.[22] However, for a skilled observer, direct observation of the horse may be more accurate than kinetic or kinematic analysis of gait when a horse is lame in more than one limb.[5]

Recognition of Hindlimb Lameness

Historically descriptions of hindlimb lameness have been confusing. An important principle in the recognition of hindlimb lameness is the concept of the *pelvic hike* or asymmetrical movement of the pelvis. This has also been termed *hip hike,* but I prefer the term *pelvic hike* because it accurately describes how the pelvis moves in a horse with unilateral hindlimb lameness. The entire pelvis, not just the lame side of the pelvis, appears to undergo elevation. Because the horse has two "hips" and only one pelvis, the term *pelvic hike* seems preferable. Pelvic hike is the vertical elevation of the pelvis when the lame limb is weight bearing. In other words, the pelvis "hikes" upward when the lame limb hits the ground and moves downward when the sound limb hits the ground. The "haunch settles downward when the sound leg touches the ground...."[1] Some clinicians find it easier to see the downward movement of the pelvis, on the side of the lame limb, rather than the pelvic hike.[5] It may be simpler to determine which side has the most movement, rather than looking for either a hike or a drop.[5] The clinician must keep in mind that the pelvic hike is the clinical impression of *the change in height of the pelvis,* not the absolute or measured height. It is the shifting of weight or load that occurs as the horse tries to reduce weight bearing (unload) in the lame limb and transfer weight (load) to the sound limb. The ease with which this can be seen depends on the horse's tail carriage; in a horse with a tail set on high and that is also carried high, this may completely obscure movements of the pelvis.

Another explanation for asymmetrical movement of the pelvis involves one of the protective or compensatory mechanisms used by the horse to assist in breakover and minimize load on the lame limb. Many horses with hindlimb lameness drift away from the lame limb toward the sound limb. Drifting may decrease the magnitude of the observed pelvic hike, but more important, it makes the lame side look lower than the sound side. This is why it is important to watch the entire pelvis as a unit rather than the individual sides of the "hips."

In most horses with hindlimb lameness, particularly those without a substantial tendency to drift away from the lame limb, the elevation of the pelvis (pelvic hike up) when the lame limb hits the ground surpasses that when the sound limb is weight bearing. This elevation can be seen readily in slow-motion videotape analysis, but it may not be as obvious during clinical examination. Observing horses with hindlimb lameness from the front as the horse trots toward you may be useful. This approach allows the pelvic hike to be seen clearly using the horse's top line as a frame of reference. Subtle pelvic elevation is best seen from this perspective. The use of markers on a fixed part of the pelvis can help to identify asymmetry. Stride length characteristics, height of foot flight, sound, and fetlock drop are also helpful (see following text).

Horses with bilateral hindlimb lameness may have a short, choppy gait that lacks impulsion, but they may have no pelvic hike. Other methods to exacerbate the baseline lameness should be performed, such as circling the horse at a trot in hand or while on a lunge line. Lameness may be accentuated when the lame or lamer limb is on the inside or outside of the circle (see following discussion).

Hindlimb Lameness Confused with Forelimb Lameness

It is important to understand how a horse with unilateral hindlimb lameness modifies its gait so that *hindlimb lameness can mimic forelimb lameness at the trot.* When the lame hindlimb hits the ground, the horse shifts its weight cranially to transfer load away from the lame limb. This causes the head and neck to shift forward and nod down at the same time. The contralateral forelimb bears weight simultaneously with the lame hindlimb and the head nod coincides, thus mimicking lameness in the forelimb ipsilateral to the lame hindlimb. I find it difficult to distinguish clinical characteristics of a head and neck nod caused by forelimb lameness from that caused by ipsilateral hindlimb lameness. Some clinicians have suggested that the head and neck nod caused by ipsilateral hindlimb lameness is less vertical in nature and more forward and downward. Head and neck movement in horses with hindlimb lameness is not always observed. Horses generally must have prominent (>3 out of 5, see later grading discussion) hindlimb lameness before compensatory head and neck movement develops. However, two horses with very similar severity of hindlimb lameness may have different characteristics of movement, which will result in an associated head nod in one, but not in the other. At the pace, a lateral gait, LH lameness mimics RF lameness and RH lameness mimics LF lameness. Evaluation of the horse moving in circles may help to determine if a head nod is related to primary forelimb or hindlimb lameness. If a head nod is exacerbated but a hindlimb lameness is less obvious, then there is probably coexistent forelimb and hindlimb lameness. However if the head nod and hindlimb lameness remain similar or both appear worse, it is more likely that the head nod reflects a primary hindlimb lameness.

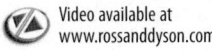
Horses can have a head and neck nod at the trot caused by singular forelimb lameness, singular ipsilateral hindlimb lameness, or concurrent forelimb and ipsilateral hindlimb lameness. A prominent head nod is seen in horses with simultaneous LF and LH lameness. The examiner first must determine whether both limbs are affected. Problems arise because occasionally a horse with only LF lameness may shorten the LH stride at the trot, leading the veterinarian to question whether LH lameness also exists. More commonly, however, horses with only lameness in a single forelimb shorten the cranial phase of the stride of the contralateral hindlimb. Horses with only LH lameness can have a rather pronounced head nod, and thus the veterinarian may question the existence of LF lameness. Although a horse with LF lameness may have a compensatory shortened stride of the LH, in the absence of lameness a marked pelvic hike should not be present. A head nod consistent with LF lameness may be inappropriately severe to be caused by mild LH lameness. If a horse has simultaneous LF and LH lameness, it is essential to perform diagnostic analgesia in the hindlimb first, because moderate-to-severe hindlimb lameness produces head and neck nod that is not abolished unless the hindlimb lameness is resolved. Resolution of the pelvic hike and reduction in the head nod should be expected with resolution of the hindlimb lameness.

Simultaneous lameness of a diagonal pair of limbs is less common than simultaneous ipsilateral lameness, except in trotters, because many horses perform at gaits that appear to induce compensatory lameness in the ipsilateral limbs. With simultaneous LH and RF lameness the head nod reflects the forelimb component, a mandatory clinical sign for perception of RF lameness. The horse may drift away from the LH with shortening of the cranial phase of the stride. The horse may have a short, choppy stride in the forelimbs and hindlimbs. The horse may have a rocking gait. It cannot shift weight or compensate from stride to stride in the usual manner and thus tends to rock back and forth from the hindlimbs to the forelimbs.

Reasonable agreement generally exists between clinical recognition of hindlimb lameness and that found experimentally. The use of markers placed on each tuber coxae of 13 horses with unilateral hindlimb lameness showed a consistent increase in vertical displacement of the pelvis during early weight bearing of the lame limb.[23] Although the rise and fall of the pelvis was readily apparent and occurred consistently with weight bearing of the lame and sound limbs, respectively, the absolute height of the pelvis on the lame side did not rise above that of the sound limb.[23] These findings are consistent with my clinical impressions. A head nod down when the diagonal forelimb was bearing weight further confirmed clinical observations that hindlimb lameness can mimic lameness of the ipsilateral forelimb.[23] In a kinematic study using a three-dimensional optoelectronic locomotion system, hip acceleration quotient increased in horses with hindlimb lameness.[24] Vertical displacement corresponded to the pelvic hike up on the lame limb, with a simultaneous forward movement of the head and neck during the stance phase of the lame limb.[24] Pelvic height differed significantly between sound and lame limbs in an experimental study using a custom-made heart-bar shoe to induce transient hindlimb lameness.[25] Pelvic height was reaffirmed as an important indicator of hindlimb lameness, but

exaggerated pelvic hike seen on the lame side was proposed to be caused by push-off from the sound limb and occurred immediately before weight bearing of the lame limb.[25] The importance of weight support and asymmetrical dorsoventral hindlimb movement (pelvic hike) was reaffirmed in a study using continuous three-dimensional kinematic monitoring of movement of the tubera coxae.[26] The hip (pelvic) hike seen on the lame side was found to be a rapid upward movement that led to an increased dorsoventral displacement.[26]

GRF has been measured in normal horses and those with forelimb and hindlimb lameness.[27-30] GRF is reduced in the lame forelimb or hindlimb with compensation by the other limbs. In horses with unilateral forelimb lameness, decreased horizontal GRF in the lame limb is compensated for by increased GRF in the contralateral forelimb and ipsilateral hindlimb.[31] Decreased vertical GRF in the lame limb is compensated for by increased vertical GRF in the contralateral forelimb during the swing phase of the lame limb, and increased vertical GRF in both the ipsilateral and contralateral hindlimbs during the stance phase of the lame limb.[31] During unilateral hindlimb lameness the decreased GRF in the lame limb is compensated for by increased GRF in the contralateral hindlimb and the contralateral and ipsilateral forelimbs.[31] These experimental data support the clinical impression that a lame horse adapts by shifting load to the contralateral limb or by shifting load in a caudal direction for forelimb lameness and in a cranial direction for hindlimb lameness. Kinetic gait analysis in horses with hindlimb lameness or spinal ataxia was recently studied using a force plate mounted in an examination aisle, a setup that may prove useful for clinical use during lameness examination.[32] Horses with hindlimb lameness had significant differences from normal and ataxic horses and their own contralateral hindlimbs in vertical peak force, vertical force impulse, and coefficient of variance of vertical force peaks.[32] Uniquely, investigators examined ataxic horses at the trot and found significant differences in lateral force peaks (lateral hindlimb movements) between normal horses and those affected with spinal ataxia.[32]

Bilaterally Symmetrical Forelimb or Hindlimb Lameness

Bilateral lameness is a common cause of poor performance and may go unrecognized without additional movement, such as circling, lunging, or riding. Horses with bilaterally symmetrical forelimb lameness may have a short, choppy gait when trotted in straight lines. Horses with hindlimb lameness may lack lift to the stride, have a subtle change of balance, or have reduced hindlimb impulsion.[5] If bilaterally symmetrical lameness is suspected, the veterinarian should select one limb and begin diagnostic analgesia. Horses often show pronounced lameness in the contralateral limb when the source of pain is eliminated.

THE LAMENESS SCORE: QUANTIFICATION OF LAMENESS SEVERITY

I believe it is important to have a standardized lameness scoring system that allows the clinician to quantify lameness within and between horses. Ideally it should be consistent worldwide, but currently a scale from 0 to 5 generally is used in North America, and a scale from 0 to 10 is often used in Europe. Definitions vary within the grading systems. The system adopted by the American Association of Equine Practitioners (AAEP) provides a framework.[33]

- Grade 1 lameness: difficult to observe and not consistently apparent regardless of circumstances (such as weight carrying, circling, inclines, hard surfaces)
- Grade 2 lameness: difficult to observe at a walk or trotting a straight line but is consistently apparent under certain circumstances (such as weight carrying, circling, inclines, hard surfaces)
- Grade 3 lameness: consistently observable at a trot under all circumstances
- Grade 4 lameness: obvious lameness with marked nodding, hitching, or shortened stride
- Grade 5 lameness: characterized by minimal weight bearing in motion or at rest and the inability to move

The AAEP system is potentially confusing because it grades lameness at both the walk and trot. It does not account for a horse that has a shortened stride at walk but trots soundly. In my experience, many lame horses show consistently observable lameness at a trot and therefore would have to be given a score of at least 3, leaving only grades 3 and 4 for use in the majority of lame horses. Horses with bilateral lameness and a shortened stride but no obvious head nod or pelvic hike are difficult to score based on this system.[5] It does not permit grading under different circumstances, such as straight lines, circles on the soft in each direction, and circles on the hard.[5]

An alternative lameness scoring system is listed in Box 7-1. Lameness is scored only with the horse at a trot, and the grading system is used most often to describe lameness at a trot in hand. The system is useful for both forelimb and hindlimb lameness and is based on a range of 0 (sound)

to 5 (non–weight bearing). In this system, a horse with unilateral hindlimb lameness of grade 3 or worse would have a head nod that mimics ipsilateral forelimb lameness. This system has limitations because as discussed previously a horse with a moderately severe hindlimb lameness may or may not have an associated head nod, depending on the gait characteristics caused by the source and degree of pain.[5] There is a practical difference between this scoring system and that put forth by the AAEP. A horse with lameness grade 1 in this modified scoring system would have a lameness grade of 2 to 3 in the AAEP system. The modified scoring system is more flexible and allows clear differentiation among most lameness conditions. However, it does not account for a bilaterally symmetrical gait abnormality and may be difficult to apply in a horse with lameness in more than one limb. Many horses evaluated for subtle lameness or poor performance have a score of 0 to 1 because consistent lameness is not observed. Use of half grades provides greater flexibility and supports adoption of a scoring system from 1 to 10, assuming 0 denotes soundness. A third system is to grade lameness independently at both the walk and trot and under different circumstances— straight lines, circles on the soft, circles on the hard, and ridden—using a relatively simple 9-point scale in which 0 is sound, 2 represents mild lameness, 4 represents moderate lameness, 6 represents severe lameness, and 8 represents non–weight-bearing lameness.[5] This system takes account of the fact that a horse may appear lamer at the walk than at the trot.

LAMENESS DETECTION
Fetlock Drop
Assessment of fetlock drop, or extension of the metacarpophalangeal and metatarsophalangeal joints, may be helpful in recognition of the lame limb. In general, *the fetlock joint of the sound limb drops farther when this limb is weight bearing than does the fetlock joint of the lame limb,* because the horse is attempting to spare the lame limb by increasing load in the sound limb. This may be easier to detect by video analysis than in a clinical situation and may be more recognizable at the walk than at a trot. However, in some horses with moderate or severe unilateral suspensory desmitis or tendonitis, the fetlock drops markedly on the lame limb when the horse is walking, but at a trot fetlock drop usually is more pronounced in the sound limb. With bilateral suspensory desmitis or severe tendonitis the fetlock may drop further in the lamer limb. In horses with chronic hindlimb suspensory desmitis excessive fetlock excursion on the affected side may falsely reduce pelvic excursion (hike) and make hindlimb lameness less obvious and more difficult to detect.

Use of Sound
Sound can be useful in lameness evaluation. *A lame horse usually lands harder on the sound limb, resulting in a louder noise.* For this sound to be appreciated, the horse must be trotted on a firm or hard surface such as pavement or concrete. However, the sound a horse makes while landing depends greatly on symmetry of the front or hind feet, and the loss of one shoe, different shoe types, or disparity in foot size confounds interpretation. Listening for regularity of rhythm and sound of footfall are important, especially

---

BOX 7-1

Lameness Scoring

Lameness grades from 0 to 5 are based on observation of the horse at a trot in hand, in a straight line, on a firm or hard surface.

0 Sound.

1 Mild lameness observed while the horse is trotted in a straight line. When the lame forelimb strikes, a subtle head nod is observed; when the lame hindlimb strikes, a subtle pelvic hike occurs. The head nod and pelvic hike may be inconsistent at times.

2 Obvious lameness is observed. The head nod and pelvic hike are seen consistently, and excursion is several centimeters.

3 Pronounced head nod and pelvic hike of several centimeters are noted. If the horse has unilateral singular hindlimb lameness, a head and neck nod is seen when the diagonal forelimb strikes the ground (mimicking ipsilateral forelimb lameness).

4 Severe lameness with extreme head nod and pelvic hike is present. The horse can still be trotted, however.

5 The horse does not bear weight on the limb. If trotted, the horse carries the limb. Horses that are non–weight bearing at the walk or while standing should not be trotted.

when evaluating the response of lame horses to diagnostic analgesia, particularly in horses with subtle lameness.[5]

Drifting

Horses with hindlimb lameness generally *drift away from the lame limb.* Drifting is one of the earliest adaptive responses of a horse with unilateral hindlimb lameness, allowing the horse to break over more easily or to reduce load bearing. Drifting may alleviate the need for extensive pelvic excursion (hike). It may make pelvic drop on the lame side more obvious. The horse may mask the lameness by reducing pelvic excursion. In some horses a pelvic hike is undetectable or subtle, but consistent drifting away from the lame side indicates the presence of hindlimb lameness. Many driven STBs with hindlimb lameness drift away from the lame limb or are "on the shaft." Horses with LH lameness have a tendency to be on the right shaft and vice versa. Drifting away from the lame limb may be most evident when horses have pain from the tarsus distally, although some clinicians have different experiences.[5] Drifting may result in the horse moving on three tracks.

Horses with severe forelimb lameness also tend to drift away from the lame limb, but this tendency usually is less obvious than in horses with hindlimb lameness. Drifting is most common with carpal lameness when the horse tends to abduct the limb during the swing phase of the stride and appears to push off with the limb, forcing the horse away from the lame side. Abduction seen in horses with carpal lameness should not be confused with swinging the limb or a swinging limb lameness. During protraction abduction seen in horses with carpal region pain appears to involve the horse carrying and placing the limb lateral to the expected site of limb placement. Racehorses with either forelimb or hindlimb lameness tend to drift away from the lame limb while training or racing at speed. This finding is an important piece of the lameness anamnesis.

Drifting toward the lame hindlimb is an unusual but important clinical sign. In horses that drift toward the lame limb, I suspect weakness and lameness exist simultaneously, suggesting a neurological component to the gait abnormality. However, a jumping horse at takeoff may push off more strongly with the nonlame hindlimb and drift across the fence toward the lame limb.[5]

EVALUATION OF LIMB FLIGHT

Observation and characterization of limb flight can be useful in determining the lame limb or limbs and possibly the location of pain within the limb. Abnormal limb flight also may predispose to lameness, especially in horses with faulty conformation. In my opinion, it is impossible to predict the site of pain causing lameness accurately based solely on limb flight and other characteristics, although some abnormalities lead to a high index of suspicion. I believe strongly that the location of pain should always be confirmed by using diagnostic analgesic techniques whenever possible. Some abnormalities are consistently associated with specific lameness conditions, whereas others are general patterns of limb flight seen with many different conditions.

Cranial and Caudal Phases of the Stride

Changes in limb flight in the cranial and caudal phases of the stride can be seen only when the horse is evaluated

from the side. In a normal horse the length of the stride of the paired forelimbs and hindlimbs, measured from hoof imprint to hoof imprint, is nearly identical from side to side. Extension and flexion of the limbs is also similar. From a clinical perspective the length of the stride of the affected limb cranial to the stance position of the contralateral limb is called the *cranial phase* of the stride, and the length of the stride caudal to the stance position of the contralateral limb is called the *caudal phase* of the stride. Obviously in a normal horse these individual parts of the stride are symmetrical. In a lame horse the overall stride length does not appear to change. If stride length changed, the horse could not trot in a straight line. Drifting is associated with lameness and could be explained by a change in stride length, but shorter stride length would be expected in the lame limb, causing the horse to drift toward the lame side, in contrast to the usual observation, drifting away from the lame limb. In racehorses, some of the tendency to drift away or toward the inside of the track could be easily explained by mild differences in stride length or strength (power). However, with the horse at a trot in hand we can assume that total stride length does not change.

In most lame horses the cranial phase of the stride of the affected limb is shortened. The caudal phase is lengthened to maintain a near equal overall stride length side to side. Shortening of the cranial phase of the stride appears to be a learned response of the horse to reduce the time spent during the stance phase and to help during breakover. Loss of propulsion, or an unwillingness to push off with the lame limb, could also explain reduction in the cranial phase of the stride. Because most lame horses have a shortened cranial phase of the stride, this finding, although quite useful in determining in which limb the horse is lame, is not particularly useful in localizing or classifying lameness and is not synonymous with swinging limb lameness. It is also important to recognize that pain causing lameness results in altered proprioceptive responses, to protect the painful area, and these responses may persist for some time after pain has resolved.[5] A classic example of attenuation of the cranial phase of the stride in the hindlimbs occurs mechanically in horses with fibrotic myopathy. This authentic swinging limb lameness causes a marked abrupt change in the later portion of the protraction phase of the affected hindlimb, shortening the cranial phase and causing a sudden downward and backward action of the limb.

The caudal phase of the stride is lengthened in most lame horses because for overall equal stride length to be maintained, this portion of the stride must compensate. I generally have not found evaluation of the caudal phase of the stride at the trot in hand clinically useful, but it is sometimes a useful observation in horses at a walk (see following text). Some horses with severe palmar foot pain have a shortened caudal phase of the stride at both walk and trot.[5]

Contrast of the cranial and caudal phases of the stride in the lame limb at a walk and a trot is useful. In most horses with forelimb lameness the cranial phase of the stride is slightly shortened at a walk but markedly shortened at a trot. Obviously, in horses with subtle lameness, this clinical sign is absent at the walk and only mildly apparent at the trot. Horses with pain in the dorsal aspect of the foot, such as hoof abscessation or laminitis, may have a shortened caudal phase of the stride at a walk. This response is an attempt to protect the painful area and to shorten during breakover. These horses walk with a marked camped-out appearance in the forelimbs. At the trot, however, the cranial phase of the stride is likely to be shortened, a clinical contrast useful in localizing lameness to the dorsal aspect of the hoof.

Most horses with hindlimb lameness have a reduction in the cranial phase of the stride at the walk and the trot. Horses with pelvic fractures involving the acetabulum prefer to keep the lame limb ahead of the contralateral limb at the walk and have marked shortening of the caudal phase of the stride, but at the trot the horse has a shortened cranial phase of the stride. Horses with hoof abscessation, most commonly of the dorsal aspect of the hoof, walk similarly, only to trot with a pronounced shortening of the cranial phase of the stride. An explanation for disparity at walk and trot in the phases of the stride in horses with pain at either end of the hindlimb is not readily apparent, but recognition of this phenomena has been quite useful, and consistent. Unilateral or bilateral laminitis and other severe causes of pain in the digit are rare in the hindlimbs and can cause similar clinical signs.

Shortening of the cranial phase of the stride does not always indicate that lameness is present in that limb. At speed a trotter with forelimb lameness shortens the cranial phase of the stride in the ipsilateral hindlimb to avoid interference with the lame limb. This observation sometimes is also made in horses being trotted in hand. This compensatory movement gives the impression that the horse may be lame in the ipsilateral hindlimb, with a subtle pelvic hike. Lameness of the foot and carpus in trotters most often causes this compensatory ipsilateral hindlimb pelvic hike. Once lameness has been abolished in the ipsilateral forelimb, the subtle pelvic hike and shortened cranial phase of the stride in the hindlimb abate. In trotters a shortened cranial phase of the stride and a pelvic hike may be related to faulty weight distribution and interference problems and not to lameness at all.

ABNORMALITIES OF LIMB FLIGHT

Abnormalities of limb flight can cause interference of one limb with another, particularly in trotters and pacers (Figure 7-2). However, horses performing at speed at any gait and those with faulty conformation also are at risk to develop interference injuries. In some horses, interference is of no consequence, but in others, especially trotters, it causes gait deficits. Skin lacerations, bruising, and underlying bone and soft tissue damage (interference injury) may occur. Various boots and other protective devices have been developed to protect the limbs from potential trauma. It is important to assess the presence and location of interference injuries. In some horses, only mild evidence of hitting is found, but other horses may have many painful areas. Chronic interference can be the sole reason for lameness or poor performance.

Front Foot Interference

Front Foot Hitting the Contralateral Forelimb

Horses with toed-out conformation tend to wing in during movement, predisposing to interference injuries.

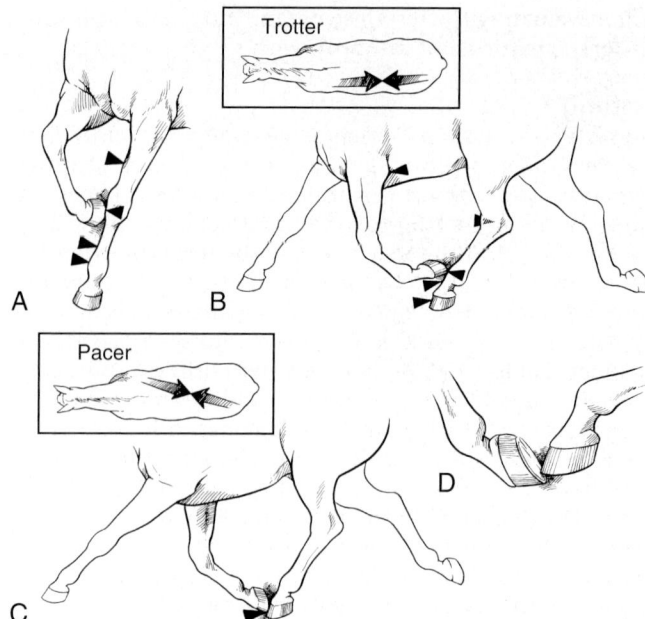

Fig. 7-2 • Types of interference. **A,** Horses at any gait can be injured by interference of a forelimb with the opposite side. **B,** Interference is common in the trotter and usually involves the ipsilateral forelimb and hindlimb. Interference within a forelimb can be seen in horses that hit the elbow of the same limb. This usually occurs because of high action, excessive weight of the shoes, or a combination of these factors. **C,** Interference in the pacer can involve the forelimb and diagonal hindlimb, commonly called crossfiring. **D,** Forging occurs during trotting when the toe of the hind foot strikes the bottom of the ipsilateral front foot.

Horses with base-narrow conformation or those with a combination of base-narrow and toed-out conformation also are at risk. However, many horses with these conformational abnormalities do not interfere. Some horses walk very closely but widen out at faster gaits. Interference injury from one hind foot hitting the medial side of the contralateral hindlimb occurs infrequently.

All types of horses, especially STB racehorses, are at risk for interference. Interference can involve any level of the limb from the foot to the proximal antebrachium. Mild interference of this type is called *brushing*. STBs often "hit their knees," which causes swelling, bruising, and lacerations of the skin on the distal medial aspect of the radius. In some horses, large, chronic swellings develop; these consist of mostly fibrous tissue. In others, osteitis of the distal radius or abscessation occurs. Even with protective gear, horses may be reluctant to perform at maximal speed to avoid injury or disruption of gait, or pain caused by interference induces the horse to go off stride.

Interference within the Same Limb

Horses can develop interference injuries within a limb when the hoof or shoe hits the ipsilateral elbow. This type of interference sometimes is seen in trotters with high action (excessive carpal flexion) and is common in gaited horses that perform with heavy shoes intended to cause high action of the forelimbs (see Figure 7-2, *B*).

Front Foot Hitting the Ipsilateral Hindlimb

Interference in trotters usually involves the toe of a forelimb interfering with (hitting) the dorsal aspect of the ipsilateral hindlimb (see Figure 7-2). Various names are given to the type of interference based on the location in which the injury occurs. Interference injury at the dorsal aspect of the hind foot or coronary band is called *scalping;* in the pastern region it is called *speedy cutting;* in the metatarsal region (shin) it is called *shin-hitting;* and in the dorsal or medial aspect of the tarsus, it is called *hock-hitting.* Because interference is common in trotters, it is important not to overinterpret signs of pain on palpation. Speedy cutting results in pain over the dorsal aspect of the proximal phalanx that should not be misinterpreted as pain associated with a midsagittal fracture.

Front Foot Hitting the Contralateral (the Diagonal) Hindlimb
Cross-firing, or the striking of the contralateral (diagonal) hindlimb by the front foot, usually occurs only in pacers (see Figure 7-2, *C*).

Hind Foot Interference
Interference as a result of a hind foot hitting the foot of the ipsilateral forelimb *(forging)* is common and usually does not result in injury. Many horses forge at a trot in hand or while being ridden. In horses with shoes the sound is unavoidable but may not be a sign of a pathological condition. Forging is most common in horses that are trotted in deep footing. Forging may reflect imbalance, lack of strength, incoordination, or poor foot trimming.[5]

Forelimb: Common Abnormalities of Limb Flight
Winging In and Winging Out
Common limb flights observed during lameness examination include winging in and winging out movement of the front feet and are often related to conformation (see Figure 4-13). Horses that are toed out tend to wing in, whereas those that are toed in tend to wing out. Such abnormalities do not necessarily compromise performance. However, such movement may result in uneven loading of the soft tissue structures and uneven hoof wear, leading to chronic imbalance. Horses that wing in tend to develop interference injuries and wear the medial aspect of the shoe excessively. Horses that wing out tend to develop lateral branch suspensory desmitis and wear the lateral aspect of the shoe excessively.

Lateral Placement of the Foot during Advancement (Abduction)
Horses normally advance the forelimbs straight ahead. When advancing the limb, horses with articular carpal pain, and some horses with pain in the proximal metacarpal region, place the foot lateral to the expected foot position. This action has been described as *abduction* of the limb, but this term may infer swinging the limb, and horses with carpal lameness seem to place the limb laterally rather than swinging the limb. However, ankylosis associated with severe osteoarthritis or arthrodesis of the carpus does necessitate swinging the limb during advancement, a much different movement from that seen in horses with more mild carpal region pain.

Horses with this abnormality of flight almost always have a shortened cranial phase of the stride. They tend to push off with the affected limb from the lateral location, resulting in a wide or peg leg type of motion at walk, and sometimes at trot. With bilateral carpal lameness the horse appears to move widely bilaterally. Not all horses with

carpal pain move widely, and this gait change is seen more often in horses with middle carpal or carpometacarpal joint pain than in those with pain in the antebrachiocarpal joint. Some horses with upper limb lameness may carry the limb widely while walking, although this characteristic is not typical of horses with shoulder pain. A horse with a humeral stress fracture sometimes may travel widely, similar to a horse with carpal lameness, but the latter is more likely. A horse with pain in the lateral aspect of a foot may move widely in the affected limb to reduce load laterally. This characteristic is seen in STB and TB racehorses with subchondral bone trauma or early stress fractures of the distal phalanx.

Plaiting
The verb *to plait* means to braid or pleat, or to make something by braiding.[3] The term is used to describe horses that walk or trot by placing one foot directly ahead of the other foot. Plaiting in the forelimbs is not nearly as common as in the hindlimbs and usually is the result of base-narrow, toed-out conformation. Old horses (usually broodmares) with severe carpus osteoarthritis and carpus varus limb deformities occasionally may swing the limb laterally and place the foot far enough medially to end up in front of, or lateral to, the opposite foot. Some horses with shoulder region lameness guard the limb and travel very closely in front. Plaiting in the forelimbs can be seen in horses with recent fractures of the thoracic dorsal spinous processes at the withers.[5] Horses with neurological disease occasionally plait.

Limb Flight in Horses with Shoulder Region Lameness
I include this section principally because the shoulder often is erroneously incriminated as the source of pain. Horses with moderate-to-severe lameness of the scapulohumeral joint or bicipital bursa have a marked shortening of the cranial phase of the stride. They also have an unusual motion of the shoulder joint that is difficult to describe. Because the cranial phase of the stride is shortened, during breakover the affected shoulder joint seems to drop or buckle forward, more so than the opposite side (assuming lameness is unilateral). There may be prominent lifting of the head and neck. Limb flight is either straight ahead or somewhat close to the opposite forelimb. Horses with shoulder region pain *do not consistently* travel widely, or abduct the affected limb. However, racehorses with humeral stress fractures may occasionally travel widely in front. With mild lameness there are no typical gait characteristics.

Hindlimb: Common Abnormalities of Limb Flight
Stabbing or "Stabby" Hindlimb Gait
A common abnormality of limb flight seen in horses with hindlimb lameness is described as a *stabbing* or "*stabby*" *gait.* During protraction of the lame hindlimb or hindlimbs, the limb travels medially, close to the opposite hindlimb, and then moves laterally during the later portion of the swing phase and is placed lateral to the expected foot placement. This motion results in excessive wear of the lateral or dorsolateral aspects of the shoe. Although this gait often is seen in horses with distal hock joint pain, it can be seen with many other sites of pain from the distal tibia to the

foot. Therefore diagnostic analgesia is required to localize the pain. However, horses with the most marked shoe wear consistent with this abnormality of limb flight are most likely to have tarsal lameness. Exaggerated stabbing hindlimb motion often is seen in horses with neurological disease.

Abduction of the Hindlimbs during Advancement

In some horses with hindlimb lameness the limb is carried forward in a position lateral to the expected position (i.e., abducted). In some horses with this limb flight the limb swings outside the expected line of limb flight, only to strike the ground near the expected position. Lateral swinging of the limb begins immediately after the lame limb leaves the ground. I have observed this abnormality most consistently in horses with stifle lameness, but it also occurs with some other upper limb lameness conditions. Care must be taken when evaluating horses that normally travel widely behind, such as trotters.

I have recognized lateral swinging of the hindlimb most commonly in pacers with articular lesions of the stifle, because the normal gait in these horses is to swing the hindlimb more than would be expected from other horses. Many horses with stifle lameness carry the limb forward lateral to the expected position, but just before impact may actually stab laterally. Therefore the veterinarian must pay close attention to limb flight directly after the lame limb leaves the ground and while it is passing the contralateral limb. Another common characteristic of horses with stifle lameness is a shortened cranial phase of the stride. The stifle joint also may appear unusually prominent and be carried somewhat away from the flank and slightly externally rotated.

Plaiting

Plaiting is more common in the hindlimb than in the forelimb and usually results from lameness rather than faulty conformation, although plaiting can occur in a horse with severe base-narrow conformation. Plaiting can be seen in horses with unilateral or bilateral lameness. In horses with unilateral lameness, it appears that limb flight actually may be altered in both hindlimbs, resulting in both hind feet being placed ahead, or in some horses, lateral to the opposite foot. In horses with severe hindlimb lameness, it appears that the affected foot is being swung around and placed directly in front or lateral to the unaffected foot. Alternatively, the horse may be trying to support most of its weight on the unaffected limb and moves this limb inside to support the lame side. In horses with bilateral lameness, it is equally difficult to determine what exactly is causing the plaiting. The horse may be reluctant to bring either hindlimb along the expected line of flight, leaving the limb medially and forcing the opposite limb to the outside to avoid interference. A horse may swing each hindlimb around the other, ultimately ending placing one foot ahead or lateral to the other. An unusual rocking type of gait is observed in horses with bilateral hindlimb lameness and plaiting. I have observed plaiting most commonly in horses with osteoarthritis of the coxofemoral joint or pelvic fractures, but I also have seen it in horses with bilateral distal hock joint pain or suspensory desmitis. Plaiting also is observed in some horses with sacroiliac joint pain.[5]

Mechanical Lameness of the Hindlimb and Limb Flight

Mechanical conditions of the hindlimb can cause profound abnormalities of limb flight (see Chapter 48). These are termed *lameness conditions* because of the gait abnormality exhibited, although in many horses pain is not characteristic.

Stringhalt

Stringhalt, an ill-defined neuromuscular disorder of the hindlimb, causes mild-to-severe hyperflexion of the tarsus. The condition can be unilateral or bilateral and usually is most obvious at a walk but can also be seen at the trot. In horses with severe stringhalt the dorsal aspect of the hoof comes close to or hits the ventral aspect of the abdomen. Horses may exhibit the clinical signs more prominently during backing or when initially moved after previous standing.

Fibrotic Myopathy

Fibrotic myopathy is characterized by a sudden downward and backward motion of the limb (slapping motion) that occurs during, and restricts the length of, the cranial phase of the stride. Hyperflexion of the hock is not a clinical feature of this gait deficit, but the restriction of the cranial phase of the stride and the slapping motion and sound can be confused with the clinical signs of stringhalt. It is most obvious at a walk.

Upward Fixation of the Patella

Upward fixation of the patella is a classic hindlimb gait deficit and one that displays the function of the stay or reciprocal apparatus. It can be intermittent or permanent and unilateral or bilateral. When the patella is locked in position over the medial trochlear ridge of the femur, the stifle and hock joints are held in extension, whereas the digit is held in partial flexion.

Shivers

Shivers is an ill-defined neuromuscular disease and is most common in Warmbloods and draft breeds; it can occur unilaterally or bilaterally. Clinical signs usually are most obvious when a horse is backed or first moves from the stall. Horses elevate and abduct the limb, and the limb may actually shiver or shake. The tail often is elevated. Signs may be accentuated if the horse is tense.

Other Hindlimb Gait Deficits

Other unusual unexplained gait deficits affecting one or both hindlimbs are observed occasionally, and they often have characteristics similar to those seen with stringhalt, fibrotic myopathy, upward fixation of the patella, and shivers. However, some distinction usually prevents easy recognition and diagnosis. A gait deficit characterized by marked hindlimb abduction seen most prominently at the walk has been recognized. This is most similar to fibrotic myopathy, because a consistent abduction of the limb is observed, and signs tend to abate when the horse is trotted. It may be related to scarring, abnormal function of the biceps femoris and gluteal muscles, or neurological disease.

Neurological disease can cause many different gait deficits, most commonly recognized in the hindlimbs but also in forelimbs. A complete neurological evaluation usually is not performed during lameness examination unless certain abnormalities are observed. Abnormal or excessive circumduction of the hindlimbs, a bouncy, stabby hindlimb gait noticed when the horse is trotted, knuckling over behind or crouching, stumbling, and lethargy are signs that should prompt further investigation.

EVALUATION OF FOOT PLACEMENT

It is important to critically evaluate foot placement. Ideally, both the front and hind feet should land flat and level on a firm surface. Foot strike patterns change on soft footing. Evaluation of foot strike is most important in horses with lameness localized to the foot, but it can also give clues regarding other causes of lameness. Abnormal foot placement can be the result of a current lameness problem but may also cause lameness.

In the forelimbs, horses commonly land on the lateral side of the foot first before rocking medially. This can be the result of abnormal conformation or hoof imbalance and can predispose to lameness in the digit and suspensory branch desmitis. Landing abnormalities in the dorsal-to-palmar direction are common but are difficult to recognize unless severe. Horses with profound pain in the toe caused by laminitis or hoof abscessation land heel first, giving a camped-out appearance, and have a shortened caudal phase of the stride. Horses with palmar foot pain may compensate by landing toe first, causing abnormal stress on the dorsal structures of the foot, but this characteristic is difficult to see except in slow motion.

In the hindlimbs, several patterns of abnormal landing or motion are recognized, not all of which are a cause or result of lameness. Landing on the toe is commonly considered the result of heel pain, but many horses with severe hindlimb lameness land on the toe. This tendency is particularly prominent when the horse is first moved, and most horses warm out of the lameness. Horses may land on the toe when walking up an incline or at the walk on the flat but generally place the heel on the ground when trotted. The most consistent lameness I see in horses that land on the toe is distal hock joint pain, but any cause of lameness from the tarsus to the foot can cause a horse to exhibit this abnormal landing pattern. Horses with lameness of the metatarsophalangeal joint region, including osteoarthritis, tenosynovitis of the digital flexor tendon sheath, or desmitis of the accessory ligament of the deep digital flexor tendon have a tendency to land on the toe. Horses with adhesions within the digital flexor tendon sheath may have severe mechanical restriction that causes toe-first landing. Old Western performance horses with deep digital flexor tendonitis have severe toe-first landing and may stand on the toe and even rise up in the heels during the examination. The condition can be bilateral or unilateral and is difficult to manage. Mild or moderate tendency to land on the toe also has been attributed to stifle lameness.[5]

Abnormal movement of the lower or entire hindlimb occasionally is noted when horses are watched from behind. Horses may place one or both hind feet in an axial position and collapse or break over the lateral aspect of the fetlock region.[5] Another uncommon hindlimb motion is characterized by excessive rotation of the hindlimb. The horse plants the hind foot and rotates the heel laterally, causing abnormal loading or twisting of the distal limb.[5]

Although this movement can lead to lameness, it sometimes is seen in horses that are successful in various sporting endeavors. I have seen this type of hindlimb motion most often in TB racehorses.

ADDITIONAL MOVEMENT DURING LAMENESS EXAMINATION

Further information about the character of lameness often can be obtained by observing the horse as it moves in circles and is ridden or driven. Some lameness conditions are apparent only under these circumstances.

Hard and Soft Surfaces
Comparison of movement on hard and soft surfaces is valuable. Foot lameness usually is worse when the horse is trotted on hard surfaces and better on a soft surface, such as grass or sand. Horses with suspensory desmitis or digital flexor tendonitis are more likely to show lameness on a soft surface. Deep sand may accentuate some lameness conditions, but an extended lameness examination under these conditions could cause proximal suspensory desmitis.[5] A slight downward incline or an uneven, rough surface may make subtle lameness more apparent.[5]

Circling
Lameness often is much more pronounced when a horse is circled. Horses should be circled in both directions: to the left (counterclockwise, LF and LH on the inside) and to the right (clockwise, RF and RH on the inside). Lameness may be more pronounced when circling at either the walk or the trot. In some horses with incomplete fractures, baseline lameness at a trot in straight lines in hand may be subtle or absent. Lameness may be readily apparent during circling, even at the walk. The additional forces of torsion and bending during circling are added to those of compression and tension. In horses with incomplete fractures, such as those involving the proximal or distal phalanges, torsion or bending forces during circling likely cause mild separation of the fracture fragments and exacerbate lameness. In horses with other lameness conditions, exacerbation of lameness may be caused by a change of load on the affected soft tissue structure or bone, redistribution of the forces of compression and tension in a medial-to-lateral direction, or additional forces of bending and torsion.

From a clinical perspective the force of compression may be dominant to other forces in determining a horse's response to circling, but it is not the only factor. Extension of the limb is also influential.[5] When the lesion is in the outside limb while the horse is circling and undergoing compression, exacerbation of the lameness occurs. For instance, lameness in horses with medially located lesions of the distal phalanx or of the third carpal bone is worse when the limb is on the outside of the circle and the lesion is being compressed. For some soft tissue injuries, tension forces may be more important. Lameness in horses with proximal suspensory desmitis often is worse with the limb on the outside of the circle, suggesting that tension is important in the expression of lameness. The same observation is not seen in horses with more distally located suspensory desmitis.

Is the lameness seen in a horse that is moving in a circle the same lameness that is seen while the horse is walking or

trotting in straight lines? In most instances, circling exacerbates the primary lameness seen in straight lines. If lameness is subtle or nonexistent when the horse is evaluated in
a straight line, the lameness seen during circling becomes
the baseline lameness. The clinician must recreate the same
conditions of circling when evaluating the results of diagnostic analgesic techniques. There is always the possibility
that lameness seen during circling may be different from
the baseline lameness seen in straight lines. For example,
a horse has grade 1 RF baseline lameness when it moves in
a straight line that increases to grade 3 when trotted in a
circle to the left, but still has grade 1 lameness when trotted
to the right. Lameness in a straight line and when trotting
to the right is absent after palmar digital analgesia but still
is rated grade 3 when the limb is on the outside of the circle.
This horse has two problems in the RF: palmar foot pain
and an additional carpal lameness that becomes evident
when the horse is trotted to the left (RF on the outside of
the circle). With bilateral forelimb or hindlimb lameness,
primary lameness often is seen in a single limb in straight
lines, but during circling the lameness is seen in whichever
limb is on the inside (or outside) of the circle. Circling is
useful in exacerbating the primary lameness problem and
identifying an additional cause of lameness not previously
noted. This additional lameness must be recognized and
treated separately from the baseline lameness.

Good correlation usually exists between the cause of
lameness seen on the straight and that seen while circling
the horse; thus it is helpful to circle the horse to try to
exacerbate lameness. Circling can be done at the walk and
trot in hand and while lunging or riding the horse. Horses
often move more freely and naturally when lunged than
when being led.[5] However, lunging is not possible in some
horses, particularly racehorses, and circling while being led
is better than no circling. The surface should be nonslip
because horses may be hesitant to move freely on slippery
surfaces and shorten or alter the stride even when lameness
is not present.[5] Soft footing is best when the horse is first
being lunged, because the horse can buck and play without
risk of injury. Hard or firm surfaces are best to exacerbate
many lameness conditions, but the surface must be nonslip
to avoid possible injury.

That lameness of the upper forelimb or hindlimb is
worse when the limb is on the outside of the circle is a
common misconception. This is true in some horses, but
a generalization cannot be made (see following text).
Shortening of the cranial phase of the stride may appear
more obvious with the limb on the outside of the circle,
but exacerbation of lameness judged by the degree of head
nod may not be observed. Another misconception is that
horses with lameness of the foot are lamest when the limb
is on the inside of the circle. Although a majority (65%) of
those with lameness localized to the foot are lamest when
the limb is on the inside of a circle, lameness can be worst
with the lame limb on the outside of a circle. This depends
in part on the location of pain within the foot.

Forelimb
Lameness Worsened with Limb on the Inside of the Circle
In many horses, lameness originating from the fetlock
region to the foot is worse with the affected limb on the
inside of the circle. Comparison of circling on hard and
soft surfaces is useful. Baseline lameness associated with

foot pain usually is dramatically increased when the horse
is circling on a hard surface, but a less obvious response is
seen when circling on softer surfaces. However, lameness
in horses with medially located lesions can be worse with
the limb on the outside of the circle.

Horses with lameness of the metacarpal region vary in
response to circling. Lameness related to metacarpal bony
injury and distally located lesions in the suspensory ligament or digital flexor tendons tends to be worse with the
limb on the inside of the circle, whereas lameness in those
with proximal suspensory desmitis is worse with the limb
on the outside. Horses with suspensory branch desmitis
may show a different response depending on lesion severity and whether the injured branch is undergoing tension
or compression.

In my experience, the degree of lameness in horses with
pain originating from the forearm, elbow joint, arm, and
shoulder joint region tends to be worse with the limb on
the inside of the circle, but opinions and experiences do
vary.[5] Observations may differ if horses are examined while
led in hand as opposed to being lunged or ridden. Lameness
in some horses with mechanical restriction of movement
that dramatically decreases the cranial phase of the stride
may be worse with the limb on the outside of the circle.

Lameness Worsened with Limb on the Outside of the Circle
Horses with medially located lesions of the lower limb,
especially foot lameness, proximal metacarpal lesions
(proximal suspensory desmitis or avulsion injury to the
McIII at the suspensory origin), or carpal pain often are
more lame with the limb on the outside of the circle.
Horses with lesions in the antebrachiocarpal joint are less
consistent in response to circling compared with those
with middle carpal joint lesions, because most of the
common injuries involve the medial aspect of the latter.
Upper limb lameness is accentuated in some horses.[5]

Lameness Improved When Circling
Lameness that appears better on a circle than in straight
lines is uncommon. Lameness in horses with medially
located lesions in the foot or carpus may improve when
the limb is on the inside of a circle. Baseline lameness in
horses with middle carpal disease involving the third and
radial carpal bones improves with the limb on the inside
of the circle. A STB racehorse with grade 2 or 3 RF baseline
lameness in a straight line that increases to grade 3 or 4
when circled to the left, but is only grade 1 or 2 when
circled to the right, may have lameness associated with the
middle carpal joint, but pain in the medial aspect of the
foot also is possible.

A horse with bilateral forelimb lameness (e.g., a horse
with grade 3 RF baseline lameness in straight lines) may
show grade 3 to 4 RF lameness when trotting to the right
but grade 1 LF lameness when trotting to the left. The
primary lameness is in the RF, and lameness is worse when
the limb is on the inside of the circle. Circling to the left
induced lameness in the LF, masking the RF lameness,
because bilateral lameness existed that was not recognized
when the horse was trotting in a straight line.

Hindlimb Lameness and Circling
In my experience, baseline lameness in most horses with
any hindlimb lameness is worse when the limb is on the

inside of the circle. Exceptions do exist, and some have different experiences and thus opinions.[5] Lameness associated with proximal suspensory desmitis often is worse with the affected limb on the outside of the circle, and the horse may stumble or take bad steps. Lameness in some horses with stifle lameness appears worse with the affected limb on the outside of a circle, but in others it appears similar to the left and the right. Many conditions of the stifle involve the medial femorotibial joint, a location that would be compressed with the limb on the outside. Lameness in any horse with a medially located lesion involving the distal hindlimb could be worse with the limb on the outside of the circle. Circling may be useful in exacerbating a primary lameness but generally is not helpful in localizing pain causing lameness.

Observation during Riding

Lameness may not be apparent when the horse is evaluated in hand in straight lines and circles but is obvious when the horse is ridden. This lameness becomes the baseline lameness for further investigation. The additional weight of a rider can exacerbate both forelimb and hindlimb lameness. Gait abnormalities and performance in horses with primary back pain or those with substantial muscle pain secondary to hindlimb lameness usually are worse when they are ridden. Hindlimb gait restriction can occur in horses with back pain but may be apparent only when a horse is ridden.[5] Problems related to an ill-fitting saddle or girth, behavioral problems, head shaking, abnormal posture or carriage of the head and neck, and refusal to take a lead or bend in certain directions may be evident only when a horse is ridden.

A horse may be easier to control when ridden than when in hand or on the lunge. Performance of specific maneuvers by the horse may accentuate lameness. A collected trot that forces more weight onto the hindlimbs may exacerbate hindlimb lameness. An extended trot may reveal the horse's inability to extend one limb compared with another and reveal lameness that was completely imperceptible under all other circumstances. The primary complaint, such as poor-quality flying changes of lead at canter, may require a riding assessment regardless of whether baseline lameness is evident under other circumstances.

However, it is important for the veterinarian to separate his or her observations from those perceived by the rider. Identification of the lame limb may be difficult for a rider, although he or she may have a very strong opinion. If the veterinarian's observations differ, the rider may be difficult to convince. It is also essential to recognize that bad riding can actually induce a false lameness that is completely unapparent if the horse is ridden well. Nonetheless, an experienced rider, trainer, or driver can be quite helpful in assessing the horse's response to diagnostic analgesia or therapy, particularly in horses with thoracolumbar pain, subtle hindlimb lameness manifested only when ridden, and poor performance related to a musculoskeletal problem. Working regularly with a skilled, experienced, and reliable rider can be very helpful.

Subtle differences in weight distribution of the rider may exacerbate or mask the presence of forelimb and especially hindlimb lameness. When the horse is performing the posting (rising) trot, lameness may be more or less prominent depending on which diagonal the rider is using. In the rising trot the rider sits on either the left or right diagonal. On the left diagonal the rider is sitting when the LF and RH are bearing weight and rising during the swing phase of these limbs. On the right diagonal the rider is sitting when the RF and LH are bearing weight. The correct diagonal is the outside diagonal (i.e., left diagonal on the right [clockwise] rein). Hindlimb lameness often is worse when the rider sits on the diagonal of the lame limb.[5] Therefore if the horse is lame in the RH, the lameness appears and feels worse when the rider sits on the left diagonal. Horses with hindlimb lameness may try to force or throw the rider to sit on the more comfortable (for both horse and rider) diagonal.[5] A horse with bilateral hindlimb lameness may appear lame in the RH when the rider sits on the left diagonal and lame in the LH when the rider sits on the right diagonal.[5] Forelimb lameness is influenced less by the diagonal on which the rider sits, but a similar pattern exists. RF lameness is worse with the rider sitting on the right diagonal.[5] This difference in lameness expression may be perceptible only by an experienced rider. Mild hindlimb lameness may become most obvious when a horse is ridden in small figure eights (two 10-m–diameter circles linked), especially when the horse changes direction from left to right or from right to left.

Observation of Inclines

Walking or trotting a horse uphill or downhill may exacerbate lameness or identify previously unapparent lameness. Lameness in horses with suspensory desmitis may be worse when they walk uphill or downhill. Lameness associated with palmar foot pain may be worse when the horse walks downhill, and the horse may show a tendency to stumble. Horses that tend to stumble or knuckle behind while walking downhill may have loose stifles (inability to maintain the position of the patella, usually caused by lack of muscle tone). Horses with neurological disease usually show more pronounced clinical signs when walking uphill or downhill.

A superficially flat, hard surface may actually slope; this can influence lameness because the horse's feet will be tilted with one side lower than the other. Thus the horse may appear different when trotting away from the observer than when returning.

EVALUATION OF LAMENESS WITH A TREADMILL OR GAIT ANALYSIS

The use of a treadmill for poor performance evaluation is well recognized, and its use in lameness assessment is discussed in detail in Chapter 98. The clinical relevance of lameness apparent only on a treadmill is open to debate. I do not find lameness examinations on a treadmill at high speed particularly useful unless slow-motion videotape is available. I prefer to assess the horse while training or performing. A horse may modify its normal gait on a treadmill. Good correlation was demonstrated between gait regularity in horses exercised on a track and a treadmill, but treadmill strides and steps were shorter, and the swing phase of the stride was reduced.[34] Horses require at least two training sessions on a treadmill before the gait becomes consistent.[35] Stride characteristics of horses galloping on a treadmill change as the slope of the treadmill increases from 0% to 8%; horses reduced the suspension phase to maintain overall stride length.[36]

Gait analysis is discussed in Chapter 22. To date in the clinical setting, assessment by an experienced, skilled observer has been more reliable in the identification of the lame limb or limbs than other, more sophisticated methods of gait analysis.

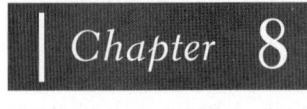

Manipulation

Mike W. Ross

Flexion or other manipulative tests often are used to induce or exacerbate lameness during lameness or prepurchase examinations.

INDUCED AND BASELINE LAMENESS

It is important to understand the concept of *induced lameness* and the possible difference between lameness seen at this stage and baseline lameness. During lameness examination, baseline lameness is established before any form of manipulation is performed. This may be difficult if more than one limb is involved, if lameness is subtle or subclinical, or if lameness is bilaterally symmetrical, which causes a gait abnormality without overt lameness. Lameness provocation is performed to exacerbate the baseline lameness or to provoke a hidden gait abnormality and attempt to localize the source of pain within a limb or limbs.

Provocative tests create induced lameness that may not have any clinical relevance to the baseline lameness observed during initial movement. These tests are not sensitive or specific and often result in false-positive and false-negative findings. Many horses with palmar foot pain respond positively to the "fetlock flexion test" (or lower limb flexion test, see following text) and could erroneously be thought to have lameness of the metacarpophalangeal joint. Similarly, a horse with proximal suspensory desmitis (PSD) may show exacerbation of lameness after distal limb flexion. A racehorse with baseline lameness as the result of a carpal chip fracture may have preexisting low-grade osteoarthritis of the metacarpophalangeal joint and respond positively to lower limb flexion but response to carpal flexion may be equivocal. Diagnostic analgesia is essential to localize the source or sources of pain. In the hindlimb, hock flexion, the so-called "spavin test," causes many false-positive reactions.

FLEXION TESTS

Flexion tests were first described early in the twentieth century, but information regarding the degree of flexion, force, or duration of the tests was lacking.[1] Variations in technique persist and produce variable responses that can be misleading. There appear to be more false-positive reactions to flexion than there are false negatives, but the

latter do occur. Flexion tests are useful during prepurchase examinations because the horses being examined usually are relatively sound, and the tests are useful at uncovering hidden sources of pain. Flexion tests may be useful in exacerbating lameness, particularly when the primary or baseline lameness is in the region being flexed, but sensitivity is doubtful. Horses judged to be clinically sound underwent a "normal" and then a "firm" lower limb flexion test (fetlock flexion).[2] Of the 50 horses tested, 20 had a positive response to normal flexion, and 10 of these horses were judged to be lame while trotting for about 15 m (50 feet) or more. Forty-nine of 50 horses had a positive response to firm flexion, and 35 of these remained lame for a minimum of 15 m. In this study the force applied was not calibrated, 7 of the 50 horses developed lameness within 60 days of completion of the study, and 24 horses had radiological abnormalities that could have contributed to a positive response to flexion.[2] Although there may be an explanation for a positive response in some horses, the high percentage of positive results in the study is in agreement with my clinical impression. In a study using the Flextest (Krypton Electronic Engineering NV, Leuven, Belgium), an apparatus designed to control traction force and time during a lower limb flexion test, the optimal force and time for flexion were 100 N and 1 minute, respectively. There was a positive response to flexion in many horses that were considered sound, and a positive response in sound horses was more likely in those in active work than in horses that had been rested or turned out on pasture. Horses were more likely to manifest a positive response to flexion as the force used in the test was increased.[3] A false-positive response to flexion can be observed in clinically normal horses and in those with unimportant low-grade problems. Lameness induced by flexion in these horses may have little clinical relevance.

However, other evidence suggests that a positive response to lower limb flexion in sound horses may be useful to predict future lameness. In a retrospective study, 151 initially sound horses were followed for 6 months. Twenty-one percent of horses with a positive forelimb flexion test result developed lameness in the area being flexed, whereas only 5% of horses with a negative flexion test result subsequently developed lameness. In young Swedish Warmbloods there was a positive correlation between a positive response to flexion and a subsequent insurance claim related to lameness.[4]

In a more recent study the predictive value of the lower limb flexion test was debated.[5] Sixty percent of sound horses responded positively to the flexion test. There was no influence of body weight, height, or range of motion, but outcome of the flexion test increased significantly with age and in mares. Over a 6-month period the number of horses responding positively decreased significantly, a finding that casts doubt on the possible predictive value of the test.[5]

Flexion tests lack specificity because it is nearly impossible to flex a single joint without flexing other joints or nearby tissues, particularly in any hindlimb or distal forelimb flexion tests. Elevation of a limb without flexion in severely lame horses may exacerbate the baseline lameness, because horses guard the limb or need to warm out of the lameness for a number of steps while trotting, thus complicating interpretation. Hindlimb flexion tests are less specific than forelimb tests because the reciprocal apparatus prevents flexion of any joint without concomitant flexion of other joints. Hindlimb flexion tests are useful in exacerbating baseline lameness, but positive responses to individual lower limb and upper limb tests, in my opinion, only localize pain causing lameness to the entire hindlimb. I believe that flexion tests are useful in exacerbating lameness, and in some horses it is the baseline or relevant lameness that is being worsened. In general, unless the horse's response is clearly pronounced and different from that of other manipulation, lameness cannot be localized based on response to flexion alone. Diagnostic analgesia should always be used, when possible, to localize pain.

Order, Duration, Force, and Venue during Flexion Tests

Consistency in technique is essential. Although force exerted by individuals varies, the flexion technique of experienced practitioners is sufficient to objectively assess response to flexion.[6] Response to flexion can and should be compared with response in the contralateral limb. Ideally the flexion test should be performed in the contralateral sound limb first before being performed in the suspect limb, to determine the horse's response. Accurate assessment of response to flexion in the contralateral nonlame limb may not be possible if the horse is severely lame after flexion of the lame limb and lameness persists. In some instances, baseline lameness is actually increased by forcing the horse to stand for the contralateral flexion test, a useful observation seen most commonly in horses with forelimb lameness (see following text). Horses with nearly bilaterally symmetrical lameness may have a similar positive test result in the less-lame contralateral limb.

Duration of flexion is somewhat controversial and may be an individual choice. In a study evaluating lower limb flexion, duration of 1 minute was considered ideal, because normal horses that underwent flexion at 100 N for 1 minute had few false-positive responses.[3] Maintaining firm flexion for 1 minute while performing all flexion tests and repeating the tests in the contralateral limbs can make this portion of the lameness examination time-consuming. On the other hand, if the clinician takes the time to perform these tests, optimum chances of success are improved. A false-positive result is more useful than a false-negative test result. Some clinicians prefer to perform flexion tests with more force but for a shorter duration. This technique works well for lower limb flexion tests. Seldom is it possible to maintain some upper limb manipulative procedures for 1 minute. Thus some latitude is necessary. I believe that duration of flexion of 45 seconds to 1 minute is enough to elicit an accurate response in most horses.

Force used during flexion varies considerably, but excessive force induces lameness in most normal horses.

Forces in the range of 100 to 150 N represent a moderate degree of force for lower limb flexion tests. In studies using a dynamometer, the maximum amount of force that could be used without a consistent withdrawal response in normal horses was 150 N.[7] The amount of force also depends on the size of the horse or the joint being flexed. The amount of force used in adult horses cannot be used in foals. Horses with obvious osteoarthritis or articular fracture, or those with substantial soft tissue injury likely to be affected by the flexion test, do not tolerate the same force as horses with more mild conditions. In a study of healthy and injured Thoroughbred (TB) racehorses, a positive correlation existed between decreased range of motion and joint injury.[8] Loss of joint motion was most likely caused by joint capsule fibrosis, but pain associated with increased intraarticular pressure from effusion or flexion also may have limited joint motion.[8] I recommend flexing a joint as much as possible with an amount of force just slightly less than the force that consistently causes a withdrawal response. Consistency should be applied between horses, paying attention to how the horse reacts; obvious resistance to sustained passive flexion may be clinically significant.

Proper evaluation of the results of flexion tests requires that the horse be observed while trotting in a straight line on a firm, nonslip surface. Evaluation during trotting is important to differentiate those horses resistant to static flexion from those with an authentic positive flexion test result. Horses usually are trotted in hand, although occasionally a horse's response to flexion is evaluated while it is being ridden. The horse should be trotted immediately after the limb is placed to the ground, with care taken to avoid scaring the horse or providing any excessive encouragement to trot, because many horses will slip initially, gallop off, or balk, all of which necessitate test repetition. If possible, the horse should be trotted away from the examiner for a minimum of 12 to 15 m.

Causes of Pain during Flexion and Positive Flexion Test Results

Forced flexion of a joint can induce pain in many potential sites. Force is being applied to both articular structures and surrounding soft tissues. The tissues on the flexion side of the joint are being compressed, whereas tissues on the extension side are under tension. During flexion, intraarticular pressure and intraosseous pressure in subchondral bone are increased.[3,8] Stretching or compression of the joint capsule, vascular constriction, and activation of pain receptors in the joints and surrounding soft tissues also can occur during flexion.[3] It is rarely possible to attribute pain on static flexion or during movement after flexion to an individual articular surface. The "fetlock flexion test" is a misnomer because as it is commonly performed it includes the interphalangeal joints and stresses surrounding soft tissue. Thus the names *lower limb flexion test* or *fetlock region flexion test* are more appropriate.

Positive Responses to Flexion

Positive responses to flexion can be seen with static flexion (see Chapter 6) and when movement follows flexion. A positive flexion test result is defined as obvious lameness or an increase over baseline lameness that is observed for more than three to five strides while the horse trots in a straight line after flexion. A mild response, even in sound horses, often is seen in the first few strides, a finding that should be compared with the contralateral limb. Sound horses warm out of this mild response quickly. Of 100 sound horses 50% had a slight response, 35% had mild lameness and 15% had distinct lameness after a lower limb flexion test.[5] A persistent, one- to two-grade increase over baseline lameness for several steps is a positive response. In horses with hindlimb lameness a marked positive response often is accompanied by reluctance to place the heel on the ground, and the horse may land only on the toe for several strides.

Forelimb Flexion Tests

Lower Limb Flexion Test

The lower limb flexion test often has been equated erroneously with the fetlock flexion test. The fetlock region can be flexed independently of interphalangeal joints (see following text). The lower limb flexion test is the most common test performed in the forelimb and involves placing a hand on the toe and forcing the fetlock and both interphalangeal joints into firm flexion (Figure 8-1). A positive response to flexion can be observed with any condition of the distal interphalangeal, proximal interphalangeal, and metacarpophalangeal joints or the navicular bone or bursa; other causes of palmar foot pain; digital flexor tenosynovitis; any soft tissue problem in the palmar pastern region; and lameness associated with the branches or proximal aspect of the suspensory ligament (SL) or proximal sesamoid bones (PSBs). Horses with lesions of the PSBs usually have markedly positive responses to this test. *This test is not specific for lameness of the metacarpophalangeal joint.* I have seen marked responses in horses with navicular disease or osteoarthritis of the interphalangeal joints. However, horses with osteoarthritis, fractures of the metacarpophalangeal joint, or tenosynovitis usually also show

a marked positive response. In a recent study of clinically sound horses in which lameness could consistently be induced by flexion with 250 N for 1 minute, lameness was alleviated by intraarticular analgesia of the metacarpophalangeal joint, but not by intraarticular analgesia of the proximal interphalangeal or distal interphalangeal joints or intrathecal analgesia of the navicular bursa.[9] Exacerbation of lameness associated with pain arising from the SL after lower limb flexion is probably caused by relaxation of the SL during flexion and then sudden loading of the ligament when the horse starts to load the limb.

The limb should be held as close to the ground as possible, and forced carpal flexion should be avoided (see Figure 8-1). All soft tissue and bony structures in the palmar aspect of the distal limb are severely compressed, resulting in low specificity for the metacarpophalangeal joint. Some people use a hand as a fulcrum or grab the toe with both hands (Figure 8-2), but this technique may result in application of excessive force, although it otherwise produces similar results.

Fetlock Flexion Test

The specificity of the lower limb flexion test can be improved by applying force to the metacarpophalangeal joint and avoiding forced flexion of the interphalangeal joints. The fetlock flexion test is performed by placing one hand along the dorsal aspect of the pastern region and one hand along the dorsal aspect of the metacarpal region, while avoiding flexion of the carpus (Figure 8-3). When compared with lower limb flexion this test is more difficult to perform because it requires more force and the clinician's effort to maintain a similar degree of flexion. The test is not specific

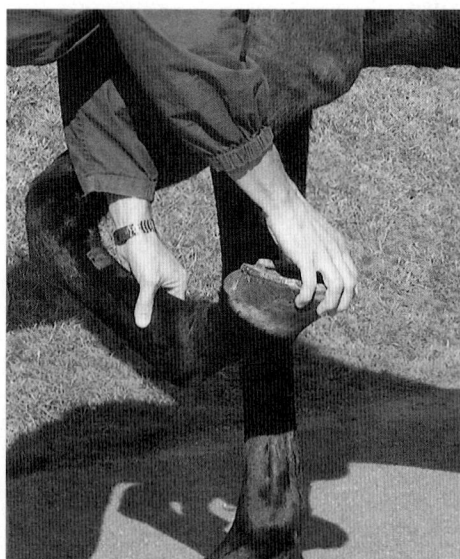

Fig. 8-1 • The lower limb flexion test is often erroneously called the *fetlock flexion test.* During the lower limb flexion test the fetlock, proximal interphalangeal, and distal interphalangeal joints are flexed; the palmar pastern and fetlock region soft tissue structures are compressed; and the dorsal structures are stretched.

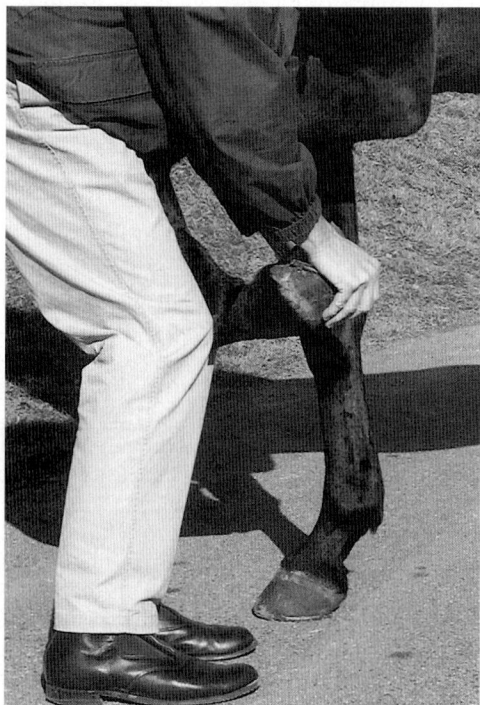

Fig. 8-2 • Extreme lower limb flexion can be achieved by using both hands on the toe with the limb cradled between the clinician's legs. With such extreme flexion even normal horses may manifest a positive response.

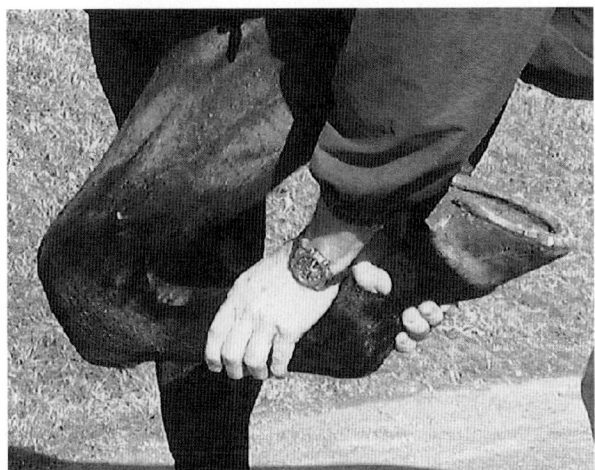

Fig. 8-3 • A true fetlock flexion test can be performed by carefully flexing only the fetlock joint. The clinician's hand grasps only the pastern and not the toe of the hoof while avoiding forced flexion of the proximal and distal interphalangeal joints (see Figure 8-1).

for articular lameness of the metacarpophalangeal joint, and horses with soft tissue problems respond positively.

Flexion of Interphalangeal Joints

In my opinion, flexion of either the proximal interphalangeal or distal interphalangeal joint without concomitant flexion of the other, or of the metacarpophalangeal joint, is impossible. Varus or valgus stress can be applied to the interphalangeal joints, and when followed by trotting, this stress can be a suitable provocative test in horses with osteoarthritis or soft tissue injuries of these joints.

Carpal Flexion Test

The carpal flexion test is the most specific of all forelimb flexion tests, and a positive response usually reflects baseline lameness associated with the carpal region. Few false-positive results occur. A positive response may reflect intraarticular pain, but a positive response also is seen in horses with carpal tenosynovitis, accessory carpal bone fractures, proximally located superficial digital flexor (SDF) and deep digital flexor (DDF) tendonitis, PSD, or avulsion fracture of the third metacarpal bone (McIII) at the SL origin. Rarely, a horse with a problem in the scapulohumeral and cubital joints or the antebrachium responds positively. A negative response does not preclude an articular lesion of the carpus, including incomplete fractures or sclerosis of the carpal bones.

The limb is elevated, and the carpus is forced into full flexion by pushing the metacarpal region directly underneath the radius (Figure 8-4). The distal limb can be pulled laterally to place the carpal joints in valgus stress or torsion.

Horses sometimes trot off lame on the contralateral limb after the carpal flexion test is performed. I have seen this most commonly in young Standardbred or TB racehorses with subchondral bone pain in the middle carpal joint and call it the "Ross crossed-extensor phenomenon." I believe that this reflects bilateral lameness, and flexion of the ipsilateral carpus causes less pain than making the horse stand for 1 minute on the contralateral limb. I have observed this response most commonly in horses with bilateral carpal lameness, but exacerbation of contralateral

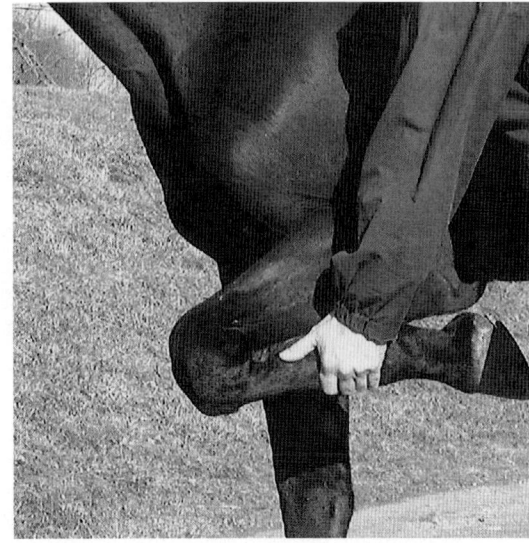

Fig. 8-4 • The carpal flexion test is the most specific of all flexion tests, but it applies concomitant mild flexion of the elbow and shoulder joints. Although false-negative results are possible, a positive carpal flexion test result usually means that lameness originates from the carpal region.

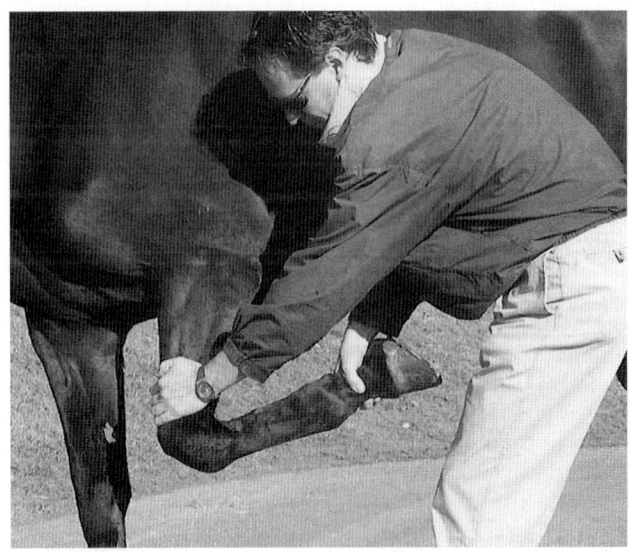

Fig. 8-5 • Upper forelimb flexion is performed by grasping the antebrachium and pulling the entire limb caudally and slightly proximally. This maneuver flexes the shoulder joint and extends the elbow joint. Horses with shoulder region lameness often respond positively to this manipulative test.

lameness is not restricted to carpal lesions. Dyson[10] has called this a "paradoxical response to flexion" and has observed exacerbation of contralateral lameness in horses with navicular syndrome, DDF tendon lesions in the digit, and distal hock joint pain.

Upper Limb Manipulation

Because of the inverse but simultaneous movement of the elbow and shoulder joints, it is difficult to accurately name the flexion tests of these joints. For instance, when the limb is pulled in a caudal direction, the shoulder joint is flexed but the elbow joint is extended. I call this manipulation *upper limb flexion* (Figure 8-5). This maneuver requires both

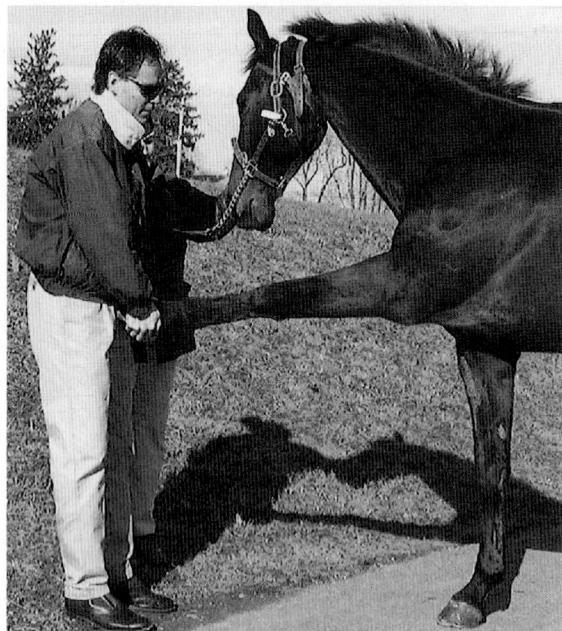

Fig. 8-6 • The upper limb extension test is performed by pulling the fore-limb out in front of the horse and forcing it proximally. This places the elbow joint in flexion and the shoulder joint in extension. In my experience, lameness of the elbow region is exacerbated by this technique, but occasionally shoulder joint lameness also is worsened.

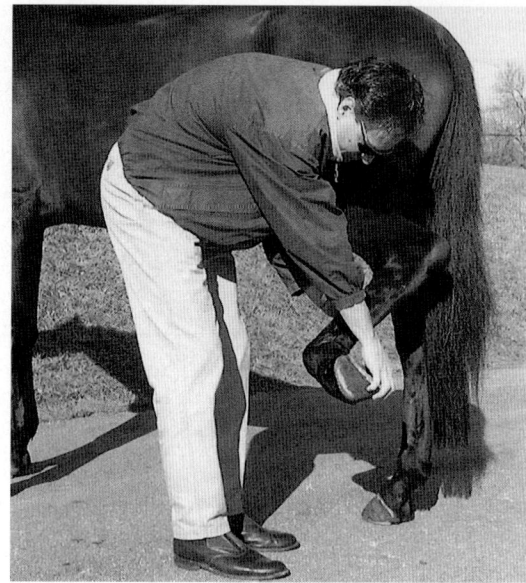

Fig. 8-7 • The lower limb flexion test in the hindlimb is performed with the limb as close to the ground as possible. Flexion of one portion of the hindlimb is impossible without flexing the entire limb, a finding that explains many false-positive hindlimb flexion test results.

hands, one hand grasping the pastern region and one grasping the cranial aspect of the antebrachium to force the entire limb in a caudal direction. When the limb is pulled in a cranial direction, resulting in *upper limb extension,* the shoulder joint is extended, but the elbow joint is flexed (Figure 8-6). Both hands are placed around the pastern region while forcing the entire forelimb into maximal extension. Maintenance of upper limb extension or flexion for even 45 seconds is difficult, so I try to maintain this position for as long as possible and then evaluate the horse while trotting. Many normal horses resist upper limb manipulation, and an alternative is to force the limb into hard flexion or extension in a rhythmical fashion six to eight times and then trot the horse. Even though the entire limb is being manipulated, there are few false-positive test results. A horse with a positive response to carpal flexion may have a similar response to upper limb manipulation because it is difficult to perform upper limb flexion without simultaneously flexing the carpus. False-negative test results can occur, probably because of the inability to place either the shoulder or the elbow joints in hard flexion. In my experience, horses with lameness originating from the elbow region are more likely to respond to upper limb extension, whereas those with lameness originating from the shoulder region are more likely to respond to upper limb flexion.

Hindlimb Flexion Tests

Hindlimb flexion tests are not specific, but they may be useful to exacerbate the baseline lameness or detect hidden sources of potential lameness. I do not believe that hindlimb flexion tests are useful in differentiating the source of pain causing lameness in most horses unless the response is dramatic, and diagnostic analgesia usually is required in all horses.

Lower Limb Flexion Test

The lower limb flexion test is performed similarly to the forelimb flexion test, but with similar force the metatarsophalangeal joint can be flexed more extremely. The veterinarian should try to keep the limb as low as possible to avoid placing hard flexion on the upper limb, although all joints are flexed to a degree. The lower limb flexion test also affects the proximal interphalangeal and distal interphalangeal joints and the surrounding soft tissues (Figure 8-7). Horses with digital flexor tenosynovitis or DDF tendonitis show a marked response to the lower limb flexion test. False-positive results can occur, but these are less common in a hindlimb than in a forelimb, even in horses in active work. Horses with pain in the upper limb may show a mild or moderate response to lower limb flexion. This test is not specific for pain located in the lower limb, and lameness in horses with stifle pain often is worse after the lower limb flexion test.[10] Horses with subchondral bone pain from maladaptive or nonadaptive bone remodeling of the distal aspect of the third metatarsal bone (MtIII) or those with incomplete fractures of the MtIII or incomplete midsagittal fractures of the proximal phalanx may show little response to this test (false-negative result). Coupled with lack of effusion of the metatarsophalangeal joint, a false-negative response to lower limb flexion may sidetrack the clinician into thinking pain originates elsewhere. Diagnostic analgesia is required to determine the source of pain.

Fetlock Flexion and Interphalangeal Joint Tests

The metatarsophalangeal joint region can be flexed independently of the interphalangeal joints in the hindlimb, or the interphalangeal joints can be flexed independently, but these tests are difficult to perform and of limited value.

Upper Limb Flexion Test

The so-called "spavin test" or "hock flexion test," misnomers for the upper limb flexion test, *is not specific for*

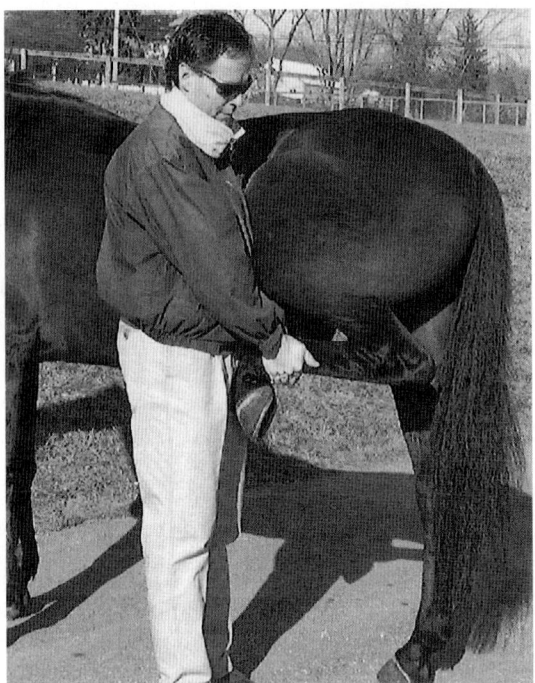

Fig. 8-8 • The hindlimb upper limb flexion test is demonstrated. This test has been called the *spavin test* or *hock flexion test,* but it is not specific for lameness of the hock. The hock and stifle joints are in forced flexion, the lower limb joints are flexed, the metatarsal region is compressed, and a small amount of forced flexion of the coxofemoral joint is induced.

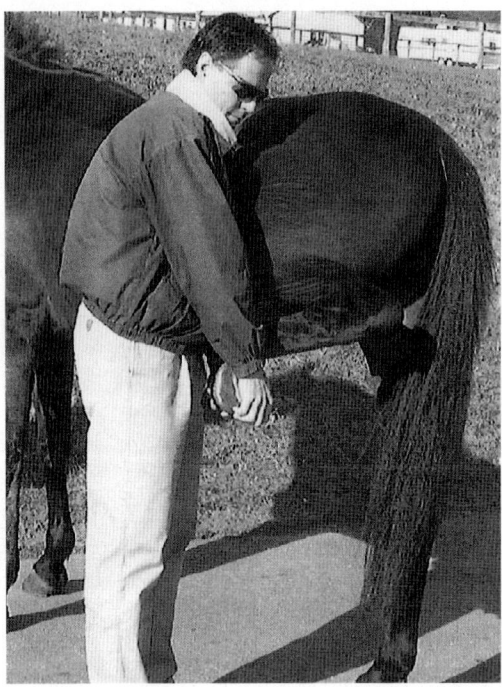

Fig. 8-9 • A hindlimb flexion test is a combination of the lower limb flexion and upper limb flexion tests.

lameness of the hock because the stifle and coxofemoral joints also are stressed hard, and mild flexion of the lower joints is inevitable. The terms *spavin test* and *hock flexion test* are deep-rooted in our profession but it is important to recognize that a positive response is *not* synonymous with distal hock joint pain.

The limb is held in hard flexion for at least 1 minute, but additional time for this test may improve its clinical value (Figure 8-8). It may be necessary to have an assistant place a hand on the contralateral hip to steady the horse, because proper performance of this test requires that the limb be elevated substantially, and the horse may lose its balance. The position of the hands in the metatarsal region is important to consider, because the force required to hold the hindlimb in this position may cause compression and pain in structures along the plantar aspect, potentially contributing to a false-positive response.

Hindlimb Flexion Test

Alternatively, the entire hindlimb can be flexed simultaneously. This test is useless in differentiating potential sources of pain in a limb, but it is quite useful in exacerbating baseline lameness or uncovering occult lameness conditions. The clinician's hands are placed on the toe and the entire limb is held in extreme flexion (Figure 8-9). An assistant may be necessary to steady the opposite hip while the limb is elevated.

"Hock" Extension Test

Hock extension may be useful in placing selective stress on the hock, independent of the stifle. Forced extension causes tension on the soft tissue structures on the dorsal, medial,

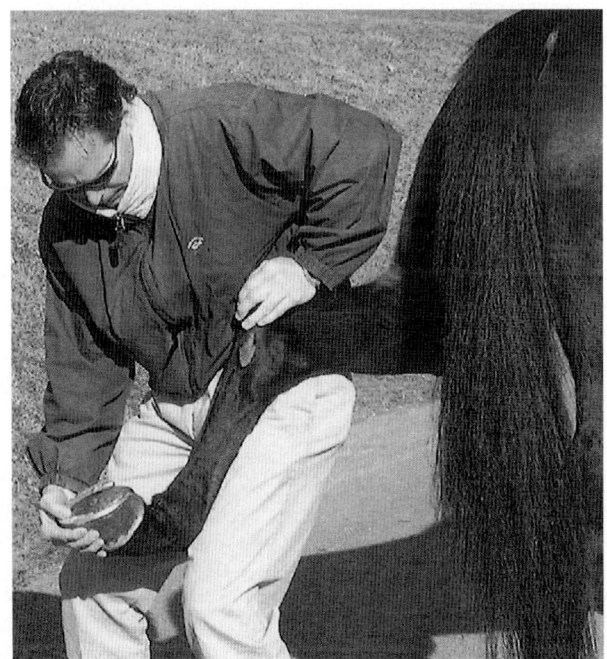

Fig. 8-10 • During the hock extension test the clinician forces the hock into extension by pushing down on the calcaneus while pulling up on the distal limb by using both the right arm and left leg. Pain from hock lameness can be exacerbated, but false-positive results from pain in other locations also can occur.

and lateral aspects of the hock. Seldom is it possible to perform this test for 1 minute; six to eight attempts at forced extension followed by trotting the horse can be substituted for more lengthy manipulation (Figure 8-10). False-positive and false-negative responses occur, which are caused mostly by the inelastic reciprocal apparatus. This

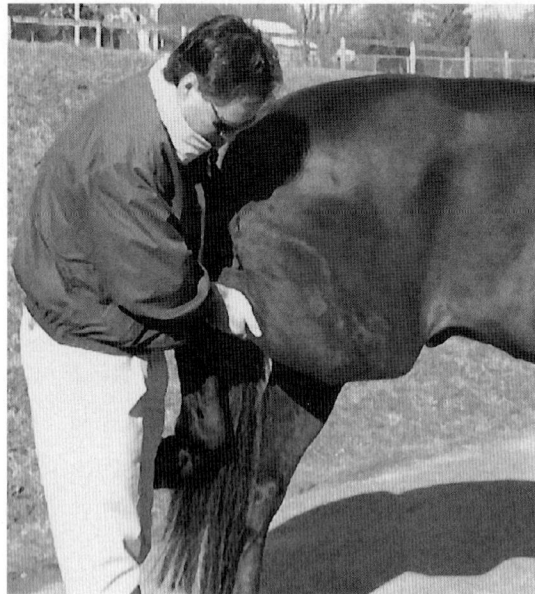

Fig. 8-11 • A seldom-used test is the stifle flexion test. This test can be difficult and dangerous to perform in fractious horses. The forced flexion of the stifle joint used in this test attempts to differentiate stifle and hock joint pain.

maneuver can reveal laxity of a damaged fibularis (peroneus) tertius.

"Stifle Flexion" Test

A modification of the upper limb flexion test can be used to place hard flexion on the stifle, independent of the hock (Figure 8-11). This test can be somewhat difficult to perform but may exacerbate lameness in horses with osteoarthritis or other conditions of the stifle. Other proximal limb joints are also in flexion; therefore some false-positive results occur. See page 87 for other manipulation of the stifle.

DIRECT OR LOCAL PALPATION FOLLOWED BY MOVEMENT

Static palpation, in which the horse's response to compression during palpation while standing is assessed, reveals useful information (see Chapter 6). Additional information can be gained by evaluating movement after palpation and dynamic provocation to induce lameness. Dynamic provocation usually is performed by digital palpation or use of hoof testers. Many horses manifest a positive response during static palpation, but the primary pain is located elsewhere. However, if lameness can be induced or baseline lameness can be increased by one or two grades by deep palpation, then the area may be relevant to the current cause of lameness. False-positive results do occur, but in my opinion these are less frequent than with most flexion tests. There are few false-negative results.

Digital Compression of a Painful Area

The veterinarian should elevate the limb and compress the painful or otherwise inflamed area for 15 to 30 seconds and then evaluate the horse at a trot in hand. Exacerbation of the baseline lameness by one or more grades is considered

a positive response. This procedure is useful in differentiating the cause of lameness in both the forelimb and hindlimb. In the forelimb, I find it useful to compress the dorsal proximal aspect of the proximal phalanx (if a midsagittal fracture is suspected), the dorsal cortex of the McIII (for bucked shins or a dorsal cortical fracture), exostoses involving the small metacarpal bones (for splints), the suspensory branches or digital flexor tendons, and the proximal palmar metacarpal region (for PSD or longitudinal or avulsion fracture of the McIII). In horses with mild SDF tendonitis, baseline lameness usually is mild or nonexistent, but obvious lameness after digital compression suggests tendonitis as a clinically significant problem.

In the hindlimbs, compression of the dorsal proximal aspect of the proximal phalanx can increase lameness from midsagittal or dorsal frontal fracture, but trauma from interference injury (of particular importance in trotters) or other forms can lead to a false-positive response. A *dynamic Churchill test*, compression followed by trotting (see Chapter 6), is useful in the diagnosis of lameness of the proximal metatarsal region and tarsus. In the hindlimb, compression of the proximal aspects of both the second and fourth metatarsal bones puts indirect pressure on the origin of the SL, and a positive response may indicate PSD. False-positive results to this provocative test are common because the entire hindlimb is in flexion, similar to upper limb flexion without compression. Compression of a "curb" followed by trotting may increase lameness.

In some horses with tibial stress fractures, an induced lameness can be seen after deep palpation of the caudal tibial cortex. With the limb elevated, the veterinarian should apply deep pressure to the caudal cortex by wrapping the fingers around the tibia from the medial aspect (see Figure 6-27). Most horses object to this maneuver, but in those with tibial stress fractures, the positive static response is followed by an exacerbation of the baseline lameness.

Axial Skeleton

Application of direct local pressure to many parts of the axial skeleton is difficult, but in some instances this procedure can lead to the detection of pain both statically and while the horse is trotting (see Chapters 6, 93, 95, and 97). In the cervical area, forced lateral bending followed by walking or trotting may exacerbate neurological signs or gait deficits in horses with cervical instability or proliferative changes. Deep palpation over the thoracolumbar spine followed by trotting can induce hindlimb stiffness or other mild gait abnormalities. Direct and deep palpation over the tubera sacrale and tubera coxae can induce hindlimb lameness in horses with stress fractures or those with chronic lameness as a result of pelvic asymmetry from old fractures. Sacroiliac compression, or manipulation of the sacrum or tail head, can induce hindlimb stiffness or lameness in horses with injuries in these areas.

INDUCED LAMENESS AFTER HOOF TESTER EXAMINATION

The hoof testers are applied in a suspected area for 15 to 30 seconds and the horse is evaluated for lameness while trotting. False-positive test results are quite common, but a marked difference between limbs can be an important clinical sign. Shoes and pad combinations may preclude complete hoof tester examination of the sole, so I often apply pressure across the heel. I have found this position to yield the most useful information in horses with palmar foot pain from most causes, but it also induces a positive response in horses with nonspecific foot pain (sore feet). Most normal horses object to firm pressure placed across the heel using hoof testers, particularly in a hindlimb, and mild lameness on the initial few steps is common, but severe lameness after this test is a useful indication that the foot is the source of baseline lameness.

THE WEDGE TEST

The *wedge test* is a form of manipulation similar to the flexion or other varus or valgus stress tests, but it is used specifically to evaluate the digit and associated soft tissues. The wedge can be used to dramatically change the dorsal-to-palmar (heel) or medial-to-lateral hoof angles. Collateral ligaments, joint capsules, subchondral bone and articular surfaces, and surrounding soft tissues can be stretched or compressed when the horse stands on the wedge. Changes in hoof angles of this magnitude can greatly change the stress placed on the DDF tendon, SDF tendon, and SL. Raising the heel reduces stress on the DDF tendon but increases stress on the SL. Raising the toe reduces stress on the SL but increases stress on the DDF tendon, navicular bone, and associated ligaments and bursa. The number of tissues affected by the wedge accounts for the lack of specificity of this test, and it likely accounts for many false-positive results. The wedge is placed in the desired position, and the horse is made to stand in this position for 30 to 60 seconds with the contralateral limb elevated (Figure 8-12). The horse is then trotted in a straight line on a firm surface. The test can be used in any limb but is performed most commonly in the forelimbs. In some horses, it is difficult to attain the desired duration regardless of whether they are lame. The horse's response to simply standing on the wedge may not give an accurate indication of how lame it will be when it is trotted. In horses content to stand in such an abnormal position, a dramatic lameness may be seen at the trot. Horses with navicular syndrome or sore feet from many causes of palmar foot pain are most likely to manifest a positive response. In my experience and that of others, the direction of the wedge that elicits the most positive response from horses with palmar foot pain is with the apex (low end) directed medially (see Figure 8-12).[11] This substantial change in the medial-to-lateral hoof angle is likely to cause stretching of the suspensory apparatus of the navicular bone and collateral ligaments of the distal interphalangeal joint or compression on articular structures. Horses with palmar foot pain may show severe lameness, but diagnostic analgesia is required to confirm the foot as a source of pain. Horses with injuries of the DDF tendon, SDF tendon, and SL may show a milder response.

VARUS OR VALGUS STRESS TESTS

Evaluation for lameness after placing varus or valgus stress on an individual joint may incriminate this area as a potential source of pain and is used most commonly in the stifle.

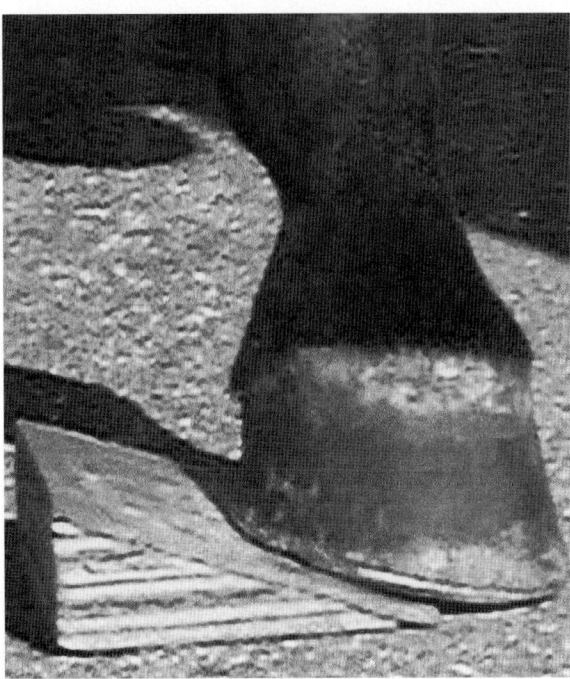

Fig. 8-12 • A 15- to 20-degree wedge can be used to manipulate the joints and soft tissue structures of the digit. The most consistent response is elicited by directing the apex (low end) of the wedge medially (as shown). The wedge also can be used to raise the heel and toe. (Wedge courtesy Norman G. Ducharme, Ithaca, New York.)

To perform the stifle valgus stress test, the clinician's shoulder (or hand) is used as a fulcrum against the distal femur, and the distal limb is pulled laterally several times before the horse is trotted (see Figure 6-25). False-positive results can be obtained because the entire distal extremity is manipulated during this test. Valgus or varus stress tests can be used in many joints in the distal limb, particularly the interphalangeal joints.

Patellar manipulation followed by trotting (see Figure 6-26) may be helpful but can be difficult to perform when horses resist forced proximal movement of the patella (frequently, the veterinarian's wrist is forced into hyperextension). Although cranial and caudal draw tests can be used to exacerbate stifle lameness, I have not found them particularly helpful, and they are dangerous to perform.

FLEXION TESTS AND DIAGNOSTIC ANALGESIA

I do not generally recommend combining the results of flexion tests and diagnostic analgesia (called "blocking the flexion test"). I often hear that baseline lameness abated after a block, but the horse still had positive flexion test results. My usual comment is, "Why bother to flex the horse if baseline lameness has been abolished?" Flexion tests induce lameness that may be unrelated to the baseline lameness, a concept that is confusing to the inexperienced and to lay people. Thus it is not unusual that a horse might have residual lameness after flexion, even if the baseline lameness has been eliminated.[4] I usually do not recommend further investigation once baseline lameness has been eliminated.

If baseline lameness is not obvious but a low-grade gait deficit is present, or if a horse has bilaterally symmetrical lameness, flexion tests or other forms of manipulation or provocation may be the only way of "seeing" lameness. In this instance, induced lameness from manipulation can be assumed to be the baseline lameness, and diagnostic analgesia can proceed. All involved parties should be well informed about the potential for misdiagnosis, but in certain circumstances this pathway may lead to a successful diagnosis.

Chapter 9

Applied Anatomy of the Musculoskeletal System

Matthew Durham and Sue J. Dyson

References on page 1257

It is beyond the scope of this book to describe all aspects of musculoskeletal anatomy in depth, yet a detailed knowledge of anatomy is fundamental to a lameness diagnostician, as highlighted in the chapters on observation and palpation (see Chapters 5 and 6). Some aspects of anatomy are considered in depth in individual chapters dealing with conditions of specific areas. This chapter considers some philosophical aspects of the importance of anatomical knowledge and describes some basic principles. It also provides illustrations that we hope will help the reader to understand better the three-dimensional aspects of anatomy.

Accurate interpretation of what we see and feel during an examination requires knowledge of what structures we are looking at and palpating. For example, a swelling is noted over the dorsal aspect of the carpus. Is the swelling diffuse and possibly related to a hygroma, periarticular edema, or cellulitis, or is there a discrete swelling, horizontally oriented, reflecting distention of the middle carpal joint? Or is it a longitudinal swelling reflecting distention of the common digital extensor tendon sheath or the tendon sheath of the extensor carpi radialis? If the swelling is longitudinal, are any compressions in the swelling caused by normal retinaculum or adhesions within the sheath (Figure 9-1)? If we examine the sheath by ultrasonography, is the echogenic band extending from the sheath wall to the enclosed tendon normal mesotendon, or is it an adhesion? If diffuse swelling is present around the dorsal aspect of the carpus associated with lameness, how can we tell if the middle carpal joint capsule is distended? We need to know that there is a palmar outpouching of the middle carpal joint on the palmarolateral aspect of the carpus, just distal to the accessory carpal bone. Thus during visual inspection and palpation the clinician should be constantly asking, "What structure am I seeing or palpating, what are its functions, and what would be the consequences of loss of function?" If it has abnormal contour or size, is this the result of swelling of that structure or of an adjacent or underlying structure? Having established what structure is abnormal, the clinician then must consider the best imaging modality. If it is a tendonous or ligamentous structure, ultrasonography probably will provide the most information, but we must remember that it has bony attachments, and damage at those attachments might best be assessed by either radiology or nuclear scintigraphy. So we need to know not only what each structure is, but also the structures to which it is attached.

During visual inspection and palpation, we also need to think logically. We know that the superficial and deep digital flexor tendons (SDFT, DDFT), the accessory ligament of the DDFT (ALDDFT), and the suspensory ligament (SL) lie on the palmar aspect of the third metacarpal bone (McIII) (Figure 9-2). Swelling confined to just the medial aspect of the metacarpal region is far more likely to reflect direct trauma to the medial aspect of the limb than sprain or strain of any of the ligamentous or tendonous structures. We need to know that the proximal aspect of the SL lies between the bases (heads) of the second and fourth metacarpal bones and therefore is inaccessible to direct palpation, and that desmitis often may be present without discernible soft tissue swelling (Figure 9-3).

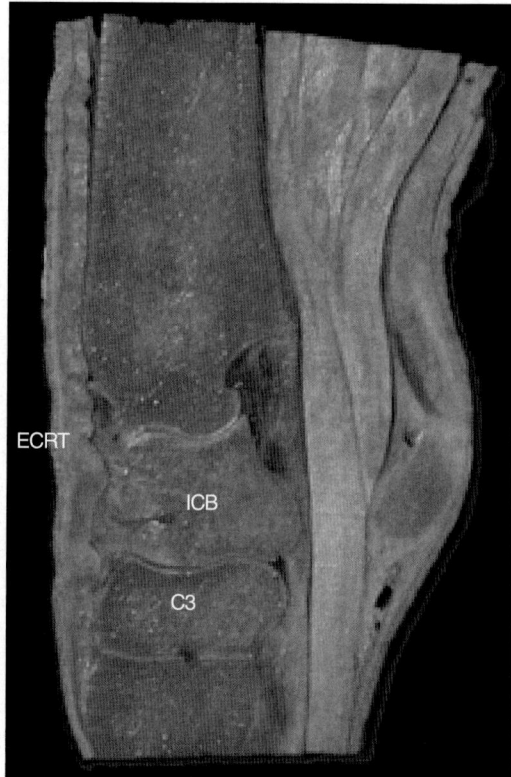

Fig. 9-1 • Sagittal anatomical section through the carpus, transecting the extensor carpi radialis tendon *(ECRT)*. *C3,* Third carpal bone; *ICB,* intermediate carpal bone.

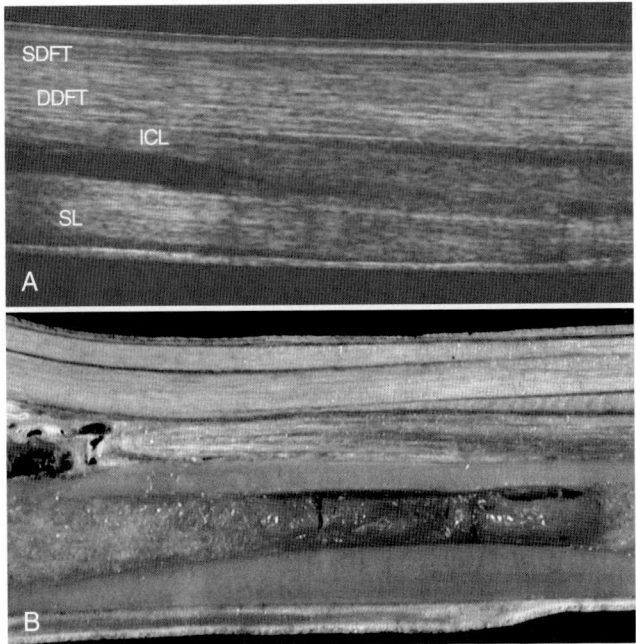

Fig. 9-2 • Sagittal views of the palmar metacarpal region. Proximal is to the right. **A,** FreeStyle Extended Imaging (Sequoia model, Acuson, Mountain View, California, United States) ultrasonographic image of the palmar metacarpal region. **B,** Corresponding anatomical section. *DDFT,* Deep digital flexor tendon; *ICL,* accessory ligament of the DDFT (inferior check ligament); *SDFT,* superficial digital flexor tendon; *SL,* suspensory ligament.

We must be aware of anatomy to realize the possible consequences of trauma to an area. The paucity of soft tissues over the cranial aspect of the stifle makes the patella and the tibial tuberosity vulnerable to direct trauma, hence the risk of fracture after hitting a fixed fence. The lack of soft tissues also means that if the horse hits a thorn hedge, the possibility of a thorn penetrating the femoropatellar joint capsule, resulting in contamination and infection, is quite high. We also need to think about how structures move relative to one another while the horse is in motion. If a steeplechase horse sustains an interference injury on the palmar aspect of the metacarpal region while galloping, the position of the skin laceration probably will not coincide with the level of the laceration in the SDFT (Figure 9-4). We also need to know the relative positions of the laceration and the digital flexor tendon sheath to be aware of the likelihood that the sheath may have been traumatized, and thus the risk of infectious tenosynovitis. Faced with a contaminated wound on the dorsal aspect of a hind fetlock and severe lameness, and the possibility of infection of the metatarsophalangeal joint, we need to know where to expect to see distention of the plantar pouch of the joint capsule and to know that this site is safely accessible for arthrocentesis.

A fundamental principle of lameness investigation is the identification of the source or sources of pain. Although this may be possible through detailed clinical examination, in many instances it is essential to perform diagnostic analgesia (see Chapter 10). A detailed knowledge of the anatomy of nerves, joint capsules and the various outpouchings, tendon sheaths, and bursae is fundamental to

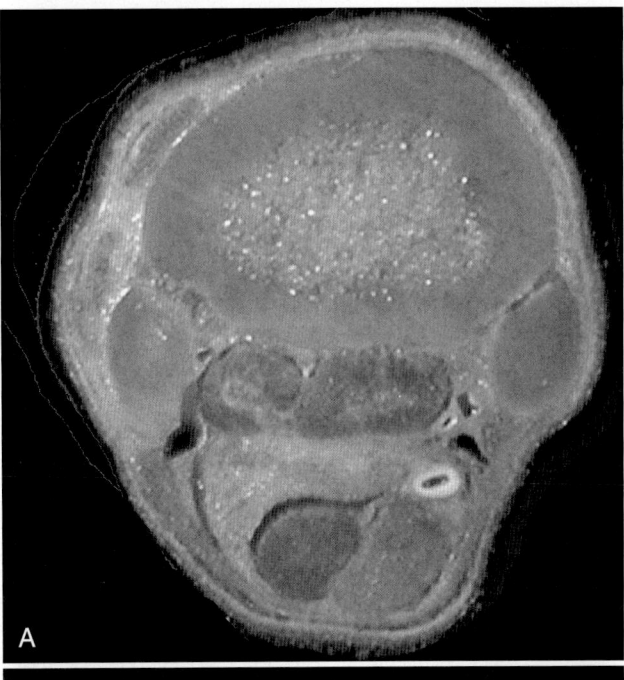

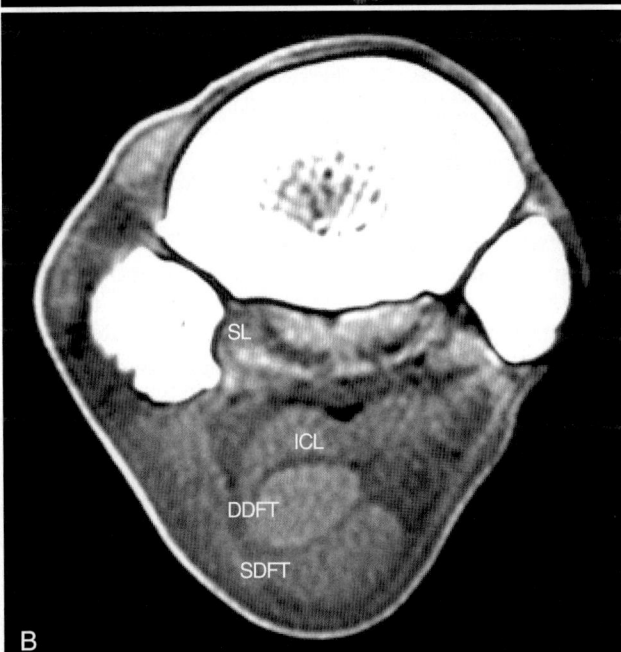

Fig. 9-3 • Transverse sections through the proximal metacarpal region. Dorsal is to the top and lateral is to the left. **A,** Anatomical specimen. **B,** Computed tomographic scan using soft tissue windowing. *DDFT,* Deep digital flexor tendon; *ICL,* accessory ligament of the deep digital flexor tendon (inferior check ligament); *SDFT,* superficial digital flexor tendon; *SL,* suspensory ligament.

safe, accurate performance of perineural and intrasynovial injections.

Given the knowledge of the close relationship among the distal interphalangeal joint capsule, the distal sesamoidean impar ligament, the collateral sesamoidean ligaments and the distal phalanx, and the close proximity of branches of the palmar digital nerve, it is not surprising that intraarticular analgesia is not specific and that other structures

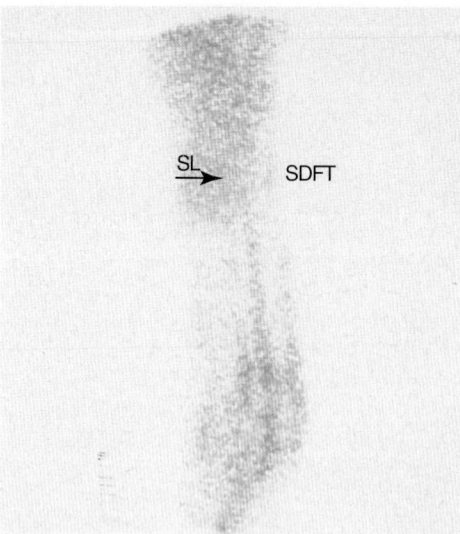

Fig. 9-4 • Lateral scintigraphic image of the metacarpal region acquired before the end of the flow (vascular) phase and at the beginning of the pool phase. This jumper had a history of low-grade chronic desmitis of the proximal aspect of the suspensory ligament *(SL)*, and mild diffuse superficial digital flexor *(SDFT)* tendonitis. An acute interference injury to the midmetacarpal region was evident on the skin. Note the proximal location of the acute injury to the SDFT. The linear area of uptake between the SL and SDFT is vascular artifact related to the time of acquisition.

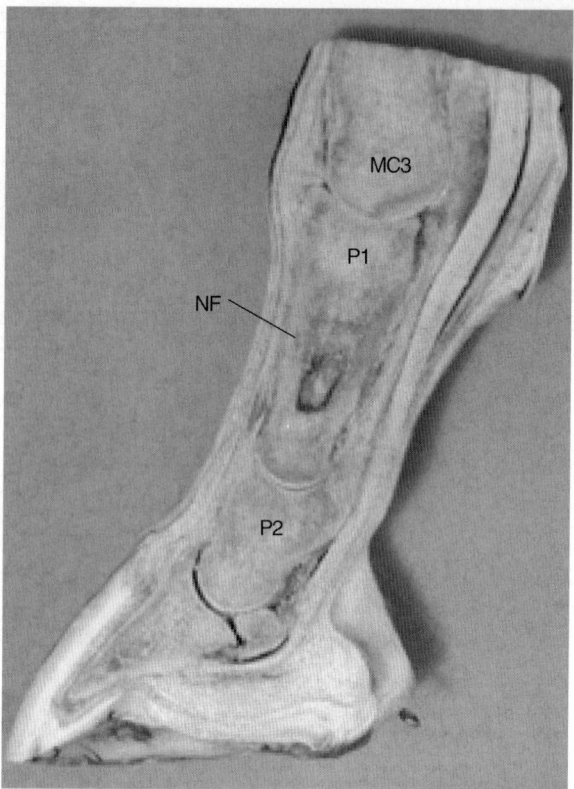

Fig. 9-5 • Sagittal anatomical section through the pastern demonstrating a common location for the nutrient foramen *(NF)* entering the proximal phalanx *(P1)*. MC3, Third metacarpal bone; *P2*, middle phalanx.

can be affected, especially if interpretation of the response is delayed or an excessively large volume of local anesthetic solution is used. Knowledge that the medial and lateral femorotibial joints do not normally communicate and that the cruciate ligaments usually are extraarticular structures is crucial for an understanding of why these joint compartments must be injected separately, and why the response to intraarticular analgesia may be both incomplete and delayed if a cruciate ligament is damaged.

Knowledge of functional neuroanatomy also is important for interpretation of specific gait abnormalities. Inability to bear weight on a hindlimb after general anesthesia may be the result of myopathy, but in the absence of marked pain and distress, it is more likely that the horse has lost extensor function and is unable to extend any of the hindlimb joints because of femoral nerve paresis. Loss of ability to extend the elbow may result from loss of triceps function associated with a fracture of the olecranon but may also be caused by radial nerve paresis.

Vascular anatomy is important because many nerves lie close to vessels. With superficial nerves and vessels, identification of the vessel may facilitate palpation of the nerve and thus aid accurate perineural injection. Avoiding penetration of the vessel and causing hematoma formation also is desirable. With regard to deeper nerves the veterinarian may benefit by knowing that the needle must be in close proximity to the nerve if blood appears in the needle hub. This information can be helpful when performing perineural analgesia of the deep branch of the fibular nerve.

Assessment of digital pulse amplitudes is an integral part of palpation. Increased pulse amplitude usually signifies a site of inflammation at, or distal to, the region of palpation, especially in association with inflammatory conditions of the foot, such as subsolar abscessation or laminitis. Palpation of the pulse in the dorsal metatarsal artery and assessment of saphenous vein filling can be helpful in the evaluation of a horse with suspected aortoiliac thrombosis.

Knowledge of the sites of major vessels is important when considering the consequences of major laceration to an area and possible avascular areas, and in planning a surgical approach to an area. All bones have one or more nutrient foramina through which major vessels enter. These usually are in standard locations (Figure 9-5). Knowledge of these sites is critical for accurate radiological interpretation because a nutrient foramen appears as a radiolucent area, which should not be confused with a pathological lesion. The position of these intraosseous vessels also has important consequences in considering repair of major long bone fractures.

Thermography relies on the detection of surface heat and is obviously greatly influenced by the position of superficial vessels. Interpretation may be misleading without knowledge of location. Thus it should be absolutely clear that anatomy is a dynamic subject and is not merely a function of knowing the origins and insertions of numerous structures.

We also need to know some fundamentals of biomechanics. What is the biomechanical function of the SL? What are the implications of loss of function? For example, how may function be altered by a change in foot angle after application of a heel wedge? How is load in the distal limb

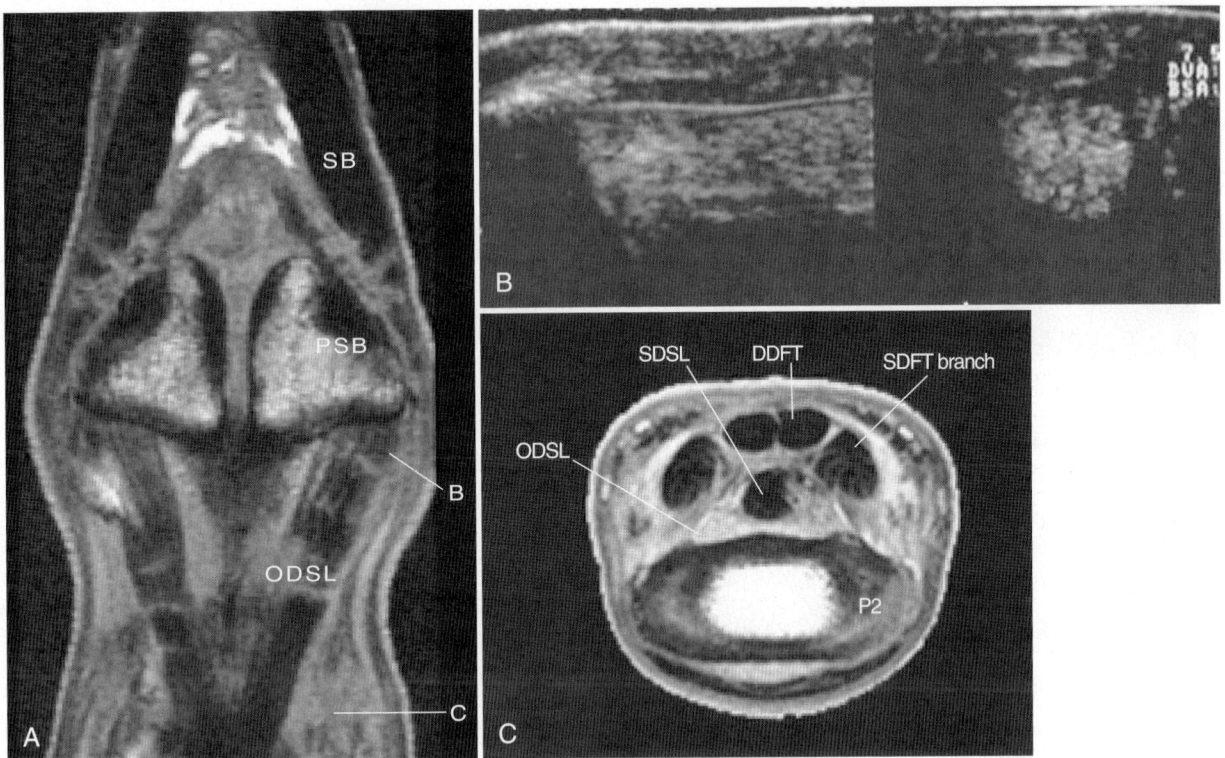

Fig. 9-6 • The oblique distal sesamoidean ligaments. **A,** Frontal magnetic resonance image (MRI) of the pastern showing the origins and insertions of the oblique distal sesamoidean ligaments *(ODSL)*. **B,** Frontal *(left)* and transverse *(right)* ultrasonographic images of the ODSLs obtained at point *B* in **A.** Proximal and dorsal are to the left. **C,** Transverse MRI scan obtained at point *C* in **A.** *DDFT,* Deep digital flexor tendon; *P2,* middle phalanx; *PSB,* proximal sesamoid bone; *SB,* suspensory branch; *SDFT,* superficial digital flexor tendon; *SDSL,* straight distal sesamoidean ligament. (**A** Courtesy Alexia L. McKnight, University of Pennsylvania, Philadelphia, Pennsylvania, United States.)

joints affected by mediolateral foot imbalance? If the accessory ligament of the SDFT is cut (superior check desmotomy), how does this alter the function of not only the SDFT but also other tendonous and ligamentous structures? Does consequent overload of the SL predispose to an increased risk of suspensory desmitis? When orthopedic surgery is being considered, which is the tension side of the bone, to which a bone plate should be applied to take advantage of the tension band principle?

In more general terms, how will lameness in the left hindlimb alter forces in the other limbs, and does this vary with the gait? Given the reciprocal apparatus of the hindlimb and the inability to flex and extend the limb joints independently, it is not surprising that the gait characteristics of hindlimb lameness are so similar, irrespective of the source of pain causing lameness. Understanding the reciprocal apparatus in addition to the results of loss of its function (e.g., after damage to the fibularis tertius) is hugely important for an understanding of hindlimb lameness.

After the source of pain causing lameness has been isolated, then it is necessary to establish what is causing pain; this requires one of a number of imaging modalities: radiography, ultrasonography, nuclear scintigraphy, magnetic resonance imaging (MRI), computed tomography (CT), and exploratory arthroscopy, bursoscopy, or tenoscopy. Accurate interpretation of the findings from any of these techniques requires specialist anatomical knowledge.

With radiographic images, various structures are superimposed, resulting in potentially confusing radiolucent lines that can mimic a fracture (e.g., in the relatively complex carpus and tarsus). A frog shadow superimposed over the navicular bone may mimic a fracture. We must be cognizant of anatomical variations, for example, the shape and size of the crena of the distal phalanx. We have to know how best to image a specific anatomical location, such as the sustentaculum tali of the calcaneus (fibular tarsal bone) using a skyline projection. For interpretation of the clinical significance of periosteal or entheseous new bone, detailed knowledge of the soft tissue structures that do (or do not) attach in that area is vital. Particularly in the fetlock and pastern areas, numerous ligamentous structures have discrete areas of attachment (Figure 9-6).

Radiography requires the awareness that we are looking at a three-dimensional structure in two dimensions, and thus images of the area must be obtained from several different angles. With ultrasonography, and more particularly with MRI and CT, structures can be imaged in three dimensions; this requires detailed knowledge of the shape, size, and relationships among structures. In the proximal metatarsal region the DDFT lies more medial than the SDFT and SL, and thus these structures cannot be imaged adequately by ultrasonography at the same time from the plantar aspect of the limb (Figure 9-7). The transducer must be moved to a plantaromedial site to evaluate the DDFT in its

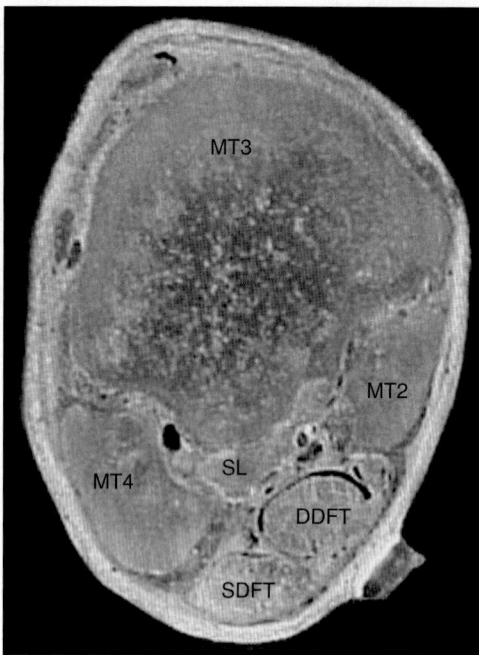

Fig. 9-7 • Transverse anatomical section of the proximal metatarsal region demonstrating the lateral position of the superficial digital flexor tendon *(SDFT)* relative to the deep digital flexor tendon *(DDFT)*. Lateral is to the left and dorsal to the top of the image. This arrangement is the opposite of that seen in the forelimb (compare with Figure 9-3). *MT2, MT3,* and *MT4,* Second, third, and fourth metatarsal bones, respectively; *SL,* suspensory ligament.

entirety. A large vessel on the plantarolateral aspect of the SL can cause shadowing artifacts in the SL.

The internal architecture of the joint becomes important during exploratory arthroscopy. What are the normal variations in cartilage thickness? Where do you expect to see a synovial fossa? Which parts of the synovial membrane are usually more vascular? Is it normal that the cranial cruciate ligament can be seen without synovial covering from the medial femoral tibial joint?

A textbook of this type cannot possibly provide detailed descriptions of all aspects of anatomy, functional anatomy, and biomechanics, nor answer all of the questions posed earlier in this chapter. It is hoped that this overview will stimulate readers to have a thirst for more knowledge of these subjects, in the understanding of their huge importance.

Lameness clinicians are encouraged to acquire a set of boiled-out bones for reference and perform detailed dissections of cadaver limbs to improve knowledge of anatomy. Practicing nerve block techniques on cadaver limbs is very important for inexperienced clinicians or those performing a new block for the first time. If a lame horse must be humanely destroyed, clinicians should take the opportunity, whenever possible, to perform a postmortem examination to correlate clinical findings with the actual lesions and revise anatomy at the same time. Each time a dissection is performed, new anatomical detail becomes apparent that previously may have been missed.

The remainder of this chapter provides some basic definitions of anatomical terms used elsewhere in the book, describes the reciprocal apparatus of the forelimb and

hindlimb, and presents correlative illustrations of anatomical specimens and images of those areas to assist in the understanding of three-dimensional anatomy.

THE LANGUAGE OF ANATOMY

The system described in the *Nomina Anatomica Veterinaria* (NAV) according to the guidelines of the International Committee on Veterinary Anatomical Nomenclature has been used so that anatomical terminology is universal. English translations of NAV terms have been used whenever possible according to these guidelines.

FORCES

The interaction of anatomical structures allows for the conversion of chemical energy into purposeful movement. It is often useful to think of complex anatomical structures in terms of interactions between simplified structural units. The interaction of forces within these anatomical units dictates the abilities and the potential weaknesses of the equine athlete. In simple terms, the stresses acting on the body are compression, tension, shear, torsion, and bending.

Compression is the force applied between two points to move them together. Examples of compression are seen in joints, such as within the middle carpal joint at the interface between the radial and third carpal bones, or the compression sustained by the digital cushion between the sole, frog, and the distal phalanx. Compression also is sustained within most bones, such as the third carpal bone or the dorsal cortex of the McIII.

Tension is the force that tends to stretch or elongate a structure. Examples of tension are most obvious in tendons and ligaments, but bones such as the olecranon or within the palmar cortex of the McIII also sustain tensile strain.

Shear is a stress at the interface between two structures moving in opposite directions. Examples of shear are seen in the femoropatellar and tarsocrural joints, within bone, and within the hoof capsule.

Torsion is the stress produced when a twisting motion is applied to an object. Examples of torsional stress are seen within joints, such as the distal hock joints, or within individual bones, such as the McIII.

Bending is a combination of compression on one side of a structure and tension on the other side. Structures subjected to bending are long bones such as the McIII, where the dorsal cortex is subjected to compression, whereas the palmar cortex is subjected to tension.

SPECIALIZED STRUCTURES
Synovial Structures
Synovial bursae, tendon sheaths, and joints have a similar function and generally similar structure. All are sacs containing synovial fluid produced by the lining of the sac. In simple terms, synovial structures facilitate the movement between independent structures by providing a hydraulic cushion of viscous fluid that limits the effects of friction to help dissipate compressive and shear forces. (For a more complete discussion on synovial structures, see Chapters 61 to 67 and 74 to 79.)

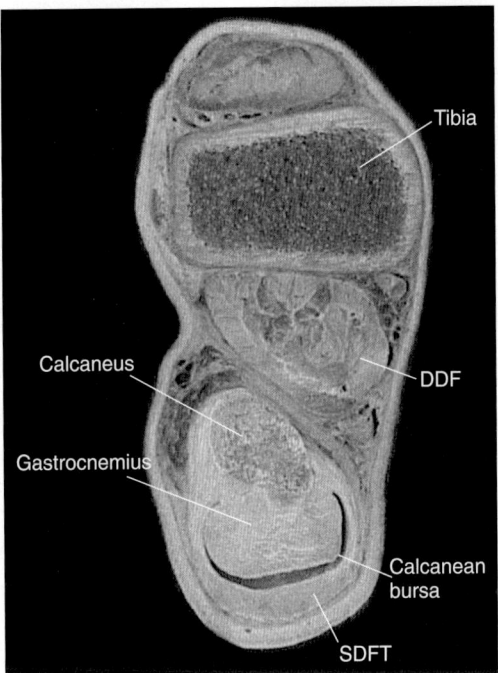

Fig. 9-8 • Transverse anatomical section through distal aspect of the tibia and proximal aspect of the calcaneus demonstrating the distinct calcanean bursa bounded by the collateral ligaments of the superficial digital flexor tendon *(SDFT). DDF,* Deep digital flexor muscle.

A diarthrosis is a mobile joint containing a synovial membrane. This membrane is flexible enough to allow for movement of the joint. The synovial fluid lubricates, hydraulically equalizes pressure between cartilage plates, and nourishes the articular cartilage.

A synovial sheath is a sac that completely surrounds a tendon, forming a synovial lining on the surface of the tendon and the lining of the sheath. The synovial reflection between these visceral and parietal layers is termed the *mesotendon.* This structure is similar to the mesentery in the abdominal cavity. Nerve and blood supply to the tendon is found within the mesotendon. In areas of great mobility within the synovial sheaths, the nerve and blood supply to the tendons is through a vinculum, which is a modified mesotendon in the form of a narrow band connecting visceral and parietal layers.

A synovial bursa is a simple sac lying between a tendon or muscle and an adjacent bony prominence. A bursa does not surround the tendon but acts as a cushion at the interface where pressure is concentrated (Figure 9-8).

Intercalated Bones

Intercalated bones are bones that arise within tendons or ligaments allowing for the interface between the tendonous structure and the underlying bone at an area of focal pressure, typically at the level of a joint. The interface between these bones is within a synovial sac. The navicular bone, proximal sesamoid bones (PSBs), and patella are intercalated bones. These bones allow for smooth movement and dissipation of focal pressure between the tendon or ligament and the underlying joint (Figure 9-9).

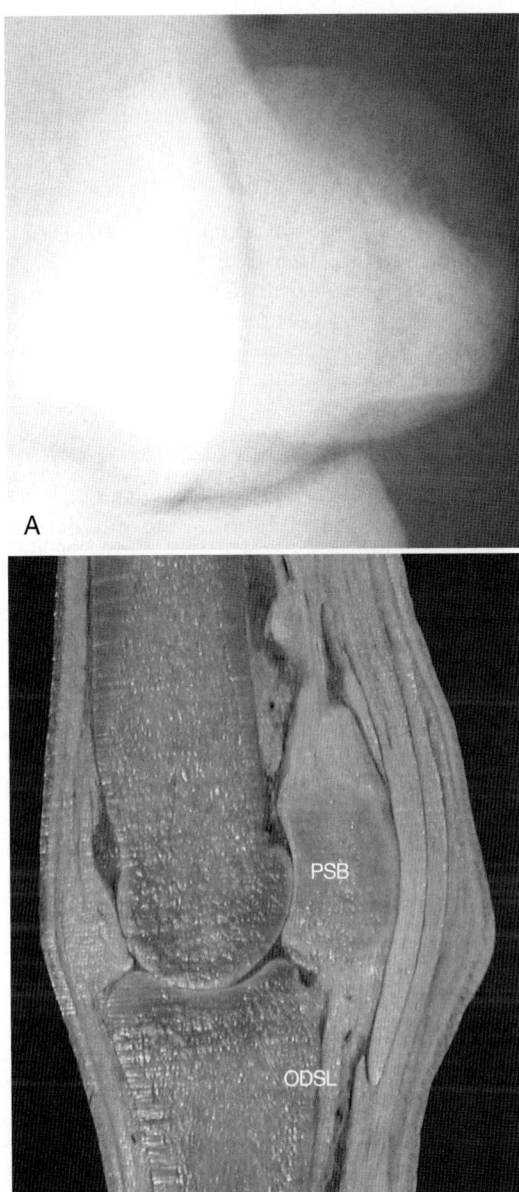

Fig. 9-9 • A, Oblique radiographic image of a normal proximal sesamoid bone *(PSB)*. **B,** Parasagittal anatomical section through suspensory branch, PSB, and oblique distal sesamoidean ligament *(ODSL)*.

Fibrocartilaginous Structures

In general terms, there are four functional arrangements of fibrocartilage: interarticular, connecting, circumferential, and stratiform.

Interarticular Fibrocartilage

Menisci are fibrocartilaginous structures located between the articular cartilages of a diarthrosis. Menisci are not directly attached to the joint surfaces but are held in place by ligaments immediately adjacent to the articular surfaces. They provide congruency between the condyles, allow for a greater range of movement of the joint, and absorb concussion. Menisci are found in the stifle and temporomandibular joints of the horse.

Connecting Fibrocartilage

A symphysis is a fibrocartilaginous joint that allows minimal movement. The pelvic symphysis and interster-nebral and intervertebral joints are examples of fibrocartilaginous joints.

Circumferential Fibrocartilage

In the coxofemoral joint the acetabular lip (labrum acetabulare) is a fibrocartilaginous ring extending the articular surface in a firm, semiflexible manner. The transverse acetabular ligament is the portion of the labrum crossing the acetabular notch. The glenoid labrum seen in other species is a poorly developed fibrous band in the shoulder of the horse.

Stratiform Fibrocartilage

Stratiform fibrocartilages arise within ligamentous structures at an interface with high focal pressure between soft tissue and bone, either within a ligament or as an extension of a bony surface. These structures are similar to intercalated bones in that they typically provide rigidity to help dissipate compressive forces, but the moderate elasticity allows for some flexibility of the structures.

The parapatellar fibrocartilage on the medial aspect of the patella, portions of the biceps brachii tendon of origin within the intertubercular (bicipital) bursa, the manica flexoria, and portions of the DDFT adjacent to the proximal aspect of the middle phalanx are examples of stratiform cartilage formation within tendonous structures. The proximal, middle, and distal scuta are stratiform fibrocartilaginous structures associated with the intersesamoidean ligament, the palmar aspect of the middle phalanx, and the collateral sesamoidean ligaments, respectively. These structures serve as semirigid pulleys primarily for the DDFT.

PASSIVE STAY APPARATUS

Distal Limb

The horse is uniquely equipped to be able to stand at rest while expending minimal muscular effort. In the forelimb and hindlimb the fetlock is prevented from overextension by a combination of structures providing passive resistance. The suspensory apparatus is the main contributor, forming a sling that maintains the fetlock in extension. In addition, the SDFT, DDFT, and the associated accessory (check) ligaments (in the forelimb) act as tension bands providing passive support. The suspensory apparatus consists primarily of the SL and branches, PSBs, and distal sesamoidean ligaments. The intercalated PSBs provide a broad face at the point where focal pressure is high at the palmar or plantar aspect of the fetlock joint, enabling the ligamentous tension band to support the fetlock. Dorsal branches of the SL join with the common or long digital extensor tendon, helping to stabilize the dorsal aspect of the digit. The axial and abaxial palmar and plantar ligaments of the proximal interphalangeal joint, the SDFT branches, and the straight sesamoidean ligament support the palmar or plantar aspect of the proximal interphalangeal joint. The navicular bone and its suspensory apparatus, in combination with the distal sesamoidean impar ligament, stabilize the palmar or plantar aspect of the distal interphalangeal joint.

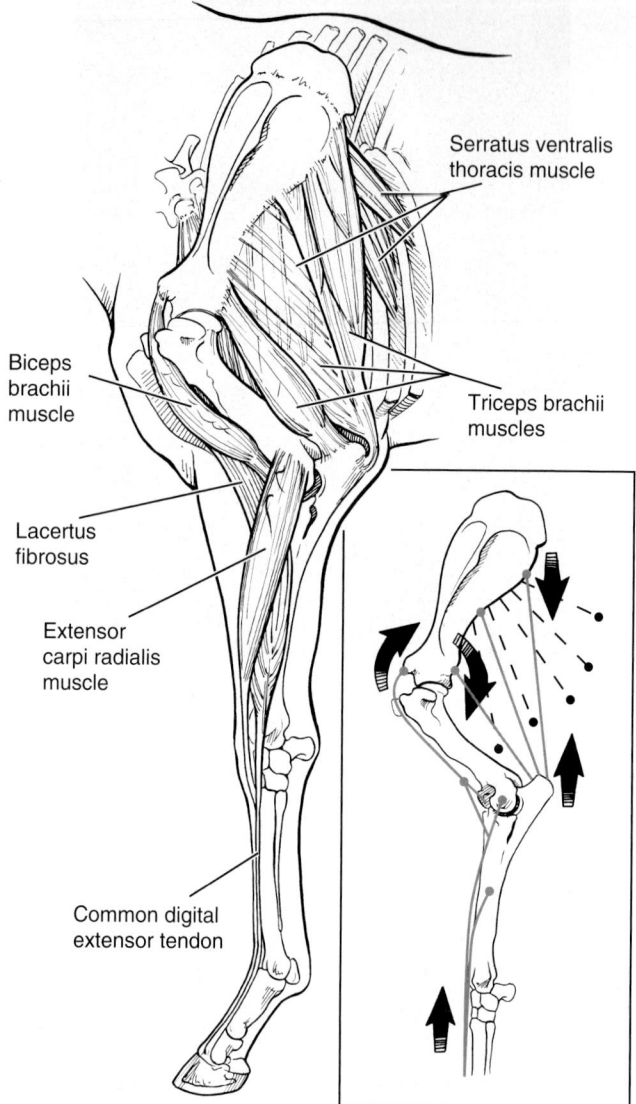

Fig. 9-10 • The passive stay apparatus of the forelimb.

Forelimb

In the forelimb the fibrous portion of the serratus ventralis thoracis acts as a sling suspending the thorax from the forelimb by its attachment to the scapula. The downward force applied by the serratus ventralis on the caudal aspect of the scapula causes slight flexion of the scapulohumeral joint, applying tension to the biceps brachii. A fibrous band of the biceps brachii extends from the supraglenoid tubercle of the scapula and continues as the lacertus fibrosus, which joins with the extensor carpi radialis to passively extend the carpus. Minimal muscular effort by the triceps on the olecranon maintains the elbow in extension (Figure 9-10).

Hindlimb

The stifle is maintained in extension by the patellar locking mechanism with minimal muscular effort. Slight muscular effort by the quadriceps and tensor fasciae latae rotates the patella medially, where the cartilaginous process of the

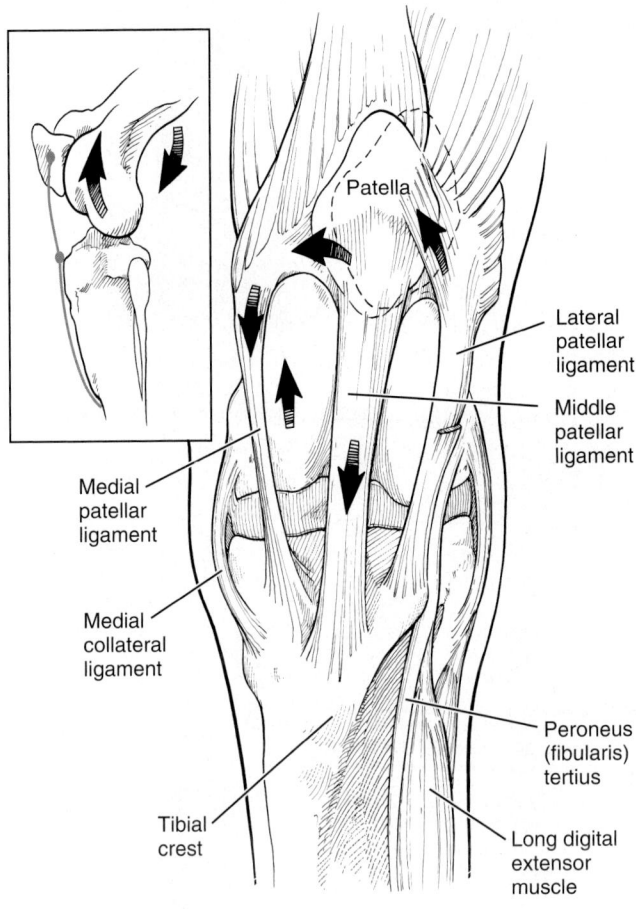

Fig. 9-11 • The patellar locking mechanism.

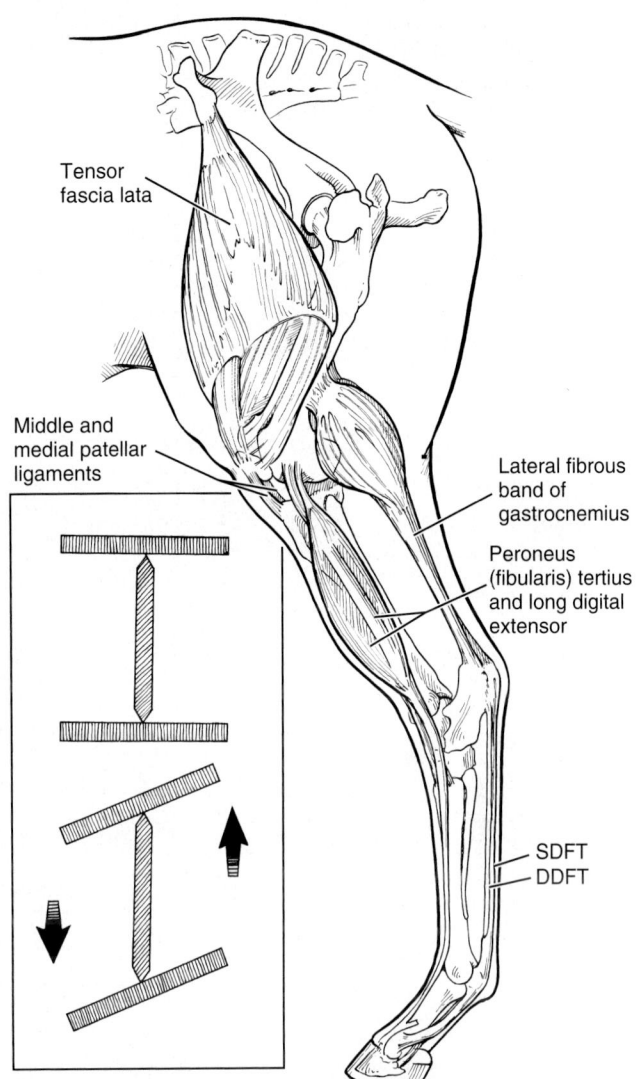

Fig. 9-12 • The reciprocal apparatus. *DDFT,* Deep digital flexor tendon; *SDFT,* superficial digital flexor tendon.

patella is caught caudal to the large prominence of the medial trochlear ridge of the femur. Slight relaxation of the quadriceps as a whole allows slight flexion of the stifle, which "locks" the patella in place by applying tension primarily to the medial and middle patellar ligaments (Figure 9-11). When the stifle is extended, the hock is passively extended by the superficial digital flexor and the fibrous component of the lateral head of the gastrocnemius muscles, which extend from the femur to the tuber calcis.

The reciprocal apparatus forces the hock to flex and extend in unison with the stifle. The reciprocal apparatus transfers mechanical energy to the distal aspect of the limb from the massive muscular structures of the upper limb without adding mass to the lower limb. The superficial digital flexor and the fibrous portion of the gastrocnemius muscles serve as the caudal component of the reciprocal apparatus, along with the long plantar ligament, which acts as a tension band to make the calcaneus, distal aspect of the tarsus, and metatarsal region a single functional lever arm. The fibularis (peroneus) tertius serves as the cranial component of the reciprocal apparatus, extending from the femur to the dorsal and lateral aspects of the tarsus (Figure 9-12). Although the fibularis tertius is important as part of the reciprocal apparatus, it is not essential for function of the passive stay apparatus, because its function is flexion of the tarsus.

A second reciprocal mechanism has been described for the lower hindlimb, where the fetlock and digit are flexed at the same time as the stifle and hock. The long digital extensor tendon and DDFT were the dorsal and plantar components suggested, but the SDFT probably also contributes.

THREE-DIMENSIONAL ANATOMY

Major advances in lameness diagnosis are being made with the assistance of advanced imaging techniques. Radiography, nuclear scintigraphy, and ultrasonography are well established, whereas CT and MRI are growing in importance. CT and MRI in particular require a detailed knowledge of three-dimensional anatomy. It is beyond the scope of this text to provide detailed correlative images of the entire musculoskeletal system. Figures 9-13 through 9-18 give a flavor of what is possible. Figures 9-13 through 9-16 highlight the complex anatomy of the navicular

Text continued on p. 100

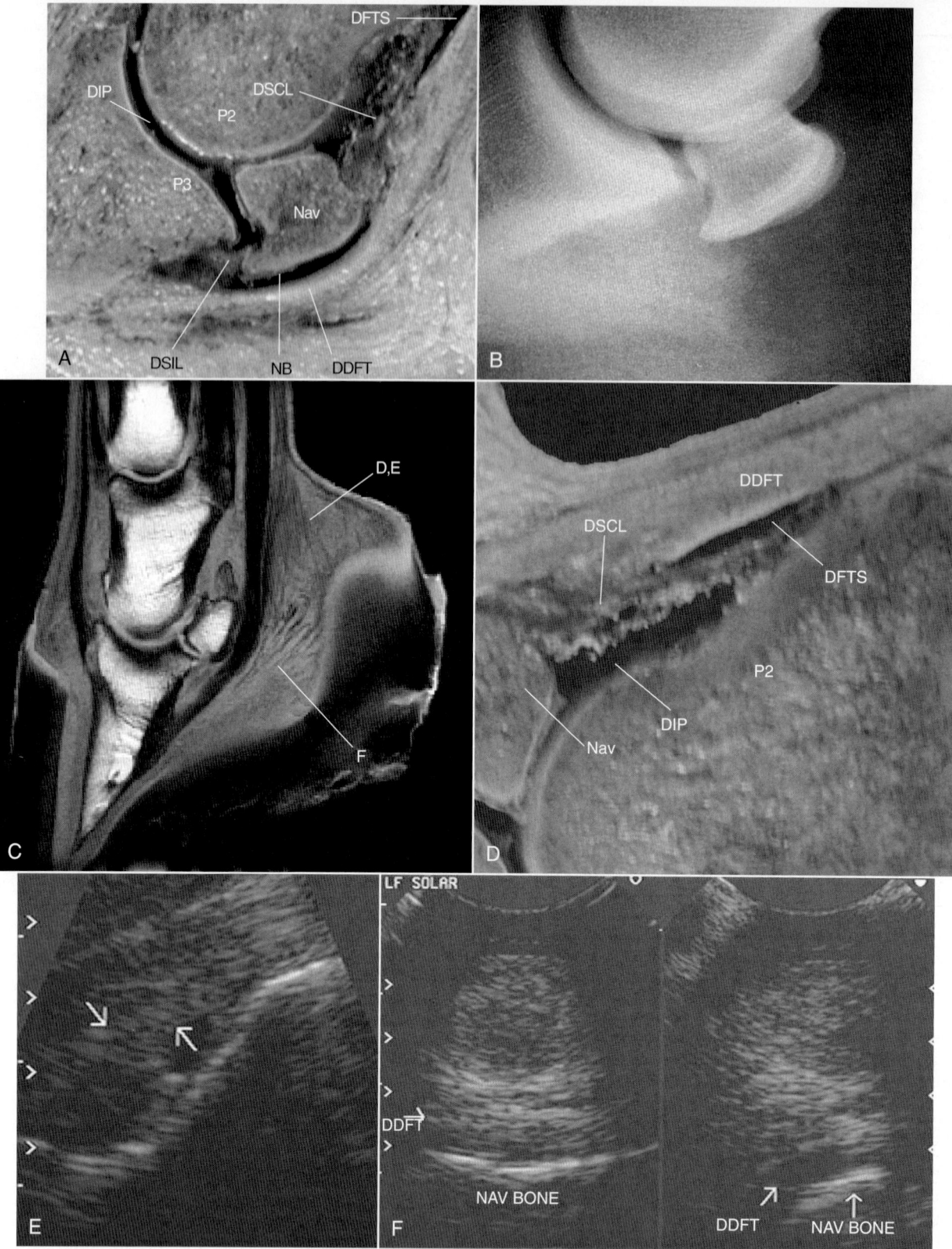

Fig. 9-13 • Comparisons of the lateral view of the navicular bone and its relationship to neighboring structures. **A,** Sagittal anatomical section showing the digital flexor tendon sheath *(DFTS)*, navicular bursa *(NB)*, and distal interphalangeal *(DIP)* joint surrounding the navicular bone. **B,** Lateromedial radiographic image centered on the navicular bone. **C,** Sagittal magnetic resonance imaging scan of the foot. **D** and **E,** Sagittal anatomical section and corresponding ultrasonographic image of the palmar aspect of the distal aspect of the pastern obtained at points *D* and *E* in panel **C.** Proximal is to the right. The arrows outline the distal sesamoidean collateral ligament. **F,** Frontal *(left)* and sagittal *(right)* ultrasonographic images obtained through the frog at point *F* in panel **C.** The hypoechoic appearance of the portion of the deep digital flexor tendon *(DDFT)* is caused by the off-incidence artifact because the fibers are not perpendicular to the line of the ultrasound beam. Lateral and proximal are to the right. *DSIL,* Distal sesamoidean impar ligament; *DSCL,* distal sesamoidean collateral ligament (axial union forming fibrous portion of T ligament); *Nav,* navicular bone; *P2,* middle phalanx; *P3,* distal phalanx. (**B** Courtesy Alexia L. McKnight, University of Pennsylvania, Philadelphia, Pennsylvania, United States.)

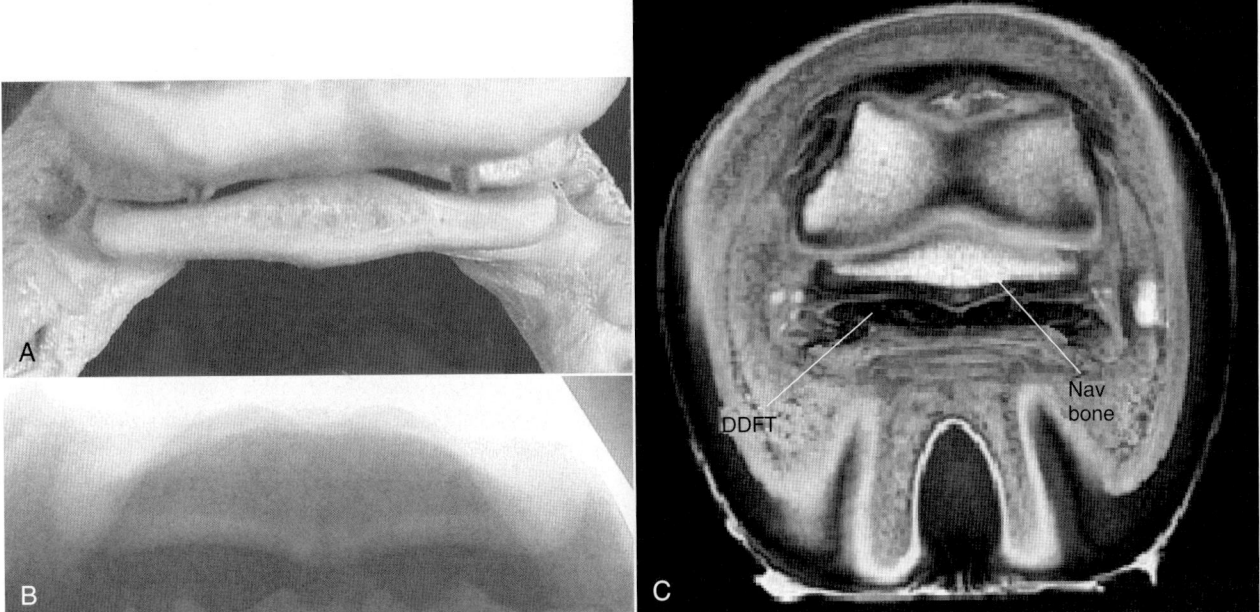

Fig. 9-14 • Transverse sections through the navicular bone. **A,** Anatomical specimen, palmar view. **B,** Palmaroproximal-palmarodistal oblique radiographic image of a normal navicular bone. **C,** Transverse magnetic resonance image. The deep digital flexor tendon *(DDFT)* is nearly as broad at this point as the navicular bone. (Courtesy Alexia L. McKnight, University of Pennsylvania, Philadelphia, Pennsylvania, United States.)

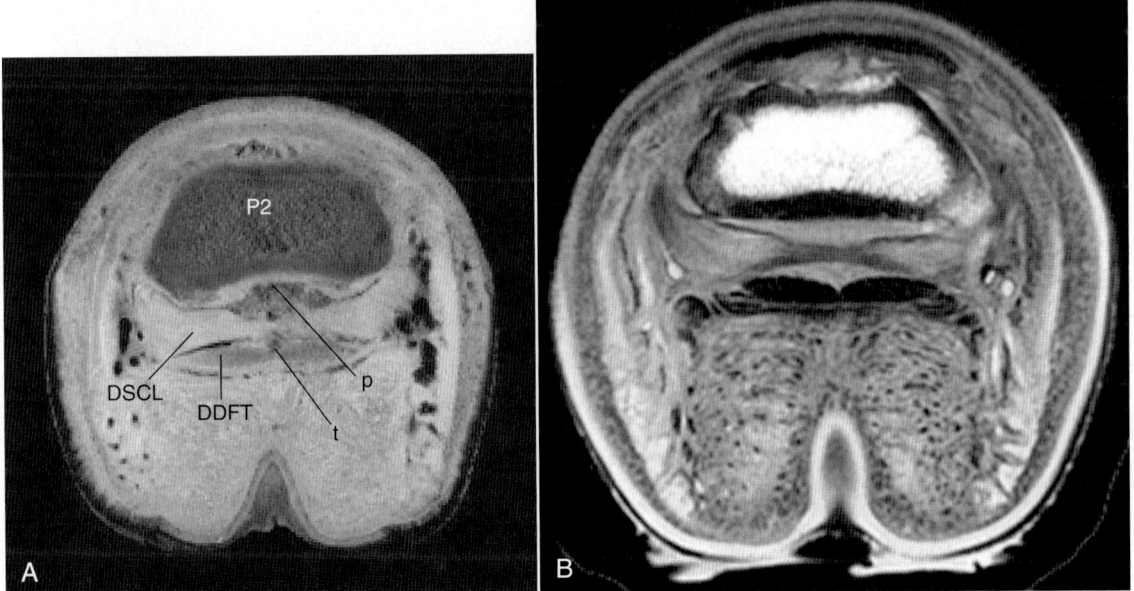

Fig. 9-15 • Transverse sections through the foot at the level of the distal sesamoidean collateral ligaments *(DSCL)*. **A,** Anatomical section showing the attachments of the DSCL to the deep digital flexor tendon *(DDFT)* marked at point *t*, and to the middle phalanx *(P2)* at point *p*. These attachments form the so-called "T ligament," which forms the boundaries between the navicular bursa, distal interphalangeal joint, and digital flexor tendon sheath. **B,** Corresponding magnetic resonance image. (Courtesy Alexia L. McKnight, University of Pennsylvania, Philadelphia, Pennsylvania, United States.)

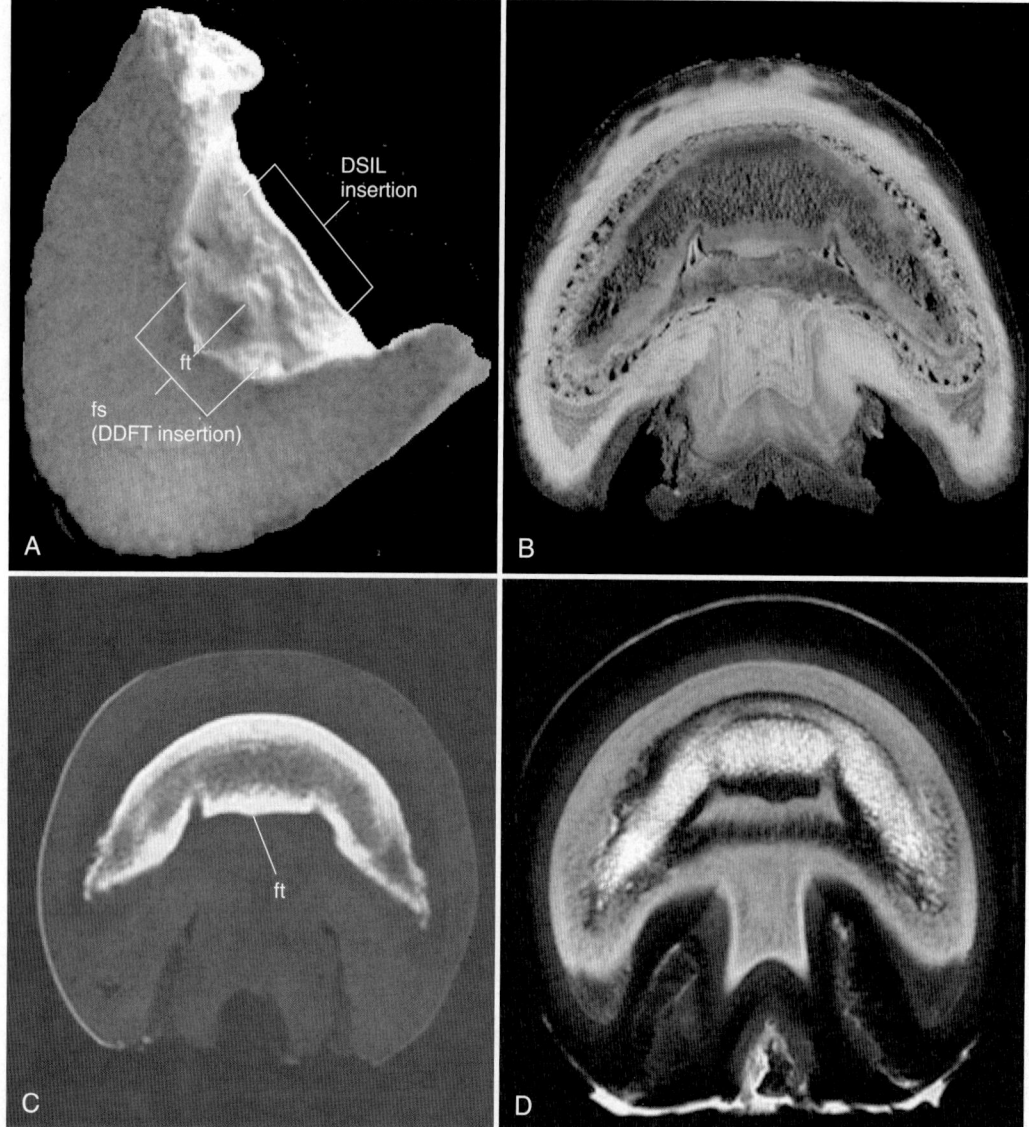

Fig. 9-16 • The insertions of the deep digital flexor tendon *(DDFT)* and distal sesamoidean impar ligament *(DSIL)*. **A,** Isolated distal phalanx solar view, showing the point of insertion of the DDFT on the flexor surface *(fs)*. The flexor tubercle (see *ft* in panel **C**) is relatively smaller than in other species but should be recognized as a normal structure as seen on computed tomographic (CT) imaging. **B,** Transverse anatomical section through the insertion of the DDFT. This slice is slightly distal to the site of insertion of the distal sesamoidean impar ligament. **C,** Transverse CT image showing a normal flexor tubercle *(ft)*. Avulsions here are difficult to demonstrate radiologically. Nuclear scintigraphy and ultrasonography can be helpful, but this area is best imaged using CT or magnetic resonance imaging (MRI). **D,** Transverse MRI scan. (**D** courtesy Alexia L. McKnight, University of Pennsylvania, Philadelphia, Pennsylvania, United States.)

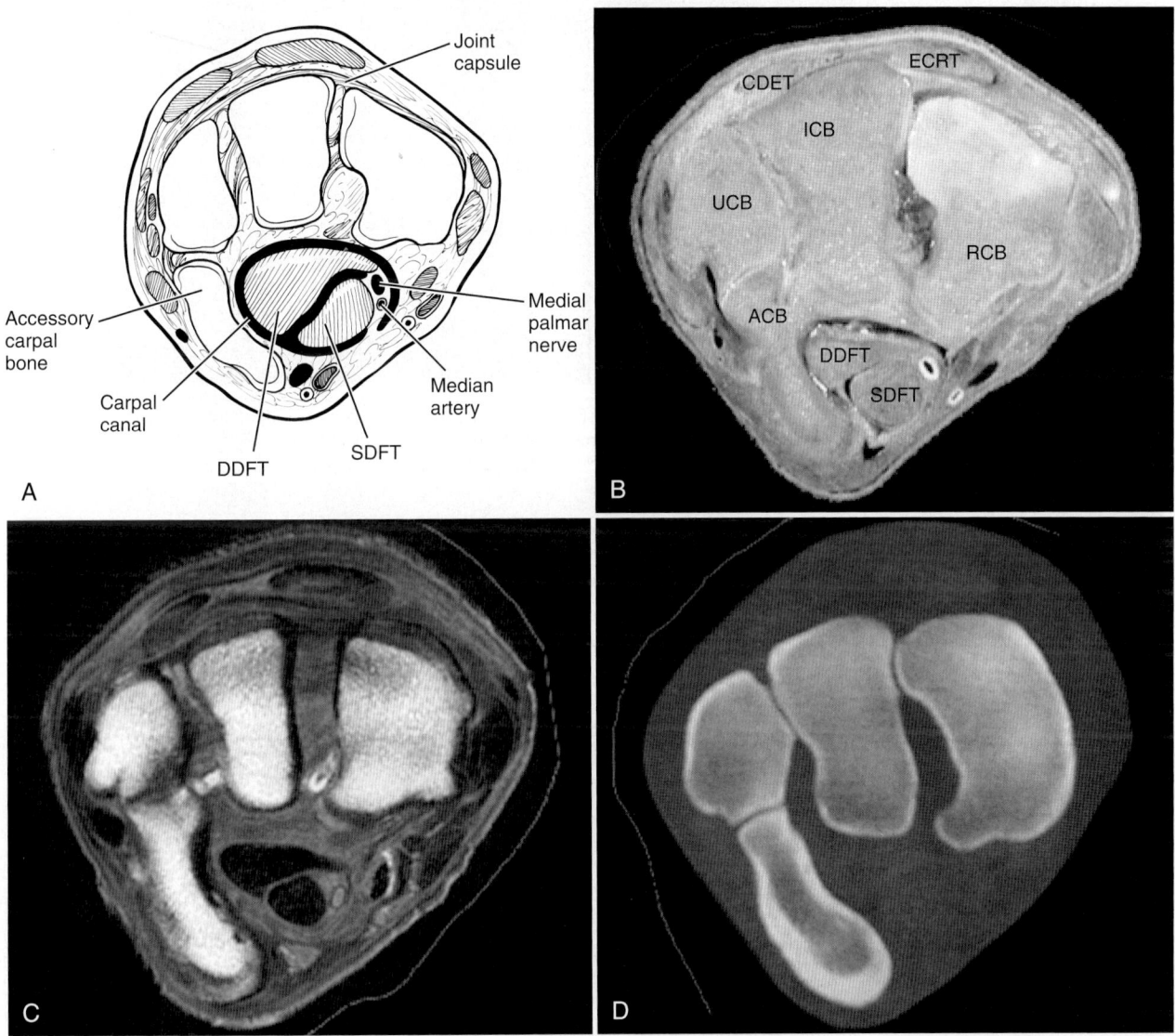

Fig. 9-17 • Transverse slices through the proximal row of carpal bones. All images are oriented with dorsal to the top and lateral to the left. **A,** Diagram of carpal bones. **B,** Anatomical section. **C,** Magnetic resonance imaging image. **D,** Computed tomographic image. *ACB,* Accessory carpal bone; *CDET,* common digital extensor tendon; *DDFT,* deep digital flexor tendon; *ECRT,* extensor carpi radialis tendon; *ICB* intermediate carpal bone; *RCB,* radial carpal bone; *SDFT,* superficial digital flexor tendon; *UCB,* ulnar carpal bone. (**C** Courtesy Alexia L McKnight, University of Pennsylvania, Philadelphia, Pennsylvania, United States.)

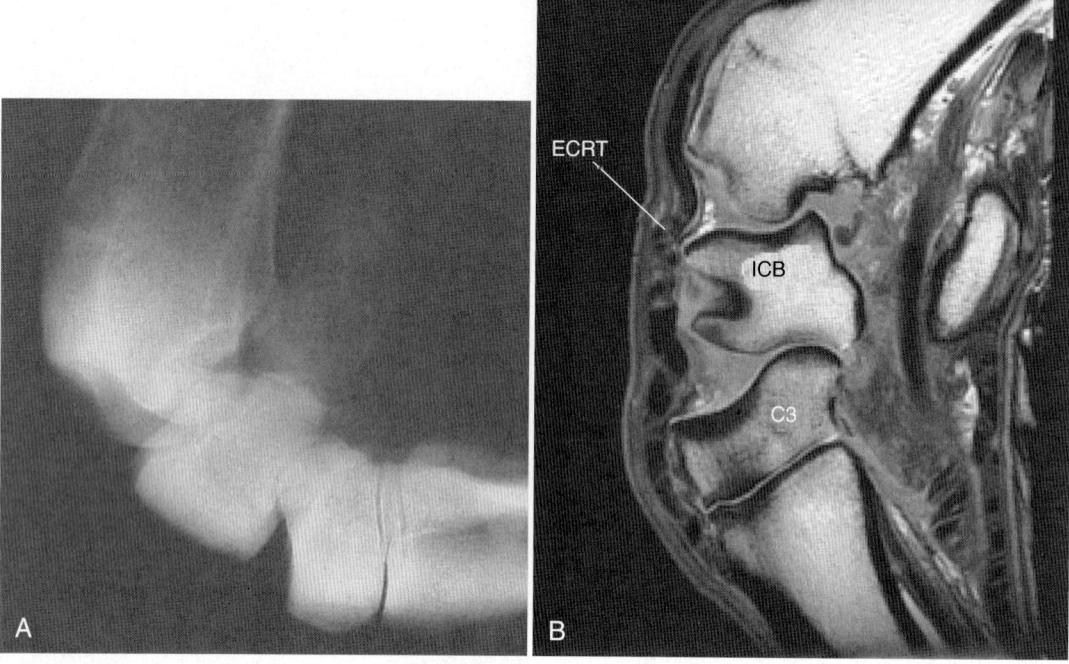

Fig. 9-18 • Lateral views of the carpus. Compare with Figure 9-1. **A,** Flexed lateromedial radiographic image. **B,** Flexed sagittal magnetic resonance imaging image through the extensor carpi radialis tendon *(ECRT). C3,* Third carpal bone; *ICB,* intermediate carpal bone. (Courtesy Alexia L McKnight, University of Pennsylvania, Philadelphia, Pennsylvania, United States.)

bone region, showing the close relationship between the collateral sesamoidean ligaments, the distal sesamoidean impar ligament, the DDFT, and the navicular bursa and distal interphalangeal joint capsule. Figures 9-17 and 9-18 demonstrate the relationship among some aspects of the complex anatomy of the carpal region.

Chapter 10

Diagnostic Analgesia

Lance H. Bassage II and Mike W. Ross

Despite the many technological advances in equine sports medicine over the past three decades, diagnostic analgesia arguably remains the most valuable tool in the equine clinician's arsenal to localize pain causing lameness. Although the technique requires a thorough understanding of anatomy, basic technical skill, and clinical experience, the equipment and expense are minimal. In addition, diagnostic analgesia can be performed on site, with the outcome immediately obvious. Any lingering concern that a suspected "shoulder problem" exists is convincingly erased when the response to perineural analgesia of the digit is observed. This chapter reviews the various perineural, intrasynovial, and local (regional) infiltration techniques for application of local analgesia in the diagnosis of lameness in horses.

LOCAL ANESTHETICS: PHARMACOLOGY AND TISSUE INTERACTIONS

Pain is transmitted specifically in the small, lightly myelinated, A delta and nonmyelinated C nerve fibers.[1] All commonly used local anesthetic solutions, regardless of the specific molecular structure, share the same basic mechanism of action—specifically, the ability to block or inhibit nociceptive nerve conduction by preventing the increase in membrane permeability to sodium ions.[2] These agents consist of a lipophilic and a hydrophilic group, connected by an intermediate chain containing a carbonyl group of an amide or ester linkage, and have traditionally been categorized as either amide- or ester-type local anesthetics.[3] Common local anesthetic solutions used in horses—2% solutions of lidocaine, mepivacaine, and bupivacaine—are of the amide type.

Compared with most local anesthetics, lidocaine and mepivacaine are considered relatively fast-acting and have a reported duration of action of 1½ to 3 hours and 2 to 3 hours, respectively. In contrast, bupivacaine is intermediate in onset but has a much longer duration of action (3 to 6 hours).[4] Bupivacaine is most suited for providing therapeutic rather than diagnostic analgesia. The results in

References on page 1257

clinical practice vary, because in *severely* lame horses the degree and duration of local analgesia are decreased, regardless of the agent used.

When local anesthetic solutions are injected, tissue damage can occur but is extremely rare.[3,4] Soft tissue swelling occurs occasionally and is likely caused by needle trauma or hematoma formation and not from a direct drug-tissue interaction. We suggest that alcohol and a clean wrap be applied to the injection sites when the diagnostic evaluation is complete to prevent or minimize swelling at injection sites. Cellulitis or other forms of infection are rare potential complications.

Acute synovitis, or *flare,* is a rare complication that can occur after intrasynovial (most commonly intraarticular) injection of local anesthetic solutions. Synovitis from intrasynovial injection of local anesthetic solution is much less common than from injection of other medications. Mepivacaine is thought to be less irritating than lidocaine when administered intraarticularly, but we have not recognized this difference.[3] However, Dyson reported that lidocaine may be considerably more irritating than mepivacaine, and clinical data documenting differences were used successfully in the licensing of mepivacaine in the United Kingdom.[5] Like cellulitis after perineural injections of local anesthetic solutions, infectious synovitis is a rare but possible sequela. To mitigate the possibility of contaminated solution, we use a new vial of local anesthetic solution when performing intrasynovial analgesic procedures.

Systemic side effects from diagnostic analgesic techniques are exceedingly rare. Cardiovascular or central nervous system signs, including muscle fasciculation, ataxia, and collapse, were reported.[3] Systemic intoxication would require a dose much higher than is commonly used, even for an extensive diagnostic evaluation. For example, the maximum single infiltration dose of lidocaine that can be safely administered to a 500-kg horse is about 6.0 g, or 300 mL of a 2% solution.[6]

Strategy, Methodology, and Other Considerations

A few basic principles must be followed to ensure success. A thorough working knowledge of regional anatomy is required. Even for seasoned veterans a review of anatomy may be required before less common techniques are performed. A most important principle when performing perineural analgesia is to *start distally in the limb and work proximally* (Figures 10-1 to 10-4). If possible, sequential blocks from distal to proximal should always be used, but in certain circumstances a different strategy can be successful. Sequential blocking requires a fair amount of time, and in certain horses, selective intraarticular or local blocks can be performed without following this "golden rule." However, in most situations, blocking a large portion of the distal limb at a proximally located site may preclude accurate determination of the source of pain causing lameness and may require an additional visit to perform additional diagnostic procedures.

It is important to test the efficacy of a perineural block before reevaluating the horse's degree of lameness. If any question exists, the block should be repeated rather than assuming deep pain has been abolished, when skin sensitivity persists. If a horse shows *partial* improvement only minutes after injection, an additional few minutes should be allowed for complete analgesia to be achieved before proceeding with the next block. Alternatively, the block can be repeated. In so doing, the clinician minimizes the potential for misinterpretation and the tendency to ascribe the residual lameness to a "second problem" that does not exist.

During this portion of the examination, we are attempting to eliminate baseline rather than induced lameness, and care must be taken when adopting the practice of "blocking out a positive flexion test" (see Chapter 8). Once baseline lameness has been eliminated, we rarely perform additional flexion tests or attempt to eliminate all induced lameness.

How is the efficacy of the block assessed? Several methods are available, but the following points should be considered. Individual horses react differently to noxious stimuli applied to the skin. Therefore it is helpful to test the contralateral (unblocked) limb to establish the horse's baseline response to the test. Similarly, covering a horse's eye or feigning a few gestures with an instrument (pen tip, hemostatic forceps) without actually contacting the skin can help differentiate between a random or anticipatory response by an apprehensive horse and a true painful response. Positioning oneself on the contralateral side of the horse when testing for sensation also can help in making this determination. The clinician should avoid using sharp instruments that can penetrate the skin and cause hemorrhage, a situation not well understood by a concerned horse owner. Hemostatic forceps, used to pinch the skin, are ideal, because they are blunt and appear to consistently induce an appropriate amount of pain. Forceps are only useful in assessing superficial or skin sensation, however.

Perineural blocks must be assessed for the amelioration of deep and not just superficial pain. To assess whether deep pain in the hoof has been ameliorated after palmar digital analgesia or other techniques, hoof testers can usually be applied with enough force to cause a painful response, even in the most stoic of horses. Physical strength of the operator must be considered. Extreme or hard joint flexion (combined with varus or valgus stress) can be used to assess whether deep pain has been abolished in more proximal locations. In some instances, however, it is impossible to avoid contacting the skin proximal to the site of local anesthetic administration, leading the clinician to assume that the block has not worked. The application of firm digital pressure in the blocked area may be a viable alternative to flexion or manipulation to help avoid these potentially confounding factors.

It is important to understand that the region of the limb that is *actually* desensitized may, in fact, differ from the region the clinician *intended* to desensitize.[7] Proximal diffusion of local anesthetic solution appears to be the most likely cause, but other, intangible factors may play a role. Using a small volume of local anesthetic solution (1 to 5 mL for most perineural blocks) can minimize but not abolish this phenomenon. To further minimize the potential for diffusion of local anesthetic solution, the horse should be reevaluated no more than 10 minutes after the injection (exceptions apply in certain situations). A recent study using 2 mL of radiopaque contrast medium injected perineurally around the palmar nerves at the level of the proximal sesamoid bones demonstrated proximal diffusion extending 2 to 3 cm within 10 minutes of injection, irrespective of whether horses stood still or walked.[8]

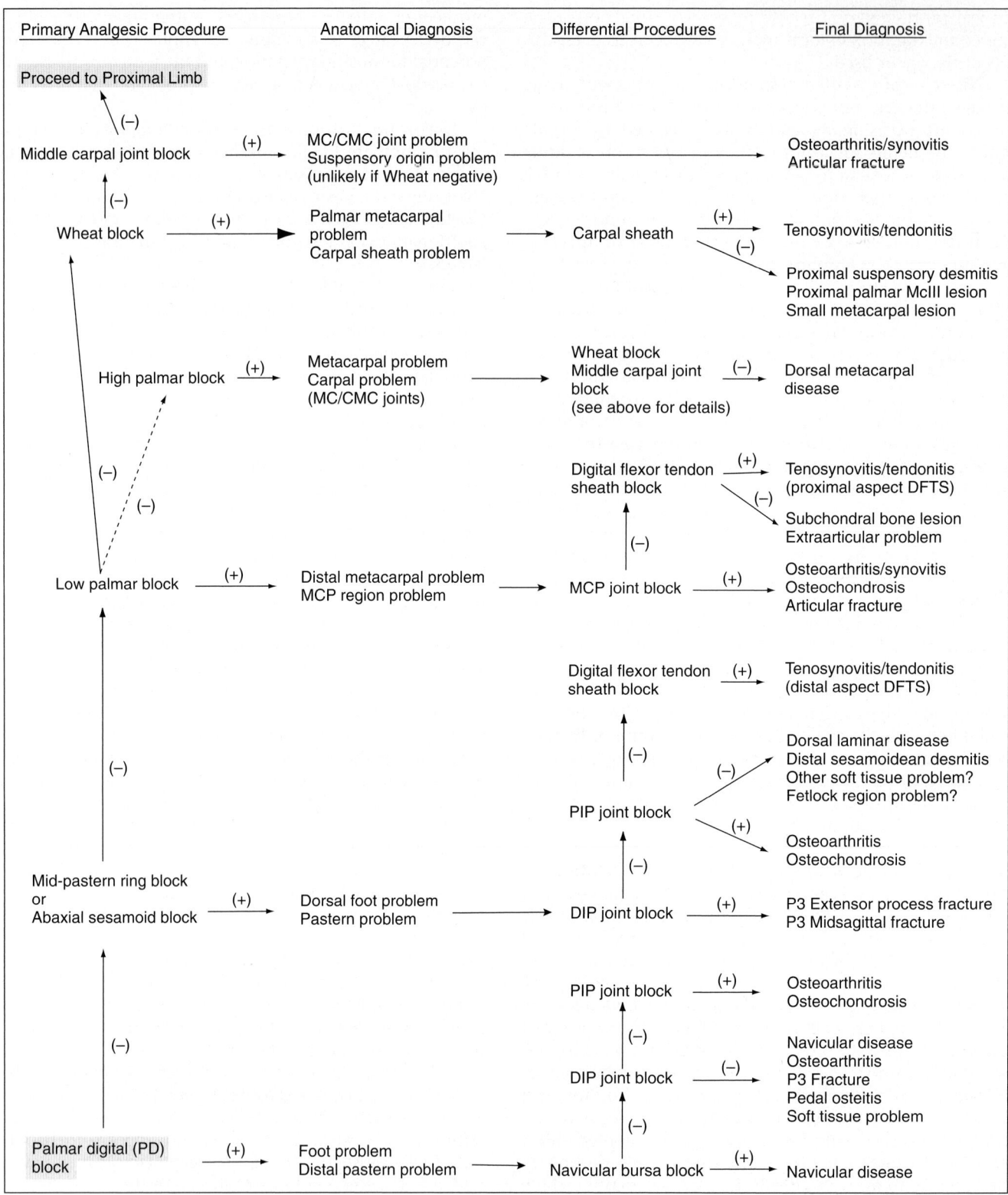

Fig. 10-1 • Blocking strategy in the forelimb: foot to carpus. *CMC,* Carpometacarpal; *DFTS,* digital flexor tendon sheath; *MC,* middle carpal; *McIII,* third metacarpal bone; *MCP,* metacarpophalangeal; *P3,* distal phalanx; *PIP,* proximal interphalangeal.

Complete analgesia, and thus 100% improvement in lameness score, is the goal when performing diagnostic analgesia, but in many horses this level of pain relief is never achieved. Improvement in degree of lameness greater than 70% to 80% after most perineural or intraarticular techniques should be considered a positive response in most horses. The quintessential response is that the horse "switches lameness" to the contralateral limb, indicating that now pain arising from the opposite limb is greater than the pain that caused the baseline lameness. However,

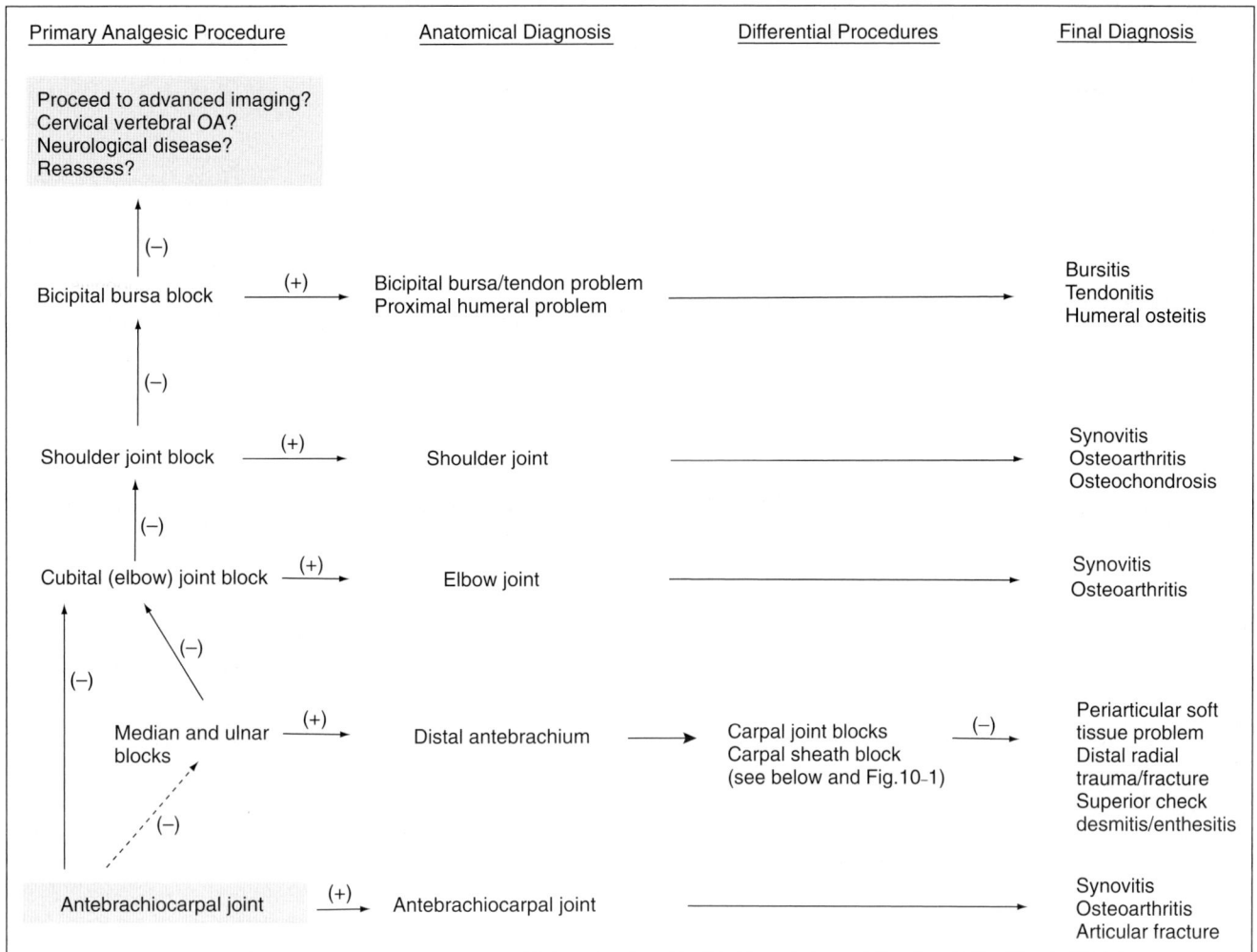

Fig. 10-2 • Blocking strategy in the forelimb: antebrachium to shoulder joint. *OA*, Osteoarthritis.

complete response may not occur, and the clinician must decide when to stop sequential blocks or when the horse has "blocked out." The clinician hopes for an obvious difference in lameness score when the horse is blocked, but in some horses, serial improvement occurs with each successive block, a situation that makes assessing the primary source of pain difficult.

Incomplete response to local analgesia in some horses may be explained by the fact that chronic pain, particularly deep bone pain, may remain resistant to complete analgesia when perineural techniques are used. For example, horses with laminitis tend to remain lame despite blocking many times at the appropriate level, probably because of neuropathic pain.[9] Mechanical gait deficits do not improve after diagnostic analgesia because pain is minimal. Horses may continue to show lameness even with pain abolition, a situation that appears to be caused by habit. These horses tend to show mild residual lameness initially, only to warm out of it quickly during examination. Other factors affecting response to diagnostic analgesia include individual variation in neuroanatomy, the intermittent nature of certain lameness conditions, and the inherent difficulty in assessing and abolishing pain in horses with subtle lameness.[10] Articular and subchondral bone lesions may not be desensitized by

intraarticular analgesia, and pain may be more effectively abolished using perineural techniques.

Sensory innervation of joints is complex and involves three classes of neurons that transmit information from four receptor types, each of which has a specific distribution throughout the joint.[11-13] Articular pain can arise from several sources, including the synovium (inflammation, effusion), fibrous joint capsule (increased intraarticular pressure), articular and periarticular ligaments, periosteum, and subchondral bone (injury, osseous vascular engorgement).[10,12,14,15] Other than small branches in the perichondrium, articular cartilage is devoid of innervation. In osteoarthritic joints, however, erosion channels, formed in the calcified layer of cartilage, are invaded by subchondral vasculature.[12] Putative nociceptive neurotransmitters were identified in these areas, and therefore it is plausible that in horses with advanced osteoarthritis, pain could be emanating from the deep cartilage layers.[16,17]

On occasion, lameness from an articular lesion abates after perineural analgesia but shows minimal or only partial response after intraarticular analgesia. In some horses, this can be explained by the fact that pain is originating from articular and periarticular tissues.[8] Subchondral bone pain—caused by maladaptive bone remodeling, cystic or erosive lesions, incomplete fractures, and

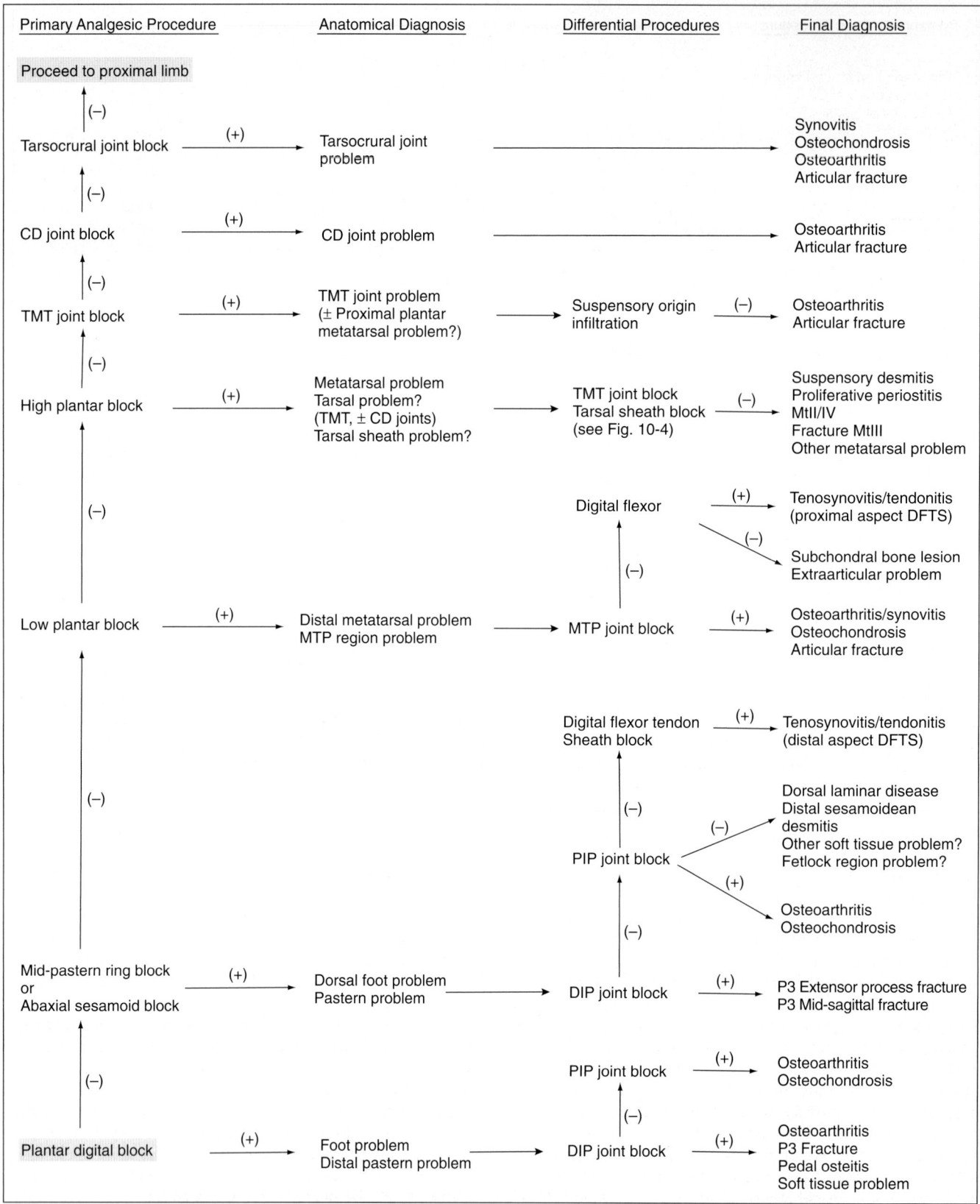

Fig. 10-3 • Blocking strategy in the hindlimb: foot to hock joint. *CD,* Centrodistal; *DFTS,* digital flexor tendon sheath; *DIP,* distal interphalangeal; *MtII, MtIII, MtIV,* second, third, and fourth metatarsal bones, respectively; *MTP,* metatarso-phalangeal; *P3,* proximal phalanx; *PIP,* proximal interphalangeal; *TMT,* tarsometatarsal.

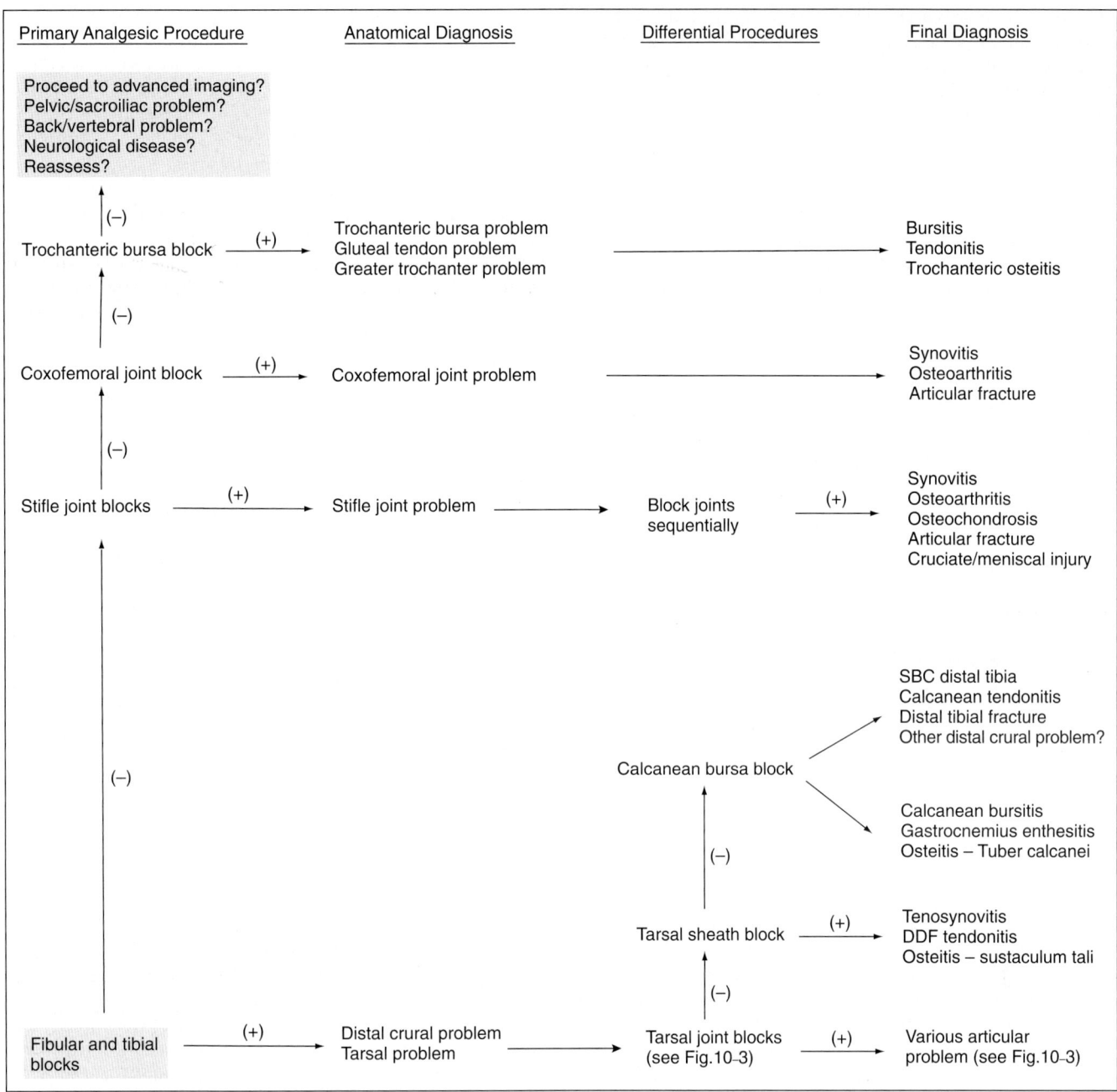

Primary Analgesic Procedure   Anatomical Diagnosis   Differential Procedures   Final Diagnosis

Proceed to advanced imaging?
Pelvic/sacroiliac problem?
Back/vertebral problem?
Neurological disease?
Reassess?

(−)

Trochanteric bursa block — (+) → Trochanteric bursa problem / Gluteal tendon problem / Greater trochanter problem → Bursitis / Tendonitis / Trochanteric osteitis

(−)

Coxofemoral joint block — (+) → Coxofemoral joint problem → Synovitis / Osteoarthritis / Articular fracture

(−)

Stifle joint blocks — (+) → Stifle joint problem → Block joints sequentially — (+) → Synovitis / Osteoarthritis / Osteochondrosis / Articular fracture / Cruciate/meniscal injury

Calcanean bursa block → SBC distal tibia / Calcanean tendonitis / Distal tibial fracture / Other distal crural problem? ↘ Calcanean bursitis / Gastrocnemius enthesitis / Osteitis – Tuber calcanei

(−)

Tarsal sheath block — (+) → Tenosynovitis / DDF tendonitis / Osteitis – sustaculum tali

(−)

(−)

Fibular and tibial blocks — (+) → Distal crural problem / Tarsal problem → Tarsal joint blocks (see Fig.10-3) — (+) → Various articular problem (see Fig.10-3)

Fig. 10-4 • Blocking strategy in the hindlimb: crus to coxofemoral joint. *DDF,* Deep digital flexor; *SBC,* subchondral bone cyst.

osteoarthritis—is inconsistently abolished by intraarticular analgesia. In fact, subchondral bone pain is abolished much more consistently by perineural techniques. Subchondral bone receives innervation from endosteal branches of peripheral nerves that enter the medullary cavity through the nutrient foramen.[10,11,18,19] Intraarticularly administered local anesthetic solutions may not penetrate subchondral bone sufficiently to completely block these nerves. This shortcoming is presumably even more likely in situations in which the cartilage is intact.

Unfortunately, intraarticular analgesia, although easier to perform, inconsistently abolishes pain from many of the common articular problems. This fact, however, is either overlooked or misunderstood by many practitioners.

Whenever possible, perineural analgesia should be performed, particularly in the distal aspect of the limbs, because this type of analgesia more consistently abolishes pain from all aspects of the joint and surrounding soft tissue structures.

Lameness Is Worse after Diagnostic Analgesia

Two uncommon situations arise when performing diagnostic analgesia. The first occurs during a blocking session. After performing palmar digital analgesia in a horse with forelimb lameness, lameness score may worsen by one or two grades. In fact, lameness may occasionally be considerably worse, prompting concern by the lameness diagnostician. Why? This unusual response occurs most commonly in horses with proximal, palmar metacarpal pain caused by proximal suspensory desmitis, avulsion fracture of the proximal palmar aspect of the third metacarpal bone (McIII), or proximally located superficial digital flexor tendonitis. Horses normally shorten the cranial phase of the stride to protect a source of pain, a common response by any lame horse. We reason that after palmar digital analgesia a lack of proprioception in the digit prompts the horse to take a somewhat longer stride, increasing the cranial phase. Compared with before the block an exaggerated load causes the horse to display a higher lameness score. Temporary exacerbation of lameness after palmar digital analgesia can be a useful characteristic to help determine the genuine source of pain.

The second situation is more ominous. A horse will occasionally be very lame, sometimes non–weight bearing, once a block wears off. This unusual, but important and sometimes difficult situation occurs when incomplete fractures become separated, displaced, or comminuted. Horses with fractures of the distal phalanx that are incomplete or have healed partially by a fibrous union or those with incomplete fractures of the proximal phalanx appear most at risk. Horses at risk are candidates for imaging before blocking, but in some this complication is unforeseen (see following discussion).

Perception of Diagnostic Analgesia by Laypersons

One of the intangible factors that can complicate the lameness examination is the layperson's perception of diagnostic analgesia or nerve blocking. In many instances the opportunity for an owner or trainer to observe the outcome of diagnostic analgesia provides the concrete evidence that finally convinces him or her of the diagnosis. The classic example is the suspected acute shoulder injury that is actually chronic navicular disease. However, for many reasons, misunderstanding about diagnostic analgesia can lead to frustration for everyone involved. Many laypersons are not fully able to recognize the baseline lameness and therefore may not be capable of seeing that the horse's lameness improves after the block. Another difficulty is trying to explain why lameness in a horse with an articular problem is better after a perineural block but no better when local anesthetic solution is placed directly into a joint. Similarly, many laypersons do not understand why a horse with an articular lameness may "block sound" but does not respond satisfactorily to therapeutic injection. This finding that a horse blocks sound but does not "inject sound" is quite common in young racehorses with subchondral bone pain. Most experienced practitioners have learned to deal with these issues, but the new graduate may need fortitude and ingenuity when explaining the results of diagnostic analgesia.

Role of Chemical Restraint

Whenever possible, use of physical (nose or shoulder twitch) rather than chemical restraint is best when diagnostic analgesia is performed. This is particularly important in horses with low-grade lameness. The analgesic properties of α_2-agonists (e.g., xylazine, detomidine) and synthetic opiates (e.g., butorphanol) are well recognized and may lead to false-positive results. Ataxia after sedation can complicate lameness interpretation. However, in some horses mild sedation or tranquilization may be necessary for performance of diagnostic analgesia and may improve the clinician's ability to evaluate the baseline lameness. Acetylpromazine (0.02 to 0.04 mg/kg intravenously) can calm a highly strung horse and facilitate the lameness examination. Extra care must be taken when performing hindlimb procedures, and the safety of everyone involved and the horse must be considered. In horses with moderate or severe lameness, xylazine (0.15 to 0.30 mg/kg intravenously) may not interfere appreciably with lameness interpretation. Similarly, extremely fractious horses can be sedated with an α_2-agonist, which then is reversed with the prescribed α_2-antagonist (e.g., yohimbine) before reevaluation. Alternatively, sedation can simply be allowed to wear off before the horse is evaluated, but diffusion of local anesthetic solution may occur or the effect may wear off, both of which may potentially cause misinterpretation of results.

Horse Preparation

Before perineural analgesia is performed, the skin and hair should be cleaned of any gross debris such as mud, bedding, feces, or poultice. Clipping usually is not necessary unless the hair coat is long and prohibits accurate palpation of anatomical landmarks or adequate cleaning of the site. The site should then be scrubbed with an antiseptic, such as povidone-iodine or chlorhexidine, using clean gauze sponges or cotton. If the clinician has any concern about inadvertent penetration of a synovial cavity, a 5-minute aseptic preparation should be performed. This is followed by isopropyl alcohol administration over the site using cotton or gauze sponges.

Aseptic preparation should always be performed before any intrasynovial injection. Considerable debate and variation exists among clinicians regarding the need to clip the hair over the site. Some clinicians always clip the hair, whereas others never do. Still others shave the hair in a small area directly over the injection site. The results of a study indicated no significant difference in the number of postscrub colony-forming units (bacterial flora) between clipped and unclipped skin over the distal interphalangeal (DIP) and carpal joints.[20] Nonetheless, we still clip the hair over all proposed intrasynovial injection sites before undertaking a 5-minute aseptic preparation. The only time we deviate from this policy is when we are specifically asked not to clip the hair, a situation that arises in some sports horses actively competing, in claiming horses, or in those being sold.

Similar variation among clinicians exists regarding wearing of sterile latex gloves when performing an intrasynovial injection. However, we recommend wearing sterile gloves during these procedures. Science aside, clipping hair and wearing sterile gloves project a positive impression to all in attendance.

How does, or should, the practitioner attempt perineural or intrasynovial analgesia in a horse with contact or chemical dermatitis (scurf) over the proposed injection site? A superficial wound or abrasion with a localized infection presents a similar quandary. For obvious reasons, these areas are difficult, if not impossible, to clean effectively. If possible, an alternative site, away from the area of dermatitis, should be used. If not, then the procedure should be delayed until the skin condition (or wound) has resolved. In many instances, dermatitis can be treated with topical medications (medicated sweats such as nitrofurazone-dimethylsulfoxide) for a few days to facilitate resolution of the problem.

Injection Techniques

Perineural injections are typically performed using needles ranging in size from 25 gauge, 1.6 cm (⅝ inch) to 20 gauge, 2.5 or 4 cm (1 to 1½ inches). Small needles cause less pain but carry the risk of breaking off within tissues if the horse kicks out or otherwise misbehaves. For this reason, we recommend using 18- or 19-gauge needles for injections or blocks within the proximal metatarsal or plantar tarsal regions. In the distal aspect of the limb the needle is inserted subcutaneously directly over and parallel to the nerve. We generally direct the needle proximally rather than distally, although this portion of the procedure differs among clinicians. One of the Editors (SJD) always inserts the needle distally; if a fractious horse throws the limb to the ground the needle is more likely to stay in situ, and the remainder of the procedure may be completed with the limb on the ground. Directing the needle distally also ensures more distal placement of the local anesthetic solution, which may be important at distal sites. The needle is inserted before the syringe is attached. To avoid excessive manipulation once the needle is inserted, a slip-type syringe hub is preferred. Syringes with screw-on hubs can be difficult to attach, requiring additional manipulation in a sometimes fractious horse, and are not generally used. However, when dense tissue requires that additional force be used for injection, the seal between the hub and the needle can be broken, a complication minimized by using a screw-on hub (see the following discussion of lateral palmar block).

Volume of local anesthetic solution varies, but for a majority of blocks in the distal limb, 1 to 5 mL is injected at each site. Larger volumes are used to perform the median and ulnar or fibular (peroneal) and tibial techniques and when infiltrating the proximal palmar (plantar) metacarpal (metatarsal) region. After injection, we briefly massage the sites with gauze sponges or clean cotton soaked in alcohol. Skin sensation and deep pain are assessed 5 to 10 minutes after injection. More time is allowed under certain circumstances (see specific comments throughout the chapter). At the completion of the examination an alcohol wrap should be applied to minimize swelling, a common sequela resulting from local irritation and bleeding from nearby vessels.

For "ring" blocks, circumferential subcutaneous infiltration of local anesthetic solution, and other local or regional infiltration techniques, we most commonly use 20- to 22-gauge, 4-cm needles. For performance of a ring block, the needle is inserted perpendicular to the long axis of the limb, and local anesthetic solution is injected as the needle is advanced, leaving a clearly visible wheal or subcutaneous bleb in most locations. The needle then is reinserted at the leading edge of this wheal, a practice that minimizes the number of injections and the horse's discomfort. However, most horses object to needle insertion even when it is performed well within the bleb. The injection is continued around the limb in this manner. For most ring blocks in the distal limb, 10 to 15 mL of local anesthetic solution is used, but larger volumes may be preferred for surgical procedures. Ring blocks can be done as a

substitute for or in combination with perineural injections (see the specific blocking techniques discussed in the chapter). However, simply placing local anesthetic solution in a subcutaneous location is not a substitute for the preferred approach, direct perineural injection.

To block a local area such as a splint or curb, the needle is typically inserted in one or two locations, and local anesthetic solution is deposited in a fan-shaped pattern. As with the perineural analgesia, the sites are massaged briefly and the horse is reevaluated in 5 to 10 minutes.

Intrasynovial injections typically are performed using needles ranging in size from 22 gauge, 2.5 cm to 18 gauge, 4 cm. If marked effusion is present, drainage of synovial fluid is advised, either by allowing the fluid to drip from the hub of the needle or by aspirating with a sterile syringe before proceeding with injection. We prefer the former procedure unless fluid analysis is necessary. The manipulation required to attach the syringe may cause the horse discomfort and potentially dislodge the needle but if successful may hasten withdrawal of synovial fluid. Brief evaluation of the color and viscosity of synovial fluid can shed some light on the disease process within and is expected practice among most racehorse trainers. Volume of local anesthetic solution varies considerably between synovial cavities, but the clinician should keep in mind that small volumes might contribute to a false-negative result. False-negative results are common in horses with severe osteoarthritis, and larger volumes of local anesthetic solution should be used. We routinely spray or wipe antiseptic solution over the injection site. After the examination a light bandage is applied over the injection sites from the metacarpophalangeal or metatarsophalangeal joint, distally. Initial reevaluation is done 5 to 10 minutes after injection. Additional evaluations may be necessary depending on the response during the initial time period. General practice is to have the horse walked in hand or with a rider after perineural or intrasynovial analgesia is administered, a procedure thought to hasten distribution of local anesthetic solution and potentially improve success. Excessive diffusion of local anesthetic solution is a potential drawback to this practice, particularly with techniques such as DIP or middle carpal analgesia (see the following discussion), although it would be a complication difficult to quantify.

Another issue to consider when performing diagnostic analgesia is whether riding or driving a horse after blocks have been performed is safe. In general, riding on the flat or driving a horse at slow speed after any of the common blocks have been performed is safe. Stumbling or knuckling can be a concern after upper limb perineural techniques, such as the median and ulnar and fibular (peroneal) and tibial techniques. Common sense should prevail, however, with regard to the horse and rider negotiating fences or performing at high speed. Horses at risk for lameness from stress or incomplete fracture are candidates for imaging before evaluation at speed after diagnostic analgesic techniques have been performed. Moreover, horses suspected of having incomplete fractures but with negative or equivocal radiological findings may best be managed conservatively without use of analgesic techniques and should undergo either follow-up radiographic examination in 10 to 14 days or scintigraphic examination.

PERINEURAL ANALGESIA IN THE FORELIMB

Palmar Digital Analgesia

Palmar digital analgesia (or palmar digital block) is the most common diagnostic analgesic procedure performed. The medial and lateral digital neurovascular bundles, consisting, in a dorsal to palmar direction, of the digital vein, artery, and nerve, course in an abaxial location to the digital flexor tendons. With the exception of small breeds or draft horses with remarkably long-haired pasterns (feathers), the palmar digital nerve is easily palpable between the proximal sesamoid bones and the cartilages of the foot. The palmar digital block can be performed with the horse in a standing position or with the limb held off the ground. We prefer the latter. If held by an assistant, the limb should be grasped in the midmetacarpal region, with the fetlock and digit hanging in neutral position. The palmar digital nerve is easily palpated in this extended position on the lateral aspect of the deep digital flexor tendon (DDFT). Alternatively, the clinician performing the block can hold the limb, a technique that requires practice. The clinician can stand facing backward with a hand grasping the midpastern region or can stand behind the limb and clutch the hoof between both legs.

A 25-gauge, 1.6-cm needle is inserted subcutaneously, directly over the nerve, just proximal to the cartilages of the foot (Figure 10-5). One of us (LHB) directs the needle in a distal direction, whereas the other (MWR) directs the needle in a proximal direction to avoid deeper penetration or laceration of digital vessels if the horse withdraws the limb. Alternatively, a 22-gauge, 4-cm needle can be inserted on the palmar midline in the midpastern region, and local anesthetic solution is then infiltrated in a V-shaped pattern. This modification of the palmar digital block is quite difficult to perform in the hindlimb but when done in the forelimb provides maximal analgesia to the bulbs of the heel and minimizes the potential for depositing local anesthetic solution dorsal to the nerve. Loss of skin sensation in the midline between the bulbs of the heels should be assessed, because this area seems most recalcitrant to palmar digital analgesia. Deep pain is assessed using hoof testers. However, if skin sensation persists, it is still worth reevaluating lameness, because in some horses deep pain and lameness may be abolished despite the persistence of skin sensation.

Traditionally the palmar digital block was felt consistently to desensitize only the palmar (plantar) one third to one half of the foot.[21] However, in clinical practice, this block desensitizes 70% to 80% of the foot. Most of the DIP joint is affected, with the exception of the proximodorsal aspect. Horses with fractures of the extensor process of the distal phalanx or injury of a collateral ligament of the DIP joint may show partial improvement after palmar digital analgesia, however. Our clinical observations have been substantiated in a recent study. Setscrews were placed near the medial and lateral aspects of the toe to simulate pain from the sole. Lameness in these horses was abolished using palmar digital analgesia performed just proximal to the heel bulbs.[22]

Classically, most horses that responded positively to palmar digital analgesia were thought to have navicular syndrome, but this block desensitizes many lameness conditions within and outside the hoof capsule (Table 10-1).

This is an important and common misconception. Lameness in horses with proximal interphalangeal joint pain, midsagittal fracture of the proximal phalanx, or other conditions involving the fetlock joints can be abolished using palmar digital analgesia.[7,23] Although using small volumes of local anesthetic solution and performing the block just above the cartilages of the foot may help to minimize the area of analgesia, these procedures do not prevent inadvertent diagnosis in some horses. Diffusion of local anesthetic solution is the most likely explanation, and even a small volume can readily spread in a proximal direction, but the normal anatomy of the digit prevents distal placement of local anesthetic solution (Figure 10-6).

The concept that palmar digital analgesia abolishes lameness in an area considerably more than the palmar (plantar) one third of the foot appears to be difficult for many to accept. Although results of studies are widely published and this finding has been emphasized at international meetings, most veterinary students still graduate today armed with this common misconception. Diffusion of local anesthetic solution easily explains why lameness conditions in the proximal aspect of the pastern or fetlock regions are desensitized by palmar digital analgesia. But what about the innervation of the hoof itself? Skeptics should consider the anatomy of the palmar digital nerve. Most practitioners have severed the palmar digital nerve while performing neurectomy. Can the clinicians recall any instance of having identified a large dorsal branch, or for that matter, any branching of the nerve at all? The lack of nerve branches in the midpastern region is circumstantial evidence that important innervation to the structures located dorsally within the hoof capsule occurs farther proximally (ill-defined dorsal branches) or after the nerve courses deep to the cartilages of the foot. It makes little sense that ill-defined dorsal branches would innervate the dorsal two thirds of the foot, leaving the robust palmar digital nerve to innervate only the palmar one third. When carefully dissected the palmar digital nerves can be seen branching extensively deep to the cartilages of the foot, sending branches dorsally to innervate the dorsal portions of the foot.

Accurately quantifying the contribution of the palmar digital nerve to the innervation of the foot or, for that matter, the exact percentage of structures desensitized by palmar digital analgesia may be impossible. Clinical experience will undoubtedly convince practitioners of the broad nature of palmar digital analgesia. Finally, it is imperative to develop expertise in diagnostic imaging of the entire digit, because the many lameness conditions affected by palmar digital analgesia require detective-like differential diagnostic skills.

Midpastern Ring Block

Traditionally the diagnostic blocks performed after palmar digital analgesia are the basisesamoid or abaxial sesamoid techniques. The basisesamoid block provides little additional information compared with palmar digital analgesia, unless, of course, the dorsal branch, originating from the digital nerve at the level of the proximal sesamoid bones, is blocked. If, however, the dorsal branch is blocked, then the basisesamoid block is in reality an abaxial sesamoid block. For this reason, we rarely perform the basisesamoid block. When performing the abaxial sesamoid

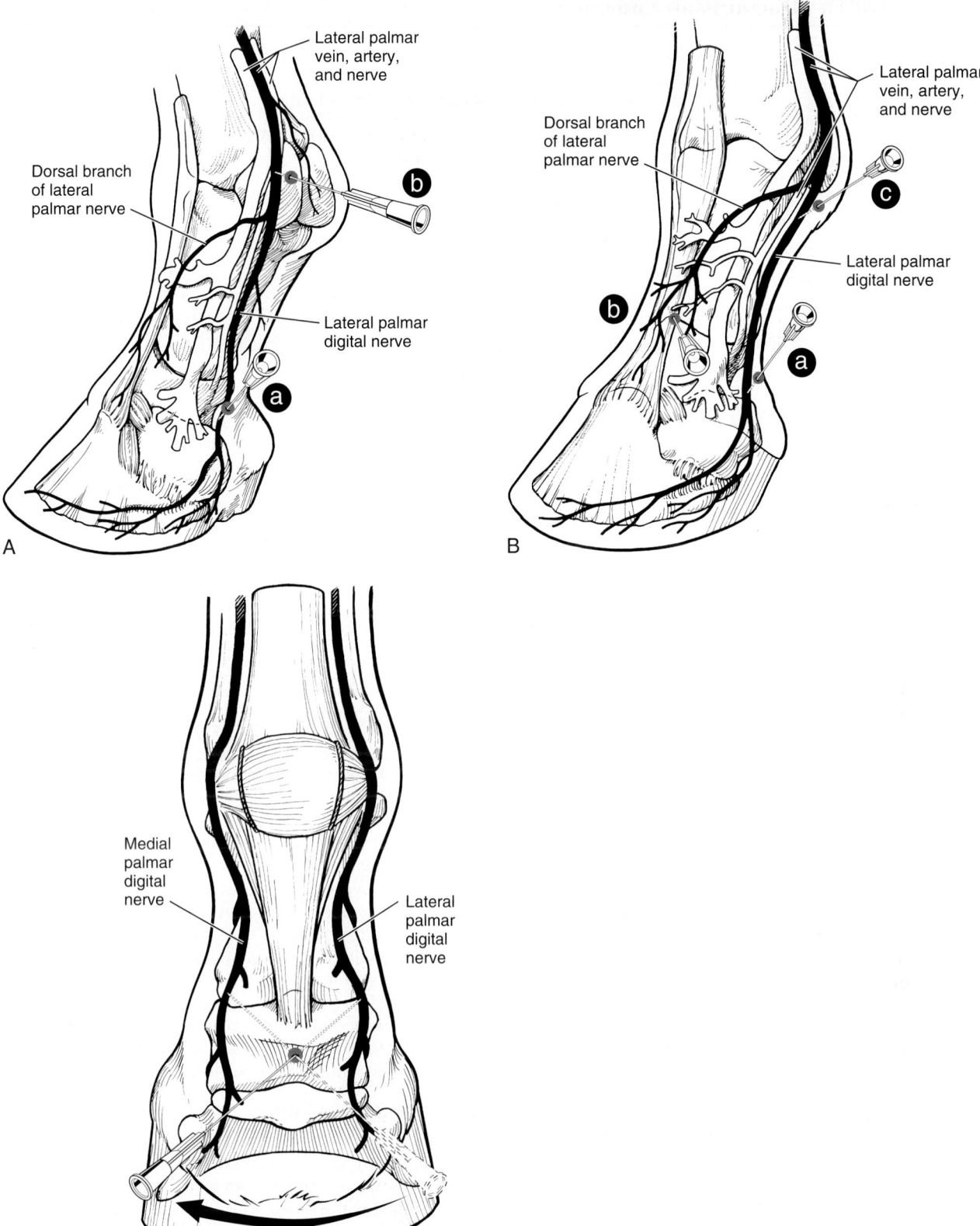

Fig. 10-5 • A, Palmarolateral view of the distal aspect of the limb showing site for needle penetration for palmar (plantar) digital analgesia *(a)*. The clinician directs the needle as shown or in a proximal direction. The palmar (plantar) digital nerve is blocked more proximally at the level of the abaxial surface of the proximal sesamoid bone *(b)*. At this level the palmar (plantar) digital nerves and dorsal branches are both blocked. **B,** Dorsolateral view of the distal aspect of the limb demonstrating needle positions for palmar (plantar) digital analgesia *(a)* with an additional dorsally directed subcutaneous ring block to desensitize the dorsal aspect of the pastern region and foot *(b)*. A block at the base of the proximal sesamoid bone *(c)* likely desensitizes the palmar (plantar) digital nerves and dorsal branches of the digital nerve (note close association of both branches to the site of the block) and provides the same region of analgesia as does the palmar digital block with the dorsal ring, or the abaxial sesamoid block. **C,** Alternative technique used for the palmar digital nerve block. The clinician inserts the needle on the palmar midline and places a line of local anesthetic solution in a proximal dorsal direction to the level of each of the medial and lateral palmar nerves in an approximately V-shaped pattern. This technique confines local anesthetic solution to the palmar aspect of the limb. This blocking technique is difficult to perform in the hindlimb.

TABLE 10-1

		Differential Diagnostic Analgesia of the Equine Foot	
DISEASE	PALMAR DIGITAL NERVE BLOCK	DISTAL INTERPHALANGEAL JOINT BLOCK	NAVICULAR BURSA BLOCK
Navicular disease	+	±	+
Synovitis DIP joint	+	+	+
Osteoarthritis DIP joint	+	+	+
Subchondral bone DIP joint	+	±	±
P3 fracture (wing)	+	+	—
P3 fracture (midsagittal)	±	+	—
Extensor process fracture (P3)	±	+	—
Pedal osteitis	+	±	±
Subsolar abscess	+	±	±
Solar pain (heel, quarter)	+	±	±
Solar pain (toe)	+	±	+
DDF tendonitis	+	—	—
DDF enthesitis (P3 insertion)	+	±	—
Sheared heel	+	—	—
Quittor	+	—	—
Laminitis (toe)	—	—	—
Laminitis (quarter, heel)	+	±	—
Toe crack	—	—	—
Quarter crack, heel crack	+	±	—
Distal sesamoidean desmitis	±	—	—
PIP joint problem	±	—	—
DFTS problem	±	—	—
P2 Fracture	±	±	—
P1 Fracture	±	—	—

DDF, Deep digital flexor; *DFTS,* digital flexor tendon sheath; *DIP,* distal interphalangeal; *P1,* proximal phalanx; *P2,* middle phalanx; *P3,* distal phalanx; *PIP,* proximal interphalangeal.

technique in racehorses, or, for that matter, in any sport horse with a propensity to develop lameness of the metacarpophalangeal or metatarsophalangeal joints, the veterinarian runs the risk of an additional misdiagnosis. When local anesthetic solution is deposited in a location abaxial to the proximal sesamoid bones, pain from the metacarpophalangeal or metatarsophalangeal joints can be inadvertently blocked, explained most likely because of diffusion of local anesthetic solution, leading the clinician to assume the horse has a problem in the foot or digit, but in reality the pain originated from these joints. For these reasons, we prefer to use a blocking sequence as follows: palmar digital nerve, followed by a dorsally directed subcutaneous ring block, followed by the low palmar or plantar block.

The midpastern ring block affects the dorsal branches of the digital nerves and desensitizes any remaining areas of the foot and pastern region that were not affected by palmar digital analgesia. In most horses this includes the dorsal 20% of the foot (dorsal laminar and extensor process regions of the distal phalanx) and the dorsal pastern region (dorsal aspects of the middle phalanx and proximal interphalangeal joint, and distal portions of the proximal phalanx). Although desirable, performing the dorsal ring block just above the cartilages of the foot usually is not possible. Instead the block is performed at the level of the midpastern region.

A 20- to 22-gauge, 4-cm needle is used to deposit subcutaneously 10 to 12 mL of local anesthetic solution, beginning near the injection site used for palmar digital analgesia over the lateral neurovascular bundle and continuing dorsally and medially, ending over the medial neurovascular bundle (see Figure 10-5). Resistance to needle advancement and injection of local anesthetic solution will invariably be encountered dorsally, if the block is done just proximal to the coronary band, because of the dense tissue (proximal interphalangeal joint capsule, extensor branches of the suspensory ligament, and extensor tendons). Performing the block in the midpastern region minimizes this problem and mitigates the potential for inadvertent penetration of the proximal interphalangeal joint.

Abaxial Sesamoid Block

Desensitizing the medial and lateral palmar nerves at the level of the proximal sesamoid bones is commonly referred to as the *abaxial sesamoid block* but may provide the same information as the basisesamoid block, if the dorsal branch of the palmar digital nerve is blocked. To avoid redundancy, we rarely perform the basisesamoid technique before progressing to the abaxial sesamoid block (see previous comments). A block done at this level essentially provides analgesia of the entire digit, because the block is performed at the level of or just proximal to the origin of the dorsal branch of the palmar digital nerve. Response to this block may vary, however. Some horses retain skin sensation in the dorsoproximal aspect of the pastern region. In others, pain arising from lesions involving the fetlock joint or periarticular tissues is abolished. In part, these phenomena can be explained by proximal diffusion

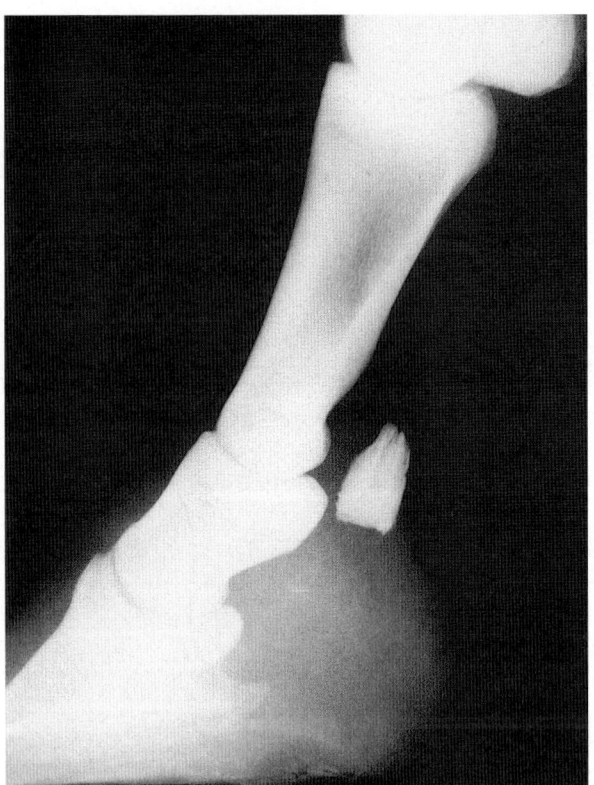

Fig. 10-6 • Radiograph showing palmar digital analgesia performed with positive contrast material. The clinician performed palmar digital analgesia as far distal as possible, but the injection site is still at the level of the proximal interphalangeal joint, explaining why palmar digital analgesia desensitizes most of the foot and the pastern region in some horses.

of local anesthetic solution, affecting the palmar digital nerves proximal to the fetlock joint. Branches of the palmar digital nerves supplying the proximal sesamoid bones, the sesamoidean nerves, could easily be blocked using an analgesic technique in this abaxial position.[24] One of the Editors (SJD) regularly performs palmar nerve blocks at the base of the proximal sesamoid bones as a first block if, on the basis of clinical examination, it is considered unlikely that the horse has foot-related pain and there is also no evidence of likely fetlock joint pain.

The abaxial sesamoid block can be performed in the standing horse or with the limb held by the clinician or an assistant. The assistant grasps the foot, facing forward. The assistant should be warned that a fractious horse may kick backwards with the limb, so he or she should stand slightly to one side, outside the plane of the limb. The palmar digital nerve can easily be palpated over the rigid proximal sesamoid bones and in fact is in its most superficial position in this location. A 25-gauge, 1.6-cm needle is directed in a proximal or distal direction and typically 1 to 3 mL of local anesthetic solution are used for each of the medial and lateral injections. Deep pain is assessed by hard flexion of the interphalangeal joints. False-negative or delayed results can arise because of deposition of local anesthetic solution outside the fascia that surrounds the neurovascular bundle.[8]

Low Palmar Analgesia

Analgesia of the metacarpophalangeal joint region and distal aspect of the limb is induced using the low palmar block or low palmar analgesia (low four-point). This technique blocks the medial and lateral palmar nerves and the medial and lateral palmar metacarpal nerves. In the forelimb a subcutaneous, dorsally directed ring block and block of the dorsal branch of the ulnar nerve completely abolishes skin sensation. Disagreement exists about whether abolishing skin sensation is necessary when performing perineural techniques. Abolition of skin sensation independently from nerves contributing to deep pain sensation, as in the case of the low palmar technique, does not necessarily mean deep pain is abolished, which is particularly relevant when a nerve responsible for skin sensation is blocked. When using these techniques for diagnostic purposes, it may be best to avoid blocking nerves that contribute only skin sensation, thus minimizing the number of needle insertions For therapeutic interventions, however, these nerves need to be blocked.

The low palmar block is performed at the level of the distal end (bell or button) of the second and fourth metacarpal bones (splint bones), with the limb in a standing position or held off the ground (Figure 10-7). A 20- or 22-gauge needle is used to inject 1.5 to 5 mL of local anesthetic solution at each injection site. To block the palmar metacarpal nerves, the needle is inserted perpendicular to the skin, just distal to the end of the splint bones, to a depth of 1 to 2 cm. It is important to deposit local anesthetic solution deep in the injection site, rather than simply in a subcutaneous location. While local anesthetic solution is continuously injected, the needle is slowly withdrawn, leaving a visible bleb in the subcutaneous space. To block the medial and lateral palmar nerves, the needle is inserted subcutaneously, in the palmar aspect of the space between the suspensory ligament and DDFT at the level of or slightly more proximal to the distal end of the splint bone. To improve the accuracy of the injection, using a fan-shaped injection technique is helpful. If the digital flexor tendon sheath (DFTS) is distended, the injections must be performed more proximally. Inadvertent penetration of the DFTS is possible even if it is not distended, so careful skin preparation is mandatory. To complete this block, local anesthetic solution is placed in the subcutaneous tissues from the bleb at the distal end of the splint bone to the dorsal midline. One of the Editors (SJD) does not do this last step.

An alternative technique to abolish pain associated with maladaptive or nonadaptive bone remodeling or other causes of subchondral bone pain of the distal aspect of the McIII is to block the lateral and medial palmar metacarpal nerves separately from the lateral and medial palmar nerves. In some horses suspected of having this injury, use of abbreviated low palmar analgesia will avoid additional injections of local anesthetic solution. With this technique the lateral or medial palmar metacarpal nerve, or both, can be blocked individually or together, and the horse's gait assessed. In many horses with this cause of lameness, contralateral forelimb lameness will then be seen. If lameness does not abate, the clinician then completes low palmar analgesia using the technique described previously (see the following discussion).

Alternatively, some clinicians prefer to use a longer needle first to deposit local anesthetic solution over the palmar metacarpal (metatarsal) nerves. The needle is then pushed subcutaneously to deposit local anesthetic solution over the palmar nerves (see Figure 10-7). When this

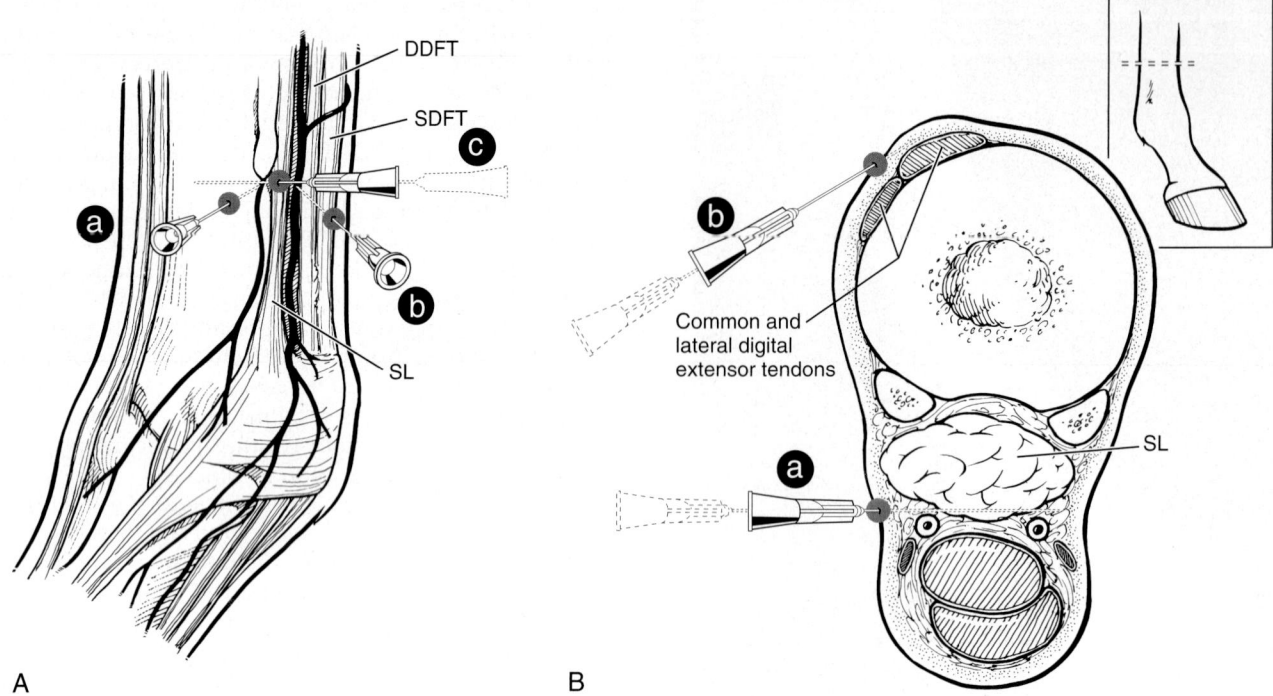

Fig. 10-7 • A, This lateral view shows needles positioned for a low palmar (plantar) nerve block. The clinician inserts a needle *(a)* just distal to the distal aspect of the fourth metacarpal or metatarsal bone and directs it axially to block the lateral palmar (plantar) metacarpal (metatarsal) nerve. The clinician then inserts a needle *(b)* between the suspensory ligament *(SL)* and deep digital flexor tendon *(DDFT)* to block the lateral palmar (plantar) nerve. The clinician repeats the two injections on the medial side. A subcutaneous ring block from the first injection site around to the dorsal midline *(c)* completely abolishes skin sensation. **B,** Transverse view of the distal left metacarpal region demonstrating an alternative technique for low palmar (plantar) analgesia. The clinician inserts a needle *(a)* in a lateral-to-medial direction between the DDFT and the SL to block the lateral and medial palmar (plantar) nerves. The palmar (plantar) metacarpal (metatarsal) nerves are blocked as depicted in **A** (not shown in this diagram), which also shows the subcutaneous ring block. The clinician inserts a needle *(b)* in a lateral-to-medial direction dorsal to the digital extensor tendons to block the dorsal metatarsal nerves of the hindlimb.

modification is performed, incompletely blocking the palmar metacarpal (metatarsal) nerves or lacerating the digital vessels is possible. The lateral and medial palmar nerves can be blocked using only the lateral injection site by advancing the needle in a medial direction, palmar to the DDFT. Although each of these modifications may theoretically decrease the number of injections needed to perform this technique, they have the disadvantages of potential hemorrhage and incomplete analgesia.

High Palmar Block
To provide analgesia to the metacarpal region, the high palmar block (high four-point, subcarpal block) is the most common technique, but a modified block (lateral palmar or Wheat block) can be performed. Inadvertent penetration of the carpometacarpal joint is a potential complication with the high palmar block. A similar complication can occur in the hindlimb but is less frequent (see the following discussion). Inadvertent penetration of the carpometacarpal joint occurred in 17% of specimens, in which a conventional high palmar block was performed, because of extensive distopalmar outpouchings (Figures 10-8 and 10-9). However, when the high palmar block was performed within 2.5 cm of the carpometacarpal joint, inadvertent penetration of this joint occurred in 67% of specimens. The carpometacarpal joint always communicates with the middle carpal joint, and therefore penetration of the carpometacarpal joint during high palmar analgesia would lead the clinician to diagnose a metacarpal problem, when in reality the authentic lameness condition exists in the carpus. Moving the injection site in a distal direction decreases the possibility of entering the carpometacarpal joint but also narrows the scope of the technique and may result in a false-negative response in a horse with proximal suspensory desmitis. Two ways around this likely complication are these: first, the clinician could perform middle carpal analgesia before performing high palmar analgesia; second, the clinician could perform a lateral palmar block in lieu of the conventional high palmar technique. In an experimental study, the carpal joints were unlikely to be entered inadvertently during performance of the lateral palmar block, although in every specimen, local anesthetic solution would have entered the carpal canal.[25] Unless the clinician is familiar with the lateral palmar block, the most straightforward approach to reduce the possibility of misdiagnosis in this region is to perform middle carpal analgesia before proceeding to the high palmar block. When local anesthetic solution is placed in the middle carpal joint, not only is the carpometacarpal joint blocked, but also the possibility exists of providing local analgesia to the proximal palmar metacarpal region. With this approach, abolishing pain associated with proximal suspensory attachment

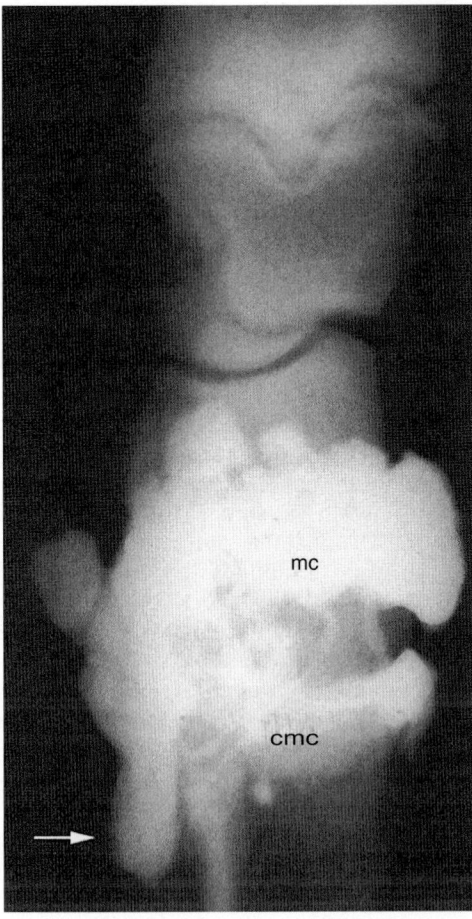

Fig. 10-8 • Positive contrast arthrogram of the middle carpal *(mc)* and carpometacarpal *(cmc)* joints (dorsal is to the right). Contrast material injected into the middle carpal joint flows freely distally into the carpometacarpal joint and fills the extensive distopalmar outpouchings of the joint *(arrow)*.

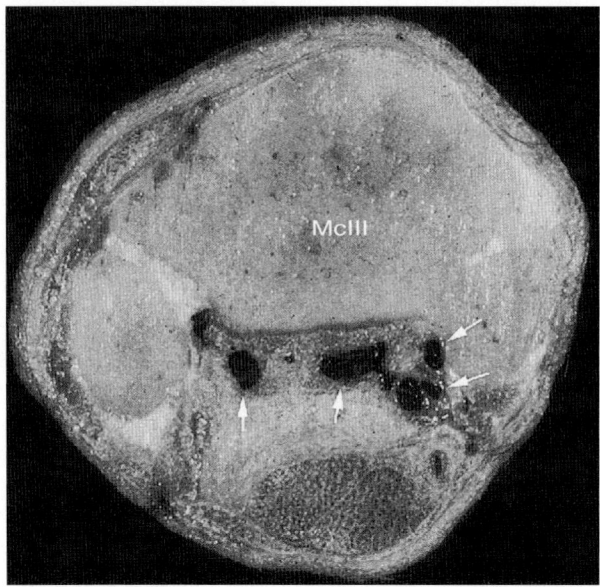

Fig. 10-10 • Transverse section of the proximal metacarpal region just distal to the carpometacarpal joint after latex injection into the middle carpal joint showing primary and secondary distopalmar outpouchings of the carpometacarpal joint *(dark areas, arrows)* interdigitating with the proximal aspect of the suspensory ligament (dorsal is up; lateral is left). This anatomical arrangement explains inadvertent analgesia of the carpus and proximal palmar metacarpal region during high palmar and middle carpal analgesia, respectively. *McIII,* Third metacarpal bone.

avulsion injury (desmitis, fracture), stress remodeling, and longitudinal fracture is possible (see Chapter 37). The palmar metacarpal nerves and suspensory branches from the lateral palmar nerve are closely associated with the distopalmar outpouchings of the carpometacarpal joint, and diffusion of local anesthetic solution from this area could explain in part this clinical finding (Figure 10-10).

It is important for the clinician to understand that interpretation of analgesic techniques in the proximal palmar metacarpal region or carpus can be somewhat complex. Correct diagnosis is always the key, and comprehensive evaluation using multiple imaging modalities is a must in differentiating lameness in this region. From the clinical perspective, one is more likely to assume incorrectly that one is dealing with a carpal problem when the authentic lameness condition resides in the proximal palmar metacarpal region than vice versa. Numerous techniques are used to perform high palmar analgesia; some provide partial and others provide complete analgesia to the metacarpal region. For complete analgesia, blocking the following nerves is necessary: the medial and lateral palmar nerves, the medial and lateral palmar metacarpal nerves, the suspensory branches, and nerves providing skin sensation along the dorsum (dorsal branch of ulnar nerve and musculocutaneous nerve). To block these nerves effectively, one must use a site close to the carpometacarpal joint, at the level where the splint bones begin to taper (Figure 10-11). If the block is done at a lower level, the region of the suspensory attachment will be missed. A 20- or 22-gauge needle at least 2.5 cm long is necessary to reach the palmar metacarpal nerves in this location. The needle is inserted axial to the splint bones just abaxial to the suspensory ligament and then guided to the palmar

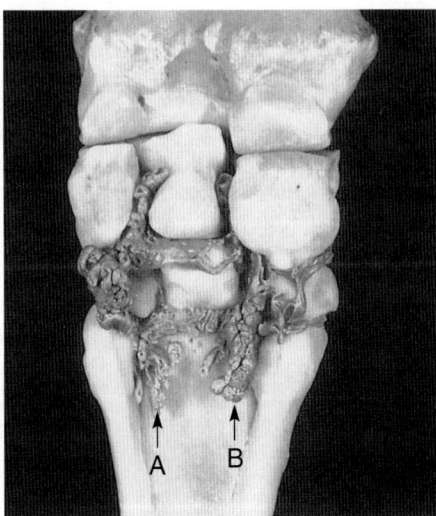

Fig. 10-9 • Liquid acrylic injected into the middle carpal joint and allowed to harden created this specimen showing the lateral *(A)* and medial *(B)* distopalmar outpouchings of the carpometacarpal joint. Secondary finger-like outpouchings ramify in the proximal palmar metacarpal region.

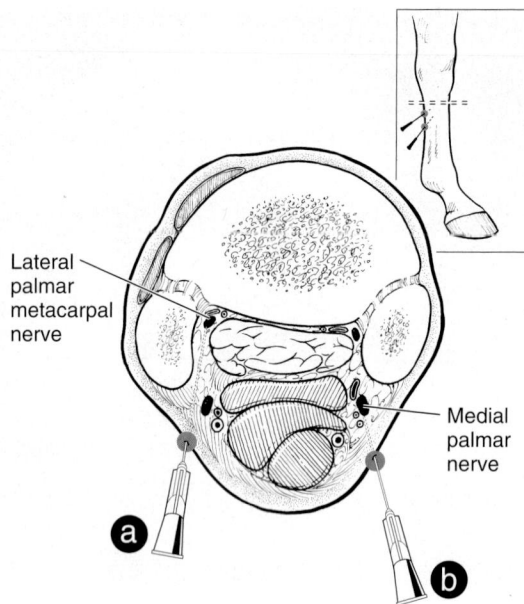

Fig. 10-11 • Transverse view of the left metacarpal region showing the technique for high palmar analgesia. The clinician inserts a needle *(a)* axial to each second and fourth metacarpal bone and uses two separate injections *(b)* to block the medial and lateral palmar nerves. The location of the high palmar technique appears in the lateral view *(inset)*.

cortex of the McIII. Five milliliters of local anesthetic solution are deposited, first deep within the tissues, and continued as the needle is withdrawn, ending with a bleb in the subcutaneous tissues. To block the medial and lateral palmar nerves between the suspensory ligament and DDFT, a smaller-gauge needle can be used to deposit 3 to 5 mL of local anesthetic solution at each of two sites. To complete this block, a circumferential subcutaneous ring block is performed to abolish skin sensation dorsally. Alternatively, the subcutaneous nerves can be blocked on either side of the common digital extensor (CDE) tendon, but small zones of sensation may persist when this technique is used. It is only necessary to complete the dorsal portion of this block to provide complete analgesia when performing procedures in the dorsal metacarpal region, such as laceration repair or standing osteostixis.

A modification of the high palmar block is performed by locally infiltrating the suspensory origin from a lateral injection site in a fan-shaped pattern. This procedure, along with one specifically to block the medial and lateral palmar metacarpal nerves, improves specificity of this complex block, because pain from only a limited number of structures is eliminated. The medial and lateral palmar nerves can also be blocked from a single lateral injection site. One of the Editors (SJD) regularly blocks just the palmar metacarpal nerves (using only 2 to 3 mL of local anesthetic solution per site) and only adds perineural analgesia of the palmar nerves if the first block is negative, in order to facilitate differentiation of suspensory ligament or McIII pain from pain arising from the more palmar soft tissue structures. A dorsal ring block is never used.

Lateral Palmar Block

An alternative method of providing analgesia to the metacarpal region is to perform what is known as the *lateral*

palmar (high two-point) or *Wheat block*.[26] For complete analgesia, however, combining this block with an independent injection over the medial palmar nerve and with a dorsal subcutaneous ring block is necessary. Originally proposed as an alternative method for analgesia of the suspensory ligament origin, this technique involves blocking the lateral palmar nerve just distal to the accessory carpal bone (Figure 10-12). The lateral palmar nerve is formed as the median and deep ulnar nerves join, proximal to the accessory carpal bone (see Figure 10-12).[27] At the level of the block, just distal to the accessory carpal bone, the lateral palmar nerve is blocked before it branches to form the medial and lateral palmar metacarpal nerves and the suspensory branches and continues distally (see Figure 10-12). The high two-point block is completed with the separate but concurrent block of the medial palmar nerve.

This technique has at least three advantages compared with conventional high palmar analgesia. Inadvertently penetrating the distopalmar outpouchings of the carpometacarpal joint is virtually impossible, although local anesthetic solution will likely enter the carpal canal.[25] Lateral palmar analgesia requires fewer needle penetrations than does conventional high palmar analgesia. Finally, only a small volume of local anesthetic solution is necessary to desensitize a number of nerves and the origin of the suspensory ligament. Pain associated with the carpal canal is abolished, however, and can be present without palpable effusion.

The lateral palmar block can be performed in the standing position or with the limb held off the ground, with the carpus in 90 degrees of flexion. The nerve cannot be palpated because it courses in the accessorial-metacarpal ligament, dense connective tissue distal to the accessory carpal bone. A 25-gauge, 1.6-cm needle is inserted to the hub, perpendicular to the skin, just distal to the accessory carpal bone, and 5 mL of local anesthetic solution are deposited within this dense tissue. Injection can be difficult to perform, and breaking the seal between the needle and syringe is common, so a screw-type hub should be used. The medial palmar nerve is then blocked as described previously. If desired, a dorsal, circumferential subcutaneous ring block provides complete analgesia to the dorsum. An alternative technique for lateral palmar nerve block has recently been described.[28] The primary advantage of this technique is that it mitigates the risk of inadvertent penetration of the carpal synovial sheath (carpal canal). The block is performed with the limb in extension. The primary landmark is a palpable groove in the flexor retinaculum just dorsal to its insertion on the palmaromedial aspect of the accessory carpal bone. A 1.5-cm, 25-gauge needle is inserted in the distal third of the groove in a mediolateral direction, and when contact is made with the medial surface of the accessory carpal bone, local anesthetic solution is injected. However, it is quite easy for the needle to hit the nerve, which results in the horse striking out, and a difficult horse may become even more fractious to block.

Median, Ulnar, and Medial Cutaneous Antebrachial Blocks

Analgesia of the distal aspect of the antebrachium and carpus can be induced by blocking the median, ulnar,

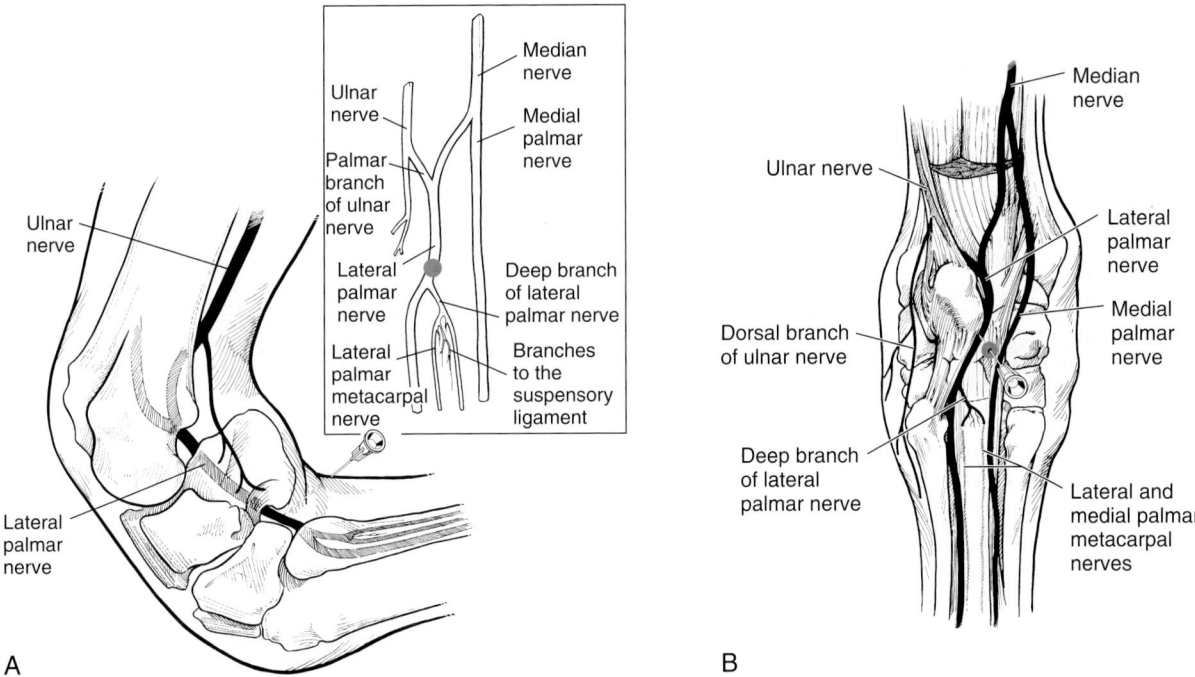

Fig. 10-12 • A, This diagram of the left carpus in a flexed position shows the location of the lateral palmar nerve block and parent nerves *(inset)* contributing to the origin of the lateral palmar and other important nerves. **B,** Palmar view of the limb showing nerves in situ and the site for needle penetration for lateral palmar nerve block.

and medial cutaneous antebrachial (musculocutaneous) nerves.[21] Because the last nerve supplies only skin sensation, for diagnostic purposes it does not need to be included in the technique. In our practices these blocks are most commonly performed to facilitate lavage of the carpal joints or carpal canal or to perform regional limb perfusion of antibiotics in standing horses. We generally default to intrasynovial analgesia in these structures, however. However, one of us (MWR) has recently evaluated several horses with subchondral bone pain in the middle carpal joint in which intraarticular carpal analgesia failed to abolish clinical signs of pain. Lameness was abolished using the median and ulnar blocks. One Editor (SJD) finds these blocks extremely valuable in horses that do not respond to subcarpal or intraarticular carpal analgesia and employs median and ulnar blocks routinely. Although the median and ulnar blocks remain infrequently used in the United States, perhaps they should be considered routine. Median, ulnar, and medial cutaneous antebrachial nerve blocks are useful in diagnosing subchondral carpal bone pain or lameness involving the carpal canal. Although the prevalence of lameness in the distal aspect of the antebrachium is low, these blocks can be used to diagnose distal radial bone cysts or enthesitis at the origin of the accessory ligament of the superficial digital flexor tendon (SDFT) (superior check ligament). These blocks can be used to eliminate the entire distal aspect of the limb as a potential source of pain. Alternatively, these blocks can be used alone to eliminate pain distal to the injection site, or the median and ulnar nerves can be blocked independently to improve specificity of the technique.

The ulnar nerve is blocked about 10 cm proximal to the accessory carpal bone on the caudal aspect of the antebrachium (Figure 10-13). A 20- or 22-gauge, 4-cm needle is inserted to the hub, perpendicular to the skin, in the groove between the flexor carpi ulnaris and the ulnaris lateralis muscles. Needle contact with the ulnar nerve may cause the horse to strike forward.[5] Ten milliliters of local anesthetic solution are injected as the needle is slowly withdrawn. Skin sensitivity along the lateral aspect of the limb from the carpus to the metacarpophalangeal joint will be eliminated.[21]

The median nerve is blocked 5 cm distal to the cubital (elbow) joint on the medial aspect of the antebrachium. At this level, the nerve lies along the caudal aspect of the radius, just cranial to the flexor carpi radialis muscle. A 20- or 22-gauge, 4-cm needle is inserted into the hub, in a lateral direction, along the caudal aspect of the radius, just distal to the superficial pectoral muscle, and 10 mL of local anesthetic solution are used (see Figure 10-13). Rarely in large horses, a 9-cm (3½-inch) spinal needle may be necessary to reach the median nerve. Often the needle hits the median nerve, a useful indicator that the tip is in the proper location.[5] In any event the needle should be kept close to or against the caudal cortex of the radius to avoid inadvertent puncture of the median artery or vein, which lies caudal to the nerve.[21,27] However, inadvertent puncture determines that the needle is close to the correct site and is highly unlikely to cause any adverse reaction. To facilitate these deep injections, the skin can be first desensitized by using a small volume of local anesthetic solution. A more distal injection site for the median nerve may eliminate the possibility of inadvertently eliminating elbow joint pain using the suggested approach.[5]

Finally (for therapeutic applications), to block the cranial and caudal branches of the medial cutaneous antebrachial (musculocutaneous) nerve, 3 mL of local anesthetic solution are injected, subcutaneously, on the cranial

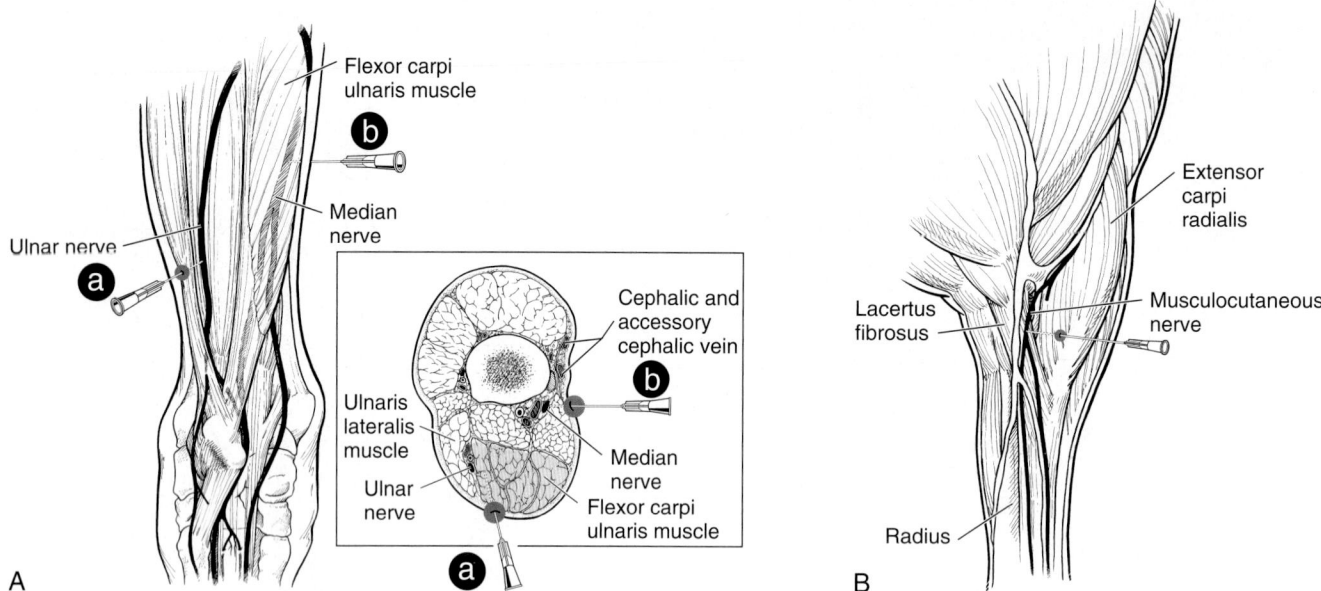

Fig. 10-13 • A, This caudal view of the left antebrachium shows the sites of needle insertion for the median and ulnar nerve blocks. A needle placed between the ulnaris lateralis and flexor carpi ulnaris muscles *(a)*, about 10 cm proximal to the accessory carpal bone, blocks the ulnar nerve. A needle inserted along the caudal aspect of the radius about 10 cm distal to the elbow joint *(b)* blocks the median nerve. The inset shows the orientation between the radius, median artery, vein, and nerve at the site of needle insertion *(b)* and shows the orientation of the needle for the ulnar nerve block *(a)*, which is performed distally. **B,** This medial view of the proximal left antebrachium shows the technique for a musculocutaneous nerve block. The nerve is blocked as it crosses the lacertus fibrosus on the cranial aspect of the proximal antebrachium. This block abolishes skin sensation on the medial and dorsal aspects of the antebrachium.

and caudal aspect of the accessory cephalic and cephalic veins, about halfway between the carpus and elbow (see Figure 10-13).[21] Alternatively, this nerve can be blocked before it branches, as it courses across the lacertus fibrosus. At this location, the nerve is easily palpable in most horses. A third method to completely abolish skin sensation is using a circumferential subcutaneous ring block, a technique that can effectively block all four cutaneous antebrachial nerves but requires a large volume of local anesthetic solution.

INTRAARTICULAR ANALGESIA IN THE FORELIMB
Distal Interphalangeal Joint
The assumption is that analgesia of the DIP joint is specific for intraarticular pain, but clinical experience and the results of recent clinical and anatomical investigations have convinced us otherwise (see Figure 10-1). Of great clinical interest is the comparative accuracy of analgesia of the DIP joint and navicular (podotrochlear) bursa in the diagnosis of navicular syndrome. Overall, analgesia of the navicular bursa is likely the most specific technique to diagnose navicular syndrome. However, results of two studies suggest that this block may not be as specific as once thought (see the section on analgesia of the podotrochlear bursa).[29,30] Analgesia of the DIP joint lacks specificity for intraarticular pain and in fact can eliminate pain associated with many conditions of the foot.[29-32] For instance, when high-performance liquid chromatography was used to study the effects of 8 mL of mepivacaine Injected into the DIP joint, there was local anesthetic solution in the synovium of the navicular bursa in all horses and in the

medullary cavity of the navicular bones in 40% of horses.[33] Similarly, a recent in vitro study showed that 15 minutes after injection of 5 mL of 2% mepivacaine into either the navicular bursa or the DIP joint, mepivacaine was detected in the alternate (uninjected) synovial structure in all specimens. In 48% of navicular bursae after DIP joint injection, and in 44% of DIP joints after navicular bursa injection, mepivacaine was present in clinically effective (analgesic) concentrations (>100 to 300 mg/L).[34] Anatomical studies showed that nociceptive neurofibers are present in the dorsal and palmar aspects of the collateral sesamoidean ligaments, within the distal sesamoidean impar ligament, and directly innervating the navicular bone, in the periarticular connective tissues of the DIP joint and proximal intramedullary portions of the distal phalanx.[35,36] The close anatomical relationship among all of these structures and the palmar digital neurovascular bundles to the DIP joint capsule makes them susceptible to desensitization by local anesthetic solution injected into the DIP joint.[36]

In a study using a setscrew model to create solar pain at the toe, DIP intraarticular analgesia abolished lameness, leading to the conclusion that pain in distant sites can be abolished using this technique.[22] Therefore a positive response to DIP intraarticular analgesia could mean lameness is caused by an articular problem, navicular syndrome, or, for that matter, solar pain. Close juxtaposition between the palmar synovial extensions of the DIP joint and digital nerves at this level was theorized as the reason that these nerves were blocked, secondary to diffusion of local anesthetic solution from the joint.[22] Therefore a protocol to examine a lame horse no longer than 5 minutes after intraarticular analgesia of the DIP joint may theoretically

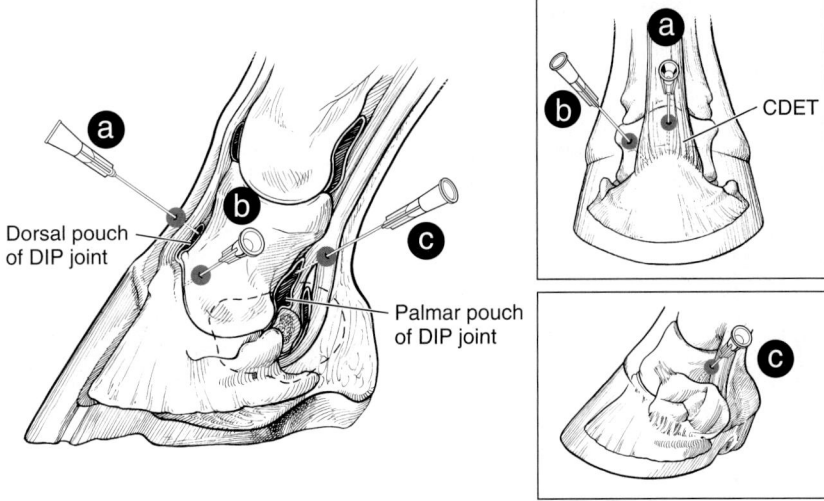

Fig. 10-14 • Lateral view of the foot showing our preferred approach for arthrocentesis of the digital interphalangeal joint using a dorsal midline needle insertion site *(a)* and directing the needle slightly distally through the common (long) digital extensor tendon. Alternatively, the clinician approaches the digital interphalangeal joint using a site medial or lateral to the extensor tendon *(b)*. The top inset shows the needle positions from the dorsal aspect. The clinician may use a palmar (plantar) approach by positioning the needle between the distal palmar (plantar) border of the middle phalanx and a palpable notch in the proximal border of the cartilage of the foot. The clinician directs the needle *(c)* in a palmaroproximolateral to dorsodistomedial direction. The lower inset shows the notch into which the needle is inserted. *CDET,* Common (long) digital extensor tendon; *DIP,* distal interphalangeal.

minimize diffusion and improve accuracy. However, in one of the Editor's (SJD) experience, pain associated with the navicular bone, navicular bursa, or DDFT has frequently been substantially improved within 5 minutes of injection of the DIP joint. Because diffusion of local anesthetic solution may be hastened by moving the horse, some clinicians prefer the horse to stand until the results of the block are evaluated.[5]

Traditionally, arthrocentesis of the DIP joint has been performed in the dorsal pouch, either medial or lateral to the CDE tendon. A 20-gauge, 2.5- to 4-cm needle is inserted about 1.5 cm proximal to the coronary band, abaxial to the CDE tendon, and directed in a distal and axial direction (Figure 10-14). An easier approach, however, is to insert the needle, angled just slightly distal from horizontal, on the dorsal midline, *through the CDE*. Synovial fluid is consistently obtained using this approach. One of the Editors (SJD) angles the needle more vertically, inserting it in the palpable dip in the distal dorsal aspect of the pastern. For the dorsal aspect of the DIP joint to be opened up, the limb should be positioned slightly ahead of the contralateral limb, and the horse should be in a standing position. Five to 10 mL of local anesthetic solution have been used traditionally, but a maximum of 6 mL may prevent leakage from the joint. Use of a lower volume of local anesthetic solution *may* also improve the specificity of the block, as was shown in a similar study using setscrews to create solar pain. Decreasing the volume of local anesthetic solution in the DIP joint from 10 mL to 6 mL resulted in a significant reduction in lameness caused by pain at the dorsal margin of the sole, but *not* at the angles of the sole.[37] The horse is examined after 5 minutes.

Alternatively, a lateral approach to the DIP joint can be used (see Figure 10-14). Landmarks include the distal palmar border of the middle phalanx dorsally and the palpable notch in the proximal border of the lateral cartilage of the foot distally. A 4-cm needle is inserted laterally and directed in a dorsodistomedial direction. This technique, however, is less reliable than the dorsal approach, because contrast material entered exclusively the DIP joint in only 13 of 20 specimens and in 7 specimens inadvertently entered the navicular bursa or DFTS.[38]

Proximal Interphalangeal Joint

Arthrocentesis of the proximal interphalangeal joint is most commonly performed in the dorsal pouch. Effusion is rarely present even in horses with severe lameness, a situation that makes arthrocentesis challenging. The injection site is just lateral (or medial) to the CDE tendon at a level of or just distal to the distal, palmar process of the proximal phalanx, located and easily palpable on the distopalmar aspect of this bone. With the horse in the standing position, a 20-gauge, 2.5-cm needle is directed slightly distally and medially (using the dorsolateral approach) and inserted until articular cartilage is encountered (Figure 10-15). Although a desirable sign, synovial fluid appearing in the hub of the needle is an unusual occurrence. Local anesthetic solution, 5 to 10 mL, is injected, and the horse is examined after 5 minutes.

An alternative approach that one author (MWR) finds much easier to perform is approaching the proximal palmar pouch of the proximal interphalangeal joint from the lateral aspect. The injection location is a V-shaped notch, located dorsal to the neurovascular bundle and between the distal palmar process of the proximal phalanx and the insertion of the lateral branch of the SDFT (see Figure 10-15). The limb is held off the ground with the digit in flexion, and a 2.5- or 4-cm needle is directed distomedially (and slightly dorsally) at an angle of about 30 degrees from the transverse plane until fluid is collected (generally at a

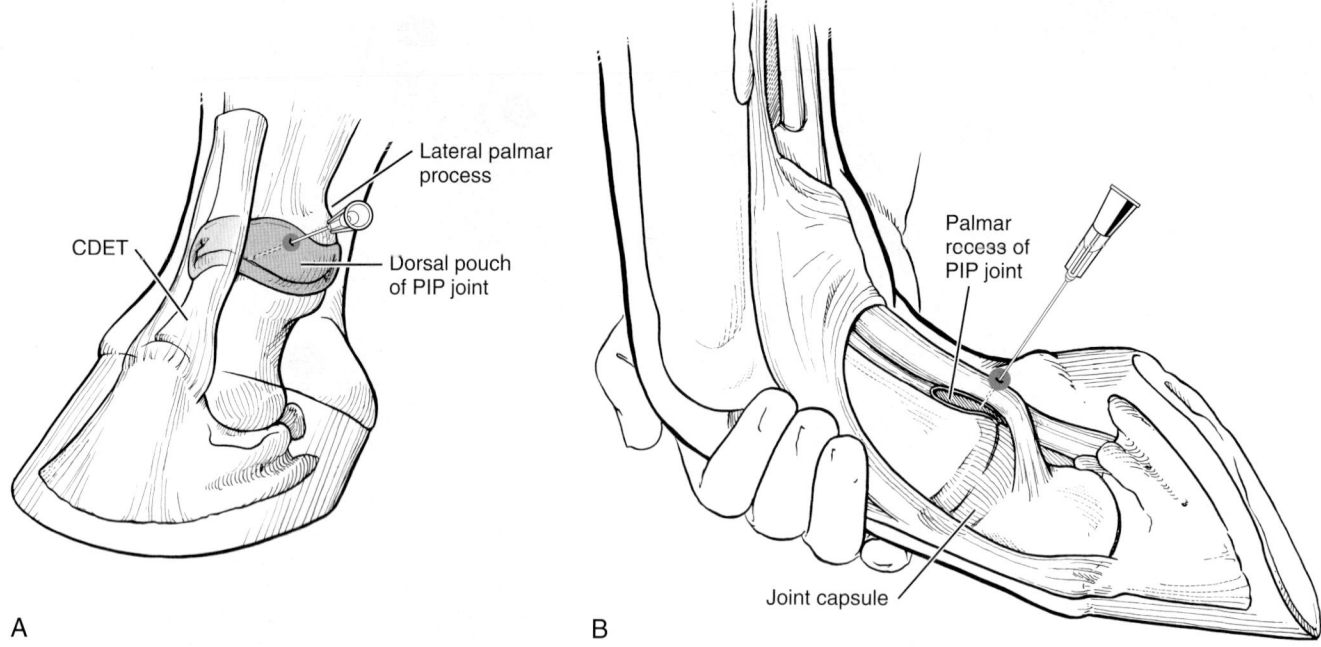

A   B

Fig. 10-15 • A, Dorsolateral view of the digit showing the site for arthrocentesis of the dorsal pouch of the proximal interphalangeal joint. The clinician inserts the needle just abaxial to the common digital extensor tendon at a site level with the palpable distal palmar (plantar) process of the proximal phalanx. **B,** Flexed lateral view of the digit indicating the site for arthrocentesis of the palmar (plantar) aspect of the proximal interphalangeal joint. The clinician inserts the needle into the V-shaped notch formed by the distal palmar (plantar) aspect of the proximal phalanx dorsally, the bony eminence associated with the attachment of the lateral collateral ligament to the distal aspect of the proximal phalanx and proximal aspect of the middle phalanx distally, and the insertion of the lateral branch of the superficial digital flexor tendon palmarodistally (plantarodistally). The clinician directs the needle distomedially (in a slightly dorsal direction) at an angle of about 30 degrees from the transverse plane until fluid appears. *CDET,* Common (long) digital extensor tendon; *PIP,* proximal interphalangeal.

depth of 2 to 3 cm).[39] Advantages of this compared with the dorsal approach include less needle manipulation, a larger injection volume, and more frequent recovery of synovial fluid. The technique is difficult to perform with the limb in an extended weight-bearing position, because the palmar or plantar aspect of the proximal interphalangeal joint is compressed. Furthermore, diffusion of local anesthetic solution into palmar soft tissue structures can confound interpretation of results.[5]

Metacarpophalangeal Joint

Four sites commonly used for arthrocentesis of the metacarpophalangeal joint include the dorsal, proximopalmar, and distopalmar sites and the approach through the collateral ligament of the proximal sesamoid bone. The two most commonly used, the dorsal and proximopalmar sites, have potential disadvantages compared with the less commonly used sites. The dorsal pouch can be prominent in horses with effusion, but inadvertently stabbing articular cartilage repeatedly is common when this approach is used. The proximopalmar pouch or recess is large and easily identified, but prominent synovial villi often occlude the needle end, complicating retrieval of synovial fluid, even in horses with severe effusion. Hemorrhage associated with large intracapsular vessels is also a common complication with the proximopalmar approach. The palmar pouch is located dorsal to the suspensory branch, palmar to the McIII, proximal to the collateral sesamoidean ligament, and distal to the bell of the splint bone (Figure 10-16).

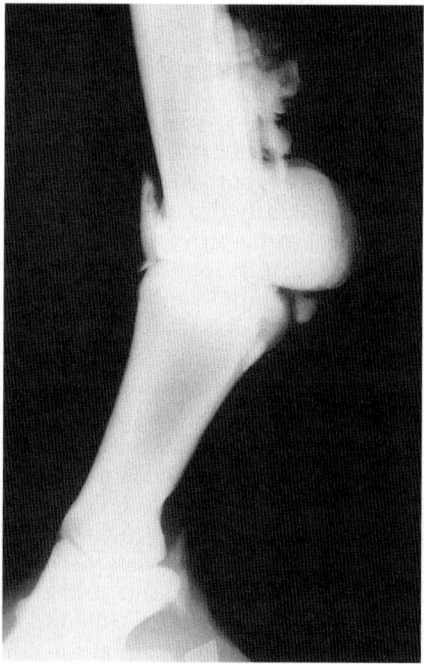

Fig. 10-16 • Positive contrast arthrogram of the metacarpophalangeal joint showing the extensive nature of the palmar pouch that extends proximally to the level of the distal end of the splint bones. The distopalmar outpouchings are reliable sites for retrieval of synovial fluid and injection.

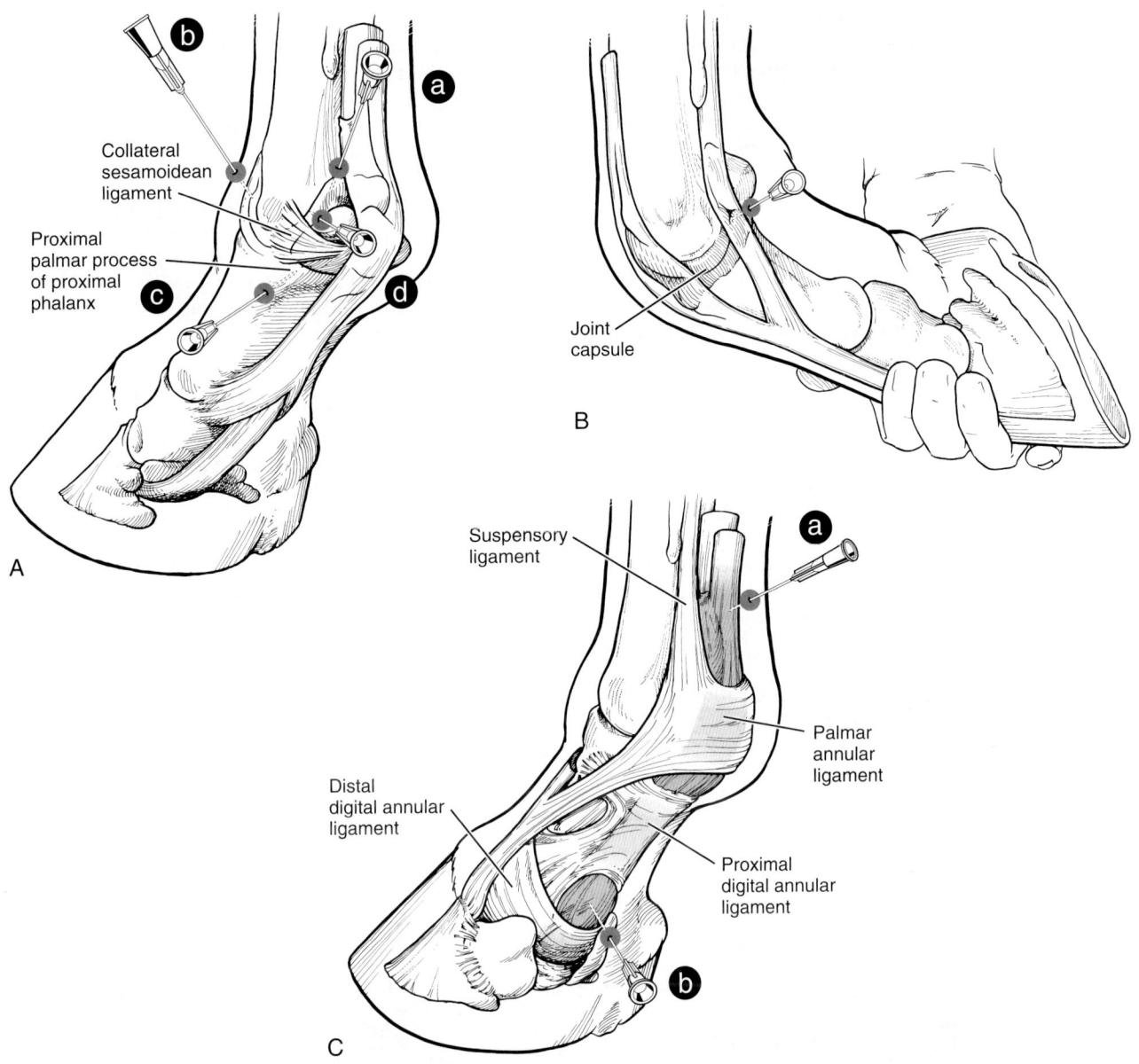

Fig. 10-17 • A, Palmarolateral (plantarolateral) view of the left metacarpophalangeal (metatarsophalangeal) joint and digit showing the sites for arthrocentesis of the proximal palmar (plantar) pouch *(a)*, the dorsal pouch *(b)*, the distal palmar (plantar) pouch *(c)*, and the palmar (plantar) pouch through the collateral ligament of the proximal sesamoid bone *(d)*. **B,** Our preferred site for metacarpophalangeal (metatarsophalangeal) joint arthrocentesis, the distal palmar (plantar) approach, using a site just proximal to the lateral palmar (plantar) process of the proximal phalanx, is easily located in the standing or flexed position. **C,** Palmarolateral (plantarolateral) view of the digit indicating sites for synoviocentesis of the proximal *(a)* and distal *(b)* aspects of the digital flexor tendon sheath. Proximally, the clinician inserts the needle proximal to the palmar (plantar) annular ligament, and distally inserts the needle on the palmar (plantar) midline into an outpouching of the digital flexor tendon sheath between the proximal and distal digital annular ligaments.

Arthrocentesis using the proximopalmar approach can be performed with the limb in the standing position or being held. An 18- to 22-gauge, 2.5- to 4-cm needle is inserted in the center of the pouch and directed slightly distally in the frontal plane until synovial fluid is recovered (Figure 10-17). It may be necessary to aspirate synovial fluid if the joint capsule is not distended.

Dorsally, arthrocentesis is performed medial or lateral to the CDE tendon (see Figure 10-17). With the limb in a standing or flexed position, the clinician can insert a needle in the distal aspect of the palmar pouch, through the collateral sesamoidean ligament, a less common but effective approach for arthrocentesis of the metacarpophalangeal joint. The technique is more easily performed with the joint held in flexion. This approach for arthrocentesis was shown to be associated with less subcutaneous and synovial inflammation than was the proximopalmar approach[40] and is the technique routinely used by one of the Editors (SJD).

Under most circumstances we prefer to perform arthrocentesis of the metacarpophalangeal joint using the distopalmar approach. The injection site is in a small but reliable recess bounded by a triad of structures. Just proximal to the readily palpable proximal, palmar process of the proximal phalanx is a distinct depression. The dorsal aspect of the proximal sesamoid bone and the palmar condyle of the McIII complete the triad but are not readily palpable. The injection site is *dorsal* to the neurovascular bundle. Synovial fluid is consistently retrieved because the injection site is in the most distal aspect of the joint, and hemorrhage is rare. A large volume of fluid can be collected, if desired, because this area is devoid of the large synovial villi that complicate the proximopalmar approach. With the horse in a standing position, a 20-gauge, 2.5-cm needle is inserted, parallel to the ground, in a dorsomedial direction until fluid is obtained (see Figure 10-17). The needle can be advanced to the hub, but the joint is quite superficial in this location. This technique can also readily be performed with the limb being held in a flexed position.

Ten mL of local anesthetic solution are injected, and the horse is reexamined in 5 to 10 minutes. In horses with subchondral bone pain, additional time may be necessary, but perineural analgesia may be necessary to abolish lameness in these horses. Diffusion of local anesthetic solution may account for partial or complete improvement in lameness in horses with suspensory branch desmitis, sesamoiditis, or injury of the straight, cruciate, or oblique sesamoidean ligaments. Therefore timely evaluation of horses after metacarpophalangeal analgesia is necessary.

Carpal Joints

Arthrocentesis of the middle carpal or antebrachiocarpal joints is one of the easiest and most straightforward of all joint injection techniques. With the carpus in flexion, injection sites are easily identified, and large portals exist through which to access the joints. Portals can be found either medial to the extensor carpi radialis (ECR) tendon or between the ECR and the CDE tendons (Figure 10-18). The middle carpal and carpometacarpal joints always communicate, but a communication between the middle carpal and antebrachiocarpal joints rarely exists. A communication between the middle carpal joint and carpal sheath only rarely is encountered clinically, but was not seen in a study using cadaver limbs. Analgesia of the middle carpal and antebrachiocarpal joints should be performed separately to differentiate lameness between these independent cavities. However, even though gross anatomic communications rarely exist between these joints, a recent in vitro study revealed the potential for diffusion of mepivacaine from one joint to the other by 15 minutes after either was injected with 10 mL of 2% mepivacaine. In only a small percentage were the concentrations of mepivacaine in each joint at levels thought to produce clinical analgesia. How this translates to the live horse also remains unknown. Nonetheless, the clinician is reminded of the importance of prompt reevaluation to minimize misinterpretation of the results, but also to keep an open mind if results of diagnostic imaging do not seem compatible with the results

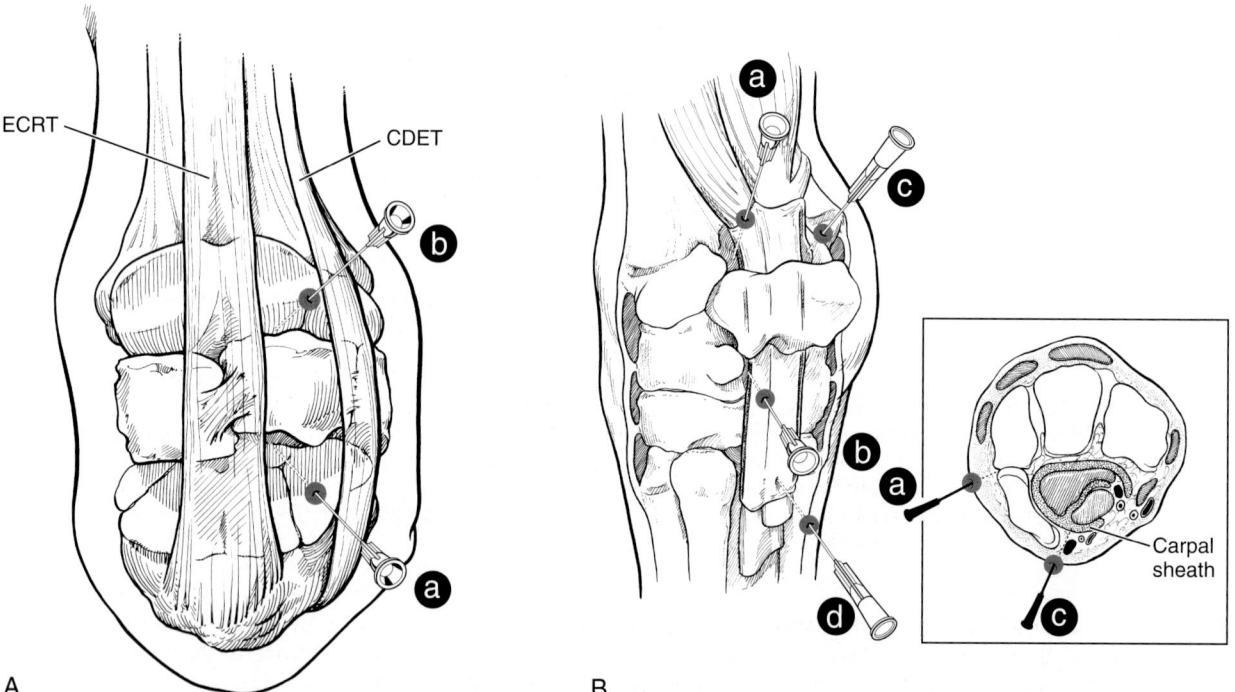

Fig. 10-18 • A, Dorsal view of the left carpus in a flexed position showing the sites for arthrocentesis of the middle carpal *(a)* and antebrachiocarpal *(b)* joints. Needles are usually positioned between the extensor carpi radialis and common digital extensor tendons (as shown), but sites for injection of both joint cavities located medial to the extensor carpi radialis tendon can be used. **B,** Lateral view of the left carpus demonstrating sites for arthrocentesis of the proximal palmar pouch of the antebrachiocarpal joint *(a)*, the palmarolateral pouch of the middle carpal joint *(b),* and the proximal *(c)* and distal *(d)* pouches of the distended carpal sheath. The inset shows the relative needle positions to enter the palmar pouch of the antebrachiocarpal joint and the carpal sheath. *CDET,* Common (long) digital extensor tendon; *ECRT,* extensor carpi radialis tendon.

of diagnostic analgesia.[34] Distopalmar outpouchings of the carpometacarpal joint complicate interpretation of analgesic techniques, because these extend a mean distance of 2.5 cm distal to the carpometacarpal articulation and are closely associated with the suspensory ligament origin and the palmar metacarpal nerves (see Figures 10-8 to 10-10).[41] Careful differential analgesic techniques and comprehensive imaging are necessary for accurate diagnosis of lameness in the carpal and proximal metacarpal regions.

Typically, a 20-gauge, 2.5-cm needle is used to inject 5 to 10 mL of local anesthetic solution into the middle carpal and antebrachiocarpal joints. If the skin can be prepared aseptically on the dorsal aspect, the injections are most commonly performed with the joint in 90 to 120 degrees of flexion. The clinician can maintain flexion, but having an assistant hold the limb securely is easier.

If the dorsal aspect of the carpus cannot be prepared aseptically, as occurs commonly in racehorses with chemically induced dermatitis (scurf), or if an additional site is needed for thorough lavage, the palmarolateral pouches of the middle carpal and antebrachiocarpal joints can be used. The palmar pouch of the antebrachiocarpal joint is bounded by the lateral digital extensor tendon dorsally and the ulnaris lateralis tendon palmarly. In horses with substantial effusion, this pouch is easily identified but must be differentiated from the lateral outpouching of the carpal sheath. Arthrocentesis can be performed either proximally or distally in the palmar pouch (see Figure 10-18). The distal injection site is located in a shallow recess between the distal lateral radius (ulna) and the ulnar carpal bone, just distal to the V-shaped convergence of the lateral digital extensor and ulnaris lateralis tendons. With the horse in a standing position, a 20-gauge, 2.5-cm needle is inserted perpendicular to the skin and advanced until synovial fluid is recovered.

The palmar pouch of the middle carpal joint is similarly accessed in a shallow depression between the ulnar and fourth carpal bones, located 2 to 2.5 cm distal to the recess palpated to access the antebrachiocarpal joint in the palmar aspect (see Figure 10-18). The shallow depression in the middle carpal joint is difficult to palpate, but in horses with severe effusion an outpouching of the joint is palpable. This approach is undertaken with the limb in a standing position, decreases the potential for iatrogenic cartilage injury, and is less dangerous to the clinician because the procedure is performed on the side rather than in front of the limb.[42] The injection is more difficult and less commonly used, however.

Cubital (Elbow) Joint

Two sites are used for arthrocentesis of the elbow joint. The cranial pouch is accessed at the level of the radiohumeral articulation, just cranial to the lateral collateral ligament. The lateral collateral ligament courses between the palpable lateral tuberosity of the radius and the lateral epicondyle of the humerus (Figure 10-19). An 18- or 20-gauge, 6- to 9-cm needle is directed medially and slightly caudally to a depth of 5 to 6 cm, beginning in the adult horse, about 3.5 cm proximal to the lateral tuberosity of the radius and 2.5 cm cranial to the lateral collateral ligament.[19] To account for differences in horse size, the injection site is generally located two thirds of the distance between the humeral epicondyle and the lateral tuberosity of the radius.

This block may be more easily performed closer to the lateral collateral ligament, and at this site the joint is penetrated in a more superficial location.[5] Before injection, every effort should be made to verify that the needle is actually in the joint. Periarticular deposition of local anesthetic solution in this location can induce temporary radial nerve dysfunction, and horses may lose the ability to extend the carpus and digit.[43] Twenty to 25 mL of local anesthetic solution are used. An older approach relied on injection of local anesthetic solution into the ulnaris lateralis bursa, once universally thought to communicate with the elbow joint. The frequency of communication between the elbow joint and ulnaris lateralis bursa was determined to be 37.5%, and therefore this approach is no longer recommended.[44]

We prefer to perform arthrocentesis in the proximolateral aspect of the caudal pouch in the palpable depression cranial to the olecranon process and caudal to the lateral epicondyle of the humerus. In most horses the site of needle penetration is 3 to 3.5 cm caudal to the lateral epicondyle (see Figure 10-19). In small horses and ponies, an 18- or 20-gauge, 4-cm needle is sufficient, but in large horses a 9-cm spinal needle is often necessary because the injection site is at the distal extent of the lateral head of the triceps muscle. The needle is advanced for 5 to 7 cm in a distal, slightly cranial, and medial direction until synovial fluid is recovered. However, this technique is often less well tolerated by difficult horses compared with the cranial pouch technique.

Elimination of skin sensitivity at the site of needle insertion by depositing a small volume of local anesthetic solution may facilitate elbow arthrocentesis, because numerous attempts may be necessary. Synovial fluid is consistently retrievable from the joint with proper needle positioning.

Scapulohumeral (Shoulder) Joint

The shoulder joint is frequently blamed for lameness in many horses but, based on the results of diagnostic analgesia, is an uncommon source of pain. Arthrocentesis of this joint is most commonly performed at a site between the cranial and caudal prominences of the greater tubercle of the humerus, just cranial to the infraspinatus tendon. This tendon is easily palpated in most horses and serves as the primary landmark. Firm, careful palpation between the cranial and caudal prominences reveals a depression or notch, which is the point of needle insertion (see Figure 10-19). Identification of landmarks is easier in horses with muscle atrophy resulting from chronic lameness.

In most horses an 18- to 20-gauge, 9-cm spinal needle is preferred, although using the entire length is not necessary. Elimination of skin sensitivity is usually not necessary. The needle is inserted in a caudomedial direction (about 45 degrees from lateral), and directed slightly distally. Attaching a syringe to aspirate synovial fluid is sometimes necessary, because in joints with minimal effusion, confirming intraarticular position of the needle may be difficult. A total of 25 to 30 mL of local anesthetic solution is used, and the horse is assessed 10 and 30 minutes after injection, because severe pain associated with osteochondrosis may resolve slowly. Analgesia of the suprascapular nerve and subsequent supraspinatus and infraspinatus muscle paralysis were reported after attempts at intraarticular shoulder

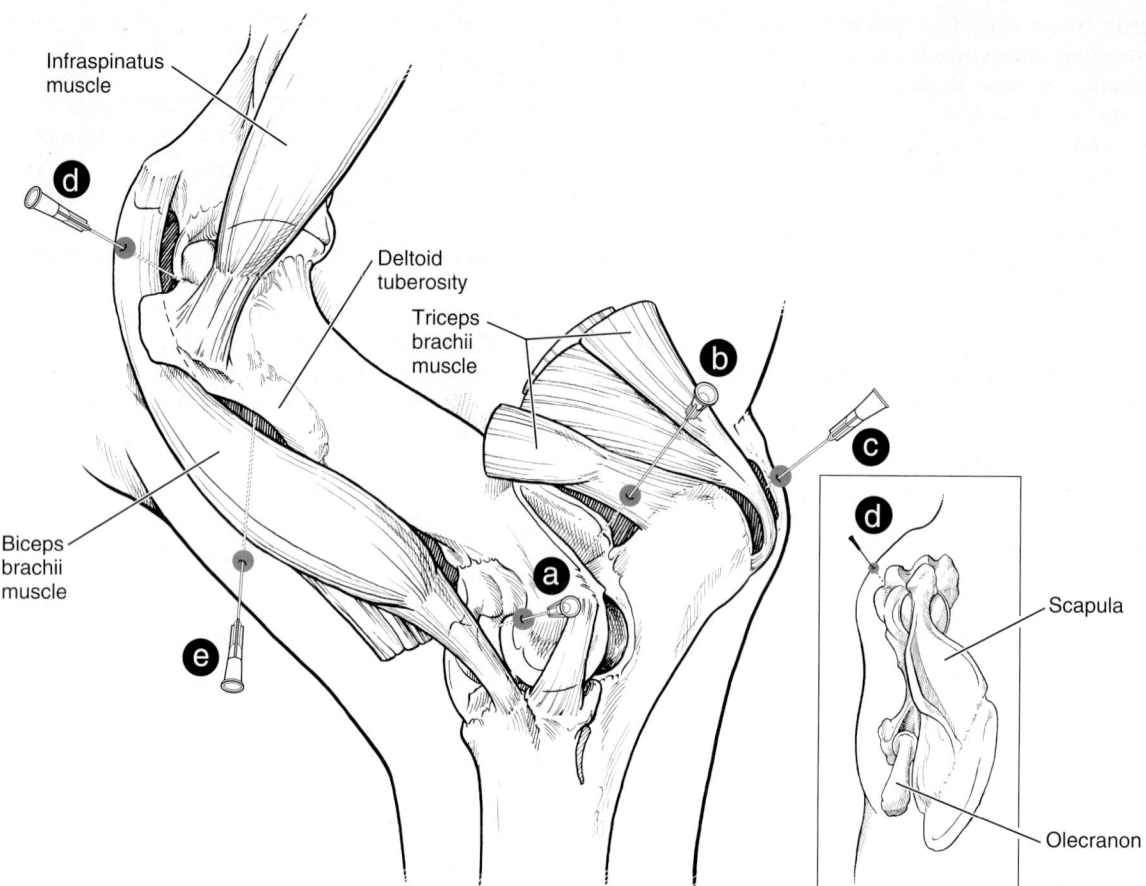

Fig. 10-19 • Lateral view of the left elbow and shoulder regions. For arthrocentesis of the cranial pouch of the elbow (cubital) joint, the clinician directs the needle (a) medially and slightly caudally to a depth of about 5 to 6 cm at a point about 3.5 cm proximal to the lateral tuberosity of the radius and 2.5 cm cranial to the lateral collateral ligament. Arthrocentesis of the proximal, caudal pouch (b) is performed at a site in the palpable depression between the cranial aspect of the olecranon and the caudal aspect of the lateral epicondyle of the humerus. One injection site is for the rarely performed technique of synoviocentesis of the olecranon bursa (c). Proximally is the site for arthrocentesis of the scapulohumeral joint (d). A needle is inserted cranial to the infraspinatus tendon in the notch between the cranial and caudal eminences of the greater tubercle of the humerus and advanced in a caudomedial direction, roughly parallel to the ground and about 45 degrees to the long axis of the body (inset). For the bicipital bursa (e), the clinician inserts the needle at a point about 4 cm proximal to the palpable distal aspect of the deltoid tuberosity of the humerus (or alternatively, a point about 3 to 4 cm distal and 6 to 7 cm caudal to the palpable aspect of the cranial process of the greater tubercle) and directs it proximally and medially, and in some patients slightly cranially.

analgesia.[43] This complication is uncommon, in our experience, and may result from proximal periarticular injection of local anesthetic solution. An alternative explanation is anesthetic solution diffusion to nerves of the brachial plexus.[5] Trauma from numerous needle insertions or injection of large volumes of local anesthetic solution (>30 mL) may increase the likelihood of this complication. In fact, some have recommended using only 8 to 10 mL, but false-negative results from the block would likely occur.[43] Our opinion is that the most likely cause of this rare complication is malposition of the needle or iatrogenic trauma. Rarely, a communication between the bicipital bursa and the shoulder joint occurs.[45] Thinking a horse has shoulder joint pain is possible then, but in reality the diagnosis is bicipital bursitis or tendonitis. Rather than a communication between the structures, the most likely explanation is inadvertent penetration of the bicipital bursa from a misdirected needle.

ANALGESIA OF FORELIMB BURSAE AND TENDON SHEATHS

In most instances, analgesia of bursae and tendon sheaths is achieved using perineural techniques, but in some horses, selective intrasynovial analgesia is indicated. Pain sensation from bursae and sheaths is likely complex, and lameness after intrabursal or intrathecal (within a sheath) analgesia may improve but not completely resolve. In fact, horses with severe lameness resulting from bursitis or tenosynovitis often have other associated soft tissue damage, a fact that explains partial improvement after intrasynovial analgesia. Extra time is usually given, after blocking, to reassess the horse's clinical signs.

Podotrochlear (Navicular) Bursa

As was noted previously (see DIP joint analgesia), analgesia of the navicular bursa has generally been regarded as the most specific block for diagnosis of navicular syndrome. Although likely still true, the results of at least two studies suggest there is potential for misinterpretation of the results of analgesia of the navicular bursa, and we question the specificity of the block. With a setscrew model used to induce solar pain, it was shown that injection of 3.5 mL of local anesthetic solution into the navicular bursa significantly reduced lameness scores in horses with pain at the dorsal aspect of the sole (but not the palmar aspect) within 15 minutes.[29] In a complementary study using endotoxin-induced synovitis of the DIP joint, injection of the navicular bursa with 3.5 mL of local anesthetic solution had no effect on lameness score at 10 minutes, but lameness was substantially decreased 20 minutes after injection (though not to a statistically significant degree [$P = .07$]).[30] Nonetheless, the clinical experience of one of the Editors (SJD) indicates that intrathecal analgesia of the navicular bursa is reasonably reliable in improving pain associated with lesions of the navicular bone, navicular bursa, and distal aspect of the DDFT, whereas pain associated with the collateral ligaments of the DIP joint is not affected.

A palmar midline approach is most commonly used for analgesia of the navicular bursa. Because needle position is difficult to assess and fluid recovery varies, radiographs should be used to confirm proper needle position. Alternatively radiodense contrast medium can be injected together with the local anesthetic solution, and a lateromedial radiographic image can then be obtained to determine that the injection was into the navicular bursa. Positioning the foot on a wooden block can minimize the problems of manipulation at the bulbs of the heel and helps to maintain aseptic technique. Subcutaneous deposition of a small volume (1 to 2 mL) of local anesthetic solution can improve horse compliance during this procedure. An 18- to 20-gauge, 9-cm

spinal needle is inserted on the palmar midline, just proximal to the hairline, and directed parallel to the sole until the needle contacts bone (Figure 10-20).[25,27,46] Others describe a similar approach, although they direct the needle parallel to the coronary band.[21,47,48] Because redirection of the needle proximally or distally often is necessary, these approaches differ little. Success depends most on personal experience, but radiographs can be critical in confirming successful entry into the navicular bursa. The direction in which the needle is inserted is often dictated by the shape of the horse's foot and the projected position of the navicular bone.[5] Plotting and marking the navicular position on the hoof wall can be helpful in determining needle direction and depth of insertion. The navicular position is located at a site 1 cm distal to and halfway between the dorsal and palmar aspects of the coronary band.[48,49] However, with experience and after identifying the navicular position, the procedure can be done blindly. In most horses the flexor surface of the navicular bone will be contacted at a depth of 4 to 5 cm. The needle is likely improperly positioned if resistance is encountered at a depth of less than 3 to 4 cm or if the needle can be advanced more than 6 to 7 cm. Spontaneous retrieval of synovial fluid is rare and usually indicates that the needle is in the DIP joint capsule or the DFTS. To avoid penetrating these structures, the needle should be placed in the middle of the flexor surface of the navicular bone.[5] Three to 5 mL of local anesthetic solution are used. If navicular syndrome is suspected, some clinicians combine injection of local anesthetic solution with a corticosteroid. Alternatively, navicular bursography[50] can be performed in combination with diagnostic analgesia by adding 1 to 2 mL of sterile, iodinated contrast material (see Chapter 30). Because in the standing horse the navicular bursa is under compression by the DDFT, suspending the

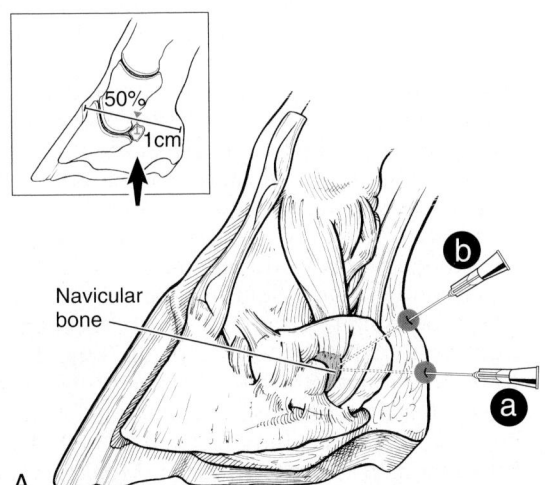 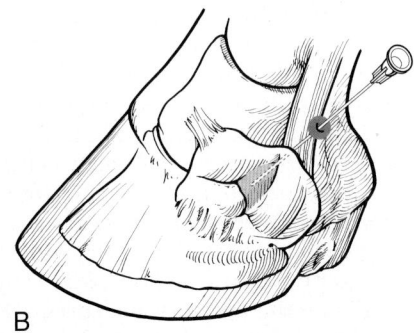

Fig. 10-20 • A, Lateral view showing two techniques for synoviocentesis of the navicular bursa of the foot. In the palmar (plantar) approach *(a)* the needle is placed just proximal to the hairline between the bulbs of the heel and inserted to the navicular bursa using the navicular position as a guide. The navicular position *(arrow)* is located by determining the point on the outside of the hoof wall that is 50% of the distance from the dorsal to the palmar (plantar) extent of the coronary band and 1 cm below *(inset)*. An approach slightly more proximal *(b)* requires placing the needle in the depression between the heel bulbs and advancing the needle in a dorsodistal direction, about 30 degrees from horizontal toward the navicular position. **B,** Palmarolateral (plantarolateral) view of the digit showing the lateral approach for synoviocentesis of the navicular bursa. The needle is inserted just proximal to the cartilage of the foot between the digital neurovascular bundle and the digital flexor tendon sheath and directed axially, distally, and slightly dorsally.

foot or placing the toe in a "navicular block" as if for radiography, with the foot in partial flexion during actual injection, are useful. Without using radiographs, being confident of accurate needle placement is difficult.

A proximal, palmar injection technique has been described. A needle is inserted into the deepest part of the hollow between the heel bulbs and advanced dorsodistally, about 30 degrees from horizontal, until contact with the bone is made.[45,51] A lateral (or medial) approach is also described. A needle is inserted just proximal to the cartilage of the foot, between the neurovascular bundle and the DFTS and directed axially, distally, and slightly dorsally until contact with bone is made (see Figure 10-20).[46,48,52] These five techniques were compared in an in vitro study. The most reliable technique was determined to be the distal palmar approach, with the needle being directed to the navicular position and the limb in a non–weight-bearing position.[53]

Digital Flexor Tendon Sheath

Two sites for intrasynovial injection of the DFTS are just proximal to the palmar (plantar) annular ligament (PAL) or in the palmar aspect of the pastern region in an outpouching of the sheath located between the proximal and distal digital annular ligaments (see Figure 10-17). Effusion facilitates identification of these sites, and rarely would an intrathecal injection be contemplated without the presence of effusion. Proximal to the PAL, villous hypertrophy of synovial membrane can complicate the procedure, because even with severe distention of the sheath, synovial fluid may be difficult to retrieve. For this reason we favor the palmar pastern approach. In some horses the sheath appears to be compartmentalized and distended proximal to the PAL but not below, and therefore injections are easier to perform proximally. A 20-gauge, 2.5-cm needle and 10 to 15 mL of local anesthetic solution are used (see also Figure 124-1). In contrast to intrasynovial analgesia in other locations in the digit, analgesia of the DFTS appears to be quite specific for lameness associated with pain arising from structures contained within it.[54] In other words, unless local anesthetic solution is inadvertently injected outside of the DFTS or leaks from it after injection, analgesia of nearby digital nerves and structures appears unusual. However, local diffusion may result in alleviation of pain from the oblique or straight sesamoidean ligaments.[55]

Alternatives to these approaches for intrasynovial injection of the DFTS are described. The procedure can be performed at a site just distal to the PSBs, between the distal aspect of the PAL and the proximal aspect of the proximal digital annular ligament (see Figure 10-17). A palmar axial sesamoidean approach has been described. With the metacarpophalangeal joint held in flexion (225-degree angle between the McIII and the proximal phalanx), a 20-gauge, 2.5-cm needle is inserted at an angle of 45 degrees, 3 mm axial to the palmar border of the PSB (midbody) and just palmar to the neurovascular bundle. Putative advantages included more reliable access to the DFTS when effusion is absent and reduced time required for successful entry.[56]

Carpal Sheath

The carpal sheath (carpal flexor sheath) envelops the SDFT and DDFT in the carpal canal. Distention of the carpal sheath is most easily recognized laterally, just proximal to

the accessory carpal bone, between the lateral digital extensor and ulnaris lateralis tendons (see Figure 10-18). Effusion of the carpal sheath must be differentiated from that of the antebrachiocarpal joint. Concurrent distention of the dorsal aspect of the antebrachiocarpal joint or distention of the distal aspect of the carpal sheath (lateral or medial, distal to the flexor retinaculum on the palmar aspect of the metacarpal region) is a sign that is helpful in determining this. Ultrasonographic evaluation or positive contrast radiography can be useful adjunct diagnostic techniques. Synoviocentesis can be performed in either the proximal or the distal aspect of the sheath, using a 20-gauge, 2.5-cm needle and 10 to 15 mL of local anesthetic solution.

Olecranon Bursa

This technique is mentioned to be complete, but we have never found an indication to perform analgesia of this bursa (see Figure 10-19). If distended, this bursa could be entered using the same techniques described for other bursae. Rarely, local analgesia over implants used to repair olecranon process fractures is necessary to investigate whether implant removal is indicated.

Bicipital Bursa

Bicipital bursitis and shoulder lameness are frequently diagnosed but in reality are uncommon causes of lameness, if the clinician religiously adheres to the principles of diagnostic analgesia. However, bicipital bursitis and tendonitis and proximal humeral osteitis, fractures, or osseous cystlike lesions can cause lameness and are diagnosed using analgesia of the bicipital bursa. The bicipital bursa is located between the greater and lesser tubercles of the humerus and the overlying tendon of origin of the biceps brachii muscle. Synoviocentesis of the bicipital bursa is routinely performed from a lateral approach, but if severe effusion exists, the bursa can be accessed medially. The injection site is located just cranial to the humerus, 4 cm proximal to the distal aspect of the deltoid tuberosity.[46] Alternatively, the site can be located by finding a point 3 to 4 cm distal and 6 to 7 cm caudal to the cranial process of the greater tubercle (see Figure 10-19).[19] Subcutaneous infiltration of local anesthetic solution at the site can be used but is rarely needed. An 18-gauge, 9-cm needle is directed in a proximal, medial, and slightly cranial direction and can be "walked off" (shaft of the needle in contact with the bone) the cranial cortex of the humerus. A change in resistance is felt, and synovial fluid may be seen in the needle hub or can be aspirated. Ten to 20 mL of local anesthetic solution are used. If injection is difficult, synovial fluid cannot be retrieved, and retrieving local anesthetic solution already injected is not possible, the bursa likely has not been entered. A recent study showed a high failure rate of injection with either technique.[57] Moreover, false-negative results also occur, despite retrieval of synovial fluid, in association with severe lesions of the tendon of biceps brachii or in the presence of dystrophic mineralization or ossification.[58] An alternative is to use an ultrasound-guided technique, which may be more accurate.

PERINEURAL ANALGESIA IN THE HINDLIMB

Perineural analgesia in the distal aspect of the hindlimb is similar to that described for the forelimb. Minor differences in innervation and anatomy must be taken into consideration, however. Technical differences in whether, or how, the limb is held and other intangible differences exist. Most clinicians are not as familiar, or frankly as comfortable, with performing hindlimb analgesic techniques, and this is particularly true with perineural analgesia. It takes a dedicated lameness detective to be enthusiastic about hindlimb analgesia, particularly in fractious or highly strung horses. Obviously, safety for the veterinarian and assistants is paramount, and physical and chemical restraint become important. Performing intraarticular analgesia is far easier, but the clinician must keep in mind that perineural techniques are much more effective in abolishing subchondral bone pain. Therefore false-negative results will likely be obtained if one is limited to only intraarticular procedures. We generally recommend that most perineural techniques distal to the tarsus be performed with the limb held off the ground by an experienced assistant, but personal preference can of course prevail. In some instances, such as when plantar digital analgesia is performed, the anatomy is much easier to identify when the limb is bearing weight. One of the Editors (SJD) routinely performs the majority of hindlimb local analgesic techniques with the limb bearing weight, and with the horse restrained in wooden stocks. The hindlimb can be positioned behind or just in front of the back wooden post; the clinician is then protected by the post if the horse kicks.

To limit the number of hindlimb injections in horses that lack clinical signs referable to the digit, starting with the low plantar block (low 4 point or 6 point block) may be reasonable, in lieu of performing sequential blocks starting with plantar digital analgesia. Of course, performing blocks distal to this site at another time may be necessary if baseline lameness is discovered using this approach. The clinician should take care when testing the efficacy of hindlimb blocks, and using a pole or similar device may be safer than using forceps.[5] Complete abolition of skin sensation in the hindlimb is less likely than in the forelimb because the distribution of cutaneous innervation varies.

Plantar Digital Analgesia

The technique for plantar digital analgesia is essentially the same as in the forelimb (see Figure 10-5). The prevalence of lameness abolished by plantar digital analgesia in the hindlimb is considerably lower than palmar digital analgesia in the forelimb but is not zero, and therefore this block should still represent a good starting point for a horse with undiagnosed hindlimb lameness. Because of the reciprocal apparatus, the digit is constantly flexed when the limb is held off the ground, and this block can be slightly more difficult to perform in this position. However, just as in the forelimb, results can be misleading with abolition of pastern or fetlock region pain.

Dorsal Ring Block of the Pastern

The section on the dorsal ring block of the pastern in the forelimb describes this technique (see Figure 10-5). This block requires several needle insertions and can be difficult to perform if the limb is held off the ground, because the dorsal aspect of the pastern is constantly flexed, making subcutaneous injection difficult.

Basisesamoid and Abaxial Sesamoid Blocks

Basisesamoid and abaxial sesamoid blocks present no essential differences between the forelimbs and hindlimbs (see Figure 10-5). Our philosophical points about the basisesamoid block (see forelimb) hold true in the hindlimb as well. The abaxial sesamoid block is avoided, if possible, in racehorses, because the high prevalence of lameness involving the metatarsophalangeal joint may lead to inadvertent misdiagnosis (a positive response to the block will be interpreted as lameness in the foot, when in reality lameness involves the metatarsophalangeal joint).

Low Plantar Block

Analgesia of the metatarsophalangeal joint region is achieved using the low plantar block, a procedure similar to the low palmar block (see Figure 10-7). This block is one of the most overlooked but most useful of all perineural techniques. It is essential to block the medial and lateral and plantar and the medial and lateral plantar metatarsal, and in some horses the dorsal metatarsal nerves. For routine diagnostic analgesia we do not block the dorsal metatarsal nerves, but for therapeutic analgesia they should be blocked. Anecdotal information suggests that some practitioners may not include the plantar metatarsal nerves when performing this block. The plantar metatarsal nerves supply innervation to the subchondral bone of the distal aspect of the third metatarsal bone (MtIII), and to provide analgesia to this important area, these nerves need to be blocked. In fact, a modification of this technique can be used in horses suspected of having subchondral, maladaptive, or nonadaptive remodeling of the MtIII, a common diagnosis in Standardbred and Thoroughbred racehorses (see Chapters 106 to 109). A positive response to an independent block of the lateral plantar metatarsal nerve can help establish this syndrome as the cause of lameness. Other causes of pain arising from the lateral aspect of the metatarsophalangeal joint, including fractures of the lateral condyle of the MtIII or of the PSBs, can be abolished using this modified technique.

The only difference between the low palmar and low plantar blocks involves the dorsal aspect of the limb (see Figure 10-7). Skin sensation laterally and medially is retained after this block, unless a circumferential, subcutaneous ring block is used. In the forelimb, it is necessary to use subcutaneous infiltration only to the dorsal midline. Alternatively, the dorsal metatarsal nerves can be blocked individually.

High Plantar Nerve Block

The high plantar or subtarsal block is one of the most important but often overlooked perineural analgesic procedures in the horse. This block is used to diagnose suspensory desmitis, arguably one of the most important lameness conditions in the hindlimb. However, suspensory desmitis can be a catchall diagnosis in some horses with occult hindlimb lameness, and the high plantar block must be done to confirm the authentic location of pain. The high plantar block should be done after completion of lower limb blocks such as low plantar analgesia to rule out other common sources of pain. Practitioners should be wary of a recent trend to complete only a subtarsal block to diagnose, erroneously in some horses, proximal suspensory desmitis, when sequential distal-to-proximal analgesic

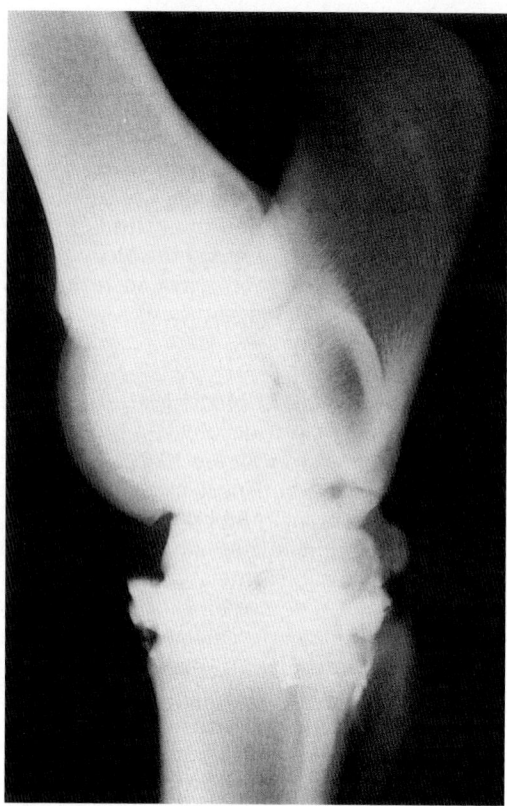

Fig. 10-21 • Positive contrast arthrogram of the tarsometatarsal joint showing short, distoplantar outpouchings extending distally toward the origin of the suspensory ligament. Inadvertent penetration of these pouches occurs during subtarsal or high plantar analgesic techniques.

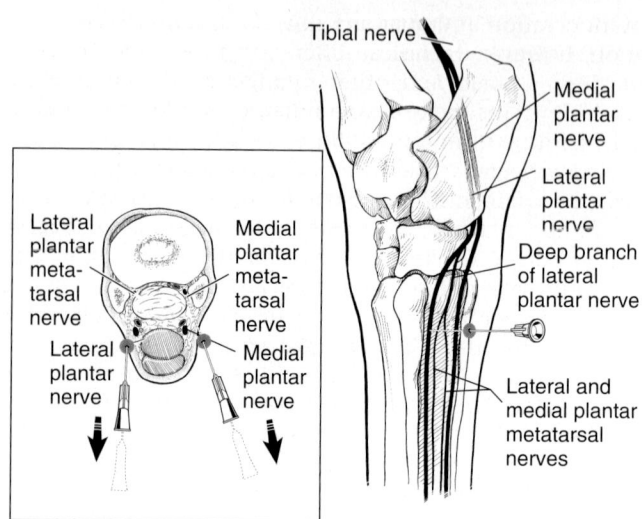

Fig. 10-22 • The high plantar block is performed at a level 4 cm distal to the proximal aspect of fourth metatarsal bone and on the medial side 3 cm distal to the proximal aspect of second metatarsal bone. The needles are inserted axial to the respective splint bone and advanced deep to contact the plantar surface of the third metatarsal bone. Local anesthetic solution is deposited in this location to block the lateral (medial) plantar metatarsal nerves and in a more superficial position as the needle is withdrawn blocks the lateral (medial) plantar nerves (inset).

techniques may have revealed an alternative source of pain. The tarsometatarsal joint has distoplantar outpouchings (similar to but less extensive than the distopalmar outpouchings of the carpometacarpal joint) that may complicate tarsometatarsal intraarticular or high plantar analgesic techniques (Figure 10-21). However, this is certainly less of a problem in the hindlimb than in the forelimb. For example, inadvertent penetration of the tarsometatarsal joint occurred in only 5% of limbs in which high plantar analgesia was performed, at a level of 1.5 cm distal to the tarsometatarsal joint. However, contrast material was found in the tarsal sheath in 40% of limbs, adding yet another dimension to this already somewhat difficult blocking technique. False-negative results have been attributed to inadvertent injection into blood or lymphatic vessels.[59] The clinician should take care in preparing the limb for this procedure and interpreting the results. It is possible, although not likely, that when a high plantar block is performed, local anesthetic solution could be inadvertently placed in the tarsometatarsal joint. A good chance also exists, however, of inducing analgesia of the tarsal sheath. Comprehensive evaluation using numerous imaging modalities is needed when attempting to differentiate causes of lameness in this important area.

The medial and lateral plantar and the medial and lateral plantar metatarsal nerves are blocked, and a circumferential dorsal ring block provides complete analgesia to the metatarsal region. Blocking only the plantar metatarsal nerves can abolish pain associated with the suspensory ligament. Most clinicians do not include the dorsal ring block, but it is necessary to do so to eliminate lameness resulting from injury of the dorsal cortex of the MtIII or to suture lacerations in this area. This block is performed most commonly and safely with the limb held off the ground. Although uncommon to rare, needle breakage is a complication during high plantar analgesia, and for this reason we prefer to use needles no smaller than 18 to 20 gauge and 4 cm long. At this level on the plantar aspect of the limb, it is impossible to palpate nerves, and unlike with the high palmar block, only one injection site exists for each, on the medial and lateral aspects of the limb. The needle is placed just distal to the tarsometatarsal joint and axial to the fourth metatarsal bone (MtIV) and inserted until contact is made with the MtIII (Figure 10-22). A minimum of 5 mL of local anesthetic solution is deposited at this deep location, and an additional 5 mL are deposited as the needle is withdrawn, leaving a definite bleb in the subcutaneous tissues. Some clinicians prefer lower volumes of local anesthetic solution. Additional local anesthetic solution can be used without risk, and a common modification is flooding the origin of the suspensory ligament with an additional 5 to 10 mL of local anesthetic solution. The procedure is then repeated medially, and the needle is inserted axial to the second metatarsal bone (MtII). To complete the block, a circumferential subcutaneous ring block is performed. The clinician must take care not to lacerate the dorsal metatarsal artery or the saphenous vein during this procedure.

An alternative technique to alleviate pain from the proximal aspect of the suspensory ligament is to block the deep branch of the lateral plantar nerve. This can be performed with the limb bearing weight or lifted, according to personal preference. A 20-gauge needle is inserted perpendicular to the skin just plantar to the MtIV at the junction where its contour changes from oblique to vertical. The needle is inserted to a depth of approximately 1 cm, and 3 mL of local anesthetic solution are deposited. This block is quick and easy to perform and is generally well tolerated but may not remove pain associated with entheseous reaction.[5] See the following text for a discussion of alternative techniques to block the suspensory origin.

Fibular (Peroneal) and Tibial Nerve Blocks

Analgesia of the distal crus and tarsus or entire distal aspect of the hindlimb is induced using the fibular and tibial nerve blocks. These blocks are used most commonly in horses with distal hock joint pain, in which intraarticular analgesia is difficult or impossible to perform. The fibular and tibial nerve blocks, when completed successfully, are more effective in eliminating pain from the complex hock joints than is intraarticular analgesia. The fibular and tibial nerve blocks also are useful in eliminating pain associated with subchondral trauma of the distal aspect of the tibia and talus, distally located tibial stress fractures, the tarsal sheath, the distal aspect of the common calcaneal tendon, the calcaneal bursa, and the plantar aspect of the hock. The clinician should keep in mind that if the high plantar block has not already been performed, the fibular and tibial nerve blocks eliminate pain associated with proximal suspensory desmitis.

The deep fibular nerve is blocked at a site located laterally, 10 cm proximal to the point of the hock (tuber calcanei), in the groove between the long and lateral digital extensor muscles (Figure 10-23). In this groove the superficial fibular nerve is easily palpated and can be rolled against the fascia of the crus. An 18- to 22-gauge, 4-cm needle is inserted to the hub or until it contacts the lateral tibial cortex, and 10 to 15 mL of local anesthetic solution

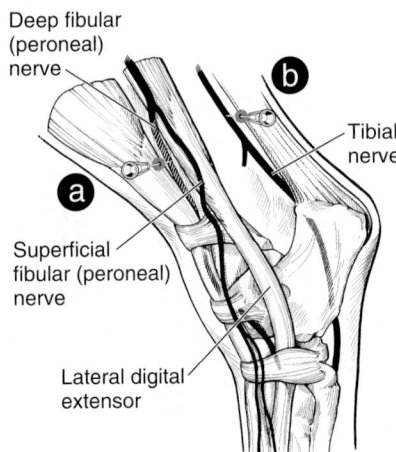

Fig. 10-23 • Lateral view of the left crus and tarsus showing the fibular (peroneal) and tibial nerve block. The deep and superficial fibular nerves are blocked by finding the groove between the long and lateral digital extensor muscles, 10 cm proximal to the tarsus, in which the superficial fibular nerve is palpable. The needle *(a)* is advanced deep to block the deep branch and withdrawn to a more superficial position to deposit local anesthetic solution subcutaneously to block the superficial branch. The tibial nerve block *(b)* is performed by palpating the nerve just cranial to the common calcaneal tendon (from either a lateral or a medial approach) in a location about 10 cm proximal to the tuber calcanei.

are injected, beginning deep and continuing as the needle is withdrawn. The needle can be redirected in a fan-shaped pattern if desired to ensure complete block of the deep branch of the fibular nerve. Seeing blood in the needle hub is common, a reliable sign of accurate needle placement, because the cranial tibial vein and artery are located close to the deep fibular nerve.[60] Performing the tibial block first is therefore preferable, as is warning the client that blood may appear.[5] The superficial fibular nerve is blocked as the needle is withdrawn from deep within the injection site. Additional local anesthetic solution (5 to 10 mL) is placed in this subcutaneous location.

The tibial nerve is blocked at a site 10 cm proximal to the tuber calcanei, cranial to the common calcaneal tendon, and caudal to the DDFT (see Figure 10-23). The nerve can be palpated as a firm cordlike structure with the limb in a flexed position. For this reason, performing this block may be easier with the limb not bearing weight. Although the tibial nerve is slightly more superficial medially, the injection can be performed either medially or laterally. A 20-gauge, 2.5-cm needle is inserted laterally, and 15 mL of local anesthetic solution are injected over the nerve. The needle tip should be palpated under the skin, medially, to ensure the proper depth of penetration. Local anesthetic solution can be placed using a fan-shaped injection technique, but the horse will object if the tibial nerve is penetrated. Although deep pain will be abolished if these nerves are successfully blocked, superficial sensation persists on the medial aspect and occasionally in the caudal (plantar) aspect of the limb. To use the fibular and tibial nerve blocks therapeutically, it is necessary to perform a circumferential subcutaneous ring block to completely abolish skin sensation. After the fibular and tibial nerve blocks, paradoxically, preexisting toe drag may persist or increase, despite resolution of weight-bearing lameness.[5] Some horses stumble or knuckle, indicating loss of extensor muscle function, but this is not common and certainly not a necessary sign to suggest that complete analgesia has been obtained. However, exercising a horse at speed or over fences should be avoided. Because of nerve size and depth, we suggest that additional time be given, as much as 20 to 30 minutes, to evaluate the effect of this block before a final conclusion is reached. Dyson has recognized improvement in horses up to 1 hour after blocking and warns that proceeding with a stifle block too soon leads to false-positive results.[5] The fibular and tibial nerve blocks are not commonly performed in practice, at least in the United States, and at best may result in only 50% to 80% improvement in lameness score, particularly in those horses with severe distal hock joint pain, although in some horses lameness is abolished completely. Allowing more time for maximal response and taking a realistic approach to the percent improvement expected are warranted when using the fibular and tibial nerve blocks. Intrasynovial analgesic techniques are certainly more specific than are the fibular and tibial nerve blocks, and although the fibular and tibial nerve blocks have limitations, the lameness diagnostician should become familiar and comfortable with this procedure. Proficiency in performing these blocks is a must for accurate diagnosis of hindlimb lameness. Performing the fibular and tibial components can independently improve specificity of the fibular and tibial nerve blocks.

INTRAARTICULAR ANALGESIA IN THE HINDLIMB

Analgesia of the DIP and proximal interphalangeal joints in the hindlimb is exactly the same as that described for the forelimb. Performing intraarticular analgesia of the metatarsophalangeal joint is the same as that described for the metacarpophalangeal joint. Perineural analgesic techniques should be used whenever possible, because subchondral bone pain is more completely abolished with these techniques, and false-negative results are less likely.

Tarsus

Tarsometatarsal Joint

The most reliable site for arthrocentesis of the tarsometatarsal joint is a lateral approach, just proximal to the MtIV. At this site is a subtle but consistent depression that can reliably be palpated. A 20-gauge, 2.5-cm needle is inserted in a dorsomedial and slightly distal direction (Figure 10-24). The needle can usually be inserted to the hub, but occasionally it hits articular cartilage. Synovial fluid is consistently retrieved, but we find it interesting that even in horses without lameness of the tarsometatarsal joint, the fluid is generally watery, lacking what is thought to be normal viscosity. In most horses, up to 4 mL of local anesthetic solution can usually be injected without encountering elevated intraarticular pressures and horse discomfort. Be aware that beyond 2 mL the horse may start to feel uncomfortable, raise the limb, or even kick. Anecdotal reports of a subtle pop or sudden decrease in pressure have been attributed to communication between the tarsometatarsal and centrodistal (distal intertarsal) joints. In reality, this most often results from rupture of the tarsometatarsal joint capsule and subsequent deposition of local anesthetic solution (or medication) extraarticularly into the tarsal space and not the centrodistal joint. We recommend using no more than 4 mL of local anesthetic solution or injecting only that amount of local anesthetic solution necessary to develop moderate intraarticular resistance to avoid inadvertent deposition into the intertarsal space. Periarticular extravasation of local anesthetic solution from excessive volume may inadvertently block the nearby lateral plantar nerve and deep branch, potentially alleviating pain associated with the suspensory ligament attachment or other structures. An alternative site for tarsometatarsal arthrocentesis is a medial approach, similar to that described for the centrodistal joint.

The issue of communication between the distal tarsal joints is important from diagnostic and therapeutic standpoints. Studies have shown that the tarsometatarsal and centrodistal joints communicate in 8% to 35% of normal horses.[59,61,62] Communication between the tarsometatarsal joint (and presumably the centrodistal joint) and the talocalcaneal-centroquartal (proximal intertarsal) and tarsocrural joints was shown to be about 4% in an in vivo study, after injection of latex in the tarsometatarsal joint.[62] Some concern and confusion exist regarding whether or not a single injection into the tarsometatarsal joint also provides analgesia or treats the centrodistal joint. Some clinicians even preferentially inject a large volume of local anesthetic solutions or drugs, hoping to block or medicate the

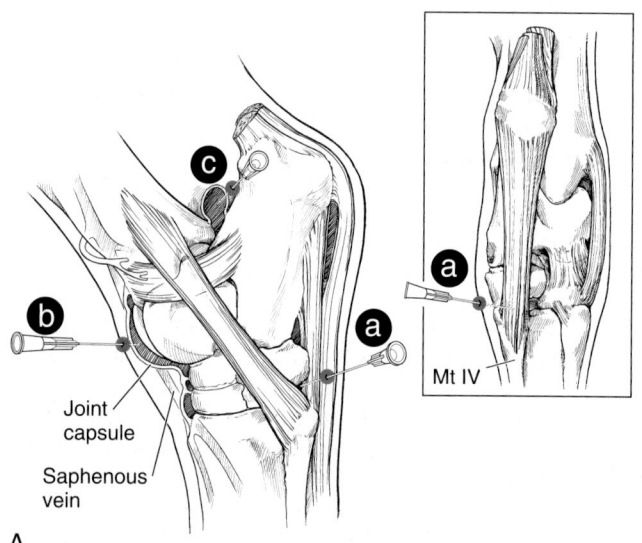

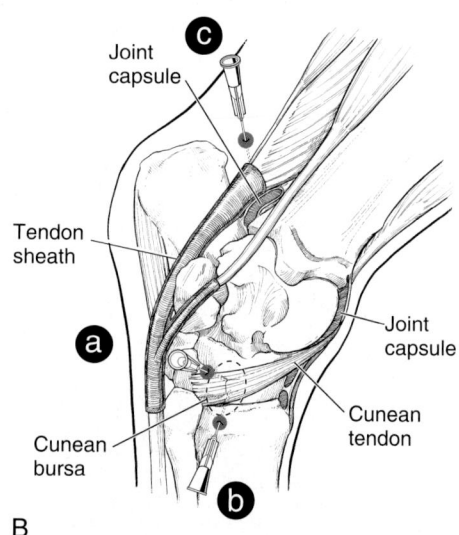

Fig. 10-24 • A, Lateral and plantar (inset) views of the left tarsus showing sites for tarsal arthrocentesis. The tarsometatarsal joint is entered by locating the depression just proximal to the proximal aspect of the fourth metatarsal bone (Mt IV) and inserting a needle (a) in the plantar aspect of this depression, directing it dorsomedially. The dorsomedial pouch of the tarsocrural joint (b) is entered either just lateral or medial to the dorsal branch of the saphenous vein or, alternatively, using the plantarolateral pouch (c). **B,** Medial view of the left tarsus. The centrodistal joint is entered by placing the needle (a) in the depression formed between the fused first and second tarsal bones, the third tarsal bone, and the central tarsal bone, which is at the proximal edge or just slightly distal to the proximal edge of the cunean tendon. The cunean bursa (dashed ellipse) is entered by locating the distal border of the cunean tendon and inserting the needle (b) under the tendon from the distal aspect or placing it directly through the tendon. The distended tarsal sheath (c) can be entered proximal, just caudal to the tarsocrural joint capsule or distal (not shown) to the tarsus.

tarsometatarsal and centrodistal joints. A recent in vitro study found that, although gross anatomic communications exist in only a minority of horses, diffusion of mepivacaine between the distal tarsal joints (as well as between the distal tarsal joints and the tarsocrural joint) occurs with a much higher frequency. Fifteen minutes after injection of 5 mL of 2% mepivacaine into either the tarsometatarsal or the centrodistal joint, mepivacaine was detected in the alternate joint at concentrations >300 mg/L in 64% and 60% of specimens, respectively.[63] Whether or not this holds true in the live horse remains undetermined. For that reason, and based on our clinical experience, we believe the clinician should still consider *the tarsometatarsal and centrodistal joints to be separate synovial cavities*. However, it is clear that in some horses analgesia or treatment of the tarsometatarsal joint will relieve centrodistal joint pain. Because the tarsometatarsal joint has distoplantar outpouchings, abolishing pain associated with the proximal suspensory attachment or lesions involving the proximal aspect of the MtIII is also possible when performing tarsometatarsal analgesia. Accurate differential diagnosis for pain involving the lower hock joints and proximal metatarsal region depends on careful interpretation of response to diagnostic analgesia and evaluation of ancillary images.

Centrodistal Joint

Compared with the tarsometatarsal joint, arthrocentesis of the centrodistal joint is relatively difficult. The centrodistal joint is small, and in fact inserting a needle any larger than 22 to 25 gauge into this joint is difficult, even in horses with normal width of joint space. We have tried several alternative sites, including dorsomedial and dorsolateral approaches. Anecdotal reports suggest that the dorsomedial approach, about 1 cm distal to the distal end of the medial trochlear ridge, is a consistent, reliable injection site, but we often enter the proximal intertarsal joint from this approach. An outpouching of the centrodistal joint exists dorsolaterally, but we reasoned that the perforating tarsal artery precluded use of this site in vivo. A recent study described the use of this dorsolateral approach. The site is identified as a point 2 to 3 mm lateral to the long digital extensor tendon and 6 to 8 mm proximal to a line drawn perpendicular to the long axis of the MtIII at the level of the proximal aspect of the MtIV. The success rate for arthrocentesis at this site was equal to that for the traditional medial approach, with purported advantages being improved safety for the clinician and easily identified landmarks. In vivo, iatrogenic injury to the dorsal pedal artery or penetrating tarsal artery was not encountered.[64]

We still preferentially use a medial approach at the distal aspect of, or through, the cunean tendon (medial tendon of insertion of the tibialis cranialis muscle), a structure that can be readily palpated. With a fingertip, the distal edge of the cunean tendon is moved proximally to reveal an ill-defined concavity, the articulation of the fused first and second tarsal bones, with the third and central tarsal bones (see Figure 10-24). This depression is sometimes located in a slightly more proximal location. This injection technique is one of the few commonly performed by standing on the opposite side of the horse. A skin bleb is useful because in most horses inserting a needle directly into the joint is difficult, and numerous attempts may be necessary. A 22- to 25-gauge, 2.5-cm needle is inserted

directly in a lateral direction, horizontally, roughly parallel to the central and third tarsal articulation, perpendicular to the skin. Slight redirection of the needle may be necessary, and in many horses joint fluid is not obtained. If the needle can be inserted to a depth of 1 to 1.5 cm, it is likely properly positioned even if synovial fluid cannot be retrieved. Fluid retrieved in a more superficial location likely indicates penetration of the cunean bursa. In horses in which diagnostic information or therapeutic injection is critical and any question of needle placement exists, radiographs are warranted. A maximum of 4 to 5 mL can be injected. If a larger volume can be comfortably injected, the needle tip is likely in the tarsal space or in the proximal intertarsal joint, or a communication with the tarsometatarsal joint exists. If the injection is difficult to perform, the needle is likely malpositioned in the subcutaneous tissues, or the needle tip is touching articular cartilage. Most clinicians attempt injection of the centrodistal joint after first injecting the tarsometatarsal joint, and in some instances, medication or local anesthetic solution readily flows from the needle. The typical response is, "There must be a communication between the tarsometatarsal and centrodistal joints." However, this clinical finding most often results from inadvertent penetration of the distended medial pouch of the tarsometatarsal joint. Fluid accumulation in the tarsal space from the tarsometatarsal joint injection can cause the same result, if the needle enters the tarsal space rather than the centrodistal joint space.

In horses with advanced osteoarthritis or even in horses with early distal hock joint pain, it may be difficult or impossible to be confident that intraarticular analgesia has been achieved. An alternative approach for providing tarsal analgesia is first to perform sequential, intraarticular analgesia of the tarsometatarsal and tarsocrural joints, and then to perform the fibular and tibial nerve blocks if lameness persists. If lameness abates after the fibular and tibial nerve blocks, a presumptive diagnosis of centrodistal joint pain can be made, assuming other sources of pain abolished by this block can be ruled out.

Tarsocrural Joint

Arthrocentesis of the tarsocrural joint is straightforward and easy compared with some joints, because of extensive and multiple dorsal and plantar outpouchings. In horses with moderate to severe effusion, identifying four distinct outpouchings—the dorsolateral, dorsomedial, plantarolateral, and plantaromedial pouches—is easy. The clinician must keep in mind that the tarsocrural and proximal intertarsal joints communicate through a large fenestration at the dorsal aspect of the joints in adult horses, although in weanlings and yearlings the fenestration often cannot be seen during arthroscopic examination. Any one of the tarsocrural joint pouches can be used, but the most common site of entry is on either side of the saphenous vein, in the dorsomedial pouch (see Figure 10-24). This particular site is preferred in horses without obvious effusion. An alternative site is the plantarolateral pouch. The most consistent site to use is the distal aspect of the dorsomedial pouch, just distal to the medial malleolus of the tibia and medial to the saphenous vein. An 18- to 20-gauge, 2.5- or 4-cm needle is used to deposit 20 to 30 mL of local anesthetic solution into the tarsocrural joint. In horses with severe osteoarthritis of the tarsocrural joint or those with subchondral bone pain, use of as much as 30 to 50 mL of local anesthetic solution is necessary to abolish pain. In these horses, a false-negative result is common if only 10 to 20 mL of local anesthetic solution is used.

The plantar pouches can be useful alternative sites for arthrocentesis if the dorsomedial pouch is unsuitable, as sometimes occurs with a wound, swelling associated with trauma of the fibularis (peroneus) tertius, or superficial dermatitis. The plantar pouches must be differentiated from distention of the tarsal sheath or other forms of thoroughpin. Although the dorsal and plantar pouches freely communicate, anatomically, flushing from one aspect of the tarsocrural to the other when the horse is in a weight-bearing position may be difficult. Fluid flow between articular surfaces and joint spaces under collateral ligaments is likely restricted when horses are in a weight-bearing position. This same phenomenon occurs in other joint spaces.

Stifle Joint

The three compartments of the equine stifle joint are the medial femorotibial, lateral femorotibial, and femoropatellar joint compartments. Most consider that the femoropatellar and medial femorotibial joints communicate in almost all horses and that the lateral femorotibial compartment is solitary, but recent anatomical studies have shed new light on this time-honored concept. The frequency of communication between the medial femorotibial and femoropatellar compartments was found to be 60% to 74% in normal horses when the injection was performed from the femoropatellar compartment.[65,66] The frequency of communication was higher (80%) when the injection was performed in the medial femorotibial compartment.[65] It is important to realize, however, *that the medial femorotibial and femoropatellar compartments did not communicate in all horses.* Inconsistency in communication depending on which compartment was injected was attributed to directionality in the normal foramen or slit between the two compartments (flow easier *from* the medial femorotibial *to* the femoropatellar compartment).

The time-honored assumption that the lateral femorotibial joint is a solitary compartment was also challenged. The lateral femorotibial joint communicated with the femoropatellar joint in 3% to 18% of horses but was indeed solitary in the majority of normal horses.[65,66] Communication may be more frequent after trauma and certainly after arthroscopic surgical procedures.

Similar to the digit, carpus, and tarsus, there is clinically important evidence that mepivacaine diffuses between the compartments of the stifle joint. The proportion of synovial compartments with mepivacaine concentration >300 mg/L 15 minutes after injection of an adjacent compartment with 10 mL of 2% mepivacaine ranged from 5% to 40%.[63] Of note, functional (diffusion) communication between the medial femorotibial and femoropatellar joints was lower than previous estimates (25% to 40% versus 60% to 80%). Volume of local anesthetic solution (10 mL) was considerably lower than is commonly used in clinical practice for intraarticular analgesia of the stifle joints, and it remains undetermined if results of in vitro studies translate to actual clinical relevance.

We recommend that each compartment of the stifle joint be injected independently, either sequentially or simultaneously, to avoid confusing results during stifle analgesia. The variable degree of communication will obviously cause some degree of uncertainty in diagnosis. The same principle is recommended for therapy as well. Needle insertion in the stifle joints is complicated by a natural tendency of horses to react inappropriately to manipulation compared with other areas of the limbs. Horses seem to object to simple palpation of the stifle and may become fractious during arthrocentesis. To avoid excessive manipulation during injection, we have found it useful to attach an extension set to the needle, a procedure that obviates the need to touch the needle or skin when attaching the syringe. If necessary, the extension set may be useful for many diagnostic procedures, particularly in the hindlimbs. In general, 20 to 30 mL of local anesthetic solution are used in each of the medial femorotibial, lateral femorotibial, and femoropatellar compartments. A common misconception is that long needles are needed to perform arthrocentesis of the stifle joint compartments. In fact, some racehorse trainers will insist that "the long needles, Doc" are necessary to achieve success in medicating the femoropatellar joint. If arthrocentesis is performed with the limb in a weight-bearing position, the joint capsules can easily be penetrated with needles no longer than 4 cm. In the flexed position, use of a spinal needle when performing femoropatellar arthrocentesis is necessary. We prefer to have the horse in a weight-bearing position, with the limb slightly ahead of the contralateral limb, a position that allows the clinician to palpate landmarks readily without undue tension on patellar and collateral ligaments.

Arthrocentesis of the medial femorotibial joint is performed at a site located just caudal to the medial patellar ligament, cranial to the medial collateral ligament, and 1 to 2 cm proximal to the medial tibial plateau (Figure 10-25). In a normal horse a distinct depression occurs at this location, but in horses with effusion, a considerable bulge in the joint capsule can be present. An 18-gauge, 4-cm needle is inserted perpendicular to the skin and can be redirected or rotated if synovial fluid is not immediately retrieved. A common mistake is to insert the needle too far distally, and in this position the needle tip enters ligaments or the medial meniscus.

Arthrocentesis of the lateral femorotibial joint is more challenging than for the other two compartments, because the lateral joint pouch is small and located deep within tissue. The site is caudal to the long digital extensor tendon and cranial to the lateral collateral ligament, just proximal to the lateral tibial plateau (see Figure 10-25). These landmarks are easily palpated, but distention of the joint capsule is not, in contrast to the medial femorotibial joint. An 18-gauge, 4-cm needle is inserted horizontally and directed in a slight caudomedial direction. Retrieval of synovial fluid varies, and redirecting or rotating the needle is often necessary. An alternate site can be used, located caudal to the lateral patellar ligament and cranial to the long digital extensor tendon, and just proximal to the tibial plateau.

Arthrocentesis of the femoropatellar joint is most commonly performed at a sub-patellar site and either lateral or medial to the middle patellar ligament. The joint capsule can be easily palpated even in most normal horses, if the horse is in a weight-bearing position. With the horse in a weight-bearing position, an 18-gauge, 4-cm needle is inserted perpendicular to the skin, or directed slightly

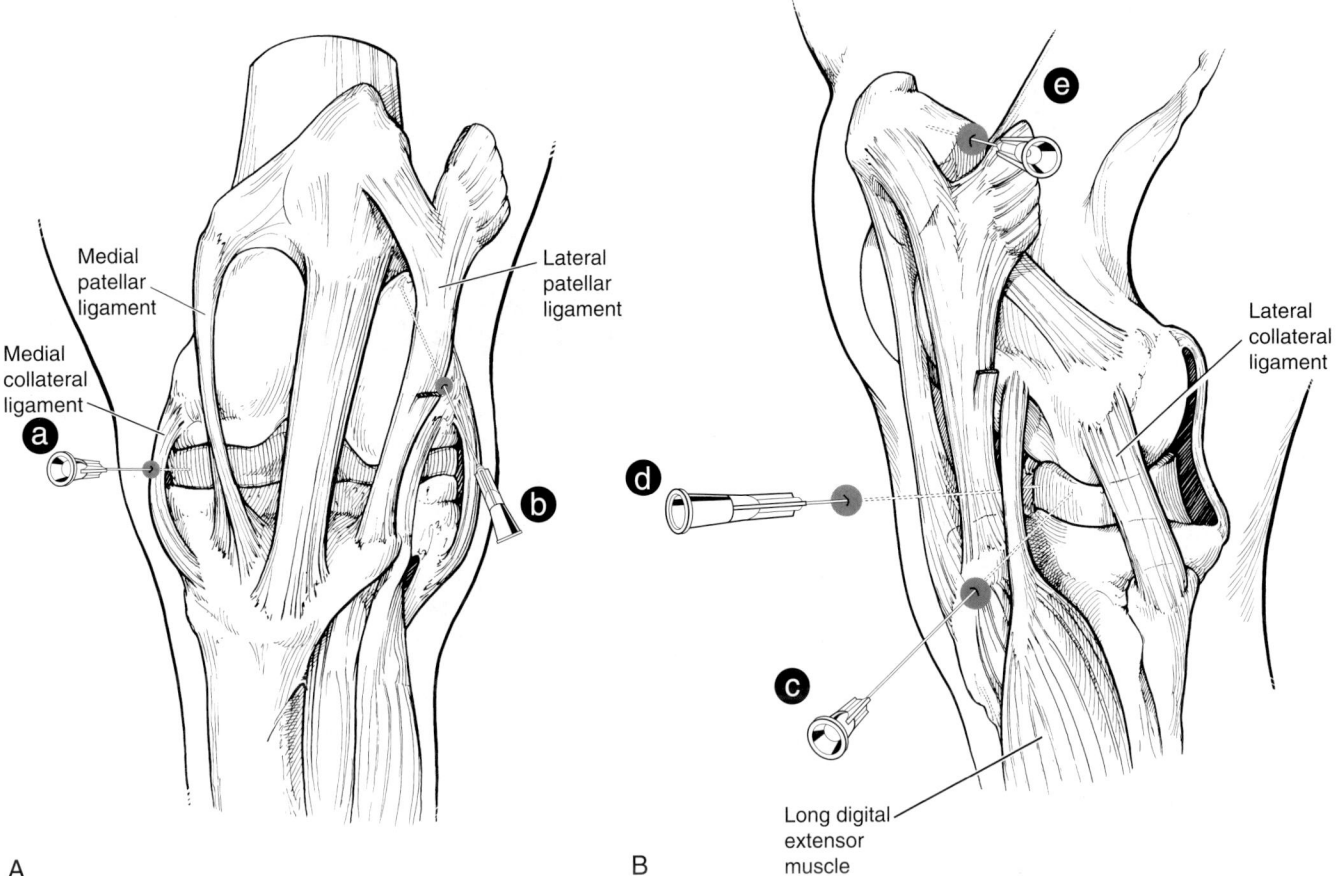

A

B

Fig. 10-25 • A, Cranial view of the left stifle. The medial femorotibial joint *(a)* is approached from a site between the medial patellar and medial collateral ligaments, about 2 cm proximal to the proximal aspect of the tibia. The femoropatellar joint *(b)* most commonly is injected either between the lateral and middle patellar ligaments or between the middle and medial patellar ligaments (not shown). The needle is directed proximally in this subpatellar position. **B,** Lateral view of the left stifle. The lateral femorotibial joint can be approached by placing the needle caudal to the long digital extensor tendon and cranial to the lateral collateral ligament *(c)* or inserting it between the lateral patellar ligament and the cranial edge of the long digital extensor tendon *(d)*. An alternative site for arthrocentesis of the femoropatellar joint *(e)* can be used by passing the needle through the lateral femoropatellar ligament.

Labels in figure: Medial patellar ligament, Lateral patellar ligament, Medial collateral ligament, Lateral collateral ligament, Long digital extensor muscle.

proximally, until joint fluid is obtained or the needle tip contacts articular cartilage of the distal femur (see Figure 10-25). The clinician does not need to angle the needle sharply proximally using this technique. What is sometimes frustrating is that even in horses with obvious femoropatellar effusion, a steady flow of synovial fluid cannot be obtained, and attempting aspiration of fluid with a syringe is seldom helpful, because synovial villi readily plug the needle, making aspiration impossible. Some clinicians perform femoropatellar arthrocentesis with the limb in a non–weight-bearing position, in which case a 9-cm spinal needle is used and the needle is directed proximally, between the patella and distal aspect of the femur. An alternative lateral approach to the femoropatellar joint has been described.[67] An 18-gauge, 4-cm needle is inserted into the lateral cul-de-sac of the femoropatellar compartment, located about 5 cm proximal to the lateral tibial plateau, caudal to the lateral patellar ligament and the lateral trochlear ridge of the femur. The needle is directed perpendicular to the long axis of the femur until bone is contacted (about 1.5 to 2 cm in most horses) and then is withdrawn slightly until synovial fluid is collected.

Proposed advantages of this approach are a reduced potential for iatrogenic injury to the articular cartilage and more reliable recovery of synovial fluid compared with the subpatellar approach.[68]

Coxofemoral (Hip) Joint

Although the coxofemoral joint is relatively large and the landmarks for needle insertion are consistent, injection is considered to be a daunting task. Few of us perform this injection technique on a regular basis, and depth of penetration makes accurate needle placement difficult. An 18-gauge, 15-cm (6-inch) spinal needle is adequate for all but the largest of draft horses. A needle of this length should be inserted carefully, and if the horse is moving or fractious, it may be necessary to provide sedation. The site is in the angle formed between the long caudal and short cranial processes of the greater trochanter of the femur (Figures 10-26 and 10-27). This site can be difficult to palpate in heavily muscled horses, and ultrasonographic evaluation can be useful to identify the injection site. The most difficult landmark to palpate consistently, but an important one nonetheless, is the cranial process. The site

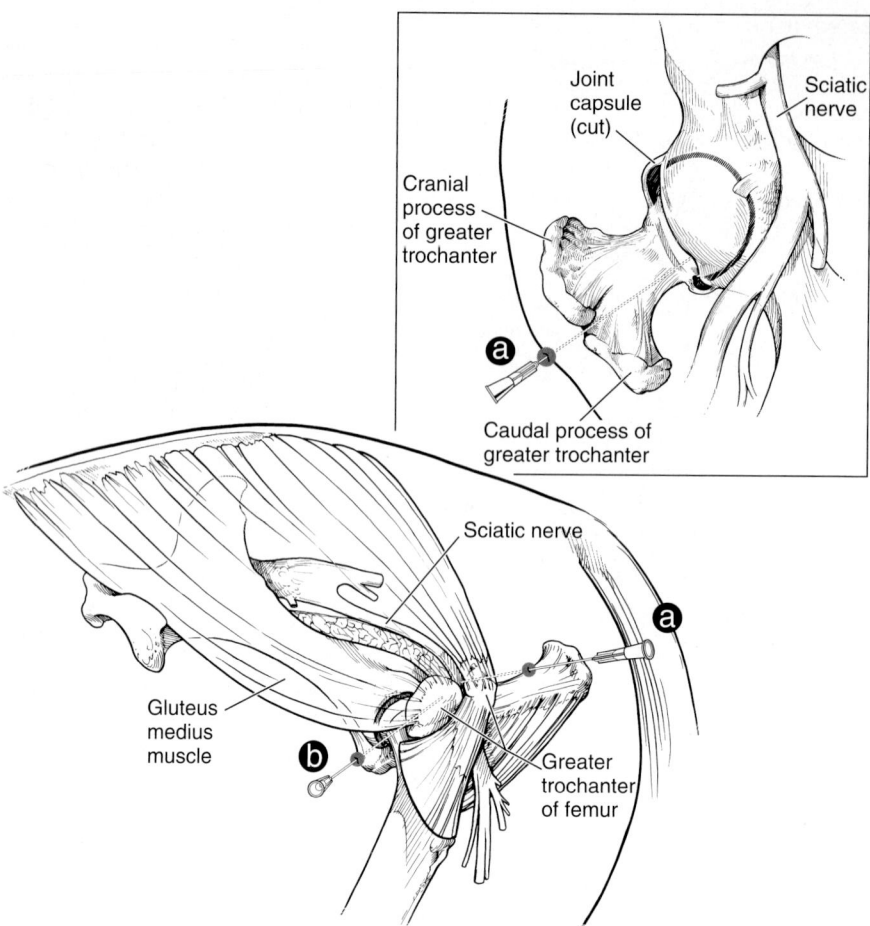

Fig. 10-26 • Lateral and dorsal *(inset)* views of the left coxofemoral joint. Arthrocentesis of the coxofemoral joint is performed by inserting the needle *(a)* in the angle formed between the caudal and cranial processes of the greater trochanter of the femur. The needle is inserted slightly cranially, distally, and medially just dorsal to the shaft of the femoral neck *(inset)*. This view *(b)* shows the seldom used diagnostic technique of synoviocentesis of the trochanteric bursa.

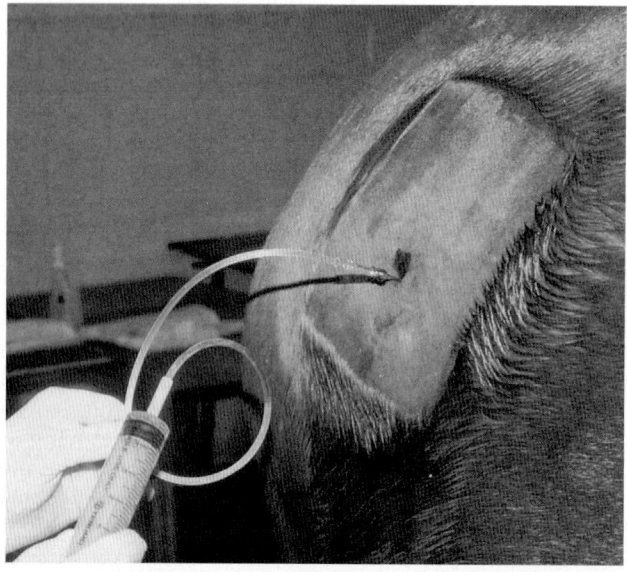

Fig. 10-27 • Arthrocentesis of the right coxofemoral joint. Using an extension set between needle and syringe, a technique that reduces the amount of manipulation necessary during the procedure, facilitates arthrocentesis of this and other joints.

is *between* the two processes, closer to the cranial process and not *caudal* to the trochanter.

Before the needle is inserted, blocking the injection site may be useful. Because the shaft of the needle is handled, sterile gloves are recommended. Needle direction is important. The needle is inserted in a slightly craniomedial direction and slightly distally and directed just dorsal to the femoral neck, until the joint capsule is penetrated. In most horses, a subtle pop can be felt as this occurs. "Walking" the needle off the femoral neck may be useful, using the bone as a guide to the coxofemoral joint. In most adult light-breed horses, this occurs within 3 to 5 cm of the hub of the needle. Synovial fluid is reliably retrieved from the coxofemoral joint, spontaneously or by aspiration. A large volume of local anesthetic solution should not be injected if synovial fluid is not readily obtained, but injecting a small volume and attempting retrieval with a syringe is useful. It is possible inadvertently to inject local anesthetic solution around the sciatic nerve, causing temporary paresis, if the needle is caudally malpositioned, and therefore local anesthetic solution should not be injected if any doubt exists that the needle is correctly positioned. The amount of local anesthetic solution used is 25 to 30 mL.

Most horses are evaluated in 20 to 30 minutes, but in horses with fractures of the acetabulum the clinician should expect only 50% improvement in lameness score, and improvement may be short-lasting (15 to 30 minutes). An alternative ultrasound-guided technique has been described and is particularly valuable in large overweight horses in which the landmarks are difficult to palpate.[69]

ANALGESIA OF HINDLIMB BURSAE AND TENDON SHEATHS

Analgesia of the navicular bursa and DFTS in the hindlimb is the same as in the forelimb.

Cunean Bursa

Occasionally, injecting the cunean bursa is necessary to assess the role of the cunean bursa and tendon in horses with distal hock joint pain, to perform cunean tenectomy, or to medicate the structure. The cunean bursa is seldom the sole source of distal hock joint pain but can play a role, so analgesia or medication of this structure is sometimes combined with other injections.

The cunean bursa is between the distal tarsal bones and the medial branch of the cranialis tibialis tendon (called the *jack tendon* or *cord*) but is seldom palpable (see Figure 10-24). The distal aspect of the cunean tendon is usually easily palpated, however, by starting at the distal aspect of the hock and sliding the fingertip in a proximal direction. Retrieving synovial fluid is unusual but possible, but during injection the clear outline of the bursa can be seen as it distends. A 20- to 22-gauge needle is inserted deep to the distal edge of the cunean tendon and directed in a proximal direction, and 3 to 5 mL of local anesthetic solution is injected. We prefer this approach, but alternatively the needle can be inserted perpendicular to the skin and directly through the tendon itself until bone is contacted.

Tarsal Sheath

Analgesia of the tarsal sheath is performed to confirm the structure as a source of lameness associated with traumatic and infectious tenosynovitis (although the response may be limited in the face of infection) and various osseous lesions, such as those involving the sustentaculum tali, or unusual exostoses (osteochondroma). The tarsal sheath surrounds the DDFT from a point approximately level with the tuber calcanei and extends to a point 2 to 3 cm distal to the tarsometatarsal joint. Distention of the tarsal sheath is commonly called *thoroughpin,* but occasionally thoroughpin appears as fluid swelling proximal to the tarsus that does not involve the tarsal sheath. The DDFT is located medial to the calcaneus as it crosses the sustentaculum tali. The heavy tarsal retinaculum medially and the calcaneus laterally restrict outpouching of the tarsal sheath to the proximal and distal aspects. The clinician should take care to differentiate tarsal sheath effusion from distention of the plantar pouches of the tarsocrural joint. A 20-gauge, 2.5-cm needle is used to inject 10 to 15 mL of local anesthetic solution.

Calcaneal Bursa

Indications for analgesia of the calcaneal bursa include traumatic and infectious bursitis, tendonitis of the gastrocnemius or SDFT at this level, and osseous lesions of the tuber calcanei. The bursa is located between the SDFT and tuber calcanei. Proximal to the tuber calcanei, the bursa is interposed between the SDFT and the gastrocnemius tendon. When distended, an unusual clinical finding, the bursa is palpable as medial and lateral outpouchings just proximal to the tuber calcanei. Smaller outpouchings are often discernable just distal to the tuber calcanei but are inconsistent. The bursa can be accessed for injection at any of these outpouchings. A 20- to 22-gauge, 2.5- or 4-cm needle is used to inject 10 mL of local anesthetic solution, after retrieval of fluid for analysis if indicated. Pain may take 20 to 30 minutes to abate in horses with osseous lesions or with severe lameness.

Trochanteric Bursa

Seldom does an indication exist to block the trochanteric bursa, although injections in this region are commonly performed to manage bursitis and muscle pain (see Chapter 47). The trochanteric bursa is located between the tendon of insertion of the gluteus accessorius muscle and the cranial process of the greater trochanter of the femur (see Figure 10-26; see also Chapter 47). In normal horses this bursa is small and likely has minimal synovial fluid. Synoviocentesis is performed using an 18- to 20-gauge, 4-cm needle, although in larger, more heavily muscled horses, a longer needle may be necessary. The needle is inserted perpendicular to the skin, directly over the cranial aspect of the greater trochanter until contact with bone is made. We have had difficulty retrieving fluid even in lame horses that have a positive response to analgesia. Generally, 5 to 10 mL of local anesthetic solution are injected until pressure is felt. If local anesthetic solution can be aspirated, the needle was likely in the bursa, but if not, the injection was likely performed in the surrounding tissues.

LOCAL INFILTRATION IN THE FORELIMB AND HINDLIMB

Local infiltration of local anesthetic solution in painful soft tissues or over painful bony swellings can be performed at any location, although some areas deserve special mention. Any localized area of pain, into which a needle can be inserted safely, is fair game for local analgesia.

The clinician must be aware, however, that local infiltration may not provide total analgesia to the region, mostly because the entire nerve supply to the region cannot be blocked. Incomplete analgesia is common in horses with bony lesions, such as bucked shins, because deep pain from the cortex of the McIII is difficult if not impossible to eliminate using subcutaneous infiltration of local anesthetic solution. In most instances, perineural analgesia for this particular condition is preferred. Local infiltration is performed in many horses in lieu of perineural technique, or in horses in which perineural analgesia has localized pain to a general region, but conflicting or numerous clinical problems exist. An advantage of local infiltration is that proprioception is not lost, and horses can be moved at speed for reevaluation after this form of analgesia. Efficacy can be assessed by deep, direct digital palpation, to confirm that the previously identified source of pain was eliminated by local analgesia.

Splints

A common suspected cause of lameness in many horses are exostoses associated most commonly with the second (McII) and fourth (McIV) metacarpal bones or the MtII or MtIV, or in combination with the McIII or MtIII. A 20- to 22-gauge, 2.5- to 4-cm needle is used to deposit 5 mL of local anesthetic solution subcutaneously over the painful exostosis. The needle is slid directly alongside the proliferative lesion, between skin and bone. For splints involving the McII or MtII and the McIV or MtIV, it is important to deposit local anesthetic solution abaxial and axial (between the suspensory ligament and splint bones) to the lesion. In some horses proliferative changes involve only the axial aspect of the McII, MtII, McIV, or MtIV (blind splints), and it is critical to block in this location. In others with primary proliferation between the McII or MtII, McIV or MtIV, and the McIII or MtIII, subcutaneous injection will suffice. When local anesthetic solution is infiltrated on the axial aspect of the splint bones, the palmar or plantar metacarpal or metatarsal nerves are likely blocked, making it possible to abolish pain from a more distal site and leading to misinterpretation of results. In horses with extensive adhesions between the axial aspects of the McII or MtII and the McIV or MtIV, the suspensory ligament pain may be incompletely abolished using a local infiltration technique, and the palmar or plantar nerves and palmar or plantar metacarpal or metatarsal nerves above the site may need to be blocked individually for pain to be abolished.

Suspensory Ligament Origin

Local infiltration or flooding the palmar metacarpal or plantar metatarsal regions at the origin of the suspensory ligament is often done in lieu of perineural analgesia, as described previously. This is also referred to by some as a *subtarsal* or *subcarpal block*. An 18- to 22-gauge, 2.5- to 4-cm needle can be used to distribute 5 to 15 mL of local anesthetic solution in a fan-shaped pattern, usually from a lateral injection site just axial to the McIV or MtIV. It is important to use adequate restraint and have the limb in a flexed position when performing this technique. In the hindlimb an 18- to 19-gauge needle should be used to minimize the potential for needle breakage, should the horse kick during the procedure.

False-positive results, attributed to inadvertent analgesia of palmar metacarpal or plantar metatarsal nerves, penetration of the distal outpouchings of the carpometacarpal and tarsometatarsal joints, or penetration of the tarsal sheath can occur.[25,56] Compared with high palmar analgesia, the incidence of inadvertent injection of the distal palmar outpouchings of the carpometacarpal joint was highest when local infiltration of the suspensory origin was performed.[25] A single injection technique was recently developed for diagnostic analgesia of the suspensory ligament origin in the hindlimb that should both limit the incidence of the previously mentioned complication, and also may be more specific for pain originating from the origin of the suspensory ligament. The technique involves blocking the deep branch of the lateral plantar nerve. The clinician holds the limb with the stifle and tarsus at 90 degrees of flexion and with the digit fully flexed. While the SDFT is deflected medially, a 2.5-cm needle is inserted to the hub, perpendicular to the skin, at a site 15 mm distal to the proximal aspect of the MtIV on the plantarolateral aspect of the limb. The needle is advanced between the lateral aspect of the SDFT and MtIV, at which point local anesthetic solution is injected.[70] It is important to understand that from the deep branch of the lateral plantar nerve originate the lateral and medial plantar metatarsal nerves that continue distally, axial to the MtIV and MtII, to provide important innervation to the fetlock joint (see previous discussion). Failure to eliminate fetlock region pain by first performing low plantar analgesia could lead to erroneous interpretation of the results of analgesia of the deep branch of the lateral plantar nerve. If only the deep branch of the lateral plantar nerve is blocked, a diagnosis of proximal plantar metatarsal pain could be made even though fetlock region pain could be the true source of pain causing lameness.

Curb

Curb, the term used for swelling of the distal, plantar aspect of the tarsus, is a complex condition involving SDF tendonitis, long plantar desmitis, subcutaneous swelling, or various combinations of these soft tissue injuries (see Chapter 78). Local infiltration can partially abolish pain associated with curb and usually involves depositing local anesthetic solution subcutaneously. Completely blocking deep pain associated with the long plantar ligament or SDFT is not possible without using the fibular and tibial nerve blocks. A tibial nerve block may be more specific.[5] A 20-gauge, 2.5- to 4-cm needle is used to inject 15 to 20 mL of local anesthetic solution with the limb in a flexed position. Adequate restraint and the help of an assistant are mandatory. Local anesthetic solution is infiltrated subcutaneously along the plantar, medial, and lateral aspects of the swelling, but deep injection into or between the SDFT and long plantar ligament is avoided. The medial injection is most comfortably and safely performed by standing on the opposite side of the horse.

Dorsal Spinous Process Impingement

Infiltration of local anesthetic solution around impinging dorsal spinous processes is a technique that is performed when attempting to confirm or rule out lameness or poor performance associated with back pain caused by impingement or other pain originating from the dorsal spinous processes of the thoracolumbar vertebrae.[71] The horse is usually evaluated under saddle or in harness or on a lunge line, because lameness associated with this condition may be subtle and only manifested under these conditions. The hair along the dorsal midline is clipped, and the site or sites are prepared aseptically. We prefer to use 22-gauge, 9-cm spinal needles, although in most instances shorter needles can easily reach the tops of the dorsal spinous processes. Needles are inserted on the dorsal midline and directed ventrally to the dorsal spinous processes or the interspinous space. Markers placed after scintigraphic or radiographic examination are helpful to determine the precise location for blocking or to administer medication. The interspinous space can be located by redirecting the needle in a cranial or caudal direction. If impingement of the dorsal spinous processes exists, it may be impossible to infiltrate between them, but placing local anesthetic solution around the processes is satisfactory.[5] Seven to 10 mL (per site) of local anesthetic solution are deposited as the needle is slowly withdrawn, and the horse is reevaluated 10 to 15 minutes later.

Using ultrasound guidance, intraarticular or periarticular injections of the cervical, thoracic, or lumbar facet joints can be performed using a 9-cm spinal needle. Injection techniques for the sacroiliac joints are described in Chapters 50 and 51.

Orthopedic Implants

Occasionally, pain associated with orthopedic implants is suspected to cause lameness. This is most commonly seen in horses after distal McIII or MtIII condylar fracture repair but can occur after repair of proximal phalanx or olecranon process fractures. Low-grade lameness is most common. Differentiating pain arising from negative interaction of implants with bone or surrounding soft tissue is nearly impossible based on the results of any diagnostic analgesia technique, because innervation to the joint or surrounding tissues is complex. Local anesthetic solution can be injected around screw heads, next to pins and wires or bone plates, and the horse is then reevaluated. Because lameness is often subtle, improvement is often difficult to judge. A combination of clinical findings and those from ancillary diagnostic techniques is used to determine the role of implant pain.

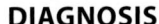

Chapter 11

Neurological Examination and Neurological Conditions Causing Gait Deficits

William V. Bernard and Jill Beech

Differentiating neurological gait deficits from lameness can sometimes be a dilemma for the clinician. Many repeated examinations and ancillary testing may be necessary, and even then experienced clinicians may give varied opinions about the same horse. Lack of definitive diagnostic tests to identify the origin of subtle gait changes, which in some horses may be perceived only by a rider or driver and not visible, promotes diagnoses that are based purely on opinions and individual prejudices. This chapter discusses the examination of a horse with gait deficits caused by disease of either the spinal cord, the most frequently documented cause of neurological gait deficits, or peripheral nerves. The chapter does not consider neurological syndromes characterized by signs of brain dysfunction, such as vestibular, cerebral, and cerebellar disorders. We also refer readers to a review on the equine spinal cord.[1]

eferences
on page
1258

DIAGNOSIS

History is important but depends not only on asking the appropriate questions but also on many uncontrollable factors, such as how closely, impartially, and astutely the horse has been observed. The time of onset of signs and rate of progression, whether the gait deficit waxes and wanes or is affected by exercise or rest, whether one or more limbs are affected, whether the affected limb varies, what the horse was doing before onset of signs occurred, whether exercise or management has changed, whether the horse has been moved geographically, whether signs occurred after transport, what medications may have been given and any observed effects, and whether other horses

on the farm or in the stable have had any recent illnesses or fever should be determined. It is also important to know if other horses on the same farm have similar clinical signs. For instance, a history of fever, respiratory disease, or abortions in horses in contact with the affected horse would make one suspect equine herpesvirus–1 (EHV-1) infection.

Clinical Examination

The clinician should observe whether the horse displays cranial nerve dysfunction; muscle hypertrophy, atrophy, or asymmetry; muscle trembling; abnormal hoof wear; or abnormal posture. Muscle atrophy may be caused by disease of the ventral horn cells of the gray matter of the spinal cord, peripheral nerve, or the muscle itself; it also can occur with disuse. Palpation can reveal abnormalities such as altered skin temperature, sweating, muscle fasciculations, abnormal sensitivity, or soreness. The horse should be observed on a flat surface, at a walk and trot, and in straight and curving lines. The horse should be evaluated on a surface that allows detection of abnormal hoof flight and placement, toe dragging, or excessive force when landing. The sound of the feet landing should be noted for consistency and loudness. Hard surfaces also may enhance abnormal hyperflexion in horses with stringhalt. Evaluation on a soft surface may be necessary if the horse is unstable or if the clinician is trying to determine whether the horse could have sore feet. Any abnormal head or neck movement associated with limb movement should be noted. It is important to permit normal neck and head movement when the horse is being led. The person leading the horse should hold the horse as loosely as is safely possible. Collapsing or sinking on a limb, knuckling, hyperflexion, spasticity, hesitance in any part of the stride, dragging of a toe, landing excessively hard, leaning to one side, or failing to track straight can indicate a neurological deficit. Various manipulations are used to diagnose whether proprioceptive or motor deficits exist and to localize the lesion. While being led, the horse should be evaluated while stopping and starting from a walk and trot, backing up, circling tightly in both directions, walking while sideways traction is applied and released on the tail, being pushed sideways from a standstill, and walking with its head elevated. Some clinicians also evaluate repositioning of the foot after placing the horse's hoof in an abnormal position. We do not find this particularly helpful because a horse's disposition, age, training, and distractions can affect its response. A horse with a normal gait may stand with its feet placed in an abnormal position for what seems an abnormally long time. Some clinicians also use wheelbarrowing and hopping reactions.[1] We do not use these tests in mature horses because we believe responses may be inconsistent and difficult to evaluate accurately and safely. Observation of the horse walking or trotting up and down inclines can be helpful in revealing whether the horse "knows where its limbs are" (proprioception) and can adjust limb movement appropriately. It may be helpful to observe the horse while it is being ridden or lunged, and in some horses while it is loose in an enclosure. Watching the horse stop and start, turn, back up, and maintain its balance during many postural maneuvers allows detection of neurological deficits that may not be obvious when the horse is being led. Consider the following:

- Are errors in range of movement of the limb (dysmetria) apparent?
- Is the horse extending its limbs to the full extent, or is the range decreased (hypometria)?
- Does the horse lift its limbs excessively high (hypermetria)?
- Is spasticity or stiffness of movement apparent?

In some horses it is necessary to observe the horse performing its usual activity, providing it is capable. However, gait deficits may be much less apparent at speed than when the horse is walking or trotting slowly. Basically, the clinician is trying to determine whether the horse moves symmetrically and smoothly with normal stride length and height of foot flight appropriate to the breed and use, whether it appears strong and consistently places its feet in the appropriate positions, and whether it moves in balanced harmonious fashion. It is sometimes difficult to determine whether certain postural or gait changes are a result of pain or weakness or are associated with motor or proprioceptive deficits. Is the horse flexing its hindlimbs excessively and holding its croup more ventrally and flexed because of pain or weakness? If the horse is shifting weight between the hind feet, is it because of weakness, as seen, for example, in lower motor neuron disease, or because of pain? When both limbs are affected, manipulation of a limb to try to localize pain may not be possible. Gaited horses can be extremely difficult to evaluate, especially if one is unfamiliar with the specific gaits. Conformation also can confound interpretation of clinical signs. It may be necessary to observe the horse on many occasions and compare its gait before and after exercise. Is the deficit consistent, or does it vary? If it worsens with exercise, is it because of pain or inability to compensate for a neurological deficit as the horse tires? Perineural analgesia may be helpful. Is there palpable evidence of muscle cramping with exercise or an increase in creatine kinase (CK) level, indicating rhabdomyolysis? A variable gait deficit and inconsistent alterations in foot flight or placement are more likely to represent a neurological deficit than lameness; single limb lameness may vary in intensity but usually remains similar in character. Painful and neurological conditions could coexist but may be difficult to differentiate even with use of commonly used analgesics such as phenylbutazone.

If the horse buckles in a limb, especially on turns, is easily pulled sideways by the tail when standing or walking, or trembles its limb, weakness of the extensor muscle groups should be suspected. When the flexor muscles are weak, the horse is unable to lift its limb normally, and the toe may be worn from dragging. Pushing the horse sideways or trying to pull on the halter and tail simultaneously can reveal weakness. If the horse is weak or has pain in one limb, it is not able to bear weight normally when the contralateral hoof is lifted from the ground. Neck flexion sideways and vertically should be evaluated for ease and range of movement. Skin sensation and the cutaneous trunci reflex and cervical reflexes should be evaluated. Tapping the trunk should elicit contraction of the cutaneous trunci muscle. Abnormalities can delineate a thoracic spinal cord lesion, because afferent input is through the dorsal thoracic nerves and cranially through the spinal cord white matter, and the efferent pathway involves the cranial thoracic motor neurons in the first thoracic and eighth cervical segments and the lateral thoracic nerve. Hypalgesia of the cutaneous trunci as assessed by response to a two-pinch test with a hemostat is rare and occurs only with severe thoracic spinal cord disease.[1] Lack of a cervicofacial reflex (failure of the facial muscles to twitch when the ipsilateral side of the cranial aspect of the neck is tapped) can suggest a lesion in the cervical cord or a branch of cranial nerve VII. If tapping the side of the neck fails to elicit contraction of the cutaneous coli muscle, a cervical cord lesion could exist. If any abnormal response to skin stimulation is detected, the test should be repeated because the horse's disposition can influence its responses. Limb reflexes usually are not used, although patellar reflexes can be elicited in horses. We do not consider the thoracolaryngeal reflex (slap test) to be helpful. Response is inconsistent in horses with cervical spinal cord lesions and may be absent in normal horses. Blindfolding the horse usually is not part of our routine neurological examination unless vestibular disease is suspected. A complete physical examination should always be conducted. In some horses with hindlimb gait deficits, palpation per rectum of the pelvic bones, lumbar region, caudal aspect of the aorta, and iliac vessels may be necessary. Simple observation may not differentiate hindlimb weakness caused by spinal cord disease from that caused by partial aortoiliac thrombosis. Horses that do not "feel right" to the rider yet show no obvious deficits to the observer whether observed saddled or in hand are problematic. It may be necessary to observe a horse from a jog cart or carriage if the gait deficit about which a driver complains is not visible to the bystander. In attempting to differentiate between a musculoskeletal and neurological condition causing a gait deficit in a limb, diagnostic analgesia may be necessary. Obviously, this does not help differentiate pain from lameness emanating from a lesion proximal to the coxofemoral or scapulohumeral joints. A course of nonsteroidal antiinflammatory drugs (such as moderate doses of phenylbutazone for days or even several weeks) may be helpful in determining whether a gait deficit is caused by pain.

Hematology and Serology

In most horses serum chemistry screens and hematological tests are not particularly helpful; however, in horses with a gait deficit caused by an underlying muscle disease, evaluation of aspartate transaminase (AST) and CK levels may be helpful. Stage of training, exercise pattern, and whether the blood specimen was obtained after exercise preceded by a day of rest must be considered in evaluation of enzyme levels. If a horse consistently has abnormally elevated enzyme levels, then the horse has rhabdomyolysis, and the clinician must decide whether the condition is causing or contributing to the horse's abnormal gait. Plasma CK and AST levels do not increase simply because of muscle atrophy; rhabdomyolysis must occur to increase the enzyme levels in the blood (see Chapter 83). Elevated plasma concentrations of CK and AST in horses that are not being exercised suggest a primary muscle disorder, such as (but not limited to) polysaccharide storage myopathy (see Chapter 83). An elevation in white blood cell count and fibrinogen level indicates inflammation. In our experience, elevation in fibrinogen level is a more consistent indicator of inflammation in the adult horse than is elevation in white blood cell count.

If clinical signs suggest equine lower motor neuron disease, serum levels of vitamin E (α-tocopherol) should be measured; levels of vitamin E have consistently been low in horses with confirmed equine motor neuron disease, unless the horse has been given supplements.[2] Thus low vitamin E levels may be suggestive of, but are not specific for, equine lower motor neuron disease. Tocopherol concentrations can decrease during winter when horses lack access to green pasture.[3] Daily variations in plasma levels may occur.[4] Low levels also have been reported in clinically normal horses[5-7] and in one horse with chronic gastrointestinal disease.[8] The laboratory that performs the test should be contacted for any specific requirements for submission of samples and to ensure they have an established normal range for vitamin E levels.

Serological testing for antibodies to various infectious agents may be indicated. In EHV-1 infection, detection of an increase in antibody titer is considered diagnostic of the disease. A horse that shows signs of neurological disease secondary to EHV-1 should have an elevated serum antibody titer, and single high titers have been the basis for initial diagnosis in individual horses. Recent vaccination confounds interpretation. Rarely, high titers may be measured in horses with no history of recent vaccination and no obvious clinical signs of EHV-1 infection.

Antibody titers for *Borrelia burgdorferi,* the cause of Lyme disease, sometimes are measured in serum from horses with ill-defined gait deficits. High titers, or rising titers, have been used as a basis for treatment of the disease. A positive titer, however, does not mean the horse has active disease. Because of the geographical variation in exposure to *B. burgdorferi,* titers may vary greatly. Serological surveys in the United States have demonstrated positive test results in 1% of samples from nonendemic areas and up to 68% in endemic areas.[9-11] Reports of horses "responding" to treatment exist,[12,13] but to date we are unaware of any horses with Lyme disease in which neurological deficits mimic primary lameness. Currently the importance of Lyme disease as a cause of equine gait deficits is unclear.

A Western blot test for the evaluation of equine protozoal myelitis (EPM) was first made commercially available at the University of Kentucky by Dr. David Granstrom.[14] Serological testing for the presence of antibodies to *Sarcocystis neurona* can be used only to indicate exposure to the organism. Through exposure to *S. neurona,* many horses develop antibodies in the absence of clinical disease Serological surveys in certain areas of the United States have shown that a high percentage of horses have positive

antibody titers. A positive test result does not mean the horse has EPM. A negative test result could theoretically occur in horses with peracute disease or perhaps in severely immunocompromised animals. However, a negative test result usually indicates that disease caused by *S. neurona* is highly unlikely. The test result also could be negative in a horse with signs of EPM if another protozoan, such as *Neospora,* causes the spinal cord lesions. In a U.S. study of several hundred horses with neurological disease, test sensitivity was 89%, but specificity was only 71%, because 30% of horses with other neurological diseases also had antibodies to *S. neurona*. Although the positive predictive value was only 72% in horses with neurological diseases, the negative predictive value was almost 90%, indicating that a negative test result is useful in this population.[14] In one study of 44 horses on a farm sampled for more than 1 year, all horses were seropositive for at least 50 weeks yet showed no neurological signs (see following discussion).[15]

Cerebrospinal Fluid Aspiration and Analysis

Cerebrospinal fluid (CSF) can be obtained from either the atlantooccipital or the lumbosacral space. The advantage of lumbosacral centesis is that it can be performed in the standing sedated horse, whereas atlantooccipital centesis requires general anesthesia. Fluid from the atlantooccipital site is considered easier to obtain and not as likely to be contaminated with blood. The atlantooccipital site is identified by palpating the cranial edge of the wings of the atlas. The hair is clipped and the site prepared aseptically. Atlantooccipital centesis is performed at the intersection of the median plane and a line drawn across the cranial edge of the wings of the atlas. In an adult horse, a 9-cm ($3\frac{1}{2}$-inch), 18- or 20-gauge spinal needle is directed toward the horse's lower lip with the head held in a flexed position. It is important that the needle remain on the midline as it is advanced, because otherwise it will be too far lateral to enter the subarachnoid space. The needle is initially inserted to a depth of approximately 2.5 cm (1 inch) and then gradually advanced. While the needle is gradually advanced to the subarachnoid space, it should be held carefully to prevent penetrating the spinal cord when advancing through the atlantooccipital membrane and the dura mater. Usually a "pop" is felt as the needle advances through the dura; however, this finding is not consistent and the stylette should be frequently removed to observe for flow of CSF. CSF usually flows from the needle once the subarachnoid space is entered; however, once a substantial depth has been reached (about 5 to 8 cm [2 to 3 inches] in an average-size horse), some clinicians advise gentle and frequent aspiration with a small syringe.

In preparation for aspiration from the lumbosacral space the type and degree of restraint is guided by the horse's behavior, the horse's stability, and the clinician's personal preference. A nose twitch, stocks, sedation, or a combination of physical and chemical restraint are options. We prefer to use light sedation with xylazine, sometimes combined with butorphanol. However, lumbosacral CSF pressure can be transiently decreased up to 15 minutes after administration of a high dose of xylazine (1.1 mg/kg intravenously).[16] The puncture site for lumbosacral centesis is identified by combining several landmarks, realizing that individual variation exists. A line drawn between the caudal edge of the tubera coxae and the intersection with the midline can be used to locate the lumbosacral space. The lumbosacral space is bordered cranially by the caudal edge of the sixth lumbar vertebra, caudally by the cranial edge of the sacrum, and laterally by the medial rim of the tubera sacrale. The dorsal spinous process of the last lumber vertebra is lower than the dorsal spinous process of the fifth lumbar vertebra. The V formed by the medial rim of the tubera sacrale is one of the more useful landmarks, and the appropriate site for puncture is within this V. The site should be prepared aseptically, and local anesthetic solution is placed subcutaneously. A small skin stab incision is usually made. The needle is inserted on the midline, at the depression palpated just caudal to the last lumbar vertebra, in the middle of the V formed by the tubera sacrale. A 15-cm, 18-gauge spinal needle is generally adequate for a horse that is 16 hands or less. A 20-cm needle may be necessary in a horse greater than 16 to 17 hands. While the clinician advances the needle, it is critical to remain on the midline. The needle can be advanced until a pop indicates it is advancing through the dura or until the horse responds as the needle stimulates nervous tissue. These responses can be unreliable and occasionally dangerous for the horse, the handler, and the individual performing the centesis. Because horses can react unpredictably (including rearing, bolting, collapsing, or kicking), it is safer to advance the needle gradually until it is near the spinal canal, approximately 12.5 cm (5 inches) in a 15- to 16-hand horse. Once the needle is near the canal, it should be advanced slowly with repeated frequent removal of the stylette and aspiration with a small syringe. The horse may move its tail when the dura is penetrated, but usually minimal reaction occurs. If fluid is obtained but the amount is small, the needle can be rotated 180 degrees. Jugular vein compression for at least 10 seconds (Queckenstedt's test) is thought to elevate intracranial CSF pressure and aid fluid collection, provided flow is not obstructed. If a hemorrhagic sample is thought to be from iatrogenic causes, the syringe can be changed frequently until subsequent aliquots are clear. If fluid is not obtained on the first attempt, the needle is withdrawn and the procedure is repeated slightly cranial or caudal to the original location. CSF samples should be placed in sterile tubes and rapidly processed after collection.

Normal CSF is clear and colorless, and red discoloration indicates hemorrhage. However, normal fluid can sometimes appear mildly hazy when grossly examined, especially in a tube with ethylenediamine tetraacetic acid. Hemorrhage can be iatrogenic or caused by underlying disease. Fluid may appear clear even with red blood cell contamination, and studies indicate that subjective evaluation of spinal fluid is sensitive in detecting blood only when the red blood cells number more than 1200/mcL.[17,18] Centrifugation of a bloody sample should produce a clear fluid with a pellet of red blood cells on the bottom of the sample tube. If hemorrhage occurred before collection and lysis of cells occurred, the supernatant may be slightly pink or xanthochromic (orange/yellow or yellow). Lysis of red blood cells reportedly can occur within 1 to 4 hours.[19] Xanthochromic CSF results from red blood cell breakdown products (bilirubin) and suggests hemorrhage or vasculitis. A centrifuged xanthochromic sample does not become clear. Turbid CSF may appear with hypercellularity or epidural fat contamination. The latter is not uncommon with lumbosacral aspirates. Formulas used to differentiate between white cell or protein elevations caused by iatrogenic blood contamination of CSF versus pathological increases have been shown to be unreliable. Contamination with a few thousand red blood cells results in minimal increase in white blood cell count or protein content.[18]

The normal reported range for leukocyte counts has been variable; usually a range of 0 to 6/mcL is cited,[20] but higher values have been reported.[21,22] Diversity in techniques can account for different values in normal CSF. Undiluted fluid can be assayed in a hemocytometer, or acidified crystal violet can be added to accentuate the cells.[20] It is important that equine reference values be determined in the laboratory the practitioner uses. As previously stated, the cell quality rapidly deteriorates in CSF, and samples for cytological testing should be processed rapidly or a portion fixed in 40% ethanol if processing must be delayed. For morphological and differential evaluation, cytocentrifugation or filtration through a glass fiber membrane filter is the preferred method of processing spinal fluid. In our experience, cell and differential counts are often normal in horses with spinal cord disease. Small lymphocytes and monocytes are normally seen. Neutrophils may be seen with blood contamination or inflammation. Eosinophilia is rarely seen in equine CSF but could occur secondary to parasite migration. Rarely, eosinophils have been seen in samples from horses with protozoal encephalomyelitis,[21] but frequently spinal fluid from horses with EPM is normal. A relative neutrophilia, with or without an increase in cell count, indicates inflammation, and intracellular bacteria may be seen in horses with bacterial meningitis.

Reported values for protein content of CSF vary considerably among laboratories, probably because of diversity in measurement techniques. A range of 10 to 120 mg/dL is generally acceptable, although some authors consider 100 to 105 mg/dL the high end of normal range.[20,23] Protein may increase because of vascular leakage (vasculitis), inflammatory lesions, trauma, iatrogenic blood contamination, or intrathecal globulin production. High-resolution protein electrophoresis of CSF has been reported in a small number of horses, but its value as a diagnostic test remains to be determined. Compared with normal horses (n = 18), horses with cervical cord compression (n = 14) often had a decreased β fraction and post-β peaks.[24] However, divergent findings have been reported. Because CK is abundant in neural tissue (and in skeletal tissue and cardiac muscle) and is a large macromolecule that does not cross the blood-brain barrier, measurement was suggested to be a sensitive index of central nervous system lesions. Horses with EPM were reported to frequently have increased CSF CK concentrations, unlike horses with cervical vertebral malformation.[25] However, another study showed that the sensitivity and specificity of CSF CK activity are inadequate for diagnostic use. Also, CSF simultaneously collected from the atlantooccipital and lumbosacral sites had disparate values for CK activity, which was not associated with site or other CSF parameters. Contamination of CSF with either epidural fat or dura, which is possible during collection, increases CK activity.[26]

Albumin is the predominant protein in normal CSF. Elevated albumin concentration can indicate hemorrhage or altered blood-brain barrier integrity. To eliminate serum albumin as a source of increased CSF protein and albumin, the following albumin quotient (AQ) has been suggested[27]:

$$AQ = \frac{CSF\ albumin}{Serum\ albumin} \times 100$$

The AQ cited for normal equine CSF is 1.4 ± 0.04,[23,27] and it was suggested that an increase above reference range indicated blood contamination during sample collection or compromise of the blood-brain barrier. The immunoglobulin G (IgG) index

$$\frac{CSF\ IgG\ concentration}{Serum\ IgG\ concentration} \div \frac{CSF\ albumin\ concentration}{Serum\ albumin\ concentration}$$

was suggested to be useful for differentiating intrathecal IgG production from an increase secondary to blood contamination or increased blood-brain barrier permeability. Normal reference range has been reported to be 0.14 to 0.24.[27] However, we do not consider these to be specific, and blood contamination can increase the IgG index without a concomitant change in AQ.[18]

Although CSF cell count, cytological examination findings, and total protein concentration often do not represent the extent or type of spinal cord or brain tissue disease, when abnormal, the values can be useful. For example, in central nervous system (CNS) disease caused by EHV-1 infection the fluid may be xanthochromic with a high protein level but normal cell count. This disassociation between elevation in protein level and normal cell count may help differentiate EHV-1 infection from EPM. Also, xanthochromic CSF indicates an alteration in the blood-brain barrier and could explain false-positive CSF immunoblot findings for *S. neurona* in a horse with positive serological test results. Unfortunately, except for EHV-1 infections and meningitis, CSF analysis with currently available tests frequently is not helpful in diagnosing spinal cord disease in horses.

In the United States, the frequency of performing CSF aspiration increased with the introduction of a Western immunoblot test for detecting *S. neurona* antibodies. Although limited data are available, the specificity and sensitivity of the immunoblot test on CSF from horses with clinical signs consistent with EPM were reported to be approximately 90%.[14] However, positive test results have been found in clinically normal horses and in horses with neuropathological lesions other than EPM. Even minute amounts of contamination of CSF with blood can cause the test result to be positive in a horse with high serum antibody levels.[19] When CSF was contaminated by even minute amounts of strongly immunoreactive blood (10^{-3} mcL of blood per milliliter of CSF), the fluid was falsely positive even though the AQ was normal.[18] This small amount of blood contamination is grossly undetectable and can correlate with as little as eight red blood cells/mcL of CSF. Also, blood contamination, without increasing the AQ, can increase the IgG index. The IgG index is not specific for intrathecal IgG production. Although the red blood cell count may be a more sensitive indicator of blood contamination than the AQ, it does not correlate with the amount of antibody contamination. Minute amounts of highly immunoreactive blood may have a greater impact on CSF Western blot analysis than a greater amount of contamination with blood with low immunoreactivity.[18]

Any compromise to the blood-brain barrier regardless of cause allows antibodies to leak into the CSF from the serum, causing a false-positive test result. Although the test for immunoblot *S. neurona* antibodies was reported to have 85% positive predictive value in a study of horses with neurological disease,[14] in the general equine population the test has poor positive predictive value. Many normal horses have positive antibody test results.[28] In contrast the negative predictive value for the test is high. With what is currently known, interpretation of positive Western blot results must be made with caution. Negative Western blot test results are generally useful to rule out EPM.

Since the introduction of the original CSF Western blot analysis detecting antibodies to *S. neurona,* other tests have been developed. These tests include a modified Western blot, an enzyme-linked immunosorbent assay (ELISA), and an immunofluorescent antibody test. Large scale critical evaluation of these tests has not been performed. However early indications suggest that all of these tests may have some limitations. The immunofluorescent antibody test cross-reacts with *Sarcocystis fayeri,* therefore resulting in false-positive diagnosis of *S. neurona* infection.[29] The ELISA is based on a surface antigen that is missing in some strains of *S. neurona;* therefore, false-negative results may occur.[30] For the reasons discussed previously, both the original and modified Western blot tests may produce false-positive results. In conclusion, antibody testing for *S. neurona* infection must be used cautiously and in conjunction with other diagnostic tests in attempts to rule out other causes of neurological disease.

Polymerase chain reaction (PCR) testing detects DNA of infectious organisms and has been applied to CSF. Its value in the diagnosis of EPM is controversial, especially when positive results have been reported on CSF samples that were negative for *S. neurona* antibodies and from horses that did not exhibit overt neurological deficits. We do not find PCR testing for the diagnosis of EPM useful. Use of the PCR technique on CSF has been helpful in diagnosing neuroborreliosis in a horse. Similar to some human cases, the PCR test result was positive yet the CSF had a negative antibody titer.[12]

Radiography

The use of radiographs in evaluating traumatic or infectious injuries, congenital lesions, and developmental malformations of the spinal column is limited by the size of the horse. Radiographs are useful in diagnosing congenital abnormalities of vertebrae, narrowing of intervertebral disk spaces, stenosis of the cervical spinal canal, osteoarthritic changes, osteomyelitis or osseous cysts, vertebral neoplasia, malalignment, and fractures. However, in most mature horses, except for the cervical spine, general anesthesia may be required for adequate radiographs of the spine. Computed tomography (CT) and magnetic resonance imaging have tremendous potential for evaluating the equine central nervous system but also are limited by the size of the horse. At present, except in foals, CT is available only for evaluating the head and cranial midcervical regions. The primary use of radiology in evaluating horses with neurological disease is localization of cervical vertebral lesions or cervical vertebral malformation and diagnosis of cervical compressive myelopathy or stenotic myelopathy (see Chapter 60).

Survey radiology is useful in the diagnosis of cervical vertebral malformation and cord compression but can be misleading. Standing lateral radiographic images of the cervical vertebrae are routinely evaluated to detect vertebral malformation and to measure spinal canal diameter and can suggest the likelihood of cervical compressive myelopathy.[1,31,32] In horses with cervical compressive myelopathy, malformations that characteristically may be identified include flare of the caudal epiphysis of the vertebral body (vertebral endplate modeling), caudal extension of the dorsal laminae, vertebral nonalignment, and osteoarthritis of articular facets. Modeling of the articular processes of the caudal cervical vertebrae is a common malformation identified in horses with cervical compressive myelopathy and in horses that do not have cervical compressive myelopathy. Radiological interpretation of changes is more difficult in older horses, because obvious changes may be seen, without impingement on the spinal canal. Subjective evaluation of articular facet abnormalities can result in a false-positive diagnosis of cervical compressive myelopathy. Identification of characteristic vertebral malformations supports but does not confirm the diagnosis of cervical compressive myelopathy, and subjective radiological evaluation of a malformation does not reliably differentiate between horses with or without cervical compressive myelopathy. Objective assessment of vertebral canal diameter is a more reliable indicator of cervical compressive myelopathy than the subjective evaluation of vertebral malformation. The minimum sagittal diameter (MSD) is the first described method of assessment of canal diameter based on lateral cervical radiographs.[31] Determination of canal diameter using the sagittal ratio improves on the original measurements by adjusting for magnification and providing a more accurate adjustment for body size.[32] The sagittal ratio measurements were developed using a population of affected (confirmed by myelogram or histopathological studies) versus nonaffected horses.[32] The sagittal ratio is determined by dividing the MSD by the width of the corresponding vertebral body. Although a sagittal ratio percent at any cervical vertebra from the third to seventh cervical vertebrae less than 50% is a strong predictor of spinal cord compression, a few horses with no pathological evidence of spinal cord compression have had sagittal ratios of less than 50%. Recently intervertebral measurements of canal diameters were shown to improve diagnosis of cord compression, and addition of intervertebral sagittal ratio measurements was recommended to increase accuracy of plain radiographs.[1]

A semiquantitative scoring system for evaluating cervical radiographs in horses younger than 1 year of age has been published. This scoring system used neurological examination alone to determine affected versus nonaffected foals and combined subjective determination of radiographic vertebral malformation and objective determination of canal diameter.[31] Vertebral canal stenosis is determined by measurement of intervertebral and intravertebral MSD. Dividing the MSD by the length of the vertebral body corrects for magnification. Malformation is determined by the subjective assessment of five categories. The most discriminating factors in the semiquantitative scoring system in differentiating affected from nonaffected foals are canal stenosis and the angle between adjacent vertebrae. The disadvantage of the semiquantitative scoring system is the inclusion of subjective determinations.

Myelographic examination is advised to obtain the best evidence of compression.[1,33-35] Myelograms also can demonstrate compression from soft tissue masses, which are not evident radiologically, and suggest transverse compression. However, myelography may not be definitive and occasionally is misleading. A study to evaluate myelography critically and compare the results with necropsy findings in a large number of horses has not been done. A diagnosis of cord compression is assumed if a 50% reduction in the width of the dorsal dye column exists. However, the diagnostic criterion of 50% decrease in width of the dorsal dye column is not well documented[34] and has been found in horses with no histological evidence of cord compression at the site of dye column decrease. Iohexol is currently the preferred contrast medium for myelography. It is important that the owner understand the advantages and disadvantages (including risks) of a myelogram before the procedure is undertaken.

Electromyography and Nerve Conduction Studies
Recording electrical activity of muscles can indicate whether evidence of denervation or a myopathy exists, although the distinction is not always clear-cut. Electromyographic examination findings in the early stages of disease or injury may be normal. Certain abnormal patterns can indicate denervation. However, depending on the specific areas to be examined, electromyography may require anesthesia or heavy sedation. It may be helpful in identifying abnormal muscles and indirectly the affected nerves. In a standing, awake horse, spontaneous muscle movement can hinder interpretation.

Values for sensory and motor nerve conduction velocities in horses and ponies were reported.[36-39] Differences in speed of conduction occur in different nerves and horses' sensory nerve conduction velocities are slower than those of ponies.[39] However, similar motor nerve conduction velocities were reported for the median and radial nerves of ponies and horses.[37] Location of the segment being measured may be important, because distal tapering of nerves may be associated with slower velocity. Skin temperature significantly affects nerve conduction velocity,[39] and variability in technique can alter findings. Slower motor nerve conduction velocities were reported in horses older than 18 years of age.[36] The procedure usually requires that the horse be anesthetized and, similar to electromyography, should be performed by a skilled person. The technique mainly has been used in research.

Nuclear Scintigraphy
Nuclear scintigraphy has been helpful in identifying lesions in the cervical, thoracic, and lumbar spinal column and pelvic areas not readily evaluated by radiography. It also has been used to evaluate vertebral changes identified radiologically, to determine whether active bone change has occurred. It has revealed hairline fractures and other unsuspected bone lesions in the appendicular skeleton as the cause of gait deficits, which sometimes had been suspected to be caused by spinal cord disease. Scintigraphic imaging from both sides of the horse can differentiate which side may have a lesion. The role of nuclear scintigraphy in diagnosing equine spinal cord disease is limited.

Ultrasonography

Ultrasonography has been used to diagnose aortoiliac thrombosis and to identify soft tissue masses near the spine or deep within muscles. It has also revealed bony proliferation or fractures of the pelvis in horses with obscure gait deficits that were originally suspected to be a result of spinal cord disease.

Virus Isolation

If horses die or are euthanized with neurological signs thought to be caused by viral disease, the spinal cord, brain, or both should be sent for virus isolation. In horses with acute disease, nasal swabs and whole blood samples can be collected.

Immunohistochemistry and Polymerase Chain Reaction Testing

Immunohistochemistry and PCR testing can be used to detect the antigen of certain infectious organisms and are applied most commonly to tissues collected at necropsy but can also be used on affected tissues obtained by biopsy.

SPECIFIC DISEASES AND SYNDROMES

Equine Protozoal Myelitis (EPM)

EPM was first reported in 1974[40-43] and appeared to be the same condition originally reported as segmental myelitis of unknown cause.[44] It is caused by infection with *S. neurona*. EPM currently appears to be limited to the Western hemisphere. It is particularly of concern in the United States, where in some regions high percentages of horses are infected. The actual number of horses confirmed as having neurological disease from EPM is much lower than the actual number of horses infected, but the disease does have a substantial and serious impact. EPM has not been confirmed in horses younger than 6 months of age, although antibodies were detected in serum from a 2-month-old foal.[45] A recent comprehensive review of this disease should be consulted for details.[46] *Neospora* species have been identified as a cause of EPM in horses from the western United States.[47-50] CSF testing was positive for *S. neurona* antibodies by Western blot test, and no antemortem features distinguished *Neospora* infection from *Sarcocystis* infection.

The disease caused by *S. neurona* tends to occur in warm, temperate, nonarid areas with resident opossums. The horse is a "dead-end" host, and the disease is not contagious. The life cycle is not completely understood, although opossums have been identified as the definitive host. The proportion of infected horses that show clinical signs is low. This disease can cause gait deficits affecting one or all limbs and may be difficult or impossible to differentiate from musculoskeletal or other neurological diseases. Signs ascribed to EPM by veterinarians in the United States have been seen in horses in the United Kingdom, where horses have no known exposure to the organism.[1] Infected horses and horses with confirmed EPM seen in Europe, Asia, or South Africa have been imported from the Western hemisphere.[46] Horses frequently show asymmetrical deficits and may have focal or multifocal muscle atrophy or cranial nerve deficits. Horses may have profound or mild motor or proprioceptive gait deficits, and onset of signs can be acute or chronic, with slow or rapid progression. It may

be difficult or impossible to differentiate subtle neurological deficits from those caused by subtle lameness or musculoskeletal pain. Behavior may change. Focal sweating may occur. Diagnosis is based on clinical signs and history, by eliminating other potential causes by radiography and other diagnostic tests, and by testing of serum or CSF for antibodies to *S. neurona*. No definitive antemortem test exists, although absence of serum antibodies to *S. neurona* makes it highly unlikely that a horse has EPM. If a horse demonstrates classic signs (e.g., asymmetrical motor deficits and muscle atrophy in the hindlimbs, asymmetrical motor deficits in one or more limbs, a limb deficit combined with cranial nerve deficits not deemed caused by peripheral nerve trauma) and has no other organ dysfunction, we would treat the horse for EPM if it has been in the United States and serological findings are positive. We would forgo CSF testing for reasons outlined earlier.

To date, drugs used to treat EPM have been a combination of trimethoprim-sulfa (sulfadiazine or sulfamethoxazole) and pyrimethamine, or sulfas and pyrimethamine, diclazuril, toltrazuril, and nitazoxanide. Because no definitive antemortem test exists to confirm the disease, evaluation of response to therapy is problematic, especially because the clinical syndrome as treated is so variable and often poorly defined. To date, no treatment trials of experimental infections have been reported. Confounding assessment of drug response is the fact that experimentally infected horses develop clinical signs that decrease over time, despite receiving no treatment.[51] Numbers of organisms ingested, virulence factors, and the horse's own immune status (which depends on heredity, previous exposure to *S. neurona*, stresses such as transport and parturition, lack of adequate nutrition, and other factors) all presumably can affect development of and recovery from the disease. In the United States the most widely used drug combination is one of the sulfa drugs and pyrimethamine. Because pyrimethamine reaches higher concentrations in the CSF and neural tissue, it is considered superior to trimethoprim. The usual dosage regimen is 20 mg of sulfadiazine per kilogram once or twice daily and 1 mg of pyrimethamine per kilogram once daily, both by mouth for at least 2 to 3 months. Diarrhea occasionally occurs in horses treated with trimethoprim-sulfamethoxazole, and anemia and leukopenia have been observed in some horses receiving 1 mg of pyrimethamine with sulfas per kilogram twice daily. Whether horses require such a prolonged course of treatment or continued high levels of pyrimethamine is unknown. Earlier treatment regimens used a lower dose, but to our knowledge no observations comparing dosages have been reported. A syndrome of bone marrow aplasia and hypoplasia, renal nephrosis or hypoplasia, and epithelial dysplasia was reported in three foals born from mares given sulfonamides, trimethoprim, pyrimethamine, vitamin E, and folic acid during gestation. The authors of that report suggested that administration of the folic acid reduced absorption of active folic acid and, combined with the folic acid inhibitors (trimethoprim and pyrimethamine), induced folic acid deficiency and lesions in the foals.[52] We do not routinely add supplements for horses being treated with trimethoprim or pyrimethamine, but if sequential blood tests indicate anemia or leukopenia, the horse should be given folinic acid, a form of bioactive tetrahydrofolate. Folic acid should not be used because it is poorly absorbed in the horse, conversion to its active form is prevented by the dihydrofolate reductase inhibitors pyrimethamine and trimethoprim, and it can competitively decrease absorption of the active form of folic acid.[46,52]

Diclazuril, a coccidiostat, has anti–*S. neurona* activity in cell cultures infected with *S. neurona*[53] and has been used to treat horses with suspected EPM.[54] It is absorbed quickly after feeding. Dosage and therapeutic efficacy are being evaluated. Toltrazuril, like diclazuril, is a triazine-based anticoccidial drug. Because the drug has good lipid solubility and oral absorption and is absorbed into the CSF, it has potential for treating EPM.[55] Ponazuril, a metabolite of toltrazuril, has in vitro activity against *S. neurona*.[56] Ponazuril appeared to have favorable clinical results in a multicenter treatment study.[46] The drug has undergone U.S. Food and Drug Administration (FDA) testing, has been approved, and is marketed under the trade name Marquis. Label recommended dosage is 5 mg/kg administered once per day orally. Studies have shown that Marquis has a wide range of safety. The lack of complicating side effects has led to numerous nonlabel dosage regimens. Some of these dosage regimens include double doses for the first 3 to 5 days of therapy, loading doses of 7 times the recommended dose followed by twice the recommended dose for the duration of therapy, and high doses given once weekly or monthly. These nonlabel uses have not been critically evaluated and should be used with caution.

Nitazoxanide kills *S. neurona* in cell cultures and has been tested in a field trial. Safety studies showed lethargy at twice the recommended dose and illness and death at four times the recommended dose. Gastrointestinal upset can be a complication of nitazoxanide therapy. Concurrent administration of a vegetable oil (corn oil) with nitazoxanide appears to increase small intestinal absorption and reduce gastrointestinal upset. Manufacturers have also recommended starting therapy with a reduced dose for several days. In seven horses with clinical signs compatible with EPM and positive immunoblot results for *S. neurona* antibodies in the CSF, clinical signs improved in six horses by the end of the trial (85 to 140 days).[57] Clinical signs recurred in two horses when treatment was stopped, but signs improved when treatment was reinitiated. Another report described two horses with a diagnosis of EPM that improved after 28 to 42 days of treatment with 50 mg of nitazoxanide per kilogram once daily.[58] Anorexia and depression were reported as side effects.[58] The CSF remained positive for *S. neurona* antibodies. Until more information is available about this drug, we do not recommend its use. Although nitazoxanide received FDA approval and was marketed as Navigator, recently the drug was taken off the market presumably as a result of gastrointestinal complications.

To our knowledge, no evidence shows that concurrent use of immune stimulants, oral antioxidants, and antiinflammatory drugs has any beneficial effect. The use of corticosteroids is controversial, because some clinicians claim corticosteroid administration can exacerbate infection. Severity of neurological signs in horses infected with *S. neurona* reportedly was increased by corticosteroids,[59] but in another study of induced disease, signs were less severe in horses given corticosteroids.[60]

Providing an accurate prognosis is difficult, given the inherent diagnostic problems. Some horses that recover or respond to treatment may not have EPM, and others may recover spontaneously. Economic factors influence duration of treatment and time allowed for convalescence. Even when a severely affected horse improves dramatically, if recovery of function is not complete, a return to previous performance levels is not possible. Signs also may recur in the same horse; whether this is caused by recrudescence of infection or reinfection is unknown. We usually give a guarded prognosis for full recovery of horses showing moderate gait deficits compatible with EPM.

Because the exact life cycle and natural intermediate hosts are unknown, definitive recommendations for control of the disease are difficult. Because the opossum is the definitive host and sheds sporocysts, which the horse ingests, fecal contamination of feedstuffs or water sources by this animal should be prevented. The role of other intermediate mammalian hosts is unclear. The efficacy of a recently introduced vaccine remains to be determined.

Cervical Spinal Cord Compression

Cervical vertebral malformations of various types have been described as the cause of cord compression and neurological signs.[1,61,62] Occasionally it may be difficult to decide if a horse is mildly affected by cervical cord compression or is bilaterally lame in the hindlimbs. Mildly affected horses may show only a slightly stiff, stabbing gait at a walk and trot, only mild circumduction of the outside hindlimb when turning, and equivocal hindlimb dysfunction at a canter. Horses with bilateral osteochondrosis dissecans of the hocks or stifles may show similar signs but usually also have joint capsule distention. Thorough lameness and neurological examinations and radiographs are needed. With more severe compression, the gait deficits increase. Circumduction may be severe, and the horse may strike the distal aspect of the limb with the opposite hoof, causing hair loss or wounds from interference. A horse may lose balance or fall, especially when backing up or turning. If the caudal cervical spinal cord is compressed, thoracic limb motor deficits and hypometria, frequently asymmetrical, may occur. The horse may severely scuff or drag its toes and have abnormal hoof wear. Occasionally, substantial bony proliferation at the synovial articular facets can result in neck stiffness and decreased ability to turn in one direction. Cervical muscle atrophy is rare but can occur if the nerves or lower motor neurons are affected. An affected horse usually lacks hindlimb impulsion and may have a somewhat stiff, bouncy canter. The horse frequently is imprecise when stopping, and the hindquarters may sway or bounce. When compression of the cranial cervical spinal cord occurs, the horse may hold its neck and head higher than normal, in an extended position, and in horses with severe clinical signs all limbs may be affected. Signs may occur suddenly or have a more gradual onset, and progression is variable.

Various vertebral abnormalities have been reported in young horses, but clinical signs can be delayed, even when radiographs reveal chronic lesions. We suspect that trauma may cause a preexisting lesion to become clinically relevant. If a horse with vertebral malformation falls, acute spinal cord compression can occur. Acute cervical spinal cord compression caused by trauma can cause tetraparesis or recumbency, but signs may be delayed in the initial stages after injury and may become apparent only when muscle spasms subside, the unstable fracture displaces, or progressive hemorrhaging is present. In the neck the occipitoatlantoaxial and caudal cervical regions are predilection sites for spinal cord injury.[1] Synovial cysts may also cause severe sudden signs of spinal cord compression, often asymmetrical and sometimes intermittent.[1] The diagnosis of synovial cysts is usually made at necropsy.

Diagnosis of cervical cord compression is based on radiography and myelography. Numerous types of vertebral abnormalities have been described. Management depends on the nature of the lesion, severity of clinical signs, intended use of the horse, and financial considerations. Horses affected by cervical vertebral malformation and cord compression at less than a year of age may improve when exercise and energy intake are restricted.[63] Although no controlled studies of a paced diet and restricted exercise program have been conducted, clinical experience supports its use in young horses with radiological evidence of cervical vertebral malformation.[1,63] This treatment is not helpful for young horses with very severe stenosis, for defects such as occipitoatlantoaxial or other cranial cervical malformations, or for older horses. Prognosis with conservative management is poor. Surgical fusion of vertebrae is indicated in some horses and has been used successfully.[62,64,65] This subject is discussed in Chapter 60.

Equine Degenerative Myeloencephalopathy and Neuroaxonal Dystrophy

Horses mildly affected by equine degenerative myeloencephalopathy and neuroaxonal dystrophy may be misdiagnosed as being lame. Clinical signs may be somewhat similar to those of cervical spinal cord compression. Because no definitive antemortem test exists, clinical diagnosis is based on clinical signs, sometimes supported by the presence of other affected horses on the same farm or in the same family.

Equine degenerative myelopathy is thought to be a vitamin E deficiency, with a likely genetic predisposition.[66,67] Neuroaxonal dystrophy appears to have a genetic basis in Morgan horses.[68] Various breeds and also Przewalski's horses and zebras can be affected, and no geographical restriction is apparent. When horses are affected at a young age (i.e., <6 to 12 months old), signs are more severe and progressive than when signs are first noted in horses 2 years old or older. However, because signs can be mild and only slowly progressive, owners may not be aware of the abnormality. When a severely affected horse is identified on an individual farm, other, more mildly affected horses are often found on the same premises or among relatives. Signs tend to be most noticeable in the hindlimbs. Affected horses usually lift the hind feet too high and slap them down on the ground and frequently lift the hoof toward the midline and then place it more laterally. The gait is jerky and asynchronous and sometimes ataxic, with excessive sideways sway of the hindquarters. Interference may occur, with a hind hoof hitting the opposite hind fetlock or pastern region. The horse may have a jerky foot placement when stopping and may pivot on the hindlimbs when turning. Severely affected horses may show forelimb ataxia and weakness of all limbs. The gait lacks impulsion. Occasionally, middle-aged horses are examined because of inability to perform at collected gaits with impulsion and precision. No musculoskeletal cause is found, but the hindlimb gait is characteristic of mild equine degenerative

myeloencephalopathy or neuroaxonal dystrophy. Mildly affected mature horses appear to function without substantial progression of signs. No ancillary diagnostic test confirms the disease. Vitamin E supplementation (5000 to 6000 units by mouth daily) has been used to treat affected horses, with some, but not total, improvement reported.[69] Horses at risk for the disease should be given vitamin E supplements. Supplementation on farms with a number of affected horses was associated with a subsequent decrease in the incidence of disease.[66] Mares and foals should have access to grass pasture, because lack of access to green pasture has been identified as a risk factor.

Equine Lower Motor Neuron Disease

Equine lower motor neuron disease has been diagnosed in many countries.[70] Older horses and those lacking access to green pasture appear to be at risk to develop equine lower motor neuron disease. The disease is thought to be caused by deficiency of antioxidant activity in the central nervous system, leading to degeneration and loss of lower motor neurons in the brainstem and spinal cord.[71] Affected horses lose muscle mass and have generalized muscle trembling, which may be more severe in the triceps and quadriceps and is exacerbated by transport. Other clinical signs include stiffness, shifting of weight between the hindlimbs, standing with all feet excessively under the body, excessive sweating, holding the tail elevated and trembling, long periods of recumbency, and sometimes excessively low head carriage. Trembling disappears when the horse lies down. Although the gait may be choppy, the horse has no lameness or ataxia. Horses move better than they stand, and therefore the condition is unlikely to be confused with lameness. Muscle atrophy may be profound. Ophthalmoscopic examination of horses with chronic equine lower motor neuron disease may reveal abnormal pigment deposition in the tapetum with a horizontal band of pigment at the tapetal-nontapetal junction.[72] Diagnosis is based on clinical signs and low serum vitamin E concentrations in unsupplemented horses or biopsy of the sacrocaudalis dorsalis medialis (dorsolateral coccygeal) muscle. Affected horses that have not been given vitamin E usually have serum vitamin E concentrations less than or equal to 1 mcg/mL.[73] Biopsy of a branch of the spinal accessory nerve, which had a high specificity and sensitivity in diagnosis of equine lower motor neuron disease, has been replaced by the muscle biopsy, which is technically much easier, can be performed in the standing horse, and has a similar diagnostic specificity and sensitivity.[74] However, false-positive test results can occur in horses that have had "tail blocks."[74] The dorsolateral coccygeal muscle is ideal for biopsy because it contains a high percent of type I oxidative fibers, which are the main muscle fibers affected by the disease. Other muscles with a high proportion of type I fibers are not accessible for biopsy. Most limb muscles have high percentages of type II fibers and are not suitable for diagnosis of the disease.

Oral vitamin E supplementation (6000 to 10,000 units by mouth daily) improves horses, and green pasture is also helpful. However, athletic ability may remain impaired.[71]

Equine Herpesvirus 1 Infection

Neurological disease caused by EHV-1 can occur in individual horses or as an outbreak. Ataxia is variable but usually symmetrical. The hindlimbs are more severely affected, and recumbency can occur. Signs occur acutely and usually stabilize within 24 to 48 hours. Because this condition is unlikely to be confused with lameness, it is not discussed further and readers are referred to a review.[1]

Miscellaneous Diseases of the Spinal Cord

Spinal cord disease from migrating parasites could manifest as an asymmetrical gait deficit. Incidence appears to vary geographically, and clinical signs reflect the path of migration. Antemortem diagnosis is usually not possible, although eosinophilia in the CSF supports the diagnosis. Various parasites including *Setaria* species, *Halicephalobus (Micronema) deletrix*, *Hypoderma*, and *Strongylus* species have been identified. Treatment includes antiparasitic and anti-inflammatory drugs.

Vertebral osteomyelitis, neoplasia, and diskospondylitis are rare causes of spinal cord disease. Signs reflect location of the lesion, which may be confirmed by radiography or scintigraphy. CSF may reflect the disease condition if it extends through the dura. Traumatically induced diskospondylitis has been described and may be difficult to differentiate from bacterial diskospondylitis.[1,75] Spinal cord traumas may occur directly or from instability of intervertebral joints. External trauma can affect any horse, and clinical signs reflect the site of the lesions. Three predilection sites for injury are the occipitoatlantoaxial region, the caudal cervical region (the fifth cervical to the first thoracic vertebrae) and midthoracolumbar region.[1] Clinical signs may initially be mild or peracute, and some horses develop severe progressive signs. It is often not possible to perform an adequate or accurate neurological examination on, or form a prognosis for, an acutely injured horse. Initial treatment includes first aid care, sedation if needed, and the administration of analgesics, antiinflammatory drugs, and mannitol. Radiographs can be useful, depending on site of injury and size of the horse. Repeated neurological evaluations are used for prognosis.

Peripheral Nerve Injuries

Except for stringhalt and radial nerve injury, peripheral nerve diseases affecting the gait are rarely diagnosed. Suprascapular nerve injury *by itself* does not alter the gait but results in atrophy of the supraspinatus and infraspinatus muscles (Sweeny; see Figure 6-20).[76-78] However, injury to the nerve usually occurs with more general trauma to the region such as a collision or fall. This type of injury frequently can lead to damage to other nerves of the limb and soft tissue structures. If other nerve roots of the brachial plexus are simultaneously damaged, the shoulder joint may be unstable and may subluxate laterally. The horse may circumduct the limb during protraction. Rest and antiinflammatory drugs are usually used. Several surgical procedures have been advocated for suprascapular nerve injury.[79]

Radial nerve paresis or paralysis is recognized, usually secondary to trauma. Horses with radial nerve paralysis cannot flex the shoulder joint or extend the elbow, knee, fetlock, or interphalangeal joints (see Figure 5-14). The dorsum of the toe rests on the ground, and the elbow is dropped. Severely affected horses have difficulty rising and often collapse on the limb if it bears weight. More mildly affected horses may advance the leg by flinging or jerking it forward from the shoulder. Evaluation of skin sensation

may not be helpful. Atrophy of the triceps and other limb extensor muscles occurs after 2 weeks, and denervation potentials can be found on electromyographic examination 3 to 4 weeks, or sooner, after radial nerve injury.[79,80] Because of the difficulty of knowing whether the gait deficits result solely from radial nerve injury or muscle damage, an accurate prognosis can be difficult in horses with acute clinical signs. Signs of radial paralysis occurring after recumbency or general anesthesia are probably caused by ischemic myopathy, with possible ischemic neuropraxia, and these horses generally recover. Prognosis depends on the cause and extent of radial nerve injury, neither of which may be identified. Prognosis is obviously better in horses that are less severely affected and those that show early signs of improvement. However, some severely affected horses completely recover. Prognosis is worse if rapid severe atrophy of extensor muscle occurs. Signs of radial nerve dysfunction may be associated with trauma to caudal cervical or cranial thoracic nerve roots secondary to an injury to the head of a rib; other nerves and muscles may also be affected. Signs of radial nerve dysfunction can also occur from lesions in the caudal cervical and cranial thoracic ventral gray matter, but other signs of spinal cord disease usually coexist, especially in EPM. Physical therapy, including splinting to avoid flexural deformity, is very important, and electrical stimulation of muscles may also help prevent atrophy. Irreversible fibrosis and contracture are likely without intervention.

Lesions in the nerves supplying the flexor muscles of the thoracic limb are extremely rare, although signs of dysfunction can accompany brachial plexus or spinal cord lesions.[77] If the ulnar nerve is sectioned, the horse may move its foot in a jerking fashion with decreased flexion of the fetlock and carpal joints. When the median nerve is cut, the horse drags the toe because of decreased flexion of the fetlock and carpus. Hypalgesia of the medial aspect of the pastern occurs, whereas with ulnar neurectomy, hypalgesia of the lateral metacarpal region occurs.[77,79] After neurectomy of the proximal musculocutaneous nerve, the horse drags its toe because of decreased elbow flexion. Because natural disease syndromes affecting these nerves are not described, prognosis is difficult because gait deficits improve with time after neurectomy.[79]

If the femoral nerve is damaged, the horse cannot extend its stifle and rests the leg in a flexed position. The hip is lower than the opposite limb, and the horse cannot support weight normally or at all when walking. When both limbs are affected, the horse will appear crouched and have great difficulty rising. The patellar reflex is absent or depressed, and with time the quadriceps muscles atrophy. Damage to the nerve has occurred during general anesthesia with horses positioned in dorsal or lateral recumbency (usually with the affected limb having been positioned uppermost) or after overextension of the limb, after pelvic or femoral fractures, or in association with space-occupying masses impinging on the nerve.[79,81,82] Lesions in the spinal cord ventral gray matter or nerve roots at the L5 or L6 lumbar vertebra can also cause signs of femoral nerve paralysis. Horses with patellar fractures and subsequent inability or reluctance to bear weight on the affected hindlimb may mimic those with femoral nerve injury.[82] Complete neurological evaluation to detect other deficits may be difficult if signs of femoral nerve paralysis are severe. Because the condition is rare and rhabdomyolysis and postoperative myopathy can mimic the signs of femoral nerve damage, giving a prognosis is difficult. Antiinflammatory drugs are usually used. Most horses with postanesthetic femoral nerve paresis make a complete recovery.[82]

Signs of paresis or paralysis of the sciatic nerve can occur in horses with pelvic fractures, with deep muscle injections in foals, or with spinal cord lesions affecting the ventral gray matter or nerve roots of the fifth lumbar to third sacral nerves. Signs reflect flexor muscle weakness. The horse can support weight on the limb if the hoof is placed flat on the ground under the pelvis. Otherwise, the horse stands with the hock and stifle extended and the dorsum of the hoof on the ground behind it. When the horse walks, it drags or jerks the limb forward. With time all muscles distal to the stifle and those of the caudal aspect of the thigh atrophy. The prognosis is very poor if the nerve is severed. If the fibular (peroneal) nerve is damaged (usually because of blunt trauma), the horse cannot extend the fetlock and interphalangeal joints or flex the tarsus normally. At rest it stands with the hoof behind it, resting on its dorsal surface. If the hoof is placed flat on the ground under the horse, the horse can support weight. When the horse moves, it drags the foot cranially, then jerks it caudally, sliding it on the ground. Skin sensation is decreased over the dorsal and lateral aspects of the tarsus and metatarsal region. With time, muscle atrophy in the craniolateral aspect of the crus can occur. Treatment involves support and protection of the distal limb. Electrical stimulation of muscles might help prevent muscle atrophy. Many horses recover with time. Gait had returned to virtually normal within 3 months of experimental transection of the fibular nerve.[79] Tibial nerve injury is uncommonly diagnosed, but a stringhalt-like gait has been described. When walking, the horse overflexes the limb and drops the foot straight to the ground when it reaches the end of the cranial phase of the stride. The gastrocnemius muscle reportedly atrophies. The horse stands with the fetlock flexed or partly knuckled, the tarsus flexed, and the hip lower than that of the unaffected leg.[81] Obturator nerve damage, which can occur after foaling, results in signs varying from abduction or circumduction and stiffness of the affected limb when walking to paraplegia. Prognosis depends on severity of signs, whether both limbs are affected, and whether adequate supportive care can be provided.

Stringhalt is easily recognized from its exaggerated flexion of the hock, which can result in a bizarre hopping, jerking, and propulsive gait when both hindlimbs are affected (see Chapter 48). Horses may be so severely affected that they "freeze" in the abnormal position or are very reluctant or unable to move, particularly in those with bilateral stringhalt. They may strike the ventral abdomen with the hoof. The gait usually is worse when the horse is walking on a hard surface and when it is anxious or frightened. Horses with mild signs may show the exaggerated hock flexion only when backing up or turning or during the first few strides after walking from a standstill. Atrophy of the distal limb muscles may occur in horses with chronic stringhalt. Spasticity, toe scuffing, and stumbling of the thoracic limbs and left laryngeal hemiplegia have been described in some affected horses.[83,84] A distal axonopathy of peripheral nerves has been described.[85,86] The condition can be sporadic or occur in outbreaks. The cause frequently is unknown, especially when only one horse is affected. Outbreaks have been associated with particular pastures, and mycotoxins are a suspected cause.[83,84] Lathyrism can also be a cause. Phenytoin and baclofen have been used with some success to decrease clinical signs.[87,88] Tenectomy of the lateral digital tendon has also been used. The course is variable, and some horses recover spontaneously. However, because it is difficult to predict which horses will recover, the prognosis is guarded, especially in horses with severe clinical signs or in single horses unassociated with a pasture outbreak.

Shivers is somewhat similar to stringhalt, and the origin and pathogenesis are unknown (see Chapter 48). Affected horses tremble one or both pelvic limbs, primarily when backing up or lifting a hoof, and they elevate the tail. Some affected horses cannot stand to have the hooves trimmed, even though the hindlimb gaits are relatively normal and otherwise functional. The clinical course seems variable, and the disease is thought to be progressive, at least in draft breeds.[79] However, we have seen affected horses remain relatively static and functional, although hoof care can be difficult because of the inability to stand for the farrier. A group of horses exists with mild hindlimb deficits resembling a combination of stringhalt and shivers. Although these horses may continue to be functional for riding, the gait disability impairs dressage performance. The cause usually is undiagnosed.

| Chapter **12**

Unexplained Lameness

Sue J. Dyson

Lameness diagnosis is a never-ending challenge, even for an experienced clinician, because despite a logical and thorough investigation it still may prove difficult to reach a satisfactory conclusion. This chapter discusses some of the reasons why a definitive diagnosis may remain elusive. In some horses it may be possible to isolate the source of pain reasonably accurately, but it may not be possible to determine the cause of pain. In other horses the source of pain cannot be determined (see Chapter 97).

FALSE-NEGATIVE RESPONSES TO DIAGNOSTIC ANALGESIA

A false-negative response to local analgesic techniques may occur for a variety of reasons, including the following:

- Inaccurate injection
- Inadequate time for the local anesthetic solution to be effective
- Failure to appreciate improvement in the lameness
- Very severe pain
- Failure to alleviate subchondral bone pain after intraarticular injection
- Extraarticular pain
- Aberrant nerve supply
- Failure, in an unshod horse, to appreciate the extent of foot soreness contributing to lameness
- Failure to appreciate the degree of lameness fluctuation within an examination period
- Failure to abolish pain associated with a neuroma
- Neuropathic pain

The following are common case examples:

1. It is misleading to conclude that pain does not arise from the centrodistal and tarsometatarsal joints and the central and third tarsal bones after a negative response to intraarticular analgesia of the centrodistal and tarsometatarsal joints. Intraarticular analgesia has only a limited ability to alleviate subchondral bone pain. In moderate to advanced osteoarthritis, subchondral bone pain is a clinically significant contributor to pain. Hock pain may be missed if it is concluded that a negative response to intraarticular analgesia precludes the existence of hock pain and if there is a failure to desensitize the hock region using regional analgesia. It should also be recognized that perineural analgesia of the fibular and tibial nerves may result in only partial improvement in lameness associated with moderate-to-severe osteoarthritis of the centrodistal and or tarsometatarsal joints.

2. Laminitis, a fracture of either the distal phalanx or the navicular bone, and a subsolar abscess are all common causes of severe foot pain. Desensitization of the foot by perineural analgesia of the palmar (plantar) nerves at the level of the proximal sesamoid bones may have a negligible effect or result in only mild improvement in lameness. Foot pain in a hindlimb is often more difficult to alleviate than in a forelimb. If clinical signs point to foot pain, but apparent desensitization of the foot fails to markedly alter the lameness, further investigation of the foot should be performed with other means (e.g., radiographic examination).

The horse in Figure 12-1 was admitted with suspected back pain but showed obvious bilateral forelimb lameness, with right forelimb lameness predominating. Digital pulse amplitudes were increased in the right forelimb, but there was no response to hoof testers. Nonetheless, the horse appeared clinically to have foot pain typical of laminitis. Apparent desensitization of the foot, performed to convince the owner that the horse had foot pain, produced absolutely no change in the lameness. The horse responded rapidly to treatment for laminitis.

3. Inadvertent intrasynovial injection may result in misleading results. For example, accidental injection into the tarsal sheath when attempting to deposit local anesthetic solution around the plantar metatarsal nerves distal to the hock may result in proximal suspensory lesions being missed.

4. Failure to allow sufficient time for local anesthetic solution to be effective may result in a false-negative response in some circumstances. Premature assessment of the response to intraarticular analgesia of the femorotibial joints may result in a false-negative result in association with a cruciate ligament injury. These ligaments have an extrasynovial location, and it may take up to an hour after injection for cruciate ligament pain to be clinically significantly improved.

5. Subchondral bone pain in the condyles of the third metacarpal (metatarsal) bones, associated with extensive sclerosis, in young Thoroughbred and Standardbred racehorses is difficult to abolish in some horses,

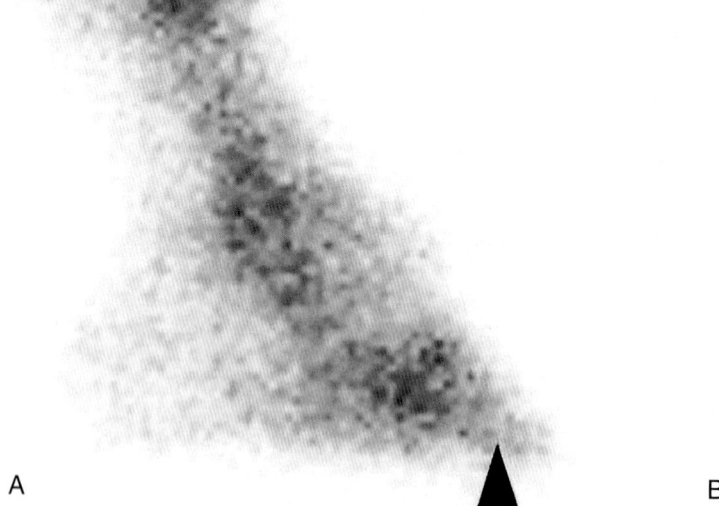
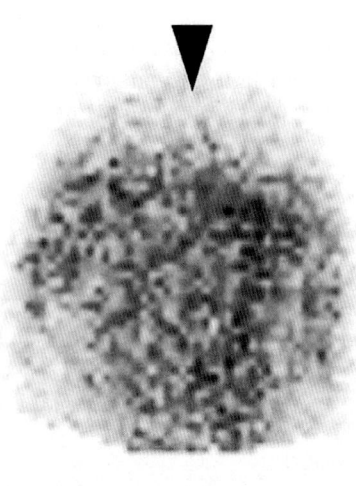

Fig. 12-1 • **A,** Lateral and **B,** solar scintigraphic images of the front feet of a horse with suspected back pain but clinical signs of laminitis. There is reduced radiopharmaceutical uptake in the toe region *(arrowheads)*. The horse showed no improvement in lameness after apparent desensitization of the lamer right front foot by palmar (abaxial sesamoid) nerve blocks, despite the firm focal pressure applied with artery forceps around the coronary band. However, the horse responded well to symptomatic treatment for laminitis.

erences
1 page
1260

and responses to distal limb nerve blocks may add confusion.[1] There may be no localizing clinical signs suggestive of fetlock region pain. Improvement in lameness is sometimes seen after either palmar digital or palmar (abaxial sesamoid) nerve blocks; a "low four-point block" may further improve but not abolish lameness. The horse may be sound only after addition of a subcarpal block of the palmar metacarpal nerves. However, there may negligible response to intraarticular analgesia of the fetlock joint.

Failure to allow sufficient time may in some circumstances result in a false-positive response and then confusion. The tibial and fibular nerves are relatively large, and it takes time for the local anesthetic solution to diffuse into them and to take effect. This time requirement, combined with the deep location of the deep fibular nerve and thus difficulty in precisely locating the site for injection, may result in a response delayed for up to an hour after injection. Testing the efficacy of these blocks through evaluation of cutaneous sensation is unreliable. If the response is deemed to be negative after 30 minutes, and intraarticular analgesia of the compartments of the stifle is then performed and the lameness improves, it may be wrongly inferred that pain originated in the stifle. However, the improvement in lameness may reflect alleviation of pain arising from the hock region. Much wasted time and money may then be spent trying to establish a cause of stifle pain.

Blocking each compartment of the stifle joint separately (e.g., the medial femorotibial joint) may not result in substantial clinical improvement in the lameness, despite the presence of stifle pain. A considerably better response is frequently seen after blocking the medial and lateral femorotibial joints and the femoropatellar joint in combination.

The importance of the clinical examination and repeated observations of a horse cannot be overemphasized. Each clinician has to learn how much to trust nerve blocks. This depends on experience and the frequency of performing blocks. An inexperienced clinician is far more likely to encounter false-negative responses. The results of nerve blocks must be compared with the clinical signs, and if the interpretation is doubtful, the block should be repeated or the area desensitized with a different technique. The clinician must develop experience in the interpretation of improvement in lameness compared with complete alleviation of pain and lameness. This contrast depends to some extent on the degree of the baseline lameness and whether the forelimbs or hindlimbs are involved.

Failure to Perform the Appropriate Nerve Blocks

Failure to perform nerve blocks in a logical and complete sequence can lead to confusion. If the response to a low six-point block in a hindlimb is negative and is followed by a positive response to tibial and fibular nerve blocks, the clinician may conclude that pain arose from the hock. Lesions of the proximal aspect of the suspensory ligament (SL) may be completely overlooked.

Blocking the Wrong Limb

Failure to appreciate that a head nod reflects hindlimb lameness and is not always a sign of forelimb lameness may result in a blocking a forelimb with negative results, when the primary source of pain is in the ipsilateral hindlimb.

Sources of Pain That Cannot Be Desensitized by Nerve Blocks

Many regions of the limbs proximal to the carpus and tarsus cannot be satisfactorily desensitized. In young horses, stress fractures are now well-recognized causes of lameness that pain from which in many circumstances cannot be blocked out. In young or older horses, fractures of the deltoid tuberosity of the humerus (Figure 12-2), the proximal aspect of the fibula (Figure 12-3), the third trochanter of the femur,

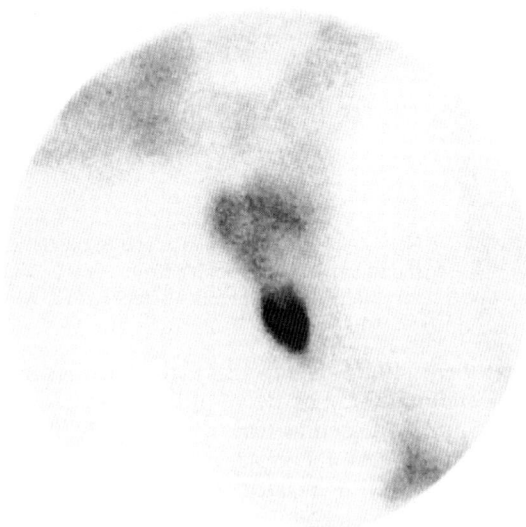

Fig. 12-2 • Lateral scintigraphic image of the shoulder region of a 6-year-old Warmblood with acute onset of moderate left forelimb lameness. Note the marked focal increased radiopharmaceutical uptake in the region of the deltoid tuberosity of the humerus. There was a slightly displaced fracture of the deltoid tuberosity of the humerus, which healed satisfactorily with conservative management.

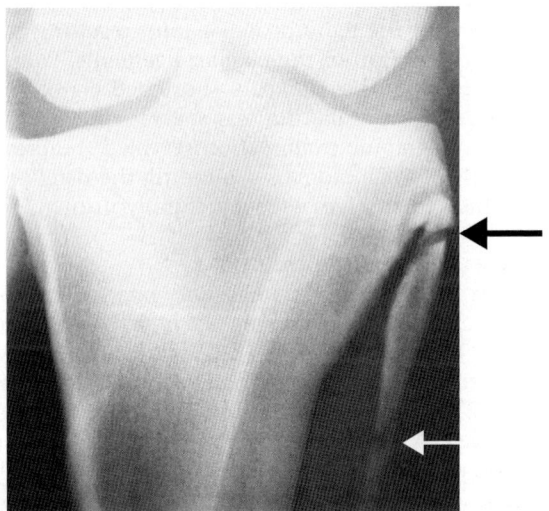

Fig. 12-3 • Caudocranial radiographic image of the left stifle of a general purpose riding horse with recent-onset, episodic, and transient severe left hindlimb lameness. There is a fracture of the proximal aspect of the fibula *(large arrow)*. The lucent line separating the different centers of ossification further distally *(small arrow)* should not be confused as a fracture. There was little evidence of bony union after 6 weeks, but after 12 weeks the fracture healed satisfactorily.

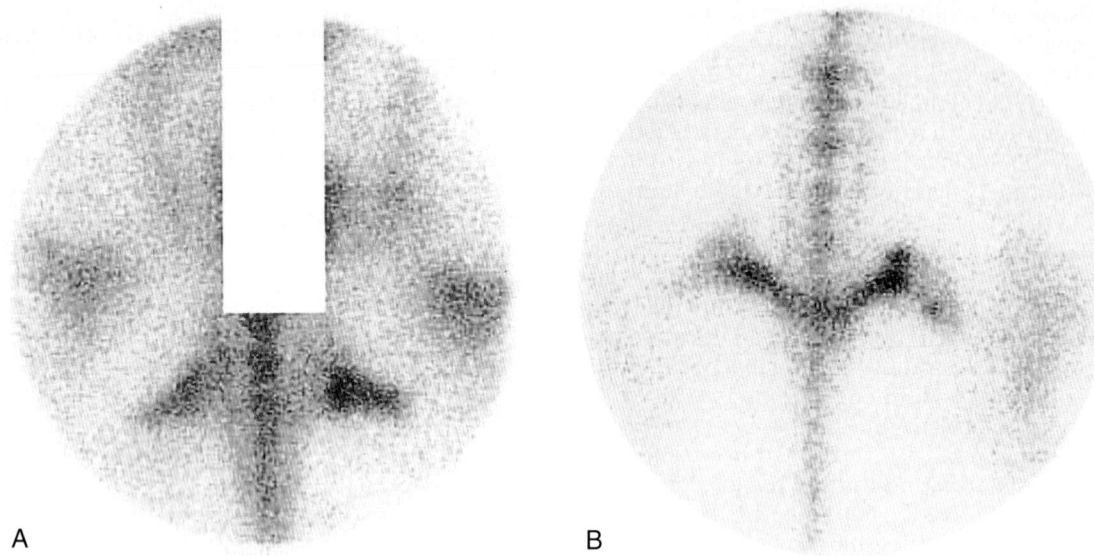

Fig. 12-4 • A, Dorsal oblique and **B,** caudal scintigraphic images of the tubera ischii of an 8-year-old Grand Prix show jumper with loss of hindlimb power and a tendency to jump to the right. There is increased radiopharmaceutical uptake in the right tuber ischium and a change of contour compatible with a fracture.

and the tuber ischium (Figure 12-4) are all causes of lameness that are unaffected by nerve blocks.

Muscle injuries, such as tearing or fibrosis of brachiocephalicus or the pectoral muscles, may have no localizing signs (see page 152). Associated lameness cannot be influenced by nerve blocks. Atypical equine rhabdomyolysis can cause hindlimb lameness without any other clinical signs typical of tying up.

Periarticular lesions of the otifle such as collateral ligament injury are usually associated with detectable soft tissue swelling, but injuries of the patellar ligaments can occur with no localizing clinical signs, and associated pain is often unresponsive to intraarticular analgesia (see Chapter 46). I have also examined five horses with acute onset of severe lameness and mild swelling on the craniomedial aspect of the femoropatellar joint resulting in loss of palpable definition of the patellar ligaments. Lameness was characterized by a markedly shortened cranial phase of the stride at the walk, but less severe lameness at the trot. Ultrasonographic examination revealed the presence of a periarticular hematoma surrounding the patellar ligaments, which themselves were structurally normal.

Pain Associated with a Neuroma

A neuroma may develop secondary to external trauma to a nerve, after abnormal stretching of a nerve, or subsequent to surgery. There is usually intense focal pain on pressure applied directly over the neuroma. However, perineural analgesia of the area may fail to abolish or improve associated lameness. A much better response may be achieved by infiltration of local anesthetic solution directly around the neuroma.

POTENTIALLY CONFUSING RESPONSES TO LOCAL ANALGESIC TECHNIQUES

Improvement without complete alleviation of lameness after perineural analgesia is not always easy to interpret. It may reflect failure to completely alleviate pain from a

single source, or there may be additional sources of pain. Sometimes lameness improves with each successive block (e.g., palmar digital, palmar [abaxial sesamoid], low four-point, and subcarpal nerve blocks). However, the lameness is not associated with any detectable radiological, ultrasonographic, or scintigraphic abnormalities. Sometimes additional useful information can be obtained by performing intraarticular analgesia of the interphalangeal and metacarpophalangeal joints, but if the response is negative the diagnosis remains inconclusive.

Isolation of pain to a region but failure to define the cause is particularly frustrating. For example, intraarticular analgesia of the femorotibial joints may be positive, but no radiological or ultrasonographic abnormalities may be detectable. Nuclear scintigraphy may reveal a generalized increased uptake of the radiopharmaceutical in the distal aspect of the femur and proximal aspect of the tibia compared with the contralateral limb. Medication of the joints may result in no improvement. Exploratory arthroscopy may reveal minor findings (e.g., mild fibrillation of the cranial meniscal ligaments) of questionable relevance, but evaluation of all the joint surfaces and meniscal cartilages is impossible. The definitive diagnosis for the cause of pain remains elusive. Computed tomography (CT) and magnetic resonance imaging (MRI) may permit the identification of subchondral bone injuries and meniscal and ligamentous injuries not accessible to arthroscopic inspection.

The importance of subchondral bone pain as a cause of lameness must not be overlooked. Such pain frequently is present without associated radiological change. A comparison of the responses to intraarticular analgesia and perineural analgesia (and the response or lack thereof to intraarticular medication) may be helpful. With subchondral pain, intraarticular analgesia may have a limited effect. Nuclear scintigraphy is a sensitive indicator of increased modeling in the subchondral bone. MRI has the potential to show subtle structural changes in the subchondral bone.

Until recently, soft tissue lesions within the hoof capsule have proved elusive to definitive diagnosis. Diagnostic ultrasonography, although possible, has marked limitations. Pool-phase scintigraphic images sometimes are helpful. Examination of the navicular bursa may yield useful information about the bursa, the deep digital flexor tendon, and the distal sesamoidean impar ligament. Advanced imaging techniques such as CT and particularly MRI have the best potential to demonstrate soft tissue pathological conditions, although determining the clinical significance of lesions is not necessarily easy.

False-positive results may be obtained if the horse is only mildly lame at investigation but has a history of a more obvious lameness. The detectable mild lameness may not necessarily reflect the original cause. Lameness that is induced when a horse is lunged in small circles on a concrete surface may not reflect the primary cause of lameness. Thus eliminating this lameness by nerve blocks may be misleading. Lameness induced by flexion also may not reflect the principal cause of lameness. Blocking the flexion response does not necessarily identify the primary cause of lameness.

A pony had moderate forelimb lameness that was markedly accentuated by lower limb flexion. The response to flexion was eliminated by either regional or intraarticular analgesia of the fetlock joint. However, the baseline lameness was unchanged and did not respond to any of the nerve blocks that were repeated on several occasions. Surgical removal of a large osseous fragment from the fetlock joint did not improve the lameness.

False Positive Results of Intrasynovial Analgesia
Lameness may be abolished or substantially improved by intraarticular analgesia of the metacarpophalangeal (metatarsophalangeal) joint with no intraarticular pathology. Pain associated with proximal lesions of the cruciate, straight, or oblique sesamoidean ligaments or the insertions of the suspensory branches may be substantially improved by intraarticular analgesia of the fetlock. Therefore in the absence of both clinical signs suggestive of fetlock joint pain (e.g., synovial effusion, joint capsule thickening, pain on manipulation) and radiological abnormalities it is suggested that the distal sesamoidean ligaments and suspensory branches be evaluated ultrasonographically. Intrathecal analgesia of the digital flexor tendon sheath has the potential to remove pain from injured distal sesamoidean ligaments; it may also relieve pain from the deep digital flexor tendon within the hoof capsule. Therefore the distal sesamoidean ligaments should be included in ultrasonographic examination of the palmar soft tissues of the pastern.

Multiple Sources of Pain in a Limb and More than One Lame Limb
Problems can arise in interpretation of nerve blocks in a horse that is lame in more than one limb, especially if there is more than one source of pain in a limb. Perineural blocks usually last for up to 2 to 3 hours unless a long-acting local anesthetic agent, such as bupivacaine, is used. If a horse is lame in several limbs it is usually easiest to start with the lamest limb and block it first. Interpretation becomes difficult if there is a failure to desensitize all the lame limbs simultaneously. If the blocks in one limb are wearing off, then lameness in the least lame limb becomes less apparent. The horse's tolerance for nerve blocks may

also compromise how much can be done. It may be necessary to start again on another occasion using bupivacaine. If simultaneous lameness of the ipsilateral forelimb and hindlimb is suspected, blocking should begin in the hindlimb. In this situation a substantial amount of the head nod probably originates from the hindlimb component. Because elimination of head nod is vital to improvement after blocking, forelimb diagnostic procedures cannot be fairly evaluated.

Very-Low-Grade Lameness
Nerve blocks, especially in hindlimbs, often result in improvement rather than complete alleviation in lameness. Assessing improvement in subtle lameness is nearly impossible. If the horse has a history of more severe lameness previously, delaying further investigation often is worthwhile. The horse should be worked to accentuate the lameness and simplify interpretation of the response to diagnostic analgesic techniques.

Improvement of Lameness in Some Situations, but Unrelieved Lameness under All Situations: Which Is the Baseline Lameness?
Sometimes a horse has lameness that appears different in nature under different circumstances. Such findings may be related to more than one cause of lameness, and it is important to recognize this fact. For example, a dressage horse had left forelimb lameness that was apparent to the rider only when the horse was ridden on the right rein (to the right). Clinical examination revealed left forelimb lameness on the right rein on the lunge on a hard surface. This was alleviated by desensitization of the foot. However, desensitization did not alter the lameness that was apparent when the horse was ridden. The cause of the lameness could not be identified. It is vitally important to relate the results of the investigation to the history.

CHALLENGES TO LAMENESS DIAGNOSIS
Very Intermittent or Sporadic Lameness
Sometimes lameness is intermittent, and the horse may be perfectly normal between episodes. Lameness may be provoked only by maximal exercise in competition. It is very important to carefully assess the history and get the owner to pay great attention to any clinical features of the lameness when present. For example, mild, transient diffuse swelling in the midmetacarpal region medially may reflect axial impingement of a splint on the SL (Figure 12-5) (see Chapter 72). Spontaneous resolution of hindlimb lameness after standing still is suggestive of aortoiliacofemoral thrombosis (see Chapter 50). Ask the owner to assess the reaction to manipulation of specific joints when the horse is lame. Pain on manipulation may suggest a joint problem such as hemarthrosis.

If it is not possible to examine the horse when it is lame, nuclear scintigraphic examination can be helpful but also has the potential to mislead (see page 153). For example, an Arab endurance horse had episodic right forelimb lameness that was present only immediately after rides longer than 30 miles. Comprehensive clinical evaluation revealed no evidence of lameness and no suggestions of the cause of previous lameness. Scintigraphic examination

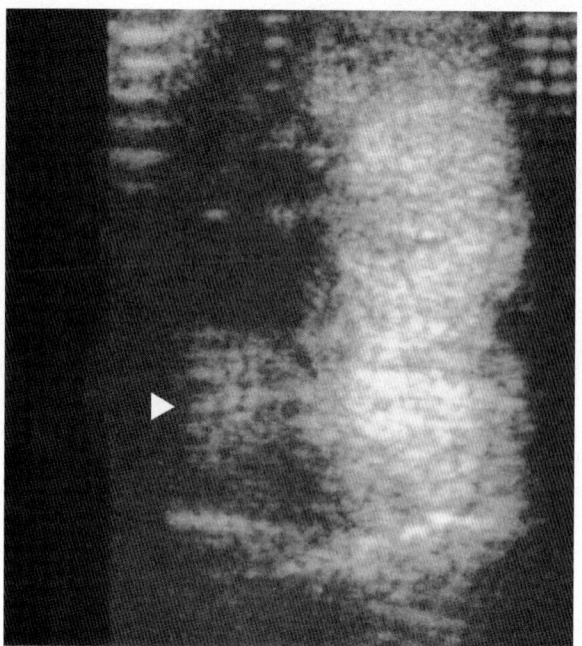

Fig. 12-5 • Transverse ultrasonographic image of the palmar metacarpal soft tissues of the right forelimb of an endurance horse at 10 cm distal to the accessory carpal bone. Medial is to the left. The horse had low-grade lameness at the end of endurance rides that resolved completely within 24 hours. Note the echogenic tissue *(arrowhead)* next to the suspensory ligament (SL). This was a granulomatous reaction between an exostosis on the second metacarpal bone (McII) and the SL. The distal half of the McII was excised and the granulomatous tissue removed. The horse made a complete recovery.

revealed increased radiopharmaceutical uptake (IRU) in the third carpal bone of the lame limb (Figure 12-6). Radiographic examination revealed marked increased radiopacity ("sclerosis") of the third carpal bone in the lame limb only, an unusual finding in an endurance horse and thought likely to be of clinical significance. Another Arab endurance horse had an acute-onset, severe right hindlimb lameness that resolved within 48 hours, but mild, extremely transient, and episodic lameness persisted over the next 3 weeks. Clinical evaluation revealed no suggestion of the cause and no current lameness. Nuclear scintigraphic examination revealed focal intense IRU in the medial plantar process of the distal phalanx, and radiographic examination confirmed a recent fracture (Figure 12-7).

Lameness associated with a distal caudal radial exostosis may be severe but extremely sporadic and often resolves rapidly. There may or may not be detectable distention of the carpal sheath at the time of lameness. With such a history of episodic severe lameness, it is worthwhile to examine the carpal sheath ultrasonographically, paying particular attention to the contour of the caudal distal aspect of the radius and the architecture of the deep digital flexor tendon (see page 162).

If nuclear scintigraphic and ultrasonographic findings are negative, it is necessary to try to recreate the circumstances under which the horse exhibits lameness. For example, hemarthrosis can cause a very severe but extremely transient lameness. The horse may be completely normal between episodes. Although hemarthrosis is unusual to rare, the joints most likely affected are the

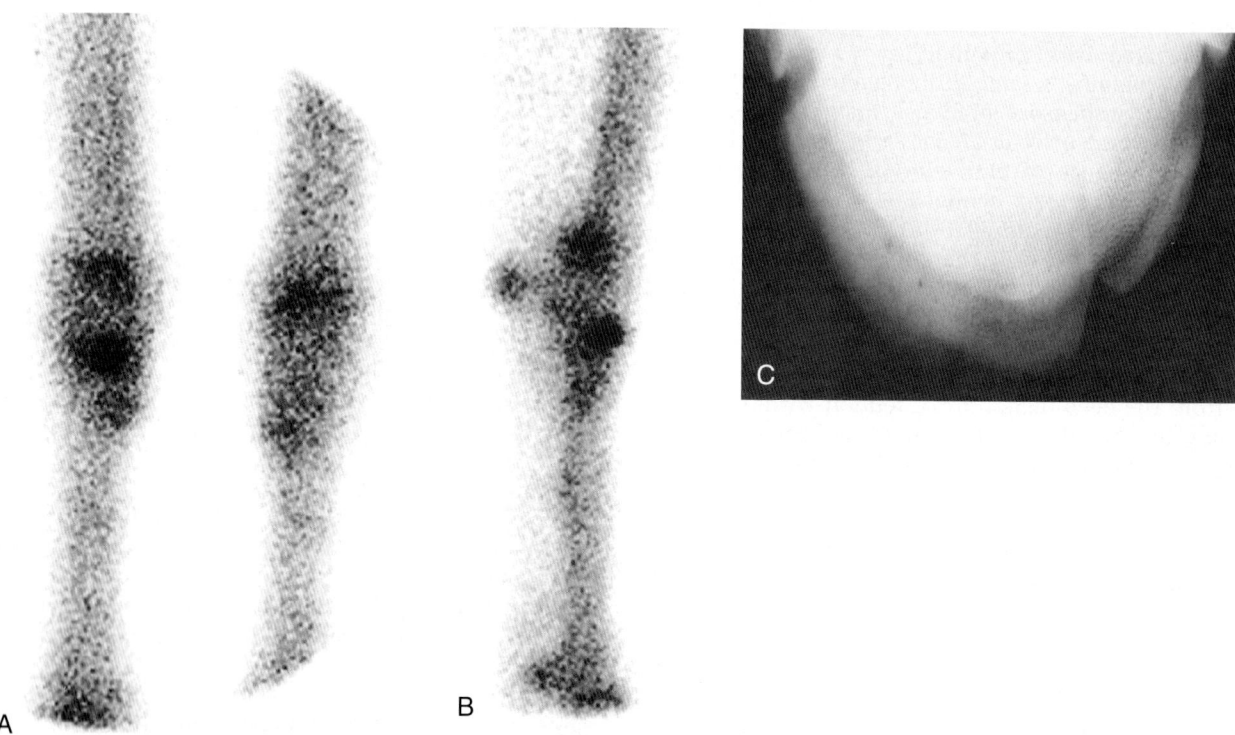

Fig. 12-6 • **A,** Dorsal scintigraphic image of the carpi of an endurance horse with episodic lameness that occurred only during endurance rides. The right forelimb is on the left. There is a focal increased radiopharmaceutical uptake in the middle of the distal row of carpal bones in the right forelimb. **B,** Lateral scintigraphic image of the right carpus. There is increased radiopharmaceutical uptake in the dorsal aspect of the third carpal bone. **C,** Dorsoproximal-dorsodistal oblique radiographic image of the right carpus showing marked increased radiopacity of the radial facet of the third metacarpal bone.

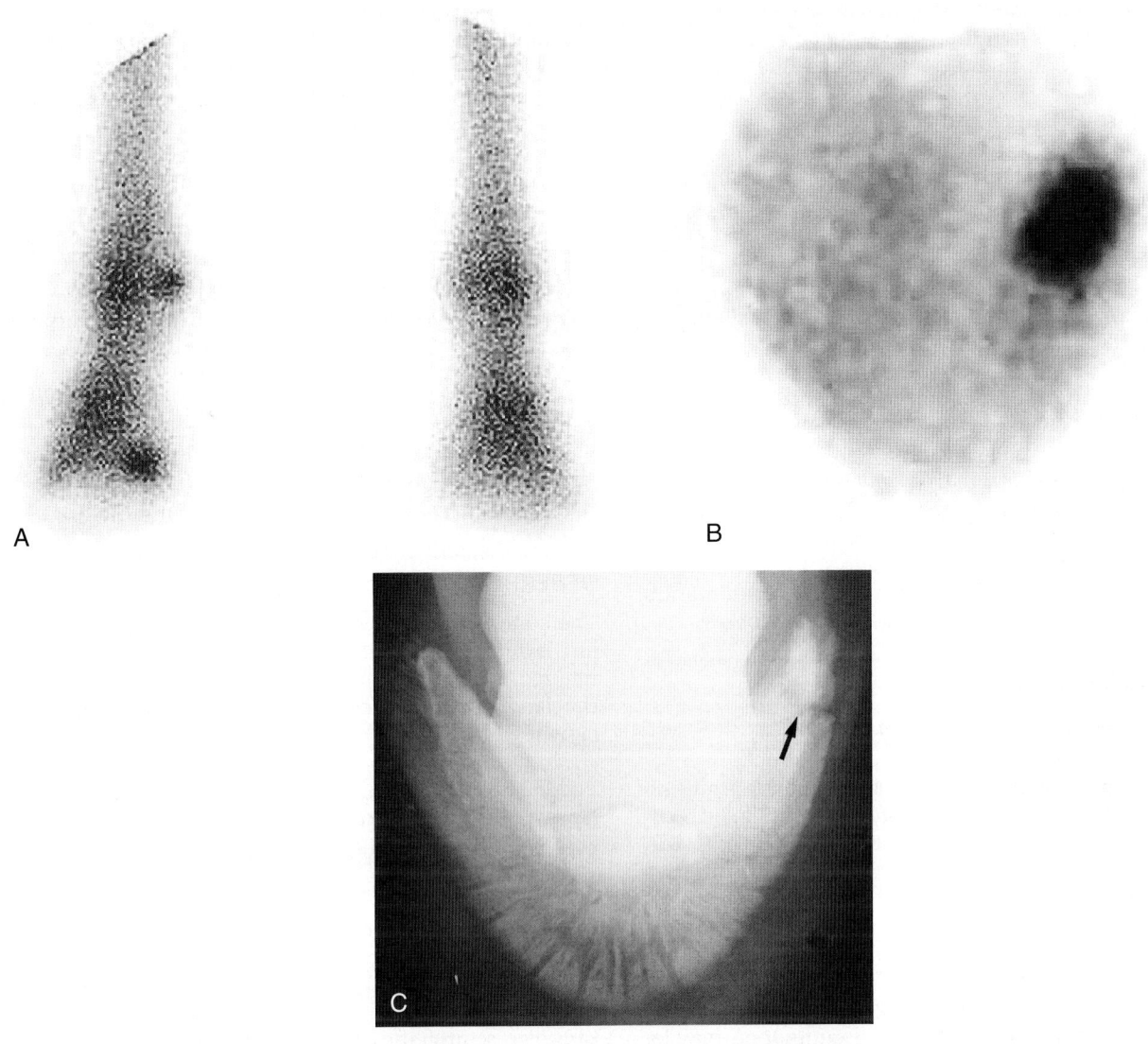

Fig. 12-7 • A, Plantar scintigraphic image of the hind feet of an endurance horse with recent onset of left hindlimb lameness that was apparent only after an endurance ride. The horse appeared clinically normal at the time of the examination. There is moderate focal increased radiopharmaceutical uptake in the medial aspect of the left hind foot *(left).* **B,** Solar scintigraphic image of the left hind foot. Medial is to the right. There is markedly increased radiopharmaceutical uptake in the medial plantar process of the distal phalanx. **C,** Plantarodorsal radiographic image of the left hind foot. There is a fracture of the medial plantar process *(arrow).* The horse was treated conservatively and made a complete recovery.

antebrachiocarpal and tarsocrural joints. Diagnosis can be reached only by arthrocentesis at the time of an acute episode, when there is usually some degree of joint capsule distention and pain on manipulation of the affected joint. Working the horse on a treadmill sometimes is helpful (see Chapter 98).

Lameness That Varies within and between Examinations

Sometimes lameness varies considerably in degree both within an examination period and between examinations. This variation makes interpretation of the response to nerve blocks potentially difficult, unless the veterinarian is aware of the fluctuation. It is important to watch a horse move for a sufficient length of time to appreciate any spontaneous changes in the degree of lameness. Horses with a subchondral bone cyst in either the distal aspect of the scapula

or the medial femoral condyle may behave in this way. Within a single examination period the horse may appear sound or lame. In such circumstances it is vital to compare the response to nerve blocks with the clinical signs exhibited. For example, if the characteristics of the lameness are suggestive of shoulder pain, but the lameness is apparently improved after desensitization of the foot, consider the possibility of spontaneous improvement in the lameness that is unrelated to the nerve block. This is, however, an unusual clinical situation, and generally it is best to rely on the results of the diagnostic blocks. A combination of nerve blocks, scintigraphic examination, and radiographic examination may enable a conclusive diagnosis to be reached. Any concurrent clinical signs must not be ignored, even if the owner thinks that swelling may have predated the onset of lameness. Core lesions in the deep digital flexor tendon within the digital flexor tendon sheath may cause episodic hindlimb lameness that may be difficult to reproduce. Presence of distention of the digital flexor tendon sheath should prompt ultrasonographic evaluation.

The Dangerous Horse and Nerve Blocks

Some horses do not tolerate needle placement and cannot be restrained safely. Nuclear scintigraphic examination sometimes indicates a diagnosis, but the results may be negative. Under such circumstances the horse can be sedated for each block. This approach obviously is time-consuming and may be of low specificity, because time must be allowed for the sedative to wear off adequately before the response to the block can be assessed. During this time the local anesthetic solution has the potential to diffuse away from the site of injection and influence more remote pain. Sedation may result in a rather sloppy gait, which can hinder interpretation, especially with mild hindlimb lameness characterized only by a toe drag. Therefore horse selection is important. However, bearing in mind these limitations, it may be the only way to proceed. Xylazine is the shortest-acting α_2-agonist available and is the drug of choice, but with a difficult horse, combination with an opioid such as butorphanol is usually necessary.

NEGATIVE RESPONSES

Negative Response to All Nerve Blocks: Where Next?

Occasionally a horse is evaluated for forelimb or hindlimb lameness that is not influenced by any local analgesic technique. Clinical signs may be suggestive of a source of pain (e.g., the foot). The reason for failure to eliminate or improve pain by nerve blocks that should result in desensitization of a region is not understood, but such results do occur occasionally.[2] If the results of the clinical examination suggest foot pain, the foot should be examined radiographically. Alternatively, there may be no clinical clues for the source of pain. Nuclear scintigraphic examination may be helpful in either situation if the pain is bony in origin but is likely to be less helpful for soft tissue injuries.

Negative Responses to Nerve Blocks, No Clinical Clues, and Negative Scintigraphic Findings

In horses with negative or equivocal scintigraphic findings consideration may be given to systematic radiographic examination, bearing in mind that not all bony lesions are sufficiently active to yield positive scintigraphic findings. However, comprehensive radiographic examination is time-consuming, expensive, and frequently unrewarding and potentially results in unnecessary exposure to radiation. Thus it is usually discouraged. In the forelimb, unusual causes of lameness such as neurological disease (usually lower motor neuron diseases, such as equine protozoal myelitis), cervical nerve root pain (radiculitis), spondylosis of the cranial thoracic vertebrae, and pectoral, sternal, or rib pain may be considered. Pain associated with advanced osteoarthritis of the scapulohumeral joint or lesions of the tendon of the biceps brachii is not reliably abolished by intraarticular analgesia of the scapulohumeral joint or intrathecal analgesia of the intertubercular bursa, respectively. Therefore radiographic examination of the cervical and cranial thoracic vertebrae, the scapulohumeral joint, and the cranial ribs may be justified, together with ultrasonographic examination of the shoulder region. In the hindlimb, neurological disease and thoracolumbar or pelvic soft tissue injuries visible neither on pool nor bone phase scintigraphic images should be considered. Keep in mind that horses with forelimb or hindlimb lameness could potentially have a distant source of pain, and comprehensive imaging (whole body bone scan, for instance) may be necessary.

NECK LESIONS AND FORELIMB LAMENESS

Forelimb lameness that is unassociated with primary limb pain has been recognized in association with bony lesions of the midcervical and caudal cervical vertebrae and the cranial thoracic vertebrae (see Chapters 52 and 53).[2,3] There are not necessarily any detectable clinical signs that can be related to the neck. In horses with confusing forelimb lameness, evaluation of the neck with radiography, scintigraphy, or both modalities is certainly indicated.

REFERRED PAIN

The concept of referred pain is well recognized in people but is more difficult in the horse. We must accept that referred pain originating from a lesion far removed from the lame limb may contribute to pain and thus cause lameness.

PREVIOUSLY UNRECOGNIZED CAUSES OF LAMENESS PROXIMAL TO THE CARPUS AND TARSUS

I think it is naive to consider that all potential causes of lameness proximal to the tarsus and carpus have been recognized. Injuries that primarily involve bone usually can be identified with nuclear scintigraphic examination. However, scintigraphy is rather insensitive in the identification of soft tissue injuries, although it may help identify some muscle injuries (Figure 12-8). Muscles can be examined ultrasonographically, but we need to know where to look for damage. Acupuncture trigger point sensitivity may provide information. Use of muscle stimulators may help to identify superficial muscles that are damaged. We know that the horse can tear the fibularis tertius, resulting in pathognomonic clinical signs. We do not know if minor injuries to this modified muscle could cause lameness. Tendonous and ligamentous pain without palpable abnormalities and therefore without a specific indication for ultrasonographic examination must always be considered. We must remain open-minded and search for other means of diagnosis.

MISINTERPRETED IMAGING FINDINGS THAT RESULT IN MISDIAGNOSIS

In horses in which the results of local analgesic techniques are equivocal or negative, it may be tempting to rely on the results of other diagnostic techniques, such as radiography, ultrasonography, and nuclear scintigraphy, without necessarily relating them to the initial clinical signs. Although these imaging modalities may help to confirm a

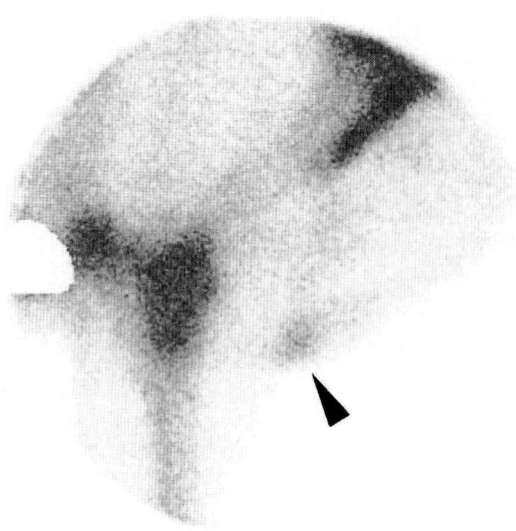

Fig. 12-8 • Lateral scintigraphic image of the right elbow region of a 4-year-old Warmblood stallion with right forelimb lameness evident only at the walk, which was unaltered by any local analgesic technique. Radiopharmaceutical uptake was increased in the biceps brachii muscle *(arrow)*, which corresponded to an area of increased echogenicity compatible with fibrosis.

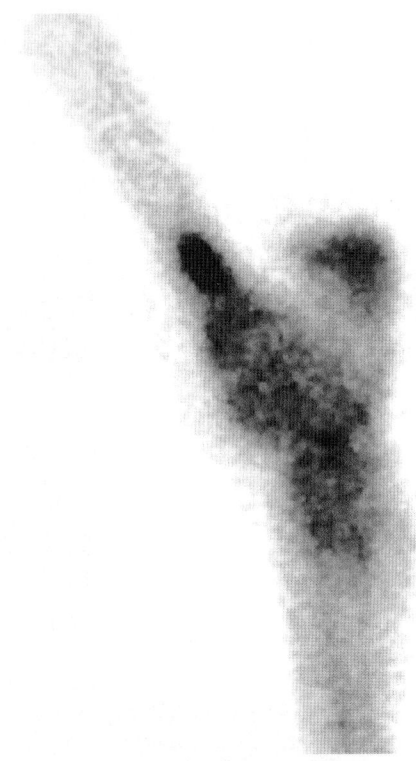

Fig. 12-10 • Lateral scintigraphic image of the tarsus and tibia of a 12-year-old advanced event horse with bilateral forelimb lameness associated with distal interphalangeal joint synovitis. The horse had no history or evidence of hindlimb lameness and competed successfully thereafter. Note the intense increased radiopharmaceutical uptake in the tibia. The horse was reexamined approximately 8 months later with similar results. The horse had been competing successfully but had recurrent forelimb lameness.

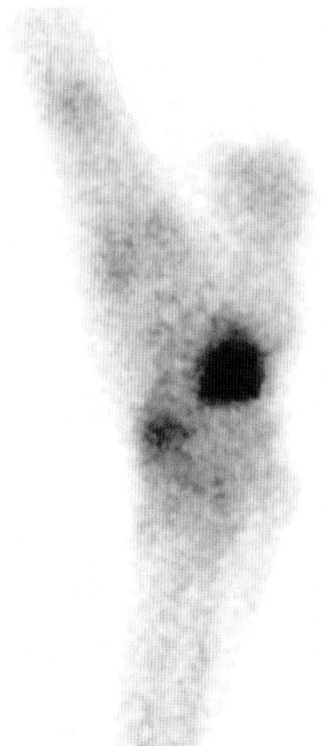

Fig. 12-9 • Lateral scintigraphic image of the tarsus of a 7-year-old riding horse. Note the marked focal increased radiopharmaceutical uptake in the hock. Lameness was completely alleviated by desensitization of the fetlock region. There was no radiological abnormality of the hock.

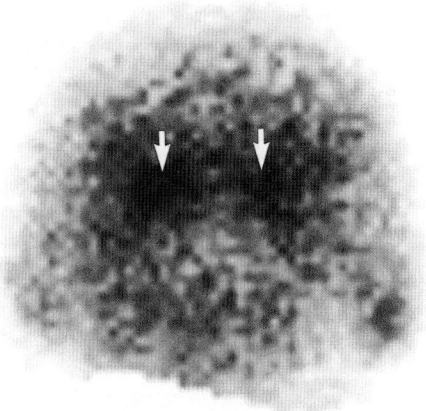

Fig. 12-11 • Solar scintigraphic image of the right front foot of a 6-year-old Warmblood. There is increased radiopharmaceutical uptake in the region of insertion of the deep digital flexor tendon on the distal phalanx. The gait characteristics were typical of proximal limb lameness, and lameness was unaltered by desensitization of the foot. The horse had a fracture of the deltoid tuberosity of the humerus.

clinical diagnosis, they also have the potential to mislead, especially if interpreted in isolation.

The horse illustrated in Figure 12-9, with focal IRU in the hock, was admitted with left hindlimb lameness that was alleviated by desensitization of the fetlock region. The horse illustrated in Figure 12-10, which has IRU in the distal tibia, was admitted with forelimb lameness. No hindlimb lameness was observed at any time, even after alleviation of the forelimb lameness. The horse in Figure 12-11, with IRU in the region of insertion of the deep

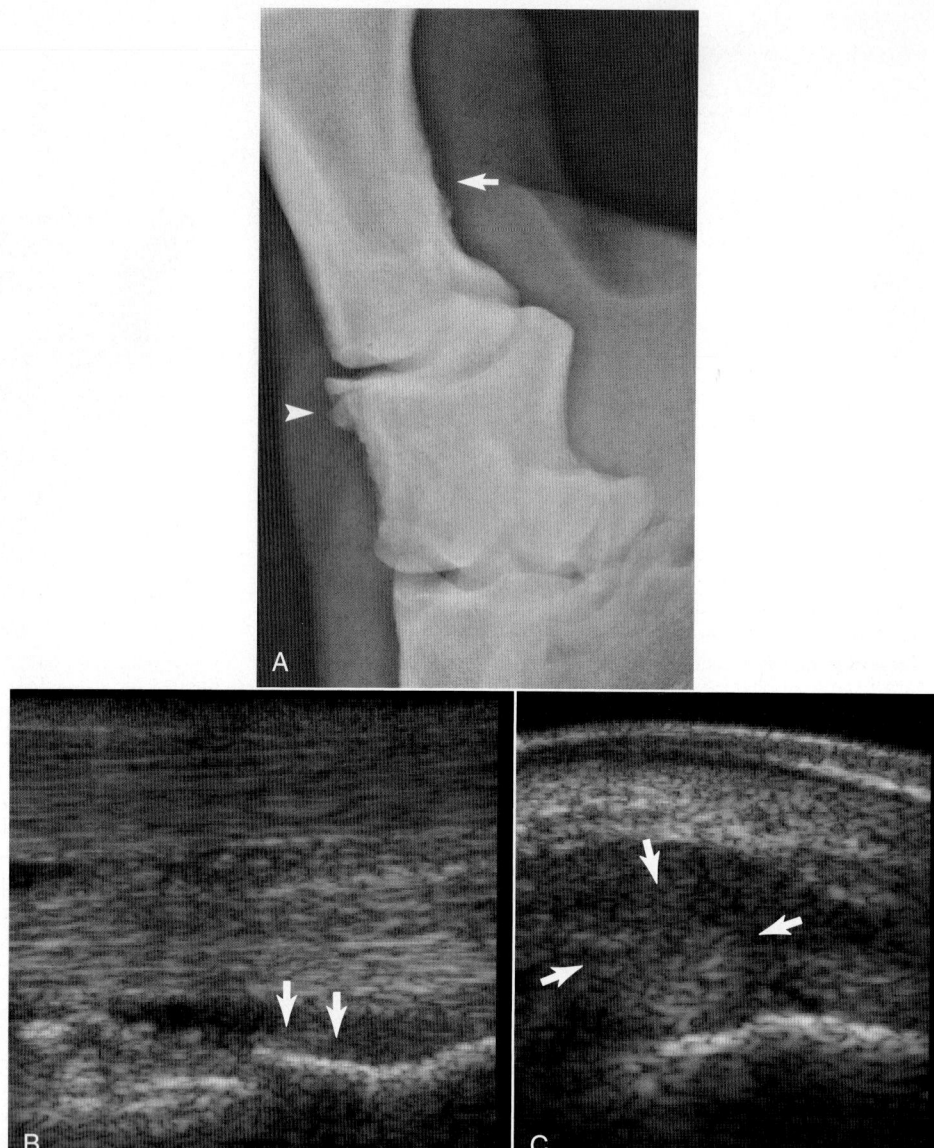

Fig. 12-12 • A, Flexed dorsolateral-palmaromedial oblique radiographic image of the right front proximal interphalangeal (PIP) joint of a 14-year-old advanced event horse with acute onset lameness, which was worst on the left rein on hard or soft surfaces. Lameness was improved by palmar digital analgesia and abolished by palmar (abaxial sesamoid) nerve blocks. There was no response to intraarticular analgesia of the PIP or distal interphalangeal (DIP) joints. There is extensive periarticular modeling of the dorsoproximal aspect of the middle phalanx *(arrowhead),* effectively increasing the effective PIP joint surface area. There is also mild enthesophyte formation at the insertion of the oblique sesamoidean ligaments on the proximal phalanx *(arrow).* **B,** Longitudinal ultrasonographic image of the pastern of the same horse as **A.** Proximal is to the left. There is enthesophyte formation at the insertion of the oblique sesamoidean ligaments *(arrow),* which appeared structurally normal. This is another coincidental finding but is an observation commonly made in conjunction with dorsal extension of the PIP joint. **C,** Transverse ultrasonographic image of the medial aspect of the coronary band of the same horse as **A** and **B.** There was subtle soft tissue swelling palpable dorsomedially. The medial collateral ligament of the DIP joint is diffusely mildly hypoechogenic, especially dorsally, but is not enlarged, and there is considerable periligamentous hypoechogenic fluid. The skin surface is abnormally convex. Diagnosis: acute desmitis of the medial collateral ligament of the DIP joint.

digital flexor tendon, had lameness associated with a fracture of the deltoid tuberosity of the humerus.

Not all radiological abnormalities are of clinical significance. Extensive periarticular modeling is sometimes seen on the dorsal aspect of the proximal interphalangeal joint, effectively increasing the joint surface area, probably to increase stability (Figure 12-12). These radiological abnormalities are not necessarily associated with intraarticular

pathology or pain. The horse in Figure 12-12 had lameness improved by palmar digital analgesia and abolished by palmar (abaxial sesamoid) nerve blocks. Lameness was not altered by intraarticular analgesia of the proximal interphalangeal joint. Right forelimb lameness, which was worst on the right rein on a circle, was caused by an acute injury of the medial collateral ligament of the distal interphalangeal joint.

ODD LAMENESS APPARENT ONLY DURING RIDING

Some causes of lameness are apparent only when the horse is ridden. Some of these are easy to block, but a minority fail to respond to local analgesic techniques. Consideration must always be given to rider-induced lameness (see page 157 and Chapter 97), discomfort caused by tack, and gait abnormalities arising through thoracolumbar (see Chapter 52), sacral, and sacroiliac pain (see Chapters 50 and 51). The possibility of the rider's weight compressing muscles in the saddle and caudal neck region and nerve compression should be considered as potential causes of forelimb pain.

Stepping short on one forelimb at the walk, a feature that may be more easy to feel than to see, is a characteristic of pain in the ipsilateral brachiocephalicus muscle. Palpation of the muscle is usually strongly resented. Lameness may be inapparent at the trot. Horses respond well to physiotherapy treatment.

Lesions of the tendon of the biceps brachii within the intertubercular bursa may result in lameness at the walk characterized by a variable degree of shortening of the cranial phase of the stride; however, at the trot lameness may be absent or slight.

Stepping short on one hindlimb at the walk but having no detectable lameness at the trot is a poorly understood syndrome that may be sudden in onset and tends to be persistent, despite prolonged rest, with or without physiotherapy, osteopathy, chiropractic manipulation, or acupuncture treatment. Such horses usually are worst when ridden at the walk but perform well at all other gaits. There is no response to antiinflammatory analgesic drugs or any analgesic technique. Comprehensive radiographic, scintigraphic, and ultrasonographic examinations are unrewarding.

There is a syndrome of forelimb lameness that is apparent only when a horse is ridden (bareback or with a saddle), which at worst often appears as a hopping-type gait, often most severe with the lame limb on the outside of a circle. Affected horses may try to break to canter in preference to trotting. This lameness is not responsive to any analgesic technique, and radiographic, ultrasonographic, and scintigraphic examination of the forelimbs, neck, ribs, sternum, and thoracolumbar region usually results in no detectable abnormality. There is a poor response to prolonged rest, with or without physiotherapy, osteopathy, chiropractic manipulation, or acupuncture treatment. There is no response to nonsteroidal antiinflammatory medication. A potential possible cause may be muscle or nerve injury axial to the scapula.

IDENTIFIABLE LESIONS: WHICH CONTRIBUTE TO THE CURRENT LAMENESS?

The presence of radiological lesions is not necessarily synonymous with pain, or the pain may be low grade and not compromise the horse's gait sufficiently to be recognized by the rider. For example, a horse may have an acute lameness referable to the stifle. Several lesions may be identified radiologically (e.g., smooth flattening of the middle of the lateral trochlear ridge of the femur, modeling of the medial articular margin of the tibial plateau, and a complete fracture of

the proximal aspect of the fibula [see Figure 12-3]). It is likely that acute lameness is related to the fibular fracture. The horse in Figure 12-3 had been coping despite radiological evidence of both osteochondrosis of the femoropatellar joint and osteoarthritis of the medial femorotibial joint.

OTHER CAUSES OF LAMENESS

Lacerations and Occult Spiral Fractures

Acute-onset, moderate-to-severe lameness sometimes develops within 2 to 3 weeks of trauma to, or laceration over, a long bone (see Figures 3-3 and 3-4). Sometimes lameness is first observed when the horse is still restricted to box rest and controlled exercise while the wound heals. There may or may not be any detectable focus of pain. Consideration must always be given to the possibility of an occult spiral fracture of, for instance, the radius that was obviously sustained at the time of the initial injury. Occult spiral fractures are most common in the radius but can involve the third metacarpal or metatarsal bones and tibia. Radiographic examination should be performed to eliminate this possibility.

Rib Lesions

A fracture of one or more cranial ribs is a rather unusual cause of forelimb lameness that usually is a sequel to direct trauma, such as a collision with another horse or a gate post, or a fall. There are usually no localizing clinical signs, although secondary neurogenic muscle atrophy may develop within the next 10 to 14 days. The lameness may suggest an upper limb problem. Diagnosis is dependent on radiographic, ultrasonographic, or scintigraphic identification of the fracture.

Sternal Injury

Sternal injury usually causes a change in behavior, such as a tendency to buck when first tacked up and mounted (i.e., extreme cold back behavior) rather than lameness. Frequently it is not possible to elicit pain by deep palpation.

Fracture of the Summits of the Dorsal Spinous Processes in the Withers Region

Acute fractures of the withers usually result in a very shortened forelimb stride and a tendency to move very closely in front ("the miniskirt walk"). There is usually obvious palpable deformity of the withers region. Diagnosis is confirmed radiologically.

Temporomandibular Joint Pain

Pain associated with one or both temporomandibular joints may cause reluctance for the horse to take the bit properly, crookedness in the head and neck carriage, and secondary gait irregularities. The joints can be assessed by applying firm pressure over each joint, which may cause pain, and by opening the mouth and moving the upper and lower jaws relative to one another and assessing mobility. Thermography may be a sensitive indicator of local inflammation. If temporomandibular pain is suspected, further investigation can be performed using nuclear scintigraphic examination and diagnostic ultrasonography.[4] Radiography is relatively insensitive unless major bony changes are present.[5] The use of a rostral 35-degree lateral 40-degree ventral-caudodorsal oblique view is recommended.[6]

Neurological Problems and Lameness or Stiffness

Early compressive lesions of the cervical spinal cord can cause an apparent low-grade hindlimb lameness that is characterized by slight toe drag and asymmetrical movement of the hindquarters. Signs of weakness or ataxia may not be evident unless a comprehensive neurological examination is performed, especially if the horse is quite fit and fresh. Neurological signs may be seen only when the horse is tired and not compensating for its gait deficits.

Equine protozoal myelitis can cause rather bizarre forelimb or hindlimb gait abnormalities, either unilaterally or bilaterally. It should be considered in the differential diagnosis of odd gait abnormalities in horses that reside or have spent time in North America (see Chapter 11).

Damage to the branch of the radial nerve that results in an innervation of the extensor muscles of the carpus and digits may cause a subtle gait abnormality that is characterized by a tendency to stumble and is associated with slight knuckling of the carpus and distal limb joints.

Stiff horse syndrome[7-9] and equine motor neuron disease[10] are unusual neurological conditions in which the horse moves better in the trot and canter than at a walk and may stand abnormally.

Shivering behavior often is seen in one or both hindlimbs in association with hindlimb lameness. The two conditions generally are unrelated. Shivering behavior may be more apparent when the horse is stressed. The behavior can make it difficult to assess whether any manipulation of the limb causes pain, or whether the horse is uncomfortable with one hindlimb picked up.

Stringhalt, or exaggerated flexion of a limb, usually a hindlimb, results in a gait abnormality most obvious at the slower speeds of walk and trot. It is not usually directly associated with any other form of lameness. It may be sudden or insidious in onset.

Congenital abnormalities of the first ribs in association with abnormalities of the adjacent brachial plexus have been seen as a cause of persistent forelimb lameness (Figure 12-13).

Acute-onset, severe, and persistent forelimb lameness has been seen in association with a mediastinal abscess that encroached on the nerve roots of the seventh cervical and first thoracic vertebrae, the stellate ganglion, and the first rib (Figure 12-14). Measurement of fibrinogen may help to identify the presence of an infective or inflammatory process.

Lyme Disease

Lyme disease has frequently been incriminated as a cause of shifting lameness that involves several limbs, but confirmed cases are extremely rare.[11] Many horses that are in areas where there are many ticks have relatively high antibody titers to *Borrelia burgdorferi*,[11,12] but this is not diagnostic of clinical disease. Lyme disease may be suspected in adult horses in endemic areas when unusual synovitis develops in absence of any known injection history or presence of a wound (see Chapter 66).

Immune-Mediated Polysynovitis

Immune-mediated polysynovitis is relatively uncommon but may result in generalized stiffness associated with transient synovial distention of several joint capsules. It is frequently not possible to identify the underlying cause,

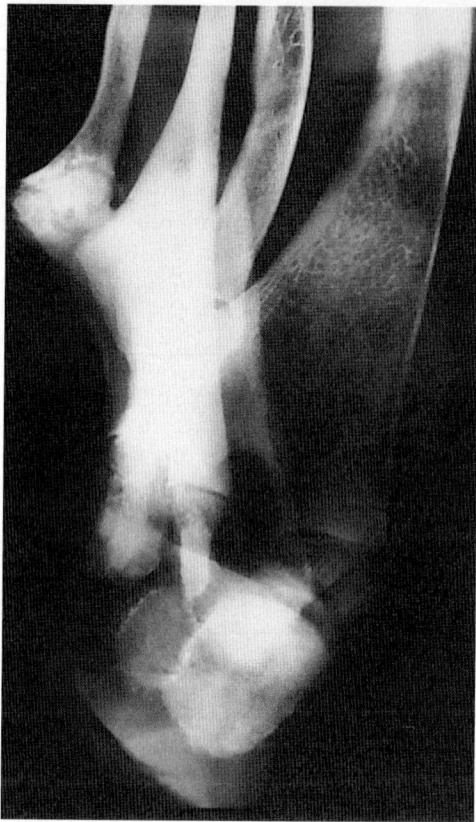

Fig. 12-13 • Postmortem specimen showing an anomalous first rib from a 3-year-old Thoroughbred with right forelimb lameness that was not altered by any local analgesic technique. There was an abnormal web of fibrous tissue that extended from this anomalous rib to incorporate part of the brachial plexus on the right side.

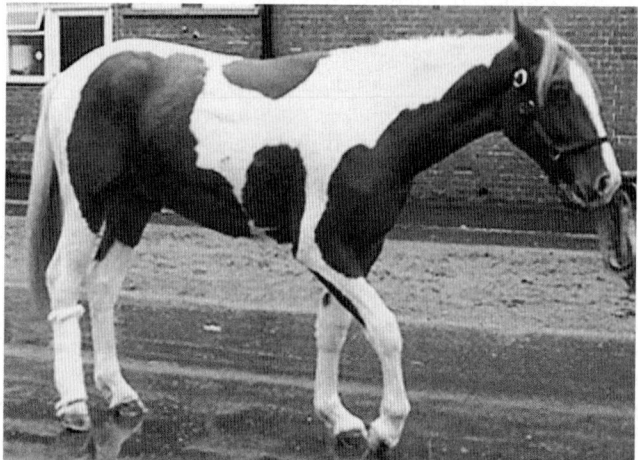

Fig. 12-14 • A 7-year-old pony with severe right forelimb lameness that progressively deteriorated. The pony had an increased fibrinogen level and intermittent pyrexia. There was a mediastinal abscess that encroached on the roots of the seventh cervical and first thoracic nerves, the stellate ganglion, and the first rib.

but this condition usually responds to corticosteroid medication (see Chapter 66).

Tack-Induced Pain

An ill-fitting saddle can induce back pain and restricted action or poor performance. The bit can induce pain through poor fit (too narrow or too wide), being too low in the horse's mouth, banging on the canine teeth, pinching the corners of the horse's mouth, or being too severe. Any oral pain related to the bit, sharp teeth, or lacerations of the tongue, cheeks, or corners of the horse's mouth may cause reluctance to accept the bit properly and gait irregularities.

Rider-Induced Problems

The rider has a potentially huge influence on the gait of the horse. If a horse is not going forward properly, either because the rider is restricting it or because the rider is not asking it to go forward properly, the forelimb and hindlimb gaits may appear irregular, mimicking pain-induced lameness. An overweight rider who is too heavy for the horse may induce hindlimb lameness. A rider who constantly sits crookedly may induce back pain and hindlimb lameness. (Rider-related problems are discussed further in Chapter 97.)

Physical Limitations of the Horse, Temperament, and Confidence

With appropriate handling and training, most horses are cooperative. However, a previously compliant horse can very rapidly change if regularly handled and ridden by someone who lacks confidence, technique, or strength. Such a horse can quickly develop evasions, such as not going forward properly, rearing, bucking, or taking off. These problems may be, but are not necessarily, pain-related. A horse that has never been trained properly may be very difficult and even potentially dangerous to the rider. Horses home-bred by amateur enthusiasts are high-risk candidates. Some horses are innately lazy and unwilling to go forward. Others are very exuberant and excessively forward going and "fizzy." The veterinarian may be asked to investigate any of these behavioral features as a potentially pain-related problem.

It is important to establish a horse's previous performance. It may be useful to see a video. Determine if there has been a change in rider or management. Establish what the horse is being fed and how much work it is getting: there is a tendency for people to overfeed and underwork horses. A comprehensive clinical evaluation may need to be repeated on several occasions before you can determine if it is a pain-related problem. Nuclear scintigraphic examination of selected areas may be useful to eliminate the presence of any underlying problems and to convince the owner that there is not a physical problem. A change of rider or work pattern may be necessary. The use of high doses of nonsteroidal, antiinflammatory drugs (e.g., 2 to 3 g of phenylbutazone, twice daily for at least 7 to 10 days) can be helpful to determine if the problem is pain related, but be aware that there may be a placebo effect. Not all pain responds to phenylbutazone, so a negative response does not preclude a pain-induced problem (see Chapter 97).

Reproductive Problems*

Some mares become more difficult to handle and ride when in season. Mares with coliclike discomfort, hindlimb lameness, or back pain when the rider is in the saddle may have painful ovaries, especially in the periovulatory period.[13,14] Indeed, pressure applied to the ovaries per rectum can elicit a pain response.[15] Palpation of a large ovulatory follicle or a follicle that has recently ovulated, other genital tract characteristics of estrus, and concomitant behavioral signs of estrus may support this diagnosis. The discomfort should subside shortly after ovulation, but it may recur with future cycles.[14]

Periovulatory discomfort is thought to be caused by a combination of extremely enlarged follicles that affect neighboring tissues and the release of follicular fluid during ovulation, some of which may leak into the peritoneal cavity and cause localized inflammation. These factors may result in localized pain that lasts approximately 24 to 48 hours.

The estrous cycle is also characterized by changes in the hormonal profile. Specific balances between gonadotropins and sex steroids are necessary for smooth transitions between phases of the reproductive cycle. It has been proposed that any alteration in the ratios between luteinizing hormone and follicle-stimulating hormone; androgens, estrogens, and progestins; or both results in erratic behavior that leads to poor performance. The judicious use of a synthetic progestagen such as altrenogest (Regumate, Intervet, Millsboro, Delaware) to stop the mare's cycling can sometimes be helpful. Ovariectomy is a treatment of last resort and does not reliably influence performance-related problems. Keep in mind that the mare's behavior when out of season will be the end result if ovariectomy is performed. Some Thoroughbred fillies appear to be predisposed to exertional rhabdomyolysis and have been successfully treated with anabolic steroids such as testosterone and boldenon undecylenate (Equipoise).

Although some stallions can be used successfully for both competition and breeding, especially if the management is good and a very clear distinction is made with handling routines, others cannot focus adequately and thus perform athletically below expectations. Performance may be enhanced by castration. However, although malorientation of testicles is frequently blamed for lameness or poor performance, in the Editors' experience this is highly unusual.

A scirrhous cord in a gelding or mastitis in a mare can cause loss of hindlimb action and hindlimb stiffness. Chronic episodic, transient hindlimb lameness associated with strenuous work (jumping) has been seen in a stallion with large internal inguinal rings.[16] The lameness resolved after herniorrhaphy.

Other Medical Problems

Muscle tumors are a rare cause of lameness, but usually there is localized soft tissue swelling, which should prompt ultrasonographic evaluation and muscle biopsy. Gastric ulceration is usually not a cause of overt lameness but may compromise performance, such as causing difficulties in jumping large spread fences.

Atypical Equine Rhabdomyolysis

Occasionally, equine rhabdomyolysis occurs without any of the typical signs of tying up, generally in event horses

*The Editors acknowledge the contribution of J. Jorgensen and R. Mansmann, who contributed a chapter entitled "Estrous Cycle and Performance in Athletic Mares" to the first edition of *Diagnosis and Management of Lameness in the Horse.*

or endurance horses. Most commonly this is recognized during competition, but it can occur at other times. A horse may pull up with an unexplained unilateral or bilateral hindlimb lameness, which may be mild to severe. The horse does not show any distress, and there are no localizing clinical signs. This may resolve, only to recur in association with exercise. Measurement of serum muscle enzymes will reveal elevated creatine kinase and aspartate transaminase concentrations. The relative degree of rise in concentration of the two enzymes will depend on whether this is a single episode or if recurrent, how frequently the horse is experiencing abnormal muscle stress, and the recent work history. Alternatively, a horse may be performing suboptimally, with reduced quality of paces and reduced scope when jumping, sometimes becoming more restricted during a work period. Affected horses may have focal or diffuse, linear regions of IRU in affected muscle groups in bone phase scintigraphic images, sometimes varying in intensity in different muscle groups. Aspartate transaminase concentration will be elevated.

Vascular Lesions

Venous obstruction in the axilla has caused episodic lameness associated with extensive soft tissue swelling in the antebrachium. Diagnosis was confirmed by a vascular scin-

tigraphic study. Brachial thrombosis has also been associated with severe forelimb lameness.[17]

Bone Fragility Disorder

A bone fragility disorder of unknown cause has been described in a small number of horses in the western United States.[18] It is characterized by an acute or chronic multilimb lameness, with no localizing clinical signs in some horses. In a small proportion there is bowing of the scapulae, lordosis, or cervical stiffness. The source of pain cannot be identified using diagnostic analgesia. Numerous sites of IRU are identified in the axial skeleton and proximal aspects of the forelimbs and hindlimbs. The condition may be progressive.

Panosteitis-like Lesions

Panosteitis is a well-recognized condition in dogs but has not been documented in the horse. However, I am aware of three horses that have had clinical and radiological signs consistent with this condition. In the dog the cause is unknown, but the relatively high frequency of occurrence in young German shepherd dogs suggests some heritable predisposition. It results in a lameness that waxes and wanes in severity, with episodic severe non–weight-bearing lameness. In the horse this condition has been recognized in mature sport horses and has been characterized by a lameness varying in severity from mild to non–weight

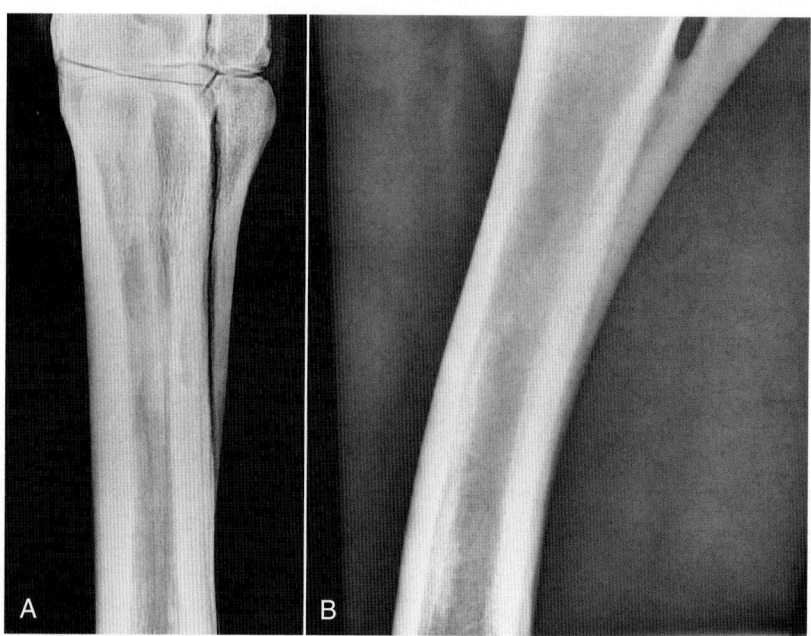

Fig. 12-15 • A, Dorsomedial-palmarolateral oblique radiographic image of the metacarpal region of the left fore-limb of a 9-year-old advanced event horse with left forelimb lameness that varied in severity from mild to severe. Perineural analgesia of the palmar and palmar metacarpal nerves in the proximal metacarpal region, performed when lameness was relatively mild, resulted in improvement and the development of right forelimb lameness. There are patchy increases in radiopacity in the medulla of the third metacarpal bone, thickening of trabecula, and endosteal new bone consistent with a panosteitis-like condition. Lesions were associated with multifocal regions of intense increased radiopharmaceutical uptake (IRU). **B,** Lateromedial radiographic image of the left radius of an 8-year-old Thoroughbred event horse with sporadic severe lameness that was unresponsive to local analgesic techniques. Cranial is to the left. Extensive endosteal new bone is present, especially cranially, along with patchy increased opacity in the medulla, consistent with a panosteitis-like condition. Lesions were also present in the right forelimb and were associated with multifocal regions of intense IRU.

bearing, with no localizing clinical signs. The response to perineural analgesia has varied depending on the site of the lesions, which may be multifocal. All three horses had a unilateral or bilateral forelimb lameness, two with the most severe lesions in the radius and one with the most severe lesion in the third metacarpal bone. The lesions are typified radiologically by a patchy increase in medullary

opacity, especially near the nutrient foramen, coarse trabeculation, and endosteal thickening (Figure 12-15). The lesions are associated with moderate to intense IRU. Lesions may be identified in more than one limb, although not all appear to be symptomatic. In the dog the condition is managed by systemic administration of nonsteroidal anti-inflammatory drugs and is usually self-limiting.

Chapter 13

Assessment of Acute-Onset, Severe Lameness

Sue J. Dyson

FIELD DIAGNOSIS OF THE INJURED HORSE

The assessment of an acutely lame horse presents a challenge in diagnosis and in dealing with the people associated with the horse, particularly if lameness occurs at a competition. The horse may have fallen and been lame immediately or may have pulled up lame, and the veterinary surgeon may be called to examine the horse on course in full view of the public.

Ideally the horse should be transported to an examination area for comprehensive evaluation, but the veterinary surgeon must establish whether the injured limb requires support before the horse is moved. Although the horse may be very lame, establishing a definitive diagnosis for the cause of the lameness at this stage may be difficult.

This may surprise riders, trainers, and owners, and maintaining their confidence in what is an emotionally charged situation can be quite difficult. If a fracture is suspected, pressure to destroy the horse humanely without delay may be felt. Although some fractures are catastrophic and merit immediate destruction of the horse on humane grounds (e.g., a spiral fracture of the humerus), other serious fractures can be repaired. Therefore as much information as possible about the site of the fracture and its configuration should be obtained before a decision is made. The limb should be supported appropriately before the horse is moved for radiographic examination. If a horse must be destroyed on humane grounds at a competition, this should be done off the course.

Although a diagnosis may be obvious in some horses immediately after the onset of lameness, the veterinarian must recognize that severe lameness may occur without an evident cause. Serial reexaminations over the following hours or days may be required before a diagnosis can be reached. Sometimes the lameness resolves spontaneously within 12 to 18 hours and its cause is never established.

The clinician must be aware of the most common causes of acute-onset, severe lameness, which include the following:
- Subsolar abscess
- Fracture
- Laminitis
- Intrasynovial sepsis
- Periarticular cellulitis

When lameness occurs during training or competition, a spectrum of other injuries must be considered. However, a history of acute-onset, severe lameness during exercise must not mislead the clinician into thinking that lameness must be caused by internal or external trauma associated with exercise. Lameness may still be caused by pain from a subsolar abscess.

This chapter describes a systematic approach to management of a horse with sudden-onset, severe lameness and focuses particularly on injuries that occur during work.

ASSESSMENT
Medical History
While performing an initial visual appraisal of the horse, establishing a history is useful. The examiner must determine the following:
- Any previous lameness, tendon or ligament injury, or history of tying up.
- Date of last shoeing.
- Circumstances of lameness: whether the horse was performing normally, fell, hit a fixed fence, or collided with a fixed object such as a guide rail or a tree. The horse may have reared in the starting stalls or reared and fallen over backward. Another horse may have kicked it. If the horse fell, could it have fallen into stinging nettles? Stinging nettles may cause both an urticarial reaction and inability to bear weight on the affected limb for several hours.

The clinician should also be aware of common injuries in the discipline in which the horse is competing.

The horse may be distressed because of the severity of pain and excited because of the atmosphere of a competition and thus difficult to restrain and examine adequately. Sedation with romifidine or detomidine, with or without butorphanol, may be necessary to facilitate examination of the horse. A horse with an acute hindlimb muscle tear or hemorrhage may show evidence of pain mimicking signs of colic.

The horse's posture should be observed while it stands still and walks a few steps. If the horse bears weight only on the toe, it may be inapparent that the horse has lost some support of the fetlock because of rupture of the superficial digital flexor tendon (SDFT) in the metacarpal region or at the musculotendonous junction in the antebrachium, unless it walks a few steps.

Limb Examination

The veterinarian should establish whether the horse is able and willing to bear weight on the limb, bearing in mind that after a fall a neurological component may contribute to the lameness, in addition to the pain. The horse's demeanor should be assessed; the degree of pain and distress usually but not invariably reflects the severity of the injury. The horse may be greatly distressed, shifting weight constantly between limbs, and may be reluctant to move. Reluctance to move may be caused by a bilateral problem (e.g., bilateral severe superficial digital flexor [SDF] tendonitis) or a more generalized problem such as equine rhabdomyolysis (tying up).

The horse should be carefully appraised visually to identify areas of swelling or a laceration. If the horse's limbs are covered in mud or grease (commonly applied to the limbs during the speed and endurance phase of a Three Day Event), this should be washed off before one proceeds with the evaluation. Boots, bandages, and the saddle and martingale should also be removed. Temporary studs in the shoes should be removed because they may be more difficult to remove later if the injury is severe.

The horse may be obviously lame on a hindlimb or forelimb, but this may mask a similar, less severe injury in a contralateral limb or a different injury; therefore all limbs should be assessed carefully. For example, a racehorse may develop a lateral condylar fracture of the third metacarpal bone in one limb and SDF tendonitis in the contralateral limb. Although the former injury results in a more severe lameness, the latter may be more important to the horse's long-term prognosis.

Occasionally, forelimb and hindlimb lameness are concurrent. Each limb should be palpated systemically with the horse bearing weight and not bearing weight. The examiner should pay careful attention to heat, swelling, abnormal muscle texture, pain on firm pressure, pain induced by manipulation of a joint, restriction of flexibility of a joint, an abnormal range of motion of the joint, audible or palpable crepitus, and the intensity of the digital pulse amplitudes.

The position of the shoe should be assessed carefully. A shoe that has moved slightly may result in nail bind. Hoof testers should be systemically applied across the wall and sole, gently at first and then firmly. Percussion should also be applied to the sole of the foot with the limb picked up and to the wall with the limb bearing weight. The clinician should not forget that if the sole is very hard, eliciting pain with hoof testers may not be possible, despite the presence of a subsolar abscess.

The limbs should be carefully assessed for lacerations. Serious damage to underlying structures may have occurred if the laceration was sustained while the horse was moving at speed, and the position of the laceration and the site of damage to underlying structures may not coincide.

Shoulder and Chest

Injuries to the shoulder region usually result from a fall or collision, which may result in severe bruising only or a fracture. A fracture of the supraglenoid tubercle of the scapula

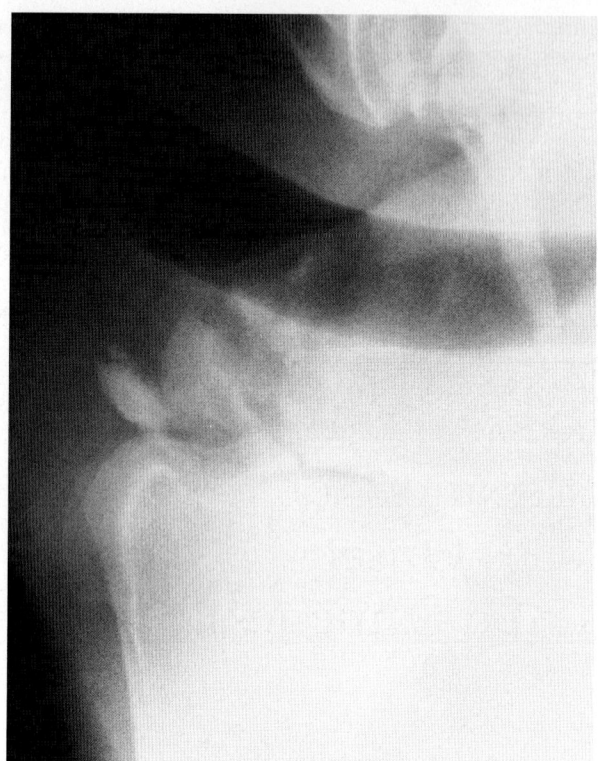

Fig. 13-1 • Mediolateral radiographic image of the left shoulder of an advanced event horse that had fallen during competition 3 days previously and developed severe left forelimb lameness from a displaced comminuted fracture of the supraglenoid tubercle of the scapula.

results in severe lameness (Figure 13-1). Slight soft tissue swelling may develop, usually without audible or palpable crepitus, and pain on palpation may be difficult to differentiate from that caused by severe bruising alone. Articular fractures of the scapula may be associated with audible crepitus on manipulation of the limb. Fractures of the body of the scapula or the humerus are usually associated with severe lameness, soft tissue swelling, and pain in that area.

After collision with a fixed object, or occasionally a fall, the scapulohumeral joint may become luxated or subluxated, with or without a fracture of the glenoid cavity of the scapula. The horse bears weight on the limb reluctantly, soft tissue swelling develops rapidly, and the distal aspect of the scapular spine may become more difficult to palpate. The limb may appear straighter than usual. A collision also may result in collateral instability of the shoulder, so-called *shoulder slip*, usually caused by trauma to nerves of the brachial plexus. The horse may have pain-related lameness because of bruising, together with mechanical lameness caused by neurological dysfunction (Figure 13-2).

Although major fractures of the scapula and humerus are usually readily evident by clinical signs, most other shoulder injuries require radiographic and sometimes ultrasonographic examination for a diagnosis to be reached.

Pectoral muscle tears may result in similar clinical signs, with severe lameness and distress. Repeated clinical examinations may reveal the site of muscle rupture, with increasing evidence of hemorrhage, inflammatory effusion, and edema.

Rib fractures can also result from direct trauma or from falls and occur most commonly in steeplechasers and polo

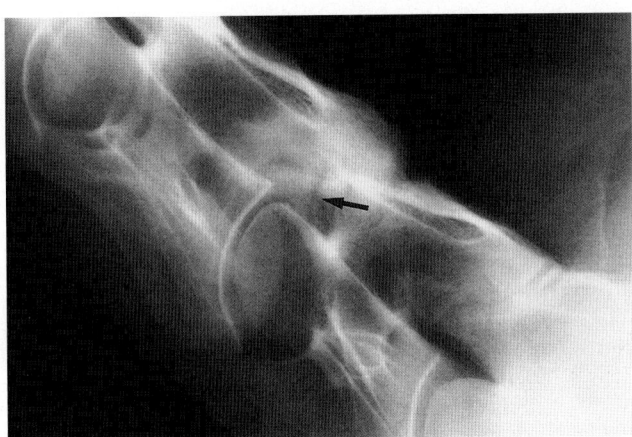

Fig. 13-2 • Lateral radiographic image of the midcervical region of a 6-year-old event horse that fell on a cross-country course. The horse was not bearing weight on the left forelimb and showed moderate hindlimb ataxia. The synovial facet joints were fractured between the sixth and seventh cervical vertebrae *(arrow)*. A cause of the forelimb lameness was not identified, and the lameness resolved within 24 hours. The horse had a complete functional recovery but had some residual neck stiffness.

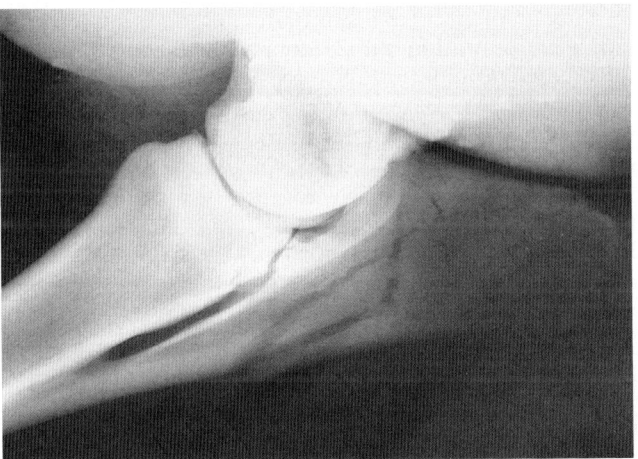

Fig. 13-3 • Mediolateral radiographic image of left elbow of an event horse that was very lame after a fall and stood with the elbow dropped. The olecranon of the ulna sustained a displaced, comminuted fracture.

ponies. Fractures in the region of the scapula and triceps result in acute, severe forelimb lameness. More caudal fractures may result in extreme stiffness and may cause severe respiratory embarrassment.

Lameness associated with the upper forelimb may also be caused by strain of the biceps brachii or brachiocephalicus muscles or hematoma formation. Careful, deep palpation of these muscles is required to identify focal pain and possibly swelling or abnormal muscle texture.

Elbow and Carpus

Acute-onset lameness associated with pain arising from the elbow region is rare, except as the result of a fall or kick. Fracture of the olecranon process of the ulna is the most common injury (Figure 13-3). If the fracture is nondisplaced, the horse may stand normally but with severe pain; or if the fracture is complete with loss of triceps function, the horse stands with a dropped elbow.

Acute-onset lameness associated with the carpus occurs most commonly in racehorses, both flat racehorses and steeplechasers, and usually is associated with a chip or slab fracture or less commonly with hemarthrosis. Synovial effusion within the antebrachiocarpal or middle carpal joint usually develops rapidly. The horse may resent maximal flexion of the carpus, and direct palpation of the carpal bones may elicit pain. Fracture of the accessory carpal bone usually results from a fall and occurs most commonly in steeplechasers; such fractures may be associated with effusion within the carpal sheath. Acute tears of the accessory ligament of the SDFT sometimes occur in polo ponies and rarely in trotters, with associated distention of the carpal sheath. Tenosynovitis caused by hemorrhage most often causes acute, severe lameness, but pain can be transient and intermittent.

Forelimb Soft Tissue Injuries

Injuries of the forelimb suspensory ligament (SL) (proximal, midbody, and branch lesions) and of the forelimb SDFT occur most commonly in racehorses and event horses, whereas desmitis of the accessory ligament of the deep digital flexor tendon (ALDDFT) occurs more commonly in show jumpers, older steeplechasers, and polo ponies.

Severe, apparently acute-onset lesions of the SDFT occasionally occur in show jumpers, especially those of international standard. Evaluation of the posture of the limb and the presence of heat, pain, and swelling are important for accurate diagnosis. Clinical signs associated with these injures can vary markedly. Substantial lesions of the SDFT can develop without detectable lameness, whereas a large tear can result in acute, severe, non–weight-bearing lameness. Bilateral tears may result in extreme distress, a reluctance to move, and a laminitic-like stance. In event horses, lameness can develop after the speed and endurance phase of a Three Day Event, associated with SDF tendonitis, but no clinical signs may suggest the injury. Swelling or localized heat and pain may take several days to develop despite improvement or resolution of the lameness. Therefore careful reappraisal of the horse over the next few days is strongly recommended if an event horse develops an acute-onset, forelimb lameness for which no diagnosis can be identified.

Rupture of the SDFT results in hyperextension of the fetlock with normal foot placement. Elevation of the toe with normal angulation of the fetlock indicates disruption of the deep digital flexor tendon (DDFT). Hyperextension of the fetlock and elevation of the toe reflect laceration or rupture of the SDFT and the DDFT. Sinking of the fetlock to the ground indicates disruption of the suspensory apparatus, with or without the flexor tendons.

Severe lameness and distress, with hyperextension of the fetlock, without obvious swelling in the metacarpal region suggest rupture of the SDFT at the musculotendonous junction. This injury occurs most commonly in steeplechasers. Rupture of the SDFT usually is a sequela to a previous injury; therefore the tendon is generally chronically enlarged. Detection of the rupture is easiest at the peracute stage, before exudate and hemorrhage fill the deficit. The site of rupture is usually in the midmetacarpal region.

Desmitis of the ALDDFT usually causes acute-onset, moderate-to-severe lameness with rapid development of soft tissue swelling in the region of the ligament. However, recurrent injuries can develop with no detectable alteration of a chronically enlarged ligament. The degree of lameness associated with a SL injury varies from mild to moderate but may be worse if a concurrent fracture of the second or fourth metacarpal bone or of the apex of a proximal sesamoid bone exists, and these structures should be evaluated carefully. Some severely lame horses with proximal suspensory desmitis have no palpable abnormalities.

Each of the tendons and ligaments in the metacarpal region should be palpated carefully, from proximally to distally, with the limb bearing weight and picked up. The size, shape, and consistency of the tendons and ligaments and any pain on palpation should be carefully assessed. With severe SDF tendonitis, the horse may be distressed, and peritendonous edema rapidly develops, which makes accurate palpation of the tendon difficult. Partial rupture may be associated with a palpable soft defect in the tendon. Bilateral SDF tendonitis sometimes occurs, with the only detectable palpable abnormality being slight enlargement of each tendon and rounding of its margins. The clinician must be aware of this, because these lesions may be missed if one assumes that because the limbs feel symmetrical, the tendons are normal.

A caudal radial osteochondroma or exostosis may cause episodic acute severe lameness associated with dorsal tearing of the DDFT. When lameness is apparent there may be distention of the carpal sheath and/or pain on passive flexion of the carpus. Lameness and other associated clinical signs may resolve rapidly.

Fractures of the Distal Aspect of the Limbs

A fracture of the lateral, or more rarely the medial, condyle of the third metacarpal or metatarsal bone results in acute-onset, severe lameness. If the fracture is incomplete and nondisplaced, no palpable abnormality may be detectable, although some effusion in the metacarpophalangeal joint usually develops within 12 to 24 hours. The horse may resent fetlock flexion; however, some horses become so distressed that in the acute phase, determining whether pressure or joint manipulation causes pain is impossible. The same can apply for a fracture of the proximal phalanx.

Subluxation of the metacarpophalangeal joint occasionally occurs, with disruption of a collateral ligament, with or without an associated fracture. The horse may be very lame, but during normal load bearing the joint may appear to be aligned normally. Instability of the joint may be detectable only with the joint stressed with the limb not bearing weight.

Feet

Trauma to the palmar aspect of the pastern may result in an innocuous skin wound but severe damage to the underlying soft tissue structures. The branches of the SDFT, the DDFT, and the digital flexor tendon sheath are particularly vulnerable. Posture of the limb should be carefully assessed to determine which structure or structures may be involved.

An overreach injury on the bulb of the heel can result in severe, deep-seated bruising and lameness, especially on hard ground. Injuries of the foot are common, especially in event horses. The differential diagnosis should include subsolar hemorrhage (especially corns), nail bind, a subsolar abscess, and a fracture of the distal phalanx.

If the horse shows any reaction to percussion of the foot or pressure applied with hoof testers, the shoe should be removed for further exploration of the foot. If the horse is very lame, removal of each nail individually using nail pullers may be preferable to levering off the shoe. The absence of reaction to hoof testers and normal digital pulse amplitudes does not preclude the existence of either laminitis or a subsolar abscess.

Hindlimb Injuries

When one examines a horse with acute hindlimb lameness that developed during exercise, consideration should always be given to tying up, even if the hindlimb musculature feels soft, local pain cannot be elicited, and the horse is not unduly distressed. The clinical manifestations of tying up vary considerably from acute, severe bilateral or unilateral hindlimb lameness with obvious firmness of the muscles of the hindquarter, with or without swelling, to a moderate unilateral hindlimb lameness that developed after the horse was not moving as freely as normal, with no detectable palpable abnormality. This lameness may persist for several hours but usually resolves within 12 to 18 hours. Occasionally, tying up can affect forelimbs, alone or together with the hindlimbs.

Measurement of substantially raised serum creatine kinase concentration 3 to 24 hours after the onset of lameness may be the only way to reach a definitive diagnosis. Alternatively, a horse may not be moving as freely as normal during a competition and subsequently may be withdrawn; further clinical signs may not develop.

Major hindlimb muscle rupture of quadriceps, semimembranosus, gastrocnemius, adductor, gracilis, or abdominal muscles results in severe lameness and distress, but diagnosis may be difficult. Careful palpation may reveal a site of rupture. Detection of acute muscle strains may be possible when superficial muscles are involved. Pain on palpation and sometimes swelling may be present; however, this is not always the case, and evaluation of deep muscles is limited. Swelling may become more apparent over the next several days.

Stifle trauma is common in horses that jump fixed fences at speed, even if the rider cannot recollect the horse hitting a fence. Lameness caused by a fracture may be sudden and severe in onset, and the horse may pull up, but in some horses it does not become apparent until the horse has finished.

Because the cranial aspect of the stifle is relatively poorly covered with soft tissues, the bones are particularly susceptible to bruising or fracture (Figure 13-4). The degree of pain on palpation does not necessarily reflect accurately the severity of the injury. Development of femoropatellar or femorotibial effusion or marked periarticular soft tissue swelling suggests a fracture. Sometimes a displaced fragment of bone can be palpated. The superficial location of the femoropatellar joint capsule also makes it vulnerable to puncture and the introduction of infection, and effusion and severe lameness may develop rapidly.

Most horses with stifle injuries require radiographic examination to establish or confirm the presence of a fracture. Although lameness associated with bruising may initially be severe, the horse generally rapidly improves within 24 to 48 hours, whereas with most fractures the lameness usually persists unchanged. The horse may be reluctant to

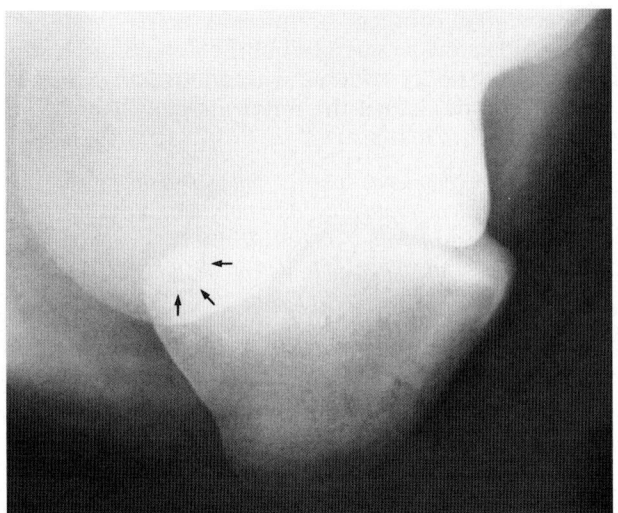

Fig. 13-4 • Cranioproximal-craniodistal oblique radiographic image of right stifle of an event horse that hit the penultimate fence at the World Equestrian Games. The horse completed the course, pulled up slightly lame, and was very lame within a few hours. The arrows show an articular fracture of the medial pole of the patella.

extend the stifle and tends to stand with the limb semi-flexed and the weight on the toe, a posture also typical of severe foot pain. Occasionally, severe ligamentous injury that cannot be detected radiologically occurs in the stifle.

Periarticular hemorrhage around the patellar ligaments can result in acute pain and lameness characterized by a shortened cranial phase of the stride at the walk, but less severe lameness at the trot. Swelling may be subtle, resulting in loss of definition of the patellar ligaments; diagnosis is dependent on ultrasonographic examination.

Rupture of the fibularis tertius usually results from a traumatic episode, with the limb getting trapped in an extended position, and results in a severe lameness with the horse unwilling to load the limb fully. Passive extension of the hock is pathognomonic.

Acute injuries to the hock are uncommon, unless the horse has a severe fall resulting in damage to the hock joint capsules and the collateral ligaments or a lateral malleolar fracture of the distal aspect of the tibia. The horse usually is severely lame and rapidly develops distention of the tarsocrural joint capsule and periarticular soft tissue swelling. Radiographic examination is indicated to determine the extent of the damage. Less commonly, slab fractures of the central or third tarsal bone or incomplete sagittal fractures of the talus cause acute, severe lameness, often with no localizing clinical signs. Kick injuries may result in a fracture. Whereas intuition would suggest that kick wounds should most likely involve the lateral aspect of the tarsus, often the medial tarsal or proximal metatarsal region is involved. Careful interpretation of radiographs may be necessary to detect small fragments displaced from the sustentaculum tali, on the distal medial aspect of the calcaneus.

Displacement of the SDFT from the tuber calcanei may occur suddenly, resulting in marked distress, especially if the tendon continues to move on and off the tuber calcanei. The tendon may slip laterally, or less commonly medially, and occasionally splits. Peritendonous soft tissue swelling develops rapidly. The horse is reluctant to bear weight on the limb and characteristically shows extreme distress,

caused by pain or instability. Careful palpation usually confirms the diagnosis, although acute soft tissue swelling may make this difficult in the initial period after injury.

Periarticular cellulitis of the tarsal region results in an extreme lameness associated with the rapid development of extensive soft tissue swelling, which is exquisitely sensitive to touch (see Chapter 107). The horse is often lamer than with a fracture, and swelling is more extensive than with synovial infection.

Injuries to the soft tissue structures of the metatarsal and pastern regions are less common than those of the metacarpal and forelimb pastern regions. Suspensory branch injuries are the most common injuries resulting from direct blunt trauma. Acute tears of the DDFT may occur within the digital flexor tendon sheath, with rapid development of effusion. Fractures of the third metatarsal bone and phalanges are also less common than in the forelimbs, except in barrel racing or cutting horses or polo ponies. Plantar process fractures of the proximal phalanx are rare but do occur in racehorses and result in moderate-to-severe lameness, with pain on manipulation of the fetlock, effusion, and in some horses periarticular soft tissue swelling, especially on the plantar aspect. Stability of the fetlock should be assessed carefully.

Stress Fractures

In young Thoroughbred racehorses the possibility of a fatigue or stress fracture must always be considered. The most common sites are the humerus, radius, ilial wing, tibia, third metacarpal bone, and tarsus. With the exception of ilial wing fractures, in which asymmetry of the tubera sacrale and pain on palpation in this area may be obvious, localizing clinical signs may otherwise be absent. A definitive diagnosis can rarely be made by clinical examination alone.

Hemarthrosis

Hemarthrosis may occur in any joint and results in acute-onset, non–weight-bearing lameness associated with distention of the joint capsule. Lameness often improves rapidly within the following 48 hours. Diagnosis is based on ultrasonography and synoviocentesis. Draining blood from the joint produces rapid relief of clinical signs.

TRANSPORTATION

In any horse with severe lameness in which making a tentative diagnosis based on a preliminary but thorough clinical examination is not possible, a decision has to be made about whether the horse is fit to travel, whether any risks are involved in travel, and whether the horse should be stabled as close as possible and be reassessed later or the following day (if this is practical). Whether the horse is insured should be established, together with the terms of the insurance policy.

The majority of horses can be taken safely to the nearest adequate diagnostic facility, which ideally should have a loading ramp, a veterinarian experienced in orthopedics, facilities for hospitalization, and high-standard radiographic, ultrasonographic, and possibly nuclear scintigraphic equipment.

Facilities for orthopedic surgery are not necessarily essential, although they are desirable, because the first step must be to reach an accurate diagnosis. When a diagnosis has been reached, the limb may then be appropriately supported to minimize risks of exacerbating the injury, if the horse is to be treated conservatively; during induction of general anesthesia; or for transfer to a suitable surgical facility. If a hindlimb fracture is suspected, the horse should be tied up (cross-tied). For transport for further diagnostic investigation or surgical treatment the injured limb should usually be supported using a Robert Jones bandage,[1] with or without splints, or an appropriate commercial splint, bearing in mind the proposed site of injury[2] (see Chapters 86 and 104). For forelimb injuries the horse should ideally travel facing backward, although some low-loading ambulances are not designed for loading from the front.[3] When possible a low-loading trailer should be used, but if this is not available, the ramp of the vehicle should be placed on a slope to minimize the gradient for loading and unloading. If a diagnosis has been made for a horse with an injury that requires rapid surgical treatment, the limb should be supported in the most appropriate way and the horse referred to the nearest surgical facility, or to the best surgical facility in close proximity to the horse's place of origin, or to the person with the most expertise and experience dealing with that kind of injury. Provided that the limb is adequately immobilized and adequate pain relief is possible, the horse should be fit to travel several hours safely and humanely.

GUIDELINES FOR HUMANE DESTRUCTION OF AN INJURED HORSE

If the horse is insured for all risks of mortality, owners, trainers, and other interested people may request humane destruction. The American Association of Equine Practitioners (AAEP) and the British Equine Veterinary Association (BEVA) have issued guidelines indicating the requirements that should be fulfilled to satisfy a claim under a mortality insurance policy. Nonetheless, the decision to advise an owner to destroy a horse on humane grounds must be the responsibility of the attending veterinary surgeon, based on the assessment of clinical signs at the time of the examination or examinations, regardless of whether the horse is insured. The veterinary surgeon's primary responsibility is always to ensure the welfare of the horse. On occasion the attending veterinary surgeon will advise euthanasia, but such a decision may not necessarily lead to a successful insurance claim. It is important that all parties be aware of

these potential conflicts of interests before a horse is destroyed. The owner's responsibility is to ensure compliance with any policy contract with an insurer.

The AAEP has issued the following guidelines for recommending euthanasia:

The AAEP recommends that the following criteria should be considered in evaluating the immediate necessity for intentional destruction of a horse. It should be pointed out that each case should be addressed on its individual merits and that the following are guidelines only. Not all criteria must be met in each case.
1. *Is the condition chronic, incurable and resulting in unnecessary pain and suffering?*
2. *Does the immediate condition present a hopeless prognosis for life?*
3. *Is the horse a hazard to itself or its handlers?*
4. *Will the horse require continuous medication for the relief of pain for the remainder of its life?*
   Justification for euthanasia of a horse for humane reasons should be based on medical grounds, not economic considerations; and further the same criteria should be applied to all horses regardless of age, sex or potential value.

The BEVA guidelines for compliance for a mortality insurance policy are as follows:

That the insured horse sustains an injury, or manifests an illness or disease, that is so severe as to warrant immediate destruction to relieve incurable and excessive pain, and that no other options of treatment are available to that horse, at that time.
   If immediate destruction cannot be justified, then the attending veterinary surgeon should provide immediate first aid treatment before:
1. *Requesting that the insurance company be contacted, or, failing that*
2. *Arranging for a second opinion from another veterinary surgeon.*

It is essential that the attending veterinary surgeon keep a written record of the injuries sustained by the horse, its identification, and the date, time, and place. The owner or agent should whenever possible sign a form consenting to euthanasia. Insurance companies frequently require some form of examination after death and may request an independent postmortem examination, and this must be borne in mind when arranging for disposal of the carcass.

References on page 1260

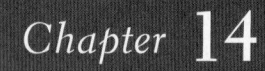

Chapter 14

The Swollen Limb

Sue J. Dyson

The development of diffuse or more localized swelling in one or more limbs can present a diagnostic challenge, requiring a systematic approach to identify the cause. Although the metacarpal, metatarsal, and pastern regions

are most commonly affected, an entire limb may be swollen, or swelling may initially be restricted to the antebrachium or crus or the carpus or tarsus, with swelling subsequently spreading distally. This chapter discusses an approach to diagnosis and management but does not provide exhaustive differential diagnoses and treatments. Some conditions are discussed in more detail in other chapters.

DIAGNOSIS

Many stabled horses develop some degree of enlargement of the distal limbs, especially the hindlimbs, that dissipates with work. Termed *filled legs* or *cold edema* (stocked-up, stoved-up), this swelling may be controlled by applying stable bandages and is of no consequence.

History

Accurate diagnosis of the cause of limb swelling requires knowledge of the history.

- Was the problem sudden or gradual in onset?
- What is the duration of the swelling?

It may be pertinent to establish when the owner last thought that the horse was normal, especially in horses that are not inspected regularly while kept at pasture. The actual duration of swelling may be longer than the owner recognized. The veterinarian also should bear in mind that some owners are remarkably unobservant, despite maintaining that they look at and groom the horse thoroughly daily.

- Were any swellings preexisting?
- What was the initial distribution of the swelling, and has this changed?
- Has similar swelling appeared previously? Lymphangitis may be a recurrent problem.
- Does any history of trauma exist?
- Has the limb been bandaged, or have boots or bandages been used for exercise? Overly tight bandages can rapidly result in severe cellulitis, skin excoriation, and hair loss. Sand or grit inside a boot can provoke severe skin inflammation and diffuse soft tissue swelling.
- Has the horse had tendonitis or desmitis? Recurrent injury may be much more severe and result in diffuse swelling, prohibiting accurate palpation of the injured structure.
- Has the horse had any other recent clinical problems? Strangles may predispose to purpura hemorrhagica.
- Does the horse show any other clinical signs, and could the limb swellings reflect systemic disease?
- Is the horse lame, and when did lameness develop relative to the recognition of swelling? If swelling preceded the lameness, more than one problem may exist.
- Have there been any recent injections?
- Has the horse received any treatment, and what was the response? Has anything topical been applied to the limb that may be irritant?

Swelling in a single limb usually reflects a local problem, whereas swelling in several limbs may be caused by systemic disease or a primary skin problem. The differential diagnosis should include the following: subsolar abscess (see Chapter 28); mud fever or scratches; scabby skin lesions on the palmar aspect of the fetlock; other bacterial pyodermas; hemorrhage or thrombosis (see Chapter 37); desmitis or tendonitis (see Chapters 69 to 72); cellulitis associated with superficial digital flexor tendonitis (see Chapter 69); skin necrosis and cellulitis after topical application of proprietary products; infected tendon or tendon sheath; cold edema; cellulitis caused by trauma or infection; fracture; hypertrophic osteopathy (see Chapter 37); muscle rupture (see Chapter 13); muscle trauma resulting in compartment syndrome (see Chapter 83); lymphangitis; photosensitization; equine viral arteritis; heart failure; and hypoproteinemia.

Clinical Examination

A systematic clinical examination should be performed by careful observation and palpation. The veterinarian should assess the horse's posture, demeanor, and attitude. Depression may reflect pain or infection.

- Is the horse febrile? The clinician should determine whether one or more limbs are involved.
- What is the distribution of the swelling? Is it localized or more diffuse? Swelling associated with a subsolar abscess is usually diffuse and involves the pastern and metacarpal or metatarsal region, extending a variable degree proximally, and is symmetrically distributed around the limb. In contrast, swelling associated with direct trauma may be restricted to the metacarpal region in the acute phase and only later spread distally, and may be most extensive on one aspect of the limb.
- Does the swelling relate to a joint or to a long bone and the surrounding soft tissues?
- Where is swelling maximal? Is swelling predominantly on one side of the limb, which may reflect trauma, because of the horse becoming cast?
- Does the metacarpal (metatarsal) region have a straight palmar (plantar) contour? Diffuse swelling in the metacarpal region is unlikely to reflect superficial digital flexor tendonitis if the palmar aspect of the limb is straight.
- Is the swelling cool, warm, or hot? Hot swelling is most likely to be associated with infection.
- Is the swelling tense, often reflecting infection, or soft?
- Is evidence of pitting edema present?
- Does light digital pressure or firm pressure elicit pain? Pain caused by only light pressure is often associated with cellulitis caused by infection (e.g., peritarsal cellulitis) or less commonly by intratendonous infection.
- How does the location of pain relate to the site of maximal swelling?
- How easily can underlying anatomical structures be palpated, and does palpation cause pain? The veterinarian should note that scabby skin lesions overlying soft tissue swelling can in themselves be remarkably painful.
- Does a draining tract suggest an abscess, cellulitis, or infectious osteitis or osteomyelitis?
- Does joint manipulation cause pain?
- Do any skin lesions exist through which infection may have entered? This may not be readily apparent in a horse with a long hair coat, and clipping may be necessary. In a horse kept at pasture the limb may be caked in mud, and thorough cleaning may be necessary before an accurate clinical examination can be made.
- Do any other skin lesions reflect a primary dermatological problem? The clinician should try to categorize any lesions identified.

The digital pulse amplitudes should be assessed: any increase highly suggests a primary foot problem. The response to pressure and percussion applied with hoof testers should be evaluated. Pulse rate, the quality of the peripheral pulses, capillary refill time, and careful auscultation of the heart and lungs should reveal whether a primary cardiac problem exists.

The mucous membranes should be examined for evidence of petechial hemorrhages, which can be seen with purpura hemorrhagica. The veterinarian should relate the swelling to the color of the limbs; swelling confined to white limbs may result from photosensitization.

The clinician should establish the degree of lameness and bear in mind that mild stiffness may result from extensive limb swelling and mechanical restriction. Extremely severe lameness often reflects infection—periarticular (e.g., peritarsal cellulitis; see Chapters 44 and 107), intraarticular, intrathecal, intratendonous, or subsolar. A horse with a fracture may be less lame. Severe lameness may also be associated with an acute muscle tear or hemorrhage. Although there may be no obvious swelling in the acute stage, diffuse filling of the affected limb may develop over the following 24 to 48 hours distal to the site of injury.

The results of this clinical examination should suggest the likely causes of the swelling, but definitive diagnosis might not be possible without further investigation. This may include radiography, ultrasonography, routine hematological testing, measurement of total protein and fibrinogen, and liver enzyme levels if indicated. Paired serum samples may be required to confirm equine viral arteritis. Treating the horse symptomatically to reduce the soft tissue swelling may be helpful to facilitate more accurate palpation. This may include the use of nonsteroidal antiinflammatory drugs (NSAIDs), hydrotherapy, poulticing or leg sweats, bandaging, and walking, with or without antimicrobial medication. Without evidence of a primary infectious process the response to corticosteroids may be helpful diagnostically, because limb filling may be an immune-mediated response. The clinician should be prepared to make repeated examinations if a primary diagnosis is not readily apparent.

Early periosteal new bone associated with hypertrophic osteopathy is readily overexposed, and greatly reduced exposure factors are required for its radiological detection. On the first day of examination the results of radiographic and ultrasonographic examinations may be misleading, and repeated examinations may be necessary. After trauma, laceration, or both to the antebrachium, crus, and metacarpal or metatarsal regions, delayed-onset lameness caused by an occult spiral fracture of the radius, tibia, or third metacarpal or metatarsal bones is possible. Many oblique radiographic images or follow-up examination may be necessary to identify the fracture. If extensive cellulitis occurs around a joint or tendon sheath, but intraarticular or intrathecal infection is suspected, the examiner should be cautious about performing synoviocentesis through infected tissues, because iatrogenic intraarticular or intrathecal infection may ensue. If skin lesions are identified as a possible primary cause of limb swelling, but these fail to respond to topical or systemic treatment, obtaining skin biopsies for culture and histological examination or seeking specialist advice from a dermatologist may be necessary.

MANAGEMENT
Mud Fever
Mud fever (scratches or pastern dermatitis) is associated with bacterial or fungal skin infection and usually is restricted to the palmar or plantar aspect of the pastern but sometimes extends farther proximally if severe. Mud fever is associated with many excoriated skin lesions, which may

develop severe crusting. Deep fissures may develop in the skin, especially if the condition goes unrecognized or in horses with many skin folds in the pastern region. Extensive edematous swelling often extends up the metacarpal and metatarsal regions. If the condition is mild, no associated lameness may occur, but severe lesions are associated with marked stiffness. The condition can occur in horses kept out in wet, muddy conditions or in horses that are stabled but work in a muddy environment. Certain soil types seem to be associated with a higher occurrence. Some horses seem prone to recurrent episodes, although this may in part reflect management practices. The condition is difficult to manage if the horse is left in wet, muddy pasture, and it must be stabled. The affected areas should be clipped and thoroughly cleaned with chlorhexidine solution. The scabs should be softened to facilitate removal. If the condition is mild, no further treatment may be required, but if the condition is more severe, daily topical application of lanolin-based emollient cream with trimethoprim and sulfadiazine and dexamethasone is indicated, sometimes combined with systemic antimicrobial treatment. Alternatively, a proprietary topical preparation can be used. The limbs should be carefully cleaned and dried after exercise.

Scabs on the Palmar Aspect of the Fetlock
Some horses seem prone to develop many small skin scabs on the palmar or plantar aspects of the fetlock. The scabs appear to be related to work on specific surfaces, which presumably cause skin irritation and subsequent bacterial infection. These skin lesions are often associated with diffuse swelling and can be exquisitely painful. The lesions rarely resolve spontaneously but usually respond to penicillin therapy.

Cellulitis Caused by Trauma
Direct trauma to a limb may result in extensive edematous soft tissue swelling unassociated with infection. If skin abrasion is concurrent, the site of the wound relative to synovial structures susceptible to infection must be evaluated carefully. Lameness may vary in degree, but if severe, the possibility of fracture must be considered. If little soft tissue covers the underlying bones, radiographic examination is prudent to eliminate the possibility of a fracture. With primary cellulitis, treatment with NSAIDs, rest, and controlled exercise is usually all that is required. A variety of commercial boots and wraps are available that provide hot and cold therapy combined sometimes with pulsed pressure, which may be beneficial in reducing soft tissue swelling. The limb should be bandaged between treatments.

Cellulitis Caused by Infection
Cellulitis associated with infection may result from blunt trauma, a penetrating wound, previous injection, or recent surgery, but in many horses no underlying cause is identified.[1,2] Thoroughbred racehorses may be most susceptible.[2,3] It usually results in fairly extensive soft tissue swelling, which tends to be warmer and more painful than swelling from noninfectious cellulitis (see Figure 5-8). Associated lameness may also be severe, depending in part on the location of infection. If the infection is untreated, abscessation may develop in muscular areas and may require surgical drainage. Cellulitis may also be concurrent with

Reference on page 1260

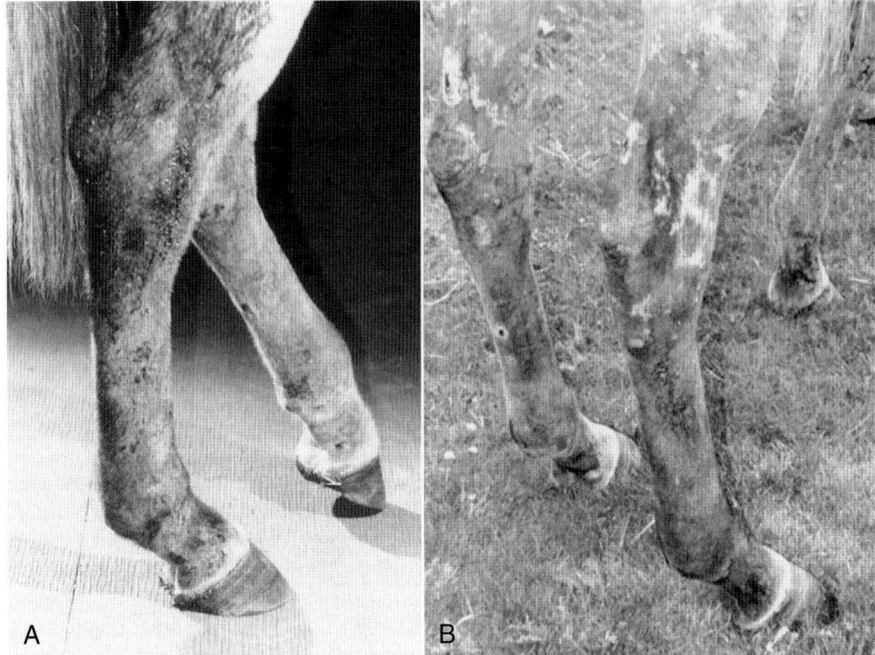

Fig. 14-1 • Photographs before **(A)** and after **(B)** antibiotic and corticosteroid therapy of an aged Thoroughbred broodmare with suspected purpura hemorrhagica. Before therapy all four limbs were edematous and erythematous, and there was diffuse crusting and with serum discharge. Signs were not limited to the distal limbs; the mare had intermittent gastrointestinal pain and hyperemia of mucous membranes. (Courtesy Mike W. Ross.)

infectious osteitis or osteomyelitis (see Chapter 37). Horses with acute infectious cellulitis usually respond well to systemic broad-spectrum antimicrobial treatment (e.g., crystalline penicillin and gentamicin), unless clostridial organisms are involved (see Chapter 83). The most common bacterial isolates are *Staphylococcus aureus* and *Streptococcus* species. Analgesia may be necessary and should be used to try to prevent secondary laminitis in the contralateral limb.

Lymphangitis

So-called lymphangitis occurs more commonly in hindlimbs than forelimbs and is often unilateral but may be bilateral. Diffuse soft tissue swelling occurs throughout the limb, often extending to the distal aspect of the limb from immediately below the stifle. The superficial lymphatic vessels may appear more prominent than usual. Serum may ooze through taut skin. The degree of swelling usually results in mechanical stiffness that improves with progressive walking. Careful inspection may reveal some small skin lacerations, often in the more distal part of the limb. Once a horse has had a severe attack of lymphangitis, it seems prone to recurrence, often after seemingly innocuous skin abrasions. Although the condition appears to be triggered by infection, antimicrobial treatment alone is inadequate and usually must be combined with long-term corticosteroid treatment (dexamethasone 0.05 to 0.2 mg/kg once daily intravenously or intramuscularly, using the lowest dose necessary to control edema, and replacing with prednisolone 0.5 to 1 mg/kg intramuscularly or by mouth twice daily, when the dexamethasone dose is <0.04 mg/kg), together with aggressive hydrotherapy and walking exercise, with or without bandaging and topical application of leg sweats. Bandaging the metatarsal region in the face of more proximal limb swelling tends to result in persistent proximal limb swelling that cannot move distally. Although prompt aggressive treatment may resolve clinical signs, persistence of marked filling for more than a week may result in chronic enlargement of the limb. Ulcerative lymphangitis occurs much less frequently and is caused by bacterial or fungal infection.

Purpura Hemorrhagica

Purpura hemorrhagica usually occurs as a sequela to previous streptococcal respiratory infection but occasionally follows other antigenic stimuli. Purpura hemorrhagica results in extensive submucosal petechial hemorrhages, evident clinically in the mucous membranes but actually more widespread, including muscle and viscera. Facial swellings and limb edema may be extensive (Figure 14-1). The horse is usually depressed, inappetent, and pyrexic. Purpura hemorrhagica is an acute, probably immune-mediated, necrotizing vasculitis. Aggressive treatment with penicillin and corticosteroids (see the previous discussion) is required.

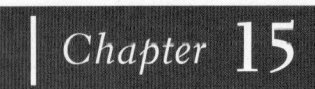

Radiography and Radiology

Sue J. Dyson

Radiography is the acquisition of radiographic images; radiology is the study and interpretation of those images. Radiography is an important part of the diagnostic armamentarium in the evaluation of lameness. Its most important role is to give information about bones and joints. However, it also can provide information about soft tissues, most particularly tendon, ligament, and joint capsule insertions. If radiography is to be used properly, then the area under investigation must be evaluated comprehensively and appropriately. A sufficient number of views, all which have been appropriately centered and exposed, should be obtained.

Obtaining high-quality radiographic images requires attention to detail. The horse must be correctly positioned and adequately restrained or sedated. For most weight-bearing examinations the horse should stand with the cannon bone of the limb to be examined in a vertical position. The horse should be standing on all four limbs, not resting a limb. The area under investigation should be cleaned to remove any surface dirt. For examinations of the foot, the shoe should be removed (if possible) to facilitate proper paring of the sole and frog, to ensure it is adequately clean, and to avoid superimposition of a radiodense shoe over the distal phalanx and navicular bone. The tail should be tied to facilitate correct positioning of the cassette or imaging plate when the stifle and hock regions are examined.

RADIOGRAPHIC DETAIL

The aim is to obtain as highly detailed radiographic images as possible. The detail that can be obtained is influenced by a number of factors, including those listed in Box 15-1.

Image Resolution

Image resolution is the objective measurement of how much detail can be provided by a film-screen combination and is measured in line pairs per millimeter. Resolution indicates the size of the smallest object that the system will record (i.e., the smallest distance that must exist between two objects before they can be distinguished as two separate entities). Image definition cannot be quantified but is the subjective impression of the amount of detail that can be seen on a radiograph.

Image Contrast

Contrast is the degree of definition on a radiographic image between adjacent structures of differing radiopacities. Opacity or radiopacity is the degree of whiteness of the object being radiographed. The denser the physical structure, the greater the degree to which the tissue absorbs x-rays, and the more opaque it appears on a radiograph.

Exposure Factors

Exposure factors affect the opacity and contrast of the radiographic image. The kilovoltage governs the quality and intensity of x-rays and affects both contrast and opacity. The quantity of x-rays reaching the x-ray film or imaging plate is the product of milliamperage and time and is also influenced by the focus-film distance (FFD), according to the inverse square law. The following equation is used to calculate the exposure of a change in distance:

$$\text{Old mAs} \times \frac{(\text{New FFD})^2}{(\text{Old FFD})^2} = \text{New mAs}$$

The milliampere-seconds and FFD affect the opacity of the image, not the contrast.

Exposure Latitude

Exposure latitude is the degree of overexposure or underexposure that can be tolerated in a correctly developed film and still produce an image of acceptable radiographic quality. A low kilovoltage yields high contrast with low latitude, whereas a high kilovoltage results in low contrast but has wide latitude. For good bone detail the kilovoltage should be less than 70 kV. Attenuation of the x-ray beam depends heavily on the atomic number of the tissues, and it is desirable that photoelectric absorption predominate. Increasing the kilovoltage also results in more forward scatter. The use of computed or digital radiography potentially results in greater latitude for a single exposure.

To obtain a radiographic image with the same opacity as the original but with decreased contrast, the milliampere-seconds are halved and the kilovoltage is increased by 15% (approximately 10 kV). To increase the contrast but maintain the opacity, the milliampere-seconds are doubled and the kilovoltage is reduced by approximately 15%.

Image Sharpness and Resolution

Lack of image sharpness can be caused by a number of factors, including movement of the horse. Short exposure times help to reduce the risk of movement blur. Reducing the FFD can increase the amount of x-rays reaching the horse, and therefore the exposure time could be reduced. However, reduction of FFD results in an increase in geometric indistinctness or *penumbra*. Image blur also may be the result of poor screen-film contact. Contact can be tested by placing a wire mesh on top of the cassette and making an exposure using a large FFD. Any loss of image sharpness is the result of poor film-screen contact.

BOX 15-1

Factors That Influence Radiographic Images

- **Film screen combination** (with conventional radiography). High-definition screens for use with single-emulsion and relatively slow film provide the best definition in the distal limbs. When higher exposure factors are required to gain adequate penetration of the more proximal parts of the limb, rare earth screens are required to minimize exposure times and thus reduce the risk of movement blur.
- **Proper contact between the film and the screen.** Old screens become warped, which results in loss of image quality. Damaged imaging plates result in artifacts.
- **Cleanliness of the screens.** Dust and hair accumulate easily within cassettes and imaging plates, resulting in radiopaque artifacts and lines on the films. Screens or imaging plates must be cleaned regularly. Careful technique is essential to reduce the risk of dust buildup.
- **Power of the x-ray machine.** The use of high-definition screens is possible only with x-ray machines capable of an output of 100 kV and 100 mAs. Otherwise, exposure times are too long, resulting in movement blur.
- **Choice of appropriate exposure factors.** This step is less critical with digital radiography when postprocessing can be used.
- **Use of the correct focus-film distance (FFD).** X-rays obey the inverse square law, so that an alteration in the FFD potentially has a big effect. Single-emulsion film and computed or digital radiographic imaging plates are particularly sensitive to a slight change in the FFD.
- **Exposure time.** The exposure time should be as short as possible to reduce movement blur.
- **Use of grids.** Grids are required in areas with a large amount of soft tissue, which results in scattered radiation.

    The use of a grid requires a higher exposure factor. If a focused grid is used, the x-ray beam must be perpendicular to the grid and centered on it, and the correct FFD should be used. Parallel grids have slightly more latitude when an FFD of more than 120 cm is used. The higher the grid ratio and lines per centimeter, the more effective the grid is in reducing scattered radiation, but the higher the grid factor. The grid factor denotes how much an exposure must be increased from nongrid values for comparable opacity. For example, if the grid factor is 2, then the milliampere-seconds (mAs) should be doubled.
- **Lead.** Lead is placed behind the cassette when large exposures are used to reduce the amount of backscatter.
- **Collimation of the x-ray beam.**
- **Use of stationary cassette holders when possible and practical to reduce movement of the cassette.**
- **Size and shape of the horse.** These factors become particularly important when the thoracolumbar region is examined. The amount of muscle mass and fat influence the exposure factors; with very large horses there is a risk of the radiographic images becoming flat as the exposure is increased. The shape of the horse's barrel also influences how closely the cassette can be placed to the back and thus influences magnification. The use of an aluminum wedge filter allows the intensity of the beam to be reduced in specific areas and is of particular value for examining areas with a marked change in soft tissue thickness from one side of the film to the other (e.g., the dorsal spinous processes in the thoracolumbar region, the shoulder, and the stifle).
- **The physics of computed and digital radiography** makes it more difficult to obtain high-quality images where there are very big differences in opacities of adjacent structures; this problem seems to be magnified in the caudal thoracic and lumbar regions of large horses.
- **Amount of soft tissue swelling.** If marked periarticular soft tissue swelling is present, higher exposures are required to achieve adequate penetration. The use of a grid in these circumstances helps to reduce scattered radiation.
- **Cooperation of the horse.**

Image resolution also can be influenced by the focal spot size of the x-ray machine. High-output x-ray machines usually have different size focal spots. A small focal spot (e.g., 0.6 mm) usually results in better image resolution, but an increased exposure time is required to achieve the same milliamperes. When movement is likely to be a problem (e.g., proximal limb examinations), a larger focal spot (1.5 to 2.0 mm) is preferable to reduce exposure times.

Film and Screen Factors

Relative speed ratings of screens and distance factors must be considered when exposure factors are being selected. Speed classification of film-screen combinations allows comparison of systems from different manufacturers. Some manufacturers use 100, 200, 400, and so on, and others use 2, 4, 8, and so forth, but the interrelationship is the same. Speed 8 screens require half the exposure (milliampere-seconds) needed for speed 4 screens; speed 200 requires twice the exposure (milliampere-seconds) of speed 400. Although the same exposures are required to provide the same image opacity using similar film-screen speeds, the detail and resolution may vary. Generally when only one screen from a pair is used (when using single-emulsion film), the speed of the system will halve. Thus if one screen from a pair rated 400 is used, the speed will be 200.

RADIATION SAFETY

Radiation safety (i.e., ensuring that personnel around the horse do not receive doses of radiation) is essential. Different codes of practice apply in various countries, but the basic principles are summarized in Box 15-2.

RESPONSE OF BONE TO STIMULI: WOLFF'S LAW

Correct interpretation of radiographic images requires knowledge of the ways in which bone responds to various stimuli. Bone models according to Wolff's law: it models according to the stresses placed on it so that it can be functionally competent with the minimum amount of bone tissue. The use of the terms *modeling* and *remodeling* creates considerable confusion because usage differs in histology and radiology. Histologically, *bone remodeling* refers to resorption and formation of bone that is coupled and occurs in basic multicellular units. This regulates the microstructure of bone without altering its shape and is a continuous process, replacing damaged bone with new bone. Thus remodeling cannot be appreciated radiologically. Radiologically, the term has been used to describe reshaping of bone to match form and function (e.g., after fracture repair). Strictly speaking, the term *modeling* should be used to describe the change in the shape of a bone as it adapts to the stresses applied to it.

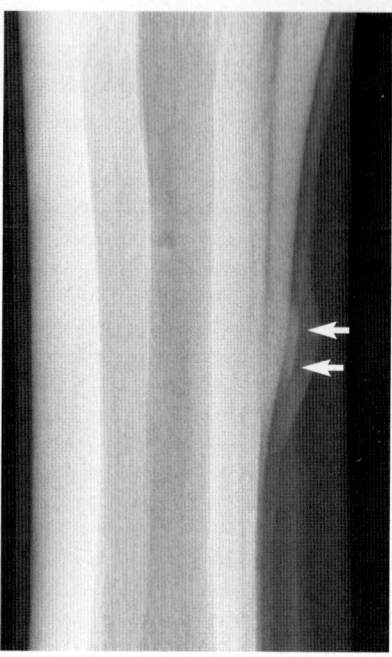

Fig. 15-1 • Dorsomedial-palmarolateral oblique radiographic image of the metacarpal region. Soft tissue swelling overlies periosteal new bone *(arrows)* on the middiaphyseal region of the second metacarpal bone.

Bone is a dynamic tissue, constantly reacting to the stimuli that it receives both internally and externally. However, it takes time to respond, and a 40% change in bone density must occur before changes are evident radiologically. Therefore radiographic images, although anatomically accurate, are relatively insensitive in the early stages of a disease process. This is known as the radiographic *latent period*. It is critical to appreciate these limitations when interpreting radiographic images. Bone can be undergoing abnormal modeling without identifiable structural change. Once radiological abnormalities have developed, some will persist over the long term without necessarily being associated with ongoing pain. Thus in effect these changes remain as scars reflecting previous injury. Aging of such lesions is impossible, and assessing clinical significance must be evaluated in the light of the clinical signs.

Bone can react to stimuli in only a limited number of ways. Bone can produce new bone, such as periosteal new bone, endosteal new bone, cortical thickening, increased thickness of trabeculae, callus formation, osteophyte and enthesophyte formation, and the palisading periosteal new bone typical of hypertrophic osteopathy. New bone often results in what has been described radiologically as *sclerosis*: increased opacity of the bone, caused by either new bone being laid down within the bone or superimposition of new bone on the surface of the bone. More than one radiographic image usually is required to determine why a structure appears to have increased opacity (i.e., is sclerotic). Strictly speaking, however, sclerosis is a localized increase in opacity of the bone caused by increased bone mass within the bone. Unless this can be determined with certainty it is preferable to use the term *increased radiopacity*.

Osteolysis is resorption of bone resulting in a radiolucency. Again, a lag period, usually of at least 10 days, occurs between the onset of osteolysis and its radiological detection. Osteolysis occurs for a variety of reasons, including pressure, infection, as part of early fracture repair, and as

part of the disease process in osteoarthritis, osteochondrosis, osseous cystlike lesions, and subchondral bone cysts. Bone destruction and resorption usually are seen more easily in cortical bone rather than cancellous bone because of the greater contrast.

Generalized demineralization, or osteopenia, of bone throughout the body rarely occurs in the horse. Localized demineralization in a single limb usually is the result of disuse and is characterized by thinning of the cortices and a more obvious trabecular pattern. The proximal sesamoid bones are particularly sensitive indicators of disuse osteopenia in the horse.

Focal demineralization and loss of bone may be caused by pressure—for example, as seen in chronic proliferative synovitis in the fetlock—resulting in erosion of the dorsoproximal aspect of the sagittal ridge of the third metacarpal bone (McIII). It may be the result of infection, invasion by fibrous tissue, or a neoplasm.

Cortical thickness changes (models) according to Wolff's law as an immature athlete develops into a mature, trained athlete. The dorsal cortex of the McIII and the third metatarsal bone becomes thicker. If a horse has marked conformational abnormalities, such as offset or bench knees, the bones model accordingly, with the lateral cortex of the distal limb bones becoming thicker.

Periosteal New Bone

Blunt trauma to bone can lead to subperiosteal hemorrhage, resulting in lifting of the periosteum away from the bone. This process may stimulate the production of periosteal new bone (Figure 15-1). Some bones, such as the second and fourth metacarpal and metatarsal bones, seem particularly prone to such reactions. There is individual variation among horses in susceptibility to such reactions. Usually a lag period of at least 14 days occurs between trauma and the radiological detection of periosteal new bone. Such bone usually is much less dense than the parent bone; therefore soft exposures (or low kilovoltages) are essential for detection of this bone, which initially has a rather irregular outline. As the bone gradually consolidates and then models, it becomes more opaque and more smoothly outlined. Curiously, although a well-established splint exostosis would be expected to become inactive, many have increased radiopharmaceutical uptake (IRU) compared with the parent bone if examined scintigraphically.

Periosteal new bone can also develop as a result of fracture, infection, inflammation, and neoplasia. Inflammation of the interosseous ligamentous attachment between the second metacarpal bone and the McIII or the fourth metacarpal bone and the McIII caused by movement and loading can result in periosteal new bone formation and a splint exostosis. It is curious that some of these formations develop rapidly without associated pain, whereas others can cause persistent pain and lameness for many weeks, despite a similar radiological appearance. The bony protuberances that develop on the proximolateral aspect of the metatarsal regions, often bilaterally, are even more enigmatic. They are rarely associated with clinical signs, although they often have IRU despite having been present for several years.

Endosteal New Bone

Endosteal new bone may develop as a result of trauma (e.g., a cortical or subcortical fracture or trauma at an enthesis) or inflammation, infection, or, less commonly, a tumor (Figure 15-2). Stress fractures of the dorsal cortex of the McIII are accompanied by the development of endosteal new bone, which may be more readily detected than the fracture itself.

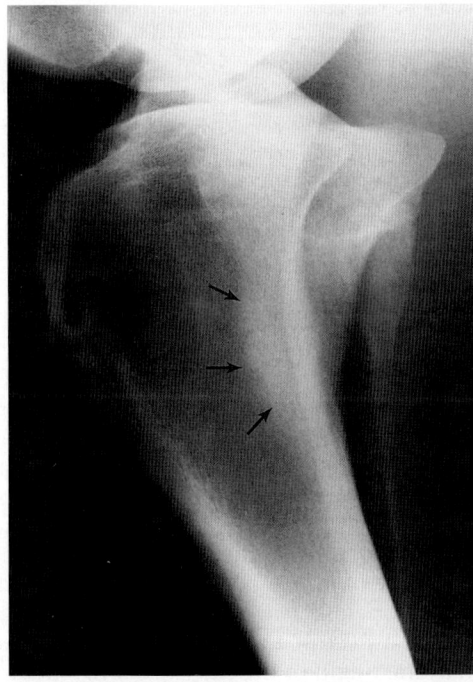

Fig. 15-2 • Lateromedial radiographic image of the proximal tibia. There is increased opacity of the subcortical bone of the proximocaudal aspect of the tibia. Endosteal new bone *(arrows)* is associated with a fatigue (stress) fracture.

Sclerosis

Sclerosis is the localized formation of new bone within bone and results in increased bone mass. It is most easily identified in trabecular bone (Figure 15-3) and occurs in response to several stimuli, including the following:

- Stress (e.g., subchondral sclerosis in osteoarthritis and sclerosis of the medulla of the navicular bone in navicular disease)
- Protection of a weakened area (e.g., sclerosis surrounding an osseous cystlike lesion or a subchondral bone cyst)
- Walling off infection (e.g., adjacent to a sequestrum or in the medullary cavity adjacent to an area of osteomyelitis)

Enostosis-like lesions are the development of bone within the medullary cavity or on the endosteum, resulting in a relatively opaque (sclerotic) area of variable size. They frequently occur adjacent to the nutrient foramen, and the origin is unclear. They may develop as a focal or multifocal lesion. They vary in size and generally are seen in the diaphyseal regions of long bones in the horse. These lesions have been seen most frequently in the humerus, the radius, the tibia, the McIII, the third metatarsal bones, and the femur. When these lesions develop, they have focal intense IRU and may be associated with pain and lameness. However, they also are seen as incidental findings.

Small focal opacities in the proximal metaphyseal region of the tibia have been seen. The origin and clinical significance are not known. Care must be taken in the fetlock region not to misinterpret the radiopacity caused by the ergot as an opaque lesion within the proximal phalanx.

Osteophyte Formation

An osteophyte is a spur of bone on a joint margin that develops as a result of a variety of stimuli, including joint instability, or in association with intraarticular disease, particularly osteoarthritis. Not all periarticular modeling changes at the junction of the articular cartilage and periarticular bone are associated with ongoing joint disease, but radiological differentiation between a subclinical osteophyte and a clinically significant one is difficult. Small spurs frequently are seen on the dorsoproximal aspect of the third metatarsal bone close to the tarsometatarsal joint. Some are quiescent, unassociated with articular pathological findings, whereas others are progressive. Small spurs on

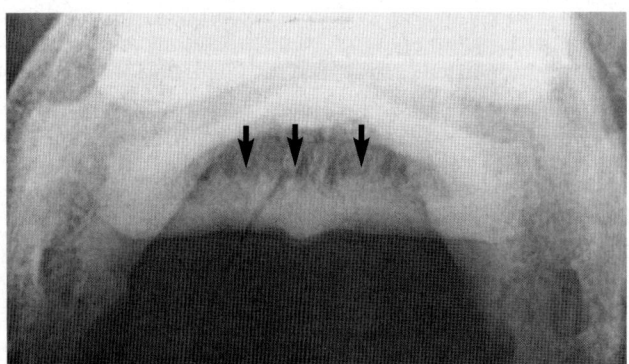

Fig. 15-3 • Palmaroproximal-palmarodistal oblique radiographic image of a navicular bone. The flexor cortex is thickened, and there is extensive endosteal new bone *(arrows)* resulting in increased radiopacity of the spongiosa.

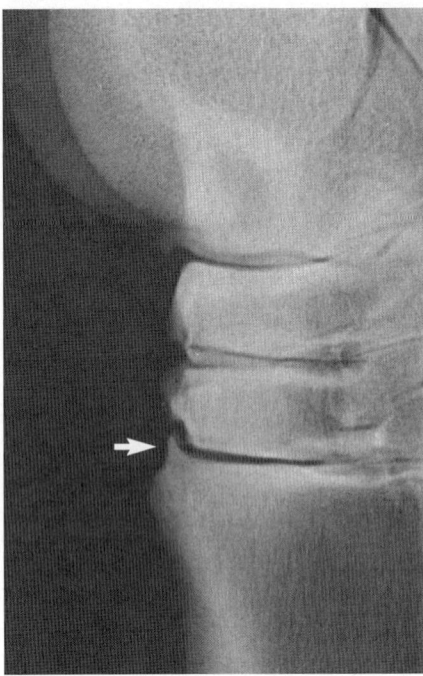

Fig. 15-4 • Lateromedial radiographic image of a hock. There is a moderately sized periarticular osteophyte on the dorsoproximal aspect of the third metatarsal bone, close to and traversing the tarsometatarsal joint *(arrow)*.

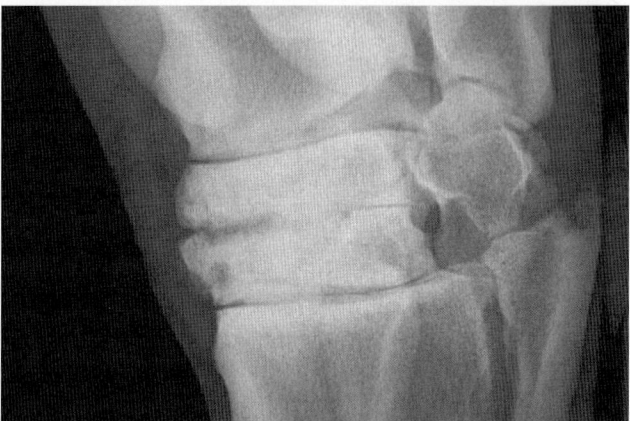

Fig. 15-5 • Dorsolateral-plantaromedial oblique radiographic image of a hock. There is narrowing of the centrodistal joint space. Radiolucent regions are seen in the subchondral bone of the central and third tarsal bones dorsomedially. There is loss of trabecular architecture because of medullary increased radiopacity in the central and third tarsal bones. Note also the osseous cystlike lesion in the distal dorsomedial aspect of the third tarsal bone.

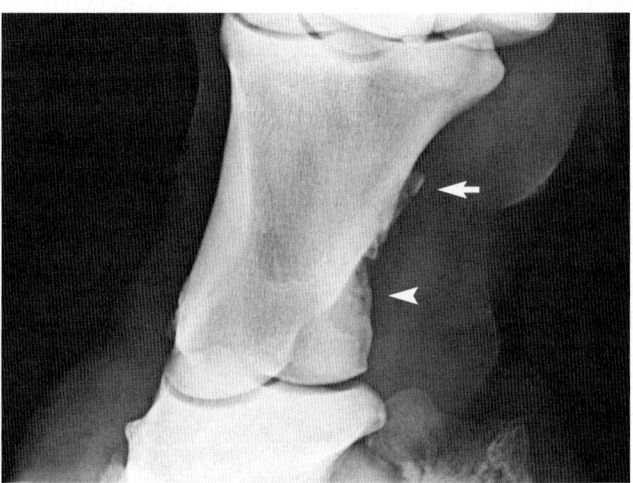

Fig. 15-6 • Dorsolateral-palmaromedial oblique radiographic image of a pastern. There is entheseous new bone *(arrow)* on the middiaphyseal region of the proximal phalanx at the site of insertion of the oblique sesamoidean ligament. There is entheseous new bone further distally *(arrowhead)* at the origin of the ligament between the proximal phalanx and the cartilage of the foot, the chondrocompedal ligament.

the dorsoproximal aspect of the middle phalanx are frequent incidental findings in Warmblood breeds. Mature horses with offset- or bench-knee conformation frequently have spurs on the lateral aspect of the antebrachiocarpal joint without associated clinical signs.

The time of development of an osteophyte after stimulus varies depending on the inciting cause and individual variation. Two weeks to several months may pass before an osteophyte may be identified radiologically. A smoothly marginated osteophyte of uniform opacity is more likely to be long-standing, whereas a poorly marginated osteophyte with a lucent tip is likely to be active.

Some joints seem to have a greater propensity than others for the development of periarticular osteophyte formation. The reason for this tendency is unknown and may in part reflect the ease with which osteophytes can be detected radiologically. Even within what is currently considered a single disease process, osteoarthritis of the distal hock joints (bone spavin), some horses develop predominantly periarticular osteophytes (Figure 15-4), whereas others have narrowing of the joint space and subchondral sclerosis. A third group develops extensive radiolucent areas (Figure 15-5).

Enthesophyte Formation
Enthesophyte formation is new bone at the site of attachment of a tendon, ligament, or joint capsule to bone. Entheseous new bone reflects the bone's response to stress applied through these structures, such as ligamentous tearing or capsular traction (Figure 15-6). Like osteophytes, enthesophyte formations take several weeks to months to develop and may or may not be associated with clinical signs. Knowledge of ligament, tendon, and capsular insertions is essential to determine which soft tissue structure

may have been damaged. In some locations, such as the hock, differentiation between enthesophyte and osteophyte formation is not easy. The attachments of the cranialis tibialis, fibularis tertius, and dorsal tarsal ligament are close to the joint margins of the tarsometatarsal joint, and differentiation between entheseous new bone at these attachments and periarticular osteophyte formation may be difficult. Entheseous new bone may take the form of spur formation, such as at the site of attachment of the common digital extensor tendon on the distal phalanx or the site of attachment of the oblique sesamoidean ligament on the palmar aspect of the proximal phalanx. At other sites, such as the origin of the suspensory ligament (SL) on the plantar aspect of the third metatarsal bone, new bone formation may be more diffuse. Diffuse new bone formation on the caudal aspect of the occiput reflects tearing of the attachment of the nuchal ligament. New bone on the dorsal aspect of the radial, intermediate, ulnar, or third carpal bones may reflect entheseous new bone at the site of attachment of intercarpal ligaments or the joint capsule. Such new bone does not necessarily reflect osteoarthritis, but it may reflect slight joint instability, which itself may predispose to the development of osteoarthritis. Similarly, joint trauma resulting in sprain of periarticular ligaments and subsequent entheseous new bone may ultimately also result in osteoarthritis.

Fracture of an enthesophyte and mineralization within the tendon or ligament attachment also may occur. A relatively common site is the radial tuberosity at the attachment of biceps brachii. Small linear opacities may be seen dorsal to the summits of the spinous processes in the thoracic region, which are associated with tearing of the attachment of the supraspinous ligament.

Spondylosis
Ossifying spondylosis occurs in the caudal half of the thoracic region in the horse. Spondyles (osteophytes) arise from the ventral aspect of the vertebral bodies near the intercentral articulations. The osteophytes extend across the intercentral articulation toward similar osteophytes on adjacent vertebrae. Usually a lucent line persists between the two spondyles, although sometimes complete bridging does occur. Spondylosis may be progressive in cranial and caudal directions, although in some horses it remains static.

New Bone of Unknown Origin
New bone sometimes develops on the dorsal aspect of the diaphysis and distal metaphyseal region of the middle phalanx. The cause of this is unknown. It may be asymptomatic.

Hypertrophic Osteopathy
Hypertrophic osteopathy (Marie's disease) is typified by palisading periosteal new bone, which appears to be perpendicular to the cortices and irregular in outline in the acute stage. It affects principally the diaphyseal and metaphyseal regions of long bones and spares the joints. In the early stages, very soft exposures must be used to avoid overexposing this relatively radiolucent bone. Later the margins of the new bone become more opaque and smoother, and the distinction between the original cortex and the new bone becomes less obvious. These bony lesions develop secondary to a tumor, abscess, or other lesion in the thorax or abdomen, or in association with diffuse granulomatous disease. The bony lesions may regress and model if the primary lesion can be identified and successfully treated.

Osteitis
Osteitis is inflammation of bone. It may be noninfectious or infectious. Noninfectious osteitis usually is the result of trauma or inflammation of the adjacent soft tissues. It is characterized by new bone formation and, less commonly, bone resorption.

Infectious Osteitis and Osteomyelitis
Infectious osteitis is inflammation of bone as a result of infection. In bones with a myeloid cavity the term *osteomyelitis* is used if the myeloid cavity is affected. Infection

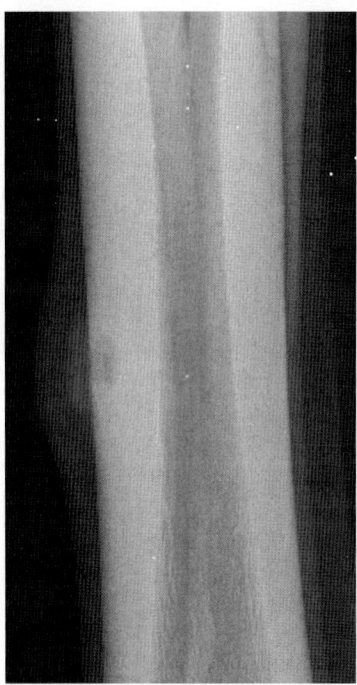

Fig. 15-7 • Dorsomedial-palmarolateral radiographic image of a metacarpal region of a 5-year-old Warmblood that had been kicked 2 months earlier. There is soft tissue swelling overlying ill-defined periosteal new bone. There is a radiolucent defect in the lateral cortex of the third metacarpal bone with an acentric, more radiolucent area. These abnormalities are consistent with infectious osteitis.

results in soft tissue swelling, new bone formation, and bone resorption. In the distal phalanx and the distal sesamoid (navicular) bone, bone lysis predominates with little new bone formation. In other bones a combination of loss of bone and new bone formation usually occurs. A piece of dead radiopaque bone, or a sequestrum, may develop, surrounded by an area of lucent granulation tissue, the involucrum (Figure 15-7). An area of more radiopaque bone may be laid down surrounding the infected area to wall off infection. A radiolucent tract, a sinus, may develop between the infected tissues and the skin. In the early stages, diagnostic ultrasonography may be more sensitive than radiography for detecting infection.

Osseous Cystlike Lesions and Subchondral Bone Cysts
Osseous cystlike lesions are solitary, circular, or semicircular lucent areas in a bone; they usually develop in the subchondral bone. Sometimes a neck can be identified connecting the cyst to the joint cavity. Cystlike lesions may be unicameral (single chambered) or, less commonly, multicameral. A sclerotic rim frequently surrounds osseous cystlike lesions. Those that develop before skeletal maturity often appear to migrate away from the joint surface as normal endochondral ossification occurs. These single osseous cystlike lesions, which are not associated with any pathological changes in the articular cartilage, should be differentiated from the more poorly defined lucent zones that develop in the subchondral bone in osteochondrosis.

The cause of osseous cystlike lesions is probably multifactorial. Some are true subchondral bone cysts and have a fibrous cystic lining. There is increasing evidence that some of these lesions develop as a response to trauma to the articular cartilage and subchondral bone. They tend to occur most commonly in the medial condyle of the femur and in the center of the glenoid cavity of the scapula. Other osseous cystlike lesions may have a different histological appearance, despite similar radiological appearance. Osseous cystlike lesions in the proximal medial aspect of the radius tend to be associated with periosteal new bone in the region of insertion of the medial collateral ligament. Other common locations include the distal aspect of the McIII and the proximal, distal, and middle phalanges.

Care should be taken when evaluating some bones, especially the phalanges, not to confuse the myeloid cavity with an osseous cystlike lesion.

The development of some osseous cystlike lesions can be followed radiologically. Some start as a small, elliptical depression in the articular surface that progressively enlarges into the subchondral bone. A sclerotic margin develops.

Osseous cystlike lesions may be associated with lameness. Lesions deep in the bone, such as those seen in the first, second, and ulnar carpal bones, are rarely associated with lameness. Cystlike lesions that are close to an articular surface are more likely to be associated with lameness. However, the lameness may be remarkable in its variable nature and severity. Lameness may resolve spontaneously or after surgical intervention, despite persistence of a lesion, radiologically.

The incidence of the development of osseous cystlike lesions is higher in young horses than older horses. Some horses develop a subchondral bone cyst early in life that remains clinically quiescent, only to cause clinical signs later in life. However, subchondral bone cysts and osseous cystlike lesions can develop in skeletally mature horses.

It can be difficult to determine the likely clinical significance of a subchondral bone cyst or an osseous cystlike lesion based purely on radiological appearance. Scintigraphic evaluation may be helpful, because many have IRU, but it can also be confusing because a long-established cystlike lesion that has been clinically quiescent can suddenly become a source of pain without evidence of active bone modeling. It is always important to evaluate radiologically the joint in its entirety, because evidence of secondary osteoarthritis warrants a more guarded prognosis.

Osteochondrosis

Osteochondrosis is considered a disorder of endochondral ossification, although there is increasing evidence that primary subchondral bone lesions also may occur. Osteochondrosis can cause osseous cystlike lesions and osteochondritis dissecans. Osteochondritis dissecans may be generalized although it is evident clinically and radiologically only in certain joints. The femoropatellar, tarsocrural, fetlock, and scapulohumeral joints are most commonly affected. Radiological abnormalities vary depending on the joint involved and include the following:

- Discrete osteochondral fragments
- Flattening or depression in the articular surface
- Subchondral lucent zones
- Increased radiopacity in the subchondral bone, surrounding lucent zones, or parallel with the joint surface
- Secondary osteoarthritis

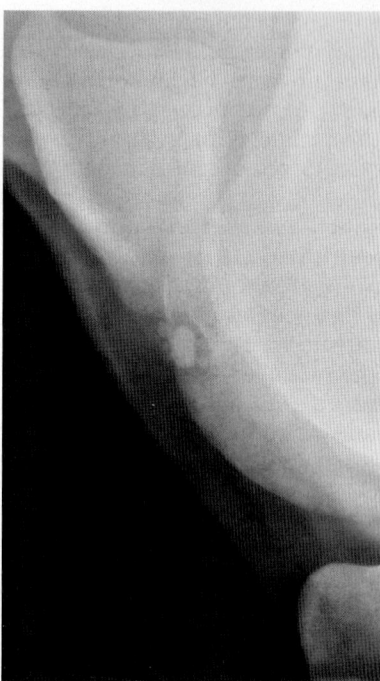

Fig. 15-8 • Caudolateral-craniomedial oblique radiographic image of a stifle of an 8-year-old Warmblood show jumper with no history of lameness, undergoing a prepurchase examination. There is a concave depression in the middle of the lateral trochlea of the femur, with mild subchondral increased radiopacity and ill-defined lucent areas. In addition, there are one large and several small radiopaque bodies visible in the concave depression. This is osteochondrosis.

Radiological changes are not always clinically significant but must be interpreted in the light of clinical signs. Flattening of contour of the lateral trochlear ridge of the femur, with sclerosis of the subchondral bone, may be seen in the absence of lameness in mature horses. However, identical changes may be present in horses with poor hindlimb action referable to pain associated with the femoropatellar joints (Figure 15-8). Flattening of contour or the presence of elliptical depressions in the trochleas of the talus with normal subchondral bone opacity is rarely associated with clinical signs. The more change in the subchondral bone, the more likely that clinical signs will be present. Small osteochondral fragments may become lodged in the synovial membrane and become progressively larger. Trauma may result in such lesions becoming dislodged and mobile and result in clinical signs.

FRACTURE

A fracture is a discontinuity of bone that may be seen radiologically as one or more lucent lines. Mach lines, or bands, should not be confused with a fracture. A Mach line or band is a radiolucent line created by edge enhancement when one bone edge is superimposed over another bone. Superimposition of the second and fourth metacarpal bones on the McIII commonly results in Mach lines. In a caudocranial view of the proximal tibia, a Mach line is created by superimposition of the tibial crest on the tibia.

Large exostoses involving the second or fourth metacarpal bone or fourth metacarpal or fourth metatarsal bone often result in confusing lucent lines, apparently within the bone, which must not be interpreted as fractures. Likewise, some bony exostoses in these locations incorporate some fibrous tissue, resulting in a persistent lucent line that should not confused with a fracture. A nutrient foramen that traverses a bone should also not be interpreted as fracture. Most nutrient foramina are broader than a recent fracture would be expected to be. A notable exception is the vertically orientated nutrient foramen in the second metacarpal or second metatarsal bone and the fourth metacarpal or fourth metatarsal bone. It is important not to misinterpret lucent lines in the foot created by the frog clefts as fracture lines. Despite careful packing of the frog clefts and sulcus (with, for example, Play-Doh), complete packing is impossible if these are very deep and will result in narrow lucent lines. Care should be taken to see if such a lucent line (e.g., apparently in the navicular bone) extends beyond the bone margins. If the angle of projection is altered slightly, does the position of the line change relative to the medial and lateral borders of the bone? Can the same lucent line be seen in a dorsopalmar image? Care must also be taken not to confuse the lucent bands between separate centers of ossification with fracture lines. The cartilages of the foot and the fibula frequently develop as separate centers of ossification, and bony union may never develop between the different ossification centers, which results in lucent gaps within each bone that persist over the long term. A long, thick hair coat that is wet sometimes can result in the appearance of a lucent line or lines superimposed over bone, which must not be interpreted as a fracture.

Some stress or fatigue fractures are never detectable radiologically. Some can be seen as one or more lucent lines, or, if fractures are chronic, there may be endosteal new bone or increased medullary opacity. If a chronic stress fracture traverses a cortex, there may be periosteal callus, although the fracture line itself may not be detectable.

Ideally, the postulated radiolucent fracture line should be detectable on more than one radiographic image to confirm the presence of a fracture. However, this is not always possible, especially if the fracture is incomplete and nondisplaced. This is particularly true for fractures of the distal phalanx and incomplete dorsal cortical fractures of the proximal phalanx. For best results, the x-ray beam must be perpendicular to the plane of the fracture line. Many different views that differ by only 5 degrees in angle of projection may be required for detection of a fissure fracture. With a complete fracture, many different views may be required for determination of the precise configuration of the fracture.

Some fractures are not detectable in the standard radiographic images of the area under examination. A fracture of the lateral palmar process of the distal phalanx may not be detectable in lateromedial, dorsopalmar, and dorsoproximal-palmarodistal oblique images. Dorsolateral-palmaromedial oblique or sometimes a palmaroproximal-palmarodistal oblique image, or a dorsal 60° proximal 45° lateral-palmarodistal medial oblique view, is required. Sagittal and some slab fractures of the third carpal bone are visible only in dorsoproximal-dorsodistal oblique images of the flexed carpus (the skyline projection). Similarly, fractures of the medial pole of the patella are only detectable in cranioproximal-craniodistal oblique images of the flexed stifle.

The normal healing process of a fracture involves osteoclasis along the fracture line within 5 to 10 days, resulting in initial broadening of the fracture line. Therefore if a fracture is suspected but cannot be seen in the acute stage, radiography should be repeated after 5 to 10 days. Care should be taken not to underexpose the radiograph, because a faint lucent line may be missed. Paradoxically, early callus formation, which develops within 14 to 21 days, will be missed if the radiograph is overexposed or not viewed over high-intensity illumination or if a computer screen is viewed in excessively bright light.

A fracture should be evaluated to determine whether it is complete or incomplete and simple or comminuted, whether fracture fragments are displaced, whether articular involvement is present, and whether any other concurrent pathological condition is present that may influence the prognosis. An apical proximal sesamoid bone fracture may be accompanied by severe desmitis of the branch of the SL, which prognostically is the more severe injury. Biaxial transverse fractures of the proximal sesamoid bones result in disruption of the suspensory apparatus and severe risk of compromising the blood supply to the distal part of the limb. An avulsion fracture of the proximal phalanx at the attachment of the lateral collateral ligament of the metacarpophalangeal joint will result in loss of joint stability.

It is important to be aware that with a single, complete fracture, two lucent lines representing the fracture traversing, for example, the dorsal and palmar cortices, may be seen. These lines should not be confused with two fractures. However, care must always be taken to make sure that there is not more than a single fracture line. For example, a common fracture in steeplechasers that fall is a vertical fracture through the body of the accessory carpal bone. These horses have a good prognosis with conservative management. Rarely, one or more chip fractures involving the articular margins of the bone occur; such injuries warrant a much more guarded prognosis. An event horse that hits a fixed fence during cross-country jumping may fracture the medial trochlear ridge of the femur. Fracture fragments may readily be seen in a lateromedial image of the stifle. Such fractures also can be accompanied by a fracture of the medial pole of the patella, which can be seen only in a skyline image. Therefore it is essential to obtain a complete radiographic series and interpret each radiograph in its entirety.

Intraarticular fractures occur when a break in the articular surface occurs. Unless some degree of displacement is present, damage to the articular cartilage may not be seen but is assumed to exist. A small degree of displacement is indicated by the presence of a slight step in the two sides of the articular portion of the fracture line. Comminution at the joint surface sometimes occurs. This may not be evident in standard radiographic images. For example, lateral condylar fractures of the McIII may be accompanied by a Y fragment at the articular margin that is detectable only in dorsodistal-palmaroproximal oblique images.

Fractures on an articular margin are called *chip fractures*. In some locations, such as the antebrachiocarpal and middle carpal joints, it is important to assess the radiographs carefully for evidence of preexisting osteoarthritis, which would have predisposed to the fracture and may influence the prognosis. The veterinarian should bear in mind that more than one chip may exist.

Chip fractures of the articular margins should be differentiated where possible from separate centers of ossification, avulsion fractures that occurred in the neonatal period, and ectopic mineralization. The position of the mineralized body relative to the articular margin, the size and shape of the body, and the contour of the articular margin should all be assessed carefully. A recent chip fracture may have a sharp edge, and a detectable fracture bed from which it originated may be seen. Separate centers of ossification usually are well rounded and uniformly opaque with no discernible fracture bed. It is important to recognize that such pieces may be clinically silent, but some are associated with lameness. The clinical significance must be interpreted in the light of clinical signs and the response to diagnostic analgesia. Ectopic mineralization may be present within the joint capsule.

Osteochondral fragments, the result of osteochondritis dissecans, should not be confused with a fracture. Osseous fragments may be seen, for instance, distal to the trochleas of the talus at the entrance to the talocalcaneal-centroquartal (proximal intertarsal) joint. These fragments may have originated from the distal (cranial) aspect of the intermediate ridge of the tibia and usually are of no clinical significance. Well-rounded, smoothly marginated osseous opacities may be seen on the proximoplantar aspect of the proximal phalanx. These may be the result of avulsion fractures of the short, deep cruciate sesamoidean ligaments that were sustained early in life; they are not always clinically significant but may compromise performance at maximum levels. The variably present first and fifth carpal bones should not be mistaken for fractures.

In some joints, it may not be possible to determine radiologically the origin of a fracture fragment. For example, fragments in the femorotibial joint frequently are not associated with any detectable disruption in bone outlines, and only arthroscopic evaluation of the joint allows determination of the origin. It also may not be possible to determine whether an accompanying soft tissue pathological condition exists. A fracture of the medial intercondylar eminence of the tibia may occur alone. The prognosis is good with surgical removal. Sometimes, however, concurrent cranial cruciate ligament damage exists at its insertion cranial to the eminence, resulting in a much more guarded prognosis.

A slab fracture is a fracture that extends from one joint surface to another (e.g., from the proximal to the distal aspect of the third carpal bone or central or third tarsal bones). These fractures can be extremely difficult to detect in the acute stage if not displaced.

In some locations, determination of the origin of a fracture fragment is facilitated by ultrasonographic examination. For example, a fragment on the palmar aspect of the fetlock may be an avulsion fracture of the insertion of the palmar annular ligament on the proximal sesamoid bone, and this is readily confirmed ultrasonographically.

Fracture healing depends on many factors, including the age of the horse, its nutritional and metabolic status, the site and stability of the fracture, the presence or absence of periosteum or infection, and the blood supply to the bone. After initial mineral resorption along the fracture line and formation of fibrous callus, calcified periosteal and endosteal callus develop. The amount and quality of callus that develops depends on the degree of stability at the fracture site and the presence or absence of infection. If a fracture is stable, either because it is incomplete or because it has been stabilized by internal fixation, healing is predominantly by primary union and endosteal reaction with minimal periosteal callus. Instability results in the development of periosteal callus.

The fracture may become stable long before the fracture line disappears radiologically. Healing may be complete within 6 to 12 weeks, with progressive narrowing and ultimate disappearance of the fracture line. However, healing of some fractures takes considerably longer. A horse may be sound and able to withstand full work despite the persistence of a radiolucent fracture line. In some locations (e.g., lateral condylar fractures of the McIII) a persistent lucent line may be associated with recurrent and persistent pain.

Some bones tend to heal by fibrous union, resulting in a persistent lucent line. These include the accessory carpal bone, the proximal and distal sesamoid bones, and the distal phalanx. Unless a fracture of the navicular bone is stabilized by internal fixation, lucent areas tend to develop in the adjacent bone along the fracture line. These indicate a chronic fracture of the navicular bone of at least 6 to 8 weeks' duration.

If a fracture line persists beyond 6 months, it can be considered to be a delayed union. Sclerosis of the bone adjacent to the fracture line may be present, and the ends of the bone may be slightly flared. Delayed union is not uncommon, but nonunion is unusual in the horse except in those bones that tend to heal by fibrous union.

Aging of a fracture is not easy to determine radiologically with any accuracy. The presence of periosteal callus (Figure 15-9) indicates a fracture of at least 14 days' duration and often substantially longer. An acute fracture has very clearly

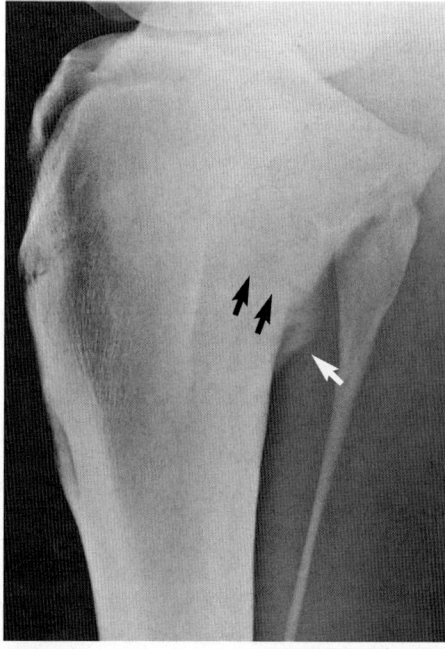

Fig. 15-9 • Craniolateral-caudomedial oblique radiographic image of the proximal aspect of the tibia of a 3-year-old Thoroughbred filly. Periosteal callus formation *(arrows)* on the caudoproximal aspect of the tibia is associated with a stress fracture. The oblique lucent line in the proximal aspect of the tibia is a nutrient foramen.

defined margins, which become less distinct as resorption occurs along the fracture line during early healing.

DEGENERATIVE JOINT DISEASE: OSTEOARTHROSIS OR OSTEOARTHRITIS

Arthritis means inflammation of a joint. The term *osteoarthritis* or *osteoarthrosis* indicates that bone has become involved and that a soft tissue component may *(-itis)* or may not *(-osis)* be present. The term *secondary joint disease* sometimes is used to denote that the degenerative changes are secondary to a known condition, such as infection or osteochondrosis. Any condition that damages cartilage, causes joint instability, or places abnormal forces on the joint may result in osteoarthritis. It may develop as a result of abnormal conformation or be the result of wear and tear on an athletic horse. However, advanced osteoarthritis sometimes is seen in relatively young horses with no identifiable predisposing cause.

Radiological abnormalities associated with osteoarthritis include the following:

- Periarticular osteophyte formation
- Narrowing of the joint space
- Subchondral lucent zones, either well or poorly defined
- Increased subchondral bone opacity (sclerosis); loss of trabecular pattern
- Thickening of the subchondral bone plate
- Joint capsule distention

However, it is important to recognize that in some joints advanced osteoarthritis may be present without any detectable radiological change. Periarticular osteophytes are not necessarily synonymous with clinically significant osteoarthritis. It is relatively unusual to see subchondral lucent zones in high-motion joints. These occur more commonly in the low-motion joints, such as the distal hock and proximal interphalangeal joints.

A relatively poor correlation exists between the degree of radiological change associated with osteoarthritis and the degree of pain and thus lameness. Advanced radiological change may be present when lameness is first recognized, which clearly must have predated the onset of recognizable clinical signs. In contrast, obvious lameness associated with joint pain may be present without detectable radiological change. Widespread wear lines may be present on the articular cartilage without associated radiological change.

Therefore dating the likely onset of clinical signs based on the radiological appearance of a joint can be difficult. It also can be difficult to predict the likely progression of minor radiological changes, such as small periarticular osteophytes, which may be present without clinical signs at, for example, a prepurchase examination.

LUXATION AND SUBLUXATION

Luxation is the complete loss of contact between articular surfaces. Subluxation is partial loss of contact between joint surfaces and may be intermittent. Both are usually the result of trauma, although congenital luxation of the patella occurs occasionally. Subluxation of the proximal interphalangeal joint may occur without any obvious cause, especially in hindlimbs. Subluxation is easy to identify radiologically, but the radiographs must be evaluated carefully to identify any concurrent fracture that will adversely influence prognosis.

Subluxation may not be obvious radiologically, and stress radiographs obtained with the limb not bearing weight, with pressure applied in a mediolateral or dorsopalmar direction, may be necessary to determine if the bones can be moved relative to each other.

DYSTROPHIC AND METASTATIC MINERALIZATION

Soft tissue mineralization is classified as metastatic or dystrophic. Metastatic mineralization is the deposition of mineral in normal tissues and is associated with hypercalcemia, hyperphosphatemia, or hypercalciuria and is unusual in the horse. Dystrophic mineralization is the deposition of mineral in injured, degenerating, or necrotic tissue and occurs quite commonly in the horse in, for example, a damaged SL. It can occur secondary to any injury to soft tissue subsequent to infarction, hemorrhage, or inflammation. Dystrophic mineralization may ultimately become ossified.

RADIOGRAPHIC EXAMINATION

For each joint or region to be examined there is a standard radiographic technique that includes a basic minimum number of views for routine evaluation of the region. This usually includes a minimum of four images for joints distal to the elbow and stifle. However, radiographic technique must be flexible. For example, if a fracture is suspected, various images differing only slightly in angle of projection may be required. Some fractures are visible only on special projections. For example, a fracture of the medial pole of the patella may be detected only in a cranioproximal-craniodistal oblique image. Exposure factors need to be altered depending on the size of the horse and the area being evaluated. Exposure factors ideal for assessing trabecular structure within medullary bone result in overexposure of immature periosteal new bone. Underexposure may result in a fracture line or alterations in corticomedullary demarcation and trabecular structure being missed.

It is also important to realize how position sensitive some radiological abnormalities are and how easily artifacts can be created. For example, the accurate evaluation of corticomedullary demarcation and trabecular structure within the navicular bone in a palmaroproximal-palmarodistal oblique image depends highly on the position of the limb and the angle of the x-ray beam. The optimum angle of the x-ray beam depends on the shape of the foot. Inappropriate positioning of the foot or use of an x-ray beam that is not tangential to the flexor surface of the navicular bone will result in artifacts.

The x-ray beam should be coned down on the area of interest as much as possible and centered on the area of interest. Lesions will be missed if an attempt is made to evaluate too much in a single image (e.g., the fetlock, pastern, and foot). It frequently is helpful to obtain comparative images of the contralateral limb. These should be obtained with identical exposure factors and similar positioning of the limb and angulation of the x-ray beam for accurate evaluation. Comparison of radiographs with a known normal example of similar age can also be helpful. It is thus useful to compile an image library of normal examples.

INTERPRETING RADIOGRAPHS

Radiographs should be evaluated in a systematic way. First, the quality of the radiographs should be assessed. Is the horse positioned appropriately? Are the radiographs of adequate quality? Are there any artifacts? The films should be viewed on a proper viewing box, both close to and from far away. The veterinarian should view the films under both normal and high-intensity illuminations, should interpret the entire film, and should follow all the bone margins and then evaluate the internal architecture. For computed or digital radiography the computer screen should be of high resolution and should be viewed in low-intensity light. The image should be windowed if necessary (i.e., alteration of brightness and contrast). The veterinarian should avoid lesion or disease spotting but aim to describe the radiological abnormalities and then deduce potential causes of the abnormality.

If a lesion is suspected but further information is required, the clinician should consider coning down, altering the exposure factors, slightly changing the angle of projection, or using special views. The radiographs should be compared with normal bone specimens, with an awareness that not all radiological abnormalities are necessarily of clinical significance. Knowledge of normal anatomy and normal variations is essential, together with knowledge of the sites of ligament, tendon, and joint capsule insertions.[1,2] Recognition of breed differences also is important.

References on page 1260

Radiological abnormalities must be interpreted in the light of clinical signs. It is also important to recognize that there are discipline differences in the potential clinical significance of some lesions. For example, mild osteoarthritis in the antebrachiocarpal or middle carpal joint may compromise the performance and career of a flat racehorse but be of little clinical significance for a show horse or low-level show jumper. It must also be recognized that it is often not possible to predict the future development of lesions. A horse with a small osteophyte on the dorsoproximal aspect of the third metatarsal bone may look identical in a later year, but a different horse may have developed extensive periarticular osteophytes involving both the centrodistal and tarsometatarsal joints.

Determining the Age of a Lesion

It is often not possible to accurately determine the age of a lesion that is identified radiologically. Periosteal new bone usually takes at least 14 days to be visible radiologically after trauma. Once new bone is well consolidated and smoothly marginated, it is impossible to determine how long it might have been present. A nondisplaced fracture may take up to 10 days to become evident radiologically; loss of clarity of the fracture margins may indicate that it has been present longer. Radiological changes compatible with osteoarthritis can precede the onset of clinical signs and may be relatively advanced when lameness is first recognized. It is not possible to determine when the changes first developed.

RADIOGRAPHIC TECHNIQUE

Standard radiographic projections are outlined in Table 15-1. For detailed descriptions of radiographic technique for all regions of the musculoskeletal system, readers are

TABLE 15-1

Standard Radiographic Projections and Suggested Extra Images		
REGION	NOTES ON RADIOGRAPHY	NOTES ON RADIOLOGY
	Front Feet	
LM	Center on position of navicular bone Angle the x-ray beam at a tangent to the bulbs of the heels Position the foot on a block so that the cassette can be placed lower than the solar surface of the foot Place a radiodense marker on the dorsal hoof wall with the proximal aspect at the coronary band to determine any possible deviation of the distal phalanx Soft exposures needed to see remodeling of distal phalanx	Variable shape of extensor process Small osseous opacities on the proximodorsal aspect of the distal phalanx may be clinically insignificant Smoothly outlined depression in sagittal ridge of navicular bone is normal
DPa	Place foot on a block Horizontal x-ray beam centered midway between the coronary band and the ground and aligned perpendicular to a tangent to the bulbs of the heels	Useful for assessing mediolateral balance and joint space width Mineralization of the cartilages of the foot (sidebone) rarely significant Mineralization of cartilages may be from separate centers, resulting in permanent lucent lines that are not fractures

TABLE 15-1

	Standard Radiographic Projections and Suggested Extra Images—cont'd	
REGION	**NOTES ON RADIOGRAPHY**	**NOTES ON RADIOLOGY**
DPr-PaDiO	Remove shoe and clean thoroughly Pack the frog clefts Different exposures needed for distal phalanx and navicular bone Avoid excessive flexion of the fetlock Dorsal hoof wall should be just in front of the vertical	Variable shape and size of crena of distal phalanx Variable smoothness of solar margins of distal phalanx Enthesophyte formation on proximolateral aspect of navicular bone a common finding in normal horses Seven or fewer small radiolucent zones along the distal border of navicular bone often normal
Pa 45° Pr-PaDiO	Remove shoe and clean foot Angle the x-ray beam according to heel height: if the heels are low, reduce the angle to 35-40° Position the foot to be examined behind the contralateral limb Center the beam between the bulbs of the heel	Artifacts (e.g., reduced corticomedullary demarcation) easily created by poor technique
Extra Views		
Flexed oblique images of interphalangeal joints (D 60° L-PaMO) or of palmar processes of distal phalanx (D 45° L-PaDiO)	Remove shoe and clean foot Pack frog clefts	Useful for detection of modeling changes of articular margins of DIP joint Essential for diagnosis of some distal phalangeal fractures
Hind Feet		
As for front feet, but easier to obtain PIPr-DDiO images of distal phalanx and navicular bone		
Pasterns		
LM		Entheseous new bone on the palmar aspect of the proximal phalanx is often seen without associated clinical signs A small spur on the dorsoproximal aspect of the middle phalanx is commonly seen in Warmblood breeds
DPa	Angle the x-ray beam downward, perpendicular to the pastern	Best view for evaluation of joint space narrowing
Flexed DL-PaMO and DM-PaLO	Flexed oblique images open up the proximal interphalangeal joint, allowing much better appreciation of the joint margins than in weight-bearing views	
Fetlocks		
LM or flexed LM	Flexed LM gives more information about the distal aspect of the sagittal ridge of the third metacarpal bone, supracondylar region, and articular margins of the proximal sesamoid bones For LM of hindlimb fetlock, angle the x-ray beam from 10 degrees plantar to a tangent to the bulbs of the heel	Well-rounded osseous fragments may be seen distal to the proximal sesamoid bones, which may be previous avulsions from either the palmar or the plantar aspect of the proximal phalanx or from the sesamoid bones
DPa or DPl	Angle the x-ray beam proximodistally at least 10° to avoid superimposition of the proximal sesamoid	The ergot is seen as a radiopaque area superimposed over the proximal bones over the joint phalanx
D 45° L-PaMO D 45° M-PaLO	Make sure the horse is standing with the cannon bone vertical, or in front of the vertical, so that the sesamoid bones are not superimposed over the proximal phalanx	Prominent lucent zones within the proximal sesamoid bones or entheseous new bone may reflect suspensory branch desmitis

Continued

TABLE 15-1

	Standard Radiographic Projections and Suggested Extra Images—cont'd	
REGION	NOTES ON RADIOGRAPHY	NOTES ON RADIOLOGY
Extra Views		
L 45° Pr-MDiO	Highlights the abaxial surface of the medial proximal sesamoid bone	
M 45° Pr-LDiO	Highlights the abaxial surface of the lateral proximal sesamoid bone	
D 30° Pr 70° L-PaDiMO	Useful for evaluation of the proximal articular margins and lateral palmar process of the proximal phalanx and projects the lateral proximal sesamoid bone distal to the medial proximal sesamoid bone	
D 30° Pr 70° M-PaDiLO	Useful for evaluation of the proximal articular margins of the proximal phalanx and medial palmar process of the proximal phalanx and projects the medial proximal sesamoid bone distal to the lateral proximal sesamoid bone	
D 45° Pr 45° L-PaDiMO	Useful for evaluation of the subchondral bone in the lateral condyle of the third metacarpal bone	
D 45° Pr 45° M-PaDiLO	Useful for evaluation of the subchondral bone of the medial condyle of the third metacarpal bone	
DPr-DDi (flexed)	Useful for evaluation of lesions of the subchondral bone of the condyles and sagittal ridge of the third metacarpal bone	
Tangential dorsopalmar views	Place foot flat on block and angle x-ray beam distoproximally at approximately 125° to the metacarpal region to highlight the palmar aspect of the condyles of the third metacarpal bone. Flexed dorsopalmar view moves proximal sesamoid bone further proximal; useful for detection of axial lesions of the sesamoid bones and some third metacarpal bone condylar fractures	
Metacarpal or Metatarsal Regions		
LM	Select images depending on region of interest	Variable degree of ossification of interosseous ligament
DL-PaMO	Several similar views with slightly different angles of projection may be useful	Nutrient vessels in second, third, and fourth metacarpal bones
DM-PaLO	Soft exposures needed for evaluation of periosteal new bone	Exostoses on second and fourth metacarpal bones common
DPa		
Carpus		
LM or flexed LM	Flexed LM opens up the intercarpal joints; the radial carpal bone drops down	Entheseous new bone on the dorsal aspect of the carpal bones common in horses that have raced
DL-PaMO		Lucent zones in the ulnar and second carpal bones are quite common
PaL-DMO		Presence of first and fifth carpal bones variable
Extra Views		
Flexed D 85° Pr-DDiO	Highlights the distal aspect of the radius	
Flexed D 55° Pr-DDiO	Highlights the proximal row of carpal bones	
Flexed D 35° Pr-DDiO	Highlights the distal row of carpal bones	
Radius		
LM		
CrL-CdMO	Views dictated by region under investigation	
CrM-CdLO		
CrCd		
Elbow		
ML	Protract the limb to be examined so that the olecranon is cranial to the contralateral pectoral muscles	

TABLE 15-1

Standard Radiographic Projections and Suggested Extra Images—cont'd		
REGION	**NOTES ON RADIOGRAPHY**	**NOTES ON RADIOLOGY**
CrCd	Rotate the cassette so that it can be held as high up under the thorax as possible	
Extra Views		
CrM-CdLO		

Shoulder

ML	Protract the limb to avoid superimposition of the scapulohumeral joints Use a grid	
Cr 45° M-CdLO		
Extra Views		
Skyline views of the humeral tubercles		

Hock

LM	Center at the level of the centrodistal joint and angle the x-ray beam 10° proximodistally to cut through the centrodistal joint space	The distal aspect of the medial trochlea of the talus has a protuberance that varies greatly in size, shape, and opacity
	Position the limb with the metatarsal region vertical	Small spurs on the dorsoproximal aspect of the third metatarsal bone are common
D 45° L-PlMO		
D 45° M-PILO		Best view for evaluating the distal (cranial) intermediate ridge of the tibia; small osseous fragments may not be of clinical significance
DPI	Because of the undulations of the centrodistal joint, a horizontal x-ray beam may not cut through all the joint space, and one side may look narrowed; repeat the view, angling the x-ray beam 5° proximodistally to determine if narrowing is real	The best view to assess joint space narrowing

Stifle

LM or flexed LM	Flexed LM image allows better evaluation of the patella and cranioproximal aspect of the tibia	Slight flattening of the lateral trochlear ridge of the femur in a mature horse may not be of clinical significance
Cd 15° Pr-CrDiO	Position the limb to be examined slightly caudal to the contralateral limb	The radiolucent lines between separate centers of ossification of the fibula should not be mistaken for fractures
Extra Views		
Flexed CrPr-CrDiO	Essential for identification of some patellar fractures	
CdL-CrMO	May provide more information about the trochleas of the femur	

Pelvis

VD in standing horse	Provides acceptable images of the ischium, caudal ilium, acetabulum, and femoral head and neck for detection of gross fractures	
VD with horse under general anesthesia		

Cervical Vertebrae

Lateral views only in standing horse	Keep the head and neck as straight as possible Use a grid	

Thoracolumbar Vertebrae

Lateral views	Horse should stand squarely, bearing weight evenly on all four limbs Evaluate the dorsal spinous processes, facet joints, and vertebral bodies separately	

Cd, Caudal; *Cr,* cranial; *D,* dorsal; *Di,* distal; *Pr,* proximal; *L,* lateral; *M,* medial; *O,* oblique; *Pa,* palmar; *Pl,* plantar; *Pr,* proximal; *V,* ventral.

referred to *Clinical Radiology of the Horse*.[3] Throughout this text, radiographic images are described using the technique advocated by the American College of Veterinary Radiology.[4]

All radiographs should be permanently labeled photographically on the film, by use of special tape attached to the cassette when the film is exposed, a labeling light box system in the darkroom, or a computer. Labels should include at least the identity of the horse, the date, the limb examined, and medial or lateral when appropriate. The following facts also are preferable on the label: the name of the owner or agent of the horse, the name of the veterinary practice, and the identity of the view (e.g., PaL-DMO). For ease of identification, it can be helpful if the horse's label is always positioned on the lateral aspect of the cassette or imaging plate; if a medial marker were omitted, it would then still be possible to differentiate between the medial and lateral sides.

Radiographs are part of the horse's permanent medical and legal record and should always be retained by the veterinary practice for future reference unless the owner of the horse gives permission for the radiographs to be transferred to another veterinary practice. Electronic or copy radiographs are easily produced if a client wishes to have his or her own copy.

Digital radiography generally uses imaging plates with a larger exposure latitude compared with traditional film-screen combinations. Therefore it is potentially easier to obtain good-quality images with a single exposure. With a computerized system the images can be manipulated to enhance contrast and magnify areas of interest; therefore lesions that might previously have been missed may be more readily identified. With an appropriate archiving system, all images can be stored digitally rather than printed. It is crucial that an adequate backup system be in place to protect against data loss. Digital radiography is not a substitute for good radiographic technique but offers the advantage of providing images that may be of superior quality and can be stored and transmitted electronically.

Chapter 16

Ultrasonographic Evaluation of the Equine Limb: Technique

Norman W. Rantanen, Joan S. Jorgensen, and Ronald L. Genovese

References on page 1260

Diagnostic ultrasonography was introduced in the early 1980s as a practical imaging modality to evaluate soft tissue injuries of the equine limb.[1] It continues to be used extensively for evaluation of tendonous and ligamentous structures to identify, confirm, and monitor soft tissue injury (Box 16-1).[2-8] Ultrasonography is now the imaging modality of choice for most soft tissue evaluation, but in the digit magnetic resonance imaging (MRI), if available, is most useful to evaluate soft tissues. However, it is user specific, and diagnostic information relies heavily on adequate equipment, limb preparation, and the scanning skills of the ultrasonographer. This chapter describes terminology and techniques and provides advice about interpretation based on our collective experiences. We describe our systematic approach, which includes both qualitative and quantitative ultrasonographic analysis of distal limb injuries. The resulting data can be used to categorize the severity of the injury and compare with subsequent examinations. The technology is still developing, and changes will evolve to improve the clinician's ability to identify and substantiate clinical findings, leading to improved management of soft tissue injury in the horse.

EQUIPMENT

Ultrasound machines used for musculoskeletal imaging require a range of transducer frequencies to examine superficial and deep structures. Soft tissues within 5 to 7 cm of the skin surface should be examined using a transducer with a frequency of at least 7.5 MHz or higher. Tissues within 7 to 15 cm of the skin surface are best evaluated with a 5.0-MHz transducer, whereas deeper tissues require a transducer in the 2.5- to 3.5-MHz range.

Sound is attenuated at 1 dB/cm depth per megahertz. Higher frequencies are attenuated at higher rates, thus limiting penetration. Conversely, lower frequencies, attenuated at lower rates, have greater penetration. The highest frequency possible should be used to obtain maximum resolution.

Claiming that one instrument is the only one to perform musculoskeletal examination is naive at best and totally inaccurate. All state-of-the-art machines have similar focusing capabilities and resolving power. Image appearances made by different machines at the same frequencies have subtle differences; however, resolution is about the

---

BOX 16-1

Indications for Ultrasonographic Evaluation of Limbs

- Diagnosis of soft tissue injuries, including muscular, vascular, tendon, tendon sheath, ligament, joint capsule, or bursal defects
- Assessment of fluid accumulation
- Evaluation of bony surfaces
- Monitoring of the healing progress
- Monitoring of the effect of training on soft tissue structures, especially tendons and ligaments

same. Images may appear more crisp from transducers with a greater number of elements. Operator proficiency (or lack of it) largely determines image quality.

Large muscle masses or bone surfaces, such as the pelvis, are more effectively scanned with phased array, convex array, annular array, or sector transducers. The small skin surface imprints and divergent beam are advantageous when tissues are imaged at greater depths. However, annular array and sector transducers have focal zones that usually favor the central portion of the beam and have beam divergence, which causes far-field, lateral beam width artifact. Convex and phased array transducers have electronic focusing, and the examiner can control focal zone number and placement. It is common for these transducers to penetrate up to 30 cm.

Linear array transducers are the most popular for tendon and ligament scanning because they facilitate anatomical recognition of structures and evaluation of longitudinal tendon and ligament fiber alignment parallel to the skin surface. Convex array and sector transducers, if used properly, work equally well. However, they are more difficult to use because it is easier to change the beam direction because of the smaller contact area. It is necessary to keep the beam at 90 degrees to the tendon or ligament fibers. Anatomical features may be more difficult to recognize. Standoff pads are essential with any transducer to image the most superficial structures.

Sector and microconvex array transducers are preferable for use on contoured skin surfaces. For instance, scanning between the heel bulbs is difficult with a flat-face, linear array transducer but simple with convex or sector transducers. It is easier to steer a divergent beam and look around from a smaller contact area compared with the flat-face, linear array transducer's broad contact area and rectangular sound beam.

Multiple frequency scanheads are available from most manufacturers; these scanheads allow operators to change frequencies relative to tissue depths without changing transducers. Newer broadband scanhead technology ensures quality, and there are no disadvantages in using these scanheads for musculoskeletal scanning, provided that basic ultrasound principles are practiced.

HORSE PREPARATION

The horse should be adequately restrained, because an anxious, fidgety horse may cause a hurried or inadequate examination, resulting in poor-quality images and interpretive errors. One author (RLG) prefers to sedate most horses that are not entered in drug-tested competition to ensure that the horse stands quietly during the examination. The horse should be held by a person who has responsibility for the safety of the ultrasonographer and the equipment. A calm, well-positioned horse allows a thorough, tension-free evaluation.

Hair, air, scurf, scabs, and dirt induce artifacts and reduce image quality. The hair should be clipped with a No. 40 or No. 50 blade then cleaned with an antiseptic scrub, followed by a generous rinse with water, taking care to follow the growth pattern of the hair. In some horses an additional close shave with a disposable razor may improve image quality. Acoustic coupling gel is applied to improve transducer contact. Excessive application of gel

causes a lateral image artifact that may impair assessment of the structures being examined, especially if peritendonous or periligamentous neural, vascular, and connective tissue structures are being evaluated. Removal of the excess gel from the transducer head or the limb corrects the artifact.

If the hair coat is fine and clipping or shaving is not possible or desired, then the limb can be washed. The examiner should spend some time wetting and soaking the hair to improve transducer contact. Topical application of alcohol while stroking the hair along its growth path may improve transducer contact,[5] but *alcohol can be harmful to some transducers*. The operator should contact the manufacturer of the equipment to ensure that it is safe to use the transducer with alcohol.

MEDICAL RECORDS

Ultrasonographic images should be recorded using thermal prints, video recording, or digital recording. Thermal images were used most commonly in the past, but digital recording is rapidly superseding them.

Thermal Print Storage Envelope

Practical hints and suggestions for medical record documentation that can simplify case records, enhance clinical information for serial studies, and improve documentation are provided in the following text. We recommend a simple form stamped on the outside of a storage envelope. The information on the envelopes can be quickly filled in using symbols or checkmarks and should include the following data: horse identification, date, owner, trainer, limb or limbs examined, and structure or structures evaluated (superficial digital flexor tendon [SDFT], deep digital flexor tendon [DDFT], accessory ligament of the DDFT [ALDDFT], main body of the suspensory ligament [SL], SL branch, pastern, hock, antebrachium, crus, and other). It is also useful to record exercise level, the reason the examination was performed, and a brief summary of clinical findings. This checklist indicates which structures have been targeted and assists in interpretation of an actual lesion versus an off-incidence angle artifact. This is especially helpful if the images are reassessed at a later time.

We have developed an alphanumerical system for ranking exercise levels (Box 16-2). The current exercise level may have an important impact on diagnosis, treatment, future exercise control, and prognosis. For instance, if a horse at pasture injured a SDFT, advising pasture rest would be contraindicated. A chart for ranking exercise levels can be duplicated easily, laminated, and taped to equipment for easy reference.

Clinical findings may be recorded concisely as follows:

Leg	Which Limb
S	Subcutaneous swelling on a scale of 0 to 5. This does not refer to tendonous or ligamentous enlargement.
L	Lameness on a scale of 0 to 5.
T	Thickening of a tendon or ligament on a scale of 0 to 5. This is independent of subcutaneous swelling.
Sen	Response to digital palpation of a tendon or ligament on a scale of 0 to 5.

H	Heat or skin temperature on a scale of 0 to 5.
TS	Distention of the digital flexor tendon sheath (DFTS) (tenosynovitis) on a scale of 0 to 5.
AS	Fetlock sinking (hyperextension of the metacarpophalangeal joint), either at rest or during movement, on a scale of 0 to 5.
Qualitative diagnosis	Comments on preliminary qualitative ultrasonographic interpretation.
New	Whether this is the first time this horse has been examined ultrasonographically for this complaint.
Re-Ck	A recheck of a previous injury.
Normal leg	This indicates which is the clinically normal limb, which may not be normal ultrasonographically. It is strongly recommended that both limbs be examined routinely.
Both abn	Both limbs are clinically abnormal.

Image Labeling

All ultrasonographic images should be labeled with the date of examination, the horse's name, the owner's or trainer's name, the limb being examined, and the location of the image. In addition, it is helpful to include the age, breed, and use of the horse and the current exercise level. Most machines automatically record the frequency of the transducer and the focal zone. If digital recording is used, a system of image backup is essential.

EXERCISE LEVELS

One of the basic concepts in the management of horses with tendon and ligament injuries is to relate increasing levels of exercise to increases in tendon and ligament loading. For instance, walking a Thoroughbred (TB) racehorse in hand results in far less SDFT loading (stretching) than racing at 35 mph. Understanding the current exercise level is important in interpretation of ultrasonographic information and advising management programs for controlled exercise during rehabilitation from an injury (see Box 16-2).

For example, if a TB racehorse with a SDFT injury of 4 months' duration were reexamined and the SDFT showed little improvement, despite box or stall rest, the veterinarian would conclude that the repair was of poor quality with a poor prognosis for a return to racing. However, if the horse had been turned out for 6 hours a day with other horses that ran around, the delayed healing would be interpreted as being caused by too much tendon loading and the lack of improvement would be attributed to low-level ongoing injury. The client would be advised to reduce the exercise level and would be given a somewhat more positive outlook for future racing soundness.

In the rehabilitation of a tendon or ligament injury, the odd exercise level numbers result in the most salient changes in tendon or ligament loading. Exercise level 1 is limited to walking, resulting in little structure loading, whereas exercise level 3 is a major step up in exercise and structure loading because it allows free movement of the horse. Exercise level 5 signals the return to active training. Finally, exercise level 7 is the ultimate goal of rehabilitation and is the return to maximal athletic use. During rehabilitation the ultrasonographer assesses the current

morphological status of a structure and advises changes in exercise levels consistent with those findings. Readily available and definable exercise levels make exercise decisions more efficient and consistent.

SCANNING TECHNIQUE

The basic objective of an ultrasonographic evaluation is to characterize the morphological characteristics of the soft

---

BOX 16-2

Exercise Level Grading Scale

Exercise Level	Type of Exercise Allowed
0	Complete stall rest.
1A	Handwalk for 15 to 30 minutes once a day.
1B	Handwalk ≥30 minutes a day or walk on a mechanical walker. We believe horses usually are more active walking on a mechanical walker than in hand.
2A	Thoroughbred (TB) and Standardbred (STB) racehorse, event horse (EV), and sports horse (SH): exercise level 1A/B plus trotting in hand for 5 to 10 minutes a day.
2B	TB racehorse, SH, and EV: trot under saddle 10 to 15 minutes once a day or swim.
	STB racehorses: walk only in the bike or swim.
	This level also includes 10 to 15 minutes of trotting on a treadmill.
3A	Small paddock turnout for all horses. Small paddock implies small enough not to be able to work up to a sustained canter or gallop.
3B	Large paddock turnout for all horses.
4A	TB and SH: 15 to 20 minutes a day of walk, trot, and canter under saddle, 3 days per week, plus any of the above levels. This level does not apply to most STBs.
4B	TB: 20 to 30 minutes a day of walk, trot, and canter under saddle, 3 to 4 days a week.
	TB racehorse: "ponying" (being led from another horse) on the racetrack. This level does not apply to most STBs.
5	TB racehorse and EV: all of the above plus normal galloping.
	STB racehorse: all of the above plus jogging.
	SH: all of the above plus normal arena flat work with limited low fence jumping where applicable.
	Dressage horses: normal work minus lateral movements and special gaits.
6	TB racehorse: all of the above plus faster gallops.
	EV: all of the above plus jumping.
	STB racehorse: all of the above plus training miles ≥2 : 10.
	SH: all of the above plus unlimited low fence jumping where applicable.
	Dressage: all of the above plus lateral movements and special gaits.
	Contest horses (reiners, cutters, and so on): all of the above plus practicing specific turns and movements.
7	In essence, this is the maximal work level for any type of athletic horse.
	TB and EV: racing, fast works, and competing.
	STB racehorse: training miles <2 : 10 and racing.
	SH: showing, jumping, hunting, and so on.
	Dressage and contest horses: competing.

tissue structures and bony surfaces of each designated anatomical area. Although physical examination findings may direct the clinician's attention to a specific structure, a thorough examination of all soft tissue and bone surface structures is imperative. In many instances, lesions in more than one anatomical region may be identified and often result in a completely different recuperation regimen. To avoid off-incidence artifacts, the ultrasound beam must be perpendicular to the target structure. Although more than one structure may be perpendicular to the ultrasound beam simultaneously in either transverse or longitudinal images, often it is necessary to redirect the ultrasound beam to adequately examine all structures at each level. Initially the limb should be systematically examined from proximal to distal to assess the morphological features of the vasculature, periligamentous and peritendonous tissue, tendons, and ligaments. Once specific abnormal or normal structures are identified, each tendon or ligament is analyzed systematically by ultrasonographically targeting the transducer to the structure at each zone and simultaneously documenting the scan on tape, on print record, or by electronic storage.

ARTIFACTS

Artifacts can cause major problems with any imaging modality but are especially prevalent with ultrasonography because the operator steers the ultrasound beam and sets the instrument parameters. Three primary artifact sources are common with diagnostic ultrasonography: operator error, ultrasound–tissue interaction, and inherent instrument design artifacts. Nothing can be done about the limitations of the imaging system except to recognize the artifacts in special scanning situations. Sound–tissue interaction creates myriad artifacts, some of which are useful and help with diagnosis. Others are annoying and can be difficult to overcome. Readers are referred to several publications that address the majority of artifacts peculiar to ultrasonography.[9-14] Operator error and ultrasound–tissue interactions are discussed further.

Operator Errors

Inadequate Skin Preparation

Excessively long or dirty hair and unclean skin attenuate the ultrasound beam and produce image artifacts. Improper scanhead coupling to the skin caused by a lack of gel or the presence of scabs or scurf is common (Figure 16-1). Artifacts created by improper skin preparation result from poor contact. Images may be dark even though gain settings may be set at the highest limits. The tendons do not have a fine texture and are more grainy or mottled than normal. Tendon margins may not be seen, and reverberation artifacts caused by trapped air within the hair may appear within images, especially if standoff pads are used. Hypoechogenic streaks may be present in the images.

Ultrasound Beam Angle

Reflection of the ultrasound beam is dependent on the sound-interface and tissue-interface geometry. Ideally the ultrasound beam should strike tissue interfaces at 90 degrees to produce the best echo reflection back to the transducer crystals, which also act as receivers. If the beam

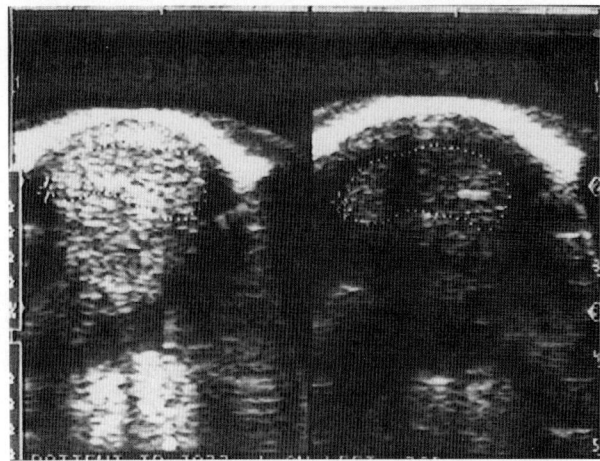

Fig. 16-1 • Transverse ultrasonographic images of the palmar metacarpal region. Improper skin preparation causes artifacts within the image on the right.

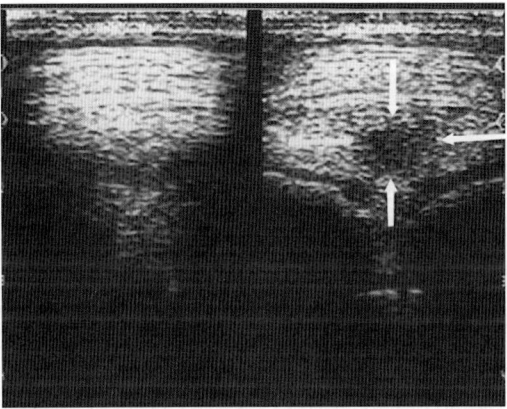

Fig. 16-2 • Transverse ultrasonographic images of the distal palmar aspects of the metacarpal region. The left deep digital flexor tendon image has a normal tendon fiber pattern. The right image has an apparent central core artifact *(arrows)* that was produced by slightly changing the angle of the ultrasound beam.

strikes a tissue interface at a smaller angle, a portion of the ultrasound is reflected away from the primary beam direction, and the interface is not seen as well or at all. This is especially important in the evaluation of tendons and ligaments in the metacarpal and metatarsal regions because the fibers usually are parallel to the skin. If the ultrasound sound beam is not perpendicular to a tendon in a transverse image, information is lost, and hypoechogenic areas, which mimic lesions, are created (Figure 16-2). The problem is not seen in longitudinal images of the metacarpal or metatarsal region obtained using a linear array transducer because its surface is parallel to the fibers. However, with convex array and sector transducers that have divergent ultrasound beams, there are only small areas within longitudinal tendon fiber images in which valid information is found (Figure 16-3). In the divergent area of the beam, sound is reflected away from the beam path and is lost to the image. It is important not to confuse these areas with pathological conditions of the tendon or ligament. The ultrasound beam must be positioned parallel to the tendon fibers. Normal tendon or ligament fibers should be seen as

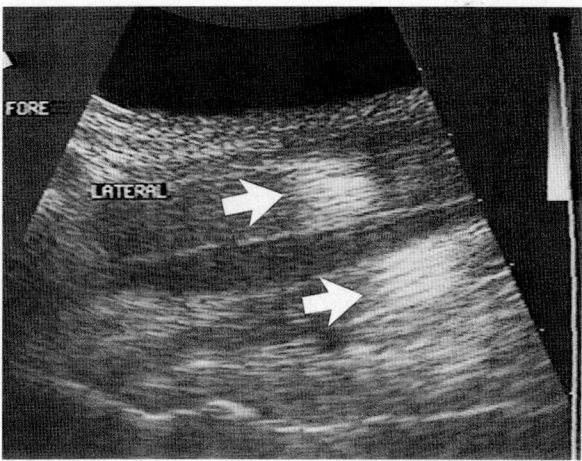

Fig. 16-3 • Longitudinal ultrasonographic image of the proximal metacarpal region. The arrows point to tendon and ligament sections where the ultrasound beam is at 90 degrees, which allows the fibers to be seen. The remaining parts of the image provide no diagnostic information.

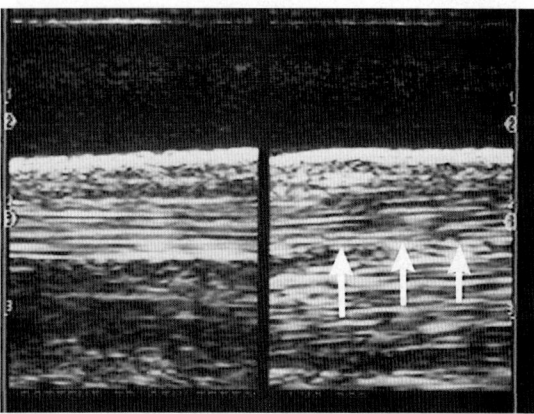

Fig. 16-4 • Longitudinal ultrasonographic images of the palmar metacarpal region. The left image was obtained with a linear array transducer parallel to the tendon fibers. The right image was obtained with the transducer slightly oblique to the tendon fibers, causing them to appear as short segments instead of continuous fiber strands *(arrows)*.

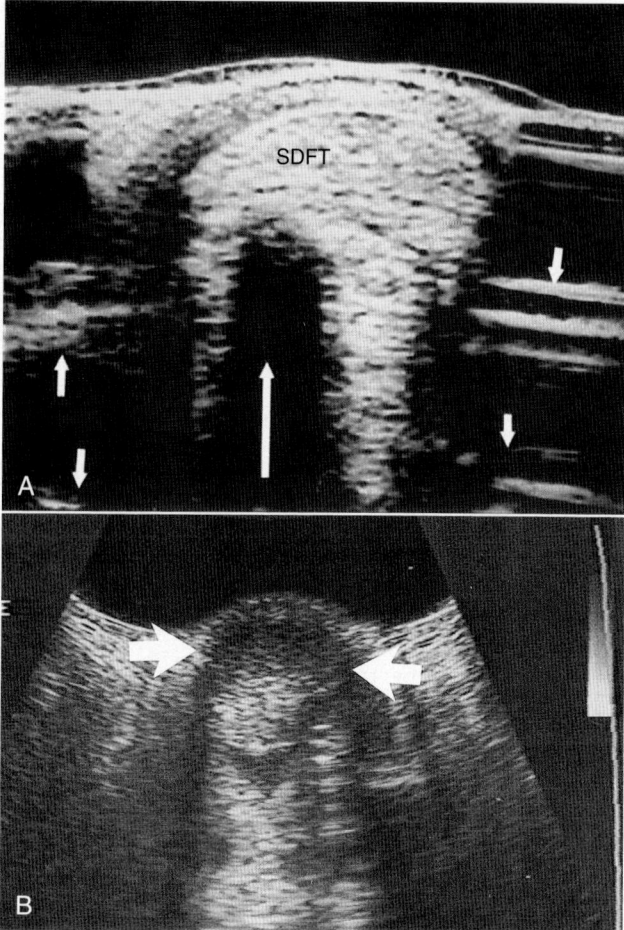

Fig. 16-5 • **A,** Transverse sector scan ultrasonographic image of the palmar metacarpal region with the near gain set too high. The superficial digital flexor tendon (SDFT) echoes are too bright and cannot be differentiated. Acoustic shadowing *(large arrow)* is caused by flexor tendon and reverberation artifacts caused by the standoff pad *(small arrows)*. **B,** The near gain was set too low, so the SDFT cannot be seen *(arrows)*.

continuous linear echogenic structures across the image (Figure 16-4). If the transducer is turned slightly, the fibers appear as short linear segments as the beam cuts obliquely across the longitudinal axis. Because fiber alignment is an important criterion to assess in diagnosis and rehabilitation of tendon and ligament injuries, care must be taken to not create this artifact.

Improper Gain Settings

Ultrasound machines have gain settings referred to as *overall, near,* and *far gain*. As ultrasound penetrates normal soft tissues, it is attenuated at the rate of 1 dB/cm of tissue thickness per megahertz. Obesity and dehydration cause greater attenuation and can limit penetration. Because energy is lost from the ultrasound beam as it passes into the tissues, the instrument gain must be increased to allow echo detection from the deeper tissue depths. Overall gain changes the brightness and darkness over the entire image. The near-gain adjustment affects the echoes closest to the

transducer. Increasing the near gain brightens the echoes, and decreasing it darkens them. The far gain affects the deeper aspect of the image. Some machines display a time-gain compensation curve at the side of the screen. Adjustment of the gain settings should produce an image in which the gray scale is similar over the entire image. Bright whites in the near field should prompt decreasing the near gain; conversely, if echoes are difficult to see, increase in the gain is necessary (Figure 16-5). Improper near-gain settings are the most common error in settings. Visibility of far-field echoes is enhanced by far-gain increases.

Improper Focal Zone Use

Before the advent of moveable and multiple focal zones, transducers had fixed focal points and well-defined focal zones. The ultrasound beam was narrowest in the focal zone in which the lateral resolution produced the best image quality. If the tissues of interest were outside the focal zone, image quality was not ideal. Use of transducers with appropriate focal zones became necessary. If a sector transducer is used to image the SDFT, a standoff pad is necessary to place the tendon in the focal zone. Variable focal zones have eliminated this problem and allow focal

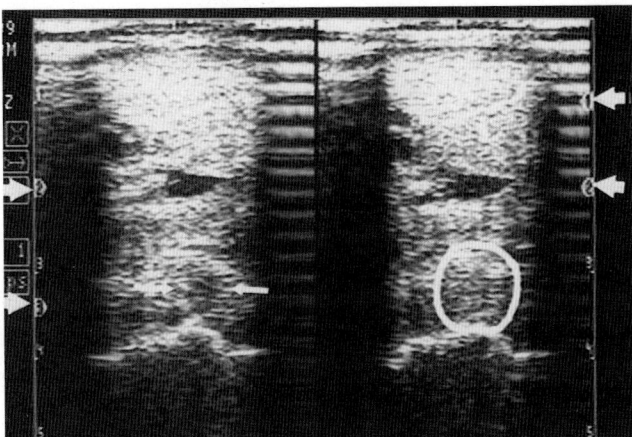

Fig. 16-6 • Transverse ultrasonographic images of the proximal metacarpal region. A focal lesion in the suspensory ligament *(arrows)* is visible on the left image. The lesion disappears *(circle)* in the right image because the focal zones are improperly placed. Arrows in the left and right margins point out the focal zone levels.

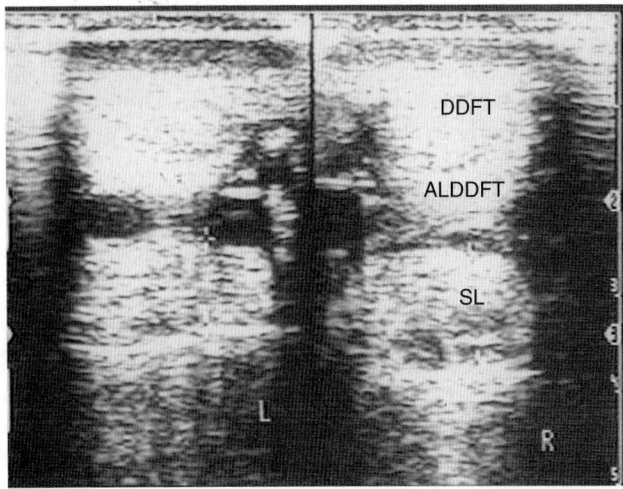

Fig. 16-7 • Transverse ultrasonographic images of the metacarpal region obtained without a standoff pad showing the deep digital flexor tendon (DDFT), accessory ligament of the DDFT (ALDDFT), and the suspensory ligament (SL). The brightness is set too high, causing tendon fiber detail loss.

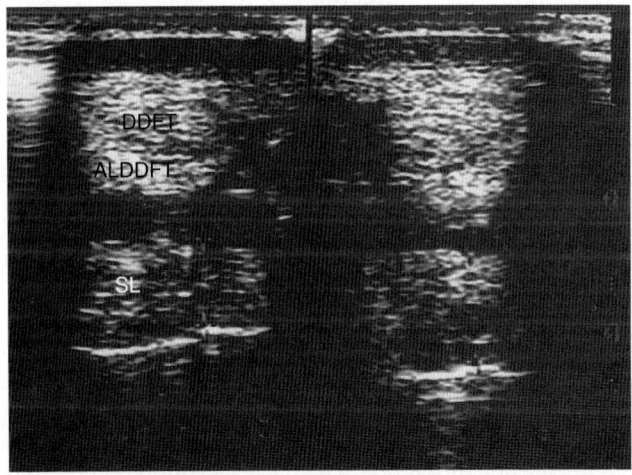

Fig. 16-8 • Transverse ultrasonographic images of the metacarpal region obtained without a standoff pad showing the deep digital flexor tendon *(DDFT)*, accessory ligament of the DDFT *(ALDDFT)*, and the suspensory ligament *(SL)*. The brightness is set too low, causing the image to be too dark.

zone placement throughout the image depth. Modern linear array and convex array transducers have multiple and moveable focal zones. However, they need to be set in the proper locations to investigate the areas of suspected abnormality. If the focal zones are not placed properly, clinically significant tendon and ligament fiber damage can be overlooked (Figure 16-6).

Incorrect Frequency Transducer

Tissue depth dictates the optimal transducer frequency. Tissues within 5 to 7 cm of the skin surface should be examined with a 7.5-MHz or higher-frequency transducer. A 5.0-MHz transducer is required to examine tissues from 7 to 12 and up to 15 cm (depending on the instrument), and a 3.0-MHz or lower-frequency transducer is necessary for tissues 15 to 30 cm deep.

Imaging the digital flexor tendons or SL with a transducer of 5.0 MHz or less results in major compromise of image quality because of lateral beam width artifact. Two types of resolution are peculiar to ultrasound. Resolution along the beam axis, or axial resolution, is frequency dependent; the higher the frequency, the better the axial resolution. Resolution in the transverse plane, or lateral resolution, is dependent on the width of the ultrasound beam; the better the focusing or sound beam narrowing, the better the lateral resolution. Smaller crystals produce narrower sound beams, hence increased lateral resolution. A transducer with a minimum frequency of 7.5 MHz should be used for superficial tendons and ligaments for best axial and lateral resolution.

Recording Images

Thermal printers were the most popular method for recording ultrasonographic images, and some are still in use. Brightness may be set too high, causing echoes to have no differentiating characteristics (Figure 16-7), or set too low, causing the image to be too dark (Figure 16-8). The same problem occurs with contrast settings; too high a setting causes excessive contrast, and too low a setting causes the image to be washed out and too dark.

It is important to consult the instruction manual to ensure that the image parameters are set properly. Proper settings also are necessary for the paper type. Interpreting improperly recorded (suboptimal) images causes substantial diagnostic error. Images must be assessed for photographic quality to preclude overlooking of lesions or overinterpretation. Suboptimal images should be repeated to preclude inaccurate interpretation and misdiagnosis. Images should always be frozen before capture.

Recording digital images on floppy disks was an effective way to capture all of the information. Depending on the system, images were recorded in bitmap (BMP) or Joint Photographic Experts Group (JPEG) formats. These were archived on hard drives and could be sent by e-mail if desired. External image capture devices functioned well, and some instruments with internal floppy drives are still in use. Digital archiving is now becoming routine. Various video formats, including video home system (VHS), 8-mm, S-Video, cineloop, and videodisk formats, are used to record motion. Recording static tissue (e.g., tendon) studies while moving the scanhead during recording can produce errors if the transducer is moved too rapidly for the frame rate to keep pace. Tendon examinations should be performed at relatively slow frame rates, as low as 7 per second, if multiple focal zones are activated. Moving the scanhead too fast causes ghosting of the image that blurs the anatomy. Activating multiple focal zones and the resultant slow frame rate can cause a similar problem with minimal scanhead movement.

Standoff Pads

Standoff pads are necessary when scanning structures near the skin, such as the SDFT and SL branches. Artifacts are produced each time they are used and can compromise image quality. It is important to recognize them. Transducers with built-in fluid standoff devices are no different. The artifacts are caused by reverberation within the standoff material and occur at a depth equaling the pad thickness (see Figure 16-5), which may obscure detail. For instance, examination of SL branches with a standoff pad can place artifacts in or near the axial border of the SL. This technique can obscure small axial border tears that are fairly common in horses. If the standoff pad thickness produces interfering artifacts, the SL branch should be examined with and without a standoff pad.

Ultrasound Tissue Interaction Artifacts (Horse-Produced Artifacts)

Ultrasonographic images are composed of returning echoes from many tissue interfaces, regardless of whether they are real or artifact. Some artifacts are useful in diagnosis and provide clues to tissue composition. Others are annoying and do not contribute to the diagnosis. Echoes are generated at tissue interfaces because of differences in acoustic impedance. Acoustic impedance is the product of tissue density (grams per cubic centimeter) and sound propagation velocity (meters per second). Substantial changes in either parameter produce acoustic barriers proportional to the magnitude difference, which causes sound reflection at the interface. Higher (brighter) amplitude echoes are created by greater acoustic impedance differences at tissue interfaces.

Skin Surface Contact

Debris and air trapped in the hair create large acoustic impedance differences and do not allow adequate sound penetration (see Figure 16-1).

Acoustic Enhancement

Whenever ultrasound passes through nonattenuating tissues, such as fluid with few or no interfaces, a slight increase in ultrasound intensity occurs in addition to less attenuation. The adjacent tissues attenuate the ultrasound normally. This causes brighter (enhanced) echoes deep to the less attenuating tissues. A good example is the enhancement seen deep to the metacarpal and metatarsal blood vessels. The SL has brighter echoes deep to the blood vessels, whereas between the blood vessels it is less echogenic (darker); it is tempting to interpret such results as abnormal (Figure 16-9). This is an inherent, tissue-produced artifact that can lead to interpretation errors but may help identify less attenuating areas within tissues such as muscle.

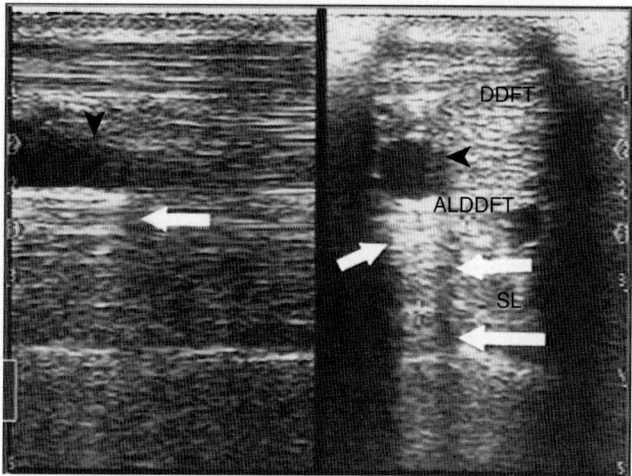

Fig. 16-9 • Longitudinal ultrasonographic image *(left)* and transverse ultrasonographic image *(right)* of the metacarpal region obtained without a standoff pad showing the deep digital flexor tendon *(DDFT)*, accessory ligament of the DDFT *(ALDDFT)*, and the suspensory ligament *(SL)*. The tissue brightness *(short arrows)* increases deep to the blood vessels. An anechoic line *(arrows)* extends deep to the blood vessels *(arrowheads)*.

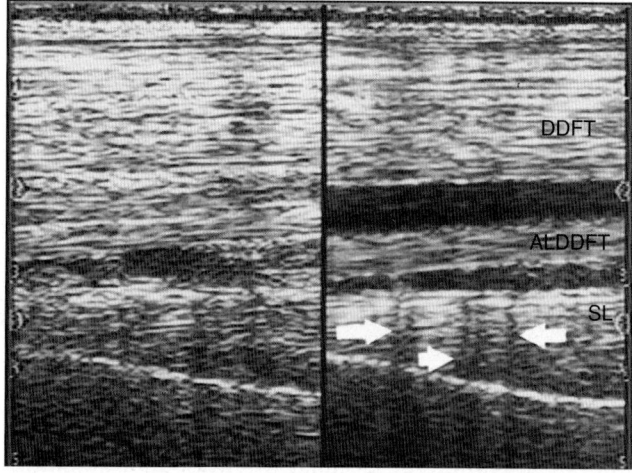

Fig. 16-10 • Longitudinal ultrasonographic images of the proximal palmar metacarpal region. Proximal is to the left. Refractive scattering *(arrows)* caused by the veins between the origin of the suspensory ligament *(SL)* and the accessory ligament of the deep digital flexor tendon *(ALDDFT)*. *DDFT,* Deep digital flexor tendon.

Refractive Scattering

If the ultrasound beam is not perpendicular to a tissue interface, hypoechogenic artifacts are caused by refraction. These artifacts can be a major problem in assessing the origin of the SL because of the anastomotic veins between it and the ALDDFT (Figure 16-10). The curved blood vessel walls create hypoechogenic lines that extend deep to the vessel walls in transverse images (see Figure 16-9). This is called *refractive scattering* and should not be misinterpreted as a lesion.

Acoustic Shadowing

A high acoustic impedance difference blocks the ultrasound beam and causes an anechogenic shadow deep to the reflecting interface. Bone and other mineralized tissue are much denser than soft tissues, and the sound propagation velocity is much faster. This creates an impenetrable acoustic barrier, and characteristically the reflector surface has bright echoes and the deeper tissues cannot be seen. These artifacts are useful because they identify soft tissue mineralization (see Figure 16-5). Bone surfaces are easily recognized because of shadowing. Dense scar tissue may create incomplete shadowing.

Reverberation
Reflection of ultrasound back and forth to the transducer from high acoustic impedance interfaces produces reverberation artifacts. The classic example is an air-filled lung surface that produces characteristic concentric reverberation echoes. Reverberation artifacts are not a major problem in tendon and ligament scanning; however, they can be important in certain circumstances. Gas production by anaerobic bacteria and air accidentally injected during diagnostic analgesia are two examples in which reverberation can be found in soft tissues. Standoff pads also create reverberation artifacts (see Figure 16-5).

Mirror Image Artifacts
Mirror image artifacts are not common problems in musculoskeletal ultrasonography and are more common in thoracic and abdominal scanning. They usually are found deep to interfaces that are highly reflective, such as air-filled lung.

Future Technology
Speckle reduction software, cross-beam scanning techniques, and the use of tissue harmonics are changing the appearance of ultrasound images. The images are smoother and lack the historically present "grainy" appearance that is common to ultrasound images. These innovations are gradually being accepted in medical imaging but are still relatively new. Some machines allow viewing the cross-beam imaging in a split-screen format with the original "grainy" images. This allows users to compare the two and to become familiar with the newer innovations. Off-axis or off-incidence scanning techniques that help to differentiate fluid from scar tissue within connective tissue structures have recently been introduced into veterinary imaging as well. With these newer technologies, artifacts peculiar to them will be defined as they find their place in medical and veterinary imaging.

TERMINOLOGY AND QUANTITATIVE MEASUREMENTS
The basis of diagnosis is to determine the morphological variation from normal, which is not always easy. The goal is to determine the size, shape, echogenicity, fiber pattern, and surrounding inflammatory reaction of any structure. These findings should be considered carefully in conjunction with clinical impressions and the current athletic use of the horse. Box 16-3 lists parameters used for characterizing tendon and ligament lesions.[15]

Echogenicity
Echogenicity refers to the whiteness or brightness of a structure. Each tendon and ligament has a characteristic

---

BOX 16-3

Parameters Used for Characterizing Tendon and Ligament Lesions

- Region or location of the lesion
- Length of the lesion
- Alteration in echogenicity
- Pattern of altered echogenicity (i.e., homogeneous, heterogeneous, focal, and diffuse)
- Alteration of fiber pattern in longitudinal images
- Percent of cross-sectional area of tendon injury
- Changes in the character of the lesion over time

BOX 16-4

Type Scores

Score	Description
0	Isoechogenic
1	Slightly hypoechogenic; mostly echogenic
2	Mixed echogenicity (50% echogenic and 50% anechogenic)
3	Mostly anechogenic or anechogenic

---

echogenic pattern at specific anatomical sites. Lesions vary in echogenicity depending on morphological consistency at the time of the examination. A scoring system can be used to improve objectivity when assessing the severity of an injury or the response to therapy (Box 16-4). Such a system may improve case management and illustrate to the client the changes in echogenicity that correlate with repair of an injury.

The following terms are used to describe ultrasound images (bear in mind that a tissue creates/generates echos and is echogenic; a normal tendon is isoechogenic; a lesion on an ultrasonographic image may appear anechoic because the damaged tendon tissue is anechogenic):

Isoechoic	The echogenicity of the structure is normal and is scored as 0.
Hypoechoic	The lesion is less than isoechoic. There are two categories of reduced echogenicity defined under the term *hypoechoic*. The first is gray or slightly off-white. This is a type 1 lesion (Figure 16-11). If the lesion is of mixed black and white tones, it is scored as a type 2 hypoechoic lesion (Figure 16-12).
Anechoic	The lesion is mostly black, a type 3 lesion.
Hyperechoic	Denoix[8] grades hyperechoic lesions as hyperechoic 1, which indicates that the lesion is brighter than isoechoic and represents dense scar tissue without an acoustic shadow. Hyperechoic 2 lesions (see Figure 16-5) represent soft tissue mineral deposition, which is characterized by casting an acoustic shadow. These echo patterns are uncommon and are generally seen in long-standing and repetitively injured tendons and ligaments.

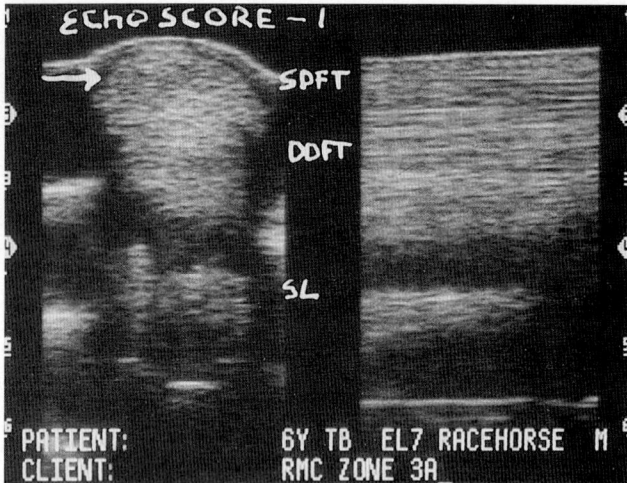

Fig. 16-11 • Transverse *(left)* and longitudinal *(right)* ultrasonographic images of zone 3A of the metacarpal region obtained using a standoff pad. A type 1 hypoechoic lesion is present in the superficial digital flexor tendon (SDFT) *(arrow)*. (See text for zone descriptions.) *DDFT,* Deep digital flexor tendon; *SL,* suspensory ligament.

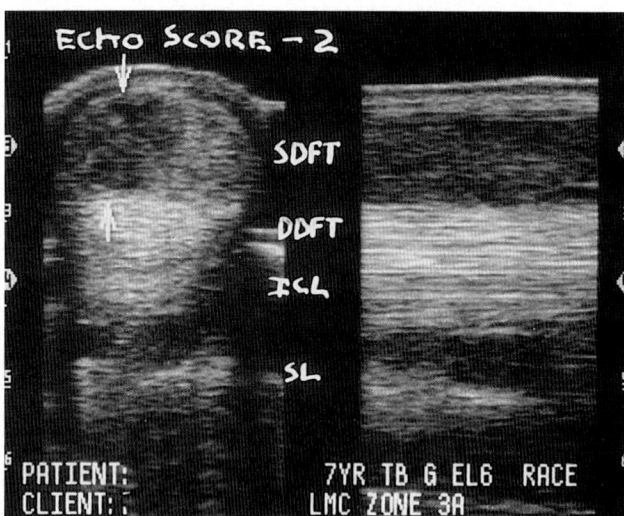

Fig. 16-12 • Transverse *(left)* and longitudinal *(right)* ultrasonographic images of zone 3A of the metacarpal region. A type 2 hypoechoic lesion is present in the superficial digital flexor tendon *(SDFT; arrows)*. *DDFT,* Deep digital flexor tendon; *ICL,* inferior check ligament (accessory ligament of the deep digital flexor tendon); *SL,* suspensory ligament.

Fiber Alignment Pattern Assessment

Assessment of fiber bundle alignment in longitudinal images determines the nature of a tendon's or ligament's fiber arrangement. Normally the fibers are aligned in parallel except in some anatomical areas, such as the origin of the hindlimb SL. When injury occurs, the expected parallel fiber pattern is disrupted. During healing of an injury, random orientation and cross-linking of new collagen fibers may create scar tissue that results in a substantial improvement in echogenicity but constitutes a poor scaffold for parallel alignment of fibers. Parallel alignment is more physiologically advantageous than random orientation of a scar, because randomly oriented scar tissue is susceptible to reinjury, especially during increased exercise. In a new injury or reinjury, longitudinal images are used

BOX 16-5		
Fiber Alignment Scoring		
Score	**Definition**	
0	Target path ≥75% parallel	
1	Target path 50% to 75% parallel	
2	Target path 25% to 50% parallel	
3	Target path ≤25% parallel	

to confirm the presence of a lesion identified in transverse images. When monitoring repair, fiber alignment can be assessed.

The longitudinal image must be obtained through the area of fiber bundle compromise to accurately assess the lesion. This is easy if a large proportion of the cross-sectional area (CSA) is involved. If a lesion is small or located on the margins of a tendon or ligament, it is more difficult. It is important to remember that fiber alignment, *not* echogenicity, is being assessed. In some instances, such as new injuries or reinjuries in the SDFT, the echogenic and fiber alignment scores (FASs) may be the same. This is rarely true for SL injuries.

An arbitrary scoring system for fiber alignment has been reported (Box 16-5).[6,8] In this system, a score is assigned to semiquantitate fiber alignment of the target path. The veterinarian should bear in mind that the target path is wide with large lesions, but in small lesions it is quite narrow.

During repair the echogenicity score usually improves at a more rapid rate than the scar remodeling and FAS. The difference in these scores may be important for tailoring an appropriate controlled exercise program. A delay in fiber alignment improvement suggests that scar remodeling must continue and prompts conservative progression in exercise management.

It is more difficult to identify the target path of fiber bundles during healing once echogenicity has improved. Printed or electronically stored images of the initial examination can be reviewed to identify the exact location of the lesion. If the original scans are not available, one author (RLG) prefers to scan each zone from medial to lateral (or vice versa) and document the longitudinal image with the most abnormal fiber alignment. FAS (see Box 16-5) has been useful in predicting the prognosis for return to racing.[16] A horse with mean FAS of less than or equal to 0.5 at 4 months after treatment of SDFT was more likely to return to racing than a horse with a mean FAS greater than 0.5. An improvement in total FAS of greater than 75% was associated with a greater chance of returning to racing.[17]

Cross-Sectional Area

CSA measurements of transverse images of a ligament or tendon are useful, especially in assessing a subtle injury or determining the clinical significance of a localized, focal hypoechogenic fiber bundle path. When assessing the proximal aspect of the SL, it is useful to determine whether a focal hypoechogenic fiber bundle is likely to be a lesion or the remains of muscle fibers. An injured tendon or ligament usually is enlarged, and although this finding may not be obvious subjectively, measurements of CSA confirm structural thickening.

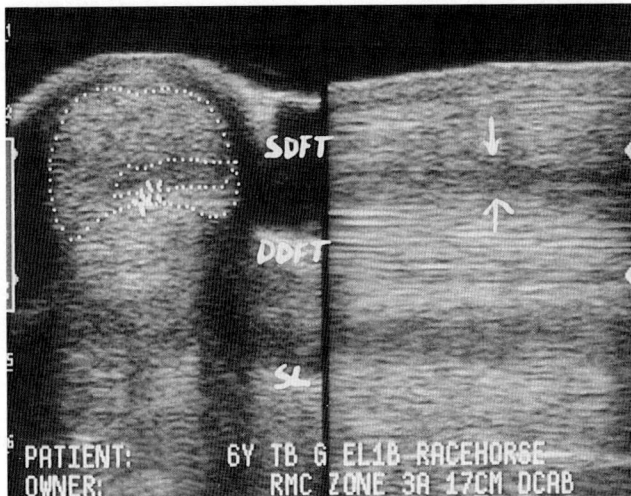

Fig. 16-13 • Transverse *(left)* and longitudinal *(right)* ultrasonographic images of zone 3A of the metacarpal region. The cross-sectional area (CSA) of the superficial digital flexor tendon *(SDFT)* is 3.05 cm². A dorsolateral type 1 hypoechoic lesion is present; the lesion is 43 mm² and represents 14.1% of the CSA of the tendon. The fiber alignment score of the targeted fiber path is 3 *(between arrows)*. *DDFT,* Deep digital flexor tendon; *SL,* suspensory ligament.

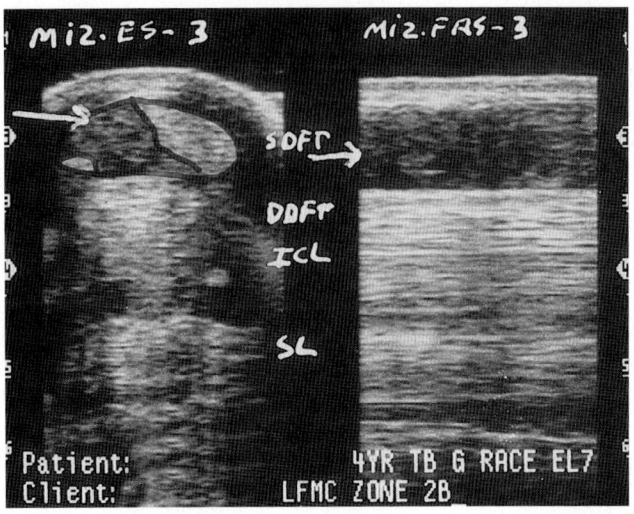

Fig. 16-14 • Transverse *(left)* and longitudinal *(right)* ultrasonographic images of zone 2B, obtained using a standoff pad. There is a large lateral border type 3 lesion of the superficial digital flexor tendon *(SDFT; horizontal arrow)* confirmed on longitudinal scan *(horizontal arrow)*. *DDFT,* Deep digital flexor tendon; *MIZ-ES,* maximal injury zone echo score; *MIZ-FAS,* maximal injury zone fiber alignment score; *SL* suspensory ligament.

CSA is also a useful parameter to evaluate the quality of repair, because decreasing size during rehabilitation indicates resolution of the inflammatory component of healing or may indicate favorable scar remodeling. Randomly oriented scars usually form in a rounded fashion and occupy more space. As the scar remodels into a more parallel alignment, less space is necessary, resulting in a reduction in CSA.

The transducer must be perpendicular to the structure to obtain accurate CSA data; otherwise the CSA may be falsely enlarged. The most common technique is to trace the structure on the monitor and the computer software automatically calculates the size. This technique also can be used to calculate lesion size and the proportion of the CSA involved (Figure 16-13). Initially this method of quantifying CSA may be time-consuming, especially when several structures are being assessed. Eventually the veterinarian can become extremely proficient at producing accurate measurements.

One author (RLG) uses a computer-assisted method that is not commercially available. Transverse images are traced with a microfine-point felt pen after the ultrasonographic study. With a digitizing pad and software program, surface area data are produced from the tracings of structures and lesions. This method is equally accurate but saves time because scans can be traced more quickly and at a more convenient time. The disadvantage is that the final quantitative information is not immediately available, but it does allow the clinician time to review the images before giving a conclusion to the owner. An alternative method is to save images on a computer disk using commercially available software (Metron-V, EponaTech, Creston, California).

Another simple and inexpensive method to determine structure and lesion CSA is creation of thermal images at all zones, and then at a convenient time, use of handheld calipers to make structures and lesions into two-dimensional squares or rectangles. This is done by measuring the palmar- or plantar-to-dorsal length and the medial-to-lateral length. These measurements are multiplied to determine the CSA. CSA obtained with handheld calipers is likely larger than the actual size. However, absolute values are less important than the relative difference between normal and suspected abnormal values. Thus if measurements are performed in a consistent manner, handheld calipers provide valid relative CSA data.

Relative sizes are best obtained by comparing the injured limb with the normal contralateral limb, but this is not possible if the injury is bilateral. The veterinarian must rely on the expected values for the age, size, and breed of the horse and level or zone of the image based on personal experience and previous images if available. Normal values for various structures are difficult to determine, and few studies have been published. Normal values for tendon and ligament sizes for TB and STB horses have been reported.[18] It is essential to measure both limbs at the same depth setting on the ultrasound machine.

In summary, quantifying the ultrasonographic image using echogenicity and FASs, along with CSA of the lesion, provides a powerful resource to aid in interpreting lesions (Figure 16-14). When an injury is assessed from proximal to distal, these scores can be summed to estimate the volume of the injury. These values can be used to categorize the injury and to monitor repair objectively.

ZONE DESIGNATIONS

The anatomical location of an ultrasonographic image can be designated by measuring the distance from a fixed landmark, such as the accessory carpal bone, or dividing the limb into zones.

Distal Aspect of Forelimbs

The palmar metacarpal and metacarpophalangeal regions may be separated into seven zones, or eight zones if the

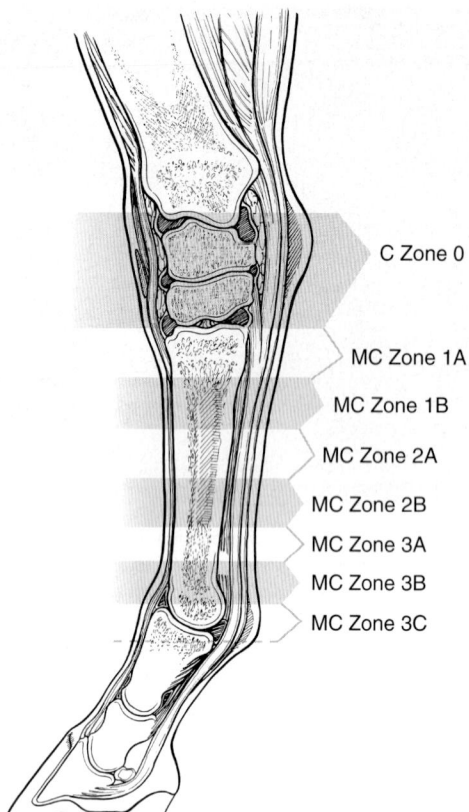

Fig. 16-15 • Ultrasonographic zone designations for the carpal *(C)* and metacarpal *(MC)* regions.

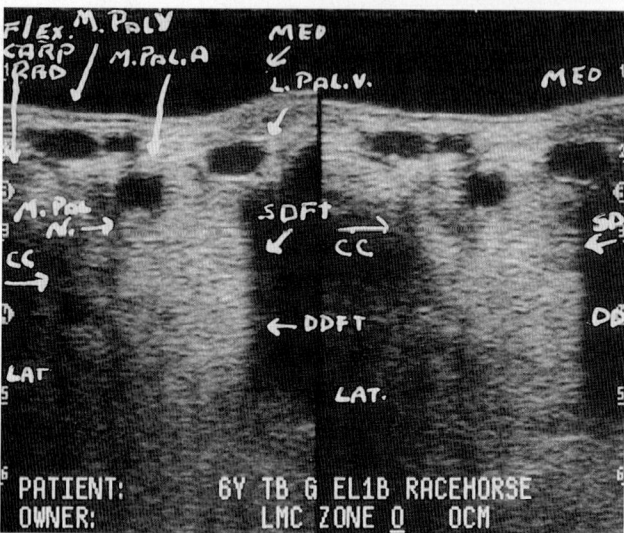

Fig. 16-16 • Transverse ultrasonographic images of a forelimb zone 0 obtained along the medial aspect of the accessory carpal bone with a standoff pad. The left image is focused on the superficial digital flexor tendon *(SDFT),* and the right image is focused on the deep digital flexor tendon *(DDFT). CC,* Carpal canal; *Flex Carp Rad,* flexor carpi radialis; *Lat,* lateral; *L Pal V,* lateral palmar vein; *M Pal A,* medial palmar artery; *M Pal N,* medial palmar nerve; *M Pal V,* medial palmar vein; *Med,* medial.

medial aspect of the carpus is included (Figure 16-15). The pastern also may be divided into zones (see page 198). Many of these zones have unique anatomical features. The measurements outlined in the following text refer to a 16.1-hand TB horse.

Zone Definitions
Zone 0
Zone 0 (approximately 5 cm in length) is located along the medial aspect of the carpus adjacent to the accessory carpal bone (Figure 16-16). Off-incidence angle artifacts may be present on the dorsal border of the DDFT, and rarely, hypoechogenic muscle bundles are seen (Figure 16-17). At this level the SDFT is uniform in echogenicity, but further proximally are hypoechogenic muscle bundles that should not be mistaken for lesions. The carpal sheath, common digital artery, and palmar carpal fascia are visible.

Zone 1A
Zone 1A extends from approximately 0.5 to 4 cm distal to the base of the accessory carpal bone. The SDFT is slightly medially placed, oval, and readily visible on the midline. The carpal retinaculum covers its palmar border proximally. The common digital artery lies close to the medial border of the SDFT. The DDFT is triangular, and the lateral border is more rounded (Figure 16-18). The ALDDFT and SL are rectangular. The medial and lateral borders of the ALDDFT and SL may not be visible from the palmar midline; therefore the transducer should be moved medially and laterally. However, to measure CSA of these

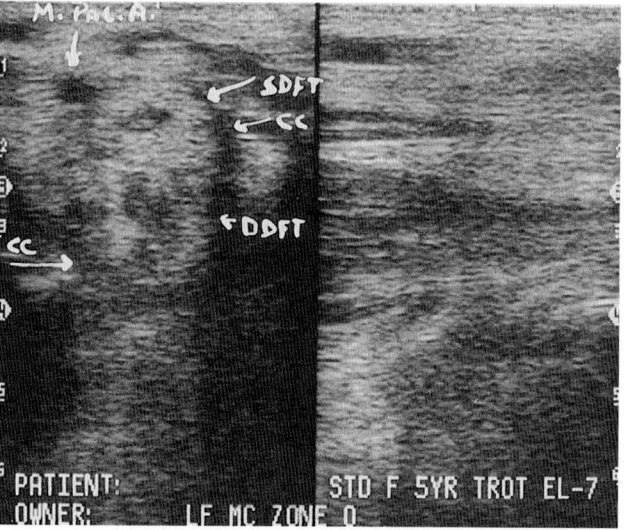

Fig. 16-17 • Transverse *(left)* and longitudinal *(right)* ultrasonographic images of the forelimb zone 0 obtained from the medial aspect of the carpus, immediately proximal to the accessory carpal bone, without a standoff pad. Note the centrally located muscle bundles of the superficial digital flexor tendon *(SDFT)* and the deep digital flexor tendon *(DDFT).* This is normal and should not be confused with a lesion. *CC,* Carpal canal; *M Pal A,* medial palmar artery.

structures, the veterinarian should use what can be seen from the palmar aspect. In most horses, anechogenic fluid in the carpal sheath is seen between the dorsal border of the DDFT and the palmar border of its accessory ligament. The medial aspect of the rectangular carpal sheath is wider than the lateral border.

The origin or enthesis of the SL is approximately 3 to 4 cm long. The SL rapidly increases in thickness from palmar to dorsal as it descends distally. In contrast, the

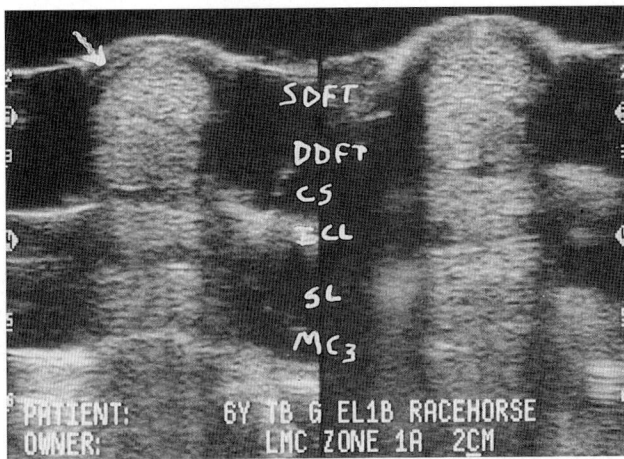

Fig. 16-18 • Transverse ultrasonographic images of the forelimb zone 1A. Carpal retinaculum *(arrow)*. *CS,* Carpal sheath; *DDFT,* deep digital flexor tendon; *ICL,* accessory ligament of the DDFT; *MC₃,* palmar border of the third metacarpal bone; *SDFT,* superficial digital flexor tendon; *SL,* suspensory ligament.

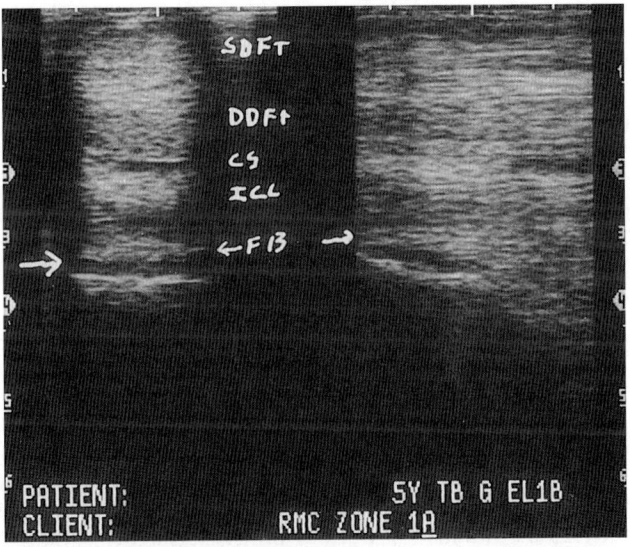

Fig. 16-19 • Transverse *(left)* and longitudinal *(right)* (proximal is to the left) ultrasonographic images from zone 1A of a forelimb obtained without a standoff pad. There is a ligamentous band (ligamentous segment of origin of suspensory ligament that originates from the palmar carpal fascia *[FB; small arrows]*) extending from the palmar aspect of the suspensory ligament, passing palmarly over the anechogenic joint recess of the carpometacarpal joint *(large horizontal arrow)* and inserting proximally on the dorsal surface of the accessory ligament of the superficial digital flexor tendon. *CS,* Carpal sheath; *DDFT,* deep digital flexor tendon; *ICL,* accessory ligament of the DDFT; *SDFT,* superficial digital flexor tendon.

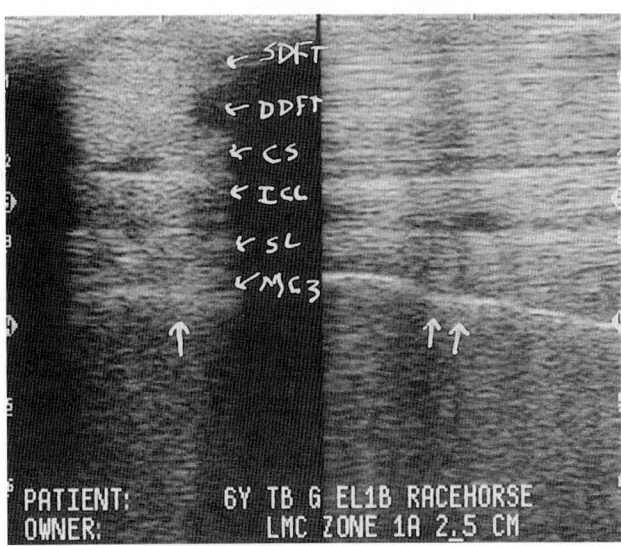

Fig. 16-20 • Transverse *(left)* and longitudinal *(right)* (proximal is to the left) ultrasonographic images from zone 1A, 2.5 cm distal to the base of the accessory carpal bone, without a standoff pad. There is a firm attachment of the suspensory ligament *(SL)* to the third metacarpal bone *(MC₃)* on the transverse *(single vertical arrow)* and the longitudinal *(double vertical arrows)* views. *CS,* Carpal sheath; *DDFT,* deep digital flexor tendon; *ICL,* accessory ligament of the DDFT; *SDFT,* superficial digital flexor tendon.

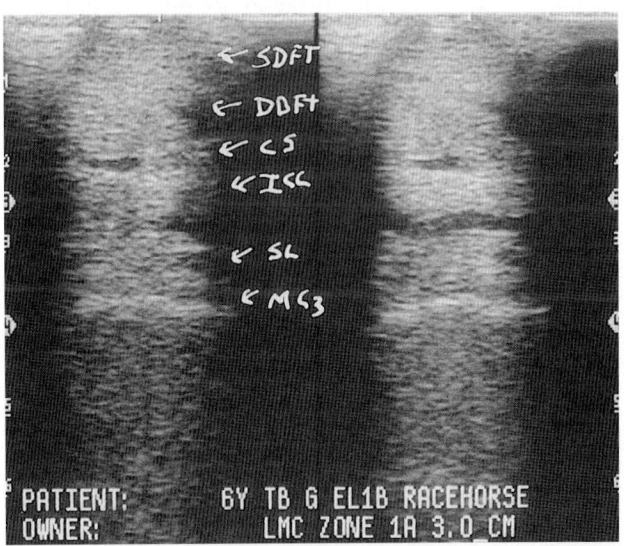

Fig. 16-21 • Transverse ultrasonographic images at the distal extent of zone 1A (3.0 cm distal to the base of the accessory carpal bone), without a standoff pad. The palmar-to-dorsal dimension of the suspensory ligament *(SL)* is the greatest for this zone in a normal horse. *CS,* Carpal sheath; *DDFT,* deep digital flexor tendon; *ICL,* accessory ligament of the DDFT, *MC₃,* third metacarpal bone; *SDFT,* superficial digital flexor tendon.

ALDDFT rapidly decreases in thickness from palmar to dorsal. Comparative CSA measurements in each forelimb should be done at precisely the same distance distal to the accessory carpal bone in zone 1A.

In the proximal metacarpal region a ligamentous band often extends proximally from the origin of the SL to insert on the palmar carpal fascia of the distal row of carpal bones (Figure 16-19). It is located between the dorsal border of the ALDDFT and the palmar recess of the carpometacarpal joint, which lies between the fibrous band and the third metacarpal bone (McIII). Anechogenic fluid in the carpometacarpal joint should not be confused with a lesion of the SL. The proximal aspect of zone 1A is proximal to the enthesis of the SL on the McIII.

At 2.5 cm distal to the accessory carpal bone the origin of the SL is firmly attached to the McIII (Figure 16-20). Entheseal fiber tearing usually occurs 1 to 3 cm distal to the accessory carpal bone. The oblique orientation of the McIII at the origin of the SL attachment can be seen on a longitudinal view (see Figure 16-20). Figure 16-21 is at the distal extent of zone 1A and the distal extent of the enthesis of the SL. Note the palmar to the dorsal width at this point in zone 1A and the firm bony attachment of the entire dorsal surface of the SL. In this example, there is complete dorsal attachment of the SL. However, in many normal horses the origin of the SL has a bilobed appearance (medial and lateral attachments), with a rounded or triangular hypoechogenic area dorsally in the midline. Clinicians must be cautious not to interpret this as a focal tear. Rarely the origin of the SL can be injured in this central location, but generally the size and shape of the hypoechogenic region are changed.

Zone 1B

Zone 1B extends from approximately 4 to 7 cm distal to the accessory carpal bone. At this level the slightly crescent-shaped SDFT is on the midline over the oval DDFT. There are no unique anatomical features of this zone that identify it, and its location is determined by measurement. In all midmetacarpal zones, as in zone 1A, the medial and lateral borders of the SL and ALDDFT may not be visible from the palmar midline. The transducer must be moved medially or laterally to identify a focal peripheral lesion of one of these structures. At times, the dorsal border of the SL can be difficult to identify because of the density of the periligamentous, fibrous connective tissue. To assist in defining that border, it can be helpful to split the screen and place the longitudinal image adjacent to the transverse image. This technique clearly demarcates the dorsal and palmar borders (Figure 16-22).

Zone 2A

Zone 2A extends from approximately 7 to 10 cm distal to the accessory carpal bone. The same comments apply for this zone as for zone 1B.

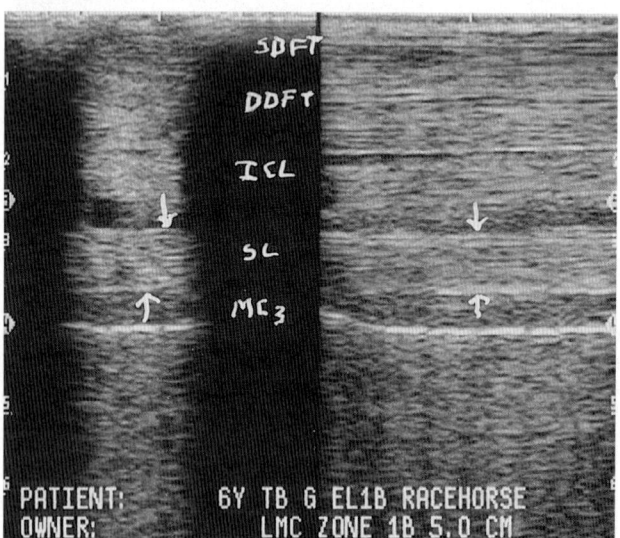

Fig. 16-22 • Transverse *(left)* and longitudinal *(right)* (proximal is to the left) ultrasonographic images of zone 1B (5 cm distal to the base of the accessory carpal bone) obtained without a standoff pad. The down arrows mark the palmar border of the suspensory ligament *(SL)*, and the up arrows mark the dorsal border. *DDFT,* Deep digital flexor tendon; *ICL,* accessory ligament of the DDFT, *MC₃,* third metacarpal bone; *SDFT,* superficial digital flexor tendon.

Zone 2B

Zone 2B extends from approximately 10 to 14 cm distal to the accessory carpal bone. One unique feature of this zone is an obliquely coursing nerve located subcutaneously on the palmar surface of the SDFT. This nerve (the communicating branch of the medial palmar nerve) and associated small vessels are a common site for a bandage pinch or "cording" swelling that suggests a primary tendon injury. Overall the anatomical relationships of tendons and ligaments are similar to zones 1B and 2A. The SDFT and ALDDFT are more crescent shaped and smaller from palmar to dorsal. At this level the carpal sheath still can be identified ultrasonographically.

Zone 3A

Zone 3A extends from approximately 14 to 18 cm distal to the accessory carpal bone. Several anatomical features characterize this zone. The first is that in many horses with tenosynovitis, this is the initial zone that incorporates the origin of the DFTS.

The SDFT is crescent shaped and smaller from palmar to dorsal but wider from medial to lateral. The ALDDFT inserts into the DDFT. In transverse images normal crescent-shaped hypoechogenic fiber bundles are seen between the dorsal surface of the DDFT and the palmar surface of its accessory ligament. The carpal sheath generally is not appreciated in this zone.

At the region of the ALDDFT insertion onto the DDFT, the two structures can clearly be separated ultrasonographically, although grossly they are conjoined. When measuring the CSA of the DDFT, the ALDDFT can be separated from the DDFT, which results in a reduced DDFT CSA, or included with it, which yields a more correct CSA determination of the DDFT. The method used is personal preference and results in valid information, provided it is consistent.

Zone 3A is just proximal to the bifurcation of the SL. In zone 3A the SL is still a single structure, but the medial and lateral borders become more rounded and the central region may be less echogenic. This is a common site of injury, especially in STB racehorses. At times it can be quite difficult to establish structural borders in acute injury. A longitudinal image viewed adjacent to a transverse may be helpful (Figure 16-23).

Zone 3B

Zone 3B is larger (approximately 5 cm in the average adult horse) than more proximal zones and is the region in which the SL bifurcates into medial and lateral branches. The zone extends from 18 to 23 cm distal to the accessory carpal bone. Anatomical structures include the DFTS; the manica flexoria, a fibrous band extending from the medial and lateral borders of the SDFT and encompassing the DDFT that is associated with a thecal space; and the intersesamoidean space and ligament with associated connective tissue and vasculature. The SDFT decreases in size from palmar to dorsal and widens from medial to lateral. The DDFT becomes ovoid. CSA measurements should be made at identical sites distal to the accessory carpal bone for accurate comparisons between limbs.

The SL branches must be examined individually from palmaromedial and palmarolateral aspects of the limb with a standoff pad. If the ligament is enlarged, no standoff pad is required. The length of a metacarpal SL branch is about

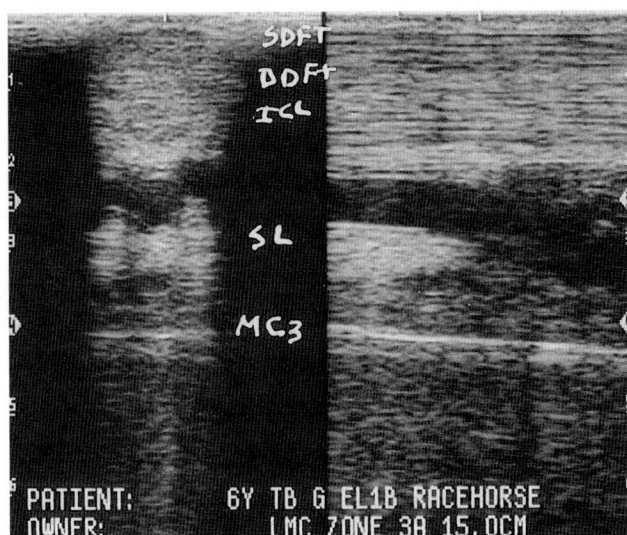

Fig. 16-23 • Transverse *(left)* and longitudinal *(right)* (proximal is to the left) ultrasonographic images from zone 3A (15 cm distal to the base of the accessory carpal bone), in which the suspensory ligament *(SL)* bifurcates. *DDFT,* Deep digital flexor tendon; *ICL,* accessory ligament of the DDFT, *MC₃,* third metacarpal bone; *SDFT,* superficial digital flexor tendon.

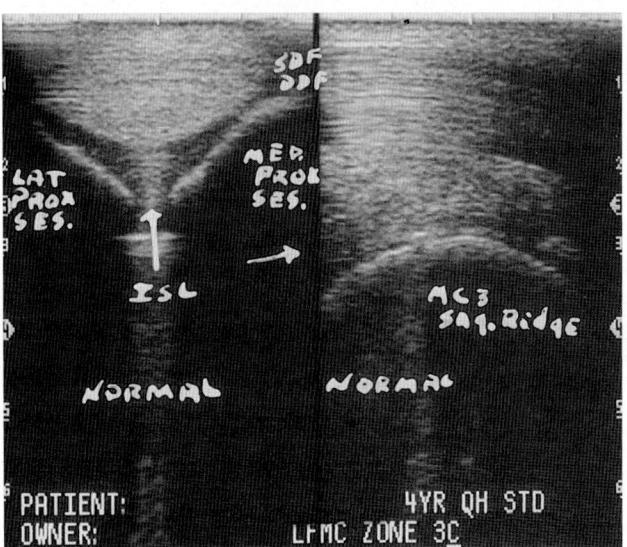

Fig. 16-25 • Transverse *(left)* and longitudinal *(right)* ultrasonographic images of zone 3C obtained without a standoff pad. Vertical and horizontal arrows indicate a normal intersesamoidean ligament. *DDF,* Deep digital flexor tendon; *ISL,* intersesamoidean ligament; *Lat Prox Ses,* lateral proximal sesamoid bone osseous shadow; *MC₃ Sag Ridge,* sagittal ridge of third metacarpal bone; *Med Prox Ses,* medial proximal sesamoid bone shadow.

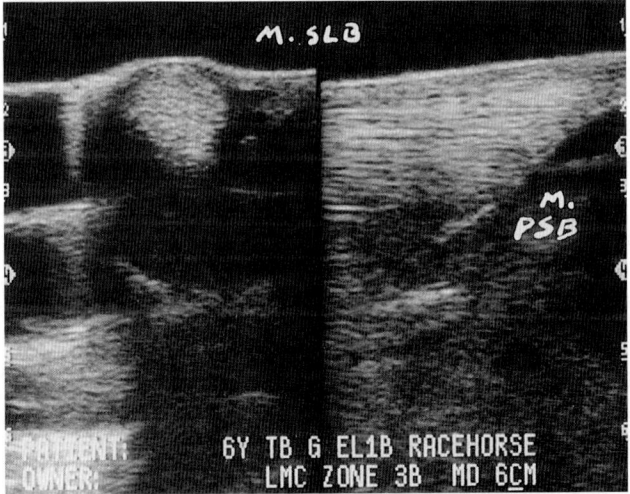

Fig. 16-24 • Transverse *(left)* and longitudinal *(right)* (proximal is to the left) ultrasonographic images of zone 3B-MD (medial placement of the transducer at the distal extent of the insertion of the medial branch of the suspensory ligament onto the medial proximal sesamoid bone). *M PSB,* Bone border of the abaxial medial proximal sesamoid bone; *M SLB,* medial suspensory ligament branch.

6 cm. To increase data points for CSA comparison, each branch is divided into three 2-cm subzones within zone 3B. For the medial branch, the zone designations are 3B-MP (medial proximal), 3B-MM (medial middle), and 3B-MD (medial distal) (Figure 16-24). For the lateral branch the zone designations are 3B-LP (lateral proximal), 3B-LM (lateral middle), and 3B-LD (lateral distal). The proximal and middle segments of each branch are oval, and the distal segment is more triangular.

Zone 3C
Zone 3C extends from 23 to 28 cm distal to the accessory carpal bone and basically includes tissues on the palmar

aspect of the metacarpophalangeal joint. The characteristic features of this zone are the presence of the bony shadows of apices of the proximal sesamoid bones (PSBs), the presence of the palmar annular ligament (PAL), and the intersesamoidean ligament (Figure 16-25).

Distal Aspect of Hindlimbs
The anatomical location of an ultrasonographic image can be designated by measuring the distance from a fixed landmark, such as the tuber calcanei or tarsometatarsal joint, or reference to a numbered zone. Most distal limb anatomical features are the same as in the forelimb. However, because of the added length of the SDFT or DDFT and the existence of the plantar ligament (long plantar tarsal ligament), the metatarsal zones move up one number.

In the hindlimb, zone 1 includes the plantar aspect of the tarsus (see Figure 78-3). In an adult horse, this is approximately 16 cm in length. Zone 1 is subdivided into two 8-cm zones, 1A and 1B. The most proximal zone of the metatarsal region is zone 2, which is subdivided into 2A and 2B; the middle third is zone 3, which is subdivided into zones 3A and 3B; and the distal aspect is zone 4, which is subdivided into zones 4A, 4B, and 4C (Figure 16-26).

Hindlimb Zones
Zone 1A
Zone 1A extends to 8 cm distal to the tuber calcanei (Figure 16-27; see Chapter 78). The SDFT is slightly crescent shaped and located subcutaneously. Deep to the SDFT is the origin of the plantar ligament. Occasionally the subcutaneous bursa or the subtendonous calcanean bursa or both bursae may be seen. The entire width of the SDFT may not be observed on a single midline view, but useful CSA data can be obtained. The extreme medial and lateral borders of the SDFT and the retinacular attachment to the calcaneus may be more visible with slight medial and lateral placement of

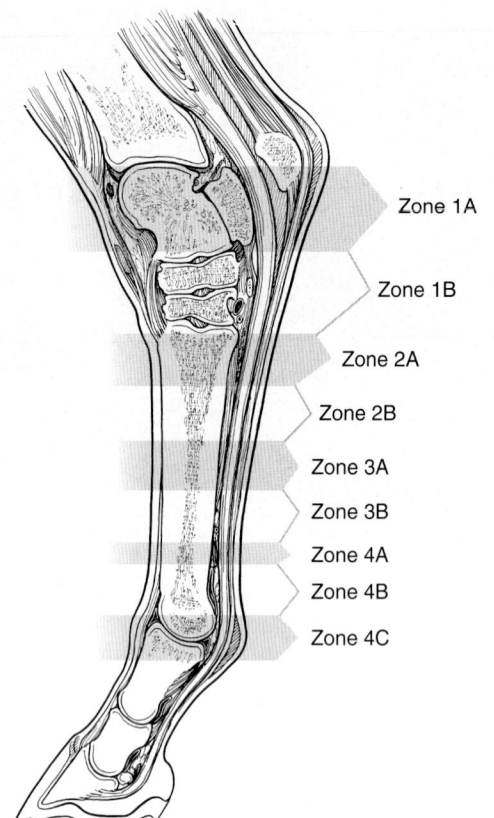

Fig. 16-26 • Ultrasonographic zone designations for tarsus and metatarsus.

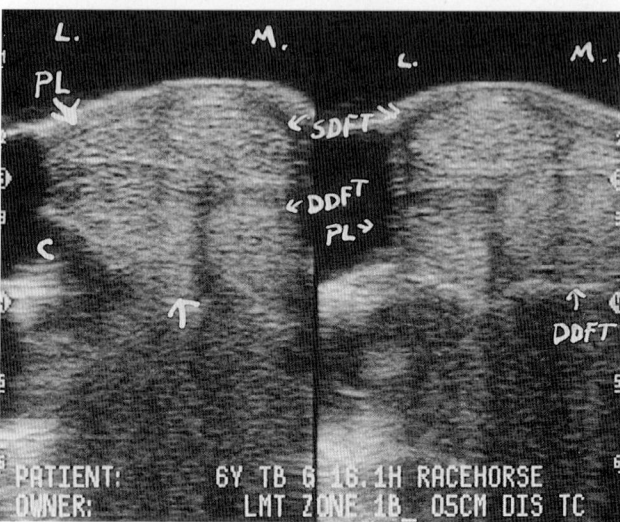

Fig. 16-28 • Transverse ultrasonographic images from zone 1B, 5 cm distal to the tuber calcanei, obtained using a standoff pad. Medial is to the right. The left image is slightly lateral of midline to highlight the plantar ligament (PL; between arrows), and the right image is slightly medial of midline to highlight the superficial digital flexor tendon (SDFT) and the deep digital flexor tendon (DDFT). C, Osseous border of the calcaneus; L, lateral; M, medial; PL, plantar ligament or long plantar tarsal ligament.

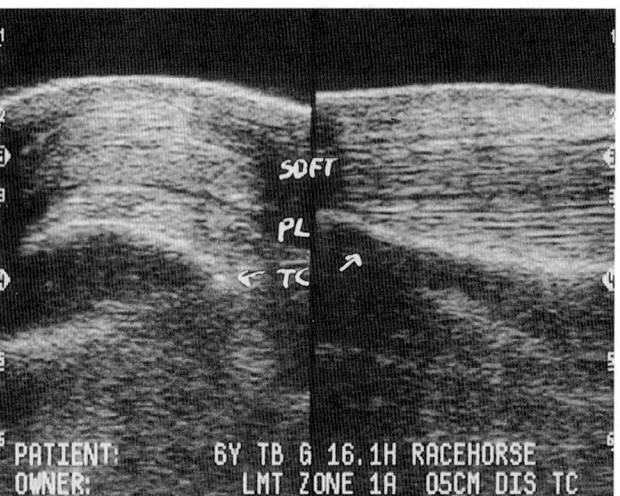

Fig. 16-27 • Transverse (left) and longitudinal (right) (proximal is to the left) ultrasonographic images of the plantar tarsus (zone 1A, 5 cm distal to the tuber calcanei) obtained using a standoff pad. PL, Plantar ligament or long plantar tarsal ligament; SDFT, superficial digital flexor tendon; TC, plantar border of the calcaneus.

the transducer. The plantar ligament is located on the midline, firmly attached to the calcaneus, with its origin approximately 3 cm distal to the tuber calcanei. The DDFT and tarsal sheath must be viewed individually by medial positioning of the transducer. The origin of the plantar ligament widens in a plantar-to-dorsal plane rapidly in this zone. Accurate comparative CSA data require precise anatomical positioning on both hindlimbs. Usually at this level, no visible muscle bundles of the DDFT are seen, but clinicians must be aware of this possibility and not interpret them as a core lesion. At 5 cm distal (zone 1B) to the tuber calcanei, the plantar ligament is roughly triangular and has multiple septated bundles that are all included in measurement of the CSA (Figure 16-28).

Zone 1B

Hindlimb zone 1B includes the distal half of the tarsus, extending from 8 to 16 cm distal to the tuber calcanei. Numerous images must be obtained from the plantar midline to assess the SDFT, from plantaromedial to assess the DDFT, and from slightly lateral to the midline to assess the plantar ligament. A wedge-shaped fibrous band emanates from the medial border of the SDFT and the fascia of the fibrous tarsal sheath and surrounds the DDFT (see Figure 16-28). There is a narrow anechoic space representing fluid in the tarsal sheath separating the DDFT and the plantar ligament. The plantar ligament decreases in plantar to dorsal size as it courses distally; it has a firm enthesis to the plantar aspect of the fourth tarsal bone and inserts onto the head of the fourth metatarsal bone (MtIV).

Zone 2A

Zone 2A is the first metatarsal zone and includes the origin of the SL (approximately 16 to 21 cm distal to the tuber calcanei) and the ALDDFT, which is a rudimentary structure in many horses. The transducer must be slightly medial to midline for complete examination of the DDFT. The SDFT can be assessed from the plantar midline. The origin of the SL can be somewhat confusing on ultrasound images, and this may create a dilemma in detecting subtle injury. The SL is firmly attached to the third metatarsal bone (MtIII) (approximately 4- to 5-cm enthesis) and

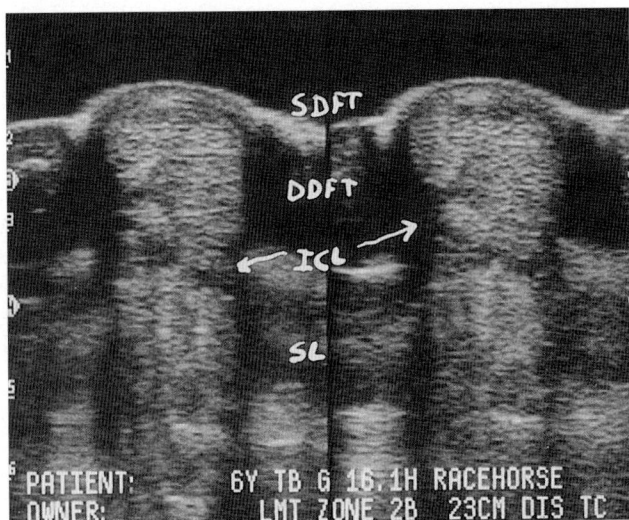

Fig. 16-29 • Transverse ultrasonographic images of zone 2B, 23 cm distal to the tuber calcanei, obtained using a standoff pad. *DDFT*, Deep digital flexor tendon; *ICL*, accessory ligament of the DDFT; *SDFT*, superficial digital flexor tendon; *SL*, suspensory ligament.

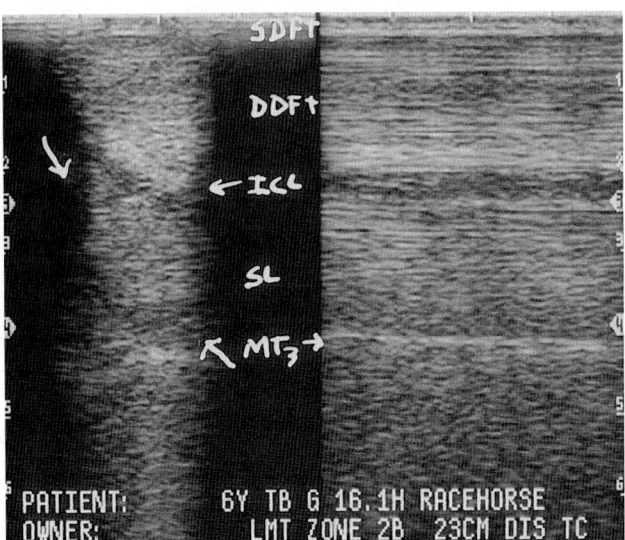

Fig. 16-30 • Transverse *(left)* and longitudinal *(right)* ultrasonographic images of zone 2B obtained without a standoff pad. The suspensory ligament *(SL)* is located between the large oblique arrows. *DDFT*, Deep digital flexor tendon; *MT₃*, plantar border of third metatarsal bone; *SDFT*, superficial digital flexor tendon.

rapidly increases in size from plantar to dorsal within zone 2A. Therefore care must be taken when measuring comparative CSAs to do so at exactly the same level within zone 2A. In longitudinal images the origin of the SL often does not have a tight parallel fiber pattern, which results in an FAS of 1. The large bony surfaces of the second metatarsal bone (MtII) and the MtIV obstruct a clear view, and often a linear anechoic artifact is created by more superficial blood vessels. The origin of the SL begins slightly lateral to midline and thus is not parallel to the plantar surface of the MtIII. The SL appears rhomboid from the plantar midline, but if viewed from slightly medial of midline, it appears more rectangular. CSA measurements should be obtained from one view or the other, but not mixed. Comparison of the longitudinal and transverse views of the SL may help in identifying the plantar and dorsal borders.

Zone 2B

Hindlimb zone 2B extends approximately 21 to 24 cm distal to the tuber calcanei. The SDFT, DDFT, ALDDFT, and SL can be viewed adequately from a midline and slightly medial positioning of the transducer (Figure 16-29). At this level the SDFT is slightly crescent shaped, and the DDFT is ovoid and slightly medially placed. The ALDDFT is visible on the dorsal border of the DDFT. The SL is roughly rectangular with an apex toward the plantar lateral aspect (Figure 16-30). No unique anatomical features identify this zone; it is identified only by measurement.

Zone 3A

Zone 3A ranges from 24 to 32 cm distal to the tuber calcanei. The SDFT is slightly crescent-shaped and is positioned directly over the DDFT. The SL at this level is roughly rectangular with an apex on the plantar lateral border. Zone 3A has no unique anatomical features.

Zone 3B

Hindlimb zone 3B extends from 28 to 32 cm distal to the tuber calcanei. The SDFT is crescent shaped and narrower

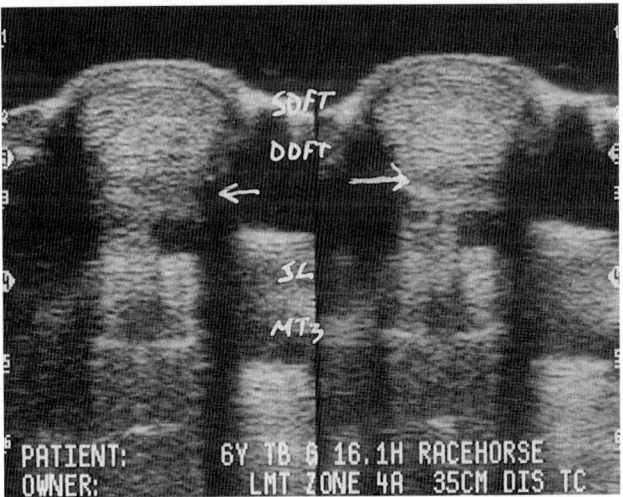

Fig. 16-31 • Transverse ultrasonographic images from zone 4A, 35 cm distal to the tuber calcanei. There is an artifactual hypoechogenic zone between the dorsal aspect of the deep digital flexor tendon *(DDFT)* and the plantar border of the accessory ligament of the DDFT insertion *(horizontal arrows)*. *MT₃*, Plantar border of third metatarsal bone; *SDFT*; superficial digital flexor tendon; *SL*, suspensory ligament.

in the plantar-to-dorsal plane and wider in a medial-to-lateral plane, whereas the DDFT is ovoid. This zone has no unique anatomical features.

Zone 4A

Hindlimb zone 4A extends from 32 to 36 cm distal to the tuber calcanei. In this zone the ALDDFT inserts into the DDFT, and a normal hypoechoic artifact may be seen on the dorsal border of the DDFT (Figure 16-31). This is the most distal zone in which the SL is a single unit. The proximal aspect of the DFTS may be seen.

Zone 4B

Hindlimb zone 4B extends from 36 to 43 cm distal to the tuber calcanei and has the same anatomical features as forelimb zone 3B. The hindlimb branches of the SL tend to be longer (approximately 10 cm) and a little larger than the forelimb branches.

Zone 4C

Zone 4C extends from 43 to 47 cm distal to the tuber calcanei and has the same anatomical features as forelimb zone 3C.

Palmar and Plantar Pastern Zones and Descriptions

Qualitative assessments are more critical in pastern ultrasonography because some lesions are not accompanied by clinically significant changes in CSA. If DFTS tenosynovitis is coupled with a subtle primary tendon injury, the tendon may be mildly enlarged. Marginal longitudinal tears of the DDFT require precise qualitative inspection of the lateral and medial borders of the DDFT and the vincula. Fibrous adhesions of the sheath may be identified but may not be accompanied by an increase in DDFT CSA.[19] It also is more difficult to obtain accurate FAS for the branches of the SDFT and oblique sesamoidean ligament (or middle distal sesamoidean ligament). The distal metacarpal or metatarsal regions should also be examined when assessing the DFTS in the pastern.

The pastern is a complex anatomical structure including many ligaments, joint recesses, vasculature, fibrocartilaginous insertional attachments, entheses, joint surfaces, and two major tendons.[20] The major structures of practical and common clinical concern are the DFTS, SDFT and branches, DDFT, oblique sesamoidean ligament (middle distal sesamoidean ligament), and straight sesamoidean ligament (or superficial distal sesamoidean ligament). The pastern can be arbitrarily divided into four zones, each with unique anatomical features. The pastern is divided into three palmar or plantar zones along the proximal phalanx (P1) and one zone at the proximal interphalangeal joint (Figure 16-32).

Pastern Zone Designations and Descriptions

Zone P1A

Zone P1A extends approximately 1 to 3 cm from the base of the ergot. Anatomical landmarks, such as the ergot, can be used to identify this zone. The SDFT is viewed from the midline and is a crescent-shaped, single-unit structure with very slight enlargement and rounding of the medial and lateral borders. The entire SDFT is included for CSA data. The palmar or plantar surface of the SDFT is covered by the thin proximal digital annular ligament. Dorsal to the SDFT on the midline view lies the ovoid DDFT. Anechogenic fluid in the DFTS is interposed between the DDFT and the triangular straight sesamoidean ligament. Occasionally a fibrous bridge of the oblique sesamoidean ligament or a small portion of the cruciate sesamoidean ligament (or deep distal sesamoidean ligament) may be identified dorsal to the straight sesamoidean ligament. Dorsal to the SDFT on the midline view is a hypoechogenic or anechogenic rounded joint recess of the metacarpophalangeal or metatarsophalangeal joint. The medial and lateral origins of the oblique sesamoidean ligament are seen as two distinctly separate structures and are more adequately viewed by medial and lateral parasagittal placement of the transducer.

Zone P1B

Zone P1B extends from 3 to 5 cm distal to the base of the ergot (Figure 16-33). The SDFT is still a single unit starting to form rounded medial and lateral branches, which are evaluated by moving the transducer medially and laterally. The DDFT has a bilobed appearance, and unless the transducer is perpendicular to the DDFT, central hypoechoic areas are seen in each lobe. The DFTS is seen on the dorsal surface of the DDFT, dorsal to which is the square or rectangular straight sesamoidean ligament. The oblique sesamoidean ligament is seen as a single structure in close

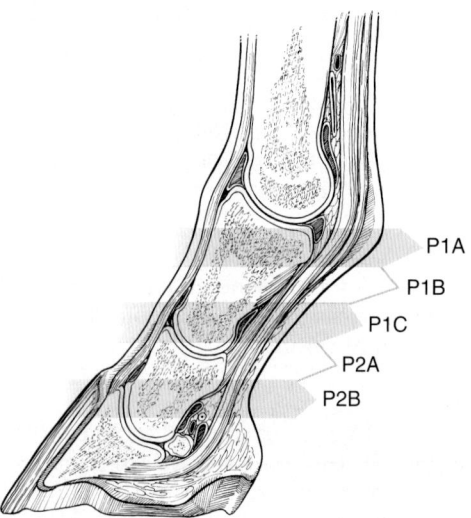

Fig. 16-32 • Ultrasonographic zone designations for the pastern. See text for zone descriptions.

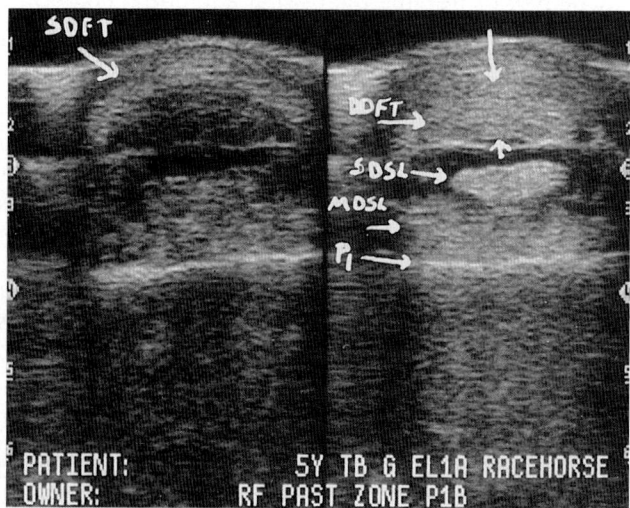

Fig. 16-33 • Transverse ultrasonographic images of zone P1B obtained using a standoff pad. The left image targets the superficial digital flexor tendon *(SDFT)*. The right image targets the deep digital flexor tendon *(DDFT)*, straight sesamoidean ligament *(SDSL)*, and middle distal sesamoidean ligament or oblique sesamoidean ligament *(MDSL)*. P_1, Palmar border of the proximal phalanx.

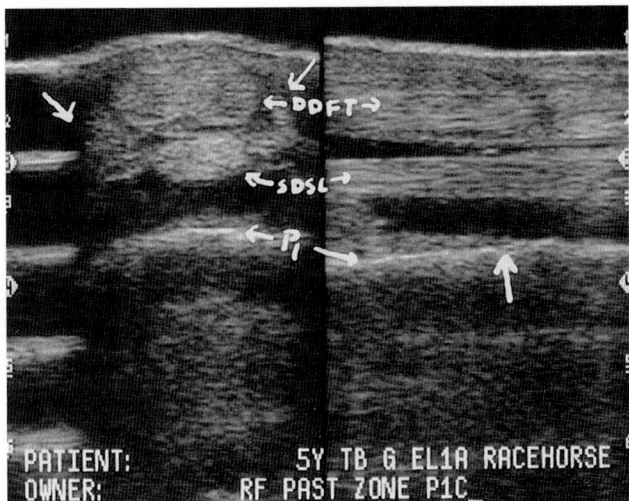

Fig. 16-34 • Transverse *(left)* and longitudinal *(right)* ultrasonographic images of zone P1C obtained using a standoff pad. The *oblique arrows* indicate the untargeted medial and lateral branches of the superficial digital flexor tendon. The vertical arrow indicates the insertion of the middle distal sesamoidean ligament *(MDSL)*. *DDFT,* Deep digital flexor tendon; P_1, palmar border of the proximal phalanx.

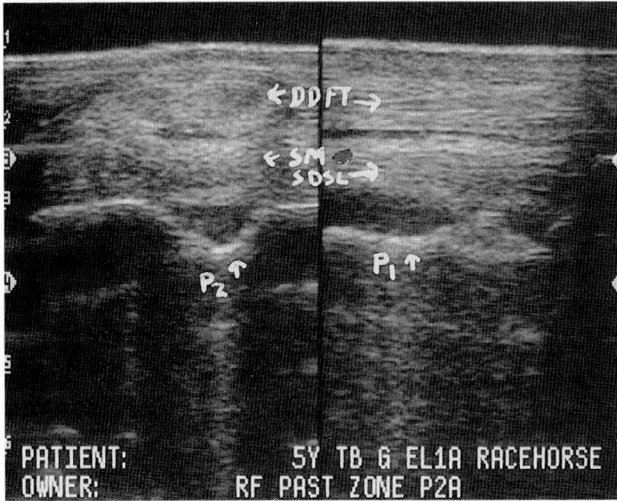

Fig. 16-35 • Transverse *(left)* and longitudinal *(right)* ultrasonographic images of zone P2A obtained using a standoff pad. *DDFT,* Deep digital flexor tendon; P_1, palmar border of the proximal phalanx; P_2, the palmar border of the middle phalanx; *SDSL,* superficial distal sesamoidean ligament or straight sesamoidean ligament; *SM,* scutum medium.

proximity to the palmar or plantar surface of P1, dorsal to the straight sesamoidean ligament.

Zone P1C

Zone P1C extends approximately 5 to 7 cm distal to the base of the ergot (Figure 16-34). The bilobed DDFT lies subcutaneously. The square or slightly rectangular straight sesamoidean ligament is on the dorsal surface of the DDFT. The oblique sesamoidean ligament is not visible because zone P1C is distal to its insertion. The teardrop-shaped medial and lateral branches of the SDFT are viewed by moving the transducer medially and laterally.

Zone P2A

Zone P2A extends approximately 6 to 9 cm distal to the base of the ergot. A thin distal digital annular ligament is closely associated with the palmar or plantar border of the DDFT. The DDFT has a bilobed appearance but is narrower from palmar or plantar to dorsal and wider from medial to lateral. Deep to the DDFT is the middle scutum, the fibrocartilaginous insertion of the straight sesamoidean ligament, which may have a heterogeneous echogenicity (Figure 16-35). Deep to the middle scutum is the proximal interphalangeal joint recess. The medial and lateral branches of the SDFT insert onto the distal aspect of the proximal phalanx and the proximal eminence of the middle phalanx.

Ultrasonography of Proximal Parts of the Limbs

Quantitative ultrasonographic evaluation can be applied to other anatomical areas and the lower limb areas described. These areas do not have zonal designations, and all are identified by measurement from a bony eminence. Many structures contain some muscle fiber bundles that are hypoechogenic, which makes detection of lesions more difficult. Whenever possible, we compare echogenicity, fiber alignment, and CSA between the limbs to

determine some quantitative data to support a qualitative diagnosis.

CLINICAL ULTRASONOGRAPHY

With these suggested fundamental principles in terminology and a systematic concept of data collection, the clinician is prepared to examine the horse. A 7-year-old TB gelding racehorse that had raced for 5 years, with 80 lifetime starts, 14 wins, and $74,568 in earnings, raced poorly 4 days previously. The next day, the trainer noted peritendonous swelling but no lameness. The horse had never had swelling in this area previously. The horse had received 2 g of phenylbutazone intravenously 24 hours before the race and 2 g immediately after the race. There was heat, slight subcutaneous swelling, and sensitivity and slight enlargement of the SDFT. A core lesion of the SDFT was detected ultrasonographically (Figure 16-36). This scenario raises several questions. How serious is the injury? Can the horse be treated symptomatically and continue to race? If the horse is rested, will it be able to race again? If the horse is rested, which therapy should be used? How will the degree of healing be determined? Each horse is assessed by subjective evaluation of the ultrasonographic images and quantitative analysis.

Quantitative Analysis

The weakest link, or maximal injured zone, is the level at which the biggest proportion of tendon CSA is reduced in echogenicity, or the zone with the largest increase in CSA when compared with a normal contralateral limb. Total structural size is obtained by summing the CSA from each zone. To obtain the percentage of total extent of injury, add the lesion CSA from all levels with a lesion. The total lesion CSA is divided by the total structure CSA and multiplied by 100. The resulting number provides an estimate of structural compromise. It is this percent of total lesion

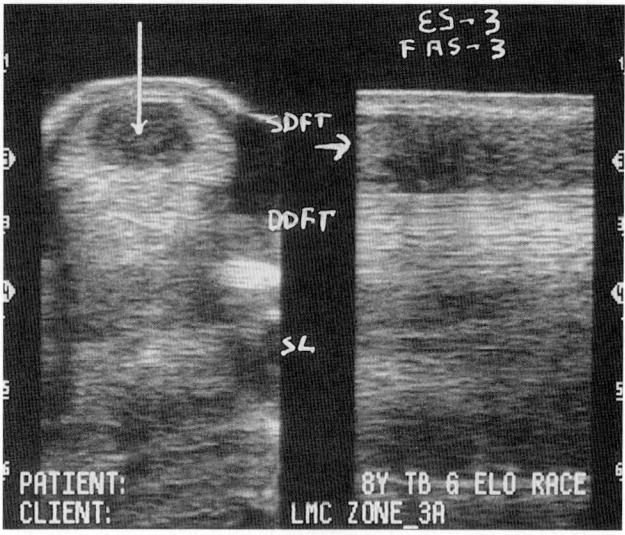

Fig. 16-36 • Transverse *(left)* and longitudinal *(right)* ultrasonographic images from zone 3A obtained using a standoff pad. The vertical arrow indicates a type 3 core lesion of the superficial digital flexor tendon *(SDFT)*. The *horizontal arrow* indicates the target path on the longitudinal image, with a fiber alignment score of 3 *(FAS-3)*. *DDFT,* Deep digital flexor tendon; *ES-3,* echo score 3; *SL,* suspensory ligament.

(% T-lesion) that is used to categorize injury and relates the severity of structural injury to the client.

Quantitative Terms

The following terms are used in reference to injuries:
1. Maximal injury zone (MIZ)
2. Maximal injury zone cross-sectional area (MIZ-CSA)
3. Maximal injury zone lesion cross-sectional area (MIZ-LCA)
4. Maximal injury zone type or echo score (MIZ-TS) (MIZ-ES)
5. Maximal injury zone fiber alignment score (MIZ-FAS)
6. Total cross-sectional area (sum of included levels; T-CSA)
7. Total lesion cross-sectional area (sum of all levels with a lesion; TL-CSA)
8. Total type or echo score (sum of all levels with a score; T-TS or T- ES)
9. Total fiber alignment score (sum of all level scores; T-FAS)
10. Average fiber alignment score (total divided by number of levels included; A-FAS)
11. Percent total lesion: ([TL-CSA ÷ T-CSA] × 100 = % T-lesion)

In a normal horse, typical measurements of T-CSA in the forelimb include the following:
- 8 zones of the SDFT = 886 mm^2
- 8 zones of the DDFT = 1001 mm^2
- 5 zones of the ALDDFT = 449 mm^2
- 11 zones of the SL = 1156 mm^2
    Main body of the SL (5 zones) = 614 mm^2
    Lateral branch (3 zones) = 258 mm^2
    Medial branch (3 zones) = 284 mm^2

We find that this quantitative assessment provides practical, useful information that can be used routinely and that lesions can be placed in one of six categories.

Lesion Categories

Category I

Category I implies no substantial qualitative or quantitative abnormality. No tendon or ligament fiber bundle lesions are detected, and all zones have lesion and FASs of zero. No single zone has a CSA measurement greater than 39% compared with the contralateral limb. This percentage of tolerance more than adequately allows for method error, especially in zones 1A and 3A. However, with precise technique, a variation greater than 25% indicates substantial structural enlargement. Assessment of T-CSA depends on the number of zones included. The larger the number of zones included, the less difference there should be between limbs:

    6/7 zones: <15%
    11 zones: <12%
    5 zones: <17%
    3 zones: <20%
    2 zones: <25%

A 9-year-old TB mare competing as a hunter developed new swelling in the right proximal metacarpal region and slight, intermittent lameness. The client was concerned that the tendon was injured, and if so, did not want to continue athletic use of the horse, which would risk further injury. Palpation revealed swelling (2/5), increased skin temperature (2/5), and a painful response to direct digital pressure of the proximal aspect of the right fore SDFT. Both forelimbs were examined ultrasonographically. No qualitative abnormalities were detected in the normal limb. Subcutaneous fluid was accumulated in the affected limb, indicating edema with or without hemorrhage, but echogenicity of the SDFT was normal. CSA was measured for seven zones of each limb. Zone 1B was determined the maximal injured zone, and the CSA of the SDFT was 25% larger than the normal limb (i.e., category I) but suggestive of tendon enlargement. The T-CSA difference was only 3%. The SDFT was considered normal, although two zones had slightly enlarged CSA (1B was +25% and 2A was +23%). It was recommended that exercise be restricted to walk and trot for 7 days with daily icing, daily bandaging with alcohol and thick standing bandages be used, and phenylbutazone (2 g once daily for 5 days) be administered. If the swelling was 100% reduced after this time, then the horse could return to normal athletic use. If no improvement occurred within 7 days or return to work caused a relapse, repeat ultrasonographic evaluation would be indicated. This horse returned to normal use.

Category II

No hypoechoic or anechoic lesions are detectable, but the affected limb has MIZ-CSA measurements greater than 39%, with or without T-CSA for six or seven zones greater than 14% of the normal limb (i.e., measurable focal or diffuse thickening of the tendon or ligament). Causes of category II injuries may include an unusual developmental difference, a new low-grade tendonitis or desmitis, or an older, currently stable healed tendon or ligament injury. Although generalized thickening may not cause great concern initially, there is evidence that continued use will eventually lead to greater injury. For example, 29% of TB racehorses (n = 13) that continued to train and race with a *new* category II SDFT injury eventually developed a clinically bowed tendon.[21]

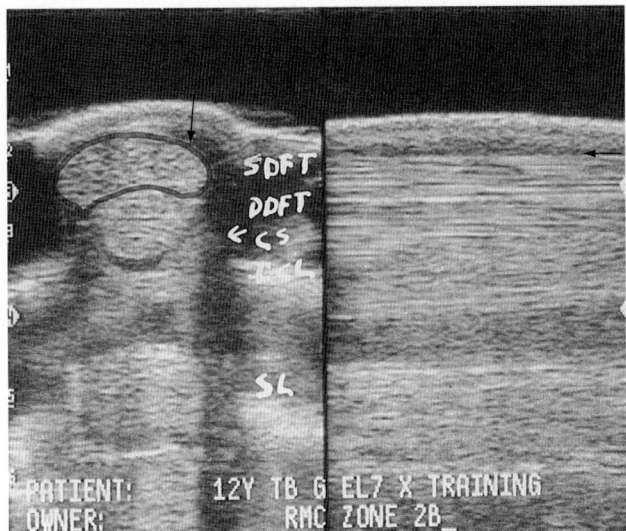

Fig. 16-37 • Transverse *(left)* and longitudinal *(right)* ultrasonographic images of zone 2B obtained using a standoff pad. The arrows indicate subcutaneous fluid accumulation. *CS,* Carpal sheath; *DDFT,* deep digital flexor tendon; *ICL,* accessory ligament of the DDFT; *SL,* suspensory ligament.

A 12-year-old TB gelding competing cross-country had recurrent swelling of the SDFT in the midmetacarpal region that reduced with rest and antiinflammatory treatment but returned if work was resumed. The horse had a long toe and was shod in smooth-toed, heavy steel shoes. There was slight, diffuse thickening (2/5) of the SDFT with increased skin temperature and marked sensitivity to direct digital pressure in zone 2B (4/5). Ultrasonographic examination revealed subcutaneous fluid and possible SDFT enlargement (Figure 16-37) in zone 2B. Inflammation of the communicating branch of the palmar nerves was noted, indicating a malpositioned bandage. However, quantitative evaluation indicated a substantial generalized tendon thickening, which is unusual for a focal bandage pinch. The T-CSA was 15% larger than the normal limb (i.e., category II). It was recommended that exercise be restricted to walking with little trotting under saddle for 3 to 4 days a week for 1 month with daily icing and use of a thick stall bandage with alcohol. Foot length was to be shortened and the horse shod with a fully grooved or creased, lighter steel shoe to decrease the strain on the tendon. Five weeks later marked clinical improvement was noted. Ultrasonographic examination revealed that the subcutaneous fluid accumulation had resolved with no qualitative abnormalities of the SDFT. Substantial reduction in the T-CSA measurements indicated a resolution of intratendonous inflammation. These findings add credence to the initial diagnosis of low-grade tendonitis. It is difficult to make this diagnosis qualitatively with any confidence. Only use of quantitative analytical techniques allows the clinician to truly appreciate these changes and be confident in a category II diagnosis.

Category III

In category III lesions, type 1 or 2 focal hypoechogenic fibers bundles are present, with or without clinically significant MIZ-CSA or T-CSA enlargement. To qualify as a category III lesion, the T-TS (T-ES) cannot exceed 3 (i.e., <

2). This abnormality may be an incidental finding, represent minimal tendon or ligament injury, or be the end result of a healed and clinically stable tendon or ligament injury. In these horses, clinical history, physical examination, and serial monitoring help to determine the clinical significance of the ultrasonographic abnormalities.

A 16-year-old Trakehner gelding, used for upper-level dressage, was examined to assess healing of desmitis of the ALDDFT. The horse had been in controlled exercise for many months, and the client was anticipating a progressive return to normal athletic use, assuming the ultrasonographic findings were favorable. Moderate thickening of the ALDDFT (3/5) was confirmed ultrasonographically, including a focal area of compromised fiber bundles along the dorsal lateral border of zone 2A (TS = 1), and a generalized alteration in fiber bundle alignment (T-FAS = 4). Given the knowledge that this horse had been rested for many months, a slow return to training was recommended. The ultrasonographic images can be used as a benchmark for evaluation of the stability of the repair as gradual increases in ligament loading commence. The horse eventually returned to upper-level dressage and has been asymptomatic for 2 years.

Even though category II and III injuries do not seem to represent a very serious compromise to a tendon or ligament, they do alert the clinician, trainer, and owner to a subtle problem that requires medical management and that with early diagnosis is more easily managed. If the decision were made to continue athletic use while performing symptomatic therapy, serial ultrasonographic monitoring would be indicated to monitor stability. In this manner, early clinically significant regressions may be detected before overt clinical signs of reinjury occur. These two injury categories are not easily diagnosed with qualitative assessment alone. Quantitative analysis identifies these low-grade abnormalities. However, these two categories often represent a dilemma for a practitioner. The clinical signs are slight, seldom associated with lameness, and often respond quickly to symptomatic therapy. Therefore it is difficult to persuade trainers to rest horses. However, category II and III tendons and ligaments often represent the earliest of ultrasonographically identifiable injury and have the best chance of full recovery with extended rest. Quantitative evidence may help a client appreciate the significance of the injury. Ultimately, regardless of whether the horse is rested or treated symptomatically for a category II or III injury, periodic comparative data will greatly assist a practitioner in advising clients and help the clients to understand the injury.

Category IV

A category IV lesion is characterized by focal hypoechoic or anechoic lesions with the T-S ≥3, with a specific % T-lesion (Table 16-1). The range of % T-lesion to qualify for category IV varies depending on the number of zones included for determining the "total." The MIZ-CSA or T-CSA may or may not be substantially enlarged. Although this category includes a wide range of injuries, it can be used to document slight injury or an important compromise of tendon or ligament fiber bundles.

A 5-year-old TB racehorse gelding had a right fore SDFT injury of 6 months' duration. The horse had been galloping daily (exercise level 5) for 2 weeks, but the last time the

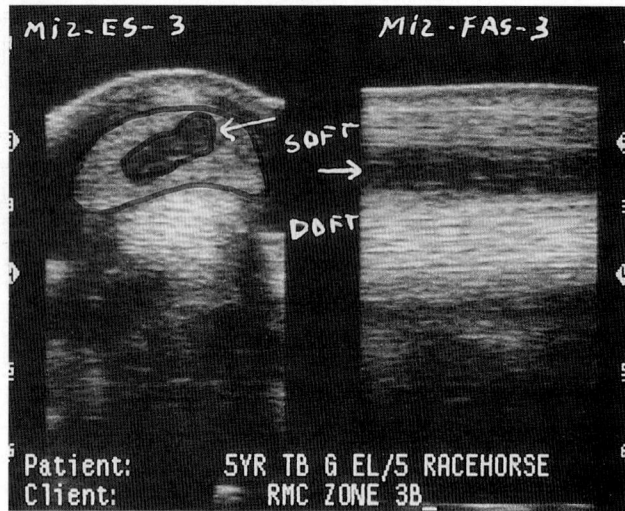

Fig. 16-38 • Transverse *(left)* and longitudinal *(right)* ultrasonographic images of zone 3B, obtained using a standoff pad. The arrows indicate a type 3 core lesion (traced on the transverse image) of the superficial digital flexor tendon *(SDFT)* on both views. The fiber alignment score of the target path of injury is 3. *DDFT,* Deep digital flexor tendon; *MIZ-ES-3;* maximal injury zone type or echo score of 3; *MIZ-FAS,* maximal injury zone fiber alignment score of 3.

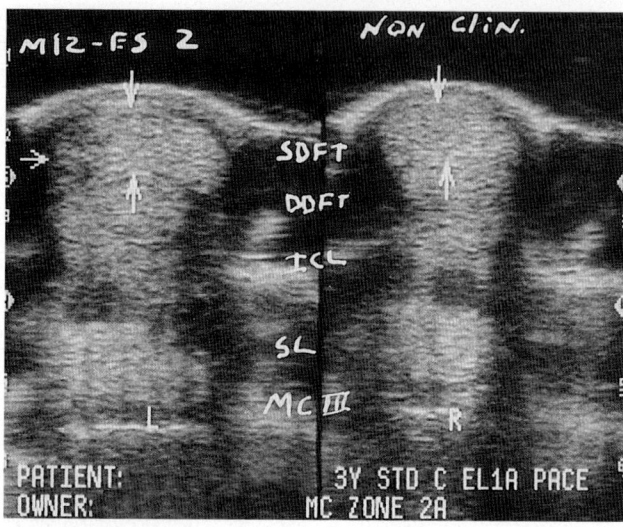

Fig. 16-39 • Transverse ultrasonographic images of zone 2A obtained using a standoff pad; the clinically abnormal limb is on the left and the clinically normal limb *(non-clin)* is on the right. The left *(L)* image (lateral to the left) demonstrates a type 2 lateral border lesion of the superficial digital flexor tendon *(SDFT; horizontal arrow).* Vertical arrows mark the palmar and dorsal borders of the SDFTs. The lateral border of the right *(R)* forelimb is to the right. *DDFT,* Deep digital flexor tendon; *ICL,* accessory ligament of the DDFT; *MIZ-ES 2,* maximal injury zone type or echo score of 2.

TABLE 16-1

Category IV T-Lesions	
ZONES USED FOR TOTAL (NO.)	**T-LESION (%)***
11	1%-10%
6 or 7	1%-15%
5	1%-20%
3	1%-25%

*All have a total type or echo score ≥3.

TABLE 16-2

Category V T-Lesion	
ZONES USED FOR TOTAL (NO.)	**T-LESION (%)***
11	11%-20%
6 or 7	16%-25%
5	21%-30%
3	26%-35%

*All have a total type or echo score ≥3.

horse galloped, right forelimb lameness and tendon swelling developed. Physical examination revealed slight swelling (1/5), low-grade lameness (2/5), moderate SDFT thickening (3/5), slight sensitivity to direct digital pressure, and localized heat (2/5) of the right forelimb. Ultrasonographic analysis of the right SDFT in zone 3B displayed a large type 3 anechoic core lesion (Figure 16-38). Quantitative data documented a T-CSA of 1243 mm². CSA was 67% larger than the left fore SDFT in zone 3B. In addition, bundles of compromised tendon were noted in six of the seven zones. These localized lesions of mixed echogenicity, mostly type 1, probably were the result of the previous injury. The new injury was localized to zones 3B and 3C, with echo scores of 2 and 3. In this analysis of reinjury, all areas of reduced echogenicity were included in the total lesion summation. Additional measurements include % T-lesion of 12%, T-TS of 11, T-FAS of 8, and A-FAS of 1.1.

Category V

Category V injuries typically have substantial MIZ-CSA or T-CSA enlargement with focal hypoechoic, anechoic, or both types of lesions. T-TS is greater than 3. This category has been arbitrarily associated with moderate tendon or

ligament injury. The range of % T-lesion to qualify for category V varies depending on the number of zones included in arriving at the "total" (Table 16-2).

Many horses with category V or VI injuries or reinjuries exhibit lameness in the early stages, but many category III and IV injuries are not associated with lameness.

A 3-year-old STB pacer, colt, developed swelling of the left fore SDFT after racing 1 week earlier and had previously sustained injury as a 2-year-old. The midmetacarpal region was slightly swollen (1/5) with moderate SDFT thickening (3/5), sensitivity to direct digital palpation (2/5), slight heat (1/5), and slight lameness (2/5). Ultrasonographic examination revealed a type 2, focal, hypoechoic lesion in the lateral border of the SDFT in zone 2A (Figure 16-39). Computer analysis of the left fore SDFT documented hypoechoic or anechogenic lesions along the lateral border in six of the seven zones (Figure 16-40). Zone 2A was designated the maximal injured zone because it had the lesion with the largest CSA (37%). The MIZ-CSA of 166 mm² was 47% larger than the same zone of the contralateral normal SDFT. T-CSA of the seven zones was 1179 mm², 31% greater than the contralateral SDFT. Additional measurements included T-TS of 11, T-FAS score of 8, and % T-lesion of 22% (i.e., category V). Unlike many newly injured tendons

FAS	Zone	Structure Size (mm²)	Lesion Size (mm²)	Type/Echo Score
0	1A	115	5 (3.86%)	1
1	1B	127	17 (12.60%)	1
2	2A	166	61 (36.57%)	2
3	2B	238	83 (34.88%)	3
1	3A	201	1.64 (32.34%)	3
1	3B	173	1.28 (16.24%)	1
0	3C	159	—	
Total 8		1179 (11.79 cm²)	258 (2.53 cm²)	11

Maximal injury score (MIZ)	2A	STAGE	Initial exam
MIZ-cross-sectional area (MIZ-CSA)	166 mm² (+41%)	SWEL	1/5
MIZ-lesion cross-sectional area (MIZ-LCA)	61 mm² (37%)	SEN	2/5
MIZ-echo (type) score (MIZ-TS)	2	ANK. SINK	0/5
MIZ-fiber alignment score (MIZ-FAS)	2	L	2/5
Total (7 levels) cross-sectional area (TCSA)	1179 mm² (+31%)	H	1/5
Total lesion cross-sectional area (TLCSA)	258 mm²	THIC	3/5
Percent total lesion (% T-Hypoechoic)	22%	T.SH	0/5
Total echo (type) score (TTS)	11	FLEX	Neg.
Total fiber alignment score (TFAS)	8		
Average fiber alignment score (AFAS)	1.1		
Present category	V		

Fig. 16-40 • A computer graphic of the left metacarpal region of the same horse as Figure 16-39 shows seven data points for quantitative evaluation. The superficial digital flexor tendon is 31% larger than the normal limb, has a 22% T-lesion, a T-echo or type score of 11, a T-fiber alignment score of 8, and an average fiber alignment score of 1.1. The maximal injury zone is 2A. The overall category of fascicle compromise is V. *ANK. SINK;* Ankle sinking; *FLEX,* flexion; *H,* heat; *L,* lameness; *SWEL,* swelling; *THIC,* Thickening; *T.SH,* tendon sheath.

or ligaments with similar T-TS and T-FAS scores, this reinjured SDFT had a difference in these scores. This may serve as a means to identify newly injured versus reinjured structures ultrasonographically.

Category VI

Category VI injuries have substantial MIZ-CSA or T-CSA enlargement with more extensive hypoechoic or anechoic lesions than category V. The range of % T-lesion to qualify for category VI varies depending on the number of zone used to determine the "total" (Table 16-3).

A 4-year-old TB racehorse gelding developed swelling of the left fore SDFT after a race 6 days earlier. Physical examination revealed slight swelling (2/5), moderate SDFT thickening (3/5), slight sensitivity to direct digital palpation (2/5), slight heat (2/5), and low-grade lameness (2/5). A large type 3 anechoic lesion of the lateral half of the SDFT was seen in zone 2B, the maximal injured zone (MIZ-LCA 92 mm² representing 54% of the tendon CSA). The MIZ-CSA was 114% larger than the contralateral normal zone 2B SDFT (see Figure 16-15). Six of the seven zones had hypoechogenic or anechogenic contiguous fiber bundles, with a 65% increase compared with the contralateral SDFT. T-LCSA was 300 mm², resulting in a 28% T-lesion. T-TS (14) and T-FAS (14) were the same, a common

TABLE 16-3

Category VI T-Lesions	
ZONES USED FOR TOTAL (NO.)	**T-LESION (%)***
11 zones	>20%
6 or 7 zones	>25%
5 zones	>30%
3 zones	>35%

*All have a total type or echo score ≥3.

finding in newly injured tendons, although not acute SL injuries.

Summary

Tendon and ligament injuries can be graded from 1 to 6 to reflect the severity of injury. Advantages of using quantitative assessment in conjunction with clinical findings and qualitative evaluation include the following:

1. Confirmation or addition to a qualitative diagnosis.
2. Improved detection of subtle structural enlargement not accompanied by detectable echogenicity abnormalities, thus reducing interpretive errors.

3. Establishment of an objective means to categorize the severity of an injury, which can be used to determine prognosis for intended use and whether continued use or extended rest is the optimal choice. It also provides baseline information that can be compared with follow-up examination findings.

4. Enhanced veterinary participation in the rehabilitation of a horse with a tendon or ligament injury.

5. Improved client appreciation of the injury and improved compliance with suggested exercise restraint and treatment.

6. Creation of a common ultrasonographic interprofessional language and provision of a valid tool for research purposes to evaluate treatment responses.

Exceptions

As with most attempts to categorize medical injuries, exceptions almost always are possible. The following are three common exceptions to quantitative categorization of tendon and ligament injuries:

1. Diffuse tendonitis or desmitis. This is an uncommon clinical manifestation of SDFT thickening and is seen mostly in 2-year-old TB racehorses and older event horses and show jumpers. The T-CSA measurements indicate substantial enlargement if the contralateral SDFT is normal. However, injury may be bilateral; therefore CSA measurements are compared with normal values for the breed, size, and age of the horse. Two-year-old TB racehorses in training tend to have larger T-CSA values than similar, older horses. In these horses, not only is the SDFT enlarged, but the entire CSA has a subtle reduction in echogenicity that extends through several zones. Although the % T-lesion is high, it does not necessarily indicate severe tendon fiber disruption because the echogenicity score for each zone is type 1 or 2 and the FAS score is 1 or 2. This indicates a diffuse tendonitis with little loss of tensile strength. Given time and restricted exercise, documentation with serial ultrasonography indicates that most 2-year-old horses generally do well (see Figure 16-33).

2. If the SDFT or SL is totally disrupted, fiber bundles in adjacent zones may appear artificially more hypoechoic or anechoic because of the loss of tension in the structure, which is otherwise known as *relaxation effect*.[22] Clinically, tension is lost and the structure can be moved medially and laterally with ease. Ultrasonography shows a loss of parallel fiber alignment and a decrease in echogenicity. Measurement of CSA is difficult and can even be decreased at the maximal injured zone (Figure 16-41). The diagnosis of complete rupture of a tendon or ligament is usually readily made clinically.

3. Total collapse of the SL is characterized clinically by an extreme extension of the metacarpophalangeal or metatarsophalangeal joint (4/5 ankle sink), with little swelling or clinically significant thickening of the SL or SL branch, and no sensitivity to direct palpation. Rupture cannot be palpated, and it appears as though the entire suspensory system has lost its cross-links and stretched, although ultrasonography shows little evidence of fiber tearing. Ultrasonographic images do not reflect the severity of the clinical signs.

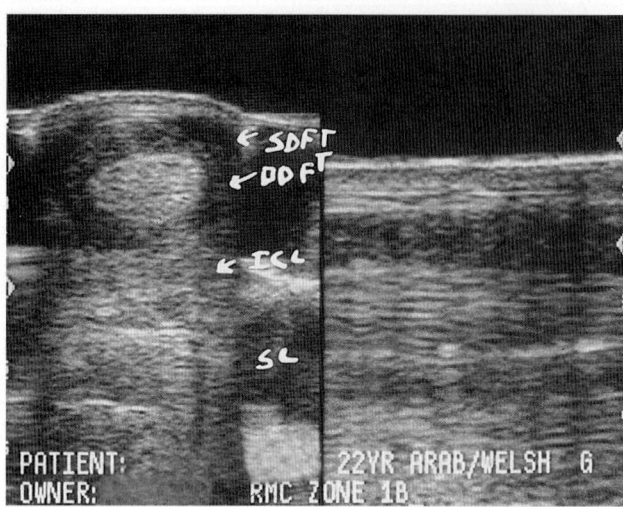

Fig. 16-41 • Transverse *(left)* and longitudinal *(right)* ultrasonographic images of zone 1B obtained with a standoff pad. The borders of the superficial digital flexor tendon *(SDFT)* are not defined, and most of the echoes present represent hematoma. The SDFT was completely ruptured. *DDFT,* Deep digital flexor tendon; *ICL,* accessory ligament of the DDFT; *SL,* suspensory ligament.

CLINICAL APPLICATIONS

If clinical evidence of swelling or thickening, with or without lameness, is present, the basic objective of an ultrasonographic evaluation is to determine the cause. Every effort must be made to determine whether tendons and ligaments are normal or abnormal and whether the lameness can be directly attributed to a soft tissue abnormality. Lameness may be visible only at high speeds in a racehorse or during special gait movements in a high-level dressage horse. In some instances the ultrasonographic data are insufficient to confirm the suspected cause, especially in subtle injury, although thorough evaluation and serial ultrasonographic examinations may provide clues.

Incidental abnormalities may be identified that have no bearing on the lameness or represent old, stable injuries of no clinical significance. Careful identification of these abnormalities and serial ultrasonographic monitoring may determine their clinical significance. Sometimes other imaging techniques, such as radiography, nuclear scintigraphy, or MRI, also are required to completely characterize an injury process. For example, evaluation of SL insertion injuries should also include radiological assessment.

Timing of Ultrasonographic Examinations: When to Scan

Timing of the initial ultrasonographic examination is critical. A clinician may be requested to examine a limb within hours of an injury. Peritendonous edema may obscure fiber damage because of acoustic enhancement, and the continued release of destructive enzymes may result in further ongoing fiber injury. Thus an examination shortly after an injury may not reveal the true extent of fiber damage. Ideally, an ultrasonographic evaluation should be delayed until at least 48 to 72 hours after the injury. If an ultrasonographic examination is performed before this time, the time after injury should be recorded, exercise restricted to walking, and symptomatic therapy instituted. Physical and ultrasonographic evaluations should be repeated after an additional 72 hours.

Clinically significant hypoechoic, anechoic, or both types of lesions may be seen in an injury less than 72 hours old. The areas of reduced echogenicity may represent a combination of hemorrhage (seroma), edema, and fiber bundle injury. The diagnostic dilemma at this stage is that the clinician cannot accurately determine the relative contribution of each. It should not necessarily be assumed that the hypoechogenic areas only represent fiber bundle injury. In most horses this assumption is true, but not always. We administer symptomatic antiinflammatory treatment and advise complete stall rest (exercise level 0) or limited hand walking (exercise level 1A) for 14 to 30 days, followed by an ultrasonographic reevaluation. (The exception to this advice would be if tendon splitting surgery were the treatment of choice to attempt to decompress a core lesion.) When the horse is reexamined, persistent hypoechogenic areas represent fiber bundle compromise, because most inflammatory edema and hemorrhage will have resolved. The severity of the injury can now be determined, and we refer to this as the *baseline evaluation*. The baseline evaluation often reveals the same or increased severity of injury compared with the initial scan (especially in core lesions caused by enzymatic degradation of damaged fiber bundles or pressure necrosis).

As an example, we can compare ultrasonographic images of a SDFT injury after 24 hours and after 22 days. The initial examination determined that the SDFT was 32% larger than the normal contralateral limb and had a 17% T-lesion (category V), a T-TS of 17, and a T-FAS of 16. After symptomatic therapy and a reduction of exercise to exercise level 1A, the baseline scans (22 days later) revealed a 12% increase in size of the SDFT compared with the normal limb, a 13% T-lesion (now category IV), a T-TS of 10, and a T-FAS of 12. The apparent decrease in severity was from resolution of the inflammatory response and absorption of the seroma. The baseline data represent the actual severity of fiber bundle compromise and serve as the starting point for rendering prognosis for intended use, treatment programs, and long-term rehabilitation exercise regimens.

Serial Ultrasonographic Examinations as Part of Case Management

Serial ultrasonographic examinations are best performed when it is anticipated that the exercise level may be increased. This justifies the examination to an owner or trainer. In addition to the ultrasonographic assessment, a clinician must always consider the physiological principles of tendon and ligament healing and the necessary physiological time for healing for the severity of an injury before advising exercise level increases. With time and as quantitative ultrasonographic analysis is more commonly used to evaluate tendon and ligament repair, more definitive recommendations will develop concerning convalescent time based on the severity and location of an injury and the intended athletic function of the horse. The same applies to the quality of the repair. Horses destined for light work will be able to perform with a less than perfect repair, but racehorses and other high-level athletes will require optimal repair and a reasonable time to give the best chance for return to athletic use without reinjury.

During rehabilitation a qualitative ultrasonographic evaluation of the clinically injured tendon is done to detect obvious lesions, evidence of reinjury, restricting peritendonous tendon sheath fibrosis, or restriction by the PAL. Objective, or quantitative, ultrasonographic assessments should also be determined. Guidelines for an optimum chance to return to racing include the following[23]:

1. At least a 60% decrease in category IV % T-lesion and <12% total lesion cross-sectional surface area (T-LCSA) for all categories of severity of injury.
2. At least a 10% to 15% decrease in T-CSA from baseline for all categories of injury (a relatively greater decrease in more seriously injured tendons).
3. At least a 70% decrease in the T-TS (ideally <4; the closer to 0, the better).
4. At least a 75% decrease in the T-FAS (ideally <4; the closer to 0, the better) before advancing to exercise level 5.
5. The horse should meet at least three of the above requirements with only minimal failure of the other criterion.

Nonetheless, even a perfectly healed tendon or ligament injury can be reinjured. Reinjury is especially common in TB racehorses. However, if the repair is of poor quality, reinjury is likely, and these horses should be held back from active training until healing has improved. Decision making is more accurate when it is based on ultrasonographic evaluation and consideration of necessary physiological time for intended use than when relying on clinical inspection.

The advantages of veterinary intervention and using quantitative ultrasonographic parameters in case management provide a means to optimize the chances of returning an injured horse to athletic usefulness and are reviewed in this clinical example. A 4-year-old TB racehorse with a left fore SDFT injury was examined 3 days after a race. The maximal injured zone was zone 2B (59% lesion), T-CSA was 1206 mm^2, T-TS was 11, and T-FAS was 16. This was a 49% T-lesion (i.e., category VI). The horse was treated with a series of three external blisters and 6 months' pasture rest, a typical theory in the early 1990s. The horse was reassessed 8 months after injury to determine whether it could return to training (exercise level 5). The tendon was tight and cold. Qualitative ultrasonographic examination indicated improvement, although abnormalities persisted, which were interpreted to be the end result of repair. Thus the trainer was wrongly advised to return to training.

In light of current knowledge, the ultrasonographic data at the time of reevaluation provided clear indication of an unstable repair. The T-CSA had increased 15% and % T-lesion decreased by only 50%, and therefore was still quite high at 22%. In addition, neither T-TS nor T-FAS met a target decrease of 75%. After 4 weeks of galloping, the horse worked at race speed (breezed) once and became lame again. An ultrasonographic evaluation identified extensive reinjury to the same tendon (i.e., category VI). Thus quantitative analysis of injuries is an extremely beneficial tool to monitor progress of tendon healing.

References on page 1261

Chapter 17

Ultrasonographic Examination of Joints

Jean-Marie Denoix

Ultrasonography has become an essential imaging technique for assessing joint lesions.[1-6] It provides information complementary to radiography but does have some limitations. Ultrasonography requires a precise knowledge of anatomy, not only bone anatomy,[4] and a systematic approach. Examining the joints of the distal part of the limb is physically uncomfortable for the imager and is time-consuming: complete examination of a joint may take up to 30 minutes. Quick examination of joints requires several years of daily practice.

The indications for ultrasonographic examination of equine joints include synovial fluid distention, local swelling, pain on passive manipulation of the joint, improvement in lameness after intraarticular or perineural analgesia, and positive radiological or scintigraphic findings. The area to be examined should be clipped, not shaved, and washed with hot water. High-resolution transducers (7.5- to 13-MHz linear probes) and a standoff pad are used for superficial structures. Convex array 2.5- to 5-MHz transducers are preferable for deeper structures. Both left and right joints should be examined to improve sensitivity and specificity. The image quality depends not only on the frequency of the transducer but also on the quality of the machine (from treatment of the signal to display on the monitor) and the skill of the operator in placing and orienting the transducer.

A comprehensive description of all joints cannot be given in this book. The fetlock joint is a model for a general approach to ultrasonography of joints because of its simple anatomy. Some aspects of examination of the stifle and hock also are presented.

FETLOCK

Each aspect of the joint should be examined systematically using 7.5- to 13-MHz linear transducers and a thin standoff pad.

Dorsal Aspect

Figure 17-1 shows normal ultrasonographic anatomy.[4,5] In normal fetlock joints the articular capsule is echogenic (except if too relaxed), and the articular margins of the proximal phalanx and the condyles of the third metacarpal bone (McIII) are smooth.

Ultrasonography is a useful technique for the differential diagnosis of soft tissue injuries on the dorsal aspect of the fetlock joint. These lesions include subcutaneous swelling or abscess, bursitis of the subtendonous bursa of the extensor tendons, extensor tendonitis, capsulitis, synovial

fluid distention of the dorsal recess of the metacarpophalangeal joint (Figure 17-2), and chronic proliferative synovitis of the proximodorsal synovial fold of this joint (Figure 17-3). Thinning, fibrillation, and fissures of the articular cartilage of the dorsal and distal aspects of the condyle of the McIII can be identified with high-resolution transducers. Subchondral bone lesions can sometimes be detected before they are visible radiologically. Ultrasonography may

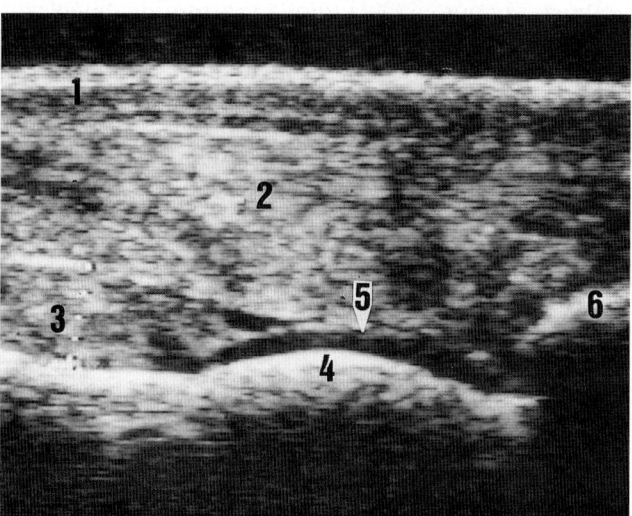

Fig. 17-1 • Sagittal ultrasonographic image of the dorsal aspect of the fetlock, normal appearance. Proximal is to the left. *1,* Skin; *2,* dorsal joint capsule; *3,* proximal synovial fold; *4,* subchondral bone of the condyle of the third metacarpal bone; *5,* articular cartilage of the condyle of third metacarpal bone; *6,* proximal phalanx.

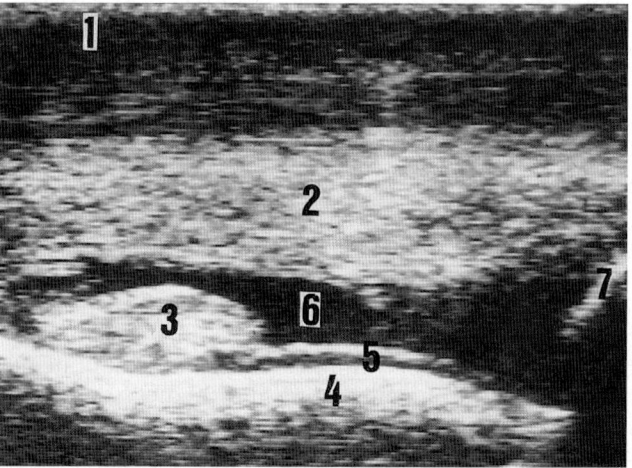

Fig. 17-2 • Sagittal ultrasonographic image of the dorsal aspect of the fetlock joint. An abnormal synovial fluid accumulation appears between the joint capsule and the articular surface. The diagnosis is synovial fluid effusion, indicative of synovitis. Proximal is to the left. *1,* Skin; *2,* dorsal joint capsule; *3,* proximal synovial fold; *4,* subchondral bone of the condyle of the third metacarpal bone; *5,* articular cartilage of the condyle of the third metacarpal bone; *6,* synovial fluid; *7,* proximal phalanx.

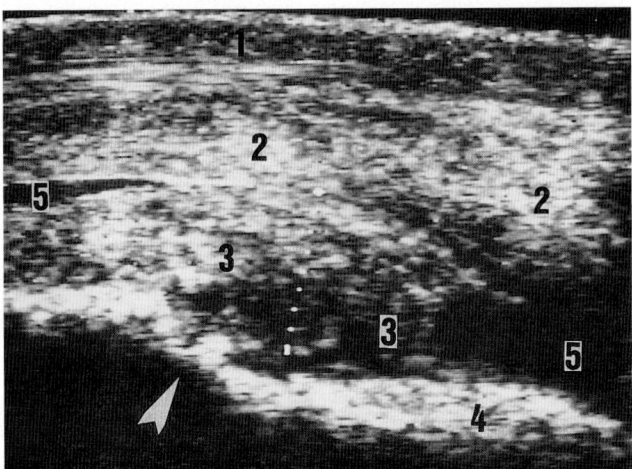

Fig. 17-3 • Sagittal ultrasonographic image of the dorsal aspect of the fetlock joint. An abnormal hypoechogenic mass appears between the capsule and the condyle of the third metacarpal bone. The proximal aspect of this condyle is irregular, indicating bone lysis *(arrowhead)*. The diagnosis is chronic proliferative synovitis. *1*, Skin; *2*, dorsal joint capsule; *3*, proximal synovial fold tremendously thickened and echogenic; *4*, condyle of the third metacarpal bone; *5*, synovial fluid.

be more sensitive than radiography for detection of the site and number of osteochondral fragments.[7]

Dorsomedial and Dorsolateral Aspects

Examination of the dorsomedial and dorsolateral aspects of the joint is especially useful for complete evaluation of the articular margins, which are smooth in a normal joint. The most common abnormal finding is the presence of periarticular osteophytes. Other injuries are subcutaneous lesions (fibrosis, swelling) and capsulitis.

Medial and Lateral Aspects

The medial and lateral collateral ligaments have superficial and deep layers.[4] If the transducer is parallel to the skin (the ultrasound beam is perpendicular to fiber interface), the superficial layer of the collateral ligament is echogenic and the deep layer is hypoechogenic. Either layer may be damaged (Figure 17-4). If both layers are affected, joint instability, subluxation, or luxation occurs.

Palmar Aspect

A normal fetlock joint has a small amount of anechogenic synovial fluid in the proximopalmar recess of the fetlock joint. Abnormal findings observed in affected horses include

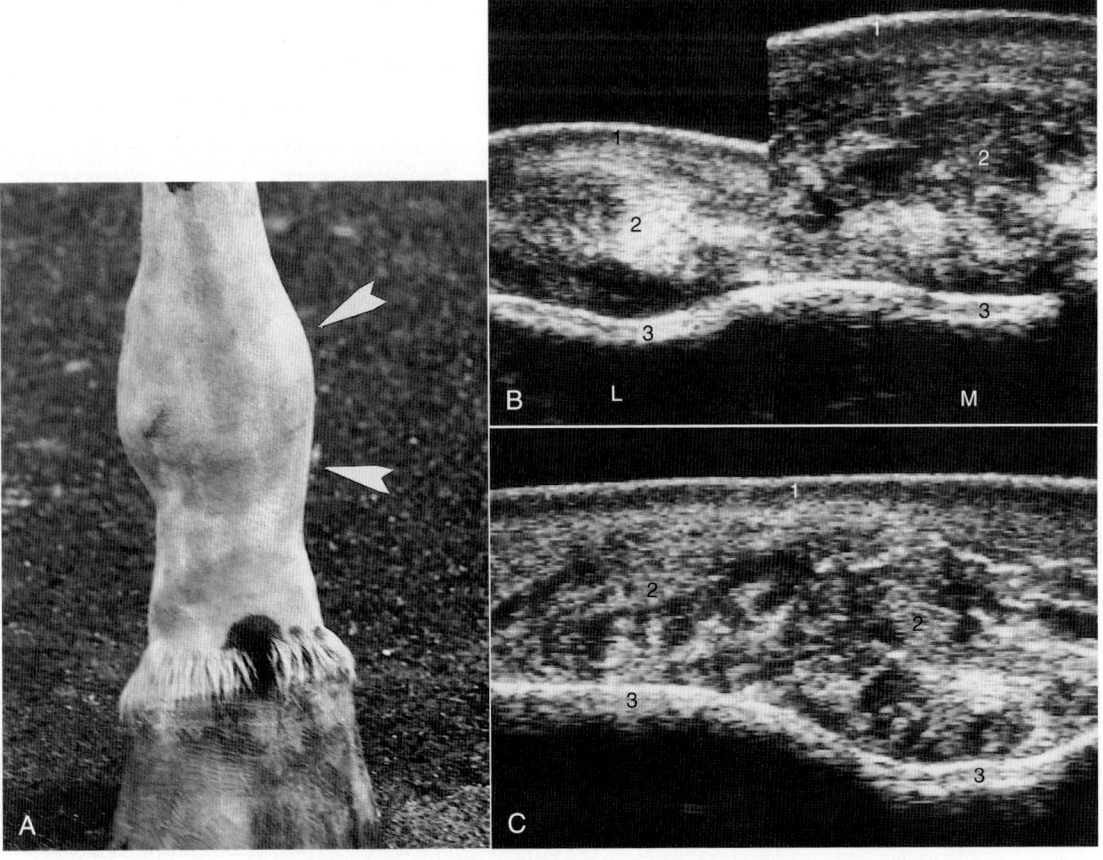

Fig. 17-4 • A, Physical appearance of an injured right hind fetlock joint (arrowheads show medial enlargement). Radiography found no bony abnormalities. **B,** Transverse ultrasonographic images of the lateral *(L)* and medial *(M)* aspects of the injured fetlock. The size and architecture differ greatly between the normal lateral collateral ligament and the injured medial ligament. **C,** Longitudinal ultrasonographic image of the medial aspect of the fetlock shows the thickening and architectural alterations of the medial collateral ligament. The diagnosis is chronic desmopathy of the medial collateral ligament. *1*, Skin; *2*, collateral ligament; *3*, condyle of the third metatarsal bone.

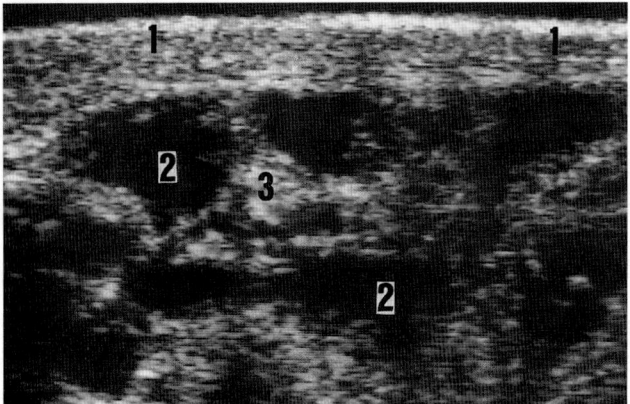

Fig. 17-5 • Longitudinal ultrasonographic image of the palmarolateral aspect of the fetlock demonstrating a marked fluid distention of the palmaroproximal recess of the fetlock. The diagnosis is synovial fluid effusion indicative of synovitis. *1*, Skin; *2*, synovial fluid; *3*, synovial membrane and villi.

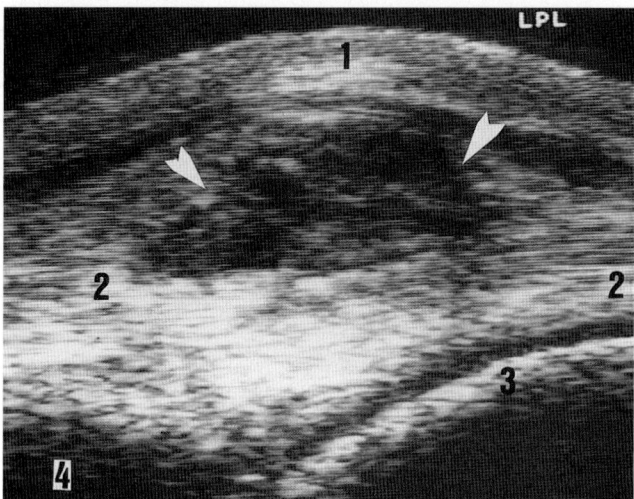

Fig. 17-6 • Longitudinal ultrasonographic image of the lateral patellar ligament demonstrating localized enlargement. At the site of the lesion *(arrowheads)* the ligament is hypoechogenic and shows severe architectural changes. Diagnosis is traumatic lateral patellar desmopathy. *1*, Skin; *2*, lateral patellar ligament; *3*, lateral ridge of the femoral trochlea (subchondral bone surface); *4*, patella.

synovial fluid distention, often associated with enlarged synovial folds, indicative of synovitis (Figure 17-5).

Echogenic material may be observed in the synovial fluid in any view. Small echogenic spots may represent fibrin or cartilaginous debris. Larger echogenic masses are compatible with osteochondral fragments. These abnormal findings are more easily seen after movement of the joint. A homogeneous increase in echogenicity of the fluid is compatible with hemarthrosis or infectious synovitis.

STIFLE

Ultrasonography has considerably improved the knowledge and the diagnosis of soft tissue injuries of the femoropatellar and femorotibial joints.

Femoropatellar Joint

The femoropatellar joint is examined using 5- to 10-MHz linear transducers with a thin standoff pad. The normal patellar ligaments are homogeneously echogenic.[1-3] The articular cartilage is thicker over the lateral trochlear ridge compared with the medial. Each femoral trochlea has a regular hyperechogenic subchondral bone surface.

Medial patellar desmopathy usually is iatrogenic (i.e., caused by medial patellar desmotomy or desmoplasty). Desmopathy of the intermediate (middle) patellar ligament is an injury that occurs in athletic horses.[8] Lateral patellar desmopathy often is caused by trauma (Figure 17-6).

Osteochondrosis of the trochlear ridges is easy to diagnose, and ultrasonography provides information on the extent of the lesion (especially in a lateromedial direction), the size and location of the osteochondral fragments, and the severity of alteration of the subchondral bone.[9] Evaluation of the synovial fluid and membrane may also be useful to assess the consequences of ligamentous and osteochondral lesions in the joint.

Medial and Lateral Femorotibial Joints

Examination of the femorotibial joint requires 5- to 10-MHz linear transducers and a thin standoff pad.[10-13] In normal joints the medial recess of the medial femorotibial joint is less than 3 cm long in a craniocaudal direction, and the

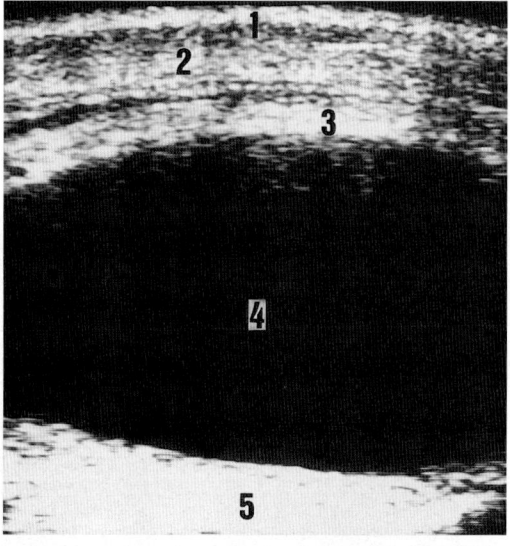

Fig. 17-7 • Transverse ultrasonographic image of the medial recess of the medial femorotibial joint. Anechogenic synovial fluid has distended this recess. The diagnosis is synovial effusion compatible with synovitis and other potential injuries of the femorotibial joint. *1*, Skin; *2*, medial femoral fascia; *3*, synovial membrane; *4*, medial recess of the medial femorotibial joint; *5*, medial aspect of the distal femur.

synovial fluid is totally anechogenic. The normal medial collateral ligament and medial meniscus are homogeneously echogenic,[1-3] provided that the ultrasound beam is perpendicular to the orientation of the fibers. The normal articular margins of the medial femoral condyle and tibial plateau are smooth and regular.

The medial recess of the medial femorotibial joint can be considered a mirror of the joint, because its size and content are influenced by all joint lesions. Abnormalities include synovial effusion (Figure 17-7); chronic

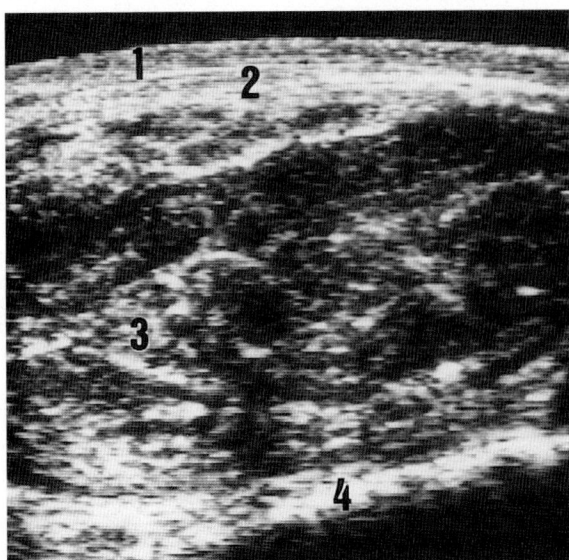

Fig. 17-8 • Transverse ultrasonographic image of the medial recess of the medial femorotibial joint. Echogenic material distends the recess. The diagnosis is hemarthrosis compatible with other potential ligament or bone injuries of the femorotibial joint. *1,* Skin; *2,* medial femoral fascia; *3,* medial recess of the medial femorotibial joint; *4,* medial aspect of the distal femur.

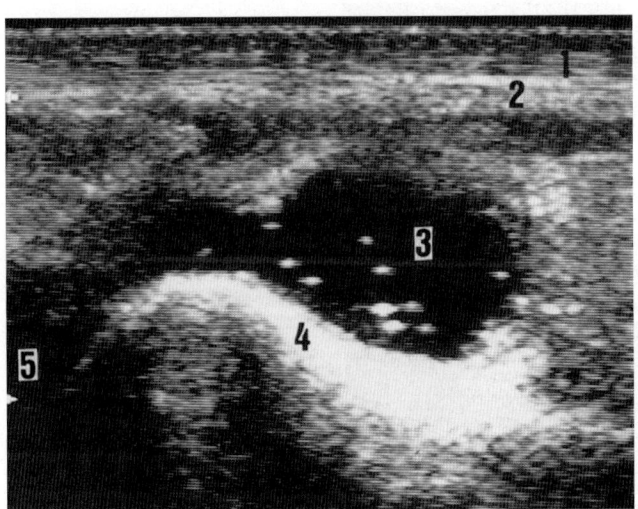

Fig. 17-9 • Longitudinal ultrasonographic image of the medial recess of the medial femorotibial joint. Echogenic material floats in the synovial fluid. These echogenic spots represent fibrin, cartilaginous debris, or meniscal debris. Proximal is to the right. *1,* Skin; *2,* medial femoral fascia; *3,* medial recess of the medial femorotibial joint; *4,* medial femoral condyle; *5,* medial meniscus (anechogenic because of the orientation of the ultrasound beam).

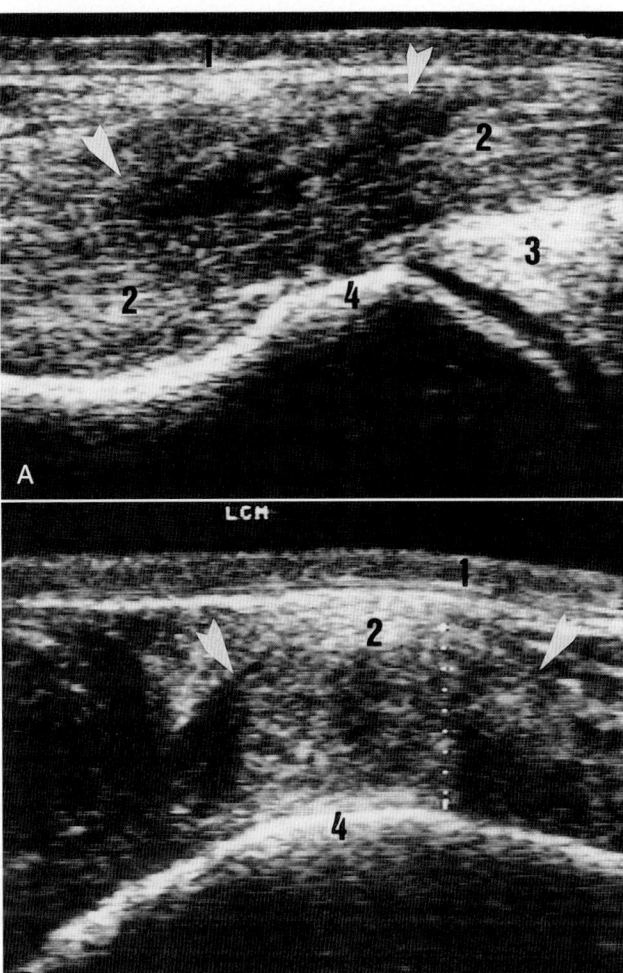

Fig. 17-10 • **A,** Longitudinal ultrasonographic image (proximal is left) of the medial collateral ligament of the femorotibial joint. This ligament is enlarged and hypoechogenic *(arrowheads).* Diagnosis is traumatic medial collateral desmopathy. **B,** Transverse ultrasound scan of the medial collateral ligament. *1,* Skin; *2,* medial collateral ligament; *3,* medial meniscus; *4,* medial femoral condyle.

proliferative synovitis; hemarthrosis (Figure 17-8); echogenic spots compatible with fibrin, cartilaginous, or meniscal debris (Figure 17-9); osteochondral fragments; and calcinosis circumscripta. The caudal recess of the medial femorotibial joint can be examined with 2.5- to 5-MHz sector or convex array probes. Distention of this recess always indicates severe femorotibial disease. Distention of the subextensorius recess on the craniolateral aspect of the lateral femorotibial joint can be observed in lateral femorotibial arthropathy or femoropatellar joint lesions.

Desmopathy of the medial collateral ligament may be identified as disruption in the normal parallel fiber pattern (Figure 17-10).

Meniscal injuries can be observed alone or with other ligamentous or bone injuries (Figure 17-11). In horses, approximately 75% of these lesions are found in the medial meniscus and 25% in the lateral meniscus. A wide range of type and severity of medial meniscal injuries may be seen (see Figures 17-11 and 17-12).

If a transducer is held vertically and moved in a caudocranial direction, complete examination of the articular margins of the femoral condyles is possible. Ultrasonography may be more sensitive than radiography in detecting periarticular osteophytes. If the stifle is examined in flexion, the cartilage and subchondral bone surface of the femoral condyles can be imaged.[1-3] Alterations of the subchondral bone surface and echogenicity may be detected.

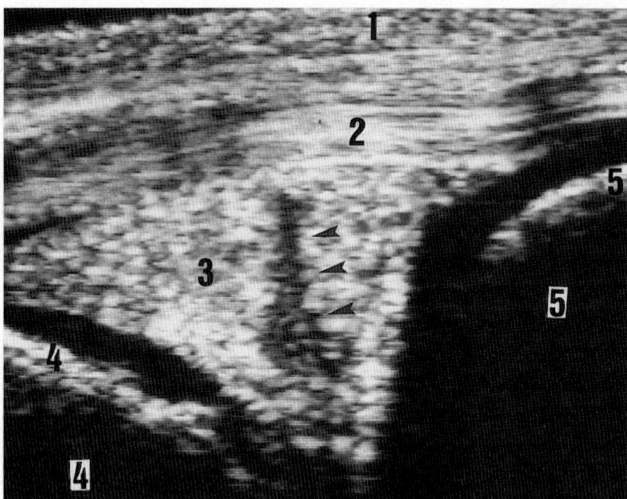

Fig. 17-11 • Proximodistal ultrasonographic image of the medial aspect of the medial femorotibial joint showing a transverse section of the body of the medial meniscus. An obvious hypoechoic defect *(arrowheads)* is seen. The diagnosis is medial meniscal lesion. *1,* Skin; *2,* medial collateral ligament; *3,* medial meniscus; *4,* medial femoral condyle (with anechoic articular cartilage); *5,* medial tibial condyle (with anechogenic articular cartilage).

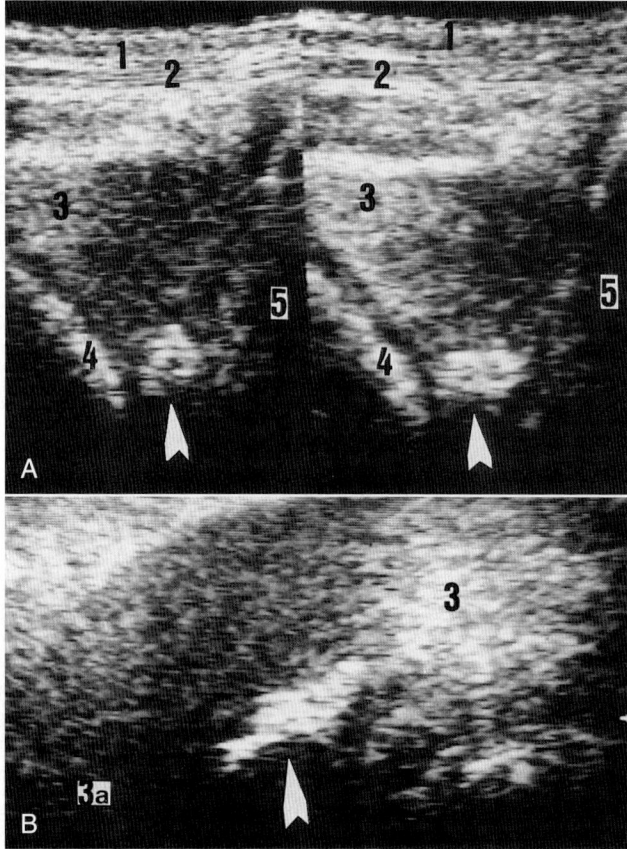

Fig. 17-12 • **A,** Proximodistal ultrasonographic image of the craniomedial aspect of the medial femorotibial joint showing transverse sections of the cranial horn of the medial meniscus. Hyperechogenic material is present in the deep (axial) part of this horn *(arrowheads)*. **B,** Transverse ultrasonographic image of the craniomedial aspect of the medial femorotibial joint showing a horizontal section of the cranial horn of the medial meniscus. This scan confirms presence of hyperechogenic material in the horn. The diagnosis is that hyperechogenic material is a focal site of mineralized metaplasia in a meniscus. *1,* Skin; *2,* medial femoral fascia; *3,* medial meniscus; *3a,* cranial attachment; *4,* medial femoral condyle; *5,* medial tibial condyle.

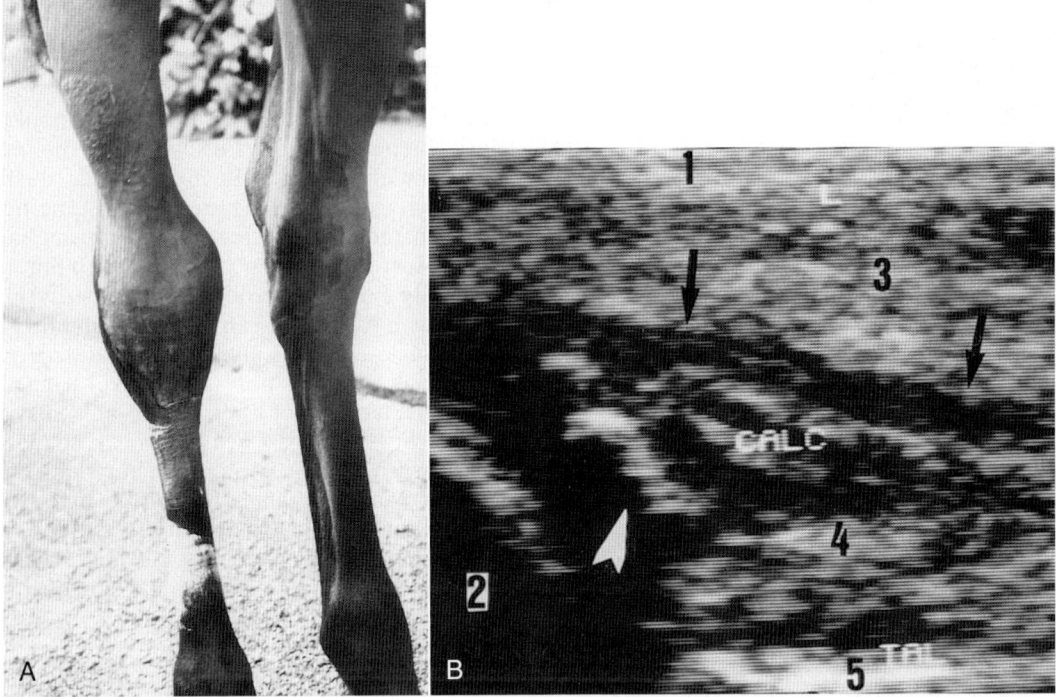

Fig. 17-13 • **A,** Acute medial collateral desmopathy in a 15-month-old filly. Physical appearance of the hock with a medial swelling. **B,** Longitudinal ultrasonographic image of the calcanean fasciculus of the medial collateral ligament. This structure is thickened and hypoechogenic with evidence of fiber disruption. An echogenic osteochondral fragment *(arrowhead)* appears close to the medial malleolus of the tibia. The diagnosis is severe desmopathy with avulsion fracture involving the calcanean fasciculus of the medial collateral ligament. *1,* skin; *2,* medial malleolus of the tibia; *3,* long medial collateral ligament; *4,* short medial collateral ligament—calcanean fasciculus *(CALC); 5,* medial aspect of the talus *(TAL).*

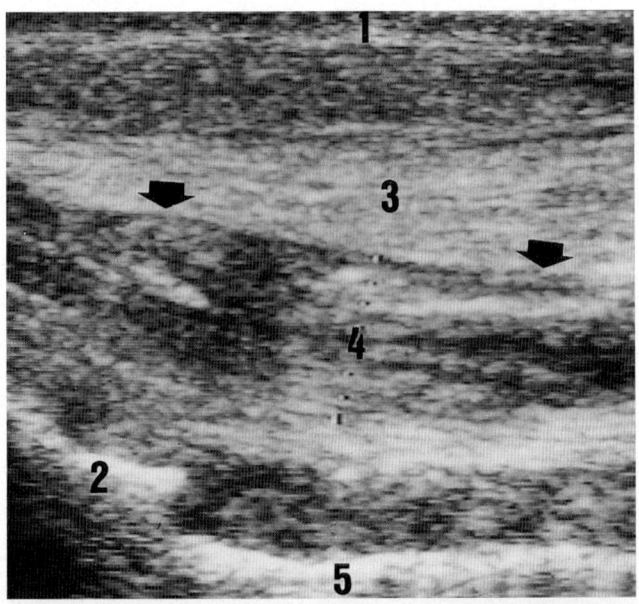

Fig. 17-14 • Longitudinal ultrasonographic image of the calcanean fasciculus of the medial collateral ligament of a 9-year-old Three Day Event gelding after injury 3 months previously. This structure *(black arrows)* is thickened and has architectural changes. The diagnosis is desmopathy of the calcanean fasciculus of the medial collateral ligament. *1,* Skin; *2,* medial malleolus of the tibia; *3,* long medial collateral ligament; *4,* short medial collateral ligament—calcanean fasciculus *(arrowheads); 5,* medial aspect of the talus.

COLLATERAL LIGAMENTS OF THE HOCK

The causes of soft tissue enlargement of the hock may be difficult to assess clinically and radiologically. The medial and lateral collateral ligaments of the hock are highly echogenic fibrous structures.[14] Each is divided into a long collateral ligament, which inserts distally on the distal aspect of the tarsus and the proximal aspect of the metatarsal region, and a short collateral ligament with two fasciculi: a calcanean fasciculus and a talien one.

Proximal avulsion fracture of the calcanean fasciculus of the medial collateral ligament has been identified (Figure 17-13). Lesions of this ligament also can be identified in hocks with no radiological abnormality (Figure 17-14). In old lesions the long medial collateral ligament remains thickened and may have focal echogenic sites associated with mineralization.

Several types of injury of the lateral collateral ligament have been identified, including desmopathy of the long lateral collateral ligament, avulsion fracture of the short lateral collateral ligament at the proximal insertion on the lateral malleolus of the tibia (distal portion of the fibula), and desmitis of the short lateral collateral ligament associated with sudden synovial distention of the tarsocrural joint capsule.

Chapter 18

Ultrasonography and Orthopedic (Nonarticular) Disease

Virginia B. Reef

The use of diagnostic ultrasonography for evaluation of tendons, ligaments, tendon sheaths, bursae, and joints is discussed in Chapters 16, 17, and 82, and horse preparation for other musculoskeletal uses is similar.

SKELETAL MUSCLE

References on page 1261

Normal skeletal muscle appears heterogeneous, with hypoechogenic muscle fibers laced with and surrounded by echogenic fascia, connective tissue, and fat. In transverse section a normal muscle has a marbled or speckled appearance, which is unique for each individual muscle, as is its striated appearance in longitudinal section.[1,2] A non–weight-bearing muscle appears more echogenic than the same muscle when the horse is fully weight bearing.[1,2] Therefore comparisons between contralateral muscles should be made when the horse is bearing weight evenly.

Traumatic muscle injuries, myositis, and masses infiltrating the muscles usually can be differentiated from one another by ultrasonography.[1] Muscle tears in horses most frequently are seen in the hindlimb and shoulder musculature. In neonatal foals, muscle tears are most commonly seen in the hindlimb.[3] The affected muscle or muscles can be identified by tracing the involved muscle from its origin to insertion. Fluid-filled anechogenic areas with hypoechogenic loculations are located within the muscle belly, associated with areas of hemorrhage and muscle fiber tearing (Figure 18-1).[1,3-6] As the muscle injury becomes more severe, large areas of interfascial and subcutaneous hemorrhage are detected. The free edge of a completely disrupted muscle may be imaged floating in the anechogenic loculated fluid in the hematoma. Echogenic areas of clot are often imaged within the intramuscular, interfascial, or subcutaneous hematoma. As these echogenic clots become more organized, they may cast an acoustic shadow from the far surface. Rupture of the gastrocnemius muscle should be considered as a cause of recumbency in neonatal foals that are unable to rise and have soft tissue swelling in the hindlimb. Rupture of the gastrocnemius muscle has been reported as a complication of dystocia.[3] Partial muscle tears are more difficult to diagnose because the ultrasonographic abnormalities are more subtle.[1] The normal striated muscle pattern is lost with increased echogenicity of the injured muscle.[1] Swelling of the affected muscle usually is present. Tears in the muscle fascia or thickening of the muscle fascia or fasciitis also may be detected ultrasonographically.[1]

Ultrasonography is an excellent tool for monitoring the resolution of the hematoma and the healing of the muscle.[1,5] The affected horse's exercise should be restricted until the hematoma has resolved and the muscle tear has filled in with tissue. As the muscle heals, the fluid becomes more echogenic and the area fills in. The healing muscle may become more heterogeneous. Hyperechogenic areas of muscle scarring are seen associated with fibrotic myopathy, especially in the semitendinosus (primarily) and semimembranosus muscles, but can also occur in other muscles such as the biceps femoris and gracilis (rare).[1,5,7] As these areas of fibrosis become more organized, acoustic shadowing from the far side of the fibrotic area may be detected. Hyperechogenic areas casting acoustic shadows are seen in horses with an ossifying myopathy and frequently are found adjacent to areas of fibrotic myopathy.[1] Areas of mineralization develop as scattered, pinpoint hyperechogenic areas that progressively become linear and result in acoustic shadowing from the near side of the areas.

Postanesthetic myopathy results in increased echogenicity of the affected muscle, with loss of the normal muscle striations.[1,2] Muscle edema may result in the muscle appearing less echogenic than normal if the lesion is evaluated early in the course of the disease. Once a large influx of inflammatory cells has occurred, the affected muscle becomes more echogenic. A necrotizing myositis usually results in a more heterogeneous ultrasonographic appearance associated with the inflammatory cell infiltrate and bacterial infection.[1] Cavitation of a severely affected muscle is associated with liquefactive necrosis. Hyperechoic echoes, associated with the local production of gas by bacteria, may be seen with an anaerobic necrotizing myositis.[1]

Muscle tumors are rare; the most common muscle tumor is hemangiosarcoma. Discrete echogenic masses in the muscle or anechogenic loculated, more heterogeneous masses may be detected.[1] Central anechogenic or

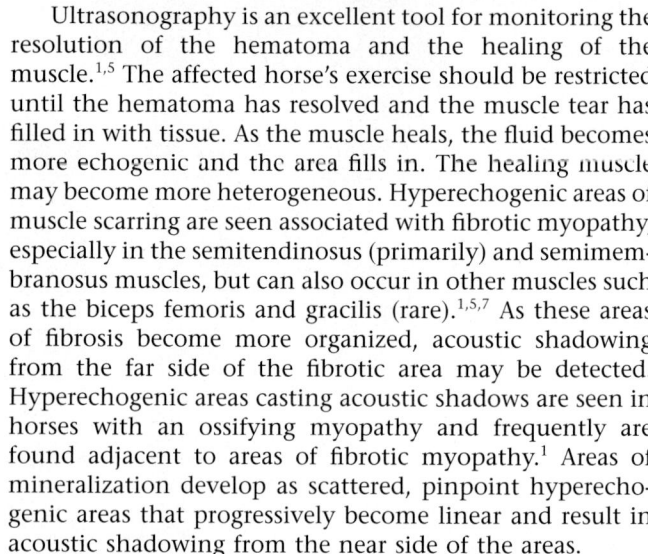

Figure 18-1 • Longitudinal ultrasonographic image of a torn semimembranosus muscle showing large, anechogenic fluid-filled areas, hypoechogenic amorphous areas, and more normal striated muscle at the periphery of the images. The anechogenic areas and hypoechogenic amorphous area are consistent with a hematoma replacing the muscle. The anechogenic area is the fluid component of the hematoma, whereas the hypoechogenic areas *(arrow)* represent the fibrin and clot.

hypoechogenic areas representing tumor necrosis are identified in large or rapidly growing tumor masses. Primary muscle tumors such as rhabdomyosarcomas are extremely rare but can be a cause of lameness.[8] Accurate identification of tumor type in muscle necessitates obtaining an ultrasound-guided biopsy and histopathological evaluation of the tissue obtained.

NERVE

Distinguishing peripheral nerves requires high-resolution images because the majority of nerves are small. Accurate knowledge of the locations of the nerves and the surrounding landmarks is important for identification. The nerves usually are slightly more echogenic than the surrounding soft tissue structures and are round to oval in transverse section.[1] Deep nerves usually appear as two tubular structures with parallel, straight, sharply hyperechogenic borders and a hypoechogenic center.[9] Superficial nerves have linear internal echoes that parallel the straight hyperechogenic borders.[1,9] Enlargement of the nerve with an increase or decrease in its echogenicity, with or without heterogeneity in its ultrasonographic appearance, is consistent with neuritis,[1] which may be a primary cause of lameness (see Chapter 82).

PENETRATING INJURIES

Ultrasonographic examination may be helpful in assessing penetrating injuries. The examiner should start at the site of the puncture wound and follow the path left by the penetrating object, a hyperechogenic tubular tract extending into the soft tissues.[10,11] The tract appears hyperechogenic from gas lining the tract. Any foreign material usually is hyperechogenic and casts acoustic shadows in two mutually perpendicular planes. Foreign material is usually irregular in shape, differs in size when imaged in two mutually perpendicular planes, and typically has high acoustic impedance relative to soft tissue. This examination can be done under aseptic surgical conditions when indicated.

DRAINING TRACTS

The cause of draining tracts should be determined systematically using ultrasonography before a contrast radiographic examination is performed. Usually the source of drainage can be confirmed by ultrasonography if a thorough ultrasonographic examination is performed, eliminating the need to perform a contrast study. The injection of contrast material into the tract also results in the injection of air. This air may limit or prevent evaluation of foreign bodies within the tract because air is a nearly perfect reflector of ultrasound waves. The air that is injected with the contrast material may mix with the fluid within the tract, surround the foreign body, and obscure it from view.

A draining tract should be scanned systematically, keeping in mind that more than one factor may cause drainage. The clinician should start at the skin surface and follow the tract,, which usually appears as hypoechogenic tissue that is oval to round in transverse section and somewhat tubular in longitudinal section. The draining tract usually is easiest to follow in transverse section, unless the tract is short and straight.[1] The draining tract should be kept in the center of the ultrasound screen as it is followed into the deeper tissues. The tract may be single, or multiple tracts may be present. Often the tract is tortuous, and each branch of the tract should be followed to its source.[1] The source of the drainage at the end of the tract or tracts should be identified. Chronic draining tracts can originate from an area of osteitis or osteomyelitis; a sequestrum, foreign body, or necrotic tissue acting as a foreign body; an abscess; or a synovial structure.[1,11] Once the source or sources of the drainage have been identified, appropriate decisions can be made regarding medical or surgical management.

FOREIGN BODIES

Foreign bodies vary in ultrasonographic appearance.[10-19] The most commonly detected foreign bodies include suture material, wood, plant material, lead, and glass. Sequestered pieces of bone, hoof that becomes embedded in the soft tissues, and necrotic tissue also can create a foreign body reaction. Suture material usually is linear or tubular, is hyperechogenic, and casts an acoustic shadow. Wood usually appears as a linear hyperechogenic structure casting a strong acoustic shadow from its near surface.[10,11,19] Plant material tends to appear as small echogenic material that casts either a weak acoustic shadow or no acoustic shadow. Embedded hoof appears as a hypoechogenic to echogenic structure that often casts no acoustic shadow, or only a weak acoustic shadow is visible. The tubular composition of the hoof wall can sometimes be appreciated during the examination.

The ultrasonographic examination can be used to substantially shorten surgical time by accurately identifying the foreign body locations and identifying the relevant adjacent structures.[10-18,20-22] The surgical approach can be made directly over the foreign body. The foreign bodies should be measured ultrasonographically in two mutually perpendicular planes preoperatively and then compared with the foreign bodies removed at surgery, helping the surgeon to confirm that all foreign material has been removed. Intraoperative localization of the foreign body also can be performed, if localization of the foreign body proves difficult at surgery, aiding the surgeon in its rapid removal.[10,11,14,15,21]

BONE

A bone surface appears as a smooth, uniform-thickness hyperechoic line that casts an acoustic shadow from its near surface.[1,4,11,12,18] Normal bony protuberances appear as bony shelves that are continuous with the parent portion of the bone. The continuity of an irregular bony surface echo can be followed ultrasonographically in at least one plane, differentiating this irregularity from a fracture. Vascular channels create breaks in the normal bony surface echo at the site of vessel penetration.

Fractures

Ultrasonography is useful in the diagnosis of fractures in areas that cannot be assessed radiologically, such as the withers, scapula, humerus, ribs, pelvis, femur, and tibia, and in finding fractures that are suspected but have not

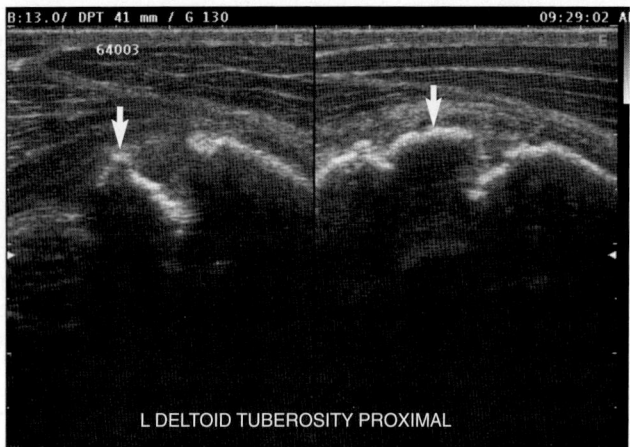

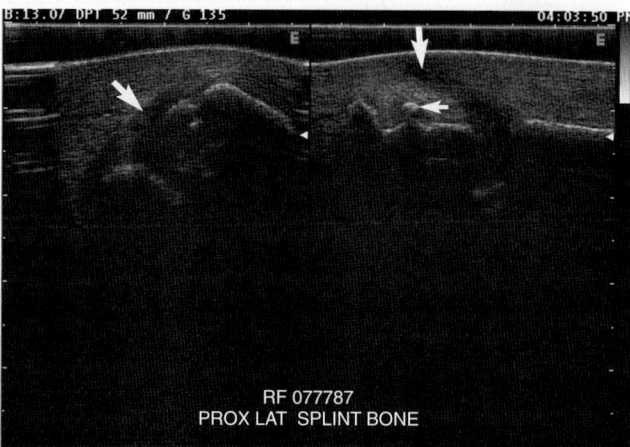

Figure 18-2 • Transverse *(left)* and longitudinal *(right)* ultrasonographic images of a healing deltoid tuberosity fracture. The original fracture *(large arrows)* was comminuted and displaced, with two of the cracks clearly visible in the bone in two mutually perpendicular planes. There is bony irregularity associated with early bridging of the fracture fragments with the underlying bone and echogenic tissue surrounding the fragments associated with fibrous tissue at the fracture site.

Figure 18-3 • Transverse *(left)* and longitudinal *(right)* ultrasonographic images of the distal metacarpal region of a horse with an acute onset of swelling, fever, and lameness associated with osteitis of the fourth metacarpal bone (McIV) and third metacarpal bone (McIII). A hypoechogenic fluid-filled tract in the subcutaneous tissues extends down to the McIV and McIII in the distal metacarpal region. A small hypoechogenic fluid layer overlies the McIV and the McIII and is indicative of osteitis *(arrows)* communicating with the tract extending out to the skin surface. There is a small fragment imaged distracted away from the underlying bone in the longitudinal view *(small arrow)*. The echo from the McIV and the McIII is slightly thinner than normal, consistent with lysis associated with the infection of the bone.

been detected with routine radiography.[11,21,23-29] The ultrasonographic diagnosis of fractures depends on imaging the fracture line or fracture fragment in two mutually perpendicular planes.[1] A nondisplaced fracture is seen as a break in the normal hyperechogenic bone surface. Detection of a hyperechogenic bony structure distracted from the underlying parent bone in two mutually perpendicular planes is consistent with a displaced fracture fragment (Figure 18-2). In an acute fracture, anechogenic fluid with hypoechogenic to echogenic loculations in the surrounding soft tissues is present. Echogenic masses of all shapes (frequently oval) within the loculated fluid are consistent with clot. These masses usually cast an acoustic shadow from the far surface as they become more organized. Disruption of the surrounding musculature frequently is seen if a fracture is displaced.

Osteitis and Osteomyelitis

The detection of an extraarticular fluid layer immediately adjacent to bone and without an intervening soft tissue layer is diagnostic of osteitis or osteomyelitis, unless the area has sustained recent trauma[1,18] (Figure 18-3). This ultrasonographic sign can be detected in horses with acute osteitis or osteomyelitis and precedes the detection of radiological changes by 10 to 14 days. Soft tissue swelling often is present in the tissues adjacent to the osteitis or osteomyelitis. In horses with early osteitis and osteomyelitis the bony surface echo immediately adjacent to the fluid layer usually has a normal ultrasonographic appearance. With increasing chronicity, irregularities are detected in the bony surface echoes that are also detectable radiologically. Thinning of the bony surface echo with scooped-out areas in the underlying bone is consistent with lysis. Irregular hyperechogenic bony spicules correspond to areas of bony proliferative change. Irregular bone has been imaged in lame horses with osteitis of the tuber calcanei.[30,31] Osteitis occurs at the insertion of the gastrocnemius tendon in horses with a concurrent infectious or noninfectious calcaneal bursitis and can occur in horses

with infectious tarsal tenosynovitis.[30,31] Sequestra are imaged as hyperechogenic fragments that cast an acoustic shadow, are surrounded by anechogenic to hypoechogenic fluid, and are distracted from the parent bone.[1,11,18] A linear wooden foreign body can mimic the ultrasonographic appearance of a sequestrum.

Ultrasonography is useful for the diagnosis of osteitis or osteomyelitis in horses with fractures where the radiological signs of fracture healing can be difficult to distinguish from those of infection.[1,11,18] Bony lysis is a component of both fracture healing and infection. Immediately after trauma, or in the immediate postoperative period, fluid is detected adjacent to the bone for several days or longer until the local hemorrhage associated with the original injury or surgical trauma has resolved. A soft tissue layer should then cover the bone in all extraarticular locations.

The detection of a fluid layer directly overlying the bone in horses with suspected osteitis or osteomyelitis should prompt ultrasound-guided aspiration of the fluid, with or without biopsy of the area, and submission of the fluid or tissue obtained for culture and susceptibility testing and histopathological examination (tissue). If surgical curettage of the affected area is chosen, this can be performed at the time of surgery. Horses that receive long-term antimicrobial drugs for osteitis or osteomyelitis should be reevaluated ultrasonographically before the treatment is discontinued. A soft tissue layer should be present over the affected bone without any intervening fluid.[1] If treatment is discontinued while a fluid layer remains overlying the bone, recurrence of the osteitis or osteomyelitis is likely.

Bone Abscess

A bone abscess may be imaged ultrasonographically as a hypoechogenic, scooped-out area in the cortical and medullary regions of the bones[1] and usually is seen in foals, often associated with *Rhodococcus equi* infections. Large adjacent subcutaneous abscesses may communicate with the bone abscess. A dynamic ultrasonographic examination displacing the fluid within the subcutaneous abscess may help to identify the defect in the underlying cortical bone.

Implants

The cause of a worsening lameness in horses with implants may be difficult to determine from the physical examination and radiological findings. Ultrasonographic examination can provide valuable information about the implant, bone, and surrounding soft tissue structures. In horses with surgical implants the detection of a fluid layer immediately adjacent to the implant, without an intervening soft tissue layer, is diagnostic of infection (Figure 18-4).[1] Infection of the implant, infection of the adjacent synovial structures, or problems associated with the implant itself often can be differentiated ultrasonographically. In horses in which fetlock or pastern arthrodesis was performed, worsening of lameness may be caused by infectious tenosynovitis of the digital flexor tendon sheath, which can be diagnosed ultrasonographically as hypoechogenic effusion within the sheath. Problems with screw placement can be identified as a probable cause of lameness, such as when a screw is inadvertently located within the deep digital flexor tendon, causing fiber disruption and tendonitis. The various implant materials (plate, screw, wire, or

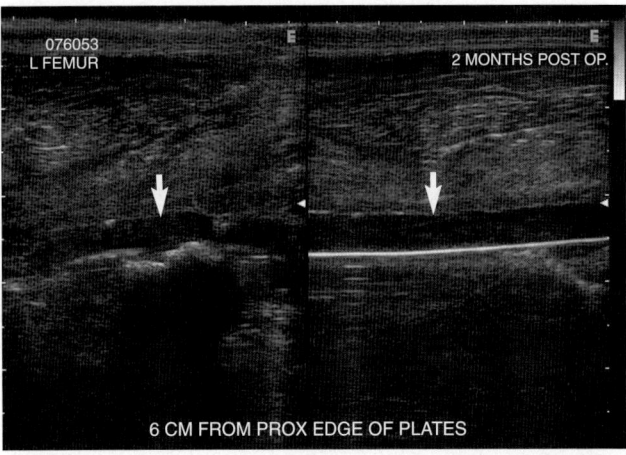

Figure 18-4 • Transverse *(left)* and longitudinal *(right)* ultrasonographic images of the left femur from a foal with a plate and screw repair of a fractured femur with an infected implant. Notice the large hypoechogenic fluid layer *(vertical arrows)* against the hyperechoic echo from the metal plate. This image was obtained 2 months postsurgery, when all of the hemorrhage associated with the fracture and its repair should have been resolved.

antimicrobial-impregnated polymethylmethacrylate bead) can be differentiated ultrasonographically by characteristic appearances. Thus the most likely cause of the horse's deterioration can be identified, and treatment can be targeted appropriately.

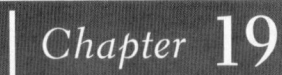

Chapter 19

Nuclear Medicine

Mike W. Ross and Vivian S. Stacy

GENERAL CONSIDERATIONS

 References on page 1262

Nuclear medicine is a relatively recent advance in diagnostic imaging of the horse, pioneered by Ueltschi[1] in Europe and Twardock and Devous[2,3] in the United States. Seeherman and colleagues[4] and Lamb and Koblik[5] further demonstrated the value of bone scintigraphy in the evaluation of sports horses. For detailed description of procedures and interpretation of scintigraphic images, the reader is referred to *Equine Scintigraphy.*[6]

Bone scintigraphy is a way to reach within the horse and extract clinically useful and relevant information and helps to answer many lameness questions that we previously could not answer. Scintigraphy is used to assess the current status of known radiological abnormalities, pursue diagnosis in horses with negative or equivocal radiographs, screen horses with obscure forelimb or hindlimb lameness, and evaluate horses with poor performance. Scintigraphy can be useful to corroborate functional information gained with other advanced imaging modalities such as magnetic

resonance imaging (MRI). However, a gamma camera is not an answer machine, and it is critically important to correlate scintigraphic findings with clinical lameness examination findings. Scintigraphy can play an important role as a screening tool but should never replace diagnostic analgesia. In fractious or highly strung horses with hindlimb lameness, scintigraphic examination may be used to provide a diagnosis, but clinical relevance still should be confirmed.

Nuclear medicine involves the in vivo or in vitro use of radioisotopes in the diagnosis and management of clinical disease. Several terms are used synonymously with *nuclear medicine,* including *nuclear scintigraphy, bone scintigraphy,* and *gamma scintigraphy,* and although these terms differ slightly, for horses most clinicians refer to *bone scintigraphy,* the technique most commonly performed. Bone scintigraphy is highly sensitive compared with radiography. It can detect as little as 10^{-13} g of radiopharmaceutical in bone, whereas changes measured in grams must occur before a lesion can be detected using radiography.[3] Important factors that decrease sensitivity include time from radiopharmaceutical administration to image acquisition, body part–to-camera distance, shielding, motion, time from injury to image acquisition, ambient temperature and peripheral perfusion, and amount of background radiation. For example, the combination of negative factors including high background radiation, motion, endogenous shielding, and distance reduce the sensitivity of pelvic and other axial skeletal scintigraphic imaging and that of upper limb imaging in both the forelimb and hindlimb. High sensitivity (94.4%) in horses with extremity fractures was found, but a lack of sensitivity in pelvic imaging was suggested.[7] Specificity is low compared with other modalities because disparate diseases can similarly alter blood flow and binding sites in bone. Direct trauma (osteitis) and fracture; stress-related bone injury, including fracture and osteoarthritis (OA); infection (infectious osteitis and less frequently osteomyelitis); osteochondrosis; enostosis-like lesions; and neoplasia are in theory difficult to differentiate scintigraphically. Accuracy can be improved by acquiring several images from different perspectives, minimizing factors affecting sensitivity, and knowing the history. For example, a focal area of increased radiopharmaceutical uptake (IRU) in the caudolateral tibial cortex of a 2-year-old Thoroughbred (TB) filly would undoubtedly represent stress-related bone injury rather than a rare bone tumor.

Radiographs depict activity in bone that has already occurred in the past several days to years. Scintigraphy is a *functional* evaluation of bone at the time of imaging. Scintigraphic evidence of bone activity means active bone formation, bone *modeling,* is occurring that might take weeks to be visible radiologically. Therefore a major advantage of scintigraphy is *early detection* of bone injury. Scintigraphy will unlikely accurately reflect changes in bone that occurred longer than 3 to 4 months before imaging. Horses given substantial rest before examination are not good candidates unless the examination is a follow-up to assess healing.

SCINTIGRAPHY AND OTHER IMAGING MODALITIES: WHERE DO THEY FIT?

Recent advances in imaging such as digital radiography (Chapter 15), computed tomography (CT; Chapter 20) and MRI (Chapter 21) have led to questions about the role of scintigraphy in lameness diagnosis. We are often asked questions such as, "Would you use scintigraphy or MRI for diagnosis?" and "Should I put MRI or scintigraphy into my practice?" We would not choose to be without the ability to use scintigraphy in lameness diagnosis. We believe that the combined and concurrent use of scintigraphy and MRI yields the most useful and relevant information and that seldom, given strict case selection, is information redundant. At the origin of the suspensory ligament in the proximal aspect of the third metacarpal and metatarsal bones, a complex area from which pain commonly originates, a combination of imaging modalities is most useful to characterize soft tissue and bony injury. Likewise, lameness abolished with palmar digital analgesia is complex, and the concurrent use of advanced imaging modalities provides complementary information. Nuclear scintigraphy has proved useful in the investigation of foot pain, specifically from the podotrochlear apparatus, and has helped determine clinical significance of lesions discernible with MRI, because a positive correlation between scintigraphy and MRI grades in lesions of the navicular bone was found.[8,9] We believe that both scintigraphy and MRI are critical for addressing complex lameness questions.

RADIOISOTOPES AND RADIOPHARMACEUTICALS

A radioisotope emits radiation (particles) that is captured using a scintillation camera. Radioisotopes such as indium-111 (^{111}In) are used occasionally, but the most common and useful radioisotope is technetium-99m (^{99m}Tc). ^{99m}Tc, a short-lived (metastable) radioisotope with a half-life of 6 hours, is ideal for radiation safety and horse retention. ^{99m}Tc is excreted almost entirely through the kidneys, so containing and monitoring urine is extremely important. ^{99m}Tc is produced when molybdenum-99 (^{99}Mo) decays to ^{99}Tc. The metastable (^{99m}Tc) radioisotope gives off a gamma ray (140 keV) that is used for imaging. Commercially, ^{99}Mo and ^{99m}Tc generators can be purchased for use in large hospitals, but an alternative, cost-effective method is the daily purchase of individual doses, a practice that obviates the need to house generators. Directly from the generator, ^{99m}Tc is in the ionic form of sodium ^{99m}Tc pertechnetate (Na^{99m}TcO$_4$) that can be injected or mixed with a bone-seeking agent or pharmaceutical. Radiation is measured in curies (Ci) or millicuries (mCi); becquerels (Bq), megabecquerels (MBq), and gigabecquerels (GBq) are also used. One millicurie is equal to 37 MBq. The recommended dose of ^{99m}Tc is 0.4 to 0.5 mCi (14.8 to 18.5 MBq)/kg, totaling 150 to 200 mCi (5.5 to 7.4 GBq) per horse. Low doses reduce radiation exposure but prolong acquisition time or may result in inadequate image quality if insufficient counts are obtained. High doses may actually reduce overall radiation exposure by limiting exposure time.

Na^{99m}TcO$_4$ can be injected intravenously directly, but only flow and pool phase studies can be performed. For most equine studies, Na^{99m}TcO$_4$ is mixed with a pharmaceutical. For bone, ^{99m}Tc is bound to methylene diphosphonate (MDP), or hydroxymethane or hydroxymethylene diphosphonate (HDP, HMDP). MDP is slightly less expensive and is the most common pharmaceutical used worldwide, but we prefer HDP because the kidneys clear it slightly faster, allowing early acquisition of delayed phase images. Henceforth MDP and HDP are used interchangeably.

The exact mechanism of binding of ^{99m}Tc-MDP to bone remains unclear. ^{99m}Tc-MDP is thought to bind to exposed sites on the inorganic hydroxyapatite crystal. Binding sites are exposed under normal and pathological conditions in areas of actively remodeling bone or in soft tissues undergoing mineralization.[10,11] ^{99m}Tc-MDP uptake occurs by the processes of chemical adsorption onto, and by direct integration into, the crystalline structure.[12] Other possible mechanisms to account for increased uptake include incorporation into the organic matrix or local hypervascularity.[11] In rat models, ^{99m}Tc was found to be incorporated into the organic matrix rather than the inorganic portion of newly formed bone.[13,14] Radiopharmaceutical may dissociate with incorporation of ^{99m}Tc and MDP individually into the organic and inorganic phases, respectively.[15] ^{99m}Tc-MDP adsorption might depend on pH and the presence of phosphates, calcium compounds, and other cations.[16]

Accumulation of ^{99m}Tc-MDP is not simply the result of changes in local blood flow, although blood flow is likely increased in sites of actively remodeling bone. Although increased blood flow does not significantly affect a bone scan,[10] *adequate* blood flow is necessary to deliver radiopharmaceutical to available binding sites in bone. Poor correlation was found between perfusion index and radiopharmaceutical uptake (RU) in delayed images when evaluating people undergoing distraction osteogenesis.[17] This study suggested that blood flow is not closely linked to bone metabolism and that delayed images most accurately predicted osteogenesis.[17] Rather than measuring blood flow, delayed images reflect changes in bone metabolism. When three-phase bone scintigraphy was used in people with osteonecrosis of the jaw secondary to bisphosphonate administration, delayed images were all positive, but increased perfusion (and increased blood pool) was found in 9 of 12 patients.[18] A three-phase bone scan can detect increased perfusion and soft-tissue inflammation if present, but it is metabolic activity of bone that influences delayed phase images. Decreased blood flow, caused by infarction or ischemia, can greatly affect a bone scan but is an unusual clinical problem (see discussion of photopenia, page 226). However, decreased peripheral blood flow in old horses or those imaged in cold weather or on days with high diurnal temperature change can adversely affect image quality (see discussion of poor-quality bone uptake, page 222).

The most important aspects of ^{99m}Tc-MDP binding relate to timing of the scan and the stage of modeling (formation). In actively remodeling bone, osteoclastic activity predominates during bone resorption, whereas osteoblastic activity dominates during bone modeling. Modeling occurs independently or in conjunction with remodeling in cancellous and cortical bone. Histological and scintigraphic findings were evaluated in a rat tibial evacuation model, and ^{99m}Tc-MDP was found to bind to sites of *active* calcification, most prevalent 12 days after injury.[19] ^{99m}Tc-labeled phosphonates were identified during bone formation, and ongoing resorption was not necessary for increased uptake to occur.[12] ^{99m}Tc-MDP accumulated in areas of calcification or in fixed bone fragments,[12,20] and accumulation was mediated by osteoblastic activity.[12] The high sensitivity of bone scintigraphy is attributed to increased osteoblast activity that precedes morphological changes visible radiologically.[21] Other mechanisms may exist, however, because positive bone scan results may be seen in people with diseases such as osteomalacia, in which high bone matrix turnover and failure of calcification occur.[19]

Site and stage of binding are important from a clinical perspective. Binding sites for ^{99m}Tc-MDP are created by osteoblast activity during bone modeling, and maximal IRU occurs 8 or 12 days after bone injury.[19,22] An acute fracture caused by direct trauma may not be scintigraphically evident for several days. Acute, traumatic injury differs from stress-related bone injury, because the latter, particularly common in racehorses, results from a continuum of bone changes that might lead to stress or catastrophic fractures and OA. Microfracture, periosteal callus, and subchondral bone damage precede the development of stress or complete fracture in the dorsal cortex and distal articular surface of the third metacarpal bone (McIII), the third metatarsal bone (MtIII), the humerus, the tibia, and the pelvis.[23-25] In horses with acute lameness from stress-related bone injury, bone scan findings usually are immediately positive because bone modeling is ongoing. In horses with stress-related bone injury a bone scan result is likely to be positive long before catastrophic fracture occurs, an important advantage of scintigraphy compared with radiography. In horses with traumatic injury, such as an acute pelvic or other upper limb fracture, a false-negative scan result may occur from lack of modeling. Other factors resulting in false-negative results include

distance, shielding, high background activity, and motion. For example, a horse developed acute hindlimb lameness during hospitalization, and, suspecting a pelvic fracture involving the acetabulum, clinicians performed scintigraphic examination on day 2, but the scan result was negative. On day 9 faint IRU appeared, consistent with fracture.

In horses with stress-related bone injury and traumatic injury a considerable decrease in RU occurs within 6 to 8 weeks after injury. Decreased intensity after fracture varies with the specific bone and fracture type. The ideal time to image, particularly in horses with pelvic or other axial skeletal trauma, is 10 days to 8 weeks after injury, although positive bone scan findings are often obtained in horses with distal extremity fractures 72 to 96 hours after known trauma.

Given the short half-life of ^{99m}Tc, it is the most widely used and versatile radioisotope when imaging a lame horse and for most nuclear medicine procedures in horses and people. The same radioisotope injected intravenously, ^{99m}Tc, can be combined with different drugs (pharmaceuticals) to target different tissues. For example, for lung perfusion images to be obtained, macroaggregated albumen is labeled with ^{99m}Tc; for brain imaging, glucoheptanate is labeled with ^{99m}Tc. Standard ^{99m}Tc-HDP is used for sinus, dental, and temporomandibular joint imaging and can be used to evaluate peripheral vasculature in first-pass studies after intravenous injection or by injection directly into distended peripheral veins for evaluation of venous return. To obtain high levels of radiopharmaceutical in the distal extremities for specific imaging or to perform experimental studies, Na^{99m}TcO$_4$ can be administered using intraosseous or intravenous regional limb perfusion techniques.[26] Our preliminary results with this technique show uneven distribution within distal limb tissues and persistence of radioisotope in large, distended veins. Peripheral lymphatic fluid dynamics can be studied using ^{99m}Tc-sulfur colloid injected directly into distended lymphatics or subcutaneous tissues.[27] Soft tissues are most commonly imaged using three-phase bone scintigraphy with ^{99m}Tc-HDP (MDP), but recently, radiolabeled biotin was found to be safe and useful to detect soft tissue inflammation without concurrent uptake of the radiopharmaceutical in bone.[28] We have limited experience using radiolabeled white cells to image osteitis, osteomyelitis, and cellulitis in horses, and although the technique is occasionally useful, our results do not appear as promising as those previously reported.[29] Briefly, white blood cells harvested from affected horses or foals are labeled with ^{99m}Tc and hexamethylpropyleneamine oxime (^{99m}Tc-HMPAO) and then reinjected to allow accumulation at sites of infection. Infection imaging is an important topic in human medicine, and advances in equine imaging using novel agents such as antibodies or antimicrobial agents may hold promise.[30]

IMAGING EQUIPMENT

Scintigraphy can be performed in two ways, but the most common and useful method is acquisition of two-dimensional images with a gamma camera. Alternatively, a handheld probe is used to acquire count density computer-generated charts, or graphs are created to determine IRU. Known as *probe point counting*, this form of

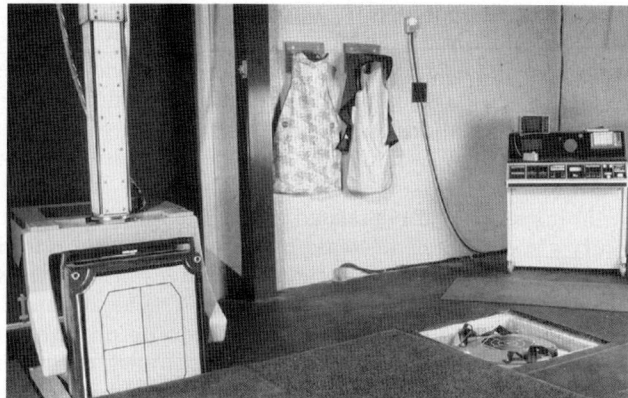

Figure 19-1 • The nuclear medicine facility at New Bolton Center, University of Pennsylvania, has large field of view and small field of view cameras. A custom-made central column overhead gantry holds the rectangular large field of view camera, which can be lowered below floor level to image the distal extremities.

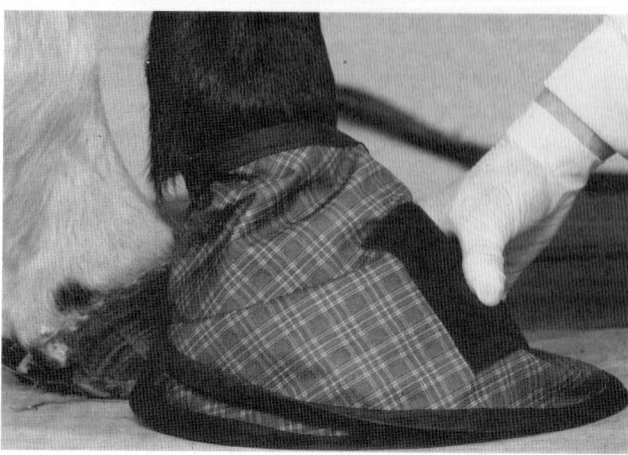

Figure 19-2 • The small field of view camera in the floor allows easy acquisition of solar images of the foot. After a wooden cover is applied, the horse stands over the small field of view camera for the solar image. A lead-lined wrap placed around the coronary band region shields the foot and camera from radiation emanating from the more proximal aspects of the affected limb.

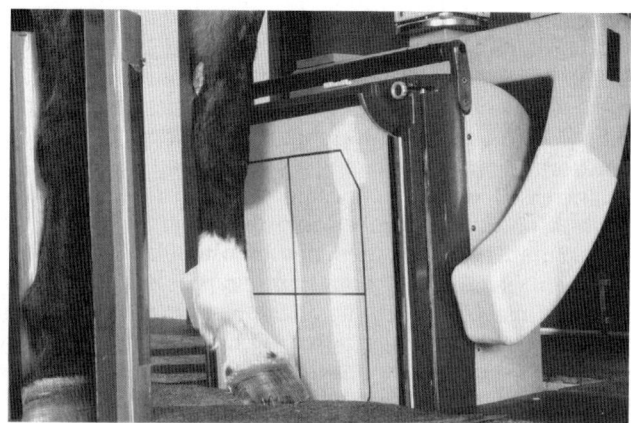

Figure 19-3 • Construction of a recess or pit into which the large field of view camera can be lowered allows imaging of the distal extremities with minimal movement of the horse. The lateral aspect of the hoof touches the face of the camera (clear polycarbonate protects the collimator). This position minimizes distance and improves resolution, improves image quality, and decreases acquisition time. A curved, lead-lined shield protects the camera and left forelimb from radiation emitted by the right forelimb.

scintigraphic examination was first introduced in 1984.[31,32] Some probes are like miniature gamma cameras built with a single photomultiplier tube. Crystal probe detectors are more expensive than the photomultiplier detectors, but they are small and easily used on the body surface, or per rectum in horses with suspected pelvic fracture.[32] Probe point counting is done with a substantially lower radioisotope dose, minimizing cost and radiation exposure. Probe point equipment is inexpensive. Because the probe is placed directly on the skin surface, body part–to-probe distance is minimal. A gamma camera is often difficult to get close to the body surface, a problem that can prolong acquisition time and decrease image quality. A good correlation appears between results of probe point counting and gamma camera imaging in acute injuries in young horses, but in older horses the technique has limited sensitivity. However, quantitative information is available only as a histogram, and an actual image allowing qualitative assessment is not obtained.

Gamma camera images are obtained in analog or digital form, and permanent hard copies of a two-dimensional scintigraphic image are generated. In people, one or several gamma cameras operating simultaneously can be used to generate a cross-sectional image similar to a CT or MRI scan. This is known as *single photon emission CT* (SPECT) and *photon emission tomography* (PET). Although SPECT and PET imaging are theoretically possible in anesthetized horses, we are not aware that the techniques have been performed.

A reconditioned gamma camera is perfectly satisfactory, less expensive than new equipment, and durable, often being useful for at least 15 to 20 years or more, with proper maintenance. Gamma cameras are either large field of view (LFOV) or small field of view (SFOV), based simply on the size (Figures 19-1 to 19-3). LFOV cameras can be rectangular or circular in shape, but crystals for rectangular cameras are more costly. In adapting equipment for use in horses, an important consideration is how to move the camera safely and easily to the horse and vice versa. Most standard gantry (support structure of the gamma camera) designs are unsuitable for equine imaging, because good-quality images can be obtained only by having the body part close to the camera. Resolution is inversely proportional to the distance between the body part and camera. To quickly obtain dorsal and lateral, and lateral and plantar, images of the forelimbs and hindlimbs, respectively, the camera must be able to be lowered below floor level (see Figure 19-3). Alternatively, the horse must be positioned on an elevated platform. Limbs can be held manually near the camera, but this practice increases radiation exposure to personnel and should be avoided whenever possible. Suitable gantries are commercially available or can be custom made. A lead collimator is also required.

IMAGE ACQUISITION

For flow and pool phase images, horses are sedated and positioned in front of the camera, and ^{99m}Tc-HDP (or MDP) is injected intravenously. Delayed phase images are then

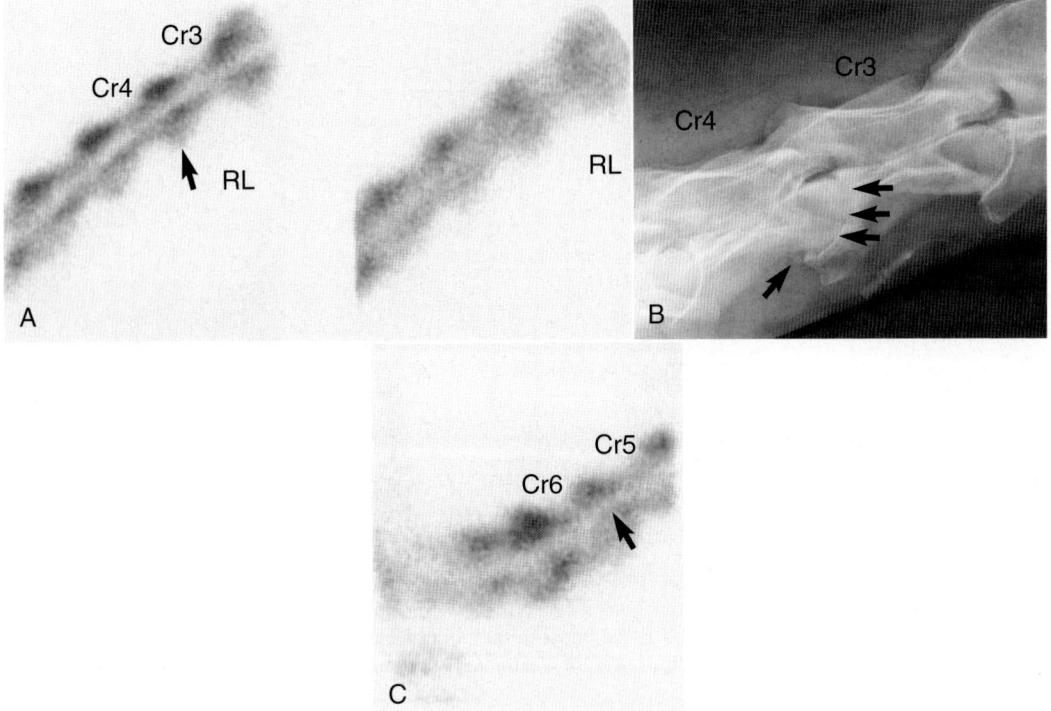

Figure 19-4 • Delayed phase scintigraphic images of an 8-year-old Thoroughbred with neurological signs consistent with compression of the cervical spinal cord. **A,** Corrected *(left)* and uncorrected *(right)* right lateral images (cranial is to the right) showing marked improvement in image quality using motion correction techniques. Note there is normal radiopharmaceutical uptake in the intervertebral joint between the third (Cr3) and fourth cervical vertebrae. **B,** Laterolateral digital radiographic image (cranial is to the right) of the cervical spine showing marked osteoarthritis in this intervertebral joint *(arrows)*. Based on lack of cervical stiffness or pain and normal scintigraphic activity, this radiological change was considered old and inactive. **C,** Right lateral scintigraphic image of the caudal cervical spine showing narrowing *(arrow)* of the vertebral canal between the fifth and sixth cervical vertebrae, a finding validated using myelography. Useful anatomical information can be obtained from scintigraphic images.

obtained 2 to 4 hours later. Scintigraphic images are produced when the horse, now the radiation source, emits gamma rays from normal and abnormal bone. The gamma rays must pass through overlying tissues and traverse the distance between the body part and the camera. An area of IRU emits more gamma rays than does adjacent normal bone and contributes more counts to the scan. Sites farther from the camera, those being shielded by overlying soft tissue or adjacent bone, or those in areas of high background activity may not be visible, because they may not contribute enough gamma rays. Gamma rays strike a sodium iodide crystal, and scintillations produced are detected and amplified by photomultiplier tubes that subsequently transmit information through electronic circuits. The image is displayed on an oscilloscope or sent directly to a film processor, called *analog imaging*. Alternatively, information is transmitted to a computer, stored digitally, manipulated, and subsequently sent to a film processor or printer.

An important recent advancement is the ready availability of user-friendly computer programs to acquire, analyze, store, and process images. Systems based on Apple, Windows, and Unix are currently available and are straightforward. Motion correction software is the latest, exciting advance; it improves upper limb and axial skeleton image quality by negating the effects of motion and allowing higher count numbers than with conventional software

(Figure 19-4). Modern software also allows postprocessing of images—for example, masking out the bladder, which might otherwise steal counts.

Images are obtained in either static or dynamic mode. Static images, most commonly obtained, are acquired using a predetermined number of counts per image. For example, because motion and soft tissue covering are limited in the distal limbs, good-quality images can be obtained using 100,000 to 150,000 counts per image. In general, increasing counts per image improves image quality, but for more counts to be acquired, time and motion become factors. Motion correction can add flexibility.

A fundamental principle of image interpretation is comparing images of one limb with those of the contralateral limb, but the clinician should keep in mind that both limbs, and for that matter all limbs, can be abnormal. To compare limbs accurately using this technique, body part–to-camera distance and camera position relative to the limb must be standardized between limbs. Time to acquire each image ranges from 30 to 90 seconds depending on radioisotope dose, type and age of horse, and ambient temperature. Time rather than count number can be standardized, assuming that limb perfusion is adequate and symmetrical. For example, lateral images of both metacarpal regions are obtained for 90 seconds and compared.

The number of images to obtain is based on the body part being examined, but usually at least two images are

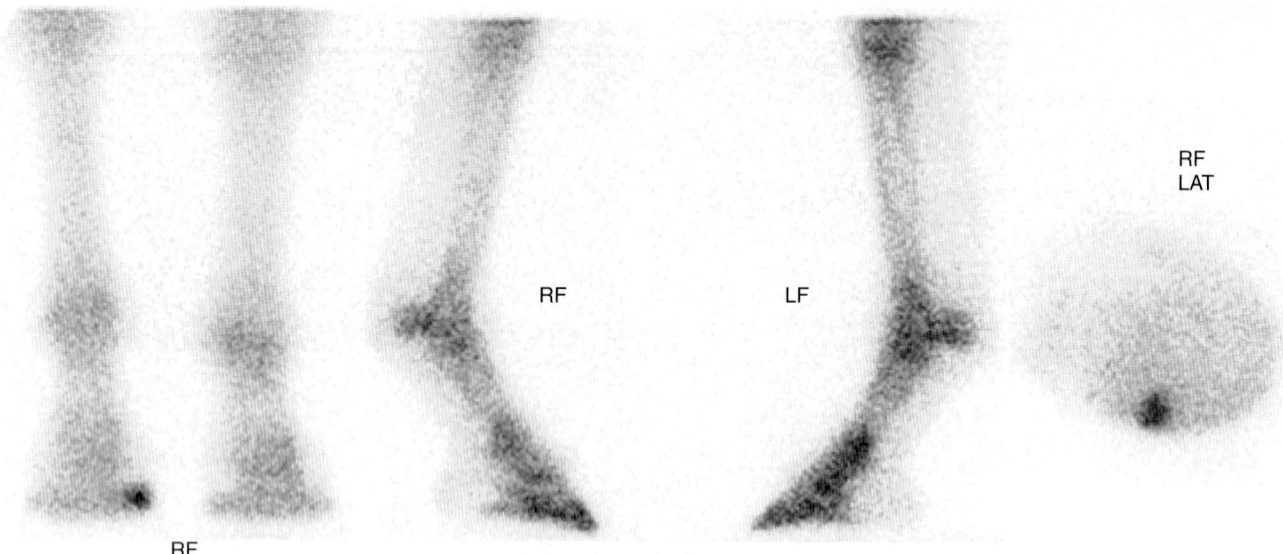

Figure 19-5 • Delayed phase scintigraphic images of a horse with a fracture of the medial aspect of the right fore-limb *(RF)* distal phalanx. The lateral *(LAT)* image of the right forelimb does not show the area of increased radiophar-maceutical uptake, and little difference is noted between both front feet. The dorsal and solar images, however, clearly show increased radiopharmaceutical uptake. It is extremely important to obtain more than one scintigraphic image. *LF,* Left forelimb.

required. In some areas this may not be possible, but the clinician should be aware that false-negative results can occur. A dorsal scintigraphic image gives detailed information about only the dorsal aspect of the limb, and abnormal palmar regions might be missed. The image and information are not the same as depicted in a dorsopalmar radiographic image. Similarly, areas of IRU on the medial side of the limb might not be visible on a lateral image. Areas more distant from the camera contribute substantially less radiation than those closer because of the inverse square law. Bone interposed between a medial lesion and the camera can effectively shield the site. A lateral image of a right forelimb failed to reveal a fracture of the medial aspect of the distal phalanx (Figure 19-5). Radiographic examination and dorsal and solar scintigraphic images, however, revealed an incomplete fracture that we completely missed in the lateral scintigraphic image. Additional images may be necessary for accurate diagnosis.

We prefer to localize lameness, because this allows for detailed examination of a specific area. For instance, routine screening images of the front digit include lateral and dorsal delayed images, but in horses in which lameness is abolished using palmar digital analgesia, pool phase images and lateral, dorsal, solar, and occasionally medial, palmar, and flexed delayed images are obtained. Diagnostic accuracy can be improved by acquiring many different images, and pinpointing a lesion using scintigraphy can allow a focused radiographic, ultrasonographic, CT, or MRI study to be performed. Combined imaging can yield additional useful information.[8,9] When augmenting the routine dorsal and plantar images of the metatarsophalangeal joint with flexed lateral and sometimes flexed dorsal and medial images, instead of saying, "There is IRU in the fetlock joint," the diagnostician can say, "There is focal IRU involving the distal, plantarolateral aspect of the MtIII," a much more accurate description (Figure 19-6).

Dynamic acquisition can be used before motion correction in delayed images or to evaluate blood flow. One- or 2-second per frame images are generated sequentially and can be evaluated individually or combined into a single composite image, with or without motion correction. First-pass angiography can be used to assess blood flow in the aorta, iliac, and femoral arteries[33] in horses with suspected thromboembolism (Figure 19-7) or to assess blood flow in the distal limb.

Image Quality

Factors that contribute to poor image quality are related to the horse and to processing. Analog (old way) and digital (new way) processing provide good-quality images provided the equipment is working properly. Regular quality control is absolutely essential to maximize image quality and avoid artifacts. A cracked or poor-quality collimator, sodium iodide crystal damage, malfunction or incorrect tuning of photomultiplier tubes, electric circuit malfunction, age, and poor general condition of refurbished equipment can cause artifacts or gradual deterioration in quality or can completely shut down the process. The dose of radioactivity administered, the number of counts acquired, image distance (distance from body part to camera surface), motion, and background radiation are most critical. As many gamma rays as possible from the affected bone must reach the crystal without motion for image quality to be maximized.

Number of Counts

Image acquisition, the principles of using count numbers as opposed to time, and the importance of standardizing images between limbs were discussed earlier. One limb may overall be more active than the contralateral limb and count faster in individual images or contribute more counts when combined in images of both limbs. Horses with

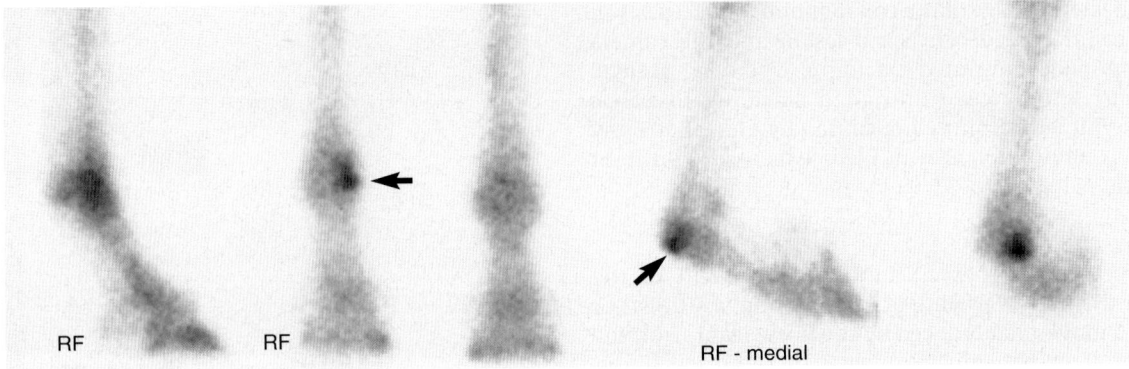

Figure 19-6 • Lateral *(left)*, dorsal *(second from left)*, flexed lateral *(second from right)*, and flexed dorsal delayed phase scintigraphic images of the right forelimb *(RF)* of a 2-year-old trotter with subchondral bone injury. The flexed lateral and dorsal images best show the focal area of increased radiopharmaceutical uptake involving the distal, medial aspect of the third metacarpal bone. Although increased radiopharmaceutical uptake appears in other images, the flexed dorsal image allows differentiation of increased radiopharmaceutical uptake involving the third metacarpal bone and the proximal phalanx.

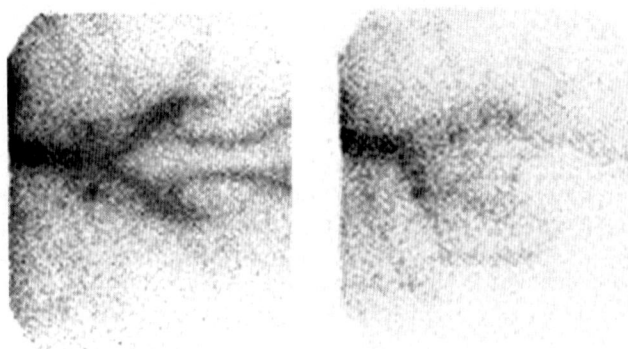

Figure 19-7 • Composite scintigraphic image generated after dynamic acquisition of 32 sequential images (2 seconds per frame) with the gamma camera positioned over the terminal aorta and branches. Imaging started 20 seconds after administration of ^{99m}Tc-hydroxymethane diphosphonate in the external jugular vein (cranial to the left, right is to the top). **A,** In a normal horse the external iliac arteries show a V-shaped divergence and a linear caudal course of the internal iliac arteries is seen. **B,** In this horse with aortoiliac thromboembolism, the direction and contour of the external iliac arteries is disrupted and the internal iliac vessels lack recognition.

unilateral lesions in the digit, such as those with distal phalanx fractures and soft tissue injuries, appear to have compensatory IRU normally in the rest of the limb. Our experience suggests that horses with distally located lesions in the affected limb often have more prominent normal uptake in delayed images in that entire limb, but others suggest that the nonlame contralateral limb may be more active because of increase in weight bearing.[34] An area of intense IRU present with a condylar fracture or stress-related bone injury may overwhelm the contribution of normal bone, making it difficult to see, a phenomenon called *count stealing*.

Distance

Having the affected body part too far from the camera is likely the most important factor contributing to false-negative bone scan findings. The ability of the camera and imaging system to resolve lesions is inversely proportional to distance. OA and subchondral bone cysts involving the

medial femorotibial joint can be completely missed unless a caudal image is obtained, simply because the lesions cannot contribute enough counts to the scan to be visible. Distance is too great. Pelvic images are dramatically and negatively affected by distance. Even if the camera is resting on the skin of the rump, some bones are still many centimeters away.

Shielding

Shielding is important in radiation safety, but it can be a negative factor in image quality and interpretation. Shielding helps or harms image quality and interpretation. High background radiation reduces image quality, because unwanted tissues steal counts. Pool phase images of the thoracolumbar spine and pelvis are rarely informative because within 1 to 2 minutes after injection, radiopharmaceutical in the kidneys and urinary bladder creates such high background levels of radiation that soft tissue lesions are missed. Delayed pelvic images are similarly affected by urine retention in the bladder. Bladder uptake causes poor image quality by creating high background levels of radiation and by superimposition on the sacrum in dorsal images. To avoid this problem, the bladder should be catheterized or a diuretic should be given. Lead shields can be placed on the skin between the bladder and camera, and count subtraction techniques can be used to take away bladder counts, but maximizing image quality by initially limiting radioactive urine is best.

Internal shielding can be a problem for interpretation. Gamma rays originating from a lesion distant to the camera must traverse bone, interposed soft tissue, and air before striking the camera. In a lateral image of the stifle, gamma rays originating from subchondral bone of the distal medial aspect of the femur must traverse the thick lateral condyle, dense ligaments, and other soft tissues, all while competing with gamma rays from other sources. Intuitively it would seem that counts would be additive, meaning a lesion medially would add to the counts normally originating from the lateral aspect, clearly showing the abnormal area. Acquiring images with sufficient counts reduces the risk of false-negative scan results. *Bone stacking,* when bones are superimposed, may explain normal areas of greater RU visible in a lateral image of the coxofemoral joint. However, often bone interposed between a lesion and the camera seems to provide unwanted shielding. Overlying skeletal muscle may also provide unwanted shielding in pelvic images. Asymmetrical muscling caused by gluteal atrophy can explain mild differences in RU between left and right sides of the pelvis.

Motion

Two sources generate excess motion: movement of the camera or the horse. Swaying of cameras hung by hoists or chains and movement induced by the horse leaning on the camera result in poor image quality. In the distal limbs, horse movement is usually not a factor and acquisition times are short. Horses sway minimally when the distal limbs are scanned, but sway excursion is large in the upper limbs because of a longer pendulum effect from the anchor point (feet). Sedation may accentuate the effect. Motion detracts greatly from upper limb and axial skeleton image quality. We use detomidine (0.008 to 0.01 mg/kg) and butorphanol (0.006 to 0.075 mg/kg), a combination that allows optimal acquisition while minimizing motion. Manual support on each side and resting the horse's head on a stationary object partially negate the tendency of the horse to sway and drift. Motion correction software is useful in improving image quality but cannot compensate for all movement.

Background Radiation

High background radiation contributing to count stealing and handling bladder interference have been discussed. Shielding the limb or body being imaged with custom-made lead-lined barricades (see Figure 19-3) or placing drapes on the horse or around the body part (see Figure 19-2) helps isolate the region being examined. Old horses, large-breed horses, and fat horses and those with extensive swelling or fibrosis in the distal limbs often have high background activity in soft tissues, which inevitably results in poor-quality delayed images.

Poor-Quality Bone Uptake

Image quality in large breed horses such as TB crosses, Warmbloods, and draft horses or in old horses may be poor despite following accepted protocol. Average image quality in large-breed horses may be worse than in young race-horses for many reasons, but age and type of exercise might explain some differences. Large-breed performance horses tend to be older than the racehorse population, lack normal physeal activity, and often have dense soft tissues and large bones in the distal limbs. Exercise type and level in this type of horse are much different from those in racehorses. A relative lack of stress-related bone injury in subchondral and cortical bone limits the number and type of scintigraphic changes seen.

Image quality in all types of horses may be compromised in areas with cold weather or great diurnal temperature differences, especially in fall, winter, and early spring.[35-37] Reduced radiopharmaceutical uptake generally occurs distal to the antebrachium and crus, either bilaterally symmetrical or asymmetrical. Delayed phase images acquired above the carpus and tarsus have high background radiation but can be adequately interpreted. A compensatory area of intense IRU may occur in the distal aspect of the

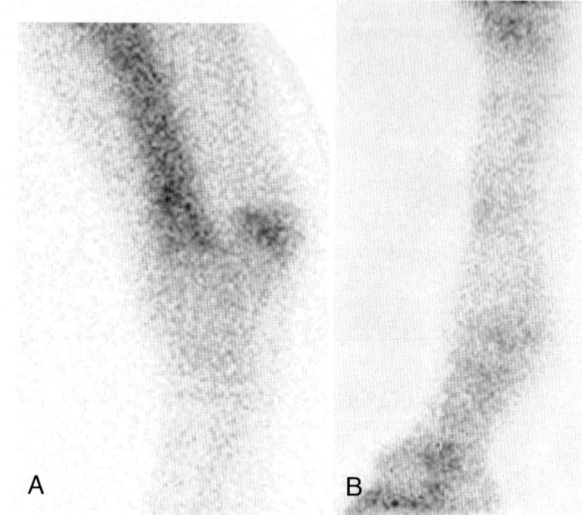

Figure 19-8 • A, Delayed phase scintigraphic image of an aged Warmblood gelding shows reasonable quality bone uptake in the proximal aspect of the limb and diffuse moderate increased radiopharmaceutical uptake in the distal aspect of the tibia. **B,** This delayed phase image is consistent with a pool phase scan of the tarsus and distal extremity. This abnormal pattern of poor bone uptake commonly appears in horses imaged in cold weather or in large breed horses.

radius and tibia. Distally, from the carpus and tarsus to the sole of the foot, images resemble pool phase images even when acquired 3 hours after injection (Figure 19-8). Occasionally a different pattern appears, with compensatory focal intense IRU in the distal radius and tibia, relative photopenia of the carpal and tarsal bones, and reduced to normal or interspersed (spotty) uptake in the metacarpal or metatarsal regions and digit. This phenomenon is not related to renal clearance, radiopharmaceutical affinity, or dose of radioisotope but appears to be caused by poor peripheral perfusion.[37] Normal horses appear to be able to shunt blood away from the periphery, presumably a homeostatic mechanism involving high sympathetic tone during times of abrupt drop in ambient temperature. Other related factors that might increase sympathetic tone are dehydration, stress, and transportation of the horse shortly before injection of radiopharmaceutical. High sympathetic tone may reduce blood flow in the distal extremity, and the radioisotope may be unable to reach available binding sites in bone. Blood supply must be *adequate* to ensure distribution of radiopharmaceutical to sites of osteoblast activity. Persistence of radiopharmaceutical in soft tissues and vessels in the distal extremity and occasional photopenia of the carpal, tarsal, or other bones cannot be explained.

We prefer that all horses be hospitalized the night before examination to avoid the problem of poor-quality bone uptake and to maximize image quality. This may reduce stress and improve hydration status. Keeping the distal limbs warm with bandages and, when the temperature is cold, applying a body blanket to maintain core temperature may help. In a recent study, Dyson and colleagues[37] found that exercise, but not the use of bandages to create warming, before injection was most important in improving peripheral blood flow and maximizing image quality in all types of horses. Horses are lunged or trotted on a treadmill for 15 to 20 minutes before injection. When we suspect poor-quality scans may result, we administer acetylpromazine (15 to 20 mg per adult horse) before injection, a practice we feel helps ensure good-quality delivery of radiopharmaceutical to peripheral tissues. In a recent study acetylpromazine caused vasodilatation, increased blood flow, and count density in flow phase images and caused earlier onset of the flow phase in normal horses but did not influence count density in delayed phase images.[38] However, effects of acetylpromazine in horses with poor peripheral perfusion and abnormal bone uptake of radiopharmaceutical are unknown. If poor-quality images result despite following these procedures, the procedures should be repeated the next day after exercise, if possible.

RADIATION SAFETY

Rules for radiation safety and licenses to obtain and house radioactive materials differ for each state and country. In Pennsylvania, as of March 2008, a license to use radioactive materials must be obtained from the state Department of Environmental Protection, whereas before, a license was obtained directly from the federal Nuclear Regulatory Commission (NRC). Pennsylvania rules for use of radioactive materials agree with and match (are said to be "in agreement" with) those issued by the NRC. Horses are quarantined for 24 hours after injection and can then leave with instructions to avoid unnecessary contact with them for an additional 36 hours. Radiation levels at the horse's body surface range from 0.4 to 0.7 mR/hr at 24 hours after injection, well below the trigger level of 2.0 mR/hr established by the NRC. Horses are kept in defined stalls in which solid waste removal is used (stall drains are plugged; shavings or straw are used for bedding). Waste is kept for 60 hours, at which time radiation levels do not differ from background.

We practice the concept of ALARA (as low as reasonably achievable) and attempt to maximize distance from horse to handler and minimize total imaging time. Persons handling radioactive materials wear body and ring badges, and all those in contact with horses wear body badges. Total yearly radiation exposure for full-time technicians is approximately 500 mR/yr (450 horses scanned each year). Most radiation exposure occurs during image acquisition, throughout which time a handler is in close proximity to the horse being imaged (radiation exposure is inversely proportional to the square of the distance). Ninety percent of total exposure has been shown to occur during image acquisition; there was no difference in exposure between persons drawing up the radiopharmaceutical and those holding the horse during its administration, but the person holding the horse during image acquisition received twice the exposure as the person operating the equipment.[39] Lead aprons, although not commonly worn, have been shown to significantly reduce radiation exposure in people performing equine scintigraphy.[40] Daily monitoring of selected sites and weekly wipe tests are performed. Nuclear medicine techniques in horses can be done safely, within NRC or other supervisory guidelines, without undue contamination or exposure.

BONE SCAN PHASES

The bone scan is divided into three phases named for the tissues in which the majority of radiopharmaceutical resides at that time. Flow phase (phase I, vascular phase) images are obtained for 1 to 3 minutes after injection, during which time radiopharmaceutical resides in blood vessels. First-pass studies of the heart and major central and peripheral vessels can be performed (see Figure 19-7). The flow phase appears to last longer in horses than in people, because radiopharmaceutical persists in distal limb veins often for greater than 10 to 15 minutes, a finding that can complicate interpretation and potentially decrease sensitivity of pool phase images. Pool phase (phase II, soft tissue phase) images are classically obtained 3 to 15 minutes after injection, during which time radiopharmaceutical resides in the extracellular fluid pool. Pool phase images are used to evaluate soft tissues such as tendons, ligaments, tendon sheaths, and bursae. A common misconception is that many distant soft tissues can be evaluated, but the short time interval dictates careful selection of sites for pool phase imaging. Delayed phase (phase III, bone phase) images are obtained 2 to 4 hours after injection, during which time radiopharmaceutical resides in bone and unbound drug has cleared the kidneys. Although information gained in flow or pool phase images is useful, delayed images are the mainstay of equine imaging. A three-phase bone scan involves acquisition of flow, pool, and delayed images, but most commonly only delayed images, or delayed and selected pool phase images, are obtained. An area of IRU visible in all three phases could indicate bone trauma, fracture, or infection, but in horses it generally indicates trauma or fracture. Pool phase and delayed phase images should be carefully evaluated to determine if areas of IRU are the same or different. In our experience, early pooling of radiopharmaceutical usually represents early bone uptake. Pool phase and delayed phase images can be superimposed, or region of interest (ROI) analysis can be used to determine size and position of IRU. In the proximal palmar metacarpal or plantar metatarsal regions, uptake of radiopharmaceutical can occur in only bone, only soft tissue, or both, and prognosis in horses with suspensory desmitis or bony injury can vary with tissue involved. Fractures are evident in delayed images, but sometimes they are visible as early as 20 to 30 seconds after injection or as progressive IRU in all phases. In horses with suspensory desmitis without bony involvement, pool phase images may indicate positive findings in horses with acute injuries but are often negative, whereas delayed phase images are often negative or equivocal. Scintigraphy is often castigated for its inability to detect proximal suspensory desmitis, but keep in mind that most horses have only soft tissue and not bone pain. In a recent study of proximal suspensory desmitis most horses had normal subjectively and objectively determined RU, and poor correlation between bone scan and radiological abnormalities was found.[41] Abnormal ultrasonographic findings in conjunction with diagnostic analgesia remain hugely important in diagnosis of proximal suspensory desmitis. Differentiating soft tissue injury from that of bone is particularly important in the foot. Bruises, laminar tearing, and subsolar abscesses should cause positive results on pool phase images, but negative or equivocal delayed phase images. In horses with long-standing infection or inflammation, osteitis of the distal phalanx can cause IRU in delayed images, complicating differentiation of involvement of the two tissues. Conversely, early bone uptake in horses with osteitis or fracture of the distal phalanx may prompt suspicion of soft tissue involvement as well. Although scintigraphy is considered highly sensitive, negative scan findings occur in horses thought to have severe soft tissue injury in the foot. In pool phase images, areas of intense IRU at the dorsal and palmar or plantar aspects of the coronary band are normal, making interpretation of uptake in important structures such as the deep digital flexor tendon (DDFT), navicular bursa, and distal interphalangeal joint difficult.

Pool phase images of the shoulder, thoracolumbar, and pelvic regions are often requested, but we have found them unrewarding. Radiopharmaceutical retention in large vessels, early (within 1 minute) intense uptake in the renal pelvis and urinary bladder, and problems such as distance, shielding, and motion all reduce probability of finding inflamed soft tissue. Pool phase images may be useful in evaluating *acute inflammation* of the DDFT, navicular bursa, superficial digital flexor tendon, suspensory ligament, and digital flexor tendon sheath but may provide negative or equivocal findings if disease is chronic and active inflammation is only mild. Images should be obtained within 4 to 6 weeks after injury to identify lesions within these structures accurately. Pool phase scintigraphic images appear to be less sensitive and specific than ultrasonographic images.

SCAN INTERPRETATION

Qualitative assessment is the most common and useful method for interpreting scintigraphic images. Quantitative assessment such as ROI analysis (comparing the region of one limb with another after considering background values), first-pass, or gaited studies and linear profile studies are easily performed but are time-consuming. However, in mature competition horses quantitative assessment may be essential to confirm relatively small differences in radiopharmaceutical uptake that can be clinically significant. Profile and ROI analyses were useful in determining differences between normal horses and those with clinical signs associated with sacroiliac (SI) joint pain, but considerable overlap in range of RU was seen.[42,43] An inverse relationship was found between RU in the tubera sacrale and age, and marked left-right asymmetry in quantitative assessment was found in horses with SI joint pain.[42] Differences in conformation of the sacrum, however, may cause alterations in RU seen both qualitatively and quantitatively, and RU in the tubera sacrale was significantly higher in males.[44] Images are qualitatively evaluated for *location, intensity,* and *character* of RU, and areas of increased uptake (hot spots) or decreased uptake are noted.

Location of Increased Radiopharmaceutical Uptake
Areas of IRU should be accurately identified and located. Is the area of IRU located in cortical or subchondral bone? Cancellous (subchondral) bone located in the epiphyses is normally more active than is bone in the diaphyses, because these regions of bone are larger and have more active bone turnover. A small area of mild IRU in subchondral bone may not be relevant, whereas the same area in the mid-diaphysis of the tibia or the McIII would indicate stress-related bone injury. Any area of IRU, even if small (1 to 2 pixels in width or length), in the cortex of a long

bone is abnormal, but not all areas of IRU are clinically significant.

Is the area of IRU on one or both sides of the joint? Scintigraphic evidence of early OA appears as a focal area of IRU on one side of a joint (see Figure 19-6). Involvement of opposing articular surfaces, determined by evaluating several views, is a negative prognostic sign. If located in the diaphysis, is the area of IRU in cortical or medullary bone? At least two orthogonal images are needed to determine location in the diaphysis. Enostosis-like lesions can appear similar to stress-related bone injury (see Chapters 12, 15, 37, 39, 40, 43, 45, and 47), but prognosis and management decisions differ (Figure 19-9). Focal IRU in horses with well-defined tibial stress fractures can be differentiated from the extensive bicortical involvement seen in horses with severe lameness and potentially catastrophic spiral fractures (Figures 19-9 and 19-10). A rare finding, an authentic fibular fracture, can be differentiated from enostosis-like lesions, soft tissue mineralization, or tibial stress fractures using lateral, caudal, and oblique images. Incidental findings such as an area of IRU associated with calcinosis circumscripta can be spectacular.

Intensity of Increased Radiopharmaceutical Uptake
Areas of IRU are described as mild, mild-moderate, moderate, moderate-intense, or intense. When analyzed using ROI analysis, areas of IRU must have 10% to 15% increased count density to be visually recognized as abnormal compared with surrounding bone or the contralateral limb. When both limbs are abnormal, an obvious difference may not be visible. Experience is critical for accurate image interpretation. In normal horses epiphyseal and metaphyseal areas of bones are more prominent than diaphyseal bone in delayed phase images, because bones are larger and there is generally more bone turnover in cancellous bone. In sound sports horses, demonstrable quantitative variations have been found in RU.[45] In the front fetlock joint, peak activity was found in the proximal aspect of the proximal phalanx, but in hindlimbs peak activity was found evenly distributed between the distal aspect of the third metatarsal condyles and the proximal aspect of the proximal phalanx.[45] Comparison using ROI analysis demonstrated that the distal condyles of the MtIII were more active than the distal aspect of the McIII; there were mild differences between right and left limbs, and age had no effect on RU.[45] In the TB racehorse, qualitative and ROI analysis have shown that in both the front and hind fetlock joints of normal horses there is greater RU in the distal aspect of the McIII or MtIII condyles than elsewhere in the fetlock. In horses with lameness localized to the region there is moderate to intense IRU.[46] IRU is more common in the medial forelimb and lateral hindlimb condyles.[46] Because time from injury to imaging is inversely proportional to intensity, IRU associated with fracture may be not intense but only mildly abnormal. Scintigraphic examination in horses suspected of having pelvic fractures may be critical for diagnosis, but expecting to see intense IRU is unrealistic, because background radiation, distance, shielding, and motion compromise image quality. Pelvic fractures are usually not as obvious as fractures in the distal aspect of the limb until muscle atrophy is pronounced. Cursory examination of images or placing undue importance on changes in intensity of RU, without considering

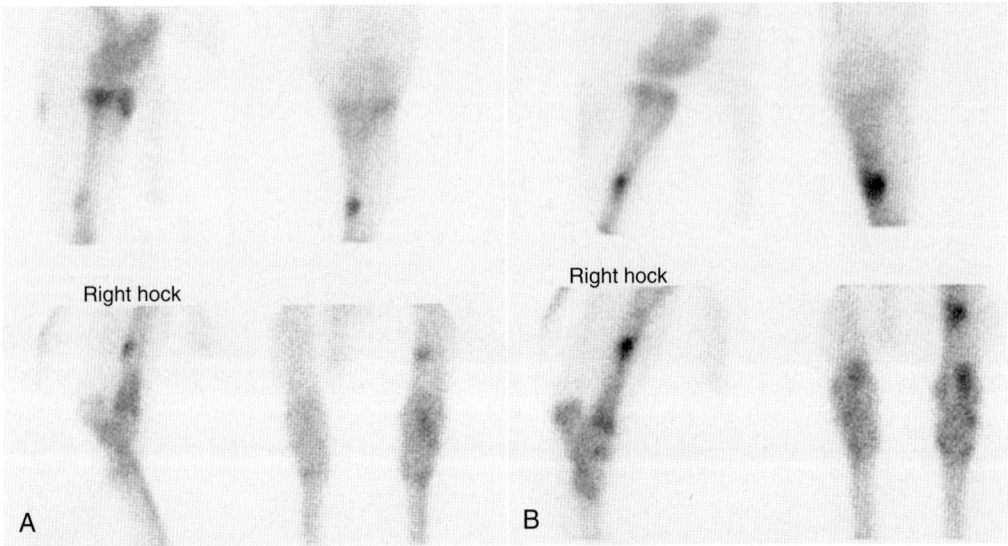

Figure 19-9 • A, Lateral (left upper and lower images) and caudal delayed phase scintigraphic images of a 2-year-old Standardbred trotter with acute, severe right hindlimb lameness and **B,** lateral (left upper and lower images) and caudal delayed phase images of a 3-year-old Thoroughbred racehorse with acute right hindlimb lameness. Note that in each horse there is focal, intense increased radiopharmaceutical uptake (IRU) in the tibia. In **A,** IRU involves the caudal tibial cortex and is caused by a tibial stress fracture, whereas in **B,** IRU is in the medullary cavity of the tibial diaphysis associated with an enostosis-like lesion. With only one image it would be impossible to differentiate these lesions, but with two images, cortical **(A)** and medullary **(B)** location can be determined.

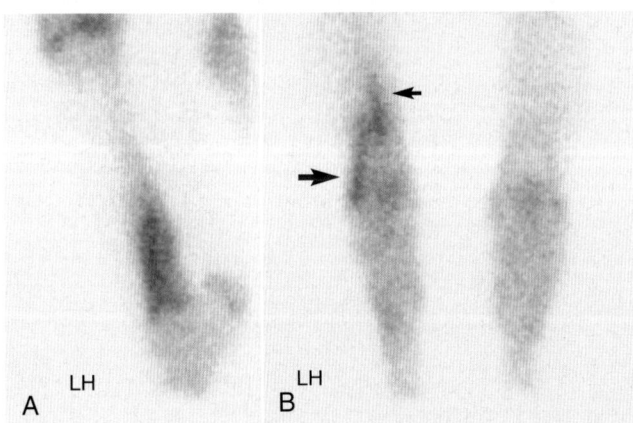

Figure 19-10 • Lateral *(left)* and caudal *(right)* delayed phase scintigraphic images of a Thoroughbred racehorse with severe, nearly non–weight-bearing left hindlimb lameness as a result of a distal spiral tibial fracture. Diffuse moderate-intense increased radiopharmaceutical uptake of the entire distal tibia can be seen in the lateral image, and the spiral nature of the fracture can be seen involving the lateral and medial tibial cortices *(arrows)* in the caudal image. Radiological findings were negative. Five weeks after imaging, this horse developed a catastrophic fracture of the left tibia and was euthanized. A distinct difference in scintigraphic appearance between this tibia and that shown in Figure 19-9, *B* demonstrates the versatility of scintigraphy. Detection of involvement of both cortices of the tibia is a grave scintigraphic finding, and horses are at profound risk for developing a comminuted, displaced fracture.

bone when IRU is only mild, whereas negative or equivocal radiological changes appear in bone when IRU is intense. Radiological evidence of fracture often lags behind scintigraphic changes, an important advantage of using scintigraphy for early diagnosis. Conversely, scintigraphic activity may abate long before radiological changes subside. Scintigraphy measures bone metabolism and can be useful in assessing the current activity of existing radiological changes. Results of all imaging modalities must be interpreted in conjunction with other clinical information. The clinician may judge radiological changes as inactive, or incidental, if a bone scan shows minimal or normal RU (see Figure 19-4).

Character of Increased Radiopharmaceutical Uptake

Focal IRU means well-localized bone modeling exists, such as that seen with fracture or other substantial bone injury. Even without radiological confirmation, focal IRU should be considered consistent with fracture, particularly in horses in which lameness has been localized to the specific region. In any horse, focal IRU indicates active bone modeling, but intensity of IRU varies with time between injury and scan. Differentiation between focal and diffuse IRU is important. For example, the dorsal cortex of the McIII of TB racehorses undergoes a spectrum of bone changes caused by high-strain cyclic fatigue that can be seen scintigraphically and radiologically. Periostitis (bucked shins) can be differentiated from dorsal cortical fracture scintigraphically, even if accompanying radiological findings are negative (Figure 19-11). Fracture or traumatic osteitis accounts for most focal areas of IRU, but infectious osteitis or osteomyelitis can look similar. Labeled white blood cell studies using ^{111}In or ^{99m}Tc can be useful to differentiate infectious

the nature of uptake, is dangerous. Even if mild and small, focal IRU should always pique the examiner's interest. Images should be evaluated before horses leave the imaging area, because additional 90-degree or 180-degree flexed or other images of the area might give important information. Commonly, advanced radiological changes may be seen in

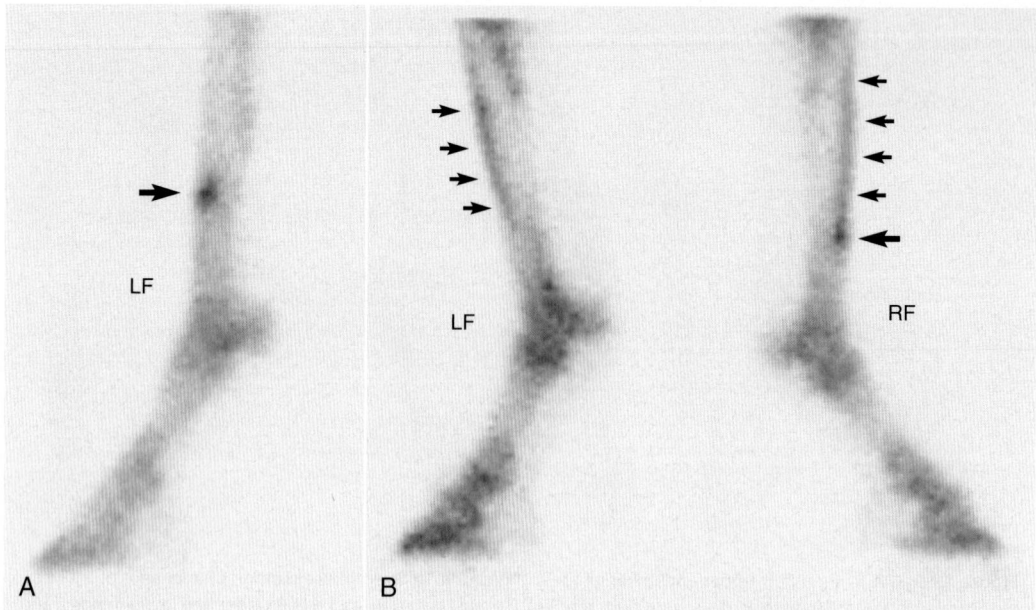

Figure 19-11 • Delayed phase scintigraphic images. **A,** Lateral image of a 4-year-old Thoroughbred (TB) colt with left forelimb lameness as a result of a dorsal cortical fracture *(arrow)* of the third metacarpal bone (McIII), and **B,** lateral images of both forelimbs of a 3-year-old TB colt with right forelimb (RF) and right hindlimb (RH) lameness after a recent race. Focal increased radiopharmaceutical uptake (IRU) must be differentiated from diffuse IRU and indicates the presence of fracture. Note the continuum of scintigraphic changes in the RF in the horse shown in **B.** Diffuse IRU is diagnostic of periostitis *(small arrows)* and distally, focal IRU *(large arrow)* indicates the presence of a dorsal cortical fracture. RH lameness was caused by another stress-related bone injury, an ilial stress fracture (not shown).

processes from other bone injury and are particularly useful when evaluating potential infection after surgery.[29] *Diffuse IRU* appears when a large area of cortical, subchondral bone or soft tissue is abnormal, but in horses with diffuse IRU, radiological changes usually are not found. *Generalized IRU* is another term used synonymously with *diffuse IRU.* A moderate, generalized greater RU associated with both sides of a joint than the metaphyseal and diaphyseal regions of long bones may be an incidental finding.

Photopenia is an unusual scintigraphic finding. Theoretically, if blood supply is not adequate during flow and pool phases, radiopharmaceutical concentrations sufficient to delineate normal or abnormal bone are not achieved. Bone infarct, abscess, intense resorption, or sequestration might cause photopenia. Resolution of scintigraphic equipment is not sufficient to see small areas of resorption in dense cortical or subchondral bone, and even if possible to resolve technically, modeling in surrounding bone would obscure, or steal, counts. No known equine disease involves only bone resorption without modeling. Photopenia is seen rarely when portions of bone are surgically removed or displaced out of view. In flow phase images of horses with lameness abolished with palmar digital analgesia there is often reduction of blood flow in the affected limb, recognized as a photopenic region between the coronary band and distal aspect of the foot on dorsal images (Figure 19-12). A relative reduction in blood flow when compared with the contralateral limb may reflect chronic reduction in weight bearing. This finding does not persist in pool phase or delayed images. Although unusual, we have seen a horse with a subperiosteal abscess of the olecranon process of the ulna with photopenia in pool phase images that was thought to be caused by fluid accumulation and

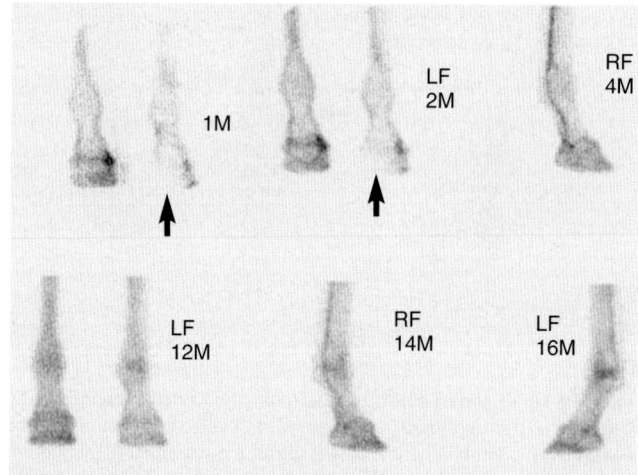

Figure 19-12 • Flow and pool phase scintigraphic images of a 2-year-old Standardbred pacer with acute left forelimb lameness as a result of a suspected subsolar bruise or abscess, but the cause was not confirmed. Note the marked photopenia *(arrows)* in the flow and early pool phase images that abates later in the scan. Delayed phase images were negative. Photopenia in flow and pool phase images can indicate the presence of infection or ischemia.

compression of nearby vessels, and a horse with photopenia of the proximal aspect of the tibia in delayed phase images caused by severe effusion of the overlying lateral femorotibial joint compartment. In addition, we have seen photopenia in delayed phase images caused by infectious osteitis, bone sequestration, and distal limb ischemia.[47]

General information can be obtained from scintigraphic images and includes an assessment of symmetry, lengths, and conformation. An assessment of the axial

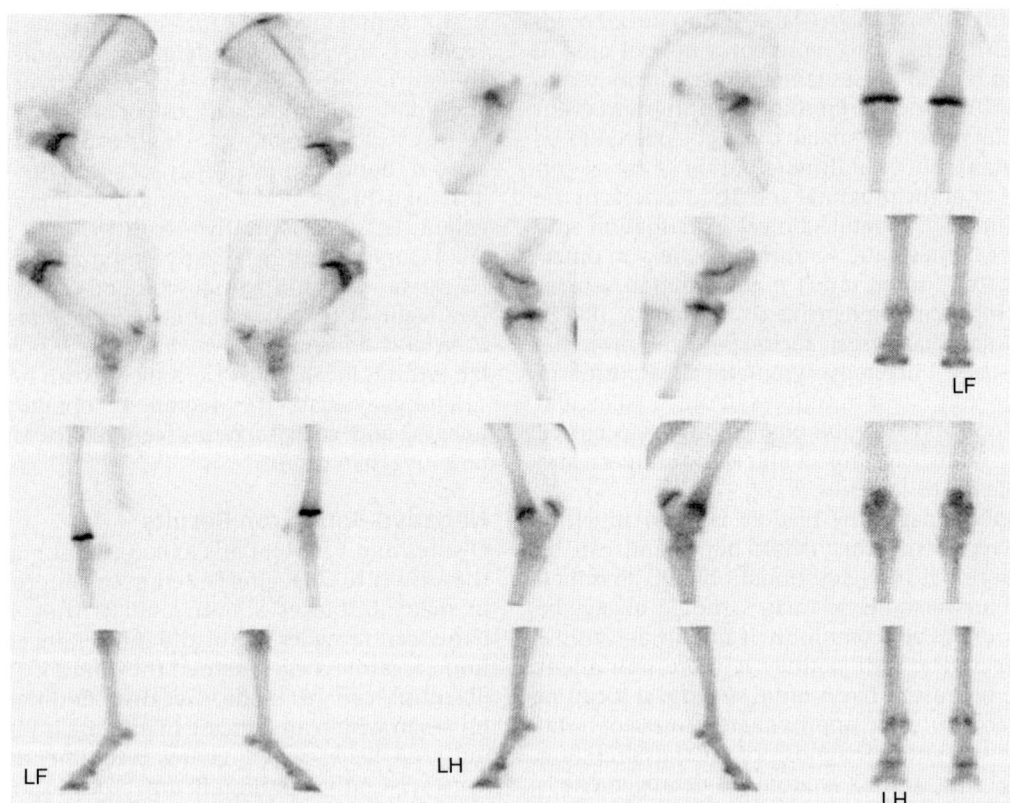

Figure 19-13 • Normal delayed scintigraphic images showing intense physeal uptake in a 2-year-old Thoroughbred in early race training. These areas are normal but may erroneously be interpreted as abnormal (false positive) or may obscure nearby lesions, causing false-negative scans.

skeleton is easily obtained from horses in a standing position, particularly the pelvis, but anatomical information is far inferior to that gained from other imaging modalities (see Figure 19-4). Pelvic asymmetry (shortened midline-to-lateral pelvic width; position, size, and angulation of the tubera sacrale, tubera coxae, or tubera ischii) can easily be measured even if RU is normal. Obvious abnormalities such as angular deformities, joint hyperflexion or hyperextension, and chronic tenosynovitis of the digital flexor tendon sheath (persistence of IRU in soft tissues seen in delayed phase images) can be documented.

False-Positive Findings

Few false-positive bone scan results occur if the clinician is aware of normal areas of greater RU and if background radiation (bladder, large vessels) is considered. Normally, cortical bone is less apparent than cancellous bone (subchondral), but both are adequately visible in good-quality images. Physeal activity in young horses is pronounced, but normal and many variations exist (Figure 19-13). Physeal activity decreases with age, but greater RU at the distal radial and tibial physes persists for years. In a study of distal radial physeal closure, radiological closure (24 to 32 months) preceded decrease in scintigraphic activity by several months (mean, 42 months).[48] In lateral pelvic images the coxofemoral joint (bone stacking of proximal femur and acetabulum) and tubera coxae are always prominent. Additional normal areas of greater RU include the lateral aspect of the metatarsophalangeal joint in plantar images, a bilobed area in the proximal aspect of the tibia in a lateral

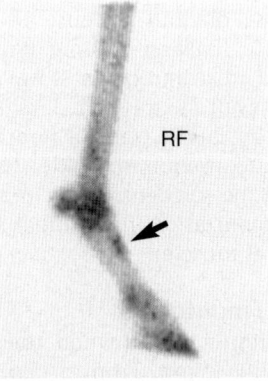

Figure 19-14 • Delayed scintigraphic image of the distal part of a fore-limb of a 7-year-old Thoroughbred jumper showing focal moderate increased radiopharmaceutical uptake in the dorsal cortex of the proximal phalanx *(arrow)*. This is a normal finding in nonracehorses and may involve one to four limbs.

image of the stifle, the distal lateral aspect of the femur and the proximal aspect of the tibia in a caudal image of the stifle, the proximal aspect of the humerus, the proximal lateral aspect of the radius (radial tuberosity), the pastern joints, the dorsal articular facets of the sixth and seventh cervical vertebrae, the dens, and many places in the skull, such as the temporomandibular joint. In some sports horses such as jumpers, hunters, dressage horses, event horses, timber horses, and driving horses, focal mild to intense IRU is found on the dorsal (most common) or palmar cortex of the proximal phalanx in one to four limbs (Figure 19-14).

We have been unable to attribute lameness to dorsal cortical IRU and feel it is likely to represent a normal area of modeling, but in 6 of 23 horses lameness was attributed to this site.[49] In another study of jumping, hunting, and event horses, IRU in the proximal phalanx was considered to be clinically important, but clear differentiation of dorsal cortical IRU from that of the proximal and distal aspects of the bone was not made.[50] Careful clinical examination and infiltration of local anesthetic solution may help to differentiate this site from other, much more common sources of pain. In the most comprehensive study to date, IRU in the dorsoproximal diaphyseal region of the proximal phalanx was usually bilaterally symmetrical, occurred in 17% of forelimbs and 7% of hindlimbs in older, taller, and heavier Warmblood and Warmblood-cross horses, occurred most commonly in dressage horses and show jumpers, and was not associated with lameness.[51]

In dorsal pelvic images the bladder is often superimposed on the sacrum or other pelvic bones and can be mistaken for abnormal IRU. Additional oblique, hemipelvic, or caudal transverse pelvic images should always be obtained. The kidneys are commonly if not always visible in delayed images. The right kidney is more prominent than is the left, because it has a more superficial location and normally accounts for approximately 60% of total glomerular filtration rate.[52] Diagnosis of renal dysfunction should be made only if gross anatomical derangement is seen and should be confirmed using specific renal function studies and ultrasonographic evaluation. In horses with long-standing hindlimb lameness and muscle atrophy, RU may appear greater in the lame compared with the nonlame limb, a possible false-positive bone scan result.

Perivascular injection or extravasation of radiopharmaceutical can cause obvious, intense IRU in soft tissues at the injection site. If a large volume of radiopharmaceutical is sequestered, distribution is slow, and poor-quality delayed images result. Extravasated radiopharmaceutical can be taken up by caudal cervical lymph nodes, causing interesting but inconsequential IRU. Other nonosseous areas of IRU may be incidental (calcinosis circumscripta, other sites of mineralization, nerve block sites) or clinically important (skeletal muscle).

False-Negative Findings

A false-negative result occurs when the image(s) fails to identify an existing lesion. From a clinical standpoint a false-negative result could be important, particularly in racehorses in which missing a stress-related bone injury could be problematic. In racehorses, in which anamnesis suggests the presence of a stress fracture, a conservative recommendation is prudent even if a negative bone scan finding is obtained. False-negative findings usually result from failing to obtain appropriate images, obtaining poor-quality images, or incorrectly interpreting images. Failure to perform diagnostic analgesia and interpret the clinical relevance of scintigraphic changes may lead to apparent but not authentic false-negative results. Problems with distance, shielding, and motion likely account for many false-negative findings. A false-negative result is possible if a horse with acute pelvic fracture is imaged within 7 to 10 days after injury. False-negative scan results rarely occur in horses with stress-related bone injury, because bone changes are long-standing and resorption and modeling

occur simultaneously. False-negative results have been reported in people undergoing chronic corticosteroid therapy and in those with disseminated metastatic disease, the elderly, and those with osteomalacia or renal osteodystrophy.[53] Bone resorption, high osteoclastic activity, and slowed bone turnover may occur with these diseases, although bone modeling usually is present to a certain extent, ensuring a positive result.

Accuracy can be greatly improved by obtaining as many standard and special scintigraphic images as possible (see Figure 19-5). *A medial lesion cannot be adequately seen using only a lateral scintigraphic image.* Knowledge that the lameness is localized to a specific site can help the clinician carefully evaluate this region by obtaining all possible images, and such targeting can reduce the chance of a false-negative result.

Negative Bone Scan Results

Owners and veterinarians look for scintigraphy to provide the answer to a nagging lameness or performance issue, but in many instances a scan result is truly negative. Every bone scan provides useful and interesting clinical information, regardless of whether the finding is positive or a diagnosis can be made. Negative findings are useful in horses in which an increase in exercise is planned, but care must be taken when giving recommendations in racehorses. Negative findings in any type of sports horse examined for poor performance or a suspected obscure lameness can help clarify the picture. Negative findings on delayed images support clinical information that pain is likely originating from soft tissues. In horses with hindlimb lameness, negative scan findings often lead us to suspect that the stifle may be a source of pain, because delayed images of this region may not be highly sensitive. Findings in horses with chronic proximal suspensory desmitis also are often negative.

Osteochondrosis in Delayed Images

We have identified areas of IRU in weanlings, yearlings, and older horses with osteochondritis dissecans or osseous cystlike lesions, but scintigraphic evidence of bone modeling can be difficult to detect, or it is missed. We have heard anecdotally that some believe osteochondrosis cannot be successfully identified scintigraphically, but our experience suggests otherwise. Intense physeal uptake in weanlings and yearlings is the most important factor in correctly identifying osteochondrosis. Count stealing is certainly important, but so is the possibility that bone modeling around osteochondritis dissecans or osseous cystlike lesions is either minimal or is present at only certain stages. Subchondral bone cysts of the distal aspect of the femur are generally scintigraphically active, but images must be interpreted carefully, and a caudal image of the stifle is mandatory. Osteochondritis dissecans of the shoulder joint involving the glenoid or proximal humeral head usually is scintigraphically active. We have identified several 2- and 3-year-old Standardbreds (STBs) and Warmbloods with large abaxially located extraarticular or small intraarticular plantar process osteochondritis dissecans fragments, or both, of the proximal phalanx in which bone modeling could be seen scintigraphically. Interestingly, in TB racehorses focal IRU in this region is common but does not usually result from plantar process fragmentation.

Osteochondritis dissecans of the lateral trochlear ridge of the femur and the cranial aspect of the intermediate ridge of the tibia is rarely scintigraphically evident.

Artifacts

Urine contamination is particularly prominent in the caudal and plantar aspects of the hindlimbs in fillies and mares. Urine contamination of the bottom of the feet is common, unless boots are applied to the horse before imaging, a procedure that is mandatory if the feet are of specific interest. Alternatively, urine can be washed away and horses can be rescanned. Damage to the collimator or crystal, maladjustment of the photopeak for ^{99m}Tc, deterioration in flood quality, and electrical problems can produce artifacts. Incidental scintigraphic findings have been discussed.

Nerve Blocks

It is reasonable to assume that injections of any type may interfere with interpretation of scintigraphic images. Local or intraarticular injections likely produce short-lived inflammatory changes that may be visible on pool or delayed phase images, but we have found this to be an overrated problem. Low and high palmar analgesic techniques have resulted in IRU seen in pool phase images for up to 17 days after injection, but little effect was seen after palmar digital and palmar (abaxial sesamoid) techniques. No effects of injections were seen in delayed phase images. The authors concluded that although effects were mild, pool phase images should be delayed for 3 to 4 days after palmar digital blocks and 2 weeks after "low" and "high" palmar local analgesic techniques.[54] We have not found it difficult to interpret pool phase images obtained 24 hours after blocking, if we are aware the horses have been blocked. By using at least two scintigraphic images it will clearly be shown that IRU is at the subcutaneous injection sites and not at important, deeper soft tissues. In most horses, little to no IRU can be seen in pool phase images and no effect occurs on delayed images with one exception. After fibular (peroneal) and tibial and median and ulnar nerve blocks, pool and delayed images show focal RU at the fibular block site and both median and ulnar block sites, respectively, and it is extremely important to know the blocking history and to obtain at least two scintigraphic images. Increased RU is likely caused by local myositis and bleeding (Figure 19-15). Intraarticular injections do not affect delayed images, but they may interfere with pool phase imaging. If pool phase images are critical, evaluation of a joint should be delayed for at least 2 weeks.

INDICATIONS AND CASE SELECTION

Bone scintigraphy is a valuable clinical tool but, like all other modalities, has limitations. Scintigraphy is useful in *early diagnosis* before injuries become radiologically apparent, a finding especially true in horses with subchondral stress-related bone injury, because scintigraphy may identify the problem months or years before radiological findings are positive. Once familiar with scintigraphy the clinician can become comfortable diagnosing fracture without adjunct radiological confirmation. Although fractures are common, scintigraphic findings of other, less obvious lesions must be differentiated and defined. The

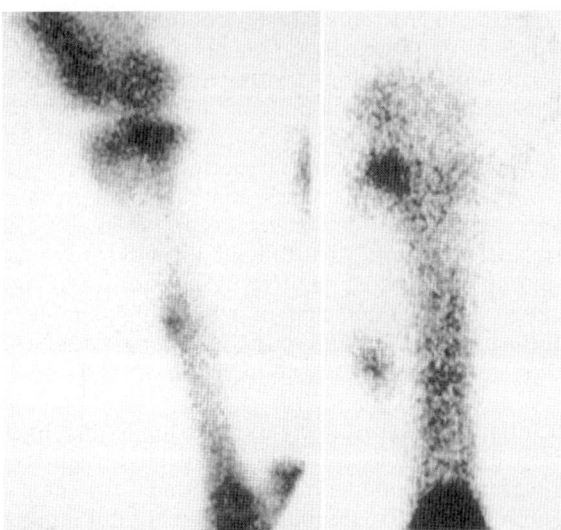

Figure 19-15 • Lateral *(left)* and caudal *(right)* delayed phase scintigraphic images showing focal increased radiopharmaceutical uptake in what appears in the lateral image as the cranial tibial cortex. In the caudal image, increased radiopharmaceutical uptake clearly involves soft tissue. Cranial tibial stress fractures are not known to occur, but this horse had a fibular and tibial nerve block the day before these images were acquired.

high expectations placed on scintigraphy to provide the lameness answer can be partially met by careful consideration of clinical characteristics of lameness and case selection. We have listed, in decreasing order, the types of clinical situations in which scintigraphy is likely to provide the most information to optimize the chance of answering that tough lameness question. Most important, horses should be lame at the time of the examination, and, when possible, lameness should be localized to a defined region in one or more limbs. Targeted imaging is invariably much more productive than whole-body screening.

Scintigraphy is most valuable in horses with unilateral or multiple limb lameness that has been localized using diagnostic analgesia but in which radiological findings are negative, equivocal, or confusing. In this group of horses, lameness at the time of scintigraphic examination allows for the distinct possibility that bone modeling subsequent to injury will be detected, if indeed bone is the source of pain. Key to accurate interpretation and obtaining all necessary views is localizing the source of pain. Scintigraphy then is most useful in horses that are *lame at the time of examination and for which lameness has been localized*.

Horses that are lame at the time of examination but in which lameness has not been localized comprise the next best group. The importance of lameness at the time of examination cannot be overemphasized. We often scan horses after periods of rest or on returning to training, but if lameness is not apparent, determining clinical relevance of findings is difficult. A subset of horses in which the lower limb has been ruled out by careful diagnostic analgesia makes even better candidates. These are horses in which an upper limb problem such as a humeral, tibial, or pelvic stress fracture may be suspected. These horses are *lame, but although the definitive source of pain has not been identified, the lower limb has been ruled out*.

Horses with an accurate history of high-speed lameness but that are not currently lame are in the next category. These are usually racehorses with stress-related bone injury and strong histories to support that lameness is indeed the cause of poor performance. Performing whole-body scans is most useful in these horses, because compensatory lameness is often present. Lameness may be subtle or difficult to detect during routine lameness examination, and diagnostic analgesia would be difficult to perform. However, this group consists of young, light horses undergoing intense training and racing in which high-strain cyclic fatigue is maximal. In this group then are *racehorses without obvious baseline lameness but in which stress-related bone injury is suspected.*

Scintigraphy is *least* likely to yield a diagnosis in show horses with nebulous histories of gait abnormalities and poor performance and with problems that can be perceived only by the rider. These horses usually are not lame, may have equivocal or negative manipulative test results, and may be difficult horses with which to work. Diagnostic analgesia may be difficult to perform or interpret. In some horses, selective analgesic techniques may improve the feel of the horse, and in some, bilaterally symmetrical lameness may be diagnosed by abolishing pain in one limb and observing lameness in the contralateral limb. Whole-body scintigraphic screening can be frustrating and unrewarding for the clinician and referring veterinarian, but it is occasionally helpful. High-quality images are essential for recognizing subtle abnormalities—for example, in the proximal palmar metacarpal or plantar metatarsal regions, in the foot, thoracolumbar spine, or pelvis. A negative scan result can help direct attention to soft tissues and adjunct evaluation using chiropractic techniques or can result in recommendation of conditioning and exercise intensity changes.

Scintigraphic examination has been used as part of a comprehensive purchase examination, but results must be carefully interpreted and clinical relevance established. Although unusual, this adjunct imaging procedure usually is requested in high-profile, expensive, upper-level sports horses, and results can often be confusing. Finding an upper-level horse of any type without any scintigraphic changes would be unusual, mirroring radiological findings in these horses. Scintigraphy has been found to be useful in establishing clinical relevance of mineralization of the cartilages of the foot, and when present, intense IRU has been associated with radiological changes that could be differentiated (wider and more irregular) from unimportant areas of mineralization or separate centers of ossification,[55-57] a possible benefit to clinicians performing examinations before purchase has been proposed.[55]

KNOWLEDGE GAINED FROM SCINTIGRAPHIC EXAMINATION OF THE LAME HORSE

Scintigraphy is a powerful tool for examining a lame horse by which we have been able to give answers, pinpoint diagnoses, study disease progression, and learn about pathogenesis of many lameness conditions. Although we cannot discuss every scintigraphic finding in the lame horse, a few select issues and areas should be reviewed.

Stress-Related Bone Injury in Cortical and Subchondral Bone

Recent studies using scintigraphy and clinical and pathological findings support the concept of a continuum of adaptive and nonadaptive (maladaptive) responses of bone leading eventually to fracture (stress or complete) and OA (see Chapter 100).[23-25,56,58] Microfracture and callus formation in pelvic bones and the humerus, and prodromal lesions and microfracture in ipsilateral and contralateral limbs of horses with condylar fractures, indicate that pathological changes preceded fracture.[23-25] Pathological changes have appeared histologically in subchondral bone of the distal aspect of the McIII, the MtIII and the third carpal bone that preceded overlying cartilage damage, indicating a continuum of changes leading to fracture or OA in racehorses.[58] Scintigraphic examination of the metatarsophalangeal joint of STBs indicated that the existence of focal IRU in the distal aspect of the MtIII was a common finding in horses in which lameness was localized to this region but in which radiological findings were negative or equivocal.[59] A continuum of subchondral bone changes has been proposed to account for the later development of fracture or OA, but early changes could be seen only scintigraphically, not radiologically (see Figure 19-6).[59] Common areas for stress-related bone injury in subchondral bone include the distal aspect of the McIII, the MtIII, the proximal sesamoid bones, and the third carpal bone (Figure 19-16), but we also feel strongly that a continuum of stress-related bone injury could account for development of fractures of the distal phalanx and OA of the distal interphalangeal joint.[60] Abnormal IRU is common in the lateral aspect of the distal phalanx in the left forelimb and medial aspect of the distal phalanx in the right forelimb, the same sites in which fracture of the distal phalanx is most common in racehorses in North America (Figure 19-17).[60,61] We know of at least two horses that subsequently developed articular palmar process fracture in these locations.[60] In nonracehorses, a common finding in those in which lameness is abolished using palmar digital analgesia is focal IRU in subchondral bone of the distal phalanx, corresponding to radiolucent defects and other radiological evidence of OA of the distal interphalangeal joint (Figure 19-18). Observations in racehorses and nonracehorses led us carefully to evaluate medial to lateral hoof balance, because many of these horses were high (longer heel length) on the affected side, strongly suggesting that mechanical forces may be involved in early stress-related bone injury.

Scintigraphic examination has allowed us to demonstrate clinically that a continuum of cortical and subchondral bone changes exists before the development of fracture or OA. This process is better understood and accepted in cortical bone but also occurs in subchondral bone and explains why horses can show lameness without obvious signs of synovitis, because pain originates from subchondral bone without obvious overlying cartilage damage. Cortical and subchondral bone undergo *stress remodeling*, the term used to describe the process by which exercised bone is modeled (new bone) and remodeled (resorption and replacement). Bone adaptation is triggered by changes in number of strain cycles and the magnitude, rate of change, and distribution of strain.[62-64] Adaptive bone remodeling is normal, but exercise may lead to nonphysiological strains,

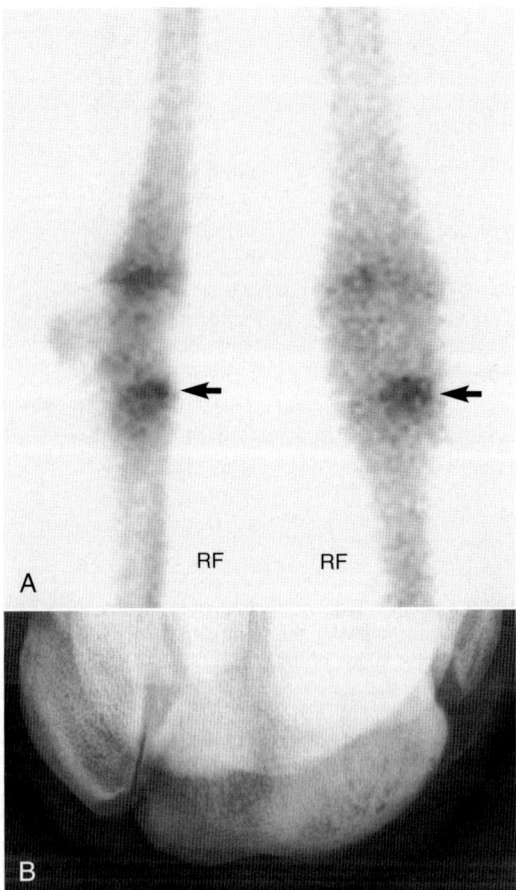

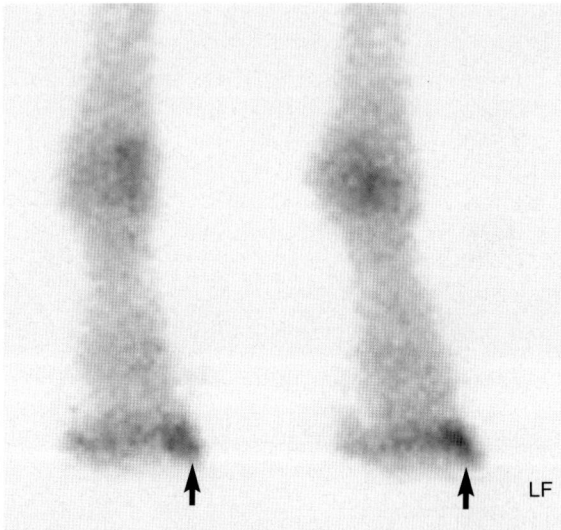

Figure 19-17 • Dorsal delayed phase scintigraphic image of the distal forelimbs in a racehorse showing a common finding of increased radio-pharmaceutical uptake in the lateral aspect of the left forelimb *(LF)* and medial aspect of the right forelimb distal phalanx. Stress-related bone injury in these locations likely leads to later development of fracture or osteoarthritis.

Figure 19-16 • **A,** Lateral *(left)* and dorsal delayed phase scintigraphic images of the right carpus of a Standardbred with stress-related bone injury of the radial facet of the third carpal bone. Focal increased radio-pharmaceutical uptake in the radial facet is a common scintigraphic finding in horses with lameness abolished by middle carpal analgesia but in which other clinical findings are equivocal. **B,** Proximodorsal-distodorsal (skyline) radiographic image of the same horse showing increased radiopacity of the radial fossa of the third carpal bone with mild radiolucent defects within the sclerotic area, a finding consistent with maladaptive or nonadaptive subchondral remodeling (medial is to the right and palmar is uppermost).

or during remodeling, resorption may outpace replacement, and both situations may lead to a nonadaptive response in which damage to cortical or subchondral bone occurs, eventually leading to fracture or OA.[4,58,60,65] Lameness appears to develop long before radiological evidence of bone damage exists, but during this time scintigraphic examination often reveals focal areas of moderate or intense IRU.

In summary, many common equine lameness conditions, including catastrophic and stress fractures and many forms of OA, result from a continuum of cortical and subchondral bone changes occurring in response to exercise. Scintigraphic examination is the only way to provide early, accurate diagnosis. Single-event injuries occur from direct trauma or acute overload of bone and soft tissue material properties, but they are in the minority in most sports horses with stress-related bone injury. We find it interesting that in the forelimb, with the exception of the distal phalanx, most stress-related bone injuries involve the medial aspect, whereas in the hindlimb most changes

involve the lateral aspect of the limb. This finding is consistent in TB and STB racehorses and must reflect loading of the limb and commonality of movement rather than the expected effects of counterclockwise racing.

Confusing or Equivocal Radiological Changes

We have often been able to pinpoint diagnosis in horses with confusing or equivocal radiological changes using scintigraphy. Although racehorses with commonly seen areas of stress-related bone injury fall into this category, we have been able to accurately identify sources of pain in other types of sport horses. Navicular disease formerly was a common default diagnosis in horses in which lameness was abolished by palmar digital analgesia. However, scintigraphic examination has allowed us to define 15 to 20 different possible sources of pain in horses with this blocking history. Navicular disease is still a common finding and has been observed to account for part or all of lameness in 65% of nonracehorse sports horses.[60] Central areas of IRU are most common, and often conventional radiographic images yield negative or equivocal findings. The palmaroproximal-palmarodistal oblique (skyline) view is most useful in identifying subtle radiological changes and should be obtained routinely (see Chapter 30). However, navicular disease should not be the default diagnosis, because OA of the distal interphalangeal and proximal interphalangeal joints, stress remodeling or stress reaction of the distal phalanx, soft tissue pain, and myriad other diagnoses can be made. We recommend the concurrent use of MRI and three-phase scintigraphic examination to help elucidate etiology in horses that have lameness abolished with palmar digital analgesia.[8,9] Differentiation of lameness in the proximal palmar metacarpal region from that of the carpus can sometimes be difficult from overlap of diagnostic analgesic techniques, but scintigraphy has proved valuable in correctly identifying horses with avulsion injury at

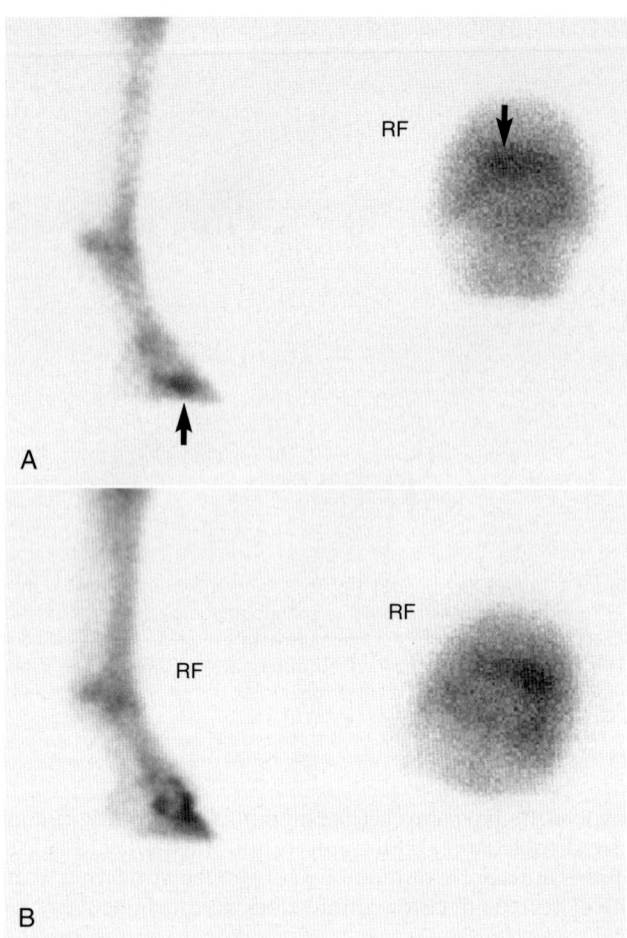

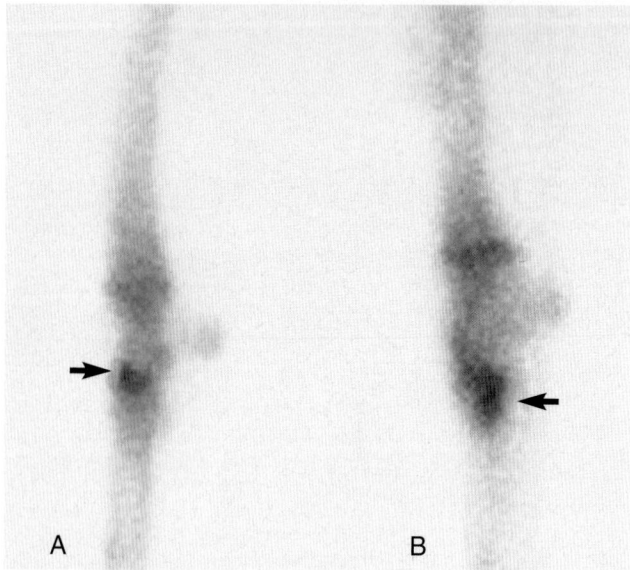

Figure 19-19 • A, Lateral delayed scintigraphic image of the carpus of a horse with a lesion involving the third carpal bone *(arrow).* **B,** Lateral delayed scintigraphic image of the carpus of another horse with an avulsion fracture of third metacarpal at the origin of the suspensory ligament *(arrow).* High palmar and middle carpal joint analgesic techniques improved lameness in both horses.

Figure 19-18 • A, Lateral *(left)* and solar delayed phase scintigraphic images of an 8-year-old large pony with moderate, focal increased radiopharmaceutical uptake (IRU) in the subchondral bone of the distal phalanx *(arrows)* and early evidence of osteoarthritis (OA) of the distal interphalangeal (DIP) joint. Areas of IRU in subchondral bone can be confused with those at the attachment of the deep digital flexor tendon. Radiographs in this pony revealed an ill-defined radiolucent defect. **B,** Lateral *(left)* and solar scintigraphic images of a 5-year-old reining Quarter Horse with similar findings in the solar image, but with scintigraphic evidence of advanced OA of the DIP joint in the lateral image. Note the moderate IRU of the dorsal and palmar aspects of the DIP joint in the lateral image. Radiographs revealed extensive changes in both the dorsal and palmar aspects of the DIP joint.

the origin of the suspensory ligament from those with lameness of the middle carpal joint (Figure 19-19). Similarly, lameness associated with the tarsus can be clearly differentiated from that of the proximal metatarsal region. Scintigraphic examination has identified horses with incomplete fractures of the talus, distal tibial subchondral bone injury, fractures of the central and third tarsal bones, and OA of the centrodistal and tarsometatarsal joints. In young racehorses the predominant scintigraphic and radiological changes are seen involving the dorsolateral aspect of the tarsus, unlike what was once thought, that the dorsomedial or medial aspect was most commonly involved (see Figure 44-1). Focal or diffuse areas of IRU are found in the thoracolumbar dorsal spinous processes and may account for clinical signs of back pain, poor performance, or gait restriction but occur only in horses that are ridden

(Chapter 52). However both false negative and false positive results may be obtained. A wide spectrum of scintigraphic and radiological changes in the thoracolumbar spine in horses without back pain has led to the conclusion that IRU in the dorsal spinous processes should be interpreted carefully and in light of other clinical signs; only 7 of 33 horses without back pain had no radiological or scintigraphic abnormalities, and in some horses IRU was pronounced.[66] We have not identified areas of IRU in the thoracolumbar spine in the STB racehorse, but these are common in young TBs in race training and in most are incidental scintigraphic findings. However, in sports horses scintigraphy may be helpful in the assessment of the clinical significance of radiological evidence of OA of the thoracolumbar facet joints[67] or spondylosis.[68] A rare scintigraphic finding in horses with acute forelimb lameness or with acute back pain and respiratory distress is fracture or other injury to a single or two adjacent vertebrae in the midthoracic region.

Confusing Clinical Signs and Unexplained Lameness

Scintigraphic examination has been useful to help explain pain in horses with confusing clinical signs and results of diagnostic analgesia. Lack of localizing clinical findings and negative or equivocal response to intraarticular analgesia prompts scintigraphic examination of numerous TB and STB racehorses each year; the most common scintigraphic abnormality found in these horses with unexplained lameness or poor performance is subchondral bone injury of the McIII or the MtIII condyles (Figure 19-20). Horses with early OA with pain originating primarily from subchondral bone do not consistently improve with intraarticular diagnostic analgesia. Likewise, horses with advanced OA do not

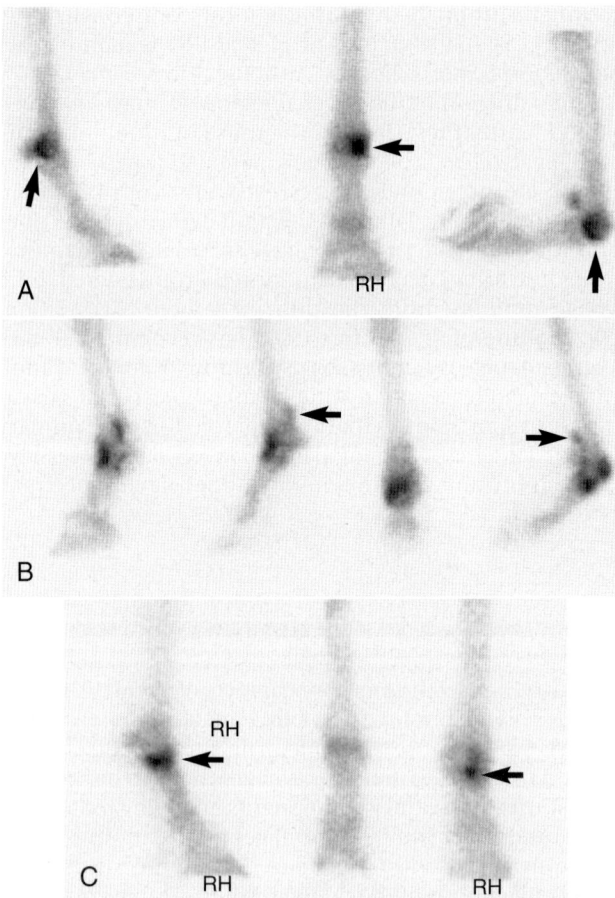

Figure 19-20 • A, Lateral *(left),* plantar, and flexed lateral delayed phase scintigraphic images of a 4-year-old Thoroughbred racehorse with maladaptive or nonadaptive subchondral bone remodeling of the distal aspect of the right third metatarsal (MtIII) condyle. Note the focal, moderate-intense increased radiopharmaceutical uptake (IRU) of the distal lateral aspect of the MtIII. **B,** Pool phase *(left)* and delayed phase lateral *(second from left),* dorsal, and flexed medial *(right)* scintigraphic images of an 11-year-old Arabian sports horse with severe osteoarthritis of the left metacarpophalangeal joint (MCPJ). Note the unusual but ominous IRU *(arrow)* in the palmar pouch of the MCPJ in pool phase images that persists in delayed phase images. **C,** Lateral *(left)* and plantar delayed phase scintigraphic images of a 5-year-old Standardbred pacer with right hindlimb lameness abolished with plantar digital analgesia. Expecting to find a lesion in the foot, we saw focal, intense IRU in the proximal aspect of the proximal phalanx consistent with a midsagittal fracture. Pain in the metatarsophalangeal joint can be abolished with plantar digital analgesia.

reliably improve with intraarticular analgesia, a finding that has prompted referral of a small number of horses in which an unusual and consistent scintigraphic abnormality of the fetlock joint was found (see Figure 19-20). Accumulation of radiopharmaceutical in subchondral bone (most commonly the distal aspect of the McIII or the MtIII and the proximal phalanx) in combination with areas of IRU in the palmar or plantar pouch of the fetlock joint is diagnostic for end-stage OA, an ominous scintigraphic finding. We have imaged racehorses in which forelimb or hindlimb lameness was abolished using palmar or plantar digital analgesia and that were suspected of having a lesion in a foot. Radiological examination of the feet was negative. Three-phase scintigraphic examination revealed IRU in the fetlock joint demonstrating clearly that palmar or plantar

analgesia can indeed abolish pain in more proximal locations in the limb. Midsagittal fracture of the proximal aspect of the proximal phalanx (see Figure 19-20), fracture of the distal condyles of the McIII or the MtIII, and fracture of the proximal sesamoid bones are most commonly found. We have examined 20 horses with IRU in the rib(s) and in some, clinical signs of forelimb lameness (ribs 1 to 3), resistance to saddling, or poor performance could be explained by fracture, anomaly, or injury of ribs, clinical answers that could not have been provided without scintigraphy.[69] We examined two horses with IRU in distal or proximal diaphyseal and metaphyseal bone and radiological evidence of periosteal new bone formation and diagnosed hypertrophic osteopathy, but the primary cause was never found. It is possible these horses had bone fragility disorder, a recently described syndrome of horses in California.[70,71] Unexplained lameness and numerous sites of IRU of the axial and proximal portion of the appendicular skeleton were found in 16 horses, particularly the scapula (13) and ribs (11), and horses had unusual clinical signs such as scapular bowing, but the cause remains undetermined. Pulmonary silicosis was incriminated in one report but affected only 4 of 16 horses in another.[70,71] Scintigraphy provided vital clinical information.

Lameness Related to the Pelvis

Good-quality scintigraphic images of the pelvis can obviate the need to obtain radiographs with horses under general anesthesia. Image quality can further be improved using motion correction software (see Figure 19-4). Horses with IRU of the coxofemoral joint often have distant areas of IRU, a scintigraphic finding that worsens prognosis for future soundness. In two horses in which scintigraphy identified single or multiple areas of IRU, fracture of the pubic symphysis, not identified in either horse scintigraphically, was found at necropsy examination in addition to those areas properly identified.[72] Although horses seemingly have one predominant source of lameness, with pelvic injury scintigraphic identification of additional sites is an important negative prognostic sign. False-negative results are also possible. Pelvic stress fractures, fractures or enthesopathy of the third trochanter and tubera ischii, sacroiliac injury, direct trauma to the tubera coxae, and fractures of the tail head and caudal aspect of the sacrum have been identified as causes of obvious to subtle signs of hindlimb lameness (see Chapters 50 and 51). We have seen very few horses with authentic abnormalities of the sacroiliac joints, but Dyson and colleagues have documented the importance of careful scintigraphic and clinical examinations of this region.[42,43]

Damaged Skeletal Muscle

Damaged skeletal muscle behaves like damaged bone. Areas of IRU in skeletal muscle appear in *delayed images* and rarely in pool phase (soft tissue) images. We have observed two distinct patterns of IRU in skeletal muscle. Most commonly, generalized IRU in the gluteal and epaxial muscles appears in racehorses, but can also be seen in sports horses, and is thought to be consistent with previous exertional rhabdomyolysis. Occasionally, IRU appears concomitantly in the latissimus dorsi muscle and rarely in the triceps muscle. In these horses, creatine kinase and aspartate transaminase enzyme concentrations usually are only mildly elevated. In the original report, IRU in skeletal muscle was seen 24 hours after horses underwent strenuous exercise on a high-speed treadmill, and the authors suggested that imaging should be performed within 24 to 48 hours of exercise.[73] Our experience is different, however, because we have seen generalized IRU of skeletal muscle in horses that have trained at least 7 to 10 days before scintigraphic examination. Of 129 horses with scintigraphic abnormalities of the pelvis, 34 had IRU in skeletal muscle.[72] Lameness associated with IRU in skeletal muscle was not apparent, but abnormal IRU in muscle was thought to explain a portion of the horse's poor performance.[72] However, not all horses with previous exertional rhabdomyolysis have scintigraphic abnormalities.

In the less common second form, IRU appears in individual muscles or portions of muscles. The hindlimb is most commonly affected, and individual portions of the biceps femoris, semitendinosus, or gluteal muscles are abnormal. Although this form is most common in racehorses, occasionally epaxial or gluteal IRU is identified in nonracehorse sports horses. Although horses may show pain on palpation of the affected region, we have not been able to identify these areas as the cause of hindlimb lameness. Elevated levels of creatine kinase and aspartate transaminase are not found. Horses with this form of IRU in muscle usually are lame in the ipsilateral hindlimb but from a distally located site. We have speculated that muscle strain or tearing may have occurred from altered limb carriage resulting from the primary lameness condition. However, one of the Editors (SJD) has recognized IRU in the gluteal, biceps femoris, or psoas muscles in association with elevated levels of creatine kinase and aspartate transaminase in sports horses that was believed to be the primary cause of lameness or poor performance. Rarely, we have identified IRU in a forelimb involving subclavius, pectoral, or triceps muscles.

Chapter 20

Computed Tomography

Sarah M. Puchalski

PHYSICS

Computed tomography (CT) is a well-established diagnostic imaging modality that has been in clinical use in medicine for several decades but only recently has become commonly used in veterinary medicine. The essential concept of a CT scanner is that an x-ray–generating tube is positioned across from a row of digital x-ray detectors in a circular gantry. The tube and detectors spin around the outside of a horse, creating a continuous radiographic image through 360 degrees. The detectors are linked to a computer system that manipulates the imaging data by a process called *back projection,* thereby generating cross-sectional images based on the subject density.[1]

References
on page
1263

EQUIPMENT

CT hardware, like most imaging technology, has undergone extensive revision since its inception. One of the most important advances in CT hardware was the advent of the slip ring, allowing for helical scanning. With helical scanning, the x-ray tube and detectors continuously spin around the horse while it translates or moves through the center of the gantry. The resultant path of the x-ray tube relative to the horse is helical, giving the technique its name. Another, equally important, major advance is the advent of multislice technology. Multislice CT is a modification of the aforementioned basic configuration whereby multiple detector rows are positioned opposite the x-ray generator. The x-ray generator exposes the subject, and the transmitted x-rays are detected by several rows of detectors on the opposite side of the gantry. Since the first appearance of a dual-slice CT scanner, this technology has burgeoned, and now up to 256-slice scanners are available. The number of detector rows determines the number of images that can be acquired per rotation of the gantry components, meaning that a four-slice scanner can acquire four images per rotation.

In order for horses to be imaged, careful consideration must be given both to the design of the CT table and to the size of the CT gantry opening. The CT table must not only support the weight of the horse but also move with speed and great precision. For a single-slice helical scanner acquiring 1-mm–thick images, the horse must move 1 mm per rotation of the gantry, which generally occurs in about 0.8 seconds. In order to accomplish this, equine CT tables have been custom-designed to work with those manufactured for scanning people. More recently, commercially available equine CT tables have come onto the market (Figure 20-1). An alternative style of CT scanner has recently resurfaced as

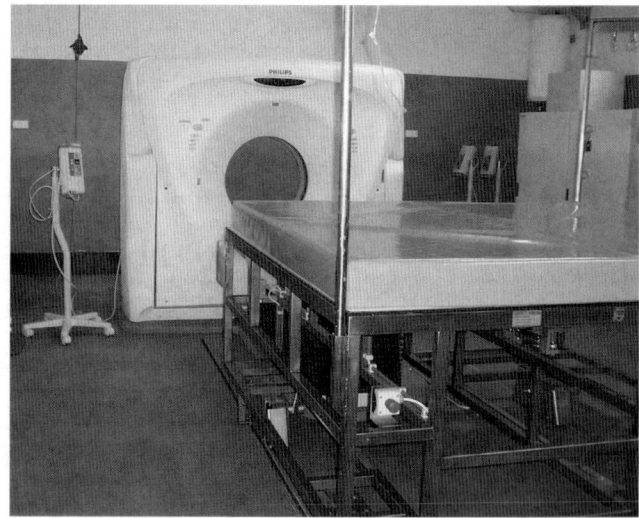

Figure 20-1 • Commercially available equine table attached to a four-slice helical computed tomography scanner. (Philips, the Netherlands.)

an option for horses. This type of CT gantry can be equipped with multislice capabilities and is portable. The gantry translates around the outside of the horse with the requisite precision and speed. CT scanners have been built for human applications and as such typically have a circular gantry opening of around 70 cm, which determines the maximum size of the patient or area to be scanned. Currently scanners with 30- to 35-cm openings are commercially available and are appropriate for equine extremity work. There is a movement toward larger gantry sizes that will likely result in machines with >80-cm openings becoming available in the near future, which should increase the clinical utility of equine CT to include larger anatomical regions.

IMAGE DISPLAY AND PROCESSING

Image Display

CT images map tissue density in the subject. Each pixel in the two-dimensional CT image actually represents a volume of tissue or volume element (voxel) defined by the pixel size in two dimensions and slice thickness in the third dimension. Typical slice thickness ranges from 1 to 10 mm, and now with multislice scanners, images less than 1 mm thick can be obtained. For each voxel, a value is recorded in Hounsfield units (HU) or CT units. This numerical value represents the density of the tissue within the voxel relative to water, which is arbitrarily set to equal zero. Density values of common tissues are listed in Box 20-1. Lesions can be described as hypodense or hyperdense.

The viewer, using routinely available image review software, can reversibly manipulate the displayed grayscale value of the tissues. Using a wide "window width" is appropriate for the evaluation of tissues with a wide density range such as bone (approximately 400 to 1500 HU). Viewing with a narrow window produces higher image contrast and is appropriate for the evaluation of tissues with a narrow density range such as soft tissue (approximately 40 to 120 HU). "Level" is to the midpoint of the grey shades that are displayed. Changing the level increases or decreases the brightness of the image. In order to perform a complete and thorough evaluation of CT images, the viewer should actively manipulate both window width and level to view all tissues (Figure 20-2).

Image Processing

Image processing refers to mathematical manipulation of the images and is most often performed in the background at the time of acquisition. Processing is used to improve the appearance of an image or help the viewer to better evaluate one type of structure such as soft tissue versus bone (see Figure 20-2).[2]

Image Reconstruction

Image reformatting and reconstruction are routinely used to manipulate the imaging data to appear differently. Image reformatting is the simplest form of reconstruction and is the process by which the viewer can "reslice" the imaging information into a different orientation (Figure 20-3). The resultant images are two-dimensional cross-sections of anatomy. The quality of the reconstructed images is highly dependent on the original slice thickness and the slice interval. Thinner slices that overlap result in better images than thicker slices or slices that do not overlap. Helical scanners are capable of producing overlapping slices, and multislice scanners can acquire images that are less than 1 mm in thickness.

Three-dimensional (3D) reconstructions use the voxel density value (HU) to create models that represent anatomy in a completely different format. Two commonly used types of 3D reconstructions are termed *surface rendering* and *volume rendering*. In a surface-rendered image, the viewer selects a minimum density threshold so that only tissue of higher density than the threshold is displayed. This technique can be useful to create a topographical impression of a fractured bone. Volume rendering uses the same principle, but a color scheme is used to depict tissues within a specific density range. The resultant image depicts the color-coded structure from whichever external viewpoint the viewer chooses. Figure 20-4 shows an intraarterial CT angiogram, viewed from the palmaromedial aspect, in which the operator has progressively increased the minimum threshold so that all tissues of lower density are removed. The final image has a threshold of about 550 HU, and only the surface of the bone and the contrast medium within the major vessels are visible.

Contrast Media

Contrast media are available for all diagnostic imaging modalities and are used to better identify or more thoroughly characterize either normal or abnormal structures. Routine radiographic contrast media (barium or iodine based) can be used to augment the clinical utility of CT. Most commonly, iodine-based injectable contrast media are given by the intravascular route to identify regions of increased blood flow or vascular permeability, as expected with injured or inflamed soft tissues. Regional intraarterial administration with concurrent CT scanning has been described to aid in the identification of soft tissue lesions of the foot.[3,4] This technique is also useful for regions higher in the limb—for example, to evaluate the suspensory ligament of both forelimbs (see Figure 20-2) and hindlimbs and the structures within the carpal canal. In the early phases of tendon and ligament injury, contrast medium is present in increased quantity because of extravasation from abnormally permeable blood vessels. As a lesion heals, neovascularization develops; contrast medium is seen within small-caliber blood vessels.[5] Alternatively, nonionic iodine-based contrast media can be injected into synovial spaces to surround and improve margin visibility of structures in or around joints, sheaths, and bursae. This

---

BOX 20-1

Density Values of Different Tissues

Tissue	Density (Hounsfield Units [HU])
Gas	−1000
Fat	−120
Water	0
Muscle	40
Equine DDFT	90-120
Medullary bone	400-600
Cortical bone	1500

DDFT, Deep digital flexor tendon.

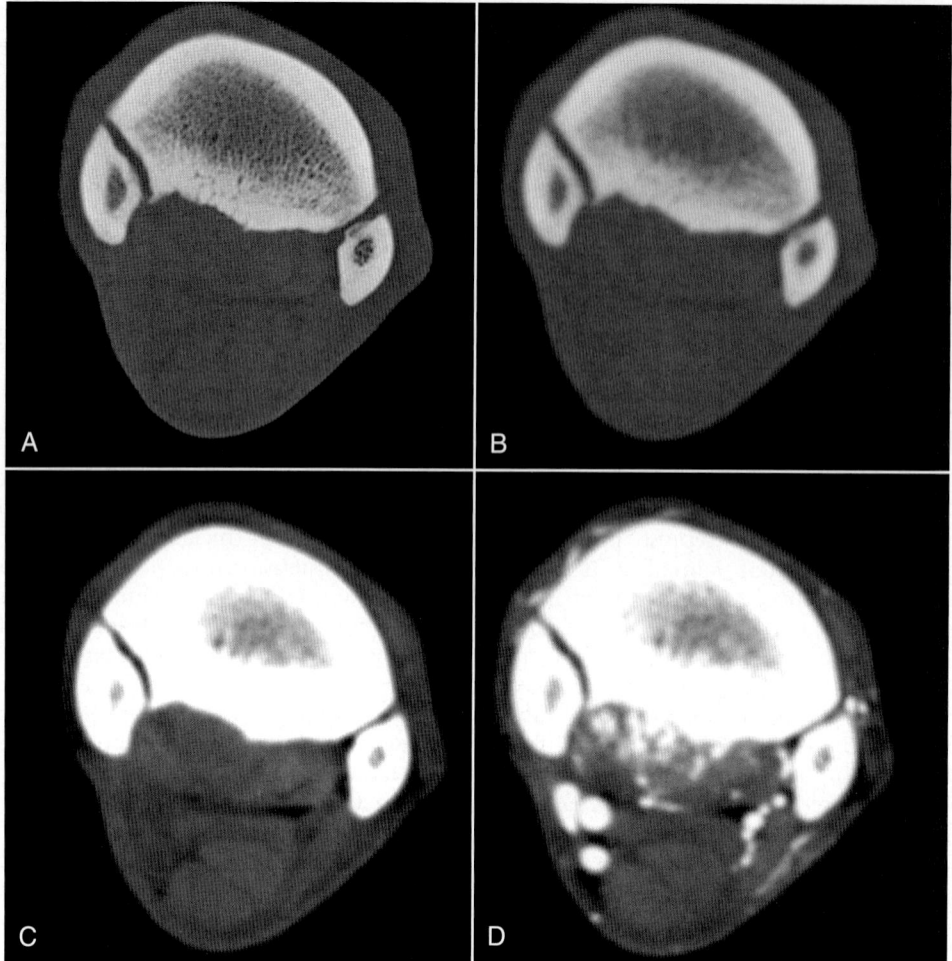

Figure 20-2 • Transverse computed tomography images all acquired at the same location in the proximal metacarpal region, but processed and displayed differently. Medial is to the left. **A** has a wide window width and has been processed with an edge-enhancing algorithm to enable accurate assessment of bone. **B** has the same window, but a smoothing algorithm has been applied for evaluation of the soft tissues. **C** is a soft tissue algorithm with a narrow window width. **D** is the same location after the regional administration of contrast medium. This horse has suspensory ligament injury that is moderately contrast enhancing with associated entheous and endosteal new bone at its origin. Note the irregular contour of the palmar cortex of the third metacarpal bone, seen best in **A** and **B,** and the periarticular osteophyte bridging the articulation between the second and third metacarpal bones. In **C,** note the hypodense areas in the suspensory ligament corresponding to areas that show contrast enhancement in **D.** The superficial and deep digital flexor tendons and the accessory ligament of the deep digital flexor tendon have uniform density.

allows for the evaluation of intraarticular ligaments (stifle, carpus) or the identification of adhesions (navicular bursa) or cartilage lesions. The systemic use of contrast medium in horses is impractical because of the large dose required and time-consuming administration.

CLINICAL APPLICATIONS
Fracture Assessment
CT's greatest strength is the detailed evaluation of osseous structures. The elimination of superimposition allows the viewer to detect small changes in bone density caused by osteolysis or proliferation that would go unnoticed on routine radiographs. This also applies to the detection of small fragments or comminuted fracture lines. These characteristics make CT an ideal choice to accurately characterize fractures, in order to establish prognosis or for preoperative planning. CT is particularly useful in evaluating fractures

when they occur in complicated anatomical regions such as the carpus or tarsus (Figure 20-5). CT intraarterial angiography of the extremity can be performed to identify concurrent soft tissue and blood vessel trauma.

Lameness Diagnosis
The goal of diagnostic imaging is to accurately identify and thoroughly describe pathology. All diagnostic imaging techniques should be considered in the light of these goals. In some horses, it is difficult to identify lesions and to thoroughly describe underlying pathology using radiography and ultrasonography, the more routinely available imaging techniques. Advanced imaging should be used when either one of these goals is not met. In lameness diagnosis, advanced diagnostic imaging techniques will usually augment a clinical workup by providing additional or different information. The clinician must carefully evaluate each horse, weigh the cost-benefit ratio, and decide if

additional diagnostic techniques are necessary to solve the clinical problem. Although CT scanning is rapid, limitations exist. CT should be used once the source of pain causing lameness is established, because it is largely impractical to "screen" numerous anatomical regions. Furthermore, general anesthesia, with its associated risks, is necessary in most horses to obtain high-quality diagnostic images.

At the Veterinary Medical Teaching Hospital of the University of California, Davis, the most common indication for using CT is the evaluation of lameness caused by

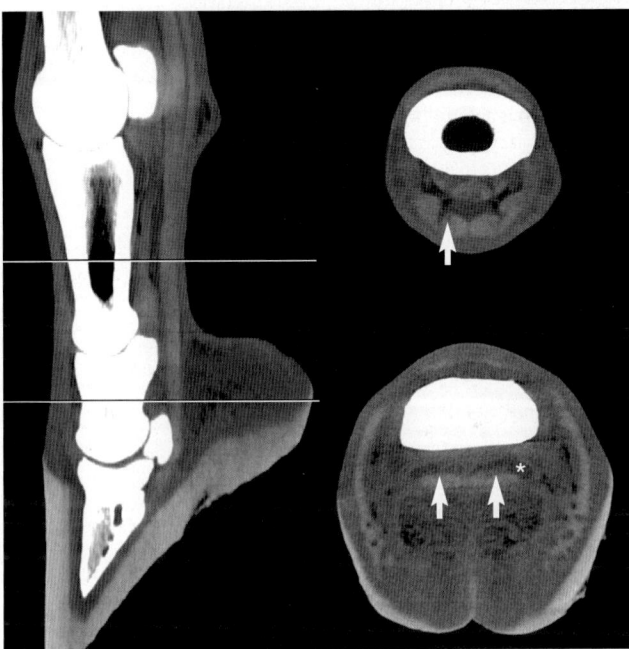

Figure 20-3 • Tranverse computed tomography images on the right (medial to the left) correspond to the levels shown by the white lines on the sagittal plane image on the left, which is reformatted from the original series. A medial lobe lesion is present in the deep digital flexor tendon (DDFT) in the pastern *(arrow)*, and biaxial dorsal lesions are present in the DDFT in the heel region, characterized by hypodense foci *(arrows)* and navicular bursa effusion laterally *(*)*.

foot pain. The addition of regional contrast medium improves the ability of CT to detect some of the commonly reported soft tissue injuries that occur deep within the hoof capsule. Lesions of the deep digital flexor tendon (DDFT) (Figure 20-6), and collateral ligaments of the distal interphalangeal joint, navicular bursa, collateral sesamoidean ligaments, and distal sesamoidean impar ligament are identified with similar frequency as those identified using magnetic resonance imaging (MRI).[6,7] Only a few equine studies exist that directly compare CT with MRI in horses with foot pain.[8,9] Recent studies show that contrast-enhanced CT compares favorably with MRI and pathology for the identification of DDFT lesions within the hoof capsule.[10,11]

CT is useful to identify conditions of bones and soft tissues, and its use is limited only by the physical configuration of the gantry and the size of horses. Most 70-cm gantry scanners are able to image up to the level of the distal diaphysis of the radius and tibia. CT is invaluable when routine diagnostic techniques are unable, because of inherent limitations of the technique, to thoroughly investigate an anatomical region. Valuable clinical information is gained from CT evaluation of subchondral bone, particularly the fetlock joint (Figure 20-7), the carpus and tarsus, and the origin of the suspensory ligament in both the forelimbs and hindlimbs (see Figure 20-2) and for evaluation of intracapsular soft tissue injury in the stifle. Contrast medium given through an intravascular route provides additional information about the underlying physiology of soft tissue structures. Tendon and ligament lesions appear hypodense, heterogeneous, and enlarged on plain CT, similar to other imaging modalities. After the administration of contrast material, soft tissue lesions typically enhance and appear hyperintense, thus helping the viewer to identify and characterize the abnormalities. CT is useful in regions where ultrasonographic evaluation is restricted by regional anatomy, such as the foot, carpal canal, or distal sesamoidean ligament attachments. Contrast medium administered into a synovial structure outlines the structures in contact with the synovial fluid. This has been particularly useful in the evaluation of

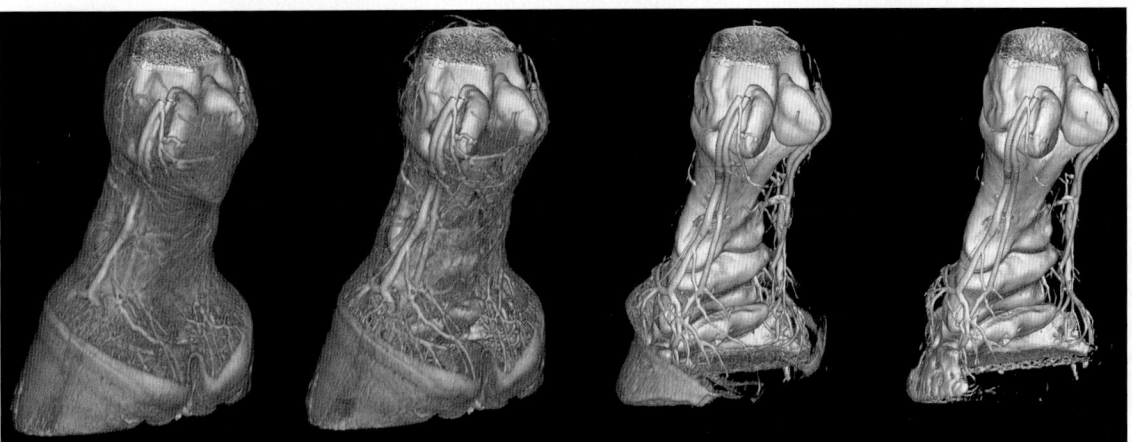

Figure 20-4 • Three-dimensional volume-rendered images of a computed tomography angiogram. The operator has progressively increased the threshold from left to right. On the left, most of the soft tissues including the hoof capsule can be identified. Extending to the right, the soft tissues disappear first, followed by the hoof capsule and then the small-caliber laminar blood vessels. On the image on the right, only the larger blood vessels containing contrast media and bone surface are visible. This horse has erosion of the flexor cortex of the navicular bone.

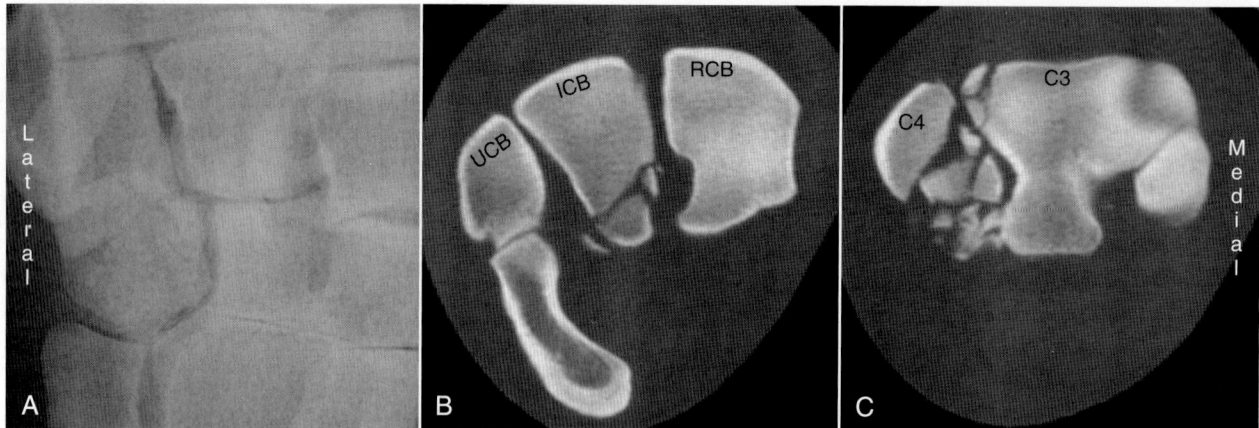

Figure 20-5 • Three images from a horse that sustained carpal fractures. **A** is a dorsal 15-degree lateral-palmarome-dial oblique radiographic image cropped to show fractures with mild displacement in the fourth carpal bone. **B** is a transverse computed tomography image at the level of the proximal row of carpal bones showing palmar, commi-nuted fractures of the intermediate carpal bone (ICB). **C** is obtained through the distal row of carpal bones. Marked fragmentation of the fourth carpal bone (C4) and a fracture of the lateral and dorsal aspects of the third carpal bone (C3) are present.

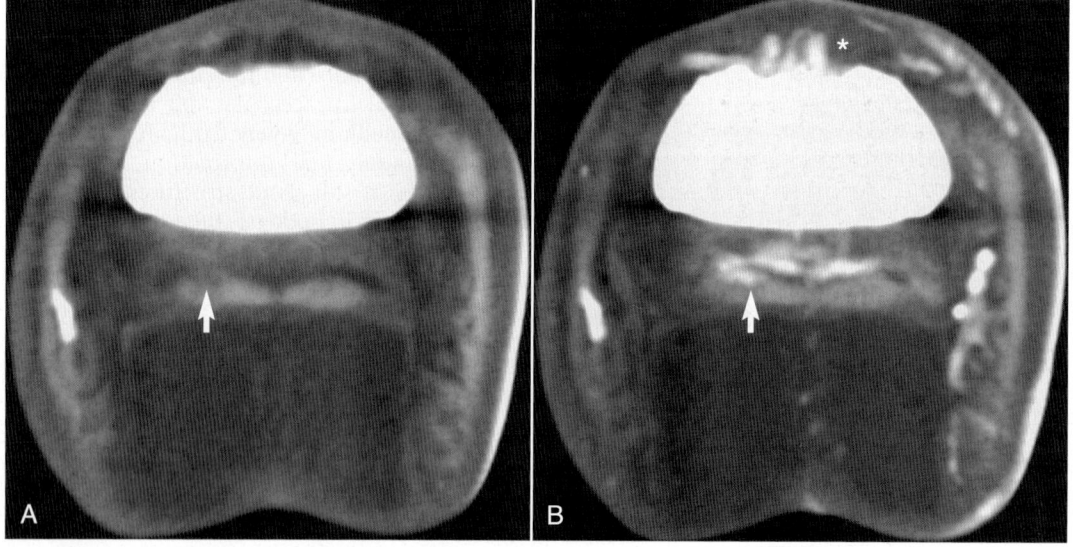

Figure 20-6 • Transverse computed tomography (CT) images obtained at the level of the middle phalanx. **A** is a precontrast CT image, and **B** is an image obtained during an intraarterial infusion of contrast medium. A lesion *(arrows)* is present in one lobe of the deep digital flexor tendon. It is heterogeneous and hypodense on precontrast images *(arrow)* but has new vessel formation resulting in contrast enhancement of the lesion after contrast medium has been administered *(arrow).* There is also irregular enhancement of the synovium of the dorsal aspect of the distal interphalangeal joint *(*).*

intraarticular soft tissue structures such as the cruciate and meniscal ligaments and the menisci of the equine stifle.[12] Arthrography also permits an indirect evaluation of the overlying articular cartilage. This can be effective in locations inaccessible to direct observation using arthroscopy.

Laminitis Evaluation
The role of CT in evaluating horses with laminitis has yet to be defined. The addition of intravascular contrast medium provides an unobstructed view of regional vasculature (see Figure 20-4). High bone detail provides an excellent way to evaluate the distal phalanx and its response to laminitis. Furthermore, quantitative techniques using dynamic contrast-enhanced CT for the measurement of

blood flow have been developed and may play a role in evaluating horses with laminitis and in research studies.[13]

Interventional Computed Tomography
CT is able to accurately image metallic structures and can therefore be used to guide procedures. Most commonly this technique is used to guide the needle placement for tissue or fluid sampling or in therapeutics, such as for the delivery of medication. Intralesional medication can be accurately delivered to those structures inaccessible to ultrasonographic guidance such as the DDFT within the hoof capsule. CT is used to guide surgical procedures such as debridement of the distal phalanx, partial hoof wall resection, and subcapsular mass removal from the hoof.

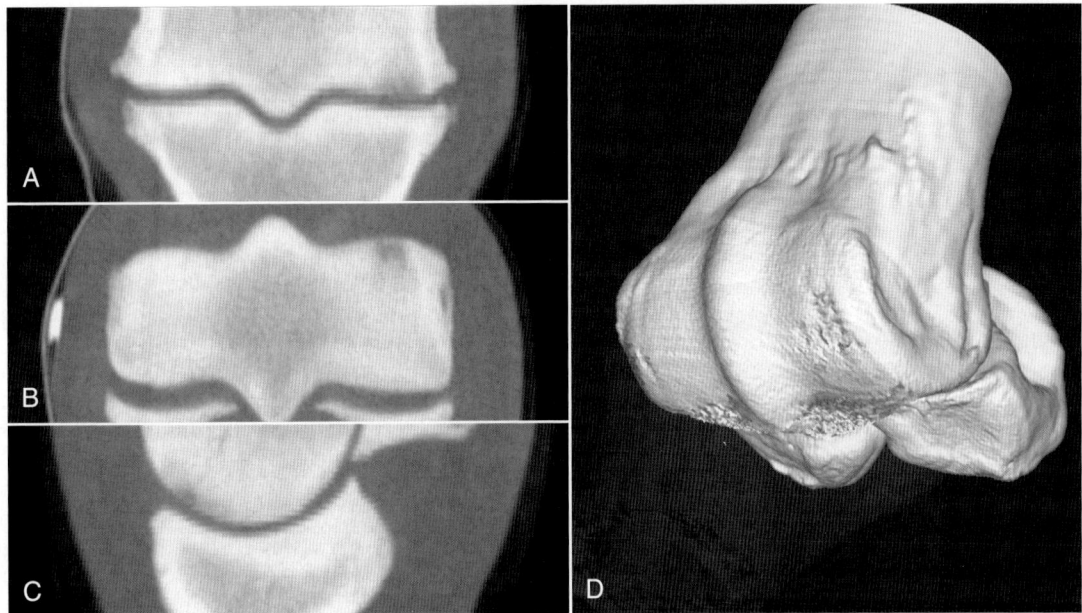

Figure 20-7 • Computed tomography images from a horse with subchondral bone injury of the distal aspect of the third metacarpal bone and periarticular osteophyte formation of the metacarpophalangeal joint. **A** is in a dorsal plane, **B** is in a transverse plane, and **C** is in a sagittal plane. **D** is a three-dimensional reconstruction with the opacity of the proximal phalanx reduced to show the articular surface of the distal aspect of the third metacarpal bone (McIII). In **A**, **B,** and **C,** note the hypodense areas in the subchondral bone of the dorsal aspect of the medial condyle of the McIII.

ADVANTAGES AND DISADVANTAGES

Advantages

CT scanning is more rapid than high- and low-field MRI. This has several benefits. General anesthesia time is minimized, and imaging sequences can be performed during a breath hold to prevent image degradation by respiratory motion. Rapid scanning allows for the concurrent administration of contrast medium. Contrast medium allows the clinician to evaluate the soft tissues and underlying pathophysiology. The contrast-enhancing pattern of tendons and ligament lesions changes over time, and it is possible that this characteristic can be exploited to monitor lesion progression or regression. The ability to characterize bone morphology using CT far exceeds that achieved using planar modalities such as radiography and nuclear scintigraphy. Metal can be imaged using CT, so interventional procedures can be guided, thereby extending CT from a

diagnostic to a therapeutic technique. Lastly, CT scanners are more affordable than high-field MRI scanners, yet provide high-quality images.

Disadvantages

CT does not provide information regarding bone activity or bone fluid accumulation, unlike nuclear scintigraphy and fluid-sensitive MRI sequences (STIR). This information can be inferred by evaluation of the imaging characteristics such as irregular bone margination that likely represents a higher level of activity. CT images of soft tissue structures have less image contrast when compared with high-field MRI, making small lesions of tendons and ligaments more difficult to identify. CT does require special facilities and trained personnel, and although the availability of CT is increasing, it still is available only in referral and university hospitals.

Magnetic Resonance Imaging

Rachel C. Murray and Sue J. Dyson

Magnetic resonance imaging (MRI) is a method of imaging that can allow examination of both osseous and soft tissues

with detailed anatomical resolution and also provides some physiological information. Advances in technology during the past 10 years have made it possible for MRI to become a practical diagnostic tool in both anesthetized and standing horses (Figures 21-1 and 21-2).[1] Use of MRI has revolutionized our understanding of foot pain in the horse and has considerably improved understanding of other types of lameness further proximally in the limb.[2-5] As a result, MRI is increasingly being used for diagnosis of orthopedic disorders in equine practice and can add considerable information to a diagnostic investigation. However, as with any imaging technique, MRI is only useful in the context of the entire clinical picture and

References on page 1263

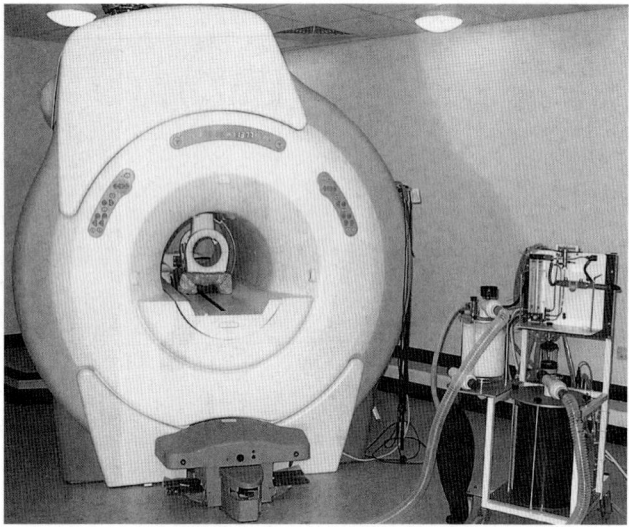

Fig. 21-1 • The 1.5-T GE Echospeed (General Electric Medical Systems, Milwaukee, Wisconsin, United States) magnet at the Animal Health Trust (Newmarket, United Kingdom) is used for MRI of horses under general anesthesia. Located in the bore of the magnet is a radiofrequency coil suitable for use on the equine distal limb. Both limbs are placed into the magnet bore. A specially shaped pad allows the coil to be placed only over the limb being imaged and in the center of the magnet.

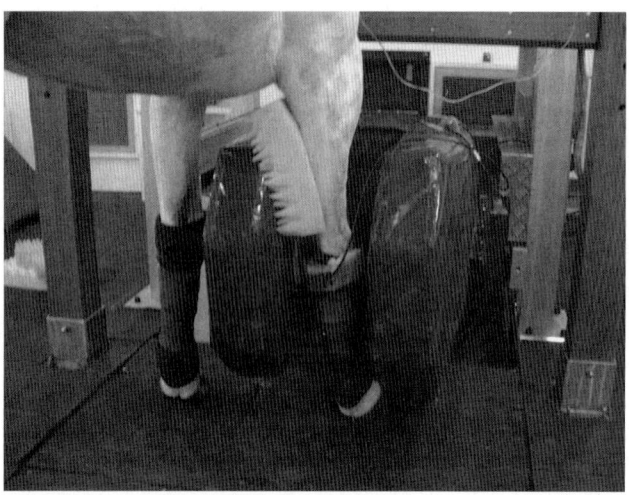

Fig. 21-2 • The Hallmarq (Hallmarq Veterinary Imaging, Guildford, United Kingdom) 0.29-T MR system at the Animal Health Trust (Newmarket, United Kingdom) is used for MRI of horses under standing sedation. This horse is undergoing MRI of the carpus.

needs to be interpreted in light of other diagnostic findings. Terminology is sometimes confused: magnetic resonance (MR) refers to the absorption of energy exhibited by particles (as atomic nuclei or electrons) in a static magnetic field when the particles are exposed to electromagnetic radiation of certain frequencies. MRI refers to a noninvasive diagnostic technique that produces computerized images of internal body tissues and is based on nuclear magnetic resonance of atoms within the body induced by the application of radio waves.

PRODUCTION OF MAGNETIC RESONANCE IMAGES

MR images are produced through interactions between a strong magnet, a radiofrequency (RF) coil, magnetic field gradients, and powerful computing facilities. MR images are based on the spinning motion of MR active nuclei (nuclei with an odd number of protons). Hydrogen nuclei are used in clinical MRI because they are abundant in the body and are particularly mobile in fat and water. When a horse (or body part) is put into the magnet, the MR active nuclei align parallel or antiparallel to the static magnetic field. To produce an image, an RF wave at a specific frequency (dependent on the magnet field strength and the MR active nuclei selected) is applied at 90 degrees to the static magnetic field, B_0. This gives energy to the hydrogen nuclei, which then spin faster and alter the net magnetization vector away from the static magnetic field. When the RF wave terminates, energy is lost from the excited hydrogen nuclei, either to the surrounding environment (spin-lattice or T1 relaxation) or to adjacent nuclei (spin-spin or T2 relaxation), and the net magnetization vector returns to zero. This energy loss is detected by the receiver as MR signal. The signal is then converted to a digital image using complex computer software. Each pixel within the matrix has a particular signal intensity, and the accumulated pixels make up the final image.

Magnets may be considered high-, mid-, and low-field strength, with field strength measured in Tesla. Magnetic field homogeneity is important in production of good quality images. RF coils are made to surround the region of interest with as little space between the coil and the area of interest as possible to maximize signal detection. They may be both a transmitter (transmits the RF waves) and receiver (detects the MR signal produced). The magnetic field gradients are used to place the MR signal in space. This is achieved by generating short-term spatial variation in magnetic field strength across the horse (or body part). There are three sets of gradient coils, each oriented in a different direction. Repeated application of large electrical current pulses results in the gradient coils making a loud noise during scan acquisition, especially at higher field strengths.

A pulse sequence includes a defined series of RF waves, gradient maneuvers, and signal detection. The repetition time (TR) defines the time between repetitions, and the echo time (TE) defines the time between the RF pulse and detection of the echo (MR signal). Selection of pulse sequence determines the image contrast and appearance of particular tissues.

Images are produced in a gray scale with the contrast defined by the particular pulse sequence used for image acquisition, the imaging parameters, and the properties of the tissue being imaged. Information is acquired as tomographic slices, so the orientation and thickness of slices (or three-dimensional [3D] volume datasets) can be varied and defined.

Generally a pilot scan with wide slice thickness is performed in three planes, and further image sequences are oriented and positioned relative to the pilot scan. It is normal practice to acquire images in three planes: sagittal, dorsal (coronal), and transverse (axial).

A complete MRI scan of a horse usually includes a series of different pulse sequences, the choice of which is determined by the operator. The tissues being examined, the suspected pathology, and the type of MRI system influence the selection of pulse sequences. For horses, the choice of sequence is also influenced greatly by time constraints to minimize risk of movement in a standing horse and limit time under general anesthesia.

Various manipulations during image acquisition can be used to look at particular features of tissues, such as fat suppression techniques to identify pathology in medullary bone. Intravenous administration of gadolinium contrast medium can be used to demonstrate blood flow, perfusion of a suspect area, or to investigate damage to the blood–brain barrier. Postprocessing manipulations can be used to reorient images acquired in an oblique orientation; to measure size, area, or volume; for motion correction; or to further understand signal intensity patterns.

EQUIPMENT FOR MRI IN HORSES

MRI can be performed in horses using various different types of systems. High-field closed systems are similar to those used in many human hospitals. These units have a superconducting, helium-cooled magnet in a cylindrical configuration into which the area of interest of the horse has to be squeezed; thus the horse needs to be under general anesthesia, and a team of operators is required to position the horse (see Figure 21-1). There are low-field open MRI systems that also require horses to be imaged under general anesthesia but have fewer restrictions on space; therefore it may be easier to position the horse into the imaging portion of the magnet. A low-field MR system for the standing horse has been developed specifically for the equine market, which has allowed images to be acquired with horses under sedation (see Figure 21-2). Use of motion-insensitive imaging sequences helps to account for slight sway that may occur during sedation. Time for image acquisition is generally longer in low-field units for the same or less resolution and image quality as a high-field system; thus horses may require sedation or general anesthesia for more prolonged periods to acquire images of the entire region required.

For the MRI systems available, in general the areas that can be imaged in the adult horse are limited to the head and cranial aspect of the neck, the forelimb up to and including the carpus, and the hindlimb up to and including the tarsus, although images of the stifle can also be obtained in a few systems in horses of suitable size and conformation.[6] In a foal, it may be possible to place the entire body into the magnet in a high-field closed or low-field open system.

ADVANTAGES AND DISADVANTAGES COMPARED WITH OTHER IMAGING TECHNIQUES

Advantages

MRI is more versatile than most other imaging modalities because of its ability to provide images sliced in many planes and 3D images in a variety of orientations. Like ultrasonography and radiography, MRI has the ability to provide anatomical information, but MRI also has a physiological sensitivity like that of nuclear scintigraphy.

MRI is the only method presently available that can assess all tissues during a single examination. Ultrasonography is extremely useful for imaging soft tissues but is impractical in a number of areas and cannot be used to assess the internal structure in bones. MR technology allows imaging of those soft tissue structures that are inaccessible with ultrasonography. Radiography shows mineralized tissues but is less sensitive than MRI because each image is obtained through the full thickness of the area, and only the orientation selected can be assessed; therefore small abnormalities may be missed. In contrast, MR images can be obtained in multiple planes without loss of image quality, and data can be assessed in slices so that the image is not limited to a summation through the entire structure. MRI has been shown to be more sensitive to pathological conditions of bone and tendons than radiography and ultrasonography, respectively.

Like MRI, computed tomography (CT) can be used in horses for accurate assessment of the 3D distribution of pathological conditions of the bone, particularly in relation to fracture configurations. Some soft tissue detail is also demonstrated with CT but generally with inferior contrast. In contrast to CT, articular cartilage can generally be assessed using MRI without use of invasive arthrography, and bone pathology without fracture may also be better evaluated with MRI. Arthroscopy is the standard of reference for the evaluation of articular cartilage, but it cannot assess deep chondral lesions and lesions of the subchondral bone.

Disadvantages

Initially the greatest disadvantages of MRI were the expense of the equipment and the requirement for general anesthesia. However, as advances in technology have reduced the costs and made it possible to obtain images in a standing horse, these problems have increasingly been resolved. Unfortunately, MRI remains limited to areas that can be placed within the magnetic field; thus the caudal aspect of the neck, the trunk, and the proximal aspects of limbs of adult horses cannot yet be imaged, but it is possible that with advances in technology, these problems may also be overcome. Until recently, unlike CT, MRI could not be used for image-guided injections because ferrous metal cannot be used within the magnet; however, MR-compatible needles have now become available.

INTERPRETATION OF MAGNETIC RESONANCE IMAGES

An understanding of MRI, a detailed knowledge of anatomy, and considerable experience are required to interpret MR images reliably. The wide range of normal anatomy within the horse population means that experience in reading equine images and use of concurrent clinical diagnostic evaluation are crucial for determining the clinical significance of a potential lesion. Lesions that may be detectable using MRI but are difficult to detect with other imaging modalities include ligament and tendon injuries (within the hoof capsule), occult fractures, articular cartilage damage, bone trauma and necrosis, osseous cystlike lesions, subchondral bone modeling, and space-occupying lesions.[7] Interpretation is improved by assessing T2-weighted, T1-weighted and/or proton density, and fat-suppressed images at each site.

Image contrast is determined by tissue proton density, T1 and T2 relaxation, and by pulse sequence and imaging parameters, which also determine the T1 and T2 weighting of the image. Clinical MRI uses hydrogen nuclei as the MR active nuclei that create the signal; thus the appearance of a tissue on MRI is determined by the density and mobility of the hydrogen nuclei it contains and their relaxation properties after excitation (when the signal is created). Images of tissues can be weighted to show proton density and T1 and T2 relaxation properties of the tissues. Tissues where the hydrogen nuclei are tightly bound have low signal intensity (black) on proton density, T1-, and T2-weighted images; for example, cortical bone or tendon. In contrast, water and fat contain highly mobile hydrogen nuclei and can produce considerable signal. However, water has high signal intensity (white) on T2-weighted images but low signal intensity (black) on T1-weighted images. Therefore each tissue has a characteristic signal intensity pattern on MR images, so with experience, normal tissues can be clearly identified (Figures 21-3 and 21-4).

The MR properties of a tissue are altered by damage, and the stage of damage and healing may be determined by differences in signal intensity patterns and the shape and size of different structures. This makes it possible to use MR images to evaluate tissue normality and the type, severity, and stage of injury in tissue damage.

Pathological processes are frequently associated with increase in free water within and around the affected tissues, which can be easily detected with MRI. These changes generally lead to an increase in signal intensity on T2-weighted images and a decrease in signal intensity on T1-weighted images. These changes may be most easily seen on T2-weighted images. However, the combined information from T2-, T1-weighted, and fat-suppressed images is most useful for interpretation. T1-weighted

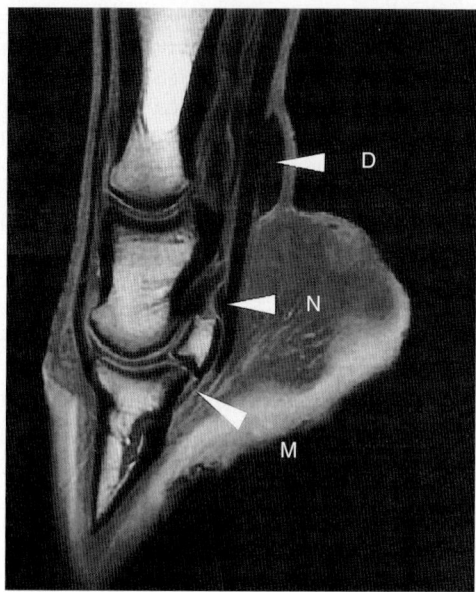

Fig. 21-3 • Sagittal magnetic resonance image of the distal aspect of a limb using a T1-weighted spoiled gradient echo sequence. The high signal intensity in the medullary cavity of the phalanges and navicular bone is caused by fat. No signal appears in the deep digital flexor tendon, straight sesamoidean ligament, and cortical bone. Higher signal intensity in the most distal portion of the deep digital flexor tendon is probably a magic angle effect (*M*). Synovial fluid is dark (low signal intensity) in the navicular bursa (*N*), distended digital flexor tendon sheath (*D*), and proximal and distal interphalangeal joints, but cartilage has a relatively higher signal intensity.

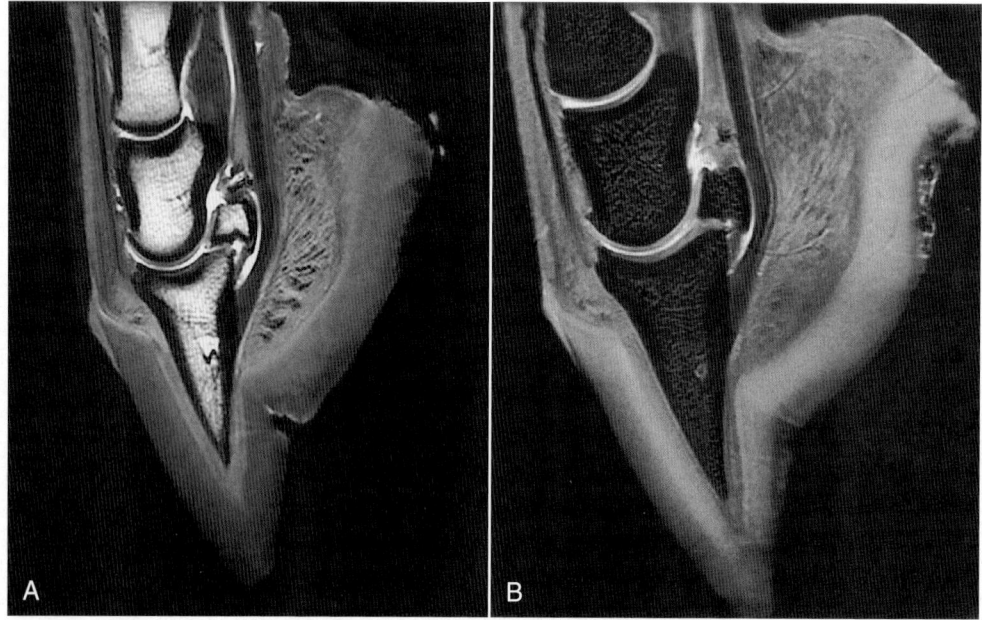

Fig. 21-4 • Sagittal magnetic resonance images of the distal aspect of a limb using a T2* gradient echo sequence. **A,** 3D T2* gradient echo image shows a relatively high signal intensity associated with medullary fat of the phalanges and navicular bone, but on this sequence fluid has high signal intensity (compare with Figure 21-3). Synovial fluid in the navicular bursa and joints has high signal intensity, but cartilage has relatively low signal intensity. **B,** Fat-saturated, 3D T2* gradient echo shows the absence of fat signal in the medullary bone and improved contrast between articular cartilage and surrounding structures.

images are often best for evaluation of tissue contours and anatomy, and fat-suppressed techniques are required for evaluation of bone medullary tissues.

In general, fluid (and edema) is hypointense on T1-weighted and hyperintense on T2-weighted images, but increased protein content in fluid also leads to increased signal intensity on T1-weighted images. On T2-weighted images, presence of blood results in a relative decrease in signal intensity compared with edema. Immature granulation tissue has high signal intensity on T2-weighted images, whereas mature fibrotic tissue has a low intensity on T2-weighted images.

Bone

Although cortical bone has low signal intensity, MRI is extremely useful for detecting bone pathology. Alterations in periosteal or endosteal surface contour may indicate bone disruption, osteophytes, or enthesophyte formation (Figure 21-5). Appearance of adjacent tissues should also be evaluated (Figure 21-6). Trabecular architecture can be seen using MRI, and alterations can be monitored. Bone pathology is frequently detected as an increase in signal intensity in T2-weighted and fat-suppressed images and a decrease in signal intensity in T1-weighted images and may represent bone necrosis, inflammation, trabecular microdamage, hemorrhage, fibrosis, and bone edema (Figure 21-7). Very small focal lesions in the cortical or subchondral bone may be associated with large areas of signal abnormality in the local cancellous bone. Residual changes on MR images may be present for months after clinical recovery. Bone abnormality may also be reflected by increased bone density (mineralization, sclerosis), seen as low signal intensity on both T1- and T2-weighted images.

Tendon

Like cortical bone, tendons and ligaments generally have low signal intensity on both T1- and T2-weighted images, thus appearing nearly black except where muscle tissue is present. Increased signal intensity indicates tendon or ligament damage. In acute stages, with inflammatory change, or tissue necrosis, damage is detected as swelling and increased signal intensity on T1- and T2-weighted images (Figure 21-8). At later stages of healing and fibrosis, the lower inflammatory fluid component results in lower signal

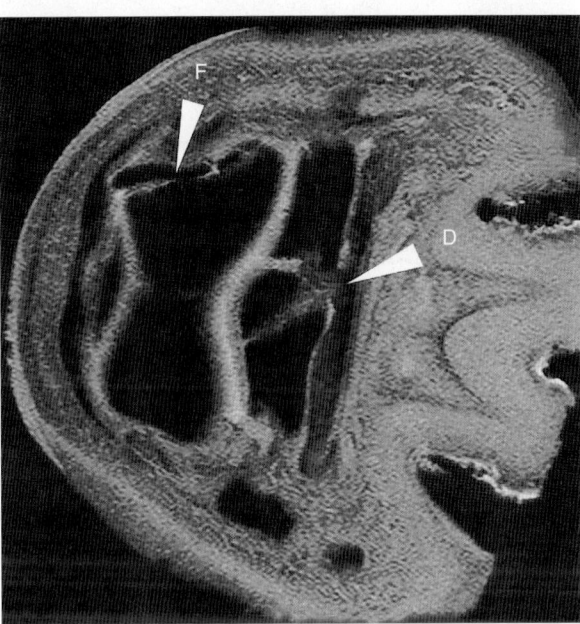

Fig. 21-6 • A transverse 3D T2* gradient echo magnetic resonance image of the distal aspect of a limb showing a comminuted fracture of the navicular bone and fracture of the middle phalanx that had been detected radiologically *(F)* and laceration of the medial branch of the deep digital flexor tendon *(D)*, which is interposed between the fracture fragments of the navicular bone.

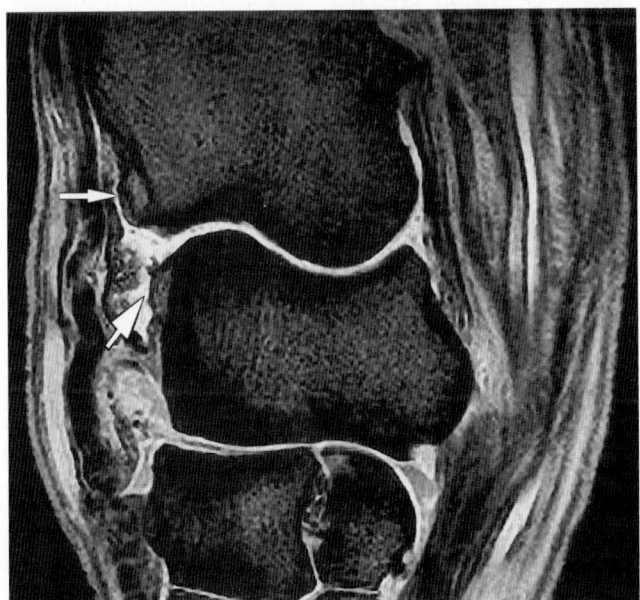

Fig. 21-5 • A sagittal T2* gradient echo magnetic resonance image of a carpus demonstrating osteophyte formation on the distal aspect of the radius and the proximal aspect of the radial carpal bone in the antebrachiocarpal joint *(arrows)*. There is synovial effusion of the antebrachiocarpal and middle carpal joints with synovial proliferation on the dorsal aspect of the antebrachiocarpal joint.

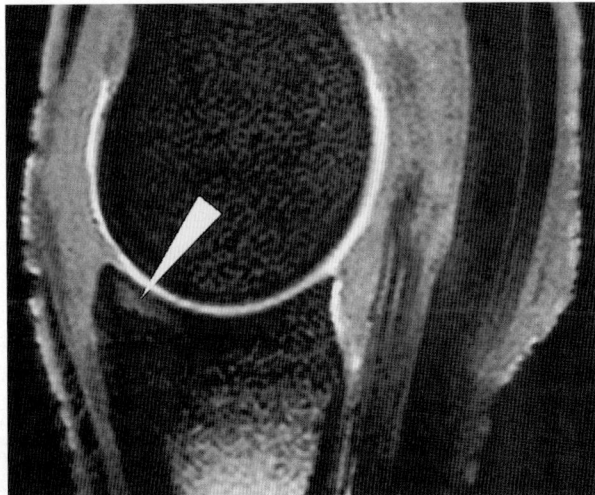

Fig. 21-7 • Sagittal fat-saturated, T2* gradient echo magnetic resonance image of a metacarpophalangeal joint showing an area of high signal intensity in the subchondral bone of the proximal phalanx *(arrow)*, representing a pathological condition of the bone. Histopathological examination revealed subchondral bone edema, inflammation, and trabecular microdamage.

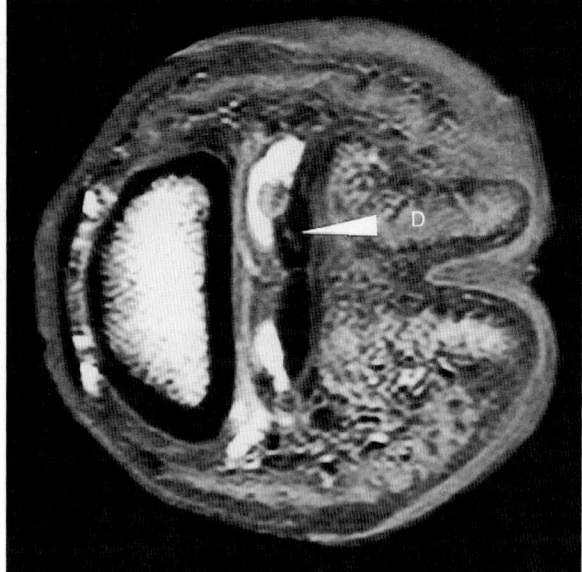

Fig. 21-8 • A transverse 3D T2* gradient echo magnetic resonance image of the distal limb of a horse with lameness that was alleviated by intrathecal analgesia of the navicular bursa. There is an area of increased signal intensity within the medial branch of the deep digital flexor tendon *(D)*, with adjacent granulation tissue protruding into the navicular bursa.

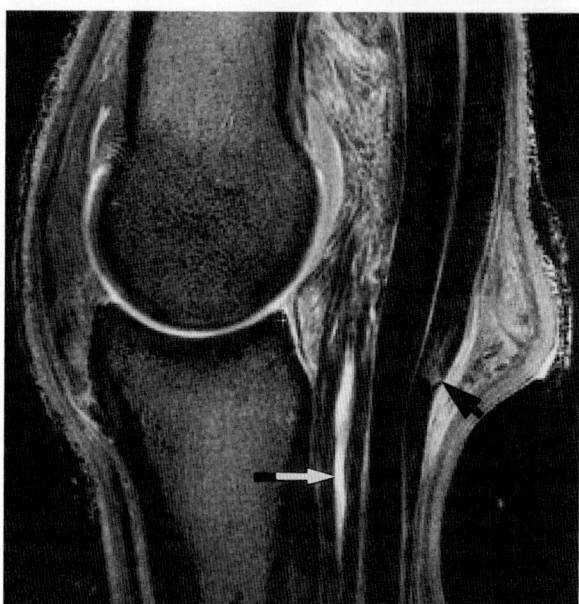

Fig. 21-9 • A sagittal T2* gradient echo magnetic resonance image of the fetlock of a horse with lameness that was alleviated by intraarticular analgesia of the metacarpophalangeal joint. There is a linear area of high signal intensity in the straight sesamoidean ligament *(white arrow)*. Increased signal intensity within the superficial digital flexor tendon *(black arrow)* corresponds to an area of cartilage metaplasia.

intensity on T2-weighted images, but signal intensity on T1-weighted images remains higher than that of normal tendon. Changes to the peritendonous tissues should also be considered.

Ligament

Mild ligament damage can be detected by the presence of periligamentar signal alteration (increased on T2-weighted images), intraligamentar increase in signal intensity (either focal or diffuse), and ligament enlargement (Figure 21-9). Tears can be represented by thinning or discontinuity. There may be evidence of damage at the ligament origin or insertion. Damage to the bone at the origin or insertion of the ligament may be seen as increased signal intensity on fat-suppressed or T2-weighted images and with decreased signal intensity on T1-weighted images. Enthesophyte formation, endosteal reaction, or osseous cystlike lesions at the origin or insertion of a ligament may also reflect ligament abnormality.

Articular Cartilage

Cartilage damage can be seen directly using MR images as changes in signal intensity and/or alterations in contour. Use of fat-suppressed images not only improves contrast in the cartilage itself but also highlights subtle areas of increased signal intensity in the subchondral bone, which may draw attention to a defect in the overlying articular surface. Likewise, focal alteration in the endosteal contour of the subchondral bone in T1- and T2-weighted images may also highlight a region of cartilage pathology.

Synovial Fluid, Synovium, and Joint Capsule

Displacement of the capsular margin represents synovial distention, and damage to the capsular tissues may be seen as thickening or discontinuity of the margin. Using

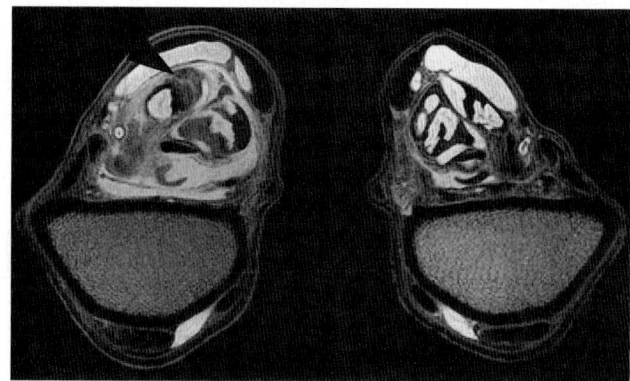

Fig. 21-10 • Transverse T2* gradient echo magnetic resonance images at the level of the musculotendonous junction of the superficial digital flexor tendon of the left *(shown on the left)* and right forelimbs. There is enlargement of the left superficial digital flexor tendon and its accessory ligament. Normal muscle tissue *(areas of high signal intensity)* is replaced by an area of low signal intensity consistent with scar tissue *(arrow)*.

MRI, it is possible to differentiate acute from chronic synovial hyperplasia and to determine the chronicity in hemarthrosis.

Muscles

Muscular inflammation appears as increased signal intensity on T2-weighted images, whereas lower signal intensity on T2-weighted images may represent fibrosis (Figure 21-10).

ARTIFACTS

As with any imaging technique, MRI is prone to artifacts that may confuse the interpreter. Ghosting (repeated picturing of a structure throughout the image) originates from movement during the acquisition of data. This can cause problems in anesthetized horses because respiratory chest movement causes large displacements of the upper forelimb during imaging. Ghosting can also occur if there is sway in a standing horse. Motion can be minimized in an anesthetized horse by weighting the limb with sand bags or reducing respiratory excursion by avoiding mechanical ventilation. In a standing horse, use of motion correction techniques has made it possible to obtain good quality images of the distal aspect of the limb even in the presence of some degree of sway. However, to minimize movement, the level and type of sedation are important, and padding or stabilizing the limb may be helpful, as well as supporting the horse's head. Acquisition of high-quality images of the carpal and tarsal regions in a standing horse presents more of a challenge because sway is magnified compared with the relatively static foot.

Anything that disturbs the homogeneity of the magnetic field can severely distort the image, resulting in a magnetic susceptibility artifact. These artifacts are more prominent in gradient echo sequences and are particularly induced by the presence of metal. Therefore shoes and residual nails must be removed from feet, and dirt must be cleaned from the sulci of the frog. Chemical shift artifact occurs when fat and water that are adjacent in the horse are shown farther apart on the image. If part of the horse is just outside the field of view but produces a signal detectable by the receiver coil, this may be shown incorrectly within the field of view, known as aliasing. The Gibbs effect (truncation artifact) results from undersampling of data and occurs when bright or dark lines appear parallel and adjacent to borders of abrupt intensity change. For example, a line of low signal intensity is incorrectly shown running through a high signal intensity area.

Partial volume effects result when structures passing obliquely through the slice of tissue are imaged; these are important when either the shape or signal intensity of tissues is assessed. Reducing the slice thickness and improving resolution minimize this effect.

The magic angle effect appears when collagen fibers are located at an angle of approximately 55 degrees to the static magnetic field. This is most important in ligaments and tendons, although it has been reported to occur in cartilage and results in an artifactual increase in signal intensity, which may mimic injury. Structures that are most likely to be affected depend on the direction of the magnetic field. In high-field–strength magnets where the magnetic field is parallel to the long axis of the limb, the magic angle effect is most likely at the insertion of the deep digital flexor tendon. However, in low-field–strength magnets with the magnetic field perpendicular to the long axis of the limb, there is more likelihood of a magic angle effect in the collateral ligaments of the distal interphalangeal joint and the oblique distal sesamoidean ligaments.[8,9] The magic angle effect is less evident on T2-weighted compared with T1-weighted images. Increasing the TE as in fast spin-echo sequences reduces the magic angle effect.

INDICATIONS FOR MRI IN EQUINE LAMENESS

MRI is most useful when pain causing lameness has been localized to a region of the limb but where a definitive diagnosis has not been made with other diagnostic imaging techniques. If abnormalities have been identified, these may be insufficient to explain the degree of lameness or a more accurate prognosis may be required; thus MRI may be justified. In a horse with foot pain with a suspected penetrating injury MRI may be chosen instead of radiography.

MRI can be invaluable for diagnosis and monitoring of orthopedic conditions in the equine limb. However, it is important that an interpreter is aware of the limitations of MRI to avoid overinterpretation or misinterpretation of signal intensity changes observed on MR images. Therefore findings should be interpreted in light of clinical findings and other diagnostic information.

| *Chapter* 22

Gait Analysis for the Quantification of Lameness

Kevin G. Keegan

Evaluation of lameness in horses is a skill first learned by training and then sharpened with experience over time. The standard of practice is an initial subjective evaluation of the horse while moving to detect and then localize the source of pain causing lameness to the affected limb or limbs. It is a difficult endeavor in horses with mild lameness, when only subtle changes in movement from normal are present. There is substantial disagreement, even between experienced clinicians, in the identification and localization of the lame limb(s) in horses with mild lameness.[1-3] There is also disagreement between experts in the amount of improvement in lameness after nerve blocks,[4] and equine veterinarians, because they are human, have been shown to be biased. The amount of disagreement between veterinarians on the results of subjective evaluation of lameness in horses is what would be expected for any difficult diagnostic test.

A contributing source of disagreement is the limited sensitivity of the human eye, which has an estimated time resolution of about 10 to 15 samples per second.[5,6] Events in stride of a horse trotting at 4 meters per second, which is about 1.5 strides per second, occur at a frequency of twice the stride rate, or about 3 times per second.[7] To prevent significant errors in detection of signal amplitude, the sampling frequency should be, at a minimum, 5 times the frequency of the event being detected.[8] Therefore the

References on page 1264

natural capability of the human eye is below or just at the minimum required to detect important asymmetry in motion events used to judge lameness in horses. All the objective methods of lameness evaluation discussed in this chapter sample data at frequencies higher than that of the naked eye, and thus are theoretically capable of higher accuracy. An objective, precise, and accurate method of lameness detection and quantification in horses is certainly justifiable.

The purpose of this chapter is to introduce and summarize the gait analysis methodology currently being studied or used. Emphasis is given to those that could be used by private practitioners. To be effective, any such system has to be easy to use, and data collection and analysis must be quick. It must be affordable and capable of providing the veterinarian with adequate return on investment. It may be most useful to veterinarians as an aid in detecting and evaluating horses with subtle lameness and lameness in several limbs. Natural stride-to-stride variability must be overcome, so that small differences in subtle lameness can be detected. For example, to detect subtle differences after diagnostic analgesia or after treatment, any such system must be capable of collecting data from multiple contiguous strides. Lameness over ground may be different from lameness on a treadmill; therefore any system must be capable of collecting data when the horse is moving over ground. Also, ideally, any system should be capable of detecting and evaluating lameness in all limbs simultaneously.

There are two general approaches to using gait analysis to detect and measure lameness in horses: kinetics and kinematics. A kinetic technique measures ground reaction forces. A kinematic technique measures motion of the body. There are advantages and disadvantages for each general approach.

KINETICS

Kinetics can rightly be considered a more direct method (compared with kinematics) for detecting and measuring lameness in horses. If a horse has pain during the weight-bearing portion of the stride because of lameness, it bears less weight on that limb, resulting in lower peak vertical ground reaction forces (GRFs) on that limb. Certain lameness conditions may decrease horizontal or transverse GRFs, but the effect on the vertical GRFs is usually most prominent.

Kinetic methods to measure GRFs include a stationary force plate, pressure-measuring pads, instrumented horse shoes, and force-measuring treadmills. A stationary force plate is the most commonly used and cited method, but each method is briefly discussed. A stationary force plate, because of its widespread use in lameness research centers around the world, is discussed in more detail.

Pressure-measuring pads are force or pressure distribution measurement systems consisting of force sensor elements installed between matting surfaces. A horse is led over the pressure-sensitive pad to collect data from single or, if the pad is long enough, a few consecutive strides. Pressure-sensitive pads can be cut and customized to fit the bottom of a horse's foot then placed between the bottom of the foot and a shoe in an attempt to collect data from multiple contiguous strides.[9,10] This technology is ideal for mapping the force or pressure profile of a surface, but peak force or pressure can also be quantified. With further development and marketing this technology may become useful for routine evaluation of shoeing techniques designed to alter force distribution within the foot. Currently there are only a few equine practices in the United States using this technology clinically to evaluate lame horses.

Instrumented horse shoes are custom-built systems designed to either directly, with force transducers, or indirectly, with strain gauges, measure vertical GRFs to the hoof during weight bearing.[11-14] Their main advantage is the ability to collect data from multiple contiguous strides in an overground, field-like setting. The main difficulties and disadvantages of instrumented horse shoes include the complexity, size, and weight of the instrumentation, which affect normal hoof and limb movement and gait. Although there are several recent reports of force-measuring horse shoes used successfully in research investigations, currently there are no commercially available systems for a practicing veterinarian to use. Strain gauges glued to the hoof wall, with the resulting strain to the hoof during weight bearing estimating GRF, can act as a surrogate for an instrumented horse shoe. Disadvantages of any hoof-mounted system for measuring GRFs to detect lameness include the need to instrument all four feet simultaneously and, more importantly, the extreme dependence of results on surface characteristics. Because of these disadvantages and the technical and design expertise required for development, it is unlikely that such a device will quickly become adopted for use during routine lameness evaluations.

A force-measuring equine treadmill is a unique piece of equipment consisting of piezoelectric load-sensitive sensors in a treadmill platform (Figure 22-1).[15,16] The only working system in regular use is at the University of Zurich in Switzerland. The force-measuring equine treadmill is exceptional for detecting small changes in lameness between treatments because of its ability to collect data from multiple, contiguous strides. It is also exceptional for determining severity and location of compensatory lameness because it is capable of measuring vertical GRFs in all four limbs simultaneously.[17] It is a one-of-a-kind, custom-built, installed piece of equipment, and as such is unlikely to be adopted for use as a lameness diagnostic aid in any but the most sophisticated equine private practices or research centers.

A stationary force plate is the most widely used and available kinetic technique for objective evaluation of lameness in horses.[18,19] Under controlled conditions of constant speed the coefficient of variation of vertical GRF between strides in both lame and sound horses is remarkably low.[20-22] Thus a lesser number of stride repetitions are required to achieve repeatable results, and small differences between treatments can be detected. A stationary force plate is also sensitive to subtle lameness detection, with some studies suggesting that force plate detection of lameness (decreased vertical GRF) is more sensitive than the human eye in subjective evaluation of lameness.[23,24] A stationary force plate, unlike the aforementioned other kinetic techniques, is also capable of measuring horizontal GRFs, which may be helpful in further differentiating type of lameness, that is, acceleratory or deceleratory. There are several force plates worldwide that are used, at least

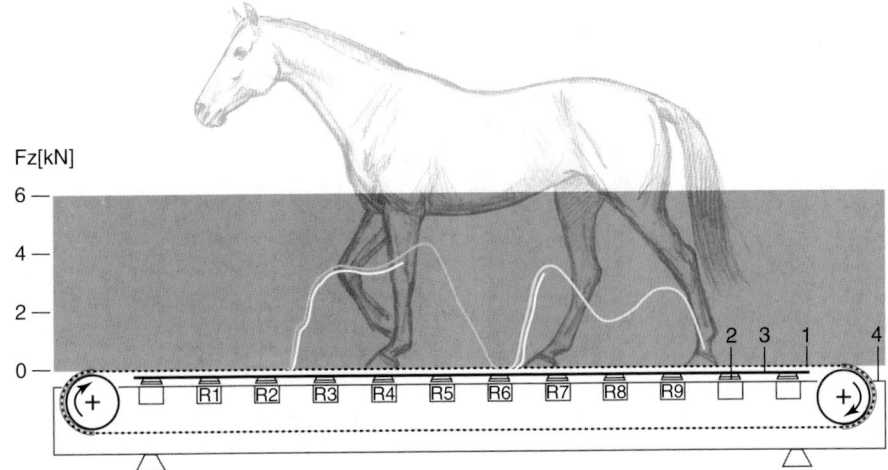

Fig. 22-1 • Treadmill-integrated force-measuring system capable of determining the vertical ground reaction forces and the hoof positions during stance phase of all limbs simultaneously. *Fz*, vertical ground reaction force in kilo-Newtons. *1*, Traction belt; *2*, shock absorber; *3*, treadmill platform; *4*, treadmill frame. *R1* through *R9*, piezoelectric force sensors of the right side of the treadmill. (Drawing courtesy Dr. Michael Weishaupt, University of Zurich, Switzerland.)

occasionally, for evaluation of lame horses. Despite the high accuracy and precision of a stationary force plate, most experts agree that five or six strikes on the force plate are needed for acceptable results.[10,20-22] Because a horse does not always strike the force plate on every attempt, the process is time consuming. Also, the size of commercially available force plates is too small, such that data from only one hoof (occasionally two hooves) are collected at one time. Collection of data from contiguous strides and simultaneous measurement of all four limbs to detect and evaluate compensatory or secondary lameness is not possible. Therefore a stationary force plate has not been readily accepted as a tool for routine, clinical evaluation of lameness.

KINEMATICS

Using kinematics is an indirect method of detecting and quantifying lameness. Pain of lameness causes the horse to bear less weight on the affected limb. The decreased vertical GRF during weight bearing perturbs, in some way, the normal, expected motion of the torso, head, neck, and limbs, usually by increasing asymmetry of movement between the right and left strides. However, motion of the torso, head, neck, and limbs is perturbed by causes other than lameness as well; for example, conscious movement of the head in a curious or anxious horse. Thus in lame horses motion perturbation is more variable than change in GRF. Therefore kinematic techniques must be able to collect numerous (more than is required for a stationary force plate), contiguous strides to attain the sensitivity required to detect and evaluate mild to moderate lameness. However, because most veterinarians observe changes in motion in a horse's gait during their subjective evaluation, kinematic techniques generate results that are generally more intuitive and well understood. Important findings in kinematic studies can be easily applied by a practicing veterinarian in a standard lameness evaluation.

Until only very recently the most commonly used kinematic technique consisted of filming the horse in motion with cameras and then analyzing the collected motion with software on a remote station. The horse is not instrumented except for possibly attaching lightweight reflective markers for easier identification of the body parts of interest. There are many different commercially available, camera-based systems for kinematic evaluation of lameness in horses. These systems use different types of cameras with different capabilities and various, custom-designed software packages with varying capabilities for data analysis. They all depend on unobstructed, line-of-sight light transmission.

I have used camera-based kinematic gait analysis to study and evaluate lameness in horses since the early 1990s and have come to the following conclusions.[1,25-38] Camera-based techniques are reliable, accurate, and sensitive for detecting and evaluating lameness if two conditions are met: (1) multiple, contiguous strides must be collected to overcome the natural stride-by-stride variability, so that small differences can be detected; and (2) the size of the field of view compared with the size of the subject must be controlled and kept as small as possible for constant and precise spatial resolution. These limitations can be relaxed somewhat for lameness in the moderate to severe range but are absolutely vital for detection and evaluation of mild lameness. Essentially these limitations confine the use of this technique for evaluation of lameness to a treadmill. Adequate data can be acquired with the horse moving over ground in front of the camera, but to capture the movement from enough strides with reasonable spatial resolution, multiple passes are required. Because of these limitations it is unlikely that camera-based kinematic gait analysis technique can be used in clinical practice. However, it is a useful investigative tool, and there are many camera-based kinematic studies of lameness from which practical information for an equine practitioner can be extracted.[1,25-80]

The long list of motion parameters that may have some association with lameness posed a problem in early studies attempting to develop objective kinematic techniques. There was always the question of what parameters were best at differentiating a sound from a lame horse? Many investigators used a shotgun approach, measuring many different variables, on small numbers of horses, calculated from a relatively small number of contiguous strides. Under these conditions, moderately severe lameness was necessary to find significant differences between sound and lame horses or between lameness grades. Results were frequently conflicting, with studies using different models of induced lameness finding different motion parameters as the most sensitive for lameness detection and quantification. Most kinematic studies of lameness involve evaluations of horses trotting on a treadmill, where assumptions about torso acceleration and deceleration or the biomechanics of limb impact and push-off are not the same as in the natural overground state. Despite these limitations, there are numerous motion parameters that have been shown to be useful for detecting and quantifying lameness in horses.

In horses with unilateral lameness, fetlock extension and distal interphalangeal joint flexion are less during weight bearing of the lame limb compared with the sound contralateral limb.* This is true for both forelimb and hindlimb lameness. These kinematic measures are considered to be two of the most sensitive indicators of weight-bearing lameness. Fetlock extension during the lame limb stance phase was 8 degrees less than in the nonlame limb stance phase in a sole pressure model of induced grade 1 (of 5) lameness.[76] However, whether 8 degrees of difference in fetlock extension can be detected by the unaided human eye in a horse at a trot is a matter of conjecture. Carpal extension during stance is reduced, but only in horses with moderate to severe lameness.[27,56,76] Proximal limb joints become more flexed during weight bearing of the lame limb, resulting in an overall limb shortening during stance,[47,76] a compensatory mechanism to reduce peak vertical GRF. Because of the competing opposite mechanisms of increased proximal joint flexion and decreased fetlock extension during lame limb stance, overall limb shortening during lame limb stance is probably not a very sensitive indicator of lameness.

In weight-bearing lameness of mild to moderate intensity, stance duration of the lame limb is increased compared with the sound limb.[16,17,25-27,81] This may seem counterintuitive but is an effective method to reduce peak vertical GRF by spreading the entire vertical GRF impulse over a longer time. The difference between lame and sound limbs is small at the trot even when lameness is of moderate intensity.[27,43,82] It is unlikely to be seen by an unaided human eye but can be measured by expanding the time domain with slow motion review of high sampling-rate video. Length of forelimb retraction, or the extent to which the horse will keep the forelimb on the ground between full weight bearing at midstance and end of breakover, has also been reported to change with forelimb lameness.[27,48,76] In a sole pressure-induced lameness model, forelimb retraction was shortened in the lame forelimb at the walk.[27] Sound forelimb retraction has also been reported to be reduced in forelimb lameness.[76] Results reported for the association of forelimb retraction with lameness are not clear enough for forelimb retraction to be considered a sensitive indicator of forelimb lameness.

The length and shape of the limb flight arc during the swing phase of the stride are commonly perceived to be associated with both forelimb and hindlimb lameness. Forelimb protraction, or the extent to which the horse swings the limb forward before impact, has been reported to increase or decrease with lameness, depending on the location of pain within the limb.[27,57,76] Heel pressure-induced forelimb lameness, similar to navicular disease, causes decreased forelimb protraction, and toe pressure-induced lameness, like laminitis, causes increased forelimb protraction.[27] Hindlimb protraction, by contrast, seems to be a sensitive indicator of most causes of weight-bearing hindlimb lameness.[28,48] It can also be easily appreciated when looking from the side of the horse as it passes by the evaluator. Comparing the space between the retracting forelimb and protracting hindlimb during each half of the stride during the walk and especially the trot is easy to do and can be a highly productive exercise for detecting difficult hindlimb lameness in the horse.

The association of other swing phase parameters with lameness and their sensitivity for detection of lameness are less clear. Stride length of the lame limb is usually less than the sound limb, but significant differences are not seen until lameness severity is of moderate intensity.[41,43] Step length, or the distance between placement of opposite limbs, is less between placement of the lame and then sound limbs than between placement of the sound and then lame limb.[76] Height of foot flight arc may be increased or decreased in a lame forelimb compared with the sound forelimb, and the shape may be different, depending on the cause of lameness.[1,21,48,60] Although it is commonly perceived that horses with hindlimb lameness drag the toe on the affected side because of low hoof flight arc, this is not always the case. In a hindlimb, height of hoof flight arc is determined by two competing factors, with the strongest determining the overall effect. Decreased propulsion during push-off of the lame hindlimb causes the hind torso to rise less. To bring the affected limb forward during the swing phase of the stride without dragging it on the ground, the proximal limb joints flex more. The comparative extents of the decreased torso rise and increased limb flexion determine the height of the hoof flight arc. Anecdotally, limb abduction or adduction during the swing phase of the stride is thought to be helpful for determination of forelimb and hindlimb lameness in horses, and the direction of horizontal swing has been associated with lameness in specific locations; for example, forelimb abduction (swing out) for carpal lameness, hindlimb adduction (swinging in) for distal tarsal lameness, and hindlimb abduction for stifle lameness. The specificity of forelimb or hindlimb abduction to detect and locate lameness has not been studied adequately. In one study of amphotericin-induced carpal lameness, carpal abduction during swing was not increased in the lame limb.[43]

There is substantial evidence from numerous studies indicating that the most sensitive kinematic measures for detecting lameness in horses are the motion parameters associated with asymmetry of vertical torso movement; more specifically, vertical displacement, velocity, and acceleration of the head and neck for forelimb lameness and of the pelvis for hindlimb lameness.* In sound horses, asymmetry of trunk and proximal limb movement is less than that of the distal limb.[51] In horses with weight-bearing

---

lameness, asymmetry of trunk and proximal limb movement is greater than that of the distal limb.[60] Thus if using asymmetry between movement of the right and left sides of the body as the metric for detecting and quantifying lameness, one should concentrate on movement of the torso and put less credence in movement of the limbs. In a directed attempt to determine the best indicators of forelimb lameness, vertical movement of the head provided the best classification between sound and lame limbs than any movement in the forelimbs.[31] As stated by one prominent equine veterinarian with experience using kinematics to determine lameness in horses, "Load redistribution in lameness is possible only by altered vertical movements of the trunk, head, and neck."[76]

Asymmetric vertical torso movement in forelimb lameness is best expressed in movement of the head and neck.* Asymmetric vertical movement of the head amplifies asymmetric vertical movement of the body's center of mass because of the long moment arm of the neck.[34,47,76,82,83] In contrast, asymmetric vertical movement of the withers was shown to be less sensitive for detecting forelimb lameness.[43,84] Asymmetric vertical movement of the head was shown in many studies to be one of the most sensitive kinematic indicators of forelimb lameness.† This, of course, is what many equine practitioners see when they evaluate horses for forelimb lameness, and it is routinely known as the "head bob." "Down on sound" and "up on bad" are both used to describe the vertical asymmetric motion of the head in horses with forelimb lameness. Simply put, the head is supposed to move down more and to a lower height when the sound forelimb is in stance, and it is supposed to move up more and to a higher height after push-off of the lame limb. It is not as simple as this because both of these statements are not mutually exclusive. In addition, whether one is interpreting total vertical head excursion or the end maximum or minimum heights of the head during the strides of right and left forelimbs, neither is correct in every horse. Minimum head position was proposed to be most diagnostic of impact forelimb lameness, the most common type of forelimb lameness in the horse, with the head moving down to its lowest position during the stance phase of the sound limb.[37] Additionally, maximum head position after push-off of the lame limb when the pain of lameness occurs in the second half of stance (lameness likely of lower incidence in the forelimb) is higher than after push-off of the sound limb.[37] This description of head movement associated with forelimb lameness has not been sufficiently proven experimentally and is solely based on hypothetical mathematical modeling of the head and torso acting as free bodies moving in opposite directions during the trot. If this description is true, then a careful study of vertical head motion may give the equine practitioner valuable information for localizing lameness within the affected forelimb.

The best indicators of asymmetric hind torso movement for detection of hindlimb lameness in the horse are (1) differential vertical movements of the tubera coxae, the "pelvic rotation" or "hip hike" technique,[28,39,84] and (2) asymmetric vertical movement of the entire pelvis between left and right hindlimb stance phases, paralleling the "head

bob" technique for detection of forelimb lameness.* The first method is easier to see in most horses with hindlimb lameness but has been criticized as misleading in the occasional horse with asymmetric pelvic anatomy and insensitive to rapid alleviation of lameness after nerve blocks. The second method, because the overall vertical movement is less, is more difficult to appreciate in horses with mild hindlimb lameness. However, because whole pelvic fall better mimics the association of vertical GRFs, it is probably more sensitive and accurate. The "pelvic rotation" or "hip hike" method centers on the fact that vertical displacement of the lame-side hemipelvis is greater than of the sound-side hemipelvis. The pelvis appears to rotate toward the side of lameness. Easily visible markers fixed to the right and left tubera coxae may help to detect this asymmetric movement. The best position for the evaluator using this method is behind the horse moving away from the evaluator. The vertical displacement method detects the whole pelvis moving down to a lower height during the stance phase of the sound hindlimb or the pelvis moving up to a greater height after push-off of the sound limb. An easily visible marker fixed to the most dorsal aspect of the pelvis between the tubera sacrale may help to detect this asymmetric movement. Using this method the evaluator can be either behind the horse as it moves away or beside the horse as it passes by. Horses with an impact type of lameness, that is, greatest pain in the deceleratory phase of stance, should primarily display asymmetric downward movement in the pelvis. Horses with an impulsive type of lameness, that is, greatest pain in the acceleratory phase of stance, should primarily display asymmetric upward movement of the pelvis.[37]

Body-mounted inertial sensors are the best for an objective kinematic system of lameness evaluation in horses.[30,32,84,85] Body movement can be detected from multiple contiguous strides and wirelessly transmitted to a remote hand-held computer in a field situation. To be clinically useful, a body-mounted inertial sensor system must satisfy several criteria, including (1) the inertial sensors must be small and light enough so that normal movement is not affected; (2) data from sensors must be sampled at a rate greater than the sampling rate of the human eye using digital transmission of sufficient bit size for accurate signal representation; (3) range of data transmission should be far enough to allow measurement of movement in the environment normally used by the veterinarian; (4) data collection and analysis should be quick; and (5) the reported measures must be valid for quantification of lameness and easy to understand.

Size of the actual sensing element is not the limiting factor in the end size and weight of the entire apparatus attached to the horse's body. Micromachined accelerometers and gyroscopes are very small. Apparatus size is dictated by the size of commercially available radio components and batteries needed for adequate transmission range and power usage. True, vertical movement, the measure of most importance for lameness detection, requires multiple, simultaneously collected sensing elements (accelerometers, gyroscopes, and magnetometers). The power requirement for transmission, and coincidentally the size and weight or "footprint" of the sensor, increases with increasing number

---

*References 7, 29, 31, 43, 50, 76.
†References 7, 31, 37, 41, 43, 47, 50, 63, 76.

*References 28, 33, 35, 37, 42, 47, 76.

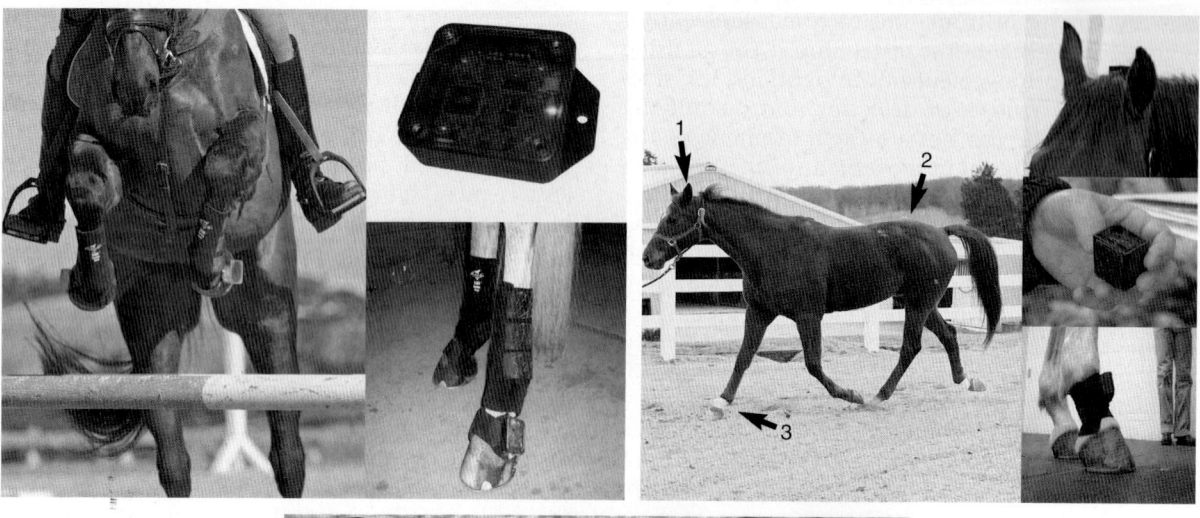

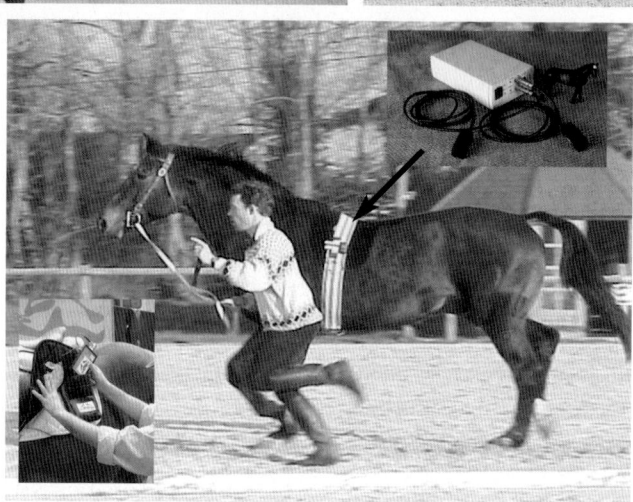

Fig. 22-2 • Currently available inertial sensor systems for field detection and evaluation of lameness in horses. *Top left:* EquuSense system from EquuSys. *Clockwise from left:* sensor nodes on forelimbs during jump; bare sensor node; closeup of sensor node on left forelimb. *Top right:* Lameness Locator from Equinosis. *Clockwise from left:* position of *1,* head accelerometer; *2,* pelvic accelerometer; and *3,* right forelimb pastern gyroscope during live field data collection; head accelerometer attached with 3M (St. Paul, Minnesota, United States) Dual Lock tape to felt head bumper; bare sensor; right forelimb pastern sensor in pastern wrap pouch. *Bottom:* Equimetrix system from Centaure-Métrix. Live horse data collection. *Insert top right:* sensors and data logger attached to girth strap. *Insert bottom left:* placing data logger in saddle pad. (Top photos courtesy Michael Davies, EquuSys. Bottom photos courtesy Dr. Eric Barrey, Centaure-Métrix.)

of sensors sampled. Higher sampling (e.g., 200 Hz over 50 Hz), increased bit size (e.g., 12-bit transmission over 8-bit), and range of transmission (e.g., 100 m vs. 30 m) also increase demands for power usage, which translates into bigger and less ideal body-mounted sensors. Using data-logging equipment attached to the horse to circumvent this size-transmission tradeoff is not convenient for a veterinarian. A veterinarian does not want to instrument the horse, collect data, stop the horse, take equipment off the horse, or download data after data collection, and then do data analysis. The veterinarian wants results quickly while performing the normal lameness evaluation, without watching computer screens or worrying about whether data are being collected properly. The end result or completed analysis should be accomplished, if not in real time, in as little time as possible. The results should be understandable to practicing veterinarians, some of whom may

not have much experience in computers, mathematics, statistics, or biomechanics and who may not have the luxury of spare time to gain such.

At the time of the writing of this chapter there are a few private companies and university laboratories around the world investigating and developing a body-mounted inertial sensor-based kinematic evaluation system for use in horses (Figure 22-2). The remainder of this chapter briefly describes some of these systems.

EquuSys Inc. (Sudbury, Massachusetts, United States) is marketing EquuSense Equine sensor systems for analysis of equine performance, including lameness. EquuSense Equine sensor systems are composed of sensors with multiple sensing units (e.g., accelerometers, gyroscopes, and magnetometers) and telemetry capability (WiFi, GPS, and Bluetooth) that are attached to the horse, and accompanying hardware (a laptop computer) and software. Each sensor provides objective and accurate information on its position, velocity, acceleration, orientation, and rotation relative to the horse or to a global reference frame. The software can track from 8 to 18 sensors, depending on the product platform selected, at up to 2000 frames/s in real time. The sensors weigh less than 100 g and can be attached to the horse with specially designed boots and pouches. The data are analyzed to give the user a graphical output of sensor trajectories. This system is a more practical, field-ready replacement for the more familiar camera and marker kinematic systems. The user determines what trajectory variables should be measured and how measured values are analyzed.

Lameness Locator is a wireless, body sensor-based lameness evaluation system developed by equine veterinarians and engineers at the University of Missouri in collaboration with engineers at the Hiroshima Institute of Technology in Japan. It is licensed to Equinosis in Columbia, Missouri for further development and commercialization to equine veterinarians only. Lameness Locator consists of three inertial sensors (two accelerometers and one gyroscope) attached to the head, right forelimb, and pelvis. Each sensor is 4 cm by 3 cm by 2 cm in dimensions and weighs less than 30 g. Vertical accelerations of the head and pelvis and angular velocity of the right forelimb are measured and wirelessly transmitted in real time to a hand-held tablet computer up to 150 m away. Custom algorithms are then implemented to detect and measure forelimb and hindlimb lameness when the horse trots or walks. The algorithms were developed from previous kinematic research at the University of Missouri using camera and markers attached to sound and lame horses. Best sites for motion detection to measure lameness were determined using a data-mining approach to analysis of large datasets. Random motion, unassociated with lameness, as a result of a misbehaving or uncooperative horse, which may interfere with detection and quantification of lameness, is extracted from the raw signals. Lameness detection and quantification results are presented to the user in a graphical interface that shows impact and propulsion asymmetry in each stride, with thresholds between what is expected for soundness and lameness. Trend and variability of collected data are also presented. Because forelimb and hindlimb lameness are measured simultaneously, compensatory or multiple-limb lameness patterns can be evaluated. The developers of Lameness Locator claim that it will be most useful to equine veterinarians evaluating horses with mild, subtle, or multiple-limb lameness and in objectively evaluating partial improvements after using diagnostic analgesia. At the time of this writing, Lameness Locator is being field-tested at 25 private practice and university teaching hospital sites in North America and Europe.

Equimetrix is a multidimensional, accelerometer system attached to the girth of an exercising horse. It is marketed by Centaure-Métrix (Evry, France) primarily in France and the Benelux countries (Belgium, the Netherlands, and Luxembourg). Three-dimensional torso acceleration is collected and logged as the horse exercises. The data are then analyzed, and output is used to measure characteristics of performance, including stride parameters (e.g., regularity, frequency, length, and timing) and "propulsion power." Although the output of Equimetrix is directed primarily toward assessing performance in exercising horses, existing algorithms could be adapted or new algorithms could be developed to more specifically evaluate lameness in horses.

Chapter 23

Arthroscopic Examination

Mike W. Ross

Arthroscopic surgery is arguably the most important advance in management and one of the most important in diagnosis of equine joint disease. Arthroscopic surgery has been a mainstay in managing joint disease since the early 1980s and has mostly replaced arthrotomy. An effective equine surgeon cannot lack extensive arthroscopic surgical experience, and lameness diagnosticians must understand indications and limitations of the technique. Innovators have used the same instruments for bursoscopy and tenoscopy (see Chapter 24). For a complete description of procedures, instrumentation, and principles of arthroscopy, the reader is referred to *Diagnostic and Surgical Arthroscopy in the Horse*.[1]

ADVANTAGES AND DISADVANTAGES OF ARTHROSCOPIC SURGERY COMPARED WITH ARTHROTOMY

Arthroscopic surgery offers several advantages compared with arthrotomy; however, this type of surgery also has some disadvantages. Both are discussed in the following text.

Advantages

Improved Visibility
Improved visibility during arthroscopic examination allows for evaluation of most of the joint compared with the limited view provided by arthrotomy. Even long arthrotomy incisions rarely provide added visibility because overlying capsule, retinaculum, and sheaths make retraction difficult. During arthroscopic examination, cartilage at locations distant to the primary lesion site, synovium, and intraarticular soft tissue structures such as ligaments can be examined. For example, newly described disease conditions involving intercarpal ligaments were not known before arthroscopic examination existed.

References on page 1265

Reduced Trauma and Morbidity

Arthroscopic examination is less traumatic and causes less morbidity. Arthroscopic examination allows surgery to be performed through small incisions and requires less surgical exposure and damage to overlying soft tissues, upholding a time-honored principle of limiting trauma. Little pain is observed in horses after arthroscopic surgery compared with arthrotomy, and many horses appear to ambulate normally. However, in an unblinded study of horses after arthroscopy under general anesthesia, horses showed mild but significant increases in discomfort compared with pain-free controls.[2] Complications such as wound dehiscence and seroma formation are minimal. Horses often show pronounced lameness for several days after arthrotomy. After arthroscopic examination and surgery, owners and trainers expect horses to return to full work soon after surgery, an idea that is fueled by widespread reports of human athletes returning to professional sports quickly after arthroscopic surgery. A general misunderstanding is that incision size is the limiting factor. Although arthrotomy does cause short-lived lameness after surgery, the fear that it will delay onset of training is unfounded because the underlying lesion dictates recovery time. Although not recommended, horses with mild conditions such as osteochondritis dissecans, effusion but no lameness, and those that receive prophylactic arthroscopic surgery can resume training a few weeks after arthroscopic examination or arthroscopic surgery. Arthroscopic surgery can be performed within weeks before a sale, and if hair was not clipped, surgical sites are barely noticeable.

Better Cosmetic Results

Improved cosmesis is a definite advantage. Small incisions cause less fibrous tissue formation, and incisions are difficult to identify 2 to 3 months after surgery. Generally the instrument portal (incision), the site through which the arthroscopic instruments are passed and lavage is performed, suffers more trauma than does the arthroscopic portal, and swelling, reactions, and fibrous tissue production are more common.

Earlier Functional Capability

Earlier return to function was once believed to be an advantage of arthroscopic surgery. However, incision size has little to do with lameness except within the first few weeks after surgery. Lameness observed in horses returned to work 4 to 6 weeks after arthroscopic surgery for substantial articular lesions has nothing to do with incision size. When horses undergoing arthroscopic surgery were given only a brief rest, results were unsatisfactory. Incisions heal from side to side, not end to end, and incision size has no effect on articular healing. Lesions must heal as completely as possible before full work can begin—a process that often takes several months. Type and location of lesions are important because horses with osteochondritis dissecans not involving weight-bearing surfaces can start training within 2 to 3 weeks of surgery, if necessary, whereas those with lesions in critical sites, such as the typical carpal osteochondral fragment, must be given 3 to 4 months of rest.

More Versatility

Improved versatility is a definite advantage because joints considered inaccessible, such as the coxofemoral joint, can be evaluated. Techniques such as repair of third carpal slab fractures, distal third metatarsal (MtIII) or third metacarpal (McIII) fractures, fractures in other joints, and resurfacing techniques can be done using arthroscopic surgery.

Fewer Complications

Arthroscopic surgery results in fewer complications. Arthrotomy of the scapulohumeral, femorotibial, femoropatellar, cubital, and tarsocrural joints has been associated with dehiscence, seroma formation, and infection, but arthroscopic surgery of these joints is safe.

Disadvantages

Expensive Instrumentation

Expense of surgical instrumentation is a disadvantage because start-up costs are high, but basic instrumentation is no more costly than routine surgical instruments. Although arthroscopic surgery can be done without video equipment, video arthroscopy is valuable for archiving images. It is much more comfortable than direct-view arthroscopy (looking directly through the eyepiece) because surgery is performed using a comfortably positioned monitor. It allows the procedure to be viewed by others and is valuable in maintaining aseptic technique because breaks in technique often occur during direct-view arthroscopic surgery.

Lack of Surgical Experience

Experience necessary to learn arthroscopic surgery is a disadvantage. Arthroscopic surgery requires skill in stereotactic techniques and orienting and operating without looking at the surgical site, and surgeons must be able to use instruments properly and safely while looking at a monitor. Preoperative planning must be done to ensure that the horse is positioned properly on the operating table and the surgeon has ready access for triangulation. Poor technique may result in iatrogenic damage or extravasation of large amounts of lavage fluid that can severely compromise distention of the joint capsule and thus ability to see adequately within the joint. Experience cannot be gained by simply attending a weekend course but rather by working long hours with cadaver specimens and observing experienced surgeons. Initially arthroscopic surgery can be time consuming until experience is gained, but with experience arthroscopic surgery is faster than arthrotomy.

Equipment Problems

Equipment failures can be a disadvantage, and because arthroscopic examination depends on electricity, a generator should always be available. Instruments are not made to withstand forces applied to cut, grasp, and debride equine bone and, along with the arthroscope, may break.

Improper Case Selection

Case selection is the most important disadvantage. Poor case selection can make arthroscopic surgery difficult and disappointing. Although much information can be gained by arthroscopic examination of any joint, prognosis should be carefully considered when operating on joints in which extensive osteoarthritis exists. Inadequate communication before surgery may leave owners and trainers with too high expectations of results. Often they have little appreciation

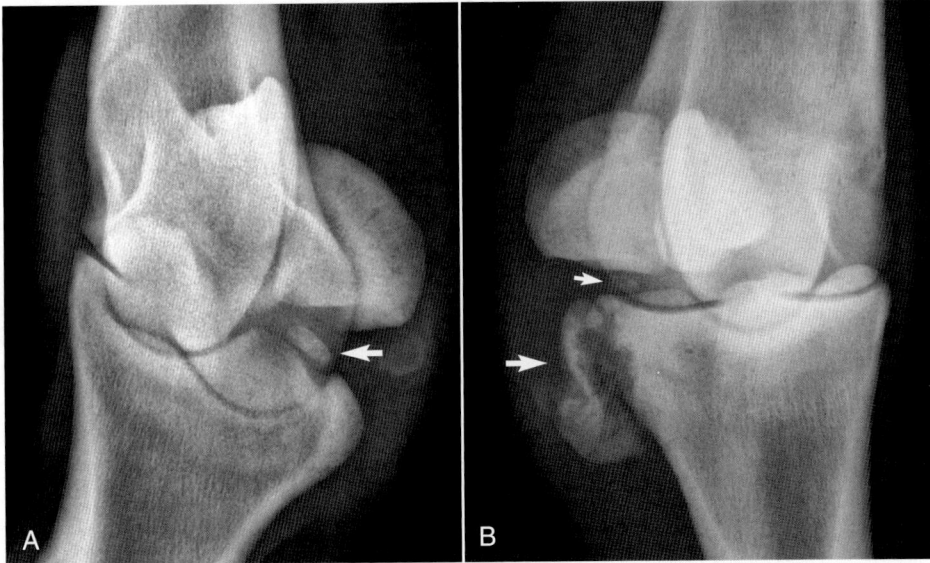

Fig. 23-1 • A, Dorsal 25° proximal medial-plantarodistal lateral oblique digital radiographic image of the right hind (RH) metatarsophalangeal joint *(MTPJ)* in a 2-year-old Standardbred (STB) trotter showing a typical intraarticularly located plantar process fragment *(arrow)* easily removed using arthroscopic techniques. This "down angled" oblique radiographic image is useful to evaluate the region between the base of the medial proximal sesamoid bone and the proximal aspect of the proximal phalanx to see these fragments. **B,** Dorsolateral-plantaromedial oblique digital radiographic image of the RH MTPJ in a 2-year-old STB pacing filly with large nonarticular *(large arrow)* and small articular *(small arrow)* plantar process fragments, which were all removed using arthroscopic techniques. To remove fragments outside the joint, a combination of sharp and blunt dissection and use of a synovial resector are necessary.

for the magnitude of cartilage damage and osteoarthritis (OA), and they only see or hear about the chip fracture(s) visible radiologically. Owners and trainers tend to want to do something, but removal of osteochondral fragments from a carpus or fetlock joint with hopeless OA can be time consuming, cause instrument failures, and, worse, often results in a poor outcome. Poor prognosis associated with some conditions must be well communicated to owners before surgery. For example, we recently reviewed the results of surgical and conservative management of scapulohumeral osteochondrosis and found that overall, prognosis was poor.[3] Prognosis varied inversely with the severity of radiological changes, and only 15% of potential racehorses started a race. Four of six nonracehorses were sound for intended use. Surgery did not improve prognosis.[3]

The fragment size that can be easily removed during arthroscopic surgery is limited, and the instrument portal must be enlarged to accommodate such fragments unless ostectomy is performed. The fragment must be located in the joint or at least close to it, a decision that must be made before surgery because arthroscopic surgery is of little benefit if the fragment is not in the joint or close enough to make the approach reasonable and safe. In the metatarsophalangeal joint, large plantar process fragments from the proximal phalanx are often located extraarticularly, and although they may still be best removed using conventional surgical techniques, I have removed large fragments with arthroscopic instrumentation; surgery is facilitated by use of a motorized synovial resector (Figure 23-1). Differentiation should be made preoperatively between fragments free in a joint, which are accessible to surgical removal, and those embedded in the joint capsule and therefore not readily removed. In the stifle joint,

fragments in the distal aspect of the femoropatellar joint may appear radiologically as if they are in the femorotibial joint. Rare fragments in the caudal pouches of the medial and lateral femorotibial joints can be difficult to retrieve, especially if the precise location cannot be determined radiologically before surgery. The approaches to the difficult caudal pouches of the medial and lateral femorotibial joints were recently refined.[4] Highly mobile fragments in a large joint such as the femoropatellar joint can prove challenging to locate. There is still a limited role for arthrotomy in equine surgery. For example, I still prefer to use a small, medial, middle carpal arthrotomy to repair sagittal slab fractures of the third carpal bone (C3) because I believe I can more accurately place the screw in the medial aspect of the C3, between the C3 and the second carpal bone.[5] Others prefer a technique using arthroscopic guidance.[1]

PRINCIPLES, INSTRUMENTATION, AND TECHNIQUE

Surgical technique, basic and advanced instrumentation, and approaches are well described elsewhere,[1] and in-depth discussion is beyond the scope of this textbook. The basic principle of arthroscopic surgery is to use a rigid 4-mm endoscope to evaluate and perform intraarticular surgery through small incisions. Smaller endoscopes (2.9 mm and smaller) facilitate surgery in smaller joints or to view lesions between joint surfaces. Limited arthroscopic surgery was previously performed through a single incision, and instruments were passed through a second slot in the arthroscopic cannula. Versatility was severely compromised. Triangulation, a versatile technique in use today, uses two distant portals so that the arthroscope and instruments create two sides of a triangle. For example, during routine tarsocrural arthroscopy the arthroscopic portal is dorsomedial and the instrument portal is dorsolateral. This allows the tips of the instruments to be in the surgical field from distant points and obviates the need for the arthroscope to be close to the lesion. The end of the arthroscope is angled 25 to 30 degrees, and a different view is obtained by simply rotating it. Endoscopes with angles of 70 and 120 degrees can be used to obtain different views and are useful when triangulation is done with incisions close together. The image must be positioned on the screen to optimize special orientation and facilitate stereotaxis.

Arthroscopic surgery can be performed with basic instruments, the most important of which are rongeurs (Ferris-Smith), grasping forceps, bone curettes, lavage cannulae, intraarticular blades, and probes. Arthroscopic surgery depends on the availability of a suitable light source and monitor, digital camera, and recording devices. A fluid delivery system is mandatory, and pumps or other methods to pressurize fluid are preferred to gravity flow systems. Many common lesions removed by arthroscopic surgery are located on the joint margin, and visibility often is compromised when joint capsule and synovium collapse or when bleeding is excessive. Carbon dioxide insufflation is sometimes used and is preferred by some surgeons.[6] Carbon dioxide insufflation was effective at maintaining distention of the metacarpophalangeal and metatarsophalangeal joints and gave excellent visibility of lesions, but fluid lavage was necessary when bleeding precluded optimal visibility.[7] Lasers are used rarely. Controlled ablation (coblation), using a form of radiofrequency energy to dissolve tissue, is used intraarticularly and in tendon sheaths and bursae (see Chapter 24). Using a new radiofrequency prototype probe, researchers were able to control cartilage cell death significantly better compared with manual debridement and use of a commercially available probe.[8] Motorized equipment is useful but expensive. Abrasion arthroplasty units include various motorized burrs to remove and smooth cartilage and bone surfaces and are used in horses with large lesions such as osteochondritis dissecans lesions of the lateral trochlear ridge of the femur. Synovial resectors are alternating, motorized, rotating blades that are helpful in removing synovium and fibrous tissue and are particularly valuable for removal of osteochondral fragments from the dorsal aspect of the distal interphalangeal joint, apical proximal sesamoid fracture fragments, large abaxial fragments originating from the proximal aspect of the proximal phalanx, and fragments from the lateral malleolus of the distal aspect of the tibia, as well as when synovectomy is indicated.

The division between diagnostic and surgical arthroscopy is now artificial because the same instruments are used for both. Diagnostic arthroscopy, that is, arthroscopic examination, generally refers to evaluating cartilage, bone, and soft tissues to gain information for diagnosis and prognosis. The client must be warned that although valuable information is always learned, arthroscopic examination may provide little therapeutic benefit. However, I believe a tendency exists to undersell arthroscopic examination because a positive intervention cannot be made unless the joint is evaluated, and much can be learned about lesions with early arthroscopic examination. This is particularly

true in the stifle, carpus and fetlock joints. Arthroscopic examination is indicated in horses with lameness localized to a joint, but in which radiological findings are negative or equivocal. Scintigraphic evidence of subchondral bone injury is common in these horses, and defects, if present, in overlying articular cartilage can be debrided and attempts at resurfacing performed arthroscopically. In young racehorses with early subchondral bone injury, arthroscopic evaluation usually reveals little to no overlying cartilage damage in those portions of the joint visible from conventional arthroscopic approaches (Figure 23-2). In these horses lack of cartilage damage likely explains the lack of obvious clinical signs such as effusion. Management of horses with novel surgical techniques such as subchondral forage or using drugs targeting subchondral bone modeling/remodeling in combination with rest is recommended.

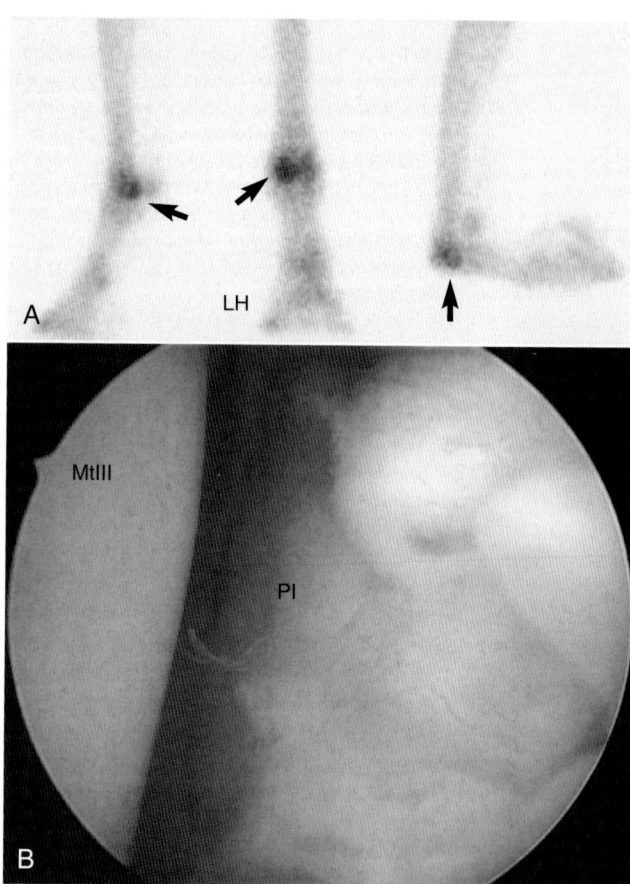

Fig. 23-2 • **A,** Delayed-phase scintigraphic images of a 3-year-old Thoroughbred colt with subchondral bone pain localized to the lateral aspect of the left metatarsophalangeal joint using lateral plantar metatarsal analgesia. Focal increased radiopharmaceutical uptake of the distal, lateral condyle of the third metatarsal bone (MtIII) (arrows) can be seen. Radiographs revealed sclerosis but no radiolucency. **B,** Intraoperative view of the plantar aspect of the left hind fetlock joint (dorsal is to the left and medial is uppermost) from an arthroscopic portal in the proximal, lateral plantar pouch showing normal-appearing articular cartilage of the lateral condyle of the MtIII overlying subchondral bone injury as depicted scintigraphically. The proximal phalanx (PI) can be seen just distal to synovial membrane between the PI and the base of the lateral proximal sesamoid bone. The entire articular surface cannot be evaluated, but visible articular cartilage appears normal. A subchondral forage technique (three 3.5-mm holes drilled from the lateral condyle into subchondral bone) was used.

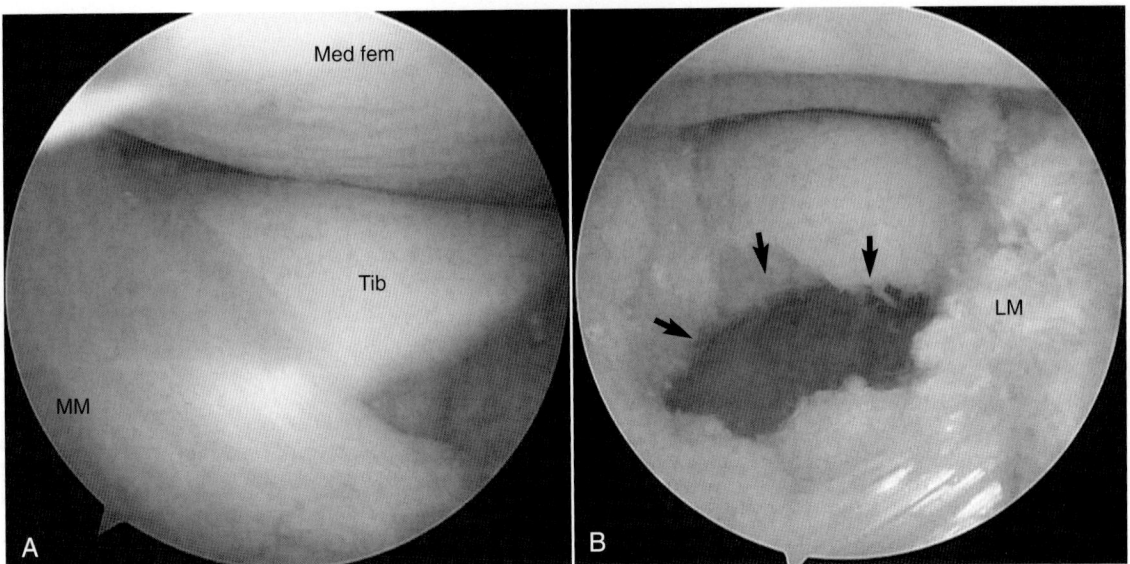

Fig. 23-3 • Intraoperative arthroscopic images of the cranial aspects of the medial femorotibial joint *(MFTJ)* (**A** [medial is to the left and proximal is uppermost]) and lateral femorotibial joint *(LFTJ)* (**B** [lateral is to the right and proximal is uppermost]) in a 3-year-old Standardbred gelding with an unusual subchondral bone cyst in the proximal lateral aspect of the tibia *(arrows)* and enlarged, frayed lateral meniscus *(LM)*. A cranial approach to the femoropatellar joint *(FPJ)* was used to evaluate the stifle and the septae between the FPJ, and the MFTJ and LFTJ were removed to allow examinations through a single approach. In this horse with left hindlimb lameness, clinical signs of stifle pain were not detected, and the horse was referred for scintigraphic examination, which revealed focal, moderately increased radiopharmaceutical uptake in the proximal, lateral aspect of the tibia. Notice the normal medial meniscus *(MM)* and articular cartilage of the proximal aspect of the tibia *(Tib)* in the MFTJ and mild undulation of articular cartilage of the distal femur *(Med fem)*. The subchondral bone cyst and torn edge of the lateral meniscus have been debrided (**B**). Prognosis is guarded at best because of subchondral bone, cartilage, and meniscal injury in the LFTJ.

Scintigraphy and ultrasonography have low sensitivity in the complex stifle joint, and arthroscopic examination should be encouraged. Walmsley et al.,[9] in a large case series, found that 47% of horses returned to full use, and prognosis was inversely proportional to severity of meniscal tearing, degree of cartilage damage, and radiological abnormalities (Figure 23-3) (see Chapter 46). Arthroscopic examination may uncover proliferative synovitis, intersesamoidean ligament injury, and intercarpal ligament injury. Intercarpal ligament injury often is associated with OA or osteochondral fragments and can cause hemarthrosis and presumably joint instability (Figure 23-4).[10,11] Lesions in difficult locations can be successfully evaluated and manipulated arthroscopically. Ten of 11 horses that had subchondral bone cysts of the distal phalanx returned to athletic use after arthroscopic debridement.[12] The distal interphalangeal joint can be difficult to evaluate, but a combination of careful manipulation and flexion can improve visibility (Figure 23-5).

Changes in articular cartilage are the most important information gained from arthroscopic examination. Prognosis was found to worsen in proportion to the extent of articular cartilage damage in the carpus,[13] but all joints are similarly affected. Surface area and depth of damage are important. Widespread damage affecting many cartilaginous surfaces is usually worse than well-defined lesions extending into subchondral bone. Cartilage damage is graded as mild (<20% damage to cartilage and subchondral bone at the primary lesion site), moderate (involvement of apposing bone, but <30% total cartilage and subchondral

bone damage of primary and apposing sites), severe (≤50% of cartilage and subchondral bone damage of primary and apposing sites), and global (extensive cartilage damage visible on most articular surfaces) (Figures 23-6 to 23-8). If cartilage lesions do not extend past the zone of calcified cartilage, healing after surgery will likely be minimal (see Microfracture discussion below).

Occult (not radiologically apparent) osteochondral fragments may be identified by arthroscopic examination. Recognition requires inspection and probing, if necessary, after synovial resection. Common sites include the medial aspect of the intermediate carpal and lateral aspect of the radial carpal bones and small fragments involving the proximodorsal aspect of the proximal phalanx. Unexplained tarsocrural effusion (bog spavin) is commonly caused by osteochondritis dissecans fragments of the distal medial malleolus of the tibia, and although fragments may be suspected radiologically, the presence is confirmed and they are removed arthroscopically. Occult or radiologically suspicious subchondral defects of the third carpal bone, the distal aspect of the medial femoral condyle, and the distal aspect of the MtIII and McIII can be confirmed and debrided.

Most arthroscopic surgery is performed to remove radiologically apparent osteochondral fragment(s). Grading cartilage damage and subchondral bone damage, along with removing one or more osteochondral fragments, is important in assessing prognosis. Discovery of severe cartilage damage in horses with few radiological changes is common, especially in the carpus and fetlock joints. Whenever possible, all aspects of the joint should be evaluated.

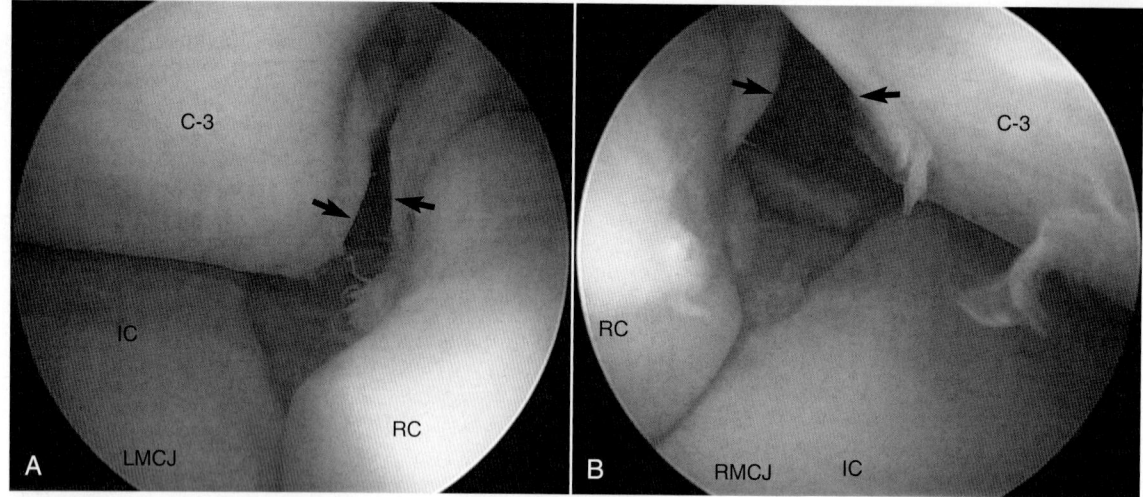

Fig. 23-4 • Intraoperative arthroscopic images of the left **(A)** and right **(B)** middle carpal joints *(MCJs)* showing complete tearing of the medial palmar intercarpal ligaments *(arrows)* in a 2-year-old Thoroughbred filly in race training. The horse was positioned in dorsal recumbency, and distal is uppermost; medial is to the right in **A** and to the left in **B**. The arthroscope has been inserted through a dorsolateral portal between the extensor carpi radialis and common digital extensor tendons in both MCJs. Tearing of the medial palmar intercarpal ligament appears as it courses from the third carpal bone *(C3)* to the radial carpal bone *(RC)*. The intermediate carpal bone *(IC)* can be seen. Tearing of the medial palmar intercarpal ligament causes hemarthrosis, a condition previously thought to be idiopathic without arthroscopic examination, and can occur in conjunction with osteochondral fragmentation and associated cartilage damage. When the intercarpal ligament is torn, the palmar aspect of the MCJ can be examined, a finding that is impossible if the ligament is intact.

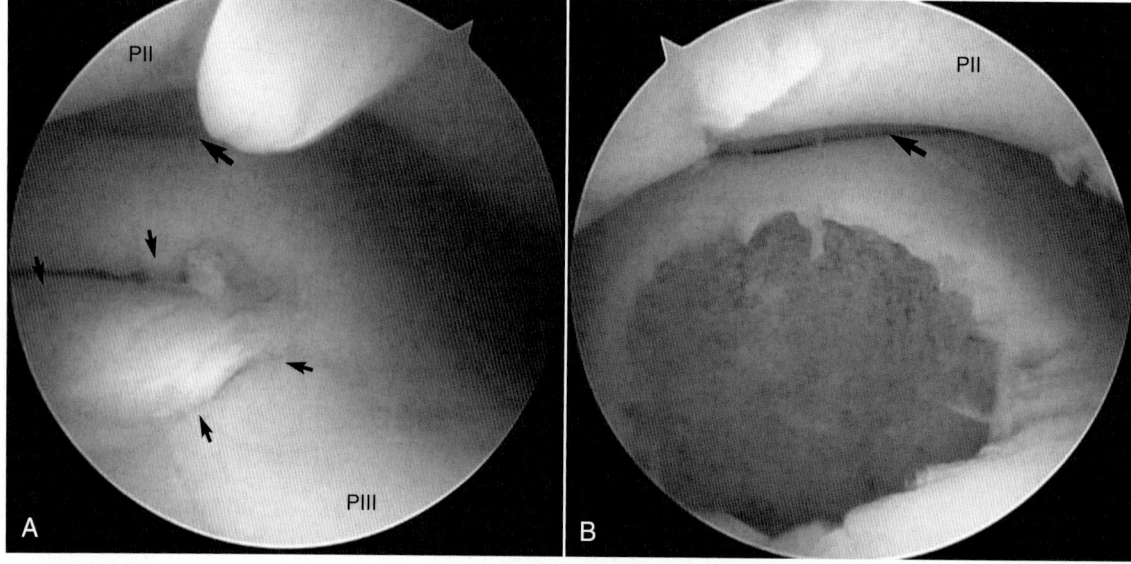

Fig. 23-5 • Intraoperative arthroscopic images before **(A)** and after debridement **(B)** of the right hind distal interphalangeal joint *(DIPJ)* in a yearling Standardbred filly with a history of acute lameness and a small wound at the dorsal aspect of the coronary band. Hair was found in the dorsal aspect of the joint and was removed. With the joint in moderate flexion and the joint surfaces retracted using an arthroscopic elevator, this lesion involving the plantar aspect of the articular surface of the distal phalanx *(PIII)* can be seen *(small arrows)*. Notice the articulation between the plantar aspect of the PIII and the navicular bone *(large arrow)*. The distal articular surface of the middle phalanx *(PII)* can be seen.

In racehorses, although cartilage damage and osteochondral fragmentation are often seen dorsally, the palmar/plantar aspect of the metacarpophalangeal joint or metatarsophalangeal joint often has extensive cartilaginous score lines or large, full-thickness areas of cartilage loss on the medial aspect of the McIII and the medial articular surface of the proximal sesamoid bone (PSB) and on the lateral aspect of the MtIII and the lateral PSB. In nonracehorse sports horses, changes are most prominent dorsally. Lesions of the patella, sometimes with fragmentation,

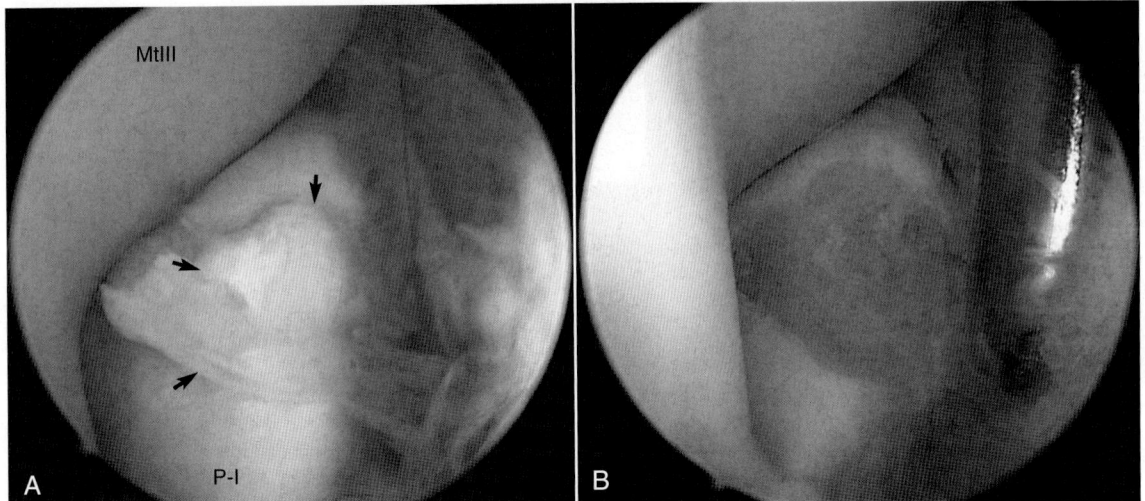

Fig. 23-6 • Intraoperative arthroscopic images of the dorsomedial aspect of the right metatarsophalangeal joint of a 3-year-old Thoroughbred filly with right hindlimb lameness (dorsal is right, proximal is top). **A,** A small osteochondral fragment (chip fracture, *arrows*) of the dorsomedial aspect of the proximal phalanx (*P-I*) is surrounded by mild cartilage damage. A small partial-thickness "score" line can be seen on the overlying medial condyle of the third metatarsal bone *(MtIII)*. **B,** The chip fracture has been removed and surrounding mild cartilage damage debrided. This horse returned to successful racing 6 months after arthroscopic surgery.

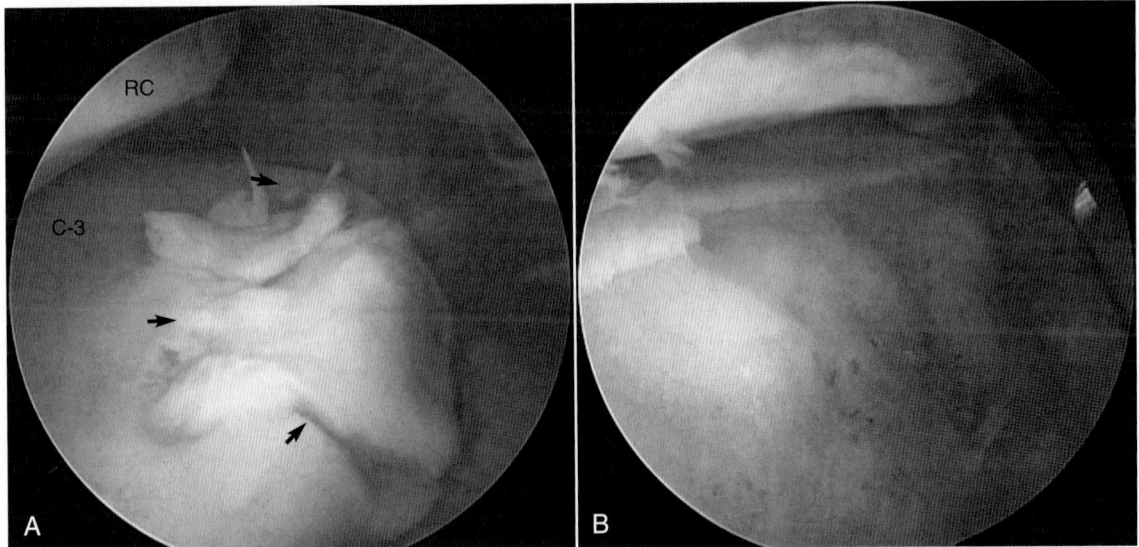

Fig. 23-7 • Intraoperative arthroscopic images of the right middle carpal joint of a 3-year-old Standardbred colt (dorsal is to the right and proximal is uppermost). **A,** A small osteochondral fragment (chip fracture, *arrows*) of the third carpal bone *(C3)* can be seen; minimal cartilage damage was found on the radiocarpal bone *(RC)*. **B,** The chip fracture has been removed, and surrounding moderate cartilage damage has been debrided. This horse has a good prognosis for racing soundness.

found during arthroscopic examination explain why some horses with large osteochondritis dissecans lesions of the lateral trochlear ridge of the femur perform poorly. Arthroscopic examination is useful in horses with infectious arthritis to evaluate articular surfaces and synovium, identify and remove foreign material (see Figure 23-5), facilitate removal of fibrin, and perform much more effective and complete lavage than is achieved by through-and-through lavage. Arthroscopic examination usually is reserved for horses with long-standing infections and those

with extensive fibrin accumulation, but the Editors strongly promote its use for acute infection as well. I have not found a good correlation between arthroscopic and ultrasonographic identification of fibrin early in the disease process (the amount of fibrin is overestimated by ultrasonography). Arthroscopic examination can facilitate drain insertion, synovectomy, and debridement or removal of osteochondral defects. Arthroscopic portals can be left open to facilitate drainage after surgery, but this procedure should be used only in horses with refractory infections.

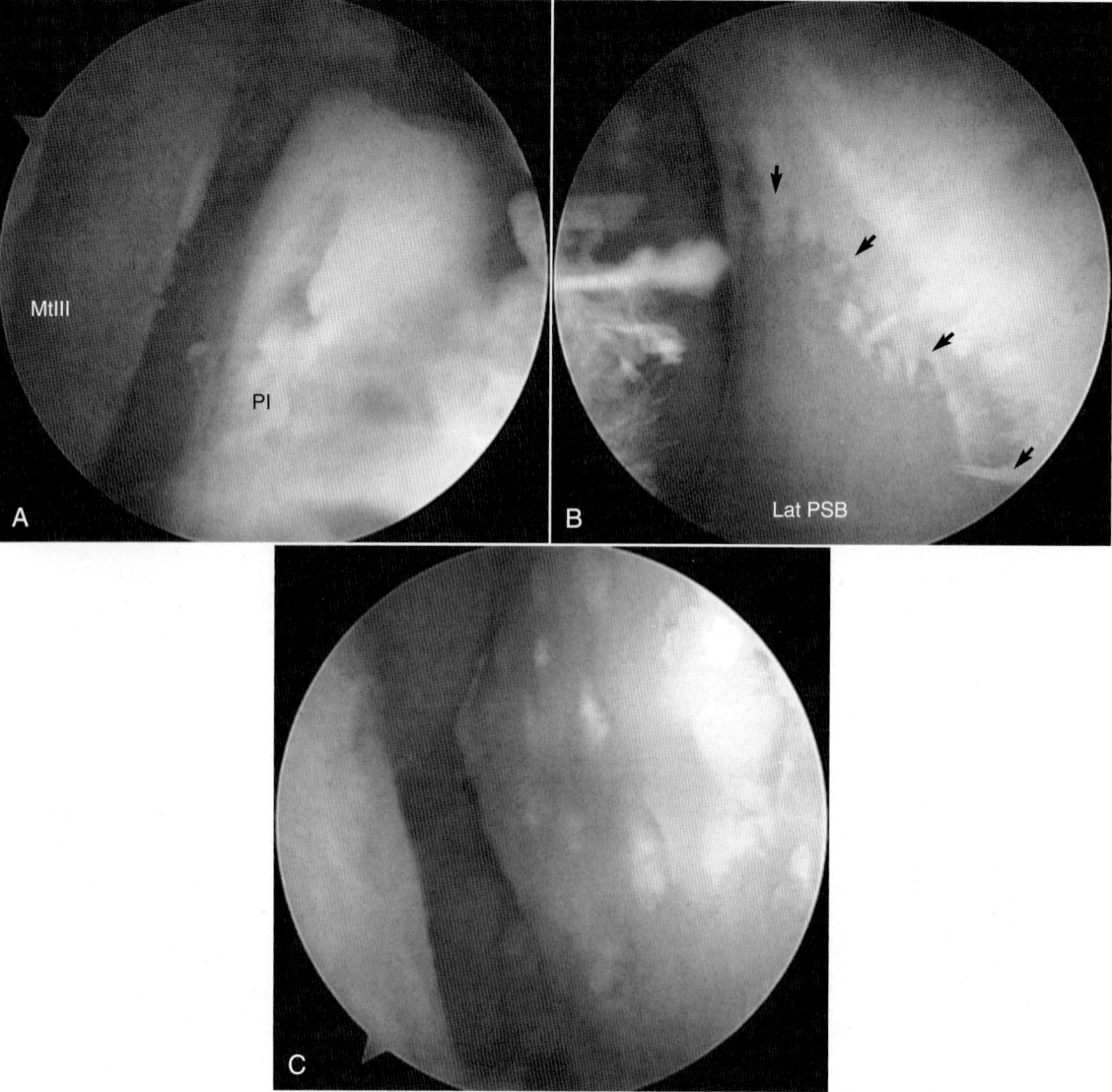

Fig. 23-8 • Intraoperative arthroscopic images of the plantar aspect of the left metatarsophalangeal joint in a 7-year-old Standardbred stallion showing severe cartilage and subchondral bone damage from end-stage osteoarthritis that developed from maladaptive bone remodeling. **A,** A large erosive lesion of the lateral condyle of the third metatarsal bone *(MtIII)* has been debrided (dorsal is to the left and proximal is uppermost). This area is difficult to see, and the arthroscope is positioned between MtIII and the lateral proximal sesamoid bone with the joint in as much extension as possible. The proximal, plantar aspect of the proximal phalanx *(P-I)* can be seen. **B,** Severe loss of articular cartilage with exposed subchondral bone *(arrows)* can be seen on the lateral proximal sesamoid bone. **C,** The technique known as microfracture has been performed in the area of complete cartilage loss on the lateral proximal sesamoid bone, but prognosis is hopeless for racing soundness.

SURGICAL PROCEDURES

The specific indications and surgical procedures are discussed in other chapters. Dorsal and palmar/plantar, medial and lateral, and cranial and caudal approaches have been described; the approach, choice of portals, fluid delivery, and instrumentation vary among joints and surgeons. Positioning the horse on the operating table is important to allow access to the involved joint(s), and repositioning may be necessary. Both lateral and dorsal recumbency are used successfully, and choices are based on the surgeon's experience and the number of joints affected. Although standing arthroscopy of the fetlock and

other joints has been described,[14] I prefer to use general anesthesia.

Minimally invasive surgery such as arthroscopic surgery continues to be developed in horses. Standard procedures include fragment removal, debridement and curettage, partial synovectomy, and incision of adhesions. Reduction, fragment removal, and screw placement in horses with condylar fractures of the McIII or the MtIII can be done using arthroscopic surgery, obviating the need for arthrotomy. A technique to insert one or more cortical bone screws to repair frontal slab fractures of the third carpal bone was an early advance that has led to use of a similar technique to repair radial carpal bone and ulnar carpal bone slab fractures, PSB fractures, and other unusually located articular fractures.[15] An alternative to arthroscopic debridement of subchondral bone cysts of the medial femoral condyle—injection of the cyst lining with corticosteroids under arthroscopic guidance—appears to give similar clinical results.[16] Thirty-five of 52 horses (67%) were considered successful. Horses with unilateral subchondral bone cysts did better than those with bilateral cysts, and the existence of osteophytes on preoperative radiographs had a negative impact on success.[16]

Cartilage Resurfacing

Recently cartilage resurfacing techniques have been used in experimental horses and in a limited number of clinically affected horses. Repair strategy involves creating access to stem cells, growth factors, and blood in subchondral bone to assist in cartilage repair or transplantation (grafting) of tissues, osteochondral grafts, or cells (chondrocytes). Partial- or full-thickness cartilage defects that do not penetrate the subchondral plate heal incompletely or not at all. An important principle in cartilage repair is to curette through the layer of calcified cartilage and perforate the subchondral plate to allow influx of healing elements. Extensive curettage seems to be self-defeating because exposure of large areas of denuded subchondral bone is associated with poor prognosis and often is found in horses with naturally occurring OA. Unfortunately, many defects already involve complete erosion into subchondral bone, at least around and apposing the primary lesion site. A technique known as *microfracture* of the subchondral plate has been introduced and involves using a 45- or 90-degree orthopedic awl (micropick) to create small perforation sites into subchondral bone in the area of cartilage damage.[17,18] Studies have shown that removal of the calcified cartilage layer alone, or perforation of the layer with the microfracture technique, improves the amount and quality of repair tissue, but this tissue lacks the biomechanical and histological character of hyaline cartilage.[19] The procedure is currently being used, but objective results compared with routine procedures have not been published.

Nixon[20] has considerable experience in transplantation resurfacing techniques and is focusing current efforts on using autogenous fibrin laden with insulin-like growth factor–1 and chondrocytes harvested from neonatal foals. An arthroscopic technique using a two-component system was used to implant the graft in experimental and clinically affected horses with defects in the carpus and subchondral cystic lesions of the medial femoral condyle and in the fetlock joint. Early results appeared promising. More recently mesenchymal stem cell grafts improved early healing of full-thickness cartilage lesions; however, there was no significant long-term difference between stem cell–treated and control defects.[21] In an osteochondral fragment model evaluating articular cartilage and subchondral bone healing and synovitis, injection of either adipose-derived or bone marrow–derived stem cells had similar results to controls.[22] It was suggested that the use of stem cells might be beneficial in joints with soft tissue injuries.

A technique called *mosaic arthroplasty* involves using arthroscopic procedures to harvest osteochondral pegs (grafts) from the trochlear groove or the medial border of the medial trochlear ridge of the femur and implant them in distant recipient sites.[23-26] Grafts harvested and implanted using special instruments have better congruence than previously reported osteochondral grafting techniques, most using donor sites in the sternum. Mosaic arthroplasty has been used to manage osteochondral defects and subchondral bone cysts in the medial condyle of the femur, the fetlock joint, and the C3 and was proposed to be useful when conservative management failed.[23-26] Seven of 10 horses returned to the previous level of performance after surgery.[26] However, in an experimental study the technique was questioned because although there was good incorporation of bony portions of the grafts into recipient subchondral bone, there was substantial cartilage degeneration.[24] Large osteochondral flaps (osteochondritis dissecans) in the stifle, tarsocrural, and fetlock joints have been successfully reattached, rather than removed, using polydioxanone pins.[27]

Postoperative Care

Aftercare instructions differ depending on the joint(s) involved, severity of cartilage damage, surgeon's experience, economic factors, and competition schedules. Bandage and wound care, administration of antiinflammatory, analgesic, and antimicrobial therapy, and suture removal are routine. Decisions about rehabilitation time should be based on the extent of the damage and its location, but often are made based on the perceived need for a quick return to training and performance. Intraarticular therapy with hyaluronan and polysulfated glycosaminoglycans (PSGAG) is often recommended, and although such therapy may be beneficial to reduce inflammatory changes in joints early after surgery, little evidence exists that repair is augmented. I generally recommend intraarticular hyaluronan 14 and 28 days after surgery in horses with mild or moderate cartilage damage and PSGAG, administered intraarticularly 3, 5, and 7 weeks after surgery, for horses with severe or global cartilage damage. Treatment with PSGAG given intramuscularly beginning 2 weeks after surgery (once weekly for 8 weeks) is recommended.

COMPLICATIONS

The infection rate after arthroscopic surgery is low, but not zero, and is generally less than other soft tissue and orthopedic procedures performed in the same hospital. Poor case selection and failure to remove the intended fragments are the most common important complications. Intraoperative radiographs should be obtained if any doubt exists about fragments (number and size) removed. Extravasation of fluid, most commonly at the instrument portal but occasionally at the arthroscopic portal, occurs frequently and is of little concern. Fibrous tissue formation at the instrument portal is common if a large amount of cartilage and bony debris is flushed from the joint or removal of several osteochondral fragments required extensive manipulation. Prolonged drainage from any portal should be managed as potential infectious arthritis. Synovial fistulae occur rarely, but they may require repair. Damage to overlying tendons may cause aesthetically unpleasing tenosynovitis that usually responds to injections, but occasionally repair of synoviosynovial fistulae is necessary.

Chapter 24

Tenoscopy and Bursoscopy

Eddy R.J. Cauvin

References on page 1266

The advantages of arthroscopy as a diagnostic and therapeutic approach to joints[1] have prompted the development of applications for other synovial cavities (see Chapter 23). *Tenoscopy* is the term used to describe endoscopy of synovial tendon sheaths, usually using a rigid arthroscope.[2] *Bursoscopy* is used for endoscopy of bursae.

Tenoscopy has many advantages. Traditional approaches to tendon sheaths, requiring long incisions over highly mobile areas, are associated with substantial postoperative risks, including wound dehiscence and ascending sheath infection.[3] These techniques are invasive, time consuming, and offer limited visibility of tendovaginal structures.[2,3] Endoscopic approaches to the carpal tunnel in people have been described[4,5] and have provided substantial improvements in terms of decreased morbidity, scarring, and loss of function compared with open techniques.[4,6] Tenoscopy in the horse was first described for the examination of the digital flexor tendon sheath (DFTS).[1,2] Since the early 1990s, other applications have been described.[7-11]

GENERAL PRINCIPLES OF TENOSCOPY AND BURSOSCOPY

Equipment

Standard arthroscopic equipment is used, including arthroscope, sleeve, and obturators; arthroscopic cannulae; probes; grasping forceps; and Ferris-Smith rongeurs. Sharp tenotomes, curettes, and meniscectomy scissors should also be available. A standard 4.0-mm, 25- to 35-degree forward angle arthroscopic endoscope is adequate for most sheaths and bursae, although thinner endoscopes may be useful for extensor sheaths. Light source and video camera apparatuses are as for arthroscopy. Motorized synovial resectors are particularly useful because debridement or synovectomy using hand-operated instruments can be tedious in large tendon sheaths.

Coblation technology (ArthroCare Corporation, Austin, Texas, United States) is a new technology that uses radiofrequency to vaporize soft tissues. I now use radiofrequency probes (Arthrowands, ArthroCare Corporation) to remove proliferative synovial tissue and masses, and a hook radiofrequency blade (Saber 30, ArthroCare Corporation) to carry out annular or retinaculum desmotomy. An added advantage is improved hemostasis.

Surgical Principles and Techniques

The basic principles of arthroscopy are also valid in tendon sheaths and bursae (see Chapter 23). The sheath usually is distended with fluids to facilitate insertion of the cannula. However, this is not necessary for the carpal and tarsal sheaths, which are not approached through distended pouches.[9,10] It is generally recommended that the portal be created with a scalpel and the cannula inserted using a blunt, conical obturator to avoid damaging the tendons. A thorough knowledge of the normal endoscopic anatomy of the sheath is paramount for several reasons. First, all the surfaces are covered by synovium and look alike, making identification of the structures difficult. Second, normal anatomical structures such as vinculae and plicae (adhesion-like formations carrying blood vessels to the tendon from the parietal sheath), endotendon (reflection of the synovial membrane, which forms a continuous band attaching the tendon to the sheath along its length), and synovial folds are apparent. These should not be damaged because they participate in the blood supply of tendons within the sheathed portion.[12-14]

Triangulation techniques are applied for instruments using separate portals. These should be created as close as possible to the lesion, although the shape of the sheath often dictates the position of the portals. The longitudinal arrangement of the sheaths and tunnel-like enclosures within retinacula often make triangulation difficult; therefore it may be useful to perform retinaculum desmotomy to improve access to some lesions, or to create instrument portals so that instruments are inserted opposite and toward the endoscope lens.

TENOSCOPY

Tenoscopy of the Digital Flexor Tendon Sheath

The DFTS is the most common site of tenosynovitis. Endoscopy is indicated as a diagnostic procedure to examine lesions of the surfaces of the deep digital flexor tendon (DDFT), superficial digital flexor tendon (SDFT), and parietal surface of the sheath. High-definition ultrasonography allows noninvasive examination of the sheath, its contents, and peripheral tissues, and provides more accurate information about the internal architecture of tendons.[15] However, differentiating some adhesions, tears, and superficial fraying of the tendons may be difficult ultrasonographically.[16-19] Tenoscopy is useful for debridement of masses, such as proliferative (villonodular) synovitis-like lesions and other lesions within the sheath, adhesiolysis, removal of debris, and synovectomy in infectious tenosynovitis.[2,19,20] A technique for desmotomy of the palmar annular ligament under endoscopic control has been described to avoid inadvertent damage to the tendons, manica flexoria, and other peritendovaginal structures.[21]

The advantages of tenoscopy over traditional open surgery are similar to those recognized for arthroscopy over arthrotomy. They include decreased morbidity and more rapid return to normal function of the sheath and reduced risks of complications, such as wound breakdown, infection, fibrosis, and ankylosis.

Anatomy

The DFTS is organized primarily around the DDFT, which it completely surrounds from the junction between the third and distal quarters of the metacarpal or metatarsal region to the level of the proximal interphalangeal joint, before tapering dorsally to the DDFT to the proximal border of the distal sesamoid bone.[12,13,15,22] At the level of the metacarpophalangeal joint, the DFTS also surrounds the SDFT, except for a wide mesotendon over the palmar/plantar aspect of the tendon. At this level the DFTS is bound dorsally by the proximal scutum, a fibrocartilage covering the palmar (plantar) surfaces of the proximal sesamoid bones (PSBs) and intersesamoidean ligament, and palmarly by a tough transverse ligament, the palmar (plantar) annular ligament (PAL), thus forming a nonelastic canal through which both digital flexor tendons run independently. In the pastern region the SDFT separates into two branches and is no longer within the DFTS. The DFTS is bound dorsally by the distal sesamoidean ligaments and palmarly (plantarly) by two broad digital annular ligaments.

The proximal pouch bulges when distended proximal to the PAL and PSBs and contains a number of long villi in normal horses. Several small, subcutaneous pouches appear between the insertions of the PAL and digital annular ligaments abaxially and over the palmar (plantar) aspect of the DDFT in the midpastern region. A number of vascular structures are found, including two large vinculae forming a V-shaped adhesion-like structure between the dorsal surface of the DDFT and the dorsal sheath wall in the proximal pastern. Densely packed villi often are found in that area. The wide palmar mesotendon prevents examination of the palmar aspect of the SDFT in the fetlock region. Immediately proximal to this level, the manica flexoria forms a smooth, thin membrane originating from the axial surfaces of the SDFT and surrounding the DDFT dorsally.

Surgical Technique

The technique for tenoscopic exploration of the DFTS has been described in detail.[2] The term *palmar* is used in the following description for either palmar or plantar. The horse may be placed in lateral recumbency with the affected limb uppermost for a lateral approach or lowermost for a medial approach. The choice of a lateral or medial portal is dictated by the site of the suspected lesion. However, if no definite lesion has been observed ultrasonographically and if a potential tear is suspected, the horse is best placed in dorsal recumbency with the limb attached to a frame or hoist so that the digit is in slight flexion. This decreases hemorrhage during the procedure. An Esmarch bandage and tourniquet may also be used.

The DFTS is distended with 10 to 20 mL of physiological solution through a needle inserted in the palmar aspect of the midpastern region. Overdistention of the DFTS is avoided because it causes flexion of the digit. A 5-mm longitudinal incision is made through the skin, immediately distal to the PAL, lateral or medial to the DDFT, and 0.5 to 1 cm palmar to the neurovascular bundle, which must be carefully avoided. A stab incision is made into the DFTS, taking care to avoid damaging the DDFT, and the cannula, with a conical obturator inserted in a proximal direction, between the DDFT and dorsal sheath wall (Figure 24-1). The DFTS is lavaged through an 18-gauge needle inserted in the proximal pouch. The obturator is replaced with the endoscope, and examination is carried out from proximal to the level of the portal by rotation and gradual

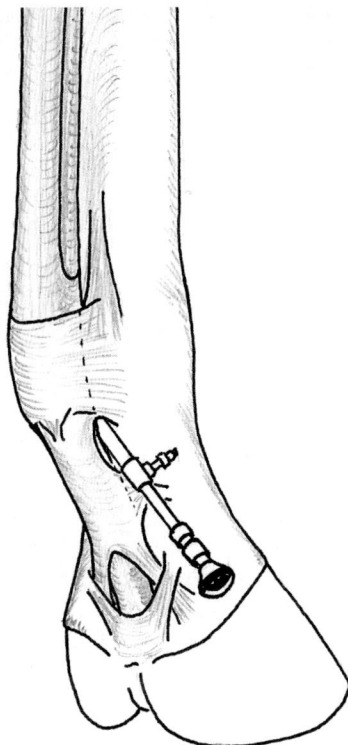

Fig. 24-1 • Digital sheath tenoscopy. The arthroscope is inserted lateral to the deep digital flexor tendon, immediately distal to the palmar annular ligament.

withdrawal. The proximal pouch is examined, followed by the abaxial aspects of the two tendons. Flexion of the fetlock joint allows insertion of the endoscope between the SDFT and DDFT without damage to the manica flexoria. The endoscope is finally rotated around the SDFT on the side of the portal to inspect the mesotendon. Examination of the opposite side is made possible by flexion of the fetlock and rotation of the arthroscope window palmarly.

The endoscope is then pushed across the DFTS, between the DDFT and dorsal sheath wall, to avoid exiting the DFTS. The endoscope is then redirected distally. The distal part of the DFTS is examined by gradual withdrawal of the endoscope. The vinculae are visible in the proximal pastern region, between the dorsal surface of the DDFT and dorsal wall (Figure 24-2). Palmarly and farther distally, bifurcation of the SDFT branches forms a manica-like ring around the DDFT (Figure 24-3).

Debridement of potential lesions is carried out through separate instrument portals made as close as possible to the lesion to allow for adequate triangulation. At the end of surgery the DFTS is lavaged through a large-bore cannula, and the skin incisions are closed. It is recommended that a pressure bandage be applied for 2 weeks postoperatively. In horses with infection with substantial debris accumulation, it is possible to place a drain, exiting in the distal palmar recess through a separate incision. A drainage portal may also be created in the distal palmar aspect of the DFTS to allow for continuous drainage postoperatively. The incision is then left to heal by contraction and epithelialization.

A technique for transection (desmotomy) of the PAL under endoscopic guidance was described,[18,20] using a

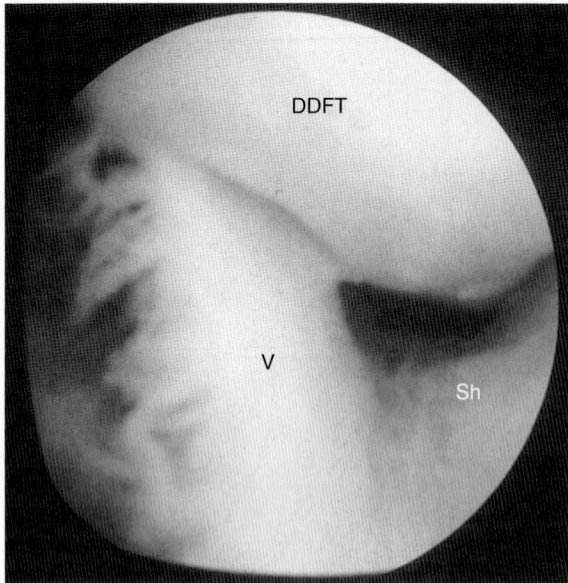

Fig. 24-2 • Tenoscopic view of the dorsal aspect of the deep digital flexor tendon *(DDFT)* in the proximal pastern region, showing one of the vinculae *(V)* between the DDFT and dorsal wall *(Sh)* of the digital flexor tendon sheath.

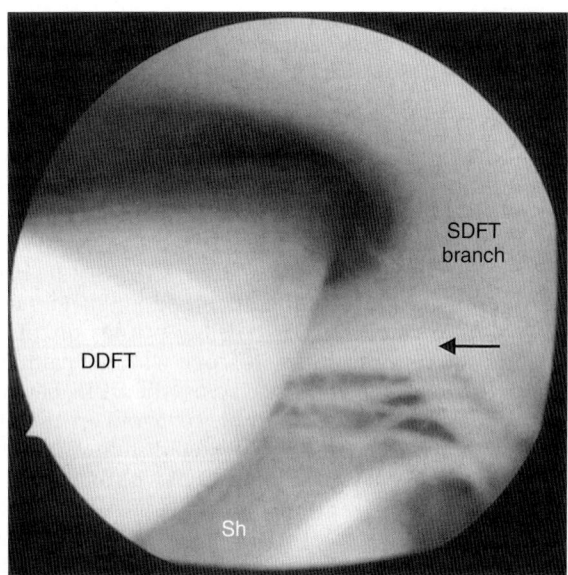

Fig. 24-3 • Tenoscopic view of the palmar aspect of the deep digital flexor tendon *(DDFT)* in the proximal pastern region, showing the manica-like ring *(arrow)* surrounding the DDFT, between the two superficial digital flexor tendon *(SDFT)* branches (within the abaxial sheath walls). The dorsal wall *(Sh)* of the digital flexor tendon sheath is rich in long villi.

desmotomy kit designed for palmar carpal ligament transection in people.[4,5] This permits adequate examination of the DFTS before PAL transection and prevents inadvertent damage to the tendons and manica flexoria. Although the use of a specific cannula facilitates the procedure, I use a grooved director for the same purpose. A radiofrequency hook blade (Saber 30, ArthroCare Corporation) facilitates the technique because there is minimal hemorrhage and less risk of inadvertent damage to peripheral structures and tendons during insertion and manipulation of the knife.

I have used an alternative technique for digital tenoscopy using an endoscopic portal made proximal to the PAL and dorsolateral to the DDFT. This technique allows adequate examination of the entire DFTS, is useful to examine lesions in the proximal phalangeal region, and provides improved triangulation when surgically treating such lesions. Using a wound as an initial endoscopic portal is often possible, although creating a new endoscope portal and using the wound for instruments is usually preferable after examination is completed.

Postoperative Care
At the end of surgery the DFTS is emptied of fluid and the skin portals are closed with staples or sutures of the surgeon's choice. Damage to the neurovascular bundle by needles and sutures is carefully avoided. The horse recovers with the limb in a pressure bandage from the foot to the distal aspect of the carpus (or tarsus) to prevent DFTS swelling and to reduce motion. Postoperative antibiotics are only necessary in horses with infectious tenosynovitis, but systemic nonsteroidal antiinflammatory drugs (NSAIDs) should be given for several days after surgery. The horse should be restricted to box rest for 3 days, and then it may be walked out in hand to decrease restrictive adhesion formation. Box stall rest with controlled exercise should be continued for 2 weeks until the sutures are removed, and then at the surgeon's discretion exercise is increased progressively. Hyaluronan has been advocated as an adjunctive therapy[2,17] but should be avoided if infection is present. Passive limb motion with repeated flexion/extension of the fetlock helps reduce stiffness in the initial stages. Cold hosing of the limb is useful to decrease potential swelling and hemorrhage after handwalking.

TARSAL SHEATH
Injuries to the tarsal sheath are relatively common (see Chapter 76). Open surgery has been associated with a high rate of postoperative complications,[3,10,24] but early results indicate that the morbidity may be greatly reduced with tenoscopy.[10]

Anatomy
The tarsal sheath is the sheath of the lateral digital flexor tendon (LDFT), the largest of the two tendons (lateral and medial digital flexor tendons), the fusion of which in the proximal metatarsal region forms the DDFT (see Chapter 76).[10,22,25] It is paramount to recognize the anatomical location of the plantar nerves and vessels that pass within the plantar flexor retinaculum and the presence of a continuous mesotendon, passing longitudinally along the plantaromedial aspect of the LDFT. However, accidental damage to these structures does not appear to have major consequences.

Surgical Technique
A technique allowing examination of the entire tarsal sheath has been described.[10] Previous distention of the tarsal sheath is not necessary. The medial edge of the sustentaculum tali and medial insertion of the retinaculum are located, and an 8-mm vertical incision is made in the skin and underlying fascia, 8 mm plantar to the edge of the bone at the point where the tendon changes direction

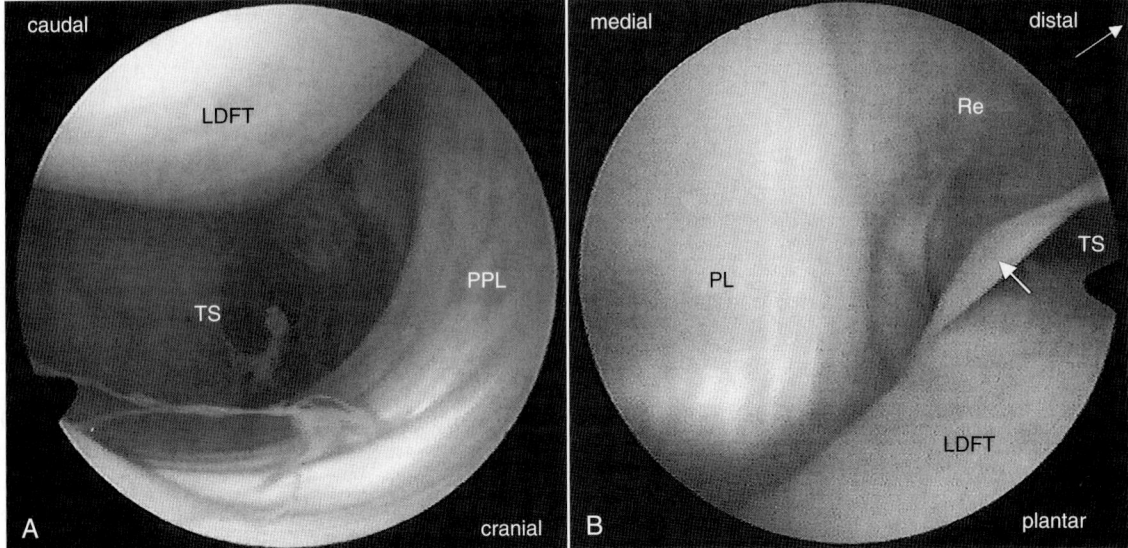

Fig. 24-4 • Tenoscopic views of the tarsal sheath. **A,** Proximal pouch of the tarsal sheath *(TS)* showing the cranial aspect of the lateral digital flexor tendon *(LDFT)* and the proximal plantar ligament *(PPL)* thickening of the plantar capsule of the tarsocrural joint. **B,** Distal recess of the tarsal sheath *(TS)*. At the tarsometatarsal joint, the end of the plantar ligament *(PL)* is visible. A synovial fold *(white arrow)* forms a small recess dorsomedially *(Re)*.

over the sustentaculum tali. The absence of blood vessels in the retinaculum deep to the incision is ascertained using hypodermic needles before making a 5-mm stab incision through the retinaculum. Care is taken to avoid damage to the underlying LDFT. The endoscope sleeve and conical, blunt obturator are inserted dorsal to the LDFT in a proximal direction. The obturator is replaced with an endoscope; the tarsal sheath is distended moderately with fluid; and examination is carried out as described for the DFTS by rotation of the window of the arthroscope and gradual withdrawal. After examination of the proximal half of the tarsal sheath, the endoscope is redirected into the distal pouch. The proximal pouch is large and lined by a thin wall (Figure 24-4, *A*). Muscle fibers from the lateral digital flexor muscle and separate head of the tibialis caudalis muscle may be seen by transillumination through the synovial membrane. Within the tight, rigid canal formed by the sustentaculum tali and retinaculum, the fibrocartilage appears glistening white, and small vessels are seen within the parietal membrane plantarly and in the mesotendon. In the distal half of the tarsal sheath, a fold of synovial membrane forming a small, blind pouch medially is seen dorsomedial to the LDFT at the level of the tarsometatarsal joint (Figure 24-4, *B*). Distal to this fold, the tarsal sheath continues as a cylindrical, blind recess dorsal to the tendon and contains small villi. The separate sheath of the medial digital flexor tendon is not visible from the tarsal sheath.

If a wound exists, most commonly at the plantaromedial edge of the sustentaculum tali, it may be used as an endoscope portal. Instruments may be inserted as required close to lesions to allow for triangulation. Needles are used to determine the optimal location for the instrument portal.

Carpal Sheath

Tenosynovitis of the carpal flexor tendon sheath (carpal sheath) is relatively rare in horses but can cause severe lameness associated with carpal canal syndrome (see Chapter 75). Wounds leading to contamination of the carpal sheath are rare but possible. Common causes of non-infectious tenosynovitis include lesions of the SDFT in the carpal region, fractured accessory carpal bone, osteochondromata of the caudal distal aspect of the radius, exostoses of the caudal perimeter of the distal radial physis, and sprain injuries to the carpal sheath,[26-28] although other causes may exist.[29] Effusion may be secondary to lesions outside the carpal sheath, such as desmitis of the accessory ligament of the DDFT (ALDDFT), accessory ligament of the SDFT (ALSDFT), limb edema, and unassociated wounds. Ultrasonography is the technique of choice for investigating carpal sheath distention, but adhesions and subtle fraying of the tendons may not be visible.[28,30] Radiography is also mandatory to rule out fractures, exostoses, and osteochondromata.[27-29,31]

Tenoscopy may be useful as a diagnostic tool if lameness is associated with pain localized to the carpal sheath by intrathecal analgesia but where no lesions are visible with other imaging methods. The main indication for tenoscopy of the carpal sheath is debridement and repair of structures within the sheath or transection of the ALSDFT.

Anatomy

The anatomy of the carpal sheath has been described elsewhere in detail.[14,21,30] Briefly, the carpal sheath is organized around the DDFT from the distal caudal aspect of the antebrachium, 4 to 7 cm proximal to the accessory carpal bone, to the metacarpal region. The carpal sheath extends around the DDFT and SDFT in the carpal region, where it is enclosed within a tight canal (the carpal canal) formed by a thick palmar carpal flexor retinaculum palmarly and medially, the accessory carpal bone laterally, and the palmar carpal ligament dorsally. At this level the SDFT is attached palmarly to the sheath wall by a thick mesotendon that contains the median artery and medial palmar nerve. A thinner mesotendon links the DDFT to the SDFT medially. Proximal to the carpal canal a large pouch occurs dorsal to the flexor muscles, bulging laterally and medially caudal to the radius if distended. Distal to the carpometacarpal joint the carpal sheath continues as a blind sack between the DDFT and ALDDFT and bulges dorsolaterally to the DDFT in the proximal third of the metacarpal area. The lateral palmar nerve and palmar veins pass within the retinaculum.

Surgical Technique

Several techniques have been described depending on the lesions identified before surgery. Removal of osteochondromata from the caudal distal aspect of the radius has been described using a lateral approach through the distended proximal pouch.[8,33] The horse is anesthetized and placed either in lateral recumbency with the affected limb uppermost or in dorsal recumbency with the foot attached to a hoist, so that carpal position may be altered during the procedure. This latter position decreases hemorrhage, which may substantially decrease visibility. The carpal sheath is distended with 40 to 60 mL of balanced electrolyte solution, and the endoscopic portal is made between the lateral digital extensor and ulnaris lateralis tendons, 3.5 cm proximal to the distal radial physeal scar. The cannula and blunt obturator are inserted proximomedially into the carpal sheath. The instrument portal is made on the same side as the arthroscope portal, 2 cm distal to it. A medial approach has also been described but appears less practical because of the presence of the ALSDFT and the median nerve and artery.[7]

This lateral proximal approach is generally recommended for desmotomy of the ALSDFT and removal of osteochondromata or caudal radial physeal exostoses. Desmotomy of the ALSDFT is carried out easily via tenoscopy.[32,33] This approach offers several advantages over the standard "open" medial approach: postoperative swelling is decreased, and the incidence of wound breakdown or seroma is nearly abolished. Intrathecal hemorrhage seems to be better tolerated than with the standard approach. Hence return to training is dramatically shortened (4 to 6 weeks). After insertion of the cannula through a portal 2.5 to 3 cm proximal to the distal radial physeal scar as described above, an instrument portal is created immediately proximal and caudal to the palpable physeal scar. The ALSDFT is easily identified by palpation with a blunt arthroscopic probe. In some horses, I use intraoperative ultrasonographic guidance to place needles at the proximal and distal borders of the ligament at the level of the flexor carpi radialis tendon. This also permits identification of the median artery and the small transverse artery, which are best avoided to reduce perioperative hemorrhage. The needles are used as landmarks for desmotomy. I use a radiofrequency hook blade (Saber 30, ArthroCare Corporation) as described for annular desmotomy, but the technique may also be performed using an arthroscopic hook blade, a tenotomy knife, or a No. 15 scalpel blade on a long No. 3 handle. After identifying the distal edge of the ligament, section is commenced at that level in a proximal direction and through the ligament until the sheath of the flexor carpi radialis tendon is entered. The section is continued proximally. The proximal quarter to third of the ligament is located outside the proximal boundaries of the carpal sheath, and this is where the transverse artery may

be inadvertently severed. The radial head of the DDFT is reclined dorsally with the endoscope, and the desmotomy is continued until all identifiable fibers are severed. Using the coagulation setting on the coblation device during the procedure helps avoid hemorrhage. When the section is completed, the cut ends of the ligament separate, showing the large communication with the flexor carpi radialis sheath. There may be tremendous postoperative swelling of the carpal sheath and the flexor carpi radialis sheath; therefore it is recommended that a pressure bandage be placed over the carpal area (see below).

These techniques do not permit examination of the distal half of the carpal sheath. Therefore another technique has been developed to facilitate endoscopic examination of most of the carpal sheath.[9] The horse may be placed in lateral recumbency with the affected limb uppermost or in dorsal recumbency with the affected limb suspended loosely, so that the carpus is slightly flexed. An 8-mm longitudinal skin incision is made without previous distention of the carpal sheath 1.5 to 2 cm distal to the distal border of the accessory carpal bone along the lateral aspect of the DDFT. A medial approach is not recommended because examination is restricted by the mesotendons and the risk of injury to the median artery and medial palmar nerve. A needle is used to ensure that no vessels are present in the fascia deep to the incision. The incision is extended with a scalpel through the fascia into the carpal sheath. The arthroscope is inserted proximally, between the DDFT and dorsal wall of the sheath. The proximal pouch is large and contains small villi. The radial head of the DDFT forms a conical prominence in the medial aspect of this pouch. Rotation of the endoscope and manipulation around the tendons allow examination of the DDFT and SDFT surfaces, caudal surface of the distal radius, and fibrocartilaginous sheath wall in the carpal canal. Minimal fluid pressure should be used to avoid flexion of the carpus. The endoscope may be inserted between the tendons to view the surfaces and the lateral aspect of the mesotendon, covered by short, thin villi. Redirecting the endoscope distally permits examination of the distal recess. A normal, longitudinal synovial fold appears dorsomedially in the carpal sheath in the distal carpal region. Instrument portals are made where necessary to allow for adequate triangulation.

Improved triangulation is obtained for removal of osteochondromata of the distal caudal radius with this method, although the endoscope may occasionally be too short.

Desmotomy of the carpal palmar retinaculum has been advocated for carpal canal syndrome associated with constriction syndrome or functional carpal ankylosis. The technique may be performed using tenoscopy.[35] I use electrosurgery because hemorrhage is often marked, particularly because there is frequently substantial concurrent synovial swelling.

Postoperative care is similar to that described for other sheaths, but postoperative hemorrhage and swelling are very common in the carpal sheath. It may not be practical to apply a pressure bandage for any length of time over the carpus. I usually apply a pressure bandage for recovery from general anesthesia and then replace it after the horse stands. The limb remains bandaged for only 48 hours because of the risk of pressure sores. The horse must be restricted to stall rest for at least 2 to 3 weeks.

Other Tendon Sheaths

Most tendon sheaths may be examined by tenoscopy, including extensor tendon sheaths in the dorsal carpal and tarsal regions. However, no published reports indicate the use of tenoscopy for these smaller synovial cavities, possibly because acceptable results have been obtained with traditional surgical exposure.[36] I have attempted tenoscopy of the carpal extensor sheaths experimentally in isolated limbs, using a 4-mm, 30-degree forward endoscope inserted medially or laterally to the tendons, proximal to the carpus. This technique provides acceptable examination of the sheath and tendon surfaces, but little movement is possible because of the tight extensor retinacula.

BURSOSCOPY

Reports of bursoscopy in horses are limited,[11,37] but it is probable that the technique would yield similar advantages to tenoscopy in horses with masses or infection in normal or acquired bursae. Surgical exposure and debridement of hygromas, capped hocks, and metacarpophalangeal subtendonous bursae are often associated with wound dehiscence and chronic infection.[38] However, I am unaware of published data describing bursoscopic examination in these locations. A technique for bursoscopy of the calcaneal bursa of the SDFT has been described and advocated for diagnosis and treatment of injuries to this structure and is probably most useful in horses with infectious bursitis.[37]

Bursoscopy of the Intertubercular Bursa

Bursoscopic surgery has been used for the management of infectious intertubercular (bicipital) bursitis,[39] and a report describes its use as a diagnostic method in a horse with traumatic bicipital bursitis.[11] The horse is placed in lateral recumbency with the affected limb uppermost. The endoscope is introduced through a craniolateral skin portal, made over the point of the shoulder, immediately cranial to the lateral (greater) tubercle of the humerus. The bicipital bursa is distended with 40 mL of fluid. The skin incision is continued through the brachiocephalicus muscle and into the bicipital bursa, and the endoscope sleeve and conical obturator are inserted in a caudoproximal direction. A technique using two separate portals has been described to improve visibility.[40] The first portal is made into the distal recess through an incision immediately proximal to the deltoid tuberosity. For the second portal, an incision is made cranioproximal to the lateral humeral tubercle to view the proximal half of the bicipital bursa. Experience with these techniques is currently limited, but they should provide similar advantages to tenoscopy, including easier access to the bicipital bursa, improved visibility, and decreased postoperative morbidity. This needs to be confirmed by more extensive reviews.

Bursoscopy of the Navicular Bursa

Endoscopic examination of the navicular bursa (bursa podotrochlearis)[41] recently has been described as an alternative to the traditional street-nail procedure.[42,43] It is the technique of choice for treating infectious navicular bursitis.

The main indication for navicular bursoscopy is for management of a contaminated or infected bursa.[41] Other indications include diagnostic examination in horses with pain localized to the palmar aspect of the foot but with no lesions identifiable using other imaging modalities and the debridement of adhesions between the navicular bone and the dorsal surface of the DDFT.[44]

Surgical Technique

The technique has been described elsewhere.[41,44-46] Standard arthroscopic equipment is used, although a thinner, 4-mm diameter or less, endoscope is more practical. The horse is placed in lateral recumbency with the metacarpal or metatarsal region supported and the digit moving loosely. A medial approach with the affected limb lowermost or a lateral approach with the limb uppermost may be used. A vertical, 5-mm skin incision is made along the abaxial border of the DDFT, 1 cm proximal to the cartilage of the foot, and palmar/plantar to the neurovascular bundle. The cannula, with a conical obturator, is inserted distally and slightly axially, dorsal to the DDFT. The obturator is replaced with the endoscope. Rotation of the endoscope allows examination of the entire proximal recess of the navicular bursa and sometimes the distal recess, including the smooth dorsal aspect of the DDFT and palmar fibrocartilage of the navicular bone. The collateral sesamoidean ligaments, blending over the proximal surface of the navicular bone into the fibrocartilage and the distal sesamoidean impar ligament, in the distal recess of the navicular bursa, are covered by synovium with thin villi. The larger proximal pouch and the T-ligament are also covered by synovium.

A wound in the sole, sulci, or frog can be used for insertion of cannulae or instruments into the navicular bursa. Some enlargement of the tract using curettes or a motorized synovial resector may be required but should be minimal to limit damage to the DDFT. If access through the wound is difficult, or to reach a lesion that cannot be accessed this way, a similar approach to that used for the endoscope may be made on the opposite side of the limb.

The navicular bursa is lavaged, and any lesions are debrided sharply. Partial synovectomy may be carried out if necessary. The use of motorized synovial resectors is recommended. At the end of the procedure the opening of a sinus tract on the solar surface of the foot may be enlarged and debrided to avoid abscess formation. Debridement of the defect through the DDFT should be minimal. An aminoglycoside antibiotic may be placed in the navicular bursa, and the skin incisions are closed routinely. A bandage including the whole hoof and extending to the proximal metacarpal or metatarsal region is applied.

Postoperative Management and Results

Postoperative use of antibiotics and NSAIDs is at the surgeon's discretion. The horse can be walked out in hand after 2 or 3 days, and exercise can be gradually resumed after healing of the wound is complete, in the absence of complications.

Complications of infection include recurrence, extension of the infection into adjacent synovial structures, and osteitis or fracture of the navicular bone.[41,43] Contamination of the distal interphalangeal joint or DFTS may be treated during the initial surgery by an endoscopic approach using the same skin portal.[41] If infection recurs, lavage through needles or bursoscopy may be performed, and an open approach through the solar surface may be used, but the prognosis should then be considered graver.

The prognosis for horses with infectious navicular bursitis using this approach[41] appears to be greatly improved compared with the more invasive street-nail procedure.[43] Seventy-five percent of horses returned to the initial use after bursoscopy versus 31.5% using the open technique, although the criteria used to judge success may be slightly different.[41] Bursoscopy is considered to be the technique of choice for infectious navicular bursitis, although I recommend using a street-nail approach for the salvage of horses with chronic bursitis with extensive damage to the podotrochlear structures.

Chapter 25

Thermography: Use in Equine Lameness

Andrew P. Bathe

References on page 1267

Infrared thermography has been used in equine orthopedics for a number of years.[1] Improvements in imaging quality and technology now yield images that are easier to interpret. The systems are also more cost effective. Thermography pictorially represents the surface temperature of an object and is a noninvasive method of detecting superficial inflammation and thus can have a role in lameness diagnosis. It is a physiological imaging modality, as is gamma scintigraphy, and thus has a lower reproducibility than anatomical imaging modalities such as radiography and ultrasonography. Superficial blood flow is a dynamic system and is likely to be variable and is also prone to artifacts, which has led some people to doubt its clinical applicability. Others consider it useful in the diagnosis of a large number of diverse conditions.[2] With experience and care in interpretation, thermography can be a useful adjunct to lameness evaluation, as part of an integrated clinical and imaging approach. Eddy and co-workers reported a 63% correlation among thermographic findings in 64 horses and ultrasonography, nuclear scintigraphy, and radiography.[3]

Heat is lost through the skin by radiation, convection, conduction, and evaporation.[4] Thermal cameras assess infrared radiation from an object; this is optically focused, collected, and transformed by detector arrays into an electronic signal that in modern systems then generates a real-time video image. The skin and hoof derive their heat from tissue metabolism and local circulation, and because the former is generally constant, variation in superficial temperature normally relates to changes in local tissue perfusion. Radiation from the equine foot and limb is more important than reflection, and lighting levels are not a major concern. Thermographic evaluation of the foot and distal aspect of the limb is complicated by the thermoregulatory role of the distal aspect of the limb, whereby the blood supply can be dramatically reduced to conserve heat in cold conditions.[5] Thus an understanding of the physiology of the distal aspect of the limb is essential for optimal image interpretation.

Several different thermal imaging systems are available. Older systems were primarily developed for military or industrial applications and are relatively cumbersome and have poor image quality. The top-end systems have a cooling system to ensure temperature stability of the detector, and this increases the fragility of the system and the maintenance costs. Uncooled camera technology is preferable in a veterinary environment because it is cheaper, lighter, and more robust. These systems have become more available recently, and the system cost for diagnostic-quality thermographic imaging is no longer prohibitive. There is still wide variation in the image quality among different systems, and it can be difficult to compare different systems, but the user becomes used to the particular thermal patterns produced by each machine. Some systems are also radiometers and allow an accurate temperature measurement to be obtained, whereas other systems do not measure the absolute temperature but are able to determine the difference between two areas within the same image. Although a radiometer is not essential, it does assist in comparisons among different examinations. Higher image quality leads to a greater ease of interpretation of the image. The quality of image processing software is also improving, but the majority of interpretation is carried out in real time. Images can be stored in a variety of digital formats for archiving and later comparison. Infrared thermographic instrumentation is far more sensitive than human hands in detecting temperature changes in an object. There may be variability of up to 1° C attributed to the camera in clinical imaging,[6] and differences of over 1° C are normally deemed as being potentially clinically significant in image interpretation.

IMAGE ACQUISITION

Imaging should be performed in a relatively bare room without radiant heat sources, drafts, or sunlight. Some clinicians recommend allowing the horse to thermally equilibrate in the environment in which it is to be imaged. Equilibration can take up to 1 hour, but although the absolute temperature changes, there is little change in the relative thermal pattern.[6] Thus equilibration is not necessary for clinical imaging. The optimal ambient temperature for imaging is 20° to 25° C. Below this temperature the distal aspect of the limbs are more prone to thermal cutoff,[5,7] and above this range the contrast between the horse and the background is lost. Thus in colder temperate climates it can be advantageous to have a "hot box" to raise the ambient temperature if thermal cutoff prevents diagnostic imaging. It can also be advantageous to image the feet after the horse has been trotted and lunged, which increases the

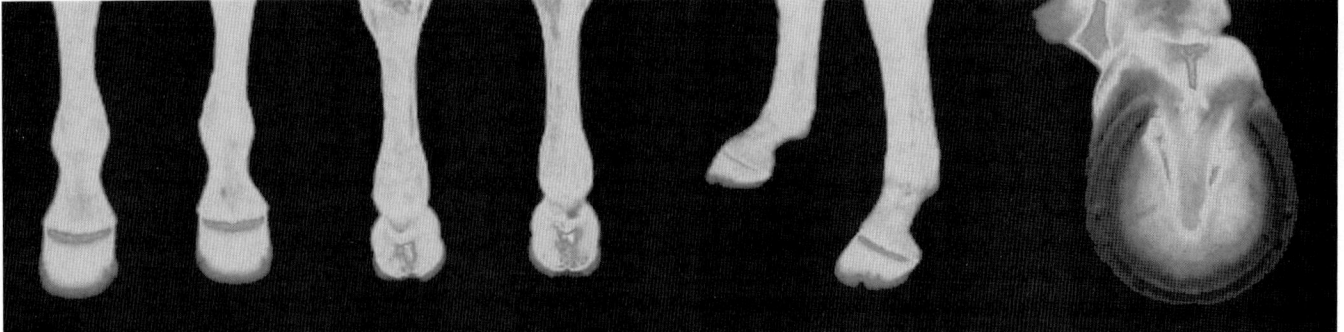

Fig. 25-1 • Normal dorsal, palmar, left lateral, and solar thermographic images of the distal aspect of the forelimbs of a horse. There is good symmetry between the limbs. The coronary band is the warmest area, and the rest of the hoof becomes colder in a regular pattern closer to the ground surface. The palmar image shows a normal increase in heat between the heel bulbs. On the solar image there is a V-shaped pattern of increased heat representing the sulci of the frog.

blood supply to the limbs and hence increases the inherent contrast of the digit relative to the background.

A long hair coat acts as an insulator and reduces the contrast within the image. Irregular patterns of clipping, topical applications, and dirt can complicate interpretation of images. Bandages and rugs should be removed at least 20 minutes before imaging. The feet should be clean for thermographic imaging of the digit and should be picked out and brushed to remove external contamination.

The distal aspect of the limb should be imaged from a dorsal position, from a palmar or plantar direction, and from the left and right sides. The limbs are then lifted, and a solar view is obtained of the feet (Figure 25-1; Color Plate 1). The joints of the proximal aspect of the limbs should be imaged cranially and laterally. The neck is imaged from the side. The back and hindquarters should be imaged as dorsally as is possible. Close-up images of regions of interest can then be performed if necessary. Comparisons should be made between sides; it can be helpful to repeat the imaging on another occasion if the results are uncertain.

It is normally most intuitive to image using a rainbow color palette, with as great a range of color depth as the system allows. There is variability in the absolute temperature of the distal aspect of the limb; therefore the thermal range should be adjusted for each individual horse. The coronary band is normally the warmest area within the image, reflecting its high vascularity. The temperature level and span of the camera are adjusted to use the whole color range for the image. The coronary band normally appears white, and the coldest part of the image is blue or black, thus maximizing the visual contrast within the image. Some cameras have an automatic setting that constantly readjusts the image in this way. This does not allow comparison of left-to-right symmetry and thus is not useful clinically.

The camera should be carefully focused, and a series of still images obtained. The absolute temperature of points of interest can be determined using a radiometer so that absolute temperature differences can be calculated. Some systems allow more detailed analysis of the images on a computer, including calculation of mean temperature within regions of interest or graphically along lines of interest. The software tends to be expensive, and there is a greater need for such images in research than in a clinical setting.

CLINICAL IMAGING

Figure 25-1 demonstrates a series of normal images of the distal aspect of the limb and digit. The coronary band is the warmest part of the image, and the hoof becomes progressively cooler toward the ground surface. The bulbs of the heel are also warm. On the solar image, the frog sulci appear warmest, as there is less tissue depth in this area. Heat generally follows the pattern of blood vessels so the medial metacarpal region is normally warmer than the lateral. Ideally the limbs appear symmetrical, but there can be variation in normal horses, especially at low ambient temperatures.[4,5] Thermoregulatory cutoff is variable, and there are intermittent periods of vasodilatation, which is not necessarily symmetrical between left and right[4] nor front and hind feet. Reevaluation of the horse some hours later may yield a different image. Exercising the horse for approximately 20 minutes or administering vasodilators such as acepromazine can increase the temperature to allow diagnostic imaging. Thermoregulatory cutoff in the distal aspect of the limb dramatically reduces the temperature and thus the contrast; therefore, subtle lesions may be missed. However, severe inflammation causes a sufficiently increased blood flow to be detectable.

Thermography is sensitive at detecting the presence of superficial inflammation within the foot, and in my opinion this is one of the more useful areas to image clinically.[8] Conditions such as subsolar or coronary band infections result in a marked increase in temperature; corns and subsolar bruising may also be associated with increased temperature. Horses with chronic palmar foot pain and navicular syndrome do not show superficial inflammation and have either normal thermographic patterns or a colder pattern than normal, especially in the heel region. The temperature in the heel does not increase after the horse is exercised,[6,7] probably because of a decrease of loading in this area rather than inherent ischemic disease. Superficial foot inflammation can obviously be diagnosed clinically without thermographic imaging in the majority of horses. Thermography is helpful in horses for which there is the suspicion of deep pathology, but also for those with mild signs of inflammation and response to hoof testers. Thermography can be helpful in optimizing the efficiency of a lameness evaluation, especially close to competition and in an extremely fractious horse, where it is advantageous

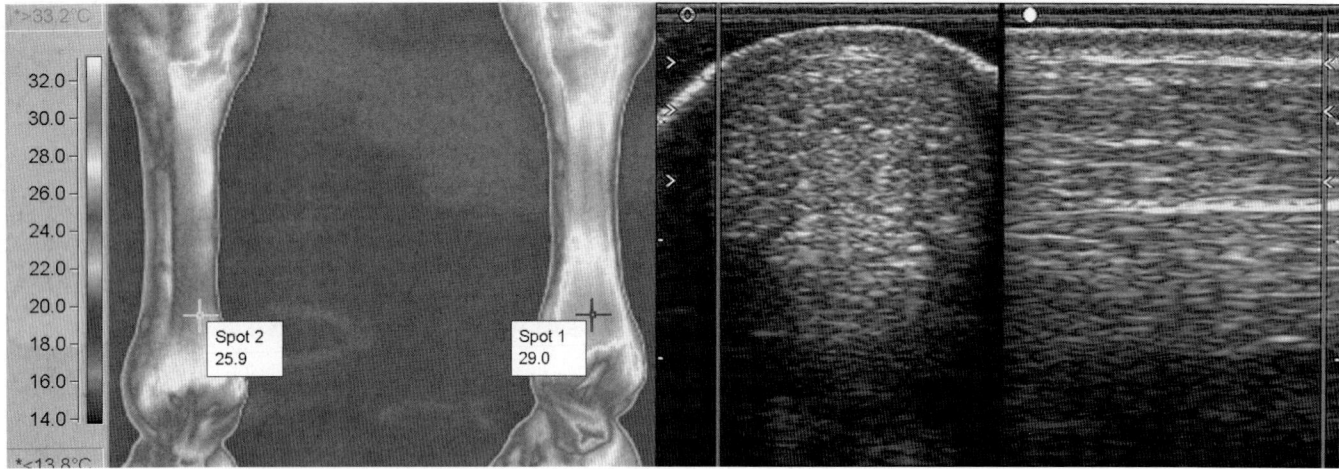

Fig. 25-2 • An advanced event horse with previous history of midbody superficial digital flexor tendonitis of the right forelimb. More recently peritendonous edema had developed distally in the right forelimb. Ultrasonographic images show increased cross-sectional area of the superficial digital flexor tendon, and areas of hyperechogenicity and hypoechogenicity. It was not possible to determine if there was active pathology or if this was the level of healing that had been reached from the previous injury. The palmar thermographic image shows rectangular clip artifacts on both limbs. There is a clinically significant increase in temperature of the distal palmar aspect of the right forelimb compared with the left, indicating inflammation, and thus the image suggests recurrent tendon injury.

to minimize the amount of diagnostic local analgesia employed. Thermography can also be used to assess foot balance. When a horse with metal shoes is trotted on a hard surface and immediately imaged, the side taking the greatest load appears warmer when the shoe is imaged. In horses with substantial mediolateral imbalance that land lateral wall first and roll over to the medial side during weight bearing, there can be an increased temperature over the coronary band medially, rather than on the side that lands first.

Thermographic evaluation can also be useful in monitoring laminitis. In acute laminitis there is increased heat within the foot.[4] The normal gradation of temperature from the coronary band to the sole is lost as the temperature on the dorsal hoof wall approaches that of the coronary band. On solar images there may be an increased temperature in the region of the tip of the distal phalanx. In chronic laminitis there may be areas of decreased temperature in the dorsal aspects of the coronary band and the hoof wall, indicating decreased perfusion and laminar separation. This is a poor prognostic indicator.

Joints are best evaluated from the dorsal aspect and tend to be cool in comparison to surrounding tissues except where there are superficial vessels. Acute inflammation can occasionally give an increased heat pattern, but chronic pathology is not normally detectable. Early signs of joint inflammation can reportedly be detected 2 weeks before lameness resulting from osteoarthritis in Thoroughbred racehorses,[9] allowing modification of training regimens to decrease the risk of serious injury.

The superficial digital flexor tendon (SDFT) can be usefully imaged thermographically. The midportion of the tendon is bilaterally symmetrical, whereas the proximal and distal portions are reduced in temperature. The majority of horses with tendonitis have localizing clinical signs and ultrasonographic abnormalities. Thermography can be useful as a routine screening procedure when dealing with a large number of horses in training, to help identify

subclinical pathology (see Figure 117-5). It can also be useful in a horse with recurrent tendonitis, with preexisting ultrasonographic abnormalities, in which it is important to determine if there is inflammation and recurrent injury (Figure 25-2; Color Plate 2).

Ligaments are more difficult to image. The proximal aspect of the suspensory ligament is positioned deeply, and in my experience there is no characteristic thermal pattern associated with desmitis. The midbody of the suspensory ligament may have increased temperature if it is inflamed, and thermography can be useful to accurately localize inflammation in horses with complex pathology affecting the splint bone and/or suspensory ligament. Active suspensory branch desmitis may be detected thermographically.

The majority of long bones are covered in muscle and cannot be imaged thermographically. However, the dorsal aspect of the third metacarpal bone can be evaluated in horses with sore shins. Thermography may be useful for screening and for grading of severity of injury.[2]

Muscle inflammation can be identified as areas of increased temperature, although some acute injuries with edema appear cool[10] (Figure 25-3; Color Plate 3). This is clinically useful, as the clinical localization of muscle strains can be difficult. Look for a consistent left-right asymmetry.

The neck should be bilaterally symmetrical, with care taken that the camera settings are not altered between the two sides. It can be helpful to reevaluate the first side after assessing the contralateral side, to ensure that any differences are genuine. Some horses with cervical pathology have interference with the sympathetic outflow and may show increased superficial blood flow at the affected dermatomes (Figure 25-4; Color Plate 4). The back has a normal, central stripe of increased temperature. Imaging laterally is prone to artifacts, and the images should be obtained as far dorsally as possible from an elevated position behind the horse. Some people image using the reflection from a stainless steel mirror positioned at an angle above the horse. The diagnosis of neck and back lesions is controversial.

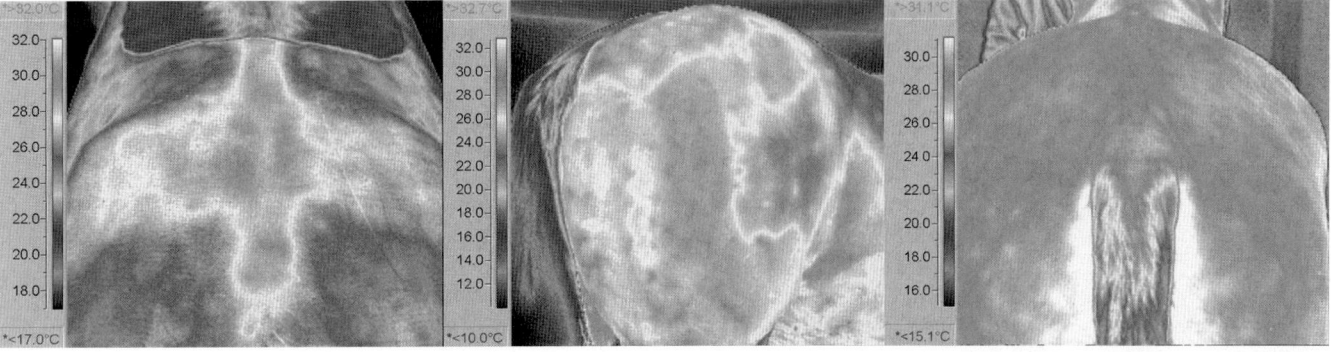

Fig. 25-3 • Three examples of muscle injury. The left thermographic image shows a left gluteal injury with increased heat signature. The middle image shows an increase in heat over the biceps femoris muscle. The right image is of a chronic gluteal injury with fibrosis, which has a cooler thermal pattern.

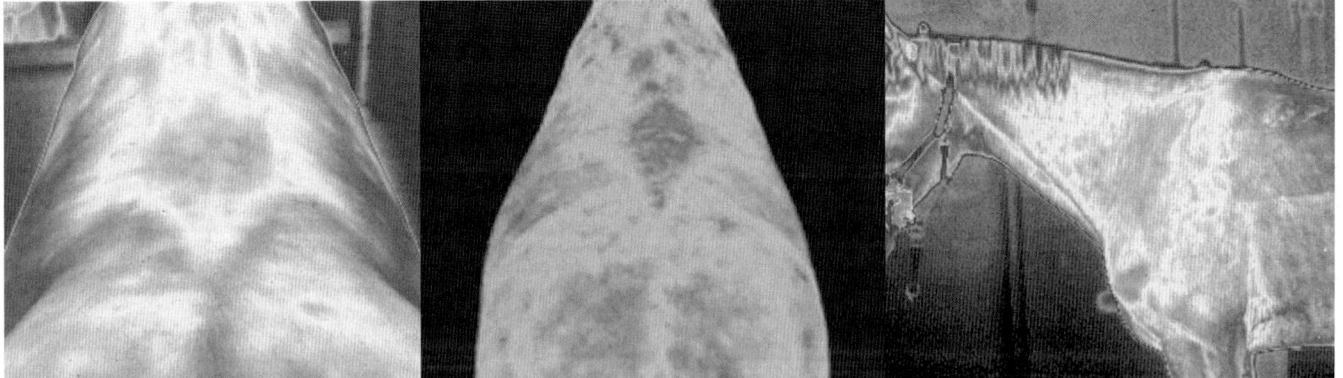

Fig. 25-4 • The left and middle thermographic images are caudodorsal views of the back, showing areas of increased heat associated with clinical signs of back pain and impinging dorsal spinous processes evident radiologically. The lateral view of the neck is from a horse with marked caudal cervical facet joint osteoarthritis. There is an increase in superficial blood flow in this region.

Some use thermography to guide acupuncture or osteopathic treatment[11] and consider that back pain can be a sympathetic associated pain syndrome. I tried sympatheticolytic drugs in a number of horses with back pain and saw improvement neither in the thermographic nor the clinical signs. In my experience thermography can detect areas of back inflammation associated with muscle injuries, impinging dorsal spinous processes, or supraspinous ligament injuries (see Figure 25-4), although the sensitivity and specificity are poor. It may be useful as part of a combined imaging approach. Thermography may also be helpful in assessment of saddle fit.

Thermography has also been used to detect methods of counterirritation[12] and is being employed by the Fédération Equestre Internationale at competitions as an adjunct to medication control.

CONCLUSION

Thermographic imaging can be a useful adjunct to a standard lameness and orthopedic evaluation. It requires a considerable investment of time to gain the necessary experience to differentiate between normal variation and patterns suggestive of pathology. Improvements in technology have brought high-quality imaging within the reach of the equine practitioner, which consequently makes image interpretation much easier. A standard protocol for imaging is important for obtaining accurate results, as is critical evaluation of the findings to integrate them into the total clinical picture. Although not necessary in the vast majority of horses with lameness, there are some horses in which thermography can be helpful. It has roles in screening populations of horses in training to pick up early signs of disease.

PART II

The Foot

Chapter	26

The Biomechanics of the Equine Limb and Its Effect on Lameness

Alan Wilson and Renate Weller

Biological structures (and sometimes those engineered by man) break, as a result of either a one-off (single event) load that exceeds their mechanical capacity or, more commonly, chronic fatigue overload, in which repeat micro-failures over time lead to failure of the whole structure. Biological tissue has the unique ability to adapt to mechanical demands and to repair itself given an appropriate mechanical stimulus and sufficient time. Complete failure of a structure happens only if the damage over time exceeds adaptation and repair.

Like man-made structures (e.g., elevators, bridges), biological designs have an inherent safety factor, defined as the ratio of the maximum stress a structure could withstand until breakage and the stress it is most likely to undergo during its lifetime. It is rather comforting that most engineered devices have a safety factor of up to 10 (so next time you read that an elevator has a maximum capacity of 18 people, know that it would actually hold 180!). Unfortunately, the safety factors[1] of equine bones and tendons are approximately 1.5 to 2.

Box 26-1 provides short definitions of biomechanical terms used in this chapter.

References on page 1267

WHEN DO MUSCULOSKELETAL STRUCTURES FAIL?

The parameters that influence failure of a musculoskeletal element are the force (magnitude, frequency and number of cycles, speed and duration of loading) the structure experiences and its ability to withstand it. The force on an individual part is related to the force that the whole limb experiences. Force is determined by body mass, speed of locomotion, and the leverage that force has on the specific part. A structure's ability to withstand force is determined by its structural properties, which in turn depend on its material properties and its dimensions. These reflect the magnitude and direction of the forces acting on it. Forces causing deformation include tension, compression, bending, and shear. Most structures are subjected to and are optimized for one predominant force, but they also have to be able to withstand other forces in normal use and even more so in exceptional circumstances. Tendons experience predominantly tensile forces, whereas joints are subjected to mainly compressive and some shear forces. Bones experience bending, with compressive forces on the concave side and tensile forces on the convex side. Bones have to withstand not only compressive forces from the horse's weight, but also the forces exerted by muscles and tendons that attach to them.

Failure in a live horse is much more complex than simple mechanics, because adaptation, repair, and compensatory mechanisms must be considered. Lameness may be not only a response to pain but also a compensatory mechanism, because it often results in an unloading of the affected limb or structure.

Elements of the musculoskeletal system have to fulfill four main requirements: force transmission without excessive deformation and fracture; use of the least amount of material to keep the metabolic costs for maintenance, transport, and regeneration down; and enough reserve of strength to cope with overload in the case of an accident.[2] Thus there is a trade-off between safety factors and energy costs. In horses the balance is shifted in favor of keeping the energy costs low while accepting a relatively high risk of musculoskeletal injury. Tendons (such as the equine digital flexor tendons or the human Achilles tendon) need to stretch to store energy in locomotion; to perform this role they need to reach high strains, which places them at a high risk for mechanical overload and damage.

In the following sections we describe the functional anatomy of the horse's limb and the material properties of its components. We discuss the influence of locomotion and the effects of conformation and farriery intervention on the loads acting on the musculoskeletal elements, such as bones, tendons, and joints. We also consider how the loads acting on the musculoskeletal system are changed with certain musculoskeletal disorders.

FUNCTIONAL ANATOMY OF THE HORSE LIMB

Horses have the ability to run fast over short distances (racing speeds reach 21 m/sec [75 km/hr]) and also to cover long distances at slower speeds with a low energy cost of locomotion. This was of evolutionary advantage because it enabled them not only to outrun predators but also to migrate to forage on the rather sparsely vegetated prairie land they originally inhabited. To achieve two

BOX 26-1

Definition of Common Terms in Biomechanics

Duty factor: Ratio of stance time and stride time. Expressed as either a fraction (between 0 and 1) or a percentage (between 0% and 100%).

Ground reaction force: Reaction force exerted from the ground onto the limb of a horse as a reaction of the force exerted by the horse onto the ground. Often split into three components: vertical (weight support), craniocaudal (acceleration and deceleration), and mediolateral (turning and balancing).

Kinetics: Study of the forces acting on bodies.

Kinematics: Study of the movement of bodies.

Safety factor: Ratio of a structure's strength to the maximum stress that the structure is likely to experience over its lifetime.

Stance phase (contact phase): Time the limb is in contact with the ground, from initial contact (foot on) to liftoff (toe off).

Stiffness: Force required to achieve a certain change in length. Slope of the force-length curve; the stiffer the structure, the higher the stiffness and the steeper the force-length curve.

Strain: Length change of a structure in relation to its starting length (e.g., through compressive or tensile load), often expressed as a percentage of the original length of the structure.

Stress: Force per unit area; also called *pressure*.

Stride time (duration): Time taken for a full stride cycle—for example, between foot contact of a limb to the following foot contact of the same limb. In general, the stride time decreases with increasing speed.

Swing phase (protraction): Time the limb is not in contact with the ground.

Stride frequency: Number of strides taken per second, measured in strides per second or Hz.

---

diverse locomotive requirements, the horse developed anatomical features that promoted energy efficiency (after all, it would not do the horse any good if it had to spend more energy to get to the food than could be gained by eating the food, or to get eaten in the process).

Although most veterinarians are familiar with some energy-saving mechanisms, such as the unguligrade stance of the horse, the patellar locking mechanism, and the stay (reciprocal) apparatus, from standard textbooks, there are many more features that play a major role in ensuring energy-efficient locomotion. This section concentrates on the musculoskeletal adaptations of the equine limb; however, a more comprehensive overview of general anatomical features is given elsewhere.[3]

Horse Limbs Function Like Pogo Sticks

If you tried to build a horse limb with children's blocks, the limb would collapse, because it would be impossible to build the fetlock joint in a hyperextended position. However, in a live limb the digital flexor tendons and ligaments on the flexor side of the limb prevent failure. Tendons have elastic properties and act like rubber bands or springs, providing resistance against which the limb presses when it comes under load, thus resisting further hyperextension and preventing collapse (Figure 26-1). The tendons are stretched at the same time, thus storing elastic strain energy, which can be returned in elastic recoil. During each step energy is stored, and it is returned when the limb leaves the ground. Energy is carried forward from one step to the next, thus reducing work the muscles have to do and saving metabolic energy. Indeed, the muscles associated with the main contributors of this system—the suspensory ligament

(SL), deep digital flexor tendon (DDFT), and superficial digital flexor tendon (SDFT)—either are not present at all (the SL and the accessory ligament of the DDFT [ALDDFT]) or are very short in relation to the tendons (e.g., the average length of the deep digital flexor muscle-tendon unit in a Thoroughbred is 77 ± 5 cm, more than 60% of which is tendon. The flexor muscles, being highly pennate and having short muscle fibers (1 cm in length), have limited capacity to change the length of the muscle-tendon unit when contracting. Approximately 7% of the energy stored in the tendons is released as heat, and during gallop the tendons of a galloping horse reach about 45°C.[4] We have reasoned that increase in temperature may account for core lesions in equine SDFTs but found that although 45°C resulted in death of some cells, tendon cells may be resistant.[5] Core lesions may result from hyperthermic damage of matrix components.[5]

Like any springlike structure, the limb itself has a certain stiffness, which is a measure of how much it shortens for a given load. A whole equine limb changes length mainly as a result of fetlock extension and length changes in the digital flexor tendons.[6] People can adjust their leg stiffness by muscle contraction to suit the softness or hardness of the ground on which they are walking or running.[7] Horses cannot adjust their leg stiffness because of the limited ability of the flexor muscles/tendons to change length, and this may be the reason why some horses cope better than others on different goings (footings). The flexor muscles do, however, damp vibrations, which otherwise would be likely to cause injury to musculoskeletal tissues.[8]

Bones

To enable a pogo-stick design, the bones in the equine limb are reduced compared with other animals: the radius and ulna are fused, and the horse bears weight only on the third metacarpal bone (McIII) or third metatarsal bone and the digit. Fewer bones allow lengthening of the limb and tendons and reduction of the mass of the distal aspect of the limb. This increases the energy storage capabilities of the digital flexor tendons and also results in a lighter limb that can be swung more rapidly and with less energetic cost, which is of benefit in locomotion. Fewer bones is thus an adaptation for maximum strength with minimum weight, because the bending strength is much higher for one large bone than for the same amount (and hence weight) of material arranged as several smaller bones.[2] However, a reduction in bone mass for energy efficiency results in an increase in fracture risk, and this is reflected in the fact that the distal limb bones are at higher risk for fracture than the proximal limb bones.[9]

Synovial Joints

Joints fulfill two main mechanical functions: they allow the movement of limb segments in relation to each other, and they act as shock absorbers. Limb movement is limited to the sagittal plane by anatomical adaptations of the phalanges and the fusion of bones, and only small, out-of-plane movements, such as adduction and abduction or rotation, are possible. Movement is further limited by the anatomical features of some of the articular surfaces, such as the interlocking configuration of trochlear and sagittal ridges and matching grooves, and is enforced by collateral ligaments. Without the need for muscular control, these

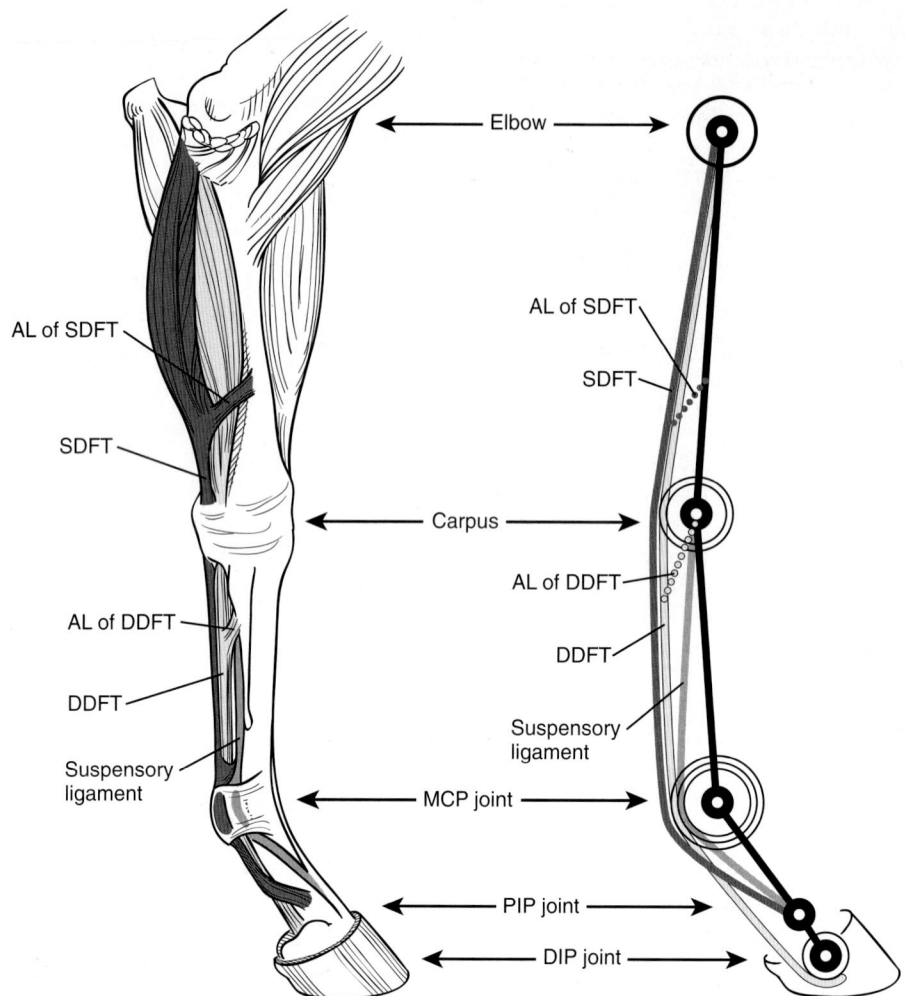

Fig. 26-1 • Anatomical drawing of an equine forelimb *(left)* and the equine forelimb modeled as a spring-system *(right)*; superficial digital flexor tendon (SDFT); deep digital flexor tendon (DDFT); accessory ligament (AL) of the DDFT; and AL of the SDFT. Limbs function like pogo sticks: the hyperextended fetlock joint is kept from collapsing by the springlike digital flexor tendons on the palmar aspect of the limb. When the limb comes under load during the stance phase of the stride, it compresses by further extending the fetlock joint while stretching the digital flexor tendons. This enables the digital flexor tendons to store elastic energy, which is released for propelling the limb into the swing phase. *MCP*, Metacarpophalangeal; *PIP*, proximal interphalangeal; *DIP*, distal interphalangeal.

features restrict joint movement to the sagittal plane, thus further decreasing metabolic costs.

Although all joints provide movement and shock absorption to a certain degree, some joints allow only a small range of movement and have the primary function of shock absorption, whereas other joints have a large range of movement and a primary function of movement. These joints can be functionally classified as low-motion or high-motion joints, respectively. The fetlock joint, a good example of a high-motion joint, goes through 90 degrees of movement during the stance phase of gallop, whereas the proximal interphalangeal joint has a range of motion of only 5 to 10 degrees. In complex joints such as the carpus and tarsus, there is a division in function: both the antebrachiocarpal and tarsocrural joints are high-motion joints, but in the more distal joints of the carpus and tarsus there is less movement; the least movement is in the carpometacarpal and tarsometatarsal joints. There is also a difference in occurrence and clinical severity of

skeletal disorders between high- and low-motion joints. Osteochrondrosis is much more common in high-motion joints, and osteoarthritis (OA) is usually of greater clinical significance than in low-motion joints.

The Foot as Interface to the Ground

The foot provides the interface between the horse and the ground. It is a complex modification of integument surrounding, supporting, and protecting structures in the distal limb of the horse. The hoof capsule encases within a confined space three bones, a series of ligaments and tendons, two synovial structures, a digital cushion, cartilages of the foot, blood vessels, and nerves. Although the horny hoof capsule provides protection of the internal structures, it does not allow for expansion through swelling; therefore any swelling that does occur as a result of injury leads to an increase in pressure and thus stimulation of pain receptors. Mechanically the foot has three main functions: shock absorption when the foot comes into

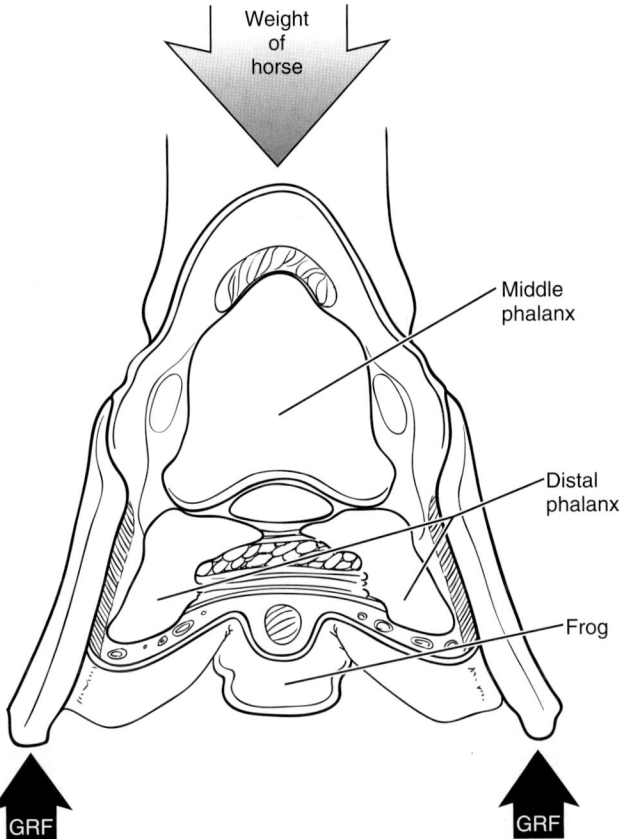

Fig. 26-2 • Schematic drawing illustrating two of the shock-absorbing features of the equine foot. First, the shape of the solar surface with the frog in the middle and the frog grooves on either side allows the heels to move sideways and distally on ground contact, while the toe retracts. Second, the suspension of the distal phalanx within the horn capsule allows forces to be transferred from the distal phalanx across the laminar junction to the hoof and to the ground via the distal border of the hoof wall. *GRF*, Ground reaction force.

contact with the ground, support and grip when the limb is bearing weight, and propulsion when the limb leaves the ground. It must also resist excessive abrasion and protect sensitive structures lying internally, while, in wild horses, allowing sufficient natural wear of the wall to maintain hoof shape.[10]

The foot has a series of "built-in" protective mechanisms that absorb part of the concussive forces and damp vibrations during impact (Figure 26-2):

1. The shape of the solar surface with the frog in the middle and the frog sulci (grooves) on either side allows the heel to move sideways and distally on ground contact while the toe retracts.
2. The suspension of the distal phalanx within the horn capsule allows forces to be transferred from the distal phalanx across the laminar junction to the hoof and to the ground via the distal border of the hoof wall.
3. The digital cushion located under the frog and sole between the cartilages of the foot is a wedge of elastic subcutaneous tissue, consisting of collagen, elastic fibers, islands of cartilage, fat, and modified skin glands; this cushion aids in shock absorption by deforming and permitting the frog to move. The

equine digital cushion, however, is small in comparison to that in other species—for example, the elephant limb, which relies heavily on its large digital cushion for shock absorption.

4. The hoof has the ability to slide along the ground surface.
5. The distal interphalangeal (DIP) joint can move by rotation and translation.

ABILITY OF STRUCTURES TO COPE WITH MECHANICAL DEMANDS

Structural and Material Properties

When a force is applied to a structure, the structure usually responds by deforming. The greater the force applied to a structure, the greater the deformation. The ability of a structure to resist deformation is expressed as stiffness and represents the slope of a structure's force-length relationship. The force-deformation relationship of biological structures behaves in a roughly linear elastic manner until the applied load causes nonreversible deformation and ends in failure. The force-deformation relationship describes the structural properties and depends on the material properties of a tendon and on its dimensions. Larger structures are able to cope with larger forces: imagine two ropes made of the same material, but double the cross-sectional area (approximately 1.41 times the diameter): the thicker rope will be able to withstand double the force of the thinner one.

It is often of interest to know about the properties of the material per se, independent of size. This is achieved by dividing the force acting on a structure by its cross-sectional area. When normalized for cross-sectional area, a force is called *stress* (σ; common units would be mega Newtons per square meter [MN/m^2] or Newtons per square millimeter [N/mm^2]). The resulting deformation of an applied stress is expressed as strain (ε), the ratio of the change in size to the original size. Being a ratio, strain does not have a dimension; however, it is often expressed as a percentage—for example, $\varepsilon = 0.1 = 10\%$. If we are interested in the property of a material rather than structure, we can express this relationship as a stress-strain curve. The slope of this curve is the ratio between the tensile stress and strain and is called the *elastic modulus* or *Young's modulus (E)*. The elastic modulus defines whether a material is "rigid" or "compliant." Rigid materials have a very high elastic modulus and deform very little under load, whereas compliant materials have a low elastic modulus and require less load to deform. Bone, for example, is relatively rigid, whereas articular cartilage is more compliant and thus is able to act as an excellent shock absorber by undergoing considerable deformation when under load. Figure 68-1 shows the stress-strain curves for the digital flexor tendons of a Thoroughbred racehorse.

The ability of structures to deform when loaded and return to their original length when the load is removed allows them to store energy. The amount of energy per unit volume is the area under the linear portion of the stress-strain curve. The capacity of a material to absorb and release energy is often referred to as *elastic resilience*. The energy a material can absorb before failure defines whether it is "brittle" or "tough": tough materials are able to absorb considerable elastic energy before failing, whereas brittle materials absorb very little. The digital flexor tendons of a horse are able to store and return a considerable amount of energy during locomotion. Load-deformation curves of tendons are different between loading and unloading, forming a "hysteresis" loop. The area of the loop presents the loss of energy, largely in the form of heat, that occurs during stretch and release (see Figure 68-2). It has been shown that the heat produced by repetition of this mechanism leads to an increase in core temperature, which may contribute to the pathogenesis of tendon injury through thermal damage.[4] A detailed description of the pathobiology of tendon injuries is given in Chapter 68.

From an injury perspective, stress is probably the most informative mechanical measure in addition to strain. Equine digital flexor tendons, for example, have different elastic moduli and experience different strain rates in vivo, but they also have different cross-sectional areas. Both the SL and the SDFT experience high strains (up to 16%) during locomotion, but the stress in the SDFT is much higher than in the SL because its cross-sectional area is only about a third of that of the SL.[11] This corresponds to the fact that the SDFT is the most commonly injured tendon or ligament (see Chapter 68).

Changes in Structural Properties

Structural properties change constantly (within limits) either through changes in dimensions or material properties, and this is likely to have an effect on the risk of musculoskeletal injury. Structural properties change with age, in response to loading, and through pathological processes. Changes in dimensions are most obvious for muscle, where exercise leads to an increase in muscle volume. Change in the external dimensions of bones, tendons, and ligaments is limited. These tissues, especially bone, respond predominantly by modifying internal structure. Most biological materials have a variety of components, each of different stiffness—for example, in the case of bone, collagen fibers, and minerals. Mechanical properties can be altered by changing the relative quantity of the components. For example, bone becomes stiffer with higher mineral content, which makes it stronger but diminishes its capacity to absorb energy on impact, making it more brittle. This suggests that there is a trade-off among stiffness, strength, and energy absorption. Chapter 68 summarizes how an equine digital flexor tendon responds to external stimuli.

Not all biological tissues react to stimuli in the same way. Tissue-specific responses play a role both in the pathogenesis of musculoskeletal injury and in how training and rehabilitation programs are designed. Problems can develop when a regimen designed to increase, for example, bone strength may be counterproductive for tendons or joints.

Locomotion and Its Effect on Musculoskeletal Tissues

For quantification purposes, locomotion can be divided into strides: a complete cycle of footfalls (e.g., from the time the left front foot hits the ground to the next time it hits the ground). Each stride can be subdivided into the time the foot spends on the ground (stance phase) and the time the foot is in the air (protraction or swing phase). The ratio between these two is often calculated as a

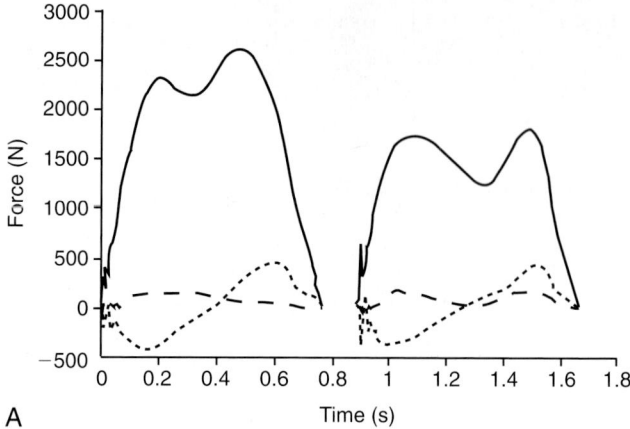

A

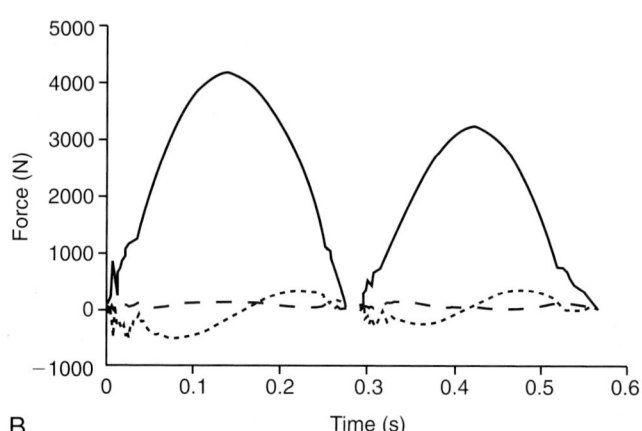

B

Fig. 26-3 • Ground reaction forces (GRFs) for subsequent forelimb (left "humps") and hindlimb (right "humps") stance phases in walk **(A)** and trot **(B)** for a 420-kg horse. Solid lines represent vertical force, short-dashed lines craniocaudal force, and long-dashed lines mediolateral force. For walk and trot, vertical peak force and impulse (area under the curve) are higher in the forelimb than in the hindlimb. Craniocaudal force shows the typical sinusoidal shape with decelerative (negative) force in the first half of stance and accelerative (positive) force in the second half. Mediolateral force is generally low in value and often more variable than the other two components of GRF. **A,** Walk: typical double-humped shape of the vertical force can be seen in both limbs. Here, vertical force reaches a maximum of approximately 62% body weight in the forelimb and approximately 45% body weight in the hindlimb. **B,** Trot: typical single-humped shape of the vertical force can be seen in both limbs. Here vertical force reaches a maximum of approximately 100% body weight in the forelimb and approximately 75% body weight in the hindlimb.

dimensionless parameter for gait characterization and is called the *duty factor*. In relation to (distal-limb–related) lameness, the stance phase is of more interest than the swing phase because the load on the limb is highest during that time. The stance phase can be divided into three main parts: impact, loading, and propulsion.

When the limb is on the ground it experiences a force, the ground reaction force (GRF) (Figures 26-3 and 26-4). The GRF is a function of mass and gravitational force ($F = $ mass $\times$ acceleration), has a magnitude and direction, and is usually described as a vector. The point underneath the foot where the force is applied is called the *point of zero moment* (PZM). The PZM and the direction and magnitude of the force vector change during the period of the stance phase. Depending on the PZM and the direction of the GRF vector, the force vector does not necessarily go straight

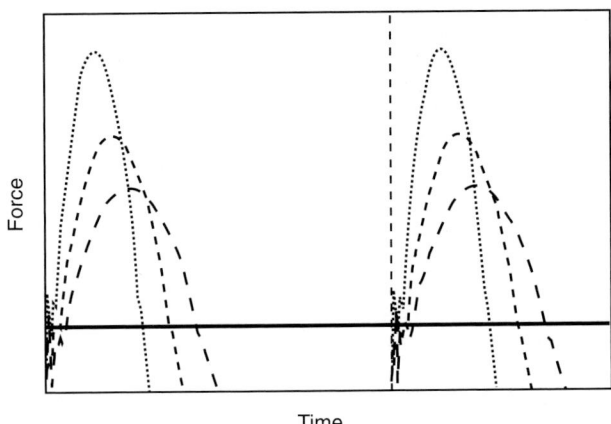

Fig. 26-4 • Schematic drawing of vertical ground reaction force (y-axis) over time (x-axis) of an individual limb in a trotting horse. Each of the three graphs represents a first stance phase followed by a swing phase and a second stance phase of the same limb. Different lines indicate different speeds (long dashes, slow; short dashes, medium; dotted line, fast) and thus different stance times (for simplification purposes, stride time (indicated by the vertical line at the beginning of the second stance phase) is assumed to be constant. With increasing speed, a decrease in stance time is observed, which results in an increase in peak vertical force (the maximum force achieved during midstance) that is inversely proportional to duty factor (ratio of stance time over stride time). The black horizontal line represents the average vertical force produced by the limb, which needs to be sufficiently large to support the body of the horse against the effect of gravity (i.e., approximately 30% body weight for each individual forelimb or approximately 20% body weight for each individual hindlimb).

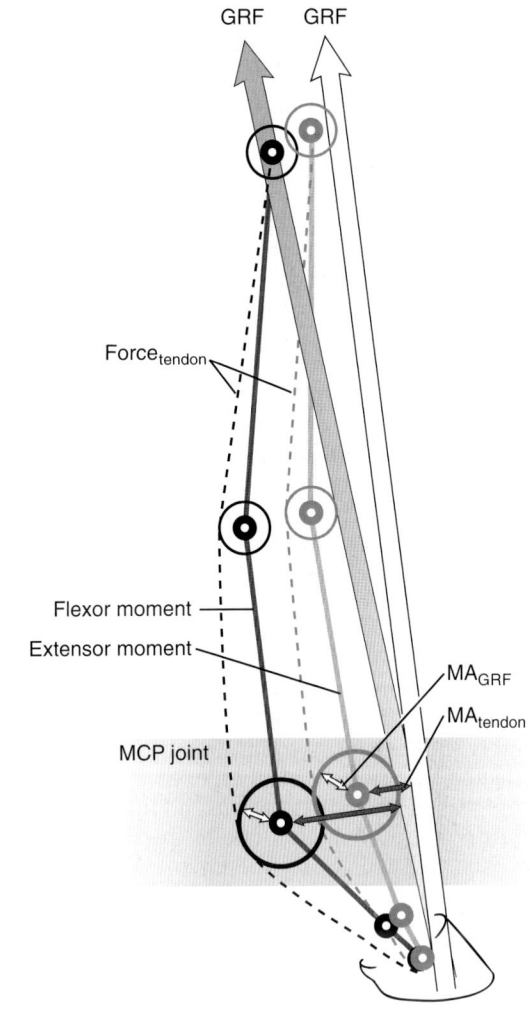

Extensor moment = Flexor moment
GRF x MA$_{GRF}$ = Force$_{tendon}$ x MA$_{tendon}$

Fig. 26-5 • Schematic drawing of the equine forelimb with the direction of the ground reaction force (GRF) vector and its moment arms around the metacarpophalangeal (MCP) joint. To prevent the limb from collapsing, the extension moment is counteracted by a flexor moment created by the digital flexor tendons (here limited to the deep digital flexor tendon) and their moment arm (MA) on the palmar aspect of the limb. As the limb comes under load, the GRF moment arm around the MCP joint increases *(shaded arrow)*. Changes in moment arms of the flexor tendons around the MCP joint are largely determined by the size of the proximal sesamoid bones and remain relatively constant *(MA tendon)*. Hence an increase in extensor moment results in an increase in the force in the digital flexor tendons. This holds true for static conditions, but the situation during movement is more complex.

through the center of rotation of the joints but might be located dorsally or cranially to it. This creates a lever for the GRF (commonly referred to as the *moment arm*) acting on the joint. The resulting rotational force (also called *torque*) causes the joints in the distal aspect of the limb to extend. This extension moment is counteracted by a flexor moment created by the digital flexor tendons and their moment arms on the palmar or plantar aspect of the limb (Figure 26-5). To prevent the limb from collapsing, the extensor moment has to equal the flexor moment:

$$Fext = GRF \times Moment\ arm\ GRF = Fflex = Force\ tendons \times$$
$$Moment\ arm\ tendons$$

where Fext is force of the extension moment and Fflex is force of the flexion moment. The moment arm of the digital flexor tendons is the distance from the center of rotation of the joint to the line of action of the tendons. The length of the tendon moment arm is largely determined by the size of the proximal sesamoid bones at the level of the fetlock joint and the distal sesamoid bone at the level of the DIP joint. Because the size of these bones remains constant, any change in the magnitude and/or direction of the GRF will have an effect on the force the flexor tendons experience. As the DDFT wraps around the distal sesamoid (navicular) bone, it exerts a compressive force on the bone that is proportional not only to the force the tendon experiences but also to the angle of the path of the DDFT.[12,13]

Impact

The foot of a galloping horse hits the ground at about 5 m/sec. On first contact with the ground the leg decelerates rapidly, which is reflected in the early increase in GRF (see Figures 26-3 and 26-4).[14] This energy is dissipated by the foot sliding through and penetrating into the surface and by muscles within the limb. The forces at impact are lower than those experienced in the rest of the stride, but the load is applied very quickly, which appears to be important in eliciting musculoskeletal injury. The impact "shock" also causes the limb to vibrate at about 35 Hz, somewhat like the plucking of a violin string. This vibration is predominantly in a horizontal direction and is caused by the large amount of elastic tendon tissue contained in the equine limb and the pogo stick–like lever system. Vibration is apparent in both forelimbs and hindlimbs, but the vibration amplitude and duration are greater in the fore-limbs. The vibration may, in itself, cause damage through increasing loading rate and the number of loading cycles experienced by the tendons. It also has a potent remodeling stimulus on bone and perhaps other tissues.

The magnitude of the vibration is dependent on several factors. Surfaces that allow the foot to slip at impact (or on hard surfaces, a shoe that slips at contact) dissipate the impact energy and reduce the impulse that causes the vibration. Surfaces with good damping characteristics absorb the vibration energy rapidly. This feature is different from the stiffness of a surface, and it is possible to have a surface that is relatively stiff (firm) but has good damping characteristics. The foot as the interface between the body and the ground has several built-in damping mechanisms (see earlier), but the other important damping system is the muscles. Active muscles absorb energy during small-amplitude, high-frequency oscillations. The digital flexor muscles have extremely short fibers and a large physiological cross-sectional area, which means that they can develop high forces but only over a length change of a few millimeters. This arrangement makes them ideal for absorbing the energy associated with a small-amplitude vibration.[8]

Impact characteristics differ among gaits, speeds, surfaces, and shoes.[14-17] The absolute length of the hoof-braking period is 30 to 50 milliseconds, independent of speed,[14] but is affected by the type of surface. In a comparison of all-weather waxed tracks to crushed-sand tracks, the former was found to reduce the amplitude of the shock at impact and the associated vibrations in French trotters.[18]

Peak Force

After initial ground contact the limb is loaded in a disto-proximal manner,[19] with the whole limb shortening toward the ground, largely because of further extension of the fetlock joint[6] but aided by rotation and translation of other segments. This prolongs the impact time and extends the period of braking, which makes the limb an effective shock absorber.[20]

The peak GRF increases with the body mass of the horse. The damage a force can cause depends not only on its magnitude, but also on how quickly it is applied. Force over time is called *impulse* and represents the area under the force/time curve (see Figure 26-4). The shape of the force/time curve is different between forelimbs and hindlimbs and varies for different gaits (see Figure 26-3) and speeds (see Figure 26-4). Impulses are highest during gallop and increase with speed within a gait. At top speed a racehorse's front foot is on the ground for only about 80 milliseconds or 17% of the stride, and the limb experiences a peak force of about 2.5 times body weight. This load is applied in only 40 milliseconds. The load on a hindlimb is considerably lower at about 1.5 times body weight. This difference in peak load may explain, in part, why hindlimbs experience a lower incidence of tendon and ligament injuries.

Speed is a function of stride frequency and stride length. An increase in speed can be achieved by increasing either of these factors; however, neither of these can be increased endlessly. Maximum running speed is constrained by the speed at which the limbs can be moved and by the GRF they can withstand. People sprinting bends change the duration of foot contact to spread the time over which the load is applied to keep limb force constant. Racing greyhounds do not change their foot-contact timings, and so have to withstand a 65% increase in limb forces; thus in this species limb force does not limit running speed.[21] It is currently not known if limb force limits running speed in horses as in people or if horses are more like greyhounds.

It is known that individual horses adopt different loco-motor strategies to achieve the same speed—for example, horses with longer limbs have lower stride frequencies than horses with shorter limbs.[22] An increase in stride frequency can be achieved by reducing the time that either the foot is off the ground (protraction time) or the limb is on the ground (stance time). Protraction time accounts for approximately 80% of the stride time and remains relatively constant during gallop.[23] Changes in stride frequency must be largely achieved through minimizing stance time. It has been shown in people that the forces a limb experiences increase with decreasing stance time, and it is reasonable to assume that the same is true in horses. This may suggest that horses that increase speed by reducing stance time are at higher risk of musculoskeletal injury. However, with an increased stance time comes an increase in the angle a limb sweeps through while the limb is on the ground and the body continues moving over it. This is probably related to an increase in the moments acting on musculoskeletal structures. However, the potential effect of this on musculoskeletal injury has not yet been investigated.

The tissues of the distal aspect of the limb function within a narrow safety margin; this is partly the result of minimizing distal limb mass but also a prerequisite of having tendons that function as elastic energy stores (because energy stored is a direct function of the square of the elongation of a tendon). The force acting through the limb is multiplied by the lever system of the distal limb to impose much higher forces on the bones and tendons of the distal aspect of the limb. These forces approach the mechanical capacity of these tissues, and a small increase in peak load results in a substantial reduction in the number of cycles to failure for the tissue. The relative load distribution between the individual digital flexor tendons also varies by, for example, the angle of the foot to the ground (resulting from either shoe design or the way the foot penetrates into the surface). Elevation of the heel results in a transfer of load from the DDFT to the SDFT and the SL (Figure 26-6).

Number of Loading Cycles

Large volumes of high-speed exercise may exceed the fatigue life of the high-stress tendons and bones. The fatigue life of these tissues (in number of cycles to failure) depends on the peak strain (deformation) experienced; a small increment in strain results in a substantial reduction in the fatigue life of a tissue. The volume of high-speed exercise applied to a horse is therefore critical. High-speed exercise is also the most potent stimulus for eliciting changes in structural properties, so there is a trade-off between providing this stimulus and exceeding the mechanical capacity of these tissues. A galloping horse imposes about 220 loading cycles per mile (strides) on its bones and tendons at a fast gallop and about 360 strides per mile at a canter. These structures have been estimated to have a fatigue life of as little as 10,000 cycles. The relationship between speed and number of cycles to failure is

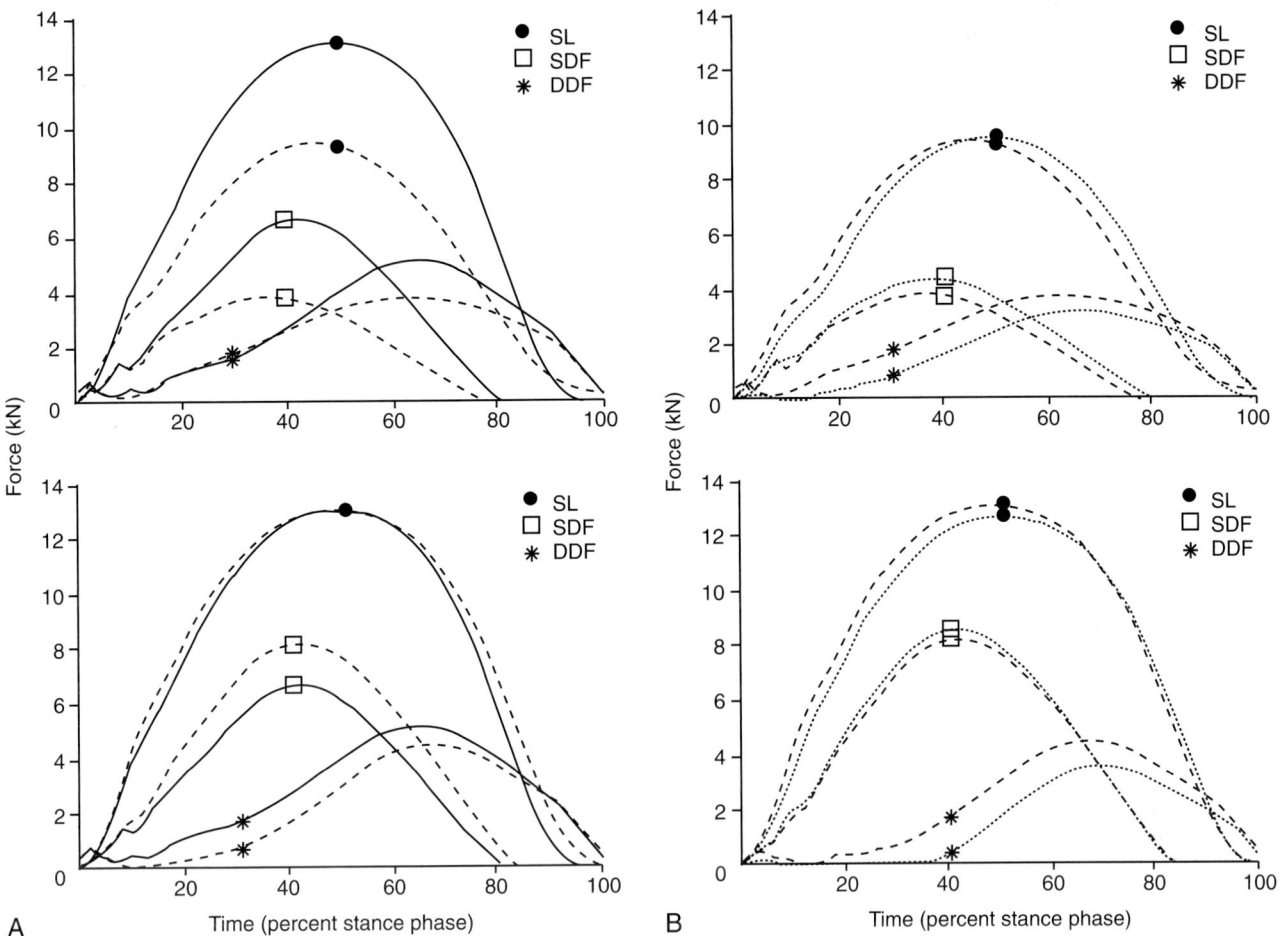

Fig. 26-6 • A, Calculation of mean digital flexor tendon and suspensory ligament (SL) forces in the affected *(top)* and contralateral *(bottom)* forelimb of five trotting horses before *(solid line)* and after *(dashed line)* experimentally induced unilateral superficial digital flexor (SDF) tendonitis. **B,** Calculation of mean digital flexor tendon and SL forces in the affected *(top)* and contralateral *(bottom)* forelimb of five trotting horses with experimentally induced unilateral SDF tendonitis before *(dashed lines)* and after *(dotted lines)* bilateral application of heel wedges. *DDF,* Deep digital flexor, including accessory ligament of the DDF tendon (ALDDFT); *SDF,* superficial digital flexor. (From Meershoek LS, Lanovaz JL, Schamhardt HC, Clayton HM: Calculated forelimb digital flexor tendon forces in horses with experimentally induced superficial digital flexor tendinitis and the effects of application of heel wedges, *Am J Vet Res* 63:432, 2002.)

of interest in the development of appropriate training programs. The time course of structural adaptations may be as long as 6 months, and there is the potential for a training program to accumulate damage (because of the exercise volume) before such protective responses occur.

What Happens to the Individual Musculoskeletal Element during Locomotion?

Foot

On contact with the ground the foot must withstand the high forces at impact. During locomotion a forelimb of a horse experiences forces of one half of body weight at a walk, approximately 1 times body weight at a trot, and up to 2.5 times body weight at a canter.

Forces act on the foot primarily in two ways: the GRF acts on the solar surface of the hoof, and tensile forces are applied by the DDFT to its insertion site on the distal phalanx. Forces acting on the foot are transferred between the distal phalanx and the hoof capsule through the laminar junction (see Figure 26-2). In effect the limb force

is transferred to the distal phalanx, and it is "hung" from the hoof wall by the laminae. This is why in laminitis, with disruption of the dorsal laminae, the dorsal aspect of the distal phalanx drops. Movement of the distal phalanx and deformation of the hoof wall have secondary effects on vascularization, the whole process being termed the *hoof mechanism*.[10]

As the hoof capsule comes under load, the main force moves from the palmar or plantar aspect of the hoof dorsally to the toe,[24] and the dorsal hoof capsule compresses. The heel expands during the first three quarters of the stance phase and contracts for a short time just before the foot leaves the ground. Heel expansion is greater in trot than in walk, but the timings are similar. Initially the middle phalanx rotates palmad or plantad, causing the heel, frog, and wall to deform under pressure. There is a direct relationship between hoof pressure, particularly in the frog, and heel expansion. However, heel expansion occurs even without ground contact with the frog, and there is no direct pressure from the ground acting on the sole or frog.[25]

The strain patterns and peak strains of the hoof capsule are complex and are influenced by numerous factors such as gait, hoof shape, shoeing, and surface and pathological conditions.[10,26,27] Generally strains are lower in walk than in trot and gallop; turning increases the strain on the medial hoof quarter.

Tendons

Accurate measurement of tendon strain is a challenge, especially in live horses, and numerous in vitro and in vivo experiments using a variety of invasive and noninvasive techniques have been conducted to assess tendon strain in horses.

The time-related pattern of loading and the magnitude differ between the digital flexor tendons (see Figure 26-6) and are influenced by surface, conformation, farriery, and pathology.[28-32] Tendon strain in vivo increases significantly from walk to trot for all digital flexor tendons with the exception of the ALDDFT. The highest strains are experienced by the SL (3.4% at walk, 5.8% at trot), followed by the SDFT (2.2% at walk, 4.2% at trot) and DDFT (1.2%, 1.7%). Strains in the ALDDFT and SL were significantly higher on pavement than on sand, but this was not found for the SDFT and DDFT.[31] At a gallop, tendon strain can reach 12% to 16%,[33] a level close to failure strain found experimentally (see Figure 68-1), suggesting that a narrow safety margin exists for tendon tissue. A similar distribution of tendon forces has been seen during landing after fences.[34] Peak forces were highest in the SL, lower in the SDFT and lowest in the DDFT. Increase in fence height resulted in a substantial increase in SDFT force, whereas forces in the SL increased only slightly, and forces in the DDFT and ALDDFT remained the same. The loading pattern of the digital flexor tendons over time differs between tendons. Force in the SL increases in the first 30% of the stance phase, remains nearly constant at 30% to 70%, and decreases between 70% of stance and foot-off. Force in the DDFT and ALDDFT increases more gradually until its peak at 75% of the stance phase and decreases rapidly thereafter, whereas the SDFT starts loading at 10% of stance and reaches its peak at midstance.

Surface characteristics were related to the incidence of tendon injuries in epidemiological studies[35,36] and had a significant influence on tendon load in two French trotters: when an all-weather track was compared with a crushed-sand track, the maximum force experienced by the SDFT was higher and was reached earlier in the stance phase on the crushed-sand track than on the all-weather track.[37] This corresponds to differences in joint kinematics and foot-surface interaction between the two surfaces. However, more studies are necessary comparing the effect of surfaces on other tendons, bones, and joints before recommendations regarding the most suitable surface can be made.

Bones

The McIII is one of the most commonly fractured bones in racehorses. The stress and strain patterns this bone experiences during locomotion[33,38,39] are complex, involving compression, shearing, bending, and twisting. Strains exceeding 3000 microstrain have been recorded for the dorsal cortex of the McIII during fast exercise, and the peak compressive strain of this bone at a speed of 16 m/sec was found to be around 4800 microstrain.[40] These high strain values are thought to stimulate bone modeling, but they can also cause simultaneous bone damage. However, the peak axial load may be unlikely to cause a fracture in this bone.[41] Axial stress, about 90 N/mm^2, can be calculated from the measured strain values by taking into account the material properties and average cross-sectional area of the McIII.[42] This corresponds to about 50% of the ultimate strength.[43] It has been shown that the force required to break a bone through bending is only about $\frac{1}{60}$ of the force required to fracture a bone in compression.[44] Therefore the bending forces are much more likely to cause overload in the McIII. Horizontally directed accelerations and hence the bending forces acting on the McIII are highest during impact, and it has been suggested that any measures interfering with this phase have an effect on the McIII stress.[41] This is supported by the fact that a shorter period of hoof braking after foot contact has been shown to result in higher amplitudes and more rapid oscillation transmitted to the McIII in horses at trot than a longer period of braking.[16]

A more detailed description of bone loading is given in Chapter 102.

Joints

Joints are mainly subjected to compressive and shear forces. Direction and magnitude of the force follows the GRF and is influenced by joint angle and conformation of the joints and limb segments. Stress relates to the size and shape of the articular surfaces and therefore differs among joints, but also within a joint. In the metacarpophalangeal (MCP) joint, for example, the stress follows the biphasic GRF pattern during walk at most articular sites, but not the sagittal groove of the proximal phalanx, where stress has been shown to continue to rise after midstance in a majority of horses.[45] This may contribute to the pathobiology of this specific area. In this joint the stress experienced by the medial part of the joint was significantly higher than the stress acting on the lateral part, which corresponds to the progression of osteoarthritic changes from medial to lateral in this joint.[46]

THE EFFECTS OF CONFORMATION ON EQUINE DISTAL LIMB MECHANICS

The effect of conformation, especially with regard to the relationship among heel height, toe length, and angulation of the phalanges, is commonly discussed by veterinarians and farriers; however, scientific evidence is scarce.

Effect of Toe Length and Angle

Toe length and angle influence the point of force application and hence the moment arm of the GRF around the joints, but also the relative timing of events during the stance phase.

A change in dorsal hoof wall angle of 3.5 degrees over an 8-week shoeing interval resulted in a shifting of the point of force in a dorsal direction and an increase in the moment around the DIP joint, which leads to an increase in stress exerted by the DDFT on the navicular bone.[47,48] This, however, was lower than expected from predictive calculations, and a compensatory mechanism involving a decrease in extension of the fetlock joint and hence an unloading of the DDFT has been suggested.[49] An additional compensatory mechanism has been suggested in the hindlimb, where a shift of the point of force laterally has been observed in late stance, resulting in a shortening of the GRF moment arm around the DIP joint.

When the heel leaves the ground, the body weight acts at the toe, producing a long lever arm on the DIP joint and hence loading the DDFT and the navicular bone. Attempts to reduce the length of this lever arm have been made by fitting a shoe with quarter clips rather than a toe clip and a shoe designed along the lines of the four-point trim (natural balance shoe). Comparing toe clip, quarter clip, and natural balance shoes, pulling the toe back made breakover (heel off to toe off) start earlier and shortened the duration of breakover. The moment arm of the GRF on the DIP joint during breakover was reduced, but because breakover started earlier and hence at a higher GRF, the peak moment and force on the navicular bone were similar with the three shoe types.[50]

Effect of Mediolateral Imbalance

The horse's limb has evolved to function in the sagittal plane, with the GRF vector ideally going through the middle of the limb column to ensure even load distribution in a mediolateral plane. Any out-of-plane conformation results in a change in direction of the GRF vector and its moment arm in relation to the musculoskeletal structure, thus resulting in their uneven loading and hence potential overloading of structures that have low safety factors. Mediolateral imbalance leads to an increase in joint pressure, as well as changes in articular contact area, as demonstrated for the DIP joint after application of medial or lateral wedges.[51] Six-degree lateral or medial wedges resulted in a significant increase in joint pressure and moved the articular contact area toward the elevated side.

One aim of veterinary and farriery intervention is to ensure mediolateral balance through foot trimming or addition of extensions. The effect of such treatments on limb mechanics in sound horses and in horses with OA of the distal hock joints (bone spavin) has been demonstrated. In one study a 6-mm–thick wedge shoe was applied to alter mediolateral foot balance in sound horses of good conformation.[24] This wedge moved the PZM toward the elevated side of the foot by about 5 to 10 mm. In a second study a 20-mm-wide lateral extension was applied to the front and separately to the hind feet of sound horses. These extensions had no apparent effect on the position of the PZM. This lack of an effect may demonstrate, however, that "if it ain't broke, you can't fix it." In addition, on soft ground an extension sinks into the ground less than the narrow side of a shoe, creating a wedge effect. In a separate study lateral extensions and trailer shoes were applied to the hind feet of horses with OA of the distal hock joints. These horses attempted to unload the dorsomedial aspect of the distal tarsal joints by redistributing their weight to the plantarolateral aspect of the foot. The lateral extensions (20 mm wide) and trailers (20 mm long on lateral heel) are assumed to act by helping the horse to redistribute its weight in a more comfortable manner either by rotating the foot or by helping the horse bear weight on the lateral side of the foot. An alternative explanation is that the corrective farriery forces the horse to move "normally" and prevents it from unloading the painful tissues and eliciting the repair process. Both extension and trailer shoes had little consistent effect on the position of the PZM through stance or on the clinical lameness score of these horses, questioning their efficacy as a treatment technique. The Editors question the assumption that pain is focused dorsomedially.

Effect of Heel Height

It is common to change heel height through the application of heel wedges to manage orthopedic disease in horses. The effect of wedges on joint angles, tendon strains, and joint pressure has been the subject of numerous studies and the mechanical effects in the following sections have been described.

Joint Angles, Tendon Strain, and Navicular Force

Heel wedges move the PZM toward the heel and therefore reduce the moment arm of the GRF at the DIP joint and unload the DDFT. The DDFT passes around the navicular bone and exerts a compressive force on the navicular bone. When the DIP joint is flexed, the angle of tendon deviation around the bone is reduced. Angular change and a reduced force in the tendon (because it has shortened) mean that the compressive force on the bone is reduced. Force on the navicular bone is reduced nearly 24% for a 6-degree heel wedge and double that for a 21-degree wedge.[12]

When the heel is unloaded toward the end of stance, there is leverage on the DIP joint, the DDFT, and the navicular bone. With wedge elevation the heel is supported until later in the stride. Vertical force on the limb is reduced when forward displacement occurs, and in turn the moment on the DIP joint should be lower.[12]

These changes are supported by another study in horses with experimentally induced superficial digital flexor (SDF) tendonitis. After bilateral application of 6-degree heel wedges, ALDDFT and DDFT force decreased in both limbs; SDFT force stayed the same in the affected limb, but increased in the contralateral limb. These findings suggest that heel wedges may not be beneficial in horses with SDF tendonitis and in fact may contribute to the high secondary injury rate in contralateral forelimbs.[34]

Experiments using heel wedges have concentrated on the immediate effects of changes in heel height, but there are long-term, repetitive effects and possible compensatory mechanisms that may be important. In a study investigating foot conformation in sound horses there was a strong negative correlation between DDFT strain and navicular bone stress and the ratio of heel and toe height. With elevation of the toe, there is an increase of the GRF moment arm around the DIP joint because of movement of the PZM toward the toe. To counteract the increased extensor moment of the GRF on the DIP joint, the flexor moment has to increase accordingly, which leads to an increase in force in the DDFT. As the DDFT wraps around the navicular bone it exerts a force on the navicular bone, and any increase in DDFT force leads to an increase in the force acting on the navicular bone.[13] The results of this study support the findings seen after heel wedge application as discussed earlier.

Joint Pressure and Articular Contact

Elevating the heel by 5 degrees has been shown to significantly increase DIP joint pressure, and lowering the heel had the opposite effect. Articular contact area shifted dorsally with elevation of the heel and palmarly when the heel was lowered.[51] An increase in intraarticular pressure may directly cause pain, and indirectly could change both vascularity of the synovium and cartilage function, triggering a cascade of detrimental events.

Hoof Capsule

The horn of the hoof capsule is arranged in tubules, which is the ideal design to withstand high compressive forces, but which can be highly susceptible to excessive bending forces (comparable to a drinking straw, which is almost impossible to squash by compressing straight from either end but is very easy to bend). The compression strength of a material diminishes rapidly with increasing length, because the buckling limit of a material is proportional to the square of the length. This is why it is a mechanical necessity to maintain tubule length by natural wear or trimming. In horses with a collapsed or underrun heel, the tubules have started to bend once they have grown distal to the distal phalanx. This impairs hoof deformation and associated blood flow to and from the hoof. Application of thin, flexible carbon fiber patches to the medial and lateral sides of the heel is beneficial in maintaining horizontal loading of hoof tubules by preventing bending and restoring hoof deformation and blood flow to more physiological levels.[52]

EFFECT OF SHOEING

Application of a Shoe

Application of a shoe changes the mass of the distal limb, alters hoof deformation, and influences foot-surface interaction.

A shoe changes the reaction of the distal limb to forces by increasing mass and changing inertia. This has numerous effects, mainly noticeable in the protraction phase of the stride.[53] Of more importance with regard to injury are the effects of shoes on the stance phase of the horse, such as a slight increase in loading of the limb, slightly faster rotation of the hoof, less vertical lifting of the hoof,[54] and an increase of up to 14% in force exerted on the navicular bone by the DDFT.[12] Shod horses also show less heel expansion during stance and more contraction of the heel at the end of stance than unshod horses.[25] There is evidence that shoes change ground contact area and load distribution.[55] These and other mechanisms may account for observed changes in shock-absorbing capabilities observed with shoes,[56,57] resulting in an increase of load during impact. This increase in impact, however, does not extend much beyond the distal phalanx, and changes between shod and unshod horses are minimal at the fetlock level.[12]

The Influence of Shoe Material

There is anecdotal evidence that some horses are "more comfortable" or "go better" in plastic or rubber shoes. This has been attributed to reduction of "jarring" after impact. Shoe grip varies among shoe types, and various techniques are commonly used to enhance shoe grip, such as studs or high-friction material such as rubber. Time and slide distance of a foot at impact are not significantly altered by shoe application regardless of the material used (steel, plastic, rubber). However, decelerating forces after impact and dynamic friction are significantly lower with plastic shoes compared with rubber or steel shoes.[58] Horses may compensate for different shoe-ground interaction by altering gait to maintain a constant slip time and distance.

The Influence of Shoe Type

Egg bar shoes have been shown to have no effect on the force on the navicular bone in sound horses[12] but have had a significant unloading effect in some horses with navicular disease, particularly those with a collapsed heel.[59] Clinical experience is similar: egg bar shoes may be beneficial in some horses but not others. The mechanism of action is unclear. Egg bar shoes may redistribute load over a larger area of the heel, reinforce or couple the flexible palmar regions of the foot, and/or reduce heel pain. Redistribution of load to make a horse more comfortable also results in a reduced force on the navicular bone. Why egg bar shoes help some horses more than others is unclear but may relate to the exact location of pain, the type of pathology, and/or the degree of heel collapse.

Shoes with toe clips, shoes with quarter clips, and natural balance shoes were compared. Pulling the toe back made breakover (heel off to toe off) start earlier and shortened the duration of breakover. The moment arm of the GRF on the DIP joint during breakover was reduced, but because breakover started earlier and hence at a higher GRF, the peak moment and force on the navicular bone were similar in the three shoe types.[50]

ALTERATIONS IN MECHANICS WITH SPECIFIC ORTHOPEDIC DISORDERS

Changes in kinematics and kinetics are mainly pain induced and rarely pathognomonic in horses. Chapter 22 provides an overview of locomotor changes and compensatory mechanisms associated with lameness in horses and how these can be assessed objectively.

Studies on changes in mechanics with specific orthopedic disorders are rare. These studies are scientifically challenging for a variety of reasons, not the least of which is difficulty in standardizing subjects.

Mechanics of Palmar Foot Pain and Navicular Syndrome

In a study investigating the mechanics of the distal limb in normal horses and horses with palmar foot pain, there was a significant difference in the load distribution through the stride. A combination of force plate analysis, motion analysis, and radiography was used to determine the limb forces, the weight distribution under the foot, the force in the DDFT, and the compressive stress on the navicular bone during the stance phase of trot. These data show that in normal horses the force on the navicular bone rises through stance to a peak at around 85% of stance just before the heel leaves the ground.[59] This force profile is caused by passive loading of the DDFT via its accessory ligament: as the DIP joint extends in late stance the tendon is stretched, increasing the force in the tendon and hence the compressive force it exerts on the navicular bone. In horses with palmar foot pain, the force on the navicular bone peaks early in stance and again just before the heel leaves the ground. The late peak is similar in magnitude in normal and diseased horses, but the early peak, present only in horses with navicular disease, results in a much higher loading rate on the bone, which may be responsible for the pathological remodeling observed in horses with the disease.[8] After palmar digital analgesia the tendon force and hence the force on the navicular bone dropped in early stance and midstance.[60] The observed changes were thought to be caused by the phenomena discussed in the following paragraphs.

The horse perceives general pain in the navicular or heel region rather than pain specific to the navicular bone. This pain could be the result of a variety of pathologies. The horse compensates for this pain in the heel region by landing toe first. The heel is unloaded at the beginning of stance to reduce concussion. After landing the PZM is moved dorsally, increasing the GRF moment arm on the DIP joint, hence increasing force in the DDFT and increasing the force exerted by the DDFT on the navicular bone. Palmar digital analgesia reverses this response to some extent, and the load on the navicular bone is reduced.[59] These data suggest there may be a positive feedback mechanism in which navicular region pain elicits a compensatory mechanism that increases the compressive force on the navicular bone. This may explain why some horses with chronic heel pain develop radiological changes in the navicular bones. Whether such an increase in loading would actually cause navicular disease is unproven. This mechanism can also provide an explanation for the reported susceptibility of horses with a broken-back hoof-pastern axis to the development of navicular disease and the tendency of some horses with long-standing navicular disease to develop boxy, upright feet. A horse with collapsed heels will tend to exert a higher force on its navicular bones (because the DDFT is stretched further; see earlier) so it will be more susceptible to develop navicular disease. A long toe increases the moment arm on the DIP joint and thus the force on the navicular bone during toe-first landing and possibly also at breakover. Some horses that are attempting to unload their heels are presumably so successful that they will develop contracted heels and upright feet.

Changes in Mechanics in Horses with Laminitis

A change in foot mechanics is also apparent in horses with laminitis. The laminar junction is weakened, and the normal force transfer from the hoof wall to the distal phalanx via the laminar junction is disrupted. In sound horses the laminae deform elastically under load; in a laminitic horse the laminae change plastically, which, together with detachment of the laminae, results in rotation and/or sinking of the distal phalanx within the hoof capsule, which further disrupts the normal mechanical behavior of the hoof with subsequent consequences to its vascularization.

Laminitic horses land heel first, which is assumed to be to protect the painful dorsal laminae (laminar detachment occurs predominantly in the dorsal region of the foot). Laminar detachment destabilizes the distal phalanx and results in rotation and/or sinking of the distal phalanx, depending on the extent of detachment with respect to the position of the PZM. Rotation occurs when there is weakening of the laminae in the dorsal region, yet the laminae at the heel remain mechanically competent. The distal phalanx pivots about this point so that the toe moves palmad and distad following the "pull" of the DDFT. Rotation of the distal phalanx causes shortening of the DDFT and reduction of the force in the DDFT. The reduction in DDFT force results in a reduced flexor moment in the DIP joint during stance. Because the moments on the DIP joint must balance, this reduces the extensor moment created by the GRF. This reduction in moment is reflected in the PZM moving toward the heel. The dorsal laminae are unloaded and the proportion of the load transferred through the intact palmar laminae is increased.[61] Rotation can thus be regarded as a self-limiting event, the magnitude (angle) of which depends on the degree of laminar detachment. If extensive laminar detachment occurs, then the forces exerted on the remaining laminae will exceed their mechanical capacity, and the distal phalanx will sink rather than rotate further.

Changes in Mechanics in Horses with Osteoarthritis of the Distal Hock Joints

Horses with OA of the distal hook joints (bone spavin) are described as having a characteristic gait. The gait is characterized by a shortened cranial phase of the stride; the limb is moved medially during the flight phase and then swung laterally just before ground impact ("stabbing"). This gait is believed to be the result of the horse attempting to reduce the load on the painful medial aspect of the tarsus. In a study comparing normal horses and horses with bone spavin and the position of the PZM in the hind feet, the PZM was found to be more plantar and lateral than in normal horses, confirming that they change their gait to unload the painful medial aspect of the tarsus.[62] The Editors have observed a similar gait associated with many other sources of hindlimb pain and debate the existence of pain on only the dorsomedial aspect of the distal hook joints.

Changes in Mechanics in Horses with Superficial Digital Flexor Tendonitis

In horses with experimentally induced SDF tendonitis, trotting speed slowed and therefore forces decreased. In the affected limb, however, force in the SL decreased more than that in the SDFT and DDFT, thus changing load distribution between the flexor structures (see Figure 26-6).[34] More information about the role of mechanics in the pathobiology of tendon injury is given in Chapter 68.

CONCLUSION

Biomechanics is an ever-changing field, the progress of which is closely linked to the evolution of new techniques and computational power. Horses do not get injured standing still, and musculoskeletal injury is strongly related to exercise. The quantification of locomotor parameters at high speed under field conditions is relatively new and will lead to more insights in the future. The horse's musculoskeletal system is finely tuned by millions of years of evolution, and changes in one structure inevitably lead to changes in others. Understanding the complex interactions among the individual musculoskeletal structures, how they are influenced by the surface, and how these interactions vary among individual horses is a prerequisite to understanding not only the development of musculoskeletal disorders, but also how to best treat them and, even better, how to prevent them.

Chapter 27

The Foot and Shoeing

◼ FOOT BALANCE, CONFORMATION, AND LAMENESS

Andrew H. Parks

Athletic injury usually results from imposition of repetitive stresses that exceed the capacity of the tissues. The magnitude of stresses and hence the likelihood of injury frequently depend on balance and conformation. Therefore balance and conformation are extremely important in maintaining optimal limb function and limiting athletic injury.

Conformation describes shape—in this case, the shape of the distal aspect of the equine limb—and conveys the size and relative proportions of the limb. Balance embraces both the conformation and function of the hoof—conformation because it describes the shape of the hoof, and function because it describes the way the hoof relates to the skeletal structures of the limb and the ground at rest and at exercise. Balance is divided into geometric (static) balance and functional (dynamic) balance.

Balance and conformation are both three-dimensional concepts. Balance usually is divided into three planes: frontal (dorsal), sagittal, and transverse. Balance in the frontal plane is called *mediolateral balance* and in the sagittal plane is called *dorsopalmar (plantar) balance*.

To understand how balance and conformation affect stresses that cause injury, it is necessary to consider the function of the distal limb and then examine how it changes with conformation and balance. Therefore consideration must be given to the musculoskeletal system, the hoof and the ground, and the interfaces. There are some substantial differences between the front and hind feet. Because almost all research and documented clinical observation are related to the front feet, all discussion in this chapter refers to the front feet unless specifically stated otherwise.

The hoof is the interface between the musculoskeletal system and the ground. The hoof functions both as an extension of the distal phalanx, as a lever about the distal interphalangeal (DIP) joint, and as an entity in itself. As part of the integument the hoof behaves differently to the structures of the musculoskeletal system, both in its manner of constant growth and its biomechanical properties. As the hoof capsule is constantly worn at the ground surface, it is replaced by the germinal epithelium of the coronary band and the sole. In nature and in an appropriately trimmed foot, there is an approximate balance between growth and loss of the hoof capsule so that the growth rings are parallel.[1-3] The exact mechanism by which hoof growth is regulated is unknown, but several factors are known to influence it: season, inflammation, nutrition, and topical irritants.[4] Growth of the wall also is inversely related to pressure on the coronary band. Hoof wall growth proximal to a hoof wall resection or horizontal grooving of the hoof wall appears accelerated, whereas the immediately adjacent hoof wall growth may be retarded.[5] This effect may be mediated by an effect on the vasculature of the coronary band.

During normal hoof growth the hoof wall migrates distally in relation to the distal phalanx by active separation and reformation of desmosomes as the primary epidermal lamellae move past the secondary epidermal lamellae.[6] The distal growth of the hoof wall under normal loading patterns is approximately even around the circumference of the hoof, and the position of the coronary band in relation to the distal phalanx is static. However, in response to locally increased and decreased loads within the hoof wall, migration of the coronary band proximally and distally in relation to the distal phalanx is superimposed on the normal pattern of hoof wall migration, suggesting that a whole segment of the wall can displace distally and even proximally by movement within the lamellae.

The stiffness of the hoof wall changes radially, and the outer stratum medium is stiffer than the inner stratum medium but is much less stiff than bone throughout. The stiffness of the hoof wall at the toe and quarters is similar, but the difference in thickness indicates that the quarters are more flexible.[7] The hoof wall sustains strains greater than bone, but under normal circumstances it operates within its elastic range at a fraction of its yield capacity.[8] The stiffness of the hoof wall increases with increased strain rate.[9] The hoof wall is viscoelastic. It responds to a rapidly applied force in an elastic deformation so that it returns to its original form rapidly; however, to a slowly applied force, it deforms in such a manner that when the force is removed, the hoof wall returns to its original form slowly.[10] Because of its physical properties the hoof wall is more fracture resistant than bone,[11] but because it is a much less stiff material than bone, it will bend and shear more readily. The biomechanical properties of the soft tissues between the hoof capsule and distal phalanx are less well understood, but the periosteum of the distal phalanx fails before the junction between the epithelial and dermal lamellae.[8] The lamellar junction is much less stiff than the hoof wall[12]; dorsally the lamellae are oriented perpendicular to the tangent to the hoof wall, but at the quarters they are in a more palmar direction.[13]

FOOT FUNCTION

At Rest

At rest a horse bears approximately 28% to 33% of its body weight on each forelimb. The exact roles of the wall, sole, and frog in weight bearing are undetermined. Weight bearing has traditionally been viewed with a horse on a flat, firm surface so that the weight-bearing surface is the full circumference of the wall and the immediately adjacent sole, although the weight is not evenly distributed around the perimeter of the foot. Studies on feral horses indicate that the toe and quarters are worn so that if the horse stood on a flat, firm surface, the weight would be transmitted through the wall at the heel and the junction of the toe and quarter biaxially, although there is

References on page 1268

some variation related to the terrain on which the horse has lived.[14] The dorsal aspect of the toe and midquarters would not bear weight. Domestic horses that were allowed to wear the feet "naturally" at pasture and then stood on different surfaces showed remarkably different loading patterns.[15] When stood on a firm surface, greatest contact was at the medial and lateral aspects of the heel and just medial and lateral to the dorsal aspect of the toe, comparable to feral horses. When stood on sand, the greatest contact was with the central aspect of the sole, and the total contact area was approximately four times greater for horses standing on sand than on a flat, firm surface.

Any part of the ground surface of the foot is potentially weight bearing. Each point of contact that bears weight transmits that force to the ground, although the pressure at each point varies. The sum of all the forces from all points of contact is called the *ground reaction force* (GRF). It is represented as a vector, with a magnitude and direction, and a location or point of force, which is also called *the point of zero moment*. In the stationary horse this force is almost vertical and located slightly medial to the dorsal third of the frog. Therefore the GRF is dorsal to the center of rotation of the DIP joint, with a resultant moment about the joint. This moment is opposed by an opposite moment created by tension in the deep digital flexor tendon (DDFT). The GRF acting through the phalanges creates a moment about the metacarpophalangeal joint that is opposed by tension in the digital flexor tendons and the suspensory ligament (SL).

At Exercise

Stride Phases

The stride is divided into flight and stance phases.[16] The stance phase of the stride is further subdivided into initial contact, impact, support, and breakover. The foot should move in a sagittal plane parallel to the longitudinal axis of the horse.[5] In an exercising horse the GRF changes in magnitude, point of force, and direction with and within the phases of the stride. The GRF is separated into components in three axes: x-axis (mediolateral), y-axis (dorsopalmar), and z-axis (vertical).

Initial Contact

At a walk, trot, or gallop the initial contact most frequently is heel first,[17,18] usually the lateral side first, or both sides simultaneously.[19,20] Medial first landing is uncommon. However, some horses may land flat-footed, and the propensity to do so increases with increasing speed.[19] When the heel does strike first, the foot is flat within 1% to 2% of the stride duration.[21] Toe-first landing is rare.[19,21] It has been suggested that the position of the foot at landing is determined by proprioceptive reflexes that optimally orient the position of the distal phalanx before impact, regardless of the length of toe or angle of the foot.[22]

Impact Phase

The impact phase is characterized by oscillations in the GRF centered on the heel that last for approximately 50 ms.[16] The oscillations are associated with the highest rate of loading during the stride; thus the greatest likelihood of injury is during the impact phase. The vertical velocity and acceleration are greater in the forelimbs than in the hindlimbs, which explains the greater concussion and likelihood of lameness in the forelimbs.[21] Significant damping of the impact oscillations occurs within the hoof, the two most distal phalanges, and the associated articulations.[23-25]

Support Phase

The support phase extends from the end of impact until the onset of breakover. At a walk the vertical GRF is biphasic, with peaks at either side of the middle of the stride, but at the trot there is a solitary peak approximately halfway through the stride.[26,27] For most of the stance phase the GRF is slightly medial to the dorsal third of the frog.[28] The force is absorbed and energy is stored by the digital flexor tendons and SL as the metacarpophalangeal joint extends[29] so that the maximal GRF coincides with maximal extension of the metacarpophalangeal joint.[17,30] At the walk, forces in the superficial digital flexor tendon (SDFT) and DDFT peak before the peak in the GRF, but the force in the accessory ligament of the DDFT (ALDDFT) peaks during the second half of the stride as the DIP and metacarpophalangeal joints extend.[31,32] The GRF in the dorsopalmar direction is negative during the first half of the stride as the limb decelerates. The foot continues to slide forward after initial impact until arrested, at 6% of the stride duration in the forelimb[33] and 23% in the hindlimb[34] in trotters on a dirt track. The fore foot bounces more on impact, whereas the hind foot slides more.[21] During the second half of the stride the horizontal GRF becomes positive as the limb accelerates to provide propulsion. The balance of propulsion and retardation is such that the forelimbs contribute more to retardation and the hindlimbs to propulsion.[27] Faster gaits create higher GRFs and greater strains in the hoof wall,[8] DDFT, SDFT, and SL.[35] Under in vitro loading conditions, hoof wall strains increase with load as strain field epicenters develop around the circumference of the hoof, at the junction of the middle and distal thirds of the hoof, regardless of load.[36]

The distal phalanx is loaded during the stance phase. It was initially thought that the palmar processes rotate palmarly during loading,[37] but recent finite element analysis indicates that the toe rotates distally and that the palmar processes move proximally; the findings of the finite element analysis, though not yet verified in vivo, are consistent with observations of hoof wall deformation and strains.[38] The sole flattens and spreads as the heel expands,[2,39] more so distally than proximally.[8] At the same time, the dorsal hoof wall flattens and rotates palmarly to parallel movement of the distal phalanx. Frog contact with the ground during exercise appears to be variable.[25,39] The role of frog pressure in hoof expansion is undetermined; there is evidence that indicates it is not involved, yet other evidence suggests that frog pressure is not the sole determinant of hoof expansion but may enhance it.[25,40] Either way, the frog must function as an effective expansion point to permit movement of the sole ventrally and the heel abaxially. It is hypothesized that the digital cushion, in conjunction with the cartilages of the foot, participates in dissipating energy during impact through a hydrodynamic mechanism.[41,42] The DIP joint passively flexes[43] and the metacarpophalangeal joint extends. During the second half of the stride the DIP joint extends[43] and the tension in the ALDDFT increases.[32] Tension in the collateral sesamoidean and distal sesamoidean impar ligaments also increases,[43] and pressure on the navicular bone increases.[44] The metacarpophalangeal joint flexes. The point of action of the GRF moves toward the toe toward the end of the stance phase.[16]

Breakover Phase

Breakover begins when the heel starts to lift off the ground and ends when the toe leaves the ground. The point of breakover is the most dorsal part of the hoof or shoe in contact with the ground as the heel begins to lift off the ground. From the instant the heel and sole have left the ground, the GRF is concentrated at the toe. Tension in the ALDDFT peaks,[31] and increased strain in the dorsal hoof wall[8] causes the distance between the medial and lateral aspects of the heel to be narrower than at rest. The horizontal forces between the ground and the hoof at the toe during the latter part of the stance phase and breakover are associated with the final stages of propulsion.

Flight Phase

The flight phase begins at maximal retraction of the limb and the foot reaches maximal height soon thereafter. A second peak in height occurs just before maximal protraction. The limb retracts slightly before impact to decelerate the limb as the distal phalanx is optimally aligned for impact. The deceleration of the forward movement of the foot is important in reducing the stresses of impact.[45] The stresses on the distal aspect of the limb during the flight phase are low, because the distal joints flex and extend passively following movement of the upper limb during protraction.[16]

Stride Characteristics

The time and motion characteristics of the stride are important in determining the animation qualities of the gait and the speed of the horse. Higher movement of the foot and greater flexion and extension of the joints represent greater animation. Long retraction with a high starting point is considered desirable, and longer strides are associated with greater speed. Maximum stride frequency is inversely related to speed index.[46-48]

The ground surface affects the angle of the hoof to the ground during the stride, the duration of the stride, and the absorption of impact energy. On a flat, firm surface the plane of the hoof is the same as that of the ground, but on a surface such as sand, the angle of the hoof with the ground increases gradually during the stance phase of the stride.[35] This rotates the plane of the sole so that it is more perpendicular to the vector of the GRF, which appears to aid traction and propulsion. Ground footing has been divided into three types: dense hard surfaces, surfaces with friction damping such as sand, and structural damping surfaces such as wood chips.[49] Friction damping occurs through displacement of small particles, whereas structural damping occurs through viscoelasticity of the particles. The duration of impact oscillations is related to the hardness of the surface. Harder surfaces are associated with a longer duration of impact oscillations than soft surfaces and less energy absorption.[50] A loose cushion on the surface reduces the peak impact force.[51] Racetracks with a hard surface result in faster race times, but horses are more likely to sustain injury associated with the increased energy of

impact.[51] Ground footing also affects stride and swing duration, which are both longer on an elastic, softer surface than a hard, firm surface.[52] At a walk, strain in the DDFT and ALDDFT is lower on sand than on a hard, flat surface,[35] such that it resembles the effect of a heel wedge.

OPTIMUM BALANCE AND CONFORMATION

Optimum function should intuitively demand optimum conformation and balance. Practitioners have inherited many empirical notions that often are based on what types of conformation and balance do not work and cause problems. Generally these ideas predate modern motion analysis and therefore relate to conformation and static balance. Modern techniques that allow dynamic evaluation of function have supplemented and sometimes contradicted the geometric approach.

Static Balance and Conformation

Viewed from the lateral aspect, the foot-pastern axis should be straight; that is, the dorsal hoof wall should be parallel to the dorsal surface of the pastern, and the angle of the heel should approximate that of the dorsal hoof wall (Figure 27-1). The angle of the dorsal hoof wall and the foot-pastern axis to the ground is variable, but it frequently is cited as 50 to 54 degrees in forelimbs and approximately 3 degrees steeper in hindlimbs.[53] Other studies report higher or lower means and variable relationship between the angles of the dorsal hoof wall of the forelimbs and hindlimbs.[54,55] In domestic horses the length of the hoof wall has been approximately linked to the weight of the horse (7.6 cm for 360 to 400 kg; 8.25 cm for 430 to 480 kg; 8.9 cm for 520 to 570 kg).[53] In feral horses the toe length ranges from 6.7 to 8.9 cm[14,54] but is independent of weight.[54] In domestic horses with either trimmed or shod hooves, the length of the heel should be approximately one third that of the toe,[2,55] but in feral horses it varies with

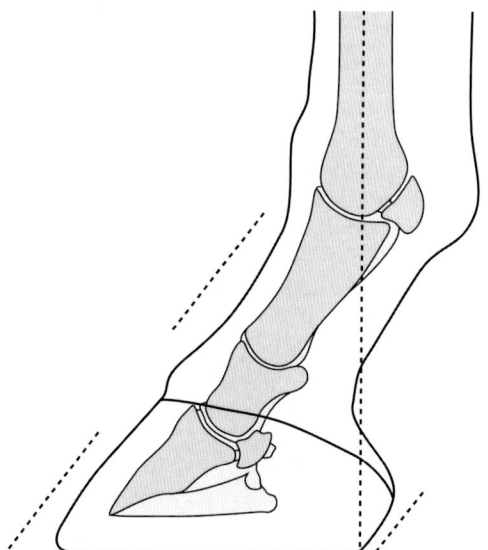

Fig. 27-1 • Traditional guidelines defining normal dorsopalmar static or geometric balance. The dorsal hoof wall should be parallel to the dorsal aspect of the pastern and to the hoof wall at the heel. A line bisecting the third metacarpal bone should reach the ground at the weight-bearing parts of the heel.

the terrain.[14] An imaginary line that bisects the third metacarpal bone (McIII) should intersect the ground at the most palmar aspect of the weight-bearing surface of the heel.[56,57]

On a lateromedial radiographic image the dorsal hoof wall should be 14 to 20 mm thick depending on breed[58-60] and parallel to the dorsal surface of the distal phalanx. The angle made by the distal solar border of the distal phalanx with the ground ranges from 2 to 10 degrees.[58,60,61] The center of rotation of the DIP joint is palmar to the center of the ground surface of the foot. Viewed from the dorsal aspect, a line bisecting the metacarpal region should bisect the phalanges and foot, so that the foot is approximately symmetrical, including the mass of foot on either side of the line and the heights and angles of the walls.[1,3,57,61] The medial quarter is frequently steeper so that the medial wall is shorter than the lateral wall.[2,62,63] A line drawn between any two comparable points on the coronary band should be parallel to the ground, and a vertical line bisecting the McIII should be perpendicular to a line drawn across the coronary band or the ground surface of the foot[62] (Figure 27-2).

On a dorsopalmar radiographic image the center of the DIP joint should be centered over the ground surface of the foot. Ideally, the articular surface of the distal phalanx should be parallel to the ground, but it is more important that the interphalangeal joint spaces be even.

Viewed from the ground surface the width and length of the hoof capsule of the fore foot should be approximately equal, although the hoof capsule may be slightly wider than it is long.[54,62] The hind foot is invariably slightly longer than it is wide. The point of breakover is best assessed from the ground surface and should be located near the center of the toe. Dynamic studies of the location of the GRF during breakover show that it deviates laterally

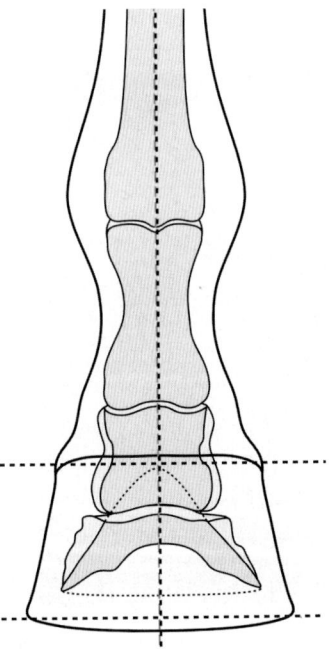

Fig. 27-2 • Traditional guidelines defining normal mediolateral static or geometric balance. A single line should bisect the metacarpal region and phalanges. A line drawn across any two comparable points on the coronary band, or on the weight-bearing surface of the foot, should be perpendicular to the axis of the metacarpal region.

during breakover, returning toward the dorsopalmar axis of the limb before the foot leaves the ground[20]; this suggests that breakover normally occurs lateral to the dorsopalmar axis of the foot. The ideal location for breakover in the dorsopalmar axis is disputed. In a traditionally trimmed and shod horse, breakover is positioned where the line of the dorsal hoof wall intersects the ground, although it may ideally be located more palmarly. With the position of the hoof wall used as the reference point, breakover is between the dorsal margin of the hoof and the white line.[64] Alternatively, breakover is 2.5 to 3.8 cm dorsal to the apex of the frog or 0.6 cm dorsal to the dorsal margin of the distal phalanx.[14,65] The relationship of the longitudinal axis of the frog to the underlying distal phalanx is relatively constant compared with the rest of the ground surface of the hoof. The medial and lateral aspects of the ground surface of the foot are symmetrical about the central axis of the frog,[3,57,64] although slight asymmetry, the lateral sole being about 5% wider than the medial sole, may be beneficial.[62] The latter is compatible with an even coronary band and a steeper medial wall. The size of the foot should be proportional to the weight of the horse.[54,55] The sole should be concave. The frog width should be at least 50% to 67% of frog length,[55,62] and the weight-bearing surface of the heel should coincide with the widest part of the frog.[55]

Dynamic Balance

Current definitions of dynamic balance describe the placement of the foot at initial impact. Traditionally, the foot is said to be in dynamic mediolateral balance when the medial and lateral aspects of the heel contact the ground simultaneously[3,63] and breakover occurs near the center of the toe.[63] The foot is said to be in dynamic dorsopalmar balance when either the heel lands slightly before the toe or the toe and the heel contact simultaneously.[3] However, both these observations are a function of observation frequency. The fewer observations made per unit time, the more likely the foot is to appear in balance. The more frequently the observations are made, the less likely the foot is to appear in dynamic balance. With increased frequency of observation, it appears that the lateral aspect of the heel or quarter commonly lands first or that the lateral and medial aspects of the heel land simultaneously, but that medial first landing is rare.[19,20] It is likely that the scope of dynamic balance will expand in the future to incorporate the magnitude, location, and direction of the GRF; distribution of stresses within the hoof capsule during the stride; and dynamics of breakover.

IMBALANCE AND POOR CONFORMATION

Balance and conformation cannot be considered in isolation, because poor conformation predisposes a horse to developing imbalance, and an imbalanced foot may cause a horse to stand as if it had poor conformation.[1] The effects of imbalance have been examined by experimentally inducing imbalance and by clinical observation. To understand the effects of imbalance it is simplest to consider the consequences of deliberately unbalancing the foot. Poor conformation cannot be readily altered under experimental conditions, and its effects must be assessed by comparison between horses with different conformations.

Mediolateral Imbalance

Mediolateral imbalance is caused by either poor trimming of a horse with good conformation or poor conformation causing excessive stress on one side of the foot so that it grows more slowly than the other side. Inappropriate shoe placement can promote imbalance. If a shoe is set too much to one side or the other, or if the shoe is rotated so that the shoe covers less of the medial or lateral aspects of one heel than the other, it alters the mediolateral stress on the hoof capsule.[66] A single heel calk causes elevation of one side of the foot; the foot tilts and rotates and may contribute to interference.[66]

Mediolateral imbalance can be induced by applying a wedge pad to elevate the medial or lateral side of a foot or trimming a foot unevenly. The coronary band is no longer parallel to the ground or perpendicular to the sagittal axis of the limb. The horn tubules of the dorsal hoof wall are no longer oriented in the sagittal plane. Dorsopalmar radiographic images demonstrate that the DIP joint space is narrower on the side of hoof elevation, and the middle phalanx slides to the lower side.[43] In addition, the condyle of the middle phalanx on the elevated side of the foot moves palmarly, in effect causing the distal phalanx to rotate on the middle phalanx so that the dorsal margin of the distal phalanx rotates away from the elevated side[43] (Figure 27-3), but the horse has the appearance of being toed toward the elevated side.[1]

The GRF shifts toward the elevated wall.[67] In foals, compressive strains were immediately increased in the lateral cortex of the McIII and decreased in the medial cortex by elevation of the lateral wall with a wedge.[68]

The immediate dynamic effects of mediolateral imbalance result in a greater frequency of mediolateral asymmetrical footfall, the lengthened side landing first.[19] The location of the GRF displaces abaxially toward the lengthened side of the foot.[19,69,70]

Prolonged mediolateral imbalance affects the relationship between the hoof capsule and the distal phalanx, causes distortion of the hoof capsule, and alters hoof wall growth.[71] If a foot is trimmed unevenly, so that one wall is longer than the other, the longer wall grows more slowly than the shorter wall. The longer wall develops a flare, and the shorter wall becomes underrun.[1,71] In more severely affected horses the coronary band bulges abaxially to create a lip at the proximal margin of the hoof wall on the elongated side. The horse breaks over on the shorter side of the toe. It is my impression that the solar margin of the distal phalanx partially realigns with the ground surface, either because the wall actually migrates proximally or because distal movement of the hoof wall is inhibited, resulting in a net proximal displacement of the coronary band in relation to the distal phalanx. Ultimately, prolonged mediolateral imbalance causes remodeling of the phalanges because of redistributed stresses according to Wolff's law.

Rotational deformities and angular deformities may mimic each other. In most rotational deformities, it appears as if the metacarpophalangeal joint is the most proximal joint to be rotated, but it is not uncommon for the carpus to appear rotated. With rotational deformities, the McIII is vertical and the observer can rotate around the limb until the metacarpal and phalangeal axes are correctly aligned unless the rotation occurs within the phalangeal axis. In

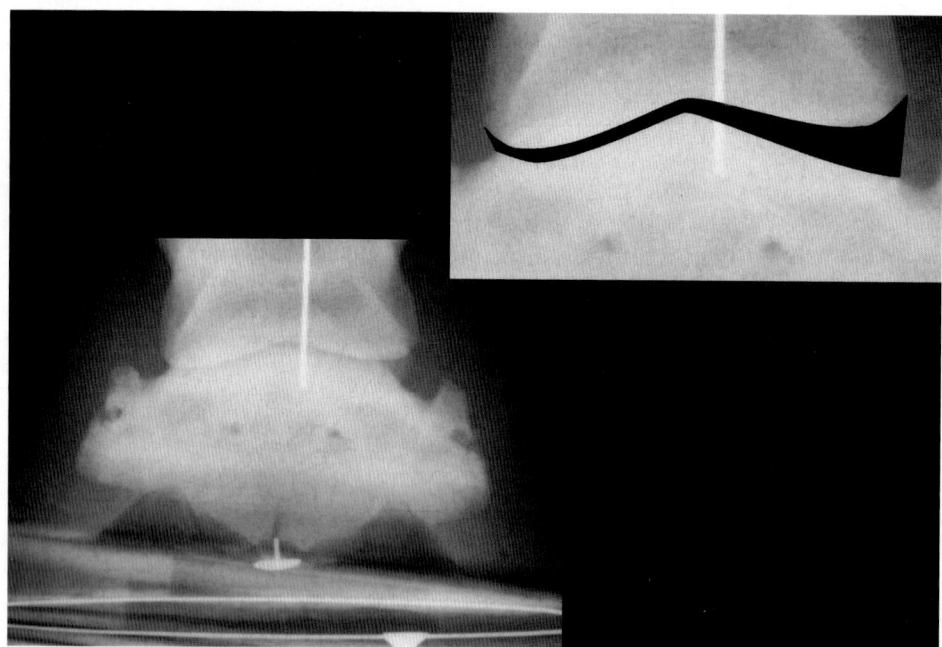

Fig. 27-3 • Mediolateral imbalance causes misalignment of the articular surfaces and rotation of phalanges in relation to each other. Deliberate elevation of one wall causes the articular surface of the distal phalanx to tilt, but it does not tilt as much as the ground surface of the foot, indicating that there is accommodation within the viscoelastic structures of the foot. The distal articular surface of the middle phalanx is displaced from the elevated side of the foot. The inset in the upper right corner shows that the joint space (outlined in black) on the elevated side of the foot *(left)* is narrower than on the lower side *(right)* of the foot, caused by compression of the distal interphalangeal joint surface on the left side.

horses with angular deformities that occur proximal to the fetlock, including base-wide or base-narrow conformation, the McIII may not be vertical and there may not be a viewpoint from which the metacarpal and phalangeal axes are correctly aligned.

Rotational deformities, such as toe-in and toe-out conformation, alter the position of the ground surface of the foot in relation to the midsagittal vertical axis of the limb. Toe-in conformation causes the foot to wing out during the flight phase of the stride,[1] and if the limb does not deviate from a vertical axis, the foot lands on the lateral heel quarter and breaks over at the lateral toe. Toe-out conformation causes the foot to wing in during the flight phase of the stride. The foot lands most frequently on the lateral heel quarter, as with toe-in conformation (see Figure 4-13). Breakover is less consistently directed than breakover in horses with toe-in conformation. Angular deformities, including base-wide and base-narrow conformation, and varus and valgus deformities also alter the position of the ground surface of the foot in relation to the ideal vertical axis of the limb. If an angular deformity (e.g., varus) is severe enough that the distal aspect of the wall at the quarter is axially directed, it will become underrun. Rotational and angular deformities may occur in combination, complicating the picture.

Dorsopalmar Imbalance

Dorsopalmar imbalance has several causes. A broken-back foot-pastern axis may follow poor trimming, either leaving the toe too long or trimming the heel too short. A shod horse wears its heels against the shoe whereas the toe wears very little, so the hoof angle changes up to 3 degrees over 8 weeks.[2,72] This change must be allowed for by trimming the toe slightly more than the heel, because even trimming around the foot causes a gradual decrease in the hoof angle.[3] Using too small a shoe or leaving a shoe on too long causes the palmar ground contact to move dorsally, imposing greater stresses on the heel, which then is prone to collapse.[63,66] Toe grabs and heel calks alter the foot axis and concentrate stress.[66] Thoroughbred horses may have a genetic predisposition for a broken-back foot-pastern axis; galloping causes the angle of the dorsal hoof wall to decrease, and removing the horse from training causes it to increase.[73]

At rest, elevation of the heel causes the DIP and pastern joints to flex and the metacarpophalangeal joint to extend.[74,75] The effect is greatest at the DIP joint.[74,75] In addition, elevation of the heel increases DIP joint pressure and localizes the contact dorsally between the middle and distal phalanges; toe elevation localizes articular contact to the palmar aspect of the joint.[76] In vitro, elevation of the heel with a wedge decreases the strain in the DDFT, the extensor branches of the SL, and the medial hoof wall[77] and decreases the moment about the center of rotation of the DIP joint.[78] The horizontal distance between the center of rotation of the DIP joint and the toe decreases with heel elevation. In addition, the horizontal distance between the toe and an imaginary vertical line bisecting the McIII dropped to the ground is decreased. The clinical consequence of heel elevation is decreased heel growth indicative of increased stress within the wall of the heel.

Lowering the heel or raising or lengthening the toe to create an acute hoof angle or long toe increases the likelihood of toe-first landing.[19,22] Heel wedges increase the

maximum flexion of the DIP joint during the support phase of the stride and decrease the maximal extension of the DIP joint during breakover.[79] Elevating the heel increases the likelihood of heel-first landing.[19] The overall impulse (force × time) on the foot is least when the foot-pastern axis is straight, indicating that a straight foot-pastern axis is least injurious to the foot.[19] At a walk, elevating the heel decreases the strain in the DDFT and its AL[32,78] with little effect on the SDFT and SL. The decreased strain in the DDFT is reflected in decreased pressure on the navicular bone.[44] Elevating the toe results in a marked increase in strain in the ALDDFT and a lesser increase in strain in the DDFT at the end of the stride as a result of increased extension of the DIP joint.[32] Strains in the SDFT and SL are either reduced or unchanged.[32,78] Horses with small hoof wall angulation have a prolonged breakover, but the length of stride, duration of the stance, and swing phases are unchanged.[19,22] When hind feet are trimmed with more acute hoof wall angulation, breakover is delayed but the timing of impact is unchanged as normal coordination is restored during the swing phase of the stride. There is an increase in overreach distance, the distance between the print of the front foot and the landing point of the hind foot.[80] Heel wedges delay the dorsal shift in the GRF and decrease the maximum torque about the DIP joint during the second half of the stride. Toe wedges have an opposite effect.[32,70] However, neither toe nor heel wedges alter the dorsopalmar position of the point of force during midstance of the stride, indicating that the heel is not unloaded. Both toe and heel wedges cause medial displacement of the point of force.[70] Increasing the length of the toe prolongs breakover but does not alter stride length; however, it increases maximal flexion of the metacarpophalangeal joint during the swing phase.[81,82]

The position of breakover in the sagittal plane appears to influence the angle of the dorsal hoof wall and the distal phalanx. Moving the point of breakover palmarly from the most dorsal margin of the hoof wall increases the angle of the dorsal hoof wall and the ground and increases the alignment between the middle and distal phalanges.[65,83] Whether this effect is related to the biomechanical properties of the dorsal hoof wall or relief of pain within the foot is undetermined. The effect of increased hoof angle on hoof wall strain is inconsistent. In an in vitro model, hoof wall strain did not change with increased hoof wall angle.[77] In contrast, in an in vivo experiment, increased hoof wall angle increased hoof wall strain more at the lateral quarter than at the toe and not at all at the medial quarter.[84]

The effect of pastern length and the angle of the foot-pastern axis are less well established. The angle of the hoof-pastern axis to the ground is a feature of a horse's conformation. It cannot be changed experimentally, but comparing horses with different conformations shows that the point of force in horses with a small hoof-pastern axis angle is more palmarly positioned than in horses with a larger axis angle.[28]

Prolonged dorsopalmar imbalance also has delayed effects because of the nature and growth of the hoof capsule. In barefoot horses, trimming the feet to reduce the dorsal wall angle by leaving the toe long causes the ground surface of the foot and the frog to become narrower, and the shape of the ground surface tends to skew away from a circular shape.[85] As might be expected, the heel appears to grow much faster, but curiously, the wall at the toe also grows faster. Neither the area of the sole nor the length of the frog change. Interestingly, when the foot is trimmed with a short toe to increase the dorsal wall angle, neither the width nor the shape of the frog or hoof changes.[85] Clinically, the same appears to occur in shod horses. In horses with extremely long toes the foot becomes "hoof bound." The heel of long-toed horses is predisposed to become underrun because the heel bends dorsally. Both of these phenomena are seen in Tennessee Walking Horses or American Saddlebreds intentionally shod with long hooves.

Other Forms of Imbalance

Many horses with imbalanced feet have a combination of mediolateral and dorsopalmar imbalance. For example, a foot with a sheared heel has one bulb of a heel longer than the other, which is frequently associated with a flared toe quarter on the opposite side of the foot.[86] Diagonal imbalance has been described dynamically. The hoof lands on one corner of the hoof capsule and then loads the diagonal corner, with consequent distortion of normal hoof capsule shape and alignment with the rest of the distal limb.[87] Other local deformations of the hoof wall occur, either uniaxially or symmetrically, that do not fit the classical description.

IMBALANCE AND POOR CONFORMATION AS A CAUSE OF LAMENESS

Poor conformation and imbalance of the distal aspect of the limb are common, as is pain causing lameness that can be isolated to the distal aspect of the limb. However, demonstrating the correlation is not always straightforward. In some horses an obvious disease process and obvious imbalance coexist, and when the imbalance is treated the lameness improves. In other lame horses, imbalance is evident with no other clinical, radiological, or scintigraphic evidence of disease, and treating imbalance also improves the lameness. In yet other lame horses, there is evidence of imbalance, with or without other evidence of disease, but treating the imbalance does not improve the lameness. To my knowledge, only one study thoroughly investigated the effects of hoof balance on injury. The odds of catastrophic musculoskeletal injury and suspensory apparatus failure were lower when the lateral sole area was greater than the medial sole area.[62] Suspensory apparatus failure was more likely the greater the difference between the angles of the dorsal hoof wall and the heels. McIII condylar fractures were less likely with a steeper toe angle.

Mediolateral imbalance is associated with a shift in the point of force of the GRF, distortion of the hoof capsule, induced asymmetry of the articulations of the distal limb, and rotation of the DIP joint. With increased compressive stresses the following problems are clinically presumed to follow imbalance: subsolar bruising, hemorrhage in the white line from laminar tearing, pain from shearing heel bulbs, quarter or heel cracks, thrush in narrow frogs, pedal osteitis, fractures of the palmar process of the distal phalanx, sidebone, synovitis, osteoarthritis, and more proximal fractures.[1,57,63,66]

The effects of dorsopalmar imbalance should be separated into the effects of broken-forward and broken-back foot-pastern axes. A broken-back foot-pastern axis increases the load on the palmar aspect of the foot during weight bearing and increases the stresses in the toe at breakover. It causes hyperextension of the DIP joint and increases the tension in DDFT and pressure on the navicular bone. Therefore it can be expected to be associated with heel bruising, lamellar tearing at the toe, osteitis of the palmar processes of the distal phalanx, navicular disease, tendonopathy at the insertion of the DDFT, and more proximal injuries of the tendons or suspensory apparatus.[3,57,63,66] In the hindlimb a broken-back foot-pastern axis appears to be associated with tarsal and back pain.

A broken-forward foot-pastern axis (upright) appears to be less pernicious.[3,57] It increases the load on the dorsal half of the foot and decreases tension in the DDFT. The principal findings are subsolar bruising distal to the dorsal distal margin of the distal phalanx and subsequent osteitis of the distal phalanx.[57]

An upright foot-pastern axis has traditionally been considered to predispose toward concussive injuries of the weight-bearing structures in the limb, whereas a foot-pastern axis with an acute angle to the ground predisposes toward strains and sprains of the flexor apparatus. Similarly, a long pastern has been considered to predispose toward strains and sprains.

Any angular deformity located more proximal in the limb that increases the mediolateral symmetrical loading of the foot can be expected to have effects similar to mediolateral imbalance. Rotational deformities do not seem to be a frequent cause of problems. Toe-out conformation is more likely to cause interference, but anecdotally, toe-in conformation is considered more likely to cause lameness.

Undoubtedly, technological advances in diagnostic imaging and pain localization will help identify other combinations of disease and structure. Epidemiological studies will confirm the relationships between the different features of poor conformation and imbalance and disease.

CLINICAL IDENTIFICATION OF HOOF IMBALANCE

The horse must be observed while it is standing squarely to assess each limb in relation to the whole and in motion on a flat, level surface. Each foot must be examined on and off the ground.

Mediolateral Imbalance

Visual inspection should note the position of the entire limbs to identify angular or rotational deviations more proximally in the limb that may have repercussions for the foot (Figure 27-4). Visual inspection of the foot on the ground should note rotational deformities of the metacarpophalangeal joint and placement of the foot in relation to the sagittal axis of the limb. The hoof capsule should be inspected closely for asymmetry of the coronary band. This is frequently a strictly visual inspection, but graphing the height of corresponding medial and lateral points on the coronary band provides objectivity that can highlight an imbalance and provide a record for future comparison.[55,88] The medial and lateral walls should be inspected for flares and evidence of an underrun heel, lipping at the coronary band, and even spacing between the growth rings.

The ground surface of the foot reflects changes elsewhere in the hoof capsule. The foot should be approximately symmetrical about the center of the frog. In

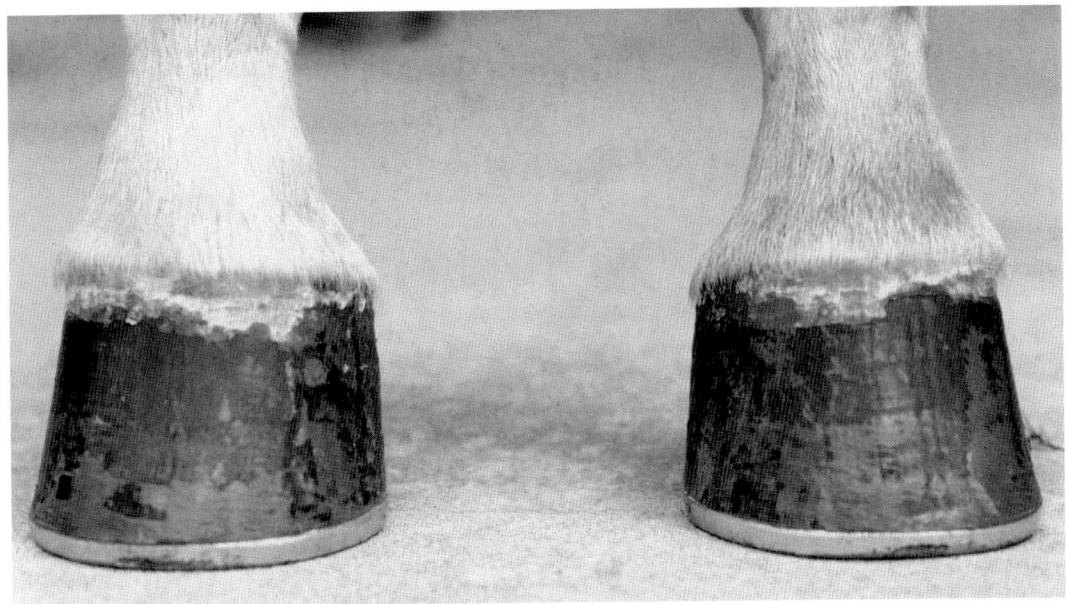

Fig. 27-4 • Feet of a yearling with bilateral mediolateral static imbalance. The lateral wall of both front feet reaches higher than the medial wall so that the lateral coronary band is higher than the medial coronary band; consequently, the dorsal aspect of the coronary band is sloping distally and medially. The growth rings are also tilted in the same direction as the coronary band. The imbalance creates the impression that the pastern is no longer centered in the foot but is displaced laterally.

mediolateral imbalance, the sole may appear wider on the side with a flare in the wall and narrower on the side with an underrun wall. Dorsal displacement of the ground surface of one heel bulb in relation to the other accompanies proximal displacement of the coronary band at the heel commonly associated with sheared heel. Wear of the shoe or wall at the toe indicates the point of breakover. Alternatively, the breakover point may be identified by lifting the antebrachium cranially, allowing the metacarpal region and pastern to hang passively, and then lowering the foot; the point of breakover is the first part of the foot to touch the ground[57]; however, this assumes that breakover occurs at the same point regardless of the gait and speed of the horse. Breakover frequently occurs slightly lateral to the center of the toe in horses with normal balance, but any marked asymmetry in breakover may indicate mediolateral imbalance. It also may follow angular or rotational deformities of the limb. Asymmetrical bruising adjacent to the wall at either quarter may signify excessive concussion caused by mediolateral imbalance or laminar tearing in a wall with a flare.

Examination of the distal aspect of the limb for rotational or angular conformation by viewing the limb on the ground from the dorsal aspect may be misleading because it is influenced by weight bearing. The ground surface of the foot automatically aligns with the surface of the ground regardless of the relative lengths of the medial and lateral hoof wall. This causes secondary rotation within the phalangeal axis. To circumvent this rotation, to find the point of breakover the limb can be examined off the ground by lifting the limb by holding it forward from under the carpus; the angulation or rotation within the distal limb is observed by sighting down the metacarpal region, pastern, and hoof.[57]

The traditional way to assess mediolateral balance is to sight across the ground surface of the foot with the leg off

the ground, holding the proximal metacarpal region and allowing the digit to hang downward in the sagittal plane with the metacarpophalangeal and interphalangeal joints in passive extension. A line drawn across any two corresponding points on the circumference of the ground surface of the wall should be perpendicular to the axis of the limb as judged by the metacarpal region. If the limb is perfectly symmetrical about the axis of the limb, without angular or rotational deformities, and the observer is directly above the limb, this technique is probably satisfactory within the limits of the observer. I question the accuracy of this technique because most distal limbs are not symmetrical but have at least some element of rotation about the metacarpophalangeal joint. A smaller number of horses have true angular deformities at the metacarpophalangeal joint. For reliability, there must be consistency in the extension of the metacarpophalangeal joint and in the position of the observer. T-squares have been used to improve the reliability of this observation,[4,57] but misalignment of the T-square with the axis of the metacarpal region decreases accuracy.

Dynamic mediolateral balance is assessed by observing the horse from in front and from behind at a walk and at a trot. Because the degree to which symmetry of landing can be detected is a function of the frequency of observation and speed of the horse, only more severe imbalances can be detected at a trot compared with a walk, and more subtle differences in timing remain undetected unless a video recorder or more sophisticated measuring equipment is used. During the flight phase of the stride, movement of the foot, phalangeal axis, and more proximal limb is observed in relation to the plane of travel to correlate with previously noted rotational and angular deformities.

A dorsopalmar radiograph is the only means to assess the relationship between the hoof capsule and the phalanges (Figure 27-5). Overt imbalance can be detected on

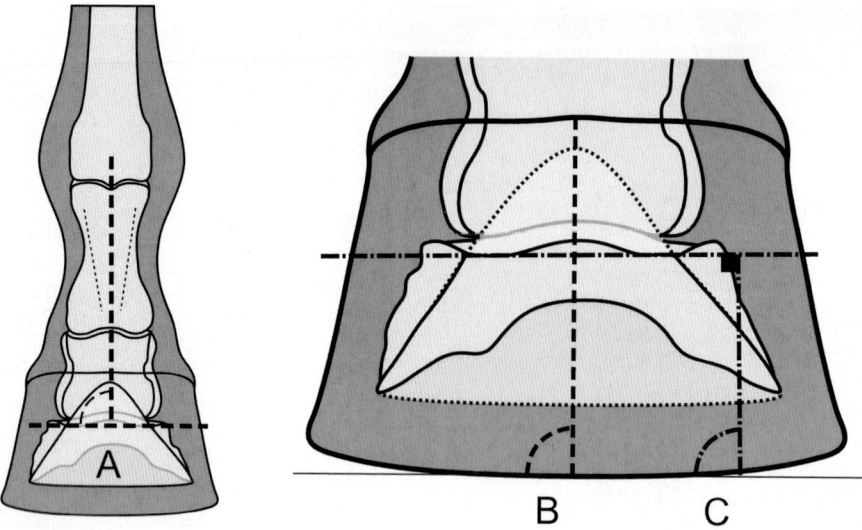

Fig. 27-5 • Radiological assessment of balance has been described by Caudron and colleagues.[89] **A,** Rotation between the phalanges is indicated when a line bisecting the distal phalanx is not perpendicular to the articular surface of the distal phalanx. **B,** A tilt in the axis of the hoof capsule is determined radiologically when a midsagittally placed wire marker is not perpendicular to the ground surface of the foot. **C,** Tilting of the distal phalanx is evident when a line drawn perpendicular to a line drawn across the articular surface of the distal phalanx is not perpendicular to the ground. All measurements presuppose that the radiographic beam bisects the foot (the dorsal wire marker bisects the apical process of the distal phalanx and the central sulcus).

routine dorsopalmar radiographs, but detection of more subtle changes requires strict technique because apparent radiological imbalance can be readily induced artificially. Both feet must be weighted equally, because unilateral weight bearing induces mediolateral asymmetry and rotation of the interphalangeal joints.[43] The foot must be allowed to assume its natural orientation to the rest of the limb, most reliably achieved if it is placed on a swiveling block. Deformation of the hoof capsule may be induced by rotation within the limb, which may change the angulation of the distal phalanx with the ground.[89] The metacarpal region must be within 10 degrees of vertical in the frontal (dorsal) plane. The x-ray beam must be horizontal and centered on the midsagittal plane so that a wire marker centered on the dorsal hoof wall bisects the central sulcus of the frog on the radiographs. Neither toe-in nor toe-out conformation alters the radiological measurements of mediolateral balance if assessed in this manner.[90,91] Interpretation of balance from dorsopalmar radiographs is usually based on examining either the relationship between the articular surface of the distal phalanx and the ground, which are ideally parallel, or the symmetry of the phalangeal joints, which should be of even width medially and laterally. When these appear to be in disagreement, I consider joint asymmetry to be more important because it is difficult to envisage a circumstance under which it is not harmful. In addition, interpretation of imbalance is more complex in horses in which the imbalance is chronic because the imbalance is associated with compensatory changes in hoof wall growth and also appears to be associated with movement of the hoof capsule in relation to the distal phalanx.

Although mediolateral imbalance can unquestionably cause lameness, the hoof capsule is not necessarily or even likely to be the site of pain that is associated with lameness. Rather the pain is associated with the effects of imbalance,

that is, stress on the deeper structures of the hoof and the musculoskeletal structures of the distal aspect of the limb. Therefore it is not surprising that the lameness may improve with perineural or intraarticular analgesia of the distal aspect of the limb in a similar manner to osteoarthritis of the DIP joint or navicular disease.

Dorsopalmar Imbalance

The limb is examined for angulation at the carpus and metacarpophalangeal joint. The foot-pastern axis is visually inspected to determine whether the axis is straight or broken forward or back. This method provides only a rough guide. Visual examination can be improved by using a gauge, one limb of which is aligned with the pastern and one with the dorsal hoof wall. However, deciding exactly what landmarks to use on the pastern for alignment introduces irregularity. In addition, the axis changes as the horse shifts its weight or posture. Similarly, concavity of the dorsal hoof wall in the sagittal plane raises the issue of with what to align the pastern. If the dorsal hoof wall is concave, usually the top third of the hoof wall is the most closely aligned to the dorsal surface of the distal phalanx.

The length of the toe from the proximal aspect of the coronary band to the ground surface in the midsagittal plane of the hoof is readily measured with a tape and compared against reference values or previous measurements for the same horse. This information is greatly underused. The length and angle of the heel also are evaluated. Only the wall at the heel distal to the bulb should be evaluated, because inclusion of the heel bulb causes the angle to be underestimated. A heel that is angled more acutely to the ground than the dorsal hoof wall is longer than a heel that is parallel to the dorsal hoof wall. Interestingly, it is the angle of the distal phalanx to the ground, and not the angle of the heel, that correlates well with the force on the navicular bone.[92]

A long toe is associated with elongation and narrowing of the ground surface of the foot. The frog width decreases in a comparable manner with the width of the foot. The length of the frog should remain almost constant, so that an increase in the length of the ground surface of the foot is reflected in an increase in the distance between the apex of the frog and the most dorsal aspect of the toe or break-over point. The ground surface of the heel should be adjacent to the base of the frog. If the ground surface of the heel projects dorsally to the base of the frog, the heel is either too long, angled too acutely, or both. Hemorrhage in the white line at the toe caused by lamellar tearing may be a secondary indicator that the toe is too long.

In a horse with a broken-forward foot axis, a flexural deformity of the DIP joint must be distinguished from heel contraction secondary to pain. In a foot with a flexural deformity the heel and frog are more likely to be wide and the ground surface of the foot is triangular, resembling a hind foot. In contrast, a contracted foot has a narrow heel and frog.

The relationships between the individual phalanges and between the phalangeal axis and the hoof are determined radiologically. The phalanges are closest to alignment when the foot-pastern axis is straight. However, the proximal interphalangeal joint usually appears slightly extended (dorsiflexed), even with a straight foot-pastern axis.[74] The dorsal hoof wall should be parallel to the distal phalanx. The angle of the solar margin of the distal phalanx with the ground, the thickness of the sole at the dorsal distal margin of the distal phalanx, and the distance from the dorsal margin of the distal phalanx to the toe should be evaluated. The center of rotation of the DIP joint is assessed in relation to the weight-bearing surface of the toe and heel. Normally, the center of rotation should be slightly palmar to the center of the ground surface of the foot. Dorsopalmar imbalance is likely if the solar margin angle is less than 2 degrees, the center of rotation of the DIP joint is markedly shifted toward the heel, and the horizontal distance between the toe and dorsal margin of the distal phalanx is elongated.

In hind feet, dorsoplantar imbalance associated with hyperextension of the DIP joint appears to take a slightly different form compared with the fore feet. The dorsal hoof wall is not necessarily long when viewed from the side. The toe frequently has been dubbed back, and it acquires a marked convexity. Viewed from the ground surface the concavity of the sole is exaggerated, and if the foot is shod, the frog lies between the branches of the shoe. This may be from descent of the frog, or proximal displacement of the heel. In my experience, these horses almost invariably are shod.

Evaluation of dynamic dorsopalmar balance suffers from the same limitations as evaluation of dynamic mediolateral balance. However, gross imbalances can be observed with the horse at a walk or trot. Normally, when viewed from the side the foot is expected to land flat or slightly heel first.

TREATMENT OF IMBALANCE AND POOR CONFORMATION

Treatment of imbalance provides at least two challenges. The first is to have a clear objective of what ideal balance is for any given horse because, although there are some hard and fast rules, other areas are unclear. For example, a straight foot-pastern axis is beneficial, but the exact length of toe that is optimal for the same foot is not clear.

The second challenge is interpreting the measured indicators of balance. For example, the measures of mediolateral imbalance, symmetry of the coronary band, sighting along the axis of the metacarpal region and across the ground surface of the foot, footfall, and dorsopalmar radiographs may not agree on whether the foot is imbalanced or the direction of the imbalance or may provide varying degrees of imbalance. Radiography appears to be the most accurate and is substantiated scientifically.[91]

Difficult balance problems may not have easy solutions, and judicious experimentation that can be both time-consuming and expensive may be necessary. Balance may be corrected, but long-standing problems may not be correctable. Poor conformation can be compensated for but can never be corrected with trimming or shoeing in an adult horse. The ability to compensate for poor conformation is inversely related to the height in the limb from which the defect originates. Major imbalances should be corrected gradually over time, or lameness may result from the correction.[4,57,63]

Rebalancing the foot can be performed by visual assessment of the hoof and foot-pastern axis before and after trimming, repeating until a satisfactory result is obtained. Rebalancing may be facilitated by radiological assessment of balance. Radiographs, with markers to indicate the angle of the dorsal hoof wall, the location of the apex of the frog, and the position of the coronary band, obtained before trimming are used as a baseline on which to base the trim. Deformation of the hoof capsule in the pretreatment radiographs may result in underestimation of the imbalance,[90] and radiographs obtained after trimming may be helpful to assess the accuracy of treatment.

Treatment of imbalance is complicated by the necessity to consider both the immediate and delayed effects. The reversal of the immediate effects of imbalance is the most straightforward, because it requires nothing more than restoring the normal length of the wall around the circumference and ground surface of the foot. The effects of viscoelastic deformation of the hoof wall caused by uneven pressure should correct spontaneously if the force is removed and sufficient time is allowed before the horse is reshod. Other deformation of the hoof wall caused by contraction or aberrant hoof growth may have to wait for new hoof wall to grow from the coronary band to the ground surface after the biomechanical forces have been optimized by trimming and shoeing.

Horses with mediolateral and dorsopalmar imbalance may respond to trimming and allowing them to go barefoot.[66] Application of poultices to the foot has been advocated to encourage hoof realignment.[88] This allows the effects of prolonged imbalance from the viscoelasticity of the hoof and misdirected hoof growth to adjust without the influence of the shoe. However, the quality of a wall that is usually shod may deteriorate over several weeks before it improves, and flat-footed horses may become more lame.

In foals, trimming, shoeing, or surgery corrects poor conformation associated with abnormal angulation in either the sagittal or frontal (dorsal) planes. Conformation in adult horses is fixed, but changing foot balance or shoeing sometimes can compensate for poor conformation. However, when the stresses are realigned to benefit a musculoskeletal structure, they become less than optimally aligned for the hoof capsule and predispose to a different problem. For example, in a horse with a long pastern at a normal angle or with a sloping pastern of normal length, the foot is further dorsal than is ideal. This creates a greater moment about the metacarpophalangeal joint. This can be compensated for in part by extending the heels of a shoe further past the heel of the foot than normal. This technique moves the most ground support palmarly, but it also moves the point of application of the GRF further palmarly, increasing both the stresses on the heel and the propensity to deform. Treatment of poor conformation is almost always a compromise.

Mediolateral Imbalance

Uncomplicated mediolateral imbalance is corrected by decreasing the length of the wall on the side of the foot in which it is longest, or lengthening the wall on the side that is shortest. If the horse has sufficient foot, it is always preferable to correct the imbalance by trimming the longer wall. However, when the hoof is insufficient to permit trimming the longer wall sufficiently to restore the equilibrium, then the shorter wall must be lengthened. A wall can be lengthened in several ways. However, care must be taken because alteration of the balance may actually cause lameness. The simplest method is to add a pad, either a shim or a full wedge pad. The shim pad is riveted to the branch of the shoe so that it is interposed between the foot and the shoe, or a full wedge pad is positioned so that the thickest portion of the pad is on the shortest side of the foot. Alternatively, the shorter wall can be lengthened by addition of acrylic. This can be allowed to set and a shoe nailed to the hoof and composite, or the shoe can be attached to the foot with the acrylic so that the position of the shoe in relation to the hoof capsule is adjusted as the acrylic dries.[93] A shoe with branches of different thickness can be used. This makes the thinner branch lighter. The width of the web can be increased to compensate for the thinner branch so that the asymmetrical effect of uneven weight distribution is minimized.

Flares and underrun walls that accompany mediolateral imbalance are frequently addressed at the time of shoeing through appropriate flare removal and shoe positioning. The longitudinal axis of the frog is a good guide to the location of the center of the ground surface of the foot in the sagittal plane. The shoe should be positioned symmetrically about the frog so that the flare that extends abaxially to the shoe is dressed back and the shoe extends abaxially past the underrun wall.[1] However, if there is distortion in the hoof wall, seen as displacement of the coronary band proximal to the flare, and there is exaggeration of the normal convexity of the wall where it is flared, then the flare is likely to return over one or more shoeing cycles. This distortion is most likely to resolve if the horse is allowed to go barefoot or, if feasible, the wall is floated at the point of the flare. If the hoof wall convexity and coronary band are not distorted, then the flare and underrun wall should correct as new hoof wall grows distally.

The most controversial issue in balancing a foot is restoring mediolateral imbalance in the following circumstances: (1) when the coronary band is asymmetrical with one heel bulb or quarter higher, usually the medial quarter or heel bulb, which is obvious with the horse standing; (2) when the ground surface of the shorter wall appears farthest from the metacarpophalangeal joint when the axis of the limb is sighted with the foot off the ground; and (3) when the shorter wall contacts the ground first at a walk. This is typical with a sheared heel. Should the long wall be shortened, potentially increasing the discrepancy in footfall, or should the long wall be lengthened, exacerbating an already imbalanced appearance? I cannot see any benefit in lengthening an already long wall or determine how this might improve the wall. Radiological evidence of joint asymmetry may resolve the dichotomy. If this fails, the horse can be shod with a shoe positioned perpendicular to the axis of the limb with the long heel floated and extra support provided by a heart bar shoe.

Compensation for angular or rotational deformities in the limb of adult horses is seldom attempted because they are not the cause of pain, and attempts to compensate for them may increase the asymmetry of stresses imposed on the hoof capsule. However, if an angular limb deformity causes a secondary mediolateral imbalance, this may need correction whenever the horse is trimmed.[63] If a rotational deformity causes either the lateral or medial heel to land long before the other, aligning the shoe branches perpendicular to the axis of the metacarpal region rather than the pastern may be beneficial.[57] A medial or lateral extension may be used to extend the ground surface of the foot or shoe under the axis of the limb to improve the distribution of forces in the more proximal parts of the limb.[3,57] However, these corrections improve function in one part of the limb at the expense of another. When angular or rotational deformities cause limb interference, it may be necessary to change shoeing to change the flight of the limb to reduce the likelihood of injury.

Dorsopalmar Imbalance

An imbalanced foot usually is related to a toe that is too long or a heel that is underrun, less frequently to a heel that is too long, and seldom to a heel or a toe that is too short. The toe or heel is trimmed until the horse has a straight foot-pastern axis. Because dorsopalmar imbalance starts to develop immediately after shoeing because of disparate growth of the toe and heel, deliberately trimming the foot 1 to 2 degrees broken forward may be useful.

Correction of a broken-back foot-pastern is more complicated after secondary changes have occurred. If excessive toe length has caused the sole to change shape so that it is longer and narrower than normal, the breakover should be brought back to a more natural position. The angle of the dorsal hoof wall should be reevaluated to determine whether it has improved before other measures are taken. In a barefooted horse the breakover is set by the trim, and in a shod horse by both the position and roll of the toe of the shoe. The foot width should increase naturally in time, and the shoe should be set full at the quarters to accommodate the abaxial movement of the quarters. An extended period may be required to regain the optimal ratio of the length to width of the ground surface of the foot. If an underrun heel is a result of a long-toe conformation, the weight-bearing surface of the heel can be moved palmarly (backed up), but the angle of the heel often is too acute to allow alignment of the foot-pastern axis regardless of toe length. This can be corrected immediately by raising the heel. The heel can be raised with a wedge pad, either a full pad or shim, with a shoe with wedged heels, or by building up the heel with acrylic.[3,94] However, this process increases the pressure on the coronary band at the heel and may decrease the rate of heel growth. Alternatively, a bar shoe may be used to limit the heel from digging into the ground.[4] Allowing the horse to go barefoot may result in the fastest improvement in conformation, but this often precludes the horse working, and flat-footed horses may become more lame. Contraction of the width of foot often accompanies dorsopalmar imbalance, and grooving or thinning the heel has been recommended.[1,65] For long-term soundness, I believe it is preferable to realign the foot-pastern axis as well as possible and then allow a wider, straighter heel to grow from the coronary band. This may require time out of work. Raising the heel is frequently the fastest way to return a horse to work; thus the manner of treatment may depend on the immediate athletic demands placed on the horse.

A broken-back hoof-pastern axis in the hind limbs is treated by trimming the toe, using radiography to assess the improvement. Frequently the solar margin of the distal phalanx is tilted by several degrees, with the dorsal margin farther from the ground than the plantar processes. In my experience, it may not be initially possible to improve the angle of the solar margin of the distal phalanx beyond parallel to the ground. It frequently is ideal to allow the hind feet to go bare. When the foot must be shod, in contrast to the fore foot, I recommend setting the toe of a rim shoe in line with where the wall at the toe should meet the ground and provide no more coverage of the heel than is necessary. It may be necessary to provide support to the ground surface of the plantar half of the foot.

Treating a broken-forward foot-pastern axis caused secondarily by pain or a flexural deformity by decreasing the dorsal hoof wall angle may exacerbate pain. A broken-forward axis resulting from pain must be addressed by treating the primary problem. Correction of a broken-forward foot-pastern axis associated with a flexural deformity is not always necessary, but when it is, it should be accompanied by desmotomy of the ALDDFT.

Compensation for a long pastern or a low foot-pastern axis when the weight-bearing surface of the foot is too far dorsal in relation to the limb may be achieved by extending the heels of the shoe.[88] This correction is directed at reducing the moment about the metacarpophalangeal joint by moving the palmar aspect of the foot or shoe farther palmarly, usually by using an egg bar shoe, but any heel extension that is not likely to result in the shoe being pulled by the hind foot will work. Compensation for an upright conformation is not readily feasible and fortunately is seldom necessary.

◼ HORSESHOES AND SHOEING

Andrew H. Parks

An equine veterinarian must be able to assess the way a horse is shod in relation to the current use of the horse and make recommendations for shoeing to improve the function of the distal aspect of the limb. This necessitates

an understanding of the basic construction and fit of a shoe and its use. Determining how a shoe affects the horse's performance requires an understanding of how the elements of a shoe function. To understand how to change the function of the distal aspect of the limb, it is necessary to know which modifications to form and fit of a shoe can achieve the desired result. It is more important to consider how a basic shoe may be modified to achieve a given result than list a variety of different shoes for specific conditions. Farriery developed as an art guided by individual and collective experience and has recently been supplemented by scientific studies. Some guidelines are derived empirically and others have a scientific basis, but the skill of the individual is a vital third element.

HORSESHOES
Foot Preparation
Shoeing cannot be considered in isolation from foot trimming. The foot is trimmed to remove the excess length of wall that accrues because the distal aspect of the wall is protected from wear by the shoe. After the foot has been cleaned, the exfoliating sole and ragged margins of the frog are debrided with a hoof knife. The wall is trimmed with nippers and then leveled with a rasp.

In addition to maintaining optimal balance in a sound horse by trimming the foot to restore the length of the foot, several other modifications to the hoof capsule may be performed, usually with the intent of improving hoof capsule shape, and often in conjunction with specific shoeing practices. *Floating the hoof wall* refers to trimming part of the hoof wall short so that the hoof will not touch the shoe at that point. The shoe supports the wall on either side of the floated area dorsally and palmarly unless the heel is floated. Floating the hoof wall is used to relieve that section of the wall from weight bearing. This encourages faster growth at the coronary band, permits proximally displaced wall to descend, relieves stress in the wall so that new wall growth may redirect itself, and relieves pain. The heel is floated to treat an underrun heel. This is most effective when the palmar aspect of the foot is given additional support (e.g., with a heart bar shoe).

Grooving of the hoof capsule is designed to mechanically dissociate the capsule on one side of the groove from the other. The groove is made through the full thickness of the stratum medium. The grooves may be created parallel or perpendicular to the horn tubules. The use of several grooves parallel to the horn tubules between the quarters and heel of the hoof capsule has been advocated to encourage expansion of the heel by increasing the flexibility of the wall but is of dubious value. Grooves perpendicular to the horn tubules usually are made around part of the circumference of the hoof capsule immediately distal to the coronary groove, typically at the toe or heel. These grooves relieve the pressure on the coronary band from the stresses in the weight-bearing wall. This increases the speed of new wall growth proximal to the groove and allows the new wall to grow independent of distracting forces in the distal aspect of the wall.

Resection of the hoof capsule involves removal of the stratum medium, usually starting at the weight-bearing surface and extending a variable distance proximally, typically involving no more than 20% to 40% of the circumference of the hoof capsule. Because this creates instability of the hoof capsule, it is used only for managing horses with laminitis, white line disease, and hoof wall avulsion injuries. Thinning the hoof wall at the heel so that partial thickness of the stratum medium is removed has been recommended to increase the flexibility of the wall and encourage expansion of the hoof capsule, but it is seldom performed.

The Horseshoe Form

In its most basic configuration a horseshoe is a curved steel bar, rectangular in cross-section, that is shaped to conform to the contour of the ground surface of the hoof wall and wide enough to cover the ground surface of the hoof wall and the immediately adjacent sole. The shoe has four surfaces: the foot and ground surfaces and the inner and outer edges, called *rims*. The parts of the shoe are named after the corresponding section of the hoof, that is, the *toe*, *quarter*, and *heel*. Each shoe has two branches, medial and lateral, that extend from the center of the toe to the medial and lateral heels, respectively. The substance of the branches is called the *web*, which has a width and thickness. The shoe is punched with nail holes, three or four in each branch, three of which are usually used. This shoe is described as *flat* because the ground surface of the shoe is level, *stamped (punched)* because it has nail holes, and *open* because the bar of metal forming the shoe does not form a continuous loop across the heel.

The shoe should fit flush with the outer margin of the dorsal half of the hoof wall from one quarter to the other. From the quarter palmarly or plantarly the shoe should incrementally extend further abaxial to the wall until it extends approximately 0.3 cm abaxial to the wall at the heel to allow for expansion and contraction of the hoof capsule as the foot alternates between weight bearing and non–weight bearing. The shoe branches extend marginally palmar or plantar to the heel to allow for growth of the hoof capsule during the shoeing cycle. This basic shoe pattern and fit may suffice for many horses but frequently is altered to suit the exercise performed by a horse or the ground surface on which the horse is worked and for therapeutic purposes.

Materials and Size

Horseshoes may be made of metal, synthetic polymers, or a composite of the two materials. Altering the material of a shoe alters the weight of a shoe for a given size, the durability of a shoe against wear and other damage, shock absorption, workability, and cost. Most horseshoes are made of steel for reasons of effectiveness, cost, wear, and workability. Aluminum also is used frequently because it is lighter and easier than steel to cold forge, but it wears faster than steel and is not as stiff. Shoes recently have been made from various synthetic polymers and composites of more than one material and are used in specialty situations, but shoe status is in constant flux as new products appear on the market and others disappear.

Metal shoes may be hand forged from bar stock or manufactured. Hand-forged shoes offer the advantage of being customized to the individual foot. However, manufactured shoes are used far more frequently than hand-forged shoes because they save time and a wide range of shoes is suitable for most feet. Bar stock is usually rectangular in cross-section and is available in different sizes varying from 0.6 to 1.2 cm thick and 1.2 to 3.1 cm wide, although the most commonly used size is 0.8 × 1.9 cm. Concave stock is frequently used in Europe. Manufactured shoes, also called *keg shoes*, are sized. However, although sizing within and usually among product lines is consistent for a given manufacturer, there is no universal standard for sizing horseshoes. Manufactured shoes may be generically shaped to the general shape of a horse's foot or specifically designed for a fore or hind foot. The former require more shaping but are cheaper and require less stock on hand. The dimensions of the stock of either manufactured or hand-forged shoes affect the weight of the shoe, stiffness, coverage of the ground surface of the foot, height the shoe elevates the foot off the ground, and rate at which the shoe wears out.

Shoe weight influences biomechanics of movement. The heavier the shoe, the more energy is expended accelerating and decelerating the limb at the beginning and end of each stride. Therefore the lightest shoe is used that is compatible with protecting the wall and adjacent sole and providing the stiffness and wear required. Shoes made from concave stock are lighter than shoes made from regular bar stock. The width and thickness of the shoe usually are uniform around the circumference of the shoe so that biomechanical influence of shoe weight and the stresses imposed are usually balanced about the axis of the limb. Occasionally a shoe may be unevenly weighted to alter the animation or balance of a gait. The increased weight may be at the toe, in one branch, or at one or both heels. Increasing the weight at the heels is done to increase animation but has not been scientifically tested. Increasing the weight of the toe has been used to encourage the horse to reach farther at the beginning of the stride. Toe weights do not increase stride length but do increase flexion in the limb of horses with poor limb flexion during protraction of the limb. They have no impact on horses that already have good limb flexion.[1]

Although the width of the web of a shoe is related to the thickness of the hoof and, at least in part, the size of the foot, it is common to increase the width of the web of the shoe to provide increased protection to the margins of the sole. The thickness of the shoe is related to the rate at which it is expected to wear and to a lesser extent the rigidity needed to prevent the shoe from bending out of shape. The height the shoe raises the foot off the ground also is influenced by the thickness of the shoe, but this is usually a secondary consideration to wear and rigidity.

Cross-Sectional Profile of Shoe Stock

The cross-sectional profile of the shoe may be modified by altering the ground surface, the solar surface, either rim of the shoe, or a combination and may affect the whole shoe or part of the shoe, such as the toe, the branch, or a heel (Figure 27-6).

Several common modifications are made to the ground surface of the whole shoe. Softening the 90-degree angles at the junction of the ground surface of the shoe and the inner and outer rims by beveling or rounding, called *rolling*, increases the ease of breakover. A shoe with a rounded outside rim is called a *roller motion shoe* and improves the ease of breakover in any direction. A similar effect is achieved with a *half round shoe*, so called because it is made from half round stock that resembles a semicircle in cross-section. The toes of flat shoes frequently are rolled or beveled only at the toe to improve the ease of breakover (Figure 27-7). A similar effect is achieved by rockering the toe, that is, bending the full thickness of the shoe

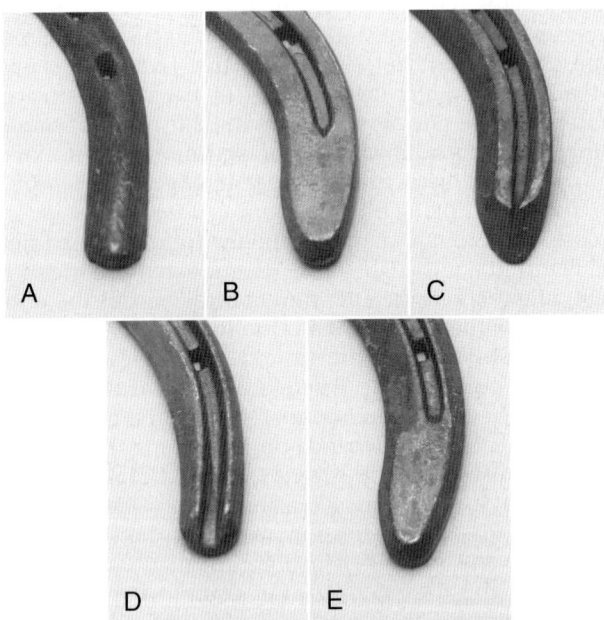

Fig. 27-6 • The cross-sectional profile of the shoe branch can be modified to vary traction and breakover. **A,** Half round. **B,** Flat shoe incompletely creased or fullered. **C,** Concave stock. **D,** Fully creased rim shoe. **E,** Incompletely creased rim shoe. (Eventer, St Croix Forge, Forest Lake, Minnesota, United States.)

proximally. Less commonly, a flat shoe may be asymmetrically beveled or rounded to improve the ease of breakover toward one side or other of the shoe to encourage a horse to breakover toward that side and direct the flight of the foot. Rounding the margin of a shoe to prevent interference is called *safing.*

There is little traction between smooth steel and the ground. Grooves in the ground surface of the shoe, called *fullering* or *creases,* increase traction. The fullering fills with dirt; the friction between dirt in the fullering and the dirt on the ground is greater than steel on dirt. In addition, the crease provides two additional edges that may bite into the ground. The full circumference of the shoe may be fullered, or it may be limited to the branches of the shoe and less frequently just the toe. Fullering a single branch of the shoe enhances traction uniaxially and delays breakover on that side of the foot. When the branches of the shoe are fullered, the nail holes are centered in the groove, which is formed to conform with the inside and outside of the nail heads.

Fullering and modifying the shoe edges frequently are performed in conjunction with each other. Rim shoes are fully fullered, and the ground surface of the rims is beveled toward the fullering of the shoe. More specialized rim shoes have a higher inside or outside rim, hence the names *inside* or *outside rim shoes* (Figure 27-8). A polo plate is a specialized form of inside rim shoe. Because the higher rim is on the inside, the horse is less likely to cause severe injury to another horse in competition yet still benefits from the additional traction of the rim. A barrel racing shoe is a form of outside rim shoe that provides greater traction than an inside rim shoe, although ease of breakover is sacrificed. A similarly modified profile of racing or training plates is termed *swedging.* A classic example of a shoe that

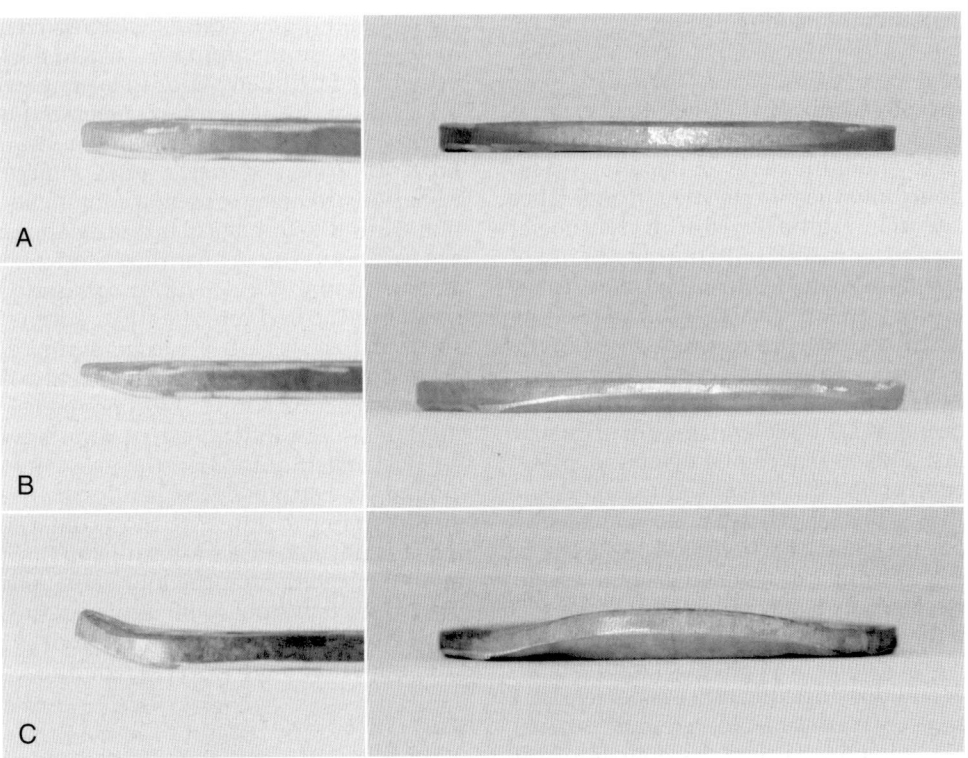

Fig. 27-7 • The toe of a shoe frequently is modified to move the point of breakover palmarly compared with a flat shoe. **A,** Flat shoe. **B,** Rolled-toe shoe. **C,** Rocker toe shoe.

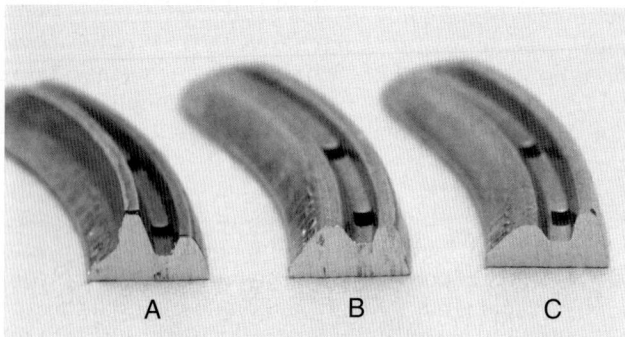

Fig. 27-8 • Cross-section of the branch of three shoes. **A,** A high inside rim. **B,** Rims of equal height; **C,** A high outside rim.

uses all these techniques is a half round, half-swedge shoe worn on the hind feet by harness horses. The inner branch is half round in cross-sectional profile, and the lateral branch of the shoe is swedged. Thus the medial branch, enhanced by the half round, breaks over rapidly, whereas the breakover of the lateral branch is delayed by the swedge.

The only common modification to the solar surface of the shoe is gentle beveling of the inner half of the web toward the inside, called *seating out* or *concaved inner surface*. Horses with flat soles are shod with seated-out or concaved shoes to decrease pressure on the sole adjacent to the wall. Less frequently the heels of the shoe are beveled to the outside margin of the shoe to encourage heel expansion, that is, abaxial movement of the wall during weight bearing. This practice is of questionable benefit, and if the shoe is beveled severely, it causes undue stress in the white line. Beveling the part of the heel of the shoe that extends abaxial to the quarters and heels, called *boxing*, decreases the likelihood of the shoe catching on another object or being trod on by another foot and pulled off.

Extensions

An *extension* is any projection of the shoe that extends outward from the normal outline of the shoe in the horizontal plane (i.e., away from the center of the sole). Extensions may be positioned anywhere around the circumference of the foot. An extension can be forged with the shoe at the time of manufacture or welded onto the outside rim of the shoe. A similar effect is obtained by using an oversized shoe positioned either forward or backward or by setting one branch of the shoe wide. Every extension has the potential to cause the shoe to act as a lever, and this lever action may be either static, when the horse is stationary and the foot bearing weight, or dynamic, particularly during the landing and breakover phases of the stride. When force is exerted on the extension by the ground, the stresses are increased in the adjacent wall and decreased in the opposite wall as the point of action of the GRF shifts. Because the digit is approximately symmetrical in the sagittal plane, the effect of medial or lateral extensions is similar. However, the absence of dorsopalmar symmetry means that dorsal and palmar or plantar extensions function differently. In addition to acting as levers, extensions increase the surface area available for ground contact, which decreases the amount the shoe descends into soft footing at that point in the circumference of the foot. If the surface area of one part of the shoe is altered, it causes

the foot to be supported by a soft ground surface more than the opposite side so the interaction between shoe and ground becomes more complex because the foot is tilted.

Abaxial extensions may be used to either force the opposite wall of the hoof capsule to the ground or support the wall adjacent to the extension. In doing so, the lever decreases the compression in the opposite wall and increases the compression in the ipsiaxial wall, which imposes a moment in the frontal plane. This effect is used in foals with angular deformities. The extension is placed on the opposite side of the limb to the side of the deviation to increase the load in the side of the limb with the extension, to slow growth, and to apply an angular force across the midsagittal plane of the limb.

Toe extensions usually are applied to foals with a flexural deformity of the DIP joint. The toe extension increases the moment about the DIP joint at breakover, as the point of action of the GRF moves dorsally, and during weight bearing if the heel is off the ground. This increases tension in the DDFT and muscle. Therefore the toe extension acts to stretch the musculotendonous unit of the deep digital flexor (DDF). Success depends on the severity of the flexural deformity. In more severely affected foals the pain generated by the increased tension in the DDFT, with or without increased compression at the toe, becomes counterproductive. The change in location of the GRF places the wall at the toe under greater compression, and it is prone to deform.

Heel extensions frequently are used uniaxially or biaxially. In performance horses, extensions frequently take the form of short continuations of the heel that are called *trailers*. Trailers are used almost exclusively on the lateral branch of hind shoes. Front shoes with trailers are likely to be removed by interference from a hind foot. Egg bar shoes project palmar or plantar to the heel of the hoof capsule and act as heel extensions. They are most commonly used on the front feet, where they are less likely to be removed by interference than shoes with trailers. Force on a biaxial heel extension decreases the moment about the DIP joint and the tension in the DDFT. Therefore horses convalescing from a DDFT injury benefit from heel extensions, frequently used in conjunction with heel elevation. Horses with navicular disease appear to benefit from egg bar shoes. The egg bar shoe acts as a palmar extension, and when the horse is on a soft surface it reduces the sinking of the heel into the surface at the beginning of the stride and acts as a heel wedge during the support phase of the stride.[2] Heel wedges are known to decrease the force on the navicular bone.[3] The consequence of this benefit is that the heel is under greater compressive stress.

Heel extensions alter the way the foot strikes the ground. If, as happens frequently, the heel is closer to the ground at impact, the extension contacts the ground first. A lateral uniaxial extension, either in line with or diverging up to 45 degrees from the midsagittal plane of the foot, is used to force the foot to pivot toward the side of the trailer as the foot lands. The toe of the foot is directed laterally after impact and breakover is redirected.

Bars

A *bar* is any part of a shoe that extends from one branch of a shoe toward the other. A *complete bar* extends from one branch to the other; a *partial bar* extends part of the way across the shoe. Most bars extend from one heel bulb to the other to form a closed shoe. A bar may extend from one quarter to the other, or even diagonally across the shoe. There are several patterns of complete bar shoes in common usage, including the straight bar, egg bar, heart bar, and heart bar–egg bar (or full-support shoe). Bar shoes offer several benefits: increased stability and ground contact surface area, local protection, and recruitment of additional weight-bearing area of the foot.

Closing the shoe is considered to make the shoe more stable by decreasing movement between the branches of the shoe and is frequently used, often in conjunction with other shoeing techniques, for instability within either the hoof capsule or distal phalanx. Bars that extend palmar or plantar to the normal position of the heel of the shoe act as a palmar or plantar extension. Bars that set under the ground surface of the foot can be adjusted to protect that part of the foot from ground contact, apply pressure to that part of the foot, or recruit that part of the foot for weight bearing. A straight bar shoe may decrease pressure on the palmar or plantar third of the frog and protect the underlying navicular bone. The heart bar shoe is used to recruit or increase the role of the frog in weight bearing, particularly in the treatment of horses with laminitis. However, heart bar shoes also may be used to support the palmar or plantar aspect of the foot to reduce the stress in the adjacent wall and permit floating of the heel.

An incomplete bar extends part of the way across the ground surface of the foot, most commonly from one heel bulb onto the frog, which supports or reduces weight bearing on a single heel bulb. Alternatively, a full bar across the full width of the foot may be used in conjunction with an incomplete shoe so that the bar covers both heel bulbs, but the shoe is incomplete between one quarter and heel bulb. The bar of a Z bar shoe is shaped with two 90-degree bends that are incorporated into a three-quarter shoe, so that one leg of the Z is attached to the heel bulb of one branch and the other is attached to the quarter of the opposite branch. This shoe also relieves one heel bulb from weight bearing.

Calks, Grabs, and Other Devices Added to the Ground Surface of the Shoe

Various devices are added to the ground surface of a shoe to increase traction. Shoe additives also influence the speed and direction of landing and breakover. Calks are projections of almost any size and shape, although most are round, square, or rectangular, on the ground surface of a shoe (Figure 27-9). The terminology to describe the different types is confusing and at times inconsistent. Different types are called *blocks*, *stickers*, and *studs*. They are made of steel or steel with a tungsten carbide core. Toe grabs and bars welded to the shoe are, in essence, greatly elongated calks. Borium, tungsten carbide crystals in a flux, is welded onto the surface of a shoe in an incremental manner so that any shape or sized projection can be formed. Some calks are permanent, whereas others are temporary. Permanent calks are forged with the shoe, molded in the case of aluminum shoes, at the time of manufacture, or welded or brazed onto the shoe at the time of fitting. Drive calks are semipermanent and are driven into a hole drilled into the shoe. Temporary calks, also called *screw-in calks* or *studs*, are screwed into tapped holes so they can be attached and

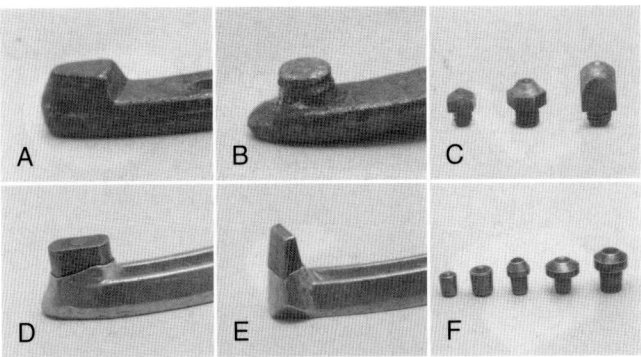

Fig. 27-9 • Calks may be forged with the shoe at the time of manufacture or added later. **A,** Calk of a "heeled" shoe formed at the time of manufacture. **B,** Calk formed by addition of borium. **C,** Various sizes of screw-in calks. **D,** A block inserted into an aluminum shoe at the time of manufacture. **E,** A sticker inserted into an aluminum shoe at the time of manufacture. **F,** Drive-in calks.

removed as needed. Cotton wool is used to plug the hole when not in use. The size and shape of the studs may be changed with the ground conditions.

Calks may be positioned at any point around the circumference of the shoe. The choice of whether to use calks, what type of calks to use, and where to position the calks follows no dogmatic guidelines but usually is based on the preference of the farrier. However, although square and round calks probably offer equal resistance to both mediolateral and dorsopalmar motion, rectangular calks offer greater resistance to motion against movement perpendicular to the long axis. Bilateral heel calks typically are used on jumpers and event horses. Racehorse shoes may be equipped with toe grabs, with or without one or two heel calks (blocks or stickers). Draft horses usually have shoes with biaxial heel calks and, less frequently, a large toe calk.

Projections from the surface of the shoe, in addition to providing traction, inevitably alter the balance of the foot by altering the way the foot contacts the ground. The harder the ground surface, the greater the effect. The taller the calk, the greater the effect. A single calk at either the heel or toe alters mediolateral and dorsopalmar balance. Two heel calks of equal height alter dorsopalmar balance. The addition of a toe calk of equal height restores dorsopalmar balance. The addition of calks to the shoe concentrates stress in the wall immediately proximal to the calk. Therefore the lowest broadest calk compatible with adequate traction is recommended.

The effect of calks on breakover and landing is a secondary consideration, because other methods usually are applied to achieve the same objective. A single heel calk acts in much the same way as an extension, causing the foot to turn toward the side with the calk as the foot lands. Symmetrical placement of two pairs of calks, one pair on either side of the toe and one pair at the heels, encourages the foot to break over in the center of the toe.

Pads

A pad is a layer of material inserted between the hoof capsule and the shoe (Figure 27-10). Pads may provide protection, diminish concussion, and alter the effective angle, length, or both of the foot and shoe. Traditionally

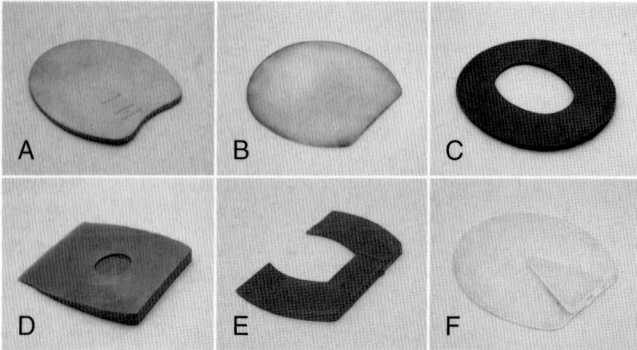

Fig. 27-10 • Pads are inserted between the shoe and the foot and take various forms. **A,** Full leather pad. **B,** Full plastic pad. **C,** Oval plastic rim pad. **D,** Full wedge pad. **E,** A bar wedge pad. **F,** A full plastic pad formed with a molded heart bar. (Cushion Frog Pad, Castle Plastics, Leominster, Massachusetts, United States.)

they have been divided by form into full and rim pads, and by composition into leather and synthetic. However, in the last two decades an imaginative range of products has become available, a range too great for comprehensive discussion. Pads may be riveted to the shoe, which is then nailed to the foot. However, shoes are available that are manufactured with a rim pad bonded to the shoe. Full pads are fitted between the foot and the shoe and cover the entire ground surface of the foot. The cavity between a full pad and the sole usually is filled with pine tar and oakum, or a synthetic equivalent such as silicone, to prevent the cavity filling with dirt. In contrast to full pads, rim pads are fitted to the contour of the shoe so that the sole is not covered.

Pads that cover the sole protect the ground surface from direct trauma. However, efficacy has been questioned because the pad and packing effectively lower the contact point with the ground. Pressure on the pad can then be transmitted to the sole, although in a more diffuse pattern. Any pad interposed between the shoe and the wall has the potential to diminish concussion on the wall. However, products vary greatly.[4] Wedge pads, either full pads or bar wedges, change the angulation of the hoof capsule to the ground. Wedge pads most commonly are used to raise the heel. Wedge pads also are used to raise either the medial or lateral wall to improve the mediolateral balance when this is not feasible by trimming. This can be achieved with a full pad, but it is more common to use a uniaxial wedged shim.

More novel pad designs include extension of the ground surface of the pad between the branches of the shoe to fill part or all of the cavity between the ground and the sole to form a flexible heart bar, or to recruit more weight-bearing surface area and support the ground surface of the foot. Similarly, silicone putty and pour-in polyurethane can be applied to form a pad in situ after the horse has been shod. Once set, these materials can be trimmed to selectively apply or relieve pressure.

Pads have several disadvantages. All pads compress, which causes the nails to loosen sooner than they otherwise would. Full pads trap moisture against the sole and frog. The underlying sole and frog are softer, and the horse is predisposed to developing thrush.

Miscellaneous Changes in Shoe Form or Fit

A shoe shape is not limited to covering the entire ground surface of the wall. Partial shoes cover part of the circumference of the hoof wall. Tips that cover just the toe are used to prevent wear at the toe in young horses. A three-quarter shoe extends from one heel to the opposite quarter and limits weight bearing in the uncovered heel bulb. A shoe may be reversed so that it is open at the toe but closed at the heel. This functions as an egg bar shoe palmarly with a shortened breakover at the toe.

Hot versus Cold Shoeing

In cold shoeing a previously manufactured shoe is shaped cold and applied to the trimmed foot. In hot shoeing a newly forged shoe or a manufactured shoe is heated in the forge and applied to the ground surface of the foot while the shoe is still hot. The heat sears and levels the trimmed surface of the foot. It should cause no discomfort to the horse. Cold shoeing is quicker and requires less equipment and less skill. Hot shoes are easier to shape than cold shoes because the steel is softer. Hot shoeing produces a better fit, because the searing levels any minor irregularities in the trim and highlights any overtly unleveled areas. This is no substitute for correct trimming of the foot beforehand. The searing also aids seating of clips. It is also considered to seal the ends of the horn tubules.

Attachment of the Shoe to the Hoof

The large majority of horseshoes are attached to the hoof capsule with nails. Horseshoe nails are available in a variety of styles and sizes, but all share a similar pattern. Each has a head, a shank (blade), and a point beveled at the tip. There are several types of head that vary in size and the angle of bevel. Heads with less bevel, such as European head nails, are suited for thicker webbed shoes. Other nails with thinner or narrower shanks, such as race and slim blade nails, minimize damage to the wall. The size and style of nail are chosen based on experience to provide secure attachment of the shoe to the hoof capsule, without unnecessarily damaging the hoof capsule. The shape of the crease and nail hole should be stamped to fit the shape of the nail head, which provides the greatest support to the nail. The heel nail is located at the bend in the quarter, the toe nail at the junction of the toe and quarter, and the quarter nail(s) evenly spaced in between. In North America, three nails are usually used in each branch of the shoe. In the United Kingdom, three nails are usually used in the medial branch and four nails in the lateral branch.

The nail should be driven into the ground surface of the foot at the outside of the white line and exit the wall approximately 1.9 cm proximally. The bevel at the point of the nail is always directed toward the sole to limit the likelihood of the nail entering the underlying sensitive structures. Once the nail is driven, only the flat head of the nail should extend distal to the shoe. Because there is some variability in thickness of hoof wall for a given sized foot, the position of the nail hole in relation to the thickness of the web should be adjusted so that it is immediately distal to the white line. When the nail holes are positioned more toward the inner rim than normal, the shoe is coarse punched; when they are toward the outer rim, the shoe is fine punched. Because the slope and thickness of the wall change between the toe and quarter, the angle at which the nail is driven decreases from toe to heel. This should be reflected in the stamping of the nail holes. These adjustments to the position, shape, and angle of nail holes are easier to accommodate on hand-forged shoes, although modern manufactured shoes are available in sufficient variety and made to such stringent specifications that most situations can be addressed satisfactorily. The number of nails, the size of the nails, the congruency of the nail holes to the shoe, and the skill with which the nails are applied determine the security of attachment of the shoe to the hoof. Small nails may not adequately attach the shoe to the foot. Large nails may split the hoof capsule.

Recently the use of various adhesives to attach shoes has become more popular. The shoe can be affixed with an adhesive by either tabs or cuffs that are attached to the circumference of the shoe and extend proximally. The cuffs are made of semirigid plastic or synthetic cloth. Alternatively, the adhesive may be directly interposed between an aluminum shoe and the ground surface of the wall and immediately adjacent to the sole. Attachment of the shoe with adhesives offers several advantages over nailing: (1) it can be used when nailing is too painful; (2) it can be used when there is insufficient wall for nailing the shoe; and (3) depending on the specific application, it permits greater expansion of the foot. However, there are disadvantages. The glue-on shoes or the adhesive are more expensive, and application of some adhesives to the side of the wall decreases the quality of the underlying wall over time. There is also a perception that glued-on shoes do not stay on as well as nailed-on shoes, but this impression is in part the result of poor case selection or poor application.

Clips are triangular-shaped projections that extend proximally from the periphery of the solar surface of the shoe. Clips may be forged from the shoe at the time of fitting, or shoes with preformed clips may be purchased. When a shoe is fitted, the outer surface of the clip is congruent with the surface of the hoof wall. Clips reduce movement between the shoe and the hoof capsule, which decreases the shear stress on the hoof nails. A single clip usually is used in the center of the toe of fore shoes, and two clips are placed near the toe quarter junction of hind shoes. A toe clip is not used on hind feet in case it should injure the fore foot, but there is no reason why side clips should not be used on fore feet. For additional stability of the hoof capsule, clips may be positioned elsewhere around the periphery of the shoe to constrain expansion of the hoof capsule. Optimally, two or more clips should be located at 180 degrees to one another around the circumference of the shoe so that the flat surfaces of the clips are aligned perpendicular to the direction of expansion.

Horseshoe Functions

The principal objective of shoeing a horse is to provide protection to the hoof wall from excessive wear. More far-reaching goals include improving balance, providing traction, modifying breakover, increasing animation, providing support or stabilization, and limiting interference.

Balance

Mediolateral and dorsopalmar balance are discussed elsewhere (see pages 288 to 293).

Protection

Shoes and accessories can provide protection from excessive wear, trauma, and excessive concussion. Protection from excessive wear is primarily required for the ground surface of the wall and is provided by any shoe that is interposed between the foot and the ground around the full circumference of the hoof wall and the adjacent sole. Protection of the rest of the ground surface of the foot, namely, the sole and the frog, may be achieved by interposing a layer between the ground and the ground surface of the foot. If a specific area needs protection, frequently this can be provided by modifying the shoe. For example, a seated-out wide-web shoe protects more of the sole adjacent to the wall than a shoe with a narrower web. A bar added to the shoe protects the underlying sole or frog. For more extensive protection to the ground surface of the foot or alleviation of concussion, a pad may be inserted between the shoe and the foot (see page 297). Some shoes are manufactured with a composite of a metal backbone to provide rigidity and synthetic polymers to provide protection against concussion.[4]

Traction

Traction is required to facilitate optimal, confident movement of a horse over the ground as the limb decelerates at the beginning of the stride, as the horse propels itself forward and around turns, and as the foot breaks over. There is an indirect inverse relationship between traction and ease of breakover. Many modifications to a shoe that increase traction delay breakover and vice versa. The amount of traction required depends on the horse, the type of exercise, and the ground surface. Decreased duration of deceleration at the beginning of the stance phase of the stride, as the foot slides before it becomes stationary, has been associated with an increase in the amplitude of horizontal shockwaves associated with initial ground contact.[5] However, it appears that the horse adjusts its gait for different shoe materials so that the duration and distance associated with deceleration are similar, despite demonstrable differences in dynamic friction between different shoes types and the ground.[6]

Increased traction is provided by decreasing the ground surface area of the shoe, creasing or fullering the shoe, adding ridges to the cross-sectional profile of the shoe, or using calks, grabs, and nail heads that project below the surface of the shoe. Increasing the ground surface area of the shoe or rounding the outer rim or both rims of the shoe reduces traction.

Breakover Modification

The speed of breakover is related to the moment created about the DIP joint by the dorsal hoof wall at the end of the stride. This is determined by the anatomical relationship between the center of rotation of the DIP joint and the most dorsal point of ground contact, termed the *breakover point,* and the shoe's resistance to being elevated off the ground. The moment about the DIP joint is dictated by the direct distance between the center of rotation of the joint and the breakover point and the angle this line forms with the ground. These are in turn influenced by the length and angle of the dorsal hoof wall. Breakover can be enhanced by shortening the toe, moving the breakover point palmarly and increasing the angle of the dorsal hoof wall. Breakover is delayed by lengthening the toe[7] and decreasing the angle of the dorsal hoof wall.[8] Shortening the toe is accomplished by trimming the foot and is limited by the underlying sensitive structures. Toe length can be increased by letting it grow out or addition of pads or a thicker webbed shoe. The breakover point can be moved palmarly by trimming a barefooted horse or rolling or rockering the toe of the shoe, squaring the toe of the shoe, or setting the shoe back. The use of rolled or rockered toes does not influence the timing of breakover.[9,10] However, rolling the toe does smooth out the hoof-unrollment process and decreases peak load during breakover.[11] The angle of the dorsal hoof wall may be increased by elevating the heel with wedge pads or using shoes with wedged heels. These practices are both preferable to leaving the heel long. The degree to which the shoe adheres to the ground is directly related to modifications made to the shoe to enhance traction.

The direction and the point on the circumference of the hoof at which breakover occurs are related to the conformation of the limb, namely, the presence of angular or rotational deformities. To change the breakover point, either the orientation of the shoe on the ground before breakover or the ease of breakover between the two branches can be changed. The direction the foot is oriented on the ground is influenced by the way it lands, and the way it lands is influenced by the path of the foot during the flight phase of the stride, which is in turn influenced by the way the foot breaks over to complete the full phase cycle. Uniaxial trailers and heel extensions turn the foot ipsilaterally at landing, which directs breakover toward the opposite side of the toe at the end of the stride.

Breakover may be redirected by changing the relative ease with which the branches leave the ground, the relative length of the lever arm, adherence of the two branches of the shoe to the ground, or a combination of these factors. Adherence is increased by use of traction devices or decreased by using a nonfullered branch. The length of the lever arm of a shoe branch may be increased by setting it more dorsal to create a small extension between the center of the toe and the toe/quarter junction or decreased by setting it back. In essence, this is what happens when the toe is squared. Increasing the ease with which one branch lifts off the ground, while decreasing the ease as the other branch lifts off, shifts the breakover point toward the side with slower breakover. Any maneuver to change the direction of breakover is accompanied by increased torsional stress in the limb.

Animation

Gait animation indicates increased range of joint movement with exaggerated temporal characteristics. Animation is primarily a cosmetic change created because such characteristics are considered esthetically desirable in certain equestrian disciplines. It may be improved by shoeing.[12] Increased animation of gait is achieved by increasing the weight of the foot and shoe and increasing the length of the foot, shoe, or both.[7] These manipulations delay breakover, which is then followed by an exaggerated response both in distance moved and joint angulation. Animation obtained by increasing the length of the foot creates imbalance and increases stresses associated with moments about the DIP joint. Animation obtained through increased

weight of the foot is accompanied by greater energy expenditure by the horse, fatigue, and a greater chance of injury. Interestingly, egg bar shoes decrease animation compared with flat shoes.[3]

Support

Support is a term widely used, seldom defined, and often ambiguous. Support usually means to hold a structure up or prevent it from collapsing. This can be interpreted in at least two ways. First, it can refer to the relationship between the foot and the ground. Second, it can refer to supporting a structure within the foot. On occasion, support may fit both of these circumstances. Specifically, supporting the foot in relation to the ground implies keeping the whole or part of the foot from descending into a ground surface that gives, or keeping the foot level. Increasing the ground surface area of the shoe at any juncture around the periphery of the foot will support that area. Typically, the palmar aspect of the foot is most likely to be supported by the use of a straight bar or an egg bar shoe.

Support as a concept applied to structures within the foot is not always straightforward. Collapse of the hoof wall under excessive compressive strain is a simple example. However, in horses with laminitis or rupture of the DDFT, the distal phalanx displaces from its normal position; the concepts behind providing support, though, are quite different. In a horse with a ruptured DDFT the relationship between the distal phalanx and the hoof capsule is intact, whereas in a horse with laminitis it is disrupted.

An injured tissue may require stress relief. The clinician should determine whether the tissue is stressed under tension (tendons, ligaments, lamellae) or compression (bone, hoof wall), at what point in the stride the stress is greatest, and whether the stress is associated with weight bearing, moments about the DIP joint, or a combination of these two factors. The stresses that are greatest during the weight-bearing phase of the stride are redirected by altering the balance of the limb by trimming the foot, applying wedges, using shoe extensions as levers, or recruiting additional parts of the ground surface of the foot to bear weight. For example, in a horse with laminitis with uniaxial damage to the lamellae, the distal phalanx displaces distally on one side of the foot only, and the DIP joint becomes correspondingly asymmetrical. Support of the DIP joint requires an extension to the side of the displacement, but this would further increase the strain in the damaged lamellae and cause further displacement. To protect the lamellae, contralateral extension, used with other measures to support a laminitic foot, would load the contraaxial lamellae and protect the damaged lamellae by reducing the load. An ipsilateral extension would be appropriate to treat a strain of a collateral ligament of the interphalangeal joints. However, redistributing the stress from one structure inevitably increases the stress on others.

Decreasing the moment about the joint reduces stresses that are greatest during extension of the DIP joint. For example, in a horse with acute laminitis, the already damaged lamellae have a greater propensity to separate with the stress associated with breakover. To reduce this stress, shortening the toe decreases the length of the lever arm, and elevating the heel decreases the tension in the DDFT.

A strain of the insertion of the DDFT is under stress during both weight bearing and breakover. A heel extension with elevation decreases the stress during weight bearing by moving the point of action of the GRF palmarly. Moving the breakover point palmarly decreases the tension in the DDFT at breakover by decreasing the torque about the DIP joint. If the DDFT were severely strained, a heel elevation and extension would prevent the toe of the foot from lifting off the ground and subluxation of the DIP joint.

It is important that the practitioner understands which tissue to support, how to achieve this support, and what side effects must be anticipated. In addition to the immediate benefits of the support provided, the clinician must contend with the changes within the hoof capsule and changes in the relationship between the hoof capsule and the distal phalanx from movement between the epidermal and dermal lamellae, the viscoelasticity of the hoof capsule, and the altered pattern of growth of the hoof.

Prevention of Interference Injury
Interference occurs when the foot of one limb contacts another limb during the stride cycle, which frequently results in injury (see Figure 7-2). Interference can be divided into two types. *Brushing* occurs when a forelimb or hindlimb interferes with the contralateral limb between the coronary band and the carpus or hock. When a limb interferes with the ipsilateral limb, the hindlimb strikes the forelimb (forging, overreaching) or, less frequently, the forelimb strikes the hindlimb (scalping, speedy cutting). *Cross-firing* occurs when a forelimb and contralateral hindlimb interfere. The causes of interference include poor balance, poor conformation, fatigue, and lameness. When poor balance, or lameness, is identified as the cause, correction of these problems should resolve the interference. Increasing the fitness of the horse or using a lighter shoe may reduce interference from fatigue in unfit horses. However, the conformation of a horse cannot be changed. For example, a horse that is toed out will wing in during the flight phase of the stride, increasing the likelihood of interference with a contralateral limb. A horse with a short back in relation to the length of its limbs has an increased tendency for interference between a forelimb and a hindlimb. Treatment of interference that cannot be eliminated by removing the cause is directed at preventing interference by influencing the flight pattern of the feet and reducing the severity of injury when interference does occur.

Contact between ipsilateral limbs occurs as the forelimb is breaking over and the hindlimb is landing. Traditionally, prevention has been aimed at encouraging the forelimb to break over faster so that it moves out of the way of the hindlimb and delaying breakover of the hindlimb so that it lands later. Forelimb breakover has been discussed previously. Delaying breakover in the hindlimbs has been accomplished by lowering the heel of the hoof or thinning the branches of the shoe at the heel. However, although this does delay breakover, limb coordination is restored during the swing phase of the stride.[13] It also creates a dorsoplantar imbalance, which may cause other problems.

Contact between contralateral forelimbs occurs because the path of the limb in the swing phase is too close to the position of the weight-bearing limb, which is most likely to occur in base-narrow, toed-out horses. Prevention aims to redirect breakover laterally away from the medial aspect of the toe so that the phalanges do not diverge as far medially from the midsagittal plane of the limb as the metacarpophalangeal joint flexes.

Contact between a hind foot and the contralateral forelimb in pacers occurs between strides as the horse is suspended. Prevention of cross-firing is aimed at encouraging the hindlimb to stay further lateral so that it does not contact the forelimb. This is accomplished by encouraging the foot to move laterally as it lands, adding a trailer to the lateral branch of the shoe, and encouraging the foot to break over toward the outside of the foot by using a half round–half swedge shoe.

To decrease the severity of injury when impact between the limbs is unavoidable, the clinician should reduce the likelihood of the shoe itself, particularly sharp edges, from contact of the limb likely to be injured and directly protect the injured limb. To limit injury caused by sharp edges at the periphery of the shoe, the margin of the shoe can be safed in the area of contact, or a shoe with a curved contour, such as a half round shoe, can be used. To limit contact between the shoe and the injured limb, the shoe can be fitted so that it is set back from the margin of the hoof wall by moving the toe of the shoe back, reversing the shoe, or moving the medial branch axially. Alternatively, the shoe is forged so that the part of the shoe making contact is set back from the wall. Boots can be worn during exercise to directly protect the part of the limb likely to be injured.

THE PRACTICE OF SHOEING
Effects of Shoeing on Foot Function
A horseshoe is not simply an extension of the hoof capsule. By interposing a shoe that has markedly different physical characteristics from the hoof capsule between the foot and the ground, a single interface is replaced by two interfaces—that between the foot and the shoe, and that between the shoe and the ground. This inevitably has consequences for foot function.

A flat shoe nailed onto the hoof decreases movement of the hoof during the impact phase of the stride,[14] although the heel is still able to expand.[15] It increases the maximum deceleration of the foot,[4] increases the frequency of vibrations within the foot as it strikes the ground,[16] and maximizes vertical GRF.[17] This influence of shoeing on the shock caused by foot impact decreases proximally to the point where the influence is minimal at the metacarpophalangeal joint.[17] Shoeing does not change the principal compressive forces within the hoof wall, although it does cause slight reorientation and decreases the variability of the stresses within the wall.[18] In addition, shoeing increases the pressure on the navicular bone by the DDFT[3] and accentuates the decrease in tissue pressure within the digital cushion that occurs soon after impact.[16] Shoeing increases stride duration, but not stride length, in young horses shod for the first time.[12] Shoeing and the addition of weight to a shod foot increase the animation of the gait.[7,12] Shoeing has minimal effect on the point of force during the stride.[19] It has been suggested that the rigidity of the shoe alters the way the hoof capsule accommodates to irregularities on the ground surface.[20] A rigid shoe causes the whole foot to tilt or twist, whereas the viscoelastic hoof capsule might permit local distortion of the hoof capsule with less displacement of the whole foot. Finally, shod horses do not wear the feet naturally. Although virtually no wear of the distal hoof wall occurs between the toe and the middle of the quarter, because there is no movement of the hoof wall against the shoe, the heel does wear against the shoe as it expands and contracts.[20] Therefore during the course of a shoeing cycle, the angle of the dorsal hoof wall decreases.[21]

It is my impression that shoeing over a prolonged period results in a thinner hoof wall. The quality of the wall adjacent to the shoe is not as good as that of the same horse barefoot. It is also my impression that the distal phalanx may change shape as the result of certain shoeing practices and imbalance. Mediolateral imbalance may change the shape of the distal phalanx.[22] Of greater importance is the effect of shoeing on the development of the feet of young horses. The feet finish growing when a horse is 4 to 6 years of age. If abaxial movement of the hoof is restricted by shoes before that age, it may affect the growth of the hoof and potentially the shape and size of the distal phalanx. I prefer to allow young horses to go barefoot until they are mature if the intended use of the horse permits.

The deleterious effects of shoeing have led to a resurgence of interest in maintaining horses barefoot with routine trimming as necessary. Although there are unquestionable benefits to keeping a horse barefoot, maintaining a horse under modern management conditions so that its feet are in a condition to withstand the demands of work without becoming lame can be challenging.

Shoeing Sound Horses for Performance

Routine shoeing is directed at maintaining optimal balance and foot function and then addressing any specific needs that are related to the nature of work the horse performs. Balance is discussed elsewhere (see pages 284 to 285). The specific needs of a horse for a given type of work often have an established tradition. Observation of how other horses competing in the same discipline are trimmed and shod is a good starting point. Farriers who specialize in shoeing horses competing at high levels are a valuable resource. Fads are as much a part of the present history of shoeing as they are of many other disciplines and should be viewed with circumspection. However, although most fads disappear, a few become part of the standard armamentarium. In addition to traditional guidelines, there are rules regulating certain trimming and shoeing practices set by the governing bodies of different branches of equine sports and competitions. These frequently regulate the type of traction devices, weight of shoe, or length of toe that may be used. These rules generally are aimed at limiting excessive injury to the horses. For example, the use of toe grabs is prohibited in racehorses in certain states in the United States because of the established association between use and severe musculoskeletal injuries. Polo ponies are allowed to compete with inside rim shoes on the fore feet but not outside rim shoes.

Corrective Shoeing

Modification of a shoe in the pursuit of one objective almost inevitably has other consequences, which may be untoward. For example, to alter the mediolateral imbalance of a foot by decreasing the thickness of the web of one branch, either the width of the web can be maintained with loss of weight or the weight of the web can be maintained but the width must be increased. Changing the weight of the web alters the inertia about the distal aspect of the limb. Changing the width of the web potentially changes the traction between the ground and the shoe and the depth the shoe sinks into the ground surface.

Corrective shoeing is directed at preventing lameness in a horse with poor conformation or balance (see pages 285 to 293) or treating a horse that has become lame. Therapeutic shoeing of lame horses requires knowledge of the cause of the problem and how to treat it. Lameness usually is related to pain that is often the response to inflammation after low-grade repetitive injury or to insult from stresses within tissues or at the interface between tissues. These stresses may be compressive, tensile, bending, torsional, shearing, or a combination of these. For example, compressive strains within the sole result in bruising and, in some horses, osteitis of the distal phalanx. Bending or shearing stresses in the wall may result in hoof cracks. Long-toe, low-heel conformation increases tension in the DDFT, compression of the navicular bone, and tension within the dorsal lamellae.

Accuracy of the diagnosis may be the first impediment. Sometimes pain causing lameness can be isolated to a specific tissue with a combination of physical examination, local analgesia, radiography, scintigraphy, and magnetic resonance imaging, but frequently the pain can be isolated to only part of the foot, and sometimes simply to the foot. The precipitating factor may not be within the tissue or structure exhibiting pain but may be a conformational change elsewhere. The more accurate the diagnosis, the more closely localized the source of pain, and the more knowledge of any underlying stresses, the more appropriate treatment is likely to be and the greater the chance of success.

The less specific the diagnosis, the more symptomatic the therapy. This is most likely to be directed at the balance of the foot and conformation of the limb, not necessarily an easy task. However, if lameness and pain persist after optimal balance is restored, the pain is most likely to be related, directly or indirectly, to the concussive forces associated with impact and weight bearing or flexion and extension of the distal aspect of the limb. The ground surface of the foot can be protected from direct impact with the ground, and the maximal deceleration and frequency of vibrations within the structures between the ground surface of the foot and the metacarpophalangeal joint can be decreased. Extension of the DIP joint can be decreased by reducing the extent that the heel sinks into a soft ground surface and the moment about the DIP joint at breakover. Torsional stresses within the distal aspect of the limb may be reduced by encouraging the foot to break over in the most natural position.

Lameness Associated with Shoeing

Although the incidence of lameness associated with shoeing is unknown, poor trimming, shoe selection, and shoe attachment are well-recognized causes of lameness. Trimming that leaves a hoof too long or imbalanced, either mediolaterally or dorsopalmarly, predisposes the distal aspect of the limb to abnormal stresses and lameness. Similarly, trimming the wall and adjacent sole too short causes undue pressure on the sole, bruising, and lameness.

Shoe selection includes size, weight, and traction devices. If the shoe is too small or short for the foot, the heel is unlikely to have adequate coverage. Pressure is concentrated in the wall and adjacent sole, which leads to bruising, hoof cracks, and an underrun heel. Shoes that are too long or wide are at greater risk of being pulled off. If the ends of long branches are redirected axially to prevent the shoe from being pulled off, the angle of the sole may bruise. If the web of the shoe is narrow, the adjacent sole is unprotected. Conversely, a wide-web shoe may impinge on a dropped sole.[23] Shoe size influences its weight. A heavy shoe may cause fatigue, decreased agility, and predispose to interference.[23] The size of a shoe also affects the effective surface of the foot. Too small a ground surface area concentrates the stresses of weight bearing.

Inappropriate use of traction devices predisposes to injury. The use of calks and toe grabs alters the balance of the limb and concentrates stress wherever they are applied. Too much traction may cause shearing within the limb as the horse places the limb on the ground because the limb decelerates too rapidly. Traction devices that anchor the limb in the ground once the foot is planted may cause fractures of the McIII or the proximal and middle phalanges as a horse pivots on the limb. An inside rim shoe provides a good compromise among traction, ability to pivot, and ease of breakover. Too little traction at least decreases a horse's confidence as it works and at worst may cause a horse to slip and injure itself.

If a shoe is unintentionally set eccentrically, so that one branch extends further abaxially than the other, greater stresses occur in the wall proximal to that branch. If the shoe is unintentionally rotated, the coverage of the heel is uneven and the heel bulb with the least coverage responds as if the foot were shod short on that branch. If the shoe is to be rotated intentionally, a larger shoe should be used.

Inappropriate attachment of the shoe to the foot may cause direct injury to the underlying sensitive tissues, damage the hoof capsule, and impair expansion. The use of larger nails than needed displaces more tissue as they are driven and therefore is more likely to fracture the hoof wall or impinge on the underlying sensitive structures. Nails that directly injure the sensitive tissues when driven, called *nail prick*, cause an instantly recognizable problem that is immediately corrected. More insidiously, a nail that is close to but not within the sensitive structures, a condition called *nail bind*, applies pressure to the lamellae or may cause the inner hoof wall to fracture toward the lamellae. This creates a tract through which infection may become established. Nail prick and nail bind may occur because the nail was driven too high or was started too far axially. The angle at which the nail holes are punched and the location of nail holes in the web of the shoe may contribute to the problem. Nails set behind the middle of the quarter adversely affect the expansion of the foot and should be avoided.

◼ NATURAL BALANCE TRIMMING AND SHOEING

Gene Ovnicek

The feet of wild and domestic horses have the same anatomy, function similarly, and require stimulation to develop and perform optimally. The equine foot is a product of its environment, and the foot modifies and changes so that the basic requirements for health, function, and soundness can be met. This works well when the horse is roaming free in an area that is large enough for optimal foot maintenance or, if used aggressively, barefooted. The sole, bars, and frog become callused and durable, with the wall chipping and wearing so that the wall at the toe is worn to the same level as at the sole. Feet managed in this self-maintaining manner are of the highest quality and generally are trouble free and healthy.

APPEARANCE OF A SELF-MAINTAINED FOOT

The wall of a self-maintained foot is worn down to the level of the sole callus in the toe region. The quarters are broken away at the widest part of the foot in horses that live in soft and sandy areas. This allows dirt to compact only in the palmar region of the foot, in the area of the bars. The heel grows beyond the height of the frog, which helps to form a trap for the dirt. The wall is worn to the level of the sole dorsal to the frog apex. The frog apex is generally in contact with the ground when the foot is loaded and is often enlarged and callused as a result of its use. Radiology shows that this area is in the center of the distal phalanx. Support for the distal phalanx is provided by the dorsal wall and sole callus, frog apex and frog buttress, bars, heel, and dirt compaction.

Horses that are ridden or live in areas with more abrasive surfaces, such as pavement or dry gravel, frequently wear the heel shorter than the level of the frog. The wall is always worn equal in height to the sole in the front part of the foot (Figure 27-11). The thickness of the live sole callus (recognized as the functional epidermal sole tissue that extends beyond the dorsal distal border of the distal phalanx) at the toe, and the thickness of the live sole at the heel are a consistent distance from the distal border of

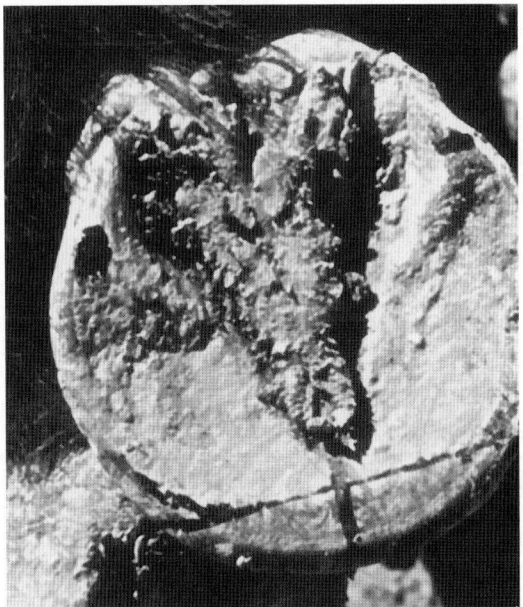

Fig. 27-11 • This imprinted feral foot shows the wall is worn to the same level as the sole at the toe. This is typical of self-maintained feet of both feral and domestic horses.

the distal phalanx.[1] Therefore the sole is a reliable reference for mediolateral balance. The wall can be trimmed or rasped to the same distance from the live sole on each side of the foot so that the distal aspect of the distal phalanx is level, parallel with the sole.

The quality of the frog and digital cushion plays a major role in dorsopalmar balance of the foot. The natural, healthy frog is designed to hold dirt between the bars and frog, and dirt seldom exceeds the level of the frog. The frog, along with the dirt compaction, is partially responsible for the alignment of the distal phalanx and the pastern. The frog, bars, and sole are all important in weight bearing.

The hoof wall breaks away while the sole and frog become callused and durable for the horse to walk on. With shod feet there is little control of the natural hoof wall trimming that occurs by wear and chipping. If the wall of a shod hoof is not prepared to a depth equal to that of the live sole plane medially and laterally, the coronary band distorts and quarter cracks and toe cracks may develop. Horses that break and crush the heel and those that develop toe cracks and quarter cracks all experience a natural but crude, deliberate way of trimming the foot so that the distal phalanx maintains a parallel medial to lateral orientation to the ground. Breaking and cracking of the wall allow the frog, bars, and sole to contact the ground to fulfill the natural function.

To maintain a horse barefooted without availability of a large, free-roaming area, owners should try to keep the horse's living area and exercising area the same. If a horse is kept in a soft, sandy pasture or large, sandy paddock, then it should be ridden daily in that same type of sandy terrain. The same is true for horses kept in dry, rocky pastures. In addition to a consistent environment, regular activity also is required, with exercise for 5 to 25 miles daily.

Most horses are housed in small, confined stalls or paddocks that are often soft, wet, and nonabrasive. The feet do not wear at all and adapt to that environment. These horses are reluctant to work barefoot on a more abrasive surface. Some horses have poor-quality, substandard feet that need some type of protection for any form of work.

NATURAL BALANCE TRIMMING FOR A BAREFOOTED HORSE

Natural balance trimming is maintaining the feet of domestic horses consistent with self-maintained feet. These instructions are for *domestic horses that are left barefoot.*

The majority of horses' feet can be separated into four types: (1) normal feet, (2) feet with an underrun heel and long toe, (3) clubbed or upright feet, and (4) unusually flat feet. In all types the sole callus, the apex of the frog, and the callused portion of the frog buttress are the support structures of the foot (Figure 27-12).

Normal Feet

The following trimming sequence is used for horses that have normal feet and are left barefooted without suitable activity to wear the feet to the natural hoof shape. After removal of dirt, the clinician should identify the sole callus in the toe area. This is the functional epidermal tissue that extends beyond the dorsal, distal border of the distal phalanx and is seen as the raised area just inside the hoof

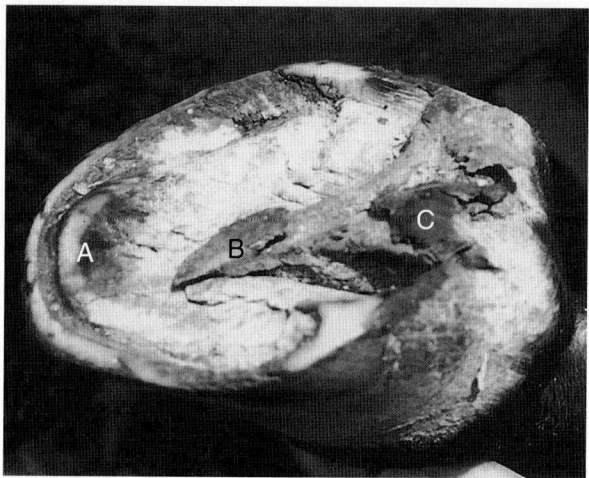

Fig. 27-12 • Important support structures of the equine digit. **A,** Sole callus. **B,** Apex of the frog. **C,** Callused portion of the frog buttress.

wall. The sole callus maintains its relationship with the distal phalanx at the 10-o'clock and 2-o'clock positions, also commonly termed the *pillars.*[2] A line across the leading (dorsal) edge of the pillars is approximately 2.5 cm (1 inch) dorsal to the true, well-identified frog apex on medium-sized feet (feet from a large size #0 to a small #2). The *live sole* is the functional epidermal sole tissue that extends beyond the distal border of the distal phalanx and has a waxy surface appearance. The clinician should remove only enough of the loose, flaky, chalky sole material so that the live sole and the sole callus are clearly seen. Most horses left barefooted have little or no sole that needs to be exfoliated or removed.

The point of breakover occurs in the self-maintained foot at a line drawn across the toe at the back edge of the sole callus (leading edge of the pillars), or approximately 2.5 cm (1 inch) dorsal to the well-identified frog apex. With a normal foot the wall in this region is firmly attached to the sole callus at ground level. The sole callus on most normal bare feet is narrow and well defined, but not in flat or clubbed feet, because in these horses the toe of the distal phalanx is closer to the ground. The hoof wall should be conservatively rasped or nipped to the back edge of the sole callus. The rocker or roll should not exceed 10 to 15 degrees from the flat plane of the sole (i.e., what is normally found on a well-worn shoe). Next, the wall is trimmed and left slightly taller than the sole callus on each side of the toe, behind the rockered portion. The finished height of the wall should be approximately 1 to 2 mm closer to the ground than the sole callus. The length of that flattened, raised area of the wall depends on the size and type of the foot and sole callus (approximately 2.0 to 2.5 cm).

The wall behind the toe callus is trimmed to the level of the live sole through the quarters. The heel that remains is flattened so that the medial and lateral aspects of the heel are equal in height to each other and at the same level as the frog buttress or slightly shorter. This generally means that the quarters at the widest part of the foot are floated.

Only the cleft of the central sulcus of the frog is routinely trimmed to lessen the chance of bacterial colonization in less active horses. The rest of the frog should not be trimmed at all, unless parts are hanging by a small attachment from the live frog structure. The bars are trimmed only if they start to turn, roll over, and become flat to the sole, or if cracked or diseased. If flares exist on the outer hoof wall, the clinician should find the most prominent growth ring near the middle of the dorsal hoof wall and remove only the amount necessary to make the wall straight from top to bottom. Rasping should not exceed half the original wall thickness, and the wall should have a fairly uniform thickness all the way around when finished. Finally, the outer rim of the hoof wall that is closest to the ground is rounded (the rim is chamfered).

Flat Feet

Horses with flat, sensitive feet that are used for trail riding and multiterrain activities often are unsuitable to leave barefoot. Many horses with flat feet have a thin sole that separates from the wall at ground level, causing laminar tearing at the distal aspect of the distal phalanx. With the sole callus used for weight bearing, the outer wall is removed in a dubbed, vertical manner to lessen the pull on the wall. The wall is brought back very close to the edge of the sole on the ground side so that no dirt will pack under the wall next to the sole. The sole of the foot is never touched with the knife or rasp. Feet of this type never need exfoliating. They need more sole thickness below the distal phalanx, which may develop if the wall is reattached closer to the ground surface of the sole. When the distal 3 to 4 cm of the wall is left to full thickness, the distal phalanx is supported proximally by stable wall. The sole callus may become more durable and develop dense protective tissue once the laminae are not torn by the wall pulling away from the sole.

The heel is rasped back to a solid horn structure, and the frog is left untouched. The clinician should not rocker the toe until the wall attaches more normally to the sole at ground level. With repeated trimming the gap between the sole and wall disappears, and eventually the callus at the toe quarters bonds tightly with the wall, and the solar surface may become concave.

Clubfeet

An upright or clubfoot often is smaller. The practitioner should not try to change it but should treat it separately, using the same guidelines as for a normal foot. The sole callus at the toe is located to determine the point for breakover. The live sole in the heel region is used as a guide for trimming the heel, leaving the sole full thickness to protect the distal border of the distal phalanx. In my opinion, the most fragile part of the horse's foot is the distal border of the distal phalanx; in an upright foot, it may be more susceptible to trauma. However, if the heel is lowered excessively while the toe is left to improve the digital alignment, damage to the distal border of the distal phalanx is more likely.

A normal foot has an even curve to the outer hoof wall at the heel buttress and an even arch to the bars, with the heel buttress terminating slightly ahead of the back of the frog. The heel buttress (end of heel) of an upright foot has an abrupt curve with bars that are quite straight. The heel ends close to the back of the frog. Excessive removal of the heel of a clubfoot does not allow the horse to land heel first and increases the chances of distal phalanx trauma from landing toe first.

The sole callus on a clubfoot is slightly different from that of normal feet. There is usually a broad, raised formation to the sole, seen just ahead of the frog apex. The callus on each side of the frog apex is more prominent and extends well behind the tip of the frog. The natural place for breakover is closer to the frog apex because of the position of the sole callus. Therefore the wall is rockered ahead of the sole callus just as in a normal foot. The live sole in the back part of the foot is deeper. The hoof wall at the heel should not be trimmed equal to the live sole. The sole callus continues palmarly to the widest part of the foot and beyond, giving the appearance of a flat, thick sole from the medial to lateral aspects of the heel. If the dorsal hoof wall is severely flared and resembles a foot with chronic laminitis, the flare should be removed.

Feet with Long Toes and Underrun Heels

An underrun heel grows forward under the foot with a sharp curve in the heel. The underrun heel ends ahead of the frog buttress with bars that are curved similarly. The frog apex is often elongated. This heel conformation is abnormal and often is painful. Natural balance trimming helps to restore the foot to a near natural shape, with alleviation of pain. The sole callus is broad and looks more like a small mound around the sole ahead of the frog apex. If the horse can be kept in a dry, soft area for 1 to 2 weeks, the toe can be aggressively rockered ahead of the callus, leaving the sole callus and medial and lateral walls to walk on. The heel needs to be trimmed back below the level of the frog if the bars and heel are severely curled and appear to end in front of the back of the frog. However, the heel should never be trimmed down past the live sole at the heel or any other part of the foot. The wall is finished normally. This aggressive trimming rapidly starts to repair the deformed feet and can be done quickly and successfully as long as the bottom of the foot is hardened and protected with hoof and sole hardeners. Alternatively, more wall can be left at the medial and lateral sole callus to not overload the sole callus. The foot will respond well with each trimming.

NATURAL BALANCE SHOEING

When preparing the sole surface for a shoe, the frog, bars, and sole are prepared conservatively, similar to feet that are left bare. Feet that are shod do not exfoliate effectively, and sole material that is showing cracks in the sole and is chalky and crumbles when it is cut with a knife should be removed. When the sole and frog material changes from a chalky, crumbly state to a waxy-appearing surface, the live or functional sole and frog has been reached, and absolutely no more cutting should be done. The live, functional sole at the toe quarters (where the sole callus is) and the live sole at the heel quarters (behind the widest part of the foot) are references to the distal border of the distal phalanx. Trimming the wall to these live, functional structures offers the best guide to attain accurate mediolateral and dorsopalmar balance.

The bottom surface of the foot is finished flat when the foot is prepared for shoeing (not relieved in the quarters as when trimmed to be left barefoot) and is hot seated if possible. Vigorous hot seating helps to dehydrate and strengthen the sole callus. It also pulls the sole proximally from the ground level to eliminate sole pressure.

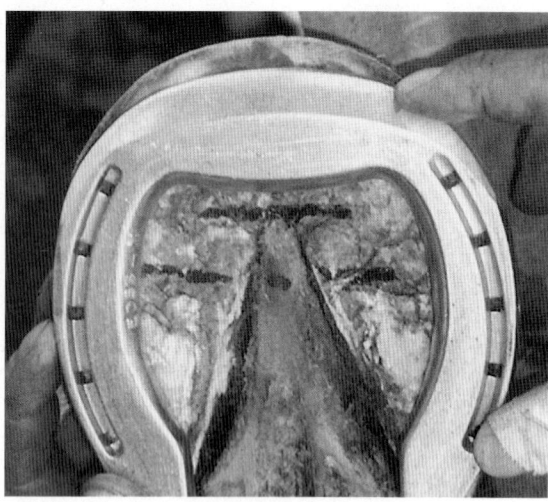

Fig. 27-13 • The aluminum Natural Balance shoe is designed to be applied 0.3 to 0.9 cm (depending on foot size) from the frog apex to the inside edge of the shoe at the toe. This placement closely meets breakover requirements with respect to the sole callus. The seated-out reverse arch on the inside border of the shoe at the toe helps to protect the distal border of the distal phalanx from sole pressure.

Shoe Placement and Application

Shoe selection is important, and wide-web rim type shoes work best for easy modification. The outer rim is normally tapered-in to the nail groove, which is helpful and somewhat mimics the way the bare foot naturally wears. That same feature is equally helpful at the toe when the shoe is squared somewhat and positioned on the foot so the breakover point of the shoe fits directly over the back edge of the sole callus at the center of the toe. The heel of the shoe should extend to the full length of the frog. A good reference for that position is the back of the crease in the central sulcus. Radiographs can be used to determine the natural position for breakover.

When premade aluminum (Thoro'Bred Racing Plate Company, Anaheim, California, United States) or steel (Malaysian Horseshoe Company, Malaysia) Natural Balance shoes are used, the same criteria of shoe placement for breakover and heel length should be followed. A wide-web rim shoe is broadened at the toe and tapered from the inner rim to the toe between the toe quarters. The shoe is placed on the foot so that the inner rim (part of breakover) is over the inside edge of the sole callus. The Natural Balance shoe is positioned a variable distance from the frog apex to the inside edge of the shoe for placement (Figure 27-13). That distance is regulated with the heel position. If a line is drawn across the widest part of the foot where the bars end, one third of the foot mass is ahead of this line to the point of breakover.

◼ HOOF RECONSTRUCTION MATERIALS AND GLUE-ON SHOES

Robert Sigafoos and Patrick T. Reilly

Advancements in adhesive technology have substantially improved the dependability of adhesive-bonded shoes. The incorporation of these materials into horseshoeing techniques allows for structural reform and external reinforcement of the hoof, with potential benefits in both therapeutic shoeing and performance enhancement of the equine athlete.

ADHESIVE TYPES

Most adhesives used to bond hoofwear to hooves evolved from use in hoof reconstruction.[1] Important features include impact resistance, type of adhesive joint loads, speed of polymerization, heat production, surface sensitivity, and environmental compatibility.

Impact resistance is particularly important because of factors such as horse's weight, speed, and high level of cyclic loading of the feet. Adhesives that remain flexible once polymerization is complete (elastomeric adhesives) perform better than rigid adhesives with similar tensile strength characteristics. When the bonding is applied directly to the hoof wall (as opposed to bonding individual components of a shoe together), at least one surface (the hoof) is always flexible. The primary load will be in peel, for which elastomeric adhesives are preferable.

Speed of polymerization is critical because the horse needs to bear weight and ambulate immediately after shoeing. The cure profile of an adhesive involves a "green" phase when the adhesive has solidified but not reached full strength. Challenging the bond in the early portion of the green phase can cause irreversible bond line failure. However, very fast polymerization may be at the expense of reduced impact strength.

The polymerization reaction produces heat that increases with the speed of the reaction. It is surface area dependent for a given volume of polymer. In concentrated volumes that are not allowed sufficient surface area to dissipate heat, temperatures can exceed 120° C in volumes typically used for hoof reconstruction or bonded shoes. Spreading the adhesive to provide increased surface area relative to volume allows dissipation of heat. Some adhesive manufacturers add fillers to very fast systems to dissipate heat, resulting in a temperature reduction of as much as 25%. Submural temperatures underlying reacting exothermic resins vary depending on the hoof wall thickness but generally do not achieve dangerous levels. However, dermal layers underlying thin hoof walls (such as those found at the quarters or in foals) may be at risk for substantial thermal trauma.

Surface sensitivity affects the ability of an adhesive to bond to a contaminated surface. Adhesives that solvate surface contaminants into the bond line are preferable. The adhesive must be resistant to moisture and microbial degradation. The adhesives commonly used for hoof reconstruction and bonded shoes are polymethyl or cyclohexyl methacrylate, cyanoacrylate, polyurethane, and, to a far lesser extent, epoxy resins. Each has distinct advantages.

Polymethyl methacrylate (PMMA) or cyclohexyl methacrylate (CHMA) systems are commonly referred to as *acrylic* adhesives. The newest elastomeric acrylic adhesives offer good impact resistance, rapid cure, minimal surface sensitivity, and excellent wetting characteristics for hoof wall and other substrates commonly used with hoof care applications. However, they have an intense odor, relatively high exothermic temperatures, and a high vapor pressure that limits shelf life in opened containers. As with all elastomeric adhesives subjected to high peel loads, the acrylic adhesives should be used with a thick bond line.

Polyurethane adhesives produce low-modulus adhesive joints. These joints exhibit excellent impact strength and perform remarkably well under high cyclic loads. Polyurethane has the best abrasion resistance and shock attenuation of all the adhesives commonly used. However, these adhesives require extensive substrate cleaning and preparation to ensure good bonds, which are often beyond the scope of practical field applications. These adhesives also do not form effective bonds with many of the plastics commonly used with hoof care, including acrylonitrile butadrene styrene (ABS), polyvinyl chloride (PVC), and acrylic-PVC copolymers.

Thermoplastic adhesives are principally dependent on mechanical bonding for adhesion, limiting structural use in horses. Cyanoacrylate adhesives are thermoplastic, single-component systems that are cure inhibited through acid stabilization. Ambient surface moisture increases constituent pH and allows the polymerization process to begin. The principal advantage of these adhesives is the ability to form bonds with substrates that are difficult to bond for most adhesives. Cyanoacrylates are the only adhesive for many types of glue-on shoes that have polyurethane as a structural bonding substrate. They have excellent strength when loaded in sheer, but poor peel and impact strength. Cyanoacrylate adhesives also are highly susceptible to post-cure moisture degradation. Because cyanoacrylates become rigid after curing, the bond line rapidly develops a "mosaic" fracture pattern when exposed to impact. This allows capillary intrusion of water into the bond line, further subjecting the bond to environmental degradation. They also have limited gap-filling characteristics. The ideal surface for successful cyanoacrylate bonding is a virtually polished surface. The bond line must be very thin.

Epoxy resins offer excellent environmental resistance, have very good sheer characteristics, and are the adhesive of choice when assembling shoe components that involve engineered fabric lay-ups and when an extended or elevated temperature curing is acceptable. These systems are not useful when bonding directly to the hoof wall, because the hardeners that are commonly used markedly increase the rigidity of the cured polymer. Polyester resins have some value in cosmetic repair of hoof wall, but they lack tensile strength and environmental resistance and have limited use.

GLUE-ON HORSESHOES

Currently four principal types of glue-on shoes are available. These include the "direct-glue" method using PMMA or CHMA adhesive, the molded polyurethane "tab type" shoes that use a cyanoacrylate adhesive, the flock-lined plastic cuff that uses an epoxy adhesive, and the fabric cuff that uses a PMMA or CHMA adhesive.

Two techniques have been used for direct-glue shoes. The first method involves the use of a PMMA or CHMA adhesive without fillers, with the bond line between the distal aspect of the hoof wall and the shoe.[2] The hoof side of the shoe is cleaned and sanded. The hoof is prepared by cleaning the dirt and loose debris from the wall and sole. The adhesive then is applied directly to the shoe and hoof, and the shoe is positioned on the hoof so that the bond

line is continuous between each bulb of the heel and incorporates an increasing percentage of the sole toward the heel. The hoof must be held non–weight bearing through the green phase of the adhesive cure cycle, approximately 3 to 5 minutes depending on ambient temperature. Given the extended cure profile of this type of adhesive, the bond should be challenged as little as possible for 12 hours. A modification of this system has been developed using staple fiberglass fibers as a filler for the adhesive.[3] The primary disadvantages are the need to keep the hoof non–weight bearing until the adhesive has green cycled and the need to bond the heel securely to the shoe.

Polyurethane "tab type" shoes use a cyanoacrylate adhesive to bond a component of the shoe (the polyurethane tab) to the hoof wall. These shoes require careful substrate preparation, including solvent cleaning and finish sanding with extremely fine sandpaper. Because cyanoacrylates have limited gap-filling properties, the prepared hoof wall must match the profile of the tab precisely. These adhesives have limited moisture and impact resistance, so shoe retention for competitive horses may prove difficult.

Plastic flock-line cuffs (Dalric Glue on Shoes, Advance Equine, Versailles, Kentucky, United States) are not actually shoes, but they act as a conjoining device to attach shoes to the dorsal aspect of the hoof wall. These devices use an epoxy (or a PMMA or CHMA adhesive) to attach the shoe to the hoof wall through a mechanical lock of the adhesive to the flock lining and rivets to attach the shoe to the cuff. This system is considerably more robust than the polyurethane tab system described previously. However, fitting the cuff to oddly configured hooves can be difficult.

The fabric cuff (Sigafoos Series Adhesive Bonded Shoes, Sound Horse Technologies, Unionville, Pennsylvania, United States) system uses a PMMA or CHMA adhesive to bond a braided fabric cuff that is an integral part of the shoe to the dorsal aspect of the hoof wall. This system comes as a fully assembled shoe (Series One) or a modular system (Series Two) that allows the farrier to assemble any type of pattern configuration desired. The use of the Sigafoos Series shoe has been shown to reduce distortion of the dorsal aspect of the hoof when used continually over an extended period of time when compared with nail-on shoes.[1] The primary disadvantage of this system is the limited choice of types of shoes currently available in the Series One system.

Glue-on shoes offer distinct advantages over mechanically attached shoes because of the noninvasive and nondestructive nature of the attachment. They are expensive, but this cost usually is recouped if the actual cost of lost shoes and the resultant hoof loss are considered. If the widespread acceptance of adhesives in other industries is any reflection on the potential for their use in the farrier industry, adhesives will become the dominant method of attachment of shoes for horses in the foreseeable future.

Many maladies of the equine hoof—from laminitis to hoof abscesses to quarter cracks—are complicated by a loss of integrity to the hoof capsule. Traumatic incidents such as the loss of a shoe can result in an interruption to the training or performance of an equine athlete. Although it is impossible to replace the exact characteristics of a compromised hoof, advances in reconstruction techniques have proven invaluable in both therapeutic horseshoeing as well as in prevention of secondary traumatic injuries associated with loss of hoof. Hoof capsule distortion has been identified as a precursor to lameness, and the ability to externally reinforce the hoof through glue-on shoes, adhesives, and composite materials has been shown to reduce distortion of the hoof.

HOOF WALL RECONSTRUCTION

Traditionally, the repair of hoof defects has been accomplished through invasive stabilizing methods, such as drilling into healthy hoof around a quarter crack and lacing the disjointed hoof together with stainless steel wire. PMMA and CHMA have been used to accomplish the same result without further invasion of the hoof through the external buildup of material on either side of a defect, and the subsequent lacing through the adhesive rather than through the hoof wall. External methods provide the same level of stabilization as the invasive method.

A limiting factor in any wire technique is that the resulting stabilization is achieved only in tension as the defect is pulled together. Predicting the forces exerted on a hoof capsule is difficult, as each foot deforms under loading forces in a unique manner. Some defects are in compression instead of tension, and various shear forces

are also exerted. The adhesion of solid metal plates provides better overall mechanical stabilization of a defect; however, these repairs are often difficult to conform to the hoof and are bulky in design. The use of fabrics saturated in adhesives has provided an alternative method of hoof wall reconstruction, affording a lightweight stabilization of the hoof to various directional forces while easily conforming to the shape of the hoof.

Composite Materials and Hoof Repairs

In considering the structural capacity of adhesives, an analogy can be made to concrete. By itself, concrete has limited structural strength, but the structural capacity is greatly increased through the incorporation of metal rebar. In much the same way, the incorporation of fabrics into adhesives greatly increases the structural capacity of hoof wall repairs. Carbon fiber resists compression very well, and Kevlar is excellent at resisting tensile forces. Ultra-high–molecular weight fabrics (such as Spectra) impart excellent abrasion resistance to a repair. Liquid crystal polymers such as Vectran impart lesser characteristics of all three materials.

The orientation and weave of the fabric should also be considered in the design of a repair, because the optimal

TABLE 27-1

Fabric Characteristics for Hoof Repairs					
FABRIC	ADHESION	WEAR	TENSILE	IMPACT	BENDING	RECOMMENDED FOR THESE TYPES OF REPAIRS
Fiberglass	4	2	1	1	1	None
Carbon fiber	4	2	4	2	1	Repair of extremely palmar heel cracks; additional reinforcement (when used with other fabrics) for repairs in very large or active horses. This fabric should never be used when tight bends are required. **Care must always be used when grinding carbon fiber as the dust is hazardous to breathe.**
Polyester	4	3	3	4	4	Recommended for most repairs. Very good (even when used alone) for most types of horses.
Kevlar	3	2	4	4	3	Excellent reinforcement for carbon fiber (markedly improves impact resistance of repairs). Good to use in heavy horses such as draft horses. Repairs done with Kevlar should be covered with polyester or Spectra in highly abrasive environments.
Spectra	1	4	4	4	4	Because of poor adhesion, Spectra should be used only for added abrasion resistance, as the outermost layer over other fabrics in extremely abrasive environments.
Vectran	3	3	4	4	3	Vectran is in the same chemical family as Kevlar, with somewhat higher abrasion resistance.
Kevlar–carbon fiber hybrid (Cobrasox)	3-4	2	4	4	2	Good for repairs on heavy horses when tight bends are not required. Repairs done with Cobrasox should be covered with polyester or Spectra in highly abrasive environments.
Vectran-polyester hybrid	3-4	3-4	3	4	3-4	Excellent replacement for polyester for highly competitive horses or heavy horses. Somewhat better abrasion resistance than Kevlar or Cobrasox.
Carbon fiber–fiberglass hybrid	4	2	3	1-2	1	None

Key: 1 = poor, 4= best. (Values are only comparative to the nine materials listed and are subjective.)

structural plane is along the directional plane of the fibers.

The most commonly used adhesives (PMMAs and urethanes) are exothermic, with a total energy release that is dependent on the quantity and thickness of the repair. The temperature at the surface of the foot is approximately 50° C, with an increase of 4 to 7° C in the dermal tissues, depending on the type of adhesive used and the thickness of both the repair and the hoof wall. Any adhesive composite repair should avoid direct contact with the dermal tissues of the hoof to avoid thermal damage. To avoid bacterial or fungal infection, an inert material, such as polystyrene foam, modeling clay, or silicone molding material, is required to separate the composite repair from the dermal tissues.

There are several considerations when choosing which fabric to use for repairing a hoof. These include adhesion,* wear resistance,† tensile strength, impact resistance, and bending.‡ The types of materials commonly used for fabric hoof repairs include fiberglass, polyester, carbon fiber (care must be used when grinding or rasping carbon fiber because the dust is hazardous to breathe), Kevlar, Spectra, and Vectran (Table 27-1).

Other considerations include the weave pattern and thread count. *Basket weave* is the simplest and least expensive type of weave available for most types of repair fabrics.

It is important to realize, however, that the cost of any of the fabrics is minimal given the small amount used for each repair. However, the basket weave has the poorest "drape" characteristics (the ability of a fabric to wrap around and conform to different shapes).

Braid has significantly better handling and drape characteristics at a slightly higher cost.

Nonwoven roving is a type of fabric usually supplied in a "tape"§ form. It is not woven. Instead, all the yarns lie parallel to one another and are lightly stitched together every few centimeters. For any given type of fabric material, the nonwoven roving is the strongest in tensile strength. Nonwoven roving (particularly carbon fiber nonwoven roving) is excellent for repairs where a great deal of strength is needed and where very little repair area is available, such as extremely caudal heel repairs. However, the drape with nonwoven roving fabrics tends to be rather poor.

Thread count refers to the number of threads per linear inch, and is sometimes called the *pick*. Tighter thread counts (i.e., more threads per inch) tend to be more abrasion and snag resistant. Lower thread counts tend to have better drape characteristics. An important consideration with hoof repair fabrics is that the adhesives typically used with hoof repair tend to have high viscosity and are difficult to saturate into many fabrics. As a result, thread counts higher than 17 threads per inch should be avoided for hoof repair.

---

*The adhesion of the hoof repair adhesive to the fabric.
†The resistance of the fabric (bonded to the hoof with hoof-repair adhesive) to abrasion from ground surfaces such as sand as well as resistance to abrasion from the opposite foot.
‡Some types of repair require the fabric to bend tightly around the hoof wall (such as when the fabric is wrapped around the heel) or an appliance (such as a wire when doing a fabric-reinforced wire suture repair).

§The term *tape* (when referring to fabrics) means that the fabric is supplied in a long, narrow (usually less than 8-inch–wide) strip. Unlike other types of tape, there is no pressure-sensitive material applied to these fabric tapes.

| Chapter 28

Trauma to the Sole and Wall

Robin M. Dabareiner, William A. Moyer, and G. Kent Carter

PROBLEMS ASSOCIATED WITH HORSESHOE NAILS

Nail Bind

History and Clinical Signs

A *close nail* or *nail bind* refers to placement of a horseshoe nail not necessarily in the sensitive structures of the hoof, but close enough that the nail exerts sufficient pressure on these structures to cause discomfort. A horseshoe nail is designed to be driven obliquely through the hoof wall. When the nail is driven, the tip is placed at the inner edge of the white line with the bevel of the nail tip facing inward. When driven, the bevel contacts the hard hoof wall and curves outward and exits 1 to 2 cm above the level of the shoe. The tip of the nail is removed and the remainder is bent over to form a clinch to hold the shoe firmly to the hoof. Correct nail placement is important because if the nail is placed too shallow (superficial), the hoof wall will weaken and possibly split; if is it placed in too far, the sensitive structures of the hoof may be entered (pricked) (Figure 28-1). Overzealous clinching of the nails causes inward bending of the nail that can result in pressure on sensitive tissues, which may result in immediate or delayed pain and lameness. Slight displacement of a shoe also can result in nail pressure on sensitive tissues.

Diagnosis

Diagnosis of nail bind is difficult and often determined by eliminating other causes of foot pain. Lameness varies from subtle to severe. Sometimes a horse exhibits a change or lack in performance. The problem may not arise until several days after shoeing. Sometimes a horse is sound when trotted in a straight line, but it shows lameness when pulled in a tight circle or when it makes a turn. It is important to realize that nail bind is not always associated with poor farriery. A good nail can become a problem nail days or weeks after shoeing if the shoe shifts, causing abnormal nail pressure, or if the horse had a poor-quality hoof wall and hoof wall loss occurs. This is a common problem in Thoroughbred (TB) racehorses and usually involves the medial heel nail (the medial quarter and heel wall usually is the thinnest

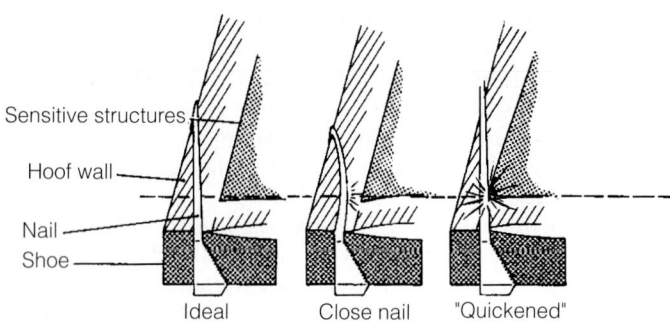

Fig. 28-1 • Schematic of ideal, close, and pricked (quickened) horseshoe nail placement.

aspect of the hoof wall). Hoof tester evaluation using both pressure and percussion on the outer hoof wall capsule may cause a painful response over the offending nail. Heat and increased digital pulse amplitudes may not be present, depending on the duration of the close nail. Often diagnosis is determined by pulling single nails one by one from the shoe and evaluating the horse for lameness after each nail is removed. Paradoxically, lameness is sometimes transiently accentuated after removal of the offending nail.

Treatment and Prognosis

The treatment of nail bind is removal of the offending nail; usually lameness resolves within a few days. The empty nail hole may be flushed with a disinfectant solution, such as dilute povidone-iodine solution, dimethyl sulfoxide, or an antiseptic solution such as thimerosal (Merthiolate, Eli Lilly, Chicago, United States). No additional treatment is usually needed. Prognosis is good once the nail has been removed, provided infection does not ensue.

Nail Prick

History and Clinical Signs

Nail prick or *quicking* refers to penetration of the sensitive hoof structures, usually the sensitive laminae, by a driven horseshoe nail (see Figure 28-1). The horse usually reacts as the farrier drives or clinches the nail by jerking the foot from the farrier.[1] Sometimes blood appears on the nail or leaks from the nail hole. Nail pricks occur for many reasons and are not always caused by a misdirected nail. Poorly made shoes, misdirected nails, selection of a nail that is too large, poorly placed nail holes, and faulty nails can result in a nail prick. Horses with poor hoof quality, thin hoof walls, or flaring hoof walls can be very difficult to nail and thus are at greatest risk. Fractious horses and young horses that have not been previously shod may lean on the farrier or repeatedly pull the foot from the farrier, making driving a nail difficult. A rushed farrier predisposes to nail pricking, but it can also happen to the best of farriers. Damage from an improperly driven nail can vary from minimal to serious infection.

Diagnosis

Diagnosis of a misdirected nail warrants great diplomacy from the veterinarian, because many owners become unjustifiably upset with the farrier. Some horses repeatedly stomp the affected foot or paw the ground immediately after shoeing. Others point the affected limb after shoeing.

References on page 1270

Lameness may not be apparent immediately but may occur days after shoeing when the nail hole becomes infected and the trapped pus begins to exert pressure. The horse usually becomes acutely lame, and the lameness worsens over time unless it is treated. An infection may migrate up the lamellae (white line) and create an abscess or soft spot at the hairline of the coronary band. The abscess is directly aligned with the hoof wall tubules leading to the infected nail hole, which is an important diagnostic aid. Hoof tester examination, using both pressure and percussion over each nail, is essential to locate the offending nail. Increased digital pulse amplitudes and heat may be present.

Treatment

Pricks from nails can be potentially serious and require immediate treatment. If the nail prick is discovered by the farrier at the time of shoeing, the nail is removed. The nail should be examined for moisture or blood. The nail hole can be irrigated with dimethyl sulfoxide, povidone-iodine solution, or hydrogen peroxide. The nail hole is packed with iodine-soaked cotton and left open. Often the nail is redirected and no further treatment is needed. Tetanus prophylaxis is essential for an unvaccinated horse.

If the offending nail cannot be localized or the nail hole is infected, the shoe is removed. Hoof testers then are used to localize the painful nail hole. Many times the pressure from the hoof testers causes black, malodorous liquid exudate to exit from the hole. This may not be obvious immediately, but if the foot is replaced to the ground and the horse walks a few steps, exudate may become obvious. The basis of treatment is to establish drainage. The infected nail hole often requires enlargement with a loop hoof knife or curette. Ideally a cone-shaped hole is made, with the larger opening at the bottom of the hoof. The hole is irrigated or the entire foot is soaked in an Epsom salt and povidone-iodine foot bath for 20 to 30 minutes twice daily until the infection is resolved. It is important to protect the foot from the environment (mud, dirt) by keeping the foot bandaged between foot soaks. Alternatively, a poultice can be applied to the foot for several days. Additional medications usually are not necessary unless infection is widespread. Antiinflammatory medication may be beneficial to decrease pain. Once the infection has cleared, the shoe is replaced. The affected nail hole can be packed with iodine-soaked cotton, and the horse reshod with a plastic pad covering the sole. Alternately, a hole can be drilled into the shoe over the affected nail hole and the shoe can be replaced, leaving access to the infected area for daily irrigation and povidone-iodine packing.

Prognosis

Prognosis after nail prick usually is good, provided that minimal damage occurs to vital structures of the foot. Establishing drainage for infection is important to avoid potential complications, such as infectious osteitis of the distal phalanx or infection of the distal interphalangeal (DIP) joint.

Solar Bruising

History and Etiology

A *bruise* is a contusion or impact injury that causes focal or generalized damage with subsequent hemorrhage of the solar corium. Sole bruising occurs commonly in all types and breeds of horses, especially in racing TBs and Standard-breds (STBs).[2] The degree and severity of lameness vary from acute, severe lameness to chronic mild or intermittent pain, depending on location and degree of damage. It is important to determine the cause of the bruise, because this dictates proper treatment and prevention. The general cause is abnormal focal weight bearing on the solar surface of the foot. The location of the bruise is helpful in determining the cause of the injury. The most common location is the junction between the bars and the walls at the heel, termed a *corn*.[3] Corns occur most frequently on the medial side of the front feet. Heel bruising may be the result of improper shoeing or trimming. Some farriers bend the medial branch of the shoe toward the frog to prevent the horse from stepping on and pulling the shoe. This shoe position causes direct pressure to the sole at the heel angle, instead of the heel wall, resulting in continued concussion and bruising. A shoe that is too small or does not extend far enough back under the heel can lead to heel bruising.[4] The ends of the shoe should extend to the widest aspect of the frog for proper heel protection. Horses with long-toe–low-heel hoof conformation are susceptible to heel bruising. Toe bruising can be caused by excessive impact or weight bearing on the toe region secondary to another cause such as heel pain. An improperly positioned horseshoe that rests on the sole instead of the hoof wall also causes toe bruising. Horses with long toes and those shod with toe grabs concentrate impact at the toe region.[4] Sole bruising occurs often in horses with flat feet because the sole repeatedly strikes the ground surface. A flat foot can be congenital, can be created by trimming the hoof wall too short, or can be caused by excessive wall breakage at the quarters. Thin-soled horses or excessive trimming of the sole reduce the sole protection and predispose to sole bruising. Loose shoes can shift position, and improperly balanced feet cause excessive impact forces to specific regions of the foot and cause bruising.[4] Riding on hard and rocky ground can result in stone bruises. A shod foot that has overgrown to the point where the shoe is riding on the sole is at risk of bruising.[4]

Clinical Signs

The degree of lameness from sole bruising can change daily, and lameness varies among horses. Removal of the shoe usually increases the degree of lameness. The bruising can be acute or chronic depending on the cause. Digital pulse amplitudes are increased after exercise, and careful hoof tester evaluation often reveals a focal painful response. Discoloration is common, but if the bruise is chronic or deep or if the horse's sole is pigmented, it may be difficult to identify. Bruising often affects several feet. In most horses, lameness will improve after perineural analgesia of the palmar digital nerves. Radiological changes are rare but may include a serum pocket (fluid line) between the distal phalanx and external sole abscess. Such lesions are easier to detect with digital or computed radiography than with conventional radiography. Persistent, chronic bruising may lead to osteolytic lesions or solar margin fractures of the distal phalanx.

Treatment

Initial treatment with phenylbutazone (2.2 mg/kg bid) and soaking the feet in Epsom salts help decrease

inflammation. Corrective or proper shoeing is imperative to shift the weight-bearing forces away from the damaged area of the foot. Sole paint consisting of a combination of equal parts of phenol, iodine, and formalin can be applied to toughen the solar surface. Hoof balance problems and shoeing causes, such as heel calks, toe grabs, or tucked heels, should be eliminated. One of many different shoeing techniques then is used to decrease impact and protect the bruised area. One method is use of a rim pad that is cut out over the bruised area so that the affected heel or quarter is "floated" and thus receives minimal weight-bearing forces. Another method is application of a bar shoe with a deeply concaved solar (inner) surface to stabilize the foot and alleviate any sole pressure from the shoe itself. A wide-web shoe may provide relief by covering and providing protection over a larger surface. It is important that this shoe be properly positioned on the hoof wall so that it does not increase sole pressure. Application of full pads packed with silicone or oakum may provide temporary relief by distributing weight-bearing forces over a wider area but often leads to a weakened and softer sole, causing recurrent problems.[5]

Prognosis

The prognosis is good if the inciting cause of the bruising can be corrected. Corrections may be difficult in horses with flat feet or long-toe–low-heel conformation, and such horses often have recurrent solar bruising.

Thrush

Thrush is a bacterial infection characterized by an accumulation of black, malodorous, necrotic material, usually originating within the central or collateral sulci of the frog of the hoof. This degenerative condition may spread to involve deeper structures of the foot, such as the digital cushion, hoof wall, and heel bulb region, causing inflammation and breakdown of these structures.[6] Many keratolytic organisms may be present, but *Fusobacterium necrophorum* is often isolated. Thrush is most often caused by poor environmental conditions; horses standing in soiled stalls, deep mud, swampy land, or wet pastures are at risk, especially if the feet are not cleaned daily.[7] Poor hoof conformation also predisposes to thrush. Saddlebreds, Tennessee Walkers and other gaited horses, and some Warmblood breeds have long feet with naturally deep frog sulci and are at risk of thrush.[7] Horses with a sheared heel or acquired frog deformity also are predisposed. Horses shod with full pads may develop thrush secondary to moisture and dirt collection under the pad. Other well-kept, clean horses can develop thrush for no apparent reason. Horses with severe thrush need to be differentiated from those with canker (see Chapter 125 and page 319). Lameness in horses with mild thrush is often blamed on the presence of thrush, but a careful lameness examination will reveal a primary source of pain elsewhere, coexistent with mild thrush.

Clinical Signs and Diagnosis

Lameness often is not apparent, but if present, the severity can vary. With severe thrush lameness can be obvious, but in most horses thrush is an additional finding and the primary source of pain is elsewhere. Diagnosis is based on the presence of black, malodorous discharge located most commonly within the frog sulci. The central frog sulcus often is malformed and very deep. A painful response may occur when the affected sulci are cleaned, because the degenerative process may extend to sensitive structures of the foot. If structural damage has occurred, the bulbs of the heel may move independently of each other, causing pain on manipulation.

Treatment

The predisposing cause should be identified and, if possible, removed. The horse should be moved to a clean, dry environment, and the feet should be cleaned daily. Any necrotic debris and undermined tissue are carefully debrided and cleaned using a hoof knife. Foot bandages may be necessary if the debridement is extensive. Systemic antimicrobial drugs may be necessary if deep or more proximal tissues are affected, but infection is usually managed by topical medication. Several caustic materials have been recommended, including a combination of phenol, tincture of iodine, and 10% formalin, Kopertox solution (Fort Dodge, Fort Dodge, Iowa, United States), or methylene blue. Initially, when the frog is very sensitive, the caustic materials may be too harsh and actually cause more tissue damage. We recommend to begin treatment by trying to dry the sensitive tissue with a mixture of sugar and povidone-iodine solution; make a paste consistency and apply that over the affected area until the tissue is dry and less sensitive. Once the frog begins to harden and keratinize, then the more caustic materials can be used. Others have recommended foot soaks in chlorine bleach (30 mL of bleach in 5 L of water). Corrective trimming and farriery may be necessary. If heel instability is present, a bar shoe may be necessary to stabilize the palmar aspect of the foot. Exercise is important to strengthen the palmar aspect of the foot and will naturally clean the feet.[7] The best treatment for thrush involves prevention by educating the client on proper hoof hygiene.

Prognosis

The prognosis for horses with thrush is favorable if the cause can be identified and eliminated and if the condition is treated before extensive hoof damage has occurred.

Sheared Heel

History and Clinical Signs

Sheared heel refers to instability between the medial and lateral bulbs of the heel. Mediolateral foot imbalance may be a predisposing cause. It is frequently but not invariably associated with distortion of the hoof capsule. The medial bulb of heel often is displaced proximally, with a steep medial wall and flaring of the lateral wall (see Figure 6-3). However, instability between the bulbs of the heel can also occur in a more normally conformed foot, and distortion of the hoof capsule as previously described is not synonymous with sheared heel. It is also important to recognize that sheared heel can be present without causing lameness, although sheared heel may be a cause of lameness.

Sheared heel may be present in one or several feet and may be associated with mild to moderate lameness. Lameness is usually worst on firm or hard footing. There may be distortion of the coronary band, which usually is higher medially. There may be a deep cleft dissecting between the medial and lateral bulbs of the heel. Sheared heel may predispose to thrush.

Diagnosis

Instability of the bulbs of the heel is detected by grasping each bulb of the heel with the left and right hands and twisting each bulb in opposite directions in a shearing motion. In a normal horse the bulbs of the heel cannot be moved independently. Considerable independent motion can be associated with pain, causing lameness. However, if the lameness is severe, another coexisting cause of lameness should be considered. Lameness associated with sheared heel is removed by perineural analgesia of the palmar digital nerves.

Treatment and Prognosis

Any mediolateral or dorsopalmar foot imbalance should be corrected. The affected foot should be floated by trimming the high heel bulb shorter than the rest of the hoof wall such that it does not bear any weight. This allows the coronary band to drop down into the correct position. The foot with the floated heel bulb should be shod with a bar shoe to provide stability to the heel region. This may need to be continued for many months, and occasionally indefinitely, until some physical attachment between the heel bulbs has become established. If the hoof capsule is distorted in shape as previously described, the medial branch of the shoe should be set slightly wide to encourage the medial wall to grow down to it and prevent it from collapsing axially. Any excess flare on the lateral wall should be removed. The prognosis is generally good.

Hoof Wall Separation (White Line Disease, Seedy Toe)

History and Clinical Signs

The white line, visible at the sole, is created by the junction of the insensitive laminae of the hoof wall and the horn of the sole. *White line disease* has historically been a term to describe the separation of the hoof wall from its laminar attachments. A crack or opening occurs within the white line, allowing a bacterial or fungal infection to invade the stratum medium, with proximity to the laminae causing cavities to develop between the laminae and outer hoof wall.[8] Environmental conditions of either too much moisture (continuous wet pastures) or drought conditions producing excessively dry feet predispose to development of a crack or opening in the white line. Horses with poor-quality hoof walls that split or crack or those with chronic laminitis and a thickened or stretched white line in the toe region may develop white line disease. The term *seedy toe* has been used differently in North America and Europe. In North America it is most often used to describe thickened or widened white line at the toe in horses with chronic laminitis, whereas in Europe it is used to describe separation at the white line, filled with crumbly material, that is not associated with laminitis. The hoof wall separation usually is a chronic condition beginning weeks or months before veterinary advice is sought, because there usually is no associated lameness. Hard ground may exacerbate any lameness seen.

Diagnosis

The degree of lameness varies, but if severe, white line disease can cause clinical signs of pain. However, the clinician should resist the temptation to incriminate this disease as the primary source of lameness until a thorough lameness examination has been completed. Because lameness is abolished after palmar digital analgesia or a dorsally directed ring block, this disease can easily be confused with many other conditions of the foot. Visual examination of the white line, assisted by a probing instrument, reveals a cavity with separation of outer hoof wall from the laminae. Radiological evaluation determines the full extent of hoof wall separation. Often the cavity is either dry or filled with necrotic debris, which may involve a bacterial or fungal infection. The cavity is usually not painful to probing.

Treatment

If the cavity is small (extends <2 cm proximally), placement of a cotton ball soaked in tincture of iodine in the cavity, with the shoe keeping the cotton in place, may be enough to stop the progression of the problem. However, if the cavity is extensive, then the separated outer hoof wall is removed using hoof nippers, hoof knife, and motorized tools. The aim is to remove cracks or crevices that could harbor bacteria. A Dremel tool burr (Dremel, Racine, Wisconsin, United States) is useful to smooth any cracks in the insensitive laminae that are exposed after hoof wall removal. Large defects in the hoof wall require protection. A heart bar shoe redistributes weight-bearing forces to the frog and palmar region of the foot and away from damaged and weakened areas. The hoof wall defects prevent normal nailing procedures; therefore clips or support bars (Figure 28-2) can help to secure the shoe to the hoof. After hoof wall removal the exposed laminae may still have an active infectious component. The horse should be kept in a clean, dry stall; the exposed laminae are treated topically with iodine or thimerosal (Merthiolate) daily for 10 days or until they are dry. The horse may then be a candidate for prosthetic hoof wall repair using a product such as Equilox (Equilox International, Pine Island, Minnesota, United States). The plastic acrylic is trimmed and shaped to the horse's natural hoof wall at the next shoeing. The hoof to which the acrylic is applied should be kept dry to avoid losing the acrylic patch. The horse may return to normal activity once the prosthetic patch is in place. It is very important to keep the patch dry, including preventing the horse from going out in the pasture when the morning dew is still present on the grass. The owner should be cautioned

that 50% of prosthetic patches may result in infection and abscessation under the patch, which will necessitate removing the patch and topically treating the exposed laminae again. It can be very difficult to sterilize the exposed laminae given the horse's barn environment.

Prognosis

Prognosis depends on response to treatment and cause of the original problem. Horses with poor hoof quality or primary laminitis often have recurrence. If the horse responds to original treatment and if environmental conditions improve, prognosis is good.

Poor Hoof Wall Quality

Poor hoof quality plagues many horses. Many factors determine hoof quality, including the environment, farrier management, hoof conformation, owner management, and use of the horse. Drought conditions may result in dry, brittle hooves that are prone to hoof wall splitting, cracking, and bruising. Foot growth slows during hot, drought conditions. Excessive moisture creates a weakened hoof wall that may flatten or collapse under normal weight-bearing forces. The heel may collapse, which leads to corns and heel bruising. In addition, the weak hoof wall will not hold nails, and the hoof wall separates in layers similar to wet plywood. A muddy environment may increase the risk of development of a secondary hoof abscess. Even worse is a fluctuation of wet-dry-wet-dry environments. Four problems that contribute to the wet-dry environment require owner education. The first is the growth of spring grass that gets high. Horses that are on pasture are exposed to the morning dew on the grass (wet), then the dry heat during the days (dry), and this morning wetness and afternoon dryness cause hoof wall separation, nails that loosen, and shoes that will not stay on. The second problem occurs when horses are allowed access to a pond or stream during the hot summer months. The horse's feet are dry until they wade into the water and then get wet; this causes brittle and cracking hoof walls. Another potential problem is daily washing of the horses after exercise during the hot summer months, or if an owner lets a water trough overflow to create a mud hole for a horse to step into. The wet-dry fluctuation causes poor hoof wall quality. Improper trimming and shoeing methods can cause substantial hoof wall damage. Horseshoe nails that are placed too far outward in the hoof wall, or exit too low in the hoof wall, weaken the hoof wall and cause splitting and cracking. Many TB horses with long-toe–low-heel hoof conformation often have collapsing heels and thin, weak hoof walls that make proper nail placement and farrier management difficult. The most common cause of weak, poor-quality feet is lack of exercise and stall housing.

Diagnosis

Diagnosis is somewhat subjective, as poor hoof quality is usually in the eye of the beholder. There are no objective criteria for determining hoof quality. Diagnosis is usually made by visual examination of the foot. Communication with the farrier is imperative for the diagnosis and future treatment plan. Horses with poor hoof wall quality often have palmar foot pain or are prone to sole and heel bruising. They are prone to losing shoes, which can accentuate the problem.

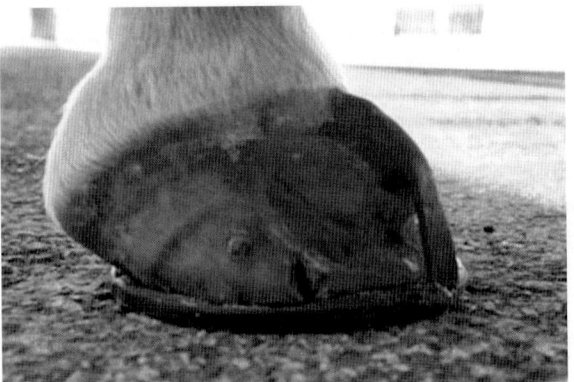

Fig. 28-2 • Extensive hoof wall removal requiring a support bar attached to the remaining hoof capsule to secure the bar shoe to the hoof.

Treatment

If possible, the cause of the poor hoof wall quality should be corrected if identified. In drought conditions, painting the entire hoof and coronary band daily with a lanolin-based hoof dressing is sometimes beneficial. We prefer the product Hoofmaker (www.manentail.com). In an excessively wet environment, confining the horse to a stall and avoiding standing water or wet pastures may improve hoof wall quality. Educating the owner concerning causes of wet-dry fluctuation is very important. If a horse is going to be in wet conditions, instruct the owner to paint the hoof wall with a hoof sealant to seal the moisture out of the feet. We have used a product called "Hoof Shield" (www.monettafarrier.com) with good success. Poor farriery can be addressed, but in many horses poor hoof conformation and poor environment are more difficult to manage. Unbalanced long-toe–low-heel hoof conformation should be corrected as much as possible with proper trimming of the heel back to the widest portion of the frog. The toe of the foot is shortened as much as possible, and a rockered, round, or square-toed shoe is used to further decrease toe length and ease breakover. Egg bar shoes are used if more heel support is needed. Access to the outdoors and being able to move about are helpful but often difficult to achieve.

Hoof quality also is a function of proper diet and exercise. The horse's nutrition should be evaluated, paying particular attention to protein quantity. Biotin supplements may be beneficial.

Prognosis

Poor hoof quality usually is not corrected but managed. Prognosis is generally unfavorable unless a specific cause can be identified and eliminated.

PENETRATING INJURIES OF THE SOLE
Subsolar Abscess

History and Clinical Signs

Subsolar abscess (gravel) is one of the most common causes of acute lameness in all horses. Subsolar abscesses may originate from a penetrating wound in the white line, nail hole, or deep subsolar bruise. A cause may not be identified. Lameness is usually acute and severe (grade 3 to 4 of 5) and may worsen over time until drainage is established. Lameness that develops during work or when a horse is turned out may falsely lead to the suspicion of a traumatic injury. The horse often points and may not bear full weight on the affected limb. Distal limb swelling often accompanies a subsolar abscess that has not drained, leading the owner to suspect tendon injury. Systemic signs of infection (fever, lethargy) may be present if deeper structures are involved. The infected tract may migrate and open at the coronary band. Before breaking open, a soft, painful area can be located by digital palpation of the coronary band.

Diagnosis

Digital pulse amplitudes are usually, but not always, increased, and the hoof capsule may have heat. A focal painful area can usually, but not always, be located with careful hoof tester examination. If the sole is extremely hard, it may be difficult to locate a subsolar abscess. Careful paring of the sole and frog may be helpful in locating the

abscess, assuming that the horn is not too hard, but the clinician must be careful not to damage good, healthy tissue while looking for the infection site. Unnecessary, aggressive paring may lead to large painful areas that take months to heal. Foot poultices and hot water foot baths with Epsom salts help to soften the horn and eventually localize the affected area, especially in horses with hard horn. Grey or black, malodorous liquid leaks from the infected tract (see Figure 6-10). Firm digital palpation of the surrounding area can help to determine the extent to which adjacent tissues are underrun. Similar clinical signs can also be seen in weak-footed TB horses, especially in the palmar aspect of the foot, associated with frank subsolar hemorrhage. Radiography sometimes is useful to identify a gas or fluid pocket (see Figure 129-1). In horses with no localizing clinical signs, it may be necessary to use local analgesic techniques to determine the site of pain causing lameness. Severe lameness associated with a subsolar abscess may be only partially improved by apparent desensitization of the foot.

Treatment

Treatment is aimed at establishing adequate drainage. If the tract is open at the sole surface, it should be enlarged just enough for good irrigation and drainage. This may require sedation or perineural analgesia of the foot. If pink tissue or blood is encountered, debridement should be discontinued. Large holes should not be used, to avoid solar corium protrusion, which can be a painful sequela to overzealous hoof paring. If drainage occurs at the level of the coronary band and solar surface, through-and-through lavage is beneficial. Debridement at the coronary band level should be minimal to prevent iatrogenic DIP joint contamination. Once drainage is established, the foot is protected from the environment and recontamination with a foot bandage or poultice. Continued foot soaks in warm water povidone-iodine and Epsom salt foot baths should be continued until infection and inflammation are eliminated. The shoe is replaced when the affected area is dry and cornified. A small cotton ball soaked in tincture of iodine is often placed in the defect before reapplication of the shoe to prevent recontamination of the site. Large areas may require a plastic pad under the shoe for solar protection. Antimicrobial drugs and nonsteroidal antiinflammatory drugs (NSAIDs) are rarely needed, unless infection is severe or deeper structures have been penetrated. Many practitioners consider antibiotics contraindicated because administration may prolong clinical signs. However, if swelling and infection of the coronary band and subcutaneous tissues of the pastern region occur, antimicrobial therapy is indicated. Because lameness can be severe in horses with this type of disseminated infection, involvement of the DIP joint is often suspected but usually not present. Tetanus prophylaxis is mandatory.

Prognosis

Prognosis in horses with a simple subsolar abscess is excellent but decreases if complications develop in which deeper structures of the foot are involved.

Deep Penetrating Injuries to the Sole

History and Clinical Signs

A horse's environment is filled with sharp objects that can penetrate the sole, causing severe damage to structures deep within the hoof capsule. All puncture wounds should be considered potentially serious, but those in the solar white line or palmar frog area require special attention because of the potential for navicular bursa, digital flexor tendon sheath (DFTS), deep digital flexor tendon (DDFT), DIP joint, or distal phalanx involvement.

The clinical signs vary with anatomical structure involved and chronicity of the injury. Lameness may be mild at the time of injury but moderate to severe once inflammation and infection occur. Penetrating wounds of the navicular bursa or DDFT result in severe lameness and a reluctance to bear weight on the heel.

Diagnosis

If a foreign body is found in the bottom of the foot, the owner should usually be instructed to leave the object in the foot, unless there is danger of further penetration. Radiography is performed immediately to determine depth of penetration and orientation, and orthogonal images are mandatory. In many horses, little superficial evidence of penetrating injury is present. Digital pulse amplitudes are increased, and the foot is usually warm to touch. Hoof testers are useful to determine a focal point of pain, but often the entire surface of the foot is reactive. If necessary, the horse should be sedated and the foot desensitized to facilitate further examination. Light paring of the sole and frog areas with a hoof knife may reveal a black spot indicating the penetration site. Often, however, the entry is not discovered, because the elastic nature of the hoof structures causes the site of penetration to collapse. If an entry wound is discovered, the foot is scrubbed thoroughly before insertion of a sterile, flexible probe. Care must be used so that inadvertent force and horse movement do not cause the probe to penetrate previously unaffected structures. A less invasive and preferred method is to place a sterile teat cannula into the hole and inject sterile radiodense material to determine the affected structures (Figure 28-3). It is important to obtain a true lateromedial radiographic image to determine the dorsal spread of the contrast media.

If infection of the navicular bursa (see later), DIP joint, or DFTS is suspected, paracentesis, synovial fluid cytological studies, and culture and antimicrobial susceptibility tests should be performed. Comprehensive radiographic examination should be performed to assess the distal phalanx and the navicular bone. Initial radiographs may appear normal, but radiolucent defects or new bone formation may become apparent within 10 to 14 days. Magnetic resonance imaging can be extremely useful to identify the extent of soft tissue injury in the face of a known penetrating injury[9] and to provide evidence of a previous penetrating injury in horses with lameness with no known history of such injury. The identification of a hemosiderin tract leading to an area of damaged tissues is pathognomonic.[10,11]

Treatment

If penetration of deep hoof structures is suspected, broad-spectrum systemic antimicrobial drugs, NSAIDs, and tetanus prophylaxis should be administered. During the initial 3 to 4 days, distal limb regional limb perfusion with an antibiotic (1 g amikacin or 2 g cefotaxime diluted in 30 mL saline) is also recommended, to achieve high local tissue concentrations of antibiotics. Systemic antibiotic

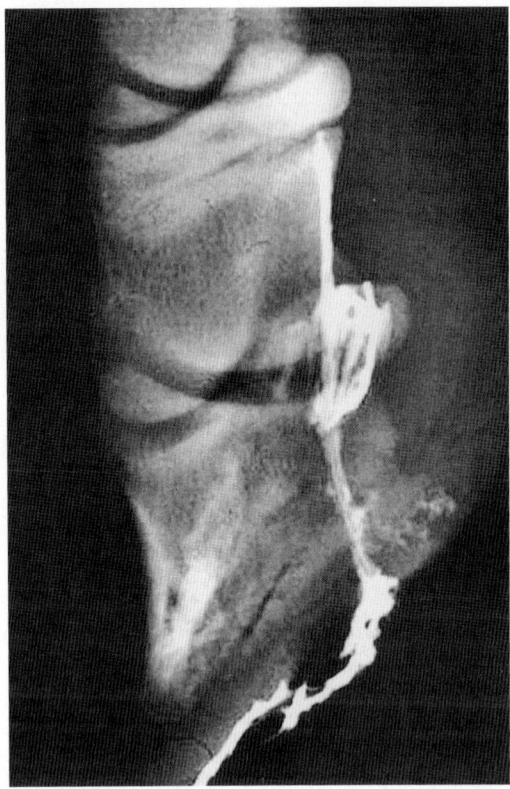

Fig. 28-3 • Oblique radiographic image of a foot; radiodense contrast material has been injected into a hole through the sole, the result of a penetrating injury. The contrast media extends proximally. A lateromedial image is also required to define better which structures may be involved.

therapy usually should be continued for 2 weeks after resolution of clinical signs of infection. Establishment of drainage, copious lavage with sterile ionic fluid, and debridement of all necrotic tissue are indicated. Management of infection of the navicular bursa is discussed later (page 316).

If the DDFT is involved (infectious tendonitis), debridement and removal of frayed and infected tendon fibers may be performed in a standing, sedated horse using a tourniquet and perineural analgesia, or with the horse under general anesthesia depending on horse temperament and owner financial constraints (see later). After debridement, use of a 4- to 8-degree wedge shoe decreases forces on the DDFT and provides some pain relief. The wedge shoe angle is gradually decreased over several months as the DDF tendon begins to heal and strengthen. The bottom of the foot requires protection with a bandage or hospital plate until the surgical site granulates in and cornifies.

Infectious Osteitis of the Distal Phalanx

Deep penetrating wounds to the sole, especially the solar–white line junction, can result in infectious osteitis of the distal phalanx. Usually a chronic, recurrent draining tract is located at the coronary band or solar surface of the foot, associated with variable lameness. Infection of the distal phalanx also can result from undetected soft tissue infection, from dissection of subsolar abscesses, or as a sequela to laminitis secondary to recurrent abscessation and ischemia at the toe. As the bone infection progresses, blood supply to the area is compromised, and the area of avascular

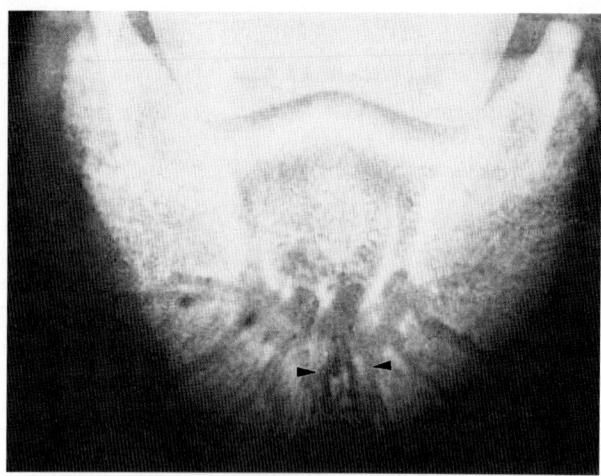

Fig. 28-4 • Dorsoproximal-palmarodistal oblique radiographic image of the distal phalanx demonstrating infectious osteitis with a sequestrum (arrowheads).

bone separates from the parent bone, forming a sequestrum.[12] Radiological abnormalities may not be detectable for weeks after a penetrating injury.[12] Radiography reveals a radiolucent area in the margin of the distal phalanx, with or without sequestrum formation (Figure 28-4). Debridement and curettage of all soft and necrotic bone often can be performed in a standing, sedated horse, but general anesthesia may be required. The foot is desensitized using perineural analgesia, cleaned with a hoof knife and steel brush, and prepared for aseptic surgery. Hemostasis is achieved by wrapping a roll of elastic bandage firmly around the fetlock joint to compress and occlude the palmar digital arteries. The infected bone is accessed by removal of sequential layers of the sole using either a motorized Dremel tool or a Galt trephine (Miltex, Bethpage, New York, United States) with a retractable pilot bit.[13] The infected bone usually is discolored and soft and should be curetted to healthy bone margins. Culture of the infected bone and microbial sensitivity testing should be performed. A postoperative radiograph should be obtained to ensure complete debridement. After surgery the surgical site is packed with sterile gauze sponges soaked in antiseptic or antimicrobial solutions, and then the foot is bandaged. Disposable diapers and duct tape are inexpensive materials used to make a waterproof foot bandage. The bandage is changed at 1- to 2-day intervals for the initial few weeks. A bar shoe and hospital plate provide solar protection. A plastic pad secured with duct tape also works well. The bolts and metal plate are removed from the hospital plate, and the surgery site can be cleaned and treated; the plate then is bolted back in place. After surgery the horse is confined to a small area until the hole granulates and cornifies, which usually requires 4 to 6 weeks. If granulation tissue becomes excessive at the surgery site, application of 2% tincture of iodine speeds healing. If severe infection is present, the surgery site can be packed lightly with antibiotic-impregnated beads for continued antibiotic release at the infected site. Regional limb perfusion with antibiotics may also be beneficial.

Prognosis

Prognosis depends on whether the infection is severe and chronic. Horses with acute penetrating wounds that receive immediate and aggressive treatment have a good chance of returning to athletic use. Horses with penetration injuries that have an established infection involving the navicular bursa (see later),[14] DFTS, or DIP joint have a poorer prognosis. Prognosis for horses with infectious osteitis of the distal phalanx is good if the cause of infection is not laminitis. In one study, up to 24% of the distal phalanx was removed with successful results.[15]

PENETRATING WOUNDS TO THE NAVICULAR BURSA (BURSA PODOTROCHLEARIS), INFECTIOUS (SEPTIC) NAVICULAR BURSITIS, "STREETNAIL"

Mike W. Ross and Sue J. Dyson

Penetration of a nail or other sharp object into the solar surface of the foot is classically referred to as "streetnail," and the historically important procedure to establish drainage of the navicular bursa is the "streetnail procedure." The term *streetnail* and the surgical procedure are largely obsolete, but the clinical significance of penetrating wounds to this region of the foot cannot be overemphasized, particularly those involving the region of the frog. Of 50 horses with puncture wounds to the hoof, only 50% of horses with wounds in the region of the frog became sound after treatment, whereas 95% of horses with puncture wounds outside the frog were sound.[16] Furthermore, 35% of horses with puncture wounds to the frog were dead at the time of follow-up.[16] Infectious navicular bursitis and sequelae were the most common reason for euthanasia.[16] Early recognition and prompt management of horses with puncture wounds to the hoof, and specifically those involving the frog and deeper tissues such as the DDFT, navicular bursa, navicular bone, and DIP joint are equally important. Ninety-three percent of horses that received surgical management within 7 days became sound, compared with only 62% of horses that were treated after 7 days.[16] Horses with infectious navicular bursitis that received surgical management within 1 week of injury had a significantly better outcome than those with delayed recognition and management (8 to 60 days after injury).[14] Horses with hindlimb infectious navicular bursitis were significantly more likely to have a successful outcome than those with forelimb involvement.[14] Of 38 horses with infectious navicular bursitis managed using the conventional open streetnail procedure of debridement and drainage of the navicular bursa, only 12 (31.6%) had a satisfactory outcome, but when results were carefully evaluated, five of these horses were used as broodmares, leaving only seven (18.4%) horses used for riding after injury.[14] Similarly, 31.6% (six of 19 horses) of horses with infectious navicular bursitis managed with open drainage and debridement became sound enough for work.[16]

Because of these disappointing results the conventional surgical procedure of creating a "window" in the frog, digital cushion, and DDFT[17] to establish distal drainage of the navicular bursa has largely fallen from favor and cannot be recommended. Currently, endoscopic examination of the navicular bursa and other synovial structures such as the DIP joint and DFTS, if necessary, is the procedure of choice. Endoscopic examination is less invasive, causes fewer complications, and provides superior visual appraisal of the navicular bursa, navicular bone, and DDFT when compared with the conventional open approach. Of 16 horses with contaminated and infected navicular bursae that underwent endoscopic examination and debridement, 12 (75%) became sound, and complications such as ongoing necrosis of the DDFT seen in horses managed with the conventional streetnail procedure did not occur.[18] There were fewer complications and shorter hospital stays, and horses appeared to be immediately more comfortable after surgery compared with previous reports; three horses with concurrent infection of the DIP joint were managed successfully.[18]

Although actual results may vary among horses and surgeons, it appears that success in managing horses with infectious navicular bursitis using minimally invasive techniques is superior to that described in the previously published results and our own experience using the conventional approach to drainage and debridement of the navicular bursa. It is important to note that early recognition and management are critical. It is also important to establish the location and depth of penetration, and a minimum of two orthogonal radiographic images are necessary, if possible with the nail or penetrating object in place. After the puncture site has been cleaned, a sterile radiodense probe can be inserted, but in some horses the depth of penetration cannot be accurately determined using this method, and there is a risk of pushing foreign material deeper into the foot. Positive contrast radiographic studies should be considered, but these may not clearly show the depth of penetration. Magnetic resonance imaging can provide rapid, accurate information about the direction and depth of penetration, the presence of foreign material, and the extent of soft tissue and osseous trauma. Synoviocentesis of the navicular bursa, DIP joint, and DFTS should be performed to determine if a deep-seated contamination or infection is present. With use of general anesthesia and aseptic technique, endoscopic examination of the involved synovial structures should then be performed. The navicular bursa and palmar surface of the navicular bone and DDFT can be evaluated endoscopically and debrided. Debridement can be performed through the original penetrating tract and by creating an additional instrument portal if necessary. Samples for bacterial culture and susceptibility testing (aerobic and anaerobic) should be collected, and the tract and frayed and damaged edges of the DDFT should be debrided. Although liberal debridement can be performed, no attempt is made to make a wide incision of the DDFT. During the procedure, lavage of the navicular bursa is performed. In thick-skinned cob-type horses direct surgical access to the navicular bursa may not be possible and entry may have to be performed via the DFTS. Thorough lavage of the DFTS is mandatory to try to prevent spread of infection. Occasionally in horses with long-standing infections and concomitant osteitis of the navicular bone, or in those in which the navicular bone was directly damaged by the original trauma, the navicular bone is curetted. If necessary the DIP joint can be evaluated, but timing of examination should be preplanned because using a contaminated endoscope after evaluating a penetrated navicular bursa to evaluate a potentially uninvolved DIP joint is contraindicated. The application of a hospital plate, use of broad-spectrum intravenous antibiotics, NSAIDs, and daily regional limb perfusion of an aminoglycoside antibiotic are recommended. Once infection is fully resolved, medication of the navicular bursa with corticosteroids may be beneficial. Although emphasis on early management is important, we have had success in horses with long-standing infectious navicular bursitis, some with radiological evidence of osteitis and fragmentation of the navicular bone, and in horses with initially severe forelimb lameness. However, when owners are spoken to initially, a guarded prognosis for future soundness should always be given, although using this approach to management of horses with penetrating wounds into the navicular bursa and surrounding structures can lead to success. Once infection is resolved, prognosis for return to full athletic function often depends on the degree of concurrent traumatic damage to tendonous and ligamentous structures within the hoof capsule incurred at the time of original injury.

HOOF WALL CRACKS

History and Clinical Signs

Hoof wall cracks occur from improper foot balance; coronary band defects; excessive hoof growth; and thin, dry, or wet hoof walls. The horny hoof wall often fails internally before being visible on the external hoof surface.[19] Central toe cracks are often associated with rotation of the distal phalanx and clubfeet. Hoof cracks are characterized by location (toe, quarter, heel, or bar), length (complete or incomplete), depth (superficial or deep), site of origin (ground surface or coronary band), and whether hemorrhage or infection is present.[19] Hoof cracks are usually obvious on visual examination of the foot, except those originating at the hairline, which may be only 1 to 2 cm long and difficult to see. Lameness may be present, depending on whether the hoof crack involves the sensitive laminae and whether infection is present.

Diagnosis

Hoof wall cracks are diagnosed by visual assessment of the hoof capsule. The depth of the hoof crack, pain, and associated instability surrounding the crack are determined by careful hoof tester examination. Pain associated with a hoof crack is usually determined by digital pressure and hoof tester manipulation over the crack. Purulent material may exude during hoof tester pressure. Radiology is useful to evaluate rotation of the distal phalanx in horses with central toe cracks. Bleeding from a hoof crack after exercise indicates that the sensitive laminae are involved.

Treatment

Treatment varies with hoof crack location, depth, horse use, and presence of exposed sensitive laminae and infection. Superficial hoof cracks do not extend into laminar tissue and therefore are not painful. These may be the result of improper foot balance or basic neglect regarding trimming. Treatment involves balancing the foot and providing stability by application of a full bar shoe. If the horse is shod correctly and restricted from strenuous activity, most hoof cracks will resolve.[20]

Treatment of horses with deeper hoof cracks varies somewhat with location of the crack. If lameness exists, diagnostic analgesia should be performed to confirm that the hoof crack is the source of pain. Careful observation of the affected foot as the horse walks slowly often shows that the defect is unstable and actually closes and pinches the underlying sensitive laminae as the foot strikes the ground, causing pain. The hoof crack is explored and debrided with a hoof knife or motorized burr (Dremel tool) to remove all necrotic and infected tissue. Any undermined hoof wall is also removed. The area is treated for 24 to 48 hours with an antiseptic such as thimerosal (Merthiolate) or tincture of iodine until the crack is dry and free of infection. The hoof wall must be stabilized so that it can regrow. Previous recommendations have suggested grooving or burring the proximal extent of the crack, but this is rarely successful.[19] Many techniques for hoof wall stabilization use a combination of frog support with a heart bar shoe and clips combined with a fiberglass patch,[20] drill and lace technique,[19] metal plate technique, or a technique using composite hoof wall repair with acrylic materials (see Chapter 27). The heart bar shoe is essential to oppose the forces causing collapse of the crack during weight bearing. The toe must be trimmed short and squared before application of the shoe. The drill and lace technique is used if the deep crack does not extend to the coronary band, and the metal plate technique is used if it does. In the metal plate technique, two drill holes are placed 1 to 2 cm on either side of the trough directly opposite each other. Care is needed to ensure that drilling too deeply does not affect deeper hoof structures. The foot should *not* be desensitized, to allow the farrier and veterinarian to assess if there is inadvertent iatrogenic penetration of deeper tissues with the screws. One or two plates are cut that are longer than the exposed hoof crack and about 0.6 cm wide. With the foot held in a non–weight-bearing position, the metal plate is drilled and bolted in place to stabilize the crack. The hoof wall adjacent to the toe crack is trimmed shorter than the remaining hoof wall to minimize weight-bearing forces on the damaged area and decrease potential bending forces on the plate. The crack is treated for several days with thimerosal (Merthiolate) or tincture of iodine until the sensitive structures begin to cornify and infection has resolved. The hoof crack can then be filled with an acrylic material (e.g., Equilox, Equilox International, Pine Island, Minnesota, United States). Adhesion of the acrylic to the hoof wall is enhanced by sanding the hoof wall, applying acetone to dry the area, and using a hair dryer at the external hoof surface before acrylic application.

Quarter and heel hoof cracks often are incomplete, and low-heel–long-toe conformation with an underslung heel may predispose horses to develop them.[19] After the crack has been debrided and infection eliminated, the foot is balanced and a heart bar shoe applied. Two holes are drilled, using a 0.24-cm drill bit, approximately 1 to 2 cm apart on either side of and parallel to the crack. The holes begin at the ground surface and extend up the hoof wall. A shoelace or synthetic multifiber suture is laced in a far-near-near-far suture pattern to stabilize the crack.[19] Another technique is to trim the hoof wall behind the quarter crack shorter than the remaining hoof wall such that it does not touch the shoe while weight bearing, applying a bar shoe and stabilizing the proximal extent of the crack after it has been debrided (Figure 28-5). After the crack is dry and free of sensitive tissue and infection, it is filled with acrylic material. Readers are also referred to Chapter 27.

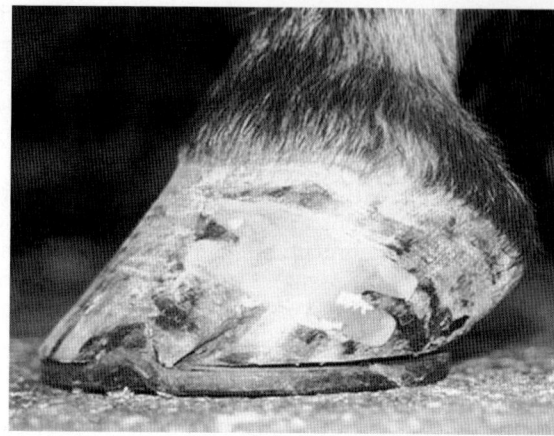

Fig. 28-5 • A quarter crack that has been debrided; the hoof wall on the palmar aspect of the crack has been "floated" and a plastic patch glued to the proximal extent of the crack for stability

Prognosis

The prognosis for horses with both superficial and deep hoof cracks is good, and lameness usually resolves as soon as the hoof is stabilized, but recurrence is common. Success is improved if the mechanical cause of the hoof crack can be identified and eliminated.

CORONARY BAND AND HOOF WALL LACERATIONS
History and Clinical Signs
The hoof wall is thicker and stronger at the toe region and becomes thinner through the quarters and heel, where the younger hoof has a greater moisture content.[20] The quarter and heel regions of the foot are susceptible to traumatic injuries. Coronary band and hoof wall lacerations usually occur from the horse catching a segment of hoof on an object as it steps down or kicking or stepping on a sharp object. Hoof avulsion injuries also can occur when the foot is entrapped between fence boards or in a cattle guard. Continued hoof imbalance, improper shoe removal, and repetitive trauma to the coronary band region result in a chronic hoof avulsion or spur—a fibrous bed of scar tissue beneath a displaced segment of hoof wall. Horses that overreach are predisposed to coronary band spurring or heel avulsion injuries. Steeplechase horses and horses racing on grass often slip and lacerate the heel region of a front foot.

Hoof avulsions are described as acute (lacerations) or chronic (repetitive trauma and spur formation) injuries. Avulsions can be complete, with total tissue loss, or incomplete in that a border of hoof remains intact. Hoof wall, coronary band, sole, distal phalanx, laminae, and the DIP joint may be involved in deep lacerations. The degree of lameness varies with duration, depth, and location of the injury. Horses with acute, superficial injuries may show mild lameness, and horses with deeper structure involvement may be non–weight bearing. If degree of lameness does not seem appropriate for severity of the laceration, the integrity of the palmar digital vein, artery, and nerve should be investigated.

Diagnosis

Diagnosis is straightforward, but involvement of deeper structures can be difficult to identify. Careful manipulation of the foot causes a painful reaction if deep structures are involved and provides valuable information regarding the integrity of the supporting hoof structures. Instability of the DIP joint may indicate the presence of collateral ligament damage. If manipulation produces a sucking noise, the DIP joint or DFTS may be involved. Before further evaluation the coronary band hair should be clipped, the outer hoof wall rasped, and the sole trimmed to eliminate any superficial contamination. The area should be scrubbed with antiseptic solution, and lavage performed. The wound then is digitally explored by the veterinarian using sterile gloves. Radiography is recommended for all deep lacerations, because fractures of the distal or middle phalanges may be present. Contrast radiographic studies may be necessary to identify openings in synovial structures. Alternately, a site far removed from the wound is clipped and prepared in a sterile manner, and the DFTS and/or DIP joint is distended with sterile saline to determine if it communicates with the laceration. Ultrasonographic examination may help to determine the extent of soft tissue damage. Bear in mind that foreign material such as wood may become trapped axial to the hoof wall, and such material may be inapparent on radiographs. The DIP joint was the most common synovial structure involved in a recent study of 101 heel bulb lacerations.[21]

Treatment

The equine foot heals primarily by epithelialization and reformation of the corium.[22] Decreasing motion at the affected site and hoof stabilization are essential for a successful outcome. Treatment varies with duration, severity, and type of injury. Incomplete, superficial hoof wall lacerations without coronary band involvement are treated by excision of the separated hoof wall and bar shoe application until healing occurs. The goal of shoeing is to eliminate weight-bearing forces at the damaged site and provide hoof stability.

Horses with incomplete, clean, acute hoof avulsions involving the coronary band can be treated by cleaning and debriding the displaced flap of tissue and suturing it back in place. This generally requires general anesthesia. Interrupted vertical mattress sutures with No. 1 or No. 2 monofilament suture are recommended.[21,22] Any undermined or contaminated hoof wall is removed. Immobilization is essential and is provided by applying a foot cast. The cast is usually left in place for 2 to 3 weeks. When applying the foot cast, the clinician should ensure that the proximal extent of the cast is located at midpastern level and does not impinge on the fetlock joint during movement. Administration of systemic antimicrobial drugs and NSAIDs may be necessary if contamination of deeper structures is suspected. If deeper structures are involved, cast application should be delayed until infection is eliminated. Open synovial structures can be lavaged daily, and the foot is protected with a sterile foot bandage. Antibiotic-impregnated beads and regional limb perfusion with antibiotics may be necessary with severe contamination.

Horses with compete avulsion injuries that appear stable during movement are treated by daily cleaning and bandaging until healing occurs. Bar shoe application is required if the hoof is unstable and contaminated. A foot cast can be used if infection is not a problem.

Repair of a chronic avulsion injury, or spur, usually requires surgical excision with the horse under general anesthesia. The hoof is rasped and prepared for aseptic surgery. The hoof wall distal to the avulsed segment should be thinned with a rasp to allow placement of the sutures through the hoof wall. The excessive cornified tissue growing from the displaced coronary band is trimmed to a level just distal to the coronary band. The fibrous tissue under the avulsed segment, which lies in the bed of the defect created by the hoof avulsion, is resected. This provides a vascularized area and room for replacement of the avulsed segment back to its original location. The displaced coronary band and hoof wall are replaced and sutured in the correct anatomical position using No. 2 monofilament suture in a simple interrupted or vertical mattress suture pattern. The surgery sites are covered with a light bandage, and the foot is immobilized in a foot cast for 2 weeks.

Prognosis

Treatment is usually prolonged and often takes 3 to 5 months for complete healing, which can be costly to the owner.[22] Incomplete superficial avulsion injuries or injuries that can be sutured usually heal by first intention, with a good functional, and sometimes cosmetic, end result. A roughened or thickened hoof wall distal to the defect often occurs at the site of avulsion, but it usually does not create a clinical problem. Prognosis decreases if deeper structures or synovial structures are involved. Complications such as infectious arthritis, fractures, and potential osteoarthritis can occur often with a guarded prognosis. In a retrospective study involving 101 horses sustaining a heel bulb laceration, 90% survived but 18% developed a hoof wall defect.[21]

CANKER

Mike W. Ross and Sue J. Dyson

Canker, a proliferative pododermatitis of the frog that may extend to undermine the sole and heel bulbs, is common in draft horses (and is discussed in detail in Chapter 125) but occurs in light horses as well. Differentiating this form of infection from the more common infection, thrush, is important. Canker is characterized by a foul odor (necrotic) and the presence of granulation-like tissue that bleeds easily when manipulated (see Figure 125-5). The principles of management are debriding, using a hospital plate and packing to maintain pressure on the healing solar wound, keeping the area clean, and applying topical antiseptic solutions or antimicrobial agents such as metronidazole (see Chapter 125). Alternatively, 53 of 54 horses with canker and in which long-term follow-up information was available were successfully managed using liberal debridement, topical cryotherapy, and the application of benzoyl peroxide on packing under a hospital plate.[23]

Reference
on pa
127

Chapter 29

Functional Anatomy of the Palmar Aspect of the Foot

Robert M. Bowker

The palmar portion of the foot consists of several important structures functioning to support the foot and the limb of the horse, as well as being an integral part of the energy dissipation mechanisms present within each limb. These palmar foot structures include the cartilages of the foot (also called the *lateral collateral* or *ungual* cartilages), the digital cushion, the frog, and an extensive vascular network. Although each of these structures is present in every foot, morphological features and tissue composition vary widely among horses, which may be responsible for differing efficiencies in ability to dissipate energy. Furthermore, such differences may in part account for differences between the feet of a sound horse and the feet of a horse with chronic lameness associated with the foot. Awareness of how these tissues interact and relate to one another during foot impact is important for understanding how the foot dissipates energy and how potential problems may arise to produce lameness when energy dissipation is not efficient and the concussive forces are transmitted to the bones and other connective tissues. The domestic horse spends considerable time standing, so the structure of the palmar aspect of the foot is important for support to the weight of the horse shifted dorsally toward the connective tissues at the toe of the foot.

The medial and lateral cartilages of the foot extend from the palmar surface of the distal phalanx to the bulbs of the heel as large vertical sheets, whereas the digital cushion lies between the medial and lateral cartilages of the foot and extends dorsally toward the solar surface of the distal phalanx distal to the deep digital flexor tendon (DDFT). Associated with each cartilage of the foot is a venous network that connects with the venous vessels under the distal phalanx and the vessels associated with the dermis of the hoof wall. The venous microvasculature forms a hydraulic system that is hypothesized to provide the mechanism for how the ground impact energies are dissipated, before these forces are transmitted to and damage the bone and other connective tissues within the foot. Horses with good or excellent hydraulic systems should be more efficient in dissipating the impact energy compared with horses with feet with less-well-developed hydraulic networks.

The cartilages of the foot lie beneath the skin and dermis and the coronary venous plexus and have previously been described as rhomboid-shaped, with a convex surface abaxially and a concave surface axially. Several ligaments secure the cartilages of the foot to the digital

bones.[1-4] However, these descriptions are overly simplistic and appear to have been obtained from examination of horses with underdeveloped structures of the palmar aspect of the foot. The morphological features of the cartilages of the foot vary greatly, with a range of shapes and thickness, the presence of an axial projection from its distal edge, and the extent of vascularity.[5] The structure of the cartilages of the foot is best determined by viewing the foot in transverse sections (Figures 29-1 and 29-2). In frontal (dorsal)

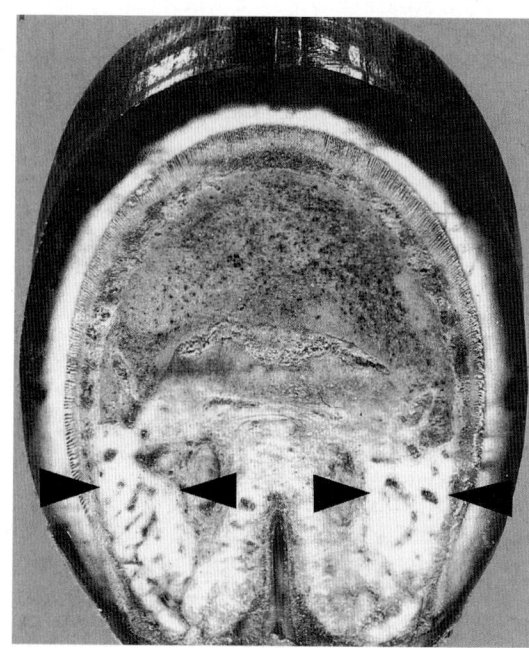

Fig. 29-1 • Transverse section through the distal aspect of a foot of a Quarter Horse 25 years of age, with no history of foot problems. Arrows show the thick cartilages of the foot. Axial projection composed of fibrocartilage extends between each cartilage of the foot.

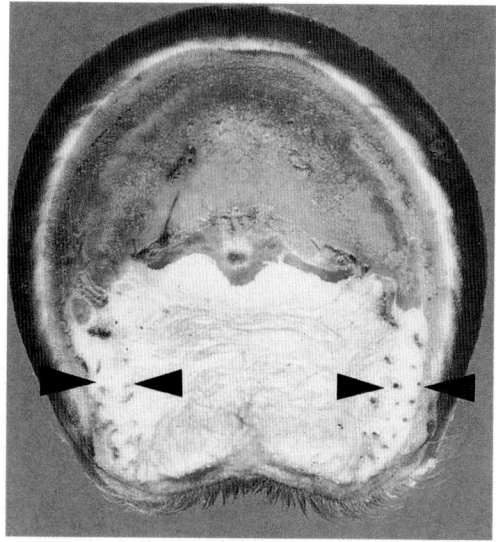

Fig. 29-2 • Transverse section of the foot of a horse with chronic foot pain with thin cartilages of the foot *(arrows)*. The digital cushion is primarily composed of fat and elastic tissue, with little fibrocartilage.

sections cut perpendicular to the ground, beginning at the bulbs of the heel, the cartilages of the foot have a C- to L-shaped configuration. Both the upright and the base parts of the L-shaped cartilage vary in thickness among horses. The mean thickness of the upright part at the level of the navicular bone ranges from 0.5 to 2.0 cm in an adult horse (450 to 550 kg body weight). The base part or axial projection of the L-shaped cartilage varies in its thickness and the distance that it extends toward the midline of the foot overlying the bars and the frog. The cartilages of the foot are thinnest in the heel region (0.45 to 1.3 cm) but become thicker closer to the distal phalanx (0.6 to 1.5 cm) and thin slightly as they attach onto the distal phalanx (0.5 to 1.0 cm). The cartilages of the foot are thicker in forelimbs than hindlimbs.

Overlying the abaxial surface of the cartilages of the foot are a plexus, the laminar dermis, and the hoof. Loose connective tissue extends from each cartilage to the DDFT. On the axial surface the axial projection of the cartilage extends toward the midline of the foot. In most feet, this axial projection extends from the dorsal half of the cartilage; the palmar half of the cartilage has virtually no, or very small, extension into the substance of the digital cushion. However, in some feet it extends the entire dorsal-palmar extent of the cartilages of the foot. This axial projection extends to overlie the epidermal ridges of the bars, with many fingerlike projections extending into the substance of the digital cushion, and may extend across the midline of the palmar aspect of the foot under the digital cushion to fuse with that of the opposite side of the foot. These white bundles of fibrous and fibrocartilaginous tissues are easily discerned from the surrounding yellow elastic, adipose, and collagen fibers of the digital cushion. The relative thickness of the axial projection in a distal-proximal orientation varies. In horses younger than 4 to 5 years of age the axial projection usually is not fully developed along the entire length of the cartilage, and in young foals there is only a thin sheet of fibrous tissue.

The cartilages of the foot contain primarily hyaline cartilage, but in many horses from 4 to 5 years of age the medial border of the cartilage develops fibrocartilage. A fibrocartilaginous ligament of variable thickness develops between the cartilage and the DDFT; this is consistently larger in forelimbs than hindlimbs. In some horses the cartilages of the foot can ossify. This may be genetically controlled, but any stress on the foot, that accentuates vibration and results in higher energy forces being transmitted through the foot, may promote ossification.

Several ligamentous attachments connect the cartilages of the foot to the distal and middle phalanges, as well as to the navicular bone.[3,4] The chondroungular ligaments attach the cartilage to the distal phalanx along the palmar process, whereas the medial and lateral chondrocoronal ligaments attach the cartilage to the proximal half of the middle phalanx. The medial and lateral ligaments of the cartilages of the foot (collateral chondroungular ligaments) attach the cartilage to the angle of the distal phalanx. The paired chondrosesamoidean ligaments attach the axial surface of the cartilage to the navicular bone. A pair of elastic ligaments extends between the proximal phalanx and the proximal surface of the cartilages of the foot; these ligaments are most prominent in larger horses, such as draft breeds. Cruciate ligaments of the cartilages of the foot

(cruciate chondroungular ligaments) connect the axial surface of the cartilage to the palmar process on the opposite side of the foot. Within the digital cushion are fiber tracts radiating from the connective tissue ventral to the attachment of the DDFT (digital torus), through the digital cushion, to the axial surface of the cartilages of the foot.

Each hoof cartilage is perforated by numerous vascular foramina, the number of which varies depending on the thickness of the cartilages of the foot. Within the vascular channels is a large central vein, with a rich network of microvessels termed *veno-venoanastomoses*.[5-7] These microvessels exit the large central vein and, after a variable course within the vascular channels, reenter the same vein. More of the vascular channels are present at the distal level of the cartilages of the foot, but in feet with relatively thicker cartilages of the foot, there are more vascular channels proximally compared with feet with much thinner cartilages. The veins coalesce proximal to the cartilage into a venous plexus before uniting to form the medial and lateral palmar digital veins.[7,8]

DIGITAL CUSHION

The digital cushion consists of a meshwork of collagen and elastic fiber bundles, with small areas of adipose tissue, and lies between the cartilages of the foot, extending dorsally as a wedge-shaped tissue attached to the DDFT and the solar surface of the distal phalanx, near the distal attachment of the DDFT.[1-4] It overlies the frog and its dermis and the axial projection from the cartilages of the foot. Proximally and dorsally the digital cushion fuses with the distal digital annular ligament and bulges into the bulbs of the heel, which are separated superficially by a central shallow groove. Some horses have areas of fibrocartilage in the digital cushion, and, if present, these extend between the cartilages of the foot and the DDFT. Two arteries pass through the digital cushion to the area distal to the digital cushion but proximal to the axial projection of the cartilages of the foot, and then branch extensively to supply the frog.[2-6] Only a few vessels ramify through the digital cushion from these two arteries.

ENERGY DISSIPATION

The function of the digital cushion is controversial. The structural organization of the cartilages of the foot, the digital cushion, and the vasculature suggests a role in energy dissipation.[5] The pressure theory suggests that at ground contact the frog stay is pushed upward into the digital cushion, forcing the cartilages of the foot outward. The depression theory emphasizes a downward movement of the pastern into the digital cushion during ground impact, forcing the cartilages of the foot to move outward. However, neither theory is consistent with measurement of negative pressure within the digital cushion during stance and locomotion.[9] The hemodynamic hypothesis provides a hydraulic mechanism during ground contact, so that impact energy is transmitted to the fluid within the blood vessels.[5] During ground impact the outward expansion of the cartilages of the foot probably occurs through the bars contacting the axial projections and the downward movement of the bony column within the hoof capsule. This creates a negative pressure within the digital cushion. At this brief moment of impact the venous blood within the vessels of the palmar aspect of the foot is forced into the microvenous vasculature within the vascular channels of the cartilages of the foot. Hydraulic resistance to flow through the microvasculature dissipates the high frequency energy waves, which are potentially deleterious to bone and other tissues. Negative pressure in the foot enables refilling of the vasculature before the next footfall. In feet with thick cartilages of the foot, enclosing more microvessels within the vascular channels, more energy is dissipated on ground contact compared with feet with thin cartilages of the foot. The fibrocartilage content of the digital cushion also is crucial to energy dissipation, because the fibrocartilage has its own energy-absorbing mechanisms. The elastic tissue acts only like a spring and absorbs little energy on ground contact, serving to return the foot to its original position as the foot leaves the ground.

The shape of the foot appears to influence the development of the cartilages of the foot and the structure of the digital cushion. In well-balanced feet, with the frog on the ground along with the bars, cartilages of the foot tend to be thick with fibrocartilage in the digital cushion.[5] In feet with a low heel and long toe, the site of ground contact of the hoof wall at the angle of the wall and the bars usually is beneath the bony part of the distal phalanx rather than underneath the cartilages of the foot. Therefore more of the energy of impact is transferred to the bone and hoof wall laminae, as the cartilages of the foot and the digital cushion are in essence bypassed during ground impact.

NAVICULAR SUSPENSORY APPARATUS

The navicular suspensory apparatus consists of several ligaments functioning to suspend the distal sesamoid bone (navicular bone) on the palmar surface of the distal interphalangeal (DIP) joint.[1-4] Proximally, paired collateral suspensory ligaments of the navicular bone (or the collateral sesamoidean ligament) arise from the distal surface of the proximal phalanx and pass in a distopalmar direction, attaching along the abaxial surface of the middle phalanx,[10] to insert on the extremities of the navicular bone. In addition, small branches attach to the axial surface of the cartilages of the foot and the distal phalanx. The attachment along the middle phalanx is important biomechanically during forward movement of the limb, because high loads are created on the joint surfaces between the navicular bone and the middle phalanx and between the navicular bone and the distal phalanx.[11] These ligaments are composed of collagen fibers with an abundance of elastic tissue fibers. Distally the distal sesamoidean impar ligament extends from the distal border of the navicular bone to the entire flexor surface of the distal phalanx adjacent to the insertion of the DDFT.[1-4] At its insertion the distal sesamoidean impar ligament contains an extensive network of microvessels containing arteriovenous complexes and nerve fibers within loose connective tissue septae.[10] The arteriovenous complexes are innervated by many peptidergic nerve fibers, including substance P, neurokinin A, and

calcitonin gene-related peptide, which are present in the many sensory fibers innervating the foot.[12] The neuropeptides substance P and neurokinin A also have pharmacological receptors, located on the small isolated microvessels and the arteriovenous complexes within the distal sesamoidean impar ligament, to control blood flow through this intricate vascular network. When these peptides are released from the sensory nerve fibers in the foot, they promote an active vasodilatation of these small vessels, presumably through a nitric oxide pathway. The locations of these arteriovenous complexes suggest that they may have two possible functions, including providing a protective mechanism for detection of high-pressure differences within the region during movement, and maintaining the hydration status of the distal sesamoidean impar ligament and other nearby connective tissues for optimal function.

The distal border of the navicular bone has a narrow, elongated facet for articulation with the distal phalanx. Between this and the attachment of the distal sesamoidean impar ligament is a fossa containing foramina for blood vessels. The proximal border also has several small foramina. The dorsal articular surface of the navicular bone and the articulation between the navicular bone and the distal phalanx create a substantial palmar extension of the articular surface of the DIP joint. During extension of the DIP joint, with fixation of the foot on the ground and the movement of the body over the distal limb, the middle phalanx contacts the dorsal articular surface of the navicular bone, and the navicular bone becomes a weight-bearing structure. Loads transmitted through the navicular bone are supported by the proximal and distal suspensory ligaments. The role of the DDFT is discussed further in Chapter 32.

DISTAL INTERPHALANGEAL JOINT

The distal articular surface of the middle phalanx, the articular surface of the distal phalanx, and the articular surfaces of the navicular bone form the DIP joint. The relatively short medial and lateral collateral ligaments of the distal DIP joint arise from the distal ends of the middle phalanx to insert on the distal phalanx and the dorsal part of the cartilages of the foot. The joint capsule has a small dorsal pouch and an extensive palmar pouch, and blends with the collateral ligaments and common digital extensor tendon. The palmar pouch of the DIP joint is greatly expandable (25 to 30 mL in volume) and is subdivided into a proximal palmar pouch and a small distal palmar pouch extending between the navicular bone and the distal phalanx. In the midline the palmar pouch extends proximally beyond the two small secondary tendons of the DDFT, which attach to the distal end of the middle phalanx. The proximal palmar pouch almost surrounds the collateral sesamoidean ligaments.[13,14] The DIP joint cavity also has several small abaxial, dorsal projecting outpouchings that are in close proximity to the sensory nerves of the medial and lateral palmar digital nerves. The DIP joint capsule therefore has a large surface area through which local anesthetic solution may diffuse. The comma-shaped navicular bursa is much smaller (approximately 3 mL in volume). Proximally it can extend over the proximal border of the navicular bone to protrude dorsally.

INNERVATION

The innervation of the equine distal forelimb is crucial to the horse because this is how the horse interacts with the environment. Thus the foot can be considered to be a neurosensory organ; touch, pressure, and proprioception, as well as nociception, are sensations conveyed in the nerves of the foot. The main innervation to the foot is via the medial and lateral palmar nerves and the medial and lateral palmar metacarpal nerves.[1-4] The distal continuations of the palmar nerves course parallel to the accompanying artery and then obliquely across the abaxial surface of the ligament of the ergot to supply most tissues of the palmar half to third of the foot (see Chapter 10). The Editors point out that, according to their clinical experience and current research results, diagnostic analgesia of the digital nerves results in analgesia of most of the foot, including the solar surface. Several small nerves branch from the medial palmar digital nerve to course with the artery of the digital cushion and to supply the palmar aspect of the foot, including the dermis of the overlying skin and frog, parts of the digital cushion, laminae of the bulbs of the heel, cartilages of the foot, and portions of the quarters. A small branch of the lateral palmar nerve may supply the ligament of the ergot. The dorsal branches of the palmar nerve continue with the palmar digital vein to innervate the dorsal aspects of the foot, including the DIP joint, the laminar and solar dermis, and the dorsal part of the cartilages of the foot. An intermediate branch from this nerve occurs in approximately a third of horses. In some horses a branch of the medial palmar metacarpal nerve supplies the coronary band. No communication occurs between the palmar metacarpal nerves and the dorsal branches of the palmar digital nerves. Variable branches occur, including one from the lateral palmar nerve in the metacarpal region extending obliquely to the coronary band, and one from the medial palmar digital nerve to the navicular bursa. In the hindlimbs an additional nerve supplies the coronary and laminar dermis of the dorsal foot, provided by the medial and lateral dorsal metatarsal nerves (terminal branches of the deep fibular nerve). Rarely branches from the plantar metatarsal nerves course under the distal ends of the second and fourth metatarsal bones to supply the dermis of the periople and coronet. The widespread distribution of these nerves provides a broad sensory and sympathetic autonomic innervation pattern to the tissues and vasculature of the foot.

The sensory nerves have many diverse functions in addition to conveying consciously perceived sensations, including touch, proprioception, and pain. The palmar digital nerves are composed of both small, unmyelinated nerves and larger, myelinated nerves in a ratio of nearly 4:1. Approximately 25% of the unmyelinated fibers are sympathetic nerves, and 75% are afferent fibers. Much of the sensory information from the foot and the activity of the sympathetic autonomic nerves is conveyed to the spinal cord through the unmyelinated fibers, which are the more slowly conducting nerve fibers. Many neurochemicals are present within the nerves including noradrenaline and adrenaline, substance P, neurokinin A, calcitonin gene-related peptide, neuropeptide Y, peptide histidine isoleucine, vasoactive intestinal peptide, and the enkephalins. These are released locally from the peripheral processes of the sensory nerves, and the effect on surrounding tissues depends on which neurochemical(s) is emitted.

Most of these peptides have been identified in the foot, usually in close association with blood vessels and other microvasculature. Within the dorsal hoof wall the sympathetic fibers containing noradrenaline and neuropeptide Y are present along the small arterioles within the dermal laminae and form dense plexuses around the arteriovenous anastomoses.[15] The same neurotransmitters are present in the navicular region, including the arteriovenous complexes.[13] Noradrenaline and neuropeptide Y promote vasoconstriction, whereas vasoactive intestinal peptide is a prominent dilator of the smooth muscle of the microvessels.[16] The other peptides, such as substance P, calcitonin gene-related peptide, and peptide histidine isoleucine, are present in the sensory nerve fibers of the dorsal hoof wall and the distal aspect of the distal sesamoidean impar ligament[10,12] and also promote vasodilation by means of an endothelial-dependent mechanism and the activation of a nitric pathway.[17,18] Activation of these sensory nerves, either directly or indirectly through pain mechanisms, produces a measurable increase in the concentration of these peptides in joints and tissues as they interact with tissue elements, such as inflammatory cells and macrophages, and controls edema formation.[19]

Other sensations, such as touch and proprioception, are mediated to the spinal cord through the larger myelinated fibers. The receptors of these nerve fibers are present in the bulbs of the heel and in association with the collateral sesamoidean ligaments.[20-22] The locations of these lamellated receptors appear to be critical for the perception of proprioceptive stimuli by the horse during movement when heel-first landing occurs. Activation of these receptors at ground impact and the rapid conduction to the spinal cord through these thickly myelinated fibers enable this sensory information to become incorporated into the spinal cord reflex mechanisms controlling locomotion. During toe-first or flatfooted landings, activation of these sensory receptors is presumably less. If a horse is shod with a pad, it may shorten its stride because the pacinian receptors are not adequately stimulated. If a finger-sized piece of rubber is attached temporarily to the pad, within one or two steps the stride extends forward maximally, as the horse "realizes" the importance of this area of the foot, by activation of the sensory receptors. If the rubber is removed after several days, the gait does not revert. Together the unmyelinated and the myelinated nerves enable the horse to smoothly negotiate the varying surfaces of the terrain during locomotion and provide a means for monitoring changes in the peripheral tissues and controlling the physiological and pathological environment within the foot. In addition to these pain-related sensory nerves, the foot also contains numerous myelinated nerves involved in touch and pressure sensation, permitting the horse to realize where its feet are during stance. Their importance is realized when riders of barefooted horses often remark that their horses are able to "feel" the ground surface and more carefully place the foot than when peripherally loaded devices (shoes) are present. Further research suggests that the active engagement of the neural elements of the foot may be critically important in determining the overall health of the foot.

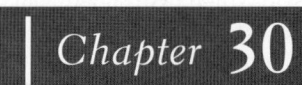

Chapter 30

Navicular Disease

Sue J. Dyson

PATHOPHYSIOLOGY OF NAVICULAR DISEASE

Navicular disease is a chronic forelimb lameness associated with pain arising from the distal sesamoid or navicular bone. It is well recognized that in association with advanced navicular disease, fibrillation of the dorsal aspect of the deep digital flexor tendon (DDFT), with or without adhesion formation between the tendon and the navicular bone, is a common feature. Recent clinical studies using magnetic resonance imaging (MRI)[1] and post mortem studies[2,3] have demonstrated that there may also be abnormalities of closely related structures, including the collateral sesamoidean ligaments (CSLs), the distal sesamoidean impar ligament (DSIL), and the navicular bursa. These structures and the navicular bone are called the podotrochlear apparatus. For the purposes of this chapter, this complex of degenerative changes will be referred to as navicular disease. Primary injury of the DDFT is considered to be a separate condition,[4] which may have a different etiopathogenesis (see Chapter 32).

Although historically considered to be a single disease, given the variety of clinical presentations it is likely that there are a number of different clinical conditions, of different etiologies, that give rise to pain in the podotrochlear apparatus. It is difficult to conceive a single disease that can result in an insidious onset, slowly progressive bilateral forelimb lameness, or an acute onset, relatively severe unilateral forelimb lameness, each with a variety of different radiological manifestations and with some horses never developing radiological changes. It is curious that sometimes clinical signs become apparent in young horses just commencing work, whereas more typically lameness is seen in mature riding horses. It is also seen in horses with vastly different distal limb conformation. It is a common condition in Quarter Horses, which tend to have narrow, upright, boxy feet, small relative to their body size, as well as in European Warmblood horses, many of which have relatively tall narrow feet. It is also common in Thoroughbred horses, which frequently have rather flat feet, with low collapsed heels, often associated with dorsopalmar foot imbalance. Recent evidence suggests there is a heritable tendency toward the development of navicular disease in Dutch and Hanoverian Warmblood horses.[5-7]

The factors causing pain in the navicular apparatus, and therefore lameness, are poorly understood. Experience with both radiography and MRI suggests that lesions in both the navicular bone and closely related structures are likely to predate the onset of lameness in some horses.[8] In some horses, a trigger factor apparently promoting pain and lameness has been a period of enforced rest for an unrelated cause.

There are no good epidemiological studies investigating risk factors for the development of navicular disease. Therefore information is largely anecdotal. The frequency of occurrence of navicular disease appears to vary between breeds. Quarter Horses,[9] Warmblood horses,[10] and Thoroughbred cross horses[11] have a relatively high incidence, whereas the occurrence and/or recognition in some breeds, such as the Finnhorse, Arab,[12] and Friesian, is relatively low.

Biomechanical Considerations

From a biomechanical perspective the podotrochlear apparatus comprising the navicular bone, the CSLs, the DSIL, and the navicular bursa, together with the DDFT, and the distal digital annular ligament are integrally related. The navicular bone, which articulates with the middle and distal phalanges, provides a constant angle of insertion and maintains the mechanical advantage of the DDFT, which exerts major compressive forces on the distal third of the bone. Contact studies between the phalanges in isolated limbs have demonstrated that the greatest forces are applied in the propulsion phase of the stride. This occurs during extension of the distal interphalangeal (DIP) joint, with increased pressure of the DDFT on the palmar aspect of the navicular bone, increased contact between the navicular bone and the middle phalanx, and increased tension in the CSLs.[13,14] Tension in the DDFT and the distal digital annular ligament promotes stability of the DIP joint. Forces may be altered by foot conformation: in a horse with "weak" heels there is greater extension of the DIP joint compared with a horse with "strong" heels, which results in increased pressure concentrated on the distal aspect of the navicular bone.[15]

Compressive forces and stress on the navicular bone were compared in clinically sound horses and horses with navicular disease.[16] Although the mean peak force and stress were similar, the force and stress in the horses with navicular disease were approximately double early in the stance phase of the stride. This early peak stress resulted in a much higher loading rate of the navicular bone in the navicular disease group. The difference in loading patterns was associated with an increased force in the DDFT in the early and mid-stance phases, probably because of increased contraction of the deep digital flexor (DDF) muscle. Contraction of the DDF muscle may result in toe-first ground contact, seen in some horses with navicular disease. It is suggested that pain associated with the navicular bone may result in a positive feedback by increasing the force in the DDFT to avoid heel-first landing, and hence paradoxically increasing the compressive force on the navicular bone. This hypothesis is supported by reduction in peak forces on the navicular bone throughout the stance phase in horses with navicular disease after perineural analgesia of the palmar digital nerves.[17]

Although low, collapsed heel conformation has anecdotally been associated with navicular disease, a recent study[18] in Irish draught cross-type horses showed no correlation between the peak force exerted on the navicular bone by the DDFT and the conformation of the hoof capsule, contrary to the earlier results.[15] However, a 1-degree decrease in angle of the solar border of the distal phalanx

References on page 1271

resulted in a fourfold increase in peak force on the navicular bone.[18] There was no correlation between the angle of the solar border of the distal phalanx and the degree of heel collapse.

The shape of the navicular bone may be determined at birth, and this may influence the biomechanical forces subsequently applied to the bone (Figure 30-1) and hence influence the risk of development of navicular disease.[6,19] Finnhorses and Friesian horses tend to have a straight or convex contour of the proximal articular border of the navicular bone and rarely develop navicular disease. There is a much higher incidence of navicular disease in the Dutch Warmblood breed, and horses in which the proximal articular margin is concave or undulating appear to be at highest risk of development of the disease.[5,6]

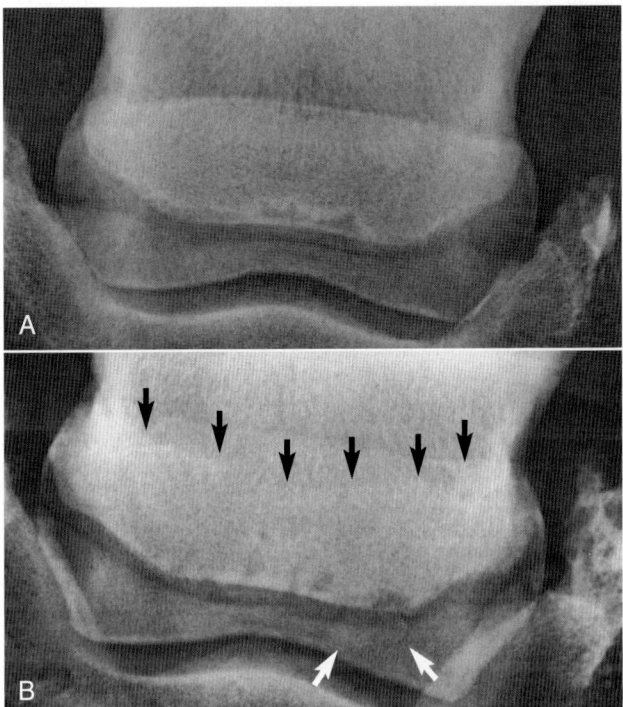

Fig. 30-1 • Dorsoproximal-palmarodistal oblique radiographic images of the navicular bone to show differences in shape of the proximal articular margin. **A,** Straight. There is an axial cluster of radiolucent zones along the distal border of the bone. **B,** Concave *(black arrows)*. There are variably shaped lucent zones along the distal border of the bone and a large distal border fragment laterally *(white arrows)*.

Histopathological Studies

Navicular disease has not been reproduced experimentally; therefore all proposed etiologies remain speculative. Earlier theories suggesting a vascular etiology with arteriosclerosis[20] or thrombosis, resulting in ischemia within the navicular bone,[21] have largely been rejected because of failure to identify ischemic bone or thrombosis, failure to reproduce clinical signs or pathological changes by occluding blood supply to the bone, and expanding evidence demonstrating increased bone modeling.[22-25] Post mortem studies to date have focused principally on horses with long-term, chronic disease, generally with advanced radiological abnormalities, reflecting the end stage of a disease complex. These studies identified striking similarities between the pathological features of navicular disease and osteoarthritis (Figure 30-2) in both people and horses.[24,25]

Studies of aging changes in the navicular bone of normal immature and mature horses suggested that there is a degenerative aging process similar to that seen in joints.[24] However, a more recent study investigating not only the navicular bone but also the DDFT, CSLs, DSIL, and navicular bursa demonstrated no age-related differences between mature horses with no history of foot-related lameness ranging from 4 to 15 years of age.[2,3] This suggests that there may be an individual susceptibility to degenerative change. Nonphysiological biomechanical factors may promote this susceptibility to degenerative change.[16,24,26]

The explanation for pain and lameness in horses with no detectable radiological change has been poorly investigated by post mortem studies. However, recent

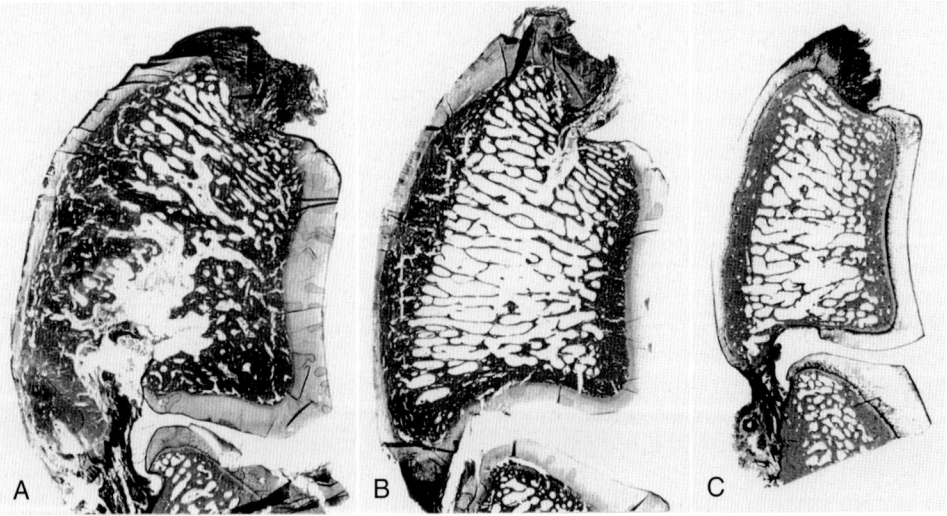

Fig. 30-2 • Sagittal sections of the navicular bones of a horse with navicular disease **(A)**, an age-matched control **(B)**, and an immature control horse **(C)**. The subchondral bone has an increased area and porosity in **A** compared with **B** and **C**; the trabecular area is decreased, but the trabeculae are thickened. (From Wright IM, Kidd L, Thorp BH: Gross, histological and histomorphometric features of the navicular bone and related structures in the horse, *Equine Vet J* 30:220, 1998.)

clinical experience with MRI has indicated that many horses with evidence of increased modeling of the navicular bone based on increased radiopharmaceutical uptake (IRU) detected using nuclear scintigraphy do have pathological abnormalities of the navicular bone detectable using MRI, with or without concurrent changes in the DDFT, CSLs, DSIL, and navicular bursa.[27,28]

Degenerative changes in the fibrocartilage on the palmar aspect of the navicular bone occur principally in the distal half of the bone, especially centered around the sagittal ridge in both sound and lame horses.[2] In horses with navicular disease there is a greater degree of fibrocartilage damage, which may extend into the subchondral bone. Partial-thickness loss of fibrocartilage in this location was one of the most common lesions significantly associated with navicular disease in one study.[25] It is likely to represent some of the earliest pathology of one form of this disease but remains difficult to identify in vivo, even with the use of MRI.[8] Degenerative change of the spongiosa is generally only seen dorsal to extensive fibrocartilage damage. Physiological forces result in adaptive remodeling of the subchondral bone in immature horses, with cortical thickening.[24] Nonphysiological forces may result in focal fibrocartilage and/or flexor cortex damage, with adjacent subchondral sclerosis dorsal to it, associated with thickening of trabeculae and focal areas of lysis. There may also be edema, congestion, and fibrosis of the marrow stroma within the medullary bone, which may result in a cystlike lesion.

Concurrently there may be fibrillation of the dorsal surface of the DDFT, which may predispose to adhesion formation between the DDFT and regions of partially or fully eroded fibrocartilage on the palmar aspect of the navicular bone. Whether lesions in the DDFT are primary or secondary to preexisting damage of the fibrocartilage currently remains open to debate. However, recent post mortem evidence suggests that there may be non–age-related degenerative vascular and matrix changes in the dorsal aspect of the DDFT in both lame and clinically normal horses.[3] Although it has been suggested that vascular occlusion and matrix changes in the DDFT may be age-related,[25] the results of a recent study showed that the severity of these changes was greater in horses with palmar foot pain than in age-matched control horses.[3] Minor fibrillation of the dorsal aspect of the DDFT was seen in both lame and control horses, whereas deep sagittal splits were only seen in lame horses. Complete occlusion of blood vessels, replacement of normal tendon architecture by focal fibroplasia, and areas of fibrocartilaginous metaplasia were common in the lame horses. As these changes are predominantly seen in the intratendonous septa, there is a strong possibility that they predispose to the development of sagittal splits in the dorsal surface of the tendon along these septal planes. Sharp edges of splits in the DDFT extending from the dorsal surface may cause ulceration of the fibrocartilage of the navicular bone and thus predispose to lesions extending into the medulla.

There is an association between changes of the flexor aspect and distal and proximal borders of the navicular bone.[2] Similar types of change occur at the proximal and distal aspects but tend to be more extensive distally. Enlarged synovial invaginations are the result of recruitment and activation of osteoclasts following the course of the nutrient vessels into the spongiosa. This may be associated with local medullary osteonecrosis and the presence of foci of fibrocartilaginous metaplasia and/or entheseous new bone close to the interface between the DSIL and the navicular bone.

Aging changes were described in the articular cartilage of the navicular bone and the opposing face of the distal phalanx.[29] There was loss of proteoglycan and tidemark advancement, which was thought to reflect excessive shear stress in the zone between the calcified and noncalcified articular cartilage. A greater number of tidemarks were seen in horses with clinical signs of navicular disease than normal horses of similar age. However, a more recent study failed to identify significant age-related changes, and low-grade degenerative changes in the articular cartilage were common in both control horses and those with navicular disease.[2]

Observations from Nuclear Scintigraphy and MRI

Previous studies using tetracycline labeling of bone[22] and scintigraphic studies[27,30] have indicated that there is evidence of increased bone turnover in association with some forms of navicular disease, even in the absence of radiological abnormalities of the bone. IRU predominantly reflects increased osteoblastic activity[31] but is not synonymous with either pain or lameness.[32] IRU may reflect a functional adaptation to foot conformation and the biomechanical forces on the navicular bone. Comparison between scintigraphy and MRI has demonstrated that many horses with focal moderate or intense IRU have abnormalities of the navicular bone detectable using MRI.[27] However, scintigraphy can also produce false-negative results, indicating that pathological abnormalities of the navicular bone are not always associated with increased osteoblastic activity.

A comparison of MRI findings in control horses with no history of foot-related pain and horses with chronic palmar foot pain showed significant alterations of the podotrochlear apparatus in the lame horses.[33] A comparative MRI and post mortem study showed good correlation between the lesions identified using MRI and histopathological findings.[34] Clinical experience with MRI in horses with foot pain provides support for the progression of lesions as outlined above and has demonstrated some earlier lesions than those investigated post mortem.[8]

However, a group of horses has also been identified with no detectable abnormalities of the flexor fibrocartilage or cortex but with diffuse abnormalities of the medulla characterized by increased signal intensity in fat-suppressed magnetic resonance (MR) images. Post mortem examination of several such horses revealed evidence of early fat necrosis with a moth-eaten appearance of the trabeculae, with necrosis of bone edges. This may have a different etiopathogenesis.

Hyperintense signal in the medulla of the navicular bone has been ascribed to the presence of edema in the marrow spaces,[35] but this was not validated post mortem. Further research is required to determine the true causes of this phenomenon. In our studies, mild or moderate focal or generalized increased signal intensity in fat-suppressed MR images was associated with trabecular thinning and widened intertrabecular spaces.[34] High-intensity increased signal associated with irregular decreased signal intensity in T1- and T2-weighted images was associated with generalized osteonecrosis and fibrosis, with irregular trabeculae, adjacent adipose tissue edema, and prominent capillary infiltration. A recent post mortem study of feet with advanced radiological abnormalities of the navicular bone demonstrated that increased signal intensity in fat-suppressed images correlated with areas of degenerate adipose tissues, hemorrhage or replacement by fibrocollagenous material, or fluid-filled cystic spaces.[36]

In some other horses, fluid-filled osseous cystlike lesions were seen in the distal aspect of the bone, apparently separate from synovial invaginations, and not associated with any detectable abnormality of the flexor aspect of the bone. Such lesions have not yet been characterized histologically, and their etiology remains speculative, although they may be associated with lesions of the DSIL.

Occasionally horses have been identified with new bone on the palmar aspect of the navicular bone, centered on the sagittal ridge. The cause of this is currently unknown.

Entheseous Changes

The presence of entheseous new bone on the proximal border of the navicular bone, reflecting previous insertional desmopathy of the CSL, is well documented radiologically[37,38] and at post mortem examination[25,37] in both clinically normal horses and horses with navicular disease. Its clinical significance remains uncertain, although more extensive new bone in this location tends to be associated with other signs of navicular disease.[37,38] Recent experience with MRI has confirmed these findings.[1] Rarely, an avulsion fracture is identified at the insertion of the CSL into the navicular bone.[8,39] Mineralized and osseous fragments (Figure 30-3) in the DSIL have also been recognized in both normal horses and in horses with navicular disease, and their clinical significance remains difficult to determine. Fragments were unusual in sound horses undergoing

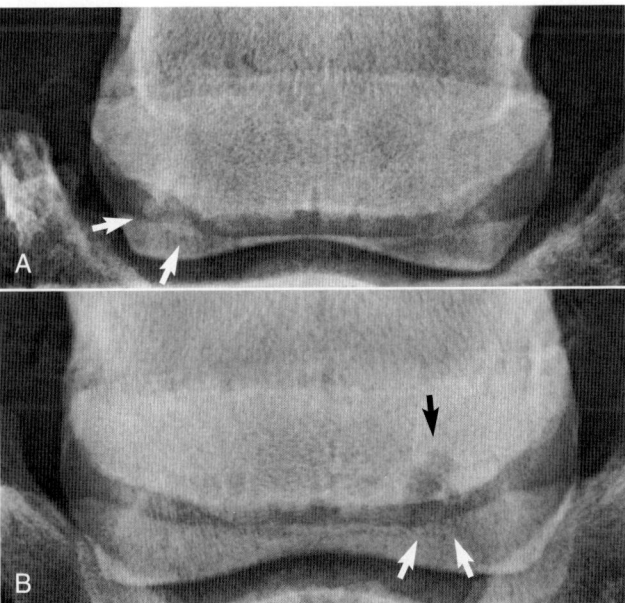

Fig. 30-3 • Dorsoproximal-palmarodistal oblique radiographic images of two navicular bones showing a large discrete mineralized fragment on the distal medial sloping border of the bone *(arrows)* **(A)** and a distal border fragment *(white arrows)* located distal to the lateral angle of the navicular bone **(B)**; there is a large radiolucent zone in the adjacent navicular bone *(black arrow)*.

prepurchase radiographic examination,[40] although their true incidence may be underestimated by radiographic examination compared with MRI or computed tomography (CT). In two post mortem studies, fragments associated with a defect in the distal margin of the navicular bone were more common in horses with navicular disease than in age-matched controls.[2,25] This has also been my clinical experience.

Fibrocartilaginous metaplasia in the body of the DSIL was more extensive in horses with navicular disease compared with age-matched control horses.[2] However, no significant differences between groups were seen in the CSLs.

Aging changes have been seen in the region of insertion of the DSIL and DDFT, with a change in fibroblast shape and an increase in proteoglycans.[14] The functional significance of this is not yet known. Evidence of inflammation was recently recognized histologically at the intersection of the DSIL and DDFT in horses with clinical signs of navicular syndrome.[29,41] Changes reflecting "abnormal stress" at the insertion of the DSIL and DDFT have been demonstrated in horses with poor foot conformation.[29] This region is rich in sensory nerve endings, with many arteriovenous complexes that are damaged in horses with navicular disease.[42]

Clinical experience with MRI has demonstrated that structural abnormalities of the DSIL are often seen in association with abnormal modeling of the distal palmar aspect of the navicular bone, with focal increased signal in fat-suppressed MR images.[1,28] It has been suggested that this focally increased signal in the distal aspect of the navicular bone at the origin of the DSIL on fat-suppressed images may represent an important early event in the etiopathogenesis of navicular disease.[33] Increased signal intensity may also be seen in the navicular bone close to the insertion of the CSLs in fat-suppressed images.[1,28] In some horses there is a linear band of increased signal intensity in fat-suppressed images, extending through the middle third of the navicular bone, from the insertion of the CSL to the origin of the DSIL. Abnormalities of the CSL have also been associated with concurrent abnormalities of the navicular bone. Based on clinical experience, it seems that these lesions may be the result of abnormal stresses at the attachments of the CSL and DSIL on the navicular bone, and this may reflect a different mechanism of navicular disease development.[8]

Although endosteal irregularity at the insertion of the DSIL on the distal phalanx may be seen in both horses with and without foot pain,[33,34] in some lame horses there is evidence of insertional desmopathy, characterized by enthesophyte formation, axial cortical disruption, osseous cystlike lesions, and/or increased signal intensity in the bone at this site in fat-suppressed images, reflecting bone edema or necrosis.[8]

The Navicular Bursa

The incidence and etiology of primary bursitis of the navicular bursa are not known, nor is the relationship to the development of navicular disease. Villous hypertrophy, hyperplasia of synovial lining cells, and venous congestion have been described in association with navicular disease, whereas the synovial membrane appeared uniform in six normal horses of undetermined age.[43] However, in another study comparing immature horses, horses with navicular disease, and age-matched controls, 3 of 25 age-matched controls had evidence of asymptomatic chronic synovitis. In both the navicular disease group and the age-matched controls, mild hyperplasia and hypertrophy were seen compared with immature horses up to 3 years of age.[25] In a more recent study, there was no evidence of acute inflammation within the navicular bursa in horses with palmar foot pain or age-matched control horses[2]; however, lame horses had marked chronic synovial proliferation compared with control horses.[2,33] There was a positive association between abnormalities of the bursa and lesions of either the dorsal aspect of the DDFT or the flexor aspect of the navicular bone. Clinical experience with MRI has indicated that abnormal distention of the bursa is a frequent finding in lame horses but is rarely seen in isolation.[1]

Associations between Injuries

It is clear from our recent post mortem study, as well as from clinical experience using MRI, that frequently several structures are affected concurrently. It is common to see various combinations of abnormalities of the navicular bone, DDFT, DSIL, CSL, and the collateral ligaments (CLs) of the DIP joint. Clinical MR examination of 263 horses with forelimb foot pain revealed 6 with abnormalities of the navicular bone alone; 29 with concurrent DDFT and navicular bone abnormalities; 60 with various combinations of abnormalities of the navicular bone, DSIL, DDFT, or CSL; 46 horses with CL injury of the DIP joint combined with lesions of the DDFT, CSL, DSIL, or navicular bone; and 25 horses with abnormalities of five or more structures.[28] The sequence of injury occurrence remains speculative. It is possible that degenerative changes in several structures may predispose to concurrent injury. The navicular bone, CSL, and DSIL act as a unit and so presumably undergo similar biomechanical stresses. Alternatively, injury to one structure may cause low-grade instability, predisposing to injury of closely related structures.

What Causes Pain?

Pain associated with navicular disease may be caused by venous congestion of the navicular bone. Dilated venules and sinusoids entrapped in fibrous marrow have only been identified in horses with navicular disease.[24] Increased intraosseous pressure has been measured in horses with navicular disease.[44,45] Distention of the navicular bursa may cause pain. The contribution of other causes or sources of pain remains open to speculation, although many sensory nerve endings have also been identified in the CSLs and the DSIL,[46,47] and given the high frequency of occurrence of concurrent abnormalities in these structures, it is likely that these nerve endings may be important in pain mediation.

The Future

It is clear that degrees of adaptive and reactive change occur in the podotrochlear apparatus and DDFT of all horses. We need to understand better both the factors that stimulate their progression and what causes pain. Identification of genetic and biomechanical risk factors would be useful. Study of horses with early navicular disease should help to establish better the interrelationship between abnormalities of the DDFT, navicular bone, CSL, and DSIL. We need to determine what factors lead to vascular and matrix changes in the DDFT. Further research into the sensory nerve supply to the podotrochlear apparatus and DDFT may help in understanding what causes pain—and therefore lameness—and how it may be treated.

DIAGNOSTIC CONSIDERATIONS

History

Most horses are presented with a history of an insidious onset of loss of performance, shortening of stride, or intermittent shifting bilateral forelimb lameness that usually is worst on firm ground. The complaint from the owner may be loss of action, stiffness, unwillingness to jump, especially drop fences, and inability to lengthen stride. Less commonly a horse may have acute-onset, moderate to severe, usually unilateral but sometimes bilateral, forelimb lameness. The condition is rare in ponies compared with horses, and although hindlimb lameness associated with navicular disease is unusual, it does occasionally occur in both ponies and horses.[48,49]

Clinical signs often are first apparent when the horse is approximately 7 to 9 years of age, although the disease can occur in young horses of 3 to 4 years of age, which may have fairly advanced radiological abnormalities. Lameness may first become apparent after a period of enforced rest because of some other unrelated problem or after a change in management. Development of lameness soon after change of ownership, associated with a change in trimming and shoeing, different work patterns, and altered periods of turnout, is not uncommon.

Clinical Signs

Pain when the horse is standing at rest may be a feature of navicular disease; however, this is a variable finding, and some clinically normal horses habitually point one or both front feet. A horse that has resting pain associated with navicular disease may stand pointing one front foot, sometimes alternating between feet. This is also a feature of horses with primary lesions of the DDFT. Alternatively, an affected horse may pack bedding under the heel or have a tendency to sit on a manger to relieve pressure on the palmar aspect of the foot. Navicular disease is recognized in horses with a wide variety of foot shapes: narrow, boxy upright feet of the Quarter Horse and low, collapsed heels typical of many Thoroughbreds. Navicular disease often is seen in association with poor mediolateral or dorsopalmar foot balance. If lameness is consistently worse on one forelimb, the feet may become asymmetrical in shape, with the lamer foot narrower with a taller heel.

The digital vessels sometimes are palpably enlarged, but this is an inconsistent, nonspecific finding. The response to hoof testers applied to the frog region is often negative,[22,49,50] although other authors[51] have described a positive response as a fairly consistent feature of navicular disease. Pain may be elicited at the toe if the horse has been repeatedly overloading the toe, resulting in subsolar bruising. Differences in clinical signs observed by different clinicians may reflect genuine differences in horse populations in different geographical locations. Distention of the DIP joint capsule is sometimes seen in association with navicular disease but not invariably so. Increased intraarticular pressure (>40 mm Hg) is said to be associated with navicular disease,[52] although in my experience there is considerable variability in the degree of DIP joint distention and pressure in both normal and lame horses.

Lameness is sometimes apparent when the horse is moving on a hard surface in straight lines. It may fluctuate in degree within an examination period or between examinations performed on different days. The horse may show a tendency to stumble associated with an altered foot placement. Overt unilateral lameness may be evident, but in some horses there is only marginal shortening of stride and reduced lift to the stride, which may be difficult to detect if the horse was not previously known to the observer. The horse may move better on a soft surface, even in circles. No clinical signs are detectable in some horses when examined moving in hand on a hard surface. Lameness generally is accentuated if the horse moves in circles on a hard surface, especially with the lame limb on the inside of the circle. In some horses, lameness is apparent only under these circumstances. Less commonly lameness is accentuated when the lame limb is on the outside of a circle. Sometimes lameness cannot be detected unless the horse is ridden, when it may move in a slightly stiff, "flat," and restricted fashion. Recognition of this requires previous knowledge of the horse, knowledge of the expected quality of movement of a horse of that type, or respecting the opinion of the rider that the horse has "lost some action." A vast difference may be detected by desensitizing both front feet. This may be easier to appreciate when riding the horse than watching it.

The response to distal limb flexion is extremely variable. Many horses with navicular disease show a transient, mild increase in lameness.[22,49,50] Resistance to flexion or marked accentuation of lameness after flexion is unlikely to reflect navicular bone pain. Distal limb flexion of one forelimb may result in increased lameness in the contralateral forelimb because of increased loading of the podotrochlear apparatus, but the same response can also be seen in horses with primary injuries of the DDFT. Elevation of the toe of the foot on a wedge or wooden board, with the contralateral limb picked up, resulting in extension of the DIP joint, may increase lameness, but this response is neither consistent nor pathognomonic for navicular disease.

If the horse's foot conformation is poor and the feet are not trimmed and shod optimally, it is worthwhile improving the trimming and shoeing and reassessing the lameness after several weeks. If the lameness has markedly improved, it is unlikely to reflect navicular disease.

Response to Local Analgesic Techniques

Perineural analgesia of the palmar digital nerves, using 1.5 to 2 mL of mepivacaine hydrochloride (2%) per site, performed immediately axial to the cartilages of the foot usually results in improvement in lameness. However, lameness often is not alleviated fully.[50,53] Occasionally there is no response. Lameness is generally alleviated completely after perineural analgesia of the palmar nerves, performed at the base of the proximal sesamoid bones, unless there is another concurrent source of pain. Horses should always be reevaluated in both straight lines and circles to determine whether lameness becomes apparent or is accentuated on the contralateral limb.

Intraarticular analgesia of the DIP joint using 4 to 6 mL of mepivacaine can alleviate or improve pain associated with the navicular bone within 5 minutes of injection.[53,54]

A negative response does not preclude navicular pain because approximately 20% of horses have a negative response to intraarticular analgesia of the DIP joint and a positive response to intrathecal analgesia of the navicular bursa[53]; this has been correlated with both radiological and post mortem abnormalities of the navicular bone. A positive response to intraarticular analgesia of the DIP joint is a nonspecific result (Figures 30-4 and 30-5) because this technique can alleviate solar pain[55] and pain associated with the palmar processes of the distal phalanx, the DSIL, the DDFT, and the joint itself.[46,53,54] Misleading positive results are more likely to occur with larger volumes of local anesthetic solution and evaluation of the response more than 10 minutes after injection.[56]

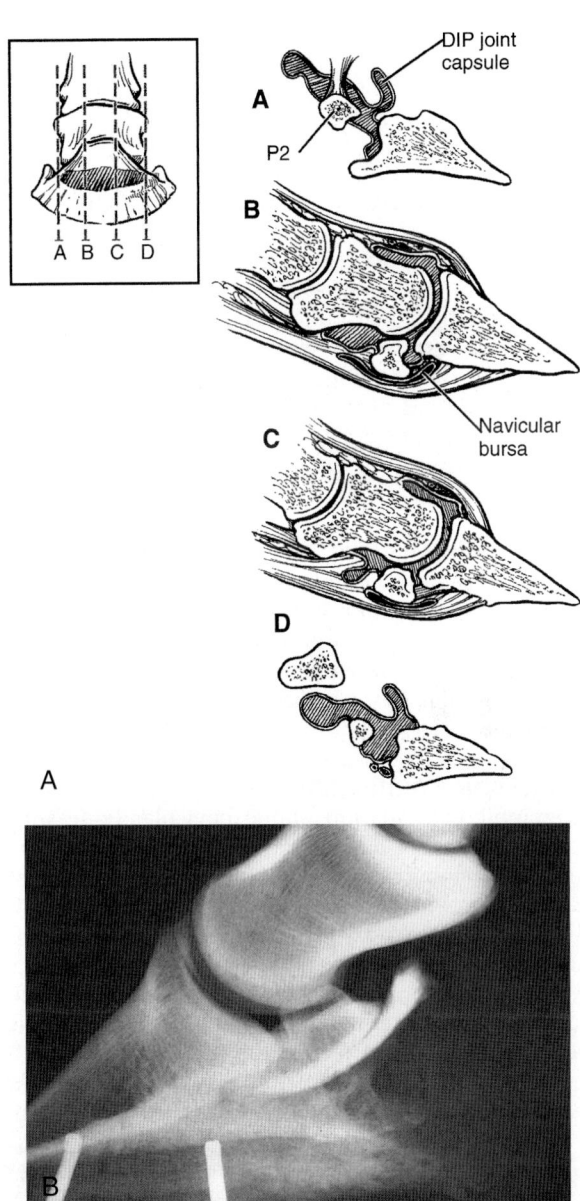

Fig. 30-4 • A, Diagram of the relationship between the distal interphalangeal *(DIP)* joint capsule, the collateral ligaments of the navicular bone, and the distal sesamoidean impar ligament. The four sagittal sections through the foot are denoted with lines *A, B, C,* and *D.* **B,** Lateromedial radiographic image of a foot. Three milliliters of radiodense contrast medium has been injected into the navicular bursa to show its proximodistal extent.

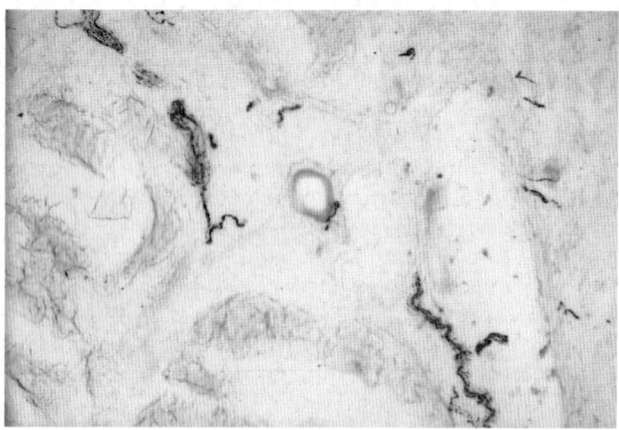

Fig. 30-5 • Histological sample stained to show substance P, a small peptide, within thinly myelinated sensory nerves in the collateral ligaments of the navicular bone, appearing to innervate microvessels and pass toward the navicular bone. (Courtesy Dr. R. Bowker.)

A positive response to analgesia of the navicular bursa (3 to 4 mL of mepivacaine) usually reflects primary navicular bone pain, primary bursal pain, or a primary lesion of the DDFT. For accurate injection into the navicular bursa, the needle should be sited in the middle of the flexor surface of the navicular bone. Placement of a needle into the navicular bursa is best performed under radiographic control or should be followed by injection of a radiographic contrast agent to check the accuracy of injection. If the needle is positioned too far proximally, there is danger of injection into the proximal palmar outpouching of the DIP joint or the digital flexor tendon sheath. If the needle is too far distal, it may enter the distal palmar outpouching of the DIP joint. If synovial fluid appears spontaneously in the needle hub, it is unlikely that the needle is positioned correctly. Improvement in lameness is usually seen within 5 minutes of injection of local anesthetic solution. A negative response to analgesia of both the DIP joint and the navicular bursa makes it unlikely that the horse has navicular disease.

Radiographic Examination

Radiographic examination of the navicular bone should be performed after removal of the shoes and appropriate preparation of the feet, and should include lateromedial (LM), dorsoproximal-palmarodistal oblique (DPr-PaDiO), and palmaroproximal-palmarodistal oblique (PaPr-PaDiO) images (Figure 30-6). Flexed oblique images of the DIP joint also are useful for evaluation of its articular margins. Appropriate positioning of the feet is critical for high-quality images. Correct angulation of the x-ray beam for PaPr-PaDiO images is crucial for diagnostic images. Artifacts can be created unless the x-ray beam is tangential to the palmar surface of the navicular bone.[8,57] The correct angle can vary between 35 and 50 degrees, depending on the shape of the foot.

The proximal border of the navicular bone has two margins: the flexor surface, which is always convex in a DPr-PaDiO image, and the articular margin, which is variable in shape. It can be categorized as concave, undulating, straight, or convex. In the Dutch Warmblood an enhanced risk of the development of navicular disease has been

suggested if the articular margin is concave or undulating rather than convex.[6]

The following features should be evaluated in all images[57] (Figures 30-6 through 30-9): the presence, number, shape, size, and location of radiolucent zones along the distal borders of the navicular bone; the presence of radiolucent zones along the proximal border of the navicular bone; radiolucent zones within the medulla of the bone; trabecular pattern within the medulla; enthesophyte formation on the proximal or distal aspects of the bone; presence of mineralization within a CSL; presence of articular osteophytes; thickness of the flexor cortex; regularity of outline of the flexor cortex; radiolucent areas in the flexor cortex; new bone formation on the flexor surface; corticomedullary definition; and presence of mineralized fragments distal to the navicular bone.

A grading system for evaluation of the navicular bone in LM and DPr-PaDiO views was devised by Dik.[58] An adapted version is presented in Box 30-1. The degree of lameness and the degree of radiological abnormality often are poorly correlated. Some horses with navicular bone pain have no detectable radiological change. Some horses, especially young horses, have relatively advanced radiological changes when lameness is first recognized. In many horses with suspected navicular disease the radiological abnormalities are equivocal. The ability to document the progression of radiological change over time (years) is relatively unusual, although the development of a cystlike lesion penetrating the flexor cortex has been noted within 21 days of the onset of acute lameness.[59]

The interpretation of distal border radiolucent zones, which represent synovial invaginations from the DIP joint,[60,61] has long been subject to controversy. It is generally accepted that the larger the number of radiolucent zones (>7), of variable size and shape, the more likely they are to be of clinical significance. Such radiolucent zones may be seen in association with localized increased radiopacity. Radiolucent zones positioned on the medial and lateral sloping borders of the bone are considered more likely to be of clinical significance. Clusters of axially positioned radiolucent zones, combined with distal elongation of the flexor border of the navicular bone, may reflect abnormal stress at the origin of the DSIL. Comparison between DPr-PaDiO and PaPr-PaDiO views helps to determine the dorsopalmar extent of the radiolucent zones. Proximal border radiolucent zones are occasionally seen and are not normal. They have been seen in association with lesions of the CSL.

Large radiolucent zones close to, but apparently discrete from, the distal border of the navicular bone may occur alone or in association with distal border synovial invaginations. Such radiolucent zones usually extend from the palmar to dorsal cortices when assessed in a PaPr-PaDiO view and are not normally seen in clinically sound horses.

Osseous fragments on the distal border of the navicular bone usually occur at the distal medial and lateral angles of the navicular bone, although less commonly involve the medial or lateral sloping border. Several studies have shown that such fragments occur more commonly in lame horses with other abnormalities of the navicular bone than in clinically normal horses.[2,25,38,62] Prevalence was low in a group of clinically normal horses undergoing a prepurchase examination.[40] Such fragments may reflect ectopic

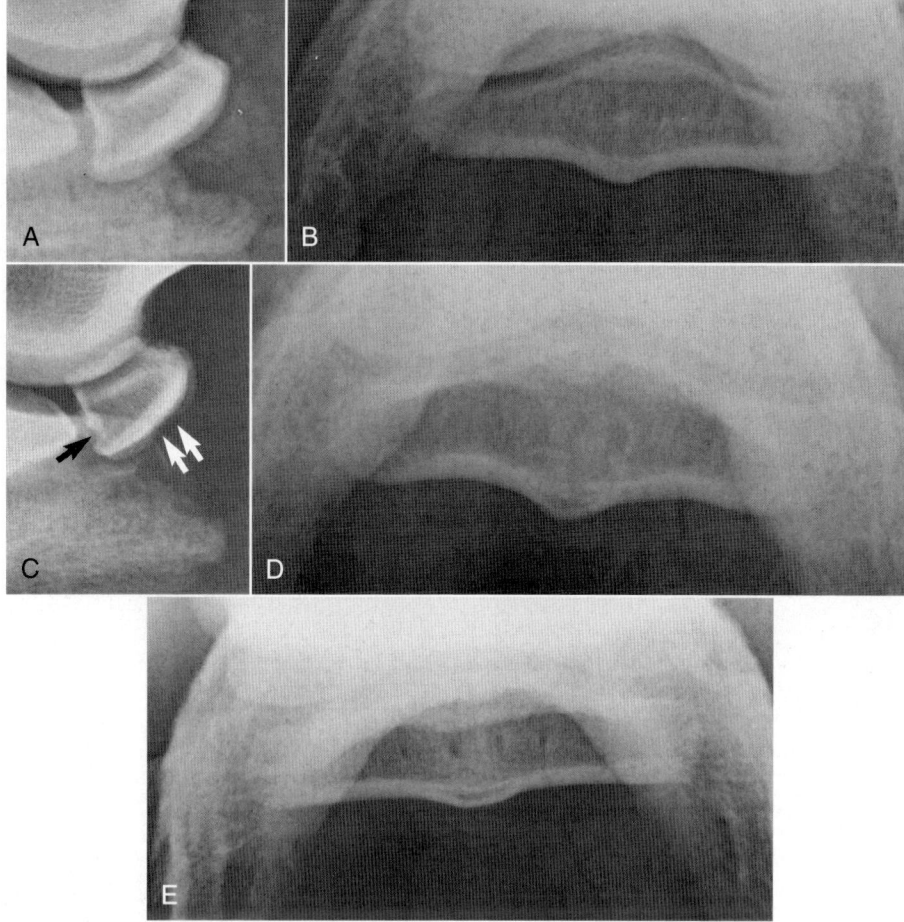

Fig. 30-6 • A, Lateromedial radiographic image of a normal navicular bone. **B,** Palmar 45° proximal-palmarodistal oblique radiographic image of a normal navicular bone. **C,** Lateromedial radiographic image of a normal navicular bone; note the smoothly outlined concave depression in the sagittal ridge (*white arrows*) and the concavity in the distal border, a normal fossa (*black arrow*). **D,** Palmar 45° proximal-palmarodistal oblique radiographic image of a normal navicular bone with a well-defined, crescent-shaped radiolucent zone in the central eminence of the flexor cortex. **E,** Palmar 50° proximal-palmarodistal oblique image of a normal navicular bone in a horse with upright foot conformation. The flexor cortex is flatter and thinner compared with **C.**

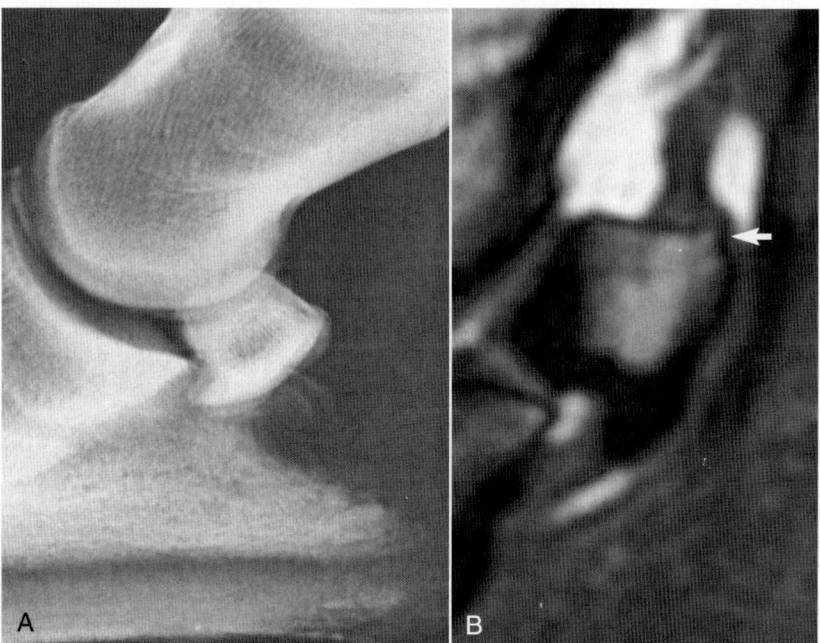

Fig. 30-7 • A, Lateromedial radiographic image of the left front foot of a 6-year-old Warmblood dressage horse with bilateral foot pain. The flexor cortex is abnormally thick. **B,** Sagittal T2*-weighted spoiled gradient-echo MR image of the same foot as in **A.** The dorsal, distal, and palmar cortices are thickened, and there is a small enthesophyte proximally (*arrow*) at the insertion of the collateral sesamoidean ligament.

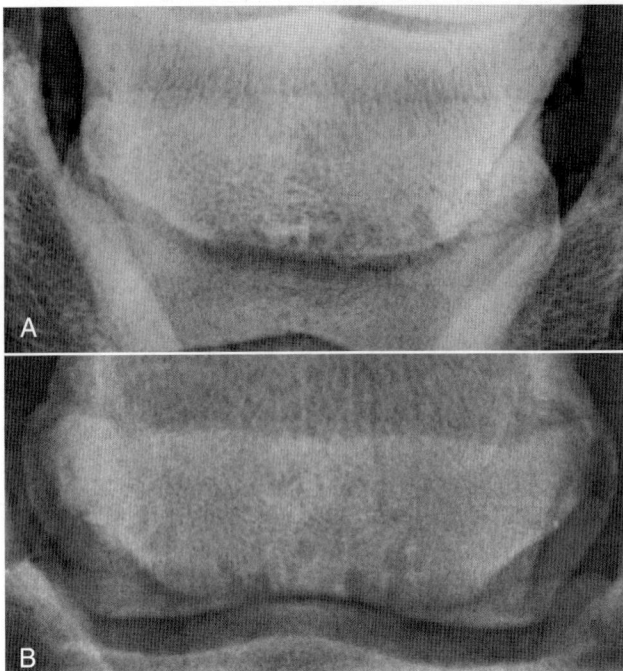

Fig. 30-8 • A, Dorsoproximal-palmarodistal oblique radiographic image of a navicular bone of a horse with clinical signs of navicular disease. Note the variably shaped and sized radiolucent zones along the distal aspect of the bone. There is proximodistal elongation of the bone. **B,** Dorsoproximal-palmarodistal oblique radiographic image of the navicular bone of a horse with clinical signs of navicular disease. Lateral is to the right. There are multiple variably shaped and sized radiolucent zones along the distal border. The modeling of the proximal medial and lateral margins of the bone is the result of enthesophyte formation.

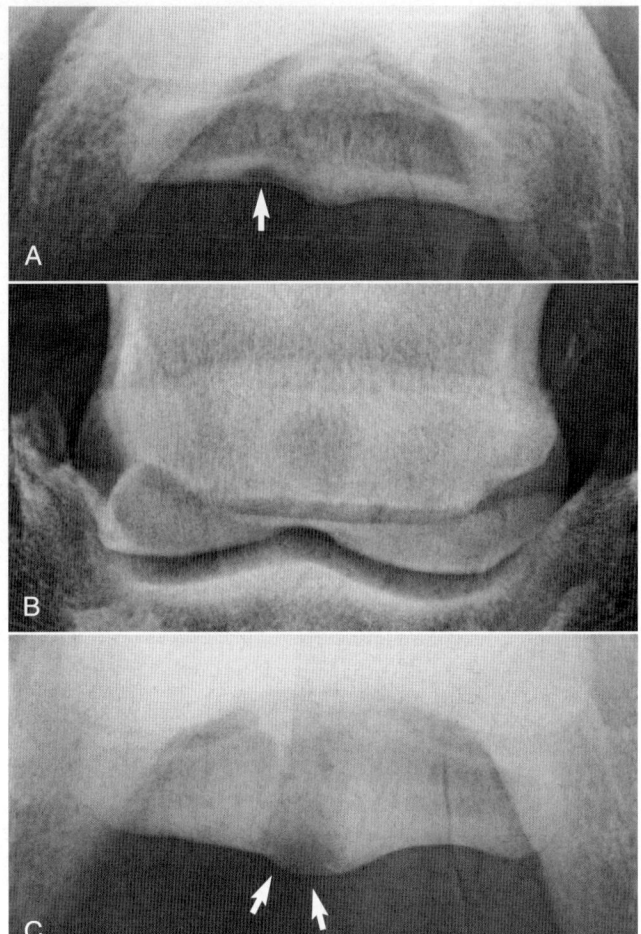

Fig. 30-9 • A, Dorsoproximal-palmarodistal oblique radiographic image of a navicular bone with a radiolucent defect in the flexor cortex of the navicular bone medially *(arrow)*. The bone appeared normal in all other radiographic projections. The horse had a bilateral forelimb lameness, which was improved by analgesia of the distal interphalangeal joint or navicular bursa. **B,** Dorsoproximal-palmarodistal oblique radiographic image of a navicular bone with a large cystlike lesion within the spongiosa of the bone, which penetrated the flexor cortex of the bone (see **C**). The horse had a bilateral forelimb lameness that was worse on soft ground with the lamer limb on the outside of a circle. Lameness was improved by palmar (abaxial sesamoid) nerve blocks. **C,** Palmaroproximal-palmarodistal oblique radiographic image of the same navicular bone as in **B,** with a large lucent area penetrating the flexor cortex of the bone. There were extensive adhesions between this defect and the deep digital flexor tendon.

mineralization in the DSIL, a fracture of the distal border of the navicular bone, or a fracture of an enthesophyte at the origin of the DSIL. The presence of a radiolucent area at the medial or lateral angle of the distal border of the navicular bone suggests the presence of a fragment, which can be present uniaxially or biaxially. Fragments can be seen as an incidental abnormality, especially if the opacity of the adjacent navicular bone is normal, but if seen in association with a radiolucent area, they are more likely to be associated with lameness. Such fragments have been associated with marked reactions in the adjacent navicular bone seen in MR images, presumably the result of chronic movement, or associated with adhesions to the DDFT and/or associated lesions of the DSIL. Fragments are most easily detected in a DPr-PaDiO image, but the ease with which they can be seen is somewhat position dependent. In some horses the presence of a fragment can be verified in a PaPr-PaDiO image, in which an opacity representing the fragment is usually seen superimposed over the spongiosa of the navicular bone. Fragments displaced from the proximal border of the navicular bone are rare and in my experience have been associated with lameness and presumably reflect an avulsion at the insertion of the CSL.[39]

A crescent-shaped lucent zone in the flexor cortex of the navicular bone in the sagittal ridge (see Figure 30-6, *D*) seen in a PaPr-PaDiO image is considered to be a normal variant, representing a reinforcement line.[63] The crescent-shaped lucent zone in the sagittal ridge of the navicular bone is rarely seen in very young horses. It represents early

navicular bone modeling in response to stress and is of unknown clinical significance. A relatively sclerotic reinforcement line develops in the subchondral bone parallel with the flexor cortex in the region of the sagittal ridge. The intervening bone is relatively radiolucent and is projected in the PaPr-PaDiO image as the crescent-shaped lucent zone in the sagittal ridge. If the bone between the reinforcement line and the flexor cortex becomes compacted, then the radiolucent zone becomes less clear and may be obliterated. An ill-defined loss of opacity at the most palmar aspect of the sagittal ridge has been seen as an incidental finding, with no other pathological change, but may be a precursor to the development of clinically significant degeneration.

Central or acentric radiolucent zones, cystlike lesions, in the spongiosa of the navicular bone seen in DPr-PaDiO

BOX 30-1

Radiological Findings of the Navicular Bone in Normal and Diseased Horses

Grade	Condition	Radiological Findings
0	Excellent	Good corticomedullary demarcation; fine trabecular pattern. Flexor cortex of uniform thickness and opacity. No radiolucent zones along the distal border of the bone, or several (<6) narrow conical radiolucent zones along the horizontal distal border. Right and left navicular bones symmetrical in shape.
1	Good	As above, but radiolucent zones on the distal border of the navicular bone more variable in shape.
2	Fair	Slightly poor definition between the palmar cortex and the medulla as a result of subcortical increased radiopacity. Crescent-shaped radiolucent zone in the central eminence of the flexor cortex of the bone. Several (<8) radiolucent zones of variable shape along the distal horizontal border of the navicular bone. Mild enthesophyte formation on the proximal border of the navicular bone. Navicular bones asymmetrical in shape. Proximal or distal extension of the flexor border of the navicular bone.
3	Poor	Poor corticomedullary definition resulting from increased medullary radiopacity. Thickening of the dorsal and flexor cortices. Poorly defined radiolucent areas in the flexor cortex of the bone. Many (>7) radiolucent zones along the distal horizontal or sloping borders of the navicular bone. Radiolucent zones along the proximal border of the bone. Large enthesophyte formation on the proximal border of the bone. Discrete mineralization within a collateral sesamoidean ligament. Radiopaque fragment on the distal border of the navicular bone.
4	Bad	Large cystlike lesion within the medulla of the navicular bone. Radiolucent region in the flexor cortex of the navicular bone. New bone on the flexor cortex of the navicular bone.

images are almost invariably of clinical significance (see Figure 30-9, *B* and *C*). They usually involve the middle third of the bone from proximal to distal, but not invariably so. In some horses such lesions can be seen to involve the flexor cortex of the bone in PaPr-PaDiO images. However, not all such lesions involve the flexor cortex. Moreover, some lesions penetrate the flexor cortex, but this cannot be verified radiologically. This depends on which part of the flexor cortex is tangential to the x-ray beam, the location of the lesion, and its size. A large radiolucent area in the flexor cortex of the navicular bone is invariably of clinical significance, and in some horses is the only detectable radiological abnormality. Such lesions usually occur at the sagittal ridge or abaxial to it. The lesion usually reflects erosion of the overlying fibrocartilage and adhesions of the DDFT. There may be associated increased radiopacity of the trabecular bone dorsal to the lesion.

New bone formation on the flexor border of the navicular bone is usually only detectable in a PaPr-PaDiO image and is usually centered around the sagittal ridge. It has only been seen in association with lameness and has not necessarily been seen in conjunction with other abnormalities of the navicular bone.

The thickness of the cortices of the navicular bone varies within and between horses. The thickness of the flexor cortex is easiest to evaluate in a well-positioned LM image (see Figure 30-6). Like any bone, shape is influenced by Wolff's law. In a sound horse with one foot that is much more upright than the other, the flexor cortex of the more upright foot is often thinner than the contralateral foot. In one form of navicular disease there is progressive thickening of the cortices of the bone (see Figure 30-7) and the trabeculae of the spongiosa.[25] Abnormal thickness of the flexor cortex of the navicular bone probably reflects pathological change.

A normal navicular bone has a regular trabecular architecture in the spongiosa that is clearly defined from the dorsal and palmar cortices in both LM and PaPr-PaDiO images. In one form of navicular disease there is generalized increased radiopacity of the spongiosa, involving particularly the middle third of the bone from laterally to medially. This can also develop as a sequel to acute trauma to the bone. However, a thick overlying frog can create increased radiopacity in this region, and this should be differentiated from genuine increased radiopacity. Alternatively, increased radiopacity may be localized toward the palmar aspect of the bone, affecting the endosteal aspect of the flexor cortex. This can be seen in association with abnormal thickness of the cortices of the bone and may be associated with a defect in the flexor cortex not detectable radiologically.

Demarcation between the spongiosa and the flexor cortex of the navicular bone must be assessed from both LM and PaPr-PaDiO images. However, it must be borne in mind that positioning of the foot during image acquisition may influence the appearance of the navicular bone in the skyline projection, and give a false impression of increased radiopacity of the spongiosa. The two views should be compared carefully.

The shape of the navicular bone should be assessed carefully in a LM image.[37] Distal extension of the flexor border of the navicular bone may reflect chronic stress at the origin of the DSIL. Proximal extension of the flexor border of the navicular bone may reflect chronic stress at the insertion of the CSLs.

Enthesophytes at the proximal medial and lateral aspects of the navicular bone are best identified in DPr-PaDiO or dorsopalmar images. Small lateral enthesophytes are a common incidental abnormality and presumably reflect asymmetrical stress at the insertion of the lateral and medial CSLs. However, the presence of a large lateral enthesophyte, or a medial enthesophyte, is more likely to reflect abnormal stress on the podotrochlear apparatus and potentially to be associated with lameness.

The position of the navicular bone in a LM radiograph relative to the middle and distal phalanges is partly influenced by the position of the limb during image acquisition. However, occasionally the bone is abnormally close to the distal phalanx. This has been seen in young horses with lameness recognized soon after the introduction of work and has generally been associated with advanced pathological changes of the navicular bone and the DIP joint. This may reflect a congenital abnormality.

Generally the larger number of radiological changes that are present in all radiographic projections, the more

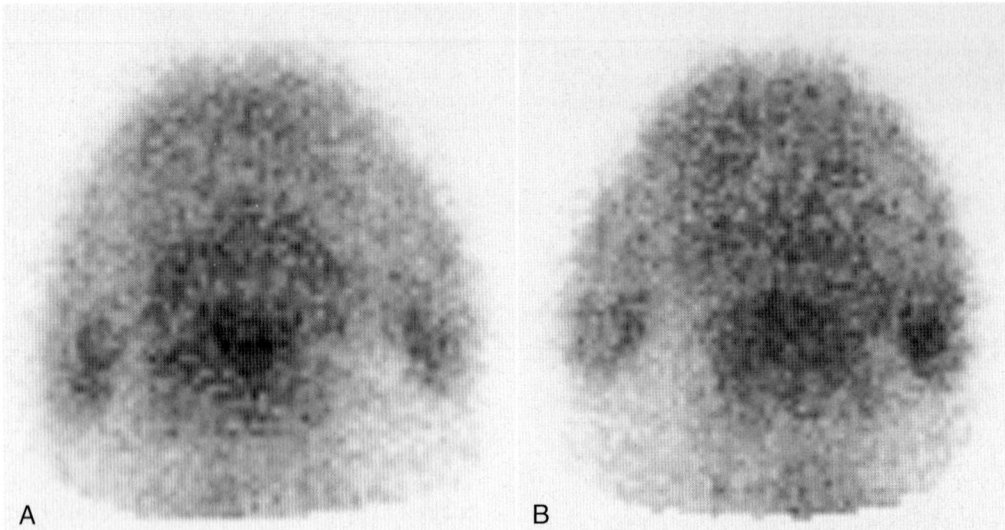

Fig. 30-10 • Solar scintigraphic bone phase images of the left **(A)** and right **(B)** front feet of a 7-year-old Warmblood with left forelimb lameness. There is focal moderate increased radiopharmaceutical uptake (IRU) in the left front navicular bone, with mild diffuse IRU in the region of insertion of the deep digital flexor tendon on the distal phalanx and mild focal IRU in the medial and lateral palmar processes of the distal phalanx. In the right forelimb there is mild diffuse IRU in the navicular bone, mild focal IRU in the lateral palmar process, and moderate IRU in the medial palmar process of the distal phalanx.

likely it is that the horse has clinical navicular disease. The most clinically significant radiological changes likely to reflect navicular disease include cystlike lesions within the medulla (see Figure 30-9, *A*) that are discrete from distal border lucencies, generalized increased radiopacity of the medulla, reduced corticomedullary demarcation, new bone on the flexor surface, and erosions of the flexor cortex of the bone (see Figure 30-9, *B* and *C*).

In some horses, concurrent degenerative changes of the DIP joint are also seen, with modeling* of the proximal dorsal articular margin of the navicular bone, the dorsal and palmar articular margins of the middle phalanx, and the extensor process of the distal phalanx.

In some horses the development of advanced radiological changes precedes the recognition of clinical signs. However, the absence of radiological abnormalities of the navicular bone does not preclude the presence of pain associated with the navicular bone and scintigraphic evidence of increased bone modeling.

Contrast Radiography of the Navicular Bursa

Contrast radiography of the navicular bursa may reveal a number of abnormalities not detectable on plain radiographs, including thinning or erosion of the flexor fibrocartilage of the navicular bone, loss of the radiopaque

contrast layer thought to be caused by adhesion formation between the DDFT and the navicular fibrocartilage, and filling defects on the palmar aspect of the bursa perhaps associated with surface fibrillation of the DDFT.[49,64] The clinical significance of these findings is currently questionable because it has been well recognized that thinning of the flexor fibrocartilage is a normal aging change, and the clinical significance of surface fibrillation of the DDFT is still open to debate.

Nuclear Scintigraphy

Tetracycline labeling of bone has revealed increased bone turnover in the navicular bone in navicular disease.[22,23] Nuclear scintigraphy offers a sensitive method of detecting increased bone turnover; however, this is not necessarily synonymous with either pathological change or pain.

Lateral pool (soft tissue) and lateral and palmar (solar) bone phase images of the front feet are required for accurate diagnosis of navicular disease (Figures 30-10 and 30-11).[27,28,30,32,65] In solar images of normal horses, uptake of the radiopharmaceutical in the navicular bone and the distal phalanx is approximately similar. However, uneven uptake in various regions of the distal phalanx can complicate interpretation. Care must be taken when interpreting lateral images not to confuse uptake in the cartilages of the foot with uptake in the navicular bone. In solar images, radiopharmaceutical uptake associated with the proximal interphalangeal joint can potentially be superimposed over the navicular bone, unless the foot is well extended during image acquisition and the pastern region is masked with a lead shield. Interpretation can also be difficult because some horses with unilateral lameness have IRU in both the left and right front navicular bones while apparently experiencing pain in only one limb.

---

*There is confusion between the histological and radiological usage of the terms *remodeling* and *modeling*. Histologically, *remodeling* refers to resorption and formation of bone that is coupled and occurs in basic multicellular units. This regulates the microstructure of bone without altering its shape and is a continuous process, replacing damaged bone with new bone. Thus it cannot be appreciated on radiographs. The term has been used with regard to radiographs to describe the reshaping of bone to match form and function (e.g., after fracture repair), but strictly speaking, the term *modeling* should be used.

Histologically, *modeling* refers to resorption and formation of bone that is not coupled and occurs at anatomically different sites (bone drift). It is a continuous process that regulates the macroscopic appearance of bone according to Wolff's law. In terms of radiography, *modeling* has been used to describe the formation of bone relative to the cartilage model that is being replaced (i.e., the normal formation of bone). Thus the two definitions do not agree; to avoid confusion, strictly speaking the term *modeling* should be applied to describe the change in shape of a bone as it adapts to the stresses applied to it.

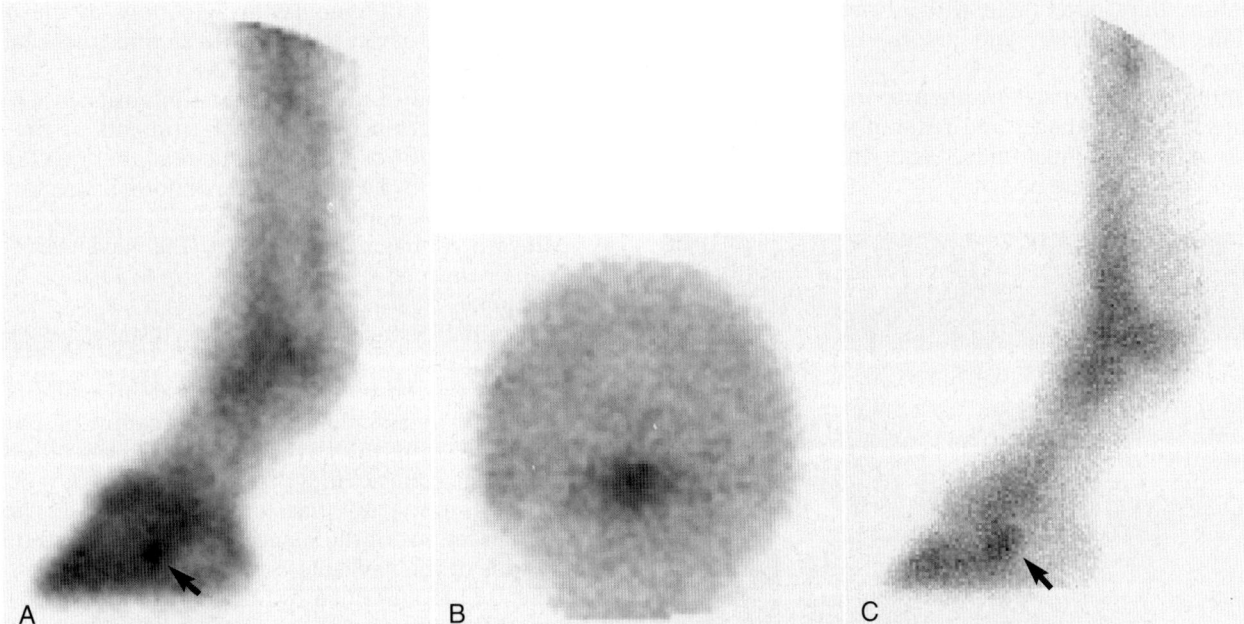

Fig. 30-11 • Scintigraphic images of the left front foot of a 5-year-old Warmblood dressage horse with acute-onset left forelimb lameness abolished by palmar digital analgesia and intraarticular analgesia of the distal interphalangeal joint. **A,** Lateral pool phase image. **B,** Solar bone phase image. **C,** Lateral bone phase image. There is focal intense increased radiopharmaceutical uptake in the navicular bone *(arrow)* in all images.

IRU in the navicular bone, with or without IRU at the region of insertion of the DDFT, has correlated well with a positive response to intrathecal analgesia of the navicular bursa[32] and with abnormalities of the navicular bone detected using MRI.[27,28] False-positive results can be found in clinically normal horses, although a relatively high percentage have subsequently developed lameness associated with palmar foot pain.[32,49]

There is a relatively high incidence of horses with clinical signs compatible with navicular disease and a positive response to intraarticular analgesia of the DIP joint or intrathecal analgesia of the navicular bursa that have no detectable radiological abnormalities of the navicular bone but have IRU in the navicular bone.[27,28,32] Thus nuclear scintigraphy offers a sensitive method of diagnosis of navicular disease, although if bone necrosis is the principal abnormality or the disease is end stage, radiopharmaceutical uptake may be normal.[28]

Computed Tomography and Magnetic Resonance Imaging

CT[66,67] (see Chapter 20) and MRI* (see Chapter 21) are potentially more sensitive than radiography in determining structural lesions of the navicular bone (Figures 30-12 through 30-15) and identifying degenerative changes in the articular cartilage of the DIP joint and primary lesions in the DDFT, the DSIL, and the CSLs. A number of different pathological changes have been identified in the navicular bone that were not detectable with high-quality computed radiography and that may have a different etiopathogenesis. These include:

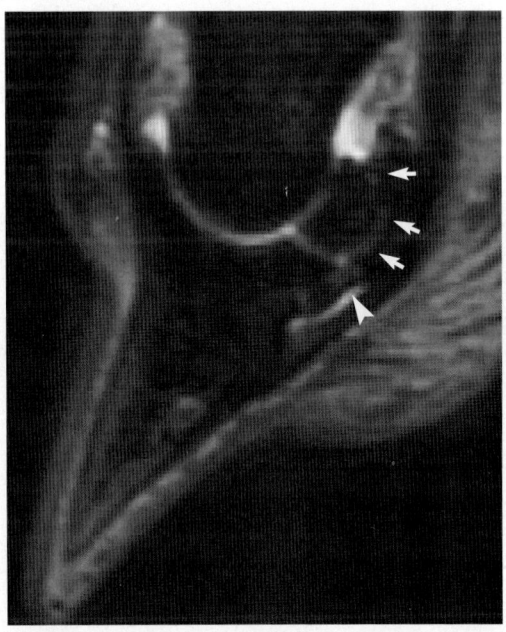

Fig. 30-12 • Sagittal short tau inversion recovery (STIR) MR image of an 8-year-old dressage horse with loss of forelimb action. There is linear increased signal intensity extending through the navicular bone between the insertion of the collateral sesamoidean ligament and the origin of the distal sesamoidean impar ligament (DSIL) *(white arrows)*. There is also increased signal intensity in the DSIL *(arrowhead)*.

• Thickening of the flexor cortex with or without endosteal irregularity, sometimes with proximal or distal extension of the flexor cortex, with or without abnormalities of the CSL or DSIL

• Degenerative ulcer-like lesions of the flexor cortex of the navicular bone, often in the distal third, centered

*References 1, 8, 28, 33, 67-71.

around the sagittal ridge, with advanced disease, adhesions of the DDFT, and lesions extending into the spongiosa

- Diffuse increased signal intensity in the spongiosa in fat-suppressed images and reduced signal intensity in T1- and T2-weighted images associated with trabecular and adipose tissue necrosis

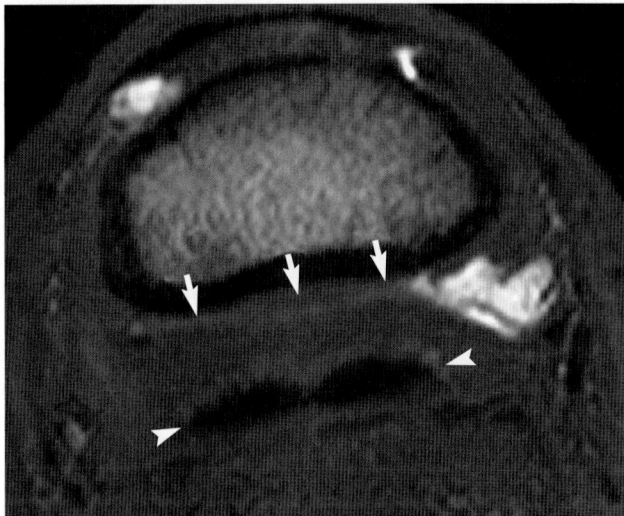

Fig. 30-13 • Transverse T2* gradient-echo magnetic resonance (MR) image of the left front foot at the level of the middle phalanx of a 7-year-old pleasure riding horse with some structural abnormalities of the navicular bone seen on MR images. The collateral sesamoidean ligament *(arrows)* is substantially thickened and is in close apposition to the deep digital flexor tendon *(arrowheads)*, which has a rather irregular dorsal border. Fluid can only be seen in the navicular bursa to the right of the image.

- Axial clusters of synovial invaginations at the distal border of the navicular bone with architectural changes of the DSIL
- A linear band of increased signal intensity in fat-suppressed images between the attachments of the CSL and DSIL, with or without structural abnormalities of the CSL and/or DSIL, reflecting abnormal stress in the podotrochlear apparatus
- Mineralized fragments distal to the navicular bone, with or without osseous reaction in the adjacent navicular bone
- Fluid-filled cystlike lesions in the distal third of the navicular bone

It must also be borne in mind that in a substantial proportion of horses there is a combination of injuries involving not only the navicular bone but also the CSL, DSIL, navicular bursa, and DDFT. In a U.K. study of 347 horses with foot pain that underwent MRI, 12 horses (3.5%) had lesions of the navicular bone alone, 40 horses had lesions of the navicular bone and DDFT (11.5%), and a further 184 (53.0%) had combinations of lesions of the podotrochlear apparatus, navicular bursa, and DDFT.[70] In a U.S. study of 151 horses in which Quarter Horses predominated, there was a much higher incidence of primary navicular bone lesions.[71] However, horses with more chronic lameness (>6 months' duration) were more likely to have concurrent soft tissue lesions, especially in the CSL.

Endoscopic Evaluation of the Navicular Bursa

Endoscopic examination of the navicular bursa (see Chapter 24) permits evaluation of the fibrocartilage on the flexor surface of the navicular bone, the navicular

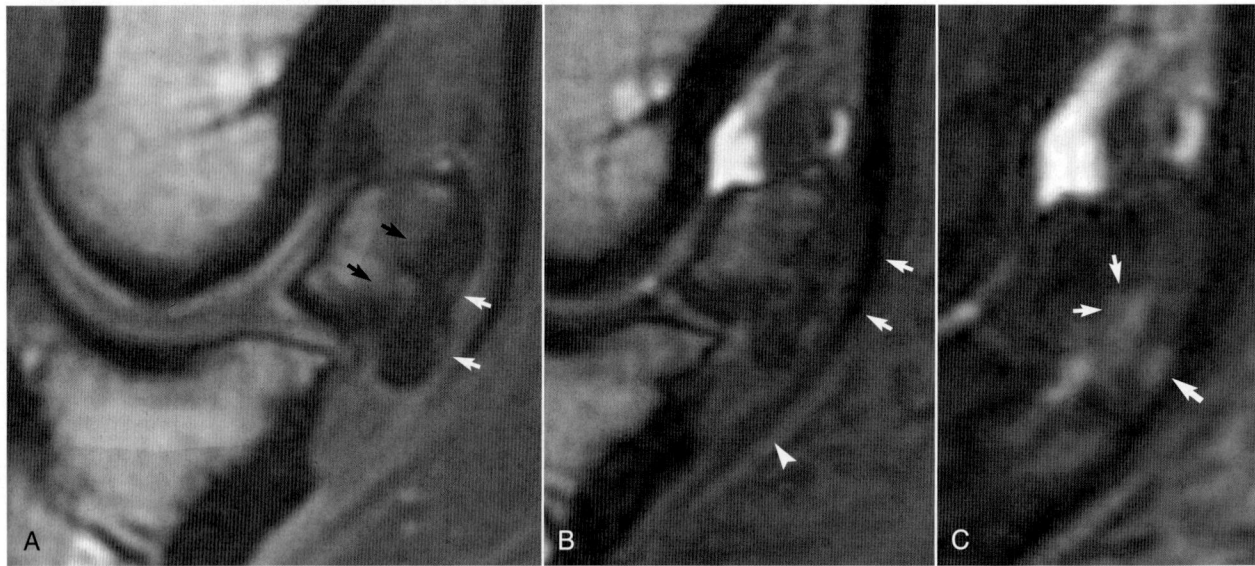

Fig. 30-14 • **A,** Sagittal T1-weighted spoiled gradient-echo magnetic resonance (MR) image; **B,** three-dimensional T2* gradient-echo MR image; and **C,** short tau inversion recovery (STIR) MR image of a Grand Prix show jumper with lameness improved by analgesia of the navicular bursa. There were no detectable radiological abnormalities, but there was focal intense increased radiopharmaceutical uptake in the navicular bone. **A,** There are two focal areas of increased signal intensity in the flexor cortex of the navicular bone; the flexor cortex is thickened, and there is marked endosteal irregularity *(black arrows).* **B,** There is loss of separation between the deep digital flexor tendon *(arrows)* and the palmar aspect of the navicular bone and close apposition of the tendon and the distal sesamoidean impar ligament *(arrowhead).* **C,** There is increased signal intensity in the flexor cortex of the navicular bone and in the spongiosa *(arrows).*

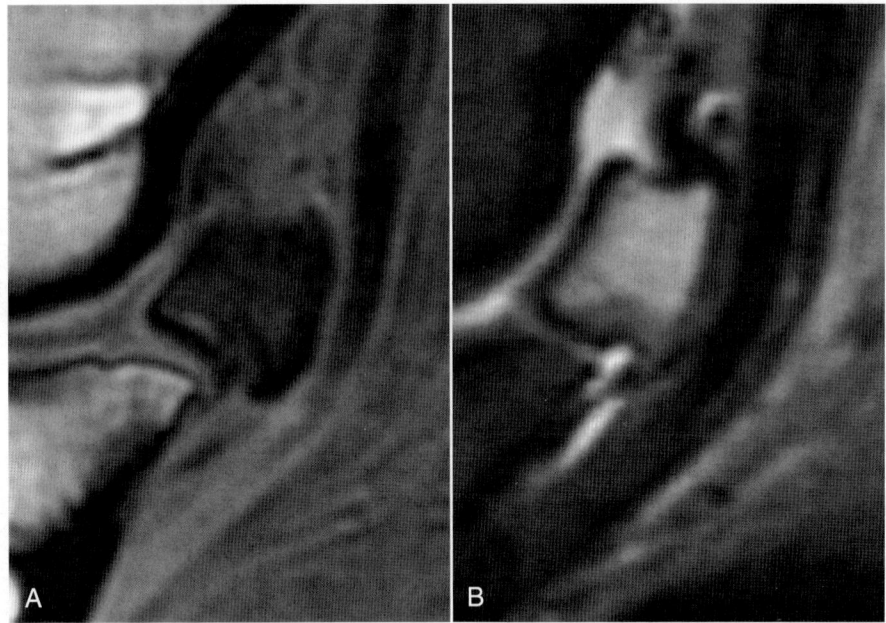

Fig. 30-15 • A, Sagittal spoiled gradient-echo magnetic resonance (MR) image; and **B,** sagittal short tau inversion recovery (STIR) MR image of the left front navicular bone of a 8-year-old Warmblood show jumper with recurrent lameness alleviated by palmar digital analgesia. There is diffuse decreased signal intensity throughout the spongiosa of the navicular bone in the T1-weighted image and diffuse hyperintense signal in the STIR image. Radiopharmaceutical uptake was normal. Post mortem examination revealed trabecular and adipose tissue necrosis of the spongiosa of the navicular bone.

bursa itself, the overlying dorsal surface of the DDFT, and a limited view of the distal sesamoidean impar ligament.[49,72] Thus it is possible to definitively identify adhesions between the DDFT and the palmar aspect of the navicular bone, thinning or full-thickness erosion of the flexor fibrocartilage of the bone, fibrillation of the dorsal aspect of the DDFT, and synovitis of the bursa. Tears in the DSIL have also been identified,[49] but these are thought to be of traumatic origin rather than part of the navicular disease complex. It is important to differentiate between age-related changes and pathological abnormalities.

OTHER SOFT TISSUE CAUSES OF PALMAR FOOT PAIN

Our understanding of soft tissue pain associated with the palmar aspect of the foot has been limited until recently to identification of pain seen in association with poor foot balance, poor shoeing, or both factors that responded to corrective trimming and shoeing (see Chapter 27). Horses that respond satisfactorily to trimming and shoeing alone are unlikely to have chronic navicular disease, and although navicular bone pain may be present, the precise source of pain cannot be determined. A hemodynamic function for the cartilages of the foot and associated vascular system may contribute to force dissipation (see Chapter 29).[73] Peptidergic sensory nerve endings also have been identified in the vascular channels of the cartilages of the foot, close to pacinian-like corpuscles, indicating that this part of the foot may respond to sensory and proprioceptive stimuli. In horses with long toes and underrun heels, the cartilages of

the foot and associated vasculature are less well developed than in a better conformed foot. This may result in less effective force distribution, predisposing to the development of palmar foot pain. In addition, morphological differences have been identified in the digital cushions between "healthy" and "weak" feet, so the digital cushion also may be involved in force dissipation.

With the advent of MRI other soft tissue causes of palmar foot pain were confirmed. These horses usually have no detectable radiological abnormalities. Primary lesions of the DDFT are discussed in detail in Chapter 32. Other injuries that should be considered include the following:

- Desmopathy of the DSIL (see Chapter 33)
- Desmopathy of the CSLs (see Figure 30-13)
- Injury of the distal digital annular ligament
- Navicular bursitis
- Synovitis or osteoarthritis of the DIP joint
- Collateral desmopathy of the DIP joint
- Lesions of the distal phalanx
- Combination injuries

Definitive diagnosis of most of these conditions requires MRI, although ultrasonography performed via the bulbs of the heel or the frog may give some information. Inflammation of the navicular bursa or the DIP joint is rarely seen as single disease entities but accompanies many other causes of foot pain. Injury of the CSL is usually seen in conjunction with other soft tissue injuries or lesions of the navicular bone and rarely alone. Lesions of the DSIL are principally degenerative in nature, although a focal tear in the DSIL has been identified by endoscopic examination of the navicular bursa in an event horse with acute-onset severe lameness that improved after perineural analgesia of

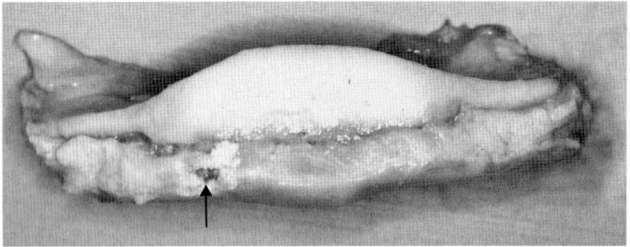

Fig. 30-16 • Gross post mortem specimen of the distal aspect of the navicular bone and the distal sesamoidean impar ligament (DSIL). There is a focal tear in the DSIL *(arrow)*, which had been identified by endoscopic evaluation of the navicular bursa. Surface fibrillation of the deep digital flexor tendon had also been seen.

the palmar digital nerves or intraarticular analgesia of the DIP joint (Figure 30-16).[74]

TREATMENT OF PRIMARY NAVICULAR DISEASE*

Navicular disease is managed because there currently is no cure for this complex condition (Figure 30-17). Rest may not be a useful strategy in the long-term management of many horses with pain in the navicular region because although lameness improves somewhat in most horses after a period of rest, it often returns shortly after the horse resumes exercise. A period of rest for some other cause often precedes the onset of clinical signs of navicular disease. When reviewing literature related to the management of navicular disease it should be borne in mind that much of it relates to palmar foot pain with no definitive diagnosis. The work of Wilson et al[16] suggests that relief of pain is vitally important to alleviate a potentially vicious circle. The horse should be encouraged to land normally, rather than toe first, to avoid increased forces on the navicular bone from the DDFT. However, it must be acknowledged that in some horses with acute lameness in which the principal pathological abnormality is increased signal intensity in fat-suppressed MR images in the spongiosa of the navicular bone, which may reflect bone trauma, the most appropriate treatment may be rest.

In horses with early navicular disease without major radiological abnormalities, medical management using nonsteroidal antiinflammatory drugs (NSAIDs), isoxsuprine, tiludronate, and careful trimming and shoeing may be effective. The aim of medical management is to attempt to return the horse to regular work as soon as possible, starting initially with work predominantly in straight lines. Horses should be exercised as much as possible daily, combining ridden exercise with either turnout or walking on a horse walker. In some horses, use of corrective trimming and shoeing combined with isoxsuprine is sufficient, whereas in others additional analgesia is required using an NSAID. In horses with marked increased radiopacity of the medulla, lesions involving the flexor surface of the navicular bone, or central osseous cystlike lesions, the response to medical management often is unsatisfactory, and surgical treatment may be indicated.

---

*The author acknowledges John B. Madison who contributed to this section in the previous edition.

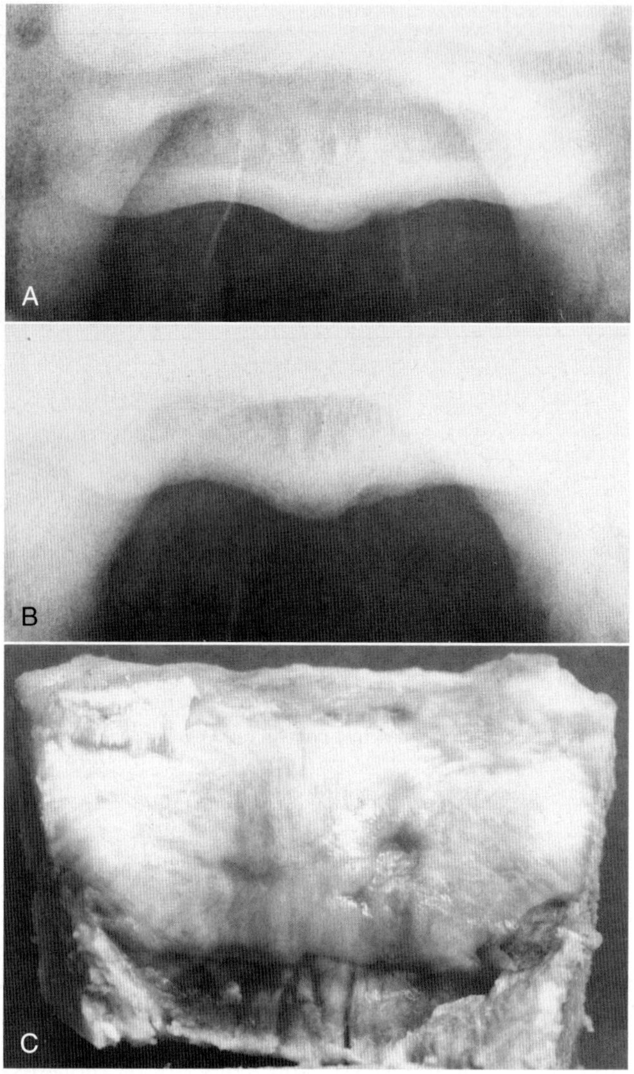

Fig. 30-17 • A, Palmar 45° proximal-palmarodistal oblique image of a navicular bone with an irregular contour of the lateral aspect of the flexor cortex. Lateral is to the right. The horse had bilateral forelimb lameness, which was improved by intraarticular analgesia of the distal interphalangeal joint or analgesia of the navicular bursa. **B,** Palmar 35° proximal-palmarodistal oblique image of the same navicular bone as in **A.** The irregularity of the flexor cortex is more obvious. Apparent reduction in corticomedullary demarcation is an artifact, the result of the angle of projection. Lateral is to the right. **C,** The same horse as in **A.** The gross pathological specimen has a defect in the flexor surface, lateral to the sagittal ridge. Lateral is to the right.

MANAGEMENT STRATEGIES
Trimming and Shoeing

Successful management depends on a good relationship with an accomplished, reliable farrier. There is an art and science to farriery, and finding the right combination of the method of trimming and the selection of an appropriate shoe for a given horse often requires some trial and error. Each foot and each horse must be examined individually with regard to the distal limb and foot conformation, limb flight, foot placement, and the intended use of the horse. Both the farrier and the veterinarian must agree, and both must also agree to alter the initial approach if it does not work. Some degree of compromise is always involved. However, some principles apply for all horses with navicular disease. The degree to which lameness can be improved by trimming and shoeing alone depends on the horse's hoof-pastern angle and the previous suitability of trimming and shoeing. If the horse already had a well-conformed foot, little will be achieved.

Care must be taken either to correct or preserve dorso-palmar and lateromedial foot balance whenever possible. This depends to some extent on the natural shape of the horse's foot and its distal limb conformation. Ideally, the hoof-pastern axis should be straight, but whether this can be achieved depends on the horse's conformation. Radical changes in foot trimming may temporarily result in increased lameness; therefore it may be necessary to achieve correct foot balance in stages. The foot should be trimmed to maintain heel mass and shorten the toe to facilitate breakover. Sufficient shortening of the toes usually requires trimming the horn from the solar and dorsal aspects of the foot. The use of the so-called four-point or natural balance trim has recently been favored in some quarters, but the same principles of breakover can probably be achieved with more traditional trimming, provided that the toe is shortened sufficiently (see Chapter 27). Although the four-point trim results in clinical improvement in some horses, in others lameness has been increased, possibly caused by excessive trimming, resulting in altered hoof wall strain,[2] or by excessive sole pressure.

Elevation of the heel may relieve pressure from the DDFT on the palmar aspect of the navicular bone, with subsequent pain relief. In a short-term study of 12 horses with navicular disease, elevation of the heel using a 3-degree wedge-heel aluminum shoe resulted in significant gait improvement as assessed by force plate analysis.[75] In a study of normal Dutch Warmblood horses, elevation of the heel using a 6-degree wedge reduced the maximal force on the navicular bone by 24% compared with flat shoes.[3] However, not all horses with palmar foot pain need to have the heel elevated, and in many the response is only temporary. A hoof angle between 50 and 55 degrees is considered ideal. Achieving a straight foot-pastern axis is also a goal, but poor foot conformation may prohibit this. Many horses with a low, collapsed heel have a natural angle of no more than 35 degrees, and it is impractical to achieve an angle of 50 to 55 degrees. Lateromedial radiographic images may be helpful to demonstrate to a less-skilled farrier whether a horse needs more or less heel. If the horse's lameness is worsened after elevating the toe using the wedge test, some degree of heel elevation may be beneficial. Elevation of the heel can be achieved by using a wedge heel shoe or a rim or complete wedge pad.

A variety of shoes have been used successfully in the management of horses with navicular disease, including egg bar, egg bar–heart bar, straight bar shoes, and the so-called Tennessee shoe, which moves the point of breakover to just in front of the apex of the frog by placing rails on the palmar aspect of the branches of the shoe. Success has also been achieved in some horses using the natural balance shoe.[76]

The strategy of using shoes that move the weight-bearing axis in a palmar direction in horses with a low, collapsed, and underrun heel is reasonably successful. However, a recent study has shown that using egg bar shoes in clinically normal Dutch Warmblood horses with well-conformed feet did not reduce force on the navicular bone compared with flat shoes.[77] The forelimb gait was also described as less animated with egg bar shoes compared with flat shoes. However, these findings cannot necessarily be translated to lame horses with less than ideal foot conformation. Many top-level show jumpers and dressage horses have been shod with egg bar shoes with no apparent detriment to the quality of the gaits. Egg bar shoes provide a greater surface area through which forces are transmitted and clinically seem to help reduce pain associated with either navicular bone pain or the DIP joint. Of 55 horses with clinically diagnosed navicular disease, 53% had permanent relief of lameness after application of egg bar shoes in a follow-up period of 12 to 40 months.[78] In some horses, clinical improvement took many weeks. Resolution of lameness was seen despite the persistence of a low, collapsed heel. In another study, treated horses showed histomorphometric evidence of altered navicular bone modeling compared with untreated controls.[79] The shoes should be made-to-measure and of sufficient size and length to provide adequate support to the heel region (Figure 30-18).

Fitting an egg bar shoe is not necessarily easy and depends on the shape of the horse's foot. If the quarters are very wide it can be difficult to "pick up" the heel bulbs. In such horses a traditional open shoe fitted long and wide at the heel or a straight bar shoe may be more appropriate. A correctly fitted egg bar shoe should project beyond the ground-bearing surface of the foot. It is more likely to be pulled off than a standard shoe, and the use of over-reach boots should always be considered, at least when the horse is worked or turned out. These shoes are not suitable for a horse that is going to work in deep mud because they are readily sucked off. In summary, the following principles may aid in the selection of a shoe: correction and then maintenance of dorsopalmar and lateromedial balance, ease of breakover achieved by rolling the toe of the shoe, maintenance of foot (and especially heel) mass, and protection of the palmar aspect of the foot from concussion.

Screw-in studs are used in many competition horses to enhance traction. Some riders just use studs in the lateral branch of the shoe to avoid the risks of tread injuries created by a medial stud in the contralateral limb. This inevitably creates mediolateral imbalance, and therefore care should be taken either to use studs in both branches or to avoid the use of studs. The studs should be positioned as far palmarly as possible to avoid shortening the effective length of the shoe. When the ground is hard, small, pointed studs are preferable to large, square-shaped studs.

Nonsteroidal Antiinflammatory Medication

A wide variety of NSAIDs are used in horses. In general, these drugs should be administered at the lowest dose necessary to achieve the desired effect. There are anecdotal reports that certain NSAIDs are better for horses with foot pain (e.g., meclofenamic acid [Arquel, Pfizer, New York, New York, United States]), but there are no controlled studies to support these claims. Phenylbutazone is widely used, and many, but not all, horses with navicular pain respond to this drug. To determine the lowest effective dose of phenylbutazone, the horse is given a dose of 4 mg/kg

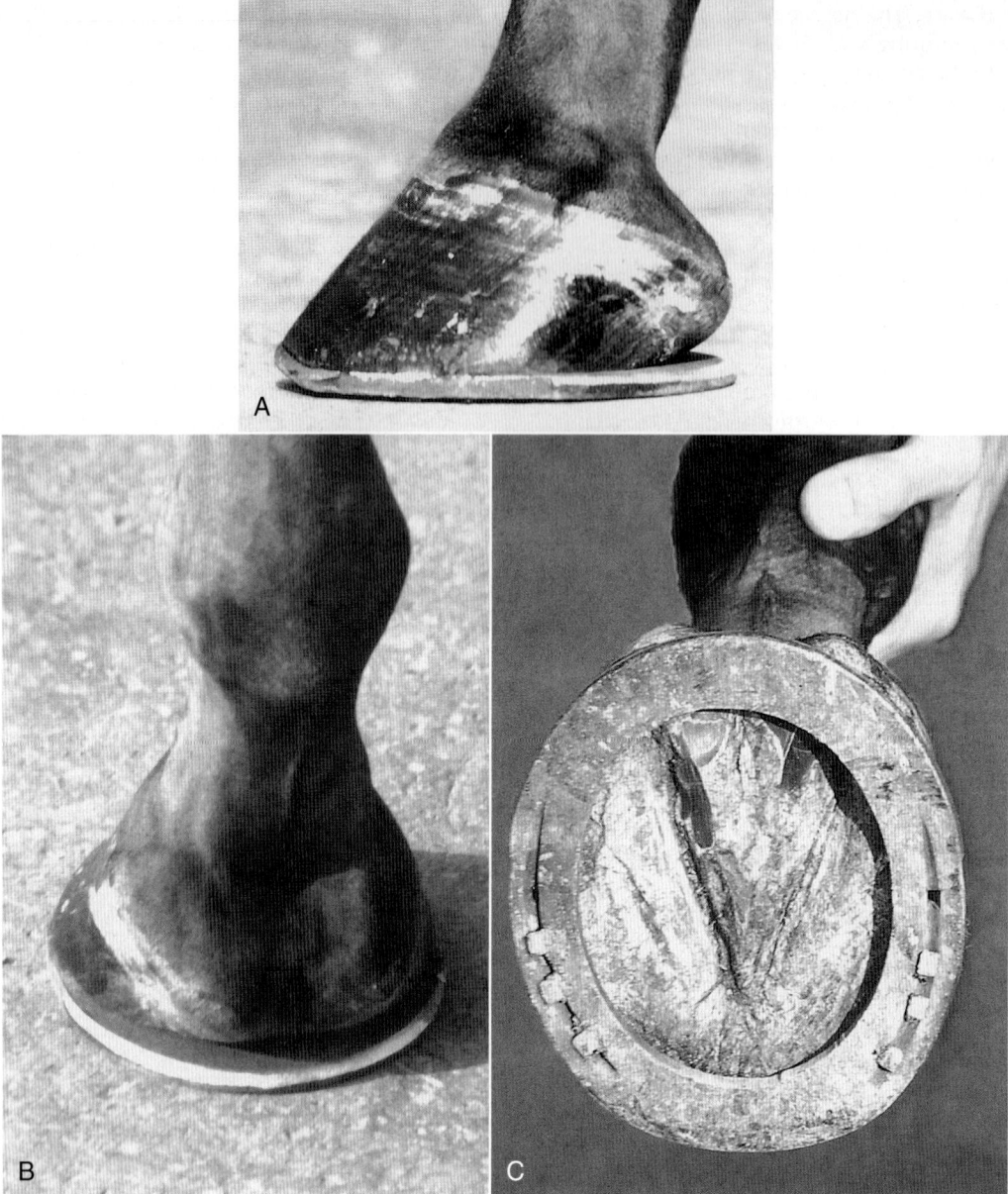

Fig. 30-18 • Lateral **(A)**, palmar **(B)**, and solar **(C)** photographs of a correctly fitted egg bar shoe. The shoe projects beyond the ground-bearing surface of the foot to cover the bulbs of the heel.

twice daily for 3 days, and the dose is then gradually decreased until the lameness returns. Depending on lameness severity, NSAID treatment may only be necessary when the horse is being used. It should be borne in mind that it has been demonstrated that phenylbutazone may influence bone turnover.[80] After bone biopsy of the tibia, mineral apposition rate was significantly decreased in horses treated with phenylbutazone (4.4 mg/kg twice daily) compared with untreated, control horses. The clinical significance of this finding in the management of navicular disease is unknown. For horses that are intolerant of phenylbutazone, carprofen ([Rimadyl; Pfizer] 1.0 to 1.5 mg/kg once daily) may be a useful alternative. A short-term study using etodolac, a COX-2 inhibitor, demonstrated significant gait improvement based on force plate data in horses with chronic navicular disease (23 mg/kg orally, once

daily)[81]; however, the horses were not in work, and its effectiveness in a clinical setting is unknown.

Isoxsuprine

Isoxsuprine is a β-agonist that causes peripheral vasodilation in people. Its mode of action in the treatment of navicular disease is unknown. It has been suggested that there are no measurable cardiovascular effects of isoxsuprine given orally in the horse.[78,79] However, orally administered slow-release isoxsuprine resin was absorbed and resulted in thermographic evidence of increased skin temperature of the distal aspect of the forelimbs for about 8 hours after administration.[80] Isoxsuprine also binds strongly to α-adrenoreceptors[81] and therefore may be active despite insignificant measurable levels in plasma.[80] The drug also may have some antiinflammatory or hemorheological properties that could explain why some horses with navicular disease appear to respond to isoxsuprine therapy. A double-blind clinical trial evaluating the response to isoxsuprine in the treatment of navicular disease demonstrated a decrease in lameness in the treated horses.[82]

If the horse responds to a trial dose of 0.6 mg/kg twice a day for 30 days, then continued treatment at the same dose given once or twice a day indefinitely may be indicated. Some horses have been treated for 12 weeks and responded satisfactorily and have then shown remission of clinical signs for up to 9 months without treatment. If no response is seen within 30 days, it is unlikely that further treatment will be beneficial. However, some horses that had no response to a dose of 0.6 mg/kg twice daily responded satisfactorily to 0.9 mg/kg twice daily. If lameness is moderate to severe, then treatment should be combined with an NSAID for the first 3 to 4 weeks of treatment. The response to treatment in horses with major radiological abnormalities is generally very poor.

Intraarticular and Intrathecal Medication

It has been demonstrated that potentially therapeutic concentrations of methylprednisolone acetate or triamcinolone acetonide can be achieved in the navicular bursa after injection of the DIP joint.[83] However, although lameness associated with navicular disease may be improved by intraarticular analgesia of the DIP joint, the intraarticular administration of hyaluronan with or without corticosteroids (e.g., triamcinolone acetonide, 10 mg) does not usually result in a similar degree of improvement, unless there is concurrent synovitis of the DIP joint. In a study of 128 horses in which lameness was improved by intraarticular analgesia of the DIP joint, the presence of radiological abnormalities of the navicular bone (mild to moderate in degree) resulted in an 18 times lesser likelihood of a successful response to intraarticular medication of the DIP joint with either polysulfated glycosaminoglycan (PSGAG) or methylprednisolone acetate compared with horses without radiological abnormalities.[88] Intrathecal injection of corticosteroids into the navicular bursa is often more effective clinically and may provide transient relief of clinical signs for up to 2 to 5 months.[89-92] In my experience, this treatment is effective only in horses with low-grade radiological abnormalities but can result in very substantial, although temporary, improvement. Repeated treatment may result in the development of dystrophic mineralization. However, the response in horses with radiological[91] or MRI evidence[91,92] of ulcers (erosions) on the palmar aspect of the navicular bone has been poor.

Other Drugs

Warfarin previously was used to treat horses with "navicular disease," and in one series an 80% success rate was claimed.[93] However, these were predominantly pleasure horses and low-level competition horses. Experience in higher-level competition horses produced disappointing results.[49] Warfarin therapy requires careful adjustment of the dose guided by monitoring of prothrombin time at least at monthly intervals. This, combined with the drug's limited efficacy, has largely resulted in the abandonment of this treatment.

Pentoxyfylline and propentofylline are hemorheological drugs that alter the deformability of the red blood cell membrane and inhibit platelet aggregation.[83,94] These drugs are advocated by some clinicians for the treatment of navicular disease, although clinical efficacy to date is largely unknown. No measurable effect on digital and laminar blood flow was seen in healthy horses after oral administration of pentoxifylline.[83] A small clinical study using propentofylline resulted in improvement but not alleviation of lameness associated with navicular disease during a 6-week treatment period.[94] A long-term clinical trial using metrenperone found similar efficacy to isoxsuprine; only 27% of horses had long-term resolution of lameness.[96]

The pathological similarities between navicular disease and osteoarthritis have prompted the use of drugs used for the management of osteoarthritis. Systemic administration of a PSGAG (Adequan, Novartis Animal Health, Basel, Switzerland; 500 mg intramuscularly every 4 days for 7 treatments) resulted in clinical improvement in lameness in treated horses compared with controls during the treatment period.[96] In my experience, PSGAG treatment has not had any long-lasting benefit on lameness associated with navicular disease.

Tiludronate

Tiludronate is a bisphosphonate that inhibits osteoclastic activity. In a placebo-controlled clinical trial, horses with navicular disease treated by intravenous infusion of tiludronate showed significantly improved lameness scores, but in no horse was lameness completely abolished.[97] I have treated approximately 20 horses in which increased signal intensity in the spongiosa of the navicular bone in fat-suppressed MR images was the principal abnormality, but the results were disappointing.[91] There is anecdotal suggestion that regional perfusion with tiludronate may be more effective.

Shockwave Therapy

There is anecdotal information that shockwave therapy may temporarily alleviate pain associated with palmar foot pain. In an uncontrolled clinical trial in 42 horses with chronic (>3 months) foot-related lameness, the effect of transcuneal shockwave therapy or therapy applied between the bulbs of the heel was compared. The latter was more efficacious, although improvement was observed with both treatments.[98]

Chemical "Neurectomy": Cryoneurectomy

Temporary resolution of palmar foot pain can be achieved by chemical ablation of sensory fibers in the palmar digital nerves. Several products are capable of causing a temporary loss of sensation when injected over the nerves. These include Sarapin (a plant alkaloid that is thought to alter transmission in type C fibers; High Chemical Company, Levittown, Pennsylvania, United States), P block, and cobra venom. The product usually is injected over, or directly into, the nerve with a corticosteroid. Injection of absolute alcohol into the perineurium may also be used. Any of these products may result in localized perineural fibrosis, which makes subsequent surgical neurectomy more complicated. Alternatively, the digital nerves may be frozen percutaneously using liquid nitrogen. Both methods result in 2 to 3 months of clinical improvement when successfully applied. In the Editors' experience, these methods work well on occasion but are unreliable. Return of sensation in most horses is accompanied by a return of the lameness.

Desmotomy of the Collateral Sesamoidean Ligaments

Desmotomy of the CSLs has been described as a treatment for navicular disease.[99,100] In an initial report from the United Kingdom, 13 of 16 horses treated with this technique were able to work without lameness,[99] and in a subsequent report, 76% of 118 horses were sound at 6 months, but only 43% remained sound 3 years later.[101] Diehl[100] from Germany reported clinical improvement in 50% of 57 horses. In a study from New Zealand, 12 of 17 horses were sound at least 6 months postoperatively.[102] In my experience there is often only short-term (6 to 12 months) improvement in lameness. It was originally suggested that this surgical procedure resulted in alteration of the biomechanical forces on the navicular bone, but clinical improvement may also be the result of sectioning the sensory nerve fibers that run in the CSLs. The original surgical technique described transecting the ligaments near the origin through oblique skin incisions, but the proximal interphalangeal joint capsule can be penetrated by this approach. Better results have been achieved via vertical skin incisions further distally, centered over the CSLs.

Desmotomy of the Accessory Ligament of the Deep Digital Flexor Tendon

Desmotomy of the accessory ligament of the DDFT was described as a treatment for navicular disease in horses with markedly upright foot conformation.[103] Long-term follow-up results are not available.

Periarterial "Sympathectomy"

Litzke et al[104] described a technique for cutting the sympathetic nerve supply to the lateral and medial digital arteries, either alone or with palmar digital neurectomy. This technique is still practiced in Germany, but the results have not been well documented.

Palmar Digital Neurectomy

If lameness associated with navicular disease is completely eliminated by perineural analgesia of the palmar digital nerves, then palmar digital neurectomy may be considered as a treatment of last resort.[106-110] The technique has been associated with a clinically significant number of complications, including failure to alleviate lameness, recurrence of lameness, complete or partial rupture of the DDFT, subluxation or luxation of the DIP joint, neuroma formation, and failure to recognize either subsolar infection or penetrating injuries of the palmar aspect of the foot. Case selection is very important. Horses with preexisting pathology of the DDFT are probably at highest risk of subsequent rupture of the DDFT. If there is radiological evidence of a substantial

defect in the flexor surface of the navicular bone, DDFT lesions are likely, and these horses should not be treated by neurectomy. A variety of techniques of palmar digital neurectomy have been described. Recent work suggests that the simple guillotine technique results in the longest period of desensitization and less neuroma formation compared with epineural capping and carbon dioxide laser division.[107] Surgery should be delayed for at least 7 days after perineural analgesia. For neurectomy, I use two long (3- to 4-cm) incisions just dorsal to the medial and lateral edges of the superficial digital flexor tendon starting just below the base of the proximal sesamoid bone. The nerve is gently stretched and transected using a scalpel blade as far distally and proximally as possible. Approximately 50% of horses have one or more (up to five) accessory branches that must be divided to achieve complete desensitization of the heel region. In most instances the accessory branches are located abaxial to the palmar digital nerve and run in a palmar direction and parallel to the ligament of the ergot. If an accessory branch is located at one surgical site, there are invariably accessory branches associated with the remaining palmar digital nerves. The incision is closed in a single layer, and the horse is confined to a box stall with handwalking only for 30 days. Phenylbutazone (2.2 mg/kg twice daily) is administered for 10 days. This limited exercise, combined with minimal handling of the nerve(s) intraoperatively, seems to reduce the risk of neuroma formation.

The horse is shod in the manner that was most successful before surgery. This procedure usually provides relief of clinical symptoms in approximately 65% to 70% of horses for approximately 12 to 18 months postoperatively.[108,109] Individual horses may have recurrence of lameness sooner.

With careful handling of the nerve intraoperatively, followed by conservative postoperative management, neuroma formation is uncommon. A painful neuroma, which may occur several months after surgery, may be successfully managed with perineural injections of Sarapin and/or triamcinolone acetonide. Occasionally a second neurectomy done proximal to the neuroma is required.

If lameness occurs because of reinnervation, surgery may be repeated, assuming that perineural analgesia of the palmar digital nerves still results in relief of pain. However, reinnervation may be caused by axons sprouting from the proximal nerve stump and anastomosing with other local nerves. Therefore repeated surgery may be less successful.

Decompression of the Navicular Bone by Surgical Drilling

A technique for drilling cystlike lesions in the navicular bone through an endoscopic approach was recently described, but long-term follow-up results are not available.[111,112] The rationale is to provide decompression to reduce intraosseous pressure.

References
on page
1273

Chapter 31

Fracture of the Navicular Bone and Congenital Bipartite Navicular Bone

Sue J. Dyson

Fractures of the navicular bone occur in a variety of configurations. The most common is a slightly oblique parasagittal fracture, medial or lateral to the midline. Y-shaped fractures and other comminuted fractures are less common. Avulsion of the entire distal border is rare. Distal border fragments are discussed elsewhere (see Chapter 30). Fractures occur more commonly in forelimbs than hindlimbs. In a series of 40 horses with navicular bone fractures, 28 (70%) occurred in a forelimb.[1] Fractures usually are traumatic in origin, although it is not always possible to identify the cause. Some fractures in hindlimbs have been the result of kicking a wall. Bipartite and tripartite navicular bones have also been described and should be differentiated from a fracture.[2] These may occur unilaterally, bilaterally or sometimes in 3 or 4 limbs in forelimbs or hindlimbs. It has been suggested that many fractures are pathological secondary to severe navicular disease,[3] but this confusion probably arises because lucent zones adjacent to the fracture line and along the distal border of the navicular bone develop rapidly, within months of fracture occurrence.[4] Palmar (plantar) displacement of fracture fragment(s) may result in laceration of the deep digital flexor tendon (DDFT).[5] Other fractures of the middle or distal phalanx occasionally occur concurrently.

HISTORY

Lameness associated with a fracture is usually acute in onset and severe. However, sometimes a horse may develop less severe lameness, and radiographic examination reveals evidence of an old fracture, which presumably healed by fibrous union but has recently become unstable. Instability between separate ossification centers can cause unilateral or bilateral mild to moderate lameness or occasionally lameness in three or four limbs.

CLINICAL EXAMINATION AND DIAGNOSIS

A horse with a fracture may be reluctant to bear full weight on the limb. Digital pulse amplitudes may be increased, and in some horses, pain can be elicited by application of hoof testers to the heel or frog regions. Percussion of the frog may be resented. Lameness usually is severe with an acute fracture and may be accentuated as a horse turns. Lameness is usually substantially improved by perineural analgesia of the palmar digital nerves, although it sometimes is unaffected. Diagnosis depends on radiological identification

of the fracture(s). Most fractures are best identified in a dorsoproximal-palmarodistal oblique image (or an "upright pedal" plantarodorsal image in a hindlimb) (Figure 31-1). It is important that frog cleft artifacts not be confused as a fracture. The clinician should examine any radiolucent line carefully to see whether it extends beyond the bone margins or changes position relative to the medial and lateral margins of the bone if the x-ray beam is reoriented 5 degrees medially or laterally. The frog clefts should be well packed with a moldable compound (e.g., Play-Doh, Hasbro, Pawtucket, Rhode Island, United States) and, if necessary, repacked. If doubt persists, a weight-bearing dorsopalmar view and a palmaroproximal-palmarodistal oblique image of the navicular bone should determine whether a fracture is present. The palmaroproximal-palmarodistal oblique image is also useful for determining the presence of comminution or displacement. The presence of radiolucent zones along the fracture line indicates that it is not of recent origin but rather is likely to have been present for at least several months (Figure 31-2). With fractures of unusual configurations occasionally radiological findings are equivocal or negative and magnetic resonance imaging (MRI) or computed tomography is required for diagnosis.

A bipartite, or less commonly a tripartite, navicular bone is usually characterized by a wider gap between the ossification centers than an acute fracture. There may or may not be radiolucent zones adjacent to the radiolucent gap between the bone fragments. Occasionally this is an

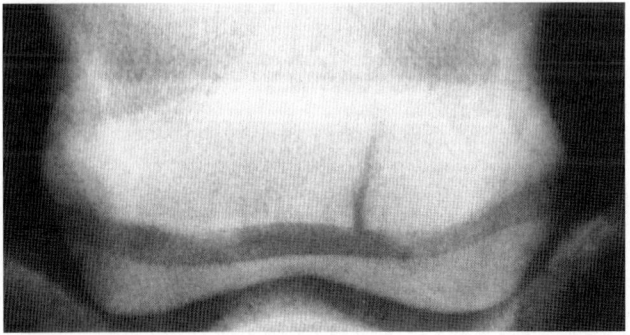

Fig. 31-1 • Dorsoproximal-palmarodistal oblique radiographic image of a navicular bone. There is an acute parasagittal fracture lateral to the midline. Lateral is to the right.

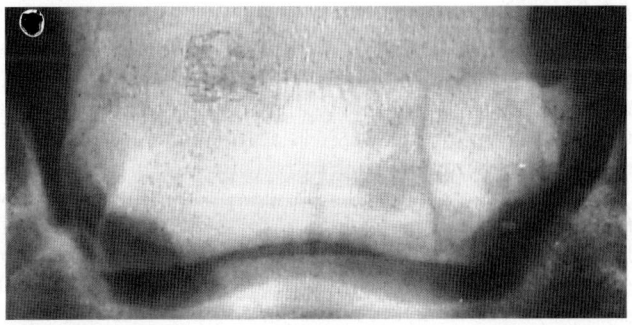

Fig. 31-2 • Dorsoproximal-palmarodistal oblique raidographic image of a navicular bone with a chronic fracture involving the lateral aspect. There are large radiolucent areas adjacent to the fracture line and modeling of the lateral proximal margin of the navicular bone.

incidental finding unrelated to current lameness. Alternatively, it may be seen in association with foot pain resulting from another related cause, such as a DDFT lesion in the same parasagittal plane. In such horses there is no increase in radiopharmaceutical uptake in the navicular bone, whereas in horses with fractures or bipartite navicular bones contributing directly to pain and lameness there is increased radiopharmaceutical uptake in the navicular bone. Bipartite navicular bones may be present in more than one limb, and if lameness is unilateral, it is recommended that the contralateral limb is also examined radiographically.

Proximal displacement of a hindlimb navicular bone secondary to complete rupture of the distal sesamoidean ligament has been reported in a steeplechaser.[6] The navicular bone was displaced proximally in a lateromedial radiographic image. The horse was managed conservatively and did return to racing.

TREATMENT

Lameness associated with a simple sagittal fracture usually improves progressively with rest, but the prognosis for complete resolution of lameness or return to full athletic function is guarded. Some horses do become sound enough for light hacking, but lameness may be recurrent.[3,7] Better results have been described in a limited number of horses by trimming the foot to establish a normal hoof-pastern

axis followed by application of four 3-degree wedge pads and a flat shoe to reduce the weight-bearing function of the navicular bone.[8] The horse is confined to box rest for 60 days and then starts walking exercise for an additional 2 months. The shoe is refitted every 4 weeks with 3 degrees less elevation at each shoeing. However, healing probably is only by fibrous union. Treatment by palmar digital neurectomy may provide symptomatic relief in some horses, but a substantial proportion develop osteoarthritis of the distal or proximal interphalangeal joints and associated lameness.[7] Internal fixation using a lag screw technique with a specially designed limb jig and radiographic control offers the best prognosis for simple, oblique sagittal fractures.[1,9] Twenty-three (68%) of 40 horses resumed work. The prognosis was significantly better for horses with fractures of less than 4 weeks' duration than for those with older fractures. Potential complications include splitting the fragment, inability to reduce the fracture resulting in a step deformity, and poor stabilization of the fracture. Experience with MRI has shown that in association with an acute fracture there may be concurrent lesions of the DDFT, which may influence prognosis. The prognosis for horses with more complicated fractures is guarded.

Palmar digital neurectomy has been used successfully in horses with lameness associated with a bipartite navicular bone; however, it is important to be aware that there may also be a related DDFT injury.

Chapter 32

Primary Lesions of the Deep Digital Flexor Tendon within the Hoof Capsule

Sue J. Dyson

ANATOMY

Within the hoof capsule the deep digital flexor tendon (DDFT) is molded to the palmar (plantar) surface of the navicular bone and separated from it by the navicular bursa. Proximally the DDFT is intimately related to the distal digital annular ligament on its palmar aspect. The distal recess of the navicular bursa separates the DDFT and the distal sesamoidean impar ligament (DSIL). The DDFT has a terminal fanlike expansion containing cartilage that occupies the entire space between the medial and lateral palmar processes of the distal phalanx. It inserts on the facies flexoria and semilunar crest of the distal phalanx. The dorsal portion of the DDFT joins with the DSIL immediately before insertion on the facies flexoria of the distal phalanx. There are parallel fibers of dense connective

tissue, separated by loose connective tissue, within which are many sensory nerves and numerous blood vessels.[1] A prominent line (tidemark) indicates the transition from nonmineralized tendon and ligament to mineralized regions of the DDFT and DSIL before attachment to the distal phalanx.[2]

Within the digit the DDFT induces axial compression of the articular surfaces of the proximal and distal interphalangeal joints.[2,3] It has an important role in stabilizing the distal interphalangeal joint. The anatomical arrangement of the collateral ligaments of the navicular bone facilitates compression of the articular surfaces of the navicular bone into those of the middle and distal phalanges.[2] The DDFT has a dorsal fibrocartilaginous pad that supports pressure of the tuberositas flexoria, the transverse prominence on the proximopalmar aspect of the middle phalanx.[3]

The relationship of the DDFT to the navicular bone varies with the phase of the stride. During the full weight-bearing stance of the stride the DDFT is only in contact with the distal aspect of the bone, whereas in the propulsion phase the DDFT bends over the distal scutum (the fibrocartilaginous insertion of the straight sesamoidean ligament on the middle phalanx) and comes into full contact with the navicular bone. Tension in the DDFT is maximal, and active muscle contraction and the elasticity in the tendon and in its accessory ligament result in extension of the distal interphalangeal joint.[3] At the beginning of the swing phase of the stride the tension in the DDFT contributes passively to induce flexion of the interphalangeal joints. During extension of the distal interphalangeal

References on page 1273

joint, which is maximum at the propulsion phase of the stride, pull on the DDFT creates a shear force between the DDFT and the DSIL.[2]

PATHOPHYSIOLOGY

Primary lesions of the DDFT have only recently been recognized clinically, and only limited information concerning pathophysiology is available. A progressive increase in proteoglycans with age was seen in the distal aspects of the DDFT and DSIL, which may be an adaptation to stress.[2] It was suggested that horses with low, weak heels may be more susceptible to these changes. Similar but more extensive changes were seen in two horses with navicular disease. Lesions within the DDFT within the foot were identified in fewer than 10% of horses with unknown history in a post mortem study of superficial digital flexor tendon and DDFT lesions in the metacarpal region and digit.[4]

In a post mortem study of 38 horses with suspected navicular disease, one horse had a core lesion of the DDFT with no associated pathological condition of the navicular bone[5]; four additional horses had histological evidence of focal regions of necrosis within the tendon concurrent with other pathological conditions of the navicular bone. Surface fibrillation was a common finding in horses with navicular disease but not in age-matched controls. No lesions of the DDFT were described in the age-matched controls. Pool et al[6] considered lesions in the DDFT to be secondary to navicular disease. Inflammation at the intersection of the DDFT and DSIL was recognized in the Quarter Horse in association with other signs compatible with navicular disease.[7] It was considered that these lesions may be involved with the pathogenesis of navicular disease.

A variety of different types of lesions of the DDFT have been identified using magnetic resonance imaging (MRI) and confirmed post mortem.[8-11] These include partial or full-thickness sagittal plane splits, dorsal abrasions, fibrillation, and core lesions. Core lesions within the tendon or on the dorsal surface, full-thickness parasagittal splits can be seen alone and are considered primary lesions of the DDFT, whereas fibrillation and small isolated incomplete parasagittal splits are commonly seen in association with other lesions of the podotrochlear apparatus.[12-14] Core lesions or full-thickness splits usually occur extending proximally from the proximal aspect of the navicular bursa or distal to the navicular bone. Isolated incomplete parasagittal plane splits, minor dorsal abrasions, and fibrillation are seen most commonly from the proximal level of the navicular bursa distally.

In recent studies comparing MRI and histopathology in groups of horses with chronic foot pain and age-matched control horses, the incidence of DDFT lesions was considerably higher than previously recognized.[8-11] Degenerative changes of the DDFT were seen in both groups but were of greater severity in the lame horses. Thickening of septae, with ghosting and occlusion of blood vessels, and fibrocartilaginous and chondroid metaplasia were characteristic findings, which may predispose to fibrillation and dorsal splits of the tendon. Such changes have also been identified in the proximity of necrotic core lesions. The presence of degenerative changes within the DDFT was not age related. With all types of lesions of the DDFT there was a notable absence of acute inflammatory reaction.

Primary deep digital flexor (DDF) tendonitis may be the result of repetitive overstress or an acute-onset traumatic tear, possibly superimposed on preexisting degenerative change. The identification of severe core lesions in young horses that have done relatively little work suggests that some horses may have an inherent predisposition to injury.

Rupture of the DDFT secondary to previous neurectomy of the palmar digital nerves is considered a separate condition; however, it is likely that a preexisting, unrecognized pathological condition of the DDFT predisposes to rupture (see Chapter 70).

Dystrophic or ectopic mineralization within the DDFT was identified radiologically, at the level of the navicular bone and immediately proximal to it, but its clinical significance has been speculative.[15] Entheseous new bone at the site of insertion of the DDFT on the facies flexoria and semilunar crest of the distal phalanx was described associated with lameness and unassociated with navicular disease.[16] Nuclear scintigraphic examination of horses with palmar foot pain has revealed horses with linear increased radiopharmaceutical uptake (IRU) in the DDFT in pool phase images or focal regions of IRU in the region of insertion of the DDFT on the distal phalanx,[17,18] either alone or in association with a region of increased uptake in the navicular bone. This has correlated well with lesions identified using MRI.

HISTORY AND CLINICAL SIGNS

Lameness associated with primary DDF tendonitis within the hoof capsule has been identified most commonly in horses that jump,[12-14] but it has also been seen in general-purpose riding horses. Lameness usually is unilateral, acute in onset, and moderate to severe in intensity. In horses with severe lameness, the horse may point the affected limb at rest. In mild to moderate injuries, lameness may resolve with rest but recur with work and progressively worsen.

There are generally no clinically significant palpable abnormalities of the limb, unless the lesion extends proximally into the pastern region. There is also no response to pressure applied to the foot with hoof testers. Lameness is often worse on a soft surface, especially on a circle, and in some horses is apparent only under these circumstances. A core lesion in the lateral lobe results in lameness worst with the lame limb on the outside of a circle, whereas a medial lobe lesion usually results in lameness worst with the lame limb on the inside of a circle. The response to distal limb flexion is variable; flexion of the nonlame limb may exacerbate lameness in the lame limb. Extension of the distal interphalangeal joint using the board or wedge test may accentuate the lameness.

LOCAL ANALGESIA

Perineural analgesia of the palmar digital nerves immediately proximal to the cartilages of the foot usually, but not invariably, improves lameness; however, rarely is lameness fully alleviated. Perineural analgesia of the palmar nerves at the level of the base of the proximal sesamoid bones usually abolishes the lameness. Intraarticular analgesia of the distal interphalangeal joint results in rapid improvement in lameness in some horses, but in others lameness persists unchanged. There has been no correlation between the analgesic response and the proximodistal site of the lesion.[12] Analgesia of the navicular bursa often results in improvement in lameness but rarely alleviates it fully. Intrathecal analgesia of the digital flexor tendon sheath may result in improvement in lameness, but this technique is not specific for DDFT lesions and does not reliably alter lameness associated with lesions confined to the insertion.

DIAGNOSTIC IMAGING

Radiography

In some lateromedial radiographic images of the foot a faint outline of the DDFT can be seen; the clinical significance of this finding is unknown. Occasionally a focus of mineralization is seen within the DDFT, at the level of or proximal to the navicular bone, and usually reflects chronic DDFT injury. In a well-positioned, high-detail lateromedial image, entheseous new bone or a radiolucent focus may be identified on the facies flexoria of the distal phalanx. This finding has been seen more commonly in heavier Warmblood breeds[16] than in Thoroughbred and cross-bred horses and has been correlated with increased bone activity identified by nuclear scintigraphy.

Ultrasonography

Diagnostic ultrasonographic imaging of the DDFT within the hoof capsule is not easy because of the horny hoof capsule and the difficulties in orientating the ultrasound transducer perpendicular to the line of the tendon fibers. Thus it is easy to create artifacts. The proximal part of the DDFT may be imaged using a 6.5-MHz transducer positioned between the bulbs of the heel, unless the heel is very contracted. The region of the DDFT overlying the navicular bone and close to its insertion is potentially seen by a solar approach, placing the transducer (7.5 MHz) on the frog. The frog must be sufficiently soft; this generally is achieved by soaking the foot by bandaging a water-soaked sponge on the foot for several hours. If the horn is exceptionally hard, soaking may have to be continued for several days. The horn must also be pared to provide a relatively flat site for placement of the ultrasound transducer. This is difficult to achieve if the horse has a very narrow foot with a deep frog cleft and sulci. Only the region of the DDFT in the midsagittal plane can be successfully imaged. Orientation is achieved most easily in longitudinal images.

A normal DDFT has linear, parallel echoes, and its margins are well defined.[20] An anechoic region representing fluid in the navicular bursa is interposed between the DDFT and the echoic line of the palmar aspect of the navicular bone. Lesions are characterized by enlargement of the tendon and thus loss of its parallel margins. Fiber pattern cannot be assessed, but the presence of mineralization can be detected. Lesions extending into the pastern region may be seen as core lesions, but false-negative results may occur. However, identification of a core lesion in the pastern is generally associated with a lesion that extends further distally.

Nuclear Scintigraphy

Pool and bone phase nuclear scintigraphic lateral and solar images of the foot have been used to identify a region of IRU either at the site of insertion of the DDFT on the facies flexoria of the distal phalanx or further proximally within the DDFT[12,18] (Figures 32-1 and 32-2). Superimposition of a lateromedial radiographic image and a lateral scintigraphic image helps to accurately locate the site of increased

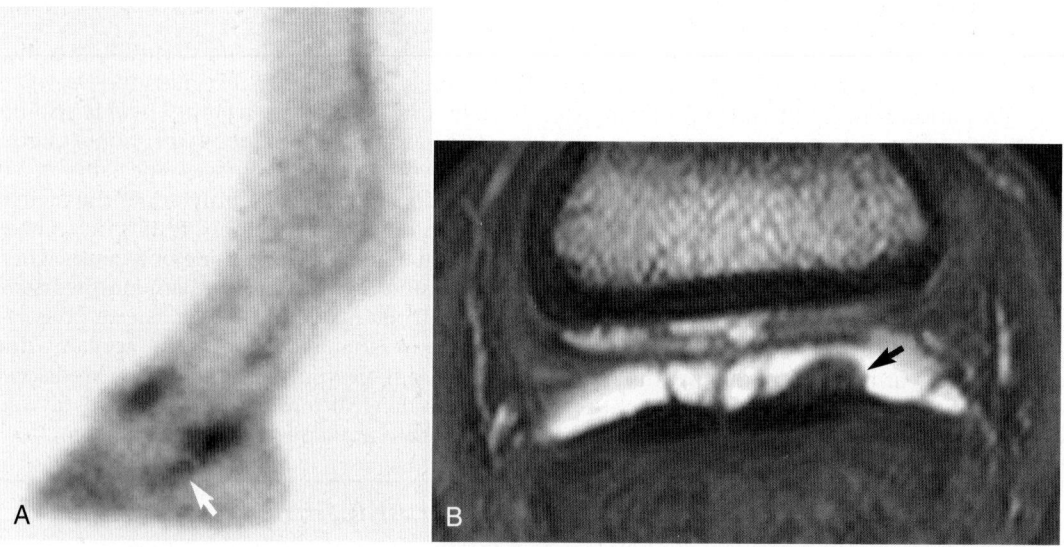

Fig. 32-1 • **A,** Lateral pool phase scintigraphic image of the left front foot of a 9-year-old event horse with a history of acute-onset severe lameness after competing. Lameness had persisted despite rest for 3 weeks. Lameness was improved by perineural analgesia of the palmar digital nerves or intraarticular analgesia of the distal interphalangeal joint, but it was not affected by analgesia of the navicular bursa. There is linear increased radiopharmaceutical uptake *(arrow)* in the region of the deep digital flexor tendon (DDFT). Magnetic resonance imaging demonstrated multifocal lesions of the DDFT. **B,** Transverse three-dimensional T2*-weighted gradient-echo magnetic resonance image of the same foot in **A,** at the level of the middle phalanx. Medial is to the left. There is a lesion of the dorsal aspect of the lateral lobe of the DDFT, with granulation tissue *(arrow)* protruding into the distended navicular bursa.

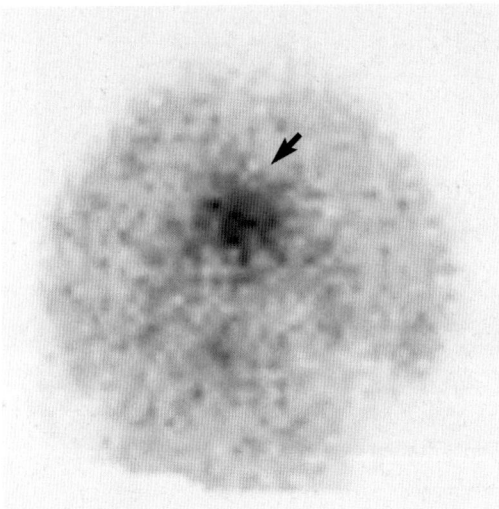

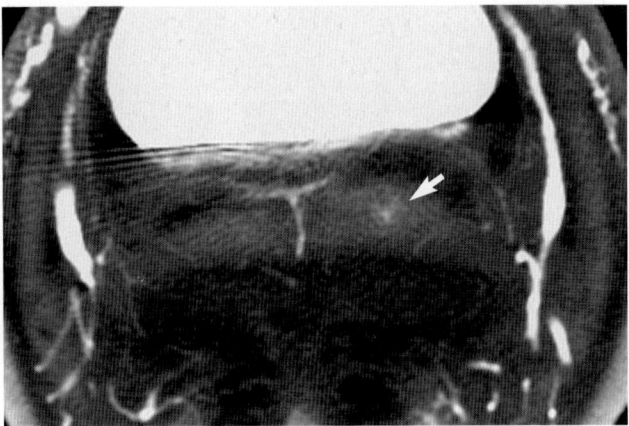

Fig. 32-3 • Transverse, contrast-enhanced computed tomographic image at the level of the middle phalanx *(MP)*. Medial is to the left. The lateral lobe of the deep digital flexor tendon is enlarged and has a central focal increase in signal density *(arrow)*.

Fig. 32-2 • Solar (palmar) bone phase scintigraphic image of the left front foot of a 7-year-old show jumper with acute-onset, chronic left forelimb lameness that was alleviated by perineural analgesia of the palmar digital nerves. There is a focal region of intensely increased radiopharmaceutical uptake in the distal phalanx at the site of the insertion of the deep digital flexor tendon (DDFT) *(arrow)*. Post mortem examination revealed focal bone necrosis and reactive bone at this site associated with the insertion of the DDFT.

radiopharmaceutical uptake. Although the bone phase solar (palmar) view may be more sensitive for identification of abnormal modeling associated with insertional stress, false-positive results may occur.[17]

The results from pool phase lateral images have correlated well with findings using MRI, arthroscopic evaluation of the DDFT through the navicular bursa, and post mortem studies. However, the presence of IRU at the DDFT insertion on the distal phalanx does not necessarily reflect an insertional injury; tendon lesions may be restricted to proximal to the navicular bone.[18]

Computed Tomography

Computed tomography (CT) can only be performed with the horse under general anesthesia but has the potential to give information about the size, shape, and internal architecture of the DDFT within the hoof capsule. Therefore it is an accurate method of diagnosis of primary DDFT lesions. Lesions have been identified in one or both of the two lobes of the DDFT and were seen as an enlargement of the DDFT with an increase or decrease in density[21,22] (Figure 32-3). Thirteen of 78 horses examined using CT had abnormalities of the DDFT within the hoof.[21] Correlation of an abnormal CT scan result with abnormalities verified at post mortem examination has been described without clinical details.[21] The use of a contrast agent can facilitate identification of relevant lesions and may be helpful in determining the chronicity of the lesion. CT also provides the opportunity to perform image-guided intervention, such as injection of a core lesion.[22]

Magnetic Resonance Imaging

MRI can be performed either with the horse under general anesthesia or in a standing sedated horse, and offers the optimal method of diagnosis of primary DDFT lesions[12-14,23] (Figures 32-4 and 32-5). Lesions are seen best in sagittal and transverse planes. Most core lesions are visible in T1- and T2-weighted images and fat-suppressed images and are characterized by increased signal intensity extending a variable distance proximodistally, often associated with enlargement of a cross-sectional area of the affected lobe. Fat-suppressed two-dimensional fast spin-echo or three-dimensional gradient-echo sequences also are useful for detection of bone pathology at the insertion. Dorsal core lesions within the navicular bursa are often covered dorsally by granulation-like tissue.

Most primary DDFT lesions have been identified immediately proximal to the navicular bone, extending a variable distance proximally, to as far as the proximal aspect of the proximal phalanx.[14] Such lesions are often not detectable using ultrasonography. A smaller proportion of lesions have been identified at the insertion of the DDFT. Lesions usually are restricted to either the medial or the lateral lobe, but occasionally they occur in both lobes. Core lesions or dorsal fiber disruption, sometimes with herniation of fibers and granulation tissue into the navicular bursa, are most common. Focal, full-thickness, sagittal plane splits have also been seen at the level of the navicular bone in association with abnormal signal intensity in the palmar cortex of the bone. Seventy-five of 347 horses (21.6%) with palmar foot pain of previously undetermined cause had primary DDFT injuries diagnosed using MRI.[19] A further 40 horses had combined lesions of the navicular bone and DDFT.

Correlation of the results of MRI examination of cadaver specimens from horses with clinically suspected DDFT lesions and post mortem examination has been good[9-11] (see Figure 32-5). Collagen necrosis and chondroid metaplasia within the DDFT have been seen in regions of increased signal intensity.[9-11] Care must be taken in the interpretation of sagittal plane images in the region of insertion of the DDFT in T1- and T2-weighted high-field magnetic resonance images because there is increased signal intensity in normal horses. This is related in part to the composition of the tendon but also to the magic angle effect, which results from orientation of fibers at approximately 55 degrees to the static magnetic field (see Figure 32-5).

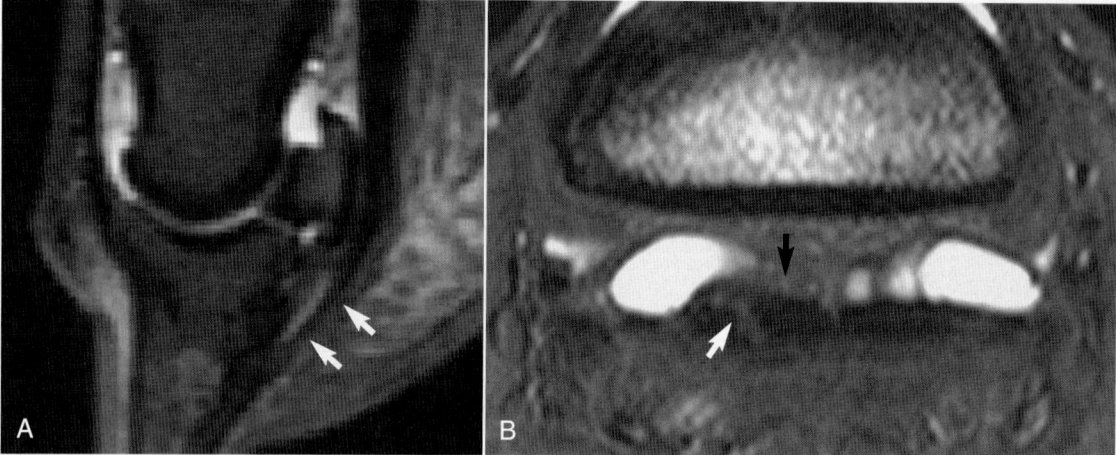

Fig. 32-4 • A, Sagittal short tau inversion recovery magnetic resonance image of a left front foot. There is swelling of the distal aspect of the deep digital flexor tendon (DDFT), which has diffuse increase in signal intensity. **B,** Transverse three-dimensional T2*-weighted, gradient-echo magnetic resonance image of the left front foot of a 9-year-old medium-level dressage horse, with lameness improved by palmar digital analgesia and abolished by perineural analgesia of the palmar (abaxial sesamoid) nerves. There is a core lesion of the DDFT characterized by increased signal intensity *(white arrow)* and some soft tissue proliferation within the navicular bursa *(black arrow)*.

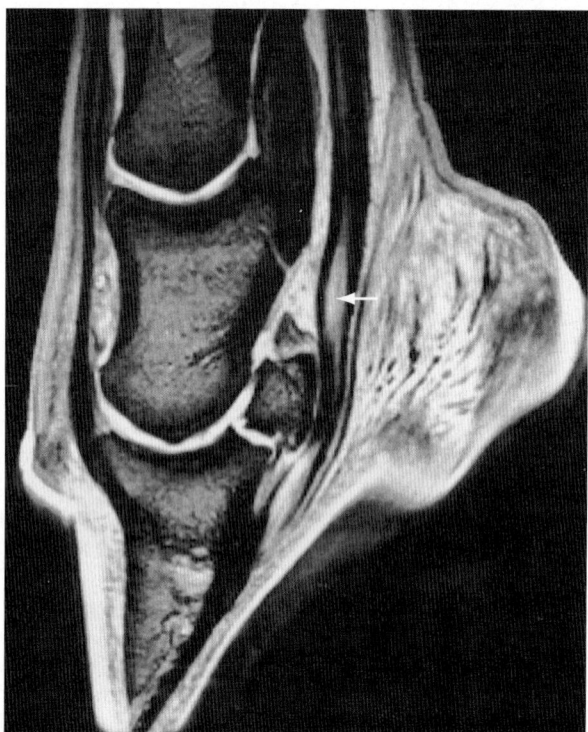

Fig. 32-5 • Sagittal spoiled gradient-echo magnetic resonance image of the right front foot of an advanced event horse with acute-onset severe lameness that was alleviated by perineural analgesia of the palmar digital nerves and improved by intraarticular analgesia of the distal interphalangeal joint. The deep digital flexor tendon (DDFT) is enlarged and has increased signal intensity proximal to the navicular bone *(arrow)*. This correlated with an extensive core lesion at post mortem examination. Increased signal intensity in the DDFT and distal sesamoidean impar ligament distal to the navicular bone reflects the magic angle effect.

SURGICAL EXPLORATION

Endoscopic examination of the digital flexor tendon sheath and the navicular bursa allows visual evaluation of the surface of the DDFT and assessment of its integrity by probing (see Chapter 24). Some dorsal core lesions of the DDFT are associated with extensive surface fibrillation of the tendon and inflammation of the synovial lining of the navicular bursa with villous proliferation. However, this technique is invasive and provides only limited information about the internal architecture of the tendon, although it does offer the option of surgical debridement of dorsal lesions.

TREATMENT

Successful treatment of horses with core lesions of the DDFT remains a challenge. Core necrosis can ultimately repair by fibroplasia; however, long-term follow-up studies to date indicate a high rate of recurrent lameness after prolonged periods (6-12 months) of box rest and controlled exercise and corrective trimming and shoeing.[19,24] Lesions often reduce in size, but usually there is persistent high signal intensity on T1-weighted magnetic resonance images. Twenty-nine per cent of 84 horses returned to full athletic function for a period of more than 6 months and up to 4 years.[24] In a separate study 25% of 55 horses returned to full athletic function. Lesion type or proximodistal location did not appear to influence prognosis.[25] Longer-term follow-up evaluation indicates that rest for a minimum of 12 to 18 months may result in an improved outcome.[26,27] Surgical debridement of dorsal core lesions within the navicular bursa was successful in 54% of 63 horses,[28,29] but with relatively short follow-up time. This technique is only of use for dorsal lesions, not central core lesions or large splits in the DDFT. Complications have included recurrent lameness associated with adhesion formation within the navicular bursa. CT-guided injections of the DDFT have been performed using a variety of preparations (A cell, platelet-rich plasma, stem cells), but long-term follow-up information is not yet available. Short-term improvement may be seen after medication of the navicular bursa and/or digital flexor tendon sheath with corticosteroids, but repeated injections may predispose to progression of lesions.

ferences
on page
1274

Chapter 33

The Distal Phalanx and Distal Interphalangeal Joint

Sue J. Dyson

◼ PRIMARY PAIN ASSOCIATED WITH THE DISTAL INTERPHALANGEAL JOINT

FUNCTIONAL ANATOMY

The distal interphalangeal (DIP) joint is a complex structure comprising not only the articulation between the middle and distal phalanges, with supporting collateral ligaments, but also the articulation with the navicular bone. It has a close relationship with the distal sesamoidean impar ligament (DSIL) and the collateral sesamoidean ligaments. The DSIL consists of bundles of longitudinally orientated collagen fibers, interspersed by synovial invaginations from the DIP joint and penetrating blood vessels.

The DIP joint can move in three planes with flexion and extension movements in the sagittal plane, lateromedial movements in the frontal plane, and rotation and sliding in the transverse plane.[1,2] During normal load bearing and propulsion on a flat, level surface, DIP joint movement is principally flexion and extension. On an uneven surface and a circle, or if the foot is unbalanced, passive movements result in the distal phalanx sliding and twisting relative to the middle phalanx. Movement is restricted by the collateral ligaments of the DIP joint, the deep digital flexor tendon (DDFT), the distal digital annular ligament, the DSIL, and collateral sesamoidean ligaments. The degree of sliding and axial rotation within the DIP joint[3] may predispose the horse to DIP joint injury and may explain why lameness associated with the DIP joint frequently is accentuated on a circle.

HISTORY

Lameness associated with the DIP joint may be acute or insidious in onset and unilateral or bilateral. It is more common in forelimbs than in hindlimbs but does occur in both. Lameness in horses with unilateral disease tends to be sudden in onset, but those with bilateral lameness may be evaluated because of poor performance (e.g., shortened stride, unwillingness to jump drop fences, or unwillingness to land with one forelimb leading).

CLINICAL SIGNS

The DIP joint capsule often is distended unilaterally or bilaterally. Distention of the joint capsule also can occur in clinically sound horses; therefore this finding is not pathognomonic for DIP joint pain. However, chronic distention does reflect synovitis, and treatment may reduce the risk of future problems. It is possible that chronic distention can predispose to low-grade instability of the joint. The dorsal proximal outpouching of the joint capsule can be palpated on the distal dorsal aspect of the pastern. Distention may result in obvious swelling, but it may be difficult to appreciate unless the horse has a fine hair coat. When distention of the joint capsule is present, ballottement of fluid from medial to lateral of the dorsal midline should be possible. The degree of distention may vary according to the recent work history.

Pain may be present on flexion or rotation of the distal limb joints. However, a marked reaction to distal limb flexion more likely reflects metacarpophalangeal joint pain. Mediolateral, dorsopalmar, or both types of foot imbalance are frequent findings and are considered important predisposing factors for the development of DIP joint pain. The degree of lameness varies depending on the nature of the underlying pathological change, recent work history, and whether lameness is unilateral or bilateral. With bilateral DIP joint pain the horse may move just a bit "flat" with a slightly shorter than normal stride. Severe lameness may reflect trauma to one of the supporting soft tissue structures of the joint. Lameness may be accentuated by distal limb flexion or rotation of the distal limb joints, but the response is variable. Lameness often is worse on a circle, especially on a hard surface, with the lamest limb either on the inside or outside of the circle.

DIAGNOSIS

Local Analgesia

Pain associated with the DIP joint often improves after perineural analgesia of the palmar digital nerves and sometimes is alleviated fully. However, in some horses perineural analgesia of the palmar nerves at the level of the base of the proximal sesamoid bones is required to completely eliminate lameness.

Intraarticular analgesia of the DIP joint is not specific for pain that affects the joint itself. The potential exists for relief of pain from the navicular bone, the DSIL and the DDFT and their insertions on the distal phalanx, the palmar processes of the distal phalanx,[4] and the sole, even at the toe.[5,6] A standard approach is suggested to aid in interpretation of the response. A maximum volume of 6 mL of local anesthetic solution should be used. After injection through a dorsal midline approach, the horse should stand still until reassessment 5 minutes after injection. The clinician should ascertain whether sensation remains around the coronary band and whether any response to hoof testers has been eliminated to determine the specificity of the block. Lameness caused by primary DIP joint pain usually improves rapidly and substantially after intraarticular analgesia. If the lameness persists, the veterinarian should reassess the horse after an additional 5 minutes. If lameness is still apparent, the DIP joint is not a likely primary source of pain. However, after this time the block still could result in further improvement in lameness as the local anesthetic solution diffuses to adjacent structures, thereby potentially confounding the response to any other block performed at this stage.[4,7] Intraarticular analgesia of the DIP joint can substantially improve lameness associated with navicular disease within 5 minutes of injection,[8,9] although 20% of horses with navicular bone pain had a negative response to intraarticular analgesia of the DIP joint.[8] Therefore the result of intraarticular analgesia of the DIP joint is best interpreted compared with the response to analgesia of the navicular bursa.[7,8] Intraarticular analgesia of the DIP joint may not relieve pain associated with a primary injury of one of the collateral ligaments, although improvement may be seen if there is concurrent synovitis or osteoarthritis (OA).

A slight or negative response to intraarticular analgesia of the DIP joint does not eliminate completely a response to treatment of the joint, especially if the joint capsule is distended. For example, medication of the joint with hyaluronan and triamcinolone acetonide (10 mg) sometimes may resolve lameness that was not altered by intraarticular analgesia.

Retrieval of synovial fluid from the DIP joint depends on the synovial fluid pressure and position of the needle. Using a dorsal approach to the joint and a 20-gauge needle, synovial fluid usually appears spontaneously in the needle hub and, if the joint capsule is distended, may flow out under pressure. Relief of this pressure may help to resolve lameness. However, not all horses with considerable pressure within the DIP joint respond to intraarticular analgesia or medication. The pressure within the DIP joint also increases if the contralateral limb is picked up; therefore if the contralateral limb is picked up to aid restraint of the horse for injection of the DIP joint of the ipsilateral limb, a tendency for backflow through the needle puncture site may occur until the contralateral limb is placed on the ground.

Imaging Techniques
Radiography
Comprehensive radiographic examination of the DIP joint should include weight-bearing dorsopalmar, lateromedial, dorsoproximal-palmarodistal oblique, and flexed dorsolateral-palmaromedial and dorsomedial-palmarolateral oblique images of the interphalangeal joints.[10] Because intraarticular analgesia may influence pain associated with the palmar processes of the distal phalanx and the navicular bone, these structures also should be evaluated carefully.

The shape of the extensor process of the distal phalanx varies considerably among horses on lateromedial images (Figure 33-1), but the shape usually is bilaterally symmetrical.[10] Modeling changes of the extensor process can be present without associated lameness. Care should be taken in interpretation of the bony prominences on the distal

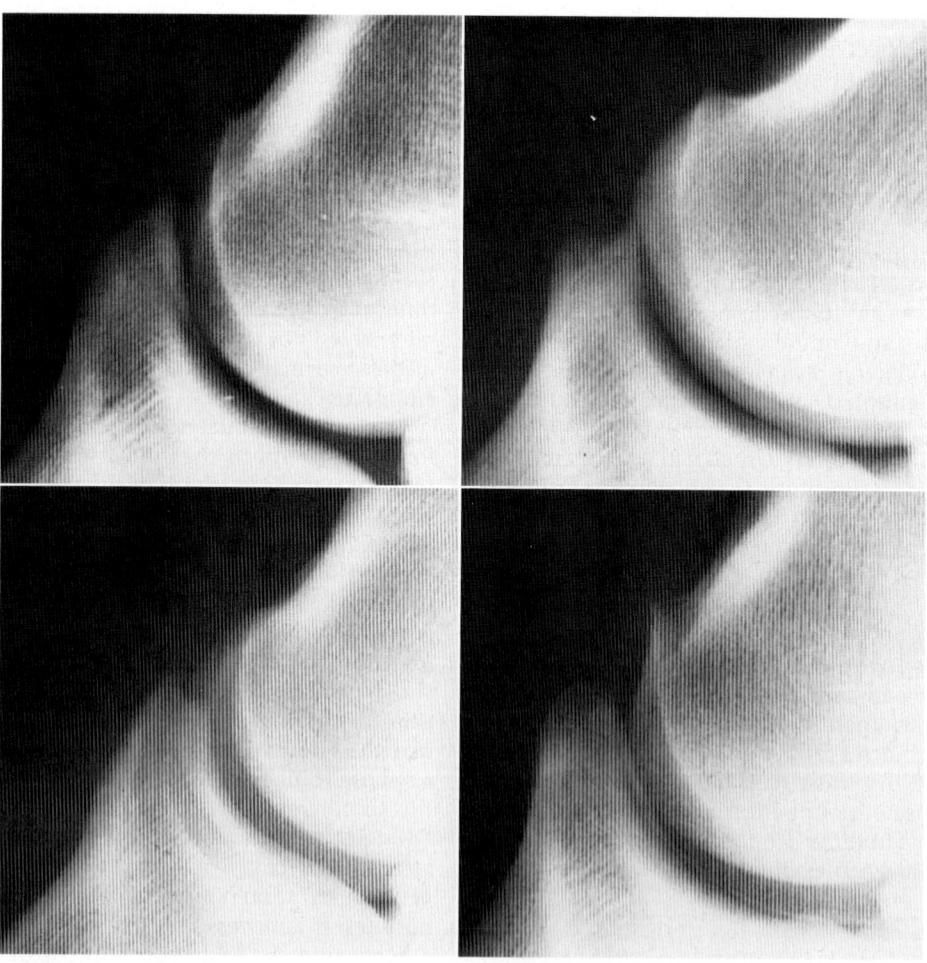

Fig. 33-1 • Lateromedial radiographic images of the extensor process of normal distal phalanges. Note the variability in shape.

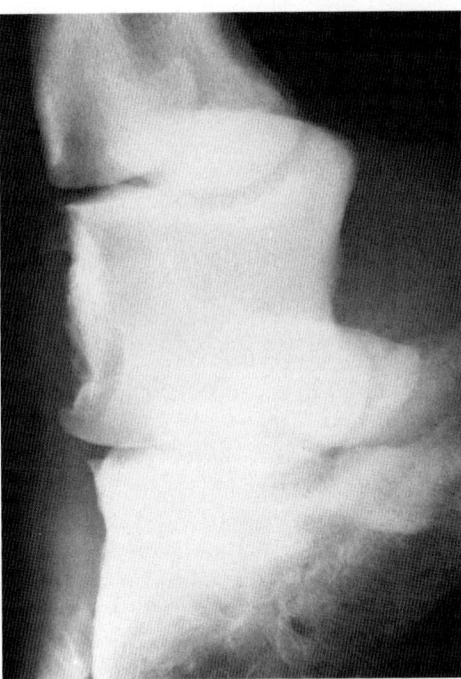

Fig. 33-2 • Flexed dorsal 60° lateral-palmaromedial oblique radiographic image of the distal interphalangeal joint. There are modeling changes of the articular margins of both the distal interphalangeal and proximal interphalangeal joints.

medial and lateral aspects of the middle phalanx, which always appear larger in bigger-boned horses. Entheseous new bone at the origins of the collateral ligaments can be seen as an incidental finding. The DIP joint should be inspected carefully for recognition of small osteophytes on the distal palmar aspect of the middle phalanx and the dorsoproximal aspect of the navicular bone. Joint space congruity and the shape of the proximal articular surface of the distal phalanx should be assessed carefully. A smoothly outlined depression sometimes is seen in the middle of the proximal articular surface of the distal phalanx in clinically normal horses.

The flexed oblique radiographic images—dorsal 60° lateral-palmaromedial oblique and dorsal 60° medial-palmarolateral oblique—enhance detection of periarticular new bone (Figure 33-2) modeling of the distal aspect of the middle phalanx and entheseous new bone at the origin of the collateral ligaments of the DIP joint. Care is needed to differentiate between periarticular osteophytes and entheseous new bone at the insertion of the digital extensor tendon. Evaluation of the integrity and thickness of the subchondral bone plate of the middle and distal phalanges is important. Discontinuity of the subchondral bone plate may be the first radiological sign of the development of an osseous cystlike lesion. Increased thickness of the subchondral bone plate may occur with OA.

New bone also may develop on the dorsal aspect of the diaphysis of the middle phalanx. Smoothly outlined new bone usually is subsynovial and clinically insignificant, whereas active-appearing, pallisading new bone usually is associated with lameness. Palisading is one of the earliest radiological signs but often is missed. The dorsal cortex of the middle phalanx may develop increased radiopacity (thicker), and early proliferative new bone may be seen.

Small, well-rounded mineralized opacities on the dorsoproximal aspect of the distal phalanx are not uncommon and may be present unassociated with clinical signs. Large mobile pieces are more likely to be associated with lameness.

The distal border of the navicular bone also should be evaluated carefully because the radiolucent zones along the distal border represent synovial invaginations from the DIP joint. An increase in size and number of these lucent zones has been observed with chronic synovitis of the DIP joint.

Ultrasonography

Diagnostic ultrasonography with a 7.5- to 13-MHz transducer and a standoff is invaluable for assessment of the dorsal pouch of the DIP joint, the amount of fluid within the joint, and the presence of synovial proliferation. Assessment of the palmar pouch is much more difficult, and evaluation of the articular cartilage is extremely limited. The structure of the proximal aspect of the collateral ligaments of the DIP joint proximal to the hoof capsule can be assessed,[11,12] as well as the chondrocompedal, chondrocoronal, and distal digital annular ligaments. Using a transcuneal approach, the insertion of the DSIL can be assessed.[13]

Nuclear Scintigraphy

Nuclear scintigraphy has been useful in the identification of horses with DIP joint capsule and subchondral bone trauma. It appears to be rather insensitive to the identification of OA unless the disease is advanced.[14] Increased radiopharmaceutical uptake (IRU) is best detected in lateral images.

Diagnostic Arthroscopy

The dorsal and palmar pouches of the DIP joint may be inspected arthroscopically; however, the view of joint surfaces is limited, and complete assessment of the integrity of the articular cartilage is not possible (see Figure 23-5). Access may be enhanced after joint trauma with resultant instability of the joint. Affected horses usually develop long-term lameness problems. Lavage of the joint may be beneficial therapeutically in some horses with chronic DIP joint pain without joint instability. A limited view of the DSIL can be seen from the navicular bursa.

Magnetic Resonance Imaging

Sagittal, frontal, and transverse magnetic resonance (MR) images of the DIP joint permit excellent evaluation of the articular cartilage and subchondral bone of the joint and the dorsal and palmar pouches of the DIP joint capsule (Figure 33-3). The DSIL, DDFT, collateral sesamoidean ligaments, and the navicular bone and bursa also may be assessed. Magnetic resonance imaging (MRI) is the imaging modality of choice for horses with chronic DIP joint pain that does not respond adequately to medical treatment.

DIFFERENTIAL DIAGNOSIS OF PRIMARY DISTAL INTERPHALANGEAL JOINT PAIN

Synovitis

The most common cause of DIP joint pain is synovitis, which may occur unilaterally or bilaterally. Lameness is mild to moderate in degree, and palpable distention of the

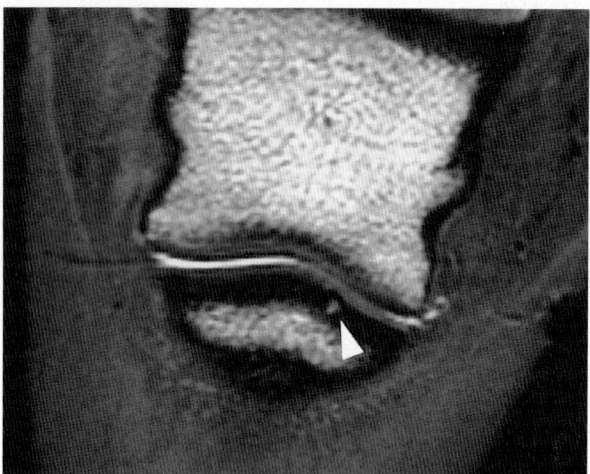

Fig. 33-3 • Dorsal three-dimensional T2* gradient-echo magnetic resonance image of the left hind foot of a riding horse with lameness of 3 months' duration. The lameness was completely resolved by intraarticular analgesia. Radiological examination was negative; scintigraphy revealed focal increased radiopharmaceutical uptake in the proximal aspect of the distal phalanx. A focal lesion is present in the subchondral bone plate of the distal phalanx (arrow).

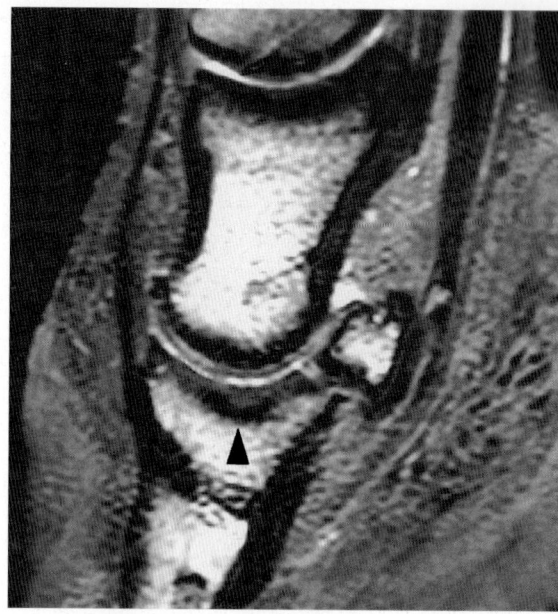

Fig. 33-4 • Sagittal three-dimensional T2* gradient-echo magnetic resonance image of the foot of a Grand Prix show jumper. There is loss of the normal homogeneous signal in the cartilage of the distal interphalangeal joint and irregularities in the subchondral bone in the center of the distal phalanx (arrow). Mild periarticular osteophyte formation was evident on radiographs. Scintigraphic examination was unremarkable.

DIP joint capsule usually is present. Intraarticular analgesia generally resolves the lameness. Treatment should be directed to identification of any predisposing causes. Corrective trimming to restore correct foot balance and appropriate shoeing are essential for successful management. Horses with a collapsed heel usually benefit substantially from properly fitted egg bar shoes (see Figure 30-18). The timing of trimming and shoeing can be crucial: if the feet are allowed to get too long, soreness may return.

In my experience, systemic administration of hyaluronan is generally of limited benefit in the initial treatment of horses with acute or chronic lameness, but it may have a role in longer-term management. Intraarticular medication using hyaluronan, with or without short-acting corticosteroids (e.g., triamcinolone acetonide) or polysulfated glycosaminoglycans (PSGAG), is the most effective treatment method. In horses with acute synovitis with only mild lameness, a single treatment with hyaluronan alone may be sufficient, but if the lameness is more severe or chronic, better results may be achieved with a combination of triamcinolone acetonide and hyaluronan. Improvement usually is evident within 5 days of treatment. If lameness persists, better results may be achieved by two additional injections using hyaluronan alone at weekly intervals. Intraarticular treatment with PSGAG is contraindicated if acute inflammation is present, but in horses with more chronic lameness, good results have been achieved using serial (up to five) weekly treatments.[15,16] PSGAG used systemically may be useful for longer-term management. Treatment is followed by walking for 7 days and then a progressive resumption of work after the final treatment. In some horses, intraarticular therapy results in long-term resolution of the problem. Others require repeated treatments at intervals as needed.

Care is necessary during injection of the DIP joint to avoid puncturing the large vessels on the distodorsal aspect of the pastern. Puncture tends to cause localized fibrosis, and future injections are more difficult. With excellent technique, the DIP joint will tolerate well many injections, and the prognosis for future soundness is good.

Osteoarthritis

Osteoarthritis without Radiological Abnormalities

Scintigraphy may be useful in the diagnosis of early subchondral lesions associated with OA. The definitive diagnosis of OA without radiological abnormalities is possible premortem only by MRI (Figure 33-4). Horses may have signs similar to those of primary synovitis, but the degree of lameness may be more severe, especially if the horse is exerted maximally, and the response to intraarticular medication tends to be shorter and less complete. MRI may show a reduced signal intensity within the articular cartilage of the DIP joint, in addition to irregularity in the cartilage surface, with or without concurrent abnormalities in the subchondral bone. The prognosis for sustained future soundness is guarded.

Osteoarthritis with Radiological Abnormalities

Correlation is lacking between modeling in the region of the extensor process of the distal phalanx and lameness associated with the DIP joint. Enthesophytes at the site of insertion of the common digital extensor tendon should be differentiated from osteophytes. Enthesophytes may not be associated with current lameness, but may reflect chronic instability of the joint. The presence of periarticular osteophytes on the distodorsal and palmar aspects of the middle phalanx and the proximal articular surface of the navicular bone is more likely to be associated with lameness (Figures 33-5 and 33-6). Radiological evidence of OA of the DIP joint can be seen with other causes of lameness, such as navicular disease. Horses with primary OA of

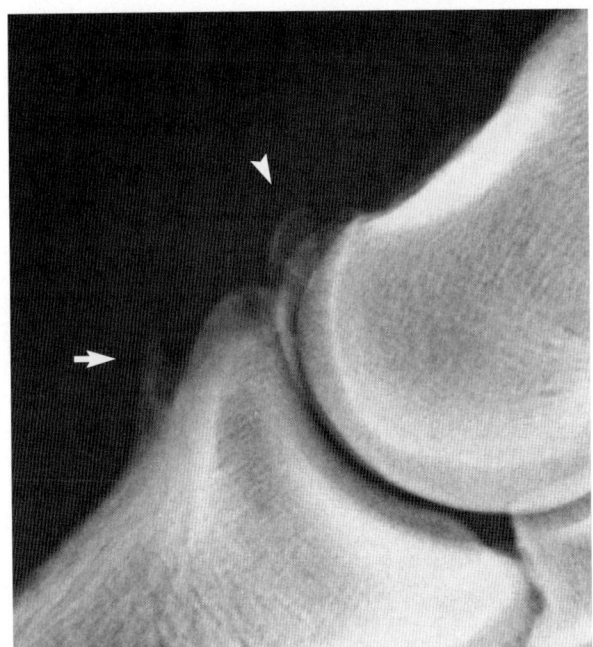

Fig. 33-5 • Lateromedial radiographic image of the distal interphalangeal joint of a 7-year-old pleasure horse. Marked enthesophyte formation is present on the dorsoproximal aspect of the distal phalanx at the insertion of the common digital extensor tendon *(arrow)*. In addition, there is a well-rounded fragment on the dorsal aspect of the distal interphalangeal joint *(arrowhead)* and modeling of the extensor process of the distal phalanx.

the DIP joint may respond better to serial treatments with PSGAG than treatment with hyaluronan and corticosteroids.[15,16] However, if concurrent severe synovitis is present, primary treatment with triamcinolone acetonide and hyaluronan, followed by intraarticular PSGAG, may yield the best results. In my experience, better results are achieved in horses that are sound after intraarticular analgesia compared with horses that show partial improvement in lameness. Prognosis usually is inversely related to the severity of the radiological abnormalities.[7]

Traumatic Damage to Articular Cartilage

Sudden onset of unilateral lameness may be related to traumatic damage to the articular cartilage of the DIP joint, with or without other concurrent soft tissue damage. Definitive diagnosis is possible only with MRI. Intraarticular medication may provide temporary relief of clinical signs, but the long-term prognosis is guarded.

Joint Capsule Trauma

Traumatic damage to the joint capsule, with or without subchondral bone trauma, usually results in sudden-onset, severe lameness that persists despite rest. Lameness may be accentuated markedly when the horse turns. In the acute stage, no abnormalities are detected on radiographic examination. However, periarticular new bone may develop after several weeks (Figure 33-7). Nuclear scintigraphic examination may show generalized increased radiopharmaceutical uptake in the region of the DIP joint (Figure 33-8). Arthroscopic evaluation in these horses has been

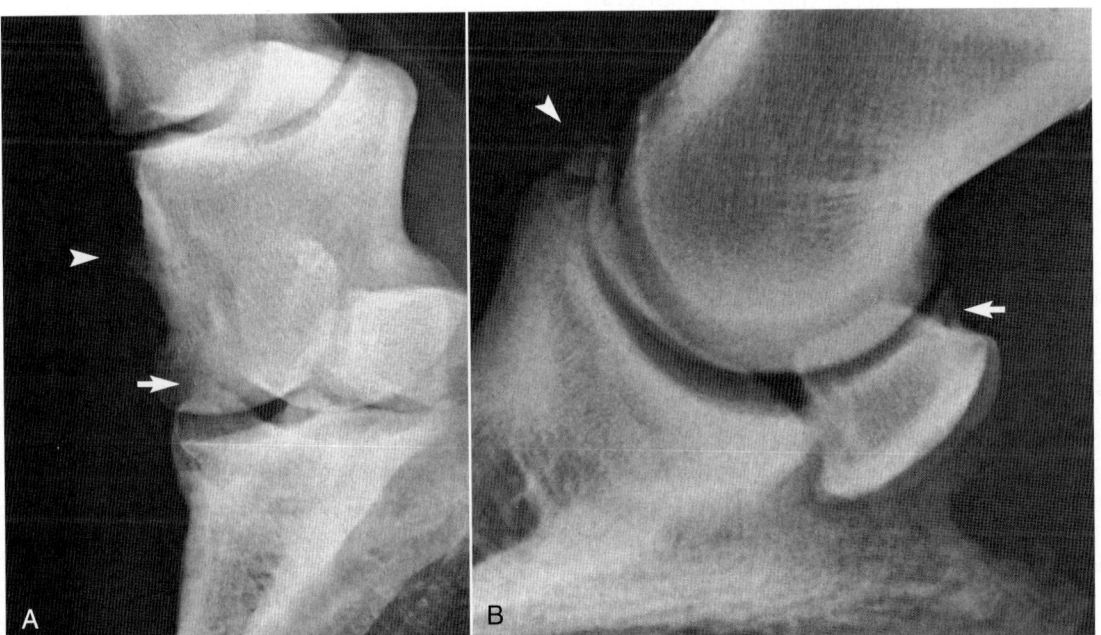

Fig. 33-6 • **A,** Dorsolateral-palmaromedial oblique radiographic image of a flexed distal interphalangeal joint of an 8-year-old show jumper with bilateral forelimb lameness improved by intraarticular analgesia of the distal interphalangeal joints. There is modeling of the proximal articular margin of the distal phalanx *(arrow)*, radiological evidence of osteoarthritis (compare with Figure 33-2). There is also enthesophyte formation on the dorsomedial aspect of the middle phalanx at the origin of the medial collateral ligament of the distal interphalangeal joint. No radiological abnormalities were seen in lateromedial or dorsopalmar radiographic images. **B,** Lateromedial radiographic image of the left front foot of a riding horse with lameness improved by intraarticular analgesia of the distal interphalangeal joint. An articular osteophyte is seen on the dorsoproximal aspect of the navicular bone *(arrow)*, and there is a fragment on the dorsal aspect of the distal interphalangeal joint *(arrowhead)*.

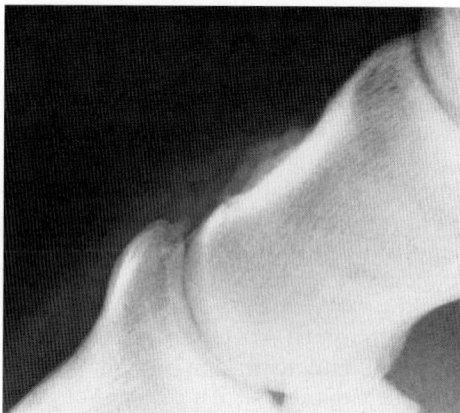

Fig. 33-7 • Lateromedial radiographic image of the left front foot of a 3-year-old Thoroughbred filly with severe lameness that improved substantially after intraarticular analgesia of the distal interphalangeal joint. Entheseous new bone is seen on the dorsal aspect of the middle phalanx, in addition to the small fragment at the extensor process of the distal phalanx. Nuclear scintigraphic examination had revealed a similar pattern of uptake of the radiopharmaceutical to that seen in Figure 33-8.

unrewarding. The response to intraarticular medication has been poor, and the prognosis for return to athletic function despite prolonged rest is guarded.

Subchondral Bone Trauma

Subchondral bone trauma may be focal or more generalized and usually is associated with unilateral lameness, which responds poorly to intraarticular medication and short periods of rest. No detectable radiological abnormalities may be apparent in the acute stage, although Ross[14] described subtle proliferative changes on the distal aspect of the middle phalanx and the proximal aspect of the distal phalanx and a variable degree of subchondral lucency in the proximal aspect of the distal phalanx. Nuclear scintigraphy may be helpful.[14] Several horses have been examined with acute-onset severe and persistent lameness, which was partially improved by intraarticular analgesia of the DIP joint. MRI has revealed a focal lesion in the proximal subchondral bone plate of the distal phalanx, usually axial and toward the palmar or plantar aspect (see Figure 33-3). Response to conservative management, with or without intraarticular medication or systemic treatment with tiludronate, has been poor.

Osseous Cystlike Lesions

Osseous cystlike lesions occur most often in the center of the proximal aspect of the distal phalanx, midway dorsal to palmar and axial.[17,18] They vary in size and the presence of visible communication with the DIP joint. Not all are detectable radiologically; some have been identified only either using MRI or at postmortem examination after a poor response to medical treatment of the DIP joint.[16] Horses with large osseous cystlike lesions may be asymptomatic but be lame at a later date. Lameness usually is unilateral, sudden in onset, and moderate to severe. Occasionally lameness is sporadic, but when present it is severe. Osseous cystlike lesions may occur in young immature horses and mature athletes. Not all osseous cystlike lesions that cause pain have active bone turnover; therefore nuclear scintigraphy may not be helpful in determining

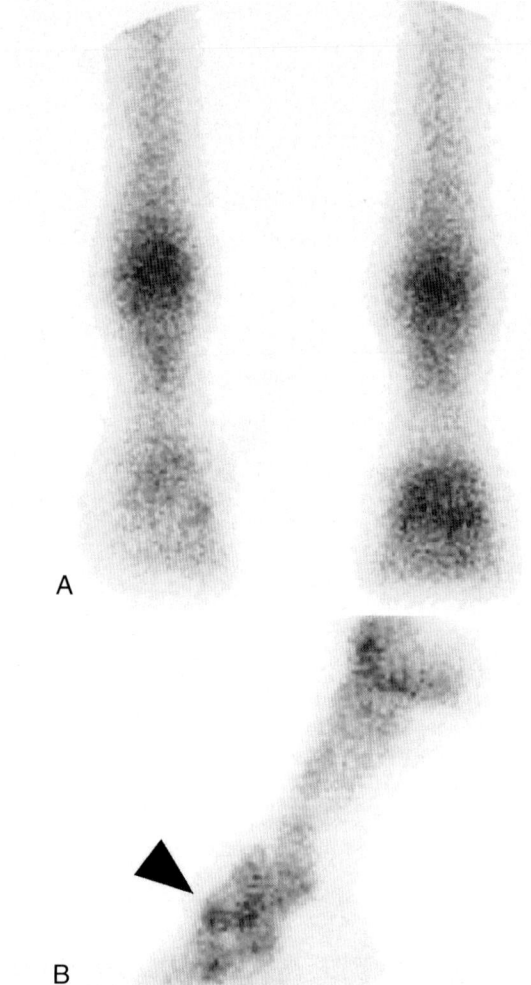

Fig. 33-8 • **A,** Dorsal nuclear scintigraphic image of the front feet of a 6-year-old show jumper with sudden-onset, severe lameness markedly improved by intraarticular analgesia of the distal interphalangeal joint. The left forelimb is on the right. Radiopharmaceutical uptake is increased in the subchondral bone of the distal interphalangeal joint. **B,** Lateral scintigraphic image of the left front foot shows increased uptake of the radiopharmaceutical centered on the distal interphalangeal joint *(arrow).* Slight periarticular new bone formation was evident radiologically. Arthroscopic evaluation revealed synovial proliferation. The horse remained lame.

whether a long-standing osseous cystlike lesion is the current cause of lameness. However, currently or recently developing osseous cystlike lesions usually are associated with marked increased bone activity and may be evident on nuclear scintigraphic scans before radiological evidence is evident. Conservative treatment may result in spontaneous resolution of the lameness, with or without resolution of the cyst, but in some horses lameness persists, with or without enlargement of the cyst. Arthroscopic access to a cyst usually may be limited if it is in the central portion of the distal phalanx. Therefore surgical debridement of a well-defined osseous cystlike lesion usually is performed through the hoof wall. Less commonly small osseous cystlike lesions are seen on the dorsoproximal aspect of the distal phalanx, palmar to the extensor process. Such cysts located more dorsally can be debrided arthroscopically. Prognosis depends in part on the integrity of the overlying articular cartilage, and lameness persists in some horses.[19,20]

Palisading New Bone on Dorsal Aspect of Middle Phalanx

Pain associated with the DIP joint occasionally is associated with new bone formation on the dorsal aspect of the middle phalanx. The origin of this new bone is unknown. Arthroscopic evaluation of the joint may reveal crumbly bone, which is easily debrided, with resolution of lameness in some horses.[21]

Osseous Fragments on the Dorsal Aspect of the Distal Interphalangeal Joint

Small osseous fragments on the dorsoproximal aspect of the extensor process of the distal phalanx may be seen in clinically normal horses. Some are pointed proximally with a flat base and look like the tip of the extensor process, whereas others are well rounded. These fragments may represent separate centers of ossification or may be a manifestation of osteochondrosis and can be incidental radiological findings. If the fragments are seen in association with DIP joint pain, the clinical significance should be interpreted with care. Arthroscopic removal should be considered only if medical therapy of the joint fails.

Fracture of Extensor Process of Distal Phalanx

Fractures of the extensor process of the distal phalanx are discussed in the next section.

Articular Chip Fracture of the Middle Phalanx

Articular chip fractures of the medial or lateral condyle of the distal aspect of the middle phalanx occasionally cause acute-onset lameness.[16] Such fractures can be detected only by flexed oblique radiographic images of the DIP joint. The prognosis after surgical removal is favorable provided joint stability has not been compromised. Surgical repair with arthroscopic guidance also is possible.

Injury of the Distal Sesamoidean Impar Ligament

Focal tears in the DSIL have been seen occasionally in association with sudden-onset, severe lameness that improves after intraarticular analgesia of the DIP joint. In horses with acute lameness, the synovial fluid may be hemorrhagic. Usually no radiological abnormalities are present. Definitive diagnosis is possible with MRI or arthroscopic evaluation of the navicular bursa.[4] The prognosis for athletic function is guarded. Rupture of a hindlimb DSIL with proximal displacement of the navicular bone has been described in a French steeplechase horse.[22] This horse was managed conservatively and did return to racing but then sustained an identical injury in the contralateral hindlimb.

More commonly, architectural changes of the DSIL reflecting chronic degenerative injury are seen in conjunction with other lesions of the podotrochlear apparatus, the navicular bursa, and sometimes the DDFT.[23,24] There may be an axial cluster of abnormally shaped and sized radiolucent zones in the distal border of the navicular bone. Distal border fragments of the navicular bone may also be associated with DSIL pathology.[25-28] Definitive diagnosis requires MRI. In low-field MR images the DSIL is difficult to evaluate because of thick slices and inferior resolution compared with high-field images. The presence of a cystic lesion in the distal third of the navicular bone, a distal border fragment, entheseous new bone at the insertion on the distal phalanx, or increased signal intensity at the insertion on the distal phalanx are good indicators of DSIL pathology.[26]

◼ FRACTURES AND FRAGMENTATION OF THE EXTENSOR PROCESS OF THE DISTAL PHALANX

HISTORY

Osteochondral fragments of the extensor process of the distal phalanx are classified as type IV fractures.[1-3] Small fragments may be traumatically induced or represent a separate center of ossification or may be a manifestation of osteochondrosis. Medium-sized fragments are considered as traumatically induced or separate centers of ossification[2] or a variation of the traumatically induced, nonunion fracture osseous bodies often observed in other locations on the distal phalanx in foals.[4] Very large pieces involving the dorsal quarter to third of the articular surface may be developmental,[5] although it has been suggested that such a fragment may be a sequela to an osseous cystlike lesion.[6]

These fragments involve predominantly the front feet, and lameness may be present. Small fragments can be seen as incidental radiological abnormalities. The fragments almost always are intraarticular, but they usually are nondisplaced to minimally displaced. Large fragments are most commonly seen in young horses, resulting in sudden-onset lameness soon after work commences. However, lameness may be unilateral despite the presence of fragments bilaterally.

CLINICAL AND IMAGING FINDINGS

Low-grade lameness may be present in horses with small fragments. Lameness alleviated by intraarticular analgesia of the DIP joint was present in 16 of 21 horses with osteochondral fragments.[3] Lameness may not develop until the horse is in full work when the presence of the fragment induces synovitis. The fragment is seen readily on a lateromedial radiographic image. Many fragments are removed prophylactically.[3]

Lameness associated with large fragments may be sudden in onset, although radiological abnormalities often appear chronic when lameness is first recognized. A strong fibrous union may maintain stability of the fragment until trauma causes minor fragment loosening. There is often marked increased radiopacity of the parent bone and extensive enthesophyte formation at the insertion of the common digital extensor tendon on the distal phalanx, reflecting chronic joint instability. In some horses the hoof shape becomes triangular or pyramidal; this clinical appearance has been described as *pyramidal disease* or *buttress foot.*[2]

TREATMENT AND PROGNOSIS

Removal of small fragments under arthroscopic guidance is a well-accepted treatment with a highly favorable prognosis.[3] Lameness resolved in 14 or 16 horses with lameness associated with a small fragment, and 5 of 5 horses remained sound after the fragment was removed prophylactically.[3] Horses can return to work within 2 weeks of fragment removal if surgery is prophylactic and at 10 weeks later if preoperative lameness was present.

Guidelines for treatment of horses with medium-sized fragments are less clear. Full recovery after internal fixation of these fragments was reported for two horses in four reports (six horses).[1,3-5] At least one horse had an acute fracture.[7] Fragment removal by dorsal midline arthrotomy has been reported in 14 horses with a successful outcome in 8 (57%).[1] Of the six horses with unfavorable results, preoperative duration of lameness exceeded 2 years in three horses, suggesting more favorable results might be expected if preoperative lameness duration were shorter. Horses usually return to full work by 4 months after surgery. Prognosis for large fragments is guarded.

◼ INJURIES OF THE COLLATERAL LIGAMENTS OF THE DISTAL INTERPHALANGEAL JOINT

Desmitis or desmopathy of the medial and/or lateral collateral ligament of the DIP joint results in a variable degree of unilateral or bilateral lameness in forelimbs or, less commonly, hindlimbs.[1-6] The injury is believed to be caused by the biomechanical forces of sliding and rotation of the joint (e.g., lateral sliding of the distal phalanx and medial rotation, which causes the medial collateral ligament to undergo great strain), sometimes superimposed on a primary degenerative lesion.[7,8] Degenerative changes are more prevalent toward the insertion of the ligament than farther proximally and include chondroid metaplasia and a unique fissuring necrosis, with cleft formation at the bone ligament interface. There may be osseous resorption at the insertion on the distal phalanx.[7] Medial injuries are more common than lateral, probably reflecting biomechanical loading. Severe damage to the body of the ligament results in obvious periligamentous soft tissue swelling and pain immediately proximal to the coronary band, but with many injuries there are no palpable abnormalities. Detection of joint instability is occasionally possible with severe injury. There is an association between extensive ossification of one or both cartilages of the foot and collateral ligament injury.[9]

In horses with severe lameness the caudal phase of the stride is shortened at the walk; at the walk the stance phase is longer than at the trot, resulting in increased extension of the DIP joint and greater stress on the collateral ligaments. At the trot lameness is generally much worse on a circle compared with straight lines, especially on a firm surface. In some horses lameness is improved by palmar digital nerve blocks, but in others palmar (abaxial sesamoid) nerve blocks are required to abolish the lameness. Intraarticular analgesia of the DIP joint may improve lameness if there is associated synovitis or secondary OA. In some horses desmitis of the body of the medial or lateral collateral ligament can be identified ultrasonographically and is characterized by enlargement in the cross-sectional area of the ligament and a diffuse reduction in echogenicity or a hypoechogenic core lesion, with or without thickening of the periligamentar soft tissues (Figure 33-9). Enthesophyte formation at the origin on the middle phalanx may also be seen ultrasonographically or radiologically (see Figure 33-6, A). However, only a limited length of the ligament can be evaluated using ultrasonography, and there are many false-negative results. Placing a wedge under one side of the foot may enable a greater length of the contralateral ligament to be evaluated than if the foot is bearing weight uniformly. In a few horses a well-defined osseous cystlike lesion has been identified in the distal phalanx at the site of insertion of a collateral ligament and rarely an osseous cystlike lesion at the origin in the middle phalanx.

Focal IRU in the distal phalanx in the region of insertion of a collateral ligament is a good indicator of the presence of an injury, although not necessarily involving the insertion.[10] However, in many horses MRI is required for definitive diagnosis. Care should be taken when

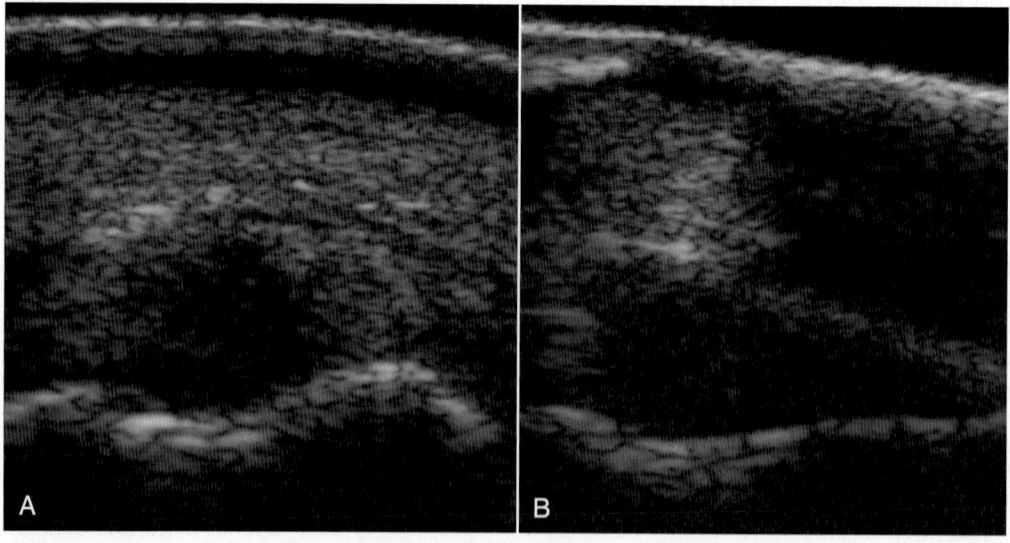

Fig. 33-9 • Transverse **(A)** and longitudinal **(B)** ultrasonographic images of the lateral collateral ligament of the distal interphalangeal joint of a 10-year-old show jumper with acute-onset, severe lameness, worst on a circle. The ligament is enlarged, and a large proportion of the ligament is anechogenic.

interpreting low-field images obtained in a standing horse because the magic angle effect may result in artifactual increased signal intensity in the lateral collateral ligament.[11,12] Magic angle effect may also influence the appearance of high-field MR images in the most proximal aspect of the collateral ligaments.[13] Confirmation of genuine injury requires identification of changes in size, shape, and signal intensity in T1- and T2-weighted images, and also in fat-suppressed images in acute injury. There may be entheseous and/or endosteal reaction at the origin and/or insertion. In some horses there is also evidence of bone trauma of the ipsilateral side of the middle or, more commonly, the distal phalanx characterized by diffuse decreased signal intensity in T1-weighted images and increased signal intensity in fat-suppressed images.[14,15] Osseous cystlike lesions may develop at the origin, or more commonly the insertion, many of which are not detectable radiologically and are only seen using MRI.

Treatment is box rest for a minimum of 2 months followed by at least 4 months of walking exercise, predominantly in straight lines. Longer convalescence may be preferable.[16] In horses with very severe injuries, consideration should be given to application of a foot cast. OA of the DIP joint is a potential sequel if there is instability of the joint. When the medial collateral ligament is damaged, a shoe with a wide medial branch and narrow lateral branch is recommended. For lateral collateral desmopathy, a shoe with a wide lateral branch with a lateral extension and a narrow medial branch is preferred. Medication of the DIP joint is indicated if there is evidence of synovitis or OA. Shock wave or radial pressure wave therapy is popular, although efficacy is questionable.[16] A nonsignificant improvement in treatment success was seen in horses treated by either shockwave therapy or radial pressure wave therapy compared with horses managed conservatively.[16] Surgical treatment of radiographically evident osseous cystlike lesions has been disappointing.[17] Palmar neurectomy has resulted in resolution of lameness in horses that had failed to respond to conservative management, and to date no untoward side effects have been seen.[16]

The prognosis for return to athletic function is guarded to fair for horses with injuries that affect primarily the body of the ligament. Horses with acute injuries probably have a more favorable prognosis than those with chronic injuries.[6,15,16] Overall 47.8% of 69 horses with primary injuries of one or both collateral ligaments returned to full athletic function; 51% of horses with increased signal intensity in fat-suppressed images returned to full function.[16] In a different study 60% of 20 horses, all with increased signal intensity in fat-suppressed images in the injured ligament, returned to full athletic function.[6] The presence of osseous abnormalities associated with collateral ligament injury did not influence outcome overall, although there was an association between excellent outcome and the presence of entheseous new bone at the insertion on the distal phalanx.[16] The coexistence of other injuries within the digit resulted in a much poorer prognosis.[16] The prognosis for horses with joint instability, or radiological abnormalities consistent with OA of the DIP joint, is also more guarded. There are anecdotal reports of treatment by stem cell injection, but no reports of clinical efficacy. Although primary traumatically induced injuries unquestionably occur, there is evidence of degenerative pathological change, especially

toward the insertion of the ligament in horses that have failed to respond to treatment.[7]

▣ OSSEOUS CYSTLIKE LESIONS IN THE DISTAL PHALANX

HISTORY

Osseous cystlike lesions in the distal phalanx usually are unilateral, solitary, and range in location from the extensor process to deep within the weight-bearing surface. Debate continues on whether the lesions have a traumatic or developmental origin. When large bilateral lesions are present in a young horse, a developmental component is strongly suggested.[1-3]

CLINICAL AND IMAGING FINDINGS

Affected horses often are young but mature, and acute-onset, moderate to severe lameness frequently is present. Less commonly the history includes low-grade, intermittent lameness. Occasionally osseous cystlike lesions are identified as incidental radiological findings. Osseous cystlike lesions sometimes are seen in older horses with pain localized to the foot. Such lesions may be clinically significant. Lameness may be exacerbated by distal limb flexion, but results of hoof tester examination usually are negative. Lesions are seen more commonly in the forelimbs, although the hindlimb was affected in 3 of 15 horses in one report.[1] Effusion of the DIP joint occasionally is present, and large bilateral lesions sometimes are associated with a buttress foot appearance.

Lameness often is unaltered by perineural analgesia of the palmar digital nerves, but it is resolved by palmar (abaxial sesamoid) nerve blocks. Intraarticular analgesia of the DIP joint improves lameness associated with osseous cystlike lesions that communicate with the joint. Small articular lesions may not be detectable radiologically, but large osseous cystlike lesions usually are readily identifiable on dorsoproximal-palmarodistal (upright pedal) images. Lesions involving the extensor process are seen readily on lateromedial images. Smaller osseous cystlike lesions located in a very medial or lateral location within the more weight-bearing aspect of the joint are best identified in weight-bearing dorsopalmar images. Nuclear scintigraphic examination may identify small osseous cystlike lesions that are not identifiable radiologically. Osseous cystlike lesions may be associated with IRU, depending on the stage of lesion development and activity of the surrounding bone. However, an osseous cystlike lesion that is scintigraphically silent still may be a cause of lameness. Some lesions can only be identified using MRI.

TREATMENT AND PROGNOSIS

Reports documenting results after either conservative or surgical treatment are limited. In one study, conservative treatment resulted in clinical improvement in approximately 30% of horses, but the prognosis for full recovery was guarded.[1] One report documented favorable results in a horse with bilateral extensor process fragmentation through what were presumed to be preexisting cystic lesions in the extensor processes.[4] Anecdotally, arthroscopic debridement of smaller extensor process lesions can be associated with full return to function.[5] Many lesions are not accessible by arthroscopy or arthrotomy through a dorsal approach. Debridement of distal phalanx lesions through the hoof wall has been described,[6] but this approach has not gained universal acceptance. However, good results have been achieved in a limited number of horses.[7] Arthroscopic debridement of centrally located lesions was successful in 10 of 11 horses (91%) 16 to 33 months of age.[8] Intraarticular medication can be useful in the ongoing management of selected horses; occasionally conservative treatment results in a horse suitable for a limited amount of riding activity.

◼ OSSEOUS TRAUMA OF THE DISTAL AND MIDDLE PHALANGES

Osseous trauma of the middle or distal phalanges usually results in acute-onset, moderate to severe lameness.[1,2] There are usually no localizing clinical signs. The response to perineural analgesia depends on the location of injury. Diagnosis usually requires MRI, although there may be IRU at the site of injury. Lesions are characterized by an area of increased signal intensity in the cancellous bone in fat-suppressed images, with a corresponding region of low signal intensity in T1-weighted images and sometimes T2* = weighted images (Figure 33-10). The most common site is the distal dorsal aspect of the middle phalanx.[3] However, lesions also occur in the distal phalanx, involving especially the palmar aspect, with or without involvement of the navicular bone. These injuries may occur alone or in association with related soft tissue injuries, such as collateral ligament injury. Extensive ossification of a cartilage of a foot may be a risk factor for osseous trauma of the ipsilateral aspect of the distal phalanx.[4-6] Lameness is often very slow to resolve, but in horses with uncomplicated injuries the prognosis is usually favorable, unless there was associated damage of the subchondral bone plate. There are anecdotal reports of beneficial effects of treatment by intravenous infusion of tiludronate.

◼ KERATOMAS AND NEOPLASTIC AND NONNEOPLASTIC SPACE-OCCUPYING LESIONS IN THE HOOF

Keratomas are classified as aberrant, possibly hyperplastic, keratin masses originating from epidermal horn-producing cells of the coronary band.[1] They also have been defined as benign neoplasms originating from the coronary dermis.[2] As the abnormal horn tubules grow distally toward the toe, hoof wall deformation may occur with disruption of the white line, which may permit entry of infection. Expansion of the mass results in pressure necrosis of the adjacent distal phalanx. Keratomas occur most often in the dorsal half of the foot.[3] A keratoma is the most common space-occupying lesion in the hoof, but other neoplastic conditions occur occasionally and result in similar clinical signs, although they usually can be differentiated radiologically.[4-8] Other nonneoplastic space-occupying lesions, such as epidermal inclusion cysts and fibrous dysplasia, have been identified that can be differentiated from a keratoma only by histological examination.[9]

HISTORY

Often mild intermittent forelimb or hindlimb lameness exists, or more severe episodes of lameness associated with recurrent subsolar abscessation may have occurred.[2,3,10-12] Neoplastic conditions may be associated with more severe lameness. Distortion of the hoof capsule may have been noted.

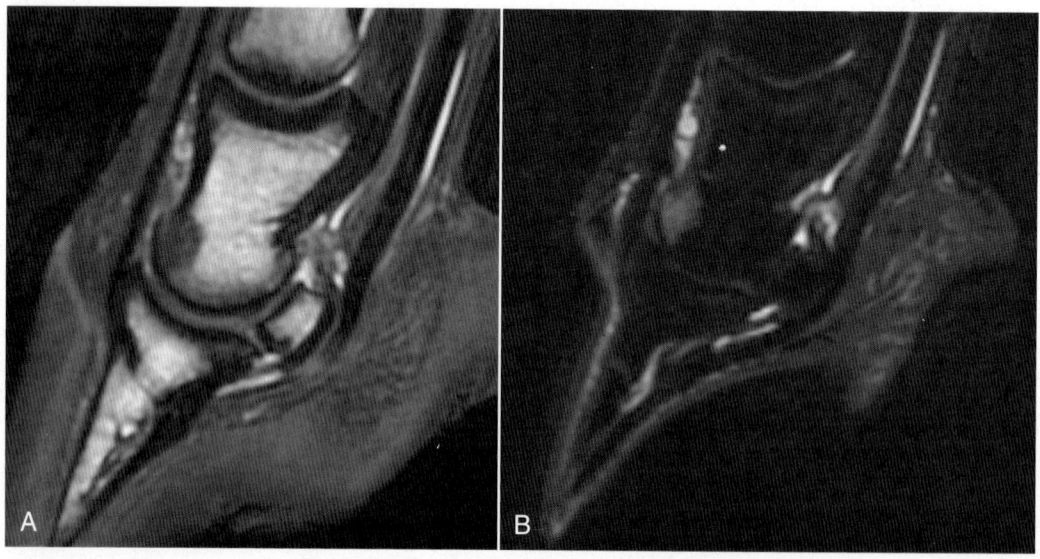

Fig. 33-10 • Sagittal T2*-weighted spoiled gradient-echo **(A)** and short tau inversion recovery (STIR) **(B)** magnetic resonance images of a 6-year-old show jumper with acute-onset left forelimb lameness abolished by palmar digital analgesia. Radiographic and ultrasonographic examinations revealed no detectable abnormality. There is reduced signal intensity in the dorsal distal aspect of the middle phalanx in the T2*-weighted image and increased signal intensity in the STIR image, consistent with bone trauma.

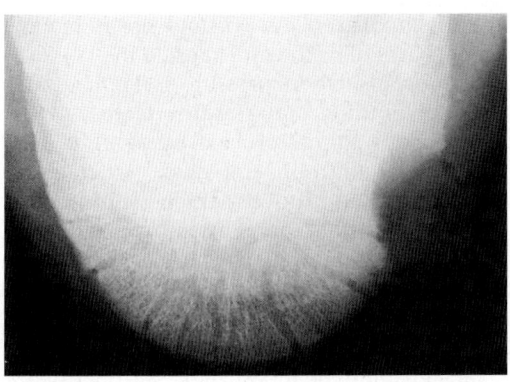

Fig. 33-11 • Slightly oblique dorsoproximal-palmarodistal oblique radiographic image of a foot. A smoothly outlined semicircular defect is present in the lateral aspect of the distal phalanx, typical of a keratoma. Lateral is to the right.

CLINICAL SIGNS AND DIAGNOSIS

The hoof capsule, the white line, or both may be distorted but not invariably. Pressure applied with hoof testers may elicit local pain. A variable degree of lameness is present that is alleviated by desensitization of the foot or unilateral palmar block on the side of the lesion. Radiographic examination may reveal a smoothly demarcated radiolucent defect in the margin of the distal phalanx (Figure 33-11). This characteristic is typical of keratomas or other nonneoplastic space-occupying lesions, whereas neoplastic lesions tend to have more irregular margins and may be associated with new bone formation.[8] Infectious osteitis of the distal phalanx may have a similar appearance, although if the osteitis is chronic, marginal sclerosis with or without new bone formation may be present. The crena at the toe of the distal phalanx should not be confused with a space-occupying lesion. Lesions are best detected in dorsoproximal-palmarodistal oblique, dorsolateral-palmaromedial oblique, or dorsomedial-palmarolateral oblique radiographic images. A keratoma also may be present in the absence of radiological change with only distortion of the hoof capsule.[3] If the clinical significance of such a radiological lesion is in doubt, nuclear scintigraphy may be helpful because such lesions usually are associated with focal IRU. Diagnostic ultrasonography also has been used to identify a keratoma at the coronary band.[13] Small keratomas that were not detected radiologically have also been identified using MRI, although not all are of clinical significance.[14] Occasionally other space-occupying lesions in the more palmar aspect of the foot are only identified in a palmaroproximal-palmarodistal oblique radiographic image of the palmar processes of the distal phalanx.

TREATMENT

Horses with keratomas and other benign space-occupying lesions respond well to surgical excision and have a good prognosis,* but those with neoplastic lesions have a more guarded prognosis. It is best to excise keratomas and other space-occupying lesions through a hoof wall rather than solar approach, if possible. Partial hoof wall resection for keratoma removal was associated with fewer postoperative complications and a more rapid return to athletic function compared with complete hoof wall resection.[16]

◼ FRACTURES OF THE DISTAL PHALANX

Fractures of the distal phalanx are a relatively common cause of lameness in horses from all disciplines and often are the result of trauma, through a misstep or high-speed impact, or kicking a fixed object.[1-13] Fractures have been classified into six types,[1,2] but other configurations also occur. Fractures of the extensor process of the distal phalanx (type IV) are discussed elsewhere (see page 355). Fractures of the solar margin of the distal phalanx (type VI), which may occur in foals or adults, are considered separately from fractures of the body of the bone. The latter may be articular or nonarticular and may comprise sagittal (type III), oblique (extending from the midline to the lateral or medial solar margin) (type II), and comminuted fractures (type V), fracture of a palmar process (type I), and, less commonly, fractures of other configurations.

FRACTURE OF THE SOLAR MARGIN OF THE DISTAL PHALANX

Foals

Fractures of the palmar-most aspect of the palmar process of the distal phalanx occur commonly in foals.[3,4] These fractures originate at the incisure (which normally separates the proximal and distal palmar process angles), continue dorsally toward the toe for 1 to 3 cm, and then extend to the solar margin. They are believed to be caused by shear forces generated by tension of the DDFT or by compression of the solar cortical surface and tension on the dorsal cortical surface during weight bearing. One hypothesis is that excessive trimming of the heel, thus increasing tension in the DDFT, or excessive trimming of the sole of the frog, thus increasing concussion on the distal phalanx and forces on the palmar processes, may be predisposing factors to these fractures, but this was not substantiated in a clinical study, perhaps because of the high overall incidence of fractures (34%).[5]

Clinical Signs and Diagnosis

Lameness usually is mild and extremely transitory, lasting only 1 to 2 days, and may precede radiological identification of a fracture. No consistent response to pressure applied with hoof testers at the heel is present. Diagnosis is based on radiological identification of a discrete osseous body at the palmar process. Fractures may be identified on lateromedial radiographic images, but dorsal 65° proximal-palmarodistal oblique radiographic images are more sensitive. Not all fractures are detectable radiologically.

Treatment and Prognosis

Even with normal management, lameness is only transitory, and spontaneous healing occurs within 4 to 8 weeks with an excellent long-term prognosis. Any type of shoe should be avoided because shoe application in foals can quickly cause contracted feet.

Adult Horses

Fractures of the solar margin of the distal phalanx in adult horses occur from the quarters toward the more dorsal aspect of the distal phalanx; these fractures also are referred to as *cracking off*.[2,6] These fractures may heal, be resorbed, or persist without signs; therefore radiological identification of solar margin fragmentation is not necessarily synonymous with identification of the source of pain causing lameness. Solar margin fractures occur almost exclusively in forelimbs. A geographical influence on the incidence of solar margin fractures is apparent, which may reflect the footing on which the horses work or other undefined factors. In the Editors' experience, these fractures are rare, whereas a study in California of distal phalanx fractures in 274 horses identified 132 (48%) horses with solar margin fractures. However, these fractures frequently occurred in association with radiological evidence of laminitis or another potential cause of lameness, such as navicular disease.[6] Solar margin fractures as the sole potential cause of lameness were identified only in 25 horses. Irregularity and reduced opacity at the solar margin, with widening of the vascular channels, may be a predisposing factor.

Clinical Signs and Diagnosis

Horses with solar margin fractures often have a history of foot soreness. With an acute solar margin fracture, there may be increased sensitivity to hoof testers at the toe, provided that the sole is not excessively hard. Lameness is removed by perineural analgesia of the palmar nerves in the proximal pastern region or at the level of the proximal sesamoid bones. Diagnosis depends on radiological identification of the fracture or fractures, which may be single or multiple and may affect a variable extent of the solar margin. Primary solar margin fractures usually are single, whereas those that occur in association with laminitis or radiological evidence of demineralization of the solar margin are more likely to be multiple, comminuted, or both. Fractures are identified readily in an appropriately exposed dorsoproximal-palmarodistal oblique radiographic image, but they are overlooked easily if the radiograph is overexposed. The radiographs should be inspected carefully to detect evidence of any other potential cause of lameness that may influence treatment and prognosis.

Treatment

Horses with lameness associated with a solar margin fracture usually require prolonged rest, especially if radiological evidence of preexisting demineralization of the solar margin is present; healing is assessed by periodic radiographic examination. The use of a broad web shoe with a concave solar margin, with or without pads, is recommended. Limited documented long-term follow-up information is available for horses with primary solar margin fractures, but the prognosis generally is favorable.

FRACTURES OF THE BODY OF THE DISTAL PHALANX

Fractures of the body of the distal phalanx occur more commonly in forelimbs than hindlimbs, but they are not uncommon in either limb.[1,2,7-13] A fracture of the body of the distal phalanx usually results in acute-onset, severe lameness, but nonarticular fractures of a palmar process of

the distal phalanx can occur without severe lameness.[13] If the fracture is articular, the DIP capsule may be distended. Pain usually occurs when pressure is applied with hoof testers, but this finding may not be a feature of a nondisplaced fracture of a palmar process, especially if it has been present for more than several days. Articular fractures invariably result in continuous lameness, but a nonarticular fracture of a palmar or plantar process of the distal phalanx may be associated with intermittent lameness, especially in a hindlimb. Clinical signs of an articular fracture usually reflect foot pain, and thus regional analgesia often is not required; however, with nonarticular fractures the clinical signs may be less specific, and perineural analgesia is usually required to determine the source of pain. Some palmar process fractures heal only by fibrous union and not osseous union. The radiological identification of a fracture that has healed by fibrous union, which does not have the appearance of a narrow, clearly defined line, should be interpreted with care. Although such a fracture may be unstable and therefore a potential source of pain, the pain causing lameness may not necessarily be related to the fracture.

Fractures of the distal phalanx are a common racehorse injury in North America. Fractures occur most often in the lateral aspect of the left front foot and the medial aspect of the right front foot in association with the counterclockwise direction of training and racing.[12] Fractures of the distal phalanx in the hindlimb in racehorses occur most commonly in the medial aspect of the foot.[12] In sports horses and general purpose horses, fracture of the medial palmar process of the distal phalanx occurs most commonly.[13]

Diagnosis

Diagnosis is based on radiological identification of a fracture (Figures 33-12 and 33-13). A very recent nondisplaced fracture may be difficult to identify radiologically unless the x-ray beam is completely parallel to the fracture line, and many oblique images may be required. The foot should be cleaned thoroughly before radiographic examination to avoid artifacts. The frog clefts may create confusing lucent lines across the distal phalanx; therefore the foot should be packed with a moldable modeling compound (e.g., Play-Doh, Hasbro, Inc., Pawtucket, Rhode Island, United States).

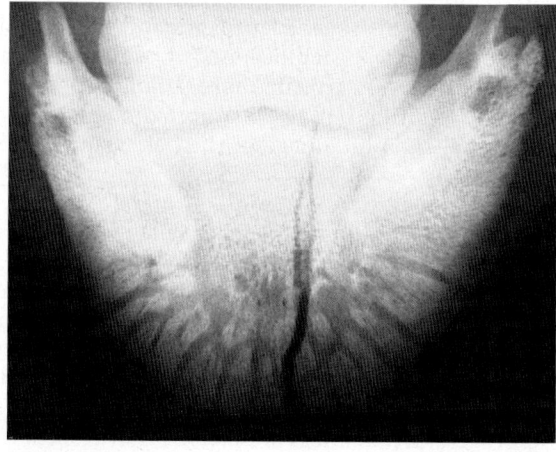

Fig. 33-12 • Dorsoproximal-plantarodistal oblique radiographic image of a left hind foot. The distal phalanx has a complete, articular, parasagittal fracture.

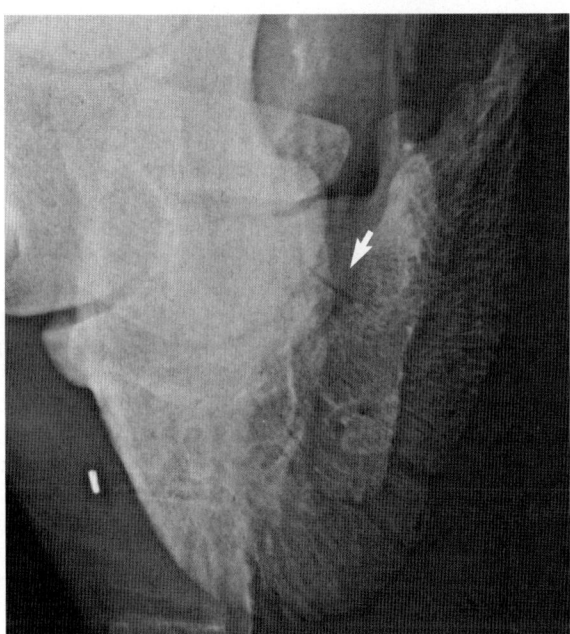

Fig. 33-13 • Dorsomedial-plantarolateral oblique radiographic image of a left hind foot. There is an incomplete, nondisplaced, nonarticular fracture of the medial plantar process of the distal phalanx *(arrow)*. This was not seen on standard radiographic images.

Many articular fractures are seen readily on dorsoproximal-palmarodistal oblique radiographic images, but fractures of the palmar processes and other less common configurations of fracture may not be apparent. A fracture of a palmar process may be evident on a lateromedial radiographic image, but oblique radiographic images of the palmar process are required in many horses. Most of these fractures can be detected in dorsal 30- to 45° lateral (or medial)-palmarodistal oblique radiographic images with the foot either bearing weight or in the upright pedal position, but occasionally oblique views are required with the horse standing on the x-ray cassette (e.g., dorsal 45°/proximal 45° lateral-palmarodistal medial oblique radiographic images). Separate centers of ossification at the palmar aspect of the palmar process should not be confused with a fracture.[10] Rarely a palmar process fracture is seen only in a palmaroproximal-palmarodistal oblique radiographic image. Occasionally obscure incomplete, nonarticular fractures of the body of the distal phalanx are identified in a palmaroproximal-palmarodistal oblique view.

Nuclear scintigraphic examination usually is unnecessary for the identification of most acute fractures, except those causing episodic lameness, but can be helpful in confirming the likely clinical significance of older fractures.[14] Scintigraphy also is useful for identification of subchondral bone trauma unassociated with detectable radiological abnormalities (see following text).

Although the majority of fractures of the distal phalanx are radiologically detectable, occasionally unusual configurations or locations have only been identified using MRI (e.g., an incomplete nondisplaced fracture on the axial aspect of a palmar process of the distal phalanx).[15]

Treatment and Prognosis

Conservative treatment of horses with nonarticular palmar process fractures, by box rest and use of a bar shoe with five clips or bar rim shoe, has a good prognosis. Complete healing of the fracture may not be evident radiologically for several months, but most fractures eventually do heal. Horses with fractures extending into the medial or lateral extremity of the DIP joint also have a good prognosis with conservative management. The horse should continue to be shod with a bar shoe when work is resumed to reduce the risks of reinjury. If a bar shoe is replaced by an open shoe, avoidance of maximum work intensity may be preferable until the hoof capsule and distal phalanx have had time to adapt to altered concussive forces. Although sagittal and oblique articular fractures of the distal phalanx often heal well if treated conservatively in horses younger than 3 years of age, the prognosis for adult horses is more guarded, and internal fixation using a lag screw technique is recommended.[1,7,9,12] Prognosis depends on whether displacement at the articular margin exists; displacement inevitably results in OA and associated lameness. Potential complications include postoperative infection and screw irritation or rejection. The use of a headless titanium Herbert cannulated screw (Zimmer Corp., Warsaw, Indiana, United States) may result in fewer complications.[16] Complete fracture healing requires 6 to 12 months of convalescence with surgical management.

COMMINUTED FRACTURES

Comminuted fractures of the distal phalanx are not common[1,2,7] but do occur occasionally. Many radiographic images may be required to establish the precise configuration of the fractures and determine possible articular involvement, which results in a more guarded prognosis. The configuration of the fracture determines whether internal fixation is a viable option.[7,12]

FRACTURES OF THE DISTAL PHALANX ASSOCIATED WITH PENETRATING INJURY

A penetrating injury of the foot (see Chapter 28) may result in a fracture of the distal phalanx of any configuration. Treatment is dictated by the fracture configuration. The primary aim is to control infection. Removal of small bone fragments that otherwise may sequestrate may be preferable.

SUBCHONDRAL TRAUMA OF THE DISTAL PHALANX

Some horses have forelimb lameness, usually unilateral, associated with pain localized to the foot but no clinically significant detectable radiological abnormality. Nuclear scintigraphic examination reveals a focal round or semicircular area of IRU, seen in a solar image, either medially or laterally, far removed from the DIP joint, or on a lateral image in the center of the bone in a similar location to fractures.[17] This lameness is believed to reflect subchondral bone trauma and is an injury that occurs particularly in racehorses in North America but also in other types of horses. Lameness usually is unaffected or, less commonly, only partially affected by intraarticular analgesia of the DIP joint. In some horses, mediolateral foot balance may be a predisposing factor. Less commonly the onset of lameness is associated with trauma. The failure to identify a fracture radiologically may reflect the inherent limitations of radiography. Alternatively, such reactions may indicate that distal phalangeal fractures, especially in racehorses, may not be single-event episodes but rather the result of stress remodeling. Treatment comprises rest and correction of any mediolateral foot imbalance. Floating the heel of the affected side may be helpful. The prognosis is favorable given sufficient time, which is proportional to the duration of lameness before diagnosis and treatment. In horses with acute lesions a period of 6 to 8 weeks of box rest and controlled walking exercise usually is sufficient, with a progressive increase in work intensity thereafter; however, in those with more chronic lesions a longer period may be necessary, and repeated scintigraphic evaluation may be helpful to determine when the lesion is no longer active.

■ PEDAL OSTEITIS: DOES IT EXIST?

Pedal osteitis strictly means inflammation of the distal phalanx and has long been suggested as a cause of forelimb lameness. However, it is a poorly defined condition, previously diagnosed radiologically, characterized by focal or general demineralization around the solar margin of the distal phalanx and widening of the vascular channels, with or without abnormal lucent areas in the palmar processes. It is now recognized that considerable variation exists in the radiological appearance of the distal phalanx in normal horses.[1-3] No good studies correlate foot conformation and the radiological appearance of the distal phalanx. It is my impression that those horses with a particularly thin sole, especially in association with a horizontal orientation of the solar margin of the distal phalanx, seem prone to foot soreness if worked regularly on hard ground, but the source of pain has been poorly defined. Radiological changes of the distal phalanx, once established, often persist over the long term and therefore are not synonymous with active inflammation. Radiographs represent a historical record of previous activity or injury. Scintigraphic examination of a large number of horses with foot pain occasionally has revealed evidence of abnormal bone turnover around the solar margins of the distal phalanx or confined to the palmar processes (see page 363).[4] In those horses with IRU around the solar margin of the distal phalanx in solar views, correlation with other clinical signs and radiological findings frequently is poor unless the condition is localized to the toe, when it often reflects laminitis. The relevance of this finding in the absence of localizing clinical signs remains open to question because it also is seen in clinically normal horses. Pedal osteitis tends to have been used to describe a cause of lameness, when frequently the cause is actually undetermined.[5] The cause of pedal osteitis has not been defined, although abnormal concussion has been suggested.

Therefore I suggest that the term pedal osteitis is inappropriate and should not be used to describe a cause of lameness on the basis of radiological findings alone. Nonetheless, a variety of radiological changes of the margins of the distal phalanx can be identified, the causes of which are poorly defined. With our current state of knowledge, attribution of lameness to these radiological changes seems inappropriate unless localizing clinical signs, or concurrent evidence of ongoing inflammation with or without abnormal bone turnover, are documented scintigraphically or using MRI. Abnormalities of one or both palmar processes of the distal phalanx have been identified using MRI (see Osteitis of the palmar processes of the distal phalanx), with irregularity of the cortices and alteration of signal intensity, but only rarely have these been considered to be the primary source of pain causing lameness.[6,7] There is an association between extensive ossification of the cartilages of the foot and trauma of the distal phalanx, usually involving the palmar processes.[8,9]

Chronic laminitis may be associated with modeling of the toe of the distal phalanx and bone resorption with or without new bone on the dorsal aspect at the toe. Mineralization also has been identified on the dorsal aspects of the distal phalanx, midway between the coronary band and the solar margin; mineralization is seen best on lateromedial or slightly oblique radiographic images. This may represent mineralization in the dermal laminae or formation of new bone on the dorsal cortex of the distal phalanx. Extensive mineralization has been associated with lameness, but some roughening of the dorsal cortex in the region of the parietal sulci may be an incidental finding. Some horses with a clubfoot conformation develop focal loss of bone around the solar margin at the toe of the distal phalanx, as well as new bone on the dorsal aspect of the bone, associated with chronic lameness on hard ground. I suggest that in these conditions the radiological changes should be described and attributed to the primary cause rather than labeled as pedal osteitis. Many horses with poor foot conformation suffer chronic lameness, probably associated with abnormal concussion to both the soft tissue and bony elements of the hoof. Identification of the primary cause of the problem and admission that the precise source or sources of pain cannot be defined are preferable to use of the term pedal osteitis, which implies a definitive diagnosis.

■ OSTEITIS OF THE PALMAR PROCESSES OF THE DISTAL PHALANX

ANATOMY

The palmar processes or angles of the distal phalanx are prism-shaped masses that project backward on the medial and lateral aspects of the bone. Each is divided into upper and lower parts by a notch or is perforated by a foramen that leads to the dorsal groove of the distal phalanx. The cartilages of the foot attach to the proximal border of each palmar process. In a normal horse, the solar and abaxial surfaces of the palmar processes are relatively smooth.

Osteitis of the palmar processes of the distal phalanx may be part of what has been called the "pedal osteitis complex," related to the long toe–low heel syndrome. Its origin is poorly understood. It occurs almost exclusively in the forelimbs and may result in irregular roughening of the bone surface (Figure 33-14, *A*).

HISTORY AND CLINICAL FINDINGS

Lameness often is bilateral, insidious in onset, and tends to be worst on hard ground, similar to navicular disease. Affected horses often have poor conformation of the feet,

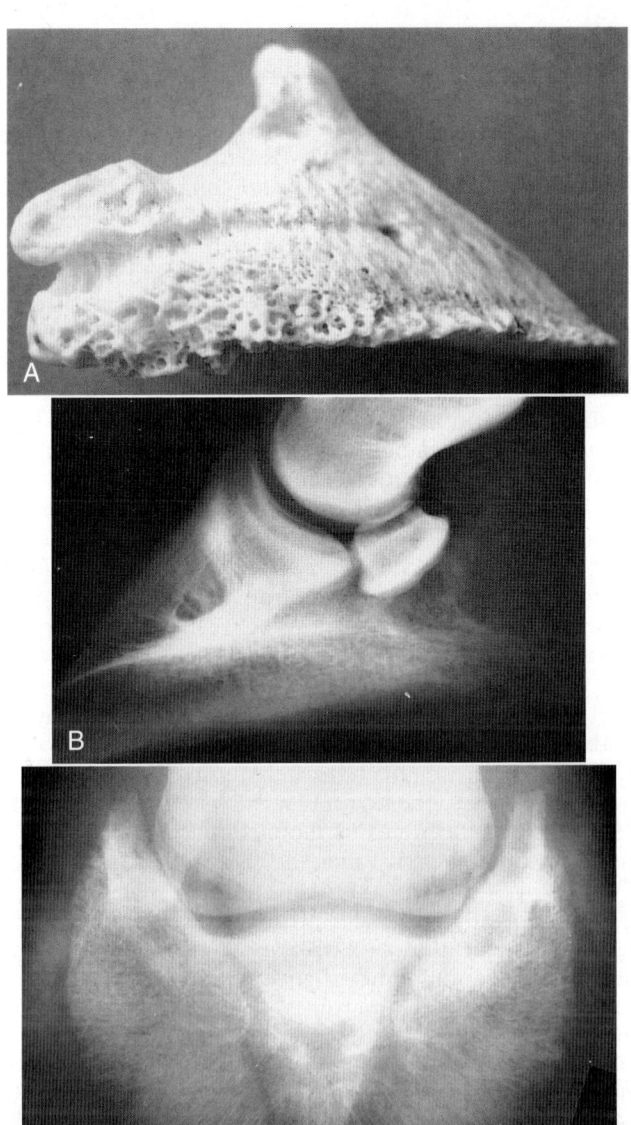

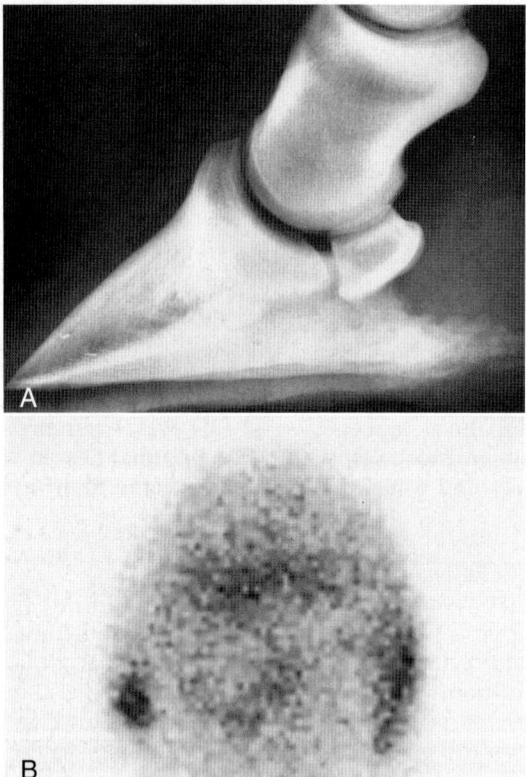

Fig. 33-15 • **A,** Lateromedial radiographic image of a front foot of a 9-year-old Warmblood. Features include the abnormally elongated shape of the palmar processes, the horizontal orientation of the distal phalanx, and the thin sole. **B,** Solar scintigraphic image of the same foot in **A**. There is intense increased radiopharmaceutical uptake in the palmar processes of the distal phalanx.

Fig. 33-14 • **A,** The distal phalanx of a horse that had chronic heel pain. The palmar process has a roughened surface, and new bone is evident on the solar surface. **B,** Lateromedial radiographic image of a foot of an 8-year-old Selle Francais with recurrent heel pain. Note the orientation of the solar surface of the distal phalanx: the palmar process is lower than the toe, and the solar aspect of the palmar processes has an irregular contour. **C,** Dorsoproximal-palmarodistal oblique radiographic image of the same foot as shown in **B**. There is a very distinct trabecular pattern in the palmar processes, with many small lucent areas.

with low, collapsed heels. The sole may be very flat, thin, and readily compressible. If the sole is readily compressible, pressure applied with hoof testers may be resented, but this usually is not a localized response.

DIAGNOSIS

Diagnosis requires a combination of response to nerve blocks, radiography, and, ideally, nuclear scintigraphy and MRI.[1-7]

Local Analgesia

Lameness is improved by perineural analgesia of the palmar digital nerves but generally is unchanged after intraarticular analgesia of the DIP joint or analgesia of the navicular bursa.

Imaging Techniques

Radiography

The orientation of the distal phalanx should be assessed in a lateromedial image. In a normal horse, the solar margin is smooth in outline and at a 5- to 10-degree angle to the sole, sloping proximally toward its palmar aspect.[1] In some affected horses the palmar processes are at the same level or lower than the toe of the distal phalanx (see Figure 33-14, *B*). The solar aspect of the palmar processes may have a fluffy appearance. The shape may change with elongation of the palmar processes; this change also is seen in dorsal 60-degree lateral-palmaromedial oblique or dorsal 60-degree medial-palmarolateral oblique images (Figure 33-15, *A*). In a dorsoproximal-palmarodistal oblique image, discrete circular radiolucent areas, 2 to 3 mm in diameter, may be visible in the palmar processes, or the trabecular pattern may be more obvious as a result of generalized demineralization (see Figure 33-14, *C*).

So-called *inversion* of the distal phalanx in hindlimbs, with the plantar processes lower than the toe, also has been seen in association with more proximal sites of pain causing hindlimb lameness, such as proximal suspensory desmitis.[2,3] I have not recognized this as a primary cause of hind foot pain.

Nuclear Scintigraphy

If the bony changes are active, nuclear scintigraphic evaluation may reveal IRU in the affected palmar processes to substantiate the relavance of the clinical and radiological findings (see Fig. 33-15, *B*). However, this is sometimes an incidental finding, and its clinical significance should be interpreted in light of other clinical observations. In a comparative radiographic, scintigraphic, and MRI study in 258 lame horses, IRU was more commonly seen in the medial palmar process of the distal phalanx than in the lateral palmar process.[4] Focal IRU was overrepresented in palmar processes with MR abnormalities in signal intensity and was more prevalent in lame than nonlame limbs.

Magnetic Resonance Imaging

MRI may reveal increased signal intensity in one or both palmar processes in fat-suppressed images, sometimes with cortical irregularity and disruption of the adjacent laminar architecture. This is evidence of active osteitis and may be a cause of primary pain and lameness. However, it is common to see mild to marked reduced signal intensity in both T1- and T2-weighted images in the medial palmar process consistent with mineralization as either an incidental finding in a nonlame limb or coexistent with one or more other lesions that are more likely to be the primary cause of lameness.[4]

TREATMENT AND PROGNOSIS

Effective treatment depends on early recognition and corrective trimming and shoeing to try to restore more normal foot conformation. The response to treatment often is slow, and during the convalescent period, work on hard ground should be avoided. Horses with chronic lameness with a markedly distorted hoof capsule have a guarded prognosis. Some horses may benefit from removal of the shoes for 6 months and unrestricted exercise at pasture, provided that the hoof wall quality permits this approach and the ground is not excessively hard.

◼ DISEASE OF THE CARTILAGES OF THE FOOT

ANATOMY

The cartilages of the foot, also referred to as the *collateral cartilages of the distal phalanx, ungular (ungual) cartilages,* and *lateral cartilages,* originate as hyaline-type cartilage and become fibrocartilage in adults.[1] They attach to the proximal border of the palmar processes of the distal phalanx. The size and shape vary, as does the degree of ossification. The cartilages have axial extensions, and they seem to provide an internal support structure for the palmar (plantar) aspect of the foot.[2] An extensive network of venovenous anastomoses is present within the cartilages. Marked differences in the thickness and tissue composition exist in the front and hind feet. The cartilages of the foot

tend to be thicker in forelimbs than in hindlimbs, perhaps reflecting the greater weight-bearing capacity of the forelimbs.[2] The digital cushion has more fibrous or cartilaginous tissue in forelimbs than in matched hind feet, which have more adipose and elastic tissues. There may also be breed differences. An extensive and complex relationship exists between the cartilages of the foot and the digital cushion. The combined role is thought to be energy dissipation, which depends on hemodynamic flow.[2]

The cartilages of the foot are joined to adjacent structures by a variety of ligaments that vary in size and definition. The chondrocompedal ligament attaches the palmaroproximal aspect of the cartilage with the proximal phalanx, with an axial branch to the distal phalanx.[1] The chondrocoronal ligament connects the dorsal part of the cartilage with the middle phalanx.[1] Ossification of the lateral cartilage of the foot may be more extensive than the medial cartilage.[3,5] The term *sidebone* has been used to describe extensive ossification of one or both cartilages of the foot. Ossification may occur from more than one center of ossification. Radiolucent lines between separate centers of ossification may persist throughout life (Figure 33-16).[4,5] The degree of ossification is greater in mature horses than in horses younger than 2 years of age.[3] Ossification tends to be more extensive in heavier breeds of horses than in lighter-weight horses. Extensive ossification is unusual in Thoroughbred and Warmblood breeds.[5] Among Finnhorses, ossification was more common and extensive in mares compared with male horses,[3] but no gender predilection was seen in a British study of mixed breeds.[5] There is generally reasonable mediolateral symmetry in the degree of ossification of cartilages of the foot, with the lateral cartilage sometimes slightly more ossified than the medial. Marked asymmetry in ossification is unusual and may be a predisposing factor for lameness.[6] There is generally greater radiopharmaceutical uptake at the base of the ossified cartilages than farther proximally, reflecting greater bone modeling, probably because of biomechanical stress.[7]

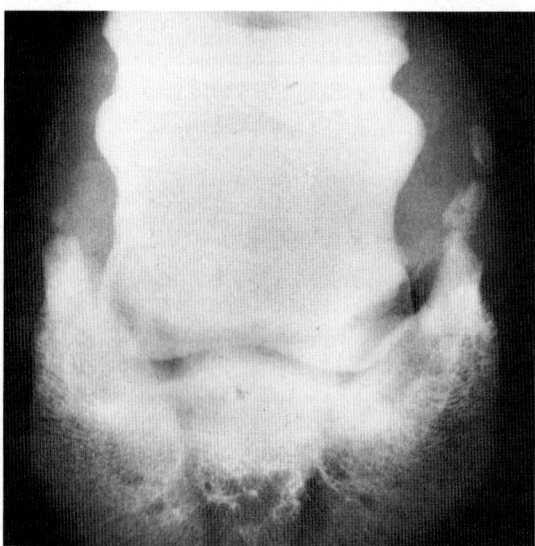

Fig. 33-16 • Dorsoproximal-palmaromedial oblique radiographic image of a foot of a mature riding horse. Lateral is to the right. Several centers of ossification of both the cartilages of the foot are present, more obvious laterally.

CLINICAL SIGNS AND DIAGNOSIS

The proximal aspect of the cartilages of the foot can be palpated proximal to the coronary band. However, palpation is an unreliable indicator of both the size of the cartilages and the degree of ossification. The degree of ossification can be established only by radiology. Lateromedial and weight-bearing dorsopalmar radiographic images are the most useful (Figure 33-17); however, additional information about modeling of the cartilages of the foot can be obtained from dorsoproximal-palmarodistal oblique and flexed dorsolateral-palmaromedial and dorsomedial-palmarolateral oblique radiographic images.[8]

Historically ossification of the cartilages of the foot has rarely been directly associated with lameness, although extensive ossification extending to the level of the proximal interphalangeal joint has been associated with a short-striding gait. However, there is now evidence that moderate to severe ossification of a cartilage of the foot may predispose to a fracture usually at the base of the ossified cartilage[8-10] or osseous trauma of the distal phalanx distal to the ossified cartilage.[6,8,9] Trauma at the junction between separate centers of ossification can also be associated with lameness.[6, 8,9]

There are usually no localizing clinical signs. Lameness is generally worse on a circle compared with straight lines, especially on a firm surface. Lameness is abolished by perineural analgesia of the palmar (abaxial sesamoid) nerves but is usually not substantially improved by intraarticular analgesia of the DIP joint.

Care should be taken not to confuse a radiolucent line between separate centers of ossification as a fracture. Nuclear scintigraphy may facilitate a definitive diagnosis of a fracture (Figure 33-18), trauma to the union between separate centers of ossification, and bone trauma of the distal phalanx.[6-9] Diagnosis of bone trauma or some fractures at the base of an ossified cartilage is confirmed using MRI.[6,8,9] These injuries can occur alone or together with injury of the ipsilateral collateral ligament of the DIP joint[6,11,12] and/or the chondrocoronal ligament or the chondrosesamoidean ligament.[8,9] There is an association between extensive ossification of the cartilages of the foot and injury of the collateral ligaments of the distal phalanx and distal phalanx trauma.[8,9,12]

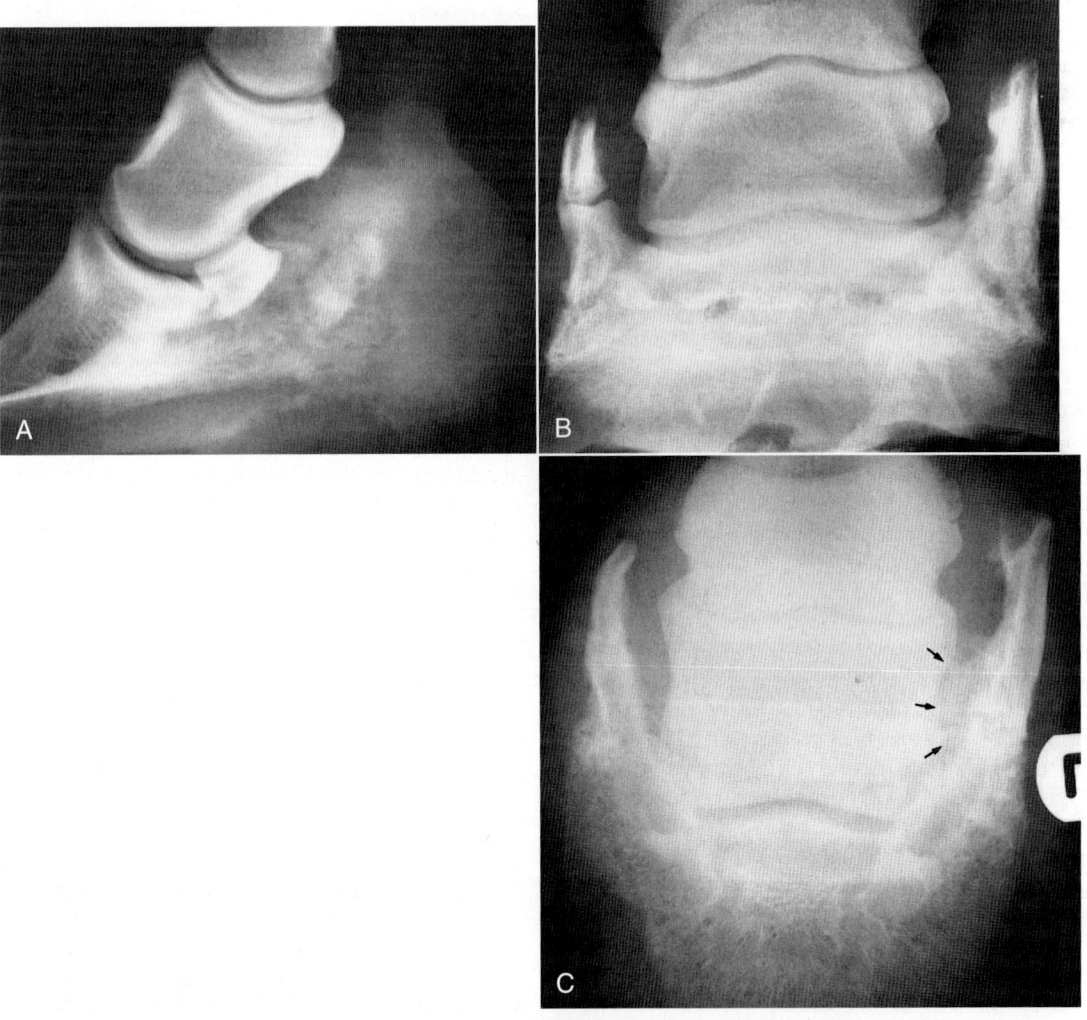

Fig. 33-17 • Lateromedial **(A),** dorsopalmar **(B),** and dorsoproximal-palmarodistal oblique **(C)** radiographic images of a foot of a 7-year-old cob gelding. There is extensive ossification of the cartilages of the foot. Medial is to the left. A separate center of ossification of the medial cartilage of the foot is seen in **B**. The horse had a previous fracture at the base of the lateral cartilage of the foot with smoothly outlined callus axially (*arrows,* **C**).

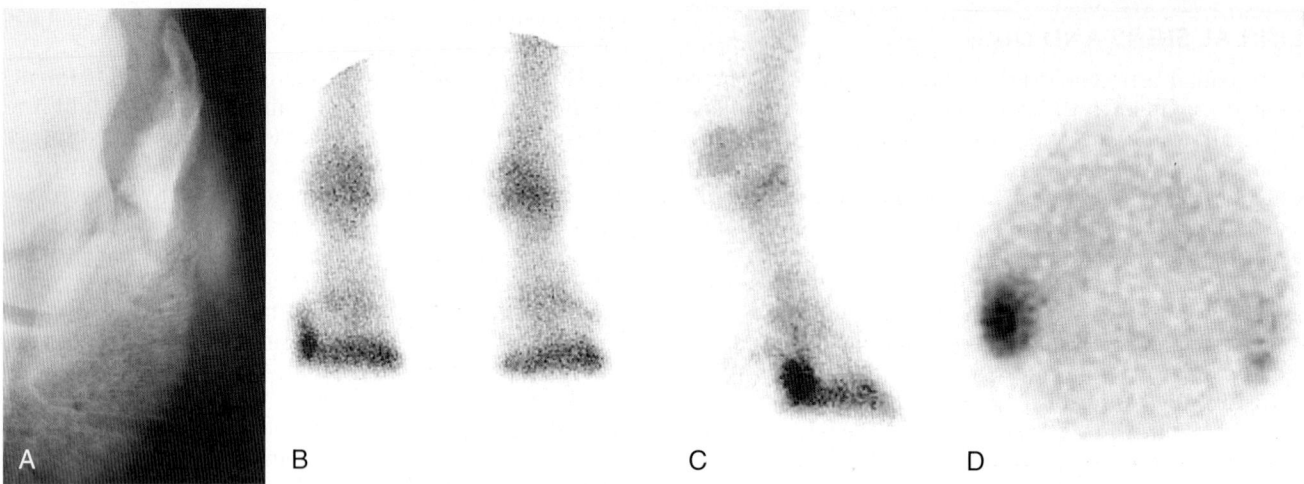

Fig. 33-18 • A, Dorsoproximal-palmarodistal oblique radiographic image of the right front foot of a Warmblood mare with severe lameness that partially improved with perineural analgesia of the palmar nerves at the base of the proximal sesamoid bones. The lateral cartilage of the foot is fractured. Dorsal (the right front foot is on the left) **(B),** lateral **(C),** and solar **(D)** scintigraphic images of the same foot in **A.** There is increased radiopharmaceutical uptake in the lateral cartilage of the right front foot.

Desmitis of the chondrocompedal, chondrosesamoidean, and chondrocoronal ligaments occasionally has been recognized in association with lameness.[8,9,13] There are no localizing clinical features and MRI is usually required for diagnosis. Entheseous new bone on the distal diaphyseal region of the proximal phalanx reflects abnormal stress at the origin of the ligament between the apex of the cartilage of the foot and the proximal phalanx and has been seen in association with extensively ossified cartilages.

Occasionally lameness has been associated with marked thickening of an unossified cartilage, hypervascularity, irregularity of the margins (especially abaxially), and increased signal intensity throughout the cartilage in fat-suppressed MR images, extending into the ipsilateral aspect of the distal phalanx.[9]

Chapter 34

Laminitis

■ PATHOPHYSIOLOGY OF LAMINITIS

Christopher C. Pollitt

A tough, flexible, connective tissue suspensory apparatus suspends the distal phalanx (DP) to the inside of the hoof wall. The surface of the inner hoof wall is folded into leaf-like lamellae (laminae) to increase the surface area of attachment between the hoof and the DP. A horse has laminitis when this attachment apparatus is compromised. Without the DP properly attached to the inside of the hoof, the weight of the horse and the forces of locomotion drive the DP down and away from the hoof wall. Arteries, veins, and nerves are sheared and crushed, and secondary to the lamellar pathology, the corium of the coronet and sole is damaged. Eventually even the DP itself may suffer deterioration and lysis of its dorsal margin. Unrelenting pain in the feet (bilateral forelimb usually) and a characteristic lameness occur. In acute laminitis the lamellar tissue suspending the DP from the inner hoof wall is affected at the junction between the connective tissue of the dermis or corium (the bone side) and the basal cell layer of the epidermal lamellae (the hoof side). This junction, the basement membrane zone or dermal/epidermal interface, appears to be the weak link in an otherwise robust and reliable structure. Wholesale epidermal cell detachment from and lysis of the lamellar basement membrane may occur,[1,2] leading to disruption of lamellar anatomy and ultimately compromise (to varying degrees) of the suspensory attachment between the DP and hoof. Associated with basement membrane lysis and dysadhesion are changes to lamellar epidermal cell morphology that result in lamellar stretching and attenuation. Thus whether by loss of basement membrane attachment or by lamellar stretching (or both), the DP draws away from the inner hoof wall and sinks downward. The degree of separation and sinking varies between horses affected with laminitis, ranging from barely detectable (mild) to catastrophically severe ("sinkers"). Ponies and small horses are usually less severely affected than their heavier cousins. A good correlation exists between the severity, as seen with the microscope (histopathology), and the degree of lameness (using the Obel grading system[3]) shown by the horse.[1] When a horse first shows laminitic pain, the anatomy of the hoof wall lamellae is already compromised. The higher the lameness grade, the more severe the microscopic damage. Any activity that places stress on an already weakened lamellar

References on page 1276

attachment apparatus (such as forced exercise) exacerbates damage and is contraindicated. The use of nerve blocks to eliminate pain encourages locomotion and does more damage. Favorable outcomes are associated with effective preventive and early therapeutic strategies.

PATHOPHYSIOLOGY

Pathological deformation of the lamellar attachment apparatus begins during the developmental phase of laminitis. Tightly controlled metabolic processes are targeted, causing lamellar-specific pathology. One mechanism behind lamellar deformation involves lamellar enzymes. Enzymes are normal constituents of lamellar cells and respond to the stresses and strains of equine life and to constant growth. Sufficient enzyme is manufactured locally to release epidermal cell-to-cell and cell-to-basement membrane attachment as required, maintaining the correct shape and orientation of the lamellae. From time to time injury to the basement membrane requires its lysis and reconstruction. The controlled release of matrix metalloproteinases (MMPs) and specific tissue inhibitors of MMP (TIMPs) keeps repair and modeling in equilibrium.[4,5] Normally the hoof lamellae slowly migrate distally past the stationary basement membrane that is firmly attached to the connective tissue covering the dorsal surface of the DP. Distal movement occurs because the hoof wall[6] continually proliferates at the coronet and moves downward past the stationary DP by a process of controlled enzymatic modeling of the lamellar epidermis and the basement membrane zone. Accumulating evidence suggests that during developmental laminitis, compromise of the basement membrane zone occurs when production of constituent lamellar enzymes is increased and they are activated out of control. The enzymes known to be involved are metalloproteinase-2 (MMP-2), metalloproteinase-9 (MMP-9), membrane-type metalloproteinase (MMP-14), and aggrecanase (ADAMTS-4), and singly or together they destroy key components of the lamellar suspensory apparatus.[7-10] A second, newly discovered lamellar deformation mechanism is seen in hyperinsulinemic horses. Experimental hyperinsulinemia is profoundly laminitogenic in ponies and horses, inducing clinical signs in 40 to 72 hours.[11,12] Limited basement membrane dysadhesion occurred in insulin-affected horses but not to the extent seen in experimental carbohydrate-induced laminitis and was virtually absent in ponies. Mitosis, normally infrequent among lamellar epidermal cells, was a feature of hyperinsulinemic lamellar histopathology possibly contributing to lamellar lengthening.[13] In laminitis induced by dosing horses with extract of Black walnut (*Juglans nigra*) heartwood, there was no evidence of basement membrane breakdown.[14,15]

HISTOPATHOLOGY OF ACUTE LAMINITIS

Most descriptions of laminitis histopathology derive from laminitis induced experimentally with a single large dose of carbohydrate of either grain starch or oligofructose.[3,16,17] The sequences of microscopic events that lead to clinical laminitis follow a consistent temporal pattern,[18] and the stages of histological laminitis can be identified by the degree of severity of these changes. Making the lamellar basement membrane clearly visible is important and

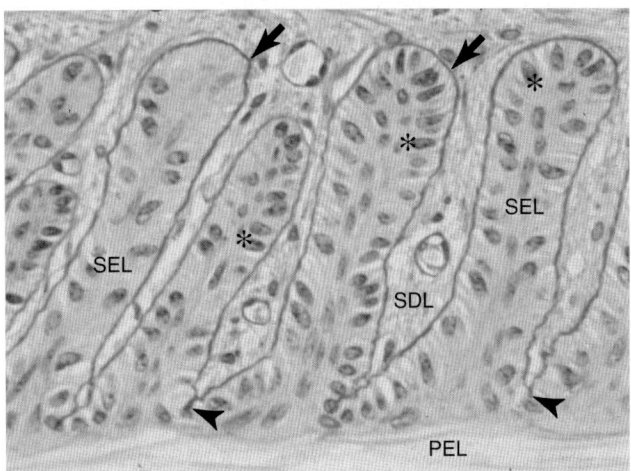

Fig. 34-1 • Micrograph of normal hoof lamellae stained to highlight the basement membrane. The basement membrane *(arrows)* of each secondary epidermal lamella *(SEL)* is a magenta (black in the figure) line closely adherent to the SEL basal cells. At secondary dermal lamellae *(SDL)* tips, between the bases of each SEL, the basement membrane *(BM)* penetrates deeply *(arrowheads)* and is close to the anuclear, keratinized, primary epidermal lamella *(PEL)*. The SEL tips are rounded (club-shaped). The basal cell nuclei are oval in shape *(stars)* and positioned away from the BM at the apex of each cell. The long axis of each basal cell nucleus is at right angles to the long axis of the SEL. The SDL are filled with connective tissue even at their very tips, between the SEL bases. These parameters of hoof lamellar anatomy form the basis of the histological grading system of laminitis histopathology. Stain, Periodic acid–Schiff; bar, 10 μm.

requires staining lamellar tissues with periodic acid–Schiff (PAS) stain or with immunohistochemical methods using basement membrane–specific antibodies.[1,2]

Normal lamellar anatomical characteristics, assessed before allocating a laminitis grade to a section of lamellar hoof tissue, are as follows (Figure 34-1):

- The tips of the secondary epidermal lamellae are always rounded (club-shaped) and never tapered or pointed.
- The basal cell nucleus is oval, with the long axis of the oval perpendicular to the long axis of the secondary epidermal lamellae. These parameters can be satisfactorily assessed using routine hematoxylin and eosin staining of sections.
- The basement membrane penetrates deeply into the crypts between the secondary epidermal lamellae and outlines the wafer-thin, but connective tissue–filled, secondary dermal lamellae.
- The basement membrane tightly adheres to the basal cells of each secondary epidermal lamella. The PAS or immunohistochemical stains show this best.

Grade 1 Histopathology

The earliest change attributable to laminitis is loss of shape and normal arrangement of the lamellar basal and parabasal cells. The basal cell nuclei become rounded instead of oval and take an abnormal position in the cytoplasm of the cell. The secondary epidermal lamellae become stretched, long, and thin, with tapering instead of club-shaped tips. These changes were present at 12 hours in serial lamellar biopsies taken after oligofructose dosing.[18] First noticeable at the tips of the secondary epidermal lamellae, teat-shaped bubbles of loose basement membrane form. PAS staining shows this best (Figure 34-2).

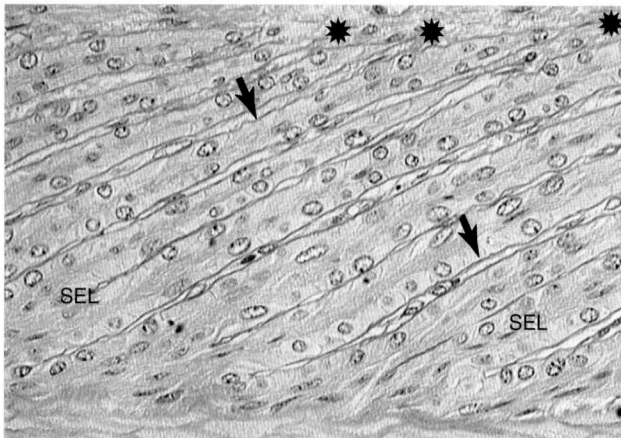

Fig. 34-2 • Grade 1 histological laminitis (periodic acid–Schiff stain). Micrograph showing hoof lamellar tissues stained to highlight the basement membrane. The basement membrane *(arrows)* is stained dark magenta (black in the figure). At the now-tapered tips of the secondary epidermal lamellae *(SELs)*, the basement membrane has lifted away *(stars)* from the underlying basal cells. Between the SEL bases the basement membrane *(BM)* is in its normal position, close to the primary epidermal lamellae; bar, 10 μm.

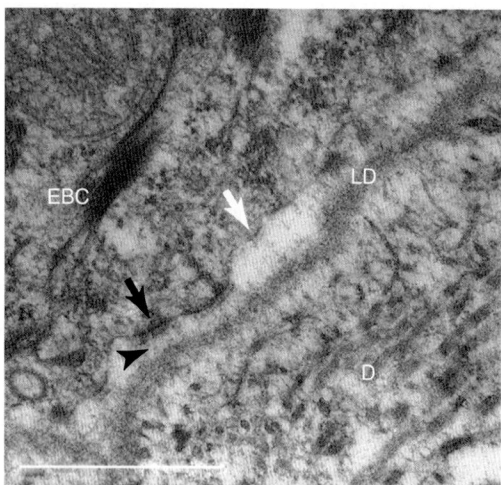

Fig. 34-3 • Electron micrograph of hoof lamellar tip developing laminitis. The lamina densa *(LD)* of the basement membrane is separating from the plasmalemma of the lamellar basal cell *(EBC)*. Some hemidesmosomes *(black arrow)* appear undamaged, but others *(white arrow)* have faded, are losing their anchoring filament attachments, and are drawing away from the basement membrane. Normally anchoring filaments *(arrowhead)* bridge the lamina densa firmly to the EBC. *D,* Dermis.

Examination of laminitis tissues with the electron microscope confirms lysis and separation of the lamellar basement membrane.[19] Importantly, the greater magnification shows widespread loss of basal cell adhesion plaques (hemidesmosomes) and contraction of the basal cell cytoskeleton away from the inner cell surface. Electron microscopy shows why the basement membrane separates from the feet of the basal cells. The filaments that anchor hemidesmosomes to the lamina densa of the basement membrane no longer bridge the dermal/epidermal interface (Figure 34-3).[13]

Grade 2 Histopathology

Because the basement membrane is no longer completely tethered to the basal cells, it slips farther away with each

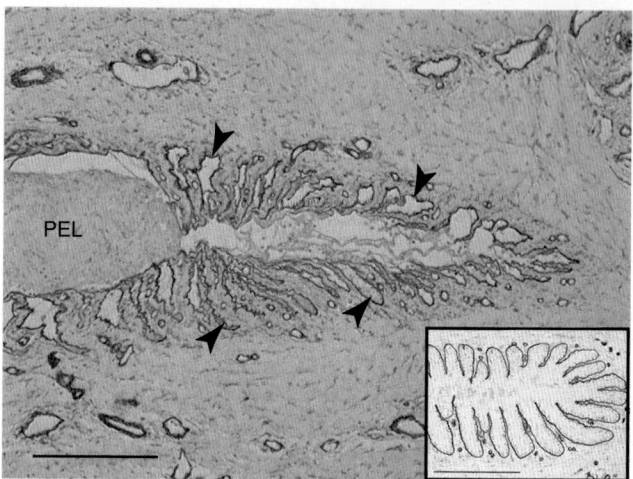

Fig. 34-4 • Grade 3 histological laminitis *(immunostain).* The basement membrane of a lamellar tip is highlighted by type IV collagen immunostaining. The tip of the primary epidermal lamella *(PEL)* has completely detached from its basement membrane. The PEL basal cells are now an unattached, amorphous mass. Collapsed tubes of basement membrane, now empty of epidermal cells, are still attached to connective tissue *(arrowheads).* The PEL has already moved 0.03 mm from its dermal compartment, and soon the distance will be measured, using a tape measure, on a radiograph. The inset shows a normal lamellar tip immunostained the same way. Type IV collagen immunostain; bars, 10 μm.

cycle of weight bearing by the horse. Portions of the lamellar basement membrane are lysed initially between the bases of the secondary epidermal lamellae (see Figure 34-2). The basement membrane retracts from the tips of secondary epidermal lamellae, taking the dermal connective tissue with it. The basement membrane–free epidermal cells appear not to be undergoing necrosis, at least initially, and clump together to form amorphous, basement membrane–free masses on either side of the lamellar axis.[1]

Grade 3 Histopathology

In laminitis the worst-case scenario is a rapid and near-total basement membrane separation from all the epidermal lamellae of the hoof toe, quarters, heel, and bars. Sheets of basement membrane peel away to form aggregations of loose, isolated basement membrane in the connective tissue adjoining the lamellae. The epidermal lamellar cells are left as isolated columns with little viable connection to the dermal connective tissue still attached to the DP. The hoof lamellar tips slide away from the basement membrane connective tissue attachments, at first microscopically, but as the degree of separation increases, the distance between hoof and DP becomes measurable in millimeters (Figure 34-4) and can be detected radiologically.[20] This manifests clinically as a sinker. Because the basement membrane is the key structure bridging the epidermis of the hoof to the connective tissue of the DP, wholesale loss and disorganization of the lamellar basement membrane follow and inexorably lead to the pathology of hoof and bone that characterizes the chronic stage of laminitis.

The laminitis process also affects the lamellar capillaries. As the basement membrane and the connective tissue between the secondary epidermal lamellae disappear, so do the capillaries. They become obliterated, compressed against the edges of the primary dermal lamellae. Without a full complement of capillaries in the lamellar circulation, blood probably bypasses the capillary bed through dilated arteriovenous shunts,[21] changing the nature of the foot circulation. A bounding pulse becomes detectable by finger palpation of the digital arteries. Furthermore, epidermal cell necrosis, intravascular coagulation, and edema are not universally present in sections made from tissues in the early stages of laminitis. The vessels in the primary dermal lamella, even the smallest, are predominantly open, without evidence of microvascular thrombi. The gross anatomical appearance of freshly dissected laminitis tissue is dryness. Sometimes the lamellae just peel apart.

Leukocytes, Inflammation, and Laminitis

It is rare to detect leukocytes in the lamellar tissues of normal horses.[14] However, extravasation of leukocytes into the perivascular lamellar dermis occurs in carbohydrate-,[1] Black walnut extract–,[14,22] and hyperinsulinemia-induced[13] forms of laminitis. Because leukocytic infiltration of tissues is associated with inflammation, the discovery that leukocytic infiltration is common to most, if not all, forms of laminitis has reemphasized an inflammatory pathway to laminitis development. There is molecular evidence that inflammatory mediators may activate many of the processes known to damage the lamellar interface.[23,24] Polymorphonuclear leukocytes are rich in MMP-9, and their presence within lamellar epidermal compartments in grade 3 histopathology[1] suggests that this basement membrane–degrading enzyme may have a pathological role in disease development. Also neutrophils produce reactive oxygen species and proinflammatory cytokines that probably contribute to cellular damage within the lamellar milieu.[15] Lamellar damage and leukocyte infiltration are readily detected by calprotectin immunostaining,[14,25] and because leukocyte infiltration precedes the expression of calprotectin in the lamellar epidermis, a role for leukocytes in initiating lamellar pathology has been suggested.[22,23] However, carbohydrate-induced laminitis studied at the 12-hour postdosing time point shows basement membrane degradation occurring in advance of leukocyte infiltration, thus downplaying an initiating role for leukocytes in lesion development.[25]

LAMINITIS THEORIES

The enzymatic theory of laminitis, based on the triggering of lamellar MMP activity,[26,27] challenged the alternative view that laminitis was caused by ischemia and ischemia/reperfusion injury damaging epidermal lamellae because blood flow was impeded.[28] Evidence against ischemia/reperfusion involvement in Black walnut extract–induced laminitis came from studies measuring xanthine oxidase, a reactive oxygen intermediate that increases in tissues affected by ischemia and ischemia/reperfusion. Xanthine oxidase was absent in tissues with Black walnut extract–induced lamellar pathology, suggesting that a global lamellar hypoxic event had not occurred.[29] Furthermore, there is evidence from three independent international laboratories that the foot circulation during the developmental phase of both carbohydrate- and hyperinsulinemia-induced laminitis is vasodilated.[30-33] Laminitis did not occur if the foot was in a state of vasoconstriction during the

developmental phase, suggesting that the trigger factors only cause laminitis if they reach the lamellar tissues at a high enough concentration and over a long enough time.[30] In current laminitis therapy there is a consistent lack of efficacy of drugs addressing ischemia, suggesting other pathogenic processes, such as inflammation, may be more important.

The actual trigger factors of laminitis remain unidentified. Gram-negative bacterial endotoxin has been detected in the circulation of horses with carbohydrate-induced laminitis[34] and is presumed to play a role in initiating lamellar pathology. Horses with colic, colitis, pleuropneumonia, and retained fetal membranes, the conditions often associated with laminitis development,[35] develop pyrexia and appear "endotoxic," but this is usually inferred from clinical signs rather than confirmed by endotoxin assay. Tumor necrosis factor and interleukin-6 (IL-6) along with other cytokines are expressed by mononuclear phagocytes within minutes of exposure to endotoxin.[36-38] Decreases in digital blood flow and lamellar perfusion, secondary effects mediated by the platelet-derived vasoconstrictors 5-hydroxytryptamine and thromboxane, follow intravenous endotoxin administration.[37] However, laminitis or even foot pain has never been elicited by the experimental administration of endotoxin into either the bloodstream or the peritoneal cavity.[39,40] Gram-negative bacteria disappear early, before the onset of clinical signs, from hindgut samples taken from horses developing carbohydrate overload-induced laminitis, suggesting no role for endotoxin in laminitis pathogenesis.[41] Instead a plethora of absorbed microbial toxins may affect lamellar compromise, including gram-positive exotoxins from the explosive proliferation of hindgut streptococci after carbohydrate overload.

Lamellar disintegration of laminitis occurs well before clinical signs. The molecular conformation of the lamellar basement membrane is altered 12 hours after dosing with oligofructose, and a major constituent of the basement membrane, collagen IV, begins to disappear. Previously, damage to the lamellar basement membrane was attributed to MMP release and activation, but new evidence places MMP activation many hours later than other molecular events.[25] An enzyme capable of modifying the proteoglycan components of lamellar basement membrane is ADAMTS-4 (A Disintegrin And Metalloproteinase with ThromboSpondin motifs), the gene for which has the greatest fold increase of any thus far discovered in laminitis development.[10,25,42] ADAMTS-4 gene expression occurs early in laminitis development, and the gene product may play a central role in the pathophysiology of the disease.

Metalloproteinase Inhibitors

The activity of tissue MMPs correlates strongly with the degree of malignancy and invasiveness of lethal human tumors, such as malignant melanoma, breast cancer, and colon cancer.[43] Research in this field has generated a wide range of chemical agents capable of inhibiting MMP activity in vitro and in vivo. BB-94 (Batimastat, British Biotech, Oxford, England) blocks the activity of the laminitis MMPs in vitro and has the potential to be a useful tool in preventing and managing acute laminitis. Whether MMP inhibitors can prevent or ameliorate naturally occurring laminitis has yet to be established.

NATURAL TRIGGER FACTORS

Insulin

To test the hypothesis that hyperinsulinemia triggers laminitis, normal, lean ponies with no previous history of insulin resistance or laminitis were subjected to prolonged hyperinsulinemia and euglycemia.[44] All the ponies developed laminitis within 72 hours of hyperinsulinemia, a finding supporting the importance of insulin in the pathogenesis of endocrinopathic laminitis. Standardbred horses subjected to the same hyperinsulinemia/euglycemia clamp protocol also developed clinical laminitis but sooner (<48 hours) and with histopathology notable for lamellar basement membrane separation.[33] Hyperinsulinemia causes profound changes in the peripheral microcirculation,[45] and a vascular (ischemic) pathogenesis for laminitis has long been sought.[46] However, hoof wall surface temperature, measured continuously in the hyperinsulinemic and control horses, showed hyperinsulinemia induced early-onset, prolonged vasodilation. Lamellar insulin receptors are located within blood vessels (but not elsewhere) and in the presence of insulin activate vascular nitric oxide synthase to produce the potent vasodilator nitric oxide. Perhaps unregulated vasodilation results in excessive cellular uptake of glucose, lamellar glucotoxicity, and oxidative stress similar to that involved in the pathogenesis of atherosclerosis and the associated up-regulated MMP-9 activity in human diabetes.[47]

Trigger Factors of Bacterial Origin

Equine lamellae, cultured in vitro, have tested resistant to virtually all known cytokines, tissue factors, and prostaglandins. Gram-negative bacterial endotoxin, extract of Black walnut (*J. nigra*), and even anaerobic culture conditions fail to induce lamellar separation or significant MMP activation.[48] Equine IL-6 added to cultured lamellar explants fails to activate lamellar MMPs or cause basement membrane disruption at the lamellar interface.[25] Some notable exceptions occur, however. Factors present in the supernatant of cultures of *Streptococcus bovis (S. bovis)* isolated from the equine cecum activate equine hoof MMP-2 and cause lamellar separation.[48] During carbohydrate overload, rapidly proliferating species of hindgut streptococci, predominantly *S. bovis* (now *Streptococcus lutetiensis*), ferment carbohydrate and produce large quantities of lactic acid.[41,49,50] In the presence of virtually unlimited substrate, the population of *S. bovis* increases exponentially and then dies and lyses en masse. The liberated cellular components of lysed hindgut streptococci may cross the mucosal barrier of the damaged hindgut and reach the hoof lamellae hematogenously to initiate laminitis. Microbial and other factors probably associate with basement membranes throughout the body but probably only cause damage to lamellar basement membranes because of their uniquely equine involvement in weight bearing.

Equine Metabolic Syndrome

The term *equine metabolic syndrome* refers to horses with a history of laminitis, insulin resistance, cresty necks, and increased adipose tissue deposits in the withers, dorsal area of the back, and rump.[51] Elevated serum insulin concentrations distinguish ponies that are susceptible to dietary pasture-associated laminitis.[52-55] Furthermore, insulin concentrations are markedly elevated in ponies that develop laminitis after grazing high carbohydrate pasture, whereas glucose, free fatty acid, and cortisol concentrations remain normal.[53,56] In contrast to people, insulin-resistant horses rarely develop pancreatic exhaustion and hyperglycemia and are capable of producing exceptionally high serum insulin concentrations.[56,57] Insulin toxicity appears to be a key factor in triggering equine laminitis. The onset of laminitis is associated with plasma insulin that exceeds 100 µIU/mL (normal range = 8 to 30 µIU/mL).[58]

Horses and ponies at risk of laminitis should be blood tested for the early detection of hyperinsulinemia, and grain or other soluble carbohydrate should be withheld for 3 hours before testing. A single blood sample showing elevated insulin predicts that laminitis will occur or may become worse.[58] Techniques should be used to lower insulin concentrations and restore insulin sensitivity. A weight-reducing diet with a low glycemic index and physical exercise reduce insulin resistance in horses.[59] Insulin-sensitizing drugs of the type given to people with type 2 diabetes have been trialed in insulin-resistant horses. Metformin, at a higher dose than previously reported (15 mg/kg body weight per os [PO] every 12 hours), reversed insulin resistance during the first 6 to 14 days of treatment, but this effect diminished by 220 days.[60] Pharmacokinetic and epidemiological studies and placebo-controlled trials may further define the potential applications of this drug in the treatment of insulin resistance and prevention of laminitis.

Equine Cushing's Disease

Older ponies and horses sometimes develop a problem with their pituitary gland, which enlarges, becomes dysfunctional, and results in the development of equine Cushing's disease (ECD). Pituitary enlargement is sometimes described as a tumor (pituitary adenoma), but most affected horses have simply pituitary hyperplasia (an increase in size for unexplainable reasons). The region of the pituitary involved is the pars intermedia, giving the condition its common medical name: pituitary pars intermedia dysfunction (PPID). The dysfunctional pituitary produces an excess of hormones and peptides that control other hormones. A sign that horses are affected by PPID is hirsutism; the hair coat grows unnaturally long and is not shed at the usual times.

The hormone imbalance is associated with hyperinsulinemia that disturbs hoof lamellar metabolism, promoting an insidious, relentlessly developing, chronic laminitis. Affected horses and ponies often have higher than normal concentrations of glucose, adrenocorticotropic hormone (ACTH), cortisone, and insulin in their blood. The levels of these substances vary throughout the day (diurnal or circadian rhythm), and care has to be taken with the interpretation of blood analysis. The clinical signs of ECD are pot belly and wasted top line, bulging supraorbital fat, polyuria and polydipsia, susceptibility to infections, and laminitis. Insulin status is a powerful prognostic indicator in horses with ECD, and insulin-resistant animals with a basal serum insulin concentration of greater than 188 µIU/mL are much more likely to develop laminitis and survive less than 2 years after diagnosis.[56] Laminitis that develops in association with ECD is usually refractory to treatment.

However, promising results have been obtained after the administration of pergolide mesylate (Permax, Valeant Pharmaceuticals International, Costa Mesa, California, United States), a drug registered for use in people. Doses in the range of 1 to 2 mg/horse/day have been recommended. The drug mechanism is to reduce production in the pituitary gland of the hormone (ACTH) that controls cortisol production in the adrenal gland. With cortisol under control, insulin responsiveness in hoof lamellae returns, and the laminitis stabilizes. Using pergolide mesylate, the ACTH concentration in horses with ECD decreases within 1 week.[58]

Exogenous Corticosteroids and Laminitis

Although not proven experimentally, an association was made between systemic or intraarticular administration of corticosteroids, including triamcinolone acetonide (TMC) and methylprednisolone acetate, and the development of laminitis in otherwise apparently healthy horses.[61] A single dose of TMC (0.05 mg/kg) given intramuscularly was cleared slowly and induced hyperglycemia and hyperinsulinemia for at least 3 days.[62] Larger intramuscular doses (0.2 mg/kg) prolonged this hyperinsulinemic effect, and serum insulin concentration of around 130 µIU/mL persisted for 6 days.[62] However, none of the treated horses developed laminitis, although a "laminar" ring, coincident with the time of injection, grew down the hoof wall. In a retrospective clinical trial only 1 of 205 horses treated with TMC developed laminitis, and it had a previous episode of laminitis in its history.[63] Nonetheless, clinicians must be aware of the risks associated with exogenously administered corticosteroids. As Bailey and Elliot[61] warn, "Glucocorticoids might only increase the risk of developing laminitis when other causative factors are present, or when the lamellar tissues are somehow 'primed' to undergo changes leading to cell damage and dysfunction." A risk factor may be the preexisting hyperinsulinemia associated with metabolic syndrome or ECD. Because hyperinsulinemia alone will precipitate clinical laminitis,[11] injecting glucocorticoid into already insulin-resistant, hyperinsulinemic horses may elevate serum insulin concentrations into the laminitogenic range.

Supporting Limb Laminitis

Laminitis in the lamellae of a single hoof can occur whenever a horse's limb is forced to bear weight unilaterally for prolonged periods. This can occur when an injury (bone or joint fracture) or disease process (infectious arthritis) in the contralateral limb is so painful that weight bearing is impossible. After days to weeks of unrelieved weight bearing, the supporting limb develops lamellar pathology, often to a severe degree. Presumably the immobile limb lacks adequate lamellar perfusion and glucose delivery that eventually trigger a lamellar pathology indistinguishable from that initiated by other causes. Development of this form of laminitis may be delayed or prevented by supporting the limb by a firmly applied elastic support bandage and shoeing with an effective support shoe. The horse should be provided with a deep bed of wood shavings or sand so that it can lie down comfortably and allow blood to circulate through its feet. Deep, compliant bedding also allows the horse to find a foot position that promotes foot circulation. The injured limb should be treated promptly and fitted with a cast or splint so that it can begin to take its share of weight bearing. Pain should be controlled with analgesics for the same reason. An exercise regimen of walking every 6 hours to encourage circulation of the contralateral foot has reduced the incidence of supporting limb laminitis in an equine hospital, but this practice may not be possible or advisable in all horses.[64]

▣ DIAGNOSIS OF LAMINITIS

Sue J. Dyson

Laminitis is characterized by an acute-onset lameness of variable severity involving one or more feet. Most often both front feet are affected, with or without the hind feet, but unilateral laminitis does occur, usually caused by excessive load bearing because of severe contralateral limb lameness. Occasionally the hind feet are affected, without involvement of the front feet. The horse may be extremely reluctant to move and, if persuaded to move, tends to land heel first, with a short, pottery gait, with the hindlimbs placed unusually far underneath the body. There is a marked shortening of the caudal phase of the stride at the walk. Lameness may be accentuated as the horse turns. Lameness is worse on hard ground than on soft ground. Although many horses show severe lameness, in those with milder lameness the lameness may be less typical, although suggestive of foot pain. When standing still the horse may position the hindlimbs unusually far underneath the body and may constantly shift weight between the limbs. A horse with severe primary lameness that has developed laminitis in the contralateral limb may start to load the originally lame limb, shifting weight between the two limbs.

Usually, but not invariably, a clinically significant increase in digital pulse amplitude occurs; however, in a thick-skinned cob-type horse this may not be palpable. In the acute phase the affected feet may be hot. Pressure or percussion applied to the feet, especially in the toe region, usually causes pain, but if the horn is excessively hard, the horse may not react. Careful palpation around the coronary band may reveal an unusual depression associated with sinking of the distal phalanx (DP). An area of unusual softness may herald infection tracking proximally in association with laminitis complicated by submural abscessation.

Clinical signs are usually diagnostic, except in less severely affected horses or those with involvement of only the hind feet, when the characteristics of the lameness may suggest foot pain, but not necessarily pathognomonic for laminitis. The response to perineural analgesia varies and is not associated necessarily with the degree of pain and lameness. Apparent desensitization of the foot with palmar (abaxial sesamoid) nerve blocks may have absolutely no effect on the lameness in some horses, although some improvement may occur in others.

Because laminitis frequently develops secondarily to a primary disease process, it is critical to evaluate the entire horse and to identify any predisposing factors that require treatment, such as endotoxemia, septic metritis, equine metabolic syndrome, or equine Cushing's disease. If equine metabolic syndrome is suspected, serum insulin concentrations and the response to an intravenous glucose tolerance test should be assessed. It has been suggested that the presence of three or more of the following may increase the risk of laminitis development tenfold: insulin resistance, compensatory β-cell response, hypertriglyceridemia, and obesity (body condition score, >6/9).[1] Recent administration of corticosteroids may also be a risk factor; in a survey of 36 European sports horse practitioners, 12 had experienced the development of severe laminitis within 7 to 10 days of administration of corticosteroids in 22 horses.[2] Corticosteroids incriminated included dexamethasone, triamcinolone, and betamethasone administered either systemically or intraarticularly for treatment of recurrent airway obstruction, joint disease, or back pain, at what would be considered to be normal dose rates. The majority, but not all, of the horses were considered overweight. Approximately 50% of affected horses were humanely destroyed because of uncontrollable sinking of the DPs.

Radiographic examination is critical for establishing a treatment protocol and prognosis. Although rotation of the DP often can be managed successfully, sinking warrants an extremely guarded prognosis. Lateromedial images help to determine whether the condition is acute or an exacerbation of a more chronic problem. Abnormal thickness of the dorsal hoof wall, with or without modeling of the toe of the DP, implies previous disease. Lateromedial images are also important to establish the baseline position of the DP within the hoof capsule. Dorsopalmar images may be useful for assessing mediolateral balance in horses with chronic, unstable laminitis and to detect radiolucent lines indicative of lamellar separation (Figure 34-6, B). If the foot is grossly misshapen, trimming it first is preferable; otherwise, a false impression of severe rotation of the DP, which merely reflects the abnormal hoof wall growth and the development of a lamellar wedge, may occur.

Standardizing the procedure (positioning, film-focus distance, and exposure factors) is essential to make meaningful comparisons between examinations. If using conventional radiography, use soft exposures or radiographic film with a large gray scale to enhance soft tissue detail. A grid is usually unnecessary. A horizontal x-ray beam should be perpendicular to the sagittal plane of the digit, centered between the toe and the heel, about 2 cm distal to the coronary band. Radiodense markers are placed on the dorsal aspect of the hoof wall and on the sole at the apex of the frog. The marker on the dorsal hoof wall should extend from the coronary band distally. This helps to establish the orientation of the DP and its position relative to the coronary band. Radiological abnormalities include rotation or sinking of the DP, increased thickness of the dorsal hoof wall, and radiolucent lines in the dorsal hoof wall, reflecting serum, necrotic tissue, or gas caused by infection or hoof wall separation.

■ MEDICAL THERAPY OF LAMINITIS
Christopher C. Pollitt

Laminitis often develops because disease is occurring in a body compartment other than the foot. Thus it is of paramount importance that the primary disease is treated urgently and effectively. If the duration and severity of the primary disease can be reduced by intensive therapy, a strong chance exists that the severity of lamellar pathology also may be reduced, thus improving the prognosis for the horse. Severe laminitis is sometimes the outcome despite

the best of current therapy, but some horses can exhibit early, mild clinical signs of laminitis yet recover with no long-term ill effects.

Currently no drug regimen is able to arrest or block the triggering of laminitis, and the severity of the initial lamellar damage is what influences the outcome.[1] An effective laminitis preventive may emerge when the mechanism behind the disintegration of the anatomy of the hoof wall lamellae is fully understood. The discovery that enzymes appear to be involved in the lamellar failure of laminitis[2-5] offers hope that proteinase inhibitor therapy, specifically targeted at hoof wall metalloproteinases, may arrest laminitis development. Horses that were able to keep the feet cool during the laminitis developmental period did not develop laminitis,[6] an observation that was the basis for developing distal limb cryotherapy as a useful preventive, first-aid measure. Bacteria are a source of laminitis trigger factors[7]; therefore effective antimicrobial therapy is a treatment priority.

Horses diagnosed with toxemia during enteritis, colitis, strangulating colic, pleuropneumonia, retained placenta, infectious metritis, and grain overload are at high risk of developing laminitis, and medical therapy and mechanical support for the distal phalanx (DP) ideally should be initiated before the clinical signs of foot pain appear. Addressing laminitis as soon as it appears in a sick horse should always be regarded as an emergency procedure. Even then, treatment may be too late. Antiendotoxin hyperimmune serum (Polymmune J, Veterinary Dynamics Inc., Templeton, California, United States) should be included in the intravenous fluid therapy for horses with, or at risk of developing, endotoxemia.

Nonsteroidal antiinflammatory drugs (NSAIDs) are given to reduce inflammation and foot pain. Flunixin meglumine (0.25 mg/kg thrice daily intravenously [IV] or 1.1 mg/kg twice daily IV) has a proven antiendotoxin effect by reducing prostaglandin production via cyclooxygenase inhibition[8,9] and is valuable. Horses receiving flunixin meglumine that subsequently were given endotoxin had significantly lower blood prostaglandin and lactate concentrations and reduced clinical signs than control horses. However, the effectiveness of flunixin meglumine or any NSAID as an antilaminitis agent has never been tested. A proven cause-and-effect link between endotoxemia and laminitis has never been established.[9]

Phenylbutazone (4.4 mg/kg IV or PO every 12 hours) appears to be a potent NSAID for the control of foot pain and is popular with most clinicians. Phenylbutazone and flunixin meglumine at the lower dose rate can be used concurrently, the former to control severe foot pain and the latter to control the effects of endotoxemia. Intravenously administered ketoprofen (2.2 mg/kg twice daily) can be used interchangeably with flunixin meglumine. Horses with acute laminitis usually require NSAID therapy for at least 2 weeks, and because of its low cost, phenylbutazone (2.2 mg/kg) is the best choice for maintenance therapy. Care must be taken not to overdose small ponies.

However, NSAIDs were administered to horses during experimental induction of laminitis without altering the outcome; laminitis still occurred.[10] When the laminitis process is triggered, virtually nothing by way of drug therapy stops its progress. The administration of phenylbutazone during the developmental and acute stages reduces foot pain and creates a more comfortable-looking horse, but the disease continues unabated. This creates an ethical dilemma: balancing the need to alleviate pain and suffering against the realization that most of what is administered is only palliative. When NSAIDs are in use, the horse should be confined to a stall with deep bedding. Exercise is contraindicated while the horse is under the influence of analgesics.

CRYOTHERAPY

Distal limb cryotherapy to cool the feet, reduce lamellar tissue metabolism, and induce digital vasoconstriction is a proven preventive strategy when administered early in the developmental phase of laminitis. Cold-induced, digital vasoconstriction during the laminitis developmental phase may limit exposure to and impact of circulating trigger factors on lamellar anatomy. Cryotherapy may bestow additional protection by slowing the kinetics of lamellar enzyme activity below a threshold that causes damage. Nuclear scintigraphic studies showed cold therapy significantly decreased perfusion of the soft tissues of a horse's foot within 30 minutes of the application of external cold.[11] An ice water footbath was used successfully to treat a pony in the developmental stage of acute laminitis after experimental cecal catheterization.[12]

Two controlled studies testing the efficacy of cryotherapy for the prevention of laminitis were completed. In the first study,[13] laminitis was induced in six horses using the oligofructose overload model. Each horse had one forelimb immersed in ice and water (mean temperature, 0.5 to 1.7°C) for a 48-hour experimental period, achieving a mean internal hoof temperature of 3.5 to 0.9°C. All horses developed clinical and histological laminitis in one or more of the untreated limbs. Laminitis did not develop in the treated limbs, and there was significantly reduced lamellar histological damage. In cooled limbs there was significantly less up-regulation of lamellar MMP mRNA compared with untreated limbs. Although cryotherapy markedly reduced the severity of laminitis, it did not completely prevent minor histological changes in four of the six horses. In the second study, cryotherapy was applied to all four limbs of six horses for 72 hours.[14] Laminitis was induced as before, and the observation period was extended until 7 days after oligofructose dosing. The horses showed either no or very mild clinical signs of laminitis, and histological examination of lamellar tissues collected 7 days postinduction showed no evidence of laminitis. Control horses were lame at 7 days and had moderate to severe laminitis histopathologically.

Cryotherapy was instigated immediately after administration of the carbohydrate induction bolus in these studies. In a horse with grain overload or acute colitis such prompt initiation of cryotherapy may not be possible. It is unclear whether such a potent prophylactic effect would occur if cryotherapy was initiated later in the course of the disease when lameness was already present. However, the potential value of cryotherapy to prevent laminitis was demonstrated, and further clinical evaluation of the technique is justified.

Cryotherapy for laminitis requires maintaining the limbs from the proximal metacarpal region and distad in a slurry of crushed ice or a circulating cold water (1 to 4°C) apparatus continuously for 24 hours or even longer if the period of septic shock, pyrexia, and digital vasodilation persists. Cryotherapy is safe, well tolerated, and economical. Unlike people, horses do not find cold therapy noxious. We have kept the forelimbs of normal horses in circulating, very cold water continuously for 3 days, with no immediate or long-term ill effect. Initial experiments support the effectiveness of cryotherapy for halting laminitis onset.[13,14] Keeping a horse with its feet in ice and water requires an extraordinary amount of time and dedication but can be done and, if laminitis is prevented, is worth the effort.

DIGITAL BLOOD FLOW THERAPY

Vasodilatory therapy and hot water footbaths during the developmental phase of laminitis are contraindicated. Drugs with vasodilator action, such as isoxsuprine hydrochloride, acepromazine, and glyceryl trinitrate (applied as patches to the pastern), may be beneficial after lamellar damage has occurred, when healing is required, but should be administered with caution during the developmental phase of laminitis. However, neither orally administered isoxsuprine nor pentoxifylline produced significant improvement in digital or lamellar blood flow when tested under controlled conditions using ultrasound and laser Doppler flowmetry.[15-17] Intravenously administered acepromazine maleate, long held to be effective at increasing lamellar microcirculatory blood flow, had no significant effect when tested by laser flowmetry.[17] Glyceryl trinitrate tested in the same way, using a Black walnut extract laminitis induction model, had no effect on lamellar blood flow.[16] The continued veterinary use of these drugs in the therapy of laminitis is questionable.

Exercise of an intensity that increases core temperature and local analgesia of the palmar or plantar nerves result in hoof wall heating (and by implication, vasodilation) and are contraindicated during the developmental stage of laminitis. Local analgesia of the foot to reduce foot pain and encourage the horse to walk may result in greater lamellar damage than in a rested, confined horse. Forced exercise of any horse with acute laminitis is strongly contraindicated.

FREE RADICAL SCAVENGERS

Dimethyl sulfoxide (DMSO) may be given intravenously for its free radical scavenging and antiinflammatory effects. DMSO (90% solution) mixed with polyionic solutions and 5% dextrose is best administered slowly at about 8 L/h. The concentration of DMSO must remain below 20% to avoid the risk of intravascular hemolysis. However, despite the potential value of DMSO, its promise as an effective laminitis therapy has not been fulfilled. Evidence exists that ischemia, reperfusion injury, and generation of free radicals are not involved in the pathogenesis of horses with laminitis induced with extract of Black walnut.[18]

RECOMMENDED TREATMENT STRATEGY

Cryotherapy is the frontline of defense against laminitis and should be instituted early, preferably before clinical signs of foot pain appear. Cryotherapy has a proven preventive effect when applied throughout the developmental period of carbohydrate-induced laminitis.[13,14] Applied to all four limbs during the developmental phase of laminitis, distal limb cryotherapy is an effective means of ameliorating the disease and is recommended in horses at risk of developing acute laminitis. Clinically, distal limb cryotherapy has been applied for up to 5 days and successfully prevented clinical laminitis in horses affected by acute colitis.[19]

The list of pharmaceuticals that have been administered to horses with laminitis is long, and, apart from the NSAIDs, none have achieved particular prominence. Aggressive treatment of the primary disease using fluids and electrolytes, antibiotics and NSAIDs, and uterine lavage for horses with infectious metritis or retained placenta is recommended.

The administration of 4 L of mineral oil four times a day may be beneficial in horses with laminitis developing from grain overload. Mineral oil has a laxative effect and is said to block the absorption of toxins in the large intestine.[20] Activated charcoal is an effective adsorbent of a range of toxins and may be useful in horses with grain overload if administered promptly. In Australia, doses of 1 to 5 g/kg/day have been used to treat plant toxicoses in large animals. The higher dose is indicated if a large quantity of grain has been consumed. However, activated charcoal has not been tested against alimentary laminitis; thus its true effectiveness is unknown. The application of cold therapy to all feet, strict confinement to a stall with a deep bedding of sand or shavings, and mechanical support for the DP are also recommended.

Laminitis developing secondary to equine Cushing's disease (pituitary pars intermedia dysfunction) is usually refractory to treatment unless horses are given pergolide mesylate (1 to 2 mg/horse/day) to reduce adrenocorticotropic hormone (ACTH) production in the pituitary gland.[21] Within 7 days of commencing pergolide treatment, plasma ACTH concentration and adrenal cortisol levels are significantly decreased and probably so is the associated hyperinsulinemia.[22] Metformin (15 mg/kg body weight PO every 12 hours) reverses insulin resistance and decreases serum insulin concentration during the first 6 to 14 days of treatment, but the effect diminishes by 220 days.[23] Responses to insulin reduction strategies may be disappointing if substantial lamellar pathology already exists. Preventive use of pergolide and metformin, before or shortly after the first laminitis episode, may be more efficacious.

Some horses that show the clinical signs of acute laminitis recover completely if treated promptly using a combination of rational medical therapy and mechanical support. However, horses recovering from even the mildest form of laminitis should be observed closely and allowed to rest. If no radiological evidence of palmar displacement of the DP within the hoof capsule is apparent, and the digital pulse amplitude is not palpably exaggerated 48 hours after treatment has ceased, the horse can be returned to its usual function with caution.

If radiographs show displacement of the DP, then the prognosis must be more guarded. Horses with a mild increase in the distance between the DP and the dorsal hoof wall, with or without rotation of the DP, often make an apparent recovery and remain sound indefinitely. However, horses with marginally greater displacement and rotation of the DP make only partial recoveries and often have a history of intermittent lameness, especially after exercise. Histopathological examination of the hoof

lamellae of partially recovered horses showed a reduction in the number of secondary epidermal lamellae. Many of the secondary epidermal lamellae had distorted and abnormal shapes even several years after the initial episode of laminitis. Some secondary epidermal lamellae become isolated from the attachment to the primary epidermal lamellae and exist as isolated, unattached islands adrift in the lamellar connective tissue. If the surface area of the lamellae of the inner hoof wall is reduced after laminitis, the effectiveness of the lamellar-DP suspensory mechanism must also be reduced. Horses developing laminitis associated with substantial initial lamellar destruction, as manifest by radiological displacement of the DP, appear never to make a complete anatomical recovery and are prone to recrudescent episodes of laminitic foot pain.

Ultimately the prognosis is directly proportional to the severity and extent of lamellar pathology. Horses with more than 15 degrees of rotation, accompanied by distal displacement of the DP within the hoof capsule, within 4 to 6 weeks of the initial episode of laminitis have a poor prognosis. Prolapse of the DP through an already necrotic sole, accompanied by subsolar and sublamellar infection, usually occurs. Discharge of purulent exudate from the coronet and the heel is common. Osteitis and radiological evidence of lysis of the distal margin of the DP develop. Such horses require months of expensive supportive care and surgery, and although occasionally a horse does make a surprisingly good recovery, most suffer months of crippling foot pain and recumbency and eventually require euthanasia on humane grounds.

The road to recovery after a serious episode of laminitis is a rocky one. The extent of lamellar pathology lies hidden beneath the hoof wall, and we can only guess at what is really going on. Radiographs and the initial degree of pain expressed by the horse, often masked by analgesics such as phenylbutazone, give valuable clues. However, relentless sinking of the DP in the hoof capsule and involvement of all four feet make recovery unlikely.

■ CHRONIC LAMINITIS

Christopher C. Pollitt and Simon N. Collins

Following the acute phase of laminitis a horse may recover fully, with no long-term adverse effects on foot function, or can progress into chronic laminitis characterized by displacement of the distal phalanx (DP) within the foot.[1,2] This occurs because the damage to the lamellar interface is so extensive that the suspensory apparatus of the distal phalanx (SADP) can no longer maintain the normal anatomical relationship between the hoof capsule, dermis, and DP, resulting in lameness (Figure 34-5).[2-7]

Continuous supportive foot management is necessary to minimize the debilitating effects.[7] Affected horses are either chronic remissive laminitics (CRLs) or refractory exacerbative laminitics (RELs).[8,9] Although CRLs are responsive to palliative treatment with nonsteroidal antiinflammatory drugs (NSAIDs), RELs are minimally responsive, and euthanasia is often the only option to relieve unrelenting pain. CRLs remain highly susceptible to recrudescent episodes of acute intense pain.[7,9] Epidemiological estimates suggest that 50% of all acutely laminitic horses become chronic, and that 50% of these remain permanently lame.[10]

The anatomical dislocation of the DP, which can be detected radiologically as "rotation" or "sinking" (Figure 34-6), depends on the extent and localization of the lamellar pathology, the magnitude of the loads placed on the foot, the effect of treatment modalities used, and disease duration.[2,7]

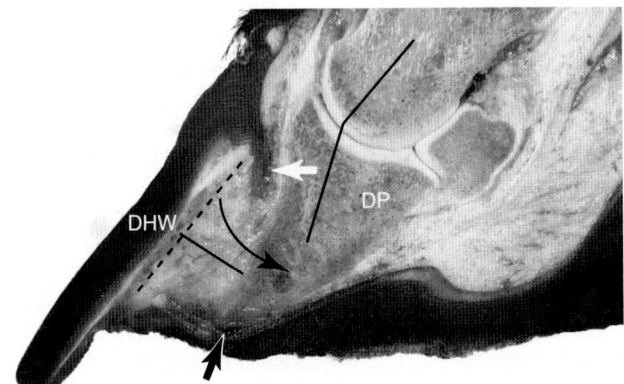

Fig. 34-5 • Sagittal section of a foot with severe chronic laminitis showing presence of a large lamellar wedge. The attachment between the distal phalanx *(DP)* and the dorsal hoof wall *(DHW)* has failed, and hoof and bone are now widely separated. The dotted line shows the original position of the DP. The angled black line shows that the DP has rotated around the distal interphalangeal joint (in the direction of the *curved black arrow*) and is no longer in alignment with the pastern axis (longitudinal axis of the proximal and middle phalanges), that is, phalangeal rotation. The material now between the inner aspect of the hoof wall and the DP is abnormal and consists of hyperplastic epidermal tissue that forms a weak, pathological structure called the lamellar wedge *(straight black line)*. The distal descent of the unsupported DP within the hoof capsule has affected the normal alignment of the dermal papillae, resulting in distorted growth of the proximal hoof wall tubules, and has caused the sole to become convex instead of concave (dropped sole). Two dark hemorrhagic zones *(white and black arrows)* show the sites of greatest pressure and trauma.

Disease progression and exacerbation are associated with the initiation of a number of changes, including lamellar wedge formation (see Figure 34-5), bone modeling and lysis (particularly at the apex of the DP), and abscessation within the solar dermis.[2,5,7,11,12] DP dislocation results in the development of vascular deficits within the coronary and solar plexi, as well as within the sublamellar and lamellar dermis.[14] There is also alteration to the normal pattern of hoof horn production from the coronary, lamellar, and solar regions of the foot, which leads to the development of a distorted hoof capsule.[2,7]

It is important to assess the nature and extent of DP dislocation because it relates directly to the degree of lameness,[13,15] the likelihood of return to former performance levels,[13,15,16] and survival outcome.[13,16,17] The following anatomical variations in DP dislocation occur, relating to the site and extent of lamellar pathology[2,7,18]:

1. Angular deviation between the dorsal aspect of the DP and the dorsal aspect of the hoof wall—ambiguously referred to elsewhere as capsular rotation
2. Phalangeal rotation—angular deviation between the dorsal aspect of the DP relative to the phalangeal axis
3. Distal displacement of the DP—distal displacement of the proximal aspect of the extensor process of the DP relative to the proximal aspect of the hoof wall (called sinking)
4. Combined phalangeal rotation and distal displacement of the DP
5. Asymmetrical distal displacement of the DP—occurring mainly on the medial or lateral aspect of the foot

With sinking of the DP there may be a depression palpable at the coronary band,[2,7] which is focal or extends around the circumference of the coronary band.

Radiological examination is essential to determine the position of the DP. Extreme changes are readily appraised by visual inspection alone. However, subtle and modest changes require objective evaluation, especially when

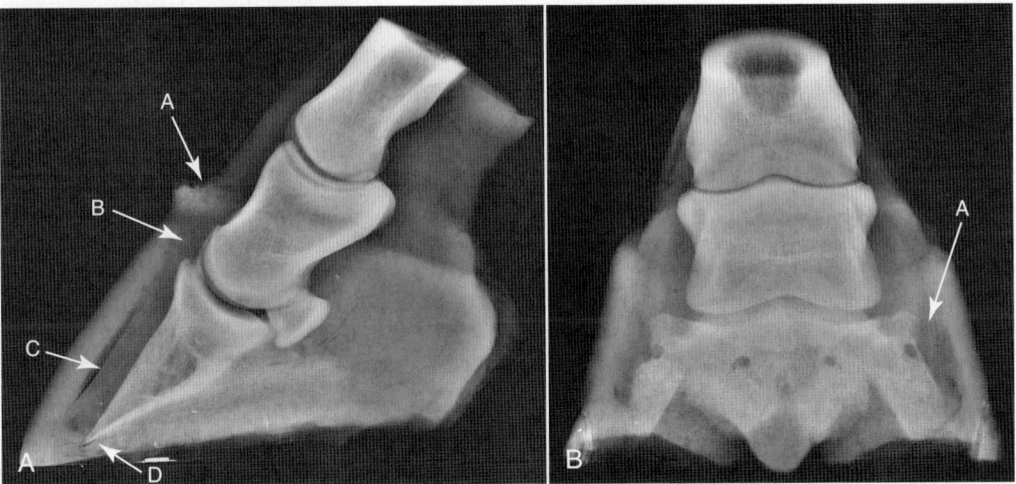

Fig. 34-6 • **A,** Lateromedial radiograph of a catastrophic "sinker" foot, showing a visible and palpable supracoronary depression *(A)*, and compression and distortion of the coronary dermis between the hoof wall and the extensor process *(B)*, following distal displacement of the distal phalanx *(DP)*. A visible airline *(C)* provides evidence of failure of the suspensory apparatus of the DP and physical separation of the dermal and epidermal lamellae. The distal displacement of the DP has resulted in penetration of the apex of the bone into the solar dermis *(D)*. **B,** Dorsopalmar radiograph of the sinker foot seen in **A,** showing a fine near-parallel array of radiolucent lines *(A)* indicating failure of the suspensory apparatus of the DP, as well as physical separation of the dermal and epidermal lamellae.

distal displacement of the DP occurs. Two parameters are of diagnostic importance: the hoof–DP distance and the coronary band extensor process distance.

In a normal foot, the perpendicular distance between the middorsal aspect of the hoof wall and the dorsal aspect of the DP (hoof–DP distance) is up to 18 mm,[19,20] and the vertical distance between the proximal aspect of the hoof capsule and the proximal aspect of the extensor process of the DP is approximately 4 mm.[21] These measurements do not take into account breed variation in foot size, and a better determination of DP dislocation may be if the hoof–DP distance exceeds 25% of the length of the palmar cortex of the DP.[20]

Dislocation results in compression and shear within the solar dermis, as well as the development of foot pain detectable clinically as a positive response to the application of hoof testers.[2,7] Recent work[22] suggests that these events, combined with inflammatory responses, can induce neuropathic changes characterized by allodynia (pain from stimuli that are not normally painful) and hyperalgesia (lowering of the pain threshold). This results in a chronic pain state that is nonresponsive to traditional NSAID treatment.

DP dislocation may also be associated with vascular trauma occurring within the solar dermis, which subsequently becomes evident as hemorrhage within the sole horn directly beneath the solar margin of the DP.[2,7] Lamellar pathology can result in the development of a "seroma" between the apical tips of the primary dermal lamellae and the basal region of the primary epidermal lamellae (adjacent to the inner hoof wall).[2] This seroma can be discerned as a mild linear reduction in radiopacity along the dermo-epidermal junction on lateromedial radiographic images optimized for evaluation of soft tissue (see Figure 34-6, A).

Progressive lamellar separation and inspissation of a seroma results in the appearance of a radiolucent airline seen in a lateromedial radiographic image[7,11,23] or as a series of fine, near-parallel radiolucent lines in a dorsopalmar radiographic image (see Figure 34-6, B). The appearance of the airline indicates that extensive lamellar separation has occurred, and supportive foot management is required to stabilize the DP and protect the surviving lamellae. This may prevent further mechanical failure of the SADP and progressive dislocation of the DP. With continued hoof growth, the airline moves distally and eventually becomes evident at the weight-bearing border of the foot, providing a potential portal for secondary, opportunistic bacterial and fungal infection.

DP dislocation initiates a number of distinct secondary changes that further compromise foot function and alter the normal pattern of hoof horn production.[2,7,11] Most notable is the development of a lamellar wedge (see Figure 34-5). The precise etiopathophysiological mechanisms that lead to its formation are not fully understood, and considerable variation in the histological appearance of this structure is reported.* This presumably reflects the progressive nature of the pathological processes that contribute to its formation over time, and the severity of the underlying lamellar pathology.

In mild laminitis, where lamellar separation is minimal, the lamellar wedge is characterized by elongation and

attenuation of the normal lamellar architecture.[2,5] More extensive separation results in lamellar fragmentation and a permanent reduction in the SADP surface area of attachment.[2,7] Hyperplastic epidermal proliferation occurs, and the resultant tissue has been described as "ectopic" white line[13] because its histological appearance, a mixture of tubular and lamellar horn, resembles that of the white line.

The dislocation of the DP within the hoof capsule triggers a series of events that alter the physical appearance of the hoof capsule.[2,7,8,22] These changes include a flattening of the sole in direct response both to the anatomical dislocation of the DP and from excessive movement of the DP occurring within the hoof capsule during weight bearing. This can cause vascular trauma of the solar dermis and lead to abscessation and the production of a false sole (Figure 34-7). In severe laminitis, the sole becomes convex, and the DP may eventually prolapse through it, which results in severe unrelenting pain and prolonged recumbency. Solar prolapse of the DP often results in the development of proliferative granulation tissue and associated subsolar abscessation at the site of the prolapse.

Elongation, attenuation, and separation of the lamellar interface become apparent on the solar surface of the hoof as a progressive "widening" of the white line,[2,7,8] which may be accompanied by hemorrhage. Dislocation also leads to pathological alterations in the coronary band. A combination of compression, vascular deficits, and reorientation of the dermal papillae alters the normal pattern of hoof horn production. There is reorientation of the dermal papillae of the coronary band,[7,28] which results in a realignment of the direction of horn growth at the midline of the hoof and leads to differential rates of proximodistal hoof horn growth around the circumference of the hoof capsule. As a result, the growth rings diverge circumferentially from the dorsal aspect of the hoof wall to

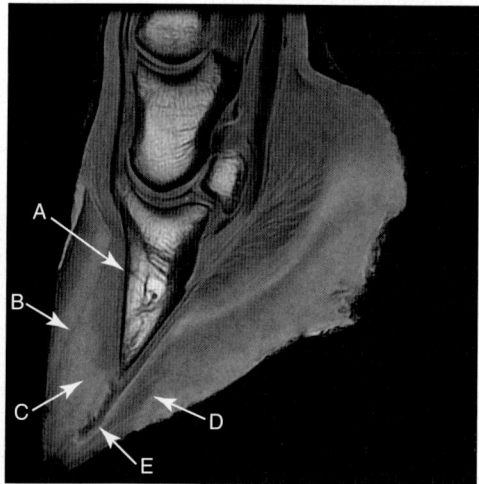

Fig. 34-7 • High-resolution sagittal three-dimensional T1-weighted spoiled gradient-echo magnetic resonance image of a chronic laminitic foot, showing angular deviation between the dorsal surface of the hoof wall (viewed proximally) and the dorsal aspect of the distal phalanx (A); a linear hypointense area at the margin of the lamellar interface, indicating lamellar separation and/or seroma formation (B); ectopic white line of the lamellar wedge (high signal intensity within the lamellar interface) and the widened sublamellar dermis proximally (intermediate signal intensity) (C); double (false) sole (D); and track of solar abscessation passing through the widened white line at the hoof wall–sole junction (E).

*References 2, 5, 11, 13, 24-26.

the heel. If left unattended this leads to the development of a distorted hoof capsule, characterized by both an excessive buildup of heel horn and dorsal concavity of the hoof wall. With advanced lesions there is a physical separation, or shear lesion, of the hoof capsule from the underlying coronary dermis,[2] and if extreme this results in complete avulsion of the hoof capsule.[2,7]

DP dislocation is often accompanied by progressive demineralization of the distal margin of the DP.[2,7,11] Radiological abnormalities vary from low-grade demineralization and slight modeling of the apex of the DP (a "ski tip") to extensive radiolucent defects on the distal, dorsal, and palmar cortices, as well as DP solar margin fractures. Extensive new bone formation may occur along the middorsal aspect of the DP, interpreted as a reactive response to increased levels of tensile stress occurring within the SADP.

There are also specific hidden dangers associated with DP dislocation that are only now being fully understood.[7] The solar dermis may become distorted around the distal margin of the DP, causing a reorientation of the dermal papillae of the sole dermis in this region. This distortion changes the direction of sole horn production and leads to the development of an in-growing mass of sole horn that progressively impinges on the distal dorsal aspect of the DP and is often associated with pronounced bone lysis. In addition, a similar change in orientation can occur in the coronary papillae, and similarly leads to an in-growing mass of hoof horn, which further compresses the coronary dermis. Foot treatments should be instigated to reduce the risk posed by altered in-growing horn production. Timely resection of the proximal and distal dorsal hoof wall overlying the in-growing zones promotes reorientation of the dermal papillae, leading to normal hoof horn growth. Treatment shoes and sole inserts should support the palmar/plantar aspect of the feet and spare (relieve) any sole pressure beneath the dorsal margin of the dislocated DP. Shoe breakover should align with the DP dorsal margin to minimize strain within the lamellar interface.

DP dislocation can also adversely alter the normal pattern of blood circulation within the foot[2,7] and thus affect foot metabolism, and is therefore of prognostic importance.

◼ VENOGRAPHY

Christopher C. Pollitt, Simon N. Collins, and Greg Baldwin

Venography is an additional method of assessing the damaged anatomical interrelationships within a chronic laminitic foot and the associated alteration to the digital circulation. The lack of valves in the digital veins distal to the midpastern region enables near-complete retrograde filling of foot veins with 20 to 25 mL of radiodense contrast media (Figure 34-8). The technique for venography is described elsewhere.[1,2] Serial venography has diagnostic and prognostic value because it may detect the progressive soft tissue pathology associated with DP rotation, and it provides objective monitoring of the response to remedial foot management.

In venograms acquired before onset of laminitis the mean perpendicular distance between the dorsal aspect of the hoof wall and the dorsal aspect of the distal phalanx

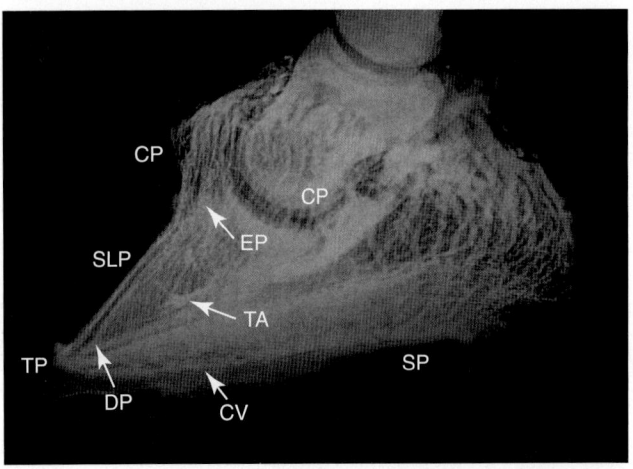

Fig. 34-8 • Lateromedial venogram of a normal foot. Most of the vessels are large veins. Veins in the solar and terminal papillae are visible but not the lamellar veins and capillaries. The dorsal margin of the distal phalanx is proximal to the circumflex vein. *CP,* Coronary venous plexus; *EP,* extensor process of the distal phalanx; *SLP,* sublamellar plexus; *TA,* terminal arch vessels *(arrow); DP,* distal phalanx (distal margin *arrow); TP,* terminal papillae; *CV,* circumflex vein *(arrow); SP,* sole papillae. (Venogram from Homestead Equine Hospital, Pacific, Missouri, United States.)

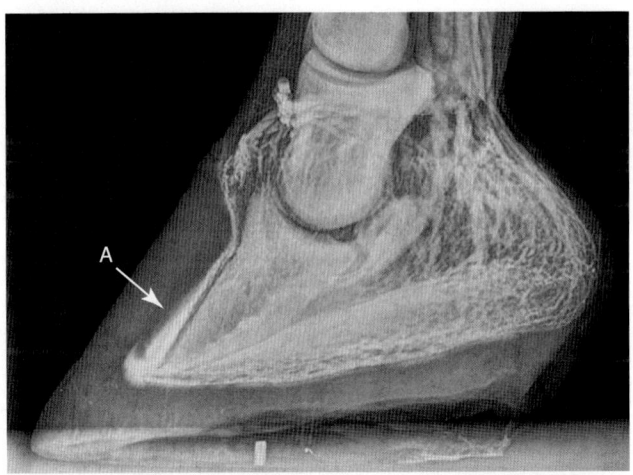

Fig. 34-9 • Lateromedial venogram of a chronic laminitic foot, showing the presence of diffuse contrast agent *(feathering)* within the sublamellar dermis distally *(A)*. Note the apex of the distal phalanx is at the level of the circumflex vessels dorsally.

(DP) (hoof–DP distance) is approximately 18 mm, and the width of the sublamellar venous plexus is 3.0 mm with a linear distance between the apex of the DP and the circumflex vessels of 8.0 mm. The apex of the DP is proximal to the level of the circumflex plexus.[3]

Chronic laminitis is associated with alteration of the venographic appearance that correlates to disease severity and progression (Figures 34-9 through 34-11). Within 7 days of the onset of experimentally induced laminitis, there is an increase in the hoof–DP distance of less than 2 mm. This is associated with a corresponding increase in the width of the sublamellar vascular plexus, with evidence of contrast media penetration into the sublamellar dermis. The apex of the dislocated DP is level with the circumflex plexus. There is reduced contrast medium filling within the coronary plexus as a result of compression of the dermal

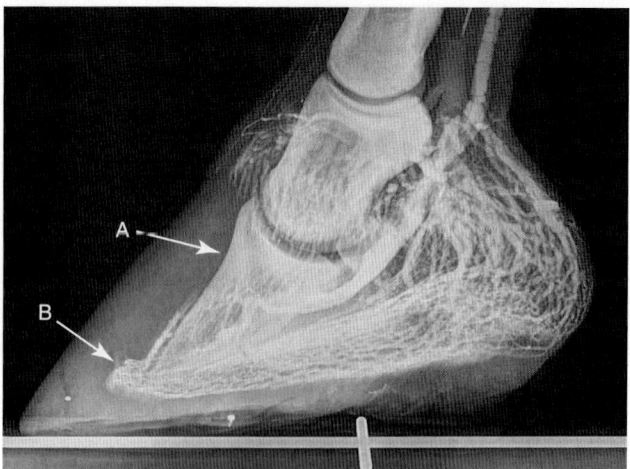

Fig. 34-10 • Lateromedial venogram of a foot with recent-onset laminitis and mild rotation of the distal phalanx, showing complete venous deficit within the coronary plexus dorsally and the proximal region of the dorsal sublamellar plexus (A). The circumflex vessels dorsally have been distorted substantially around the apex of the distal phalanx (B), which is indicative of the hidden danger of an inward-growing solar horn. (Venogram from Davide Zani, University of Milan, Italy.)

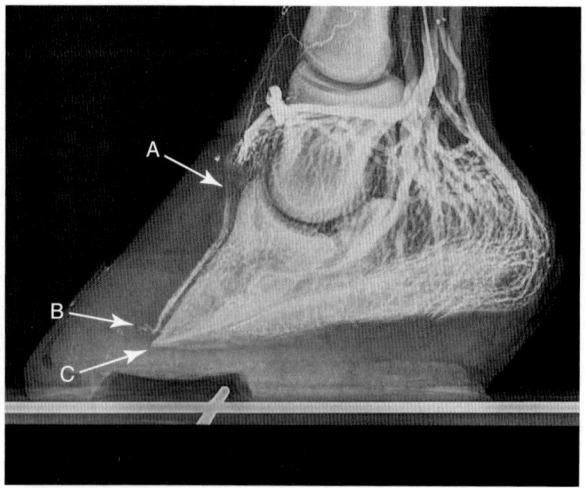

Fig. 34-11 • Lateromedial venogram of the same laminitic foot as shown in Figure 34-10 following supportive farriery intervention. Foot trimming and remedial shoeing have resulted in the partial restoration of venous filling within the coronary plexus dorsally and the proximal region of the dorsal sublamellar plexus (A). However, a venous deficit has developed in the circumflex vessels dorsally (B), and the apex of the distal phalanx (C) has descended below the level of the circumflex vessels, resulting in a pronounced venous deficit in the solar plexus dorsally. (Venogram from Davide Zani, University of Milan, Italy.)

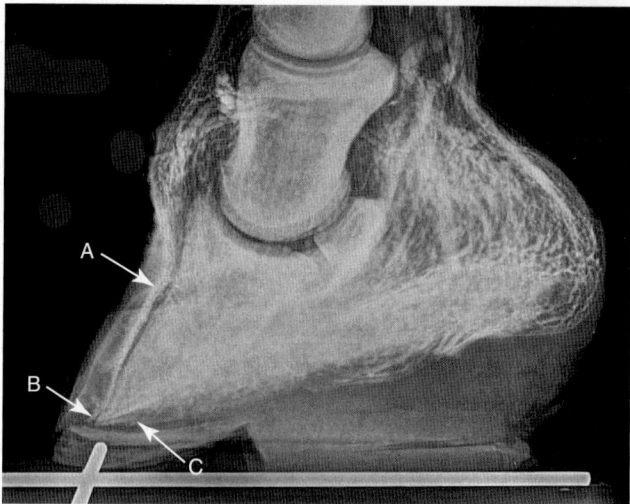

Fig. 34-12 • Lateromedial venogram of the same laminitic foot as shown in Figures 34-10 and 34-11 following coronary band peeling and removal of the dorsal aspect of the hoof wall. This has resulted in restoration of venous filling within the coronary and sublamellar plexus (A). In addition, there has been realignment of the circumflex vessels at the apex of the distal phalanx (B) and a modest improvement of venous filling of the solar plexus (C). (Venogram from Davide Zani, University of Milan, Italy.)

tissues between the extensor process of the DP and the proximal aspect of the hoof wall.

There may also be distortion of the circumflex plexus as pathological abnormalities of the solar dermis around the apex of the DP develop. Inward-growing lamellae (lamellar wedge) and distorted inward-growing tubular horn of the proximal hoof wall and dorsal sole further alter patterns of contrast media distribution.

With more severe DP dislocation, the increase in hoof–DP distance is greater than 4 mm, and the magnitude of the filling deficit in the coronary plexus increases. The apex

of the DP is distal to the circumflex plexus (see Figure 34-11). These events are associated with widening and distortion of the sublamellar and circumflex vascular beds. The sublamellar vascular bed increases in width with contrast medium penetration throughout the sublamellar dermis. The distance between the tip of the DP and the circumflex vessels also increases. Vascular filling deficits may also be evident within the distal, dorsal sublamellar plexus, evidence of an encroaching lamellar wedge and a prelude to DP lysis in this region.

Treatment of a chronic laminitic horse is aimed at stabilizing the foot, preventing further DP dislocation, and crucially restoring the circulation (Figures 34-11 and 34-12). Various treatment approaches have been suggested. These include rasping of the distal portion of the dorsal hoof wall and the dorsal aspect of the sole to relieve pressure on the circumflex vessels of the toe and to allow realignment of the solar plexus at the apex of the DP. The concurrent application of beveled, rocker, or reversed shoes may also help by reducing weight-bearing pressure in this region of the foot. Shoe breakover should be aligned with the dorsal distal margin of the DP to reduce strain within the lamellar interface. Complete or partial hoof wall resection, as well as paring of the lamellar wedge, is advocated to aid reinstatement of the sublamellar circulation (see Figure 34-12). Finally, coronary band hoof wall peels or deep coronary band grooving[4] may be beneficial to relieve compression of the coronary dermis, and hence reestablish the coronary plexus circulation. In addition, this treatment option aids realignment of the dermal papillae and restoration of normal patterns of hoof wall growth.

Serial venography gives important information on the progression of chronic laminitis pathology that is not detectable by standard radiology. The venographic changes, detectable early in the chronic phase, are a reference point for assessing the success of supportive therapy or subsequent clinical deterioration (see Figures 34-10 through

34-12). If no contrast medium filling deficits develop and the width of the sublamellar plexus remains stable, a guarded prognosis is justified. Deficits in venous filling with contrast media reflect focal dermal compression by distorted, aberrant lamellar and tubular hoof growth. This can potentially be corrected with judicious, timely hoof capsule resections. Filling deficits may reverse if hoof capsule modification is successful.

◼ HOOF CARE OF A LAMINITIC HORSE

Frank A. Nickels

Hoof care in all phases of laminitis is extremely important. The goal is to reduce stress to the damaged lamellae by minimizing the distracting forces affecting the displacement of the distal phalanx (DP) (rotation or sinking). These distracting forces are the weight of the horse, the constant pull of the deep digital flexor tendon (DDFT), and the leverage on the toe of the hoof capsule. Nothing can be done about the horse's weight, but absolute stall rest can reduce the increased stress associated with movement. Some of the weight of the horse can be partially redirected away from the hoof wall in the resting horse by removing the shoes. Recruiting other parts of the ground surface of the hoof to bear weight can also reduce stress on the hoof wall with the use of particular bedding or sole pads. Elevating the heel reduces the stress on the DDFT. In horses with rapid rotation or penetration of the corium through the sole, a tenotomy of the DDFT[1,3,4] was recommended to eliminate any pull on the DP. Finally, beveling (unweighting) the toe with a rasp helps increase ease of breakover, thereby decreasing the stress created by the leverage of the toe. Baseline radiographic examination is important to establish the relationship between the DP and the hoof capsule. I place both feet on two 8 × 13 × 18-cm wooden blocks that provide comfort to the horse, evenly weight the digits, and eliminate radiological distortion. There are linear radiodense markers embedded in the surface of the blocks. I also place small spherical radiodense markers at the dorsal aspect of the coronary band and at the apex of the frog and a linear marker on the dorsal aspect of the hoof capsule (Figure 34-13).

In the developmental phase of laminitis the goal is to recognize the possibility of disease and be prepared if the disease occurs. The goal is to prevent and/or minimize the distal displacement of the DP. This can be partially accomplished by transferring weight from the wall to the solar surface of the foot and by reducing the pull of the DDFT. If the horse is shod, the shoes should be removed carefully by rasping off each nail clinch, then removing each nail separately with a creased nail puller. This helps to reduce mechanical trauma, pain, and discomfort associated with shoe removal. The only hoof care necessary in this phase is to bevel (unweight) the toe with a rasp back to a point 2.5 to 4 cm in front of the true apex of the frog, depending on the size of the hoof (see Figure 34-13). In a normal horse, the frog can serve as a reference point for the tip of the DP, which is located approximately 1.9 to 2.5 cm dorsal to the apex of the frog (see Figure 34-13). Soft bedding materials such as wet sand or damp peat provide good support and relief, but they may be difficult and expensive to maintain.

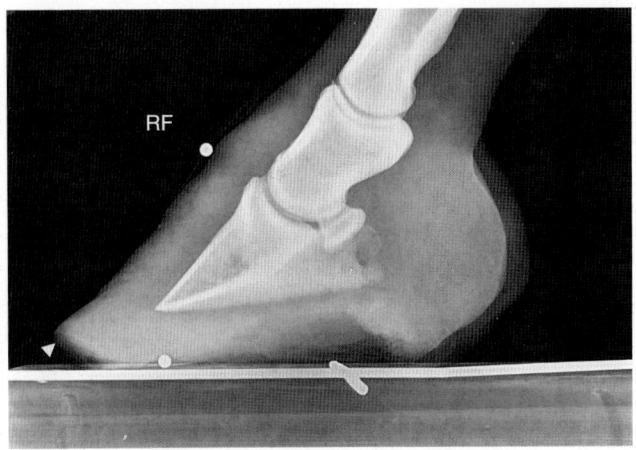

Fig. 34-13 • Lateromedial radiographic image showing small, spherical radiodense markers at the apex of the frog and dorsal aspect of the hoof. There also is a wire imbedded on the surface of the wood block on which the foot is resting. Note that the toe of the hoof capsule has been unweighted *(white arrowhead)*.

Alternatively, frog or sole pads can be used. Frog support using Lily pads (Nanric, Inc., Lawrenceburg, Kentucky, United States) or roll gauze taped to the frog was commonly used in the past but is being replaced by pads that adapt to the entire solar surface, providing more support and comfort to the entire foot. High-density foam is one of the most practical and economical methods for providing solar support. Sheets of 5-cm extruded foam, used for house insulation (Styrofoam Scoreboard, Dow Chemical, Midland, Michigan, United States), can be purchased at home centers or building supply companies. For foam application, stand the horse on small precut rectangular blocks of the foam insulation, and then cut and shape the block to the foot using a serrated bread knife, leaving 1.3 to 2.5 cm extending in front of the toe to prevent it from being pushed back as the horse walks. Attach the shaped pad to the foot with duct tape (Figure 34-14). The 5-cm extruded foam may be too thick for some horses or ponies with small feet, and sheets of 2.5- and 3.8-cm foam are more appropriate. In the developmental phase only one layer is usually necessary. Closed cell foam is also useful and is commercially available. These pads can be attached with duct or elastic tape (Elastikon, Johnson & Johnson Consumer Companies, Inc., Skillman, New Jersey, United States).

In the acute phase of laminitis the goal is to recognize the disease early and take appropriate actions to relieve the pain and provide support and comfort to minimize the effects of the disease. If the shoes have not been previously removed it is important to remove the shoes as atraumatically as possible, as outlined above, to provide solar support. In some horses it may not be possible to remove the shoes or it may aggravate the condition. Solar support can be accomplished with the shoe left in place in these situations. The only hoof care necessary is to unweight the toe if possible. Soft bedding materials such as wet sand or damp peat provide support and relief, especially for those horses from which the shoes cannot be removed.

In the acute phase of laminitis two layers of foam are used to provide support and elevate the heel. One layer is applied and is then removed after 24 hours when it becomes compressed. Ideally, this layer will compress evenly to

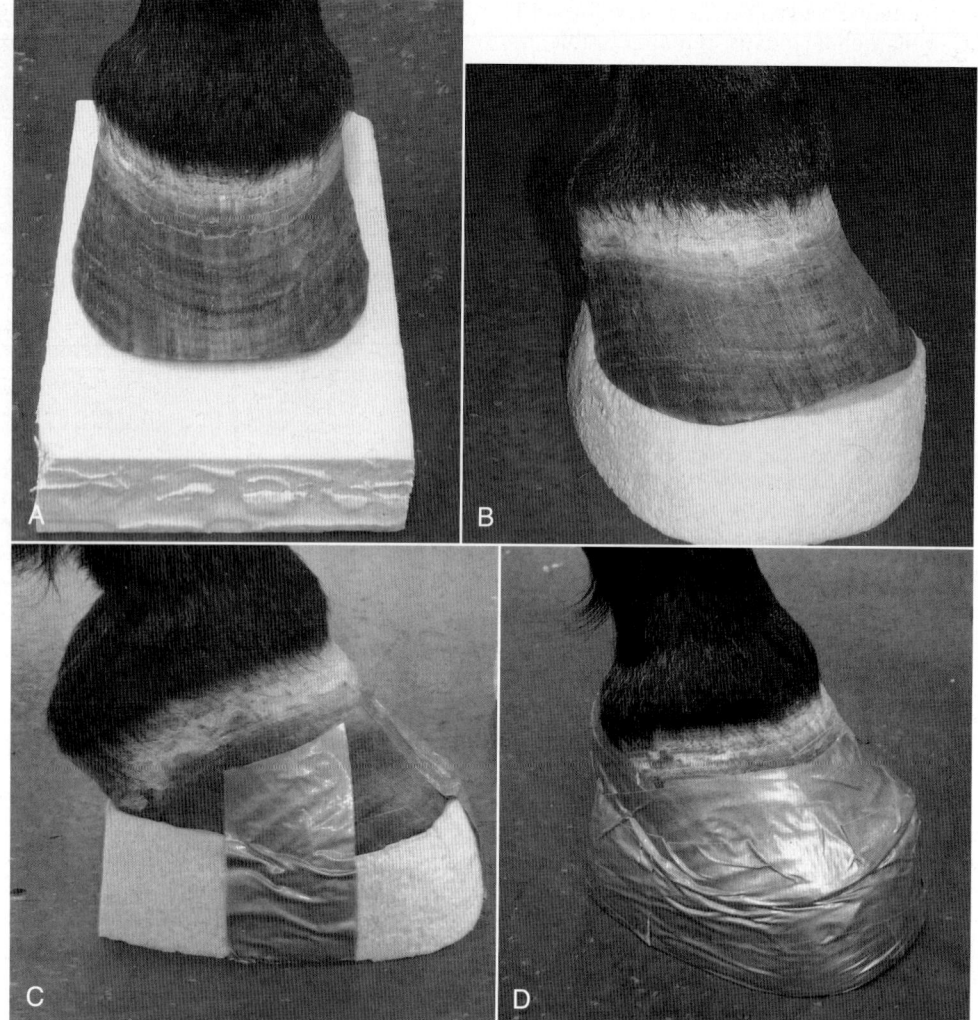

Fig. 34-14 • These four pictures show a horse standing on a precut block of foam **(A)**, the foam pad trimmed **(B)**, duct tape applied to the bottom of the pad **(C)**, and the pad attached to the foot with duct tape **(D)**.

approximately 2 cm. Remove the dorsal portion (from the apex of frog to the toe) of this pad to reduce the pressure over the most painful area of the sole. This trimmed pad and another foam layer are then attached to the foot with duct tape to raise the heel and provide more cushion to an area of the foot that can tolerate weight bearing (Figure 34-15). The foam pads should be replaced every 4 to 5 days or as needed. A commercial therapeutic boot system, Soft-Ride (Soft-Ride, Inc., Vermilion, Ohio, United States), which has a variety of orthotic inserts, provides support, relief from pain, and is relatively easy to apply. A commercial wedge pad system (Redden Ultimate, Nanric, Inc.) using rubber impression material (Advanced Cushion Support, Nanric, Inc.) is available and works very well in horses not getting adequate support from the foam insulation or other types of solar support (Figure 34-16). These commercial pads are taped or glued to the foot. The system combines a cuff with two attached, 5-degree wedge pads with a built-in dorsal to palmar breakover. The bottom wedge also has beveled edges for ease of medial to lateral breakover; this bottom wedge can be removed separately.

The goal of hoof care in the chronic phase of laminitis is to minimize further rotation of the DP. The following principles should be used when preparing the hoof and selecting a therapeutic horseshoe: (1) the palmar aspect of the hoof should be supported using all structures (sole, bars, and frog, including the central and lateral sulci); (2) the sole should be protected by not removing any portion of the sole dorsal to the apex of the frog; (3) the hoof wall should be trimmed from the quarters to the heel only to realign the solar surface of the DP and the weight-bearing surface of the hoof; (4) the dorsal aspect of the hoof capsule should be protected by bringing the point of breakover back to a point 2.5 and 3.8 cm (depending on the size of the hoof) in front of the true apex of the frog; and (5) the heels should be raised to reduce the tension of the DDFT. Two of the goals of hoof care—realignment of the solar surface of the DP and raising the heel to reduce tension of the DDFT—seem counterintuitive. In a chronic unstable laminitic horse these two principles are necessary to reduce the tension of the tendon and provide comfort. In a chronic stable laminitic horse with only mild misalignment of the solar surface of the DP, raising the heel after trimming is not necessary. Specific hoof care management in the chronic phase depends on whether the condition is stable or unstable. In horses maintaining a stable

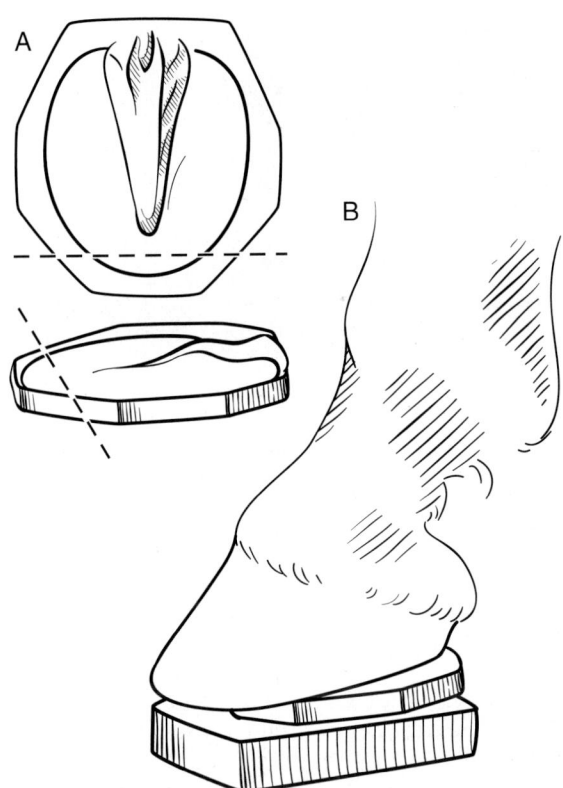

Fig. 34-15 • The drawing illustrates the trimming *(dashed line)* of a compressed foam pad **(A)**, which is then added to new layer of foam **(B)** before attaching the two to the hoof with duct tape.

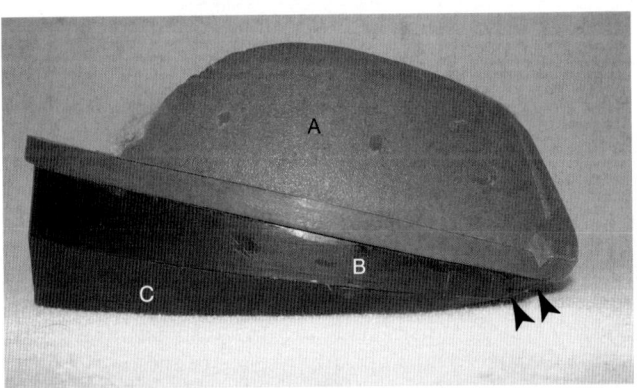

Fig. 34-16 • Redden Ultimate (Nanric, Inc., Lawrenceburg, Kentucky, United States) is a wedge system that can be attached to the hoof by a cuff *(A)* with special glue or adhesive tape. There are two 5-degree wedge pads *(B* and *C)* attached to each other with screws. The bottom pad *(C)* has round edges for ease of lateral to medial breakover. The arrowheads show how the system eases the dorsal to palmar breakover.

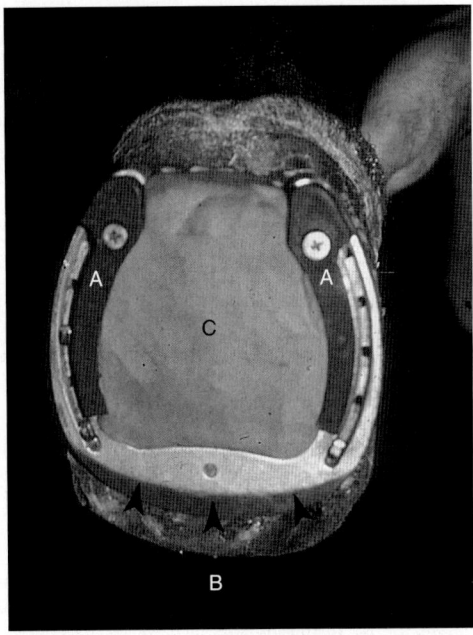

Fig. 34-17 • The Ovnicek aluminum shoe (EDSS, Penrose, Colorado, United States) has interchangeable plastic rails *(A)*. The shoe is specially machined to pull the point of breakover *(small arrows)* back. It is designed to set back from the toe of the hoof *(B)*. Sole support is provided with rubber impression material *(C)*.

condition, trimming alone may be all that is necessary, carefully following the stipulated principles. Generally, the traditional therapeutic horse shoes (heart bar shoe, reverse shoe with a wedge, reverse shoe with frog support, and the egg bar shoe with a treatment plate) advocated for chronic laminitis may be beneficial only if the condition is reasonably stable. Horses with instability of the DP require horse shoes that are adaptable and more compatible with the goals of hoof care. There are a number of commercially made, aluminum rail shoes (EDSS, Penrose, Colorado, United States; Aluminum 4 Point Rail Shoe, Nanric, Inc.)

(Figure 34-17) that provide the additional requirements for support. The new design of these shoes automatically pulls the breakover back, raises the heel, and provides palmar support. Ideally, the breakover should be close to the tip of the DP. A rubber impression material (Advanced Cushion Support, Nanric, Inc.) is used between the palmar structures of the sole and the shoes to provide support of the entire foot.

Horses with severe rotation and/or penetration of the sole usually have insufficient heel to realign the DP and the weight-bearing surface of the hoof by removing the heel alone. I have used a special shoeing technique to reestablish this relationship. A rubber impression material (Advanced Cushion Support, Nanric, Inc.) is used to provide the sole support and acts as a spacer between the weight-bearing surface of the hoof wall and the therapeutic shoe (Figure 34-18). These shoes cannot be attached to the hoof conventionally but rather are fastened to the hoof using an acrylic adhesive and fiberglass cloth (Equilox and Equilox Composite Cloth, Equilox International, Pine Island, Minnesota, United States). Routine clinical and radiological evaluations provide useful information to determine the horse's progress every 5 to 6 weeks when the shoes are reset. This is a difficult technique to perform and to keep the foot balanced without placing undue stress to the hoof capsule. An alternative to this technique is to apply synthetic polymer (Steward Clogs, EDSS) (Figure 34-19) or wooden fabricated shoes[3] (Figure 34-20). The wooden shoe can be easily adapted to complement the realignment of the DP. The same principles for treating a chronic laminitic horse are applicable for the wooden shoes.

In horses with an unstable foot or feet exhibiting progressive rotation or penetration of the corium through the sole, a deep digital flexor tenotomy[1,3,4] is recommended to reduce the active forces influencing separation of the

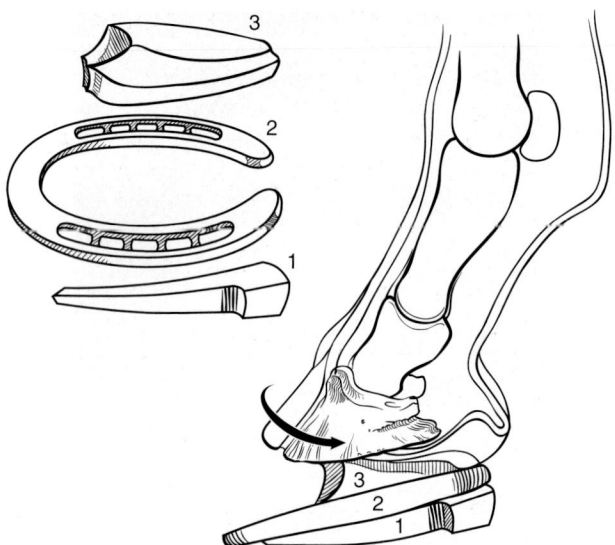

Fig. 34-18 • This drawing illustrates the special shoeing technique for realigning the foot when there is penetration of the sole by the corium. The components of this technique are plastic rails *(1)*, the EDSS shoe *(2)*, and cushion elastomer *(3)*. The cushion elastomer is used as a spacer to keep the contact surface of the shoe parallel to the solar surface of the distal phalanx. The shoe is attached with a hoof acrylic and fiberglass cloth because it cannot be attached to the hoof conventionally (not shown).

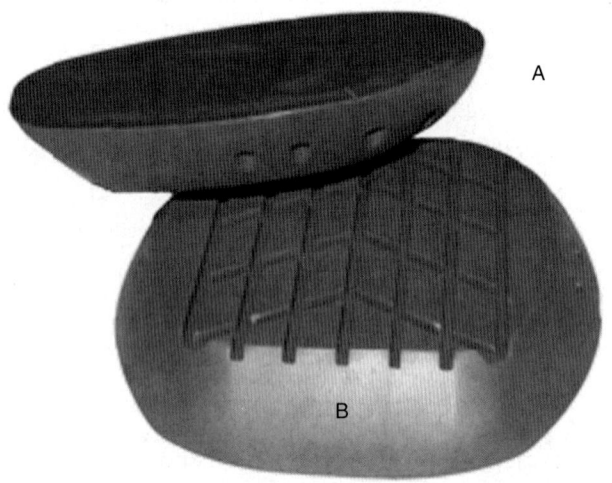

Fig. 34-19 • The Steward clog. **A,** The toe of the shoe. **B,** The heel.

lamellae and DP on the sole in the next section. This procedure relieves pain, prevents or minimizes rotation, and allows reestablishment of the normal relationship between the solar surface of the DP and the weight-bearing surface of hoof. Severing the DDFT causes partial luxation and hyperextension of the distal interphalangeal (DIP) joint, as well as overloading of the superficial digital flexor tendon (SDFT). This abnormal joint position may cause palmar foot pain and usually results in osteoarthritis of the DIP joint. Severe overloading of the SDFT may result in damage to the tendon, ultimately resulting in a flexural deformity of the metacarpophalangeal joint. Postoperative management of these horses is important to prevent or minimize

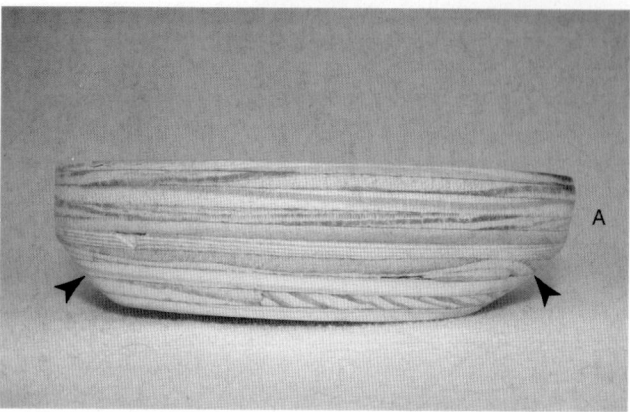

Fig. 34-20 • An example of a wooden fabricated shoe. The front of the shoe is labeled **A**. The black arrowheads show how the system eases the dorsal to palmar breakover. The sides of the wooden shoe are beveled approximately the same as the dorsal aspect.

these complications. Shoeing is crucial for protecting the DIP joint and reducing the load on the tendons. The horse is shod with a slight flexion of the DIP joint with a shoe in which the heels are raised and extend palmarly about 1 to 1.5 cm. The treatment of these horses with complicated laminitis may take months or years to resolve, takes perseverance and a team commitment, and can be an emotional roller-coaster for the owners. Owners should be made aware of these realities.

■ DEEP DIGITAL FLEXOR TENOTOMY FOR MANAGING LAMINITIS

Robert J. Hunt

Transection of the deep digital flexor tendon (DDFT) has been advocated in treatment of horses with chronic refractory laminitis.[1-4] The procedure initially appeared to have merit when used in horses with acute laminitis, but the long-term results were poor because of the severe and unstable nature of the laminitis.[2] The procedure attenuated pain, but most horses had ongoing displacement of the distal phalanx (DP) and suffered recurrent abscessation, and ultimately humane destruction was necessary.

The rationale for surgery is based on the biomechanical forces in the foot, which include the attachments of the dermal lamellae between the DP and the hoof wall, the downward vertical load through the bony column of the limb, the proximal palmar traction of the DDFT on the DP, the proximal pull of the common digital extensor tendon, and the digital cushion. The balance of these forces maintains a functional unit.

During a non–weight-bearing state, minimal force is imposed on the digit by the DDFT. When the limb is placed under load, the DDFT serves as a tension band and places shearing forces on the dorsal lamellae of the digit from its proximal palmar pull. The predominant force on the digit is the vertical load produced by the weight of the horse. Neither of these forces is necessarily detrimental under normal conditions; however, with compromise of the dorsal lamellae during laminitis, these forces result in distraction of the DP from the hoof capsule. The type and extent of displacement of the DP are determined by the degree of laminar damage and the load placed on the foot.

The rationale for tenotomy is to reduce the proximal palmar pull of the DDFT on the DP and therefore to decrease the shearing forces on the lamellae of the dorsal aspect of the foot. Transecting the tendon also permits lowering the heel if indicated to allow more normal alignment of the DP. The procedure generally is considered a salvage procedure for breeding horses or horses not intended for athletic endeavors, although some horses have returned to successful athletic careers. The degree of damage associated with the laminitis, rather than the surgery, limits future soundness.

No clear-cut guidelines dictate when and if surgery should be performed. In general, surgery is reserved for horses with chronic recurring laminitis that suffer from periodic hoof abscesses and show distal phalangeal rotation and contraction of the hoof wall, minimal to no sinking (distal displacement), and can produce a reasonable dorsal hoof wall. Horses with acute laminitis with instability of the DP–hoof wall unit are not good surgical candidates. If tenotomy is performed, additional measures, such as transfixation casting, must be provided.

Tenotomy may be repeated with recurrence of clinical signs or with the development of a metacarpophalangeal joint flexural deformity subsequent to a midpastern tenotomy. Performing repeat tenotomy is easier after a mid-metacarpal tenotomy, although repeat tenotomy is also possible to perform following a midpastern tenotomy. I have performed repeat tenotomy of the DDFT numerous times in horses with chronic recurring pain associated with laminitis. Clinical improvement was seen after each procedure, although subjectively the effects were not as beneficial or prolonged as in the previous tenotomy. This may have been associated with progressive deterioration of the digit associated with laminitis or from adhesions of the DDFT preventing tension relief after transection.

Deep digital flexor tenotomy is performed in the mid-metacarpal or midpastern region (Figures 34-21 and 34-22). When performed in the midmetacarpal region, the tenotomy may be done with the horse standing, under local analgesia, or under general anesthesia. An audible pop often occurs once transection is complete. A 1- to 2-cm gap in the transected tendon ends is immediately palpable. The stab incisions do not require closure, but a firm pressure bandage is applied.

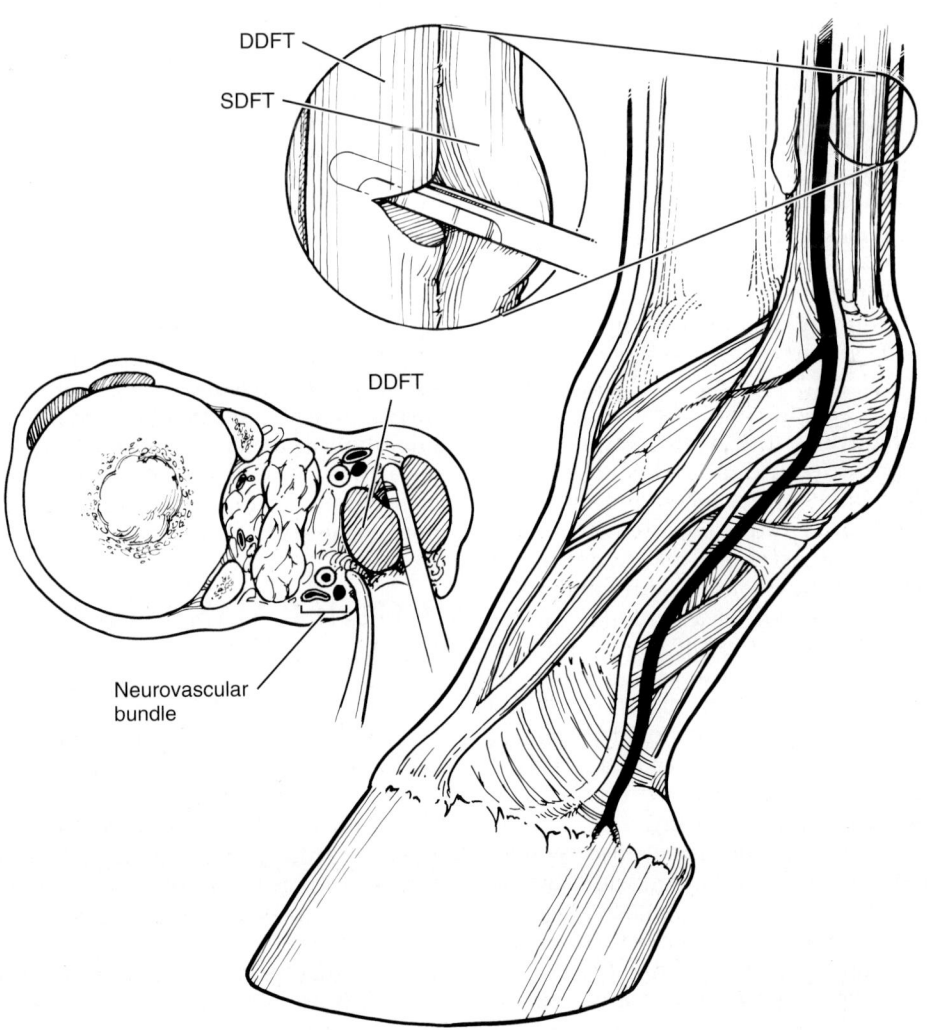

Fig. 34-21 • Deep digital flexor tenotomy can be performed in the metacarpal region in a standing horse or with the horse under general anesthesia. *DDFT,* Deep digital flexor tendon; *SDFT,* superficial digital flexor tendon.

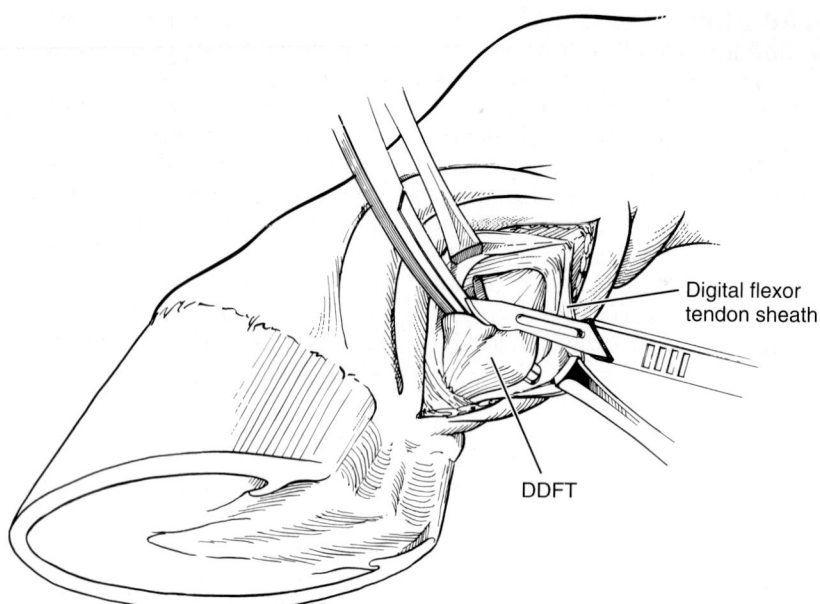

Digital flexor
tendon sheath

DDFT

Fig. 34-22 • Deep digital flexor tenotomy can be performed in the midpastern region with the horse under general anesthesia. *DDFT,* Deep digital flexor tendon.

A modification of this technique involves the use of self-fashioned "butter knife" malleable retractors. A 3-cm skin incision is made over the DDFT on the lateral aspect of the metacarpal region. Using blunt dissection along the dorsal and palmar borders of the DDFT, two planes are created for insertion of the butter knife retractors. Care is taken to exclude the neurovascular bundle from potential transection. The DDFT is sharply transected using a No. 10 scalpel, and the skin is closed in routine fashion.

Midpastern tenotomy is almost always performed with the horse recumbent, with the limb flexed to relax the DDFT (see Figure 34-22). Performing the procedure in a standing horse is possible if general anesthesia is prohibited, such as in a late-term pregnant mare. However, in a standing horse there is a higher risk of contamination of the surgical site, with possible involvement of the digital flexor tendon sheath (DFTS); therefore extreme caution should be taken.

It is mandatory to apply an extended and optimally elevated heel shoe in horses with midpastern tenotomy before or during surgery; an exception may be for horses with severe contraction of the hoof and surrounding soft tissues. The shoe should be worn for a minimum of 8 to 10 weeks to prevent luxation of the DIP joint. Although this shoe is not mandatory for all horses with midmetacarpal tenotomy, if clinical evidence exists of DIP joint luxation, an extended and elevated heel shoe should be applied. After tenotomy a horse should be confined to a restricted stall-size area. Bandages should be changed every 2 to 4 days for 8 to 10 weeks to minimize swelling.

Depending on the solar angle of the DP, the heel may be lowered to facilitate alignment, but in feet with extreme contraction, changes should be made gradually. Relative "unloading" of the dorsal aspect of the foot may be accomplished by shifting the breakover in a palmar direction.

The amount of tension release is greater after midpastern tenotomy because of the anatomical approximation to the insertion of the DDFT on the DP and unrestricted separation within the DFTS. The tendon may separate 6 to 10 cm after transection in this region. In contrast, separation after midmetacarpal tenotomy is limited by peritendon attachment to the subcutaneous tissue.

Clinical improvement is generally seen within 2 to 3 days of surgery. In general, clinical effects after tenotomy appear to be beneficial for several months. A flexural deformity of the metacarpophalangeal joint may develop from chronic pain, resulting in unweighting of the limb and contracture of scar tissue at the tenotomy site. Chronic pain may result from overloading the superficial digital flexor tendon before healing, osteoarthritis of the DIP joint, or chronic infections of the digit. Chronic infection may be a major complication, especially if infectious osteitis of the DP develops. Systemic antibiotics, local debridement, topical antimicrobial drugs, and bandaging are important in resolving infection. Treatment of such complicated conditions may take many months to resolve at great emotional and financial cost, and everybody involved must be aware of this.

■ OTHER MANAGEMENT ASPECTS OF LAMINITIS

Sue J. Dyson and Mike W. Ross

Medical management of laminitis (see page 372) and some aspects of hoof care focused on a horse with progressive rotation of the distal phalanx (DP) (see page 379) are discussed elsewhere. This section discusses some additional aspects of management, routine care, monitoring of the horse, and prevention of recurrence. It must be acknowledged that in equine practice, ideal management is not always possible, and compromises must sometimes be made to adapt to the prevailing circumstances.

In a horse with acute laminitis, some clinicians favor removal of the shoes, assuming that the horse can stand on soft bedding. However, in our experience, removal of the shoes often results in increased discomfort, and in the acute stages of laminitis, we prefer to leave the shoes in place. Alternatively, the normal shoes may be replaced with glue-on heart bar shoes, foam pads, frog pads, or custom-made boots,[1] which seem to enhance comfort. Not all affected horses develop rotation or sinking of the DP; however, even if baseline radiographs reveal no evidence of rotation, each horse should be monitored carefully. If there is any evidence of increased discomfort, the feet should be reexamined radiologically. The client must be instructed carefully about observing the horse's stance and the frequency of shifting weight between limbs, mobility, and the amount of time spent lying down, as well as advised that veterinary advice should be sought if there is any evidence of deterioration.

Ideally a horse with acute laminitis should be restricted to stable rest, but this is not always possible, especially for a child's pony that lives outdoors throughout the year. In these circumstances, a small area of the field should be fenced off using electric fencing. This area should be tightly mown, and the grass clippings should be removed. Spreading a thick layer of wood shavings over the entire surface may be beneficial.

Many horses and ponies that develop laminitis are grossly overweight, and reduction of body weight is crucial for successful management. Owners are often reluctant to admit that the horse is overweight and find it difficult to restrict the diet adequately. It is helpful to weigh the horse or make an estimate of body weight using a height-specific weight tape[2] and then set a target for the expected weight loss with monitoring at intervals. Strict instructions concerning dietary management should be made, stipulating the amounts of food, preferably by measured weights, that should be fed. Horses should receive a maximum of 7 MJ/kg dry matter equivalent to poor quality hay. Hay should be soaked for a minimum of 12 hours to reduce soluble carbohydrates. Concentrate foods and other glycemic foods, such as apples and carrots, should be eliminated; however, supplementation with vitamins C (5 mg/kg) and E (4 IU/kg) is potentially beneficial for their antioxidant effects. Low-energy chaff or small quantities of nonmolassed sugar beet pulp is acceptable. If a pony lives outdoors and cannot be stabled, then a strip grazing system should be established; each strip should be finely mown before the pony has access to it. A grazing muzzle may also be useful. If a horse has clinical evidence suggestive of equine metabolic syndrome, combined with increased serum insulin concentrations and an abnormal response to an intravenous glucose tolerance test, then oral administration of metformin (15 to 17.5 mg/kg PO twice daily), an insulin-sensitizing drug, is recommended, although clinical efficacy is not yet proven, and there are questions concerning bioavailability.[3] Serum insulin levels should be measured episodically.

In horses with chronic laminitis, even if rotation of the DP occurred previously, the position of the DP may actually be stable. The heel tends to grow more quickly than the toe, and regular trimming of the heel and shortening the toe are imperative to try to reestablish correct alignment of the DP within the hoof capsule and relative to the phalangeal axis. It will take weeks to months to reestablish these alignments, and it is critical that this is a slow, deliberate process without using aggressive angle changes. The heart bar shoe recruits part of the frog to share load bearing, and if correctly fitted, it shifts weight-bearing load away from the toe, thus sparing the dorsal structures of the foot. This approach, combined with removal of the lamellar wedge, often results in improved comfort and alignment of the hoof wall and DP. Correct positioning of the frog support plate is critical so that even, mild pressure is applied over the length of the frog. Reverse shoes or W shoes (open toe shoe with a heart bar) nailed on with one or two nails both medially and laterally, or glued or taped in place, may provide comfort in some horses. Often what works in one horse may not work in another, and a different strategy must be used. It may be necessary to obtain follow-up radiographs at 2-week intervals to determine whether additional trimming is necessary.

The term *derotation* of the DP has become popular; however, we believe that this is an inappropriate term. Although lowering the heel changes the angle of the DP with respect to the middle phalanx, it cannot acutely change the position of the DP relative to the hoof wall. The position of the DP within the hoof capsule often appears improved after removal of excessive toe.

It is critical for the farrier and veterinarian to work together closely. Although in general a slow deliberate approach to trimming is used, if the veterinarian believes that the farrier is not trimming the foot sufficiently aggressively, obtaining lateromedial radiographs may be helpful to demonstrate excess toe, heel, or both, as well as the position of the DP relative to the dorsal hoof wall and the phalangeal axis. Lateromedial radiographs are also useful for demonstrating excessive separation of the dorsal hoof wall or accumulation of fluid, as well as for determining when limited dorsal hoof wall resection may be indicated. If sinking of one or more of the DPs is evident radiologically, the owner must be advised that the prognosis for recovery is extremely guarded.

If pain is not adequately controlled by systemic analgesics, daily monitoring of the horse, preferably by a veterinarian, is crucial to identify signs of impending penetration of the sole, such as increased softening of the sole dorsal to the apex of the frog and red discoloration. The coronary bands of all feet should be assessed carefully; depression at the coronary band may herald sinking of the DP. Increased lameness may be associated with a subsolar abscess that requires establishment of drainage. A horse that has developed or is at risk of development of mechanically induced laminitis because of a painful condition in the contralateral limb must be monitored particularly vigilantly. In these horses, subtle evidence of mechanical laminitis is easily missed and usually occurs between 4 and 6 weeks after injury to the contralateral limb. However, in some horses, usually racehorses, mechanical laminitis occurs early, even within the first few days, and is inexplicable. Often the first sign of contralateral mechanical laminitis is increased weight bearing on the injured limb, or treading. Increased weight bearing on the injured limb may be a sign of improved comfort, but the clinician should investigate the contralateral limb carefully for the development of mechanical laminitis. Chronic laminitis may be associated with neuropathic pain, which responds poorly to nonsteroidal antiinflammatory drugs.[4] Treatment with gabapentin (2.5 to 5 mg/kg PO twice daily) may improve comfort[5,6]; however, the horse is likely to appear constantly drowsy, and to date there are no long-term data that document any long-term efficacy of this treatment.

Careful assessment of digital pulse amplitudes and foot temperature may be useful for detecting the development of laminitis or deterioration of preexisting laminitis. In older horses in which laminitis cannot be stabilized, consideration should always be given to the existence of primary equine Cushing's disease, which must be treated appropriately.

It is critical that clients be kept well informed of the likely outcome and are well appraised of the long convalescent periods that often are required after substantial rotation of the DP occurs. They must be warned that unexpected relapses may occur despite steady progress. Clients must be aware that the prognosis is hopeless in some horses, and euthanasia may be required. Humane decisions for euthanasia can be difficult. Nonetheless, it is important to recognize that with early aggressive treatment some horses can make a complete recovery to athletic function despite marked rotation of one or more DPs. The prognosis is generally more favorable in ponies than in horses. Clients must be advised that continued long-term dietary management may be crucial to prevention of recurrent laminitis.

The prognosis in heavy breeds of horses with sinking of the DPs is generally hopeless. These horses seem particularly prone to the development of laminitis secondary to retention of the placenta, and although with aggressive management they can be salvaged until the foal is weaned, longer-term treatment is invariably unsuccessful.

PART III

The Forelimb

Chapter 35

The Proximal and Middle Phalanges and Proximal Interphalangeal Joint

Alan J. Ruggles

erences n page 1279

ANATOMICAL CONSIDERATIONS

The term *pastern* originated from the shackle that was secured below the metacarpophalangeal or metatarsophalangeal joints to tether a horse to the pasture.[1] The proximal interphalangeal (PIP) joint or pastern joint is a diarthrodial joint, which is formed from the distal aspect of the proximal phalanx and the proximal aspect of the middle phalanx. The pastern region is bounded dorsally by the common digital extensor tendon and on the palmar/plantar border by the distal sesamoidean ligaments, digital flexor tendons, digital flexor tendon sheath (DFTS), and the proximal and distal digital annular ligaments. The superficial digital flexor tendon (SDFT) inserts on the distal palmar/plantar aspect of the proximal phalanx and the proximal palmar/plantar aspect of the middle phalanx. The straight sesamoidean ligament arises from the base of the proximal sesamoid bones (PSBs) and extends distally to insert on the proximal palmar/plantar aspect of the middle phalanx. The oblique (middle) sesamoidean ligaments arise from the base of the PSBs and attach to the triangular region on the palmar/plantar region of the middle portion of the proximal phalanx. The medial and lateral collateral ligaments of the PIP joint provide support in the sagittal plane and attach to the collateral tubercles of the distal aspect of the proximal phalanx and proximal palmar/plantar aspect of the middle phalanx. The paired smaller abaxial and axial ligaments are located just palmar/plantar to the collateral ligaments. The neurovascular bundle of the digit runs just abaxial to the deep digital flexor tendon on the medial and lateral sides.

The palmar/plantar eminence of the middle phalanx extends proximal to the horizontal axis of the joint surface and blends proximally with a fibrocartilaginous cap at the most proximal extent of the middle phalanx. In the adult horse this is dense, and it is important to engage this portion of the bone during internal fixation of fractures or arthrodesis procedures.

The proximity of the pastern region to the ground, the paucity of soft tissue coverage over the dorsum and sides, and the important soft tissue structures on the palmar/plantar surfaces make it especially vulnerable to external trauma. Wounds in this region may involve the DFTS and warrant careful investigation. Angular deformities from growth disturbances at the pastern are uncommon but do occur. More commonly, deformities arise from physeal abnormalities of the distal aspect of the third metacarpal/metatarsal bones affecting the metacarpophalangeal/metatarsophalangeal joints. Radiological closure of the proximal physis of the proximal and middle phalanges occurs by 6 to 9 months of age, but functional closure is earlier, usually by 8 weeks of age. Radiological closure of the distal physis of the proximal phalanx occurs by 1 month of age. Radiological closure of the distal physis of the middle phalanx occurs by the time of birth.[2]

LAMENESS EXAMINATION

Physical derangements usually are obvious because of minimal soft tissue coverage of the pastern. Phalangeal fractures usually are associated with soft tissue swelling and focal pain. Effusion of the DFTS is typical of penetrating wounds of the sheath, damage to the enclosed digital flexor tendons, or injury of the sesamoidean ligaments located dorsal to the sheath. In horses with osteoarthritis (OA), new bone formation on the dorsomedial and dorsolateral aspects of the PIP joint often occurs, causing obvious swelling around the joint. Angular deformity of the digit with limb shortening often is present in horses with complex fractures of the proximal or middle phalanx. Effusion in the metacarpophalangeal or metatarsophalangeal joint is common in horses with fractures of the proximal articular surface of the proximal phalanx.

Lameness from the pastern region ranges from severe to subtle depending on the injury. Generally, disorders involving the PIP joint or DFTS cause obvious lameness, but lameness from early OA of the PIP joint may be mild, and the clinical signs and blocking pattern may be confused with foot or occasionally fetlock lameness. Pain in the pastern region may be exacerbated by distal limb flexion. There is often a weight-bearing lameness that is worse if a horse is lunged or trotted with the affected limb on the inside of a circle.

Response to intraarticular analgesia varies depending on the injury, but improvement of lameness by 50% or more implicates the PIP joint as an important source of pain. Entry into the PIP joint can be difficult, especially if new bone is present as a result of OA. Techniques for intraarticular and perineural analgesia are described in

Chapter 10. Complete analgesia of the PIP joint is not always accomplished by perineural analgesia of the palmar nerves at the level of the PSBs, and a low four-point (palmar and palmar metacarpal nerves) block may be necessary. However, in some horses lameness improves with palmar/plantar digital analgesia. Intraarticular analgesia of the PIP joint should be considered in a horse with suspected metacarpophalangeal or metatarsophalangeal joint pain that has not responded to treatment. Complete analgesia of the DFTS requires intrasynovial or a low four-point block. Localization by perineural analgesia to the pastern joint does not limit the source of the lameness to the joint itself. Injury to the soft tissue structures should be carefully evaluated if radiological examination reveals no clinically significant abnormalities.

IMAGING CONSIDERATIONS

Standard radiographic examination for evaluation of the proximal phalanx includes lateromedial, dorsopalmar (plantar), dorsal 45° lateral-palmaromedial oblique, and dorsal 45° medial-palmarolateral oblique images. Oblique radiographs that are angled distally are helpful to identify osteochondral fragments on the proximal palmar/plantar aspect of the proximal phalanx.[3] If a sagittal plane fracture of the proximal phalanx is suspected, dorsopalmar/plantar radiographs that are 5 degrees medial or lateral to the mid-sagittal plane are useful. Slight underexposure of a lateromedial image helps to identify callus on the proximodorsal aspect of the proximal phalanx associated with chronic, short, incomplete fractures. Radiographic examination of the PIP joint includes lateromedial, dorsopalmar/plantar, and oblique images. Flexed oblique images are particularly helpful for evaluation of the articular margins.[3] A well-positioned and exposed dorsopalmar/plantar image may reveal subtle joint space narrowing and increased radiopacity of the subchondral bone consistent with early OA. Comparative views of the contralateral limb may be helpful.

Contrast radiography may be used to determine the course of fistulous tracts or to identify communication between wounds and the DFTS or areas of proliferative synovium within the DFTS. Contrast radiography is performed by placement of a 50% solution of diatrizoate preglumine and diatrizoate sodium (Hypaque-76, Nyromed, Princeton, New Jersey, United States) within a draining tract or directly into the synovial structure after aseptic preparation. Standard radiographs are obtained to identify communication with draining tracts or filling defects.

Computed or digital radiography is helpful in detecting subtle changes in trabecular bone architecture and opacity and is the present state of the art for radiographic examination. Computed tomography (CT) of the distal aspect of the limb offers detailed information regarding structural injury to the bony column of the digit that may not be apparent on radiographic examination.

Ultrasonographic evaluation of the pastern region is helpful in identifying abnormalities associated with the soft tissue structures[4] and is discussed in detail in Chapters 16 and 82.

Magnetic resonance imaging (MRI) of the pastern region is indicated in horses that have pain localized to the pastern region without radiological or ultrasonographic evidence of disease and may reveal soft tissue, bone, and/or cartilage

pathology.[5] A more detailed discussion of MRI is found in Chapter 21. Benign osseous cystlike lesions are identified more commonly with MRI than with radiology in the proximal and middle phalanges but are frequently not associated with pain and lameness, and their significance should not be overinterpreted.

Nuclear scintigraphy is useful in identifying incomplete fractures of the proximal phalanx. Incomplete fractures of the proximal articular margin of the proximal phalanx can occur in all breeds, but they are most commonly seen in Standardbred (STB) and Thoroughbred (TB) racehorses. Clinical signs and response to perineural analgesia vary. Nuclear scintigraphy should be considered to eliminate fracture in horses with lameness referable to the fetlock and clinical signs consistent with an incomplete fracture of the proximal phalanx. Nuclear scintigraphy can be helpful to identify bone modeling in the early phases of OA of the PIP joint. Other bone-related abnormalities in the pastern region often are evident radiologically, and scintigraphy is unnecessary.

BREED PREDILECTION

Differential diagnoses of disorders of the pastern region of all breeds include OA, osteochondrosis, fractures, and infection. The types of fractures tend to be specific to breed or use. Fractures of the proximal phalanx occur most often in racing breeds, with the STB most often affected. Fractures of the middle phalanx occur most commonly in horses used for Western-type activities, such as reining, but are seen in all breeds during lunging or after kicks. Osteochondrosis of the proximal aspect of the proximal phalanx is common in yearling and 2-year-old TB and STB horses. Osteochondrosis of the distal aspect of the proximal phalanx and proximal aspect of the middle phalanx is less common with no breed predilection. OA of the PIP joint occurs most often in older horses used for riding or Western-type activities. It may be seen in young horses secondary to osteochondrosis.

FRACTURES OF THE PROXIMAL PHALANX

Fractures of the proximal phalanx are important causes of lameness in all breeds. Racing breeds are particularly prone. Clinical signs vary from subtle to obvious. In horses with complete fractures, lameness is severe, and limb swelling and deformity may be present. In horses with incomplete fractures, lameness may be subtle, and careful clinical and radiographic examination may be necessary to define the fracture. Serial radiographs may be needed to detect radiolucency and callus formation associated with short incomplete fractures of the proximal phalanx. Nuclear scintigraphy may be helpful.

Fractures of the proximal phalanx include the following types:
- Short and long incomplete sagittal fractures
- Complete fractures that exit the lateral cortex
- Simple complete fractures
- Moderately comminuted fracture
- Severely comminuted fracture
- Dorsal frontal
- Proximal palmar/plantar avulsion fractures associated with the collateral ligament
- Fracture of the proximal physis

Incomplete fractures of the proximal phalanx occur most commonly in racing breeds, but are also seen in sports and endurance horses. Clinical signs include mild to severe lameness. Fetlock joint effusion and mild swelling and pain over the dorsal aspect of the proximal phalanx are common but may not be present. Most fractures are readily identified radiologically, but in some horses dorsopalmar/plantar images that are slightly oblique to the sagittal plane are useful. In addition, obtaining follow-up radiographs 7 to 10 days after the fracture allows time for osteoclastic resorption along the fracture line to occur so that the fracture line becomes more obvious. However, there are some incomplete sagittal fractures that occur midway between the dorsal and palmar cortices of the proximal phalanx that may never be detectable radiologically and can only be identified using MRI or CT. Treatment of horses with incomplete sagittal fractures includes stall rest or internal fixation, depending on the degree of lameness, concern about catastrophic fracture of the bone, and economic factors. The advantages of surgical repair are well documented, but horses with incomplete short fractures of the proximal aspect of the proximal phalanx can often be managed with rest alone. In some circumstances a bone screw is placed to provide compression for short fractures to reduce the risk of fracture recurrence. Indications for internal fixation of incomplete fractures include fractures that extend more than 15 mm from the proximal articular surface, those with potential for catastrophic failure, and those that occur in horses with severe lameness. Internal fixation is accomplished by placement of 4.5- or 5.5-mm cortex bone screws in lag fashion. Although 4.5-mm screws generally are used and provide ample compression, 5.5-mm cortex screws have greater pull-out strength compared with 4.5-mm cortex screws in dense bone.[6] However, the 5.5-mm cortex screws can be used to replace a stripped 4.5-mm thread. In a nondisplaced fracture, open reduction is not required, and the screws can be placed through minimal incisions. Arthroscopic examination of the dorsal and palmar/plantar aspects of the joint is recommended to evaluate articular cartilage and identify and treat additional abnormalities if present. Although most incomplete sagittal fractures of the proximal phalanx are simple, occasionally there is a transverse component, and radiographs should be examined carefully, especially when lameness is severe. Horses with incomplete fractures are reported to have a 67% to 89% chance to return to racing soundness after treatment. However, STBs returned to racing with slower racing times and reduced performance indices.[7-9]

Horses with complete fractures of the proximal phalanx are candidates for internal fixation to provide anatomical reduction and compression of the articular surfaces, improved comfort, reduced risk of OA, and early return to use. In horses with acute, minimally displaced fractures, reduction may be achieved by percutaneous placement of bone reduction forceps under radiographic or arthroscopic guidance. Open reduction, arthrotomy, or both may be required in horses with moderately to severely displaced fractures, chronic fractures, or fractures in which fragments of bone prevent reduction of the fracture fragments. After debridement of the fracture bed and reduction of the fracture, compression of the fracture fragments is accomplished using 4.5- or 5.5-mm cortex bone screws. External coaptation with a half-limb cast may be required for recovery

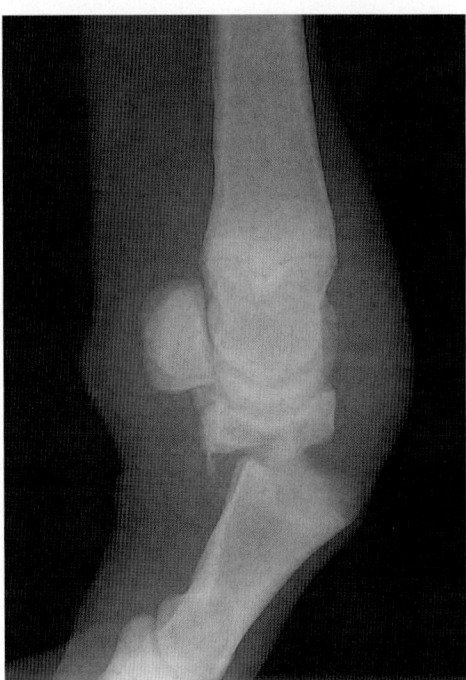

Fig. 35-1 • Lateromedial radiographic image of a Thoroughbred weanling with a Salter-Harris type II fracture of the proximal physis of the proximal phalanx. The horse was treated by application of a cast for 6 weeks; follow-up radiology after cast removal revealed healing of the fracture and normal alignment of the digit.

from general anesthesia or the immediate postoperative period. Prognosis for horses with noncomminuted complete fractures depends on whether the PIP joint is involved. Horses with fractures that enter the PIP joint had an approximately 50% chance to return to racing. Of those with complete fractures that exited the lateral cortex, 71% returned to racing.[7-9]

Salter-Harris type II fractures of the proximal aspect of the proximal phalanx occur in foals and weanlings (Figure 35-1). Reduction of the fracture is accomplished with the horse under general anesthesia. Methods of coaptation include bandaging alone, bandaging with splinting, or half-limb cast application. I prefer to use a cast for 4 weeks, but it is important that the cast be changed at 2 weeks. Other clinicians prefer less aggressive coaptation because of concerns of flexor laxity and osteoporosis of the PSBs. One of the Editors (MWR) prefers internal fixation of Salter-Harris type II fractures in foals because of this concern. Techniques include the placement of 3.5- or 4.5-mm bone screws in lag fashion from the metaphyseal component (usually palmarolateral/plantarolateral) in a dorsomedial direction or use of a small bone plate applied to the dorsomedial aspect of the proximal phalanx, using the tension band principle for repair. Rigid internal fixation mitigates the need to use prolonged external coaptation (see Figure 41-7).

Dorsal frontal fractures of the proximal aspect of the proximal phalanx occur in three general types: incomplete proximal dorsal articular fractures, complete proximal dorsal articular fractures, and fractures that originate in the midportion of the proximal articulation and extend distally into the proximal phalanx. Incomplete proximal dorsal frontal fractures occur most commonly in STB racehorses. The right hindlimb is most commonly affected.

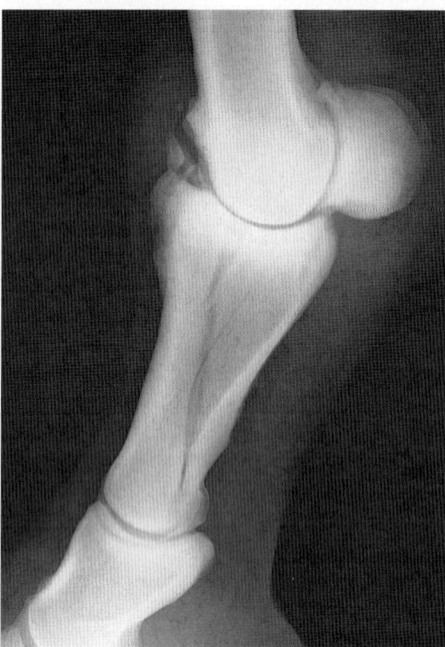

Fig. 35-2 • Lateromedial radiographic image of a 12-year-old Thoroughbred mare with a large frontal plane fracture of the proximal phalanx of a forelimb. There is advanced preexisting osteoarthritis of the metacarpophalangeal joint. The fracture was repaired with 5.5-mm cortex screws in lag fashion and a cast applied for 6 weeks.

Proximal dorsal articular fractures can be treated with rest alone or internal fixation with a 3.5-mm cortex bone screw. The prognosis for horses with proximal fractures is good.[10] Horses with large fractures that originate in the central portion of the metacarpophalangeal or metatarsophalangeal joint need internal fixation to preserve joint integrity, even if intended for only pasture or breeding soundness. In my experience, OA tends to be preexisting or develops despite anatomical reduction and internal fixation of the fracture, and the prognosis for athletic soundness is poorer (Figure 35-2).[11] The 5.5-mm cortex screws, which have a greater resistance to bending, are recommended because there may be larger bending forces in these fractures compared with sagittal plane fractures.

Horses with comminuted fractures of the proximal phalanx have acute, non–weight-bearing lameness and often limb deformity. Appropriate first aid is required to prevent further injury to the soft tissues and the digital arterial blood supply. A half-limb cast with a dorsally incorporated splint is appropriate to realign the bony column for transport to a surgical facility. Comminuted fractures can be divided into two categories for treatment: those with and those without an intact column (strut) of bone extending from the proximal to distal articular surfaces. An intact strut of bone allows reconstruction of many comminuted fractures of the proximal phalanx by lag screw fixation of the fracture fragments to the strut.[12] Treatment strategies include the following:

• Complete reconstruction via bone screws, plates, or both by open reduction
• Partial reconstruction and transfixation cast or external fixator
• Transfixation cast alone
• Use of external skeletal fixation (see Chapter 87)

In my opinion, the use of half-limb casts alone is not the best method of sole treatment for most horses with comminuted fractures of the proximal phalanx, although successful outcomes have been reported. Half-limb casts significantly reduce axial loading in the intact skeleton, but the risks of fracture compression, skin injuries leading to open fractures, and contralateral limb laminitis are substantial.[13,14] The use of transfixation casts for management of these fractures has been reported. Based on the relatively poor outcome for comfort, some attempt at reconstruction of the fracture is recommended when possible.[15]

Horses with comminuted fractures with an existing strut of bone are candidates for open reduction and reconstruction with bone screws. An initial study reported an unacceptably high risk of infection after open reduction and internal fixation,[16] but a more recent report described a good prognosis for pasture soundness.[12] If the strut has a transverse fracture but enough bone stock proximal and distal to the transverse fracture, then reconstruction of proximal phalanx fractures with two 4.5-mm narrow dynamic compression or locking compression plates and bone screws is advised. With both screw fixation alone and plate and screw fixation, external coaptation with a half-limb cast is required. Partial reconstruction of the articular surfaces and placement of a transfixation cast or external fixator is elected in horses with severely comminuted fractures to reduce degenerative changes, improve short- and long-term comfort, and reduce the requirement for subsequent arthrodesis. A transfixation cast is used when comminution is severe enough to prevent anatomical reconstruction and protection of the fracture from collapse is required. Transfixation casts have been shown to significantly improve axial stability compared with standard casts in an osteotomy model.[17] External fixators are used in place of transfixation casts if the fracture is open to allow direct access to the injury site (see Chapter 87).[18] The use of transfixation casts and external fixators carries the risk of catastrophic failure of the third metacarpal (metatarsal) bone and prolonged healing; the overall prognosis for salvage is only fair.[15]

Palmar/plantar avulsion fractures of the proximal phalanx usually occur after kicks, falls, or stall injury (Figure 35-3). Lameness is variable, and fetlock effusion is usually present. Differential diagnosis includes fracture and osteochondritis dissecans fragmentation. Because this region is the distal attachment for the collateral ligaments, surgical treatment is recommended to improve bony union and prevent OA. Treatment options include lag screw fixation, with one or preferably two 3.5-mm cortex bone screws. Surgical removal is also possible for chronic or small fractures or those that cannot be properly reduced. After removal or repair, external coaptation for recovery from general anesthesia and then for an additional 4 weeks is recommended. The prognosis is considered good with either treatment in the absence of OA.

DORSAL OSTEOCHONDRAL FRAGMENTS IN THE METACARPOPHALANGEAL/ METATARSOPHALANGEAL JOINT

See Chapters 36 and 42 for a discussion of dorsal osteochondral fragments in the metacarpophalangeal/metatarsophalangeal joint.

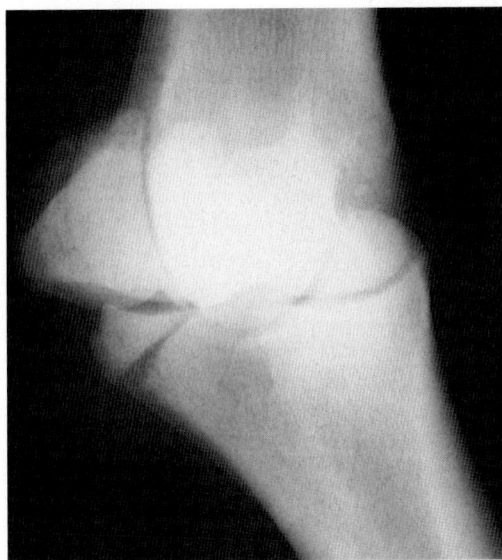

Fig. 35-3 • Dorsolateral-plantaromedial oblique radiographic image of a metatarsophalangeal joint of a 2-year-old Standardbred colt. There is an avulsion fracture of the proximal plantarolateral aspect of the proximal phalanx. The fracture was stabilized with two 3.5-mm cortex screws placed in lag fashion.

OSTEOCHONDROSIS OF THE PROXIMAL INTERPHALANGEAL JOINT

Osteochondrosis of the PIP joint is less common than that of the metacarpophalangeal or metatarsophalangeal joints. As with other sites, osteochondrosis involves fragmentation (osteochondritis dissecans) or osseous cystlike lesions. Sites include the distal aspect of the proximal phalanx and proximal aspect of the middle phalanx. The radiolucent area at the distal central aspect of the proximal phalanx is a normal finding and represents the space between the lateral and medial condyles of the distal aspect of the proximal phalanx. Radiolucent areas or fragmentation in the condylar regions of the distal aspect of the proximal phalanx tend to cause clinical signs. In the most severe circumstances, these subchondral radiolucencies in weight-bearing portions of the joint may cause substantial OA and lameness requiring arthrodesis of the PIP joint. Osseous cystlike lesions are more common in the hindlimb than in the forelimb and can occur bilaterally. Osseous cystlike lesions can communicate with the PIP joint, and if lameness is present, radiological evidence of OA can be substantial. Subtle clinical signs often are seen in horses with osseous cystlike lesions that do not communicate with the PIP joint. Although unusual, sudden-onset severe lameness can occur as a result of osseous cystlike lesions even though the radiological abnormality was present for several months or years. Clinical relevance of osseous cystlike lesions must be established using diagnostic analgesia, and in some horses scintigraphy is required. Management of horses with osseous cystlike lesions may include intraarticular injections or arthrodesis of the PIP joint in some horses. Arthrodesis of the PIP joint can yield a good prognosis for soundness in Western performance horses or other types of sports horses that are not expected to perform at advanced levels. A periarticular drilling procedure can be used in horses with osseous cystlike lesions that do not

communicate with the PIP joint. A small drill bit is used under radiographic or fluoroscopic guidance to approach the cystic cavity. Methylprednisolone acetate, expanded stem cells, or liquid bone marrow can be injected. Alternatively, cancellous bone can be packed into the cyst cavity. Radiological evidence of healing of the cyst cavity is variable, and in some horses residual lameness remains.

Osteochondral fragments associated with osteochondrosis tend to occur at the palmar/plantar eminence of the proximal aspect of the middle phalanx and cause variable lameness. They often are an incidental finding found on radiographs acquired before sale, but they certainly can complicate the sales process. Prognosis is difficult to assess in yearlings that have not been trained. Osteochondrosis fragments are more common in hindlimbs than in forelimbs. In adult horses there may be radiological evidence of advanced OA, even if lameness is mild. Because these fragments can be difficult to remove, it is important to document the true source of lameness before surgery is considered. Arthroscopic techniques for the pastern have been described and are most commonly used for dorsal fragments. Palmar/plantar fragments can be accessed arthroscopically or removed via arthrotomy, which may be preferable for large fragments (see Chapter 23 and Figure 23-1).[19,20]

OSTEOARTHRITIS OF THE PROXIMAL INTERPHALANGEAL JOINT

OA of the PIP joint is also known as *high ringbone.* Horses used for jumping, dressage, and Western-type activities seem to be prone to high ringbone. It can also be a consequence of articular fracture, infection, or osteochondrosis. The clinical signs of OA of the PIP joint include mild to severe lameness. Lameness is exacerbated by distal limb flexion. Obvious bony formation or angular deformity may be present in horses with advanced lameness. Diagnosis is based on clinical signs, response to perineural or intraarticular analgesia, and radiological findings. Radiological abnormalities commonly include periarticular new bone formation, subchondral bone increased radiopacity, and loss of joint space typically on the medial aspect of the PIP joint. However, small dorsal periarticular osteophytes are a frequent incidental radiological abnormality and are not necessarily of clinical significance. Angular deformity is typically only present in horses with advanced OA resulting from collapse of the joint surface typically on the medial side. Comparative radiographs of the contralateral limb should also be obtained because the condition may be bilateral. Pain associated with the PIP joint may be present without any radiological signs of OA, and scintigraphic examination is useful in documenting active bone modeling. On the other hand, horses may develop acute severe lameness with radiological evidence of existing OA that predated any clinical evidence of pain. Lameness improves after perineural or intraarticular analgesia.

In horses with mild OA of the PIP joint that is unrelated to fracture, conservative treatment includes therapeutic shoeing aimed at reducing the toe length and elevating the heel and easing breakover in some horses. Nonsteroidal antiinflammatory drugs are useful. The therapeutic value of administering intramuscular glycosaminoglycans and intravenous hyaluronan is questionable. Intraarticular injections are of considerable value. A combination of hyaluronan and corticosteroids or corticosteroids alone are most effective in horses with mild or moderate OA. However, in horses with advanced OA, particularly those with extensive periarticular new bone proliferation and extensive loss of joint space, arthrodesis should be considered. The surgical procedure is invasive and expensive but is generally considered a better solution over the long term. Natural ankylosis of the PIP joint can occur, but it is a long, painful process and one that is not necessarily complete. Surgical arthrodesis is best. Tibial neurectomy can be helpful in horses with advanced hindlimb proximal interphalangeal OA that are not meant to resume athletic careers.[21]

ARTHRODESIS OF THE PROXIMAL INTERPHALANGEAL JOINT

Arthrodesis of the PIP joint is indicated in horses with advanced OA or an articular fracture. Lag screw fixation of simple fractures can be performed, but because of difficulty in obtaining anatomical reduction of the PIP joint surface and resisting tension forces at the palmar/plantar eminences, lag screw fixation alone is usually unsuccessful in preventing OA and returning horses to athletic soundness. Therefore I recommend PIP joint arthrodesis in horses with articular fractures.

Many methods of arthrodesis of the PIP joint are described, and opinions vary as to which is preferred. Current preferred methods involve the insertion of three parallel 4.5- or 5.5-mm screws or dorsally applied plate or plates with additional transarticular screws. I have used both methods and prefer the plating technique because when compared with screws alone it improves comfort in the immediate postoperative period as a result of increased biomechanical stability and reduces the necessity for prolonged cast application. This method requires cast coaptation for 2 to 3 weeks to protect the incision site. The plating technique provided improved stability compared with the three 5.5-mm parallel screw technique in fatigue testing.[22] After arthrodesis of the PIP joint with screws alone, approximately 80% to 89% of horses with hindlimb and 46% to 80% of horses with forelimb lameness returned to athletic soundness.[23-25] Long-term follow-up data for the plate/screw technique revealed 81% of horses with forelimb and 95% of horses with hindlimb arthrodesis were able to resume performance careers.[26] The locking compression plate (LCP) has been recently advocated for arthrodesis of the PIP joint, and its new design with the Combi hole at one end avoids the long pointed end interfering with the extensor process of the distal phalanx. Long-term follow-up data regarding the use of LCP/screw technique for pastern arthrodesis are not yet available.

Horses with comminuted middle phalanx fractures (Figure 35-4) or those that involve the distal interphalangeal (DIP) joint should undergo arthrodesis of the PIP joint with single or double plating and potentially transfixation casts or external skeletal fixation (see Chapter 87). Comminuted fractures of the middle phalanx should be repaired if possible to preserve the DIP joint surface and, if possible, the PIP joint surface. Displacement of the distal articular surface considerably worsens prognosis. Single or double

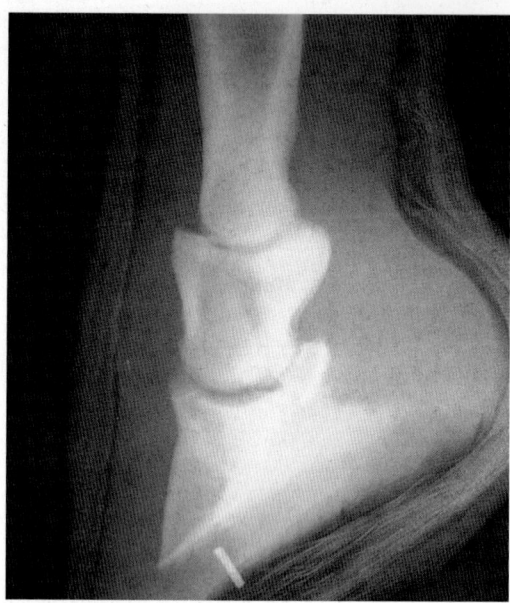

Fig. 35-4 • Lateromedial radiographic image of the left hindlimb of a 7-year-old Thoroughbred-cross gelding with a comminuted articular fracture of the middle phalanx. The radiograph was obtained through a distal limb cast. The fracture was repaired using two 4.5-mm narrow dynamic compression plates and 5.5-mm cortex screws, with arthrodesis of the proximal interphalangeal joint. The gelding returned to competitive jumping.

plating can be used depending on the configuration of the fracture. The use of additional screws placed in lag fashion is usually required to reduce large fragments and reconstruct the articular surface. Another plate technique using a Y-plate has been tested experimentally and shows similar biomechanical properties to the double-plate technique.[27] Cast coaptation is required for 6 to 8 weeks after surgery. Transfixation pins are used to prevent collapse of the fracture in horses with severely comminuted fractures. This technique may be combined with plate and screw fixation. Prognosis after double-plate fixation of 10 horses with comminuted fracture of the middle phalanx was good for pasture soundness, and 5 horses were able to be ridden or shown, but mild lameness persisted.[28]

BONE TRAUMA

Since the advent of MRI, one of the Editors (SJD) has recognized horses with acute-onset severe lameness associated with pain in the pastern region in the absence of detectable radiological abnormality in the acute stage. These horses have had evidence of primary osseous pathology characterized by focal or diffuse areas of increased signal intensity in fat-suppressed images and reduced signal intensity in T1-weighted images, consistent with bone edema, fibrosis, or necrosis. Some horses have made a slow but spontaneous recovery, whereas others have subsequently developed radiological evidence of OA of the proximal or DIP joints associated with persistent lameness.[29-31]

SOFT TISSUE INJURIES

Soft tissue injuries in the pastern are discussed in Chapter 82.

SUBLUXATION OF THE PROXIMAL INTERPHALANGEAL JOINT

Subluxation of the PIP joint is uncommon and can occur in the palmar/plantar direction or dorsally. Palmar/plantar subluxation usually is seen after severe, traumatic soft tissue injury, such as complete tearing of the distal sesamoidean ligaments, SDFT branch injury, or a combination of soft tissue injuries or fracture. Treatment options for palmar/plantar subluxation include both conservative and surgical management. External coaptation can be successful in adult horses managed acutely. The application of a Kimzey splint (Kimzey Leg Saver Splint, Kimzey, Inc., Woodland, California, United States) is an excellent method of first aid for this injury. Cast immobilization can be successful, but instability of the PIP joint may preclude successful realignment with this method. Arthrodesis of the PIP joint is always an option. Dorsal subluxation can occur after traumatic disruption of the suspensory apparatus and arthrodesis of the fetlock joint to manage this problem, but it most commonly occurs in horses with progressive, severe suspensory desmitis. This is particularly true in the STB or TB racehorse, in which suspensory desmitis is common. Swelling along the dorsal aspect of the pastern region is the first clinical sign recognized, but progressive hyperextension (dropping) of the fetlock joint is usually present. The appearance of dorsal subluxation in any horse with chronic suspensory desmitis is a negative prognostic sign. Dorsal subluxation may also occur in association with transection of a branch of SDFT, severe injuries of the oblique sesamoidean ligaments, or rupture of the straight sesamoidean ligament. In these horses there is usually no associated hyperextension of the fetlock.

Chronic injuries of the oblique or straight sesamoidean ligaments may be associated with dorsal extension of the dorsal articular margins of the PIP joint, presumably a response to low-grade instability of the joint.[3,29] This is not synonymous with OA. Although radiological abnormalities may be obvious, such changes are not necessarily associated with pain and lameness.

Dorsal subluxation of the PIP joint can occur without any identifiable structural abnormality of the pastern or metatarsal soft tissue structures. This occurs primarily in the hindlimbs in young horses, and lameness is usually absent or mild. Dorsal subluxation is most often dynamic in nature and resolves during full weight bearing. The presence of changes consistent with OA worsens prognosis. Dorsal subluxation of the PIP joint as a result of mild flexor deformity was reported in three horses. In these horses, ranging in age from 5 months to 4 years, subluxation was believed to be caused by mild contraction of the deep digital flexor tendon (DDFT) without compensatory contraction of the SDFT. Subluxation was seen primarily during early weight bearing, but the condition resolved during full weight bearing. Tenotomy of the medial head of the DDFT in the proximal metatarsal region resolved dynamic dorsal subluxation.[32]

WOUNDS AND INFECTION IN THE PASTERN REGION

Lacerations and puncture wounds in the pastern region have a high propensity to involve the PIP joint or DFTS.

Careful inspection of the wound, radiography, ultrasonography, and analysis of synovial aspirates are often required to determine the extent of the wounds. Wounds that involve the PIP joint or DFTS require aggressive management to prevent synovial infection. Treatments include synovial lavage, wound debridement, drain placement, and systemic and regional antimicrobial therapy with or without tenoscopic examination. Intrasynovial, systemic, and regional perfusion of antimicrobial agents can be used. Sequelae of PIP joint infection include OA. Sequelae of infection of the DFTS include intrasynovial adhesion formation and infectious osteitis of the PSBs (see Chapters 72 and 74).

Infectious disorders of the pastern region can be caused by injuries or hematogenous spread of bacteria, particularly in young horses. Although this chapter is not meant to be a discussion of the treatment of infection, it is important to point out some things of note. Serial radiography, ultrasonography, and MRI are useful for determining the location and extent of the infectious process. Determination of the actual structure involved can be challenging in the pastern region. Regional perfusion of antimicrobial agents is particularly useful in the pastern region to combat infection. Tissue levels can reach as high as 30 times and synovial levels up to 100 times the minimum inhibitory concentration for up to 24 hours after regional perfusion.[33] Even horses with obvious bone involvement from infectious phystis/arthritis can be treated successfully with systemic and regional antimicrobial agents and lavage (Figure 35-5).

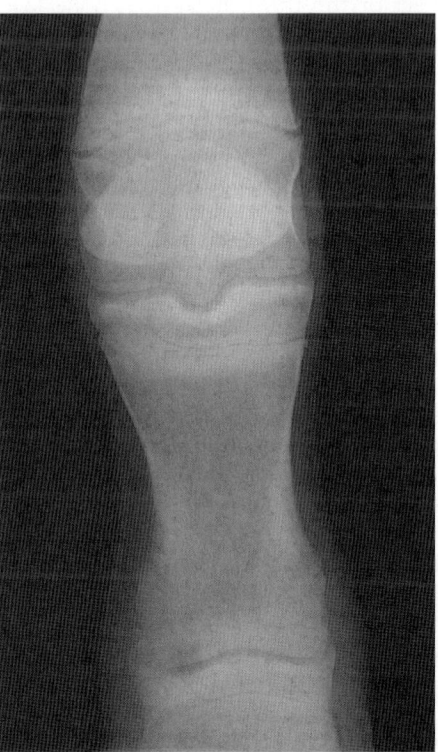

Fig. 35-5 • Dorsoplantar radiographic image of a 3-month-old Thoroughbred colt with infectious arthritis/epiphysitis of the proximal aspect of the middle phalanx. Medial is to the left. Note the well-circumscribed radiolucent area in the proximomedial aspect of the epiphysis. The foal was treated with joint lavage and regional perfusion of the digit with antimicrobial agents and made a complete recovery. Presale radiographs obtained 1 year later revealed no detectable radiological abnormality.

Chapter 36

The Metacarpophalangeal Joint

Dean W. Richardson and Sue J. Dyson

ANATOMICAL CONSIDERATIONS

The metacarpophalangeal (fetlock) joint is an intensely loaded, high-motion joint that is frequently injured in athletic horses. Fetlock region lameness can occur in horses of any occupation, but the joint is at particularly high risk in horses performing at maximal speed. Countering the high load experienced by the joint is the elastic suspensory apparatus that constrains the range of extension. Both the superficial and deep digital flexor muscle tendon units additionally serve to actively support the fetlock joint because of their position on the palmar aspect of the joint. Loss of this active support by the digital flexor tendons may lead to overload of the suspensory apparatus support and some degree of hyperextension. Extreme extension of the metacarpophalangeal joint results in impingement of the proximal rim of the proximal phalanx against the dorsal aspect of the third metacarpal bone (McIII), high compressive forces on the distal, palmar aspect of the McIII opposing the proximal sesamoid bones (PSBs), and both tensile and bending forces on the PSBs intercalated within the suspensory apparatus.[1] Complex forces of torsion on the loaded fetlock joint result in a myriad of injuries.

The metacarpophalangeal joint is anatomically composed of the distal aspect of the McIII, the proximal phalanx, and both PSBs. A single synovial space extends on its palmar aspect at least 3 cm proximal to the apex of the PSBs. Dorsally, a bilobed synovial "pad" is located on the proximal dorsal articular rim of the distal aspect of the McIII; this pad presumably functions to help cushion the impingement of the McIII and proximal phalanx. The ligamentous elements of the fetlock joint are complex and important. Well-developed medial and lateral collateral metacarpophalangeal and metacarposesamoidean ligaments constrain the almost purely sagittal motion of this joint, but both abduction and rotation occur.[2] The suspensory branches insert on the proximal, palmar abaxial margins of the PSBs and functionally continue through the distal sesamoidean ligaments to attach the distal portion of the PSBs to the proximal phalanx (cruciate or deep and oblique or middle) and the middle phalanx (straight or superficial). The intersesamoidean ligament attaches the axial aspects of the PSBs.

The digital flexor tendon sheath and its contents are described elsewhere (see Chapter 74). The common digital extensor tendon is unsheathed as it passes over the dorsal aspect of the joint. Branches of the medial and lateral palmar and metacarpal nerves primarily supply innervation to the fetlock joint,[3] but small subcutaneous branches of the ulnar nerve supply a minor amount of dorsal sensory innervation.

References on page 1280

DIAGNOSIS

Careful physical examination to detect heat, swelling (effusion with or without periarticular fibrosis), and pain with palpation or manipulation is critical for diagnosis of lameness of the metacarpophalangeal joint. However, physical findings may be subtle or seemingly nonexistent, whereas diagnostic analgesia often pinpoints the joint or region as the source of pain. Interpretation of fetlock flexion test results should be made with caution because many horses have false-positive responses to forced flexion of this joint, especially if the toe is used to increase leverage. Pain originating in the limb distal to the fetlock joint often is exacerbated by fetlock or lower limb flexion tests. False-negative responses to fetlock joint flexion also are common, especially in horses with subchondral bone injury and chip fractures. Flexion tests are discussed further in Chapter 8. Increased fluid in the fetlock joint can also be a false localizing sign. The presence of an effusion in the absence of heat and pain may indicate some derangement in synovial function but not necessarily point to the source of a clinically relevant lameness. Lameness characteristically occurs with weight bearing and usually, but not always, is worse with the limb on the inside of a circle. If clinical signs do not adequately localize lameness, perineural or intrasynovial analgesia can specify the region relatively easily. In the absence of localizing clinical signs, the foot and pastern regions should first be eliminated as sources of pain by a midpastern digital nerve block with a dorsal subcutaneous ring. Ideally this is followed by intraarticular analgesia of the metacarpophalangeal joint. If the lameness does not improve within 15 to 20 minutes of intraarticular analgesia, the clinician should perform a low palmar block or palmar and palmar metacarpal nerve blocks. In most horses with intraarticular chip fractures, synovitis, capsulitis, and osteoarthritis (OA), lameness improves after intraarticular analgesia. Horses with major fractures, nonarticular fractures, subchondral bone injuries, and tendon and tendon sheath lesions usually are only markedly improved with perineural analgesia. Perineural techniques are superior to definitively abolish pain associated with the fetlock joint. Pain in horses that do not respond to intraarticular analgesia should not necessarily be presumed to originate elsewhere. False-positive results to intraarticular analgesia can also be obtained; lameness associated with a suspensory branch injury or injury of the proximal aspect of the oblique, cruciate, or straight sesamoidean ligaments may be substantially improved or abolished. Subchondral bone pain will not always, or completely, be eliminated with intraarticular analgesia.

Several techniques are used for intrasynovial analgesia of the fetlock joint. One author (DWR) prefers to inject the local anesthetic solution with the horse's limb on the ground. The dorsal aspect of the fetlock is readily accessible when the horse is bearing weight. As the clinician faces forward and presses the back of his or her arm against the horse's carpus, a 22-gauge, 2.5-cm needle attached to a 75-cm extension set is inserted horizontally into the dorsal aspect of the joint just proximal to the margin of the proximal phalanx and deep to the common digital extensor tendon. One of us (DWR) uses 10 to 15 mL of 2%

mepivacaine, but many practitioners use no more than 6 to 10 mL. One author (SJD) prefers to inject into the palmar pouch through the metacarposesamoidean ligament, with the limb flexed, using a 21-gauge, 3.8-cm needle, injecting 6 to 10 mL of 2% mepivacaine depending on the size of the horse. Other techniques are described in Chapter 10.

IMAGING CONSIDERATIONS

The fetlock joint is easy to image accurately because of the size and accessibility. Numerous flexed and oblique radiographic images to specifically silhouette or separate structures help to identify subtle lesions. The same advantages apply to scintigraphic and ultrasonographic imaging. For example, flexed lateral scintigraphic images can help determine whether a lesion in the palmar aspect of the fetlock involves the base of a PSB or the palmar surface of the McIII. A minimum set of radiographs should include dorsopalmar, lateromedial, flexed lateromedial, and both oblique images. The size of the region and absence of overlying soft tissues results in excellently detailed radiographs, even with portable x-ray machines, if suitable screen–film combinations are used or computed or digital radiography is available. A number of specific radiographic images should be obtained if certain lesions are suspected. For example, if a subchondral injury involving the distal palmar aspect of the McIII is suspected, the oblique images should be taken in a more proximal to distal direction than usual. If a lateral condylar fracture is identified, a partially flexed dorsopalmar image should be used to help identify comminution along the distal palmar aspect of the fracture line.[4,5] Osteochondrosis of the sagittal ridge of the McIII and incomplete sagittal fractures of the proximal phalanx are lesions that can be difficult to identify in overexposed lateromedial images or underexposed dorsopalmar images, but digital radiography has largely eliminated the need to obtain numerous exposures with different techniques. Reference to the location of soft tissue attachments in the fetlock region is necessary for accurate interpretation.[6]

Nuclear scintigraphy has proven to be an exceptionally valuable tool to evaluate the fetlocks of active racehorses because so many injuries involve those joints, especially the distal metacarpal/metatarsal condyles. Flexed lateral images and dorsopalmar/plantarodorsal images allow excellent anatomic discrimination of which specific structures in the fetlock region have increased radiopharmaceutical uptake (IRU).[7] In particular, flexed lateral and dorsal scintigraphic images can be very helpful to separate palmar metacarpal and PSB uptake. Scintigraphy is also useful for detection of subchondral and trabecular bone injuries in sports horses.[8,9]

Ultrasonographic evaluation of the fetlock can be valuable for evaluation of tendon and ligament injuries around the fetlock, especially the digital flexor tendons, the palmar annular ligament (see Chapter 74), and the dorsal synovial pad/plica, as well as the bone margins.[10,11] Ultrasonography (96%) was more accurate than radiology (44%) in predicting the number and location of osseous fragments on the dorsal aspect of the metacarpophalangeal and metatarsophalangeal joints identified using arthroscopy.[12] Three-dimensional imaging modalities such as computed tomography (CT)[13-15] (see Chapter 20) or magnetic resonance imaging (MRI) (see Chapter 21) can also be very valuable in the fetlock, especially in areas like the distal palmar McIII condyle, the axial aspect of the PSBs, and the periarticular soft tissues.[16-19]

TYPES OF FETLOCK JOINT LAMENESS

Most fetlock joint lamenesses can be categorized into one of three types:
1. Acute or repetitive overload injuries without specific fracture or fractures: capsulitis/synovitis, chronic proliferative (villonodular) synovitis, OA, subchondral bone injury without obvious fracture, and sesamoiditis
2. Articular fragments/lesions that can be removed (traumatic and developmental lesions) from the dorsal or palmar aspects of the proximal phalanx; apical, abaxial, and basilar PSB fractures; and fragments from the sagittal ridge of the McIII
3. Major articular fractures (i.e., those that should be repaired), including sagittal and frontal/near frontal (dorsal) plane fractures (mostly seen in the hindlimbs); collateral ligament avulsion injuries (mostly foals and yearlings) of the proximal phalanx; midbody, large abaxial, or basilar fragments of the PSBs; and condylar fractures of the McIII

Conditions specific to the metatarsophalangeal joint and a detailed description of sagittal fractures of the proximal phalanx are discussed elsewhere (see Chapters 35 and 42). Injuries of the digital flexor tendon sheath, superficial and deep digital flexor tendons, the palmar annular ligament, and the proximal digital annular ligament are discussed in Chapter 74. Suspensory ligament (SL) branch injuries are discussed in Chapter 72. Injuries of the distal sesamoidean ligaments are discussed in Chapter 82. Traumatic disruption of the suspensory apparatus is discussed in Chapter 104.

ACUTE OR REPETITIVE OVERLOAD INJURIES
Capsulitis/Synovitis

Clinical Signs
Virtually every young racehorse has one or more episodes of metacarpophalangeal capsulitis or synovitis that is characterized by heat, effusion, and pain with flexion. Overt lameness usually is mild and often not evident after the horse warms up. Signs typically manifest as the horse increases the speed and distance of its exercise regimen. If the typical localizing signs are missed, the major indication may be a decrease in performance. In horses with chronic disease, visible thickening of the periarticular tissues usually is noticeable, with decreased range of motion of the joint. In mature sports horses, capsulitis and/or synovitis is less common as a primary condition but is more likely to be associated with sudden-onset moderate to severe lameness.

Diagnosis
A diagnosis of primary capsulitis or synovitis usually is made by clinical observations and the absence of radiological or scintigraphic bony abnormalities. Synovitis and capsulitis may also accompany other causes of fetlock joint lameness, such as chip fractures. Synovial fluid analysis has not

been particularly useful in diagnosis or prognosis for most fetlock joint injuries except to help identify infection.

Treatment

In most young horses the condition resolves with nonsteroidal antiinflammatory drugs (NSAIDs), adjustments in training, and increased fitness. Intraarticular hyaluronan (20 mg) is helpful in horses with acute, mild to moderate synovitis, but a combination of hyaluronan with a low dose of a corticosteroid (e.g., 3 to 5 mg of triamcinolone acetonide or 20 to 30 mg of methylprednisolone acetate) is more consistently effective in resolving the clinical signs of inflammation. Injection should be followed by a decrease in exercise intensity for at least 1 to 2 weeks. Postexercise icing of the involved fetlock joints can be helpful. Generic OA treatments, including oral glucosamine with or without chondroitin sulfate, intramuscular polysulfated glycosaminoglycans (PSGAGs), and intravenous hyaluronan merit consideration, but they do not usually yield the consistent response seen with intraarticular therapy. Topical application of 1% diclofenac sodium (Surpass, IDEXX Pharmaceuticals, Inc., Greensboro, North Carolina, United States) appears to reduce inflammation.

Chronic Proliferative (Villonodular) Synovitis

Clinical Signs

Chronic capsulitis/synovitis is caused by repetitive injury of the dorsal aspect of the fetlock joint. The lesion is defined by a thickening of the normally dorsally located bilobed synovial pad that hangs down on either side of the sagittal ridge of the McIII. With extreme extension of the fetlock joint, the dorsal rim of the proximal phalanx impinges on the synovial pad, and repetitive trauma results in its inflammation and subsequent fibrosis. The tissue can become so thick that the dorsal profile of the joint is visibly disfigured. The characteristic swelling is asymmetrical on the midproximodorsal aspect of the fetlock (Figure 36-1) rather than simply spherical in outline as in a typical osteoarthritic fetlock joint (this is called an *osselet*). Exercise inflames the tissue further, and clinical signs of lameness or diminished performance can result.

Diagnosis

The diagnosis of proliferative synovitis is based on physical examination, radiography, ultrasonography, or a combination of these modalities. The most common radiological sign of the lesion is a crescent-shaped, radiolucent "cutout" on the dorsal aspect of the McIII at the level of the joint capsule attachment (Figure 36-2). The proliferative lesion may undergo dystrophic mineralization and be radiologically visible. Radiographic contrast studies can be used, but ultrasonography is simpler and more reliable (Figure 36-3). Normal thickness on ultrasonographic examination has been described as less than 2 mm,[10,11] but mere identification of a slightly thicker than average structure is certainly not an indication for surgical excision. Many older racehorses have a substantially thicker synovial pad without any associated discomfort. Horses with severe OA have proliferative synovitis in the palmar pouch, and a large concave outline of the distal palmar aspect of the McIII is seen proximal to the PSBs (Figure 36-4 and Figure 34-17), which is associated with a poor prognosis.

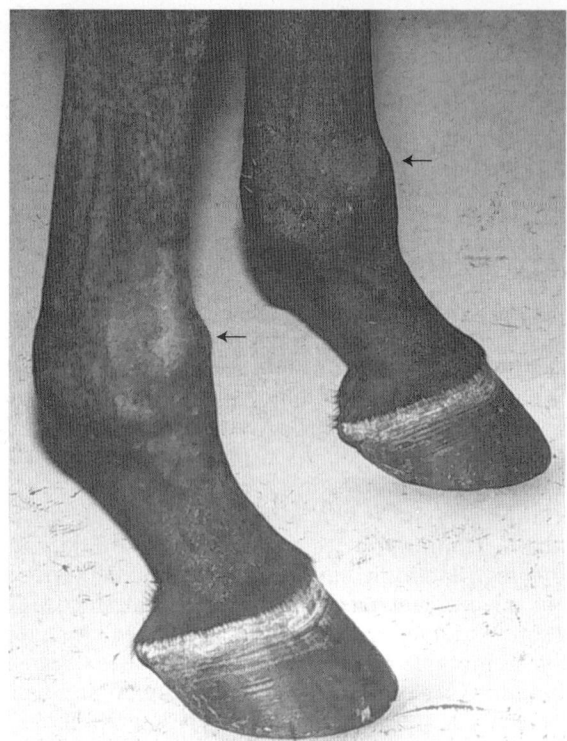

Fig. 36-1 • An older Thoroughbred racehorse with chronic proliferative synovitis. The dorsal swellings are firm and localized in the proximodorsal aspect of the joints *(arrows)*.

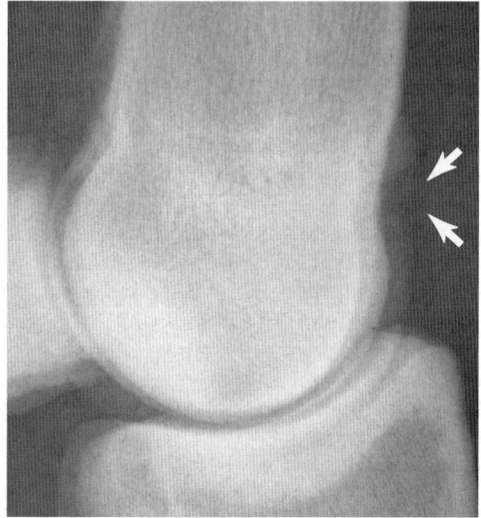

Fig. 36-2 • Chronic proliferative (villonodular) synovitis of the metacarpophalangeal joint with a typical erosive lesion *(arrows)* along the proximal dorsal margin of the sagittal ridge of the third metacarpal bone seen in a lateromedial radiographic image. The fibrotic tissue may have small fragments of bone and cartilage or dystrophic mineralization.

Treatment

Treatment for proliferative synovitis usually consists of aggressive intraarticular therapy (e.g., hyaluronan and corticosteroids), rest, and alterations in training. Many horses require frequent medication until the joint becomes stiff enough to prevent dorsal impingement. Horses appear to be able to work through this problem as they develop increasing strength and fitness. If the horse does not

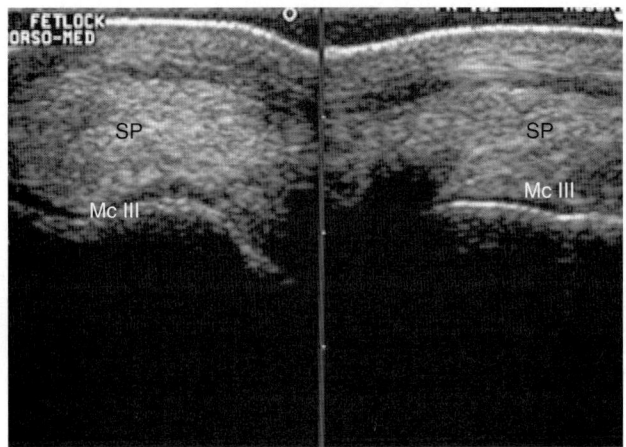

Fig. 36-3 • Transverse *(left)* and longitudinal *(right)* ultrasonographic images of the distal dorsal metacarpal region. Ultrasonographic examination can confirm a thickened synovial pad, but the diagnosis usually is made based on physical examination and radiological findings. *McIII,* Third metacarpal bone; *SP,* synovial pad.

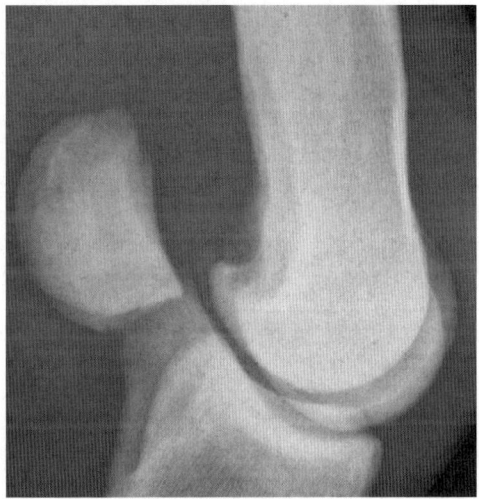

Fig. 36-4 • Flexed lateromedial radiographic image of a Thoroughbred racehorse with severe chronic synovitis and osteoarthritis that led to the development of a large erosive lesion of the distal palmar aspect of the third metacarpal (McIII) bone. There is a large concave outline of the palmar cortex of the McIII just proximal to the proximal sesamoid bones.

respond to medical treatment, surgical excision using an arthroscopic technique is recommended.[20,21] Surgical debridement must be followed with continued medical treatment and careful attention to the training regimen. It is important to recognize that the thickening of the proximal dorsal synovial pad may be just one part of a chronic, osteoarthritic joint. In such horses, any therapy such as surgery directed solely at this lesion probably will fail.

Osteochondral Fragments in the Synovial Pad

Well-rounded osteochondral fragments in the synovial pad on the dorsoproximal aspect of the fetlock have been described in Warmblood horses in both forelimbs and hindlimbs, either as an incidental finding in presale radiographs obtained at 2 and 3 years of age (n = 102) or in association with fetlock joint pain in mature horses (n = 2).[22] Radiological differentiation between these fragments and those that are a manifestation of osteochondrosis may not be possible. However, ultrasonographic examination has confirmed their presence within the synovial pad, and this has been verified at arthroscopic examination and by histology. Histological examination revealed that these fragments consistently comprised an osseous center covered with cartilage on one side and surrounded by fibrous tissue. In a study of 127 joints, multivariable analysis of variance showed a significant association between the presence of a fragment more than 10 mm in length and severe synovial proliferation, wear lines on the dorsal aspect of the McIII, and cartilage erosions. The long-term clinical significance of such lesions has not been determined. The etiology of these fragments has not been established.

Osteoarthritis

Clinical Signs

OA of the metacarpophalangeal joint is common, especially in racehorses, endurance horses, polo ponies, event horses, and show jumpers. There is usually a progression of disease from medial to lateral, reflecting the biomechanical loading of the joint.[23] The degree of lameness varies from mild to severe depending on the stage of the disease and recent work history. There is often associated synovitis and/or capsulitis, with palpable distention and/or thickening of the joint capsule. However, the absence of joint effusion does not preclude the presence of OA. There is often resentment of passive flexion of the joint and exacerbation of lameness by flexion; however, the absence of these clinical signs also does not preclude the presence of OA. The range of passive joint motion may be reduced because of increased stiffness of the soft tissues on the dorsal aspect of the joint.

Diagnosis

Lameness is usually abolished by perineural analgesia using a "low four-point block," but the response to intraarticular analgesia is variable, depending on the degree of subchondral bone pain. Increased intraarticular pressure may be a significant contributor to pain and lameness.[24] Radiography usually reveals periarticular modeling on the dorsoproximal aspects of the proximal phalanx, medially more than laterally, with or without modeling of the distal dorsal aspects of the McIII. There may be thickening of the proximal subchondral bone plate of the proximal phalanx. Subchondral radiolucent areas are rare. With advanced OA there may be supracondylar lysis of the distal palmar aspect of the McIII and modeling of the proximal and distal articular margins of the PSBs. In some horses the only radiological change is narrowing of the joint space, reflecting advanced articular cartilage loss and a poor prognosis. It is important not to overlook this and to appreciate its clinical significance.

Treatment

Intraarticular medication with corticosteroids (triamcinolone acetonide) and hyaluronan or PSGAGs is usually effective in early OA, combined with correction of any foot imbalance. Modification of the training program and selection of work surfaces may be important. Local therapy (e.g., whirlpool boots, spa therapy) can be of benefit. The value of oral nutraceuticals is difficult to quantify but may have a management role. Autologous conditioned serum (inter-leukin–1 receptor antagonist) is being used with increasing frequency with anecdotally favorable results. If the clinical signs are inconsistent with the radiological abnormalities or there is a poor response to treatment, further investigation by exploratory arthroscopy (in the presence of joint effusion) or MRI (in the absence of joint effusion) may be warranted.

Traumatically Induced Cartilage and/or Subchondral Bone Injury

Trauma to the fetlock, the result of hitting a jump, getting a show jump pole tangled between the forelimbs, falling, or stumbling, may result in sudden onset of lameness associated with effusion of the metacarpophalangeal joint.[8,25] Lameness is abolished by intraarticular analgesia. At the time of acute onset of lameness there may be no detectable radiological abnormality, and follow-up radiographs may also have no detectable lesion. Although there may be a transient response to intraarticular medication, effusion and lameness usually persist. Exploratory arthroscopy may reveal a focal area of cartilage loss usually on the dorsal distal aspect of the condyle of the McIII, with exposure of subchondral bone, and some softening of the immediately surrounding articular cartilage or peeling off of a large piece of cartilage—a "delamination" injury. Debridement of such lesions invariably results in clinical improvement. If the lesion is located dorsal to the region of maximum weight bearing, the horse may become sound, but lesions on the major weight-bearing aspect result in a guarded prognosis for return to full athletic function.

Alternatively, follow-up radiographs may reveal a radiolucent area in the subchondral bone of the distal aspect of the McIII, seen best in a dorsal 25° proximal-palmarodistal oblique image. Such osseous cystlike lesions are usually associated with an overlying area of full-thickness cartilage loss. Like the cartilage lesions described above, lesions on the weight-bearing part of the McIII usually result in persistent lameness, but some horses have returned to full athletic function following debridement of more dorsally located lesions. However, the presence of extensive wear lines in the articular cartilage reflecting concurrent OA warrants a guarded prognosis. Trauma through an accident while jumping has also resulted in osseous fragmentation of the dorsoproximal medial or lateral aspects of the proximal phalanx. High-detail radiographs may be necessary to differentiate this fragmentation from periarticular osteophyte formation. However, the immediate recognition of such radiological abnormalities soon after an accident is diagnostic of traumatic joint injury rather than OA. Such fragmentation may be associated with a traumatically induced deep groove in the opposing articular cartilage of the distal aspect of the McIII; therefore, although arthroscopic removal of the fragments is likely to result in clinical improvement, long-term repeated intraarticular medication of the joint is likely to be required to maintain soundness. Secondary OA may ensue.

Subchondral Bone Injury

Clinical Signs

Subchondral bone injury is an extremely important cause of lameness involving the metacarpophalangeal joint,

especially in racehorses.[26,27] Similar lesions are being recognized with increasing frequency in elite endurance horses and also in other sports horses. There are no specific localizing clinical signs in many horses other than variable lameness and an observable diminution in performance. Signs such as heat, swelling, or response to flexion can be absent or extremely subtle, even in horses with overt lameness. Although subchondral bone injury is far more common in racehorses, it appears that single-step overload injuries that focally damage a portion of the McIII or the proximal phalanx can occur in nonracehorses. Such injuries may result in radiologically visible increased radiopacity or radiolucency. The severity of the lameness in such horses can be surprising, and infection may be a differential diagnosis.

Diagnosis

The inconsistent response to local analgesia can make diagnosis difficult unless a reasonably high index of suspicion for these lesions is maintained. Many horses do not achieve soundness with intraarticular analgesia. Horses with full-thickness cartilage injury overlying the subchondral injury may be most likely to experience improvement in lameness because of the access of the local anesthetic agent to the site. Lameness in most horses improves dramatically with low palmar analgesia (four-point block); however, subcarpal analgesia of the palmar metacarpal nerves is sometimes required for complete resolution of lameness.

The two most common locations for subchondral injury of the fetlock in racehorses are the distal palmar aspect of the McIII and the proximal phalanx under the center of the weight-bearing portion of the medial or lateral articular surfaces. The palmar McIII lesion appears to develop as a focal overload injury where the base of the PSB impacts during maximal weight bearing.[15,16] In this location, linear or crescent-shaped lucencies are the most common indications of a major advanced subchondral bone injury (Figure 36-5). These often can be seen on a lateromedial image, but special radiographic images may improve the likelihood of seeing a lesion. A slightly flexed, horizontal beam dorsopalmar image silhouetting

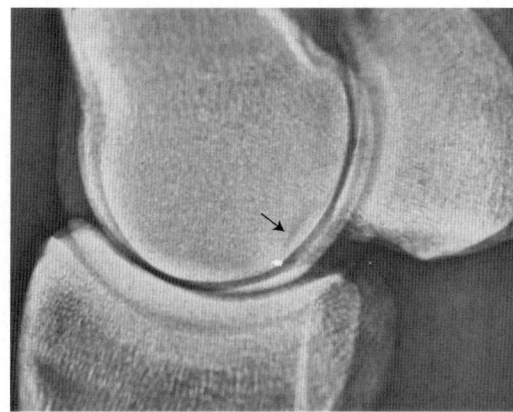

Fig. 36-5 • Lateromedial radiographic image of a metacarpophalangeal joint. Subchondral crescent-shaped *(arrow)* and linear radiolucencies in the distal palmar articular surface of the third metacarpal bone are important radiological findings. Most horses with such lesions have clinical signs of fetlock pain, especially with hard training. The cartilage overlying such lesions is damaged and often unstable.

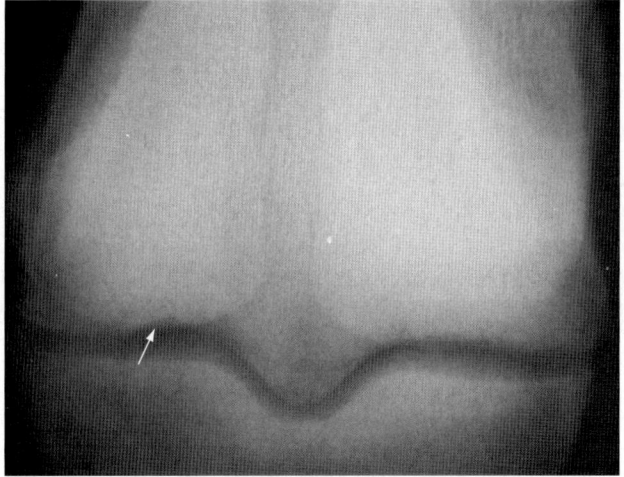

Fig. 36-6 • Slightly flexed dorsopalmar radiographic image of the metacarpophalangeal joint is helpful to define lesions *(arrow)* of the distal palmar aspect of the third metacarpal bone.

the distal palmar aspect of the McIII can help define an irregular subchondral outline (Figure 36-6).[4,5] Oblique images obtained in a slightly (25 to 30 degrees) proximal-distal direction also allow a better evaluation of the palmar aspect of the condyle and the identification of radiolucent defects (see Figure 42-1).[7] With lesions of the proximal phalanx, an increase in subchondral radiopacity may be evident before radiolucent lesions develop, but increased radiopacity in the McIII is much more difficult to recognize, and differentiation between normal adaptive modeling and injury is not easy.

Scintigraphy is the most sensitive routine diagnostic tool and can identify lesions in racehorses well before radiological lesions are evident (Figure 36-7). Scintigraphy can also be useful in sports horses (positive in 12 of 15 horses with subchondral and trabecular bone lesions detected using MRI), but if trabecular sclerosis is the principal lesion, then scintigraphy may be negative.[8] Even arthroscopic diagnosis can be difficult in the fetlock joint because the anatomical location of these lesions makes evaluation difficult. If the lesions are accessible, the overlying cartilage may be thin or discolored. The amount of cartilage fibrillation or crazing of the joint surface is variable. MRI is expensive but provides more detailed information about the precise location of injury and some information about the type of bone injury, distinguishing early phases of repetitive stress injury (see Figure 107-7).[16-19] MRI may reveal areas of reduced signal intensity in T1- and T2-weighted images consistent with mineralization (so-called sclerosis or densification) of the bone. There may also be areas of high signal intensity on fat-suppressed images and low signal intensity on T1-weighted images that may reflect bone edema, hemorrhage, fibrosis, or necrosis. High-field images may also reveal areas of cartilage pathology.

In 13 sports and pleasure horses, MRI revealed areas of thickening of the subchondral bone plate and altered signal intensity in the trabecular bone, with mild lesions of one of the collateral ligaments in 5.[16] Mediolateral distribution of injuries was similar. Six of 13 horses returned to full function with conservative management.

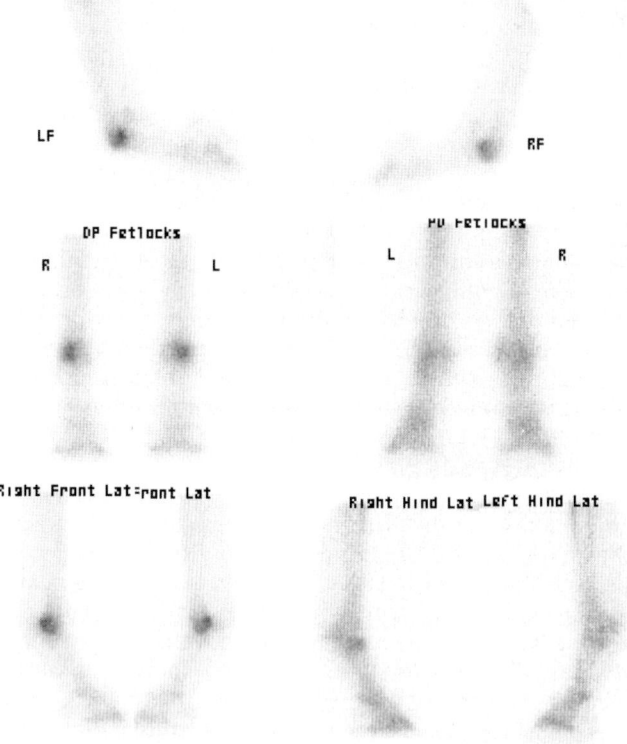

Fig. 36-7 • Typical scintigraphic appearance of repetitive stress injury to the distal palmar aspect of the third metacarpal bone. The pattern of increased radiopharmaceutical uptake is made more definitive by comparing standing and flexed lateral images.

Treatment

Rest, or at least decreased training intensity, is the most common recommendation for subchondral bone injury in racehorses. It is currently very difficult to define which horses with injury of this location are going to develop more serious problems such as condylar fractures if they continue in hard work. However, in a recent post mortem MRI study of horses (n = 47) subjected to euthanasia on a UK racecourse as a result of a lateral condylar fracture, compared with the contralateral limb (n = 46) and a limb from control horses subjected to euthanasia for unrelated reasons (n = 98), a combined thickness of the subchondral bone and trabecular mineralization of the palmar aspect of the condyle of the McIII of more than 2 cm resulted in an odds ratio for fracture of 4.23 compared with controls.[28] Medications such as bisphosphonates (tiludronate), isoxsuprine, and aspirin are frequently recommended; however, there is little information to support their efficacy. Damaged bone can heal if the horse is rested, but the prognosis depends on the amount of structural damage to the overlying cartilage and any loss in the normal architecture of this critical area.

INJURIES TO THE PROXIMAL PHALANX
Osteochondral Fragments: Dorsoproximal Aspect of the Proximal Phalanx
Clinical Signs

The most common chip fracture in Thoroughbred (TB) racehorses involves the proximal dorsal aspect of the proximal phalanx and is an important differential diagnosis in any young TB with acute swelling or heat in a metacarpophalangeal joint. Affected horses rarely are lame for more than 2 days after a fracture and may never show overt lameness. An observant groom or trainer may notice an effusion with some heat, and forced flexion usually causes a painful response. Common historical findings include diminished performance, refusal to change leads, and bearing in or out, especially in the stretch.

Dorsal chip fractures can also be seen in yearlings and nonracehorses as an incidental finding. Most presumably occur as a traumatic event during early development and simply go unrecognized until presale radiographs are obtained. Juvenile fragments occur equally in the forelimbs and hindlimbs, whereas traumatic injuries in active racehorses and sports horses are more common in the forelimbs.

Diagnosis

Chip fractures of the proximodorsal aspect of the proximal phalanx of any size are not difficult to diagnose if they are displaced, but nondisplaced fragments may require nearly perfect radiographs. Most chips occur on the prominence just medial to the median sagittal groove of the proximal phalanx. The left forelimb is slightly more commonly affected than the right forelimb in North American TBs. Bilateral chips are fairly common, and thus radiographs of both fetlocks should be obtained before surgery is performed. The fragments generally are seen best on a dorsolateral-palmaromedial oblique or lateromedial image, depending on the obliquity of the fracture line and image (Figure 36-8, *A* and *B*). Correct radiographic technique is especially important for small chips because overexposure burns out the lesion on a lateromedial image and underexposed oblique images do not have enough penetration. Although most radiologically diagnosed fractures are dorsomedial, it is important to evaluate arthroscopically the entire dorsal rim of the proximal phalanx because small chondral fractures are common. Horses in which a dorsolateral fragment is seen radiologically usually also have a lesion on the dorsomedial side. Finally, it is fairly common for fractures to be more evident on early radiographs than on follow-up images because they can become crushed into much smaller fragments pushed back down into the original fracture bed following exercise.

Treatment

Treatment for horses with these chip fractures is less controversial since the advent of arthroscopy. The previous morbidity associated with large incisions on the dorsal aspect of the fetlock to remove rather small fragments made surgical treatment much less attractive. With arthroscopic technique, however, the fragments can be easily and atraumatically removed. An excellent prognosis after a short (approximately 4 to 6 weeks) postoperative convalescence can be given if there are no other degenerative changes in the joint.[29-31] In economically unworthy animals, a period of 3 to 4 months' rest, followed by intraarticular medications as needed, also affords a favorable prognosis, especially if the fragment is not markedly displaced. In our opinion, superior conditioning when these horses return to work helps prolong careers. Injecting a horse with a corticosteroid after it develops an acute chip fracture also can achieve a favorable short-term result and is always a consideration if the horse's immediate racing demands will not allow a substantial period of rest. However, training and racing a horse with an unstable chip fracture may lead to more rapid degenerative changes in the fetlock. Such horses often have extensive score lines, thin cartilage, and more advanced osteoarthritic changes if the fragment is removed arthroscopically at a later date.

Short Sesamoidean Avulsions (Osteochondral Fragments) from the Palmar Aspect of the Proximal Phalanx

Clinical Signs

Characterization of osteochondral fragments arising from the proximal palmar aspect of the proximal phalanx is

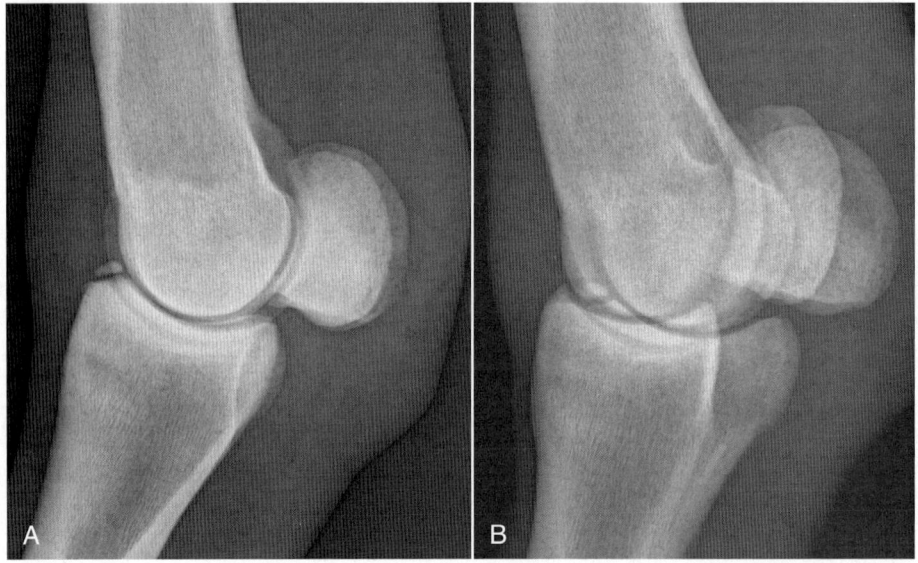

Fig. 36-8 • Proximal dorsomedial osteochondral fragments of the proximal phalanx are the most common chip fracture in Thoroughbred racehorses and can be seen on lateromedial **(A)** and dorsolateral-palmaromedial oblique images **(B)**.

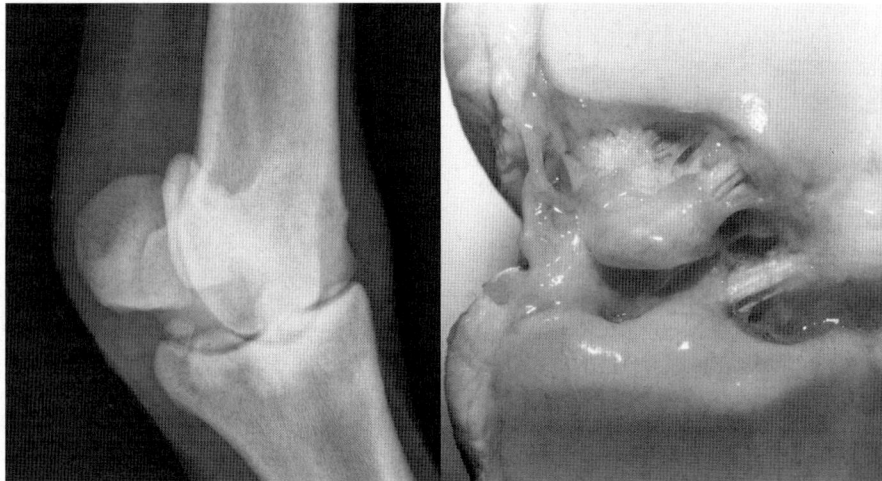

Fig. 36-9 • A typical osteochondral fragment avulsed from the proximal palmar/plantar margin of the proximal phalanx. In the dissection, the attachment of the fragment to the base of the sesamoid by the short sesamoidean ligament is evident, as is the smoothly remodeled defect in the rim of the proximal phalanx.

somewhat controversial. Many consider these fragments to be manifestations of osteochondrosis because they are recognized in very young, untrained animals. It seems most probable that the fragments result from avulsion of a portion of the incompletely ossified proximal phalanx followed by development of a traumatic secondary ossification center.[32,33] The fragments are consistently attached to the short sesamoidean ligament and there is often a small defect in the proximal aspect of the proximal phalanx (Figure 36-9). These fragments are much more common in the hindlimbs (see Chapter 42) and most common in the Standardbred (STB) racehorse. They are also commonly recognized in European Warmbloods. Medial fragments are more common than lateral, but fragments can be numerous and in several limbs. These fragments often are found on presale radiographs, and the relevance to lameness should always be questioned. Many successful athletic horses perform with these lesions. Racehorses in which the fragments affect performance rarely show overt lameness. TBs may be unable to maintain a straight path or fail to change leads properly, and STBs tend to ride a shaft or take a line. Horses in which the lesions cause clinically significant lameness usually have an effusion. Most are not painful to fetlock manipulation. It is possible for fragments in this location to be acute avulsions in older horses, and it is also possible for a fragment that was previously clinically silent to become displaced and painful.

Diagnosis

Oblique radiographic images are best for delineating fragments arising from the palmar proximal aspect of the proximal phalanx. A flexed image helps to further separate the fragment from the base of the PSBs. This separation is useful with proliferative change at the distal dorsal margin of the PSBs or small, basilar sesamoid fractures. Proximal phalangeal fragments usually are well rounded but can also have odd polygonal shapes.

Training a horse after intraarticular analgesia and recognition of improvement in gait should be diagnostic, but the subtle nature of the lameness can make this difficult. Clinical improvement after empirical intraarticular medication also supports the relevance of a radiological lesion. Scintigraphic localization of a lesion may also help confirm the diagnosis, but IRU may be only mild or increased in other parts of the joint, making diagnosis difficult in many racehorses.

Treatment

Treatment consists of arthroscopic removal of the lesion if the clinician is confident that the fragment or fragments are the source of pain causing lameness or if the horse is going to public sale. The most common situation is that the fragments are identified before a horse enters training and the fragments are removed prophylactically. Arthroscopic removal is much less traumatic than arthrotomy for this type of lesion. The prognosis is excellent if the lameness diagnosis is correct.[34] If good arthroscopic technique with minimal soft tissue trauma is used, horses require a short convalescence (4 to 6 weeks). Intraarticular injection of corticosteroids with or without hyaluronan can also improve the clinical signs, but surgery is preferable.

Larger Palmar Fragments of the Proximal Phalanx

Large fracture fragments often cause a more obvious lameness than the more common rounded fragments from the proximal palmar rim of the proximal phalanx. They must be distinguished from more palmar fragments that involve the insertions of the true distal sesamoidean ligaments because the latter are not equally good candidates for surgical removal. Very large, acute fractures of the palmar process of the proximal phalanx can be repaired with screws if recognized early (see Chapter 35). Large fragments occur in foals and weanlings, but clinical signs may abate quickly or be nonexistent. Lameness may be evident only when training or racing ensues. In foals, these fragments may be recognized radiologically if there is effusion, mild to moderate lameness, and obvious periarticular swelling. Lameness is seldom commensurate with fragment size. The lesions in foals are largely cartilaginous and can be followed over time as they develop as a separate center of ossification. These fractures should be differentiated from an avulsion fracture at the site of the medial (or, less commonly, the lateral) collateral ligament (see page 410).

Major Fractures of the Proximal Phalanx: Sagittal Fractures

The most common major fracture of the proximal phalanx is a sagittal crack propagating from the proximal sagittal groove. Horses with long sagittal, displaced sagittal, and comminuted fractures developing from an original fracture in the sagittal or frontal plane have obvious localizing signs of swelling and pain. Horses with shorter sagittal fractures may show more subtle signs. Degree of lameness with short, incomplete sagittal fractures is remarkably variable; some horses are almost unable to bear weight, whereas in others the lameness is barely perceptible (see Chapter 35). There is usually effusion of the fetlock joint, pain on manipulation (flexion and twisting), and pain with firm pressure over the middorsal aspect of the proximal phalanx. Sagittal fractures of the proximal aspect of the proximal phalanx are obvious radiologically if they extend more than a few centimeters from the joint surface, but a short, incomplete fracture is very frequently missed without good-quality radiographs. Although historically short incomplete fractures of the proximal aspect of the proximal phalanx were all thought to be dorsally located, recent information from MRI indicates that some short incomplete fractures are located midway between the dorsal and palmar cortices.[25] If a dorsal fracture is more than 10 days old, there is usually a definite periosteal change on the dorsal cortex seen on a lateromedial image just distal to the capsular attachments. Initially the change is very indistinct, but within a few more weeks, distinct periosteal new bone is obvious. Whenever proliferative change is seen in this area, the dorsopalmar images should be carefully evaluated for a sagittal fracture. Underexposure results in lesions being missed. However, a fracture midway between the dorsal and palmar cortices will not be associated with periosteal new bone formation, although in a dorsopalmar view it may be possible to detect thickening of the subchondral bone plate in the region of the sagittal groove compared with the contralateral limb. These fractures are more common in STBs than TBs but are also being recognized with increasing frequency in elite endurance horses and frequently involve more than one limb. These fractures also occur in other sports horses,[8,35,36] and as in racehorses there is some evidence that preexisting pathological modeling of the bone may predate fracture. Even though these fractures are short and indistinct, they may cause surprisingly severe lameness. The clinician should always suspect such fractures because blocking followed by lunging, high-speed training, or pasture exercise may catastrophically propagate the fracture (Figure 36-10). For management and prognosis, see Chapter 35.

Dorsal Frontal Fractures of the Proximal Phalanx

See Chapters 35 and 42 for a discussion of dorsal frontal fractures of the proximal phalanx.

CONDITIONS OF THE PROXIMAL SESAMOID BONES

Sesamoiditis

Clinical Signs

The PSBs are an integral part of the suspensory apparatus and metacarpophalangeal articulation. They are susceptible

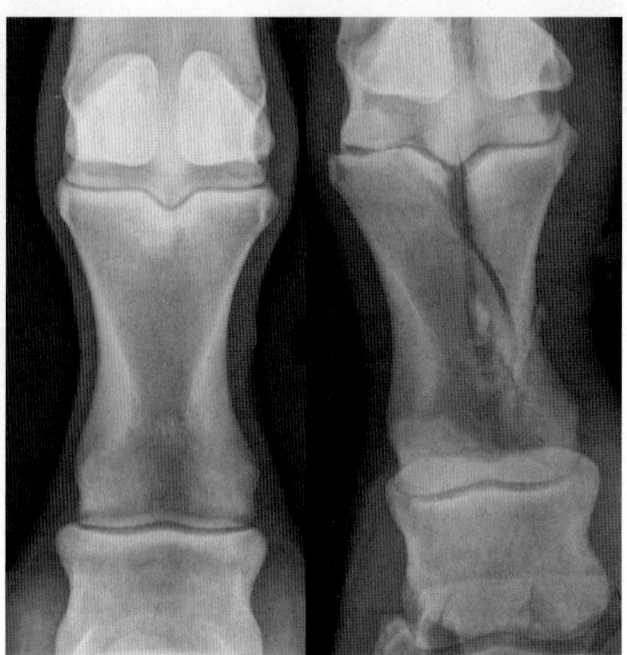

Fig. 36-10 • A subtle sagittal fracture of the proximal phalanx *(left)* that dehisced catastrophically following perineural analgesia *(right)*.

to injury in all athletic horses, but particularly in those that perform at speed. Lameness resulting from sesamoiditis in sports horses is comparatively rare. Sesamoiditis is a clinically distinctive condition, although it is poorly characterized pathologically. There is usually pain with direct, firm palpation over the abaxial aspect of the affected PSB(s) and sometimes pain with fetlock flexion. Often, however, the lameness is manifest only after hard exercise. It is important to recognize that the radiological detection of an increased number and size of vascular channels may be an incidental finding. In a study to determine prevalence of radiological changes in the repository radiographs of 1162 TB yearlings selling in Kentucky, most yearlings (98%) had radiologically apparent vascular channels in the PSBs.[37] Irregular channels (>2 mm wide or with nonparallel sides) were more common (79%) than were regular vascular channels (56%). In a second study, race performance of these yearlings was studied. Yearlings with enthesophyte formation of the PSBs in the hindlimbs placed in a significantly smaller percentage of starts and earned significantly less money per start; however, the presence of abnormal vascular channels did not appear to influence performance.[38] However, the evidence is conflicting. In a study of 487 TB yearlings, those with vascular channels with nonparallel sides and more than 2 mm in width had a reduced number of race starts at 2 years of age and reduced earnings at 2 and 3 years of age compared with normal horses. Contour of the PSBs did not influence performance.[39] In a longitudinal radiological study of 71 2-year-old STBs examined at 3-monthly intervals over 1 year, 22% had no vascular channels and 55% had one or two vascular channels less than 1 mm in width, which did not change and did not influence performance. Three or more vascular channels less than 1 mm wide were seen in 13% of horses at the start of the study; the percentage decreased with time as some horses were removed from training. If lameness was observed, it was attributed to suspensory desmitis or superficial digital flexor tendonitis. Seven horses (10%) had wide abnormally shaped vascular channels, all of which were considered to be associated with lameness during training.[40] In a radiological study of 753 STB trotters in Norway examined between 6 and 21 months of age, the presence of radiological abnormalities did not influence race earnings at 3 and 4 years of age.[41]

Diagnosis

The pain causing lameness is eliminated with perineural, but not intraarticular, analgesia. Radiological evidence of sesamoiditis involves four basic changes: marginal osteophytes, enthesophytes, enlarged vascular channels, and focal radiolucent defects (Figure 36-11). Marginal osteophytes occur at the proximal dorsal and distal dorsal extremities of the PSBs. Best seen on lateromedial images, these lesions represent later changes of generalized OA of the fetlock joint and usually can be considered a poor prognostic sign. Enthesophytes occur along the palmar aspect of the proximal half of the abaxial ridge of the PSB or the distal third of the bone at the sites of origin of the distal sesamoidean ligaments. These changes are frequently abaxial in location and therefore seen best on oblique images. Interpretation of vascular channels in the PSBs is always subjective. The direction of any linear radiolucency is important to note; vascular channels have a radial orientation, whereas hairline fractures usually extend farther and are closer to transverse (parallel to the ground) (Figure 36-12).

True radiolucent changes that are not associated with the normal trabecular pattern or vascular channels may indicate infection (see Chapters 72 and 74). Such lesions may arise after known trauma to the region, especially a penetrating injury. Such lesions are usually extremely painful on palpation. A second important differential diagnosis is an avulsion fracture at the attachment of the palmar annular ligament (see Chapter 74). Radiolucent defects of hindlimb PSBs have also been described as a sequel to routine catheterization of the dorsal metatarsal artery for the measurement of intraoperative arterial blood pressure, with the development of severe lameness within 21 days of surgery.[42] It was speculated that the lesions may be caused by ischemic necrosis or hematogenous spread of bacteria.

Nuclear scintigraphy is exceptionally useful for diagnosis of sesamoiditis and can identify early changes and help confirm whether a chronic radiological change is currently active. A complete series of scintigraphic images, including standing lateral, flexed lateral, and dorsal, can aid in exact localization of a lesion within a particular PSB.

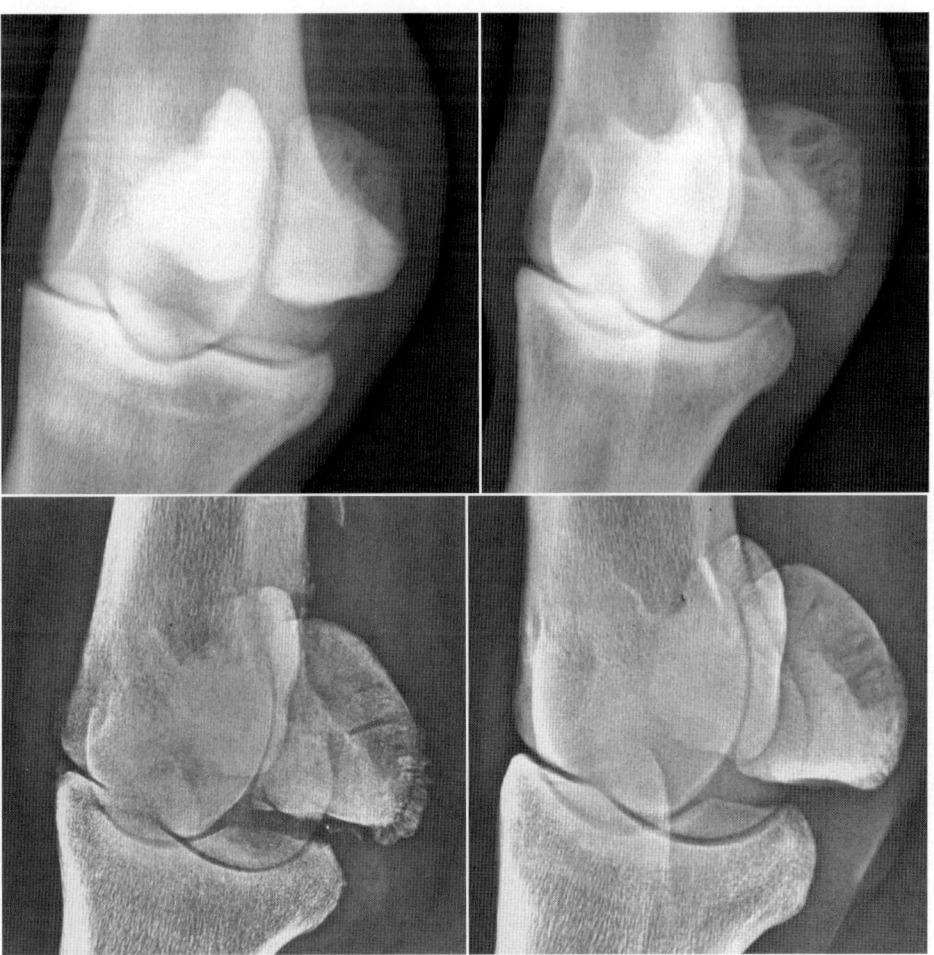

Fig. 36-11 • Sesamoiditis lesions have a range of radiological pathology, including enlarged vascular channels, radiolucency, and enthesophytes.

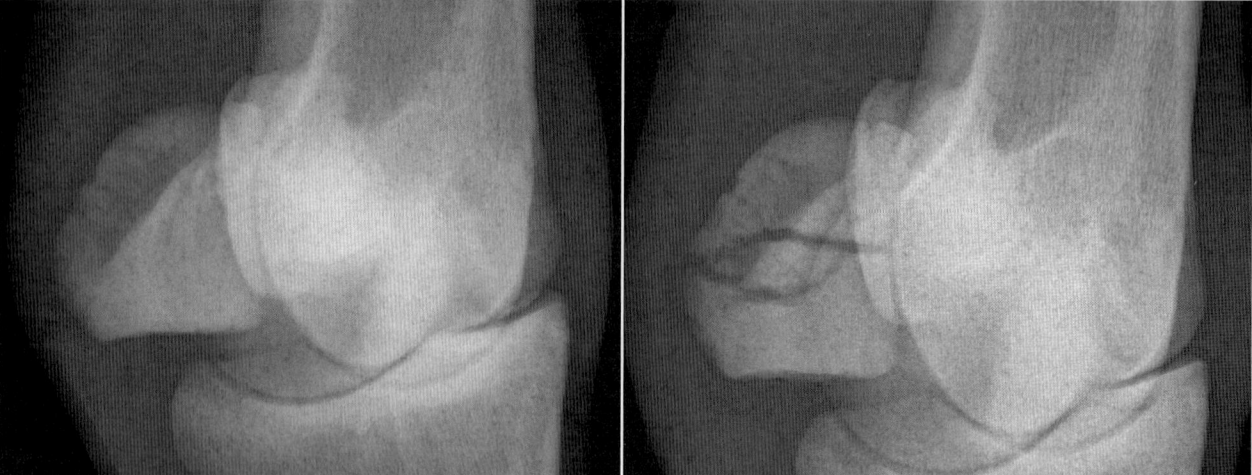

Fig. 36-12 • Very subtle transverse lucencies in a proximal sesamoid bone can be an indication of an incomplete fracture *(left)*. A midbody fracture *(right)* developed in a race a few weeks after the radiograph on the left was obtained.

Treatment

Treatment of horses with sesamoiditis is difficult and usually involves enforced rest and symptomatic treatment to counter inflammation and pain. Many racehorses with sesamoiditis are clinically helped considerably by postexercise icing and altered training regimens, such as swimming. It seems to be easier to manage older, proven racehorses with sesamoiditis by such methods than younger, unraced horses. Aspirin and isoxsuprine have been used, but there is no reliable evidence for efficacy. Shock wave therapy is probably the best current therapeutic option for horses with active sesamoiditis, although its efficacy and mechanisms of action are still debatable. Tiludronate has also been used for sesamoiditis and may have some rationale, but there is no good information about its efficacy.

Proximal Sesamoid Bone Fractures

There is anatomical variation in configuration of PSB fractures, substantially influencing clinical signs and outcome. Biaxial PSB fractures are a potentially catastrophic injury. A recent post mortem study indicated that TB racehorses with severe PSB fractures (75 of 121 fractures were transverse midbody fractures) had a higher exercise intensity in the previous 12 months compared with horses with other musculoskeletal injuries or other causes of death.[43]

Clinical Signs

Because the PSBs are such important elements in the suspensory apparatus and support of the fetlock joint, fractures are usually associated with obvious clinical signs of heat, swelling, and pain with flexion or direct pressure, as well as an obvious weight-bearing lameness.

Diagnosis

Lameness caused by most PSB fractures is eliminated or greatly reduced by intraarticular or perineural analgesia. Apical, midbody, and basilar fractures of the PSBs usually are easy to diagnose radiologically with routine views. Abaxial fractures more frequently are missed and are best demonstrated by a lateral proximal-medial distal or medial proximal-lateral distal oblique image that is tangential to the abaxial surface of the suspect PSB. This projection also is useful in determining whether the fracture is articular. Axial fractures usually are associated with displaced condylar fractures of the McIII or third metatarsal bone (MtIII). Diagnosis requires a well-penetrated dorsopalmar image that is well positioned. Even slight obliquity obscures the fracture line. Midbody fractures frequently have wedge-shaped, comminuted fragments present at the abaxial margins. They should not be confused with the overlapping lines of the palmar and dorsal cortices that occur because of fracture displacement and failure to obtain the radiograph directly through the fracture line.

Ultrasonography can be a valuable adjunct in evaluating PSB fractures because soft tissue attachments of the SL, intersesamoidean ligament, and distal sesamoidean ligaments can be simultaneously injured.

Apical Fractures

Apical fractures comprising less than 30% of the bone occur primarily in racehorses, but they can occur in all types of horses. Forelimb apical PSB fractures are much less common than hindlimb injuries in racing TBs[44,45] and STBs.[46] In sports horses this injury is most common in event horses and show jumpers. These injuries are caused by a combination of bending and suspensory tensile forces. In young STBs the fracture is particularly common in the right hind lateral PSB. Horses with apical PSB fractures are usually mildly to moderately lame unless a concomitant SL injury is present. Although lameness in some horses has been managed successfully with rest alone, arthroscopic removal of the fractured fragment generally is recommended. Both prognosis and convalescent time depend on fragment size and presence of suspensory desmitis. Horses with small, apical fragments without major SL ligament injury can resume training within 4 to 6 weeks after surgery, especially if they were fit at the time of injury. Horses with large fragments usually associated with suspensory branch injury may need 6 to 12 months of convalescence and have a poor prognosis. The prognosis for return to racing was poorer for forelimb injuries than hindlimb injuries in racing TBs. In horses less than 2 years of age, 55% of 11 horses with a forelimb fracture raced after arthroscopic removal of the fragment, whereas 86% of 139 horses with a hindlimb injury raced.[44] In horses 2 years of age or more, 67% of 30 horses with a forelimb fracture returned to racing after surgery compared with 83% of 54 horses with hindlimb injury. In both age categories, fracture of a medial PSB significantly reduced the likelihood of return to racing.[45]

Abaxial Fractures

Abaxial fractures are true avulsion injuries involving the insertion of the SL on the abaxial surface. Most involve a narrow rim of the articular surface and can be removed by an arthroscopic approach. Displaced fragments should be removed, whereas extremely large fragments can be repaired with 3.5-mm screws. Horses with nondisplaced fragments sometimes can be treated with rest. The prognosis depends on the size of the fragment and the concomitant suspensory compromise. In a study of 47 horses, predominantly TB and Quarter Horse racehorses and Western performance horses with an abaxial sesamoid fracture, 38 had a forelimb fracture, usually of the medial PSB. Nonracehorses had a better prognosis for return to full athletic function (6/6, 100%) after arthroscopic removal of the fracture compared with racehorses (25/35, 71%), with only 16 of 35 (46%) racing at the same class as preinjury.[47]

Basilar Fractures

Basilar fractures of the PSBs are seen in all athletic horses and are treated according to configuration.[48,49] Horses with smaller, wedge-shaped fragments that do not extend more than 50% to 75% of the dorsopalmar width of the PSB are clear candidates for surgical excision of the fragment (Figure 36-13). Such fragments do not heal with rest and

cause persistent lameness, presumably because of instability and incongruity at the articular surface. The prognosis with arthroscopic technique is at least 50% for return to athletic function because the distal sesamoidean ligaments are not disrupted. Horses are usually given 4 to 6 months of rest after removal of such fragments (3 months with very small pieces). Nonarticular fractures can be removed via an incision in the straight sesamoidean ligament, and 9 of 10 horses from a variety of disciplines returned to their intended use.[50]

Horses with larger, basilar PSB fractures that extend to the palmar aspect of the bone have the poorest prognosis because fractures often are substantially displaced and involve a greater proportion of distal sesamoidean ligament origin (Figure 36-14). They also are more difficult to repair than midbody fractures because of the size and shape of the fracture. The prognosis for horses with large, displaced, or comminuted basilar PSB fractures is poor for return to any reasonable level of athletic activity.

Some horses with severe OA develop small basilar fractures. These fractures typically are more rounded, irregular, or multiply fragmented than acute chip fractures (Figure 36-15). Acute chip fractures have a sharply demarcated triangular shape. Horses with these degenerate basilar fractures are very poor candidates for any surgical treatment, and horses have a grave prognosis for return to athletic activity. Radiologically evident narrowing of the joint space between the PSB and the McIII (Figure 36-16) and the development of a radiological "waist" in the distal aspect of the McIII are associated signs of severe OA (Figure 36-17).

Midbody PSB Fractures

Midbody fractures of the PSB can occur in any horse, but they usually are seen in racehorses. In North American TBs, the medial PSBs of the forelimb are most commonly affected. In the STB, hind lateral midbody PSB fractures are

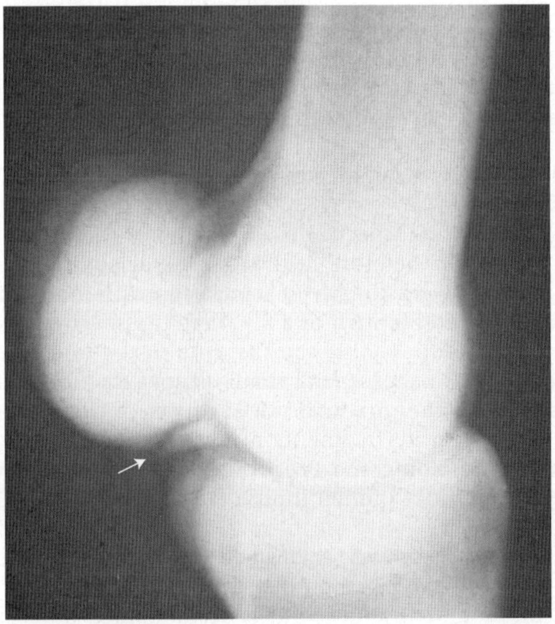

Fig. 36-13 • Lateromedial radiographic image of a metacarpophalangeal joint. There is a basilar sesamoid fracture *(arrow)*. Small, triangular, basilar sesamoid fragments that do not involve the major distal sesamoidean ligaments are appropriate candidates for arthroscopic removal.

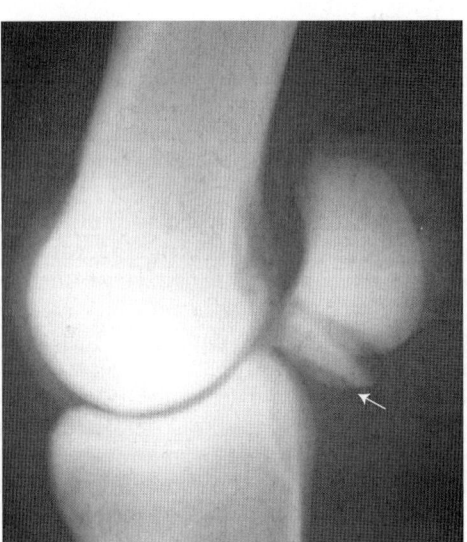

Fig. 36-14 • Flexed lateromedial radiographic image of a metacarpophalangeal joint. There is a large displaced basilar sesamoid fracture *(arrow)*. Large basilar fractures are very difficult to successfully repair. There are extensive attachments of the distal sesamoidean ligaments; therefore the prognosis associated with surgical removal is poor.

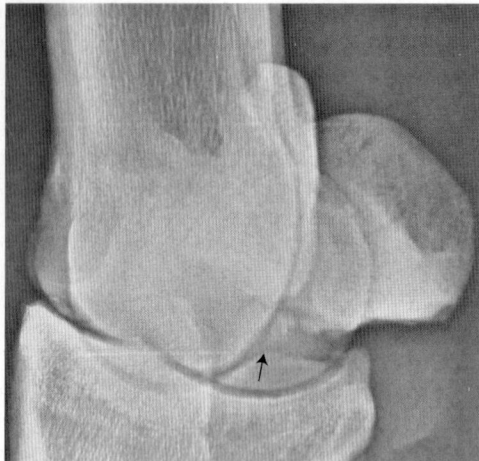

Fig. 36-15 • Dorsomedial-palmarolateral oblique radiographic image of a metacarpophalangeal joint. There are fragments distal to the proximal sesamoid bone (arrow). Irregular, "crumbled" fragments from the base of the proximal sesamoid bone usually are seen in joints with moderate to severe osteoarthritis. Note also the modeling of the articular margins of the proximal phalanx.

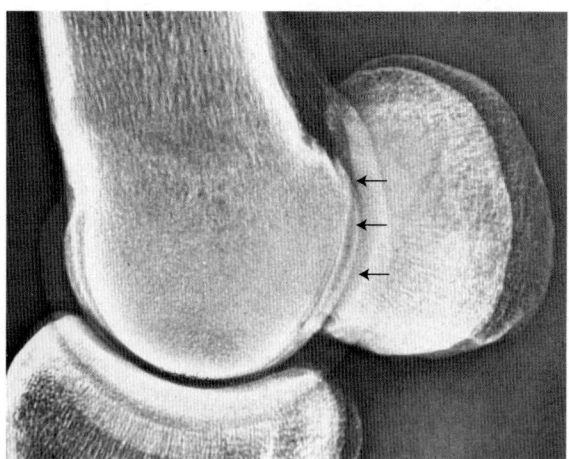

Fig. 36-16 • Lateromedial radiographic image of a metacarpophalangeal joint. Note the loss of space between the proximal sesamoid bones (PSBs) and the third metacarpal bone (McIII) (arrows). Near-complete loss of joint space between the McIII and the PSBs can precede that between the distal aspect of the McIII and the proximal phalanx. Horses with this degree of cartilage damage are often candidates for euthanasia or arthrodesis.

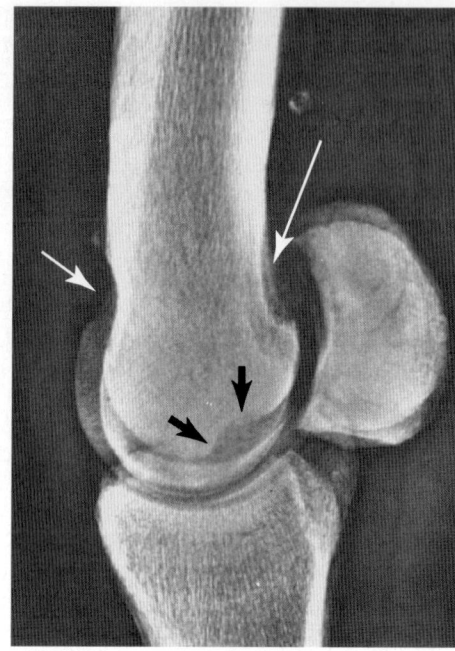

Fig. 36-17 • Slightly oblique flexed lateromedial radiographic image of a metacarpophalangeal joint. Development of a "waist" around the proximal joint margin on the third metacarpal bone, both dorsally and palmarly (white arrows), is indicative of severe, chronic osteoarthritis. There is a pronounced defect of the distal palmar aspect of the third metacarpal bone (black arrows).

most common. Numerous surgical techniques have been used to repair such fractures, including cast coaptation alone, bone grafting and casting, lag screws (distal to proximal or proximal to distal) with or without cancellous grafting, and hemicerclage wiring and graft.[51,52] Regardless of the technique used, midbody PSB fractures are serious injuries, and horses require an extended period of rest after surgery. With surgery, 60% to 70% of horses with midbody fractures can return to athletic function, but most horses drop substantially in class. The owner or trainer should be advised that almost a year of convalescence is required for horses with such injuries.

Axial PSB Fractures

Axial PSB fractures are nearly always seen in combination with displaced lateral condylar fractures of the McIII or MtIII (Figure 36-18). They are recognized radiologically only on a dorsopalmar image, and it is difficult to determine fracture depth. Some fractures involve deep gouges in the articular surface, and most are avulsions by the intersesamoidean ligament. They usually are not treated specifically because of inaccessibility and the likelihood that the condylar fracture and overall joint damage will limit return to function. Recognition of an axial PSB fracture is important primarily as an indicator of more severe trauma to the joint and a poorer prognosis. The prognosis for a horse returning to race after this injury is extremely poor.[53] Early metacarpophalangeal arthrodesis should be seriously considered in horses with a displaced axial sesamoid fracture.

Intraarticular Fragmentation Associated with Suspensory Branch Injury

The distal dorsal aspect of the branches of the SL are subsynovial and therefore intimately associated with the fetlock joint. Occasionally in association with injury of the medial or lateral branch of a SL, there is associated distention of the fetlock joint capsule; in a flexed lateromedial radiographic image, several small osseous fractures can be identified on the proximal dorsal aspect of the ipsilateral PSB. Such fracture fragments must be surgically removed for a successful outcome. Prognosis depends on the severity of the suspensory branch injury.

Intersesamoidean Ligament Injury

Intersesamoidean ligamentous injury without fracture is difficult to diagnose unless it is accompanied by radiolucency along the axial aspect of one or both PSBs (Figure 36-19). Affected horses often are extremely lame even at a walk. Scintigraphy frequently identifies an area of intense, focal IRU. The intersesamoidean ligament also can be

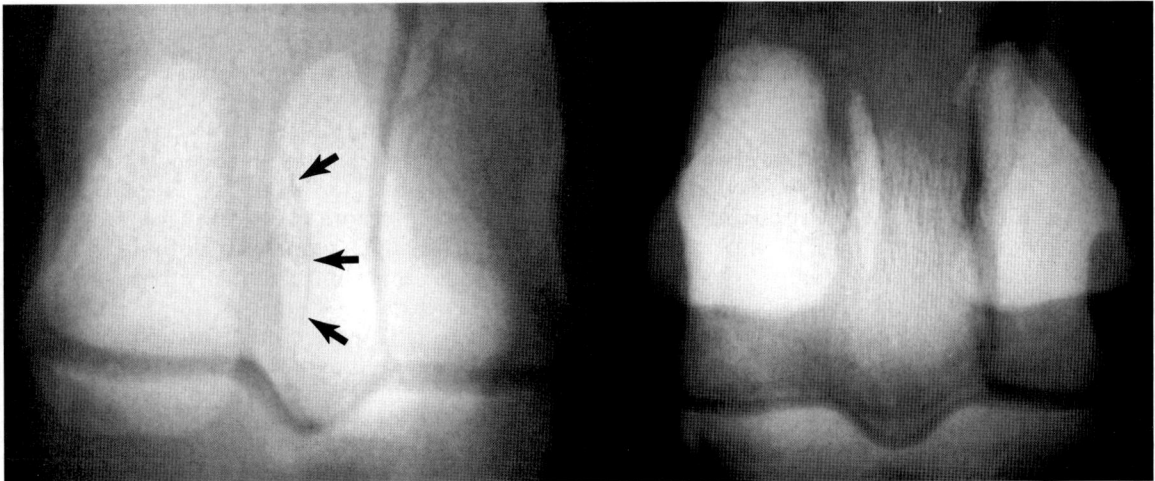

Fig. 36-18 • Displaced lateral condylar fracture of the third metacarpal bone with a nondisplaced axial fracture *(arrows)* of the lateral PSB *(left)*. In horses with very badly displaced lateral condylar fractures, the axial fragment of the PSB can become completely avulsed *(right)*. Clinicians should look for axial PSB fractures in every horse with a displaced lateral condylar fracture. This type of fracture is associated with a very poor prognosis for return to racing.

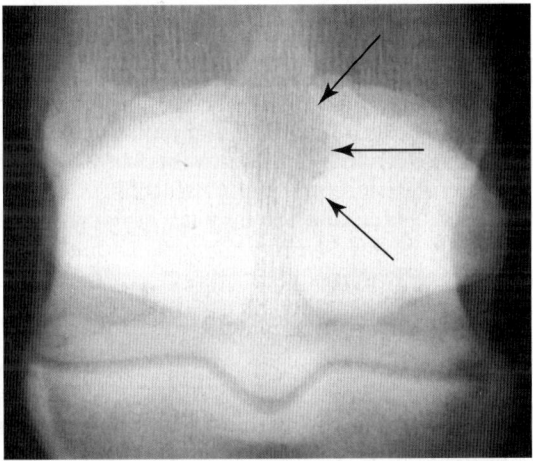

Fig. 36-19 • A good-quality dorsopalmar radiographic image is necessary to diagnose a radiolucent defect involving the axial margin of the proximal sesamoid bone *(arrows)*.

evaluated ultrasonographically to a limited extent. The ligamentous lesion may be visible and debrided arthroscopically, but it is not known if this alters the outcome. Horses generally are treated with support bandages and stall rest for several months. The prognosis for return to high-level athletic activity appears to be guarded, especially with conservative management, but a large series of horses has not been reviewed. Lameness resolved in eight horses treated by surgical debridement.[55] Differential diagnosis for radiolucent lesions in the intersesamoidean region also includes osteomyelitis.[37] If an infection is the cause of the bone loss, horses typically have more obvious localizing signs, such as joint capsule and digital flexor tendon sheath distention, and the prognosis is poor.

PSB Fractures in Young Foals

PSB fractures in young foals (apical, abaxial, midbody, and basilar) can occur at pasture and appear to be underdiagnosed because clinical signs are surprisingly subtle and foals often are not thoroughly examined for mild lameness. Because most fractures involve only one PSB and the suspensory apparatus is still functional, severe lameness does not develop. Clinicians should look for subtle clinical signs of fetlock region swelling, pain with flexion, and pain with pressure over the PSBs in any foal with mild to moderate lameness. Several bones can be affected. Signs often abate quickly, especially in young foals (<2 months of age), in which these fractures are most common. Good-quality radiographs are essential because the fractured apical, basilar, or abaxial fragments are often poorly mineralized. Unlike in older horses, PSB fractures in foals frequently progress to form a bony union (see Figures 128-6 and 128-7). If the fragments have any displacement, however, an enlarged PSB can result. These oversized PSBs often are diagnosed in yearlings or 2-year-olds on prepurchase or presale radiographs. Surprisingly, enlargement of the fetlock joint is usually difficult to detect. Although some horses have raced successfully with enlarged PSBs, this abnormality can be a source of lameness as the horse proceeds in training.

PSB fractures in foals are essentially a management problem. Avoidance of situations in which a young, weak foal has to chase its dam around a large pasture to the point of exhaustion can prevent many fractures. It is essential to slowly return foals back to pasture if they have been stall confined for any reason. Early recognition of lameness in foals can allow diagnosis before the fragments become markedly displaced. Early diagnosis improves prognosis considerably because minimally displaced fractures nearly always heal completely with rest alone. Uncontrolled exercise by the foal must be avoided because the degree of displacement dictates the eventual PSB deformity. Surgical treatment of foal PSB fractures is primarily indicated in markedly displaced fractures close to the midbody of the bone. A suturing technique with high-tensile–strength flexible fiber is probably the best current option.

FRACTURES OF THE THIRD METACARPAL BONE

Condylar Fractures

Clinical Signs

The most important fracture of the fetlock joint is that involving the condyles of the McIII. They occur almost exclusively in racehorses and elite endurance horses, usually only when horses are running at racing speeds. This is also an occasional injury in event horses. Because the fractures involve a major weight-bearing surface, most horses are overtly lame, with clear localizing signs of pain and swelling. Most are very positive to any manipulation of the fetlock. Degree of lameness often does not directly correlate with the degree of displacement. Many horses with incomplete, acute fractures are lamer than one with a clearly displaced, complete fracture. This is particularly true with incomplete medial fractures. Although it appears that many horses that develop condylar fractures have preexisting subchondral damage of the distal palmar aspect of the condyle,[27,56] the majority do not have a strong history of previous fetlock lameness (see Chapter 42 for fractures of the MtIII).

Diagnosis

Radiological diagnosis is not difficult in most horses. A dorsopalmar image should be centered over the condyle and the x-ray beam directed 15 to 20 degrees downward. If the beam is too horizontal, the PSBs may obscure the distal articular surface of the McIII. Lesions may be missed if images are underexposed. The most common fractures involve the lateral condyle and clearly propagate toward the lateral cortex. Some extend only 1 to 2 cm proximally from the joint surface, and these can be particularly difficult to see without good-quality radiographs. Lateral condylar fractures rarely spiral or extend into the middiaphysis. Medial condylar fractures, however, usually extend up the diaphysis in a spiraling fashion or have an occult Y-shaped configuration at the middiaphysis. *It is essential to remember the difference between lateral and medial fractures.* Horses with

medial condylar fractures *must* have a complete, high-quality set of radiographs that encompass the entire length of the McIII in an attempt to identify fracture configuration. Most importantly, the owner or trainer must be informed immediately of the substantial risk associated with medial fractures, especially those involving a hindlimb.

The prognosis for horses with displaced, lateral condylar fractures, regardless of treatment, is much poorer for return to function compared with those with nondisplaced fractures. This is almost certainly the result of a combination of preexisting disease of the fetlock joint and the magnitude of damage done to the joint when the fracture occurs. Accurate prognosis requires radiographic examination of the palmar distal aspect of the McIII. The radiographer should slightly flex the fetlock and use a horizontal beam to obtain a dorsopalmar image (Figure 36-20). This helps to define comminution of the condyle along the fracture margin, as well as subchondral radiolucent defects that may have preceded the fracture.

Most horses with condylar fractures are best treated with lag screws. Nondisplaced or minimally displaced fractures can be repaired through stab incisions alone, but arthroscopic evaluation of the joint should allow a more accurate assessment of the prognosis. Displaced fractures require accurate reduction of the distal articular surface, so they must be reduced under arthroscopic guidance or through an open incision. Horses with medial condylar fractures should undergo surgery with extreme caution because catastrophic failure in the middiaphysis can occur during recovery from general anesthesia or even several days to weeks after repair (see Chapter 42). Horses with spiral fractures extending the length of the diaphysis may be successfully repaired with carefully positioned lag screws alone, but those with medial fractures that disappear in the middiaphysis should be repaired with a bone plate combined with lag screws across the condyle. Most complications of condylar fractures occur because of a failure to recognize potential problems before surgery. Even if certain complications cannot be entirely avoided, forewarning the owner of the risks is advisable.

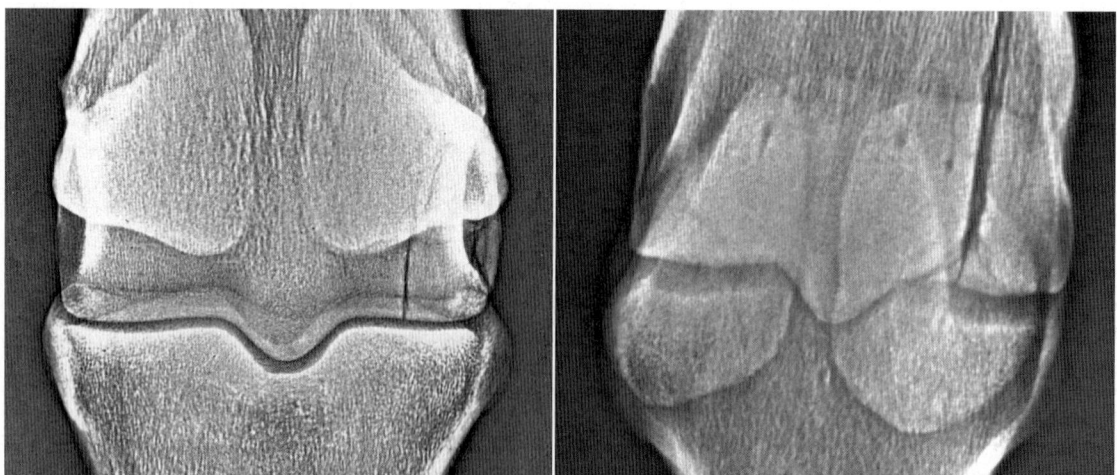

Fig. 36-20 • A standard dorsopalmar image of a lateral condylar fracture obtained at a 10- to 15-degree proximal to distal obliquity will separate the distal aspect of the third metacarpal bone from the base of the proximal sesamoid bones *(left)*, but a dorsopalmar image obtained with the fetlock slightly flexed is needed to silhouette the distal palmar margin of the bone where comminution typically occurs *(right)*.

Other fractures of the distal third of the McIII bone are discussed in Chapter 37.

OSTEOCHONDROSIS

Sagittal Ridge of the Third Metacarpal Bone

The most common site of osteochondrosis in the metacarpophalangeal joint (excluding proximal palmar lesions) is the dorsal sagittal ridge of the McIII/MtIII (Figure 36-21).[57] These lesions often are clinically silent, but mild to moderate effusion and lameness may be noted. They are often diagnosed in weanlings or on yearling presale radiographs. They are best seen on a dorsopalmar image or a slightly underexposed flexed lateromedial image. If no fragment is obvious and clinical signs are minimal, it is advisable to rest the horse for a couple of months because some healing may occur, especially in younger horses. Arthroscopic debridement is an option, but the resulting bony defect will remain evident, and thus the likelihood of a rewarding sale price is lessened. If the lesion does not fill in radiologically by the spring of its yearling year, arthroscopic evaluation may be suggested. A completely conservative (i.e., nonsurgical) approach is justified if the clinical signs are minimal. The prognosis likely depends on the size of the lesion. Horses with lesions more proximal on the sagittal ridge may have a better prognosis than those closer to its distal aspect.

In older horses, traumatic chip fractures may occur on the distal aspect of the sagittal ridge in a similar location to that of typical osteochondrosis (Figure 36-22). This injury may occur in jumpers striking an obstacle with the fetlock joint in a palmarly flexed position. These fragments usually are unstable and should be arthroscopically removed. The prognosis is favorable if the fragment is fairly small.

Osseous Cystlike Lesions of the Third Metacarpal Bone

Osseous cystlike lesions of the distal aspect of the McIII/MtIII occur on the weight-bearing surface of the condyle and may be a manifestation of osteochondrosis. Most

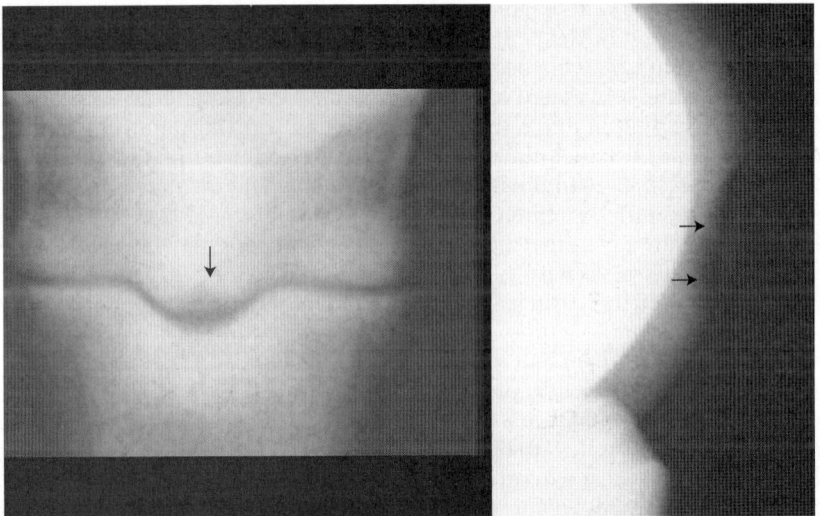

Fig. 36-21 • Dorsopalmar *(left)* and flexed lateromedial *(right)* images of a metacarpophalangeal joint. Note the radiolucent defect *(arrow)* in the sagittal image in the dorsopalmar image and the smoothly outlined defect in the dorsal aspect of the sagittal ridge *(arrows)* of the third metacarpal bone in the lateromedial image.

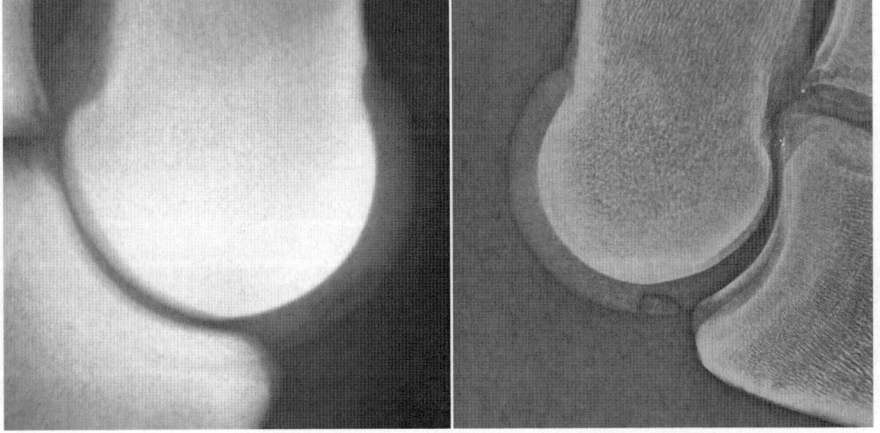

Fig. 36-22 • In adult horses some fragments involving the dorsal sagittal ridge of the third metacarpal bone are caused by direct trauma. Both of these horses struck fixed objects with the affected fetlock in flexion.

occur in the medial condyle and are diagnosed in yearlings or early in training as a 2-year-old. The lesions are easy to recognize radiologically, and horses have obvious lameness exacerbated by lower limb flexion. Perineural analgesia and scintigraphy also localize the problem. Surgical debridement has been the typical treatment, and the reported results are unexpectedly favorable.[58]

COLLATERAL LIGAMENT INJURY

The fetlock joint has strong anatomical constraints, and the equine limb and gait have a strongly sagittal orientation; therefore mediolateral instability is relatively uncommon except after severe trauma (e.g., foot in a hole or lower limb in a gate or fence). Mild forms of collateral desmitis are suspected in horses with pain on fetlock manipulation, focal pain, and swelling over the affected ligament or lameness exacerbated with valgus or varus stress. The diagnosis is confirmed by ultrasonographic examination. However, localizing clinical signs may be absent, and if a horse has pain causing lameness localized to the fetlock region by perineural analgesia and little response to intraarticular analgesia, then the collateral ligaments should be included in a routine ultrasonographic assessment of the periarticular structures. It must be borne in mind that the deep and superficial components of each collateral ligament cannot be evaluated simultaneously because of their different fiber orientations. Radiographs usually are not helpful unless there is an avulsion fracture or lack of congruency of the joint surfaces. However, radiographic examination is important if there is joint laxity because there may be concurrent intraarticular fragments. Joint instability is most likely to be demonstrated on non–weight-bearing, valgus or varus stressed dorsopalmar (plantar) radiographs.

Treatment of horses with collateral ligament injury usually consists of rest and adequate external coaptation. The fetlock is an inherently stable joint in the sagittal plane; thus minimal support is necessary unless the injury is severe. If the joint is very unstable, a cast extending to the proximal metacarpal region is maintained for 4 to 6 weeks. If the injury is not overtly unstable, a single polyvinyl chloride pipe splint applied on the side ipsilateral to the collateral injury should be adequate. The duration of rest should be based on clinical soundness, palpable stability, and the ultrasonographic appearance of the ligamentous tissues (see Chapter 17). Shock wave therapy for insertional desmopathies may be beneficial, but firm data are still unavailable. Stem cells, acellular matrices, and platelet-rich plasma are also empirically used. Eight of 16 horses with rupture of a collateral ligament of the metacarpophalangeal or metatarsophalangeal joint returned to pleasure riding after casting for a mean of 71 days.[59]

Collateral ligament avulsion injuries involving the insertion on the proximal phalanx are perhaps the most commonly recognized fetlock collateral ligament injury. These may easily be mistaken for the more common dorsal chip fractures on oblique views, but careful scrutiny reveals that the fragment is too far abaxial for a typical chip fracture (Figure 36-23). If a fracture is seen abaxial to the apex of the dorsal eminences of the proximal phalanx, the fragment is almost certainly not going to be from the typical articular margin location. In addition, the fracture can also usually be seen in an abaxial position on a dorsopalmar (dorsoplantar) image. These fragments often involve a portion of the articular margin and cause lameness. Arthroscopic removal should be performed, but it can be difficult because of the limited space on the medial or lateral aspects. The arthroscope portal should be dorsoproximal on the same side as the lesion. The instrument portal should be just dorsal to the edge of the collateral ligament. The fragments may be tightly attached along the abaxial margin, and an arthroscopic scalpel or other sharp dissection tool may be needed to separate them. The most important issue with these fragments is that the clinician accurately discriminates between them and a more typical articular margin fracture; otherwise, the surgical procedure may be very frustrating.

TRAUMATIC DISRUPTION OF THE SUSPENSORY APPARATUS

See Chapter 104 for a discussion of traumatic disruption of the suspensory apparatus and associated catastrophic injuries.

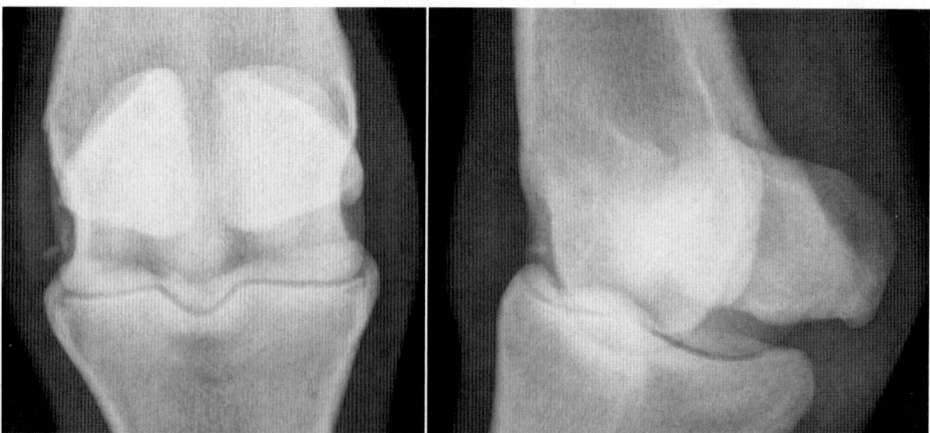

Fig. 36-23 • Collateral ligament avulsions from the proximal phalanx are usually visible on the dorsopalmar *(left)* and the oblique *(right)* radiographic images. On the oblique image, these fragments appear a long way from the third metacarpal bone and that distinguishes them from a typical dorsal proximal phalanx chip fracture.

The Metacarpal Region

Sue J. Dyson

ANATOMY

This chapter discusses the examination and diagnosis of injuries to the metacarpal region of the horse. The detailed anatomy of the deep digital flexor tendon (DDFT) (see Chapter 70), the accessory ligament of the deep digital flexor tendon (ALDDFT) (see Chapter 71), the superficial digital flexor tendon (SDFT) (see Chapter 69), and the third interosseous muscle or suspensory ligament (SL) (see Chapter 72) is discussed elsewhere.

In the metacarpal region the interosseous ligaments attach the second (McII) and fourth (McIV) metacarpal bones to the third metacarpal bone (McIII). These ligaments ossify to a variable extent during skeletal maturation. Fibrous bands extend from the distal aspect of the McII and McIV to the medial and lateral proximal sesamoid bones (PSBs).

The proximal aspect of the third interosseous muscle or SL attaches to the proximal palmar aspect of the McIII and the palmar carpal ligament and lies between the McII and McIV. Large exostoses on the axial aspect of the McII or the McIV have the potential to impinge on the abaxial border of the SL. The carpal sheath (see Chapter 75) extends through the proximal third of the metacarpal region. The amount of fluid in the carpal sheath varies between horses but is usually bilaterally symmetrical.

The digital flexor tendon sheath (DFTS) envelops the SDFT and DDFT from the distal third of the metacarpal region to the middle of the middle phalanx. Palmar to the metacarpophalangeal joint, the sheath passes through the inelastic canal created by the palmar annular ligament (PAL), the palmar fibrocartilaginous surfaces of the PSBs, and the intersesamoidean ligament. Within the DFTS, proximal to the sesamoidean canal, the SDFT forms a ring (the manica flexoria) around the DDFT. In the palmar mid-sagittal plane, a synovial reflection, the vincula, attaches the SDFT to the DFTS wall. Proximal to the manica flexoria, the DDFT is attached medially and laterally by mesotendon to the DFTS wall. The lateral mesotendon is more substantial and extends farther distally.

The palmar and palmar metacarpal nerves innervate the palmar metacarpal region. The SL is innervated by the medial and lateral palmar metacarpal nerves, branches of the deep branch of the lateral palmar nerve. This nerve receives contributions from the ulnar and median nerves. The medial palmar metacarpal nerve has fibers only from the median nerve, whereas the lateral palmar metacarpal nerve has fibers from the ulnar and median nerves.[1] The SDFT and DDFT are innervated by the palmar nerves.[2]

In the proximal metacarpal region, the palmar nerves lie beneath relatively thick fascia, whereas farther distally they are more superficial. In the proximal 5 cm of the metacarpal region, the palmar metacarpal nerves and the distal palmar outpouching of the carpometacarpal joint capsule are in close proximity.

DIAGNOSIS
Clinical Examination
The metacarpal region should be examined visually from all angles to identify any changes in contour caused by swelling. If the limb is hairy, subtle swellings may easily be missed, especially in heavier breeds of horses, and if injury to the metacarpal region is suspected, then clipping the hair to facilitate examination can be useful. Palpation of the metacarpal region should be performed systematically with the limb bearing weight and with the limb semiflexed. With the limb bearing weight, the contour of the dorsal and palmar aspects of the limb should be straight. Distention of the medial palmar vein may reflect local inflammation. The size of the SL and its branches is assessed by running both thumbs down the dorsal and palmar borders from proximally to distally, medially, and laterally; they should remain equidistant. With the limb lifted, the margins of each of the SDFT, DDFT, ALDDFT, and SL should be carefully palpated to detect rounding of the margins, enlargement, or change in texture. Each structure should be squeezed, starting proximally and working distally, gently at first and then with increasing pressure to determine whether pain can be elicited. Careful comparison should be made with the contralateral limb, bearing in mind that lesions may be present bilaterally. Assess the response in light of the horse's temperament and the recent work history. Abnormal stiffness of a structure may reflect previous injury. It is necessary to roll away the digital flexor tendons and compress the SL against the palmar aspect of the McIII to assess the most proximal part of the SL.

The axial and palmar margins of the McII and McIV should be palpated to identify any new bone formation (a splint) and to determine whether applied pressure causes pain. It is also important to assess whether the axial margin of the splint is clearly demarcated from the SL. Firm pressure should be applied to the dorsal aspects of the McIII to identify pain.

Local Analgesic Techniques
When local analgesic techniques are performed in the metacarpal region, it is important to recognize the potential for local anesthetic solution to diffuse proximally from the site of injection and thereby desensitize structures farther proximally, partially, or completely. Minimum volumes of local anesthetic solution should be used (maximum 2 mL/site and less in ponies) to minimize the risks of misinterpretation. The horse should stand still after injection before reassessment of the gait and should be reevaluated no more than 10 minutes after injection. Even then, false-positive results may be seen.

The metacarpal region seems particularly prone to development of swelling at the site of injection, which potentially may be permanent. The limb should be thoroughly scrubbed with chlorhexidine before injection to minimize the risk of adverse reaction and because of the potential for inadvertent injection into a synovial cavity (the DFTS, carpal sheath, or carpometacarpal joint capsule). The use of nonirritating local anesthetic solution (mepivacaine) is strongly recommended. It is also suggested that a stable bandage be applied to the limb for about 18 hours after injection.

Perineural analgesia of the palmar nerves at the level of the base of the PSBs desensitizes the foot and pastern regions, but in some horses it may also alleviate pain from the metacarpophalangeal joint, the proximal phalanx, PAL, SL branches, and DFTS. In horses with pain arising from the metacarpal region, lameness often appears paradoxically worse after palmar (abaxial sesamoid) nerve blocks, especially with proximal suspensory desmitis. Complete desensitization of the distal third of the metacarpal region requires perineural analgesia of the palmar nerves at the junction of the proximal two thirds and distal one third of the metacarpal region and the palmar metacarpal nerves distal to the distal aspect of the McII and McIV, the so-called low palmar or four-point block. Care should be taken to avoid inadvertent injection into the DFTS, which can occur when performing the palmar block despite no synovial fluid appearing in the needle hub. Proximal diffusion may result in partial alleviation of pain from the body of the SL in association with ultrasonographic evidence of proximal suspensory desmitis. If a unilateral lesion is suspected, the block may be performed medially or laterally alone.

Desensitization of one specific PSB can be achieved by blocking the sesamoidean nerve by introducing a needle between the insertion of the SL and the dorsal aspect of the abaxial surface of the sesamoid bone. The needle is directed toward the apex of the bone, and 0.5 mL of local anesthetic solution is injected.[3]

Elimination of pain from the entire metacarpal region requires blocking the palmar nerves immediately distal to the carpus and the deep branch of the ulnar nerve (and thus the palmar metacarpal nerves). However, often it is useful to be more specific and desensitize the deep structures (the palmar aspect of the McIII and the SL) or the more superficial structures (SDFT, DDFT, and ALDDFT). Perineural analgesia of the deep branch of the lateral palmar nerve or of the palmar metacarpal nerves by subcarpal injection should theoretically not abolish pain from the fetlock or more distal aspect of the limb, but this does sometimes occur. It is therefore important to perform the low 4-point block first. Blocking the palmar metacarpal nerves immediately distal to the carpus runs the risk of inadvertent injection into the distopalmar outpouchings of the carpometacarpal joint or spread of the local anesthetic solution by diffusion. Theoretically the risk of failure to desensitize the most proximal aspect of the SL exists, but diffusion of local anesthetic solution usually removes pain; false-negative results sometimes occur. The response should be compared with that following intraarticular analgesia of the middle carpal joint. Occasionally subcarpal analgesia of the palmar metacarpal nerves relieves pain associated with a primary middle carpal joint lesion better than intraarticular analgesia. Intraarticular analgesia of the middle carpal joint may relieve pain associated with proximal suspensory desmitis or a palmar cortical fatigue fracture of the McIII.

Perineural analgesia of the lateral palmar nerve from the lateral[4] or medial[5] approach entails less risk of affecting the middle carpal joint, but it does not eliminate it totally. The potential to remove pain from the lateral aspect of the more distal part of the limb also exists. From the lateral approach there is also a substantial risk of desensitization of the carpal sheath. This block can be particularly useful in a difficult horse, which is easier to inject with the limb bearing weight rather than semiflexed.

Theoretically, blocking the ulnar nerve should not completely remove pain associated with the proximal aspect of the SL or the proximal palmar aspect of the McIII because of the contribution of fibers from the median nerve to the medial and lateral palmar metacarpal nerves. However, in practice it generally does. The ulnar nerve block can be particularly useful to differentiate proximal metacarpal region pain from carpal pain in horses with an equivocal response to subcarpal analgesia; however, occasionally carpal pain is reduced.

Perineural analgesia of the palmar nerves (2 mL/site) should not desensitize the deeper structures (the McIII, SL) but should alleviate pain from the more superficial structures (SDFT, DDFT, and ALDDFT). Local infiltration around a painful exostosis of the McII or the McIV seems to be the most effective way of determining whether pain from the exostosis is contributing to the lameness observed. However, occasionally perineural analgesia proximal to the painful splint exostosis is necessary to abolish pain.

Intrathecal analgesia of the DFTS usually results in improvement in lameness associated with pain from within the sheath, but a better response is frequently seen after perineural analgesia of the palmar and palmar metacarpal nerves. Injection into the DFTS is most easily performed on the palmar midline of the pastern region, distal to the proximal digital annular ligament. The likelihood of inducing iatrogenic hemorrhage at this site is small, and retrieval of synovial fluid usually is easier than from the DFTS proximal to the PAL. If distention of the DFTS is only mild, compression of the proximal part of the sheath by an assistant to increase distention in the palmar pouch in the pastern can be helpful. Injection into the carpal sheath is usually only indicated if the sheath is distended (see Chapter 75).

IMAGING

Radiography and Radiology

Radiographic examination of the metacarpal region is usually tailored to each particular horse concerning the images required and the exposure factors used. With localized periosteal new bone, often finely coned-down images and use of soft exposures (low kilovolts [peak]) are required to demonstrate the lesion best. Several similar images varying slightly in obliquity may be required rather than a full series of dorsopalmar, lateromedial, dorsolateral-palmaromedial oblique, and palmarolateral-dorsomedial oblique images. Therefore a flexible approach must be used, depending on the initial clinical signs. Little soft tissue covers the metacarpal region; therefore a grid is not required. A high-definition screen with slow-speed film provides the best detail, although this may not be necessary with digital or computed radiography. Diffuse swelling in the metacarpal region makes images appear flatter, lacking contrast. Exposure factors may need to be increased slightly.

Superimposition of the McII and McIV over the McIII can create confusing radiolucent Mach lines (see page 174). The nutrient canal in the McII and McIV varies in prominence[6] and should not be confused as a fracture. Ossification varies between the McII and McIV and the McIII in normal horses.

Ultrasonography

Ultrasonographic examination of the metacarpal region is discussed in detail elsewhere (see Chapters 16 and 69 to 72). In large, cob-type horses, the skin and underlying subcutaneous tissues in the metacarpal region may be thick, making it difficult to obtain high-resolution images. Dense stubble may persist after fine clipping of the hair coat, making it difficult to maintain good contact. Deep skin folds may further complicate the issue. For these horses it may be necessary to amplify the power and gain controls of the ultrasound machine and increase the focal depth of the transducer. Image quality may be enhanced by application of copious amounts of the ultrasound coupling gel to the skin for at least 15 minutes before imaging.

Nuclear Scintigraphy

Blood pool (soft tissue phase) and bone phase (delayed) images of the metacarpal region are particularly useful in horses in which pain has been localized to the metacarpal region but in which no clinically significant radiological or ultrasonographic abnormalities have been identified. Many exostoses involving the McII and the McIV, although clinically inactive, are associated with moderately increased radiopharmaceutical uptake (IRU). Clinically silent enostosis-like lesions also may have IRU.

Magnetic Resonance Imaging

Both high-field[7-9] and low-field[10] magnetic resonance imaging (MRI) have the potential to identify both osseous and soft tissue injuries that are not detectable using conventional imaging modalities.

DIFFERENTIAL DIAGNOSIS

Bucked or Sore Shins and Saucer (Dorsal Cortical) Fractures of the Third Metacarpal Bone

See Chapter 102 for a discussion of bucked shins and dorsal cortical (saucer) fractures of the McIII.

Medial and Lateral Condylar Fractures of the Third Metacarpal Bone

See Chapter 36 for a discussion of medial and lateral condylar fractures of the McIII (see page 408).

Incomplete, Longitudinal Palmar Cortical Fatigue Fractures of the Third Metacarpal Bone and Stress Reactions

Incomplete palmar cortical fatigue fractures of the McIII are relatively common and almost invariably involve the medial aspect of the bone,[11-14] may involve the metaphyseal and proximal diaphyseal region, and sometimes extend proximally to involve the carpometacarpal joint. They are believed to be fatigue or stress fractures because increased

radiopacity may be present radiologically when lameness is first recognized, indicating previous bony reaction.

These fractures occur most commonly in young horses, but they also occur in skeletally mature horses. In some horses, a recent increase in work intensity can be identified, which may be a predisposing factor. These fractures have been identified in a variety of racehorses sports horses, including horses used for flat and harness racing, National Hunt racing, and point-to-point racing, dressage, eventing, and endurance riding.

Clinical Signs

Lameness usually is sudden in onset and may be unilateral or bilateral. In some horses with bilateral injury, lameness is insidious in onset, and the horse has loss of forelimb action. Lameness varies from moderate to severe and tends to be worst on hard ground, and often the horse appears to become lamer the farther it trots. After the horse turns at the walk, the lameness then improves and again deteriorates as the horse trots. If the lameness is bilateral and similar in degree in each limb, the horse moves with a short striding, stilted gait.

Usually no localizing clinical signs suggest the source of pain. Often the horse does not react to palpation of the proximopalmar aspect of the McIII, unless the injury is acute.

Diagnosis

Lameness is substantially improved or alleviated by palmar metacarpal (subcarpal) nerve blocks or perineural analgesia of the deep branch of the lateral palmar nerve. Lameness may be improved in some horses by intraarticular analgesia of the middle carpal joint.

Dorsopalmar radiographic images of the proximal metacarpal region may reveal increased radiopacity of the proximal medial aspect of the McIII, with or without a longitudinal radiolucent line extending a variable distance proximodistally (Figure 37-1). If present, the radiolucent line is invariably located medial to the axis of the McIII. Several slightly oblique dorsopalmar images may facilitate identification of a fracture. Generally no radiological abnormality is detectable in other images, although very occasionally periosteal callus is seen on the palmar aspect of the McIII in a lateromedial image. In some horses, no detectable radiological abnormality exists at any stage.

Diagnostic ultrasonography usually reveals no detectable abnormality. Rarely a defect in the palmar cortex of the McIII can be identified. Nuclear scintigraphic images usually demonstrate moderate to intense IRU in the proximal palmar aspect of the McIII in dorsal and lateral bone phase images (Figure 37-2). Early radiopharmaceutical uptake in the proximal palmar aspect of the McIII may also be evident in pool phase images. This pattern of uptake is indistinguishable from that associated with an avulsion fracture of the McIII at the attachment of the SL. It is not known whether horses without radiological change, but with scintigraphic evidence of an increased bone modeling in the proximal aspect of the McIII, would develop a radiologically evident incomplete palmar cortical fracture of the McIII if the horses were kept in work, or whether this is a different manifestation of the response of bone to exercise.

MRI in a small number of Thoroughbred (TB) racehorses with no detectable radiological abnormality revealed

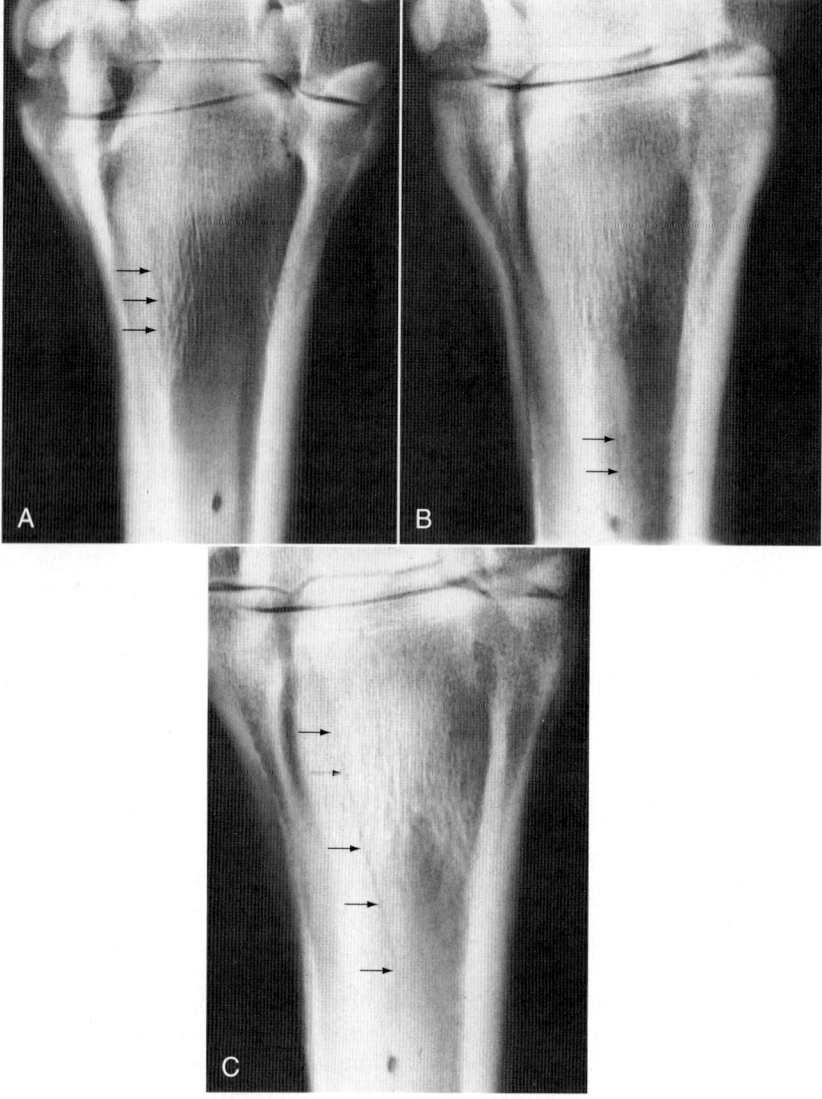

Fig. 37-1 • A, Dorsopalmar radiographic image of the right third metacarpal bone of a 6-year-old Thoroughbred hurdler with moderate right forelimb lameness recognized 7 days previously and alleviated by subcarpal analgesia of the palmar metacarpal nerves. Medial is to the left. The medial aspect of the metaphyseal and proximal diaphyseal regions of the third metacarpal bone has increased radiopacity. A poorly defined longitudinal radiolucent line *(arrows)* represents an incomplete longitudinal palmar cortical fatigue fracture. **B,** Dorsopalmar radiographic image of the right proximal metacarpal region of a 6-year-old Arabian endurance horse with a moderate right forelimb lameness of 3 weeks' duration. Lameness was alleviated by perineural analgesia of the deep branch of the lateral palmar nerve. Well-defined increased radiopacity immediately proximal to the nutrient foramen surrounds a longitudinal radiolucent line in the third metacarpal bone *(arrows).* **C,** The same horse as in **B** after 4 weeks of box rest. The radiolucent line extends further proximally *(arrows).*

diffuse areas of reduced signal intensity in the proximal palmar aspect of the McIII in T1 gradient echo (GRE) images and increased signal intensity in fat-suppressed and T2-weighted GRE images (surrounded by a hypointense rim in T2-weighted images, the result of a fluid-fat cancellation artefact), consistent with bone trauma.[15] In some horses a cortical defect consistent with a fracture was identified, usually medially. The clinical characteristics of the lameness in these horses were not described and scintigraphy was not performed. It is not clear whether these injuries are stress-related bone injuries that reflect a continuum with palmar cortical fatigue fractures. Similar abnormalities have also been seen in endurance and other

sports horses, in association with IRU, and similar lameness characteristics of those described for palmar cortical fatigue fractures.[10] Generally the entire palmar aspect of the McIII is involved, sometimes accompanied by signal alterations in the McII or the McIV, unlike the palmar cortical stress fractures described above in which radiological abnormalities are usually restricted to the medial aspect of the McIII. However, the MR signal alterations were usually most extensive medially.

Treatment

Most horses respond well to rest, with box rest for 1 month and then box rest and controlled walking exercise for

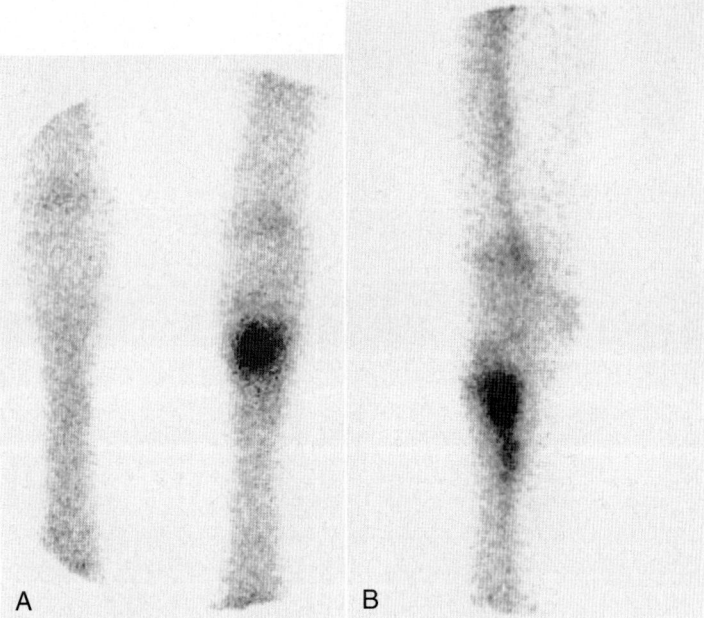

Fig. 37-2 • Dorsal **(A)** and lateral **(B)** scintigraphic images of the carpal and proximal metacarpal regions of the forelimbs of an 8-year-old advanced event horse with acute-onset moderate left forelimb lameness of 3 weeks' duration. The left forelimb is on the right in the dorsal image **(A).** Lameness was alleviated by subcarpal analgesia of the palmar metacarpal nerves. The character of the lameness was typical of a palmar cortical fatigue fracture, but no radiological or ultrasonographic abnormality was detected. Intense focal increased radiopharmaceutical uptake in the proximal, medial, palmar aspect of the third metacarpal bone is compatible with a stress or fatigue fracture.

another 2 months. Horses are then able to slowly and progressively resume normal work. The incidence of recurrent injury is small. Every attempt should be made to identify any problem with the previous training program that may have predisposed the horse to injury.

Midshaft Fractures of the Third Metacarpal Bone

See page 502 for a discussion of midshaft fractures of the McIII.

Transverse Stress Fractures of the Distal Metaphyseal Region of the Third Metacarpal Region

Transverse stress fractures of the distal metaphyseal region of the McIII are relatively uncommon.[16] I have seen this fracture in horses of 4 to 7 years of age in the first season of racing over fences, in young polo ponies, and in pleasure horses that have galloped on the beach. These fractures are believed to be stress fractures because endosteal and periosteal callus has usually been identified radiologically at the first recognition of the lameness. Acute fractures have also been identified in young TB flat racehorses, sometimes only in light work.

Clinical Signs

In young immature TB racehorses there is usually acute-onset severe lameness unassociated with work. There is rapid development of swelling in the distal third of the metacarpal region on the palmar, palmaromedial, or palmarolateral aspects, which is exquisitely painful on palpation and may mimic cellulitis. Radiographs are usually negative initially, but within 7 to 10 days a tranverse

radiopaque line becomes apparent across the distal metaphyseal region and ill-defined periosteal new bone proximally and distally, resulting in distortion of the distal aspect of the McII or the McIV. In some horses, a radiolucent fracture line may eventually be identified. Lameness takes several months to resolve, and there is slow remodeling of the periosteal callus.

In older horses, lameness is usually acute in onset after fast work, is moderate to severe, and may be unilateral or bilateral. Lameness may improve rapidly with the horse appearing sound within a few days. In horses with longstanding lameness, a change in contour of the distal dorsal aspect of the McIII is visible and is associated with periosteal callus formation. In these horses, pain may be elicited by firm pressure applied to the distal dorsal or palmar aspects of the McIII. Twisting the McIII may also induce pain. However, horses with acute lameness may have no localizing signs.

Diagnosis

If lameness persists, local analgesic techniques can be used to isolate the pain, but in some horses this is not possible because of the rapid resolution of lameness, unless the horse is maintained in full work. Lameness is eliminated by palmar (midcannon) and palmar metacarpal (distal to the button of the McII and the McIV) nerve blocks, but it is not influenced by intraarticular analgesia of the metacarpophalangeal joint.

Dorsopalmar, dorsolateral-palmaromedial oblique, dorsomedial-palmarolateral oblique, and lateromedial radiographic images of the fetlock region should be obtained. Flexed lateromedial images are preferable because this technique lifts the PSBs away from the palmar cortex of the

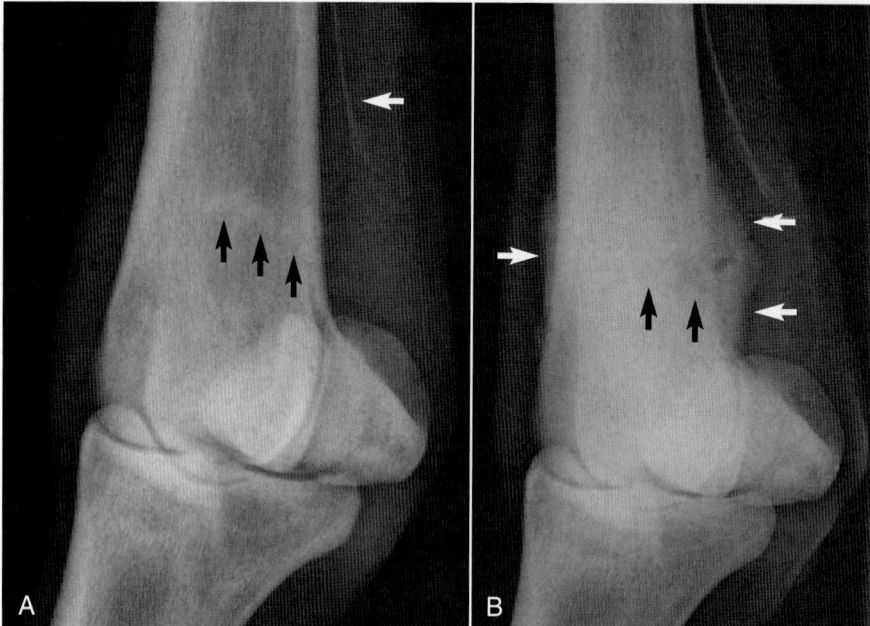

Fig. 37-3 • Dorsolateral-palmaromedial oblique radiographic images of fetlock region of a 3-year-old Thorough-bred flat racehorse obtained 4 days (**A**) and 33 days (**B**) after onset of severe lameness, associated with soft tissue swelling in the distal metacarpal region. There is a transverse stress fracture of the distal metaphyseal region of the third metacarpal bone *(black arrows)* with periosteal callus *(white arrows)*. Note the distortion of the distal aspect of the fourth metacarpal bone.

McIII, allowing better evaluation. Radiological abnormalities may include a horizontal fracture line and endosteal and periosteal callus (Figure 37-3). Some horses, in particular those with acute lameness, may have no detectable abnormality.

Nuclear scintigraphy is invaluable for determining the likely presence of a stress fracture in those horses that lack radiological abnormalities or in which lameness rapidly resolves. There is IRU in the distal metaphyseal region of the McIII.

Treatment

Most horses respond well to 3 months' rest, with 1 month of box rest and then box rest combined with walking exercise. Work intensity can then be progressively increased. The previous training program should be reviewed to try to identify any features that may have predisposed the horse to fracture. Extensive periosteal callus gradually remodels.

Dorsomedial Articular Fractures of the Third Metacarpal Bone

Dorsomedial articular fractures of the McIII have only been recorded in the Standardbred (STB) racehorse,[17] although similar fractures have been identified in the McIII of TBs. The condition usually affects horses 2 to 4 years of age and occurs most commonly in pacers.

Clinical Signs

Lameness is acute in onset, after racing or training, and severe. Lameness persists despite rest. A bony swelling may be palpable on the proximal, dorsomedial aspect of the McIII. Direct pressure may elicit pain.

Diagnosis

Lameness is generally improved by intraarticular analgesia of the middle carpal joint. Diagnosis is based on radiological identification of the fracture, best viewed in a dorsolateral-palmaromedial oblique image. The fracture is articular, nondisplaced, and usually incomplete (Figure 37-4). Active periosteal new bone invariably exists at the distal aspect of the fracture, close to the insertion of the extensor carpi radialis tendon, even in an acute injury.

Treatment

Treatment consists of rest for a minimum of 3 months. The fractures usually heal with modeling of the periosteal reaction and progressive loss of distinction of the fracture line. Lameness resolves, and horses are able to withstand training before the fracture line completely disappears radiographically.

Stress Reactions in the Condyles of the Third Metacarpal Bone

See Chapter 36 for a discussion of stress reactions (see page 398).

Subchondral Bone Trauma

Osseous trauma of the condyles of the distal aspect of the McIII is a diagnosis made using MRI.[18,19] There is usually acute-onset lameness with no localizing clinical signs. Pain is localized to the fetlock region using perineural analgesia. The response to perineural analgesia is often better than to intraarticular analgesia. Radiographic and ultrasonographic examinations usually reveal no detectable abnormality. Scintigraphy usually reveals IRU. There is increased signal intensity in fat-suppressed magnetic resonance images,

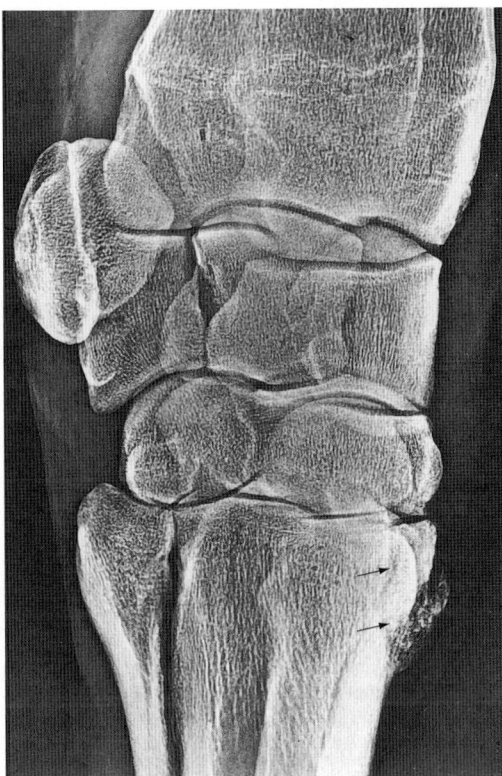

Fig. 37-4 • Dorsolateral-palmaromedial oblique xeroradiographic view of the proximal metacarpal region of a 3-year-old Standardbred male with a dorsomedial articular fracture of the third metacarpal bone. The wide oblique incomplete fracture line (arrows) and presence of proliferative new bone along the dorsomedial aspect of the third metacarpal bone indicate that bone activity in this region preceded the development of acute lameness. (Courtesy Mike Ross, Kennett Square, Pennsylvania, United States.)

with reduced signal intensity in T1- and T2-weighted images, in a variable distribution in the distal aspect of the the McIII. In young TB racehorses, subchondral bone trauma is thought to represent stress–adaptation mismatch and is a manifestation of stress-related bone injury (see page 398), often occurring bilaterally. However, in mature sports horses, it more often occurs unilaterally and may reflect single episode trauma. Lameness usually resolves with rest in sports horses, but young TB racehorses may be difficult to keep sound when returned to training.

Avulsion Fracture of the Third Metacarpal Bone at the Origin of the Suspensory Ligament

Avulsion fracture of the McIII at the origin of the SL occurs most commonly in young racehorses (STBs more than TBs).[20-24] Some fractures described as avulsions appear to occur immediately distal to the site of attachment of the SL.

Clinical Signs

Onset of lameness usually is acute, and lameness is generally moderate to severe and unilateral. In the acute stage, the horse generally resents pressure applied over the palmar proximal aspect of the McIII. Eliciting pain may be more difficult in horses with chronic lameness. Lameness generally improves but may not resolve by box rest.

Diagnosis

In horses with acute lameness, diagnosis usually can be based on the clinical signs and ultrasonographic or radiological demonstration of a fracture. In horses with more chronic lameness, local analgesic techniques may be required. Perineural analgesia of the palmar metacarpal (subcarpal) nerves or of the deep branch of the lateral palmar nerve usually improves lameness substantially. Intraarticular analgesia of the middle carpal joint, performed by palmar or dorsal approaches, may also improve the lameness.

An avulsion fracture is best detected radiologically in dorsopalmar or slightly oblique dorsopalmar images and lateromedial, or flexed lateromedial, images. The fracture may appear as an almost straight or saucer-shaped lucent line (with the base proximal or distal) (Figure 37-5) or as a punched-out lesion.

An avulsed fragment is usually easiest to detect by ultrasonography in longitudinal images and, if displaced, appears as a discontinuity of the palmar cortex of the McIII. An incomplete fracture may be more difficult to detect. Examining the limb while the horse is bearing weight and not bearing weight can be helpful. Slight periosteal callus may be seen in horses with a more chronic fracture. A small focal tear in the dorsal aspect of the SL at the site of the fracture may be visible in transverse and longitudinal images. Nuclear scintigraphy has been used diagnostically.[25]

Treatment

The horse should be restricted to box rest for 6 weeks, followed by box rest and controlled exercise for at least another 6 weeks. The horse should be monitored clinically, radiologically, and ultrasonographically. Lameness caused by avulsion fracture generally takes longer to resolve than in horses with primary proximal suspensory desmitis, sometimes up to 2 months. A fracture may remain detectable radiologically for between 2 and 4 months. Periosteal callus is best seen by ultrasonography and usually is undetectable until 4 to 6 weeks after injury. The total convalescent period is usually between 4 and 6 months. Most TBs ultimately make a complete recovery and return to full athletic function without recurrent injury. Occasionally the fracture fragment may sequestrate or suspensory desmitis may progress, which results in a more guarded prognosis. However, some STBs have long-term lameness that is refractory to treatment. Superior results may be achieved using osteostixis.[26]

Osteoarthritis of the Carpometacarpal Joint

Osteoarthritis (OA) of the carpometacarpal joint is an unusual cause of forelimb lameness. It usually occurs in mature horses used for any discipline. Clusters of Arabians with severe OA have been described[27,28] but the condition can occur in horses of any breed.[28]

Clinical Signs

Lameness may be acute or insidious in onset and ranges from mild to severe. In my clinical experience usually no localizing clinical signs are present, although sometimes there is localized swelling associated with extensive periarticular proliferative new bone, which may be a more typical clinical presentation in Arabians and Quarter Horses.[28]

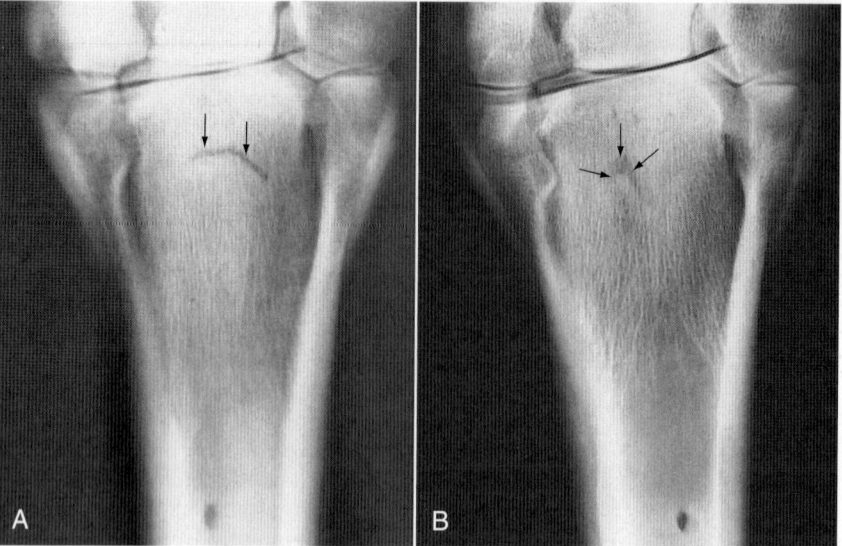

Fig. 37-5 • A, Dorsopalmar radiographic image of the proximal aspect of the left metacarpal region of a 4-year-old Thoroughbred with acute-onset moderate left forelimb lameness. Lameness was alleviated by perineural analgesia of the lateral palmar nerve just distal to the accessory carpal bone. The curved radiolucent line *(arrows)* in the proximal aspect of the third metacarpal bone represents an avulsion fracture at the origin of the suspensory ligament. **B,** Dorsopalmar radiographic image of the proximal metacarpal region of a 3-year-old Thoroughbred with lameness of 2 weeks' duration. A punched-out radiopacity distal to a crescent-shaped lucent area *(arrows)* in the third metacarpal bone represents an avulsion fracture at the origin of the suspensory ligament.

Carpal flexion is often not restricted or resented in association with mild radiological abnormalities, but when extensive new bone formation is present carpal flexion is restricted.

Diagnosis

Lameness may be improved by palmar metacarpal (subcarpal) nerve blocks, probably because of proximal diffusion of the local anesthetic solution. Intraarticular analgesia of the middle carpal joint also improves lameness. Radiological examination usually reveals that changes are restricted to the medial or lateral side of the joint, with narrowing of the joint space between the carpus and the McII or the McIV, with subchondral increased radiopacity (see Figure 3-2; Figure 37-6) and often periosteal new bone extending along the proximal metaphyseal region of the McII or the McIV. Lucent zones may appear in the base (head) of the McII or the McIV. In Arabians and Quarter Horses the majority of radiological abnormalities were medial.[28]

Treatment

Response to intraarticular medication of the carpometacarpal joint has been poor.[27,28] Palliative treatment with a nonsteroidal antiinflammatory drug (NSAID) may allow horses with mild lameness to be maintained in work. Partial carpal arthrodesis may alleviate pain (see Chapter 38).[29,30] Athrodesis resulted in 10 of 12 horses (83%) being described as sound approximately 2 years postoperatively, but only six horses (50%) returned to ridden activity.[30]

Osseous Cystlike Lesions in the Proximal Aspect of the Second Metacarpal Bone

Osseous cystlike lesions sometimes are identified in the proximal aspect of the McII (Figure 37-7) in association

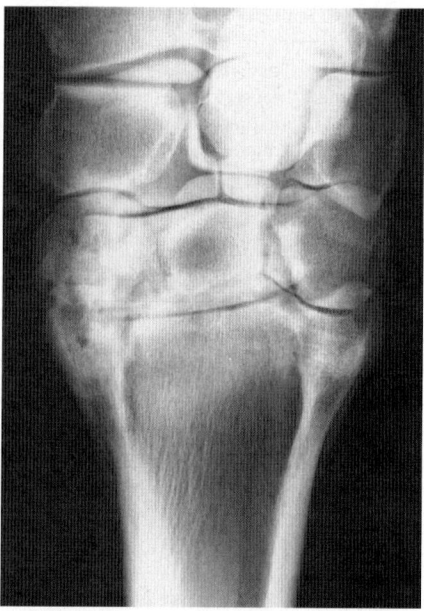

Fig. 37-6 • Dorsopalmar radiographic image of the proximal metacarpal region of a 10-year-old gelding. Medial is to the left. Narrowing of the carpometacarpal joint on the medial aspect of the joint and radiolucent areas in the subchondral bone indicate osteoarthritis of the carpometacarpal joint.

with lameness that is localized to the proximal metacarpal or distal carpal regions. These osseous cystlike lesions occur most commonly in the presence of a first carpal bone,[11] which also may have radiolucent zones. These lesions often occur bilaterally, although lameness may be unilateral. These lesions are generally considered incidental abnormalities unassociated with pain, and the clinician should search for another potential cause of lameness.

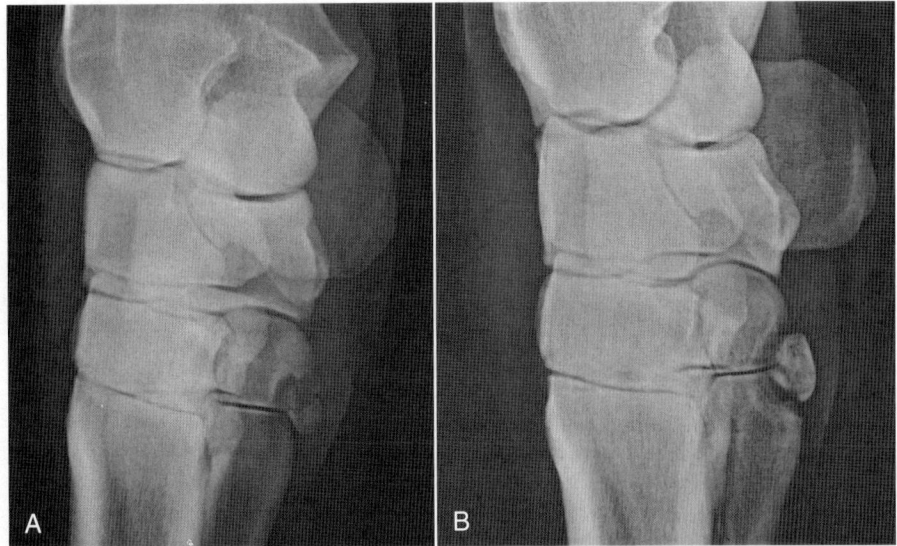

Fig. 37-7 • A, Dorsomedial-palmarolateral oblique radiographic image of the proximal metacarpal region of a 7-year-old Thoroughbred. There is an osseous cystlike lesion in the second carpal bone in association with the presence of a first carpal bone. Both forelimbs were identical. **B,** Dorsomedial-palmarolateral oblique image of the proximal metacarpal region of a 6-year-old riding horse. The radiolucent areas in the palmar aspect of the second carpal bone and proximal palmar aspect of the second metacarpal bone are associated with the presence of a first carpal bone. These were incidental radiological findings not related to lameness.

Syndesmopathy between the Second and Third or Fourth and Third Metacarpal Bones

Interosseous ligaments between the McII and the McIII and between the McIV and the McIII ossify to a variable extent. Occasionally complete osseous union develops throughout the length of the bones with internal increased radiopacity of both bones. The biomechanical implications of this are currently not understood. Inflammation of the interosseous ligament with entheseous or endosteal new bone at the ligaments' attachments was identified using MRI as the only detectable abnormality in horses with pain localized to the metacarpal region or in association with SL pathology.[10,31]

Exostoses of the Second and Fourth Metacarpal Bones (Splints)

Exostoses on the McII or the McIV (splints) may develop because of direct trauma, resulting in subperiosteal hemorrhage and lifting of the periosteum, or instability between the McII (or the McIV) and the McIII. However, many splints do not involve the interosseous space between the McII (or the IV) and the McIII and develop without evidence of trauma. Some splints develop without associated pain and lameness, with little evidence of active inflammation, whereas others result in a localized soft tissue inflammatory reaction, pain, and lameness. The reasons for these differences are not known. Splints may occur at any level but most commonly involve the proximal half of the bone. Lesions involving the McII occur most commonly.

Lesions may develop in young, immature horses or, less commonly, in older horses. Horses with bench (offset) carpal conformation seem particularly prone to develop splints involving the McII, but often these develop without associated lameness.

Clinical Signs

Lameness may be sudden or insidious in onset and tends to deteriorate with work and be worst on hard ground. There is usually an obvious palpable swelling comprising a bony exostosis, surrounded by an edematous soft tissue reaction, with localized heat and pain on firm palpation. The swelling should be palpated carefully with the limb not bearing weight because sometimes only focal areas of the swelling appear to be painful.

It is important to assess the axial aspect of the exostosis to determine whether there may be impingement on the adjacent SL. Such horses may have had a preexisting splint that was previously inactive. The horse often has a history of more extensive soft tissue swelling developing with hard work. Lameness may be provoked by hard work but rapidly improves with rest or light work. With the limb not bearing weight it may be difficult to palpate the border of the SL adjacent to the exostosis, and pain may be elicited by firm pressure applied to this localized area of the SL.

Diagnosis

Diagnosis of a straightforward splint often can be based on clinical signs, and further diagnostic procedures may not be necessary. Radiology may be useful to document the size and activity of the exostosis (Figure 37-8). Several oblique images using soft exposures are required. Care should be taken not to confuse as fracture radiolucent lines that are caused by layers of new bone being superimposed, by incorporation of fibrous tissue, or an edge effect created by the parent bone. Radiography cannot properly document the axial extent of any exostosis.

Nerve blocks or local infiltration may be necessary to prove or disprove that an exostosis is the primary cause of pain resulting in lameness and to identify any concurrent problem(s). Diagnostic ultrasonography is essential if an

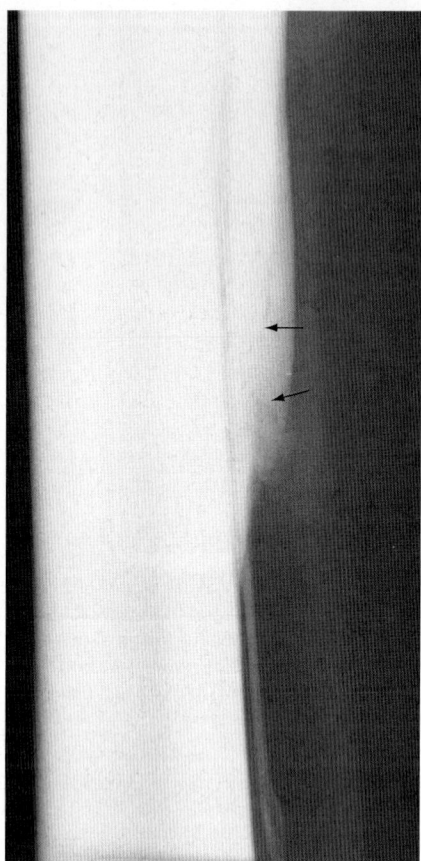

Fig. 37-8 • Dorsomedial-palmarolateral oblique image of the metacarpal region. There is smoothly outlined enlargement of the middle of the diaphysis of the second metacarpal bone, with ill-defined, irregularly outlined periosteal new bone at the distal end of the middle third of the bone. The ill-defined radiolucent lines *(arrows)* within the bone result from new bone formation and should not be confused with fractures.

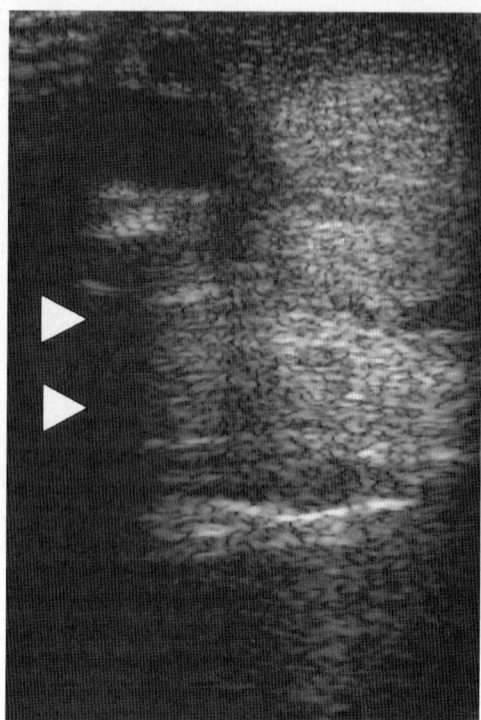

Fig. 37-9 • Transverse ultrasonographic image of the palmar metacarpal soft tissues at 14 cm distal to the accessory carpal bone. Medial is to the left. The irregular medial border of the suspensory ligament and the echogenic material *(arrowheads)* medial to it are apparent. A moderate size exostosis (splint) on the second metacarpal bone extended axially to impinge on the suspensory ligament. Granulomatous-like tissue was interposed between the splint and the suspensory ligament.

impingement on the SL is suspected. Identification of echogenic tissue axial to the exostosis and contiguous with the SL may be possible (Figure 37-9). The ipsilateral border of the SL may be irregular and reduced in echogenicity. In a small proportion of horses, adhesions between the SL and the McII or the McIV can only be identified using MRI.[8,10]

Nuclear scintigraphy is generally unnecessary, but it should be noted that even long-standing splints, which appear to be insignificant clinically, often have mild to moderate IRU compared with the parent bone. Why active bone modeling occurs is not known.

Treatment

Lameness associated with a clinically active exostosis usually resolves with rest, and the surrounding soft tissue swelling resolves. The exostosis remodels and is usually ultimately somewhat smaller. However, sometimes irregular-appearing, palisade-like new bone may persist radiologically. The time taken for the bony reaction to settle is extremely variable, ranging from 2 to 3 weeks to 2 to 3 months. This can be difficult to predict accurately and may reflect how quickly the condition was recognized and box rest instituted. Local infiltration with corticosteroids may facilitate reduction of the soft tissue reaction, but whether this alters the course of the condition is debatable. Topical application of dimethyl sulfoxide has a similar effect.

Work should not resume until firm palpation of the exostosis fails to induce pain. Premature return to work is likely to exacerbate the problem. Some degree of fitness may be maintained by swimming exercise.

Some horses seem particularly predisposed to produce large amounts of new bone. The reason for this is unknown. Large exostoses on the McII are vulnerable to direct trauma from the contralateral limb, especially if the horse moves closely in front, or dishes. Some protection may be provided by always applying protective boots when the horse is worked or turned out. In horses with severe exostoses, surgical amputation of the exostosis and more distal aspect of the metacarpal bone should be considered. Ostectomy of the exostosis and liberal removal of the surrounding periosteum from the splint bone and the McIII without removing the distal segment of the splint bone also have been cosmetically and functionally successful in some horses. Surgical technique may influence the risk of reformation of periosteal new bone.[32]

In some horses chronic pain associated with a splint persists, despite appropriate conservative management. Pin-firing is suggested if pain persists longer than 6 weeks after lameness was first recognized (see Chapter 88). An additional 6 weeks of walking is required before normal work can be resumed after firing.

If there is axial impingement of the exostosis on the SL or adhesions between the splint exostosis and SL, surgical treatment is required. Amputation of the McII or the McIV proximal to the exostosis is the treatment of choice, assuming that this leaves the proximal third of the bone intact, providing stability to the carpus. Often a granulomatous-type reaction occurs between the exostosis and the ipsilateral margin of the SL; this material should also be removed. Alternatively, segmental ostectomy can be performed. One Editor (MWR) prefers to use a different approach because instability of the proximal segment of the McII or the McIV often results in recurrence of lameness and bony proliferation at the ostectomy site. A combination of metacarpal fasciotomy, ostectomy of the exostosis on the axial aspect of the McII or the McIV, adhesiolysis, and the local deposition of antiinflammatory products such as hyaluronan is used.

Fractures of the Second and Fourth Metacarpal Bones

Fractures of the McII and McIV bones may result from direct external trauma or internal forces, frequently in association with suspensory desmitis.[33-37] The latter is particularly common in horses that race over fences, STBs, and, less frequently, event horses.

Fractures caused by internal forces usually occur at the junction between the proximal two thirds and distal one third of the metacarpal bone. The distal ends of the McII and the McIV are connected by fibrous bands to the abaxial surface of the medial and lateral PSBs. Hyperextension of the fetlock and stretching of these fibrous bands may predispose to fracture. Suspensory desmitis may precede fracture and result in modeling and progressive deviation of the distal part of the bone away from the McIII because of pressure or adhesions, thus predisposing to fracture. Fractures at this location unassociated with suspensory desmitis are relatively uncommon, but they do occasionally occur.

Fractures Caused by Internal Trauma
Clinical Signs

Lameness is acute in onset and moderate. Diffuse edematous soft tissue swelling rapidly develops in the distal half of the metacarpal region, more extensively medially if the McII is fractured and laterally if the McIV is involved. Occasionally both the McII and the McIV bones are fractured simultaneously. One or both forelimbs may be affected. Careful palpation reveals enlargement of the body and/or branch of the SL. Palpating instability of the distal piece of the fractured bone may be possible, but extensive soft tissue swelling may prevent this.

Diagnosis

Radiographic examination should include the metacarpal bone and the ipsilateral PSB because lesions may occur at both sites concurrently. Preexisting abnormalities of the McII or the McIV suggest long-term suspensory desmitis (Figure 37-10, *A*). The fracture should be evaluated to determine the degree of displacement and the presence of comminution and callus. Ultrasonographic examination is performed to assess the degree of suspensory desmitis, which is the most important prognostic factor.

Treatment

Some controversy exists concerning the optimal treatment for horses with fractures of the distal third of the McII and the McIV. Some infer that most horses can be managed conservatively, whereas others advocate surgical removal of the fracture fragment. Nondisplaced or slightly displaced fractures usually heal satisfactorily within 4 to 6 weeks if the horse is confined to box rest. Only a small amount of callus develops, which subsequently remodels (see Figure 37-10, *B*). Small radiolucent defects may persist because of

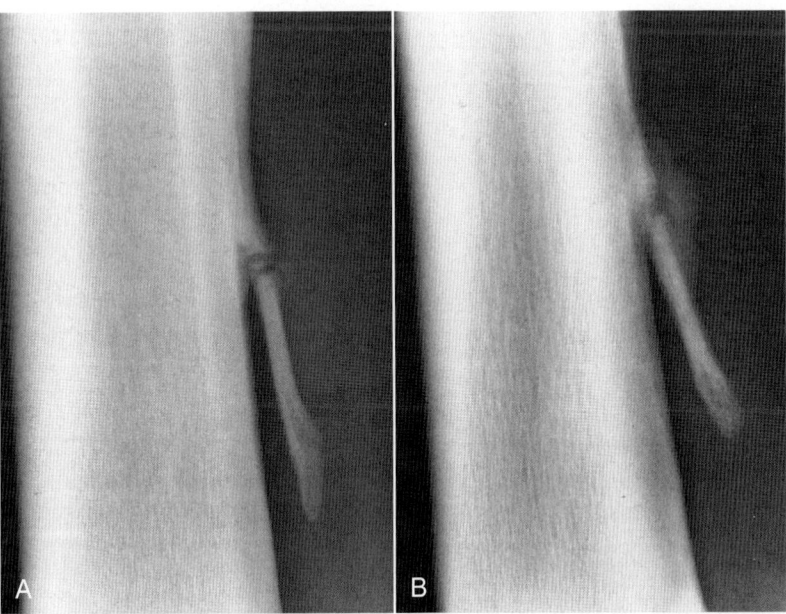

Fig. 37-10 • A, Dorsomedial-palmarolateral oblique radiographic image of the second metacarpal bone of a 7-year-old Thoroughbred steeplechaser. There is a complete, displaced fracture at the junction between the middle and distal thirds of the bone. The axial deviation of the bone indicates previous distortion of the bone in association with desmitis of the medial branch of the suspensory ligament. Some endosteal and periosteal callus is present. **B,** Dorsomedial-palmarolateral oblique radiographic image of the second metacarpal bone of an endurance pony. There is a healing fracture of the second metacarpal bone, associated with desmitis of the medial branch of the suspensory ligament.

incorporation of fibrous tissue. If a fracture is moderately displaced, a larger amount of callus may develop, or a thick layer of fibrous tissue may be laid down, which envelops the entire distal aspect of the metacarpal bone. A large exostosis may impinge on the SL. Therefore surgical removal of these fragments is recommended. The convalescent program is dictated by the degree of suspensory desmitis. Prognosis is better in STBs than in TBs.

Fractures Caused by External Trauma

Fractures of the McII or the McIV caused by external trauma may be simple or comminuted, open or closed.

Clinical Signs

Lameness is acute in onset and is associated with soft tissue swelling around the fracture site, heat, and pain. An open wound may be present. Thorough debridement, cleaning, and lavage of open wounds are important to minimize the risks of infection.

Diagnosis

Radiographic examination is essential to determine the precise position and nature of the fracture (Figure 37-11). If the fracture is chronic or associated with an open wound, the radiographs should be appraised carefully for evidence of infectious osteitis.

Treatment

Fractures involving the proximal third of the bone may require surgical stabilization of the bone to prevent carpal instability, especially if the fracture involves McII. Insertion of small plates with screws into the McII without traversing the interosseous space is the preferred method of management. Oblique fractures of the proximal aspect of the McII or the McIV can be repaired using 3.5-mm bone screws and stainless steel wire using the tension band principle in an intrabone technique (screws only engage the involved splint bone and not the McIII). Alternatively, screws placed between the McII and the McIII can be used, but fixation may be unstable, and chronic lameness could develop because of synostosis between the two bones or reaction from the implants themselves. When horses have simple displaced or comminuted fractures of the McII or the McIV, but with infection, all efforts should be made to resolve infection before surgical fixation is attempted. However, if the fracture is comminuted and the carpus appears to be stable, conservative management may be satisfactory. Simple or more complicated fractures in the distal two thirds of the bone can be treated either conservatively or by surgical removal, depending on the size of the pieces and their location.

Palmar Annular Desmitis

See Chapter 74 for a discussion of palmar annular desmitis.

Avulsion of the Attachment of the Palmar Annular Ligament from a Proximal Sesamoid Bone

See Chapter 72 for a discussion of avulsion of the attachment of the PAL from a proximal sesamoid bone.

Constriction of the Digital Flexor Tendon Sheath by the Palmar Annular Ligament

See Chapter 74 for a discussion of constriction of the DFTS by the PAL.

Tenosynovitis of the Digital Flexor Tendon Sheath: Primary and Secondary

See Chapter 74 for a discussion of primary and secondary tenosynovitis of the DFTS.

Proximal Suspensory Desmitis

See Chapter 72 for a discussion of proximal suspensory desmitis.

Desmitis of the Body of the Suspensory Ligament

See Chapter 72 for a discussion of desmitis of the body of the SL.

Desmitis of the Medial or Lateral Branch of the Suspensory Ligament

See Chapter 72 for a discussion of desmitis of the medial or lateral branch of the SL.

Desmitis of the Accessory Ligament of the Deep Digital Flexor Tendon

See Chapter 71 for a discussion of desmitis of the ALDDFT.

Deep Digital Flexor Tendonitis

See Chapter 70 for a discussion of deep digital flexor tendonitis.

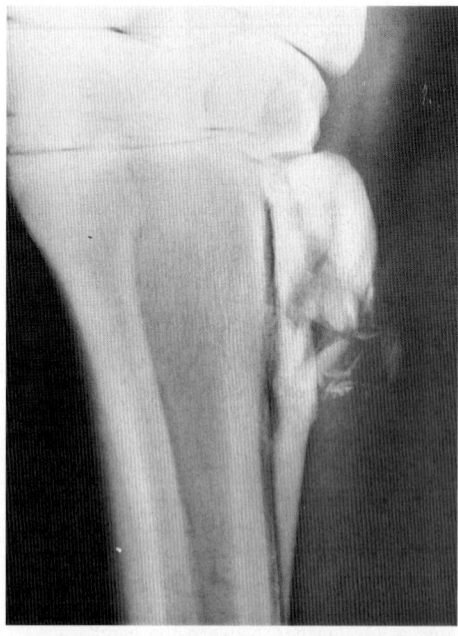

Fig. 37-11 • Dorsolateral-palmaromedial oblique radiographic image of the metacarpal region. There is a comminuted, displaced articular fracture of the proximal third of the fourth metacarpal bone. The fracture was repaired surgically using a small plate, but osteoarthritis of the carpometacarpal joint developed subsequently.

Superficial Digital Flexor Tendonitis

See Chapter 69 for a discussion of superficial digital flexor tendonitis.

Traumatic Lacerations of the Superficial Digital Flexor Tendon and the Deep Digital Flexor Tendon

See Chapter 81 for a discussion of traumatic lacerations of the SDFT and DDFT.

Distention of the Carpal Sheath

See Chapter 75 for a discussion of distention of the carpal sheath.

DIFFERENTIAL DIAGNOSIS OF DIFFUSE FILLING IN THE METACARPAL REGION

Diffuse filling in the metacarpal region, with or without stiffness or lameness, is common. The clinician makes a diagnosis of the cause through review of the history of the horse and careful clinical examination (Box 37-1).

The clinician should assess the following points:

- Is the swelling symmetrical, or does it predominantly involve only one side of the limb?
- Does swelling extend the entire length of the metacarpal region, or only part of it?
- Has any filling occurred in the pastern region, or the carpus and proximally?
- Does the palmar aspect of the limb have a straight contour?
- Is the swelling edematous?
- What are the intensities of the digital pulse amplitudes?
- Is the limb hot or cold?
- Is the horse febrile?
- Is the horse bright and alert, or depressed?
- Is more than one limb involved?
- Are any skin lesions apparent?

BOX 37-1

Differential Diagnosis of Diffuse Filling in the Metacarpal Region

- So-called cold edema
- Cellulitis
- Edema and inflammatory reaction associated with a subsolar abscess
- Scabby skin lesions on the palmar aspect of the fetlock
- Mud fever
- Lymphangitis
- Purpura hemorrhagica
- Hemorrhage
- Filling caused by direct trauma
- Tendonous or ligamentous injury
- Thrombosis
- Fracture
- Equine viral arteritis
- Infection of a tendon
- Infection of the digital flexor tendon sheath
- Photosensitization
- Hypertrophic osteopathy

- What color is the limb?
- Is the horse sound, stiff, or lame?
- What is the severity of lameness?
- Is each anatomical structure palpable?
- Is each structure intact and of normal size and shape?
- Does palpation of a specific structure elicit pain?

Hemorrhage

Hemorrhage in the proximal metacarpal region is an occasional cause of acute-onset, severe lameness during work. Extensive soft tissue swelling rapidly develops, mimicking a severe tear of the ALDDFT. The swelling makes it difficult to palpate accurately specific structures. However, ultrasonographic examination reveals no detectable structural abnormality of the digital flexor tendons and the ALDDFT. Application of a large support bandage and treatment with NSAIDs brings rapid relief. The bandage should be maintained and changed as needed for approximately 7 to 10 days. When the bandage is removed, the limb is usually of normal contour. The limb should be reexamined by ultrasonography to confirm that no structural abnormalities exist before allowing the horse to resume normal work. The cause of this condition is unknown, and the likelihood of recurrence is small.

Thrombosis

Thrombosis of the medial palmar vein is a rare cause of lameness in the horse. Partial thrombosis may result in periodic diffuse filling of the distal limb associated with lameness. Complete occlusion may result in severe lameness and distal limb swelling soon after starting any exercise. Diagnosis is based on careful palpation of the vasculature combined with ultrasonography, including Doppler. Treatment requires vascular surgery.

Infection of Tendons

Infection of the SDFT or DDFT, without any evidence of a penetrating wound, is an unusual cause of lameness, but unless infection is recognized early and treated aggressively, it can have catastrophic consequences.[38]

Clinical Signs

Sudden-onset, severe unilateral lameness involves a forelimb or hindlimb. Frequently this follows within 24 hours of strenuous exercise. The horse is usually reluctant to bear weight on the limb, and effective control of pain can be difficult. Considerable peritendonous edema develops rapidly, precluding accurate palpation of the digital flexor tendons. Palpation reveals localized heat and exquisite pain. The skin may become tight, and if the infection is unrecognized and untreated, pus may exude through defects in the skin within several days.

Diagnosis

Ultrasonographic evaluation reveals a central anechogenic defect within the infected tendon (Figure 37-12) that progresses rapidly and may extend the length of the metacarpal or metatarsal region within a few days. In the early stages, lameness may be disproportionately severe relative to the perceived amount of tendon damage. Bacterial culture has frequently yielded a coagulase-positive *Staphylococcus*.

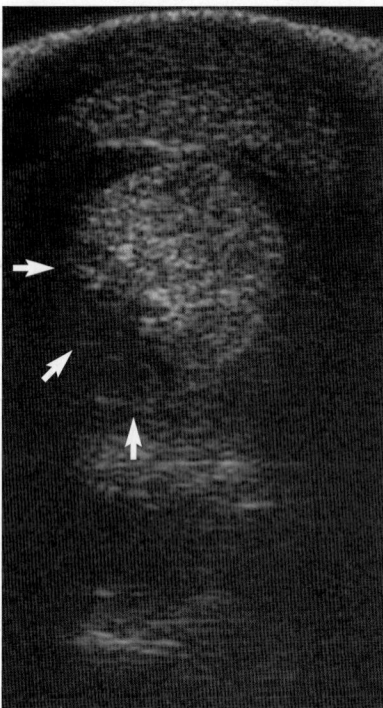

Fig. 37-12 • Transverse ultrasonographic image of the plantar metatarsal region. There is subcutaneous edema. The deep digital flexor tendon is enlarged and has a large anechogenic region dorsomedially *(arrows)* that progressed rapidly. The horse had extensive peritendonous soft tissue swelling and severe lameness associated with the infected tendon.

Treatment

Aggressive systemic antimicrobial therapy with crystalline penicillin, gentamicin, and metronidazole has usually proved inadequate, with progression of tendon destruction despite therapy. Drainage of pus and lavage combined with antimicrobial therapy has successfully controlled infection in some, but not all, horses. However, the prognosis for return to athletic function is extremely guarded.

Cellulitis, Skin Necrosis, and Necrosis of the Superficial Digital Flexor Tendon after Topical Applications

Cellulitis, skin necrosis, and subsequent necrosis of the SDFT are poorly understood conditions. The syndrome has been recognized in National Hunt racehorses.[39] After racing, many horses receive a topical application of a clay-like substance to the metacarpal regions, with or without overlying bandages.

Clinical Signs

Clinical signs are apparent within 24 to 72 hours and include peritendonous edema and serum ooze progressing to skin slough and exposure of the SDFT. The tendon may also be affected, without evidence of preexisting strain-type injury. Lameness varies from moderate to severe. The condition may be unilateral or bilateral. The horse may have had the same topical application previously but not necessarily so. Frequently other horses have been treated with the same batch of the proprietary claylike substance with no adverse effects. A variety of different

proprietary products have been incriminated. Curiously, to my knowledge, the condition has not been seen in event horses, although many receive similar treatments after competing.

Treatment

The condition usually progresses to a huge area of skin loss on the palmar aspect of the metacarpal region, with or without major damage to the underlying SDFT. No therapy has successfully halted this progression. Healing is by granulation tissue and fibrosis. If the horse survives, it has a massively thickened limb, and most horses have not returned to racing.

Cellulitis Associated with Superficial Digital Flexor Tendonitis

Cellulitis sometimes occurs with superficial digital flexor tendonitis. Clinical signs are usually recognized within 24 to 48 hours after competition. The horse has diffuse filling in the metacarpal region(s), and pinpoint pricks appear in the skin through which serum oozes within several days. The horse may be slightly lame or have a stiff gait. Symptomatic therapy usually resolves the majority of filling and lameness, and a primary tendon injury may go unrecognized without careful inspection. Careful ultrasonographic evaluation is mandatory because almost invariably primary tendonitis is present. Care should be taken in the presence of clinically significant subcutaneous edema because acoustic enhancement may mask a subtle tendon lesion. Such horses should be reevaluated after resolution of the edema.

Enostosis-like Lesions

Enostosis-like lesions are focal areas of new bone formation within the medullary cavity of a bone, occurring on the endosteal surface or close to a nutrient foramen. They occasionally occur in the McIII and may be single or multiple. They can occur as incidental radiological abnormalities or in association with lameness. Nuclear scintigraphy may reveal IRU at the site of these lesions, but this does not necessarily imply that associated pain exists. Clinical significance can only be ascribed by eliminating all other sources of pain.

Hypertrophic Osteopathy

Hypertrophic osteopathy, or Marie's disease, frequently involves the metacarpal region, resulting in localized or diffuse soft tissue swelling that overlies new bone formation.[40] Hypertrophic osteopathy has been associated with thoracic disease, a variety of vascular lesions, granulomatous enteritis, and some tumors in the thorax and abdomen. Identification of the primary lesion and successful treatment may result in resolution of the bony lesions and associated clinical signs.

Clinical Signs

The acute stage of hypertrophic osteopathy produces heat and edematous swelling overlying areas of new bone formation. Palpation of the affected bones produces pain. All the limbs should be inspected carefully to establish the extent of the lesions. Depending on the limbs affected, the horse may show overt lameness or generalized stiffness.

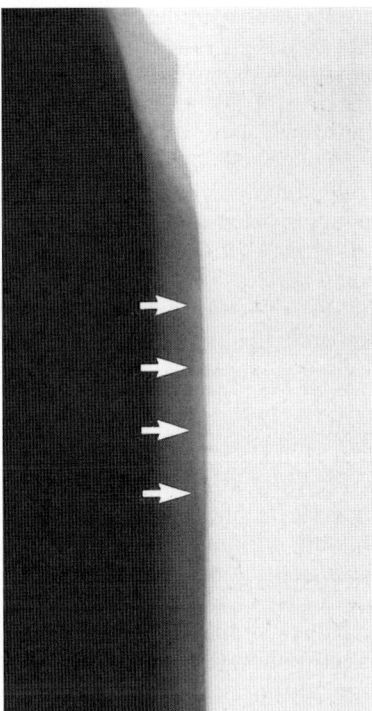

Fig. 37-13 • Dorsolateral-palmaromedial oblique radiographic image of the proximal metacarpal region using soft exposure factors to show palisading new bone *(arrows)* on the dorsal aspect of the third metacarpal bone typical of hypertrophic osteopathy. The 7-year-old breeding stallion had avian tuberculosis and was successfully treated, with the bony lesions resolving.

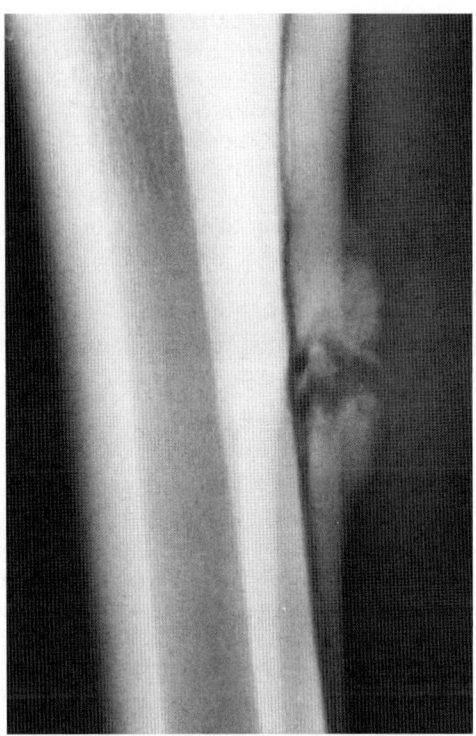

Fig. 37-14 • Dorsolateral-palmaromedial oblique image of the metacarpal region. A radiolucent zone (an involucrum) surrounds a separate radiopaque fragment within the fourth metacarpal bone (a sequestrum). Periosteal new bone appears on the diaphysis of the fourth metacarpal bone, through which is a lucent canal (a cloaca).

Although careful clinical appraisal of the entire horse may reveal clinical signs of an underlying disease process, often no clues are present. Clinical evaluation should include palpation of all lymph nodes, auscultation of the heart and lungs, and rectal examination.

Diagnosis

Radiographic examination, using soft exposures, reveals palisading periosteal new bone in the diaphyseal and metaphyseal regions of the McIII and other affected bones but usually excluding the joints (Figure 37-13). The palisading new bone, perpendicular to the cortices, is pathognomonic.

Every effort should be made to try to define the primary causal lesion. Additional diagnostic tests should include thoracic radiography and echocardiography, examination of a tracheal aspirate and peritoneal fluid, and routine hematological and clinical biochemistry testing. If weight loss is evident, an oral glucose tolerance test should be performed to assess small intestinal absorption of disaccharide sugars. A labeled white blood cell nuclear scintigraphic examination of the thorax and abdomen may be helpful. Skin biopsies may reveal evidence of vasculitis.

Treatment

If the primary cause of the condition can be identified and successfully treated, then the bony lesions will resolve spontaneously. The new bone becomes progressively more radiopaque and corticalized and gradually models to restore a more normal contour. Occasionally lesions have resolved spontaneously after treatment with phenylbutazone.

Osteitis or Osteomyelitis

Infectious osteitis or osteomyelitis occurs commonly in the metacarpal region because of the relative lack of soft tissue coverage of the bones and is usually a sequel to known trauma, with or without an open wound.

Clinical Signs

There is localized soft tissue swelling and mild to moderate lameness, and usually a draining tract is apparent.

Diagnosis

Ultrasonographic evaluation reveals an anechogenic region adjacent to the bone in the acute stage, as well as the accumulation of pus, before radiological changes are evident. Radiological abnormalities may include a radiolucent region within the cortex of the bone, periosteal new bone, and a sequestrum and involucrum in horses with advanced infection (Figure 37-14).

Treatment

Aggressive antimicrobial therapy sometimes successfully resolves the infection, but surgical debridement is indicated in horses with advanced sequestration.

USE OF BOOTS AND BANDAGES TO PREVENT INJURY

The use of stable bandages, protective boots and bandages for exercise, and proprietary clays and cooling agents after exercise is common among horse owners in their efforts to protect horses from injury and to help to manage preexisting injuries. Bandages that are applied too tightly have tremendous potential to cause local damage, not only to the underlying skin on the dorsal and palmar aspects of the metacarpal region but also to the underlying tendons. The midmetacarpal region appears to be particularly vulnerable. Transient (a few hours') application of an overly tight bandage results in a "bandage bow," localized subcutaneous edema overlying the SDFT. More prolonged application of a bandage that is too tight results in hair loss and skin necrosis. Hair that regrows is white. Excessive sustained pressure causes tendon necrosis.

Persistent bandaging at appropriate pressures does not cause damage but leaves permanent rings in the hair; if these rings are visible at a prepurchase examination, they should alert the veterinarian that the horse usually stands in bandages. Properly applied stable bandages can be used to control filled legs and in horses prone to distention of the fetlock joint capsule or the DFTS.

The use of bandages or boots during exercise is somewhat controversial. A properly applied bandage should aim to permit a normal range of motion but protect against movement in an abnormal range.[41-48] Little evidence exists that a bandage applied circumferentially around the limb reduces loads on the digital flexor tendons and thereby reduces the risk of overstretch injury. Studies on cadaver models have shown that distal limb bandages may increase the amount of energy a limb can absorb during repeated loading.[41,42] Strain on the proximal aspect of the SL may be decreased in a standing or walking horse.[43] In exercising horses, fetlock extension was reduced.[40] However, shock attenuation was unaffected.[41] The effectiveness of stabilizing support bandages in people decreases rapidly with exercise, and restriction in motion may have an adverse effect on performance in healthy athletes. Athletic taping of the fetlock of horses exercised at the trot had no effect on SDFT or SL strains; fetlock extension during stance was not affected, but there was a decrease in peak vertical force measured using a force plate.[46] In exercising horses the core temperature within the SDFT increases substantially, and although the role of temperature in tendon injury remains uncertain, bandaging has the potential to promote heating. The effects of a gamgee bandage, a neoprene boot, a three-layered bandage, and a Dalmar tendon support boot (Dalmar Ireland Ltd., Glanmire, Ireland) on fetlock extension were compared in an in vitro model. The Dalmar support boot reduced fetlock extension.[47] Moreover, kinematic studies of fetlock extension at walk and trot comparing four different boot designs showed a small decrease (0.5-1.5 degrees) in fetlock extension at the trot with all boots compared to without boots, suggesting that this may reduce tension in the SL and SDFT. However, studies at the canter, gallop, and jumping have not been performed. Therefore little current rationale exists for use of bandages or boots to prevent tendon strain injuries.

Boots and bandages have the potential to attenuate forces from direct trauma to the limb, for example, as the result of a horse hitting a fixed fence. However, without reinforcement, none properly protects against strike injuries from the hindlimb of the same horse or from strike injuries from adjacent horses. Such strike injuries can result in severe tendon injuries. The introduction of a more resilient bulletproof type of material into part of a boot, or applied as a palmar reinforcement under a bandage, can provide some protection against these devastating injuries, but the effect of such rigid material on normal movement of the flexor tendons is not known.

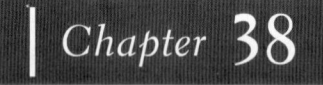

Chapter 38

The Carpus

Mike W. Ross

ANATOMY

References on page 1282

The carpus consists of the antebrachiocarpal, middle carpal, and carpometacarpal joints. The antebrachiocarpal and middle carpal joints are considered ginglymi, but they are not typical of hinge joints; the carpometacarpal joint is arthrodial.[1] Arthrodial joints also exist between carpal bones in each respective row. Effective movement of the carpus originates from the antebrachiocarpal and middle carpal joints. The carpometacarpal joint does not open, but it is subject to shear stress. The antebrachiocarpal joint lies between the distal aspect of the radius and the proximal row of carpal bones. The distal, dorsal aspect of the radius has deep grooves in which run the tendons of the extensor carpi radialis and common digital extensor muscles. In flexion the tendons compress the dorsal aspect of the antebrachiocarpal joint, limiting visibility when arthroscopic examination is performed. The proximal row of carpal bones includes the accessory carpal bone, which articulates with the distal aspect of the radius and the ulnar carpal bone. The accessory carpal bone forms the lateral border of the carpal canal. From lateral to medial, the ulnar carpal, the intermediate carpal, and the radial carpal bones complete the proximal row.

The middle carpal joint lies between the proximal and distal rows of carpal bones. The number of bones in the distal row varies but always includes, from medial to lateral, the second, third, and fourth carpal bones. A first carpal bone is present unilaterally or bilaterally in approximately 50% of horses[1] and should not be mistaken on radiographs for an osteochondral fragment. The first carpal bone articulates with the second metacarpal bone (McII) and the second carpal bone, and its presence is often associated with radiolucent areas in the McII. A fifth carpal bone is rare, but if present is small, articulates with the fourth carpal bone and the proximal aspect of the fourth metacarpal bone (McIV), and can be confused with an osteochondral fragment. The second, third, and fourth carpal bones articulate with the McII, the third metacarpal bone (McIII), and the McIV, respectively. The articulation of the second carpal bone and the McII is broader than is that of the fourth carpal bone and the McIV, and hence the McII receives greater load, an important fact to consider with fractures of the McII and the McIV. The third carpal bone, the largest bone in the distal row, has two fossae separated by a distinct ridge, the intermediate (lateral) and radial (medial). The radial fossa is largest, receives greater load, and is more commonly injured. The third carpal bone is L shaped and has a large, dense palmar portion that is rarely injured.

The carpal bones are held together by intercarpal ligaments including the dense palmar carpal ligament from which the accessory ligament of the deep digital flexor tendon arises. The strong intercarpal ligaments play a major role in stability, and the palmar intercarpal ligaments have been shown to provide more resistance to extension of the carpus than does the palmar carpal ligament.[2] When large medial and lateral corner osteochondral fragments of the third carpal bone are removed, the intercarpal ligaments and capsular attachments must be incised. These dense attachments provide stability, which can be advantageous when slab fractures are repaired. The dorsomedial intercarpal ligament courses between the medial aspect of the second carpal bone and the dorsomedial aspect of the radial carpal bone,[3] but during arthroscopic examination it appears to blend with the joint capsule. A theory was proposed that the dorsomedial intercarpal ligament became hypertrophied and impinged on the articular surface of the radial carpal bone, causing secondary modeling in young racehorses and lameness.[4] Recent studies of normal carpi found that the dorsomedial intercarpal ligament was neither hypertrophied nor impinging on the radial carpal bone. A definite relationship exists between the development of pathological conditions on the distal aspect of the radial carpal bone and the attachment of the dorsomedial intercarpal ligament, but I have not observed hypertrophy or impingement. The majority of radial carpal bone osteochondral fragments occur within or just lateral to the attachment site of the dorsomedial intercarpal ligament. Because the dorsomedial intercarpal ligament resists dorsomedial displacement of the radial carpal bone,[3] this site is prone to develop osteochondral fragments. In abnormal carpi, hypertrophy of the dorsomedial intercarpal ligament has been found to be apparent, but no correlation existed between hypertrophy and cartilage or subchondral bone damage.[5]

The medial and lateral palmar intercarpal ligaments resist displacement and dissipate axial forces by allowing abaxial translation of carpal bones.[6,7] The long and short medial and lateral collateral ligaments originate on the radius and attach to the proximal aspects of the McII and the McIV, and the abaxial surface of the carpal bones, respectively. The collateral ligaments provided the major resistance to dorsal displacement of the proximal row of carpal bones during experimental loading, but the small but important palmar intercarpal ligaments contributed 23% resistance.[2] The lateral palmar intercarpal ligament mostly attaches proximally on the ulnar carpal bone and distally on the third carpal bone and may be divided,[3] findings different from those previously reported—that the distal attachment was mostly on the fourth carpal bone.[8] The medial palmar intercarpal ligament has four bundles that vary in size, and it courses between the radial carpal bone proximally and the palmaromedial surface of the

third carpal bone and palmarolateral surface of the second carpal bone distally.[3] Tearing of the medial palmar intercarpal ligament and to a lesser extent the lateral palmar intercarpal ligament was observed in horses with carpal disease and was recently proposed to be associated with cartilage and subchondral bone damage (see the following discussion).[8,9]

The carpus has a dense joint capsule dorsally that blends with the overlying fascia and retinaculum. Synovium in young horses is often thickened or folded dorsally in the middle carpal joint and can interfere with visibility during arthroscopic surgery. This fold appears to smooth as horses age or as osteoarthritis develops. The antebrachial fascia blends with the retinaculum that functions to restrain extensor tendons. Retinaculum thickens and forms the medial and palmar borders of the carpal canal. The palmar retinaculum is sometimes severed in horses with carpal tenosynovitis and tendonitis (see Chapter 75). Anatomical considerations and flexor and extensor tendon injuries are discussed elsewhere (see Chapters 69 and 77). The sheathed extensor carpi radialis and common digital extensor tendons, located dorsally and dorsolaterally, respectively, limit carpal palpation and restrict access. Cul-de-sacs of distended antebrachiocarpal and middle carpal joint capsules can be palpated medial to the extensor carpi radialis tendon or between the extensor carpi radialis and common digital extensor tendons in a standing horse. Arthrocentesis and arthroscopic examination require careful placement of needles and instruments in these portals to avoid injury to tendons and sheaths. These portals can be easily felt as distinct depressions when the carpus is flexed. The sheathed lateral digital extensor tendon, located on the lateral aspect, should be avoided during arthrocentesis of the palmarolateral pouches. The sheathed extensor carpi obliquus tendon is small and passes obliquely over the antebrachiocarpal joint from lateral to medial to attach to the McII. This tendon can readily be seen medially during arthroscopic examination of the antebrachiocarpal joint. Extensor tenosynovitis must be differentiated from middle carpal and antebrachiocarpal joint effusion and hygroma. The antebrachiocarpal and middle carpal joints each have a palmarolateral and a palmaromedial outpouching through which arthrocentesis and arthroscopic evaluation can be performed. Unless greatly distended, the palmarolateral outpouchings are larger than the corresponding palmaromedial outpouchings. The palmarolateral outpouching of the antebrachiocarpal joint is in close proximity to the carpal sheath, and inadvertent penetration of the carpal sheath can occur during arthrocentesis or arthroscopic examination even when the palmarolateral outpouching is distended.

Knowledge of the communications and boundaries of the carpal joints is important in understanding the extent of disease processes and the results of diagnostic analgesia (see Chapter 10). The antebrachiocarpal joint is considered solitary, although in a single specimen in a cadaver study the joint communicated with the middle carpal and carpometacarpal joints.[10] In some horses a communication appears between the antebrachiocarpal joint and the carpal sheath. The middle carpal and carpometacarpal joints always communicate (see Figures 10-8 through 10-10). Communication between the middle carpal and carpometacarpal joints and the carpal sheath is rare. The carpometacarpal joint has distinct distopalmar outpouchings located axial to the McII and the McIV that have secondary pouches interdigitating within the proximal aspect of the suspensory ligament (SL). These outpouchings explain inadvertent analgesia of the carpometacarpal and middle carpal joint while performing high palmar analgesia and possibly why lameness abates during middle carpal analgesia in horses with avulsion fractures of the proximopalmar aspect of the McIII or proximal suspensory desmitis.[11]

CONFORMATION

Racehorses, especially Thoroughbreds (TBs), with offset-knee (bench-knee) and back-at-the-knee (calf-knee) conformation are predisposed to develop carpal lameness. Mild in-at-the-knee (carpus valgus) deformity is common and of little concern, but if the deformity is severe, it can predispose to carpal lameness similar to that in horses with out-at-the-knee (carpus varus) conformation (see Chapter 4).

CLINICAL CHARACTERISTICS AND DIAGNOSIS OF CARPAL LAMENESS

Carpal lameness is a common finding in many sports horses, but it is most common in racehorses. Former racehorses used in other disciplines may have chronic osteoarthritis (OA) or recurrence of osteochondral fragmentation. Primary carpal lameness in nonracehorses occurs from trauma such as from falls, kick wounds, and hitting fences; hyperextension injury resulting in fractures of the accessory carpal bone; and occasionally primary OA. Old horses, in particular Arabian horses, appear prone to develop inexplicable chronic, often severe OA of the carpometacarpal joint. Palmar carpal injury occurs in horses that fall or during recovery from general anesthesia and can result in moderate to severe lameness and subsequent OA. Palmar carpal injury most commonly involves the antebrachiocarpal joint, and clinical signs may not develop until hours or a few days after recovery from general anesthesia. Injury may result from trauma when the affected carpus is hyperextended or flexed and usually occurs in horses during rough recoveries but can occur, inexplicably, in horses with seemingly uneventful recoveries.

Few historical facts are pathognomonic for carpal lameness unless severe swelling and lameness develop acutely or a trauma is observed. TB racehorses may lug (bear) in, lug out, or fail to change leads. A Standardbred (STB) racehorse may be on a line. Horses may be racing poorly, particularly those with bilaterally symmetrical lameness. In racehorses with right forelimb carpal lameness, signs may be worse on the turns. Although most STBs are on the ipsilateral line, rarely a horse with right forelimb carpal lameness will be on the left line, presumably because the horse is bearing away from medially located pain or has a shortened stride in the right forelimb. Nonracehorses may have poor performance, fail to change leads, and hit or refuse fences. They may be uncomfortable when studs are placed in or removed from the shoes. Ponies with antebrachiocarpal joint pain may start to stumble.

Degree of lameness varies with the type and severity of carpal injury. Horses with early or mild chronic OA have mild lameness, whereas those with acute osteochondral

fragments, slab fractures, or other more serious injuries have more severe lameness. Horses with infectious arthritis and comminuted carpal or other severe fractures may not bear weight at the walk. Dynamic angular deformity, carpus valgus or varus, may be seen in horses attempting to bear weight with comminuted fractures and loss of joint integrity. Lameness may be intermittent in horses with early and incomplete osteochondral fragments and may be apparent only after training or racing. Racehorses with bilaterally symmetrical lameness may not show overt lameness but have a wide, short gait bilaterally. Advancing and placing the affected limb wide while walking or trotting (pacing) is typical of carpal lameness (see Chapter 7). Horses with severe OA and natural carpal ankylosis or surgical arthrodesis swing (abduct) the limb because the carpus cannot flex. Advancement and placement of the limb in a lateral (abducted) position is not pathognomonic for carpal lameness, and horses with proximal palmar metacarpal pain or those with pain originating laterally in the digit may manifest similar signs. However, carpal tenosynovitis does not result in this typical carpal gait. Horses with carpal lameness have a shortened cranial phase of the stride. Lameness can be worse with the limb on the inside or outside of the circle depending on whether the location of pain is medial or lateral, but, in general, lameness in most horses with carpal lameness is worse with the limb on the *outside* of the circle.

Increased temperature (heat) over the dorsal surface of the carpus is a reliable indicator of carpal disease, but false positive and negative findings occur. If horses have been clipped for painting or blistering, or effects of topical counterirritation are still present, the area can be warm and sensitive without carpal lameness. The dorsal surface of each carpus should be evaluated and compared, but differences are difficult to detect if lameness is bilateral. Effusion is usually a reliable indicator for carpal synovitis, but it is not pathognomonic for carpal lameness. Horses with subchondral bone injury without overlying cartilage damage or incomplete osteochondral fragments often have carpal lameness without effusion. Effusion is suppressed in horses that have recently had corticosteroid injections. Effusion occurs commonly in young horses with early carpitis and in horses with advanced cartilage damage, osteochondral fragments, and infectious arthritis. Swelling associated with distention of the antebrachiocarpal or middle carpal joints is orientated horizontally on the dorsal aspect of the carpus, whereas effusion in a tendon sheath results in a longitudinally orientated swelling, compressed at intervals by horizontally orientated retinacular bands. With the horse's limb in a weight-bearing position, the clinician's fingers are used to ballot fluid within a distended carpal joint capsule. Capsular swellings are located between extensor tendons and medial to the tendon of the extensor carpi radialis. Older horses with chronic carpal changes often have mild or moderate effusion but can perform satisfactorily. In some horses there may be focal dorsal herniation of the antebrachiocarpal or middle carpal joint capsules.

Horses with acute carpal lameness, especially those with synovitis, often show a marked response to static flexion of the carpus. Horses with carpal tenosynovitis or other palmar carpal lameness also respond. Horses with pain from the proximal aspect of the limb, such as myositis in the proximal aspect of the antebrachium or elbow region pain, respond to carpal flexion (false-positive response). Static and dynamic flexion can be negative in horses with carpal lameness, especially in those with subchondral bone pain. Degree of flexion is usually decreased in horses with chronic OA because of joint capsule fibrosis. Careful palpation of all bony and soft tissue structures of the carpal region should be performed with the limb in standing and flexed positions, and responses should be compared with the contralateral limb. Swellings are best felt with the horse's limb in a standing position. Swellings of nearby sheaths should be differentiated from authentic carpal effusion by location and ballottement. Horses with chronic OA often have firm, fibrous thickening at joint capsule attachments. Dorsomedial bony swelling of the radial and third carpal bones is observed and palpated in horses with chronic severe OA. The proximal aspect of the McII and the McIV should be palpated for bony and soft tissue swelling associated with fracture or exostoses. The proximal palmar metacarpal region should be palpated with the horse in the standing and flexed positions to differentiate pain in this region from carpal pain. The superficial digital flexor tendon should be carefully palpated to detect enlargement and pain, because horses with proximal superficial digital flexor tendonitis often manifest a positive response to carpal flexion. However, swelling of the superficial digital flexor tendon is easily overlooked because of compression by the extensive palmar retinaculum.

In my experience, the carpal flexion test is the most specific of any flexion test used, and if the test result is positive, carpal *region* pain is highly probable. A positive test result does not always incriminate the carpal joints, and the surrounding soft tissue structures must be kept in mind. A negative test result does not rule out carpal pain. Horses with subchondral bone pain, usually young racehorses with sclerosis of the third carpal bone, often have a negative or equivocal response to flexion. Horses with palmar metacarpal or elbow pain can respond positively.

Diagnostic Analgesia

In many horses, clinical signs and characteristic gait may allow a tentative diagnosis of carpal lameness, but in most horses diagnostic analgesia should be performed. Analgesia of the middle carpal and antebrachiocarpal joints should be performed independently and sequentially. Dorsal intraarticular techniques are most common, but in horses with scurf from previous counterirritant application or dorsal wounds, the palmarolateral pouches are used. Careful selective perineural and intraarticular analgesic techniques should be performed to differentiate between proximal palmar metacarpal pain and authentic carpal pain (see Chapter 10). Intraarticular analgesic techniques are highly specific, but false-negative results may occur.[12] False-positive results may also result because of abolition of carpal sheath pain or proximal palmar metacarpal region pain. Subchondral bone pain may not always be eliminated by intrasynovial deposition of local anesthetic solution, because nerve fibers may be located in bone or travel to the site by another extrasynovial route. The median and ulnar nerve block, although lacking specificity, is useful in horses with suspected carpal region pain that is not abolished by intraarticular techniques.

Laboratory analysis of synovial fluid is reserved for horses in which acute inflammation or infectious arthritis is suspected, but color and viscosity should be evaluated, and abnormalities may help to convince an owner or trainer of a carpal problem. In a normal flexed carpus, fluid does not readily drain from a small-gauge needle, and compression of the joint capsule at a distant site is usually necessary. Horses with effusion have thin synovial fluid that drips spontaneously without compression of the nearby capsule. Horses with true serosanguineous fluid (as opposed to contamination by penetration of capsular or synovial vessels) likely have cartilage damage with exposed subchondral bone or an osteochondral fragment. Hemarthrosis can be caused by trauma or bleeding from a torn intercarpal ligament.

Imaging
Radiography

A minimum of six well-exposed and positioned radiographic images are necessary for comprehensive examination of the carpus, including the dorsopalmar (DPa), lateromedial (LM), dorsal 45° lateral-palmaromedial oblique (DL-PaMO), dorsal 45° medial-palmarolateral oblique (DM-PaLO), and flexed LM images and the dorsoproximal-dorsodistal (tangential, skyline) image of the distal row of carpal bones. The skyline image is most important for assessing subtle radiological changes of the third carpal bone, but well-positioned images are often difficult to obtain. Evaluation of the radial fossa requires flexion of the limb in the sagittal plane with the metacarpal region beneath the antebrachium (Figure 38-1). Lateral positioning of the distal part of the limb results in overlap of the radial fossa of the third carpal bone and the radial carpal bone. The skyline image underestimates the amount of increased radiopacity of the third carpal bone and magnifies normal anatomy and lesions approximately twofold.[13] The skyline image is not a true proximal-to-distal view of the second, third, and fourth carpal bones, and therefore lesions located palmar to the dorsal edge of the radial carpal bone cannot be seen. The skyline image cannot be used to evaluate fracture lines located more than 8 to 10 mm from the dorsal edge of the third carpal bone or to differentiate large osteochondral fragments from frontal slab fractures of the third carpal bone. Additional images, such as the tangential image of the proximal row of carpal bones (used to identify osteochondral fragments and unusually located frontal or sagittal slab fractures), flexed oblique images (e.g., DL-PaMO view with the limb held in flexion for evaluation of the articular surfaces of the third and radial carpal bones), and weight-bearing, oblique images of different obliquity (e.g., off DPa views, used to identify sagittal slab fractures of the third carpal bone) are sometimes useful. Considerable confusion arises in description of oblique images, with the use of terms *lateral* and *medial oblique* instead of naming the images according to the direction of the x-ray beam. To most clinicians, the lateral oblique is equivalent to a DL-PaMO image, but to others it is just the opposite. Follow-up radiographic examination is recommended in 10 to 14 days if fracture is suspected but initial radiological findings are negative or equivocal.

Normal radiological anatomy of the carpus is difficult because carpal bones overlap considerably, bones shift during flexion, and normal radiolucent defects and aberrant carpal bones can be difficult to interpret. In the skyline

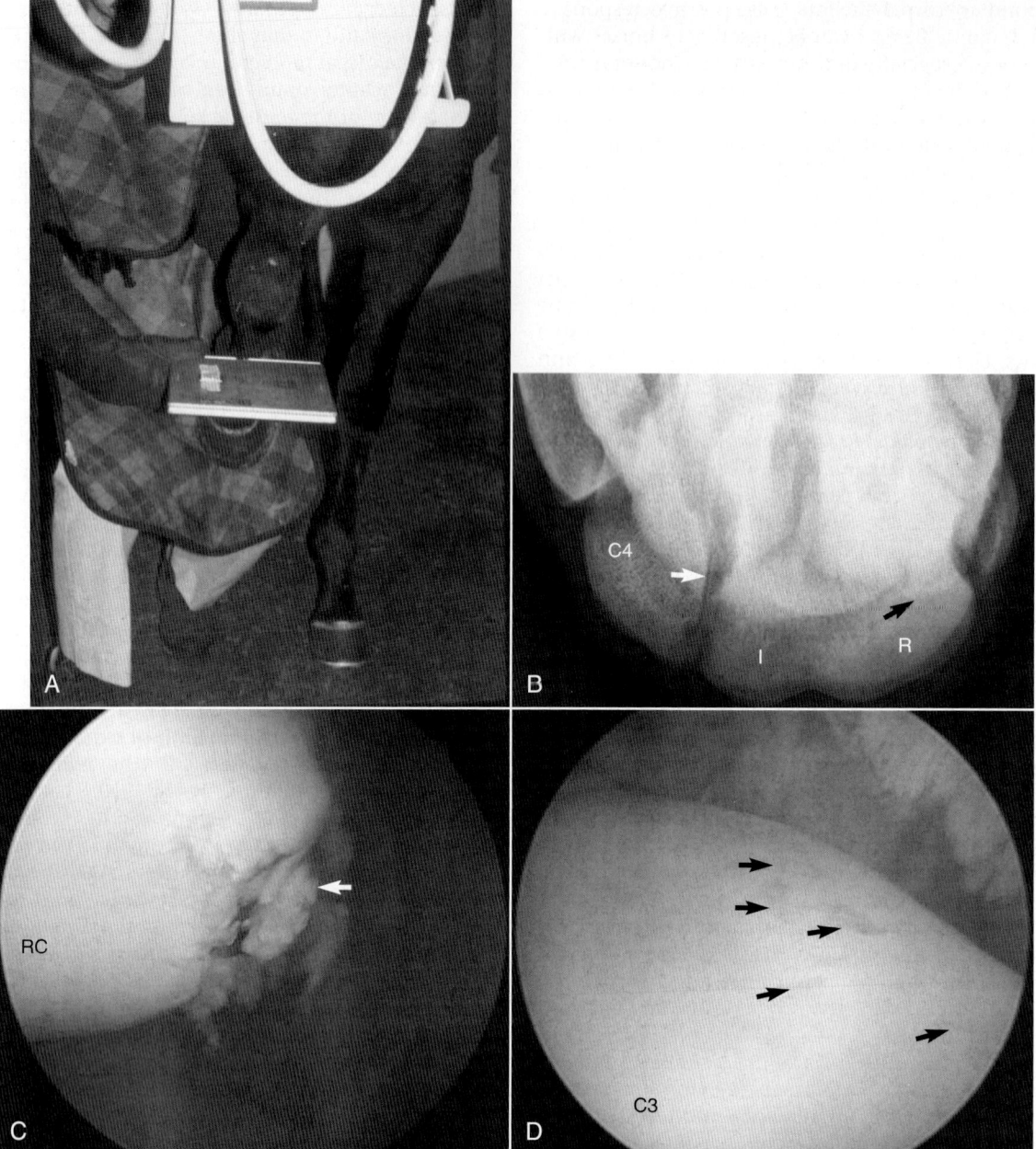

Fig. 38-1 • A, A well-positioned dorsoproximal-dorsodistal (skyline) radiographic image of the distal row of carpal bones requires that the third metacarpal bone be aligned directly under the radius. This makes the radial fossa visible. **B,** Resulting digital radiographic image shows radial (R) and intermediate (I) fossae of the third carpal bone (C3) (medial is to the right and palmar is uppermost). There is dense increased radiopacity of the radial fossa. Sometimes overlap of the normal articulation between the third and fourth (C4) carpal bones appears as a linear radiolucent defect *(white arrow)* in the lateral aspect of C3, a finding confused with sagittal fracture of that bone. Often when digital radiographic techniques are used, fracture lines not visible on conventional radiographs can be seen, such as in this 3-year-old Thoroughbred colt with a small osteochondral fragment of the radial carpal bone *(black arrow)*. The fracture fragment is superimposed on C3 but can readily be seen. **C,** Intraoperative arthroscopic photograph showing the chip fracture *(arrow)* and surrounding cartilage damage on the radial carpal bone (RC) in this horse. **D,** Intraoperative arthroscopic photograph showing thin articular cartilage and partial-thickness cartilaginous defects on C3 *(arrows)* that accompany sclerotic subchondral bone.

image of the distal row, the normal articulation between the third and fourth carpal bones can be superimposed on the lateral aspect of the third carpal bone and confused with a sagittal fracture (see Figure 38-1, *B*). On a DM-PaLO image the normal articulation between the second and third carpal bones should not be confused with a sagittal slab fracture, but this image is essential to diagnose sagittal fracture of the third carpal bone correctly, which runs parallel to this articulation. Radiolucent defects or osseous cystlike lesions are often seen in the ulnar carpal bone and are considered incidental findings, but when they appear in other bones, they can cause lameness regardless of

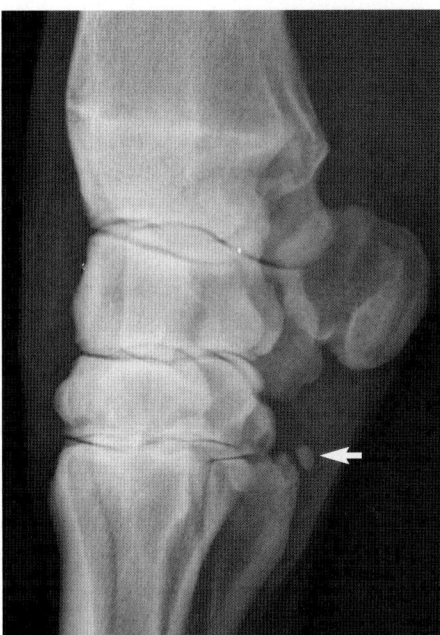

Fig. 38-2 • Dorsal 45° lateral-palmaromedial oblique radiographic image of a left carpus in a 2-year-old Standardbred colt. A fifth carpal bone is present *(arrow)*. Note the lucent area in the proximal aspect of the fourth metacarpal bone. Fifth and first carpal bones should not be confused with osteochondral fragments.

whether communication with a joint exists. In LM and oblique images, the first and fifth carpal bones can be confused with osteochondral fragments. Radiolucent defects in the McII and the McIV often occur in the presence of the first (see Figure 37-7) and fifth (Figure 38-2) carpal bones but are normal. In a flexed LM image the radial carpal bone moves distally relative to the intermediate carpal bone. This normal finding is quite useful in determining the exact positioning of osteochondral fragments or other lesions on the proximal or distal surfaces of the radial and intermediate carpal bones. The flexed LM image is also highly useful for evaluation of the distal dorsal articular surface and subchondral bone of the radial carpal bone. Xeroradiography has largely been discontinued, but computed radiography and digital radiography are available at most institutions and many private practices and yield images superior to those obtained by conventional radiography, but positioning and exposure must still be optimized. Subtle radiological changes can be readily seen in most digital radiographic images, as can fragments, radiolucent defects, and other changes not previously visible on conventional images (see Figure 38-1). Care must be taken not to confuse normal articulations for fractures.

Computed tomography (CT) is available at some institutions and private referral hospitals and can be of value to determine fracture configuration and the presence of comminution, such as that demonstrated in a recent report of an Arabian filly with carpal instability, in which comminution that was not seen when digital radiography was used was confirmed with CT.[14] Magnetic resonance imaging (MRI) has potential to be useful in the diagnosis of carpal region soft tissue and bony injuries but may have limited value because it is currently difficult to position a horse within some magnets to comprehensively evaluate the entire carpal region. Through use of ex vivo MRI, minor cartilage lesions and sclerotic subchondral bone have readily been seen in intact cadaveric specimens.[15] Magnetic resonance (MR) contrast arthrography has been compared with arthroscopy and gross necropsy examination to evaluate and define the lateral palmar outpouching of the middle carpal joint.[16] All structures of the palmarolateral outpouching including portions of the lateral collateral and lateral palmar intercarpal ligaments were visible in MR images, and information obtained compared favorably with arthroscopic examination performed after synovectomy using a motorized intraarticular blade.[16] Ultrasonographic examination of the carpus can be useful to determine the extent of soft tissue damage, to determine if wounds or fistulous tracts communicate with carpal joints, and to diagnose extensor and digital flexor tendon injury, carpal tenosynovitis, and desmitis. Using ultrasonographic examination, the body and division into medial and lateral branches of the medial palmar intercarpal ligament could be seen from a dorsal approach, and the technique may be useful to image horses suspected of having injury of the ligament.[17]

Scintigraphy

Scintigraphy is especially useful to diagnose early stress-related subchondral bone injury and differentiate carpal lesions from those of the proximal metacarpal region (see Figure 19-19). A common finding in young racehorses is carpal lameness localized by clinical signs and diagnostic analgesia with negative or equivocal radiological abnormalities. Focal areas of increased radiopharmaceutical uptake (IRU) are often found unilaterally or bilaterally, most commonly in the third carpal bone (see Figure 19-16). Scintigraphy can be used to verify or refute the importance of sclerosis in the third carpal bone. Scintigraphy is useful in diagnosing unusual fractures of the palmar aspect of the third carpal bone, corner fractures or table surface collapse of the third carpal bone or other carpal bones, and lesions that are not apparent or are located in obscure areas not depicted radiologically. Focal areas of IRU occur with many carpal injuries, and although sensitivity is high, the specificity of scintigraphic images is low and differentiation of specific types of injuries is difficult. Scintigraphy is most useful in localizing the site of injury, based on which additional radiographic images are obtained, or rest is recommended, followed by repeated radiographic examination.

In general, scintigraphic examination is used when lameness is localized but a specific diagnosis cannot be made. In racehorses referred for evaluation of poor performance and obscure high-speed lameness, comprehensive scintigraphic examination of all limbs often reveals focal areas of IRU in the carpus, even when evidence of overt lameness is lacking. Areas of IRU are in locations typical for horses to develop osteochondral fragments and signs of OA. Whether these areas of IRU represent sources of pain causing high-speed or subtle lameness is unknown, but often radiological evidence of bone modeling (increased radiopacity, marginal osteophytes) or incomplete osteochondral fragments exists. Treadmill exercise of previously untrained horses has resulted in a significant IRU,[18] a finding indicating scintigraphy can be useful to monitor skeletal response to exercise in normal horses. Mild IRU is seen as an adaptive response to bone modeling associated with exercise. In contrast, earlier work in normal horses showed exercise significantly increased subchondral bone density and uptake of radiopharmaceutical in the McIII condyles, but neither parameter increased significantly in carpal bones.[19] More recently, in horses undergoing exercise after experimentally induced OA of the middle carpal joint, scintigraphic changes (IRU) were significantly correlated with lameness and increased beyond the normal adaptive response seen in association with exercise.[20]

Diagnostic Arthroscopy

Specific diagnosis is usually made before surgery, and in most racehorses arthroscopy is interventional rather than diagnostic. When results of thorough clinical, radiographic, and scintigraphic examinations are combined, a specific site of injury is usually identified. In racehorses, lameness of the carpus without scintigraphic or radiological abnormalities is unusual. Lack of subchondral bone involvement leads the veterinarian to suspect soft tissue diseases such as synovitis and intercarpal ligament tearing. In these horses, careful examination of the proximal palmar metacarpal region and carpal canal should be performed to avoid inadvertent misdiagnosis. Arthroscopic examination then is used to eliminate primary cartilage damage or intercarpal ligament tearing, but often arthroscopic findings can be unrewarding. Without overt cartilage damage the prognosis is favorable, so information gained by arthroscopic examination is useful, even if a primary diagnosis cannot be made. In sports horses the frequency of carpal joint injury is less than in racehorses but arthroscopy has proved invaluable for identification of focal full-thickness cartilage defects in the middle carpal joint and palmar intercarpal ligament injury. Recently, arthroscopic approaches to the palmarolateral and palmaromedial outpouchings of the antebrachiocarpal and middle carpal joints were refined, and it was proposed that approaches to these pouches would be useful to remove fracture fragments and to evaluate palmar intercarpal ligaments.[21] I have used approaches to these joints to remove fragments from both the antebrachiocarpal and middle carpal joints, the results of which are discussed subsequently.

In horses with scintigraphic evidence of IRU and those with OA but without radiological confirmation of osteochondral fragmentation, arthroscopic examination usually reveals cartilage damage, the extent of which can be graded. Prognosis is inversely related to degree of cartilage damage (see Figures 23-7 and 38-1). Occult osteochondral fragments, most commonly involving the third and radial carpal bones, and intercarpal ligament tearing are found frequently in these horses (see Figure 23-4).

SPECIFIC CONDITIONS OF THE CARPUS

Osteoarthritis

OA is the most common carpal problem, but clear differentiation of OA from osteochondral fragmentation is difficult, because both problems are intertwined. Horses with osteochondral fragments often develop OA, and horses with early OA, and some with chronic OA, develop osteochondral fragments. Pathogenesis of OA and osteochondral fragmentation appears similar if not identical in some horses, but OA of the equine carpus has two forms. The most common form is seen in racehorses or ex-racehorses

that initially develop stress-related subchondral bone injury of the middle carpal and antebrachiocarpal joints that leads to, or accompanies, overlying cartilage damage and osteochondral fragmentation (see Figure 38-1). A second form of OA develops in nonracehorses and is less common. Horses are usually middle aged or older, but occasionally it occurs in younger horses. Typical clinical and radiological evidence of OA exists, but osteochondral fragments are unusual (see Chapters 61 and 84).

OA in racehorses develops from a continuum of stress-related subchondral bone injury and cartilage damage, resulting from impact loading of the carpal bones during training and racing. This process has been studied most thoroughly in the third carpal bone but also occurs in other bones of the middle carpal and antebrachiocarpal joints. Sclerosis of the dorsal aspect of the third carpal bone is an adaptive response in racehorses.[23,24] With continued loading the third carpal bone becomes densely sclerotic, and in this stage the response becomes maladaptive or nonadaptive and pathological. Subchondral changes precede those in overlying cartilage, a finding seen experimentally[25] and clinically during arthroscopic examination in horses with primary stress-related subchondral bone injury (see Figure 38-1). Sclerotic subchondral bone may induce overlying cartilage damage from abnormal shear forces existing between normal and sclerotic areas.[26] In most horses sclerosis leads to areas of resorption and necrosis, which then lead to osteochondral fragmentation and eventually to more advanced OA.[6,23,27,28] A possible explanation for bone failure is the lack of support of overlying sclerotic subchondral bone by structurally weakened underlying trabecular bone.[29] When carpal bone morphology and metabolism were studied in TB racehorses and unraced controls, racehorses were found to have a net increase in bone formation, leading to stiffer, sclerotic subchondral bone; but in addition, they had increased bone collagen synthesis and remodeling in adjacent trabecular bone that may have been structurally weakened.[29] Because many of the changes in early OA in racehorses are mechanically induced, factors such as faulty conformation, intense exercise programs, and differences between racing breeds alter the rate of development and severity of OA. The pathological process continues, and some horses develop OA without osteochondral fragments, whereas others develop osteochondral fragments initially and then OA secondarily.

In many racehorses extensive OA and osteochondral fragmentation lead to retirement, but some are able to compete in other sporting events. Progressive OA can then develop later in life. In middle-aged to old nonracehorses, primary OA develops without stress-related subchondral bone injury, high-impact loading, or development of osteochondral fragmentation. This condition can be seen in Western performance horses, other sports horses, or even in horses and ponies used for pleasure riding. Often severe radiological evidence of OA is seen on initial examination when lameness is subtle (Figure 38-3). In fact, it has been proposed that the threshold of pain in riding horses with severe OA of the antebrachiocarpal joint may be higher than in those with similar conditions of the middle carpal joint, because observation of lameness by owners of these horses was a late event.[30] Faulty conformation such as carpus valgus, back at the knee, or bench knee is seen

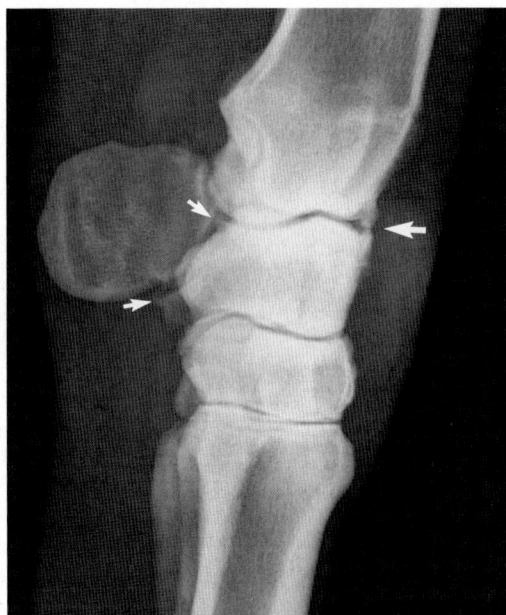

Fig. 38-3 • Lateromedial digital radiographic image of the right carpus of an aged Quarter Horse gelding with advanced osteoarthritis of the antebrachiocarpal joint. Extensive marginal osteophyte formation in both the dorsal *(large arrow)* and palmar *(small arrows)* aspects of the joint can be seen. It is often difficult to determine if osteophytes represent osteoarthritic change or are actually small osteochondral fragments, but the close interrelationship of the most common causes of carpal lameness can be seen.

in some horses, but in others neither mechanical nor training-related factors are present. OA in these horses can involve the antebrachiocarpal and middle carpal joints together or separately, but when disease involves the carpometacarpal joint, chronic and severe lameness develops (see Figure 3-2).

Clinical Signs and Diagnosis

Clinical signs of OA vary depending on age and use of horse, but they are similar to those of other carpal diseases. Classic signs of OA, such as obvious lameness, typical carpal gait, effusion, and a painful response to static and dynamic flexion, may be present, particularly in horses with advanced OA and in old horses with severe changes, but clinical signs can be subtle in young racehorses. In racehorses with early OA, historical information such as lugging in or out, being on a line, or poor performance may be present. Effusion varies, and absence of this clinical sign does not preclude the carpus as the source of pain. Carpal lameness was common in young STB racehorses, occurring in 28% of horses in training, and was attributed to subchondral bone pain and early sclerosis, because in most horses there was little to no effusion of the middle carpal joint.[31] Overall, carpal lameness was the most common cause for more than 1 month of rest (wastage) and was thought to be accentuated by speed training and poor forelimb conformation.[31] Racehorses in early training are prone to develop effusion primarily of the middle carpal joint, but the antebrachiocarpal joint can also be involved. Effusion may be most evident after work, but lameness usually is not present. Effusion usually results from strain of soft tissues, such as intercarpal ligaments or the joint

capsule, but in horses with more advanced OA, effusion represents inflammation caused by continued cartilage damage. Clinical signs resolve after a brief period of rest or reduction in training. Most commonly, racehorses with early OA manifest clinical signs later in training as a 2-year-old or when racing begins.

Diagnosis should be confirmed using diagnostic analgesia of the involved joint(s). In horses with severe OA, complete resolution of lameness may not occur until median and ulnar blocks are performed. After pain in the primary limb has been abolished, lameness may be seen in the contralateral limb, indicating bilateral carpal lameness.

Radiological evidence of OA in young horses is often lacking, but increased radiopacity of the third carpal bone may be seen in a skyline image (see discussion of small osteochondral fragmentation). Early radiological changes include mild enthesophyte formation, most common on the radial carpal bone, and subtle marginal osteophytes on the carpal bones and distal radius. In horses with advanced OA, marginal osteophytes and enthesophytes become numerous and large, sometimes causing obvious visible bony swelling (see Figure 38-3). Loss of joint space occurs late in OA, but it is not an obvious radiological sign. Osteochondral fragments may be present, can be numerous, and may have occurred earlier during a racing career or can develop when marginal osteophytes break. Radiological evaluation of the contralateral carpus should be performed.

Scintigraphic examination is an excellent tool for diagnosis of early OA in racehorses, but IRU must be differentiated from mild normal adaptive increased uptake of radiopharmaceutical.[18-20,31] Initially, focal areas of IRU are located on one side of a joint, such as in the third carpal bone, but later, subchondral IRU can be seen diffusely in one or more joints. Arthroscopic examination may be useful to establish prognosis and to evaluate possible soft tissue injury, such as intercarpal ligament tearing, and may be useful therapeutically.

Management

Management of OA is discussed in Chapter 84. Because pathogenesis involves stress-related subchondral bone injury, an important part of management of OA in racehorses involves stress relief by enforced rest or a reduction in training or racing intensity. Racehorses (STBs) without obvious radiological changes are given 2 to 3 weeks of hand walking or walking in the jog cart, nonsteroidal antiinflammatory drugs (NSAIDs), and local therapy such as cold water hosing or icing. Topical counterirritation is still a popular management technique administered to young racehorses early in training. Intraarticular administration of hyaluronan, with or without a short-acting corticosteroid, may help in horses with synovitis, but it is of limited value if the primary source of pain is subchondral bone with intact overlying cartilage. In racehorses with advanced sclerosis of the third carpal bone and early enthesophyte and marginal osteophyte formation, extended rest of 3 to 4 months is recommended. However, economic factors may dictate that these horses remain in training; thus work intensity often is decreased and horses receive a single or a series of intraarticular injections with hyaluronan or polysulfated glycosaminoglycans (PSGAGs). Horses with radiologically apparent osteochondral fragments are surgical candidates, but postoperative progression of OA and recurrence of fragmentation are common. As OA progresses in horses with or without osteochondral fragments, numerous intraarticular injections, often including methylprednisolone acetate, may be necessary to reduce inflammation, but if training and racing continue, OA progresses in an accelerated fashion. Bisphosphonate administration in combination with a modification in exercise or rest may have a beneficial effect, but more clinical study is necessary.

A syndrome has been recognized in ponies with OA of the antebrachiocarpal joint. These ponies are presented for examination because of repetitive stumbling when ridden. There is generally resentment of carpal flexion and restricted flexion, although no obvious lameness. Although the response to intraarticular analgesia may be disappointing, the response to intraarticular medication is often good. Although historically sclerosis of the third carpal bone has been considered a disease of the racehorse, it has also been recognized as a cause of intermittent lameness in both endurance horses and event horses. Focal areas of full thickness cartilage loss in the medial aspect of the middle carpal joint have been identified arthroscopically in a small number of show jumpers that had no localizing clinical signs, lameness that was improved by intraarticular analgesia, and no detectable radiological abnormality. Some sports horses with carpal OA show lameness only when ridden and not under other circumstances. In ex-racehorses or nonracehorse sports horses with primary OA, radiological changes may be advanced when lameness is first recognized, because OA is chronic and well tolerated. Conservative management is recommended and includes rest, NSAID therapy, and intraarticular injections. Horses with radiological evidence of large intact or broken osteophytes or old osteochondral fragments may be considered candidates for arthroscopic surgery, but although arthroscopic examination may be important to establish prognosis, surgical removal of osteophytes and old osteochondral fragments does not often result in long-term clinical improvement and may accelerate progression of OA (see Figure 38-3). Involvement of the carpometacarpal joint warrants a guarded prognosis.

Prognosis depends on the number of joints and limbs affected, rate of progression of clinical signs, severity of cartilage damage, presence of osteochondral fragments, and level of competition. Most racehorses with early OA and even those with radiological evidence of osteophytes and enthesophytes can race at some level, if the horses raced before diagnosis. Horses with advanced changes before racing begins, particularly those with faulty conformation, are unlikely to race but can be sound enough to perform other sporting activities. Valuable horses with severe OA, such as broodmares or breeding stallions, may be candidates for partial (intercarpal) or pancarpal arthrodesis.

Trauma to the craniodistal aspect of the radius and dorsal aspect of the carpus may result in the rapid development of periarticular new bone on the distocranial aspect of the radius and the dorsal aspect of the intermediate carpal bone. There is often associated diffuse soft tissue swelling. Lameness may be absent or mild, but there is marked resentment of carpal flexion, and flexion may induce moderate-to-severe lameness. I speculate that this occurs because of pressure mediated by the extensor tendons on this new bone.

Osteoarthritis of the Carpometacarpal Joint

Primary osteoarthritis of the carpometacarpal joint is unusual to rare but occurs primarily in old horses, especially Arabians,[32] and is insidious and progressive (see Figure 3-2 and Chapter 37).

Osteochondral Fragmentation
Small Fragments

Osteochondral fragmentation is a disease primarily of racehorses or ex-racehorses, and pathogenesis is identical to that described for OA. I prefer to use the terms *carpal osteochondral fragments* (osteochondral fragments) and *osteochondral fragmentation* instead of *carpal chip fractures* to emphasize the importance of pathogenesis. The term *chip fracture* implies a single event traumatic injury. Although trauma plays a role, osteochondral fragments are not single-event injuries but are the end result of stress-related subchondral bone injury caused by repetitive loading, initially an adaptive response but later becoming nonadaptive remodeling and pathological.[23,25,27,28] Sites located dorsally are prone to develop osteochondral fragments. Osteochondral fragments differ in size and number of joints affected. Small osteochondral fragments are those that involve one joint surface, such as either the middle carpal or the antebrachiocarpal joints. Large osteochondral fragments that involve two joint surfaces are called slab fractures. Often, advanced changes occur in subchondral bone, such as sclerosis of the third carpal bone or other evidence of modeling or remodeling that preceded development of lameness and osteochondral fragments, findings that support the concept that osteochondral fragments are not single-event injuries. The antebrachiocarpal joint is more susceptible to injury from supraphysiological loads or acute overload injury,[6] particularly in fatigued horses, but fractures still occur associated with pathological conditions of the bone. Palmar carpal osteochondral fragments, such as those involving the accessory carpal bone or other bones of the antebrachiocarpal joint, occur as single event injuries such as falls, carpal hyperextension, or recovery from general anesthesia. Palmar carpal fragments in the middle carpal joint are often seen in combination with other dorsally located small or large osteochondral fragments (see later).[22]

In my experience, faulty conformation such as back at the knee predisposes TB and STB racehorses to develop osteochondral fragments, and trotters are more at risk than pacers. However, in a study attempting to evaluate the role of back-at-the-knee conformation in the development of osteochondral fragments in 21 horses, no differences in carpal angle were found compared with 10 horses without osteochondral fragments.[33] No association between back-at-the-knee conformation and the development of carpal lameness was found in recent studies in TBs and Quarter Horses (QHs), but elite horses were studied, and those with faulty conformation may have been excluded.[34,35] Somewhat surprising, mild carpus valgus conformation was proposed to be protective against carpal lameness, and an association between increased humeral length and carpal lameness was found (see Chapter 4).[30]

Carpal osteochondral fragments occur in defined locations in all racehorses, but distribution varies depending on the type of racehorse. In the STB, osteochondral fragments occur almost exclusively in the medial aspect of the middle carpal joint and rarely in the antebrachiocarpal joint.[36] Although rare, osteochondral fragments in the STB antebrachiocarpal joint are most common in trotters and usually involve the distal aspect of the radius. In the middle carpal joint we found a nearly equal distribution of osteochondral fragments between the radial and third carpal bones, but in another study those of the third carpal bone outnumbered osteochondral fragments of the radial carpal bone by 2:1.[36,37] The preponderance of osteochondral fragments in the medial aspect of the middle carpal joint in the STB is interesting, because training involves clockwise and counterclockwise exercise, whereas racing is counterclockwise. The assumption is that counterclockwise direction of training and racing places asymmetrical and uneven load distribution on each forelimb and may predispose the lateral aspect of the left forelimb and medial aspect of the right forelimb to compression injury. In two STB studies a nearly equal distribution of osteochondral fragments was noted between left and right middle carpal joints,[36,37] but in another study osteochondral fragments of the third carpal bone occurred more commonly in the right carpus.[28] Trotters were more likely to have right osteochondral fragments and had significantly more osteochondral fragments of the third carpal bone than the radial carpal bone compared with pacers.[28]

In TBs in North America, third carpal bone fractures occur more commonly in the right carpus, but considering all small osteochondral fragments, the distribution between left and right is similar.[27,28,37] Palmar osteochondral fragments were more common in the right carpus, reflecting the preponderance of TB racehorses in that study and the fact that most fragments originated from co-existent dorsally located small or large osteochondral fragments.[22] In TB and QH racehorses, osteochondral fragments are commonly seen in the middle carpal and antebrachiocarpal joints.[37-39] These breeds in North America have a predilection for development of osteochondral fragments in the lateral aspect of the left antebrachiocarpal joint and the medial aspect of the right middle carpal joint, a distribution supporting the concept that osteochondral fragments develop on the compression side during counterclockwise training and racing. Overall, in TB and QH racehorses the most common sites for osteochondral fragments are the proximal aspect of the third and distal aspect of the radial carpal bones,[22,37,39] followed by the proximal aspect of the intermediate carpal bone and the distal lateral aspect of the radius. Osteochondral fragments often develop on apposing surfaces, supporting the concept that certain sites are biomechanically at risk. This may be evident radiologically, but in some horses apposing fragmentation is identified only at arthroscopic surgery, and both limbs should be examined radiographically routinely, even if clinical signs are absent. Osteochondral fragments can be found at numerous sites in one or both carpi. Differences between racing breeds in distribution of osteochondral fragments may be explained by gait and sites predisposed to stress-related subchondral bone injury. Almost all STB osteochondral fragments occur medially, equally in both middle carpal joints. Most forelimb scintigraphic changes in STBs occur medially, indicating that the medial aspect in both forelimbs is at risk for stress-related subchondral bone injury. Classic training programs include many miles each day of jogging (trotting or pacing) clockwise (the wrong way of the track), and training one to two times each week counterclockwise (the right way). Although all speed is performed in one direction, STBs jog many more miles in the other direction, and the number of loading cycles may be more important than speed. Direction of training and racing is not the only factor influencing fracture location because QHs and TBs have a similar distribution yet race differently. The two-beat trot and pace and a more caudal center of balance with a cart and driver result in reduced carpal loads in STBs at speed compared with galloping racing breeds. The low occurrence of osteochondral fragments in the antebrachiocarpal joint of STBs may reflect absence of supraphysiological loads. Racing speeds in the STB are lower than in the TB and substantially lower than in the QH. Fatigue rather than speed of racing may be a factor.

Clinical Signs

Lameness in horses with small osteochondral fragments varies from subtle to severe. In most horses, prominent-to-severe lameness is seen immediately after the fracture occurs, but subtle prodromal clinical signs are often present. Historically, horses may have been treated for suspected carpal lameness, may be on a line (STB), may lug in or out, or may fail to take a lead or change leads. Degree of lameness depends on location and number of osteochondral fragments and whether osteochondral fragments are present bilaterally. Horses with third carpal bone osteochondral fragments, and in particular incomplete fractures, show more pronounced lameness than those with osteochondral fragments elsewhere. Lameness is increased when the affected limb is on the outside of the circle in horses with osteochondral fragments in the middle carpal joint, but this response varies in those with osteochondral fragments in the antebrachiocarpal joint. TB and QH racehorses with osteochondral fragments of the distal, lateral aspect of the radius or proximal aspect of the intermediate carpal bone may show only mild signs of lameness. I have always thought the antebrachiocarpal joint was more "forgiving" than the middle carpal joint, with horses able to endure more substantial injury or larger osteochondral fragments, without showing overt signs of lameness, an observation shared by others.[30] Horses with bilateral osteochondral fragments may show minimal overt lameness. Horses with lameness inappropriately severe for the location, number, or size of fragment(s) present may have substantial cartilage damage.

There is generally effusion and heat over the carpus, but in horses with incomplete fractures, clinical signs can be subtle. Palpation may reveal a focal painful response over the site of fragmentation, and occasionally fragments can be palpated directly. Degree of flexion varies, but usually the response to a carpal flexion test is positive. Signs of OA including joint capsule fibrosis and enthesophyte production are common, particularly in horses with chronic lameness. Arthrocentesis usually reveals serosanguineous fluid, particularly if lameness is acute. Intraarticular analgesia usually, but not always, abolishes signs of pain.

Radiographic examination is usually diagnostic, and all views should be obtained. In STBs abnormalities are usually only detected in DL-PaMO and LM images and a skyline image of the distal row of carpal bones. All common osteochondral fragment locations should be carefully evaluated.

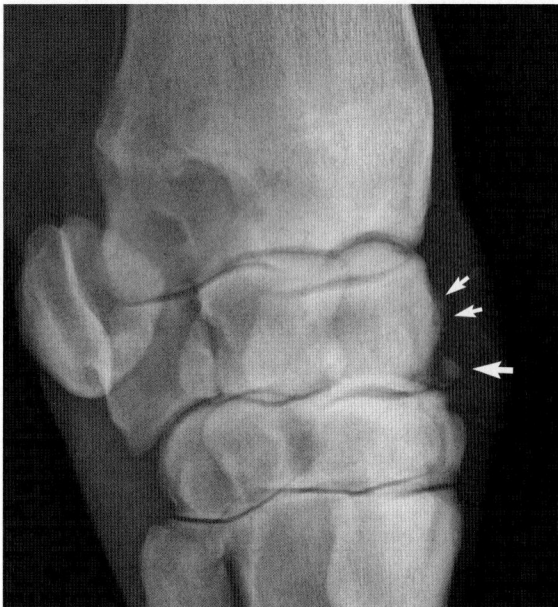

Fig. 38-4 • Dorsal 45° lateral-palmaromedial oblique radiographic image of a Thoroughbred racehorse with a typical small, displaced, distal radial carpal osteochondral fragment *(large arrow),* the most common small osteochondral fragment. The presence of entheseous new bone formation *(small arrows)* at the joint capsule attachment indicates that damage of the radial carpal bone is chronic.

Fragments involving the distal aspect of the radial carpal bone are most visible on a DL-PaMO image and can vary in size, can be displaced or nondisplaced, and may extend to the level of the joint capsule attachment (Figure 38-4). Osteochondral fragments involving the third carpal bone most commonly affect the radial fossa and can be seen on the DL-PaMO, LM, and skyline images (Figure 38-5). Small osteochondral fragments involve only the middle carpal joint surface and usually break out dorsally, near the joint capsule attachment on the third carpal bone. It is important to differentiate small osteochondral fragments from frontal or sagittal slab fractures. Third carpal bone osteochondral fragments can be singular or numerous, involve only the radial or intermediate (rare) fossa or both, can be complete or incomplete, or can involve the medial (most common) or lateral corners of the bone. Medial corner fragments of the third carpal bone may resemble subchondral lucency and sagittal slab fracture, so other views must be carefully interpreted. Authentic sagittal slab fractures must be confirmed using a DM-PaLO image. Osteochondral fragments of the distal, lateral aspect of the radius are the largest of the small osteochondral fragments and are often bipartite. The large dorsal fragment is separated from the parent radius by a small separate fragment in the interposed trough (Figure 38-6). The large dorsal fragment can extend proximal to the joint capsule attachment on the distal lateral aspect of the radius. Concomitant osteochondral fragments frequently involve the proximal medial aspect of the intermediate carpal bone. Osteochondral fragments of the proximal aspect of the intermediate carpal bone may occur alone or in combination with osteochondral fragments of the distal lateral aspect of the radius (Figure 38-7). Other, less common osteochondral fragments do occur alone but usually in combination with

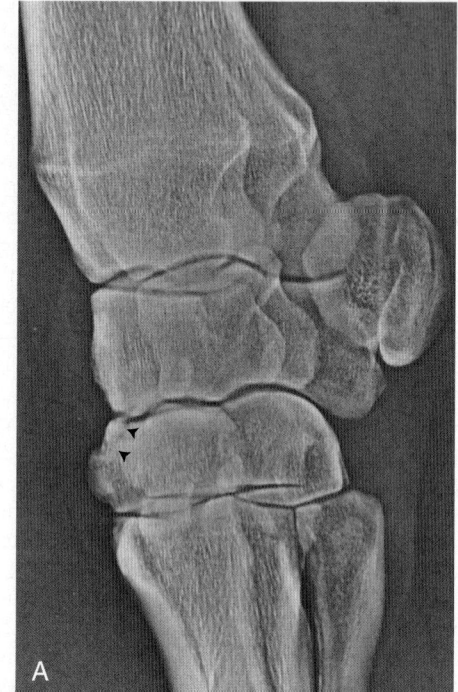

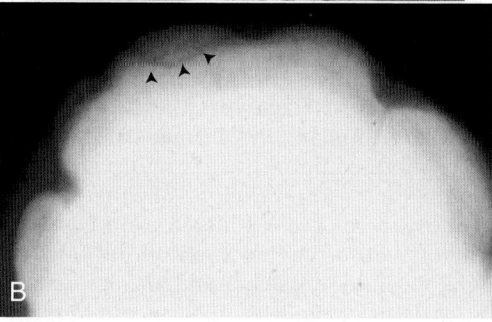

Fig. 38-5 • Dorsolateral-palmaromedial oblique xeroradiographic **(A)** and skyline radiographic **(B)** images of a horse with a third carpal bone small osteochondral fragment. The osteochondral fragment *(arrowheads)* breaks out of the dorsal aspect of the third carpal bone in the dorsolateral-palmaromedial oblique image, confirmation that it does not span both articular surfaces of the third carpal bone.

other osteochondral fragments. Evidence of OA such as enthesophytes and marginal osteophytes may be present (see Figure 38-4). Sclerosis of the third carpal bone is common in horses with osteochondral fragments of the third and radial carpal bones. Mild sclerosis is a normal adaptive response to training, and the presence of sclerosis as a solitary finding is not diagnostic of carpal lameness. Degree of sclerotic change is important, because in my experience a positive correlation exists between the degree of the third carpal bone sclerosis and the extent of cartilage damage on the third and radial carpal bones. However, a radiological study showed no significant relationship between degree of increased radiopacity and prognosis,[40] and although there was a continuous increase in the density of the third carpal bone in STB trotters in race training, increased radiopacity was of limited value in predicting carpal lameness.[41] More recently, however, carpal lameness was more likely in STBs with higher grades of third carpal bone increased radiopacity.[42]

Scintigraphic examination is an excellent method to diagnose incomplete or occult osteochondral fragments

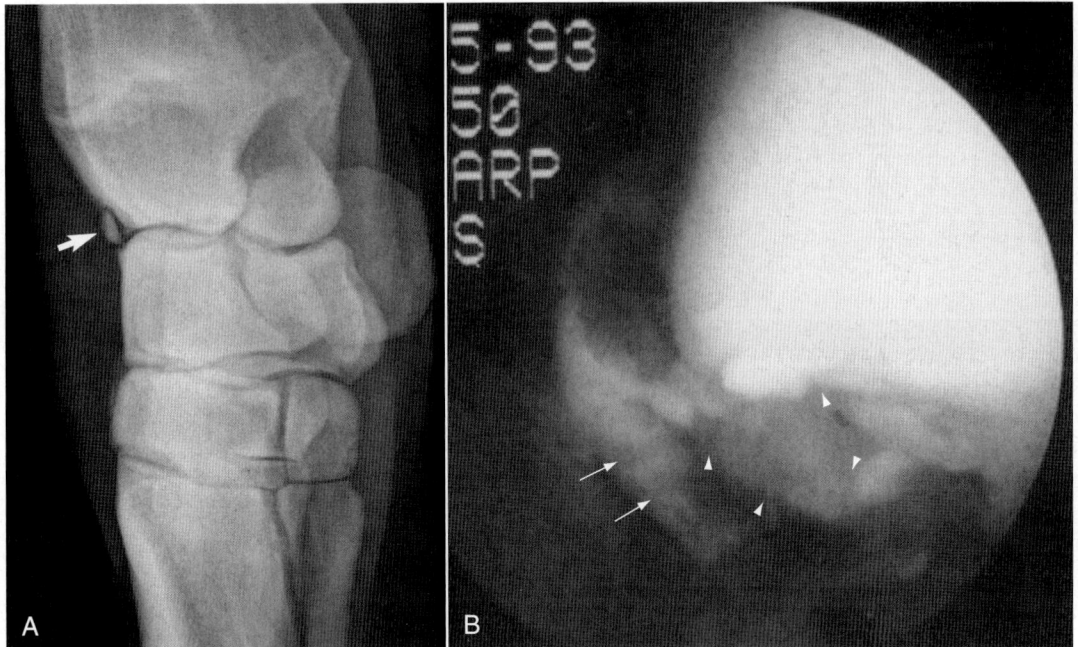

Fig. 38-6 • **A,** Dorsal 45° medial-palmarolateral oblique radiographic image of a right carpus showing typical distal lateral radius small osteochondral fragment *(arrow)* in a Thoroughbred. **B,** Intraoperative photograph (dorsal is to the left; proximal is up) shows large dorsal fragment *(arrows)* separated from the parent radius by a small, interposed wedge-shaped fragment *(arrowheads).*

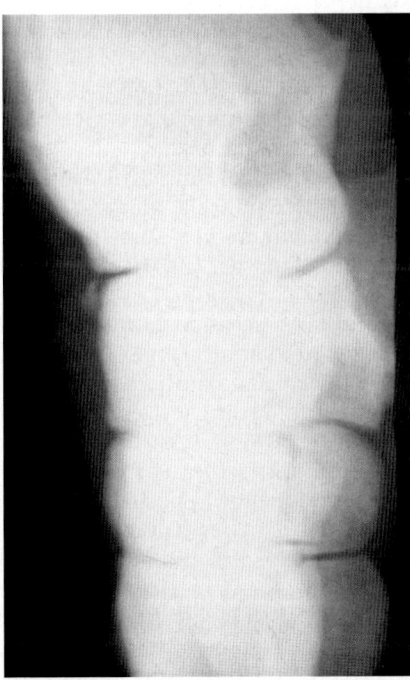

Fig. 38-7 • Dorsomedial-palmarolateral oblique radiographic image of a typical osteochondral fragment of the proximal aspect of the intermediate carpal bone. These fragments often appear in combination with osteochondral fragments of the distal lateral aspect of the radius and vary in size, but they generally occur slightly more medially than those of the distal, lateral aspect of the radius.

and to evaluate other sites of stress-related subchondral bone injury in the involved or contralateral carpus. Focal IRU on one side of a joint seen in several scintigraphic images, including a flexed dorsal image, can help pinpoint exact location of osteochondral fragments.

Management

The ideal treatment is surgical removal of osteochondral fragments, because unstable surfaces and fragment movement predispose to additional synovitis and development of osteoarthritis (see Figure 23-7). Fragments left in place to heal in displaced fashion cause uneven joint surfaces and are prone to refracture. Arthroscopic examination also allows evaluation and grading of cartilage damage and intercarpal ligament integrity and identification of occult fragments. However, factors such as economic value, racing class, and time of year relative to upcoming races and location of osteochondral fragments are relevant. Horses not worthy of arthroscopic surgery are managed with short-term rest and intraarticular injections of hyaluronan and corticosteroids, or they are given 3 to 6 months of rest. When conservative management procedures are used, fractures develop fibrous unions and become stable, but they are usually displaced and may resemble marginal osteophytes when healed. Many horses that are managed conservatively, especially those with fractures in the antebrachiocarpal joint, return to racing successfully, but recurrence of osteochondral fragments and development of OA are likely. It is difficult to convince owners and trainers to give horses long-term (>6 months) rest. However, rest, with or without arthroscopic surgery, is critical, not only for healing of incomplete fractures or, if osteochondral fragments have been removed, the fracture site, but also for healing of the surrounding cartilage and subchondral bone. Horses with incomplete osteochondral fragments are candidates for conservative management, but if horses are not given adequate time for fracture healing, recurrence is likely (Figure 38-8). Alternatively, I have recommended arthroscopic surgery and fragment removal in horses with incomplete fractures if I know the client will not opt for long-term rest without surgical intervention. Although

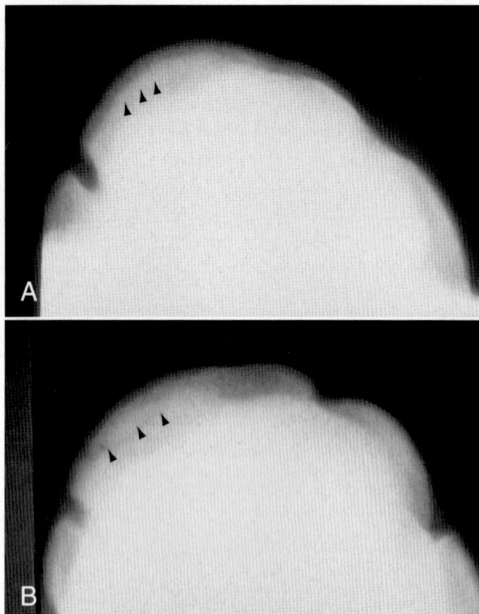

Fig. 38-8 • **A,** Dorsoproximal-dorsodistal (skyline) radiographic image of the distal row of carpal bones of a 2-year-old Standardbred colt with an incomplete osteochondral fragment of the third carpal bone. In this image there is predominantly dense increased radiopacity of the radial fossa, and the faint fracture is difficult to identify *(arrowheads).* **B,** Seven months later, when the horse was 3 years old, lameness and fracture recurred. The horse had been given inadequate rest to allow the fracture to heal completely.

carpal lameness may recur, at least the original osteochondral fragment will not refracture. During arthroscopic surgery, cartilage damage is graded as mild, moderate, severe, or global, and prognosis is inversely proportional to the extent of damage—a clinical finding substantiated in studies in STB, TB, and QH racehorses[36,39] (see Figures 23-4 and 23-7, and Figure 38-1). During arthroscopic surgery, the osteochondral fragment(s) are removed and the surrounding cartilage and bone are curetted, depending on the amount of damage seen. If partial thickness cartilage damage is seen and damage does not extend into subchondral bone past the zone of calcified cartilage, then microfracture can be performed (see Chapter 23). Damage on apposing surfaces is common, and occult osteochondral fragments are often found there or at distant locations. Bilateral carpal arthroscopic surgery is commonly performed in all racing breeds, and in the TB and QH it may be necessary to evaluate all major joints.

After arthroscopic surgery horses are given a progressively increasing exercise program, the length of which depends on severity of damage and location of osteochondral fragments. For instance, in TB racehorses with osteochondral fragments of the distal, lateral aspect of the radius and the proximal aspect of the intermediate carpal bone, I recommend 2 weeks of stall rest, followed by 4 weeks of stall rest with hand walking (or walking in a caged walker), followed by 2 to 4 weeks of turnout or swimming physiotherapy. Lameness is less pronounced initially, and horses appear able to return to work earlier when osteochondral fragments involve the antebrachiocarpal joint rather than the middle carpal joint. In horses with routine distal radial carpal bone and proximal third carpal bone fragments, I recommend 4 weeks of stall rest, followed by 4 weeks of

stall rest with hand walking, followed by 8 weeks of turnout or swimming physiotherapy. In horses with numerous fragments and severe or global cartilage damage, I recommend 4 to 6 months of total rest.

After arthroscopic surgery I recommend the use of intraarticular injections of hyaluronan at 14 and 28 days in horses with mild or moderate cartilage damage, and a series of intraarticular PSGAG injections at 3, 5, and 7 weeks after surgery. I recommend intramuscular administration of PSGAGs once weekly for 8 weeks, beginning 14 days after surgery. Little concrete evidence shows that any form or combination of intraarticular therapy is of long-term benefit for cartilage healing after surgery, although antiinflammatory effects are likely mildly beneficial. Short-term benefit of several intraarticular or parenterally administered products evaluated in an osteochondral fragment model has been shown (see Chapter 84).

Cartilage resurfacing techniques have been used experimentally and in a limited number of horses with osteochondral fragments and OA (see Chapters 23, 63, and 84). Cell-based techniques such as injection of cloned chondrocytes in autogenous fibrin loaded with growth factors appear promising. Microfracture of calcified cartilage appears promising in experimental trials, but seeing horses with partial-thickness cartilage damage is unusual. Subchondral bone is usually already exposed, obviating the need to use this.

Prognosis depends on several factors, including type and age of horse, racing class, limb(s) affected, number and location of osteochondral fragment(s), and amount of cartilage damage. Intuitively, a better prognosis would be expected in the STB than the TB and QH, because load is better shared by the hindlimbs and gait allows compensation by a lateral or diagonal limb. However, in STBs osteochondral fragments often develop later in the nonadaptive remodeling process, when OA is already well beyond that in TBs with comparable lesions. In most racehorses any damage of the third carpal bone is a major limiting factor in prognosis, and because osteochondral fragments of the third carpal bone are common in STBs, overall prognosis for STBs might be expected to be less favorable than for TBs and QHs. The prognosis for horses with lesions in the antebrachiocarpal joint is better than for those in the middle carpal joint, and because osteochondral fragments occur with similar frequency in both joints in TBs and QHs, the overall prognosis is better. The prognosis for return to racing is good to excellent, but the likelihood of racing at the preinjury level is inversely proportional to the degree of cartilage damage. Seventy-four percent of STBs with osteochondral fragments returned to racing after arthroscopic surgery, but only 61% raced at or above the preinjury level. Pacers were more likely than trotters to start a race and to have five starts before and after injury.[36] Kinematic studies show that the pace may slow forelimb fatigue and reduce forelimb load.[43] Median earnings per start decreased significantly after injury and arthroscopic surgery, but horses went significantly faster after surgery.[36]

Of 445 TB and QH racehorses, 303 (68%) raced at a level equal to or better than the preinjury level, but when grouped according to cartilage damage, only 53% of horses with the most severe cartilage damage raced at these levels. Eleven percent of horses had decreased performance and had carpal lameness, 6% developed additional osteochondral fragments, and 2% developed collapsing slab fractures while racing.[36] Prognosis was worse for horses with osteochondral fragments of the third carpal bone.

Palmar Carpal Osteochondral Fragments

Osteochondral fragments can occur in the palmar aspect of the carpus and can result from a single-event injury or can be associated with other osteochondral fragments in the dorsal aspect of the carpal joints. Trauma may result from falling, hitting a fence, or landing with subsequent hyperextension of the carpus or falling when the carpus is flexed (hyperflexion). Palmar carpal injury is one of the more common catastrophic injuries occurring in horses during recovery from general anesthesia (Figure 38-9, *A*). Palmar carpal injury after general anesthesia can be career-limiting or career-ending and often leads to severe OA of the involved carpal joints. In horses that sustain palmar carpal fragments as a result of a traumatic event, osteochondral fragments usually involve the palmar aspect of the radial and intermediate carpal bones and the articular surface of the accessory carpal bone but can involve any of the carpal bones, can be singular or numerous, and occur medially and laterally. Articular osteochondral fragments of the accessory carpal bone are usually comminuted and involve at least two or three pieces.

In horses with known chronic osteochondral fragments in the dorsal aspect of the carpus and those with OA, radiographs occasionally reveal what appear to be small fragments or mineralization in the palmarolateral or palmaromedial aspects of the middle carpal joint (see Figure 38-9, *B*). It was once thought that radiopacities in the palmar aspect of the middle carpal joint were areas of dystrophic mineralization after corticosteroid injections, but it is now known these are most likely small fragments that migrate from the dorsal to the palmar aspect of the joint and occur when training and racing continues in horses with existing osteochondral fragments, which then become macerated. When the condition is observed, cartilage damage is usually extensive, and prognosis is guarded. In a study of 31 racehorses with palmar carpal osteochondral fragments, only 48% of horses returned to racing and earned money, and only 32% had five or more race starts after injury.[22] Horses with numerous fragments had significantly lower earnings and lower performance indices after surgery than those with one fragment, and those with fragments smaller than 3 mm diameter were significantly less likely to return to racing than those with larger fragments.[22] Palmar carpal fragments were most commonly seen in the palmarolateral pouch of the middle carpal joint and in 24 horses were associated with coexistent osteochondral fragmentation in the dorsal aspect of the joint.[22] Seven horses had palmar carpal fragments without associated dorsal fragmentation, and in six of these seven horses fragments involved the palmar aspect of the antebrachiocarpal joint (all involved the proximal aspect of the radial carpal bone).[22] It has been suggested that fragment migration from the dorsal to the palmar aspect of the middle carpal joint occurs because of medial palmar intercarpal ligament injury, an association that I have not found true. No association was found between palmar carpal fragment size or number and medial palmar intercarpal ligament injury.[22]

Lameness is acute in onset, with effusion of the middle carpal or antebrachiocarpal joints. Often the response to static flexion of the carpus is profound. Careful

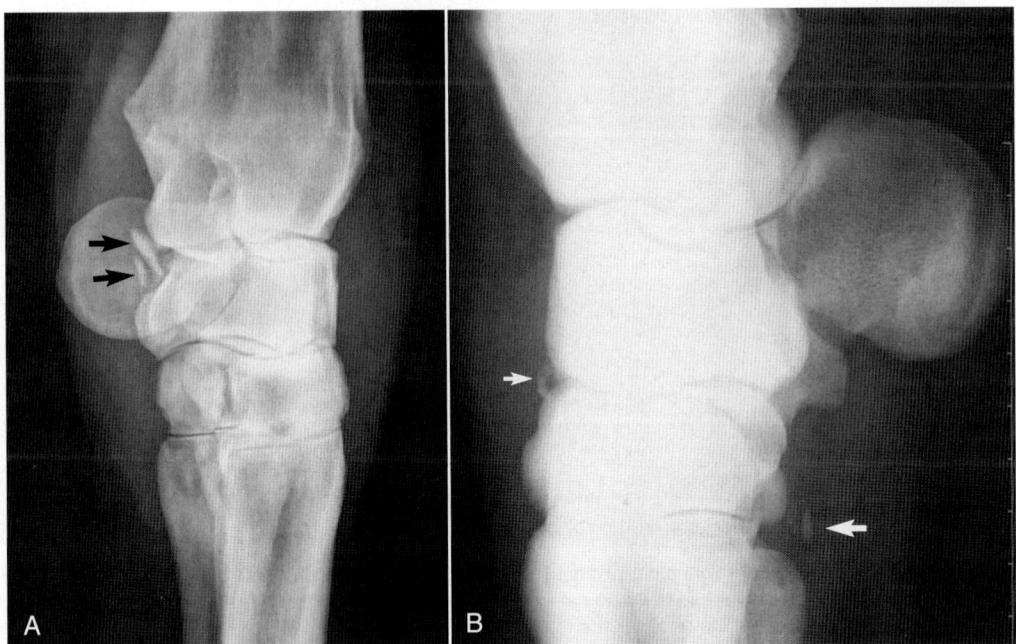

Fig. 38-9 • A, Dorsal 45° medial-palmarolateral digital radiographic image of the left carpus of a horse sustaining a comminuted palmar carpal fracture of the radial carpal bone *(arrows)* and intermediate carpal bones during recovery from general anesthesia. Because of severe lameness this horse was euthanized. **B,** Lateromedial digital radiographic image of a racehorse with palmar carpal osteochondral fragments *(large arrow)* located in the palmarolateral pouch of the middle carpal joint. Fragments have migrated from a primary site of osteochondral fragmentation, the distal dorsal aspect of the radial carpal bone *(small arrow)*. (**A** courtesy David Levine and Eric Parente, Kennett Square, Pennsylvania, United States. **B** courtesy of Liberty Getman, Kennett Square, Pennsylvania, United States.)

interpretation of radiographs is necessary to confirm the presence of osteochondral fragments, locate precisely the parent bone from which the osteochondral fragment arose, and determine the number of fragments. The clinician should recognize that osteochondral fragments in the palmar aspect of the carpus may represent only one aspect of more global damage to the joint(s). Any evidence of fragmentation dorsally, or active OA if trauma occurred at least 10 to 14 days before radiographic examination, is a poor prognostic indicator, because this reflects substantial subchondral bone and cartilage injury dorsally. OA and chronic lameness are inevitable, particularly in horses with palmar carpal injury sustained while jumping or during recovery from general anesthesia. Palmar osteochondral fragments can be removed using arthroscopic surgery or arthrotomy,[44] but access can be difficult. Recent studies have refined the surgical approaches and anatomy of the palmar pouches of the carpal joints and the value of arthroscopic examination.[16,21,22] The palmarolateral pouch of the antebrachiocarpal joint is large, and osteochondral fragments involving the accessory and intermediate carpal bones can be removed from this approach. When removing osteochondral fragments from the palmaromedial or the palmarolateral aspect of the middle carpal joint, both portals must be made within a small joint pouch, making triangulation difficult. Prognosis for future soundness is guarded to fair for racehorses (see earlier). In nonrace-horses, prognosis for horses with single fragments without substantial OA is fair, but it is guarded to poor in those

with substantial instability or bone and cartilage damage at more distant sites.

Large Osteochondral Fragments: Slab Fractures

Slab fractures are defined as fractures that involve a proximal and distal articular surface and thus traverse the entire depth (proximal-distal direction) of the bone. Size and involvement of two articular surfaces differentiate these fractures from small osteochondral fragments. Slab fractures of the third carpal bone are by far the most common form of large osteochondral fragments in the carpus, but slab fractures of the radial, fourth, and intermediate carpal bones occasionally occur. A combination of radial and third carpal bone slab fractures occurs in TB racehorses and may lead to instability and carpal collapse. In most instances, slab fractures develop as a terminal event in the cascade of maladaptive or nonadaptive remodeling changes leading to sclerosis, biomechanical weakness, and subsequent fracture. When slab fractures occur in unusual locations, the possibility of single-event injury must be considered. Slab fractures occur almost exclusively in racehorses.

Frontal (Dorsal) Slab Fractures of the Third Carpal Bone

The most common large osteochondral fragment in the carpus is a slab fracture of the third carpal bone in the frontal (dorsal) plane. A frontal slab fracture of the third carpal bone usually involves the radial fossa, but fractures of the intermediate fossa alone or in combination with fracture of the radial fossa do occur (Figures 38-10 and

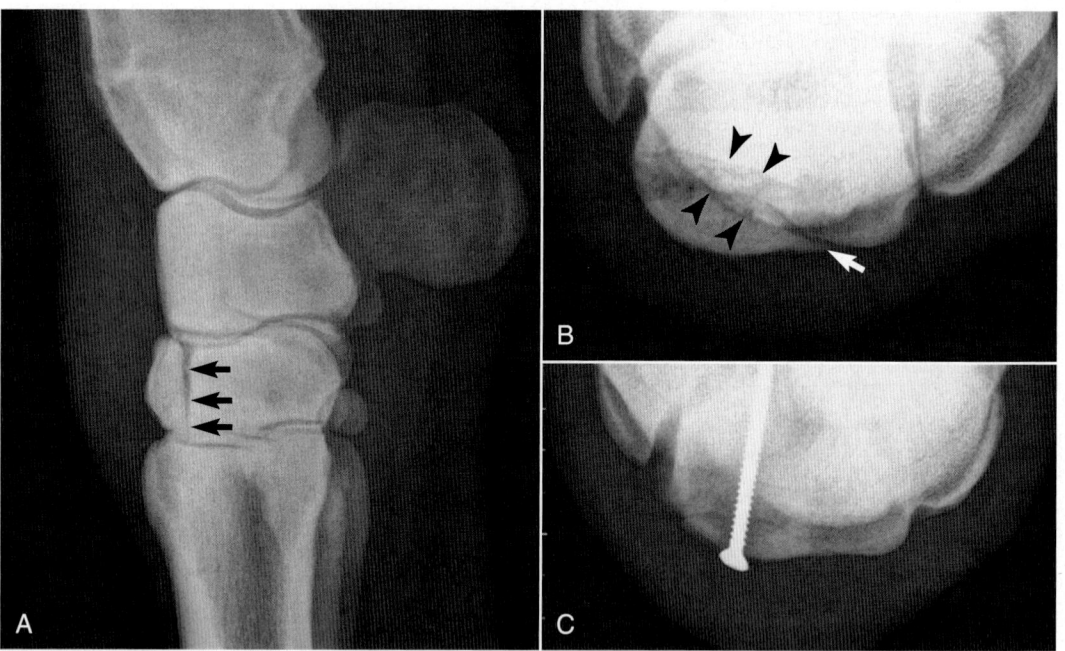

Fig. 38-10 • **A,** Standing lateromedial digital radiographic image (dorsal is to the left) showing a complete, mildly displaced frontal slab fracture of the radial fossa of the third carpal bone *(arrows)* in a 3-year-old Thoroughbred racehorse. The fracture line traverses the entire depth of the third carpal bone involving the middle carpal and carpometacarpal joints. Displacement is best seen in this radiographic image. **B,** Dorsoproximal-dorsodistal (skyline) digital radiographic image of the distal row of carpal bones showing the frontal slab fracture of the radial fossa of the third carpal bone (medial is left and palmar is uppermost). The slab fracture traverses the entire radial fossa *(arrow)*. Interposed between the fracture line and the parent third carpal bone is a wedge-shaped osteochondral fragment *(arrowheads)* that is generally removed before repair. **C,** The frontal slab fracture has been repaired using a single 3.5-mm bone screw placed in lag fashion in the center of the fracture fragment using arthroscopic guidance. The wedge-shaped fragment seen in the preoperative view **(B)** has been removed, and there is good anatomical alignment of the repair.

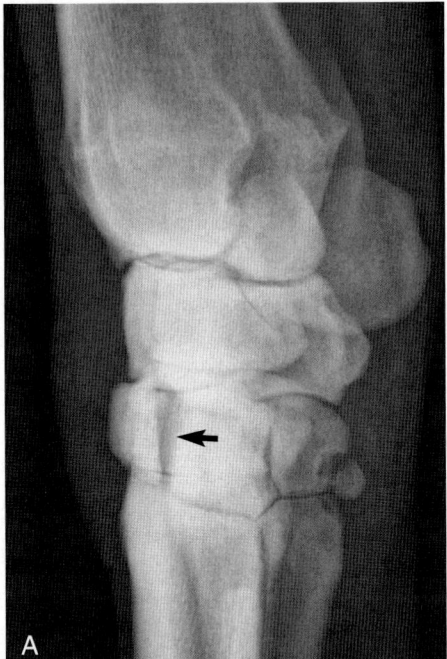

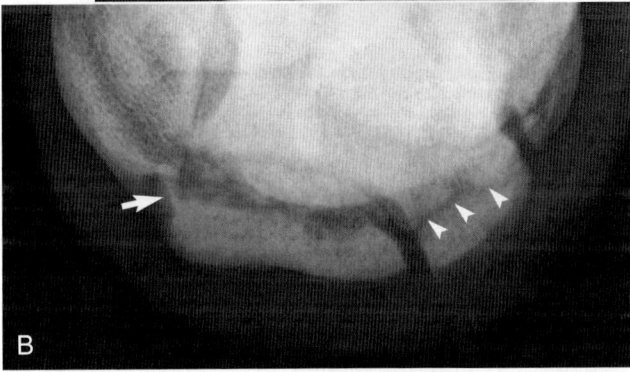

Fig. 38-11 • A, Dorsal 45° medial-palmarolateral oblique digital radiographic image showing a displaced frontal slab fracture of the intermediate fossa of the third carpal bone *(arrow)*. **B,** Dorsoproximal-dorsodistal digital radiographic image of the distal row of carpal bones (medial is to the left and palmar is uppermost) showing a comminuted frontal slab fracture of the third carpal bone involving the radial *(large arrow at fracture line)* and intermediate *(arrowheads at fracture line)* fossae.

38-11). Frontal slab fractures of the third carpal bone involving the radial fossa vary in size and can involve the entire medial-to-lateral width of the fossa, or any portion of it, and range from the common size of 8 to 10 mm in the dorsal-to-palmar direction up to 20 to 25 mm. These latter, large fragments cannot be seen on a skyline radiographic image, extend across the entire medial-to-lateral width of the third carpal bone involving both fossae, and are L shaped (Figure 38-12).

Lameness in horses with a frontal slab fracture is acute and severe and is generally worse than in those with small osteochondral fragments, but chronic, subtle prodromal lameness may have been present. A previous history of small osteochondral fragments and arthroscopic surgery is common. Lameness may be less than expected in horses recently injected with corticosteroids and in those with bilateral frontal slab fractures of the third carpal bone. Clinical signs such as heat, effusion, and response to static

and dynamic flexion are pronounced, and horses are usually lame at the walk. Horses with non–weight-bearing lameness may have unstable carpi and should be evaluated carefully for collapse from comminuted fractures. The contralateral carpus should always be evaluated and palpation should be complete to uncover compensatory lameness problems. In TB racehorses in North America the right third carpal bone is affected more commonly than the left,[45] but in STBs the distribution between right and left is similar.[46]

Frontal slab fractures of the third carpal bone are usually obvious radiologically. If they involve the radial fossa, fractures are best seen on the LM, flexed LM, and DL-PaMO images and a skyline image. Because frontal slab fractures of the third carpal bone by definition involve the middle carpal and carpometacarpal joint surfaces, if a fracture line breaks out dorsally before reaching the carpometacarpal joint, the fragment is not a true slab fracture. This is important when determining a management plan. A frontal slab fracture of the third carpal bone can be incomplete, complete but nondisplaced, or complete and displaced and may be associated with other small osteochondral fragments. Degree of displacement is worse on a standing LM image, but when the carpus is flexed, the fracture returns to near normal alignment. Flexion is a useful maneuver during reduction. In most instances a triangular, wedge-shaped fragment appears in the trough between the slab fracture fragment and the parent bone, and this accounts for the appearance of many fracture lines in a skyline view (see Figure 38-10, *B*). Careful examination of the overlying radial carpal bone is required in TB racehorses, because concomitant slab fracture of the radial carpal bone can accompany a frontal slab fracture of the third carpal bone.

Management depends on several factors, including the horse's value, age, racing class, presence of other lameness problems, and specifically whether the frontal slab fracture of the third carpal bone is incomplete, displaced, or comminuted. Long-term rest (6 months) is successful in horses with incomplete or complete nondisplaced fractures. However, surgical fixation can help preserve articular surfaces by preventing displacement. Frontal slab fracture fragments that are thin (<5 mm in the dorsal-to-palmar direction) can be removed using arthroscopic surgery or conventional arthrotomy techniques or, if the articular surface is intact, can be repaired. Arthroscopic techniques are preferred when possible, and the technique remains largely unchanged since originally described.[47] Surgical removal of small frontal slab fractures of the third carpal bone can be difficult using arthroscopic techniques and can leave a large defect radiologically but is successful. Horses with large frontal slab fragments that are displaced are usually managed with arthroscopic surgery and internal fixation, using one or two cortex screws placed in lag fashion. Either 3.5- or 4.5-mm screws can be used, but I prefer using one or two 3.5-mm screws because the screw heads are smaller and countersinking in the dorsal aspect of the third carpal bone is not necessary. Horses with large frontal fractures of the radial fossa, those with comminuted fractures involving both the radial and intermediate fossae (see Figure 38-11), and those in which fracture fragments cannot be adequately reduced should be repaired with 4.5-mm screws, because 3.5-mm screws can sometimes break. Use of needles and intraoperative radiographs to position and guide screw insertion accurately is preferred.[45]

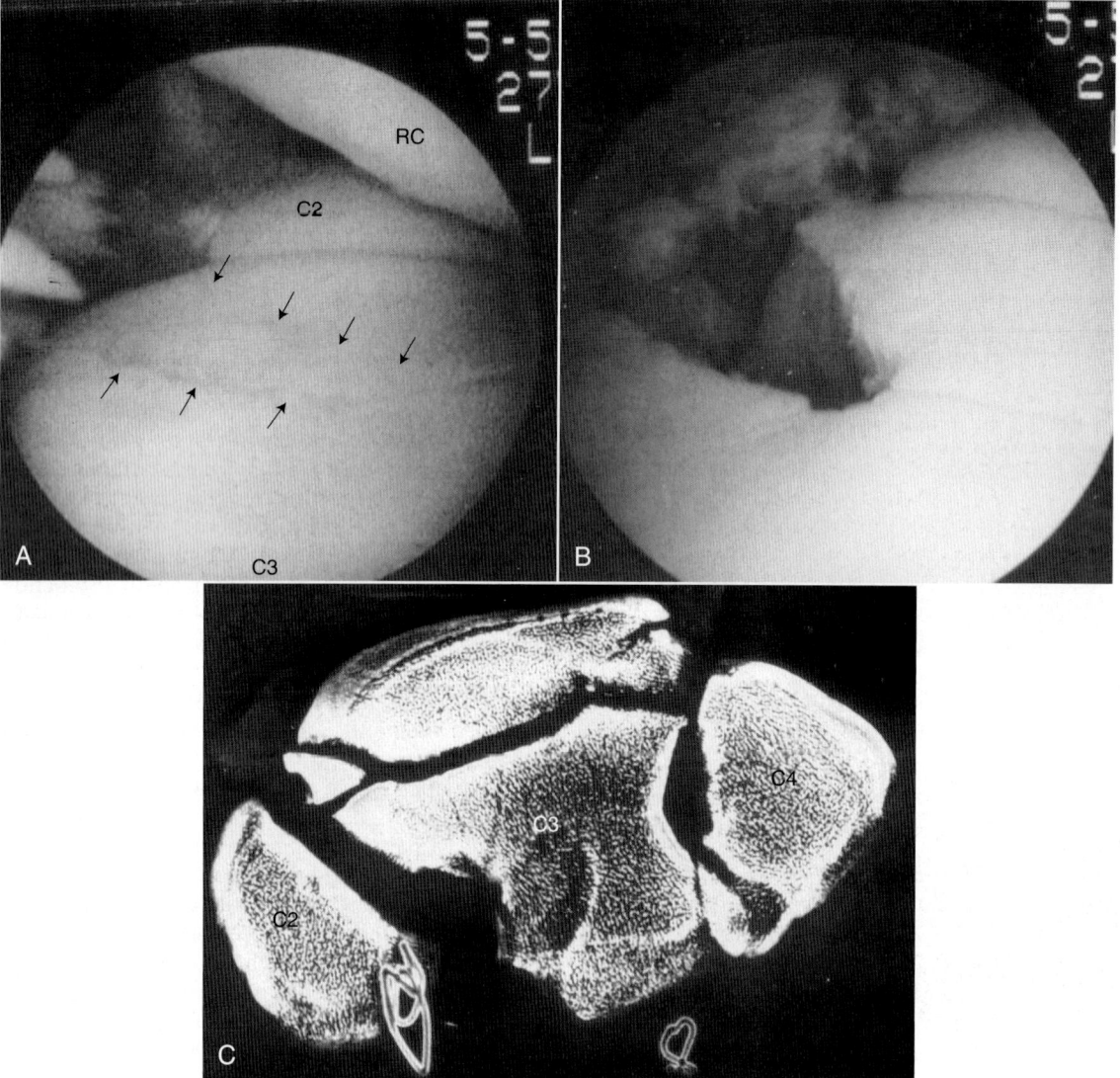

Fig. 38-12 • This pacer had an L-shaped fracture of the third carpal bone that involved a sagittal and frontal component. **A,** The initial intraoperative photograph shows the sagittal component *(arrows)* and crushed medial aspect of the third carpal bone. **B,** This area was debrided, and the fracture healed without internal fixation. The sagittal component of the fracture appears palmar to the defect. **C,** True proximal-to-distal radiographic image of a trotter obtained at necropsy shows that the large slab fracture of the third carpal bone has frontal and sagittal components. *C2,* Second carpal bone; *C3,* third carpal bone; *C4,* fourth carpal bone; *RC,* radial carpal bone.

A single bone screw provides adequate fixation in horses with most frontal slab fractures of the third carpal bone involving only the radial fossa, because capsular attachments maintain rotational stability. The fracture line is debrided, often before screw placement, and the wedge-shaped trough fragment is removed, leaving a gap at the fracture line. Loose cartilage is curetted, cartilage damage is graded, and other small osteochondral fragments are removed if present. Alternatively the proximal articular surface of the fragment may be removed, with repair of the distal aspect, leaving the portion of the fragment with capsular attachments intact. Occasionally, additional slab fractures of the third or radial carpal bones are found and repaired. In horses with more than one slab fracture, a Robert Jones bandage or cast is used for recovery from general anesthesia. In TB racehorses with a frontal slab fracture of the third carpal bone, an ominous defect in the

articular cartilage of the radial carpal bone is often seen, caused by the incongruent apposing surface of the third carpal bone, but in most horses subchondral bone fracture is not present. Horses are typically given stall rest for 4 weeks, followed by stall rest with hand walking for 8 weeks, followed by turnout in a small paddock for 2 to 3 months before beginning race training. Recommendations for intraarticular therapy are similar to those in horses with small osteochondral fragments.

In a large retrospective study of TB and STB racehorses with a frontal slab fracture of the third carpal bone, the radial fossa was involved in 87% of horses, and females of both breeds were less likely to race after injury and surgery, but treatment and fracture characteristics had no effect on outcome.[46] Fracture characteristics such as size and degree of displacement did influence treatment selection, so thin frontal slab fractures of the third carpal bone were removed, displaced fractures were repaired, and horses with incomplete or nondisplaced frontal slab fracture of the third carpal bone were managed conservatively.[46] All STBs that had raced before surgery also raced after surgery, and overall 77% raced after surgery. Sixty-five percent of TBs with frontal slab fractures of the third carpal bone raced after surgery, and although earnings per start decreased in both breeds, the decrease was more pronounced in TBs.[46] In another study, 67% of TBs with a frontal slab fracture of the third carpal bone raced at least once after surgery, but the mean claiming value in horses decreased significantly.[45] In a study in which lag screw fixation was used in horses with incomplete frontal plane fractures of the radial facet of the third carpal bone, 69% of horses were considered to have successful outcomes, and there was no difference in racing longevity or ability after surgery between principles and age-, sex-, and sire-matched controls.[48]

Sagittal Slab Fractures of the Third Carpal Bone
Sagittal slab fractures of the third carpal bone are much less common than frontal slab fractures, usually involve the medial aspect of the radial fossa (see Figures 38-12 and 38-13), and occur in a direction parallel to the articulation between the second and third carpal bones. However, sagittal slab fractures of the third carpal bone can occur in the intermediate fossa, and fractures can be bilateral. Authentic

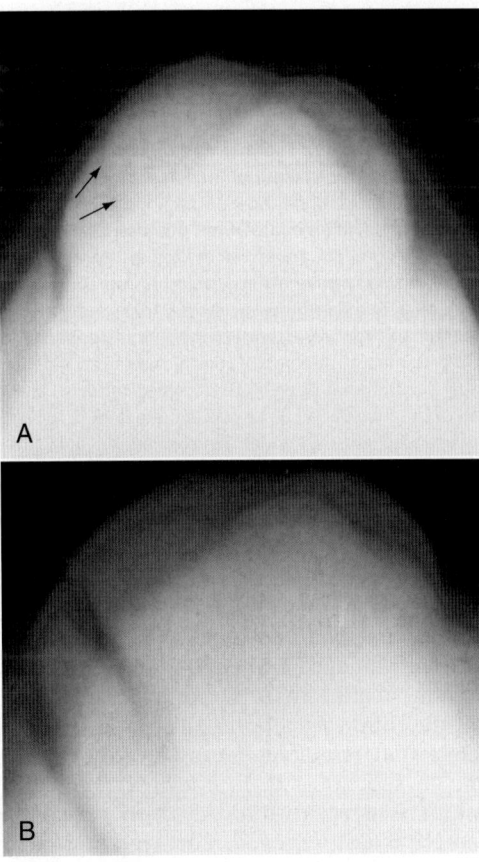

Fig. 38-13 • Initial **(A)** and 8-month follow-up **(B)** skyline radiographic images of the third carpal bone showing a sagittal slab fracture *(arrows)* that failed to heal and became a nonunion **(B).** This Standardbred trained and raced with the nonunion fracture but dropped substantially in class. Results such as this have prompted me to manage sagittal slab fractures of the third carpal bone surgically.

sagittal slab fractures of the third carpal bone involve both articular surfaces of the bone and can be best seen radiologically in skyline and DM-PaLO images. Sagittal slab fractures of the third carpal bone must be differentiated from corner fractures, subchondral lucency, and other crushing-type injuries that occur in the radial fossa. Clinical signs associated with sagittal slab fractures of the third carpal bone are similar to those of other osteochondral fragments but are usually less severe than a frontal slab fracture of the bone. Lameness is usually prominent, but in horses with bilateral fracture or substantial OA or osteochondral fragments in the contralateral carpus, diagnostic analgesia may be required. Often horses have a prominent history of chronic carpal lameness before acute lameness develops. Of 32 racehorses with sagittal slab fracture of the third carpal bone, 19 were TBs, 11 were STBs, and 2 were Arabian racehorses, and fractures were found in the right forelimb (19), left forelimb (12), and bilaterally in one horse.[49] Overall, 22 (69%) horses raced after treatment, all seven horses treated with interfragmentary compression raced, and horses that underwent interfragmentary compression had significantly higher earnings per start than those treated without surgery.[49] Eight of nine horses managed with arthroscopic debridement raced, but only 7 of 16 horses managed conservatively raced.[49]

Conservative management was recommended, but only 7 of 12 horses with a sagittal slab fracture of the third carpal bone managed conservatively raced.[50] Fracture healing takes extensive time, and a chronic nonunion often develops (see Figure 38-13, *B*). Horses can be sound enough to race with chronic nonunion fractures, but this is undesirable. I have seen one STB and one TB racehorse with bilateral lateral, nonunion sagittal slab fractures of the third carpal bone racing successfully, but with conservative management comes a risk of chronic high-speed lameness, worse if fracture involves the right forelimb, and horses drop substantially in racing class. If any doubt exists about the nature of a lesion affecting the medial aspect of the third carpal bone, arthroscopic examination can be performed to formulate a surgical plan. If an authentic sagittal slab fracture of the third carpal bone does not exist, but medial corner osteochondral fragments, necrotic subchondral bone, or other crush-type injuries are found, a combination of fragment removal and curettage is performed. I currently recommend surgical management for most horses with sagittal slab fractures of the third carpal bone. To repair a fracture, I prefer a direct view provided by arthrotomy, because positioning a screw perpendicular to the fracture line using arthroscopic surgery and stereotactic techniques is difficult and because the fracture is closely associated with the second carpal bone. A single 3.5-mm screw is placed in lag fashion. Alternatively, arthroscopic evaluation and debridement result in a better outcome than does conservative management.[49] Evaluating the joint arthroscopically and then formulating a management plan is a reasonable approach, but certainly surgical management is preferred over rest alone. Management after surgery is similar to that described for horses with frontal slab fractures of the third carpal bone.

Slab Fractures of Other Carpal Bones
Slab fractures of carpal bones other than the third are unusual. Whenever slab fractures of the radial carpal bone

or other unusual slab fractures are discovered, all radiographic images should be evaluated carefully. CT was shown to be valuable in identifying fracture lines and comminution not seen using radiography.[14] Slab fractures of the radial carpal bone can occur independent of or in combination with frontal slab fracture of the third carpal bone. When frontal slab fractures of the radial and third carpal bones occur simultaneously and carpal instability results, the fracture is called a *comminuted carpal fracture*. Repairing both bones by placing numerous screws using arthroscopic surgery may be possible. A sleeve or full-limb fiberglass cast is placed, and an assisted recovery from general anesthesia is recommended.

Slab fractures of the intermediate, fourth, and ulnar carpal bones occur rarely. In five horses with intermediate and fourth carpal bone slab fractures, outcome was poor because of delay in diagnosis, and four horses were only pasture sound.[51] Surgical repair should proceed as early as possible, but prognosis is limited by cartilage damage and other osteochondral fragments.

Subchondral Lucency of the Third Carpal Bone

Subchondral lucency of the third carpal bone[52] is an unusual condition occurring most commonly in STB racehorses, although it is occasionally seen in the TB racehorse, and is seen radiologically as single or multiple central areas of bone loss in the radial fossa of the third carpal bone (Figure 38-14). Overall, I am seeing fewer STB racehorses with this lesion. Earlier recognition and intervention may be credited. Lesions can be seen in a DL-PaMO image in horses with advanced subchondral lucency of the third carpal bone. Mild-to-severe sclerosis may surround radiolucent defects,[52] but in one study no relationship was found between radiolucency of the third carpal bone and increased radiopacity.[40] The lesion was more common in the right carpus, and, although pacers predominated, distribution was similar to the racing population in the United States.[52] Pathogenesis is identical to that described for OA, osteochondral fragments, and slab fractures of the third carpal bone, but in horses with subchondral lucency of the third carpal bone, necrosis of subchondral bone causes table surface collapse rather than osteochondral fragments or slab fractures involving the dorsal margin. Subchondral lucency of the third carpal bone is not a disease of young racehorses, because the mean age in STBs was 4.1 years (range, 3 to 7 years) and chronic stress-related subchondral bone injury is required.

There are prodromal clinical signs of mild carpal lameness and usually a history of the administration of numerous intraarticular injections before onset of acute lameness, usually graded from 2 to 4 on a 5-point scale. Heat, effusion, and a positive response to flexion may be absent, and diagnostic analgesia is usually required to confirm diagnosis. The results of initial radiological evaluation may be equivocal, and follow-up radiographic and scintigraphic examinations can help pinpoint subchondral lucency of the third carpal bone. Focal areas of IRU in the radial fossa of the third carpal bone similar to that seen with frontal or sagittal slab fracture are seen.

Surgical debridement is the treatment of choice (see Figure 38-14, *B*). During arthroscopic examination, soft crumbly necrotic subchondral bone and damaged overlying cartilage are found. In some horses only a small

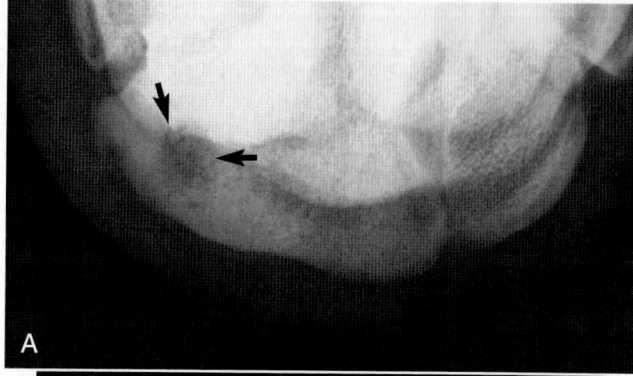

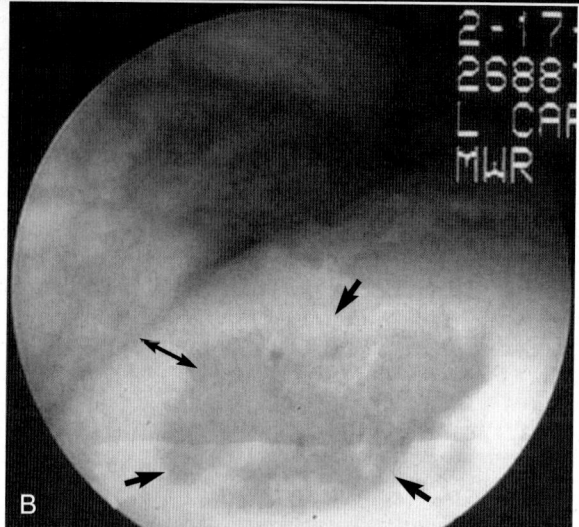

Fig. 38-14 • A, Dorsoproximal-dorsodistal (skyline) digital radiographic image of the left carpus of a Thoroughbred racehorse with subchondral lucency *(arrows)* of the radial fossa of the left third carpal bone (medial is to the left and palmar is uppermost). Subchondral lucency of the third carpal bone should be differentiated from other sagittal plane injury, such as sagittal slab fracture. This horse underwent arthroscopic debridement successfully. **B,** Intraoperative arthroscopic photograph of the left third carpal bone of a Standardbred racehorse that underwent successful debridement of subchondral lucency of the third carpal bone (dorsal is to the left and proximal is uppermost). Full-thickness cartilage damage and soft, crumbly subchondral bone were debrided *(arrows)*, and the dorsal aspect (rim) of the third carpal bone was left intact *(double-headed arrow)*. (**A** courtesy Dean Richardson, Kennett Square, Pennsylvania, United States.)

full-thickness cartilage defect can be probed, but deep extensive subchondral bone softening is later found, whereas in others, fibrin-filled, full-thickness defects resembling subchondral bone collapse or table surface fracture are found. The damaged tissue is curetted, and if the resulting lesion is smaller than 5 mm palmar to the dorsal margin of the third carpal bone, this rim is removed, creating a defect that resembles removal of an osteochondral fragment. If subchondral lucency of the third carpal bone lesions is deep within the third carpal bone, the dorsal margin is not removed. Cartilage resurfacing could be considered, but it is not necessary for a successful outcome.

Prognosis is excellent for return to racing, particularly in pacers, but horses drop in racing class. Prognosis for return to racing the next year is guarded in 3- or 4-year-old trotters, but some make useful older racehorses. Of nine

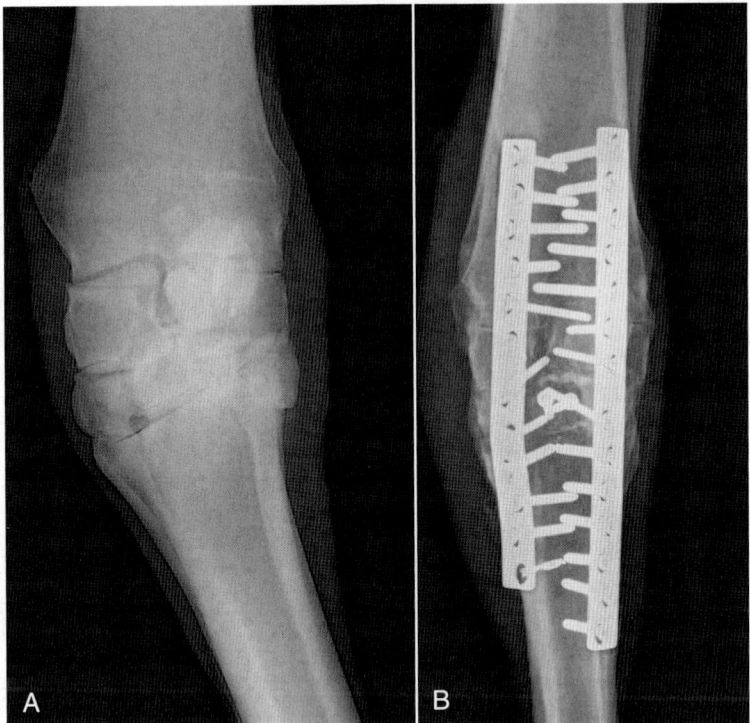

Fig. 38-15 • **A,** Non–weight-bearing dorsopalmar computed radiographic image obtained before surgery of the left carpus (lateral is to the right and proximal is uppermost) in an aged gelding riding horse that sustained a comminuted carpal fracture while turned out. Notice marked carpus valgus limb deformity caused by collapse of the lateral aspect of the middle carpal joint. There were comminuted fractures of the third and fourth carpal bones. **B,** Dorsopalmar digital radiographic image obtained 3 years after successful panarthrodesis of the carpus, showing complete fusion of the antebrachiocarpal, middle carpal, and carpometacarpal joints. Two broad dynamic compression plates and interfragmentary compression of the third carpal bone were used. Today, locking compression plates would likely be used, but successful arthrodesis was achieved with this fixation in conjunction with external coaptation with a fiberglass sleeve cast.

horses, eight returned to racing, but only six raced at the previous level.[52]

Comminuted Fractures

Comminuted fractures are unusual, but they occur occasionally in TB and QH racehorses and other horses that sustain injury while turned out in a field. *Comminuted* in this sense refers to numerous fractures in more than one carpal bone. In STB racehorses, large, comminuted fractures of the third carpal bone can occur, but I have not seen a STB with a large osteochondral fracture involving more than one bone. The most common combination of fractures in TB and QH racehorses involves the third carpal bone and either the radial or intermediate carpal bone, or both. Carpal instability, most commonly carpus varus, is usually readily apparent if horses bear weight, but they are usually non–weight bearing. These injuries occur almost exclusively in racehorses, and often horses have chronic carpal lameness before injury, but fracture can occur in other types of horses without previous lameness during turnout exercise. Effusion and edema of surrounding soft tissues occurs. Diagnosis of comminuted fracture and instability is confirmed radiologically (Figure 38-15). If fractures involve only the distal row of carpal bones, instability is minimal and prognosis is better than if the middle carpal and antebrachiocarpal joints are involved. Consideration should be given for euthanasia if the horse is a gelding or

intact male with limited breeding potential. Conservative management using sleeve or full-limb casts, or a combination of splints with a Robert Jones bandage, may give support and provide comfort, but usually instability is pronounced, horses develop extensive cast sores, and they are at profound risk to develop laminitis in the contralateral limb. Severe OA, collapse, and angular limb deformity generally result in an unacceptable outcome in horses managed conservatively. Surgical management using carpal arthrodesis is the treatment of choice.

Carpal Arthrodesis

Arthrodesis is indicated when horses have comminuted carpal fractures and instability, when they have severe lameness and OA of one or more carpal joints, or when OA is severe with collapse and angular deformity of the carpus. Partial (intercarpal) carpal arthrodesis involves fusing the middle carpal and carpometacarpal joints using bone plates applied to the proximal row of carpal bones and the McIII. Pancarpal arthrodesis involves bridging the entire carpus with bone plates applied to the distal radius, both rows of carpal bones, and the McIII, fusing all three joints. Two plates, either dynamic compression plates or, more recently, locking compression plates,[53,54] are used for either technique, and in one study allografts were used to provide axial support in some horses with collapsed carpi undergoing pancarpal arthrodesis. In one horse, I successfully used acrylic to create an artificial fourth carpal bone to maintain axial stability, in addition to two dynamic compression plates and interfragmentary repair of fractures (see Figure 38-15). Overall, prognosis for salvage is good, but complications included infection and contralateral laminitis. Of 36 horses undergoing carpal arthrodesis, 30 (83%) survived 3 months, and 24 (67%) survived at least 9 months after surgery.[55] Prognosis was similar between horses undergoing pancarpal and partial carpal arthrodesis.[55,56]

Accessory Carpal Bone Fractures

Fracture of the accessory carpal bone results from trauma, such as a fall while jumping, a hyperextension injury when landing, or an accident while turned out. Acute, severe lameness and swelling involve the palmar aspect of the carpus. Horses have severe pain during carpal flexion. Carpal tenosynovitis may occur acutely, but it is difficult to differentiate from diffuse swelling. Pronounced lameness lasts for several days, but horses are rarely non–weight bearing, and swelling resolves in 2 to 3 weeks. Horses with a chronic fracture may have little to no swelling, and diagnosis may be difficult unless carpal tenosynovitis is present, because the lameness is not typical of carpal pain.

The most common fracture of the accessory carpal bone is a vertical slab fracture that involves the palmar aspect of the bone in the frontal (dorsal) plane (Figure 38-16). Most fragments are simple, but small fragments at the proximal aspect of the fracture may occur. Fractures can be incomplete, but most are complete with mild displacement. Gross

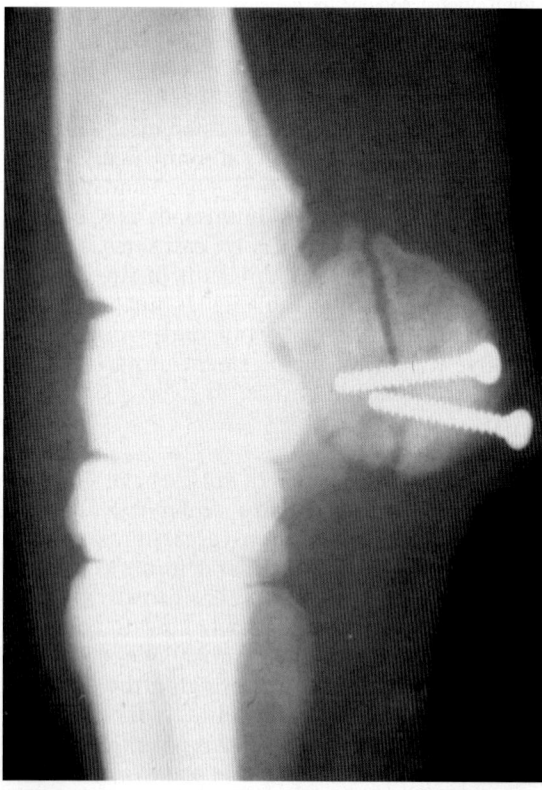

Fig. 38-16 • A lateromedial radiographic image of a horse with a failed attempt at surgical management of a frontal slab fracture of the accessory carpal bone. These fractures are best managed conservatively without attempting repairs such as this one.

displacement and large comminuted fragments are unusual. Articular fractures were discussed previously (see page 439).

Conservative management of horses with nonarticular fractures of the accessory carpal bone is recommended. The forces on the accessory carpal bone are substantial and result in failure of screw fixation, chronic instability, implant loosening, and osteitis (see Figure 38-16). Surgical fixation using the tension band principle may be successful, but I have not attempted repair because prognosis is favorable with conservative management. Horses are given NSAIDs, and a heavy full-limb cotton bandage is applied. Horses are given stall rest for 8 weeks, followed by stall rest with hand walking for 8 weeks, followed by walking with a rider up for 8 weeks. Radiographs most often reveal bony proliferative changes and fibrous rather than bony union of the fracture. Even with fibrous union, horses are usually serviceably sound. Prognosis for TB racehorses appears to be worse than for field hunters, jumpers, and other horses that may be able to perform with a mild gait restriction from chronic fibrosis. Carpal canal syndrome and carpal tenosynovitis may result (see Chapter 75).

Osteochondrosis

Osteochondrosis of the carpus is rare. In a radiological study of yearling TBs, 0.4% had either radiological changes associated with osteochondritis dissecans (OCD) or a subchondral bone cyst, other than that seen involving the distal aspect of the ulnar carpal bone (see later).[57] In experimental studies extensive cartilage lesions histologically similar to those in naturally occurring OCD have been produced. Rarely, radiographs of yearlings before or after public sales reveal rounded osteochondral fragments, usually involving the distal medial aspect of the radius or the distal medial aspect of the radial carpal bone or proximal aspect of the third carpal bone. These fragments appear as solitary osteochondral fragments and do not have associated marginal osteophytes or enthesophytes, unlike osteochondral fragments caused by trauma at a young age. At the time of surgery these unusual fragments appear intercalated in dense joint capsule attachments, are rounded, and often have a smooth defect in the distal aspect of the radius or third carpal bone, apparently the origin of the fragment. Whether these fragments represent a form of OCD or old trauma is not known, but they appear similar to forms of OCD found elsewhere.

Osseous Cystlike Lesions

Osseous cystlike lesions do occur in the carpus. Those of the ulnar carpal bone are common, appear to be incidental radiological findings, are usually nonarticular, and have sclerotic borders. Often, small bony fragments can be seen within the radiolucent defect and can be misinterpreted as acute fractures, sometimes called *avulsion injury of the lateral palmar intercarpal ligament* (see later). Ulnar carpal bone radiolucent defects were the most common radiological abnormality found in a large study of TB yearlings.[57] Abnormalities of the distal aspect of the ulnar carpal bone were found in 20% of yearlings and were exclusively unilateral, and no negative association between this radiological change and racing performance was found.[57,58] Incidental osseous cystlike lesions may also be seen in the second carpal bone, often in the presence of the first carpal bone, and also in the base (head) of the McII. Osseous cystlike lesions of the radial carpal bone and distal aspect of the radius can cause lameness.[59] Effusion, heat, and a positive response to flexion are inconsistent, and diagnostic analgesia is usually necessary. Radiological signs may be obvious, but in some horses they are subtle, and scintigraphic examination is useful to pinpoint the area of modeling. In horses with an osseous cystlike lesion that communicates with an articular surface, I have performed debridement and curettage, but results have been unfavorable to fair at best. Alternatively, I have had good success using a combination of rest (4 to 6 months) and serial intraarticular injections (two or three) of hyaluronan and corticosteroids (40 mg methylprednisolone acetate) when cysts appear radiologically to communicate with a carpal joint (see Figure 39-4).

Osteochondromatosis

Osteochondromatosis is rare but has been seen in the carpometacarpal joint.[60] Progressive enlargement of the carpometacarpal joint and numerous unusual radiopacities were seen radiologically.[60] Arthroscopic examination of the carpometacarpal joint was possible, and osteochondral fragments were removed[60] (see Chapter 67).

Infectious Arthritis

See Chapter 65 for a discussion of infectious arthritis.

Other Fractures Involving the Carpus

Avulsion Fracture of the Third Metacarpal Bone Associated with the Origin of the Suspensory Ligament

See Chapter 37 for a discussion of avulsion fracture of the McIII associated with the origin of the SL (page 417).

Incomplete, Longitudinal Fracture of the Proximal Palmar Cortex of the Third Metacarpal Bone

See Chapter 37 for a discussion of incomplete, longitudinal fracture of the proximal palmar cortex of the McIII (page 413).

Dorsomedial Articular Fracture of the Proximal Aspect of the Third Metacarpal Bone

See Chapter 37 for a discussion of dorsomedial articular fracture of the proximal aspect of the McIII (page 416).

Fracture of the Proximal Aspect of the Second and Fourth Metacarpal Bones

See Chapter 37 for a discussion of the proximal aspect of the McII and the McIV (page 421).

Articular Fracture of the Distal Aspect of the Radius

Fractures of the distal aspect of the radius rarely involve the antebrachiocarpal joint. Complete or incomplete, displaced or nondisplaced fractures of the radius in the sagittal plane and resembling condylar fractures of the McIII or the third metatarsal bone can occur.[61] Horses should be managed conservatively using full-limb bandages, NSAIDs, and absolute stall rest if fractures are nondisplaced. Some consideration should be given to cross-tying the horse for 3 to 6 weeks. Comminuted fractures of the radius, or those involving the distal radial physis and epiphysis that involve the antebrachiocarpal joint, should be repaired.

Soft Tissue Injuries of the Carpus and Carpal Region

Medial Palmar Intercarpal Ligament

Various degrees of tearing of the medial palmar intercarpal ligament have been observed during arthroscopic examination of horses with osteochondral fragments or OA and in some horses with occult carpal lameness (see Figure 23-4). The medial palmar intercarpal ligament has recently been the source of considerable study and supposition, but whether tearing of this ligament observed in horses with carpal disease is causative or simply results from other pathological conditions is not yet known. The anatomy of the medial palmar intercarpal ligament and the relationship between osteochondral fragments and the dorsomedial intercarpal ligament were previously discussed (see page 427).

Because tearing of the medial palmar intercarpal ligament is an observation during arthroscopic examination of the middle carpal joint and a diagnosis impossible currently to make before surgery, specific clinical signs cannot be described. Once MRI becomes more widely available, diagnosis in horses with occult carpal lameness suspected to originate from the medial palmar intercarpal ligament may be possible before arthroscopic examination. Tearing of the medial palmar intercarpal ligament was observed in 27 joints in 20 horses with carpal lameness.[5] No correlation was found between tearing and severity of clinical signs. Joints with more medial palmar intercarpal ligament tearing had significantly *less* cartilage and subchondral bone damage, and an inverse relationship existed between the size and number of osteochondral fragments and ligament damage.[5] Therefore, although tearing of the medial palmar intercarpal ligament occurred commonly in horses with middle carpal joint damage, tearing was not seen with severe subchondral bone damage, and what role damage plays in the development of joint disease remains questionable.

In my experience, tearing of the medial palmar intercarpal ligament is unusual without at least mild cartilage damage or osteochondral fragmentation, but I have seen a small number of horses in which the only identifiable lesion was tearing and hemorrhage of the frayed ends, resulting in hemarthrosis. Complete tearing of the medial palmar intercarpal ligament occurs more frequently in TB racehorses compared with STBs; partial tearing (fraying) of the medial palmar intercarpal ligament is quite common in STBs. In horses with a complete tear of the ligament, examining the palmar aspect of the middle carpal joint from the routine dorsal approach was possible. Rupture of the medial palmar intercarpal ligament has been seen in a small number of nonracehorse competition horses with pain localized to the middle carpal joint.[62] No other lesion was identified during arthroscopic examination. I suspect tearing of the medial palmar intercarpal ligament in horses with confirmed carpal lameness, but in which scintigraphic and radiological findings are negative or equivocal, and in those with unexplained hemarthrosis of the middle carpal joint. Because horses that fall into this category are rare, prognosis is difficult to estimate.

Lateral Palmar Intercarpal Ligament

Avulsion injury at the origin of the lateral palmar intercarpal ligament on the ulnar carpal bone has been described

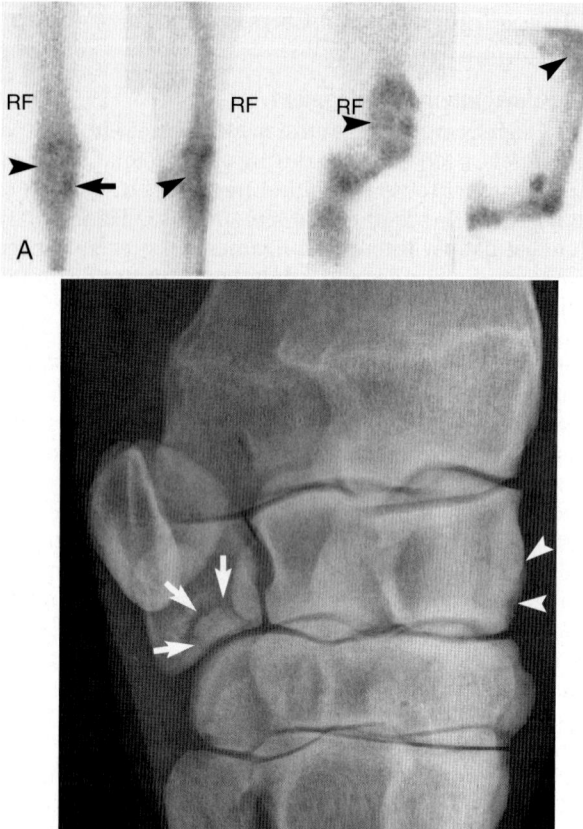

Fig. 38-17 • **A,** Delayed-phase scintigraphic images of a 3-year-old Thoroughbred colt with mild increased radiopharmaceutical uptake (IRU) in the medial aspect of the right radial carpal bone *(arrow).* There is normal radiopharmaceutical uptake in the region of the ulnar carpal bone *(arrowheads).* **B,** Dorsal 45° lateral-palmaromedial oblique digital radiographic image of the right carpus showing mild enthesophyte and marginal osteophyte formation of the dorsomedial aspect of the radial carpal bone *(arrowheads).* Note also a bony fragment at the distal aspect of the ulnar carpal bone *(arrows).* This fragment is likely an *incidental* finding because IRU was not seen.

and characterized, but I remain skeptical of this lesion as an authentic cause of lameness.[63,64] Differentiation between genuine avulsion injury and the common radiological abnormalities such as radiolucent defects and fragments that occur commonly at the distal aspect of the ulnar carpal bone is difficult. I have not been able to document IRU on scintigraphic examination of horses with radiological evidence of fracture, radiolucent defects, or radiolucent defects with fragmentation, in this location (Figure 38-17). Fragments removed from this location histologically were consistent with fracture, and the authors differentiated fracture from the common cystic lesions that occur in this location by the presence of actual fragments and the position of the fragments at the palmar transition zone at the confluence of the lateral palmar intercarpal ligament.[63] In the clinical report 26 of 37 horses underwent arthroscopic surgery to remove fragments and 20 returned to work, whereas five of nine horses managed conservatively returned to work.[64] Scintigraphic examination was not performed, and complete clinical examination including diagnostic analgesia was not included for all horses.[64] Careful

clinical examination and advanced imaging may be necessary to differentiate horses with radiological abnormalities of the distal aspect of the ulnar carpal bone. It is possible that the presence of radiolucent defects, fragments, or a combination of radiological abnormalities in young untrained horses could be associated with the future development of other carpal lameness such as OA and osteochondral fragmentation, but to establish an association would require a large prospective clinical study.

Collateral Ligament

Injury of the dense collateral ligaments of the carpus is rare (see Chapter 67). Usually fracture of the distal aspect of the radius, the carpal bones, or the proximal aspect of the McII and the McIV occurs instead of collateral ligament damage. In foals, collateral ligament laxity is seen commonly and is self-limiting but can contribute to the development of angular limb deformity. Three horses with collateral desmopathy remained lame despite prolonged rest, and ultrasonographic examination was useful to characterize the injury.[65]

Carpal Tenosynovitis and Flexor Tendonitis

See Chapters 69 and 75 for a discussion of carpal tenosynovitis and flexor tendonitis.

Exostoses of the Distal Caudal Aspect of the Radius

An unusual clustering of horses with carpal region pain as a result of carpal tenosynovitis from impingement of small exostoses of the caudal perimeter of the radial physis on structures of the carpal canal has been reported.[66] I have seen three horses with carpal tenosynovitis as a result of irritation of deep surface of the deep digital flexor tendon by exostoses from the distal, caudal aspect of the radius and acute-onset lameness as a result of hemorrhage and inflammation of the carpal sheath. Signs resolved after tenoscopy and ostectomy. Radiological evidence of small exostoses of the distal, caudal radius is common, and careful clinical examination including diagnostic analgesia should be performed to ensure a correct diagnosis. See Chapters 70 and 75 for more information.

Extensor Tendon

See Chapter 77 for a discussion of extensor tendon injury.

Proximal Suspensory Desmitis

See Chapter 72 for a discussion of proximal suspensory desmitis.

Synovial Ganglion

See Chapter 67 for a discussion of synovial ganglion injury.

Carpal Hygroma

Hygroma refers to a sac, bursa, or cavity filled with fluid. Carpal hygroma usually results from direct and blunt trauma to the dorsal aspect of the joint, including the capsule and overlying extensor tendons and sheaths. Carpal hygroma is an occasional complication after arthroscopic surgery or arthrotomy of the carpus. During arthrotomy, a distinct subcutaneous space over the dorsal aspect of the carpus is encountered, but in most instances this is a potential rather than a real space. When traumatized, this space fills with fluid, resulting in a large sac. Initially, diffuse edema may be present, and horses may be lame, particularly after flexion, but lameness soon abates. A large, fluid filled, nonpainful swelling results that must be differentiated from extensor tenosynovitis (longitudinal swellings) and herniation of the middle carpal and antebrachiocarpal joint capsules (horizontal swellings). Lameness is usually not observed in horses with chronic hygroma unless a large swelling prohibits carpal flexion. Communication with an extensor sheath or joint capsule is rare, unless previous arthroscopic surgery has been performed and a portal inadvertently was made through a tendon sheath. In naturally occurring carpal hygroma a secretory lining is present, but it must develop from cell differentiation because communication with a source of synovial cells is lacking. Diagnosis is based on clinical signs. Positive contrast radiography and ultrasonographic examination are used to determine extent and communication with nearby structures.

The swelling is usually persistent, but it often does not compromise gait, although swelling does result in a cosmetic blemish. I have heard of resolution after injection with oxytetracycline, atropine, or contrast material. Drainage, with or without corticosteroid injection, and chronic bandaging are usually unsuccessful in permanently resolving swelling. Surgical management in the form of en bloc resection is the treatment of choice for cosmetic results. Simply draining the cavity and inserting through-and-through or closed-suction drains may temporarily resolve

swelling, but recurrence is likely. I attempt resection en bloc without entering the hygroma cavity, but invariably the lining is penetrated. The lining is dissected from all overlying subcutaneous tissues and underlying capsule and tendon sheaths. Once the lining is removed, Penrose drains are placed, a light sterile bandage is applied, and horses recover with a sleeve cast-bandage that is left in place a minimum of 7 to 10 days. Drains are removed in 7 to 10 days when cast material is cut, and then the cast material can be used as a splint over a heavy padded bandage. Horses are given absolute stall confinement for 3 weeks. This treatment is successful but expensive.

Neoplasia

A rare cause of carpal region lameness is neoplasia. Lameness and progressive swelling were seen in a 20-year-old horse with chondrosarcoma of the distal aspect of the radius that caused bony proliferation and swelling of the antebrachiocarpal joint.[67] I have seen an undifferentiated sarcoma of the distal aspect of the antebrachium causing progressive swelling, mild lameness, and a reduction in carpal flexion in a TB broodmare.

Hypertrophic Osteopathy

Lameness associated with hypertrophic osteopathy (see Chapters 15 and 37) is usually mild, and the condition does not directly affect the carpus, but fibrous and bony swelling of the distal aspect of the radius may cause enlargement of the antebrachiocarpal joint region, prompting radiographic examination.

Chapter 39

The Antebrachium

Lance H. Bassage II and Mike W. Ross

ANATOMY

The antebrachium lies between the elbow and carpus and is composed principally of the radius and small vestigial portion of the ulna and the flexor and extensor muscles. The tendons of the superficial and deep digital flexor muscles, the accessory ligament of the superficial digital flexor tendon, and the carpal sheath are discussed elsewhere (see Chapters 69, 70, and 75). The medial aspect of the antebrachium is relatively devoid of soft tissue coverage, and this is important when considering fractures of the radius. Major neurovascular structures include the median artery (continuation of the brachial artery in the proximal antebrachium), vein, and nerve; the radial, ulnar, and cutaneous antebrachial nerves; and the accessory cephalic and cephalic veins.

CLINICAL DIAGNOSIS AND IMAGING CONSIDERATIONS

Lameness associated with the antebrachial region is relatively unusual. Clinical signs are obvious in horses with unstable radial fractures or in those with marked soft tissue swelling. In others diagnosis can be challenging, and ruling out other causes of forelimb lameness and then using diagnostic imaging to reach a definite diagnosis may be necessary. Perineural analgesia of the median and ulnar nerves (see Chapter 10) is performed to rule out more distal sources of pain.

Definitive diagnosis of most lameness problems of the antebrachium can be made using conventional radiography and ultrasonography, but nuclear scintigraphy is useful for diagnosing incomplete and stress fractures of the radius, enostosis-like lesions, and enthesopathy at the origin of the accessory ligament of the superficial digital flexor tendon.

Osteochondroma of the Distal Aspect of the Radius
See Chapter 75 for a discussion of osteochondroma of the distal aspect of the radius.

Physeal Dysplasia of the Distal Aspect of the Radius (Physitis)
See Chapter 57 for a discussion of physitis.

Traumatic Physitis and Closure of the Distal Radial Physis

A syndrome of vague forelimb lameness believed to be associated with inflammation or pain originating from the distal radial physis has been recognized in young racehorses in early training. Anecdotally the condition appears to be more prevalent in 2-year-old colts. Distal radial physeal closure determined radiologically occurred earlier in fillies (701 days) than in colts (748 days).[1] Presumably the condition results from repetitive trauma to an open physis. The term *open knees* is commonly used to describe the state of skeletal immaturity. This condition is distinct from physeal dysplasia (physitis), because the condition is not a developmental abnormality, is not associated with clinically apparent enlargement of the metaphyseal region, and occurs in 2-year-old horses in active training.

References on page 1283

Mild to moderate forelimb lameness is vague, without indications of a problem elsewhere in the limb. The condition is usually bilateral, but horses can show unilateral lameness, because one limb is more painful than the other. Horses often have a choppy stride, with the legs carried wide. Focal heat may be present, but swelling is usually absent or minimal, and pain may be difficult to detect. Presumptive diagnosis is made on the basis of history, clinical signs, and ruling out other causes of lameness. A positive response to median and ulnar nerve blocks can be used to confirm that the distal aspect of the antebrachium is the source of pain, but this can also abolish subchondral bone pain in the carpus. Definitive radiological abnormalities are rarely present, but a radiologically open physis supports the diagnosis. Nuclear scintigraphy is generally not helpful, because all horses of this age have moderate-to-intense increased radiopharmaceutical uptake (IRU) at the physis. However, scintigraphy is useful for identifying or ruling out other potential causes of lameness, and asymmetrical radiopharmaceutical uptake (greater in the affected physis of the more severely affected limb) may support the diagnosis.

Treatment consists primarily of rest or a reduction in exercise intensity and systemic nonsteroidal antiinflammatory drugs (NSAIDs). Duration of rest varies with the skeletal maturity of the horse and severity of the condition. Local injection of corticosteroids or other drugs, such as homeopathic remedies, and systemic treatment with anabolic steroids have been used but are of dubious value. For some horses, slow jogging for 4 to 6 weeks may be all that is required; for others, stall confinement with hand-walking exercise progressing to paddock turnout for several months may be necessary. Follow-up radiographs can be used to monitor physeal closure, which is often used to determine the appropriate time to resume harder training.

The issue of distal radial physeal closure, the role of radiographs in making this determination, and how to determine the point when training should commence are controversial. Many trainers and veterinarians customarily obtain radiographs of the distal aspect of the radius of 2-year-olds, and those with open knees (radiological evidence that bony union at the physis is incomplete) are withheld from hard training until the physes have closed. Radiological closure of the distal radial physis generally occurs by 20 to 24 months of age[2] or slightly later.[1] Scin-

tigraphic activity of the distal radial physis persists well after radiological evidence of closure is observed.[3] However, endochondral ossification ceases (biological closure) before fusion is evident radiologically, and in our experience horses with a thin or faintly visible physeal remnant visible radiologically are at low risk for traumatic physitis.

Because the diagnosis is difficult to substantiate and pain may originate from an undetermined source, giving an accurate prognosis is difficult. If other more common conditions have been ruled out and the diagnosis of traumatic physitis is accurate, the prognosis is excellent. Many horses remaining in training develop signs of carpal lameness, and traumatic physitis may simply represent a prodromal phase of early osteoarthritis and bone pain. Finally, no correlation between age or month of closure of the distal radial physes and money won, races won, fastest mile, or fastest win mile during the 2-year-old year was found in Standardbreds.[4]

Radial Fractures

Radial fractures almost always result from external trauma, often a kick from another horse in adults, or from being stepped on or kicked by a mare in foals. Stress fractures of the radius also occur,[5,6] but in our experience true stress fractures of the radius are rare, and the description of those reported by others is similar to what we have termed *enostosis-like lesions* (see the following discussion). One of us (MWR) recently evaluated images of a 4-year-old Thoroughbred colt in race training, with a history of sudden left forelimb lameness, with a genuine radial stress fracture involving the medial, middiaphyseal cortex (Figure 39-1). Cortical location of stress fractures as determined scintigraphically and radiologically differentiates this injury from enostosis-like lesions.

Clinical signs depend on the severity and location of the fracture. Horses with complete fractures (which are nearly always displaced) are severely lame (non–weight bearing, grade 5) and have marked soft tissue swelling associated with the fracture itself or the site of the original wound. The limb may have an unusual angle, and crepitus is usually audible and palpable. Often an associated wound results from the initial injury or is caused by fragment penetration, especially on the medial aspect of the antebrachium. Horses with incomplete or nondisplaced fractures have moderate to severe lameness (grade 3 to 5) shortly after the injury, but within 12 to 72 hours they are often fully weight bearing and walking with minimal lameness. However, resumption of exercise or turnout often results in the fracture becoming displaced within 1 to 2 days (see Figure 3-4). Horses with true stress fractures have moderate lameness (grade 1 to 3) at a trot.

For horses with complete, displaced (unstable) fractures of the radius the diagnosis is straightforward. Radiology is needed only to define fracture configuration and to determine if repair is possible. Radiographs are *essential* in the initial evaluation of *any* horse with a wound in the antebrachium or over the proximal aspect of the carpus that has a history of acute, moderate-to-severe lameness associated with the injury. Lameness associated with incomplete or hairline fractures of the radius may be transient, but radiographs often reveal obvious or suspicious

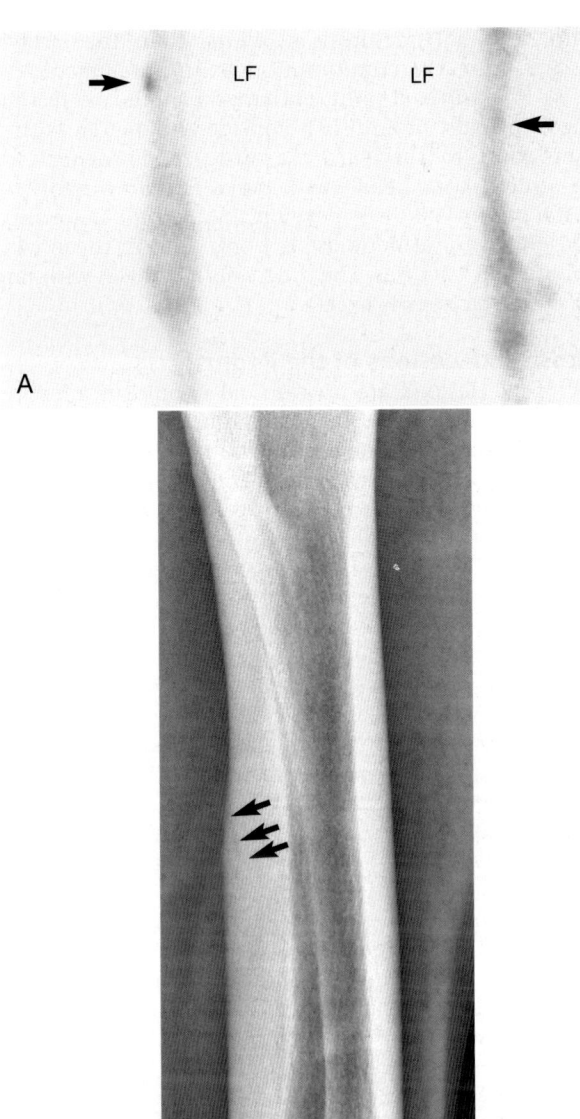

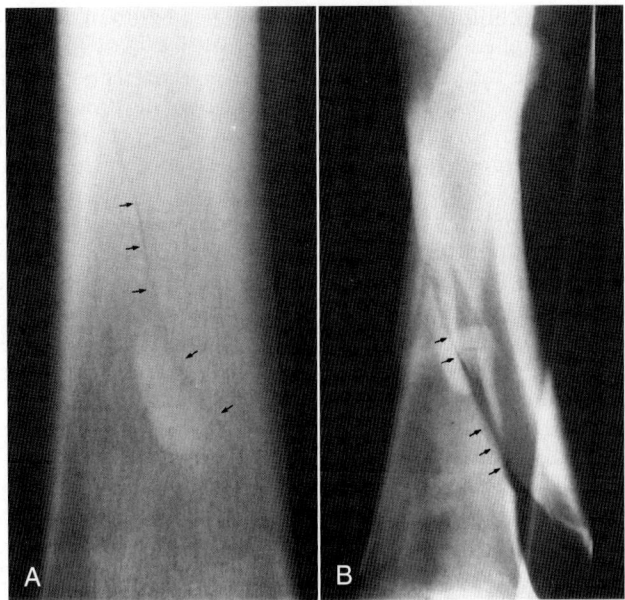

Fig. 39-2 • **A,** Craniocaudal radiographic image of the distal radius of a horse revealing a nondisplaced fracture *(arrows)*. The horse had been found acutely severely lame with a small wound over the distal cranial aspect of the antebrachium earlier that day. **B,** Craniocaudal radiographic image 1 day later. Catastrophic fracture occurred even though the horse was confined to a box stall. The original fracture line *(arrows)* and the edge of a plastic fence post used as a splint are visible.

Fig. 39-1 • **A,** Delayed-phase cranial (left image; medial is to the left and proximal is uppermost) and lateral (cranial is left) scintigraphic images of a 4-year-old Thoroughbred colt with acute left forelimb lameness. A focal area *(arrows)* of increased radiopharmaceutical uptake (IRU) involves the caudomedial cortex of the radius. In the cranial and lateral images, IRU can clearly be seen to involve the cortex rather than the medullary cavity of the radius. Cortical location is diagnostic for a stress fracture rather than an enostosis-like lesion. **B,** Cranial 45° medial-caudolateral oblique digital radiographic image of the left radius showing an oblique stress fracture *(arrows)* of the caudomedial cortex. (Courtesy Dean Richardson, Kennett Square, Pennsylvania, United States.)

fracture lines (Figure 39-2, *A*). Any radiological evidence of bone injury, often a localized cortical fragmentation or compression fracture, warrants high suspicion of an incomplete fracture, and a full series of radiographs should be obtained. Any horse that has persistent lameness after antebrachial trauma in which original radiological findings were negative should be reevaluated within 7 to 10 days, when a fracture may be evident. The horse should be confined to box rest in the interim. Diagnosis in horses with incomplete fractures or stress fractures can sometimes be difficult. Scintigraphic examination is important to differentiate fracture from other problems of the radius, such as enostosis-like lesions.

Emergency management of horses with long-bone fractures has been well described[7] (see Chapter 86). Horses with unstable fractures should be sedated, wounds should be treated, and a full-limb Robert Jones dressing with splints should be applied. A caudal splint extending from the ground to the point of the elbow (olecranon process) and a lateral splint extending to the withers are attached with tape. The bandage should have a flat surface to allow the lateral splint to be *in contact with* the skin of the upper limb and torso to prevent distal limb abduction. An oversized bandage reduces the effectiveness of the splints. Properly applying external coaptation is time-consuming and difficult, but appropriate stabilization is essential to reduce the risks of further fracture displacement and skin penetration. NSAIDs and broad-spectrum antimicrobial therapy should be administered. Horses should travel facing backward.

Confinement to a stall is *mandatory* for any horse with any radiological abnormality, including focal cortical defects, or with known trauma but with no detectable lesions. Catastrophic failure of the radius often results when small cortical defects or incomplete fractures become displaced (see Figure 39-2, *B*). We recommend conservative management in adult horses with incomplete or nondisplaced radial fractures. If possible, the horse should be transported to a surgical facility even if conservative management is chosen, because the fracture could become displaced and immediate surgical repair may be necessary. However, transport also involves risks that must be weighed against economic considerations and other factors affecting prognosis. Horses with incomplete fractures should be strictly confined to a stall for 8 weeks. External coaptation is applied as described previously for 4 to 8 weeks but can be difficult to maintain. Cross-tying is generally unnecessary, because horses tend not to lie down with bulky external coaptation in place. If radiographs reveal acceptable progression of healing after 8 weeks, the horse is restricted to box stall rest with hand-walking exercise for another 2 months. The majority of fractures are clinically healed in 4 months, although complete radiological healing may take up to 6 months or more in adult horses. Paddock turnout is generally allowed after 4 months, and horses return to work 5 to 6 months after injury.

NSAIDs are administered as needed to provide comfort and minimize the potential for contralateral limb laminitis. NSAID administration is usually necessary for only 7 to 10 days, and if pain is not adequately controlled, the horse should be reassessed carefully for fracture displacement or progression or infection associated with any wounds. Antibiotic therapy should be given to horses with wounds or deep pressure sores associated with the bandage and splints.

Horses with complete or displaced radial fractures require open reduction and internal fixation, but the prognosis in adult horses is poor to grave. The current method of choice is the application of two bone plates, one on the cranial surface and one on the lateral or medial surface, depending on fracture configuration.[8,9] In adult horses, use of the dynamic condylar screw plate can be considered and use of locking compression plates should be encouraged. Repair of fractures located at the most proximal or distal aspect of the radius or those with severe comminution is considerably more difficult, and these horses have a grave prognosis. In foals surgical repair is more successful, and a midshaft transverse or short oblique fracture with minor comminution is most common. Although infection is still a concern, implant or bone failure, seen commonly in adult horses, is less frequent. Physeal fractures result in premature closure of the physis, even if repaired surgically. Plate removal is necessary for foals intended to be used for racing.

Management of horses with rare radial stress fractures consists of rest for 4 months. Horses are given 2 months of box stall rest and 2 months of individual turnout in a small paddock before being returned to training. Follow-up radiographic and scintigraphic examinations are recommended.

Prognosis for horses with incomplete or nondisplaced fractures of the radius is good, but clients should be warned of the possible complications of fracture propagation and contralateral laminitis, if initial lameness is severe. Those that do not develop complications, and in which fractures heal uneventfully, have an excellent prognosis for return to full athletic function. Prognosis for surgical repair of radial fractures in adult horses is poor but depends greatly on fracture configuration and whether the fracture is open. Horses with open fractures have a worse prognosis, because infection is an important and frequent complication. Adult horses with long spiral or oblique fractures are the best surgical candidates, whereas those with comminution or fractures involving the proximal and distal aspects of the radius, in particular those involving the antebrachiocarpal or elbow joints, have a poor-to-grave prognosis. Overall the success rate of surgical management of an adult horse with a complete radial fracture is no better than 10% and is expensive. If severe comminution exists, the fracture is open, or it involves a joint, euthanasia should be recommended. In foals, prognosis is considerably better, with a good prognosis for survival and a fair-to-good prognosis for future athletic use.[8,9] Foals with radial fractures involving the distal physis will likely develop angular limb deformity, and prognosis for athletic use is worse than in those with middiaphyseal fractures. The prognosis for horses with rare radial stress fractures is excellent.

Enostosis-like Lesions of the Radius

Enostosis-like lesions are an unusual condition affecting many long bones, including the radius (see Chapters 12 and 19). *Enostosis* is defined as "bone within a bone," and because the cause has yet to be determined, the term *enostosis-like lesion* is used. Enostosis-like lesions are focal or multifocal intramedullary mild-to-dense radiopacities. Scintigraphically, enostosis-like lesions are associated with mild-to-intense IRU on delayed (bone phase) images (Figure 39-3, *A*). Lesions may occur in one or more bones simultaneously but are not necessarily associated with lameness.[10,11] Previously, enostosis-like lesions were described as bone infarcts or bone islands. Histological examination of specimens harvested from an enostosis-like lesion in a humerus revealed changes compatible with ischemia of cancellous bone and bone marrow.[12] Histological changes were similar to those in specimens examined from horses with medullary infarcts or those in bone adjacent to diaphyseal fractures and cortical stress fractures. However, the findings were not pathognomonic or exclusively characteristic of either of these entities.[12] We believe enostosis-like lesions may be caused by primary disruption of medullary vasculature and secondary development of bone sclerosis. Enostosis-like lesions are possibly an atypical form of bone infarct. Enostosis-like lesions are frequently found close to a nutrient foramen.[10] Because enostosis-like lesions occur in adult horses of all ages and performance categories, they are not likely to be stress fractures.

Although enostosis-like lesions can be an incidental radiological or scintigraphic finding of the radius, or most long bones, lameness apparently attributable to the condition occurs in approximately 50% of affected horses. Lameness from enostosis-like lesions is most common in horses with lesions involving the humerus and femur, whereas in other bones such as the radius and tibia, signs of lameness may be subtle or nonexistent.[13] An unusual clustering of Thoroughbred racehorses has been documented, with acute, forelimb or hindlimb lameness referable to enostosis-like lesions of the radii and tibiae, respectively, mimicking lameness seen in racehorses with stress fractures of these bones.[13] In horses with clinically relevant enostosis-like lesions, lameness is usually mild but may be severe. Although enostosis-like lesions can affect many bones simultaneously, lameness is usually restricted to a single limb.

Because completely abolishing pain originating from the radius may be difficult using diagnostic analgesia, in most horses with enostosis-like lesions diagnosis is made by ruling out other potential causes of lameness. Enostosis-like lesions must be differentiated from true stress fractures. It is imperative that two perpendicular scintigraphic images be obtained, to allow differentiation of cortical and medullary IRU (see Figure 39-1). Although treatment of

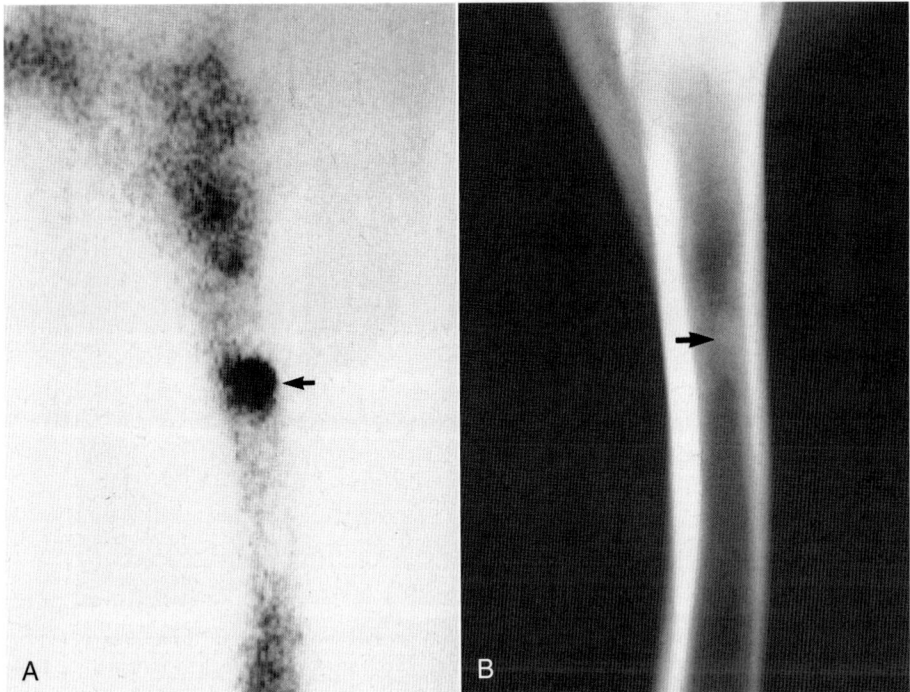

Fig. 39-3 • A, Lateral delayed (bone) phase scintigraphic image showing focal, intense increased radiopharmaceutical uptake *(arrow)* in the medullary cavity consistent with an enostosis-like lesion. Two scintigraphic images were compared, and increased radiopharmaceutical uptake was determined to involve the medullary cavity rather than the cortex. **B,** Lateromedial radiographic image reveals intramedullary increased radiopacity *(arrow)* on the endosteal surface and adjacent to the nutrient foramen, radiological signs typical in horses with enostosis-like lesions.

horses with enostosis-like lesions and of those with stress fractures is similar, cause and recurrence are different. Enostosis-like lesions are associated with mild-to-intense IRU in the medulla. In our experience enostosis-like lesions causing lameness are usually moderately to intensely active. Radiographs reveal corresponding single or multiple, focal or multifocal areas of increased radiopacity within the medullary cavity (see Figure 39-3, *B*). The lesions are frequently in contact with the endosteal surface and are most often in close proximity to the nutrient foramen. In the radius, follow-up scintigraphic and radiological evaluation 4 to 9 months after initial diagnosis often reveals resolution of the enostosis-like lesions, although resolution of radiological changes lags behind those visible scintigraphically.

Treatment of horses with enostosis-like lesions thought to be causing lameness is nearly identical to that for those with stress fractures. NSAIDs (phenylbutazone, 2.2 mg/kg, bid) are administered for 5 to 10 days or longer depending on degree of lameness. Horses are restricted to stall rest with hand-walking exercise for 2 months, followed by a minimum of 2 months in an individual small paddock. Follow-up clinical, scintigraphic, and radiographic evaluation is recommended. Prognosis for most horses with enostosis-like lesions is excellent, and recurrent lameness is rare, although occasionally longer convalescence (6 to 9 months) is required.

Osseous Cystlike Lesions of the Distal Radius

Osseous cystlike lesions occur in immature[14] and adult horses[15] and may result from osteochondrosis or trauma.

Occasionally, osseous cystlike lesions occur secondary to severe osteoarthritis of the antebrachiocarpal joint. Lameness ranges from mild to severe (grade 1 to 4) and may be sudden or insidious in onset.[14,15] Often no localizing clinical signs are present, unless osseous cystlike lesions are secondary to osteoarthritis of the antebrachiocarpal joint, when effusion may be present.

Lameness is localized to the antebrachiocarpal joint and distal aspect of the radius by intraarticular analgesia or by using median and ulnar nerve blocks. Response to intraarticular analgesia of the antebrachiocarpal joint is inconsistent; most horses show partial improvement. Scintigraphy is useful in horses in which diagnostic analgesia fails to localize lameness. Radiographs reveal a well-defined radiolucent defect in the subchondral bone, often with a sclerotic margin (Figure 39-4), with or without communication with the antebrachiocarpal joint.

Management remains controversial, and a universally accepted method is not currently available. Successful surgical management using an extraarticular approach, debridement, and cancellous bone grafting has been described.[15] Osseous cystlike lesions that enter the antebrachiocarpal joint can be debrided using an intraarticular approach, whereas those without communication are best managed using an extraarticular approach. Nonsurgical management has been successful and consisted of restricted exercise, with or without intraarticular administration of hyaluronan.[14] We treat horses conservatively. Duration of restricted exercise and number and type of intraarticular injections are determined on a case-by-case basis. Horses are given a minimum of 4 to 6 months of rest, or longer if

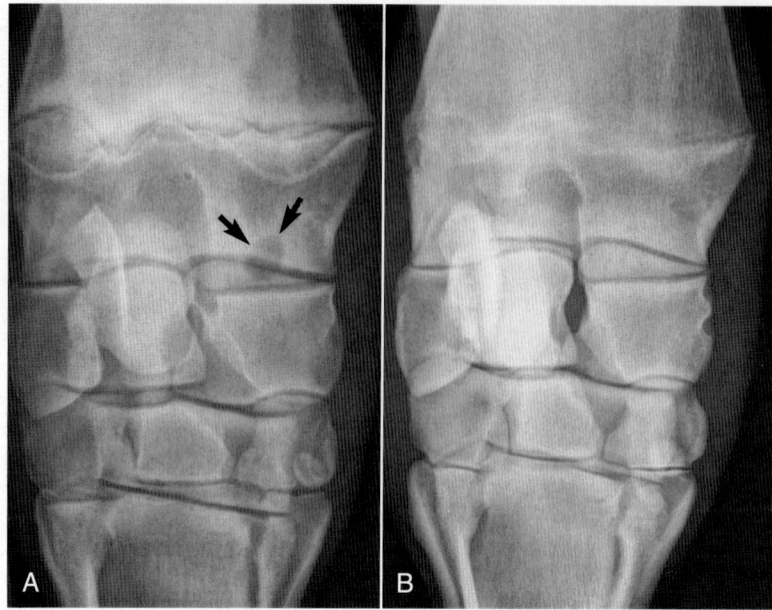

Fig. 39-4 • A, Craniocaudal digital radiographic image of the distal aspect of the right radius of a Standardbred weanling with an osseous cystlike lesion *(arrows)* of the distal, medial aspect of the radius, close to the antebrachio-carpal joint. This weanling was given stall rest for 4 months, and three intraarticular injections with hyaluronan and methylprednisolone acetate were performed. **B,** Seven-month follow-up craniocaudal image showing near complete resolution of the bone cyst.

gradual improvement in clinical signs is seen. Conservative management is the first choice in immature horses (<2 years of age). Extraarticular corticosteroid injection using a small drill bit has been successful in other sites and may be applicable for lesions involving the distal aspect of the radius. If little improvement is seen after 6 months, then surgical debridement (with or without grafting) should be considered. Limited data are available on which to base prognosis, which may be better in immature horses (<2 years of age).

Desmitis of the Accessory Ligament of the Superficial Digital Flexor Tendon
See Chapter 75 for a discussion of desmitis of the accessory ligament of the superficial digital flexor tendon.

Acute Caudal Antebrachial Myositis
Myositis and traumatic injury of the muscles in the caudal aspect of the antebrachium are relatively rare. Horses that compete over jumps at speed such as Three Day Event, timber, and steeplechase horses appear to be at risk to traumatize these muscles, presumably as a result of hyperextension of the metacarpophalangeal and carpal joints during landing. Occasionally, horses develop inexplicable myositis or injury of these muscle unassociated with a known traumatic event. Infectious myositis can result from puncture or kick wounds (see the following discussion).

Presumptive diagnosis can usually be made on the basis of history and clinical signs. The antebrachium should be carefully evaluated for even small puncture wounds. A recent but seemingly unrelated area of injury or small wound in the elbow or axillary region may be an important part of the history or physical examination. The clinician

should measure rectal temperature. Pyrexia indicates infection. Radiography should be performed to rule out bony injury, such as an incomplete fracture of the radius. Ultrasonographic examination reveals heterogeneous echogenicity within the bellies and between the fascia of the affected muscles, compatible with fiber disruption and hematoma formation.

Treatment consists of systemic NSAID administration (7 to 10 days) and hydrotherapy. Cold water hosing is administered for 15 to 20 minutes twice a day for 5 days, and then warm water hosing is initiated for 5 days. Broad-spectrum antimicrobial therapy is given if infection is suspected (see the following discussion). Horses are confined to a stall for 6 weeks, and hand-walking exercise is initiated, beginning at 5 minutes twice a day and increasing by 5 minutes each week. Passive flexion and extension of the carpus (30 to 50 repetitions daily) helps to improve range of motion and possibly fiber alignment. Clinical and ultrasonographic evaluation is recommended after 6 weeks. Work should not commence until carpal flexion is normal and the horse is sound. The prognosis for return to full athletic function is good.

Infectious Myositis and Cellulitis
Small puncture wounds in the antebrachium, elbow, and pectoral region can result in infections that cause tremendous antebrachial swelling associated with subcutaneous or deeper tissues. Small wounds may seal over quickly but result in inoculation of bacteria into deeper tissues, causing diffuse cellulitis or infectious myositis. Abrasions from equipment such as hobbles in a Standardbred racehorse can lead to deep infections of the proximal aspect of the antebrachium. Usually swelling is also present in the distal aspect of the limb, and the carpal sheath may show

sympathetic effusion. Infectious myositis may lead to deep abscess formation. Lameness is usually moderate to severe. The horse may be depressed and is usually pyrexic. White blood cell count and fibrinogen concentration are raised. Skin sloughing may develop with aggressive infections caused by *Streptococcus* or *Staphylococcus* species. Radiographs should be obtained, because a radial or ulnar fracture may occur concurrent with infection, but radiological findings are usually negative unless osteitis of the radius or ulna exists (see the following discussion).

Treatment involves administration of broad-spectrum antimicrobial drugs and NSAIDs and the application of topical warm water hydrotherapy. Full-limb bandaging is recommended to reduce swelling in the antebrachium and distal aspect of the limb. Horses with diffuse cellulitis usually respond quickly (within 3 to 5 days), whereas those with deeper infections require prolonged therapy. Horses with an abscess need surgical drainage.

Osteitis and Osteomyelitis of the Radius and Ulna

Osteitis and osteomyelitis of the radius and/or ulna can result from penetrating trauma, most commonly a kick. Clinical signs are similar to those seen with extensive soft tissue infection (see the preceding discussion), and some component of infectious myositis or cellulitis is present in most horses with osteomyelitis and in many with osteitis. Radiographs are diagnostic (Figure 39-5). Focal cortical trauma or fractures may also be present (see preceding section on radial fractures). Radiographs are indicated in all horses with infectious antebrachial myositis or cellulitis that exhibit a poor response to appropriate antimicrobial treatment and other ancillary therapy. Osteitis and osteomyelitis should be suspected in all horses with radial or ulnar fractures or focal cortical trauma associated with an open wound that subsequently develop signs of soft tissue infection. Infectious arthritis of the elbow or carpus may be present, either from direct involvement with a wound, or extension of the bone infection into the joint.[16]

Treatment is similar to that outlined for infectious myositis or cellulitis. Additional therapeutic options include surgical debridement and local antimicrobial delivery, such as intraosseous antimicrobial perfusion and use of antimicrobial-impregnated bone cement. The reader is referred to Chapter 65 for details on the diagnosis and management of infectious arthritis. Prognosis for horses with localized osteitis is generally favorable. Prognosis for those with osteomyelitis is more guarded and is dependent on the extent and severity of the infection, as well as the nature of any concurrent problems or injuries.

Swelling of the Antebrachium Associated with Other Conditions

Horses with infectious arthritis of the elbow joint, fractures of the proximal aspect of the radius or ulna, or distal

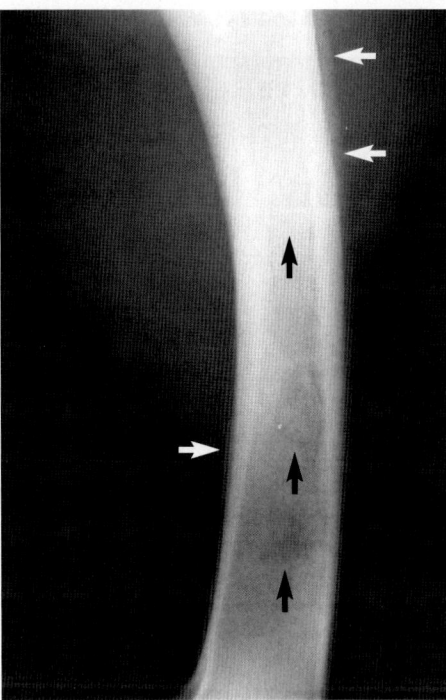

Fig. 39-5 • Lateromedial radiographic image of the right radius of a horse with extensive osteomyelitis resulting from a penetrating wound. Note the characteristic periosteal proliferative reaction *(white arrows)* and the osteolytic and osteoproliferative changes within the medullary cavity *(black arrows)*.

humeral fractures often have swelling of the antebrachium. These conditions should be kept in mind if diagnosis of a primary problem in the antebrachium cannot be made.

Hypertrophic Osteopathy

Hypertrophic osteopathy is an unusual disorder involving bilaterally symmetrical proliferation of fibrous tissue and periosteal bone in the appendicular and, less frequently, the axial skeleton, involving the metaphyseal and diaphyseal regions of several bones of all limbs.[17,18] Hypertrophic osteopathy may be associated with disease in the thorax or abdomen or with vascular abnormalities. Cause is unknown but may be neurogenic, mediated by the vagus nerve, or hormonal, leading to changes in regional blood flow. Clinical signs include soft tissue swelling and stiffness or lameness, often associated with elevated fibrinogen levels. Radiology of affected bones reveals palisading periosteal new bone. Identification of the primary lesion is important, because bony lesions may resolve with successful treatment of the underlying disease.[17-20] NSAIDs may ameliorate clinical signs.

Chapter 40

The Elbow, Brachium, and Shoulder

Sue J. Dyson

ANATOMICAL CONSIDERATIONS

The elbow joint consists of the humerus, radius, and ulna. The distal aspect of the humerus develops from three ossification centers: the diaphysis, the distal epiphysis, and the epiphysis of the medial condyle. These close radiologically at 11 to 24 months of age. The radius and ulna have a single proximal epiphysis. The radial physis closes radiologically at 11 to 24 months of age, but the ulnar physis does not close until 24 to 36 months of age. Physeal closure occurs later in non-Thoroughbred (TB) breeds.

The cranial aspect of the olecranon of the ulna has articular and nonarticular components. The anconeal process and trochlear notch articulate with the humerus. At the distal part of the trochlear notch is a distinct ridge. Distal to this is a large, non–weight-bearing synovial fossa.

The elbow is a ginglymus joint, supported medially and laterally by collateral ligaments. The medial collateral ligament consists of a long superficial part and a deeper short part. The medial collateral ligament arises from an eminence on the medial epicondyle of the humerus. The deep part inserts on the radial tuberosity; the superficial part inserts on a more distal prominence, just distal to the interosseous space between the radius and ulna. The lateral collateral ligament arises from a depression in the lateral epicondyle of the humerus and inserts on the lateral tuberosity of the radius, just distal to the joint margin. The joint capsule is extremely thin caudally, where it forms a pouch in the olecranon fossa. Cranially the joint capsule is strengthened by oblique fibers and blends with the collateral ligaments medially and laterally.

The most readily palpable landmarks are the olecranon of the ulna and the lateral collateral ligament of the humeroradial joint. Minimal soft tissue covers the lateral aspect of the elbow, making it vulnerable to the effects of direct trauma and penetrating wounds.

The humerus is surrounded by muscles, which largely protect it from the effects of direct trauma. The deltoid tuberosity on the craniolateral aspect is usually readily palpable and is potentially vulnerable to the effects of direct trauma. The deltoid tuberosity is the most useful landmark for identifying the point for needle insertion for synoviocentesis of the intertubercular (bicipital) bursa. The proximal aspect of the humerus has several centers of ossification for the humeral head and the greater and lesser tubercles, which gradually fuse at 3 to 5 months of age. Radiological closure of the proximal humeral physis occurs at 24 to 36 months of age.

The scapula has four centers of ossification: the scapular cartilage, body of the scapula, cranial part of the glenoid cavity of the scapula, and supraglenoid tubercle and coracoid process. The ossification center for the cranial part of the glenoid cavity fuses directly with the body of the scapula, and this is complete radiologically by 5 months of age. The physis between the supraglenoid tubercle and coracoid process and the body of the scapula closes radiologically at 12 to 24 months of age—earlier in TB and TB crossbreeds than in ponies. These physeal lines remain weak links, and it is through these that fractures of the supraglenoid tubercle and cranial part of the glenoid cavity of the scapula tend to occur.

The scapula is attached by the serratus ventralis muscles to the axial skeleton. Other muscles involved in attachment of the thoracic limb to the trunk and neck are the four pectoral muscles, the brachiocephalicus, and omotransversarius.

The brachial plexus lies on the axial aspect of the scapula and is derived from the sixth, seventh, and eighth cervical nerve roots and the first thoracic nerve. These nerve roots are potentially vulnerable to trauma where they exit the cervical and cranial thoracic vertebrae, and these are relatively common sites for neuroma formation after trauma. The nerves of the brachial plexus are responsible for innervation of many of the principal muscles of the shoulder region.

The scapulohumeral or shoulder joint is unusual because of the absence of collateral ligaments. Stability therefore depends on muscular support on the medial and lateral aspects by the subscapularis, teres minor, infraspinatus, and supraspinatus. Cranial support is provided by the biceps brachii and supraspinatus, and caudal support is rendered by the long head of the triceps brachii. Overlying muscles make it impossible in mature horses to appreciate distention of the joint capsule by palpation. The joint capsule attaches closely to the margins of the scapulohumeral joint, and this, together with the surrounding muscles, restricts arthroscopic evaluation within the joint. The suprascapular nerve wraps around the cranial margin of the scapula proximal to the supraglenoid tubercle and provides innervation to the infraspinatus and supraspinatus muscles.

Considering its embryological development and function, the so-called *intertubercular (bicipital) bursa* would be more appropriately called a *tendon sheath*.[1] The bursa surrounds the tendon of biceps brachii, which originates from the supraglenoid tubercle of the scapula. The craniodistal pull of the biceps brachii results in cranial and distal displacement of fractures of the supraglenoid tubercle. Communication was identified between the scapulohumeral joint capsule and the intertubercular bursa using contrast arthrography in 3 of 18 limbs (17%)[2]; thus in some horses intraarticular analgesia of the scapulohumeral joint has the potential to cause improvement in lameness caused by pain arising from the intertubercular bursa. The tendon of biceps brachii is partially cartilaginous proximally and passes over the smooth intertuberal groove of the humerus and then becomes predominantly muscular with a tendonous core.

The most important palpable landmarks in the shoulder region are the cranial and caudal eminences of the greater tubercle of the humerus. The notch between these

Reference on page 1283

eminences provides the portal for arthrocentesis of the scapulohumeral joint. The scapular spine is usually readily palpable except in exceptionally fat horses or heavily muscled individuals and becomes more prominent if the supraspinatus or infraspinatus muscles atrophy.

DIAGNOSIS
Clinical Signs
In the adult horse lameness associated with the elbow or shoulder region is comparatively rare, except after direct trauma caused by a fall, collision with a solid object such as a gatepost, or collision with another horse. In immature athletic horses, stress fractures of the scapula, humerus, and radius; osseous cystlike lesions; and osteochondrosis are quite common.

Lameness associated with the shoulder or elbow region is usually sudden in onset and generally moderate to severe. After trauma to the shoulder or elbow, or in association with severe lameness, the horse tends to stand with its weight inclined toward the contralateral limb, not fully load bearing on the lame limb. The horse may resent turning on the limb. Muscle atrophy in the shoulder region is not specific for lameness associated with the proximal aspect of the limb but is often more severe than if the pain arises farther distally. Rapid loss of the bulk of supraspinatus and infraspinatus muscles alone is likely to reflect damage to the suprascapular nerve, whereas involvement of additional muscles is more likely to reflect a brachial plexus injury. Swelling in the elbow or shoulder region usually reflects direct trauma but may be seen with subluxation or luxation of the shoulder or elbow joint. Patchy sweating is sometimes seen with a lesion of the brachial plexus. Pain elicited by deep palpation is relatively unusual and is generally associated with direct trauma. Care should always be taken to compare the reaction with that to palpation of the contralateral limb. The reaction to manipulation of the proximal limb joints should also be interpreted with care because many normal horses resent extreme flexion, extension, or abduction.

Many normal horses show some resentment of firm palpation of the brachiocephalicus muscles at the base of the neck. These muscles often become sore with a more distal source of pain causing lameness. Primary muscle pain causing lameness does sometimes occur and is associated with a more marked pain reaction on palpation and muscle spasm. It may cause a lameness most evident when the horse is ridden at the walk, characterized by lifting of the head and neck as the ipsilateral limb is protracted. Lesions of the tendon of biceps brachii are also sometimes associated with lameness that is worse at walk than trot.

If lameness is mild, then the character of the lameness is nonspecific; but if lameness is moderate to severe, it is often characterized by a shortened cranial phase of the stride, a reduced height of the arc of foot flight, and a marked head lift and nod. These gait characteristics are evident at the walk and the trot. Observation of the moving horse from the front and the side is particularly useful. The horse may pivot on the lame limb when turning. The gait characteristics of shoulder slip (see page 473) are more easily identified by observing the horse walking toward you. Lameness is frequently accentuated with the lame limb on the outside of a circle. In horses with proximal limb lameness, especially associated with muscle fibrosis, lameness may be evident only when the horse is ridden, performing specific movements. Manipulative tests of the proximal limb joints are rather nonspecific and frequently unrewarding.

Lameness may fluctuate in degree under different circumstances and within an examination period; therefore it is important to observe the horse for a sufficient length of time before proceeding with local analgesic techniques. If lameness is apparent only when the horse is ridden, the horse may be sensitive to the diagonal on which the rider sits.

Lameness caused by trauma resulting in only bruising usually improves rapidly, within a few days. Persistence of lameness merits further investigation.

Local Analgesia
It is important to recognize the potential effect of a median nerve block, performed in the proximal antebrachium, on elbow pain. Elbow lameness may be substantially improved, presumably because of local diffusion of the local anesthetic solution. Techniques for intraarticular analgesia of the elbow and shoulder and intrathecal analgesia of the intertubercular bursa are described in detail in Chapter 10. Intraarticular analgesia of the elbow and shoulder joints usually improves but rarely eliminates pain associated with either joint. The elbow and shoulder joints are relatively large; therefore use of at least 10 mL of local anesthetic solution (mepivacaine, 2%) is recommended for the elbow joint and 20 mL for the shoulder joint. Retrieving synovial fluid from each joint is usually possible. Absence of resistance to injection is not a guarantee that the needle is in an intraarticular location. Walking the horse after the block facilitates circulation of the local anesthetic solution throughout the joint. Although improvement in lameness may be seen rapidly, within 10 to 15 minutes after injection, at least 1 hour should elapse after the block before the result is considered negative. The block generally is effective for up to 2 hours. The block usually has no influence over pain associated with periarticular structures.

When performing intraarticular analgesia of the shoulder, it is important to recognize that there is communication with the intertubercular bursa in some horses. In some horses instability of shoulder, so-called *shoulder slip,* appears transiently (for up to 2 hours) after injection of local anesthetic solution. This prohibits interpretation of the nerve block. The cause is presumably diffusion of local anesthetic solution to nerves innervating the muscles responsible for maintaining stability of the shoulder. Positive-contrast arthrography has shown that injection of volumes greater than 20 mL pose a danger of pooling at the site of injection or leakage from the joint capsule.. An experimental study demonstrated that deposition of mepivacaine over the suprascapular nerve could result in transient shoulder slip, but this may be the result of diffusion to affect the brachial plexus (see page 473).[3]

Intrathecal analgesia of the intertubercular bursa may improve lameness associated with lesions of the tendon of biceps brachii, the bursa itself, or the humeral tubercles, but accurate intrathecal injection may not be reliable.[4] The bursa is large, and use of 20 mL of local anesthetic solution is recommended.

False-negative results to both intraarticular analgesia of the shoulder and elbow joints and intrathecal analgesia of the intertubercular bursa may occur, and radiological, scintigraphic, and ultrasonographic evaluation of these areas is indicated if clinical signs are suggestive of shoulder or elbow region pain. Many other potential sources of pain in the proximal limb cannot be desensitized by local analgesic techniques. If the response to distal limb analgesia and the blocks described previously is negative, nuclear scintigraphic evaluation may be warranted.

Assessment of Muscles
Electrical stimulation of muscles may help to identify muscle-related pain (see page 824).

IMAGING
Radiography and Radiology
Radiographic examination of the elbow requires a minimum of mediolateral and craniocaudal images.[5] The limb should be pulled forward sufficiently to avoid the pectoral muscle mass to evaluate the distal aspect of the humerus properly. Additional oblique images may be of value in selected horses. Routine radiographic examination of the scapulohumeral joint should include mediolateral and craniomedial-caudolateral oblique images. In some horses cranioproximal-craniodistal oblique images of the humeral tubercles are useful. Examination of the entire length of the humerus can be difficult, because often when such examination is indicated, the horse has pain and is reluctant to allow the limb to be adequately protracted. Accurate evaluation of the entire scapula is also not easy because of superimposition over the thoracic vertebrae and the contralateral limb.

Fast-speed, rare earth screens and appropriate film are essential if using conventional radiography. Use of a grid will greatly enhance image quality, especially in the shoulder region. High exposure factors are required (e.g., 100 kV, 100 mAs, for a mediolateral image of the shoulder). Underexposure will result in lesions being missed.

It is important to recognize that the cranial articular margin of the proximal radius has several lips that should not be confused with osteophytes (Figure 40-1). The cranial tuberosity of the proximal aspect of the radius may appear roughened in slightly oblique mediolateral views.

In the scapulohumeral joint a small circular radiolucent region is sometimes seen in the subchondral bone in the middle of the glenoid cavity of the scapula (Figure 40-2). A radiolucent edge effect is often seen in the proximal humerus, the result of superimposition of the lateral rim of the glenoid cavity of the scapula.

Ultrasonography
Diagnostic ultrasonography is invaluable for assessing muscle structure in the shoulder region. Normal muscle has a homogeneous echogenicity. Identification of hyperechogenic regions indicative of muscle necrosis, fibrosis, or mineralization is usually associated with lameness.

Evaluation of the elbow joint itself is limited in the weight-bearing position because of the difficulty in getting access medially. Examination of the lateral collateral ligament of the humeroradial joint is straightforward. For evaluation of the medial aspect, the limb should be pulled forward, but unless the medial collateral ligament is under tension, its echogenicity may lack homogeneity.

In the shoulder region ultrasonography is important for assessing the intertubercular bursa, humeral tubercles, tendon of biceps brachii (Figure 40-3, A and B), tendons of insertion of the supraspinatus and infraspinatus muscles (Figure 40-3, C and D), and the infraspinatus bursa (Figure 40-3, B).[6-10] Care should be taken to ensure that the horse is fully load bearing on the limb, because hypoechogenic artifacts can be created, especially in the tendon of biceps brachii, unless the musculature is under tension. The medial and lateral lobes of the tendon of biceps brachii and the isthmus between them should each be evaluated individually, because getting the entire structure into focus simultaneously is difficult.

Nuclear Scintigraphy
Nuclear scintigraphic evaluation of the proximal aspect of the forelimbs is indicated if the responses are negative to median and ulnar nerve blocks, intraarticular analgesia of

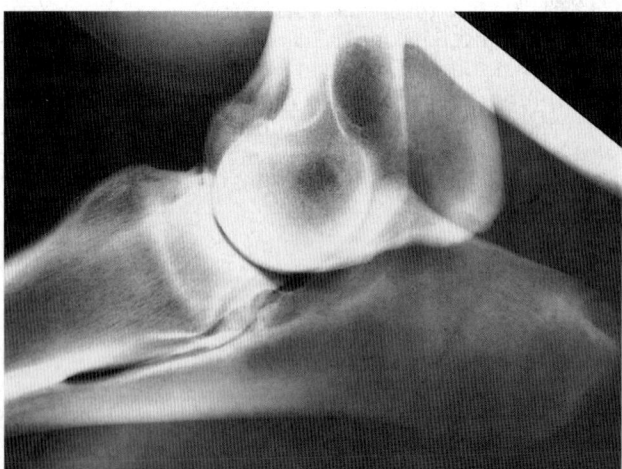

Fig. 40-1 • Mediolateral radiographic image of the elbow joint of a normal adult horse. The lips on the cranioproximal aspect of the radius are a normal radiological feature.

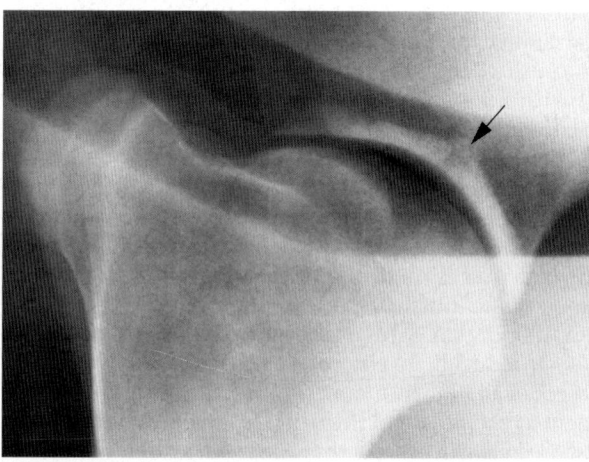

Fig. 40-2 • Mediolateral radiographic image of a scapulohumeral joint of a normal adult horse. There is a small lucent zone in the subchondral bone in the middle of the glenoid cavity of the scapula *(arrow)*. Note also the radiolucent band crossing the humeral head and the edge effect caused by superimposition of the articular margins of the scapula.

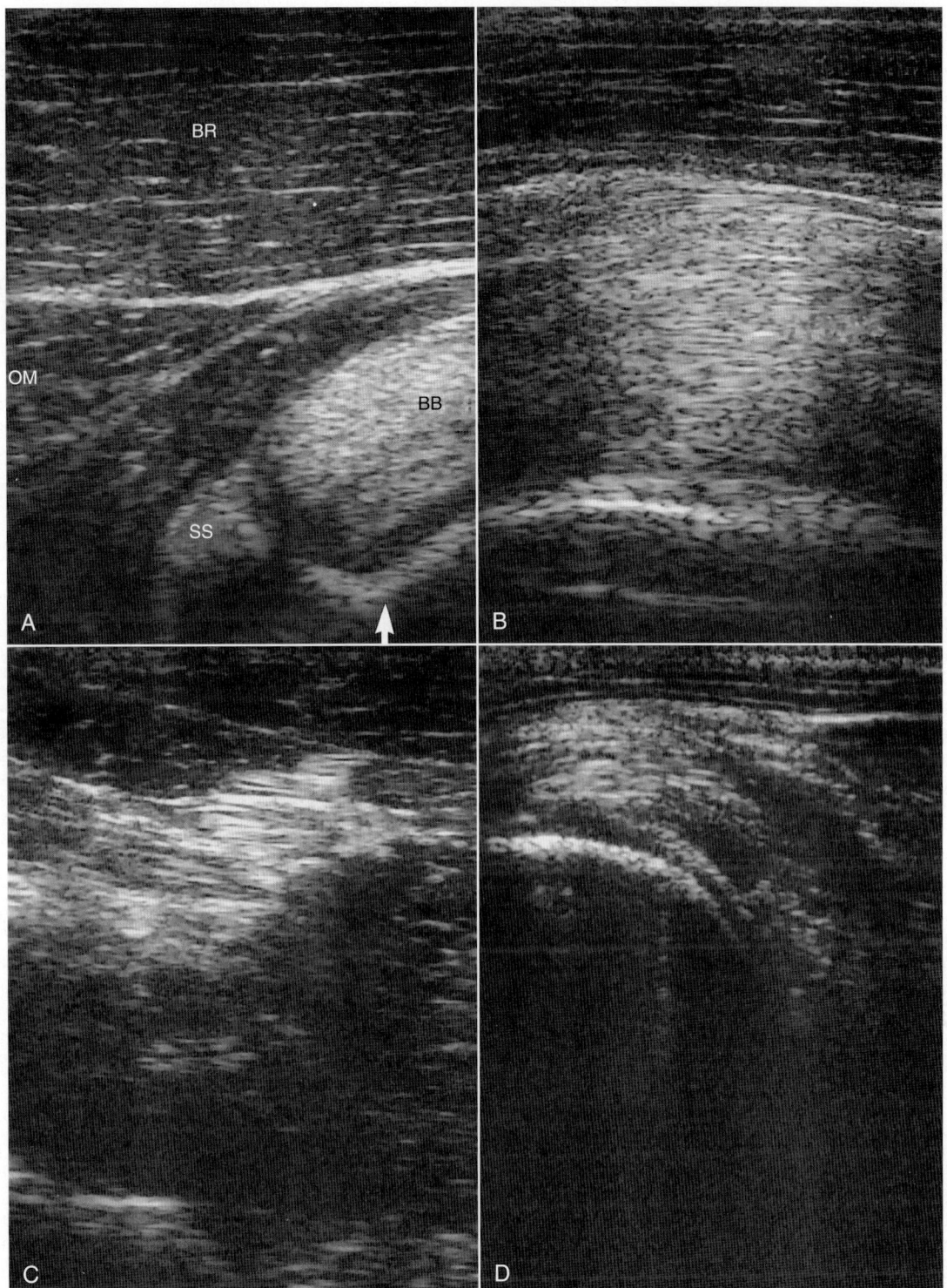

Fig. 40-3 • **A,** Transverse ultrasonographic image of the cranial proximal aspect of the humerus of a normal horse. Medial is left. There is a small amount of anechogenic fluid within the intertubercular bursa, and the contour of the humeral tubercle is smooth *(arrow)*. **B,** Longitudinal ultrasonographic image of the tendon of biceps brachii and the overlying brachiocephalicus muscle. Proximal is left. **C,** Transverse image of the tendon of infraspinatus within the infraspinatus muscle. **D,** Transverse ultrasonographic image of the insertion of the infraspinatus on the proximal aspect of the humerus. The anechogenic space, the infraspinatus bursa, appears between the tendon of insertion and the bone. *BB,* Medial lobe of the tendon of biceps brachii; *BR,* brachiocephalicus; *OM,* omotransversarius; *SS,* medial tendon of insertion of the supraspinatus.

the elbow and shoulder joints, and intrathecal analgesia of the intertubercular bursa. Scintigraphy is also indicated if history and clinical signs suggest a stress fracture. Scintigraphy has also been useful for identifying enostosis-like lesions (bone islands) in the humerus and fractures of the deltoid tuberosity of the humerus. Care should be taken to localize any region of increased radiopharmaceutical uptake (IRU) as precisely as possible to identify the likely underlying pathological condition. IRU in the first rib can easily be misinterpreted unless a cranial image is obtained to separate the scapula and humerus from the underlying rib. Examination of the scintigraphic images should include careful assessment of the soft tissues, because abnormal uptake of the radiopharmaceutical in muscle can sometimes be identified in bone phase images.

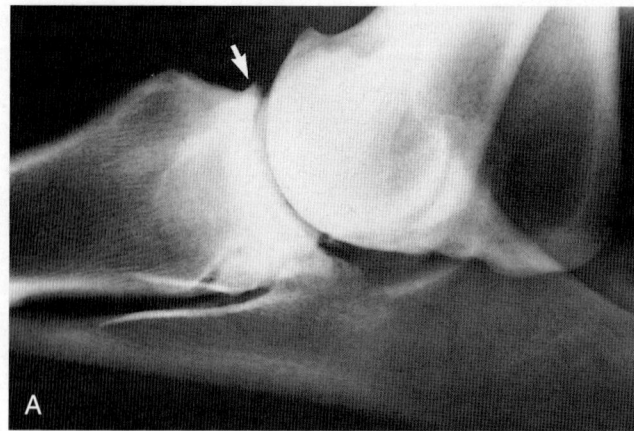

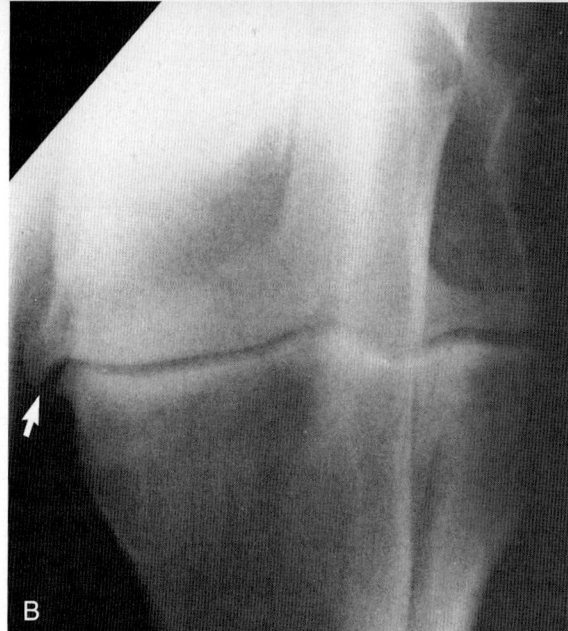

Fig. 40-4 • Mediolateral **(A)** and craniocaudal **(B)** (medial is to the left) radiographic images of the elbow joint of a 9-year-old event horse with left forelimb lameness alleviated by intraarticular analgesia of the elbow. The periarticular osteophytes *(arrows)* and subtle narrowing of the joint space medially indicate osteoarthritis. The horse failed to respond to intraarticular medication.

DIFFERENTIAL DIAGNOSIS

Elbow

Osteoarthritis

Osteoarthritis (OA) of the elbow is relatively unusual and tends to be seen in older athletic horses. Often the horse has a history of trauma. The horse may resent manipulation of the elbow, but appreciating joint effusion is usually not possible. Lameness often varies in degree, within and between examinations, and is usually worst on a hard surface, especially on a circle.

Intraarticular analgesia improves lameness. Periarticular osteophyte formation, alterations in subchondral bone opacity, and narrowing of joint space width may be seen radiologically (Figure 40-4). Care should be taken not to misinterpret as osteophytes normal bony lips on the dorsoproximal aspect of the radius in a mediolateral image.

The repeated use of intraarticular polysulfated glycosaminoglycans has been most effective in resolving lameness, but the long-term prognosis for return to full athletic function is guarded.

Osseous Cystlike Lesions

Osseous cystlike lesions occur most commonly medially in the proximal radial epiphysis (Figure 40-5) and usually result in acute-onset, relatively severe lameness in immature athletic horses.

Lameness may vary greatly in degree, within and between examinations, and is usually substantially improved by intraarticular analgesia. In addition to a well-defined osseous cystlike lesion, there is often periosteal new bone on the proximal medial metaphyseal region of the radius. Intraarticular medication with hyaluronan or corticosteroids (triamcinolone acetonide or methylprednisolone acetate) has resulted in successful resolution of lameness.[1,11] In some horses the osseous cystlike lesions have resolved radiologically. Surgical treatment by curettage of the cyst using an extraarticular approach has been successful in some horses, but fracture through the cyst has been a recognized complication.[12] Recurrent lameness after surgical treatment is also possible.[13] An ill-defined osseous cystlike lesion is occasionally seen in older horses with OA of the elbow with no known previous history of lameness; it is likely that the cystlike lesion had been present

asymptomatically before the development of pain associated with OA.

Less commonly, large, less well-defined osseous cystlike lesions have been identified in the distal aspect of the humerus in young Thoroughbreds being prepared for the yearling sales or just after entering training.[1] Lameness is acute in onset, persists despite box rest, and is generally not influenced by intraarticular analgesia of the elbow. Nuclear scintigraphic examination reveals a region of IRU in the distal aspect of the humerus, more centrally located than that associated with a stress fracture (see page 463). Careful radiological examination reveals a less well-defined osseous cystlike lesion. Conservative management has resulted in persistent lameness, and the results of surgical treatment have been disappointing. Young horses with smaller osseous cystlike lesions in the distal medial humerus have been identified and have responded to conservative management.[12]

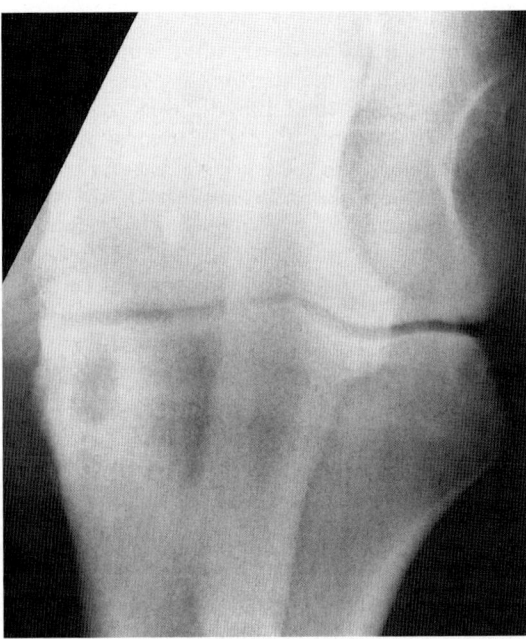

Fig. 40-5 • Craniocaudal radiographic image of the proximal aspect of the radius of a 3-year-old Thoroughbred racehorse with left forelimb lameness, which substantially improved with intraarticular analgesia of the elbow. There is a well-defined osseous cystlike lesion in the proximomedial aspect of the radius. Note also the periosteal new bone on the proximomedial aspect of the radius. Intraarticular medication with hyaluronan resolved lameness, and the horse raced successfully.

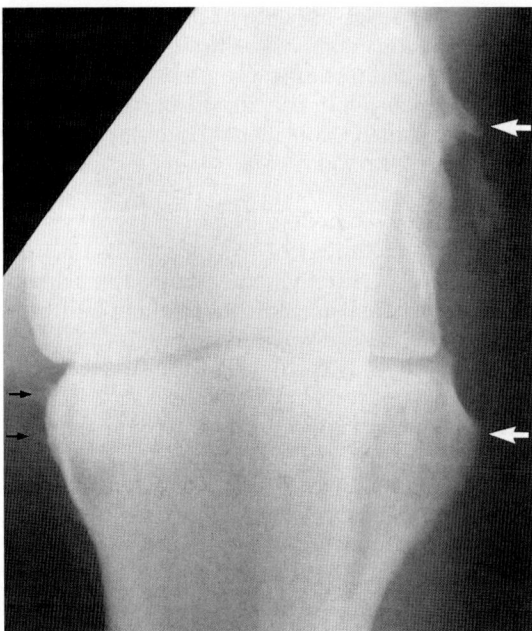

Fig. 40-6 • Craniocaudal radiographic image of the elbow of 15-year-old pony that had chronic left forelimb lameness after a fall. There is entheseous new bone at the attachments of the lateral collateral ligament of the humeroradial joint *(white arrows)* with mineralization within the ligament. There is also new bone on the proximomedial aspect of the radius *(black arrows)*. Periarticular osteophyte formation was also visible in a mediolateral image. Ultrasonographic examination revealed poor fiber pattern within the lateral collateral ligament. Postmortem examination confirmed desmitis of the lateral collateral ligament and osteoarthritis of the elbow joint.

Osteochondrosis

The elbow is a relatively rare location for osteochondrosis, but occasionally lameness is identified in young TBs and STBs in training associated with osteochondrosis lesions of the distal aspect of the humerus or the proximal aspect of the radius. Lameness is improved by intraarticular analgesia. Various radiological changes have been identified. Results of medical and surgical management have been disappointing. Osteochondrosis lesions of the anconeal process of the ulna also occur rarely,[14] but they should not be confused with a separate ossification center in young foals.[15]

Stress Reactions in Subchondral Bone

Intermittent lameness has been identified in a small number of event horses associated with an assumed stress reaction in the subchondral bone of the distal aspect of the humerus.[1] Lameness is induced by jumping but tends to resolve if the horse is not jumped. Lameness may be improved by intraarticular analgesia of the elbow (curious). No bony abnormalities have been identified radiologically. Nuclear scintigraphic examination reveals a region of IRU in the subchondral bone of the distal aspect of the humerus. Treatment with box rest and controlled walking exercise for 3 months has resulted in resolution of lameness and a normal distribution of the radiopharmaceutical. Horses have been able to return to full athletic function without recurrent injury.

Collateral Ligament Injury

Injury to the collateral ligaments of the elbow is not common and usually results from a traumatic injury such as a fall. Damage to the lateral collateral ligament has been

identified most frequently. Severe injuries may also be associated with injury to the joint capsule, and osteoarthritis may ensue. Lameness is acute in onset. Subtle soft tissue swelling may be appreciated in the elbow region, and manipulation of the elbow may induce pain. Lameness may be partially improved by intraarticular analgesia of the elbow. If damage is restricted to extraarticular structures, then the response may be negative. Nuclear scintigraphic examination may be helpful in these horses. IRU occurs at the sites of ligament attachment on the distal aspect of the humerus and proximal aspect of the radius.

Definitive diagnosis requires ultrasonographic examination and identification of disruption of the normally linear pattern of echoes within the ligament. Sometimes periosteal new bone or avulsion fractures can be identified at the region of ligamentous attachment.[16] Radiographic examination should also be performed to identify any concurrent pathological condition of the bone, such as enthesophyte formation, an avulsion fracture, or secondary OA (Figure 40-6).

Horses with minor lesions have responded well to a period of box rest and controlled walking exercise, but those with lesions that have been associated with entheseous new bone formation often have had persistent lameness and have developed OA.

Luxation

Luxation of the elbow joint is usually seen with a fracture of the olecranon or proximal aspect of the radius or separation of the radius and ulna, although luxation occasionally occurs alone. Lameness is acute in onset and severe and is associated with considerable swelling in the elbow region. Comprehensive radiographic examination is essential to determine if one or more concurrent fractures are present. Surgical repair can be considered, but the prognosis for athletic function is poor.

Enthesopathy of the Biceps Brachii

Tearing of the attachment of the biceps brachii from the cranioproximal aspect of the radius may be associated with a traumatic injury such as a fall, but frequently history does not suggest the cause. Lameness is sudden in onset and often not associated with any localizing signs, except pain on manipulation of the elbow in horses with acute lameness. The lameness has no particular characteristics. The response to local analgesic techniques is negative. Radiographic examination may reveal periosteal new bone on the cranioproximal aspect of the humerus in horses with chronic lameness[17] (Figure 40-7). Sometimes an adjacent mineralized fragment is present, an avulsion fracture or dystrophic mineralization. Some new bone formation on the cranioproximal aspect of the radius can be seen in normal horses, reflecting previous injury; therefore care should be taken in interpreting its current clinical significance. Nuclear scintigraphic examination is helpful for acute lameness before periosteal new bone develops and in horses with chronic lameness. Ultrasonographic evaluation has not been helpful. Treatment is by rest. The prognosis is guarded to fair.

Avulsion of the Origin of the Ulnaris Lateralis

The ulnaris lateralis functions to flex the carpus and extend the elbow. An avulsion fracture at the origin of the ulnaris lateralis, from a site caudal and distal to the origin of the lateral collateral ligament of the humeroradial joint, is a rare cause of lameness. Lameness is acute in onset and moderate to severe, following a fall, resulting in diffuse soft tissue swelling on the lateral aspect of the elbow. Diagnosis is based on radiography and ultrasonography. A nonarticular avulsion fragment and enlargement and marked disruption of the tendon of origin of the ulnaris lateralis are present.[18]

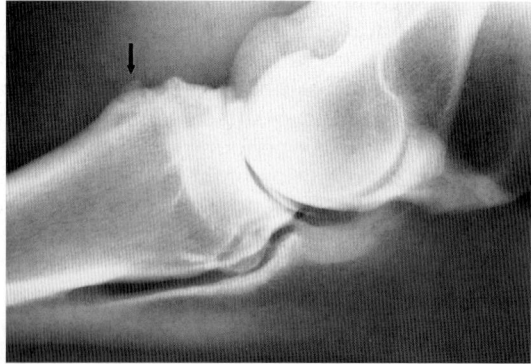

Fig. 40-7 • Mediolateral radiographic image of the right elbow of 9-year-old show jumper with chronic right forelimb lameness that no local analgesic technique influenced. There is new bone on the cranial tuberosity of the radius at the site of insertion of the biceps brachii *(arrow)*. Nuclear scintigraphy gave evidence of increased bone modeling at this site. The horse had persistent lameness despite prolonged rest.

Fracture of the Olecranon

Fracture of the olecranon of the ulna usually results from a kick or fall, resulting in acute-onset, severe lameness. The horse may stand with the elbow dropped because of lack of an effective attachment of the triceps, the principal extensor of the elbow. Soft tissue swelling may or may not be palpable. Traction on the summit of the olecranon elicits pain. Although many fractures are comminuted, detecting crepitus is unusual. Radiographic examination should include mediolateral and craniocaudal images to assess the configuration of the fracture and to identify any other bony lesions (see Figure 13-3). Fractures have been classified into five types[19]:

- *Type 1.* Fractures of immature horses that involve the growth plate and the metaphysis. These are subdivided into type 1a, a nonarticular fracture involving only the growth plate, and type 1b, a Salter-Harris type II articular fracture involving the anconeal process and proximal part of the trochlear notch.
- *Type 2.* A simple articular fracture involving the middle of the trochlear notch.
- *Type 3.* A nonarticular fracture involving the proximal metaphyseal region.
- *Type 4.* Comminuted articular fractures.
- *Type 5.* A fracture involving the distal olecranon or ulnar shaft, extending proximally and entering the distal, nonarticular part of the trochlear notch.

A fracture that enters the trochlear notch should be examined carefully to determine whether it involves the articular or nonarticular portion. Treatment by internal fixation usually warrants a fair-to-good prognosis,[20-23] provided that the fracture is identified early and unless comminution is excessive. Conservative management has also been successful if the fracture is not displaced; the best results are achieved with type 5 fractures.[24] If the horse is treated conservatively, healing should be monitored radiologically to ensure that no displacement has occurred. Potential complications of conservative management include nonunion, OA, development of a flexural deformity or contralateral laminitis, or development of an angular limb deformity in the contralateral limb.

Olecranon Bursitis

See Chapter 79 for a discussion of olecranon bursitis.

Humerus

Fractures of the Deltoid Tuberosity

Fracture of the deltoid tuberosity of the humerus occurs occasionally.[5,25] Often no cause is identifiable, although in some horses trauma has been recognized. Lameness is acute in onset and moderate to severe, depending on the configuration of the fracture. Generally no soft tissue swelling is detectable, although deep palpation in the region may cause pain in acute, but not chronic, injuries. Turning on the limb induces pain. In the absence of localizing signs, nuclear scintigraphic examination may be the best indicator of the injury (Figure 40-8, *A*).

Diagnosis is by radiographic examination. A craniomedial-caudolateral oblique image is essential (Figure 40-8, *B*), because abnormalities may not be detectable in mediolateral images. Several configurations of fracture have been

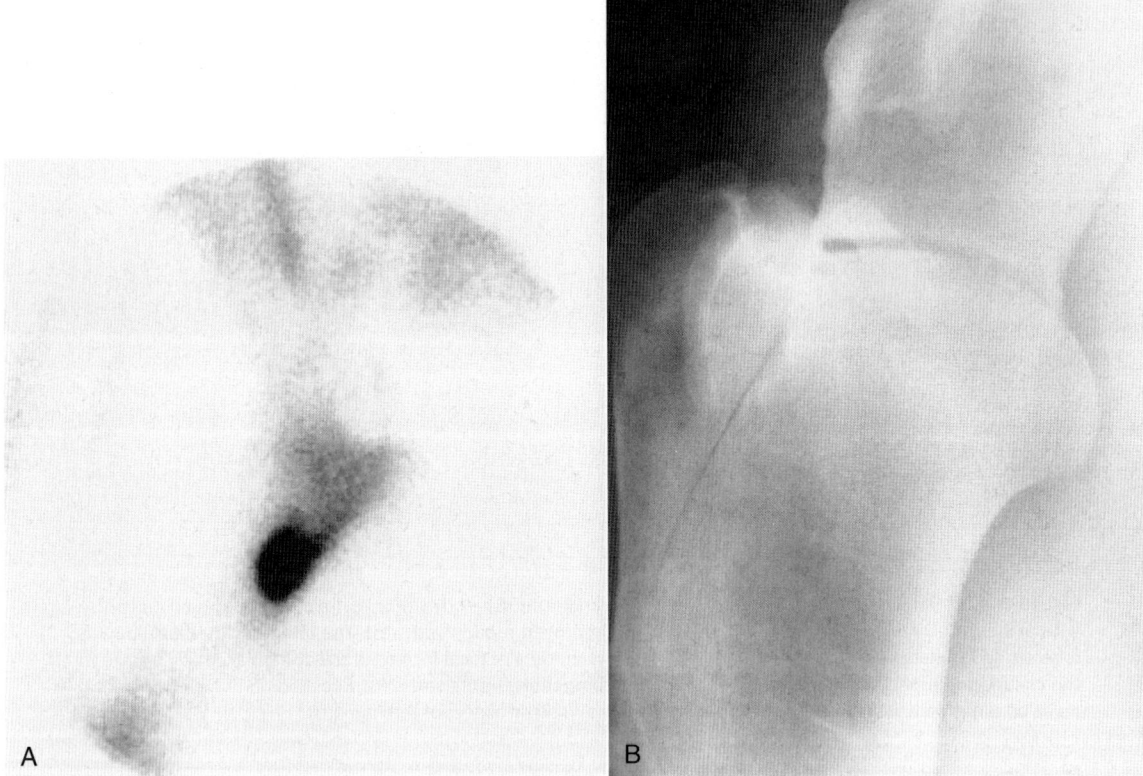

Fig. 40-8 • A, Lateral scintigraphic image of the right shoulder of 7-year-old dressage horse with acute-onset, moderately severe lameness of 2 weeks' duration with no associated localizing clinical signs. There is marked focal increased radiopharmaceutical uptake in the region of the deltoid tuberosity of the humerus. Radiographic examination revealed an incomplete fracture line through the base of the tuberosity and slight periosteal callus. **B,** Craniomedial-caudolateral oblique radiographic image of the proximal aspect of the humerus of a 3-year-old Thoroughbred broodmare with acute-onset, severe right forelimb lameness. There is an incomplete fracture of the deltoid tuberosity of the humerus. The mare made a complete functional recovery, but a radiologically visible osseous cystlike lesion developed distal to the greater tubercle of the humerus.

identified: small chip fractures, single or comminuted, a longitudinal fracture through the tuberosity itself, and an incomplete oblique fracture extending proximocaudally through the humeral diaphysis and metaphysis. Conservative management results in a favorable outcome, unless an oblique fracture is displaced, for which internal fixation is recommended. The prognosis is good.

Stress Fractures
Stress fractures of the humerus are relatively common in young Thoroughbreds in training. Humeral stress fractures occur frequently in 3-year-old and older racehorses within 4 to 8 weeks of retraining, and in North America they are often seen from February to April. The most common locations are the proximocaudal aspect of the humerus and the distal cranial and caudal aspects.[26-28] Unilateral lameness is usually acute in onset and relatively severe. This lameness often improves relatively rapidly with box rest. Despite preexisting callus formation indicative of previous ongoing bony reaction, previous lameness has often not been recognized. Usually no localizing signs are apparent, and the response to distal limb nerve blocks is negative. Nuclear scintigraphic examination is the most sensitive means of detecting a fracture and should be performed if a stress fracture is suspected on clinical grounds, because premature return to work may potentially result in a more

catastrophic fracture. A focal region of IRU is identified in the proximocaudal aspect of the humerus or the distal cranial or caudal aspects (Figure 40-9). Fractures are usually medial. Rarely there is a pattern of IRU consistent with an incomplete spiral fracture of the humeral diaphysis. Radiological examination is less sensitive, although in some horses new bone formation can be identified on the caudal aspect of the proximal epiphysis, sometimes with increased radiopacity of the subchondral bone or new bone on the cranial aspect of the distal metaphysis and physis. Identification of new bone associated with a distal caudal fracture is rare.[28] With treatment of box rest and controlled walking exercise for a minimum of 3 months, followed by a graduated return to work, the prognosis is good.

Fractures of the Greater or Lesser Tubercles
A fracture of the greater or lesser tubercle of the humerus is an occasional cause of unilateral forelimb lameness.[6,29-33] The history is often unknown, and usually no localizing clinical signs are apparent. Lameness varies in degree. Intrathecal analgesia of the intertubercular bursa may improve the lameness. Although some fractures may be suspected on a mediolateral radiographic image, craniomedial-caudolateral oblique and cranioproximal-craniodistal (skyline) oblique radiographic images are often necessary. A caudolateral-craniomedial oblique image may be useful

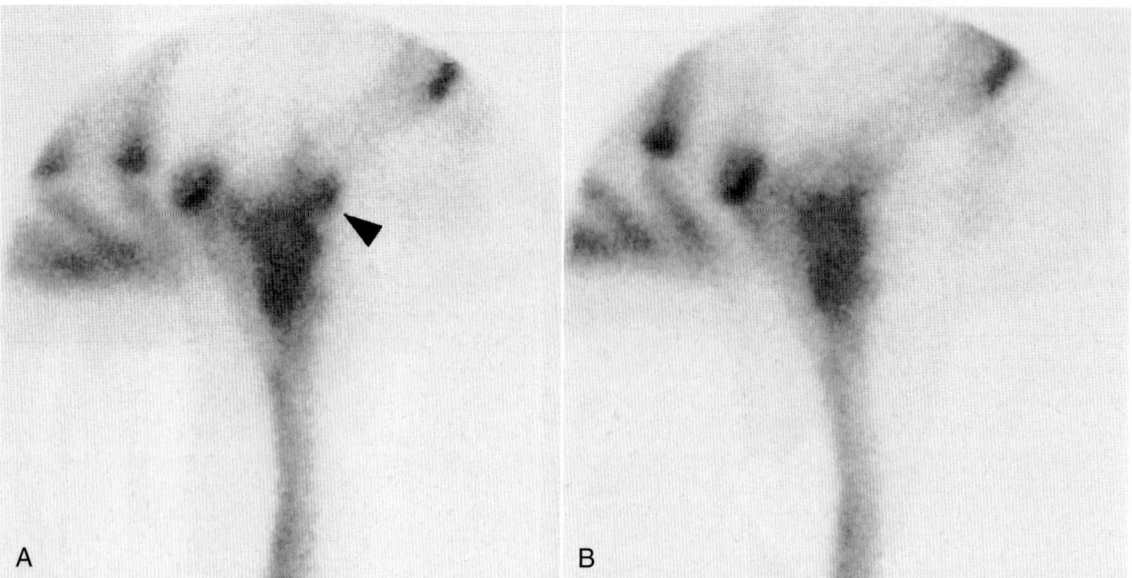

Fig. 40-9 • Lateral scintigraphic images of the left **(A)** and right **(B)** elbows of 2-year-old Thoroughbred racehorse with acute-onset, severe left forelimb lameness that improved rapidly with rest. The image of the left elbow is reversed to facilitate comparison with the right. There is moderate, focal increased radiopharmaceutical uptake in the craniodistal aspect of the right humerus *(arrow),* compatible with a stress fracture. Radiographic examination revealed slight periosteal and endosteal callus on the craniodistal aspect of the humerus.

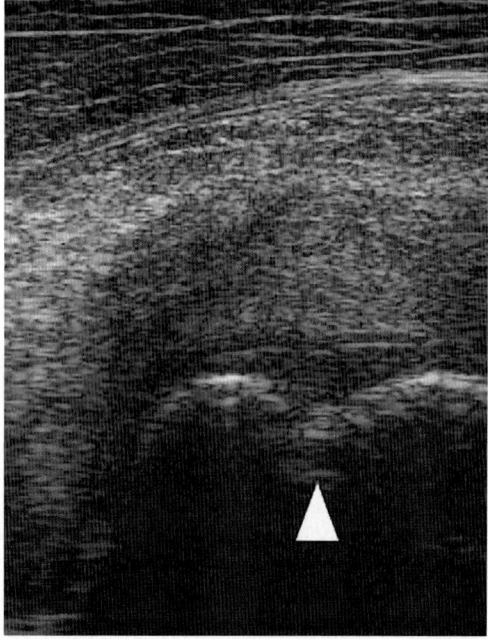

Fig. 40-10 • Transverse ultrasonographic image of the humeral tubercles and tendon of biceps brachii of a 2-year-old Thoroughbred filly with severe lameness at the walk. Lateral is to the right. There was slight soft tissue swelling in the shoulder region, but no focus of pain could be identified. Nuclear scintigraphic examination revealed marked focal increased radiopharmaceutical uptake in the humeral tubercles. There were no radiological abnormalities. Cortical disruption *(arrow)* is apparent.

to highlight a fracture of the cranial aspect of the greater tubercle.[5,30] Fracture fragments may also be accurately localized using diagnostic ultrasonography[29] and in some horses are detectable only ultrasonographically (Figure 40-10). The overlying intertubercular bursa and tendon of biceps brachii should be inspected carefully. Small fractures may be removed surgically. Endoscopy of the intertubercular bursa permits reasonable access to the greater tubercle but not the lesser tubercle.[29] Outcome is usually favorable.

Diaphyseal Fractures

Diaphyseal fractures of the humerus usually result from a fall or other traumatic incident and may be oblique, spiral, or severely comminuted. Lameness is acute in onset and severe, associated with considerable swelling, pain, and crepitus. The horse may stand with the elbow dropped, slight carpal flexion, and the weight only on the toe. Radial nerve paralysis may occur concurrently (see pages 144 and 474). The diagnosis is usually obvious, and the prognosis is poor, so humane destruction is justified.[34] Successful repair may be achieved in selected horses younger than 3 years of age.[35] Conservative management in foals with diaphyseal fractures is a reasonable choice, but breakdown of soft tissues and angular limb deformities of the contralateral limb are potential complications.

Proximal Physeal Injuries

Injuries of the proximal humeral physis are rare, but Salter-Harris type I and II fractures have been seen in horses younger than 2 years of age.[36] The prognosis with conservative management is poor.

Enostosis-like Lesions (Bone Islands)

Enostosis-like lesions, or solitary bone islands, have been recognized only since the advent of nuclear scintigraphy (see Chapters 19 and 39). An *enostosis* is defined as bone developing within the medullary cavity or on the endosteum, resulting in an area of increased radiopacity. In the horse, enostosis-like lesions have been described as focal or multifocal intramedullary sclerosis in the diaphyseal region of long bones, near the nutrient foramen, often developing on the endosteal surface of the bone. The cause of these lesions is unknown. Such endosteal reactions must be differentiated from endosteal callus secondary to a stress fracture. The presence of such radiopaque lesions is not always associated with lameness.

In the humerus, enostosis-like lesions occasionally cause acute-onset, moderate-to-severe lameness in young Thoroughbreds and older athletes, but they may be present asymptomatically. Usually no localizing clinical features are present. Lameness resolves relatively rapidly with rest, thus mimicking the behavior of horses with a stress fracture and therefore warranting nuclear scintigraphic examination. A region of intense IRU occurs in the distal caudal aspect of the humerus, distinguishable from a stress fracture because of its slightly more proximal and medullary location (Figure 40-11, *A*). Radiological examination usually reveals a relatively large, oval-shaped opacity within the medulla, adjacent to the nutrient foramen (Figure 40-11, *B*). However, initial radiological evaluation may be negative. Because lesions may be present asymptomatically, it is important to rule out other potential causes of lameness.

Treatment is similar to that for a horse with a stress fracture: box rest and controlled walking exercise for approximately 3 months. An area of increased radiopacity may persist radiologically. Follow-up scintigraphic evaluation sometimes reveals normal radiopharmaceutical uptake, although in some horses there is persistent IRU despite resolution of lameness. The prognosis is usually good, although occasionally horses have lesions in several limbs and lameness may shift from limb to limb.

Scapulohumeral Joint

Osteochondrosis

Osteochondrosis of the scapulohumeral joint is often clinically evident in the first year of life, but in some horses it is not manifested until the horse is 2 to 5 years of age, although periods of unexplained lameness may occur. Delayed-onset lameness is often associated with relatively subtle radiological changes, which are more localized compared with those in horses that have lameness evident earlier. Lameness is often acute in onset and moderate to severe and is generally characteristic of proximal limb lameness. Often the foot of the most severely affected limb rapidly becomes more upright and boxy. In young, immature athletic horses radiological changes are often present bilaterally, although clinical signs may be evident only unilaterally. Intraarticular analgesia usually results in improvement in lameness rather than complete alleviation; therefore the clinical significance of lesions in the contralateral limb can be difficult to interpret.

Radiological abnormalities involve the glenoid cavity of the scapula, the humeral head, or both and include flattening of the articular surfaces, resulting in loss of congruity of the articular surfaces, irregular lucent zones in the subchondral bone, modeling of the ventral angle of the scapula, and blurring of the normally sharp outline of

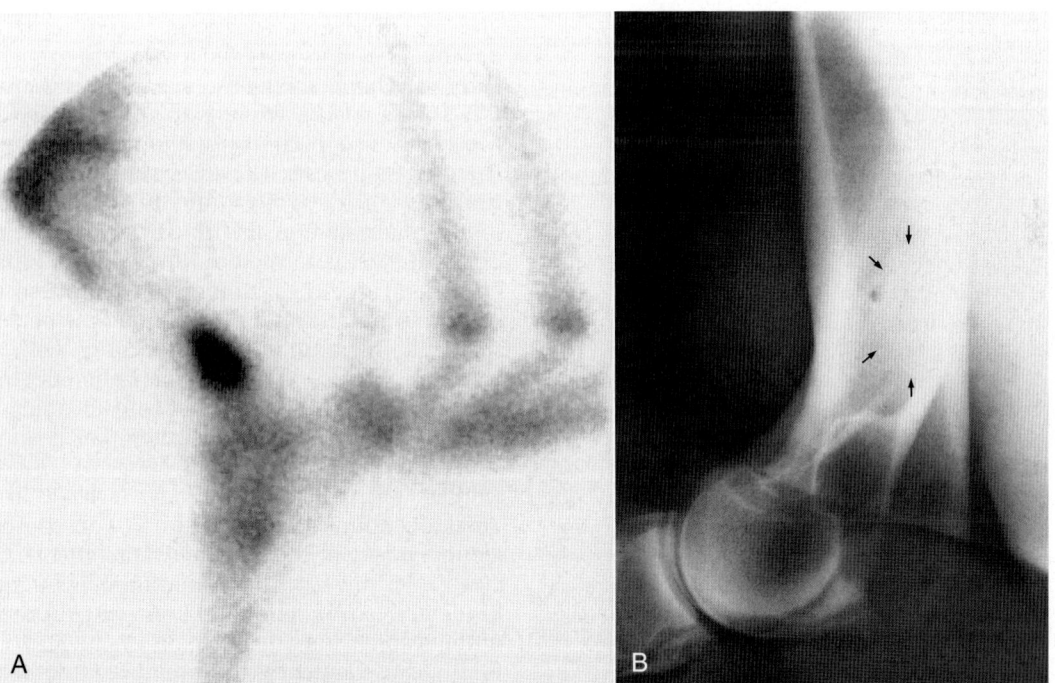

Fig. 40-11 • Lateral scintigraphic **(A)** and mediolateral radiographic images **(B)** of the left humerus of 3-year-old Thoroughbred filly in race training with left forelimb lameness of 3 weeks' duration. The lameness was not altered by local analgesic techniques. **A,** The nuclear scintigraphic image shows a region of intense focal increased radiopharmaceutical uptake in the distal diaphyseal region of the humerus, proximal to the usual site of stress fractures. **B,** There is a well-circumscribed area of increased radiopacity *(arrows)* adjacent to the principal nutrient foramen. This is an enostosis-like lesion. Lameness resolved after 2 months of box rest, and the lesion was scintigraphically silent, although there was no change in radiological appearance. The horse remained sound when returned to training.

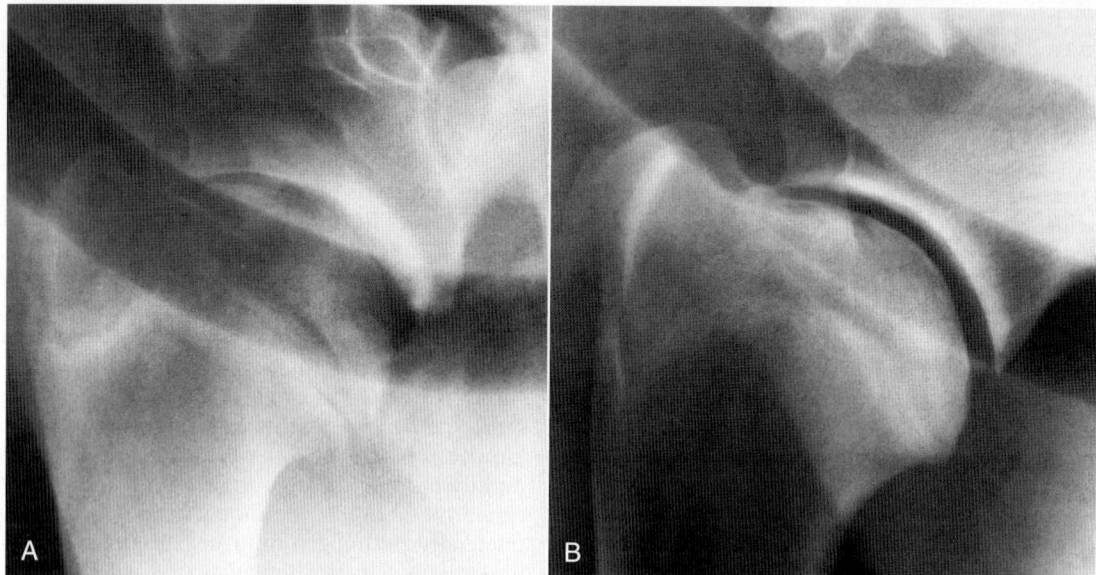

Fig. 40-12 • A, Mediolateral radiographic image of the scapulohumeral joint of an 8-month-old Thoroughbred colt with severe left forelimb lameness. Radiolucent areas in the subchondral bone of the distal scapula and increased radiopacity and modeling of the glenoid cavity and ventral angle of the scapula are compatible with osteochondrosis. The humeral head also has variable radiopacity. **B,** The same horse 15 months after surgical debridement. The horse was sound. Substantial modeling of the glenoid cavity of the scapula has occurred. The horse trained and raced.

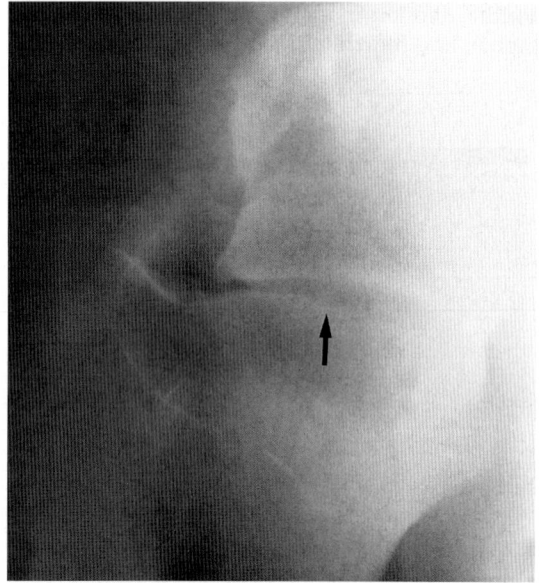

Fig. 40-13 • Craniomedial-caudolateral oblique image of the scapulo-humeral joint of a 3-year-old Thoroughbred with lameness alleviated by intraarticular analgesia of the scapulohumeral joint. A well-defined depression in the proximal articular surface of the humerus is compatible with mild osteochondrosis (arrow). This was the only detectable radiological abnormality. With repeated intraarticular medication the mare raced successfully, winning several more Group 1 races.

the glenoid cavity, because of modeling of the articular margins (Figures 40-12 and 40-13). Generally a good correlation exists between the degree of lameness and the severity of radiological abnormalities. However, radiology may underestimate the degree of lesion severity.[36]

If lameness is recognized in a horse younger than 18 months of age, conservative management usually results in persistent lameness. Surgical treatment by radical arthroscopic debridement has resulted in some young horses being able to withstand race training, although their longer-term future has been poorly documented. In one study 45% of treated horses were able to return to athletic activity.[37] However, in another study only 15.4% of 26 potential racehorses started a race.[38] In some horses treated early, the bone shows a remarkable capacity to remodel (see Figure 40-12), whereas in others there is no change. Most horses show clinically significant improvement, even if lameness persists. However, surgical treatment in older horses is much less rewarding. In horses with minor radiological abnormalities, identified when in race training, periodic intraarticular medication with sodium hyaluronan and triamcinolone acetonide has permitted the horses to remain in training and race, although lameness has tended to recur. In weanlings and yearlings with moderate-to-severe lesions, conservative management, including stall rest, intraarticular injections of hyaluronan, and periodic radiological assessment of healing, has been successful.[1]

Subchondral Bone Cysts and Other Osseous Cystlike Lesions

True subchondral bone cysts occur in the middle of the glenoid cavity of the scapula (Figure 40-14). Other osseous cystlike lesions have been identified less frequently in the humeral head. Subchondral bone cysts in the distal aspect of the scapula and other osseous cystlike lesions most commonly cause lameness in immature athletic horses, 1 to 3 years of age, but subchondral bone cysts in the distal aspect of the scapula have also been identified in much older horses with no prior history of lameness. Trauma may be an inciting cause. Lameness is usually acute in onset and moderate to severe. In some horses the lameness varies extremely, within and between examination periods, from barely detectable at any gait to obvious at the walk. Lameness is usually substantially improved by intraarticular

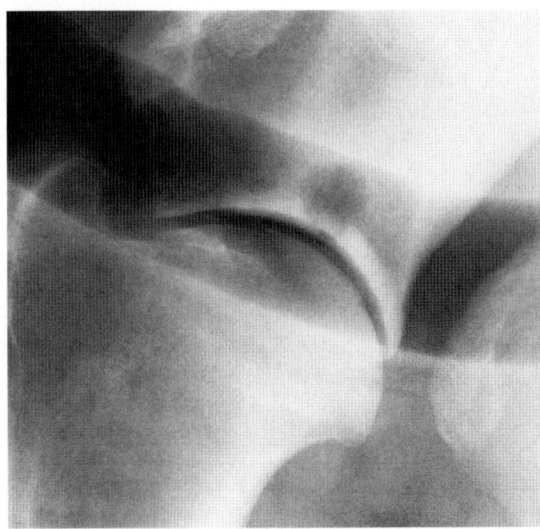

Fig. 40-14 • Mediolateral radiographic image of the scapulohumeral joint of 9-year-old hunter with episodic severe right forelimb lameness. There is a large, well-defined subchondral bone cyst in the middle of the distal scapula. The lameness responded to intraarticular medication with corticosteroids (triamcinolone).

analgesia of the scapulohumeral joint. However, interpretation can be extremely difficult in those horses that show marked spontaneous variations in lameness.

Small radiolucent zones are occasionally seen in the middle of the opaque band of subchondral bone of the glenoid cavity of the scapula in clinically normal horses and in the contralateral limb of horses with lameness associated with a large subchondral bone cyst in the distal aspect of the scapula. Lameness that is improved by intraarticular analgesia associated with such lesions but no other radiological change is seen infrequently.[1,2,39] This has been correlated with defects in the articular cartilage extending into the subchondral bone.[39] More commonly a large circular or dome-shaped radiolucent area is seen, surrounded by a narrow rim of increased radiopacity. In some older horses in which such subchondral bone cysts have been identified, the cysts have been less well defined because they are less radiolucent. In skeletally mature horses similar lesions have occasionally been identified bilaterally associated with apparently unilateral lameness.

In skeletally immature horses subchondral bone cysts have been seen to enlarge progressively, and some appear to move proximally in the bone. Those identified in skeletally mature horses seem to persist unchanged. Osseous cystlike lesions in the proximal aspect of the humerus occur as circular radiolucent regions in the middle-to-caudal aspect. Some of these have been seen to fill in radiologically with time. Solitary subchondral bone cysts in the distal aspect of the scapula are generally not associated with any other detectable radiological change, whereas other osseous cystlike lesions are sometimes seen together with remodeling of the ventral angle of the scapula.

Nuclear scintigraphic examination may be helpful in horses in which lameness varies extremely in degree within an examination period. Subchondral bone cysts are associated with active bone modeling; therefore there is intense focal IRU.

Intraarticular medication of the scapulohumeral joint using hyaluronan and methylprednisolone acetate has been successful in resolving lameness in immature athletic horses, but results have been poorer in older horses.

Surgical treatment of subtle, small lucent zones has been successful,[39] but effective debridement of large lesions is impractical.

Osseous Cystlike Lesions in the Humeral Tubercles

Osseous cystlike lesions in the humeral tubercles are discussed on page 471.

Osteoarthritis in Miniature Breeds

Sudden-onset, severe lameness is sometimes seen in Shetland and Falabella ponies and Miniature horses.[40] Dysplasia of the joint predisposing to instability may be a predisposing factor for OA in some.[40,41] Usually no known history of previous lameness or trauma exists. Lameness is typical of proximal limb pain. Manipulation of the shoulder may cause pain. Lameness is improved but rarely alleviated by intraarticular analgesia. Radiological examination sometimes reveals evidence of advanced OA, including periarticular osteophyte formation, and modeling of the ventral angle of the scapula (Figure 40-15). Occasionally, fragmentation of the ventral angle of the scapula occurs. Often new bone forms on the distal caudal border of the scapula and the proximal caudal aspect of the humerus in the regions of attachment of the joint capsule. In some ponies the contour of the glenoid cavity of the scapula appears flattened (see discussion of dysplasia on page 468), resulting in loss of congruity between the distal aspect of the scapula and the humeral head. In ponies with less severe abnormalities, radiological abnormalities may be detectable only in a craniomedial-caudolateral oblique image. In those ponies with minor radiological change at the time of onset of clinical signs, changes tend to have been rapidly progressive.

Arthroscopic evaluation of the joint reveals extensive softening of the articular cartilage, and surgical debridement has resulted in some clinical improvement, although lameness has persisted. The prognosis for athletic function is guarded. Surgical arthrodesis has been described.[42]

Osteoarthritis in Nonminiature Breeds

OA in the scapulohumeral joint is relatively uncommon,[36] except as a sequela to osteochondrosis, an intraarticular fracture, or a tear of the scapulohumeral joint capsule. Lameness is mild to moderate and is usually improved by intraarticular analgesia, but false-negative responses do occur. Radiological abnormalities include loss of congruity between the glenoid cavity of the scapula and the humeral head, because of flattening of the humeral head or modeling of the ventral angle of the scapula; periarticular osteophyte formation, most easily seen on the cranial articular margins of the scapula; and radiolucent areas in the subchondral bone. The response to intraarticular medication is usually poor, and the prognosis for athletic function is guarded.

Care should be taken when evaluating the scapulohumeral joint arthroscopically, because widespread aging changes occur in the articular cartilage, especially of the distal aspect of the scapula.[2] These include softening of the articular cartilage and extensive fissure formation

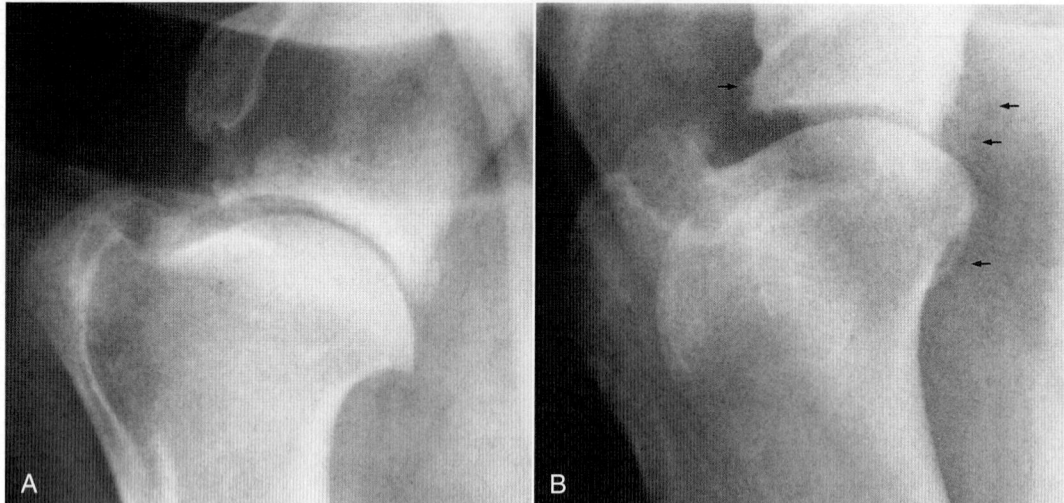

Fig. 40-15 • **A,** Mediolateral radiographic image of the scapulohumeral joint of a 4-year-old Shetland pony with acute-onset, severe lameness that improved with intraarticular analgesia. There is marked modeling of the ventral angle of the scapula, periosteal new bone formation, and generalized increased radiopacity of the distal aspect of the scapula caused by extensive new bone. **B,** Craniomedial-caudolateral oblique radiographic image of a scapulohumeral joint of 5-year-old Miniature horse. There is poor congruity between the glenoid cavity of the scapula and the humeral head. Note also the periarticular periosteal new bone *(arrows).*

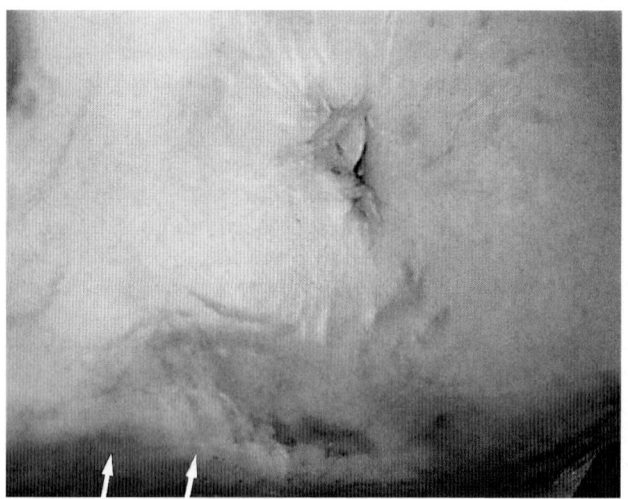

Fig. 40-16 • Postmortem appearance of the glenoid cavity of the scapula of an 8-year-old Thoroughbred with no history of lameness. There is modeling of the articular margin *(arrows),* and the articular cartilage appears irregular. This was bilaterally symmetrical and is a typical normal finding in mature horses.

(Figure 40-16). Modeling changes of the articular margins of the glenoid cavity of the scapula may also occur.

Tearing of the Scapulohumeral Joint Capsule

Localized tearing of the scapulohumeral joint capsule is an unusual cause of lameness that is improved by intraarticular analgesia. In the acute stage no detectable radiological abnormalities may be apparent, but with more chronic lameness entheseous new bone may be seen in the region of damage. Nuclear scintigraphic examination may reveal focal or more generalized IRU in the region of the scapulohumeral joint. Although ultrasonographic examination may be helpful if the lesion is lateral, medial lesions cannot

be seen. Definitive diagnosis is based on diagnostic arthroscopy of the scapulohumeral joint. The prognosis for recovery for athletic function is guarded.

Dysplasia

Dysplasia of the scapulohumeral joint has been identified in Shetland ponies[41] and Miniature horses,[1] sometimes together with subluxation of the joint or with OA (see the earlier discussion of OA in miniature breeds, page 467). Flattening of the radius of curvature of the glenoid cavity of the scapula occurs.

Luxation

Luxation of the scapulohumeral joint has been seen in ponies[2] more frequently than in horses and results in acute-onset, severe lameness associated with extensive swelling in the shoulder region (Figure 40-17, *A*). If the humerus has luxated laterally, the scapular spine is less easy to palpate than usual. The horse is reluctant to bear full weight on the limb at rest and is usually non–weight bearing at the walk. Diagnosis is confirmed by radiographic examination (Figure 40-17, *B*). Mediolateral and craniomedial-caudolateral oblique images should be obtained to determine whether a concurrent fracture is present and whether the luxation is medial or lateral. The humerus can luxate cranioproximally or caudoproximally.

A horse with simple acute luxation, without any concurrent fracture, can be treated by manual reduction of the luxation with the horse under general anesthesia in dorsal recumbency. A hobble is placed around the distal aspect of the affected limb, and the limb is maximally extended vertically. Pressure is applied to the shoulder region to reduce the luxation. An assisted recovery from general anesthesia is recommended, followed by cross-tying to prevent the horse from lying down, minimize the risks of reinjury, and allow the traumatized joint capsule to heal. Periarticular fibrosis inevitably develops, and treating the

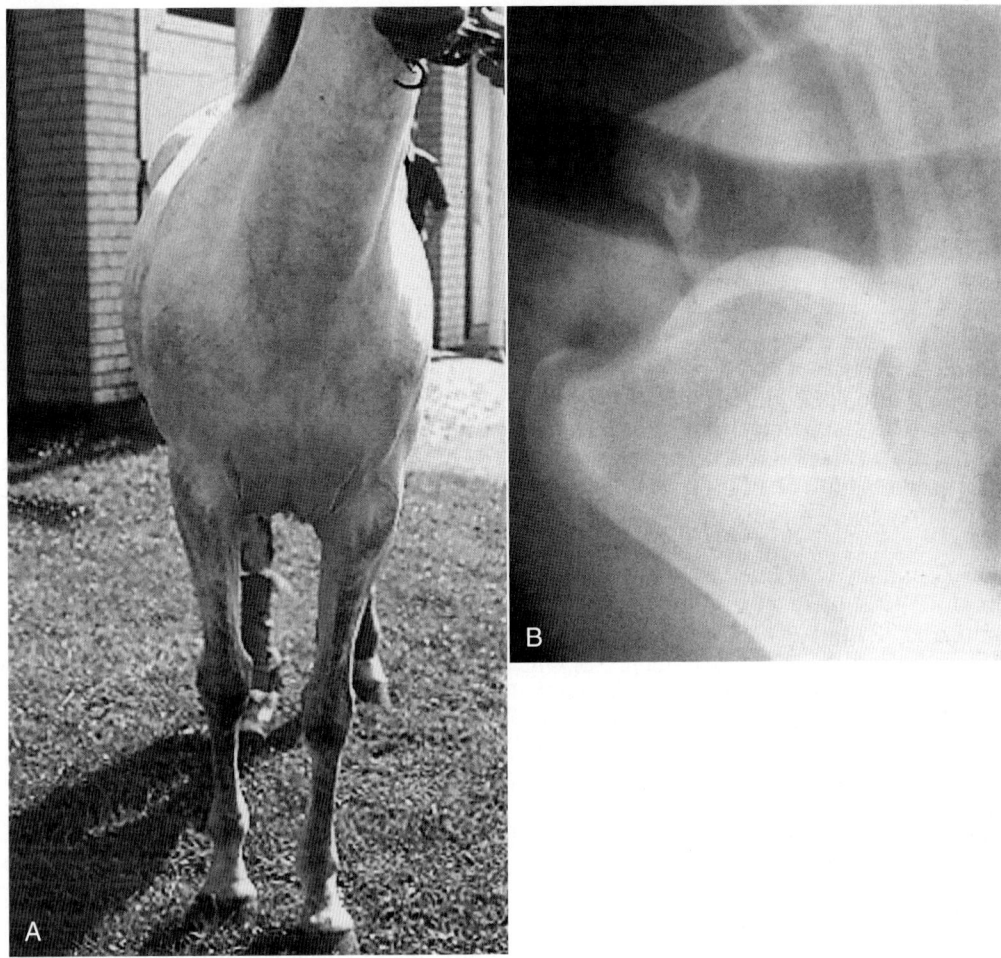

Fig. 40-17 • A, An 8-year-old pony gelding with acute-onset, severe right forelimb lameness associated with swelling in the shoulder region. **B,** Mediolateral radiographic view of the scapulohumeral joint showing cranioproximal luxation of the humerus. The luxation was successfully reduced with the pony under general anesthesia, and the pony made a complete functional recovery.

horse with nonsteroidal antiinflammatory drugs and a controlled exercise program to restore normal joint mobility may be necessary. A complete functional recovery has been achieved in a small number of ponies. The presence of any concurrent fracture predisposes to recurrent luxation and warrants an extremely guarded prognosis. Persistent luxation results in the rapid development of a deep groove in the humeral head, extending from cranially to caudally; thus the prognosis is poor.[2]

Fracture of the Articular Surface of the Scapula or the Proximal Aspect of the Humerus

Fracture of the articular surface of the scapula may result from a fall when the horse is jumping, resulting in acute-onset, severe lameness.[43] Manipulation of the joint may produce pain, and sometimes crepitus can be elicited. Periarticular soft tissue swelling occurs in the acute stage, but this resolves relatively rapidly. Diagnosis requires high-quality radiographs, because the only detectable radiological abnormality may be loss of clarity of the articular margins of the distal aspect of the scapula. Mediolateral and craniomedial-caudolateral oblique images should be obtained. Follow-up radiographs may show modeling of

the ventral angle of the scapula. The prognosis for athletic function is hopeless.

Crushing of the caudal aspect of the humeral head has been seen as a result of a fall, resulting in acute-onset severe lameness. There may be no detectable radiological abnormality, but there is intense IRU in the humeral head. Severe lameness persists, yet follow-up radiographs may reveal only modeling of the ventral angle of the scapula. Postmortem examination has confirmed the diagnosis.[44]

Periarticular Trauma

Periarticular trauma—the result of a fall, collision between two horses, or collision between a horse and a solid object—may result in sudden-onset, severe, unilateral forelimb lameness because of severe bruising. Extensive periarticular soft tissue swelling may develop rapidly, with pain on deep palpation. In the acute stage determining whether a concurrent fracture is present may be difficult, especially fracture of the supraglenoid tubercle of the scapula or the first rib, because history and clinical signs are so similar.

If damage is restricted to bruising, lameness generally rapidly improves over the following 7 days. However, if concurrent trauma to the suprascapular nerve or its branch to the infraspinatus muscle occurred, clinically significant neurogenic atrophy of the supraspinatus or infraspinatus muscles may occur within 7 days (see page 473). If moderate-to-severe lameness persists, then radiographic examination is indicated. If damage is restricted to soft tissue structures, then treatment with nonsteroidal antiinflammatory drugs combined with restriction to box rest and controlled exercise usually results in a rapid and complete recovery.

Intertubercular Bursa

Congenital abnormalities of the bicipital apparatus are a rare cause of lameness, sometimes not recognized until maturity.[45] Lameness is characterized by a shortened cranial phase of the stride at both the walk and the trot. Affected horses have generalized atrophy of the shoulder musculature or specifically of the biceps brachii, and abnormal prominence of the point of the shoulder. Contraction of the ipsilateral foot is probably a reflection of a chronic problem, despite reported acute onset of lameness. It may occur unilaterally or bilaterally. Mediolateral and cranio-proximal-craniodistal oblique radiographic images should be obtained. Abnormalities include absence of a lesser tubercle of the humerus, narrowing of the groove between the greater and intermediate tubercles, and evidence of OA of the scapulohumeral joint, probably the result of instability. Ultrasonography reveals either complete medial displacement of the tendon of biceps brachii or an abnormal shape and position of the tendon.

Rupture of the Tendon of Biceps Brachii

Rupture of the tendon of biceps brachii is a rare injury sustained as the result of a fall while jumping at speed.[46] It results in severe lameness at the walk, associated with diffuse soft tissue swelling around the shoulder. Diagnosis is based on radiographic and ultrasonographic examinations. The tendon may rupture through the isthmus between the medial and lateral lobes. The prognosis is hopeless.

Tendonitis of Biceps Brachii

Injury of the tendon of biceps brachii is a relatively uncommon cause of forelimb lameness, with no typical history. Frequently no localizing signs suggest the source of pain. In some horses forced retraction of the limb induces discomfort, but this is an unreliable finding. Lameness varies from mild to severe, and only if lameness is severe are the gait characteristics typical of proximal limb lameness. In some horses lameness is more obvious in the walk than at any other pace. Lameness is usually improved by intrathecal analgesia of the intertubercular bursa, although it may take up to half an hour. Some false-negative results occur in association with severe lesions.[44]

Diagnosis is based on ultrasonographic examination. The entire length of the tendon of biceps brachii should be examined carefully from its origin on the supraglenoid tubercle of the scapula to the musculotendonous junction. The horse should be standing fully load bearing on the limb to avoid hypoechoic artifacts within the tendon. It is important to be aware of the anatomy of the tendon, which changes in shape from proximally to distally.[8,10] Examining the medial and lateral lobes independently is often necessary, because maintaining both lobes in focus simultaneously is difficult. The tendon should be examined in transverse and longitudinal planes and careful

comparison made with the contralateral limb. Ultrasonographic abnormalities include enlargement of the tendon, loss of definition of one of its margins, hypoechoic defects within the tendon, and loss of fiber pattern in longitudinal images. The humeral tubercles should be inspected carefully for evidence of any concurrent damage. Concurrent evidence of bursitis characterized by an abnormal amount of fluid within the sheath (bursa) may also be present and results in an increased anechogenic space between the tendon and the humerus. Horses with chronic lameness may show evidence of hyperechogenic foci within the tendon, representing fibrosis, mineralization, or ossification. Adhesions may develop between the tendon and the wall of the bursa. Occasionally, echogenic bodies are seen free within the bursa.

Treatment of horses with tendonitis of biceps brachii consists of box rest and controlled walking exercise.[47] Injection of hyaluronan may be beneficial. The tendon should be monitored by ultrasonography at up to 3-month intervals. At least 6 to 9 months of convalescent time are required for horses with acute lesions, which have a fair prognosis. The prognosis for horses with chronic injuries is poor. Permanent enlargement of the tendon within the confined space between the brachiocephalicus muscle and the humerus and loss of normal gliding function cause persistent pain. Tenectomy or tenotomy has been described.[48]

Osteitis of the Humeral Tubercles

Osteitis of the humeral tubercles is a rare cause of forelimb lameness.[31] Horses show moderate-to-severe lameness and resent manipulation of the shoulder. Abnormalities of the humeral tubercles are seen radiologically as lucent areas or by ultrasonography as a roughened surface to the bone and overlying cartilage. The intertubercular bursa may contain an abnormal amount of fluid and the tendon of biceps brachii may be enlarged, with peritendonous reaction. Surgical exploration may reveal necrotic areas of bone that are readily debrided, resulting in improvement in lameness.

Fracture of the Humeral Tubercles

A discussion of fracture of the humeral tubercles appears on page 463 (see Figure 40-10).

Infection

Infection of the intertubercular bursa occasionally causes acute-onset, moderate-to-severe forelimb lameness.[49-51] Infection may be a sequela to known trauma, a previous injection, and a penetrating wound, but it has been recognized with no history of trauma or evidence of a wound, presumably infection being hematogenous in origin. Infection occurs in immature athletic horses and older horses.

The horse may stand slightly favoring the lame limb. Deep palpation in the region of the bursa may elicit pain. Retraction of the limb is resented. Lameness is often evident at the walk. Synovial fluid withdrawn from the bursa is usually grossly brown discolored and turbid, and therefore intrathecal analgesia is usually unnecessary. Diagnostic ultrasonography reveals an abnormal amount of fluid within the bursa; sometimes echogenic material is seen within the fluid, and the surface of the tendon of biceps brachii may be less well defined than normal because of fibrin deposition. Diagnosis is confirmed by measuring differential white blood cell count and total protein concentration and by cytological examination of the synovial fluid, with polymorphonuclear leukocytes dominating.

Treatment is by radical surgical debridement and thorough lavage of the bursa by open surgery[49] or endoscopy,[50] combined with long-term, broad-spectrum antimicrobial therapy (e.g., crystalline penicillin and gentamicin) and the use of nonsteroidal antiinflammatory analgesic drugs. If a penetrating wound is identified, consideration should be given to using metronidazole. When the acute inflammatory response has subsided, controlled exercise is important to try to limit adhesion formation. If the condition is recognized and treated early and aggressively, a favorable outcome can be achieved, but prolonged therapy is often required.[49]

Noninfectious Bursitis

Noninfectious bursitis does occur occasionally alone, together with tendonitis of biceps brachii (see page 470), or with osteitis of the humeral tubercles.[6,52] Lameness varies in degree and is usually substantially improved by intrathecal analgesia. Diagnosis is verified by ultrasonographic examination of the intertubercular bursa. The bursa has an abnormal amount of fluid but no abnormalities of the enclosed tendon or the humeral tubercles. Treatment by intrathecal administration of hyaluronan and triamcinolone acetonide, combined with controlled exercise, is usually successful.

Mineralization

Mineralization or ossification within the tendon of biceps brachii has been seen alone, or as a sequela to a previous fracture of the supraglenoid tubercle.[1,53] Ectopic mineralization within the bursa has been associated with substantial proliferation of the synovial membrane of the intertubercular bursa.[9] No typical history is known. Lameness varies in degree and only if moderate to severe is typical of a proximal limb lameness. Lameness may be improved by intrathecal analgesia of the intertubercular bursa. Mineralization may be identified radiologically, but it can be obscured by the humeral tubercles. Radiography is useful to identify any previous fracture. There may be associated IRU.[53] Diagnostic ultrasonography provides more accurate information about the precise site and extent of mineralization and any concurrent pathological condition of the tendon. The prognosis for return to full athletic function is guarded.

Osseous Cystlike Lesions in the Humeral Tubercles

Osseous cystlike lesions in the humeral tubercles may develop secondary to trauma such as a fall or change in biomechanics resulting from other causes of lameness, or they may arise from an unknown cause.[44,54-56] There is acute-onset moderate-to-severe lameness, usually with no localizing clinical signs. There is often no or limited response to either intraarticular analgesia of the scapulohumeral joint or intrathecal analgesia of the intertubercular bursa. Either lesions are identified using survey radiology or their presence is highlighted by scintigraphic evaluation demonstrating focal moderate-to-intense IRU. Lesions are sometimes not evident on mediolateral radiographs but may be seen in craniomedial-caudolateral oblique images.

If a lesion involves the cortex of the tubercle, osseous and cartilage defects may be identified using ultrasonography. In some horses there are also lesions in the biceps brachii tendon. Lameness has generally resolved with rest, with or without medication of the intertubercular bursa, although a radiolucent lesion may persist. Successful surgical treatment has also been described.[55]

Scapula

Fracture of the Supraglenoid Tubercle

The scapula has four centers of ossification: the scapular cartilage, body of the scapula, cranial part of the glenoid cavity of the scapula, and supraglenoid tubercle. The cranial part of the glenoid cavity of the scapula fuses with the body by 5 months of age. The physis of the supraglenoid tubercle closes at 12 to 24 months of age. Fracture of the supraglenoid tubercle of the scapula is a relatively common injury, resulting from a collision with a solid object or fall. Fractures frequently occur through the original physes.[43] The fracture may be simple or comminuted, involving only the supraglenoid tubercle, without an articular component. Alternatively, the fracture may pass through the glenoid notch of the scapula, which may result in one large fracture or separation of both original physes.

Lameness is sudden in onset and moderate to severe. Over the first week the horse may show progressive improvement, but lameness persists. Neurogenic atrophy of the supraspinatus and infraspinatus muscles may develop within 7 days if a concurrent injury of the suprascapular nerve occurred. Disuse atrophy develops more slowly.

A palpable thickening in the region of the supraglenoid tubercle exists, but crepitus is rarely appreciated.

Diagnosis is confirmed radiologically (see Figure 13-1). The fracture fragments are often displaced craniodistally, because of the pull of the biceps brachii, and if treated conservatively a nonunion develops. The radiographs should be inspected carefully to determine if the fracture has an articular component, which warrants a more guarded prognosis. Rarely, there will be concomitant luxation of the scapulohumeral joint.

The prognosis with conservative treatment is poor for return to athletic function. Surgical treatment by removal of the fracture fragment(s) has been successful in some horses, although the level of work to which horses have returned has not been well documented. Various methods of internal fixation have been attempted, but the large distracting forces of biceps brachii have to be overcome. A small number of horses younger than 2 years of age and less than 400 kg body weight have been successfully treated by complete tenotomy of the biceps brachii and internal fixation using three 5.5-mm cortical bone screws.[57] Alternatively, in foals, yearlings, and small horses, the fracture can be repaired using a tension band technique with either a small plate or screws, preserving the biceps tendon.

Stress Fractures

Stress fractures of the body of the scapula are an occasional cause of acute-onset forelimb lameness in young Thoroughbreds in training.[1,58,59] Usually no localizing clinical signs are present, although occasionally focal pain can be identified. Lameness often frequently improves spontaneously with rest. A premature return to training may result in a catastrophic fracture. Scintigraphic examination reveals IRU in the mid-to-distal aspect of the scapula. Occasionally a fracture can be confirmed using ultrasonography. Treatment requires 6 to 8 weeks of box rest and controlled walking exercise, followed by a graduated return to full work. In my experience the prognosis has been good, but in a report from North America two of seven horses (29%) that resumed training had recurrent injury.[59]

Fracture of the Body of the Scapula

Fractures of the body of the scapula usually result from the horse falling at a fence when jumping at speed. Complete fractures result in severe lameness and extensive soft tissue swelling and merit destruction on humane grounds. Diagnosis is usually obvious based on clinical signs, and radiographic examination is not necessary. Radiography or scintigraphic examination is required for the diagnosis of incomplete fractures (Figure 40-18). High-quality radiographs are required, and this may be difficult because the horse may resent protraction of the limb because of pain. Horses with fractures that enter the scapulohumeral joint have a poor prognosis. However, horses with extraarticular, incomplete fractures of the body of the scapula have a good prognosis for return to full athletic function with conservative management.

Fracture of the Scapular Spine

Fractures of the scapular spine result from a fall, collision with a solid object, or occasionally a kick. Acute-onset, moderate lameness occurs with associated localized soft tissue swelling and pain on palpation. Oblique radiographic skyline views of the scapular spine are necessary to identify a fracture. Diagnostic ultrasonography may be more helpful in identifying a fracture. Most horses with fractures heal adequately with conservative management. Occasionally a sequestrum develops, necessitating surgical

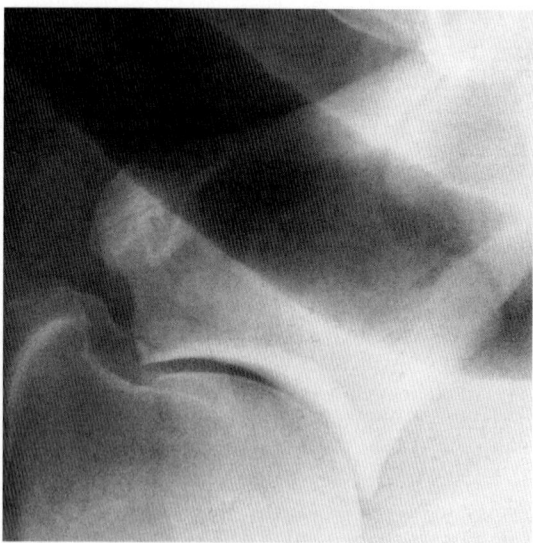

Fig. 40-18 • Mediolateral radiographic image of 7-year-old event horse with acute-onset, severe left forelimb lameness after a fall. There is an incomplete fracture of the body of the scapula. The horse was treated conservatively and made a complete recovery.

debridement. The prognosis for return to full athletic function is good.

Infection of the Infraspinatus Bursa

Injury of the infraspinatus bursa and tendon seldom occur except as a result of a penetrating injury in the shoulder region, resulting in infectious bursitis.[60] Signs include generalized swelling in the shoulder region, pain on manipulation of the shoulder, and lameness characterized by a shortened cranial phase of the stride. Ultrasonography reveals distention of the infraspinatus bursa with echogenic fluid, with thickening of the synovium if chronic. Evaluation of the greater tubercle of the humerus may reveal roughening or a fracture. Treatment includes lavage of the bursa, surgical debridement if indicated, and broad spectrum antimicrobial therapy. The prognosis is good.

Muscle

Triceps Myopathy

See Chapter 83 for a discussion of triceps myopathy.

Muscle Lesions: Brachiocephalicus, Biceps Brachii, and Pectorals

Lesions of muscles in the shoulder region have not been well documented and probably occur more commonly than recognized. However, clinical signs are rather nonspecific, and diagnosis is difficult. A number of dressage horses have been identified that have shown forelimb lameness only while performing lateral work. Palpation has revealed no detectable abnormality. Local analgesic techniques have not altered the lameness. Ultrasonographic examination has revealed hyperechogenic areas of fibrosis or mineralization within the brachiocephalicus in the lame limb only.

A dressage horse showed lameness only at the walk. Local analgesic techniques were ineffective. Nuclear scintigraphic evaluation revealed focal moderate IRU in the musculature cranioproximal to the elbow. This correlated with a hyperechogenic region within the biceps brachii.

Some horses have forelimb lameness associated with palpable soreness of the pectoral muscles, which responds well to physiotherapy. Soreness of the brachiocephalicus muscles is often seen with lameness caused by distal limb pain. Lameness is sometimes seen associated with primary brachiocephalicus muscle damage in dressage horses, show jumpers, event horses, and horses that race over fences. In most horses with acute lameness, palpation reveals muscle soreness and induces muscle spasm. However, in horses with chronic muscle injury pain can be more difficult to identify. In some horses lameness was evident only in walk and was characterized by lifting of the head and neck as the ipsilateral limb was protracted.

Rupture of Serratus Ventralis

The serratus ventralis muscles arise from the third to seventh cervical vertebrae and the first eight to nine ribs and insert on the medial proximal aspect of each scapula. They sling the thorax between the forelimbs. Rupture of one or both of these muscles is a rare injury, caused by trauma. The proximal border of the scapula moves proximally. If rupture is bilateral, the scapulae become higher than the summits of the dorsal spinous processes in the withers region. Rupture of the serratus ventralis should be differentiated from neurological disease causing loss of function of the muscle.[1]

The horse tends to stand with the forelimbs close together. Palpation of the withers region or manipulation of the forelimbs causes pain. The horse is reluctant to move, takes small steps, and nods the neck stiffly.

Radiographic examination should be performed to rule out a fracture of the scapula or the dorsal spinous processes of the cranial thoracic vertebrae. The prognosis for athletic function is poor.

Nerve

Atrophy of Supraspinatus and Infraspinatus Muscles: Damage to the Suprascapular Nerve

The suprascapular nerve wraps around the cranial aspect of the neck of the scapula and in this position is vulnerable to trauma resulting in perineural edema, stretching, and neuroma formation. Neuroma formation usually results in permanent loss of function and subsequent neurogenic atrophy of supraspinatus and infraspinatus muscles. This can occur within 7 days of injury. Atrophy results in abnormal prominence of the scapular spine, but damage to the suprascapular nerve alone does not result in any loss of stability of the scapulohumeral joint. Lameness may be the result of trauma at the time of the injury but generally resolves rapidly, unless a concurrent fracture is present.

This condition has been called *Sweeny,* but this can be confusing because this term has also been used to describe instability of the shoulder or shoulder slip resulting from loss of collateral support of the shoulder musculature. This latter condition is separate and should not be confused (see the following discussion). Experimental transection of the suprascapular nerve in two ponies and one adult horse resulted in rapid atrophy of the supraspinatus and infraspinatus muscles, which persisted over the long term but produced no gait abnormality.[2]

The injury usually results from a fall or collision with another horse or solid object. Permanent muscle atrophy may ensue, but this results only in a cosmetic defect, not a functional deficit. Electromyography can be used to determine whether any other muscles are affected, which would suggest an injury to the brachial plexus or to other nerves in addition to the suprascapular nerve. Patchy sweating indicates a lesion elsewhere.

Surgical treatment has been performed to decompress the suprascapular nerve by cutting out a notch on the craniodistal aspect of the scapula and removing fibrotic material from around the nerve.[44] Surgical treatment has resulted in restoration of more normal muscle mass.[61] Care must be taken not to traumatize the scapula unduly, because this may predispose to fracture.

Instability of Shoulder: Damage to the Brachial Plexus

Lack of collateral support to the scapulohumeral joint by loss of function of the muscles on the medial (subscapularis) and lateral aspects of the joint results in so-called *shoulder slip.* As the horse starts to bear weight on the limb, the shoulder joint bulges abaxially (Figure 40-19; see Figure 6-19). Concurrently the heel of the foot tends to rotate outward. This gait abnormality is evaluated most easily viewing the horse walking toward the observer. The gait abnormality may be slight or severe.

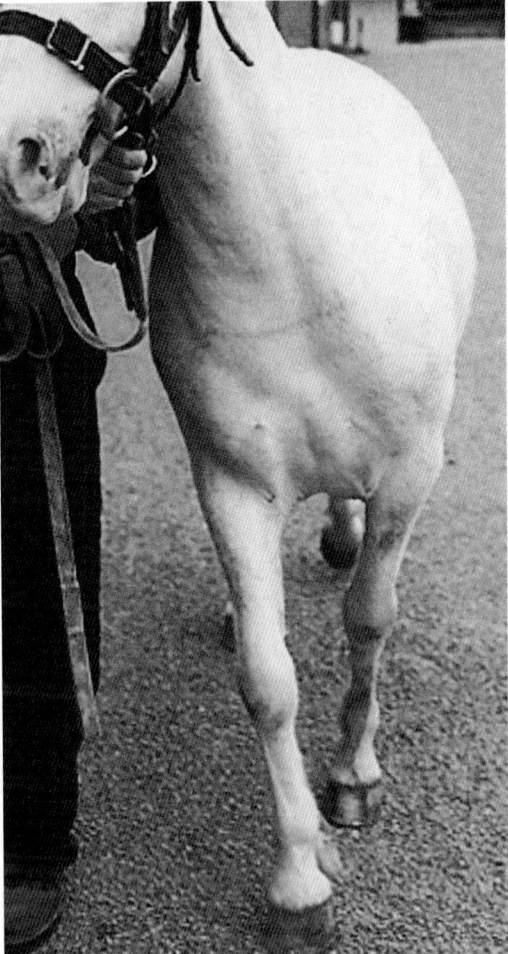

Fig. 40-19 • A 7-year-old driving pony with acute-onset instability of the left shoulder joint probably caused by a brachial plexus injury. The injury was of 12 days' duration. Note the medial placement of the left front foot. The heel rotated laterally as the foot broke over. There was moderate atrophy of the left infraspinatus, supraspinatus, and triceps muscles. The pony was treated conservatively, progressively improved, and made a complete functional recovery.

Instability of the shoulder was formerly ascribed to atrophy of the supraspinatus and infraspinatus nerves secondary to suprascapular nerve damage, but profound atrophy of these muscles can be present with no detectable gait abnormality.[2,11] Experimental transection of the suprascapular nerve has resulted in profound atrophy of supraspinatus and infraspinatus muscles but no detectable gait abnormality.[2] Seven horses with persistent instability of the shoulder that were humanely destroyed and examined post mortem had atrophy of at least the supraspinatus, infraspinatus, and subscapularis muscles. All horses had neuroma formation involving nerves of the brachial plexus or the ventral nerve roots of the contributing nerves. The suprascapular nerve appeared normal as it passed over the cranial aspect of the scapula.

Instability of the shoulder invariably results from trauma, usually the horse colliding with a solid object. Pain-related lameness may also be present initially, but this generally resolves within 1 to 2 weeks, provided that a concurrent fracture does not exist. Similar clinical signs occasionally occur transiently (for 1 to 3 hours) after intraarticular analgesia of the scapulohumeral joint, presumably because of extraarticular leakage of local anesthetic solution. Instability of the shoulder has also been seen in a Miniature horse with dysplasia of the scapulohumeral joint and advanced OA.

After trauma, initially no muscle atrophy is detectable, but atrophy of several muscles is usually detectable within 7 to 10 days. Patchy sweating may develop in the caudal neck region or over the scapula, depending on which nerves have been damaged. Electromyography can be used to determine accurately which muscles are affected.

Prognosis depends on the nature of the nerve damage and the ability to achieve reinnervation of the affected muscles. Nerve regeneration occurs at approximately 1 mm per day. Progressive improvement in gait is a good prognostic sign. A normal gait may be restored despite persistence of atrophy of the supraspinatus and infraspinatus muscles.[2,62] However, a persistent gait abnormality 6 months after injury warrants a guarded prognosis. Surgical treatment is impractical because of the inaccessibility of the brachial plexus or the ventral nerve roots. Scapular notch resection is not indicated, because nerves in addition to or other than the suprascapular nerve are involved. This procedure also risks secondary fracture of the scapula.

Radial Nerve Paralysis

Radial nerve paralysis is an occasional cause of lameness.[63,64] The clinical signs depend on the site or sites of damage. Complete radial nerve paralysis is most common, with loss of function of the extensor muscles of the elbow, carpus, and digit, and results in inability to stand on the limb. The elbow is dropped, and the horse tends to stand with the affected limb forward, with the antebrachium at an angle of approximately 45 degrees to the ground, with the carpus and fetlock semiflexed (see Figure 5-14). Less commonly only the extensor muscles of the elbow are affected, so although the limb may be advanced forward, the elbow will drop during weight bearing. Occasionally only the extensor muscles of the carpus and digit are affected, so that the limb is advanced and placed normally, but then the carpus or fetlock may slightly knuckle forward. The horse has a tendency to stumble.

Lameness is usually sudden in onset. The horse may have a history of trauma. Paralysis occurs most commonly in young horses turned out together. Although damage to the radial nerve itself may be the cause of lameness,[63,64] many injuries are probably caused by compression of the brachial plexus between the scapula and the ribs or can be associated with a fracture of the dorsal aspect of a rib involving the eighth cervical nerve. An electromyogram may demonstrate involvement of more than the radial nerve. Equine protozoal myelitis should be considered in older horses, especially if evidence of other lower motor neuron pathological conditions exists (see page 140).

Many horses make a slow progressive recovery. Electrical stimulation of the affected muscles may help to maintain muscle mass. Problems may arise in young horses with overload of the contralateral limb, unless symptoms resolve quickly. An improvement within 2 to 4 weeks warrants an optimistic prognosis. Persistence of clinical signs for more than 6 months warrants a guarded prognosis.

Fracture of the First Rib

Occasionally, acute-onset, severe lameness follows trauma from a fall or collision with a solid object associated with a fracture of the first rib. The lameness is typical of a proximal limb injury, but no other localizing signs are present. Atrophy of the infraspinatus alone has also been recognized in some horses. Diagnosis is by radiographic examination. Nuclear scintigraphic examination may facilitate diagnosis. The prognosis is good after rest.

PART IV

The Hindlimb

Chapter 41

The Hind Foot and Pastern

Mike W. Ross

References on page 1284

The contribution of the hind foot and pastern to hindlimb lameness is considerably less important than that of the digit to forelimb lameness. Extensive information regarding lameness of the foot and pastern in the forelimb is found in Chapters 26 to 35 and 82. This information is directly applicable to the hindlimb. During lameness examination, the hind foot and pastern are easily overlooked because they are in a potentially dangerous place to examine. Other regions of the hindlimb have been presumed to be more important, and, historically, little has been taught about the distal part of the limb. Without a commitment to performing diagnostic analgesic techniques in the distal aspect of the hindlimb, there is little way to discover whether the digit is the authentic source of pain unless the problem is severe or obvious. Subtle primary or compensatory lameness problems of this region are likely to go unnoticed daily. However, in certain sports horses, such as the draft horse, lameness of the hind foot and pastern is so common that this region cannot be overlooked. I am curious as to why infectious osteitis of the distal phalanx is more common in the hind feet. Of 26 affected limbs in 21 lame foals with infectious osteitis of the distal phalanx, most likely hematogenous in origin, 18 (69%) were hindlimbs.[1] Infectious arthritis in foals occurs more commonly in hindlimb joints, specifically the femoropatellar and tarsocrural joints, than in forelimb joints, a finding that is equally difficult to explain.[2]

ANATOMY AND INNERVATION OF THE HIND FOOT AND PASTERN

The bones are essentially the same as in the forelimb. The hind distal phalanx is narrower compared with the forelimb and has a steeper dorsal angle. The plantar surface is more concave, and the plantar processes are closer together.[1] In external appearance, the hind foot usually is more upright than the fore foot, but abnormal wear and shoeing practices can produce a common pathological condition of a low, underrun heel (see Chapter 6). The hind middle phalanx is narrower and longer, and the hind proximal phalanx is slightly shorter than the corresponding bones in the forelimb.[3] The ligaments, tendons, digital flexor tendon sheath (DFTS), and distal interphalangeal and proximal interphalangeal joints are the same as in the forelimb. Innervation of the foot is derived primarily from the medial and lateral plantar nerves, which originate from the tibial nerve (see Chapter 10). The medial and lateral plantar metatarsal nerves, which originate from the deep branch of the lateral plantar nerve, become superficial just distal to the "bell" of the second and fourth metatarsal bones. Unlike the palmar metacarpal nerves, the hindlimb medial and lateral plantar metatarsal nerves supply sensation to the pastern region and coronary band, a fact that can complicate interpretation of perineural analgesia in the hind digit.[4]

EXAMINATION, CLINICAL SIGNS, AND DIAGNOSIS

The clinical examination of the hind foot and pastern was described in Chapter 6, and a detailed description of the clinical investigation of the foot and shoeing is found in Chapters 27, 28, and 30 to 34. A conscientious effort must be made during every lameness examination to evaluate the hind foot with the limb in both the standing and flexed positions. The type of shoeing and shoe wear are important in understanding potential lameness conditions of the foot, but perhaps more important, study of hind foot balance and shoeing can provide important clues in the diagnosis of lameness located more proximally in the limb. Dramatic abnormalities in balance and shoe additives, such as calks, grabs, trailers, and bars, can place added forces of shear and torsion on hindlimb bones and joints. Therapeutic recommendations cannot be made unless the clinician is aware of the type of shoes that are currently in place. Hoof imbalance has not been studied extensively in the hindlimb, but dorsal to plantar and medial to lateral hoof imbalance is a likely contributor to lameness in the proximal interphalangeal and metatarsophalangeal joints. Palpation for signs of inflammation, such as increased digital pulse amplitude, heat, swelling, and pain, must be performed but can be difficult in fractious horses. Palpation is difficult in the hindlimb because of the stay apparatus, which causes the digit to flex involuntarily. Palpation of the plantar pastern soft tissue structures is difficult, and subtle swelling and pain associated with the distal sesamoidean ligaments or other structures can be easily overlooked. In draft horses, signs of inflammation can be obscure (Figure 41-1).

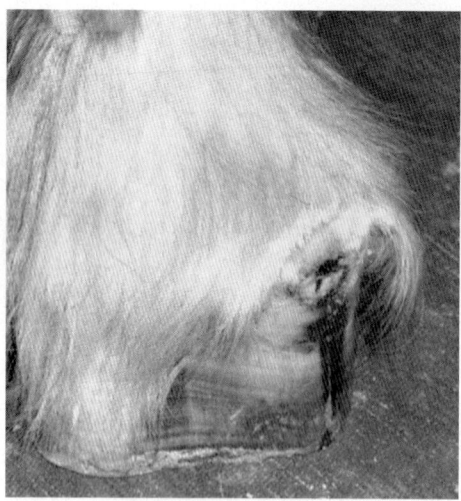

Fig. 41-1 • The defect in the coronary band of this draft horse was not detected until the long hair (or feathers) was shaved. Hoof tester examination yielded negative findings, but investigation of the foot was prompted by a positive response to perineural analgesia.

Examination with hoof testers is important, but normally horses show considerable sensitivity across the heel (see Chapter 6). Because the foot is incorporated in the rigid hoof capsule and swelling may not be apparent, even severe lameness conditions, such as abscesses or fractures, can go unnoticed. Commonly lameness of the hind foot is misinterpreted as originating high up in the limb, because clinical signs are not prominent and are easy to overlook.

Degree of lameness varies greatly. Most recognized problems of the hind foot cause obvious, often severe lameness, but occasionally subtle or insidious problems occur. Horses with the most common problems, such as a hoof abscess and penetrating wounds, may not bear weight. If they are bearing weight, horses usually are severely lame at the trot. Horses with severe hind foot lameness, particularly of the toe region, may walk with a shortened *caudal* phase of the stride, similar to horses with pain in the coxofemoral region (see Chapter 7). Horses with most lameness conditions typically have a shortened cranial phase of the stride at both the walk and trot. Observing a paradoxical shortened caudal phase of the stride at the walk and the more typically seen shortened cranial phase of the stride at the trot can be an indication of hind foot pain. The horse may bear weight only on the toe. Turning may accentuate pain. At the trot, horses with hind foot and pastern lameness travel like horses with pain that originates anywhere distal to the distal aspect of the crus, and no typical alteration in limb flight is observed. When the horse is viewed from behind, limb flight is characterized by moving the foot straight ahead or slightly medial to the line of expected limb flight and then stabbing laterally during the later portion of the stride, just before impact.

Lameness associated with many conditions in this region worsens with a lower limb flexion test. Horses with osteoarthritis of the distal interphalangeal and proximal interphalangeal joints or tenosynovitis of the DFTS and tendonitis of the deep digital flexor tendon (DDFT) respond prominently. In general, hindlimb flexion tests have low specificity, and in horses that respond markedly to lower limb flexion, a source of pain located more proximal in the limb cannot be dismissed without using diagnostic analgesia.

Lameness must be localized using perineural or intraarticular analgesic techniques. Differentiation of sources of pain in the hind foot and pastern can be problematic because the same difficulties in interpretation of plantar digital and distal interphalangeal analgesic techniques occur as in the forelimb. When the plantar digital block is done with the limb elevated, it is difficult to inject local anesthetic solution just above the cartilages of the foot, so this block is usually performed in a more proximal location than in the forelimb. It may be difficult to remove all pain in horses with severe lameness. Pain associated with the proximal aspect of the proximal phalanx, such as from midsagittal fractures, or from other causes of pain in the metatarsophalangeal joint can easily be removed inadvertently during performance of plantar digital analgesia.[5] Careful interpretation of analgesic techniques is necessary, particularly in racehorses, in which metatarsophalangeal joint region lameness is common (Figure 41-2).

Imaging considerations are similar to those described in the forelimb. It may be preferable to obtain plantarodorsal rather than dorsoplantar radiographic views of the foot. Many horses are reluctant to stand on a block with the foot bearing weight for lateromedial views. Satisfactory images can readily be obtained with the foot bearing weight only on the toe, provided that the foot is not rotated.[6]

SPECIFIC LAMENESS CONDITIONS

Overall the most common conditions of the hind foot and pastern involve hoof abscesses and bruises, penetrating wounds into the hoof capsule and soft tissues of the pastern region, and cellulitis. Scratches can cause horses to appear lame at a walk and when severe, lame also at the trot. Management of these conditions is well described elsewhere.

Fractures of the Distal Phalanx

Fractures of the distal phalanx occur in any type of sports horse as the result of direct trauma from kicking a wall or trailer. Occasionally horses step on a hard object while turned out or during competition. In racehorses, fractures of the distal phalanx can occur as a result of maladaptive or nonadaptive remodeling, but this is much less common than in the forelimb. Because many fractures are the result of direct trauma, the distribution varies. Of 72 racehorses with fractures of the distal phalanx, only nine fractures involved a hindlimb, but eight involved the medial aspect of the distal phalanx.[7] Distribution of hindlimb distal phalangeal fractures differs markedly from that seen in the forelimb of racehorses, in which left front (LF) lateral and right front (RF) medial fractures are most common.[7] Medial location seems counterintuitive if hindlimb distal phalangeal fractures share a common cause with those seen in the forelimb. In the forelimb it is proposed that many distal phalangeal fractures are stress fractures that occur as a result of chronic repetitive bone injury, and the distribution reflects a counterclockwise direction of racing, making the lateral side of the LF and medial side of the RF (compression side of bone) prone to the development of fracture.[7] It is the distal lateral aspect of the hindlimb that appears prone to the development of other stress-related

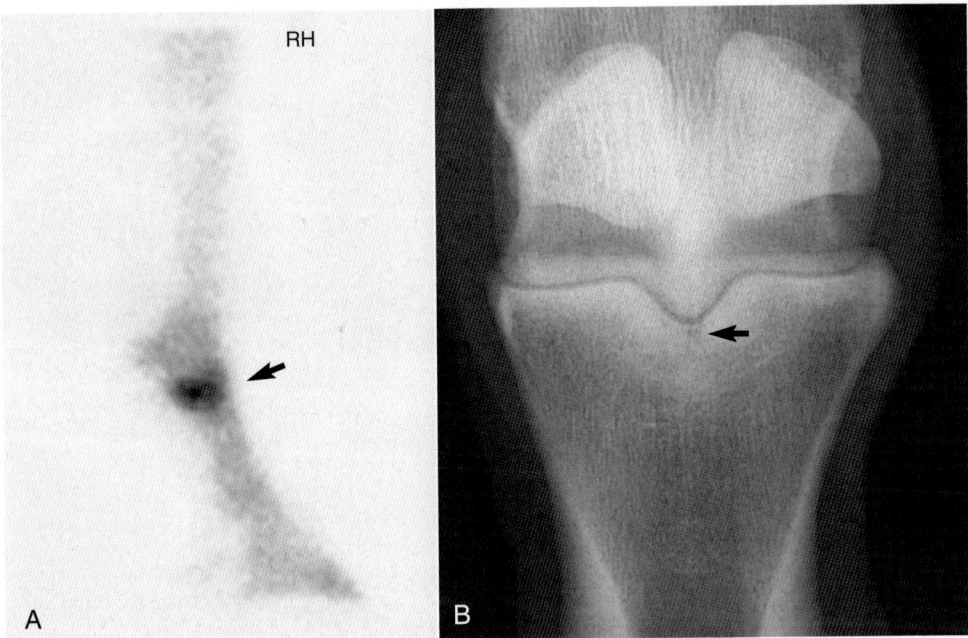

Fig. 41-2 • A, Lateral delayed phase scintigraphic image of a 4-year-old Standardbred pacer with right hindlimb lameness thought to originate in the foot because the horse was sound after plantar digital analgesia. However, focal, intense increased radiopharmaceutical uptake of the proximal aspect of the proximal phalanx *(arrow)* is diagnostic for fracture. **B,** Dorsoplantar digital radiographic image documenting the presence of a short, midsagittal fracture of the proximal phalanx *(arrow)*. Pain originating from the metatarsophalangeal joint can be desensitized by plantar digital analgesia.

subchondral bone injury (see Chapters 19, 42, and 106 to 109), and why the distribution of distal phalangeal fractures is different is unknown. Articular plantar process fractures are most common, but incomplete (stress) fractures and midsagittal fractures also occur. Lameness is variable in degree, and it is important to recognize that lameness may be episodic in horses with a nonarticular plantar process fracture. Fractures often can be seen in lateromedial radiographic images, but special oblique images may be required. Comminuted fractures are rare but develop as the result of direct trauma. An unusual fracture near the insertion of the DDFT was found in a 2-year-old Thoroughbred colt referred for scintigraphic examination for undiagnosed right hindlimb lameness (Figure 41-3). This horse raced successfully with conservative management and corrective shoeing. Conservative management in most horses with fracture of the distal phalanx is quite successful. The decision to perform neurectomy is often made earlier than for injuries in a forelimb.

Laminitis

In horses with enterocolitis, pleuritis, metritis, or other systemic diseases, laminitis can develop in all four limbs, but rarely is the condition seen in only the hindlimbs. Even when hind feet are involved, clinical signs usually are most prominent in the front feet. Laminitis restricted to the hind feet has been seen only in overweight cob-type horses and ponies.[8] Traumatic laminitis can occur from intense exercise on hard ground in unshod horses, but it most commonly develops in the contralateral limb of horses with severe unilateral hindlimb lameness. In the latter form, called *orthopedic laminitis*, distal displacement or rotation

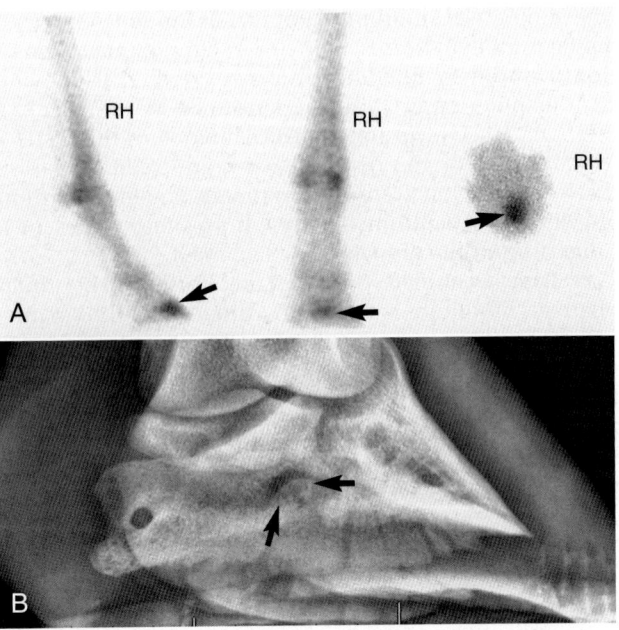

Fig. 41-3 • A, Lateral *(left image)*, plantar *(middle image)*, and solar *(right image)* delayed phase scintigraphic images of a 2-year-old Thoroughbred colt in race training referred because of undiagnosed right hindlimb lameness. Lameness improved but did not abate completely after plantar digital and low plantar analgesia. Focal, intense increased radiopharmaceutical uptake *(arrows)* is seen in an unusual location, near the insertion of the deep digital flexor tendon on the distal, central aspect of the distal phalanx. **B,** Dorsal 45° lateral-plantaromedial oblique digital radiographic image showing an unusual lesion thought to be a small fracture fragment *(arrow)*.

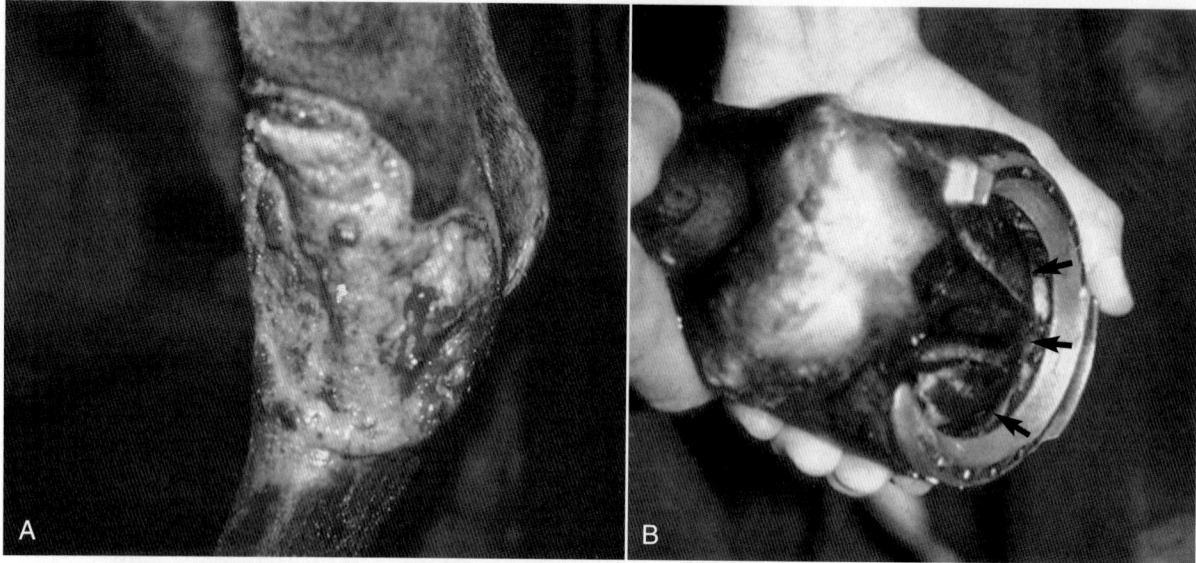

Fig. 41-4 • A, Large wound in the left tarsal region as a result of inappropriate application of a topical counterirritant that caused chronic, severe lameness and eventually caused infectious arthritis of the distal hock joints. **B,** Photograph of the contralateral hind foot showing a noticeable convexity of the sole *(arrows),* the result of rotation and distal displacement of the distal phalanx (orthopedic laminitis).

of the distal phalanx generally takes considerable time to develop (5 to 8 weeks) and can go unrecognized for several weeks (Figure 41-4). Often the first clinical sign that a problem is developing in the contralateral (laminitic) limb is that the lameness is observed to be inexplicably considerably improved in the original limb, or the horse starts to constantly shift weight between the two hindlimbs. Rarely, I have observed hindlimb laminitis as an apparently incidental finding in horses referred for scintigraphic examination for primary forelimb lameness or when whole-body scintigraphic examinations are performed. Marked increased radiopharmaceutical uptake (IRU) involving the distal or dorsal aspect of the distal phalanx and radiological evidence of rotation were seen. Primary lameness is found elsewhere, but laminitis in these horses may represent an unusual form of compensatory lameness.

I have examined two pleasure horses with primary bilateral hindlimb laminitis (without forelimb involvement) in which an unusual hindlimb gait was observed. At the walk horses had a goose-stepping gait like that seen in horses with fibrotic myopathy. The horses appeared to be attempting to land with an exaggerated heel-to-toe hoof strike. Both horses had a marked shortening of the caudal phase of the stride. At the trot horses had a short, choppy gait, but because lameness was bilateral, overt unilateral signs could not be seen.

Keratoma
Keratoma involving the hind feet is rare. An unusual radiolucent defect thought to be a keratoma that caused lameness and poor racing performance and was associated with IRU has been seen in the distal phalanx of a Thoroughbred racehorse.[9]

Navicular Syndrome
Navicular disease, osseous cystlike lesions, fractures, and malformations of the navicular bone are unusual in the hindlimb but do occur in all types of horses and ponies

(see Chapters 30 and 31). In fact, in young racehorses, odd conditions of the navicular bone seem more common in the hindlimb than in the forelimb. The foot should never be discounted as a potential source of lameness (Figures 41-5 and 41-6). Degree of lameness is variable; lameness is usually unilateral and improved by perineural analgesia of the plantar digital nerves. Lesions are usually readily detectable radiologically. Lesions may occur bilaterally; therefore radiographic examination of both hind feet is recommended. It may be more difficult to obtain a skyline image of the navicular bone in a hindlimb than in a forelimb. Scintigraphy can be helpful in some horses, particularly in those suspected of having pain originating more proximal in the limb and fractious horses in which diagnostic analgesia to properly localize pain is dangerous.

Distal Interphalangeal Joint
Primary osteoarthritis of the hind distal interphalangeal joint is rare. Osteophytes involving the extensor process of the distal phalanx are commonly seen but are usually incidental radiological findings. Osteoarthritis occurs as a result of instability or incongruity caused by articular fractures of the distal phalanx. Occasionally subchondral bone damage of the articular surface of the distal phalanx occurs and is recognized as radiolucent defects and secondary osteoarthritic changes; this damage usually is seen in older nonracehorse sports horses. Chronic, undiagnosed hindlimb lameness is followed by acute, prominent lameness. Diagnosis may be difficult, thus prompting scintigraphic examination. Focal areas of IRU in the subchondral bone of the distal phalanx should be differentiated from those in horses with incomplete fracture.

Extensor process fragments or fractures are rare. Osseous cystlike lesions as a result of osteochondrosis of the distal phalanx are seen occasionally. Some small lesions restricted to the subchondral bone of the distal phalanx are difficult to identify radiologically but usually result in intense, focal IRU scintigraphically. Definitive diagnosis may be possible

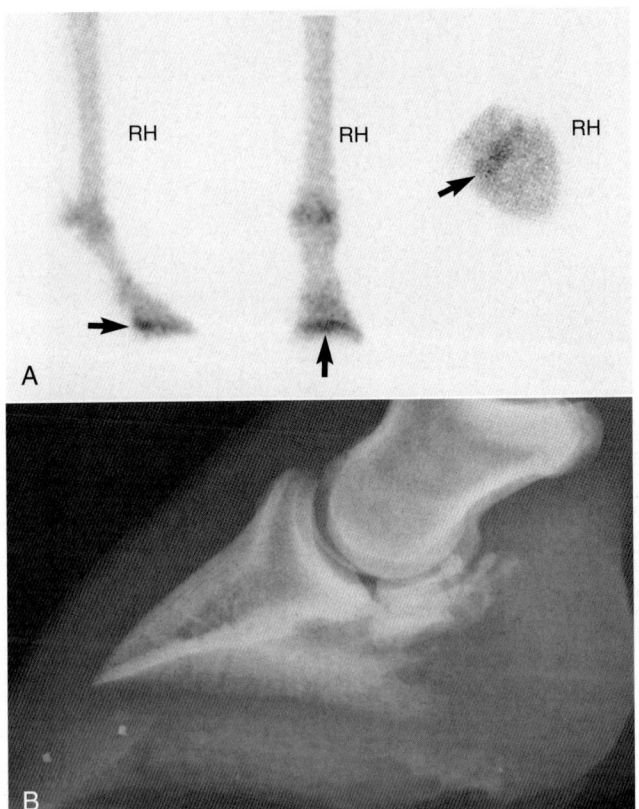

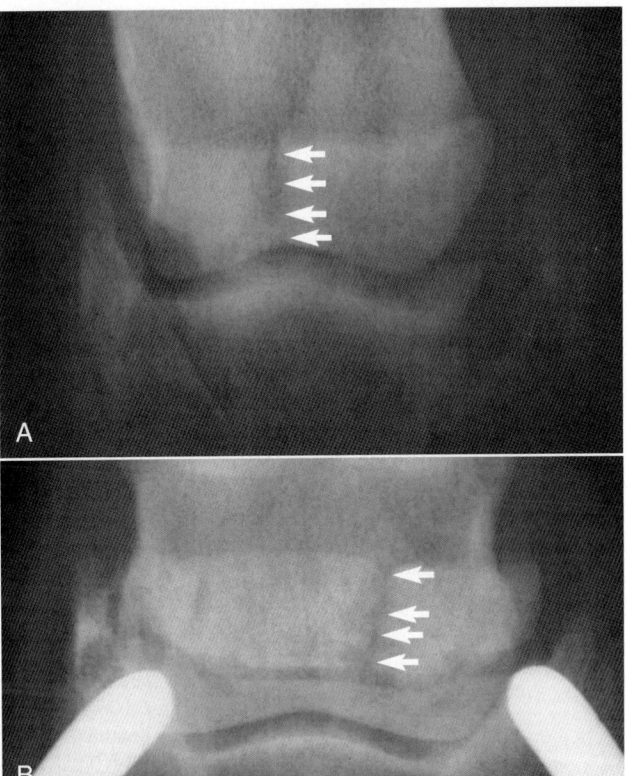

Fig. 41-5 • A, Lateral *(left image),* plantar *(middle image),* and solar *(right image)* delayed (bone) phase scintigraphic images showing focal, moderately increased radiopharmaceutical uptake of the navicular bone in a 2-year-old, unraced Thoroughbred filly, admitted for examination of chronic right hindlimb lameness. **B,** Corresponding lateromedial digital radiographic image showing extensive degeneration of the navicular bone, with both bony proliferation and radiolucent defects present. There was no history of a penetrating wound or other traumatic incident, and an unusual malformation of the navicular bone was diagnosed. Note the close proximity of the distal aspect of the navicular bone to the distal phalanx, the abnormal orientation of the distal phalanx, and the abnormal shape of the hoof capsule.

Fig. 41-6 • Dorsal 65° proximal-plantaro(palmaro)distal oblique digital radiographic images of the left hind (LH) **(A)** and left fore (LF) **(B)** feet showing unusual, coexistent navicular bone fractures in a 3-year-old Standardbred filly pacer. Baseline 3 to 4 out of 5 LH lameness resolved after plantar digital analgesia, but the filly then showed marked LF lameness. Acute LH navicular bone fracture *(arrows)* with mild displacement and chronic LF navicular bone fracture or bipartite navicular bone anomaly *(arrows)* were diagnosed.

only with magnetic resonance imaging (MRI) or at postmortem examination.[8] Other fractures involving the distal aspect of the middle phalanx and comminuted fractures of this bone occur. Involvement of the distal interphalangeal joint in horses with comminuted fractures of the middle phalanx is a negative prognostic finding.

Collateral ligament injury of the distal interphalangeal joint is an uncommon cause of hindlimb lameness but does occur, usually with no localizing clinical signs. Although occasionally lesions can be identified using ultrasonography, diagnosis usually requires MRI.

Deep Digital Flexor Tendonitis

Primary injuries of the DDFT are an unusual cause of hindlimb lameness but have been identified in show jumpers and event horses. There has been an acute onset of moderate-to-severe unilateral lameness, usually with no localizing clinical signs. Diagnosis usually requires MRI.

Infectious Osteitis in Foals

See Chapter 128.

The Hind Pastern

Lameness of the hind pastern region includes osteoarthritis of the proximal interphalangeal joint, osseous cystlike lesions of the distal aspect of the proximal phalanx, osteochondral fragmentation of the proximal interphalangeal joint, subluxation of the proximal interphalangeal joint, tenosynovitis of the DFTS, tendonitis of the DDFT and the branches of the superficial digital flexor tendon, injury of the distal sesamoidean ligaments, penetrating wounds, and cellulitis (see Chapters 35, 70, 74, and 82). Fractures of the proximal and middle phalanges are discussed in detail in Chapter 35. One fracture type, Salter-Harris type II fractures of the proximal aspect of the proximal phalanx, occurs most commonly in the hindlimb. Because physeal fractures are inherently more stable than those of the diaphyseal region of long bones, it is compelling to simply apply external coaptation such as a fiberglass cast incorporating the foot. However, prolonged cast immobilization quickly causes flexor laxity in foals and can predispose to osteoarthritis and sesamoiditis. Invariably, even with inherent stability, fracture displacement occurs. The metaphyseal component is usually plantaromedial, and even with external coaptation the proximal fracture fragment shifts distally and plantarolaterally and a gap opens on the dorsomedial aspect. Internal fixation using screws placed from

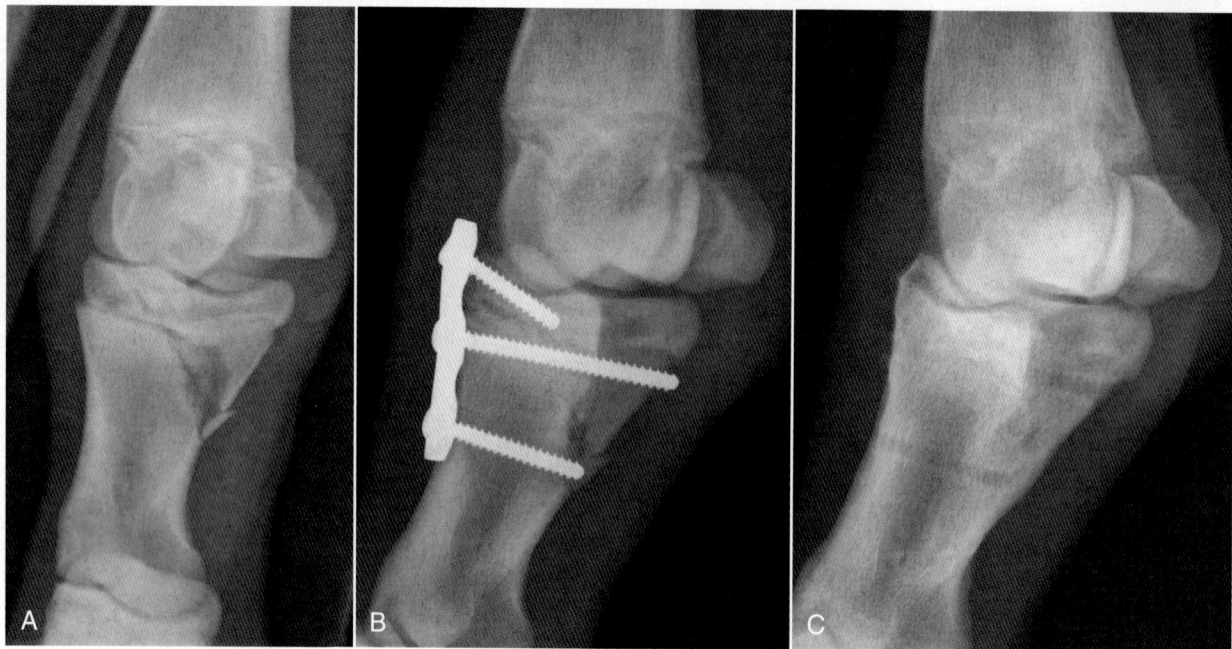

Fig. 41-7 • Dorsal 45° medial-plantarolateral oblique digital radiographic images before (**A**) and immediately after (**B**) repair and 3 months after repair and implant removal (**C**) in a weanling Warmblood foal with a Salter-Harris type II fracture of the proximal aspect of the right hind proximal phalanx. Using the tension band principle, a three-hole, limited-contact dynamic compression plate was applied to the dorsolateral aspect of the proximal phalanx; the middle screw was placed in lag fashion through the metaphyseal component. Rigid internal fixation obviated the need for prolonged external coaptation and maintained fracture alignment.

the plantaromedially located metaphyseal portion improves stability, but alignment of the fracture is hard to maintain. An alternative approach is to apply a dorsolateral dynamic compression plate, a technique that takes advantage of the tension band principle, because the tension side of the proximal phalanx appears to be dorsolateral when this fracture occurs (Figure 41-7). Rigid internal fixation obviates the need to maintain foals in external coaptation. Because the epiphysis is narrow, care must be taken when placing the proximal screw.

Chapter 42

The Metatarsophalangeal Joint

Mike W. Ross

References on page 1285

Lameness of the metatarsophalangeal (MTP) joint is similar to that of the metacarpophalangeal joint, but historically it has largely been ignored and was mentioned only twice in a leading lameness textbook.[1] With fastidious use of both intraarticular and perineural analgesia, the MTP joint is now known to contribute substantially to hindlimb lameness.[2]

ANATOMY

The MTP joint is nearly identical to the metacarpophalangeal joint and is composed of the distal articular surface of the third metatarsal bone (MtIII), its sagittal ridge, and the medial and lateral condyles; the medial and lateral proximal sesamoid bones (PSBs); and the proximal articular surface of the proximal phalanx, which has a prominent axially located sagittal groove (see Chapter 36). Minor differences exist in the shape and length of the proximal phalanx between the forelimbs and hindlimbs but are not clinically relevant. The MTP joint normally is more upright than the metacarpophalangeal joint and can achieve a greater degree of flexion. The lateral-to-medial width of the lateral condyle of the MtIII is less than that of the medial condyle. In racehorses, based on the results of scintigraphic examination, stress-related bone injury occurs predominantly in the lateral aspect of the hindlimb, which may be related to the smaller surface area of the lateral condyle. The joint capsule, intersesamoidean and collateral sesamoidean ligaments, suspensory ligament (SL) attachments, and digital flexor tendons all function to move and support the MTP joint. The dense collateral ligaments have short deep, and long superficial components. In the hindlimb the lateral digital extensor tendon joins with the long digital extensor tendon in the proximal dorsal metatarsal region. Therefore only the long digital extensor tendon is encountered during arthrocentesis or surgical procedures performed in the dorsal aspect of the MTP joint.

CONFORMATION

Fetlock valgus and varus deformities affect the MTP joint in foals, but fetlock varus deformity is of most concern and needs to be corrected early (see Chapter 58). Most normal horses are slightly toed out in the hindlimbs, but in some horses toed-out conformation may play a role in uneven load distribution and affect hindlimb gait. Horses with toed-out conformation tend to travel close behind and stab laterally during limb advancement, a gait that may cause excessive lateral shoe wear and hoof imbalance. Such gait and hoof imbalance may predispose the lateral aspect of the MTP joint to stress-related bone injury. Horses that are excessively straight behind have an abnormal degree of extension (or dorsiflexion) of the MTP joint. This conformation is undesirable because it places abnormal load on the SL and predisposes to suspensory desmitis, stifle joint lameness, and secondary osteoarthritis (OA) of the MTP joint. Horses with bull-nose foot conformation and long, weak hind pasterns may be predisposed to injury (see Chapter 4, Figure 4-34). When viewed from behind when walking and trotting, some horses—especially those with a base-narrow conformation—appear to collapse laterally over each hind fetlock.

CLINICAL CHARACTERISTICS AND DIAGNOSIS OF METATARSOPHALANGEAL JOINT LAMENESS

Lameness of the MTP joint occurs in most sports horses and is common in the racehorse. Both Standardbred (STB) and Thoroughbred (TB) racehorses are prone to injury of this joint, but MTP joint lameness is more common in the STB, because gait and load distribution predispose to hindlimb lameness in this breed (see Chapter 2). Lameness of the MTP joint should never be discounted in the TB racehorse, and in both the STB and TB racehorse in my referral practice, conditions of this joint are the most common cause of undiagnosed hindlimb lameness. Curiously, MTP joint lameness is apparently uncommon in Western performance horses despite the predominant use of the hindlimbs for many maneuvers and thus tremendous forces applied to the MTP joint (see Chapter 120). With Western performance horses, sporting activity may play a role because in barrel horses and team roping heading horses, lameness of the distal aspect of the hindlimb including the MTP joint was uncommon, but in team roping heeling horses, the MTP joint contributed substantially to lameness and poor performance.[3,4] There is no pathognomonic historical information that incriminates the MTP joint more than other sources of hindlimb lameness, but racehorses are usually worse in turns. Absence of palpable abnormalities and clinical signs incriminating other areas of pain in the hindlimb, particularly in a racehorse, would make me consider the MTP joint region, because it is the most commonly overlooked area in my practice. In horses with bilateral MTP joint lameness, poor performance may be the only historical finding and overt signs of lameness may not be present, but a short, choppy gait or intermittent, shifting hindlimb lameness is seen. A gait typical of bilateral stress-related bone injury of the distal aspect of the MtIII in TB racehorses being trotted in hand is described as an "exaggerated pelvic excursion" in a dorsoventral direction (see Chapter 107).

Clinical signs of MTP joint lameness vary from subtle to overt and depend on the nature and severity of injury. Signs of inflammation may be absent in horses with stress-related bone injury but severe in horses with displaced or comminuted fractures. At the trot limb flight is similar to lameness originating from the metatarsal region and hock. As the limb moves forward, it deviates medially and is then stabbed laterally at the end of the cranial phase of the stride. The cranial phase is shortened commensurately with the degree of pain. Lameness is more pronounced with the affected limb on the inside of a circle. I find it useful to characterize clinical signs into three categories: severe, unrelenting lameness; intermittent, severe lameness; and chronic, low-grade lameness. TB racehorses often have bilateral MTP joint pain and show poor hindlimb action and a tendency to bunny-hop behind in canter.

Severe, Unrelenting Lameness

The severe, unrelenting form of MTP joint lameness is associated with intraarticular fractures or severe, end-stage OA. Horses are obviously lame at the walk, cannot be trotted, and may be non–weight bearing. Deformity of the MTP joint may be obvious, as in horses with comminuted fractures of the proximal phalanx. Effusion is obvious and diffuse; periarticular soft tissue swelling may be present. Horses with acute, displaced condylar fractures of the MtIII may have acute, progressive edema of the diaphyseal region, and those with comminuted fractures of the proximal phalanx often have severe soft tissue swelling. Palpation and flexion elicit severe pain and, in horses with comminuted or displaced fractures, crepitus. Radiographs are usually diagnostic. This category includes severe, complete, or comminuted fractures (e.g., spiral fractures of the MtIII); comminuted or complete fractures of the proximal phalanx; midbody fractures of the PSBs; complex fractures involving the MtIII, the proximal phalanx, and the PSBs; luxation or subluxation; and end-stage OA. Horses with acute tendonitis of the deep digital flexor tendon (DDFT) with tenosynovitis can be severely lame, and intrathecal analgesia of the digital flexor tendon sheath (DFTS) may only partially remove pain. Ultrasonographic examination is required. However, some sports horses with DDFT lesions show lameness that is challenging to diagnose because of its sporadic nature.

Intermittent, Severe Lameness

Horses with intermittent, severe lameness of the MTP joint may be able to train and perform at some level but develop severe lameness afterward. When exhibiting clinical signs, horses are lame at the walk, even toe-touching lame, and are obviously lame at the trot (grade 3 or 4 of 5), but after resting and receiving nonsteroidal antiinflammatory drugs (NSAIDs), horses are often able to gallop, jog, or train within 1 to 5 days. In some instances horses may be able to race, only to become lame once again. When walking in hand, horses often show marked lameness while turning, even if they are sound while walking in a straight line. Obvious signs of inflammation usually are not present, but horses generally respond positively to the lower limb flexion test and may show a painful response to deep palpation. Horses with incomplete midsagittal or dorsal (frontal) fractures of the proximal phalanx often manifest a painful response when firm digital pressure is placed on the proximal, dorsal aspect (see Figure 6-37). Effusion may be present, but it is often absent or minimal even in horses with incomplete fractures. Because clinical signs may be difficult to detect, diagnostic analgesia is often necessary. Radiographs are usually diagnostic, but if findings are equivocal or the radiographs are obtained before radiological changes develop, scintigraphic examination or follow-up radiographic examination in 10 to 14 days is required. Digital and computed radiography can be helpful. Conditions such as incomplete fractures of the MtIII, the proximal phalanx, and the PSBs and moderate OA are in this category.

Chronic, Low-Grade Lameness

Diagnosis of chronic, low-grade MTP joint lameness is difficult. Specific signs that localize lameness to the MTP joint are lacking, and lameness may be only subtle to mild (grade 1 of 5) at the trot in hand. Horses examined at the track and carrying a rider may show only mild lameness. In racehorses, effusion and the response to lower limb flexion varies, but it can be negative. There is often mild increase in temperature, a subtle but useful sign of subchondral bone injury. In nonracehorses there may be effusion of the MTP joint and often the DFTS, but effusion is often longstanding and may be easily overlooked if reported by the handler as preexistent. Palpation may reveal mildly suspicious areas (e.g., pain over the abaxial aspect of the PSBs) in horses with sesamoiditis, but in most horses no abnormalities are noted. Concomitant lameness of the MTP joint and stifle region, called intralimb compensatory lameness, occurs most often in racehorses but is recognized in nonracehorses, and clinical signs may not abate until both sites are blocked or treated. The association between the stifle and MTP joint is difficult to explain. In young horses with "loose stifles," knuckling of the MTP joint occurs when horses, particularly STBs, are jogged or worked slowly. Perhaps stretching of MTP joint capsule attachments or early subchondral bone trauma occurs during knuckling. Horses with "loose stifles" are thought to have patellar ligament and muscular instability and laxity and may benefit from counterirritant injection and simultaneous management of the MTP joint problem.

Diagnostic analgesia is required to localize pain causing lameness to the MTP joint, but in many horses lameness is difficult to accurately assess with the horse at a trot in hand. It is extremely important to recognize the need to employ perineural diagnostic analgesic techniques in addition to or in lieu of intraarticular analgesia in order to abolish all pain associated with the MTP joint. Radiological findings may be normal and horses are referred for scintigraphic examination, which often reveals stress-related bone injury. Special radiographic images may be needed to evaluate the distal aspect of the MtIII or for accurate identification of osteochondral fragments located in the dorsal and plantar aspects of the joint. In this category are conditions such as stress-related bone injury of the MtIII, early OA, osteochondral fragments that occur traumatically or as the result of osteochondrosis, and sesamoiditis.

Diagnostic Analgesia

Articular pain originating from the MTP joint can usually be abolished or at least partially alleviated by intraarticular analgesia. Because only one injection is required, intraarticular analgesia is easier and safer to perform than perineural techniques, but pain originating from subchondral bone may not abate or may be only partially alleviated by intraarticular analgesia. Therefore, it is extremely important to recognize that the low plantar perineural technique or a variation must be used, because it is more effective in alleviating pain from all sources (see Chapter 10).

A variation of the low plantar block, the lateral plantar metatarsal block, can be performed in horses with stress-related bone injury of the distal plantarolateral aspect of the MtIII (see Chapter 107).[5] This block is particularly valuable in horses with bilateral lameness, because after one limb is blocked, the horse becomes obviously lame in the other. Other sources of pain located laterally in the MTP joint, such as sesamoiditis, small fractures of the PSBs, can be blocked by this technique, but the most common reason horses improve after lateral plantar metatarsal analgesia is alleviation of subchondral bone pain of the distal aspect of the MtIII.

In horses with chronic, low-grade lameness it may be necessary to perform analgesia and watch the horse train. Resolution of subtle signs, such as bearing in or out, not feeling right behind, performing dressage maneuvers, or, in STB racehorses, being on a shaft or a line, may be the only sign of a positive response to diagnostic analgesia. Although perineural analgesia may result in slight loss of proprioception, it is generally preferable, because intraarticular analgesia may result in a false-negative response. If pain is elicited by firm palpation of the dorsoproximal aspect of the proximal phalanx, suspect a midsagittal fracture. Nerve blocks are contraindicated because of the risk of creating a complete or comminuted fracture.

The clinician should be aware that it is possible to inadvertently block pain associated with subchondral bone of the MTP joint when performing plantar digital or plantar perineural analgesia. This occurs most frequently in racehorses with midsagittal fracture of the proximal phalanx but can occur in horses with OA or other conditions (see Chapters 10 and 41).

IMAGING CONSIDERATIONS
Radiography and Radiology

Examination should include dorsoplantar (DPl), lateromedial (LM), dorsolateral-plantaromedial oblique (DL-PlMO), and dorsomedial-plantarolateral oblique (DM-PlLO) images. A flexed LM image is useful to evaluate the sagittal ridge for the presence of osteochondrosis lesions and to see dorsal frontal fractures of the proximal phalanx. Vacuum phenomenon can occur because the MTP joint can be placed in extreme flexion. Sudden decompression of the joint during stress flexion is believed to cause what appears to be an air artifact in the distal plantar aspect of the MtIII.[6]

Horizontal oblique images are useful to evaluate the proximal-dorsal aspect of the proximal phalanx for the presence of osteochondral fragments, but overlap between the base of the PSBs and the proximal aspect of the proximal phalanx can hide lesions associated with the

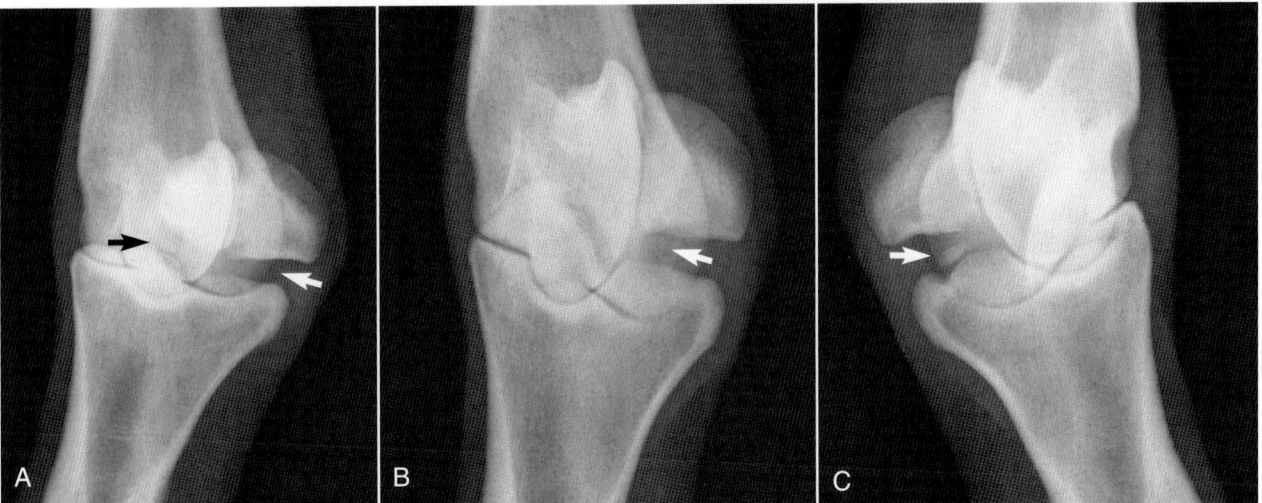

Fig. 42-1 • A, Dorsal 45° lateral-plantaromedial oblique digital radiographic image of a 3-year-old Standardbred filly with maladaptive subchondral bone remodeling obtained using a horizontal x-ray beam. Often, there is overlap between the base of the proximal sesamoid bones (PSBs) and proximal aspect of the proximal phalanx *(white arrow)*, but in this well-positioned view no overlap exists. A medial, plantar osteochondral fragment can be seen *(black arrow)*. **B,** Dorsal 20° proximal, 45° lateral-plantarodistal medial oblique digital radiographic image of the same filly showing a large radiolucent lesion in the distal aspect of the lateral condyle of the third metatarsal bone (MtIII) that was not seen in a conventional oblique image **(A).** A proximodistal (down-angled) radiographic image opens up the space between the PSBs and the proximal phalanx. **C,** A similar down-angled oblique image of the plantaromedial aspect of the joint allows complete visibility of the plantar osteochondral fragment *(arrow)*.

distal-plantar aspect of the joint. Overlap in the plantar aspect of this joint is more common than in the metacarpophalangeal joint and occurs when the distal hindlimb is not vertically positioned. The x-ray beam should be angled down 15 to 20 degrees to separate the PSBs and proximal phalanx (Figure 42-1).

Using a horizontal x-ray beam in a DPl image, the PSBs are superimposed over the distal aspect of the MtIII and the MTP joint. To better evaluate these areas, dorsal 15° proximal-plantarodistal oblique (D15° Pr-PlDiO), flexed DPl, and standing 125-degree DPl images should be used. Proximolateral (medial)-distolateral (medial) and proximoplantar-distoplantar tangential images of the PSBs are occasionally used to evaluate the abaxial and plantar surfaces of the PSBs, respectively.

Approximately 5% to 10% of normal horses have a small unilateral or bilateral radiolucent notch (<1 mm in length) in the sagittal grove of the proximal phalanx that is seen in a DPl image and should not be confused with a midsagittal fracture. I have seen this "notch" most commonly in the DPl image of the STB racehorse. If clinical signs are consistent with midsagittal fracture, scintigraphic examination is recommended. Flattening of the plantar distal aspect of the MtIII condyles is not as common as in the metacarpophalangeal joint, but increased radiopacity of the plantar aspect of the MtIII can be seen in horses with stress-related bone injury and early OA if well-exposed LM and flexed LM images are obtained. I question the clinical significance of flattening of the condyles of the MtIII in most horses. Digital and computed radiographs are useful in the evaluation of horses with stress-related bone injury and incomplete fractures. Computed tomography (CT) and magnetic resonance imaging (MRI; see later) are also useful, but availability is limited.

Scintigraphic Examination

Scintigraphic examination is the best way to establish a diagnosis in many horses with intermittent, severe, or chronic low-grade lameness of the MTP joint. The most common scintigraphic findings in the MTP joint of STB and TB racehorses are focal areas of increased radiopharmaceutical uptake (IRU) that involve the distal plantarolateral aspect of the MtIII (see Figure 19-20, *A*; Figures 42-2 and 42-3).[7] This IRU is a form of stress-related bone injury and early OA that is found in many racehorses with chronic, low-grade lameness, bilateral hindlimb lameness, and poor performance. Special radiographic images may then reveal increased radiopacity or radiolucent defects (see Figures 42-1 and 42-3). Similar scintigraphic findings are seen in horses with lateral condylar fractures of the MtIII. Focal areas of IRU are seen in horses with midsagittal or dorsal frontal fractures of the proximal phalanx (see Figure 19-20, *C*), sesamoiditis (Figure 42-4), and osteochondrosis of the plantar process of the proximal phalanx (see Figure 23-1; Figure 42-5). Often areas of IRU are found in unusual sites, such as those associated with the medial PSB (osteochondral fragments of the abaxial border and sesamoiditis), intersesamoidean ligament injury with radiolucent defects in one or both PSBs, incomplete fractures of the PSBs, and medial condylar fractures of the MtIII. Any focal area of IRU located medially in the MTP joint should be investigated, because incidental findings are unusual in this location.

Scintigraphic changes are usually less pronounced in nonracehorses, and negative or equivocal results often occur. The most common scintigraphic findings in jumpers and dressage horses with MTP joint lameness are diffuse mild areas of IRU in all bones or focal mild or moderate IRU in the dorsal or central aspects of the joint that involve

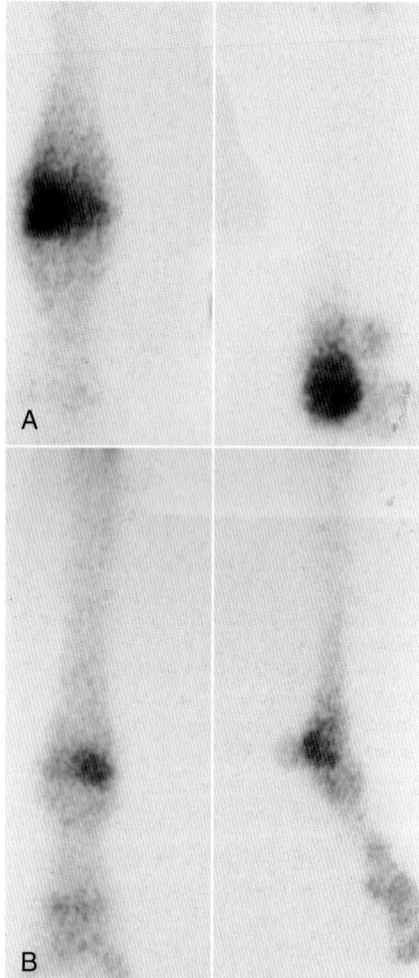

Fig. 42-2 • **A,** Plantar (lateral to the left) and flexed lateral (on the right) left hindlimb and **B,** plantar (lateral to the right) and lateral (on the right) right hindlimb delayed (bone) phase scintigraphic images of the metatarsophalangeal (MTP) joint in two Standardbred racehorses. All images show focal increased radiopharmaceutical uptake of the distal, plantarolateral aspect of the third metatarsal bone, which is the most common scintigraphic finding in the MTP joint of racehorses.

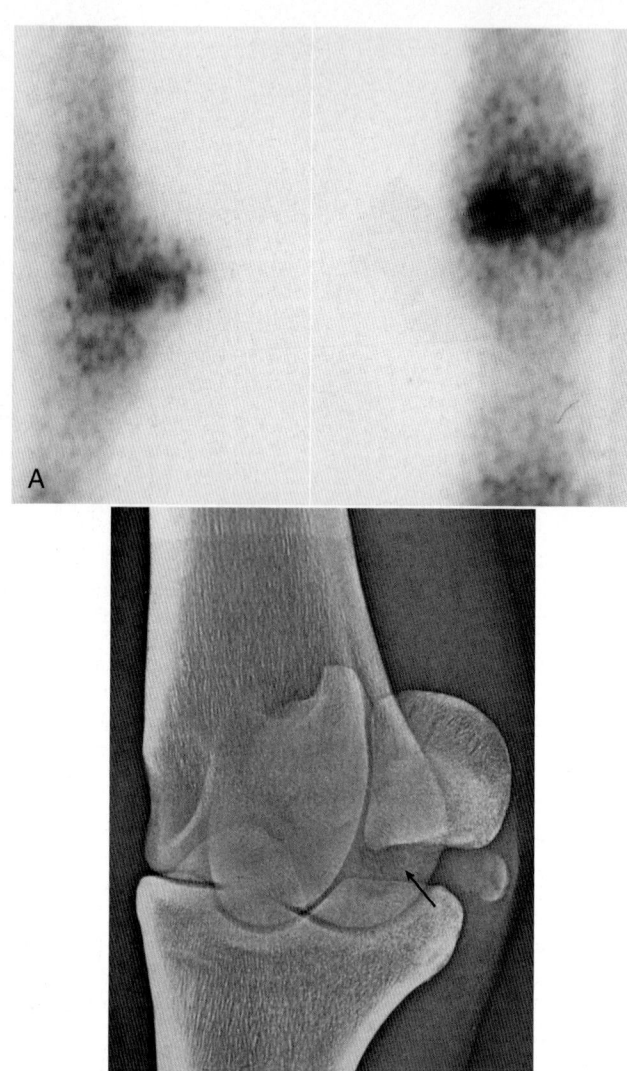

Fig. 42-3 • **A,** Lateral (on the left) and plantar (lateral is to the left) bone phase scintigraphic images of a metatarsophalangeal joint. There is increased radiopharmaceutical uptake in the plantar aspect of the lateral condyle of the third metatarsal bone. **B,** Dorsolateral proximal-plantaromedial distal oblique xeroradiographic image showing a radiolucent defect *(arrow)* of the same area. This defect can easily be missed on routinely positioned images, but the increased radiopharmaceutical uptake seen in this area scintigraphically **(A)** prompted further investigation.

the distal aspect of the MtIII and proximal aspect of the proximal phalanx and are associated with radiological evidence of marginal osteophytes and enthesophytes. There is a distinct difference in the scintigraphic and radiological appearance of the MTP joint of nonracehorses and racehorses, because in racehorses IRU is generally focal in nature and IRU and radiological changes involve the plantar aspect of the joint. In a 2004 study of clinically sound horses, generalized, even radiopharmaceutical uptake across the distal aspect of the MtIII and the proximal aspect of the proximal phalanx was found.[8] Radiopharmaceutical uptake was significantly higher in the condyles of the MtIII of hindlimbs than in forelimbs, there was no effect of age, and there was a trend for region of interest ratios to be higher in the right hind MTP joint when compared with the left.[8] In some nonracehorses arthroscopic examination has revealed full-thickness cartilage damage that primarily involves the distal dorsomedial aspect of the MtIII (medial condyle) and is consistent with OA. Focal IRU in the proximal aspect of the plantar pouch is seen in

horses with severe OA (an ominous finding) (see Figure 19-20, *B*). I believe this finding is caused by accumulation of subchondral bone fragments in this location or modeling of the distal plantar aspect of the MtIII.

Magnetic Resonance Imaging

MRI is useful to evaluate bone and soft tissue abnormalities in the MTP joint and nearby structures (see Chapters 21, 107, and 108). In fact, in some horse-dense locations such as Newmarket, England, examination of the metacarpophalangeal and MTP joints using standing low-field MRI has become as commonplace as scintigraphic examination and is often preferentially requested by TB trainers.[9] In TB and STB racehorses with maladaptive or nonadaptive bone remodeling of the distal aspect of the MtIII, MRI

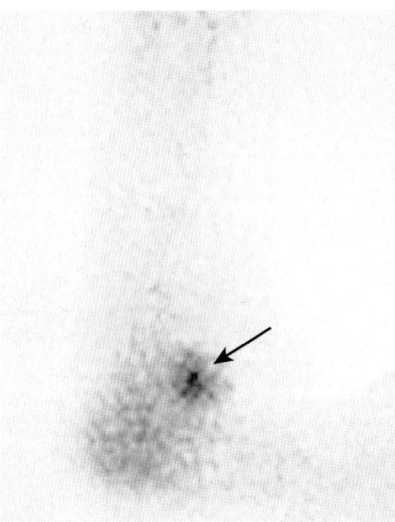

Fig. 42-4 • Flexed lateral delayed (bone) phase scintigraphic image of a 2-year-old Standardbred racehorse with lateral sesamoiditis. There is focal moderate increased radiopharmaceutical uptake in the proximal sesamoid bones *(arrow)*. When these findings were combined with those of the plantar image, the increased radiopharmaceutical uptake was localized to the lateral proximal sesamoid bone.

examination reveals extensive subchondral bone damage characterized predominately by low signal intensity of the plantar aspect of the lateral condyle of MtIII on T1- and T2-weighted images, a finding supporting the existence of chronic, sclerotic subchondral bone (Figure 42-6, *A* and *B*). Within the areas of low signal intensity is often a small area of high signal intensity near the articular cartilage (see Figure 42-6, *A* and *B*). In fat-suppressed short tau inversion recovery (STIR) image sequences, small, focal areas of high signal intensity within sclerotic bone are often found, indicating the presence of necrotic, and perhaps ischemic, bone, but widespread areas of high signal intensity consistent with bone edema from acute trauma are not often seen (Figure 42-6, *C*). Although numerous authors or speakers have characterized these lesions as bone bruises, bone edema (fluid accumulation) characteristic of bone bruises found in subchondral bone in people is not a hallmark of this common lesion in horses. Large areas of increased signal intensity likely indicated the presence of a fracture of the MtIII. Areas of increased signal intensity within sclerotic subchondral bone in horses with repetitive stress injuries could represent proteinaceous fluid, but likely represent regions of necrotic bone or granulation tissue.[9] Areas of necrotic bone seen on magnetic resonance (MR) images correspond to radiolucent defects. Areas of bone loss, necrotic subchondral bone, or areas of intense resorption within sclerotic bone may warrant consideration when trying to manage horses with this lesion (see later). In horses with acute-onset clinical signs consistent with acute subchondral bone injury or fracture, bone edema can be more prominent. In 13 horses, most of which were non-racehorses, with lameness of metacarpophalangeal or MTP joints and without radiological abnormalities, the most common finding was decreased signal intensity in T1-weighted images, indicating the presence of sclerotic subchondral bone.[10] In nine horses, decreased signal intensity

in T-2*-weighted images was consistent with sclerosis, but five had increased signal intensity in fat-suppressed STIR images consistent with what was described as fluid accumulation within the sclerotic regions.[10] Importantly, MRI abnormalities and subchondral bone lesions were found not only in racehorses but in horses used for show jumping and general purpose riding.[10] Lesions similar to those described for racehorses were seen in the MTP joint of sports horses.[11] Focal areas of IRU seen scintigraphically appeared in MR images as areas of low signal intensity on T1- and T2-weighted images with or without small areas of increased signal intensity in STIR images, indicating the presence of chronic, repetitive stress injuries of the distal aspect of the MtIII in sports horses in addition to acute, traumatic injuries.[11] In an earlier study of 11 horses (eight racehorses), subchondral bone damage was identified using MRI, although there were no or equivocal radiological abnormalities.[12] Four horses had lesions in the metacarpophalangeal or MTP joints. Horses with acute-onset lameness had subchondral bone injury characterized by increased signal intensity in STIR and T2-weighted images.[12] In two horses, decreased signal intensity in proton density images (similar to T1-weighted images) indicated the presence of sclerotic subchondral bone of the distal aspect of the MtIII, but dense bone was surrounded by areas of increased signal intensity in STIR sequences.[12] Only two horses had bone scintigraphy performed, and areas of IRU in the damaged subchondral bone were seen.[12] Horses with acute subchondral bone injury should improve with rest, whereas those with chronic, sclerotic, and osteoarthritic subchondral bone may improve temporarily with rest but long-term prognosis is guarded. MRI was useful in the evaluation of horses with oblique and straight distal sesamoidean desmitis in 27 horses with lameness localized to the metacarpophalangeal or MTP joint region, of which 17 had lameness and injury in the hindlimb.[13] Careful examination of soft tissue structures associated with the MTP joint, including use of diagnostic ultrasonographic examination, is necessary, because in some horses the results of diagnostic analgesia will be ineffective at differentiating authentic sources of pain in the region.

Ultrasonographic Examination

Ultrasonographic examination of the MTP joint region is indicated for suspensory branch desmitis (see Chapter 72). The abaxial aspect of the PSBs should be examined carefully to identify tearing and small avulsion fractures. Proliferative synovitis (villonodular synovitis) is unusual in the MTP joint. The DDFT should be evaluated carefully if tenosynovitis of the DFTS is present[14] (see Chapter 74). Ultrasonographic examination is useful in horses with intersesamoidean and collateral ligament injuries or those with wounds and draining tracts to look for foreign material or communication with the articular surface. The distal sesamoidean ligaments should also be examined carefully, because intraarticular analgesia of the MTP joint has the potential to resolve lameness associated with injury to these ligaments, which can be present with no localizing clinical signs.

Computed Tomography

CT (see Chapter 20) is useful to characterize complex fractures of the MTP joint, to aid in preoperative planning for

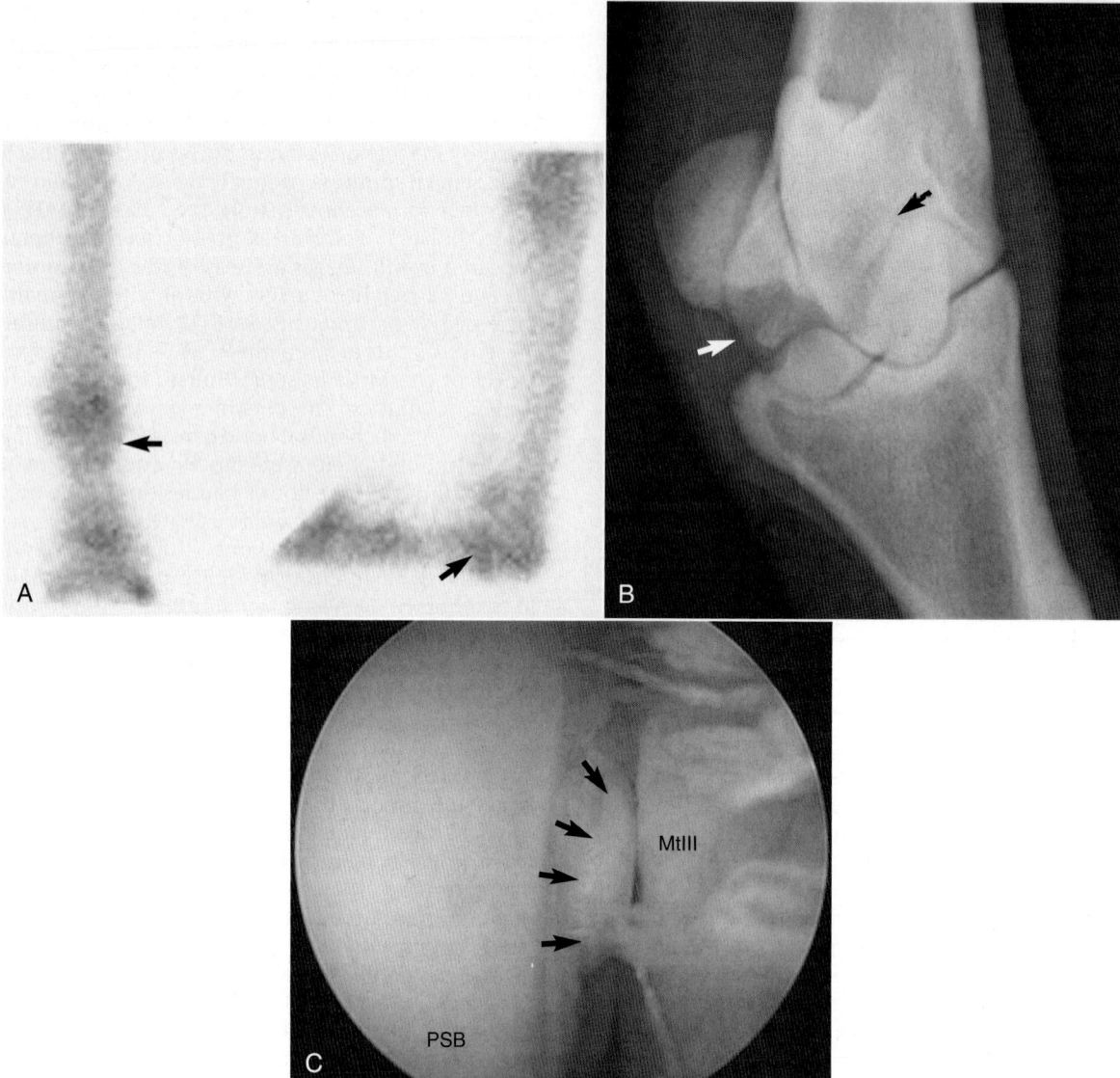

Fig. 42-5 • A, Plantar (left, lateral is to the right) and flexed lateral delayed (bone) phase scintigraphic images of a 3-year-old Standardbred trotter. There is focal mild increased radiopharmaceutical uptake (IRU) involving the proximal aspect of the proximal phalanx *(arrows),* evidence of mild bone modeling associated with lateral and medial axial articular osteochondral fragments of the plantar process of the proximal phalanx. IRU of the lateral aspect of the distal phalanx in the hindlimb is a common incidental scintigraphic finding. **B,** Dorsal 20° proximal lateral-plantarodistal medial oblique digital radiographic image of the same horse showing the presence of lateral *(white arrow)* and medial *(black arrow)* articular osteochondral fragments. Osteochondrosis lesions occur in this region more commonly on the medial aspect of the proximal phalanx but can be biaxial. **C,** Intraoperative arthroscopic photograph (plantar is to the left and proximal is uppermost) showing the medial fragment interposed between the base of the medial proximal sesamoid bone (PSB) and the proximal phalanx. The medial condyle of the third metatarsal bone (MtIII) is immediately dorsal to the fragment. The arthroscope was positioned in the lateral plantar pouch, and separate instrument incisions were used to remove both the medial (shown) and lateral fragments.

surgical repair, and to study other defects of articular surfaces. CT has been found to be superior to radiology in detecting articular comminution, small cracks and lucencies in the MtIII condyles, and fractures of the PSBs.[15] However, orthogonal radiography has been found to be superior to CT in detecting fractures of the dorsal aspect of the proximal phalanx, and both imaging modalities were poor at detecting plantar fractures of the proximal phalanx and coalescing cracks in the subchondral bone of the MtIII.[15]

CT is not as useful as scintigraphy and MRI in the evaluation of subchondral bone injury.

Arthroscopic Examination

Arthroscopic surgery is used frequently for removal of osteochondral fragments and fractures of the PSBs, assistance in fracture reduction and screw placement in horses with condylar fractures of the distal aspect of the MtIII and fractures of the proximal phalanx, and lavage and

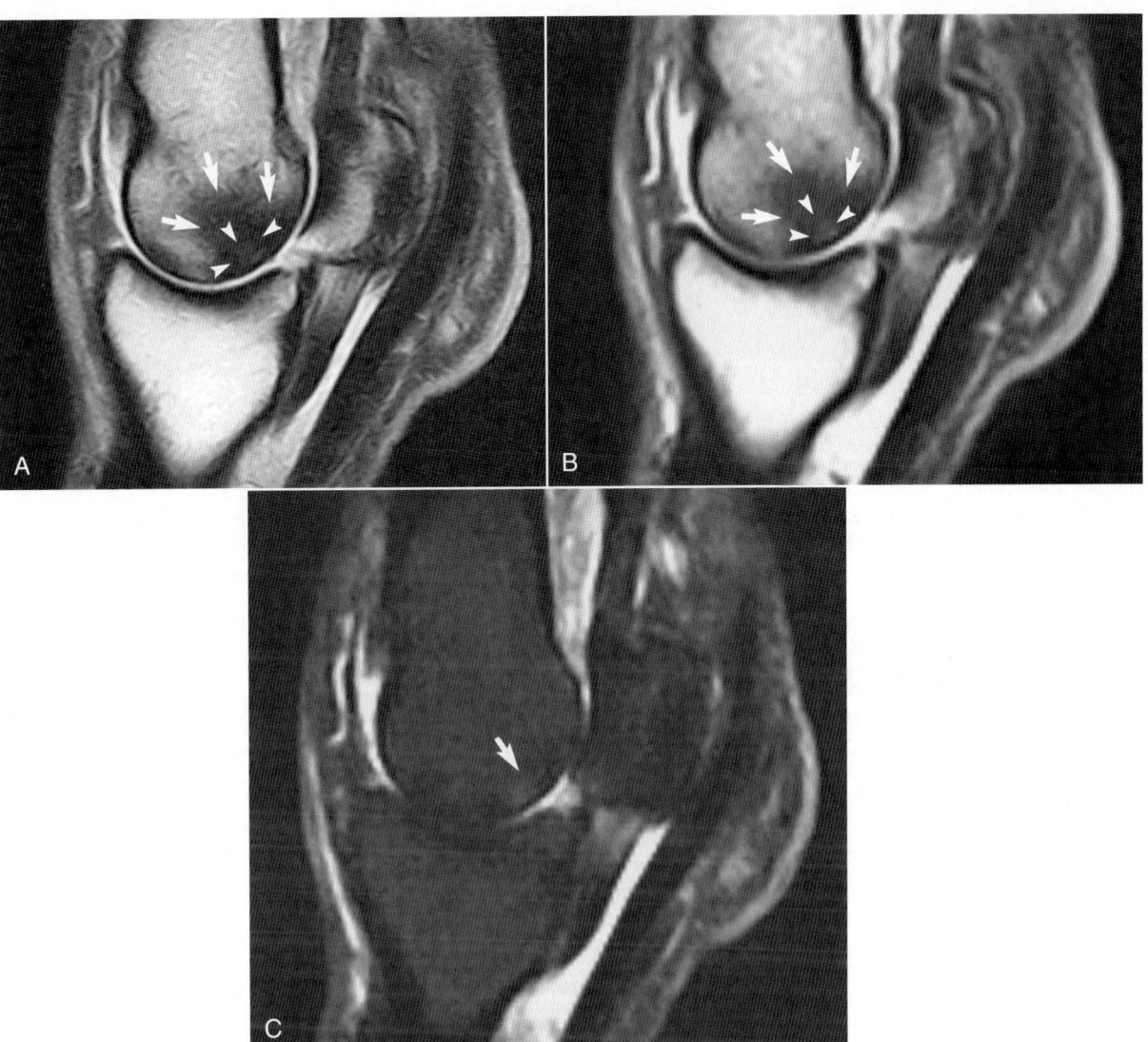

Fig. 42-6 • Sagittal, low-field (0.25T) magnetic resonance images, obtained with the horse under general anesthesia, of a 4-year-old Thoroughbred racehorse with lameness localized to the lateral aspect of the right metatarsophalangeal joint by using lateral plantar metatarsal analgesia. **A,** T1-weighted image showing decreased signal intensity *(arrows)* surrounding an area of increased signal intensity *(arrowheads).* **B,** T2-weighted image showing the same signal distribution, indicating there is dense, sclerotic subchondral bone surrounding an area of necrotic, ischemic subchondral bone or fluid accumulation. **C,** Short tau inversion recovery (STIR) image showing increased signal intensity *(arrow),* confirming the presence of an area of necrotic subchondral bone within dense, sclerotic bone typical of a horse with stress-related subchondral bone damage.

debridement in horses with infectious arthritis. Diagnostic arthroscopic examination is indicated if lameness is localized to the MTP joint but radiological findings are negative or suggestive of occult osteochondral fragments, but such examination should be undertaken after evaluating the results of advanced imaging such as scintigraphic imaging and MRI. Before I was able to routinely use scintigraphy I often elected to evaluate the articular surface of the MTP joint arthroscopically, only to be disappointed in my inability to substantiate obvious abnormalities. Using scintigraphy and more recently MRI, I can often characterize injury of the joint without the need for diagnostic arthroscopy. The most common diagnosis is subchondral bone injury without obvious overlying cartilage damage, findings that obviate the need to examine the joint arthroscopically.

Diagnostic arthroscopy is indicated if cartilage damage or osteochondral fragments are suspected, and to confirm the extent of cartilage damage in horses with OA. Occult fragments involving the proximodorsal aspect of the proximal phalanx are occasionally found. Cartilage damage, sometimes full thickness, is found on the distal-dorsal aspect of the MtIII and the proximal aspect of the proximal phalanx in nonracehorses. In racehorses with OA, cartilage lesions are usually most pronounced in the plantar pouch, with extensive scoring or large areas of full-thickness damage and exposed subchondral bone on the PSBs. Although stress-related bone injury and later overlying cartilage damage is seen on the distal plantarolateral aspect of the MtIII, this area is difficult to evaluate during arthroscopic examination (Figure 42-7).

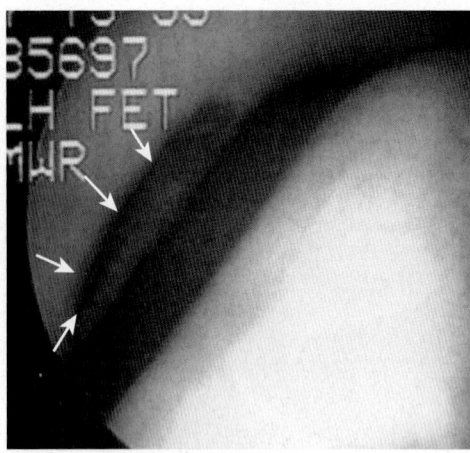

Fig. 42-7 • Intraoperative photograph of a 5-year-old Standardbred trotter with severe stress-related bone injury of the distal plantarolateral aspect of the third metatarsal bone *(arrows)*. This area was debrided and the horse raced, but it dropped substantially in race class and was retired.

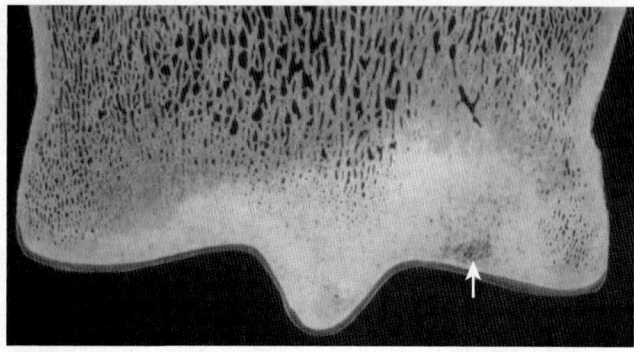

Fig. 42-8 • Dorsal plane microradiograph (100 μm) of the distal aspect of the third metatarsal bone (lateral is to the right) showing dense subchondral sclerosis and an area of intense resorption or necrosis of bone *(arrow)*. Cartilage overlying this area is intact. Severe subchondral modeling and remodeling and later osteoarthritis develop in the metatarsophalangeal joints of racehorses.

SPECIFIC CONDITIONS OF THE METATARSOPHALANGEAL JOINT

Stress-Related Subchondral Bone Injury and Osteoarthritis

The term *OA* implies disease of both the supporting bone and the articular surface of the MTP joint. The concept that the earliest lesion in OA of the MTP joint in racehorses begins in subchondral bone is essential to understanding clinical signs, successful use of diagnostic analgesia, progression of bone and cartilage loss, and the horse's response (or lack thereof) to therapy. There are two syndromes of MTP joint OA; one is seen in racehorses and the other in nonracehorse sports horses.

In racehorses, OA begins as a maladaptive or nonadaptive stress-related bone injury in subchondral bone. Subchondral maladaptive or nonadaptive bone injury is the most common reason I examine TB and STB racehorses with hindlimb lameness or poor performance. Although the overlying cartilage may be biomechanically and biochemically inferior, obvious clinical signs such as synovitis and a positive response to lower limb flexion are not seen until later. Low-grade unilateral or bilateral lameness is present, which is localized best by low plantar or lateral plantar metatarsal analgesia. Often, horses have a short, choppy gait, mimicking what would be expected if horses had bilateral or, in some, quadrilateral foot pain. Most often, blocking one hindlimb produces obvious contralateral hindlimb lameness in horses with bilateral subchondral bone injury. Horses are often thought to have something "up high" and usually have been unsuccessfully treated for other suspected sources of hindlimb pain. Early stress-related bone injury is best substantiated using scintigraphic examination. Focal areas of IRU are present in the MtIII; the PSBs and the proximal aspect of the proximal phalanx also can be affected (see Figures 19-20, 42-2, and 42-3). Initial radiological findings either are negative or reveal subtle increased radiopacity, but later radiolucent defects develop in subchondral bone, which are best revealed in a DPrL-PlDiMO image (see Figure 42-3). Increased radiopacity is most obvious in the LM, flexed LM, and DPrL-PlDiMO images.

Later, overlying full-thickness cartilage damage develops (see Figures 19-20, *B*, 23-8, and 42-7; Figure 42-8). Stress-related bone injury can continue to the point where severe OA or fracture of the MtIII develops; this type of severe injury is most common in racehorses 4 to 6 years old (see Figures 19-20 and 23-8). However, in some STBs the process causes lameness when horses are 2- or early 3-year-olds and then subsides or stabilizes. The condition is rarely seen in STBs until training speeds faster than 2 minutes, 20 seconds for a mile are achieved. In TB racehorses, this remodeling process is common in later 2- and 3-year-olds but can also be seen in older horses. Older horses given time off because of undiagnosed lameness or other conditions are at risk to develop stress-related bone injury in the MTP joint 6 to 8 weeks after returning to training, when signs of poor gait or lameness develop and a focal area of IRU can be identified. In my experience, subchondral lucency occurs later in the TB than in the STB and is uncommon. Differences between the racing breeds related to gait, speed, and load distribution may account for this difference in progression of OA. End-stage OA develops in STB racehorses that have continued racing for many years and can be progressive in broodmares and breeding stallions.

In nonracehorse sports horses OA is an insidious process usually without marked subchondral bone involvement. Bone and cartilage gradually deteriorate. Some horses affected may be ex-racehorses, but most are not. I have observed OA of the MTP joint mostly in upper-level jumpers and dressage horses. In these horses lameness is often chronic and low grade (grade 1 or 2 of 5), but it can progress to severe or intermittently severe. Effusion and a positive response to lower limb flexion are common findings. Concomitant tenosynovitis of the DFTS and previous lameness caused by suspensory desmitis and distal hock joint pain are common. Lameness is more consistently abolished using intraarticular analgesia in jumpers and dressage horses than in racehorses, but in some horses low plantar analgesia is required. Marginal osteophytes and enthesophytes are often detectable radiologically. Scintigraphy may reveal focal IRU in the central or dorsal aspect of the joint, diffuse IRU, or equivocal findings, and scintigraphic abnormalities are usually much less obvious than those found in racehorses. Occasionally, acute-onset lameness associated with focal IRU of the distal aspect of the MtIII occurs that is similar to that found in racehorses. This lameness may indicate acute subchondral overload trauma from landing wrong after jumping a fence, stepping on uneven ground, or sustaining a fall or other accident in a paddock. In nonracehorse sports horses, arthroscopic examination often reveals cartilage damage most extensive in the dorsal aspect of the joint, marginal osteophytes on the apices of the PSBs, and occasionally osteochondral fragments of the proximal dorsal aspect of the proximal phalanx.

Shoeing and hoof balance may play a role in development or expression of clinical signs of OA in all horses but may be more important in racehorses. In the STB racehorse clinical signs often develop within 2 to 3 weeks of a shoeing change, usually with the application of aluminum shoes with a low toe grab. Aluminum shoes are light and generally applied to pacers that are close to qualifying speed, but they are often used in trotters as well. Shear stress associated with these shoes may exacerbate existing disease or cause further trauma to subchondral bone. Aluminum shoeing is common in TB racehorses in North America, where these shoes are associated with other fetlock joint lameness and catastrophic breakdown. An aluminum shoe with a toe grab and with turned-down heels has been commonly used in recent years, and I have observed this shoe in many TBs with subchondral bone injury of the distal aspect of the MtIII, severe suspensory branch desmitis, and other catastrophic injuries of the MTP joint. Abnormal hoof wear caused by gait, the presence of concomitant distal hock joint or metatarsal region pain, or hoof imbalance may cause asymmetrical loading of the MTP joint and add to subchondral bone trauma.

Management of Stress-Related Bone Injury and Osteoarthritis

Reducing bone stress is key to initial management in racehorses with early OA characterized primarily by stress-related bone injury, because high-impact loading or high-strain cyclic fatigue of subchondral bone is the primary lesion. In STBs I previously recommended 4 to 6 weeks of light jogging (<2 miles per day), but results were poor even if recommendations were followed. I reassessed several horses after 6 weeks of light jogging, and although scintigraphic changes subsided, the horses were still as lame or slightly worse. I now recommend 3 weeks of walking and light jogging followed by reevaluation. Although 3 weeks' reduction in training may allow early healing or remodeling of damaged subchondral bone and microfractures, bone and muscle undergo detraining and horses need several (i.e., 3 to 6) weeks of slow return to normal exercise intensity. If lameness resolves, horses are returned to training, but if lameness persists I recommend 3 to 4 months of rest. In TBs, recurrence is quite high if horses are given only 6 to 8 weeks of rest. I recommend either 3 to 4 months of turnout or a program of 3 weeks of handwalking, followed by 3 weeks of walking with a rider up, followed by 3 weeks of trotting either with a rider up or using an exercise pony. Longer periods of rest would likely be beneficial to allow complete healing of subchondral bone, but most often owners and trainers are reluctant to agree. A gradual return to normal exercise intensity is then recommended if horses are sound and moving well.

Hoof balance and shoeing characteristics should be evaluated and in most instances changed. A simple change in shoeing to an easier shoe, such as a flat steel or aluminum shoe, may reduce shear and torsion of the MTP joint. Toe grabs and any other shoe additives must be removed. Perhaps the best change, if possible, is to leave the horse barefoot for several weeks. If medial-to-lateral hoof imbalance is poor, it should be corrected. The relationship of track and training surface to the development of subchondral bone injury is currently unknown, but this type of injury is quite common in TB racehorses training and racing in Europe and other countries, in which grass and all-weather (synthetic) surfaces are used (see Chapter 107). Although incidence of race-day injuries may change from a change in track surface, it is the track surface on which the horse trains, and thus the surface that cancellous and cortical bone "sees" day to day, that likely influences bone modeling and remodeling. In an unpublished preliminary study, we found that areas of IRU of the distal aspect of the MtIII or the third metacarpal bone (McIII) were the most common scintigraphic abnormality in horses training on grass and a synthetic surface, and although MTP or metacarpophalangeal lameness was common, the prevalence of stress fractures of long bones was markedly reduced compared with a cohort of TB racehorses training on dirt.[16] These results differ from anecdotal reports of injuries being discovered in TB racehorses being trained and raced on synthetic surfaces. Sporadic or clustering of injuries appears common, ranging from numerous horses developing unusual muscle injuries in the upper hindlimbs to an overabundance of stress fractures. Stress-related subchondral bone injury has been a predominant finding by some practitioners evaluating horses training on synthetic surfaces but not by all. In some racing jurisdictions, high toe grabs and turned-down shoes cannot be worn by horses racing on synthetic surfaces, a fact that may complicate epidemiological studies of injuries because this type of shoeing has been linked to substantial and sometimes fatal injuries of the metacarpophalangeal or MTP joints. In my opinion a change of shoeing philosophy to flat racing plates and, from the therapeutic standpoint, training horses without hind shoes may reduce negative forces acting on the MTP joint.

Because the initial lesion is in subchondral bone, intraarticular injections appear to have limited therapeutic benefit but may make theoretical sense. Active treatment may help in persuading trainers to follow the recommended work program. A series of three intraarticular injections of polysulfated glycosaminoglycans (PSGAGs) are given every other week. Alternatively, if horses are currently racing but have mild unilateral or bilateral lameness or scintigraphic evidence of stress-related bone injury and poor performance, I recommend intraarticular injection with hyaluronan and methylprednisolone acetate (80 mg). Intramuscular administration of PSGAGs (once weekly for 8 weeks) is recommended, but therapeutic benefit is difficult to assess. NSAIDs such as phenylbutazone (2.2 to 4.4 mg/kg bid) are recommended. NSAIDs may help horses in modified exercise programs "get over the hump" when lameness persists after scintigraphic evidence of stress-related bone injury subsides. Because pathogenesis involves sclerotic subchondral bone, the roles of ischemia and increased intraosseous pressure in causing bone pain or necrosis and subsequent collapse of weakened areas of subchondral bone have been questioned. I used to recommend the administration of isoxsuprine (400 mg bid orally) in an attempt to improve peripheral blood flow. However, research evidence supports neither the achievement of adequate blood levels nor increased blood flow by use of the drug, and I do not currently recommend its use. Other drugs, such as aspirin (17 mg/kg bid orally), may be useful in improving blood flow, but half-life is short and therapeutic benefit has yet to be established. If increased intraosseous pressure and early ischemia lead to pain and subchondral bone damage, a procedure such as subchondral bone drilling, which is used to manage stress-related bone injury in cortical bone of the McIII, may be beneficial, but it is currently only experimental. Topical counterirritation has historically been used and makes theoretical sense in horses with stress-related bone injury if increased blood flow occurs. The time-honored treatment of blistering and turning out may be the best method of management. I have used focused shock-wave therapy in some STB and TB racehorses with stress-related bone injury by aiming the shock waves at the plantarolateral aspect of the MtIII. Early results appear promising, but horses are given concurrent modified exercise programs and other therapy.

Bisphosphonate Therapy for Management of Subchondral Bone Pain

The bisphosphonate drug tiludronate has received considerable attention in recent years for management of numerous lameness problems, but although there are many anecdotal reports there is scant scientific evidence to support its use in the horse. Bisphosphonate drugs are largely antiresorptive and work by reducing osteoclastic activity. In maladaptive or nonadaptive bone remodeling and in horses with more advanced OA the predominant process is one of bone accumulation; dense sclerotic bone develops in the subchondral plate and adjacent cancellous bone, so in theory a drug to reduce osteoclastic resorption might have a net effect of *increasing* bone formation. How and why would antiresorptive drugs work in predominantly sclerotic subchondral bone? Bisphosphonate compounds may help to normalize metabolism in bone injuries characterized by abnormal resorption and formation, such as what is seen with navicular disease, a disease with similarities to maladaptive or nonadaptive remodeling of the MtIII and other bones. Based on this theory, in a double-blind, placebo-controlled study, there was improvement in lameness scores of horses with navicular disease given tiludronate at 1 mg/kg intravenously (IV) once daily for 10 days and horses returned to a normal level of activity 2 to 6 months after administration.[17] Furthermore, horses with OA of the thoracolumbar vertebral column given the same dose of tiludronate showed significant improvement in dorsal flexibility compared with untreated controls.[18] In horses, adaptive response to high-strain cyclic fatigue in the subchondral plate and adjacent subchondral bone occurs in response to race training. In a histological study of TB distal MtIII and McIII condyles, site-specific increases in microcrack density in calcified cartilage and resorption spaces in the adjacent subchondral plate were interpreted as evidence of mechanical failure of the joint surface from progressive endochondral ossification and modeling or remodeling of subchondral bone.[19] Propagation of

microcracks into subchondral bone may be critical to the subsequent development of condylar fractures or OA.[19] In sclerotic subchondral bone, osteocyte morphology was abnormal and numbers were reduced, but site-specific microdamage, targeted remodeling of adjacent subchondral bone, and multiple pathways of mechanotransduction of the McIII were thought to be important in adaptation to exercise.[20] In a study of 25 distal McIII condyles of TB racehorses, extensive microcrack formation leading to microfracture was found in sclerotic subchondral bone close to the calcified cartilage layer, and the presence of osteoclastic resorption along microfracture lines was proposed to have caused previous weakening.[21] In these studies the presence of resorption and bone weakening in calcified cartilage and adjacent subchondral bone may lend evidence to justify the use of bisphosphonate compounds, primarily for reduction in resorption and potentiation of healing of microdamage. In people with OA of the knee, joint space narrowing and sclerosis of the nearby subchondral plate occurs, and sclerotic bone may act to stress-protect adjacent cancellous bone, called *subarticular bone,* because vertical and horizontal trabeculae number were reduced, resulting in bone loss.[22] Through use of fractal signature analysis to measure differences of cancellous bone density in osteoarthritic medial knee compartments in people, increased trabecular number associated with thinning and fenestration of trabeculae in subarticular regions confirmed that overall, cancellous bone was osteoporotic.[23] Osteoporosis, although not known to be found in horses with OA, could potentially be managed using bisphosphonate therapy. Bisphosphonate therapy alone[24] and in combination with estrogen therapy[25] slowed early changes in subchondral bone architecture and reduced the prevalence of osteoarthrosis-related subchondral bone lesions. Given the presence of intense resorption at various sites and the presence of osteoporotic subchondral bone, a case could be made for the administration of bisphosphonate drugs. Long-term studies and more double-blind, placebo-controlled studies[17] need to be done.

Anecdotally, there may be benefit from use of tiludronate in horses with OA and subchondral bone injury, but it makes most sense to combine the drug with rest or a modification in exercise to allow healing of microdamage. Although lameness scores improved in horses with navicular disease,[17] my limited experience in horses with subchondral bone pain of the distal aspect of the MtIII suggests that amelioration of lameness is subtle and that long-term evidence of benefit cannot be established. The drug can be used IV, at a dose of 1 mg/kg in a single infusion or divided over 10 days for a total dose of 1 mg/kg, because both dosage regimens resulted in similar plasma exposure and pharmacologic effects.[26] There has been a trend to administer the drug to horses with single distal limb lesions using intravenous regional limb perfusion techniques, but this technique would be impractical in horses with numerous abnormalities involving more than a single limb and has not been studied. Use of the drug and continued training and racing may potentially lead to condylar fracture or other further injury, particularly in TB racehorses, a sequela that should be strongly considered. Anecdotal reports suggest that there may be immediate improvement in lameness scores after bisphosphonate administration, indicating that an analgesic effect may occur that could potentially lead to further training and racing. Currently I believe that targeting areas of bone resorption or necrosis and relative osteoporosis and attempting to normalize subchondral bone formation and healing using bisphosphonate therapy in combination with a reduction in exercise intensity comprise a reasonable approach, particularly in horses with bilateral hindlimb subchondral bone pain (or more numerous abnormalities). I prefer a single slow, IV infusion (1 mg/kg) while warning owners and trainers about the limited collective knowledge of complications in the horse, such as signs of colic during or immediately after drug administration, and of the known complication of osteonecrosis of the jaw associated with bisphosphonate use in people.[27]

Surgical Management of Subchondral Bone Injury

I have used the surgical technique of subchondral perforation (forage) in three horses—two TB and one STB racehorses—with unilateral hindlimb lameness in which lateral plantar metatarsal analgesia abolished lameness (horses did not show lameness in the contralateral hindlimb after blocking of the principal limb), and bone scintigraphy identified focal IRU of the distal, plantarolateral aspect of the MtIII. In one horse (Figure 42-9) MRI showed typical subchondral bone injury of the lateral MtIII condyle (see Figure 42-6). Arthroscopic examination of the plantar aspect of the MTP joint in all horses revealed normal-appearing articular cartilage, and by means of a combination of needles preplaced along the plantar aspect of the

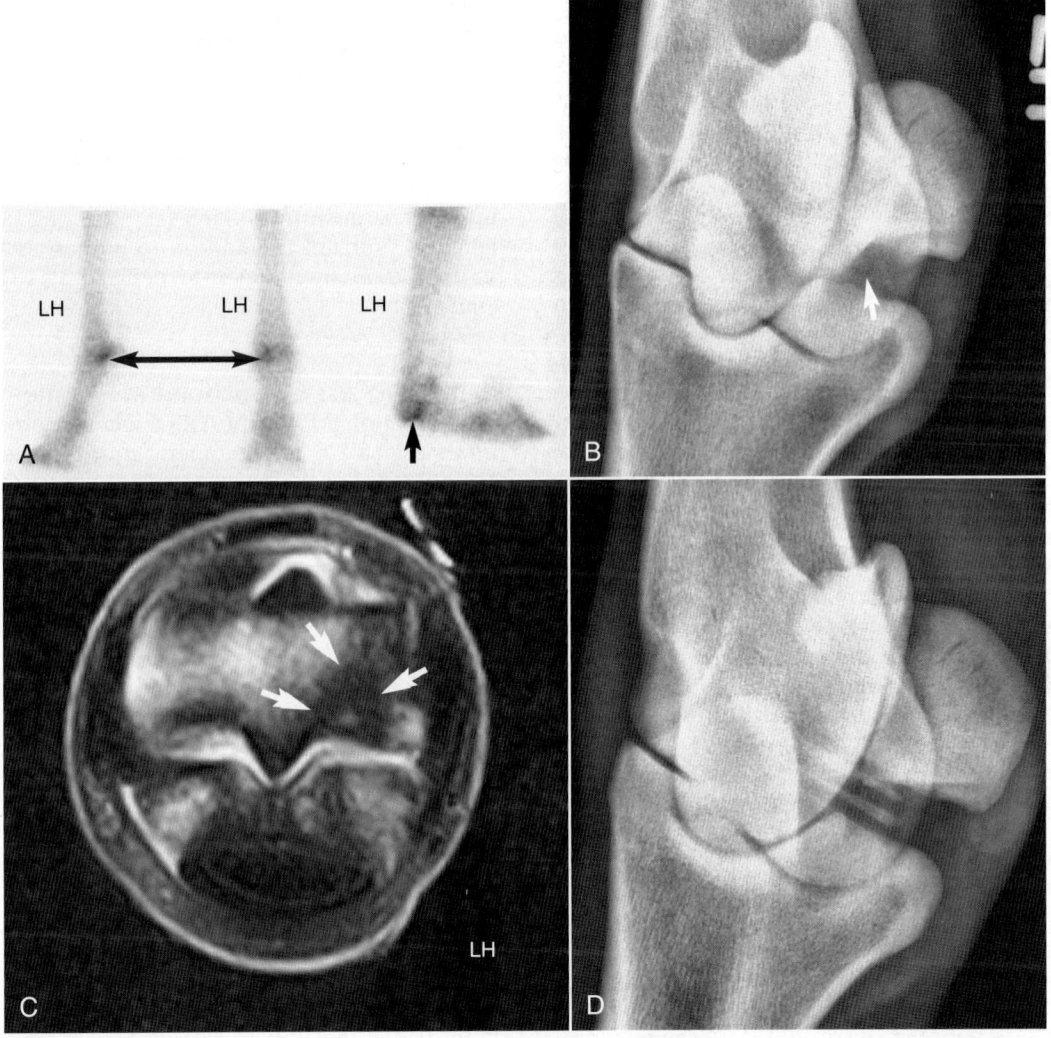

Fig. 42-9 • A, Lateral (dorsal is to the left), plantar (lateral is to the left), and flexed lateral delayed-phase scintigraphic images of an unraced, 2-year-old pacing colt with left hindlimb lameness abolished with lateral plantar analgesia. Focal, moderate increased radiopharmaceutical uptake (IRU; *arrows*) of the distal, plantarolateral aspect of the third metatarsal bone (MtIII) is diagnostic for maladaptive or nonadaptive subchondral bone injury. **B,** Dorsal 20° proximal, 45° lateral-plantarodistal medial digital radiographic image showing a small radiolucent defect in the plantar aspect of the lateral condyle of the MtIII *(arrow).* **C,** T2-weighted magnetic resonance image of the left metatarsophalangeal joint (lateral is to the right; dorsal is uppermost) showing dense, sclerotic subchondral bone *(arrows)* surrounding an area of increased signal intensity in the region in which the radiolucent defect can be seen. An area of necrotic subchondral bone is present. **D,** Dorsal 20° proximal, 45° lateral-plentarodistal medial digital radiographic image obtained after three 3.5-mm holes were drilled from the lateral aspect of the lateral condyle through the damaged subchondral bone. This horse raced successfully as a 3-year-old.

MtIII under arthroscopic guidance and intraoperative fluoroscopy, three 3.5-mm holes were drilled in a lateral-to-medial direction through the plantar aspect of the lateral MtIII condyle. Drill holes extended past the axis of the MtIII into but not through the medial condyle. Horses were given 4 months of rest before returning to training. The rationale for this approach is similar to what is done in horses with dorsal cortical fractures of the McIII, in which osteostixis is performed. Subchondral forage may allow marrow components from the medial condyle and adjacent lateral condyle to repopulate and heal damaged subchondral bone, and there may be immediate decompression of painful, sclerotic subchondral bone. All three horses raced after surgery, but in one TB lameness recurred after two race starts. An alternative surgical approach of inserting a positional or set cortex bone screw may make theoretical sense.

In racehorses with more advanced OA the therapeutic value of intraarticular injections becomes greater, because overlying cartilage damage and synovitis become prominent. However, horses generally drop substantially in race class and eventually are retired. In TB racehorses, intraarticular injections have little benefit in horses in training but may have limited value in horses actively racing. The disease process appears to be self-limiting in TBs, because horses with continued chronic, low-grade lameness are often retired before the disease process advances, or horses develop compensatory lameness in the forelimbs. Although a putative relationship exits between horses with maladaptive or nonadaptive remodeling and the subsequent development of condylar fractures, this is difficult to substantiate. In three TB racehorses that subsequently developed condylar fractures, a previous bone scan showed IRU of the distal aspect of the McIII but radiographs were negative, lending some clinical evidence of a cause-and-effect relationship. I have seen numerous racehorses, most of which were STBs, that developed extensive OA of the MTP joint after earlier diagnosis with maladaptive or nonadaptive bone remodeling. It is possible that lameness from subchondral bone pain in numerous limbs may limit exertion, power, or race speed and cause poor performance, but not fracture. In essence, horses may not race fast enough to develop fractures. STB racehorses often go off stride or develop compensatory lameness problems, in the same limb or other limbs, that may lead to poor performance rather than fracture. In the TB racehorse subchondral radiolucency is unusual in my experience, but others have recognized progression of OA and the development of changes similar to those seen in STBs (see Chapter 108). Why some horses are able to race with persistence of IRU, radiolucency, and sclerosis whereas others cannot is not easy to answer. Prognosis for both racing breeds appears to be guarded to fair at best. Of 19 STBs with lameness and IRU of the plantarolateral aspect of the MtIII, 18 raced, but only 13 remained at the same racing class or improved.[7] When radiolucent areas become prominent, arthroscopic examination and debridement may be an option, but it is difficult to manipulate instruments in the distal plantar pouch because manipulation must be done with the joint in flexion (see Figure 42-8). It is impossible to reach these lesions using a dorsal approach, because they are located approximately 8 mm plantar to the middle of the condyle. In horses with end-stage OA (i.e., loss of joint space, tilting of the sagittal

ridge and groove, and severe proliferative and radiolucent changes), arthrodesis must be considered in broodmare or stallion prospects (see Figure 23-8). Humane destruction may be necessary.

Nonracehorses often respond favorably to intraarticular injections of PSGAGs, hyaluronan, and short-acting corticosteroids (e.g., triamcinolone acetonide, isoflupredone acetate) or long-acting corticosteroids (e.g., methylprednisolone acetate). Exercise level is reduced for a period of 2 to 3 weeks, and horses are given NSAIDs. Topical therapy using cold water hosing, poulticing, and bandaging is recommended. When lameness persists and scintigraphic examination reveals focal IRU in the dorsal aspect of the joint, or in horses with chronic lameness, long-term rest is necessary. Arthroscopic examination in these horses reveals areas of partial- or full-thickness cartilage damage that can be managed by debridement and microfracture into subchondral bone. However, the therapeutic value of arthroscopy is limited. If osteophytes are removed, they generally reform. If surgery is combined with rest, horses usually become sound, but lameness often returns when competition resumes. Prognosis for horses performing at the previous level of competition is guarded to poor. Rehabilitation of upper-level performance horses is quite difficult, because most have at least one compensatory lameness problem in addition to primary OA of the MTP joint. Horses may be able to perform at a lower level of competition.

Plantar Process Osteochondral Fragments

Fragmentation of the proximal plantar processes of the proximal phalanx is a common finding in young STBs and Warmbloods but is also seen in TBs, Arabians, and Western performance horses. This condition has become more frequently recognized since presale and postsale radiography has become common.

There are four distinct manifestations of decreasing frequency: axial articular fragments; abaxial, nonarticular fragments; nonarticular fragments originating from the base of the PSBs; and true acute fractures. (I prefer an anatomical description rather than reference to different types.[28]) The condition is much more common in the hindlimbs, except for nonarticular fragments from the base of the PSBs, which occur almost exclusively in forelimbs (see Chapter 36). Combinations of axial and abaxial fragments often occur. The condition can be unilateral or bilateral and can be biaxial (involving both sides of the same joint).

Axial Articular Fragments

Axial articular fragments are most important and are most often medial, but can be lateral, biaxial, and bilateral. Of 119 horses with axial articular fragments, 92% were STBs; 95% of fragments were in the hindlimbs, most commonly the medial aspect of the left hindlimb (44%).[29] The incidence of axial articular fragments in 1- and 2-year-old STBs ranges from 5.6% to 28.8% but in TBs has been estimated at 2%.[30] The etiology remains controversial, but because STBs and the hindlimbs are clearly predisposed and fragments are recognized at an early age, osteochondrosis is the most likely explanation. Heritability estimates of axial articular fragments in STBs using a nonlinear model were

0.21, and fragments were seen in 11.8% of foals.[31] I feel it is implausible that a large number of STB foals develop traumatic fractures at this site, whereas other breeds do not. I believe hereditary factors are most important. A traumatic cause has been suggested in some studies, because portions of the fragments were irregular, were entrapped by mature fibrous tissue, and contained spicules of bone not covered by fibrocartilage, which gave the histological appearance of a fracture healed by fibrous union.[30,32,33] Evidence of short distal sesamoidean ligament insertions was not found and fragments were old.[30] Unfortunately, axial articular fragments examined were taken from horses with a mean age of 3.4 years and after horses had trained and raced, rather than from weanlings and yearlings, so degeneration and remodeling of fragments could have occurred. With only capsular attachments, how do alleged avulsion fractures occur? Etiology is most important when dispute or arbitration ensues after horses have been sold at public auction (see Chapter 99).

Chronic low-grade, high-speed MTP joint lameness can occur. Horses often have a previous history of other ipsilateral hindlimb lameness, such as distal hock joint pain. Effusion and a positive response to lower limb flexion are lacking or inconsistent. Lameness is alleviated most consistently with low plantar analgesia, but differentiation from early stress-related bone injury and OA can be difficult without scintigraphic examination. Stress-related bone injury or other bony abnormalities, such as midsagittal fracture of the proximal phalanx and occasionally condylar fractures of the MtIII, are commonly found simultaneously with axial articular fragments. Many horses with axial articular fragments never develop lameness, and fragments are detected only on survey radiographs. If and how axial articular fragments cause lameness is not well understood. Axial articular fragments may vibrate at speed or become interposed in the joint surface during flexion, but synovitis does not play a role. These fragments may affect mechanics of the ipsilateral PSB or impinge on distal sesamoidean ligaments.[28] Nociceptive fibers have been found in soft tissue attachments, and stretching during full extension may cause pain.[30] In older horses, evidence of full-thickness cartilage damage on the MtIII and the PSBs suggests that axial articular fragments may contribute to the development of OA.

Radiological examination reveals one or more fragments seen best in down-angled oblique views (see Figure 23-1, 42-1, and 42-5). If surgery is considered, both limbs should be examined radiographically. Scintigraphic examination may reveal mild abnormal bone modeling, but IRU is more commonly seen in horses with abaxial, nonarticular fragments (see Figure 42-5).

Axial articular fragments should be removed using arthroscopic surgery. In recent years I have advised removal of fragments before horses begin training, because "down time" associated with arthroscopic surgery is less than if surgery is performed in the middle of a racing year. Subjectively it appears that horses that undergo surgery earlier have fewer problems with stress-related bone injury and OA. In breeds such as the TB and Warmblood, axial articular fragments may complicate sales and can be removed prophylactically. During arthroscopic surgery fragments are carefully trimmed free of capsular attachments with a specially designed intraarticular blade and are removed.[34]

If arthroscopic surgery is performed before training begins, horses are given 7 days of stall rest, followed by 7 days of stall rest with handwalking, then 7 to 14 days of walking in the jog cart (STBs) or walking and light trotting with an exercise pony (TB). If lameness develops when horses are in advanced stages of training or are racing, I recommend at least 2 to 3 months of rest before training resumes. The prognosis is good for future soundness if the fragment(s) caused the lameness. In one study 63% of racehorses and 100% of nonracehorses had performance similar to preinjury levels after surgery, but the presence of cartilage damage or synovial proliferation was significantly associated with an adverse outcome.[28]

Abaxial, Nonarticular Fragments

Abaxial, nonarticular fragments can be single or multiple and may occur in combination with axial articular fragments, either on the same side or the opposite side of the joint. Abaxial, nonarticular fragments usually are lateral and can be bilateral. Abaxial, nonarticular fragments can be large and involve the entire lateral, plantar process (see Figure 23-1), including a small articular portion, but most are nonarticular. These fragments resemble old fractures radiologically, but I believe they are manifestations of osteochondrosis.[31,33] Fragments are often seen in weanlings or yearlings without clinical signs of lameness, and when seen in older horses, lameness is rarely acute. Abaxial, nonarticular fragments have been described as ununited proximoplantar tuberosities, and in some horses fragments identified at a young age subsequently reunited with the parent bone.[35] In my experience, union of abaxial, nonarticular fragments in older horses is rare but does occur.

Lameness is mild (grade 1 of 5 with the horse in hand), usually present at high speed, and worse around turns. Pain is abolished by low plantar analgesia. Palpation may reveal mild bony enlargement, but this enlargement is easily missed. Once horses are clipped, bony swelling is obvious. Response to lower limb flexion is inconsistent. Occasionally a weanling or yearling develops acute lameness with obvious soft tissue swelling that involves the fetlock joint. Radiographs reveal an old abaxial, nonarticular fragment, but generally lameness resolves quickly and is not related to the fragment.

Radiographs reveal one or more abaxial, nonarticular fragments, which are occasionally accompanied by axial articular fragments (see Figure 23-1). Fragments are old and rounded, and radiolucent changes of the parent plantar process of the proximal phalanx are common. A clear separation exists between the fragment and proximal phalanx that is filled by dense, fibrous tissue. Scintigraphic examination may reveal mild IRU.

Abaxial, nonarticular fragments may or may not cause lameness, and clear differentiation between sources of pain can be difficult. The decision of whether to perform surgery is often difficult, because often conventional surgery is required to remove these nonarticular pieces.[34] Although the procedure is tedious and best done by using a motorized synovial resector, large abaxial fragments can be removed arthroscopically (see Chapter 23 and Figure 23-1). After surgery horses are given 4 weeks of stall rest, followed by 4 weeks of stall rest with handwalking, then 4 to 8 weeks of turnout in a small paddock or light jogging or galloping.

Prognosis is excellent for future soundness, but among STB racehorses, pacers have a better prognosis than trotters. In yearlings with a combination of axial articular fragments and abaxial, nonarticular fragments, I usually recommend arthroscopic surgery to remove axial articular fragments and leave abaxial, nonarticular fragments in place unless clinical signs develop at a later date.

Although I strongly believe that axial articular fragments and abaxial, nonarticular fragments cause lameness and I recommend surgery both therapeutically and prophylactically, others question the clinical significance of these fragments. In a study evaluating radiological findings in STBs before beginning training and subsequent race performance, there was no significant association between the presence of axial articular fragments, abaxial, nonarticular fragments, and other forms of osteochondrosis and either race performance or racing longevity.[36]

Nonarticular Fragments Originating from the Proximal Sesamoid Bones

Nonarticular fragments originating from the PSBs, the most unusual form of fragmentation, are discussed in conjunction with plantar process fragmentation of the proximal phalanx since radiological findings can be similar to those associated with articular or nonarticular plantar process fragments. Nonarticular fragments originating from the PSBs occur almost exclusively in the forelimb and are rare in the hindlimb. Horses with this form of fragmentation have high-speed lameness and clinical signs are similar to those seen with the other, more common forms of plantar/palmar fragmentation. Radiologically, nonarticular fragments originating from the PSBs are best seen in LM radiographic images, are intercalated in the distal sesamoidean ligaments, can be singular or numerous, and are located plantar/palmar to the articular surface of the PSBs, usually midway between the PSBs and the proximal aspect of the proximal phalanx. These fragments may result from osteochondrosis or from avulsion injury that occurred when horses were sucklings. Nonarticular fragments originating from the PSBs can be removed by using a ligament-separating approach with conventional surgical techniques or by using arthroscopic techniques; a motorized synovial resector is required to debride capsular and distal sesamoidean ligament attachments. Damage to the distal sesamoidean ligaments is unavoidable and I question the value of surgical removal of these fragments. Horses generally return to racing or training at a level similar to that achieved before surgery and high-speed lameness often recurs.

Acute Fractures of the Proximal Plantar Process

True fractures of the proximal plantar process of the proximal phalanx occur, usually are recognized after known or suspected trauma, but are rare. Acute lameness and soft tissue swelling are present. Radiology reveals an acute fracture with a narrow, well-defined fracture line. The margins of the fracture are not rounded, nor are there radiolucent changes in the proximal phalanx. Internal fixation and fiberglass cast application are recommended. Prognosis depends on duration of the fracture before repair and fracture size. OA is a potential complication.

Osteochondrosis of the Sagittal Ridge of the Third Metatarsal Bone

A discussion of osteochondrosis of the sagittal ridge of the MtIII is presented in Chapters 36 and 56.

Osteochondral Fragments of the Dorsoproximal Aspect of the Proximal Phalanx

Osteochondral fragments of the dorsoproximal aspect of the proximal phalanx are common and occur in two forms. Well-rounded osteochondral fragments often occur in young horses, may be a manifestation of osteochondrosis, and are asymptomatic (Figure 42-10). In a recent study of 117 Warmblood horses with fragments in this location, histopathological examination of fragments removed arthroscopically revealed smooth hyaline cartilage surrounding a bony center, and fragments were thought to be a component of developmental orthopedic disease.[37] Acute osteochondral fragments result in mild lameness or change in performance and are associated with an effusion and a positive response to lower limb flexion (see Figure 23-6). Arthroscopic surgery and removal of these osteochondral fragments is recommended. In older STB and TB racehorses, osteochondral fragments can be large and numerous, and after surgery a minimum of 8 weeks' rest is given. Cartilage damage on the opposing surface of the MtIII is common, and the amount is commensurate with size and duration of osteochondral fragments.

Other Osteochondral Fragments

Osteochondral fragments may be identified dorsal or plantar to the collateral ligaments, usually laterally. These osteochondral fragments are usually traumatically induced and may originate from the distal dorsal aspect of the

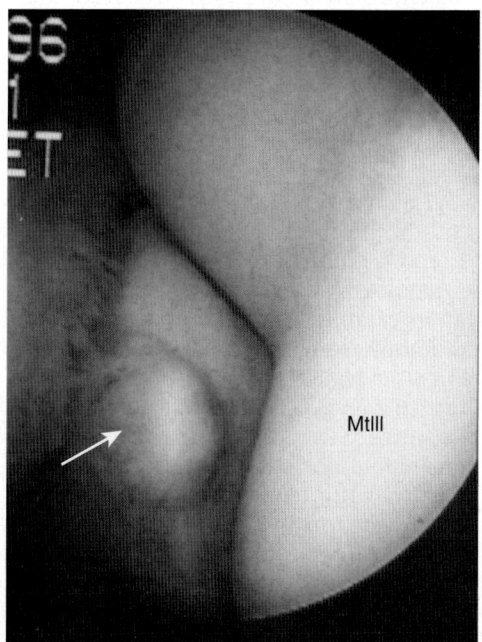

Fig. 42-10 • Intraoperative photograph of an osteochondral fragment (*arrow*) of the proximal dorsomedial aspect of the proximal phalanx. *MtIII,* Third metatarsal bone.

MtIII, but they are not avulsion fractures. Proliferative changes often develop. Treatment is by surgical removal, but prognosis is guarded in racehorses.

A rare finding in the MTP joint is a loose fragment located in the distal aspect of the plantar pouch. In some horses, small defects in the dorsal aspect of the sagittal ridge of the MtIII can be seen radiologically. A small fragment may have detached and migrated to the plantar pouch. Large, loose fragments may exist for some time in the plantar pouch without causing lameness.

Fractures of the Proximal Phalanx

One of the most common major fractures in the MTP joint is midsagittal fracture of the proximal phalanx or other fractures with a midsagittal component. These fractures occur most often in racehorses but also occur in other sports horses. In racehorses, midsagittal fractures of the proximal phalanx occur in STBs equally in hindlimbs and forelimbs, but in TBs, forelimb fractures are most common. These fractures are discussed in Chapters 35 and 36. Horses with moderately comminuted fractures of the proximal phalanx, in which an intact fragment of bone (strut) spans the distance between the proximal and distal articular surfaces of the proximal phalanx, can be managed successfully and salvaged for breeding purposes using open reduction and internal fixation. Those with massive comminution without an intact strut can be salvaged, but use of transfixation pin casting or external skeletal fixation to maintain axial alignment is necessary. In a study of 64 horses with comminuted fractures of the proximal phalanx, 26 fractures involved the hindlimbs, and overall, 33 of 36 (92%) horses with moderately comminuted fractures managed by open reduction and internal fixation were considered to have successful outcomes (salvaged for breeding, pasture soundness, or light riding).[38] Twelve of 26 horses (46%) with severely comminuted fractures managed with external skeletal fixation or transfixation pin casting survived, but management was complicated and hospitalization was prolonged.[38]

Dorsal Frontal Fractures of the Proximal Phalanx

Dorsal frontal fractures of the proximal phalanx occur much more commonly in the hindlimbs than in the forelimbs, and large osteochondral fragments in the forelimb may cause similar clinical signs. Size and depth of fracture appear different between forelimbs and hindlimbs; in the forelimbs, when dorsal frontal fracture occurs it is usually a long fracture beginning deep within the articular surface and extending distally, well into the diaphysis of the proximal phalanx, as compared with the typical fracture in the hindlimbs, which is 7 to 10 mm deep (from dorsal to plantar) and approximately 20 mm in length. They occur in both TB and STB racehorses. Dorsal frontal fractures may be more common in the right hindlimb. Although these fractures are reported to be more common in TBs,[39] in my experience the fracture is near equally as common in STBs and can be unilateral or bilateral. If a dorsal frontal fracture of the proximal phalanx is diagnosed scintigraphically, contralateral IRU of the dorsal proximal aspect of the proximal phalanx is commonly seen (Figure 42-11). IRU associated with a dorsal frontal fracture of the proximal phalanx must be differentiated from a midsagittal fracture. Midsagittal fractures are single-event injuries, but a dorsal frontal

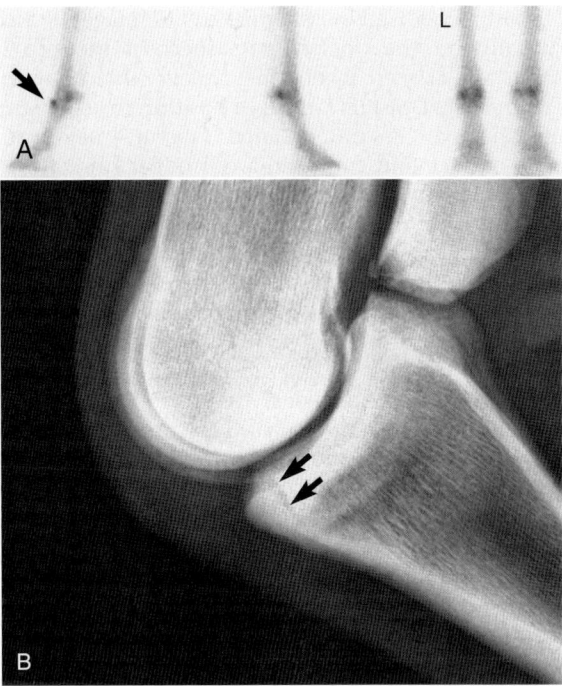

Fig. 42-11 • A, Delayed (bone) phase lateral and plantar scintigraphic images of a metatarsophalangeal (MTP) joint of a 3-year-old Thoroughbred filly showing focal, intense increased radiopharmaceutical uptake (IRU) associated with the proximal dorsal aspect of the proximal phalanx *(arrow)* in the left hindlimb (LH) Mild-moderate IRU is seen in the right hindlimb, associated with early maladaptive or nonadaptive bone remodeling of the distal plantarolateral aspect of the third metatarsal bone. **B,** Flexed lateromedial digital radiographic image of the LH MTP joint showing the typical configuration of a nondisplaced dorsal frontal fracture of the proximal phalanx *(arrows)*. Because the fracture is nondisplaced and there are no interposed fragments in the fracture line, this horse can be managed conservatively with an excellent prognosis.

fracture of the proximal phalanx may be caused by stress-related bone injury, because gradations of IRU are seen in the proximal phalanx and concomitant contralateral IRU occurs. Although bilateral fracture or evidence of stress-related bone injury can be seen bilaterally simultaneously, horses may develop contralateral fracture the next year. TB racehorses appear to be able to tolerate pain associated with dorsal frontal fractures better than STB racehorses; I have seen many that have raced with this fracture. There may be chronic proliferative changes and a displaced fracture in a TB horse that raced within the prior 10 days. Displaced fractures do not occur in STBs, and lameness may be noticed earlier than in the TB racehorse. Pacers are most likely to have an obvious fracture, whereas fractures in trotters may be scintigraphically active with only subtle radiological changes.

A dorsal frontal fracture of the proximal phalanx usually results in intermittent, severe lameness, but bilateral fractures may cause poor performance without causing obvious signs of lameness. Effusion is present but may be only mild unless fractures are displaced. The response to lower limb flexion is positive. Intraarticular or low plantar analgesia abolishes lameness in horses with complete or displaced fractures, but the low plantar technique should be used in those with stress-related bone injury or incomplete fractures. Radiographs reveal a single fracture line that is best recognized in LM or flexed LM images. Fractures are usually on the dorsolateral aspect of the proximal phalanx, and if seen in oblique radiographic images, are best seen in the DM-PlLO image, a position to keep in mind if surgical repair is contemplated. Fractures begin at the articular surface and course in a dorsodistal direction (see Figure 42-11). In TBs with displaced fractures an osteochondral fragment often is interposed between the main fracture fragment and the parent bone.

If fractures are nondisplaced, conservative management provides a good-to-excellent prognosis in both TBs and STBs. Horses are given 4 weeks of stall rest, followed by 4 weeks of stall rest with handwalking, then 4 to 8 weeks of turnout in a small paddock. Two treatment options are available for horses with displaced fractures. In those with large fragments and interposed osteochondral fragments, arthroscopic surgery is recommended to remove small osteochondral fragments and to repair the dorsal frontal fracture using one or two 3.5-mm screws. If the fracture cannot be reduced or is broken or small, the fragment should be removed. Prognosis is good to excellent for future racing, but horses may drop in class, particularly those with compensatory or numerous lameness problems. Long dorsal frontal fractures, such as those that occur in the forelimbs, cause acute, severe lameness and should be repaired (see Chapter 36).

Fractures of the Proximal Sesamoid Bones

Overall, fractures of the PSBs appear to be near equally distributed between the metacarpophalangeal and MTP joints, but distribution depends on fracture configuration. In STB racehorses, distribution of all PSB fractures likely favors the hindlimbs. In a study of TB racehorses less than 2 years old, 92% of apical fractures of the PSBs occurred in the hindlimbs, and overall 84% of horses raced after arthroscopic surgical removal of the fracture fragments, a prognosis similar to racing performance of maternal siblings.[40] In another study, in TB racehorses that were 2-year-olds or older, 64% of apical fractures of the PSBs occurred in the hindlimbs, and prognosis for racing after arthroscopic removal of hindlimb fractures was 83%.[41] In both studies, prognosis for racing was better when fractures occurred in a hindlimb than in a forelimb.[40,41] Apical fractures of the PSBs are more common in the hindlimb of STBs and most often involve the lateral PSB. Fractures of the abaxial aspect of the PSBs, sometimes including an apical component, occur most commonly in the medial PSB in the forelimb. Midbody and basilar fractures of the PSBs appear to be more common in the forelimbs. Fractures of the PSBs can be traumatic or pathological. Young racehorses develop acute lameness and fracture without preexisting disease of the PSB or SL. However, the PSB undergoes extensive remodeling similar to the MtIII, and it is possible, perhaps even likely, that these fractures represent a form of stress-related bone injury. In older racehorses and in some nonracehorse sports horses, preexisting radiolucent and proliferative sesamoiditis and suspensory branch desmitis are present, and fractures of the PSB appear to develop as a pathological, secondary, end-stage injury. In some nonracehorse sports horses, fracture occurs as a single event without preexisting injury. Prognosis depends on the size of the fracture fragment and the degree of suspensory desmitis. In STB racehorses, prognosis is better in pacers than in trotters, and prognosis is poor in horses developing fractures early in training before racing begins (see Chapter 36). The prognosis is good in nonracehorse sports horses without preexisting injury. Arthroscopic surgical removal of apical, abaxial, and small basilar fracture fragments and repair of large basilar and midbody fractures are recommended (see Chapter 36).

Fractures of the Distal Aspect of the Third Metatarsal Bone

Condylar fractures of the distal aspect of the MtIII occur less frequently than those of the McIII (see Chapter 36). In a study of 135 horses with condylar fractures, 81% and 85% involved the forelimbs and lateral condyles, respectively.[42] Lateral and medial condylar fractures of the MtIII occur, but lateral fractures are most common. Lateral condylar fractures can be short and incomplete, long and incomplete, or long and complete. Bilateral fractures occasionally occur simultaneously. Condylar fractures are primarily racing injuries. In a study of TB, STB, and Arabian racehorses, TBs were overrepresented and STBs underrepresented; TBs had significantly more lateral and forelimb fractures than STBs.[43] Clinical signs are commensurate with the length and degree of displacement. Medial condylar fractures can be short, incomplete, and difficult to diagnose. However, most commonly lameness is severe and radiographs reveal that the fracture is long and incomplete but goes straight proximally to end abruptly in the diaphysis, forms a Y-shaped pattern (Figure 42-12), or spirals proximally to end near or at the tarsometatarsal joint (Figure 42-13). Occult fissure lines and spiraling should always be suspected, and it is critical to know the location of the fracture before horses are transported and prognosis is discussed. Horses with medial condylar fractures are at extreme risk for fracture propagation or comminution. Even after surgical repair, horses are at risk during recovery from general anesthesia and early in the postoperative period. In 15 horses with medial condylar fractures of the MtIII, the fractures of 12 horses were repaired, two horses suffered catastrophic fracture during recovery from general anesthesia, and three horses developed complete fracture within 4 days after surgery.[44] Recovery from general anesthesia should be assisted and may best be performed using a pool recovery system, if available.

Horses with short, incomplete lateral and medial condylar fractures can be managed conservatively or can undergo surgical repair. Those with longer spiral or medial condylar fractures with a Y shape should undergo surgical repair. This repair can be accomplished by use of a combination of open observation of the fracture line and either screw fixation (see Figure 42-13) or a combination of screws and a dynamic compression plate or locking compression plate (see Figure 42-12). Prognosis depends on whether fractures are medial or lateral, whether they are displaced or nondisplaced, and whether a plate or numerous screws are used for repair. If fractures heal and plates (if used) are removed, prognosis for racing is favorable, but horses will often drop in race class or fail to reach full potential.

Sesamoiditis

In the STB, hindlimb sesamoiditis is most common in the lateral PSB but can occur medially and be a source of occult

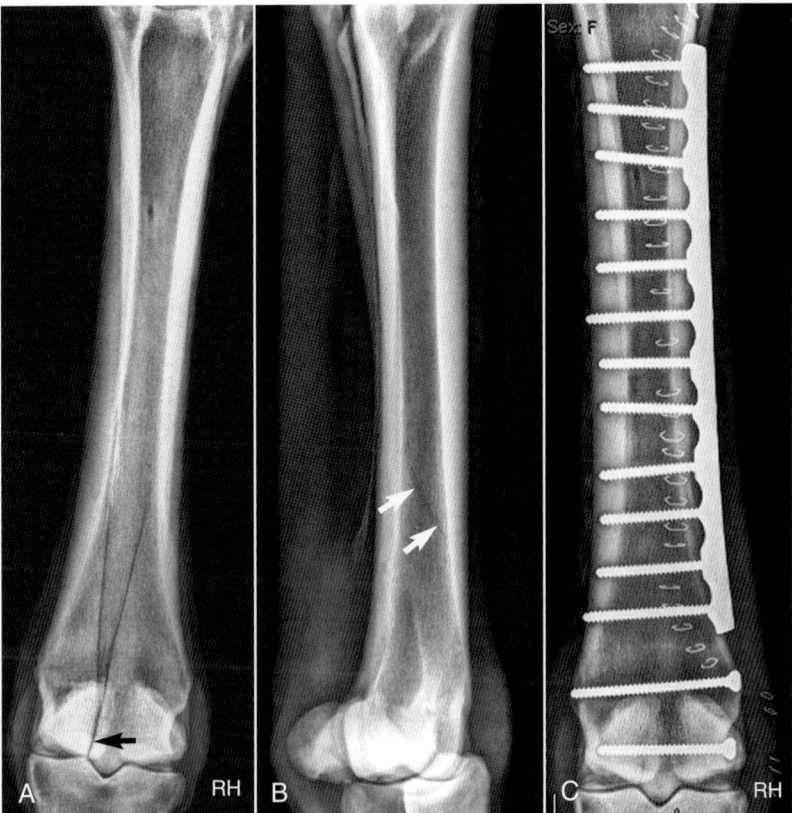

Fig. 42-12 • Digital radiographic images before and after surgery of a 2-year-old Thoroughbred filly with a nondisplaced, spiral fracture of the third metatarsal bone (MtIII) beginning at the medial condyle. **A,** Dorsoplantar radiographic image (lateral is to the right) showing the fracture line *(arrow)* beginning from the medial condyle and propagating proximally in a slight spiral fashion. Both dorsal and plantar cortical lines can be seen. **B,** Dorsal 45° medial-plantarolateral radiographic image showing that the fracture line abruptly becomes oblique *(arrows)* and stops in the middiaphyseal region. This horse would be at risk for catastrophic injury without repair, and during or immediately after surgery if repair were performed with bone screws alone. **C,** Postoperative dorsoplantar radiographic image showing repair of the fracture using screws placed in lag fashion and a 12-hole limited-contact dynamic compression plate applied to the lateral aspect of the MtIII, using a dorsal, transtendonous approach. The distal two screws and the first four distal screws in the plate have been placed in lag fashion. The plate was later removed at 3 months after surgery, and the filly raced successfully as a 3-year-old.

MTP joint lameness. In TBs sesamoiditis is most commonly observed in the forelimb. TBs can have obvious radiolucent lines in the PSBs in hindlimbs that are often asymptomatic. Disparity between limbs, rather than size or number of radiolucent lines, was found in a study to be most important in determining clinical significance in TBs; horses with three or more channels were less likely to race as 2-year-olds and had decreased earnings per start.[45] In another study, in the STB racehorse the presence of one to three or more radiolucent defects less than or equal to 1 mm in width was not associated with lameness referable to the PSBs, but horses with wide, abnormally shaped defects developed lameness from sesamoiditis.[46] Conversely, Grøndahl and colleagues reported that of 753 young STBs that underwent radiographic examination before training, 21 horses had severe sesamoiditis, fractures, or enlarged PSBs, but a correlation between sesamoid pathology and lameness or decreased racing performance and earnings could not be made. In that study hindlimb PSBs were affected in only six horses, and lameness developed in 14 horses.[47] Although lameness could not be directly attributed to

changes in the PSBs, in some horses MTP joint lameness was diagnosed, and perhaps compensatory lameness developed as a result of chronic, low-grade or high-speed lameness in these trotters. Seven of 21 horses had concomitant osteochondral fragments of the plantar/palmar process of the proximal phalanx, although a clear relationship could not be established.[47]

Radiolucent Defects of the Axial Border of the Proximal Sesamoid Bones
See Chapters 72 and 74 for a discussion of radiolucent defects of the axial border of the PSBs.

Flexural Deformity of the Metatarsophalangeal Joint
Dorsal subluxation of the MTP joint (buckle or knuckle forward) occurs in horses with flexural deformity. Intermittent subluxation occurs in those with mild deformity, but some horses with more severe deformity maintain the MTP joint in partial flexion. Horses with chronic, severe tenosynovitis of the DFTS with extensive adhesions may

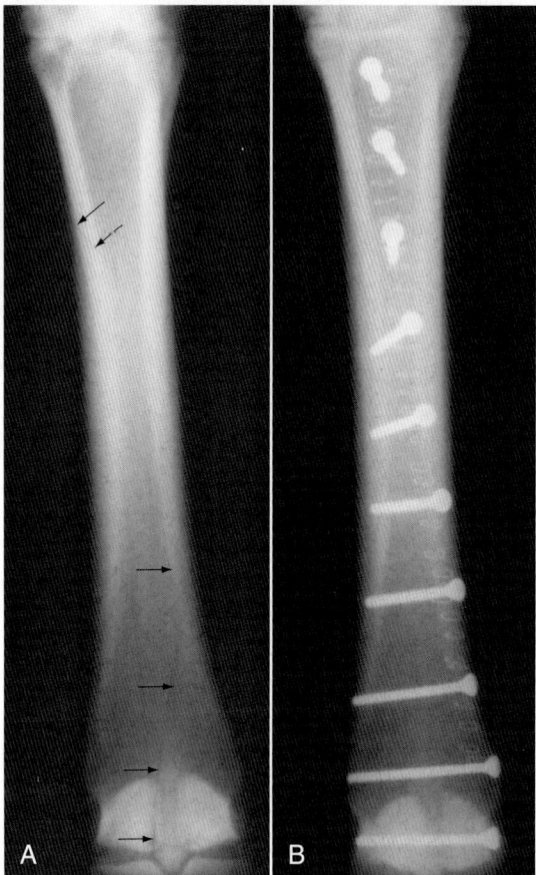

Fig. 42-13 • Dorsoplantar radiographic images of the metatarsophalangeal (MTP) joint and the entire metatarsal region. There is a spiral fracture of the third metatarsal bone *(arrows)* beginning at the medial condyle of the third metatarsal bone (medial is the left) in the MTP joint and extending to near the tarsometatarsal joint (confirmed at surgery after subperiosteal dissection) before **(A)** and after **(B)** surgery.

develop progressive, severe flexural deformity. Desmopathies of the accessory ligament of the DDFT may cause flexural deformity (see Chapter 71). In some horses, application of an extremely elevated heel shoe (e.g., 5 to 8 cm) may help alleviate pain (see Chapter 59).

Dropped fetlock or plantar subluxation (hyperextension) occurs in horses with severe chronic suspensory desmitis or those with severe, acute tearing of the superficial digital flexor tendon (SDFT), the DDFT, or both the SDFT and DDFT.

Soft Tissue Injuries of the Metatarsophalangeal Joint and Fetlock Region

Proliferative Synovitis
Proliferative synovitis (i.e., enlarged synovial pad or villonodular synovitis) occurs in the dorsal aspect of the MTP joint in horses with chronic OA. However, it is much less

common than in the metacarpophalangeal joint and is a rare primary cause of pain (see Chapter 36).

Luxation and Subluxation: Tearing of a Collateral Ligament
Complete disruption of a collateral ligament causes luxation and results in severe, non–weight-bearing lameness and usually obvious valgus or varus deformity. This injury is more common in adult horses, because physeal fractures of the distal aspect of the MtIII and proximal phalanx are more likely in foals. Initially little swelling occurs, but within a few hours soft tissue swelling can be prominent and manipulation of the joint reveals instability. Diagnosis is confirmed radiologically using DPl and stressed DPl images. Radiographs should be examined carefully for the presence of concurrent fractures on the contralateral or plantar aspects of the joint. Ultrasonography is used to identify the injured portion of the collateral ligament and extent of injury. After manual reduction with the horse under general anesthesia, a fiberglass cast should be applied. The cast should be changed within 7 to 10 days, because swelling resolves and the cast loosens. Cast coaptation should be maintained for 8 to 10 weeks, and then a heavy bandage should be applied. If crushing of the opposite side or plantar aspect of the joint did not occur, prognosis for soundness is guarded to fair. OA and chronic desmitis of the collateral ligament are possible. In a study, eight of 17 horses with rupture of the collateral ligaments of the metacarpophalangeal or MTP joints had hindlimb injury, and the lateral collateral ligament was more commonly affected. The presence of avulsion fracture fragments did not negatively affect prognosis. Ultrasonographic examination was useful in characterizing injury. Eight of 16 horses managed with external coaptation returned to some form of rider exercise.[48]

Collateral Desmitis
Primary injury of the collateral ligament without luxation is rare in my experience. Clinical signs include firm soft tissue swelling and ultrasonographic evidence of desmitis in horses with lameness that is abolished by low plantar analgesia. Avulsion fractures may occur as a result of trauma.

Suspensory Desmitis
See Chapter 72 for a discussion of suspensory desmitis.

Distal Sesamoidean Ligament Injury
See Chapter 72 for a discussion of injury of the distal sesamoidean ligaments.

Tenosynovitis of the Digital Flexor Tendon Sheath
See Chapter 74 for a discussion of tenosynovitis of the DFTS.

Deep Digital Flexor Tendonitis
See Chapters 70 and 74 for a discussion of deep digital flexor tendonitis.

Chapter 43

The Metatarsal Region

Mike W. Ross

The metatarsal region, like most of the distal hindlimb, has received little attention in previous lameness textbooks. However, it is a common source of lameness problems and should not be overlooked, especially in view of the high incidence of suspensory desmitis in sports horses.

ANATOMY

The metatarsal region is bordered by the tarsometatarsal joint proximally and the metatarsophalangeal joint distally. The large third metatarsal bone (MtIII) provides all structural support and weight bearing and articulates predominantly with the third tarsal bone proximally and the proximal phalanx and proximal sesamoid bones (PSBs) distally. A prominent nutrient foramen in the MtIII should not be mistaken for a fracture and is usually located slightly higher than that of the third metacarpal bone (McIII).[1]

The second metatarsal bone (MtII) and fourth metatarsal bone (MtIV) are commonly referred to as the *medial* and *lateral splint bones*, respectively. The MtII articulates with the combined first and second tarsal bones proximally and ends distally with an enlarged "bell." The MtIV articulates with the fourth tarsal bone proximally but transmits less load than the MtII. The dorsal metatarsal artery runs obliquely, in a distoplantar direction, in the proximal lateral aspect of the metatarsal region and then parallel and close to the dorsal aspect of the MtIV as it courses distally in the midmetatarsal region. The dorsal metatarsal artery then courses deep to the MtIV and must be avoided during distal splint ostectomy. I examined one horse in which the dorsal metatarsal artery coursed through a bony and fibrous ring-like foramen in the distal aspect of the MtIV and was inadvertently severed during ostectomy of the MtIV. Because the dorsal metatarsal artery is superficial, it can be lacerated from wounds in the lateral metatarsal region. Bleeding can be profound, and the ends of a lacerated dorsal metatarsal artery should be ligated unless anastomosis is performed with the horse under general anesthesia. Collateral circulation develops if ligation is necessary. The long plantar ligament attaches to the proximal aspect of the MtIV.

The orientation of the metatarsal bones is clinically important. The proximal aspect of the MtIV is large and is located in a more plantar location than its counterpart, the fourth metacarpal bone (McIV). This orientation makes it impossible to palpate the normal proximal and midbody portions of the suspensory ligament (SL). Therefore unless it is grossly enlarged, the SL cannot be palpated, and conditions such as mild-to-moderate suspensory desmitis can easily be missed, particularly if lameness is chronic and signs of acute inflammation are not present.

Dense metatarsal fascia attaches to the abaxial margins of the MtII and the MtIV and encircles the SL, deep digital flexor tendon (DDFT), and superficial digital flexor tendon (SDFT). A thinner fascia, the suspensory laminar fascia, lies superficial to the SL, deep to the DDFT. The metatarsal and laminar fascial layers appear confluent at the attachment on the MtII. Swelling of the SL within these fascial compartments can cause pain by compression of the adjacent metatarsal nerves.[2] The SL has a broad origin on the proximal, plantar surface of the MtIII and a small attachment to the distal tarsal bones. The hind SL is slightly longer and thinner than the front SL, and muscle content may be higher in hindlimbs compared with forelimbs, which can complicate ultrasonographic examination.[3] It has been suggested that the higher incidence of suspensory desmitis in Standardbreds (STBs) than in Thoroughbreds (TBs) is related to higher muscle content, but this is unproven.[3]

The plantar surface of the MtIII and the origin of the SL are oblique and not parallel to the dorsal surface of MtIII. During ultrasonographic examination, care should be taken to account for obliquity and to position the transducer perpendicular to SL fibers (see Chapter 72). The SL is bordered by the MtII and the MtIV and is thus trapped within a bony and dense soft tissue encasement. In the midmetatarsal region the body of the SL can be palpated as it emerges from this bony encasement and courses distally to divide into the medial and lateral branches that attach to the abaxial border of each PSB. The accessory ligament of the DDFT (ALDDFT) is usually present and is a variably sized structure ranging from thin to thick and occasionally has two or three parts; in a small proportion of horses (10 of 165, or 6.1%) there was no identifiable ALDDFT.[4] Although the ALDDFT is anatomically present in most horses, injury is rare (see Chapter 71). Desmotomy to manage flexural deformity is rarely performed and generally would be ineffective because of the small size of the ALDDFT. I examined an aged Quarter Horse gelding with enlarged ALDDFTs with unusual flexural deformity characterized by intermittent, dynamic heel elevation; during walking the heels would land flat, but during standing the heels elevated bilaterally (see Chapter 71). I severed the ALDDFT in each hindlimb, and although improvement was seen temporarily, flexural deformity recurred. The DDFT is located plantar to the SL for most of the metatarsal region, but in the proximal metatarsal region it is positioned plantaromedially. The SDFT is located plantar to both the SL and DDFT. Because the tarsal sheath ends in the proximal metatarsal region, distention can sometimes be palpated (see Chapter 76). The digital flexor tendon sheath (DFTS) begins in the plantar, distal third of the metatarsal region and encompasses the DDFT and SDFT (see Chapter 74).

In the proximal third of the metatarsal region the lateral digital extensor tendon joins with the long digital extensor tendon, and the combined tendons course distally. The fibularis tertius and cranialis tibialis attach to the proximal, dorsal, and medial aspects of the MtIII. Osseous proliferation and fracture can occur at these locations.

Distal continuation of the superficial fibular and saphenous nerves provides dorsal skin sensation. The tibial nerve divides to form the medial and lateral plantar nerves in the plantar tarsal region. The lateral plantar nerve, which courses plantar to the origin of the SL, gives off a deep

erences
n page
1286

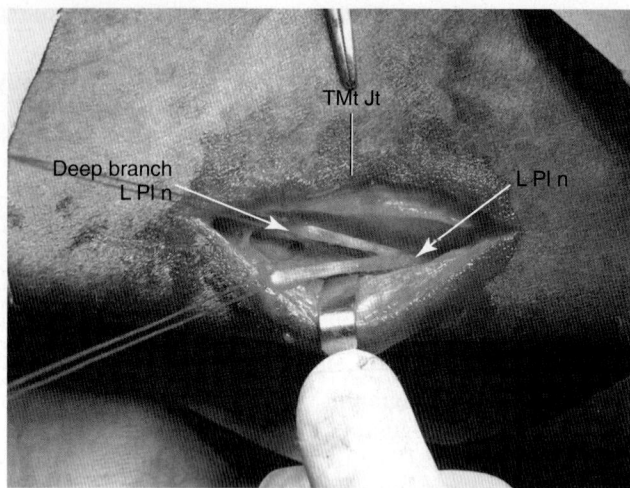

Fig. 43-1 • Intraoperative photograph of a Warmblood gelding with chronic, recurrent proximal suspensory desmitis of the left hindlimb after a surgical approach to sever the deep branch of the lateral plantar nerve (L Pl n). The horse is in right lateral recumbency (proximal is to the right and dorsal is uppermost), the Kelly forceps is positioned at the level of the tarsometatarsal joint (TMt Jt), and the Senn retractors are positioned deep to the metatarsal fascia and superficial digital flexor tendon, both of which are retracted in a plantar direction. The parent lateral plantar nerve (L Pl n) coursing distally originates from the tibial nerve proximal to the tarsus and divides into a deep branch, a segment of which is removed during neurectomy, and then continues distally as the lateral plantar nerve. The deep branch further divides within the suspensory ligament and proximal metatarsal region to innervate the proximal aspect of the suspensory ligament and the plantar cortex of the third metatarsal bone; it then divides into lateral and medial plantar metatarsal nerves, which continue distally to innervate the fetlock joint (not shown, deep to the suspensory ligament).

branch that innervates the proximal aspect of the SL and gives off branches, which continue distally as the lateral and medial plantar metatarsal nerves that course on the axial aspects of each respective splint bone (see Figure 10-22; Figure 43-1). Neurectomy of the deep branch of the lateral plantar nerve provides analgesia of the origin of the SL and the plantar cortex of the MtIII and partial analgesia of sites more distal to the level of and including the metatarsophalangeal joint. Accurate interpretation of diagnostic analgesia is critical when planning this surgical procedure. Neurectomy has received considerable attention recently as a surgical approach for management of proximal suspensory desmitis (PSD; see later).[5,6] Histological changes consistent with nerve compression have been identified in horses undergoing neurectomy of the deep branch of the lateral plantar nerve, and nerve compression was proposed as a possible cause of residual pain in horses even after desmitis resolved.[6] In that study, 62% of horses returned to soundness after neurectomy,[6] whereas in a different study 19 of 20 horses treated by neurectomy and laminar fasciotomy returned to the previous level of performance.[5] The deep branch of the lateral plantar nerve that was examined histologically[6] lies within the dense metatarsal but outside the laminar fascial planes. Recognition of neuritis in this segment indicates that compression of the deep branch may be occurring within this fascial compartment. The lateral plantar nerve and its counterpart, the medial plantar nerve, continue distally between the SL and DDFT.

Conformation

Sickle-hock and more important straight hindlimb conformation predispose to metatarsal region lameness (see Chapter 4).

CLINICAL CHARACTERISTICS AND DIAGNOSIS OF LAMENESS IN THE METATARSAL REGION

There are no pathognomonic historical findings related to metatarsal region pain causing lameness. Palpation of the metatarsal region should be done with the horse in standing and non–weight-bearing positions. The metatarsal region cannot be adequately palpated when the horse is standing, because soft tissue structures in the proximal metatarsal region are not readily palpable in this position. Careful palpation for signs of inflammation and bony swelling should be performed with the limb in both positions. Even when the limb is flexed, it is still difficult to define the SL and DDFT proximally. However, it is possible to apply pressure over the proximal aspect of the SL to check for a painful response. In some horses with PSD, edema may be present or the area may feel full or slightly thickened, but dense fascia covering the SL and DDFT prevents expansion, and swelling may go undetected. A painful response to deep palpation over the proximal aspect of the medial splint bone and distal aspect of the tarsus, referred to as the *Churchill test*, may indicate the presence of referred pain and primary distal hock joint lameness, but in my experience this is a nonspecific test. Many horses with hindlimb lameness originating from sites other than the distal hock joints manifest a positive response to compression of both the medial and lateral splint bones and distal, medial aspect of the tarsus. Palpation of the dorsal cortex of the MtIII may reveal pain in trotters or other horses that interfere and may be an important finding, but palpation may not necessarily localize the primary source of pain that is causing lameness. Careful palpation of the abaxial and axial aspects of both splint bones is necessary to uncover hidden splint exostoses. Even subtle enlargement of the SL body, as it emerges from the bony encasement of the splint bones, that is accompanied by a painful response can indicate early suspensory desmitis. Both branches of the SL and attachments to the PSBs should be carefully palpated. Horses with a history of curb may develop progressive SDF tendonitis in the proximal metatarsal region, but this can easily be overlooked unless the area is carefully palpated (see Chapters 6, 69, and 78).

Diagnostic Analgesia

The high plantar perineural block (see Chapter 10) should be used to localize pain to the metatarsal region. Medial and lateral plantar nerves and medial and lateral plantar metatarsal nerves are blocked just distal (approximately 1.5 cm) to the tarsometatarsal joint (see Chapter 10). Variations of this block are often used, but it is important to recognize that subtarsal analgesic techniques targeting the lateral plantar nerve, or its deep branch, will not block the medial plantar nerve, and false-negative results could be obtained. More important, false-positive results incriminating the proximal aspect of the SL as a source of pain can occur. Subtarsal analgesia should be performed only after results of low plantar analgesia are observed, because most injection techniques in the subtarsal region are likely to desensitize the plantar metatarsal nerves, important contributors to innervation of the metatarsophalangeal joint. An injection technique was recently described for the diagnosis of PSD; the lateral plantar nerve is blocked approximately 15 mm distal to the head of the MtIV, just axial to the MtIV, at a depth of 25 mm.[7] Although in theory this block is done in close proximity to the deep branch of the lateral plantar nerve, it is within the same fascial compartment as the parent branch, leading to the possibility of blocking this important contributor to distal limb innervation. If completed as a stand-alone technique without first performing low plantar analgesia, subtarsal analgesia may lead the clinician to the erroneous impression that pain is emanating from the proximal aspect of the SL. Management of horses with PSD by desmoplasty and fasciotomy was recently described, but criteria for inclusion of cases suggested that pain was localized to the proximal metacarpal or metatarsal region by use of only subcarpal or subtarsal analgesia without first blocking the distal aspect of the limb.[8]

In the forelimb, distal palmar outpouchings of the carpometacarpal joint complicate interpretation of diagnostic analgesic techniques. In the hindlimb, distal plantar outpouchings of the tarsometatarsal joint can potentially be penetrated when high plantar analgesic techniques are performed, but outpouchings of the joint were not seen in magnetic resonance images of cadaver specimens in a study comparing imaging modalities in the plantar metatarsal region.[9] In an in vivo radiographic contrast study in only 5% of limbs was the tarsometatarsal joint inadvertently penetrated when injection mimicking high plantar analgesia was performed at a level of 1.5 cm distal to the tarsometatarsal joint, although in the same study inadvertent penetration of the tarsal sheath occurred in 40% of limbs.[10] Care must be taken when interpreting diagnostic analgesia.

Imaging Considerations

Routine radiographic examination includes the dorsoplantar (DPl), lateromedial (LM), dorsolateral-plantaromedial oblique (DL-PlMO), and dorsomedial-plantarolateral oblique (DM-PlLO) images. In a DPl image of the proximal aspect of the MtIII, there is a normal area of mild increased radiopacity that should not be interpreted as modeling that is associated with stress reaction of the origin of the SL (Figure 43-2). Accurate assessment of the proximal aspect of the MtIII for the presence of increased radiopacity or avulsion fracture requires that radiographic views be centered at this level.

Pool and delayed (bone) phase scintigraphic examination is quite useful to differentiate bone from soft tissue injury in horses with proximal plantar metatarsal pain and osteoarthritis. It is also useful to differentiate other conditions of the tarsometatarsal joint from those involving the proximal aspect of the MtIII. Focal increased radiopharmaceutical uptake (IRU) seen in delayed (bone) phase images involving the proximal plantar aspect of the MtIII is the most important scintigraphic finding in the metatarsal region. In TB and STB racehorses there is normally mild to mild-moderate IRU of the dorsal cortex of the MtIII, from the most proximal aspect to the mid-to-distal diaphysis. This finding was originally proposed to be age dependent

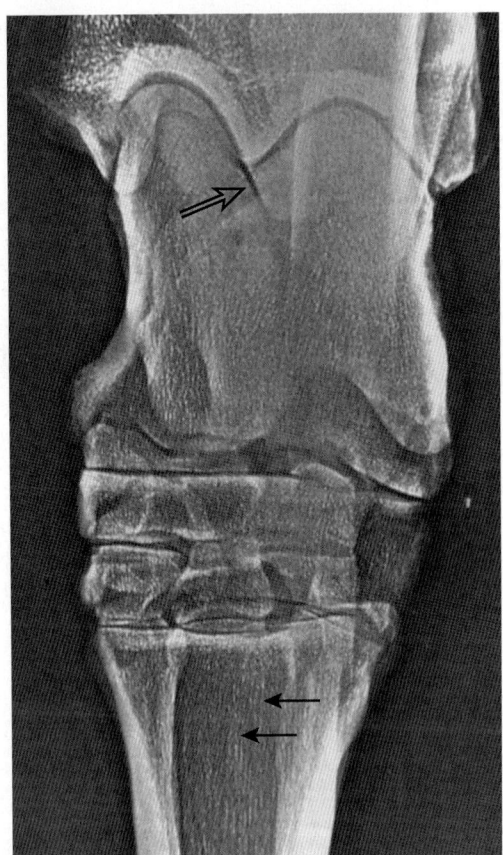

Fig. 43-2 • Dorsoplantar radiographic image showing the normal coarse trabecular pattern *(arrows)* seen in the proximal aspect of the third metatarsal bone, which can be mistaken for increased radiopacity associated with the suspensory attachment. This Standardbred racehorse had a sagittal fracture of the talus. Note the radiolucency of the talus *(open arrow)*.

because the dorsal cortex of the McIII could be "seen" scintigraphically as a normal finding in young but not older TB racehorses.[11] In a population of predominantly sports horses and few racehorses the dorsal cortex was evident visually and with use of profile analysis in all horses regardless of age.[12] When normal plantar scintigraphic images of the proximal metatarsal region are evaluated, there is usually asymmetrical radiopharmaceutical uptake (RU), with greater RU of the lateral aspect involving the lateral aspect of the MtIII and the MtIV. A central area of increased radiopacity seen radiologically (see Figure 43-2) does not appear to be active scintigraphically in normal horses. Asymmetrical RU was confirmed in a recent scintigraphic study of the proximal metacarpal and metatarsal regions in normal horses.[13] Using region of interest analysis there was significantly higher RU in the lateral aspect of the metatarsal region compared with the medial aspect in plantar images, and significantly higher RU in the right proximal metatarsal region compared with the left. In lateral images there was maximum RU in the central and plantar aspect of the proximal metatarsal region. There was no effect of age on RU.[13] In horses with PSD, visual appraisal and profile analysis of scintigraphic images failed to reveal abnormalities in most of 126 horses with forelimb or hindlimb lameness, but quantitative analysis using region of interest analysis revealed greater RU ratios in plantar images of lame limbs compared with nonlame limbs.[14] Given that PSD is primarily a soft tissue injury, the lack of scintigraphic findings is easily understood; that many horses have chronic or recurrent hindlimb PSD could explain mild scintigraphic abnormalities found in plantar metatarsal images.

Ultrasonographic evaluation should be performed to evaluate the plantar soft tissue structures, the most important of which is the SL (see Chapters 16, 72, and 78). Computed tomography (CT) can be useful to evaluate complex fractures in the metatarsal region, the plantar cortex of the MtIII, and bony exostoses of the metatarsal bones (see Chapter 20). CT was useful in imaging new bone formation on the proximal plantar aspect of the MtIII in three horses with PSD that were successfully treated by ostectomy and osteostixis of the MtIII.[15] Magnetic resonance imaging (MRI) is quite valuable in the diagnosis of PSD and for identifying adhesions between the MtII or the MtIV and the SL (see Chapters 21 and 37). In a study comparing the results of ultrasonography, MRI, and histology of the SL in the forelimb and hindlimb, the heterogeneity of the SL including the presence of muscular and adipose tissue, artifacts, and variable size were thought to be limitations of ultrasonographic examination.[9] In the hindlimb the SL had a single large area of origin on the MtIII with a few fibers originating from the distal row of tarsal bones, was mildly bilobed in appearance, and was located slightly more laterally on the MtIII than at the corresponding position in the forelimb; significantly more muscular tissue was found laterally and similar sizes of the lateral and medial lobes were found.[8] There was good correlation in morphology between MRI and histology, but cross-sectional area measurements were significantly higher with MRI than with either ultrasonography or histology, and histological cross-sectional area measurements were significantly higher than those obtained with ultrasonography.[9] At the origin of the SL in the hindlimb, ultrasonographically determined cross-sectional area measurements were less than half of those determined using histology and MRI. Although relative measurements between limbs obtained using ultrasonography may be comparable, measurements between horses must be interpreted with caution.[9] Measurement of plantar-to-dorsal thickness, however, was similar using all three modalities and may be the most useful measurement with which to compare sizes within and between horses.[9] Ultrasonographic examination of the proximal aspect of the SL will likely underestimate cross-sectional area, and heterogeneity must be interpreted carefully. MRI was useful in characterizing injury and formulating management options in the proximal metacarpal and metatarsal regions of 45 horses, of which 13 horses had hindlimb PSD.[16]

SPECIFIC CONDITIONS OF THE METATARSAL REGION

Bucked and Sore Shins: Dorsal Cortical Fractures of the Third Metatarsal Bone

Modeling and remodeling of the dorsal cortex of the MtIII occur similarly to that of the McIII, but differences in load distribution between forelimbs and hindlimbs account for the relative lack of clinical signs associated with this process in the hindlimbs. Scintigraphic examination often reveals mild, diffuse IRU in the dorsal cortex of the MtIII in TB

racehorses (see earlier discussion), but clinical signs of bucked shins are rare. In trotters common findings are pain on palpation, wounds and abrasions, and in some horses bony swelling that is associated with interference injury in the dorsal or dorsal medial metatarsal region. Although these areas are painful to palpation, most sites are a sign rather than the cause of a high-speed gait deficit. Finding evidence of interference injury, however, is quite important, because interference is often a sign of ipsilateral forelimb lameness and can be a cause of horses making breaks (going off stride). Dorsal cortical fractures are rare but can occur in TB and STB racehorses.

Medial and Lateral Condylar and Spiral Fractures of the Third Metatarsal Bone

Medial and lateral condylar and spiral fractures of the MtIII are discussed in Chapter 42.

Midshaft, Simple, or Comminuted Fractures of the Third Metatarsal Bone

Diaphyseal fractures of the MtIII can result from propagation and displacement of medial condylar fractures. Direct trauma is the most common cause, often from kicks by other horses. Complete fracture of the MtIII occurs in foals and adult horses. Critical prognostic factors are degree of comminution; proximity of the fracture to the metatarsophalangeal joint and tarsometatarsal joints; integrity of the vascular supply; whether the fracture is open or closed; degree of contamination if open; and the horse's age, value, performance level, and intended use. Prognosis for adult horses with open, comminuted fractures of the MtIII is poor, but in those with closed, mildly comminuted or oblique fractures, repair is possible and prognosis is guarded to fair. Often, financial considerations are paramount in determining success with fractures of the metatarsal region in adult horses, because even if fractures are open and comminuted, advanced methods of repair and use of techniques such as intravenous regional limb perfusion may improve prognosis. The locking compression plate, designed with locking screws to provide a fixed-angle construct not dependent on the plate-bone interface being in compression, is ideal to use in horses with comminuted fractures and can be thought of as an internal-external fixator. This advanced system was successfully used in two horses recently and would be my choice if internal fixation was to be used in repair of a MtIII fracture.[17] Horses with open fractures with gross contamination have a grave prognosis, regardless of age and degree of comminution, but those with small areas of skin loss and minor contamination can be successfully managed. Repair in horses with comminuted fractures involving the tarsometatarsal joint is difficult, but transfixation pin casts using the distal tibia and distal aspect of the MtIII could be considered. In foals, vascular supply of the limb distal to a fracture is a concern and should be assessed clinically or by using angiography or Doppler ultrasonography. Prognosis in foals with simple or mildly comminuted midshaft MtIII fractures repaired using one or two dynamic compression plates is fair to good (Figure 43-3). In foals, external coaptation often causes profound flexor tendon laxity and should be avoided. External skeletal fixation by using pins and

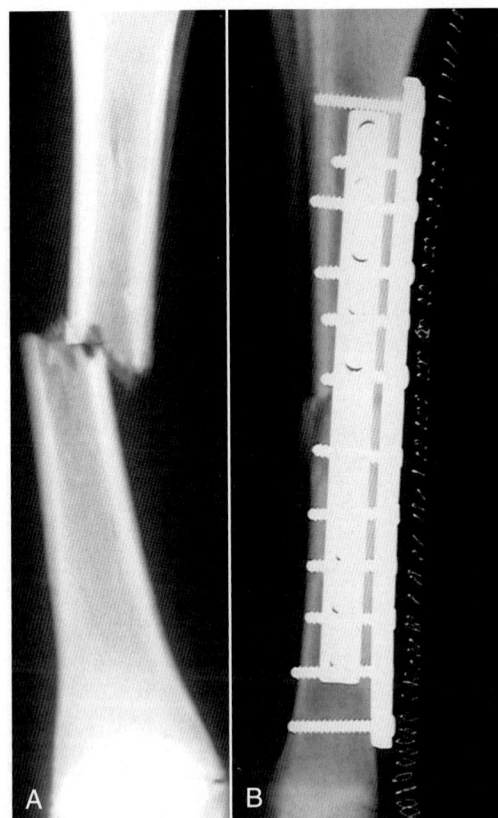

Fig. 43-3 • This open (mildly contaminated) midshaft fracture of the third metatarsal bone in a 4-month-old Thoroughbred colt was successfully managed using two dynamic compression plates and a half-limb bandage. **A,** The preoperative and **B,** postoperative appearance of the third metatarsal bone are shown. The plates were removed 4 months later.

sidebars of casting material or acrylic is possible in a foal. In adult horses, methods of stabilization and repair include internal fixation using two bone plates, locking compression plates or a combination of limited-contact dynamic and locking compression plates, transfixation pin casts in combination with internal fixation, and casts alone.

Of 25 horses with MtIII or McIII fractures that were managed with internal fixation, external coaptation, or both, age, sex, weight, and the limb affected were not related to outcome, but affected horses were younger than the general hospital population. Seventeen horses had open fractures, and infection was the most common complication after surgery.[17] Nonunion in an infected fracture was the most common reason for failure (seven horses). Of 24 horses in which outcome was determined, 16 (67%) had healed fractures and 12 (50%) horses were sound for the intended use.[17] Intended use was not defined; therefore prognosis in foals for future racing could not be determined. Of 37 horses and foals undergoing transfixation pin casting for management of difficult fractures, 10 of 15 horses (67%) in which fractures involved the McIII or the MtIII survived, a prognosis level similar to that seen with internal fixation.[18,19] Five of six horses, including both foals, managed with transfixation pin casting of the MtIII fractures survived.[19] Transfixation pin casting is often chosen when fractures are difficult or open, when there is gross contamination, and when financial constraints preclude use of expensive implants such as the locking compression plates and screws.

Physeal Fractures of the Distal Aspect of the Third Metatarsal Bone

The most common fracture of the distal MtIII physis is a Salter-Harris type II fracture, but various other fractures can occur. These fractures are usually quite stable, but perfect reduction is difficult to achieve. Fracture reduction and external coaptation are usually successful, but insertion of one or two 3.5- or 4.5-mm bone screws in the metaphyseal component may help stabilize the fracture and reduce the time necessary for external coaptation. Even short periods of cast immobilization in foals can cause rapid onset of flexor tendon laxity. Cast-bandage and bandage-splint combinations are preferred in young foals that are only several weeks old.

Incomplete Longitudinal Fractures of the Plantar Aspect of the Third Metatarsal Bone and Stress Reactions

Incomplete longitudinal fractures of the plantar cortex of the MtIII occur considerably less frequently than those of the McIII. Stress reactions of the MtIII, defined as focal areas of IRU without radiological confirmation of fracture, occur as part of a continuum of stress-related bone injury at the origin of the SL. Combined MtIII injury and PSD worsens prognosis, and it is important to establish whether injury involves bone, soft tissue, or both (see Chapters 37 and 72).

Transverse Stress Fractures of the Distal Aspect of the Third Metatarsal Bone

Transverse stress fractures of the distal aspect of the McIII are described in Chapter 37. I have not recognized this specific fracture type in the MtIII.

Avulsion Fractures of the Third Metatarsal Bone Associated with the Origin of the Suspensory Ligament

Avulsion fractures of the MtIII that are associated with the origin of the SL are frequently seen and can be solitary injuries or associated with PSD. Horses can have acute-onset or chronic mild-to-moderate hindlimb lameness, depending on size and duration of fracture. Fractures occur most commonly in dressage horses, jumpers, and STB racehorses. Local signs of swelling are usually absent, and diagnostic analgesia is essential for localization of pain. Focal areas of IRU are seen that are roughly triangular and involve the proximal plantar aspect of the MtIII (Figure 43-4). It is important to differentiate IRU from that seen in the tarsometatarsal joint, but concomitant IRU in both areas is not unusual. A well-defined fracture is often not detectable radiologically, and usually only suspicious areas of radiolucency and increased radiopacity are seen. Bilateral avulsion fractures or stress reactions occur. Conservative management using a progressive increase in exercise without turnout is usually successful. Recurrence is common and most likely in horses that have associated PSD (see Chapter 72).

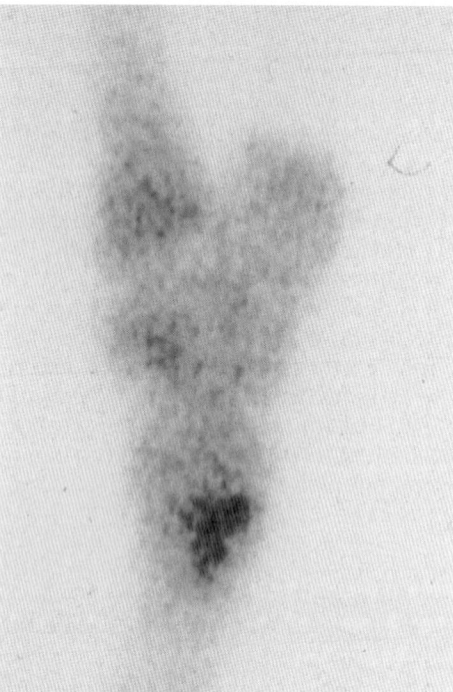

Fig. 43-4 • Delayed (bone) phase, lateral scintigraphic image showing focal, triangular increased radiopharmaceutical uptake typical of an avulsion fracture of the third metatarsal bone that is associated with the origin of the suspensory ligament.

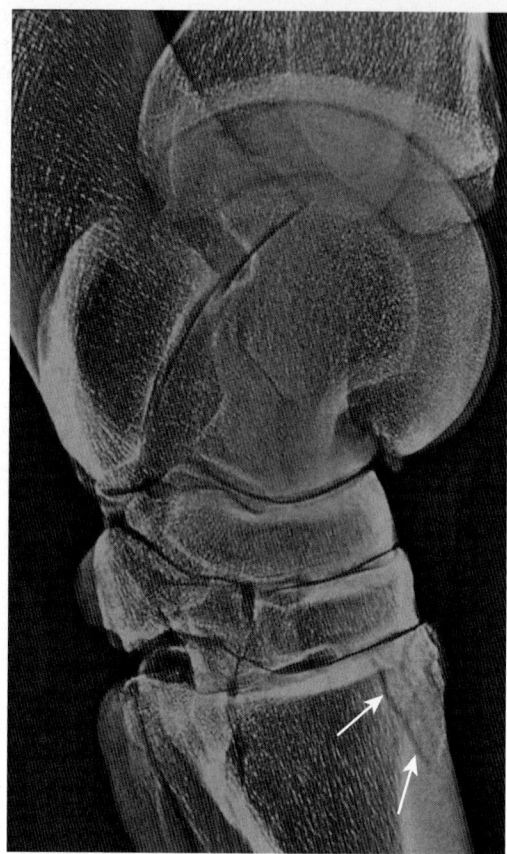

Fig. 43-5 • Dorsomedial-plantarolateral xeroradiographic image of the hock and proximal metatarsal region of a Standardbred racehorse. There is an articular fracture of the dorsoproximolateral aspect of the third metatarsal bone (MtIII) *(arrows)*. Note the bone modeling of the proximal aspects of the MtIII that preceded the fracture.

Articular Fracture of the Dorsoproximolateral Aspect of the Third Metatarsal Bone

Articular fracture of the dorsoproximolateral aspect of the MtIII occurs primarily in STB and TB racehorses.[20,21] Acute onset of lameness is common, but a history of either chronic, undiagnosed hindlimb lameness or lameness referable to the distal hock joints is usually uncovered. This fracture occurs most commonly in horses with sickle-hock conformation, a conformational abnormality that predisposes to dorsal and plantar tarsal and proximal metatarsal injury, and may worsen prognosis. This fracture occurs most frequently in horses in the later stages of training, but often before racing, a clinical characteristic that may worsen prognosis. Acute soft tissue swelling is rare. A small bony enlargement is often palpable but is easy to miss. Horses exhibit a positive response to upper limb flexion and to focal, deep pressure over the dorsolateral aspect of the MtIII. Lameness partially resolves after intraarticular analgesia of the tarsometatarsal joint or perineural analgesia of the fibular and tibial nerves. Initial radiological examination reveals the presence of bony proliferation, indicating that bone modeling preceded acute fracture (Figure 43-5). Incomplete fractures are most common, but complete and mildly displaced fractures also occur. Scintigraphic examination is useful in differentiating this fracture from other conditions involving the tarsometatarsal joint and those involving the proximal plantar aspect of the MtIII. Radiographs and scintigraphic images of the contralateral hindlimb often reveal similar but less pronounced changes.

Because proliferative changes precede fracture, it is presumed that the cause involves chronic fatigue and stress-related bone injury. Attachment of the tendons of the fibularis tertius and cranialis tibialis muscles likely contributes substantially to bone stress and may play a role. Concomitant radiological evidence of osteoarthritis involving the dorsal aspect of the tarsometatarsal and centrodistal joints and dorsoproximolateral fracture of the MtIII is common.

Conservative management is advised in horses with incomplete fractures, but in those with displaced fractures, internal fixation using one or two 3.5-mm bone screws placed in lag fashion is advised. If horses raced before fracture, the prognosis for future racing is good but only fair to guarded for returning to or sustaining racing in the same class. Horses that develop this fracture before actual racing begins have a poor prognosis. When horses return to training or racing, progressive osteoarthritis of the tarsometatarsal and centrodistal joints appears to be a limiting factor even when the fracture heals and proliferative changes on the MtIII smooth.

Exostoses of the Second, Third, and Fourth Metatarsal Bones

Exostoses of the metatarsal bones (splint exostoses, splints) occur considerably less commonly than those involving the metacarpal bones, but they can cause lameness, or in racehorses, high-speed soreness. However, it is common to find large exostoses involving the proximal lateral aspect of the MtIII or MtIV as an incidental finding that is usually not associated with lameness, although the lesion is scintigraphically active. Splint exostoses can be caused by direct trauma or instability between the metatarsal bones. There is a common misconception that splints arise from tearing of the interosseous ligaments between the MtII or MtIV and the MtIII, but many splints do not involve the space between bones, and it is difficult to believe that instability and primary desmitis adequately explain the cause of splints. Many splints in the hindlimb involve the MtIII alone (and not the MtII or the MtIV), although the MtII and the MtIV can be affected. Axially located exostoses (blind splints) do occur and are most important proximally, where bony proliferation could crowd or impinge on the proximal aspect of the SL and lateral and medial plantar metatarsal nerves. Adhesions may occur between the axial aspect of the exostosis and the SL and other nearby soft tissue structures, but lameness from adhesions and encroachment into the region of the SL appears to involve the McII or McIV most commonly. Direct trauma from interference injury is the most likely cause of most medially located splints. Faulty conformation does not appear to play a prominent role. Mature distal splint exostoses may predispose the MtII and MtIV to fracture in horses with progressive enlargement of the SL.

Lameness associated with splint exostoses is usually mild (grade 1 to 1½ of 5). Direct palpation elicits a painful withdrawal response, and lameness is exacerbated. Infiltration of local anesthetic solution alleviates pain and a majority of observed lameness, but perineural analgesia of the lateral plantar metatarsal and lateral plantar nerves, or medial plantar metatarsal and medial plantar nerves proximal to exostoses involving the MtIV and the MtII, respectively, may be required. Radiographs should be obtained when a fracture is suspected but otherwise yield little useful information unless there is drainage associated with bony proliferation.

Management of horses with splint exostoses includes local cold therapy, including cold water hosing and icing, the application of a poultice and bandaging, and the administration of nonsteroidal antiinflammatory drugs (NSAIDs). Injections of methylprednisolone acetate (80 mg) and Sarapin, an extract of the pitcher plant (6 mL), subcutaneously and axially if needed for each exostosis reduce inflammation and pain. Repeat injections are often necessary. Cryotherapy is popular in racehorses, but clinicians should be aware that superficial skin pain persists for several weeks afterward, which leaves few ways to monitor improvement other than to monitor performance. Surgical removal of persistently painful exostoses by periostectomy, ostectomy of exostoses without removing the parent MtII or MtIV, adhesiolysis, and fasciotomy can be performed if exostoses involve the axial aspects and encroach on or are adhered to the SL. Surgery is usually not required for abaxially located splint exostoses.

Fractures of the Second and Fourth Metatarsal Bones

Fractures of the MtII and MtIV occur primarily as a result of direct trauma from either a kick from another horse or kicking into or through a stationary object. The MtIV is injured most commonly. Simple, comminuted, and displaced fractures occur, and often wounds extend directly into the fracture site. The MtIV bears little load and appears to have remarkable recuperative ability. Diagnosis is usually straightforward, particularly if a wound is involved, but in some horses the presence of chronic lameness or drainage several weeks after injury prompts later radiographic examination, and only then is fracture diagnosed. Radiographs often reveal extensive comminution, but in many horses, basic axial alignment of fragments is maintained. When fractures of either the MtIV or MtII involve the tarsometatarsal joint, and particularly if fractures are open, infectious arthritis and osteoarthritis are possible but may be amenable to treatment.

The majority of MtIV fractures heal with conservative management, despite comminution and infectious osteitis, with appropriate antimicrobial administration and wound care. Loose subcutaneously located fragments can be removed with ease and deep tissue samples should be collected for bacterial culture and antimicrobial susceptibility testing. Although internal fixation,[22] total ostectomy of the MtIV,[23] and segmental ostectomy[24] have been described, I have rarely found it necessary to contemplate surgery, with the exception of removing loose bone fragments from wounds or persistently draining tracts (Figure 43-6). Comminuted fractures with an intact column of bone will heal satisfactorily in most horses, although delayed unions or nonunions requiring surgical intervention occur infrequently. Horses may need 4 to 6 months of rest, and long-term antimicrobial therapy (4 to 8 weeks) may be necessary in horses with open or infected fractures. Impingement on

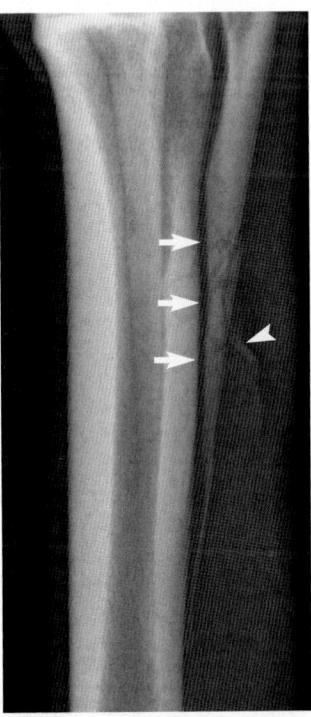

Fig. 43-6 • Dorsal 45° lateral-plantaromedial oblique digital radiographic image of a horse with an open, comminuted fracture of the fourth metatarsal bone (MtIV) *(arrows)*. As long as an intact column of bone is present, fractures of the MtIV will often heal without major surgical intervention except for removal of loose fragments *(arrowhead)* through the original wound. Long-term management with antimicrobial agents and rest is necessary.

the SL function by callus from fracture healing is a possible complication but is unusual. Fractures of the mid and distal aspects of the MtII and MtIV are caused by chronic suspensory desmitis involving the body or branches. Suspensory desmitis is primary and MtII and MtIV fractures are secondary, resulting from a bowstring effect of the enlarging SL. Occasionally, axially located callus from an old splint bone fracture may cause mild lameness from local irritation of the nearby SL. Local injections of antiinflammatory agents resolve pain in most instances, but occasionally exostoses and the distal aspect of the splint bone are removed.

Ostectomy of distal fragments of the MtII and MtIV can be performed in combination with SL splitting and, in some horses, with ostectomy of apical or abaxial fracture fragments of the PSBs. A triad of clinical problems involving the SL, splint bone, and PSBs (called the *three Ss*) is often seen, and all three structures should be evaluated before management and prognostic recommendations are made.

Enostosis-like Lesions of the Third Metatarsal Bone

During scintigraphic examination, single or multifocal areas of IRU within the medullary cavity of the MtIII are occasionally seen, and intensity can range from mild to intense. Subsequent radiological examination reveals one or more round to irregularly shaped radiopacities within the medullary cavity. Lameness in horses with enostosis-like lesions of the MtIII is unusual, particularly if there are small, focal areas of IRU involving only the area around the nutrient foramen. Of 17 enostosis-like lesions (in 10 horses), four lesions were identified in the MtIII, but in only one horse was lameness localized to the metatarsal region.[25] Lameness, if present, should abate with a high plantar block and resolves with rest and the administration of NSAIDs.

Hypertrophic Osteopathy

Hypertrophic osteopathy is discussed in Chapter 37.

Suspensory Desmitis

Suspensory desmitis, including PSD, suspensory body desmitis, and suspensory branch desmitis and associated bony injury, is the most important cause of lameness in the metatarsal region (see Chapter 72).

Hindlimb proximal and proximal and body desmitis are career-threatening injuries and horses should be managed aggressively. Managing horses with hindlimb suspensory desmitis is exceedingly more challenging than managing those with similar forelimb injuries—the proverbial apples and oranges comparison. One of the Editors (SJD) has written extensively on the subject and aptly points out that the prognosis in horses with acute forelimb PSD approaches 90%, whereas prognosis in those with acute hindlimb desmitis managed conservatively is 14%.[26] I have managed 23 horses, 13 nonracehorses (dressage horses, jumpers, event horses) and 10 STB trotters, with confirmed proximal and body suspensory desmitis by using autogenous bone marrow injection[27] and proximal metatarsal fasciotomy. Horses are placed under general anesthesia, and a medial approach is used to gain access to the proximal aspect of the SL (Figure 43-7). A large volume, 30 to 60 mL, of liquid bone marrow is harvested from the sternum and injected directly into the proximal aspect of the SL and body as determined by ultrasonographic evaluation. The dense,

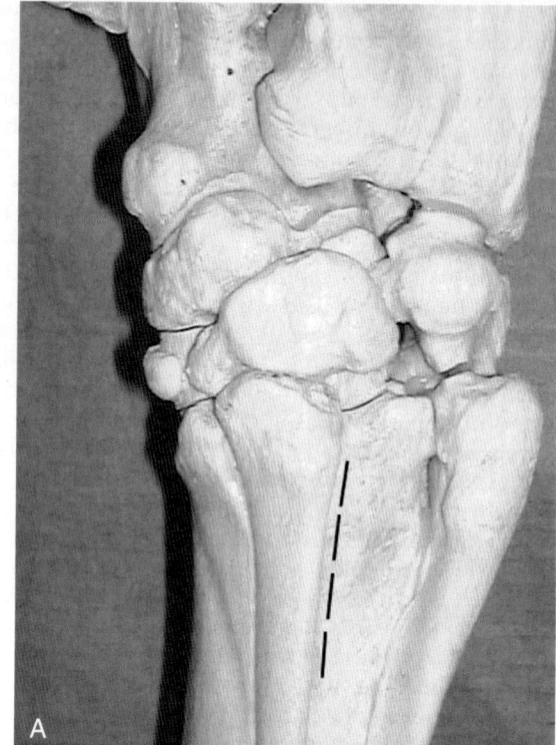

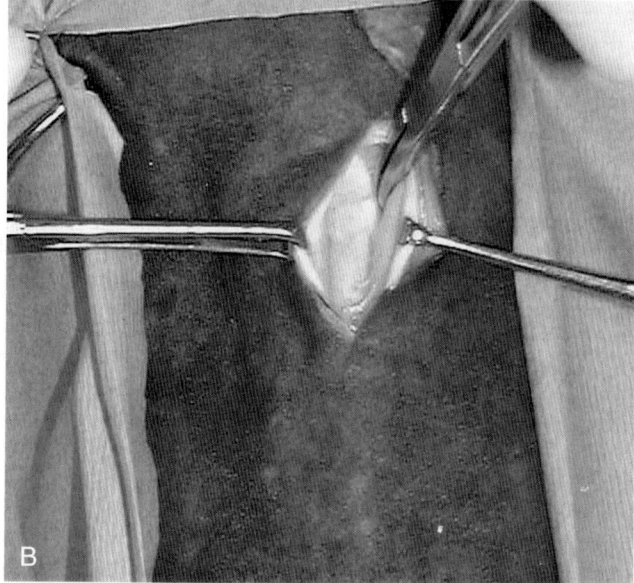

Fig. 43-7 • An anatomy specimen **(A)** and a cadaver specimen **(B)** showing the location and approach *(dotted line)* for bone marrow injection and fasciotomy used in management of horses with proximal suspensory and body desmitis. Dense metatarsal fascia is being retracted using Allis tissue forceps, exposing the origin of the suspensory ligament (curved Kelly forceps is positioned plantar to the suspensory ligament).

overlying medial metatarsal fascia is transected from the level of just proximal to the tarsometatarsal joint to the midbody region. Although no attempt was made to separately incise the laminar suspensory fascia, this fascial layer is confluent with the overlying metatarsal fascia along the axial aspect of the MtII. The subcutaneous tissues and skin are closed. Horses should be given 4 to 6 months of progressive increase in exercise, including 4 weeks of stall rest, followed by 4 weeks of stall rest with handwalking, 4 weeks of walking with a rider up or in the jog cart, and then 4 weeks of walking and light trotting. Turnout exercise is forbidden. Of 13 nonracehorses, eight (62%) returned to full work, three of these to elite competition; one horse returned to a lower level of competition, but lameness persisted or recurred in four horses. Of 10 trotters, eight raced but only two raced more than five starts without recurrence of desmitis. Hindlimb suspensory desmitis in the trotter is a substantial cause of lameness and is career-limiting. Whether improvement in some horses may result from reparative processes accelerated by the transfer of stem cells, the injection of growth factor–rich substrate into damaged SLs (see Chapters 72 and 73), fasciotomy and relief of compartment syndrome, or a combination of factors is unknown. In an experimental study, acellular bone marrow was significantly better than platelet-rich plasma and growth factors in stimulating cartilage oligo-meric matrix protein production in an in vitro study using cultured SL fibroblasts.[28] See Chapters 72 and 73 for a complete discussion regarding alternative approaches to healing, reparative and regenerative healing, and other aspects of management of suspensory desmitis. Numerous other management options are available including stem cell therapy (see Chapter 73), a combination of desmo-plasty (splitting) and fasciotomy,[8] fasciotomy and neurec-tomy of the deep branch of the lateral plantar nerve,[4] and radial pressure wave therapy.[29] Realistically, prognosis is only guarded to fair for return to the same level of competi-tion, particularly in elite horses and STB trotters, and to date, a method of management suitable for all horses is not available. Accurate diagnosis and imaging must be per-formed to authenticate location and source of pain. Prog-nosis is particularly guarded in older Warmblood horses with desmitis extending into the body of the SL with pal-pably thickened metatarsal regions, in those with straight hindlimb conformation and with hyperextension of the metatarsophalangeal joints (dropped fetlock joints), and in those in which desmitis is chronic and recurrent. A particu-larly severe form of suspensory desmitis is seen in some Warmblood horses, and may possibly be associated with pathological accumulation of proteoglycans in connective tissues, and resembles the degenerative suspensory disorder known to occur in the Peruvian Paso and related breeds.[30,31] Horses can have severe unilateral or bilateral desmitis with severe lameness and hyperextension of the hock and fetlock joints and are most often refractory to treatment.

Tenosynovitis of the Digital Flexor Tendon Sheath
Tenosynovitis of the DFTS is discussed in Chapter 74.

Desmopathy of the Accessory Ligament of the Deep Digital Flexor Tendon
Desmitis of the ALDDFT is discussed in Chapter 71.

Deep Digital Flexor Tendonitis
Deep digital flexor tendonitis is discussed in Chapters 70, 76, and 78.

Superficial Digital Flexor Tendonitis
Tendonitis of the superficial digital flexor (SDF) is an unusual-to-rare cause of lameness, but it occurs in race-horses with chronic, progressive curb and in any type of

sports horse as a result of direct trauma (see Chapter 78). SDF tendonitis may be obvious clinically or may be more subtle and requires careful palpation and ultrasonographic examination for confirmation of diagnosis. STB and TB racehorses with spontaneous SDF tendonitis invariably have sickle-hock conformation. The points of the hock should be compared, because in some horses loss of support accompanies SDF tendonitis and is a negative prognostic sign. Long-term rest has been successful in pacers, but trot-ters and TB racehorses have a poor prognosis for returning to racing. Most horses, regardless of breed or gait, drop in race class.

Undiagnosed Metatarsal Region Lameness
In a small proportion of horses, lameness can be localized to the metatarsal region by high plantar analgesia, but comprehensive imaging fails to identify a source of pain. I believe most of these horses have PSD and pain from subtle swelling of the SL. Measurement of the cross-sectional area and comparison with the contralateral limb are useful. Horses with lameness inappropriate for the degree of injury confirmed using radiographic and ultrasonographic exami-nations should be referred for scintigraphic examination and are likely candidates for MRI or CT examination. Pain associated with the distal tarsal joints and tarsal sheath occasionally can be abolished using high plantar analgesic techniques, a fact that must be kept in mind in horses in which a diagnosis in the metatarsal region cannot be made.

Wounds of the Metatarsal Region
Wounds involving the metatarsal region are common and can be simple and involve the skin and subcutaneous tissues, but they are often complex and involve bone and deep soft tissue structures. Lacerations often involve the extensor and digital flexor tendons (see Chapter 81), and those involving the digital flexor tendons have serious implications for future performance and salvage. Lacera-tion of the long digital extensor tendon often delays healing of overlying wounds because movement of tendon ends exacerbates granulation tissue formation and delays wound contraction and epithelialization. Horses with long digital extensor tendon lacerations knuckle initially, but func-tional healing of the tendon most often results. A common wound is a distal-based flap wound that exposes the dorsal cortex of the MtIII and often is associated with extensor tendon lacerations. Because the skin base is distal, much of the proximal, triangular section of skin becomes necrotic. The skin should not be removed prematurely. Osteitis of the MtIII from direct trauma, drying from exposure, super-ficial infection, and loss of blood supply may prolong healing. Occasionally, large areas of the dorsal cortex of the MtIII have radiological characteristics of sequestra, but in many horses surgical removal or curettage is not required. In my experience, many horses have received unnecessary surgery to remove damaged areas of the MtIII cortex that if left in place would likely have healed unevent-fully. However, horses that develop extensive proliferative changes of the MtIII usually have adhesions to the long digital extensor tendon and often have chronic lameness.

Small puncture wounds may result in localized osteitis of the MtII or MtIV. Removal and curettage should be reserved for those with purulent drainage refractory to management with antimicrobial therapy. Horses without drainage but with radiological evidence of fragmentation within a radiolucent defect can be managed conservatively unless expedient resolution of the problem is mandatory. Horses with wounds and evidence of MtIII cortical crushing or obvious fractures should be managed with caution because catastrophic fracture could develop. Of substantial risk are those with acute, cortical fractures that resemble true saucer fractures. If horses are placed under general anesthesia to remove what is misinterpreted as devitalized pieces of cortex, there is a risk for catastrophic fracture during recovery from general anesthesia.

Acquired or secondary stringhalt is an unusual complication from metatarsal region wounds involving the long digital extensor tendon and sometimes the lateral digital extensor tendon. Horses at risk are those with extensive proliferation of the MtIII and adhesion formation with the overlying long digital extensor tendon. Mechanisms to account for the development of stringhalt include adhesion formation and interruption of the normal myotactic reflex.[32] Of 10 horses that developed stringhalt after dorsal metatarsal trauma, six horses developed stringhalt within 3 months, three developed stringhalt after 3 months, and in one horse time of injury to development of stringhalt was undetermined.[32] Of four horses managed with rest and progressive exercise, stringhalt resolved in one, improved in two, and remained the same in one horse.[32] Of five horses that received surgical management using lateral digital extensor myotenectomy, stringhalt resolved in two, improved in two, and remained the same in one

horse.[31] In my limited experience with this condition, prognosis is guarded to poor for complete resolution of the gait deficit.

Diffuse Swelling in the Metatarsal Region
Diffuse swelling in the metacarpal region is discussed in Chapter 37, and this also applies to the metatarsal region.

Severe Cellulitis of the Metatarsal Region
Cellulitis of the hindlimb occurs frequently from kick wounds or other trauma. In many horses obvious signs of trauma are lacking, but severe lameness and signs of infection in the metatarsal region occur. A severe form of cellulitis occurs primarily in TB racehorses in which severe lameness, swelling, and fever develop, apparently from a very small skin wound or excoriation, because an obvious wound is most difficult to find. This condition is similar to focal, peritarsal cellulitis (see Chapters 44 and 107). Initially it is difficult to differentiate cellulitis from infection of the tarsal sheath, SDFT, DDFT, and the DFTS, because swelling is diffuse and horses are severely lame. Within 48 to 72 hours, skin necrosis and sloughing can occur, which exposes an underlying and sometimes infected SDFT. *Staphylococcus* and occasionally *Streptococcus* species are cultured. Laminitis in the contralateral limb is a risk initially. Skin sloughing can be pronounced and requires weeks to months of wound care and, in some horses, grafting. Involvement of the underlying SDFT and other soft tissue structures is a poor prognostic sign.

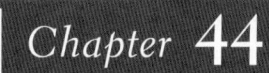

Chapter 44

The Tarsus

*Sue J. Dyson and Mike W. Ross**

ANATOMICAL CONSIDERATIONS

The tarsus consists of the tarsocrural, talocalcaneal, talocalcaneal-centroquartal (proximal intertarsal), centrodistal (distal intertarsal), and tarsometatarsal joints. The bones include the talus and calcaneus and the central, first and second fused, third, and fourth tarsal bones.[1] The tarsocrural joint is a ginglymus joint based on the shape of deep grooves on the cochlear articular surface of the distal end of the tibia with the extensive surface of the trochlea of the talus. The articulation of these joints is at an angle of 12 to 15 degrees dorsolateral to the sagittal plane of the limb. The talocalcaneal-centroquartal (proximal intertarsal), centrodistal, and tarsometatarsal joints are plane joints and are capable of only small amounts of gliding (shear) movement.

References on page 1286

The tibia follows an almost circular path along the talar ridges, and most movement occurs in the tarsocrural joint; however, there are translations and rotations at other sites.[2] Hock flexion is associated with abduction of the distal part of the limb caused by an oblique axis of motion.[3] There is outward rotation of the third metatarsal bone (MtIII) during the swing phase, followed by a small inward rotation during stance, when the hock is compressed. Thus at the gallop the hindlimbs swing outside the forelimbs as the tarsus flexes and then move back toward the midline as the tarsus extends before landing. Excessive rotation leads to visible wobbling of the tarsus. There is a locking mechanism among the talus, the central and third tarsal bones, and the MtIII.[4] A process on the distal plantar aspect of the talus fits into an indentation on the proximal aspect of the central tarsal bone; a ridge on the distal aspect of the central tarsal bone engages with a fossa on the proximal aspect of the third tarsal bone. A triangular plantar process of the third tarsal bone prevents the third tarsal bone from sliding across the proximal aspect of the MtIII. The oblique dorsal ligament extends distally from a small origin on the talus, spreading across the central and third tarsal bones, limiting motion.

Biomechanical studies have shown greatest compression on the distal medial aspect of the tibia and the proximal lateral aspect of the MtIII, suggesting that compressive load is transferred from medial to lateral through the tarsus. Radiopharmaceutical uptake (RU) in normal horses is greatest dorsally and laterally in the distal aspect of the

*The authors acknowledge and appreciate the work of Robin M. Dabareiner and G. Kent Carter, who contributed to this chapter in the previous edition of this text.

tarsus, suggesting increased adaptive bone modeling in response to high load.[5] There are differences in subchondral bone and cartilage thickness in the central and third tarsal bones from medially to laterally, varying dependent on intensity and type of exercise history, reflecting loading.[6,7] The distal tarsal joints function to absorb energy in the early stance phase and contribute to propulsion in the late stance phase. Conformation influences tarsal function.[8] Horses with large tarsal angles (>165.5 degrees) have been shown to have less flexion and less energy absorption in the impact phase at the trot compared with horses with intermediate (155.5 to 165.5 degrees) or small (<155.5 degrees) angles.[8] Horses with large hock angles generated less vertical impulse than horses with small angles, and net extensor force was lower.[8] Thus large tarsal angles may result in less propulsion and less absorption of concussion, which may influence both performance and soundness. However, horses with small hock angles had greater flexion during the stance phase, which may compress the dorsal aspects of the bones. Abnormal tarsal conformation can lead to lameness. Anecdotally, horses with small hock angles (sickle hocks) often develop osteoarthritis (OA) of the distal hock joints, curb, and soft tissue injury in the distal, plantar aspect of the hock and may be prone to the development of fracture of the central and third tarsal bones. Horses with large hock angles (straight-hock conformation), surprisingly, may be less prone to the development of tarsal pain, but they appear predisposed to the development of suspensory desmitis and stifle region pain.

Flexion of the stifle and hock is synchronous because of the reciprocal apparatus; there is rapid flexion of the tarsus at the beginning of the stance phase of the stride and maximal extension at the end of the stance phase. There is a peak of flexion in the middle of the swing phase. There is also coupling of movement of the tarsus and fetlock in flexion and extension because of passive action of the superficial digital flexor tendon and the long digital extensor tendon, respectively.

The fibrous part of the combined tarsal joint capsule surrounds all synovial compartments and attaches proximally to the tibia and distally to the distal tarsal bones, blending with the collateral ligaments (CLs), and to the metatarsal bones.[2] The dorsomedial aspect of the joint capsule is thin and uncovered by any tendons or ligaments and forms a fluctuant swelling over the medial trochlea of the talus. The proximal aspect of the plantar fibrous joint capsule is also thin and extends proximally about 5 cm caudal to the distal aspect of the tibia.[2] The plantar distal aspect of the joint capsule consists of the plantar and tarsometatarsal ligaments, which are thick and tightly adherent to the distal tarsal bones. The tarsus is composed of four synovial compartments. The tarsocrural compartment lubricates the tarsocrural joint and the dorsal aspect of the proximal intertarsal joint. The tarsocrural compartment is the largest compartment and is composed of four pouches: the dorsomedial, dorsolateral, plantaromedial, and plantarolateral. This provides several sites at which arthrocentesis can be performed. The proximal intertarsal synovial sac lines the talus and calcaneus proximally and the plantar aspect of the central and third tarsal bones distally and communicates dorsally with the tarsocrural joint. The large fenestration between the tarsocrural and the proximal intertarsal joints allows loose osteochondral fragments to

move freely between the conjoined joints. Disease of one joint obligatorily involves both compartments, because they function as one. In horses <1 year of age this opening appears small or slitlike or is not readily apparent when evaluated arthroscopically. The centrodistal joint lubricates the articulation between the central and third tarsal bones and the bones on each side, and the tarsometatarsal joint lubricates the third and fourth tarsal bones with the second metatarsal bone (MtII), the MtIII, and the fourth metatarsal bone (MtIV). The superficial location of the joint capsules makes them susceptible to penetration and the introduction of infection in association with trauma to the tarsus.

There is communication in 8% to 39% of the centrodistal and tarsometatarsal joints, but not necessarily in both hocks of the same horse,[9-11] although substances may spread between them by diffusion even in the absence of frank communication.[12,13] Communication between the distal tarsal joints and the tarsocrural joint was demonstrated in 3% of horses after injection of radiodense contrast medium into the tarsometatarsal joints in live horses[10]; however, in a cadaver study mepivacaine injected into the centrodistal or tarsometatarsal joints spread to the tarsocrural joint within 15 minutes of injection in 88% and 92% of limbs, respectively.[12]

Anatomical aspects of the gastrocnemius and calcaneal bursae and the tarsal sheath are discussed elsewhere (Chapters 76, 79, and 80). The distal tendon of the long digital extensor muscle is enclosed within a synovial sheath as it passes over the dorsolateral aspect of the tarsus. This sheath is compressed by transverse retinacular bands, resulting in a loculated appearance if the sheath is distended. Such longitudinal swelling is a quite common incidental finding in both sound and lame horses either unilaterally or bilaterally and is only rarely associated with pain and lameness. Focal lesions of the long digital extensor tendon have been identified ultrasonographically, but usually unassociated with lameness.

Numerous ligaments surround the hock. Both the lateral and medial CLs have one long and three short components.[14] The long lateral CL is superficial; originates at the caudal aspect of the lateral malleolus of the distal tibia; inserts on the distal lateral aspect of the calcaneus with additional fibers to the fourth tarsal bone, the MtIII, and the MtIV; and forms a canal for the tendon of the lateral digital extensor muscle. The short lateral CLs lie deep to the long lateral CL and originate from the cranial aspect of the lateral malleolus, pass plantad, and attach to the lateral surface of the calcaneus and the proximolateral plantar aspect of the talus. The long medial CL originates from the caudal aspect of the medial malleolus, attaches distally to the MtII and the MtIII, and also attaches to the medial aspect of the distal tarsal bones. The short medial CLs lie deep to the long medial CL and extend from the medial malleolus to the medial aspect of the calcaneus and sustentaculum tali. The long plantar ligament is a strong, flat band that originates at the proximal plantar surface of the calcaneus, extends distally, and attaches to the fourth tarsal bone and the MtIV. The dorsal tarsal ligament spreads out distally from the distal tuberosity of the talus and attaches to the central and third tarsal bones and proximal aspect of the MtIII and the MtIV. Numerous short intertarsal ligaments connect adjacent bones of the tarsus and have connections between tarsal and metatarsal bones.

The suspensory ligament (SL) also has an accessory ligament that extends proximally to originate from the plantar aspect of the fourth tarsal bone and the calcaneus.[15] This anatomical relationship between the SL and the tarsus may explain why distal hock joint pain and suspensory injury may coexist, why some horses with primary SL pain show a positive response to tarsal flexion, and why there may be confusion with diagnostic analgesic techniques used to differentiate distal hock joint pain from proximal suspensory desmitis.

Diagnosis

Clinical Signs

Swelling is a variable feature of hock-related lameness. There are numerous common swellings of the tarsus, but the presence of swelling is not pathognomonic for tarsal region pain (see Chapter 6, page 58, and Figures 6-28 through 6-32). Swellings include capped hock, which must be differentiated from lateral dislocation or luxation of the superficial digital flexor tendon and swelling of the calcaneal bursae; tarsal sheath–associated or, less commonly, non–sheath associated thoroughpin; bog spavin (effusion of the tarsocrural joint); bone spavin (bony prominence of the dorsal and medial aspects of the distal tarsal region); curb (see Figure 78-1), a collection of soft tissue injuries involving the distal plantar aspect of the hock; and diffuse soft tissue swelling in the distal aspect of the crus and dorsal aspect of the tarsus associated with injury of the fibularis (peroneus) tertius. Rapid development of diffuse periarticular swelling may follow trauma of the tarsus or may herald periarticular cellulitis. Distention of the tarsocrural joint can be an incidental finding but may reflect primary joint pathology. Distention of the distal hock joint capsules is rarely detectable clinically, but if it occurs in association with OA, there may be firm enlargement on the medial aspect of the limb reflecting periarticular new bone and overlying fibrous tissue. The presence of this swelling, bone spavin, is neither required for horses to be lame as a result of distal hock joint pain nor pathognomonic for distal hock joint pain in horses in which it is found. Swelling restricted to the medial or lateral aspect of the tarsus may reflect CL injury and malleolar fractures of the distal aspect of the tibia.

Some horses with tarsal region pain resent passive flexion, but exaggerated lifting of the limb to avoid maximal flexion is more likely to reflect stifle pain. Although there are many advocates of the Churchill test for the detection of distal hock joint pain (see Chapter 6), we do not find this test particularly useful because there are many false-positive and some false-negative responses. This may reflect the degree of pressure applied, because one author (SJD) is rarely able to induce pain, whereas the other (MWR) frequently does elicit a pain response. Some horses with distal hock joint pain do manifest a positive reaction to palpation of the medial soft tissue structures and the proximal medial metatarsal region, likely reflecting the presence of periarticular soft tissue pain associated with OA. Horses often manifest a positive response to compression of the distal medial aspect of the tarsus and proximal medial aspect of the metatarsal region statically, and lameness can often be exacerbated with compression of this region followed by trotting, a dynamic test; yet pain in these horses is localized

with diagnostic analgesia to the distal portion of the hindlimb. Proximal suspensory desmitis and lameness associated with the metatarsophalangeal joint are common diagnoses in these horses. It is possible that horses with distal hindlimb pain move abnormally and have coexistent pain in the region compressed using the Churchill test (see Figures 6-33 through 6-35). The absence of a positive Churchill test result should not lead the examiner to conclude the horse does not have tarsal region pain, a false-negative response. Unless clinical signs are diagnostic or a horse is suspected to have a fracture, diagnostic analgesia should always be used to confirm the presence of tarsal region pain.

Shoe wear can be excessive in horses with chronic tarsal region pain. Shoes are often worn on the toe or, most commonly, on the dorsal and lateral aspects (see Figure 6-38). Often, the fullering and toe grab, if present, are worn completely through, a finding that is most prominent in horses shod in aluminum shoes. Horses with pain causing lameness from other sources in the distal aspect of the hindlimb can manifest similar shoe wear, so this finding is not pathognomonic of distal hock joint pain. Horses with chronic tarsal region pain often have coexistent signs of pain on palpation of the gluteal and thoracolumbar area. Concurrent back and gluteal pain is likely secondary to chronic abnormal limb carriage causing muscle pain.

Lameness can range from mild to severe. Horses often warm out of lameness and are often able to perform with low-level distal hock joint pain. In racehorses, particular the Standardbred (STB), trainers often comment that the "horse throws away the lameness at speed." There are no pathognomonic clinical signs or gait deficits associated with tarsal region pain. Gait abnormalities associated with hock-related lameness are very variable both in degree and in character, depending on the underlying cause of lameness. A reduction in the cranial phase of the stride at the trot is a consistent finding but is a common finding in horses with any source of pain causing hindlimb lameness. When observed from behind, a trotting horse with tarsal region pain during protraction swings the affected hindlimb medially toward the midline and then stabs laterally while landing, often called a "stabby" hindlimb gait. This is particularly noticeable when horses have bilateral hindlimb lameness. Based on the clinical observation of a stabby hindlimb gait and positive response to upper limb flexion (see later) a diagnosis of distal hock joint pain is made, particularly in Western performance horses or gaited breeds, and empirical treatment is undertaken and is successful. However, this stabby hindlimb gait is not pathognomonic for tarsal region pain, and horses with lameness as a result of pain originating anywhere in the distal aspect of the hindlimbs can manifest this type of gait abnormality. Diagnostic analgesia should be used if horses do not respond to initial treatment. Some horses with severe tarsal region pain and swelling carry the limb wide, avoid flexion, and swing the limb laterally during protraction. These horses are often reluctant to flex the hock while standing during the palpation and manipulation portions of a lameness examination.

Kinematic gait measurements were recorded after endotoxin-induced lameness of the distal tarsal joints.[16] Both fetlock and tarsal joint extension during stance phase decreased, fetlock joint flexion and hoof height during swing phase increased, limb protraction decreased, and vertical excursion of the tuber coxae became more asymmetrical. These observations are not entirely consistent with the observations made in natural disease.

More recently, three-dimensional kinematic gait analysis was performed before and after experimental induction of synovitis of the centrodistal and tarsometatarsal joints resulting in mild lameness.[17] There were significant decreases in tarsal joint flexion and in dorsal translation (sliding) of the metatarsal region relative to the tibia during the stance phase.[17] Measurement of ground reaction forces with subtle lameness indicated reduced weight bearing on both the lame hindlimb and the contralateral forelimb but no change in the opposite hindlimb. Thus the gait may appear to have less bounce, rather than overt lameness being detectable. With mild increase in lameness there was reduced tarsal flexion in the stance phase and decreased forward sliding of the distal joints. This results in reduced propulsion, influencing quality of the gait, and less absorption of concussion. Movements that require maximum tarsal flexion are likely to be most painful, and resistance to perform such movements may be apparent before lameness is observed.

Horses with tarsal region pain often respond positively to an upper limb flexion test (see Chapter 8, page 84 and Figure 8-8). This test has erroneously been called the *spavin test* and a positive response should not be interpreted as pathognomonic for tarsal region pain. When it is suspected that a horse has tarsal region pain, this test often gives false-positive results. The most marked response to an upper limb flexion test may indeed be observed in horses with tarsal region pain, but a positive response can be seen with pain originating from the stifle, the hip region, and even the distal aspects of the limb. The upper limb flexion test is not specific, nor is the "hock extension test" (see Figure 8-10), a test used to exacerbate lameness in horses with tarsal region pain. There is no substitute for accurate diagnostic analgesia.

Diagnostic Analgesia
Analgesia of the hock region can be accomplished by perineural analgesia of the fibular (peroneal) and tibial nerves or by intraarticular analgesia. Although the latter is theoretically more specific, there are a number of important limitations. False negative results can occur in the presence of subchondral bone pain and/or extensive cartilage pathology. Horses with incomplete fractures of the talus or central tarsal bone often show little response to intraarticular diagnostic analgesia but do show a marked improvement after perineural analgesia of the fibular and tibial nerves. Lameness may be improved rather than abolished, and although this may be easy to appreciate in a moderately lame horse, it is less easy in a horse with a subtle lameness. Intraarticular analgesia has limited ability to influence periarticular soft tissue structures that may be contributing to pain causing lameness. The capacity of the centrodistal and tarsometatarsal joints is relatively small, and injection of too large a volume of local anesthetic solution results in leakage; the close proximity of the plantar outpouchings of the tarsometatarsal joint to the SL means that intraarticular analgesia of the tarsometatarsal joint may remove pain from the SL. With advanced joint space loss or periarticular new bone formation, intraarticular analgesia may not be physically possible.

Perineural analgesia of the fibular and tibial nerves is well tolerated by most horses (see Chapter 10). One of us (SJD) deposits a subcutaneous bleb of local anesthetic solution at both injection sites using a 25-G needle before performing the blocks. Although a 3.7-cm needle is adequate for most horses, to reach the deep branch of the fibular nerve requires a 5-cm needle in large (700 kg) horses. These nerves are large, and it takes longer for analgesia to develop than with more distal limb blocks. Do not be in a hurry to move proximally in the limb and perform intraarticular analgesia of the stifle or hip joints, because these blocks may take a full hour to work. We usually first evaluate the horse 20 minutes after injection and for up to an hour. It is important to recognize that successful blocks may increase or create a toe drag; improved stride length, rhythm, and symmetry of the hindquarters must therefore be used to evaluate improvement in lameness. Occasionally a horse will stumble slightly after fibular and tibial nerve blocks, but we commonly see horses ridden before and after and do not believe there are undue risks.

When performing intraarticular analgesia of the distal tarsal joints, we routinely block the tarsometatarsal joint first, because this is relatively easy and safe to perform, and commonly find that horses with centrodistal joint pathology are improved. If there is partial or no response, then the centrodistal joint is blocked. In a study using 66 cadaver limbs, mepivacaine (5 mL) was injected into either the tarsometatarsal or centrodistal joints; synovial fluid samples were collected from the tarsocrural, centrodistal, and tarsometatarsal joints 15 minutes later.[12] Concentrations of mepivacaine that were potentially analgesic were found in the centrodistal and tarsocrural joints after injection of the tarsometatarsal joint in 64% and 4% of limbs, respectively. After injection of the centrodistal joint, analgesic concentrations of mepivacaine were found in the tarsometatarsal and tarsocrural joints in 60% and 24% of limbs, respectively. Despite these results we have never clinically recognized improvement in tarsocrural joint pain after intraarticular analgesia of the centrodistal and/or tarsometatarsal joints. We use a maximum volume of 3 to 4 mL of mepivacaine and evaluate the response 5 to 10 minutes after injection. Larger volumes will leak out of the injection site, increasing the likelihood of inadvertent analgesia of the proximal SL and other metatarsal structures. False-negative results may occur even in the absence of detectable radiological abnormalities, and the response to intraarticular medication may be substantially better. However for the much larger tarsocrural joint we use at least 20 mL of mepivacaine and will wait up to 30 minutes before declaring that the response is negative. One of us (MWR) has found that volumes of local anesthetic solution of up to 40 to 50 mL may be required to abolish pain associated with severe OA of the tarsocrural joint, and often the examiner needs to wait 45 to 60 minutes for the full effect of the intraarticular block to work.

DIAGNOSTIC IMAGING
Four radiographic images of the tarsus are required: lateromedial, dorsolateral-plantaromedial oblique, dorsomedial-plantarolateral oblique (DM-PILO), and dorsoplantar.[18] Lesions may be detectable only in a single view; thus in our opinion all four views should be obtained routinely.

To cut through the centrodistal and tarsometatarsal joint spaces, it is important that the horse be standing with the metatarsal region vertical and bearing weight evenly on each hindlimb. Because the centrodistal and tarsometatarsal joints slope distally from laterally to medially, to reliably cut through the joint spaces in a lateromedial image, the x-ray beam should be angled 10 degrees distally. If a horizontal x-ray beam is used, it can be difficult to cut through the entire centrodistal joint space in a dorsoplantar projection, and it may appear that one side of the joint is narrowed. An additional dorsal 5° proximal-plantarodistal oblique image helps to determine whether there is genuine joint space narrowing.

Some lesions may be missed in dorsoplantar images, such as an axial osteochondrosis lesion of the medial malleolus of the tibia or a parasagittal fracture of the talus. Additional views obtained by angling the x-ray beam slightly obliquely (dorsal 10- to 20° lateral-plantaromedial oblique image) may be required in selected horses. A flexed lateromedial image and a flexed skyline image can give important additional information in some horses, particularly those with lesions involving the proximal and plantar aspects of the talus, those with osteochondral fragments involving the plantar pouch of the tarsocrural joint, and those with radiolucent defects on the calcaneus. A flexed dorsoplantar image can be useful to evaluate the proximal aspect of the talus in horses with incomplete fractures of this bone but is difficult to obtain.

Nuclear scintigraphy is most useful when pain causing lameness has been localized to the tarsus but no radiological or ultrasonographic abnormalities are detected to explain the lameness.[19] The identification of increased radiopharmaceutical uptake (IRU) may prompt acquisition of additional radiographic images that yield a diagnosis. Scintigraphy may also be useful in horses that are difficult to nerve block or those that are examined for poor performance rather than overt lameness. It is important to recognize that RU in the distal tarsal bones can be influenced by the type of work history. For example, there is greater RU in the dorsal aspect of the central and third tarsal bones in elite show jumpers compared with horses from other disciplines.[5] In a plantar scintigraphic image of the tarsus it is common and considered normal to have greater RU in the subchondral bone of the lateral aspect of the tarsometatarsal joint and the proximal aspect of the MtIV compared with medially.[20] This finding should not be interpreted as supportive of a diagnosis of distal hock joint pain. In young racehorses with early OA of the centrodistal and tarsometatarsal joints, focal moderate-to-intense IRU is found most often in the dorsal and lateral aspects of these joints, corresponding to radiological abnormalities detectable on the dorsomedial-plantarolateral radiographic image.[21] The most common location for fractures of the central and third tarsal bones is on the dorsolateral aspect, and fractures can most reliably be seen in the dorsomedial-plantarolateral oblique radiographic image (Figure 44-1). These findings differ somewhat from most anecdotal reports, suggesting that it is the medial aspect of these joints that show early radiological changes and may be a reflection of a difference between racehorses and sports horses. In older racehorses with advanced OA and sports horses, scintigraphic and radiological evidence of OA is commonly found on both the medial and lateral aspects of the distal hock joints.

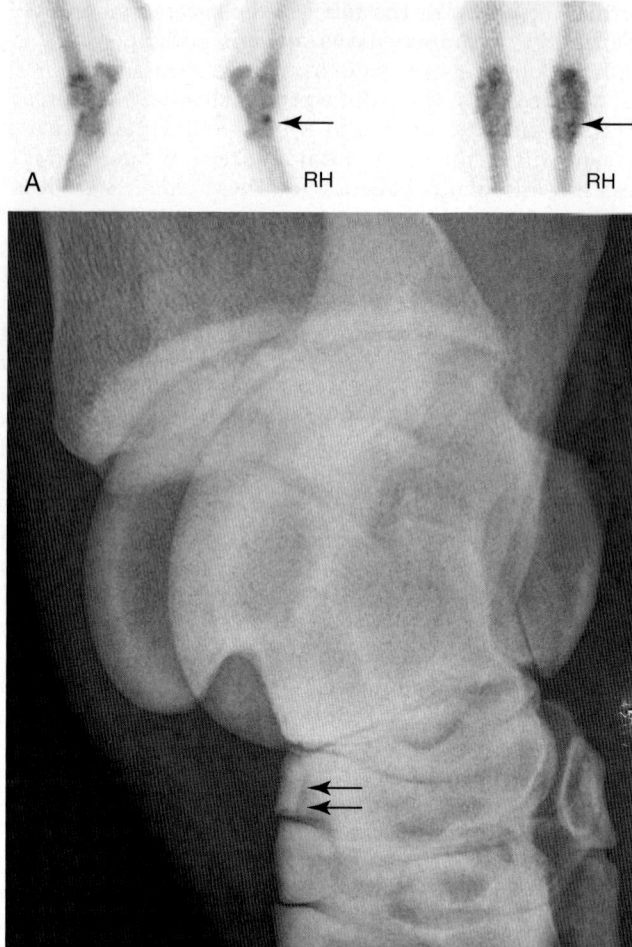

Fig. 44-1 • A, Lateral (left two images) and plantar scintigraphic images of a 2-year-old Standardbred pacing filly with right hindlimb lameness as a result of a central tarsal bone fracture. Focal, moderate increased radiopharmaceutical uptake can be seen involving the dorsolateral aspect of this bone (arrows), a common location to find fractures or early osteoarthritis in racehorses. **B,** Dorsomedial-plantarolateral (DM-PILO) digital radiographic image showing an incomplete fracture of the central tarsal bone (arrows). Fractures of the central and third tarsal bones and early signs of osteoarthritis can be seen most commonly in a DM-PILO radiographic view, indicating disease in young racehorses is found in predominantly the dorsal and lateral aspects of the distal hock joints.

Ultrasonography is invaluable for the assessment of both periarticular soft tissues and the tarsocrural joint. An excellent review of normal anatomy and examples of abnormality are published elsewhere.[22] Magnetic resonance imaging (MRI) and computed tomography (CT) have the potential to yield valuable additional information when a diagnosis cannot be reached by other means. Normal MRI and CT anatomy references are available.[23-25]

ARTICULAR DISEASES OF THE TARSUS

Osteoarthritis of the Distal Hock Joints and Distal Hock Joint Pain

Distal hock joint pain is common in horses from all disciplines and is often associated with OA. Distal hock joint pain is known colloquially as *bone* or *jack spavin* or *occult* or *blind spavin* in the absence of radiological abnormalities. The term *juvenile spavin* has been used to describe early OA that had a prevalence of 20% in a group of horses younger than 2 years of age.[26] Although it is usually seen in mature horses used for sport or pleasure, distal hock joint pain can occur in young Thoroughbred (TB) and STB racehorses and Western performance horses (see Chapter 120). Distal hock joint pain may be a sequela to incomplete ossification of the central and third tarsal bones (see page 517). Certain conformational abnormalities (such as sickle-hock, in-at-the-hock, or cow-hock conformation) or excessive straightness of the hindlimbs may predispose to distal hock joint pain, although this condition frequently occurs in normally conformed horses. Traditionally it has been proposed that OA of the distal hock joints is caused by excessive compression and rotation of the distal tarsal joints as the horse jumps or stops, which results in abnormal tension on the intertarsal ligaments. However, this theory is not consistent with the common recognition of distal hock joint pain in pleasure horses or its high incidence in Icelandic horses, a breed in which OA is thought to be a heritable condition.[27] Distal hock joint pain is classically thought to begin on the dorsomedial aspect of the joints and to progress dorsally. However, it is our experience that in OA, scintigraphic or radiological abnormalities are frequently first identified only on the dorsolateral aspect of the joints, a region of high compressive strain. Previous exercise history and thus loading of the joints may be influential.[28] Nuclear scintigraphic studies of clinically normal mature horses in active work has shown mild greater uptake of radiopharmaceutical on the lateral aspect, which is consistent with increased modeling, presumably the result of a relative increased loading laterally compared with medially.[7]

The centrodistal and tarsometatarsal joints are most commonly affected, either individually or together, but OA of the proximal intertarsal joint does occur, usually in association with OA of the more distal joints. The condition may be unilateral but is often bilateral. Occasionally OA of the talocalcaneal joint occurs either in isolation[29,30] or together with OA of the centrodistal and tarsometatarsal joints[31] (see page 516).

History

Clinical signs of distal hock joint pain vary considerably among horses, ranging from a moderate-to-severe unilateral lameness to subtle changes in performance without overt lameness (see Chapters 97 and 106 to 129). These signs include the horse becoming disunited in canter, being unwilling to canter with a particular lead, and being reluctant to turn or decelerate with proper engagement of the hindlimbs. The owner may comment that the farrier has experienced difficulties when shoeing the horse. Frequently a horse with bilateral distal hock joint pain has low-grade stiffness that wears off (warms out of pain) with work. Lameness frequently improves or resolves with rest but recurs when work is resumed. Treatment with nonsteroidal antiinflammatory drugs (NSAIDs) usually results in an improvement in lameness unless it is severe.

Clinical Signs

In many horses no abnormalities are detectable by visual inspection or palpation of the hock region. In horses with more chronic distal hock joint pain there may be enlargement over the medial or dorsomedial aspects of the distal hock joints, which is the result of periarticular soft tissue thickening. Distention of the tarsocrural joint capsule may occur either coincidentally or reflect involvement of the proximal intertarsal joint. Frequently there is secondary soreness of the epaxial muscles in the lumbar region and sometimes caudal gluteal muscle soreness. The toe and branches of the shoe of the lame limb, or both limbs, may wear abnormally. In our experience, shoe wear in this location, however, is not pathognomonic of distal hock joint pain. Some horses, if not properly trimmed, develop lateral flare of the hoof and mediolateral foot imbalance, with the foot higher medially. Lameness may worsen when shoe additives such as toe grabs and heel calks are applied, an observation that can be useful in therapeutically shoeing a horse with distal hock joint pain (see later). Flexion of the limb may be resisted slightly, but marked lifting of the limb during flexion is more likely to reflect stifle pain. The Churchill test (see Chapter 6) is helpful in identifying distal hock joint pain in some, but by no means all, horses. Soreness associated with specific acupuncture points (see Chapter 92) can also be suggestive of distal hock joint pain.

Lameness varies greatly in degree and is not necessarily correlated with the degree or type of osteoarthritic change detected radiologically. The horse should be assessed moving from the side, from behind, and from in front to appreciate all gait abnormalities. These abnormalities may include asymmetrical movement of the tubera coxae and tubera sacrale; reduced arc height of foot flight, with or without toe drag; shortening of the cranial phase of the stride; reduced extension of the fetlock; and a tendency for the limb to swing medially during protraction and slide laterally at ground contact. Lameness may be accentuated on a circle, in some horses with the lame or lamer limb on the outside, and in others with it on the inside. Gait abnormalities may be accentuated if the horse is ridden. However, none of these characteristics is pathognomonic for distal hock joint pain.

Proximal (upper) limb flexion tests (i.e., the so-called *spavin test*) are useful in accentuating lameness in some, but not all, horses with distal hock joint pain. The hindlimb should be held with the metatarsal region parallel to the ground for 60 to 90 seconds before the horse is trotted away. The limb may be held either by the toe of the foot or by cupping the hands behind the fetlock. Applying pressure to the digital flexor tendons should be avoided. The response to flexion should be interpreted in light of the discipline of the horse, current work history, the degree of accentuation of lameness, and its duration. Flexion of the nonlame or least lame limb should be performed first and the response compared with the contralateral limb. In some horses there is a paradoxical increase in lameness in the weight-bearing limb, presumably because of joint compression or increased subchondral bone pressure. Because of the reciprocal apparatus of the hindlimb, a positive response to proximal limb flexion is not specific for distal hock joint pain. The response to flexion may be recorded as none (0), mild (+1), moderate (+2), or severe (+3). A severe response is unusual in horses with distal hock joint pain.

Diagnostic Analgesia

Diagnostic analgesia is important to confirm the source(s) of pain. Although intraarticular analgesia is potentially

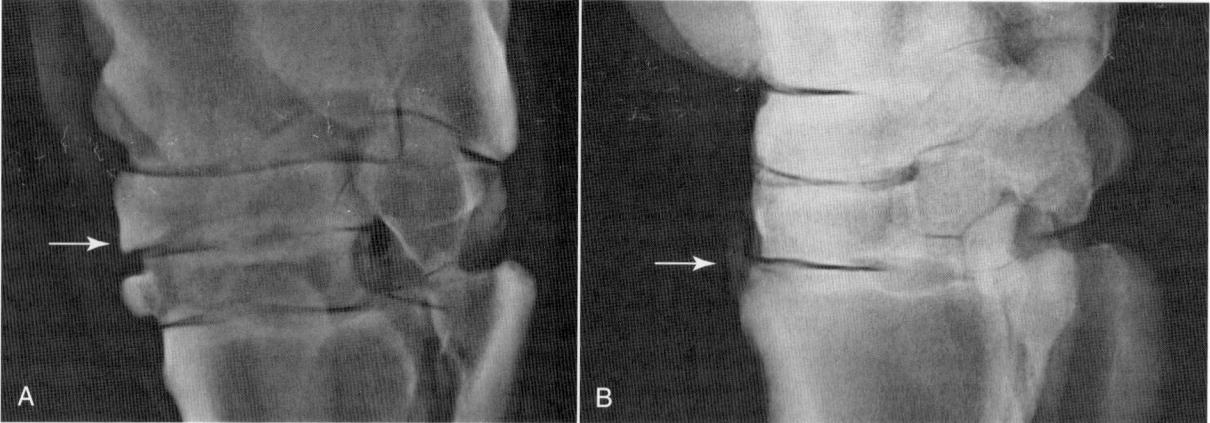

Fig. 44-2 • A, Dorsolateral-plantaromedial oblique radiographic image of the tarsus of a horse with mild periarticular osteophyte formation *(arrow)* on the distal dorsomedial aspect of the central tarsal bone and increased radiopacity of the adjacent trabecular bone. **B,** Lateromedial radiographic image of the distal tarsal joints. There is a large periarticular osteophyte on the dorsoproximal aspect of the third metatarsal bone *(arrow)*, traversing the tarsometatarsal joint.

more specific than perineural analgesia, the results can be misleading. A negative response to intraarticular analgesia does not preclude distal hock joint pain. Narrowing of the centrodistal joint space or periarticular new bone can prohibit intraarticular injection. In the presence of extensive subchondral bone damage the response to intraarticular analgesia is very poor. Even in the absence of radiological change the response to intraarticular medication is sometimes substantially better than that to intraarticular analgesia, but the converse is also true in some horses.

However, intraarticular analgesia is very useful in many horses. The degree of communication between the centrodistal and tarsometatarsal joints is variable.[9,10] The techniques for intraarticular analgesia are described in Chapter 10. Improvement in lameness by 50% or more is considered a positive response. In our experience, lameness is often substantially improved within 10 minutes, although some practitioners reassess lameness after 30 minutes.[32] We find reassessment of the response to flexion potentially misleading, although some practitioners routinely repeat flexion tests.[32] Perineural analgesia of the superficial and deep fibular (peroneal) and tibial nerves (see Chapter 10), although not specific for distal hock joint pain, can be very helpful in confirming hock pain, assuming that pain arising from the more distal aspects of the limb has already been excluded. With practice these blocks are reliable and safe and often result in a much greater degree of improvement in lameness than intraarticular analgesia. Improvement is generally seen within 20 minutes, but occasionally the response is delayed, and it is preferable not to proceed with further blocks until at least 1 hour has elapsed. Horses with specific performance problems associated with distal hock joint pain, rather than overt lameness, may respond better to intraarticular medication than either intraarticular or perineural analgesia.

Radiography and Radiology

Both hocks should be examined radiographically because the condition is often bilateral, although at the time of examination lameness may be unilateral. Radiological abnormalities consistent with osteoarthritis include periarticular osteophyte formation (Figure 44-2), subchondral

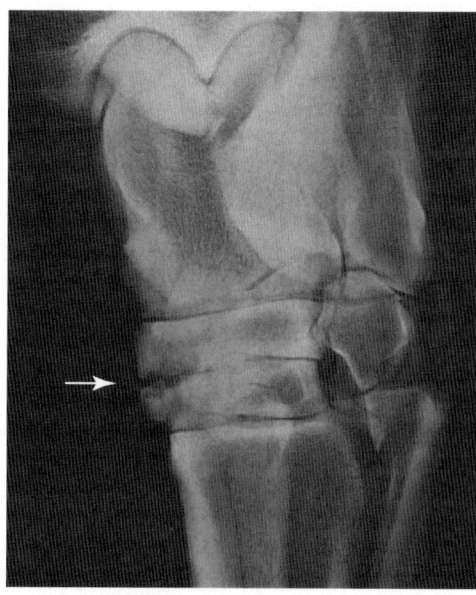

Fig. 44-3 • Dorsolateral-plantaromedial oblique radiographic image of the tarsus of a horse with osteoarthritis of the centrodistal joint. There is subchondral radiolucency involving the subchondral bone of the medial aspect of the centrodistal joint *(arrow)*. There is also increased opacity in the region of the interosseous ligament between the central and third tarsal bones.

lucent areas (Figure 44-3), increased opacity of subchondral and trabecular bone, periosteal new bone, and narrowing of joint spaces. The correlation between the degree of lameness and the extent of radiological abnormalities is poor.[33,34] Some horses show profound lameness initially, with no detectable radiological abnormality but with rapidly progressive lesions. Other horses respond to intraarticular analgesia but never develop radiological abnormalities. However, extensive changes may be present when lameness is first recognized. Some horses predominantly develop periarticular changes, whereas others have abnormalities confined to the central and third tarsal bones and the proximal aspect of the MtIII. The reason for these differences is currently unclear. Small osteophytes or enthesophytes on the dorsoproximal aspect of the MtIII can be incidental radiological abnormalities; they were found to occur in 25% of 455 horses, in 13% of which they were bilateral.[35] Osteophytes and enthesophytes could not be reliably distinguished. There was no significant difference in frequency of occurrence in lame and nonlame horses; nor was there any significant difference in frequency of occurrence among horses with distal hock joint pain, proximal suspensory desmitis, or other causes of lameness unassociated with the hock.[35] However, there was an association between the presence of a spur and the radiological grade of OA in the centrodistal and tarsometatarsal joints. Horses with severe subchondral radiolucency tend to be lamer and respond poorly to intraarticular analgesia and intraarticular medication. Involvement of the talocalcaneal-centroquartal (proximal intertarsal) joint merits a more guarded prognosis.

Nuclear Scintigraphy
In many horses nuclear scintigraphy is unnecessary, but it can be very helpful in difficult horses and those with performance problems rather than overt lameness.[19,36] A region of IRU may be focal or more diffuse. Very focal IRU may reflect intertarsal ligament enthesopathy rather than OA.[37] Intense IRU may be present in the absence of radiological abnormality, and these horses tend to respond poorly to intraarticular medication, despite a positive response to intraarticular analgesia. In young racehorses and in some sports horses, focal IRU can indicate the presence of a fracture of the central or third tarsal bone (see Figure 44-1), explaining the lack of response to intraarticular medication. Because IRU may occur in association with primary lameness originating from pain elsewhere in the limb, results should be interpreted cautiously, unless supported by radiological abnormalities.

Treatment
The aim of treatment is to provide pain relief so that the horse can remain in work. Traditionally it has been suggested that if the horse is maintained in work, the affected joints will fuse. However, progressive radiological ankylosis is rarely observed, although radiological examination tends to underestimate the degree of joint fusion. Horses with involvement of the talocalcaneal-centroquartal joint and extensive radiolucent defects of subchondral bone have a more guarded prognosis.

Treatment options include a combination of palliative therapy with NSAIDs; intraarticular medication with corticosteroids, hyaluronan, or polysulfated glycosaminoglycans (PSGAGs); with or without systemic treatment with PSGAGs, oral nutraceuticals, or both, combined with corrective trimming and shoeing[38]; and adaptation of the work program. Extracorporeal shock wave treatment has recently been described, but long-term results are lacking.[39] Intravenous infusion of a bisphosphonate, tiludronate, may reduce the severity of lameness in some horses but rarely results in resolution of lameness.[40] If medical therapy fails, surgical treatment, including cunean tenectomy, subchondral forage to reduce intraosseous pressure,[41] drilling of the affected joints to promote arthrodesis,[42] chemical induction of ankylosis using sodium monoiodoacetate[43-51] or ethyl alcohol,[46] and neurectomy[47] are options.

Selection of treatment depends on the degree of lameness, extent of radiological abnormalities, use of the horse, regulations for competition, response to previous treatment, time available, and financial constraints. Resting the horse usually is not beneficial. Palliative treatment with NSAIDs such as phenylbutazone is useful in pleasure horses; the lowest dose that alleviates lameness should be used. Long-term use of phenylbutazone, 1 g twice daily for a 500-kg horse, is generally well tolerated. Any treatment should be combined with corrective trimming and shoeing to ensure correct mediolateral balance and to facilitate breakover by shortening the toe, squaring and rolling the toe of the shoe, or setting the shoe back from the toe. A lateral trailer[14] or a lateral extension of the shoe provides symptomatic relief in some horses and tends to stop excessive twisting of the limb. However, these devices may be contraindicated in horses that have to stop and turn quickly, because the extension may dig into the footing and stop the distal limb abruptly, causing abnormal torque on the distal limb joints. Removing toe grabs and heel calks and using a flat shoe may reduce shear stress on the distal hock joints.

Intraarticular medication with corticosteroids, such as methylprednisolone acetate or triamcinolone acetonide, with or without hyaluronan, is extremely useful for management of horses with distal hock joint pain. However, horses with extensive radiological abnormalities, especially diffuse radiolucent regions in the subchondral bone, often have a limited response. Horses with scintigraphic abnormalities in the absence of radiological change also respond poorly. Some veterinarians routinely treat both the centrodistal and tarsometatarsal joints of both hocks by using 60 to 80 mg of methylprednisolone acetate in each joint.[29] If the competition schedule allows, the horse is turned out for 3 to 4 days, followed by 3 to 4 days of light riding before resumption of normal activity. Phenylbutazone (2.2 mg/kg sid) is also recommended for 7 days to decrease the possibility of postinjection joint flare. Most horses are sound enough to resume work within 7 to 10 days and stay serviceably sound for 3 to 6 months, depending on severity of disease and level of horse use.

Similar results have been achieved using triamcinolone acetonide, 6 mg per joint (SJD). One of us (SJD) does not routinely combine intraarticular therapy with NSAIDs and usually treats only the tarsometatarsal joint. A study by Serena and colleagues demonstrated that therapeutic concentrations of methylprednisolone acetate were achieved in the centrodistal joint within 6 hours of injection of 80 mg into the tarsometatarsal joint in eight of nine horses (in the ninth horse concentrations were similar in both joints, indicating direct communication between the two joints).[13] However, higher concentrations can be obtained by direct injection. There are no controlled clinical trials assessing the relative efficacy of different corticosteroids or the use of a combination of corticosteroids and hyaluronan, although some clinicians believe that combination therapy lasts longer. Hyaluronan alone is of dubious value. There are also no large-scale, long-term follow-up studies. However, in a retrospective study of 42 horses that were examined at a referral hospital and used predominantly for general purposes or amateur-level competitions and that showed a positive response (>50% improvement in lameness) to intraarticular analgesia of the tarsometatarsal or centrodistal joints, 38% became sound enough to resume full work after intraarticular medication with either triamcinolone acetonide or methylprednisolone acetate.[48] In a different study with similar inclusion criteria, 52% of 46 horses were able to return to their former athletic function.[49] The choice of drug did not influence outcome in either study. Both studies showed no relationship between the severity of radiological abnormality and outcome. However, we believe that this reflects one of the inclusion criteria that horses had to respond to intraarticular analgesia. In our experience horses with extensive subchondral radiolucent areas respond poorly to both intraarticular analgesia and medical treatment.

Corticosteroid injections can be repeated two or three times per year without promoting progressive radiological change. In some horses it is possible to predict when lameness will recur, and repeated treatment before this recurrence can maintain soundness. Although cunean bursitis is rarely recognized as a primary cause of lameness, some horses respond better if intraarticular treatment is combined with treatment of the bursa. In young racehorses with distal hock joint pain, one of us (MWR) uses a combination of intraarticular injection (tarsometatarsal and centrodistal joints) of a combination of corticosteroids (methylprednisolone acetate [40 to 80 mg/joint] and isoflupredone acetate [2 mg/joint]) and infiltration of this combination of corticosteroids and Sarapin into the cunean bursa and subcutaneously over the proximal aspect of the MtII. It is in this area on the medial aspect of the tarsus and proximal aspect of the metatarsal region that these horses show a positive response to deep palpation (see earlier). A series of intraarticular injections of PSGAG (three injections given every 2 weeks) can be useful in competition horses and racehorses with distal hock joint pain.

Systemic medication with PSGAG (500 mg intramuscularly [IM] once weekly for 6 weeks), hyaluronan (4 mg intravenously [IV] monthly), or oral nutraceuticals may be beneficial as adjunctive therapy. A small-scale study showed reduced frequency of intraarticular medication after the introduction of oral nutraceuticals.[50] Anecdotally, treatment with PSGAG 3 to 4 days before an event may be useful. In some horses, increasing the dose of PSGAG to 1 g weekly gives better results. Clinical trials with intravenous administration of tiludronate have shown mixed results; overall there was a positive effect on the degree of lameness, but lameness did not resolve in the majority.[40]

In a small-scale study shock wave treatment that was performed with horses under general anesthesia, followed by 5 weeks of rest, resulted in an 80% improvement in lameness in horses 90 days later,[39] but long-term results are not available.

A variety of techniques for surgical arthrodesis of the distal hock joints* and subchondral forage[41] exists. Subchondral forage, which aims to reduce intraosseous pressure and therefore pain, can provide rapid pain relief in some horses, enabling return to work. However, this technique has not found widespread favor. Techniques aimed at achieving arthrodesis are more popular, but effective arthrodesis and resolution of lameness often takes up to 12 months using either drill or laser techniques. Careful surgical technique is essential to avoid the development of extensive periarticular new bone, which can itself cause pain. With use of the three-drill tract procedure,[42,51] a 66%

success rate has been reported.[51] However, the results in upper-level competition horses have been less favorable.[32] In Western performance horses a success rate of approximately 70% has been achieved.[56] Generally both the centrodistal and tarsometatarsal joints are treated. Cunean tenectomy alone may result in temporary improvement in clinical signs but is unlikely to restore soundness.[57] Chemical fusion with sodium monoiodoacetate has had excellent results in some horses,[43,45] with reported success rates of 27 of 29 horses (93%) and 41 of 50 (82%) horses 12 months after treatment. However, even if positive radiographic contrast studies do not show physical communication between the centrodistal and talocalcaneal-centroquartal joint, it is likely that in some horses sodium monoiodoacetate can spread to these joints and result in progressive OA. Ethyl alcohol can also be used to achieve arthrodesis,[46] but there are currently no long-term follow-up results, although anecdotally the results are favorable. Arthrodesis of the centrodistal and tarsometatarsal joints can be followed by either fracture of the central or third tarsal bone or the development of OA in the talocalcaneal-centroquartal joint. Once OA of this joint has developed, there is obligatory involvement of the tarsocrural joint, and chronic, severe lameness ensues. Neurectomy of the deep fibular nerve and a partial neurectomy of the tibial nerves relieves the pain associated with OA of the distal hock joints,[47] and approximately 60% of treated horses return to full athletic function.

Osteoarthritis of the Talocalcaneal Joint

OA of the talocalcaneal joint is unusual and may occur in isolation[29,30] or together with OA of the centrodistal and/or tarsometatarsal joints.[31] There are frequently no localizing signs, although in a retrospective study there was distention of the tarsocrural joint in six of 18 horses.[31] Lameness is resolved by perineural analgesia of the fibular and tibial nerves and may be improved by intraarticular analgesia of the tarsocrural joint. Radiological abnormalities are best identified in lateromedial or dorsomedial-plantarolateral oblique images, or in some horses a flexed proximoplantar-distal plantar image, and include subchondral lucency or increased radiopacity and narrowing of the joint space (Figure 44-4). Scintigraphy reveals focal, moderate-to-intense IRU in the subchondral bone of the talocalcaneal joint and can be differentiated from enthesopathy of the attachment of the lateral CL and lesions involving the sustentaculum tali (see later) by acquiring lateral, plantar, and, if necessary, medial and flexed lateral scintigraphic images. Occasionally lesions that are not evident radiologically can be identified using MRI or CT. The prognosis with conservative management is guarded to poor. Surgical arthrodesis has resulted in improvement in, but not resolution of, lameness.[31]

Osteoarthritis of the Tarsocrural Joint

OA of the tarsocrural joint may occur as a primary disease, may develop secondarily to osteochondrosis (see Chapter 56) or OA of the distal hock joints (see page 512), or may be a sequela to trauma. There may be distention of the tarsocrural joint capsule, but this is a variable feature. The joint capsule may feel thickened, more so than observed in horses with idiopathic effusion or a bog spavin as the result of osteochondritis dissecans (OCD). Initially horses

*References 17, 21, 22, 41, 51-56.

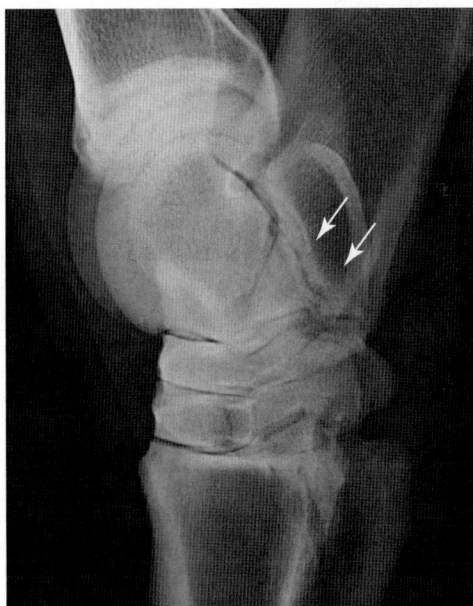

Fig. 44-4 • Lateromedial radiographic image of a tarsus of a horse with osteoarthritis of the talocalcaneal joint. Some loss of joint space and irregular subchondral radiolucency *(arrows)* are present.

respond favorably to intraarticular injections into the tarsocrural joint. There is controversy regarding the association of corticosteroid injections and the subsequent development of OA of this joint. Although in most horses with end-stage OA there is a history of numerous injections including corticosteroids into the tarsocrural joint, this is not always the case. We both believe that there is an association between the presence of OCD and the subsequent development of severe OA in older horses (6- to 8-year-old racehorses and sports horses), whether or not the affected horse had arthroscopic surgery to remove the fragments at a young age.

Lameness varies from mild to severe. Horses with longitudinal wear lines on the trochleas of the talus secondary to OCD of the cranial intermediate ridge of the distal aspect of the tibia often have only mild lameness. However, horses with focal partial- or full-thickness cartilage erosions on weight-bearing parts of the trochleas of the talus may have severe lameness (see Figure 56-11). The response to proximal limb flexion is variable. Lameness usually is partially improved by intraarticular analgesia, but occasionally there are false-negative results. A large volume (up to 50 mL) of local anesthetic solution may be necessary, and often it takes 45 to 60 minutes for lameness to improve in horses with severe OA of the tarsocrural joint. Perineural analgesia of the fibular and tibial nerves results in substantial improvement in lameness. In horses with primary OA of the tarsocrural joint, usually there are no detectable radiological abnormalities, or only subtle evidence of subchondral sclerosis and narrowing of the tarsocrural joint space, and scintigraphic examination is often inconclusive. Diffuse mild IRU may be all that is seen, sometimes localized to the cranial and caudal distal aspect of the tibia. In racehorses, scintigraphic examination often reveals IRU involving the distal aspect of the tibia and proximal aspect of the talus and must be differentiated from subchondral trauma or fracture of the distal tibia and talus.[58] A flexed lateral

scintigraphic image reveals that IRU involves both sides of the tarsocrural joint, unlike focal uptake, which remains associated with either the talus or the distal tibia. Ultrasonographic examination may reveal synovial proliferation even in the absence of detectable joint effusion. Definitive diagnosis is dependent on arthroscopic examination of the joint. The prognosis for resolution of lameness and return to full athletic function is generally poor to grave. Response to intraarticular medication is often disappointing.

Incomplete Ossification of the Central and Third Tarsal Bones
Incomplete ossification of the central and third tarsal bones is most common in premature or twin foals, but it can occur in full-term singles and is characterized by a sickle-hocked appearance. It may occur unilaterally or bilaterally. Radiologically the bones are smaller and more rounded than usual. Early recognition and treatment are essential to avoid crushing of these bones with resultant progressive OA. Foals with this condition must be rested in a stall or turned out in a small paddock with only their mare. However, many owners or farm managers are loath to give foals rest, and the condition becomes progressive, often leading to collapse and OA and fracture. Cylinder tube casts can be used effectively with good results. In some horses the condition goes unrecognized until a young horse increases work intensity, although the horse may have a preexisting curblike appearance of the hock. Lameness may be sudden in onset despite the existence of advanced radiological changes. Radiological examination reveals a wedge shape of the central and third tarsal bones, which are narrower dorsally (see Figure 128-4). One or more bones may be fractured. There is often advanced OA. Although affected horses may be used for pleasure riding, the prognosis for competition use is guarded.

Distention of the Tarsocrural Joint Capsule
There are many causes of acute or chronic synovitis of the tarsocrural joint (also known as *bog spavin*) including osteochondrosis, OA, trauma, poor conformation, hemarthrosis, infection, and idiopathic causes. There are case reports of eosinophilic synovitis[59] and ectopic cartilage of unknown origin.[60] Signalment varies and depends on origin. Clinical signs are excessive tarsocrural joint fluid, which is most easily recognized on the dorsomedial and plantarolateral aspects of the joint. Lameness may or may not be present and is dependent on the cause. Excessive distention of the joint capsule may result in mechanical lameness. Diagnosis is made on the basis of clinical appearance and the response to intraarticular analgesia if the horse is lame. Arthrocentesis may reveal hemorrhage. Oddly, the tarsocrural and antebrachiocarpal joints are the most common joints in which we have diagnosed intermittent severe lameness as a result of hemarthrosis.[21] Large vessels that traverse the dorsal aspects of the joint capsules in both joints may be at risk for injury and cause subsequent bleeding into the joint. Radiographic examination should include four standard images, but if no radiological abnormality is detected, flexed lateromedial and flexed dorsoplantar (skyline) images may be helpful. Slightly oblique dorsoplantar images may be necessary to identify OCD of the medial malleolus of the tibia (see Chapter 56). The radiographs should be

inspected carefully for evidence of previous surgery for removal of an osteochondral fragment from the cranial intermediate ridge of the distal aspect of the tibia or other common locations associated with OCD. Occasionally, small fragments remain at previous sites from which OCD lesions were removed, and it is possible that these small fragments or repair tissue at the site may be loose, causing persistent effusion. Lameness in these horses is usually minimal, and the decision to reoperate should be made on a case-by-case basis and reserved for those horses with pain that can be abolished with diagnostic analgesia. Effusion often persists even after removal of OCD fragments from the tarsocrural joint, and persistent effusion is usually not a cause of lameness but may be of concern cosmetically.

Ultrasonography is useful for characterizing the appearance of the fluid within the joint; synovial fluid is anechogenic, whereas blood is echogenic. Ultrasonography is also useful for assessment of the thickness of the joint capsule, the presence of synovial hyperplasia, and the thickness of the articular cartilage and may be more accurate than radiography for identification of osteochondral fragments.[61] In the absence of radiological or ultrasonographic abnormalities, a diagnosis of idiopathic synovitis is made.

Treatment of horses with idiopathic synovitis involves fluid drainage and intraarticular injection of either 80 mg of methylprednisolone acetate or 12 mg of triamcinolone acetonide. Combining hyaluronan with the corticosteroids may provide joint protection, but the strong antiinflammatory effect of the corticosteroids seems most beneficial. Pressure bandages should be applied to help maintain joint decompression. Phenylbutazone (2.2 mg/kg) once daily for 7 days and confinement to a small area for 2 weeks is recommended. Approximately 50% of horses have resolution or decrease in effusion, although some horses may require retreatment. Intraarticular injection of atropine (8 mg) is sometimes successful. If joint effusion returns and the horse is not lame, the owner is advised that the horse has a cosmetic blemish that will probably not resolve completely. Horses that are lame and block to the tarsocrural joint but have no radiological lesions are candidates for scintigraphic examination and diagnostic arthroscopy (see discussion of OA of the tarsocrural joint, page 516). Hemarthrosis is discussed in Chapter 66.

Osteochondrosis of the Tarsocrural Joint
See Chapter 56 for a discussion of osteochondrosis of the tarsocrural joint (page 635).

Subchondral Bone Trauma
With the advent of MRI and CT there is increasing recognition of the role of subchondral bone trauma and pain in causing lameness.[62] There are anecdotal reports of lesions involving the talus, calcaneus, and central and third tarsal bones, but as yet these lesions have been rather poorly defined, and risk factors and response to treatment have not been documented.

Osseous Cystlike Lesions
Occult osseous cystlike lesions, detected using CT but usually not by radiography, have been recorded in the medial malleolus of the tibia (five horses), intertrochlear groove of the talus (four horses), lateral malleolus (two horses), and cranial intermediate ridge of the distal aspect

of the tibia (one horse).[63] We have also seen single or multiple lesions in the distal subchondral bone plate of the tibia and the trochleas of the talus that were detectable scintigraphically and radiologically.[64] There are usually no localizing clinical signs. Lameness is moderate to severe. In some but not all horses lameness is substantially improved by intraarticular analgesia of the tarsocrural joint. These lesions are associated with focal intense IRU. These lesions are believed to be of infectious or traumatic origin. Conservative management has resulted in persistent lameness in most but not all horses. Surgical curettage may offer a more favorable prognosis, but lesions involving the subchondral bone of the distal aspect of the tibia in the trochlear grooves are not accessible to arthroscopic evaluation and curettage. To access these lesions an extraarticular approach may be necessary. Four of six horses (67%) managed surgically returned to athletic function.[63]

Fragments in the Talocalcaneal-Centroquartal (Proximal Intertarsal) Joint

The tarsocrural joint communicates directly with the proximal intertarsal joint in immature horses through a slitlike opening and in adult horses through a broad opening in the dorsal reflection of the synovium that is located at the distal dorsal aspect of the talus (see Chapter 56). The proximal intertarsal joint is approached through this synovial fenestration during arthroscopic exploration of the tarsocrural joint. A report describes 17 horses with either a free-floating fragment, which was suspected to have originated and been dislodged from an associated OCD lesion in the tarsocrural joint, or a fragment located at the distal end of the medial trochlear ridge with attachment to the synovial reflection that separates the tarsocrural and proximal intertarsal joints.[65] However, such fragments can be seen as incidental abnormalities and unassociated with lameness.[18] Fragments associated with the distal aspect of the medial trochlear ridge of the talus can be seen in only a lateromedial radiographic image, whereas loose fragments within the proximal intertarsal joint most often can be seen on numerous radiographic images. Careful examination of the cranial intermediate ridge of the distal aspect of the tibia is necessary, because loose fragments within the proximal intertarsal joint most often dislodge from this location, and a depression will often be seen from which original fragment originated. Fragments associated with the distal aspect of the medial trochlear ridge are often enveloped in the joint capsule separating the tarsocrural and proximal intertarsal joints, medial to the fenestration between the joints. Sharp dissection is necessary to incise capsular attachments, and care must be taken to avoid damage to the articular surface of the central tarsal bone. Fourteen of 17 horses returned to racing or intended performance activity after arthroscopic removal of the fragment.[65]

TARSAL BONE FRACTURES AND LUXATIONS
Fractures of the Distal Tarsal Bones
Fractures of the central and third tarsal bones occur most frequently in STBs, cutting horses, or TB racehorses,[66-70] but they occasionally occur in other horses, sometimes secondary to previous fusion of the centrodistal and tarsometatarsal joints. These fractures cause an acute onset of a

moderate-to-severe hindlimb lameness that is usually most noticeable when the affected limb is on the inside of a circle.[32] Despite acute onset of lameness, these fractures in young racing TBs may be the result of stress-related bone injury.[69] The lameness is exacerbated by upper limb flexion. The degree of lameness diminishes after 1 to 2 weeks of rest, but lameness returns if the horse returns to work. Some horses with incomplete fractures of the central tarsal and third tarsal bones can race a number of times before lameness becomes pronounced. On initial diagnosis, some fractures appear chronic in both the TB and STB racehorse. Horses with bilateral third tarsal bone fractures may be examined for poor performance rather than overt unilateral hindlimb lameness. Within STB racehorses in North America, central and third tarsal bone fractures are more common than expected in pacers compared with trotters, even if the normal 3:1 pacer/trotter ratio is considered. Heat, soft tissue swelling, and pain on digital palpation of the distal tarsal bones usually accompany the fracture. Synovial effusion of the tarsocrural joint may occur in horses with central tarsal bone fractures but is not usually seen in horses with third tarsal bone fractures. Intraarticular analgesia is used to diagnose central and third tarsal bone slab fractures, but in some horses, particularly those with incomplete or complete, nondisplaced fractures, fibular (peroneal) and tibial nerve blocks are needed to abolish pain.

Diagnosis is made by radiography or scintigraphy, but a fracture may not be radiologically apparent until up to 10 days after injury, when demineralization of the fracture line occurs. Scintigraphy is useful in horses with mild or bilateral hindlimb lameness. Incomplete or bilateral fractures may be seen. Many fractures can often be identified on a lateromedial radiographic image but most consistently can be seen on a DM-PlLO image. If no radiological abnormality is detectable in standard images, additional oblique images, including a plantar 25° lateral-dorsomedial oblique image, should be obtained (or D65° M-PlLO image) (Figure 44-5). However, the precise location and orientation of fractures seem to vary between disciplines and

between the central and third tarsal bones. Thus if a fracture is suspected, additional oblique images may be required. CT can be useful to determine the exact location and configuration of a fracture and to pinpoint screw location if surgical repair is elected. In STBs, two types of central tarsal bone fractures are seen. Authentic frontal (dorsal) plane slab fractures extending from the proximal-to-distal articular surfaces of the central tarsal bone are most common and are best seen in either a DM-PlLO or lateromedial image (see Figure 44-1). Another type of central tarsal bone fracture courses distodorsally from the proximal aspect of the central tarsal bone in the dorsal plane and breaks out of the dorsal cortex of the bone just proximal to the distal articular surface of the central tarsal bone (Figure 44-6). This second type of fracture can best be seen in a lateromedial radiographic image, and because the fracture line does not appear to extend to the distal articular surface, this fracture may not be an authentic slab fracture. Lameness is pronounced, and horses exhibit identical clinical signs to those with larger fragments. In Western performance horses the fracture line is generally located in a more plantar region of the third and central tarsal bones than is seen in racehorses. Third tarsal bone fractures are most commonly dorsal or dorsolateral. In TB racehorses a wedge-shaped conformation of the dorsolateral aspect of the third tarsal bone may be a risk factor for fracture.[71] Comminuted fractures are more common in the central tarsal bone and may be difficult to identify radiologically.[67] If comminution occurs, it is usually at the proximal aspect of the fracture, and fragments can be seen and removed using arthroscopic surgical techniques through the tarsocrural joint. Nuclear scintigraphy is invaluable for identifying the likely presence of a fracture if it cannot be determined radiologically.

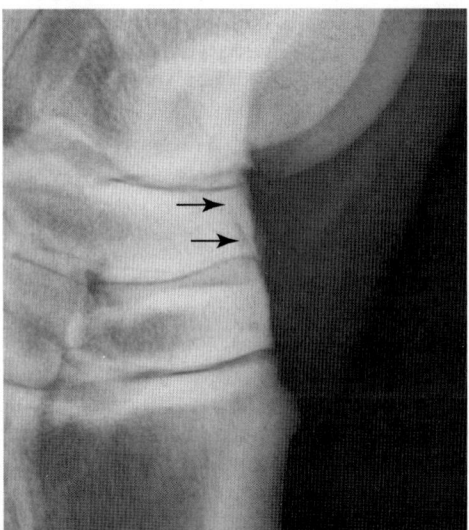

Fig. 44-6 • Lateromedial digital radiographic image of the right tarsus of a 3-year-old Standardbred filly with pronounced lameness abolished by perineural analgesia of the fibular (peroneal) and tibial nerves. Lameness did not change after intraarticular analgesia of the tarsocrural joint. There is an oblique dorsal plane fracture of the central tarsal bone *(arrows)* that courses distodorsally from the proximal articular surface of the central tarsal bone and to the dorsal cortex, just proximal to the centrodistal joint. Mild proliferative changes can be seen, indicating that at the time of diagnosis the fracture was chronic.

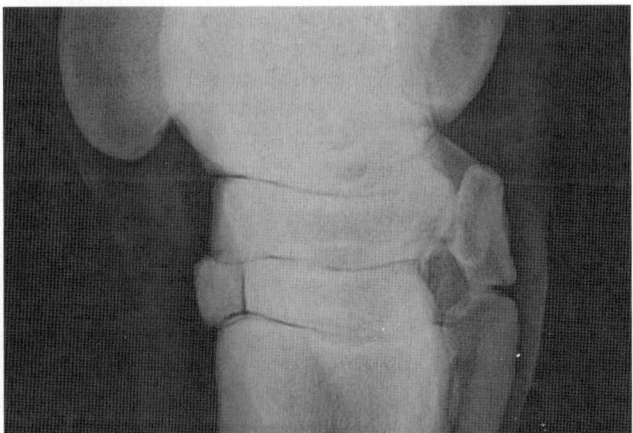

Fig. 44-5 • Plantar 25° lateral-dorsomedial oblique radiographic image of a tarsus. There is a complete slab fracture of the third tarsal bone. This radiographic image is the same projection as a dorsomedial-plantarolateral oblique image showing that the fracture is located on the dorsolateral aspect of the third tarsal bone.

Horses may be treated conservatively[69,70,72,73] or surgically.[67,68,70,71] Seven horses with fractures of the third tarsal bone that were treated conservatively remained lame for 12 months after injury,[67,68] whereas three horses treated by lag-screw compression returned to racing within 6 months.[67] Six racehorses with central tarsal bone fractures remained lame, whereas six Quarter Horses treated surgically made a complete recovery.[68] However, conservative management resulted in return to training within 8 months for 73% of 45 TB racehorses with fractures of the central or third tarsal bone,[69] and this corresponds with our experience. In a retrospective study 20 of 24 horses with slab fractures of the central tarsal bone were STBs, and of these 82% raced after injury with conservative management.[70] Of 28 horses with third tarsal bone slab fractures managed conservatively, 25 had unilateral and three had bilateral fractures, and there were 12 TBs, 15 STBs and one Quarter Horse.[70] After conservative management, 87% of the STBs and 71% of the TBs raced after injury.[70] During the study period five STBs with slab fractures of the central (one horse) and third (four horses) tarsal bones underwent surgical management with interfragmentary compression, and three raced after surgry.[70] Ten of 14 STBs (71%) and two of six TBs (33%) returned to racing and started at least five races after injury, and four of five Quarter Horses (80%) returned to previous athletic function with conservative management.[72] The prognosis in STBs appears satisfactory when conservative management is used, but there appears to be room for improvement in the TB racehorse. We do not know the long-term prognosis of a large group of TB racehorses managed surgically, however. If surgical treatment is performed, case selection is important, because many horses with central tarsal bone fractures have hidden fracture lines that could be inadvertently displaced during screw placement. The large head of a 4.5-mm cortex bone screw may cause soft tissue inflammation and a periosteal reaction. For third and central tarsal bone fractures, 3.5-mm cortex bone screws are preferred. One or two screws should be placed through stab incisions by using radiographic or fluoroscopic guidance, or by using CT. The use of a Herbert cannulated compression screw has been reported.[68] Horses with fragments that are too small to allow lag-screw fixation, or those with chronic fractures of the third tarsal bone causing OA of the centrodistal or tarsometatarsal joints, can be managed by surgical drilling to facilitate arthrodesis of the joints.

Sagittal Fracture of the Talus

Sagittal fractures of the talus are rare, usually nondisplaced, can be difficult to diagnose, and have been recorded most frequently in STB and TB racehorses,[74,75] but they can occur in any type of horse. Twelve racehorses had a history of chronic, mild hindlimb lameness that became acutely severe during a race.[74,75] One of us (SJD) has also seen two endurance horses with acute-onset severe lameness after an endurance race.[64] Lameness in other types of horses may be associated with trauma. Lameness is moderate to severe and is sometimes associated with distention of the tarsocrural joint capsule. The horse may stand with the limb somewhat protracted and show accentuation of lameness when turning. Intraarticular analgesia may improve lameness but rarely removes it completely, and negative results may also occur. Horses show marked improvement after

fibular (peroneal) and tibial perineural analgesia. Fractures in racehorses usually originate at the proximal aspect of the sagittal groove of the talus and are often incomplete. Nondisplaced fractures can be difficult to identify radiologically; extra images, including a dorsal 10- to 20° lateral-plantaromedial oblique and a flexed dorsoplantar (skyline) image, can be helpful. Fractures caused by trauma are frequently comminuted, and the degree of damage may not be apparent radiologically. Nuclear scintigraphy can be helpful in confirming the presence of a fracture; there is usually intense focal IRU in the proximal aspect of the talus.[74]

Eleven racehorses with incomplete sagittal fractures of the talus were managed conservatively with a minimum of 1 month of stall rest followed by small paddock turnout. Seven returned to racing performance within 7 to 8 months after injury; approximately 50% had the same or improved performance.[74] Both endurance horses were managed conservatively and returned to full athletic function.[59] Horses with complete sagittal fractures have been managed by lag-screw compression using two 4.5-mm cortex bone screws.[70] Prognosis may be favorable in horses with simple acute fractures, but the prognosis for horses with comminuted fractures is poor.

One of us (MWR) has seen two foals that had complete, nondisplaced slab fractures of the talus that healed well with conservative management.[64] Acute lameness and moderate tarsocrural effusion were found in both foals; the fracture line could best be seen coursing from the proximal-to-distal articular surface of the talus in a dorsal 15° lateral-plantaromedial oblique radiographic image (Figure 44-7).

Fractures of the Fibular Tarsal Bone

Fractures of the fibular tarsal bone (or calcaneus) are uncommon and usually the result of trauma. Physeal fractures in foals and fractures through the body of the bone are easily diagnosed because of the obvious loss of gastrocnemius muscle function, which results in a dropped-hock appearance. Chip fractures involving the plantar aspect of the calcaneus can be difficult to diagnose unless soft tissue swelling is present or a draining tract secondary to sequestra formation exists. Surgical removal of small fragments may be necessary, depending on size and location of the fragment (intraarticular or extraarticular). Diagnosis is confirmed radiologically. Flexed lateromedial and skyline images of the calcaneus are recommended in addition to standard views (Figure 44-8). Complete body and physeal fractures can be difficult to reduce and stabilize, but horses can be managed successfully with bone plates, screws, and wires by using the tension-band principle. It is not possible to place a bone plate directly plantad because of the presence of the superficial digital flexor tendon, but the plantarolateral or lateral surface of the calcaneus has been used successfully. One of us (MWR) has used a combination of interfragmentary compression and figure-eight tension band wiring to successfully repair fractures of the calcaneus in two miniature horses.[64] Conservative therapy using casting methods alone has been unrewarding and is not recommended. Horses with open, comminuted fractures have a grave prognosis, and humane destruction should be advised. Prognosis for future performance activity in horses with physeal or full-body fractures is considered poor.

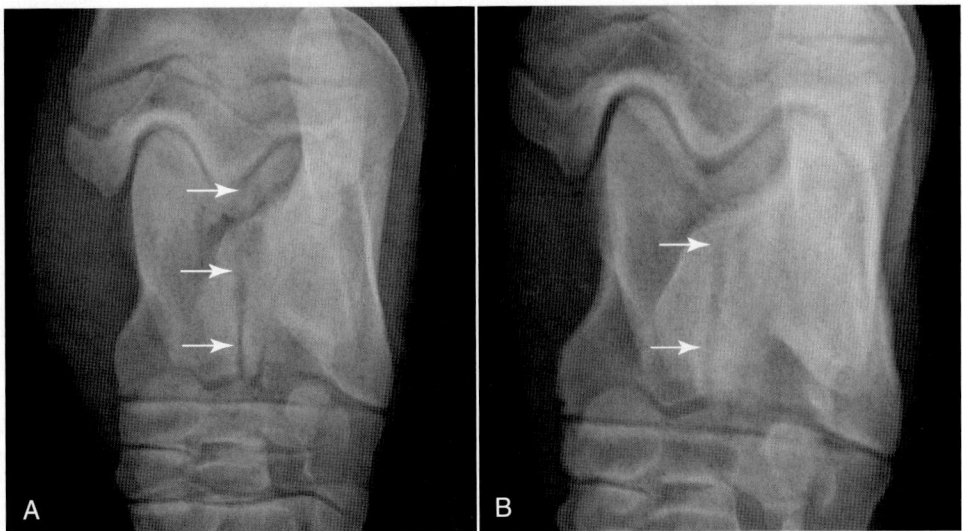

Fig. 44-7 • Initial **(A)** and 6-week follow-up **(B)** digital dorsal 15° lateral-plantaromedial oblique radiographic images of a suckling Standardbred foal with acute hindlimb lameness and moderate tarsocrural joint effusion. **A,** A non-displaced sagittal fracture of the talus can be seen (arrows) coursing from the proximal-to-distal articular surfaces. **B,** Six weeks later the fracture line appears blurred and cannot be seen at the proximal aspect of the talus but can still be seen at the distal aspect (arrows). This foal made a complete recovery using conservative management consisting of 10 weeks of box stall rest. (Courtesy Dr. Jan Henriksen, Walnridge Equine Clinic, Creamridge, New Jersey, United States.)

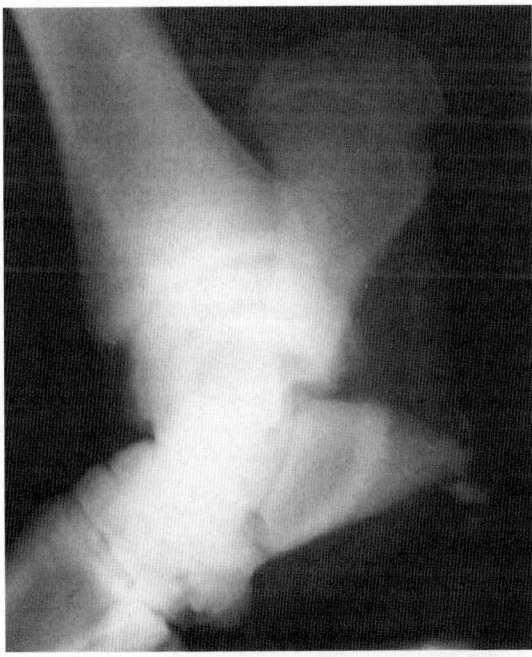

Fig. 44-8 • Flexed lateromedial radiographic image of a tarsus. There is a complete, comminuted articular fracture through the calcaneus.

Fracture of the Lateral Malleolus of the Tibia

The lateral malleolus is considered to be the distal end of the fibula and develops as a separate center of ossification that fuses to the distal tibial epiphysis by 1 year of age. The long lateral and deeper short CLs originate on the lateral malleolus of the tibia, just plantar to the groove for the tendon of the lateral digital extensor muscle. Only a small portion of the lateral malleolus is intraarticular; therefore most fracture fragments are located within the joint capsule

and CLs. The lateral malleolus is mostly covered by soft tissue attachments; therefore careful dissection and the use of a motorized synovial resector are necessary for successful removal of fracture fragments using arthroscopic techniques.

Lateral malleolar fractures are usually traumatic in origin. Small, well-rounded fragments, probably a manifestation of osteochondrosis, occur occasionally and should be differentiated because horses are often asymptomatic. Clinical and radiological signs and results of surgical removal of the fragments have been reported in 16 horses.[76] All were TBs with injuries incurred either during a fall in a race over fences or from being kicked. All horses had a moderate degree of lameness and tarsocrural effusion. Approximately 50% of the horses had periarticular swelling, thickening of the CL, and pain on digital palpation of the lateral malleolus. All fractures were visible on a dorsoplantar radiographic image (Figure 44-9). Fourteen fractures were unilateral and two bilateral, with nine simple and nine comminuted. Thirteen of 16 fragments were displaced distally and rotated 90 degrees.

Ultrasonographic evaluation is useful to determine the location of the fracture in a dorsoplantar plane and to identify a concurrent collateral desmitis.[22] Horses with small or minimally displaced fractures have been successfully managed conservatively. Surgical removal may result in a quicker recovery. The tarsocrural joint should be inspected arthroscopically to remove any debris, and surgical removal of most fragments is possible; use of a motorized synovial resector facilitates debridement of the joint capsule and CL attachments to the fracture fragment. In some horses the fragment can be easily removed via an incision through the lateral CL of the tarsocrural joint, depending on fragment orientation. Thirteen of 16 horses treated by fragment removal returned to full athletic function.[76] If the fracture fragment is of adequate size or if there

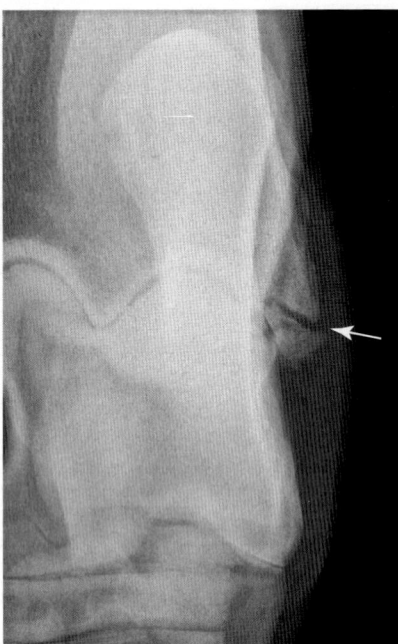

Fig. 44-9 • Dorsoplantar radiographic image of a tarsus. There is a fracture of the lateral malleolus *(arrow)*.

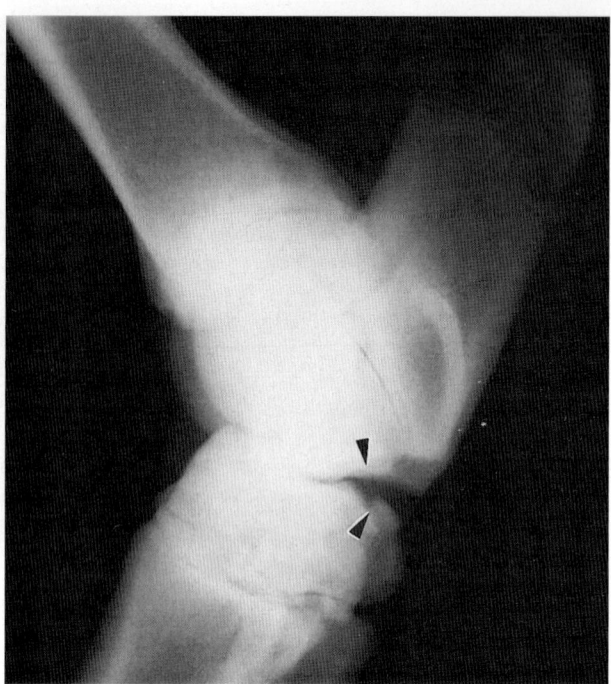

Fig. 44-10 • Flexed lateromedial image of a hock. There is widening of the plantar aspect of the talocalcaneal-centroquartal joint *(arrows)*, which is indicative of luxation.

is instability of the tarsocrural joint, lag-screw fixation and tension band wiring should be considered. One of us (MWR) examined a horse with lateral and medial malleolar fractures; repaired the larger, comminuted, displaced lateral malleolar fracture using a single 4.5-mm cortex bone screw placed in lag fashion augmented by a figure-eight tension band wire; and repaired the nondisplaced medial fracture using interfragmentary compression.[64] The repair was performed using conventional surgical techniques, and small fragments originating from the lateral malleolus were removed. With conservative or surgical management the prognosis is good.

Fractures of the Medial Malleolus of the Tibia

Fractures of the medial malleolus of the distal tibia are rare. Similar to fractures of the lateral malleolus (see earlier), occasionally, small rounded fragments are displaced distal to the medial malleolus, intercalated in the medial CL. These fragments may be a manifestation of osteochondrosis and are distinct from the more common OCD fragments originating from the cranial, articular component of the medial malleolus (usually axially), in the tarsocrural joint. Alternatively, these rounded fragments may be the result of an old fracture. Authentic fracture of the medial malleolus occurs rarely alone, or in combination with lateral malleolar fractures (see earlier).[64,77,78]

Tarsal Joint Luxation

Complete luxation or subluxation of the tarsocrural, talocalcaneal-centroquartal (proximal intertarsal), and tarsometatarsal joints may occur, with or without concurrent tarsal bone fractures.[79,80] Tarsal luxations are the result of severe trauma from kicks from other horses or limb entrapment in fixed objects, such as a fence or cattle guards. Proximal intertarsal and tarsometatarsal luxations are most common. Luxation causes severe, non–weight-bearing lameness, and there may be abnormal deviation of the limb

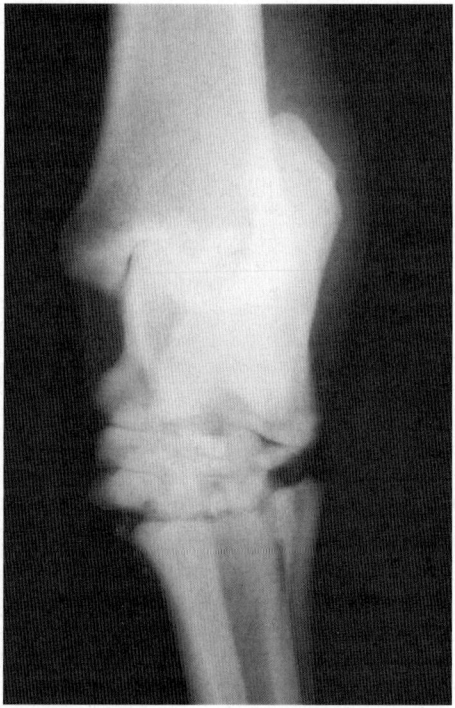

Fig. 44-11 • Stressed dorsoplantar image of a hock. There is luxation of the tarsometatarsal joint, which is associated with fracture of the third and fourth tarsal bones.

at the tarsus. Crepitus may be present with a fracture, and palpation reveals tarsal joint instability. Diagnosis is confirmed by radiological examination. Dorsoplantar radiographic images obtained with medial or lateral limb traction are recommended to determine the extent of CL damage (Figures 44-10, 44-11, and 44-12). Treatment consists of

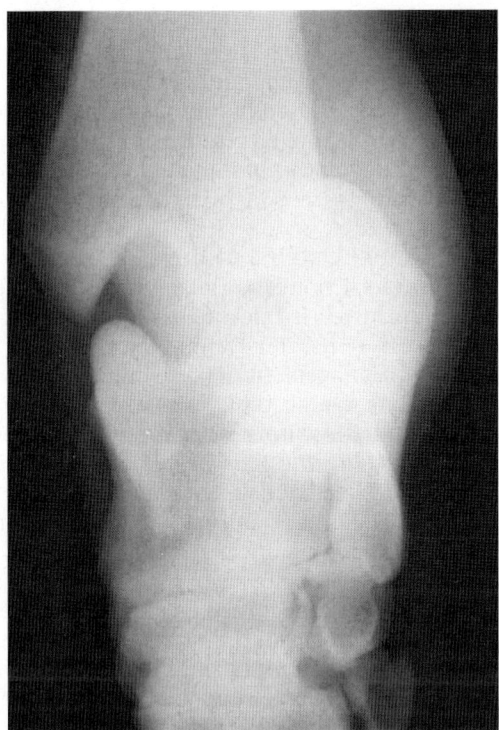

Fig. 44-12 • Stressed dorsoplantar image of a hock. There is luxation of the tarsocrural joint.

reduction of the luxation with the horse under general anesthesia and stabilization with the application of a full hindlimb cast extending from the foot to a point level with the tibial tuberosity. Alternatively, external coaptation consisting of a Robert Jones bandage with splints (custom-made) or external cast material (cast, bandage) can be applied to a standing, sedated horse. Although reduction will be less than ideal and invariably an angular deformity will persist, a successful outcome can be achieved.[64] Internal fixation is rarely indicated but may be necessary with concurrent tarsal bone fracture. Double plating techniques using conventional or locking compression plates applied proximal to the fracture or luxation using the plantarolateral aspect of the calcaneus and the medial aspect of the hock and ending distally in the metatarsal bones, in combination with external coaptation, could be used. Tarsocrural or tarsal luxation with functionally intact CLs can be difficult to reduce, but manipulation of the tarsus with the limb in a flexed position may facilitate reduction. The limb should be maintained in a cast or other external coaptation constructed to be as rigid as possible for 4 to 6 weeks if the CLs are intact and 6 to 8 weeks if the CLs are ruptured.[79,80] After the cast has been removed, the hindlimb is placed in a heavy cotton bandage with rigid splints for an additional 4 to 6 weeks before turnout in a small area is allowed. Of the seven reported horses with tarsal joint luxation (three proximal intertarsal, three tarsometatarsal, and one tarsocrural), all were treated with closed reduction and external coaptation, and all returned to either light riding, pasture soundness, or breeding activity. The presence of tarsal bone fractures did not affect outcome. All horses had a reduction in range of motion of the tarsus and OA that prevented the return to athletic soundness. Prognosis for horses with

proximal intertarsal and tarsometatarsal joint luxations is reasonably good for pasture soundness.[79] A guarded prognosis is warranted for horses with tarsocrural joint luxation because of the difficulty in reducing the luxation.

SOFT TISSUE INJURY OF THE TARSUS

Various soft tissue injuries of the tarsus are discussed elsewhere: calcanean bursitis (see Chapter 79), cunean tendon bursitis-tarsitis (see Chapter 108), curb (see Chapter 78), subcutaneous calcaneal bursitis (capped hock; see Chapter 79), distention of the tarsal sheath (thoroughpin; see Chapter 76), and dislocation/luxation of the superficial flexor tendon from the tuber calcanei (see Chapter 80). Distention of the long digital extensor tendon sheath is discussed previously (see page 509).

Collateral Ligament Damage
Complete extension of the tarsocrural joint is prevented by tension in the CLs. CL injury is usually the result of trauma or a fall; however, it is not a common injury. CL injury was identified in only 23% of 133 horses that underwent ultrasonographic evaluation of the tarsus because of suspected soft tissue injury.[22] Lameness varies from mild to severe, depending on the degree of damage. There is often distention of the tarsocrural joint capsule and periarticular soft tissue swelling. Flexion is usually resented. Analgesic techniques are usually not required, but lameness may be improved in some horses by intraarticular analgesia of the tarsocrural joint. In an acute injury there often are no radiological abnormalities unless there is an avulsion fracture[81]; however, 4 to 6 weeks after injury, enthesophytes develop at the origin or insertions of the injured CLs. Nuclear scintigraphy is helpful in horses with mild injuries because it demonstrates intense, focal IRU at the ligament attachment sites.[82] Ultrasonographic evaluation is used to identify the injured structure(s) and assess the severity of the injury (see Chapter 17).[22] In a series of 23 horses, 18 sustained medial CL injury, including three with both medial and lateral CL injury, and five horses had lateral CL injury alone, with injury to the superficial components being most common either alone or together with injury to the deep component. Initial treatment involves stall rest, cold water therapy, topical dimethyl sulfoxide with or without corticosteroids, and NSAIDs. Long periods of rest (e.g., 6 months) followed by a controlled exercise program have been recommended.[81] Prognosis depends on the severity of injury, but horses with very extensive periosteal new bone have been able to return to full athletic function, although some residual enlargement of the hock has persisted.[21,64]

Old avulsion fractures at the insertion of the lateral and less commonly the medial short CL are sometimes detected in horses with pain causing lameness localized to the hock with no other explanation for the cause of lameness. There is no associated IRU, and the clinical significance of such fractures is difficult to determine accurately. It is conceivable that low grade motion may cause pain.

Enthesopathy of the Lateral Collateral Ligaments of the Tarsocrural Joint
Enthesopathy of the long, and less commonly, the short lateral CLs is a rare condition that is recognized most often

in STB racehorses, especially pacers, but does rarely occur in TBs. It results in lameness that is improved by analgesia of the tarsocrural joint. There may be distention of the tarsocrural joint capsule, and subtle, localized soft tissue swelling may be present. Diagnosis usually depends on scintigraphic findings[83] with focal, intense IRU on the lateral aspect of the calcaneus. Entheseous new bone is usually detectable radiologically. Local injections with methylprednisolone acetate and Sarapin, an extract of the pitcher plant, may result in improvement, but rest is the treatment of choice.

Rupture of the Fibularis Tertius
See Chapter 80 for a discussion of rupture of the fibularis (peroneus) tertius.

Stringhalt
See Chapter 48 for a discussion of stringhalt.

MISCELLANEOUS TARSAL INJURIES
Osseous Cystlike Lesions in the Tuber Calcanei
Osseous cystlike lesions in the tuber calcanei have been identified as a cause of moderate to severe lameness either with no localizing clinical signs (Figure 44-13)[64] or in association with distention of the calcaneal bursa.[83] It has been suggested that such lesions may be a reaction at the enthesis of the gastrocnemius tendon, but no associated lesions of the gastrocnemius tendon have been seen.[84] In two horses lameness developed after known trauma (a kick and a fall),[84] but in other horses there was no known potential cause. In the latter horses lameness was abolished by fibular and tibial nerve blocks. Lateromedial, dorsolateral-plantaromedial oblique and skyline images of the calcaneus are required for accurate localization of the lesion. Treatment of two horses with associated distention of the calcaneal bursa by either conservative management or surgical debridement resulted in persistent lameness.[84] The horses

with no associated soft tissue swelling did not respond to rest, but intralesional injection of corticosteroids has resulted in resolution of lameness in two horses.[64] Calcaneal bursitis is rarely caused by primary injury of the gastrocnemius tendon at the attachment to the calcaneus or a combined injury of the gastrocnemius and superficial digital flexor tendons (see Chapters 79 and 80).

Infectious (Septic) Osteitis of the Calcaneus
Osteitis of the tarsal bones is uncommon. However, the enlarged end of the tuber calcanei has minimal soft tissue protection and is at risk for traumatic injury and subsequent infection. Management of these injuries can be complicated if the tarsocrural joint, calcaneal bursa, or tarsal sheath is involved. Most horses sustain a traumatic injury from kicking a fixed object or being kicked by another horse.[85,86] Osteitis usually causes moderate-to-severe lameness, cellulitis, and tarsal tenosynovitis. The severity of lameness often decreases once drainage has been established. Twenty-two of 28 horses had a wound or draining tract over the plantar aspect of the calcaneus.[85] Lateromedial, flexed lateromedial, and plantaroproximal-plantarodistal (skyline) radiographic images are the most helpful (Figure 44-14). Radiological signs of calcaneal osteitis or sequestra formation may take several days or weeks to appear, and thus sequential radiological evaluation is recommended. Rarely is the medullary cavity of the calcaneus involved; hence the term *osteitis* rather than *osteomyelitis* is preferred. Ultrasonography is useful to assess calcanean bursa or tarsal sheath involvement. If tarsal sheath involvement is suspected, cytological evaluation of the tendon sheath fluid with aerobic and anaerobic microbial culture and susceptibility testing is recommended (see Chapter 76). Treatment is based on resolving the infection and debriding any bony lesions. Debridement can often be done using bursoscopic techniques, but if wound revision is needed a conventional surgical approach to the infected bone can be used. One of us (MWR) has had success in

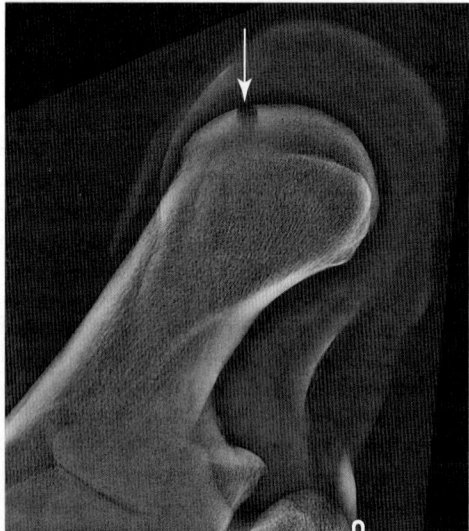

Fig. 44-13 • Flexed plantaroproximal-plantarodistal radiographic view of the calcaneus. There is a well-defined focal osteolytic lesion in the plantarolateral aspect of the tuber calcanei (arrow). Compare with Figure 44-14. There were no localizing clinical signs.

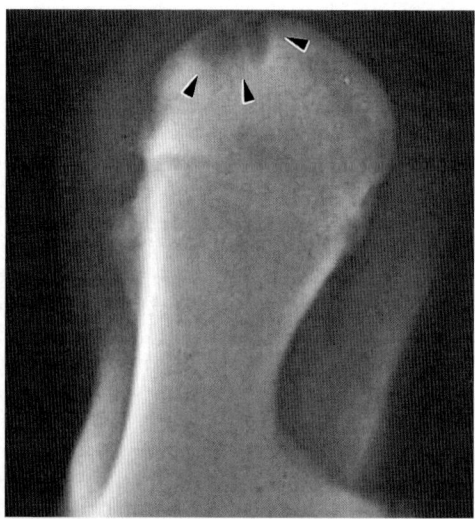

Fig. 44-14 • Flexed plantaroproximal-plantarodistal radiographic view of the calcaneus. There is an osteolytic lesion in the tuber calcanei (arrows), the result of infection. There is also new bone on the lateral aspect (to the left) of the calcaneus.

managing horses with infectious calcaneal bursitis and calcaneal osteitis, using liberal debridement and primary wound revision and closure, closed suction drainage, and external coaptation using a full-limb or sleeve cast or bandage to immobilize the tarsus after surgery. External coaptation appears important in overall management because limiting motion improves the horse's comfort and allows early healing of revised wounds in this region. Although debridement of all infected bone and soft tissue is an important principle in management of horses with infectious osteitis of the calcaneus, aggressive debridement of the calcaneus to remove large amounts of bone should be avoided. Broad-spectrum antimicrobial drugs such as penicillin (22,000 IU/kg q12h IM) and gentamicin sulfate (6.6 mg/kg q24h IV) are recommended until culture results are known. Pure bacterial cultures were isolated in 14 of 28 horses in one report,[85] but mixed bacterial isolates do occur. The most common pure bacteria colonies isolated were *Escherichia coli, Streptococcus zooepidemicus, Staphylococcus aureus,* and *Enterobacter cloacae.* All isolates were susceptible to penicillin, gentamicin, or trimethoprim sulfamethoxazole. With acute infection, antimicrobial medication alone may be satisfactory, but surgical intervention to remove infected soft tissue and damaged bone or sequestra is usually required. Resection of the infected soft tissues and curettage of the bony lesion can resolve calcaneal lesions that do not involve the tarsal sheath. Infections involving the tarsal sheath require flushing the sheath and establishing drainage (see Chapters 24 and 76). Duration of antimicrobial therapy depends on clinical response, but therapy should continue for at least 7 days after resolution of the lameness and wound drainage. Phenylbutazone (2.2 mg/kg orally [PO]) should be used as needed for pain relief.

The prognosis for horses with calcaneal osteitis depends on the structures involved, duration of infection before treatment, type and susceptibility of isolated bacteria, and the ability to get the original wound to heal. Long-term management (several weeks to months) is often needed, and an important but often limiting factor is the owner's financial commitment. Chronic persistent drainage, persistent severe lameness, or contralateral laminitis can negatively influence prognosis, and aggressive, expensive therapy is often needed. Quick and aggressive medical and surgical treatment improves the chances of horses returning to athletic function. In one study, nine of 18 horses were used as broodmares and nine returned to athletic function.[85,86]

Osteitis of the Sustentaculum Tali

The sustentaculum tali is on the plantaromedial aspect of the calcaneus. Injuries involving the medial aspect of the hock often involve the sustentaculum tali and adjacent tarsal sheath. Injury usually occurs from direct trauma, most commonly from a kick wound. Lameness is often severe. Diagnosis can be difficult because of the severe soft tissue swelling that accompanies this injury, especially when acute. Although unusual, there can be communication of the site of infection or fragmentation of the sustentaculum tali with the tarsocrural joint. Radiographic examination should include dorsomedial-plantarolateral oblique, dorsoplantar, and plantaroproximal-plantarodistal images. Ultrasonography is useful to assess the deep digital

flexor tendon (DDFT) and tarsal sheath. Infection of the tarsal sheath as a result of sustentaculum tali fragmentation (see Figure 76-3) or lysis requires surgical curettage of the sustentaculum tali and lavage and flushing of the tarsal sheath. Horses with bony irregularities in the tarsal groove of the sustentaculum tali can be severely lame, even without infection, because of motion of the DDFT against the roughened bone, which results in severe tendonitis. The tarsal retinaculum can become constrictive if the tendon is inflamed and swollen, which causes further tendon damage and pain. Surgery with the horse under general anesthesia is recommended to transect the tarsal retinaculum, explore and curette necrotic bone involving the sustentaculum tali, and drain and flush the tarsal sheath.[87] The tarsal groove should be smoothed with a curette to avoid abrasion to the DDFT after surgery. Endoscopic examination of the tarsal sheath may be difficult in horses with severe swelling from concomitant infection. In horses with mild swelling, with drainage localized to the region of the sustentaculum tali, and without substantial tarsal tenosynovitis, a small incision should be made directly over the fragments. The fragments should be removed and the site curetted; the incision is closed primarily. In these horses, prognosis for future soundness is favorable. Horses should be treated with systemic antibiotics based on culture and susceptibility results. Antimicrobial therapy is continued for at least 7 days after resolution of clinical signs and may require 4 to 6 weeks of treatment. After surgery, horses should be confined to a stall or small run for 8 weeks with daily handwalking, followed by 6 more weeks of pasture turnout before returning to normal activity. Prognosis is good for returning to athletic activity. Seven of nine horses returned to previous use (three barrel racing, one cutting, and three pleasure riding) after surgery.[87]

Lesions of the Sustentaculum Tali

Lesions of the sustentaculum tali of the fibular tarsal bone may occur as a result of known direct trauma, such as a kick injury to the medial aspect of the hock,[88] or in association with chronic injuries of the DDFT. Eight of eight horses with proliferative new bone on the plantar and/or medial aspect of the sustentaculum tali had marked distention of the tarsal sheath and lameness. Four had a history of a kick injury. Conservative or surgical management resulted in persistent lameness. Postmortem examination revealed marked fibrillation of the DDFT and adhesions to the tarsal sheath and/or the sustentaculum tali.

Chronic lesions of the DDFT may be associated with the development of dystrophic mineralization within the tarsal sheath and osseous irregularity of the sustentaculum tali. Distention of the tarsal sheath and lameness are present. The prognosis is poor.

Congenital Deformations of the Tarsus

Congenital dysplasia of the sustentaculum tali is rare and has been documented in TBs[89] and Saddlebreds characterized clinically by a tarsal valgus conformation and a broader plantar profile than usual. The DDFT is positioned more dorsally and medially than usual because of flattening of the proximal aspect of the sustentaculum tali.

A complete fibula may be present in Shetland ponies.[90,91] This results in an abnormal swelling on the distal lateral aspect of the tibia and outward splaying of the limbs distal to the hocks.

Infectious Arthritis
See Chapter 65 for a discussion of infectious arthritis.

Periarticular Cellulitis (see also Chapter 107)
Peritarsal infection results in acute-onset, very severe non–weight-bearing lameness associated with localized swelling that is usually but not invariably on the dorsal aspects of the hock. The swelling is hot and exquisitely painful to palpation. These signs are associated with an elevated rectal temperature, neutrophilia, and hyperfibrinogenemia. In some horses, skin abrasions can be identified somewhere in the more distal part of the limb.

Prompt, aggressive treatment with oxytetracycline (5 mg/kg IV sid) or other antimicrobial agents and phenylbutazone (4.4 mg/kg) for at least 5 days, combined with forced walking exercise for as much as possible daily, usually results in rapid resolution of lameness. Horses can often start trotting within 3 days of the onset of clinical signs and should be trotted for 10- to 15-minute periods repeatedly through the day. The prognosis is usually favorable; 1 of 10 horses developed osteomyelitis of the third tarsal and fourth tarsal bones, although this horse ultimately made a complete recovery.[92]

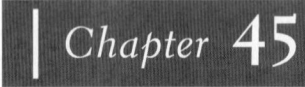

Chapter 45

The Crus

Mike W. Ross

ANATOMY

The crus is located between the stifle and hock joints. Anatomy of the hock and stifle are discussed in Chapters 44 and 46. The medial aspect of the tibia lacks muscle covering and is easily palpated, but muscles and tendons cover the cranial, lateral, and caudal aspects. The tibia has proximal and distal physes and a separate center of ossification for the tibial tuberosity.

The fibula is lateral, does not share axial load, and fuses with the tibia to form the lateral malleolus. The proximal aspect of the fibula may develop from two or more separate centers of ossification, and fibrous union may persist throughout life. The result of this union is transverse radiolucent lines that are evident radiologically and should not be mistaken for fractures (see discussion of rare fibular fractures later).[1,2]

References on page 1288

Muscles and tendons of the crus are important in locomotion and support of the hindlimb. The long digital extensor muscle originates from a common tendon with the fibularis tertius from the extensor fossa of the femur and is located cranially and laterally in the crus. The fibularis tertius courses distally to divide into dorsal and dorsolateral tendons of attachment. Avulsion injury of the tendon of origin of the fibularis tertius and long digital extensor causes a classic disruption of the hindlimb reciprocal apparatus. The tibialis cranialis muscle is deep to the long digital extensor muscle and distally splits into two parts, the medial of which is called the *cunean tendon* (jack tendon) and may play a minor role in distal hock joint pain. The lateral digital extensor muscle originates proximally, and its tendon courses laterally over the tarsus and joins the long digital extensor muscle in the proximal metatarsal region. Myotenectomy of the lateral digital extensor tendon and muscle is often performed for management of stringhalt.

The paired gastrocnemius muscles originate from the distal, caudal aspect of the femur and share a single, strong tendon that courses distally and inserts on the calcaneus. The superficial digital flexor and deep digital flexor muscles and tendons arise caudally. The superficial digital flexor tendon (SDFT) begins medial to the gastrocnemius tendon and courses from medial to caudal to attach to the calcaneus before continuing distally. The deep digital flexor tendon (DDFT) is deep to both the SDFT and the gastrocnemius tendons and courses distally over the plantaromedial aspect of the calcaneus, the sustentaculum tali. The combined SDFT and gastrocnemius tendons form the common calcaneal tendon, the major extensor of the hock, and injuries can cause partial or complete loss of hock support. The tarsal sheath begins in the distal, caudal aspect of the crus and surrounds the DDFT.

The fibular (peroneal) nerve originates from the sciatic nerve and branches in the proximal aspect of the crus to become the superficial and deep fibular nerves that run between the long digital extensor and lateral digital extensor muscles and tendons. The tibial nerve is palpable in the distal, caudal aspect of the crus, cranial to the common calcaneal tendon.

CLINICAL CHARACTERISTICS AND DIAGNOSIS OF LAMENESS OF THE CRUS

Degree of lameness can vary from a subtle, high-speed lameness seen in horses with early stress-related bone injury to an acute, non–weight-bearing lameness, swelling, and deformity seen in horses with complete tibial fractures. Horses with tearing of the gastrocnemius tendon, musculotendonous junction, origin, and insertion have varying degrees of hyperflexion of the tarsocrural joint and partial loss of the reciprocal apparatus. Because the hock drops during weight bearing, the degree of pelvic hike is less than expected and the degree of lameness may be underestimated. Foals with fibularis tertius and long digital extensor avulsion injury lose integrity of the reciprocal apparatus and have swelling on the lateral, proximal aspect of the crus. Rarely, foals can injure the fibularis tertius distally near the tarsus. Fibularis tertius injury in adult horses may cause swelling of the distal, cranial aspect of the crus near the tarsocrural joint, but lesions in the midcrus are not associated with swelling. In calcinosis circumscripta, round-to-oblong, nonpainful mineralized masses are attached to the distal aspect of the lateral patellar ligament and lateral femorotibial joint capsule or collateral ligament.

No gait characteristics are pathognomonic for pain associated with the crus. Lameness of the crus is similar to that seen in horses with pain originating anywhere from the tarsus to the hind foot. Horses with tibial stress fractures have a shortened cranial phase of the stride and, most often, a stabbing type of hindlimb gait when viewed from behind. Injuries of the crus should be suspected when lameness is pronounced, but sites in the rest of the limb are eliminated by using diagnostic analgesia. In Thoroughbreds (TBs), in which the risk of tibial stress fractures is high, a tentative diagnosis of stress fracture is made when lameness is pronounced and recurrent after work.

Palpation of the crus should be done with the limb in both the standing and flexed positions, but this often yields no information. The medial side of the tibia is most easily felt, and occasionally in horses with tibial stress fractures, mild swelling is present and pain is elicited by deep compression (see Figure 6-27). Unfortunately, most tibial stress fractures involve the caudolateral cortex, and it is difficult to compress this area during palpation. Digital tibial percussion sometimes elicits a painful response in horses with tibial stress fractures, but there are many false-positive and false-negative responses. Forced tibial torsion with the limb in a flexed position may elicit pain in horses with tibial stress fractures (see Chapter 107), but I have found the results of this test to be inconsistent.

Diagnostic Analgesia

There is no practical method to use diagnostic analgesia in the entire crus. The distal portion is blocked when fibular and tibial nerve blocks are performed, and pain from injuries involving the distal aspect of the tibia and caudal soft tissues may be abolished, but this block is unreliable for abolition of crus-related pain. Lameness of the crus becomes more likely in horses in which perineural and intraarticular techniques for the rest of the limb have been exhausted. In at least three TB racehorses, pain associated with tibial stress fractures has been abolished or diminished by intraarticular analgesia of the femorotibial joint. An explanation is not readily apparent.

Imaging Considerations

Large cassettes or imaging plates (35 × 43 cm) should be used to obtain radiographs of the entire length of the tibia. There are normal areas of modeling involving the cranial proximal cortex of the tibia that appear as layers or a mound of bone, but stress fractures do not occur here. Occasionally, an obvious bony proliferation is seen involving the caudal or caudolateral tibial cortex, under the fibula in normal horses. Periosteal and endosteal proliferation of the caudal and lateral (medial is unusual) cortex and oblique linear radiolucency are changes that may be seen in horses with tibial stress fractures. Enostosis-like lesions appear as single or numerous medullary radiopacities. In some horses the fibula has one or more transverse radiolucent lines through the proximal third of the bone that should not be mistaken for fractures. Stress-related bone injury of the tibia is most easily imaged and diagnosed using scintigraphic examination. Without scintigraphy the diagnosis can be easily missed radiologically. Enostosis-like lesions may be

associated with single to numerous areas of increased radiopharmaceutical uptake (IRU) in the medullary cavity and should be differentiated from the cortical uptake associated with tibial stress fractures. Numerous scintigraphic images are used to differentiate enostosis-like lesions, tibial stress fractures, and rare authentic lesions of the fibulae.

Ultrasonographic examination is useful in evaluating the gastrocnemius muscle and tendon. Patellar desmitis at the attachments can be diagnosed by using ultrasonographic and scintigraphic examinations. Ultrasonographic examination is useful in horses with fibularis tertius injury or thoroughpin or "false" thoroughpin and to evaluate the tarsal sheath.

SPECIFIC CONDITIONS OF THE CRUS

Tibial Stress Fractures

Tibial stress fractures are the most common lameness condition of the crus and occur most commonly in TB racehorses. In my experience, tibial stress fractures are rare in other sports horses, including the Standardbred (STB) racehorse. In an 8-year period, of 1020 STBs in which scintigraphic examination was performed, only three horses (two of which were trotters) had tibial stress fractures.[3] Thirteen STB racehorses, 11 pacers, and two trotters with tibial stress fractures were reported in one study,[4] but based on my experience this is a highly unusual clustering of horses. In that study pacers were overrepresented, and factors such as breeding, track size, training methods, and referral bias may have played a role. In my experience and practice area tibial stress fractures occur more commonly in trotters than in pacers. The caudal tibial cortex appears prone to stress-related bone injury because it is under compressive forces when loaded. The highest compressive forces were recorded in the middiaphysis at the walk, but loading at the gallop, pace, and trot was not determined.[4-6]

Tibial stress fractures usually occur in 2- and 3-year-old TB racehorses. In one study, tibial stress fractures occurred most commonly in 2-year-olds or unraced horses.[7] In my experience tibial stress fractures occur later in training than stress fractures of the humerus, can occur when horses are racing, and also occur in older horses. Lameness in horses with humeral stress fractures often occurs within 4-8 weeks of returning to training in the early 3- or 4-year-old racing year. In horses with tibial stress fractures usually lameness is unilateral. Stress-related bone injury is more advanced in the lame limb, but scintigraphic evidence of stress-related bone injury can be bilateral. Typically TB racehorses with tibial stress fractures usually become acutely lame after training or racing, only to become reasonably sound within 3 to 5 days. Lameness recurs after another work session or race, but overt clinical signs other than lameness are subtle or lacking. Horses with pelvic stress fractures and those with stress-related bone injury of the distal aspect of the third metatarsal bone manifest similar clinical signs. Lameness may be severe initially, but within a few days horses can be trotted and show grade 2 to 4 lameness (of 5). Lameness may be worse in horses with caudal or caudomedial stress fractures than in those with caudolateral stress fractures. Horses with spiral tibial fractures involving the medial and lateral cortices and often the cranial cortex of the distal aspect of the tibia can be nearly non–weight bearing (see Figure 19-10).

Tibial stress fractures are seen as focal areas of IRU in the caudal or caudal lateral tibial cortex in the middiaphysis and are usually singular but can be multiple and bilateral (see Chapter 19). Tibial stress fractures must be differentiated from enostosis-like lesions, which can cause similar clinical signs but scintigraphically are located in the medullary cavity (see Figure 19-9). Caudomedial tibial stress fractures occur but are unusual. In horses in North America, tibial stress fractures are usually located from middiaphysis to the distal aspect of the tibia, but occasionally a fracture is seen in the proximal, caudal metaphyseal region. In TBs racing in Europe the proximal caudal site is affected more commonly than is seen in TBs from North America.[8] Of 42 TB racehorses with tibial stress fractures examined in England, 52% had middiaphyseal fractures, 29% had distal tibial fractures, and 19% had proximal caudal fractures.[9] In Australia fracture distribution mimics that seen in North America.[7] Occasionally a spiral fracture of the distal tibial cortex is seen scintigraphically, but fractures are usually initially not detectable radiologically (see Figure 19-10). Horses with this configuration of fracture are at risk for catastrophic failure of the tibia, even while being stall rested. In general, intensity of IRU is inversely proportional to the amount of radiological change. In a U.K. study in Newmarket, no correlation was found between scintigraphic and radiological grades in TB racehorses.[9] Curiously, there was no relationship between scintigraphic grade and degree of lameness, a finding that differs from my clinical experience.[9] This may reflect the rapidity with which horses undergo scintigraphic examination in a first-opinion racehorse practice, compared with the delay before horses are referred to my second-opinion practice. In horses with stress-related bone injury a continuum of bone changes occurs; these bone changes precede and eventually lead to fracture. If radiographs show proliferative changes and an oblique fracture line, IRU is usually mild to moderate. In horses that develop sudden, severe lameness, focal or spiral intense IRU is seen, but radiological changes are equivocal or mild. Authentic tibial stress fractures do not occur in the cranial cortex (except distally in horses with spiral fractures), but IRU from a previous fibular nerve block can produce an artifact resembling fracture (see Figure 19-15).

Most horses are given 4 weeks of stall rest, followed by 4 weeks of stall rest with handwalking, then 8 weeks of turnout in a small paddock before returning to race training. In North America it is difficult to enforce a 16-week rest period, but earlier return to race training predisposes to recurrence of stress-related bone injury and fracture. Trainers are often content with a 45- to 60-day period of rest but balk at giving longer rest periods; however, fractures heal neither clinically nor scintigraphically in 60 days. Because stress fractures occur as a result of accumulated bone stress from race training, early return to training on the very surface on which the horse was training when the fracture occurred and in the same training regimen predisposes to reinjury. Fracture of the contralateral limb the next racing year is possible, but recurrence of ipsilateral fracture is unusual, unlike recurrence seen early in training in horses with humeral stress fractures. Horses with severe lameness may have difficulty rising in the stall and should be bedded on good footing or kept in the standing position for several weeks by the use of crossties or other suitable restraints. Clients should be warned that even while horses are resting, spiral tibial fractures can become comminuted.

Tibial Diaphyseal Fractures in Adult Horses

Tibial fractures in adult horses occur from trauma from falling, from spills (falls) sustained while performing, from being kicked, or during attempts to rise after general anesthesia. Horses with tibial stress fractures, usually those with severe initial lameness or spiral fracture, can develop comminuted fractures if turnout exercise is given too soon or if a horse struggles to rise in a stall. One of the only reported successful repairs of an adult horse with a displaced tibial fracture was performed after the horse had been anesthetized for radiographs of the pelvis and coxofemoral joint only to develop a displaced, closed tibial fracture as a result of displacement from a tibial stress fracture. The injury was repaired using two dynamic compression plates and bone screws.[10] In general, however, prognosis is grave for adult horses with displaced, comminuted tibial fractures, because comminution is severe, additional fracture lines often propagate proximal and distal from the fracture site, fractures are often open, and implant failures are common (Figure 45-1). Prognosis for horses with comminuted fractures involving the distal aspect of the tibia and tarsocrural joint is hopeless. A horse with a closed, simple, or mildly comminuted midshaft oblique or transverse fracture may be a candidate for an attempt at internal fixation. With newly developed implants such as the locking compression plate, and with the use of sling assistance to protect the contralateral limb from the development of laminitis and to add stress protection of the repaired limb, it may be possible to successfully repair simple, mildly comminuted or oblique midshaft tibial fractures in adult horses. However, prognosis is poor to grave, because even with double-plating or triple-plating techniques, implant or bone failure is common and fixation usually fails during anesthetic recovery even with a pool recovery system. Given the extremely poor prognosis,

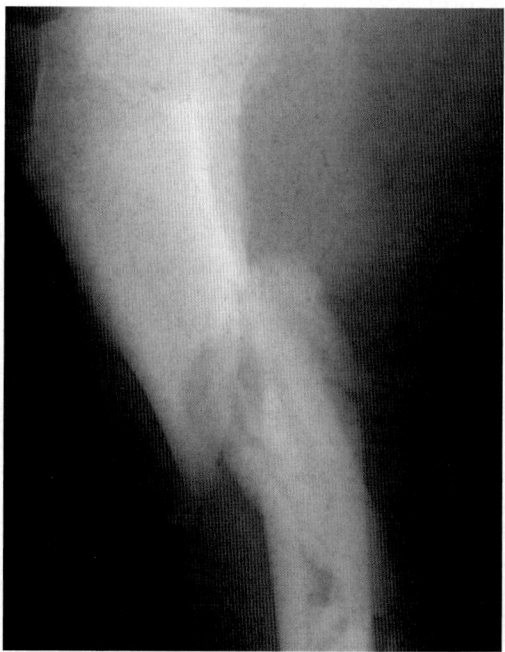

Fig. 45-1 • Lateromedial radiographic image of an adult equine tibia. There is a typical comminuted tibial fracture. The prognosis is grave and the horse should be humanely destroyed.

transportation of a horse with a flail leg should be avoided. Most horses should be immediately destroyed.

Tibial Fractures in Foals

Suckling and weanling foals with displaced, comminuted tibial fractures have a reasonable prognosis for salvage, and some become performance horses and racehorses. The size of the foal is critical, and complications in those heavier than 225 to 325 kg may be similar to those in adult horses. Most foals with tibial fractures sustain kick trauma from mares or have other accidents.

Proximal Physeal Tibial Fractures

Salter-Harris type II fractures occur in sucklings, weanlings, and rarely in yearlings. These fractures result in acute-onset lameness and swelling of the proximal, medial aspect of the crus and stifle. Within 1 to 3 days, foals are often weight bearing and may be surprisingly comfortable. Radiographs reveal a simple Salter-Harris type II fracture with a lateral metaphyseal component (Figure 45-2). Occasionally, mild

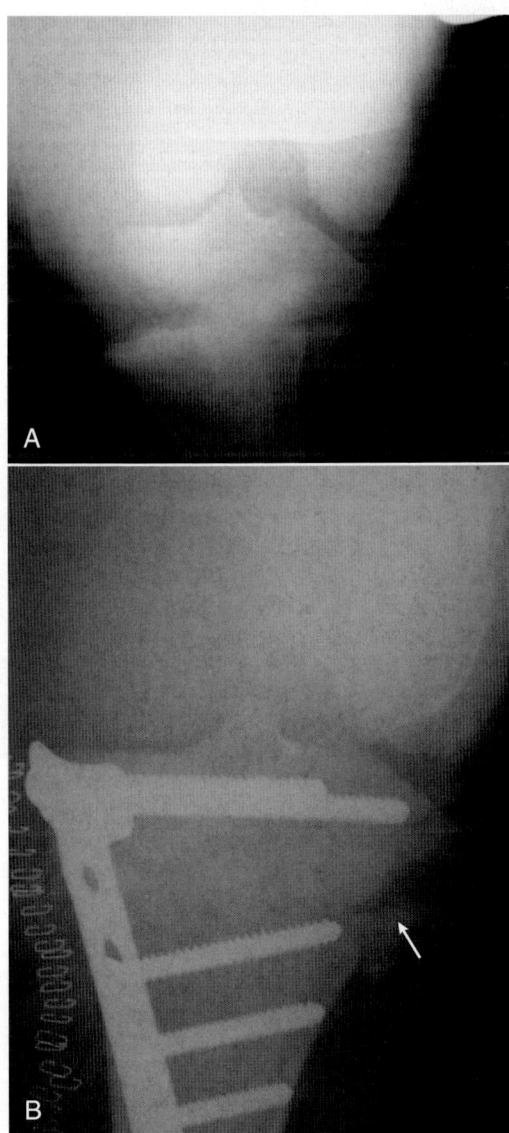

Fig. 45-2 • Caudocranial radiographic images of a foal with a Salter-Harris type II fracture of the proximal tibial physis before **(A)** and after **(B)** surgery. Note the lateral metaphyseal component *(arrow)*.

comminution exists laterally. Foals with minimal displacement can be managed conservatively, but progressive displacement, as evidenced by valgus deformity, usually occurs. Foals should be treated surgically. Many methods have been used, but the most stable repair is a medial approach in which either a T plate or two short dynamic compression plates are applied by using 5.5-mm cortex bone screws in the epiphyseal component. A long metaphyseal component can be engaged using screws placed in lag fashion. The tension side of the proximal aspect of the tibia is medial, and the T plate should be applied in this location. Because the soft tissue covering is minimal, chronic drainage from the wound is common until the plate(s) is removed. Prognosis for life is good to excellent and for soundness is fair to good. Prognosis for racing is not established, and sequelae from differences in limb length are unknown, but racing is not out of the question.

Middiaphyseal Tibial Fractures

Similar considerations for degree of comminution, location of fracture, and whether the site is open or closed apply to foals and adult horses, but in foals prognosis associated with repair is considerably better than in adults. Foals with closed, midshaft, transverse, or oblique fractures with minimal comminution are the best surgical candidates, but successful repair of those with comminution has been achieved (Figure 45-3). Foals with open fractures that are associated with a small wound and minimal contamination are also surgical candidates. A cranial approach is used to place two dynamic or locking compression plates on the craniolateral and craniomedial aspects, and additional screws are used to repair loose fragments. In a retrospective study of nine foals whose injuries were repaired in this manner, results were considered excellent in six and good or fair in two.[11] Additional stability can be achieved using locking compression plates, but success was reasonable with older style of implants. If fractures heal, implants should be removed, and if contralateral angular deformity does not develop, prognosis for racing should be fair to good.

Distal Physeal Fractures of the Tibia

Distal physeal fractures of the tibia do occur but are rare. Acute severe lameness, swelling, and angular and rotational deformity of the limb are present. Salter-Harris type II fractures are most common, but the small size of the epiphysis complicates surgical repair. Substantial tibial shortening can be expected, and prognosis is poor.

Tibial Malleolar Fractures

Medial malleolar fractures are rare but occasionally occur from trauma and may be associated with substantial collateral ligament injury. When collateral ligament injury is minimal, fragments can be removed arthroscopically, but visibility can be difficult without proper instrumentation. After fragments are removed, the arthroscope can usually be advanced to the plantar pouch. Prognosis is good in horses without substantial collateral ligament damage and tarsocrural instability. However, if there are additional loose fragments within the joint, this may indicate further damage of the tarsocrural joint.

See Chapter 44 for a discussion of lateral malleolar fractures.

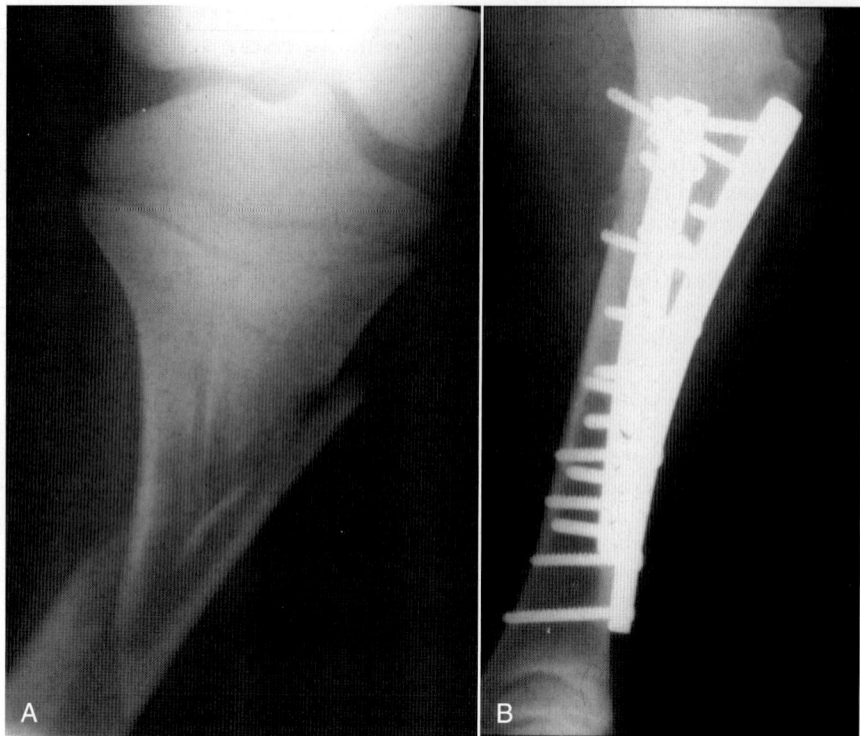

Fig. 45-3 • **A,** Preoperative and **B,** postoperative radiographic images of a 2-month-old Standardbred foal with a diaphyseal tibial fracture.

Tibial Tuberosity Fractures

Direct trauma causes tibial tuberosity fractures, which occur most often in field hunters and jumpers. Fractures are usually nonarticular and can vary in length, width, and depth. In most horses with injuries that are managed conservatively, fractures heal functionally but without radiological evidence of union. In a retrospective study surgical repair of nonarticular fractures in six horses resulted in a successful outcome.[12] Large fractures involving the femorotibial joint surfaces can be repaired, but surgical repair is not necessary in most horses and can be associated with catastrophic fracture of the tibia if occult fracture lines are not recognized and implant failure occurs[13] (see Figure 46-12). In one study, 10 of 14 horses with nonarticular tibial tuberosity fractures that were managed conservatively were sound, and horses performed at the expected level[14] (Figure 45-4). If fractures are repaired rather than simply having screws placed across the fracture line, a tension band technique such as a short plate and screws or a combination of screws and wire should be used.

Enostosis-like Lesions of the Tibia

Enostosis-like lesions of the tibia are diagnosed by scintigraphic and radiological examinations. These lesions can be a cause of chronic, mild hindlimb lameness, or in the TB (rarely STB) racehorse they occasionally cause acute pronounced lameness mimicking that seen with a tibial stress fracture.

Osteochondroma of the Tibia

Osteochondroma of the tibia is a rare radiological finding in the distal, caudal aspect of the tibia and may be incidental or may cause tarsal tenosynovitis. I have seen one adult horse with osteochondroma that as a foal had

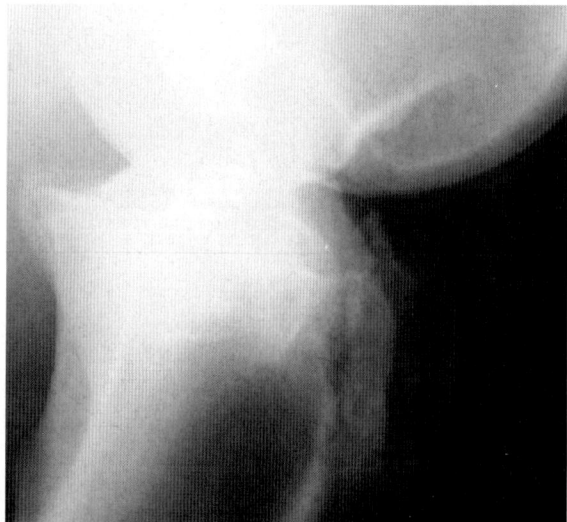

Fig. 45-4 • Lateromedial radiographic image of the proximal aspect of the tibia in a horse with chronic lameness and fracture of the tibial tuberosity. Conservative management of this horse resulted in a successful outcome, although radiological evidence of fracture union was never achieved.

repair of a tibial fracture. The condition has rarely been reported.[15]

Osseous Cystlike Lesions of the Proximal Aspect of the Tibia

Osseous cystlike lesions of the proximal aspect of the tibia are unusual, may be the result of osteochondrosis, and frequently communicate with the lateral femorotibial joint (see Figure 23-3) (Figure 45-5). There may be concomitant osteochondrosis lesions involving the distal aspect of the

55a

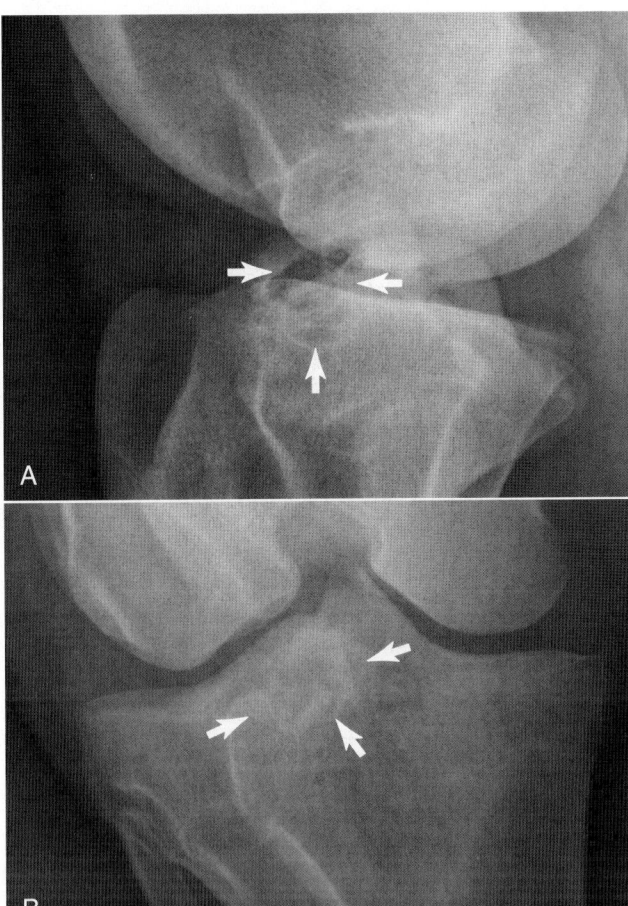

Fig. 45-5 • Lateromedial (**A**) and caudocranial (**B,** lateral is to the left) digital radiographic images of a 3-year-old Standardbred gelding with a multiloculated osseous cystlike lesion and increased radiopacity of the proximal lateral tibial epiphysis *(arrows)*. Intraarticular photographs are shown in Figure 23-3. This horse underwent arthroscopic surgical debridement using a cranial approach through the femoropatellar joint and septectomy.

lateral femoral condyle. Some adult horses develop radiolucent changes caused by osteoarthritis, but in these horses osseous cystlike lesions are acquired, not developmental. Some adult horses develop sudden-onset lameness associated with a well-established osseous cystlike lesion that was previously asymptomatic with no evidence of primary osteoarthritis. Clinical signs are similar to those in horses with other subchondral bone cysts or osseous cystlike lesions of the femorotibial joint, but lameness is often pronounced in adult horses with osteoarthritis. In most horses with osseous cystlike lesions involving the lateral femorotibial joint, curettage is difficult without elevating or severing the lateral meniscus. Some of these horses respond to conservative management and intraarticular injections of hyaluronan and corticosteroids. Intralesional injection with corticosteroids has also been reported. In horses with acquired osseous cystlike lesions related to osteoarthritis, the lesion is usually medial and prognosis is poor because cartilage damage of the proximal tibial condyle and distal medial femoral condyle is usually severe. One study described 12 horses with osseous cystlike lesions. In six the lesions were believed to be the result of osteochondrosis, and three of the six horses that received surgical debridement became athletes. Only two of six horses in which osseous cystlike lesions

were caused by osteoarthritis returned to work after surgery.[16] Often, location precludes complete surgical debridement because cysts most commonly occur in the midportion of the proximal aspect of the tibia under the lateral meniscus. Prognosis worsens when the cyst cannot be completely debrided, there is concomitant involvement of the distal aspect of the femur, there is deterioration or tearing of the lateral meniscus, or there is substantial osteoarthritis.

Osseous Cystlike Lesions of the Distal Aspect of the Tibia

Osseous cystlike lesions of the distal aspect of the tibia are rare injuries and appear to be acquired as the result of trauma or stress-related bone injury. I have seen osseous cystlike lesions in this location in a jumper and a STB racehorse. In both horses, there was acute-onset lameness and tarsocrural effusion. However, such lesions can be present in the absence of effusion. Scintigraphic examination revealed focal, moderate-to-intense IRU of the distal aspect of the tibia. Horses were rested and later performed at a level similar to preinjury level. Computed tomography was useful in elucidating the lesion in other horses (see Chapter 20).

Physitis of the Distal Tibia

Physitis of the distal tibia is discussed in Chapters 57 and 128.

Fibular Fractures

Authentic fibular fractures occur rarely and are often fortuitously diagnosed scintigraphically or radiologically when images are obtained in horses with undiagnosed hindlimb lameness or in those with suspected tibial stress fractures. Fractures occur either proximally or in the mid-diaphyseal region and can appear as a chronic nonunion fracture with bulbous proliferation on each side of the fracture. There can be numerous apparent fibular fractures, and the condition can occur bilaterally. Proliferation likely existed before onset of clinical signs. Horses with midshaft fibular fractures have a large, nearly intact fibula that may predispose to fracture, but a causal relationship between this anatomical finding and fracture has not been established. Often, scintigraphic examination reveals focal IRU at the fracture site and sometimes diffuse IRU in the fibula peripheral to the fracture (Figure 45-6). The entire limb should be evaluated carefully to exclude another site of pain causing lameness. In a Warmblood jumper I observed a focal area of intense IRU of the midfibula that appeared radiologically like a large, chronic nonunion, but moderate hindlimb lameness abated after high plantar analgesia, and suspensory desmitis was the bona fide source of pain. Occasionally there is focal IRU involving both the most proximal aspect of the fibula and the immediately adjacent tibia that may reflect trauma to their articulation. Verification of this as a cause of pain and lameness is difficult. I have seen horses—three TB racehorses and one STB racehorse—with authentic fibular fractures that were discovered during scintigraphic examination. Horses were examined for poor racing or training performance or undiagnosed or high-speed hindlimb lameness and were sound with rest (see Figure 45-6).[17] Four months' rest is recommended, but in horses in which lameness persists, segmental fibular ostectomy remains a potential surgical approach. The entire limb should be evaluated carefully to exclude another site

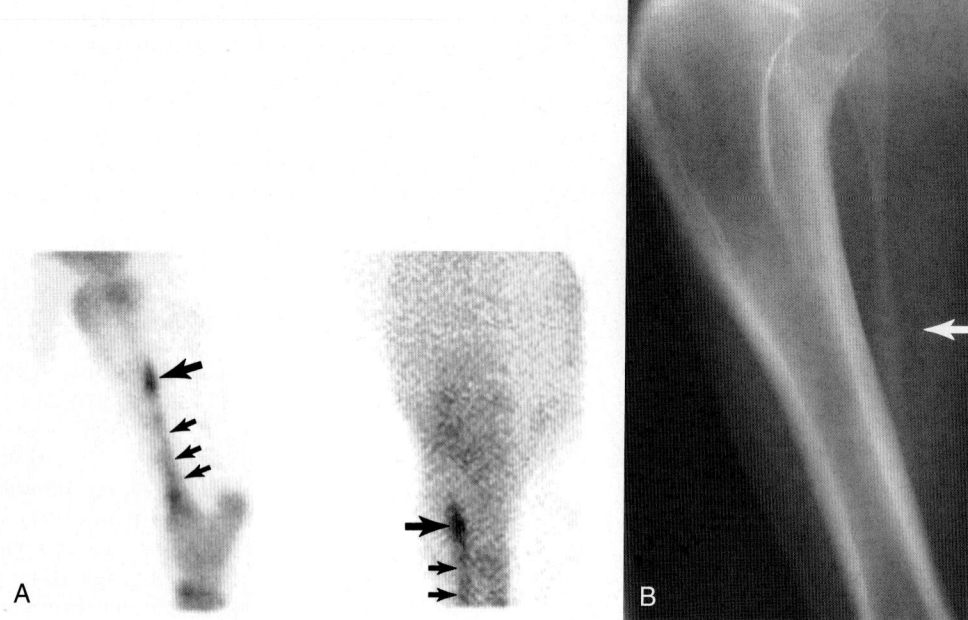

Fig. 45-6 • A, Lateral (left) and caudal (lateral is to the left) delayed phase scintigraphic images of a 4-year-old Standardbred racehorse that underwent bone scintigraphy for undiagnosed left hindlimb lameness. Focal, intense increased radiopharmaceutical uptake (IRU) of the left fibula *(large arrows)* is diagnostic of fracture. In the lateral image, focal IRU could easily be confused with a tibial stress fracture, but in the caudal image IRU is clearly in the fistula. There is diffuse mild-to-moderate IRU in the fibula distal to the fracture site *(small arrows),* indicating that abnormal bone modeling exists peripheral to the fracture site. **B,** Craniolateral-caudomedial oblique plain radiographic image showing a midshaft fibular fracture *(arrow)* and bony enlargement of the fibula proximal and distal to the fracture site. A large, nearly intact fibula is present.

of pain causing lameness. Six horses with proximal fibular fractures made complete functional recoveries; horses were sound within 3 months, but a fracture line persisted radiologically until 4 to 6 months after the injury.[8]

Nonossifying Fibromas of the Proximal Tibia

A yearling TB filly with rare, nonossifying fibromas of both tibias was examined because of kyphosis of the lumbar spine and a stilted hindlimb gait.[18] Radiographs revealing radiolucent defects and sclerosis of the proximal tibial epiphyses and scintigraphic images published in the case report[18] look similar to those of horses I have seen with multiloculated proximal tibial osseous cystlike lesions thought to be a form of osteochondrosis (see Figure 45-5).

Tumors

Hemangiosarcoma occurs rarely in the proximal aspect of the crus. Firm, slow-growing, subcutaneous, soft tissue masses without bone involvement are composed of multiloculated areas of hemorrhage and can be excised without recurrence. It was reported that a fibrosarcoma of the distal, caudomedial aspect of the crus just above the tarsus was resected and recurrence was not seen at 1½ years after surgery.[19]

Soft Tissue Injuries of the Crus

Fibularis tertius injury in foals and adult horses is discussed in Chapter 80, and gastrocnemius tendonitis is discussed in Chapter 80. Stringhalt is discussed in Chapter 48.

Chapter 46

The Stifle

John P. Walmsley

ANATOMY

Developmental Anatomy

The seven centers of ossification in the stifle of the foal are the metaphyses of the femur and tibia, the distal femoral epiphysis, the proximal tibial epiphysis, the patella, the tibial tuberosity (the apophysis), and the fibula. The proximal tibial physis closes at about 2½ years of age. The tibial apophyseal-epiphyseal physis closes by 1 year of age. The apophysis does not fuse with the metaphysis until 3 years of age. This apophysis is an important radiological feature in a young horse and can be mistaken for a fracture. The distal femoral physis closes by about 2½ years of age. In young foals, the margins of the femoral trochleas and the patella are irregular for the first 3 months of life because of incomplete ossification. The fibula is not evident radiologically until about 2 months of age, and a high percentage of adult horses have one and occasionally up to three horizontal radiolucent lines in the fibula distal

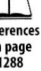

to its head. These should not be confused with fracture lines.[1]

Reciprocal Apparatus

The reciprocal apparatus has an important influence on the action of the stifle. Extension of the joint exerts a pull on the superficial digital flexor tendon, which originates in the supracondyloid fossa of the femur and is mostly tendonous. Because this flexor tendon has an insertion on the calcaneus, the hock must extend simultaneously with the stifle. On the cranial aspect of the stifle, the fibularis (peroneus) tertius, also a tendonous structure, originates in common with the long digital extensor tendon between the lateral trochlea and the lateral condyle of the femur.[2] The fibularis tertius passes through the extensor sulcus in the lateral part of the tibial head, associates closely with the deeper tibialis cranialis muscle, and inserts on the third tarsal and third metatarsal bones and the fourth tarsal bone and calcaneus. Flexion of the stifle necessitates flexion of the hock because of the action of the fibularis tertius.[2] Weight bearing is achieved without much muscular effort by the parapatellar fibrocartilage of the medial patellar ligament hooking over the medial femoral trochlea by contraction of the quadriceps femoris. The patella is released by contraction of the quadriceps femoris, combined with the lateral pull of the tensor fascia latae and biceps femoris.

Femoropatellar Joint

The articulation between the patella and the trochleas of the femur forms the femoropatellar articulation. The patella has three straight ligaments. The medial patellar ligament attaches to the medial border and the distal aspect (apex) of the patella through the parapatellar fibrocartilage. Arthroscopically the ligament can be viewed beneath the joint capsule. Distally the medial patellar ligament attaches medial to the groove on the cranial aspect of the tibial tuberosity. The middle patellar ligament originates on the cranial part of the patella just proximal to the apex and inserts in the distal part of the groove of the tibial tuberosity. The lateral patellar ligament extends from the lateral aspect of the patella to the lateral part of the tibial crest. The biceps femoris has a tendon of insertion on this ligament.[3] Femoropatellar ligaments also reinforce the joint capsule medially and laterally, the lateral ligament being the more distinct.

The medial trochlear ridge of the femur is larger and more rounded than the lateral trochlear ridge and articulates with the medial part of the patella and the fibrocartilage of the medial patellar ligament. The joint capsule has a large suprapatellar pouch and inserts abaxially on the trochlear ridges forming lateral and medial recesses, the lateral being the smaller. A large fat pad is cranial to the joint capsule, proximal and distal to the patella. In my experience, most horses have a slitlike opening into the respective femorotibial joints at the distal end of the medial trochlear ridge and frequently the lateral trochlear ridge as well. Latex passed from the femoropatellar to the medial femorotibial joint in 60% to 65% of horses and in the reverse direction in 80% of horses.[3] Diffusion of mepivacaine between all the compartments may occur in about 75% of horses.[4]

Femorotibial Joints

The medial and lateral femorotibial joints are separate compartments, which are divided by an intact median septum in a healthy joint. However, they may communicate after trauma.[5] The crescent-shaped, fibrocartilaginous medial and lateral menisci lie between the respective femoral and tibial condyles to form a congruent articulation.[2] Both are attached to the tibia, cranial to the intercondylar eminences, by cranial ligaments. The medial ligament wraps around the cranial aspect of the medial intercondylar eminence before inserting on the tibia. The medial meniscus is also attached caudally to the medial intercondylar eminence by the caudal ligament, which can be seen arthroscopically in the caudal part of the medial femorotibial joint. The lateral meniscus attaches caudally to the popliteal notch of the tibia and through the strong meniscofemoral ligament to the caudal part of the intercondylar notch of the femur. Only the cranial and caudal poles of the menisci can be viewed arthroscopically because of the close apposition of the tibia and femur, but the respective cranial ligaments are clearly visible. During flexion the menisci slide caudally, and during extension they slide cranially.

The cranial cruciate ligament has its tibial attachment cranial to the medial intercondylar eminence and its femoral attachment in the lateral part of the intercondylar notch. The cranial cruciate ligament lies beneath the median septum and usually cannot be directly viewed arthroscopically without removing the septum. A better view is often gained from the lateral compartment. The caudal cruciate ligament originates in the popliteal notch of the caudal aspect of the tibia and runs proximally, medial to the cranial cruciate ligament, to insert cranially in the intercondylar notch of the femur.[6] The ligament can be viewed beneath the septum in the cranial and caudal medial compartment of the femorotibial joint. In the dog, the cranial cruciate ligament is under tension during extension of the femorotibial joint,[7] and this may be so in the horse.

The collateral ligaments both originate proximally on the respective epicondyles of the femur. The medial collateral ligament inserts distally on the tibia distal to the medial condyle and has attachments to the medial meniscus. The lateral collateral ligament lies over the popliteal tendon and inserts distally on the head of the fibula. The popliteal tendon originates close to the lateral collateral ligament on the femur and courses distally and caudally, in close apposition to the femoral condyle, to a triangular area of insertion on the proximal caudal aspect of the tibia. The tendon is viewed arthroscopically in the cranial aspect of the lateral femorotibial joint and also in the caudal part, which it effectively divides, limiting the arthroscopic accessibility. The tendon of origin of the long digital extensor muscle can be followed arthroscopically in the cranial compartment of the lateral femorotibial joint from its origin on the extensor notch of the femur and is usually invested within the joint capsule, although in some traumatized joints, the tendon appears separate.[5]

DIAGNOSIS
General Considerations

The history may give an important lead to diagnosing the cause of lameness. For example, a young horse is a candidate for osteochondrosis or subchondral cystic lesions.

Acute-onset stifle lameness in a horse at pasture or during work is more likely to be a traumatic injury involving ligaments or bone. Sudden reduction of work or poor condition may predispose to upward fixation of the patella. Palpation of the patellar ligaments and the outline of the patella, collateral ligaments, long digital extensor tendon, tibial crest, and medial and lateral tibial condyles should be possible. Many horses with stifle injuries manifest no abnormalities on physical examination of the joint. If severe trauma has occurred, the whole region may be swollen, making palpation of the individual structures difficult. The horse may guard the limb so strongly that instability may not be obvious. Because of the ligamentous structures around the joint, distention is only readily palpable over the cranial aspect of the femoropatellar joint and over the medial femorotibial joint cranial to the medial collateral ligament.

Gait and Manipulative Tests

Differentiating stifle lameness in the horse by studying the gait is difficult because the reciprocal apparatus coordinates the movement of the whole limb. In my view, attributing the cause of certain gait changes to stifle pain is not possible. Some horses with stifle pain may carry the stifle slightly abducted, but this is not specific. A careful analysis of the whole limb is required to establish the site of pain causing lameness. Other gait changes that may be seen with stifle lameness, but which are also not specific, are a reduced cranial phase of the stride and a reduced flexion of the limb in flight. Many horses with stifle pain dislike going downhill. Horses with delayed release or upward fixation of the patella tend to avoid fully extending the limb and appear to have a crouching gait. Flexion of the upper limb exacerbates lameness in horses with stifle pain, and abduction of the limb may be resented. When performing proximal limb flexion tests, holding the limb at midmetatarsal level, rather than by the foot, helps to differentiate between upper and lower limb pain.

Three specific manipulative tests have been described for the stifle. These are the cruciate test, collateral ligament test,[8] and patellar displacement test. Most horses with clinically significant stifle pain resent these tests, which makes the tests difficult to perform and to interpret. All manipulation or flexion tests should be done on the contralateral limb first. For the cruciate test, the affected limb should be weight bearing. The head of the tibia is pushed caudally and then released 5 to 10 times before trotting the horse. Laxity is supposed to be appreciated and lameness exacerbated if severe cruciate injury exists. I have never found this test effective. Pain in the affected joint provokes strong guarding by the horse so that the procedure is impossible to perform. The medial collateral ligament test involves abducting the distal limb against shoulder pressure exerted on the femorotibial joint 5 to 10 times before trotting the horse. Horses with ruptured medial collateral ligaments are so painful and instability is so great that this test is inappropriate, but it can be useful for a sprain of the ligament. The lateral collateral ligament is less often affected, but it can be tested by pulling the distal aspect of the limb medially. Lameness associated with problems with patella release may be worsened by pushing the patella proximally several times with the horse weight bearing before trotting, but again this is often an unrewarding test.

DIAGNOSTIC ANALGESIA

In many horses with low-grade stifle lameness, positive diagnostic analgesia is the only way to localize the site of pain, so it is an important test. Because diffusion of local anesthetic solution between the three joint compartments is so variable,[4] all three must be blocked to ensure a valid test. Alleviation of lameness after analgesia of one compartment does not necessarily infer that that compartment is definitely the source of pain.

I use a 5-cm, 19-gauge needle for each joint compartment and up to 30 mL of local anesthetic solution because experience has shown that 20 mL in each compartment might be incompletely effective in a 600-kg horse. Strict aseptic procedure should be followed. Arthrocentesis of the femoropatellar joint is well tolerated and performed first. An intradermal bleb is usually unnecessary. However, an inexperienced veterinarian may find one helpful for the medial femorotibial compartment because some horses are sensitive to injection at this site. My preferred approach for the femoropatellar joint is between the middle and medial patellar ligaments. Synovial fluid is infrequently retrieved from this site unless the joint capsule is distended. If a synovial fluid sample is required, it may be retrieved more easily through a lateral approach.[9] The lateral cul-de-sac is entered caudal to the caudal edge of the lateral patellar ligament and 5 cm proximal to the tibial condyle. The medial femorotibial compartment is entered over the medial tibial condyle between the medial patellar ligament and the medial collateral ligament. A small outpouching of the joint capsule may be palpated. The lateral femorotibial compartment is best approached just cranial or caudal to the long digital extensor tendon and close to the tibial plateau. Less space is available between the meniscus and the joint capsule in the latter approach, so the former is preferred. An improvement in lameness can be expected in 30 minutes, but the clinician is wise to allow at least 1 hour for the final assessment.

Horses with a number of conditions causing lameness in the stifle respond incompletely or not at all to intraarticular analgesia. Horses with medial or lateral collateral ligament or patellar ligament injuries may be unaffected. Horses with subchondral bone cysts in the medial femoral condyle show a variable response, ranging from resolution of lameness to little change, and analgesia can take a long time to take effect. Horses with conditions that cause severe lameness are often only partially improved by analgesia; these conditions include infections; fractures, particularly patellar and tibial crest fractures; advanced osteoarthritis (OA); and severe cruciate and meniscal tears.

IMAGING CONSIDERATIONS

Radiography

Although many stifle injuries are not associated with detectable radiological changes, radiography is usually the first imaging mode to be used once the site of pain causing lameness has been established as the stifle, or if the distal aspect of the limb has been excluded as a potential source of pain. An x-ray machine capable of producing at least 90 kV and 20 mAs is required. In larger horses, adequate definition will only be achieved with even higher-powered x-ray generators. Fast-screen film combinations can be used particularly for caudocranial images. Using as slow a combination as possible is always worthwhile, commensurate with safe practice, to achieve the best definition on the radiograph. Large cassettes are necessary and should be held in a cassette holder with a long handle. Because of the difficulty of aligning the cassette perfectly in the standing horse, using a grid is impractical, although one can be used if the horse is under general anesthesia. Many horses dislike having cassettes placed close to the stifles, so great care must be taken with this procedure. If any doubt exists about the horse's temperament, the horse should be sedated.

Five standard images are most commonly used: lateromedial, flexed lateromedial, caudocranial, caudolateral-craniomedial oblique, and cranioproximal-craniodistal oblique (skyline). The radiographic anatomy of the soft tissue attachments of the stifle is well described.[10]

Lateromedial Image

The horse should be standing naturally for this image. The x-ray beam is directed perpendicular to the stifle. The stifle is naturally rotated slightly laterally in most horses, which predisposes to the beam being directed from too far cranially. The x-ray beam should pass just proximal to and parallel to the tibial plateau. The landmark on which to target the x-ray beam is the lateral condyle of the tibia. The cassette has to be pushed as far proximal as possible, which can be difficult in a well-muscled horse or a stallion. In a well-positioned radiographic image, the femoral condyles are superimposed on each other.

Flexed Lateromedial Image

The limb is held in the farrier's position with the tibia parallel to the ground. If the stifle is held with its axial plane vertical, directing the x-ray beam perpendicular to the joint is easier. The same landmarks are used as for the standing lateromedial image. When the x-ray beam is correctly positioned, the femoral condyles are superimposed. When compared with the standing lateromedial radiographic image, the flexed image reveals a greater area of the medial intercondylar eminence of the tibia and the cranial part of the femoral condyles and also allows more complete imaging of the patella.

Caudocranial Image

The caudocranial image requires relatively high exposure factors. A key feature for correct positioning is the angle of the tibia because the x-ray beam should be perpendicular to the tibia. Placing the horse in its natural stance or with the limb slightly caudal to the contralateral limb facilitates correct alignment. The x-ray beam should divide the limb in the caudocranial plane and pass just proximal to the level of the lateral tibial condyle. The natural lateral rotation of the stifle should also be taken into account. Thus the x-ray beam is usually aimed craniodistally and craniolaterally and meets the caudal musculature of the thigh surprisingly proximally. The correct image defines the femorotibial joint spaces and clearly images the intercondylar eminence of the tibia within the supracondylar fossa of the femur.

Caudal 30° Lateral-Craniomedial Oblique Image

For the caudal 30° lateral-craniomedial oblique image, the x-ray beam is directed 30 degrees from the caudocranial plane and slightly from proximal to distal, so that it crosses parallel to the tibial plateau, which it should bisect. The main value of this image is imaging the lateral femoral trochlea, with the advantage of highlighting the medial femoral condyle, and it can be used to screen for osteochondrosis lesions and subchondral cystic lesions.

Cranioproximal-Craniodistal Oblique Image

The cranioproximal-craniodistal oblique image is a skyline image of the patella and femoral trochlear ridges and may be the only view on which a patellar fracture may be seen. In a standing horse, the limb is held in the farrier's position with the tibia horizontal. The x-ray beam is aimed along the articular surface of the patella, but it may be impeded by the horse's flank. Twisting the metatarsal region medially, which rotates the stifle laterally, sometimes allows better access to the patella. The cassette is held along the cranial proximal aspect of the tibia, and the x-ray beam is directed almost vertically. Checking the position of the patella on a previous flexed lateromedial image helps to decide on the correct beam angle. In an anesthetized horse, the leg is flexed with the horse in dorsal recumbency, and the x-ray beam is directed from distal to proximal.

The contours of the femoral trochlear ridges and the patella are irregular in young foals. In most foals this irregularity is present up to 11 weeks of age, and in 45% of foals, up to 25 weeks.[11] In foals older than 5 months of age, irregularity of the femoral trochleas is abnormal. Irregularity of the femoral or tibial condyles is abnormal at any age.

Ultrasonography

A substantial proportion of stifle lameness is caused by soft tissue damage; therefore ultrasonography has a potential diagnostic role in defining the injury and has several advantages over other imaging diagnostic techniques. At present, ultrasonography is the only method of assessing soft tissue injury in the stifle in a standing horse. The disadvantages are that ultrasonography requires experience to be used effectively and a good-quality ultrasound scanner with a sector and a linear array transducer is necessary. Transducer frequencies of 7.5 and 5 MHz are needed to image the cranial aspect of the stifle, but a 3-MHz transducer is required to image the caudal part of the stifle.[12-15] When it becomes available, magnetic resonance imaging (MRI) is likely to be a superior imaging technique for soft tissues of the equine stifle.[16] Computed tomography (CT) has already proven useful for evaluation of meniscal tears and for detection of cartilage and subchondral and trabecular bone injury.[17]

Ultrasonography can be valuable for differentiating joint capsule distention from extraarticular swelling. Soft tissue structures that can be imaged include the patellar ligaments, the menisci and the respective cranial ligaments, the collateral ligaments, the cranial and caudal cruciate ligaments, the meniscofemoral ligaments, the origin of the long digital extensor tendon, and the popliteal tendon. The articular cartilage and bony outline of the femoral trochlear ridges and the cranial and caudal third of the femoral condyles may also be imaged.[12-15]

The patellar ligaments and the collateral ligaments can be imaged longitudinally and transversely with a 7.5- to 10-MHz linear array transducer with the horse weight bearing. The middle patellar ligament is the most obvious of the three and is a useful landmark. The femorotibial collateral ligaments can be imaged from the attachments on the distal lateral or medial femoral epicondyles to the attachments on the proximal medial or lateral aspects of the tibia, and they lie over the respective menisci.[18] The menisci can also be imaged with this transducer from caudal to the medial and the lateral patellar ligaments. They appear as wedge-shaped structures of moderate echogenicity with the base of the wedge closer to the transducer. The cranial ligaments of the menisci are more easily imaged with a small convex array or sector transducer, which can be aimed more perpendicular to the meniscal ligaments and which can be more easily positioned between the patellar ligaments. The cruciate ligaments are difficult to image because aligning the transducer perpendicular to the fibers of the ligament is difficult. Only a small length of ligament can be imaged at a time, which can make interpretation equivocal. Cruciate ligaments can only be viewed with the stifle in a flexed position using a convex array or sector scanner. Useful information on the surfaces of the femoral trochlear ridges and condyles can be obtained. The condyles are imaged with the stifle in a flexed position, and this can be helpful in diagnosing subchondral bone cysts.[19] From caudal, a sector transducer is preferable for imaging the caudal cruciate ligament and the meniscofemoral ligaments, and a 3-MHz transducer is necessary in large horses.[13]

Scintigraphy

Scintigraphy has been used on horses for more than 30 years, but little published evidence assesses its specificity and sensitivity for conditions of the stifle. A recent study of 16 horses indicated moderate to high sensitivity of scintigraphy for detection of meniscal damage, cruciate ligament injury, or articular cartilage pathology in the stifle using arthroscopy as the gold standard, but specificity was low, indicating a high risk of false-negative results.[20] For most stifle conditions, scintigraphic findings are variable, and although positive findings are obviously helpful, negative findings can also add useful information. The clinical significance of any scintigraphic result should be confirmed as exhaustively as possible by other tests, particularly diagnostic analgesia because false-positive results also occur. In the normal adult stifle, the caudal aspect of the tibial epiphysis often has highest uptake of radiopharmaceutical.[21]

Nuclear scintigraphy is most consistently valuable in diagnosing incomplete avulsion fractures associated with the stifle.[22,23] However, although positive results may be obtained within 24 hours of injury, in some horses at least 3 days must elapse before clinically significant increased radiopharmaceutical uptake (IRU) occurs. Subchondral cystic lesions that cause lameness may be scintigraphically positive or negative (Figure 46-1). The lesions are more likely to be detected in older horses, using a caudal image, than in an immature horse with high background activity. Absence of radiopharmaceutical uptake was thought to be the result of osteoclasts being the dominant cells in certain stages of the condition.[24,25] However, in the Editors' experience the majority of subchondral cystic lesions do have focal IRU. Although scintigraphy has been used to assess osteochondrosis in people,[26] bone scan findings are not well documented in horses. I have seen positive and negative scintigraphic results associated with clinically

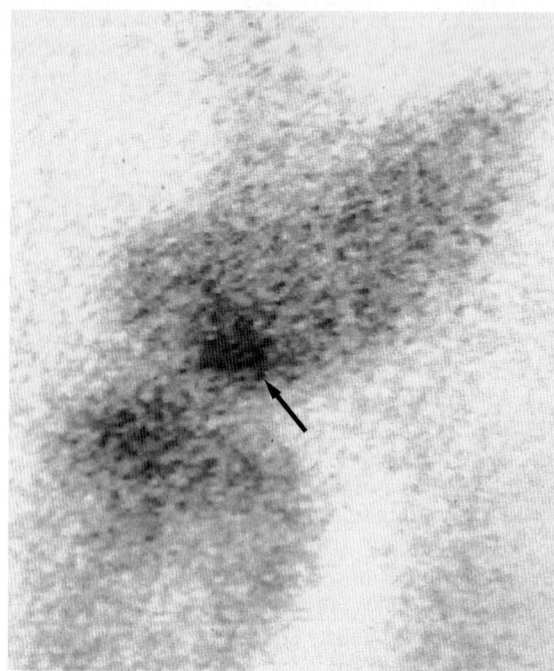

Fig. 46-1 • Lateral delayed (bone) phase scintigraphic image of the right stifle of a 9-year-old Thoroughbred cross gelding. There is focal increased radiopharmaceutical uptake in the distal femoral condyle (*arrow*). A subchondral bone cyst in the medial femoral condyle thought to be causing lameness was seen radiologically.

significant osteochondrosis of the lateral femoral trochlea. Soft tissue injuries of the stifle are often scintigraphically negative, but in my experience IRU can occasionally be encountered in these horses, especially in association with enthesopathy.

Scintigraphy is certainly a useful tool as a diagnostic aid for lameness in the stifle and can be useful for evaluating the bone activity of lesions. Occasionally horses may respond positively to intraarticular analgesia, but no clinically significant abnormalities are found on radiography, ultrasonography, and arthroscopy. IRU in the stifle may be the only finding. Making a definitive diagnosis in these horses is difficult, although conceivably subchondral bone pain may be a possible cause of the lameness. One should bear in mind that many stifle conditions are negative scintigraphically. Conversely, the joint may be scintigraphically positive when the cause of lameness is elsewhere in the limb.

ARTICULAR DISEASES

Femoropatellar Joint

Osteochondrosis

Osteochondrosis has been recognized in horses for more than 50 years and is an important cause of stifle lameness in young horses. The exact cause of the disease is still not well defined, but several factors are known to influence its development. Adequate dietary copper is important. Mare's milk is relatively low in copper, and because the foal relies on copper stored in its liver during late pregnancy, it will be deficient if the mare's diet contains insufficient copper. The zinc/copper ratio is also important because zinc inhibits the absorption of copper.[27] Foals on high-energy diets are more prone to the disease.[28] Insufficient or excessive exercise and trauma may be factors that influence the development of the disease. Genetic factors may predispose to osteochondrosis in the hock of Swedish Standardbreds (STBs).[29] Large, fast-growing males are more susceptible. Osteochondrosis is most frequently seen in Thoroughbreds (TBs) and Warmbloods. The lesions probably develop in the first 7 months of life,[30] but sometimes clinical signs may not be manifest until the horse is brought into work. In the sports horse this may be as late as 5 years of age or even older when a mild to moderate lameness may develop as the horse begins more serious work. In my experience, surprisingly severe lesions can remain undetected until this time. Lesions are most commonly seen on the lateral trochlear ridge of the femur[31] but do occur on the medial trochlea, intertrochlear groove, and patella and are often bilateral.

Signs and Diagnosis

Osteochondrosis may be present asymptomatically. Lameness is often acute in onset and varies from a subtle gait deficit to marked lameness. Lameness is often more acute in onset and more severe in foals and young yearlings than in older horses. Distention of the femoropatellar joint capsule is often present and can be severe, especially in foals and yearlings. Gluteal muscle atrophy is seen in horses with severe lesions. Flexion tests are mostly positive. Synovial fluid may be hemorrhagic, but it is often normal. Intraarticular analgesia of the femoropatellar joint should improve lameness. However, in mature horses lameness may be mild, with no effusion and a poor response to intraarticular analgesia. In such horses arthroscopic evaluation often reveals an extensive area of cobblestone-like cartilage, with extensive fibrillation over a large portion of the lateral trochlea of the femur. This cartilage is often well adherent to the subchondral bone and little clinical benefit is derived from surgery.

Radiological changes include the following: no detectable signs, slight loss of contour or loss of outline of the lateral trochlear ridge, irregular defects in the trochlear ridge, radiodense fragments within the defect (Figure 46-2), round radiopaque bodies loose in the joint, and more rarely, irregularities on the patellar apex or the medial trochlear ridge.[1,32,33] Lateromedial and caudolateral-craniomedial oblique images are the most useful projections. Horses with radiological lesions do not always show lameness.[25,27] Some horses have no detectable radiological abnormalities, but osteochondrosis lesions are diagnosed on arthroscopic examination. Lesions without fragmentation in young foals may resolve with time,[32,33] but many progress.[34]

Treatment

Conservative management, with confinement and correction of dietary imbalances, and arthroscopic debridement of the lesions are the main treatment options. Conservative management is appropriate for horses with mild lesions. Because of the insensitivity of radiological evaluation of osteochondrosis lesions, an argument can be made for arthroscopic examination of most horses with lesions seen radiologically or persistent femoropatellar effusion and lameness that fails to respond to conservative treatment.[35]

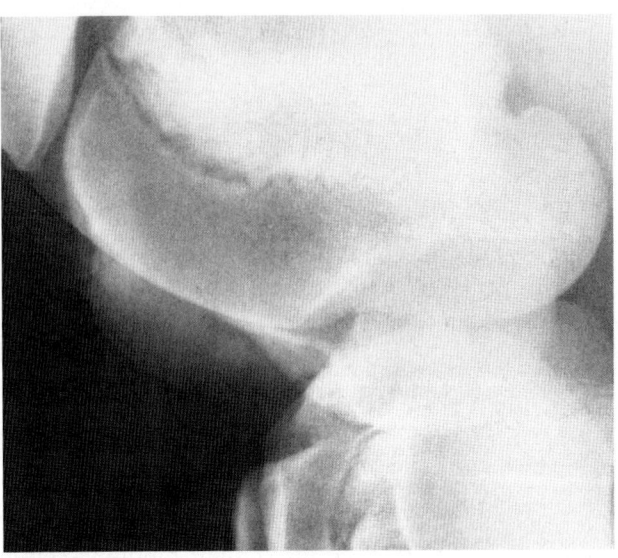

Fig. 46-2 • Lateromedial radiographic view of the femoropatellar joint of a yearling Thoroughbred colt. There is a large irregular defect in the subchondral bone of the lateral trochlear ridge containing several radiodense fragments.

Arthroscopic examination would ensure that horses with radiologically silent cartilage lesions are treated effectively. OA can also be evaluated. For horses with fragmentation and clinically significant radiolucent defects of subchondral bone, arthroscopic surgery is probably the treatment of choice.[31] In my opinion, more caution is required when treating foals arthroscopically because some foals with large lesions seen radiologically are found to have intact cartilage at arthroscopy. Debridement of such lesions can leave unacceptably large deficits in the lateral trochlear ridge. Reattaching these cartilage flaps with polydioxanone pins may be a more appropriate treatment and has shown good results with seven of nine foals achieving athletic use.[36]

A variety of lesions are seen arthroscopically. The articular cartilage may appear intact, but if probed, large flaps may lift from the subchondral bone. Large defects on the lateral trochlear ridge may contain nodules of mineralized cartilage, which are readily removed, and often large tufts of fibrillated cartilage are associated with the lesion. The exposed subchondral bone is frequently soft and crumbly. Extensive areas of fibrillated cartilage over the adjacent lateral trochlear ridge and the opposing patella are often present in older horses.[5] Loose cartilage should be removed, and the lesion should be curetted to healthy subchondral bone, which is a source of pluripotential cells. The cartilage perimeter should be vertical to allow better attachment of tissue regrowth.[37] Thorough lavage to remove all debris, particularly of the suprapatellar pouch, at the completion of surgery is essential. Six weeks of stable rest with daily handwalking after 2 weeks is recommended postoperatively. The horse should then be left for another 4 to 5 months at pasture before returning to work.

Prognosis

Mild lesions in foals were shown to heal with conservative management.[32,33] For foals with more severe lesions, better results were reported with arthroscopic debridement.[31] Sixty-four percent of 161 horses were able to perform athletically. In this series, treatment of older horses and those with mild to moderate lesions was most successful, which has also been the experience in my practice. The presence of extensive secondary articular cartilage fibrillation did not have a significant effect on the outcome in horses more than 2 years of age.[5]

Upward Fixation of the Patella and Delayed Patellar Release

Upward fixation of the patella occurs when the stifle subtends an angle of approximately 145 degrees and the medial patellar ligament hooks over the medial trochlea of the femur, thus locking the reciprocal apparatus with the limb in extension. The condition is more common in horses with a straight hindlimb conformation with a stifle angle nearer 140 degrees (in the normal horse the angle is about 135 degrees), so that only a small degree of extension is required for upward fixation to occur.[38] Upward fixation is not a luxation of the patella, despite being commonly described as such. Predisposing straight hindlimb conformation or the condition itself may be hereditary.[39] Upward fixation of the patella is more commonly seen in young horses and ponies, especially if they are in poor condition, when weak thigh musculature fails to release the patella. Upward fixation can occur in older horses after trauma to the stifle region, is most frequently manifest when the affected horse is stabled, and sometimes occurs in fit horses that are suddenly given box rest. Lameness may develop in horses with more severe or long-standing lesions. I recognize delayed patellar release as a condition in which delayed release of the patella occurs, without complete upward fixation, and which presumably is a less severe form of the disease.

Signs and Diagnosis

A horse with upward fixation of the patella stands with the hindlimb locked in extension with the fetlock flexed (Figure 46-3). The leg releases with a snap, usually unaided,

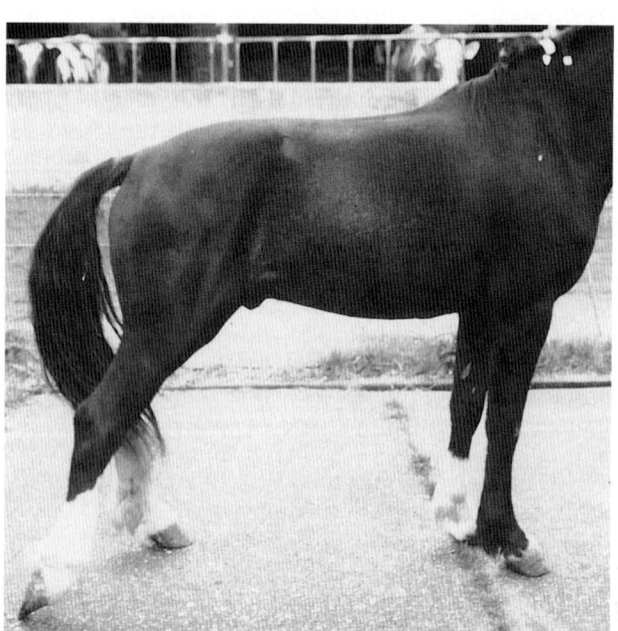

Fig. 46-3 • Three-year-old Welsh Cob gelding with the typical stance of upward fixation of the patella in the right hindlimb.

but occasionally the horse needs assistance. Some horses merely show intermittent delayed release of the patella, especially when turned toward the affected limb. This can be mistaken for stringhalt. Delayed patellar release is manifested by a catching of the patella as the limb is protracted, usually as the horse moves off. Delayed release of the patella may be evident as a rather jerky movement of the patella when the horse moves over in the stable or as it decelerates from canter to trot or trot to walk. Horses in which the condition is chronic develop stifle soreness and may be resistant to work, especially in deep going. If the condition is more serious, horses try to avoid extending the hindlimbs while walking uphill or downhill. Femoropatellar effusion may be present. Diagnosis may depend on the history and the owner's description if the horse does not lock the patella during the examination. Locking the patella manually may be possible by pushing it proximally, although this can be difficult and is resented by many horses. A careful search should be made for concurrent stifle disease such as osteochondrosis or soft tissue injury, and the site of any lameness should be confirmed by diagnostic analgesia. Radiographic examination of both stifles is prudent because any pathological condition caused by upward fixation or concurrent with it affects treatment and prognosis.

Treatment

For a horse that has the patella locked, pushing the patella medially and distally and backing the horse is recommended but difficult to do. Pulling the limb forward with a side line may provide relief. If the upward fixation of the patella is intermittent and not causing lameness, a conditioning program should be undertaken. This includes an exercise regimen, the administration of anthelmintics, an increased plane of nutrition, and dentistry as appropriate for each horse. The exercise regimen depends on the specific circumstances for each horse. Daily lunging should be instituted to a level that is appropriate for the age and type of horse. Stable rest is usually contraindicated, and turning the horse out to pasture as much as possible is preferable. Immature horses should be allowed time to outgrow the problem. Injection of counterirritants containing iodine into the medial and middle patellar ligaments has been used at this stage of the disease.[40] Horses with delayed patellar release require the same management.

Because of potential complications, which include fragmentation of the patella and lameness, surgery is only indicated when the following criteria have been fulfilled:

1. Upward fixation of the patella persists despite an appropriate conditioning program.
2. Lameness has developed because of the disease.
3. The condition in an immature horse does not resolve as the horse matures.

The surgery can be performed under local anesthesia in the standing horse.[41] A small incision is made over the distal part of the medial patellar ligament. I find that minimizing the incision length seems to reduce the incidence of postoperative swelling. A curved Kelly forceps is then advanced caudally under the ligament, developing a path for a blunt-ended bistoury. The bistoury is passed until its end can be palpated caudal to the medial patellar ligament, before the ligament is severed close to its tibial insertion.

Stringent asepsis should be observed. Once the ligament is severed, the border of the tendon of the sartorius muscle is palpable caudally. Some surgeons prefer to perform this surgery with the horse under general anesthesia, which allows for complete asepsis: the ligament can be exteriorized before severing, and the fascia overlying the ligament can be sutured before skin closure.

An alternative treatment involving numerous splitting incisions in the medial patellar ligament was described and was successful in four horses and three Shetland ponies, but only two horses were followed beyond 5 months.[42]

Postoperatively I prefer to confine the horse for 2 months to allow the patella to settle in its new position in the intertrochlear groove. Handwalking can be introduced during the second month.

Prognosis

A substantial number of horses respond to conservative treatment. Occasional recurrences happen if the horse has enforced stable rest, but many grow out of the condition. After surgery and in the absence of degenerative changes in the joint, the horse should return to normal use, although some appear to have a slightly restricted gait. Recurrence of the condition is unusual. Some fibrous thickening is palpable at the surgical site for many years in most horses and indefinitely in some horses. Clinically significant complications including lameness, local swelling, fragmentation of the patella, and fracture of the patella were reported.[43-48] Fragmentation of the patella was produced after experimental medial patellar desmotomy.[46] If fragmentation causes lameness, horses can be managed arthroscopically with good results.[33] In my experience, up to 30% of horses have minor fragmentation of the patella, without clinical signs, after medial patellar desmotomy. Injury of the middle patellar ligament can also occur secondary to medial patellar desmotomy.[49,50]

Fragmentation of the Patella

Fragmentation of the patella is generally considered to be a sequela to medial patellar desmotomy or to be associated with upward fixation of the patella, and it is manifested by fragmentation of cartilage and bone off the apex of the patella.[43,46,48,50] This condition is not chondromalacia of the patella, which could be a form of osteochondrosis, and has not been specifically reported in horses. If the condition follows desmotomy, clinical signs can appear from 3 weeks to more than 12 months postoperatively. Horses can develop fragmentation within a few weeks of surgery without clinical signs.[5] Medial patellar desmotomy was performed experimentally in 12 horses, and of these eight developed fragmentation.[46] The lesions may be caused by instability of the patella after medial patellar desmotomy.

Signs and Diagnosis

Lameness varies from a stiff hindlimb action to an obvious lameness. Flexion is resented and worsens the lameness. Synovial effusion is common, and excessive fibrous tissue reaction may be present at the surgical site. Radiologically, small bone fragments are present close to the apex of the patella (Figure 46-4), often combined with radiolucent defects of subchondral bone and roughening or spurring of the distal cranial aspect of the patella.

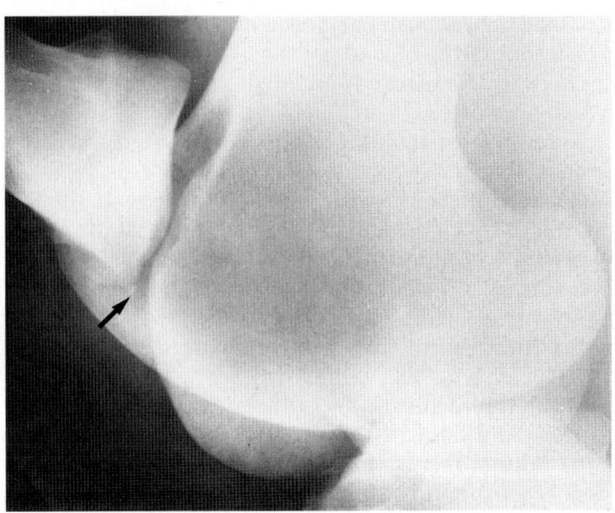

Fig. 46-4 • Lateromedial radiographic image of the stifle of a 7-year-old Thoroughbred cross gelding that had previously had a medial patellar desmotomy to treat intermittent upward fixation of the patella. The apex of the patella is fragmented *(arrow)*.

Treatment

Arthroscopic debridement is indicated. The lesions are most commonly on the lateral surface of the apex of the patella and may be partly obscured by synovial villi; therefore a careful arthroscopic examination should be performed before deciding on the site of the instrument portal. Debridement of the lesion to healthy subchondral bone is required.

Prognosis

The prognosis for athletic function is reasonable, although some horses appear to have a slightly stiff hindlimb action because of the original medial patellar desmotomy. Ten of 15 horses returned to athletic use.[43] In my experience, the incidence of the condition has decreased in the past 8 years, which may be because fewer patellar desmotomies are performed or because more care is taken during convalescence.[5] However, the condition still occurs despite appropriate rest after medial patellar desmotomy.[50]

Luxation of the Patella

Lateral luxation of the patella in the foal is considered to be an inherited condition caused by a recessive gene.[51] Luxation in an adult horse is likely to be traumatic in origin.[38] Because the medial trochlear ridge of the femur is largest, only severe trauma induces medial displacement of the patella. Hypoplasia of the lateral trochlea of the femur is often present in association with lateral luxation of the patella,[39] but the condition also occurs in foals with apparently normal conformation.[51] Luxation is most common in miniature breeds but has been reported in STBs, TBs, and an Arabian foal,[52-54] and I have seen it in a Welsh Cob.[5]

Signs and Diagnosis

The condition may be unilateral or bilateral and has been graded as follows:
- Grade 1: The patella can be manually luxated but readily reduces itself.

- Grade 2: The patella is usually in place but luxates intermittently.
- Grade 3: The patella is usually luxated but can be manually relocated.
- Grade 4: The patella is continuously luxated and cannot be relocated.[53]

Severely affected foals are unable to extend the stifle and stand in a characteristic crouching position. If less severe, the condition may not be obvious clinically, but horses are usually reluctant to flex the stifle and have a stiff gait in the affected limb. Some horses show little evidence of the disease until degenerative changes provoke lameness. I have seen a TB yearling with severe osteochondrosis of the lateral trochlear ridge, which led to a diminution of the ridge and allowed the patella to luxate laterally. One of the Editors (MWR) has seen numerous STB foals with severe osteochondrosis of the lateral trochlear ridge of the femur and patellar luxation. Lateromedial, cranioproximal-craniodistal oblique, and caudocranial radiographic images are the most useful to ascertain the position of the patella and to evaluate the trochlear ridges.

Treatment

Lateral release and medial imbrication of the femoropatellar compartment are necessary to maintain the patella in the intertrochlear groove.[52-54] Both lateral release and medial imbrication appear to be important. Recession sulcoplasty is valuable in the presence of hypoplasia of the lateral trochlear ridge of the femur.[54]

Prognosis

Poor success can be expected with surgery in the presence of OA, large osteochondrosis lesions, and in larger horses. In foals there is a moderate prospect of achieving athletic function. Aggregating the results from the three reported case series, the patella maintained its position postoperatively in eight of 11 foals.[52-54] Breeding from affected horses should be discouraged.

Osteoarthritis

Any injury to the femoropatellar joint can potentially cause OA. The injury could be simple trauma or result from any of the previously mentioned conditions if they have caused irreversible changes.

Signs and Diagnosis

The clinical signs depend on the cause and severity of the condition. Lameness is usually persistent, and chronic joint distention may be present. If osteochondrosis is responsible for OA, radiological changes typical of chronic osteochondrosis are likely to be present (see page 536). Cartilage fibrillation, ranging from focal tufting to widespread involvement of the femoral trochlear or patellar articular cartilage, may be seen arthroscopically, and full-thickness defects of the articular cartilage may be present in more severely affected horses.

Treatment

Initially treatment depends on the inciting condition and is described in the appropriate sections. However, once chronic osteoarthritic changes have developed, realistically therapy is likely only to be palliative. Intraarticular medication with small doses of corticosteroids, such as 10 mg of triamcinolone acetonide combined with hyaluronan, may give temporary relief. A controlled exercise regimen may help, and an arthroscopic debridement prolongs working life in some horses.

Prognosis

The femoropatellar joint is more forgiving than the femorotibial joints, and although OA will not resolve, if mild it may be tolerated enough for a horse to perform useful work. More severely affected horses are unlikely to return to athletic use.

Distal Luxation of the Patella

One report of distal luxation of the patella has been made.[55] The horse held the affected limb flexed and non–weight bearing. The patella was relocated with the horse under general anesthesia, and when the horse was reexamined 3 months later, no lameness was seen.

Patellar Ligament Injuries

Patellar ligament injuries are rare. Sprain of the middle patellar ligament is the most common, although lateral patellar ligament injuries also occur.[49] There may be an association between middle patellar desmitis and previous medial patellar desmotomy. Jumping horses are most commonly affected. Lesions may occur unilaterally, or less commonly bilaterally.

Signs and Diagnosis

Lameness can be moderate to severe in the acute phase but varies. The severity of lameness is usually commensurate with the degree of ligamentous damage and is most severe in horses with partial ruptures. Sometimes no localizing signs are apparent, but femoropatellar effusion, periarticular thickening, or edema may be seen in some horses. Intraarticular analgesia of the femoropatellar joint may slightly improve lameness in some horses, but in others there is no effect on the lameness. The diagnosis is confirmed by ultrasonography. Proximal, midbody, and distal lesions have been identified. Differentiation should be made between core lesions and partial-thickness tears. Radiological changes are unusual, and one should bear in mind that entheseous change on the cranial distal aspect of the patella may be seen as an incidental radiological finding. However, extensive entheseous new bone may be of clinical significance. Scintigraphy may show focal IRU in the patella or more commonly the cranioproximal aspect of the tibia in association with proximal or distal lesions of the middle patellar ligament.

Treatment

Horses with severe injuries may require rest for up to 6 months. In one Editor's experience (SJD) conservative management has yielded poor results in horses with extensive core lesions, and treatment by injection of porcine urinary bladder matrix or mesenchymal stem cells has improved the prognosis. The presence of periligamentous fibrosis is a poor prognostic finding. Horses with partial-thickness tears have also responded poorly to any form of management, including surgical debridement.

Prognosis

Lameness is often slow to resolve and is recurrent in some horses.

Femorotibial Joint

Subchondral Cystic Lesions

The cause of subchondral bone cysts and other osseous cystlike lesions is still unknown. The distal weight-bearing aspect of the medial femoral condyle is the most frequent site for subchondral bone cysts.[56] Osseous cystlike lesions were identified in the caudal aspect of the femoral condyles in foals.[57] Osseous cystlike lesions also occur in the proximal aspect of the tibia. Lesions thought to result from osteochondrosis were in the lateral aspect of the tibia, and those associated with OA were more common medially in a report of 12 horses.[58] Subchondral bone cysts and osseous cystlike lesions may be a form of osteochondrosis,[59] but trauma is also probably an important factor. Subchondral bone cysts in the medial femoral condyle have been produced experimentally after development of full-thickness defects in cartilage and subchondral bone.[24] Lesions did not form if the defects were made only in cartilage. The lining of these lesions has been shown to contain active inflammatory enzymes that cause bone resorption.[60] In the literature the syndrome in the young horse is emphasized, but in my experience subchondral bone cysts and osseous cystlike lesions occur in any age group, mostly apparent as a primary lesion but sometimes as a sequel to OA.

Signs and Diagnosis

The condition is reported to be more common in horses less than 4 years old,[56] but in my practice it is encountered in horses of all ages.[5] Lameness is mild to moderate but can be severe at first and acute in onset. Lameness may be intermittent, especially in older horses. Affected horses seem to be lamer when turning. Occasionally mild medial femorotibial effusion occurs, but often no signs are obvious on physical examination. Intraarticular analgesia of the medial femorotibial joint may be required to diagnose the site of pain causing lameness. Because the subchondral bone is probably the site of pain, local anesthetic solution must diffuse into the lesion and may not be completely effective. A 50% improvement in lameness justifies radiographic examination.

The caudocranial, caudolateral-craniomedial oblique, and flexed lateromedial radiographic images are the most useful for demonstrating the lesion. Subchondral bone cysts in the medial femoral condyle are relatively round or oval, with a variably sized base and communication with the joint (Figure 46-5). Increased radiopacity of the rim is usually seen only in horses with older lesions. Radiological signs of OA may also be apparent in some horses. The osseous cystlike lesions in the tibia have a similar morphology. Subchondral bone cysts can also occur as incidental radiological findings in sound horses. Lesions in the caudal aspect of the femoral condyles in foals may appear radiologically as localized or extensive osseous defects. Scintigraphic findings in horses with subchondral bone cysts are inconsistent,[24] but most have IRU. Flattening or indentation of the distal medial femoral condyle is sometimes seen radiologically and may be a precursor of a subchondral bone cyst. These lesions are relatively common and frequently do not cause lameness. Occasionally IRU is seen associated with these defects.[5] In my experience, positive scintigraphic findings, together with a positive response to diagnostic analgesia, are good indications that

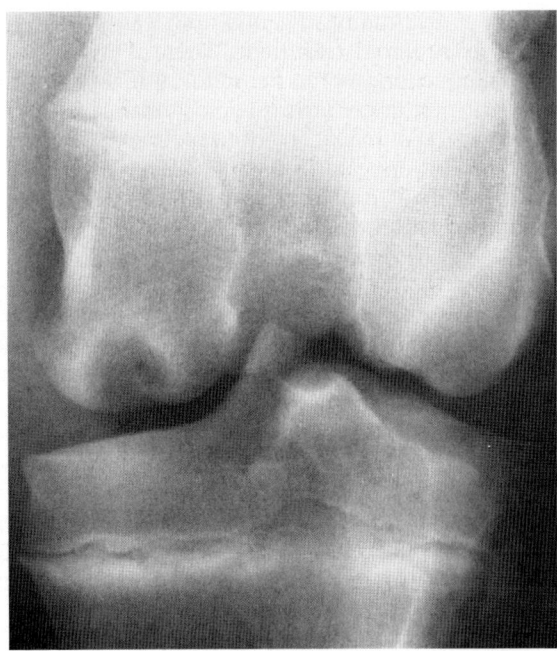

Fig. 46-5 • A caudocranial radiographic image of the right stifle of a yearling Thoroughbred colt. Medial is to the left. There is a subchondral bone cyst in the medial femoral condyle with increased radiopacity of the rim and a wide base that communicates with the medial femorotibial joint.

the defect is a cause of lameness, but some scintigraphically positive lesions do not result in clinical signs; the Editors consider this unusual. Arthroscopic evaluation of horses with subtle osteochondral defects of the medial femoral condyle detected radiologically revealed that flattening of the medial condyle or a subchondral lucent area was associated with a focal or more generalized cartilage defect in 18 of 20 and four of four limbs, respectively. Treatment by abrasion arthroplasty and microfracture resulted in seven of nine horses with focal cartilage lesions returning to full athletic function, and two of six with generalized cartilage pathology.[61]

Treatment

Conservative treatment involves stable or pasture rest, with or without nonsteroidal antiinflammatory medication or intraarticular corticosteroids.[62,63] Horses with nonarticular osseous cystlike lesions or small articular defects are probably best managed conservatively. For articular lesions and horses that do not respond to conservative management, arthroscopic debridement has been advocated.[56,59,64] Debridement of the cyst lining and removal of all debris from the joint are the goals. Experimentally the use of cancellous bone grafts did not improve the outcome.[65] Postoperative intralesional corticosteroid has been advocated to suppress the inflammatory mediators.[60] Subchondral bone forage is contraindicated because reports indicate that it may worsen the lesion.[56] Debridement of small medial condylar defects should be approached with caution because this may provoke a worsening of the lesion. Tibial osseous cystlike lesions can be debrided arthroscopically, but many of them lie beneath the cranial meniscal ligament, which must be divided to gain access. It was reported that the success rate for horses more than 3 years of age was poor (35% of 46 horses sound at follow-up evaluation),[66] and many surgeons now lean toward intra-lesional corticosteroid treatment. There is evidence that numerous injections of corticosteroids into the fibrous lining of the cyst under arthroscopic guidance is the most effective method of management in older horses, and early reported success appears to be superior to that achieved using debridement in older horses (13/18 horses sound at follow-up evaluation).[67]

Prognosis

A 50% success rate was reported with conservative treatment of horses with medial femoral condylar subchondral cysts, but remodeling of bone may be more prolonged than with surgical treatment.[62] Arthroscopic debridement carries a 70% to 75% success rate in horses less than 3 years old.[56,64] Preexisting OA results in a more guarded prognosis. Improvement of clinical signs after surgery frequently occurs without radiological resolution. Limited reports of surgical treatment of tibial osseous cystlike lesions[58] suggest that horses with lateral proximal tibial osteochondrosis-associated lesions may respond best, and this is also my experience.

Meniscal and Meniscal Ligament Injuries

The cause of meniscal injuries in horses is not well documented, but in dogs meniscal injuries are considered to be caused by crushing forces combined with tibial rotation and flexion or extension of the stifle.[7] Meniscal injuries have also been reported in horses.[68-71] I have diagnosed 126 meniscal injuries arthroscopically as the primary cause of lameness. The medial meniscus was affected in 80% of horses. The cranial ligaments of the menisci were involved in nearly all horses.[72] Concurrent injury to other structures in the stifle was frequently diagnosed, including articular cartilage damage on the femoral condyles in 96 horses and cruciate injury in 18 horses. Secondary medial collateral ligament injury was not diagnosed. Primary medial collateral ligament rupture with secondary meniscal injury was not included in the series. Twenty-seven of 79 other horses that were examined arthroscopically and that had other stifle injuries, but no evidence of meniscal damage, did have fibrillation of the axial borders of the cranial ligaments of the menisci.[68] The clinical significance of this is uncertain.

Signs and Diagnosis

Lameness is often acute and severe in onset after trauma but mostly becomes low grade and persistent. Distention of the femoropatellar or medial femorotibial joints can be expected in horses with more severe injury.[71] Lameness is exacerbated by flexion of the limb in about 90% of horses.[55] Diagnostic analgesia is usually necessary to confirm the site of pain causing lameness but may not render the horse completely sound. Radiological signs occured in 52% of horses that I have diagnosed with meniscal injury. New bone formation on the cranial aspect of the medial intercondylar eminence of the tibia was the most frequent finding (25%)[72] and appears to be more common with meniscal than cruciate ligament disease, in which it occurred in five of 71 (7%) cases treated at my hospital[72] (Figure 46-6). Dystrophic mineralization and osteoarthritic radiological changes may be seen in horses with severe lesions. Ultrasonography can be a valuable aid in diagnosis, although some lesions will not be visible

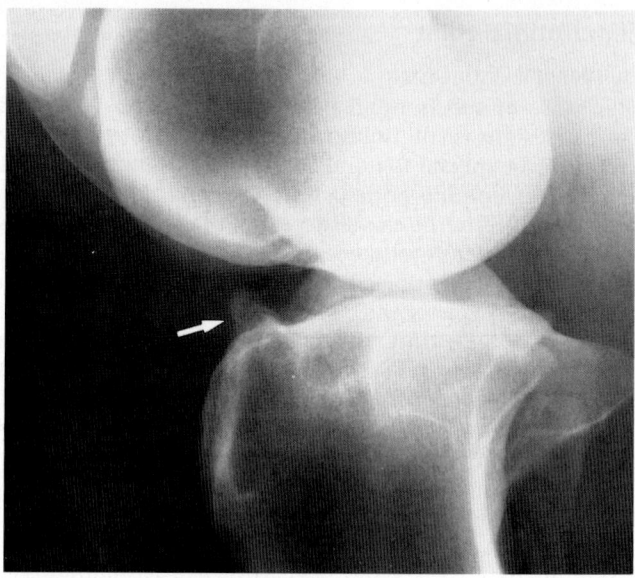

Fig. 46-6 • Lateromedial radiographic image of the left stifle of a 7-year-old Thoroughbred cross gelding. There is new bone on the cranial aspect of the intercondylar eminences of the tibia (arrow). Note also the large radiolucent zone in the proximal aspect of the tibia. There is an old osteochondrosis lesion involving the lateral trochlear ridge of the femur. Arthroscopic examination revealed a tear of the medial meniscus.

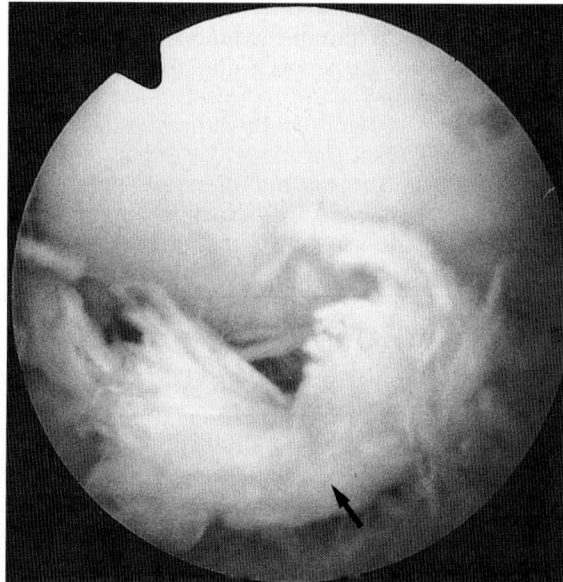

Fig. 46-7 • Arthroscopic photograph of the left lateral femorotibial joint of a 6-year-old eventer gelding. The lateral meniscus has a grade 2 tear (arrow).

ultrasonographically, and artifactual changes can be difficult to differentiate.[73,74]

Arthroscopy offers the best chance of a definitive diagnosis and an assessment of concurrent damage. Because only the cranial and caudal poles of the menisci can be seen, assessment of meniscal injury is limited. Owing to these limitations, I graded changes visible from cranially as follows:

1. Tears extending longitudinally from the cranial ligament into the meniscus, with minimal separation
2. Tears involving the cranial pole in which the extent of the injury is visible (Figure 46-7)

3. Severe tears that extend beneath the femoral condyle and that cannot be completely assessed or debrided[71]

Treatment

Horses with acute stifle injuries that have no definitive diagnosis should be managed with rest and antiinflammatory medication, followed by controlled exercise. Arthroscopy is indicated if conservative therapy is unsuccessful or for severely lame horses. Grade 1 meniscal tears can only be superficially debrided. Intraarticular suturing for some horses may be a way forward. Grade 2 and 3 tears are debrided as effectively as possible by removing all loose tissue. A careful assessment of visible concurrent damage should be made. Postoperatively controlled exercise begins at 2 to 3 weeks and can gradually be increased over 3 months, depending on progress and the extent of the injury. Free exercise at pasture should be avoided for 6 months.

Prognosis

Return to full athletic use can be expected in about 50% of horses overall, although improvement may be seen in another 10%.[71,72] Full function was regained in 60% of 67 horses with grade 1 tears, 65% of 35 horses with grade 2 tears, 10% of 24 horses with grade 3 tears, and neither of 2 horses with two menisci affected. In the Editors' experience the prognosis for return to full athletic function in upper level sports horses is guarded. Concurrent articular cartilage damage significantly worsened the prognosis,[71] and nine of 18 horses with concurrent cruciate ligament injury became sound. Horses treated arthroscopically within 2 months of injury fared 25% better than those treated later than 2 months.[72] If radiological signs of OA were present, the prognosis was also significantly worsened.[71]

Cranial and Caudal Cruciate Ligament Injuries

In the dog the cranial cruciate ligament can be injured when the stifle is in hyperextension or after sudden rotation with the stifle in flexion,[7] and this is likely to pertain to the horse. Direct trauma to the joint or degenerative change in the ligament can also lead to cruciate injury in the horse.[5,75] Experimentally[76] and in my clinical experience[5] the cranial cruciate ligament fails most frequently at midbody level, but avulsions of its tibial and less often of its femoral attachments have been reported.[75,77] Caudal cruciate ligament injuries occur less frequently.[78] Concurrent injuries, including damage to the medial collateral ligament, the menisci, and articular cartilage, are often associated with cruciate tears.[75,79]

Signs and Diagnosis

Lameness is often associated with a history of trauma and is usually acute in onset and severe at first. Distention of the femoropatellar or the femorotibial joints is sometimes present. In horses with severe injuries, crepitus may be detectable. The cruciate draw test appears to be valueless in the conscious horse, but a proximal limb flexion test is usually positive, especially with severe injury. In horses with mild injuries, diagnostic analgesia is required to confirm the site of pain causing lameness. In my series of 75 horses with cranial and caudal cruciate ligament injuries diagnosed at arthroscopy, radiological signs included the following[5]:

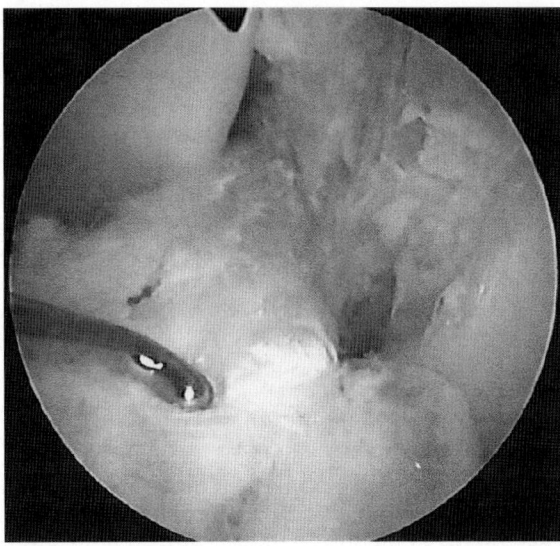

Fig. 46-8 • An arthroscopic view of the right femorotibial joint of an 8-year-old Warmblood gelding. The median septum has been removed with the motorized synovial resector to reveal a chronic, low-grade fiber disruption of the cranial cruciate ligament.

- No changes in at least 56% of horses.
- Fracture of the intercondylar eminence of the tibia; however, this can occur without clinically significant cruciate injury.
- New bone formation cranial to the intercondylar eminence of the tibia. This finding was three times more common in horses with meniscal injuries than those with cruciate ligament injuries in my series.
- Bony resorption or fragmentation at the femoral attachment of the cruciate ligaments.
- Cranial displacement of the tibia with cranial cruciate ligament rupture.
- OA, or mineralization of the ligament, associated with chronic lesions.

Ultrasonographic evaluation of the cruciate ligaments is difficult. Arthroscopy offers the best evaluation of the cruciate ligaments. The cranial cruciate ligament is covered by the median septum, which may make the ligament difficult to assess, but the septum is often disrupted in cranial cruciate ligament injury. Motorized debridement of the septum may be required to see the ligament. The caudal cruciate ligament is viewed from the cranial and caudal aspects of the medial femorotibial joint. The caudal medial aspect of the femorotibial joint can be approached cranially[80] or caudally.[81] Mild cranial cruciate ligament changes are difficult to quantify because of inflammatory changes in the median septum, but fiber disruption is seen in moderate injuries (Figure 46-8). With acute, severe injuries of the cranial cruciate ligament, inflammatory debris must be removed before the torn ends of the ligament can be seen. Concurrent articular cartilage or meniscal damage within the joint is common.

Treatment

With acute injuries the same treatment criteria apply as for meniscal injuries. The indications for arthroscopy and postoperative management are also similar. Arthroscopic debridement is best performed with a motorized synovial resector. Repair in horses with complete cruciate ligament rupture has not been reported, and the best treatment that can be offered is good debridement of loose tissue to allow less severe injuries the best chance to heal.

Prognosis

Prognosis is poor in horses with moderate to severe injuries. In one report, two of 10 horses were pasture sound and one raced,[75] and in another report two of six were pasture sound.[79] In my series, lameness persisted in four of six horses with severe injuries; 10 of 17 horses with moderate injuries became sound; and 18 of 29 horses with minor superficial changes became sound.[5]

Collateral Ligament Injuries

Injury of the medial collateral ligament is more frequently diagnosed than injury of the lateral collateral ligament. Such injury is associated with acute trauma, which, as in the dog, probably involves a medial or lateral force on the joint or distal aspect of the limb.[79] Concurrent injury of the menisci or cruciate ligaments commonly occurs in horses with severe injuries,[79,82] but not necessarily in those with more moderate injuries.

Signs and Diagnosis

The most easily diagnosed collateral ligament injuries are complete ruptures of the medial collateral ligament, which manifest as acute, severe lameness after trauma. Instability of the stifle occurs with swelling and pain over the ligament. Sprains of the collateral ligaments are less obvious. Heat and pain may be palpable, and chronic thickening develops in some horses. The collateral ligament test can be useful but is not specific. Flexion of the limb is usually painful, but intraarticular analgesia of the medial femorotibial joint may be negative. If complete rupture of the ligament has occurred, stressed caudocranial radiographs are diagnostic. Widening of the joint space occurs on the affected side (Figure 46-9). Enthesophyte formation at the origin and insertion may be seen in horses with chronic injuries. Ultrasonography can be helpful in diagnosing and assessing the injury.[18]

Treatment

Horses with mild sprains, in which no instability occurs, are treated with stall rest for 6 weeks and antiinflammatory medication until the inflammation subsides, followed by controlled exercise for another 6 weeks. One report describes the repair of a complete rupture of the medial collateral ligament using braided polyester material attached to two 6.5-mm cancellous screws in the femur and tibia to stabilize the joint.[83] Orthopedic wire was originally used, but it dislodged postoperatively. The surgery is a salvage procedure and is not well documented, and concurrent injury and horse compliance should be carefully assessed before undertaking surgery.

Prognosis

Horses with mild sprains have a moderate chance of returning to athletic use, depending on the extent of any concurrent injury. Results are not well documented, and in my view the prognosis is probably poor if entheseous change develops at the medial collateral ligament attachments. The prognosis for horses with complete ruptures is grave.

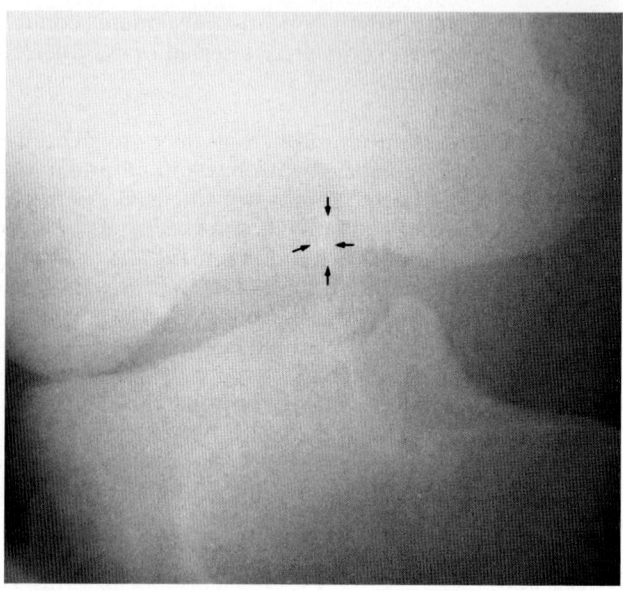

Fig. 46-9 • Stressed caudocranial radiographic image of the left stifle of a 10-year-old riding horse with rupture of the medial collateral ligament of the femorotibial joint. Medial is to the right. There is widening of the medial joint space. Note also the osseous opacity proximal to the intercondylar eminences (arrows).

The horse described above that was treated surgically was comfortable at pasture until it became lame after falling 9 months postoperatively. Because associated meniscal or cruciate injury is common, a high chance exists of OA in the long term, even if the medial collateral ligament heals.

Articular Cartilage Trauma

Articular cartilage defects on the medial or lateral femoral condyles or on the axial part of the tibial plateau are frequently encountered during arthroscopic examination. Usually they accompany other femorotibial injuries, but occasionally they are the only finding, in which case they may be considered the primary cause of lameness.[84] Cartilage lesions were diagnosed as the primary cause of lameness in 150 of 632 horses undergoing diagnostic arthroscopy of the stifle in my series.[5] Primary lesions may be seen on both the medial and lateral femoral condyles.

Signs and Diagnosis

Horses in which articular cartilage lesions are a primary cause of lameness usually have mild to moderate lameness. Diagnostic analgesia is required to define the site of pain causing lameness. Abnormalities are rarely seen radiologically. At arthroscopy, a variety of lesions may be present. These include thickening, softening, and creasing of the cartilage, widespread fibrillation, focal tufts of fibrillated cartilage, circumscribed nodules of cartilage, apparent tears of the articular surface, and areas of exposed subchondral bone.[72,84,85]

Treatment

Doubt about the long-term effect of debridement of cartilage lesions still exists.[86] Small, full-thickness lesions are probably best debrided to subchondral bone; micropicking the bone appears to improve healing to a degree.[87] The effect of smoothing partial-thickness defects is still controversial and may provoke the development of an osseous cystlike lesion.[56,86] Debris should be thoroughly lavaged from the joint. Postoperative intraarticular medication with disease-modifying OA drugs could be helpful.

Prognosis

The prognosis for return to soundness for horses with cartilage defects is generally considered guarded. Six of seven horses with focal defects returned to racing, but five horses with larger lesions remained lame.[84] In my practice, a full-thickness articular cartilage defect was diagnosed arthroscopically in 38 horses as being the primary cause of lameness. Sixteen of 24 horses (67%) for which follow-up information was available became sound.[5] Of the horses with less severe lesions, 30 of 38 (79%) of those with mild changes (mild fibrillation, mild soft creased cartilage, mild focal fibrillation, n = 77) and 17 of 22 (77%) of those with moderate changes (generalized fibrillation, shear lesions, severe thickening and creasing, partial-thickness linear defect, n = 37) returned to full use. In the Editors' experience prognosis for upper level sports horses to return to full athletic function is guarded.

Osteoarthritis

OA of the femorotibial joint can be a sequel to any injury described in this chapter that has the potential to damage the articular cartilage. OA is likely to develop when the initial tissue damage is severe, is not treated, or is treated ineffectively. OA of the medial femorotibial joint is much more common than in the lateral femorotibial joint.

Signs and Diagnosis

Many horses have a history of lameness that has already been treated or chronic lameness of varying intensity. Diagnostic analgesia may be required to identify the site of pain causing lameness, but joint effusion and thickening are palpable on the medial aspect of the joint in many horses. Flexion of the limb is painful, and some horses resent holding up the limb for shoeing. Radiological examination reveals typical changes associated with OA, including osteophytosis, flattening of the articular surfaces of the femoral condyles, increased radiopacity and radiolucent zones in the subchondral bone, narrowing of the joint space, and dystrophic mineralization of soft tissues.

Treatment

Management of OA is at best palliative. If possible, the inciting lesion should be treated appropriately in an attempt to prevent worsening of the changes. Intraarticular corticosteroids, glycosaminoglycans, or any medication designed to slow the progress of the disease, as well as arthroscopy in some horses, may give temporary relief.

Prognosis

Once radiological changes of OA are manifest, in particular, joint space narrowing, the prognosis for athletic soundness is poor. With careful management, less severely affected horses may be able to perform light work or be kept at pasture.

Subchondral Bone Trauma and "Bone Bruising"

Early experience with CT[17] and MRI is providing some explanation for horses with lameness that is improved by intraarticular analgesia of the stifle joints, but in which radiography, ultrasonography, scintigraphy, and, in some horses, exploratory arthroscopy fail to explain the cause of pain. Primary osseous lesions have been identified reflecting bone trauma.

Fractures Involving the Stifle

Fractures of the Patella

External trauma is the commonest cause of patellar fracture in the horse.[88] Contraction of the quadriceps muscles may be the cause of some avulsion fractures. The majority of horses have a history of direct trauma, such as a kick, or an impact on the stifle by hitting a fixed fence while jumping. If the trauma occurs while the stifle is in flexion, the patella is fixed against the trochlear ridge of the femur, which is thought to render it more vulnerable to fracture.[89]

A variety of fracture morphology is seen.[89,90] Sagittal fractures of the medial aspect of the patella are probably the most frequent. These are usually articular, and the fragment often involves a substantial area of the attachment of the parapatellar fibrocartilage of the medial patellar ligament. Fragmentation of the base of the patella sometimes accompanies these fractures[88] or may be seen separately. Nonarticular fractures are mostly seen as mildly displaced fragments on the cranial aspect. Complete horizontal fractures are severe injuries, and the massive forces exerted by the extensor muscles have an important bearing on their management. Complete sagittal fractures are less catastrophic because the distracting forces are not as strong. Comminuted fractures of the whole body of the patella occasionally occur after severe trauma.

Signs and Diagnosis

The history and clinical signs often strongly suggest the possibility of patellar fracture. Initially lameness may be severe and remains so in horses with midsagittal and horizontal fractures. In horses with many of the smaller avulsion fractures or fractures of the medial aspect, lameness becomes moderate to mild after a few days. Often evidence of trauma and local swelling are apparent in the stifle region. Crepitus is occasionally present, and pain may be elicited on palpation of the patella. The femoropatellar joint is usually distended. Horses with chronic, less severe fractures often have surprisingly little direct evidence of the injury. Flexion of the limb is usually painful.

Radiography is essential to confirm the diagnosis and to evaluate the fracture. Lateromedial images may give no indication of the fracture, so a cranioproximal-craniodistal image is essential (Figure 46-10). Severely injured horses greatly resent positioning for this radiographic image and may require analgesia. Occasionally general anesthesia is required, but it should not be attempted without treatment options being in place.

Treatment

Horses with open wounds must be treated with debridement and antibiotics, and it is vital to establish if joint infection exists and treat it appropriately. Horses with small nondisplaced, nonarticular fractures may be managed conservatively with stable rest. Most heal by fibrous union only. Horses may return to work in 8 weeks. Horses with fragments originating from the base of the patella need arthroscopic debridement if debris is loose in the joint.

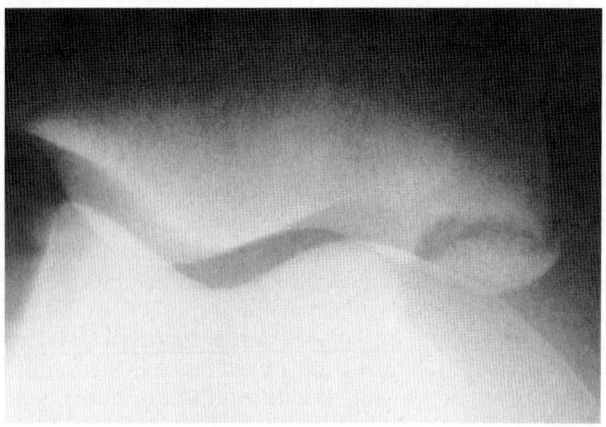

Fig. 46-10 • Cranioproximal-craniodistal radiographic image of the right patella of a 10-year-old eventer gelding that hit a cross-country fence with the right stifle. Medial is to the right, and cranial is to the top. There is a displaced fracture of the medial pole of the patella.

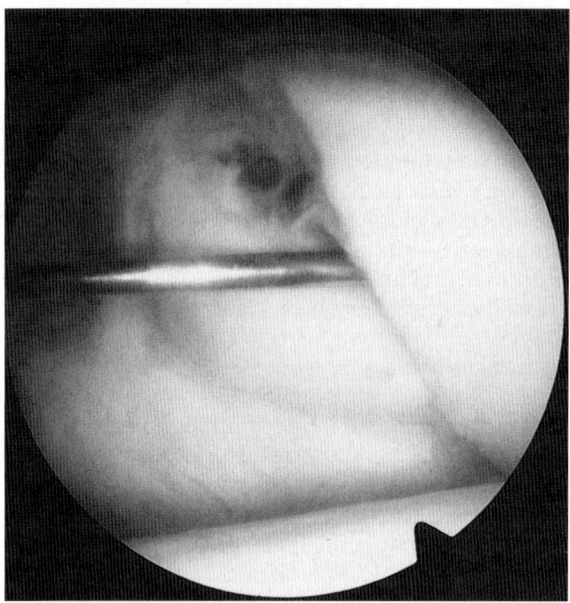

Fig. 46-11 • Arthroscopic photograph of the left patella of the horse in Figure 46-10 showing the fracture line (with probe inserted) in the medial aspect of the patella.

Small fragments at the base of the patella, which are embedded in the soft tissue attachments, may not require removal.[91] Articular fractures of the medial aspect are best removed.[88] This can be done by arthrotomy or arthroscopy (Figure 46-11) and requires careful dissection of the fragment from the medial patellar ligament. The distal end of the fracture is clearly seen arthroscopically. Concurrent joint damage should be evaluated and can have an important bearing on the outcome. Horses with complete horizontal fractures must be treated by internal fixation.[89,92,93] Lag screw fixation with 5.5-mm cortex screws or partially threaded 6-mm cancellous screws, possibly with reinforcement with tension band wiring, is necessary to combat the huge distraction forces of the extensor muscles. Recovery from general anesthesia has to be carefully controlled by delaying attempts of the horse to stand by use of sedation to avoid breakdown of the repair. Sagittal fractures can also be repaired using the lag screw principle.[94]

Prognosis

Horses with small, nonarticular fractures usually have a good prognosis with conservative management.[91] Ten of 12 horses with medial fractures without concurrent joint disease treated by partial patellectomy returned to athletic use.[88] My experience has been similar. Internal fixation of horizontal and midbody vertical fractures can be rewarding, but the risk of breakdown during recovery from general anesthesia is substantial, especially in horses with horizontal fractures. Horses with severely comminuted fractures have a poor prognosis.

Fracture of the Intercondylar Eminence of the Tibia

These fractures have been described as avulsion fractures of the insertion of the cranial cruciate ligament.[75,95,96] However, because the insertion of the cranial cruciate ligament is cranial to the eminence, they are not avulsions but are likely caused by trauma from a lateral force from the medial femoral condyle on the intercondylar eminence.[97]

Signs and Diagnosis

The history and clinical signs are similar to those seen with other acute, severe stifle injuries, and confirmation of the fracture is made radiologically. The caudocranial and flexed lateromedial images are the most useful. Once the acute inflammation has subsided, lameness can be mild to moderate in horses that do not have clinically significant injuries to vital soft tissue structures.

Treatment

An arthroscopic assessment is essential for evaluating the fracture and concurrent soft tissue damage in the joint, which is extensive in some horses. If accompanying soft tissue injuries are not severe, treatment can be rewarding. Small fragments should be removed. Horses with large fragments can be treated by internal fixation.[97] Alternatively, large fragments can be removed, but this depends on fragment configuration and the involvement of soft tissue structures, such as the cranial cruciate ligament or the cranial ligament of the medial meniscus that wraps around the cranial surface of the eminence.[95,96]

Prognosis

If soft tissue damage is reparable, the prognosis for fracture treatment can be good. The possibility always exists of articular cartilage or soft tissue damage that is not detected at arthroscopic examination[78] but that may ultimately cause chronic lameness.

Fracture Fragments Originating from the Femoral Trochlear Ridges or Femoral Condyles in Adult Horses

Fractures of the distal aspect of the femur usually result from direct external trauma, such as hitting a fence while jumping, a penetrating wound, or a kick.[91,98]

Signs and Diagnosis

Characteristically there is a sudden-onset, moderate to severe lameness, with a history of acute trauma. Effusion of the femoropatellar joint is usually present. With condylar fractures there is also effusion of the medial femorotibial joint. Crepitus may be present, and flexion of the joint causes pain. In the femoropatellar joint, fragments arise most commonly from the distal aspect of the lateral trochlear ridge and are best seen on flexed and standing lateromedial radiographic images. Caudocranial images are also important for identifying the position of fragments in the cranial or caudal femorotibial joints, and cranioproximal-craniodistal oblique images are necessary to rule out concurrent patellar fractures. The fracture site may not be obvious. Because these fractures are commonly caused by direct trauma, often the stifle region has a wound, and in these circumstances a strong chance of infection in the joint exists. Infection should be ruled out by arthrocentesis. Infection can also occur by extension into the joint, hours or even days after the injury. If a sudden increase in lameness occurs, arthrocentesis must be repeated.

Treatment

Fragments should be removed to prevent the development of OA. Most can be removed arthroscopically,[91,98] but arthrotomy may be necessary for excision of large fragments.[99] In many horses I prefer to wait a few days before examining the joints arthroscopically because the initial intraarticular hemorrhage hinders surgery. Many horses have a severely inflamed synovium in which fragments may be embedded and difficult to find. Fragments in the femoropatellar joints are often loose, whereas in the femorotibial joints they more often have soft tissue attachments, but conditions vary greatly, and intraoperative radiography to ensure removal of all fragments can be useful. Evaluation of the remainder of the stifle joint for concurrent injuries is important.

Prognosis

Horses with trochlear ridge fractures have a good prognosis after fragment removal.[91,98] If no clinically significant soft tissue damage occurred, the prognosis is also favorable after removal of fracture fragments in the femorotibial joint. One should bear in mind on the initial assessment that some of these injuries are not as catastrophic as the radiological changes suggest.

Salter-Harris Fractures of the Femur, Types III and IV

Type III and IV Salter-Harris fractures of the femur tend to occur in older foals and usually result from a fall with the limb in adduction or from an external trauma. From limited reports, type II fractures, which are not discussed in this section, are the most common physeal fracture; however, of the articular fractures, type IV fractures appear to be more common.[100-102] Type IV fractures often have a characteristic configuration in which the fracture begins in the trochlear ridges in the horizontal plane and exits through the caudal lateral diaphyseal cortex.[100]

Signs and Diagnosis

Foals with minimally displaced fractures may be weight bearing, but the others usually have acute, severe lameness, swelling, pain, and often crepitus in the affected joint. Radiology confirms the fracture and should include enough views to establish its configuration.

Treatment

Conservative treatment may be appropriate for horses with stable, minimally displaced fractures.[100] Internal fixation is indicated for horses with displaced or unstable fractures. Repairs using lag screw fixation, cobra head bone plates,

and angle blade plates have been reported.[100-103] Implanting screws through the articular cartilage of the femoral trochlea is sometimes necessary, and crossing the physis with an implant does not seem to have affected growth in the distal femoral physis in older foals.[100] The dynamic condylar screw plate may be of value.

Prognosis

The few published reports[100] indicate that foals with minimally displaced fractures have a good chance of achieving athletic use with conservative treatment. If surgery is required, the outcome is more equivocal, but good success has been achieved in some horses.

Fractures of the Tibial Tuberosity

The tibial tuberosity is a relatively exposed structure and is susceptible to fracture after direct trauma, such as a kick, or a collision with a fence. These fractures are not associated with the physis of the tibial tuberosity and may not be authentic avulsion fractures, although the lateral patellar ligament is often involved. If patellar ligaments are involved, fractures may displace proximally.[104] If proximal displacement is observed radiologically, a tension band technique should be used for surgical repair, although conservative management can be successful (see below). Traction apophysitis similar to Osgood-Schlatter disease in people has been reported in horses[105] but is rare. In the horse reported, lameness was mild, and small fragments detached from the cranial aspect of the tibial tuberosity were visible radiologically. A variety of fracture configurations occur, from small fragments on the cranial proximal aspect to large fractures extending from distal to the tibial crest to proximally into the femorotibial joint.

Signs and Diagnosis

Most horses are acutely, severely lame immediately after sustaining the fracture, but in some this may settle into a milder lameness if left untreated. Swelling and crepitus are common. Occasionally with minimally displaced fractures there is only mild lameness and no history suggestive of a fracture. A wound on the lateral aspect of the tibia may be present, and intraarticular fractures may be associated with joint effusion. Care should be taken to rule out other injuries in the stifle, such as fracture of the patella, or joint infection if an open wound exists. Infection can even develop by extension into the joint through a skin graze. Because of the lateral curvature of the tibial tuberosity, several radiographic images are often required to identify the contour of the fracture, the caudolateral-craniomedial oblique image being the most useful. The tibial tuberosity does not fuse until at least 3 years of age,[106] and its physis should not be confused with a fracture.

Treatment

Nonarticular fractures may heal with conservative treatment. Horses with large intraarticular fractures can also be treated by internal fixation. Lag screw fixation does not provide a secure enough repair, so tension band wiring,[107] a lateral narrow dynamic compression plate,[108] and a cranial narrow dynamic compression plate[85] have been used. I believe that the most secure repair is achieved with the latter (Figure 46-12). The plate should extend well distal to the distal extremity of the fracture to withstand

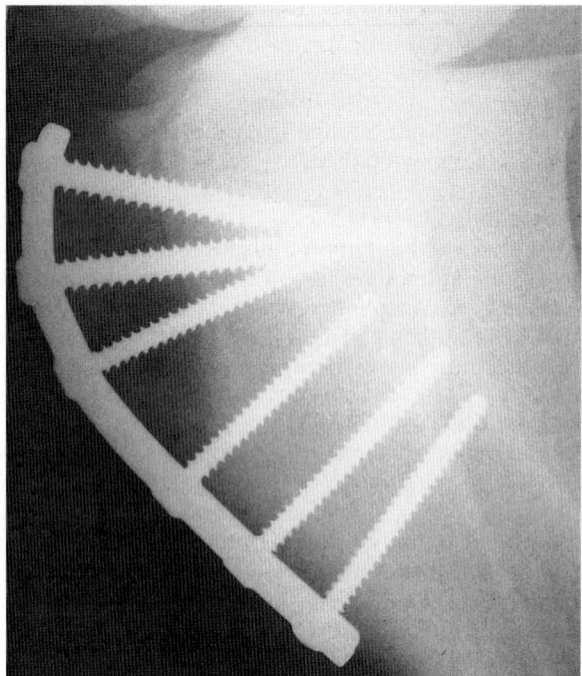

Fig. 46-12 • Postoperative lateromedial radiographic image of the right tibia of a 13-year-old pony gelding that had sustained a fracture of the tibial tuberosity. The horse has been managed using internal fixation with a narrow dynamic compression plate.

the distraction forces of the quadriceps muscles. Because of the shape of the cranial proximal aspect of the tibia, contouring of the plate demands considerable twisting and bending, but this does not seem to affect its efficacy. A technique for preoperative plate bending was reported as a way of saving surgery time,[109] but in my experience plate contouring is not especially time consuming. Most horses are substantially more comfortable postoperatively, but they should be prevented from lying down for 2 weeks.

Prognosis
Conservative treatment of horses with nondisplaced, small fragments results in a good prognosis. Horses with larger fractures may also respond to conservative treatment with complete return to soundness. Fifteen horses with nonarticular fractures were treated conservatively, and 12 returned to full use. Neither size nor displacement of the fragment affected outcome, and the horses returned to work in a mean of 6.3 months.[110] Those that remained lame had concurrent soft tissue injury in the stifle.[110] Good results for return to full athletic function have been reported after repair with a cranially applied plate,[104] and in my view this is the treatment of choice for articular fractures. A potential risk exists for failure of the repair during recovery from general anesthesia or the early postoperative period[108] or for catastrophic tibial fracture. This emphasizes the importance of adequate fixation and restriction of the horse during early convalescence.

Fractures of the Fibula
Fracture of the fibula is usually caused by direct trauma and is a rare injury (see Chapter 45). Lameness is often moderate to severe at first. Palpation of the region may not elicit obvious pain, but radiography should be diagnostic. The caudocranial image is the most useful, but great care must be taken to differentiate a fracture from persistent radiolucent lines that result from separate ossification centers in the fibula. As many as three of these lines can be present, and they may be irregular. Scintigraphy is a useful aid to diagnosis in the absence of localizing clinical signs or if one has difficulty in radiological interpretation. From limited experience, confinement of the horse for 2 to 4 months is usually long enough for reasonable healing to take place, and the prognosis is good.

Other Diseases

Avulsion of the Origin of the Fibularis (Peroneus) Tertius and Long Digital Extensor Tendon
Avulsion of the origin of the fibularis tertius and long digital extensor tendon is a relatively rare condition in horses and is usually caused by sudden, forceful hyperextension of the hindlimb. Midsubstance tears are probably more common than avulsions of the common tendon of origin of the fibularis tertius and long digital extensor muscles, but the latter have been reported in foals.[111-113] Avulsions of the origin of the fibularis tertius and long digital extensor muscle occasionally occur in adult horses,[5] although more distal injuries are commoner. Foals may be more likely to suffer avulsions because of weaker bone.[112] Minor disruption of the common tendon of origin may be seen arthroscopically.[5]

Signs and Diagnosis
The classical sign of rupture of fibularis tertius and avulsion of its origin is the ability to extend the hock while the stifle is flexed, resulting in a dimpling of the common calcaneal ("Achilles") tendon. Synchronous flexion of the hock and stifle was reported with avulsions of the origin, presumably because the avulsed bone is held by the joint capsule.[112] Horses may bear weight normally, but during the protraction phase of a stride, the distal limb appears flaccid. Lameness can be severe at first, and distention of the femorotibial and femoropatellar joints may be present. Radiological examination is necessary for diagnosing avulsion fractures. Minor disruptions of the tendon of origin manifest as nonspecific lameness associated with pain in the stifle and can be diagnosed by arthroscopic examination; they may accompany other stifle injuries.[5]

Treatment
Horses with injuries to the tendon of origin are usually best evaluated arthroscopically, which also offers the opportunity to check for concurrent injury. Small bone fragments can be removed, but large fragments embedded in the joint capsule may be better left.[112] Six weeks of stable rest followed by controlled exercise for 3 months is recommended after surgery.

Prognosis
Horses with avulsion injuries have a guarded prognosis for full soundness, but successful outcome has been reported.[112] Minor disruptions of the origin may heal but much depends on concurrent injuries.

Calcinosis Circumscripta
Calcinosis circumscripta lesions are described as calcified, granular, amorphous deposits that induce fibrous

reaction.[114] They usually lie in the subcutaneous tissue close to joints or tendon sheaths. The lateral aspect of the stifle adjacent to the fibula is the predilection site for these lesions,[114-116] but they have been reported on the dorsolateral surface of the hock,[114] the neck, and the shoulder.[114,115] Calcinosis circumscripta is an uncommon condition, more often seen in young horses. The cause is unknown.

Signs and Diagnosis

The usual reason for examination is an unsightly lesion that has been slowly increasing in size. Occasionally the lesion appears to affect the horse's gait. Lesions are usually hard, well circumscribed, and firmly attached to underlying tissue. The overlying skin is not involved. Caudocranial radiographs show a circumscribed, roughly oval lesion of mineralized tissue (Figure 46-13) lying close to the lateral aspect of the femorotibial joint, with the bulk of the lesion distal to this. These lesions may be seen incidentally on scintigraphic examination as focal areas of intense IRU on the lateral proximal aspect of the crus. The lesion is clearly visible in a caudal image in a subcutaneous location, superficial to the tibial cortex, but in a lateral image IRU could be confused with a proximal tibial stress fracture.

Treatment

Treatment is only indicated if the lesion causes clinical complications or for cosmetic reasons. Surgical excision is necessary to remove the mass. Care should be taken when embarking on excision because some lesions are attached to the femorotibial joint capsule, which may be entered inadvertently. Steps should be taken to prevent postoperative seroma formation by closing dead space, suturing a stent bandage over the wound, and preventing the horse from lying down for several days postoperatively. The mass usually has a thick fibrous capsule and contains deposits of gritty material.

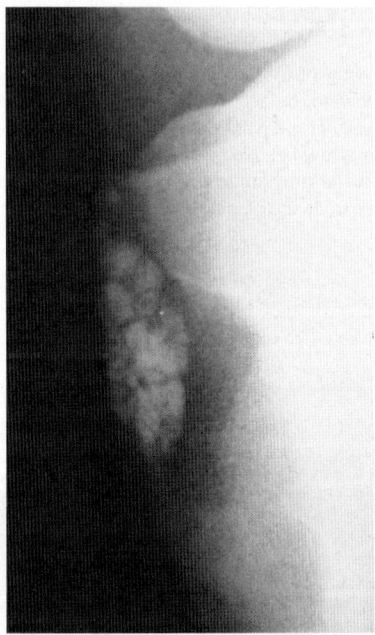

Fig. 46-13 • Caudocranial radiographic image (lateral is to the left) of the left stifle of an 8-year-old riding horse with an oval mass of mineralized tissue lateral to the head of the left tibia. The lesion is typical of calcinosis circumscripta.

Prognosis

In horses that are not treated, the mass remains but may not cause complications. A good result can be expected after surgical excision. Regrowth has not been reported, but postoperative problems with wound healing could be serious if the femorotibial joint is involved.

Injury of the Origin of Gastrocnemius
See Chapter 80.

Hematoma in the Stifle Region

The stifle region is vulnerable to external trauma, particularly when horses jump. Profound injuries to vital structures may result, but frequently external trauma causes only superficial bruising or a subcutaneous hematoma. The clinician's task is to differentiate between a swollen stifle that has a potentially career-threatening injury and one that has a superficial lesion such as a hematoma.

Signs and Diagnosis

A hematoma is manifested as a variably sized swelling, usually on the cranial aspect of the stifle, and may take several hours to reach maximum size. Smaller swellings may be difficult to differentiate from femoropatellar joint effusion. A hematoma is only painful on palpation until the initial bruising and swelling have settled. An uncomplicated hematoma does not usually cause lameness once the discomfort associated with the initial bleeding has passed. Other concurrent injury should be suspected if the horse is substantially lame, especially if lameness persists for several days. A hematoma may occasionally involve only the stifle initially but appears to spread to the inguinal and ventral abdominal areas. Huge swellings can cause oozing from the skin and skin loss. A careful search should be made for open wounds, which could lead to infection in the hematoma or cellulitis. Cellulitis usually takes at least 24 hours to form, and the swelling is firmer than a hematoma, hot, and painful. Lameness worsens as infection progresses.

Ultrasonography is a helpful tool for diagnosing hematoma, which can be confirmed by centesis of the swelling using aseptic technique. In the early stages, frank blood is retrieved, but as the blood clots, the fluid collected will be serum. Radiographic examination is indicated if lameness is severe or persists.

Treatment

In the initial phase, when hemorrhage is likely, the horse should be confined and cold applied to help to slow hemorrhage. Phenylbutazone can be given for its antiinflammatory effect. Antibiotics should be administered if the horse has an open wound. Although some clinicians believe that draining these hematomas is contraindicated, in my experience hematomas resolve better after effective drainage. Drainage should not be attempted until the hemorrhage has stopped and the free blood has clotted, usually 3 to 4 days after the injury. A 2- to 4-cm scalpel incision at the most dependent point of the hematoma ensures that drainage continues until the cavity has filled in.

Prognosis

In the absence of concurrent injury or infection and once the hematoma has resolved and is free of fluid, the prognosis for athletic use is good.

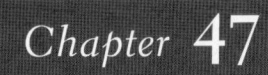

Chapter 47

The Thigh

Dan L. Hawkins and Mike W. Ross

▣ THE GLUTEAL SYNDROME

Dan L. Hawkins

References on page 1290

Pain that can be demonstrated with digital pressure along a line between the wing of the ilium and the greater trochanter of the femur was first recognized as a cause of lameness more than 50 years ago.[1-3] Various aspects of the origin, diagnosis, and management of the syndrome have been appreciated since its initial recognition by Dr. Churchill and myself.[1-5] The condition has also been referred to as *sacrosciatic lameness* or *pelvic myositis*. We prefer to use the term *gluteal syndrome* because we believe that there may be more than one abnormality that will result in this type of pain.

Gluteal syndrome has been diagnosed in most breeds and uses of horses. Standardbred (STB) racehorses seem to have the highest incidence, but it is not uncommonly seen in Thoroughbred (TB) and endurance racehorses. One risk factor for STBs is related to the more recent harness and race bike designs that tend to decrease the weight borne by the forelimbs while transferring weight to the hindlimbs. Gluteal syndrome has been diagnosed in horses that are used for hunting, jumping, and eventing.

Based on dissections of cadavers, the accessory head of the middle gluteal muscle was identified as the deep structure that best corresponds anatomically to the characteristic pattern of pain. This muscle originates on the concave surface of the wing of the ilium near a tuber coxae. At its caudal extent, the accessory head of the middle gluteal muscle forms a flat tendon that passes over the cranial aspect of the greater trochanter of the femur and inserts on the crest below it. The accessory head is directly related to other aspects of the middle gluteal and superficial gluteal muscles superficially and is important in propulsion of the hindlimbs[6] (Figure 47-1).

The pathological process associated with the accessory head of the middle gluteal muscle is uncertain. It is known that in horses with some acute injuries a hematoma may form in the area between the ilium and the greater trochanter of the femur. Small, hypoechogenic areas may be demonstrated ultrasonographically in muscle tissue in the same area. In other horses, the muscle may become partially detached from the ilium. Horses with the latter condition develop a depression in the musculature caudal to a tuber coxae after the acute stage. In horses with chronic pain, the affected muscle mass may become very firm, presumably as a result of fibrosis. Post mortem evaluation of two horses with chronic refractory gluteal syndrome did not provide any conclusive information. Other potential changes such as fasciitis, gluteal tendonitis, or injury to one or more adjacent muscles have been considered. Whatever the cause, the source of pain is consistently confined to the area described.

To date, the most reliable, practical method of diagnosis is by careful, systematic physical examination of the area between the wing of the ilium and the greater trochanter of the femur with the horse standing on the limb. More specifically, the musculature should be palpated and examined for changes in resilience, swelling, or fibrosis. The position and outline of the tuber coxae should be evaluated. Next, gentle, deep pressure should be applied along the entire area described with the tips of eight digits (Figure 47-2). Initially, light digital pressure should be applied, but then the pressure is gradually increased to firm, deep pressure. The pressure is maintained briefly to evaluate the horse's response. Finally the area caudal to the ilium, the central portion, and the caudal part of the accessory head of the middle gluteal muscle should be examined similarly. Each third of the area should be considered separately to determine whether the area is affected generally or whether

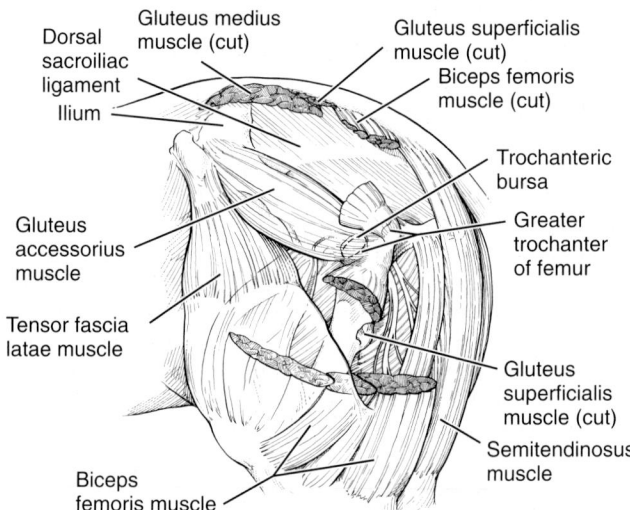

Fig. 47-1 • Drawing of the anatomy of the lateral pelvic and proximal thigh regions showing the accessory head of the middle gluteal muscle, the most likely source of pain associated with gluteal syndrome. The tendon of the accessory head of the middle gluteal passes over the cranial portion of the greater trochanter, where there is a bursa. Inflammation in this region causes trochanteric bursitis.

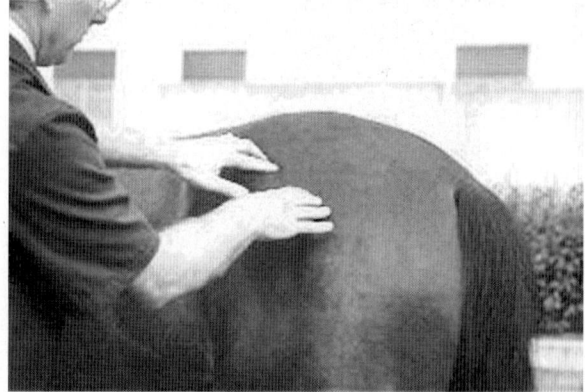

Fig. 47-2 • Careful palpation for pain is the only way to establish the clinical diagnosis of gluteal syndrome.

the injury is confined to one or more sections. An unaffected horse will not respond to the examination of any of the areas. An affected horse leans away from the pressure while showing a reluctance to voluntarily bear full weight on the limb as long as the pressure is maintained. A positive response for this syndrome as described is specific and should not be confused with that for trochanteric bursitis (see Trochanteric Bursitis section).

Most horses with acute gluteal syndrome tend to drag the toe of the affected limb on the ground at a walk. Horses with chronic gluteal syndrome do not drag the toe at a walk, but at a slow trot they break over on the inside of the toe and swing the leg medially and then laterally, finally landing on the outside branch or toe of the shoe. At this gait the lameness produced appears identical to that caused by trochanteric bursitis or tarsitis. When the horse trots, paces, or runs at high speed, the abnormality starts off as described, then the limb appears to tire and is carried more in abduction the further in the race or competition the horse proceeds. It appears that early in the race the horse is able to tolerate the gluteal pain and continue to use the limb for propulsion. However, with sustained speed or intensity of effort over distance, compensatory mechanisms within the limb fatigue as pain from the gluteal injury becomes overwhelming. At this point, a STB may make a break or freeze on a line; a TB may bolt or stop trying in the race; and a show horse may refuse to jump or crash when it tries. Many of these horses are believed to have a stifle problem because the quadriceps muscles fasciculate when they pull up. Others are believed to have exercise-induced pulmonary hemorrhage because they stopped like a bleeder, but no blood is seen endoscopically. Regardless, speed, intensity of work, and distance are key factors in how this problem affects an athletic horse. Some horses that accommodate to the injury or are treated and do not recover to total soundness can perform reasonably well at slower speeds or less intense work.

There is not a specific cause for gluteal syndrome. The onset is frequently directly associated with being cast in a stall, slipping or falling while playing in a paddock, or going down in a trailer or van and struggling to get up while the head is tied. Gluteal syndrome also develops when there is a chronic, preexisting problem in the distal aspect of the same limb, such as hock lameness, suspensory desmitis, or other problem that causes the horse to carry its weight on the toe at high speed. Slipping or losing footing on a soft racetrack or other muddy surface is also associated with development of the clinical signs.

Horses with this injury are best treated while in moderate, controlled exercise, regardless of the treatment approach. Rest alone, even for extended periods, has not been successful as a treatment. Several weeks of careful exercise management with repeated evaluations provide the best chance for a favorable response to treatment. Horses with acute injury, hemorrhage, and severe lameness should be rested until they are walking well and the seroma has resorbed before resuming exercise and treatment. Intramuscular injections of a counterirritant, acupuncture, and extracorporeal shock wave therapy are the best treatment options. At present, I still believe that injections of a counterirritant into the area of sensitivity yield the best results in the shortest time. The injection site is prepared with a surgical scrub followed by rinsing with 70% isopropyl

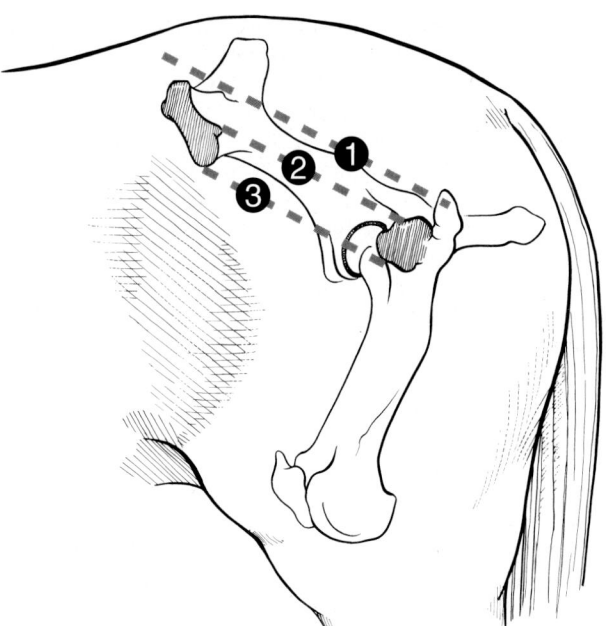

Fig. 47-3 • Diagrammatic representation of the injection pattern for intramuscular injections of counterirritant solution to manage gluteal syndrome. The dashed lines (1, 2, and 3) provide a grid to guide injection into 20 sites.

alcohol. An injection grid is marked on the horse by drawing three lines in the wet hair over the accessory head of the middle gluteal muscle (Figure 47-3). One hundred milliliters of 2% iodine diluted in sesame oil solution is injected intramuscularly into 20 sites (5 mL/site) on and between the grid lines with a 4-cm, 19-gauge needle. If the pain is concentrated in the cranial or caudal third of the area between a tuber coxae and the ipsilateral greater trochanter of the femur, the injection sites can be limited to the cranial or caudal half of the area, respectively. After injection, daily moderate, controlled exercise is recommended beginning the day after injection for all horses. After injection, horses with acute or recent gluteal syndrome are walked and jogged for 3 weeks and then reexamined. If the lameness is improved but the area is still sensitive or if there has been no improvement, the injection is repeated in the same manner. Horses with chronic gluteal syndrome are walked and jogged for only 1 week before light training is resumed. Some horses respond dramatically to the treatment and appear to be pain-free within less than a week. The injury cannot heal within that time frame; therefore the temptation to resume full training too quickly must be resisted. When the treatment is successful and horses return to full work and racing, 10% to 20% may experience a recurrence of the problem. These horses generally respond well to an additional treatment as they did previously.

Lameness that fails to improve after two or three injections at 3-week intervals is considered refractory to this mode of treatment. For these horses, I suggest that the trainer or owner try another form of treatment, such as therapeutic ultrasound, acupuncture, or shock wave therapy. Approximately 10% to 15% of horses do not respond to any mode of treatment and never recover from the injury. The prognosis is guarded initially for unilateral injury and poor if the problem is bilateral or if there is a chronic condition more distally in the same leg. In these horses with more complicated injuries, failure is related to the aggravating effect of each injury on the other.

Shoeing can be a factor in the management of the gluteal syndrome. Slipping on the racetrack, cross-country course, or show jumping arena is a major factor in development and recurrence of the injury. I recommend that TB racehorses that have or have had this condition be shod with block heels on both branches of each hind shoe. Calks applied near the end of both branches of the hind shoes during training and competition can be used in other types of horses.

◼ TROCHANTERIC BURSITIS

Dan L. Hawkins

Pain elicited by firm digital pressure over the greater trochanter of the femur and the musculature immediately caudal to it is attributed to inflammation of the trochanteric bursa and is a cause of lameness in horses.[1,2] Historically this condition has been referred to as *trochanteric bursitis*, *trochanteric lameness*, and *whorl bone lameness*.[7] Anatomically the bursa is interposed between the flat tendon of the accessory head of the middle gluteal muscle and the cranial portion of the greater trochanter, which is covered with cartilage at this point. The tendon inserts on the crest below the greater trochanter (see Figure 47-1).[7]

Although confident, positive diagnosis is achieved by physical examination in almost all horses, a technique of injection of local anesthetic solution into the bursa has been described (see Chapter 10).[8] The condition is relatively common for all breeds and uses of athletic horses and is generally considered to be a secondary problem. Trochanteric bursitis often is associated with tarsitis or other problems in the affected limb in which the horse lands on the toe. An additional cause that has been overlooked is that associated with overreaching with the hindlimbs to compensate for a chronic problem in the forelimbs. A horse that is chronically sore in front (e.g., navicular disease) will try to carry more of its weight on the hindlimbs by overextending the ipsilateral limb, which results in excessive strain on the tendon of the middle gluteal muscle. Wet, cold weather conditions appear to have a positive association with the incidence and response to treatment.

Trochanteric bursitis causes a gait abnormality that is similar to that produced by tarsitis or other sources of pain causing lameness in the distal aspect of a hindlimb. A horse with purely trochanteric lameness breaks over on the medial aspect of the toe; carries the leg medially, even crossing the midline; and then moves the leg laterally to land on the lateral aspect of the toe and branch of the shoe. The length of stride is shortened, and the hindquarters are carried toward the opposite side, which is sometimes described as "dog trotting" at a slow gait. Trochanteric lameness especially affects horses when they are racing around turns, jumping, circling, or performing precision dressage movements.

Trochanteric bursitis is generally a chronic condition that is diagnosed at the same time as a primary condition in the lower limb or ipsilateral forelimb. The more distal condition should be addressed before the bursitis is treated. Occasionally trochanteric bursitis is identified

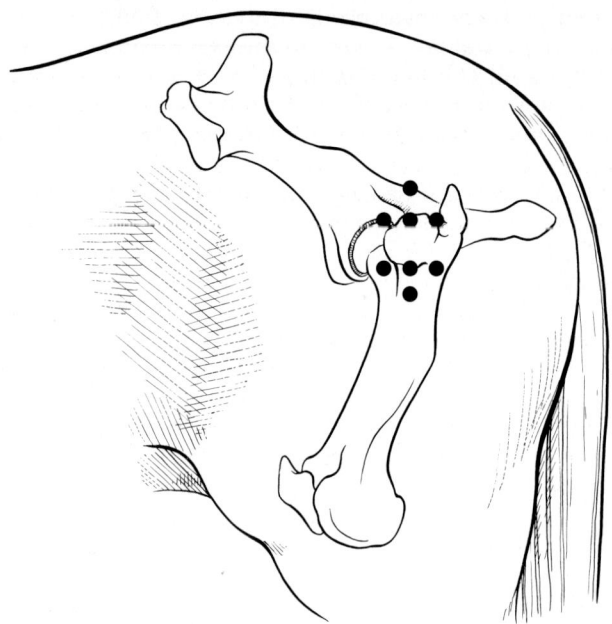

Fig. 47-4 • Diagrammatic representation of the injection pattern (black circles) to manage horses with trochanteric bursitis.

without an associated primary condition, or it may spontaneously resolve after correction of the associated primary lameness.

Rest is of no value in treating horses with trochanteric bursitis and may intensify the lameness when the horse returns to training. The most effective, practical treatment of trochanteric bursitis is injection of the soft tissues over and around the bursa with a counterirritant solution. The area for injection is prepared with a surgical scrub followed by rinsing with 70% isopropyl alcohol. Approximately 6 mL of 2% iodine diluted in sesame oil solution should be injected into eight sites with a 4-cm, 19-gauge needle (Figure 47-4). The horse should be maintained with mild, controlled exercise for 1 week before resuming normal work. Normally within 5 to 7 days after treatment the horse should become sound behind and no longer resent palpation over the bursa. Horses that require reinjection are more commonly encountered during cold, wet climatic conditions. The prognosis is good for obtaining a cure for trochanteric bursitis provided the associated primary lameness is corrected. Alternatively, solutions of a corticosteroid can be injected in the same manner. In my experience, injection of corticosteroids directly into the bursa is not necessary to alleviate the lameness.

Trochanteric bursitis has been addressed here as a performance-limiting condition in the athletic horse. Trochanteric bursitis that results from external trauma, infection associated with a wound, or a fracture of the greater trochanter of the femur is not discussed.

FRACTURES OF THE FEMUR

Fractures of the femur occur most commonly in foals and weanlings, although they may be seen in older horses. Most femoral fractures result from external trauma, such as a kick or fall with the limb in adduction or abduction. In young foals, fractures may be associated with breaking to lead. In most horses the traumatic incident is not witnessed, but the horse is found with an unstable, non–weight-bearing lameness in the affected hindlimb. Because of the energy required to fracture the femur of an adult horse, the fracture generally has a severely comminuted configuration. Although foals and weanlings most commonly acquire diaphyseal femur fractures, fractures involving the proximal or distal femoral physis are not uncommon. Salter-Harris type II distal femur fractures are most commonly seen in older weanlings and yearlings.

Diagnosis

In most horses, the diagnosis can be made after a brief physical examination. Femoral fractures result in an acute onset of severe lameness, with swelling in the area of the femur. Swelling occurs rapidly and is generally profound, particularly in adult horses with comminuted fractures. Degree of swelling can be used to differentiate fracture location (see Figure 5-12). Horses with pelvic fractures rarely develop swelling in both the medial and lateral aspects of the thigh, although horses with fractures of a tuber coxae may develop swelling of the proximal, lateral aspect of the thigh. Rotational instability is elicited when internal or external rotation is applied by grasping the proximal tibia and calcaneal tuber. Crepitation may be appreciated with manipulation of the limb. However, swelling and hemorrhage in the large muscle mass of the thigh may keep the fracture ends separated and make it difficult to elicit crepitus. The large muscle mass also makes open fractures uncommon. Swelling is most consistent with diaphyseal fractures, but it is often less obvious with proximal physeal fractures and minimally displaced distal

physeal fractures. In most horses, the distance between reference points, such as the patella and the greater trochanter of the femur, is shortened because of the overriding of the fracture fragments that is caused by contraction of the quadriceps muscles. Foals with proximal physeal fractures may be able to bear some weight on the affected limb.

Radiological evaluation is required to obtain a definitive diagnosis and determine the severity of a femoral fracture (Figure 47-5). Radiography of horses larger than young foals requires use of general anesthesia unless the fracture is located in the distal aspect of the femur. Many small foals can undergo radiography safely when recumbent under heavy tranquilization or general anesthesia. Because induction and recovery of large yearlings and adults cannot be assisted sufficiently to prevent complications and discomfort, general anesthesia is contraindicated for assessment of unstable femur fractures. Ultrasonography can be used to confirm a displaced femoral fracture in a standing horse.

Once the horse is in lateral recumbency with the affected limb down against the cassette and the opposite limb abducted, the x-ray beam should be directed from medial to lateral. Radiography of the diaphysis and proximal aspect of the femur requires a grid and high-capacity x-ray generator except for examination of small foals and the distal aspect of the femur of larger horses. Two exposures are generally required for the mediolateral images because of the variation in soft tissue mass around the distal and proximal aspects of the femur. Craniocaudal images are also required to assess the severity of the fracture and the degree of overriding. Evaluation of the proximal physis requires that the horse be positioned in dorsal recumbency with the cassette and grid under the coxofemoral area.

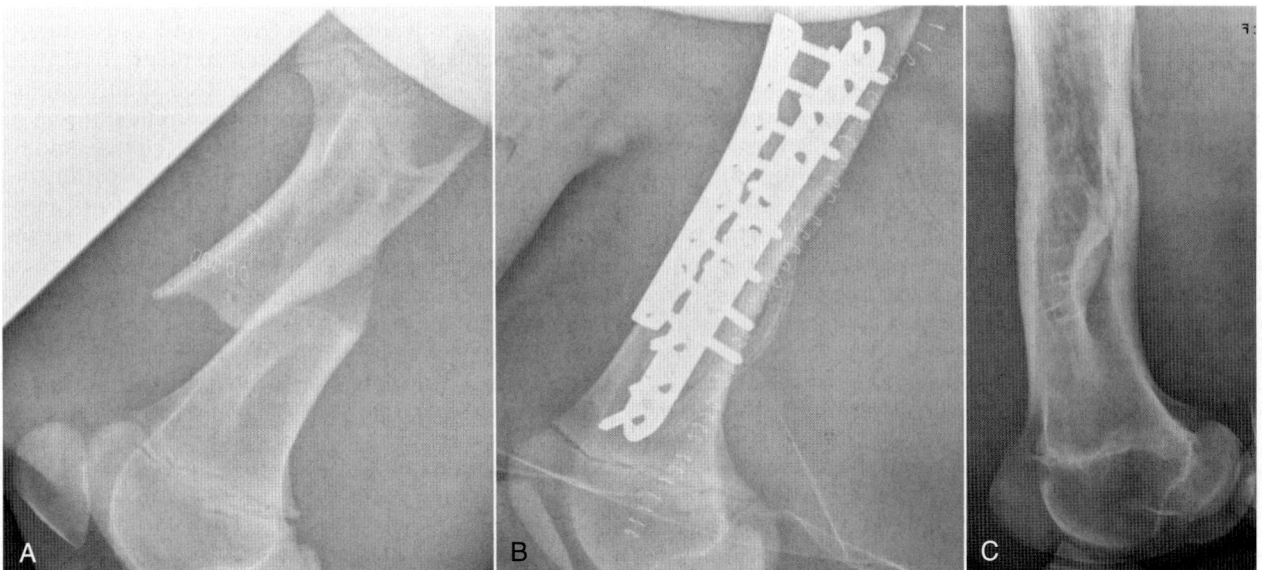

Fig. 47-5 • Lateromedial digital radiographic images of a left femur. **A,** Initial view of a 2-month-old Thoroughbred filly with a simple, short-oblique, midshaft femoral fracture showing the typical cranioproximal displacement of the proximal fragment and caudodistal displacement of the distal fragment. The fracture was considered closed because there was no obvious communication between a superficial wound from the causative kick and the fracture site; the wound was stapled (stainless steel staples are visible) before admission. **B,** Postoperative image showing internal fixation using a lateral locking compression plate and a cranial limited-contact dynamic compression plate. A closed suction drain is visible. **C,** Radiographic image of the femur 2 years after injury and repair. The now 2-year-old filly was sound. The plates were removed 5 months after surgery; the fracture healed completely; and the stifle and hip (not shown) joints were radiologically normal.

Case Selection for Treatment and Prognosis

The decision to treat horses with femoral fractures by surgical intervention depends on several variables. The size of the horse is the single most important consideration, regardless of fracture type. Successful surgical treatment of diaphyseal or proximal physeal fractures has been accomplished only in foals and small ponies.[9] Distal physeal fractures have been successfully repaired in yearlings.[10,11] However, adult horses or young horses weighing more than 200 kg (440 lb) with displaced diaphyseal fractures warrant humane destruction.[12] Fracture location and configuration, soft tissue injury, temperament of the horse, client expectations, and economic considerations are other important determinants for case selection. Compromise of the vascular supply caused by the fracture, damaged major vessels, and swelling can result in failure because of necrosis of the distal aspect of the limb.[13]

Surgical techniques, complications, and the prognosis for horses with diaphyseal and proximal and distal physeal femoral fractures were reviewed.[9,12,14] Of foals with diaphyseal fractures that were repaired with double plating, 50% of the fractures healed, and 75% of the horses were able to perform the intended use.[15] The most common complications were seroma formation and infection. Foals with a successful outcome were younger than 3 months of age (see Figure 47-5). Additionally, an intact caudal cortex was considered necessary for a successful outcome. Newly designed implants such as the locking compression plate (LCP) may improve prognosis and make possible successful surgical repair in older horses or in those with comminuted fractures because stable anatomical alignment, exact contouring of the plate to bone, and compression of the plate to bone are not needed (see Figure 47-5).[16] Successful outcome was achieved in two foals with open, comminuted femoral fractures repaired using two LCPs and a combination of locking and conventional cortex bone screws.[16] Conservative management of horses with diaphyseal fractures can result in fracture healing. However, limb shortening, rotational deformity, and serious varus deformity in the contralateral limb are common complications of this approach. The prognosis of horses with distal fractures was more guarded than that for diaphyseal fractures because of the limited amount of bone for implant purchase. Success of the condylar screw plate for repair of a distal femur Salter-Harris type III fracture in a 2-year-old horse suggests this implant has application in repair of selected distal femoral fractures in horses.[17] Conservative management of horses with distal fractures can result in a satisfactory outcome if the fracture is minimally displaced and stable.[15]

Although proximal femoral physeal fractures account for 16% of physeal fractures in the horse,[18] sufficient reported results of surgical treatment to establish good prognostic information are lacking. Currently the prognosis for successful repair is guarded at best. Conservative management is unlikely to result in a comfortable horse. Unstable fixation, necrosis of the femoral head, and osteoarthritis of the coxofemoral joint are the more common complications associated with failure of surgical or conservative approaches.

Other less common types of proximal femoral fractures that cause less severe lameness in older horses include the third trochanter (see Chapter 50) and greater trochanter.

Ultrasonography is helpful in confirming these fractures. Unless horses with these fractures have an associated wound or bone becomes sequestered, they should be managed with stall rest.[9] Stress fractures of the femur are rare but occasionally occur in the proximal cranial femoral cortex.

FIBROTIC AND OSSIFYING MYOPATHY

See Chapter 48 for a discussion of fibrotic or ossifying myopathy.

GASTROCNEMIUS MUSCLE INJURY

See Chapter 80 for a complete discussion of gastrocnemius muscle injury. Injury of the origin of the gastrocnemius can cause acute, severe hindlimb lameness in foals and adult horses. The diagnosis is straightforward when the reciprocal apparatus is disrupted, the most common clinical presentation in foals. Of six foals with gastrocnemius rupture, five had a history of dystocia and assisted delivery (three in a hip-locked position); four foals had complete disruption of the reciprocal apparatus and were unable to rise; life-threatening hemorrhage into the gastrocnemius muscle occurred in one foal, and concurrent perinatal diseases complicated management; and neither of the two foals discharged from the hospital were sound for athletic use.[19] Successful restoration of the reciprocal apparatus after rupture of the gastrocnemius and superficial digital flexor muscles was achieved in a 6-month-old Warmblood filly using a modified Thomas splint–cast combination.[20] The prognosis is grave when there is complete disruption of the reciprocal apparatus in adult horses. However, partial tearing at the origin of the gastrocnemius, musculotendonous junction, or more distally near or at the attachment on the calcaneus can occur and cause moderate hindlimb lameness that is difficult to diagnose. A peculiar gait is seen in some horses with gastrocnemius origin and tendon injury. Horses appear to have difficulty maintaining stability of the limb during late stance phase and when pushing off and exhibit marked internal rotation of the distal limb with lateral rotation of the point of the calcaneus.[21] Some horses exhibit this type of hindlimb movement normally, but it is symmetrical and not accompanied by lameness. I have seen this peculiar gait in other horses with caudal thigh pain such as fracture of the tuber ischium with avulsion injury of the caudal thigh muscles. Gastrocnemius origin injury can be challenging to diagnose, but increased radiopharmaceutical uptake and bony proliferation were found in three of four horses,[21] and ultrasonographic examination using comparative images of the contralateral limb is necessary, particularly in horses with injury of the more distal aspects of the gastrocnemius musculotendonous junction and tendon.

Gracilis Muscle Injury

Although unusual, acute severe lameness and swelling of the medial thigh occur as a result of gracilis muscle injury. Gracilis muscle injury caused substantial hindlimb lameness in two barrel racing horses; the site of injury was confirmed using local infiltration into the affected muscles, and ultrasonographic examination confirmed injury.[22] One horse developed an unusual gait consistent with fibrotic myopathy that resolved after resection of scar tissue.[22] In this report, both horses returned to athletic use.[22] Gracilis muscle injury is seen in polo horses (see Chapter 119, page 1164).

Other Thigh Injuries

Generalized muscle injury can cause acute swelling of the medial aspect of the thigh and pronounced lameness. Rarely, swelling, lameness, and fever are found in horses that develop abscesses in the medial thigh or inguinal region. Ultrasonographic examination for diagnosis, surgical drainage, and appropriate antimicrobial and antiinflammatory therapy are necessary. A horse with swelling of the thigh, fever, and sudden death was diagnosed with a dissecting aortic aneurysm.[23] Large, dissecting hematomas from direct trauma may originate near the stifle and extend into the medial and sometimes the caudal aspects of the thigh and may require surgical drainage. Fractures of the tubera ischii, tubera coxae, and rarely luxation of the coxofemoral joint can cause swelling of the thigh. These conditions are discussed in detail in Chapters 49, 50, and 126.

Mechanical and Neurological Lameness in the Forelimbs and Hindlimbs

Sue J. Dyson and Mike W. Ross*

GENERAL CONSIDERATIONS

Mechanical lameness reflects altered biomechanical forces affecting limb function. The biomechanics of limb function depend on normal functioning of peripheral nerves, muscles, tendons, and ligaments. Appropriate muscle contraction and relaxation are important factors in limb biomechanics. A muscle that cannot contract with sufficient force or a muscle that cannot relax and stretch can result in an altered gait. Mechanical lamenesses are typically most obvious at the walk and often become less evident or disappear at the trot. Gait alterations may not be evident at the canter, although a horse with a mechanical lameness may not be capable of generating a smooth canter and may appear to be hopping or "off" behind at the canter. Mechanical lamenesses include altered gaits caused by decreased and increased joint flexion.

The importance of proper functioning of the neuromuscular system for a normal hindlimb gait is exemplified by horses with chronic motor neuron disease and myopathy from equine polysaccharide storage myopathy (EPSSM). Both of these neuromuscular disorders can be associated with a fibrotic myopathy-type or stringhalt-type of gait. Horses with EPSSM may develop prolonged or intermittent upward fixation of the patella. Underlying myopathy was found in some but not all horses with shivers (shiverers).[1,2] Neuropathy is known to be a cause of stringhalt[3,4] and was found in horses with fibrotic myopathy.[5] Trauma to peripheral nerves may also cause a mechanical lameness. The possible role of altered proprioceptive input to the affected limb is intriguing and is discussed under appropriate headings.

Equine protozoal myelitis or myeloencephalitis (EPM) with involvement of motor neurons causing selective denervation may also cause mechanical lameness. In horses with EPM, lameness cannot be abolished using diagnostic analgesia. Horses with lameness from EPM should, however, also exhibit proprioceptive deficits and ataxia and usually exhibit muscle atrophy. Lameness in horses with EPM may be caused by pain arising from atrophied muscles, nerve root pain, or pain originating from peripheral nerves. EPM is unlikely to cause an obvious mechanical lameness without accompanying ataxia. It is difficult to accept that EPM could cause selective damage to motor neurons sufficient to cause a mechanical lameness without also causing concurrent spinal cord white matter damage and ataxia, but it does do so occasionally, and neurological deficits may be subtle early in the disease. Careful neurological evaluation by a clinician with expertise in equine neurological evaluation is an important part of examining a horse with mechanical lameness because distinguishing between gait abnormality caused by mechanical lameness and gait abnormality caused by neurological disease may be difficult.

Electromyography and muscle biopsy may aid in determining the cause of mechanical or neurologically mediated lameness. Concentric needle electromyography of denervated muscle often reveals abnormal spontaneous activity such as positive sharp waves, fibrillations, and myotonic bursts. Abnormal spontaneous activity may also be present in muscles of horses with myopathy, but these findings are generally mild and may be absent. Biopsy of the semimembranosus or semitendinosus muscle is useful for evaluating evidence of denervation atrophy and EPSSM. However, if denervation of a single muscle or part of a muscle causes the gait alteration, sampling error may result in a false-negative result.

Mechanical lameness does not always cause pain, and horses usually do not respond to nonsteroidal antiinflammatory drug therapy. Methocarbamol therapy is indicated only when muscle cramping from central nervous system disease is suspected. Phenytoin therapy has proved to be useful in some horses with mechanical lameness, particularly those with stringhalt.

Mechanical lameness in the horse is the result of abnormal structure or function of the musculoskeletal system or,

*The authors of this chapter acknowledge and appreciate the contribution of Beth A. Valentine, who authored this chapter in the previous edition.

erences page 291

more commonly, of the neuromuscular system. Possibly a variety of underlying problems can result in the same type of mechanical lameness. Limb dysfunction may also be caused by an imbalance of flexor and extensor muscle activity as a result of a primary neurological cause.

ANATOMICAL CONSIDERATIONS

A number of unique anatomical features in the equine hindlimb contribute to mechanical lameness. The configuration of the patellar ligaments in the stifle joint allows locking of the stifle into an extended position (see page 94). The stay apparatus minimizes the muscular effort required for a horse to stand for long periods. The reciprocal apparatus links the actions of the stifle and hock, primarily through the fibularis (peroneus) tertius and superficial digital flexor tendons, such that an abnormal action in either joint affects the action of both.

Innervation patterns to the muscles of the hindlimbs may also contribute to mechanical lameness. The semitendinosus muscle, for example, receives innervation from two different nerves: the caudal gluteal and sciatic nerves. Often more than one muscular branch innervates long muscles such as the semitendinosus and possibly the semimembranosus. Damage to one nerve or to a muscular branch can result in partial denervation of a large muscle, with resultant altered biomechanical forces leading to abnormal limb action.

UPWARD FIXATION OF THE PATELLA (LOCKING STIFLE) AND DELAYED RELEASE OF THE PATELLA

Clinical Characteristics

Horses and ponies with upward fixation of the patella are episodically unable to flex the stifle or the hock and drag the extended limb behind them on the toe (see Figures 5-18 and 48-1). The condition occurs most commonly after a period of standing still and tends to decrease with continued exercise. An intermittent form of patellar fixation, called *delayed release of the patella*, also occurs, in which the patella appears to catch briefly, sometimes followed by exaggerated flexion of the stifle and hock. Low-grade intermittent upward fixation or delayed release of the patella is relatively common, but it is often difficult to detect and is not necessarily observed daily. Affected horses have a slightly jerky movement of the patella that may be most apparent during deceleration from trot to walk and when the horse is working in deep footing, especially on turns. Affected horses may appear to be in some discomfort, may be resistant to work especially in deep footing, and can become irritable. Both upward fixation of the patella and delayed release may occur unilaterally or bilaterally. Fifty-five of 78 horses (70.5%) with upward fixation of the patella were affected unilaterally and 23 (29.5%) bilaterally.[6]

Warmbloods, Thoroughbreds, Standardbreds, and some pony breeds (e.g., Shetland and Miniature ponies) may be predisposed to upward fixation of the patella.[6] The episodic nature of intermittent upward fixation of the patella adds to the difficulty of detecting an affected horse. Careful observation while moving the horse over from side to side, turning in small circles, or walking down an incline can be particularly useful. Clinical signs of upward fixation of the

patella or delayed release of the patella are most commonly seen in young horses, especially those kept stabled, and signs may diminish or disappear if the horse becomes fitter and stronger. However, clinical signs may recur if the horse is confined to box rest for an unrelated reason. Persistent upward fixation of the patella has also been described in a foal.[7]

Cause

Upward fixation of the patella has been attributed to abnormal laxity and to increased tenseness of patellar ligaments. Decreased force of muscle contraction of the thigh muscles (quadriceps and biceps femoris) that move the patella out of the locked position may also cause upward fixation of the patella. This may be the explanation for upward fixation of the patella occurring in unfit horses, those in poor condition, or those with underlying myopathy, causing weak or stiff muscles. Horses and ponies with overly straight hindlimbs may be prone to upward fixation of the patella because such conformation can result in overextension of the stifle joint, leading to patellar locking.[6,7] Sixteen of 78 horses (20.5%) with upward fixation of the patella had straight hindlimb conformation.[6] Foot conformation may also play a role. Thirty-one of 78 horses (39.7%) had long toes and/or a higher inside wall of the hind foot of the affected limb(s).[6] Permanent upward fixation of the patella occurs rarely secondary to luxation or subluxation of the ipsilateral coxofemoral joint (see Chapters 50 and 126).

Biomechanical Basis

Upward fixation of the patella is caused by failure of the medial patellar ligament to unhook from the medial ridge of the femoral trochlea, causing the stifle to lock in extension. Abnormalities of the fibrocartilage at the medial aspect of the patella also possibly make the joint prone to locking. Once the stifle is locked in extension, the hock is also fixed in extension through the action of the reciprocal apparatus. The biomechanical basis for stifle hyperflexion after the brief period of patellar catching in intermittent upward fixation of the patella (or delayed release of the patella) is not entirely clear and may be from increased force of contraction of the biceps and quadriceps muscles during the transient locking phase. Clearly, therapy for this disorder should be directed at correcting the underlying cause. Unfortunately, for many horses an exact cause is never determined.

Medical Therapy

Exercise is an important part of therapy for horses with upward fixation of the patella. Conditioning exercise, including work on hills, may result in complete resolution of the problem in some horses. Uphill work may be more beneficial than downhill exercise. Horses that respond to conditioning exercise indicate that muscle dysfunction can play an important role in the development of upward fixation of the patella. Corrective trimming and shoeing is also important; the toe should be shortened to facilitate breakover, and mediolateral imbalance should be corrected. It has been suggested that rounding the medial aspect of the foot to promote medial breakover may be beneficial together with elevation of the lateral heel using a wedge-heel shoe.[6] Thirty-three of 64 (51.6%) horses with upward

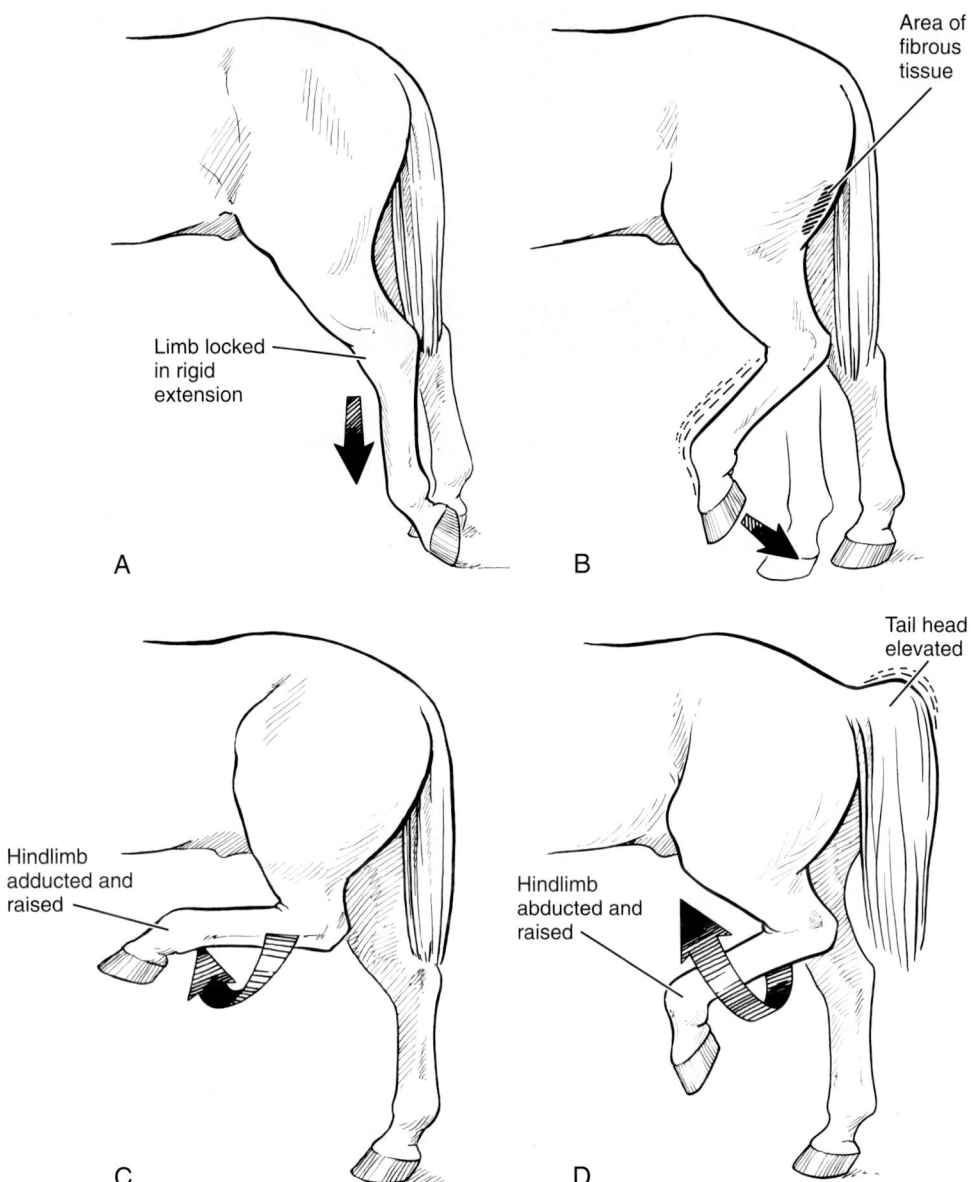

Fig. 48-1 · Diagrammatic representation of the common mechanical hindlimb gait abnormalities. **A,** In horses with upward fixation of the patella, the hindlimb is periodically held in rigid extension. The fetlock joint is flexed, and the horse walks on the toe. Horses with intermittent upward fixation can have a gait similar to shivers (see **D**). **B,** Horses with fibrotic myopathy show slapping of the affected hindlimb downward just before the end of the cranial phase of every walk stride. Hock flexion is near normal, but fibrous tissue in the caudal thigh region limits the cranial phase of the stride. **C,** Horses with stringhalt exaggerate flexion of the hock with the hindlimb in a normal (adducted) position. This gait occurs at every walk stride. Excessive hock flexion causes some horses to hit the ventral abdomen with the dorsum of the hindlimb. **D,** Horses with shivers often have abnormal tail head elevation and hold the affected hindlimb in a flexed and raised position away from the midline (abducted). This abnormal gait occurs sporadically, not at every walk step, which helps to distinguish it from stringhalt.

fixation of the patella had a successful outcome following corrective trimming and shoeing, dietary management to promote better condition, and exercise, and a further 13 (20.3%) improved.[6]

If underlying myopathy such as EPSSM is the cause, diet change to one that is high in fat and low in starches and sugars[9] and continued exercise conditioning may be beneficial. The most effective diets are those that provide at least 20% to 25% of total daily energy from fat and less than 20% of total daily energy from starches and sugars.

Another medical therapy is administration of estrogenic compounds. The rationale is presumably that estrogens can cause tendon and ligament relaxation. Whether horses with upward fixation of the patella have overly tense patellar ligaments and whether estrogen has any effect on patellar ligaments and tendons are unclear. Estrogen effects on muscle cell metabolism and muscle tone are possible. Anecdotal evidence suggests that some horses may benefit from this type of therapy. Intramuscular injection of 1 mg of estradiol cypionate per 45 kg of body weight (i.e., 11 mg/500 kg) once weekly for 3 to 5 weeks has been recommended.

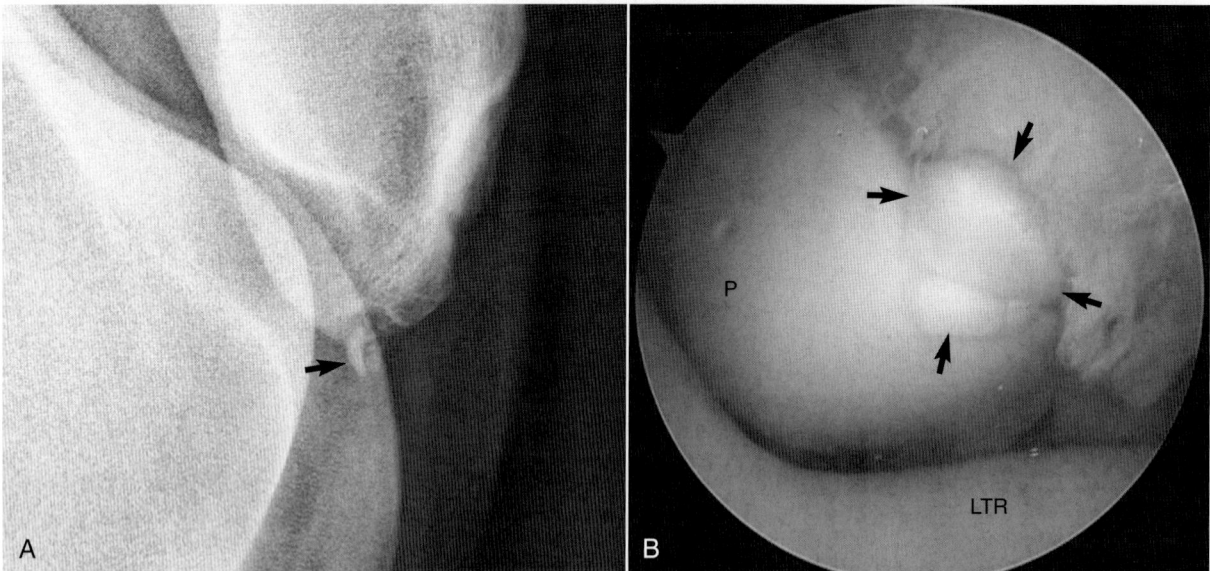

Fig. 48-2 · A, Lateromedial digital radiographic image *(cranial is the right and proximal is uppermost)* of the right stifle joint in a 7-year-old Warmblood gelding with bilateral hindlimb lameness. This horse had instability of the hindlimb characterized by knuckling after bilateral medial patellar desmotomy and the subsequent development of distal patellar fragmentation, bilaterally *(arrow).* **B,** Intraoperative arthroscopic photograph *(lateral is to the right and proximal is uppermost)* showing fragmentation *(arrows)* of the distal aspect of the left patella *(P).* The underlying lateral trochlear ridge *(LTR)* of the distal femur can be seen. The fragments were removed from both stifle joints.

Injection of iodine-containing counterirritants into and around the medial and middle patellar ligaments has also been advocated.[10] It has been proposed that maturation of a fibrous and inflammatory response may result in stiffening of the ligaments and thus relieve upward fixation of the patella.[11] Injection of a 2% solution of iodine in oil or of ethanolamine oleate has been advocated. Injection of 1 to 1.25 mL of these compounds into numerous sites in and around the distal aspect of the medial and middle patellar ligaments is recommended. However, in an experimental study in normal horses, injection into the medial and middle patellar ligaments with iodine in almond oil provoked more fibroplasia and infiltration of inflammatory cells than ethanolamine.[11]

Surgical Therapy

Medial patellar desmotomy may be necessary, although this should be considered only in horses with upward fixation of the patella that is unresponsive to conditioning exercise or medical therapy, or for horses that are persistently locked for several days. Because the transected ligament eventually heals with a fibrous union, the main benefit of surgery may be temporarily to alter the action of the stifle joint such that the horse is capable of conditioning exercise. Development of fragmentation of the apex of the patella (sometimes referred to as patellar chondromalacia) and associated lameness may occur after medial patellar desmotomy, although rest for 3 months postoperatively may reduce the risk (see Figure 46-4) (Figure 48-2).[12] Treatment of fragmentation of the apex of the patella is by arthroscopic debridement (see Chapter 46). Middle patellar desmitis is also a potential untoward sequela.[6,13] Occasionally after medial patellar desmotomy persistent lameness develops from residual desmitis, swelling and inflammation, or osteitis of the patella. One of us (MWR) has seen

horses develop instability and knuckling of the hindlimb after medial patellar desmotomy. Percutaneous splitting of the medial patellar ligament may be equally effective, with less potential for secondary fragmentation of the apex of the patella.[14,15] Twenty-three horses were treated by ligament splitting without complication,[15] whereas eight of 18 horses (45%) treated by desmotomy had secondary stifle-related lameness, despite many being rested for 3 months postoperatively.[6] A modification of the originally described technique for medial patellar splitting (desmoplasty) can be equally effective.[16,17] Briefly, in a standing horse after sedation and the injection of local anesthetic solution subcutaneously over the involved medial patellar ligament(s), a 14-gauge, 4-cm-long needle is used to perform desmoplasty. The needle is inserted through skin at three locations (proximal, midligament, distal), and four to nine desmoplasty incisions, in roughly a cranial-to-caudal direction, are made in a fan-shaped fashion.[16,17] One of us (MWR) has used 12 to 15 deep incisions, and although I was initially skeptical of efficacy, I have been impressed with resolution of clinical signs soon after the procedure, even in horses that are almost persistently locked. Horses are maintained on phenylbutazone, and the femoropatellar joint is medicated with hyaluronan and short-acting corticosteroids.

Identification of a chronically thickened medial patellar ligament at a clinical examination for an unrelated reason (e.g., a prepurchase examination) usually reflects previous medial patellar desmotomy or splitting.

FIBROTIC MYOPATHY
Clinical Characteristics
The gait of fibrotic myopathy is characterized by a shortened cranial swing phase of the affected hindlimb while

walking, with an abrupt catching of the forward swing, a slight caudal swing, and slapping of the hoof onto the ground (see Figure 48-1). This abnormal gait is present at every walk stride and has a characteristic sound, but it is often much less apparent at the trot and canter. However, an affected horse appears lame at the trot. The degree of gait impairment varies according to the severity and extent of muscle pathology. Affected horses may have a palpable thickening on the caudal aspect of the crus, which may extend distally and medially toward the tuber calcanei, but this is not a consistent finding. Osseous metaplasia may accompany fibrosis in some horses. Affected muscles may exhibit some degree of atrophy. Some horses have an obvious dimple, scar, or depression in the affected muscle. Ultrasonographic evaluation of the caudal thigh musculature can be useful[18] and may detect focal hyperechogenic areas of fibrosis when none are palpable or hyperechogenic areas with underlying acoustic shadowing associated with mineralization. The proximodistal extent of muscle abnormality can be determined.

Fibrotic myopathy may be more common in Western performance horses and gaited horses. Fibrotic myopathy is most often a unilateral problem but can occur bilaterally. Fibrotic myopathy may occur first in one hindlimb, followed by development of a similar abnormal gait in the other hindlimb months to years later. This gait abnormality does not appear to be painful or distressing to the horse, and signs do not increase from anxiety or decreased ambient temperature. Fibrotic myopathy occurs most often in adult horses but has also been described in neonates. Fibrotic myopathy in foals is not associated with palpable fibrosis of the distal aspect of semitendinosus muscle. Diagnosis is made by recognition of the typical gait abnormality. Occasionally injection of local anesthetic solution into the involved muscle bellies may partially alleviate clinical signs (see Chapter 122).

Cause

Fibrotic myopathy is usually the result of trauma of the semitendinosus muscle during activities that result in extreme tension, such as sliding stops in reining horses and struggling from catching a leg in a halter or tether. Traumatic injuries to the semitendinosus, or inflammatory processes such as abscesses at injection sites, can cause fibrotic myopathy. Less commonly, damage to the semimembranosus or gracilis muscle (see Chapter 47) is a cause.[19] Fibrotic myopathy present at birth has been speculated to be caused by trauma at or soon after birth.[20] Adhesions between the semitendinosus and the semimembranosus or biceps femoris muscles causing restriction of muscle action have been proposed.[21] Careful study of a small series of horses with fibrotic myopathy found that underlying traumatic or degenerative neuropathy causing denervation of the distal semitendinosus muscle can result in fibrotic myopathy.[5] Two horses with minimal fibrosis had bilateral fibrotic myopathy from degenerative neuropathy of unknown cause. One horse had unilateral fibrotic myopathy caused by nerve damage after fracture and scarring of the caudal aspect of the greater trochanter. This horse had characteristic fibrosis of the distal aspect of semitendinosus muscle. Underlying neuropathy is the most likely cause in horses in which fibrotic myopathy develops in one hindlimb and progresses to involve the other hindlimb.

Biomechanical Basis

Functional shortening caused by muscle scarring, adhesions to adjacent muscles, or denervation results in increased muscle tension that does not allow full extension of the stifle, and secondarily the hock, during the cranial swing phase.

Medical Therapy

No medical therapy has been shown to be consistently useful in treating fibrotic myopathy. In horses with complex muscle injury, such as those that develop fibrotic myopathy after lacerations or other traumatic injuries that involve not only the semitendinosus but the nearby semimembranosus muscle, corticosteroid injections into the fibrotic scars and nonsteroidal antiinflammatory therapy may partially alleviate clinical signs. Short-term improvement is reported in gaited horses with early fibrotic myopathy after injection of antiinflammatory drugs into involved muscles (see Chapter 122). Exercise does not appear to alleviate or exacerbate the abnormal gait.

Surgical Therapy

Surgical resection of the affected distal semitendinosus muscle (semitendinosus myotomy)[22] or affected muscle and tendon of insertion (semitendinosus myotenectomy)[19,21] and semitendinosus tenectomy at the tibial and tuber calcaneal insertions[20] have all resulted in some degree of immediate gait improvement. However, occasionally no immediate reponse has been seen, but delayed improvement has been observed following tenectomy.[23] Myotomy and myotenectomy have been associated with a relatively high degree of postoperative complications compared with simple tenectomy. If portions of muscle are excised, submission of these samples to a histopathologist with expertise in the pathology of neuromuscular disease may aid in determining the cause. Recurrence and exacerbation of clinical signs after myotomy and myectomy are the most common complications. Occasionally myotomy (fibrotomy) results in appreciable clinical improvement in horses with well-defined scars. At least partial recurrence of fibrotic myopathy after successful surgery occurs in about one third of horses, although the resultant gait deficit may not interfere with full return to function.[22] If progressive neuropathy is the cause, recurrence of signs after any type of surgery is likely.

STRINGHALT
Clinical Characteristics

A horse with stringhalt has an exaggerated upward flexion of a hindlimb or both hindlimbs that occurs at every walk stride (see Figure 48-1).[24-26] The affected limb is brought up and in (adducted) underneath the horse, such that the fetlock may contact the ventral abdominal wall. This abnormal gait often lessens considerably during the trot and usually, but not always, disappears at the canter. Affected horses may have difficulty backing, and the gait abnormality may only be apparent while backing in horses with mild disease. In such horses a diagnosis of mild shivers should also be considered. The Australian form of stringhalt is often bilateral and occurs in groups of horses on pasture containing a plant similar to dandelions known as flatweed *(Hypochoeris radicata)*.[3] The toxic principle is as yet unknown. Forelimbs may also be affected in horses with Australian stringhalt. A similar syndrome has been seen in the Pacific Northwest of North America,[24] in Europe,[26] and in South America.[27] In an outbreak in Brazil, plants containing *H. radicata* were fed to a normal horse and mild stringhalt developed, but signs abated when a similar plant from a different location was fed, leading to speculation that plants may vary in toxicity.[27] In mice, ingestion of *H. radicata* was associated with a significant increase in a metabolic biomarker, scyllo-inositol, known to be associated with other neurodegenerative diseases from neuronal and glial dysfunction.[28] Horses with stringhalt may or may not appear distressed by the gait abnormality. Similar to shivers (see the following discussion), anxiety and cold weather are reported to increase the severity of clinical signs in horses with stringhalt.[4,24]

Cause

True stringhalt and sporadic, or pasture-associated, stringhalt are most likely caused by underlying neuropathy. The Australian form of stringhalt has been clearly shown to be from underlying neuropathy.[3] Some horses with sporadic stringhalt have had evidence of neuropathy and denervation atrophy, although the cause has not been apparent. Histopathological evaluation of the lateral digital extensor muscle after lateral digital extensor myotenectomy has been particularly useful in detecting evidence of denervation atrophy. Horses with equine motor neuron disease have generalized denervation atrophy and can develop stringhalt that may be bilateral. Denervation atrophy of numerous muscles of the affected hindlimb is seen in horses with stringhalt from EPM. Careful examination of numerous nerves from horses with sporadic[24] or pasture-associated stringhalt[3] has revealed widespread neuropathy. Laryngeal hemiplegia associated with stringhalt is common, indicating a predisposition for abnormalities of long nerves. Stringhalt may be a different form of neuropathy than that seen in horses only developing laryngeal hemiplegia because clinical signs in some horses that develop stringhalt spontaneously resolve. Stringhalt may be similar to peripheral neuropathies in dogs, in which long nerves such as the recurrent laryngeal and sciatic nerves can be preferentially involved, and the cause is often not known. Lesions occur in the left recurrent laryngeal nerve in about 60% of horses with Australian stringhalt.[3] Clinical signs of laryngeal dysfunction may or may not be apparent. Development of stringhalt has been reported in horses after trauma to the dorsal tarsal and metatarsal regions in the area of the extensor tendons.[25] If proprioceptive deficits and ataxia are detected in a horse with stringhalt, peripheral neuropathy caused by EPM should be considered likely.

Biomechanical Basis

Although underlying neuropathy is well established as a cause of stringhalt, the biomechanical basis for the exaggerated flexion is still somewhat perplexing. Altered proprioception from neuropathy was suggested,[6] and this hypothesis is appealing. In stringhalt, however, the gait deficit appears to be consistently abnormal, stride to stride, unlike that seen in horses with other forms of proprioceptive deficits. Neuropathy may lead to paresthesia or altered input to or activity of muscle spindles. Given the exaggerated flexion of the hindlimbs of most horses after placement of hindlimb shipping (traveling) boots, altered sensation leading to limb hyperflexion is plausible. Other proposed causes include tendon adhesions around the tarsocrural joint or altered tendon reflexes after trauma[24] and hyperexcitability of motor neurons.[4]

Medical Therapy

For horses with stringhalt associated with plant toxicity, removal from the pasture may be curative, although recovery may take months to years and may not be complete.[4] Trauma-induced stringhalt may resolve with exercise therapy.[25] Oral phenytoin at 15 to 25 mg/kg once or twice daily may also be effective in some horses. The beneficial actions of phenytoin may include stabilization of neuronal, peripheral nerve, or skeletal muscle membrane electrical activity or decreased anxiety from sedation.[4] Botulinum toxin type B was used to reduce anal tone in horses, and it is compelling to consider its use for management of horses with stringhalt and other neuromuscular conditions.[29] Horses appear unusually sensitive to the effects of botulinum toxin; therefore caution should be used. In a recent experimental and clinical study, normal ponies (400 IU) and two Warmbloods with stringhalt (700 IU) were injected with botulinum toxin type A into the long digital extensor, lateral digital extensor, and vastus lateralis muscles.[30] Surface electromyography revealed reduced surface signals over the injected muscles; there was obvious clinical improvement in the two horses with stringhalt that lasted 12 weeks after injection, and kinematic studies confirmed a reduction in intensity of hindlimb hyperflexion.[30]

Surgical Therapy

Horses with residual gait abnormality after plant toxicity or traumatic neuropathy and horses with stringhalt caused by degenerative peripheral neuropathy may benefit from lateral digital extensor myotenectomy.[26] Horses with traumatically induced stringhalt appear to benefit most from lateral digital myotenectomy. In some horses, clinical signs may actually gradually worsen after surgery. Resolution of clinical signs after blocking the lateral digital extensor tendon may be a useful response to determine whether myotenectomy is indicated (see Chapter 122). In horses with stringhalt in which local anesthetic solution is placed directly into the lateral digital extensor muscle, both of us have observed 50% to 75% improvement in clinical signs, but clinical signs also improve if the cranial tibial and long digital extensor muscles are blocked. Selective blocking of the superficial and deep fibular (peroneal) nerves, the common fibular nerve, and the tibial nerve may help determine etiology in some horses, but the response is inconsistent. Selective peroneal (fibular) neurectomy remains a potential method of surgical management. Although some affected horses may return to full and high-level athletic performance after surgery, for many this should be considered a salvage procedure to allow a more normal gait for breeding horses, pasture pets, and horses in which the owner's expectations of performance are limited to light hacking.

SHIVERS (SHIVERERS, SHIVERING)

Clinical Characteristics

First described in draft breeds, shivering also occurs commonly in Warmbloods. Anecdotal evidence suggests a heritable predisposition. Shivers also occurs sporadically in other breeds, including Thoroughbreds, Quarter Horses, Arabians, and Morgans.

The clinical features of shivers, particularly in horses with early or mild disease, may resemble stringhalt or intermittent upward fixation of the patella. Affected horses may be described as stringy, especially by draft horse owners. Affected horses exhibit an episodic hyperflexion of the hindlimb and often abduct the limb before placing the hoof on the ground (see Figure 48-1). The affected limb may be held up in a flexed and abducted position for several seconds. This is most commonly seen when the limb is picked up. Sometimes the tail is simultaneously raised (Figure 48-3) . The horse may stretch its head up or forward during these episodes, and flickering of the eyelids and ears occurs occasionally. The muscles of the affected limb may tremble, and sometimes the tail quivers. Some horses only show clinical signs when the limbs are picked up and have a normal gait under all other circumstances. If an abnormal gait is present, unlike stringhalt it is sporadic rather than occurring at every stride and is not apparent at the trot or canter. The abnormal gait is most often seen when backing, turning tight circles, in the first walk stride after standing, and in the last walk stride before halting. The clinical signs may also be seen periodically while the horse is standing still. Anecdotally, the abnormal gait may be exacerbated by lack of exercise, cold ambient temperature, and increased anxiety in the horse. Neurological examination does not reveal evidence of postural reflex abnormalities or of ataxia.

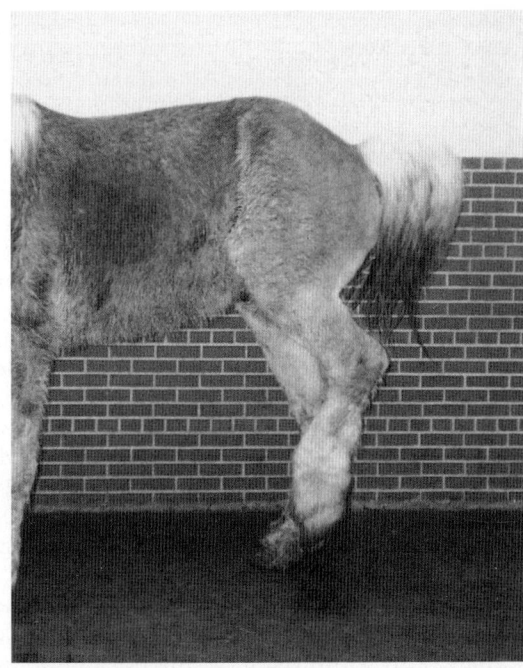

Fig. 48-3 · Belgian draft horse exhibiting the raised tail and hindlimb overflexion characteristic of severe shivers.

The farrier may first diagnose shivers because trimming and shoeing the hindlimbs is often difficult. The horse may be reluctant or appear unable to hold the affected limb up or to stand on three limbs for any length of time. When asked to lift a hind foot, the horse often hesitates, followed by an exaggerated flexion. Affected horses may appear worried when a hindlimb is picked up. They may be more comfortable if allowed to turn the head and neck toward the limb being picked up.[23]

Shivers may be a progressive disorder in some but not all horses. Severely affected horses develop generalized muscle atrophy and weakness and may exhibit periodic cramping of each leg in succession, with occasional leaning of the body such that the horse appears ready to fall. Onset is often between 2 and 4 years of age, but this varies extremely, as does the rate of progression. One of the authors (SJD) is aware of a homebred 10-year-old Warmblood mare that exhibited shivers as a neonate and has continued to show similar clinical signs throughout its life. The most severe form of progressive shivers occurs in draft horses. A somewhat milder form occurs in Warmbloods, in which sporadic abnormal hindlimb action is seen, but Warmbloods with shivers rarely exhibit a raised and quivering tail. Clinical signs in such horses are often mistaken for stringhalt or intermittent upward fixation of the patella. Affected horses can continue to compete at high levels in dressage or jumping for many years. Prepurchase evaluation of these high-performing shiverers can be particularly vexing because the expected progression of signs is completely unpredictable.

Occasionally shivering is seen in one or both forelimbs. The gait is usually not affected; however, when the limb is picked up, the limb shows muscle tremors.

A recently recognized and poorly understood syndrome known as "stiff-horse syndrome" may resemble shivers. Affected horses have a stiff gait and muscle spasms in the epaxial muscles of the lower back and in the muscles of the hindlimbs. Spasms may be precipitated by voluntary movements or by someone picking up a limb. Increased levels of antibodies to glutamic acid decarboxylase have been reported.[31]

Abnormal flexion of one or both hindlimbs mimicking shivering has also been seen as a result of chorioptic mange affecting the distal aspect of the hindlimbs of a Shire horse.[23]

Cause

Although an underlying neuropathy was proposed, careful study of two draft horses with shivers failed to reveal evidence of peripheral or central nervous system disease.[1] Examination of muscle from these and a small but growing number of horses with shivers of various breeds has revealed underlying EPSSM. Contiguous groups of glycogen-depleted skeletal muscle fibers in muscles of the proximal thigh and back have been seen in a small number of horses studied and indicate that this disorder may involve episodic muscle contracture (cramping).[1] However, a more recent study in Belgian draft horses failed to demonstrate a convincing association between EPSSM and shivers.[32]

Biomechanical Basis

Explaining the abnormal gait of shivers is difficult. The possible role of episodic muscle cramp or abnormal sensations within the affected leg is worthy of further study. Horses with an abscess in a hind hoof may show an abnormal flexing of the limb while standing that resembles shivers, and hind hoof abscesses often increase the abnormal action of the affected hindlimb in horses with shivers.

Medical Therapy

There is no reliable method of treatment. Change to a high-fat and low-starch and low-sugar diet may be beneficial in some horses after 4 to 6 months.[2,8] Whether this therapy acts by decreasing muscle cramping, decreasing anxiety in the horse, a combination of these effects, or some other mechanism is still unknown. These horses include those in which muscle biopsy revealed characteristic changes of EPSSM and horses with no apparent abnormalities in the muscle samples examined. Improvement is often only partial, but most owners have been pleased with results, and it is conceivable that dietary therapy may help to slow the progression of the disease.

Surgical Therapy

No surgical therapy is available for shivers.

HINDLIMB EXTENSOR WEAKNESS

Group outbreaks of bilateral hindlimb extensor weakness resulting in knuckling of the hind fetlocks either transiently or for longer periods, or in horses with more severe signs, such as inability to ambulate faster than a walk or paraplegia, have been associated with the consumption of big bale silage or poor quality fungal-infested hay.[33] In some horses, clinical signs were mild and nonprogressive, whereas in others severe signs developed within hours. Affected horses showed no signs of flexor weakness or ataxia, but some showed proprioceptive deficits and reduced skin sensation. In some horses, spontaneous resolution of clinical signs was observed over 6 months, whereas in others clinical signs were slowly progressive. Post mortem examination revealed consistent evidence of neuronal degeneration in the sciatic nerves and to a lesser extent in the lumbar intumescence of the spinal cord; however, other peripheral nerves were not routinely examined. Clinical signs in some of the mildly affected horses were consistent with femoral nerve paralysis (see also Chapter 11).

Unilateral or bilateral femoral nerve paralysis most commonly occurs after general anesthesia.[34] If unilateral, the horse cannot extend the stifle and rests the limb in a flexed position on the dorsal aspect of the fetlock. If bilateral, the horse is unable to stand for any length of time, except in a crouched position with the hindlimbs flexed.

Intermittent knuckling of one or both hind fetlocks when ridden may be seen alone or in association with another cause of hindlimb lameness. It may reflect a proprioceptive deficit, altered limb placement in an attempt to minimize pain, or be neurologically mediated.[23] The rider may complain that the hindlimbs sporadically "give way." Often young horses in early race training stumble or knuckle behind, a condition sometimes referred to as "loose stifles." This condition may be more common in young Standardbred racehorses and is often managed with patellar intraligamentous or periligamentous injections of counterirritants. Efficacy is questionable, but in most horses the condition resolves as training continues.

STUMBLING

Stumbling may occur in front or behind. Stumbling in front is frequently a reflection of foot pain; foot placement is altered to try to minimize pain, resulting in a more "toe first" landing pattern. Stumbling behind may be a reflection of extensor weakness (see Hindlimb Extensor Weakness section). It may also be a reflection of hindlimb lameness that results in toe drag (see Toe Drag section). Stumbling either in front or behind is often worst on uneven footing.

FLEXION OF THE FETLOCK AND INABILITY TO LOAD THE HEEL

Permanent semiflexion of a fetlock with inability to fully load the heel may be the result of chronic desmopathy of the accessory ligament of the deep digital flexor tendon (DDFT). In forelimbs, this is usually unilateral and is the result of chronic work-related injury of both the accessory ligament of the DDFT and the superficial digital flexor tendon, with associated adhesion formation. In hindlimbs the condition may be unilateral or bilateral and is associated with a chronic degeneration of the accessory ligament of the DDFT (see Chapter 71).[35]

TOE DRAG

Some clinically normal horses show a mild bilateral hindlimb toe drag, especially when worked on a soft surface, which may not be apparent under other circumstances.[23] A unilateral hindlimb toe drag is usually a reflection of a pain-related lameness. A bilateral hindlimb toe drag may reflect laziness, unfitness, long toes as a result of poor trimming, weakness, flexor weakness, bilateral lameness, ataxia, scirrhous cord, mastitis, and thoracolumbar or sacroiliac region pain.

PACING AT THE WALK

Walk is normally a four-beat gait: left hind, left fore, right hind, right fore. Occasionally a horse starts to pace at the walk, that is, the left hindlimb and left forelimb are advanced more or less simultaneously, followed by the right forelimb and hindlimb in an almost two-beat gait. This is often variable in degree within and between examinations and is usually most obvious when the horse is walking down an incline. This change in interlimb coordination is believed to be neurologically mediated, although no other gait abnormality or neurological deficit is detectable, and the mechanism has not been defined.[36] Other aspects of performance may be completely unaffected. The gait is not influenced by antiinflammatory analgesic drugs. The pace is considered a primitive gait, whereas the walk is one of the most complex because of the variability in overlap and lag time between limbs.[37] Once a horse has started to pace at the walk, it usually continues to do so. Pacing may have no clinical relevance in some horses, particularly older horses that curiously develop the condition spontaneously. However, in young horses not bred to pace (i.e., Standardbreds), pacing may be an early sign of progressive neurological disease.

STEPPING SHORT ON A HINDLIMB AT THE WALK

Stepping short on one hindlimb at the walk but with no detectable lameness at the trot is a poorly understood syndrome, which may be sudden in onset and tends to be persistent despite prolonged rest, with or without physiotherapy, osteopathy, chiropractic manipulation, or acupuncture treatment. Such horses have an obvious gait abnormality when ridden at the walk but perform normally at all other gaits. When examined moving in hand at the walk, the hindlimb gait is usually symmetrical. There is no response to antiinflammatory analgesic drugs or any local analgesic technique. Comprehensive radiographic, scintigraphic, and ultrasonographic examinations are unrewarding.

The gait may be influenced by neck position, being more obvious in a collected walk than if the horse is allowed to walk on a long rein. The cause is unknown. Continued work does not seem to have a deleterious effect.

UNUSUAL ABDUCTION OF A HINDLIMB

Rarely, a horse is observed to have excessive abduction of the hindlimb during protraction. Gait deficit is prominent at the walk but abates at the trot. No obvious source of pain can be found, and horses appear able to perform with this unusual gait deficit. Excessive abduction at the walk may be a manifestation of shivers, but we have observed this deficit rarely in light breeds as well.

OTHER MECHANICAL LAMENESSES

The biomechanical basis of mechanical lameness resulting in decreased flexion of the stifle and hock, such as fibrotic myopathy and upward fixation of the patella, is readily understood. These gaits are also characteristic and readily distinguished from other mechanical lamenesses. However, the mechanical lamenesses resulting in hyperflexion—that is, intermittent upward fixation of the patella, stringhalt, and shivers—have clinical similarities that can make them difficult to distinguish. One may also safely say that altered gaits from abnormal muscle or nerve function may not fall into one of the previously defined categories. A horse may appear stringy, locked up, have a goose waddle or stiff, stabbing hindlimb gait, or just appear off in a hindlimb because of mechanical lameness. A slight reduction in hock flexion at the walk may be considered normal for a horse, but this gait may also reflect a mechanical lameness (see Chapters 12 and 97).

In all horses with perplexing hindlimb lameness, the possibility of a form of mechanical lameness should be considered. This is especially true in breeds such as draft, Quarter Horse, and Warmblood-related breeds that are recognized to have a predilection for underlying myopathy. Because underlying myopathy or neuropathy is likely to be the most common cause of mechanical lameness, electromyography and muscle biopsy should be considered in all horses with mechanical lameness of the forelimbs or hindlimbs.

PART V

The Axial Skeleton

Chapter 49

Diagnosis and Management of Pelvic Fractures in the Thoroughbred Racehorse

Robert C. Pilsworth

References on page 1291

Injuries to the pelvis of the horse have historically been considered uncommon.[1-3] They have also previously been described as invariably resulting from external trauma.[4] Pelvic fractures are now recognized as a common cause of lameness in the racing Thoroughbred (TB). Stover et al[5] confirmed a high incidence of stress fractures in the pelvis of American racing TBs examined at post mortem. Similarly in a clinical study performed in Newmarket, England, pelvic fractures were found to be common in the young racing TB.[6,7] We now realize that pelvic fractures in the TB are most often the end stage of a cycle of bone fatigue and injury, commonly called stress-related bone injury. This has focused attention on early detection before the development of a full-blown displaced fracture. This section outlines steps to aid in early detection and management strategies subsequent to diagnosis.

PELVIC ANATOMY

The pelvis comprises the symmetrical halves and the sacrum in the midline. The left and right halves of the pelvis are joined in the ventral midline at the pubic symphysis. Although technically a joint, this becomes mineralized with age and is a bony union in most horses. A second joint occurs on each side between the pelvis and the head of the femur, forming the coxofemoral joint. The third joint is that between the ventral surface of the pelvis and the sacrum, the sacroiliac joint. Only the coxofemoral joint has any substantial degree of movement. The sacroiliac joint does have a synovial membrane, but it is largely immobile in many horses. In most horses the sacroiliac joint is spanned by dense bands of fibrous connective tissue, and despite having a cartilage surface, little or no movement takes place in the normal sacroiliac joint. Each half of the pelvis comprises three bones, which meet at the

acetabulum, the ilium cranially, the ischium caudally, and the pubis medially. The ilium has a large wing of bone extending from the tuber sacrale in the midline to the tuber coxae at the lateral extremity. The blade of the ilium narrows to form the shaft, which extends back to form the cranial segment of the coxofemoral joint. Caudal to the coxofemoral joint, and forming its caudal margin, is the ischium. Joining the two acetabula, forming the floor of the pelvis with its contralateral counterpart, is the pubis. The bones of the pelvis form a large fulcrum on which most of the gluteal muscle mass originates, to exert considerable propulsive forces on the hindlimbs. Although the pelvis can fracture anywhere as a result of external trauma or a fall, as is common with many other stress injuries, the forces involved in locomotion create predilection sites for stress fractures. These sites are associated with the concentration of forces involved in load bearing at speed and the biomechanics, innate structure, and form of the bone.

DIAGNOSTIC TECHNIQUES

Clinical Examination

A thorough working knowledge of the anatomy of the equine pelvis is essential for clinical examination to be useful. Because of the large muscle mass over the horse's hindquarters, only the bony extremities of the pelvis can be palpated. However, it is often possible to gain information about horses with pelvic injuries by studying the position of these bony landmarks. For example, the normal position and angle of the tuber coxae in the racehorse are often disturbed in horses with fracture or sacroiliac joint instability. The position of the tubera coxae can be assessed by viewing the horse from behind, with an assistant placing fingertips on the craniodorsal extremity of the tubera coxae (Figure 49-1). It is important that the horse stands completely level, with both hind feet together, for this test to be meaningful. Some horses, however, show asymmetry viewed in this way that is not linked to lameness. Similarly, careful palpation of the tubera sacrale can give information about the possible involvement of the sacral wing of the ilium or disruption of the sacroiliac joint.

Ventral displacement of one tuber sacrale is commonly encountered in ilial wing fractures, where the overlap of the fracture fragments seems to allow the tuber sacrale to move ventrally. Often a pain response is associated with palpation of a horse with tuber sacrale displacement, and sometimes movement of the bone itself may be felt if the fracture is complete. Fracture of a tuber coxae is often produced by external trauma, usually after a fall, but can also occur as a stress-related athletic injury. This usually results in a cranioventral displacement of the fracture fragment

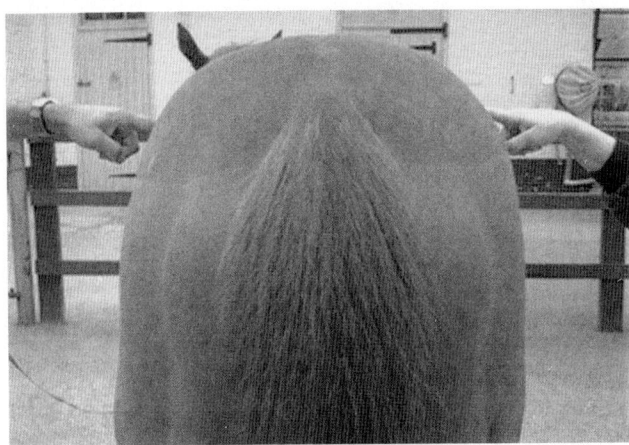

Fig. 49-1 • Assessment of the position of the bony pelvis by fingertip levels placed on the dorsal extremity of the tubera coxae on either side.

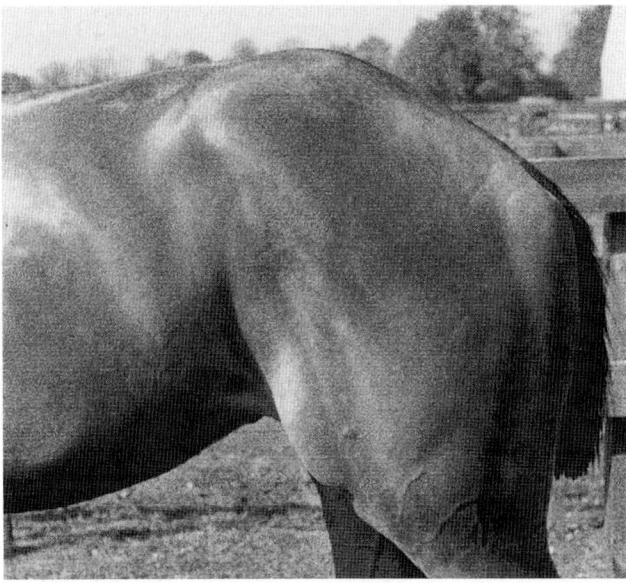

Fig. 49-2 • A horse with a sacral fracture. Note the abrupt angle change just behind the tubera sacrale, where the sacrum and coccyx have moved ventrally. The tail has complete flaccid paralysis. This filly had urine and fecal retention.

because of the distractive forces of associated musculature. The tuber coxae in these horses can often be felt situated in the sublumbar fossa, and the remnant fracture bed can be palpated at the original site. Fractures of the ischium can sometimes be felt by manual palpation, although the extensive muscle spasm and protective boarding that are associated with these fractures often preclude this examination. Usually there is hemorrhage and swelling in the acute phase, but a clear loss of muscle mass or even a "hollow" in the caudal contour of the rump may develop with time as inflammation subsides. Finally, muscle tone in the tail and anus should be evaluated because fractures involving the sacrum can involve neural elements that supply these structures and cause flaccid paralysis of the tail, rectum, anal ring, and vulva (in a filly), that is, the cauda equina syndrome (Figure 49-2). Bilateral ilial wing fractures can produce the same neurological appearance associated with severe nerve root damage consequent on movement of the pelvis in relation to the sacrum.

Rectal examination allows direct manual assessment of the integrity of the pubis, internal surface of the wing of the ilium, and ventral border of the sacroiliac joint. Sometimes an obvious, sharp discontinuity in the bone surface can be felt, particularly in horses with fracture of the pubis. Gentle rocking of the horse by an assistant, while the clinician maintains digital contact with the bone surface of the pelvis per rectum, sometimes allows an appreciation of relative movement of adjacent bones or, more commonly, a sensation of crepitus. In horses with fracture of the ilial wing, a soft asymmetrical swelling can often be felt at the fracture site, representing a subfascial hematoma. The more serious and potentially fatal hemorrhage that occurs when an iliac artery is severed by the sharp dorsal edge of the fractured ilium often cannot be detected per rectum. If not immediately fatal, this free blood often percolates ventrally to cause massive swelling and edema of the thigh musculature.

Some horses have several stress fractures identified scintigraphically, only one of which may have initially collapsed, leading to overt lameness. Progressive collapse of the pelvis may then occur during the convalescent period, as incomplete fractures become complete and displaced because of bone resorption and weakening of the fracture

site. The degree of lameness seen in these horses varies enormously, depending on the type and extent of the fracture, and is considered separately in the following discussions of each class of fracture.

Diagnostic Ultrasonography

Ultrasonography is useful for diagnosing pelvic fractures and has proved especially useful in demonstrating fractures of the ilial wing (Figure 49-3), ilial shaft, tuber coxae, and ischium. Ultrasonography is quick, easy, and within the capability of clinicians with a suitable ultrasound machine. Ultrasonography may eliminate the requirement for a horse to travel to a referral center for diagnosis, and the risk associated with radiography under general anesthesia can be avoided. Ultrasonography has obvious limitations. For example, adequate imaging of the sacral wing, sacroiliac joint, and the femoral head is not possible. Fractures with minimal displacement or poorly developed callus are also difficult to image, as are incomplete fractures involving the ventral surface of the ilium. For this reason, ultrasonography should not be regarded as a standalone imaging modality for identifying a fracture of the pelvis but should be used with a thorough clinical examination and, if available, scintigraphy. In many horses, the exact site and extent of the fracture can be determined, which allow improved prognostic and management advice to be given. The healing process can be monitored by serial examinations, allowing the management program to be tailored to the individual horse (see Figure 49-3, *B* and *C*). A longitudinal- or sector-array ultrasound transducer can be used, provided it has a deep enough penetration to see the bone surface (i.e., a 3.5- or 5-MHz transducer). The muscle mass lying above the bone structures acts as a natural "standoff," bringing the bone surfaces into the focal zone of the ultrasound beam. A separate standoff may be required to evaluate the position of the tubera sacrale and to detect any displacement. In thin-coated horses, no clipping is required,

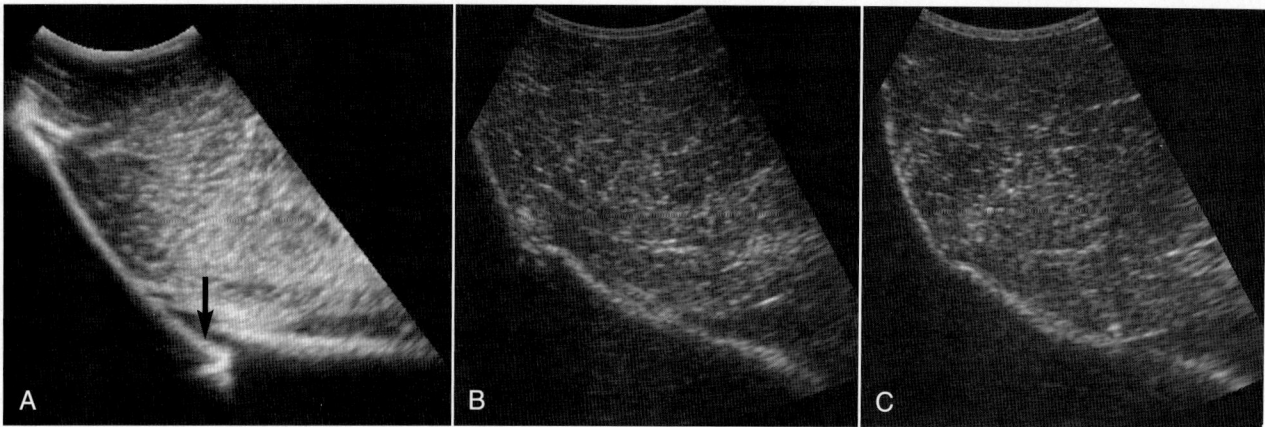

Fig. 49-3 • A, Ultrasonographic image of the right ilial wing obtained using a 3- to 5-MHz transducer. There is a stress fracture of the ilial wing *(arrow)*. The fracture appears as a discontinuity in the pelvis surface, with some comminution evident. Adjacent to the fracture is irregular echogenic material (callus), and just dorsal to the fracture is an anechogenic defect in the muscle (hemorrhage). Healing can be monitored by serial ultrasonographic examination, here at 63 days **(B)** and 109 days **(C)** following injury.

provided adequate saturation of the coat is achieved by degreasing with a detergent solution (chlorhexidine) or by soaking in surgical spirit, followed by application of a coupling gel before scanning. Horses with thicker hair coats must be clipped to obtain images of adequate quality. Images can be difficult to produce in horses with large amounts of subcutaneous fat because of the attenuating properties of this tissue. Numerous blood vessels running through the musculature can create acoustic shadows, which may be confused with a discontinuity of the bone surface. Identifying the bony landmarks such as the tubera sacrale, tubera coxae, cranial and caudal margins of the ilial wing, and greater trochanters of the femur allow anatomical orientation. A dry pelvic specimen is also useful in orientation. Both sides of the pelvis should be evaluated because the normal side can be used for comparison. However, keep in mind that bilateral ilial wing stress fractures occur and both sides may be abnormal. For recording and reference purposes, the area of the ilial wing imaged is referred to as line A, B, or C, and the distance from the tuber sacrale is measured. Scans aligned longitudinally along the ilial shaft are referred to as line D. This simple system is useful, especially in follow-up examinations. A systematic method for recording ultrasonographic findings has been published elsewhere.[8]

Radiography

Radiography of the pelvis is easily carried out in a foal when it can be performed under heavy sedation, for example, with a combination of detomidine and butorphanol, with the foal allowed to stand again shortly after the procedure. Standard projections include a ventrodorsal image with the foal lying on its back and a lateral image with the foal lying on its side on top of the cassette. A grid is mandatory to reduce scattered radiation produced by the large mass of soft tissue covering the pelvis. Radiography in adult horses is considerably more difficult. General anesthesia is required for thorough radiographic examination of the pelvis for numerous reasons, including the safety of the horse, personnel, and radiographic equipment. Administering general anesthesia to a horse suspected of having a pelvic fracture

is contraindicated because of the possibility of the horse displacing the fracture on recovery. Fracture displacement can lead to fatal hemorrhage or worsening of clinical signs, which is particularly true in horses with an incomplete fracture of the wing and shaft of the ilium. It is also difficult to get high-quality radiographs of the pelvic bones without extensive previous starvation of the horse to allow emptying of the gastrointestinal tract. Small, incomplete, pelvic stress fractures are extremely difficult to see radiologically. Three techniques for standing radiography in the horse have been described.[9-11] However, in my experience this has proved difficult, presents real risks of damage to the equipment, and is a substantial radiation hazard to attending personnel. The standing examination is also limited to examination of the acetabulum and ilial shaft, and images of the ilial wing are obscured by the sublumbar and overlying dorsal lumbar musculature. Image quality obtained in this way is also often poor; however, it may permit detection of substantially displaced fractures. Although radiography used to be the imaging technique of choice for assessing horses with pelvic fractures, it has been replaced by combined ultrasonographic and scintigraphic evaluation in many hospitals.

Scintigraphy

Scintigraphy is considered the most sensitive method of assessing acute bone damage in the horse (see Chapter 19).[3,12-17] Special techniques for examining the pelvis have also been described, including an oblique image of the ilium, which is useful in diagnosing incomplete stress fractures in this site.[16] Sacroiliac joint luxation has also been described as a scintigraphic diagnosis, the appearance of which is extremely similar to the ilial wing fractures observed by others.[3] Equine scintigraphic techniques applicable to the pelvis, as well as numerous examples of normal and most types of pathology, have also been published in detail elsewhere.[17] To examine the equine pelvis fully using a gamma camera, dorsal images of the entire pelvis are mandatory. The lateral image of the pelvis tends to be difficult to interpret because of the areas of focal greater radiopharmaceutical uptake (RU) observed at tubera coxae and the coxofemoral joints in a normal horse. The massive muscle mass interposed between the slender bones of the iliac shaft and the gamma camera results in extensive shielding and poor images. Radioactive urine in the underlying bladder contributes to extensive background radiation, further decreasing image quality. Movement is a key factor in limiting image quality, but motion correction software can be used to minimize this complication. However, the lateral oblique image described by Hornof et al[16] usually gives better images of the iliac wing and shaft. A caudal oblique image is also used by some to give better images of the coxofemoral joint and acetabulum. A method for scintigraphic examination of the pelvis using a hand-held probe has also been described.[18] If a pelvic fracture is strongly suspected and initial scintigraphic examination is performed within 3 to 5 days of injury and is negative, a follow-up examination should be performed at least 10 days from the time of injury. Early fractures, even those with associated displacement, may not be evident scintigraphically for several days after injury.

FRACTURES OF THE TUBER COXAE

Fractures of a tuber coxae are often described as a knocked-down hip. They are relatively common and fairly straightforward to diagnose by clinical examination of the bony landmarks of the pelvis. They may occur after direct trauma or a fall but also as an athletic injury in training or racing.

Clinical Signs

On the first day of injury, the horse is moderately to severely lame, even at the walk. Often the horse shows intense muscle spasm and guarding of the affected hindquarter. The horse may sweat and scrape the ground, which can mimic signs of colic. The affected tuber coxae is often displaced cranioventrally and is palpable in the region of the sublumbar fossa. The parent bed from which the fragment originated is often palpable in the original site of the tuber coxae. Lameness rapidly resolves, and many horses are walking sound after only 24 to 48 hours, but they will still trot lame. Hemorrhage often occurs, which may present as a subcutaneous hematoma. Occasionally the sharp spiculated end of the ilium wears through the overlying skin, leading to development of an open fracture, which can be extremely difficult to treat because the skin overlying the sharp fragment will not heal and infection becomes a problem.

Radiographic Examination

A technique to evaluate the tubera coxae in the standing horse was recently described, but strict attention to limiting radiation exposure to attending personnel should be followed.[11] A medial 50° dorsal-lateroventral oblique radiographic image is obtained with the horse standing, sedated in stocks with the horse bearing weight on the affected limb and resting the unaffected limb, if possible.[11]

Scintigraphic Examination

Scintigraphic examination is probably not indicated in most horses because the clinical diagnosis is straightforward. If performed, scintigraphic examination reveals clinically significant focal increased radiopharmaceutical uptake (IRU) associated with the displaced tuber coxae and also a fairly obvious distortion of the normal anatomy of the pelvis on the dorsal image. In the Editors' experience, photopenic regions associated with ventral displacement of the fracture fragments may be present.

Ultrasonographic Examination

Directly after injury, horses with a tuber coxae fracture have clinical signs similar to those with other fractures of the pelvis, and an ultrasonographic examination helps to confirm the diagnosis and to define better the limits of the fracture. The fracture is easily seen as a disruption to the normally smooth and continuous contour of the iliac wing as it approaches the tuber coxae. A standoff may be required for better imaging of the bone immediately beneath the skin. It is important to perform a thorough examination of all the bony structures in case there are fractures in other regions of the pelvis.

FRACTURES OF THE ILIAL WING

Fractures of the iliac wing appear to be among the most commonly encountered type of athletic stress fractures in the skeletally immature TB racehorse.[17-20]

Clinical Signs

A horse with a complete iliac wing fracture often shows lameness, but the initial lameness varies from lame at the walk to grade 1 to 4 of 5 at the trot. Lameness often resolves rapidly within 24 to 48 hours, and the horse then has a slight gait abnormality, walking with the back hunched up, but with no overt lameness. A horse with an iliac wing fracture often plaits with the hindlimbs at the trot and has a shortened stride. Although a complete fracture may be present on only one side, evidence of a subclinical stress fracture in the same site on the contralateral limb is common, and this may contribute to the peculiar gait shown by the horse. Obviously, pain from both sacroiliac joints considerably affects the freedom of movement of the hindlimbs. A horse with bilateral lesions may appear to have signs of exertional rhabdomyolysis, but plasma creatine kinase levels are often normal or only slightly increased (500 to 1500 IU/L).

Incomplete fractures may occur on one or both sides, and this can often show as poor propulsion and a poor hindlimb action rather than overt lameness. In a horse with a complete fracture, ventral displacement of the ipsilateral tuber sacrale is often apparent and can be detected by careful digital examination of the midline of the spine and both tubera sacrale. Firm pressure in the previous site of the tuber sacrale often evinces a marked pain response, with associated muscle spasm over the sacroiliac joint region. Palpating the tip of the tuber sacrale in its ventrally displaced position is sometimes possible. Often fairly profound muscle wastage is associated with this injury in the first 2 weeks, and this contributes substantially to the apparent asymmetry of the horse when viewed from behind. Bilateral complete fractures lead to profound stiffness, unwillingness to walk, and boarding of the muscles of the pelvis in response to digital manipulation. They can lead to collapse and inability to rise, with substantial neurological deficits in severe injuries.

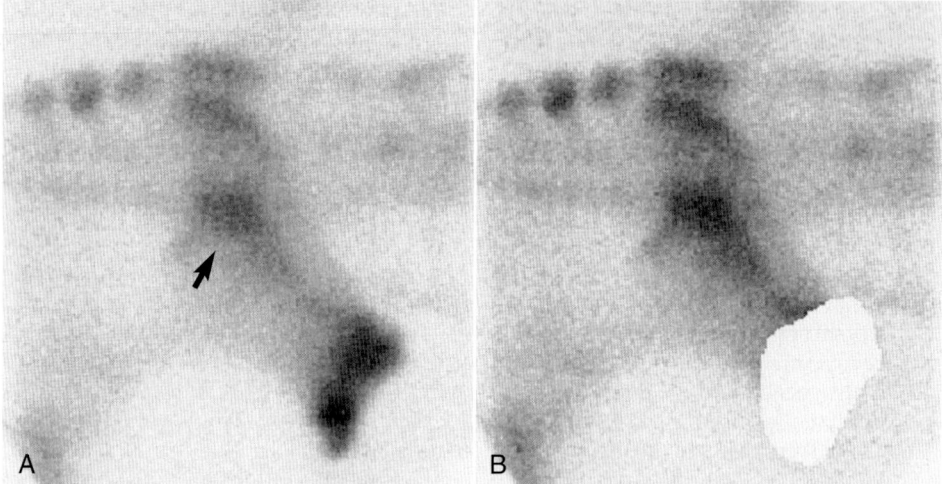

Fig. 49-4 • A, Dorsal lateral oblique delayed (bone) phase scintigraphic image over the right side of the pelvis of a horse with a stress fracture of the ilial wing. Cranial is to the right. Focal increased radiopharmaceutical uptake (IRU) *(arrow)* appears about one fourth of the way between the tuber sacrale and tuber coxae, the most common predilection site for stress fractures of the ilial wing. Masking of areas of apparent greater RU, which are the consequence of normal bone with little attenuating soft tissue cover (tuber coxae), allows better recognition of the pathology otherwise obscured by "count capture" **(B).** (Courtesy Animal Health Trust, Newmarket, U.K.)

Scintigraphic Examination

Scintigraphy usually reveals marked focal IRU associated with the ilial wing, usually 10 to 15 cm from the midline (Figure 49-4). IRU may be bilateral or unilateral. A clear fracture line and the displacement of the ilial wing are sometimes visible. The lateral oblique image[16] is particularly useful in determining whether the fracture extends to the cranial and caudal cortices of the ilial wing, although masking of the normal greater RU associated with the tubera coxae, caused by lack of attenuation of the gamma rays by overlying muscle as the bone approaches the skin surface, may be needed to highlight these changes (see Figure 49-4, *B*).

Ultrasonographic Examination

The normal ultrasonographic appearance of the ilial wing is a smooth and regular concave hyperechoic line, extending between the tuber sacrale and the ipsilateral tuber coxae. Acoustic shadowing and refraction artifacts can be created by the many blood vessels within the musculature and must not be confused with disruption to the bone contour. Ilial wing fractures appear as a disruption to the ilial wing contour, with changes ranging from a clear fracture gap to small irregular echogenic areas on the dorsal surface, representing prodromal periosteal new bone formation. The fractures normally run sagitally and involve the bone dorsal to or in proximity with the sacroiliac joint. The bone abnormalities often appear more severe toward the caudal margin of the fracture. Sometimes hemorrhage at the site of fracture appears as an anechoic defect in the normal heterogeneous echogenicity of skeletal muscle (see Figure 49-3, *A*).

FRACTURES OF THE ILIAL SHAFT

The ilial shaft is a common site for fracture after a fall or as a spontaneous athletically induced injury.

Clinical Signs

Fracture of the ilial shaft is extremely painful, producing non–weight-bearing lameness, and is often associated with shock from extreme pain and rapid blood loss. The tubera coxae often are markedly asymmetrical when viewed from behind, although encouraging the horse to bear weight equally to allow this examination to be carried out can be difficult. Sometimes with incomplete or minimally displaced fractures, no displacement of the tuber coxae is apparent initially, but in these horses the pelvis often collapses early in convalescence, at which time asymmetry becomes obvious. Collapse of the pelvis can often make the fracture less painful for the horse for reasons that are unclear. Rectal examination is often useful, and gentle rocking of the horse while the arm is inserted in the rectum often allows clear crepitus to be felt with the fingertips on the ilial shaft of the affected side. A hematoma next to the fractured ilium can also be easily palpated in many horses. Not uncommonly, horses damage the iliac arteries with the sharp edges of the comminuted fracture fragments, and this can result in severe and sometimes fatal hemorrhage.

Horses usually do not resent palpation and flexion of the distal aspect of the limb, although forced abduction of the limb, including the hock and stifle, may elicit a painful response. Palpation of the hindquarters usually results in intense muscle spasm and guarding on the affected side. Bizarre consequences of the severe lameness and change in functional anatomy after some of these fractures are not uncommon and include permanent upward fixation of the patella, contracture of the hamstring group of muscles, and spastic hyperextension of the tarsus. These complications invariably result in a grave prognosis.

Scintigraphic Examination

Many horses are too lame to allow transport to an equine clinic for scintigraphic examination, and a combination of clinical signs and ultrasonographic findings can establish the diagnosis. If scintigraphy is performed, a caudal oblique image is often extremely useful in illustrating the extent and nature of the fracture. Because pelvic anatomy is directly visible on a scintigraphic image, the displacement of the fracture fragments and ilial wing is often easily appreciated.

Ultrasonographic Examination

The ilial shaft is examined by aligning the ultrasound beam in a craniocaudal direction and following the ilial shaft from the flat surface of the ilial wing toward the greater trochanter of the femur. With ultrasonography, a displaced ilial shaft fracture is easily detected as a discontinuity to the bone surface. Passive movement of the limb may show independent movement of the fracture margins in real-time scanning. Hypoechogenic areas may be present around the fracture line and represent hemorrhage into the musculature. As with other fractures, if displacement is minimal, an ultrasonographic examination may fail to detect any pathological condition.

FRACTURES OF THE PUBIS AND ISCHIUM

Discrete fractures of the ischium are relatively uncommon. The horse usually has unilateral lameness with obvious swelling over the caudal aspect of the thigh. A fall or rearing over backward is often noted in the history, but these fractures can also develop as a spontaneous athletic injury. Often palpable crepitus and a marked pain response on firm digital pressure to the site are apparent. The tail may be held to one side because of muscle spasm associated with the painful lesion. Often focal sweating occurs on a patch of skin on the back of the thigh, presumably resulting from nerve damage. With time, the acute swelling subsides, and a "caved-in" appearance of the caudal aspect of the upper thigh may develop when viewed from the side.

Fractures of the pubis are uncommon and usually only encountered with other multiple pelvic fractures or after a fall.

Scintigraphic Examination

Scintigraphy shows focal IRU associated with the ischium and sometimes clear displacement of a segment of bone. Isolated fractures of the pubis can be difficult to see because of the mass of bone and muscle interposed between the fracture site and the gamma camera. For this reason, a hand-held probe, used per rectum, can give useful information. A bladder artifact produced by delayed excretion of urine may give the appearance of an IRU in this site.

Ultrasonographic Examination

The pubis is the least rewarding of the pelvic bones to examine by ultrasonography. A rectal probe is required, and only marked changes are detectable. The ultrasonographic examination is limited by the small degree of probe movement that is possible within the rectum, coupled with the irregular normal contour of the bone at this site.

Part of the ischium is also examined internally using a rectal transducer. This approach may be the only way to detect any ultrasonographic changes associated with an acetabular fracture. The caudal-most portion of the ischium and the ischiatic tuberosity can be examined percutaneously. Normally a smooth concave contour extends

caudally from the greater trochanter of the femur. Ultrasonographic changes similar to those described in other sites where bone damage has taken place can be seen in this area. Comparing the contralateral ischium with the fractured one is useful.

FRACTURES INVOLVING THE ACETABULUM

Horses with fractures of the ilial shaft and ischium that involve the acetabulum have the poorest prognosis of all for return to athletic function as a racehorse and normally develop osteoarthritis (OA) of the coxofemoral joint, which results in permanent and progressive lameness. Acetabular fractures commonly result from trauma, often subsequent to slipping over or being cast. This is one of the more frequent causes of lameness in a horse found not bearing weight on a hindlimb in the stable or paddock, with no obvious inciting cause.

Clinical Examination

The horse is extremely lame and is often unwilling to move. The horse has extremely short protraction of the hindlimbs at the walk and often hops rather than attempting to bear weight. Both Editors have observed that horses willing to walk with fractures or severe OA of the coxofemoral joint often have a shortened caudal phase of the stride, differentiating this area of pain from many others in the hindlimb. Pain occurs on abduction of the limb, and often firm palpation of the muscle mass around the coxofemoral joint causes muscle spasm and pain. Crepitus may be felt with displaced fractures if the hand is applied to the greater trochanter of the femur while the horse is walked, although commonly these fractures are incomplete and crepitus is not apparent. Crepitus may also be felt if the horse is rocked during rectal examination with the hand on the pelvic brim. In horses younger than 2 years of age, separation of the femoral head can occur from trauma and produces similar clinical signs to a comminuted acetabular fracture.

Scintigraphic Examination

Scintigraphic examination reveals focal IRU associated with the coxofemoral joint, greater trochanter of the femur, and ilial shaft on the affected side. The IRU is particularly visible on a caudal oblique image in which both coxofemoral joints can usually be seen using a large field of view gamma camera. OA of the coxofemoral joint contributes substantially to IRU in horses with a chronic fracture. These fractures are not associated with intense focal IRU initially, and early examination may give false-negative results. At least 1 week is required before scintigraphic abnormalities are detectable, and often this time period is necessary to allow humane transport of the horse. If the clinician is doubtful, the scan should be repeated 14 days later, when bone uptake will be maximal.[16] Separation of the femoral head, which occurs infrequently in yearlings usually after a fall, produces similar scintigraphic changes, with moderate IRU associated with the coxofemoral joint.

Ultrasonographic Examination

Because of the great depth of the acetabulum and the many changing bone contours, the acetabulum is probably the most difficult area of the pelvis to image by ultrasonography. Subtle pathological conditions may well be missed. The greater trochanter of the femur provides a good landmark by which to orient the image. The normal acetabular region is represented as a smooth and regular hyperechoic line of the acetabular rim. The greater trochanter of the femur is close to the skin surface as a hyperechoic line extending down and toward the acetabular rim. In some horses, a hypocchogenic region represents the joint space. In foals and immature animals, a hyperechoic convex line extends from the greater trochanter and represents the femoral head.

A fracture can appear as a discontinuity or irregular roughening of the acetabular rim and will be particularly obvious if greater degrees of callus are present.

PRINCIPLES OF TREATMENT OF HORSES WITH PELVIC FRACTURES

Surgical repair of pelvic fractures is not currently a realistic option in the adult horse. The period of box rest required for bony union ranges from 2 to 3 months, judged by monitoring fracture healing with ultrasonography. The end result in terms of the functional anatomy of the pelvis depends on the degree of displacement in the initial insult and the extent of subsequent distraction of the fracture fragments by subsequent muscle contracture. For example, tuber coxae fracture fragments heal by becoming adherent to the cranial wing of the pelvis through fibrous union. Despite the fact that the position of the tuber coxae often changes by several centimeters and the tuber coxae comes to rest in the sublumbar fossa, many horses make a full return to athletic function and race with success. Fractures of the sacral wing of the ilium are often nondisplaced and can make an extremely good, smooth bone union after healing (see Figure 49-3). Often an abnormal angle is apparent on the ilial surface because of distraction of the fragments by muscle contraction before healing. Although the abnormal angulation of the pelvic blade cannot help the stability of the sacroiliac joint immediately beneath the fracture, many affected horses go on to train and race successfully. In a review of 20 horses with ilial fractures, 15 horses made a full recovery to advanced race training, and 11 of these raced successfully.[6] Involvement of the ilial shaft considerably worsens the prognosis for racing, although many heal adequately to allow retirement to stud. Some general principles of the care and management of horses apply equally to the different types of pelvic fractures and can be outlined as follows:

- Pain should be controlled during the initial phase by administration of nonsteroidal antiinflammatory drugs (NSAIDs), such as phenylbutazone, until the horse appears comfortable walking around the stable.
- The risk that normal recumbency in the box will result in displacement of an already fractured pelvis is always present. Unfortunately, the proximity of the sharp edge of the fractured ilium to the iliac arteries makes this a potentially life-threatening complication. Therefore a horse suspected of major pelvic bone injury should be tied up by the head during the initial convalescent period. When doing so, it is important that the horse has enough rope to move around comfortably, without a sufficient length to encourage it to attempt to lie

down. A "break string" should always be between the rope and the head collar, so that if a horse tries to lie down, it can do so without risk. Tying the horse in a position where it can see outside events is best, so that the horse is not alarmed by things happening behind it, to avoid the horse being startled and the risk of displacement of a lesion.

Horses should remain tied up for no more than 1 month. Many horses cope with being tied up without problems, but while they are tied up, horses should be fed from the floor several times a day and be held by an attendant while they eat. This encourages drainage of bronchial secretions from the trachea and may help to prevent pleuritis and pleuropneumonia, which can develop with prolonged periods of being tied up.[21] During the period that NSAIDs are administered by mouth, any increase in rectal temperature will be masked. For this reason it is vital to take regular (every 48 hours) blood samples to assess changes in white blood cell count, serum amyloid protein A (SAA), and fibrinogen level, which may signal an early onset of pneumonia or pleuritis. Subsequent to NSAID therapy, rectal temperature should be monitored twice daily. When a horse is untied after 1 month, the fracture fragments possibly still can displace, leading to fatal hemorrhage. However, displacement is rare, and the clinician must balance the potential risk to the horse against the humanitarian aspects of keeping a horse tied up continuously for more than 1 month. Although I feel strongly about tying up horses with pelvic fractures, others feel differently, and many horses with pelvic fractures have been managed successfully without being tied up.

- Once untied, a horse requires a minimum of another 1 to 2 months of stable rest, depending on the extent and severity of the fracture, combined with daily walking exercise to encourage normal blood flow to the feet, before turnout is safe. Pasture rest for another 2 months is then advisable for horses with a severe, displaced fracture, even before contemplating covering. Pregnancy and parturition can severely test fracture healing; therefore a prolonged convalescent period is required. Often questions arise about the suitability of mares undergoing pregnancy and parturition after pelvic fractures. In my experience, the main concerns are lameness, the ability to get up and down, and maintaining weight rather than callus formation and the physical inability to deliver a foal.
- If a pelvic fracture has led to an extreme unilateral lameness, the contralateral foot is at real risk of developing laminitis. Many horses will not allow the contralateral limb to be raised long enough to fit a frog support. Therefore it is vital that the horse is bedded on deep litter (bedding), so that the bedding can pack up under the foot to give some support. A frog support should be placed as soon as possible, and the shoes should be removed. Once the horse is able to bear weight on the affected limb, short periods of walking exercise help prevent vascular stasis and lymphangitis that often accompany weight bearing on one limb for prolonged periods. Walking may also help prevent supporting limb laminitis, but only if the horse is not profoundly lame in the affected limb. Support bandaging of the

contralateral limb in horses with severe unilateral lameness is probably worthwhile and certainly helps to prevent the occurrence of lymphedema.

- Administration of acetylpromazine in small doses (25 to 50 mg orally twice daily or 0.02 to 0.04 mg/kg injected intramuscularly twice daily, judged on degree of tranquilization by the first dose) to a lame horse helps for three reasons: preventing laminitis (although the evidence for efficacy is limited; see Chapter 34); relieving some anxiety and allowing the horse to rest, which is important for recovery; and preventing upward fixation of the patella, to which the horses are prone, presumably by causing mild muscle relaxation.

- Most horses with incomplete or minimally displaced complete ilial wing stress fractures become sound rapidly. I do not normally keep these horses tied up, but nonetheless a small but real risk of fatal hemorrhage exists in these horses, even when they are apparently sound. Displacement is rare, but from the outset the risk should be explained to and understood by all involved in the management decisions. These horses will often commence walking exercise much more quickly (after 2 to 4 weeks) and return to trotting at 6 weeks, with a rehabilitation period of 8 weeks.

- Adult horses with fractures involving the acetabulum have the poorest prognosis for return to athletic function, although horses often become sound enough to be retired to pasture. Compromise of the diameter of the pelvic canal can be a complication, especially if the ilial shaft is involved and the fracture has healed with abundant callus. Even for experienced clinicians, being categorical about the ability of a mare with a narrowed pelvic canal to breed can be difficult. Often a trial mating to an inexpensive stallion is the most pragmatic management choice, if the clinician has doubts.

Careful thought should be given to each individual horse to make sure that the horse's future is worthwhile, in terms of quality of life for the horse and the economic realities of the situation, before subjecting a horse to a prolonged and, by necessity, painful convalescent period.

Prognosis in foals with acetabular fractures is considerably better than in adult horses. Treating a foal with an acetabular fracture is definitely worthwhile because at this age the pelvis appears capable of healing with much less chance of the development of OA in the coxofemoral joint when compared with adult horses. Foals are treated with 12 weeks of box rest initially and progressive turnout in a nursery paddock.

Separation of the femoral head in a young horse carries a hopeless prognosis and, if confirmed, should lead to immediate euthanasia.

- As with any horse that has had a prolonged period of box rest, the clinician must remember that although the pelvic fracture may have healed, the rest of the horse's skeleton will have demineralized substantially because of disuse. Therefore it is vital that horses are treated as "naive skeletal specimens" when training is resumed. The exercise program should increase gradually, beginning with walking only for the first 2 weeks and building up gradually through walking and trotting to slow speed cantering, eventually reattaining race speed training. Clinicians should remember that the skeleton takes approximately 1 month at each gait to adapt to the loads placed on it. Bringing a horse back from injury often takes as long as the period of box rest itself, if further orthopedic problems are to be avoided.

Chapter 50

Lumbosacral and Pelvic Injuries in Sports and Pleasure Horses

Sue J. Dyson

lumbar vertebra and the cranial articular processes of the sacrum. Movement is principally restricted to flexion and extension because of the large transverse processes.[1] Congenital variations in anatomy can be seen, including fusion of the fifth and sixth lumbar vertebrae or sacralization of the sixth lumbar vertebra resulting in lumbosacral ankylosis. These result in stress concentration on adjacent joints. The biomechanical stresses of movement of the lumbosacral joint place particular compression and traction forces on the intervertebral disk, which may predispose to disk degeneration.

References on page 1292

ANATOMICAL CONSIDERATIONS

Detailed anatomy of the ilium, ischium, pubis, sacrum, coxofemoral joint, sacroiliac joints, nerves, and major vessels is described elsewhere (see Chapters 49, page 564, and 51, page 583). The lumbosacral joint comprises five separate joints: the intercentral joint between the caudal aspect of the vertebral body of the sixth lumbar vertebra and the sacrum, between which is an intervertebral disk; two intertransverse joints; and two synovial intervertebral articulations between the articular processes of the sixth

CLINICAL SIGNS

History

Pelvic injury in a mature athletic horse is a comparatively unusual cause of lameness, except as the result of trauma from a fall, rearing and falling over backward, becoming cast in the stable, or sustaining an injury during transport. When the horse has no history of trauma, diagnosis can be difficult, and excluding all possible sources of pain in the distal aspect of the limb is frequently necessary before focusing on the pelvic region.

Horses with clinically significant pathological conditions of the lumbosacral or sacroiliac joints frequently have a history of progressive reduction in performance, difficulty engaging the hindlimbs, and poor hindlimb impulsion, especially when ridden.[2,3]

Clinical Examination

Clinical assessment of individual structures of the pelvic region by visual examination and palpation is not easy, especially in Warmblood and draft breeds, because of the large muscle mass of the hindquarters. Frequently, only the tubera coxae and tubera sacrale can be palpated. Large muscle mass may prohibit palpation of the greater trochanter of the femur. Atrophy of the hindquarter musculature is nonspecific and can reflect disuse because of pain arising anywhere in the limb, although atrophy of the muscles around the tail head often reflects injury to the tuber ischium or local nerve damage. Asymmetry of the height of the tubera sacrale is a common finding in horses in full work, free from lameness, although it may be seen along with poor performance or alterations in hindlimb gait. Apparent asymmetry may actually reflect differences in size of the dorsal sacroiliac ligaments. Alteration in muscle mass in the proximity of the tubera sacrale superficially can give a false impression of asymmetry of the tubera sacrale. Asymmetry of the tubera coxae may reflect a previous injury unassociated with ongoing pain. Poor muscle development in the lumbar region and over the hindquarters may make the tubera sacrale and the summits of the dorsal spinous processes of the lumbar vertebrae appear abnormally prominent. This should alert the clinician to the possibility of thoracolumbar or pelvic pain; however, this finding is nonspecific and may reflect the horse's work history.

The pelvic region should be appraised visually and palpated systematically, and although preliminary assessment is usually best performed in the stable, for accurate evaluation of symmetry of the musculature and bony elements of the pelvic region the horse should be standing completely squarely behind on a firm, level surface with the horse looking straight ahead. In a horse with severe lameness this may not be possible because the horse may be unwilling to load the lame limb fully. Careful differentiation should be made between muscular and bony asymmetry. Muscle atrophy can make accurate assessment of symmetry of the pelvic bones difficult. To evaluate accurately the levelness of the tubera coxae, two assistants each must place an index finger on the craniodorsal aspect of each tuber coxae and extend the finger horizontally, or the tubera coxae should be marked using tape. Elevation of the tail may be necessary to identify muscle atrophy around the tail head, which may be seen along with nerve damage, or injuries of the ipsilateral tuber ischium.

Assessment of symmetry when the horse is unwilling to bear weight evenly on both hindlimbs is not easy, but particular attention should be paid to the way in which the limb is positioned. An abnormally straight limb may reflect luxation of the coxofemoral joint and secondary upward fixation of the patella. The greater trochanter of the femur of the lame limb may appear higher than that of the contralateral limb.

The muscles of the lumbar and pelvic regions should be assessed carefully to identify any area of abnormal muscle tension, pain on palpation, or unusual firmness. Firm stroking of the muscles first with a finger and then with a blunt-ended object (e.g., artery forceps) is useful to determine whether muscle spasm or muscle fasciculation is induced. Palpation of the caudal muscles of the thigh is also important because abnormal pain or tension can reflect primary muscle injury or an injury of the ipsilateral tuber ischium.

Firm pressure should be applied to the bony prominences to see whether pain or an abnormal reaction, such as sinking on the hindlimbs when pressure is applied to the tubera sacrale, can be induced. Both tubera coxae should be grasped simultaneously and the horse rocked from side to side to determine whether crepitus can be detected by palpation or auscultation, bearing in mind that the absence of crepitus does not preclude a fracture. Pull the tail while holding one hand over the coxofemoral joint; palpable crepitus may reflect a fracture, severe osteoarthritis (OA), or subluxation of the joint.

Careful, systematic examination of the pelvic canal region per rectum is also indicated to assess the aorta and iliac arteries, psoas musculature, the lumbosacral joint, the caudal aspect of the ilial shaft, and the pubis and ischium.

Pelvic injuries should also be considered when a clinician examines a recumbent horse that has fallen over a fence. Palpation of the pelvic region is even more difficult in these circumstances. Even with a severe fracture, palpating any abnormality may be impossible. The clinician should bear in mind that in the acute phase, local reflexes such as the patellar reflex and the withdrawal reflex may be suppressed, which does not necessarily reflect a spinal cord injury. Major fractures may be associated with rupture of one or more large vessels, resulting in potentially fatal internal hemorrhage. Thus it is important to assess the recumbent horse as a whole, monitoring pulse rate, color of mucous membranes, and capillary refill time. Increased pulse rate and progressive pallor of the mucous membranes are good indicators of major vessel rupture, such as laceration of the iliac artery after fracture of the ilial shaft.

Manipulation of the limb may be resented if pain is associated with the coxofemoral joint, but generally the responses to flexion of the limb, protraction, retraction, and abduction are rather nonspecific. A horse with pain associated with the sacroiliac joints or a coxofemoral joint may be reluctant to stand on one limb, with the other limb raised, and may behave awkwardly in anticipation of discomfort. However, the reaction is nonspecific, and one must bear in mind that some horses present difficulties in picking up the hindlimbs in the absence of any sign of lameness or poor performance. Difficulties in picking up hindlimbs may be caused by reluctance to accentuate weight bearing on the lamest limb, reluctance to flex the lame limb, or may be psychological. If the horse is a shiverer, unilaterally or bilaterally, the response to hindlimb flexion can be difficult to assess.

The degree and character of lameness depend on the underlying cause. Fracture or luxation of the coxofemoral joint results in acute-onset severe lameness. Lameness associated with other lesions in the pelvic region may vary in degree, not only among horses with similar lesions but also within and between examination periods. Pain from the coxofemoral joint frequently results in the horse moving on three tracks, with the nonlame limb being placed between the two forelimbs. On the lunge the horse may be inclined to break to canter rather than move with adequate hindlimb impulsion, but this is not specific for pelvic pain and is typical of many horses with hindlimb lameness. Pain associated with the coxofemoral joint or the greater trochanter of the femur sometimes results in the horse carrying the lame limb in canter. Lesions associated with the sacroiliac joints frequently result in the horse crossing over each hindlimb at the trot (i.e., plaiting), but this is not pathognomonic, and some horses move with a base-wide hindlimb gait.[2] The horse may move with reduced hindlimb impulsion rather than overt lameness. Although acute fractures of the tuber ischium invariably cause lameness, chronic injuries may result in loss of performance (e.g., jumping to the right) rather than overt lameness.

The response to flexion tests is nonspecific. The clinician should bear in mind that increased weight bearing on one limb, caused by flexing the contralateral limb, may accentuate lameness in the weight-bearing limb. Turning the horse in small circles, inducing rotational forces on the coxofemoral joint, may accentuate lameness associated with the coxofemoral joint.

Ridden exercise is invaluable in horses with a history of poor performance, reduced hindlimb impulsion, or low-grade lameness because frequently the lameness or restriction in hindlimb gait is accentuated. This may be most obvious in deep footing. Some horses with sacroiliac joint region pain or lumbosacral region pain show extreme reluctance to go forward freely. Affected horses may feel to the rider much worse than they appear to a trained observer. However, care must be taken to differentiate these horses from those with bilateral hindlimb lameness, thoracolumbar pain, or recurrent low-grade exertional rhabdomyolysis and those performing poorly because of the rider (see Chapter 97), previous poor schooling, or a combination of boredom and an unwilling temperament.

Analgesic Techniques

In horses with chronic lameness, reduced hindlimb impulsion, or poor performance, excluding the distal aspect of the limb as a source of pain by performing perineural analgesia of the fibular and tibial nerves and intraarticular analgesia of the three compartments of the stifle joint may first be necessary. If the response is negative, intraarticular analgesia of the coxofemoral joint may be indicated. This is relatively straightforward to perform if the horse is not well muscled and the greater trochanter of the femur is readily palpable. However, in the majority of heavily muscled, mature competition horses, needle placement must be guided by ultrasonography.[4] Even if the needle is accurately positioned, retrieval of synovial fluid may be difficult. Extraarticular deposition of local anesthetic solution may result in transient paralysis of the obturator nerve and instability of the limb. The technique is described in Chapter 10.

Intraarticular injection of the sacroiliac joint cannot be achieved; however, infiltration of local anesthetic solution around the sacroiliac joint region may result in dramatic clinical improvement, presumably by alleviation of pain associated with the joint and periarticular structures. It cannot be considered an entirely specific technique and potentially could also influence pain from the lumbosacral joint and local nerve roots. The techniques are described on page 589. Infiltration of local anesthetic solution around the sacroiliac joint regions resulted in significant improvement in 95 of 108 horses with clinical signs suggestive of sacroiliac joint pain.[5] Horses were reassessed ridden 15 minutes after injection. If local anesthetic solution is placed too far caudally there is the possibility of inducing sciatic nerve paralysis either unilaterally or bilaterally. In my experience, this is extremely rare (<2%), but if bilateral, the horse will become recumbent and may remain so for up to 3 hours before returning to normality.[5]

Serum Muscle Enzyme Concentration

Measuring serum concentration of creatine kinase (CK) and aspartate transaminase (AST) is invaluable for diagnosing horses with acute and chronic rhabdomyolysis (tying up). In horses with chronic tying up, comparing resting levels with concentrations reached after maximum exercise may be necessary. Peak levels of CK are likely to occur 3 hours after exercise. If a horse has had a tying-up episode within the past 4 or 5 days, AST levels almost invariably will be increased. Some horses with chronic recurrent problems have constantly elevated levels of CK and AST. The degree of elevation of muscle enzyme concentrations may show a poor correlation with the severity of clinical signs.

DIAGNOSTIC IMAGING

Radiography

Radiographic examination of the pelvic region of a horse, anesthetized and positioned in dorsal recumbency or in the standing position, is described in depth elsewhere.[6] Since the advent of nuclear scintigraphy and diagnostic ultrasonography the indications for radiographic examination have decreased. If the source of pain has been localized to the coxofemoral joint, radiographic examination is indicated to determine the nature of the pathological condition and hence prognosis. High-quality radiographs can only be obtained with the horse positioned in dorsal recumbency under general anesthesia. Evaluation of the sacroiliac joints can be difficult because of the superimposition of abdominal viscera. Identification of new bone formation on the caudal aspect of the joint and irregular joint space width are poor prognostic indicators. Nuclear scintigraphic examination gives accurate information about bone turnover, but anatomical detail is less well defined. Therefore radiography of a horse with a suspected acetabular fracture may be indicated at least 6 weeks after the onset of lameness to determine whether a suspected fracture involves the coxofemoral joint, which merits an extremely guarded prognosis for return to full athletic function in a mature horse.

Radiographs of the coxofemoral joint, caudal aspect of the ilial shaft, and the ischium obtained in the standing position may be satisfactory for confirmation of luxation or major fractures of the joint.[6] A dorsal 50° proximal medial–ventrodistal lateral oblique image can be used to assess the integrity of the tubera coxae in a standing horse.[7]

Ultrasonography

Diagnostic ultrasonography of the pelvic region can be performed transcutaneously or per rectum.[8,9] The choice of transducer frequency depends on the structures to be imaged. Transcutaneous evaluation of the bony elements of the pelvis and the deep musculature requires a 5- or 3.5-MHz transducer, depending on the size of the horse, whereas evaluation of the dorsal sacroiliac ligaments, sublumbar musculature, ventral aspect of the lumbar and sacral vertebrae, and aorta and iliac arteries is better performed using a 5- or 10-MHz transducer. Evaluation of nerve roots per rectum may be best achieved using a 10- to 12-MHz transducer.

Diagnostic ultrasonography is useful in evaluating fractures (see Chapter 49, page 564), assessing muscles (see Chapter 83) and the sacroiliac ligaments (see page 578), determining blood vessel patency (see page 581), assessing the lumbar vertebrae and articulations, and evaluating nerve roots.

Nuclear Scintigraphy

Nuclear scintigraphic evaluation of the pelvic region is useful for identifying fractures, stress reactions in bone, increased bone modeling associated with OA and other bony lesions, and evidence of rhabdomyolysis; for evaluating blood flow in the aorta, iliac, and femoral arteries; and for assessing the sacroiliac joints.[10] Sensitivity of the technique in part depends on the angle of the gamma camera to the area of interest and the degree of overlying muscle mass. It is important to recognize that some lesions may be bilateral; therefore recognition of the normal scintigraphic appearance of the region in horses of different ages and different disciplines is important. The clinician should bear in mind that superficial bony structures such as the tubera coxae and tubera sacrale always have apparently greater radiopharmaceutical uptake (RU) than deeper structures. Unilateral muscle atrophy and shape of the pelvis may also confound interpretation.[10-14]

Radioactive urine in the bladder may complicate interpretation; therefore the judicious use of furosemide to induce urination before examination is essential.

Complete evaluation of the pelvic region requires dorsal images of the sacroiliac joints, oblique images of the ilial wings, caudodorsal and caudal images of the tubera ischii, and lateral and caudolateral images of the coxofemoral joints. Care must be taken in interpreting the appearance of the sacroiliac joints because age-related changes occur in normal horses.[10-15] Swaying movement of the horse during image acquisition can result in images that mimic abnormalities, and using motion correction software is invaluable.

DIFFERENTIAL DIAGNOSIS

Fractures

Clinical features, diagnosis, and treatment of fractures of the pelvis in the young Thoroughbred (TB) racehorse have been dealt with in depth (see Chapter 49), and this section focuses on differences in mature athletic horses. The incidence of stress or fatigue fractures of the pelvic region in the mature horse is low, except in horses that race over fences, which have a substantial incidence of ilial stress fractures. The clinical features are similar to those in the young racehorse (see Chapter 49), although there is a higher prevalence of horses with fractures extending into the ilial shaft that have a guarded prognosis. The majority of other fractures result from external trauma.

Tuber Ischium

Trauma to or fractures of the tubera ischii sometimes occur in event horses that fall when jumping up onto a bank, may also occur in any horses as a result of a fall on the flat, and also have been recognized in horses from other disciplines with no known history of trauma.[17-19] Lameness is usually acute in onset and severe. Mild localized swelling is easily overlooked unless the tuber ischium is suspected as a site of injury. The ipsilateral semimembranosus and semitendinosus muscles are usually sore to palpation. Atrophy of the muscles around the tail head often develops within 7 to 10 days. Usually crepitus is not palpable. In horses with chronic lameness, pain on palpation may not be evident, although the tubera ischii may appear asymmetrical, and the lameness may be only mild or moderate.

Diagnosis of a fracture of the tuber ischium can be confirmed using nuclear scintigraphy (Figure 50-1). Dorsal oblique and caudal images are useful. Usually increased radiopharmaceutical uptake (IRU) and an abnormal pattern of uptake are apparent.[16] In some horses determining whether the fracture is complete and whether it has become substantially displaced may be possible. It is important to recognize that IRU may persist for many years after injury, and therefore the results of scintigraphic examination must be carefully correlated with the results of clinical examination.[19] Discontinuity of the bone outline may also be confirmed using diagnostic ultrasonography. Limited radiographic examination can be performed in a standing horse, but it is most easily and safely done with the horse under general anesthesia. Less commonly there is entheseous reaction with IRU in both the tuber ischium and the ipsilateral semimembranosus and/or semitendinosus muscles. Ultrasonographic examination may demonstrate irregularity of the tuber ischium and decreased or increased echogenicity of the injured muscles depending on the acuteness or chronicity of injury.

Treatment by restriction to box rest usually results in a satisfactory outcome, although occasionally sequestration

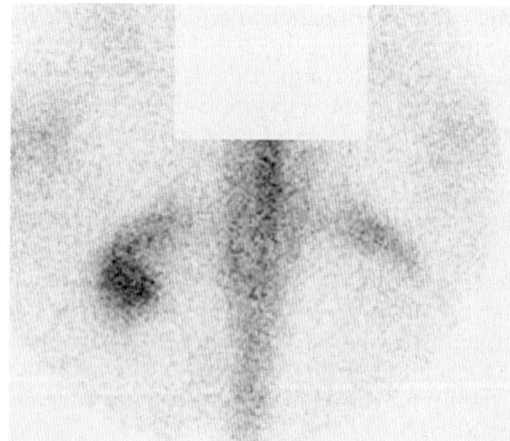

Fig. 50-1 • Caudal scintigraphic image of a 7-year-old part Shire riding horse with acute-onset left hindlimb lameness after falling over while being shod. There was no response to tibial and fibular nerve blocks or to intraarticular analgesia of all three compartments of the stifle joint. There is an abnormal pattern of radiopharmaceutical uptake and increased radiopharmaceutical uptake in the left tuber ischium consistent with a displaced fracture of the tuber ischium, which was confirmed using ultrasonography.

of the fracture fragment occurs, necessitating surgical removal.

Occasionally a horse shows no obvious lameness, but it has reduced performance and a tendency to jump drifting consistently to one side because of pushing off unevenly with each hindlimb. This symptom is associated with reduced muscle development over one of the tubera and IRU in the tuber ischium (see Figure 12-4). The outline of the tuber ischium appears irregular in an ultrasonographic image.

Ilial Wing and/or Shaft

Fractures of the ilial wing and/or shaft are unusual in mature sports horses and are almost invariably the result of a heavy fall when jumping and may be catastrophic if the fracture(s) becomes displaced and results in laceration of the iliac artery and fatal hemorrhage. Initial diagnosis is challenging because the horse is invariably recumbent and may mimic a severely winded horse, which may remain down for 30 to 45 minutes. There may be remarkably few signs of pain considering the severity of injury. If the horse is in lateral recumbency with the affected limb down, the horse may be unable to make any attempt to get up. Examination per rectum may facilitate a diagnosis. In my experience, most of such fractures have been fatal. Monitoring pulse and respiratory rates and color of the mucous membranes is the best method of diagnosing potentially fatal hemorrhage.

Tuber Coxae

Fractures of a tuber coxae in sports and pleasure horses have little difference to those in racehorses (see Chapter 49). The prognosis is usually favorable, with 27 of 29 horses (93%) returning to full athletic function.[7] Horses with partial fractures of the cranial or caudolateral aspects of a tuber coxae returned to use more quickly than horses with complete transverse, longitudinal, or oblique fractures (mean 3 months vs. 6.5 months).

Greater Trochanter of the Femur

Fracture of the greater trochanter of the femur is an unusual injury causing severe lameness. The fracture fragment is often displaced cranially because of the pull of the attachments of the deep and middle gluteal muscles.

Usually no localizing clinical signs are apparent unless the horse is poorly muscled and the greater trochanter is readily palpable. The diagnosis is based on nuclear scintigraphic examination, with or without diagnostic ultrasonography. The prognosis for return to athletic function with conservative treatment is guarded.

Sacrum

Fractures of the sacrum may be complete or incomplete and result in bilateral hindlimb lameness. If the fracture is complete, the contour of the hindquarters when viewed from the side changes, so that the rump has abnormal angulation (Figure 50-2). Associated neurological signs include flaccid paralysis of the tail, reduced sensation around the tail head, urine dribbling in a mare, and loss of anal tone. The onset of neurological signs may be delayed for several weeks after the primary fracture. The fracture may be palpable per rectum. The fracture may be confirmed radiologically and using diagnostic ultrasonography per

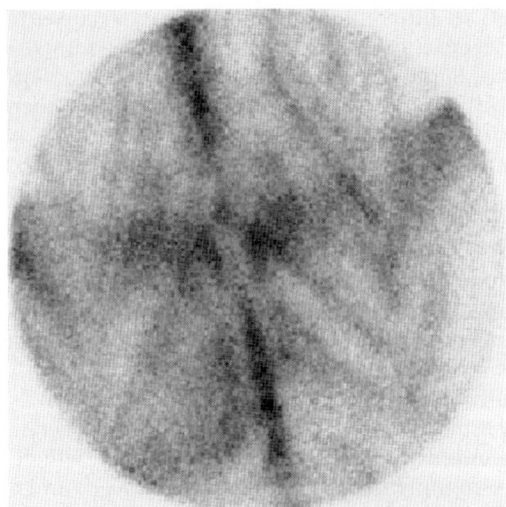

Fig. 50-2 • Dorsal bone phase scintigraphic image of the pelvic region of a 12-year-old Thoroughbred mare, a former winner of the European Three Day Event Championships. The mare had shown slight but clinically significant loss of performance with no overt lameness. She had never shown any signs typical of classical tying up. There are linear stripes of abnormal radiopharmaceutical uptake in the gluteal muscles, which also were seen in the psoas, biceps femoris, and semitendinosus and semimembranosus muscles. This is compatible with recurrent exertional rhabdomyolysis and was associated with persistently elevated levels of creatine kinase and aspartate transaminase.

rectum. The prognosis for return to athletic function is guarded, although horses with more caudal fractures have made a complete functional recovery. Fractures of the femur are considered in Chapter 47.

Equine Rhabdomyolysis (Tying Up)

Equine rhabdomyolysis is considered in depth elsewhere (see Chapter 83). This section focuses on aspects of diagnosis and differential diagnosis of lameness associated with the hindquarters and pelvic injuries in sports horses used for different disciplines and is restricted to recurrent exertional rhabdomyolysis (RER).

The spectrum of clinical signs associated with RER is enormous. A horse may have mild bilateral hindlimb stiffness or loss of freedom of action that may deteriorate slightly with work, without the horse becoming unduly distressed, but the horse sometimes requires a prolonged recovery period after work. Such horses may have no palpable firmness of the hindquarter musculature or pain induced by firm palpation and a normal pattern of sweating. The horse may be able to compete but performs below expectations. These clinical signs are not unique to exertional rhabdomyolysis and may be seen in horses with severe thoracolumbar discomfort associated with impinging dorsal spinous processes, pain associated with the sacroiliac joints, or bilateral hindlimb lameness. Some horses show progressive agitation during ridden exercise and awkwardness to ride, without recognition of a gait abnormality. Careful clinical evaluation usually reveals a progressive shortening of stride.

Alternatively, a horse may start to jump poorly during, for example, the cross-country phase of a Three Day Event and pull up with a unilateral hindlimb lameness, with no localizing clinical signs, that resolves within 24 hours. In contrast, a different horse may have recurrent acute-onset, severe episodes—often provoked by competition, for example, during the cross-country phase of a Three Day Event—that may be so bad as to result in recumbency. An endurance horse may demonstrate unilateral or bilateral hindlimb lameness at the final vet gate but show no typical signs of tying up.

The incidence of RER depends to some extent on the discipline in which the horse is involved, occurring most commonly in racehorses (see Chapters 83, 106, and 107), endurance horses (see Chapter 118), and event horses (see Chapter 117). RER is unusual in show jumpers and dressage horses but occasionally occurs in competitive TB-type ponies. In all these horses, the results of muscle biopsies usually indicate no evidence of abnormal glycogen metabolism as in polysaccharide storage myopathy, which occurs more commonly in draft and draft crossbreeds and Quarter Horses. In the TB, evidence indicates that RER may be a heritable condition, as an autosomal recessive trait with variable expression.[20] A familial trait has also been observed in some part-TB event horses. However, RER in many event and endurance horses does not become apparent until the horse is middle aged, or even older. The condition is manifest more frequently in mares than in stallions or geldings.

Diagnosis is based on measuring elevated serum muscle enzymes (CK and AST) after exercise (see page 573). The degree of muscle enzyme elevation frequently does not correlate with the severity of clinical signs. Interpretation is not always straightforward because asymptomatic endurance horses frequently have extremely high levels of CK and AST during and after a ride. Horses with low-grade RER, which occurs daily, often have constantly elevated levels of CK and AST, even if rested.

Nuclear scintigraphy can be useful in horses with low-grade hindlimb stiffness and poor performance to validate a diagnosis of suspected RER,[10,21] to evaluate blood flow to the hindlimb musculature,[22] and to exclude any other concurrent musculoskeletal lesions. In association with RER in some but not all horses, abnormal uptake of ^{99m}Tc–methylene diphosphonate occurs in the affected muscles in the bone phase of the scan, appearing usually as linear streaking (see Figure 50-2), but in horses with more severe, long-standing RER, affected muscles may show large areas of intense IRU. Lesions are not restricted to the gluteal muscle mass, but they may also affect quadriceps, biceps femoris, semitendinosus, semimembranosus, psoas, and longissimus dorsi muscles. Lesions may be symmetrical or asymmetrical. However, normal RU does not exclude RER.

Muscle biopsy is used to determine whether any evidence exists of polysaccharide storage myopathy. Feeding horses a high-fat and low-carbohydrate diet may reduce the frequency and severity of attacks after a period of 3 to 6 months.[23]

Measuring fractional excretion of electrolytes (sodium, potassium, calcium phosphorus, and chloride) can be useful to identify those horses that seem unable to absorb or to use normally specific dietary electrolytes and that might benefit from dietary supplementation.[24,25] For accurate interpretation of results, it is important that the horse is consuming its normal diet and has recovered from any recent acute attack of exertional rhabdomyolysis when blood and urine samples are collected. A midstream urine sample should be collected, preferably freely voided rather

than by catheterization. Results are only valid if serum creatinine is within the normal range and the fractional excretion of creatinine is normal. Results should be compared with the normal ranges for a horse on a similar diet because results for horses eating an oat- and hay-based diet are different than for those on a cube-based diet or a diet high in alfalfa. Fractional excretion ratios for potassium tend to be high if the horse is allowed access to pasture. Low values for fractional excretion ratios for sodium or calcium indicate that the diet should be supplemented with sodium chloride or either calcium carbonate or calcium gluconate, respectively. Appropriate dietary supplementation may help to prevent further attacks.

Management practices may also help to prevent attacks in some horses. These include daily work, with a long, slow warm-up period, turnout as much as possible, and avoiding undue stress, especially in highly strung, nervous individuals. However, some horses, especially those with daily low-grade clinical signs that are not stress provoked, prove intractable to successful management.

Muscle Injury

Muscle soreness is frequently unassociated with any recognizable histopathological changes within the muscle and is often secondary to some other cause of lameness because of the altered way in which the horse is moving. Muscle soreness can often be induced by overuse of an under-trained muscle and can result in localized soreness and stiffness for several days. Focal intense muscle spasm and pain can cause sudden-onset reduction in performance and, if primary, are usually alleviated by manipulation to relieve the muscle spasm, producing rapid amelioration of clinical signs.

Focal muscle soreness associated with localized swelling may be caused by intramuscular hemorrhage, muscle fiber tearing, or exertional rhabdomyolysis. Diagnosis of the cause may be determined by measuring serum muscle enzyme concentrations and by ultrasonographic evaluation (Figure 50-3). Hemorrhage results in an area of diffuse

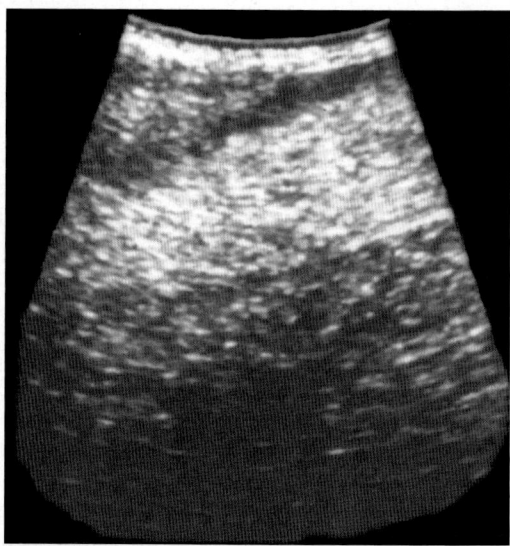

Fig. 50-3 • Ultrasonographic image of the semimembranosus muscle of a 6-year-old Thoroughbred with acute-onset, severe left hindlimb lameness. The horse had palpable enlargement of the muscle and localized soreness. The increased echogenicity reflects hemorrhage.

increase in echogenicity within the muscle. This should be differentiated from hyperechogenic regions that result from chronic muscle fibrosis. Serum muscle enzyme concentrations are usually not elevated in those horses with hemorrhage, muscle fiber tearing, or fibrosis.

Damage to deep muscles of the hindquarters is difficult to identify because localizing clinical signs are frequently not apparent to alert the clinician to the possible site of damage. Thermographic evaluation can be useful to help identify superficial muscle injury.

Some horses with reduced performance have pain on palpation of the psoas muscles per rectum. Pain may be primary or secondary to pathological conditions of the lumbosacral or sacroiliac regions and is an indication for nuclear scintigraphic evaluation of the pelvic region and ultrasonographic examination of the lumbosacral vertebrae.

Sacroiliac Joint Injury

See Chapter 51 for further discussion of sacroiliac joint injury. Detailed anatomy of the sacroiliac joints is discussed elsewhere (see page 583).

The diagnosis of sacroiliac joint disease has tended historically to be a dustbin diagnosis, frequently made by exclusion when the clinical signs could not be explained by any other condition. The high incidence of pathological degenerative lesions found in the sacroiliac joints of TB racehorses[26] and in mixed-breed horses[27] indicates that degenerative disease of the sacroiliac joint is likely to be a clinically significant problem, but definitive diagnosis remains difficult. In a study of 74 horses with sacroiliac joint pain, affected horses were older than the normal clinic population, and there was a high proportion of Warmblood horses.[2] Horses used for dressage or show jumping predominated. Affected horses were also of great body weight and height. However, the condition is seen in horses used for all sports disciplines and has been recognized in competition ponies.

I recognize six clinical manifestations of sacroiliac joint region pain[5]: an acute onset of unwillingness to go forward when ridden; sudden onset of bucking and kicking out with one or both hindlimbs when ridden; insidious onset of reduced hindlimb impulsion and engagement; sacroiliac joint region pain in association with primary thoracolumbar region pain; unilateral or bilateral hindlimb lameness and secondary sacroiliac joint region pain; and sacroiliac region pain secondary to a previous ilial stress fracture.

Pathological changes of the sacroiliac joint include lipping, cortical buttressing, and osteophyte formation, together with enlargement of the joint surfaces. These signs are thought to be a response to chronic instability of the joints, although no evidence of ligamentous laxity has been identified.[27,28] Erosion of the articular cartilage may also occur, but joint ankylosis has not been documented. A positive association has been recognized between the severity of the impingement of thoracolumbar dorsal spinous processes and lumbar transverse processes and the severity of sacroiliac lesions and also between the severity of articular process degeneration and the degree of pathological conditions of the sacroiliac region.

A separate entity of enthesophyte formation at the site of attachment of the sacroiliac ligaments has been described unassociated with pathological conditions of the sacroiliac

joints.[29] The clinical significance of this finding has not been well defined.

Subluxation of the sacroiliac joint is comparatively rare[29,30] and results from acute, traumatic disruption of the dorsal sacroiliac ligament and the sacroiliac joint capsule. Subluxation should be differentiated from an acute ilial wing fracture resulting in depression of the ipsilateral tuber sacrale (see pages 564 and 567).

The prominence of the tubera sacrale and lumbar dorsal spinous processes varies between horses and in part reflects the conformation of the back and hindlimbs and the fitness of the horse. They may appear extremely prominent in a lean, fit event or endurance horse; however, this would be unusual in a normal dressage or show jumping horse. However, abnormal prominence could also result from poor development of the epaxial muscles in the lumbar region caused by the horse not using its back and hindlimbs properly. Poor muscle development may be a reflection of pain or of the horse's previous training: if the horse has never been asked to engage the hindlimbs properly and work through its back, these muscles will not be well developed.

Many apparently clinically normal horses have some degree of asymmetry of the height and/or shape of each tuber sacrale and the overlying soft tissues. Careful clinical appraisal of a small proportion of these horses may reveal subtle hindlimb gait abnormalities and mild discomfort induced by pressure applied over the tubera sacrale or by picking up one hindlimb and swaying the horse on the other. These findings are more likely to be detected in horses that are not fully fit and are often ameliorated when the horse is fitter and has greater muscle support. They may reflect mild instability of the sacroiliac joints but are not necessarily synonymous with degenerative change. Mild secondary sacroiliac joint region pain is often seen in association with hindlimb proximal suspensory desmitis.

Pain associated with the sacroiliac joints may be present despite symmetry of the tubera sacrale, is usually a bilateral condition, and is rarely associated with unilateral hindlimb lameness.[2] Pain often manifests as reduced performance, failure properly to engage the hindlimbs, and back stiffness. Signs are often greatly accentuated when the horse is ridden. In horses with mild clinical signs, the loss of hindlimb power and lack of suppleness through the horse's back may be much easier for the rider to feel than for an observer to appreciate. The rider may feel that he or she is being thrown forward in trot. Gait irregularities may be most apparent as the horse changes direction through a tight circle. Specific lateral movements such as half pass or sequence flying changes may be difficult. The quality of the canter is often worse than the trot. The horse may become progressively more unwilling to work under saddle and start to resist.

A comprehensive clinical evaluation is essential to preclude other conditions that may present similarly, such as bilateral distal hock joint pain. Precluding the hindlimbs as a potential source of pain by performing perineural analgesia of the tibial and fibular nerves and intraarticular anesthesia of the femorotibial and femoropatellar joints of one hindlimb may be necessary to see whether lameness becomes apparent in the contralateral limb.

Using a 15-cm needle inserted on the midline at the lumbosacral space and directed approximately 20 degrees caudally, local anesthetic solution (up to 20 mL/side) can be infiltrated in the direction of the sacroiliac joints (see page 589). This may improve clinical signs in some horses and resulted in clinically significant change in 95 of 108 horses with suspected sacroiliac pain in which local analgesia was performed.[5] However, false-negative results do occur.

Nuclear scintigraphic examination may facilitate diagnosis by helping to preclude the presence of other clinically significant causes of poor hindlimb action and by giving a positive indication of abnormalities of the sacroiliac joints.[10-15,31,32] Profile analysis and quantitative evaluation using regions of interest are required for accurate diagnosis. The results ideally should be compared with horses of similar age and work history because of apparent significant age-related variability between clinically normal horses.[11] Considerable overlap in ratios of RU between each sacroiliac joint region and a standard reference site also occurs in clinically normal horses, horses with lameness unrelated to the sacroiliac joint, and horses with clinical signs compatible with sacroiliac joint disease.[32] However, RU is bilaterally symmetrical in a normal horse. Excessive motion during image acquisition can result in images that are not of diagnostic quality and may mimic abnormalities; therefore images ideally should be acquired dynamically, and motion correction software should be used.[11] Residual radiopharmaceutical in the bladder may also confound interpretation. Abnormalities are recognized as abnormal patterns of RU (Figure 50-4) and asymmetrical ratios of RU between the left and right sacroiliac joint regions.[28] Care must be taken to differentiate between uptake in the tubera sacrale and uptake associated with the region of the sacroiliac joints.

Radiographic examination requires general anesthesia and can be frustrating because superimposition of abdominal viscera can preclude evaluation of the sacroiliac

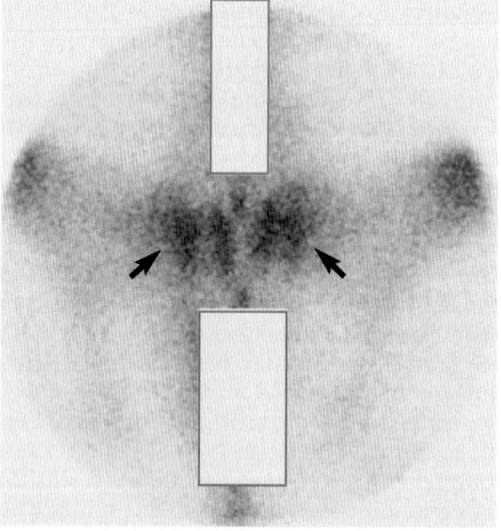

Fig. 50-4 • Dorsal delayed (bone) phase scintigraphic image of a 9-year-old Warmblood dressage horse with clinical signs compatible with chronic sacroiliac joint disease. The horse's performance was markedly improved by periarticular infiltration of local anesthetic solution around the sacroiliac joints. There is increased radiopharmaceutical uptake in the region of both the left and right sacroiliac joints. The horse failed to respond to treatment, and a diagnosis of osteoarthritis of the sacroiliac joints was confirmed post mortem.

joints.[6,33] However, detection of joint space irregularities and spur formation on the caudal aspect of the joints are poor prognostic indicators.

Ultrasonographic examination should be performed transcutaneously to evaluate the dorsal sacroiliac ligaments[8,9,34,35] and per rectum[2,8] to assess the sacroiliac joints and to eliminate as potential diagnoses pathological conditions of the lumbosacral vertebrae. Irregularities of the caudal aspect of the sacroiliac joint may be identified.

Management is essentially palliative, and prognosis is generally inversely correlated with the severity of clinical signs. Local infiltration[33] of a phenol-based sclerosing agent, P2G (phenol, glucose, glycerin), or a combination of corticosteroids (methylprednisolone acetate, 200 mg) and Sarapin (High Chemical Company, Levittown, Pennsylvania, United States) appears to provide relief in some horses. Some horses benefit from treatment with nonsteroidal antiinflammatory drugs (NSAIDs), which provide partial pain relief, enabling the horse to work better and develop increased muscle strength. Daily work on the lunge using side reins, a Pessoa or a chambon, together with exercise in a cage horse walker in which the horse is free and not tied, and no ridden exercise for several weeks may be of substantial benefit. Acupuncture therapy helps some horses. Affected horses should be maintained in work at all times to maintain muscular fitness. Horses with acute problems respond best.

Sacroiliac joint disease may occur with other conditions; therefore careful appraisal of the whole horse is essential if a successful management strategy is to be achieved.[2,5] Nuclear scintigraphic evaluation should include the thoracolumbar region. Concurrent impingement of dorsal spinous processes in the midthoracic, caudal thoracic, or cranial lumbar regions may occur with or without associated pain (see page 598). Infiltration of local anesthetic solution between or around the impinging dorsal spinous processes may be necessary to determine their contribution to the clinical problem. Careful evaluation of the synovial intervertebral articulations, especially close to the thoracolumbar junction, is also important. Occasionally sacroiliac disease has been seen together with OA of the coxofemoral joints. This warrants a guarded prognosis.

Desmitis of the Dorsal Sacroiliac Ligament

Desmitis of the dorsal sacroiliac ligament has been recognized in horses that have back pain, with or without focal pain on palpation.[31,32] Usually lesions have been restricted to one side and have been characterized by ultrasonography as enlargements of the ligament and disruption of normal architecture, with hypoechoic regions in transverse images and loss of parallel alignment of echoes in longitudinal images. Enthesophyte formation may occur on the tuber sacrale. Such lesions have been seen alone or with other causes of back pain.

New Bone on the Caudal Aspect of the Wing of the Sacrum

A few mature competition horses used for dressage or show jumping have insidious onset loss of hindlimb action, progressing to unwillingness to maintain a proper trot. These horses have appeared considerably worse when ridden compared with evaluation in hand or on the lunge. The horses have shown abnormal sensitivity to palpation in the

Video available at
www.rossanddyson.com
Chapter 50 **Lumbosacral and Pelvic Injuries** 579

general areas of the sacroiliac joints. However, careful analysis of nuclear scintigraphic images has shown relatively normal radiopharmaceutical uptake in the region of the joints themselves but increased uptake abaxial to the joints. The horses have responded poorly to treatment with NSAIDs or other analgesic drugs. Post mortem examination has revealed spurs of new bone on the wings of the sacrum just caudal to the auricular surface but not involving the sacroiliac joint itself.[26,27] This has been seen in association with fusion of the transverse processes of caudal lumbar vertebrae and osseous proliferation involving intervertebral foramina or synovial articulations.

Lumbosacral Joint

The clinical signs referable to lumbosacral pathology are difficult to differentiate from those associated with sacroiliac joint region pain and lesions in the thoracolumbar region. Moreover, lumbosacral pathology may coexist with sacroiliac or thoracolumbar lesions; therefore systematic radiographic, scintigraphic, and ultrasonographic evaluation of all areas should be performed. Lesions of the lumbosacral joint may be present in asymptomatic horses[26]; thus determination of the potential clinical significance of abnormalities is not always easy. Radiographic examination of the lumbosacral joint is only possible with the horse in dorsal recumbency under general anesthesia. Lesions of the intertransverse joints are not uncommon, but their clinical significance is unclear. Nuclear scintigraphy is not particularly sensitive for detection of lesions of the lumbosacral joint largely because of the large overlying muscle mass resulting in shielding.

The lumbosacral joint and the intertransverse joints are evaluated ultrasonographically per rectum (Figure 50-5). The transrectal ultrasonographic appearance of the lumbosacral joint was assessed in 43 horses with no history or clinical evidence of back pain or hindlimb lameness.[36] In

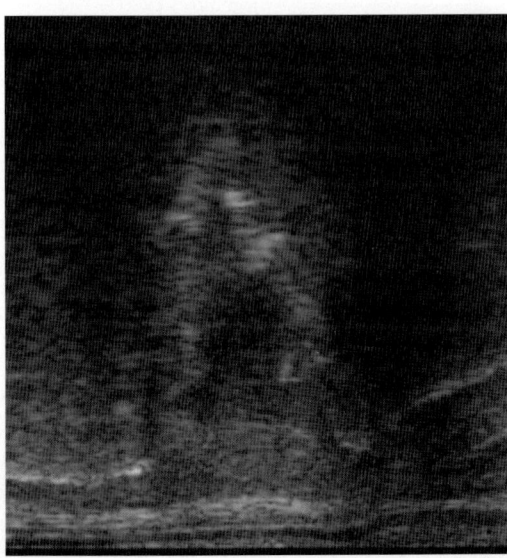

Fig. 50-5 • Ultrasonographic image of the lumbosacral joint of a 10-year-old show jumper with a history of loss of performance. Dorsal is to the top and cranial to the right. The margins of the lumbosacral joint are poorly defined, and there is a large area of reduced echogenicity within the intervertebral disk. There are also focal hyperechogenic foci. This is consistent with intervertebral disk degeneration.

the majority of horses (34/43, 79.1%) the lumbosacral disk had uniform or mildly heterogeneous echogenicity. Variations included hyperechogenic regions within the lumbosacral disk with or without an acoustic shadow, and mild or moderate irregularity of the opposing surfaces of the last lumbar and the first sacral vertebral bodies. Marked irregularity of the bony surfaces or marked disruption of the lumbosacral disk was not seen in any horse. The mean distance between the ventral aspects of the last lumbar and first sacral vertebrae was 14.2 mm (range: 7.1 to 26.5 mm). The degree of protrusion of the ventral aspect of the lumbosacral disk ranged from 0 to 5 mm (mean: 1.32 mm). The mean angle between the ventral surfaces of the last lumbar and first sacral vertebrae was 147 degrees (range: 118 to 165 degrees). There was no significant effect of the age, breed, gender, or size of the horses on either subjective findings in the lumbosacral joint or objective measurements.

Abnormalities that may be of clinical significance include:

1. Congenital lumbosacral ankylosis with reduced size or absence of the intervertebral disk
2. Focal loss of echogenicity of the intervertebral disk consistent with disk degeneration
3. Large focal hyperechogenic regions in the intervertebral disk consistent with dystrophic mineralization
4. Ventral herniation of the intervertebral disk
5. Ventral subluxation of the sacrum
6. Osseous irregularities of the intertransverse articulation(s)

Lesions of the lumbosacral joint are treated by deep paramedian injection[3,35,37,38] of corticosteroids with Sarapin (High Chemical Company) or local anesthetic solution under ultrasound guidance. The needle is inserted 4 cm from the median plane on a line connecting the cranial aspects of the tubera coxae. The needle is directed obliquely caudally and is inserted under the ilial wing until contact is made with bone in the vicinity of the axial aspect of the lumbosacral intertransverse joint. This is repeated on the left and right sides. Success of treatment is highly variable, but is often transient. Modification of the work program as discussed in Chapter 52 (see page 605) is also important.

Aortoiliacofemoral Thrombosis

Aortoiliacofemoral thrombosis is a relatively uncommon cause of exercise-induced hindlimb lameness of variable severity.[39] Clinical signs may be sudden and severe in onset or subtle initially and slowly progressive. Horses of all ages may be affected. The incidence is higher in male horses than mares. The pathogenesis is unknown.

Clinical signs vary depending on the site(s) of thrombus formation, its size, and the degree of vessel occlusion. Lesions occur most commonly at the terminal aspect of the aorta, but they may also involve the internal and external iliac arteries and the femoral arteries, unilaterally or bilaterally. Lesions restricted to the femoral artery have not been documented. With mild lesions, the horse may show poor performance, early fatigue, or slight loss of hindlimb action during a work period. If the lesion(s) is predominantly unilateral, the horse may show episodic hindlimb lameness induced by work. With more advanced lesions, progressive shortening of hindlimb stride may occur with exercise,

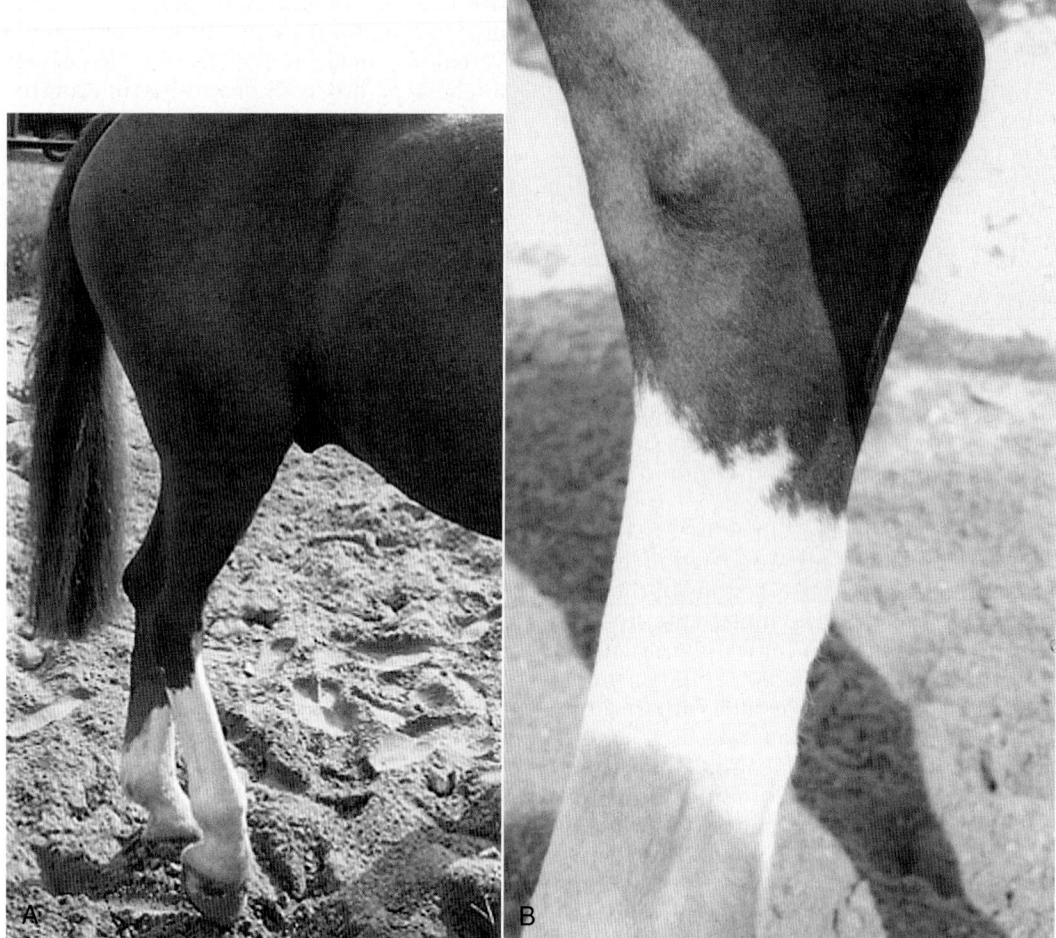

Fig. 50-6 • A 9-year-old gelding with aortoiliac thrombosis. Clinical signs were provoked by just 5 minutes of lunging exercise. **A,** The horse repeatedly flexed each hindlimb, stamping it to the ground. No evidence of sweating over the hindquarters was apparent, but the horse was sweating profusely over the neck and flanks. **B,** The saphenous vein cannot be seen because of delayed filling.

followed by development of distress and sweating, except over the hindlimbs (Figure 50-6, *A*). If the horse is allowed to stop, it may repeatedly flex its hindlimbs and stamp the feet to the ground. The affected limbs feel cool, and delayed filling of the saphenous veins may be seen (see Figure 50-6, *B*), with reduced pulse amplitudes in the dorsal metatarsal artery. Clinical signs usually resolve if the horse is allowed to stand still for a few minutes.

In horses with advanced thromboembolism, it is usually possible to palpate a thrombus per rectum in the terminal aspect of the aorta, which feels abnormally firm. Pulses in the iliac arteries may be reduced or absent. With less advanced lesions, diagnostic ultrasonography is required for identification of the lesion (Figure 50-7). Ultrasonography is also useful to determine the extent of the lesions.[40] Examination of part of the femoral artery can be performed transcutaneously on the medial aspect of the crus,[3,41] and the use of Doppler ultrasonography to measure blood flow characteristics should help to determine whether a more proximal site of obstruction exists.[40,42]

First-pass radionuclide angiography can be used to determine blood flow in the aorta and iliac arteries[22,43] and also the femoral arteries. However, the sensitivity of the technique for detecting subtle lesions has yet to be determined.

The aims of treatment are to try to prevent further thrombus formation and to promote the development of a collateral blood supply for adequate perfusion. No drugs are available that alter a preformed thrombus. Treatment rationale has been based on pain relief and the use of antiinflammatory drugs, platelet inhibitors, anthelmintics, fibrinolytic agents, and anticoagulant drugs. Those most commonly used include phenylbutazone (2.2 mg/kg twice daily for 2 months), aspirin (5 mg/kg daily for several months), and isoxsuprine (1 mg/kg twice daily for 3 months). Successful treatment presumably is based on development of an effective collateral blood supply.

I have successfully managed some mildly affected horses with long-term aspirin therapy, but horses with more severe lesions are usually refractory to treatment. Only two of 29 horses returned to former athletic function, with resolution of clinical signs, following medical treatment.[38] Surgical removal is feasible,[44,45] although the rate of complications is high. Surgery was successful in 53% of 17 horses, but four horses had postoperative myopathy, two of which were humanely destroyed, and a fifth horse sustained a fatal femoral fracture during recovery from anesthesia.[45] Reocclusion of the treated vessels may occur.

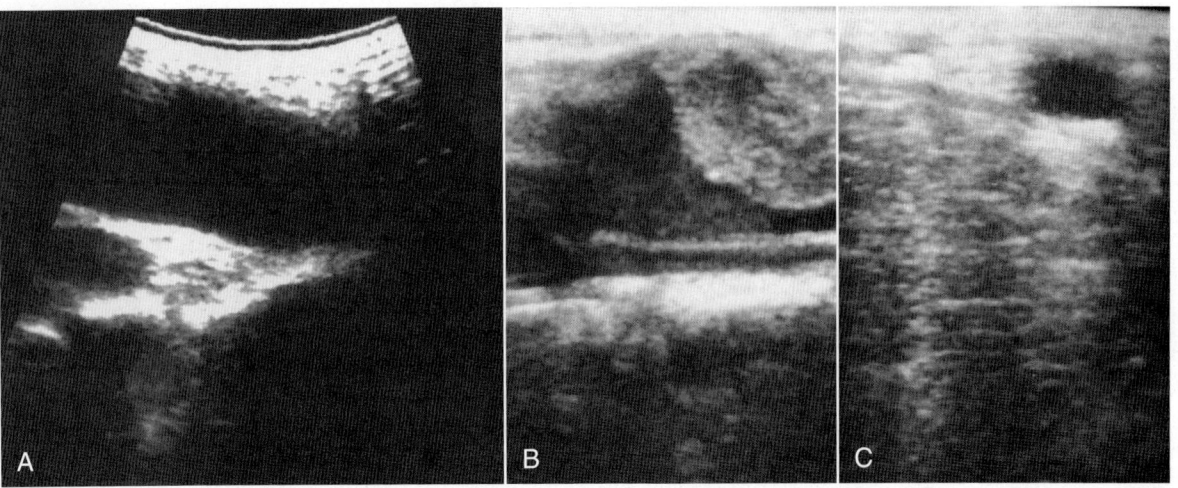

Fig. 50-7 • Longitudinal ultrasonographic images of the terminal aorta of a normal horse **(A)** and a horse with aortoiliac thrombosis **(B)**. Cranial is to the left. There is a large echogenic mass in the aorta of the clinically affected horse. **C,** Transverse ultrasonographic image of the right external iliac artery. This appears normal, but an extensive thrombus was identified farther distally at post mortem examination.

Coxofemoral Joint

The coxofemoral joint is rarely a source of pain causing lameness in the horse.

Dysplasia

Dysplasia of the coxofemoral joint is rare, usually occurs bilaterally, and predisposes relatively young horses to develop OA. The prognosis for athletic function is poor. Dysplasia may be a heritable condition in the Norwegian Dole.

Osseous Cystlike Lesions

An osseous cystlike lesion occasionally has been identified in young horses and associated with lameness.[46] The lesions have resulted in chronic lameness.

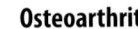

Osteoarthritis

OA of the coxofemoral joint is an unusual cause of hindlimb lameness in the horse, usually occurring unilaterally but occasionally bilaterally. OA may occur secondary to dysplasia, rupture of the teres ligament (see page 582), or trauma.

Lameness varies from moderate to severe. The horse resents flexion of the limb and is unwilling to stand on the limb for long periods with the contralateral limb picked up. The degree of gluteal muscle disuse atrophy may be more than that from pain in the more distal part of the limb. Lameness may be characterized by a tendency for the horse to move on three tracks.

Intraarticular analgesia usually, but not always, improves lameness, but it is rarely alleviated fully.

Nuclear scintigraphic evaluation may help in highlighting the coxofemoral joint as abnormal, especially if the results of intraarticular analgesia are equivocal. However, it is important to be aware that loss of muscle over the hindquarter of the lame limb may confound image interpretation. I have found it useful to evaluate ratios of RU in the region of the coxofemoral joint and another standardized location and compare this with values for normal horses. Caudal oblique images can be helpful. The clinician should be aware that RU associated with a normal coxofemoral joint is much less than that of the cranial and caudal parts of the greater trochanter of the femur.

Definitive diagnosis of OA requires radiographic examination, and high-quality radiographs can only be achieved with the horse in dorsal recumbency under general anesthesia. Abnormalities include periarticular osteophyte formation, new bone formation along the femoral neck, lucent zones in the subchondral bone of the acetabulum or femoral head, and loss of congruity between the acetabulum and femoral head (Figure 50-8). Care should be taken not to confuse the depression in the femoral head and underlying radiolucent zone at the site of insertion of the teres ligament as a lesion.

Intraarticular medication of a coxofemoral joint with radiological abnormalities has yielded disappointing results. The prognosis for return to athletic function is guarded.

Trochanteric Bursitis

Trochanteric bursitis has been described in the older literature, but the Editors have not recognized this condition. The condition is discussed elsewhere (page 552).

Luxation with or without Secondary Upward Fixation of the Patella

Luxation or subluxation of the coxofemoral joint is an unusual injury and can occur as a primary injury or secondary to an unstable fracture of the ilial shaft. The trauma causing luxation also can result in articular fractures of the acetabulum. Permanent upward fixation of the patella may develop as a sequela because of displacement of the femur. The femur is displaced proximally; therefore the greater trochanter of the femur appears higher on the lame limb. However, this can be difficult to assess because the horse is usually reluctant to bear weight on the limb. Upward fixation of the patella results in an abnormally straight hindlimb stance and an inability to flex the limb. The diagnosis can be confirmed radiologically, and with high-output x-ray machines, diagnostic radiographs can be obtained with the horse standing; however, determining whether concurrent

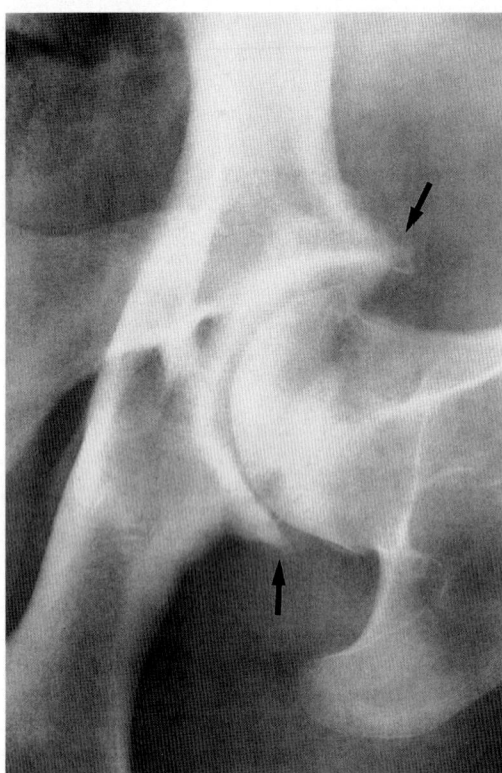

Fig. 50-8 • Ventrodorsal radiographic image of the left coxofemoral joint of a 9-year-old steeplechaser with osteoarthritis. The horse had raced successfully the previous season, but it now showed moderate left hindlimb lameness at trot and carried the left hindlimb at canter. Note the marked periarticular osteophyte formation on the pelvic acetabulum *(arrows)* and the irregular subchondral bone opacity.

fractures exist may be difficult. Ultrasonography can also be used to verify the presence of subluxation.[47] The prognosis for athletic function is hopeless.

Rupture of the Teres Ligament

Rupture of the teres ligament results from trauma. It has been seen in a horse that tried to get up prematurely from general anesthesia while the limbs were still restrained in hobbles, and in other circumstances in which a hindlimb has become trapped. Lameness is severe, with the horse being unwilling to bear weight on the limb. Secondary OA rapidly ensues. Definitive diagnosis is only possible post mortem. The prognosis for athletic function is hopeless.

Displacement of the Femoral Head

Displacement of the femoral head has been seen occasionally in young horses with severe lameness and reluctance to bear weight on the limb. Diagnosis is confirmed radiologically. The prognosis is hopeless.

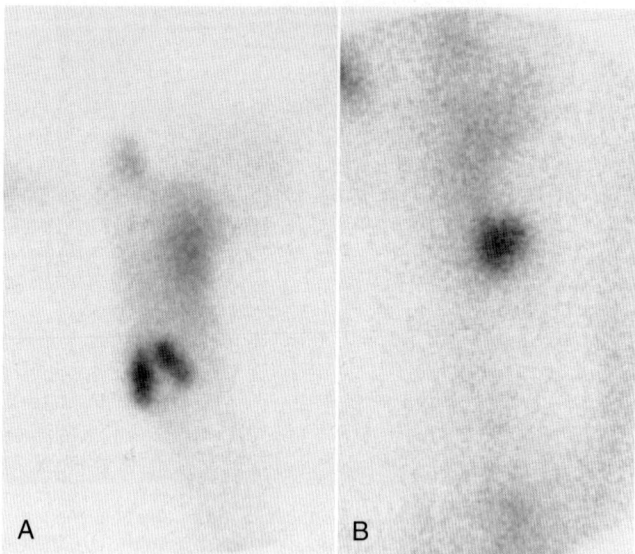

Fig. 50-9 • Lateral **(A)** and caudal **(B)** scintigraphic images of the right femur of a 7-year-old Warmblood dressage horse with sudden onset of severe right hindlimb lameness. In the lateral image **(A),** there are two areas of focal intense increased radiopharmaceutical uptake (IRU) in the region of the third trochanter of the femur; IRU is seen within the third trochanter in the caudal image. This is consistent with a fracture of the third trochanter of the femur.

Fracture (or Enthesopathy) of the Third Trochanter of the Femur

Fracture of the third trochanter of the femur is a relatively unusual injury, resulting in acute-onset severe lameness that often improves rapidly with box rest. In a lean, poorly muscled horse, eliciting pain by palpation may be possible, but in a well-muscled Warmblood type, eliciting pain is usually not possible, even in acute injuries. No particular gait characteristics are apparent. Nuclear scintigraphy is particularly valuable for tentative diagnosis of a fracture[10,16] characterized by IRU (Figure 50-9) and sometimes a change in the pattern of uptake. Diagnosis may be confirmed radiologically, but good-quality radiographs in large horses can only be achieved under general anesthesia. Oblique radiographic images can be acquired standing in small horses. Fractures are often longitudinal, occurring at the base of the trochanter, but horizontal fractures have been seen.[6,16] Displacement is usually minimal. Diagnostic ultrasonography is sometimes useful to confirm a fracture and to exclude abnormalities of the superficial gluteal muscle, which inserts on the third trochanter. Insertional tears of this muscle may be associated with a similar scintigraphic appearance. Treatment is box rest for 2 months, followed by walking exercise for another month. Healing may occur by osseous or fibrous union. Prognosis is good.

Chapter 51

Diagnosis and Management of Sacroiliac Joint Injuries

Kevin K. Haussler

ANATOMICAL AND FUNCTIONAL FEATURES

The sacroiliac joint is a synovial articulation located at the junction between the ventral aspect of the wing of the ilium and the dorsal aspect of the wing of the sacrum (Figure 51-1). The sacroiliac joint functions in pelvic attachment to the axial skeleton, providing support during weight bearing and helping to transfer propulsive forces of the hindlimb to the vertebral column. The sacroiliac joint is an atypical synovial articulation because of hyaline cartilage on the sacral articular surface and a thin layer of fibrocartilage on the ilial articular surface.[1] The articular surfaces of the sacroiliac joint are nearly flat and closely apposed to support gliding movements. The sacroiliac articular surfaces diverge cranially at about 40 degrees from a transverse plane and are angled craniodorsally to caudoventrally at about 60 degrees from the horizontal plane. The joint capsule is thin and closely follows the margins of the sacroiliac articular cartilage. The sacroiliac joint capsule is reinforced ventrally by the ventral sacroiliac ligament.[2] A small amount (<1 mL) of synovial fluid is normally present in the joint.[1] Because of articular surface remodeling, the size and shape of the sacroiliac joint margins vary considerably according to age and body weight.[3] Typically the sacroiliac joint outline is L-shaped, with the convex border directed caudoventrally.

The pelvis is firmly attached to the axial skeleton by sacroiliac and sacrosciatic ligaments, which form a strong ligamentous sling (see Figure 51-1). The weight of the caudal aspect of the vertebral column is suspended from the sacroiliac ligaments, which function similarly to the fibromuscular sling found between the proximal aspect of the forelimb and the lateral thoracic body wall. Subsequently the sacroiliac articular cartilage may never be fully weight bearing, unlike most articular cartilage. The sacroiliac joint is supported by three pairs of strong ligaments: the dorsal, interosseous, and ventral sacroiliac ligaments. The dorsal sacroiliac ligament consists of dorsal and lateral portions (Figure 51-2). The dorsal portions form two round cords that span from the dorsal aspects of the tubera sacrale to the dorsal apices of the sacral spinous processes. The lateral portion forms a sheet of connective tissue that spans from the caudal margin of each tuber sacrale and iliac wing to the lateral border of the sacrum. The lateral portion of the sacroiliac ligament is continuous ventrally with the sacrosciatic ligament. The interosseous ligament of the sacroiliac joint is robust and consists of a series of vertical fibers that connect the ventral aspect of the wing of the ilium to the dorsal aspect of the wing of the sacrum (see Figure 51-1). The interosseous sacroiliac ligament provides the major resistance to vertically oriented weight-bearing forces acting on the sacrum. The ventral sacroiliac ligament interconnects the ventral aspects of the wings of the ilium and sacrum. The ventral sacroiliac ligament is thin and closely applied to the ventral margins of the sacroiliac joint capsule.

Neurovascular structures adjacent to the sacroiliac joint include the sciatic nerve, cranial gluteal nerve, and cranial gluteal artery and vein. These structures collectively travel through the greater sciatic foramen, ventromedial to the sacroiliac articulation (see Figure 51-2). The cranial gluteal artery and vein arise from the internal iliac vessels and travel over the ventral sacroiliac ligament and the caudomedial aspect of the sacroiliac joint before emerging at the greater sciatic foramen. The cranial gluteal artery and vein

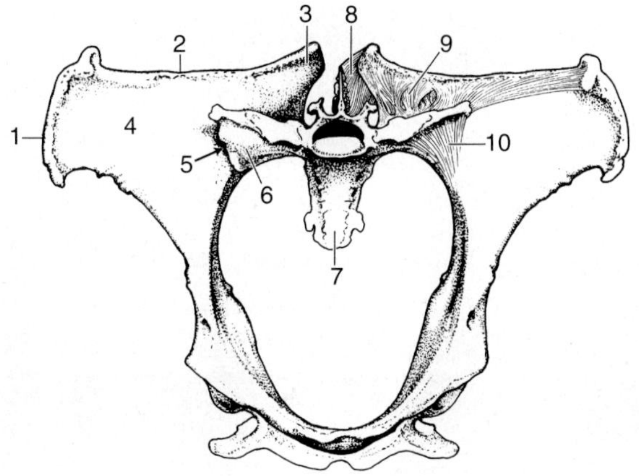

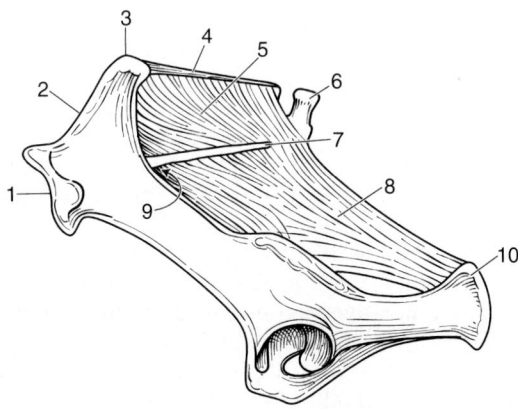

Figure 51-1 • Diagram of the pelvis, sacrum, and sacroiliac ligaments (cranial view). *1,* Tuber coxae; *2,* ilial crest; *3,* tuber sacrale; *4,* ventral surface of the ilial wing; *5,* sacroiliac articulation; *6,* sacral wing; *7,* sacrum; *8,* dorsal sacroiliac ligament; *9,* interosseous sacroiliac ligament; *10,* ventral sacroiliac ligament. (Modified from Dyce KM, Sack WO, Wensing CJG: *Textbook of veterinary anatomy,* ed 2, Philadelphia, 1996, Saunders.)

Figure 51-2 • Diagram of the pelvis, sacrum, and sacroiliac ligaments (lateral view). *1,* Tuber coxae; *2,* ilial crest; *3,* tuber sacrale; *4,* dorsal sacroiliac ligament (dorsal portion); *5,* dorsal sacroiliac ligament (lateral portion); *6,* first coccygeal vertebrae; *7,* lateral portion of sacrum; *8,* sacrosciatic ligament; *9,* greater sciatic foramen; *10,* ischial tuberosity.

continue dorsally into the gluteal musculature. The middle and accessory gluteal muscles originate from the dorsal aspect of the ilial wing and have attachments near the caudomedial aspect of the sacroiliac joint. Within the pelvic canal, a portion of the internal obturator and iliacus muscles covers the ventral sacroiliac joint margins.

The robust sacroiliac and sacrosciatic ligaments limit motion at the sacroiliac articulations.[4] Shear forces would be expected at the sacroiliac articular surfaces more than compressive forces, which are common in most limb articulations.[5] Sacroiliac joint movements are restricted to small amounts of approximately 1 degree during flexion (nutation) and extension (counternutation), with an apparent axis of rotation oriented transversely near the caudomedial aspect of the joint.[6,7] As a result of coupled sacroiliac joint motion of flexion-extension, lateral bending, and axial rotation combined with concurrent pelvic deformation, motion at the sacroiliac joints is complex.[8] Lateral movements at the sacroiliac articulations are severely restricted, primarily because of lateral attachments of the ventral sacroiliac ligaments and, to a lesser degree, the lateral portion of the dorsal sacroiliac ligaments and the sacrosciatic ligaments. The wings of the ilium overlay the sacral articular surfaces dorsally and laterally, which precludes any axial rotation from occurring at the sacroiliac joint. Dorsal displacement of the ilial wings is limited by the robust interosseous ligament, the ventral sacroiliac ligament, and lateral portion of the dorsal sacroiliac ligaments.[9] Propulsive forces of the hindlimb are transmitted dorsally and cranially to the vertebral column by the articular configuration of the overlapping and divergent ilial wings over the sacrum and by reinforcement from the dorsal and interosseous sacroiliac ligaments. The dorsal sacroiliac ligament also provides resistance against contraction of the powerful longissimus muscle and robust thoracolumbar fascia, which attach along the cranial border of the ilial wing.

PATHOLOGICAL CONDITIONS

The antemortem diagnosis of sacroiliac joint injury in horses is difficult and often based on a diagnosis of exclusion.[10] Diagnosis is complicated by anatomical inaccessibility, mild chronic clinical signs so that opportunities for correlation with necropsy findings are uncommon, and ongoing controversies over the clinical relevance and prevalence of pathological conditions of the articular surface and ligaments.[4] Terms used to describe pathological conditions of the sacroiliac joint include sacroiliac sprain or instability,[11,12] sacroiliac joint subluxation,[13] and sacroiliac arthrosis.[14,15] The prevalence of pathological conditions of the sacroiliac joint in performance horses is probably high, and many may go undiagnosed.[4,14,16] In a necropsy survey of 36 Thoroughbred (TB) racehorses with no known back or sacroiliac joint problems, we observed various degrees of degenerative sacroiliac joint changes in all specimens.[17] The clinical importance of osseous sacroiliac joint pathological conditions is difficult to determine because many presumed normal horses have osteoarthritic changes similar to horses with known back or sacroiliac problems.[1,4] Possibly the majority of sacroiliac joint pathological conditions are subclinical; however, if similar findings were noted in any other musculoskeletal location, the articular changes would be considered clinically relevant and a

likely contributing cause of lameness. A more likely scenario is that deep sclerotogenous pain (e.g., vertebral or sacroiliac joint osteoarthritis [OA]) is often poorly localized and perceived as deep aching pain, based on reports of similar pathological conditions of the sacroiliac joint in affected people. Clinically the most common reported signs of sacroiliac joint disorders in horses are poor performance, lack of impulsion, and a mild, chronic hindlimb lameness, which can easily be overlooked or dismissed as not clinically relevant.[4,18] Obvious signs of lameness and localized pain or inflammation are not typical clinical characteristics of sacroiliac joint or pelvic injuries, unless pelvic fractures or substantial joint disruption is present.

OA of the sacroiliac joints is usually a bilateral condition and may be present despite symmetry of the tubera sacrale.[19] Degenerative changes of the sacroiliac joint include (in apparent order of increasing severity) articular surface lipping, cortical buttressing, articular recession, osteophytes, and intraarticular erosions (Figure 51-3). In our survey of 36 TB racehorses, sacroiliac degenerative changes were classified as mild in 8% of specimens, moderate in 61%, and severe in 31%. Age was not associated with overall prevalence or severity of sacroiliac joint degenerative changes.[17] Osseous changes are usually bilaterally symmetrical and most commonly located at the caudomedial aspect of the articulation.[1,17] The pathogenesis of proliferative sacroiliac joint changes is uncertain, but it is thought to be related to chronic instability resulting in gradual remodeling and subsequent enlargement of the caudomedial joint surfaces. Histologically the caudomedial extensions consist of apparently normal cancellous bone.[4] Articular cartilage erosion is a lytic process of articular surfaces that presumably leads to eventual sacroiliac joint ankylosis.[17] However, ankylosis of the sacroiliac joint is rare, which is surprising based on the limited joint motion and the potential severity of osseous pathological conditions present.[1,17,20] Fibrous interconnections between the articular surfaces have also been reported in presumed normal sacroiliac joints.[1] Articular cartilage discoloration, a presumed indicator of sacroiliac joint degeneration, is

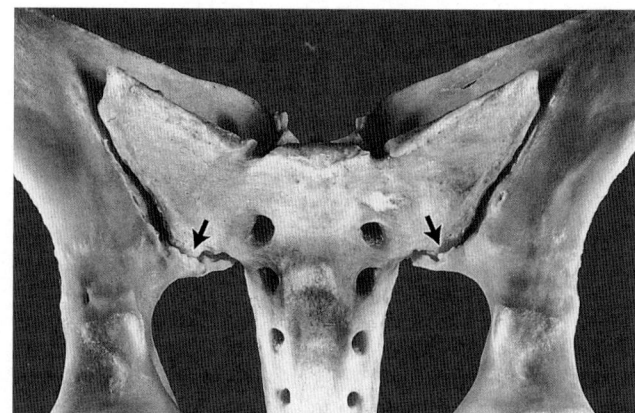

Figure 51-3 • Bilateral osteoarthritis of the sacroiliac articulations (ventral view). Severe proliferative changes of the caudomedial third of the sacroiliac joints *(arrows)* in an 8-year-old racing Thoroughbred gelding that was euthanized because of an acute colic episode. Normal sacroiliac joint margins are typically smooth and linear as represented by the cranial half of the sacroiliac articulations.

common in racehorses, but it has a reported higher prevalence in Standardbreds (STBs) compared with TBs.[14] One theory is that these changes are caused by differences in pelvic and sacroiliac joint biomechanics associated with pacing and trotting (i.e., lateral bending or shear forces) in STBs compared with galloping (i.e., flexion and extension movements) in TBs.[21] Biomechanical studies are warranted to support or refute these claims.

Sacroiliac desmitis, the most common soft tissue injury, was documented by ultrasonography in the dorsal portion of the dorsal sacroiliac ligament.[22] A diagnosis of sacroiliac desmitis is based on loss of normal echogenicity on a transverse image and a decrease in parallel fiber pattern on a longitudinal image. Sacroiliac ligament injuries usually occur because of acute trauma, but few horses with documented injury were reported.[17,23]

Complete sacroiliac ligament disruption is most likely caused by substantial trauma, such as flipping over backward, or catastrophic musculoskeletal injuries associated with race training.[17] Post mortem findings associated with traumatic sacroiliac ligament injuries include either unilateral or bilateral joint capsule disruption, avulsion fractures of the sacroiliac ligament attachment sites, and noticeable sacroiliac joint laxity. Dorsal or ventral sacroiliac ligaments can be affected, depending on the inciting mechanism of injury.[9,17,23] Complete sacroiliac ligament disruption may produce unilateral or bilateral dorsal displacement of the tubera sacrale, depending on the extent of injury (Figure 51-4).

Acute sacroiliac ligament injuries have been reported to contribute to development of chronic sacroiliac joint instability.[11,23] However, the presence and relevance of chronic sacroiliac ligament injury and sacroiliac joint laxity are controversial. Rooney et al[23,24] documented chronic sacroiliac joint injuries of the cranial portion of the ventral sacroiliac ligaments, which were found to be elongated or torn on the affected side. Desmitis of the insertion site of the dorsal portion of the dorsal sacroiliac ligament at the insertion on the tuber sacrale was reported.[9] In other studies osseous changes were found at the caudomedial sacroiliac joint margins in horses suspected of having chronic sacroiliac injury; however, no obvious sacroiliac ligament laxity was observed.[4,11,12] Radiologically some of these horses had an apparent increase in the sacroiliac joint space; however, no visible sacroiliac ligament injury, joint laxity, or subluxation was observed at necropsy.[4,12] In our necropsy survey of 36 TB racehorses, no evidence of chronic ligament injury or sacroiliac joint subluxation was observed.[17] However, this could be related to the previous removal of horses from race training with poor performance or hindlimb lameness associated with chronic sacroiliac joint injury.

The pathogenesis of apparent spontaneous or insidious differences in tuber sacrale height needs to be further researched.[4] Unilateral or bilateral dorsal displacement of the tubera sacrale is often a presumed indication of sacroiliac subluxation.[25] In my opinion, variable degrees of tubera sacrale height asymmetry occur frequently and may be caused by chronic asymmetric muscular or ligamentous forces acting on the malleable osseous pelvis and not by direct sacroiliac ligament injury.[26] Tubera sacrale height asymmetries are common in horses without documented sacroiliac joint injuries (see Figure 51-4). In only a few horses have tubera sacrale height asymmetries been associated with chronic sacroiliac ligament injuries or joint laxity.[24] In a study of 4-year-old STB trotters with tubera sacrale height asymmetries of more than 1 cm, associations were found with poor performance, but otherwise the asymmetry was of questionable clinical importance.[16] If substantial tubera sacrale height differences are identified, which side is affected is unclear and difficult to determine: the seemingly dorsally displaced tuber sacrale or the less prominent tuber sacrale on the opposite side.[4,16] Presumed sacroiliac joint subluxation produces an elevated tuber sacrale on the affected side, whereas complete ilial wing fractures (the most common type of pelvic fracture) typically produce a palpably depressed tuber sacrale on the affected side.[27]

CLINICAL PRESENTATION

Horses with sacroiliac joint injuries vary in clinical presentation, usually based on the duration and extent of injury present. The history of horses with acute sacroiliac joint injury usually includes slipping, falling, or trauma that causes pelvic rotation or induces high stresses.[25] Horses with acute sacroiliac joint injuries often have noticeable lameness and localized sensitivity to palpation of the surrounding soft tissues or tubera sacrale (Figure 51-5), which must be differentiated from other sources of back, pelvic, or hindlimb pain. Diagnosis of acute sacroiliac ligament rupture and subsequent sacroiliac joint subluxation or luxation is based on history, physical examination, and diagnostic imaging. Because the majority of horses have some degree of tuber sacrale height asymmetry, a diagnosis of acute sacroiliac joint subluxation can only be confirmed if symmetry of the tuber sacrale was documented immediately before the injury, and subsequently gross asymmetry of the tubera sacrale is noted with localized signs of pain or inflammation.

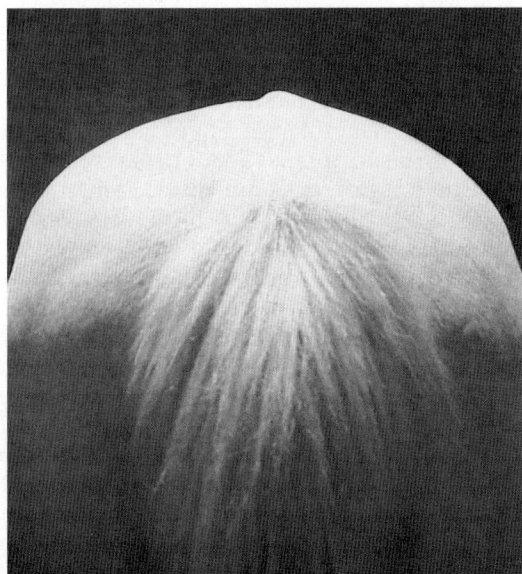

Figure 51-4 • Photograph of tubera sacrale height asymmetry (caudal view). The tuber sacrale on the right side is dorsally displaced, with apparent gluteal muscle symmetry. (Courtesy Al Kane, Ft. Collins, Colo, United States.)

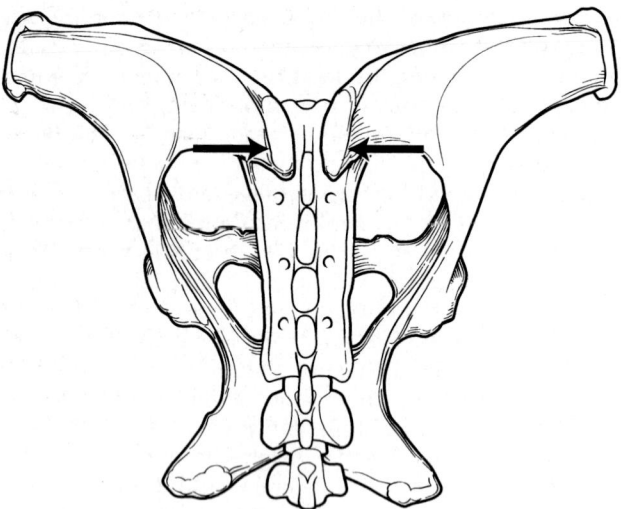

Figure 51-5 • Diagram of sacroiliac joint provocation test (dorsal view). Firm pressure is applied bilaterally with both hands, compressing the dorsal aspects of the tubera sacrale.

Important historical findings in horses with chronic sacroiliac joint injuries usually involve repetitive overuse versus a single traumatic event.[14] The most consistent clinical feature of chronic sacroiliac joint injury is a prolonged, nonprogressive history of reduced or poor performance.[4] In a recent study Warmblood horses involved in dressage and show jumping were most commonly affected.[28] Changes in performance included back stiffness, unwillingness to work, lack of impulsion from one or both hindlimbs, and refusing jumps. The duration of clinical signs varied from 1 month to more than 1 year, and to an untrained observer many of the horses appeared clinically normal.[28] Subtle gait asymmetries may be noticed at slow speeds during ground work or dressage movements and in harness horses at racing speeds.[4] Signs are often markedly accentuated when the horse is ridden, especially with changes in direction through tight circles in trot, half passes, or flying lead changes in canter.[19] Chronic sacroiliac joint injuries usually produce a low-grade or intermittent hindlimb lameness or stiffness that cannot be localized by routine lameness examination techniques and is improved only temporarily with antiinflammatory medications.[4] The affected sacroiliac joint usually corresponds to the side of lameness or reduced cranial swing phase of the affected hindlimb, but bilateral gait abnormalities can occur. Gait asymmetries involve subtle differences in pelvic movement or reduced hindlimb flexion or stride lengths. Affected horses commonly resent standing on the affected hindlimb while the contralateral hindlimb is lifted off the ground during hock flexion or shoeing.[18] Affected horses may also drag a hind foot and have mild hindlimb abduction before hoof contact (i.e., plaiting or rope walking).[4] Disuse atrophy of the gluteal musculature is an inconsistent finding; however, some horses have pelvic asymmetry with a lower tuber coxae and noticeable gluteal muscle atrophy on the affected side.[4,29] Observation of the tubera sacrale may reveal unilateral or bilateral (i.e., hunters' or jumpers' bumps) differences in height or dorsal prominence (see Figure 51-4). Unilateral or bilateral prominence of the tubera sacrale varies between horses and may be related to

conformation of the back or pelvis.[19] Poor thoracolumbar epaxial or gluteal muscle development may cause the tubera sacrale to be more visually prominent in horses that have chronic back or sacroiliac pain or lack proper collection and engagement of the hindlimbs.

Two clinical manifestations of sacroiliac joint dysfunction were proposed.[30] Horses in one category exhibit pain and poor performance that is responsive to local analgesia, tubera sacrale symmetry, and poorly defined pelvic or sacroiliac joint pathology (i.e., functional instability caused by altered neuromotor control). Those in the second category display poor performance and marked gait alterations, bony and soft tissue asymmetry, small improvements with local analgesia, and pathological changes associated with chronic joint instability (i.e., structural instability). Further research is needed to assess whether these proposed categories are clinically useful and distinct or whether they represent a continuum of sacroiliac joint dysfunction.

PHYSICAL EXAMINATION

Clinical signs of sacroiliac joint injury vary and may occur in conjunction with other sources of hindlimb lameness or poor performance. The sacroiliac joint is relatively inaccessible to direct evaluation or palpation, and the normally small amount of sacroiliac joint motion is difficult to detect clinically.[31] Horses with acute sacroiliac joint injuries may have localized sensitivity to palpation of the surrounding soft tissues in the dorsal aspect of the croup.[4] A localized region of edema may occasionally be palpated over the lumbosacral junction[32]; however, this is not a specific finding related to sacroiliac joint injury. Protective muscle spasms may be palpated in the adjacent middle gluteal musculature and the vertebral portions of the biceps femoris, semitendinosus, and semimembranosus muscles. In horses with acute sacroiliac injuries, asymmetry in gluteal muscle development is uncommon, unless pronounced osseous pelvic asymmetry is also present. Pain may be elicited by applying firm digital pressure over the dorsal aspects of the tubera sacrale or caudal lumbar and sacral dorsal spinous processes. Unilateral or bilateral prominence of the tubera sacrale may be noted, but it is not usually clinically relevant unless associated with clinical signs of localized pain or inflammation, or positive findings on diagnostic imaging are found (e.g., scintigraphy). In horses with sacroiliac joint pain, the tubera sacrale may appear grossly symmetrical despite asymmetric croup musculature.[28] Normally the tubera sacrale move in unison during pelvic movement in locomotion. A palpable or visible independent movement of the tubera sacrale at a walk or during treadmill locomotion indicates sacroiliac joint subluxation or a complete pelvic fracture. Crepitus associated with sacroiliac joint instability or complete pelvic fracture may be palpable or auscultated with a stethoscope placed over the gluteal musculature as the pelvis is repeatedly rocked laterally. Horses with acute sacroiliac joint injuries may also resent flexion of the hindlimb on the affected side or rectal palpation in the region of the sacroiliac joint.

Horses with chronic sacroiliac joint injuries often have compensatory stiffness and pain in the proximal aspect of the hindlimb.[25] Concurrent forelimb or hindlimb lameness needs to be excluded with perineural and intraarticular diagnostic analgesia.[28] Upper limb flexion is often negative.[4] Mild discomfort can be produced in some horses by picking up one pelvic limb and inducing a gentle lateral sway on the weighted limb.[19] Farriers often complain that affected horses have difficulty or refuse to stand while being shod, presumably because of strain or pain induced in the affected single weight-bearing limb.[28] Rectal examination for chronic sacroiliac joint subluxation is usually unrewarding and will not be diagnostic unless bone proliferation, excess joint motion, or joint crepitus during externally applied movements is identified.[25] A pain response or palpable muscle hypertonicity in the iliopsoas muscles may be noted during rectal examination. Serum chemistry indicators of skeletal muscle injury or inflammation (i.e., creatine kinase [CK] and aspartate transaminase [AST]) are often negative.

The apex of the second sacral spinous process is a reliable landmark used to evaluate relative unilateral or bilateral tubera sacrale displacement. The robust dorsal portion of the dorsal sacroiliac ligament spans between the tubera sacrale and the sacral spinous processes. Normally the dorsal apices of the tubera sacrale and the second sacral spinous process lie in close apposition and follow the contour of the croup. Using palpation, ultrasonography, or radiology, a physical discrepancy in height often can be identified between the dorsal profile of the sacral spinous processes (which should remain constant, unless fractured) and the potentially dorsally or ventrally displaced tuber sacrale. In this manner, unilateral (i.e., tubera sacrale height asymmetry) or bilateral tubera sacrale displacement (i.e., hunters' or jumpers' bumps) can be diagnosed, depending on whether one or both tubera sacrale are elevated relative to the apices of the sacral spinous processes. Bilateral tubera sacrale displacement has an unknown clinical relevance and may occur without clinical signs in many high-level competition horses.[32] Theoretically the hunters' or jumpers' bumps may provide a longer lever arm for the strong longissimus and thoracolumbar fascia to produce extension at the lumbosacral joint, resulting in increased impulsion and range of hindlimb motion, with subsequent improved performance.

Firm digital pressure applied to the dorsal aspect of each tuber sacrale was reported to produce a variable and inconsistent pain response.[18] The tolerance to palpation and applied pressure to soft tissues and bony landmarks of the sacroiliac joint region are subjective assessments. Pressure algometry has the potential to quantify muscle or bone pain in horses with sacroiliac joint injuries.[33] Affected horses have lower mechanical nociceptive thresholds and greater left-right differences compared with control horses. In my experience, dramatic pain responses have been produced in affected horses with specific provocation tests, which are useful to establish a presumptive diagnosis of pelvic stress fracture or sacroiliac joint injury. The first procedure involves simultaneous manual compression of the dorsal aspects of both tubera sacrale, which induces a bending moment on the iliac wing and presumably compresses the sacroiliac articulations (see Figure 51-5). Acutely affected horses may have a dramatic reaction to this manipulation and demonstrate sudden hindlimb flexion and an apparent inability to bear weight in the hindlimbs when pressure is applied. Clinicians should gradually apply increasing pressure because affected horses may actually collapse in the hindlimbs and fall to the ground if excess force is applied to the painful tubera sacrale. A negative response is characterized by minimal pain response and slight extension of the lumbosacral joint during manual compression of the tubera sacrale. This test is not specific for pathological conditions of the sacroiliac joint because horses with incomplete or stress fractures of the ilial wing may respond even more dramatically to the applied pressure.

A second procedure used to identify sacroiliac ligament injury involves rhythmically applying a ventrally directed force over the lumbosacral dorsal spinous processes to stress the supporting sacroiliac ligaments. This procedure requires the clinician to get up on an elevated surface (e.g., mounting block) so that the applied forces can be directed vertically over the sixth lumbar and second sacral dorsal spinous processes. Horses with sacroiliac ligament injuries would be expected to resent the induced movement because it specifically stresses the interosseous sacroiliac ligament (i.e., ligamentous sling of the sacropelvic junction). Horses with lumbosacral vertebral joint dysfunction (i.e., localized pain, reduced joint motion, and muscle hypertonicity without structural pathological conditions) may also resent this procedure. Rhythmically applied ventrally directed forces over the dorsal spinous processes at the sacrocaudal junction would be expected specifically to stress the dorsal portion of the dorsal sacroiliac ligament. A positive response to this test combined with positive ultrasonographic findings of desmitis of the dorsal sacroiliac ligament would be highly suggestive of clinically relevant sacroiliac ligament injury.

A similar procedure involves rhythmically applying a ventrally directed force over each tuber coxae to induce general sacroiliac and lumbosacral joint motion. A normal response to the induced movement is fluid vertical motion of the lumbosacral region, with an amplitude of 1 to 2 cm of dorsoventral movement measured over the lumbar dorsal spinous processes. Affected horses have a noticeable pain response, resent the induced movement, or have protective gluteal or sublumbar muscle spasms. The vertically directed force also induces movement at the lumbosacral junction, which must be differentiated from sacroiliac joint injury.

Additional procedures used to localize sacroiliac joint or ligament injuries involve indirectly evaluating pain and ligamentous laxity in the sacroiliac joint using laterally applied forces (Figures 51-6 and 51-7). These procedures are similar to valgus-varus stress tests used to evaluate collateral ligaments of the distal limb articulations. Caution should be taken not to apply excessive force because of the long lever arm action of the sacral apex on the sacroiliac ligaments, which can unduly stress unstable or partially torn ligaments or aggravate an acutely inflamed sacroiliac joint. The proposed mechanism of action of these tests is to use the base of the tail and sacrum as a handle to apply a lateral (horizontal plane) stress to the sacroiliac joint as the wing of the ilium is stabilized. The technique involves two parts. First, the base of the hand closest to the horse's head is placed over the lateral aspect of the tuber sacrale. The hand closest to the tail grasps the base of the tail head (the second and third coccygeal bones). The sacroiliac joints are then evaluated as firm pressure is simultaneously

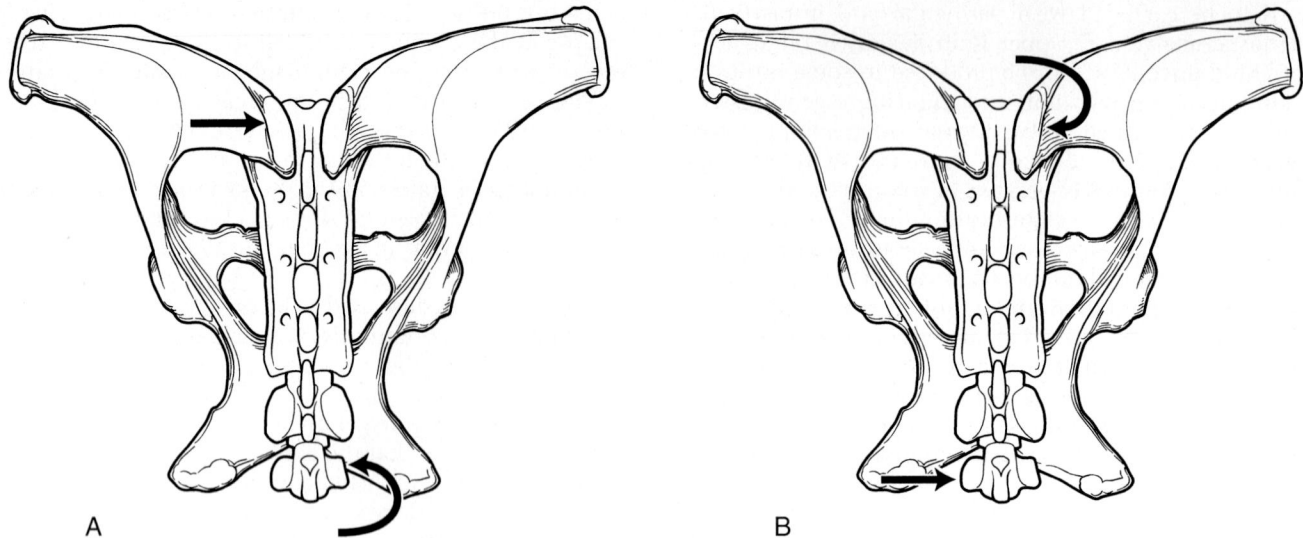

Figure 51-6 • Diagram of second sacroiliac joint provocation test (dorsal view). **A,** Firm pressure is applied by both hands, pushing with the hand at the ipsilateral tuber sacrale away from the clinician while simultaneously pulling with the hand at the tail head toward him or her. **B,** Firm pressure is applied by both hands, pulling with the hand at the contralateral tuber sacrale toward the clinician while simultaneously pushing with the hand at the tail head away from him or her.

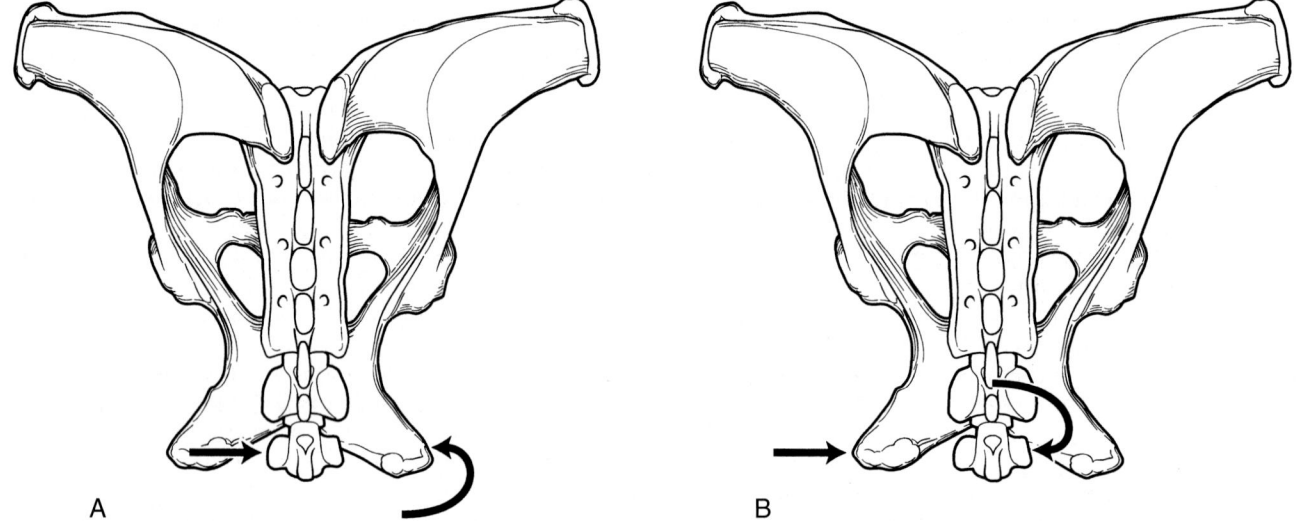

Figure 51-7 • Diagram of third sacroiliac joint provocation test (dorsal view). **A,** Firm pressure is applied by both hands, pushing with the hand at the tail head away from the clinician while simultaneously pulling with the hand at the contralateral ischial tuberosity toward him or her. **B,** Firm pressure is applied by both hands, pulling with the hand at the tail head toward the clinician while simultaneously pushing with the hand at the ipsilateral ischial tuberosity away from him or her.

applied by both hands, pushing with the hand at the tuber sacrale away from the clinician and pulling with the hand at the tail head toward him or her (see Figure 51-6, *A*). Theoretically this maneuver produces compression of contralateral sacroiliac articular surfaces and distraction of the ipsilateral sacroiliac articular surfaces.

The second portion of the technique involves repeating the procedure and reversing the direction of the applied forces (see Figure 51-6, *B*). The fingers of the hand closest to the horse's head are placed over the contralateral tuber sacrale, and the base of the hand closest to the tail is placed

against the ipsilateral base of the tail head (second and third coccygeal bones). The sacroiliac joints are again evaluated as firm pressure is applied by both hands, pulling with the hand at the tuber sacrale toward the clinician and pushing with the hand at the tail head away from him or her. Theoretically the contralateral sacroiliac articular surfaces are distracted, and the ipsilateral sacroiliac articular surfaces are compressed. A pain response to the induced movements may be identified unilaterally or bilaterally, depending on the extent of inflammation or injury present. In general, sacroiliac joint compression would be expected to aggravate osteoarthritic changes, whereas joint distraction would be expected to stress any injured or inflamed sacroiliac ligaments.

A variation of this basic technique uses repeatedly applied laterally directed forces over the ischial tuberosity instead of the tuber sacrale (see Figure 51-7). This procedure incorporates two long lever arms to stress the supporting sacroiliac ligaments. Again caution should be taken not to apply excessive force because of the long lever arm action of the sacral apex and ischial tuberosities on the sacroiliac ligaments. Lastly, proximal hindlimb manipulation is done to assess coxofemoral and stifle joint range of motion and the willingness to actively extend the hindlimb. Concurrent joint stiffness or muscle hypertonicity can be identified and localized as the proximal aspect of the hindlimb is passively protracted, abducted, flexed, and retracted.

LOCAL ANALGESIA

Intraarticular analgesia of the sacroiliac joint is nearly impossible because of its deep anatomical location and inaccessible joint capsule.[34] Experimentally, intraarticular sacroiliac injections have been accomplished by drilling a hole through the wing of the ilium, dorsal to the sacroiliac joint.[18] Regional perfusion with local anesthetic solutions or antiinflammatory drugs for diagnostic or therapeutic purposes was described.[35] Approaches from the cranial aspect of the wing of the ilium and the lumbosacral junction are typically used[32]; however, because of the wide overlying wing of the ilium, the proximity and diffusion of the medication near the sacroiliac joint are questionable.

I recommend a caudomedial approach to the sacroiliac joint region because of anatomical and pathological considerations.[34] The caudomedial portion of the sacroiliac joint is the most frequent site of pathological conditions of the sacroiliac joint.[1,4,17] Therefore diagnostic analgesia or therapeutic analgesia or antiinflammatory drugs should be directed toward the caudal aspect of the sacroiliac joint in the region of documented pathological condition. Two approaches are described, using 20- to 25-cm-long needles, depending on the depth and conformation of the gluteal musculature (Figure 51-8). Surgical preparation of the injection site is recommended, similar to other joint injection techniques. Ultrasound guidance is also recommended to allow the caudomedial aspect of the sacroiliac joint to be seen and identification of neurovascular structures that must be avoided at the greater sciatic foramen (see Figure 51-2).[34,35] The cranial gluteal artery and nerve emerge laterally around the caudal margin of the ilial wing and travel dorsocaudally, adjacent to the sacroiliac joint. Other vital structures, including the sciatic nerve, lie ventral to the sacroiliac joint and travel on or within the substance of the sacrosciatic ligament.

The first approach involves needle placement dorsally over the iliac wing, ipsilateral to the affected sacroiliac joint (see Figure 51-8, *A*). This approach is technically easier, but it potentially has a higher risk of injury to the adjacent neurovascular structures. The needle is directed ventrally, toward the region of the sacroiliac joint, and walked off the caudal border of the iliac wing in the region of the sacroiliac joint. Care must be taken to avoid the deeper neurovascular structures. The needle is not advanced once it is walked off the caudal aspect of the iliac wing.

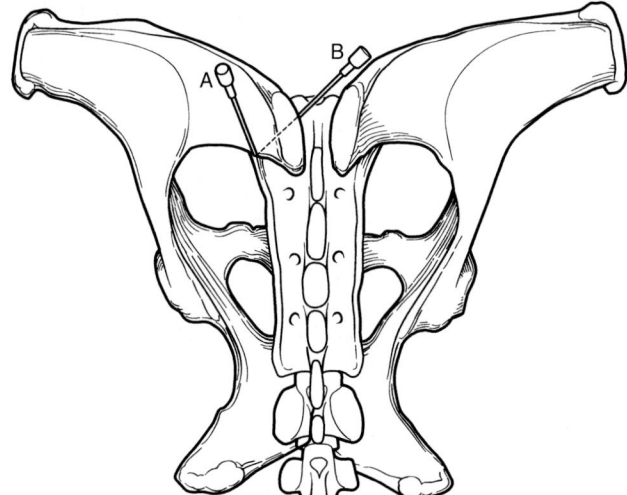

Figure 51-8 • Diagram of two approaches to the sacroiliac joint for diagnostic analgesia and therapeutic analgesia or administration of antiinflammatory drugs (dorsal view). **A,** Dorsal approach over the ipsilateral iliac wing near the caudomedial aspect of the affected sacroiliac joint. **B,** Medial approach from the cranial aspect of the contralateral tuber sacrale with the needle directed toward the caudomedial aspect of the affected sacroiliac joint.

Diffusion of the injected material occurs within the middle or accessory gluteal muscles, near the caudomedial attachments of the ventral sacroiliac ligament.

A second preferred approach involves needle placement at the cranial margin of the contralateral tuber sacrale (see Figure 51-8, *B*). This approach is slightly more technically challenging but has a lower risk of injury to the adjacent neurovascular structures. The needle is inserted along the cranial aspect of the contralateral tuber sacrale and directed toward the cranial edge of the ipsilateral greater trochanter. The needle is placed contralaterally to the affected sacroiliac joint because the needle has to be guided between the divergent sixth lumbar and first sacral dorsal spinous processes and directed into the space formed by the ventral aspect of the ilial wing and the dorsal portion of the sacrum. The needle is advanced caudolaterally along the medial aspect of the affected ilial wing toward the caudomedial portion of the affected sacroiliac joint until contact is made with bone, near the sacroiliac joint margin. Diffusion of the injected material is expected to occur within the longissimus muscle or interosseous sacroiliac ligament. The dorsal nerve branches of the sacral nerves possibly may also be affected with this approach because the nerves exit the first and second dorsal sacral foramina.

DIAGNOSTIC IMAGING

Ultrasonography has been used to evaluate the dorsal surface of the iliac wing and caudal margin of the sacroiliac articulation to identify dorsal cortex irregularities associated with incomplete and complete ilial wing fractures.[36,37] The dorsal sacroiliac ligament can be readily imaged on either side of the sacral dorsal spinous processes caudal to the tubera sacrale.[9] Abnormal ultrasound images of the dorsal sacroiliac ligament include enthesopathies at the tubera sacrale attachment sites, hypoechoic changes within the ligament, and modification of fiber orientation.[9,22,38] Increased cross-sectional area of the dorsal sacroiliac ligament was reported to cause acute lameness, whereas decreased cross-sectional area was observed in horses with chronic lameness associated with sacroiliac injuries.[38] The thoracolumbar longissimus fascia and tendon lie medial to the dorsal portion of the dorsal sacroiliac ligament and blend with its fibers as it inserts on the sacral spinous processes.[10] Longissimus tendonitis needs to be differentiated from dorsal sacroiliac desmitis because management of the two conditions may vary considerably.[39] The interosseous sacroiliac ligament has not been imaged because of its inaccessible location underneath the ventral aspect of the ilial wing. In contrast, the ventral sacroiliac ligament and the ventral joint margins of the sacroiliac joint can be seen using transrectal ultrasonography.[9] Ventral periarticular modeling of the sacroiliac joint was observed with transrectal ultrasound approaches.[39]

Primary indications for radiography of the pelvis include acute or severe pelvic asymmetries, upper hindlimb lameness, and pelvic crepitus or fractures.[40] The deep anatomical location of the sacroiliac joint and superimposition of abdominal viscera make radiographic imaging difficult at best. Ventilation-induced blurring of the abdominal viscera during general anesthesia with horses in dorsal recumbency is a simple technique to help delineate the bony structures of the sacroiliac region.[41] The radiological features of chronic sacroiliac joint disease are minimal and include nonspecific increases in the joint space and enlargement of the caudomedial aspect of the sacroiliac joint.[4] Radiography is not a sensitive indicator of sacroiliac joint disease because presumably normal horses may have dramatic differences in sacroiliac joint shape.[41] Linear tomography was used to examine the lumbosacral and sacroiliac regions of horses, but limited access to equipment has restricted its clinical usefulness.[15] Positive findings include widening of the sacroiliac joint and irregular joint outlines, with osteophyte formation at the caudal aspect of the joint. Osseous changes are common bilaterally, but they may be more pronounced on the clinically more affected side.[15]

Nuclear scintigraphy is considered by some authors to be an accurate and diagnostically useful technique for identifying acute and chronic sacroiliac joint injuries. However, ilial wing and soft tissue attenuation (from 71% to 82%), large distance between the ilial wing and camera face, horse movement, and background activity severely compromise the pelvic scintigraphic image, and only dramatic radiopharmaceutical uptake (RU) can be reliably detected.[42,43] In addition, large variations exist in RU in both affected and unaffected horses. Young horses have well-defined tubera sacrale and relatively less RU in the adjacent regions of the sacroiliac joints.[44] Older horses and horses with sacroiliac joint pathology have less distinct differences in RU between the tubera sacrale and the sacroiliac joints.[19] Subjective evaluation or quantitative analysis of bone scans typically is able to identify asymmetric RU over the affected tuber sacrale or wing of the ilium in the region of the sacroiliac joint. However, presumed normal horses, without a history of hindlimb or sacroiliac joint injuries, may have mild asymmetric RU over the tubera sacrale and sacroiliac joint regions.[19] Non–motion-corrected scintigraphic images are

often not of diagnostic quality and can be misinterpreted as abnormal.[44] Motion-corrected images are much more likely to give accurate diagnostic information. A dorsal image of the sacrum is considered the most diagnostic image for evaluating and comparing the sacroiliac joints.[18] However, RU in the relatively superficial tubera sacrale may mask RU in the sacroiliac joints in a dorsal image. Oblique images of the ilial wings are recommended to confirm left to right asymmetries in RU, especially when identifying stress fractures, and to separate the tuber sacrale dorsally from the sacroiliac joint region ventrally.[45] However, oblique images may be difficult to interpret because of inconsistent camera positioning on the left and right sides. The thick overlying gluteal musculature may also attenuate RU from an affected sacroiliac joint.[43] Any left-right asymmetry in gluteal muscle mass will produce a false-positive interpretation of RU on the side with the atrophic or reduced muscle mass.[42] Stress fractures of the ilial wing may be difficult to differentiate from sacroiliac joint injuries because of the common location and extension of the incomplete fracture line into the sacroiliac joint.[18,27,46] Increased RU (IRU) within the pelvis does not necessarily indicate a primary cause of pain.[47] A compensatory response within the osseous pelvis, insufficient pelvic pain to cause lameness, and other sources of lameness that cause more discomfort than the pelvic lesion associated with the area of IRU may all cause disassociation between a positive scintigraphic finding and the primary source of pain. Nuclear scintigraphy should also include the caudal thoracolumbar spine to rule out concurrent pathology, such as impinging dorsal spinous processes.[19]

Thermography is used to diagnose muscle strain or inflammation in the sacroiliac and croup regions. Horses with sacroiliac joint injuries are expected to have protective muscle spasms in the adjacent musculature. Palpation of muscle sensitivity has been correlated with abnormal thermographic images in most horses.[48] Thermographic imaging of horses with sacroiliac injuries demonstrates a change in the normal temperature pattern over the croup, with increased temperature associated with acute desmitis and decreased temperature over the sacroiliac area on the affected side in horses with chronic sacroiliac injury.[38] In the Editors' experience thermography may be helpful in the identification of acute desmitis of the dorsal sacroiliac ligament, but is usually of no value in the assessment of horses with chronic sacroiliac joint region pain. All diagnostic imaging modalities need to be carefully evaluated with respect to clinical signs exhibited by the individual horse.[19,49]

DIFFERENTIAL DIAGNOSIS

Causes of sacroiliac joint pain or injury were postulated to result from sacroiliac or lumbosacral arthrosis, sacroiliac desmitis or sprain, sacroiliac subluxation or luxation, pelvic stress fractures, complete ilial wing fractures, or sacral fractures.[32] Additional differential diagnoses include aortoiliac thromboembolism, exertional rhabdomyolysis, trochanteric bursitis, and impinged dorsal spinous processes in the lumbar vertebrae.[25] Horses with presumed thoracolumbar vertebral problems may also have concurrent chronic sacroiliac joint injuries. In a report on 443 horses with back problems, chronic sacroiliac joint problems were identified in 15%.[11] Clinical signs of lower hindlimb lameness may overlap and mimic signs of presumed pathological conditions of the sacroiliac joint. It is important that a thorough and complete lower limb lameness evaluation is completed before, or along with, an upper hindlimb or sacroiliac joint workup.

Based on a review of the literature, OA of the sacroiliac joint is the most prevalent disease process affecting horses with sacroiliac joint pain or dysfunction.[1,4,11,17] Sacroiliac desmitis was documented in horses and may be an important cause of pathological conditions in horses with acute sacroiliac joint injuries.[9] Documented complete rupture of the sacroiliac ligaments was only reported in a few horses with acute and chronic disease.[17,24] The presumed diagnosis of sacroiliac joint subluxation based solely on tubera sacrale height asymmetry is inappropriate.[31] Horses with chronic sacroiliac problems and presumed sacroiliac joint subluxation have not had identifiable changes in the sacroiliac ligaments at necropsy.[4] In addition, STB trotters with substantial tubera sacrale height asymmetries did not have significant increases in sacroiliac pain compared with horses with lesser degrees of asymmetry.[16] In my opinion, an antemortem diagnosis of sacroiliac joint luxation can only be supported if an acute change in tubera sacrale height caused by substantial trauma has been documented or if sacroiliac joint instability (i.e., crepitus or independent tubera sacrale movement) is evident during physical examination. Pelvic stress fractures should be ruled out in horses with sacroiliac pain or dysfunction.[50] A high prevalence of occult pelvic stress fractures was reported in TB racehorses.[46] The incomplete fracture lines extend into the caudomedial aspect of the sacroiliac joint, which could possibly produce concurrent sacroiliac joint inflammation and OA. A diagnosis of sacroiliac joint injury is often based on a diagnosis of exclusion because of difficulties in clinical evaluation and diagnostic imaging. We are hopeful future investigations into sacroiliac joint problems in horses will produce a better and more comprehensive understanding of this often misdiagnosed clinical entity.

TREATMENT

Because definitive diagnosis of pathological conditions of the sacroiliac joint is difficult, treatment recommendations are usually symptomatic. Few studies on treatment efficacy have been reported in the equine literature. In people, analgesics, antiinflammatories, intraarticular and periarticular injections of corticosteroids, and prolotherapy (i.e., injection of sclerosing agents) were advocated as sole treatments for sacroiliac joint dysfunction. However, effective treatment and long-term rehabilitation of sacroiliac joint injuries often rely on the development of specific physical therapy and training programs that stimulate neuromotor and biomechanical restoration of articular, muscular, fascial, and ligamentous function.[30] In general, rest and various forms of physical therapy are indicated for horses

with ligamentous injuries. Prolonged rest (6 to 12 months) and systemic antiinflammatory medications are prescribed for horses with acute and chronic sacroiliac joint injuries. Complete box stall rest for 30 to 45 days was recommended to support ligamentous healing in horses with acute injuries.[25] The local injection of irritants or sclerosing agents was suggested to stimulate fibrosis and subsequent sacroiliac joint stability.[25] In my opinion, no scientific support or clinical indication exists for such proposed treatments of back or sacroiliac joint problems. With such haphazard and potentially injurious treatment modalities there appears to be a better chance of inducing further injury rather than of stimulating any healing response. Treatment of horses with chronic sacroiliac joint injury typically focuses on a gradual return to a low level of exercise to maintain muscle development of the back and gluteal regions to counteract the clinical signs of poor performance and reduced hindlimb impulsion.[29] Extended rest is contraindicated because reduced muscle tone may exacerbate the injury.

Because of the deep and inaccessible location of the sacroiliac joint, intraarticular injections of local anesthetic solutions or antiinflammatory medications for diagnostic or therapeutic purposes are impractical.[18] However, local perfusion of the sacroiliac joint with local anesthetic solutions or antiinflammatory drugs for diagnostic and therapeutic purposes is a viable alternative.[32] Concurrent lameness of the ipsilateral lower hindlimb was reported in horses with signs of chronic sacroiliac joint injuries.[18] Therefore a detailed lameness examination coupled with appropriate treatment of the pathological conditions of the lower hindlimb is often indicated. Additional factors such as corrective shoeing and modifications in exercise or training programs need to be addressed concurrently. Acupuncture and chiropractic are nontraditional approaches that are used by some clinicians to assist in the diagnosis and symptomatic treatment of horses with presumed sacroiliac joint problems. Efficacy of modalities needs to be confirmed before further recommendations can be made.

PROGNOSIS

Long-term follow-up evaluation suggests that prognosis for horses with sacroiliac joint injury is poor for return to the previous level of activity.[18] Some horses may have an improvement in performance or lameness but will not be able to return to normal athletic activities because of recurring, low-grade lameness. Most horses will be pasture sound or able to function only at low levels of exercise. We hope that improvements in providing a specific diagnosis of the type of sacroiliac joint injury present will provide affected horses with better and more specific treatment options in the future.

ACKNOWLEDGMENT
I thank Michael Simmons for assistance with the illustrations.

Chapter 52

Thoracolumbar Spine

Jean-Marie Denoix and Sue J. Dyson

Back problems are a major cause of altered gait or performance (see Chapters 50, 51, and 97). Both identification and documentation of vertebral lesions are difficult in horses; therefore treating back pain is a challenge for the equine clinician. The equine back is a large area covered by thick muscles. Therefore assessment of the bony elements is limited. Every joint in the thoracolumbar region has restricted mobility; therefore detecting changes in restricted movement when the horse is working is difficult. Diagnostic imaging of the thoracolumbar region is also limited, and radiological assessment requires special equipment. Specific treatment of back pain can only be performed after complete identification of the site and nature of the lesions.

ANATOMY AND FUNCTION

Bones

The thoracolumbar spine is basically composed of 18 thoracic vertebrae (T1 to T18), six lumbar vertebrae (L1 to L6), and five fused sacral vertebrae (S1 to S5). Some horses have individual (congenital) variations at the cervicothoracic, thoracolumbar, and lumbosacral junctions. The most common is the sacralization of the last lumbar vertebra (sacralization of L6), which can be seen by ultrasonography. Transitional vertebrae, with a rib on one side and a transverse process on the other side, can be found at the thoracolumbar junction. Intervertebral ankylosis alters the biomechanical behavior of the involved part of the spine, especially at the lumbosacral junction, which in normal horses is the most mobile joint between T2 and S1. Ankylosis of this joint puts more stresses on the caudal lumbar intervertebral joints and may predispose to osteoarthritis (OA) of the facet joints and intervertebral disk lesions. Fusion of the lumbar transverse processes (see the following discussion) is also sometimes seen, and this has similar consequences on adjacent intervertebral joints, but the consequences are fewer because little movement usually occurs in these joints. Transitional transverse processes, or ribs that do not involve the vertebral body, have less biomechanical significance.

The first 10 thoracic vertebrae have long spinous processes. These have a dorsocaudal orientation and provide insertion for the strong but elastic supraspinous ligament. The anticlinal vertebra, the vertebra with a spinous process perpendicular to the vertebral axis, is usually T15. Caudal to the anticlinal vertebra the spinous processes are orientated obliquely dorsocranially. The spinous processes are higher between L2 and L5. Therefore lumbar muscular atrophy results in a kyphotic appearance of the lumbar area.

In most horses the spinous processes of L6 and S1 are divergent, allowing a range of flexion and extension movements at the lumbosacral joint. The transverse processes from L5 (sometimes L4) to S1 articulate through intertransverse synovial joints, which limit lateral flexion in this area. The lumbar vertebral bodies are bigger than the thoracic ones and have a ventral crest for the insertion of the diaphragm.

Joints

Stability of the thoracolumbar vertebrae is provided by the supraspinous and interspinous ligaments, the joints between the cranial and caudal articular processes (the facet joints), the joints between the vertebral bodies, and the dorsal and ventral longitudinal ligaments. Stability of the spinous processes is provided by the supraspinous and interspinous ligaments (Figure 52-1). These ligaments are wider and more elastic in the cranial and middle thoracic areas, permitting more movement than in the caudal thoracic and lumbar regions.

The caudal and cranial articular processes articulate via synovial intervertebral articulations (the facet joints). At the base of the spinous processes these joints are symmetrically placed on each side of the median plane (Figure 52-2). These are typical synovial (diarthrodial) joints with articular cartilage, a closed synovial cavity containing synovial fluid, a synovial membrane, and a fibrous capsule. They have a single flat articular facet in the cranial thoracic area (up to T12) and two angulated articular facets between T12 and T16. From T17 to S1 the articular facets are congruent,

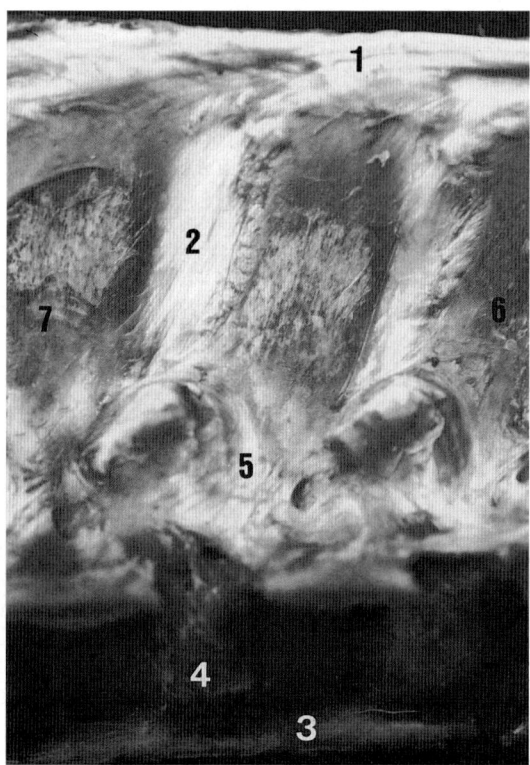

Fig. 52-1 • Anatomical specimen showing the ligaments of the thoracolumbar spine. Cranial is to the right. *1*, Supraspinous ligament; *2*, interspinous ligament; *3*, ventral longitudinal ligament; *4*, fibrous superficial part of the intervertebral disk; *5*, articular capsule of the synovial intervertebral joint; *6*, first lumbar vertebra; *7*, third lumbar vertebra.

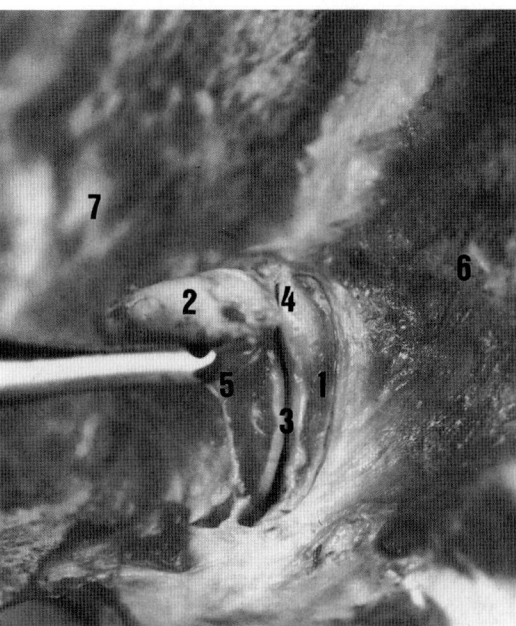

Fig. 52-2 • Anatomical specimen showing a synovial intervertebral articulation. *1,* Caudal articular process; *2,* cranial articular process; *3,* joint space; *4,* articular margin; *5,* articular capsule and synovial membrane (reflected); *6,* first lumbar vertebra; *7,* second lumbar vertebra.

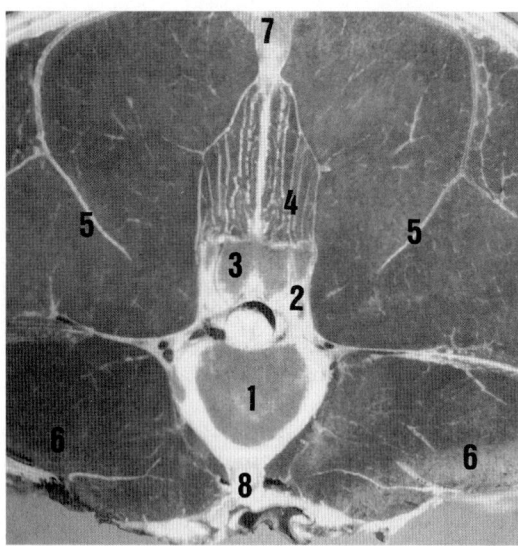

Fig. 52-3 • Transverse anatomical section of the normal lumbar region of a 6-year-old Selle Français mare. *1,* Vertebral head of third lumbar vertebra; *2,* cranial articular process of third lumbar vertebra; *3,* caudal articular process of second lumbar vertebra; *4,* multifidus muscle; *5,* erector spinae muscle; *6,* psoas muscles; *7,* supraspinous ligament; *8,* ventral longitudinal ligament.

with a cylindrical shape aligned on a paramedian axis. These regional variations are correlated with the limited mobility of the lumbar spine and the wider range of movement in the thoracic region, including flexion and extension in the median plane, lateral flexion in the horizontal plane, and rotation. The vertebral bodies are stabilized by joints composed of a fibrous intervertebral disk and two longitudinal ligaments. The ventral longitudinal ligament is replaced by the longissimus cervicis muscle in the cranial thoracic area. The dorsal longitudinal ligament is located in the vertebral canal and adherent to the dorsal border of each intervertebral disk.

Muscles

The vertebral column is moved by wide muscles (Figure 52-3). The strong epaxial muscles, located dorsal to the vertebral axis, have an extensor effect when contracted bilaterally. Unilateral contraction induces lateral flexion and contributes to rotation of the vertebral column. Electromyographic studies show that the epaxial muscles limit flexion and stabilize the vertebral column during the suspension phase at the trot.[1,2]

The epaxial muscles include the following:
1. Spinosus muscle, inserting on the spinous processes
2. Longissimus dorsi muscle, which extends to the caudal cervical spine
3. Iliocostalis muscle

The longissimus dorsi is the strongest muscle. The iliocostalis muscles are small but have a greater role in lateral flexion because of their eccentric location. Caudally, these muscles fuse to form the erector spinae muscle. The multifidus muscle lies under the spinosus muscle and is in close contact with the vertebrae (juxtavertebral muscle). This muscle plays a major role in the stability of the vertebrae and in the proprioceptive adjustment of the spine.

The hypaxial muscles, located ventral to the vertebral axis, have a flexor effect on the spine when contracted bilaterally. Unilateral contraction induces lateral flexion and contributes to rotation of the vertebral column. The hypaxial muscles include psoas minor and major, rectus abdominis, and rectus oblique.

The psoas minor and major muscles insert on the ventral aspect of the lumbar and caudal three thoracic vertebrae (juxtavertebral muscles). They act mainly at the lumbosacral junction but are also able to flex the thoracolumbar junction and the lumbar spine. The rectus abdominis muscle is an effective flexor of the complete thoracolumbar spine because of its eccentric insertions on the pubis, sternum, and ventral part of the ribs. The oblique muscles can create lateral flexion and rotation of the thoracolumbar spine because of eccentric insertions on the tubera coxae and ribs. Electromyographic studies show that the rectus abdominis muscles act to limit extension and stabilize the vertebral column during each diagonal stance phase at the trot.[1,2]

Blood Vessels and Nerves

The vertebrae, intervertebral joints, and axial muscles are supplied by segmental thoracic and lumbar arteries and veins. Innervation is provided by thoracic and lumbar spinal nerves that pass through the intervertebral foramina.

DIAGNOSIS OF BACK PAIN

The objectives of clinical examination of the horse's back[3-7] are to determine whether back pain is present, the site or sites of pain, and the potential lesions responsible for the pain. Acute back pain can arise after traumatic injuries, such as a fall, or after an awkward jump. Acute pain and muscle spasm may be identified and may be the primary lesion, but a complete radiographic examination of the thoracolumbar spine may be indicated to assess for

ferences n page 1293

vertebral fractures or long-standing bony lesions that may be responsible for the accident. These lesions may become clinically significant because of overstress on the intervertebral structures. For example, a long-standing spondylosis lesion may cause acute pain on landing after a jump.

A poor rider or an ill-fitting saddle may cause back pain, but correction of these problems may not be easy. It is important to manage these causes of back pain before proceeding with more advanced imaging techniques.

Back pain may also be manifest by abnormal behavior, for example, bucking (see page 992).

Physical Examination
Physical examination is essential in diagnosing back pain. Only the main criteria for each step or procedure are discussed. It is obviously important to perform a comprehensive evaluation of the whole horse to identify any other potential problems that may contribute to gait abnormalities or poor performance.

Inspection
The most commonly described abnormal curvatures of the back are lumbar kyphosis and thoracic lordosis. These can be seen in the same horse. Atrophy of the epaxial muscles in the lumbosacral regions results in prominence of the normal summits of the spinous processes and apparent kyphosis of the lumbar spine. Detection of atrophy of the epaxial muscles is a key finding in a horse with potential back pain because atrophy reflects the reduction of movement in the painful areas. The finding can help provide information on the possible location of the lesions. However, one should bear in mind that muscular development also reflects the horse's previous work history, and if the horse has never worked properly through its back, the epaxial muscles will be poorly developed.

Thoracic lordosis may be seen in clinically normal horses and does not necessarily imply the presence of back pain. However, a short coupled horse with lordosis is more likely to have impinging spinous processes, a reflection of the horse's normal conformation.

Abnormal swellings in the saddle area or abnormal hair loss may reflect a poorly fitting saddle or the position and balance of the rider. A rider who sits crookedly predisposes to excessive movement of the saddle and asymmetrical hair loss. However, it should be noted that hindlimb lameness may also induce abnormal movement of the saddle.

The stance of the horse may also be important; some horses with back pain may stand either camped out or camped under. However, a normal stance certainly does not preclude thoracolumbar region pain.

Palpation
Palpation of the thoracolumbar region should be performed with the horse standing quietly, bearing weight evenly on all limbs. Time should be spent getting the horse accustomed to the clinician's presence, especially with an apprehensive horse, so that the horse's true reactions to pain and pressure can be assessed. Unless approached quietly a thin-skinned Thoroughbred (TB) type may give a false impression of guarding the back and having protective spasm of the epaxial muscles.

Palpation of the superficial structures of the thoracolumbar region helps to identify supraspinous desmopathy

and deformation or malalignment of the spinous processes. Identification of localized muscle tension can be a key feature in establishing the presence of a clinically significant lesion. The thickness of the epaxial muscles prohibits accurate assessment of deeper structures.

Pressure
Pressure on the superficial structures, such as the supraspinous ligament and the epaxial muscles, is useful to assess pain. Reliably assessing the response to pressure applied to deeper structures, such as the epaxial synovial intervertebral articulation complexes, is not possible.

Mobilization
Stimulation of movement of the thoracolumbar spine (Figure 52-4) is important to assess the amount of movement tolerated by the horse and any signs of pain, such as flexion of the limbs, alteration of facial expression, tension of the back muscles, movement of the tail, and alteration of behavior (kicking, rearing, bucking, and grunting).

The following protocol is recommended:
1. Assessment of thoracic flexion, thoracic extension, thoracolumbar extension, lumbosacral extension, and complete thoracolumbar and lumbosacral flexion in the median (sagittal) plane

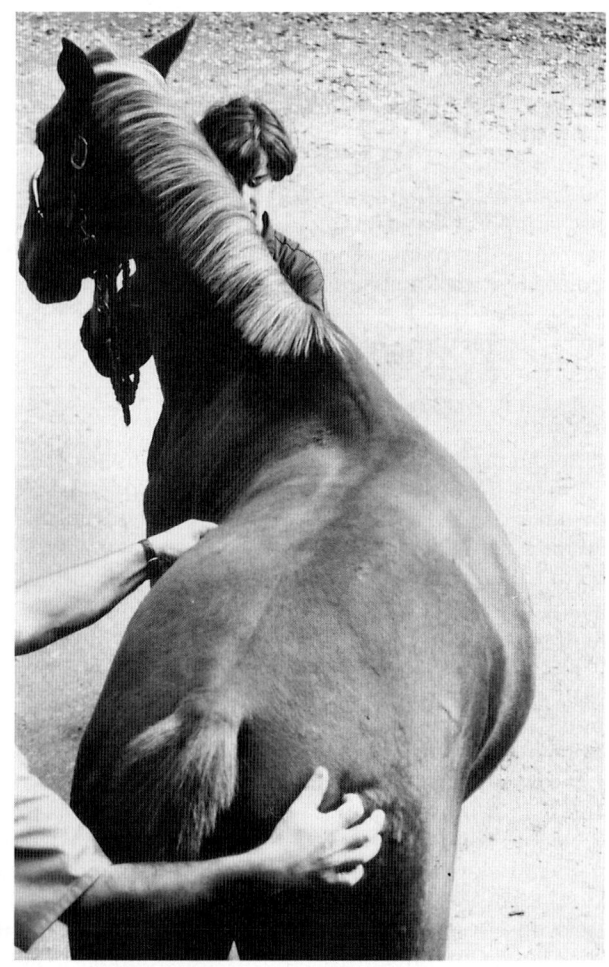

Fig. 52-4 • Physical examination by left lateral flexion of the thoracolumbar spine. The two main criteria evaluated are the amount of movement and manifestations of pain.

2. Assessment of right and left thoracolumbar lateral flexion (and rotation) (see Figure 52-4)
3. Assessment of left and right cervical (and thoracic) lateral flexion (and rotation)

The clinician should try to determine which movements are restricted or not tolerated so as to determine potential sources of pain. These movements can be induced by skin stimulation of the dorsal and lateral aspects of the trunk and hindquarters. Although some horses respond to soft digital stimulation, in others a stronger stimulus is required, for example, using the tips of a pair of artery forceps. Firm stroking with a hard instrument displaced craniocaudally and inducing spectacular wide extension and flexion movements may lack sensitivity and specificity in determining the site of back pain, but firm stroking may be necessary in extremely stoical cob-type horses to induce any movement. A normal, relaxed horse is able to flex and extend the thoracolumbar spine smoothly and repeatedly. The degree of movement reflects in part the type of horse. Cob-type horses naturally tend to have much more restricted movement than TBs or Warmbloods. The clinician will find it useful to keep one hand resting on the midback region during these maneuvers to detect induced muscle spasm or abnormal cracking of the muscles or ligaments (a crepitus-like feeling as the epaxial muscles or ligaments contract and relax). Further descriptions of assessment of thoracolumbar movement are provided in Chapter 51. Pressure algometry has been used to more objectively quantify back pain.[8,9]

Examination during Movement

Evaluation of the horse moving at walk, trot, and canter is essential to assess whether pain is present and to identify functional disorders, such as limitation of regional intervertebral mobility (Figure 52-5). The clinician should always bear in mind that impinging spinous processes can be present asymptomatically. Therefore the clinical significance of impinging spinous processes should not be overinterpreted, unless clinical signs of back pain are evident. The horse should be assessed moving in straight lines and in small circles at a walk and trot on a hard surface and moving at a trot and canter on the lunge to determine whether any reduction of back mobility is apparent (Table 52-1).

In vivo kinematic studies have quantified dorsoventral flexibility of the back in sound horses trotting[10,11] and at various gaits on the treadmill.[12] Horses with vertebral lesions showed a reduction of passive flexibility of the

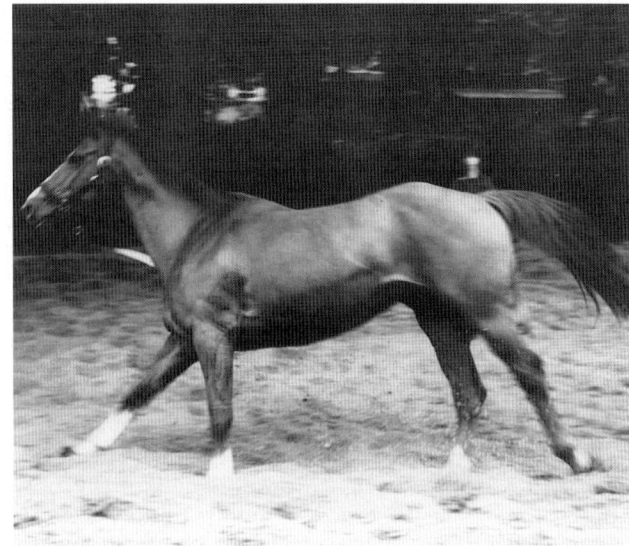

Fig. 52-5 • Dynamic examination by evaluating the active back movement at the canter on the lunge.

TABLE 52-1

Criteria Used for Evaluating Back Disorders*			
GROUND	GAIT	DIRECTION OF MOVEMENT	CRITERIA
Hard	Walk	Straight line	Rotation (tuber coxae mobility) (lateral flexion)
		Figure eight (3-m diameter)	Lateral flexion
	Trot	Left circle (7-m diameter)	Lateral flexion
		Right circle (7-m diameter)	(Passive TL flexibility)
Soft	Trot	Right circle (10-m diameter)	Passive DV flexibility (TL>LS)
			Lateral flexion
			Hindlimb propulsion
	Canter	Right circle (10-m diameter)	Active flexion and extension movements (LS>TL)
			Hindlimb protraction/propulsion
			Hindlimb placement (rotary canter)
			Coordination and balance
	Trot	Left circle (10-m diameter)	Same as above
	Canter		
Hard	Trot	Left circle (7-m diameter)	Lateral flexion
		Right circle (7-m diameter)	(Passive TL flexibility)
		Straight line	Passive DV flexibility (TL>LS): side aspect
			Rotation (tuber coxae mobility); lateral flexion: caudal aspect

TL, Thoracolumbar; *LS*, lumbosacral; *DV*, dorsoventral.
*Assessment involves a horse moving first on a hard surface, then on a soft surface, and then on a hard surface, in straight lines and circles, at walk, trot, and canter.

back at trot,[13-15] with reduced flexion and extension, lateral flexion, and rotation. Thus the horse may appear to hold its back rather stiffly. This can be caused by mechanical problems (partial or complete ankylosis) or pain. Back pain may also influence stride length and limb flight, resulting in a more restricted and less animated gait. On the lunge the horse may show loss of balance and a tendency to lean the body rather than bend the trunk toward the direction of circle. However, such clinical signs may also be seen in association with lameness, which, if bilateral, may not be obvious.

Examination of the Horse Being Ridden or in Harness

The presence and the degree of back pain may be underestimated unless the horse is evaluated under its normal working conditions, that is, ridden or in harness. The influence of a rider on mobility of the horse's back has recently been quantified.[16] The clinician should watch carefully as the tack or harness is applied, particularly as the girth is tightened. However, the clinician should bear in mind that cold-back behavior (see Chapter 97) is not necessarily a reflection of back pain, although it may be. The fit of the saddle for the horse and the rider should be evaluated. Back mobility,[3] the movements that the horse finds difficult, and the horse's attitude toward work should all be assessed (see Chapter 97). The clinician should pay attention also to the observations of the rider because the horse may feel considerably worse than it appears. The rider may describe lack of hindlimb power, lateral stiffness of the back to the left or right, unwillingness of the horse properly to take the bit, or loss of fluidity in the paces. The rider may complain of back pain induced by riding the horse.

Examination of the horse while it is ridden also gives the clinician the opportunity to assess the rider because back pain is readily induced by poor riding, a situation that may not be easy to handle diplomatically.

Local Analgesia

Diagnostic infiltration of local anesthetic solution may be useful to assess the clinical significance of impingement of spinous processes, where only the bones, ligaments, and adjacent muscles are affected by the analgesia. If impingement is severe, local anesthetic solution can only be deposited around the spinous processes and not between them. The volume of local anesthetic solution required depends on the number of spinous processes involved. Sixty to 80 mL of mepivacaine is injected at several sites using 4-cm needles if four or five impinging spinous processes exist. The response is assessed in 15 to 20 minutes and is most accurately evaluated by observing the horse while it is ridden and by the rider's feel. If kissing spines is the only clinically significant lesion, then substantial improvement should be anticipated, but if other lesions are contributing to pain, the response is limited.

If deeper injections are performed in the region of the epaxial synovial intervertebral articulations, interpretation may be confounded because the injections are effectively intramuscular injections, and the local anesthetic solution may readily diffuse to affect sites on the dorsal and ventral rami of the spinal nerves. Thus local analgesia has potentially limited value for the assessment of the clinical significance of OA of the synovial intervertebral articulations and little value for assessment of intervertebral disk disease and spondylosis.

IMAGING

Radiography and ultrasonography are essential to determine potential causes of pain or mechanical restriction. Nuclear scintigraphy is also a useful tool to detect abnormal bone activity and to help establish the clinical significance of radiological findings.

Radiography

Indications for radiographic examination of the thoracolumbar spine include owner complaints of a back problem in their horse, abnormal clinical findings, poor performance, or as part of the assessment of an obscure lameness.

The horse should stand squarely on all limbs.[17] Sedation may be necessary using detomidine (3 to 7 mg) or romifidine (12 to 25 mg). A high-output x-ray machine is necessary, with a rotating anode and an 80-kW power generator, for example.

Imaging plates or cassettes (20- × 40-cm format) with fast screens and sensitive or high-sensitive films are used to provide highly sensitive film-screen combinations. The cassettes should be placed in a vertically orientated ceiling or wall-mounted cassette holder, which can be aligned with the x-ray machine. The cassette should be placed as close to the trunk of the horse as possible. A 10:1 ratio focused grid is used to reduce radiation scatter. The focus-film distance varies between 1.15 and 1.30 m. The x-ray beam is directed perpendicular to the vertebral column axis. At least five exposures are required (Figure 52-6) to obtain a complete evaluation of the thoracolumbar spine between T10 and L4. In some horses L5 or L6 may also be imaged. The exposure parameters are summarized in Table 52-2. Additional horizontal 20° ventral oblique radiographic images are useful to assess the left and right thoracic synovial intervertebral articulations.[6] To reduce motion, the exposure is performed during the last part of expiration.

Ultrasonography

Ultrasonographic examination of all the epaxial structures is possible.[18-20] Imaging of the spinous processes and associated ligaments is performed with 7.5- or 10-MHz probes. A standoff pad is used to improve detection of the superficial structures. Imaging of the articular and transverse processes can be performed with 5- to 2.5-MHz probes. Longitudinal median and paramedian scans and transverse scans are combined to image all dorsal vertebral structures. For ultrasonographic examination the hair on the median plane over the spinous processes is removed with a No. 40 clipper blade, and the skin is cleaned. The skin is never shaved. When the hair is short (during the summer time), wetting the hair and skin with hot water for several minutes allows examination without clipping. Aqueous contact transmission gel is applied to the wet skin to couple the transducer to the skin to avoid air interference and artifacts. The lumbosacral and intertransverse lumbar and lumbosacral articulations can be assessed per rectum.[21]

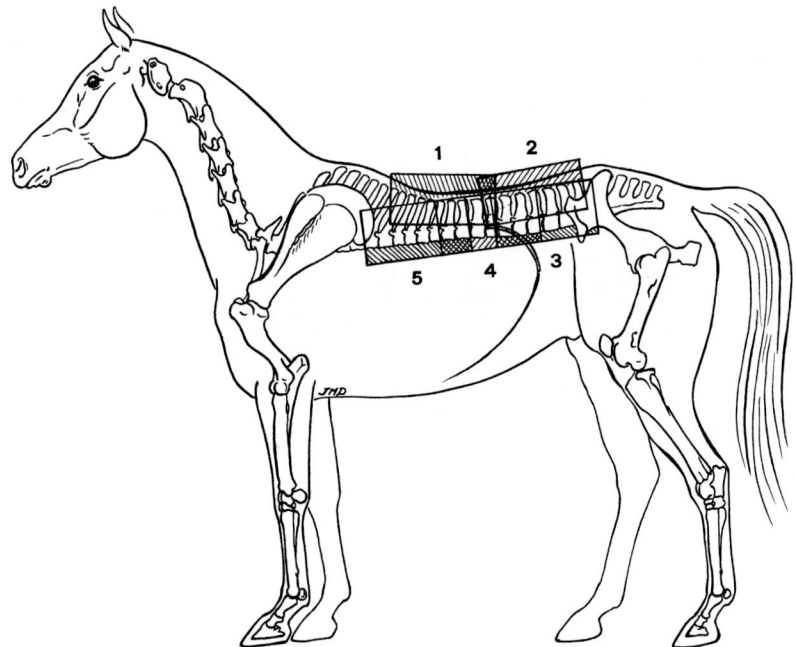

Fig. 52-6 • Position of the imaging plates for radiographic examination of the thoracolumbar spine. *1,* Thoracic spinous processes; *2,* lumbar spinous processes; *3,* lumbar vertebral bodies and synovial intervertebral articulation; *4,* thoracolumbar vertebral bodies and synovial intervertebral articulation; *5,* thoracic vertebral bodies and synovial intervertebral articulation.

TABLE 52-2

*Technical Parameters Used for the Exposure of Different Regions of the Thoracolumbar Spine**				
REGIONS	**FILM**	**KV**	**MA**	**EXPOSURE DURATION (MSEC)**
Thoracic dorsal spinous processes	Sensitive	73-77	80-110	71-107
Lumbar dorsal spinous processes	Sensitive	77-83	110-160	110-182
Midthoracic region, vertebral bodies, and facet joints (T10-T16)	High sensitive	70-77	100-140	86.5-141
Thoracolumbar junction, vertebral bodies, and facet joints (T15-L2)	High sensitive	81-85	160-250	177-344
Lumbar region, vertebral bodies, and facet joints (T18-L4)	High sensitive	85-93	280-320	406-580

*All examinations performed using a 10 : 1 grid and rare earth fast screen. Horses of 450- to 650-kg body weight.

Nuclear Scintigraphy

Patterns of radiopharmaceutical uptake (RU) in clinically normal riding horses have been described and compared with radiological findings.[22,23] In a retrospective study of 50 horses with back pain, the most common abnormal finding was increased radiopharmaceutical uptake (IRU) in the spinous processes between T12 and L2, identified in 48 horses.[24] Three horses had abnormal RU in the vertebral bodies of L3 to L6 and T11 to T14. Patterns of RU associated with OA of the synovial intervertebral articulations[25] and spondylosis[26] have been described. However, normal RU does not preclude the presence of clinically significant osseous pathology.[25,26]

Lateral or slightly oblique lateral images give the most information. Scattered radiation is a problem because of the large muscle mass overlying the vertebrae, so use of a high-resolution collimator is preferred. This requires longer acquisition times to obtain an adequate number of counts to give adequate image quality. Slight swaying movement of the horse during image acquisition and the movement of breathing detract from image quality unless motion correction software is used. The gamma camera may need to be angled slightly to avoid the kidneys being superimposed over the caudal thoracic vertebrae. At least three images are required to evaluate the entire length of the thoracolumbar spine, and comparable images from the left and right sides can be useful. If images are acquired from only one side, the right side is best because of the position of the kidney. Dorsal images are occasionally useful to clarify the anatomical position of a focus of IRU identified in a lateral image. The summits of the spinous processes in the withers region, the caudoproximal aspect of the scapula, and the kidneys may all have greater normal RU than the rest of the thoracolumbar spine and may effectively conceal lesions (Figure 52-7). Masking these areas out after image acquisition potentially results in more information. Using a high-frequency filter can also yield additional information, making a subtle focus of IRU more obvious, and

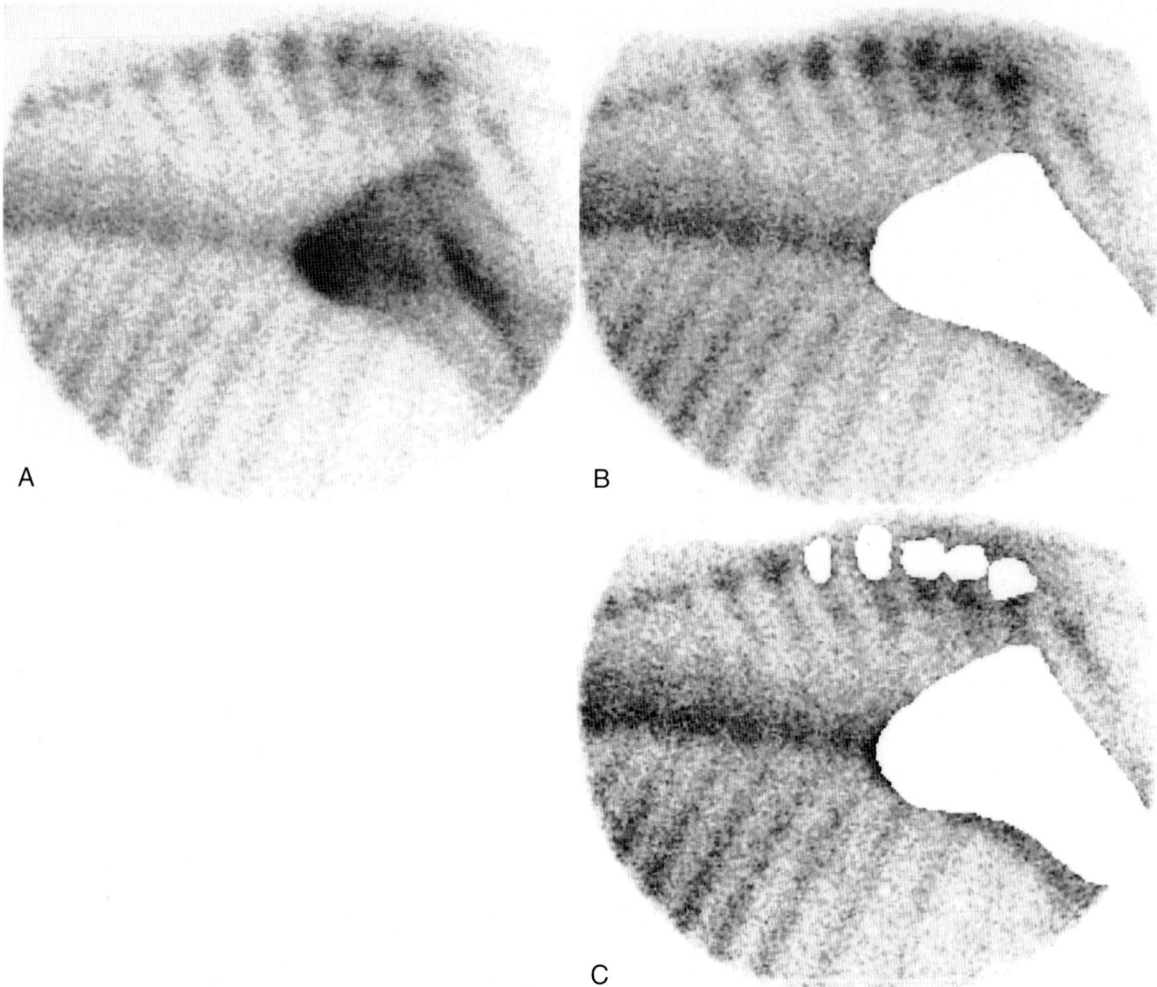

Fig. 52-7 • A, Motion-corrected scintigraphic image of the cranial thoracic vertebrae without a filter. There is greater radiopharmaceutical uptake (RU) in the summits of the spinous processes in the withers region and the scapula than elsewhere. **B,** The same image as **A** after masking the scapula. **C,** The same image as **A** after masking the summits of the spinous processes at the withers and the caudal aspect of the scapula. Masking increases the information available. These images show normal patterns of RU.

facilitating anatomical localization of IRU. Image resolution in fat horses may be compromised by scattered radiation in the soft tissues.

Thermography

Normal thermographic patterns of the thoracolumbar region have been described.[27] Thermography may be useful in identifying acute superficial muscle injuries or demonstrating to an owner the impact of a poorly fitting saddle or a rider sitting crookedly. However, in horses with chronic back pain, thermography does not usually add useful information and lacks sensitivity and specificity.

LESIONS

Spinal Processes and Associated Ligaments

Impingement of the Dorsal Spinous Processes: Kissing Spines and Overriding Spinous Processes

Impingement of the summits of the spinous processes, or kissing spines, is a well-known pathological entity of the horse's back[28]; however, it is important to recognize that

lesions may not be restricted to the summits, and the entire length of the spinous processes must be evaluated. The most common location of these lesions is the vertebral segment between T10 and T18 (Figure 52-8), although lesions also occur between L1 and L6.[17] Modeling of the dorsal aspect of a spinous process or an avulsion fracture reflects an insertional lesion of the supraspinous ligament. We grade impingement of the dorsal part of the spinous processes as follows:

- Grade 1: Narrowing of the interspinous space with mild increased opacity of the cortical margins of the spinous processes
- Grade 2: Loss of the interspinous space with moderate increased opacity of the cortical margins of the spinous processes
- Grade 3: Severe increased opacity of the cortical margins of the spinous processes, caused in part by transverse thickening, or radiolucent areas
- Grade 4: Severe increased opacity of the cortical margins, osteolysis, and change in shape of the spinous processes; overriding (overlap) of the spinous processes

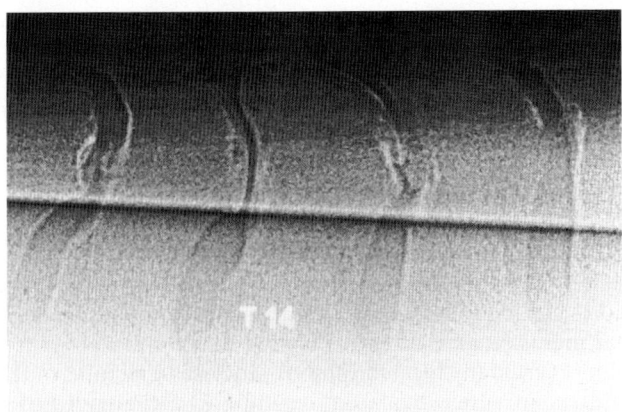

Fig. 52-8 • Lateral radiographic image of the spinous processes of the twelfth to sixteenth thoracic vertebrae. Cranial is to the left. There are radiological signs of impingement of the spinous processes between the eleventh and sixteenth thoracic vertebrae, with clinically significant marginal bone remodeling. *T14,* Fourteenth thoracic vertebra.

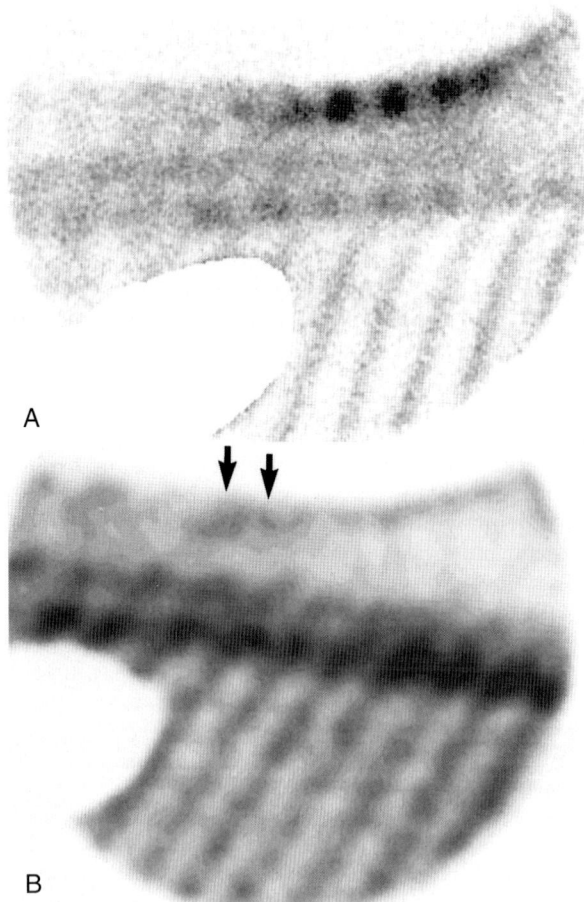

Fig. 52-9 • A, Lateral nuclear scintigraphic image of the thoracolumbar region of a 10-year-old Grand Prix dressage horse with loss of action. There is increased radiopharmaceutical uptake (IRU) in the dorsal aspects of six adjacent spinous processes. The horse showed clinical signs of restricted mobility of the back. Radiographic examination revealed impinging spinous processes. The horse's gait was dramatically improved by infiltration of local anesthetic solution around the affected spinous processes. **B,** Lateral nuclear scintigraphic image of the thoracic region of an 8-year-old show jumper gelding with stiffness of the thoracolumbar region and poor hindlimb impulsion. A high-resolution filter has been applied to the image. There is mild IRU in the summits of two spinous processes in the caudal thoracic region *(arrows).* However, five adjacent spinous processes were impinging, and infiltration of local anesthetic solution produced a profound clinical improvement. No soft tissue lesions were identified by ultrasonography.

Overriding of spinous processes is a congenital condition with abnormal orientation of the spinous processes and similar changes in the margins of adjacent spinous processes. Other congenital abnormalities include complete fusion of two adjacent spinous processes or "webs" of spinous processes, or bony bridges between one or more adjacent spinous processes. The contour of the middle part of a spinous process may be altered because of enthesophyte formation at the insertion of the interspinous ligaments. Kissing lesions may also be seen at the ventral part of a spinous process with type 4 lesions of the epaxial synovial intervertebral articulation (see page 601). Generally speaking, the more severe and extensive the radiological abnormalities, the more likely they are to be of clinical significance; however, two close spinous processes may be associated with pain in a horse with a low pain threshold.

Ultrasonographic examination can easily demonstrate contact or modeling between two adjacent spinous processes, transverse thickening of the processes, and abnormal alignment. However, ultrasonography is more useful to assess concomitant supraspinous ligament lesions, including insertion desmopathies (enthesopathies) on the summits of the spinous processes.

Nuclear scintigraphy can help identify evidence of active bone modeling of the spinous processes and other potential lesions. However, one must bear in mind that active bone modeling is not synonymous with pain. Increased modeling of the dorsal aspects of the spinous processes may reflect impingement or insertional desmopathy of the supraspinous ligament (Figure 52-9). The degree of IRU does not always appear to be well correlated with the severity of the clinical signs or the radiological abnormalities (see Figure 52-9, *A*). Obvious focal IRU can be seen in horses with neither back pain nor radiological abnormality, whereas some horses with back pain associated with impinging spinous processes have only mild IRU. Mechanical limitations may contribute to back stiffness, which may predispose to the development of other lesions.

Kissing spines can be found in performance horses with no clinical manifestations of back pain. Therefore the clinical significance of kissing spines must be carefully assessed. Kissing spines may also be present with another vertebral lesion, which may have a greater influence on prognosis; therefore a comprehensive evaluation of all structures should be performed, even if kissing spines have been identified. Radiological findings should be carefully correlated with the results of the physical examination and preferably with nuclear scintigraphic examination and the response to local analgesia.

Desmopathies: Supraspinous Ligament Injuries

Injuries of the supraspinous ligament occur most commonly between T15 and L3 and may be associated with palpable localized thickening and pain. Lesions are identified best by ultrasonography[18,19]; however, it is important to recognize that regions of altered echogenicity can be seen in some clinically normal horses.[30]

Thickening of the supraspinous ligament induces a local deformation (bump) of the dorsal profile of the thoracolumbar area, which can be measured by ultrasonography and compared with two adjacent equivalent locations. Lesions usually occur at a spinous process, sometimes extending between two adjacent spinous processes. The normal supraspinous ligament is uniformly echogenic (Figure 52-10). Hypoechogenic lesions in the deep and intermediate part of the supraspinous ligament (Figure 52-11) are compatible with recent or chronic desmopathies of the supraspinous ligament. Hyperechogenic foci, with or without acoustic shadows, may be seen in the supraspinous ligament. They reflect chronic or old desmopathy. Insertion desmopathy (enthesopathy) of the supraspinous ligament can be identified by irregularity of the surface of the spinous process, with a thicker appearance. Alteration of echogenicity and fiber orientation occurs in the supraspinous ligament.

With low-exposure radiographs, the soft tissue thickening and some focal radiopacities may be seen in horses with long-standing injuries. Avulsion fractures or bone modeling and increased opacity of the dorsal surface of the spinous processes may also be noted.[29]

Nuclear scintigraphic examination may reveal IRU in the summit of one or more spinous processes in association with insertional lesions of the supraspinous ligament.

Fractures of Spinous Processes

Fractures of the spinous processes usually occur in the withers region as the result of the horse falling over backwards. However, other traumatic episodes, such as the horse getting stuck under a dividing rail between two compartments of a trailer or lorry (van), may result in fractures of more caudally located spinous processes. Fractures of the withers are often displaced, resulting in a change in conformation. There is generally focal pain and swelling, as well as marked back stiffness. An affected horse moves in a restricted fashion, often plaiting the forelimbs. Diagnosis is confirmed by radiographic or scintigraphic examination. Although the radiological abnormalities may be dramatic, the prognosis is generally favorable with conservative management. A purpose-fitted saddle may be required to accommodate the change in the horse's shape.

Articular Processes: Synovial Intervertebral Articulations

Normal Anatomy

The articular processes' synovial intervertebral articulation complex is located dorsal to the vertebral canal and is composed of the caudal articular process of one vertebra, the joint space, and the cranial articular process of the following vertebra (Figures 52-12 through 52-14).[17]

On lateral radiographic images, in the middle of the film, the left and right synovial intervertebral articulations are superimposed. On the extremities of the film, the images of the left and right synovial intervertebral articulations are progressively dissociated because of the divergent x-ray beam. In some horses the ribs are extremely convex dorsally and are superimposed over the thoracic and the first lumbar synovial intervertebral articulations, prohibiting assessment. Oblique radiographic images from left to right and right to left permit evaluation of the left and right synovial intervertebral articulations independently.[6]

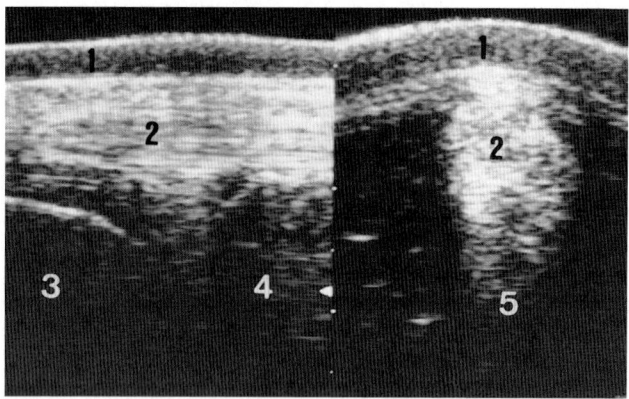

Fig. 52-10 • Median *(left)* and transverse *(right)* ultrasonographic images of the normal supraspinous ligament in the lumbar area. *1,* Skin; *2,* supraspinous ligament; *3,* second lumbar vertebra; *4,* third lumbar vertebra; *5,* interspinous ligament.

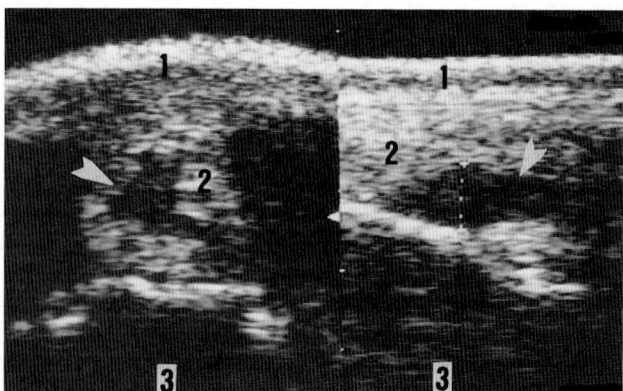

Fig. 52-11 • Transverse *(left)* and median *(right)* ultrasonographic images indicate supraspinous desmopathy. The ligament is thickened and presents a central hypoechogenic zone *(arrowheads)*. *1,* Skin; *2,* supraspinous ligament; *3,* seventeenth thoracic spinous process.

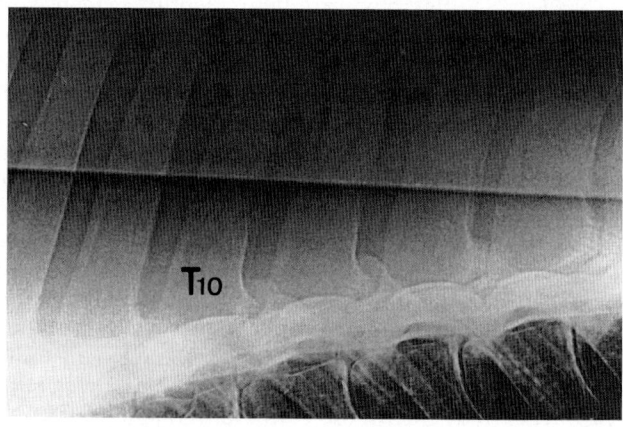

Fig. 52-12 • Normal radiological appearance of the synovial intervertebral articulations in the midthoracic area. Cranial is to the left. *T10,* Tenth thoracic vertebra.

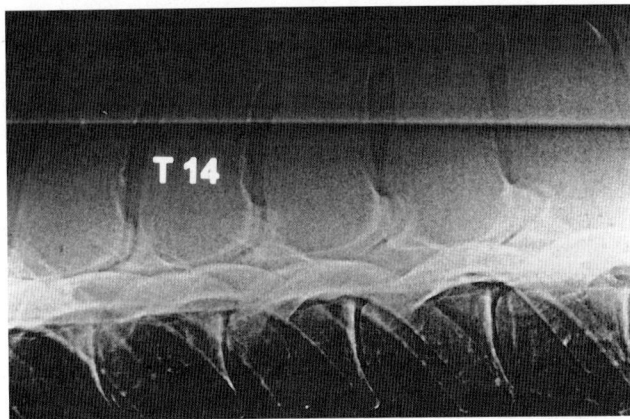

Fig. 52-13 • Normal radiological appearance of the synovial intervertebral articulations in the caudal thoracic area. Cranial is to the left. *T14,* Fourteenth thoracic vertebra.

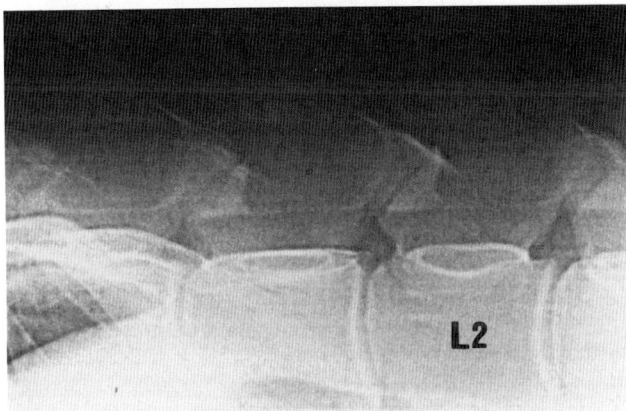

Fig. 52-14 • Normal radiological appearance of the synovial intervertebral articulations in the lumbar area. Cranial is to the left. *L2,* Second lumbar vertebra.

The radiolucent cartilaginous joint space is thin and more clearly defined in the thoracic areas, where the articular facets are flat (see Figure 52-12), than in the lumbar area because of the condylar shape. Between T12 and T16 the joint space is a wide V shape, with a cranial oblique branch and a shorter vertical caudal branch (see Figure 52-13). At the thoracolumbar junction and in the lumbar region the joint space is less well defined. Usually, the joint space is linear and makes a 40-degree angle with the horizontal (see Figure 52-14). The caudal articular process is dorsal to the corresponding intervertebral foramen and is triangular with a caudal apex in the lumbar region. The thickness of the dense subchondral bone of the cranial articular process increases caudally. The cranial articular process is extended dorsocranially by a mammillary process, which is larger in the thoracic area than in the lumbar area.

On transverse ultrasonographic images obtained using 2.5- to 5-MHz probes, the synovial intervertebral articulations can be imaged (Figure 52-15). On each side the joint space separating the cranial (lateral) and caudal (medial) articular process can be identified.[19] This joint space is limited dorsally by a thin articular capsule. Comparison of the left and right synovial intervertebral articulations of

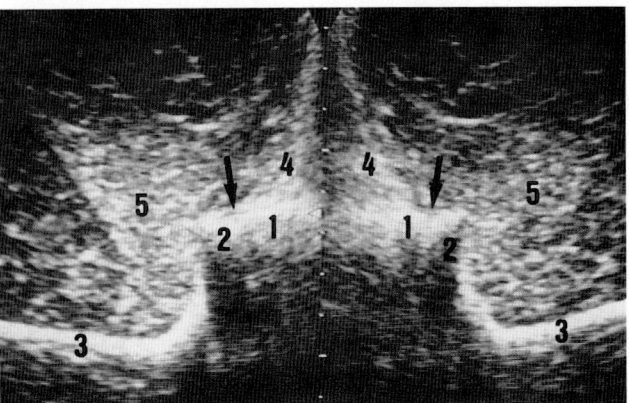

Fig. 52-15 • Transverse ultrasonographic image of the synovial intervertebral articulations between the first and second lumbar vertebrae shows normal appearance (compare with Figure 52-3). *1,* Caudal articular process of first lumbar vertebra; *2,* cranial articular process of second lumbar vertebra; *3,* transverse process of second lumbar vertebra; *4,* multifidus muscle; *5,* longissimus muscle; *arrow,* joint space of the epaxial synovial intervertebral articulation.

TABLE 52-3

	Types of Radiographic Lesions of the Thoracolumbar Synovial Intervertebral Articulations	
TYPES	**GENERAL CRITERIA**	**RADIOLOGICAL SIGNS**
1	Asymmetry	No clear joint space; double joint space
2	Modification of opacity of the articular process	Increased radiopacity of the subchondral bone Increased opacity of the synovial intervertebral articulations
3		Radiolucent areas in the subchondral bone Increased opacity of the articular process
4	Periarticular proliferation	Dorsal periarticular proliferation Increased size of the synovial intervertebral articulations Often associated with alteration in opacity of subchondral bone
5		Ventral periarticular proliferation
6	Ankylosis	Dorsal bridge between two adjacent vertebrae
7		Osteolysis of the synovial intervertebral articulations No joint space
8	Fracture	Radiolucent line on the caudal (or cranial) articular process

the same intervertebral joint is helpful to assess size and shape.

Abnormal Findings
Eight types of abnormal radiological findings associated with OA have been identified in the synovial intervertebral articulations of the equine thoracolumbar spine[6,17] (Table 52-3). These findings were mainly present at the

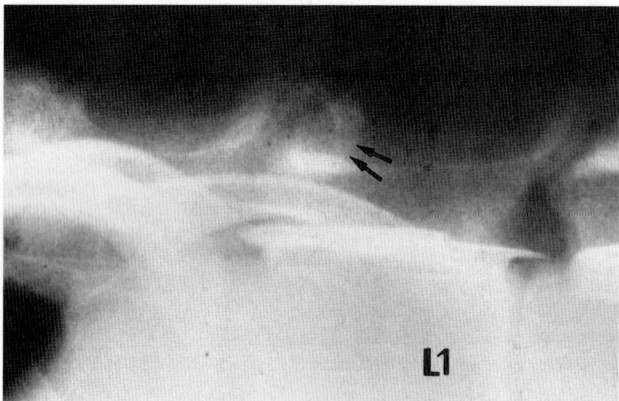

Fig. 52-16 • Lateral radiographic image of the thoracolumbar junction. Cranial is to the left. There are type 2 lesions *(arrows)* of the synovial intervertebral articulations between the eighteenth thoracic and first lumbar vertebrae in this 5-year-old French trotter male. Compare with the opacity of the cranial articular processes in Figure 52-14. *L1,* First lumbar vertebra.

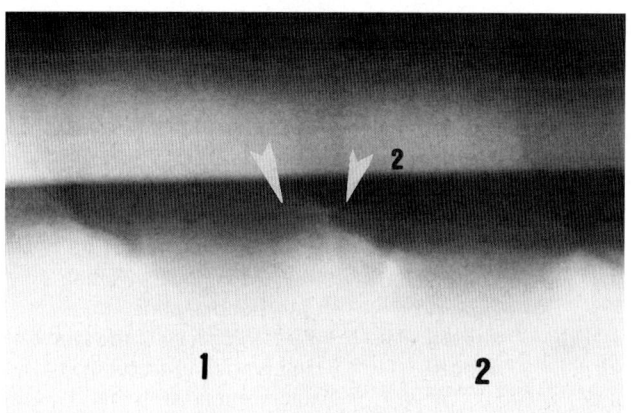

Fig. 52-17 • Lateral radiographic image of the cranial lumbar vertebrae. Cranial is to the left. There is a mild (grade 1) type 4 lesion of the synovial intervertebral articulation complex between the first *(1)* and second *(2)* lumbar vertebrae in this 8-year-old mare.

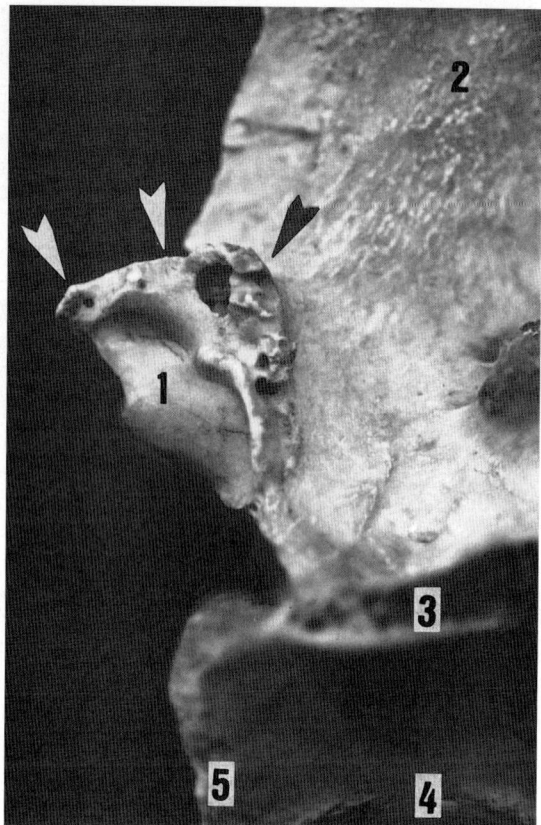

Fig. 52-18 • Bone specimen showing a moderate (grade 2) type 4 lesion *(arrowheads)* of the caudal articular process of the third lumbar vertebra. *1,* Caudal articular process; *2,* dorsal spinous process; *3,* transverse process; *4,* vertebral body; *5,* vertebral fossa.

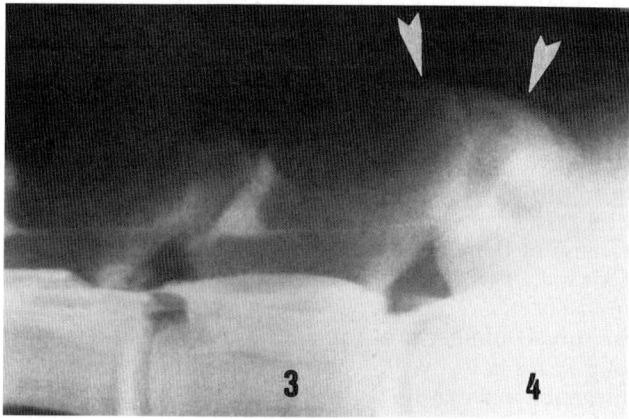

Fig. 52-19 • Lateral radiographic image of the midlumbar vertebrae. Cranial is to the left. There is a severe (grade 3) type 4 lesion *(arrowheads)* of the synovial intervertebral articulation between the third *(3)* and fourth *(4)* lumbar vertebrae in this 12-year-old mare.

thoracolumbar junction and in the lumbar area. Types 2, 4, and 6 (Figures 52-16 to 52-19) were mainly found between T16 and L3. Types 5 and 7 have mainly been found in the lumbar area. However, lesions may occur anywhere from T9 to L5.[6] Abnormalities have been found in mature riding horses and immature racehorses.

Dorsal periarticular proliferation (types 4 and 6) can be imaged with ultrasonography, and with this procedure determining whether the proliferation is symmetrical or, if not, which side is the most affected is possible (Figure 52-20).

Nuclear scintigraphy can be helpful in identifying evidence of abnormal bone modeling in the region of synovial intervertebral articulations, especially in horses where radiological appraisal is limited by the ribs. There was a strong association between the presence of moderate or intense IRU and radiological abnormalities in a study of 65 horses with back pain and radiological evidence of OA, whereas in 31 horses with no evidence of back pain RU was generally normal.[25]

In our experience, synovial intervertebral articulation lesions are much more consistently associated with back pain than are kissing spines. However, in a series of 644 horses with thoracolumbar region pain, only 77 (12%) had OA of the synovial intervertebral articulations, 47 of which had concurrent impinging or overriding dorsal spinous processes.[6]

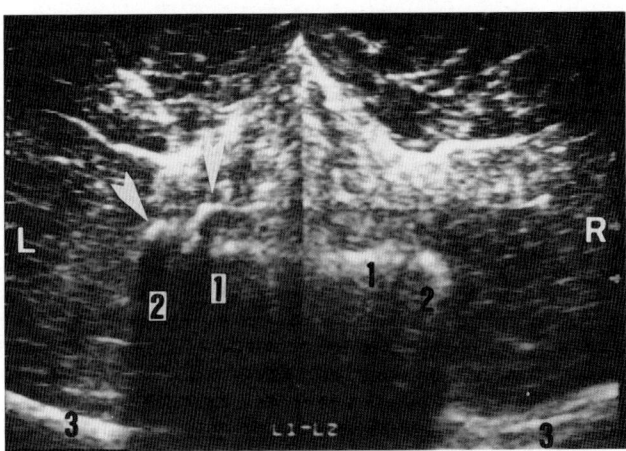

Fig. 52-20 • Transverse ultrasonographic image of the synovial intervertebral articulation between the first and second lumbar vertebrae in a 5-year-old French trotter mare: on the left side *(L)* a dorsal periarticular osteophyte is present *(arrowheads)*. *1,* Caudal articular process of first lumbar vertebra; *2,* cranial articular process of second lumbar vertebra; *3,* transverse process of second lumbar vertebra.

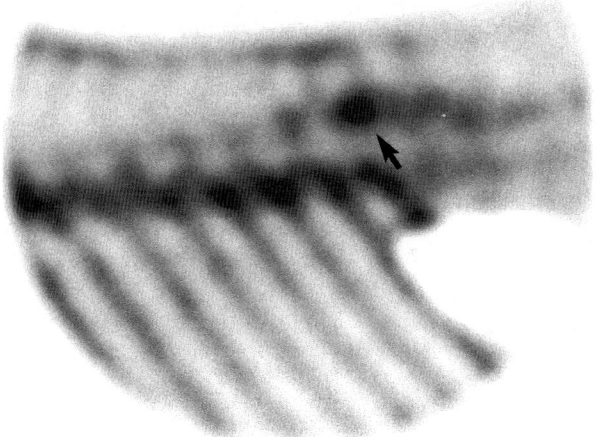

Fig. 52-22 • Lateral scintigraphic image of the thoracolumbar region of a 2-year-old Thoroughbred filly with back pain and loss of performance. There is a focal region of increased radiopharmaceutical uptake at the thoracolumbar junction *(arrow)*, compatible with a laminar stress fracture.

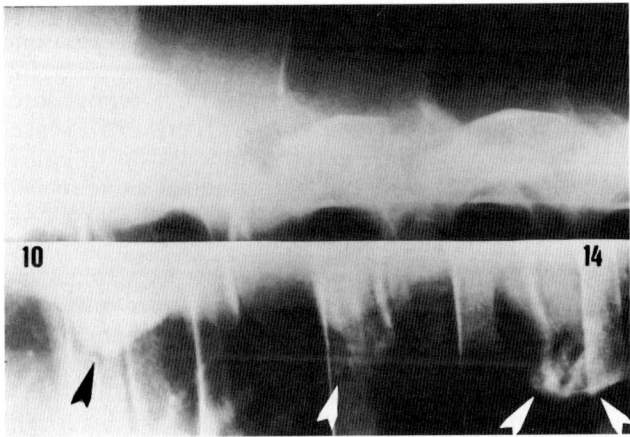

Fig. 52-21 • Lateral radiographic image of the vertebral bodies of the caudal thoracic vertebrae. Cranial is to the left. There is extensive ventral spondylosis *(arrowheads)* between the tenth *(10)* and fourteenth *(14)* thoracic vertebrae in this 13-year-old international show jumper stallion.

Vertebral Bodies and Disks of the Thoracolumbar Region

Lesions of the vertebral bodies are less commonly found in horses[28] and cannot be imaged by ultrasonography in the thoracolumbar area (except caudal to L4 with a transrectal approach). These lesions include the following[17,28,31,32]:

1. Ventral, ventrolateral, or lateral bony proliferation (often called vertebral spondylosis); these lesions are mainly found in the midthoracic area (Figure 52-21), but they can be seen in the lumbar area. Lesions range from small osseous spurs to complete bone bridges resulting in ankylosis. Although single lesions can occur, often several adjacent vertebrae are affected.[28]
2. Vertebral body deformation (trapezoid shape) of the caudal thoracic vertebrae
3. Deformation of the adjacent vertebral head and fossa (disk enthesopathy) found in the caudal thoracic area

4. Ski jump deformation (dorsal bony extension of the vertebral fossa) found in the caudal thoracic area
5. Fracture
6. Subluxation and intervertebral disk compression or protrusion

These lesions have been found in horses with a history or clinical manifestations of back pain—acute, intermittent, and chronic—and are considered to be of likely clinical significance. However, spondylosis also is an incidental finding in low-level performance horses with no history or clinical manifestations of back pain. Spondylosis was identified in 23 of 670 (3.3%) horses with back pain, usually occurring between T10 and T14.[26] There was a range of one to five lesions (mean 2.3). However, only nine of the 23 horses had spondylosis as the sole osseous lesion; the remainder also had impingement of the dorsal spinous processes and/or OA of the synovial intervertebral articulations. Nuclear scintigraphy may help to identify spondylosis and to elucidate the clinical significance of these findings in horses with back pain; however, not all lesions have IRU. In 17 of 23 horses with spondylosis that underwent scintigraphic evaluation, 64.7% had IRU associated with spondylosis, but only 33.3% of horses with lesions identified radiologically had IRU.[26] Extensive spondylosis may potentially limit back mobility, despite the absence of IRU.

Fracture and/or subluxation of a thoracolumbar vertebral body normally results in neurological abnormalities, but occasionally horses have acute severe back pain, with rapid atrophy of the epaxial musculature, but no evidence of ataxia.

Vertebral laminar stress fractures have been identified using nuclear scintigraphy in young TB flat race horses with loss of performance and clinical evidence of back pain (Figure 52-22). They have been seen most commonly at the thoracolumbar junction and in the lumbar vertebrae. In a post mortem sample of TB race horses, 18 (50%) of 36 specimens had evidence of vertebral stress fractures.[33]

The Lumbosacral Joint

The lumbosacral joint (see also Chapter 50) and the intertransverse joints are evaluated ultrasonographically per rectum. Clinically significant abnormalities include[21]:

1. Congenital lumbosacral ankylosis, with reduced size or absence of the intervertebral disk
2. Focal loss of echogenicity of the intervertebral disk consistent with disk degeneration
3. Focal hyperechogenic regions in the intervertebral disk consistent with dystrophic mineralization
4. Ventral herniation of the intervertebral disk
5. Ventral subluxation of the sacrum
6. Osseous irregularities of the intertransverse articulation(s)

Muscle Injury

See Chapter 83 for a discussion of muscle injury.

PROGNOSIS

The prognosis for horses with any back lesion depends on a number of factors, including the individual pain tolerance of the horse, the skill of the rider and trainer, the discipline in which the horse is involved, and the type, number, and severity of lesions. Vertebral lesions are tolerated better by flat race horses than by Three Day Event horses, show jumpers, and dressage horses. Racing trotters tolerate vertebral lesions poorly. The prognosis for each lesion is not influenced by the level of work but more by the rider's or trainer's ability to exploit the horse despite its problems. A horse with an acute isolated supraspinous ligament injury has a good long-term prognosis, whereas horses with restricted mobility of the back caused by extensive kissing spines or type 6 or 7 synovial intervertebral articulation lesions have a poor prognosis. Horses with grades 3 and 4 dorsal kissing spines have a guarded prognosis, as do those with ventral kissing spine lesions. The prognosis for horses with synovial intervertebral articulation lesions depends on severity and the number of joints affected. Horse tolerance of ventral thoracic spondylosis seems to vary more, but generally the larger the number of vertebrae affected, the poorer the prognosis.

SPECIFIC MANAGEMENT

The general aims of management of back problems are to remove pain and to make the horse as comfortable as possible, as soon as possible, to allow it to be exercised to avoid further muscle loss and to promote muscle function and strength. Medical treatment aims to remove pain and muscle spasm.

Systemic Treatment

Treatment of horses with back pain with nonsteroidal anti-inflammatory drugs (NSAIDs) usually has disappointing results. Many horses are brought in for in-depth investigation of the cause of back pain because of lack of response to treatment with phenylbutazone or other NSAIDs. Treatment of muscle spasm with myorelaxants is indicated and sometimes useful; for example, thiocolchicoside (2 to

4 mg/100 kg twice weekly for 4 weeks) and methocarbamol (10 mg/kg intravenously). Repeated treatments may be necessary.

Intravenous infusion of tiludronate has resulted in improvement in clinical signs associated with OA of the synovial intervertebral articulations[37] and may also be indicated for treatment of osseous abnormalities associated with the lumbosacral joint.

Local Injections

Local perispinal or interspinal injections of corticosteroids, sometimes in association with myorelaxants or Sarapin (High Chemical Company, Levittown, Pennsylvania, United States), are used to treat horses with kissing spines: flumethasone (0.5 to 1 mg/injection site with a maximum total dose of 4 mg); dexamethasone (isonicotinate, 1.5 to 2.5 mg/injection site, with a maximum total dose of 10 mg); or methylprednisolone acetate (40 to 60 mg/injection site, with a maximum total dose of 200 mg).

Horses with OA of the synovial intervertebral articulations are treated by deep paramedian injections of corticosteroids (see the previous discussion) into the multifidus muscle on each side at the level of the lesion, 2 cm apart from the median plane, using 9- to 11-cm needles. These local injections are best performed using ultrasonographic guidance (Figure 52-23). Injections are made into the multifidus muscles that provide proprioceptive information on intervertebral movements. Therefore we suggest that the use of Sarapin is contraindicated in this situation. Local infiltrations can be performed alone or with mesotherapy.

Horses with lesions of the lumbosacral joint are treated by deep paramedian injection of corticosteroids with Sarapin or local anesthetic solution under ultrasound guidance.[21] The needle is inserted 4 cm from the median plane on a line connecting the cranial aspects of the tubera coxae. The needle is directed obliquely caudally and is inserted under the ilial wing until contact is made with

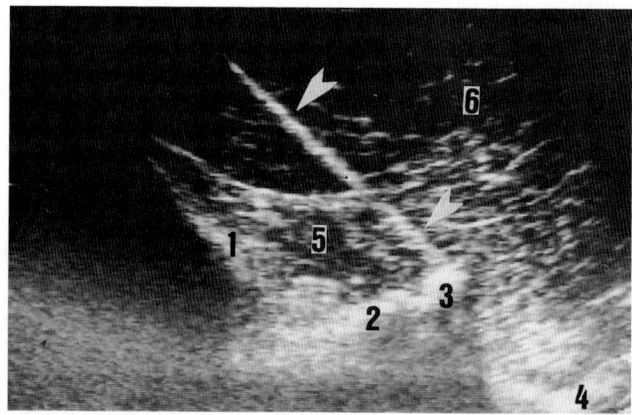

Fig. 52-23 • Transverse ultrasonographic image showing an ultrasound-guided periarticular injection for the treatment of synovial intervertebral articulation arthropathies. The probe is placed on a paramedian position; thus the image is slightly oblique. *1,* Spinous process; *2,* caudal articular process of first lumbar vertebra; *3,* cranial articular process of second lumbar vertebra; *4,* transverse process; *5,* multifidus muscle; *6,* longissimus muscle; *arrowheads,* needle.

bone in the vicinity of the axial aspect of the lumbosacral intertransverse joint. This is repeated on the left and right sides.

Mesotherapy

Mesotherapy is a technique that has been used for more than 40 years in France and consists of intradermal injections with short and thin needles (5 mm long) in the dermatomes corresponding to the site(s) of the lesion(s).

The principle is based on the theory of the gait control of pain, which takes place in the dorsal horn of the spinal cord. According to this theory, which is currently controversial, type I and II nerve fibers coming from the skin have collateral fibers that can inhibit the conduction of information in the spinothalamic fasciculus, transmitting painful information from deep structures of the same spinal segment to the thalamus and cerebrum.

After aseptic preparation of the skin, mesotherapeutic injections are usually made using a local anesthetic solution (lidocaine, 140 mg), a short-acting corticosteroid (dexamethasone, 15 mg), and a myorelaxant (thiocolchicoside, 20 mg). Injection with only saline solution may also have beneficial effects. Because most horses are sensitive to the procedure, the horse is placed in stocks, and the use of a twitch and sedation are recommended. A multiinjector (Coveto, Montaigu, France) is used. These intradermal injections are performed at the level of the lesion and caudal to it, taking into account the caudal orientation of the segmental nerves. For example, if one is treating kissing spines between T10 and T15, the treated region extends from T10 to L1. If the lesions involve the synovial intervertebral articulation between T17 and L2, the treated area should extend between T17 and the lumbosacral junction. If lesions are at the lumbosacral junction, the treated area should extend caudally to the croup. Two to three rows of injections are made on each side of the median plane.

After local injections or mesotherapy, the horse is restricted to light work on the lunge, without a surcingle, for 3 days. Normal training is progressively resumed over 5 days. A substantial improvement is anticipated within 7 to 14 days. If improvement is limited, mesotherapy should be repeated 2 to 3 weeks after the first treatment. The expected duration of action varies between 3 and more than 12 months. In horses with chronic pain, ideally a maximum of two local infiltrations should be performed each year with, or alternately with, mesotherapy.

Acupuncture

Acupuncture can be useful for treating chronic pain in some horses (see Chapter 92); however, relief of clinical signs may only be short term.[34]

TRAINING MANAGEMENT

With the medical treatment to reduce pain, modification of the training program is an essential part of the management of back problems.[35] The aims of the exercise management are to avoid further muscle atrophy and to develop the back proprioceptive control and intervertebral stability. Rest is contraindicated, except in untreatable horses that are not improved by any kind of treatment and

management. The general recommendations include the following:
- Check the saddle fitting.
- In young horses, recognize that training must be progressive.
- Use a progressive warm-up program, first on the lunge without a saddle, then on the lunge with a saddle, then with the rider at walk, and so on. The use of a Pessoa or chambon when the horse is worked on the lunge may be of benefit.
- After the warm-up period at the walk, in sports horses, first work at the canter rather than at the trot. During cantering, the vertebral column undergoes only one slow and active flexion/extension cycle per stride, whereas the vertebral column undergoes two passive flexion/extension movements per stride at the trot.
- Identify and then remove every exercise that induces discomfort. For example, do no short turns to the right for 2 weeks, and then reassess if the horse is more comfortable turning to the right.

Some physical exercises, such as lowering of the neck (flexion of the cervicothoracic junction), may have a therapeutic value because they induce an associated thoracic flexion, which provides more support to the weight of the rider. A separation of the spinous processes reduces the contact between them.[35,36] An elongation of the strong epaxial muscles reduces muscle contraction.[35]

Exercises to increase hypaxial muscle strength may also be of clinically significant benefit.

ALTERNATIVE MEDICINES

Much interest exists in using alternative therapeutic techniques to manage back pain in horses. Once a clear diagnosis is established, alternative techniques, if appropriately applied and objectively assessed for each pathological entity, may be useful adjunctively in managing horses with back pain (see Chapters 93 through 96). Collaboration with a specialized physiotherapist or chiropractor may be of major benefit.

SURGERY

Surgical treatment of kissing spines by resection of the summit of one or more spinous processes has been successful in some horses that had not responded to conservative management.[39-42] Case selection is important and should be restricted to horses with lesions only involving the dorsal aspect of the spinous processes, without other clinically significant osseous abnormalities. A postoperative convalescent period of 6 months is generally required. Twenty-seven of 50 Warmblood horses (54%) used for dressage or show jumping returned to full athletic function at the previous level of performance.[39] One hundred fifty of 209 horses (72%) used for various disciplines returned to full work after removal of the summits of one to six dorsal spinous processes, although the level of work was not specified.[40] There was no significant difference between the number of spines removed and the outcome; however, in the authors' experience, the greater the number of spinous processes affected, the more guarded the prognosis for return to full athletic function as a sports horse.

Chapter 53

The Cervical Spine and Soft Tissues of the Neck

Sue J. Dyson

This chapter discusses disorders of the neck that may give rise to lameness or poor performance or result in an abnormal neck shape, abnormal neck posture at rest or while moving, or neck stiffness. Transient neurological conditions, conditions caused by trauma resulting in other injuries, and gait abnormalities that may be confused with lameness are considered, but those associated with compression of the cervical spinal cord are discussed in Chapter 60.

ANATOMY

The neck consists of seven cervical vertebrae, which articulate both by intercentral articulations and by synovial articulations, which have large joint capsules to accommodate the degree of movement between adjacent vertebrae. Interposed between the vertebral bodies are intervertebral fibrocartilages to which is attached the dorsal longitudinal ligament, which lies on the floor of the vertebral canal. The ligamentum flavum connects the arches of adjacent vertebrae. The atlas (the first cervical vertebra) and the axis (the second cervical vertebra) have a unique shape and specialized joints. The atlanto-occipital joint is a ginglymus joint, which permits flexion and extension and also a small amount of lateral oblique movement. The atlantoaxial joint is a trochoid or pivot joint; the atlas and head rotate on the axis. The ligament of the dens is strong and fan shaped and extends from the dorsal surface of the odontoid peg (dens) to the ventral arch of the axis. The ligamentum nuchae extends from the occiput to the withers and consists of funicular and lamellar parts. The lamellar part separates the two lateral muscle groups. The atlantal bursa is interposed between the funicular part of the ligamentum nuchae and the dorsal arch of the atlas; a second bursa may exist between the ligament and the spine of the axis. The muscles of the neck can be divided into lateral and ventral groups. The neck has eight cervical nerves, the first of which emerges through the intervertebral foramen of the atlas, the second through that of the axis, and the eighth between the seventh cervical vertebra and the first thoracic vertebra. The sixth to eighth cervical nerves contribute to the brachial plexus.

REASONS FOR CLINICAL PRESENTATION

A horse may be presented for evaluation of the neck for a variety of reasons. The horse may have a history of a fall on the neck while jumping, having reared up and fallen over backward, or having collided with another horse or solid object, thus sustaining neck trauma. The horse may have neck pain from having pulled backward while being tied up. The horse may have no history of trauma but have abnormal neck posture, swelling, a stiff neck, neck pain, or difficulties in lowering and raising the head. The horse may have a performance-related problem such as unwillingness to work on the bit, an unsteady head carriage, or abnormal head posture. A neck lesion should also be considered in a horse with forelimb lameness when pain cannot be localized to the limb. Subtle hindlimb gait abnormalities, such as a tendency to stumble, may be caused by a neurological deficit without overt ataxia, reflecting a compressive lesion of the cervical spinal cord.

CLINICAL EXAMINATION

It is important to recognize that head and neck carriage depends in part on conformation: the way in which the neck comes out of the shoulder and the shape of the neck. The shape of the neck is also influenced by the way in which the horse works. If a horse carries the head and neck high, with the head somewhat extended, the ventral strap muscles tend to be abnormally well developed, resulting in a ewe-neck conformation. Many horses naturally bend more easily to the right than to the left or vice versa, and the muscles on the side of the neck, especially dorsocranially, are developed asymmetrically. Such asymmetry is particularly obvious if the neck is viewed from above by the rider. If a horse is excessively thin, then the cervical vertebrae become prominent and the caudodorsal neck region becomes dorsally concave, whereas in a fit, well-muscled horse that works regularly on the bit, this region is dorsally convex. Most stallions and many native pony breeds have a prominent dorsal convexity to the neck region, resulting in a cresty appearance. A horse that is excessively fat tends to lay down plaques of fat throughout the body, including the neck region, and this can be misinterpreted as abnormal neck swelling.

If a horse is particularly thick through the jaw, that is, has a large mandible, it is physically difficult to work on the bit (i.e., flexing at the poll so that the front of the head is in approximately the vertical position). Although neck pain can cause a reluctance to work on the bit, more common causes include rider-associated or training problems, mouth pain, forelimb or hindlimb lameness, and back pain. Some horses strongly resist the rider's aids to work on the bit, despite the absence of pain. The use of artificial aids such as draw or running reins, which give the rider a mechanical advantage, may help to break a vicious cycle and encourage the horse to become more submissive and compliant. Similarly, work on the lunge line using a chambon (a device that runs from the girth via a headpiece to the bit rings) can encourage the horse to work in a correct outline and develop fitness and strength of the appropriate musculature. Working the horse in trot over appropriately spaced trotting poles can also help to encourage a horse to work in a correct outline, with a round and supple back.

A rider may complain of neck stiffness or difficulties in getting a horse to bend correctly in a circle. Although this may be caused by neck pain, neck stiffness may be a protective mechanism by the horse to avoid pain associated with lameness, especially forelimb lameness. A horse with left forelimb lameness, for example, may be reluctant to bend properly to the left, and when unrestrained by a rider on the lunge, on the left rein may hold the neck and head slightly to the right, giving the appearance of looking out of the circle. Thus load distribution is altered and lameness minimized. Such lameness actually may not be evident during riding, although this may be the only circumstance under which the rider recognizes the problem. The lameness may be more obvious on the lunge or even in hand in straight lines. When a horse has an abnormal neck and/or head posture, a comprehensive clinical evaluation of the entire horse should be performed. Neck pain or abnormal posture may reflect a primary lesion elsewhere (e.g., central or peripheral vestibular disease, fracture of the spinous processes of the cranial thoracic vertebrae, a mediastinal or thoracic abscess, or a systemic disease such as tetanus).

Detailed examination of the neck should include assessment of the neck conformation, the shape and posture at rest, and the position of the head relative to the neck and trunk. The veterinarian should note any patchy sweating or change in hair color reflecting intermittent sweating that may suggest local nerve damage. Look carefully at the musculature to identify any localized atrophy. Palpate the right and left sides of the neck to assess symmetry and the presence of abnormal swellings or depressions and to identify any neck muscle pain, tension, or fasciculation. Deep palpation should be performed on the left and right sides of the neck to identify pain.

A series of nine equidistant acupoints (acupuncture points) exist along an arc on the crest of the neck.[1] The most cranial is in the depression just cranial to the wing of the atlas and just caudal to the ear. The most caudal point is a few centimeters dorsocranial to the dorsocranial

ferences
n page
1294

aspect of the scapula. Six intervertebral acupoints also exist between the vertebrae. An abnormal response to firm palpation of these points may reflect neck pain.

Neck flexibility should be assessed from side to side and up and down. This can be done by manually manipulating the neck, but many normal horses resist this. Holding a bowl of food by the horse's shoulder to assess lateral flexibility is helpful. Ideally the horse should be positioned against a wall, so that the horse cannot swing its hindquarters away from the examiner during this assessment. The clinician should try to differentiate between the horse properly flexing the neck and twisting the head on the neck. Compare flexibility to the left and to the right. To assess extension of the neck, the veterinarian should evaluate the ease with which the horse can stretch to eat from above head height. Observing the horse grazing is helpful to assess ventral mobility of the neck. Especially with lesions in the caudal neck region a horse may have to straddle the forelimbs excessively to lower the head to the ground to graze (Figure 53-1, A). The horse should also be observed moving in small circles to the left and the right, and loose on the lunge.

Assessing skin sensation and local reflexes, such as the cervicofacial and the thoracolaryngeal reflexes, and comparing carefully the right and left sides may be useful. The consistency and patency of the jugular veins should be evaluated.

The horse should be observed moving in hand and on the lunge, and if necessary should be ridden, to assess neck posture and the presence of neurological gait abnormalities, restriction in forelimb gait, or lameness. The clinician should note how any gait abnormality is influenced by the positions of the head and neck. Forelimb lameness occasionally is associated with a primary cervical lesion, usually, but not invariably, together with other clinical signs referable to the neck.[2]

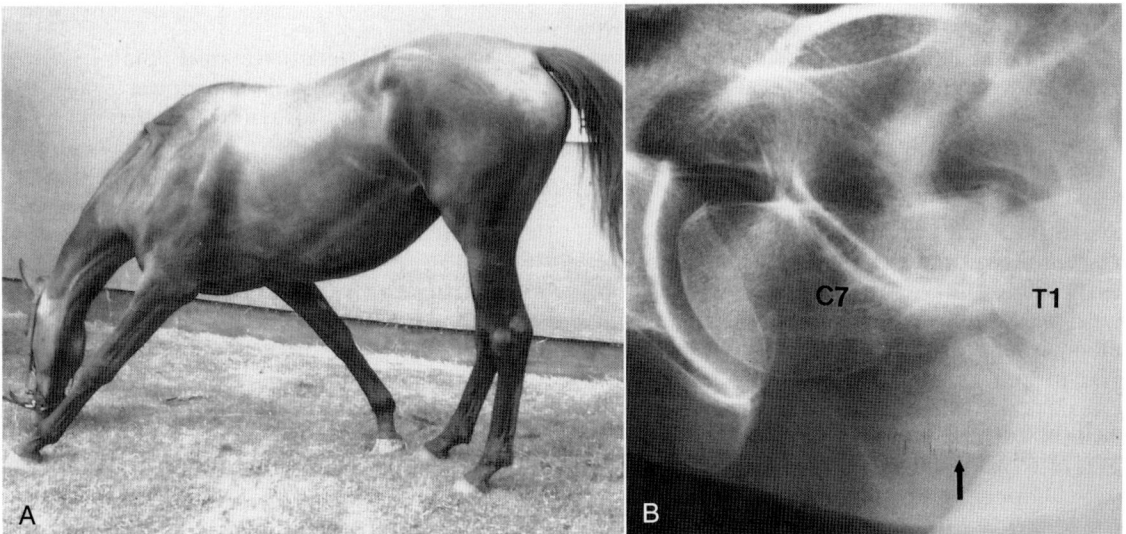

Fig. 53-1 • A, A 3-year-old Thoroughbred filly with severe neck pain and restricted forelimb gait associated with a displaced articular fracture of the ventral processes of the seventh cervical vertebra. The horse must adopt the straddled forelimb stance to lower the head to graze. **B,** Lateral radiographic image of the caudal cervical vertebrae (sixth cervical to first thoracic vertebra) of the same horse. Cranial is to the left. The ventral processes of the seventh cervical vertebra are displaced *(arrow)*. The intercentral joint space between the seventh cervical *(C7)* and first thoracic *(T1)* vertebrae is narrowed greatly, with abnormal orientation of the vertebral bodies.

IMAGING CONSIDERATIONS

Radiography and Radiology

Comprehensive radiographic examination of the neck requires at least five exposures, assuming that large cassettes or imaging plates are used, including the poll, cranial, midneck and caudal neck regions and the base of the neck to evaluate the first and second thoracic vertebrae.[3] Lateral-lateral images are obtained easily in the standing position, but ventrodorsal images are best obtained with the horse in dorsal recumbency under general anesthesia, except in small ponies and foals. Positioning of the neck is important, because any rotation of the head and neck makes evaluation difficult, in particular the synovial articulations. Relatively large exposures are required for the more caudal neck regions, so radiation safety is important, and the cassette should be supported in a holder, not held by hand. A grid is useful, especially in the caudal neck region, to reduce scattered radiation. Obtaining exposures from left to right and right to left may be useful. Lateral oblique images of the cervical vertebrae may give additional information.

A number of variations of the normal radiological appearance of the cervical vertebrae should not be mistaken for lesions. A spur on the dorsocaudal aspect of the second cervical vertebra may project into the vertebral canal. The ventral processes of the sixth cervical vertebra and occasionally other vertebrae have small separate centers of ossification. The ventral lamina on the sixth cervical vertebra may be transposed onto the ventral aspect of the seventh cervical vertebra, unilaterally or bilaterally. The seventh cervical vertebra has a small spinous process, which may be superimposed over the synovial articulation between the sixth and seventh cervical vertebrae and should not be confused with periarticular new bone. In older horses small spondylitic spurs may be seen on the ventral aspect of the vertebral bodies. Modeling of the dorsal synovial articulations between the fifth and sixth and between the sixth and seventh cervical vertebrae is common in middle-aged and older horses[3-5] (Figure 53-2).

Major radiological abnormalities such as fusion of two adjacent vertebrae can be present subclinically, in part because of the great mobility between adjacent vertebrae (Figure 53-3, *A*). The clinical significance of such lesions may also be determined by the athletic demands placed on the horse.

Nuclear Scintigraphy

Lateral and ventral scintigraphic images of the neck can be obtained. Ideally, images should be obtained from the left and right sides. In normal horses there is usually greater radiopharmaceutical uptake in the synovial articulations between the fifth and sixth and sixth and seventh cervical vertebrae, compared with the more cranial articulations reflecting the mobility of these joints and the biomechanical forces imposed on these articulations. There is often greater radiopharmaceutical uptake in the odontoid peg (dens) of the axis, compared with the surrounding vertebrae.

Increased radiopharmaceutical uptake (IRU) is not necessarily synonymous with a lesion that is clinically significant; therefore images must be interpreted with care (see Figure 53-3, *B*). The clinician should compare images obtained from the left and right sides carefully, because

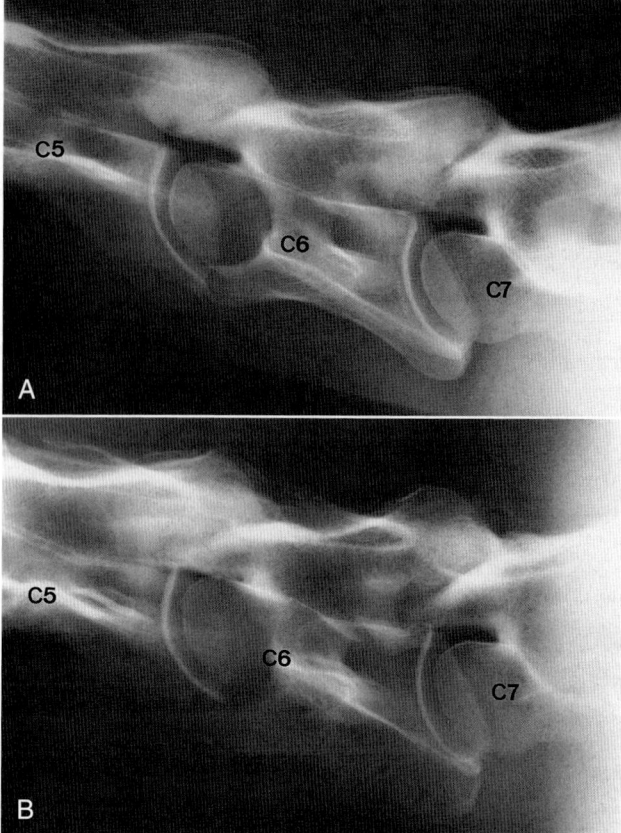

Fig. 53-2 • A, Lateral radiographic image of the caudal cervical vertebrae of normal 4-year-old Thoroughbred. The synovial articulations between the fifth (*C5*) and sixth (*C6*) cervical and sixth and seventh (*C7*) cervical vertebrae are outlined smoothly. The intervertebral foramina are distinct. Compare with part **B** and Figure 53-8. **B,** Lateral radiographic image of the caudal cervical vertebrae of 9-year-old clinically normal horse. The synovial articulations are enlarged between the fifth (*C5*) and sixth (*C6*) cervical vertebrae and particularly between the sixth and seventh (*C7*) cervical vertebrae.

disparity in radiopharmaceutical uptake may be clinically significant. The veterinarian should evaluate the actual conformation of the synovial articulations, because a change in shape even without IRU may be important. Fractures are not always associated with prominent IRU, and lesions may be missed in the caudal neck region because of the overlying muscle mass and the scapulae.

Ultrasonography

The indications for ultrasonographic examination include evaluating swellings, assessing painful muscles and lesions of the ligamentum nuchae, assessment of the intercentral and synovial vertebral articulations (facet joints), documenting jugular vein thrombophlebitis, and administering ultrasound-guided injections.[6-8]

Computed Tomography

Computed tomography (CT) has the potential to give three-dimensional information about the cervical vertebrae and with contrast-enhanced studies can give information about spinal cord and nerve compression. However, general anesthesia is required, and it is practical to image only the cranial cervical vertebrae.[9-11]

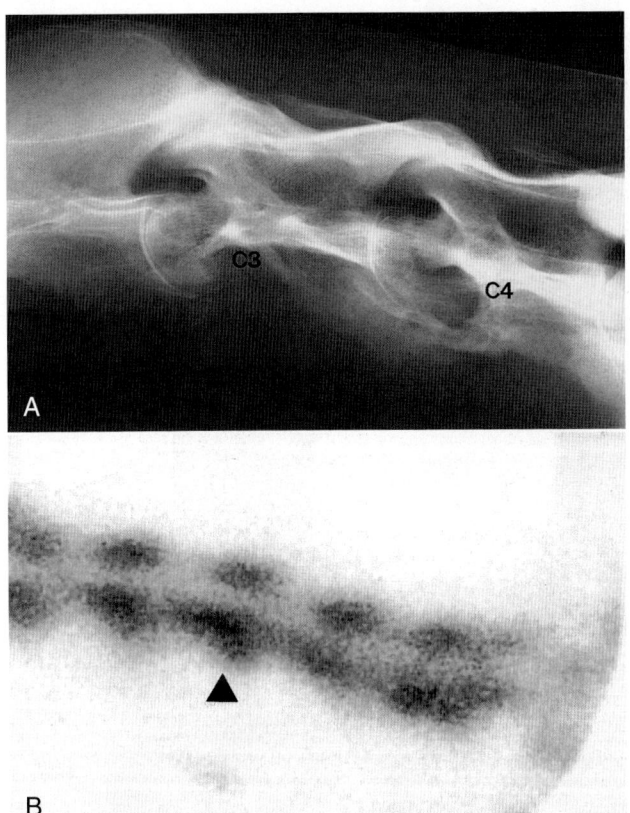

Fig. 53-3 • A, Lateral radiographic image of a 15-year-old Arabian international-level endurance horse that had been competing successfully with no clinical signs referable to the neck. There is abnormal angulation between the third *(C3)* and fourth *(C4)* cervical vertebrae. The vertebral bodies of the third and fourth cervical vertebrae are osteoporotic. Extensive new bone has formed over the ventral aspect of the intercentral articulation between the third and fourth cervical vertebrae, with narrowing of the intercentral joint space and thinning of the caudal end plate of the third cervical vertebra. The ventral profile of the more cranial aspect of the third cervical vertebra is abnormal. **B,** Lateral scintigraphic image of the midneck region of the same horse. Note the increased radiopharmaceutical uptake in the vertebral body of the fourth cervical vertebra *(arrowhead).*

Thermography

Thermographic examination of the neck is discussed in detail elsewhere (see Chapters 25 and 95). However, I have found thermography of limited usefulness, except for identifying acute superficial muscle injuries.

Electromyography

Electromyography (EMG) can be used to quantify the motor unit action potential and to identify insertional activity and pathological spontaneous electrical activity in muscle that can help to differentiate between myopathy and neuropathy and to localize the source of a lesion. It has been suggested that EMG can be used to help to determine the clinical significance of radiological abnormalities of the cervical vertebrae by detection of evidence of neuropathy.[12]

OTHER DIAGNOSTIC TESTS

In selected horses with neck pain, valuable information may be obtained from hematological and serum biochemical tests. Measuring *Brucella* titers and tuberculosis testing are occasionally useful. Bone biopsy may be valuable for determining the cause of some bony lesions.

CLINICAL CONDITIONS

Occipito-Atlantoaxial Malformation

Occipito-atlantoaxial malformation (OAAM) is a congenital abnormality,[13] and although it can occur in any breed,[14] OAAM appears to be a heritable condition in Arabian horses[15] (see Chapter 123). Clinical signs are usually recognizable within the first few weeks of life and include an abnormal neck shape in the poll region, with prominence on the left or right sides or both, and/or scoliosis (Figure 53-4, *A*). These signs are best appreciated when viewed from above. Usually no associated soft tissue swelling or pain exists, although an abnormal clicking sound may be audible because of subluxation of the atlantoaxial joint. The horse may have an abnormal limitation of movement in the poll region. The gait should be assessed carefully for neurological abnormalities; however, in many horses no neurological gait deficits are apparent.

Diagnosis is confirmed radiologically using lateral and ventrodorsal views. Bony abnormalities include fusion of the atlas to the occiput, atlantoaxial luxation, and abnormal shapes of the atlas and axis, often asymmetrical (see Figure 53-4, *B*).

No treatment is available for horses with OAAM. Prognosis for athletic function is determined by the degree of neck stiffness. Because of the heritable nature of this condition in Arabian horses, breeding of affected horses or the sire or the dam is inadvisable.

Other Congenital Abnormalities

OAAM is the most common congenital abnormality of the cervical vertebrae, but congenital torticollis is seen occasionally, caused by malformation of more caudal cervical vertebrae. Vertebral body fusion usually is seen with a meningomyelocele, resulting in neurological abnormalities, and therefore is not considered further.

Subluxation of the First and Second Cervical Vertebrae

Subluxation of the first and second cervical vertebrae is an unusual condition, probably related to trauma such as a fall, although the horse may have no recent history of such.[16-22] The condition is associated with damage of the ligament of the dens or the ventral longitudinal ligament between the first and second cervical vertebrae or occurs secondary to a fracture of the dens.[17,18] An affected horse usually has a stiff neck and a tendency for the head and neck to be somewhat extended (Figure 53-5, *A*). Differentiating between neck pain and stiffness may be difficult. An audible clicking noise may emanate from the region, and occasionally abnormal movement between the vertebrae can be appreciated. Because of the relatively wide sagittal diameter of the vertebral canal at this site, generally no associated compression of the cervical spinal cord occurs. Occasionally, neurological abnormalities are seen in horses with a displaced fracture of the dens.[22]

Diagnosis is based on radiographic examination, using lateral-lateral images with the neck in natural (neutral) and

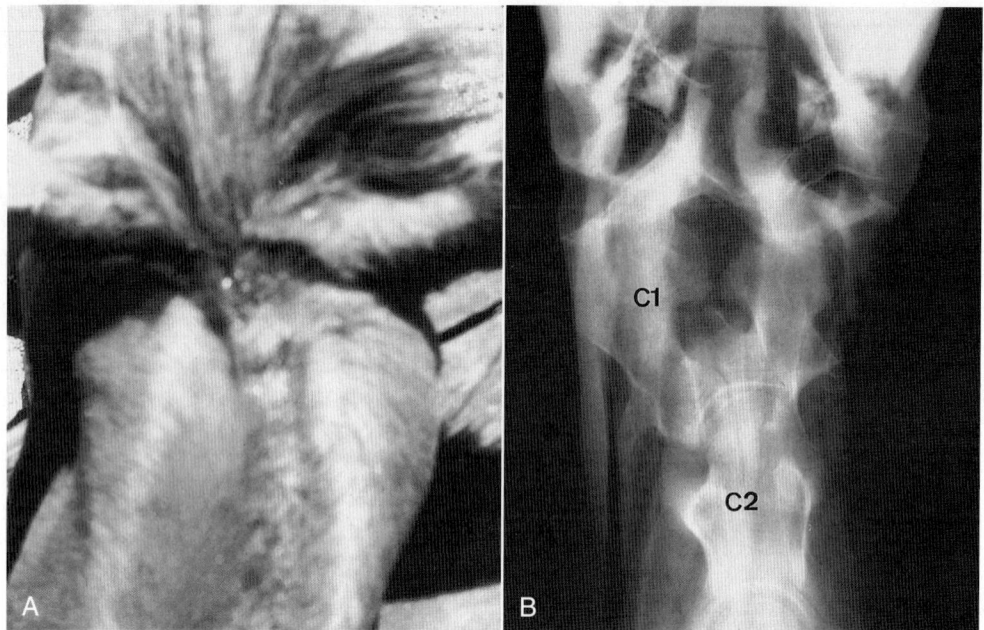

Fig. 53-4 • A, Dorsal view of the poll region of a 6-month-old Thoroughbred filly with an abnormal asymmetrical shape and scoliosis of the cranial neck region and neck stiffness associated with occipito-atlantoaxial malformation. **B,** Ventrodorsal radiographic image of the same horse. Note the distorted shape of the atlas, its fusion with the occiput, and the abnormal orientation of the intercentral articulation between the first (*C1*) and second (*C2*) cervical vertebrae.

extended positions. Radiological abnormalities may include abnormal orientation between the first and second cervical vertebrae (see Figure 53-5, *B*). The position of the dens may be abnormal, resulting in narrowing of the space between it and the dorsal lamina of the vertebral arch of the first cervical vertebra. In a study of yearling Thoroughbreds the mean minimum sagittal diameter was 34 mm and the minimum was 26 mm.[20] Narrowing of the distance between the vertebral arch of the first and second cervical vertebrae may occur in the extended versus neutral position of the neck. The shape of the dens may be altered because of secondary new bone formation. Occasionally the dens is fractured, usually at the junction between the odontoid process and the body of the vertebra.[22] The synovial facet joints between the first and second cervical vertebrae may be altered in shape.

Foals with fractures of the odontoid peg have been successfully treated by surgical stabilization, but limited information exists about long-term prognosis.[18,19,21] Foals with subluxation without neurological abnormalities have a good prognosis for life; prognosis for athletic function is fair, depending on the intended level of competition. No reports of successful management of subluxation in adult horses exist, and the prognosis for return to athletic function with conservative management is poor. However, it was reported that four of five horses with an acute fracture of the dens returned to athletic function, despite neurological gait abnormalities at the time of acute injury, although one had a tendency to trip.[22]

Subluxation of the Sixth and Seventh Cervical Vertebrae

Subluxation of the sixth and seventh cervical vertebrae is usually recognized in adult horses with a complaint of lack of hindlimb power or with difficulties in performing movements requiring collection or, if a breeding stallion, difficulties in mounting either mares or a dummy. Careful clinical examination usually reveals mild-to-moderate hindlimb ataxia. Radiographic examination reveals dorsal displacement of the head of the seventh cervical vertebra. Subluxation of the sixth and seventh cervical vertebrae has less commonly been identified as a cause of bilateral forelimb lameness.[23]

Insertional Desmopathy of the Nuchal Ligament and Injury to Semispinalis

The nuchal ligament is a bilobed structure, fans at its insertion on the occiput, and is surrounded by muscle, the semispinalis to the left and right and the rectus capitis ventrally. New bone formation at the insertion on the occiput may be an incidental finding. Examination of 302 Warmbloods from 1 to 22 years of age revealed new bone in 85%. A postmortem study of Warmbloods revealed a similar high proportion of horses with chondroid metaplasia at the insertion of the ligament and dystrophic mineralization.[24] A smaller radiological study of Thoroughbreds revealed new bone on the caudal aspect of the occiput in only 5%.[24]

Horses with insertional desmopathy of the nuchal ligament or injury to the tendon of insertion of semispinalis often have a history of trauma to the region (e.g., pulling back when tied up) or an excessive amount of lunging exercise while restricted with side or draw reins.[24-26] Horses should be examined while being lunged, with and without side reins, and ridden. Clinical signs include permanent resistance against the reins, with difficulty or unwillingness to lower and flex the head and neck when ridden and poor flexion at the poll. In contrast to horses with back pain,

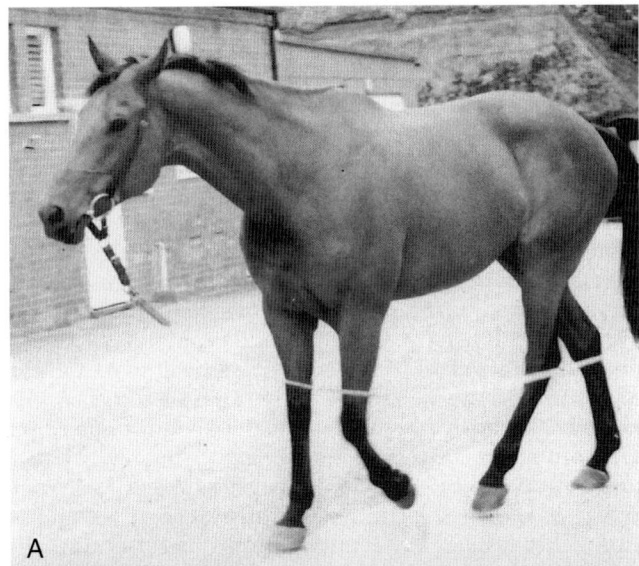

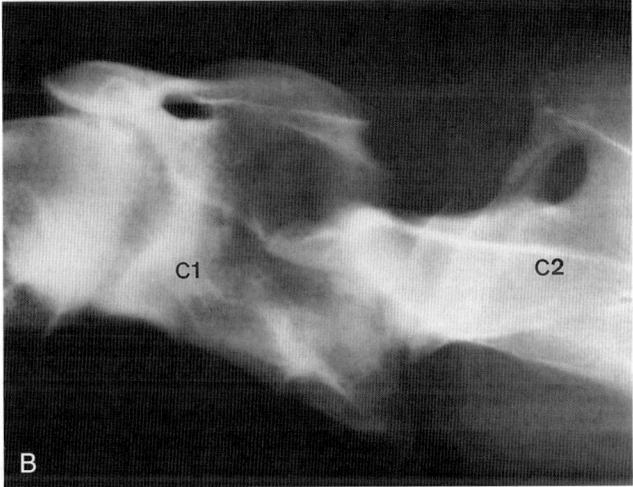

Fig. 53-5 • A, A 9-year-old advanced event horse that had shown neck stiffness since traveling from the United States to Great Britain. The head is extended somewhat, and there was significant neck stiffness or guarding. A clicking sound emanated from the cranial neck region. **B,** Lateral-lateral radiographic image of the cranial neck region of the same horse. There is an abnormal orientation between the first *(C1)* and second *(C2)* cervical vertebrae. Space between the dorsal aspect of the dens and the ventral aspect of the dorsal lamina of the vertebral arch of the first cervical vertebra is reduced. The dorsal aspect of the dens is irregular because of new bone formation. Postmortem examination confirmed partial disruption of the ligament of the dens.

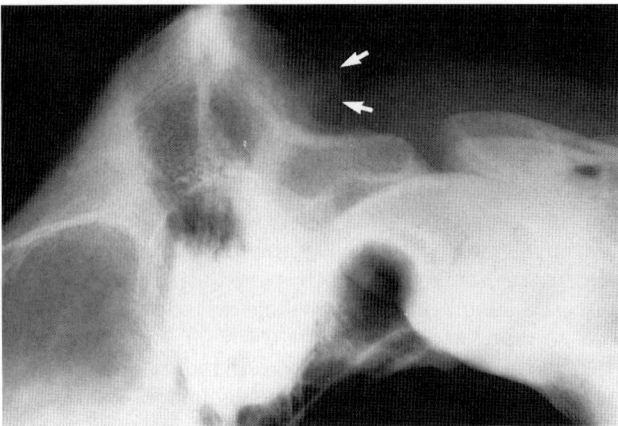

Fig. 53-6 • Lateral-lateral radiographic image of the head of an 8-year-old Warmblood show jumper with a history of reluctance to accept and go forward to the bit and stiffness. There is enthesophyte formation on the caudal aspect of the occiput at the insertion of the nuchal ligament *(arrows).* The horse responded well to local infiltration with corticosteroids and local anesthetic solution and modification of the training program.

hindlimb impulsion is usually good. The horse may have a tendency to rear or shake its head.

Pain cannot usually be elicited by palpation. Radiological examination may reveal new bone on the caudal aspect of the occiput that may extend farther ventrally and dorsally than the actual insertion of the ligamentum nuchae (Figure 53-6). Mineralization sometimes is seen dorsal to the first cervical vertebra as an incidental radiological finding, unassociated with clinical signs. Scintigraphic examination findings may be negative. Ultrasonographic examination is not easy, and interpretation is difficult. Mineralization within the ligament may cause shadowing artifacts. CT offers the most sensitive means of detecting lesions in either the nuchal ligaments or the border of insertion of semispinalis.[24] Diagnosis depends on a positive response to infiltration of local anesthetic solution. Fifteen milliliters of mepivacaine are infiltrated on the left and right sides, and the response is assessed after 15 to 30 minutes. Care must be taken not to inject into the epidural space, which will result in ataxia.

Treatment consists of repeated infiltration of corticosteroids, Traumeel (a homeopathic remedy), and local anesthetic solution and modification of the training program, with no work on the bit for 8 weeks.[26] The horse should be worked principally in straight lines. In the stable the horse should be encouraged to flex the poll region gently from side to side and up and down. The use of acupuncture or magnetic field therapy, laser therapy, ultrasound, or shock wave therapy may help some horses. The results vary. Seventy percent of 26 horses return to full work, although not all are completely normal. Extracorporeal shock wave therapy, two or three applications at 14-day intervals, in addition to 4 weeks of work without requiring flexion of the poll has been reported to be successful in resolving clinical signs in 12 of 22 horses and in improving signs in six other horses.[27] Surgical treatment by transection of the nuchal ligament and the fascia of semispinalis has resulted in improvement in a small number of horses refractory to conservative management.[24]

Disorders of the Neck Musculature

The clinical significance of localized muscle soreness and/or tenseness is poorly understood and documented. I have had experience with a number of horses with subtle performance problems, including slight neck stiffness, reluctance to work properly on the bit and to accept an even contact, and intermittent, slight gait irregularities associated with soreness around and in front of the wings of the axis. Clinical improvement has been seen after relief of this pain by rapid and sudden rotation of the head about the axis.[24]

Many horses resent firm palpation of the brachiocephalicus muscles at the base of the neck. This may be more obvious in horses with forelimb lameness, especially those with pain in the distal part of the limb. This muscle soreness is generally a secondary rather than a primary cause of lameness. Transient improvement in gait may be seen after local therapy using laser therapy, H-wave therapy, ultrasound, and/or massage.

Primary brachiocephalicus pain at the base of the neck has been seen in performance horses, causing subtle gait abnormalities at the walk when ridden, characterized by abnormal lifting of the neck as the limb was advanced and a shortened cranial phase of the stride ipsilateral to the sore muscle. Bilateral brachiocephalicus muscle pain has also been seen in association with throwing up of the head when in the air over a fence and on landing. Treatment of the sore muscles abolished this behavior.

Local muscle soreness also may be seen with a poorly fitting saddle or girth or with a rider who is unable to ride truly in balance with the horse. The primary problem must be addressed if treatment is to be successful. Some driving horses develop forelimb lameness that is seen only when the horse is pulling and may be associated with pressure from the harness. Adaptation of the harness may relieve the problem.

Some horses seem to need to learn how to use the neck and forelimb musculature to maximum advantage and have a restricted forelimb gait without appearing overtly lame. The gait is not altered by distal limb nerve blocks. Some improvement may be achieved by daily massage of the muscles at the base of the neck and manual full protraction of the forelimbs. This is combined with exercise to encourage the horse to lengthen the forelimb stride and to round the back. Lunging in a chambon, trotting over appropriately placed trot poles, and repeatedly lengthening and shortening the stride all may be beneficial. Trotting down the tramlines in a field of corn or rapeseed can also be of enormous help.

Occasionally as the result of a fall or pulling back when tied, acute severe neck muscle soreness develops. The horse is best treated initially with nonsteroidal antiinflammatory drugs (NSAIDs), rest, and local physiotherapy, followed by progressive remobilization when the acute muscle soreness has subsided. The prognosis is good.

I have examined several horses that have had episodic transient attacks of profound neck pain and stiffness, holding the neck relatively low. In some horses a severe unilateral forelimb lameness occurs, often resulting in the limb being held in a semiflexed position at rest. These attacks vary in duration (hours to days), and generally horses have been completely normal between episodes. To date, neither a definitive cause nor an effective treatment has been identified for this syndrome. However, there is usually a very marked enlargement of the caudal cervical facet joints, with narrowing of the intervertebral foramen, and it is suspected that nerve root impingement may cause episodic pain. Careful manipulation of the caudal neck region may result in instantaneous relief of clinical signs.

Dystrophic mineralization is seen sometimes as an incidental radiological finding in the neck musculature, secondary to previous intramuscular injections.

Muscle Abscess

Horses sometimes develop localized muscle soreness and swelling at the site of intramuscular injection, especially equine influenza injections, which can result in neck stiffness and a restricted forelimb gait. Signs usually resolve within 24 to 48 hours. Treatment is generally unnecessary, although hot packing and analgesia may be beneficial. More irritant drugs, such as iron injections, may result in the development of a sterile abscess.

The development of a single or multiloculated abscess cavity filled with malodorous material is usually a sequela to an intramuscular injection of a variety of drugs administered within the previous few weeks. Clinical signs include neck pain and stiffness, localized neck swelling with or without focal patchy sweating, and sometimes pyrexia. Diagnosis is based on the history and clinical signs and can be confirmed by ultrasonography. The abscess cavity is usually filled with anechogenic material surrounded by a hyperechogenic abscess wall.

Treatment is by surgical drainage, which is easily performed in the standing horse. The abscess cavity should be thoroughly lavaged. Systemic antimicrobial drugs usually are not required, unless clostridial myositis is suspected based on the fulminant nature of the condition (see Chapter 83). The prognosis for most horses with muscle abscesses is good, provided that adequate drainage is established. However, surgical removal of the entire abscess occasionally is required.

Osteoarthritis

Anatomical studies have shown that approximately 50% of normal mature horses have some unilateral or bilateral modeling of the synovial facet joints between the sixth and seventh cervical vertebrae. The modeling often is accompanied by extension of fibrocartilage across the cranial border of the dorsal arch of the seventh cervical vertebra and irregular enlargement of the articular processes.[4,5] The spinous process of the seventh cervical vertebra may become flattened or fragmented by contact with the sixth cervical vertebra when the neck is extended. Radiologically these changes result in irregularity of the normally smooth outline of the synovial articulations. Similar modeling changes also occur in the synovial articulation between the sixth and seventh cervical vertebrae.[24] A bony knob may develop on the ventral aspect of one or both cranial articular processes at the articulations between the fifth and sixth cervical vertebrae and between the sixth and seventh cervical vertebrae. When well developed, this knob forms a buttress that impinges onto the body or the arch of the more cranial vertebra and forms a false joint. The buttress partially obliterates the intervertebral foramen, but it is often of no clinical significance.[3-5] Buttresses occur at the articulation between the sixth and seventh cervical vertebrae in 18% of normal horses.[4]

The potential exists for large amounts of new bone associated with osteoarthritis of the cervical synovial articulations to encroach axially into the vertebral canal, resulting in compression of the spinal cord and hindlimb weakness and ataxia, or into the intervertebral foramen, resulting in nerve root compression with local or referred pain and possibly lameness and patchy sweating. Severe osteoarthritic change may progress to partial or complete fusion and thus neck stiffness. With enlargement of a synovial articulation also generally comes enlargement of the joint capsule, and synovial outpouchings or cysts may develop that may impinge on the spinal cord.

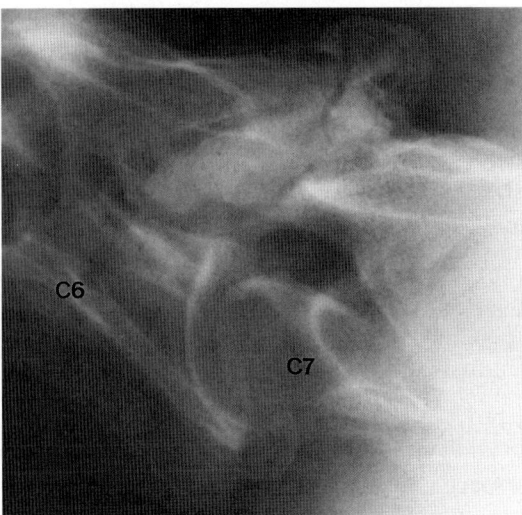

Fig. 53-7 • Slightly oblique lateral-lateral radiographic image of the caudal cervical region of a 7-year-old riding horse with mild right forelimb lameness and an abnormally low head and neck carriage. Lameness was unaltered by comprehensive diagnostic analgesia of the right forelimb. There is extensive modeling of the articular facet joints between the sixth *(C6)* and seventh *(C7)* cervical vertebrae, with a large radiodense mass with heterogeneous opacity extending dorsally. Obtaining a true lateral-lateral image was not possible. The obliquity of the radiograph makes it difficult to assess the intervertebral foramen. Postmortem examination revealed compression of the seventh cervical spinal nerve at the level of the foramen.

Radiological abnormalities associated with osteoarthritis include enlargement of one or more of the articular facets and alteration in joint space width (Figure 53-7). Widening of the joint space is usually associated with asymmetrical facet enlargement; narrowing is caused by articular cartilage degeneration. Pitted lucent zones may develop in the articular facets, with extension of the dorsal laminae between adjacent vertebrae and partial or complete obliteration of the adjacent intervertebral foramina. Sometimes fractures are seen dorsal to a joint. Abnormalities often develop on the left and right sides but are frequently asymmetrical. With substantial asymmetry of the synovial articulations the affected and immediately more cranial vertebrae may appear rotated on a lateral radiographic image, although the horse had appeared to be standing with its head and neck straight in the sagittal plane. Radiographic examination from left to right and from right to left and oblique radiographic images can help to determine on which side a unilateral lesion is present. A lesion that is close to the cassette is clearer and magnification is less than if the lesion is on the opposite side of the neck. Ultrasonography can also be used to demonstrate periarticular modeling and increased synovial fluid within a joint.

The clinical importance of osteoarthritis of one or more synovial articulations can be difficult to determine by clinical and radiographic examinations alone, except by exclusion. The greater the degree of abnormality and the larger the number of articulations involved, the more likely the condition is clinically significant. In normal horses, finding osteoarthritic change cranial to the articulation between the fifth and sixth cervical vertebrae is rare. Unilateral forelimb lameness has been seen with lesions between the fourth cervical and first thoracic vertebrae.[2] Nuclear scintigraphic examination may give further information in horses with neck stiffness or forelimb lameness apparently not referable to the limb itself. Ultrasound-guided intraarticular analgesia may help to determine the clinical significance of radiological abnormalities (Figure 60-5).

In one report, seven of eight horses with forelimb lameness associated with radiological abnormalities of the cervical vertebrae also had subtle to obvious signs of neck pain.[2] Patterns of muscle atrophy in the neck and shoulder regions varied. The character of lameness varied. Radiological abnormalities included substantial modeling of the synovial articulations in the caudal neck region in three horses; a fourth had modeling and a fracture involving the synovial articulation between the fourth and fifth cervical vertebrae. One horse had abnormalities of the intercentral articulation between the seventh cervical and first thoracic vertebrae and a discrete mineralized fragment dorsal to it. Large lucent zones were identified in a vertebral body (the fourth and sixth cervical vertebrae) in two horses. A fracture of the vertebral body of the seventh cervical vertebra was seen in one horse.

Nerve root impingement in the caudal neck region may cause radicular or referred pain and account for forelimb lameness. Neck pain itself can also cause forelimb lameness. Compression of the seventh cervical nerve was confirmed post mortem in a horse with osteoarthritis of the articulations between the sixth and seventh cervical vertebrae and between the seventh cervical and first thoracic vertebrae.[2] Nerve root compression with severe osteoarthritis has also been demonstrated using contrast-enhanced CT.[9]

In horses with mild ataxia, neck stiffness or forelimb lameness associated with osteoarthritis of cervical synovial articulations, the response to rest and treatment with NSAIDs has been limited. Local periarticular or intraarticular infiltration of corticosteroids, performed using ultrasonographic guidance, may bring temporary relief. There is limited documented evidence for the efficacy and duration of effect of medication of the synovial articulations of the caudal cervical vertebrae. In a recent study of 59 sports or pleasure horses with ataxia, neck stiffness or pain, or obscure forelimb lameness, 19 horses (32%) returned to full function and 18 horses (31%) improved more than 50%.[28] However, the effect was generally short lived, with 55% showing improvement for a duration of less than 1 month to up to 6 months. The inclusion criteria for the study were poorly defined and follow-up results were based on the owners' subjective opinions. Epidural injection of corticosteroids performed with the horse under general anesthesia has been shown to result in relief of neck stiffness in a horse with osteoarthritis of the synovial articulation between the fourth and fifth cervical vertebrae and clinical evidence of nerve root compression.[29]

Osteoarthritis, especially in the caudal neck region, may result in associated enlargement of the joint capsule(s) and subsequent pressure on the spinal cord. In horses with mild osteoarthritis obvious ataxia may not be seen, but the history may include the tendency to stumble or to knuckle behind, or lack of hindlimb impulsion. Such signs often have been attributed to lameness but are invariably unaltered by diagnostic treatment with NSAIDs. Clinical signs may be subtle and intermittent. Such horses usually show abnormal weakness if pulled to one side by traction on the tail while the horse is walking—the sway test. A normal

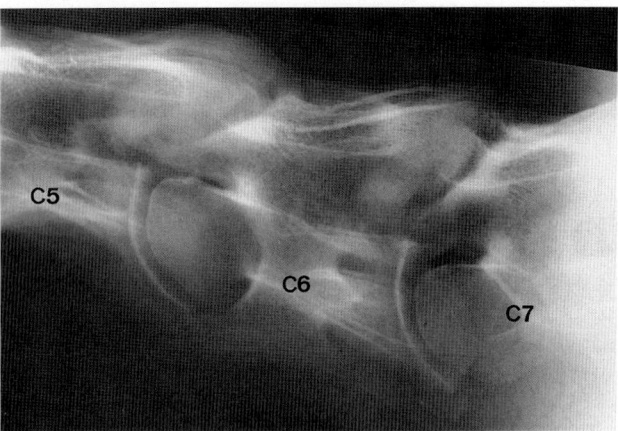

Fig. 53-8 • Lateral radiographic image of the caudal cervical vertebrae of 4-year-old dressage horse with mild hindlimb weakness and a tendency to stumble behind, especially in downward transitions from trot to walk. The synovial articulations between the fifth (C5) and sixth (C6) cervical and sixth and seventh (C7) cervical vertebrae are enlarged greatly (compare with Figure 53-2, A). The joint spaces are widened, reflecting asymmetrical modeling of the articular processes. There is a ventral buttress at the articulation of the sixth and seventh cervical vertebrae, with reduction in size of the intervertebral foramen.

horse easily may be pulled off line once, but then strongly resists. A weak horse can be pulled off line repeatedly. Weakness may also be apparent as the horse decelerates from trot to walk, with exaggerated up-and-down movement of the hindquarters and asymmetric hindlimb placement. This may result in irregular movement of each patella and may be confused with mild intermittent upward fixation or delayed release of the patella (see Chapters 46 and 48). At faster speeds the horse may look completely normal, although some affected horses demonstrate a remarkably croup-high canter when on the lunge. In a young horse, advanced osteoarthritis of one or more caudal cervical synovial articulations is strong circumstantial evidence of cause and effect (Figure 53-8). Definitive diagnosis in an older horse is much more difficult, because radiological evidence of osteoarthritis may be present without associated clinical signs. Myelography may help.[30] The prognosis is poor, and the horse may be potentially unsafe to ride. Surgical treatment can be considered and generally results in clinical improvement, but few sports horses become upper level athletes, and some develop recurrent ataxia several years later.

Diskospondylitis

A survey of the cervical intervertebral disks of 103 horses from birth to 23 years of age confirmed that they consisted solely of fibrocartilage, with no nucleus pulposus.[31] Age-related degenerative changes were identified, but even with severe disintegration of the disks, no referable clinical signs had been apparent.

Diskospondylitis is a rare cause of neck pain, forelimb lameness, or ataxia.[30,31] Although diskospondylitis is usually an infectious condition in dogs, no proven relationship occurs in the horse, and trauma may be an inciting cause. Lesions in the horse have been identified in the caudal neck region (the articulations between the sixth and seventh cervical vertebrae and the seventh cervical and first thoracic vertebrae) and between the third and fourth cervical vertebrae in association with severe neck pain and a bilaterally short, stiff forelimb lameness or episodic, unilateral forelimb lameness. Occasionally a horse may be reluctant to work "on the bit." High-quality radiographs are required for accurate diagnosis. Lesions are characterized by loss of the normal opacity of the cranial and caudal endplates of the affected vertebrae, with or without alteration in the intercentral joint space. Scintigraphic examination may help to localize the affected joint(s). Ultrasonography may be more sensitive in the identification of early bone lesions and abscess formation. The prognosis is guarded, although in one report a broodmare that was admitted with profound neck pain and periodic severe left forelimb lameness, associated with roughening of the endplates at the intercentral articulation between the sixth and seventh cervical vertebrae and narrowing of the intercentral space, after a collision with a fence, made a spontaneous recovery.[32] A second horse was treated by surgical debridement of the disc space and implantation of a cancellous bone graft, with resolution of clinical signs.[33]

Fracture

Fractures of the cervical vertebrae usually result from trauma: the horse rearing up and falling over backward or sideways; pulling back when tied up; or falling while jumping, usually at speed. Clinical signs are sudden in onset and include holding the neck in an abnormally low position, stiffness, a focal or more diffuse area of pain, with or without localized or more diffuse soft tissue swelling, and muscle guarding. Audible or palpable crepitus is sometimes detected. The horse may be unable to lower its head to the ground or may be able to do so only by straddling of the forelimbs (see Figure 53-1, A). Associated hindlimb and forelimb ataxia may be apparent, which can be transient and self-resolving, or persistent. Patchy sweating and localized muscle atrophy may develop. Occasionally an associated unilateral or bilateral forelimb lameness occurs.

Diagnosis is confirmed radiologically (see Figure 53-1, A) (Figure 53-9). Most fractures are detectable on lateral-lateral images, although ventrodorsal images give additional information about the extent of the fractures, especially those involving the atlas or axis. Lateral oblique images can also be helpful in selected horses. Care should be taken not to confuse physes and separate centers of ossification with fractures.

The prognosis depends on the site and configuration of the fracture(s), the degree of displacement, and hence the likelihood of permanent compression of the spinal cord, either by a displaced fracture or by subsequent callus formation.

Fractures of the atlas and axis, especially through the physis of the separate center of ossification of the dens, are particularly common in foals. The prognosis for complete recovery is fair with conservative management, provided that no evidence of ataxia exists. Usually no treatment is required other than confinement to a box or small pen.

Fractures of the cervical vertebrae in adults more commonly involve the vertebral body or arch in the midneck region (the third to sixth cervical vertebrae) or the synovial articular facets of the more caudal vertebrae (the fifth to seventh cervical vertebrae). Local hemorrhage and edema may result in ataxia, which usually resolves within a few

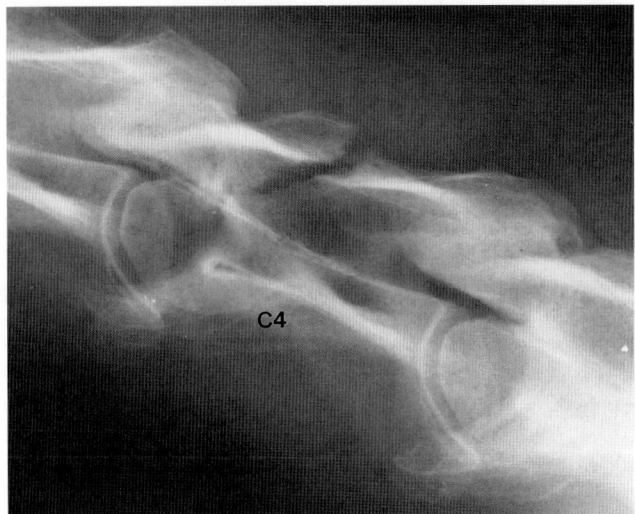

Fig. 53-9 • Lateral radiographic image of the third to fifth cervical vertebrae of a 9-year-old Dutch Warmblood dressage horse with severe neck pain, stiffness, and incoordination after a fall 12 days previously. The fourth cervical vertebra (C4) has a comminuted, slightly displaced fracture of the dorsal arch. Ataxia resolved within another 14 days, and the horse made a complete functional recovery.

days. Persistence of ataxia warrants a guarded prognosis. Most fractures heal by callus formation, and this may subsequently impinge on the spinal cord, causing later ataxia. A fracture of a vertebral body also may result in damage to the adjacent intervertebral disk and associated ligaments, which subsequently may protrude into the vertebral canal and cause ataxia. Thus in the acute stage giving an accurate prognosis may be difficult. However, many fractures of the vertebral bodies and synovial articulations do heal, and horses may be able to return to athletic function, although residual neck stiffness may be present.

In the acute stage the horse should be confined to box rest. Analgesics may be necessary to control severe pain, but they should be used judiciously to avoid encouraging excessive movement of the neck. The position of the water bucket and manger should be adjusted so that the horse can drink and eat from normal head height. The hay should be fed at a height level with the head, preferably loose, or if in a hay net, a net with large holes, with the hay well shaken first. The horse should not be tied up during the convalescent period in case it pulls back. Reappraising the horse clinically and radiologically every 6 to 8 weeks is helpful. Maximum clinical improvement may not be seen until 6 to 9 months after injury. Selected fractures may require surgical stabilization.[8]

Myeloma

Myeloma is a myeloproliferative disorder that can cause radiolucent lesions in any bone, including the cervical vertebrae, with associated bone pain.[24,34] Cervical vertebral myeloma was diagnosed in several horses of a wide range of breeds and ages.[34] Clinical signs included intermittent pyrexia, severe neck pain and stiffness, episodic forelimb lameness, weight loss, and a variety of other abnormalities. Diagnosis is based on hematological, radiographic, and bone biopsy examinations. Hematological abnormalities include anemia, leukocytosis, neutrophilia, and lymphocytosis. Total protein concentration is elevated greatly.

Protein electrophoresis shows a clinically significant monoclonal peak in the gamma region. Radiological examination of affected bones reveals clearly demarcated lucent zones, usually without a sclerotic rim. Bone biopsy is useful to confirm the diagnosis, but currently no treatment is available and the prognosis is hopeless.

Other Cystlike Lesions in Cervical Vertebrae

Occasionally, single or several well-demarcated radiolucent zones are identified in one or more adjacent vertebrae, associated with profound neck pain, with or without forelimb lameness.[35] These lesions have not been proved to be caused by osteomyelitis or myeloma, although a definitive diagnosis has not always been possible by bone biopsy or postmortem examination. One horse with extremely severe neck pain and forelimb lameness had radiolucent zones in the fifth and sixth cervical vertebrae, and bone biopsy revealed accumulation of abnormal plasma cells, but the horse made a most spectacular and complete recovery after exploratory surgery and returned to international show jumping. A show pony had a large cystlike lesion in the fourth cervical vertebra with profound neck pain and left forelimb lameness (Figure 53-10). Postmortem examination revealed a cavity filled with granulation tissue, surrounded by a large area of bone necrosis, but no suggestion of the underlying cause.

Vertebral Osteomyelitis

Cervical vertebral osteomyelitis usually occurs secondary to a systemic disease such as *Rhodococcus equi* infection in foals, *Streptococcus equi* infection (strangles), tuberculosis, or brucellosis; or as an extension of soft tissue infection[4]; or through hematogenous spread. Clinical signs may include pyrexia, neck stiffness or pain, and an abnormal neck posture, poor appetite, and weight loss. Usually leukocytosis, neutrophilia, and hyperfibrinogenemia are also present. Radiological examination of the cervical vertebrae may reveal focal radiolucent zones, with or without surrounding increased radiopacity, in one or more vertebrae.[4] Useful diagnostic tests include bone biopsy, tuberculosis skin testing, and measurement of *Brucella* titers. Aggressive antimicrobial treatment may result in amelioration of clinical signs, but the prognosis is guarded.

Jugular Vein Thrombophlebitis

Thrombophlebitis of the jugular vein is a common condition associated with intravenous injection and chemical irritation, mechanical trauma to the vessel wall through catheterization, or a coagulation disorder. The vein feels abnormally hard, but unless the left and right sides are affected, the thrombus is infected, or thromboemboli settle elsewhere, usually no other clinical signs are apparent.

Occasionally a long length of the jugular vein is occluded by a thrombus in which bacteria are seeded, resulting in infectious thrombophlebitis. Clinical signs include neck stiffness and pain, localized heat and swelling, and pyrexia. If a long length of the vessel is involved, ipsilateral swelling of the head may occur. Diagnosis is based on clinical signs and ultrasonography.[6] A heterogeneous, cavitating echogenic thrombus can be seen in the jugular vein. Usually leukocytosis, neutrophilia, and hyperfibrinogenemia are present. A horse with a localized, small infected thrombus usually responds well to prolonged

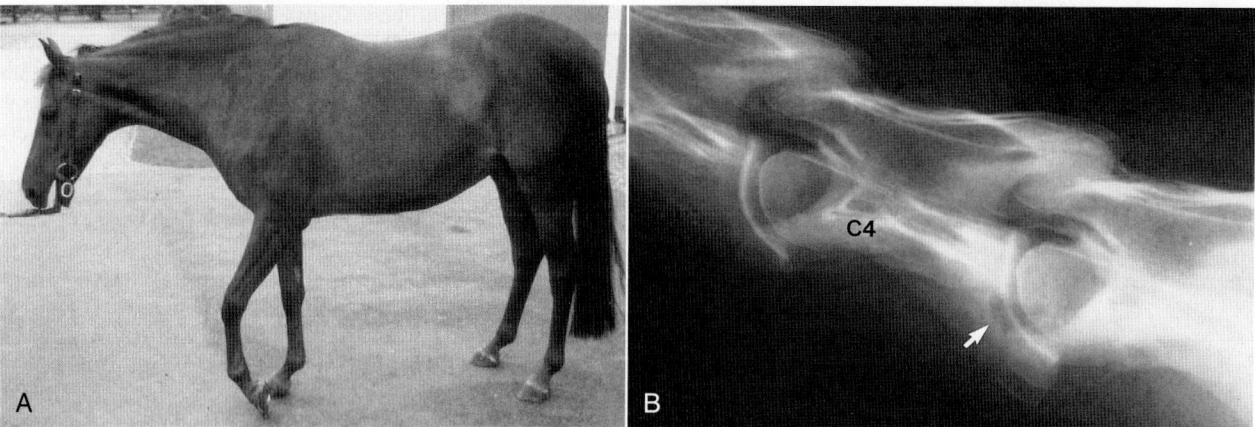

Fig. 53-10 • A, A 13-year-old show pony with exquisite neck pain, worse on the left side, and episodic severe left forelimb lameness. The pony showed a shortened cranial phase of the stride at the walk, and periodically the pony stopped, holding the limb in a semiflexed position, and was reluctant to move forward. There was hyperesthesia of the caudal half of the left side of the neck. **B,** Lateral-lateral radiographic image of the midneck region of the same pony. A large radiolucent zone *(arrow)* is visible in the caudal aspect of the vertebral body of the fourth cervical vertebra *(C4)*. There is a loss of continuity of the caudal cortex.

systemic antimicrobial therapy. Injection of antimicrobial drugs into the thrombus may be indicated if there is inadequate response to systemic therapy. The lesion should be monitored clinically and ultrasonographically. With more extensive lesions or associated toxemia or bacteremia, surgical ligation and removal of the vein may be required, combined with systemic antimicrobial treatment.

Inadvertent perivascular injection of an irritant drug, such as phenylbutazone, may result in the rapid development of localized pain and swelling caused by chemical irritation. This may be followed by an aggressive inflammatory response, leading to sloughing of the skin. If perivascular injection is suspected, then the area should be treated by local infiltration with a balanced electrolyte solution (1 L) to dilute the drug, combined with local anesthetic solution (10 to 20 mL mepivacaine) to reduce pain. Periodic hot packing seems to ameliorate clinical signs. If the condition is initially untreated and local tissue necrosis supervenes, a skin slough is almost inevitable, and prophylactic antimicrobial therapy may be indicated.

Neck Stiffness and Cervical Vertebral Mobilization under General Anesthesia

Assessment of neck flexibility has been described (see page 607). Restricted neck mobility associated with other clinical signs suggestive of neck pain, for example, reluctance to accept the bit, may be an indication for cervical vertebral

mobilization under general anesthesia (see Chapter 95). The aim is to assist in restoring normal function to soft tissue components of joints. However, horses with preexisting osteoarthritic changes are unlikely to respond. Repeated or maintained end-of-range passive joint movements may lower intraarticular pressure, inhibit reflex muscle contraction around a joint, and reduce muscle tension on the periarticular soft tissues and thus relieve pain. The manipulations are performed with the horse in left and right lateral recumbency under general anesthesia. Nine manipulations are performed in sequence to include extension of the head and neck, extension with rotation to the left and then to the right, rotation of the head to the left and to the right, flexion of the neck to the left and to the right, and flexion and rotation in each direction. For each maneuver the head and neck are moved to a position at the end of the resistance-free range. Constant pressure then is applied so that movement through the stiff and reduced range can be initiated. The pressure then is maintained until the joints and associated soft tissues move through the range of resistance. When movement ceases, a new end range is established and pressure is released. The maneuver may then be repeated. After treatment, horses are rested for 5 days and then start light work. Clinical improvement usually is appreciable within 2 weeks.[36] Repeated treatment may be necessary in selected horses. Occasionally, clinical signs deteriorate after treatment.

PART VI

Developmental Orthopedic Disease and Lameness

Chapter 54

Pathogenesis of Osteochondrosis

Janet Douglas

OSTEOCHONDROSIS: DEFINITIONS AND TERMINOLOGY

Equine osteochondrosis (OC) is characterized by focal failures of endochondral ossification that typically occur in well-defined predilection sites. Lesions that result from external trauma or infection are not generally regarded as OC.[1,2] The thickened, retained growth cartilage that characterizes typical lesions (Figure 54-1) in the articular-epiphyseal cartilage complex (AECC) may be complicated by development of fissures that extend from the deepest layers of the lesion to the articular surface. Cartilaginous or osteochondral fragments may then detach from the parent bone, forming intraarticular fragments.[3] Once lesions extend to the articular surface, thereby causing inflammation of the joint, the condition may be referred to as *osteochondritis*.[4,5] The term *osteochondritis dissecans* (OCD) is usually reserved for lesions in which a dissecting flap of tissue is present (Figure 54-2).[3] Although it has been proposed that the term *dyschondroplasia* should be used in place of OC,[3,6] the term OC remains in widespread use and is used in this chapter to refer to the primary lesion. *Dyschondroplasia* is used only when referring to work by authors who prefer this term. A condition similar to equine OC occurs in a number of other animal species, as well as in people.[1]

ENDOCHONDRAL OSSIFICATION

Endochondral ossification is the process by which growing cartilage is systematically replaced by bone to form the growing skeleton.[7] This process occurs at three main sites: the physis, the epiphysis, and the cuboidal bones of the carpus and tarsus. Chondrocytes in the physis can be divided into a series of layers or zones (Figure 54-3). The zone farthest from the metaphysis is the resting or reserve zone. Adjacent to this is the proliferative zone, in which chondrocytes divide. These cells progress to the hypertrophic zone, in which they enlarge and form ordered columns. During this stage the chondrocytes become surrounded by extracellular matrix that gradually becomes mineralized in the zone of provisional calcification. The chondrocyte columns are then invaded by metaphyseal blood vessels, and bone forms on the residual columns of calcified cartilage. This mixture of calcified cartilage and immature bone (primary spongiosa) is then gradually remodeled to produce the mature bone of the metaphysis.[7] Endochondral ossification, which continues throughout the period of growth, also occurs in the AECC at the ends of long bones (Figure 54-4).[8] The chondrocytes of the AECC that are closest to the articular surface produce articular cartilage, whereas those cells closer to the epiphysis participate in endochondral ossification in the same manner as occurs in the physis. It is generally accepted that the growth cartilages of both the physis and the AECC are susceptible to OC.[1,3,8-11]

CHARACTERISTICS OF OSTEOCHONDROSIS

Equine OC characteristically manifests as one or two lesions that occur in known predilection sites. In this so-called "typical pattern" of the disease, lesions are often bilaterally symmetrical, although only one lesion may cause clinical signs.[12] The femoropatellar (lateral and medial femoral trochlear ridges, lateral facet of patella), tarsocrural (cranial aspect of the intermediate ridge and medial malleolus of the distal aspect of the tibia, lateral and medial trochlear ridges of the talus), scapulohumeral (glenoid fossa and humeral head), and metacarpophalangeal and metatarsophalangeal joints (midsagittal ridge and condyles of the third metacarpal or metatarsal bone) are affected most commonly. OC of the elbow, hip, and cervical vertebral joints has also been described,[12,13] but lesions in these sites are less common and the etiology is more controversial.[12] This typical pattern of OC contrasts with that of the atypical pattern in which animals show numerous articular (and sometimes physeal) lesions.[12,14] Predilection and nonpredilection sites may be affected in these horses, and bilaterally symmetrical lesions are absent or infrequent. A third pattern of lesion distribution, the mixed pattern, describes horses in which both typical and atypical lesions are present.[14]

OC may manifest very early in life. For example, lesions of the cranial aspect of the intermediate ridge of the tibia have been identified in foals that are less than 1 month old.[15-17] Lesions of the lateral trochlear ridge of the femur may appear later (3 to 4 months of age),[17] but lesions at this site, on the medial femoral condyle, and in the tarsocrural and fetlock joints all develop before approximately 7 or 8 months of age.[18,19] The studies from which these conclusions were drawn were conducted in a range of breeds. In contrast, recent radiological data suggest that the

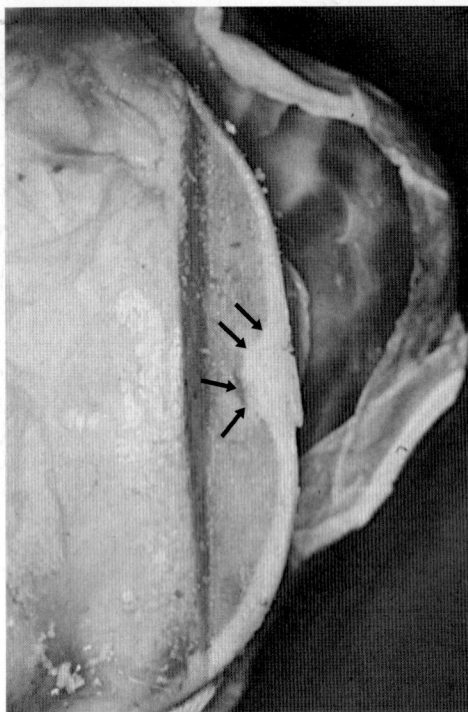

Fig. 54-1 • Section through the articular-epiphyseal cartilage complex and epiphysis showing thickened retained cartilage *(arrows)*. (Courtesy Gustavo Hernández-Vidal, Faculty of Veterinary Medicine, Universidad Autónoma de Nuevo León, Monterrey, Mexico.)

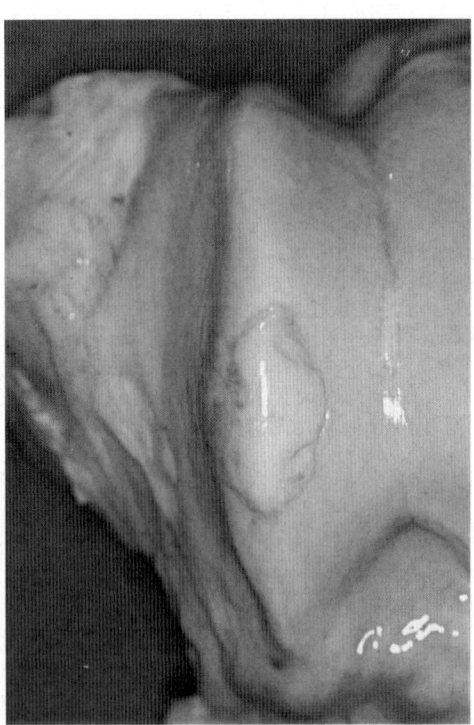

Fig. 54-2 • Dissecting flap of articular cartilage (osteochondritis dissecans lesion) on the lateral trochlear ridge of the femur. (Courtesy Gustavo Hernández-Vidal, Faculty of Veterinary Medicine, Universidad Autónoma de Nuevo León, Monterrey, Mexico.)

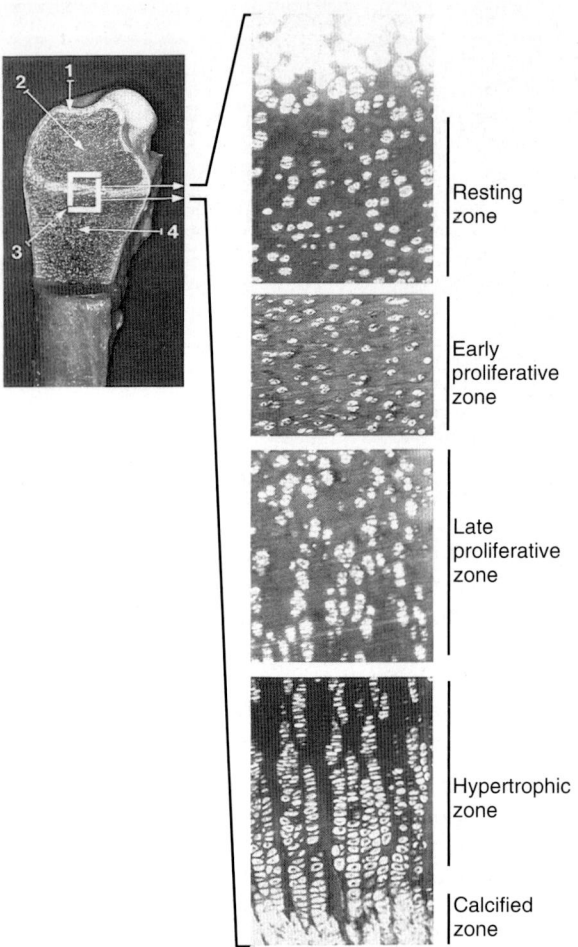

Resting zone

Early proliferative zone

Late proliferative zone

Hypertrophic zone

Calcified zone

Fig. 54-3 • Sagittal section of the epiphysis, metaphysis, and diaphysis of growing bone, with sequential histological sections showing the different zones of the physis (metaphyseal growth cartilage). *1,* Articular-epiphyseal growth cartilage complex; *2,* secondary ossification center in the epiphysis; *3,* metaphyseal growth cartilage; *4,* primary ossification center in the diaphysis. Toluidine blue stain. (Courtesy Gustavo Hernández-Vidal, Faculty of Veterinary Medicine, Universidad Autónoma de Nuevo León, Monterrey, Mexico.)

prevalence of OC may increase substantially after approximately 1 year of age in South German Coldbloods.[20] Further work is necessary to establish whether there are breed differences in the timing of lesion development.

It is important to realize that most osteochondral lesions identified radiologically in young horses heal without intervention[17,21-23] and that lesions that lead to clinical signs represent only a small fraction of the total. Thus many of the lesions identified in postmortem studies would never have become clinically relevant and may not even be evident radiologically. The age at which lesions are capable of repair appears to depend on the joint involved. A longitudinal study involving Dutch Warmbloods determined that OC lesions of the hock (the cranial aspect of the intermediate ridge of the tibia and the lateral trochlear ridge of the talus) that were still present at 5 months of age never regressed.[17] Five months was thus designated as the "age of no return" for tarsocrural lesions. In contrast, lesions of the lateral trochlear ridge of the femur did not become permanent until the animal was 8 months of age.[17]

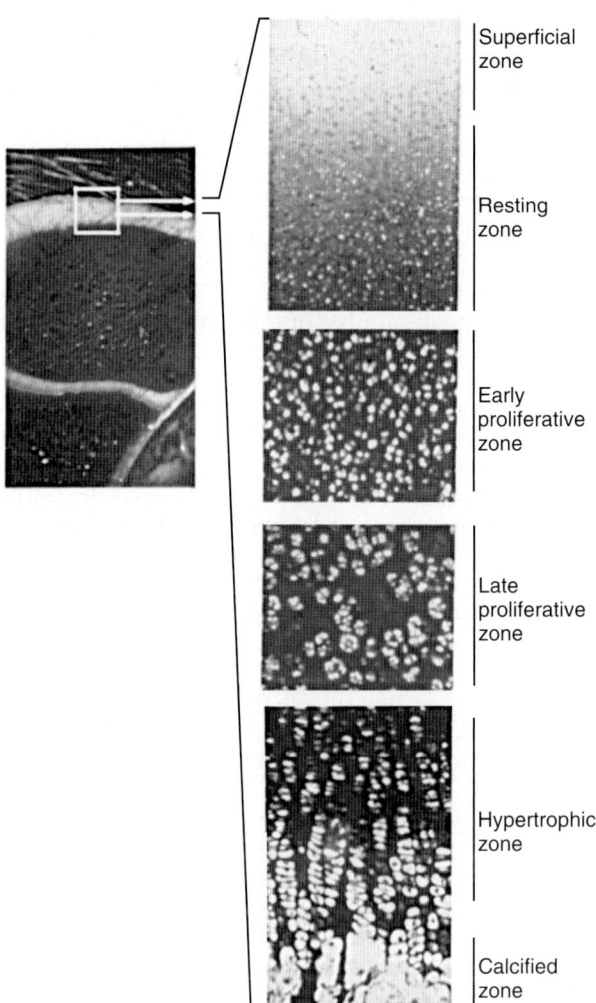

Fig. 54-4 • Sagittal section of the epiphysis with sequential histological sections showing the different zones of the articular-epiphyseal cartilage complex. Toluidine blue stain. (Courtesy Gustavo Hernández-Vidal, Faculty of Veterinary Medicine, Universidad Autónoma de Nuevo León, Monterrey, Mexico.)

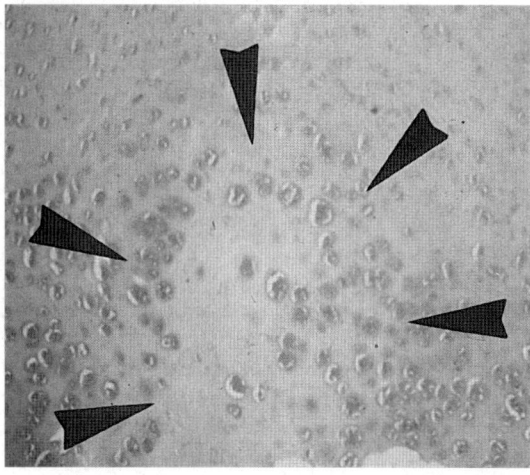

Fig. 54-5 • Chondrocyte clusters *(arrows)* surrounding an area of necrotic cartilage. Toluidine blue stain. (Courtesy Frances Henson, Department of Veterinary Medicine, University of Cambridge, Cambridge, United Kingdom.)

The features of equine OC lesions were reported as early as 1947.[9] Since then the gross and histological characteristics of the condition have been described and defined by numerous authors. Early descriptions characterized OC as a lack of chondrocyte differentiation that prevented provisional calcification of the matrix and invasion of the cartilage by blood vessels.[3] Necrosis was described as a secondary change.[3] A more recent histological study that examined AECC samples from the lateral trochlear ridge of the femur of horses ranging in age from 270 days' gestation to 4 years defined OC ("dyschondroplasia") as the presence of cartilage cores (i.e., cartilage extending into subchondral bone).[24] This study identified two types of lesion that could be differentiated on the basis of type VI collagen immunoreactivity. However, both types showed evidence of chondrocyte clusters and chondronecrosis. Lesions of one type (group A) showed disruption of the normal sequential transition of chondrocytes through the stages of proliferation and maturation and were characterized by accumulation of large numbers of small, rounded chondrocytes, apparently arrested at the prehypertrophic stage. In contrast, group B lesions showed alteration in the staining pattern of mineralized cartilage and adjacent subchondral bone and complete absence of invading capillaries into newly formed bone.[24,25] Differentiation of lesions into subcategories was not reported in a recent histological study in which necrosis of growth cartilage was described as a common feature of OC lesions.[15] This study was carried out using material from the distal tibiae of foals that were all 5 months old or younger (the age range during which the disease is initiated at this site).[17] The results suggested that chondrocyte necrosis precedes matrix change (identified histologically as relative eosinophilia and pallor in hematoxylin-eosin–stained sections and as pallor in toluidine blue–stained sections), delayed ossification, and fissure formation. Moreover, these authors considered chondrocyte clusters to be a sign of attempted repair rather than a primary change.[15]

It is obvious from this short summary that histological definitions and descriptions of OC vary, making accurate identification of lesions difficult.[24] Even chondrocyte clusters (Figure 54-5), considered by many to be one of the most consistent findings in OC lesions,[24,26] are not pathognomonic for the disease,[15,24] and, unless used to define the condition, necrosis is not a universal finding.[25,27] It is thus not surprising that the relevance to OC of some of the lesions studied has been questioned.[28] The matter is complicated further by the limited repertoire of responses that bone and cartilage can mount to injury and developmental abnormalities[12] and by the fact that many lesions are not identified until they have reached the chronic stage. The features of such chronic lesions may represent the results of secondary change and attempted repair, rather than primary osteochondrotic change. The results of studies based on such lesions may thus be misleading. This situation has resulted in a wide-ranging, heterogeneous, and somewhat confusing body of literature, in which equine OC has been ascribed to genetic, dietary, endocrine, biomechanical, traumatic, ischemic, and toxic causes.[12,18,26,29-33]

RELATIONSHIP AMONG PHYSEAL DYSPLASIA (PHYSITIS), SUBCHONDRAL BONE CYSTS, AND OSTEOCHONDROSIS

The relationship between OC and physeal dysplasia (physitis or epiphysitis) is poorly defined. Retained cartilage has long been regarded as a possible cause of physeal dysplasia,[16,34] and OC lesions of the physis have been described in clinically affected horses (thickened and irregular metaphyseal growth cartilage)[5,10] and in foals with experimentally induced dyschondroplasia (retained cartilage cores).[26,35] If OC truly is a generalized or multifocal disturbance of endochondral ossification, it would seem logical that metaphyseal growth cartilage has the potential for involvement. However, some have questioned whether articular and physeal lesions have the same cause and have proposed that physitis be regarded as a manifestation of developmental orthopedic disease but not of OC.[12] Moreover, the results of a recent study suggest that many enlargements of the distal aspect of the third metacarpal and metatarsal bones, including those with evidence of increased metaphyseal cartilage thickness, represent physiological remodeling rather than a pathological process.[36] The role of OC in the pathogenesis of equine physeal dysplasia thus remains unclear. However, it should be noted that a similar pathogenic mechanism (failure of blood supply to growth cartilage) has been proposed for both articular OC and physeal lesions in pigs.[1] Physitis is covered in more detail in Chapter 57 and is not discussed further here.

The relationship among OC, subchondral bone cysts, and osseous cystlike lesions is also controversial. In contrast to OCD lesions, which are most commonly found on the nonloaded margins of high-motion joints, bone cysts typically occur in the central, loaded areas of joints.[2] Originally interpreted as a manifestation of retained cartilage of the AECC,[10,37-39] many cysts are now thought to be traumatic in origin.[40,41] This proposed cause was demonstrated experimentally by the successful induction of cysts in the medial femoral condyle (a predilection site) after creation of a linear slit in the articular cartilage followed by normal weight bearing.[42] OC may thus be only one of several possible causative mechanisms,[12,40,43] and cysts may result from a number of nonspecific articular injuries sustained at a load-bearing site.[12]

PROPOSED CAUSATIVE FACTORS

Numerous studies aimed at determining the cause and pathogenesis of equine OC have been performed, and many of the factors investigated have been shown to influence the incidence of osteochondral lesions. However, because OC cannot yet be diagnosed on anything other than morphological grounds, it is unclear whether the lesions induced by some of these potential causative factors are the same as those that occur under "natural" conditions. A pertinent example is low copper intake, which has been shown to induce osteochondral lesions[44] but which is not believed to be a causative factor in most horses with naturally occurring OC.[1,45]

It is generally accepted that equine OC has a multifactorial cause.[1,25,45] This renders more difficult the task of unraveling the pathogenesis of the disease. Further complications are introduced by the presence of interrelationships among a number of proposed causative factors. For example, a horse's growth rate may be affected by its genetic background,[46] its plane of nutrition,[47] and possibly also by its hormonal response to carbohydrate intake,[48] all factors that have been implicated in the pathogenesis of OC.

Another topic that requires clarification is the balance between generalized or systemic and local factors. OC has historically been described as a generalized failure of endochondral ossification.[16] However, the propensity for lesions to occur in a small number of bilaterally symmetrical predilection sites argues strongly that local factors are important in the cause. It remains to be determined whether lesions can be induced solely by these local factors or whether the presence of an underlying generalized disorder (e.g., biomechanically or biochemically inferior tissue) is a prerequisite for lesion development. The following discussion summarizes major findings relating to the pathogenesis of equine OC.

Involvement of Cartilage Canals

There has been much interest recently in the role of cartilage canals in the pathogenesis of equine OC. Cartilage canals are channels that invade the epiphyseal growth cartilage from the surrounding perichondrial plexus.[49] The arterioles, venules, and capillaries that they contain assist in the nutrition of epiphyseal cartilage, much of which is too far from synovial fluid to obtain nutrients by diffusion.[1] Under normal circumstances the cartilage canals become obliterated in a regionally staggered sequence[29,49] as endochondral ossification (and therefore growth) ceases. Studies performed to date have found no evidence of cartilage canals in foals after approximately 6 or 7 months of age.[18,27,50] There is an apparent anatomical association between prolonged dependence of cartilage on a vascular supply and predisposition to OC.[29]

A number of investigations have highlighted an association between the presence of cartilage canals and development of OC. However, the proposed pathogenic mechanism differs among studies. A report published in 1995 that involved examination of tissue from 35 horses younger than 18 months of age found that cartilage canals containing patent blood vessels were present in all samples taken from OC predilection and nonpredilection sites in foals younger than 3 weeks of age.[18] Overall, 34% of the horses had lesions of OC in the medial femoral condyle, lateral femoral trochlear ridge, and/or distal aspect of the tibia, and the prevalence rose to 56% in horses 3 weeks to 5 months of age. All the lesions seen in this age group (3 weeks to 5 months) were associated with necrotic cartilage canal blood vessels. Lesions found in horses 7 months of age and older had extensive involvement of subchondral bone and bone marrow and were considered to be chronic. The authors concluded that OC lesions develop before 7 months of age and that ischemic necrosis of cartilage is involved in the pathogenesis of the condition.[18]

This conclusion is supported by the results of more recent work conducted using tissue from the distal tibiae and tarsi of foals 5 months of age or younger.[15,29,51] From the results of a histopathological study, it was concluded that early OC lesions manifest as areas of cartilage canal and chondrocyte necrosis within the proliferative zone.[15]

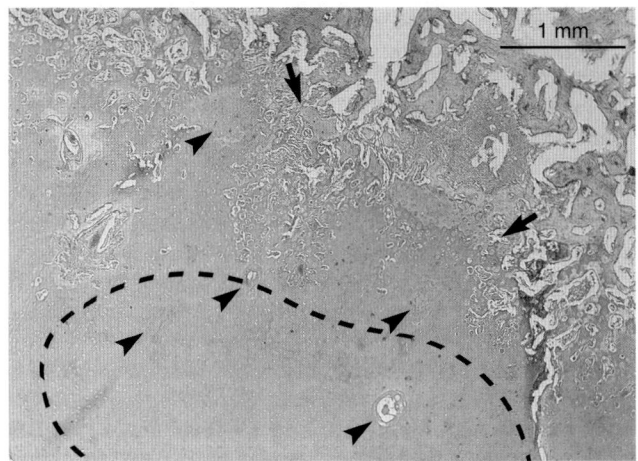

Fig. 54-6 • Histological section from the intermediate ridge of the tibia of a 3-week-old foal showing an area of chondrocyte necrosis within the proliferative zone *(stippled outline)* and a band of chondronecrosis within the ossification front *(between arrows)*. Both are associated with necrotic cartilage canals *(arrowheads)*. Toluidine blue stain. (Courtesy Osteochondrosis Research Group at the Equine Clinic, Norwegian School of Veterinary Science, Oslo, Norway.)

As the ossification front advances, these lesions become incorporated in the chondro-osseous junction where the necrotic chondrocytes and altered matrix are believed to represent conditions unfavorable for vascular invasion and replacement by bone (Figure 54-6). Vascular perfusion techniques were used to show that as foals grow the mid-portion of each cartilage canal becomes incorporated into the ossification front.[29] Anastomoses then form between canal vessels and subchondral vessels at this point.[29] As a result, tissue that is nourished by the vessels in the end of the cartilage canal farthest from the perichondrium comes to be nourished by subchondral vessels. The histological lesions identified were consistently characterized by the presence of necrotic growth cartilage in association with necrotic cartilage canal vessels located at the point where the vessels cross the ossification front, suggesting that the vessels are prone to failure at this point.[29] These results are supported by the results of micro–computed tomography analysis.[51]

An earlier study proposed a different mechanism for involvement of cartilage canals in the pathogenesis of OC. In this investigation, which involved horses that were in some cases considerably older than those in the previous study (≤15 months), nonnecrotic dyschondroplastic lesions were associated with cartilage canals containing patent vessels.[27] This finding led the investigators to propose that in some circumstances the presence of cartilage canals may be associated with failure of chondrocytes to hypertrophy and that this may be the initiating lesion. It was suggested that blood vessels within cartilage canals may expose local growth cartilage to any imbalance of systemic hormones (such as that induced by a high-energy diet) and that chronicity of lesions accounted for the difference between these findings[27] and those of studies in which necrosis is a dominant feature. It should be noted that proximity of osteochondral lesions to the remnants of cartilage canals has been reported in many studies, but is not a universal finding.[52]

Body Size and Growth Rate

The widespread anecdotal belief that OC is more prevalent in large horses and those with a rapid growth rate gained support from the results of a Swedish survey involving 77 Standardbred (STB) foals.[53] This study reported a positive relationship between radiologically evident OC of the tarsocrural joint and body weight at birth, body weight during the growth period, average daily weight gain, and skeletal frame size. Seven of the eight foals that developed tarsocrural OC were sired by the same stallion, but the relationship among OC, body measurements, and growth rate was still present when affected and unaffected foals by this sire were considered in isolation.

In postmortem studies, positive associations were reported between various measures of body size and number and severity of OC or OC-like lesions in the limbs and cervical vertebrae of 12-month-old animals of various breeds[47] and between recent average daily weight gain and tarsocrural osteochondral lesions in 5-month-old Thoroughbred (TB) foals.[54] However, this latter study found no significant association between body weight and the frequency or severity of lesions, a finding that was echoed in a recent study involving Hanoverian foals.[55]

Further evidence for a relationship among OC, body size, and growth rate comes from a study performed in Warmbloods.[56] Weight and height were measured from birth to 5 or 11 months of age in 43 foals with a presumed genetic predisposition to OC of the femoropatellar or tarsocrural joints. The foals' stifle and hock joints were evaluated radiologically, macroscopically, and histologically. Development of femoropatellar OC was associated with a higher overall rate of weight gain and greater final body weight and height. Moreover, the period during which weight gain of the OC-positive foals was significantly higher than that of the OC-negative foals coincided with the period during which femoropatellar joint lesions become visible radiologically.[17] In contrast to the previously described findings in STBs,[53] no relationship existed between tarsocrural OC and body size or growth rate in this population of Dutch Warmbloods.[56] A similar lack of correlation between surgical OC lesions and body weight has been reported in TBs.[57]

Nutrition

A number of dietary factors have been implicated in the pathogenesis of OC. These include digestible energy, phosphorus, and copper.

Digestible Energy and Protein

The results of a French study have suggested that a high plane of nutrition does not in itself predispose to development of OC, as long as the ration is balanced.[47] However, a high nutrient intake was implicated in the pathogenesis of OC for many years[10] and the topic has been explored in a number of studies. One landmark trial investigated the effects on skeletal development of feeding 129% of National Research Council (NRC, 1989)[58] recommendations for digestible energy or 126% of NRC recommendations for crude protein to foals approximately 5 months of age.[26] A control group received 100% of NRC recommendations for energy and protein. After 12 to 16 weeks on the experimental diets, all foals were euthanized, growth plates and the growth cartilage of the AECC were examined, and a definitive diagnosis of dyschondroplasia was made only when a retained core of cartilage was identified histologically. Dyschondroplasia occurred in two of 12 control foals (17%), four of six foals on the high-protein diet (67%), and all 12 foals on the high-energy diet. The lesions in the foals in the high-protein group were minor and were mainly single lesions of the growth plates, with no AECC involvement. No significant difference in incidence occurred between the control and high-protein groups. In contrast, many of the foals in the high-energy group had lesions of the AECC and the growth plates, and the difference in incidence between the control and high-energy groups was significant.

The effects of overfeeding on endochondral ossification within the growth plate have been described. Twelve TB weanlings aged 6 to 8 months were randomly assigned to receive diets containing 70%, 100%, or 130% of the National Research Council recommendations (1978)[59] for digestible energy and protein.[60] All diets contained 100% of the recommended levels of calcium and phosphorus. Biopsies of the distal radial physis obtained after 8 months showed that physeal thickness was directly proportional to digestible energy level. Moreover, the physes of the overfed horses showed many features similar to those of OC: the reserve and hypertrophic zones were enlarged, the hypertrophic cartilage had lost its normal columnar organization, and metaphyseal capillaries appeared unable to penetrate this abnormal hypertrophic cartilage. It was concluded that the lesions associated with overfeeding were similar to those caused by hypothyroidism and that the link between dietary excess and OC is mediated by endocrine factors.[60]

Subsequent work showed that ingestion of a high-energy meal is associated with accelerated insulin secretion, decreased thyroxine (T_4) secretion, and accelerated conversion of T_4 to triiodothyronine (T_3).[61] Insulin, T_3, and T_4 play a role in controlling the terminal differentiation of chondrocytes,[62,63] and it is possible that the transient postprandial hypothyroxemia induced by diets high in energy could adversely affect osteochondral development. Moreover, studies conducted on equine tissue suggest that insulin may promote the survival or depress the differentiation of chondrocytes in growth cartilage, potentially reducing the rate at which cells enter the terminal phases of hypertrophy and leading to accumulation of prehypertrophic chondrocytes.[64]

The possibility of a relationship between abnormal insulin levels and osteochondral lesions is supported by the finding that postprandial plasma glucose and insulin levels are significantly higher in young horses with OC than in unaffected animals,[57,65] an association that may be mediated, at least in part, by the glycemic index of the feed.[57] An association between feeds with a high glycemic index and increased plasma levels of insulin-like growth factor I (IGF-I) has been observed during periods of rapid growth.[66] IGF-I, which is structurally similar to insulin, is primarily involved in the control of growth and differentiation,[67] including regulation of chondrocyte growth and endochondral ossification.[64,68] However, recent data show that there is cross-talk between the insulin and IGF-I pathways, and that IGF-I participates in metabolic activities such as promotion of glucose uptake.[67] The suggestion that a high glycemic index feeding regimen and osteochondrotic risk may be linked via increased IGF-I levels is contradicted by

a study in which OC-positive foals were found to have significantly lower IGF-I activity than those without the disease.[69] The significance of the IGF-I pathway in the pathogenesis of OC thus remains unclear.

Calcium and Phosphorus

The effects of overfeeding phosphorus (388% of NRC [1989] recommendations), calcium (342%), and both calcium and digestible energy (342% and 129%, respectively) for 16 to 18 weeks was assessed in foals aged 2½ to 6½ months at the start of the study.[35] The diets containing excessive phosphorus and calcium provided 100% of NRC recommendations for digestible energy. Histologically confirmed dyschondroplastic lesions were found in numerous joints and growth plates in two control foals (17%), five foals fed excess phosphorus (83%), two foals fed excess calcium (33%), and six foals fed excess digestible energy and calcium (100%). The lesions were more numerous and severe in the foals fed high-phosphorus or high–digestible energy and high-calcium diets than in the control foals or those fed high-calcium diets only. Dyschondroplasia is thus not induced by diets high in calcium and is not alleviated by excessive calcium in foals fed excessive energy. The apparent association between excessive dietary phosphorus and abnormal endochondral ossification may be mediated by acidosis[35] or by osteoporosis-induced weakening of the subchondral bone plate.[45]

Copper

Copper is a necessary cofactor of lysyl oxidase, the enzyme that catalyzes the oxidative deamination of lysine and hydroxylysine residues to their corresponding aldehydes. This is a necessary step in the formation of pyridinoline cross-links in collagen and elastin. Low-copper diets have been associated with an increase in the soluble fraction of articular collagen, reduced collagen cross-linking of cartilage and bone, and an increased incidence of osteochondral lesions in growing foals.[44,70] A plausible mechanistic link thus exists between low copper levels and the development of OC, via the formation of biomechanically weak cartilage and bone. However, the clinical significance of this proposed pathogenic mechanism in the cause of naturally occurring OC remains unclear.

Several early studies showed an association between primary or secondary copper deficiency and equine osteochondral lesions.[70-72] However, the lesions reported—which included intrachondral splitting through the hypertrophic zone and denudation of subchondral bone—were generally much more widespread and severe than typically occur under field conditions.[70-72] Moreover, retention of cartilage was not a major pathological feature.[70] This link between copper deficiency and development of osteochondral lesions prompted investigations into the effects on equine skeletal development of copper supplementation during late gestation and the early growing period. In one such study, 21 pregnant mares were assigned to a control group (13 ppm dietary copper) or a supplemented group (32 ppm) during the last 3 to 6 months of pregnancy and the first 3 months of lactation.[32] The foals were subsequently fed diets containing 15 ppm (control) or 55 ppm (supplemented) copper for up to 6 months. The copper content of the control foals' diet was close to NRC recommendations. OC was defined as thickening of cartilage within the physis or

AECC. Compared with the supplemented foals, 6-month-old control foals had nearly twice as many lesions in the physes and more than five times as many in the AECC. The most notable lesions in the control group were cartilage thickening and separation of the cranial aspect of the intermediate ridge of the tibia.[32]

A separate study investigated the effects of feeding diets containing 8 and 25 ppm copper to 3-month-old foals for 6 months.[44] Cartilage and bone lesions were rare in the foals fed 25 ppm copper. In contrast, the majority of the foals fed 8 ppm copper were severely affected with numerous lesions. Cartilaginous flaps and cartilage thinning, erosion, and eburnation comprised the majority of the lesions, many of which were associated with microfractures within the physes and primary spongiosa of the long bones and cervical vertebrae. Biochemical analysis of tissues from four low-copper–diet foals with OCD-like lesions revealed significantly fewer pyridinoline cross-links in articular cartilage, physeal cartilage, and bone than in tissues from a group of six foals (four supplemented, two on low-copper diets) with no lesions. This study thus demonstrated a link among low dietary copper, inferior collagen quality, and OCD-like lesions.[44]

The pathological condition induced in these two studies by dietary copper levels of 8 and 15 ppm appeared similar to naturally occurring OC grossly, radiologically, and in many cases histologically.[32,44] However, the relevance to the field situation of the lesions recorded remains unknown. Foals fed the lower amount of dietary copper in these studies typically had numerous lesions, many of which were present in the cervical vertebrae.[32,44] This lesion distribution would thus be described as atypical.[12,14] Moreover, it is evident that relatively high levels of dietary copper (25 and 55 ppm) do not completely prevent osteochondral lesions,[32,44] and that relatively low levels (4 to 11 ppm) do not always result in foals with numerous osteochondral abnormalities.[26,52,73] Supplementation of foals' diets with copper is thus not a panacea, nor is it always effective.[73] Provision of copper supplements to pregnant mares has also generally been unsuccessful in reducing the incidence of osteochondral lesions at 5 to 6 months of age,[52,54] although one study did show a positive effect.[73]

Heredity

Heritability studies of equine OC have been completed in a number of breeds. The proportion of the total variation in incidence attributed to genetic factors is expressed as the heritability coefficient, and values of up to 0.52 have been reported for OC of the hock (Table 54-1).[33,74-77] Although the standard errors are in some studies substantial and the range of heritability coefficients reported is quite wide (a factor that may be attributed, in part, to variation in the mathematical approaches used),[75,77] these findings suggest that at least some manifestations of OC have a genetic component.

Recent genome-wide searches for markers associated with OC have identified significant quantitative trait loci on a number of equine chromosomes in Hanoverians and South German Coldbloods.[78,79] Further study has revealed a significant association between a single nucleotide polymorphism in the *AOAH* gene and fetlock OC in South German Coldbloods,[80] but a role in osteochondral development or repair for the protein encoded by this gene (acyloxyacyl hydrolase) has not been identified.

In spite of the success of these early genomic studies, it remains likely that OC is a polygenic disorder[81] that develops from the superimposition of environmental factors on a susceptible genetic background. Moreover, genetic factors may influence the development of disease either directly or via influences on other factors that appear to be associated with OC such as conformation, growth rate, and the hormonal response to ingestion of food.[53,56,57,65] Analysis of large numbers of genotypes will therefore be required for successful identification of the genes involved,[82] and identification of a simple set of genetic markers is a goal that may well prove elusive.

An alternative strategy for reducing the incidence of OC is to exclude affected mares and stallions from breeding programs. The results of genomic and heritability studies suggest that OC lesions at different anatomical sites may be genetically related,[75,78] and this raises the possibility that it may be possible to reduce the overall incidence of the disease by such a strategy of selective breeding. The results of mathematical modeling suggest that the incidence of OC in Maremmano horses could be reduced from 16% to 2% over five generations by active selection of both stallions and mares free of the disease.[77] Researchers who simulated the effects of various selection strategies in Dutch Warmbloods came to a similar conclusion,[83] estimating that the incidence of OC would decrease from 25% to 13% over 50 years (2.4% reduction per generation) as a result of two alternative strategies: (1) active selection for

TABLE 54-1

	Incidence and Heritability of Osteochondrosis Lesions			
SITE OF LESION	BREED	RANGE OF INCIDENCE AMONG PROGENY GROUPS (%)	HERITABILITY COEFFICIENT* (MEAN ± SE)	REFERENCE
Hock	Standardbred	3.4 to 30	0.26 ± 0.14	Schougaard et al, 1990[74]
Hock	Standardbred	0 to 24	0.24 ± 0.19 to 0.27 ± 0.08	Philipsson et al, 1993[33]
Hock	South German Coldblood	—	0.04 ± 0.07	Wittwer et al, 2007[75]
Hock	Standardbred	0 to 69	0.52	Grøndahl and Dolvik, 1993[76]
Fetlock	South German Coldblood	—	0.16 ± 0.16	Wittwer et al, 2007[75]
Stifle, hock, and fetlock	Maremmano	—	0.09 ± 0.24 to 0.14 ± 0.22	Pieramati et al, 2003[77]

SE, Standard error.

*The heritability coefficient may overestimate the true heritability if there is a high incidence of lesions in one progeny group (as occurred in the study of Grøndahl and Dolvik, 1993[76]).

OC-negative mares and stallions, and (2) progeny testing of stallions. The model output concluded that these strategies were more effective than selection of OC-negative stallions only (17% incidence at 50 years) and no active selection (21%).

Gender

Early reports suggested that the incidence of equine OC was substantially higher in males than females.[9,10] Nonsignificant relationships between male gender and OC were reported in epidemiological studies in which male/female incidence ratios of 1.6 : 1 and 1.4 : 1 were found.[84,85] However, a controlled study involving Warmbloods reported no gender predisposition for OC of the tarsocrural or femoropatellar joints,[56] and similar findings were reported in TBs.[54] In contrast, a study involving South German Coldbloods found a twofold higher risk for OC of the hock and fetlock joints in female horses,[20] and a study involving feral horses found typical OC lesions only in fillies.[86]

Exercise

The role of exercise in the pathogenesis of OC has been investigated experimentally, with conflicting results. In one study the incidence of OC was compared in foals subjected to low- and high-exercise regimens from ages 3 to 24 months.[87] All foals were housed in groups or kept in boxes and allowed paddock exercise for 2 to 4 hours per day. In addition, the low-exercise group received 15 to 45 minutes of walking exercise per day. The high-exercise group received 15 to 45 minutes of walking and trotting, plus eight to 20 gallop sprints of short duration (10 to 15 seconds). At the end of the study, hock and stifle joints were examined clinically and radiologically. OC was detected in only three (6%) of the 50 foals in the high-exercise group, but in 13 (20%) of the 66 foals in the low-exercise group, demonstrating a significant protective effect of high-intensity, short-duration exercise on the incidence of OC.

These findings were not supported by the results of a subsequent extensive investigation into the effects of exercise on musculoskeletal development. Forty-three foals with a presumed genetic predisposition to OC of the femoropatellar or tarsocrural joints were subjected to one of three exercise regimens: pasture exercise only, confinement to a box stall, and confinement to a box stall with an increasing number of gallop sprints.[23] These exercise regimens were imposed from 1 week of age to 5 months, and the incidence of OC, including subchondral bone cysts, was determined at postmortem examination in a subset of the foals at 5 months of age (eight per group). The remaining foals were subjected to the same light exercise regimen for an additional 6 months before euthanasia at 11 months of age. Lesions were found in all 5-month-old foals.[23] Frequency was highest in the tarsocrural joints (1.9 lesions per foal), with a lower incidence in the femoropatellar or femorotibial (1.0), cervical intervertebral (1.0), and metatarsophalangeal joints (0.6). Exercise did not influence the number of lesions, although there was a tendency for lesions to be more severe in the box-rested foals. Exercise also appeared to influence the type and distribution of lesions within the stifle joint: the foals subjected to box rest were more likely to develop subchondral bone cysts (femoral condyles), whereas the trained foals tended to develop OC or OCD lesions (lateral trochlear ridge of the

femur). This difference suggests an effect of mechanical loading on lesion development because the lateral trochlear ridge is loaded by the patella during exercise,[12] and subchondral bone cysts tend to develop at the point of maximum load bearing during the support phase of the stride.[23,40,43] It was concluded that exercise has no role in the pathogenesis of OC, although it may alter the appearance and distribution of lesions.[23] It should be noted that other studies conducted on tissues from these foals suggested that a regimen of box rest supplemented with short bouts of high-intensity exercise (gallop sprints) had deleterious long-term effects on chondrocyte metabolism and viability[88,89] and cannot be recommended for optimal musculoskeletal development.

Trauma and Biomechanical Force

The roles of trauma and biomechanical force in the pathogenesis of osteochondral lesions are not well established. It is generally agreed that biomechanical forces are responsible for converting an OC lesion into a dissecting OCD lesion,[5,10,16] although little solid evidence exists to support this assertion. More pertinent is establishment of the roles of trauma and biomechanical force as primary causative factors. The consistent location of typical OC lesions within joints does suggest involvement of physical factors in the pathogenesis.[90] It has been proposed that physeal dysplasia could result from excessive force on normal tissues or from the superimposition of normal force on structurally deficient tissues,[34] and a similar hypothesis has been suggested for the development of articular OC.[14,28] Many of the factors discussed previously could lead to generation of abnormal skeletal tissues, and abnormally high forces could result from excessive or inappropriate exercise, excessive body weight, or poor conformation.[34] A possible relationship between severe outward rotation of the hindlimb and tarsocrural OC was noted in a study of growing STB foals,[53] but proof of a causative effect requires further research.

The Role of Enzymes and Signaling Peptides

There is evidence that disturbances in the expression or function of a number of enzymes and/or signaling peptides may be involved in the pathogenesis of OC. Cathepsins and matrix metalloproteinases (MMPs) are proteases that are involved in the degradation of collagen and other extracellular matrix components. Cathepsin B is present in the AECC of normal growing horses, particularly in the hypertrophic zone,[52,91,92] and is abundant in the chondrocyte clusters that are commonly found in OC lesions.[52,91,93] Increased MMP activity was identified in OC lesions, particularly in the deep zone adjacent to subchondral bone, around chondrocyte clusters, and in lines that radiate from the deep zone toward the articular surface.[94] Other alterations in collagen metabolism that have been identified in association with the presence or severity of OC include changes in serum levels of biomarkers of collagen degradation and synthesis, reduced hydroxylysyl pyridinoline cross-linking (unassociated with copper deficiency), and reduced total collagen content of cartilage.[95-97]

The potential roles of parathyroid hormone–related protein (PTHrP) and Indian hedgehog (Ihh) in the pathogenesis of OC have been evaluated. These signaling molecules, which regulate chondrocyte differentiation and hypertrophy in growth cartilage via a negative feedback loop,[98] are expressed at significantly higher levels in osteochondrotic cartilage than in control tissue, and it has been proposed that this may result in retention of prehypertrophic cartilage and delayed endochondral ossification.[99,100] However, identification of reduced levels of Gli1 (the primary transcription factor for Ihh) in diseased cartilage suggests that further work in this area is necessary.[100]

Another peptide that may be involved in the pathogenesis of OC is transforming growth factor–β1 (TGF-β1), a signaling peptide that is particularly important in controlling mammalian endochondral ossification[101,102] and that has been shown to stimulate PTHrP expression.[103,104] Reduced TGF-β1 expression has been identified in the AECC of the lateral trochlear ridge of the femur in horses with dyschondroplasia at this site, and it was suggested that this may result in cessation of chondrocyte hypertrophy and an accumulation of prehypertrophic chondrocytes.[105] However, the clinical significance of these findings has not been established. In this work, as in all other investigations into the pathogenesis of OC, it is important that distinctions be made between primary and secondary change whenever possible.

Toxic Causes of Osteochondral Lesions
Foals exposed to excessive amounts of zinc and zinc and cadmium in combination have been found to develop generalized, severe osteochondral lesions.[31,106-108] The gross lesions described in these reports were characterized by separation of articular cartilage from subchondral bone. The role of cadmium in the pathogenesis of these lesions is unclear.[31,106,108] However, the effect of excessive dietary zinc is likely to be mediated by secondary copper deficiency.[109] These environmental contaminants are clearly toxic causes of osteochondral lesions and are not considered to be factors in the pathogenesis of naturally occurring OC.

SUMMARY
A range of conditions results in failure of endochondral ossification and retention of cartilage cores at the cartilage-bone interface. However, opinions regarding pathogenesis of OC still differ widely on the major factors involved in the cause of the naturally occurring condition. The situation is complicated by the apparently multifactorial nature of the condition,[1,5,8,25,45] by the fact that environmental influences and genetic susceptibility apparently combine to determine the final outcome,[53] and by the superimposition of secondary changes on primary lesions. However, it is hoped that a renewed focus on the examination of early lesions may allow development of a unified theory on the pathogenesis of the disease.

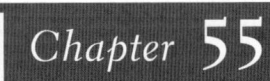

Chapter 55

The Role of Nutrition in Developmental Orthopedic Disease: Nutritional Management

Joe D. Pagan

Nutrition may play an important role in the pathogenesis of developmental orthopedic disease in horses. Deficiencies, excesses, and imbalances of nutrients may result in an increase in the incidence and severity of physitis, angular limb deformity, wobbler syndrome (wobbles), and osteochondrosis.

NUTRITIONAL FACTORS AS A CAUSE OF DEVELOPMENTAL ORTHOPEDIC DISEASE

Mineral Deficiencies
A deficiency of minerals, including calcium, phosphorus, copper, and zinc, may lead to developmental orthopedic disease. Most commonly fed cereal grains and forages contain insufficient quantities of several minerals. A ration of grass hay and oats supplies only 40% and 70% of a weanling's calcium and phosphorus requirements, respectively, and less than 40% of its requirements for copper and zinc (Table 55-1). The best method of diagnosing mineral deficiencies is through ration evaluation. Blood, hair, and hoof analysis is of limited usefulness.

Mineral Excesses
Horses can tolerate fairly high levels of mineral intake, but excesses of calcium, phosphorus, zinc, iodine, fluoride, and heavy metals, such as lead and cadmium, may lead to developmental orthopedic disease (Table 55-2[1,2]).

Mineral excesses occur because of overfortification or environmental contamination. Massive oversupplementation of calcium (>300% of required amount) may lead to a secondary mineral deficiency by interfering with the absorption of other minerals such as phosphorus, zinc, and iodine. Excessive calcium intake may be compounded by using legume hays as the primary forage source. Iodine and selenium oversupplementation occurs if supplements are fed at inappropriate levels. A ration evaluation is the best way to identify this type of mineral imbalance.

Environmental contamination is a more likely cause of developmental orthopedic disease, because contamination may result in extremely high intakes of potentially toxic minerals. If a farm is experiencing an unusually high incidence of developmental orthopedic disease or if the location and severity of skeletal lesions are abnormal, environmental contamination should be investigated. Blood, feed, and water analysis should be performed. Chemical

References on page 1297

TABLE 55-1

	NUTRIENT CONCENTRATION REQUIRED IN TOTAL DIET (90% DRY BASIS)						
Mineral Requirements for Weanlings							
MINERAL	MODERATE GROWTH	RAPID GROWTH	GRASS HAY	ALFALFA HAY	OATS	CORN	BARLEY
Calcium (%)	0.62	0.70	0.35	1.25	0.08	0.05	0.05
Phosphorus (%)	0.40	0.45	0.20	0.22	0.34	0.27	0.34
Zinc (ppm)	65	65	9	16	6	4	8
Copper (ppm)	22	22	17	28	35	19	17

TABLE 55-2

*Toxic Mineral Levels**		
MINERAL	MINERAL LEVEL NEEDED BY YOUNG HORSE (PPM)	TOXIC LEVEL (PPM)
Zinc	60-70	9000
Iodine	0.2-0.3	5
Fluoride	—	50
Lead	—	80
Selenium	0.2-0.3	5
Manganese	60-70	4000
Copper	20-30	300-500
Cobalt	0.1	400
Iron	125	5000

*Adapted from Cunha TJ: *Horse feeding and nutrition,* ed 2, Orlando, 2007, Academic Press[1]; and National Research Council: *Nutrient requirements of horses,* ed 6, Washington, DC, 2007, National Academies Press.[2]

analysis of hoof and hair samples may reveal valuable information. Farms that are located near factories or smelters are most at risk, although osteochondrosis caused by zinc-induced copper deficiency has been reported on farms using fence paint containing zinc or galvanized water pipes.

Mineral Imbalances

The ratio of minerals may be as important as the actual amount of individual minerals in the ration. High levels of phosphorus inhibit the absorption of calcium and lead to a deficiency, even if the amount of calcium present is normally adequate. The calcium/phosphorus ratio in the rations of young horses should never be below 1:1 and ideally should be 1.5:1. Too much calcium may affect phosphorus status, particularly if the level of phosphorus is marginal. Calcium/phosphorus ratios greater than 2.5:1 should be avoided if possible. Forage diets with high calcium levels should be supplemented with phosphorus. The zinc/copper ratio should be 3:1 to 4:1.

Dietary Energy Excesses

In the Thoroughbred (TB) industry, large, well-grown yearlings are desirable when offered for sale at public auction because selling price is influenced by body size. Yearlings that sold higher than the median of the session in which they were sold were heavier and taller than yearlings that sold below the session median.[3] In addition, TBs that were heavy and tall as yearlings had the most earnings, graded stakes wins, and grade-1 stakes wins.[4] Because of the premium price paid for mass, young TBs are often grown rapidly to achieve maximal size. Excessive energy intake can lead to rapid growth and increased body fat, which may predispose young horses to developmental orthopedic disease. A Kentucky study showed that growth rate and body size might increase the incidence of certain types of developmental orthopedic diseases in TB foals.[5] Yearlings that showed osteochondrosis of the hock and stifle were large at birth, grew rapidly from 3 to 8 months of age, and were heavier than the average population as weanlings.

The source of energy for young horses also may be important, because hyperglycemia and hyperinsulinemia have been implicated in the pathogenesis of osteochondrosis.[6,7] Foals that experience an exaggerated and sustained increase in circulating glucose or insulin in response to a carbohydrate (grain) meal may be predisposed to develop osteochondrosis.[8]

In a large field trial, 218 TB weanlings (average age 300 ± 40 days, average body weight 300 ± 43 kg) were studied.[8] A glycemic response test was conducted by feeding a meal that consisted of the weanling's normal concentrate at a level of intake equal to 1.4 g of nonstructural carbohydrate per kilogram of body mass. A single blood sample was collected 120 minutes after feeding to determine glucose and insulin levels. A high glucose and insulin response to a concentrate meal was associated with an increased incidence of osteochondrosis. More research is needed to determine whether the incidence of osteochondrosis can be reduced through feeding foals concentrates that produce low glycemic responses.

RATION EVALUATIONS

The best way to determine whether nutrition is a contributing factor to developmental orthopedic disease is to perform a ration evaluation, which compares the intake of several essential nutrients with the requirements of the horse. Gross deficiencies or excesses of key nutrients then can be identified and corrected. In the past, ration evaluations were time-consuming and cumbersome, because much of the mathematical calculation was done by hand. Fortunately computer programs are now available that make ration evaluations quick and easy to interpret. Kentucky Equine Research (Versailles, Kentucky, United States) has developed an equine ration evaluation program called MicroSteed (www.ker.com).

Types of Evaluations

Ration evaluations can be approached in two ways. One way is to add up what is being fed and compare it with the horse's requirements. This may not be easy because most horse owners do not know exactly what their horses are eating. Alternatively, a new ration may be developed.

Protocol

Every nutrition evaluation should include a description of the horse, definition of nutrient requirements, determination of nutrients in feedstuffs, determination of intake of feedstuffs, calculation of nutrient intake, comparison of intake with requirements, and adjustment of the ration to correct deficiencies or excesses.

Describing the Horse

Different classes of horses have different nutrient requirements, and each class may eat different amounts of forage and grain. Within each class of horse, it is important to know the horse's current body weight, its age and mature body weight if growing, and its rate of body weight gain or loss.

Defining Nutrient Requirements

Ration evaluations are intended to compare a horse's daily nutrient intake with a set of requirements to determine how well the feeding program meets the horse's nutritional needs. The National Research Council (NRC) publishes a set of requirements for horses, but NRC values generally represent *minimum* requirements for most nutrients. These are the levels of intake that are required to prevent the onset of clinical signs associated with frank deficiency. No allowances are included to account for factors that may increase the requirement of a nutrient. The bioavailability of nutrients may be different, and other substances within a ration may interfere with the digestibility or use of a nutrient.

MicroSteed includes two different sets of nutrient requirements—the NRC and Kentucky Equine Research requirements—based on a combination of NRC numbers, research conducted since publication of the most recent NRC recommendations, and experience in the field. The user has the option of selecting NRC or Kentucky Equine Research requirements or adding a custom set of requirements.

NRC values for digestible energy and protein fairly accurately describe the needs of most horses. These two requirements were primarily developed from direct measurements of growth response and energy balance. Other requirements, such as those for calcium and phosphorus, were developed using more theoretical calculations involving estimates of endogenous losses and digestibility. Still others were based on values developed for other species or from single experiments that were far from conclusive. Kentucky Equine Research requirements use values ranging from 1.25 to 3 times those recommended by the NRC for most vitamins and minerals. These nutrient requirements are not absolute, but it is assumed that they adequately reflect horses' needs under a wide range of conditions.

Determining Nutrients in Feedstuffs

The accuracy of evaluating the diet depends on proper sampling of feedstuffs. The feeds should be thoroughly mixed and a representative sample taken. Pelleted feeds are fairly uniform, but sampling is more critical for textured feeds and home mixes. If an odd nutrient value is encountered, the clinician should look to sampling error as a likely cause.

A hay core can be used to obtain a representative hay sample for analysis. Pasture analysis is more difficult. Should the entire pasture be systematically sampled or only those areas heavily grazed? Horses tend to be spot grazers; therefore sampling the heavily grazed areas is probably best.

When expressing feed intakes and nutrient composition, air dry values for hay and grain and 100% dry matter values for pasture are used, because hay and grain intakes actually are measured as fed, and pasture intakes tend to be estimated. The moisture content of the pasture is not relevant to the evaluation and only complicates intake calculations.

A number of commercial laboratories analyze forages and feeds. For a typical ration evaluation for young growing horses, the following nutrients should be analyzed or calculated for each forage and concentrate: digestible energy (megacalories [Mcal] or megajoules [MJ], typically estimated), crude protein (percent), lysine (percent, typically estimated), acid or neutral detergent fiber (percent), calcium (percent), phosphorus (percent), zinc (percent), copper (percent), and manganese (percent).

These nutrients usually are included on a standard panel analysis at a reasonable cost. Other minerals, such as selenium and iodine, usually are analyzed separately, and analysis can be expensive. Selenium and iodine are not essential for evaluations that focus on identifying nutritional causes of developmental orthopedic disease.

Determining Intake of Feedstuffs

A common flaw in many ration evaluations is measuring intake inaccurately. A weighing scale should be used to measure the amount of grain and hay offered. A certain degree of hay wastage usually occurs, and this should be taken into account when calculating intake. The amount of forage and grain consumed by young horses varies tremendously, depending on geographical location and forage availability. Typically, horses that are raised in tropical environments depend heavily on grain in the ration. Yearlings raised in temperate areas with abundant forage may eat rations that contain 80% forage.

Calculating Nutrient Intake

Determining pasture intake is the most difficult part of conducting a ration evaluation. Two methods usually are employed to estimate pasture intake. The simpler method is arbitrarily to estimate intake at about 1% to 1.5% of a young horse's body weight. The obtained value is approximate, but it is representative of most young horses at pasture for most of the day. A second and more accurate method is to calculate pasture intake energetically, by subtracting the digestible energy intake from all other feedstuffs from the horse's daily energy requirement. Dividing this number by the calculated energy density of the pasture yields daily dry matter intake. For example, a yearling that weighs 330 kg with an average daily gain of 0.55 kg/day should require 20.4 Mcal of digestible energy per day. If that yearling is eating 3.65 kg of sweet feed (10.8 Mcal of digestible energy) and 2 kg of mature alfalfa hay (3.6 Mcal digestible energy), then the yearling must be consuming around 6 Mcal of digestible energy from pasture. Most grass pastures contain about 2.2 Mcal of digestible energy per kilogram, so this yearling must consume about 2.73 kg of pasture dry matter per day. These intakes can then be used to evaluate the adequacy of the ration for other nutrients. In MicroSteed, pasture intake can be estimated automatically by first entering the other feedstuffs into the ration and then using an estimate key to perform the calculation just described. This method of calculating pasture energy intake works well, provided that the horse actually is consuming the intakes of other feedstuffs and that the correct energy requirements were selected.

Using the method described previously for estimating pasture intake often yields a negative number. If this occurs, then the digestible energy intake of the other feeds is too high, or the calculated energy consumption is too low. Sometimes horse owners report higher intakes of feeds than actually are eaten, which is particularly true for forages, because hay rarely is weighed and large quantities often are wasted. Grain intake can also be overestimated because the coffee can that is used to measure grain does not hold nearly as much grain as it does coffee. At other times the hay and grain intake may be correct, but the horse may be consuming more energy than calculated. Increased energy intake can occur if the horse is expending extra energy to work or keep warm in cold weather, or a young horse may be growing faster than assumed. For example, a yearling needs about 5 kg of additional grain (16.1 Mcal of digestible energy) per kilogram of gain. If average daily gain is higher than assumed, then the horse may be eating significantly more digestible energy than calculated.

Comparing Intake with Requirements

Rarely will the nutrients supplied by a ration exactly match a horse's requirements, and balancing rations with this type of precision is unnecessary. Instead, the key to interpreting a ration evaluation is to identify deficiencies, excesses, or imbalances of nutrients that may affect growth and skeletal soundness. For most nutrients a level of intake in excess of 90% of required is not considered deficient. What is interpreted as excessive varies tremendously among nutrients. For instance, potassium plays only a minor role in skeletal development; a young horse at pasture may consume greater than 300% of its potassium requirement. Most of this potassium comes from the pasture and is perfectly harmless. Even small excesses of other nutrients, such as energy, may play a significant role in the development of skeletal disease. Energy intakes that are 115% of required might trigger mild developmental orthopedic disease, and levels above 130% almost certainly will cause problems in rapidly growing horses.

FEEDING PRACTICES THAT CONTRIBUTE TO DEVELOPMENTAL ORTHOPEDIC DISEASE

Several feeding scenarios may contribute to developmental orthopedic disease. Once identified, most can be corrected easily through adjustments in feed type and intake. Several of the most common mistakes made in feeding young growing horses are explained.

Overfeeding

One of the most common problems of feeding young horses is excessive intake that results in accelerated growth

rate or fattening. Both conditions may contribute to developmental orthopedic disease. Unfortunately, there are no simple rules about how much grain is too much, because total intake of forage and grain determines energy consumption. Large intakes of grain are appropriate if the forage is sparse or of poor quality, as often is the case in tropical environments. For example, grain intakes as high as 2% to 2.5% of body weight may be necessary to sustain reasonable growth in weanlings that have access to no forage other than tropical pasture. Conversely, grain intakes higher than 1% of body weight may be considered excessive when weanlings are raised on lush temperate pasture or have access to high-quality alfalfa hay.

The surest way to document excessive intake is by weighing and using condition scoring in the growing horse. Based on a system developed by Henneke and colleagues,[9] condition scoring measures fat deposition. Horses are scored from 1 to 9 (1 denoting extreme thinness and 9 indicating obesity). In a Kentucky study, fillies tended to have higher condition scores than colts, and the difference was greatest at 4 months of age (fillies 6.48; colts 6.0). These condition scores are considered moderate to fleshy according to the Henneke scoring system. By 12 months of age the condition scores of the colts and fillies had dropped to 5.3 and 5.4, respectively. Both sexes increased condition score slightly from 14 to 18 months.

Managing the growth in horses becomes a balance between producing a desirable individual for a particular purpose without creating skeletal problems that will reduce a horse's subsequent athletic ability. Growing a foal too slowly results in the risk of it being too small at a particular age or never obtaining optimal mature body size. Therefore it is widely recommended to maintain a steady growth rate by regularly weighing and measuring horses during the growth period.[1,10]

If growth rate cannot be measured, excessive intake can often be assessed by ration evaluation. For example, a 6-month-old TB weanling (250 kg body mass; 500 kg mature body mass) was being fed 4 kg of a 16% protein sweet feed and 2 kg of alfalfa hay per day, with access to high-quality fall Kentucky pasture. To support a reasonable rate of growth (0.80 kg/day), this weanling required about 17 Mcal of digestible energy per day. The hay and grain intake of this foal alone would supply about 17.5 Mcal of digestible energy, which is slightly above the weanling's requirement. If a reasonable level of pasture intake were included (1% body mass or 2.5 kg dry matter), this weanling would be consuming 135% of its digestible energy requirement, a level likely to cause problems.

To reduce intake, the alfalfa hay should be eliminated, if the pasture is indeed adequate. If hay were needed when the weanling was stalled, grass hay would be more appropriate. Grain intake should be reduced to a level of about 3 kg/day. At this level of grain intake the weanling would need to consume about 3.3 kg of pasture dry matter to support a growth rate of 0.80 kg/day, and the ration would be nicely balanced.

Inappropriate Grain for Forage Provided

Occasionally the concentrate offered to a growing horse is incorrectly fortified to complement the forage that is being fed. The problem occurs particularly when the forage is mostly alfalfa or clover. Most concentrates for young horses are formulated with levels of minerals and protein needed to balance grass forage.

For example, a 12-month-old yearling (315 kg body mass; 500 kg mature body mass; 0.50 kg/day average daily growth) is raised without access to pasture, and the only forage available is alfalfa hay, which is fed at a level of intake equal to 1.5% of the yearling's body mass (4.72 kg/day). At this level of forage intake, the yearling would require only about 2.5 kg of grain per day. If a typical 14% protein sweet feed that was formulated to balance grass forage were used, the ration would be inappropriate for a number of reasons. Calcium would be 183% of the yearling's requirement, with a calcium/phosphorus ratio of 2.9:1. This would not be a problem except that phosphorus and zinc are marginal in the ration. Because calcium may interfere with the absorption of these minerals, the yearling may be at risk for developmental orthopedic disease from a zinc or phosphorus deficiency. The solution is to feed a concentrate that is more appropriately balanced for legume hay. For example, a 12% protein feed with 0.4% calcium, 0.9% phosphorus, and 180 ppm zinc would be more suitable.

Inadequate Fortification in Grain

The most common reasons for inadequate fortification are using unfortified or underfortified grain mixes, using correctly fortified feeds at levels of intake that are below the manufacturer's recommendation, or using fortified feeds diluted with straight cereal grains. These errors in feeding can be corrected by incorporating a highly fortified grain balancer supplement.

For example, a 6-month-old weanling (200 kg body mass; 400 kg mature body mass; 0.60 kg/day average daily growth) is fed 3 kg/day of a 10% protein sweet feed that is intended for adult horses. To compound matters, the weanling is also fed grass hay, with an estimated intake of 2.3 kg/day. This ration is deficient in protein, calcium, phosphorus, zinc, and copper. The foal would be prone to a rough hair coat and physitis. There are two ways to correct this problem. A properly formulated 14% to 16% protein grain mix with adequate mineral fortification could be used, or 1 kg of a grain balancer pellet could be substituted for 1 kg of the 10% sweet feed. This type of supplement is typically fortified with 25% to 30% protein, 2.5% to 3.0% calcium, 1.75% to 2.0% phosphorus, 125 to 175 ppm copper, and 375 to 475 ppm zinc. This is an extremely useful type of supplement to correct underfortified rations.

FEEDING SYSTEMS TO PREVENT DEVELOPMENTAL ORTHOPEDIC DISEASE

The nutritional requirements of a broodmare can be divided into three stages. Stage one is early pregnancy, from conception through the first 7 months of gestation. Barren mares and pregnant mares without suckling foals fit into this nutritional category. Stage two encompasses the last trimester of pregnancy, from around 7 months of pregnancy through foaling. Stage three is lactation, which generally lasts 5 to 6 months after foaling. The most common mistakes are overfeeding during early pregnancy and underfeeding during lactation.

Early Pregnancy

Proper feeding of a mare during pregnancy requires an understanding of how the fetus develops during gestation. Contrary to popular belief, the fetus does not grow at a constant rate throughout the entire 11 months of pregnancy. The fetus is small during the first 5 months of pregnancy. At 7 months of pregnancy the fetus equals only about 20% of its weight at birth. At this stage in pregnancy the fetus equals less than 2% of the mare's weight, and its nutrient requirements are minuscule compared with the mare's own maintenance requirements (Table 55-3). Therefore the mare can be fed essentially the same as if she were not pregnant. Mare owners often greatly increase feed intake after a mare is pronounced in foal, reasoning that she is now eating for two. Increased feeding is unnecessary and may lead to obesity and foaling difficulties, especially if the mare has access to high-quality pasture.

Late Pregnancy

The fetus begins to develop rapidly after 7 months of pregnancy, and its nutrient requirements become substantially greater than the mare's maintenance requirements; therefore adjustments should be made to the mare's diet. Digestible energy requirements increase about 15% over early pregnancy. Protein and mineral requirements increase to a greater extent, because the fetal tissue being synthesized during this time is high in protein, calcium, and phosphorus. During the last 4 months of pregnancy the fetus and placenta retain about 77 g of protein, 7.5 g of calcium, and 4 g of phosphorus per day. Trace mineral supplementation is also important because the fetus stores iron, zinc, copper, and manganese in its liver for use during the

TABLE 55-3

	Expected Feed Consumption by Horses				
	% OF BODY WEIGHT			**% OF DIET**	
HORSE	**FORAGE**	**CONCENTRATE**		**FORAGE**	**CONCENTRATE**
Maintenance	1-2	0-1		50-100	0-50
Pregnant mare	1-2	0.3-10		50-85	15-50
Lactating mare (early)	1-2.5	0.5-2		33-85	15-66
Lactating mare (late)	1-2	0.5-1.5		40-80	20-60
Weanling	0.5-1.8	1-2.5		30-65	35-70
Yearling	1-2.5	0.5-2		33-80	20-66
Performance horse	1-2	0.5-2		33-80	20-66

first few months after birth, mare's milk being low in these elements.

New Zealand researchers studied the effect of copper supplementation on the incidence of developmental orthopedic disease in TB foals.[11] Pregnant TB mares were divided into copper-supplemented and control groups. Live foals born to each group of mares were also divided into copper-supplemented and control groups. Copper supplementation of mares was associated with a significant reduction in the physitis scores of the foals at 150 days of age. Foals from mares that received no supplementation had a mean physitis score of 6, whereas foals from supplemented mares had a mean score of 3.7. A lower score means less physitis. Copper supplementation of the foals had no significant effect on physitis scores. A significantly lower incidence of articular cartilage lesions occurred in foals from supplemented mares. However, copper supplementation of the foals had no significant effect on physeal cartilage lesions.[11] Mares in late pregnancy often are overfed energy in an attempt to supply adequate protein and minerals to the developing foal. If a pregnant mare becomes fat during late pregnancy, she should be switched to a feed that is more concentrated in protein and minerals so that less can be fed per day. This will restrict her energy intake while ensuring that she receives adequate quantities of other key nutrients.

Lactation

A mare's nutrient requirements increase substantially after foaling. During the first 3 months of lactation, mares produce milk at a rate equal to about 3% of body weight per day. This milk is rich in energy, protein, calcium, phosphorus, and vitamins. Therefore the mare should be fed enough grain to meet its greatly increased nutrient requirements. Mares in early lactation usually require 4.5 to 6.5 kg of grain per day, depending on the type and quality of forage they are consuming. This grain mix should be fortified with additional protein, minerals, and vitamins to meet the lactating mare's needs. Trace mineral fortification is not as important for lactating mares, because milk contains low levels of these nutrients, and adding more to the lactating mare's diet does not increase the trace mineral content of the milk. Calcium and phosphorus are the minerals that should be of primary concern during lactation. Grain intake should be increased gradually during the last few weeks of pregnancy so that the mare is consuming nearly the amount that it will require for milk production at foaling. A rapid increase in grain should be avoided at foaling because it could lead to colic or laminitis. Milk production begins to decline after about 3 months of lactation, and grain intake can be reduced to maintain the mare in desirable condition.

Sucklings

If a broodmare has been fed properly during late pregnancy, giving mineral supplements to a suckling is unnecessary until it reaches 90 days of age. At 90 days, moderate amounts of a well-fortified foal feed can be introduced and gradually increased until the suckling is consuming around 0.5 kg of feed per month of age.

Birth month has a significant effect on suckling growth. Kentucky TBs born in the winter (January and February) have been found to be smaller at birth and to grow more slowly during the first 2 months compared with spring-born foals. These winter-born foals then exhibited rapid daily weight gain at 3 months of age, coinciding with a spring pasture flush.[12] This compensatory growth resulted in there being no difference in body weights between foals born in any birth month at 5 months of age. This rapid growth spurt exhibited in winter-born foals may be undesirable owing to the risk of developmental orthopedic disease, and thus growth of the suckling must be carefully managed.

Furthermore, it is critical that the suckling be accustomed to eating grain before weaning. If the suckling does not become accustomed to eating grain, there is a good chance that its growth rate will decrease dramatically at weaning. When the weanling finally starts eating grain, a compensatory growth spurt occurs that may result in developmental orthopedic disease.

Weanlings

The most critical stage of growth for preventing developmental orthopedic disease is from weaning to 12 months of age, when the skeleton is most vulnerable to disease and when nutrient intake and balance are most important. Weanlings should grow at a moderate rate with adequate mineral supplementation. In temperate regions the contribution of pasture to the diet often is underestimated, leading to excessive growth rates and developmental orthopedic disease.

Yearlings

Once a horse has reached 12 months of age, it is much less likely to develop many forms of developmental orthopedic disease than a younger horse. Many of the lesions that become clinically relevant after this age probably developed at a younger age. Proper nutrient balance remains important for the yearling, and delaying as long as possible the increased energy intakes that are required for sales preparation is best, because the skeleton is less vulnerable to developmental orthopedic disease as a yearling ages. Normally, increasing energy intake 90 days before a sale is enough time to add the extra body condition that often is expected in a sales yearling. Physitis in the carpus is often a major concern for the sales yearling. The level of trace mineral supplementation should remain high to reduce the incidence of physitis in sales yearlings, and a substantial portion of the energy normally supplied from grain should be replaced with fat and fermentable fiber. Sales preparation grain mixes can contain as much as 10% fat. Good sources of fermentable fiber include beet pulp and soy hulls.

NUTRITIONAL MANAGEMENT OF DEVELOPMENTAL ORTHOPEDIC DISEASE

The goal of a feeding program for young horses is to reduce or eliminate the incidence of developmental orthopedic disease. Unfortunately, developmental orthopedic disease still occurs in some foals. Nutritional intervention can help reduce the severity of many forms of developmental orthopedic disease, but not all of the damage resulting from the disease is reversible. However, it is important to alter the feeding programs of foals with developmental orthopedic disease. The type of alteration follows a similar pattern but depends on the foal's age and the type of developmental orthopedic disease. In almost every instance, energy intake should be reduced while adequate levels of protein and minerals are maintained. The rationale for this type of modification is that skeletal growth should be slowed, but adequate substrate should be available to promote healthy bone development.

Physitis

Grain intake should be restricted to a level supplying around 75% of the foal's normal energy requirement. This restriction, however, should not compromise protein and mineral intake, so a different type of feed formulation may be required. For instance, a 6-month-old weanling (250 kg body mass; 500 kg mature body mass; 0.8 kg average daily growth) on a decent fall pasture would normally consume around 3.5 kg of a 16% protein foal feed. If this foal were to develop physitis, it should be confined and fed grass hay (3 kg/day). Reducing the grain intake to 75% of the foal's normal digestible energy would result in shortages of protein, lysine, calcium, and phosphorus. These shortfalls could be overcome by replacing 1 kg of the 16% sweet feed with a grain balancer pellet. This ration would supply 90%

of the foal's normal protein requirement, along with a good supply of minerals. As the physitis resolves, intake of the 16% grain mix can be slowly increased and the supplement pellet intake slowly decreased, until the foal returns to its normal ration.

Cervical Vertebral Malformation

A feeding program like the one described previously is also appropriate for a horse with cervical vertebral malformation, except that the degree of exercise and energy restriction may be more severe. In this case a feeding program that combines grass hay (2 kg) with a moderate amount of alfalfa hay (2 kg/day) and 1 kg of balancer pellet would result in a reduction in energy intake equal to 65% of normal intake while maintaining adequate levels of protein and mineral intake.

Osteochondrosis

Once a foal has developed osteochondrosis that is severe enough to produce clinical signs, the effect of diet is minimal in solving the existing lesion, but reducing energy intake and body weight while maintaining adequate protein and mineral intake is advised.

Chapter 56

Diagnosis and Management of Osteochondrosis and Osseous Cystlike Lesions

Dean W. Richardson

The pathogenesis of osteochondrosis (OC), palmar or plantar osteochondral fragments of the proximal phalanx, ununited palmar or plantar eminences of the proximal phalanx, subchondral bone cysts, and other osseous cyst-like lesions is discussed in Chapters 36, 42, and 54. In this book the term *subchondral bone cyst* is used for large radiolucent areas in the subchondral bone of the medial femoral condyle; these cysts have a consistent pathological structure with a true cellular cyst lining. Osseous cystlike lesions in other locations vary more in structure. This chapter discusses the diagnosis and management of these lesions and other osseous fragments believed to be at least predominantly developmental in origin. The joints most commonly affected include the hock, stifle, fetlock, and shoulder. It is common for matching joints to have lesions but much less common to find OC lesions in different joints. This is consistent with the concept of such lesions occurring during some finite window of vulnerability during development that is specific for a given anatomical location.

Clinical signs of OC range from none to severe lameness. Moderate-to-severe joint effusion often occurs with minimal or no lameness. The clinical signs are not necessarily coincident with the development of the lesion. Most OC lesions are probably formed before 6 months of age, yet most are diagnosed at a later age. Some lesions seen radiologically heal, or they at least become stable enough never to cause a clinically apparent lameness. Lesions in racing Thoroughbreds (TBs) and Standardbreds (STBs) are usually recognized by 2 years of age, but in Warmbloods (WBLs) that are older when they begin training, clinical signs may not be seen until the horse is 5 to 6 years of age or even older. Acute, more severe lameness in older horses occurs occasionally when osteochondritis dissecans (OCD) fragments become loose.

Diagnosis is based on typical clinical signs and radiology. Most OCD flaps in horses have an osseous component and so can be identified using plain radiography. Defects in subchondral bone contours are also easily identified. Radiologically apparent defects in subchondral bone must be interpreted with caution in foals, especially in areas where endochondral ossification occurs later, such as the femoral or talar trochlear ridges and the third metacarpal or metatarsal sagittal ridge. An irregularity in the contour of subchondral bone does *not* mean that an articular defect is necessarily present; the lesion still possibly may heal. Therefore surgical intervention should be delayed until it is clear that either a loose fragment is present or the healing is progressing inadequately. Radiologically apparent lesions must always be interpreted with the clinical signs, because some do not cause clinical signs. If a lesion is identified, the contralateral joint should always be examined radiologically, because bilateral involvement (quadrilateral in the fetlock) is common. The presence of bilateral radiologically apparent lesions in a horse that is unilaterally lame is not unusual and further emphasizes the need to clinically evaluate the individual horse fully.

Decisions concerning treatment should take into consideration the age of the horse, its intended use, the severity of the lesions and anatomical location, whether the horse is intended for sale through public auction, and, if so, the timing of the sale and the conditions of sale. Prophylactic removal of OCD lesions for economic reasons may be justified in all horses intended for future sale. Most buyers are more willing to purchase horses after an OCD lesion has been removed and the horse has returned to work.

LESIONS IN THE METACARPOPHALANGEAL AND METATARSOPHALANGEAL JOINTS

Osteochondritis Dissecans of the Sagittal Ridge of the Third Metacarpal and Metatarsal Bones

Most foals and yearlings with OCD lesions of the sagittal ridge of the third metacarpal bone (McIII) or third metatarsal bone (MtIII) are not recognized as lame. A variable degree of joint effusion occurs, and the lesions are usually first identified on presale radiographs. Unstable lesions cause lameness and persistent effusion when a horse starts work. Lameness is eliminated by intraarticular or perineural analgesia.

Lesions are more common in the MtIII than in the McIII, but all fetlocks should be examined radiologically if a lesion is recognized in one, using perfectly exposed (or slightly underexposed) flexed lateromedial images (Figure 56-1). Lesions on the dorsoproximal aspect of the sagittal ridge are easiest to recognize, but lesions may occur farther distally or, less commonly, on the palmar or plantar aspect of the sagittal ridge. The latter can also be seen radiologically on the dorsopalmar (plantar) image. The larger fragments extend abaxially along the proximal margin of the articular cartilage under the dorsal synovial fold.

Conservative management should always be considered in horses younger than 18 months old, because lesions can show improvement radiologically and presumably heal. Surgery is indicated in young horses with fetlock effusion and lameness. Young horses treated surgically often do well clinically, but the long-term radiological appearance is inferior to that seen in horses in which the lesions heal spontaneously. Older horses of training age with unstable fragments are treated by arthroscopic debridement. Proximal lesions are technically easy to approach and debride, but lesions that are more distal can be exposed only by slight or moderate flexion of the joint. The arthroscope portal therefore should be made more distal than usual, and a needle should be used to identify a suitable instrument portal. Debriding a sagittal ridge lesion with a portal placed through the extensor tendon directly over the lesion is easiest. Long reaches across a flexed joint may result in undesirable iatrogenic trauma.

The prognosis depends on the size and location of the flap. Probably 90% of horses with typical lesions of the more proximal portion of the sagittal ridge go on to athletic function. Horses with distal lesions in a more weight-bearing location do not do as well as those with flaps at the proximal articular margin, and the radiological appearance does not improve spontaneously as often.

Osseous Cystlike Lesions

Osseous cystlike lesions occur on the weight-bearing surface of the condyles of the McIII and the MtIII. Most occur in the medial condyle and are diagnosed in horses 1 to 2 years of age. The lesions are easy to recognize radiologically (Figure 56-2) and result in obvious lameness, exacerbated by distal limb flexion. Lameness is improved by perineural or intraarticular analgesia. Lameness associated with an osseous cystlike lesion sometimes occurs in foals. At the time of onset of lameness no lesion may be identifiable radiologically, or only a subtle defect in the outline of the subchondral bone may be apparent. However,

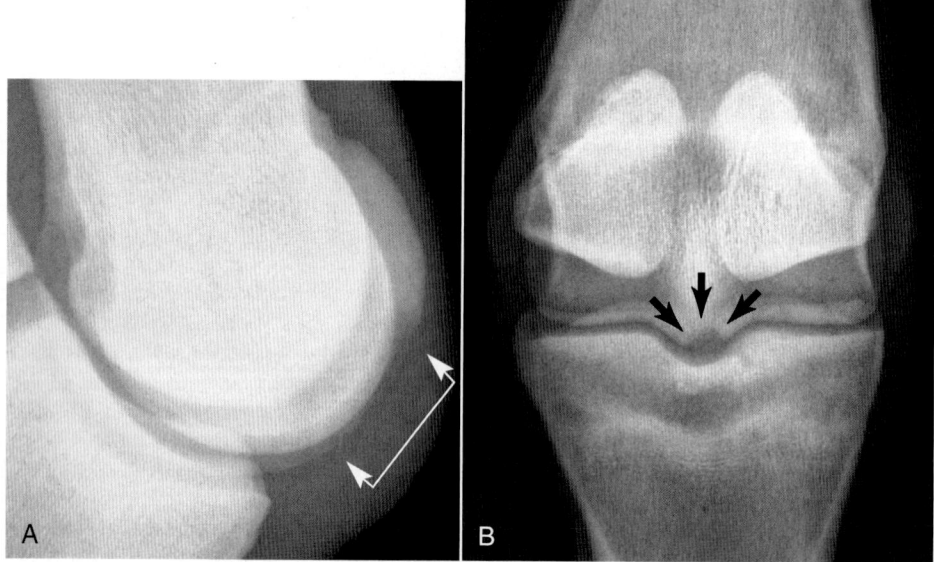

Fig. 56-1 • A typical distal sagittal ridge osteochondritis dissecans lesion (*arrows*) of the third metacarpal bone is seen best on a slightly underexposed flexed lateromedial radiographic image (**A**) and a well-exposed dorsopalmar image (**B**).

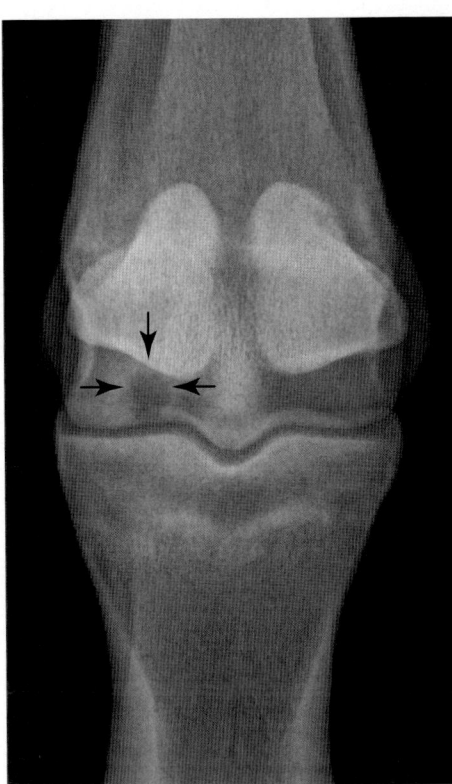

Fig. 56-2 • A dorsopalmar radiographic image of a metacarpophalangeal joint showing a typical osseous cystlike lesion involving the lateral third metacarpal condyle *(arrows)*.

eferences on page 1297

sequential radiographs obtained over the following 6 to 8 weeks may reveal development of an osseous cystlike lesion. Surgical debridement may be successful,[1] but corticosteroids administered intraarticularly or intralesionally also may result in clinically significant improvement in young horses. Although simple debridement of the McIII and the MtIII osseous cystlike lesions has been reasonably successful, the intensity of loading on the distal aspect of the McIII and the MtIII in athletic horses makes horses with these lesions good candidates for advanced joint resurfacing techniques.

Palmar or Plantar Osteochondral Fragments of the Proximal Phalanx

Osteochondral fragments arising from the proximal palmar or plantar aspect of the proximal phalanx are common radiological findings in WBLs, STBs, and TBs, especially in the hindlimbs. Palmar or plantar osteochondral fragments and ununited palmar or plantar eminences may not cause clinical signs or merely cause mild discomfort at high levels of performance. Assessment of clinical importance and management are discussed in detail in Chapters 36 and 42.

Osteochondral Fragments on the Dorsoproximal Aspect of the Proximal Phalanx

Small, well-rounded osseous opacities on the dorsoproximal aspect of the proximal phalanx are common radiological findings. Most probably occur as small chip fractures of

the developing dorsal rim of the proximal phalanx in foals that subsequently ossify. Whether a true underlying developmental defect (OCD) in this location exists is unclear. Although fragments in this location do not always cause overt lameness, they often are removed in valuable prospective athletic horses and sales horses. Many of these fragments are loosely tethered along the dorsal rim of the proximal phalanx and can cause damage to the distal aspect of the McIII or the MtIII in an intensively exercised horse. Arthroscopic removal is quick and easy, and the prognosis is close to 100% for full function. Horses can be returned to full work within 4 to 6 weeks after removal of these fragments. Often fragments in this location are removed before horses enter training or before a public auction.

LESIONS OF THE PROXIMAL INTERPHALANGEAL JOINT

Lesions in the proximal interphalangeal joint usually cause lameness at a young age, often when the horse is a weanling. Single, discrete, well-defined osseous cystlike lesions or multiple poorly defined radiolucent lesions may be identified, occurring most commonly in the distal condyles of the proximal phalanx (Figure 56-3). Surgical access to most pastern osseous cystlike lesions is difficult, and simple debridement is not usually feasible. Lesions may be advanced when lameness is first recognized, and although occasionally horses spontaneously improve without treatment, horses that are obviously lame usually develop osteoarthritis (OA). Therefore horses that do not respond adequately to corticosteroids administered intraarticularly probably should have an early arthrodesis, especially if a hindlimb is affected. Arthrodesis in young or small horses has been accomplished with one of the well-described techniques using two or three transarticular 5.5-mm screws placed in lag fashion[2-5] or a three-hole narrow plate and two transarticular screws.[6] In larger horses I currently use two to four transarticular 5.5-mm screws and a central dorsal three-hole locking pastern arthrodesis plate.[7] The prognosis for athletic function after pastern arthrodesis appears to depend highly on the desired level of activity. Little doubt exists, however, that the prognosis is far superior in a hindlimb than in a forelimb. Most retrospective studies have reported greater than 80% return to athletic function after a hindlimb pastern arthrodesis, but prognosis after a forelimb arthrodesis is likely only around 50%. The intensity of the exercise is probably critical. Few successful elite-level athletic horses (racehorses, upper-level dressage horses, jumping horses) have fused front pastern joints.

Small osteochondral fragments of the proximal interphalangeal joint occur both dorsally and palmarly or plantarly.[8-10] Like the fragments in the fetlock, many of these appear to be juvenile traumatic injuries that are diagnosed later in life, but a developmental cause cannot be excluded. These fragments do not always cause lameness, so perineural or intraarticular analgesia should be used to confirm the clinical significance of the fragments. The dorsal fragments are relatively straightforward to remove arthroscopically. The palmar fragments require a more technically demanding surgery.[8]

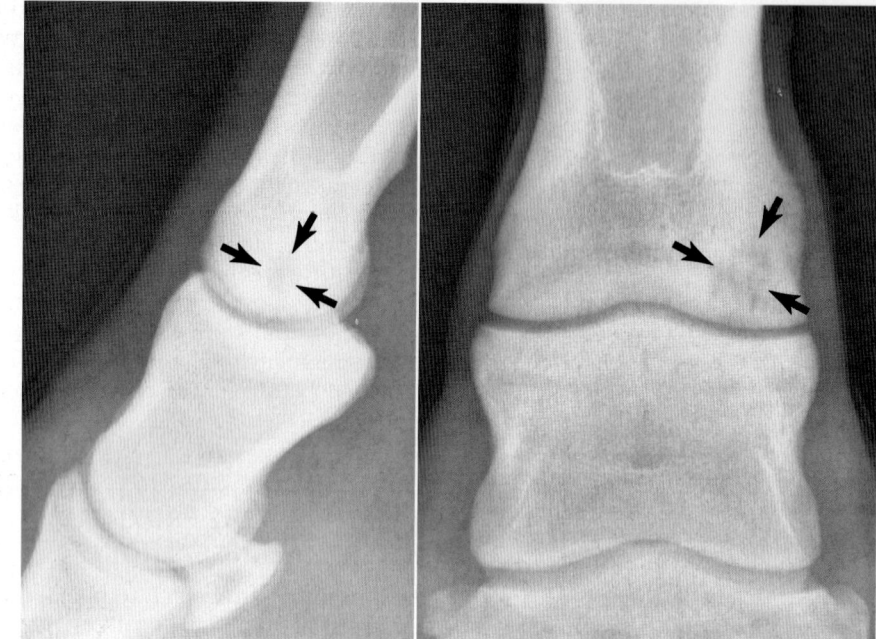

Fig. 56-3 • Lateromedial *(left)* and dorsopalmar *(right)* radiographic images of a proximal interphalangeal joint. The most common manifestation of osteochondrosis in the pastern is an osseous cystlike lesion *(arrows)* in the distal aspect of the condyle of the proximal phalanx.

LESIONS OF THE DISTAL INTERPHALANGEAL JOINT

Well-rounded osteochondral fragments on the dorsoproximal aspect of the extensor process of the distal phalanx are also believed to be developmental in origin. Small fragments are frequently incidental radiological findings, and treatment is not necessary unless associated lameness exists. Lameness should be improved substantially by intraarticular analgesia. Nuclear scintigraphy may help definitive diagnosis. Treatment of horses with lesions associated with lameness is arthroscopic removal of the fragment. The prognosis is excellent (>90%) if the fragment is removed before OA of the distal interphalangeal joint has developed. These fragments are often well embedded in the extensor tendon insertion, so not all fragments adversely affect joint function. As with many other small osteochondral fragments, removal is sometimes done prophylactically.

Osseous cystlike lesions of the distal phalanx can be large and associated with dramatic lameness (Figures 56-4 and 56-5). The pathogenesis may be similar to that of subchondral bone cysts of the distal aspect of the femur. An attempt usually is made to manage such lesions with medications administered intraarticularly. If that is unsuccessful, intralesional corticosteroid injection under fluoroscopic or computed tomographic guidance through the hoof wall is an option. Arthroscopic debridement in young horses with accessible lesions has resulted in good success.[11] Extremely large (deep) cysts can be debrided by removing the extensor process in order to provide access.

LESIONS OF THE SCAPULOHUMERAL JOINT

OC of the scapulohumeral joint may involve the glenoid of the scapula or the humeral head. Humeral head lesions can be solitary, but scapular lesions usually appear with substantial pathological abnormalities of the humeral head in young horses (<2 years old). Lameness can develop insidiously or acutely, presumably after an acute disruption of an unstable osteochondral flap. Recognizing a developing flexural deformity or clubfoot may confuse diagnosis of shoulder lameness in a chronically lame young horse. Occasionally, mild lesions are not recognized until a horse starts training. Lameness is improved by intraarticular analgesia but often is not eliminated. Radiological abnormalities may include poorly defined subchondral radiolucent areas, with or without sclerosis, flattening of the articular surfaces, and modeling of the articular margins, especially the ventral angle of the scapula (see Chapter 40).

Lameness in some young horses improves with rest, and early surgery should not be encouraged in foals younger than 8 to 10 months old unless they are intractably lame. Affected foals should be confined to a stall or small paddock and reexamined clinically and radiologically at 60-day intervals. Intraarticular medication has not been consistently helpful in weanlings and yearlings. The outcome after arthroscopic treatment of OC of the scapulohumeral joint is unpredictable, and lameness can dramatically worsen after surgery. Of 26 potential racehorses, only four (15.4%) started a race, whereas four of six non-racehorses were sound in a recent study of 32 horses that underwent management for osteochondrosis of the scapulohumeral joint.[12] There were no differences between horses managed surgically and those managed conservatively.[12] Radiography may underestimate the severity of lesions, especially those involving the humeral head. It is important to emphasize to an owner before surgery that considerable uncertainty exists about the clinical outcome in any given horse with OC in the shoulder. Solitary osseous cystlike lesions also occur, most commonly in the

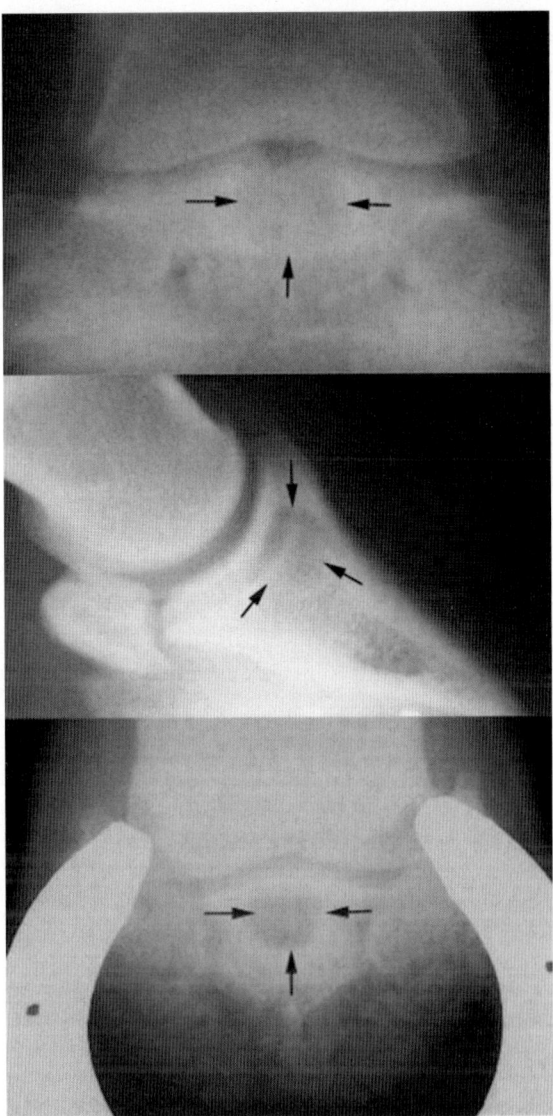

Fig. 56-4 • Dorsopalmar *(top)*, lateromedial *(middle)*, and dorsoproximal-palmarodistal oblique *(bottom)* radiographic images of a foal. There is a large osseous cystlike lesion in the distal phalanx *(arrows)*. Large osseous cystlike lesions of the distal phalanx are difficult management problems because they are relatively inaccessible to surgical debridement.

middle of the distal aspect of the scapula but sometimes in the humeral head (see Chapter 40, Figure 40-14).

OSTEOCHONDROSIS OF THE TARSOCRURAL JOINT

OC of the tarsocrural joint is common in many breeds. Obvious joint capsule distention (bog spavin) may precede recognition of any gait abnormality. Effusion may not be recognized in racehorses examined for poor performance associated with OC, but in show horses with lameness, effusion almost invariably occurs. Horses with radiologically identified lesions are not always lame; therefore diagnosis should be confirmed by intraarticular analgesia or by response to intraarticular medication with corticosteroids. At least four radiographic images should be obtained,

because numerous lesions may be present. If OC is suspected clinically but no lesion is identified radiologically, repeating the dorsoplantar image with slightly different angles of projection is worthwhile, because medial malleolar lesions can be difficult to see (Figure 56-6). Flexed lateromedial images may be necessary to identify lesions involving the plantar aspect of the tarsocrural joint.

OC of the tarsocrural joint is recognized as a common radiological finding in STBs, TBs, and WBLs, but it is not always associated with lameness. Few of the common OC lesions in the hock heal spontaneously after 5 months of age, so surgical removal in young horses, especially sales yearlings, has become commonplace. These lesions are almost always in peripheral, less than completely weight-bearing locations, and removal does not seriously compromise joint function. Prognosis is excellent. However, fragments that cause lameness at a later age are a greater problem because the loose fragments and debris often cause extensive cartilage damage. Older show jumpers in particular may dislodge distal tibial OCD lesions and develop acute clinical signs of effusion and lameness (Figure 56-7).

The cranial aspect of the intermediate ridge of the tibia is the most common site of lesions (Figure 56-8). These lesions rarely cause overt lameness unless major effusion occurs. Arthroscopic removal of the fragment is straightforward and nearly always results in reduction of the lameness and effusion. Lesions may be identified radiologically bilaterally, although only one limb is chronically affected. Loose fragments may become detached in the tarsocrural joint and can become lodged in the communicating proximal intertarsal joint (see Figure 56-8). The opening from the tarsocrural joint into the proximal intertarsal joint at the distal margin of the talar trochlear groove is small or not patent or is small in young foals or weanlings, but as the opening enlarges in older horses, large fragments can move into the proximal intertarsal joint pouches.[13] If a fragment of bone is found dorsal to (or even on the distal edge of) the central tarsal bone, the fragment is probably one loose in the proximal intertarsal joint that gravitated into that pouch. Fragments associated with lameness should be removed, but it is certainly possible for fragments to localize in this joint and remain stable, causing no clinical signs. It is important to recognize that the fragments in the proximal intertarsal joint usually are not easily seen with an arthroscope and often have to be removed blindly with a rongeurs guided arthroscopically into the joint pouch.

Lesions of the distal aspect of the lateral trochlear ridge of the talus can be enormous and if loose may cause acute severe lameness and substantial effusion (Figure 56-9). This lesion seems to be more common in heavy breeds and STBs. Horses with small, well-attached lesions can be managed conservatively, but any displaced fragment should be removed. The prognosis generally depends on how proximally and axially the lesion extends, but even large lesions can be removed with a good prognosis.

OCD lesions of the medial malleolus of the tibia are easily missed because they are always on the axial rather than the distal (more visible) part of the malleolus (see Figure 56-6). Medial malleolar OCD lesions usually cause more lameness and more effusion than the more common lesions of the cranial aspect of the intermediate ridge of

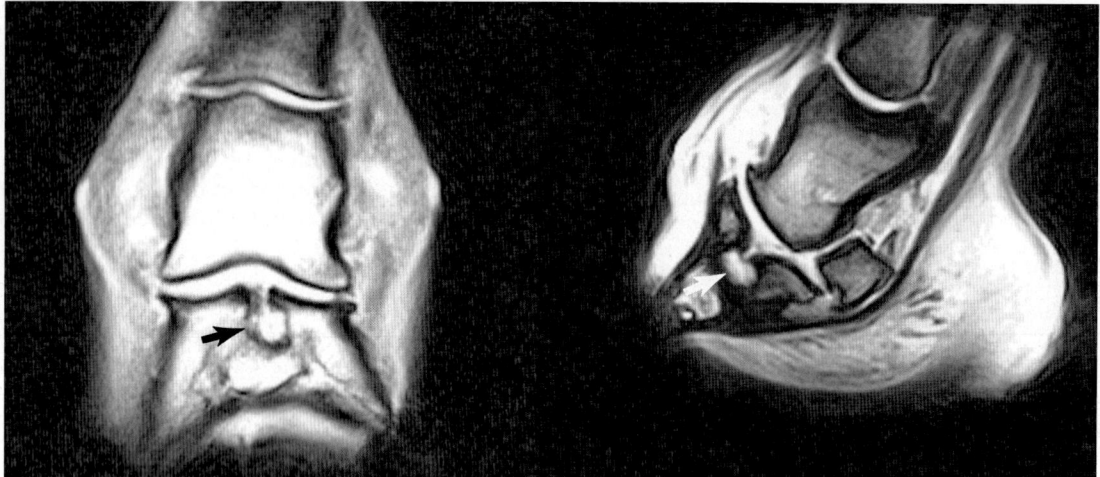

Fig. 56-5 • Dorsal (left) and sagittal plane magnetic resonance images of a large osseous cystlike lesion of the distal phalanx. There is a large round area of increased signal intensity *(arrows)* in the subchondral bone of the distal phalanx that appears to communicate with the articular surface of the distal interphalangeal joint. Intralesional or intraarticular corticosteroids are often used to treat horses with such lesions, but debridement is feasible using an arthroscopic technique.

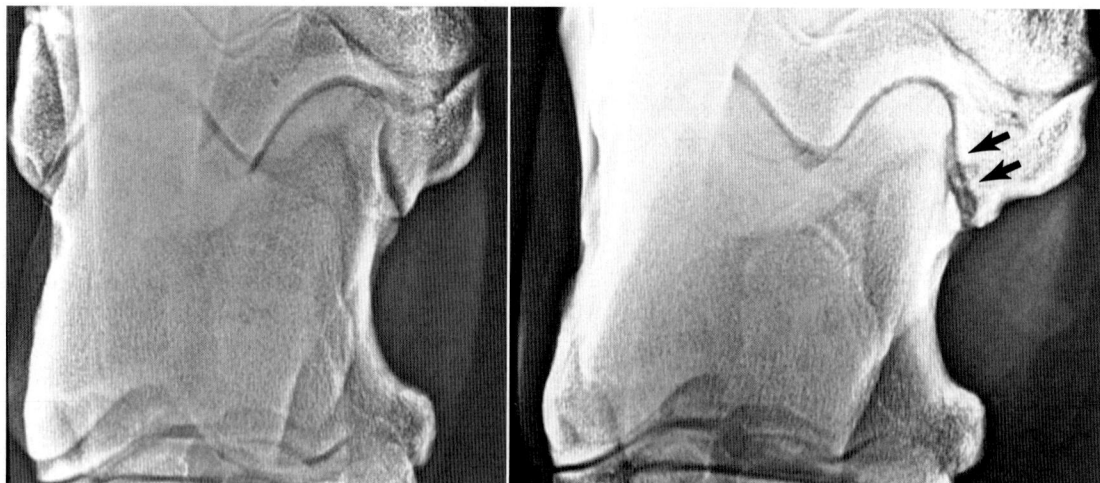

Fig. 56-6 • Dorsoplantar (left image) and dorsal 10° lateral-plantaromedial oblique xeroradiographic images of a hock. Identification of osteochondritis dissecans lesions of the medial malleolus requires well-positioned radiographic images. Identifying the lesion on the dorsoplantar image is difficult, but a slight alteration in the obliquity (right image) reveals a large defect *(arrows)*.

the tibia. Unless the lesion is unusually large, the prognosis after arthroscopic removal is excellent. Early removal is recommended, because erosive lesions on the medial trochlea of the talus can become severe over time.

Medial trochlear ridge lesions should be interpreted with caution; most distal medial trochlear ridge lesions are incidental radiological findings, and affected horses do not require treatment. Some fragments ostensibly are unstable or somehow irritating because they will be associated with clinical signs (Figure 56-10). Distal medial trochlear ridge lesions may be on the proximal or distal side of the capsular attachment separating the tarsocrural and proximal intertarsal joints. These fragments can reliably be seen only in a lateromedial radiographic image, a radiological finding that is useful to differentiate horses with distal medial trochlear ridge fragments and those with loose fragments

within the proximal intertarsal joint. The fragments wholly within the tarsocrural joint appear to be less stable and more likely to cause lameness. In all horses the decision for surgical removal should be based on a definitive response to intraarticular analgesia. The arthroscopic removal of the tarsocrural lesions is easy and can be done with minimal dissection. Lesions under the capsular attachment often require sharp dissection of the attachment to expose the fragment. Care should always be taken to dissect the minimal amount of soft tissue, especially because the attachments course abaxially.

More centrally positioned, smoothly outlined depressions in the surface of the medial trochlear ridge of the talus are common in large WBLs, draft horses, and draft-cross horses. The subchondral bone architecture is usually normal, and no associated clinical signs are apparent.

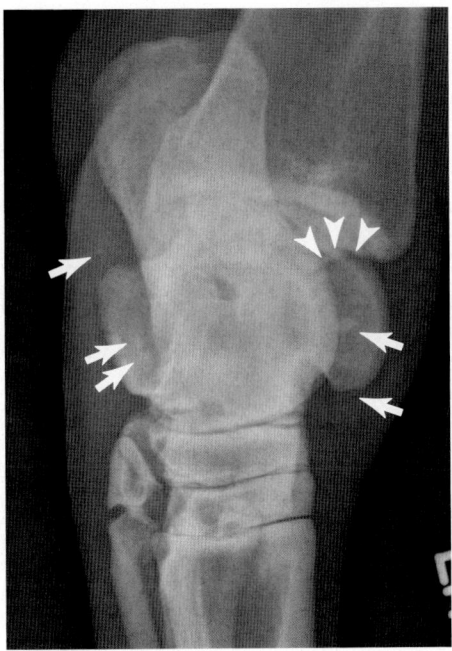

Fig. 56-7 • Dorsomedial-plantarolateral oblique radiographic image of the hock of an adult jumper. A defect *(arrowheads)* is evident in the cranial aspect of the intermediate ridge of the tibia. The osteochondritis dissecans fragment displaced from that location was crushed into numerous pieces distributed throughout the tarsocrural joint *(arrows)*.

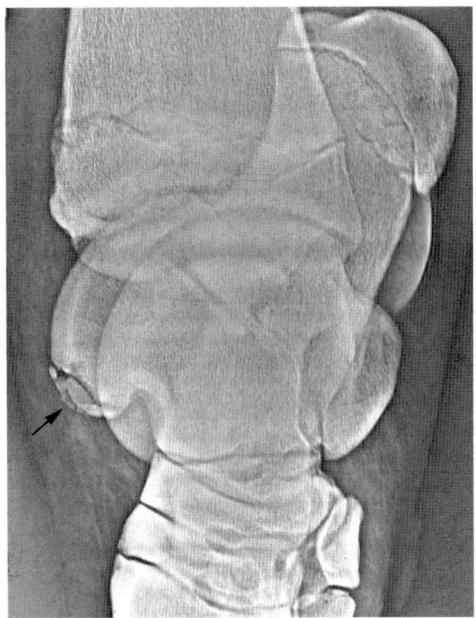

Fig. 56-9 • Dorsomedial-plantarolateral oblique xeroradiographic image of a hock. Osteochondritis dissecans fragments *(arrow)* arising from the distal aspect of the lateral trochlear ridge of the talus are often large, but after surgical removal horses have a good prognosis regardless of size of the lesion.

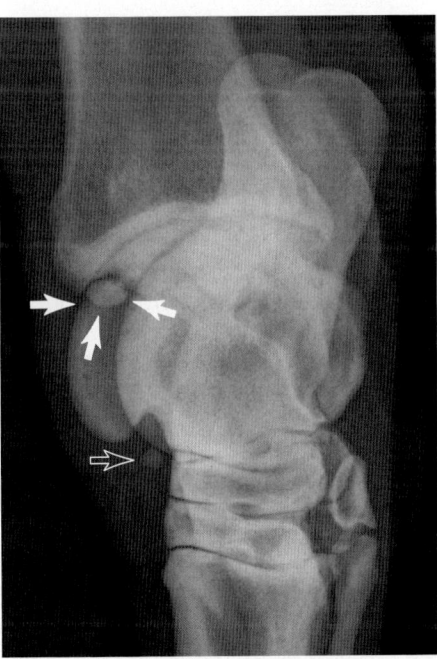

Fig. 56-8 • Dorsomedial-plantarolateral oblique radiographic image of a hock with a loose osteochondritis dissecans fragment in the proximal intertarsal joint *(open arrow)*. This fragment *(open arrow)* "dropped" from the cranial aspect of the intermediate ridge of the tibia, where a larger fragment still resides *(arrows)*.

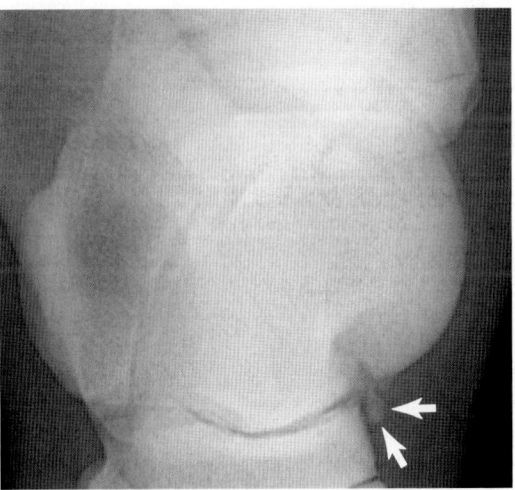

Fig. 56-10 • Lateromedial radiographic image of a hock. Small fragments *(arrows)* along the distal dorsal aspect of the medial trochlear ridge of the talus commonly do not cause lameness, but some are unstable and induce effusion and lameness, particularly fragments on the proximal side of the proximal intertarsal joint capsule.

These lesions rarely have an unstable chondral or osteochondral flap that can be removed.

Lateral malleolar fragments are usually traumatic (see Chapter 44) and are only rarely (about 1%) OC lesions. Unlike the traumatic fractures, lateral malleolar OCD lesions have irregular diffuse radiolucency within the malleolus instead of a distinctly separated fragment. Arthroscopic debridement of lateral malleolar OCD lesions is difficult because of the extensive collateral ligament attachments that obscure the structure.

Arthroscopic removal of OCD lesions from the hock usually can be followed by a short convalescence and rapid return to work or pasture exercise. Typically a horse is walked in hand for 4 to 6 weeks and then reevaluated. If the effusion has resolved and the horse is jogging soundly, the level of exercise can be increased steadily. Sodium hyaluronan is administered intraarticularly at about the time of suture removal.

Most horses with OCD of the hock have an excellent prognosis, especially if lesions are removed early, before substantial damage to the joint occurs. The specific location of the OCD lesion probably makes less difference than the size, because most hock OCD lesions occur on the peripheral, less than fully weight-bearing surfaces of the bones. Controversy remains about the need to remove all hock OCD lesions, but clearly horses have an excellent (>80%) chance of performing at the expected level after arthroscopic removal of typical lesions.[14-16]

The tarsocrural joint appears to be particularly vulnerable to a form of erosive OA that can result in extensive, full-thickness loss of articular cartilage (Figure 56-11). This occurs in the absence of known trauma or radiologically evident lesions, but most horses with the lesion have a history of intraarticularly administered corticosteroids used to manage an effusion. The exact mechanism of this process in the tarsocrural joint is not known, but corticosteroids should be used cautiously to manage effusions of this joint.

LESIONS OF THE STIFLE

Diagnosis and management of OC of the femoropatellar joint, subchondral bone cysts in the medial femoral condyle, and other osseous cystlike lesions in the stifle are discussed in detail in Chapter 46.

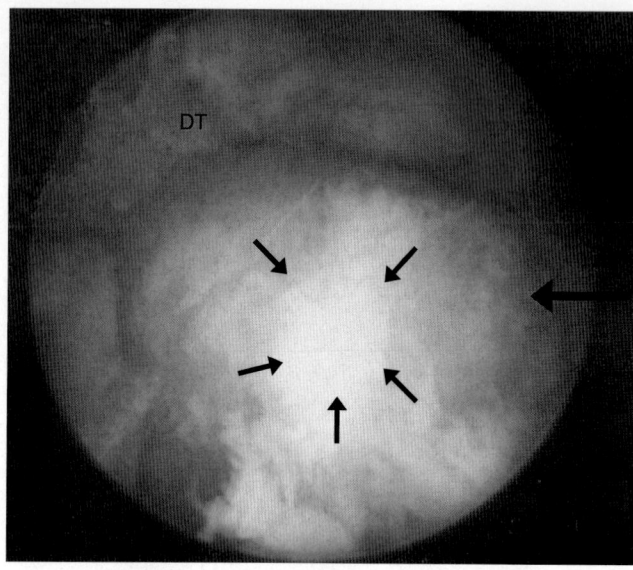

Fig. 56-11 • Unlike in most other joints in the horse, full-thickness cartilage erosion of the talus (medial trochlear ridge) *(large arrow)* and distal aspect of the tibia *(DT)* occurs with surprisingly few bony changes such as subchondral lysis or marginal osteophytes. Arthroscopy affords the best means of making the diagnosis. The medial trochlear ridge is nearly devoid of cartilage except for loose and fibrillated cartilage on its summit *(small arrows)*.

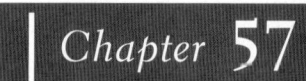

Chapter 57

Physitis

David R. Ellis

References on page 1298

Physitis occurs in the horse in three principal forms: infectious physitis and type V and type VI Salter-Harris growth plate injuries.[1] Type V growth plate injury can arise secondary to congenital but persistent angular limb deformities in foals, but these, infections, and type VI injuries are not considered in this chapter. Type V Salter-Harris injuries are considered a manifestation of acquired physitis, one of the group of disorders known as *developmental orthopedic disease*.[2] The inclusion of acquired physitis under the umbrella of osteochondrosis may be more debatable. Jeffcott[3] considered that the condition was better defined as physeal dysplasia, implying a disturbance of endochondral ossification rather than an inflammatory condition. Bramlage[4] outlined two forms of physitis based on radiological interpretation of the site at which changes were seen. The two forms were those that were seen at the periphery, usually on the medial aspect, and those that were seen in the axial or central section of the growth plate.

Physitis is largely confined to the lighter-boned, faster-growing breeds of horse, particularly Thoroughbreds and Thoroughbred crossbreeds. Milder physitis is relatively common, and rarely does experienced stud management allow the condition to develop far enough for severe lameness and conformational changes to occur. Only in horses with more extreme or persistent physitis would radiographic examination be undertaken in the United Kingdom. Clinical recognition of enlargement of the growth plate or slight change in conformation usually results in a presumptive diagnosis of physitis and indicates an immediate change of the horse's management as the first line of treatment.

PATHOGENESIS

I consider the pathogenesis of physitis to be consistent with a type V Salter-Harris growth plate injury. This implies a compression lesion that arises medially as a consequence of the greater weight being borne on the medial aspect of the forelimb. Although the medial aspect of the forelimb is the most frequent site, physitis also occurs laterally in a foal with a carpal valgus deformity. Physitis arises at a time in the most active growing phases of young horses, when endochondral ossification is at its peak in the affected physis. It also occurs in the contralateral limb after a chronic lameness, at the fetlock in a younger foal, or at the carpus in older foals and yearlings. For example, I have encountered physitis in the contralateral forelimbs of foals with severe acquired flexural deformity of the distal interphalangeal joint (Figure 57-1). Although physitis may result in an upright conformation of the fetlock joint,

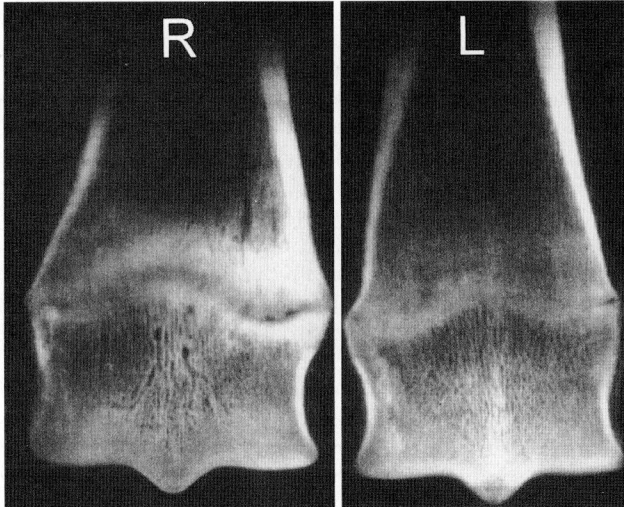

Fig. 57-1 • Dorsopalmar radiographic images of frontal sections of the distal aspect of the third metacarpal bones of a 5-month-old foal with chronic and severe flexural deformity of the left *(L)* distal interphalangeal joint and physitis in the contralateral distal metacarpal physis *(R)*. Note the more intense mineralization of the growth plate cartilage and bridging at the medial aspect (to the right of the image) of the right forelimb, typical of Salter-Harris type V growth plate injury.

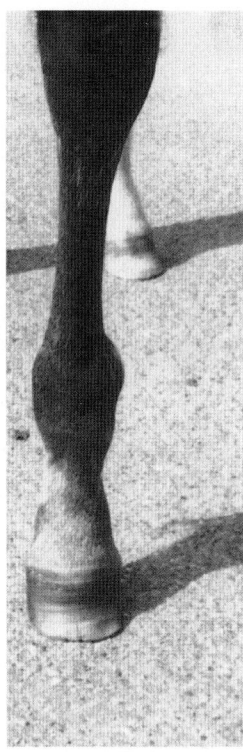

Fig. 57-2 • Physitis of the distal aspect of the right third metacarpal bone (growth plate), with some involvement of the proximal physis of the proximal phalanx, giving the fetlock an hourglass shape.

probably from off-loading the limb to relieve pain, physitis does not cause other flexural deformity.

Physitis is more common on farms that use rigorous or heavy feeding programs. Owners whose stock lives on lush pasture and is supplemented with concentrate feed have a higher incidence of physitis among their horses than those who keep their horses on leaner management. A higher incidence of developmental orthopedic disease is noted in foals and yearlings raised on young (<7 years old) pastures.

I have seen balanced mineral supplementation and withdrawal of concentrates dramatically reduce the incidence of physitis on some farms. Diet and forage analysis can be helpful when high incidence of developmental orthopedic disease is persistent (see Chapter 55), but mineral clearance ratios (creatinine phosphate in particular) are rarely necessary to adjust supplementation. Certain mares may also produce more foals with physitis compared with similarly managed mares, which implies a hereditary predisposition.

CLINICAL SIGNS

Clinical physitis is recognized at three main sites: the distal aspect of the third metacarpal or metatarsal bone, the distal aspect of the radius, and, less frequently, the distal aspect of the tibia. During lameness investigations, physitis has been noticed at other sites, such as the distal aspect of the femur and cervical vertebrae.

Physitis is seen in the fetlock region in foals aged 3 to 6 months and occurs at the distal aspect of the radius from 8 months to 2 years of age. Clinical signs are characterized by firm, warm, and painful enlargement of the growth plate, most commonly on its medial aspect. The proximal physis of the proximal phalanx also may be enlarged at

the fetlock, giving the fetlocks an hourglass shape when viewed from the dorsal aspect (Figure 57-2). Early signs at the distal radial or tibial growth plates include a convex appearance in the medial contour of the metaphysis just proximal to the physis; this should be a straight or slightly concave outline. Swelling also is located around the distal dorsomedial aspect of the radius (Figure 57-3). This dorsal component can lead the clinician to suspect that the condition has arisen from external trauma. As with the fetlock joint, warmth on palpation is present, as is tenderness when pressure is applied across the growth plate while the leg is held partially flexed. Full and forced flexion of the fetlock, carpus, or tarsus also may be resented. Most affected horses have changes at the distal medial aspect of the radius, but a few with preexisting carpus valgus conformation may develop the condition laterally. Bilateral lameness may be seen as a stilted gait. The conformation may become more upright through the pastern, and fetlock varus deformity may develop because the horse walks on the outside of the hoof to alleviate pain from pressure on the medial physis. I suspect that foals and yearlings that develop a carpus varus conformation (start to go bandy) are likely to have a subclinical form of physitis that encourages them to bear more weight on the lateral aspect of the forelimbs. If physitis continues unchecked, growth ceases on the medial side, exacerbating the carpus varus deformity, and ultimately, premature closure of the growth plate fixes the abnormal conformation. This chain of events also occurs in horses that develop physitis in the distal lateral aspect of the radius, resulting in a permanent carpus valgus conformation.

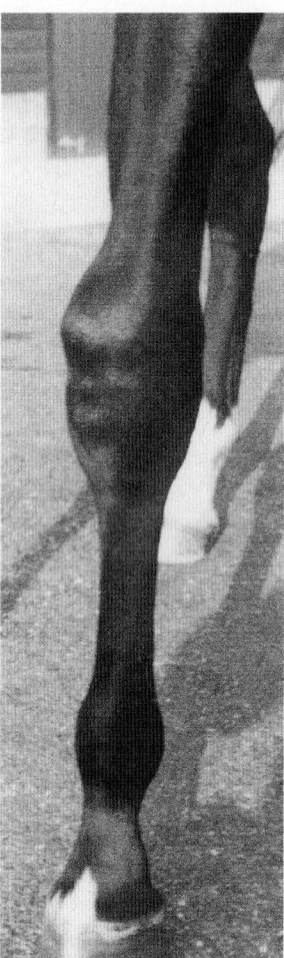

Fig. 57-3 • Dorsal view of a left forelimb; lateral is to the right. Physitis of the left distal radial growth plate with characteristic dorsomedial swelling and concavity of the outline of the medial aspect of the distal metaphysis is shown.

TREATMENT

Treatment centers on stable rest. Nonsteroidal antiinflammatory drugs can be helpful, particularly in horses that are very lame or have inflamed and painful growth plates. I have no experience of using corticosteroids or anabolic steroids in horses with physitis. Although body condition and conformation can vary, it is important to assess the nutrition of affected foals and other horses. Reduction of body weight and particularly a reduction in energy content in the diet must be made. Starving these horses completely is unwise, and it is important that mineral intake includes the correct balance of calcium and phosphorus and adequate copper and zinc. The length of rest required varies with the severity of the physitis and ranges from 2 weeks to 2 months. Corrective hoof trimming must also be undertaken, especially if the horse has developed an angular limb deformity (see Chapter 58). For varus deformity the unworn medial hoof wall must be removed (inside is lowered), and if the angulation is severe, fitting a lateral hoof extension is necessary.

Surgery usually is unsuccessful in horses that develop severe varus limb deformity resulting from physitis. This experience, coupled with the disappointing results obtained when operating on yearlings with congenital angular deformities, has led me to stop recommending periosteal elevation or physeal retardation techniques in these groups of affected horses.

The prognosis for racing or other extreme athletic activities is good, provided the condition was not so severe that the conformation is permanently affected. If carpus varus and bench-knee conformation is marked, then the animal is likely to develop lameness from splints, carpitis, sesamoiditis, or suspensory branch desmitis when more serious training is undertaken.

Chapter 58

Angular Limb Deformities

José M. García-López and Eric J. Parente

▣ DIAGNOSIS AND CONSERVATIVE MANAGEMENT

Angular limb deformities are considered lateral or medial deviations to the long axis of the limb in the dorsal (frontal) plane. A lateral deviation distal to the carpus, termed *carpus valgus,* is the most common. Tarsus valgus and fetlock varus (a medial deviation) are the next most common, respectively. The toed-in or toed-out appearance that often accompanies an angular deformity is a concurrent rotational deformity and should not be confused with the angular deformity. An outward (external) rotation is usually observed concurrently with a valgus deformity, and an inward (internal) rotation is seen with a varus deformity. No confirmed breed or sex predilection is known, but subjectively there may be some genetic predisposition. For a foal to be born with a mild bilateral carpal valgus and toed-out appearance is considered normal by most clinicians, and as the foal grows and the chest widens, the limbs straighten progressively.

Angular limb deformities usually are congenital, but they can be developmental, and have numerous causes. An acquired angular deformity is defined as worsening or failure of correction of the normal slight carpus valgus conformation in a neonatal foal. The cause and the severity and progression of the deformity are vital pieces of information that should be acquired before a treatment plan is formulated. Treatment is predicated by these factors. Foals are like molding plastic. The conformation changes slowly with growth. Genetics, nutrition, amount of exercise or weight bearing, and veterinary interventions all influence the conformation of the adult horse. Some of these factors can be influenced as a young horse matures, and small adjustments often need to be made to the treatment plan as the animal grows. The foal should always be evaluated with the amount of remaining growth in mind and not just its present status. Because the greatest impact on conformation is made during periods of rapid growth, early recognition and regular reevaluations are extremely important to achieve a positive outcome.

Growth rates are most rapid in the neonate and slow considerably within the first year. Most of the growth from the distal radial and tibial physes occurs within the first 6 months of age. Most of the growth from the distal aspect of the third metacarpal bone (McIII) and the third metatarsal bone (MtIII) occurs within the first 3 months of age. Minimal changes take place beyond these times. Radiology alone cannot be used to determine the end of bone growth, because a physis is radiologically apparent long after clinically relevant growth has abated. In a normal foal, carpus valgus should be corrected to within 5 to 7 degrees of normal by 4 months of age and should be almost straight by 8 to 10 months of age.

EXAMINATION OF THE FOAL

It is critical to determine the extent and cause of the deformity before developing a management plan. Foals should be examined while they are standing and walking and radiographically. Occasionally foals are assessed in lateral recumbency.

Deformities can be assessed subjectively by visual examination. The foal should stand as squarely as possible, with the foot directly below the proximal part of the limb. Deviations from this stance exacerbate any deformities that truly exist. Because most foals stand still only transiently, repositioning the foal several times to evaluate each limb independently is often necessary. This allows observation of how the foal stands most frequently in a relaxed position. The clinician stands directly in front of the dorsum of the long bones for evaluation of the forelimbs, not necessarily at the front of the toe. The orientation of the toe may be affected by a concurrent rotational deformity, which confounds interpretation. Hindlimbs should be evaluated similarly but directly from behind. The forelimbs can also be evaluated by standing shoulder to shoulder with the foal, looking down the limb toward the ground.

All limbs also should be evaluated with the foal walking away from and toward the clinician. Breakover is determined for each foot, which may be helpful in deciding the most appropriate way to manage the foal. The entire assessment of a foal should be graded and recorded on video or on paper for future reference.

Radiology provides an objective assessment of angular deformity, but sequential radiographic examinatoins may be unreliable if the obliquity varies. Differences in radiographic projection can result in a misinterpretation of worsening or improvement, which is particularly true when trying to quantify small differences in the angle. Long, narrow (18 × 43 cm) cassettes should be used to measure the angle of the deformity, by evaluating the intersection of a line representing the long axis of the proximal and distal aspects of the long bones from the joint in question. This is more accurate in the carpus and fetlock than in the tarsus. Radiology is essential to identify cuboidal injury or malformation. Such a deformity dramatically worsens the

foal's prognosis. Foals with angular deformity resulting from cuboidal bone abnormalities usually have compromised range of motion, but this often is detected best with the foal in lateral recumbency.

PERIARTICULAR LAXITY

Periarticular laxity is the major cause of congenital angular limb deformities and often improves dramatically within the first 4 weeks of life, without any intervention, as the periarticular tissues become less elastic. The improvement is most dramatic in a windswept foal, which has a tarsus valgus of one limb and a concurrent varus of the other. Limited exercise is all that is required for these foals to become normal.

Infrequently the deformity can be so severe, particularly in the fetlock, that the foal is unable to bear weight on the sole of its foot. Immediate treatment is required to establish normal weight bearing. Custom-made glue-on shoes are particularly useful to prevent abnormal breakover and to keep the foot flat on the ground. If the foal has excessive laxity of the lateral collateral ligaments and a tendency to break over on the lateral side of the foot, a lateral extension shoe is used to maintain appropriate alignment of the limb. The foal should initially be restricted to a stall before turnout in a small paddock or round pen with just the mare. Soft tissues become progressively stronger, and normal activity can be permitted within a relatively short time. Allowing premature excessive exercise can lead to proximal sesamoid bone fractures (see Chapter 36) and other injuries. Glue-on shoes are usually required for several weeks, but they then should be removed to prevent contracture of the foot. External coaptation also should be avoided if possible. Splints are used only to maintain joint alignment if absolutely necessary. Splints are contraindicated to try to pull or push a limb straight. Rigid support from a splint or cast usually leads to greater soft tissue laxity. Trying to support a limb results in continued laxity and soft tissue wounds from bandaging. Every foal must be managed on an individual basis with the goal of achieving normal weight bearing and function while providing the minimal amount of support necessary.

ASYMMETRICAL PHYSEAL GROWTH

Asymmetrical growth of a distal physis is a cause of angular limb deformity. Greater growth from the distal physis of the radius medially compared with growth laterally results in carpus valgus. Continued asymmetrical growth precludes the normal correction anticipated with resolution of periarticular laxity. Greater growth from the lateral aspect of the distal physes of the McIII or the MtIII results in fetlock varus. With time and limited exercise (stall or small paddock turnout, alone with the mare) substantial self-correction occurs for most foals with angular deformities. Radiology can be used to evaluate objectively the degree of deformity and the difference in physeal growth, but it is not always required.

Fetlock varus is often overlooked and affects the left hind fetlock most commonly, possibly because of in utero positioning. Because growth at the distal physis of the McIII and the MtIII terminates within a few months, early recognition of this deformity is critical.

TRAUMA-RELATED DEFORMITIES

Developmental causes of angular deformities are likely secondary to excessive or asymmetrical weight bearing and can be more serious than congenital abnormalities. Incomplete ossification of the cuboidal bones in a foal can result in cuboidal bone crush and a secondary angular limb deformity. The lateral carpal bones most commonly are affected, resulting in carpus valgus. Although the deformity is clearly apparent, the health and function of the joint is most critical. The carpi and tarsi of any premature or dysmature foal should be examined radiologically. Because ossification is incomplete, abnormal cuboidal bones appear round or in other shapes, and if crushing exists, the bones are wedge shaped, overlap opposing bones, or are fractured. If the foal's activity can be managed strictly in a hospital situation, no further support is recommended. Limited, strictly controlled exercise encourages appropriate ossification. If the foal's activity cannot be strictly managed and the foal has moderate strength, sleeve casts are recommended to prevent cuboidal bone crush. Sleeve casts should be changed or removed in 10 to 14 days in a growing foal. Radiological reevaluation every 2 weeks helps determine the length of time a cast is required.

Foals can also develop angular limb deformities secondary to lameness in the contralateral limb. If foals become non–weight bearing on a single limb, they adopt a tripod-like stance by bringing the contralateral limb more medial and toeing in. Over several weeks this results in asymmetrical bony growth of the nonlame limb and varus deformity of all joints, with internal rotation of the distal aspect of the limb. A dorsolateral toe extension can be placed on the foot of the nonlame limb to try to encourage a more abducted stance, but resolution of the primary lameness is the best way to prevent the contralateral limb deformity from occurring. Once the deformity has occurred, correction is improbable.

CONSERVATIVE MANAGEMENT

In most situations, judicious minimal intervention is all that is required to correct angular limb deformities. This includes limited small paddock exercise and careful attention to the foot. Trimming the foot and using shoe extensions can influence a foal's ability to self-correct an angular limb deformity by affecting the weight bearing and tracking of the limb. A foal younger than 4 months of age with mild carpus valgus likely requires no specific intervention. A foal with a moderate carpus valgus, toed-out appearance would benefit from shoes with dorsomedial extensions. This encourages the foal to adduct the limb and turn in more when breaking over. The result is more physiologically normal strain on the limbs, which should result in a straighter limb. A similar external appearance can be achieved by overtrimming the lateral hoof wall, but the effect is not the same. Although trimming the foot in this manner may give the appearance of an immediate benefit, it may have a negative long-term effect of an unbalanced foot, compensating for a limb with a deformity. This method has, however, been used for years with apparent success.

More aggressive intervention is infrequently required. Surgical intervention should be reserved for those foals that are not improving fast enough for the amount of growth potential remaining. Therefore frequent reevaluation to monitor progress of a foal with an angular limb deformity is critical. Surgical intervention has a greater effect on a young foal because of the more rapid growth; thus early surgical intervention should be considered for a foal with a severe deformity.

■ SURGICAL MANAGEMENT

José M. García-López

A high proportion of foals with angular limb deformities are treated successfully conservatively, but surgical intervention is warranted if a deviation is severe or if deformity persists despite adequate management, including restriction of exercise and corrective farriery. Various surgical techniques aimed at accelerating or decreasing the growth on a particular side of the growth plate have been described.[1-7] Surgical technique depends on the age of the foal, the degree of angular limb deformity, the anatomical site, and whether the deformity is varus or valgus (Figure 58-1).

Before surgery, all the limbs should be assessed from the front, from the back, and while standing next to the limbs. Good-quality radiographs, which include a substantial length of the bones proximal and distal to the deviation, should be obtained to assess bone structure (Figure 58-2) and to determine the pivot point and pivot point angle of the deviation. The pivot point is the intersection of two lines drawn parallel to the long axis of the bones proximal and distal to the articulation in question (Figure 58-3). The pivot point indicates the origin of the deviation

References on page 1298

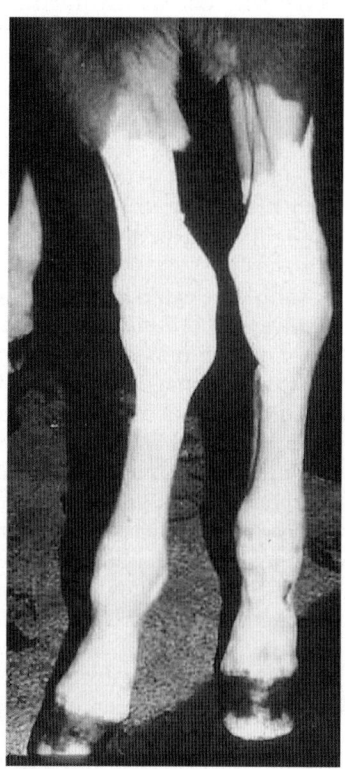

Fig. 58-1 • Dorsal view of a foal with right carpus valgus and a mild left carpal varus deformities.

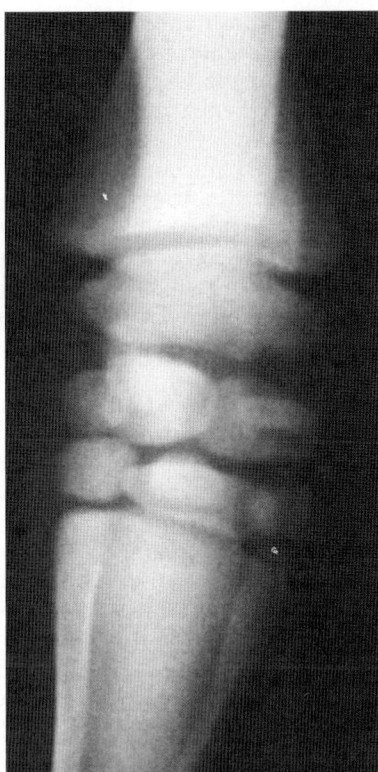

Fig. 58-2 • Dorsopalmar radiographic image of a carpus with mild incomplete ossification of the carpal bones and valgus deformity. Medial is to the right.

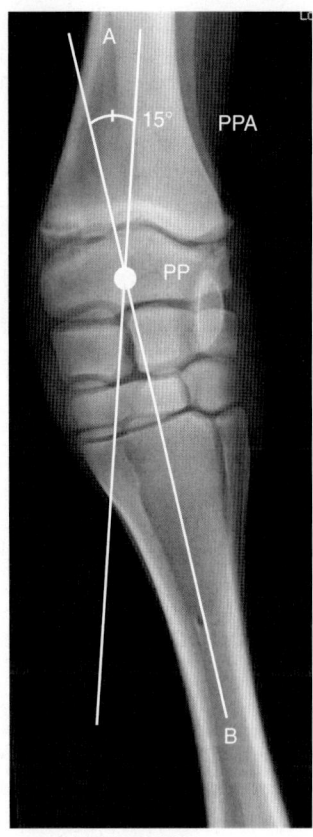

Fig. 58-3 • Dorsopalmar radiographic image of a carpus with valgus deformity. Lateral is to the right. Lines are drawn parallel to the long axis of the radius *(A)* and third metacarpal bone *(B)*. The point at which these lines intersect is known as the pivot point *(PP)*, and the angle between them is the pivot point angle *(PPA)*.

and helps to determine whether the cuboidal bones, in the case of the carpus and tarsus, are involved in the deviation, or if deviation is caused by disproportionate physeal growth only. Abnormalities in the structure of these bones can have a substantial influence on the effect of the procedure and the future athletic potential of the horse. The pivot point angle is the angle formed by the intersection of these two lines and indicates the severity of the condition.[8]

Hemicircumferential periosteal transection and elevation, or periosteal stripping, aims to accelerate growth on the concave side of the limb, laterally for valgus and medially for varus deformities.[1] Previous work on chicken radii had shown that a circumferential division of the periosteum, rather than a longitudinal one, resulted in increased bone growth. The proposal was that the periosteum functioned as a fibroelastic tube that spanned the diaphysis, provided an even tension between both epiphyses, and was responsible for the regulation of growth.[1,9] A horizontal or circumferential division of the periosteum would result in a release of tension at the level of the growth plate, resulting in the induction of new bone production on the side of the division.

The procedure has been thoroughly described.[4-6] Hemicircumferential periosteal transection and elevation is performed with the foal in lateral recumbency under general anesthesia, with the concave side of the affected limb uppermost. If the procedure is going to be performed bilaterally, dorsal recumbency is recommended. The position of the physis is identified using a 20-gauge needle. For a carpus valgus deformity, a 4- to 6-cm longitudinal incision is made between the common and lateral digital extensor tendons starting just proximal to the medial

physis. The incision is extended through to the periosteum. Using a curved scalpel blade (No. 12), a horizontal incision is made 1 to 2 cm proximal and parallel to the physis, at the distal end of the initial incision (parallel to the skin incision), forming an inverted T. The periosteal flaps are elevated with the aid of a periosteal elevator and then allowed to return to the normal position. It is important to transect the remnant of the ulna, or if the ulna is ossified, it should be removed with the aid of rongeurs. In foals with hindlimb tarsus valgus the veterinarian should bear in mind that a fibular remnant may be present. The incision is closed routinely and the area is bandaged for 10 to 14 days. The foal is kept in a large stall or small paddock until the deformity has been corrected.

Hemicircumferential periosteal transection and elevation has been reported to exert its effects for up to 2 months, but the procedure can be repeated if further correction is needed.[4] There are no reports of overcorrection of the deformity, although one of the Editors (MWR) is aware of a few foals in which transphyseal bridging techniques on the opposite of the limb were necessary after hemicircumferential periosteal transection, giving the distinct appearance that overcorrection occurred. Early reports suggested an approximately 80% success rate[1,3]; however, more recent work indicates less favorable results.[10-12] A large retrospective study in Thoroughbred racehorses investigated racing performance after hemicircumferential periosteal transection and elevation.[10] A lower percentage of treated horses were able to start a race and had a lower starts percentile ranking number compared with half-siblings. Most of the foals appeared to respond favorably to hemicircumferential periosteal transection and elevation based on external appearance of the limbs, but preexisting conditions, such as abnormal cuboidal bone formation from incomplete ossification or osteoarthritis secondary to abnormal loading of the limb before correction, may have influenced subsequent performance.

The technique of physeal stimulation, a modification of hemicircumferential transection and elevation, was reported to be successful.[13] Briefly, a needle is inserted into the physis on the concave portion of the limb (for example, the distal lateral aspect of the radial physes for foals with carpus valgus limb deformity) and numerous needle punctures are made into the physis, but deep to the periosteum, in a fan-shaped fashion.[13] I have no experience with this technique.

Angular limb deformities are probably the most common orthopedic problem affecting Thoroughbred foals.[1014] Early surgical intervention was previously recommended to take maximum advantage of the growth potential of the physis, to try to provide foals with excellent conformation, and to enhance sale value and possibly potential performance. Based on current knowledge, it now seems likely that a large number of foals with mild angular limb deformities underwent unnecessary surgery. The reported success for correction of angular limb deformities, particularly in the carpus, after hemicircumferential periosteal transection and elevation has been recently challenged. Foals with carpus valgus that underwent hemicircumferential periosteal transection and elevation were no more likely to improve than were those managed with stall rest and corrective farriery.[11,12] Although the efficacy or need to perform hemicircumferential periosteal transection and elevation when treating foals with mild to moderate carpus valgus deviations is a matter of current debate, the same cannot be said necessarily for other regions of the limb, such as the tarsus and fetlocks, without further investigation.

Transphyseal bridging is performed on the convex side of a deformity to decrease the growth rate on that side of the physis. Traditionally, transphyseal bridging has been performed in young foals with severe deformities or in foals in which most of the growth in a particular physis has subsided. Transphyseal bridging has been performed successfully using cortical screws with cerclage wire in a figure eight, with a small dynamic compression plate, or with orthopedic staples.[4-6]

The foal is positioned in lateral recumbency under general anesthesia, with the convex side of the affected limb uppermost, or in dorsal recumbency. The position of the physis is identified and checked radiologically using a 20-gauge needle inserted into the physis. Stab incisions are made for placement of cortical screws and cerclage wire; one incision is made in the center of the epiphysis and the other approximately 2 cm proximal to the physis. Once the subcutaneous tissues between both incisions have been bluntly dissected, a 4.5- or 3.5-mm cortex screw is placed through each incision, slightly angled toward the physis. Screw size depends on the size of the foal, but 4.5-mm screws are preferred. Before complete tightening of the screws, a loop of 18-gauge wire is fed through the proximal incision and positioned around the distal screw head. The wire is then tightened over the proximal screw head, forming a figure eight. Once the wire has been tightened, the screws are tightened and the incisions are closed routinely. When performing this procedure in the distal aspect of the tibia, the clinician should be aware of the contour of the tarsocrural joint, because placing the epiphyseal screw into the joint is possible. The screw should be angled more sharply toward the physis than in the distal aspect of the radius. Postoperatively the foal should be kept in a large stall and monitored closely. Follow-up radiographs are strongly recommended to assess the amount of correction. Prompt removal of the implants is essential, because overcorrection of the deformity is possible.

A surgical alternative to transphyseal bridging has been described and is currently known as the transphyseal screw technique.[4,7] A single screw, either 3.5 mm or 4.5 mm in diameter, is inserted in neutral fashion across the growth plate through a small stab incision in order to create the desired compression on the convex side of the deformity, as with transphyseal bridging (Figure 58-4). This technique has been successful in achieving adequate correction of angular limb deformities, with the advantage of a better cosmetic result. Postoperative care for horses treated with a transphyseal screw is similar to that for transphyseal bridging. Prompt removal of the screw just before correction is achieved is encouraged because overcorrection is possible and there is a lag phase between screw removal and continued growth on the operated side.

In foals and young horses with an angular limb deformity that persists after physeal closure, corrective ostectomy or osteotomy can be performed. A step ostectomy (sagittal plane) or step osteotomy (dorsal plane) is preferred

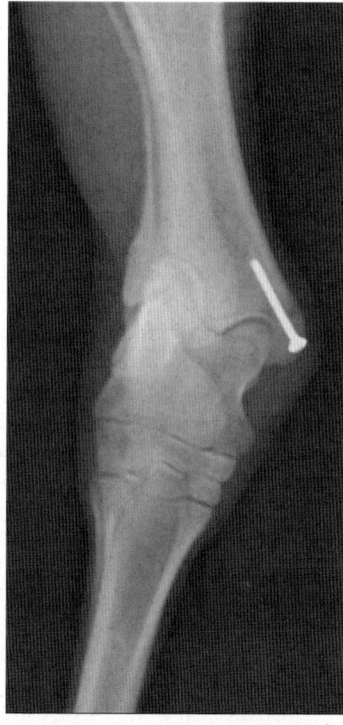

Fig. 58-4 • Dorsoplantar radiographic image of a tarsus with valgus deformity after a transphyseal screw procedure.

to a closing wedge ostectomy, because limb length is preserved and interfragmentary compression between the bone pieces is better.[4] These techniques are generally considered to be salvage procedures.

Tarsus valgus deformities frequently go unrecognized by both owners and veterinarians, possibly from lack of observation of the foal from behind and the inherent offset position of the tarsus.[15,16] Early recognition and sometimes more aggressive surgical management of tarsal angular limb deformities are critical to achieve satisfactory results. Although the distal tibial physis has a tremendous growth rate until 4 months of age, foals younger than 2 months of age responded more favorably to hemicircumferential periosteal transection and elevation than older foals. Transphyseal bridging was more effective than hemicircumferential periosteal transection and elevation, especially in foals older than 2 months of age.[15] This is a substantial change from the previous perception that hemicircumferential periosteal transection and elevation alone were adequate when managing most tarsus valgus deformities in foals 4 to 6 months of age. Early recognition of incomplete ossification of the tarsal bones (Figure 58-5) is crucial, because the condition, if unrecognized, leads to collapse of the third or central tarsal bones, resulting in osteoarthritis.[15,16] Of 22 foals with incomplete ossification of the tarsal bones, 73% had tarsus valgus deformities. Only 32% of the foals were able to achieve the intended use.[16]

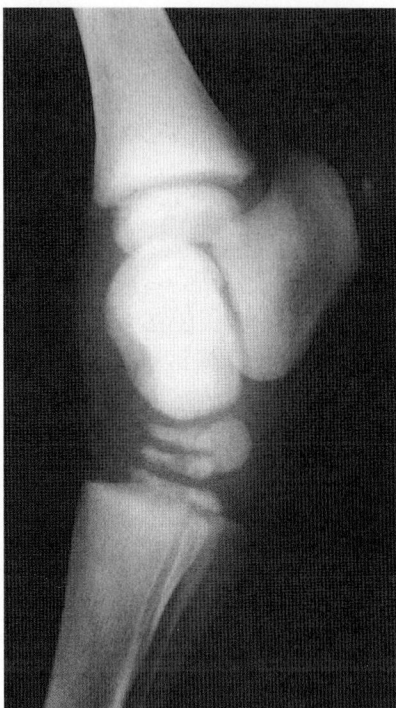

Fig. 58-5 • Lateromedial radiographic image of a neonatal tarsus with incomplete ossification of the tarsal bones. Note the heterogenous radiopacity of the third tarsal bone.

Chapter 59

Flexural Limb Deformities in Foals

Robert J. Hunt

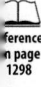

References on page 1298

Flexural limb deformity is the inability to extend a limb fully. Generally hyperflexion of a region results from a disparity in the length of the musculotendonous unit relative to the length of the bone. The deformities are categorized as congenital or acquired and may occur during in utero development or at any time after birth. Different anatomical structures may be involved, including the digital flexor tendons, suspensory apparatus, joint capsule, and surrounding fascia, skin, and bone.[1-6]

CONGENITAL FLEXURAL DEFORMITIES

Congenital deformities are present at birth, and the cause is often unknown. Although uterine malposition of the fetus is often discussed, because of the voluminous nature of the uterus and the ability of the foal to move, uterine malposition is an improbable cause of flexural deformity in most instances. Other documented causes include exposure of the mare to influenza and ingestion of Sudan grass, locoweed, or other teratogenic agents during development of the fetus.[2,3,7] Equine goiter, neuromuscular disorders, and defects in elastin formation or collagen cross-linking may be involved in the pathogenesis.

Congenital flexural deformities most commonly involve the distal interphalangeal (DIP) joints, carpus, tarsus, and metacarpophalangeal and metatarsophalangeal joints, singularly or in combination.[2] Both forelimbs are usually involved, and occasionally other variations of skeletal deformities are evident, such as hindlimb deformity (windswept), spinal deformity, rye nose, and cleft palate. Sporadically occurring deformities involving the scapulohumeral, cubital, coxofemoral, or femorotibial joints may occur in combination with other congenital skeletal anomalies. Congenital flexural deformities are a common cause of dystocia in the broodmare, resulting in loss of the foal and subsequent reproductive loss of the mare.

Treatment for congenital flexural deformities varies with the anatomical location involved and severity of the condition. Therapeutic intervention for foals with severe flexural deformities associated with arthrogryposis or gross spinal deformities should be discouraged, and humane destruction is recommended. Surgical transection of the digital flexor tendons and palmar carpal fascia generally fails to alleviate this deformity. Splinting and casting is also futile, although rarely a foal has survived with limited athletic potential.

Mild flexural deformities of the carpal, metacarpophalangeal or metatarsophalangeal, or DIP joints resolve

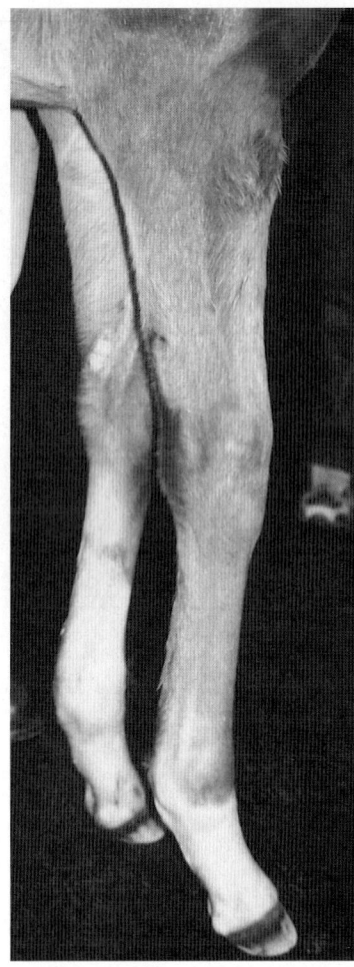

Fig. 59-1 • Mild bilateral flexural deformity of the carpus. This degree of deformity is self-limiting.

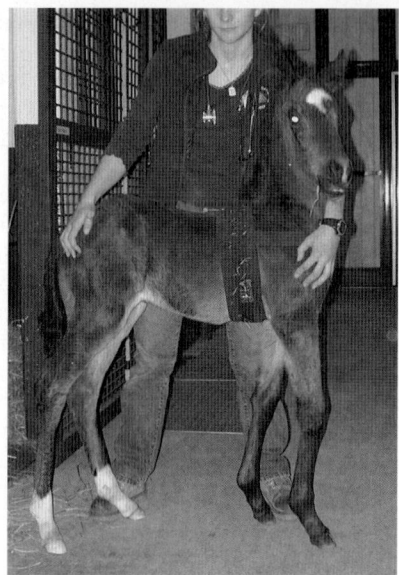

Fig. 59-2 • Moderate unilateral flexural deformity of the right carpus.

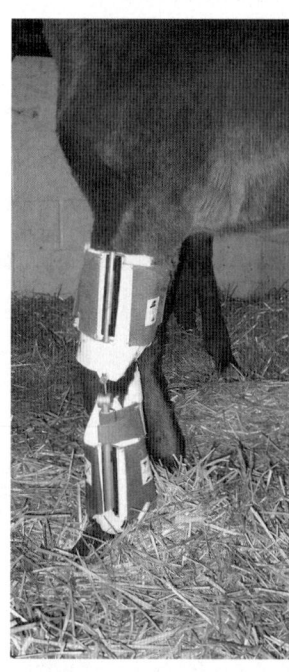

Fig. 59-3 • Articulating brace used in foals with flexural deformity of the carpus.

spontaneously if the foal has the ability to stand, nurse, and ambulate on its own. Most foals with mild and moderate deformities of these sites respond favorably to physiotherapy, by manually extending the limbs every 4 to 6 hours for 15-minute sessions, or forcing the foal to ambulate (Figure 59-1). Heavy bandaging, splinting or casting, and the administration of oxytetracycline can be helpful.[2,8] Foals with deformities advanced enough to require assistance to stand respond more rapidly after application of a cast, which should be changed every 2 to 3 days (Figure 59-2). If a carpal deformity severe enough to prevent standing is recognized at parturition, the foal should be heavily sedated, within 30 to 45 minutes, and full-leg casts should be applied with the limbs placed in extension. These should be changed within 24 hours and reset. Generally a rapid response is seen after the first or second application of casts. If the foal develops any complications with the casts or becomes distressed, casts should be removed. Commercially available articulating braces (Almanza Corrective Boot, www.redboot.com.ar/home.html; Equine Bracing Solutions, Trumansburg, New York, United States; Dynasplint Systems, Serverna Park, Maryland, United States) are available and allow adjusting the degree of extension in a specific region of the limb (Figure 59-3). As with all splints, caution must be exercised to prevent pressure sores. It is important to assist the foal in nursing and

to provide supportive care in an intensive neonatal facility, because these horses are at high risk for developing complications with other body systems.

Oxytetracycline (2 to 4 g) administered slowly intravenously is also beneficial, but it should not be used in a neonate until serum creatinine is within normal limits.[8] Oxytetracycline may be given daily or every other day for three or four treatments. Complications of oxytetracycline administration include renal failure, diarrhea, and, most commonly, excessive laxity of other, normal joints. The precise mechanism of action for tendon relaxation remains speculative.

Flexural deformity of the DIP joint is most often self-limiting if the foal can stand without buckling forward.

Bandaging of the lower limb, physical therapy, and administration of oxytetracycline hastens recovery. If the foot angle is beyond 90 degrees (i.e., the dorsal aspect of the foot is in front of the vertical), casting or splinting may be necessary. Toe extensions are generally counterproductive and hinder ambulation of the foal.

Splints may be constructed from polyvinyl chloride (PVC) material, fashioned from fiberglass cast material, or purchased commercially. When splints are used for management of flexural deformity, the clinician must exercise extreme caution to prevent rub sores or pressure sores. Splints should be applied only for brief periods, in a schedule such as 4 to 6 hours on followed by 4 to 6 hours off. Properly applied casts are more effective, require less maintenance, and result in fewer pressure sores than splints.

Prognosis for future athletic performance is good for foals with congenital flexural deformities that respond favorably in the first 2 weeks of life. In general, if the foal is able to stand, nurse, and ambulate without assistance, most congenital flexural deformities are self-limiting and warrant a good prognosis. Foals may require several months to stop buckling dorsally at the carpus. Foals with flexural deformity of the metacarpophalangeal or metatarsophalangeal joints typically respond within the first or second week of life. Prognosis for future performance is poor for foals with severe flexural deformity of the carpus, tarsus, or metacarpophalangeal or metatarsophalangeal joints that show no improvement after several days of treatment and have difficulty ambulating without assistance after 1 to 2 weeks of treatment. Foals with congenital flexural deformities involving the scapulohumeral, cubital, coxofemoral, or femorotibial joints have a poor prognosis for future athletic performance.

ACQUIRED FLEXURAL DEFORMITIES

Acquired flexural deformities develop after birth until the second year of life. Commonly involved areas include the DIP joint, metacarpophalangeal joint, and carpus. Acquired flexural deformity of the DIP joint is recognized at 3 to 6 months of age, carpal flexural deformity is seen at 1 to 6 months of age, and flexural deformity of the metacarpophalangeal joint is recognized later, during the yearling or early 2-year-old year (9 to 18 months).[9]

Common causes of flexural deformity of the metacarpophalangeal joint and carpus are believed to include a genetic propensity for rapid growth, overnutrition, and pain. Relative excess feeding or overassimilation of nutrients in foals that have an inherent potential for rapid physical development is a frequent finding in foals with acquired flexural deformity, especially involving the carpus and the metacarpophalangeal joint. During periods of rapid bone lengthening the potential for passive elongation of the tendonous unit is limited because of the accessory ligaments, and a discrepancy in the length of the bone-to-tendon unit may result. Another theory is that a pain-mediated response during physeal dysplasia results in altered load bearing on the limbs. This is believed to initiate secondary contraction and shortening of the musculotendonous unit, resulting in limited extension of a region. Any cause of pain resulting in prolonged reduced weight bearing in a limb may result in this syndrome.

Genetics may be involved with the development of acquired flexural deformity of the DIP joints (club feet). Other factors include diet and exercise. Protracted lameness from another cause such as osteochondrosis of the upper limb also predisposes to development of acquired DIP joint deformity. It is therefore important to identify an associated source of lameness.

Early clinical signs of acquired flexural deformity of the DIP joint consist of a prominent bulge at the coronary band, increase in length of the heel relative to the toe, and failure of the heel to contact the ground after trimming (Figure 59-4, *A*). Eventually the foot develops a boxy shape with a dish shape along the dorsal hoof wall. This deformity is commonly accompanied by a back-at-the-knee (calf-knee) conformation (see Figure 59-4, *B*).

Treatment for foals with acquired flexural deformity of the DIP joint initially entails exercise restriction, frequent lowering of the heel, dietary restrictions, and pain control with nonsteroidal antiinflammatory drugs such as flunixin meglumine. Weaning the foal may be advantageous. If the toe becomes excessively worn, constructing a cap over the toe with one of the commercially available hoof composites may aid in protecting the toe and dorsal aspect of the sole from bruising and may temporarily serve as a lever arm. Although elevating the heel with a wedge shoe or pad provides comfort for the foal, the deformity gradually worsens, and eventually obtaining a normal angle and shape to the hoof is difficult. Glue-on shoes should likewise be used with caution, because they tend to promote a box shape to the foot. Oxytetracycline may be used but exacerbates the back-at-the-knee conformation.

If no improvement is achieved within 1 to 2 months of conservative treatment, surgical intervention with desmotomy of the accessory ligament of the deep digital flexor tendon (ALDDFT) is recommended. When surgical treatment is combined with a trimming program, hoof conformation and function will be much improved. The owner should be made aware of the potential for a blemish at the surgical site. In a group of 23 Standardbreds treated for flexural deformity of the DIP joint, 11 foals had desmotomy of the ALDDFT, of which six raced or were sound. All foals operated on by 8 months of age had a favorable outcome. None of the 12 foals that did not undergo surgery had a favorable outcome.[10]

Foals in which the dorsal aspect of the hoof is in front of the vertical (hoof angle >90 degrees) are candidates for deep digital flexor tenotomy, although desmotomy of the ALDDFT has been helpful in some foals when combined with farriery, oxytetracycline, and phenylbutazone therapy. With deformities of this severity, contracture of the joint capsule and surrounding soft tissues often precludes successful management for an athletic future.

Early treatment of foals with flexural deformity involving the metacarpophalangeal and metatarsophalangeal joints consists of eliminating pain through the use of analgesics, exercise restriction, and correction of any underlying nutritional problems. Any extremes in hoof angle should be corrected, and the foot should be trimmed at an angle suitable for that individual. If no improvement is achieved with conservative treatment, desmotomy of the accessory ligament of the superficial digital flexor tendon or of the ALDDFT may be helpful in select instances of moderate deformity. If the underlying cause is not

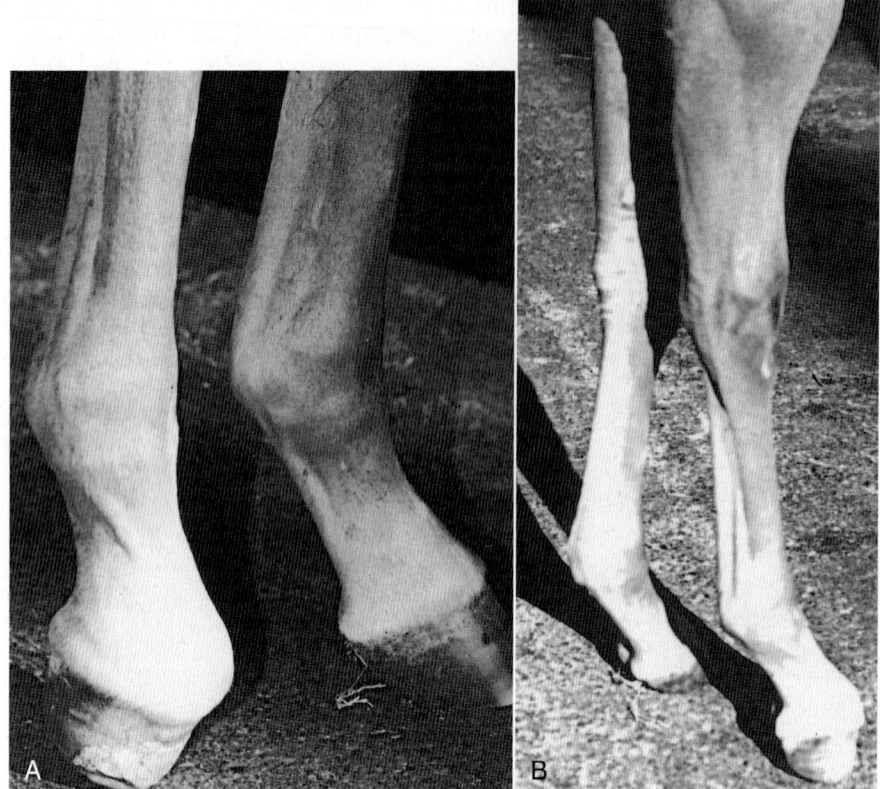

Fig. 59-4 • A, Advanced flexural deformity of the right front distal interphalangeal joint. The heel does not contact the ground, and the dorsal aspect of the hoof wall is dish shaped. **B,** Calf-kneed conformation is associated with a clubfoot.

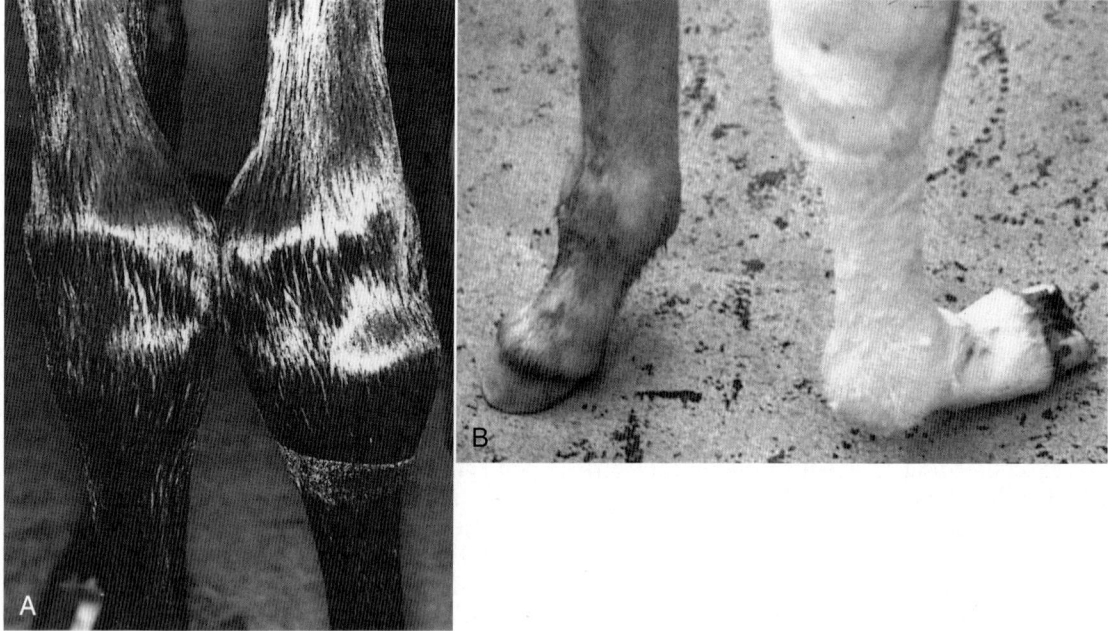

Fig. 59-5 • Rupture of the common digital extensor tendon. **A,** Note the fluctuant swelling over the dorsolateral surface of the left carpus. **B,** The fetlock buckles forward.

addressed, the benefits of surgery will be only transient. Foals with severe deformity resulting in the limb persistently buckling forward rarely respond favorably to conservative or surgical treatment. Transection of both accessory ligaments or of the superficial digital flexor tendon may

provide some improvement in horses with advanced deformity.

Treatment for acquired flexural deformity of the carpus is aimed at eliminating the underlying cause, and if the deformity is recognized early, conservative management is generally effective. The nutritional program (see Chapter 55) and growth chart for the foal should be reviewed and errors corrected if found. The nutritional program is often already balanced in some of these foals, and treatment is empirical and focused on reducing the energy intake and slowing the growth. Dietary restriction, limitation of turnout schedule and exercise, and treatment with nonsteroidal antiinflammatory drugs are currently accepted practice. Feeding of grain and other sources high in energy and protein to the mare should be restricted in an attempt to reduce the nutritional quality of the milk and to prevent the foal from ingesting grain while eating with the mare. In foals with severe deformity, limiting access to milk through muzzling the foal and stripping the mare periodically throughout the day may be attempted. However, weaning the foal from the mare to control the diet is generally easier. Acquired carpal flexural deformities may require weeks to months to correct. Splints, bandaging, and oxytetracycline may provide some benefit. These benefits are often short-lived if the underlying cause is not addressed.

Rupture of the common or lateral digital extensor tendon is often mistaken for flexural deformity of the metacarpophalangeal joint or carpus because the foal knuckles forward when walking. The disorder may be recognized shortly after birth or generally by 3 to 4 days of life; rarely it may occur in foals up to 3 weeks of age. Diagnosis is based on the characteristic gait of knuckling forward at the fetlock and the presence of a fluctuant swelling over the dorsolateral surface of the carpus (Figure 59-5). There is usually palpable laxity in the extensor tendons. The limb can be placed in a normal position when the foal is standing. There may be a greater tendency to rupture the extensor tendons in foals with flexural deformities, especially in those that are born prematurely.

Treatment consists of applying a heavily padded splint over the dorsal or palmar aspect of the lower limb to prevent knuckling forward and traumatizing the dorsum of the pastern and fetlock. Dorsally placed splints are most effective if they do not slip or rotate. Casting may be used but is generally not necessary. Stall confinement is important until the foal develops the ability to use the limb. Foals generally require 1 week to 2 months of splinting and bandaging before they learn to ambulate properly. The prognosis is invariably good.

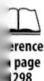

Chapter 60

Cervical Stenotic Myelopathy

Richard J. Piercy*

erences page 1298

Cervical stenotic myelopathy (CSM; wobbler syndrome), a common spinal cord disease of horses, is characterized by malformation of the cervical vertebrae, stenosis of the vertebral canal, and spinal cord compression.[1] The age of onset is typically 6 months to 3 years, although mature horses are also sometimes affected. Young horses with the disorder have commonly grown rapidly and are more likely to have developmental orthopedic disease of the appendicular skeleton than peers.[2] Male horses are more frequently affected than females.[3] CSM has been reported in most light and draft horse breeds, although Thoroughbred and Warmblood horses appear to be particularly predisposed.

CLINICAL SIGNS

The clinical signs of spinal cord compression are usually insidious in onset, although owners sometimes report a traumatic incident before recognizing any ataxia. Such traumatic incidents may occur because of mild or previously unrecognized neurological deficits (e.g., occasional tripping) that result in a fall.

Horses with CSM generally have neurological deficits that are recognizable in all limbs, characterized by symmetrical weakness, ataxia, and spasticity.[4] In most instances the hindlimbs are more severely affected than the forelimbs, probably because of the more superficial location of hindlimb tracts in the white matter of the spinal cord. At rest, severely affected horses may have a base-wide stance and delayed responses to proprioceptive positioning, whereas at the walk, weakness may be manifest by stumbling and toe dragging. Horses with prolonged clinical signs of CSM may therefore have hooves or shoes that are chipped, worn, or squared at the toe. Ataxia (a sign associated with defective proprioception) is evident as truncal sway at a walk, inconsistent and erratic foot placement, and circumduction and posting (pivoting on the inside limb) of the hindlimbs during circling. Moderately to severely affected horses sometimes have lacerations on the heel bulbs and medial aspects of the forelimbs from overreaching and interference. Spasticity, characterized by a stiff-legged gait and exaggerated movements, may be observed in moderately affected horses, especially in the forelimbs or in the hindlimbs when stepping over curbs or poles. When prompted to back, horses may stand basewide, lean backward, and drag the forelimbs. Occasionally, signs associated with the forelimbs may be more severe than those in the hindlimbs, particularly in horses with caudal cervical lesions, probably because of involvement of local spinal cord grey matter.

A grading scale (0 to 5) is often used to score horses with signs of spinal ataxia and weakness: 0, normal; 1, very mild deficits detectable only with complex movements (e.g., walking with head elevated, on an incline or when circling); 2, mild-moderate deficits that are detectable at the walk; 3, marked deficits obvious at the walk; 4, severe deficits that result in difficulty remaining standing; 5, recumbent. Some clinicians favor an approach in which

*The author acknowledges and appreciates the work of Dr. Bonnie Rush, who authored this contribution in the previous edition.

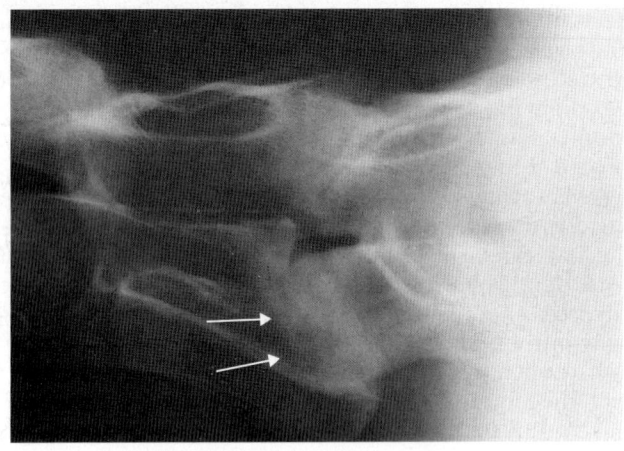

Figure 60-1 • Lateral-lateral radiographic image of the caudal aspect of the neck of a 4-year-old Paint gelding with cervical pain and spinal ataxia. Cranial is to the left. Note the abnormal intercentral articulation between the sixth and seventh cervical vertebrae *(arrows)*. This represents end-stage diskospondylosis.

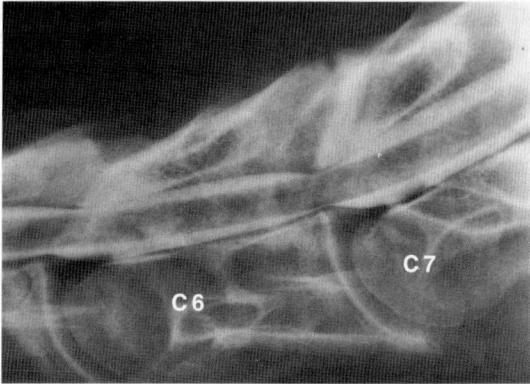

Figure 60-2 • Lateral-lateral radiographic image during myelographic examination of the fifth to seventh *(C7)* cervical vertebrae of a 3-year-old Thoroughbred colt with static spinal cord compression. The dorsal and ventral contrast columns are attenuated by more than 50% at the fifth and sixth *(C6)* and sixth and seventh cervical vertebral articulations.

individual limbs are scored separately for signs of ataxia and weakness, with a global score being used to summarize the total neurological deficit. Such an approach is helpful when evaluating disease progression and response to treatments.[5]

Asymmetrical ataxia and paresis are observed occasionally in horses with dorsolateral compression of the spinal cord caused by proliferative, degenerative articular processes and periarticular soft tissues.[6] Infrequently, signs of compressive radiculopathy, such as cervical pain, atrophy of the cervical musculature, cutaneous hypalgesia, and hyporeflexia of cervical reflexes adjacent to the site of spinal cord compression may be evident. These signs are more commonly observed in horses older than 4 years of age with moderate-to-severe arthropathy of the fifth to seventh cervical vertebrae (C5 to C7) and usually result from peripheral nerve compression by proliferative articular processes as the nerve root exits the vertebral canal through the intervertebral foramen.[7]

In some instances arthropathy of the caudal cervical vertebral articular processes may produce forelimb lameness, caused by spinal nerve root compression, without producing clinical signs of spinal cord compression.[8] Affected horses typically have a short cranial phase of the stride and a low forelimb foot arc and may stand or walk with the head and neck extended (see Chapter 53). Rarely, diskospondylosis of the cervical vertebrae produces a short-strided gait and cervical pain, with or without spinal ataxia (Figure 60-1). Horses with diskospondylosis or arthropathy of the caudal vertebrae may exhibit signs of lameness, pain, or stiffness with the neck in only certain positions or when the head and neck are manipulated or the horse is turned. For example, some affected horses may be unwilling to turn the neck laterally when offered food.

Dynamic spinal cord compression usually occurs in younger horses (<2 years of age) and is associated with instability of the cervical vertebrae, particularly between C3 and C6. Dorsal laminar extension, caudal epiphyseal flare, or abnormal ossification patterns may contribute to the problem. Static vertebral canal stenosis (type II) is characterized by constant spinal cord compression, regardless

of neck position (Figure 60-2), and is seen usually in older horses.[9] It generally results from osteoarthritis (OA) of the articular processes and proliferation of periarticular soft tissue structures. Synovial cysts, which are often associated with OA of the articular processes, may produce waxing and waning, or acute-onset asymmetrical neurological signs. In some horses with static compression, flexion of the neck stretches the ligamentum flavum and relieves spinal cord compression, whereas extension exacerbates the problem.

DIAGNOSIS

The following neurological disorders should be considered potential differential diagnoses and may produce signs similar to or indistinguishable from CSM: equine protozoal myeloencephalitis (EPM), equine degenerative myeloencephalopathy (EDM), equine herpesvirus–1 (EHV-1) myelitis, occipitoatlantoaxial malformation, spinal cord trauma, vertebral fracture, vertebral abscess or neoplasia, and verminous myelitis (see Chapter 11).

Horses with traumatic cervical vertebral disorders usually exhibit pain during manipulation or palpation of the neck, and the disorder may sometimes be differentiated from CSM by standing radiographic examination. Occipitoatlantoaxial malformation (see Chapter 53) occurs primarily in Arabian horses and is diagnosed definitively by radiological evaluation (see Figure 53-4, *B*). EDM is diagnosed by exclusion (unremarkable cerebrospinal fluid [CSF] cytological examination findings, negative immunoblot analysis for *Sarcocystis neurona,* and negative radiological findings and myelographic examination findings). A veterinarian may suspect EDM based on the age (usually less than 18 months) and during neurological examination (hyporeflexia, and similar degrees of ataxia in the forelimbs and hindlimbs), but definitive diagnosis is achieved only by postmortem examination. Although several breeds have been reported with the disease, EDM appears to have a familial predisposition in Standardbred horses.[10] Horses with EHV-1 myelitis may have urinary incontinence, poor tail tone, and hindlimb lower motor neuron weakness. Signs associated with cranial nerve involvement may occasionally be observed. In EHV-1 myelitis, CSF evaluation typically reveals xanthochromia and albuminocytological dissociation (high protein concentration, normal cell count); a rising EHV-1 serum antibody titer, virus isolation, and polymerase chain reaction (PCR) diagnosis all may be used to provide supportive evidence of EHV-1 myelitis. In areas where EPM is endemic (such as North and South America) or in horses exported from these regions, distinguishing between EPM and CSM can be difficult. Asymmetrical ataxia, focal sweating, and focal muscle atrophy should direct diagnostic efforts toward EPM; however, symmetrical spinal ataxia does not preclude a diagnosis of EPM. EPM-affected horses with symmetrical ataxia are differentiated from those with CSM on the basis of standing radiographic examination, CSF immunoblot analysis for *S. neurona,* and, in some circumstances, myelographic evaluation (see comments on equine myelography, later). Immunoblot analysis of CSF is frequently positive, however, if horses affected by CSM are in a geographical area with a high seroprevalence of EPM. Therefore differentiation of these two conditions should not be determined on the basis of CSF analysis alone. Findings of cytological analysis of CSF are usually unremarkable in horses with CSM, although mild xanthochromia or slightly increased protein concentration may be observed in affected horses, especially if signs have developed acutely, perhaps precipitated by trauma.

Plain radiography of the cervical vertebrae can be used to assess the likelihood of CSM in horses with spinal ataxia.[11] Accurate assessment of cervical radiographs requires a precise lateral-lateral radiographic image of the cervical vertebrae,[12] ensuring that the ventral prominences of the transverse processes are perfectly overlying each other. Radiographic obliquity results in indistinct margins of the ventral aspect of the vertebral canal, and in erroneous values for objective measurements. Obtaining precise lateral-lateral radiographs of the cervical vertebrae in recumbent horses is difficult, so whenever possible, plain or digital radiographs should be obtained in the standing, sedated horse.

Cervical radiographs should be evaluated subjectively and objectively. Subjective interpretation is based on examining for the presence of five characteristic malformations of the cervical vertebrae, which include (1) flare of the caudal epiphysis of the vertebral body (the so-called "ski-jump appearance"); (2) abnormal ossification of the articular processes; (3) subluxation or malalignment between adjacent vertebrae; (4) extension of the vertebral caudal dorsal lamina; and (5) OA of the articular processes (Figure 60-3). Estimating the importance of lesions identified through subjective interpretation can be difficult and is based on the clinician's experience and interpreting the balance of probability. For example, OA of (especially the caudal) vertebral articular processes is recognized commonly in normal horses.[13] Hence recognition of characteristic vertebral malformations is considered supportive in diagnosis at best.[14]

Objective assessment of vertebral canal diameter is more accurate than subjective evaluation of vertebral malformation for identifying young horses affected by CSM, but may lead to false negative diagnoses in older horses.[9] Both intervertebral and intravertebral measurements are used. The sensitivity and specificity of the intravertebral sagittal ratio for identifying horses affected by CSM are approximately 90% for vertebral sites between the fourth

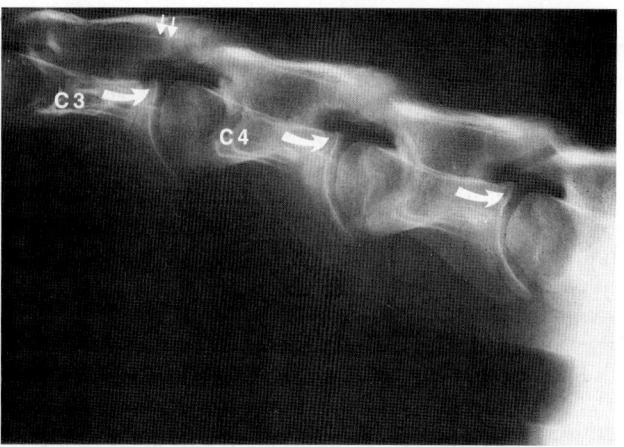

Figure 60-3 • Lateral-lateral radiographic image of the midneck region of an 8-month-old Quarter Horse colt with spinal ataxia caused by cervical stenotic myelopathy. Bony malformations consistent with cervical stenotic myelopathy include flare of the caudal epiphyses *(curved arrows),* caudal extension of the third cervical vertebra dorsal lamina *(arrows),* and malalignment of the articulation of the third *(C3)* and fourth *(C4)* cervical vertebrae.

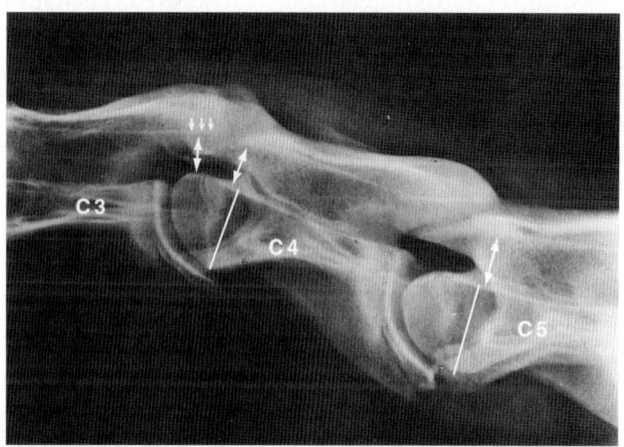

Figure 60-4 • Lateral-lateral radiographic image of the third *(C3),* fourth *(C4),* and fifth *(C5)* cervical vertebrae of a 2-year-old Thoroughbred colt with cervical stenotic myelopathy. The sagittal ratio is determined by dividing the intravertebral minimum sagittal diameter *(double arrow)* by the width of the vertebral body *(line).* The intervertebral minimum sagittal diameter is measured from the caudoventral aspect of the dorsal lamina of C3 to the craniodorsal aspect of the vertebral body of C4 *(double arrow below the smaller arrows).* There is caudal extension of the dorsal lamina of C3 *(smaller arrows),* and there is malalignment at the articulation of C3 and C4.

and seventh cervical vertebrae, suggesting that generalized stenosis of the vertebral canal may be the most important factor in the development of CSM (especially in young horses).[11] The intravertebral sagittal ratio is calculated by dividing the minimum sagittal diameter of the vertebral canal (the narrowest perpendicular distance from the dorsal aspect of the vertebral body to the ventral border of the dorsal lamina) by the maximum width of the cranial vertebral physis (from the vertebral canal) (Figure 60-4). Because the vertebral body is located within the same anatomical plane as the vertebral canal, this ratio negates effects of magnification resulting from variability in object-plate distance. In most normal horses, the sagittal ratio exceeds 52% from the fourth to sixth cervical vertebrae and

56% at the seventh cervical vertebrae in horses greater than 320 kg. The positive predictive value of such measurements is probably higher, and the negative predictive value lower, in ataxic horses from countries where conflicting diagnoses (such as EPM) are not routinely encountered (i.e., false-positive results are less likely, but false-negative results are more likely because the underlying prevalence of CSM in ataxic horses is higher). Similarly, the positive and negative predictive values of objective cervical radiography measurements in the absence of ataxia (e.g., during prepurchase radiography) have not been evaluated, but false-positive results are likely to be more common and false-negative results less common, because the prevalence of CSM in this population is much lower. Judicious use of additional diagnostic tests (e.g., CSF evaluation) to help rule out other differential diagnoses should be considered to increase pretest probability, especially in countries where other causes of spinal ataxia are common.

Some clinicians advocate use of ratiometric measurements that take into account the distance between adjacent vertebrae (intervertebral ratios) (see Figure 60-4) based on the rationale that most compressive lesions occur between, rather than within, the vertebrae.[15] Particularly high-quality radiographs are usually required for such measurements, but analysis suggests that this approach may be helpful in differentiating CSM from other conditions.[16] Further comparison of both methods in a large group of horses is needed based on a gold standard diagnosis established at postmortem examination, because myelography is problematic (see discussion later). However, available postmortem material may be skewed toward severely affected horses because these horses may more often be euthanized.

A semiquantitative scoring system developed by Mayhew and colleagues[17] is advocated in foals younger than 1 year of age for assessment of cervical radiographs for diagnosis of CSM. The scoring system combines objective measurement of vertebral canal diameter and subjective evaluation of vertebral malformation. Stenosis of the vertebral canal is assessed by determination of the intervertebral and intravertebral minimum sagittal diameter (see Figure 60-4). The intervertebral and intravertebral minimum sagittal diameters are corrected for radiographic magnification by dividing these values by the length of the vertebral body. The maximum score for cervical vertebral stenosis is 10 points. Cervical vertebral malformation is determined by subjective assessment of five categories: (1) encroachment of the caudal epiphysis of the vertebral body dorsally into the vertebral canal, (2) caudal extension of the dorsal lamina to the cranial physis of the adjacent vertebra, (3) angulation between adjacent vertebral bodies, (4) abnormal ossification of the physis, and (5) OA of the articular processes. The maximum score allotted for each category of bony malformation is 5 points. A total score of 12 or higher (maximum total score 35) confirms the radiological diagnosis of CSM. Stenosis of the vertebral canal and malalignment between adjacent vertebrae are the most discriminating parameters in this semiquantitative scoring system to differentiate normal from affected foals.

Radiology may be used to predict the likelihood of CSM, and in countries where conflicting differential diagnoses are rare (and in the absence of other signs to the contrary), radiology is often considered sufficient to make a presumptive diagnosis of cervical compression without the need for further tests. In countries where EPM or other conflicting differential diagnoses are possibilities, many clinicians favor myelography for diagnosis. Unfortunately, for most intervertebral sites, myelography results in a high number of false-positive and false-negative results.[18] Myelography remains, however, a prerequisite if surgical intervention is considered a viable option on the basis of severity of signs and the owner's wishes and expectations (see later). This is because standing radiography does not definitively pinpoint the actual site of the compressive lesion(s).[11] Typically during myelography, however, clinicians obtain additional radiographic images, such as the lateral-lateral projections in neutral, extended, and flexed positions, although the last technique in particular results in more false-positive diagnoses.[18] Radiography of the neck in different positions does, however, enable the clinician to attempt to differentiate between static and dynamic compressive lesions. Note that neck flexion and extension while horses are under anesthesia are contraindicated if there is evidence of compression on the initial neutral views. Ventrodorsal images may be attempted in small or young horses, especially in the cranial aspect of the neck, and may demonstrate an asymmetrical compressive lesion that might otherwise account for some false-negative diagnoses in larger horses.

Various techniques have been used for interpreting equine myelograms. In normal horses there should be no or minimal change to the width of the dorsal dye column, but it is common to have loss of the ventral dye column. Consequently, most commonly at intervertebral sites between C2 and C6, diagnosis of spinal cord compression is made on the basis of a 50% or greater decrease in the sagittal width of the dorsal and ventral contrast columns in comparison with the column width at the immediate cranial or caudal midvertebral site.[12] At C6-C7, a reduction of more than 20% of the dural diameter measured in the midbody region is best used to diagnose compression, because this measurement has a relatively high sensitivity and specificity.[18] Clinicians may favor use of different "cutoff" values for exclusion or inclusion of diagnosis based on the consequence of the derived decision (i.e., possible euthanasia or surgery).[16] As in interpretation of plain radiographs, the positive predictive value for myelography is likely to be higher in ataxic horses from countries without many conflicting differential diagnoses because the prevalence of true vertebral compression in ataxic horses is relatively higher.

Horses should be monitored for 24 hours after the myelographic procedure for depression, fever, seizure, or more severe ataxia. Worsening of neurological status after myelography may result from spinal cord trauma during hyperflexion or as a result of the general anesthesia or recovery, iatrogenic puncture of the spinal cord, or chemical meningitis. Administration of phenylbutazone (4.4 mg/kg orally [PO] q24h) 1 day before until 1 day after myelographic examination is recommended.

Additional techniques that have been used or proposed for evaluating horses with compressive myelopathy include electromyography of the cervical musculature (examining for presence of signs of local muscle denervation caused by grey matter or peripheral nerve disease),[19] transtentorial magnetic stimulation,[20] and kinematic gait analysis,[21] but

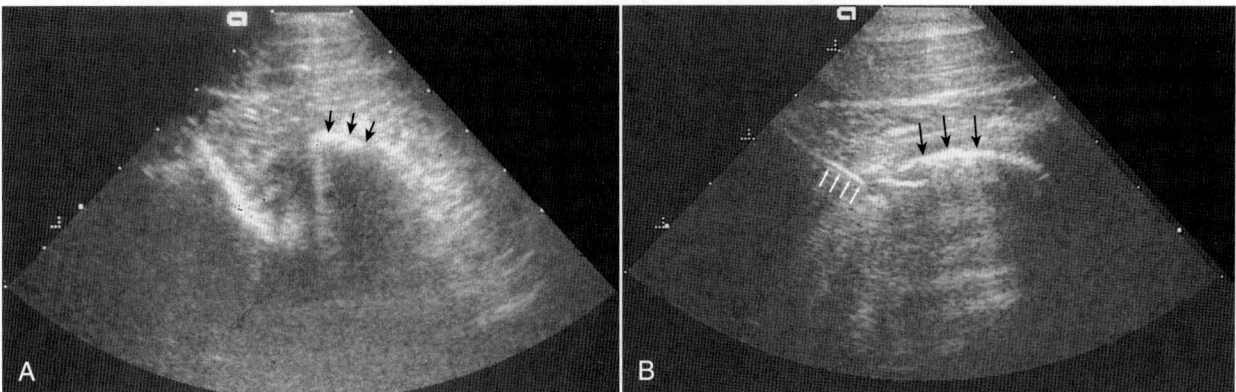

Figure 60-5 • A, Ultrasonographic examination of the articulation of the fifth and sixth cervical vertebrae (coronal image). The cranial articular process of the sixth cervical vertebra *(arrows)* is superficial to the caudal articular process of the fifth cervical vertebra. **B,** Ultrasonographic examination during arthrocentesis of the articulation of the fifth and sixth cervical vertebrae (transverse image). A 15-cm spinal needle is entering the ventrolateral aspect of the joint *(white arrows)* deep to the cranial articular process of the sixth cervical vertebra *(black arrows).*

such techniques require further validation before their widespread use is recommended. Antemortem diagnosis of CSM therefore has inherent problems and limitations, of which the clinician should be aware, but a combination of tests and methodologies taken in the context of the signalment, history, and comprehensive physical and neurological examinations likely optimizes accurate diagnosis.

CONSERVATIVE MANAGEMENT

Successful conservative management of foals younger than 1 year of age with CSM has been achieved using the paced diet program.[17,22] The goal of this dietary program is to retard bone growth, enhance bone metabolism, and allow the vertebral canal diameter to enlarge to relieve spinal cord compression. This dietary program is restricted in energy and protein (65% to 75% of National Research Council [NRC] recommendations) but maintains balanced vitamin and mineral intake (minimum 100% NRC recommendations). Vitamins A and E are provided at 3 times NRC recommendations, and selenium is supplemented to 0.3 ppm. Roughage is provided by pasture or low-quality (6% to 9% crude protein) timothy hay. Dietary regimens are individually formulated according to the age and weight of the foal. Solitary stall confinement is recommended to minimize repetitive spinal cord compression caused by dynamic instability.

Most clinicians advocate antiinflammatory therapy in all horses with CSM.[9] Administration of glucocorticoids and/or nonsteroidal antiinflammatory drugs may reduce edema and provide transient improvement in neurological signs or may reduce compression from inflamed associated soft tissues. Some clinicians advocate use of dimethyl sulfoxide, particularly in horses in which clinical signs have developed acutely. Spontaneous recovery from CSM without dietary management or surgical intervention is not reported.

Horses with cervical pain and forelimb lameness caused by cervical vertebral arthropathy may benefit from intraarticular administration of corticosteroids or chondroprotective agents. Intraarticular administration of medication is performed with ultrasound guidance using a 15-cm

(6-inch), 18-gauge spinal needle in a standing, sedated, or recumbent horse.[23] The cranial articular process of the more caudal vertebra is superficial to the caudal process of the cranial vertebra (Figure 60-5, *A*). The articular space is accessed at the cranioventral opening of the articular facet, which is angled approximately 60 degrees from the ultrasound beam. The needle should be introduced 5 cm cranial to the joint and inserted at a 30-degree angle to the skin surface (Figure 60-5, *B*). Joint penetration should be confirmed by aspiration of synovial fluid. If the neck is extended, the transverse process of the cranial vertebra may obscure the path to the articulation. Intraarticular administration of triamcinolone acetonide (6 mg per joint) or methylprednisolone acetate (100 mg per joint) has produced a reduction in cervical pain in more than 50% of horses with arthrosis of the articular processes.[24] The goal of intraarticular antiinflammatory therapy should be to improve cervical mobility, reduce cervical pain, and eliminate forelimb lameness. In my experience, intraarticular therapy rarely improves spinal ataxia presumed to be associated with articular process OA.

SURGICAL TREATMENT

Surgical intervention is the most widely reported therapeutic approach for (particularly adult) horses with CSM. Cervical vertebral interbody fusion (ventral stabilization) was first described in 1979 for horses with dynamic spinal cord compression, and it is widely performed, particularly in certain centers.[25] The procedure fuses adjacent vertebrae in the extended position, which provides immediate relief of most dynamic spinal cord compressive lesions while preventing repetitive spinal cord trauma. Dorsal laminectomy (subtotal Funkquist type B) is described for horses with static CSM and provides immediate decompression of the spinal cord.[26] Portions of the dorsal lamina, ligamentum flavum, and joint capsule overlying the site of spinal cord compression are removed during dorsal laminectomy. This procedure effectively decompresses the spinal cord. However, it has been associated with substantial postoperative complications[27] and is not widely performed. Interbody fusion is an alternative to dorsal laminectomy for horses with static compressive lesions because after cervical vertebral fusion the articular processes remodel and soft tissue structures atrophy, resulting in delayed decompression of the spinal cord over several months.[28]

Cervical vertebral fusion improves the neurological status of 44% to 90% of horses with CSM, and 12% to 62% of horses return to athletic function.[27,29] Of the horses that return to athletic function, approximately 60% are able to perform at the level of intended use, including racing, jumping, and pleasure performance activities. The anticipated magnitude of improvement is one to two neurological grades after cervical fusion. Occasionally, three grades of improvement in neurological status have been achieved. However, it is unusual for a horse with grade IV neurological deficits to become neurologically normal after cervical vertebral fusion. Rarely, a domino effect can occur in horses after vertebral fusion, wherein spinal cord compression develops at the intervertebral site adjacent to the site of fusion. This may result from added forces at the adjacent site or natural progression of the disease.[30] Subtotal laminectomy is reported to improve the neurological status of 40% to 75% of horses with static compression.[26]

Fatal postoperative complications have been reported with surgical management of horses with static compressive lesions of the caudal cervical vertebrae (subtotal laminectomy and interbody fusion). Complications directly related to the surgical procedure include vertebral body fracture, spinal cord edema, and implant failure. Seroma formation is common after cervical vertebral interbody fusion and can be minimized by use of a pressure bandage maintained over the surgical site for 2 to 3 weeks.[27]

The most important horse-related factor for determining postoperative prognosis is duration of clinical signs before surgical intervention. Horses with neurological gait deficits present for less than 1 month before surgery are more likely to return to athletic function than are horses with signs of greater than 3 months' duration.[27] The number of spinal cord compressive sites and horse age do not appear to affect the long-term outcome of horses with cervical vertebral interbody fusion. Horses with dynamic compressive lesions appear to have a better postoperative result than those with static compressive lesions. Horses with lesions involving the sixth and seventh cervical vertebrae have a less favorable prognosis than those with lesions affecting the third to fifth cervical vertebrae.

The duration of convalescence and rehabilitation after cervical vertebral interbody fusion is approximately 12 to 18 months, and a horse's neurological status may continue to improve throughout that time. An individualized exercise program dependent on capability, projected use, and neurological status should be designed to promote muscular strength and coordination. Extended exercise at slow speed, including ponying (being led from another horse), working over poles, and lunging on inclines, is recommended during rehabilitation to build muscular strength. The point at which the horse is competent to return to athletic function after cervical vertebral interbody fusion should be determined by neurological examination.

PART VII

Arthritis

Chapter 61

Osteoarthritis

John P. Caron

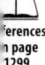
References
on page
1299

Joints are highly differentiated structures composed of a number of connective tissues including bone, articular cartilage, and periarticular soft tissues, all of which contribute to normal joint function and undergo changes in structure and metabolism in disease.[1,2] From the point of view of joint diseases, perhaps the most important of these components is articular or hyaline cartilage, composed principally of a precisely organized arrangement of collagens and proteoglycans. This tissue is responsible for the load-distributing functions of the joint, and, in health, cartilaginous surfaces glide over one another in a virtually frictionless manner, even when under substantial load. In joint trauma or osteoarthritis (OA), the normal structure and function of articular cartilage are deranged, leading to biochemical, structural, and biomechanical abnormalities in all joint tissues. If the trauma is uncorrected, the result is progressive joint destruction, a process likened to organ failure in other body systems. Joint disease is a particularly prevalent cause of lameness and as such is an expensive equine health problem.[3-5] An understanding of the biology and pathobiology of joints enables the clinician better to diagnose joint disease and to provide appropriate treatment and prevention recommendations.

STRUCTURE AND FUNCTION OF NORMAL JOINTS

Synovium and Synovial Fluid

The synovium is a vascular connective tissue lining the inner surface of the joint and consists of the cells of the synovial intima and a subsynovial stroma; the latter is composed of various amounts of fibrous, areolar, and fatty tissues. The synovium covers all articular surfaces, excluding articular cartilage and localized areas of bone. However, synovium is not uniform throughout the joint, and dense connective tissue may be found in its place in areas predisposed to trauma. Because the synovial lining bears neither true epithelium nor conventional basement membrane separating the joint cavity from the synovial vasculature, no true synovial membrane exists. Rather the intima and subsynovial tissues comprise a structural and functional continuum that acts as a macromolecular sieve.

The synovial intima is lined by a diverse population of synoviocytes, which have been classified according to their ultrastructure and with the use of specific antisera.[6-8] The three cell types are type A cells, of macrophage origin; fibroblast-derived type B cells; and type C cells, which appear to be an intermediate between A and B forms.[7,9-11] The most abundant are the type B cells, which synthesize a variety of important macromolecules, including collagen and hyaluronan.[12,13] The viscosity of synovial fluid is largely the result of the concentration and degree of polymerization of hyaluronan, which serves a vital function in soft tissue lubrication. Type A cells, comprising only 10% to 20% of the lining cells, are predominately phagocytic. However, apparently some overlap in function between the two principal cell types exists.[14,15] Importantly, synoviocytes synthesize a variety of soluble mediators implicated in the pathogenetic events of OA, including cytokines (e.g., interleukin-1 [IL-1]),[16-18] eicosanoids (e.g., prostaglandin E_2),[19,20] and proteinases.[21] That the synovial lining is capable of expressing these substances supports a role for the synovium in the pathogenesis of OA.

Deep to the synovial lining, the subsynovial region possesses a rich blood supply that is essential to generating synovial fluid, facilitates the exchange of nutrients and metabolic wastes of the synovium, and provides the sole source of nutrition to adult articular cartilage. Because of the specialized structure and functions of the synovial lining and subsynovial stroma, synovial blood flow is subject to a complex regulatory system involving extrinsic control and locally produced factors such as angiotensin II, endothelin-1, and nitric oxide.[2]

Periarticular Soft Tissues

The periarticular soft tissues include muscles, tendons, ligaments, and joint capsule. Muscles effect movement and, via complex reflexes, are vital to providing joint stability and protecting the joint from supraphysiological excursion. Muscle mass is more abundant near joints with a wide range of movement, such as the shoulder and the hip, and less so around joints that move in a single plane. Tendons serve as a bridge between muscle and bone, and ligaments provide stability between bones composing a joint. Tendons and ligaments are of similar, although not identical, composition, consisting mainly of water, an organized array of collagen bundles (predominantly type I), and a sparse population of fibroblasts. Ligaments contain more elastin fibers and have greater elasticity than tendons.[22] Importantly, the molecular composition of these tissues responds to physical stimuli, and immobilization elicits catabolic events leading to tissue weakening.[23] The composition of capsular structures parallels that of ligaments. Indeed, some ligaments can be recognized only as hypertrophied portions of the joint capsule. The fundamental role of the capsule is to provide stability; however, its specific nature varies with anatomical location and joint position. For example, the caudal capsule of the human knee is lax in flexion but exerts an important stabilizing force when the joint is in extension.[24]

Subchondral Bone

Although subchondral bone is histologically and biochemically similar to bone in other locations, the organization of the subchondral plate is specific. The plate is thinner than cortical bone found at other locations, and its Haversian systems are oriented parallel to the joint surface rather than parallel to the long axis of the bone.[25] Similarly the organization of subchondral cancellous bone varies between joints, reflecting predominant biomechanical forces and adaptation to exercise.[26,27] The deformability of the subchondral cortical and epiphyseal trabecular bone exceeds that of the diaphyseal cortical shaft by many times and has the important function of force attenuation. As such, possibly the bone stiffening (sclerosis) observed in OA contributes to disease progression.[28,29]

Articular Cartilage

Cartilage is the principal working tissue of the joint and allows simultaneous motion and weight-bearing with negligible friction. Cartilage covers the subchondral plate of bones composing the joint, to which the cartilage is firmly attached. Its thickness varies between joints and at different locations within them. Cartilage is composed of water, collagen, and proteoglycans that are present in respective proportions of 65% to 80%, 10% to 30%, and 5% to 10% of its wet weight. Chondrocytes account for less than 2% of its volume in most species. In adults, cartilage is avascular, alymphatic, and aneural; thus cartilage is nourished mainly via the synovial fluid (see the following discussion). Because articular cartilage is aneural, lesions restricted to cartilage are nonpainful, and the innervation of the underlying bone and adjacent periarticular soft tissues is responsible for providing information on joint position.

Cartilage possesses a number of zones or layers including the following:
- The superficial (tangential or gliding) zone, in which the cells are elongated and oriented parallel to the joint surface
- A middle (transitional) zone, in which the cells are rounded and appear randomly distributed
- A deep (radial) zone, containing cells arranged in columns oriented perpendicular to the surface
- A calcified zone, in which cells are heavily encrusted with hydroxyapatite crystals (Figure 61-1)

The latter two zones are separated by an irregular line, visible on standard histological preparations, called the tidemark, the specific function of which is unclear.[30] The density of chondrocytes in the matrix varies with depth from the articular surface, as does the macromolecular composition of the matrix surrounding the chondrocytes. These regional differences can be identified histologically and have been designated as the pericellular, territorial, and interterritorial regions.

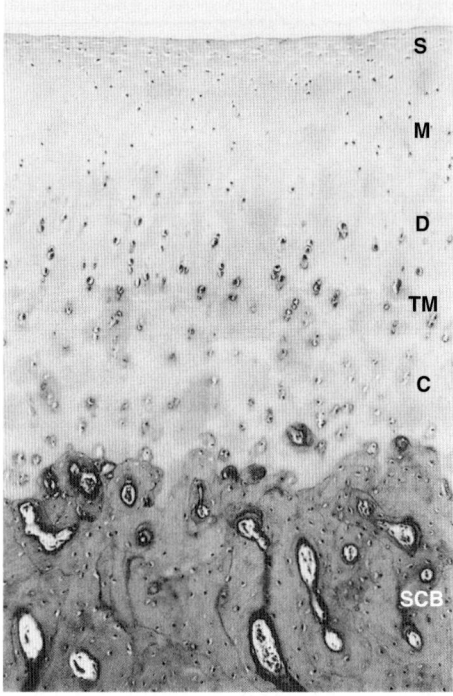

Fig. 61-1 • Photomicrograph illustrating regional organization of mammalian cartilage. The four main zones from the articular surface to the subchondral plate include the superficial (tangential) *(S)*, the middle (transitional) *(M)*, the deep (radial) *(D)*, and the calcified *(C)* zones. The deep and calcified zones are separated by the tidemark *(TM)*. Pericellular matrix regions, distinguishable by their histological and ultrastructural differences and located at progressively greater distances from chondrocyte lacunae, are the pericellular, territorial, and interterritorial regions (×50). *SCB,* Subchondral bone.

The unique functional properties of articular cartilage are reflected in its biochemistry. Articular cartilage is composed of an abundant, specialized extracellular matrix maintained by the aforementioned sparse population of chondrocytes (Figure 61-2). Its water content varies with age but may be as high as 80%.[31] This water is freely exchangeable with that in the synovial fluid and is maintained in the matrix in the form of a gel, with matrix collagens and proteoglycans. Water movement is believed to be pivotal to the capacity of cartilage to absorb and distribute compressive load and for its lubrication.

Collagens

The collagens of articular cartilage differ from those found in most other locations in the body. Several collagens, fibrillar and nonfibrillar, are present in this tissue and are thought to provide cartilage with structural support. These proteins also interact with other matrix components to contribute to cartilage architecture and function.[32-34] Collagen fibrils are oriented parallel to the joint surface in the superficial zone and act as a protective layer, whereas larger, radially oriented fibrils in the deeper layers anchor the cartilage to the underlying articular end plate.

Type II collagen is the most abundant in cartilage, accounting for about 90% of the fibrillar network and half of the dry weight of cartilage.[2,35] Type II collagen consists of three identical amino acid chains arranged in a triple helix, is less soluble, possesses a higher proportion of hydroxylysine residues, and is more richly glycosylated

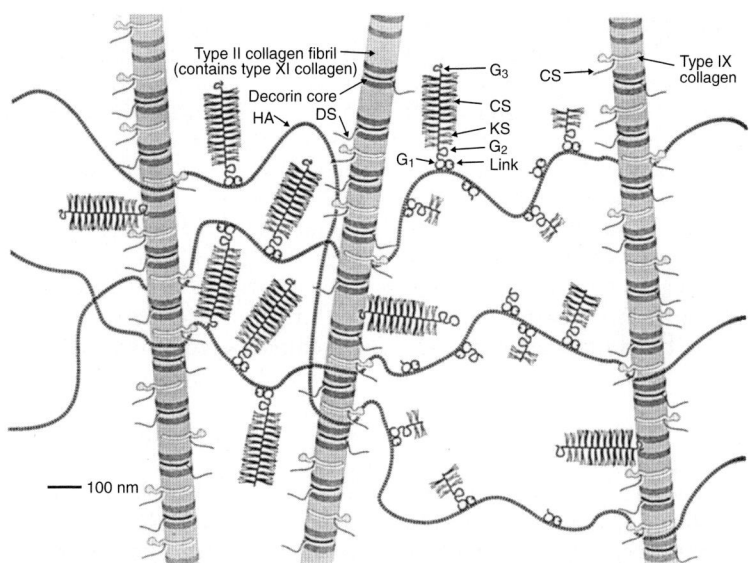

Fig. 61-2 • Organization of the major extracellular matrix components in articular cartilage. The principal collagen of cartilage is type II, and a network of these fibrils provides much of the tensile strength of the tissue. Aggrecan is composed of a linear protein with three globular domains (G_1 to G_3) to which are attached numerous glycosaminoglycan chains of chondroitin sulfate *(CS)* and keratan sulfate *(KS)* (see also Figure 61-4). Supramolecular aggregates are formed by the noncovalent interaction of aggrecan with hyaluronan *(HA)* and stabilized by link protein *(Link)*. The negatively charged glycosaminoglycans (*CS* and *KS*) attract several times their weight in water, and this proteoglycan-water composite is responsible for the compressive stiffness of cartilage. Cartilage also has a number of minor proteoglycans and collagens (e.g., decorin and dermatan sulfate [*DS*], the functions of which are not fully characterized). Fragments of aggrecan, remaining bound to hyaluronan, are depicted to illustrate the effects of proteolytic activity in cartilage. (From Koopman WJ, editor: *Arthritis and allied conditions: a textbook of rheumatology,* ed 13, vol 1, Baltimore, 1997, Williams & Wilkins.)

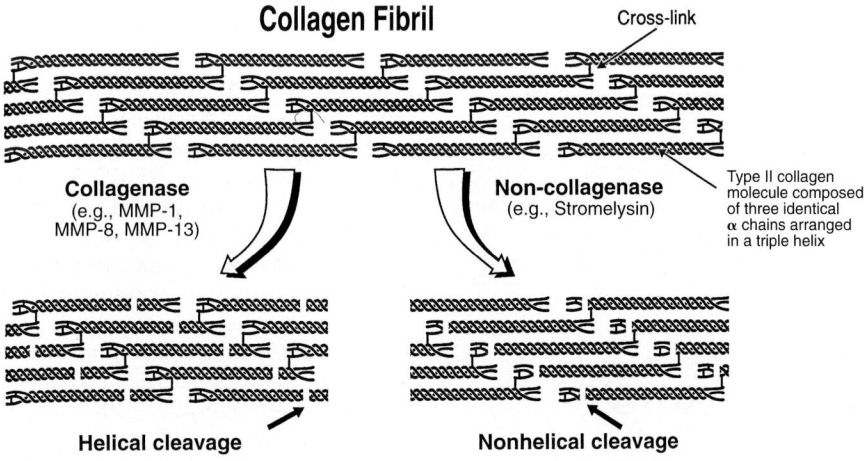

Fig. 61-3 • Schematic representation of collagen fibril organization and its proteolytic degradation in cartilage. Cartilage collagen is arranged in fibrils of cross-linked, triple-helical molecules overlapping at regular intervals. Collagenases cleave intact helical collagen and produce characteristic "$\frac{3}{4}$-$\frac{1}{4}$" fragments. Other proteases (e.g., stromelysin) degrade collagen in nonhelical regions. (From Koopman WJ, editor: *Arthritis and allied conditions: a textbook of rheumatology,* ed 13, vol 1, Baltimore, 1997, Williams & Wilkins.)

than type I collagen.[36,37] Unlike type I, which typically forms fibers, type II collagen is organized in the form of fibrils that are composed of molecules aligned with a 25% overlap or quarter stagger (Figure 61-3). This structure is stabilized by chemical bonds between specific amino acids in each chain, called hydroxypyridinium cross-links.[38] Fibrils are not uniform in size throughout the matrix; they tend to be larger in the middle and deep zones of the matrix, which reflects regional biomechanical demands.[39]

This protein is arranged in arcades, which form the three-dimensional network or skeleton of the cartilage matrix. Type II collagen is produced by the chondrocytes, and whereas significant degradation and resynthesis of fibrils occur during growth and development, limited turnover occurs in adults.[40,41]

Minor collagens are present in modest amounts in cartilage, and the specific roles of these collagens in its structure and function have yet to be defined fully. Type XI is a fibrillar collagen that is found within type II fibrils. Its function is unclear, but likely it plays a role in type II collagen fibril assembly and organization because a mutation in the type XI gene in mice leads to a disorganized matrix, with abnormally thick collagen fibrils.[42] Type VI is a microfibrillar collagen that may act as a bridge between fibrillar collagen and other matrix components.[43,44] So-called fibril-associated small collagens include collagens IX, XI, and XIV. Type IX collagen molecules bound covalently to the surface of type II fibrils may serve to stabilize the latter.[45] Types XII and XIV collagen also are associated with fibrillar collagen, but the specific functions have yet to be identified.

Proteoglycans

By definition, proteoglycans are composite molecules consisting of protein and glycosaminoglycan (polysaccharide) components. This definition is broad because some of the aforementioned minor collagens (e.g., type IX) have a single glycosaminoglycan side chain and thus can be designated as proteoglycans. A number of proteoglycans are found in articular cartilage. Aggrecan, the largest and most abundant, has a well-defined function in the extracellular matrix; however, the specific roles of the smaller proteoglycans remain to be characterized fully.

Aggrecan is the primary proteoglycan of articular cartilage that interacts with hyaluronan to form aggregates (see Figures 61-2 and 61-3; Figure 61-4). The individual or monomeric form of this molecule consists of a linear core protein interrupted by three globular domains. The first of these globular domains is designated G_1, exists at the amino-terminal portion of the molecule, and is the site at which the proteoglycan attaches to hyaluronan. As many as 100 aggrecan monomers may be attached to the same hyaluronan chain to form supramolecular aggregates of

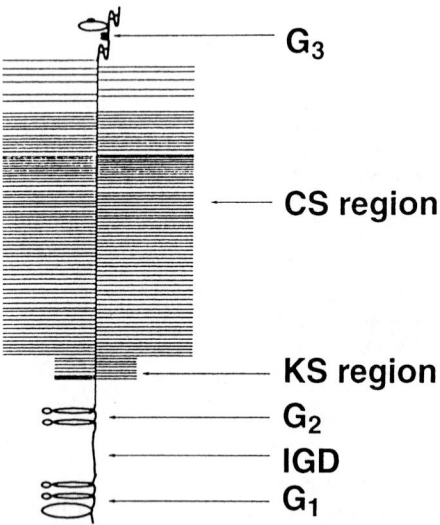

Fig. 61-4 • Schematic representation of an aggrecan monomer. Proteolytic cleavage of the molecule in vivo usually first occurs in the G_1 to G_2 interglobular domain *(IGD)*. The specific sites involved vary among the enzymes implicated in the process. Keratan sulfate *(KS)* and chondroitin sulfate *(CS)* regions are positioned on the periphery of the molecule. (From Koopman WJ, editor: *Arthritis and allied conditions: a textbook of rheumatology,* ed 13, vol 1, Baltimore, 1997, Williams & Wilkins.)

micrometer dimensions (see Figure 61-2).[46] The interaction of aggrecan with hyaluronan is noncovalent but is stabilized by a link protein that binds to the G_1 domain and hyaluronan with equal affinity.[47] Equine link protein was characterized and is similar to that found in human cartilage.[48] The specific functions of the G_2 and G_3 domains are unclear; however, because the G_3 domain is present in only about one third of the aggrecan monomers in adult cartilage, it is unlikely that it plays a pivotal role in the extracellular matrix.[49]

In the region between the second and third globular domains, glycosaminoglycan chains of variable length and composition are attached radially to the protein core (see Figure 61-4). Immediately adjacent to the G_2 domain is a region rich in keratan sulfate, and this portion of the proteoglycan, detectable by monoclonal antibodies, has served as a tissue marker of matrix turnover.[50] Farther peripherally on the core protein is the chondroitin sulfate–rich region, where up to 100 chondroitin sulfate chains may be found attached radially to the core protein. These chondroitin sulfate chains vary in length, which is the main reason for heterogeneity in the size of aggrecan. Importantly, these glycosaminoglycan chains contain numerous carboxyl and sulfate groups, so that aggrecan is highly negatively charged and can bind up to 50 times its weight in water.[46,51,52] This highly hydrated matrix gives cartilage its compressive stiffness and ability to dissipate load.

Matrix Proteins

Cartilage, like other connective tissues, contains a number of noncollagenous proteins, many of which are proteoglycans. Among the best characterized of the small proteoglycans are decorin, biglycan, lumican, and fibromodulin, all of which are similar in molecular organization. These proteins have been shown to interact with a number of matrix constituents, including cartilage collagens, and in many cases these interactions involve a number of different collagens and appear to regulate a variety of metabolic processes.[46,52] For example, decorin and fibromodulin inhibit fibrillogenesis of type II collagen, a process that may regulate the size of collagen fibrils in the matrix.[53] Some of these small matrix proteins also may contribute to the antiadhesive properties of articular cartilage.[54,55]

Cartilage also contains a number of small proteins that are neither collagens nor proteoglycans,[56,57] and most are involved in interactions with a variety of matrix molecules and chondrocytes. For example, anchorin is found on the surface of chondrocytes and within the cell membrane and has a high affinity for type II collagen fibrils. These properties suggest that anchorin may act as a mechano-receptor, providing chondrocytes with information on changes in stresses experienced by the matrix. Fibronectin is a minor component of cartilage that is thought to contribute to matrix assembly, via interactions with chondrocytes and elements of the extracellular matrix. Fibronectin fragments are present in elevated quantities in OA and may contribute to catabolic events in affected cartilage.[58,59] Cartilage oligomeric matrix protein (COMP), also known as thrombospondin-5, is abundant in articular cartilage and is formed by the association of five identical subunits. COMP is most abundant in the proliferative cell layer of growth cartilage, where it is thought to regulate cell growth.

Chondrocytes

Studies of cartilage metabolism contradict the seemingly inert histological appearance of this relatively acellular tissue. Despite the fact that chondrocytes represent a small percentage of the volume of cartilage, they are responsible for extracellular matrix synthesis, including all the collagens and proteoglycans. They are also capable of elaborating a variety of proteolytic enzymes effecting degradation of matrix macromolecules. The rate of turnover of the various matrix components is not uniform. At least a portion of the proteoglycan pool is renewed at a relatively rapid rate, whereas the rate of collagen turnover is minimal.[60-62] Chondrocyte metabolism is influenced by intrinsic and extrinsic mechanical influences. For example, cyclic loading and alterations in matrix pressure, as a result of changes in solute content, materially influence proteoglycan synthetic rates.[63,64] Thus the maintenance of the cartilage matrix involves the chondrocyte-mediated processes of synthesis and degradation, and the cartilage loss in OA appears to be attributable to a disequilibrium in favor of matrix degradation.

Nutrition

Unlike the cartilage of growing animals, in which articular cartilage receives some blood supply from subchondral vasculature, adult articular cartilage contains no blood vessels. As a result, the chondrocyte exists under relatively hypoxic and acidic conditions, with an extracellular pH typically 7.1 to 7.2.[65] Nutrients migrate from subsynovial vessels to the synovial fluid and subsequently penetrate the dense connective tissue matrix of the cartilage, while metabolic wastes are simultaneously cleared in the opposite direction. The density of the matrix appears not to hamper diffusion because molecules as large as hemoglobin (65 kDa) can penetrate normal articular cartilage.[66] The highly charged proteoglycans contained in the matrix do not inhibit the diffusion of small, uncharged molecules.[67] Entry of solutes into the matrix occurs by simple diffusion or may be facilitated by compression-relaxation cycles. Intermittent loading of cartilage is vital to its health, as is evidenced by the deleterious effects of immobilization.[68]

Joint Lubrication

Although several mechanisms for cartilage-on-cartilage lubrication have been hypothesized, two main systems are accepted: a hydrostatic or weeping system that functions at high loads, and a boundary system that functions at low loads.[69] Hydrostatic lubrication of opposing cartilaginous surfaces is effected by a thin film of water liberated from the matrix during cartilage compression. Because little movement of water can occur from cartilage to the subchondral bone, most is squeezed from the opposing cartilages onto the surface, immediately peripheral to the zone of impending contact.[70] With the release of compressive force, the cartilage expands, and water is drawn back into the matrix.

Whereas hydrostatic mechanisms function well under relatively heavy loads, boundary lubrication occurs under low-load conditions. Boundary lubrication is accomplished by specialized materials including lubricin[71] (a glycoprotein of synovial origin) and hyaluronan. These molecules bind to opposing articular cartilage surfaces and prevent the direct contact of these surfaces under low loads.

Coefficients of friction were unchanged after hyaluronidase treatment of synovial fluid, suggesting that hyaluronan has no place in cartilage-on-cartilage lubrication.[72,73] However, others have found that hyaluronan actually does function as a boundary lubricant.[74,75]

Articular soft tissues require lubrication because they contribute most of the frictional resistance to joint movement. Indeed, the energy requirement for the stretching of articular soft tissues is 100 times that of the frictional resistance of opposing cartilage surfaces.[76] The synovium is lubricated by a thin film of synovial fluid, rich in hyaluronan, its principal boundary lubricant.[77]

Intraarticular Volume and Pressure

Intraarticular volume varies and is influenced by joint position (see Chapter 66). Specifically, volume and pressure are respectively minimal and maximal near the extremes of flexion and extension.[78-81] This effect is exacerbated in horses with synovial effusion, providing a physiological rationale for diagnostic flexion tests in equine lameness examinations. Moreover, the pointing of an equine limb in which there is joint effusion likely parallels the observation that in the human knee there is a maximum of intraarticular volume (and minimum of intraarticular pressure and pain) at 30 degrees of flexion.[82,83]

Whereas intraarticular pressure varies during movement, pressure within a normal joint is subatmospheric at rest.[84,85] As a result, the normal synovial cavity is merely a potential space, the surfaces of which are coated with a thin film of synovial fluid to reduce friction during movement. Although the mechanisms by which this negative pressure occurs remain unclear, the phenomenon contributes measurably to joint stability.[86] Lack of familiarity with the physiological concept of negative intraarticular pressure in normal joints results in the common misconception that the sound of air being aspirated into a joint during arthrocentesis heralds a dry or diseased joint.

Biomechanical Considerations

Articular cartilage remains healthy despite being regularly subjected to considerable normal and shear forces during normal activities. A number of mechanisms exist to facilitate this phenomenon, including the transmission of forces to surrounding tissues by periarticular soft tissues, the incongruity of cartilage surfaces, and the inherent compliance of cartilage and subchondral bone. Indeed, the capacity for considerable elastic deformation permits normal cartilage to withstand compressive stresses considerably greater than those of body weight alone.[87,88] Nonetheless, cartilage is subject to mechanical breakdown after supraphysiological stresses, and loads exceeding 25 kg/cm^2 are reported to result in matrix damage.[89] Apparently these loads occur in specific areas of cartilage under a variety of clinical circumstances, such as the cartilage degeneration that accompanies the incongruent articular surfaces of a poorly reduced or unstable intraarticular fracture.

At the tissue level, the ability of cartilage matrix to resist compression and shear is a function of the interaction of collagen, aggrecan, and tissue fluid. Aggrecan can absorb many times its weight in water, but its complete hydration is restricted by the collagen network. Thus a balance exists between the internal swelling pressure exerted by the association of water with aggrecan (Gibbs-Donnan ionic equilibrium) and the tensile forces of the collagen fibrils. Cartilage under load undergoes a two-phase (viscoelastic) deformation.[90,91] Initially rapid bulk movement of water from the matrix and compression of collagen occur. Subsequently, a time-dependent compression occurs, known as the creep phase, in which water flows through the matrix at a slower rate.

These mechanical phenomena were studied in experiments evaluating the mechanical properties of cartilage after the selective depletion of specific matrix components. The tensile strength of cartilage is a function of its type II collagen content because strength is reduced in collagen-depleted tissues but is unaffected by proteoglycan removal.[92,93] Proteoglycans (mainly aggrecan) provide the matrix with its compressive stiffness and protect the collagen network from mechanical damage. Trypsin-treated (proteoglycan-depleted) specimens lose the ability to rebound from compressive load and have reduced stiffness.[94]

At rest, opposing articular surfaces are not completely congruent, but when loaded, articular cartilage contact increases, which serves to distribute stress and increase joint stability. This may be a physiological reason why cartilage tends to be somewhat thicker in less congruous joints, such as the hip and stifle.[95] Although cartilage is designed to withstand compressive stress, its ability to act as a shock absorber is finite, largely because it receives its nutrition by diffusion and as a result is of limited thickness. Because its ability to absorb load is limited, cartilage must transmit load to the underlying subchondral bone. As such the articular ends of most bones are flared (less force per unit area) and deform under physiological load to absorb stress.[96] Noteworthy is that the stiffness of the subchondral bone is attributable not only to the cancellous trabeculae but also to the extracellular fluid content. This was demonstrated in an experiment where subchondral stiffness of canine femoral heads was reduced by 30% after fluid decompression by drilling.[97] When the subchondral bone is unable to accommodate loading, so-called adaptive remodeling failure occurs, in which repetitive subchondral deformation causes trabecular microfractures, which may or may not be accompanied by changes in articular cartilage. Fortunately, when occurring at an acceptable rate, trabecular microfractures undergo a reparative response leading to an orientation of subchondral bone that provides improved strength and shock absorption capacity.[98] Articular surfaces are protected by stress distribution mechanisms beyond those of cartilage and bone. For example, muscles absorb a large proportion of the force experienced during impact loading, leaving the remainder to be cushioned by cartilage and bone. Fine-tuned neuromuscular reflexes are required for this system to work effectively, and small failures in these reflex arcs lead to insufficient attenuation of impact loading, which may lead to degenerative changes in cartilage and subchondral bone.[99]

OSTEOARTHRITIS

Etiopathogenesis

OA has been defined as an essentially noninflammatory disorder of movable joints, characterized by degeneration and loss of articular cartilage and the development of new bone on joint surfaces and margins.[36,100] As in people,

equine OA is probably not a single disease but reflects a common response of joint tissues to a number of potential causes. Unfortunately the specific contributions and interactions of various mechanical and biological factors contributing to development of OA lesions remain unclear.

Three pathogenetic mechanisms are hypothesized for OA.[100] The first involves a fundamentally defective cartilage, with abnormal biomechanical properties. In this pathway a biomechanically flawed matrix fails under normal loading. In people a type II collagen defect exemplifies this primary form of OA.[101,102] OA attributed to inherently defective cartilage matrix components has not yet been identified in the horse.

A second proposed pathogenetic pathway of OA involves physical changes in the subchondral bone.[28,29] Because articular cartilage is too thin to be an effective shock absorber, impact loading must be attenuated by periarticular soft tissues, muscles, and subchondral bone. Although substantially stiffer than cartilage or joint capsule, cancellous subchondral bone is considered an important shock attenuator. Thus in this hypothesis of OA pathogenesis, normal mechanical stresses result in microfractures of the subchondral and epiphyseal trabecular bone. However, when occurring at an excessive frequency, these fractures exceed the rate at which optimal healing and remodeling of the subchondral trabeculae can occur. Bone accretion with healing of these microfractures increases the density of the subchondral plate and adjacent trabeculae, with a concomitant reduction in the ability to absorb repetitive physiological loads. The resulting increase in bone stiffness leads to a state in which the bone-cartilage unit fails to deform normally under load, and the cartilage experiences supraphysiological stresses, resulting in mechanical damage. Subsequent events are those outlined in the following discussion of the third pathogenetic mechanism of OA.

To date, a cause-and-effect relationship between subchondral bone plate thickening and cartilage degeneration remains to be established. The hypothesis that subchondral bone and cartilage degeneration are related is supported by the demonstration of microfractures of the subchondral plate and more distant trabeculae in arthritic specimens.[103] Moreover, in mice with OA, cartilage degenerates over areas of sclerotic bone but remains intact over areas of normal bone density.[104] However, mathematical models predict that even with considerable increases in subchondral bone stiffness, cartilage stresses are only modestly increased.[105] Collectively these data indicate that subchondral sclerosis contributes to the osteoarthritic process but is probably not a prerequisite to initiate articular cartilage destruction.[106]

The third and most popular hypothesis of the pathogenesis of OA is based on the concept of mechanical forces causing damage to healthy cartilage.[36,52,100,107] Matricial or cellular injury by these forces results in metabolic alterations of chondrocytes, leading to the release of proteolytic enzymes that cause cartilage fibrillation and breakdown of the proteoglycan network. Cartilage is remarkably resistant to shear forces but is relatively susceptible to repetitive impact trauma. In people, repetitive trauma is an acknowledged predisposing factor to OA in athletes (e.g., metacarpophalangeal joints of boxers) and certain occupations (e.g., shoulder joints of jack-hammer operators). Of many potential causes, repeated microtrauma (use trauma) is probably the most common pathogenetic factor in equine OA, and the correlation of lesions at defined sites in horses participating in specific sports supports this hypothesis.

Role of the Synovium

Although conventional concepts of OA emphasize the direct and predominant involvement of cartilage and bone in OA development, it is increasingly recognized that the synovium contributes to the central pathophysiological event of cartilage matrix depletion. Recent investigations in several species have shown that synoviocytes are a rich source of a variety of inflammatory mediators and degradative enzymes implicated in cartilaginous degeneration, including prostaglandins,[19,20,108-111] cytokines,[112-114] and matrix metalloproteinases (MMPs).[113-116] These laboratory data are supplemented by the identification of increased levels of these and other inflammatory mediators in the synovial fluid of horses with naturally occurring or experimentally induced synovitis.[117-124] Experiments using synovially conditioned culture media, or coincubation of synovial tissues with cartilage, support a role of the synovial membrane in cartilage degradation.[125,126] Recent experiments indicate that synovial macrophages are important contributors to the inflammatory and degradative responses in affected joints, effects mediated by a combination of IL-1 and tumor necrosis factor–α (TNF-α) (see Cytokines discussion).[127] Nonetheless, determining the specific role of the synovium in OA is hampered by the fact that both chondrocytes and synoviocytes are a rich source of the pertinent mediators and enzymes. Thus precise characterization of the relative quantitative and temporal contributions of cartilage and synovium to lesion development has not yet been accomplished.

Role of the Chondrocyte

Of all joint tissues, articular cartilage shows the greatest aberration from normal during disease development, and it is generally considered that metabolic changes in chondrocytes play a primary role in the pathophysiological events of cartilage loss. In normal joints, chondrocytes are responsible for maintaining a balance between matrix degradation and repair, and this equilibrium is maintained by a complex interaction between chondrocytes, cytokines, and mechanical stimuli.[128] In OA, a disruption of this homeostatic state develops, in which catabolic processes predominate. Although proteoglycan synthesis is greater than normal early in the disease, the rate of matrix digestion is sufficient that the result is a net loss of matrix. With this imbalance toward matrix depletion, cartilage mass is progressively lost, and the viscoelastic properties of the remaining tissue become insufficient to withstand normal loads. Subsequently, cartilage fissuring and separation occur (Figure 61-5). The ultimate result is generalized cartilage loss and secondary remodeling of bone and articular soft tissues (Figure 61-6).

A number of studies indicate that an important initial biochemical change in OA is the loss of aggregating proteoglycans. Up-regulation of chondrocyte proteoglycan synthesis is insufficient to offset enhanced degradation, so that the concentration in the matrix progressively decreases. In addition to a reduced quantity of proteoglycan, the quality of molecules remaining in the matrix, and newly

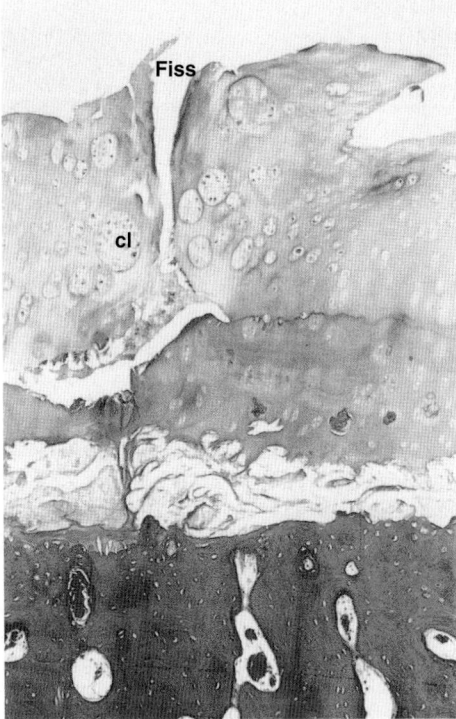

Fig. 61-5 • Photomicrograph illustrating the pathological changes associated with cartilage matrix degeneration. Loss of matrix proteoglycans alters the biomechanical properties and ultimately leads to fissures *(Fiss)* in the cartilage, in this case a full-thickness fissure. Chondrocyte clones *(cl)* represent the abortive healing attempts of chondrocytes (×50).

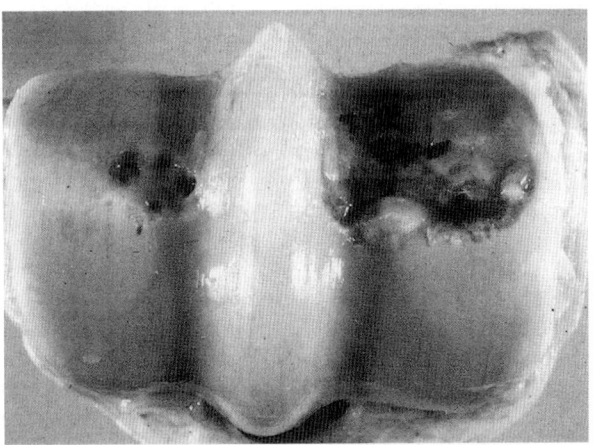

Fig. 61-6 • Post mortem specimen of the distal aspect of an equine third metacarpal bone illustrating partial and full-thickness cartilage loss. Although osteoarthritis affects all articular tissues, degeneration of extracellular matrix of cartilage and its subsequent loss are considered the central events in the disease. Note also the wear lines on the articular cartilage.

synthesized replacements, appears to be altered.[129,130] Collagen degradation accompanies proteoglycan loss and is manifested by surface fibrillation (Figure 61-7). The loss of collagen and changes in collagen fibril size contribute to weakening of the matrix and may account for the increased water content in early cartilage lesions.[131-133]

Whereas degradation of articular cartilage may occur by the action of a number of mediators, including oxygen-derived free radicals,[134-137] proteolytic enzymes synthesized

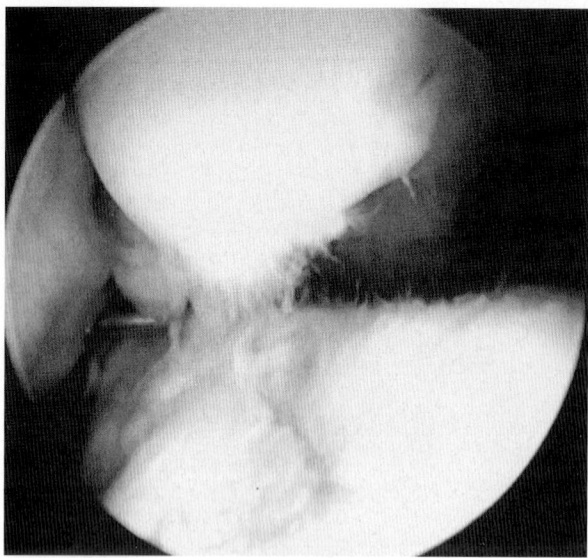

Fig. 61-7 • Arthroscopic endophotograph of the middle carpal joint of a Standardbred racehorse with a large osteochondral fragment of the third carpal bone (top) and concomitant lesions of the intermediate carpal bone (bottom). Cartilage fibrillation is substantial, and its evaluation is greatly facilitated by fluid distention of the joint. Fibrillation indicates damage to the collagenous network of the extracellular matrix.

by chondrocytes are thought to be the major mediators of matrix depletion. Proteinases are classified according to the catalytic mechanism into four main groups, including aspartic proteinases, cysteine proteinases, serine proteinases, and metalloproteinases. Members of each class are synthesized by chondrocytes or synoviocytes and may contribute to cartilage degradation. However, the MMPs and related enzymes apparently are the most active in OA.[36,52,138-140] Chondrocytes have surface receptors that respond to mechanical stress, and physical disruptions of cell-matrix associations can negatively influence chondrocyte synthetic activites.[141]

Matrix-Degrading Enzymes

MMPs are considered to play a major role in cartilage matrix degradation in OA because this group of proteinases is capable of digesting all major components of the extracellular matrix. The relative contributions of these proteolytic enzymes to the overall process remain to be firmly established; however, a wealth of evidence implicates them in cartilage loss. Specifically, MMPs are synthesized by synoviocytes and chondrocytes[21,52,142-144] and are present in increased concentrations in diseased cartilage,[145,146] and the topographical distribution and concentration of MMPs in cartilage are correlated with the histological severity of lesions.[146-148] Several types of MMPs are expressed by articular tissues, and these are classified as collagenases, stromelysins, gelatinases, membrane-type metalloproteinases, and other MMPs.[144] In addition to other substrates, collagenases degrade intact, helical type II collagen. Stromelysins cleave partially degraded collagen, proteoglycans, and other minor proteins in cartilage. The gelatinases have a diverse range of substrates, including partially degraded type II collagen and types X and XI collagen and elastin. Like collagenases, membrane-type 1 MMP is also capable of digesting fibrillar collagen and a number of other matrix components. MMPs

are secreted in an inactive or latent form and require activation through proteolytic cleavage. A variety of enzymes including trypsin, chymotrypsin, plasmin, kallikrein, cathepsin B, and certain MMPs themselves are capable of such cleavage.[52,138,148] The classification and general properties of MMPs are summarized in Table 61-1.

Several members of the ADAM (a disintegrin and metalloproteinase) family of enzymes were shown to be expressed by chondrocytes.[149,150] Many of the ADAM enzymes are proteinases and are structurally and functionally related to MMPs. Importantly, certain members of this group cleave aggrecan at a specific site in the interglobular (G_1 to G_2) domain, resulting in aggrecan fragments identical to those found in the tissues and synovial fluids of osteoarthritic animals. These proteinases have been termed *aggrecanase* and share many similarities to typical MMPs, including the inactivation with conventional MMP inhibitors and being inhibited by tissue inhibitor of matrix metalloproteinase–1 (TIMP-1).[151] Two forms of aggrecanase have been implicated in OA, and both are ADAMTS enzymes (ADAM with thrombospondin type 1 motifs).[152,153] (The thrombospondin subunits of the protein appear to be critical for the binding and digestion of aggrecan.[154]) ADAMTS4 and ADAMTS5 (aggrecanases 1 and 2, respectively) are related enzymes but demonstrate important differences in their regulation by cytokines. For example, although ADAMTS4 is induced by cytokines and ADAMTS5 appears to be constitutively expressed, both are implicated in aggrecan degradation in OA.[155] Aggrecanase is considered pivotal in proteoglycan degradation. Indeed, some contend that aggrecanase is the principal mediator of proteoglycan depletion in OA.[140]

In healthy cartilage, the activity of proteolytic enzymes is controlled by a number of mechanisms, one of which is naturally occurring inhibitory proteins. The most important of these inhibitors are the TIMPs.[52,137,144,156] Synthesized by synoviocytes, chondrocytes, and endothelial cells, TIMPs inactivate MMPs by binding to them in a 1:1 noncovalent complex,[157] and these inhibitors are hypothesized to be critical to the longevity of the extracellular matrix of cartilage.[148,158] TIMP exists in at least four forms, the first three of which (TIMP-1, TIMP-2, TIMP-3) are expressed by chondrocytes. Interestingly, each is subject to somewhat different regulatory mechanisms.[159,160] The important role of TIMPs in cartilage matrix health is supported by the observation that imbalances in the ratio of MMP to TIMP synthesis in cartilage are important determinants of the rate of matrix degradation.[148,161]

Cytokines

Cytokine is a general term to describe a broad array of small regulatory proteins produced by a variety of cells in the body. In joints, these mediators exist in a complex balance of activities that regulate the metabolism of the synovial membrane, bone, and articular cartilage in health and disease (Table 61-2).[162,163] Numerous cytokines are involved in articular metabolism, and they possess one or more proinflammatory (catabolic), antiinflammatory (regulatory), or anabolic functions. Important in OA are the proinflammatory cytokines, such as IL-1 and TNF-α. Chondrocyte receptors for IL-1 and TNF-α are up-regulated in osteoarthritic cartilage, and the activation of these receptors has several deleterious effects on chondrocyte metabolism.[164,165]

TABLE 61-1

Matrix Metalloproteinases Implicated in Cartilage Matrix Degradation		
PROTEINASE*	MMP	CARTILAGE SUBSTRATES
Collagenases		
Interstitial collagenase (collagenase)[†]	MMP-1[‡]	Collagens II and X (not IX and XI), denatured type II, aggrecan, link protein
Neutrophil collagenase[†]	MMP-8	Collagen II, aggrecan, link protein
Collagenase 3[†§]	MMP-13[‡]	Collagens II, IV, IX, X; aggrecan; fibronectin
Stromelysins		
Stromelysin 1[†]	MMP-3[‡]	Aggrecan, fibronectin; denatured collagen II; collagens IV, IX, X, XI; procollagens; link protein; decorin; elastin; laminin
Stromelysin 2[†]	MMP-10	Same as for stromelysin 1
Gelatinases		
Gelatinase A (72 kD)[†]	MMP-2[‡]	Denatured collagen II, collagens X and XI, elastin
Gelatinase B (92 kD)[†]	MMP-9[‡]	Aggrecan, fibronectin, collagens IX and XI, procollagens, link protein, decorin, elastin
MT-MMPs		
MT1-MMP[†]	MMP-14	Aggrecan, collagen II, denatured collagen II, fibronectin, laminin
Others		
Matrilysin (PUMP)[†]	MMP-7	Aggrecan
Stromelysin-3	MMP-11	Proteoglycan, denatured collagen II, fibronectin, laminin
Macrophage metalloelastase	MMP-12	Elastin
Novel MMP	MMP-19	Denatured collagen II, collagen IV, aggrecan, fibronectin, laminin

MMP, Matrix metalloproteinase, *MT(1)-MMP*, membrane-type (1) matrix metalloproteinase; *PUMP*, putative metalloproteinase.

*All except membrane-type 1 MMP are inhibited by some or all of the tissue inhibitors of metalloproteinases 1 to 3.

[†]Expressed by chondrocytes. All are expressed in synovium.

[‡]MMPs characterized in the horse.

[§]MMP-13 expression is relatively weak in equine synovium.

TABLE 61-2

General Classification of Cytokines and Their Actions on Cartilage Metabolism		
CATEGORY OF CYTOKINE	EXAMPLES	ACTIONS
Catabolic (pro-inflammatory) cytokines	IL-1, TNFα	Promote MMP synthesis Promote nitric oxide and PGE$_2$ production Inhibit collagen II and aggrecan synthesis
Modulatory (regulatory) cytokines*	IL-4, IL-6, IL-10, IL-13	Stimulate TIMP synthesis Promote IRAP synthesis Inhibit IL-1 synthesis
Anabolic cytokines (growth factors)	IGF-1, TGF-β, bFGF	Promote collagen II synthesis Promote proteoglycan synthesis

IL, Interleukin; *TNF*, tumor necrosis factor; *MMP*, matrix metalloproteinase; *PGE$_2$*, prostaglandin E$_2$; *TIMP*, tissue inhibitor of matrix metalloproteinase; *IRAP*, interleukin-1 receptor antagonist protein; *IGF*, insulin-like growth factor; *bFGF*, basic fibroblast growth factor.

*Regulatory cytokines can have mixed actions (e.g., IL-6 amplifies IL-1 effects on MMP synthesis but induces TIMP synthesis).

A wealth of recent research suggests that IL-1 is the most important of the proinflammatory cytokines in OA. Early studies using cartilage organ culture provided data supporting a role for IL-1 in cartilage matrix degradation,[166] which were supplemented by the identification of elevated levels of this cytokine in synovial fluids of affected patients, including horses.[119,120] IL-1 is involved in the destruction of the extracellular matrix and formation of the functionally inadequate repair tissue in arthritic cartilage. IL-1 decreases the synthesis of proteoglycans and type II collagen and induces the synthesis and secretion of proteolytic enzymes that degrade these matrix macromolecules.[167-177]

Decreased synthesis of matrix macromolecules occurs in cartilage exposed to IL-1 concentrations substantially less than those required to stimulate matrix degradation.[169] Catabolism is further promoted by inhibition of the synthesis of MMP inhibitors such as TIMP.[178] In addition, IL-1 stimulates the synthesis of prostaglandin E$_2$ and nitric oxide, the effects of which are outlined in the following discussion.[179-183] IL-1 may also contribute to the proliferative events in OA. Osteophytosis may be caused, at least in part, by the stimulation of osteoblast-like cells by IL-1.[184] Perhaps the most compelling evidence supporting the involvement of IL-1 in OA is the protective effect of IL-1 receptor antagonist protein, which blocks many of the catabolic events typical of IL-1 in vitro. This naturally occurring competitive antagonist of IL-1 was shown to be protective for OA-like lesions in arthritis models.[185-187]

TNF-α is another proinflammatory cytokine that was implicated in the development of osteoarthritic lesions and was found in elevated concentrations in inflamed and arthritic joints.[188-191] Like IL-1, this cytokine stimulates the synthesis of matrix-degrading enzymes[175] and inhibits chondrocyte synthesis of proteoglycan and collagen.[176] TNF-α appears to be less potent than IL-1[192]; however, the effects of IL-1 and TNF-α are potentiated when combined.[193] TNF-α appears to stimulate the synthesis of IL-1.[194] Experiments with adenoviral transfers of the gene expressing an endogenous inhibitor of nuclear factor κB (IκBα) indicate that a substantial proportion of synovially derived inflammatory mediators and degradative enzymes are regulated by the nuclear factor κB (NFκB) pathway.[195]

The degradative effects of certain cytokines, including IL-1 and TNF-α, are balanced by inhibitory cytokines (e.g., IL-4, IL-10, and IL-13). Moreover, opposing effects on matrix synthesis are induced by other cytokines, also known as growth factors (e.g., insulin-like growth factor and basic fibroblast growth factor) (see Table 61-2). Using these antiinflammatory and inhibitory cytokines to control the osteoarthritic process is an active area of research.

Nitric Oxide

Nitric oxide is another mediator of the pathophysiological events in OA. This highly reactive, cytotoxic free radical is a byproduct of the oxidation of L-arginine to citrulline, catalyzed by a group of enzymes called nitric oxide synthases (NOSs), which produce large amounts of the mediator when cells expressing this enzyme are activated by mediators such as endotoxins and cytokines.[182,183,196] Early evidence for the involvement of nitric oxide in rheumatic diseases was the observation that nitrite, a stable end product of nitric oxide, was found in elevated concentrations in the synovial fluid and serum of people with rheumatoid arthritis.[197] Subsequently, it has been shown that osteoarthritic cartilage spontaneously produces nitric oxide.[198-200] Nitric oxide may mediate the inhibition of chondrocyte synthetic activities that occur in OA. Proteoglycan and type 2 collagen synthesis are inhibited under conditions conducive to nitric oxide formation.[201-203] Thus, like other inflammatory mediators, inducible NOS is stimulated by IL-1 and TNF-α and requires NFκB for its expression.[204]

Nitric oxide also is hypothesized to mediate, in part, the augmented expression and activation of MMPs,[205,206] as well as the reduced synthesis of the natural IL-1 receptor antagonist protein,[199] and is reported to be an important inducer of chondrocyte apoptosis.[207] However, the specific role of nitric oxide in IL-1–induced cartilage matrix depletion is controversial. Early laboratory studies revealed that the MMP activity in IL-1– and TNF-α–stimulated cartilage cultures was enhanced by adding substrates favoring nitric oxide formation (nitric oxide donors), and this effect was blocked by NOS inhibitors.[205,206] Conversely, cytokine-mediated induction of MMP expression can occur independently of stimulation by nitric oxide,[208] and cytokine-stimulated cartilage explants cultured in the presence of nitric oxide inhibitors had rates of proteoglycan depletion comparable with controls.[209] Nonetheless, nitric

oxide remains an important area of study, because in animal models of inflammatory arthritis and OA, using compounds that directly or indirectly inhibit NOS activity reduces the severity of lesions.[210-213]

Prostaglandins

Prostaglandins are found in elevated concentrations in inflamed joints,[188,214] and although the specific effects of prostaglandins on joint metabolism are unclear, it is widely held that prostaglandin E$_2$ contributes to the lesions of OA. Prostaglandin E$_2$ causes synovial inflammation and may contribute to cartilage matrix depletion[215,216] and the erosion of cartilage and bone.[217] Certain data indicate that prostaglandins may actually modulate the release of metalloproteinases, such as collagenases and stromelysins.[218,219] Conversely, increasing evidence suggests that cytokine and MMP expression in articular cells is regulated by E-series prostaglandins.[20,220] The net effect of this regulation is unclear because, like corticosteroids, prostaglandin E$_2$ appears to inhibit TIMP synthesis and MMP synthesis.[221] Moreover, some of the effects of prostanoids may be indirect, acting by promoting the synthesis of other proteins that have unique influences on cartilage metabolism.[222] Thus although prostanoids are a factor in the signs and certain of the pathophysiological processes of OA, the specific role in regulating cartilage depletion and the interactions with other mediators of cartilage lesion development requires elucidation.

Clinical Evaluation of Joint Disease

Joint Pain

Traumatic arthritis and OA may be the most common cause of lameness in equine athletes of all types. Unfortunately, there is a weak correlation between the magnitude of pain and the severity of articular damage observed.[223-225] The hallmark of OA is articular cartilage degeneration, a process occurring in a tissue devoid of sensory innervation. As a result, lameness is typically attributed to involvement of periarticular soft tissues and bone, the former being relatively richly innervated. In capsular and ligamentous tissues, unmyelinated sensory nerve fibers conduct painful sensations from widely distributed free nerve endings.[226,227] With joint inflammation, these receptors exhibit increased sensitivity. Specifically the threshold for these receptors is reduced by inflammatory mediators such as prostaglandins, and increased receptor activity accompanies physiological joint excursions.[228] Although the severity of soft tissue changes and lameness are related,[229,230] horses with substantial periarticular fibrosis occasionally demonstrate less than the expected degree of lameness. Studies of joint capsule innervation in arthritic specimens revealed that with time degeneration of neurons is common, which provides a potential reason for the less than expected magnitude of pain in some horses having clearly demonstrable changes in periarticular soft tissues.

Bone and periosteum also contribute to pain observed in horses with OA. The periosteum is well innervated, and the periosteal disruption that accompanies the development of periarticular osteophytes is a source of joint pain.[231] The subchondral plate and epiphyseal trabecular bone make variable contributions to clinical signs. For example, many, but not all, horses with subchondral cystic lesions demonstrate lameness.[232-234] Inconsistent lameness among horses with similar radiological signs parallels the weak correlation between pain and radiological findings of early OA in people.[235,236] Osseous receptor stimulation often accompanies joint movements that cause elevations in intramedullary pressure. People with OA of the hip have elevated intraosseous pressure,[237] which in some people responds favorably to cortical fenestration. Elevation in intramedullary pressure occurs with flexion or extension of equine joints and is a likely source of articular pain in some horses. For example, both simulated effusion and metatarsophalangeal joint flexion increase intramedullary pressure in the third metatarsal bone.[238] The concept also is supported by the clinical observation of a favorable response to transcortical decompression in horses with lameness related to osseous cystlike lesions.

Magnetic resonance imaging (MRI) has been used to try to characterize osseous lesions associated with pain in people with OA. For example, one study demonstrated a correlation between knee pain and the presence of poorly marginated areas of increased signal intensity (T_2-weighted images).[239] These areas of increased signal intensity, corresponding to fluid, have been termed "marrow edema." Unfortunately, the fluid comprising them has not been identified in correlative histological examinations.[240-242]

Local Signs

Limited range of motion is a common feature of equine OA and is probably caused by a combination of factors, including guarding from pain, synovial effusion and edema, and progressive periarticular fibrosis. Synovial edema and proliferation and pain are probably the main causes of reduced range of motion in horses with early OA, whereas fibrosis is important in chronically affected horses. The specific mechanisms causing periarticular fibrosis are unclear. However, cytokines and neuropeptides are likely to contribute to fibrosis, given the mitogenic effects on fibroblasts of these substances.[243-245]

Effusion is a common feature of OA and is manifested in joints in the distal aspect of equine limbs as visible or palpable distention of joint pouches. Leakage of protein into the synovial space, because of increased permeability in the capillary endothelium and intercellular spaces of the synovium, which is not matched by compensatory increases in lymphatic clearance, leads to a progressively increased colloid osmotic pressure and augmented synovial fluid volume. Although mild effusion enhances nutrient exchange in the joint,[246] severe effusion results in progressively elevated intraarticular pressure that ultimately destabilizes the joint and causes pain, stiffness, and a reduced range of motion. Increased permeability of the synovium to cells and proteins varies with the degree of synovial inflammation and is reflected in cytological findings in synovial fluid samples.

Synovial Fluid Changes

Reduced viscosity of synovial fluid is a frequent finding in horses with OA, particularly in horses with active synovitis. Reduced viscosity has been attributed to a reduced concentration, or depolymerization, of synovial fluid hyaluronan. Substantial reductions in hyaluronan concentration have been documented in the synovia of horses with chronic traumatic arthritis[247]; however, considerable variability

exists. In a study comparing the hyaluronan concentration in normal horses with those having lameness that could be eliminated by intraarticular analgesia, normal horses had a mean hyaluronan concentration approximately 50% higher than that of horses with synovitis. However, the variability between horses was sufficient that this difference was not statistically significant.[248] Clinical determinations of hyaluronan concentration are not routine because of this variability and the technically involved procedures required for the quantitative determination of hyaluronan. The mucin clot test is a relatively simple, semiquantitative test of hyaluronan quantity and quality, but it is not particularly sensitive. Therefore the quality of hyaluronan is often determined clinically by assessing viscosity on gross inspection of synovial fluid obtained during arthrocentesis.

Because increases in cell numbers and protein concentration in OA are not dramatic, cytological evaluation of synovial fluid is not used routinely diagnostically. Cytological analysis of synovial fluid is most useful in identifying and monitoring infection and untoward postinjection reactions. Approximate values for cell count and total protein concentrations under a variety of clinical situations are given in Table 61-3. Total protein concentration varies between joints, tending to be considerably higher in the larger, more proximal joints, such as the scapulohumeral joint.

Role of Radiography/Radiology

Radiography has long been the traditional means of assessing the structural changes of OA (see Chapter 15). Radiography has the advantages of availability, convenience, relative safety, and economy. Indeed, it is standard practice for many veterinarians to localize lameness to a particular area of the limb and subsequently to obtain radiographs in an attempt to identify changes to support a diagnosis of OA. Despite the advantages of superior contrast resolution and options for postprocessing image enhancement that accompany advances in digital radiography, the technique still lacks sensitivity and is of limited value in identifying horses with incipient or focal lesions. Radiology does, however, have some merit in characterizing changes in bone that accompany chronic OA and can be useful in adding confidence to the diagnosis of established disease. Nevertheless, it should be recognized that radiologically undetectable performance-limiting lesions occur in horses.[257,258]

Radiological findings tend to witness past events in the pathological process and do not consistently reflect ongoing processes. Additionally, in horses, as has been long accepted in people, a lack of correlation exists between lameness or reduced performance and specific osseous structural changes evident radiologically.[259-263] A lack of correlation with arthroscopically evident degeneration and radiological findings is also common.[264-267] In addition to this underlying fundamental biological dichotomy, precise quantification of radiological findings is hampered by difficulties in precisely duplicating conditions from one radiographic examination to the next. Positioning, degree of weight bearing, and radiographic technique contribute measurably to results. Nonetheless, largely because of its aforementioned advantages, radiology remains a principal method of evaluating horses with joint disease.

The radiological features of OA mirror the pathological changes occurring in the affected joint (Figure 61-8).

TABLE 61-3

Synovial Fluid Cytology for Various Clinical Conditions and Diagnostic or Therapeutic Manipulations* [249-256]

PARAMETER	NORMAL	MILD SYNOVITIS (e.g., OCD)	OSTEOARTHRITIS	INFECTIOUS ARTHRITIS[†]	ARTHROCENTESIS[‡]	BALANCED ELECTROLYTE SOLUTION[‡]	LOCAL ANESTHETICS[‡§]	GENTAMICIN[‡]	DMSO[‡] (10% SOLUTION)
Total leukocytes (per µL)	50-500	20-250	$\leq 1 \times 10^3$	$20\text{-}200 \times 10^3$	$1\text{-}4 \times 10^3$	$6\text{-}45 \times 10^3$ (typically 20×10^3)	$2\text{-}10 \times 10^3$		$8\text{-}40 \times 10^3$
Neutrophils (%)	<10	<10	<15	>90 (variable toxic changes)	50	80	60	50	>50
Mononuclear cells (%)	>90	>90	>85	<10	50	20	40	50	<50
Total protein (g/dL)	0.8-2.5	0.8-3.0	0.8-3.5	4.0-8.0+	1.5-2.5	3.0-4.0	2.5-4.0	4.5-6.0	2.5-4.0

*Listed ranges are approximate. Considerable variability exists in published reports.

†Significant elevations in leukocyte counts and total protein concentration occur within the first 12 hours in experimentally inoculated joints. Values shown represent those observed at 24 hours.

‡Leukocyte counts and total protein concentrations correspond to the maximum values that typically occur within the first 24 hours.

§Synovial response to lidocaine and mepivacaine are comparable.

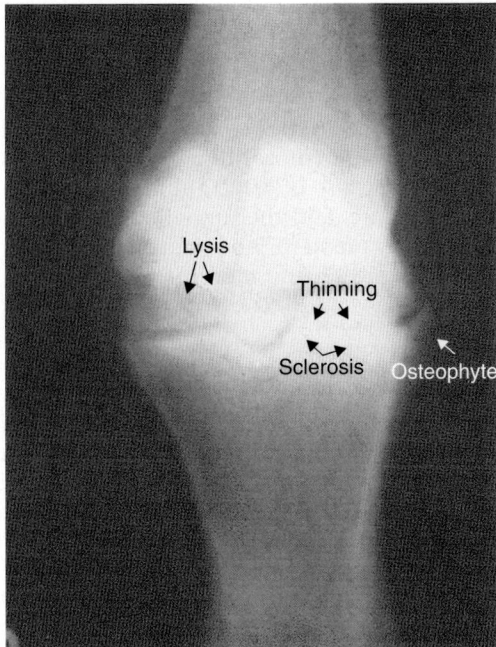

Fig. 61-8 • Dorsopalmar radiographic image of the metacarpophalangeal joint of a horse demonstrating radiological changes of advanced osteoarthritis. There is periarticular osteophytosis, joint-space thinning, and subchondral bone increased radiopacity (sclerosis) and radiolucency (lysis).

BOX 61-1

Radiological Features of Osteoarthritis

Radiological Feature	*Pathogenetic Mechanism**
Periarticular osteophytosis	Endochondral ossification occurring at bony margins of unknown cause. Possible repair attempt modulated by altered cytokine milieu.
(Asymmetrical) Joint space thinning	Cartilage degeneration and loss.[†] Usually at areas of weight bearing or high stress. May be absent when focal cartilage loss occurs.
Subchondral increased radiopacity	Deposition of new bone as a response to changes in force transmission and from healing of trabecular microfractures. Corresponds to areas of maximum stress. Clinically significant sclerosis often corresponds to full-thickness cartilage loss.
Subchondral radiolucency	Less common change of uncertain pathogenesis. Possibly pressure necrosis from synovial fluid gaining access to subchondral plate via fissures, or related to pressure necrosis from trauma to bone.
Osteochondral bodies	Disintegration of joint surfaces or fractured osteophytes. May represent inciting lesions (e.g., osteochondral fracture).
Advanced remodeling/ankylosis	Articular response to advanced degeneration. Environment more consistent with fracture than synovial joint.

*Specific pathophysiological mechanisms and reasons for disproportionate representation of changes among and between joints remain unclear.
[†]Seldom used as a marker of disease progression because of problems with technical aspects of radiographic positioning and focal-film distance.

Initially, joint space narrowing, subchondral increased radiopacity (sclerosis), and osteophytosis occur. With time, subchondral radiolucent defects (lysis), osteochondral fragmentation, and eventually ankylosis may develop (Box 61-1). In horses substantial differences appear between specific joints respecting the relative degree of these changes. For example, radiologically evident changes tend to be less dramatic and appear later in the disease process in the metacarpophalangeal and metatarsophalangeal joints than in many other articulations.

Other Imaging Modalities

Increasingly available are other imaging modalities for assessing joint diseases. Among them are nuclear scintigraphy, MRI, and ultrasonography.

Nuclear Scintigraphy

Although more commonly used to detect nondisplaced, incomplete fractures and to identify stress-related bone damage in performance horses, nuclear scintigraphy can provide useful information in selected horses with OA (see Chapter 19). Whereas radiography (and related techniques, including computed tomography) provides considerable anatomical detail of osseous changes in affected joints, nuclear scintigraphy yields current physiological information on bone metabolism. The main disadvantages of scintigraphy are its relatively poor resolution (isotopes produce much fewer gamma rays than the number of x-rays generated by a cathode tube) and a lack of specificity because bone responds to most insults by increasing turnover. Owing to the unavailability of a cartilage-specific agent, the most common approach to the scintigraphic study of OA is using the delayed bone phase images, obtained 3 to 4 hours after injection of the radiopharmaceutical. Currently used agents are the bisphosphonates, which bind to the microcrystals of hydroxyapatite in bone. Areas of increased bone modeling have enhanced localization of the radiopharmaceutical, as long as an adequate blood supply exists.

It has long been known that bone-seeking isotopes accumulate rapidly in the bone of OA joints.[268] The most intense radiopharmaceutical uptake typically occurs in the subchondral bone and at the osteochondral junctions of osteophytes, although temporal variation in the anatomical distribution of uptake may occur, as was illustrated in an animal OA model.[269] Evidence exists that scintigraphy is useful in predicting the progression of OA in the human knee,[270] and scintigraphy apparently may prove useful in diagnosing preclinical joint disease, that is, before the appearance of radiological abnormalities.[271] Conversely, bone phase images may be normal in chronic OA joints if the rate of bone turnover returns to normal.

In the equine athlete, scintigraphy has proved useful to document a number of sport-specific lesions among different types of equine athletes.[271-273] Unlike the human digit, the size of the bones in the equine skeleton is sufficient that relatively precise anatomical localization of lesions is often possible. Moreover, nuclear scintigraphy has the advantage of allowing a survey of all joints in a single examination. Importantly, as for radiography, close correlation between lameness and scintigraphic findings does not always exist.[271,274]

Magnetic Resonance Imaging

MRI involves detecting alternating electrical current produced when hydrogen protons, predominately found in fat and water, are subjected to pulsed electromagnetic fields applied in a specific manner (see Chapter 21). The rate at which protons change orientation varies among soft tissues and fluids of different composition, which allows the considerable tissue discrimination possible with MRI.

MRI is assuming a growing role in assessing joint disease in people and has a number of compelling advantages over many of the existing imaging modalities. Specifically, MRI has the capacity to provide noninvasive, high-resolution, three-dimensional (tomographic) images of all joint components. Importantly, advances in equipment and improved imaging sequences allow direct evaluation of articular cartilage, rather than the indirect assessment obtained using conventional radiography. Specifically, high-field MRI can be used to evaluate cartilage morphology, determine tissue volume, and evaluate cartilage composition. In human patients, detailed analysis of cartilage structure, including the detection of subtle cartilage lesions, is now possible using current sequences and protocols.[275] Cartilage loss is a hallmark of OA, and assessment of cartilage volume using MRI has been shown to be both sensitive and reliable.[276,277] In the future, quantitative assessments of cartilage volume and composition may prove useful to monitor disease progression and therapeutic responses. Specialized techniques, including the use of contrast agents (e.g., gadopentetate dimeglumine), enable the assessment of glycosaminoglycan content in joint cartilage. To date, the technique of delayed gadolinium-enhanced MRI of cartilage has proved useful in monitoring the influence of exercise on cartilage health and for assessing the effects of a number of interventions on matrix composition.[275] Optimizing MRI as a diagnostic and monitoring tool requires sophisticated (high-field) equipment and considerable experience for proper image acquisition and interpretation.

Developments in low-field magnets and motion correction software adaptable to the standing horse have made possible diagnostic MRI of the equine distal limb; however, these systems are unsuitable for evaluating cartilage in the manner described previously.[278-280]

To date, MRI studies of equine joints have been largely limited to anatomical and correlative studies of cadaver specimens.[281-284] In one of the few published reports of using the technique to investigate OA in the horse, post mortem magnetic resonance images of the metacarpophalangeal joint correlated well with arthroscopic and necropsy findings.[285] Widespread use of MRI in horses is limited by the availability, expense, and the tunnel configuration of currently available equipment; however, it holds considerable promise as a diagnostic and monitoring tool in the future.

Ultrasonography

Ultrasonographic evaluation of diseased joints represents an additional diagnostic tool that has enjoyed increased use lately (see Chapter 17). Ultrasonography initially was used to assess chronic proliferative synovitis in the metacarpophalangeal joint.[286,287] More recently its use has expanded to include most appendicular (and some axial) skeletal joints.

The principal benefit of ultrasonographic examination over conventional radiography is its superiority in demonstrating soft tissue abnormalities such as thickened synovial and capsular tissues and damaged intraarticular and periarticular ligaments. With experience and an appropriate knowledge of the regional anatomy and acoustic principles, it is also possible to identify and localize accumulations of synovial or other fluids. Although the ultrasound beam cannot penetrate the cortex, surface characteristics of bone can be evaluated, including periarticular osteophytes and enthesophytes, osteochondral fragments, and irregularities in the subchondral plate. Ultrasonographic features of arthritic cartilage include thinning, loss of sharp contours, and changes in echogenicity. Inherent limitations of ultrasonography preclude its use in areas where the tissue overlying the joint of interest is too voluminous and for structures having a shape or orientation that is not conducive to ultrasonographic evaluation. The basic principles and techniques of ultrasonographic examination of equine joints have been thoroughly reviewed.[288]

Chapter 62

Markers of Osteoarthritis: Implications for Early Diagnosis and Monitoring of the Pathological Course and Effects of Therapy

David D. Frisbie

Although joint disease can be diagnosed using routine clinical methods, more accurate and earlier diagnosis may lead to identification of osteoarthritis (OA) before irreversible changes occur within joint tissues. Measuring levels of molecular products of tissue turnover, known as biomarkers, from healthy and diseased cartilage and bone has the potential to achieve early diagnosis and allow a better understanding of the pathophysiology of OA. The potential also exists to monitor disease, especially in response to novel therapeutic agents. Work with biomarkers of articular cartilage and bone in people and horses with OA has yielded promising results. This chapter discusses some of the markers that currently are being evaluated in synovial fluid and serum samples, with a focus on those of potential benefit to the equine industry.

STRUCTURE AND METABOLISM OF ARTICULAR CARTILAGE AND BONE IN HEALTH AND DISEASE

Articular cartilage is a complex tissue with an extensive extracellular matrix. The two main components that define the cartilage matrix are type II collagen and aggrecan (see

Chapter 61). A balance of synthesis and degradation orchestrated by the chondrocytes maintains normal populations of these molecules within the cartilage matrix. Osteocytes, osteoblasts, and osteoclasts maintain the structural and functional integrity of bone matrix by regulating synthetic and degradative pathways. Synoviocytes also influence homeostasis in cartilage and bone. OA often is characterized by degradative changes within articular cartilage, bone, and synovium. Direct and indirect factors assault the matrix molecules of these tissues, resulting in degeneration and loss of some macromolecules.

What are direct and indirect molecular markers? Direct molecular markers specifically identify a known molecular process within a given tissue. For example, fibrillar collagens, such as types I and II, are synthesized as immature procollagens that undergo proteolytic changes before conversion to mature collagen fibrils. Peptides at either end of the procollagen molecule are cleaved before the procollagen is incorporated into a mature collagen fibril. Estimations of type II collagen synthesis were obtained from synovial fluid and serum samples by using a specific antibody that recognizes the propeptides cleaved from the carboxyl termini.[1] Conversely, an indirect molecular marker reflects more general change that is not clearly definable and may represent contributions from several events and tissues. Indirect markers are cytokines, growth factors, and matrix metalloproteinases (MMPs). OA involves changes in subchondral bone and synovium; therefore assessment of molecular markers from these tissues is relevant.

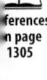

References on page 1305

INDIVIDUAL SKELETAL BIOMARKERS OF ARTICULAR CARTILAGE METABOLISM IN OSTEOARTHRITIS

Anabolic Processes

The carboxyl propeptide of type II collagen is a useful measure of the anabolic process of type II collagen synthesis. Studies have shown that levels of carboxyl propeptide of type II collagen were significantly higher in synovial fluid from people with OA compared with those without OA. Levels peaked early in the radiological progression of the disease and declined in patients with severe radiological changes.[2,3] This biomarker also has been shown to change significantly in serum samples from people with OA and rheumatoid arthritis.[4,5]

Chondroitin sulfate (CS) is a major glycosaminoglycan (GAG) of aggrecan, and measuring specific CS epitopes on newly synthesized proteoglycan (PG) molecules is a useful biomarker for aggrecan synthesis. An epitope called CS-846 that normally is found in fetal tissues, but is almost absent in healthy adult articular cartilage, has been measured in many species. Levels of CS-846 epitope were increased in synovial fluid in people after injury or primary OA compared with levels in synovial fluid from normal joints. Serum levels were elevated in joint disease but to a lesser extent than synovial fluid levels.[6,7] Other CS epitopes such as 3B3 and 7D4 were shown to be useful in assessing cartilage injury in animal models and in people with clinical disease.[8] Using arthroscopic evaluation, a negative correlation was found between synovial fluid 3B3 concentrations and gross articular damage that was thought to be caused

by decreased normal cartilage volume, or inhibition of synthesis, with increasingly severe lesions. Conversely, in people, increased levels of synovial 7D4 epitope were found in diseased knees compared with contralateral normal knees.[9]

Catabolic Processes

Measuring the degradation of type II collagen is of potential benefit in monitoring OA. Antibodies have been developed to identify exposed but previously inaccessible cleaved or denatured type II collagen fragments. Significant elevations in levels of degraded type II collagen were demonstrated in synovial fluid and serum samples from horses, dogs, and rabbits with experimentally induced OA.[10,11] Significant increases were detected in the serum of people with OA, with a correlation to disease activity.[10]

Keratan sulfate (KS), one of the GAGs found on proteoglycan molecules of aggrecan, has been evaluated extensively. In people, elevations in serum levels of KS were associated with OA in some, but not all, studies.[7,12,13] Lack of correlation of serum[14] and synovial fluid[8] KS levels with cartilage damage compromises the value of serum KS as a biomarker of joint disease in people. In dogs, a specific KS epitope (5D4) was of limited value in experimentally induced and naturally occurring cruciate ligament injury.[15,16] The usefulness of KS in serum and synovial fluid of horses with osteochondral fragmentation is also questionable.[17]

In an initial equine study of molecular markers, carboxyl propeptide of type II collagen and the GAG epitopes CS-846 and KS were measured in synovial fluid and serum of horses with and without carpal osteochondral fragments.[17] Synovial fluid and serum CS-846 epitope concentrations were significantly higher in joints with osteochondral fragments compared with normal joints and showed good correlation with grades of cartilage damage. Serum concentrations of carboxyl propeptide of type II collagen were elevated in horses with osteochondral fragments, and good correlation between carboxyl propeptide of type II collagen concentration and arthroscopic lesion grade was found. A single blood sample assayed for CS-846 and carboxyl propeptide of type II collagen levels resulted in 79% accuracy for prediction of an osteochondral fragment.

CS-846, KS, and carboxyl propeptide of type II collagen concentrations were measured in synovial fluid of horses with normal joints and those with osteochondrosis.[18] Significantly higher levels of carboxyl propeptide of type II collagen and lower amounts of CS-846 and KS epitopes were found in affected joints compared with normal joints.

Cartilage oligomeric protein (COMP) is an abundant noncollagenous protein constituent of cartilage. COMP was once thought to be cartilage specific, but it has also been localized in tendons and synovium. Serum and synovial fluid concentrations of COMP are increased in people with OA.[19,20] A positive correlation exists between COMP levels and radiological grading of OA, progression of radiological changes,[21] and results of nuclear scintigraphy in people.[22] Gene expression of COMP in synoviocytes is upregulated in OA, suggesting that this marker may be useful to indicate synovitis.

Unlike the elevation of COMP levels in people with OA, in horses initial studies demonstrated that serum and synovial fluid levels of COMP were significantly *lower* in horses with diseased joints.[23] It appears that this discrepancy was caused by the antibody used in the initial equine studies recognizing mainly intact rather than intact and breakdown products of COMP. Thus a subsequent study[24] in the horse using an antibody (14G4) recognizing both intact and breakdown fragments confirmed that COMP levels *increase* with OA.

INDIVIDUAL SKELETAL BIOMARKERS OF BONE METABOLISM IN JOINT DISEASE

Anabolic and catabolic cascades exist in bone, but specific markers in normal and disease states are not clearly defined. This section deals only with bone markers thought to be important in joint disease.

Anabolic Processes

Osteocalcin (OCa) is a small noncollagenous protein associated with bone assembly and turnover and has been measured in serum and synovial fluid samples from people with OA. Levels of OCa correlated with bone scan findings and markers of cartilage metabolism.[22,25] However, because OCa levels are higher in serum than synovial fluid, OCa in synovial fluid may be derived from peripheral blood and may not reflect local joint disease.[25]

OCa levels were measured in horses, and, as in people, they appear to vary with age and with the administration of corticosteroids,[25,26] but the effect of gender remains unclear.[26] General anesthesia affects serum OCa levels for 4 days.[27]

Bone-specific alkaline phosphatase is an isoform of alkaline phosphatase that is expressed at high levels on the cell surface of the bone-forming osteoblasts and plays an important role in bone formation. In a recent equine study, a correlation was found between synovial fluid levels of bone-specific alkaline phosphatase (BAP), KS-5D4 epitope, and total GAG, as well as between all three biomarkers, and the amount of joint damage defined arthroscopically.[28] This supports a putative role for altered subchondral bone metabolism in equine OA.

Catabolic Processes

Type I collagen C-telopeptides (CTX) may be useful markers of bone resorption. CTX levels in people with rheumatoid arthritis were positively correlated with indices of disease activity and joint destruction.[29,30] The marker was influenced by the administration of corticosteroids. CTX is present in equine serum, although its usefulness as a marker of pathological processes is unknown.[31]

Human bone sialoprotein is found only in adult bone, and levels are seven times higher at the interface of cartilage and bone compared with other locations in bone.[32] Serum levels are elevated significantly in people with clinically apparent OA and those with bone scans consistent with OA.[32,33] Equine bone sialoprotein has yet to be characterized, but development of an assay is currently underway. The hope is that this will be useful in identifying subchondral bone damage in horses with OA.

FUTURE OF BIOMARKERS IN OSTEOARTHRITIS

Limited data are available regarding the use of biomarkers to diagnose and monitor equine joint disease. Factors influencing levels of biomarkers include liver and kidney clearance, circadian rhythms, intestinal peristalsis, exercise level, age, breed, diet, sex, drug administration, surgery, and general anesthesia. Methods of sample collection and storage also may be influential.

Although biomarkers may have a role in diagnosis and monitoring equine OA, a combination of markers likely will be required, especially because so many factors influence activity. Proof-of-principle work has been completed showing that biomarkers significantly change in the face of experimentally induced OA, and this change is significantly greater than with exercise alone.[34,35] Specifically, synovial fluid concentration for eight of eight biomarkers was significantly increased in OA-affected joints of horses undergoing exercise compared with sham joints of similarly exercised horses. Likewise, serum from OA-affected horses had a significant increase in six of eight biomarkers compared with serum from similarly exercised horses. Using biomarker levels from either synovial fluid or serum, horses could be correctly categorized into the appropriate group (OA-affected or sham) 100% of the time within 14 days of OA induction using discriminant analysis, suggesting great promise for the use of biomarkers.

To date, in a clinical setting, several cross-sectional studies have looked at numerous biomarkers in both synovial fluid and serum for the potential to be useful in noninvasive prediction of disease severity. Specifically, COMP was significantly altered in serum in horses with clinical OA compared with control horses.[36] Differences in synovial fluid COMP levels were identified when making similar comparisons in horses with OA.[24,37,38] Another cross-sectional study[39] using the contralateral limb as a control demonstrated that concentrations of BAP, KS, KS/GAG ratio, and hyaluronan were all significantly different in early OA compared with contralateral joints. It was also observed that BAP and KS concentrations and the KS/GAG ratio had good correlations with articular cartilage pathology. These cross-sectional studies provide good examples for the potential use of biomarkers in equine medicine; prospective longitudinal studies are the next step for providing further proof of principle.

One such study has been completed through collaboration of the Equine Research Center at Colorado State University and equine veterinarians practicing at southern California Thoroughbred racetracks. Two- and 3-year-old racehorses were entered in the study (N = 238).[40] Horses had monthly musculoskeletal examinations, and blood was collected and stored for later biomarker examination. Horses were followed for a maximum of 10 months and were considered to have sustained an injury if they were out of training for more than 30 days. Horses with solitary musculoskeletal injuries and completion of more than 2 months in the study were analyzed for biomarker levels, along with a randomly selected control population of uninjured horses. The following were considered musculoskeletal injuries: intraarticular fragmentation, tendon or ligamentous injury, stress fractures, and dorsal metacarpal disease. Fifty-nine horses sustained a single musculoskeletal injury; 71 acted as uninjured controls. The greatest change in biomarker levels was 4 to 6 months before injury. Using sophisticated statistical modeling, it was possible, based on biomarker levels in this group of horses, to accurately predict horses that would sustain an injury 73.9% of the time. Given these promising results, another study has been instituted in Western performance horses, which have a less tightly controlled training pattern compared with Thoroughbred racehorses. Because exercise is known to affect biomarker levels, this will be an important test of the "real world" application of biomarkers in musculoskeletal disease.

Chapter 63

Gene Therapy

C. Wayne McIlwraith and David D. Frisbie

It was well stated by Anderson in *Nature* in 1998: "Despite our present lack of knowledge, gene therapy will almost certainly revolutionize the practice of medicine over the next 25 years."[1] Gene therapy has the potential to revolutionize intraarticular therapy, both for the prevention of osteoarthritis (OA) and its management.

There are two approaches to gene therapy: (1) identifying a genetic disease (e.g., OA) and then replacing the defective gene, or (2) using gene therapy to increase levels of selected therapeutic proteins, as with interleukin-1 receptor antagonist (IL-1ra). Until gene defects are clearly identified, gene therapy for OA is likely to use the second approach, promoting production of disease-modifying agents such as catabolic antagonists or anabolic promoters.

REVIEW OF COMPONENTS OF GENE THERAPY

A gene, which is a functional unit of DNA, consists of a DNA sequence that produces a single polypeptide. This gene sequence codes for a specific messenger RNA that goes from nucleus to cytoplasm to translate the amino acid sequence (protein).

Gene therapy is targeted on the production of a selected therapeutic protein to alter a disease process. This protein may enhance (e.g., insulin-like growth factor–1 [IGF-1]) or repress (e.g., IL-1ra) a specific cellular process. The essential components of gene therapy include (1) isolation of a gene (called cloning), (2) manipulation of the gene (engineering), and (3) transfer of the gene into the host cells (transfection/transduction). The gene sequence is initially isolated and characterized and is then engineered by the addition of regulatory elements (promoters) that allow control of protein production.

The essential component of gene transfer is the vector. Gene delivery vectors facilitate the transfer of the therapeutic gene into the nucleus of the target cell. Once in the nucleus, the gene is decoded (expressed) to produce a protein. Viruses, the most commonly used vectors, have the ability to transfer genes into a host cell in an efficient, logical, and easy manner. Viruses used as vectors have been rendered incapable of replicative spread by removal of viral genes and insertion of the therapeutic gene(s). Viral vectors are more efficient than nonviral vectors.

There are two potential methods of gene transfer. Ex vivo gene transfer is an indirect technique where the cells are collected from the joint and grown in the laboratory (e.g., synovial cells). The gene is then transferred (transduced) into cultured cells using a viral vector, and the transduced cells are reimplanted after testing for protein production. Ex vivo transfer is safer but less convenient than the second technique, in vivo transfer. In vivo transfer involves direct transfer of a vector to the target tissues. For example, synovial cells could be transfected by direct transmission of an *IL-1ra* gene using an adenovirus vector injected into a joint (Figure 63-1). Adenoviruses are the most common vectors proposed for use in human patients with clinical disease[2] and were used in our equine studies.[3-9] Adenoviral vectors can transduce dividing and nondividing cells and are amenable to in vivo transfer. The adenoviral vector takes up an episomal location (extrachromosomal) in the host nucleus. Second-generation vectors give protein expression for 21 to 40 days.

GENE THERAPY AND JOINT DISEASE

Our investigation of the potential value of gene therapy in the treatment of OA is partially based on limitations of traditional therapy. Currently, most therapeutic agents need to be directly administered intraarticularly, and the half-life of most commonly used agents is short.[10,11] Gene transfer provides an excellent alternative to conventional therapy because a single intraarticular injection results in the production of the specific therapeutic protein within diseased joint(s) for a prolonged period.[12] The potential for the use of gene therapy is best illustrated by our work

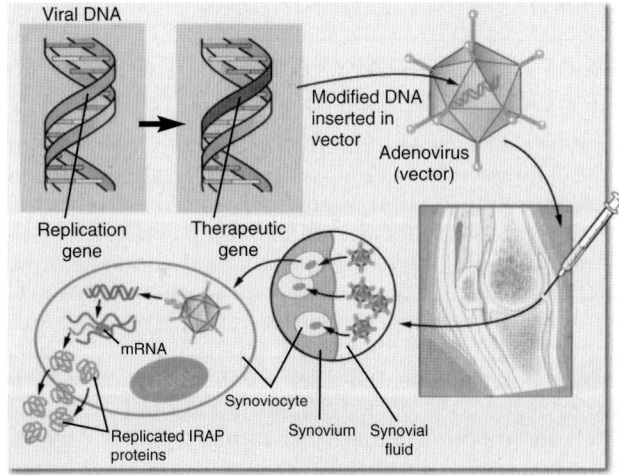

Fig. 63-1 • Schematic drawing representing in vivo gene transfer to the synovium. This is the way in which gene therapy with interleukin-1 receptor antagonist was performed. (Reproduced with permission from McIlwraith CW: Milne lecture: from arthroscopy to gene therapy—30 years of looking in joints, *Proc Am Assoc Equine Pract* 51:83, 2005.)

References on page 1306

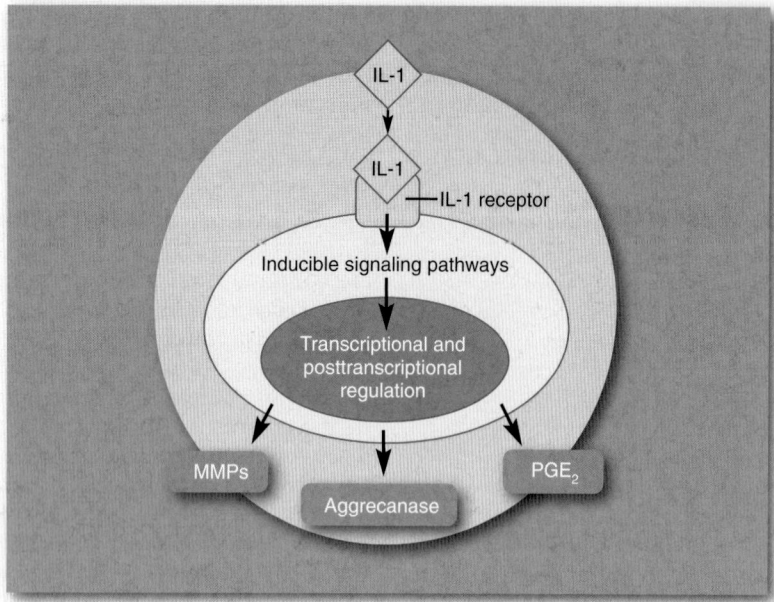

Fig. 63-2 • Diagram of interleukin-1 (IL-1) activation of matrix metalloproteinase, aggrecanase, and prostaglandin E₂ release acting through IL-1 receptors on the cell membranes. (Reproduced with permission from McIlwraith CW: Milne lecture: From arthroscopy to gene therapy—30 years of looking in joints, *Proc Am Assoc Equine Pract* 51:73, 2005.)

demonstrating that experimental OA can be suppressed by the use of gene therapy. Cytokines such as interleukin-1 (IL-1) and tumor necrosis factor (TNF) modulate the synthesis of metalloproteinases (MMPs) by synovial cells and are largely responsible for the mediation of joint disease.[13-15] The mechanism by which IL-1 causes up-regulation of deleterious mediators is illustrated in Figure 63-2.

Any of the articular tissues, including synovium, articular cartilage, and meniscus, are possible targets for gene transfer. However, the synovium is the best because of its large surface area and contact with the joint space, and has been used with IL-1ra. Synovium is also a convenient target because the gene vector can be administered intraarticularly. Extracellular matrix would limit vector penetration in cartilage cells.

USE OF GENE THERAPY TO PREVENT ARTICULAR CARTILAGE DEGRADATION IN OSTEOARTHRITIS

It is now well accepted that the IL-l "system" is important in the pathogenesis of OA and articular cartilage degradation. There are two agonists, IL-lα and IL-lβ, with IL-1–converting enzyme responsible for activation of both cytokines. There is also an IL-1ra. Both the agonists and the antagonists function through type I and type II receptors on the cell membrane of the target cell (this can be synovium or a chondrocyte) (see Figure 63-2). Up-regulators of IL-l gene transcription include IL-l itself, TNF, and IL-2. IL-1 in turn up-regulates MMP activity, prostaglandin E₂, and IL-6, which are important in articular cartilage matrix degradation. The type I IL-l receptor mediates biological responses to IL-6. The type II receptor does not deliver biological signals but tracks IL-1 and inhibits its action. Type II soluble receptors are also potential therapeutic agents. Following intraarticular administration of IL-1ra protein in the Pond-Nuki model of OA, there was a dose-dependent reduction

in the incidence of osteophytes, size and grade of tibial cartilage erosion, cartilage histological changes, and MMP-1 expression.[16] However, multiple and regular dosing of the protein is essential.

The first report of gene transfer of IL-1ra was in 1993.[17] A collaborative effort between the University of Pittsburgh School of Medicine Department of Orthopedic Surgery and Molecular Genetics and Colorado State University (CSU) Orthopaedic Research Center was successful in treating experimental equine OA using gene therapy with equine IL-1ra using an adenoviral vector. Our collaborators Evans and Robbins had previously done work in experimental animals using an adenoviral vector to transport the equine *IL-1ra* gene, and it was this adenoviral vector containing the equine gene that was used in our studies. The first step was the identification and sequencing of the gene and coding equine *IL-1ra*, previously done in our laboratory in 1998.[18]

Proof-of-principle experiments began. First, in vitro expression of an active equine IL-1ra protein after gene transfer of the equine *IL-1ra* gene sequence to cultured equine synoviocytes using an adenoviral vector was validated.[19] Synoviocytes were transfected with Ad-EqIL-1ra at 0, 1, 10, and 100 multiplicity of infection. We assayed the media for and found sufficient active protein (Quantikine human IL-1ra immunoassay; R&D Systems, Minneapolis, Minnesota, United States). Then in an in vivo dose titration study we found that our Ad-EqIL-1ra vector led to a dose-dependent increase in the concentration of IL-1ra in synovial fluid. The maximum duration of IL-1ra production (35 days) was with 10 or 20×10^{10} particles per joint. However, a higher dose of 50×10^{10} produced an undesired synovial leukocytosis.

Next we tested this regimen using our previously described equine OA model[20,21] using eight treated and eight control horses.[4] Fourteen days after surgery, horses received 20×10^{10} Ad-EqIL-1ra viral particles per joint and continued in a standardized exercise protocol. Relevant levels of IL-1ra protein were measured in the synovial fluid. At 8 weeks, treated horses showed marked reduction in full-thickness cartilage erosions in the induced OA joints and lower inflammatory scores in the synovium compared with control horses. Safranin O fast green staining was depleted in the control joints but was close to normal in the treated joints. There was increased proteoglycan synthesis in the articular cartilage of treated joints. From these data we concluded that transduction of cells with Ad-EqIL-1ra led to synthesis of biologically active equine IL-1ra and excellent suppression of experimentally induced equine OA.

To put the therapeutic benefit of this gene therapy into perspective compared with conventionally used medication, gene therapy was better at reducing the progression of experimentally created OA than were triamcinolone acetonide (Vetalog; Fort Dodge Animal Health, Overland Park, Kansas, United States)[20] and methylprednisolone acetate (Depo-Medrol; Pfizer, New York, New York, United States),[21] both of which were tested in similar fashion. This was the first study to demonstrate both clinical improvement as a result of gene therapy and significant improvements in gross and histological changes. We concluded that we may have discovered a practical and potentially effective therapy for equine OA. However, subsequent studies revealed that repeated administration of the viral vector induced substantial reactive synovitis, and now our focus has been in trying to achieve a better, nonreactive vector. Work is centered on attempts at developing an adeno-associated viral (aaV) vector, which has been difficult and frustrating. However, recent work in our laboratory has shown good green fluorescent protein expression with an equine aaV vector, and we are optimistic that we have found a better method of gene therapy with IL-1ra in the horse.[22,23]

GENE THERAPY AND PROMOTION OF CARTILAGE HEALING

There is potential value in using anabolic genes, such as IGF-1, to heal existing cartilage defects. Adenoviral-mediated IGF-1 gene transduction of equine synovium caused persistent elevations of synovial fluid IGF-1 ligand.[24] Enhancement of cartilage healing in an equine model was demonstrated with genetic modification of chondrocytes with IGF-1.[25]

Following our positive results with *IL-1ra* gene transfer in experimentally induced OA, the possibility of gene therapy with both IL-1ra and IGF-1 was explored. We reasoned that promotion of anabolism in combination with inhibition of catabolism could provide an appropriate environment for articular cartilage healing. In another collaborative effort among our laboratory, Cornell University, University of Pittsburgh, and Harvard, we have evaluated the value of the combined gene therapy protocol using IL-1ra to decrease the effect of IL-1 on cartilage repair and IGF-1, which had previously been shown to enhance cartilage healing and to reduce the deleterious effects of IL-1.[26-28] Using an osteoarthritic IL-1 coculture (synovium and articular cartilage), gene transduction with IGF-1 and IL-1ra proteins was demonstrated using an adenoviral vector with the reduction of proteoglycan loss from the cartilage.[26] There was also restoration of cartilage matrix without IL-1 being detected using the same in vitro system.[27] Combination gene therapy was then evaluated in vivo using full-thickness articular chondral defects treated with microfracture in the horse.[28] Gene therapy enhanced the quality of the repair tissue in full-thickness equine chondral defects compared with microfracture alone, resulting in increased concentration of type II collagen and aggrecan in the repair tissue.

GENE THERAPY AND BONE HEALING

The delivery of growth factors using gene therapy to enhance bone healing was reviewed.[29] Initial work at CSU was done evaluating an adenoviral-bone morphogenetic protein–2 (BMP-2) gene therapy protocol in an infected nonunion fracture model.[30] Beneficial effects were obtained, and more recently the use of adeno-BMP-2 gene therapy is being evaluated in a splint gap osteotomy model in the horse.

Chapter 64

Models of Equine Joint Disease

Chris E. Kawcak

Animals have been used extensively as models of joint disease to study clinical conditions in people. However, veterinary researchers have the luxury of using experimental animals from species that are clinically relevant. Unlike in human research, one has no need to assume similarity in findings between species. Equine models of joint disease have been used for several decades to test the effects of drugs and various treatments on joints and to evaluate the pathogenesis of certain diseases. Joint disease can be assessed in horses with clinical disease; however, large numbers are needed for each treatment group to see significant statistical differences in the face of great variation among individual horses. Owner compliance, differing treatment protocols among clinicians, and variability among horses in response to disease and treatment, as well as conformation, limb use, and size, all contribute to this variation. Furthermore, clinical studies take a long time to perform, and the effects of treatment take a long time to be seen. Consequently, in vitro and in vivo models have been developed to give researchers better-controlled studies that can be done in a relatively short time.

The model to be used should be designed to answer a question by using a testable hypothesis. Variability should be reduced as much as possible so that the question can be answered with little outside influence. However, as more and more variables are eliminated, the model becomes less representative of the clinical situation. For instance, the efficacy of oral joint supplements in reducing joint disease cannot rely solely on results from in vitro studies. The drugs must be tested in vivo to determine if and how they work. However, to determine the effects of a drug or chemical on articular cartilage matrix metabolism, a quick, relatively inexpensive in vitro test can be conducted. Therefore the type of model to be used depends on the question to be answered.

Two types of models are used to study equine joint disease. In vitro models can be used to study various treatments, using cells, cell lines, or tissues harvested from joints to test usually one specific pathological pathway or treatment scheme. In vivo systems can be used to test drugs and to determine the pathophysiological response to an insult. Unlike in vitro studies, in vivo studies involve the entire joint, allowing researchers to assess the whole organ to determine truly the clinical efficacy of a drug.

In this chapter the complexity of joint disease and the use of joint models are discussed. The difficulties in modeling joint disease, the rationale for selecting specific models, specific examples of models used for the study of the joint disease, and the current status and future use of equine models of joint disease are considered.

COMPLEXITY OF JOINT DISEASE

The joint can be considered an organ because it is composed of several different types of tissues that biomechanically and biochemically interact with each other. Joint disease can result from several factors. First, the disease has a direct biochemical effect on all tissues. For instance, with synovitis, inflammatory mediators can be released into the joint space and put the articular cartilage into a catabolic state.[1-4] Second, the pain produced by joint disease can result in a change in the character of the gait.[5,6] Consequently this change in joint loading alters biomechanical inputs on all tissues, resulting in a biochemical change in the response by tissues.[7,8] Third, disease of one tissue can result in a change in the mechanical input on another tissue. For instance, articular cartilage degeneration, which can result in increased stress to subchondral bone, can induce a sclerotic response.[9] As another example, subchondral bone sclerosis, which commonly occurs in racehorses, can lead to increased stress on overlying articular cartilage.[10] Therefore in the live horse all tissues are affected by one another.

Because several factors can influence joint disease, researchers have attempted to control these influences in experimental studies. However, not all of the factors can be controlled. For instance, several mechanical factors play a role in joint disease; specifically, mechanical input can vary with horse size, exercise intensity, conformation, neurological control, and lameness. Consequently, differences in the stress to joints can result in changes in biochemical pathways in those tissues. For instance, ponies are one third to one half the size of horses and have little naturally occurring joint disease. Therefore they may not be the best equine models of joint disease for joint healing studies and exercise studies because of lower imposed stresses. However,

References on page 1306

they are still good models if imposed stresses do not play a role in the specific disease being studied, such as induced synovitis models. Tissue material properties also have an influence on joint disease. For instance, weaker tissues undergo greater biomechanical changes than those that are stronger. Factors that control material properties of tissues include genetics, loading history, and age of the animal. The tissue remodeling status and the ability of horses to remodel articular cartilage, subchondral bone, and soft tissues can also influence joint disease, which is also affected by age, loading history, and genetics. The inflammatory response can also change the joint environment. Specifically, differences in the immune system at the time of disease can greatly influence the inflammatory response to the joint and influence the concentration of cytokines released into the joint.

Variables such as age, size, conformation, and neurological status can be controlled in experimental in vivo studies. However, loading history and the presence of subclinical disease are virtually impossible to control. With the advent of more sophisticated imaging equipment, such as computed tomography (CT) and magnetic resonance imaging (MRI), more information on loading history and subclinical disease can be obtained. For instance, subchondral bone density is indicative of loading history.[11] Therefore researchers at the Equine Orthopaedic Research Center (EORC) at Colorado State University often perform prestudy CT examinations to determine subchondral bone density as an indicator of loading history. Another benefit of CT and MRI is that some subclinical diseases may be more easily detectable. Researchers at the EORC also initiate a controlled exercise program on a high-speed treadmill before starting the study. The hope is that this can normalize the loading histories of experimental horses. Equally important as loading history and subclinical disease is the biomechanical and biochemical status of the articular cartilage, which at this time is difficult to assess noninvasively at the beginning of a project. With the advent of MRI and pressure probes, articular cartilage and bone matrix structure can be assessed more readily.

TYPES OF MODELS
In Vitro Models

Several types of models have been used to study joint disease. In vitro models have been used and are increasing in use for several reasons. Researchers in university settings are constantly driven to develop in vitro studies to reduce the use of live animals and to address the humane issues that surround live animal research. Currently, in vivo models are essential for testing new drugs. However, animal care and use committees at universities critically evaluate in vivo research projects to be sure that they are necessary. These committees are under constant pressure to ensure that research animal use falls within appropriate ethical guidelines. In vitro systems for studying joint disease can be performed on cells from the tissues of joints. Culture systems can be created for cells such as synoviocytes and chondrocytes in two-dimensional and three-dimensional matrices. Isolated cells also can be evaluated, within the individual matrices, or within artificial matrices. Isolated cells are used to evaluate cellular response to therapeutic agents. Specific outcomes are analyzed to determine cell metabolism and proliferation. Some cell cultures are allowed or stimulated to produce the matrix, and specific cell matrix interaction and matrix metabolism can be studied. Cells are often cultured within artificial matrices to evaluate cell-matrix interactions and cell proliferation within the matrix.

Tissues from living systems are also used for in vitro study of joint diseases. The advantages of such a system over isolated cells are that cells can be maintained within the natural matrix and the experiments are relatively easy to perform. However, tissues must equilibrate in the culture medium to a steady state. This metabolic state may not truly reflect the in vivo state, because no axial load exists and the tissue edges are unconfined. The change in stress patterns and bathing in artificial media then influence articular cartilage matrix metabolism, often leading to increased articular cartilage matrix degradation. Tissues that are harvested from cadavers and specimens are placed within the medium, which is changed every 24 to 48 hours. These tissues then can be manipulated for study, and the medium and tissue can be evaluated. Media collected during the study can be analyzed for release or degradation of matrix components and inflammatory mediators. Tissues can be assessed for changes in cell proliferation, matrix synthesis, and characteristics of matrix degradation. Various molecular techniques can also be performed on the tissues.

Two types of tissue cultures are available. Single tissues can be studied to determine biochemical, molecular, mechanical, and histological changes that occur with certain influences.[12,13] However, coculture systems also can be evaluated to determine interactions between tissues. Investigators in the EORC have studied synovium–articular cartilage and articular cartilage–subchondral bone coculture systems. Exposure of articular cartilage matrix to subchondral bone caused a significant reduction in articular cartilage matrix metabolism.[14] Furthermore, similar findings also were seen in the synovium–articular cartilage coculture systems, in that exposure of articular cartilage matrix to subintimal tissues and vessels led to a significant reduction in articular cartilage matrix metabolism.[15] From these studies one can conclude that exposure of various depths of synovium and subchondral bone to articular cartilage can lead to release of mediators that can change articular cartilage metabolism. Unlike the equilibration period for in vitro experiments, this change in metabolism is severe and long lasting. However, when articular cartilage is cocultured with synoviocytes, there is a protective effect on articular cartilage degradation. Therefore one can conclude that cocultured systems using pure cells can be used to measure simultaneous effects from both tissues.[16]

Examples of in vitro studies that have been performed on tissues and cells include study of enrofloxacin on articular cartilage explants,[17] glucosamine and chondroitin on explants,[18,19] glucosamine alone on cells,[20,21] the effect of single-impact injury on articular cartilage explants,[22] the effects of nonsteroidal antiinflammatory drugs and herbal preparations on tissues,[23] and evaluation of corticosteroids and growth factors on articular cartilage.[24] These studies demonstrate the robustness of in vitro systems to study various medications and pathological events.

In addition to study of specific tissues and cells, the isolated joints can be used to study various factors. For instance, Hardy and colleagues developed an isolated perfused limb to study the physiological response of inflammation on joints.[25,26] In addition, Bragdon and colleagues used the same system to evaluate drug delivery.[27] This system is shown to work well to study the physiological response of the joint to various factors. This is mostly focused on the vascular and cell permeability response. In addition, cadaver limbs can also be used to study various physical responses of joints and limbs. Easton and I used an isolated forelimb to study loading patterns and the correlation of subchondral bone density in the fetlock joint of horses.[28] Briefly, the isolated forelimb was placed in a loading system and the preparation was loaded to variable fetlock joint angles, including that corresponding to galloping. Dye staining was then used to characterize the loading pattern in the third metacarpal bone, the proximal sesamoid bones, and the proximal phalanx. It has long been established that fractures can be studied with this type of system, as illustrated by distal radial fracture repair.[29]

In vitro experiments are relatively straightforward to perform and allow large numbers of repeats. Consequently the numbers are strong for statistical analysis. However, only one small portion of the disease process usually can be evaluated. Furthermore, the more tissues are removed from the natural joint environment, the greater the change in matrix metabolism and response to treatment.

In Vivo Studies

In vivo studies have been used for decades to study equine joint disease. The advantages of in vivo systems are that the cells and matrices are kept within the native environment and can be studied without the influence of harvest and culturing, and normal interaction among tissues can be maintained. The disadvantages are that live animals are humanely destroyed, and the costs can be prohibitive. In vivo studies are used for evaluating medications and articular cartilage healing techniques and for determining pathological responses to disease. An understanding of the clinical disease and an appreciation for strict experimental design are needed to produce useful in vivo models. In vivo studies in the horse have gained popularity because Frisbie and colleagues showed that equine articular cartilage is more similar to human cartilage than is cartilage from other species.[30]

Various inciting mechanisms can be used to induce experimental joint disease. For instance, synovitis models are used to evaluate the sequence of events that occurs and the influence of various drugs and medications. Change in gait, measurement of inflammatory mediators, assessment of articular cartilage matrix metabolism, and various clinical tests have been studied. Examples of these studies include injection of lipopolysaccharide,[1,31] interleukin-1,[26] sodium monoiodoacetate,[32,33] filipin,[2,34] polyvinyl alcohol foam particles,[35] carrageenan,[36] Freund's adjuvant,[37] blood,[38] and amphotericin[6] into joints. Of these models, those that use the natural inflammatory mediators, such as lipopolysaccharide and interleukin-1, seem to be the best for promoting the natural cycle of events in inflammation. The advantages of such studies are that they are quick, relatively well investigated, and replicate a common clinical problem.

Instability models also have been studied in horses. The purposes of these studies have been to determine the sequence of events that occurs within tissues because of instability and to induce osteoarthritis (OA).[15,25,39] Once OA has been induced, various treatments can be examined. An example of an instability model includes cutting the collateral and collateral sesamoidean ligaments in the metacarpophalangeal joints of horses.[39] Unlike in the dog, complete surgical transection of the cranial cruciate ligament in horses has not resulted in progressive OA.[40] Mild osteophyte formation occurred in these joints, but no progressive articular surface changes or lameness were appreciated. The results are unlike those in horses with naturally occurring cranial cruciate ligament damage, in which some horses are lame and substantial articular cartilage damage may result. Unlike synovitis models, instability models are relatively long term and represent an example of chronic, progressive disease.[41,42]

Forced exercise can also lead to changes in joint environment. Examples include evaluation of osteochondral tissues in response to various levels of exercise. Significant changes have been found in articular cartilage matrix biochemical and biomechanical properties in exercised horses compared with horses not exercised.[43] Strenuous exercise led to significant increases in calcified cartilage thickness, significant decreases in articular cartilage mechanical properties, and significant increases in fibronectin at the sites of degradation.[43-45] Treadmill exercise led to significant increase in clinical disease in the metacarpophalangeal joints of horses. This was detected grossly and using various imaging techniques.[46] Currently several studies are ongoing to evaluate the effects of exercise to determine the level of exercise most appropriate for protecting the tissues of the musculoskeletal system. At the EORC horses with experimentally induced OA are being compared with young normal horses that are exercised, in the hope of differentiating clinical and diagnostic test results in horses undergoing exercise-induced adaptation from those in horses with joint disease. There have been recent studies on the effects of exercise on foals, weanlings, and yearlings, to investigate whether early exercise will lead to stronger musculoskeletal tissues, with generally negative results.[47-53]

The osteochondral fragment model is a blend of in vivo models and involves inducing a clinically relevant disease (Editors' note: for racehorses, but not necessarily for other equine athletes) through creation of an osteochondral fragment and imposed exercise. Researchers at the EORC have used this model extensively, which induces progressive OA yet is benign enough to induce grade 1 to grade 3 lameness.[54] In addition, osteochondral fragments have been taken from the tarsocrural joint and implanted into the carpus and metacarpophalangeal joint to induce inflammation.[55]

Using the osteochondral fragment model various medications have been studied, including betamethasone,[56] intravenous hyaluronan,[57] triamcinolone acetonide,[58] and methylprednisolone acetate,[59] as have gene therapy for joint disease,[60] change of biomarkers with exercise,[61] and the effects of exercise on imaging outcomes.[62] The response to avocado and soybean unsaponifiables,[63] intraarticular autologous conditioned serum,[64] and the interleukin-1 receptor antagonist gene[65] have also been evaluated. Mechanical nociceptive thresholds have been determined.[66]

Models of disuse also have been shown to induce osteochondral damage. Disuse is a clinically relevant problem that induces articular cartilage and subchondral bone atrophy. Examples include a significant reduction in articular cartilage matrix metabolism in horses with a lower limb cast.[67] Furthermore, application of a cast for 7 weeks, followed by treadmill exercise, has been shown to lead to a significant increase in lameness in the limb with the cast and a significant decrease in bone formation.[68-70] Disuse models are important, because casts are used clinically and can lead to substantial problems after removal. Often the race is between healing and the degradative changes caused by disuse.

Models of articular cartilage healing have been studied extensively because of the need to test various modes of treatment in vivo. These models also have been stimulated by the cutting edge research being done by several equine research laboratories around the world and the fact that the horse is becoming more accepted as a model of articular cartilage healing for people. If an implant or technique can stimulate and maintain articular cartilage healing in a horse, then the thought is that the implant or technique should work in people. Several equine models are used to study joint healing. Besides the type of treatment that is tested, the models vary in the depth and size of articular cartilage defect formation. Partial-thickness and full-thickness articular cartilage, articular and calcified cartilage, and osteochondral defects have been evaluated in vivo and treated with various techniques.

The size and location of osteochondral lesions appear to have an effect on healing.[71] Small lesions in weight-bearing areas healed better than large lesions and lesions in non–weight-bearing areas. The physical characteristics of the lesions also affect healing. For instance, subchondral cystic lesions developed in horses with linear articular cartilage lesions but not in horses with elliptical lesions.[72] The subchondral defects did not fill in with bone. Trauma to the subchondral bone led to cyst formation.[73] The presence or absence of calcified cartilage also plays a role in articular cartilage healing. Calcified articular cartilage has reduced defect filling compared with defects without the presence of calcified cartilage.[74] However, the conclusion from that study and others was that calcified cartilage may provide support for improved healing. Consequently the influence of calcified cartilage on healing is currently being investigated.[75]

Various articular cartilage resurfacing treatments have been tested in vivo, including periosteal grafts,[76,77] sternal cartilage grafts,[78,79] mosaicplasty,[80] subchondral micropicking,[74] and cell-based grafting.[77] Sternal cartilage grafts have produced short-term benefits; however, significant degradation occurred after 4 months, with subchondral cyst formation.[78,79] Mosaicplasty has shown promise; however, harvest sites are needed to obtain tissue for implantation.[80,81] Subchondral bone micropicking may improve healing of osteochondral defects and is simple to perform.[74] Cell-based grafting may be beneficial, but it requires special equipment and advanced training to perform.[82,83] Other techniques that have been assessed in the horse include radiofrequency and mechanical debridement[84,85]; various growth factors in gene therapy[86,87]; and stem cell therapy.[88] The horse may be an ideal model for evaluation of stem cell therapy for human joints.[89]

Models of infectious arthritis also have been studied (see Chapter 65). For instance, studies have aimed at identifying the ability of certain medications to potentiate infection when injected along with a subinfective dose of bacteria. This work proved the clinical impression that polysulfated glycosaminoglycans increased the chances of infectious arthritis unless given with antibiotics.[90,91] Comparisons of various treatment methods used to treat infectious arthritis have also been performed.[92,93]

Biomechanical Models

Computerized models currently are being developed to study joint disease not only in people, but also in horses and other animals. Specifically, these models are derived from the geometry of the joints, the forces imparted by limb loading and muscle force, and the material properties of tendons, ligaments, and articular cartilage. Consequently, joint disease can be imitated on a computer and the resulting change in joint forces determined. These models also can be used to determine what changes in loading may be expected in horses with clinical disease. Surgical procedures can be inserted into the program, and the resulting forces evaluated.

In vivo work will not be replaced in the near future because it is the best means of evaluating tissue response to disease and treatment. However, newer in vitro systems and computer models are becoming more precise and better accepted by the research community and clinicians. In musculoskeletal modeling to characterize the forces that surround the joint[94-99] the goal is to create a finite element model of the joint of interest and input various loading parameters that are seen during exercise and may lead to injury.

Chapter 65

Infectious Arthritis and Fungal Infectious Arthritis

Alicia L. Bertone and Jennifer M. Cohen

▣ INFECTIOUS ARTHRITIS

Alicia L. Bertone

Classic clinical signs of infectious arthritis are heat and swelling and rapid development of non–weight-bearing lameness, often in less than 24 hours. The suspicion of joint infection increases if a predisposing risk factor is evident, such as prematurity, a high sepsis score, or multi-systemic disease in a foal[1,2] or preceding joint injection in an adult horse. Fracture and nonarticular infection (cellulitis or foot abscess) need to be differentiated from infectious arthritis, because in these diseases, acute, severe lameness also develops.[3,4]

CAUSES

Musculoskeletal infection was reported to cause death in 5.2% of 2468 foals.[5] Yearly morbidity was 27.4% (677 foals), and morbidity attributed to musculoskeletal infection was 2.1%. Septicemia was the second most common cause of death, and hematogenous spread was the most common cause of infectious arthritis.[6] Bacteremia with infectious arthritis in foals decreased survival.[7] The risk of infection was highest in the first 30 days postpartum and was lowest in practices that assessed the efficacy of transfer of passive immunity. Isolation of *Salmonella* species from synovial fluid and systemic disease were associated with an unfavorable prognosis for survival.[1]

In two retrospective studies of 153 mature horses[8,9] the most common causes of synovial infection were traumatic wounds (36.5% for joints and 55% for tendon sheaths), injections (34.1% and 22%), postoperative infection (1.0% for arthroscopy,[10] 19.8% overall for joints), and idiopathic causes (9.5% and 22%).[9] Standardbreds,[9] draft breeds,[10] and the tarsocrural joint[9,10] were overrepresented in adult horses with joint infection, reflecting a greater number of joint injections in these breeds and this joint.

Of 424 bacterial isolates from 233 horses with joint, tendon sheath, or bone infection, 91% were aerobic or facultative anaerobes. The most common organisms were Enterobacteriaceae (28.8%), followed by streptococci (13%) and staphylococci (11.8%).[11] In foals, Enterobacteriaceae including *Escherichia coli* and *Staphylococcus* species[1,12] were more likely to be isolated. Staphylococci, specifically *Staphylococcus aureus,* are the most common organisms isolated from infections occurring after surgery or injections. Foals or horses with infectious arthritis secondary to penetrating wounds are likely to have multiple bacterial infections. *Clostridium* species have been isolated from foals[13] and were the most common anaerobes isolated, particularly from wounds near the hoof.[11] Fungal or mycobacterial organisms are a rare cause of infectious arthritis but can be considered pathogens if identified in pure culture more than once (see later).[14,15] Reactive arthritis in foals with septicemia from *Rhodococcus equi* or subsequent to injection reactions can be confused with infectious arthritis, but lameness usually is not prominent, and synovial fluid nucleated cell counts are often within normal limits.[16,17]

EXAMINATION AND INITIAL MANAGEMENT

Potential infectious arthritis must be considered an emergency and is treated most effectively with early diagnosis. A systematic approach should include hematological examination; measurement of plasma fibrinogen; synovial fluid analysis, including cytological examination, Gram stain, and synovial fluid culture (up to 5 mL of synovial fluid in a broth culture bottle); and radiography.[3] In foals, particularly those with abnormal sepsis scores, blood culture should be performed simultaneously. In adult horses, systemic blood examination is less rewarding than in foals, particularly in the early phases of clinical signs. In horses with experimental infectious arthritis, elevations in leukocyte count and total protein and fibrinogen concentrations have been found to take several days to develop and were changed significantly from baseline values for individual horses, but they remained in the normal range

References on page 1308

for all horses.[18] Before arthrocentesis is performed, surgical scrub materials, sterile gloves, needles, syringes, broth culture bottles, ethylenediamine tetraacetic acid (EDTA) or heparin tubes for cytological examinations, smear slides for Gram stain, and a dose of antimicrobial agents to instill directly into the joint after sampling should be available (see the following discussion).

Adult horses should be sedated. Foals can be placed in lateral recumbency with administration of an α_2-agonist and synthetic narcotic combination. Although data suggest that aseptic preparation of unclipped hair may be adequate and may significantly decrease bacterial counts on the skin,[19] clipping the site for arthrocentesis is strongly recommended. In horses with periarticular wounds, arthrocentesis should be performed well away from the wound to avoid the risk of joint contamination, if the joint is not contaminated already from the wound. To determine if a joint and wound communicate, the clinician should infuse 50 to 200 mL of balanced electrolyte solution into the joint after a synovial fluid sample has been obtained for culture and cytological examination. The clinician should watch closely for leakage of fluid from the wound. This is easier than using blue dye injections or contrast radiography. The joint should be drained and antibiotic instilled into the joint after samples have been obtained and any lavage or injection of fluid completed. Samples should be submitted immediately for evaluation.

If the joint fluid is grossly cloudy, turbid, or flocculent, broad-spectrum antibiotics initially should be given intravenously (IV), and ingress and egress or through-and-through lavage of the joint should be performed until diagnosis of infectious arthritis can be confirmed. Antibiotic should be instilled into the joint after lavage has been completed. If a wound or puncture is the inciting cause, endoscopic evaluation of the synovial cavity is recommended. In one study of 95 contaminated or infected joints, 43% had intraarticular foreign material found at endoscopy.[20]

DIAGNOSIS

Gross evaluation of the synovial fluid can be informative. If newspaper print cannot be read through the fluid sample, it probably has a cell count of at least 30×10^9 nucleated cells per liter. Fluid from infected joints is usually turbid, cloudy, and watery. Flocculence develops in chronically infected joints or joints that have been invaded with a needle or surgery. Blood contamination makes gross assessment of synovial fluid difficult, and determining if infection is present without clinicopathological analysis is often impossible. Serosanguineous fluid commonly is obtained from infected joints (Figure 65-1). An estimate of the amount of blood (packed cell volume [PCV]) or red blood cell count) can be made to correct for the number of nucleated cells contaminating the sample (hemorrhage from arthrocentesis or leakage of blood from the infection):

$$\frac{PCV\ (\%)\ of\ synovial\ fluid}{Actual\ or\ estimated\ PCV\ (\%)\ of\ blood} = \frac{X\ (WBCs \times 10^9/L\ in\ synovial\ fluid)}{Actual\ or\ estimated\ WBCs \times 10^9/L\ blood}$$

where WBCs are white blood cells.

Synovial fluid nucleated cell count, differential cell count, and total protein concentration are the most useful

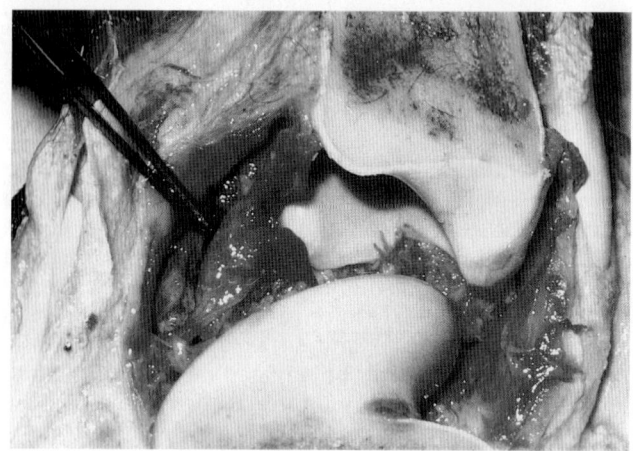

Fig. 65-1 • At postmortem examination, hemorrhagic synovitis associated with acute joint infection is seen in this tarsocrural joint.

parameters to evaluate in diagnosing infectious arthritis. Although other biomarkers, such as lactate, metalloproteinases, and myeloperoxidase activity, have been found to be increased in synovial fluid from infected joints, most correlate with the nucleated cell count.[18,21,22] Synovial fluid nucleated cell counts in excess of 30×10^9 cells/L, with more than 80% neutrophils, or total protein concentration in excess of 40 g/L are considered consistent with infection, particularly if these synovial fluid parameters correlate with clinical signs and predisposing circumstances.[3,23] The likelihood of isolating the causative organism is correlated positively to the nucleated cell count—that is, higher nucleated cell counts are associated with greater isolation rates.[23] Approximately 25% of samples from horses suspected of having infectious arthritis have bacteria on Gram stain, confirming infection and offering the added benefit of assisting with identifying the organism and the initial selection of an antimicrobial agent.[18]

For horses that do not meet obvious criteria for infectious arthritis, assessment of all parameters is necessary to conclude that the joint is infected. It is important to note that joints can be infected with nucleated cell counts lower than 30×10^9/L. Infection should be suspected if nucleated cell counts are 10×10^9/L to 30×10^9/L and fluid is not serosanguineous, clinical signs of substantial lameness exist, fluid is flocculent (coagulating cells may falsely lower the measured cell count), a predisposing cause for infection is present (septicemia, surgery, or joint injection), and protein concentration exceeds 40 g/L. Previous intraarticular treatment with corticosteroids may delay onset of clinical signs and confuse interpretation of nucleated cell counts and total protein concentration in the acute phase.[24,25]

Synovial fluid protein levels continue to increase in chronically infected joints to more than 60 g/L in some horses.[18] Few other differential diagnoses, other than infection, produce significant elevations in total protein concentration (>50 g/L). Isolation of a pure culture of a single organism, particularly a known pathogen, such as a coagulase-positive *Staphylococcus* species, almost always indicates infection is present, even if the nucleated cell count is low.

In horses with chronic infectious arthritis refractory to aggressive treatment, nucleated cell counts can be low (5 to 10×10^9/L), but organisms, usually *Staphylococcus*, can still be isolated. In these horses the synovial fluid protein values are often high (>50 g/L) and other clinical signs of infectious arthritis (lameness, effusion, and heat) persist. In my experience these are horses that developed infectious arthritis after injection with a corticosteroid, were treated with systemic antibiotics and lavage but not aggressive drainage, have a nidus of infected subchondral bone that keeps seeding the joint, or have a joint with severe cartilage erosion.

The distribution of nucleated cells in synovial fluid is an important aid to diagnosis. In horses with early infectious arthritis, nucleated cells almost always consist of more than 80% neutrophils and commonly more than 90% neutrophils. The neutrophils usually appear healthy and not degenerate, although in overwhelming or aggressive infection, degeneration of neutrophils is seen. If synovial fluid has less than 75% neutrophils, infection is usually resolving.

Techniques that may be useful clinically in the future for diagnosis include polymerase chain reaction (PCR) analysis for detecting base pairs of bacterial or viral DNA in the synovial fluid[26,27] and determining enzyme and cytokine release that may be compatible with infection.[28-30] Benefits of PCR include rapid (<24 hours), sensitive testing that can detect selected species of bacteria in the presence of antimicrobial drugs. PCR diagnostic techniques are sensitive because they amplify small quantities of bacterial DNA. Inherent in high sensitivity, however, is a possible high false-positive rate, because of skin contamination or contamination with bacteria at the time of arthrocentesis. Future clinical use and evaluation of this technique are expected.

Identification of enzyme/cytokine ratios or quantity may be specific for infection, because infection is the largest joint challenge that exists. Knowledge of the presence and interaction of mediators and inhibitors in joints is growing rapidly and is an active area of research. For further information on this aspect of joint infection, the reader is referred to other publications.[28,30]

It is important to determine whether bone or physeal involvement is concomitant, particularly in foals with refractory infectious arthritis. In most foals with bone involvement, radiolucent changes occur rapidly and are often detectable within 1 week after onset of clinical signs. In most bones, radiological changes may be apparent in 7 to 10 days, but if the small cuboidal bones of the carpus or tarsus are involved, the clinician may face an even greater diagnostic challenge. Infarction associated with infection may slow bone resorption, and evidence of radiolucency may lag for several days.

Nuclear scintigraphy may be useful to locate foci of infected bone, particularly in identifying involvement of subclinical sites of infection in polyarthritic foals, but the technique has practical restrictions. Normal bone scans or radiolabeled white cell studies can be performed (see Chapter 19). The foal becomes radioactive, and handling of the foal, blood samples, and synovial fluid samples poses a small risk to attendants. In addition, if the joints surrounding the small bones are infected, the resolution of the scan may be inadequate to identify specific bone involvement. Magnetic resonance imaging offers promise of improved identification of osteomyelitis[31,32] and has

become available at many referral hospitals. Osteomyelitis is present in up to 59% of foals with infectious arthritis, but a favorable prognosis still can be achieved with treatment,[1] although the prognosis for athletic function is reduced when adjacent bone is involved or infectious arthritis is protracted.

In adult horses with acute-onset lameness associated with a wound, radiological examination should be performed to rule out the presence of radiodense foreign material or concurrent traumatic osseous injury. In the absence of a wound, if lameness has already been present for some days, radiological examination is warranted to determine if there are any bony changes, which will prompt early arthroscopic evaluation and debridement. Radiological examination is also indicated in a horse that has failed to show progressive improvement after instigation of appropriate management. The presence of radiolucent areas is indicative of likely bone infection, which warrants a more guarded prognosis, especially if progressive.

ANTIMICROBIAL THERAPY

Systemic Therapy

Intravenous antimicrobial therapy should be initiated immediately, before bacterial culture results are available. Systemic administration of broad-spectrum antimicrobial drugs should be combined with the local administration of antimicrobial agents. Most common combinations include penicillin with an aminoglycoside or a third-generation cephalosporin such as ceftiofur sodium or cefotaxime.[33] In a retrospective study of equine musculoskeletal infections, gentamicin and amikacin were effective against 85% and 95% of equine isolates, respectively, indicating that they are good choices for initial combination therapy.[11] Antimicrobial drugs given orally should be reserved for infection that is resolving, because gastrointestinal absorption is erratic, and blood and tissue levels are lower. Oral enrofloxacin is used to treat chronic bone and synovial infections in mature horses without reported incident, but enrofloxacin is not currently approved for use in horses. Enrofloxacin (Baytril 100) administered IV at 5 mg/kg once daily is effective and safe in mature (3 years of age and older) horses.[34] Enrofloxacin may cause lameness and cartilage lesions in foals and should not be used.[35] Enrofloxacin should not be administered to lactating mares, because the milk may concentrate the drug and subject the foal to chondrotoxic doses. (Editor's note [MWR]: In several horses orally administered enrofloxacin has not been effective at managing infectious arthritis, even when testing has suggested that in vitro susceptibility is present.)

Antimicrobial drugs should be given IV and in general at a dosage interval that maximizes peak serum levels and sustains trough levels that are at or above the minimum inhibitory concentration (MIC) for the isolated organism. Serum antimicrobial peak and trough measurements should be periodically checked to maximize effectiveness and minimize toxicity (see the following discussion).

Aminoglycoside administered once daily may be most effective, producing a large serum aminoglycoside concentration and a greater bactericidal effect than more frequent administration.[36] The aminoglycoside postantibiotic effect (duration of sustained antimicrobial killing) is concentration dependent. With a single daily dose, trough levels are lower than with repeated administration, thus lowering the risk of toxicity. Using in vivo models of infectious osteomyelitis, improved efficacy of gentamicin was demonstrated using once-daily administration (6.6 mg/kg body mass IV) compared with three-times-a-day administration (2.2 mg/kg body mass IV). In normal horses, gentamicin (administered at 6.6 mg/kg body mass once daily for 10 days) did not induce signs of nephrotoxicity and prolonged the postantibiotic effect.[37] Therefore gentamicin and other aminoglycosides should be administered once daily in horses. However, the pharmacokinetics of aminoglycosides are altered in septic and premature hypoxic foals.[38] Serum drug concentrations should be measured to adjust dosage intervals. Sepsis score and creatinine concentration are inversely correlated to amikacin clearance in foals and could be useful indicators of altered drug disposition and delayed clearance.[39] The dosage interval may need to be lengthened beyond 24 hours in these foals to avoid toxicity because of higher trough concentrations. In septic neonatal foals, administration of gentamicin at 3.3 mg/kg twice daily IV produced peak serum concentrations of more than 6 mcg/mL and trough concentration less than 2 mcg/mL in all foals without toxicity or development of new sites of infection.[40]

The drug must have excellent diffusion into the joint.[8] Most antimicrobial drugs penetrate the synovium in therapeutic concentrations when administered systemically at recommended doses.[4] Concentrations of aminoglycosides actually may be greater in inflamed joints compared with normal joints.[41] If systemic blood trough levels drop below the MIC for that antimicrobial drug, synovial fluid concentrations may also drop below the MIC. Local antimicrobial drug administration (intraarticular), used to sustain high drug concentrations at the site of infection, may be most effective in both killing bacteria and penetrating organic debris.

Most positive synovial fluid cultures will be so within 24 hours after onset of infection, and a Gram stain can be immediately helpful. An additional 24 hours is usually needed to confirm the identity and susceptibility pattern of the organism. In my opinion, a broad-spectrum antimicrobial drug should be administered initially and continued at least until clinical signs begin to resolve substantially. Some joints may contain single or several organisms that were not isolated, particularly if infection was caused by a wound or by septicemia. Joints may be open, or repeatedly invaded during treatment, or a foal may be at risk for continued showers of bacteremia, thereby increasing the risk of a shift in causative organism in the middle of treatment.

Local Therapy

For years local administration of antimicrobial agents was considered taboo, because solutions varied in pH and were believed to be injurious to tissues. The deleterious effects of local antibiotic administration were greatly overemphasized, and one of the most substantial advances in the management of horses with infectious arthritis and osteomyelitis has been the implementation of local antimicrobial therapy. High tissue concentration of antimicrobial agents causes rapid elimination of joint and bone infections.[42,43] Many innovative methods are being explored to provide high local antimicrobial drug levels. Administration of

systemic antimicrobial agents remains an important adjunctive therapy, but it is recognized that tissue concentrations at the site of infection may be considerably lower than those achieved with local administration of drugs (at or below the MIC for the organism), and therefore systemic administration is less effective.[44]

Direct Local Infusion of Antimicrobial Drugs

Intraarticular injection of antimicrobial drugs into an infected joint every 24 hours is effective for early infectious arthritis. Intracarpal administration of 150 mg gentamicin has been found to maintain synovial fluid gentamicin concentrations well above the MIC for most equine pathogens (2 mcg/mL) for 24 hours.[42,45] Most antimicrobial drugs, including penicillin, the cephalosporins, and aminoglycosides, are minimally irritating.

Appropriate intraarticular doses of antimicrobial drugs are not scientifically identified, but anecdotally up to 500 mg gentamicin, 250 mg amikacin, 1×10^6 units of sodium penicillin, 500 mg cefazolin, and 500 mg ceftiofur sodium have been used without reported difficulties. Fluoroquinolones should not be used because at high concentrations the drugs are toxic to chondrocytes.[46]

Topical lavage of an infected joint or osteomyelitic bone is beneficial for the removal of infected organic debris, destructive enzymes, and neutrophils, but the inclusion of antimicrobial or antiseptic compounds in the lavage solution is still of questionable benefit. An increase in the local antimicrobial drug concentration is expected after lavage with antimicrobial drugs, but most of the drug leaves the joint with the lavage solution. Injection of antimicrobial drugs at the termination of lavage is probably more efficient. Use of antiseptics and potentiated antiseptics (EDTA and Tris buffer) in lavage may kill surface bacteria, but sustained killing is expected to be limited.[47] Even dilute antiseptic compounds such as 0.05% chlorhexidine can be irritating to equine joints.[48]

Antimicrobial-Impregnated Biomaterials

One of the most practical methods for maintaining slow but effective release of antimicrobial agents in bone and joint infections is the intraarticular insertion of impregnated polymethylmethacrylate (PMMA) beads.[49] In a study of 1085 open limb fractures in people, the postoperative infection rate was significantly reduced, from 12% to 3.7%, when aminoglycoside PMMA beads were inserted at surgery.[50] PMMA impregnated with aminoglycoside and cefazolin was used in horses with open fractures and with bone, implant, and joint infections, and survival rate was about 60%.[51,52] In 12 horses with infectious arthritis treated with gentamicin-impregnated PMMA beads and lavage, including six with osteomyelitis, 92% survived.[53] Several antimicrobial drugs were shown to elute from PMMA in active concentrations, including aminoglycosides such as amikacin and gentamicin, and fluoroquinolones such as ciprofloxacin.[43,53-55] Use of fluoroquinolones in PMMA is not currently recommended in joints, because the concentrations expected to be released with local therapy may be toxic to equine chondrocytes.[46]

Implants (beads) can be prepared in the operating room, or beads can be gas sterilized and stored for future use. The antimicrobial compound (1 or 2 g of powder or liquid) is mixed thoroughly with 20 to 40 g of PMMA (medical grade) and shaped as desired. Beads can be placed on suture material to assist with retrieval from the joint. The beads can be placed into the joint through an arthrotomy, which is usually left open to drain. If infection recrudesces, existing beads can be exchanged with fresh ones or with those impregnated with different antimicrobial agents. Small beads (4 × 6 mm) can be placed through arthroscopic portals or cannulas, thus avoiding arthrotomy. Arthrotomy, however, can also assist with joint drainage if left open to heal by contraction and epithelialization. In my experience, if infection is rapidly eliminated, the beads can be difficult if not impossible to retrieve. Beads frequently migrate to a joint pouch and become enveloped by synovium. If the arthrotomy heals quickly, the beads may need to be removed surgically. Occasionally beads well removed from articular surfaces can be left in place permanently. Long-term sequelae appear minimal, but studies to date have not been performed. Complications with PMMA implants include the use of too many or too large beads, causing soft tissue trauma and pain, failure to exchange beads in unresolving infection, and placement of beads under tendons and on articular cartilage. If osteomyelitis exists, lesions can be debrided and lavaged, and beads can be implanted directly into the bone bed. Beads placed directly into bone lesions are usually removed without difficulty.

Addition of antimicrobial compounds to PMMA alters the biomechanics of PMMA, particularly when liquid forms are used. For purposes of treating joint infection, accuracy in drug elution and biomechanical properties of the PMMA are not critical. Use of the PMMA in orthopedic implants may require more precise preparation of implant material. The elution rate of antimicrobial drugs varies with size and shape of the implant, the amount of antimicrobial agent impregnated, and the type and form of antimicrobial drug selected and depends on thorough and even mixing of the formulation.

Antimicrobial-Impregnated Biodegradable Drug Delivery Systems

Although PMMA offers advantages for local antibiotic delivery, its permanency is not ideal, particularly for certain tissue types. Many biodegradable compounds have been investigated as possible implants for antimicrobial drug delivery, most notably collagen,[56,57] DL–lactide-glycolide copolymers, polyanhydrides, polylactide, sebacic acid, tricalcium phosphate and calcium carbonate bone cement, and plaster of Paris.[58-63] Because of the ongoing degradation a greater amount and duration of antimicrobial drug release can be achieved. In a study using rabbits with infectious osteomyelitis, bacterial counts were significantly lower in those treated with gentamicin-polyanhydride implants than in those treated with gentamicin-PMMA implants.[60]

In horses, 50:50 DL–lactide-glycolide copolymers and poly(DL)lactide impregnated with gentamicin that eluted for 10 days eliminated infection of synovial explants in vitro without significant detrimental effects on synovial cell function (hyaluronan production), morphology, or viability.[58] In horses with experimentally induced *Staphylococcus* joint infection, intraarticular treatment with C44 fatty acid–sebacic acid (1:1) beads impregnated 20% with gentamicin as the sole treatment effectively eliminated joint infection in 33% of joints by day 3 and 66% of joints

by day 13.[62] Lameness significantly improved. Gentamicin concentration peaked at 82 mcg/mL at 24 hours after insertion of beads and remained higher than 10 mcg/mL for 12 days (range of 5 to 41 times the MIC for the organism).[62] Currently these implants are being investigated for clinical use, but they are not yet commercially available. Plaster of Paris beads may offer a practical option for degradable implants, but biocompatibility studies should be performed.[63]

Regional Perfusion

Regional perfusion can be used to deliver therapeutic concentrations of antimicrobial agents to a selected region of the limb, usually using the venous system for drug administration with horses under anesthesia or sedated. Drugs also can be administered using an intraosseous route.[64] In either case a tourniquet is applied proximal to the infected bone or joint for approximately 30 minutes (Figure 65-2). Concentrations of gentamicin obtained in synovial fluid rose to a peak of 589 mcg/mL immediately after regional perfusion and declined to 4.8 mcg/mL at 24 hours.[65] This technique was used to decrease WBC numbers in infected synovial fluid in experimentally induced equine arthritis and is most practical if applied when the horse is anesthetized for other treatment of infection, such as debridement and lavage, when intraosseous infusion can be performed simultaneously.[66] Advantages of this technique include the use of antimicrobial drugs that may be toxic if administered systemically (vancomycin)[67] or directly into the joint (enrofloxacin),[68] the ability to repeat daily injections, and distribution to the entire limb including bone. Limitations include the development of vasculitis, difficult identification of the vein, and the discomfort of a tourniquet and infusion of antimicrobial drugs. Perineural analgesia can be performed. Intraarticular antimicrobial drug concentrations using intravenous regional infusion are

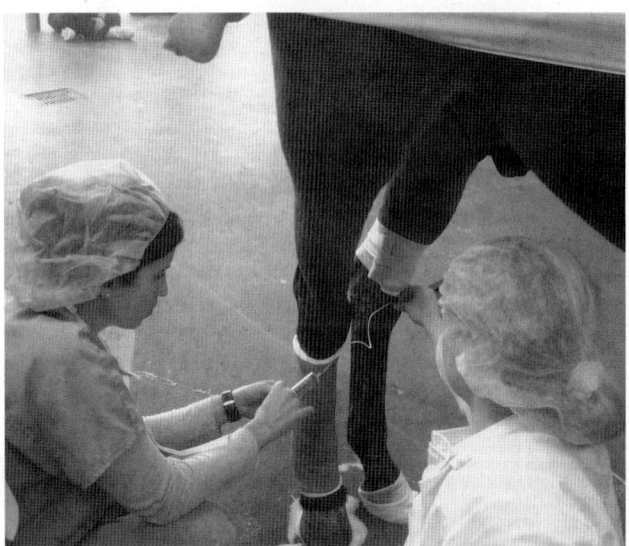

Fig. 65-2 • Use of regional limb perfusion to deliver an antimicrobial drug into an infected tarsocrural joint. The tourniquet above the joint permits retrograde infusion of the saphenous vein. Concentrations of antimicrobial drugs above the minimum inhibitory concentration for most organisms that cause musculoskeletal infection can be maintained for 24 hours. The tourniquet is maintained for 30 minutes and then removed.

not as high as those obtained with direct intraarticular injection.[45,69]

Bone concentration of antimicrobial agents is similar after intraarticular injection or regional perfusion.[69] In foals with infectious arthritis and adjacent osteomyelitis, either delivery method should effectively provide bone antimicrobial concentrations, but for foals with numerous joint or bone sites affected, regional perfusion offers an advantage. Intraarticular administration relies on drug diffusion through cartilage or local blood supply to reach bone. Caution should be used when applying tourniquets in foals, because even short durations of application can induce clinical signs of distal limb ischemia. In foals with compromised bone blood flow from swelling and toxic effects of infection, this may be detrimental. I have seen two foals develop severe osteonecrosis after repeated regional perfusion procedures, a complication attributed to tourniquet application.

Balloon Constant Rate Infusion Systems

Constant rate infusion (CRI) of antimicrobial drugs, with or without local anesthetic solution, can be administered by commercial systems designed to deliver a constant rate of a therapeutic agent. These systems typically come as kits, and tubing is placed intraarticularly, usually at the initial arthroscopic evaluation and debridement of the infected joint. The reservoir (balloon) for the therapeutic agent(s) can be secured to the limb and aseptically refilled as needed (Figure 65-3). These systems have been reported to provide a clinical response and long-term outcome similar to other techniques for treatment of equine infectious synovitis.[70] Use of local anesthetic solution in CRI systems is controversial for joints because both lidocaine hydrochloride and mepivacaine hydrochloride have demonstrated chondrocyte toxicity when in direct contact in culture.[71,72]

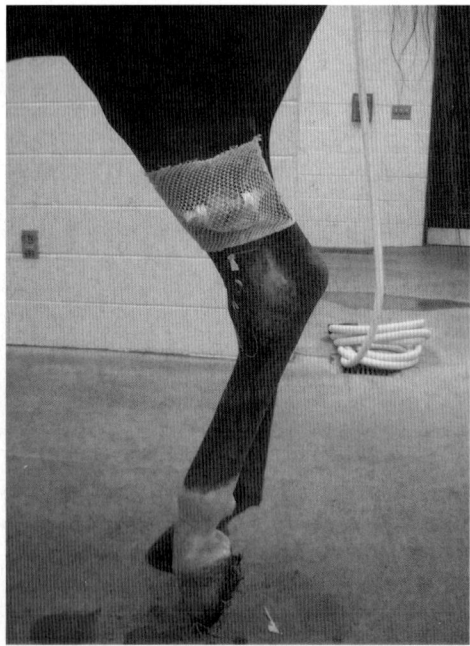

Fig. 65-3 • A horse with an infected tarsocrural joint with a constant rate infusion balloon system installed to deliver an antimicrobial drug directly into the joint. The reservoir balloon is refilled daily.

JOINT DRAINAGE AND DEBRIDEMENT

Joint lavage and drainage are vital for the effective management of infectious arthritis.[1,4,6,8,20] Ideally, arthroscopic evaluation should be performed to remove foreign material and fibrin and to assess cartilage health. Removal of angry, infected synovium may reduce bacterial count and a source of infection. Healthy synovium should not be removed, because it may help combat the infection and may normalize joint health. In horses, maximal synovectomy has been found to be no better than open arthrotomy for management of infectious arthritis.[73] After synovectomy villous structures may not be regained for many months.[73-76] Repeated through-and-through lavage using needles placed on opposite sides of a joint can be effective in eliminating infection in some horses, but the lavage fluid may completely bypass some areas of a joint, allowing the infection to persist. Arthroscopy permits more thorough lavage of the entire joint, and together with a form of continued joint drainage, provides the most complete and rapid method to remove infective material and to estimate the extent of damage.[4,8,20]

Arthroscopic portals can be enlarged to function effectively as open arthrotomy incisions for continued drainage, or closed suction drainage can be initiated. The goal of either technique is continued joint decompression and drainage. Arthrotomies usually heal without complication and with minimal scarring. With continued infection, arthrotomies stay open and may develop excessive granulation or fibrous tissue, but this complication may occur with other methods of chronic drainage as well. Open drainage in joints that cannot be bandaged, such as the stifle, can be performed by tying up the horses using crossties or an overhead wire. Adhesive bandages applied using ether can be used to cover open drainage sites. I have not seen substantial permanent complications associated with arthrotomy and open drainage. Open arthrotomy can be used to insert PMMA beads for treatment of osteomyelitis or in horses with refractory infection.

Properly managed closed suction drainage is useful for large joints such as the tarsocrural and scapulohumeral joints, using a flat, fenestrated, latex drain. The drain should be tunneled under the skin to exit at a site removed from the joint. Negative pressure is applied using a large syringe, with a large guarded needle passed through the syringe to keep the plunger retracted.[77] The syringe is evacuated several times a day, and the drain is left in place until only small volumes of fluid are collected or the fluid appears relatively normal grossly and cytologically, and lameness improves. If the suction system fails, the drain is removed.

After initial debridement, lavage, and establishment of drainage, the joint can be flushed and local antimicrobial drug therapy applied daily, usually for 3 days. If clinical improvement is dramatic, further lavage is optional, but local antimicrobial injection should continue for 3 days. If clinical improvement continues, local antimicrobial therapy is discontinued. The joint is then rested for 24 hours and the synovial fluid is reassessed. Ideally, follow-up synovial fluid contains fewer than 15×10^9 nucleated cells/L, but irritation from aggressive lavage and intraarticular antimicrobial compounds can result in higher cell counts.

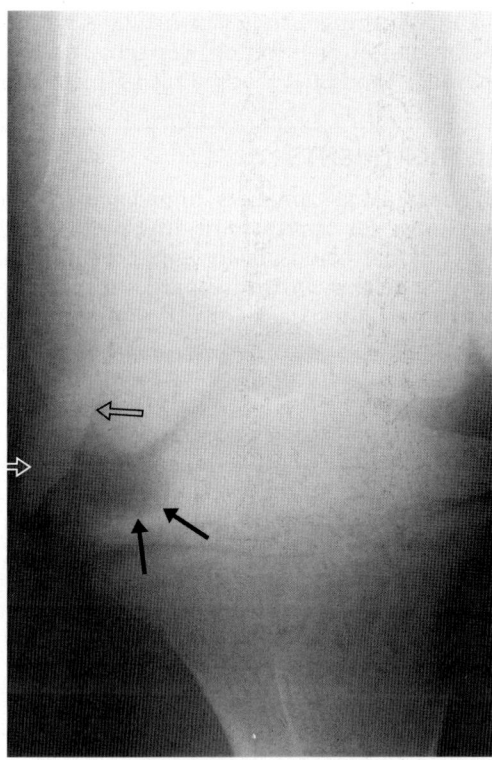

Fig. 65-4 • Craniocaudal radiographic image of a foal's stifle joint demonstrating radiolucency of the medial tibial plateau *(solid black arrows)* that was debrided arthroscopically and a singular polymethylmethacrylate bead *(open arrows)* was placed intraarticularly.

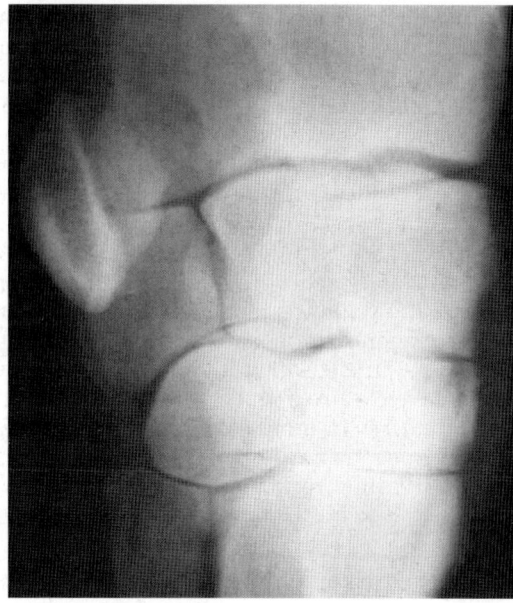

Fig. 65-5 • Dorsolateral-palmaromedial radiographic image of a carpus of a Standardbred racehorse with infectious osteomyelitis and necrosis of the dorsomedial aspect of the third carpal bone. The infection occurred subsequent to an intraarticular injection.

Clinical improvement is assessed by evaluating rectal temperature, lameness, and heat over the joint surface. The synovial fluid nucleated cell counts should decline slowly over the next 7 days if infection remains under control. If nucleated cell counts rise again or if lameness recurs, lavage and local antimicrobial therapy can be reinstituted. Having to perform two series of lavage procedures (3 days each time) in foals is typical.

Articular Osteomyelitis

Fifty percent of foals with infectious arthritis also have osteomyelitis or bone necrosis.[1,8,9,13] Usually bone is infected, but bone infarction can also occur. These foals are best treated using arthroscopic debridement, and joint infection usually clears within days of removal of infected bone. The importance of arthroscopic debridement cannot be overemphasized. In young foals with severe joint distention, lesions that would not normally be amenable to arthroscopic evaluation and debridement become accessible, such as those involving the tibial plateau (Figure 65-4), caudal aspect of the humeral head, or coxofemoral joint. In my experience infection or necrosis of the tarsal bones and some aspects of the carpal bones is the most difficult to treat, because they are not directly accessible using arthroscopy. Insertion of PMMA beads close to the distal tarsal joints and prolonged systemic antimicrobial administration may be successful.

In adult horses with articular osteomyelitis it is critical to debride the infected bone as soon as the condition is recognized radiologically (Figure 65-5). In chronic, progressive, infectious osteomyelitis in adult horses, arthrodesis,

joint resection, or stimulated ankylosis with a bone graft may be the only way to eliminate joint pain.[78-81] Infection of implants does not always occur. Bone infection can resolve with prolonged antimicrobial drug therapy, but joint immobilization is important to assist with elimination of infective organisms.

PAIN MANAGEMENT
Nonsteroidal Antiinflammatory Drugs

In a rabbit model of infectious arthritis caused by *Staphylococcus*, use of nonsteroidal antiinflammatory drugs (NSAIDs) with antimicrobial drugs significantly reduced joint swelling, prostaglandin E_2 release, and collagen joint destruction compared with the administration of antimicrobial drugs alone.[82] In mature horses phenylbutazone administration (4.4 to 8.8 mg/kg body mass daily) is commonly used to reduce pain and joint inflammation. Risk of laminitis in the supporting limbs of lame horses is an important consideration in treatment of infectious arthritis. Cyclooxygenase-2 (COX-2) inhibitors are approved for use in horses and seem promising at reducing the risk of toxic side effects, such as gastrointestinal ulcers and nephrotoxicity, seen with currently marketed NSAIDs.[83] COX-2 inhibitors reduce the production of inducible prostaglandin E_2 without suppressing the constitutive form of prostaglandin E_2 that protects epithelial mucosa homeostasis. Administration of NSAIDs in horses with infectious arthritis must be titrated to allow for the accurate assessment of joint pain as an indicator of clinical response to treatment. Most currently available NSAIDs marketed for use in horses, or used off label in horses, have been demonstrated to suppress equine synovial membrane inflammation and prostaglandin E_2 release in culture experiments.[84,85]

Dimethyl sulfoxide (DMSO) solution (10% to 40%) has been used experimentally to treat synovitis and clinically to treat infectious arthritis in horses.[4] Lavage or intraarticular injection of up to 40% DMSO does not appear to have clinically significant negative effects on articular cartilage. DMSO is a free radical scavenger, antiseptic, and analgesic and may inhibit chemotaxis of inflammatory cells. Practically, DMSO can be used in lavage fluid, particularly in the last liter of lavage. Because of the high solubility of DMSO, some residual drug probably is absorbed into the synovium during lavage.

Epidural Narcotics

Placement of indwelling epidural catheters and chronic infusion of α_2-agonists and narcotics such as morphine have been useful in alleviating hindlimb lameness and in horses with severe pain secondary to infectious arthritis (see Chapter 85).[86,87] In horses with chronic osteomyelitis or refractory infectious arthritis, this technique may be useful in preventing recumbency or supporting limb laminitis.

TOPICAL TREATMENT, BANDAGING, AND ALTERNATIVE THERAPY

Diclofenac topical medications can be directly applied to swollen and painful joints as antiinflammatory agents. DMSO applied topically to horses with experimentally induced carpal synovitis has significantly reduced synovial fluid nucleated cell counts.[88] DMSO was detectable in the synovial fluid of five of six horses and in the plasma of one of six horses, indicating its penetration of the tissues from topical application.[88] Topical application over infected joints may reduce synovitis.

Pressure bandages applied to reduce swelling also can reduce joint pain. Edema formation can be overwhelming in horses with infected joints and produce stiffness, discomfort, elevated synovial fluid production (joint pressure), and poor joint clearance of infected material through the lymphatic system. Pressure bandages should be sterile, particularly when covering open arthrotomy incisions.

Once acute inflammation has resolved, passive flexion is indicated to enhance lymph flow, improve drainage, reduce edema, and enhance joint range of motion. Capsulitis associated with infection can be a substantial complication, and physiotherapy to restore joint function can be critical to improving long-term outcome and joint motion.

PROGNOSIS

Adult horses with infectious arthritis have a good prognosis for survival and for return to athletic function, provided that infection is recognized early. In most horses infection is eliminated.[4,8,9,53] Preexisting osteoarthritis and articular cartilage damage are the most common reasons for failure to return to performance. Prompt recognition, aggressive drainage and lavage, and early treatment with local antimicrobial drugs have steadily improved prognosis to more than 80%[8] and hopefully success rates close to 100% will be possible. Aggressive surgical debridement and use of implantable elution materials for chronic administration and multiple site delivery of antimicrobial agents have improved prognoses. The prognosis in foals is more guarded. In one study septicemia, osteomyelitis, and hypogammaglobulinemia resulted in a lower prognosis for life in foals compared with adults, and infection was eliminated

in only 50%.[9] In other studies of neonates[1,13] and adult horses,[8] elimination of infection was achieved in 70%,[1,8] 50% survived,[8,13] and 30% reached racing performance.[1]

FUTURE TREATMENTS

Newer biodegradable polymers impregnated with antimicrobial drugs for direct joint insertion through an arthroscopic portal could greatly enhance the process of sustained drug delivery. Arthroscopic instrumentation can be used to insert the beads into the joints of standing horses.

Medical therapies for intraarticular drug therapy in the future may focus on prevention of *S. aureus* adhesion. A prominent feature of *S. aureus* virulence is the production of a bacterial surface marker that recognizes adhesive matrix molecules in collagen, precipitating bacterial adherence.[89,90] Monoclonal antibody, receptor antagonists, and vaccination challenges reduce the risk of acquiring infection with *S. aureus* in experimental animals.[89,91] These therapies may also be useful in the horse, because *S. aureus* is the most common cause of joint infection in adult horses.

■ FUNGAL INFECTIOUS ARTHRITIS
Jennifer M. Cohen

LITERATURE REVIEW

Unlike bacterial infectious arthritis, which occurs commonly in horses,[1-4] there are few reports in the equine literature describing infectious arthritis caused by fungi. As with bacteria, fungi can invade a synovial structure by direct inoculation from an exogenous source (secondary to trauma, surgery, or joint injection), by hematogenous spread, or by direct extension from an adjacent focus.[5] Predisposing factors to fungal infectious arthritis in people include previous (often repeated) intraarticular injection of glucocorticoids, severe systemic illness, long-term administration of systemic antibiotics, treatment with immunosuppressive agents, joint prostheses, and intravenous drug abuse.[5-7] In the equine literature there is reference to fungal infectious arthritis in only six adult horses and two foals.[8-13] Of these, four had a history of previous joint injection with corticosteroids, three were systemically ill (neonatal septicemia [both foals] and gastrointestinal disease [one]), and one horse had a history of trauma.[8-13] All horses had had previous therapy with an antimicrobial agent, and six horses had received numerous antimicrobial drugs, including systemic administration of penicillin (five), trimethoprim-sulfamethoxazole (four), amikacin sulfate (three), ceftiofur sodium (three), ticarcillin clavulanate (two), rifampin (two), gentamicin sulfate (one), chloramphenicol (one), streptomycin (one) and metronidazole (one).[9-12] Amikacin sulfate was administered intraarticularly before diagnosis of fungal infectious arthritis in two horses.[8,12] Although certain fungal diseases have a regional (geographic) distribution, including coccidioidomycosis, histoplasmosis, and blastomycosis, no geographic predilection was suspected in the horses with intraarticular fungal infection.[8-13] Rather, the development of fungal infectious arthritis appears to be the result of a combination of factors, including systemic or local immunosuppression (either secondary to systemic disease or the result of corticosteroid administration) and the use of systemic or intraarticular antimicrobial therapy. These likely create an ideal environment for fungi to thrive. Weakened local immune response and lack of competition from bacterial pathogens allow opportunistic organisms such as *Candida* to colonize a joint that would normally be inhospitable.

CLINICAL SIGNS AND DIAGNOSIS

The clinical manifestation of fungal infectious arthritis closely resembles that of bacterial infectious arthritis, including severe lameness, joint effusion, and variable degrees of periarticular edema. As is true for horses with bacterial infectious arthritis,[4] the metacarpophalangeal and the tarsocrural joints are overrepresented in horses with fungal infectious arthritis.[8-13] Although fever (body temperature >38°C) is detected in more than 50% of horses with bacterial infectious arthritis,[4] only one of eight horses (12.5%) reported to have fungal infectious arthritis was pyrexic at the time of diagnosis.[8-13] Radiological findings in seven horses with fungal infectious arthritis included the presence of focal subchondral radiolucency (six), periarticular bone proliferation (four), osteopenia (two), and joint space narrowing (two).[8-13] Nuclear scintigraphy revealed diffuse increased radiopharmaceutical uptake (IRU) of all bones of the metacarpophalangeal joint, with focal intense IRU in the distal, palmar aspect of the third metacarpal bone and the proximal aspect of the proximal phalanx in one horse with *Candida utilis* infection.[8] The reported synovial fluid nucleated cell count ranged from 15,000 to 82,000 cells/mcL (median 45,000 cells/mcL).[8-12] Synovial fluid total protein concentrations ranged from 1.8 to 5.4 g/dL (median 4.3 g/dL).[8-10,12]

Fungal organisms were observed cytologically in synovial fluid of only one of the eight horses (12.5%) in the previous reports.[8-13] Similarly, fungal organisms were identified using Gram stain in only 20% of people with fungal infectious arthritis.[5] Definitive diagnosis of fungal infectious arthritis is most frequently by fungal culture from synovial fluid.[8-13] Unfortunately, although fungi can be isolated from reduced solidified holding media and blood culture media,[8] they are generally slow growing and it frequently takes 7 to 10 days for a positive result. During this time initiation of antifungal therapy is delayed, often resulting in exacerbation of clinical signs and hospital costs. Speciation and susceptibility testing are also slow for fungal organisms, frequently taking an additional 10 to 15 days before results are obtained. Of eight horses reported to have fungal infectious arthritis, six had infections caused by *Candida* species. There were two horses with *Candida albicans* and one each with *Candida famata, Candida parapsilosis, Candida tropicalis*, and *C. utilis*. The remaining two horses had monoarticular infection with *Aspergillus fumigatus* or *Scedosporium prolificans*. A summary of the results of in vitro susceptibility testing of horses reported to have fungal infectious arthritis is provided in Table 65-1.

MANAGEMENT

Successful management of horses with fungal infectious arthritis is dependent on the attending veterinarian's ability to make a timely diagnosis and respond with aggressive medical and surgical therapy. Most horses with fungal infectious arthritis have chronic synovitis, fibrin accumulation within affected joints, and thickened periarticular tissues, making lavage in standing horses or using needles difficult. Arthroscopic debridement and lavage are mandatory in most horses; additional information about the integrity of articular cartilage and samples of synovial membrane and fibrin can also be obtained at the time of surgery. Although antiseptics such as povidone-iodine[9] or antifungal agents such as miconazole[9] are occasionally added to lavage fluids, there is no evidence that these improve outcome.

Whenever possible, medical therapy should include prolonged administration (6 to 8 weeks) of appropriate systemic antifungal agents. Antifungal drugs reported to be administered systemically in horses include amphotericin B,[9-11] fluconazole,[8-10] ketoconazole,[9,12] and itraconazole.[12] Systemic administration regimens previously used for amphotericin B, fluconazole, ketoconazole, and itraconazole and a suggested regimen for voriconazole are provided in Table 65-2. Although there is no published information regarding clinical use of voriconazole, pharmacokinetics after intravenous and oral administration have been established in the horse.[14]

Because in vitro susceptibility results may not be available for some time, initiation of empiric antifungal chemotherapy while awaiting final culture results is highly recommended. Although more fungal organisms isolated from equine joints are sensitive to amphotericin B than any other antifungal chemotherapeutic agent, use of this drug (both systemic and local) has been associated with severe undesirable side effects, making it a poor choice for initial empiric antifungal therapy. Rather, I recommend systemic administration of fluconazole or itraconazole combined with local administration of additional drugs (see later). In my experience, lameness will usually dramatically improve within 24 hours of administration of appropriate antifungal chemotherapeutic drugs even in horses with well-established infection.

Local administration of antifungal agents by intraarticular injection and regional limb perfusion are important adjuncts to parenteral therapy.[8,10] Intraarticular administration of fluconazole (20 mg)[8] and voriconazole (100 mg)[15] has been used in the successful management of fungal infectious arthritis without known complications. Although intraarticular administration of amphotericin B has been reported in at least one horse[10] and is regularly performed in people with fungal infectious arthritis,[16] the drug is a well-established model for inducing chemical arthritis in the horse and its use is questionable. In horses in which amphotericin B is deemed necessary, based on the results of in vitro culture and susceptibility testing, local administration by regional limb perfusion may be preferred to parenteral or intraarticular administration. I gave amphotericin B at a dose of 5 mg, diluted in 50 mL of 5% dextrose, by regional limb perfusion on several occasions with minimal untoward side effects. Clinical improvement in conjunction with systemic and intraarticular administration of fluconazole was achieved in a horse with *C. utilis* infectious arthritis.[8] Severe phlebitis and cellulitis were observed after regional limb perfusion with higher doses (100 mg) of amphotericin B.[17] Pharmacokinetic studies examining the synovial fluid, tissue, and plasma concentrations of

TABLE 65-1

Results of In Vitro Susceptibility Testing for Five Fungal Organisms Isolated from Horses with Fungal Infectious Arthritis										
FUNGAL ISOLATE[8-13]	AMPHOTERICIN B	CLOTRIMAZOLE	FLUCONAZOLE	1-FLUOROCYTOSINE	5-FLUOROCYTOSINE	ITRACONAZOLE	KETOCONAZOLE	MICONAZOLE	NYSTATIN
Aspergillus fumigatus	Unknown	Unknown	Unknown	Unknown	Unknown	Sensitive	Resistant	Unknown	Unknown
Candida famata	Sensitive	Unknown	Unknown	Unknown	Sensitive	Unknown	Resistant	Unknown	Unknown
Candida parapsilosis	Sensitive	Unknown	Resistant	Unknown	Unknown	Unknown	Unknown	Unknown	Unknown
Candida tropicalis	Sensitive	Resistant	Unknown	Unknown	Sensitive	Unknown	Resistant	Resistant	Unknown
Candida utilis	Sensitive	Sensitive	Sensitive	Sensitive	Unknown	Intermediate	Sensitive	Intermediate	Sensitive

TABLE 65-2

Suggested Antifungal Drug Administration Regimens[8,9,12,14]					
DRUG	DOSE	FREQUENCY	ROUTE OF ADMINISTRATION	DURATION	REFERENCE
Amphotericin B	0.33-0.89 mg/kg*	q24h	IV in 1 L D5W	30 days	9
Amphotericin B	0.1 mg/kg[†]	q24h	IV in 1 L D5W	30 days	9
Fluconazole	14 mg/kg loading dose once then 5 mg/kg	q24h	PO	8 weeks	8
Ketoconazole	10 mg/kg	q24h	PO	6 weeks	9
Ketoconazole	30 mg/kg	q12h	PO	Unknown	12
Itraconazole	5 mg/kg	q24h	PO	9 weeks	12
Voriconazole	3 mg/kg	q12h	PO	Unknown	14

IV, Intravenously; *D5W,* 5% dextrose solution.
*This dose of amphotericin B was associated with discomfort during administration, and thrombophlebitis, hyperthermia, and azotemia developed.
[†]Unwanted side effects observed after administration of higher doses of amphotericin B were not observed at this dose. Trough plasma concentrations of amphotericin B remained greater than minimum inhibitory concentration (MIC).

amphotericin B after regional limb perfusion have not been performed.

PROGNOSIS

Even with an aggressive multipronged approach to therapy, the prognosis for horses with fungal infectious arthritis must be considered guarded at best. Of the eight reported horses with fungal infectious arthritis, only five survived to discharge. Of these five horses, one returned to athletic function, three were retired and used for breeding, and one was retired to pasture. However, most surviving horses had no radiological changes in the affected joints at the time of initiation of antifungal treatment, and earlier detection and treatment may have improved prognosis for athletic function. Careful cytologic examination for fungi in synovial fluid and submission of fluid specifically for isolation of fungi early in the management of horses with refractory infectious arthritis may help to diagnose fungal infectious arthritis.

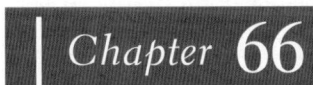

Chapter 66

Noninfectious Arthritis

Alicia L. Bertone

Noninfectious arthritis is characterized by pain, heat, swelling (effusion), erythema, and lameness. Joint structure and function, aspects of diagnosis and management of joint disease, and osteoarthritis (OA) are discussed in Chapters 61 and 84. This chapter focuses on normal and abnormal joint physiology and other specific noninfectious joint diseases.

JOINT PHYSIOLOGY

Fluid flow from the vascular space into the interstitium and joint space (third compartment space) and out into venules and lymphatics is tightly governed by Starling forces, which are a balance of arterial and venous pressures and colloid osmotic forces across the joint. The resultant fluid flow through the joint is modified by permeability of the synovium (osmotic reflection coefficient) and the vessel surface area available for fluid transport (filtration coefficient). Even in normal joints these forces are influenced by gravity (joint dependency), motion (exercise), and structure (joint compliance).[1-7]

Horses are unique in needing joint motion to maintain isogravimetric states of the joints (no fluid gain or loss), especially in peripheral joints.[1] In normal stationary equine limbs, lymphatic drainage from joints approximates zero until joint pressure exceeds 11 mm Hg for the fetlock joint (transitional microvascular pressure). In standing animals without counter forces, such as motion or external bandages to increase lymph flow forces, gravitational pressures increase arterial pressure to the joint and venous and lymphatic pressure from the joint. The result is tissue edema and joint effusion.

JOINT PATHOPHYSIOLOGY (SYNOVITIS)

The balance of these forces is altered in horses with synovitis because of the increased blood flow, altered synovial permeability, structural joint capsular changes, and loss of joint motion because of pain.[1,3,5,8,9] These factors profoundly affect joint physiology, contribute to clinical signs, and result in damage to the synovium and articular cartilage. Early signs of effusion that precede clinical detection of inflammation are related to changes in the hemodynamics of the joint, including increased blood flow and reduced joint motion.[8,9]

In chronic arthritis, capsular thickening, fibrosis, and altered synovial function likely influence fluid dynamics. Capsular fibrosis and joint enlargement produce decreased tissue compliance, and an increase in intraarticular pressure occurs, even with slight increases in joint effusion.

References on page 1311

Articular cartilage is avascular and depends on synovial fluid for nutrition, so alteration in fluid flux affects nutritional exchange between the articular cartilage and synovium. Reduced nutrition exchange to articular cartilage exacerbates articular surface fibrillation and degenerative changes.[10,11]

PATHOLOGICAL JOINT CONDITIONS ASSOCIATED WITH ARTHRITIS

Effusion

Increased blood flow and capillary leakage occur early and contribute to increased fluid volume in the joint interstitium and synovial fluid, recognized as effusion. The condition is stimulated by vascular changes and neurotransmitter release, particularly α_2-adrenergic stimulation.[2,8,9] Because of low intraarticular pressures in normal equine joints (-5 mm Hg[6]; -1.25 mm Hg[12]), effusion precedes interstitial edema, until intraarticular pressure is greater than 11 mm Hg.[1] These physiological circumstances make detection of effusion one of the most sensitive indicators of early joint stress. Effusion, although common, is not normal and alters joint function. Congruent motion of joint surfaces depends on normal negative pressure and is important in decreasing shear force (side-to-side, sloppy movement).[7] Effusion is not painful as long as capsular tension is normal. Through the phenomenon of creep-relaxation, capsular tension is reduced in distended joints. Normal joints are relatively compliant and can accommodate fairly large changes in fluid volume with minimal increase in pressure, but elastance profiles of these joints may be permanently altered.[13] Joints with high structural congruence, such as the tarsocrural joint, are less affected biomechanically by joint effusion than are less congruent joints.[7]

High synovial fluid volume becomes more important during joint motion. Joint pressure profiles are profoundly altered by joint angle.[6,7,13] With effusion, as initial intraarticular pressure is increased, the capacity to accommodate rapid changes in pressure goes down, causing a rapid rise in intraarticular pressure and capsular wall tension at extreme joint angles, resulting in sharp pain during maximal joint excursion and simultaneous reduction in synovial perfusion.[14] These effects could be present even if synovitis is not recognized clinically. The influence of intermittent synovial ischemia is not elucidated fully, but it may be important in diseases of synovial proliferation.

Inflammation

Inflammation causes a humoral (vascular) and a cellular response. In early arthritis, cells are up-regulated to produce inflammatory mediators. Gene transcriptional profiles may be unique to certain forms of arthritis and potentially could be used in the future to recognize and prevent arthritis. Up-regulation of genes causes protein production, initiation of the inflammatory cascade, and further release of inflammatory mediators. Important mediators include cytokines interleukin-1, interleukin-6, and tumor necrosis factor.[2-4,15,16] Secondary mediators such as the eicosanoids (prostaglandin E_2 and leukotrienes),[2-4,15] free oxygen radicals,[17] substance P,[3] and nitric oxide[3,4] are also proarthritic and amplify pain.

Cellular influx causes effusion and subsequent clinical recognition of synovitis. The degree of synovitis and articular cartilage damage are directly proportional to synovial fluid nucleated cell count in infectious and noninfectious arthritis. Neutrophils are highly migratory and can move into joint fluid within 3 hours after a chemotactic stimulus, such as with the introduction of interleukin-1, paclitaxel, or endotoxin.[2,8,9,15,18] These cells are damaging to surrounding tissue because they have destructive enzymes and alter the synovial fluid environment. In noninfectious arthritis, nucleated cell count is usually less than 30,000 nucleated cells/mcL,[15] but values greater than 100,000 nucleated cells/mcL occur in autoimmune arthritis,[19] in endotoxin-induced arthritis,[16,20] and early in reactive arthritis.

Ischemia

Intraarticular pressures greater than 30 mm Hg cause significant reduction in the perfusion of the synovium and fibrous layer of the joint capsule.[14] Pressures of this magnitude occur in horses with palpable effusion of the fetlock joint and are present when synovitis is prominent.[12] Pressures greater than 60 mm Hg can reduce blood flow profoundly, and pressures approximating 100 mm Hg can cause capsule joint rupture (carpus and fetlock[21]). Clinically, joint rupture is uncommon but was hypothesized to contribute to dorsal fetlock capsular thickening.[12] I have seen this as a rare occurrence in the plantar pouch of the tarsocrural joint and the palmar pouch of the antebrachiocarpal joint. Intraarticular pressure can reach high levels during maximal flexion and extension, particularly in horses with resting pressures greater than 30 mm Hg.[6] Ischemia has been hypothesized to be a component of synovitis, particularly in the proliferative form.[22] Low oxygen tension stimulates angiogenesis and granulation tissue formation, resulting in fibrosis. In chronically inflamed joints, clubbed and thickened synovial membrane often is seen during arthroscopic surgery, supporting the concept of synovial ischemia.

Synovial Fluid Lubrication: Hyaluronan

Synovial cells produce hyaluronan. A protective layer of high-concentration hyaluronan remains close to the surface of the synovium, and the remainder diffuses into the joint space, creating the unique viscosity of synovial fluid.[3,7] Adequate hyaluronan concentration is critical to provide lubrication of synovial soft tissues, particularly synovial villi. During inflammatory synovitis, lubrication of the soft tissues is reduced because of dilution of hyaluronan and a reduction in hyaluronan production. Swollen, edematous villi cause an elevated coefficient of friction. In horses with mild effusion, hyaluronan concentration can be normal because increased production by synovial cells matches elevation in synovial fluid volume.[23] When inflammation increases, synovial cell production decreases and degradation of hyaluronan increases. In horses with severe joint inflammation or hemarthrosis, hyaluronan concentration may be negligible.

Pain in Arthritis

Sensory and motor innervation help maintain joint stability, and in the absence of these protective reflexes, severe arthropathy may develop.[24] When activated, the peripheral nervous system can initiate the major features of acute inflammation, such as vasodilation and effusion, and lower the threshold for pain.[25] The C and A nerve fibers responsible for pain sensation in arthritis are activated by amines (such as serotonin) and neuropeptides (calcitonin gene-related peptide and substance P) that also act locally to exert proinflammatory effects on synovium. A role of substance P in joint pain is supported by the clinical effectiveness of the substance P–depleting substance, capsaicin. Capsaicin initially activates C fibers, resulting in substance P release and pain, but subsequently desensitizes or causes degeneration of C fibers.[26]

The contribution of neuropeptides may be different in acute and chronic inflammatory arthritis. Edema formation in denervated limbs may indicate that loss of sensory innervation could play a role in acute arthritis.[27] Increased edema formation and decreased permeability to macromolecules have been observed in denervated limbs subjected to interleukin-1 induction of synovitis.[2] The role of innervation in chronic arthritis is complex, because the neuropeptide substance P and calcitonin gene-related peptide were increased in sciatic nerve, dorsal root ganglia, and periarticular tissues but were decreased in synovium.

The therapeutic implications are intriguing. Intramuscular gold or topically applied capsaicin could selectively destroy C fibers, thus lowering substance P levels, and these have been found to be clinically useful. Nonsteroidal antiinflammatory drugs (NSAIDs) decrease prostanoid production, and intraarticular corticosteroids inhibit the arachidonic acid cascade, thus having direct and indirect effects.[28] In addition, stimulation of primary afferent nociceptive fibers causes release of glutamate and substance P from central spinal pathways. This nociceptive input can be inhibited by stimulation of proprioceptive and tactile type I and II fibers. Stimulation of these fibers can be accomplished by high-frequency, low-intensity transcutaneous neural stimulation, frequently used in physiotherapy.

AUTOIMMMUNE-MEDIATED ARTHRITIS

Rheumatoid arthritis is a steroid-responsive arthritis, associated with high synovial nucleated cell counts, progressing to bone erosion and pannus formation. For establishment of a diagnosis of rheumatoid arthritis, an autoimmune component and production of rheumatoid factor must be documented. According to these criteria rheumatoid arthritis has not been reported in horses. In human systemic lupus erythematosus (SLE), systemic disease is also present, and autoantibodies are directed toward nuclear cellular material. An SLE-like disease has been described in a young horse.[29] In horses, anti–collagen type II antibodies and immune complexes have been identified in synovial fluid of horses with OA and joint trauma. However, these immune complexes are much less common in horses with mild synovitis and have been found in sera. Relationship of cause and effect of these immunological findings is unclear, because immune complexes are found in many disease types. Although these autoantibodies may be associated with equine diseases, it is unlikely that they initiate arthritis in horses.[30] They may develop after exposure to type II collagen, after articular cartilage trauma, or with wear. Specific assays of synovial fluid for immunoglobulin

M–rheumatoid factor (a feature of rheumatoid arthritis), antibodies to heat-shock protein, and antinuclear antibodies (ANAs), a feature of SLE, reveal only modestly low levels of rheumatoid factor without correlation to disease and no ANAs.[31]

IMMUNE-MEDIATED ARTHRITIS

The presence of synovitis and immunoglobulin G complex deposition in the synovium of foals has been reported.[32-34] This form of synovitis is called *immune-mediated arthritis* and may be associated with circulating immune complexes formed as a result of systemic disease.[32] Using specific monoclonal antibody techniques, immune-mediated arthritis was diagnosed in a 6-week-old pony foal infected with equine herpesvirus–4.[33] Three horses were hyperimmunized with *Streptococcus* equine M protein vaccine and subsequently injected intraarticularly with purified streptococcal M protein. Severe suppurative synovitis developed, and synovial fluid nucleated cell counts were greater than 100,000 cells/mcL.[34] Eosinophils were prominent in the synovial fluid and synovial membrane in two horses.

A clinical syndrome of polysynovitis and vasculitis secondary to high circulating M protein (after streptococcal infection), or associated with *Rhodococcus equi* infections, is recognized and thought to be caused by immune-mediated arthritis. Seventeen (35%) of 48 foals with *R. equi* pneumonia infection had chronic active noninfectious arthritis. Pathogenesis involves immunocomplexes in the synovium. The hallmark of immune-mediated arthritis in foals is effusion in one or more joints but minimal lameness.[35] Synovitis often resolves in several weeks with or without treatment. Foals should be restricted to box rest, but no other specific treatment is necessary. Corticosteroids are contraindicated, because bacterial infection may be perpetuated.

REACTIVE SYNOVITIS

Reactive synovitis may occur after intraarticular injection of any product. Any intraarticular injection incites at least mild synovitis. The activated drug or a product in the solution may chemically induce reactive synovitis. Endotoxin contamination of multiple-dose vials or even single-dose products may cause reactive synovitis. In the case of a multiple-dose vial, a suspicion of endotoxin contamination should be high if more than one horse shows clinical signs within a short period. Horses are exquisitely sensitive to endotoxin, and concentrations above 0.125 ng per joint incite synovitis.[36] After intraarticular injection of methylprednisolone acetate, inflammatory cells surrounding vehicle crystals were identified in synovium 6 weeks later.[37] Reactive synovitis associated with methylprednisolone acetate may be most common in the distal interphalangeal joint. Although unusual, within a few hours after injection, horses can show severe lameness. Steroid arthropathy may be a form of reactive synovitis. The distal interphalangeal and tarsocrural joints appear most at risk to develop reactive arthritis after intraarticular injection of polysulfated glycosaminoglycans.[38]

Reactive synovitis must be distinguished from early infectious arthritis. Distinguishing features of reactive arthritis include early onset after injection (about 24 hours), synovial nucleated counts less than 30,000 cells/mcL, and resolution of clinical signs within 1 to 3 days. Lameness ranges from mild to severe, and in some horses distinguishing reactive arthritis from infectious arthritis may be difficult, and prompt management with intraarticular lavage, systemic and local antimicrobial drug administration, and antiinflammatory therapy should be instituted. Culture and susceptibility testing should be performed if any suspicion exists that a bacterial infection is present, if synovitis does not resolve quickly, or in horses in which lameness persists.

Eosinophilic synovitis is rare and may represent an allergic reaction to an injected product, or to parasite migration, or could be truly idiopathic.[34,39] Joint lavage to assist in removing foreign material, and the administration of NSAIDs and anthelmintic treatment are indicated.

Foreign bodies rarely may be present within a joint or tendon sheath and incite chronic reactive synovitis. Broken needles, plant or seed awns or thorns, and debris from nearby wounds can cause reactive synovitis. Radiological and ultrasonographic examinations can be helpful to identify the nature of the foreign material.[40] Cellulitis close to a joint may cause reactive synovitis that resolves with successful treatment of the primary infection.

TRAUMATIC SYNOVITIS

Primary traumatic synovitis is an early form of OA. Horses at risk are usually in active sports training. Lameness usually is managed by intraarticular and systemic medication. Early medical intervention and appropriate joint rest and physiotherapy are critical to prevent loss of glycosaminoglycan from articular cartilage and permanent joint wear. Early loss of articular cartilage proteoglycan is reversible with medication and joint rest. If training is continued, some horses will develop proliferative synovitis, chip fractures, intraarticular ligament injury, and OA. Intermittent hemarthrosis (see later) may be detected with primary traumatic synovitis, but often it indicates injury to subchondral bone, such as chip fracture or cartilage elevation.

PROLIFERATIVE (VILLONODULAR) SYNOVITIS

Chronic traumatic synovitis and continued exercise result in a painful thickening of the synovium, proliferative synovitis, particularly in areas of compression trauma.[41-45] The most common location is the dorsal fibrous pad (synovial pad) of the metacarpophalangeal joint, directly under the broad, flat common digital extensor tendon and joint capsule.[41] At maximal extension and flexion, pad compression results in intrasynovial hemorrhage, granulation tissue formation, fibrosis, and mineralization. Diagnosis and management are discussed in Chapter 36.

Chronic proliferative synovitis is a frequent finding in the carpal and tarsocrural joints during arthroscopic examination. Diffuse proliferative synovitis can be seen in horses that have had frequent intraarticular injections and have continued in exercise. Capsular fibrosis and loss of fine villous architecture occur. I do not recommend radical synovectomy, but removal of fibrotic tufts of capsule and synovium prone to pinching or demonstrating signs of internal hemorrhage and edema is warranted.

See Chapters 54 and 56 for a discussion of osteochondrosis.

IDIOPATHIC ARTHRITIS

Synovitis can occur without any known cause or associated trauma and can be truly idiopathic, although synovitis may be related to circulating toxins, including endotoxin, streptococcal cell wall, M protein, and viruses. In people, bacterial and viral deoxyribonucleic acid and bacterial peptidoglycans have been located in joints of patients with early rheumatoid and other noninfectious arthritides.[46,47] In horses synovitis can be associated with vasculitis, such as that seen with equine viral arteritis.

HEMARTHROSIS

Bleeding into a joint (hemarthrosis) causes joint capsule distention, severe pain, and lameness.[48] Draining the blood from the joint usually results in rapid relief of clinical signs. The cause of hemorrhage may be trauma to proliferative hemorrhagic synovium, an intraarticular fracture, or tearing of an intraarticular ligament. Hemorrhage may occur on a single occasion or may be recurrent. Diagnosis of hemorrhage is simple, by arthrocentesis, but identification of the primary cause can be more difficult. In the absence of radiological abnormalities, exploratory arthroscopy is warranted in a horse with recurrent episodic severe lameness associated with hemarthrosis. Hemorrhage associated with proliferative synovitis may be managed successfully by subtotal synovectomy. (Editors' note: hemarthrosis appears to most commonly affect the antebrachiocarpal and tarsocrural joints but rarely can involve other joints such as the middle carpal joint.)

LYME DISEASE

Although strictly speaking an infectious disease, Lyme disease is discussed in this section because it should be considered a differential diagnosis in tick-endemic areas in a horse with shifting limb lameness associated with synovitis in several joints.[49,50] However, many clinically normal horses have antibody titers to *Borrelia burgdorferi,* and high titers are not synonymous with clinical disease.[51] Authentic Lyme disease is poorly documented in the horse, and definitive diagnosis would require identification of substantially raised titers in paired serum samples. Tetracycline most effectively eliminated positive cultures and antibodies to *Borrelia* as compared with use of doxycycline or ceftiofur.[52]

| *Chapter* 67

Other Joint Conditions

Chris E. Kawcak

Several types of joint diseases are rare and have been presented only in case reports or small retrospective studies. This makes generalizations about these diseases difficult and searching for information a tedious process.

DISEASES OF SOFT TISSUES OF THE JOINT

Soft tissue structures serve to support the joint, and disease can result in abnormal stresses to the articular cartilage and hence chronic progression of articular cartilage degeneration and osteoarthritis (OA) (see Chapter 61). Preoperative diagnosis of some soft tissue injuries is difficult, often leaving the surgeon with little to do other than evaluate the injured area and debride fibrillated tissue during arthroscopic surgery. With the advent of newer diagnostic techniques such as magnetic resonance imaging (see Chapter 21) and increased use of ultrasonography (see Chapter 17), soft tissue injuries can be characterized better preoperatively.

Most soft tissues of joints, such as ligaments, menisci, and joint capsules, function to support joints. Joint ligaments maintain alignment of opposing and adjacent bones in joints. They form a connection between opposing bones (such as the tibia and femur in the stifle) and between adjacent bones in more complex joints (such as between the carpal bones). They function to maintain alignment and allow for movement of the joint. The meniscal cartilages function as cushions between the tibia and femur of the femorotibial joints. Proper material characteristics are necessary for maintenance of the joint environment. The joint capsule is also responsible for maintaining joint support and provides a barrier for synovial fluid. Because the capsule surrounds the entire joint, appropriate elasticity is needed to maintain joint flexibility (see Chapter 66).

Ligament Injuries

Joint ligament injury can be an incidental finding during surgery or a devastating cause of lameness. For instance, medial palmar intercarpal ligament damage can be an incidental finding during arthroscopic surgery and has been seen incidentally in necropsy specimens (see Figure 23-4 and Chapter 38).[1]

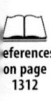

References on page 1312

Injury to cruciate ligaments and menisci of the stifle usually causes substantial pain (see Chapter 46), but cutting the cranial cruciate ligament in an attempt to create a model of OA did not lead to OA in horses. Therefore further destabilization of the joint beyond cruciate injury must usually occur, with possible damage to other soft tissue structures, including the joint capsule.

Collateral ligament injury caused by a bad step or laceration can result in subtle or severe lameness. I have seen low-grade lameness in a horse that had complete tearing of the medial collateral ligament of the metatarsophalangeal joint (Figure 67-1). Laxity of the joint was detected by manipulation and stress radiographs. The joint was immobilized in a cast for 6 weeks, followed by use of a splint for an additional 6 weeks. Reinjury occurred after splint removal, and the joint was recast. After immobilization for 16 weeks the injury healed well enough for trail riding. Others have described collateral ligament abnormalities in the carpus and its close association with OA.[2]

Ligament injuries usually heal slowly, and gradual return to function is needed to strengthen the tissues. The consequences of collateral ligament injury depend on the severity of damage to the ligament, contamination in the joint, and damage to other structures in the joint and may be difficult to predict at the time of injury. Long-term instability may place abnormal stresses on the joint and lead to progressive OA. Cutting the lateral collateral and lateral collateral sesamoidean ligaments of the metacarpophalangeal joint resulted in lameness, increased joint circumference, decreased range of motion, and osteophyte formation in 8 weeks, resulting in OA.[1]

Hygroma

A hygroma is an adventitious or acquired bursa on the dorsum of the carpus caused by trauma from falling, getting up and down, or hitting a fence or by chronically pawing and hitting the dorsum of the carpus.[3-5] Nonpainful, fluctuant, uniform soft tissue swelling occurs on the dorsal aspect of the carpus. Pressure does not induce swelling in any associated joints or tendon sheaths. Range of motion of

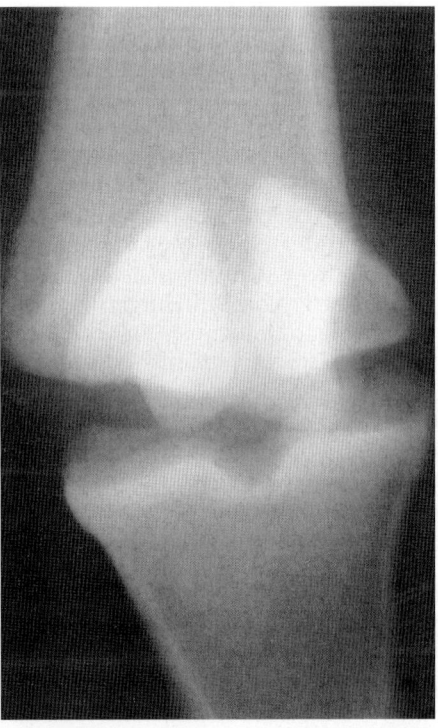

Fig. 67-1 • A 3-year-old Paint gelding had acute swelling on the medial aspect of the metatarsophalangeal joint. A stress dorsoplantar radiographic image shows subluxation of the metatarsophalangeal joint caused by complete rupture of the medial collateral ligament (medial is to the left).

the carpus may be reduced, but lameness is unusual. Injection of radiodense contrast agent into the hygroma or ultrasonographic examination confirms its extraarticular position.

Spontaneous resolution of hygromas may occur, but treatment is often necessary. Drainage and injection of antiinflammatory agents has been used with varying success; in many horses repeated injection is necessary.[4,5] I have seen spontaneous resolution after injection of a radiodense contrast agent. Injection of atropine (7 mg) may resolve the swelling. Owners should be warned that bandaging is an essential component of treatment and that long-term chronic thickening may occur.

Other treatments include incisional drainage; injection of irritants, such as iodine or Lugol's solution; and blistering,[4,5] but contrast radiography should be performed to ensure that the hygroma is an isolated structure. Although preoperative contrast radiographs may show no communication between a hygroma and a joint or tendon sheath, one might exist in the form of a one-way valve from the joint into the mass.[6] Treatment involving drainage of the mass with a Penrose drain and bandaging has been used successfully for recurrent hygromas. Drains usually are removed once drainage stops, 2 to 7 days after placement.[7] Surgical excision can be performed in horses with chronic hygroma and is best accomplished if the fluid sac is left intact and dissected from the other tissues (see Chapter 38).[8] Soft tissue and skin closure are routine, and a splint can be used to prevent flexion for better healing. Prognosis for resolution of hygroma is often good, although some degree of thickening usually persists.

Synovial Hernia

A synovial hernia is a defect in a joint capsule or tendon sheath through which the synovial membrane can protrude. The condition rarely causes lameness but is a cosmetic blemish (see Chapter 74). A well-defined, round, soft tissue mass can be palpated over a joint, and with palpation fluid often can be moved between the hernia and the underlying joint or tendon sheath (Figure 67-2). The hernia may disappear with joint flexion. Contrast agent injected into the hernial sac is detected in the underlying joint or tendon sheath, although a one-way valve may be present, limiting movement of contrast material. If the synovial hernia is of cosmetic concern, surgical excision can be performed, with a good prognosis for soundness provided no other joint diseases are present.[9]

Ganglion

A ganglion is a fluid-filled structure that connects to a joint or tendon sheath through a one-way tract from the joint into the mass.[3] Unlike a synovial hernia, the mass lacks a synovial lining and often is filled with mucin. Ganglions are rare in the horse but common in people, and they have been reported around the stifle and the carpus.[3] A ganglion adjacent to the fetlock was associated with lameness that was alleviated by regional analgesia and after surgical excision of the mass.[10] However, communication with the digital flexor tendon sheath and joint was not demonstrable by ultrasonography. Demonstrating connection between a ganglion and an adjacent joint by injection of radiographic contrast agent into the mass may or may not be possible (see Chapter 74).[7]

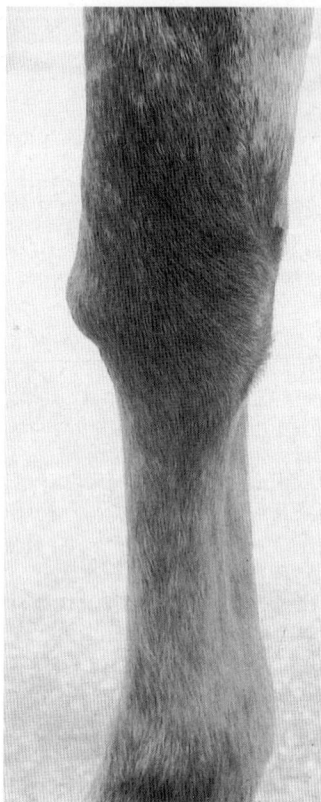

Fig. 67-2 • A synovial hernia on the dorsum of a carpus.

Synovial Fistula

Synovial fistulae are communications between two synovial structures, usually a joint and tendon sheath. They have occurred between the antebrachiocarpal joint and the common digital extensor tendon; the middle carpal joint and the extensor carpi radialis tendon sheath or the common digital extensor tendon sheath; the proximal interphalangeal joint and long digital extensor tendon sheath; and the extensor carpi radialis tendon sheath and a carpal hygroma.[6,11-13] Additional joint damage is often present in association with the fistula, causing lameness referable to the area.

Swelling in the joint and nearby tendon sheath occurs, and fluid is often movable between the structures (Figure 67-3). Radiology may reveal additional joint or tendon sheath damage, and contrast agent injected into one of the structures is visible in the other.[11]

Occasionally a fistula can be seen during arthroscopic surgery, but closure of the fistula requires an arthrotomy. However, arthroscopic surgery for treatment of a primary problem, without repair of the fistula, has resulted in resolution of lameness, without resolution of the swelling. I do not close these fistulae unless a cosmetic effect is important, or if the swelling itself is impeding performance, or if medical therapy fails to alleviate lameness.

NEOPLASIA

Joint-associated tumors in horses are rare and consequently behave unpredictably, and relying on treatment information from other species is difficult. Soft tissue tumors in horses are vascular, fibrous, or synovial in origin. Benign

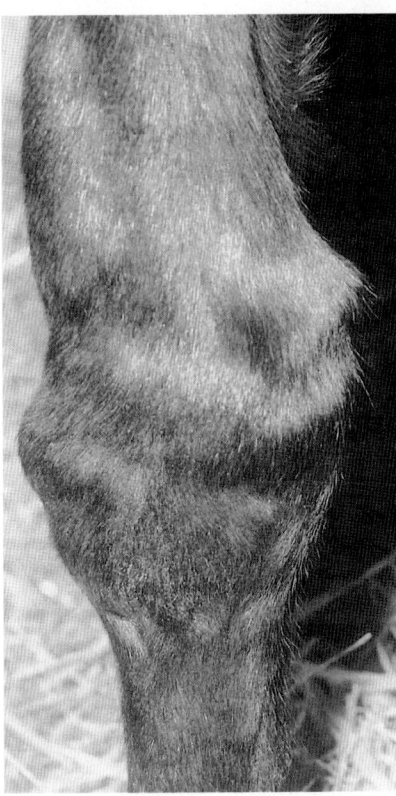

Fig. 67-3 • Dorsal view of a carpus with effusion of the antebrachiocarpal joint and common digital extensor tendon sheath. A synovial fistula was seen during arthroscopic surgery.

vascular masses such as hemangiomas have been seen in carpal and digital flexor tendon sheaths of horses.[3] The digital flexor tendon sheaths were distended with blood-stained fluid, but no associated lameness occurred, and surgical excision of the masses was curative.

Fibromas may occur as slow-growing masses near the tarsus, stifle, and distal radius. These masses are rarely erosive to associated bone. Complete surgical excision may be curative, but incomplete excision can result in recurrence.[12,14] A fibroma on the proximal lateral aspect of the tarsus was incompletely resected, and over a 4-month period the mass regrew to larger than its original size.[15]

Villonodular (proliferative) synovitis is a common traumatic injury on the proximal dorsal aspect of the metacarpophalangeal joints of racehorses and is not a tumor (see Chapters 36 and 66). Keratinization of a villonodular synovitis was associated with severe lameness.[16] It was suggested that this was a form of epidermal inclusion cyst, the result of inadvertent introduction of epidermal tissue into the joint after repeated arthrocentesis for previous infectious arthritis, resulting in a foreign body reaction. Surgical resection resulted in resolution of lameness. Pigmented

villonodular synovitis has occurred in the metatarsophalangeal and femoropatellar joints, resulting in chronic lameness in a mule.[17]

Synovial cell sarcomas have been identified in the antebrachium,[15] a digital flexor tendon sheath,[18] and the proximal interphalangeal joint associated with soft tissue swelling and variable lameness. The masses had infiltrated the soft tissues and caused localized inflammatory bone loss because of pressure. There may be recurrence after surgical excision.[19] Chondrosarcomas are rare, but they have been described in a metacarpophalangeal joint[20] and the carpal region,[21] associated with expansible radiolucent lesions. Osteosarcoma is also quite rare but has been described in the proximal aspect of the tibia and periarticular to the shoulder joint.[22] The horse with the periarticular mass was successfully managed with excision.[22] Osteosarcoma was described in the tarsus of a horse and involved the calcaneus and the proximal intertarsal joint.[23] Mast cell tumors have also been identified around joints as mineralized masses that are responsive to excision.[24] They do not appear to invade joint capsules in general. A secondary melanosarcoma in a shoulder joint that caused severe lameness has been described.[25]

A hemangiosarcoma occurred in the tarsal sheath, and surgical excision resulted in relief of lameness.[26] However, in a retrospective study of hemangiosarcoma in young horses, the investigators found masses in numerous joints that not only caused radiological evidence of pressure atrophy on surrounding bones but also were unresponsive to surgical excision.[27] A neonatal foal with unusual congenital hemangiosarcomas in numerous sites, including the fetlock and stifle joints, has been described.[28] The synovial fluid from those joints was hemorrhagic to orange in appearance.

OSTEOCHONDROMATOSIS

Synovial chondromatosis and osteochondromatosis are conditions involving pieces of uncalcified and calcified hyaline cartilage, respectively. Synovial chondromatosis is a disease in which hyaline cartilage can occur in the joint in pedunculated form, within the synovial membrane, or free within the joint. Osteochondromatosis results when endochondral ossification of the mass occurs, often making it difficult to differentiate from osteochondral fragmentation. Osteochondromatosis has occurred in the femorotibial joint.[3,29] Secondary osteochondromatosis also occurs within joints with OA. The condition is often painful in people, and surgical removal is indicated. Osteochondromatosis has occurred incidentally in horses without lameness.

Calcinosis Circumscripta

For a discussion of calcinosis circumscripta, see Chapter 46.

PART VIII

The Soft Tissues

Chapter 68

Pathophysiology of Tendon Injury

Roger K.W. Smith

FUNCTIONAL ANATOMY OF EQUINE TENDONS AND LIGAMENTS

Tendons passively *transfer force* generated by muscle to bony attachments on the opposite side of a joint, or joints, to provide movement. In contrast the function of a ligament is to resist distraction of its two bony attachments (e.g., collateral ligaments and suspensory ligament [SL]). Although this function is true for most tendons and ligaments, the horse has evolved its digital flexor tendons and SL to exhibit additional functions. These tendons and ligaments, situated on the palmar distal aspect of the equine limb (Figure 68-1), receive large weight-bearing loads because of the hyperextended metacarpophalangeal and metatarsophalangeal joints. As a result the tendons and ligaments on the palmar aspect of the distal limb act to *support* the metacarpophalangeal and metatarsophalangeal joint during normal weight bearing.

In addition, the equine digital flexor tendons exhibit considerable elasticity that is used to *store energy* for energy-efficient locomotion.[1] In the case of the superficial digital flexor tendon (SDFT), its muscle is highly pennate (the muscle fibers are arranged at an oblique angle to the line of pull of the muscle, which maximizes power and minimizes contraction distance) and is unable to contract by more than a few millimeters.[2] Therefore the action of the muscle, together with its accessory ligament, is largely passive to fix the origin of the SDFT in space. Although the muscle contracts only a short distance, its action, together with the tendon elasticity, also provides *shock absorption*.[2] The gait of a horse at speed can be compared with a weight (the horse's body) bouncing up and down on elastic springs (the digital flexor tendons and SL) in a similar fashion to a pogo stick's bouncing.[3] This arrangement allows horses to reach and maintain high speeds while minimizing energy expenditure (see Chapter 26).

References on page 1312

FUNCTIONAL CHARACTERISTICS

Biomechanical Properties

When a tendon is loaded, it stretches. The relationship between the force and the elongation defines the structural properties of the specific tendon or ligament. Because these properties depend on the size of the structure, comparison between tendons and ligaments is better made from the material properties of the tissue, which are determined by plotting the force per unit area (stress) against the percentage elongation (strain). A stylized example of such a stress-strain curve for tendon is shown in Figure 68-1. The curve has the following four regions:

1. The toe region, where stretch to the tendon is nonlinear. This is associated with the elimination of the undulating pattern of the collagen fibrils (known as *crimp*; see the following discussion).
2. Linear deformation—the area of the curve from which the modulus of elasticity, which characterizes the elasticity of the tendon, is determined. The mechanism for this elongation is unclear, but it involves elongation of the collagenous network, with the majority of the elongation arising from the movement of tendon fascicles relative to one another.[4]
3. The yield region, in which irreversible lengthening of the tendon occurs at these strains, possibly arising from covalent cross-link rupture and slippage of collagen fibrils.
4. Rupture, in which the stress falls quickly to zero as the collagen cross-links or fibrils sequentially rupture.

Biomechanical Parameters

A number of simple biomechanical parameters, which are derived from their structural and material properties, can be ascribed to tendons. Some of the values of these parameters for the palmar supporting structures of the distal limb are shown in Table 68-1. A parameter not frequently calculated, but probably more relevant to the in vivo situation, is the force or stress at the yield point, after which irreversible damage is occurring.

Structural Properties

The ultimate tensile strength is the load at which the tendon breaks. The SDFT receives in excess of 1 metric ton at maximum weight bearing in vivo and breaks at 1.2 to 2 metric tons when tested ex vivo in a materials testing apparatus. Within any population of horses, large variation occurs in the ultimate tensile force, with up to a twofold difference between the weakest and strongest tendons.[5]

Stiffness is the load required to extend a tendon by a unit length and is the parameter that has to be optimized to the weight of the horse for the tendon to act efficiently as a spring.

Material Properties

One property is the ultimate tensile stress. As the SDFT is only about 1 cm^2 in cross-sectional area, the ultimate tensile stress (force at failure per unit area) in the horse is close to 100 MPa, which is at the upper limit of previously documented figures for other species (45 to 125 MPa).[6,7] The large variation seen for the structural strength also exists for ultimate tensile stress, indicating that the variation does not result merely from differences in cross-sectional area. It is hypothesized that the horses with weaker tendons are more prone to tendon injury. Another property is the modulus of elasticity or stiffness *(E)*, which is a constant determined from the ratio of stress to strain for the linear part of the stress-strain curve. The modulus of elasticity for the SDFT is about 1000 MPa. Frequently it is correlated with ultimate tensile stress, so that the stronger the tendon, the stiffer it is.

The property, ultimate tensile strain, is the percentage extension of the tendon at its breaking point. In vitro testing of equine digital flexor tendons indicates that they usually

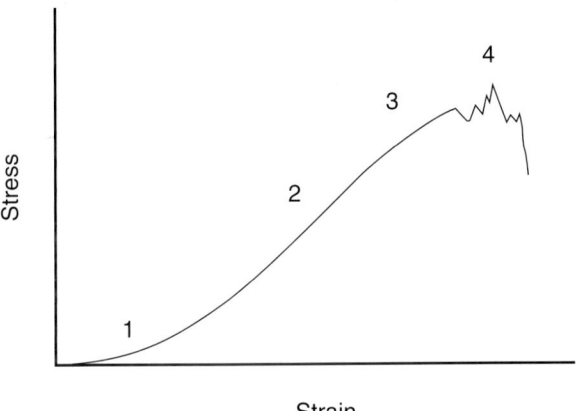

Fig. 68-1 • Simplified stress-strain curve for tendon. *1,* Toe region; *2,* linear deformation; *3,* yield, *4,* rupture. (From Goodship AE, Birch HL, Wilson AM: The pathobiology and repair of tendon and ligament injury, *Vet Clin North Am Equine Pract* 10:323, 1994.)

extend by 10% to 12% of the original length before they rupture, although values of up to 20% have been reported.[8] However, the ultimate tensile strain reflects only the final strain before rupture and includes that yield portion of the stress-strain curve that represents irreversible damage to the tendon tissue (see Figure 68-1). In addition, the ultimate tensile strain is not constant along the length of the SDFT in vitro[9]; the highest ultimate tensile strain occurs in the metacarpal region (the region most frequently injured).

In vivo, the normal strains in the digital flexor tendons (in ponies) are about 2% to 4% at the walk and 4% to 6% at the trot.[10] At the gallop in Thoroughbreds (TBs), maximum strains in the metacarpal region of the SDFT can reach 16%.[11] Such strains are far greater than usually expected in tendons from most species and reflect the highly specialized nature of the equine digital flexor tendon. If these high strains are truly representative of the strains within the tendon, they indicate that equine tendon is operating at or close to its ultimate tensile strain. This suggests little tolerance in the system, which explains the high incidence of injury in this structure. However, some caution in the interpretation of in vitro measurements is necessary, because studies have shown different results obtained between in vivo and in vitro tests.[10]

Hysteresis

Hysteresis refers to the energy loss between the loading and unloading cycles of tendon (Figure 68-2), determined from the area between these two curves. Hysteresis is usually about 5% in equine tendons.[12] Some of this energy is responsible for the rise in temperature within the tendon core associated with repeated loading (as in an exercising horse), which has been suggested as a causative factor in equine superficial digital flexor tendonitis[13] (see the following discussion).

Classification of Tendons and the Relationship to Function

Research has demonstrated that tendons possess different properties depending on function.[8,14] The tendons in the

TABLE 68-1

	In Vitro Biomechanical Parameters Quoted for the Palmar or Plantar Supporting Structures of the Equine Distal Limb				
TENDON	**ULTIMATE TENSILE FORCE (kN)**	**ULTIMATE TENSILE STRESS (MPa)**	**ULTIMATE TENSILE STRAIN (%)**	***E* (MPa)**	**REFERENCE**
SDFT	12.43	—	—	1096.5	84
	12.37	128.5	17.8	1188.9	14
	12.34	—	12.5	1189.0	9
	13.6 (range 9.5–20)	—	—	—	5
SDFT (HL)	—	—	12.3	1000–1282	12
DDFT	17.00	—	—	1585	84
	19.27	89	—	613	100
DDFT (HL)	—	—	10.0	738–1398	12
CDET	6.72	179	—	1523	14
ALDDFT	8.71	—	—	490	84
SL	17.15	—	10–12	1100	84
	17.43	78	—	510	100
SL (HL)	—	—	11.0	576–669	12

ALDDFT, Accessory ligament of the deep digital flexor tendon; *CDET,* common digital extensor tendon; *DDFT,* deep digital flexor tendon; *HL,* hindlimb; *SDFT,* superficial digital flexor tendon; *SL,* suspensory ligament; *E,* modulus of elasticity (stiffness).

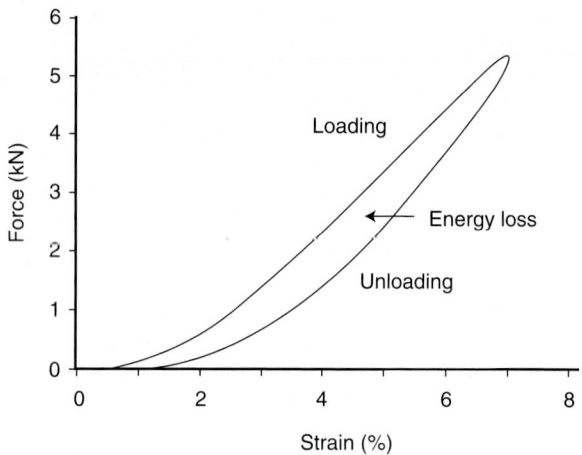

Fig. 68-2 • Hysteresis loop for tendon. (From Goodship AE, Birch HL, Wilson AM: The pathobiology and repair of tendon and ligament injury, *Vet Clin North Am Equine Pract* 10:323, 1994.)

horse, like those in people, can be divided into two broad categories: those with the primary function of withstanding the weight of the horse (weight-bearing tendons) and those with the primary function of flexing, extending, or rotating joints (positional tendons). Weight-bearing tendons, such as the equine digital flexor tendons, are more elastic than positional tendons (e.g., the equine digital extensor tendons), which reflects the function of the digital flexor tendons as elastic energy stores. Positional tendons require stiffness for accurate positioning of the limb or digit. Human finger tendons are stiff for such a purpose, and although equine digital extensor tendons are not required for accurate placement of the digit, they nevertheless resemble this category of positional tendons. [14] These differences in biomechanical properties are reflected in the anatomical features of the tendons.

ANATOMICAL STRUCTURE
Morphology of Tendons
Tendon is composed of a hierarchical structure of subunits. To the naked eye, in cross-section the tendon substance is divided into a number of fascicles, which are in turn composed of ever decreasingly sized subunits: fibers and then fibrils.

The fascicles are held together by the loose connective tissue, the endotendon, which is confluent with the outside of the tendon, the epitendon. The endotendon contains vascular and neural elements. In regions where the tendons are not surrounded by a tendon sheath, a thick fibrous layer, the paratendon, further surrounds the tendon.

Crimp
In longitudinal section, under a light microscope, the collagen fibers in tendon have a wavy appearance known as *crimp*. This pattern is responsible in part for the elasticity of the tendon, and it is eliminated in the toe region of the stress-strain curve when the mechanical behavior of the tendon is nonlinear. A generalized reduction in the crimp angle occurs with aging, with a differentially greater reduction in the central fibers. [15,16] As a tendon stretches, the central fibers straighten first and therefore receive

differentially greater load than the peripheral fibers, which may explain the site of pathological damage in those horses with centrally positioned core lesions. The reason for lesions situated peripherally in a tendon is less clear, unless these are also focal regions of the tendons that have developed atypically straightened fibers. Lesions involving the entire cross-section of the tendon represent a more generalized disruption of the tendon matrix.

Collagen Fibril Diameter
The collagen fibrils are composed of many triple helical collagen molecules arranged in a quarter stagger, which gives a characteristic banding pattern on electron microscopy. These collagen molecules are synthesized by the tenocytes within the tendon, where early events of collagen fibril formation are associated with cellular projections (fibripositors), [17,18] which are thought to be responsible for laying down the template of linearly arranged collagen fibrils during development. Subsequent enlargement of the collagen fibrils occurs extracellularly, by covalent intermolecular cross-linking (see the following discussion). Fusion of adjacent fibrils is responsible for the increasing size of collagen fibrils with age. [19,20] Soon after birth, foals develop the characteristic of a bimodal or trimodal pattern of fibril diameters in the SDFT, in which the fibrils can be grouped into two or three populations (small [40 nm], medium [120 nm], and large [>200 nm]), whereas positional tendons tend to have a more consistent unimodal distribution of larger diameter fibrils in adults. [21]

Associated Structures
Blood Supply
Tendons obtain nutrients from two primary processes: perfusion and diffusion. Diffusion of nutrients from compartments other than blood occurs predominantly where the tendon is enclosed in a sheath, the synovial fluid playing an important role in tendon nutrition.

The principal blood supply in tendon arises from three sources: proximally, the musculotendonous junction; distally, the osseous insertion; and between these two, the tendon is supplied by intratendonous and extratendonous vessels. The extratendonous supply arises from the paratendon in extrasynovial tendon and from mesotendon attachments within synovial tendon sheaths (such as the vinculum between the fetlock annular ligament and the SDFT). The predominance of either source in the midtendon region depends on the species and the tendon. In the equine SDFT, two major parallel vessels run longitudinally in the lateral and medial borders of the midmetacarpal tendon, accompanied by an extensive anastomosing network of vessels. [22] These vessels anastomose with paratendon blood vessels, although removal of the paratendon blood supply in the horse failed to produce gross pathological damage. However, ligation of the intratendonous supply in the midmetacarpal region produced ischemic pathological damage, demonstrating the importance of the intratendonous supply. The deep digital flexor tendon (DDFT) also has an anastomosing vascular network, except for its dorsal aspect as it passes over the metacarpophalangeal joint, where it has a more fibrocartilaginous phenotype to resist the compressive forces in this region. [23]

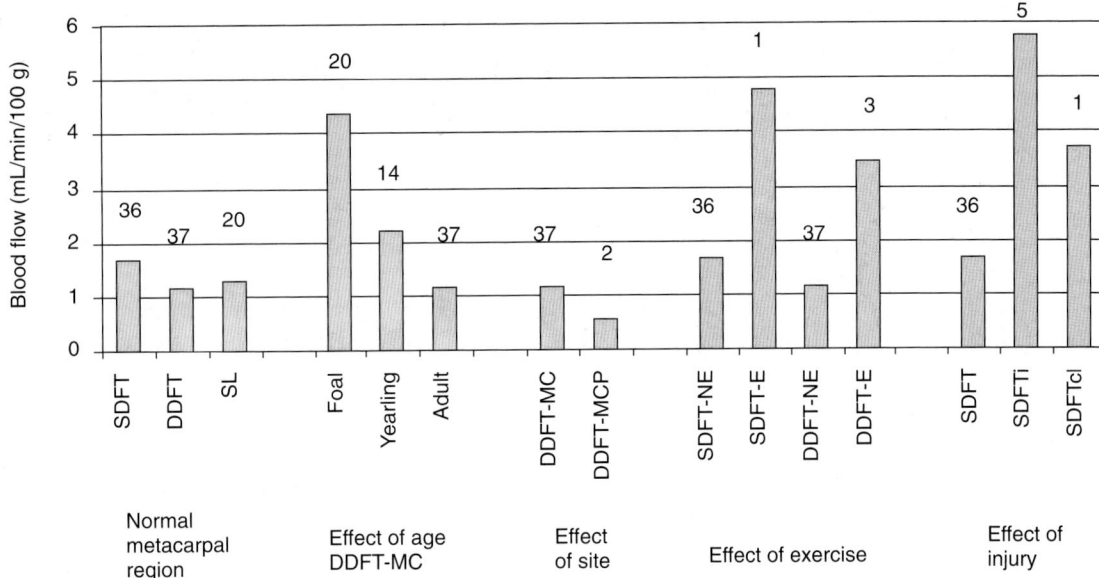

Fig. 68-3 • Absolute blood flow in equine digital flexor tendons derived from ^{133}Xe clearance half-times. Numbers above the columns indicate the numbers of tendons evaluated. *DDFT,* Deep digital flexor tendon; *E,* exercised; *MC,* metacarpal region; *MCP,* metacarpophalangeal region; *NE,* not exercised; *SDFT,* superficial digital flexor tendon; *SDFTcl,* contralateral "normal" SDFT; *SDFTi,* superficial digital flexor tendonitis. (From Jones AJ: Normal and diseased equine digital flexor tendon: blood flow, biochemical and serological studies, PhD thesis, 1993, University of London.)

Tendon has been shown to have a good blood supply based on a number of techniques, usually involving clearance measurements of various radionuclides injected intratendonously (most commonly ^{133}Xe and ^{24}Na). The SDFT appears to have good blood supply similar to that of resting skeletal muscle, although findings have been inconsistent among studies and among animals on successive measurements. The large variation in the blood flow under different circumstances may indicate that external factors, as yet undefined, influence blood flow on a day-to-day basis.

Differences in blood flow between the SDFT and DDFT are affected by age, exercise, and injury (Figure 68-3).[24] The SDFT has a slightly higher blood flow than the DDFT, which reflects its good vascular anatomy (see the previous discussion). However, studies showed similar functional blood flow throughout the metacarpal region of the SDFT, although histologically and microangiographically the middle and distal regions were less well vascularized.[25] However, not surprisingly, the DDFT in the metacarpophalangeal joint region has a significantly lower blood flow, associated with its fibrocartilaginous phenotype, with few blood vessels because of the high compressive forces in this region, which would limit any blood flow.

The blood flow appears to be considerably higher in foals than in adult horses, with a gradual decline in blood flow to the adult level by 3 years of age.

Exercise induces an increase in blood flow (about 200%), although this increase is delayed in animals not previously trained. The tendon blood supply therefore appears to exhibit a fitness memory.

Injury provokes a considerable increase in blood flow (>300%), which occurs in both clinically affected and clinically unaffected limbs, consistent with the bilateral nature of tendonitis in the horse, even though one limb is more severely affected than the other. Other measurements carried out in injured tendons have yielded variable results, which have been interpreted as representing the coexistence of fibrous tissue with low blood flow and hyperemic areas of acutely inflamed tendon.

Cellular Components

Although the biomechanical characteristics of tendon are determined by the composition and organization of the extracellular matrix, tenocytes are essential for the formation and maintenance of tendon tissue. At least three different populations of tenocytes are identifiable within the fascicles of normal equine tendon and ligament[8,26] (Figure 68-4):

- Type I: Cells with thin, spindle-shaped nuclei
- Type II: Groups of cells with more rounded, thick, cigar-shaped nuclei
- Type III: Cartilage-like cells with round nuclei and visible nucleoli

The proportion of these cells varies between tendons and ligaments, with tendon site, and with age.[27] Young tendon has considerably larger numbers of type II cells arranged between collagen bundles. With aging, type I cells predominate, whereas in the areas subjected to compressive forces, type III cells can be identified.

The activity of these different cell types is unknown. The different cell types identifiable histologically may represent different cell lines or different states of extracellular matrix production. A reasonable assumption is to suppose that type II and III cells are metabolically more active and are responsible for maintaining the tendon extracellular matrix, although the metabolic activity of the type I cells cannot be discounted. There appear to be phenotypic differences between cells recovered from different tendons maintained in vitro, which reflect the matrix of the tendon from which they were derived. Tenocytes recovered from flexor tendons exhibit high cartilage oligomeric matrix protein (COMP) synthesis (see later), whereas those

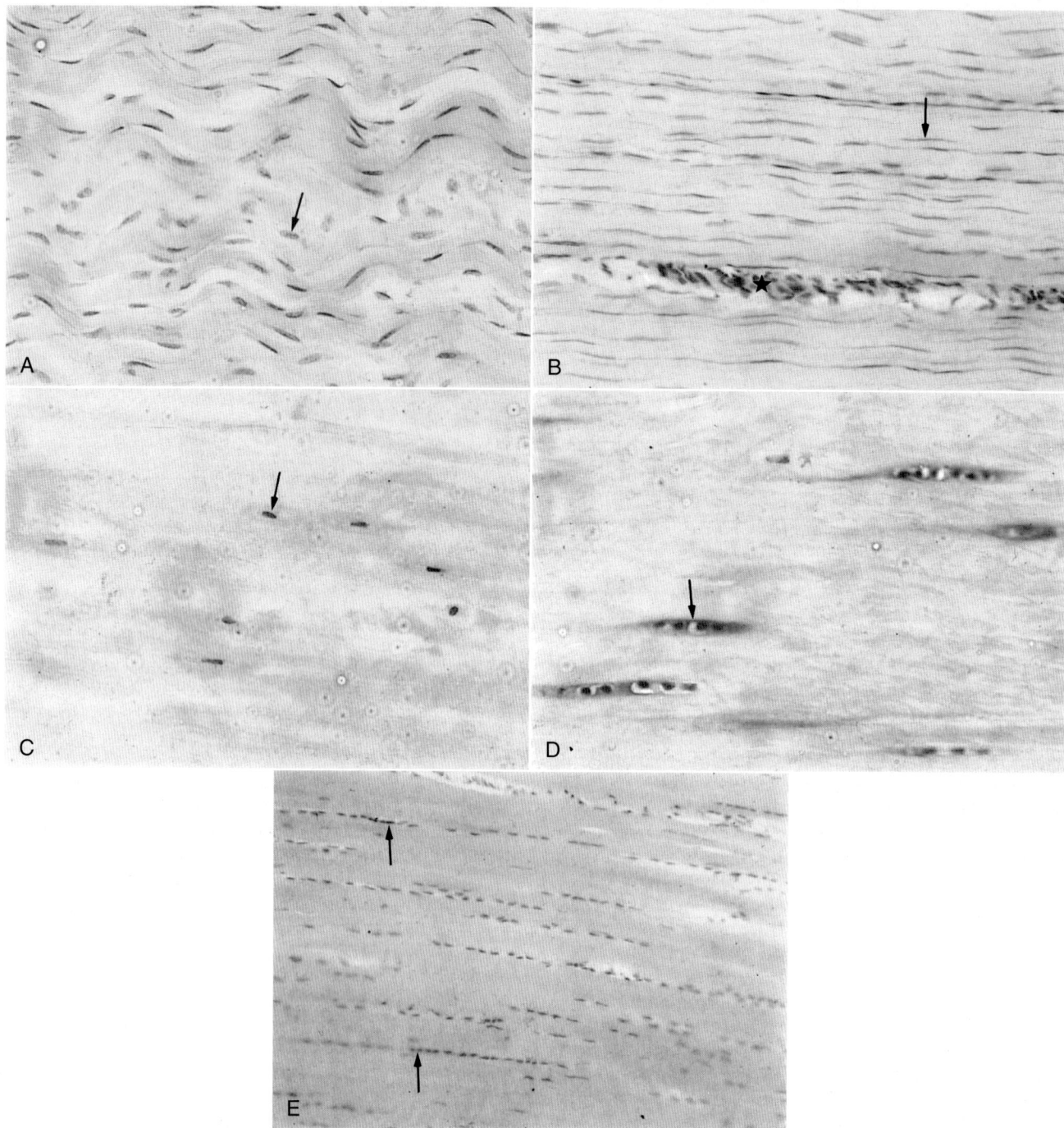

Fig. 68-4 • Histological features of equine tendon and ligament. **A,** Foal superficial digital flexor tendon (SDFT) showing obvious crimp and predominantly type II cells *(arrow)*. **B,** Young SDFT showing reduction in crimp and increased number of type I cells *(arrow)*. Note also the endotendon septa *(star)*. **C,** Aged deep digital flexor tendon from the metacarpophalangeal region showing acellular regions and type III cells *(arrow)*, resembling the chondrocyte phenotype associated with compressive loading in this region. **D,** Chondroid metaplasia *(arrow)* in an aged SDFT. The acellular areas are visible between the regions of chondroid metaplasia. **E,** Suspensory ligament branch showing the lines of type II cells *(arrows)* characteristic of ligament.

recovered from extensor tendons produce much less COMP but are metabolically more active.[28]

Ligament has a much higher cell population, with a predominance of type II cells arranged in columns. In the SDFT of the horse, which has greater numbers of cells during growth, total tendon cell numbers remain relatively constant after skeletal maturity. However, acellular areas develop, especially in the center of the SDFT in the metacarpal region, although the degree of acellularity is not particularly related to age.[29] More active, type II cells can be found surrounding the fibrils in these regions, as well as chondroid metaplasia. Other areas, typified by the DDFT in the metacarpophalangeal region, also have acellular regions associated with a fibrocartilaginous phenotype

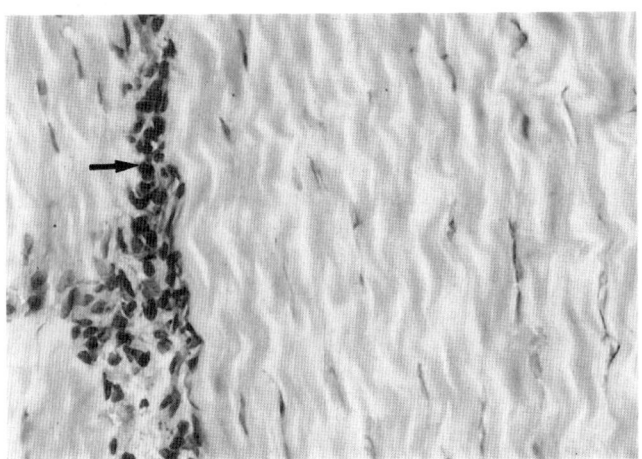

Fig. 68-5 • Immunohistochemical staining for transforming growth factor–β3 in equine superficial digital flexor tendon. Note the concentration of stain *(arrow)* in the endotendon septa. (Courtesy Eddy Cauvin, Lyon, France.)

(type III cells and cartilage-like matrix) as a result of concurrent compressive forces as the tendon wraps around the metacarpophalangeal joint. Other cells are associated with the tendon, namely the paratendon, epitendon, and endotendon fibroblasts and the synovial-like cells of the epitendon within the tendon sheaths. These cell populations may also play important roles in maintaining tendon tissue, especially because the endotendon harbors certain growth factors, such as transforming growth factor-β (TGF-β) (Figure 68-5).[30] Furthermore, as the endotendon contains the vasculature, it is also likely to contain a source of pluripotential cells, which may be responsible for intrinsic healing mechanisms,[31,32] although pluripotentiality in cells derived from tendon has showed inferior capabilities compared with cells recovered from a more conventional source, the bone marrow.[33]

The regulation of tenocyte metabolism still is not understood fully but probably relies on a combination of mechanical and cytokine stimuli. Tenocytes have been shown to sense and react rapidly to mechanical stimuli in vitro.[34] However, equine tenocytes in culture require the addition of a suitable growth factor to initiate a synthetic response to load.[28] The use of confocal microscopy has provided an insight into the relationship among tenocytes. Staining with a membrane dye revealed extensive cytoplasmic extensions from tenocytes, which form a complex meshwork around the collagen bundles. Gap junctions exist between cytoplasmic extensions, which would provide an ideal arrangement for the coordinated biosynthetic reactions to mechanical stimuli.[35]

Of the multitude of growth factors having effects on connective tissues, TGF-β and insulin-like growth factor 1 have been investigated the most in equine tendon.[30,36,37] The synthesis and distribution of TGF-β isoforms in equine digital flexor tendon vary with age. The highest levels are observed in young equine digital flexor tendon, especially within the endotendon.[30] Levels decline after skeletal maturity, especially in the tendon fascicles themselves, and this may result in a relative lack of tenocyte synthetic activity after skeletal maturity. However, it is not yet clear which are the most fundamental growth factors in equine

tendons and how the growth factor milieu acts to cause tendon matrix synthesis and repair.

Molecular Composition of Tendon Matrix

Tendons are composed predominantly of extracellular matrix, within which is a wide array of proteins, organized and interacting to produce the mechanical properties of tendon. The tendon extracellular matrix is composed predominantly of water (about 65% wet weight), collagen (about 30% wet weight), and noncollagenous glycoproteins (about 5% wet weight).

Collagen

About 80% of the dry weight of the tendon is collagen, of which the predominant collagen type is type I (>95%).[8] Type III collagen is present in the endotendon and increases as the horse ages. Type II (the collagen of articular cartilage) is likely to occur at the same sites in the horse as described in other species—namely, tendon insertions and where tendons develop fibrocartilage-like tissue associated with a change in the direction of pull around bony prominences (e.g., at the metacarpophalangeal joint).

Collagen fibrils are strong, but the bonds formed between these fibrils and the higher order subunits are more likely to determine the strength of the tissue. The major covalent cross-link of type I collagen in tendon is between hydroxylysine and lysine residues.[38] Lysine and hydroxylysine are converted to the respective aldehydes by the action of the enzyme lysyl oxidase, which is inhibited by β-aminopropionitrile fumarate, a chemical that has been used in the treatment of equine tendon injuries. These lysine and hydroxylysine aldehydes then can form a number of different types of cross-links: reducible (e.g., dihydroxylysinonorleucine and hydroxylysinonorleucine) or nonreducible (hydroxylysylpyridinoline). The reducible cross-links become reduced with age so that at maturity their level is less than 10% of the level in the foal.[39]

Noncovalent cross-links (electrostatic in nature) are provided by the proteoglycans and other glycoproteins, especially the small proteoglycan decorin, which coats the collagen fibril. Although individually these cross-links are less strong than the covalent cross-links, the high number and involvement in the higher order organization of the collagen network make them potentially major determinants of tendon mechanical properties.

Noncollagenous Glycoproteins
Cartilage Oligomeric Matrix Protein
COMP is a large molecule consisting of five subunits, bound via disulfide bonds at their N-termini to form a five-armed protein, with a bouquet of arms with globular C-terminal domains that can interact with other matrix components (Figure 68-6).[40,41] Although initially thought to be restricted in distribution to cartilage, COMP subsequently was found largely in tissues whose function primarily is to resist load. Thus COMP is found in significant amounts in tendon, ligament, cartilage, intervertebral disk, and meniscus. In equine digital flexor tendons COMP shows large variation with site and age.[42] Levels are low at birth and in the digital extensor tendon at all ages but accumulate within the digital flexors rapidly with weight bearing. Levels peak in the metacarpal region of the SDFT (at about 3% dry weight of tendon) at skeletal maturity and

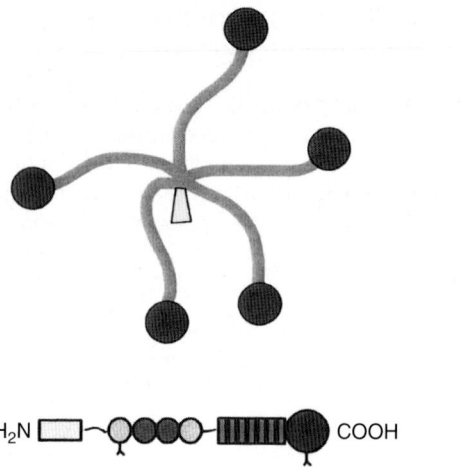

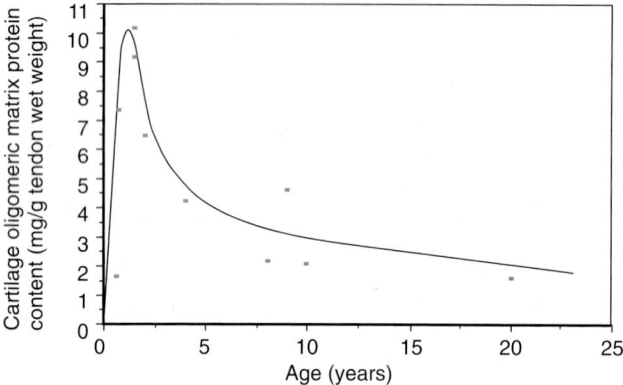

Fig. 68-6 • Illustration of the cartilage oligomeric matrix protein molecule. (Courtesy K. Rosenberg, Lund, Sweden.)

Fig. 68-7 • The variation of cartilage oligomeric matrix protein levels with age in the metacarpal region of the superficial digital flexor tendon. (Modified from Smith RK, Zunino L, Webbon PM, et al: The distribution of cartilage oligomeric matrix protein [COMP] in tendon and its variation with tendon site, age and load, *Matrix Biol* 16:255, 1997.)

subsequently decline (Figure 68-7). Levels peak at a lower level in the metacarpophalangeal regions and in the DDFT but are maintained in the former.

The function of COMP has not yet been elucidated completely, but COMP is known to bind fibrillar collagens (I, II, and IX),[43,44] and a mutation in the human COMP gene is responsible for pseudoachondroplasia, characterized by lax tendons and ligaments, short stature, and early-onset osteoarthritis.[45,46] Although COMP may have a structural role, present research data suggest that it also may act to bring collagen molecules together to form fibrils, and it may assist in the organization of the collagen network.[47] This role may explain the decline in COMP levels after skeletal maturity in the metacarpal region, because the collagen matrix has been formed and limited remodeling occurs in an adult. In the equine SDFT, a significant correlation has been shown between ultimate tensile stress and COMP levels at skeletal maturity.[48] Thus high levels of COMP during development potentially enable the formation of a high-quality tendon matrix.

Proteoglycans

Proteoglycans are a group of molecules that possess a protein core and a side chain of sugars (glycosaminoglycans, or GAGs). The sugar side chains are highly variable in type and length so that great diversity exists even within a given tissue. Work on a variety of soft tissues, especially articular cartilage, has demonstrated a large number of different proteoglycans that are vital to maintaining the structural integrity of the tissue by playing structural roles or by regulating the metabolism of the tissue.

Proteoglycans are largely divided into two broad categories, the large and small proteoglycans. The large proteoglycans are exemplified by the major proteoglycan of cartilage, aggrecan, and the fibroblast-derived large proteoglycan, versican. These molecules possess a large number of GAG side chains, and some can form aggregates with hyaluronic acid. With the repulsion of the negatively charged GAG chains, this molecule has a bottle-brush shape and can trap large quantities of water. The swelling potential for this molecule, when restrained by the collagen network of cartilage, produces a structural matrix ideally suited to resisting compression. In tendon, areas subjected to compressive forces develop a matrix rich in these large proteoglycans, such as in the DDFT and SDFT in the metacarpophalangeal region.

The small proteoglycans such as decorin, biglycan, fibromodulin, and lumican usually have only one or two GAG side chains. Many of these proteoglycans have wide tissue distribution and both structural and regulatory roles. A number of these proteoglycans bind to other members of the extracellular matrix. Thus decorin, the most common proteoglycan in tensional tendon (e.g., metacarpal region of the digital flexor tendons), has been shown to bind to fibrils of type I collagen.[49] Decorin is thought to be responsible for regulating collagen fibril diameter and, together with the other small proteoglycans, may be responsible for providing electrostatic cross-links between fibrils, thus being also an important determinant of tendon strength. Targeted disruption of the genes for some of these small proteoglycans has confirmed a suggested role in maintaining tissue structural integrity. Deleting or knocking out the decorin gene results in variably sized collagen fibrils and poor mechanical strength in skin,[50] whereas targeted disruption of the fibromodulin gene causes altered collagen fibril morphology and reduced mechanical strength in tendon.[51]

Other Noncollagenous Glycoproteins

A number of other noncollagenous glycoproteins have been described in tendon, including elastin (not thought to be important for tendon elasticity in the horse),[39] fibronectin (which is up-regulated after injury), thrombospondin-4, PRELP (*p*roline *a*rginine-rich *e*nd *l*eucine-rich *r*epeat *p*rotein), and tenascin-C. However, the functions of these, and others that have yet to be characterized, have not been determined fully.

Types of Tendon Injury

Tendons can withstand intrinsic (overstrain) or extrinsic (percutaneous) injury or displacement. The most common injury in the horse is the intrinsic injury of the SDFT in the metacarpal region. Epidemiological data have indicated a frequency of 24% in National Hunt horses in

TABLE 68-2

		Studies Aimed at Investigating the Effect of Exercise of Equine Digital Flexor Tendons				
POPULATION	STUDY NAME	AGE OF HORSE AT ONSET OF EXERCISE	DURATION OF EXERCISE	NATURE OF EXERCISE	AGE AT ANALYSIS	REFERENCES FOR PROTOCOL
Thoroughbred	Bristol, long-term study	21 months	18 months	Treadmill	3 years, 3 months	46, 49
Thoroughbred	Bristol, short-term study	19 months	4½ months	Treadmill	23½ months	49
Warmblood	Utrecht study	1 week	19 weeks high intensity followed by 6 months low intensity	Over ground	5 months (first group), 11 months (second group)	68

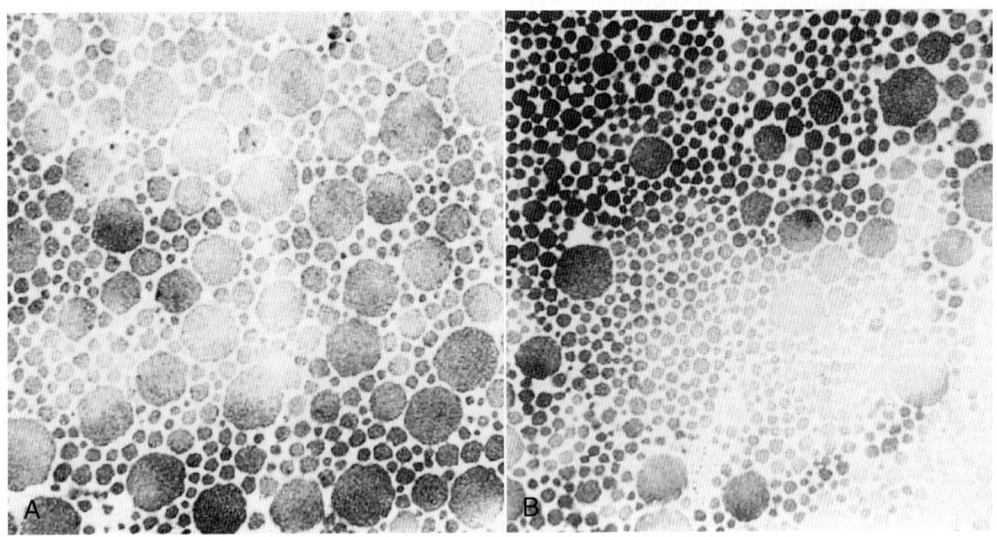

Fig. 68-8 • Difference in collagen fibril populations in control and treadmill-exercised yearlings. **A,** Control. **B,** Treadmill exercised. Note the increased proportion of small-diameter fibrils compared with the nonexercised cohort **(A)**. (From Patterson-Kane JC, Firth EC, Parry DAD, et al: Comparison of collagen fibril populations in the superficial digital flexor tendons of exercised and nonexercised Thoroughbreds, *Equine Vet J* 29:121, 1997.)

training, rising to as high as 40% in some yards.[52,53] Much of our understanding of tendon physiology (as described previously) and pathogenesis relates to the SDFT. Insertional injuries, although common in the human athlete, are rarer in the horse and more commonly are seen associated with the SL rather than the SDFT.

Clinical superficial digital flexor tendonopathy* varies in severity from individual fibril or fiber slippage to individual fibril or fiber rupture and ultimately to complete rupture of tendon with progressive involvement of more groups of fibers and fascicles. Although some overstrain injuries can be caused by simple overload of the tendon, clinical tendonopathy in many mature horses is believed to be preceded by subclinical degeneration of the tendon matrix. This is based on a number of observations. First, postmortem examination of tendons of horses euthanized for reasons other than tendonopathy revealed low-grade pathological damage ranging from acellular areas, chondroid metaplasia, and cyst formation.[29,54] Second, tendonopathy is frequently a bilateral disease, although one limb is more severely affected than the other. Although bilateral changes sometimes can be difficult to identify clinically, ultrasonography often confirms some degree of bilateral involvement.[52] Third, research has identified a number of changes that occur within tendons, associated with aging and exercise, that are believed to be the major drivers of tendon degeneration that precedes clinical injury.

Mechanisms of Tendon Injury: Effect of Aging and Exercise

Various controlled exercise studies in adult and young horses (Table 68-2) have provided considerable information on the effect of exercise on normal equine tendons. In none of these studies was there any indication of clinical tendonopathy induced by the exercise protocols.

Regional differences in collagen fibril diameter have been seen in long-term exercised older horses, but not in short-term exercised or younger horses.[55] Within the central region of the SDFT there was a higher proportion of smaller fibrils in comparison with controls (Figure 68-8).

---

*Editors' note: The terms *tendonopathy* and *tendonitis* are used in this chapter, often synonymously. Most horses with injury of a digital flexor tendon have clinical signs such as heat, pain, and swelling, and as such the term tendonitis would generally apply. However, in some a lack of clinical signs and histological changes associated with inflammation may be most consistent with chronic degeneration of a digital flexor tendon; thus, the term tendonopathy may apply.

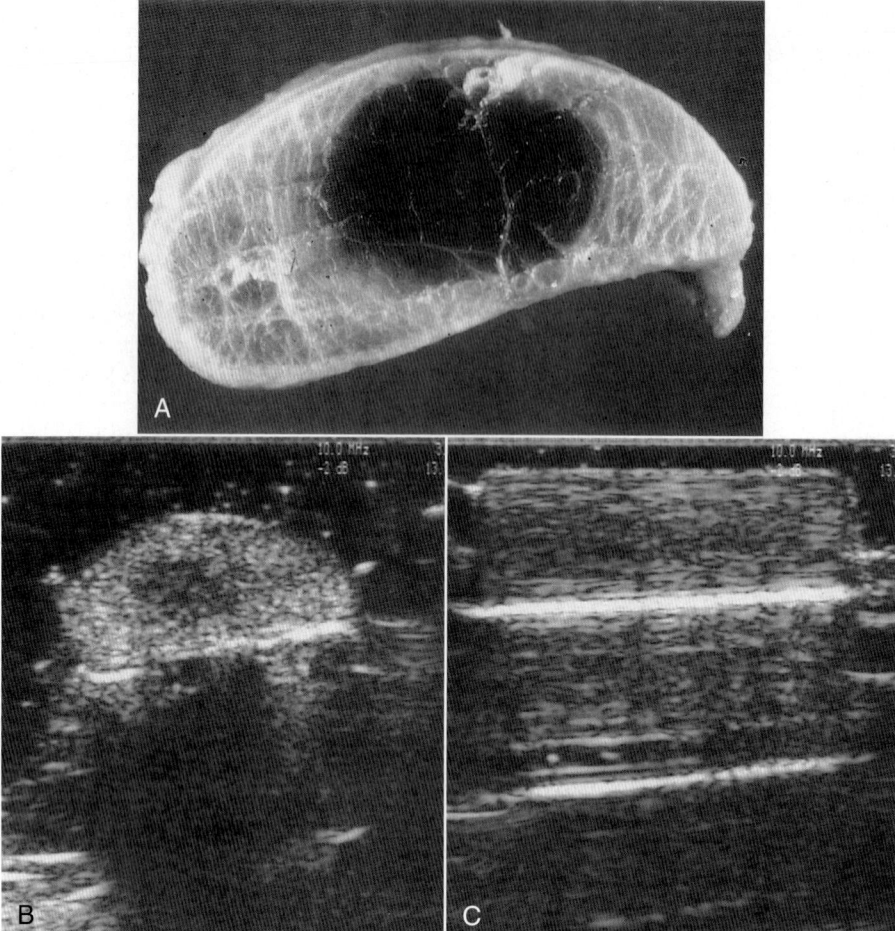

Fig. 68-9 • **A,** Transverse section of the superficial digital flexor tendon from the midmetacarpal region, showing asymptomatic central discoloration observed in some tendons at postmortem examination. **B** and **C,** Note the abnormalities demonstrated when the tendon is examined by ultrasonography in a water bath. The central hypoechoic region and increase in the tendon cross-sectional area in the transverse scans **(B)** and the central disruption of the fiber alignment pattern in the longitudinal view **(C)** resemble the changes observed with ultrasonography in clinical tendonitis. (From Goodship AE, Birch HL: Exercise effects on the skeletal tissues. In Back W, Clayton H, eds: *Equine locomotion,* London, 2001, Saunders.)

The higher proportion of small fibrils did not correlate with new collagen formation and thus may result from disassembly of the larger-diameter fibrils, rather than the formation of new collagen, which would indicate an adaptive response. Furthermore, the reduction in crimp pattern seen with aging was accelerated by the exercise protocols in adult horses.[56]

Changes in molecular composition also occurred in long-term exercise studies, with a reduction in GAG content and an accelerated loss of COMP in the center of the tendon.[57-59] In contrast, molecular analysis of tendons recovered post mortem with central discoloration but no previous diagnosis of superficial digital flexor tendonitis demonstrated an increase in type III collagen and GAG.[60] Because these tendons were enlarged substantially and had central hypoechoic lesions when examined by ultrasonography in vitro (Figure 68-9), these molecular changes probably reflect a reparative response rather than a degenerative change associated with aging and exercise.

In young growing horses, removal of load from tendon results in a lack of the normal COMP accumulation in tendon with growth, whereas removal of load after COMP has accumulated does not alter its levels in the tendon. Data have shown an association between COMP levels and tendon strength at skeletal maturity,[48] so too little exercise may inhibit the ability of the tendon to develop quality tendon matrix. However, exercise studies during skeletal development indicated that tendons are more easily damaged if the exercise level is too high.[61]

These controlled exercise studies suggest that exercise accelerates a degenerative change that occurs inevitably with aging. Thus the research data suggest that after skeletal maturity a tendon has limited ability to adapt. Instead, cumulative fatigue damage weakens the tendon matrix and allows the initiation of clinical tendonitis when loading overcomes the resistive strength of the tendon, and the tissue tears. In support of this hypothesis, epidemiological studies documented a strong association of age and exercise with the incidence of tendon injury in both horses and people.[53,62,63]

Further confirmation of cellular activity during growth, but not after skeletal maturity, has been provided by studies of matrix turnover and gene expression. The turnover of collagen was determined for experimental animals, but not for the horse. In experimental animals, collagen turnover was high in neonates and growing animals, but it declined to low levels in adults.[64,65] In bovine digital flexor tendons, matrix gene expression, as determined by in situ hybridization, was easily detectable in young, growing calves, but no gene activity was present in the metacarpal region in adults.[65] Interestingly, gene activity persisted in the metacarpophalangeal region, which may explain the relative resistance to injury of this region, because of its capability to remodel microdamage. In support of this hypothesis, COMP levels in this region of the equine SDFT and DDFT do not decline after skeletal maturity. The absence of synthetic activity in the metacarpal region appears to arise from a number of mechanisms. Research has shown that flexor tenocytes recovered from older tendons have reduced innate responsiveness[28] as well as having reduced levels of anabolic growth factors in the matrix, which act synergistically to elaborate an adaptive response. In studies investigating TGF-β in equine tendons, young equine tendon had high levels, but amounts declined after skeletal maturity.[30] Furthermore, there are reduced cell numbers in old tendon, and cells show no ability to increase with exercise,[27] reducing the cellular capacity for a response. Gap junction communication, evident in young tendon, through which a synthetic response can be coordinated, is dramatically reduced in older tendon.[66]

In contrast, young growing tendon does appear to be sensitive to the effects of loading and exercise. The adaptive response of a growing animal may not be constant, and research data suggest that any response may be most pronounced early in life and may decline with growth. The level and amount of work necessary to induce this response are unknown, although, by analogy with bone remodeling in response to load, high strain rates may be the most effective. In support of this hypothesis, epidemiological studies indicated that horses are less prone to metacarpal fracture when they begin training earlier.[67] However, as with other skeletal tissue development, such as cartilage, it is hypothesized that a window of opportunity may be exploited to optimize conditioning of tendons for athletic performance (Figure 68-10). The large variation seen in the mechanical properties within a population could be accounted for by variations in tendon development or in rate of accumulation of microdamage, both caused by environmental factors, or it could be genetically determined. Although genetic factors have been linked to Achilles tendonitis in people,[68-70] no such genetic determinants have yet been identified in horses, although one study gave a heritability coefficient for SDFT tendonopathy of 0.17.[71] Such genetic factors could act by provoking the development of a less competent matrix or giving rise to a poor conformation that may predispose to tendonitis.[72] However, the relative contributions of genetics and environment are so closely entwined that it is difficult to apportion causation specifically between the two.

Hypothesized Mechanisms of Tendon Degeneration

Mechanical Influences

Sudden overextension of the metacarpophalangeal joint may cause mechanical disruption of the digital flexor tendons. Although this may be the mechanism of certain tendon injuries, such as deep digital flexor tendonitis, direct

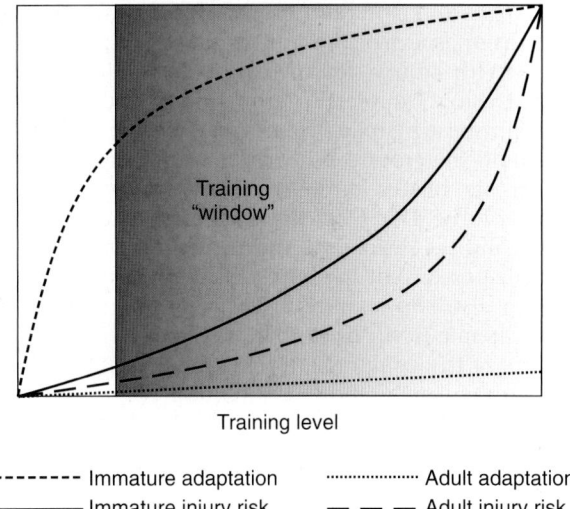

Fig. 68-10 • Hypothesized schematic representation of the adaptive response and injury risk for growing (immature) and adult (>2 years of age) equine digital flexor tendons. (Modified from Goodship AE, Birch HL: Exercise effects on the skeletal tissues. In Back W, Clayton H, eds: *Equine locomotion*, London, 2001, Saunders.)

low-grade mechanical forces, such as experienced under maximal loading, could be responsible for the cumulative fatigue microdamage of the tendon matrix. Subsequent clinical tendonitis is initiated by similar, or sudden supramaximal, loading after the accumulation of microdamage.

Physical Influences: Exercise-Induced Hyperthermia

Because of the hysteresis loop, when a tendon is loaded and unloaded, a loss of stored energy as heat results in temperature increases within the equine digital flexor tendons. Thermocouples have been placed inside the SDFT, and these have recorded temperatures of up to 45° C during periods of galloping.[13] Such temperatures are used to kill neoplastic cells therapeutically, so it was hypothesized that these temperatures would interfere with tenocyte metabolism and possibly destroy the cells. However, in vitro experiments have shown that tenocytes are much more resistant to these temperature increases in comparison with other fibroblast-like cells.[73] However, these experiments were performed on tenocytes in suspension culture, and more recent experiments in two-dimensional culture have suggested that such temperature rises can adversely influence gap junction communication between cells.[74] It is certainly possible that although the cells remain viable with such temperature increases, hyperemia may still adversely influence tendon matrix quality. An alteration in the normal balance between synthesis and resorption activity of tenocytes or a direct denaturing effect on tendon extracellular matrix may occur.

Vascular Theories

Blood flow through tendon is a complex issue, and its relevance to clinical injury is still unsubstantiated. Under maximal loading, blood flow is limited or abolished within the tendon because of the compressive forces generated by the lengthening of the tendon, and this may give rise to relative hypoxia. Indeed, color flow Doppler ultrasonography of equine tendons shows no detectable flow when a horse is standing still, and even flow in the blood vessels of the distal aspect of the limb is sluggish until the horse moves. With injury, an increase in blood flow can be detected using Doppler ultrasonography, but only when the weight-bearing load is removed from the limb when it is raised off the ground. Some areas of equine digital flexor tendons are relatively poorly perfused (e.g., the dorsal portion of the DDFT in the metacarpophalangeal joint region), and this level (but not just the dorsal surface) is a site predisposed to deep digital flexor tendonitis. However, this area also shows histological adaptation to the relatively ischemic environment, with fewer cells and increased amounts of the compression-resisting extracellular matrix components. Furthermore, the tendon may receive some of its nutrition at this site by diffusion from the digital flexor tendon sheath synovial fluid. Similar alterations in the extracellular matrix composition are seen at the corresponding positions in the SDFT, and one could assume that the forces on this tendon would be similar to those of the DDFT at the same site. Therefore a reduced blood flow would also be expected at this level, and yet clinically this region is invariably spared injury in all but the most severe tendonitis.

Equine tendon cells do rely at least in part on oxidative metabolism, although blocking aerobic metabolism does not prevent normal cell proliferation.[75] Based on studies in other species, tenocytes may be more resistant to hypoxia than other, similar fibroblast-like cells.

Laser Doppler flowmetry has suggested that a change in blood supply is not the initiating cause in human Achilles tendonitis,[76] in contrast to the previously proposed hypoxic cause for tendonitis based on electron microscopic investigations of normal and diseased Achilles tendons.[77]

Another result of poor perfusion under loading is the generation of toxic free radicals when perfusion is restored. Such reperfusion injury also was proposed as a causative factor for tendonitis through the destruction of tenocytes or tendon matrix by the free radicals, although this at present remains a speculative mechanism.

Proteolytic Enzymes

Various stimuli, including those mentioned previously, could result in the synthesis, release, or activation of proteolytic enzymes. Relatively little information is available on the constitutive or induced expression of proteases in tendon, although activity of procollagenase and aggrecanase was described in human and bovine tendon explants in vitro.[78,79] An imbalance between the matrix synthesis and degradation of various extracellular matrix proteins is a possible mechanism whereby the tendon can be weakened and predisposed to clinical tendonitis, and in vitro studies have supported this as a mechanism for the weakening of tendon by cyclical mechanical load.[80] Interestingly, the influence of cyclical loading in inducing proteolytic enzyme activity appears to be exaggerated with age, possibly explaining in part the age-related increase in injury risk.[80]

Factors Affecting the Loading of the Superficial Digital Flexor Tendon and Initiation of Clinical Tendonitis

Peak SDFT forces are responsible for initiating clinical tendonitis. When a tendon has been weakened sufficiently by a preceding degenerative change, factors that increase the peak loading of the SDFT therefore also act to increase the risk of clinical tendonitis.

The SDFT is loaded preferentially at the early stage of the stride,[8,10,81] which represents the time of highest injury risk. External factors, such as the rider's weight or hard ground, increase these peak forces, although possibly only in certain tendons. Data have suggested that landing from a jump increases the peak forces in the SDFT but not the SL.[82] The greater height and number of fences jumped at Grand Prix–level show jumping would explain the higher incidence of injury in these horses compared with those competing at a lower level (see Chapters 69 and 115).

The influence of conformation on the risk of superficial digital flexor tendonitis is not clear. Most studies have failed to find an association between conformation and an increased risk of tendonitis.[83] However, one study did identify upright metacarpophalangeal joint conformation as being associated with increased risk.[72] Foot conformation may also have an influence on the loading of the SDFT (and SL). The lowering of the toe with respect to the heel, or the raising of the heel with respect to the toe, results in reduced loading of the secondary supporter of the metacarpophalangeal joint, the DDFT, thereby increasing the loading of the primary supporter of the joint, the SL (and possibly the SDFT), often only detectable at a trot.[11,84,85] As a corollary to this, the long-toe, low-heel conformation characteristic of TBs may actually protect horses from superficial digital flexor tendonitis. However, such alterations in tendon loading may be only short-lived.

The ground surface also potentially influences the loading of the SDFT. Soft ground may predispose to increased strains in the SDFT by allowing the toe to sink. However, using sand has been shown largely to have little effect on strains of the SDFT and DDFT.[10] The effect of ground surface on the incidence of tendonitis is probably more related to determining the speed of the horse. Speed is correlated with strains of the SDFT and correlated with the incidence of SDFT tendonitis in racehorses (see Chapters 69, 106-108, and 112). Thus ground surfaces that slow the horse tend to be protective of SDFT tendonitis, whereas the driest and hardest racecourses are associated with the highest incidence of tendonitis.

Many horses develop tendonitis toward the end of a race or event when they are fatigued. Fatigue will cause greater incoordination, which can result in increased peak loads on the SDFT, thereby increasing the risk of injury.

Because tendon degeneration appears to be related to the number of loading cycles, the greater the exercise history and age, the more at risk the horse becomes. This certainly explains the strong association between age and tendonitis and may explain why older, sedentary horses still can develop tendonitis. Because the subclinical phase of tendon degeneration affects both limbs similarly, clinical superficial digital flexor tendonitis is frequently bilateral. Changes are frequently observed with ultrasonography on both limbs,[52] although one limb is usually more severely affected than the other.

Strategies for Preventing Tendon Disease

Based on the previously described influences on tendon metabolism and function, a number of preventative strategies can be proposed. First, maximizing the quality of

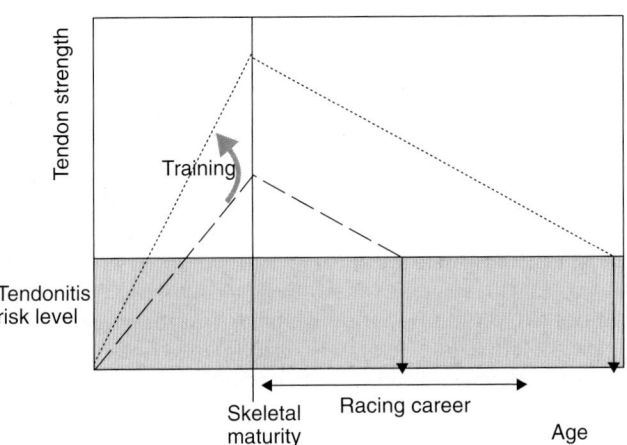

Fig. 68-11 • Strategy for the prevention of tendonitis in the horse. The dotted line refers to a horse that develops strong tendons, whereas the dashed line represents a horse with poor-quality tendons at skeletal maturity (which appears to be at about 2 years of age). The latter experiences tendonitis during its racing and competitive career because of inevitable and cumulative fatigue damage to the tendon, whereas the former, although having the same degeneration, starts from a stronger point and therefore does not develop tendonitis. The early introduction of exercise during development potentially improves tendon quality (arrow), thereby subsequently reducing the incidence of tendonitis.

tendon before skeletal maturity with the early introduction of controlled exercise may be possible, thereby reducing the incidence of tendon injury in subsequent racing and competition (Figure 68-11). To test this hypothesis for tendons, two studies have investigated the ability of early exercise regimens to induce a beneficial adaptive response in equine digital flexor tendons. However, neither treadmill exercise nor exercise over ground induced any measurable effects on the digital flexor tendons,[86,87] apart from an accelerated rate of growth in the size of the tendon.[88] This may have been because the functional ability of the tendon to withstand training and racing was not evaluated or because the additional exercise given to the exercised group of foals was insufficient. Alternatively, the natural exercise performed by foals at pasture included a large amount of jumping activity at play, which is perfectly suited to imparting high strain rates onto the digital flexor tendons, and this potentially induces maximum adaptation in both groups.

A second approach could be to identify genetic influences on the risk of tendonopathy. Certainly, the occurrence of tendonopathy in young flat racehorses may be expected to be more related to genetic factors because the injury is occurring very early in the horse's exercise history, before degeneration could have accumulated. Work is currently underway to identify any such genetic risks that could potentially be reduced by selective breeding.

Risk factors for clinical injury have yet to be fully identified, but research has indicated that certain racing surfaces (e.g., hard ground[89]) and shoe types (e.g., toe grabs in Standardbreds, which increase the risk of suspensory disease[90]) are associated with tendon or ligament disease, and hence avoiding them can reduce the frequency of injury substantially. Epidemiological research into identifying these risk factors systematically is hence warranted and currently underway.[91]

Addressing the biological basis of tendon degeneration provides a more widespread approach to preventing tendon disease in all athletic horses. The reactivation of the tenocyte synthetic machinery may be more difficult to accomplish because of the factors mentioned earlier. Therefore slowing or stopping the degenerative mechanisms is the strategy most likely to be successful.

Finally, the early detection of subtle clinical disease, or ideally in the subclinical phase of tendon degeneration, may allow an alteration of training to minimize the risk of progression to more severe disease. Although the subclinical phase is currently difficult to identify by palpation or ultrasonographic examination because it causes minimal, if any, inflammatory reaction, in the future, serological assays[92] to detect matrix proteins released from the tendon may prove useful for detecting and monitoring this phase. Results to date are not promising.

Pathological Conditions and Phases of Tendon Healing

Once load has overcome the structural strength of the tendon, the tendon tears. The extent of this damage can vary from subtle individual fiber tears, through central defects, to generalized involvement and ultimately rupture. However, even in the last situation, the paratendon usually remains intact. After this tissue failure, repair takes place by three separate but overlapping clinical phases: the acute inflammatory phase, the subacute reparative phase, and the chronic remodeling phase.

The acute inflammatory phase begins with the onset of the clinical injury and lasts usually only 1 to 2 weeks, although this is in part determined by the severity of the injury and the antiinflammatory therapy initiated. This phase is characterized by substantial inflammation, with intratendonous hemorrhage, increased blood supply and edema, and the infiltration of leukocytes, initially neutrophils, but followed by macrophages and monocytes. The pronounced inflammation, if unchecked, results in the release of proteolytic enzymes, which, although directed at removing necrotic collagen, also digest relatively intact tendon collagen, which may cause the expansion of the lesion in the few days after the onset of the clinical tendonitis.

The subacute reparative phase begins within a few days of the injury, overlapping with the acute phase, and peaks after about 3 weeks.[93,94] This phase is characterized by a strong angiogenic response and the accumulation of fibroblasts within the damaged tissue. These fibroblasts probably can be derived from a number of sources including the resident tenocytes, endotendon, and paratendon cells, and monocytes of vascular origin, although studies using transgenic rats have indicated that, at least in this species, the majority of the new cells that remain in the tendon after repair are derived from local tissues.[95] Increased levels of inflammation appear to be related to increased cellular infiltration and the amount of fibrosis occurring subsequently. The invading cells are responsible for synthesizing scar tissue (tendon tissue is not regenerated), characterized by small collagen fibrils, with an increased proportion of type III collagen,[96,97] organized into haphazardly arranged fascicles. The scar tissue formed is initially weaker than tendon tissue, and hence healing tendon is predisposed to reinjury at the injury site. Such episodes of reinjury perpetuate the first two phases and increase the amount of damaged tendon and hence the severity of the injury.

The absence of a paratendon and an externally derived blood supply within a tendon sheath may explain the relative poor response in healing in these areas. The formation of adhesions within tendon sheaths, although responsible for limiting the movement of the tendons subsequently, provides a method of allowing angiogenesis and the infiltration of cells into damaged tendon tissue within a tendon sheath. Hence, although adhesions have deleterious effects on the function of tendons, they are a normal response to encourage tendon healing in this region.

During the chronic remodeling phase, which begins several months after the injury, the scar tissue slowly remodels over a number of months. This remodeling process is associated with an increase in the proportion of type I collagen,[98] the major component of normal tendon. However, in spite of this conversion the tissue never becomes normal tendon tissue, although it is probably more functional. Controlled loading (exercise) during this phase may help promote this conversion and, even more important, may align the collagen fibrils in the direction of force, which further improves the mechanical properties of the scar tissue. This aspect of the remodeling process is followed by assessing the fiber alignment score on ultrasonographic images (see Chapter 69).

Reinjury is unfortunately common, even after healing is complete, in the same tendon, the contralateral tendon, or other supporting structures of the metacarpophalangeal joint. As the injured tendon remodels, it becomes stronger, so that fully healed tendon (15 to 18 months after injury) is frequently stronger than normal tendon.[99] However, remodeled tendon has poor elasticity, resulting in increased strain in adjacent, relatively undamaged regions of the tendon. Therefore if reinjury occurs in the same tendon, it frequently occurs at adjacent or remote sites to the original injury. Subsequent injury to the contralateral tendon is also effectively a reinjury because of the bilateral nature of the preceding degeneration and clinical tendonitis.[100] Subsequent injury to the SL may be the consequence of some loss of support of the metacarpophalangeal joint, caused by substantial lengthening of the SDFT, which can occur with severe superficial digital flexor tendonitis. The SL may also suffer cumulative microdamage, which would increase further its susceptibility to injury.

Chapter 69

Superficial Digital Flexor Tendonitis

Mike W. Ross, Ronald L. Genovese, Sue J. Dyson, and Joan S. Jorgensen

The first two sections of this chapter consider the general clinical manifestations of tendonitis and then the specific surgical management of tendonitis in racehorses. The third section discusses some of the variable clinical presentations in other competition and pleasure horses and factors influencing treatment and prognosis. In this chapter we have chosen to retain the term *tendonitis* to refer to the clinical syndrome of injury of the superficial digital flexor tendon, because clinical signs of inflammation are hallmarks and tendonitis is pertinent. We recognize that others prefer the term *tendonopathy* (see Chapter 68).

■ SUPERFICIAL DIGITAL FLEXOR TENDONITIS IN RACEHORSES

Joan S. Jorgensen, Ronald L. Genovese, and Mike W. Ross

Superficial digital flexor tendon (SDFT) injuries substantially compromise athletic performance and may culminate in a career-ending injury. The incidence of SDFT injuries in Thoroughbred (TB) racehorses ranges from 7% to 43%,[1,2] and such horses are most at risk because of high racing speeds or high speeds associated with jumping (steeplechase racing, see Chapter 112).[3] In National Hunt horses the prevalence of tendonitis of the SDFT as detected using ultrasonographic examination was found to be 24%.[4] In that study a reference range of cross-sectional area (CSA) measurement was obtained (77 to 139 mm^2), but ultrasonographic examination could not predict injury, and variation in prevalence among yards suggested that training methods may influence injury rate.[4] Tendonitis is quite common in the Standardbred (STB) racehorse, more so in pacers in North America than in trotters (see Chapter 108). Other performance horses, including upper-level event horses (see Chapter 117), have an increased risk of SDFT injury (see page 721). Horses used for dressage (see page 725), high-level show jumpers (see Chapter 115 and page 724), racing Arabians (see Chapter 111) and Quarter Horses (see Chapter 110), polo ponies (see Chapter 119), and fox hunters incur SDFT injuries less frequently.[3,5,6] SDFT injury from athletic use in racehorses commonly is seen because of repetitive speed cycles over distance and possibly genetic predisposition to SDFT injury.[7] We are aware of several TB racehorse mares and at least one TB stallion and one STB stallion that are known to have progeny with an increased susceptibility to SDFT injury compared with the normal racehorse population. Additional factors that may predispose a horse to SDFT injury include conformation (see Chapters 4 and 26), working surfaces, shoeing, training methodology, and the relationship between the level of physical fitness and the current exercise.

SDFT injury also occurs spontaneously in sedentary or lightly used horses older than 15 years of age. These tendon injuries often are severe and generally involve the proximal metacarpal region and the carpus and extend to the musculotendonous junction in the antebrachium. Many of

References on page 1314

these injuries result in overt lameness, tendon thickening, and carpal sheath effusion (see Figure 6-18). Sometimes, however, the only clinical sign is lameness, which is often pronounced to severe, with little palpable thickening of the SDFT. Subtle swelling in the proximal aspect of the SDFT is easily missed, particularly when the limb is held in flexion. These injuries occasionally can be difficult to diagnose, requiring local analgesia and ultrasonography. Although older nonracehorses appear prone to the development of superficial digital flexor (SDF) tendonitis in the proximal metacarpal and palmar carpal regions, the condition is sometimes seen in older STB racehorses, usually pacers. In a recent study, only two of 12 nonracehorses with tendonitis of the proximal aspect of the SDFT returned to previous use with medical management; horses were significantly older (mean age of 18 years, median 17 years, and range 11 to 23 years) than a comparison group with tendonitis of the SDFT in the midmetacarpal region, and prognosis was significantly worse than in the same comparison group (10 of 22 horses with midmetacarpal SDF tendonitis returned to previous use after injury).[8] In an unpublished study of 29 horses with tendonitis of the proximal aspect of the SDFT, mean age was 13 years (median 15, range 2 to 30 years), there were six racehorses and 23 nonracehorses of mixed use, lameness was generally pronounced, and ultrasonographic evaluation revealed injury that often involved the palmar carpal region from near the musculotendonous junction to the proximal metacarpal region.[9] Overall, 14 of 24 horses (58%) became sound and returned to work, and five of seven horses managed surgically (desmotomy of the accessory ligament of the SDFT [ALSDFT],otherwise known as superior check desmotomy) in combination with carpal retinaculotomy and proximal metacarpal fasciotomy, or transection of the ALSDFT in combination with intralesional injections of fresh bone marrow) returned to work.[9]

SDFT injuries from athletic use occur in the forelimb far more frequently than in the hindlimb. In one U.S. study of 143 TB racehorses, 58% of SDFT injuries occurred in the left forelimb and 42% in the right forelimb.[10] Bilateral injury is common and has been recognized more frequently since veterinarians have been examining both limbs routinely by ultrasonography.

Most injuries in the SDFT caused by athletic use occur in the midmetacarpal region (zones 2B to 3B), but injuries also occur at the musculotendonous junction of the antebrachium, in the carpal canal and subcarpal region, and in the pastern (see Chapter 82). The plantar hock region is the most common site of SDFT injury in hindlimbs, especially in the STB racehorse (see Chapters 78 and 108). SDF tendonitis in the hindlimb in the plantar tarsal region is referred to as *curb* and is one of the collection of soft tissue injuries comprising this injury (see Figure 4-30). Occasionally this injury extends into the midmetatarsal region. Infrequently, a subtle SDFT injury is associated with tenosynovitis of the digital flexor tendon sheath (DFTS) in hunters, jumpers, and dressage horses. In the STB racehorse, tendonitis often extends to the distal metacarpal region, involving the DFTS and palmar annular ligament, and there is generalized soft tissue thickening in the palmar aspect of the fetlock region.

Racehorses with SDFT injuries traditionally have been regarded as having a guarded-to-poor prognosis for return

to racing, although the prognosis for other athletic disciplines is more optimistic. Before ultrasonography was used routinely, documentation of SDFT injury was limited. Diagnosis was based on gait evaluation and palpation of a swollen or thickened tendon. The injury was referred to as a *bowed tendon,* and morphological abnormality and severity of injury were little appreciated.

Substantial progress has been made in understanding the nature of tendon injury and the mechanisms of healing (see Chapter 68). Historically, tendon injuries have healed by the process of scar tissue formation and maturation, known as *reparative healing*. During repair, injured elastic tendon fibers are replaced with modified fibrous scar tissue, resulting in a tendon repair that is never totally normal. The quality of repair can vary greatly. Some tendon injuries repair and resolve with enough mature collagen so that they return to nearly normal size, with sufficient remodeling that approximately parallel alignment of the repair tissue results. Other injuries develop a scar, with an overall increase in tendon size, poor or random fibrous tissue alignment, and peritendonous fibrosis.

Many of the proposed therapeutic approaches are directed at maximizing the chances for a more physiologically functioning tendon. Therapy requires a multifaceted approach that reduces the acute inflammatory response and hemorrhage in the acute phase and improves fiber alignment during the long rehabilitation phase. The ultimate goal of any treatment and management program is to maximize the chances for a tendon to repair with adequate strength and elasticity for a return to a similar level of performance with the lowest risk of reinjury. Recently attempts have been made to heal equine soft tissue injuries using principles of *regenerative healing*. Regenerative healing occurs in fetal tissues and involves restoration of tissue without scar formation. Regenerative techniques involve the use of freshly harvested or cultured mesenchymal stem cells (MSCs) derived from bone marrow, adipose tissue, or other sources in an attempt to heal adult tissues in a manner similar to healing seen in a fetus (see Chapter 73). Improvement was reported in nine of 12 horses with SDF tendonitis injected with undifferentiated autologous MSCs, and the technique was found to be safe and efficacious.[11] Reimplantation of autologous bone marrow-derived MSCs in 168 TB racehorses (National Hunt horses) with SDF tendonitis resulted in a substantially smaller reinjury rate (18%)[12] than that previously reported (56%[13]).

It is important to recognize the variables that may affect the ultimate prognosis when SDFT injuries are managed. Not all tendon injuries are the same, and case management depends on the specific injury, medical factors, and other nonmedical factors.

CLINICAL SIGNS

Clinical signs of SDFT injury in racehorses vary considerably depending on the location of the primary injury, type of injury, severity, and timing of the examination. Occasionally, clinical signs may be delayed by days or weeks. Furthermore, a lack of correlation may exist between the severity of the injury and the severity of tendonitis in any given individual, especially in the more common core tendon injuries experienced by TB racehorses. In contrast, STB racehorses more often experience lateral and medial border tendon injuries that result in substantial swelling but less severely injured tendon fascicles. Identification of subtle, yet important, reinjury by clinical evaluation may be difficult because of previous tendon thickening. Thus ultrasonographic imaging is essential to confirm clinical signs and to evaluate the extent of injury to the SDFT.

Lameness

Pain on direct compression of the SDFT and mild swelling are the earliest signs of SDF tendonitis. Lameness is often not present at first, a characteristic that often delays veterinary intervention. Because horses are not often overtly lame in the early stages of tendonitis, and subtle pain and swelling either are missed or respond to symptomatic therapy, lesions can progress in severity. The degree of lameness associated with a tendon lesion in the midmetacarpal region is usually correlated with the severity of the injury. Slight to high-slight (category II to IV) injuries generally are not associated with any appreciable lameness, whereas mid-moderate to high-moderate (category V) injuries cause only transient lameness. Most severely injured tendons (category VI), or a total rupture of the SDFT, result in at least transient lameness, which may be severe. In contrast, lesions in the carpal canal or proximal metacarpal region (zones 0 and 1A) consistently are associated with pronounced lameness.

Swelling

For assessing tendon injuries, swelling is defined as subcutaneous or peritendonous fluid accumulation. Digital palpation reveals a soft or semifirm, diffuse or focal fluid accumulation that may prohibit exact palpation of the SDFT. Subcutaneous swelling can be associated with tendon injury, especially in the acute stage of injury. Careful digital palpation of the limb held in a semiflexed position may reveal slight crepitus in an acutely injured tendon. However, subcutaneous inflammation or hemorrhage is not associated invariably with tendon injury. Examples of focal edema or hemorrhage without substantial SDFT injury include swelling associated with cording of the midmetacarpal region secondary to a malpositioned bandage or subcutaneous swelling in the proximal or distal metacarpal region caused by malpositioned tendon boots or stable (stall) bandages. An example of diffuse swelling is pitting edema (see Chapter 14), occasionally caused by external blistering. Diffuse filling also may reflect a subsolar abscess or cellulitis.

Thickening

Thickening or enlargement specifically indicates SDFT swelling secondary to injury or a thickened end-stage repair from a previous injury. In this context, subcutaneous swelling is not appreciable, but a palpable enlargement of the SDFT occurs. In many slightly and diffusely injured tendons, thickening may be difficult to appreciate, and careful comparison with the normal contralateral limb may be required to identify SDFT enlargement. In more severely injured tendons examined in the subacute phase, enlargement generally can be felt. Two clinical situations in which assessing SDFT thickening is difficult are a focal SDFT injury in the subcarpal region, where the tendon is enveloped by the retinaculum, especially in colder climates when limb hair is long, and instances of SDFT injury within

the DFTS that also is associated with tenosynovitis. Tenosynovitis makes distinguishing between tendon thickening and tendon sheath fibrosis difficult.

When palpating the SDFT, one should always determine if the medial and lateral borders of the SDFT can be separated clearly from the accessory ligament of the deep digital flexor tendon (DDFT) and the tendon itself. If both digital flexor tendons are slightly enlarged, detection of abnormality is more difficult; however, frequently the margins of both tendons are more rounded than normal. Assessing the flexibility of the SDFT also is useful, because abnormal stiffness usually reflects previous injury.

Heat

Increase in surface temperature often can be the earliest and most subtle clinical sign of SDFT injury or reinjury. Digital appreciation of an increase in skin temperature, or thermography, often can indicate tendon inflammation. Because extensive use of liniments and daily bandaging in racehorses also increases skin temperature, one must be careful when making this assessment.

Sensitivity to Direct Digital Palpation

A painful response to direct digital palpation is often a reliable clinical test for tendon injury and may be the earliest clinical sign detectable (see Figure 6-15). Examination is best performed by holding the limb in a semiflexed position and palpating with the thumb and forefinger systematically from proximal to distal in the metacarpal region in an effort to elicit a painful response. When a sensitive area is palpated, the horse generally flinches. The examination has many caveats. If a sensitive response is elicited bilaterally, the horse may merely be hyperresponding to increased pressure and possibly has no injury. Not all horses with tendon injury have a painful response. Horses with blistering of the skin, adverse local drug reaction, infection, or cording are also hyperresponsive and more reactive than those with a tendon injury. In addition, extreme sensitivity to direct palpation coupled with focal or diffuse swelling may indicate a problem not related to the tendon.

Tendon Profile

Evaluation of the tendon profile with the limb in a full weight-bearing position can provide valuable information. In a normal limb the metacarpal region has a straight palmar profile. A normal SDFT should be superficial and parallel to the DDFT. It is important to examine the profile from all possible angles. With a slight injury, the tendon often has a normal profile when viewed from the lateral aspect and a convex or bowed profile from the medial aspect, or vice versa. In fact, slight changes on tendon profile are often most obvious when examining the horse visually from the opposite side (Figure 69-1). It takes considerable damage to the SDFT to change the visually detected profile of the tendon, and ultrasonographic evidence of tendon injury is often much more pronounced than expected. In a horse with an acute total rupture, little swelling and thickening may be present if the leg is examined within 2 hours of the injury. However, with the limb in full weight-bearing position, one may note hyperextension of the metacarpophalangeal joint. In this case, digital palpation along the palmar aspect of the tendon reveals a

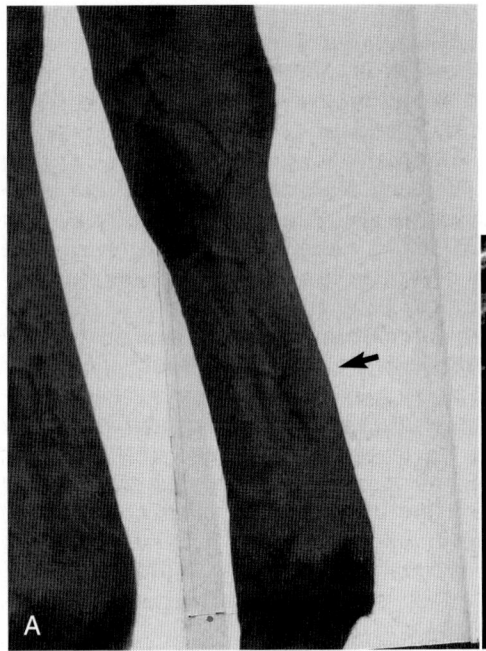
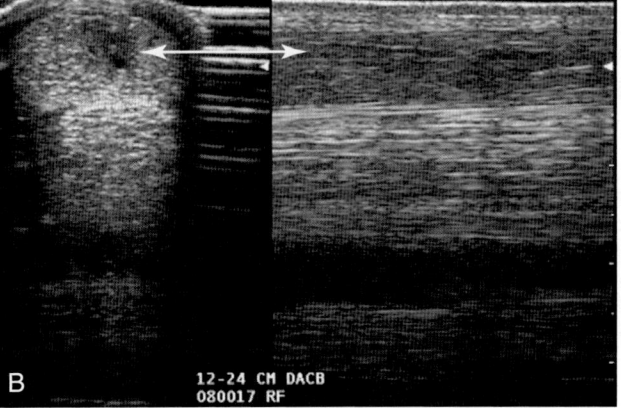

Fig. 69-1 • A, Photograph of the right front (RF) metacarpal region taken from the left side showing swelling of the superficial digital flexor tendon (SDFT) in the midmetacarpal region *(arrow)*. Often the change in profile of the SDFT is best seen from this perspective (the left forelimb can be seen in the foreground). **B,** Transverse (left) and longitudinal ultrasonographic images of the RF SDFT in this 3-year-old Thoroughbred gelding racehorse with substantial injury of the SDFT. A central core lesion (double-headed arrow) and enlargement of the entire SDFT can be seen. Ultrasonographic evidence of tendonitis is often much more extensive than is realized during visual inspection of the limb, a fact that may delay veterinary intervention. This horse underwent successful surgical management using desmotomy of the accessory ligament of the SDFT (superior check desmotomy) and desmoplasty (tendon splitting).

1- to 2-cm defect in the SDFT. Digital palpation with the limb in a semiflexed position also reveals laxity and excessive mobility of the tendon.

Swelling in the Distal Metacarpal Region

In horses with chronic tendonitis of the SDFT or in those with only tendonitis of the SDFT in the distal metacarpal region, there can be involvement of the DFTS and the palmar annular ligament (PAL). Chronic, distal metacarpal tendonitis of the SDFT in the region of the PAL is common in STB racehorses, polo ponies, and older TB racehorses (Figure 69-2). It is important to differentiate clinical syndromes in this region. In horses with chronic tendonitis of the SDFT, the primary lesion is the tendon injury with subsequent restriction of movement through the "fetlock canal" (reduced gliding function) by the PAL. Thus the PAL is not primarily involved but is merely a "passenger" in the clinical syndrome. In these horses palmar annular desmotomy is critical to restore gliding function and to decompress the swollen SDFT, but there is no actual palmar annular desmitis. Primary palmar annular desmitis, tenosynovitis of the DFTS, and deep digital flexor (DDF) tendonitis are other clinical syndromes that cause swelling in the distal, palmar metacarpal region and should be differentiated from distal SDFT lesions and compression by the PAL (see later discussion and Chapters 70 and 74).

Tenosynovitis of the Carpal Sheath or Digital Flexor Tendon Sheath

Tenosynovitis may be associated with a tendon injury or may be a clinical entity without tendon injury (see

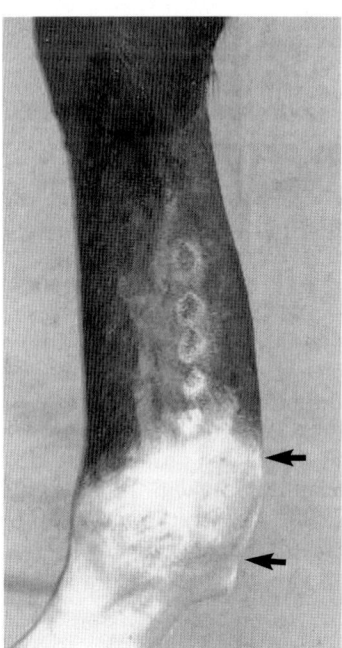

Fig. 69-2 • Photograph of the left metacarpal region of an aged Standardbred gelding racehorse with chronic, severe tendonitis of the left front superficial digital flexor tendon (SDFT). Notice that the thickened SDFT is compressed by the palmar annular ligament (PAL) *(arrows)* in the palmar fetlock region. The PAL is a secondary problem causing restriction of gliding function of the injured SDFT. Palmar annular desmotomy in combination with desmotomy of the accessory ligament of the SDFT was performed successfully. Previous cryotherapy for suspensory desmitis was performed (white hairs).

Chapters 74 and 75). Ultrasonographic evaluation is required to appreciate tendon injury in the presence of tenosynovitis.

Tendon Injury Limited to the Pastern

Injury to one or both of the SDFT branches of the pastern is generally but not always associated with branch thickening and a painful response to direct digital pressure (see also Chapter 82). This is best appreciated with the limb held in a semiflexed position and direct pressure placed on the branch with the clinician's thumb. Injury to the SDFT branch(es) may be associated with tenosynovitis. Injury to the branches of the SDFT should be carefully differentiated from injuries of the distal sesamoidean ligaments.

MANAGEMENT OF THE ACUTE PHASE OF TENDON INJURY IN RACEHORSES

In most horses with subtotal SDFT injuries in the acute phase, antiinflammatory and supportive management is instituted. A variety of treatment regimens are available. For the most part, systemic nonsteroidal antiinflammatory drugs (NSAIDs) such as phenylbutazone (4.4 mg/kg/day) for 7 to 10 days and a single dose of systemic corticosteroids such as dexamethasone (0.04 mg/kg) are included in the initial therapy. Perilesionally administered corticosteroids are considered contraindicated in horses with tendon injuries, especially long-term use, because these drugs are thought to delay collagen formation. However, some clinicians use a single perilesional dose of triamcinolone acetonide (6 to 9 mg) or methylprednisolone acetate (40 mg) (dystrophic mineralization occasionally has been associated with methylprednisolone therapy) in horses with slight, peripheral tendon injuries in STB racehorses, especially when associated with curb (see Chapter 78). Practitioners often administer a course of polysulfated glycosaminoglycans (PSGAGs; 1 vial per week for 4 weeks) in the acute stage.

Physical therapy is indicated, and we recommend icing for 1 to 2 hours once or twice a day, with application of a poultice, or simple support bandaging for horses with subtotal injuries. Casting may be indicated for horses with rupture of the SDFT. Exercise generally is restricted to stall (box) rest or limited hand walking. In horses with subtotal injuries, we prefer to keep the injured limb shod in a fully grooved bar shoe, with a straight hoof-pastern axis, so that the metacarpophalangeal joint position is normal in a standing position. We do not advocate raising or lowering the heel to an exaggerated position. We perform an ultrasonographic examination within the first few days and then again 3 to 4 weeks later. Sometimes tendon splitting is advised for horses with small core lesions.

INJURY ASSESSMENT AND GOALS FOR AN ATHLETIC OUTCOME

Qualitative assessment combines the physical findings and a subjective ultrasonographic appraisal. This gives an accurate diagnosis, but we also strongly encourage the use of quantitative ultrasonographic evaluation. This includes data such as CSA and echogenicity and fiber alignment scores (see Chapter 16).

Optimal healing of SDFT injuries depends on managing a number of variables, including the personality of the horse; its age, sex, athletic use, conformation, injury episode number, and maximal level of exercise attained; and the severity of the injury. For instance, a 4-year-old TB gelding racehorse that has an upright conformation, has never raced, and experiences a severe (category VI) SDFT injury after one gallop has a poor prognosis with any treatment. If this horse were to sustain a small core lesion of the SDFT, its prognosis would be more guarded because of its conformation and the exercise level at which injury occurred compared with a similar injury in a well-conformed, seasoned racehorse.

Athletic outcome of a racehorse may be divided into three categories: successful, meaning completion of five or more races (I); partially successful, completion of one to four races (II); and failure, meaning reinjury occurred before the first race was completed (III). Horses with successful outcomes can be further subdivided into those with reinjury and those with no reinjury. Horses with partially successful outcomes can be further subdivided into those sustaining reinjury and those injuring the contralateral SDFT or a forelimb suspensory ligament.

ULTRASONOGRAPHIC EVALUATION AND CATEGORIZATION OF INJURIES

If clinical evaluation indicates a possible SDFT injury, ultrasonography should be used to confirm the diagnosis and objectively assess the severity of injury. Sequential examinations provide a guide to controlled exercise management and are used to assess progress of repair and attempt to establish an optimal time to return to full work.

The acquisition and assessment of accurate ultrasonographic data require high-quality images, and it is important to develop a rigid, standardized technique (see Chapter 16). The ultrasonographer must take primary responsibility for image interpretation. For a second person to give an opinion on images previously obtained by someone else is often difficult.

Quantitative ultrasonographic data include CSA, percentage of CSA occupied by a lesion, grade of echogenicity of a lesion (type or echo score [TS]), and assessment of fiber bundle alignment in longitudinal images (fiber alignment score [FAS]). Each of these data points is assessed at every defined level of the limb (zone), and they are then summed to provide total scores. These scores then can be used to categorize an injury as minimal (category III), slight (category IV), moderate (category V), or severe (category VI) (see Chapter 16). The following comments apply to forelimb and hindlimb injuries, although reference is made to only the metacarpal region.

Initial Evaluation

Early examination of a suspected new injury of the SDFT may not reveal any anechoic or hypoechoic lesions. However, if the CSA of a single zone is more than 39% larger than in the contralateral limb, or if the total of six of seven zones is more than 14% larger than in the contralateral limb, then tendonitis should be suspected (category II). If tendonitis cannot be substantiated by ultrasonography, despite soft tissue swelling, then conservative management is indicated. The horse should be restricted to walking exercise for at least 72 hours and then reevaluated clinically and ultrasonographically. Symptomatic therapy includes systemic NSAIDs, daily icing, and mild leg liniments or sweats with limb bandaging. One must recognize that sometimes a lesion(s) cannot be identified ultrasonographically for at least several days or longer.

Within 7 days of injury a hypoechoic or anechoic lesion may represent tendon fascicle damage, hemorrhage, or inflammatory exudates and is most likely a combination of all three. Distinguishing the relative contributions of each or determining accurately the severity of injury, which may be underestimated or overestimated, is not possible. Initially, damaged collagen fibers may be grossly intact but nonfunctional, resulting in reflecting echoes. Ongoing enzymatic degradation and further injury caused by pressure necrosis may result in a lesion deteriorating over 3 to 4 weeks. In contrast, infrequently the hemorrhage and inflammatory exudates resolve over the following 3 to 4 weeks and result in a great improvement of the lesion, and the injury to fiber bundles may not be as serious as initially indicated.

Baseline Evaluation

If an initial examination is done within 1 to 7 days of a new injury or a reinjury, we strongly advise that a second ultrasonographic evaluation be performed 2 to 4 weeks (preferably 4 weeks) later to obtain baseline data about the severity of injury (see Chapter 16).

SUBACUTE PHASE TREATMENT AND LONG-TERM REHABILITATION

History of Treatment in Racehorses

A wide variety of short-term and long-term treatment programs for SDF tendonitis are used, sometimes implemented regardless of the severity of the injury or reinjury, and with or without prolonged rest or controlled exercise. No comprehensive reports comparing various treatments of similarly injured tendons are available, and therefore proposing specific recommendations that will give the best prognosis for return to racing is difficult.

A comprehensive retrospective study of TB and STB racehorses currently is being performed to compare the rate of return to racing among a variety of therapeutic regimens for minimal (category III), slight (category IV), moderate (category V), and severe (category VI) tendon injuries documented by ultrasonography. Therapies include pasture turnout, external blistering, internal blistering, intralesional therapies (excluding β-aminopropionitrile fumarate [Bapten]), or a combination of these. In addition, the amount of layup time is being considered for each category of injury. If all therapeutic regimens are combined (Figure 69-3), preliminary data indicate that few racehorses successfully return to racing without reinjury (athletic outcome I, completed five or more races), especially with severe injuries.[14] In addition, these data demonstrate that few racehorses are able to return to racing and not experience reinjury of the SDFT, sustain injury to the contralateral SDFT, or injure the suspensory apparatus (subcategories IB and IC). Ultimately, we hope that this research helps to determine optimum therapy for specific lesions and better equip the veterinarian to provide accurate prognostic information.

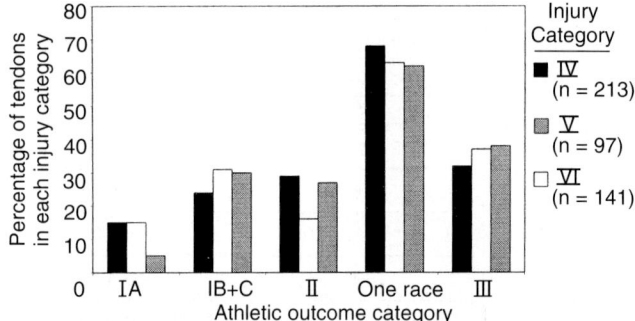

Fig. 69-3 • A successful return to racing becomes increasingly difficult as the severity of tendon injury increases. Treatments for slight (category IV), moderate (category V), and severe (category VI) superficial digital flexor tendon injuries including pasture turnout, external or internal blistering, intralesional injections (excluding β-aminopropionitrile fumarate), or a combination of these were assessed for their success in return to racing. Athletic outcome categories (AOCs) were separated into five groups. AOC IA refers to those horses that have successfully raced at least five times with no reinjury. AOC IB + C includes those that have raced at least five times but have reinjured the same tendon (group B) or the contralateral tendon (group C). AOC II includes those that have raced successfully one to four times and includes tendons that have been reinjured, whereas horses with tendon injuries in AOC III have never raced successfully. An additional group of all those that completed at least one race was included. Data are represented as the percentage of tendons in each injury category that resulted in the ultimate AOC.

Symptomatic Treatment with Continued Exercise

If the decision is made to treat a horse with an injured tendon symptomatically and continue exercise (racing), serial ultrasonographic examinations should be performed, because changes in size or echogenicity may be detected before clinical signs are obvious. If the ultrasonographic examination demonstrates progressive injury or instability and the horse is not athletically (economically) productive, stopping racing and considering long-term rehabilitation would be wise. Naturally, any racehorse racing with an injured tendon is risking more serious injury.

A retrospective study of 209 tendons from 207 TB racehorses was performed to determine if quantitative ultrasonographic assessment could aid in accurately defining an SDFT injury and provide evidence for determining a prognosis for racing in horses that underwent symptomatic treatment with continued exercise. Eighty-eight percent of horses that had no or minimal injury (categories I and III) started more than three races, whereas 12% failed. Thirty-five percent of horses with slight (IV), moderate (V), or severe (VI) injuries started more than three races, but 82% had recurrent injury.[10] Ultrasonography is therefore helpful to determine the prognosis for returning to racing. Symptomatic therapy while continuing to race is a viable therapeutic option for minimal tendon injuries.

Consider a 3-year-old TB gelding racehorse with a swollen left front SDFT after a race (Figure 69-4). Quantitative ultrasonographic analysis revealed a total lesion area of 13%, TS of 7, and total FAS of 7, indicating a mildly injured (category IV) tendon. The horse was treated symptomatically with antiinflammatory medication and continued to race. After 4½ months and six races the horse was racing well, having earned more than $34,000. After two additional races, the total lesional area increased and the

Zone	Structure Size (mm²)	Lesion Size (mm²)	Fiber Alignment Score	Type/Echo Score	Clinical Findings
1A	87	—	—	—	Lameness: 0/5
1B	82	11 (14.25%)	—	1	Swelling: 2/5
2A	88	5 (6.18%)	—	1	Thickening: 1/5
2B	108	16 (14.84%)	1	1	Sensitivity: 2/5
3A	139	14 (10.47%)	3	2	Heat: 2/5
3B	**123**	**36 (29.19%)**	**3**	**2**	Tendon sheath involvement: 1/5
					Fetlock sinking: 0/5
Totals	627	82 (13%)	7	7	Fetlock flexion: Negligible

Bold type indicates maximal injury zone.

Fig. 69-4 • Data derived from an initial computerized scan of a 3-year-old Thoroughbred racehorse actively racing with a category IV injury (<15% tendon lesion). The type (or echo) score and fiber alignment score are similar, indicating a new lesion. Zone 3B was determined to be the maximal injury zone, with a 29% increase in size compared with the contralateral limb.

Zone	Structure Size (mm²)	Lesion Size (mm²)	Fiber Alignment Score	Type/Echo Score	Clinical Findings
1A	109	—	—	—	Lameness: 0/5
1B	95	—	—	—	Swelling: 1/5 (zone 3C)
2A	122	—	—	—	Thickening: 2/5
2B	157	11 (7.38%)	1	2	Sensitivity: 0/5
3A	136	14 (9.59%)	1	1	Heat: 1/5
3B	**178**	**28 (15.68%)***	**2**	**1**	Tendon sheath involvement: 0/5
3C	164	23 (13.90%)*	3	3	Fetlock sinking: 0/5
Totals	961	76 (8%)	7	7	Fetlock flexion: Negative or no abnormality detected

Bold type indicates maximal injury zone.
*Evidence of focal instability of echogenicity near the metacarpophalangeal joint.

Fig. 69-5 • Data derived from a computerized scan of a right forelimb superficial digital flexor tendon injury 11½ months after the baseline scan and 6 weeks after galloping was resumed. Before galloping, the total cross-sectional area was 975 mm², which decreased to 961 mm². However, new hypoechogenic lesions were documented in zones 3B and 3C, indicating an unstable healing process.

horse's performance decreased. Long-term therapy with time off was instituted. STB racehorses are generally more successful than TBs in continued performance with a tendon injury.[14]

A retrospective study of pretraining (exercise level 5) ultrasonographic data from 106 injured racehorses provided four criteria that we use as a guideline for an optimum return to racing[15]:

1. At least a 60% decrease in category IV total lesional area, or fewer than 12% total hypoechogenic fiber bundles for all categories of severity of injury
2. At least a 10% to 15% decrease in total CSA from baseline for all categories of injury (a relatively greater decrease in more seriously injured tendons)
3. At least a 70% decrease in the total TS (ideally <4; the closer to zero, the better)

4. At least a 75% decrease in the total FAS (ideally <4; the closer to zero, the better) before advancement to exercise level 5

The horse should meet at least three of the four criteria, with only minimal failure of the other criterion. Horses that met all criteria or failed only one had a 50% chance to be successful as defined by completing five races. If a horse failed more than one criterion, the chance of reinjury before racing one race was 85%. All horses (100%) that failed all criteria had reinjury.

Ultrasonographic evaluation is used to monitor tendon stability during training. For example, ultrasonographic examination of a right front SDFT 11½ months after the baseline scan and after 6 weeks of galloping indicated stable total CSA values but increased hypoechogenic tendon fascicles in zones 3B and 3C (Figure 69-5). Clinically, increased

Zone	Structure Size (mm²)	Lesion Size (mm²)	Fiber Alignment Score	Type/Echo Score	Clinical Findings
1A	88	—	—	—	Lameness: 0/5
1B	116	—	—	—	Swelling: 0/5
2A	114	9 (7.71%)	1	1	Thickening: 2/5
2B	151	17 (11.27%)	1	1	Sensitivity: 0/5
3A	160	16 (10.40%)	1	1	Heat: 0/5
3B	**202**	**53 (26.37%)***	**3**	**3**	Tendon sheath involvement: 0/5
3C	191	27 (14.06%)*	3	3	Fetlock sinking: 0/5
Totals	1022	122 (12%)	9	9	Fetlock flexion: Negative or no abnormality detected

Bold type indicates maximal injury zone.
*Evidence of focal instability of echogenicity near the metacarpophalangeal joint.

Fig. 69-6 • Data derived from a computerized scan of the same limb as in Figure 69-5. After 16 days of continued exercise, clinically significant reinjury is documented by an increase in total cross-sectional area to 1022 mm², worsening type score and fiber alignment score in zones 3B and 3C, and an increase in the total percentage hypoechogenic volume of the injury. These findings illustrate the importance of quantitative analysis in monitoring tendon healing and predicting responses to an aggressive treatment program.

heat and swelling in the distal metacarpal region were found, which indicated tendon instability at the current exercise level and a high risk of reinjury with continued training. The trainer was unwilling for economic reasons to pursue another long-term treatment program and decided on an intermediate program of 30 days of ponying (leading the horse from another horse) and swimming. Six weeks later substantial reinjury of the SDFT occurred in the distal metacarpal region (Figure 69-6). Use of serial ultrasonographic monitoring is discussed in detail elsewhere (see Chapter 16).

Common Long-Term Treatment Programs

Controlled Exercise and Time Out of Training
A graded exercise program based on severity of the injury and the ultrasonographic progress during rehabilitation has been used.[16] Turnout in a large paddock was not permitted. The time out of training ranged from 9 to 12 months, depending on the initial severity of the injury and ultrasonographic progress. Twenty-eight TB racehorses were managed in this manner, and 20 (71%) of the 28 returned to racing. Only two (25%) of eight horses treated with time off and large pasture exercise had a successful outcome. The difference between horses managed in an uncontrolled fashion, using unlimited exercise while being turned out, and horses managed in a vigorously controlled exercise program is hugely important.[16] One of us (MWR) feels strongly that "turnout is the antithesis of healing," and the results of the study by Gillis emphasize the point. Currently no consensus exists on the treatment of choice for SDF tendonitis in racehorses, but most treatment regimens are combined with a controlled exercise program and serial ultrasonographic assessment. One of us (MWR) feels strongly that surgical management is important. Most horses with category II (tendonitis without lesions perceptible by ultrasonography) or III (total echogenicity score less than 3) lesions have a reasonably favorable prognosis

for successful return to racing (defined as five or more races [athletic outcome I]) if they are confined to controlled exercise for sufficient time.

External and Internal Blistering, Pin Firing, and Time Off for Long-Term Rehabilitation
One of the most common therapeutic regimens in the United States for rehabilitating racehorses with SDFT injuries includes some sort of counterirritation (see Chapter 88), plus controlled exercise or turnout into a large pasture. Many counterirritation options exist, including external blistering agents such as a variety of iodine-based liniments, internal peritendonous injection of 2% iodine in almond oil (internal blister), and pin firing. Several reasons exist for the persistent use of these treatment regimens, in spite of evidence suggesting that turnout exercise is contraindicated and the limited research suggesting that external blistering and especially pin firing have no beneficial effect on tendon injury repair.[17] No alternative therapeutic regimens result in a consistent return to racing without reinjury or injury to another soft tissue structure. Tradition is strong, and most newer surgical and medical treatment regimens are expensive, even though the prognosis remains guarded.

Counterirritation promotes angiogenesis, and, when used, exercise is restricted. In a retrospective study of 54 TB and STB racehorses treated with pin firing or external blistering and given more than 6 months out of training, 23 (43%) returned to race at least once.[18] Ten (19%) of these horses returned to racing without experiencing reinjury to the tendon. These data indicate that racehorses treated by counterirritation can return successfully to racing, and so counterirritation will continue to be used until alternative methods prove to have significant and consistent improved athletic outcomes. If counterirritation is the treatment option selected by the trainer or owner, athletic outcomes may be improved if treatment is combined with a controlled exercise program and serial ultrasonographic examinations. We recommend reexamination every 2 months to evaluate the quality of repair and to determine if the current exercise program is excessive for any given stage of healing.

Intralesional β-Aminopropionitrile Fumarate and Controlled Exercise

The following information regarding β-aminopropionitrile fumarate is included as it appeared in the first edition of this textbook, because it is historically important and lessons learned from the long-term study of the effects of the chemical are important. During study of the effects of the chemical, work by Genovese, Reef, and others demonstrated the value of serial ultrasonographic examinations and fiber score assessment in horses being managed in the various treatment protocols. They and others, including Dyson (see discussion of SDF tendonitis in nonracehorses, later) believed strongly in the value of the chemical in combination with strict rehabilitation. Currently there is no commercially available source to acquire the chemical, and use of it has largely ceased in North America (MWR).

β-Aminopropionitrile fumarate is a toxic substance found in the seeds of the plant *Lathyrus odoratus* (sweet pea). If β-aminopropionitrile fumarate is injected into an injured tendon 30 to 90 days after injury, it binds to the enzyme lysyl oxidase and inhibits the deamination of lysine. This temporarily blocks cross-linking between collagen fibers and improves the quality of repair, if combined with controlled exercise, to generate piezoelectric forces and encourage axial alignment of the repairing collagen fibers. In a naturally healing tendon the collagen fibers may be aligned randomly, whereas treatment with β-aminopropionitrile fumarate may encourage parallel alignment of the fibers, resulting in a stronger, more physiological repair. Treatment with β-aminopropionitrile fumarate combined with a controlled exercise program has resulted in superior healing, with more type I collagen fibers and improved longitudinal fiber alignment than in horses treated without exercise.[19] β-Aminopropionitrile fumarate does not increase tenocyte formation and only affects the orientation of the scar and does not hasten repair. Theoretically intralesionally administered β-aminopropionitrile fumarate is indicated for horses with moderate to severe injuries, when a large volume of the tendon will be repaired by scarring.

β-Aminopropionitrile fumarate is administered 30 to 90 days after injury and is used at a rate of 1 mL (0.7 mg) per 3% total lesional area, up to a maximum of 10 mL (7 mg). Pretreatment quantitative ultrasonographic evaluation is important for establishing the anatomical extent of the lesion to be treated and the dose required.

Several clinical trials with β-aminopropionitrile fumarate have been performed. Genovese reported an improvement in quantitative ultrasonographic morphology.[20] In a study in the United Kingdom, six of seven TB flat racehorses failed to complete one race,[3] but a trial in the United States determined that 50% of treated horses returned to racing and completed at least five races.[21] Clinical trials performed in Ohio compared the results of β-aminopropionitrile fumarate treatment (75 horses) with use of a placebo (10 horses). All horses followed a similar exercise program. In phase 1, horses were out of training for less than 6 months, but the rate of reinjury was high. In phase 2, convalescence

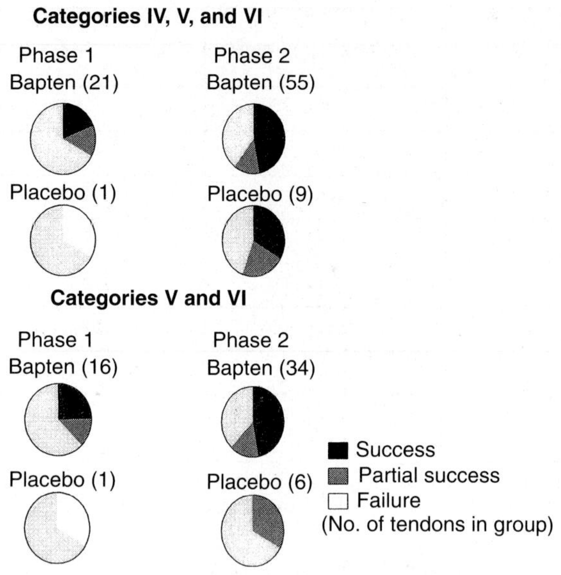

Fig. 69-7 • Superficial digital flexor tendon injuries treated with β-aminopropionitrile fumarate were compared with placebo groups in two phases of the study. Phase 1 required less than 6 months of layup time, whereas phase 2 studies increased the convalescent time to at least 6 months for category IV injuries, 8 months for category V, and 10 months for category VI injuries. The percent of the total number of tendons was divided into three groups: success (raced at least five times after injury), partial success (raced one to four times), and failure (never raced). In phase 1, injuries including mild (category IV), moderate (category V), and severe (category VI) were grouped together to determine outcome; in phase 2 only moderate and severe categories were grouped.

was increased, based on the ultrasonographic grading of the severity of the injury. Horses with a category IV lesion had at least 6 months out of training; this was extended to 8 months for horses with category V lesions and 10 months for those with category VI injuries. In phase 2 the success rate increased (Figure 69-7).

Thirty-seven percent of treated horses with moderate (category V) or severe (category VI) injuries returned to racing without recurrence of injury; 57% failed to race once. None of the placebo group returned to racing without recurrent injury, and 71% failed to race once. Although slight (category IV) and moderate (category V) tendon lesions may appear healed clinically and by ultrasonography (with qualitative and quantitative assessment) 4 to 5 months after treatment, the strength of repair is inadequate to permit return to full training, and further time is essential for collagen maturation and remodeling.

Improvements in management have resulted in increased success with the use of β-aminopropionitrile fumarate. Racehorses with career-ending category VI injuries also have been rehabilitated for low-level dressage or eventing, or as show hunters or show jumpers.

Intralesional or Perilesional Administration of Hyaluronan

Hyaluronan is a component of the tendon matrix, directly influences collagen fibril formation and aggregation, and stimulates fibrillogenesis of type 1 collagen. Hyaluronan may decrease adhesion formation during tendon repair. In a clinical field trial, treatment of horses with acute anechoic tendon lesions with a single intralesional injection of high-molecular-weight hyaluronan (Hylartin-V) was compared with use of a saline placebo. Ultrasonography showed that 60% of lesions resolved in the hyaluronan group compared with 24% resolved in the placebo-treated group, but athletic outcome results were not reported.[22] A separate long-term study comparing reinjury rate at a minimum follow-up of 2 years after treatment with intralesional high-molecular-weight hyaluronan combined with a controlled exercise program or controlled exercise alone found no significant difference in recurrence of injury. Neither study reported any adverse reaction to intralesionally administered high-molecular-weight hyaluronan.[22,23]

Corticosteroids

Repeated treatments with corticosteroids may impair tendon healing, but many veterinarians have anecdotally reported that low doses of corticosteroids combined with hyaluronan can be used successfully to manage category III or IV peripheral SDFT lesions in STB racehorses. This practice seldom is used in TB racehorses because of the concern of acute breakdown, an uncommon occurrence in the STB racehorse. A single perilesional injection of 6 to 9 mg triamcinolone acetonide with 10 to 20 mg hyaluronan is suggested. Methylprednisolone acetate is not recommended, because it may be associated with development of dystrophic mineralization. It is important to note that continued exercise during this treatment may lead to more serious injury. Therefore close clinical and ultrasonographic monitoring, modification of training schedules (downscaled), and spaced, selected races for optimal results are recommended.

Intralesional and Systemic Administration of Polysulfated Glycosaminoglycans

PSGAGs are reported to inhibit macrophage activation and collagenase and metalloproteinase activity and therefore may be useful in the acute stage of tendon injury or reinjury.[2] The suggestion has been made that PSGAG may stimulate tenocyte repair. However, in a long-term clinical study, no significant difference was found in the recurrent injury rate of horses with tendons treated with systemic or intralesionally administered PSGAGs compared with controlled exercise alone.[23,24] However, because tendon injuries are potentially career threatening, one author (RLG) often recommends weekly systemic administration of PSGAGs for 4 to 6 weeks for horses with acute injuries of less than 8 weeks' duration. This is combined with other long-term rehabilitation procedures.

Physical Therapies

Physical therapeutic approaches for long-term rehabilitation of a tendon injury, such as therapeutic ultrasound, low-frequency laser, extracorporeal shock wave therapy, cryotherapy, and electromagnetic field therapy frequently are used by owners, but no clinical studies document their therapeutic value over conservative, controlled exercise management.

Other Proposed Long-Term Treatments

See Chapter 73 for a complete discussion of alternative treatments including MSCs, growth factors, and other methods to stimulate regenerative or reparative healing. See the following discussion regarding the surgical management of SDF tendonitis.

◼ SURGICAL MANAGEMENT OF SUPERFICIAL DIGITAL FLEXOR TENDONITIS

Mike W. Ross

Surgical management remains a most useful and viable alternative to all other methods currently employed to augment reparative and regenerative healing of an injured SDFT. Time-honored principles such as decompression, improved gliding function, reduced load, and protection of inelastic scar formation are achieved with surgical management. Postoperative exercise and rehabilitation must be vigorously controlled and are optimized if a philosophy of restricted, controlled exercise without uncontrolled, unlimited turnout exercise is adopted.

TRANSECTION OF THE ACCESSORY LIGAMENT OF THE SUPERFICIAL DIGITAL FLEXOR TENDON

Since Bramlage first described transection of the ALSDFT, also known as *superior* or *proximal check desmotomy*, as a novel surgical treatment for tendonitis of the SDFT, there has been controversy regarding efficacy of the procedure.[1-6] Early, optimistic results were reported in TB racehorses and included 32 of 36 horses (89%) that returned to racing and 25 horses that competed at a level equal to or above the preinjury level.[3] The results of that study were criticized because criteria for success, defined as completing two races and starting a third, were lenient, and horses developing contralateral limb lameness, including tendonitis, were excluded. Results from a larger group of TB racehorses, using a more strict definition of success, revealed that 97 of 137 horses raced (71%) and 70 horses (51%) made more than five starts after surgery, but average earnings decreased in 58% of horses. In that study the mean time from surgery to first start was 353 days.[4] The proposal was that the ALSDFT heals after transection but in an elongated fashion, causing an increased length of the bone-ligament-tendon-bone (radius-ALSDFT-SDFT–proximal and middle phalanges) construct.[5] In a smaller, separate study evaluating the long-term effects of transection of the ALSDFT and other treatments, 53% of flat racehorses, 58% of steeplechasers, and 73% of hurdlers competed in five or more races after surgery.[6] Clearly, with more strict definitions of success, earlier results have been downgraded but do appear superior to results from unmonitored conservative therapy alone. For instance, one estimate claims that only 20% of TB racehorses will complete three or more races after injury.[7] In a separate study of TB horses treated without surgery, 52% returned to racing, but 48% had recurrent tendonitis.[8] More recently, 20 of 28 (71%) TB racehorses were managed successfully nonsurgically with careful rehabilitation (controlled exercise, no turnout), serial ultrasonographic examinations, and a minimum of 8 to 9 months of rest.[9] Clearly, controlled exercise and careful clinical and ultrasonographic examinations are important components of any rehabilitation program. In contrast to other reported results, another study found no difference in prognosis in TB racehorses treated with transection of the ALSDFT compared with conservative management and in fact found horses that underwent surgery to be at risk to develop suspensory desmitis.[10]

In the STB racehorse, results after transection of the ALSDFT are clearly superior to those achieved in the TB racehorse and published results in horses receiving only conservative management. In our study, 35 of 38 horses raced after surgery (92%), and 33 horses (87%) started more than five races, but tendonitis recurred in six horses.[11] Using a strict definition of success, 71% of horses started five or more times after surgery without recurrence of tendonitis, median earnings per start decreased significantly, and mean time from surgery to first start was 237 days. Suspensory desmitis developed in five horses, all of which had bilateral transection of the ALSDFT.[11] In a similar study, 82% of STB horses raced after transection of the ALSDFT, and 69% competed in five or more starts. In that study, horses that raced before injury had a better prognosis.[5] Published results of conservative management in STB racehorses are scant, but in one retrospective study, 31 (76%) of 41 STB racehorses completed two races and started a third, but tendonitis recurred in 43% of these horses.[12]

In summary, transection of the ALSDFT is clearly beneficial in the STB racehorse. Results of transection of the ALSDFT in other types of sports horses have not been published, but I suspect hunters, jumpers, event, and dressage horses have a prognosis somewhere between those published for TB and STB racehorses. Unpublished results in the Three Day Event horse suggest that transection of the ALSDFT may be of limited value, although reasons for this are not known.[13] In a study of 33 horses in which 22 were nonracehorses, tendon splitting under ultrasonographic guidance, combined in some horses with transection of the ALSDFT, resulted in a 68% return to previous level of competition.[14] In the TB racehorse, results of transection of the ALSDFT may be superior to those achieved with intratendonous injections and uncontrolled rehabilitation but are not as favorable as conservative management with controlled exercise.

Surgical Procedure

Currently I prefer conventional surgery using a transthecal approach through the flexor carpi radialis tendon sheath.[3] Compared with the original description of transection of the ALSDFT, this modified approach allows the surgeon to close the incision in three layers, providing a much more secure closure. Transection of the ALSDFT is performed in a caudal location where the ligament is well defined. The surgical procedure is performed using a medial approach, with the horse in lateral recumbency (repositioned if bilateral transection of the ALSDFT is performed) without tourniquet application. The initial incision is made directly over or just cranial to the cephalic vein. The vein is carefully dissected free from underlying antebrachial fascia and retracted caudally. The cranial approach to the vein is less vascular than is the caudal approach, and in most horses a vein penetrating the antebrachial fascia is clamped and ligated. It is important to sever the ALSDFT completely, because incomplete division does not allow immediate transfer of load to the muscle. Intuitively, with incomplete division, it is likely that the ALSDFT would heal faster after surgery and there is less likelihood that the ligament would heal in an elongated fashion. To sever the ligament completely, careful dissection of the proximal fibers from the nutrient artery and vein often is necessary, and in some horses these structures are cut inadvertently or division is

necessary. Division of the vessels causes no known clinical problem, but the vessel ends should be ligated to prevent edema and seroma formation.

Often the proximal aspect of the carpal canal is penetrated, because the ALSDFT is attached to this structure distally. In horses undergoing transection of the ALSDFT an occasional complication is inadvertent transection of the nutrient artery. Ligation of the vessel ends has no adverse clinical consequence. Complications with the surgical procedure are unusual, but the clinician should be aware of what normal healing of the surgical site entails. Nearly all sites develop diffuse swelling within 1 to 3 days after surgery, and in some horses hematoma or seroma formation occurs. The medial antebrachial region is highly vascular, and swelling is common and expected. If necessary, fluid can be evacuated, but this is seldom necessary. Firm, fibrous tissue forms at the surgical site by 4 to 6 weeks after surgery and may persist for several months. However, in most horses it is difficult to see residual swelling by 6 to 8 months after surgery, and cosmetic appearance is acceptable, if not normal, thereafter. I do not believe the postoperative morbidity associated with transection of the ALSDFT is sufficient to warrant a change to the tenoscopic approach.

Transection of the ALSDFT can be accomplished using an endoscopic (tenoscopic) approach through the carpal sheath. Both tenoscopic portals are made on the lateral aspect of the limb. Positioning a horse in lateral recumbency is preferred, but the surgical procedure can be done with the horse in dorsal recumbency if bilateral transection of the ALSDFT is necessary.[15] The ALSDFT can be seen through the sheath and severed, but problems with hemorrhage from transection of the nutrient vessel can be encountered, and whether the entire ligament has been transected is sometimes unclear. Some surgeons prefer the endoscopic approach to avoid swelling that occurs with conventional surgery, but I feel this concern is overrated. Although this approach may be considered more elegant than conventional surgery, I prefer the conventional approach described previously.

How Transection Works

Originally, transection of the ALSDFT was thought to reduce tendon strain, thereby reducing the risk of recurrence of tendonitis. If a gap remained in the ALSDFT after transection, one could reasonably assume load was transferred to the SDF muscle. In this case the muscle rather than the inelastic scar within the tendon could stretch, thereby protecting the healed portion of tendon. Experimental evidence in cadaver specimens suggests that after transection of the ALSDFT, load is transferred immediately to the muscle, but tendon strain increases because of a decrease in the metacarpophalangeal joint angle (hyperextension).[16] Significantly increased strains in both the SDFT and the suspensory ligament were measured in equine cadaver limbs after transection of the ALSDFT in another study, and significant changes in metacarpophalangeal and carpal joint angles had occurred.[17] Both of these studies were performed using cadaver limbs and in vivo results are unknown. Increased tendon strain after transection of the ALSDFT may promote optimal tendon remodeling and collagen cross-linking. It has been proposed that the ALSDFT likely heals after transection, but in an elongated fashion, allowing increased length of the bone-ligament-tendon-bone axis, rather than replacing this load-bearing axis with muscle. This in theory would increase elastic limit of the damaged tendon and negate the intrinsic loss of elasticity found in healed but scarred tendon.[5] I was initially skeptical of the mechanical effects of transection of the ALSDFT, but immediately after surgery horses may exhibit back-at-the-knee conformation (calf knee). Circumstantially the fact that suspensory desmitis and changes in carpal angle occur in horses after transection of the ALSDFT implicates a shift in distribution of load from the SDFT to the suspensory ligament.[10,11] These clinical observations were reinforced with data from the experimental study using cadaver limbs in which increase strain in the suspensory ligament and changes in joint angles were confirmed.[17] Although suspensory desmitis is a serious soft tissue injury and possibility of suspensory injury has altered recommendations for transection of the ALSDFT, I do not consider the risk of suspensory desmitis after surgery a reason to abandon the procedure either in racehorses or in other, nonracehorse sports horses. Based mostly on clinical impression I believe transection of the ALSDFT applies the time-honored principles of decompression, reduced load (increased strain), and protection of the inelastic scar achieved during reparative healing.

When Transection Should Be Performed

I used to perform transection of the ALSDFT with the assumption that the procedure was useful in preventing recurrence of tendonitis, and no attempt was made to perform surgery immediately after discovery of tendonitis. However, my current recommendation is that the procedure be performed as early as possible after injury. Obvious, visible reduction in tendon size occurs in the first 5 to 10 days after surgery, and although I cannot substantiate this claim, the procedure may be important in limiting or reducing inflammation and thus may improve the quality of early healing. Immediate reduction of load on the damaged tendon may explain decreased swelling, but possibly transection of the ALSDFT may function to decompress the injured tendon or may alter blood flow. Reduction in tendon swelling is most marked in horses undergoing transection of the ALSDFT and palmar annular desmotomy but occurs in those undergoing ALSDFT desmotomy alone. Ultrasonographic examination as early as 3 to 4 weeks after surgery often reveals marked improvement of anechoic or hypoechoic regions and reduced CSA measurements that compare favorably with those shown by others recommending intralesional injection of various products aimed at stimulating reparative or regenerative healing of the SDFT (Figure 69-8).

Horse Selection for Transection

Racehorses with mild, diffuse tendonitis or those with core lesions involving 10% or less of the CSA of the tendon likely will heal with conservative management and generally are not considered surgical candidates unless injury is recurrent. Racehorses with recurrent diffuse tendonitis, severe diffuse tendonitis, or core lesions involving 10% to 15% or more of the CSA of the tendon are surgical candidates. In other sports horses, transection of the ALSDFT is recommended in the affected limb in upper-level performance horses using similar guidelines as racehorses, but in lower-level horses conservative management of more severe injuries is often successful.

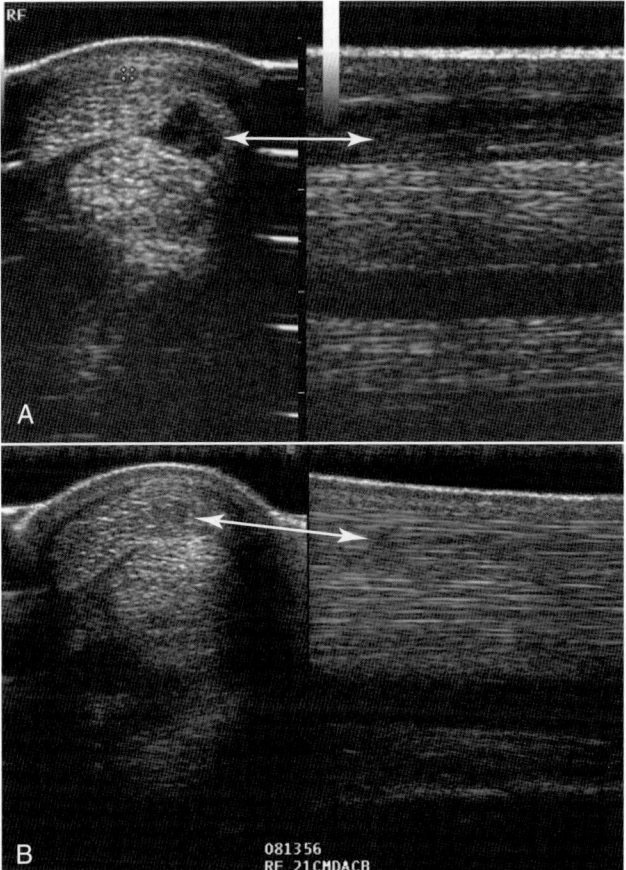

Fig. 69-8 • Transverse *(left)* and longitudinal ultrasonographic images at 21 cm distal to the accessory carpal bone of the right front superficial digital flexor tendon (SDFT) of a 4-year-old Standardbred mare, pacer, with severe superficial digital flexor tendonitis before **(A)** and 28 days after **(B)** transection of the accessory ligament of the SDFT and palmar annular desmotomy. There is marked improvement in the echogenicity of the SDFT soon after surgery, confirming the observation that the clinical appearance of the tendon improves quickly after surgical management.

Bilateral Transection

Bramlage's early results using transection of the ALSDFT in TB racehorses were complicated by the development of SDF tendonitis in the contralateral limb.[2,3] In any racehorse, bilateral tendonitis is not uncommon. Ultrasonographic evaluation of young racehorses with obvious tendonitis in one limb often reveals mild tendonitis in the contralateral limb, and I suggest that both limbs be examined carefully before surgery. These facts led me to consider performing transection of the ALSDFT in racehorses bilaterally, even when the procedure was done prophylactically. However, the horse's age, existence of concomitant suspensory desmitis in the contralateral limb, gait (in STB racehorses), type of sports horse, and cause of tendonitis play a role in decision making. Bilateral transection of the ALSDFT is recommended in horses with bilateral tendonitis; in young, unproven (unraced or early in training) 2- or 3-year-old TB or STB racehorses with unilateral tendonitis in which the contralateral limb is operated on prophylactically; and in horses with subtle ultrasonographic evidence of contralateral tendonitis. Unilateral transection of the ALSDFT (surgical procedure performed in affected limb only) is recommended in show horses; in young racehorses, particularly STB racehorses with suspensory desmitis in the contralateral limb; and in horses with tendonitis caused by direct trauma (tendonitis is unlikely to occur in the contralateral limb), such as a bandage bow. In older TB and STB racehorses I most often recommend transection of the ALSDFT in the affected limb only. In STBs, pacers are more likely than trotters to develop contralateral tendonitis, so in young, unproven pacers I will likely recommend bilateral transection more often than in trotters. In older, proven pacers, I recommend transection only in the affected limb.

Aftercare

Horses are given 2 weeks of absolute stall rest, followed by 6 weeks of stall rest with an increasing handwalking program, beginning with 10 to 15 minutes twice daily. After 8 weeks, an additional handwalking program, walking in the jog cart (STB racehorses), or swimming physiotherapy is recommended for an additional 8 weeks. Turnout exercise is not permitted. Horses then are placed back into early training by trotting and light galloping (TBs) or by walking and light jogging (STBs). Serial ultrasonographic examinations should be performed each time an incremental increase in exercise is planned or when clinical evidence of mild inflammation exists. Time to first start varies considerably but in TB and STB racehorses is 11 to 12 months and 8 to 9 months, respectively.

Large, full-limb support bandages are considered important in limiting motion and swelling at the surgical site(s) and are maintained and changed as needed for a minimum of 14 days. Once bandages have been removed, swelling inevitably occurs at the site(s) of transection of the ALSDFT. An inner, lighter bandage is covered by a heavy cotton, full-limb dressing. Concomitant systemic use of PSGAGs or hyaluronan is controversial, and clear benefits have not been demonstrated, but the use of these medications makes sense to me theoretically. Eight weekly injections of PSGAGs are recommended. Dramatic clinical improvement in tendon size occurs when transection of the ALSDFT is combined with other surgical procedures (see Figure 69-8) or in horses in which peritendonous injection of corticosteroids or a combination of corticosteroids and other antiinflammatory products is used adjunctively with surgery. Phenylbutazone (4.4 mg/kg, intravenously or orally [PO], twice daily for 10 to 14 days) administration appears useful in reducing swelling and improving comfort after surgery.

PALMAR ANNULAR DESMOTOMY

Much attention has been given to transection of the ALSDFT and to tendon splitting, but little to no recent mention has been made of palmar annular desmotomy. This procedure remains a most useful surgical treatment, usually combined with transection of the ALSDFT, to manage tendonitis of the distal aspect of the SDFT. Two distinct clinical situations occur in which palmar annular desmotomy is recommended. The most successful is adjunct use of palmar annular desmotomy in horses with SDF tendonitis. The PAL is a passenger in the disease process, which results in annular constriction of the SDFT. As the SDFT enlarges, the PAL impedes gliding function of the tendon. Further tendon enlargement and inflammation may cause thickening of the PAL, but the primary

disease process involves the SDFT, not the PAL or DFTS. The PAL often becomes thickened and adheres to underlying DFTS and SDFT. Once the PAL impedes SDFT function, lameness, continued swelling, and inflammation occur. Palmar annular desmotomy usually is combined with transection of the ALSDFT but can be a career-saving procedure when done alone. Palmar annular desmotomy provides immediate decompression and improved gliding function of the SDFT, which are important, time-honored surgical principles to follow. The decision to transect the PAL is based on clinical observations. Typically a notch appears along the palmar aspect of the limb when viewed from the side, at the location of the PAL. Even if impingement is not severe, I recommend palmar annular desmotomy. Viewed with ultrasonography the PAL may be normal to moderately thickened and adhesions may exist, but actual evidence of PAL desmitis is lacking. The SDFT is abnormal. After palmar annular desmotomy a reduction in tendon size is seen within 5 to 10 days, and clinically initial swelling appears to redistribute proximal to the PAL and distal to the level of the surgical site. The PAL likely reforms in an elongated fashion after surgery but well after tendon size has decreased. Adhesion formation between the PAL, DFTS, and SDFT may occur after surgery, and inadvertent damage to the edge of the SDFT is possible, but the benefits appear to outweigh the risks of the procedure.

The second and less successful clinical situation in which palmar annular desmotomy is used is in horses with chronic tenosynovitis without tendonitis of the SDFT. These horses may have primary tendonitis of the DDFT, injury of the manica flexoria, or rarely primary palmar annular desmitis (see Chapter 74).

I prefer a minimally invasive conventional surgical approach. A 1.5-cm stab incision is made medially (when used with transection of the ALSDFT) just proximal to the PAL through skin, subcutaneous tissues, and DFTS, but care should be taken to avoid incision of the medial (lateral) aspect of the SDFT. In horses with chronic, severe tendonitis the tissue can be quite thick and care must be taken not to incise the underlying SDFT. A curved bistoury (Sontec Instruments, Englewood, Colorado, United States) or one blade of a pair of straight Mayo scissors is inserted deep to the PAL, superficial to the SDFT. The PAL is incised in its entirety, and care must be taken to transect the distal aspect completely. Reversing the bistoury or scissors blade and transecting the remaining fibers of the PAL and thickened DFTS proximal to the incision may be necessary. The small incision then is closed using subcutaneous and skin sutures. Occasionally a larger incision is necessary in horses with severe and chronic tendonitis, because adhesions preclude accurate insertion of the bistoury or scissors. Care after surgery is the same as described for transection of the ALSDFT when the procedures are done simultaneously, but if palmar annular desmotomy is performed alone, an accelerated exercise program often is advised. Long stall rest periods after palmar annular desmotomy may promote earlier healing of the severed PAL and adhesion formation. After an initial 2-week period of stall rest, handwalking is undertaken for 2 weeks and the tendon is reevaluated. Acceleration of the exercise program at this point may be recommended depending on factors such as the horse's value, class of racing, time of season, and owner's and trainer's proposed schedule.

Other surgical approaches, including an extended open approach or an open approach without entering the DFTS, have been described, but I do not recommend them. The approach described previously can be done with horses in the standing position or while they are under general anesthesia. Endoscopic examination of the DFTS and transection of the PAL have been described elegantly (see Chapters 24 and 74).[18] This is a novel visually pleasing surgical procedure, but in my hospital it is expensive and time-consuming to perform. Complications with any approach include incisional dehiscence, delayed healing, infection, and damage to the ipsilateral edge of the SDFT. Horses with severe tendonitis in which the SDFT is severely enlarged and those with extensive adhesions and thickening of the PAL and DFTS are at greatest risk for complications.

TENOSCOPY OF THE DIGITAL FLEXOR TENDON SHEATH AND CARPAL SHEATH

See Chapter 24 for additional discussion of tenoscopy of the DFTS and carpal sheath. I perform tenoscopy of the DFTS for management of tenosynovitis primarily in non-racehorses and most commonly in the hindlimb. Tenoscopy is valuable for validation of ultrasonographic findings, to evaluate the surfaces and debride defects in the flexor tendons, to debride tears in the manica flexoria, to remove the manica flexoria in horses with complete tears of the structure, to remove soft tissue masses and perform adhesiolysis, and to perform palmar or plantar annular desmotomy under endoscopic guidance. Carpal tenoscopy is valuable to perform ostectomy of the distal caudal aspect of the radius in horses with the unusual condition of exostosis of the distal caudal aspect of the radius and accompanying tenosynovitis, to remove supracarpal exostoses, and to inspect and debride lesions associated with the flexor tendons and the ALSDFT. Occasionally a trotter develops acute tenosynovitis and lameness as a result of hemorrhage in the carpal sheath, and careful ultrasonographic examination reveals injury to the ALSDFT. Desmitis of the ALSDFT has been reported in trotters and nonracehorses and was managed conservatively.[19] However, tenoscopic examination provides additional information about the soft tissue structures and extent of injury, and, importantly the torn edges of the ALSDFT can be debrided.

PROXIMAL METACARPAL FASCIOTOMY AND CARPAL RETINACULAR RELEASE

For horses with proximally located SDF tendonitis an effective method to decompress the damaged, enlarged SDFT and improve gliding function is to transect the proximal metacarpal fascia and carpal retinaculum (desmotomy, retinaculotomy). Clinical diagnosis in horses with only proximal SDF tendonitis can be challenging because swelling and pain can be easily missed during palpation. Lameness is often inappropriately severe based on the minimal clinical signs present; horses often stand with an over-at-the-knee conformation (bucked knee), a positive response to carpal flexion is manifested, and horses may have mild

carpal tenosynovitis. Lameness may worsen after palmar digital analgesia, a clinical observation most commonly seen in horses with proximal palmar metacarpal and palmar carpal region pain. Horses with proximal SDF tendonitis have been reported to have a poor prognosis (two of 12 horses returned to full work).[20] My experience with conservative management appears to be somewhat better than in this publication, but I believe surgical management offers the best chance for full recovery.[21] Horses with severe mid-to-distal SDF tendonitis may have proximal involvement, and fasciotomy or carpal retinacular release appears beneficial. Old horses with inexplicably severe SDF tendonitis often have extension of tendonitis to the region of the carpal canal and may have moderate to severe carpal tenosynovitis (see discussion on page 707). Carpal retinacular release is described for use in horses with carpal tenosynovitis, but it can be useful in horses with SDF tendonitis in which transection of the metacarpal fascia is done concomitantly. This procedure most often is performed in combination with transection of the ALSDFT but can be combined with palmar annular desmotomy also. Prognosis in horses with SDF tendonitis in which transection of the ALSDFT and fasciotomy or carpal retinacular release are performed is guarded to good. Prognosis in old horses requiring transection of the ALSDFT, fasciotomy or carpal retinacular release, or, in some, palmar annular desmotomy is better than expected, because swelling and lameness are often severe in these horses. Substantial reduction in tendon size and lameness score after surgery can be expected, and some horses have returned to light riding or field hunting.

Fasciotomy or carpal retinacular release is done using conventional surgical techniques and usually via a medial approach, because the procedure often is combined with transection of the ALSDFT (Figure 69-9). To perform fasciotomy alone a 2- to 3-cm incision is made through skin and subcutaneous tissues just dorsal to the cephalic vein at the level of the proximal aspect of the second metacarpal bone. Because underlying tendonitis is present, bleeding can be excessive. A 1-cm incision is made in the dense, underlying metacarpal fascia, and straight Mayo scissors are used to extend the fasciotomy proximally through distal aspect of the carpal retinaculum to the level of the distal aspect of the accessory carpal bone and distally to the midmetacarpal region. No distinction is perceivable between fascia and retinaculum because the tissues blend together. Complete transection of the carpal retinaculum is often necessary and requires tedious dissection and careful ligation of vessels. The radial artery and vein run between the inner and outer lamina of the carpal retinaculum and care must be taken to avoid severing these vascular structures. It is mandatory to sever both the inner and outer lamina of the carpal retinaculum to provide decompression and improved gliding function of the SDFT (see Figure 69-9). I prefer using conventional surgical techniques but tenoscopic approaches exist. Conventional surgical incisions often are quite long since it is necessary to sever the carpal retinaculum to the level of the proximal aspect of the accessory carpal bone. Subcutaneous tissues and skin are closed routinely. Bandaging and care after surgery are the same as for transection of the ALSDFT because the procedures usually are performed in combination.

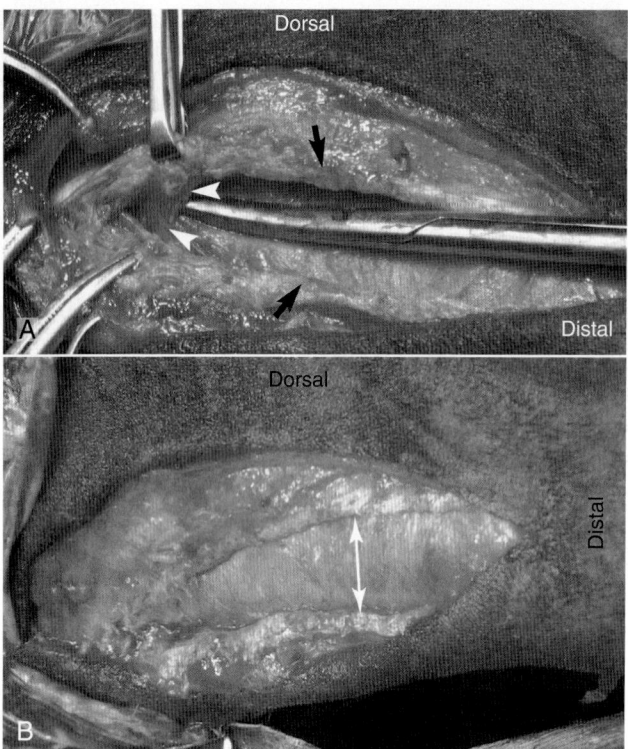

Fig. 69-9 • A, Intraoperative photograph (taken from a palmar perspective) of a 5-year-old Standardbred stallion, pacer, with pronounced lameness from tendonitis of the proximal aspect of the left front superficial digital flexor tendon (SDFT; distal is to the right and dorsal is to the top). The horse is positioned in left lateral recumbency under general anesthesia, and desmotomy of the medial metacarpal fascia (fasciotomy) and carpal retinaculum is underway. The thick, outer lamina of the carpal retinaculum *(black arrows)* is an extension of the metacarpal fascia that has been cut, but it is important to completely sever the inner lamina *(white arrowheads on top of Metzenbaum scissors)* that encircles and constricts the swollen SDFT. **B,** Intraoperative photograph (taken from a palmar perspective) of the same horse after metacarpal fasciotomy and desmotomy of the carpal retinaculum showing that the enlarged SDFT is now decompressed, expanding the cut edges of the severed fibrous tissue *(double-headed arrow).* This horse raced successfully after surgery.

TENOPLASTY—TENDON SPLITTING

Interest in tendon splitting as an adjunct method to manage SDF tendonitis has been renewed. Originally the procedure was developed to promote vascularization of the tendon in horses with chronic tendonitis, and early results showed promise.[22] Experimental studies questioned the value of tendon splitting, and the conclusion was that splitting induced excessive granulation tissue and slow healing of areas of tendon necrosis.[23,24] Clinical use of the technique then fell out of favor, but renewed interest was sparked by reports of combined use of splitting with transection of the ALSDFT in a clinical study and improved healing and revascularization of acute collagenase-induced tendon injuries in an experimental study.[25,26] The collagenase model produces severe tendonitis with extensive necrosis, and I question the value of this model in mimicking the naturally occurring disease. Various authors have reported clinical experiences with tendon splitting used with other procedures, but clinical studies using splitting alone are lacking.[4,5,11,14] Tendon splitting currently is used in horses

with core lesions early in the disease process rather than in horses with chronic tendonitis, the group for which the procedure was designed originally. Tendon splitting, done to decompress areas of hemorrhage, or to provide vascular access channels early after injury, makes theoretical sense for horses with anechoic lesions, but it is of questionable value if done once granulation tissue has formed or mature collagen fibers exist. The rationale given for use in early lesions is to decompress the area of hemorrhage and to provide vascular access channels to improve vascularization by vessel ingrowth. Soon after injury areas of hemorrhage become granulation tissue in which the value of decompression would be minimal. The surgical procedure would have to be performed before granulation tissue develops (3 to 5 days, but certainly before 2 weeks) and may be best reserved for horses with anechoic lesions. Damage caused to peritendonous tissues and surrounding intact tendon fibers must be considered and may outweigh any benefit. However, the procedure has been done apparently successfully or at least without outward harmful effects.

In clinical practice I use the procedure when requested by referring veterinarians or in TB racehorses with anechoic or hypoechoic core lesions. In fact, my best results in TB racehorses have been achieved using tenoplasty in combination with transection of the ALSDFT (see Figure 69-1). The percutaneous technique is preferred, and using a double-edged tenotome is recommended. The procedure seldom is used in the STB racehorse, and in our report detailing results of transection of the ALSDFT in this racing breed, tendon splitting was done in only one horse.[11] In STB racehorses managed with transection of the ALSDFT, I often recommend palmar annular desmotomy if tendonitis extends to the distal metacarpal region, but seldom recommend tenoplasty. In the STB racehorse, I will consider tenoplasty in horses with lesions involving the lateral aspect of the SDFT. Currently I recommend that tenoplasty be done in TB racehorses or other non-STB sports horses with transection of the ALSDFT. Needle decompression of anechoic lesions early after injury may make theoretical sense to provide early decompression, but creation of vascular access channels using this method appears implausible and I do not use the technique.

COMBINED SURGICAL PROCEDURES

Because SDF tendonitis is career-limiting in many sports horses, early and aggressive surgical management should be considered. Potentially, injection of growth factors, MSCs, fresh liquid bone marrow or bone marrow concentrate, or other substances used with surgery and strict rehabilitation may offer the best hope for a successful outcome. Combined surgical management using transection of the ALSDFT and palmar annular desmotomy; transection of the ALSDFT, annular desmotomy, and fasciotomy or carpal retinacular release; or in some horses various combinations with tenoplasty has been successful even in horses with severe tendonitis. In my experience, using transection of the ALSDFT without palmar annular desmotomy in horses with distal SDF tendonitis often results in failure, as does using transection of the ALSDFT without fasciotomy or carpal retinacular release in those with lesions involving the proximal aspect of the SDFT.

The ideal management program for horses with SDF tendonitis has yet to be discovered but should rely on the principles of tendon healing, including minimizing peritendonous scar tissue formation, minimizing the effect of hemorrhage and subsequent granulation tissue formation and disorganized fiber alignment, maximizing gliding function within and external to the SDFT, reducing load and protecting inelastic scar tissue by increasing the length of the bone-ligament-tendon-bone construct, and using an exercise regimen that allows healing and maturation of collagen fibers without deleterious effects of uncontrolled exercise. Surgical management preserves many of these time-honored principles and has proved useful in many types of sports horses.

Treatment of tendon injuries in racehorses is a challenge to clinicians and researchers. Return to racing is associated with a high rate of recurrent injury. However, much progress has been made in the past two decades in diagnostic identification and classification of injury, and the biochemical and biomechanical aspects of tendon injury. Treatment and management programs by necessity depend heavily on economics and trainer decisions relative to continued exercise or long-term rehabilitation. Of vital importance are accurate injury severity categorization, controlled exercise in long-term rehabilitation programs, and ultrasonographic monitoring at all levels of treatment. Improved athletic outcome results gradually evolve as continued basic science research and clinical investigations of past and proposed therapeutic regimens unfold.

■ SUPERFICIAL DIGITAL FLEXOR TENDONITIS IN EVENT HORSES, SHOW JUMPERS, DRESSAGE HORSES, AND PLEASURE HORSES

Sue J. Dyson

SDF tendonitis is a potentially career-limiting injury in event horses and Grand Prix–level show jumpers. Although the incidence of SDF tendonitis is much lower in dressage horses, it is also an important injury. The clinical manifestations vary considerably.

SUPERFICIAL DIGITAL FLEXOR TENDONITIS IN EVENT HORSES

Clinical Signs

Although all event horses are at risk for injury of the SDFT, the incidence of injury is highest in horses competing at advanced or international level, especially those competing in Three Day Events.[1,2] This is probably because of the combination of galloping long distances and jumping on very variable terrain and footing. The introduction of short format Three Day Events does not appear to have reduced the risk of injury. After training or competing, riders commonly apply a proprietary clay to the forelimbs and bandage the limbs at least overnight. This practice may result in early warning signs of impending tendon damage being missed. Because lesions frequently occur bilaterally, subtle changes in limb temperature may be missed except by the most astute and vigilant riders or grooms.

The clinical signs associated with tendon damage vary markedly. A horse may pull up lame after the cross-country phase of an event and rapidly develop peritendonous soft tissue swelling and pain on palpation of the tendon. In some horses the degree of pain is severe and the horse may be distressed and reluctant to bear weight on the limb. If lesions occur bilaterally, the horse may be reluctant to move and its behavior may mimic that of a horse that is tying up. These horses may require both analgesia and sedation to relieve the distress. Clinicians should be aware that a horse may appear very lame, but it may not be possible to elicit pain by palpation of the tendon, although the tendon may feel abnormally soft.

In contrast, a horse may complete the cross-country phase and appear sound, with lameness developing several hours later. Although soft tissue swelling may develop, in some horses there may be absolutely no clues as to the cause of lameness (i.e., no heat, pain, or swelling). This may persist for many days, and then suddenly enlargement, subtle or obvious, of the SDFT may be seen despite resolution of lameness. If swelling is subtle, it may be overlooked and only recognized after localization of the pain causing lameness by local analgesic techniques and clipping of the limb in preparation for ultrasonographic evaluation.

In other horses, lameness is never present. The horse initially may exhibit poor performance, and clinical examination may reveal that the SDFTs are slightly enlarged. Alternatively, the horse may have localized heat and pain on pressure applied to the SDFT, with no history of lameness. Some horses have obvious clinical signs of SDF tendonitis after the first training gallop, cross-country schooling, first event, or a period of reduced work for some months after a Three Day Event. It seems highly likely that these horses sustained damage to the SDFT(s) at the Three Day Event without associated detectable clinical signs.

Clinical signs and the severity of the tendon injury are not necessarily correlated. The clinical signs of SDF tendonitis can easily be masked. I have examined a number of horses at events when the horses have finished lame and had clinical signs compatible with SDF tendonitis. The horses were treated by application of a modified Robert Jones bandage and systemic NSAIDs. Ultrasonographic examination after 5 to 7 days was recommended. The horses were then examined by the owners' regular veterinary surgeons, who were unable to detect any palpable abnormality after removal of the bandage and therefore elected not to perform an ultrasonographic examination. Return to work was recommended by the second veterinary surgeons with catastrophic consequences. Some horses that have completed the speed and endurance phase of a Three Day Event and sustained a tendon injury can be managed to pass the final horse inspection and complete the show jumping without marked deterioration of the tendon injury. In older horses (usually >12 years of age) lesions of the most proximal aspect of the SDFT may develop, extending into the carpal sheath.[3] These can be quite difficult to palpate because heat is difficult to detect and the tight flexor retinaculum may conceal swelling, but they usually cause lameness. The lameness is variable in severity and may be inapparent following rest for several days, but recurs after fast work. Lameness is frequently accentuated by carpal flexion. Lameness may be improved by palmar and palmar metacarpal nerve blocks, but median and ulnar nerve blocks are sometimes required to abolish lameness.

SDFT injury can also arise after an overreach injury; there may also be damage to other structures. The effects of local trauma can vary from localized peritendonous edema with no evidence of tendon damage, to localized hypoechoic or anechoic lesions on the palmar aspect of the SDFT (the result of blunt trauma), to partial or complete laceration (see Chapter 81). Local traumatic injuries do not extend far proximodistally, but partial lacerations can be associated with the development of longitudinal splits extending proximally or distally, which are the result of altered shear stresses. Careful ultrasonographic examination of all adjacent structures is important to establish the severity of injury, bearing in mind that the site of a skin abrasion may not coincide with the site of tendon injury. The subsequent development of peritendonous fibrosis may influence the prognosis.

Diagnostic Ultrasonography

In my opinion, whenever unexplained lameness occurs in an event horse, the SDFTs should be examined ultrasonographically. I also recommend routine ultrasonographic examination 10 to 14 days after the horse has completed a Three Day Event. Baseline ultrasonographic images should be available for comparison, with measurements of CSA at 4-cm intervals distal to the accessory carpal bone throughout the metacarpal region (Figure 69-10). Mild asymptomatic lesions may be identified and should be monitored serially. Ultrasonographic examination should be mandatory for any horse with a history of slight heat or filling in the metacarpal region unless there is an obvious cause (see Figure 69-6). However, it is equally important to recognize the constraints of ultrasonographic examinations from both the skill of the veterinarian and the limitations of the resolution of ultrasonographic images. If an SDFT appears normal ultrasonographically but the clinical signs raise suspicion of injury, the horse should be treated as if it has a tendon injury, with repeat examination after a further 7 to 14 days.

In horses with early subtle tendonitis the only abnormality detectable may be slight, localized enlargement in CSA of the tendon; therefore area measurements and comparisons with the contralateral limb can be extremely valuable. If the injury is bilateral, subtle enlargement in both SDFTs is easily missed. It is important to examine the relative sizes of the SDFT and DDFT and to be aware of the way in which a normal SDFT changes shape from proximally to distally in the metacarpal region (see Chapter 16).

It is also important to look carefully at the echogenicity of the SDFT and compare it with the DDFT and more proximal and distal sites within the SDFT. Subtle lesions often result in a slight diffuse reduction in echogenicity of part or all of the CSA of the tendon, but only in a localized region. Such lesions are easily missed, especially if the gain controls of the ultrasound machine are set too high or if the limb is examined without fine clipping of the hair coat. Detection of these early injuries is very important, because a horse can make a relatively rapid complete recovery at this stage, whereas continued work may result in a much more severe, career-limiting injury. In these early injuries, longitudinal images of the tendon often appear normal. Both forelimbs should be examined routinely.

Because lesions may be very localized, it is important to carefully and systematically examine the tendon from proximally to distally. Although gross core lesions of the

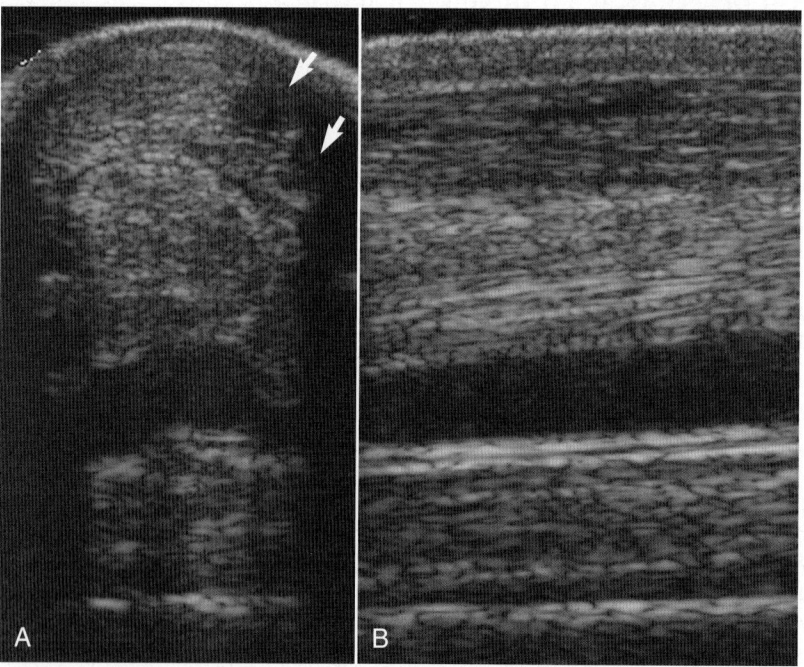

Fig. 69-10 • A, Transverse ultrasonographic image of the palmar aspect of the right forelimb of a 9-year-old advanced event horse; the scan was obtained at 17 cm distal to the accessory carpal bone. Medial is to the left. The horse initially had slight heat in the metacarpal region but no lameness. The superficial digital flexor tendon is enlarged (cross-sectional area 1.2 cm²), and there are focal anechogenic regions on the lateral border. The lesion extended from 14 to 20 cm distal to the accessory carpal bone. **B,** Lateral parasagittal ultrasonographic image of zone 2B; proximal is to the left. There is some loss of long linear echoes, with an anechoic lesion on the palmar aspect.

SDFT are relatively easily identified without fine clipping of the hair coat, image resolution is inferior. Application of mineral oil helps to improve resolution, but this can destroy the ultrasound standoff pad. Subtle lesions will be missed unless the hair is clipped, although shaving is unnecessary. Owners may be reluctant to allow the limbs to be clipped, suggesting that this may jeopardize the horse's evaluation at an inspection at a forthcoming Three Day Event if the limbs actually appear normal and the horse is able to compete. Owners must be persuaded that it may be essential to clip the limbs and that only a narrow strip is necessary; the clinician should suggest that if the horse is fit to compete, the entire horse should then be clipped.

Treatment

Management of SDF tendonitis in the event horse is difficult. Individual horses' capacities to recover from tendon injuries vary considerably. In some horses a marked improvement is seen in the clinical and ultrasonographic appearance of the tendon within 3 months of first injury, whereas little progress is seen in other horses with a similar injury. In almost all horses a convalescent period of 1 year after injury is required. In some horses, normal echogenicity is never restored, and a fairly obvious central hypoechoic area persists ultrasonographically. These horses may be able to withstand one day events but frequently sustain reinjury at a Three Day Event. Lesions in the distal one fourth of the metacarpal region (zones 3B and 3C) are particularly at risk for reinjury. Even in those horses in which relatively normal echogenicity is restored, it is relatively unusual for them to be able to complete more than two Three Day Events without reinjury unless the original injury was mild.

Most published studies of the treatment of SDF tendonitis relate to the racing TB and STB. It is generally accepted that the rate of reinjury is high, especially for horses competing in Three Day Events. Although a horse may be managed successfully to complete one Three Day Event after injury, the risk of subsequent injury is very high.

Of 23 event horses treated with a controlled exercise program alone, 57% were able to return to full athletic function without recurrent injury for a minimum of 2 years after resumption of full work,[4] compared with 56% of 25 horses that received intralesional hyaluronan and the same controlled exercise program and 58% of 31 horses that received intralesional PSGAGs administered intralesionally, systemically, or by both routes. Almost all horses with a unilateral injury reinjured the same tendon. No horses completed more than two Three Day Events without recurrent injury.

The results of intralesional treatment with β-aminopropionitrile fumarate are similar if both the treated limb and the noninjured limb are considered.[5] However, the reinjury rate in the treated limb was considerably better (16%). Of 22 advanced-level event horses, 14 have completed two to six Three Day Events, including nine that have completed three or more Three Day Events at championship level four-star FEI events without recurrent injury. An additional five horses completed two to five Three Day Events before injuring the contralateral limb; three of these horses have completed two additional four-star Three Day Events. Overall, in my experience this treatment seems to offer the best long-term prognosis for event horses with moderate-to-severe injuries of the SDFT, although a licensed product is no longer available. After treatment, horses are walked for 30 to 60 minutes daily for 4 months and are then reexamined ultrasonographically. Successfully treated horses had a remarkably good strength of fiber pattern in longitudinal ultrasonographic images 4 months after treatment. This feature appears to be a good prognostic indicator. Work intensity is slowly and progressively increased thereafter, with horses generally reaching full work by 12 months after treatment. It is premature to judge the efficacy of stem cell therapy, but early results from 109 horses from all racehorse and sports horse disciplines showed a reinjury rate of 13% 1 year after resumption of work.[6] My clinical experience with event horses has been less favorable, although some horses have responded extremely well with sustained return to full athletic function. More recent data from 83 flat racehorses and eight National Hunt racehorses (which excludes horses lost to follow-up) indicate a reinjury rate of 31% (flat racehorses 50%; National Hunt racehorses 23%) 2 years after resumption of full work.[6] A problem remains with medical management, by whatever means, of a horse with a unilateral injury, with no detectable ultrasonographic lesion in the contralateral limb. There is no doubt that despite successful management of the injured limb, the noninjured limb is at risk of subsequent injury.

Desmotomy of the accessory ligament of the SDFT has been less successful in the management of SDFT lesions in event horses than in racehorses, and the disappointing results achieved in my clinic and elsewhere in the United Kingdom have led to this technique being abandoned. It has also fallen out of favor in the United States. Tendon splitting has been used for anechoic central core lesions, combined with a controlled exercise program, with successful results, but the number of treated horses does not compare with the studies described previously.

Regardless of the method of management, serial ultrasonographic examinations during the convalescent period seem to be the most accurate predictors of the final outcome. If the echogenicity and fiber pattern have improved markedly by 4 months after injury, then the longer-term prognosis is much better than in horses in which improvement is only slight. The strength of the fiber pattern when full work is resumed is a good predictor of whether the horse will sustain reinjury.[4,5] It does appear that some horses have an innately better ability to repair tendon lesions than others. Use of Doppler ultrasonography can be helpful for monitoring repair and for identification of reinjury. Normal SDFTs usually have minimal discernible blood flow. After injury a vascular pattern is usually obvious and subsides 3 to 6 months after injury. Reappearance of blood flow indicates reinjury.

Horses with proximal lesions that extend into the carpal canal have generally responded poorly to conservative management, with a high rate of recurrent injury. Surgical release of the flexor retinaculum has enabled several horses to return to full athletic function. The results of treatment with intralesional MSCs have been disappointing.

Pastern Lesions

Injury to the medial or the lateral branch of the SDFT in the pastern region occurs most commonly in forelimbs but also occasionally in hindlimbs (see Chapter 82). Such injury can occur as an isolated acute lesion or as a sequela to previous tendonitis in the metacarpal region. There is usually acute-onset, moderate lameness. In some horses, soft tissue swelling is immediately apparent on the palmar aspect of the pastern, but in others, obvious swelling may take several days to develop. In these horses, perineural analgesia may be required in the acute stage to localize the source of pain. Lameness is alleviated by perineural analgesia of the palmar nerves at the level of the proximal sesamoid bones. Diagnosis is confirmed ultrasonographically. The affected branch is usually enlarged, with poor demarcation of its margins and diffuse or focal areas of reduced echogenicity. There may be some peritendonous hyperechogenic tissue representing fibrosis. Horses with acute lesions with no preceding tendonitis have a fair prognosis for complete recovery after adequate rest for at least 6 months. However, horses with lesions secondary to tendonitis in the metacarpal region have a more guarded prognosis.

SUPERFICIAL DIGITAL FLEXOR TENDONITIS IN SHOW JUMPERS

Injury to the SDFT is comparatively unusual in show jumping horses, except either those competing at international level,[1,7] or horses approximately 15 years of age or older. Injury to the SDFT is most commonly unilateral. There are six typical manifestations:

1. Insidious-onset peritendonous swelling and enlargement of the SDFT, but no associated lameness (Figure 69-11, A). Such horses can generally be managed, but if maintained in full work it is likely that the lesion will deteriorate.
2. Sudden onset of severe lameness while jumping, with rapid development of heat, pain, or swelling. In some horses this is a sequela to previous low-grade injury, but in others there were no previous warning signs. Injuries occur most frequently during competition and may result in an acute, severe lameness with the horse abruptly stopping during a round. Alternatively, the horse may finish lame.
3. Sudden-onset lameness in an older horse, with a lesion extending into the carpal sheath.
4. Sudden-onset lameness associated with distention of the DFTS. There may be no palpable abnormality of the digital flexor tendons, but ultrasonography will reveal a marginal lesion of the SDFT.
5. Progressive enlargement of the SDFT after a previous injury of the accessory ligament of the DDFT (ALDDFT) and lameness. There is usually adhesion formation between the SDFT and the ALDDFT.

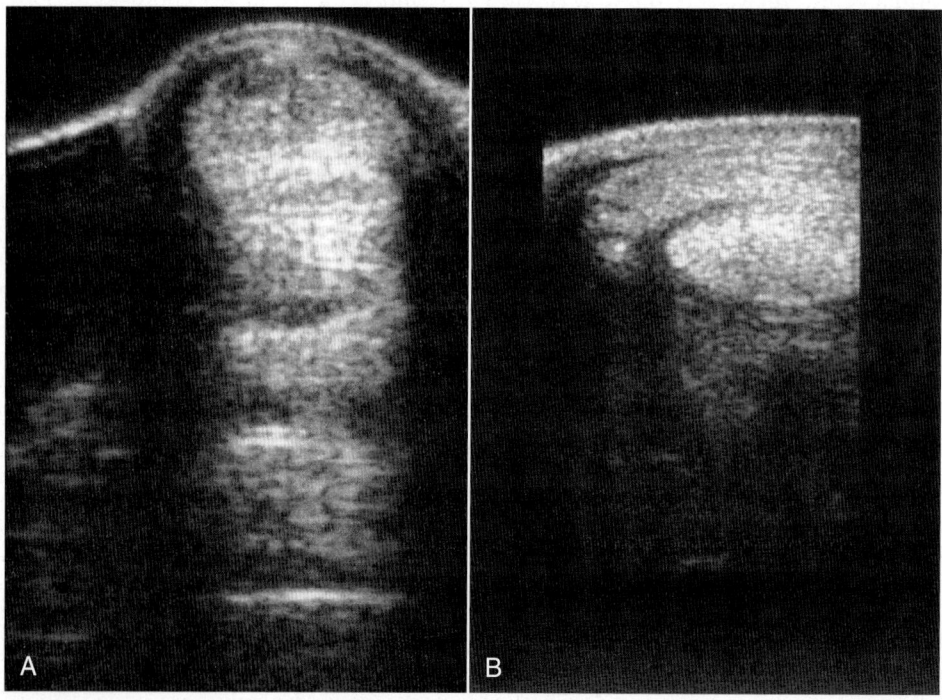

Fig. 69-11 • **A,** Transverse ultrasonographic image of the palmar aspect of the left forelimb of a 13-year-old Grand Prix show jumper; the image was obtained at 11 cm distal to the accessory carpal bone. The horse initially had localized heat and swelling but no lameness. A focal hypoechoic lesion is seen on the palmar margin of the superficial digital flexor tendon (SDFT). The lesion extended less than 1 cm proximodistally. The horse's condition was managed symptomatically, and the horse continued to compete successfully for 6 months with no change in the lesion; the horse then developed acute lameness with exacerbation of the injury. **B,** Transverse ultrasonographic image of the palmar aspect of the distal metacarpal region of a 14-year-old Grand Prix show jumper with acute-onset, severe lameness associated with distention of the digital flexor tendon sheath. Medial is to the left. The medial aspect of the SDFT is enlarged, its margin is irregular, and there are focal anechoic lesions.

6. Occasionally, traumatic injuries occur to the SDFT within the carpal sheath after the horse has sustained a fall (see Chapter 75).

Injuries restricted to the proximal one third of the metacarpal region are common, and there appears to be a tendency for the development of peritendonous adhesions and recurrent lameness. Horses with these lesions have been difficult to manage successfully, as are those with lesions that extend proximally into the carpal canal. However, horses with lesions restricted to the metacarpal region, without peritendonous adhesions, can be rehabilitated and returned to competition with judicious, symptomatic management relatively quickly compared with event horses with a comparable injury. Some horses can withstand return to full work despite persistence of quite obvious ultrasonographic abnormalities of the SDFT. However, the tendon must be monitored carefully, because some horses continue to sustain recurrent low-grade injuries, which result in the tendon becoming progressively larger and wrapping around the DDFT and becoming contiguous with the ALDDFT. Severe injuries predispose to the development of secondary desmitis of the ALDDFT (see Chapter 71).

Desmitis of the ALDDFT may occur as a primary lesion. Severe lesions predispose to the development of secondary SDF tendonitis. Horses with these injuries are difficult to manage successfully. Marginal tears of the SDFT within the DFTS occur occasionally, manifesting as an acute-onset lameness associated with distention of the DFTS (see Figure 69-11, *B*).

Fourteen (93%) of 15 show jumpers with unilateral SDF tendonitis that were treated conservatively after a controlled exercise program were able to return to full athletic function for at least 2 years without recurrent injury, compared with four (80%) of five horses treated with intralesional hyaluronan and three (75%) of four horses treated with PSGAG.[4] Five horses with severe lesions that had not responded adequately to conservative management were subsequently treated with β-aminopropionitrile fumarate, and all have withstood return to international competition without recurrent injury.[5] Horses with lesions extending into the carpal canal have been treated by carpal retinacular release with variable results.

Older horses (>15 years of age) with SDT tendonitis generally have a more guarded prognosis. Some of these injuries appear to be progressive degenerative lesions, which deteriorate despite rest.[3] Injury of the SDFT in ponies is unusual, but I have experience of several teenage event and show jumping ponies that have sustained injuries of the SDFT in the proximal metacarpal region extending into the carpal canal. Although these ponies had unilateral lameness, lesions were identified ultrasonographically bilaterally. Bilateral carpal retinacular release resulted in a favorable outcome.

SUPERFICIAL DIGITAL FLEXOR TENDONITIS IN DRESSAGE HORSES

SDF tendonitis is not a common injury in dressage horses, but it does occur occasionally (Figure 69-12). The

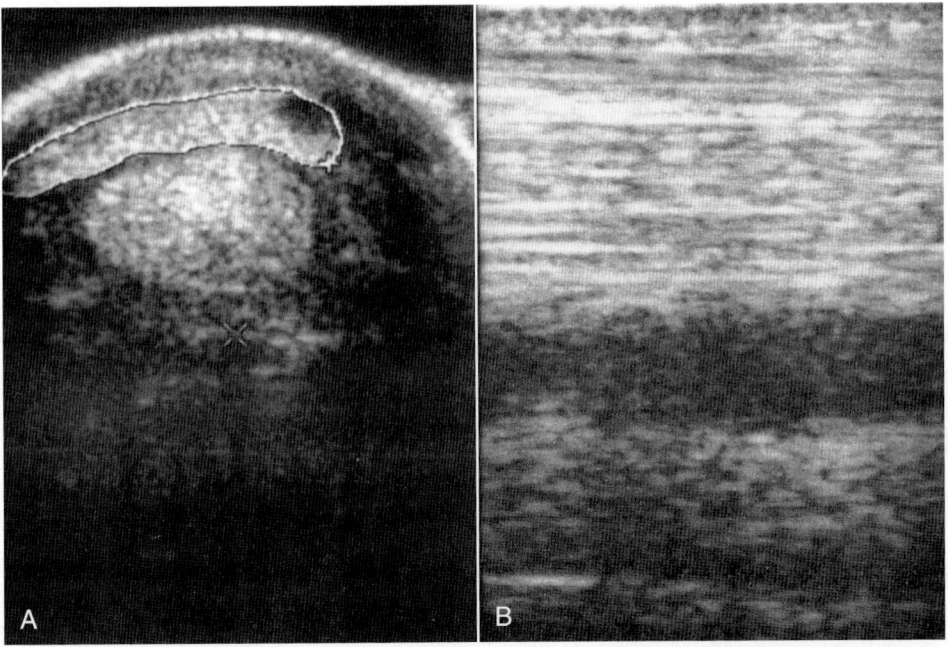

Fig. 69-12 • A, Transverse ultrasonographic image of the palmar aspect of the left forelimb of a 12-year-old Grand Prix dressage horse. The image was obtained at 22 cm distal to the accessory carpal bone; medial is to the left. The horse had exceptionally extravagant forelimb paces and acute-onset, moderate lameness. There is a focal hypoechoic lesion on the lateral aspect of the superficial digital flexor tendon (SDFT). The lesion extended from 16 to 26 cm distal to the accessory carpal bone. At this level the tendon is slightly enlarged (cross-sectional area 1.2 cm²), but at all other levels it was of normal size. **B,** Longitudinal ultrasonographic image of zone 3A obtained from the palmar midline; proximal is to the left. The SDFT appears normal. *Continued*

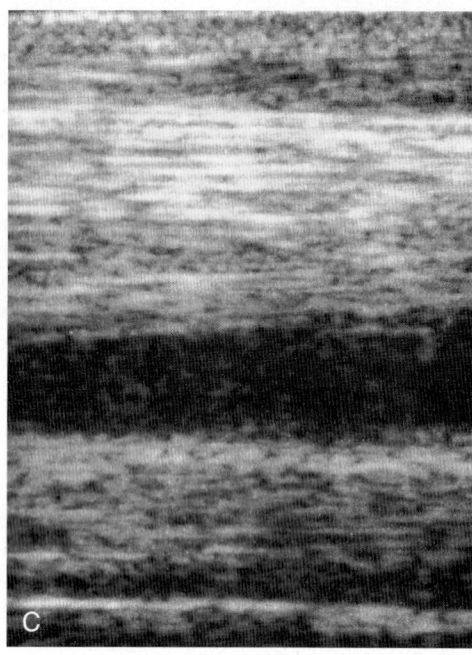

Fig. 69-12, cont'd. • C, Longitudinal ultrasonographic image of zone 3A obtained from the palmarolateral aspect of the metacarpal region shows reduced echogenicity of the SDFT.

at-risk horses appear to be young, very extravagantly moving horses and older Grand Prix horses. Lesions are often quite focal, may be marginal, and are usually associated with low-level lameness. Most lesions occur in the forelimb, but lesions also occur in the distal metatarsal and pastern regions of hindlimbs. Lesions also occur in some relatively young horses disproportionate to the quality of their paces and work history, and these are often difficult to manage and may reflect primary degenerative lesions. Young, big-moving horses with low-grade lesions are managed by restriction to stall rest and controlled exercise, and horses usually resume work after resolution of localized heat, pain, and peritendonous swelling. Horses

with lesions in the proximal one third of the metacarpal region are much more difficult to manage, and clinical signs resolve very slowly regardless of the method of management. Hindlimb lesions have been restricted to the DFTS and are sometimes bilateral. They often are associated with adhesion formation within the DFTS and tend to result in chronic lameness.

Some marginal tears of the SDFT are recognized only during exploratory tenoscopy of a distended DFTS. Concurrent tears of the manica flexoria have also been identified during tenoscopic evaluation. The results of debridement of marginal tears of the SDFT within the DFTS in dressage horses have been rather disappointing. Although lameness has often improved, minor career-limiting gait abnormalities have persisted.

RUPTURE OF THE SUPERFICIAL DIGITAL FLEXOR TENDON IN PLEASURE HORSES

SDF tendonitis is an uncommon injury in general-purpose riding horses, but spontaneous rupture occurs occasionally in old horses in the midmetacarpal region.[8] This results in acute-onset, severe lameness often identified in horses turned out in a field. There is diffuse soft tissue swelling in the metacarpal region, and hyperextension of the fetlock if the horse will bear weight on the limb. If the limb is picked up, a palpable defect can be identified in the SDFT, with the tendon flaccid both proximal and distal to the site of rupture. Ultrasonographic examination reveals complete loss of fiber pattern and an anechogenic region at the site of rupture. Treatment consists of application of a Robert Jones bandage, NSAIDs, and box rest for at least 2 months, with a progressive increase in walking exercise thereafter. Nine of nine horses aged 18 to 22 years made a complete functional recovery, returning to light work within 6 months of injury.[8] One horse subsequently ruptured the contralateral SDFT.

Rupture of the SDFT at the musculotendonous junction is discussed in Chapter 75.

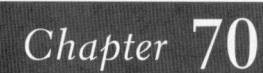

The Deep Digital Flexor Tendon

Sue J. Dyson

ANATOMY

In the forelimb the deep digital flexor tendon (DDFT) has three heads: the humeral head, the largest, and the smaller radial and ulnar heads.[1] The tendon of the humeral head

develops 8 to 10 cm proximal to the antebrachiocarpal joint, but muscular tissue persists to the level of the antebrachiocarpal joint, where the ulnar and radial heads join. The merged tendon is triangular in cross-section within the carpal canal but becomes more rounded in the metacarpal region. The accessory ligament of the DDFT (ALDDFT) merges with the DDFT in the middle third of the metacarpal region.

In the hindlimb the DDFT is formed by a large lateral digital flexor tendon and a smaller medial digital flexor tendon. The lateral digital flexor tendon incorporates the caudal tibialis tendon and passes over the sustentaculum tali within the tarsal sheath. The medial digital flexor tendon passes over the proximal tubercle of the talus, on the medial aspect of the talus, in its own synovial sheath. These two tendons fuse in the proximal metatarsal region.

In the proximal metatarsal region the DDFT is a large oval structure that becomes smaller farther distally. The ALDDFT in the hindlimb varies in size and is generally comparatively smaller than in the forelimb and may be absent; in some horses it is a bifid structure.

At the fetlock region the DDFT becomes wider, elliptical, and fibrocartilaginous and is enclosed within the digital flexor tendon sheath (DFTS). In the pastern region the tendon becomes bilobed. At the level of the proximal part of the middle phalanx the dorsal part of the tendon becomes a fibrocartilaginous pad. Distally the DDFT is molded to the palmar or plantar aspect of the navicular bone. The DDFT is broad, has a terminal fanlike expansion containing cartilage, and inserts on the facies flexoria of the distal phalanx, delineated dorsally by the semilunar line and the adjacent surface of the cartilage of the foot.

The DDFT has a high modulus of elasticity (1585 MPa) and a considerable strength to rupture (approximately 1700 daN).[1] The ALDDFT has a low modulus of elasticity (490 MPa) and a moderate strength to rupture (approximately 490 daN). The DDFT limits carpal and fetlock extension under high loads. In the fetlock region the DDFT is under tension and compression. It is therefore fibrocartilaginous in this region and in the pastern, where the tendon is under pressure from the tuberositas flexoria, a transverse prominence on the proximal palmar aspect of the middle phalanx. In the digit the DDFT facilitates flexion of the proximal interphalangeal joint during weight bearing and stabilizes the distal interphalangeal joint.

The position of the DDFT and the navicular bone varies considerably during the stance phase. In the full weight-bearing position the DDFT is in close contact with only the distal border of the navicular bone, but during propulsion it comes into full contact with the palmar aspect of the bone. The tendon is stretched maximally as active contraction of the muscle bellies and the elasticity in the tendon result in elevation of the fetlock and extension of the distal interphalangeal joint. During the swing phase of the stride the DDFT relaxes. The DFTS facilitates displacement of the digital flexor tendons during flexion and extension.

DDFT injuries occur most commonly in the fetlock or pastern regions within the DFTS or within the hoof capsule. Injuries in the metacarpal or metatarsal regions and the carpus or tarsus are less common.[2-22]

DEEP DIGITAL FLEXOR TENDONITIS ASSOCIATED WITH RECURRENT DESMITIS OF THE ACCESSORY LIGAMENT OF THE DEEP DIGITAL FLEXOR TENDON

Injuries of the DDFT in the carpal or metacarpal region, proximal to the DFTS, are rare except in association with chronic desmitis of the ALDDFT (see Chapter 71). Recurrent desmitis may be accompanied by pathological lesions of the DDFT.[2] Because of the close proximity of the DDFT and its accessory ligament, it is difficult to assess each structure accurately by palpation, especially with chronic enlargement of the ALDDFT, which may wrap around the borders of the DDFT. Ultrasonographic examination may reveal slight enlargement of the DDFT. The dorsal

border may be less well defined, and diffuse hypoechogenic regions may occur within the DDFT, extending a variable distance proximodistally. These injuries usually result in recurrent lameness.

It has also been noted that in association with substantial enlargement of the superficial digital flexor tendon (SDFT) because of chronic tendonitis, the DDFT becomes smaller in cross-sectional area.[3] With chronic enlargement of the ALDDFT, the DDFT also may reduce in size.

Primary deep digital flexor tendonitis in the proximal metacarpal region is rare. A single case was recorded by Genovese and Rantanen[4] in an 8-year-old Quarter Horse used for English pleasure riding. Lesions have been identified using magnetic resonance imaging in a small number of horses.[5,6] Occasionally, traumatic injuries of the DDFT have been seen within the carpal sheath (see Chapter 75).

DEEP DIGITAL FLEXOR TENDONITIS IN THE CARPAL SHEATH SECONDARY TO SOLITARY OSTEOCHONDROMA OR A DISTAL RADIAL PHYSEAL EXOSTOSIS

Lesions of the DDFT within the carpal sheath are an unusual cause of lameness except secondary to irritation by a solitary osteochondroma or a distal radial physeal exostosis.[7] An osteochondroma is an exostosis continuous with the cortex of the bone and is covered by cartilage. The osteochondroma develops immediately proximal to the distal radial physis, often medial to the midline. Lameness is sudden in onset and usually is accentuated by carpal flexion. There is usually distention of the carpal sheath, but some horses with physeal exostoses have severe, sporadic lameness with no localizing clinical signs. An osteochondroma is readily identifiable radiologically, but some physeal exostoses are more readily identified using ultrasonography. Ultrasonographic examination from the distal medial aspect of the antebrachium also reveals the abnormal bone contour, an abnormal amount of fluid within the carpal sheath, and an irregular dorsal contour of the DDFT. Treatment is by tenoscopic surgical removal of the osteochondroma or exostosis and debridement of any torn fibers of the DDFT. The prognosis for return to athletic function is excellent.

DEEP DIGITAL FLEXOR TENDONITIS WITHIN THE DIGITAL FLEXOR TENDON SHEATH IN THE FETLOCK REGION

Some enlargement of the DFTS is common in hindlimbs, often unassociated with lameness, but occurs less frequently in forelimbs. Sudden-onset lameness associated with distention of a DFTS in a forelimb or a hindlimb may be caused by a variety of different lesions, but deep digital flexor tendonitis always should be considered[5,6] (see Chapter 74). It is rare to identify lesions of the DDFT within a DFTS that is not distended. Some horses develop deep digital flexor tendonitis *after* long-term chronic enlargement of the DFTS.

Lameness associated with DDFT lesions within the DFTS occurs more frequently in hindlimbs than in forelimbs and in horses from a variety of disciplines. The

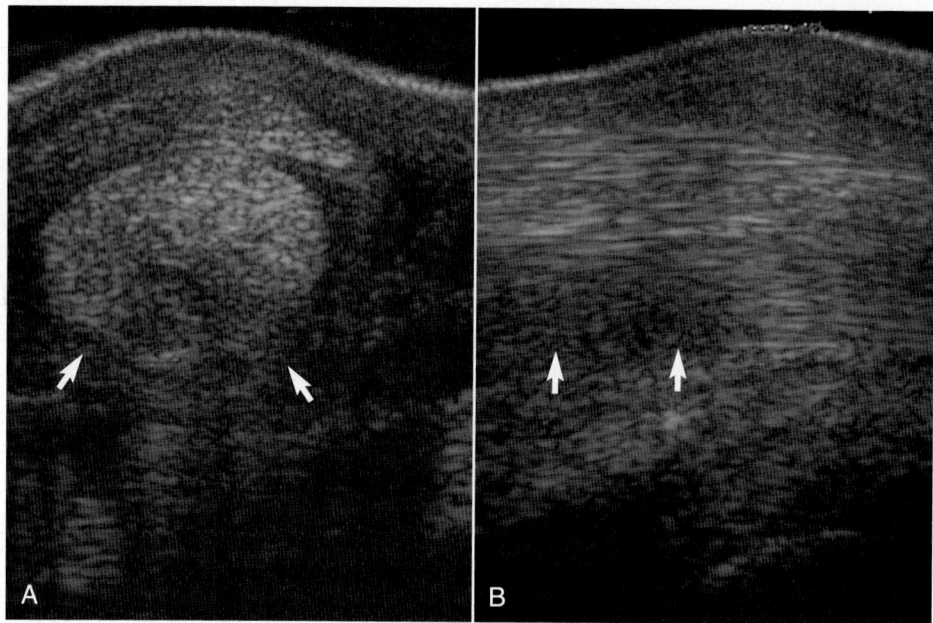

Fig. 70-1 • Transverse (**A**) and longitudinal (**B**) ultrasonographic images of the left hindlimb of a horse with sporadic left hindlimb lameness. There was chronic moderate distention of the digital flexor tendon sheath of both hindlimbs. There is diffuse reduction in echogenicity in the dorsal half of the deep digital flexor tendon (**A**, *arrows*) and loss of fiber pattern (**B**, *arrows*).

condition usually occurs unilaterally, although it has been seen bilaterally in the hindlimbs of several Warmblood dressage horses[3] and in show jumpers.

Lameness varies from mild to moderately severe. Distention and thickening of the DFTS may make accurate palpation of the DDFT difficult. In some horses pain can be elicited by palpation of the margins of the tendon or by firm pressure applied to its palmar (plantar) aspect. The tendon should be assessed throughout its length, proximal and distal to the fetlock. In the acute stage there may be localized heat. Passive flexion of the lower limb may induce pain. If forelimb lameness is only mild in straight lines, it may be exaggerated on the lunge on a soft surface, especially in medium and extended trot. Distal limb flexion often accentuates the lameness. Occasionally in hindlimbs lesions of the DDFT within the DFTS have been the cause of sporadic lameness. The intermittent nature of the lameness makes definitive identification of the cause a diagnostic challenge. Such a history seen in conjunction with distention of the DFTS should prompt ultrasonographic examination (Figure 70-1).[16]

Intrathecal analgesia of the DFTS usually results in substantial improvement but rarely alleviates lameness. Better improvement is seen after perineural analgesia of the palmar or plantar nerves and palmar metacarpal (plantar metatarsal) nerves (a so-called low 4-point block) proximal to the distended DFTS. In horses in which the metacarpophalangeal (metatarsophalangeal) joint capsule also is distended, performing intraarticular analgesia may be necessary to be sure that distention is not contributing to pain.

Definitive diagnosis requires ultrasonographic examination. Four types of lesions involving the DDFT have been identified: enlargement and change in shape of the tendon, focal hypoechoic lesions within the tendon or on its border, mineralization within the DDFT, and marginal tears.[8-14] The first three are readily diagnosed using

diagnostic ultrasonography, but the marginal tears are much more difficult to identify. Surgical exploration may be required for definitive diagnosis.[8] Acute-onset focal hypoechogenic areas generally are not seen with preexisting adhesion formation, although any of the other lesions may be.

The normal DDFT changes in its shape and cross-sectional area from proximally to distally, but it is usually bilaterally symmetrical. A normal DDFT is uniform in its echogenicity, and its margins are clearly defined. At the site at which the ALDDFT merges with the DDFT there may be a relatively hypoechogenic region, especially in the hindlimbs. This is a normal variant. Hypoechoic artifacts are induced readily in the distal fetlock and pastern regions if the ultrasound transducer is not perpendicular to the tendon, and in these regions evaluating the SDFT and DDFT simultaneously is difficult. Echogenic synovial plicae (mesotendon) extend medially and laterally from the DDFT to the DFTS wall in the proximal recess of the DFTS (Figure 70-2, *A*). These are seen much more obviously when the tendon sheath is distended and should not be mistaken for marginal tears or adhesions. With chronic tenosynovitis, these plicae may become thickened. Distal to the fetlock is an echogenic palmar (plantar) synovial fold that should not be confused with an adhesion (see Figure 70-2, *B*). The ergot on the palmar (plantar) distal aspect of the fetlock prohibits ultrasonographic evaluation at this level, and lesions of the DDFT may be missed. The size of the palmar (plantar) annular ligament (PAL) and the presence of subcutaneous fibrosis should also be evaluated because this may influence prognosis.[13]

Enlargement or Change in Shape of the Deep Digital Flexor Tendon

In horses with low-grade injuries the only detectable ultrasonographic abnormality is a change in shape or size of the

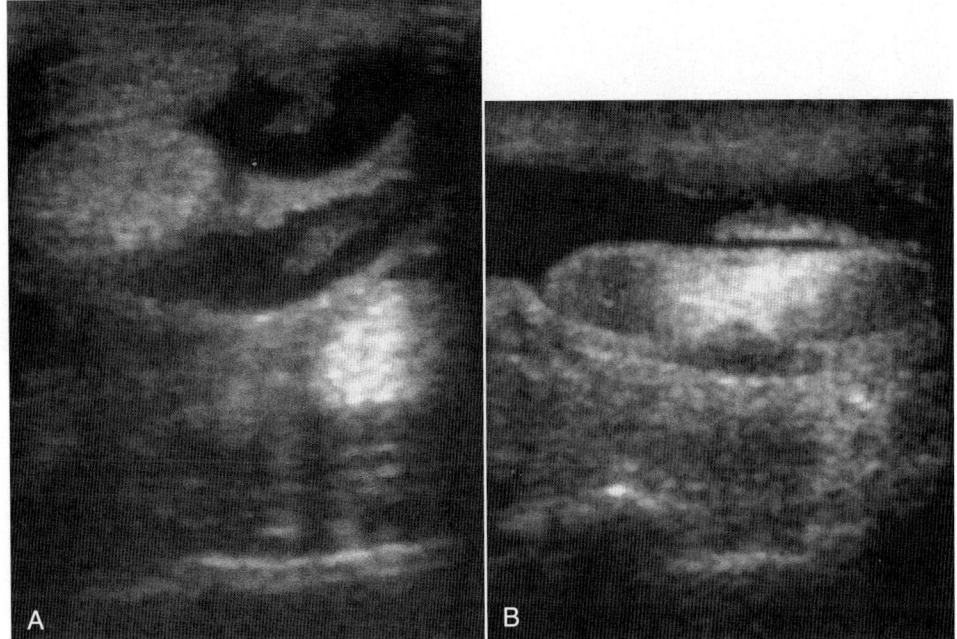

Fig. 70-2 • Transverse ultrasonographic images of the digital flexor tendon sheath (DFTS) in **(A)** the distal metacarpal region and **(B)** the pastern. Medial is to the left. **A,** An abnormal amount of fluid is within the DFTS, but the deep digital flexor tendon (DDFT) appears normal. Note the prominent synovial plica extending from the lateral aspect of the DDFT. This plica also is thickened slightly, and other echogenic material is within the anechogenic synovial fluid, but the horse had no associated lameness. **B,** Note the abnormal amount of fluid within the DFTS, and the synovial plica on the palmar aspect of the DDFT. These are normal anatomical structures that are visible most readily when the DFTS is distended.

DDFT. The echogenicity and fiber pattern may appear normal; therefore these injuries are easily overlooked. The DDFT may look rounder in cross-section, rather than elliptical. Careful comparison with the contralateral limb at the same distance distal to the accessory carpal bone is important for accurate diagnosis. Comparison of the relative sizes of the SDFT and DDFT can also be helpful. Cross-sectional area measurements of the SDFT are prone to error at this level, and therefore measurements of the dorsopalmar thickness of the SDFT and DDFT are more accurate. If the horse fails to respond satisfactorily to conservative management, then consideration should be given to the presence of a marginal tear that may not be detectable with ultrasonography.[3]

Constriction of the DFTS and its contents by an enlarged PAL may result in secondary compression of the DDFT.

Focal Hypoechoic Lesions

The cross-sectional area of the DDFT may be enlarged. Focal hypoechoic lesions vary in size and position within the cross-section of the tendon and in length. Some are small, occupying less than one tenth of the cross-sectional area of the tendon and extending less than 1 cm proximodistally, whereas others are considerably more extensive (Figure 70-3).[5] Generally, larger lesions are associated with more severe lameness. These lesions generally occur immediately proximal to, or at the level of, the fetlock joint. An abnormal amount of synovial fluid is found within the DFTS, and sometimes adhesions are identified.

In some horses, inspection of the medial or lateral border of the DDFT reveals loss of definition of the margin of the tendon and an area of reduced echogenicity, indicating major fiber disruption. These lesions are easy to diagnose. The marginal tears described subsequently (see page 730) are more difficult to detect.

Small lesions have resolved with rest, and horses have returned to full athletic function. However, large lesions tend to persist, and ultrasonographic examination may reveal no change, even if the horse has been rested for more than 1 year. Large lesions have been associated with recurrent lameness.[8] Intrathecal medication with hyaluronan, triamcinolone acetonide, or methylprednisolone acetate has resulted in only temporary relief. Desmotomy of the PAL has resulted in only temporary remission of clinical signs. The prognosis for return to full athletic function is guarded. A few sports horses have been successfully managed by intralesional injection of cultured mesenchymal stem cells, with subsequent ultrasonographic resolution of lesions and return to full athletic function, without recurrent injury for up to 3 years after treatment.[23]

Fibrosis and Mineralization within the Deep Digital Flexor Tendon

Some horses develop widespread hyperechogenic foci within the DDFT in the fetlock region. Some of these create shadowing artifacts and therefore represent mineralization (Figure 70-4). The foci generally but not invariably reflect a chronic injury.[14] If extensive, they make evaluation of the remaining tendon architecture difficult because of acoustic shadowing. The cross-sectional area of the tendon usually is enlarged. Ill-defined hypoechogenic regions

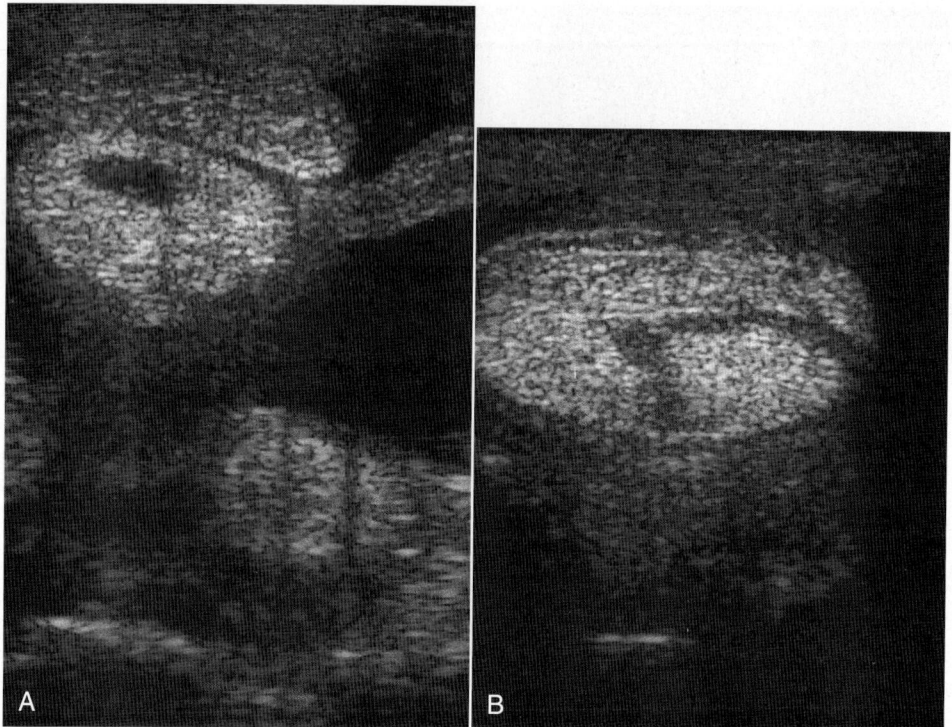

Fig. 70-3 • Transverse ultrasonographic images of the distal metatarsal region of a horse with acute-onset right hindlimb lameness associated with distention of the digital flexor tendon sheath (DFTS). Medial is to the left. An abnormal amount of fluid is within the DFTS. **A,** There is a well-defined anechogenic lesion within the deep digital flexor tendon, close to the plantar border. Note also the rather poorly defined dorsal border. **B,** Slightly farther distally the lesion can be seen to involve the dorsal and plantar borders of the tendon.

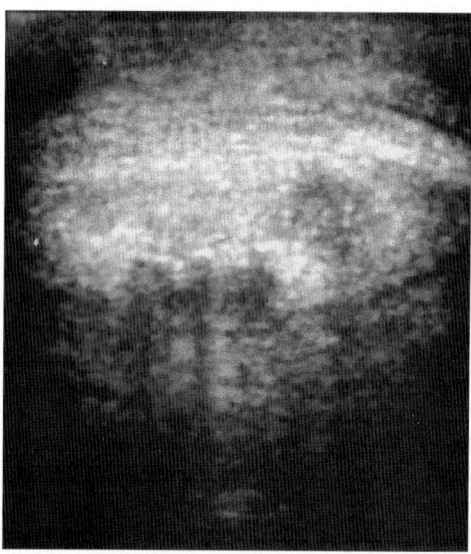

Fig. 70-4 • Transverse ultrasonographic image of the distal metatarsal region of an 8-year-old event horse with chronic right hindlimb lameness associated with distention of the digital flexor tendon sheath. Medial is to the left. The deep digital flexor tendon (DDFT) is enlarged. Many hyperechogenic foci are within the DDFT, resulting in shadowing artifacts that make accurate evaluation of the structure of the more dorsal aspects of the tendon impossible.

often extend proximally or distally from hyperechogenic foci or are remote from them. Fibrous adhesions may extend from the DDFT to the DFTS wall.

The cause of these hyperechogenic lesions is unknown, although some affected horses have a history of previous injections of corticosteroids into the DFTS. Most of the affected horses are middle-aged Warmblood-type horses used for show jumping or dressage. These lesions tend to result in persistent long-term lameness.

Marginal Tears of the Deep Digital Flexor Tendon

Marginal tears of the DDFT have been identified on the medial, lateral, and dorsal borders.[3,8] Lesions involving the lateral margin have been identified most commonly, varying in length (Figure 70-5). Frequently the proximal extent of the tear is at the level of the manica flexoria. Some lesions extend as far distally as the proximal digital annular ligament. In some horses the lesion is a frontal (dorsal) plane split in the margin of the tendon; in other horses a sagittal tear of fibers occurs. Frontal plane splits in the DDFT, which may be the result of compression of the tendon with the fetlock in extension, may not be detectable by ultrasonography, although often a detectable enlargement of the cross-sectional area of the DDFT exists. The affected margin may be slightly less well defined compared with normal findings. Occasionally a torn echogenic strand is seen partially detached from the DDFT. Care must be taken not to confuse the synovial plicae on the medial and lateral borders of the tendon with a marginal tear. It is important to recognize that lesions may occur at more than one location; therefore evaluation of all accessible regions of the DDFT is recommended.

Diagnosis is based on surgical exploration of the DFTS, which is indicated if a horse has pain associated with the DFTS along with abnormalities of the DDFT detected by ultrasonography, or no detectable changes, but a failure to

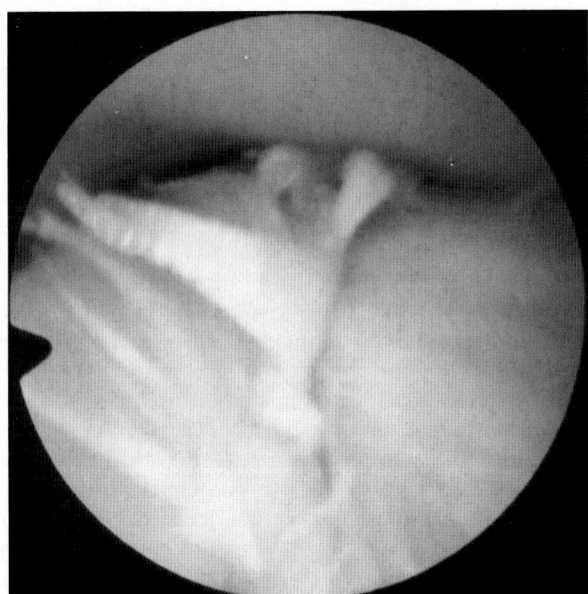

Fig. 70-5 • The lateral margin of the deep digital flexor tendon (DDFT) within the digital flexor tendon sheath in the distal metacarpal region, viewed tenoscopically. The DDFT has a marginal tear. Ultrasonographic examination revealed slight enlargement of the DDFT, but otherwise the tendon appeared structurally normal. (Courtesy I.M. Wright, Newmarket, England.)

respond to conservative management (see Chapter 74). Tenoscopic evaluation via a portal on the proximopalmar (proximoplantar) aspect of the pastern enables the most comprehensive view of the flexor tendons.[17] However, proper evaluation of the DDFT underneath the manica flexoria may not be possible unless the manica flexoria is transected. Treatment can be by debridement of the lesion, which can be done tenoscopically, or by debridement and suturing. The latter may be achieved most effectively by transection of the palmar PAL and opening of the DFTS, followed by primary closure of the PAL; however, this technique is potentially associated with some morbidity. Some horses develop thickening of the PAL and/or the proximal digital annular ligament postoperatively, together with subcutaneous fibrosis, which results in persistent lameness. Five of six horses used for dressage, show jumping, or horse trials treated by open surgery to repair defects in the margin of the DDFT had persistent lameness associated with this type of reaction.[3] Therefore tenoscopic debridement is the preferred method of management, although the prognosis remains guarded. Prognosis for horses treated by tenoscopic debridement depends in part on the length of the lesion, with 40% to 59% of horses returning to full athletic function.[10,12] Generally horses with hindlimb injuries have had a better prognosis than those with forelimb injuries.

DEEP DIGITAL FLEXOR INJURIES IN THE PASTERN REGION

The DDFT within the pastern remains within the DFTS, over which lie the thin proximal and distal digital annular ligaments. The tendon is therefore relatively close to the skin surface and so is vulnerable to the effects of direct trauma and puncture wounds.

In the pastern region the DDFT is a bilobed structure, each lobe being similar in size and shape at any level. Care must be taken when evaluating the tendon by ultrasonography because off-incidence artifacts are created readily. These may be seen as central, round hypoechogenic areas and should not be mistaken for lesions.

Deep Digital Flexor Tendonitis

Deep digital flexor tendonitis restricted to the pastern region is not a common cause of lameness and occurs less often than sprain of the oblique sesamoidean ligaments or strain of one of the branches of the SDFT (see Chapter 32). Many horses with lesions of the DDFT have lesions that extend into the hoof capsule and are discussed in Chapter 32. Tendonitis of the DDFT in the pastern region is seen most often in skeletally mature horses and occurs more often in forelimbs than in hindlimbs. Deep digital flexor tendonitis occurs in a variety of sports horses, but the incidence in racehorses is lower than in other performance horses.

Deep digital flexor tendonitis in the pastern region usually results in acute-onset, unilateral, moderate-to-severe lameness that is persistent. Less commonly lameness is detectable only after maximal exertion and has resolved with rest but has progressively worsened over 1 to 2 years.[3] Slight, firm soft tissue swelling may occur on the palmar midline of the pastern region. Often, slight distention of the DFTS occurs in the pastern region, but an obvious windgall may not be apparent. Firm palpation on, or just to one side of, the palmar midline of the pastern region may cause pain. Lameness is often worse on a soft surface compared with a hard surface and generally is improved substantially by perineural analgesia of the palmar nerves at the level of the proximal sesamoid bones.

Diagnosis is based on ultrasonographic evaluation. Careful comparison of the size and shape of the contralateral DDFT is useful. The ease with which the tendon can be evaluated distally in the pastern depends on the conformation of the pastern and foot. Evaluation is more difficult in horses with a narrow heel and a deep cleft between each bulb. A lesion may involve just one lobe of the tendon or both and is usually characterized by enlargement and alteration in shape of the tendon, with or without hypoechogenic regions within the tendon. Off-incidence imaging may be necessary to identify areas of fibrosis. The medial and lateral margins of the tendon should be carefully evaluated. In horses with chronic injuries focal hyperechogenic foci consistent with dystrophic mineralization may be seen. Occasionally a complex of injuries is identified involving not only the DDFT, but also a distal sesamoidean ligament or the distal digital annular ligament. All structures should be examined carefully and systematically. Horses with lesions restricted to the DDFT that have been recognized early usually respond reasonably to prolonged rest (6 to 12 months), with progressive resolution of hypoechoic defects as assessed by ultrasonography. Some enlargement of the tendon may persist long term. Horses with more chronic injuries or complex injuries including adhesion formation respond less favorably, with a high incidence of recurrent lameness, even with surgical intervention. There are anecdotal reports of successful treatment by intralesional injection of platelet-rich plasma or cultured mesenchymal stem cells. However, if the periphery of the DDFT is not intact, leakage of mesenchymal stem cells may result in echogenic tissue being laid down within the DFTS, with associated chronic lameness.

Lesions of the DDFT have been described in association with primary injuries of the distal digital annular ligament diagnosed using magnetic resonance imaging.[24] Such injuries have been characterized by focal thickening of the distal digital annular ligament and increased signal intensity in at least T1- and T2-weighted images. It was suggested that lameness could be successfully treated by transection of the distal digital annular ligament, but given the integral relationship between the DDFT and the distal digital annular ligament it is difficult to see how this can be achieved. In my clinical experience injuries of the DDFT and the ipsilateral aspect of the distal digital annular ligament are usually identified in association with other soft tissue injuries on the ipsilateral aspect of the foot.

Injury Caused by Blunt Trauma in the Pastern Region

Direct blunt trauma caused by, for example, a severe overreach can result in severe inflammation of the subcutaneous tissue, the digital annular ligaments, and sometimes also the DDFT. If the proximal or distal digital annular ligament becomes thickened and fibrosed, this can create undue pressure on the DDFT and chronic pain, without any structural abnormality of the DDFT. In the acute stage, generalized swelling occurs in the pastern region, and palpation elicits pain. Ultrasonographic examination is required to determine which structures have been damaged. This may need to be repeated as fibrotic reactions develop in the ensuing weeks. The prognosis is generally favorable unless the digital annular ligaments become substantially thickened or the palmar aspect of the DDFT is torn.

An overreach sometimes results in laceration of the skin and the palmar aspect of the DDFT. These lacerations may not coincide because of the mobile nature of the skin, and damage to the DDFT may be overlooked unless the tendon is examined by ultrasonography. One or both branches of the SDFT may also be damaged, so all structures should be evaluated carefully and systematically. Such lesions often heal with extensive fibrotic reactions and adhesion formation to the DFTS, which may result in chronic lameness.

Puncture Wounds of the Deep Digital Flexor Tendon and Blunt Trauma

Puncture wounds in the palmar (plantar) aspect of the pastern region, caused by sharp objects such as a flint, can cause sudden-onset, moderate-to-severe lameness and rapid development of effusion within the DFTS. Ultrasonographic examination can be used to determine whether the DDFT was penetrated. An anechoic defect may be seen in its palmar border. With prompt treatment by vigorous lavage of the DFTS combined with systemic broad-spectrum antimicrobial therapy, the outcome may be favorable. Ideally the DFTS and its contents should be inspected using an arthroscope to determine if any foreign material was embedded within the DDFT that might seriously compromise the outcome.

Alternatively, blunt trauma to the pastern region may result in an innocuous wound followed by the subsequent development of severe lameness in association with a core lesion of the DDFT. It is postulated that this may be the result of avascular necrosis of the tendon.[18] The prognosis is poor.

Rupture of the Deep Digital Flexor Tendon

Rupture of the DDFT in the pastern region or within the hoof capsule is usually a sequela to a previous neurectomy of the palmar digital nerves. Neurectomy is usually performed because of suspected navicular disease or to relieve chronic foot pain of unknown cause. Preexisting lesions of the DDFT are likely to predispose to tendon rupture. I have never examined a horse with spontaneous rupture of the DDFT that did not have a history of neurectomy. Lameness may be insidious and progressive or sudden in onset, associated with extensive swelling in the pastern region. Thickening results from enlargement of the DDFT, peritendonous fibrosis, and, in horses with long-term injuries, secondary superficial digital flexor tendonitis. Complete rupture results in the toe of the limb flipping up when the limb is bearing weight (Figure 70-6). These clinical signs are pathognomonic. In such horses the proximal end of the DDFT may retract proximally, resulting in the SDFT becoming opposed to the fibrocartilaginous scutum on the palmar aspect of the pastern region. Radiologically a variable degree of subluxation of the distal interphalangeal joint exists, depending on the degree of integrity of the DDFT. The prognosis is hopeless for athletic function. Extensive peritendonous fibrosis ultimately develops, providing adequate

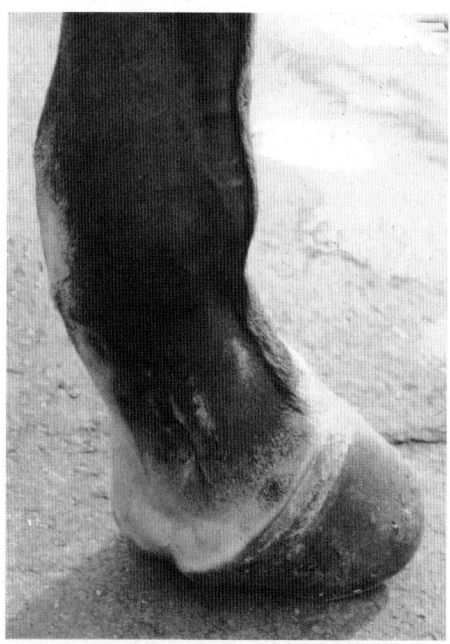

Fig. 70-6 • The distal aspect of the right forelimb of a horse with rupture of the deep digital flexor tendon 5 months after palmar digital neurectomy. The toe is flipped upward, associated with subluxation of the distal interphalangeal joint. There is considerable thickening in the pastern region caused by peritendonous fibrosis. Note the surgical scar.

support to preserve life for breeding, assuming that the contralateral limb can withstand the strain in the interim. Arthrodesis of the distal interphalangeal joint remains a management option for salvage of a horse for breeding purposes or pasture soundness.

LESIONS OF THE DEEP DIGITAL FLEXOR TENDON WITHIN THE HOOF CAPSULE

Lesions of the DDFT within the hoof capsule are discussed in Chapter 32.

LESIONS OF THE DEEP DIGITAL FLEXOR TENDON IN THE TARSAL AND PROXIMAL METATARSAL REGIONS

Primary deep digital flexor tendonitis in the tarsal or proximal metatarsal regions is an unusual cause of hindlimb lameness (see Chapter 76). Lesions in the proximal metatarsal region have been identified in young Thoroughbreds in race training, with lameness associated with mild swelling in the proximal plantar metatarsal region. Lameness was improved transiently by intraarticular analgesia of the tarsometatarsal joint in two horses, presumably because of local diffusion of local anesthetic solution.[3] Subtarsal analgesia of the plantar and plantar metatarsal nerves alleviated lameness in one horse. Ultrasonographic examination revealed enlargement of the DDFT in the proximal metatarsal region, poor definition of the margins, and diffuse hypoechogenic areas within the tendon. Rest for 3 months resulted in resolution of lameness, and the prognosis is favorable for return to racing.

Primary lesions of the DDFT in the tarsal region have been identified only in skeletally mature horses and are comparatively rare. Lameness is sudden in onset and moderate in degree. Mild distention of the tarsal sheath may occur, but localizing signs may be absent. Lameness is improved by perineural analgesia of the tibial and fibular nerves, but it is unaffected by intraarticular analgesia of the hock joints. Diagnosis relies on ultrasonographic examination. The DDFT may be examined from the plantaromedial aspect of the hock within the tarsal sheath. The DDFT is a large oval structure with well-defined margins. The dorsolateral aspect of the tendon may appear slightly less echogenic than the remainder of the tendon due to structural adaptation, and care should be taken not to misinterpret this as a lesion (Figure 70-7). Careful comparison with the contralateral limb is essential. Abnormalities include enlargement of the tendon, poor demarcation of the borders, and hypoechogenic areas. Lesions may also be identified by tenoscopic examination of the tarsal sheath (see Chapters 24 and 76).

Lesions of the DDFT also have been identified in association with bony lesions of the sustentaculum tali of the

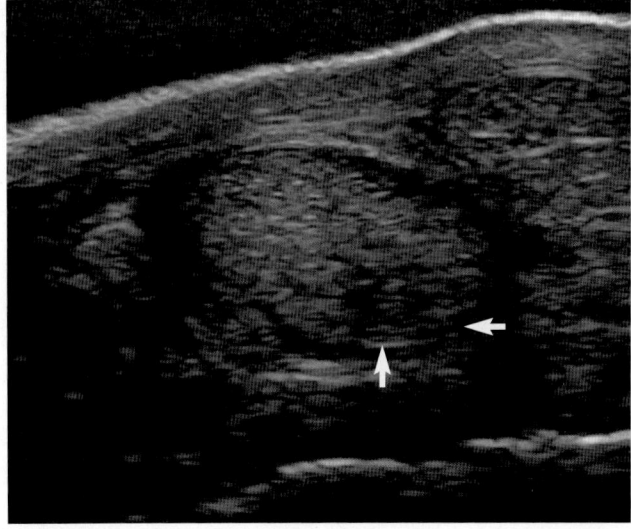

Fig. 70-7 • Transverse ultrasonographic image of the plantaromedial aspect of the distal tarsal region of a normal horse. Medial is to the left. Note the relatively hypoechogenic area dorsolaterally *(arrows)*, a normal finding.

fibular tarsal bone (calcaneus) and ectopic mineralization within the tarsal sheath.[19] These horses may have fibrillation of the DDFT and adhesion formation. These lesions generally are seen with obvious distention of the tarsal sheath and long-term lameness and probably occur secondary to primary pathological conditions of the bone. The sustentaculum tali should be evaluated radiologically using plantarolateral-dorsomedial oblique and flexed dorsoplantar images. The prognosis for athletic performance is poor with conservative or surgical management.

Dorsomedial luxation of the DDFT secondary to congenital malformation of the sustentaculum tali has been recognized in young Saddlebred horses and occasionally in Thoroughbreds.[3,20] Clinically the plantar aspect of the tarsal region appears broader than normal, with tarsus valgus. Lameness may not be obvious. Diagnosis is based on radiological examination: the sustentaculum tali appears flattened in a dorsoplantar (flexed) image.[21] This may result in a mechanical lameness. Surgical treatment has been attempted, but the horse did not race.[22] Congenital medial displacement of both the DDFT and SDFT in a hindlimb has also been seen, with a secondary valgus deformation of the metatarsal region and distal physeal trauma of the third metatarsal bone.[23]

INFECTION OF THE DEEP DIGITAL FLEXOR TENDON

Infection of the DDFT is discussed in Chapter 37 (see page 423).

Chapter 71

Injuries of the Accessory Ligament of the Deep Digital Flexor Tendon

Sue J. Dyson

References on page 1316

ANATOMY

In the forelimbs the accessory ligament of the deep digital flexor tendon (ALDDFT) is a substantial structure, similar in size to the deep digital flexor tendon (DDFT). The ALDDFT continues the common palmar ligament of the carpus, originating principally from the palmar aspect of the third carpal bone.[1] Proximally the ALDDFT is broad and rectangular in cross-section; farther distally it becomes narrower and thicker and blends with the DDFT in the middle one third of the metacarpal region. Fibrous bundles run from the lateral border of the ALDDFT to the superficial digital flexor tendon (SDFT) in the proximal half of the metacarpal region, and these predispose the horse to develop adhesions between the ALDDFT and the SDFT in horses with severe superficial digital flexor tendonitis or severe desmitis of the ALDDFT. The ALDDFT forms the dorsal wall of the carpal canal, within which is the carpal synovial sheath, which is interspersed between the DDFT and its accessory ligament.

In the hindlimbs the size of the ALDDFT varies extremely, but it is generally smaller than in the forelimb and rarely more than half the thickness of the DDFT. The ligament is usually symmetrical in the left and right hindlimbs of an individual horse. A recent postmortem study showed that the ALDDFT was absent in 6% of 165 hindlimbs and was occasionally a bifid structure.[2]

A forelimb ALDDFT has a low modulus of elasticity and a moderate strength to rupture, whereas the DDFT has a high modulus of elasticity and a strength to rupture that is more than three times that of the forelimb ALDDFT. In the forelimb the ALDDFT is loaded during the late stance phase, during extension of the digital joints,[1] or when landing over a fence.[3] The ALDDFT prevents overstretching of the DDFT by passively carrying the load during maximal extension of the distal interphalangeal and metacarpophalangeal joints. The ALDDFT also functions to facilitate carpal extension when the limb is loaded.[1] During flexion of the limb the ALDDFT is relaxed completely, and active muscle contraction results in the DDFT sliding proximally within the carpal sheath. The role of the ALDDFT in the hindlimb is less clear.

Desmitis of the ALDDFT usually occurs in forelimbs[4-9] but *occasionally* is recognized as a cause of hindlimb lameness.[4,10-13] In forelimbs desmitis may occur alone[4,7] as an acute injury or may develop secondary to previous severe tendonitis of the SDFT. In the latter case the SDFT is enlarged substantially and wraps around the medial and lateral margins of the DDFT. Adhesions develop between adjacent structures. In horses with chronic, severe desmitis of the ALDDFT, additional injury may occur to the adjacent DDFT.[7,8] A flexural deformity of the metacarpophalangeal or metatarsophalangeal joint may develop after severe injury to the ALDDFT.[4,9] Occasionally a flexural deformity of the metatarsophalangeal joint develops in one or both hindlimbs without a history of lameness, but ultrasonography reveals chronic architectural changes in the ALDDFT.[11-13] The flexural deformity may be relieved by desmotomy of the ALDDFT, provided that contracture of periarticular soft tissues has not already occurred.

PATHOGENESIS

Degenerative aging changes take place in the ALDDFT of forelimbs, and these may be a substantial predisposing factor in the development of desmitis. The amount of fibrillar collagen and number of large collagen fibers in the ALDDFT decrease with increasing age.[14] In a study of mechanical properties of the ALDDFT in relationship to age, failure forces of the ALDDFT of older horses were significantly lower than those of the ALDDFT in younger horses.[15] Fibrillar ruptures developed in the ALDDFT of old horses at forces and strains that were approximately half those of the forces inducing total failure in young horses. It has been suggested that fibrillar rupture occurs at relatively low strains in older horses and that repetitive microtrauma may lead to clinical desmitis.[14,15]

The incidence of desmitis of the ALDDFT is rather different from that of other tendonous and ligamentous injuries. Injuries occur more often in horses older than 8 years of age.[4-6] The incidence in Thoroughbreds is comparatively low (rare in the Standardbred), and therefore this is an unusual injury in event horses or racehorses, except in older steeplechasers. Desmitis is a relatively common injury in ponies (see Chapter 126) and crossbred horses, including pleasure horses.[4,5] The incidence in Warmblood horses is also high.[6] Desmitis occurs in older show jumpers (see Chapter 115), especially Grand Prix–level horses,[12] in older dressage horses,[12] and also sometimes in young, extravagantly moving dressage horses (see Chapter 116). Desmitis is generally a unilateral forelimb injury (Figure 71-1), although occasionally it occurs bilaterally, and is a rare cause of hindlimb lameness.

In hindlimbs, desmopathy of the ALDDFT has been seen most frequently in cob-type breeds[11-13] and Quarter Horses or Quarter Horse crosses,[16] even in some horses or ponies of a comparatively young age, and does not appear to have been induced traumatically in all horses. In some of these horses the condition has been bilateral, developing simultaneously or sequentially in each hindlimb. Desmopathy frequently has been associated with a tendency to stand with the fetlock of the affected limb partially flexed (Figure 71-2), resulting in the development of a flexural deformity. The condition also has been recognized together with swelling on the plantar aspect of the pastern, associated with concurrent desmitis of the straight or oblique sesamoidean ligaments.[11]

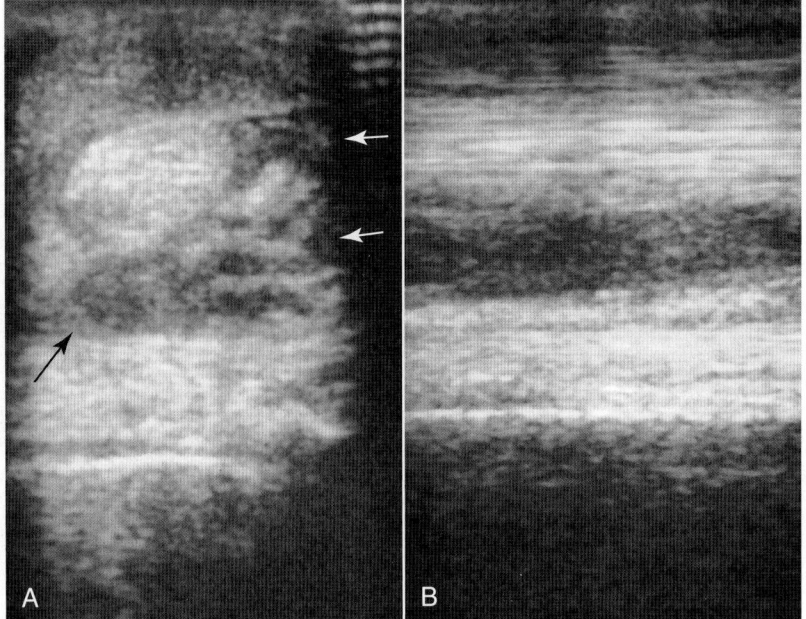

Fig. 71-1 • **A,** Transverse ultrasonographic image of the palmar metacarpal soft tissue structures, 11 cm distal to the accessory carpal bone, of an 8-year-old Grand Prix show jumper. Medial is to the left. The accessory ligament of the deep digital flexor tendon (ALDDFT) is considerably enlarged *(arrows)* and diffusely hypoechogenic, with focal anechoic areas dorsomedially. **B,** Longitudinal ultrasonographic image of the palmar metacarpal sort tissues in zone 2A of the same horse as in **A.** Proximal is to the left. There is a diffuse reduction in echogenicity of the ALDDFT and poor fiber pattern.

HISTORY AND CLINICAL SIGNS

There is usually an acute-onset moderate-to-severe lameness during exercise.[4-6] A show jumper may pull up lame after jumping a large fence or after a water jump.[12] Swelling develops rapidly in the proximal one third of the metacarpal region, dorsal to the SDFT. Determining by palpation whether the DDFT or accessory ligament is enlarged can be difficult, but injuries of the DDFT in this area are unusual. Some horses develop desmitis secondary to previous superficial digital flexor tendonitis, and in these horses separating the margins of the SDFT from the ALDDFT often is difficult.

Clinical signs include swelling, heat, pain on palpation, and lameness. The horse may stand with slight elevation of the heel and flexion of the metacarpophalangeal joint. Some degree of swelling often persists, even after long-term convalescence. In horses with reinjury, new swelling may be only slight, and careful palpation is required to identify a focus of pain. Occasionally there are no localizing clinical signs, but lameness is improved by palmar and palmar metacarpal (subcarpal) nerve blocks or abolished by median and ulnar nerve blocks. Lesions of the ALDDFT that were not detectable ultrasonographically have been identified with magnetic resonance imaging.[17,18] However, great care must be taken in interpretation because in normal horses the ALDDFT may have higher signal intensity than the DDFT or the SDFT in some image sequences.[19,20] There also may be bands of lower and higher signal intensity reflecting histological variation in infrastructure. Focal lesions have also been identified ultrasonographically at the origin of the ALDDFT on the palmar aspect of the third carpal bone.[18]

Some horses with desmitis in a hindlimb have acute-onset lameness associated with localized swelling. In sports horses injury may be localized to the proximal metatarsal region, resulting in subtle edematous swelling in the proximomedial aspect, whereas in general-purpose riding horses injury is usually further distal in the metatarsal region, with more obvious enlargement of the ALDDFT. However, some horses do not have an acute-onset lameness but have an insidious onset of stiffness and a tendency to stand with the fetlock semiflexed, progressing to inability to load the heel of the affected limb. This may be unilateral or bilateral.[11] Teenage cob-types and British native pony breeds appear particularly at risk. Careful palpation may reveal enlargement of the ALDDFT, but the thick skin of these types of horse may prohibit accurate palpation.

ULTRASONOGRAPHY

Diagnosis is usually confirmed by ultrasonography (see Figures 71-1 to 71-3). The transducer should be focused initially at the depth of the ALDDFT, which should be examined in transverse and longitudinal planes. Comparative images of the contralateral limb also should be obtained. If the transducer has a built-in standoff, this may create artifacts at the level of the ALDDFT. Some lesions are localized to the lateral or, less commonly, the medial margin of the ALDDFT, and these lesions may be missed unless the limb is evaluated from the lateral and medial aspects respectively, preferably using a standoff pad.

The ALDDFT is normally the most echogenic of the palmar metacarpal (plantar metatarsal) soft tissue structures, and its borders are well defined. In some ponies the

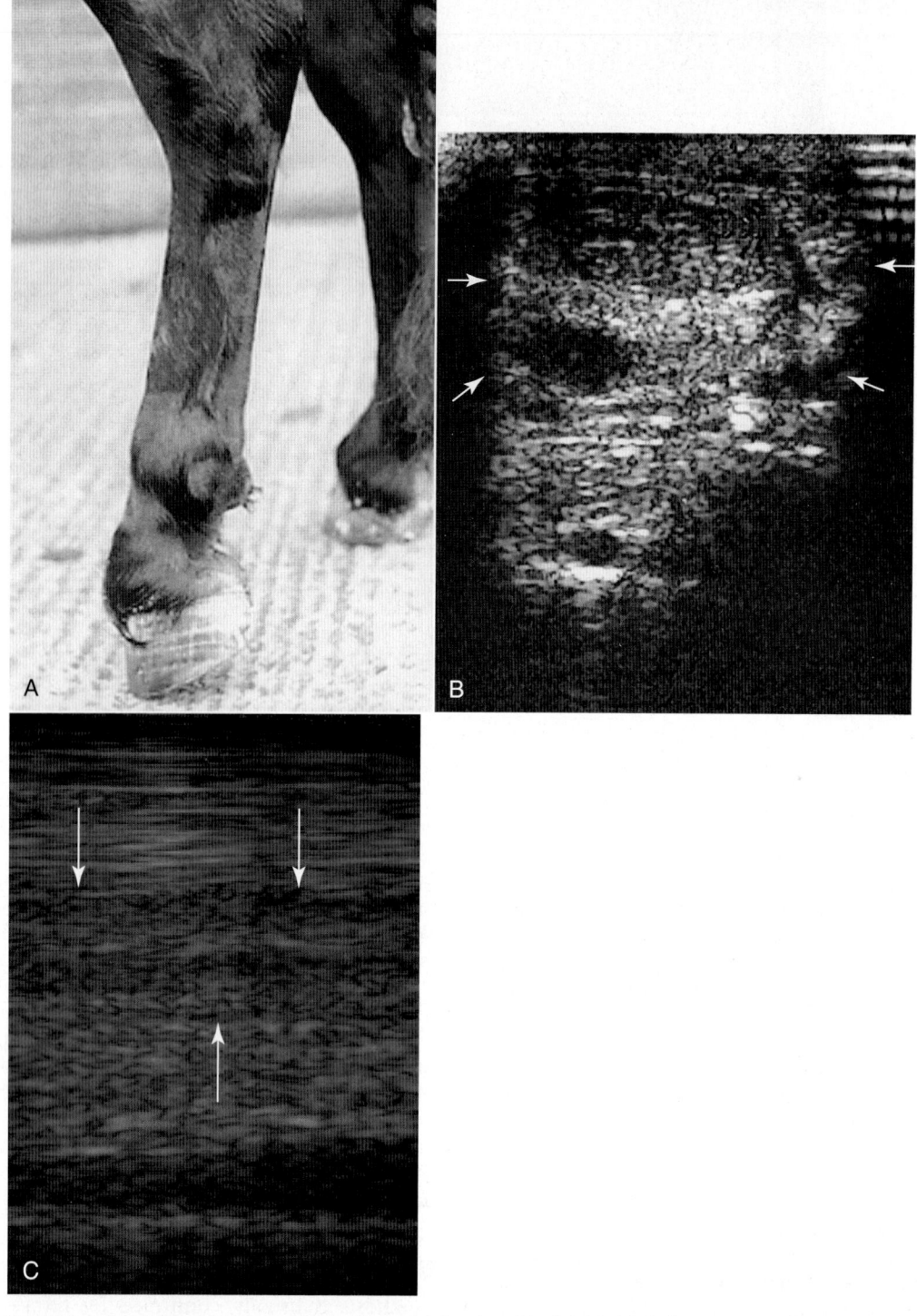

Fig. 71-2 • A, A 6-year-old Fell pony with a flexural deformity of the left hind fetlock associated with chronic desmopathy of the accessory ligament of the deep digital flexor tendon (ALDDFT). The pony was unable to place the heel of the left hind foot on the ground. Even when the pony was heavily sedated, extending the left hind fetlock was not possible. Firm enlargement on the plantar aspect of the pastern associated with desmitis of the straight distal sesamoidean ligament was also apparent. Similar abnormalities had developed in the right hindlimb approximately 12 months previously. **B,** Transverse ultrasonographic image of the plantar metatarsal soft tissues approximately 10 cm distal to the tarsometatarsal joint. Medial is to the left. The ALDDFT is enlarged considerably *(arrows),* and there is a large anechogenic lesion centrally. **C,** Longitudinal ultrasonographic image in zone 2A. Proximal is to the left. There is marked loss of fiber pattern in the ALDDFT *(arrows).*

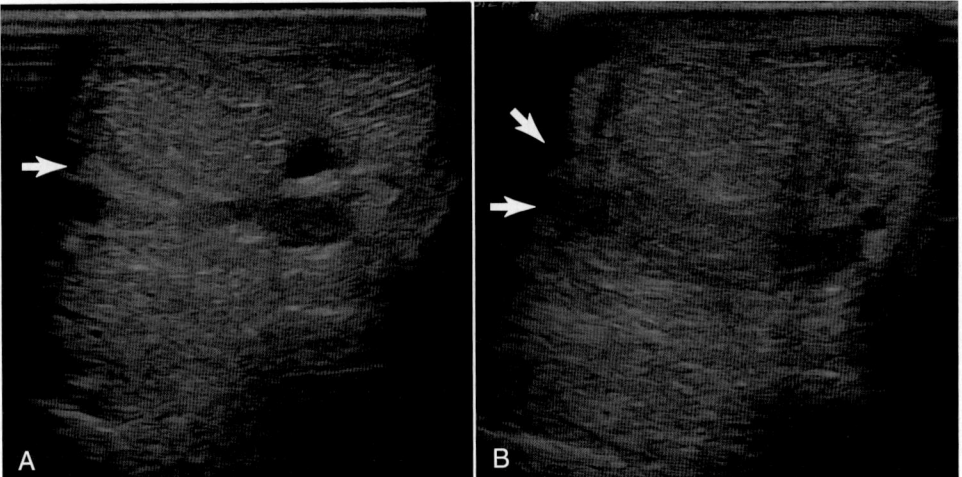

Fig. 71-3 • A, Transverse ultrasonographic image of the left hindlimb of a 12-year-old Thoroughbred–cross event horse with acute-onset right hindlimb lameness. Medial is to the left. The image was acquired from the plantaro-medial aspect of the limb at 5 cm distal to the tarsometatarsal (TMT) joint. The accessory ligament of the deep digital flexor tendon (ALDDFT) is narrow from dorsal to plantar *(arrow)*, well separated from the suspensory ligament (SL), and more echogenic than either the deep digital flexor tendon (DDFT) or the SL. **B,** Transverse ultrasonographic image of the right hindlimb obtained 5 cm distal to the TMT joint. Medial is to the left. Clinically there was palpable edematous swelling in the proximal metatarsal region, medially more than laterally, between the SL and the DDFT. The ALDDFT is enlarged *(arrows)* with diffuse decrease in echogenicity involving almost the entire ligament, with an anechogenic area medially. There is no longer space between the ALDDFT and the SL.

ALDDFT is less echogenic than the DDFT and suspensory ligament.

With forelimb injury, the ALDDFT invariably is enlarged and tends to expand around the borders of the DDFT, especially laterally. With severe injuries, it may be necessary to move the transducer medially and laterally to evaluate properly the margins of the ligament. Often definition of the borders of the ligament is lost, with a diffuse reduction in echogenicity of the ligament, sometimes with anechogenic areas. Occasionally a large proportion of the ligament is anechogenic. Central core lesions are comparatively rare, although acentric lesions restricted to the lateral border may occur, with the majority of the ligament appearing relatively normal. The dorsal border of the DDFT should be inspected carefully for evidence of concurrent injury, especially in horses with recurrent injury. In horses in which injury has been sustained secondary to previous superficial digital flexor tendonitis or in which desmitis of the ALDDFT is recurrent, the SDFT also should be evaluated for evidence of simultaneous recurrent injury or recent injury. The transducer should be focused on the SDFT, using a standoff. Adhesions between the ALDDFT and adjacent structures may be best identified in longitudinal images obtained with the limb not bearing weight. With passive flexion and extension of the fetlock it should be possible to see independent movement of the SDFT, DDFT, and ALDDFT, provided that no clinically significant adhesion formation has occurred. Concurrent injury of the suspensory ligament is seen rarely in association with desmitis of the ALDDFT. Occasionally, periligamentar echogenic tissue develops because of tearing of surrounding fascia.

In horses with chronic desmitis, when substantial enlargement of the ALDDFT occurs, with or without enlargement of the SDFT, the cross-sectional area of the DDFT often is reduced significantly.[12]

In acute hindlimb injuries in the proximal metatarsal region the ALDDFT should be evaluated from the plantaro-medial aspect of the limb (see Figure 71-3). In horses that initially had an enlarged ALDDFT and inability to load the heel of the affected limb, the ALDDFT usually is enlarged, with poorly demarcated borders, and is diffusely hypoecho-genic. Examination can be challenging in cob-types with very thick skin and a dense hair coat, especially if there are areas of dermal fibrosis. It is often necessary to use a transducer with lower frequency (e.g., 8 MHz) and to turn up the gain controls. It is important to be aware of the normal architecture of the ALDDFT because frequently the entire cross-sectional area of the ALDDFT may be diffusely hypoechoic, and if the appearance is bilaterally symmetrical such lesions may be overlooked. Other structures in the metacarpal or metatarsal regions and pastern should be examined, because lesions have been identified simultaneously in the SDFT[16] and the distal sesamoidean ligaments.[12]

TREATMENT

In horses with acute, first-time primary injuries of the ALDDFT, conservative treatment is usually satisfactory, but the prognosis is more guarded for horses with longer-term injuries when horses have continued to exercise. The horse should be restricted to box rest and controlled walking exercise for a minimum of 3 months and then should be reevaluated ultrasonographically. Nonsteroidal antiinflam-matory drugs should be given if the horse will not load the limb normally at rest to avoid development of a secondary flexural deformity of the metacarpophalangeal joint. Any foot imbalance should be corrected.

Improvement in echogenicity generally is seen more quickly than in comparable injuries of the SDFT. Box rest and controlled walking exercise should continue until the ligament is of similar echogenicity to the DDFT in transverse and longitudinal images. Progress should be monitored monthly after the first reevaluation 3 months after injury.

Horses that are allowed uncontrolled turnout in the initial 3-month period tend to have persistent clinical signs, and lesions persist ultrasonographically. Treatment with β-aminopropionitrile fumarate could be considered, especially in horses that have sustained a recurrent injury; however, no published reports of its efficacy in treating this condition are available, although successful results have been achieved, and a licensed product is no longer available.[12] There are also anecdotal reports of successful treatment with fresh bone marrow, platelet-rich plasma, or mesenchymal stem cell therapy. I have treated six horses with chronic forelimb injuries of the ALDDFT with mesenchymal stem cells and the results to date have been extremely promising.

Differences in the reported success of conservative treatment of horses with forelimb injuries of the ALDDFT have been substantial.[4-6] A number of factors, including the chronicity of the injury when therapy was first instituted and the type of horse, probably account for this disparity in success. I[4] reported complete functional recovery in 76% of 27 horses and ponies, whereas McDiarmid[5] reported only 43% success, and Van den Belt, Becker, and Dik[6] reported only 18%. Most of the horses in the series of Van den Belt, Becker, and Dik were large Warmbloods, whereas my series[4] included a large number of ponies. In my experience early recognition and aggressive treatment are key factors to a successful outcome. In a series of 13 horses with acute hindlimb injury in the mid-metatarsal region, 73% returned to full athletic function.[11] These were mostly pleasure riding horses. Proximal hindlimb lesions in sports horses have not been well documented; in my experience four of seven horses have returned to their former athletic function.

In horses with chronic, recurrent desmitis, in horses with evidence of adhesions between the ALDDFT and the

SDFT, or in those that tend to stand with the fetlock flexed, surgical treatment by desmotomy of the ALDDFT may be indicated.[4,7] The treated ligament heals by scar tissue that is inferior in strength to normal ligament, but the ligament will be longer, and this may reduce the strain on it[21] and thus reduce the risks of reinjury. Experimental removal of a full-thickness piece of the ALDDFT of 1 cm length resulted in long-term repair by scar tissue, in which orientation of the collagen was random. The healed ligaments were 1 cm longer than control ligaments and enlarged in cross-sectional area. The functional characteristics, force, and elongation at failure reached 80% of control values.[22]

The number of published long-term follow-up results for treatment of horses with chronic desmitis of the ALDDFT by desmotomy is limited. In my experience desmotomy has been successful in horses with chronic desmitis of the ALDDFT alone, but in those with concurrent superficial digital flexor tendonitis, or a flexural deformity of the metacarpophalangeal joint that cannot be corrected passively, the results have been disappointing. Horses with concurrent superficial digital flexor tendonitis have been relieved of evidence of resting pain, but restoring these horses to full athletic function has not been possible.

Horses with insidious onset of desmopathy of the ALDDFT of one or both hindlimbs have a poor prognosis with conservative treatment.[11] Treatment by desmotomy or desmectomy also resulted in persistent lameness in the majority, with preexisting contracture of the fetlock being an extremely poor prognostic indicator.

The prognosis depends on the chronicity of the injury and evidence of any concurrent injury to the DDFT or SDFT. Horses with acute injuries have a better prognosis than those with chronic injuries. Horses with recurrent injuries have a more guarded prognosis, especially if lesions are identified in the DDFT. Horses with lesions of the ALDDFT that have developed secondary to superficial digital flexor tendonitis have the most guarded prognosis, especially if any evidence of flexural deformity exists.

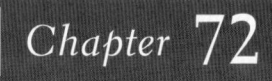

Chapter 72

The Suspensory Apparatus

Sue J. Dyson and Ronald L. Genovese

ANATOMY AND PATHOPHYSIOLOGY

The suspensory ligament (SL) is correctly called the *third interosseous muscle,* but it is referred to as the SL throughout this text. The anatomy in the forelimbs and hindlimbs is similar, and separate mention of the hindlimb is made only when substantial differences exist.

The SL can be divided into three separate regions that are subject to injury: the proximal part, the body, and the branches. For clinical purposes, in the forelimb the proximal part extends from 4 to 12 cm distal to the accessory

carpal bone, and in the hindlimb, from 2 to 10 cm distal to the tarsometatarsal joint. The distal sesamoidean ligaments are considered individually.

In the forelimb the SL originates from two differently shaped lobes that rapidly fuse. In the hindlimb this division is less obvious. The SL contains a variable amount of muscular tissue (2% to 11%), which tends to be bilaterally symmetrical.[1] In the forelimb the SL originates from the palmar carpal ligament and the proximal aspect of the third metacarpal bone (McIII), whereas in the hindlimb it originates principally from the proximoplantar aspect of the third metatarsal bone (MtIII). There is an accessory ligament of the SL that extends proximally and originates on the plantar aspect of the fourth tarsal bone. The SL in the forelimb is approximately rectangular in cross-section, but it is more rounded in the hindlimb. There are also fibers that arise from the axial aspect of the fourth metacarpal bone (McIV).

The body of the SL descends between the second metacarpal or metatarsal bone (McII, MtII) and the McIV or the

 References on page 1316

fourth metatarsal bone (MtIV) and divides into two branches at a variable site in the midmetacarpal (midmetatarsal) region. The level of division is usually bilaterally symmetrical. Each branch inserts on the abaxial surface of the corresponding proximal sesamoid bone (PSB). Each branch detaches a thin extensor branch dorsodistally that courses obliquely across the pastern to join the dorsal digital extensor tendon just above the proximal interphalangeal joint. Each extensor branch also blends with the corresponding collateral sesamoidean ligament.

The distal sesamoidean ligaments are the functional continuation of the SL in the digit and consist of the straight sesamoidean ligament, oblique sesamoidean ligaments, cruciate sesamoidean ligaments, and short sesamoidean ligaments. All attach proximally to the base of the PSBs and the proximal scutum. The straight sesamoidean ligament is a flat trapezoidal band that inserts via the scutum medium onto the proximal aspect of the middle phalanx. The oblique sesamoidean ligaments are triangular structures that converge to insert on the palmar aspect of the proximal phalanx. The cruciate sesamoidean ligaments form the palmar wall of the distal palmar synovial recess of the metacarpophalangeal joint. They consist of two thin layers of tissue that cross each other and insert on the proximal palmar tuberosities of the proximal phalanx. The short sesamoidean ligaments insert on the proximal palmar aspect of the proximal phalanx and are difficult to separate from the dorsal aspect of the oblique sesamoidean ligaments.

The palmar ligament of the fetlock, also referred to as the *intersesamoidean ligament,* is a thick collagen structure that completely covers the palmar and axial surfaces of the PSBs and is strongly attached to them. Together with the PSBs, the palmar ligament forms the proximal scutum. The concave palmar surface of the proximal scutum provides a smooth surface over which the digital flexor tendons glide.

In the forelimb the SL is innervated by the palmar metacarpal nerves, derived from the lateral palmar nerve, which receives fibers from the ulnar and median nerves.[2] The hindlimb SL is innervated by the plantar metatarsal nerves, branches from the deep branch of the lateral plantar nerve, which is derived from the tibial nerve. The proximal aspect of the SL is closely related to the distal palmar outpouchings of the carpometacarpal joint in the forelimb[3] and the plantar outpouchings of the tarsometatarsal joint in the hindlimb.[4]

The principal function of the SL is to prevent excessive extension of the fetlock joint.[5] During weight bearing the relative tension in the SL and digital flexor tendons regulates the stresses applied to different aspects of the McIII. When a limb is fully load bearing, the distal parts of the SL branches are apposed closely to the abaxial aspects of the metacarpal condyles and then move to the palmar aspect as the fetlock drops. During hyperextension the PSBs move distally and dorsally, so the branches of the SL act as articular surfaces to balance the position of the McIII. If the limb is loaded asymmetrically, so that torque is on the fetlock, the SL branches contribute to joint stability on the side opposite compression of the joint.

Some evidence exists that training increases the strength of the SL; the mean absolute load to failure in a single load-to-failure compression test was significantly higher in horses that were in race training compared with those that were confined to box or paddock rest.[6] In the trained group failure was most likely to be by fracture of a PSB, whereas in the untrained group the SL failed. However, when six 2-year-old Thoroughbred (TB) fillies underwent an 18-month controlled exercise program including galloping and were compared with six fillies that were restricted to walking exercise, no differences in the collagen fibril mass-average diameter in the body of the SL were found.[7] Mass-average diameter is correlated with ligament strength.

PROXIMAL SUSPENSORY DESMITIS IN THE FORELIMB

Proximal suspensory desmitis (PSD) is a common injury in the forelimbs[8-12] of athletic horses and may occur unilaterally or bilaterally. Some confusion has occurred about what constitutes PSD, and many clinicians have used this term for lameness that is worse with the affected limb on the outside of a circle and that is alleviated by analgesia of the proximal palmar metacarpal region but in which radiological and ultrasonographic findings have been negative. In our experience this case scenario is relatively unusual. Ultrasonographic abnormalities of the proximal SL are usually detectable, and the absence of detectable structural abnormality should alert the veterinarian to search for an alternative diagnosis. However, in a small proportion of horses abnormalities of the SL that were not apparent using ultrasonography have been identified using magnetic resonance imaging (MRI).[13,14]

PSD usually results in sudden-onset lameness, which can be remarkably transient, resolving within 24 hours unless the horse is worked hard. In horses with more chronic desmitis, lameness may be persistent. Lameness varies from mild to moderate and is rarely severe, unless the lesion is extensive. Lameness in Standardbred (STB) racehorses may be apparent only at high speeds. Bilateral PSD may result in loss of action rather than overt lameness, which occurs more commonly in flat racehorses than other sports horses, probably because of failure to recognize earlier, subtle unilateral lameness. However, dressage horses and event horses may be similarly affected. In a jumping horse the rider's complaint may be of failure of a horse to land with a specific forelimb leading. While ground reaction force is greater in the nonlead forelimb when landing from a fence, the lead forelimb has greater extension of the fetlock, resulting in potentially greater stress on the suspensory apparatus. So with SL injury the horse may be reluctant to land with the lame forelimb leading. Lameness is usually worse on soft ground, especially with the affected limb on the outside of a circle, and when subtle may be more easily felt by a rider than seen by an observer. In some horses lameness is never detectable either in hand or on the lunge and is only apparent when the horse is ridden. Lameness may not be apparent at the working trot but may be detectable at the medium or extended trot. Presumably this reflects increased stress on the SL because of increased extension of the fetlock at extended trot compared with working trot. Recognition of these features in the history may be important, because acute lameness often resolves rapidly, and working the horse hard to reproduce lameness, with the inherent risk of worsening the injury, may be undesirable. Lameness is often transiently accentuated by distal limb flexion. We believe that this is because the suspensory apparatus is relaxed during flexion and undergoes sudden stretching when the limb is loaded.

In the acute phase slight edema in the proximal metacarpal region, localized heat, and distention of the medial palmar vein may occur, but these features may be transient or absent. Pressure applied to the SL against the palmar aspect of the McIII or forced extension and protraction of the limb may elicit pain, but the absence of pain does not preclude the presence of PSD.

The feet should be evaluated carefully, because frequently foot imbalance is a predisposing factor. Back-at-the-knee and tied-in below the knee conformations also may be predisposing factors.

PSD is a common compensatory injury; therefore the whole horse should be evaluated to ensure that other causes of lameness are not missed. There is a relationship between front foot pain and PSD. PSD can occur in forelimbs and hindlimbs simultaneously.

Diagnostic Analgesic Techniques

If PSD is suspected, perineural analgesia of the lateral palmar nerve using lateral[3] or medial[15] approaches (2 mL mepivacaine) or the medial and lateral palmar metacarpal nerves (2 mL per site) is indicated (see Chapter 10). This should result in substantial improvement in, or alleviation of, lameness within 10 minutes, assuming PSD is the only cause of lameness. However, neither technique is necessarily specific. Blockade of the lateral palmar nerve also has the potential to alleviate pain associated with a lateral source of pain in the more distal aspect of the limb (e.g., a splint). The risks of influencing middle carpal joint pain are less than with the subcarpal approach, but with the lateral approach local anesthetic solution may diffuse and improve lameness associated with the middle carpal joint[16] or with the carpal canal. Perineural analgesia of the palmar metacarpal nerves may alleviate pain associated with the middle carpal or carpometacarpal joints because of local diffusion or inadvertent deposition of local anesthetic solution into the distopalmar outpouchings of the carpometacarpal joint capsule. There is no right or wrong method, but it is important to be aware of the limitations of whichever technique is used. One author (SJD) usually blocks the medial and lateral palmar metacarpal nerves using a lateral approach, with the limb non–weight bearing. In a difficult, potentially dangerous horse that strikes out, the lateral palmar nerve is blocked with the limb bearing weight. It is easy to hit the lateral palmar nerve using the medial approach, causing the horse sudden severe pain; therefore this technique is rarely used. A false-negative result may be achieved because of inadvertent injection into the carpal sheath or failure of the local anesthetic solution to diffuse proximally to the most proximal extent of a lesion. Although the SL receives innervation from fibers from the median and ulnar nerves, perineural analgesia of the ulnar nerve usually resolves or substantially improves lameness associated with PSD. However, in a minority of horses perineural analgesia of the median and ulnar nerves is required to abolish lameness completely.

Intraarticular analgesia of the middle carpal joint may result in partial improvement or complete alleviation of pain associated with the proximal aspect of the SL in some

horses (15 [60%] of 25 horses).[16] Using a dorsal approach to the middle carpal joint rather than a palmarolateral approach should theoretically reduce the risks of diffusion of local anesthetic solution to the proximal aspect of the SL and palmar metacarpal nerves; however, in practice the difference seems minor. Comparison of the relative responses to middle carpal analgesia (6 mL mepivacaine; assessed 10 minutes after injection) and perineural analgesia of the lateral palmar nerve or the palmar metacarpal nerves is potentially useful but can be highly misleading. Generally a horse with lameness caused by PSD responds better to perineural analgesia than intraarticular analgesia, but this is not universal. Similarly, primary middle carpal joint pain usually is improved best by intraarticular analgesia, but this is not always the case. Middle carpal joint pain and PSD may occur concurrently, especially in STB and TB racehorses. The clinician should evaluate the response to these diagnostic analgesic techniques in light of the following:

- The use of the horse and thus the likelihood of the site of injury, and other clinical signs
- Other clinical signs: for example, distention of the middle carpal joint capsule and pain on passive manipulation of the carpus
- The degree and character of the lameness

Perineural analgesia of the palmar nerves at the level of the base of the PSBs often results in lameness because of PSD appearing worse. We believe that this reflects some loss of proprioceptive function of the distal aspect of the limb so that the horse is less able to protect the painful SL. Perineural analgesia of the palmar nerves (at midmetacarpal level) and palmar metacarpal nerves (distal to the button of the McII and the McIV) (four-point or low palmar block) often results in some improvement in pain associated with PSD, possibly because of proximal diffusion of local anesthetic solution via lymphatic vessels or along fascial planes. However, a recent contrast study indicated that this may not occur.[17] Perhaps improvement may be due to pain extending further distally in the SL than the site of detectable injury.

More than one source of pain may be contributing to lameness. PSD and concurrent foot pain occur commonly. Hindlimb lameness also may be present, especially in the contralateral hindlimb, so it is important to assess and to reevaluate the whole horse.

Differential Diagnosis

PSD should be differentiated from middle carpal joint pain, being aware that especially in young TB racehorses and STB racehorses lesions may occur in both locations simultaneously. Osteoarthritis of the carpometacarpal joint occasionally occurs (see page 417). Horses with pain associated with palmar cortical fatigue fractures or stress reactions of the McIII[11,18-20] respond similarly to diagnostic analgesic techniques; however, in horses with fracture, lameness tends to be more severe and worse on firm ground and often deteriorates the farther the horse trots (see page 413). Avulsion fractures of the McIII at the origin of the SL (see page 417) occur less frequently and tend to be associated with more persistent and severe lameness.[1,21] Pain associated with the carpal sheath or carpal retinaculum also should be considered (see Chapter 75). Perineural analgesia of the deep branch of the lateral palmar nerve or the palmar metacarpal nerves alone should not alleviate pain associated with the deep digital flexor tendon (DDFT) or its accessory ligament (ALDDFT), the superficial digital flexor tendon (SDFT), or the fetlock region, without simultaneous blockade of the palmar nerves. However, horses with proximal lesions of the SDFT or ALDDFT may show partial improvement in lameness.

Diagnostic Ultrasonography

Diagnostic ultrasonography is essential for accurate diagnosis of PSD. The limb should be evaluated in transverse and longitudinal planes, and careful comparison should be made with the contralateral limb. High-quality images are required, because lesions can be subtle and easily missed if the gain controls are too high or if the transducer is not focused on the SL. Artifacts are readily created if the transducer is not in complete contact with the limb. The contours of the proximal palmar aspect of the metacarpal region can make obtaining longitudinal images difficult, especially because the proximal palmar aspect of the McIII slopes backward. Therefore creating hypoechoic artifacts at the enthesis of the SL on the McIII is easy. Cross-sectional area measurements may be extremely valuable, especially in horses with acute PSD, because enlargement of the ligament may be the only detectable ultrasonographic abnormality. Bear in mind that muscular tissue appears less echogenic than does ligamentous tissue and that proximally the SL originates in two halves. The entire cross-section of the SL cannot be seen from a palmar approach, and marginal lesions may be missed unless oblique images are also obtained. A convex transducer or virtual convex transducer allows a greater proportion of the proximal abaxial aspects of the SL to be evaluated in transverse images compared with a linear transducer. Previous injuries to the SL may not resolve fully to restore normal, uniform echogenicity. Be aware that poor diagnostic analgesic technique may result in aspiration of air, which creates artifacts. This usually resolves in 24 hours. A thin band of the SL passes proximally from the enthesis on the McIII to blend with the palmar carpal fascia. The anechogenic space seen dorsal to the SL at this level is fluid in the palmar recess of the carpometacarpal joint and should not be mistaken for a lesion (Figure 72-1).

Abnormalities associated with PSD include the following[22] (Figures 72-2 and 72-3):

- Enlargement of the cross-sectional area. This may result in reduction of space between the SL and the palmar cortex of the McIII or reduced space between the SL and the ALDDFT
- Poor demarcation of the margins of the SL, especially the dorsal margin
- Focal or diffuse areas of reduced echogenicity. These may extend less than 1 cm proximodistally and occupy from less than 10% to up to the entire cross-sectional area of the ligament
- Focal anechoic core lesions
- Reduced strength of fiber pattern
- Focal fibrosis or mineralization (rare in acute injuries)
- Mild increased echogenicity of the entire SL in long-term, chronic injuries
- Entheseous new bone on the palmar aspect of the McIII

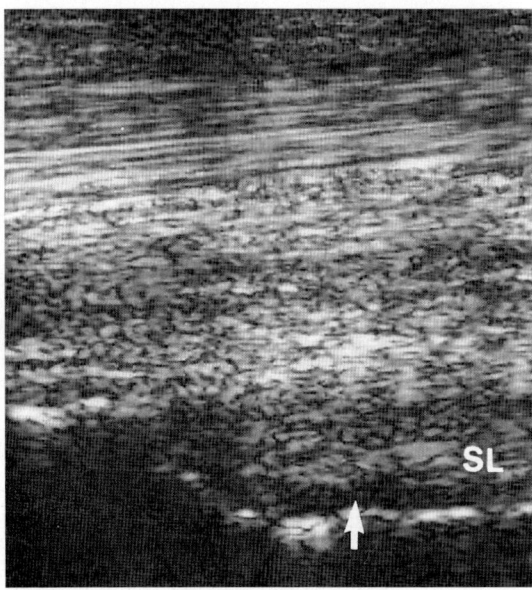

Fig. 72-1 • Longitudinal (proximal is to the left) ultrasonographic image of the proximal metacarpal region. The thin echogenic band from the suspensory ligament *(SL)* passes proximally from the enthesis of the suspensory ligament on the third metacarpal bone to blend with the palmar fascia. Dorsal to the suspensory ligament is anechogenic fluid within the palmar recess of the carpometacarpal joint capsule *(arrow)*.

In a horse with bilateral PSD an obvious lesion may be detectable in the lamer limb, but abnormalities may be much more subtle and occasionally not apparent in the less lame limb. In a 3-year-old TB that sustains PSD at 2 years of age, mild lameness may be recurrent, and discerning any structural abnormality other than enlargement of the SL may not be possible.

The degree of ultrasonographic abnormality (cross-sectional area involved and proximodistal extent of the lesion) usually reflects the severity of the lameness. In horses with acute PSD the ultrasonographic abnormalities may be subtle, although if lameness is unilateral, slight enlargement of cross-sectional area may be detectable. Care should be taken to compare measurements in the contralateral limb at the same distance distal to the accessory carpal bone. Ultrasonographic abnormalities may worsen over the next 10 to 14 days, and reevaluation may be useful to confirm the diagnosis.

In horses with an avulsion fracture of the McIII at the origin of the SL, the fracture fragment is usually readily identifiable and generally is associated with only a focal lesion in the SL itself, usually restricted to the dorsal aspect (see page 417).

Radiography and Radiology

Because of the potential nonspecificity of local analgesic techniques I recommend radiographic examination of the carpus and proximal metacarpal region using at least flexed lateromedial, dorsolateral-palmaromedial oblique, dorsomedial-palmarolateral oblique, and dorsopalmar images. In racehorses, endurance, and event horses a skyline image of the third carpal bone may also be required. Usually no detectable radiological abnormalities of the McIII occur in horses with acute PSD. With chronic PSD, a generalized area of increased opacity of the proximal aspect of the

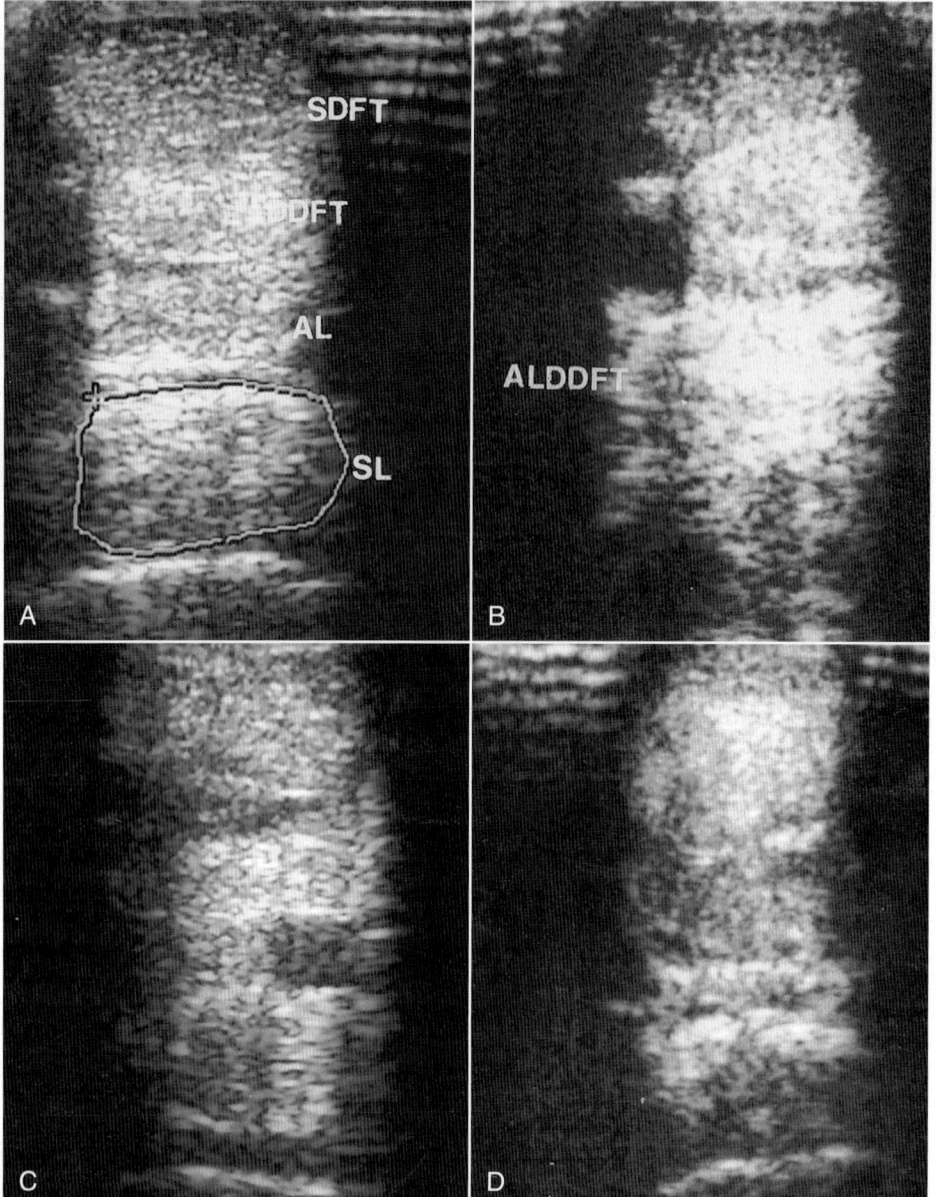

Fig. 72-2 • **A,** Transverse ultrasonographic image of the metacarpal region of a 3-year-old Thoroughbred, with mild forelimb lameness, at 9 cm distal to the accessory carpal bone. The suspensory ligament *(SL)* shows a slight overall reduction in echogenicity compatible with proximal suspensory desmitis. The ligament is enlarged (cross-sectional area 1.39 cm^2 compared with 1.25 cm^2 in the contralateral limb). The lesion extended less than 1 cm proximodistally. **B,** Transverse ultrasonographic image of the metacarpal region at 8 cm distal to the accessory carpal bone of the right forelimb of a 7-year-old medium-level dressage horse. The entire cross-sectional area of the SL is reduced in echogenicity. The lesion extended 1.5 cm proximodistally. Note also the hyperechoic appearance of the accessory ligament of the deep digital flexor tendon *(ALDDFT)*. **C,** Transverse ultrasonographic image of the proximal metacarpal region of a 6-year-old event horse with acute-onset right forelimb lameness. There is a hypoechoic lesion in the medial aspect of the SL that extends less than 1 cm proximodistally. Medial is left. **D,** Transverse ultrasonographic image of the right forelimb of a 7-year-old dressage horse with bilateral forelimb lameness. The palmar aspect of the SL is slightly increased in echogenicity, but the dorsal aspect is diffusely hypoechogenic.

McIII may be seen in dorsopalmar images. This increased radiopacity should be differentiated from that associated with a palmar cortical fatigue fracture,[23] which is invariably medial. A focal linear region of increased opacity may reflect the presence of an entheseous spike. In a lateromedial image subcortical endosteal reaction in the proximal palmar aspect of the McIII may be apparent. These secondary bony changes (endosteal and entheseous new bone) in

a forelimb reflect chronicity of the injury and are associated with a more guarded prognosis.

Nuclear Scintigraphy
Reports in the literature about the usefulness of nuclear scintigraphy for diagnosing PSD are confusing because of failure to correlate scintigraphic findings with ultrasonographic and radiological findings and because avulsion

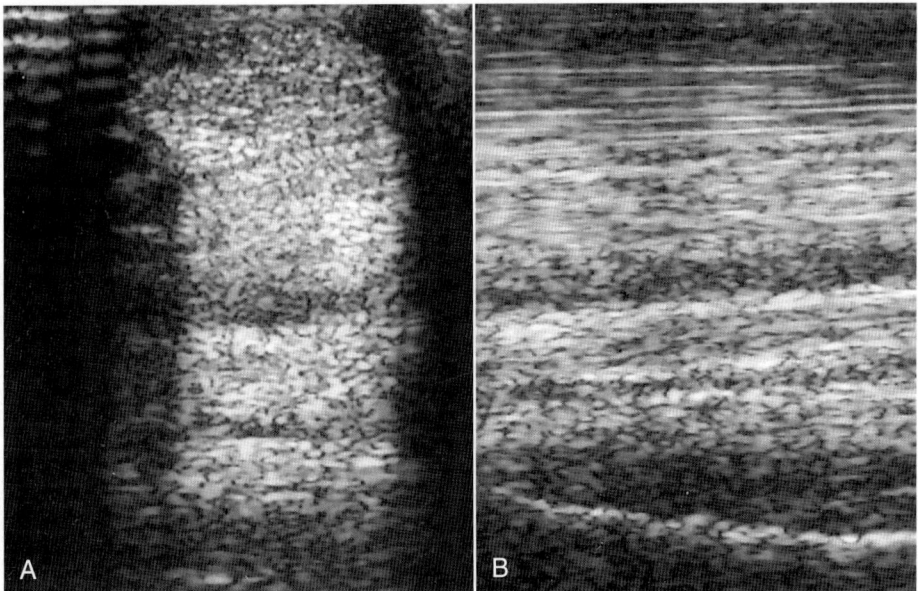

Fig. 72-3 • A, Transverse ultrasonographic image of the proximal metacarpal region at 8 cm distal to the accessory carpal bone of the left forelimb of a Grand Prix show jumper. The horse had developed acute severe lameness immediately after completing a jumping round 2 weeks previously. The dorsal half of the suspensory ligament is diffusely hypoechogenic. **B,** Longitudinal ultrasonographic image of the proximal metacarpal region of the same horse. Proximal is to the left. The dorsal aspect of the suspensory ligament is diffusely hypoechogenic.

fractures of the McIII were not considered separately.[24,25] Nuclear scintigraphy is generally unnecessary for diagnosing PSD, provided that good-quality ultrasonographic images are obtained, but may give additional information about associated bone turnover at the origin of the SL. Pool and bone phase images may be negative. Abnormal radiopharmaceutical uptake in the pool phase may actually reflect early bone uptake. Increased uptake of ^{99m}Tc-methylene diphosphonate was identified in the proximal palmar aspect of the McIII in approximately 6% of 40 horses with ultrasonographic evidence of PSD.[26] Therefore negative scintigraphic images do not preclude the presence of PSD. The presence of increased radiopharmaceutical uptake (IRU) reflecting enthesis injury is usually associated with more severe lameness that takes longer to resolve. IRU associated with either an avulsion fracture of the McIII at the insertion of the SL or a stress fracture is likely to be more intense. IRU in the bone phase, seen in the absence of ultrasonographic and radiological abnormalities, is more likely to reflect a primary pathological condition of bone.

Magnetic Resonance Imaging

MRI is usually not necessary for the diagnosis of PSD but should be considered if no ultrasonographic abnormality can be identified.[13,14] Interpretation is confounded by the presence of variable amounts of muscle and adipose tissue in the center of each lobe of the SL, which has high signal intensity.[27,28] Increased signal intensity in the surrounding ligamentous tissue reflects injury and may be accompanied by enlargement of the SL and sometimes adhesions to the McII, McIII, and McIV. However, it is important to recognize the normal fibers of the SL, which originate from the axial aspect of the McIV extending up to 7 cm distal to the carpometacarpal joint.[28] MRI may be more sensitive than ultrasonography for identification of entheseous new bone and endosteal reaction at the ligament's origin. MRI is the most accurate method of detection of syndesmopathy between the McIII and either the McII or the McIV, which is an unusual but important differential diagnosis. It is also valuable for the detection of primary bone trauma of the McIII.

Computed Tomography

Computed tomography (CT) or contrast-enhanced CT can also be useful for the diagnosis of PSD and entheseous new bone.

Treatment

Most horses with acute forelimb PSD respond well to box rest and controlled walking exercise for 3 months.[29,30] Uncontrolled turnout is contraindicated. Attention to correct foot balance is important. Elevation of the heel is contraindicated because it increases load on the SL. A premature resumption of work usually results in recurrent injury. Approximately 90% of horses resume full athletic function without recurrent injury.[1] In the early period after return to work circumstances that create hyperextension of the fetlock should be avoided. For example, dressage horses should avoid medium and extended trot. Attention should also be paid to the footing on which the horse works. Horses with chronic PSD may require more prolonged rehabilitation, and in a small proportion lameness is persistent. If low-grade residual lameness persists after 3 to 6 months but serial ultrasonographic examinations reveal no change in echogenicity, then introduction of trotting exercise sometimes stimulates further repair and resolution of lameness. Some TB racehorses with chronic lesions have been able to be maintained in training with judicious use of phenylbutazone, without clinically significant deterioration of the lesion. No fatalities associated with PSD occurred in 630 TB racehorses examined post mortem because of musculoskeletal injuries.[29] Some STB racehorses with acute lesions have been managed by slightly reducing the training schedule, administering local injections of corticosteroids and hyaluronan, using symptomatic antiinflammatory therapy (local icing, liniments such as dimethyl sulfoxide [DMSO] and corticosteroid paints, and phenylbutazone as necessary), and shortening the toes and increasing hoof angle. Although a few treated horses were able to race successfully, prognosis after rest was better.[29]

Extracorporeal shock wave treatment or radial pressure wave therapy (three treatments at 2-week intervals) was successful in some horses with chronic lesions that had failed to respond to conservative management.[31,32] Ten (50%) of 20 horses with chronic forelimb PSD with lameness of greater than 3 months' duration were in full work 6 months after treatment.[32] Repeated long-term treatments are sometimes required. Local infiltration with 4 to 6 mL of 2% iodine in almond oil has been used successfully.[8]

In some horses the lesions disappear completely ultrasonographically. In others echogenicity may increase, but uniform echogenicity is never restored. Rest should be continued until the ultrasonographic appearance remains stable.

Surgical splitting of the SL has been used in some horses with PSD with successful results in some horses; however, the results have been unpredictable.[14,33] There are currently no long-term, peer-reviewed studies of the results of injection of pigs' urinary bladder matrix, mesenchymal stem cells, or other biological agents such as platelet-rich plasma, although anecdotally successful results have been reported. In sports horses with chronic injuries that have failed to respond to conservative management, one author (SJD) has successfully used either mesenchymal stem cells or desmoplasty combined with injection of platelet-rich plasma.

PROXIMAL SUSPENSORY DESMITIS IN THE HINDLIMB

PSD in the hindlimb results in either an insidious or a sudden-onset lameness that may be mild or severe. Some horses show poor performance rather than a recognized lameness. In contrast to the forelimb, lameness may persist and remain severe, despite restriction to box rest. Such persistence probably is caused by a compartment-like syndrome and pressure on the adjacent plantar metatarsal nerves.[34,35] In view of the chronicity of some lesions when first identified and the finding of secondary radiological changes in sound horses, some lesions likely exist subclinically or are associated with a low-grade lameness that goes unrecognized. The incidence of bilateral lesions is higher than in forelimbs.

PSD in the hindlimb occurs in horses in all athletic disciplines and of all ages and is a particular problem in dressage horses.[36] There is an association between straight hock conformation and hyperextension of the metatarsophalangeal joint and hindlimb PSD (Figure 72-4). Such conformational abnormalities were identified in nine (21%) of 42 horses with hindlimb PSD but in only four (8%) of 50 horses examined consecutively with hindlimb lameness unrelated to the suspensory apparatus.[37] Straight hock conformation may predispose to PSD or develop secondarily; hyperextension of the metatarsophalangeal joint

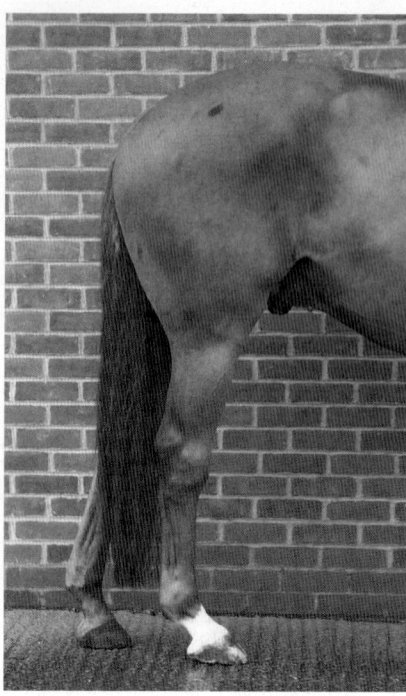

Fig. 72-4 • The hindlimbs of a 7-year-old show jumper with proximal suspensory desmitis of the right hindlimb. Note the relatively straight hock conformation and the sloping pasterns associated with hyperextension of the hind fetlocks. The horse also has rather low heels and long toes.

may develop as a sequela to PSD, probably as the result of progressive degeneration of the SL. A long-toe and low-heel conformation also may be a predisposing factor, especially if associated with abnormal orientation of the distal phalanx, with the plantar aspect lower than the toe.[29]

PSD in the hindlimb in a STB racehorse is common and usually results in an abnormal gait at high speeds, which may or may not be apparent at the trot. Unilateral left hindlimb lameness may manifest as the horse drifting to the right shaft and being on the left line and vice versa.

Horses with acute hindlimb PSD may have localized heat and swelling and pain on pressure applied to the SL, but frequently no localizing clinical features are apparent.

Lameness is often characterized by a reduced height of arc of foot flight, with or without intermittent catching of the toe. There may be reduced extension of the metatarsophalangeal joint unless the functional integrity of the SL is compromised. The cranial phase of the stride may be shortened. Lameness may be accentuated by proximal or distal limb flexion. Bilateral lesions may result in poor hindlimb action rather than obvious hindlimb lameness. Performance horses may not be overtly lame in hand, but when ridden show reduced hindlimb impulsion, difficulties in transitions, stiffness, resistant behavior, evasions such as bolting, difficulties in turning or stopping, reluctance to perform certain dressage movements, or reduced power when jumping. Lameness may be more obvious on a circle on the lunge, but unlike in forelimb PSD the lameness is not necessarily worse with the lamer limb on the outside. Approximately 50% of horses with hindlimb PSD are lamer with the affected limb on the outside or inside of a circle. As with many horses with hindlimb lameness, lameness is often more obvious when the horse is ridden, especially when the rider sits on the diagonal of the lame or lamer limb.

Diagnostic Analgesic Techniques

Perineural analgesia of the plantar nerves (midmetatarsal level) and plantar metatarsal nerves may result in slight improvement in lameness because of proximal diffusion of the local anesthetic solution or distal extension of pain in the SL, or concomitant injury of a SL branch. Lameness usually is improved substantially by perineural analgesia of the medial and lateral plantar metatarsal nerves (2 mL of mepivacaine 2% per site) or the deep branch of the lateral plantar nerve distal to the tarsus, but lameness may not be alleviated fully. Improvement is usually seen within 10 minutes of injection. Critical evaluation of the degree of improvement is considered essential if considering treatment by neurectomy of the deep branch of the lateral plantar nerve. If there is a component of entheseous pain, this may result in only partial improvement in lameness, which is further improved by deep infiltration of local anesthetic solution toward the plantar aspect of the MtIII. PSD may occur together with pain associated with the tarsometatarsal joint, and if lameness is improved but not abolished by subtarsal analgesia, addition of intraarticular analgesia of the tarsometatarsal joint may abolish the lameness. False-negative results also may be obtained because of inadvertent injection into the tarsal sheath or the tarsometatarsal joint capsule. Subtarsal analgesia can influence tarsometatarsal joint pain, and occasionally (two [8%] of 24 horses[34]), intraarticular analgesia of the tarsometatarsal (TMT) joint alleviates pain associated with PSD. It is also important to recognize that improvement in lameness after perineural analgesia of the deep branch of the lateral plantar nerve is not synonymous with PSD. There may be other causes of pain, improvement of which results in improvement in lameness. However, an improvement in lameness of 85% or more is usually associated with PSD. Nonetheless, I recommend comparing the response with the effect of intraarticular analgesia of the TMT joint. Perineural analgesia of the tibial nerve alone alleviates pain associated with PSD without substantially influencing tarsal pain. However, the tibial nerve is large; therefore 20 minutes may pass before analgesia is achieved effectively. In horses with bilateral hindlimb stiffness or lack of hindlimb impulsion, best improvement may be seen after perineural analgesia of the deep branch of the lateral plantar nerve performed bilaterally simultaneously. Some horses have secondary sacroiliac joint region pain, and the rider may complain of persistent lack of hindlimb power unless this region is also blocked.

Diagnostic Ultrasonography

High-quality ultrasonographic images are essential for accurate diagnosis, but are not always possible to achieve because of the shape of the limb, position of blood vessels, and the presence of other artifacts. The proximal aspect of the SL should be examined from the plantaromedial aspect of the metatarsal region to evaluate as much of the cross-sectional area as possible. Large vessels plantarolateral to the SL may result in broad linear anechoic artifacts within the SL (Figure 72-5). In large Warmblood horses in particular the SL is situated deeply, and the ultrasound transducer must be focused accordingly. In transverse and

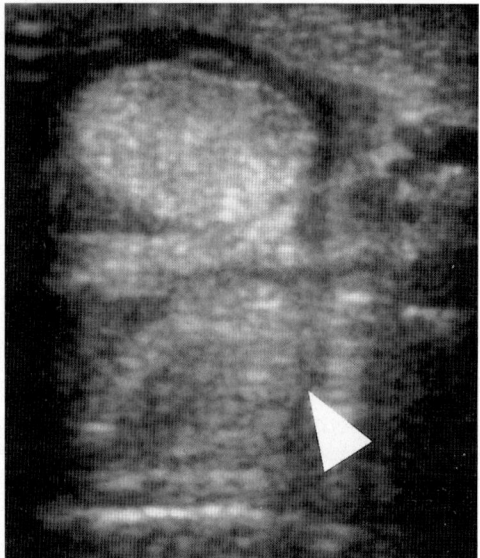

Fig. 72-5 • Transverse ultrasonographic image of the proximal metatarsal region of a horse with proximal suspensory desmitis. Medial is to the left. The narrow anechogenic band through the suspensory ligament *(arrowhead)* is an artifact caused by the overlying plantar vessel. The suspensory ligament has a diffuse reduction in echogenicity.

longitudinal images the most proximal part of the SL in a normal horse may appear slightly less echogenic than the DDFT (Figure 72-6). Detection of subtle abnormalities requires careful comparison with the contralateral limb, bearing in mind that lesions may be bilateral, and measurement of cross-sectional area or dorsoplantar thickness. Cross-sectional area measurements underestimate real size because the ligament cannot be imaged in its entirety proximally. The SL should be imaged routinely in transverse and longitudinal planes. The shape of the proximoplantar aspect of the metatarsal region influences how easy it is to obtain high-quality images. Use of a standoff pad can provide a larger contact area and thereby enhance image quality in some horses. Acquisition of transverse images using either a convex array or a virtual convex transducer may permit evaluation of more of the mediolateral extent of the SL than using a linear transducer. It is also important to recognize that injury may be localized to either the medial or the lateral aspect of the SL.

In hindlimb PSD focal anechogenic areas are relatively unusual, except in the STB racehorse. More commonly the SL is enlarged, with poor demarcation of its borders and a diffuse reduction in echogenicity of part or all of the cross-sectional area of the ligament (see Figure 72-5) (Figure 72-7). Fibrosis or ectopic mineralization occurs more often in hindlimbs than in forelimbs. An irregular contour of the plantar aspect of the MtIII may reflect enthesophyte formation. In some horses, especially those with abnormal conformation, the lesions may progress despite box rest.

Occasionally there are concurrent injuries of the SL branches, especially in horses with abnormal conformation, and consideration should be given to routine evaluation of the SL in its entirety.

Radiography and Radiology

Distal hock joint pain and PSD may coexist, so it is recommended that a comprehensive radiographic examination

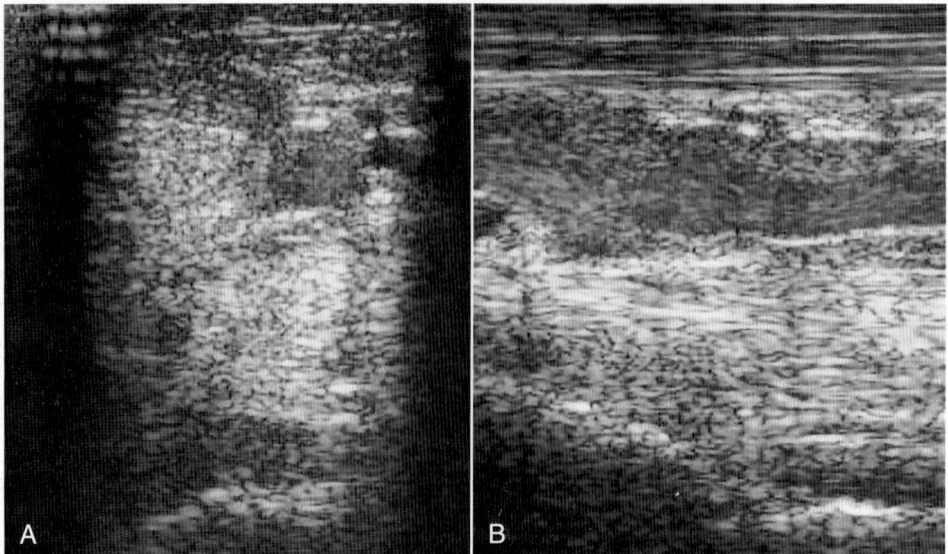

Fig. 72-6 • A, Transverse ultrasonographic image of the proximal metatarsal region of a normal horse, 4 cm distal to the tarsometatarsal joint. Medial is to the left. The suspensory ligament is similar in echogenicity to the deep digital flexor tendon. **B,** Longitudinal ultrasonographic image of the proximal metatarsal region of a normal horse. Proximal is to the left.

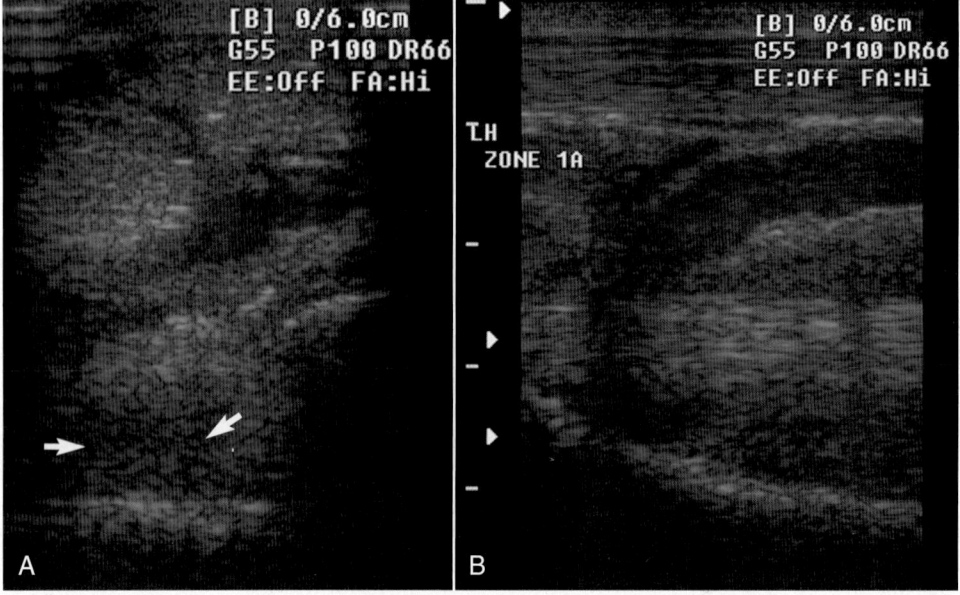

Fig. 72-7 • Transverse **(A)** ultrasonographic image at 4 cm distal to the tarsometatarsal joint and longitudinal image **(B)** of the left, proximal metatarsal region of an 11-year-old show jumper with left hindlimb lameness caused by proximal suspensory desmitis. The damaged suspensory ligament is diffusely hypoechogenic dorsomedially *(arrows)* with diffuse loss of fiber pattern in the longitudinal image. The overlying blood vessel is dilated.

of the hock and proximal metatarsal region is performed using four standard images. Diagnosis should never be based on radiology alone, because some sound horses have some increased radiopacity of the proximal aspect of the MtIII (see Figure 43-2). In horses with chronic active PSD this tends to be more extensive. In the dorsoplantar image, increased opacity of the proximal aspect of the MtIII is often more obvious laterally. In a lateromedial image subcortical increased radiopacity and alteration of the trabecular pattern of the proximoplantar aspect of the MtIII may be caused by endosteal new bone, extending up to

4 cm proximodistally (Figure 72-8). The plantar cortex may itself be thickened, and in addition enthesophyte formation may be visible on the plantar aspect. However, in some horses with acute injury no radiological abnormality is detectable. Radiology is also important to identify osteoarthritis of the distal hock joints, which may be contributing to pain and lameness.

Nuclear Scintigraphy

Nuclear scintigraphy is not a sensitive means of detecting PSD in hindlimbs.[26] Pool phase images have been found to

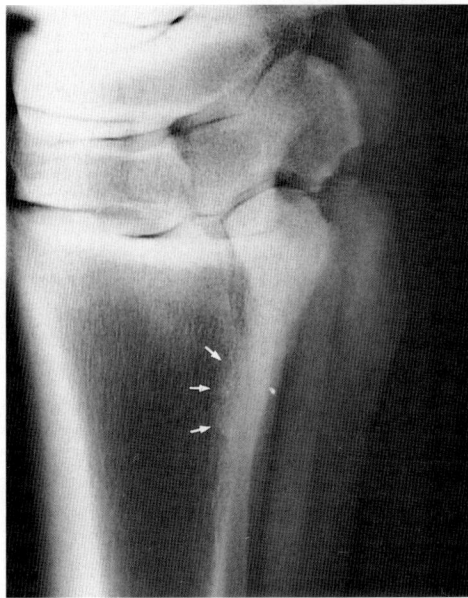

Fig. 72-8 • Lateromedial radiographic image of the right hindlimb of a 7-year-old dressage horse with chronic proximal suspensory desmitis. The proximoplantar aspect of the third metatarsal bone *(arrows)* has increased subcortical radiopacity.

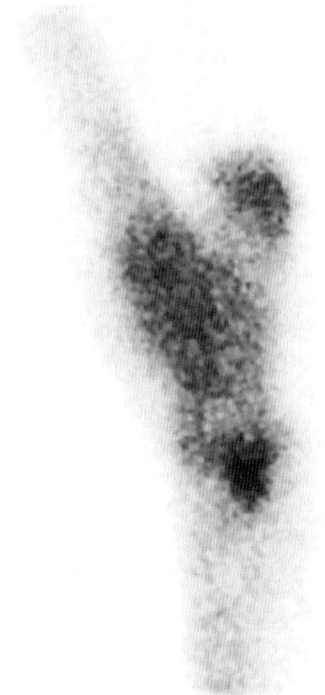

Fig. 72-9 • Lateral scintigraphic image of the left hindlimb of a 9-year-old Warmblood show jumper with proximal suspensory desmitis. There is marked focal increased radiopharmaceutical uptake in the proximoplantar aspect of the third metatarsal bone.

be positive in only 12% of 46 horses with ultrasonographic evidence of PSD. In bone phase images, IRU in the proximoplantar aspect of the MtIII was found in 12% of 82 horses (Figure 72-9). IRU was associated with more severe ultrasonographic lesions. IRU in the proximoplantar aspect of the MtIII, with no detectable ultrasonographic abnormality of the SL and no radiological change associated with

enthesopathy, may be associated with a primary pathological condition of bone, such as bone trauma or entheseous reaction at the origin of the SL, which has been demonstrated using MRI.

Magnetic Resonance Imaging and Computed Tomography

Lesions of the proximal aspect of the SL that were not evident on ultrasonography have been identified with MRI[13,14,38,39] or computed tomography. MRI has also identified adhesions to the MtII and to the MtIV (Figure 72-10, *A*) and endosteal and entheseous reactions at the ligament's origin (Figure 72-10, *B*).

Differential Diagnosis

PSD should be differentiated from pain associated with the tarsometatarsal joint, an avulsion fracture of the MtIII at the origin of the SL, primary stress reactions in the MtIII, bone trauma, and syndesmopathy between the MtIII and either the MtII or the MtIII.

A recent study compared the results of ultrasonography and MRI in 46 limbs of 38 horses in which lameness was improved at least 60% by perineural analgesia of the deep branch of the lateral plantar nerve. Using MRI as the gold standard, 21 limbs had PSD, including nine with osseous abnormalities of the MtIII; four horses had osseous injury at the origin of the SL as the only abnormality.[39] However, in nine limbs there were injuries unrelated to the SL, including OA of the distal tarsal joints, enthesopathy of an intertarsal ligament, and osseous pathology of the central or fourth tarsal bones or the MtIII in a variety of locations. No diagnosis was reached for the cause of lameness in 12 limbs. It was suggested that neuropathy of the deep branch of the lateral plantar nerve could possibly be the source of pain in these 12 horses. Ultrasonography had a moderate sensitivity (0.77) and low sensitivity (0.33) for diagnosis of PSD with MRI as the gold standard, with both false-positive and false-negative results.

Treatment

The prognosis for horses with PSD in the hindlimb with conservative management generally has been poor. Only six (14%) of 42 horses seen in a referral practice were able to resume full work without detectable lameness for at least 1 year; all six had been lame for less than 5 weeks.[37] All these horses showed substantial improvement in clinical signs within 3 months of the onset of lameness. Two additional horses resumed full work but developed lameness in another limb. Seven horses improved greatly and were able to work, despite persistent mild lameness. Twenty-four horses (57%) had persistent or recurrent lameness. Results from a first opinion practice also were disappointing, with only 10 (59%) of 17 horses resuming work.[1]

Horses with acute (less than 4 to 6 weeks' duration) hindlimb PSD respond reasonably well to local infiltration with corticosteroids, aimed at reducing inflammation and therefore swelling and thus minimizing the risk of developing a compartment syndrome (see the following discussion). Foot imbalance is corrected and egg bar shoes are used to reduce extension of the fetlock. Horses with chronic PSD have a guarded prognosis regardless of the treatment. Lameness often tends to persist unchanged, even after

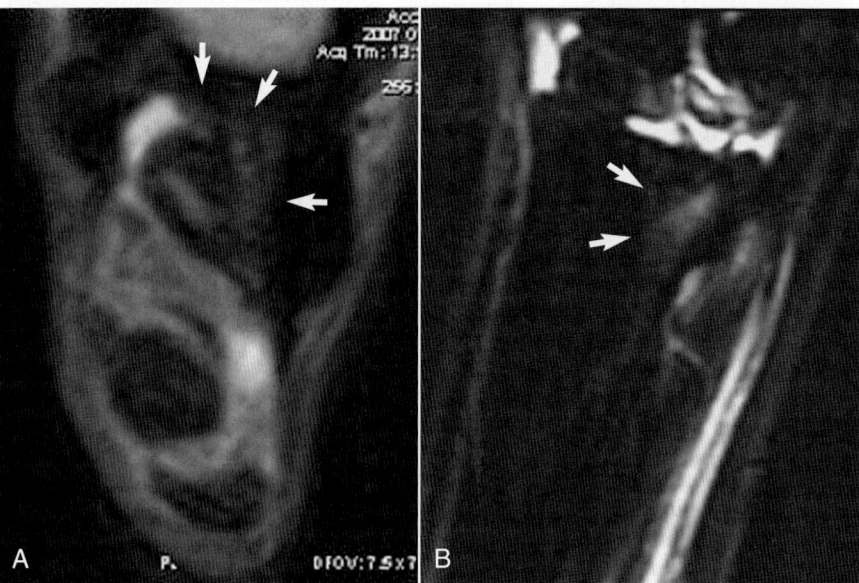

Fig. 72-10 • **A,** Transverse T2* gradient echo low-field magnetic resonance image of the proximal metatarsal region of a 6-year-old show jumper. Lateral is to the right. There are adhesions between the suspensory ligament and the axial aspect of the fourth metatarsal bone and the plantar aspect of the third metatarsal bone (MtIII) *(arrows).* **B,** Sagittal short tau inversion recovery (STIR) magnetic resonance image of the left hindlimb of a 3-year-old Thoroughbred flat racehorse with mild architectural abnormalities of the suspensory ligament origin detected ultrasonographically. The horse exhibited severe lameness. There is diffuse increased signal intensity in the proximo-plantar aspect of the MtIII at the origin of the suspensory ligament.

prolonged box rest, which is unusual for a primary soft tissue lesion. In some horses lesions are progressive. Local infiltration with corticosteroids, polysulfated glycosaminoglycans, hyaluronan, or homeopathic drugs such as Actovegin and Traumeel has given disappointing results.

In some horses an initial improvement in lameness is seen after box rest and controlled walking exercise for 2 to 3 months, and then no further improvement is seen. Increasing the exercise despite the lameness sometimes results in further improvement. Some horses have worked satisfactorily while being treated with phenylbutazone, without apparent deterioration of clinical signs or ultrasonographic abnormalities. This indicates that in some horses the SL is able to withstand load and the horse can work satisfactorily provided that pain is controlled.

Extracorporeal shock wave therapy or radial pressure wave therapy appears to be helpful in some horses.[32] Eighteen of 30 horses with PSD in forelimbs or hindlimbs were in work 6 months after treatment. Eighteen (40%) of 45 horses with unilateral or bilateral chronic (lameness of greater than 3 months' duration) hindlimb PSD were in full work 6 months after treatment[32]; however, a small proportion of these horses have experienced recurrent lameness subsequently. Horses with mild or moderate ultrasonographic lesions responded better than those with severe lesions. Injection of 2% iodine in almond oil resulted in 12 (55%) of 22 horses returning to work.[29]

Tibial neurectomy performed in eight horses enabled six to return to full athletic function (show jumping and horse trials) for at least 2 years after surgery, with no postoperative complications.[14] Neurectomy of the deep branch of the lateral plantar nerve has been combined with incising the thin fascial covering of the plantar aspect of the SL and was successful in 79% of 200 horses,[40] 91% of 84

horses,[41] and 62.5% of 16 horses.[35] It has also been combined with osteostixis.[40,42] A further 70% of 120 horses treated by one author (SJD) have returned to full athletic function after neurectomy of the deep branch of the lateral plantar nerve, but two horses experienced deterioration because of progressive lesions in the SL.[14] Both of these horses had preexisting excessively straight hock conformation and/or hyperextension of the fetlock of the lame limb. This has also been reported elsewhere,[43] and these conformational abnormalities are considered to be contraindications for surgery.

Postoperative management depends on the severity of the initial injury. Improvement in ultrasonographic appearance is generally seen by 2 months postoperatively, but this may in part reflect neurogenic muscle atrophy. Although some horses may successfully return to work at this stage, horses with severe injuries and those with osseous pain may need a considerably longer rehabilitation period. The presence of IRU associated with PSD usually indicates that a prolonged convalescence will be required. Neurectomy may result in atrophy of the muscle component of the SL, which could potentially influence its function.[44] The SL is closely related anatomically to the distal hock joints by its accessory ligament. Horses with low-grade residual lameness may respond to intraarticular medication of the distal hock joints.

Fasciotomy of the deep plantar metatarsal fascia has been successful in some horses.[14] Injection of about 30 mL of bone marrow also is claimed to be successful, especially if combined with fasciotomy, allowing 85% of horses to return to the former level of function[14] (see also Chapter 73). Injection of platelet-rich plasma or mesenchymal stem cells has also been combined with fasciotomy, but without neurectomy and anecdotally is successful.

Gross Pathological and Histopathological Findings

Postmortem examinations have been performed on both hindlimbs of eight horses, six with unilateral lameness and two with bilateral lameness.[22,34] Abnormalities of the SLs were confined to the lame limbs. The SLs were grossly enlarged, with thickening of surrounding fascia and peri-ligamentous tissues, especially on the plantar aspect. Histological changes in the SL included hypercellularity and acellular areas; hemosiderin deposition; fibrosis; hyalinization of collagen; an increased number of fibrous septae, some with blood vessels; neovascularization; and chondroid metaplasia. Although chondroid metaplasia was seen at the ligament-bone interface in lame and sound limbs, intraligamentous chondroid metaplasia was seen only in the lame limbs. These histological abnormalities are consistent with degenerative rather than inflammatory changes.

Evidence of compression of adjacent peripheral nerves was found in the lame limb of five horses.[22,34] Abnormalities of the plantar metatarsal nerves included thickening of the perineurium, perineural fibrosis, reduction or absence of nerve fibers, and Renaut bodies. Similar abnormalities have been identified in the deep branch of the lateral plantar nerve bilaterally in 11 bilaterally lame horses and unilaterally in the lame limb of five unilaterally lame horses.[35]

These changes support the theory that PSD in the hindlimb results in a compartment syndrome and some pain may possibly be neuropathic in origin.

AVULSION FRACTURES OF THE THIRD METACARPAL OR METATARSAL BONE AT THE ORIGIN OF THE SUSPENSORY LIGAMENT

Avulsion fractures of the third metacarpal or metatarsal bone at the region of the SL are discussed on page 417.

SUSPENSORY DESMITIS: BODY LESIONS

Desmitis of the body of the SL is principally an injury of horses that race, STBs and TBs (flat racehorses and jumpers). In TBs in Europe the incidence is much higher in horses that race over fences (National Hunt Racing and point to pointing; see Chapter 112) compared with flat racehorses. Although PSD and desmitis of the medial and/or lateral branches of the SL are relatively common injuries in event horses, show jumpers, dressage horses, and endurance horses, body lesions are recognized less frequently, except as associated with an exostosis of the McII or the MtIV (the splint bones) or as a sequela to a branch injury. Injuries occur in forelimbs and hindlimbs, and in STBs several limbs may be affected concurrently, whereas in TBs lesions generally are restricted to the forelimb.[29,45] There is frequently a poor correlation between the extent of the lesions and the degree of lameness. Performance, however, can be compromised despite lack of evidence of overt lameness. In STB racehorses lameness may be observed or tolerated while athletic function continues. This continued exercise may result in progressive injury or injury to other tendonous or ligamentous structures.

Soreness on palpation of the SL is not synonymous with structural damage. Event horses frequently have sore SLs for several days after fast work or competition, but rarely does this appear to be associated with a clinically significant problem. Soreness does not appear to be a warning sign of impending desmitis. Upper-level show jumpers may have a sore forelimb SL the day after competition, which often highlights overload caused by lameness in another limb.

Clinical Signs

The clinical signs associated with suspensory body desmitis vary in presence and degree and include the following:
- Localized heat
- Periligamentous edema; severe periligamentous soft tissue swelling may make accurate palpation of the SL difficult
- Rounding of the margins of the SL
- Enlargement of the body of the SL
- Pain on palpation of the margins of the SL
- Abnormal stiffness of the SL
- Pain on palpation of the distal third of the McII or the MtIV, if there is a concurrent fracture
- Lameness; absence of lameness does not preclude clinically significant desmitis
- Hyperextension of the fetlock joint (fetlock drop); in the hindlimb, straight hock conformation

Diagnosis

Diagnosis is based on clinical signs and ultrasonographic assessment. Diagnostic analgesic techniques rarely are required unless another contributory cause of lameness or recurrence of previous desmitis is suspected. In a horse with previous desmitis a previously enlarged SL may have no detectable change in size, shape, or reaction to palpation. Perineural analgesia of the palmar metacarpal nerves proximal to the site of the suspect lesion should remove associated lameness.

The body of the SL of a normal horse is not always uniform in echogenicity because of variable amounts of muscle tissue in the ligament and variations in the level of bifurcation of the SL between horses. This can make detection of subtle lesions difficult. The maximum injury zone is frequently at the region of the bifurcation of the SL, which may appear hypoechogenic in normal horses (Figure 72-11). Careful comparison with the contralateral limb may help if clinical signs are unilateral. Ultrasonographic abnormalities associated with active desmitis include the following:
- Enlargement of the body of the ligament in transverse and median planes
- Loss of definition of one or more of the margins of the ligament
- Focal hypoechoic areas, peripheral or central, extending a variable distance proximodistally
- A diffuse reduction in echogenicity of some or all of the cross-sectional area of the ligament
- In horses with chronic desmitis, focal hyperechogenic areas representing fibrosis or mineralization.

Enlargement may be the only detectable abnormality. Careful comparison with the contralateral limb can be helpful. Reference can be made to studies of sizes in normal horses of similar breed, but caution is urged because notable differences do exist between U.S. and European TBs. The extent of ultrasonographic abnormality is not always

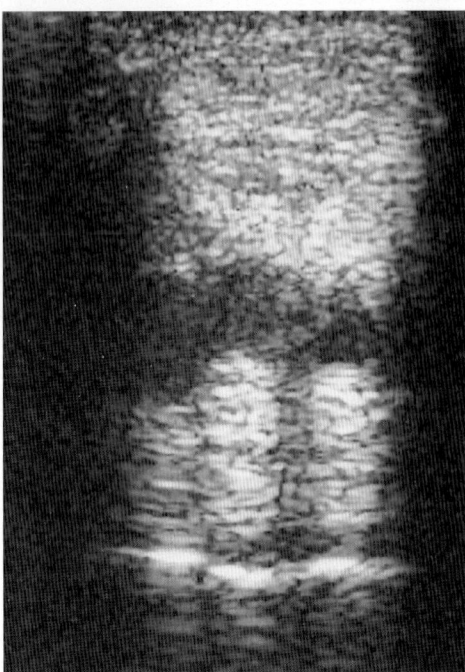

Fig. 72-11 • Transverse ultrasonographic image of a normal forelimb suspensory ligament at the level of the beginning of the bifurcation, 18 cm distal to the accessory carpal bone. The central, less echogenic region should not be mistaken for a lesion.

correlated with the severity of clinical signs. A reasonable correlation exists with the severity of the ultrasonographic grade of the injury and the prognosis; however, a diffuse reduction in echogenicity of the cross-sectional area is also associated with a poor prognosis. Lesions may extend into the branches, which should also be examined by ultrasonography.

Many lesions persist long term, although focal lesions in STBs may fill in. In TBs a readily detectable defect often persists, despite some increase in echogenicity and slight reduction in size. This can limit the value of serial ultrasonographic evaluations to determine when a horse might be able to withstand work. Determining objectively to what extent healing has taken place and the strength of the repair tissue often is not possible. This may explain the high rate of recurrence of body lesions in STBs and TBs. Racing careers of STBs can usually be extended, whereas managing TBs is much more difficult, because lameness in TBs rarely stabilizes.[29] Horses with slight lesions may be responsive to symptomatic treatment, and a horse may train and race well; however, the lesion is likely to be progressive. The risk of catastrophic breakdown of the suspensory apparatus must always be considered in a TB racehorse. In STB racehorses rest for about 3 months may confer no extra advantage to symptomatic treatment and continued training[30] with respect to racing performance. Lesions are usually progressive, and periodic ultrasonographic monitoring is recommended.

There is a high rate of reinjury to the body of the SL of the same or the contralateral limb or to a branch of the same or the contralateral limb subsequent to desmitis of the body of the SL.[29]

Radiographic examination of the McII and the McIV is indicated if clinical examination suggests abnormal modeling or a fracture, because surgical amputation may be indicated[29] (see page 421).

Management

Treatment is aimed at reducing inflammation by the administration of systemic nonsteroidal antiinflammatory drugs (NSAIDs), local or systemic corticosteroids, hydrotherapy, and controlled exercise. Cryotherapy is used by some clinicians to provide pain relief, but a real risk of progressive deterioration of the lesion exists (see Chapter 89).

Progress is monitored clinically and by serial ultrasonographic examinations. Ideally there should be progressive reduction in cross-sectional area, improvement in echogenicity and fiber alignment, no restrictive periligamentous fibrosis, and reasonable stability in all of these features as exercise is increased. In STBs handwalking exercise is advocated for the first 4 weeks.[29] Provided that some improvement in the ultrasonographic appearance of the ligament occurs and the horse is sound when jogged in hand, the horse is harnessed and walked in the jog cart for another 4 weeks. Flat shoes are preferred. The horse is reassessed by ultrasonography after 8 weeks, and if further filling in of the defect occurs, short slow jogging is reintroduced and gradually increased. A third ultrasonographic examination is performed after 8 weeks of jogging, and provided that the lesion is uniformly echogenic to the remainder of the SL and has a linear arrangement of fibers, normal jogging and speed work are resumed. Although this method is successful in some STBs, in others a longer period of convalescence is required.

Continued medical therapy includes daily hydrotherapy—for example, whirlpool boots, stable and exercise bandages, massage with emollient oils, leg sweats, and leg tighteners with or without DMSO. The aim is to stimulate circulation, reduce inflammation, and provide pain relief. The work program should be adapted so that days of light work are interspersed with hard work. Swimming is a useful method of maintaining cardiovascular fitness but should not be used alone, because the musculoskeletal system requires regular stimulation to avoid other injuries.

Intralesional treatment with β-aminopropionitrile fumarate has been used in STB and TB racehorses with moderate to severe injuries of the SL body[30]; however, a licensed product is no longer available. Eleven of 18 horses successfully returned to racing, although some dropped in class. A recent in vitro study compared the potential for various blood-based biological products to induce SL regeneration and indicated that bone marrow aspirates were potentially superior to platelet-rich plasma.[46] However, nine of nine STB racehorses treated by intralesional injection of platelet-rich plasma returned to racing, with similar performance to that of control horses for 2 years after treatment.[47] It is important to note, however, that STBs have a much higher tolerance of SL injuries than TBs.

Surgical splitting of the body of the SL usually is not advocated in STBs or TBs.[29] However, occasionally, large chronic lesions with associated McII or McIV fractures are split, combined with surgical removal of the fracture piece in STB and, less commonly, TB racehorses. Pin firing combined with rest may be of benefit in some horses with chronic desmitis[29] (see Chapter 88).

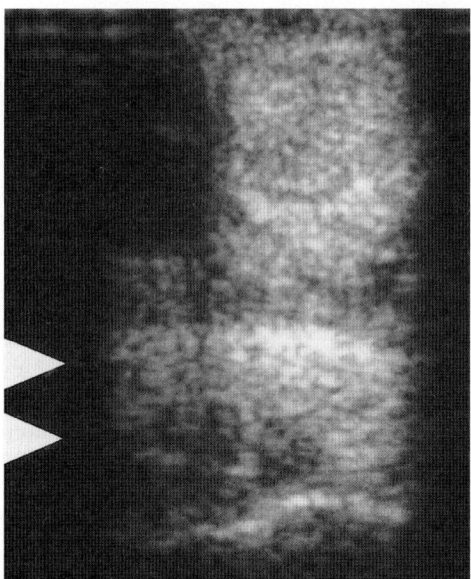

Fig. 72-12 • Transverse ultrasonographic image of the midmetacarpal region of a 7-year-old show jumper with intermittent left forelimb lameness associated with localized enlargement of the axial aspect of the second metacarpal bone (a splint). Slight pain could be elicited by pressure. Separating the axial border of the bone from the suspensory ligament by palpation was not possible. Lameness was alleviated by local infiltration of local anesthetic solution. Echogenic material *(arrowheads)* extends from the medial aspect of the suspensory ligament, which was slightly hypoechoic dorsomedially. Surgical exploration revealed a loose spicule of bone adjacent to the splint and a granulomatous reaction between it and the suspensory ligament. A focal defect was found in the medial border of the suspensory ligament.

SUSPENSORY DESMITIS ASSOCIATED WITH AN EXOSTOSIS ON THE SECOND OR FOURTH METACARPAL OR METATARSAL BONE (SPLINT)

Suspensory desmitis associated with exostosis of the McII (MtII) or the McIV (MtIV) is discussed on page 419 (Figure 72-12).

SUSPENSORY DESMITIS ASSOCIATED WITH FRACTURE OF THE DISTAL THIRD OF THE SECOND OR FOURTH METACARPAL OR METATARSAL BONE

Suspensory desmitis associated with fracture of the distal third of the McII (MtII) or the McIV (MtIV) is discussed on page 421.

SUSPENSORY DESMITIS: BRANCH LESIONS

Desmitis of the medial and/or lateral branches of the SL in forelimbs and hindlimbs is a relatively common injury in all types of sports horses. Usually only a single branch is affected in a single limb, although both branches may be affected, especially in hindlimbs. Foot imbalance often is recognized in affected horses and may be a predisposing factor. Some horses, particularly event horses, have acute-onset distention of the metacarpophalangeal joint capsule concurrent with SL branch desmitis. Detection of

radiological abnormalities (modeling or fracture of the distal aspect of the McII or the McIV or a PSB) in some horses at the time of recognition of an acute, first-time injury suggests a subclinical preexisting problem. As with PSD, there is some evidence that some suspensory branch injuries in hindlimbs may be degenerative in origin.[48]

Clinical Signs

The clinical signs depend on the degree of damage and chronicity of the lesion(s) and include localized heat and swelling. Swelling often is caused by enlargement of the branch, together with periligamentous edema or fibrosis. In some hindlimb injuries swelling may be predominantly because of periligamentous fibrosis. Associated distention of the metacarpophalangeal or metatarsophalangeal joint capsule may occur because of the subsynovial location of the axial aspect of the distal third of the ligament.[49] In hindlimbs sometimes considerable distention of the digital flexor tendon sheath (DFTS) occurs, making assessing the SL branches by palpation difficult. Mild swelling may also easily be overlooked unless a standardized method of palpation is used. A normal SL is uniform in dorsopalmar (dorsoplantar) width throughout its length. With the limb bearing full weight, place the thumbs of both hands on the dorsal and palmar (plantar) aspect of the SL body and follow the ligament distally. The thumbs should remain equidistant unless there is enlargement of the SL. The medial and lateral branches should both be assessed routinely. Pain usually is elicited by direct pressure applied to the injured branch or by passive flexion of the fetlock. Lameness varies, may be absent, usually is proportional to the degree of damage, and is related inversely to the duration of injury. A notable exception is in the hindlimbs of older dressage horses, in which occasionally both branches sustain damage, and strong adhesions develop between them. These horses experience persistent, severe lameness. Occasionally, younger horses from any discipline develop acute-onset, severe, and persistent hindlimb lameness associated with progressive stretching of a single branch and the development of periligamentous fibrosis. There is associated hyperextension of the fetlock.

Diagnosis

Diagnosis is based on clinical signs and ultrasonographic examination. Diagnostic analgesic techniques usually are required only if more than one lesion is suspected as the cause of lameness. In horses with acute branch injury with concurrent distention of the metacarpophalangeal joint capsule, we suggest that the horse be reevaluated after 2 to 3 weeks. If joint capsule distention and pain on manipulation persist, then the joint should be blocked intraarticularly.

The entire SL should be examined by ultrasonography, because lesions may extend beyond areas that are palpably abnormal. Ultrasonographic abnormalities include the following (Figures 72-13 to 72-15):

- Abnormalities of the body of the SL (see page 749)
- Enlargement of the branch
- Change in shape of the branch
- Loss of definition of one or more margins of the branch
- Well-defined or poorly defined hypoechoic areas, central or peripheral

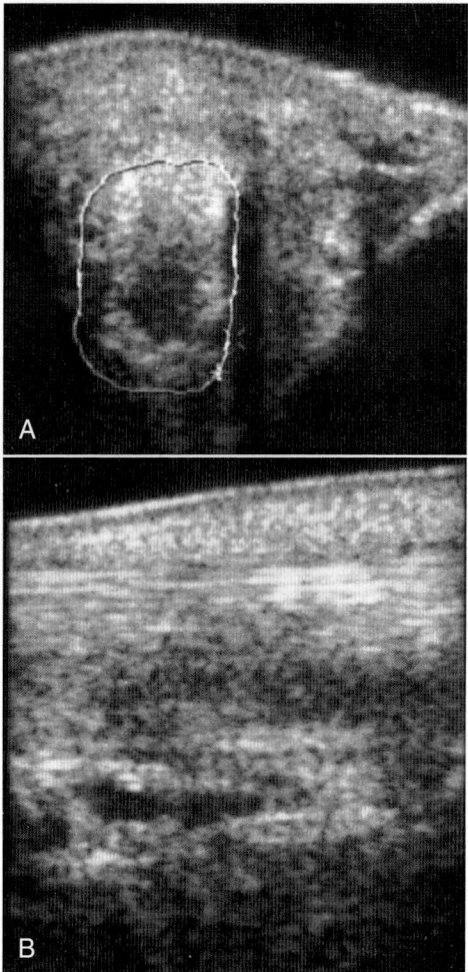

Fig. 72-13 • A, Transverse ultrasonographic image of the medial branch of the suspensory ligament of the right forelimb of a 14-year-old Grand Prix dressage horse. The suspensory ligament branch is enlarged (cross-sectional area 2.02 cm²) and has a large, almost anechoic lesion. The echogenic material subcutaneously also contributed to the soft tissue swelling. **B,** Longitudinal ultrasonographic image of the medial branch of the suspensory ligament of the right forelimb of the same horse. Proximal is to the left. There is a marked loss of fiber pattern within the suspensory ligament. Note also the subcutaneous echogenic material.

- A diffuse reduction of echogenicity involving some or all of the cross-sectional area of the branch
- Echogenic material subcutaneously; this may be uniform in echogenicity or include areas of reduced echogenicity reflecting tearing of periligamentous fibrous tissue
- Echogenic material between the medial and lateral branches
- Hyperechogenic foci or larger masses within the branch
- An irregular contour or fracture of the ipsilateral PSB
- An abnormal amount of fluid within the DFTS and/or the metacarpophalangeal (metatarsophalangeal) joint

The branches should be examined in transverse and longitudinal planes. Lesions restricted to the insertion are sometimes detectable only in longitudinal images. Sometimes horses show slight localized swelling and heat in the region of a SL branch, with a subtle alteration in gait, in which no ultrasonographic abnormality of the SL can be identified. The swelling appears to be principally periligamentous. Some of these horses can be maintained safely in work, whereas in others clinical signs deteriorate with the development of a branch lesion. Recurrent lameness may also result from tearing of periligamentous fibrous tissue. Occasionally, concurrent lesions of the oblique sesamoidean ligaments occur.

Radiological examination of the ipsilateral splint bone and PSB should be performed. Abnormalities may include the following:

- Dystrophic mineralization in the SL
- Distortion in shape of the ipsilateral splint bone
- Fracture of the distal aspect of the ipsilateral splint bone
- Fracture(s) of the ipsilateral PSB (see Figure 72-15)
- Radiating lucent lines within the ipsilateral PSB
- Modeling of the palmar aspect of the PSB
- Abnormally distal location of the PSB, reflecting stretching of the SL

Fractures influence the treatment and prognosis. However, radiological evidence of sesamoiditis is not well correlated with the outcome, although primary sesamoiditis unassociated with SL desmitis can cause recurrent lameness (see Chapter 36). Occasionally lesions cannot be identified using ultrasonography but are recognized using MRI.

Management

Treatment depends on the occupation of the horse, the breed, and the severity of the clinical signs and ultrasonographic abnormalities. There are no large-scale, peer-reviewed reports of the success of management of SL branch injuries in either racehorses or sports horses. Horses with acute central core lesions may be treated by splitting (desmoplasty), with horses returning to work within 9 months. Horses with more peripheral or poorly demarcated lesions are not suitable for splitting, but their injuries can be managed conservatively by appropriate trimming and shoeing, box rest, and a controlled increasing exercise program. Intralesional injection of β-aminopropionitrile fumarate (five 7-mg injections on alternate days) combined with a controlled increasing work program over 6 to 9 months has been successful.[30] There are anecdotal reports of the success of mesenchymal stem cell treatment or intralesional injection of platelet-rich plasma or bone marrow. Our experience to date is that the results are rather unpredictable, although some excellent outcomes have been achieved.

Dressage horses and show jumpers with minor lesions and only subtle ultrasonographic abnormalities have been managed successfully by appropriate trimming and shoeing with egg bar shoes, combined with modification of the training program for 6 to 8 weeks. Some horses can be managed successfully and maintained in work by aggressive local therapy (e.g., use of whirlpool boots, laser or ultrasound therapy, leg sweats, and cold therapy). Continued work in an event horse usually results in substantial progression of the lesion. In a TB racehorse, continued training in the face of SL branch injury runs the risk of an acute breakdown injury of the suspensory apparatus. In STB racehorses symptomatic treatment is common, with NSAIDs as required, daily icing, topical application of a

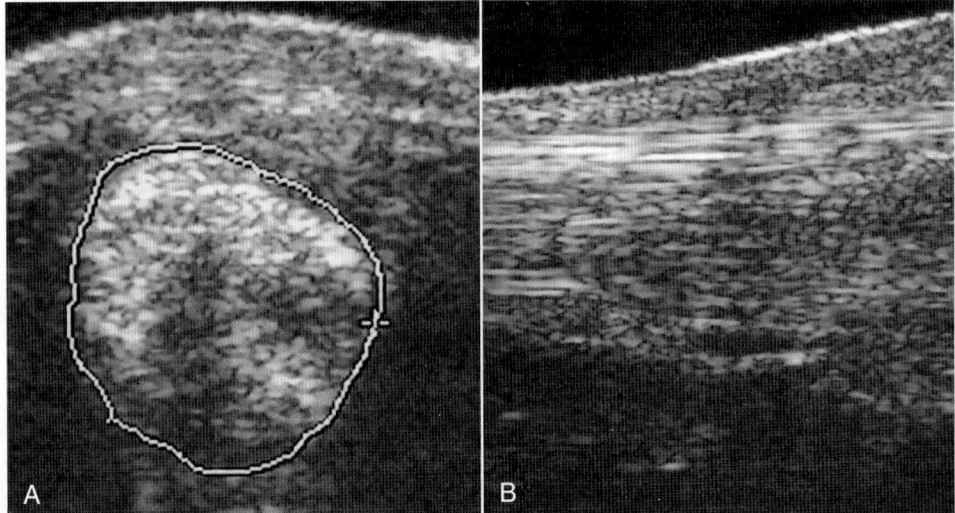

Fig. 72-14 • A, Transverse ultrasonographic image of the lateral branch of the suspensory ligament of the left hindlimb of a 7-year-old intermediate-level event horse with lameness of 2 weeks' duration. The suspensory branch is considerably enlarged (cross-sectional area 2.0 cm²). Its margins are poorly defined, and there is marked loss of echogenicity. **B,** Longitudinal ultrasonographic image of the lateral branch of the suspensory ligament of the same horse. Proximal is to the left. The ligament is hypoechoic, with loss of fiber pattern.

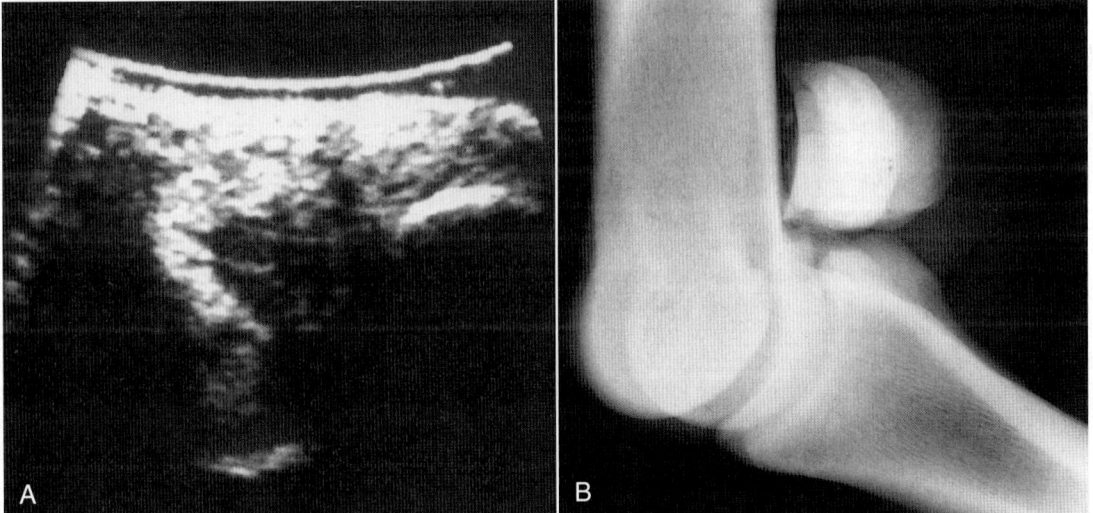

Fig. 72-15 • A, Transverse ultrasonographic image of the lateral branch of the suspensory ligament, close to its insertion on the lateral proximal sesamoid bone, of the right hindlimb of a 9-year-old advanced event horse with acute-onset lameness. The ligament has a large, almost anechoic defect. **B,** Flexed, slightly oblique lateromedial radiographic image of the right hind fetlock of the same horse. The lateral proximal sesamoid bone is positioned slightly more dorsally. Several small osseous opacities are seen dorsal to it. These were removed arthroscopically, and torn fibers at the suspensory ligament branch insertion were debrided.

DMSO-cortisone liniment, and modification of the training schedule to light jogging or swimming between races. Lesions may remain stable or progress slowly and usually ultimately compromise performance substantially. Management is more difficult in horses that race at a high level, in which training cannot be reduced enough or the speed of the race results in overload of the compromised structure. Horses seem to do less well on a slower track surface, with a deep cushion, compared with a fast track surface.

Ultrasonographically, lesions are often slow to resolve and some persist long term (longer than 18 months). Some horses are able to resume full work after a convalescent period of at least 9 months, despite the persistence of a lesion, although the incidence of recurrent injury is high. If a lesion persists as viewed by ultrasonography, knowing when to recommend resumption of work is difficult. Generally the horse should have been rested at least 6 months, and no appreciable change should be found in the ultrasonographic appearance of the SL branch between two examinations 3 months apart. With increased exercise the ligament should remain stable in size and echogenicity.

Arthroscopic examination of the palmar (plantar) pouch of the metacarpophalangeal (metatarsophalangeal) joint may be indicated if there is persistent synovial distention associated with an axial lesion of the SL branch.[49] Intrasynovial torn fibers can be debrided and, occasionally, small avulsion fractures removed. Thirteen of 18 horses (72%) with an axial branch injury that involved the fetlock joint returned to full athletic function for between 5 months and 6 years.[49]

Horses with forelimb or hindlimb suspensory branch lesions with periligamentous fibrosis, or echogenic material extending between the two branches (seen more often in hindlimbs) have a poor prognosis. This echogenic material represents firm fibrous adhesions between the branches. Periligamentous fibrosis impedes mobility of the SL branch and is often associated with a disproportionately severe lameness compared with lesions of the branch itself. There are anecdotal reports of surgical debridement, but the results have been disappointing. An abnormally low position of the PSBs is also a poor prognostic indicator, reflecting degeneration and stretching of the suspensory apparatus.

PROXIMAL SESAMOID BONE FRACTURE ASSOCIATED WITH A BRANCH INJURY

Proximal sesamoid fractures associated with SL branch injury are discussed on page 404.

AVULSION FRACTURE OF A PROXIMAL SESAMOID BONE AT THE INSERTION OF THE PALMAR ANNULAR LIGAMENT

Avulsion injuries of the palmar annular ligament (PAL) at its insertion on a PSB are not common[29,50] and must be differentiated carefully from abaxial PSB fractures (see Chapter 36, page 405). Injuries occur in forelimbs and hindlimbs. Horses with acute injury show lameness associated with diffuse soft tissue swelling palmar to a PSB.[29] Swelling does not involve the ipsilateral SL branch unless that branch has been damaged concurrently. There may also be mild distention of the fetlock joint capsule and the DFTS. It may be possible to elicit pain by firm pressure applied to the abaxial aspect of the PSB. In horses with more chronic injury no localizing clinical signs may be apparent. Radiological examination may reveal a punched-out lesion of the PSB (Figure 72-16) or a small detached fragment of bone (Figure 72-17), the origin of which cannot be determined. Ultrasonographic examination helps to determine the origin of the fragment. The PAL should be examined from the palmar aspect of the limb and then followed around to its insertion. An osseous echogenic body may be seen attached to the PAL close to the PSB. Treatment by surgical removal of the fragment or conservative management has resulted in return to full athletic function.[29,50]

DAMAGE OF THE PALMAR (PLANTAR) LIGAMENT OF THE FETLOCK (INTERSESAMOIDEAN LIGAMENT)
Focal Tears in the Body of the Intersesamoidean Ligament
Focal tears in the body of the intersesamoidean ligament are an unusual cause of lameness and can be diagnosed

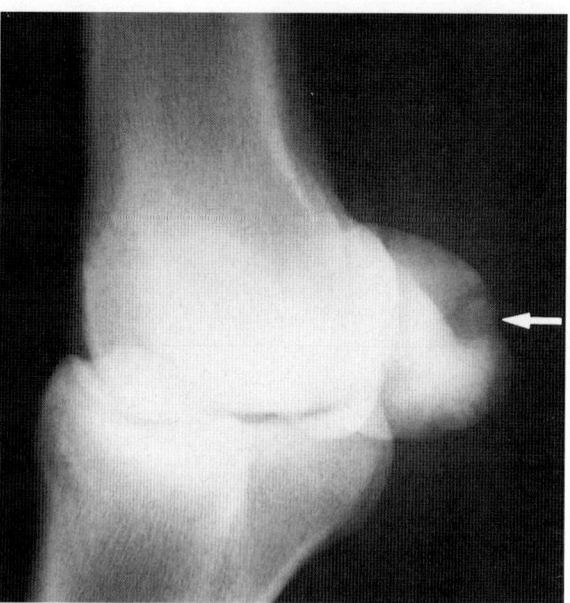

Fig. 72-16 • Dorsolateral-palmaromedial oblique radiographic image of the right front fetlock of a 7-year-old advanced event horse. A punched-out radiopacity is visible on the palmar aspect of the bone *(arrow)*. This is an avulsion injury at the insertion of the palmar annular ligament. Note also the new bone on the palmar distal aspect of the bone.

definitively only by arthroscopic evaluation of the palmar (plantar) pouch of the metacarpophalangeal (metatarsophalangeal) joint.[29] Lameness is usually acute in onset and moderate to severe. Lameness improves with rest but often persists. There may be effusion in the metacarpophalangeal (metatarsophalangeal) joint. Lameness is improved by intraarticular analgesia. Usually no identifiable radiological abnormalities occur. Small focal tears are extremely difficult to identify using ultrasonography. Nuclear scintigraphic examination of a small number of horses with small focal tears not involving the insertion of the ligament has revealed slight generalized IRU in the fetlock region but not localized to the PSBs. Horses with focal ligament tears have a poor response to surgical debridement and prolonged rest, with or without intraarticular medication, and the prognosis for return to athletic function is guarded.

Degeneration or Partial Rupture of the Intersesamoidean Ligament
Degenerative lesions and partial rupture of the intersesamoidean ligament have been seen only in older, mature athletic horses and are relatively rare.[51] The condition has been recognized in forelimbs and hindlimbs and may occur as a single injury or with other soft tissue or bony lesions.

Lameness is acute in onset and moderate to severe. Mild distention of the metacarpophalangeal (metatarsophalangeal) joint capsule or the DFTS may occur. Lameness may be improved by intraarticular analgesia, but the response to perineural analgesia of the palmar (plantar) and palmar (plantar) metacarpal (metatarsal) nerves is often better.

Diagnosis is based on ultrasonography, and a number of abnormalities have been identified:

x

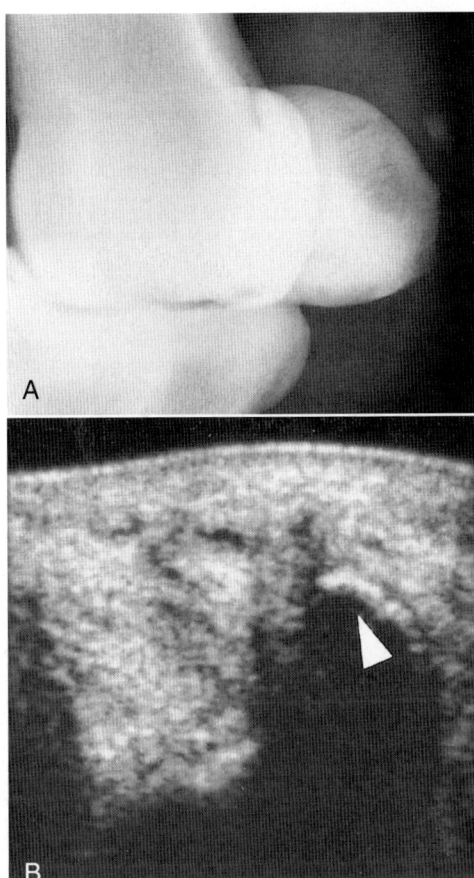

Fig. 72-17 • A, Dorsomedial-palmarolateral oblique radiographic image of the right front fetlock of a 9-year-old Grand Prix show jumper with acute-onset lameness associated with soft tissue swelling on the medial aspect of the fetlock, palmar to the medial branch of the suspensory ligament. There was also slight edematous swelling around the distal aspect of the medial branch of the suspensory ligament. There is an osseous fragment palmar to the proximal sesamoid bones, but its origin could not be determined radiologically. **B,** Transverse ultrasonographic image of the palmaromedial aspect of the fetlock. A thick hyperechoic line represents the osseous fragment *(arrow)* that was an avulsion of the insertion of the palmar annular ligament.

- An increase in the space between the PSBs
- An increased thickness of the palmar ligament
- Reduced echogenicity of the palmar ligament
- Focal hyperechogenic regions in the palmar ligament
- Dorsal displacement of the digital flexor tendons
- Thinning of the palmar ligament and reduction in the space between the ligament and the dorsal aspect of the DDFT
- Irregularity of the facies flexoria of a PSB (this may correlate with radiolucent areas in the axial aspect of the bone)

Careful examination of the digital flexor tendons, the PAL, and the distal sesamoidean ligaments should be performed to identify any concurrent injuries.

Radiological examination occasionally may reveal osteolytic lesions on the axial aspect of the PSBs (see the following discussion).

The prognosis for return to athletic function is extremely guarded.[29]

Insertional Injury of the Intersesamoidean Ligament

Aseptic necrosis of the axial aspect of the PSBs has been described as a cause of lameness in forelimbs and hindlimbs.[49,50] The condition has been characterized by the development of radiolucent zones in the axial aspect of one or both PSBs (Figure 72-18), lesions that have also been seen with infection (see the following discussion). Histological examination of two horses indicated that these lesions reflect trauma of the insertion of the intersesamoidean ligament.[29] Insertional lesions of the palmar ligament of the fetlock also may occur without radiological change and have been identified arthroscopically (Figure 72-19).

In contrast to horses with associated infection, usually no substantial soft tissue swelling occurs in the fetlock region, although distention of the metacarpophalangeal (metatarsophalangeal) joint capsule, the DFTS, or both may occur. In some horses, eliciting pain by palpation may be difficult. Lameness may vary from moderate to severe and is often worse with the horse walking in a circle compared with walking in a straight line.

Perineural analgesia by a four-point block usually results in much better improvement in lameness than intra-articular analgesia. In the acute stage radiological examination findings may be negative. Ultrasonographic evaluation may be unrewarding, but in some horses an irregular outline of one of the PSBs may be seen, with reduced echogenicity of the intersesamoidean ligament (see Figure 72-18).

Nuclear scintigraphic examination usually reveals focal, intense IRU in one or both PSBs, in contrast to the pattern of uptake that has been seen with focal lesions in the body of the intersesamoidean ligament (see the previous discussion). IRU localized to a PSB also may be caused by an incomplete fracture or subchondral trauma. Sequential radiological examination may reveal the development of lucent zones on the axial aspect of the proximal sesamoid bones.

These lesions may be associated with long-term lameness, although surgical debridement has resulted in return to former athletic function in some horses.[52,53] Arthroscopic evaluation usually reveals a defect in the palmar ligament (see Figure 72-19), through which a probe can be inserted into the bony defect. Occasionally the palmar ligament is intact and must be incised to permit access to the osseous defect. Defects usually are more pronounced in one PSB, but they can involve both PSBs. Damaged palmar ligament and bone are debrided. Occasionally, to approach lesions not involving the articular surface, it may be necessary to create a small apical fracture to gain access to the bony defect.

INFECTION OF THE AXIAL ASPECT OF THE PROXIMAL SESAMOID BONES

Aseptic necrosis[51,52] and osteomyelitis[54] of the PSBs have been described, but in one author's experience (SJD) aseptic necrosis occurs more commonly. *Aseptic necrosis* is probably an inappropriate term, because the Editors believe that lesions develop secondary to trauma of the insertion of the intersesamoidean ligament (see the previous discussion). Infection is not necessarily associated with a known route of infection, but several horses with infection have been

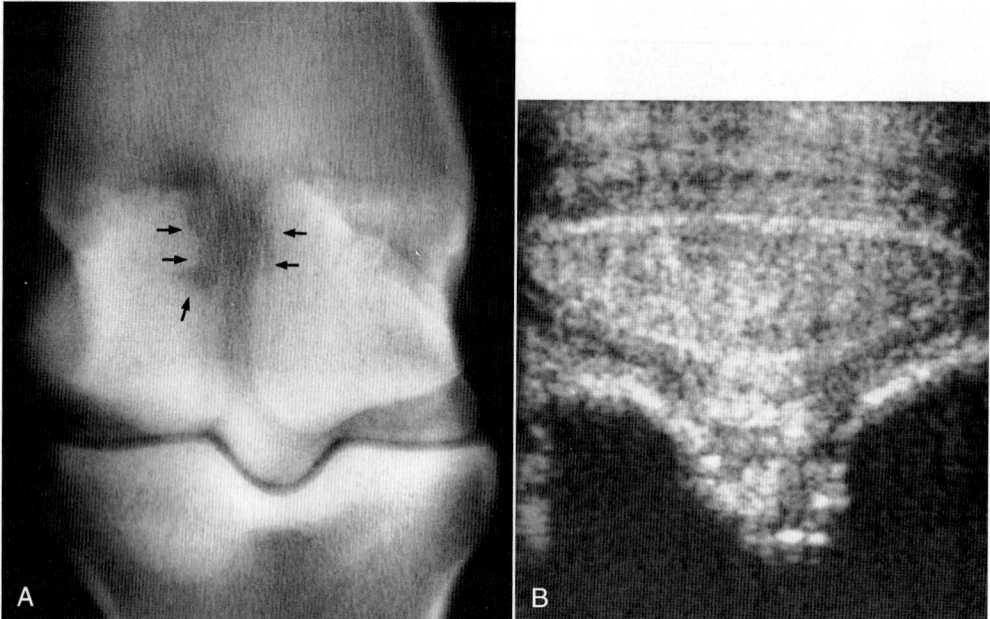

Fig. 72-18 • A, Dorsoplantar radiographic image of the right hind fetlock of a 6-year-old Thoroughbred with severe lameness associated with moderate distention of the metatarsophalangeal joint capsule and mild distention of the digital flexor tendon sheath. Medial is to the left. The axial borders of the proximal sesamoid bones are poorly defined proximally, with radiolucent areas in the bone *(arrows)*. Histological examination confirmed traumatic insertional injuries of the palmar ligament of the fetlock. **B,** Transverse ultrasonographic image of the plantar aspect of the fetlock of the same horse. Medial is to the left. Note the irregularity of the outline of the proximal sesamoid bones and the rather heterogeneous echogenicity of the intersesamoidean ligament.

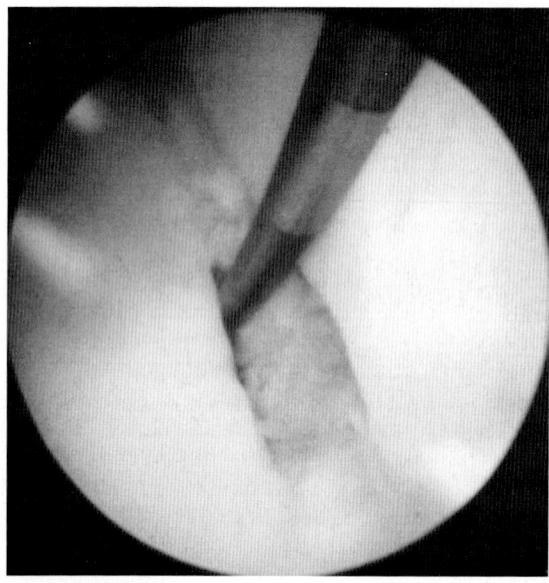

Fig. 72-19 • Arthroscopic picture of focal tear in the palmar ligament of the fetlock at its insertion on the medial proximal sesamoid bone. (Courtesy I.M. Wright, Newmarket, Suffolk, England.)

seen after puncture wounds in the pastern region or cellulitis[29] (Figure 72-20).

Infection of the PSBs may occur in forelimbs and hindlimbs and is characterized by radiolucent zones involving the axial margin of the medial or lateral PSB, or both. Pain may be elicited by pressure over the PSBs. Fetlock flexion usually is resented. Distention of the fetlock joint capsule and the DFTS and surrounding soft tissue swelling are variable features. Synoviocentesis may reveal evidence of infection in adjacent structures. In some horses a penetrating wound can be identified in the palmar aspect of the fetlock or pastern. Lameness varies from moderate to severe.

High-resolution dorsal 15- to 20-degree proximal-palmarodistal (plantarodistal) oblique radiographic images, with adequate penetration, are essential for diagnosis. If the radiographs are underexposed, lesions will be missed. Ultrasonography is useful for confirming the diagnosis and for identifying other concurrent lesions (see Figure 72-20), such as extensive tenosynovitis of the DFTS, deposition of echogenic material around the affected PSB, reduced echogenicity of the intersesamoidean ligament, and lesions of the digital flexor tendons or adhesions between them.[1]

The prognosis with conservative or surgical management is extremely guarded.

STRAIGHT SESAMOIDEAN DESMITIS

Desmitis of the straight sesamoidean ligament is an unusual cause of lameness that usually occurs in a forelimb, but it has been recognized in hindlimbs.[55-58] One of the authors (SJD) has recognized it most commonly in event horses and show jumpers. The condition may occur alone, or together with injury to either an oblique sesamoidean ligament or other soft tissue lesions in the digit. Lameness is sudden in onset, usually with no detectable swelling in the acute phase. Some swelling may develop subsequently, but this can be difficult to detect if the lesion is far proximal. Concurrent effusion may occur in the DFTS, and palpation

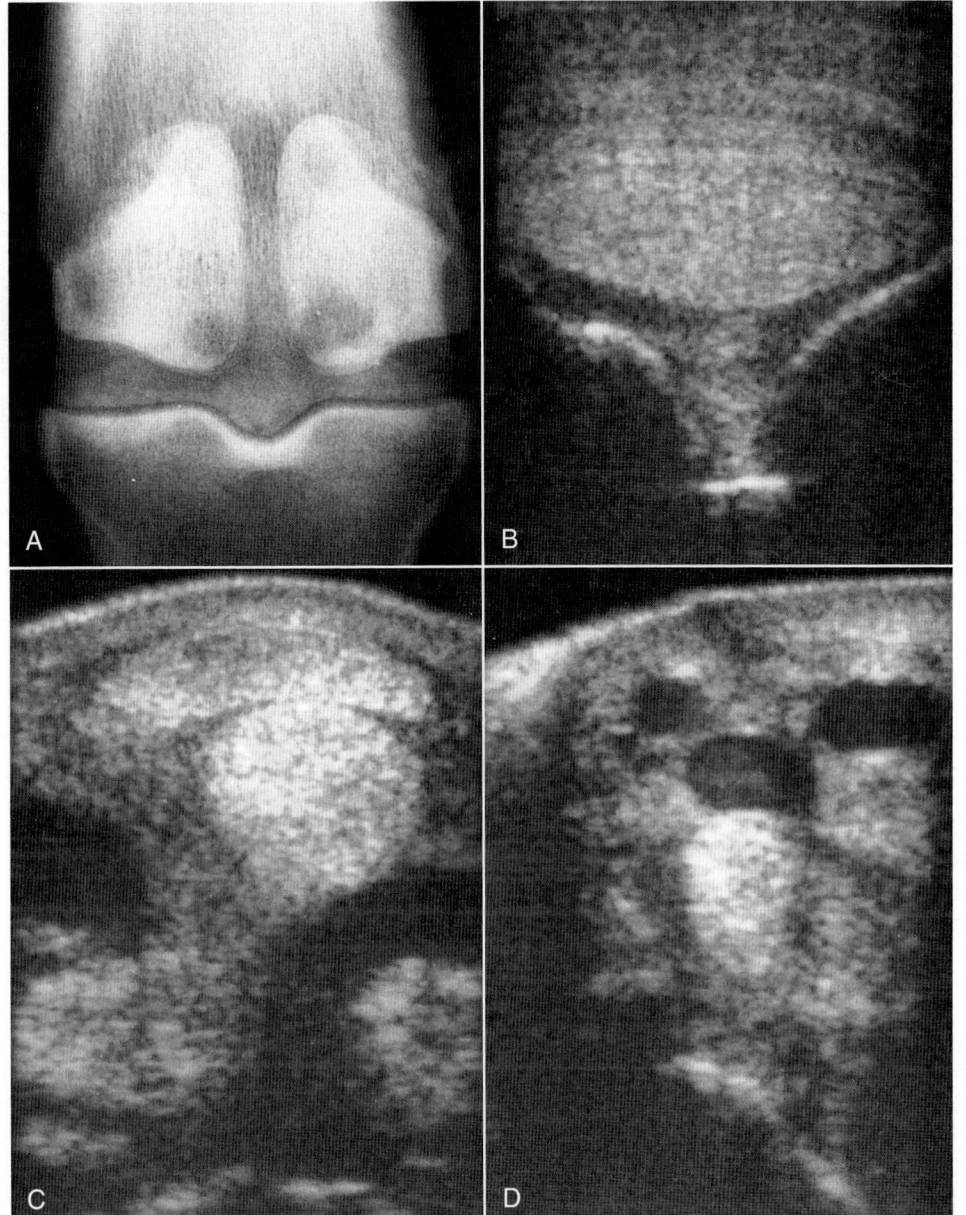

Fig. 72-20 • A, Dorsopalmar radiographic image of the right metacarpophalangeal joint of an 8-year-old Thoroughbred with massive swelling of the metacarpal region, restricted flexibility of the fetlock, and distention of the digital flexor tendon sheath. There are large radiolucent zones involving the distal axial borders of the proximal sesamoid bones. **B,** Transverse ultrasonographic image of the distal aspect of the metacarpal region of the same horse. Note the asymmetrical appearance of the proximal sesamoid bones and the difference in distance between them and the dorsal border of the deep digital flexor tendon (DDFT). **C,** Transverse ultrasonographic image of the distal metacarpal region of the same horse. Note the abnormal amount of fluid within the digital flexor tendon sheath and the echogenic material around the DDFT. **D,** Palmar oblique ultrasonographic image. Note the subcutaneous echogenic material and the distended vessels. These lesions were associated with infection.

on the palmar midline of the pastern region may elicit pain, but not invariably so. Lameness may be severe acutely and then rapidly improving but persisting. Lameness is alleviated by palmar nerve blocks at the level of the base of the PSBs. Diagnosis is based on ultrasonography or MRI. Ultrasonographic abnormalities include the following (Figure 72-21):

- Enlargement of the straight sesamoidean ligament and therefore reduction in the space between it and the DDFT

- Focal or diffuse reduction in echogenicity
- Increased fluid within the DFTS in some horses

Care should be taken not to misinterpret the normal hypoechoic area in the most distal part of the ligament as a lesion. This represents the cartilaginous scutum at the insertion.

Lesions may occur localized to the insertion, either unilaterally or bilaterally, and alone or in conjunction with other causes of palmar foot pain, such as navicular disease.

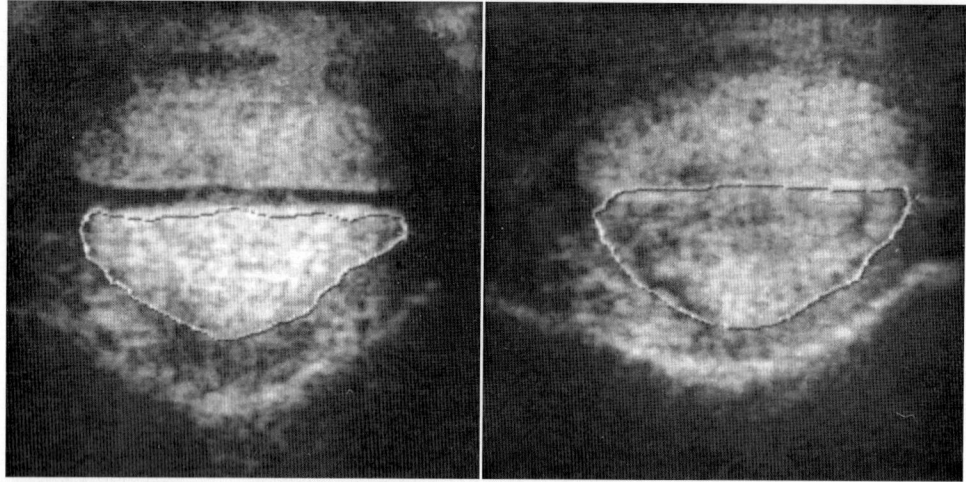

Fig. 72-21 • Transverse ultrasonographic images of the left (on the left) and right proximal pastern regions of an advanced event horse with acute-onset, severe right forelimb lameness after completion of a cross-country course. The lameness improved greatly within 24 hours. Flexion of the right front fetlock elicited pain, but no swelling or pain on direct palpation could be detected. Lameness was alleviated by perineural analgesia of the palmar nerves at the level of the fetlock joint. The right straight sesamoidean ligament is enlarged (cross-sectional area 1.46 cm²) compared with the left (1.35 cm²), resulting in loss of space between it and the deep digital flexor tendon. The ligament is also hypoechogenic.

There is often no palpable abnormality unless the injury is severe. Lameness is removed by perineural analgesia of the palmar nerves at the base of the PSBs. However, improvement may be seen after palmar digital nerve blocks if these are performed in the midpastern region or because of proximal diffusion from a more distal injection site. Although some lesions can be identified ultrasonographically, the shape of the pastern influences the ease with which these structures can be imaged accurately. Recent experience with MRI suggests that these injuries may occur more frequently than previously recognized. MRI seems more sensitive than ultrasonography for the detection of these injuries.[58,57] Improvement in lameness may also be seen after intrathecal analgesia of the DFTS, presumably because of local diffusion of local anesthetic solution.

Occasionally, concurrent lesions of the straight and oblique sesamoidean ligaments occur and have a more guarded prognosis.

Treatment has consisted of box rest, corrective trimming and shoeing, and controlled walking exercise, with periodic reevaluation with ultrasonography. Intralesional injections of bone marrow, platelet-rich plasma, or mesenchymal stem cells could be considered, although limited experience to date has not yielded good results. Usually, progressive resolution of lameness occurs over 6 to 8 weeks, with gradual improvement in the ultrasonographic appearance of the ligament over 6 months. However, the prognosis for return to full athletic function at a high level of competition is guarded because the incidence of recurrent injury is high. Severe lesions have shown poor capacity to heal, with persistent lameness.

Loss of tension (relaxation) of the straight sesamoidean ligament may occur if the SL is ruptured, resulting in instability or luxation of the proximal interphalangeal joint (palmar or plantar subluxation). Ultrasonographic abnormalities include the following:

- Apparent enlargement of the ligament cross-sectional area
- Loss of fiber alignment
- Focal hypoechoic areas caused by lack of tension

OBLIQUE (MIDDLE) SESAMOIDEAN DESMITIS

Desmitis of one or both oblique sesamoidean ligament(s) occurs in forelimbs and hindlimbs, but it is a more common source of forelimb lameness. Lameness is usually acute in onset and moderate to severe. In the acute stage often no localizing clinical signs are apparent, but in the following 7 to 10 days swelling may develop in the pastern region, and pain may be elicited by firm palpation. However, lesions may occur without detectable palpable abnormalities, alone or with another cause of lameness. Severe lesions may be associated with dorsal subluxation of the proximal interphalangeal joint, characterized clinically by an abnormal convex contour on the dorsal aspect of the pastern at the level of the joint. With chronic lesions dorsal extension of the joint margins of the proximal interphalangeal joint may be seen radiologically. Lameness, which is often worst on a soft surface, is usually alleviated by palmar (abaxial sesamoid) nerve blocks. One should note that tendonitis of the medial or lateral branch of the SDFT is a more common injury in the pastern, has a similar clinical presentation, and is more likely to be associated with detectable soft tissue swelling. Lesions of an oblique sesamoidean ligament may be localized to the origin immediately distal to the PSB, and pain associated with such lesions may be abolished by intraarticular analgesia of the fetlock joint, reflecting the close anatomical relationship between the palmar (plantar) distal outpouchings of the fetlock joint capsule. Intrathecal analgesia of the DFTS may also result in resolution of lameness, presumably because of local diffusion of local anesthetic solution.

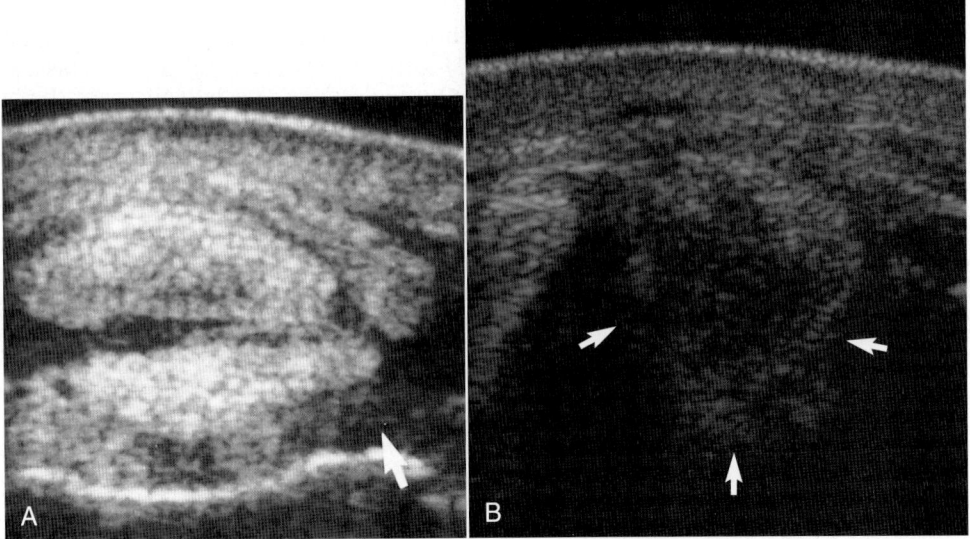

Fig. 72-22 • **A,** Transverse ultrasonographic image of a 7-year-old Thoroughbred with left forelimb lameness of 10 days' duration. Medial is to the left. The lateral oblique sesamoidean ligament is diffusely hypoechoic *(arrow).* **B,** Transverse ultrasonographic image of a 12-year-old Warmblood with left hindlimb lameness of 6 days' duration obtained immediately distal to the lateral proximal sesamoid bone. The oblique sesamoidean ligament is enlarged and diffusely hypoechogenic *(arrows).*

One also must recognize that enthesophyte formation on the palmar aspect of the proximal phalanx at the site of insertion of the oblique sesamoidean ligaments is a common incidental radiological abnormality frequently unassociated with clinical signs and often is not associated with any detectable ultrasonographic structural abnormality of the ligament. Well-circumscribed, smoothly marginated osseous bodies, possibly old avulsion fractures from the base of a PSB, are common radiological and ultrasonographic observations in mature horses in which the oblique sesamoidean ligament appears to be structurally normal.

Ultrasonographic abnormalities of the oblique sesamoidean ligament are often identified concurrently with some other cause of lameness—for example, osteoarthritis of the proximal interphalangeal joint or desmitis of a branch of the SL.

Ultrasonographic abnormalities include one or more of the following (Figures 72-22 and 72-23):

- Enlargement
- Diffuse reduction of echogenicity
- Focal hypoechoic areas
- Poor demarcation of the margins of the ligament
- Reduction in space between the ligament and the SDFT
- Enthesophyte formation on the palmar (plantar) aspect of the proximal phalanx or the base of the ipsilateral PSB
- An avulsion fracture of the base of the ipsilateral PSB or at the insertion on the palmar aspect of the proximal phalanx

Each ligament should be evaluated carefully in transverse and longitudinal planes. Occasionally lesions occur together with injuries to other soft tissues of the pastern, so all structures should be evaluated systematically. Some lesions are not detectable with ultrasonography but are identified using MRI.[57,58]

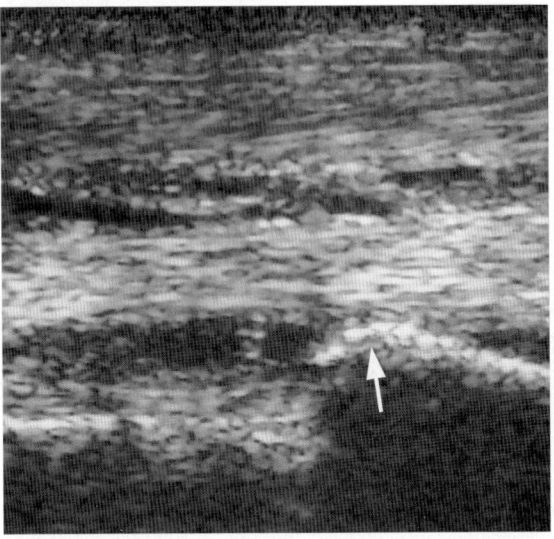

Fig. 72-23 • Longitudinal ultrasonographic image of the right front pastern of a 7-year-old pleasure riding horse with moderate lameness. Proximal is to the left. A large enthesophyte *(arrow)* is visible on the palmar aspect of the proximal phalanx. The region of insertion of the oblique sesamoidean ligament is reduced markedly in echogenicity. The horse also had osteoarthritis of the proximal interphalangeal joint.

Horses with a primary injury of the distal sesamoidean ligaments have a high incidence of recurrent injury if returned to full athletic function after conservative management. The effects of surgical splitting or of biological agents such as platelet-rich plasma or mesenchymal stem cells remain unproven. However, horses with primary lameness from another cause may have an enlarged oblique sesamoidean ligament of normal echogenicity, apparently unassociated with clinical signs.

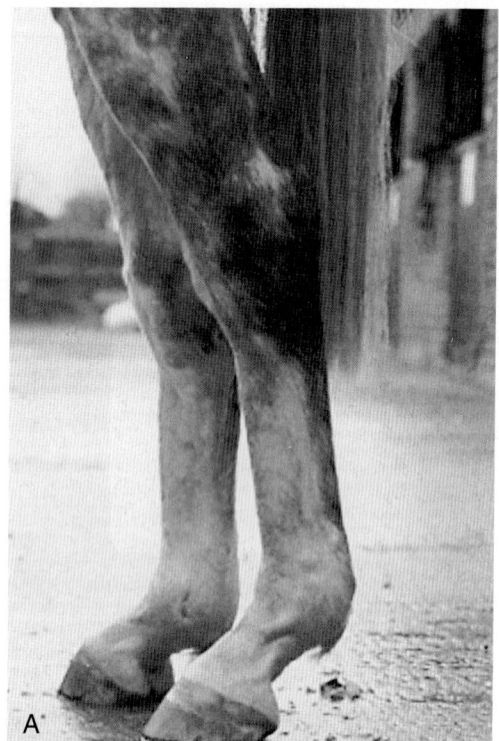

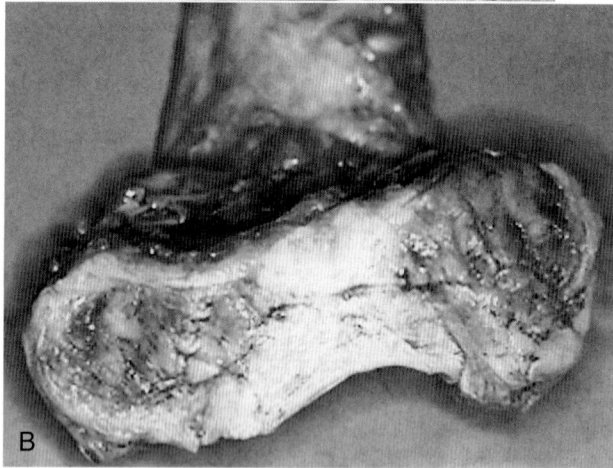

Fig. 72-24 • **A,** The hindlimbs of a 14-year-old Thoroughbred gelding with hyperextension of the hind fetlocks and soft tissue enlargement around the distal aspect of the branches of the suspensory ligaments. The superficial digital flexor tendon of the right hindlimb was subluxated laterally. **B,** The distal aspect of the suspensory ligament branches of the same horse. Considerable fibrous tissue surrounds the branches. The ligaments were discolored substantially, with no normal-appearing ligamentous tissue.

showed PSD and had straight hock conformation. These horses developed hyperextension of the hind fetlock joints (Figure 72-24). The condition has been characterized by a diffuse decrease in echogenicity of the proximal aspect of the SLs, which becomes progressively more extensive distally. A similar clinical condition has been recognized in older horses, especially broodmares, with progressive hyperextension (dorsiflexion) of the hind fetlock joints, which may result in abrasion of the plantar aspect of the fetlocks. Progressive hyperextension of the hind fetlock joints also has been seen in middle-aged performance horses with apparent lengthening of branches of the SL and periligamentous fibrous reaction. Some breeds, including the Peruvian Paso[59-61] and Andalusian horses, seem particularly at risk and may show evidence of the condition in all four limbs. The condition is generally bilateral and is usually associated with a deterioration in hindlimb gait rather than an overt lameness, although Peruvian Pasos may be more severely affected. Secondary lateral luxation of the SDFT from the point of hock occurs occasionally, probably associated with the straight angle of the hock.

Histologically the lesions are characterized by chondroid metaplasia, associated proteoglycan deposition, and acellular and fibrillated collagen fibers and merger of adjacent fascicles of fibrillated collagen to form megafascicles. Granulation tissue in interfascicular septae makes abortive attempts at repair.

The cause of these conditions is not known. They are probably complex disorders involving genetic, molecular, conformational, and biomechanical factors. It has been suggested that in the Peruvian Paso the condition is associated with a systemic disorder characterized by proteoglycan accumulation[61]; however, this conclusion has been refuted.[62] The SLs and other tissues from affected Peruvian Pasos and unaffected STBs and Quarter Horses were examined using Safranin-O staining for detection of proteoglycan. Proteoglycan deposition was not unique to the affected Peruvian Pasos, being present in the nuchal ligament, heart, muscle, and other tissues, with similar or greater amounts in the control horses. However, greater amounts were detected in the SLs of affected horses compared with control horses. It was concluded that cartilage metaplasia and associated proteoglycan deposition in affected SLs were the response to injury rather than the cause.

The condition is generally progressive. Flat shoes with plantar extensions help to lift the fetlock and may prevent secondary trauma, but the prognosis for proper athletic function is guarded.

PROGRESSIVE ATRAUMATIC BREAKDOWN OF THE SUSPENSORY LIGAMENTS

Progressive degenerative changes in hindlimb SLs have been seen in a small number of horses that originally

TRAUMATIC DISRUPTION OF THE SUSPENSORY APPARATUS

Traumatic disruption of the suspensory apparatus is discussed on page 969.

Chapter 73

Clinical Use of Stem Cells, Marrow Components, and Other Growth Factors

Lisa Fortier

References on page 1317

Scar tissue that forms after tendon and ligament injuries is architecturally and biomechanically inferior to normal tissues, rendering the structure susceptible to reinjury.[1] The goals of regenerative therapies, such as stem cells and growth factors, are to restore normal structure and function to tissues to enhance healing, restore pain-free physical activity, and avoid reinjury. Successful regenerative healing of any tissue is intended to closely mimic events of development in which there are spatial and temporal interactions between scaffold, growth factors, and cell populations. An understanding of the molecular and mechanical processes involved in the development of tendon and ligamentous injuries and between acute and repetitive overload pathologies will help guide development of target therapies for each specific disorder.

For many of the regenerative therapies presently available, technology and marketing are ahead of laboratory and clinical research. Most of the products being used to manage equine tendon and ligament injuries have been evaluated experimentally to some extent, but long-term clinical safety and efficacy data are limited. Ideally, the efficacy data would be obtained using prospective, blinded, and controlled clinical trials, although these studies are exceedingly difficult and expensive to perform. At a minimum, results of new treatments should be compared retrospectively with carefully selected historical case-matched studies. As part of a comprehensive plan, benefits from adjunctive surgical manipulations should also be evaluated. Desmotomy of the accessory ligament (superior [proximal] check ligament) of the superficial digital flexor tendon (SDFT) should be considered for horses with superficial digital flexor (SDF) tendonitis. In areas where a tendon or ligament is anatomically confined by surrounding structures and therefore susceptible to compression, such as the fetlock canal and carpal canal for horses with tendon injuries, as well as the proximal metacarpal/metatarsal regions in horses with enlargement of the proximal aspect of the suspensory ligament, surgical release of the restricting fascia should be implemented as part of a multitargeted approach to tendon/ligament healing. Critical to a successful outcome of all treatment regimens is a carefully implemented rehabilitation program. Well documented in studies of regenerative healing is the importance of mechanical stimulation and the type and quantity of the scaffold, growth factor(s), and/or stem cells.[2-6]

STEM CELL THERAPIES

The therapeutic role of stem cells in regenerative medicine is not fully understood. It is unclear whether stem cells ultimately function as a tissue-specific cell, such as a tenocyte, or whether they primarily improve tissue repair through secretion of immunomodulatory and trophic bioactive factors.[7] These questions are not purely pedantic in nature because if stem cells are truly immunomodulatory, then allogeneic transplantations should be possible. If allogeneic stem cells were efficacious and could be used safely, then "off-the-shelf" stem cell products could be developed to increase availability and rapid implementation of stem cell therapies.

The stem cell field continues to rapidly evolve experimentally and clinically. At a basic level, stem cells are broadly defined as undifferentiated cells that possess the ability to divide for indefinite periods in culture and may give rise to highly specialized cells of each tissue type (i.e., mesoderm, ectoderm, and endoderm). There are two broad categories of stem cells: embryonic and adult derived (see Hipp and Atala[6] and Tweedell[8] for recent reviews). Embryonic stem (ES) cells used to be defined as those derived from embryos, more specifically from day 8, preimplantation blastocyts. Using recent advances, ES cells can be generated from adult fibroblasts using many of the same technologies that were used to clone Dolly the sheep. These cells are known as induced pluripotent stem (iPS) cells. Adult-derived mesenchymal stem cells (MSCs) can be obtained from bone marrow, fat, umbilical cord blood, muscle, and many other tissues, including cartilage, trabecular bone, and tendon.[6] Hematopoietic stem cells (HSCs) are those cells in bone marrow, which are the basis of bone marrow transplantation, and are capable of forming all types of blood cells. Arguments can be made about the optimal source of stem cells for regenerative therapy; importantly, studies are needed to define the need for stem cells in such endeavors. Presently, stem cell therapies for tendon or ligament regeneration in horses are not regulated by the Food and Drug Administration in the United States or elsewhere.[9]

Commonly Used Stem Cell Products

Presently, there are three approaches to using stem cell therapy in horses, and all use MSCs, although equine ES, iPS, and umbilical cord blood–derived cells are beginning to be investigated. First, MSCs in a mixed cell population can be harvested from bone marrow aspirates; second, MSCs from bone marrow can be cultured; and third, a mixed cell population of MSCs can be harvested from adipose tissue. Each technique has its strengths and weaknesses.

Bone Marrow–Derived MSCs (BM-MSCs)

BM-MSCs can be easily and noninvasively obtained and compared with other MSCs, and they have a greater capacity to differentiate into other tissue types.[10-12] BM-MSCs have received the most scientific attention and hence are the best characterized. The process is straightforward. In standing sedated horses, bone marrow is collected from the sternum or the tuber coxae using local analgesia. Fresh bone marrow is either injected directly into the injured tissue, or the nucleated adherent cell population (containing the BM-MSCs) is isolated and expanded in the laboratory before injection.

Bone Marrow Aspirate and Injection of Fresh Bone Marrow

Bone marrow is aspirated from the sternum at a site where the cranial third of the girth would sit (Figure 73-1). This site is relatively safe and has large marrow spaces compared with the marrow spaces cranial and caudal to the girth. However, it must be borne in mind that several horses have died as a result of inadvertent puncture of the heart during bone marrow collection from the sternum. The horse has seven sternal marrow spaces, and they become progressively smaller toward the manubrium and xiphoid processes (Figure 73-2). Ultrasonography is used by some to locate the sternebrae to avoid inadvertent penetration of the intersternebral space and puncture of the heart. The site is clipped, surgically prepared, and a bleb of local anesthetic solution is injected subcutaneously over the aspiration site(s). Bone penetration and aspiration are facilitated by use of a bone marrow (Jamshidi) biopsy needle with a double-diamond stylet and interlocking T-handle, with a large inner diameter cannula (e.g., 11 gauge × 100 mm). Ideally, the site of injection in the tendon/ligament is aseptically prepared before obtaining the bone marrow aspirate, so that the bone marrow can be injected under ultrasonographic guidance immediately to avoid clotting in the syringe. If performed efficiently, anticoagulant is not necessary, which further simplifies the direct aspiration-injection technique. Advantages of this approach are the simplicity of the technique, ability to perform the procedure at the time of diagnosis, and the relatively low cost. The primary disadvantage is the low number of stem cells that are contained in raw bone marrow aspirates. In people and cats, the number of stem cells in raw bone marrow is reported to be 0.001% to 0.01% of the mononuclear cell population.[13,14] Using the direct aspiration-injection technique, Herthel[15] reported improved clinical outcome in horses affected with suspensory desmitis.

Culture-Expanded BM-MSCs

There is experimental evidence to support the use of isolated and culture-expanded BM-MSCs from investigations in laboratory animals, in which MSCs were implanted into surgically created lesions. Improvement in tissue organization and composition and mechanics compared with controls was seen after injection of MSCs into tendons and ligaments.[16-18] To obtain 10×10^6 cells, the recommended number for injection, approximately 3 weeks of culture is required to expand the selected cells. Implantation is performed as described using ultrasonographic guidance. After culture, the MSCs are suspended in the horse's own bone marrow supernatant or plasma to avoid injection of allogeneic antigens and to gain potential beneficial effects of rich growth factors that could be present in the supernatant. Laboratory research has demonstrated significant anabolic effects of bone marrow supernatant on tendon- and ligament-derived cells.[19-22]

In a small case-control study (n = 11), BM-MSCs resulted in less reinjury of the SDFT in racehorses compared with a control population.[23] Recently, in more than 1000 horses treated with cultured BM-MSCs, Smith[24] found a significant decrease in reinjury rate for racehorses and other sports horses of all disciplines combined compared with conventionally treated historical controls. Ectopic bone formation, a potential problem when reimplanting BM-MSCs, was not observed in either study. Interestingly, Smith[24] reported that early (<44 days from injury) implantation of cells was associated with significantly less reinjury compared with those horses in which a longer interval between injury and implantation was used. These results suggest that implantation of cells before fibrous tissue formation enhances healing.

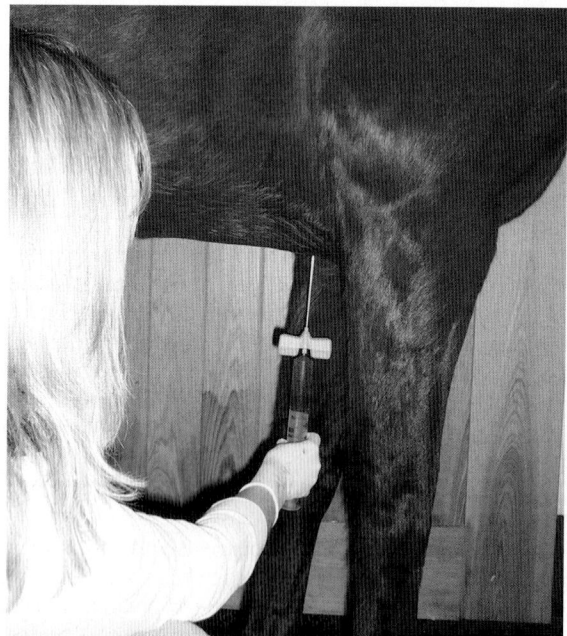

Fig. 73-1 • To obtain a sternal bone marrow aspirate, the bone marrow biopsy needle is inserted at the cranial extent of where a girth would cross the ventral aspect of the chest. Using this location, the needle would most likely enter the third sternal bone marrow space (see Figure 73-2).

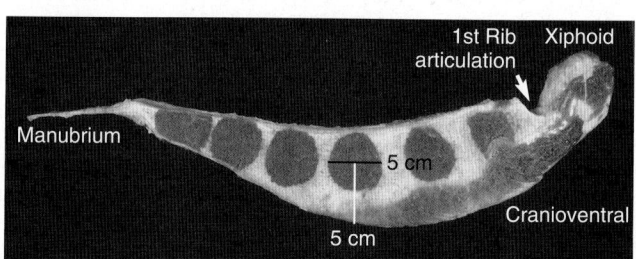

Fig. 73-2 • Sagittal section of a sternum from a 450-kg adult horse (cranial is to the right) showing the typical six marrow spaces of the equine sternum. The needle shown in Figure 73-1 most likely enters the third marrow space. This marrow space is approximately 5 cm in diameter, and there it is approximately 5 cm from the ventral aspect of the sternum to the center of the sternal space. This picture demonstrates the diminishing amount of sternal cartilage surrounding the caudal sternal spaces. Although less ventral cartilage might facilitate entry into the marrow space, there is also less room for error dorsally and thereby increased risk of inadvertent cardiac puncture if the bone marrow aspirate needle is inserted too deeply. A generally safe guideline is to insert the bone marrow aspirate needle 2 to 3 cm after initial contact with the ventral aspect of the sternal cartilage. If no bone marrow aspirate is obtained, it is safest to move 2 to 3 cm cranial or caudal on the sternum and reattempt bone marrow aspiration.

There are several commercial and private laboratories providing services for isolation and expansion of BM-MSCs. Each laboratory has distinct directions for aspiration and shipping of bone marrow aspirate to the facility and for implantation of the resultant stem cell product. Therefore the chosen laboratory should be contacted directly for specific instructions.

Adipose-Derived MSCs (A-MSCs)

The currently available technique uses a mixed population of cells derived from adipose tissue surgically excised from the tail head region. The A-MSCs are not cultured but are simply isolated and reinjected into the horse. Compared with techniques using cultured BM-MSCs, this technique supplies a greater number of nucleated cells (not necessarily stem cells) in a short period (48 hours). The cells are reimplanted under ultrasonographic guidance. There are currently no published results for the application of A-MSCs in equine tendonitis, although the results of an experimental pilot study demonstrated significant improvement in histologic score in the A-MSC–treated tendons over phosphate-buffered saline–treated control tendons.[25] Like culture-expanded MSCs, the laboratory chosen to provide the service should be contacted for detailed instructions.

The Future of Stem Cell Therapy

There are several avenues of stem cell therapy for tendon or ligament injuries presently under investigation. Equine ES cells, umbilical cord blood–derived stem cells, and tendon-derived stem cells are in use for treatment of tendonitis or desmitis. Equine iPS cells are being investigated. iPS cells could have greater differentiation capacity than other adult-derived stem cells, and iPS cells are "horse specific," which will alleviate concerns of immune rejection. Finally, genetically modified stem cells have been investigated in vitro and in vivo and show tremendous promise for enhancing organized repair of tendons and other musculoskeletal tissues.[26]

GROWTH FACTOR–BASED BIOLOGICS

Several medical treatments for equine tendonitis and desmitis have centered on delivery of single or multiple growth factors to the site of injury. Growth factors are protein signaling molecules that regulate cellular metabolism. They are temporally and spatially expressed during tendon and ligament development and repair.[27-29] Growth factors stimulate cell proliferation, increase extracellular matrix synthesis, and promote vascular in-growth. In addition to the anabolic effects, growth factors down-regulate catabolic, matrix-degrading cytokines such as interleukins and matrix metalloproteinases.

The growth factors most widely studied in tendon and ligament healing include insulin-like growth factor–1 (IGF-1), platelet-derived growth factor (PDGF), bone morphogenetic protein–12, transforming growth factor–β (TGF-β), vascular endothelial growth factor (VEGF), growth/differentiation factor, and basic fibroblast growth factor.[17,30-35] Growth factors are available individually as recombinant, purified proteins or can be injected within a less-defined milieu of a bone marrow aspirate or as platelet-rich plasma (PRP). Growth factors are delivered to a tendon or ligament using a series of intralesional injections. In the future, gene therapy techniques could be used to deliver more sustained levels of growth factor expression.[7] There are numerous animal studies demonstrating the advantages of using growth factors for enhanced healing of tendonitis, desmitis, and tendon lacerations, but despite these experimental studies, there are few long-term, multicentered, human or equine clinical data available for any of the growth factors. For example, experimentally, intralesional administration of IGF-1 enhanced return of tendon fiber pattern and improved mechanical characteristics in a collagenase-induced SDF tendonitis model.[34] Clinically, results after IGF-1 injection only appear comparable with those previously reported for flat-track racehorses treated with conservative therapy alone.

Platelet-Rich Plasma (PRP)

PRP is a fraction of venous blood with a concentrated platelet count, generally greater than two to four times normal baseline. During wound healing, platelet aggregation results in release of bioactive substances that promote tissue repair, regulate inflammation, and stimulate recruitment of stem cells.[36] Use of PRP in tissue healing is aimed at enhancing the natural biological process induced after platelet aggregation and degranulation. Platelets contain high concentrations of several growth factors, including PDGF, TGF-β, and VEGF, all of which have been shown using in vitro and in vivo animal models to enhance tendon and ligament healing.[3,19,37-39] PRP is generated through a simple centrifugation or filtration process of venous blood to concentrate platelets. The advantages of using PRP include ease of use, administration of autologous peptides, delivery of a combination of growth factors, and low cost (relative to stem cells). After contact of platelets with exposed basement membrane in damaged soft tissues, PRP clots, resulting in the formation of a fibrin scaffold to allow for cellular migration into the injury, and as a mechanism to retain the growth factors at the site of injury. The primary disadvantages are the lack of stem cells within a preparation and the variability between the various products with respect to platelet concentration and residual leukocyte content.

Several companies are marketing specialized devices designed to create PRP. Not surprisingly, when investigated, platelet concentrations are highly and positively correlated to growth factor concentrations.[38] In addition, platelet concentrations are highly and positively correlated to tendon and ligament matrix gene expression. In other words, when platelet concentrations are high, there are more growth factors, as well as more extracellular matrix expression, such as collagen type I and cartilage oligomeric matrix protein, in both tendon and suspensory ligament. In contrast, white blood cell concentration is highly and positively correlated with collagen type III, which represents scar tissue, and with matrix-degrading enzyme gene expression. Collectively, these data support the notion of selecting a device with high platelet and low leukocyte concentration to maximize tissue repair and minimize further matrix loss.

Clinical evidence for the benefit of injecting PRP in people is encouraging.[40] In horses, a case-control study in Standardbred racehorses with midbody suspensory desmitis demonstrated that a single injection of PRP resulted in an excellent prognosis for return to racing (the Editors note that the prognosis associated with the return to racing of

Standardbred racehorses with suspensory desmitis is considered favorable with rest alone).[41] Typically, PRP is injected into the affected tissue 7 to 10 days after injury when the inflammatory phase of wound healing is receding. The optimal number of platelets and frequency of injection have not been determined. A typical treatment protocol presently includes a single injection under ultrasonographic guidance using enough PRP to fill the defect

as observed ultrasonographically. Horses are reassessed every 30 days, and if substantial improvement in clinical and ultrasonographic findings is not observed, then a second injection should be considered. The majority of horses only require one injection. As with all other therapies, a controlled rehabilitation regimen is critical for successful repair, restoration of pain-free function, and prevention of reinjury.

Chapter 74

Diseases of the Digital Flexor Tendon Sheath, Palmar Annular Ligament, and Digital Annular Ligaments

Michael C. Schramme and Roger K.W. Smith

Synovial effusion of the digital flexor tendon sheath (DFTS) is common in all types of working horses. Frequently, effusion is idiopathic in origin and affects the DFTS of both hindlimbs without causing lameness. Occasionally synovial effusion is seen in a single limb along with lameness. Before the advent of ultrasonography and tenoscopy, injury to the soft tissue structures of the DFTS often remained unrecognized. The cause of chronic synovial effusion and lameness remained elusive, and a diagnosis of idiopathic tenosynovitis was made readily. Because modern diagnostic techniques have become commonplace in equine lameness practice, specific injuries of the structures of the DFTS have been identified.

ANATOMICAL CONSIDERATIONS

References on page 1318

The detailed anatomy of the DFTS and its contents was well described[1] and is similar in forelimbs and hindlimbs. Reference is made to palmar and metacarpal region throughout, but the terms *plantar region* and *metatarsal region* strictly apply to the hindlimb. The DFTS is a thin-walled structure that encompasses the superficial digital flexor tendon (SDFT) and the deep digital flexor tendon (DDFT) from the level of the distal third of the metacarpal region to the T ligament, just proximal to the navicular bursa and the palmar pouch of the distal interphalangeal joint. The DFTS is mesenchymal in cell origin and is composed of two layers: an outer fibrous layer and an inner synovial layer. The fibrous layer provides strength and vascularity to the sheath. The synovial layer provides a smooth, frictionless surface and produces constituents of the synovial fluid. The palmar wall of the sheath incorporates three annular

ligaments: the palmar annular ligament (PAL) and the proximal and the distal digital annular ligaments. These annular ligaments bind the digital flexor tendons to the palmar aspect of the digit, are effectively thickenings of the fibrous layer of the sheath wall with a transverse fiber orientation, and measure 2 mm or less in thickness.

The PAL or annular ligament of the fetlock joint inserts on the palmar border of the proximal sesamoid bones (PSBs), is continuous with the palmar (intersesamoidean) ligament of the fetlock joint, and thus converts the proximal scutum into an inelastic canal. The strong, transversely arranged fibers of the PAL bind down the digital flexor tendons into the proximal scutum. Distal to the PAL and immediately under the skin, the deep fascia forms a second, quadrilateral ligament: the proximal digital annular ligament. This ligament is a fibrous sheet that covers and adheres to the palmar surface of the SDFT and attaches laterally and medially by two bands to the proximal phalanx: one to the proximopalmar tuberosity and one that joins the insertion of the distal branch of the SDFT to the distal part of the proximal phalanx. This arrangement firmly binds the SDFT and DDFT, enveloped by the DFTS, in the palmar pastern region. The distal digital annular ligament adheres to the palmar surface of the distal part of the DDFT and binds down the terminal part of this tendon. The ligament is a crescent-shaped fibrous sheet attached by a strong band on either side of the middle of the proximal phalanx, covering the distal branches of the SDFT.

The dorsal wall of the DFTS is formed by the proximal scutum, middle scutum, and distal sesamoidean ligaments. The proximal scutum and the middle scutum are strong fibrocartilaginous pads that allow sliding of the digital flexor tendons along the palmar aspect of the fetlock and pastern regions, respectively. The proximal scutum is composed of the two PSBs and the thick intersesamoidean ligament. The latter is a thick sagittal structure made of transversely aligned collagen fibers. The intersesamoidean ligament covers and is attached strongly to the whole palmar and axial aspect of the PSBs and creates a solid union between these bones. The concave palmar face of the proximal scutum allows sliding of the digital flexor tendons in the palmar fetlock region. The proximal scutum extends proximally to the apex of each PSB between the two distal branches of the suspensory ligament (SL). Distally the proximal scutum gives origin to the distal sesamoidean ligaments, which represent the functional continuation of the SL and consist of the straight, oblique, cruciate, and short sesamoidean ligaments. The straight sesamoidean ligament inserts distally on the middle scutum, together with the distal branches of the SDFT and the palmar ligaments of the proximal interphalangeal joint. The middle scutum is a thick, fibrocartilaginous structure attached to the proximopalmar aspect of the middle phalanx. The middle scutum contacts the palmar aspect of the distal condyles of the proximal phalanx dorsally and the DDFT palmarly.

Within the DFTS, the SDFT and DDFT are intimately related. A fibrous ring (the manica flexoria) emanates from the lateral and medial borders of the SDFT and encircles the DDFT completely, from the proximal limit of the DFTS to the proximal aspect of the PSBs. The synovial lining of the DFTS adheres to the palmar surface of the SDFT in the sagittal midline proximal to the PAL, along the dorsal surface of the PAL and along the dorsal surface of the proximal digital annular ligament. The synovial lining of the DFTS also adheres to the palmar surface of the DDFT between the proximal digital annular ligament and the distal digital annular ligament, and along the dorsal surface of the distal digital annular ligament. The sagittal adhesion-like mesotendon between the SDFT and PAL is referred to as the vinculum of the SDFT. The DDFT also has a mesotendon that attaches to its palmar surface at the level of the proximal interphalangeal joint (see Figure 70-2, *B*). These mesotendon attachments contain vascular branches that contribute to the arterial supply of the intrasynovial part of the tendon.

The DFTS facilitates displacement of the digital flexor tendons during flexion and extension of the fetlock and interphalangeal joints. During metacarpophalangeal (metatarsophalangeal) joint movements, the two digital flexor tendons displace together, but during interphalangeal joint movements, displacement of the DDFT is greater than that of the SDFT.

DIAGNOSTIC TECHNIQUES

Diagnostic techniques that localize disease to the DFTS include synoviocentesis and synovial fluid analysis and intrathecal or perineural injection of local anesthetic solution. Synoviocentesis of the DFTS can be performed in one of the several recesses of the sheath. Access to the proximal pouch is possible when the sheath is distended with synovial fluid but difficult when it is not. Synoviocentesis can be achieved by introducing a 2.5-cm needle along the dorsal aspect of the DDFT, between the DDFT and the lateral branch of the SL, a few centimeters proximal to the lateral PSB. Easier access can be gained via the distal palmar pouch of the sheath, which extends between the two distal branches of the SDFT and between the two digital annular ligaments, along the palmar surface of the DDFT. One should remember that this pouch is divided sagittally by the mesotendon of the DDFT in its distal part. The needle can be introduced through the skin to one side of the midline and, to avoid iatrogenic damage to the DDFT, gently and slowly advanced at approximately 45 degrees to the skin surface until synovial fluid is seen at the needle hub. To increase distention of the distal palmar recess, it can be useful temporarily to compress the proximal pouch by firm application of an elasticated bandage (see Figure 124-1). Alternatively, the needle can be aimed to access this pouch between the lateral or medial border of the DDFT and the ipsilateral distal branch of the SDFT, which will prevent inadvertent needle penetration of the DDFT, although the palmar pouch of the proximal interphalangeal joint can be entered if the needle is introduced too

deeply. The DFTS also can be accessed through its proximal or distal collateral recesses. The proximal collateral recess is situated in the triangular space palmaromedially or palmarolaterally, between the base of a PSB, the proximal insertion of the proximal digital annular ligament, and the dorsal border of the DDFT. The space can be entered 1 cm distal to the base of a PSB and 1 cm palmar or plantar to the neurovascular bundle. The distal collateral recess is located on the lateral (or medial) aspect of the pastern, between the digital flexor tendons and the distal sesamoidean ligaments and between the proximal and distal insertions of the proximal digital annular ligament. A cadaver study showed that synoviocentesis of the DFTS using these techniques was most consistently successful when performed at the level of the proximal lateral recess on a non–weight-bearing limb.[2] In addition, a palmar-plantar axial sesamoidean approach was described where the needle was introduced axial to the PSB in the flexed limb. This technique was described as being optimal for synoviocentesis.[3] Ten milliliters of local anesthetic solution is injected for adequate analgesia of the DFTS (see Chapter 10). It is important to recognize that intrathecal analgesia of the DFTS is not specific for elimination of pain from the contained structures and can influence pain from the oblique and straight sesamoidean ligaments.[5] Moreover, in some horses with DFTS pathology, the response to perineural analgesia is better than to intrathecal analgesia.

Characteristics of synovial fluid of the DFTS do not vary from those of the distal limb synovial joints. Normal synovial fluid is clear yellow and has a nucleated cell count of 770 cells/mcL or less and a total protein concentration of 1.0 g/dL or less.[4] More sophisticated analysis of the synovial fluid for molecular markers offers the prospect of better preoperative identification of the presence of intrathecal tendon pathology.[6]

IMAGING OF THE DIGITAL FLEXOR TENDON SHEATH

Diagnostic ultrasonography is by far the most commonly used technique for evaluating the DFTS. The DFTS is first encountered at level 3A and continues distally to level P1C and beyond (see Chapter 16).[8] The PAL can be demonstrated in normal horses as a thin (1 to 2 mm) echogenic band immediately adjacent to the palmar surface of the SDFT at level 3C. The proximal digital annular ligament and distal digital annular ligament usually cannot be recognized in the palmar midline, unless they are abnormally thickened. The vinculum of the SDFT at the level of the PSB is easily identifiable by ultrasonography, but the distal mesotendon of the DDFT in the phalangeal region is only occasionally visible, usually when distention of the DFTS provides negative contrast (see Figure 70-2, *B*). A normal synovial reflection or mesotendon joins the lateral and medial borders of the DDFT in the proximal recess of the DFTS, which should not be mistaken for an adhesion (see Figure 70-2, *A*). The thickness of the DFTS can be assessed at levels 3A and 3B, where the capsule is identifiable as an echogenic band dorsal to the DDFT and the manica flexoria.

Before the widespread use of ultrasonography for examining the soft tissues of the DFTS, negative contrast radiography was described for the assessment of tenosynovitis and annular desmitis.[9] To perform this technique, a tourniquet is applied distal to the carpus in a standing or anesthetized horse; 50 to 100 mL of air is injected into the DFTS; and another 200 to 300 mL of air is injected subcutaneously. Sometimes extra air is injected between the SDFT and DDFT at the midmetacarpal level. One postinflation lateromedial radiograph obtained at half the milliampere second value of standard skeletal exposure for this region is normally sufficient to make an accurate diagnosis. Although this technique effectively demonstrates the thickness of the PAL, its use has become superseded by the widespread availability of diagnostic ultrasonography.

Survey radiography of the DFTS is performed to demonstrate evidence of intrathecal air or gas caused by a penetrating wound, the presence of metaplastic mineralization of injured soft tissue structures, or concurrent pathological conditions of the bone. Positive contrast radiography[10] may provide the most conclusive evidence of wound communication with the synovial space and may also provide additional information in the diagnosis of synovioceles associated with the DFTS. Although fistulography and filling of the intrathecal space with sterile iodine-based contrast medium is diagnostic of communication between the wound and the DFTS, we prefer to access the DFTS by placing a needle at a site remote from the wound. This minimizes the risk of forcing bacteria or foreign material present in the deeper layers of the wound into the synovial space. Using a remote site further avoids the risk of inadvertently introducing bacteria while passing the needle through an area of cellulitis into the synovial cavity. Infiltration of 10 to 20 mL of sterile contrast medium followed by manipulation of the digit should result in flow of contrast medium from the wound and can be demonstrated radiologically (Figure 74-1).

Tenoscopy is the ultimate imaging modality for evaluating the internal structures of the DFTS.[11] An endoscope is introduced routinely in the proximal collateral recess of the sheath, 1 cm distal to the base of the PSB and 1 cm palmar or plantar to the neurovascular bundle, but access to other synovial recesses is also possible (see Chapter 24). This approach allows for a complete examination of the DFTS and its contents, except for the palmar surface of the SDFT, unless substantial thickening of any of the annular ligaments or extensive subcutaneous fibrosis has occurred. Access in ponies and cob-types with very thick skin can also be difficult. The approach also facilitates therapeutic maneuvers within the DFTS, such as PAL desmotomy, adhesiotomy, synovial mass removal, and debridement of fibrillated or torn areas of the digital flexor tendons, manica flexoria, or intersesamoidean ligament.

Magnetic resonance imaging has superior soft tissue contrast and has been of use to identify occult lesions not seen radiologically or ultrasonographically such as isolated adhesions, lesions of the SDFT or DDFT, and injury of the distal digital annular ligament.

DISEASES OF THE DIGITAL FLEXOR TENDON SHEATH

Noninfectious Tenosynovitis

Etiopathogenesis

Acute noninfectious tenosynovitis is a traumatic synovitis/capsulitis of the sheath lining. As for joints, a traumatic

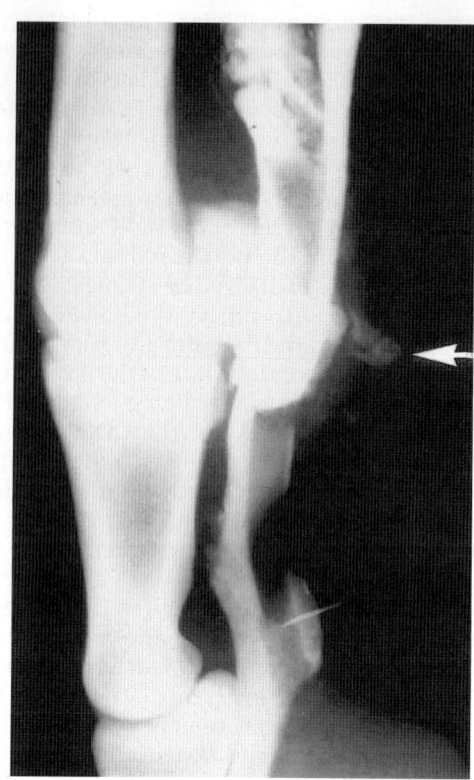

Fig. 74-1 • Lateromedial radiographic image of the fetlock region. A positive-contrast tenogram of the digital flexor tendon sheath, followed by manipulation of the digit, resulted in flow of radiodense contrast medium from a wound *(arrow)*.

synovitis/capsulitis can be caused by accumulative low-grade trauma associated with normal exercise, acute trauma associated with direct impact force (e.g., overreach), or an abnormal force outside the normal range of movement of the fetlock region (e.g., hyperextension). Synovitis/capsulitis is more frequently secondary to damage to the internal or supporting structures of the DFTS, such as disruption of the visceral or parietal synovial layers, tearing of the vincula, tearing of the sheath wall with herniation or synoviocele formation, central or marginal damage to the flexor tendons, tearing of the manica flexoria, and spraining of the PAL or proximal digital annular ligament. Each of these complicating conditions is likely to result in continuous irritation of the sheath and cause chronic tenosynovitis. Chronic tenosynovitis may be associated with villonodular thickening of the sheath lining, especially in the proximal recess; adhesion formation between the visceral and parietal synovial lining; and fibrosis with reduced elasticity of the DFTS capsule. When these conditions are present, a self-perpetuating cycle occurs of improvement with rest, followed by repeated inflammation with exercise. This results in increased inflammation and lameness, further fibrosis, and eventually thickening of the PAL and stenosis of the fetlock canal (see the following discussion of PAL syndrome). *Complex tenosynovitis* has been defined as tenosynovitis with thickening of the PAL, synovial distention, and adhesions or synovial masses, or both (Figure 74-2).[12] Windgalls, especially those occurring bilaterally in the hindlimbs, are another form of low-grade chronic tenosynovitis. Although lameness is not usually a feature of windgalls, the synovial effusion is still likely to reflect the presence of low-grade chronic synovitis of the DFTS, caused by the continuous stress of use-induced overloading.

Diagnosis

Acute tenosynovitis is characterized by a sudden onset of mild to severe lameness, accompanied by DFTS distention that can be palpated in the proximolateral and proximomedial pouches of the sheath and in the palmarodistal recess between both branches of the SDFT. The palmar or plantar region of the fetlock has increased skin temperature, and forced flexion of the fetlock is painful and exacerbates lameness. Chronic tenosynovitis produces similar signs, except for the signs of acute inflammation, although repeat injury may cause these signs to be superimposed on an established tenosynovitis. Disproportionate distention and pain in different regions of the DFTS can reflect the site of the primary pathology; pain on palpation of the proximal aspect of the DFTS is present when there is tearing of the digital flexor tendons in this location.

Ultrasonographic examination is essential for identifying any primary pathology responsible for the tenosynovitis, such as adhesions and complicating injuries of the digital flexor tendons (see Figure 69-8, *A*), the intersesamoidean ligament, or annular ligaments, and to document the staging of the condition.[13] DFTS effusion may also accompany injury to the intrathecal part of the SDFT associated with a classic bowed tendon (see Chapter 69). However, intrathecal tendon injuries occur more commonly as focal core lesions in the DDFT (see Chapter 70) or as longitudinal tears of the SDFT, DDFT, or manica flexoria. DDFT tears usually involve the lateral or medial borders of the tendon in the forelimb; hence oblique ultrasonographic views can sometimes identify defects on these borders, although they are easily missed. Oblique images are also required to image the abaxial margins of the SDFT. Manica flexoria tears are more frequently seen in hindlimb tenosynovitis and are also easily missed using transverse ultrasonographic images because the tears are usually incomplete and located at the site of attachment of the manica flexoria to the SDFT. Recently, we have found that a midline longitudinal scan immediately proximal to the PSBs provides the best image for identifying instability and/or thickening of the manica flexoria that accompanies tears (Figure 74-3). However, negative ultrasonographic findings do not preclude a tear in the manica flexoria.

Ultrasonographically, tenosynovitis has three progressive stages.[14] Symmetrical distention of the DFTS without

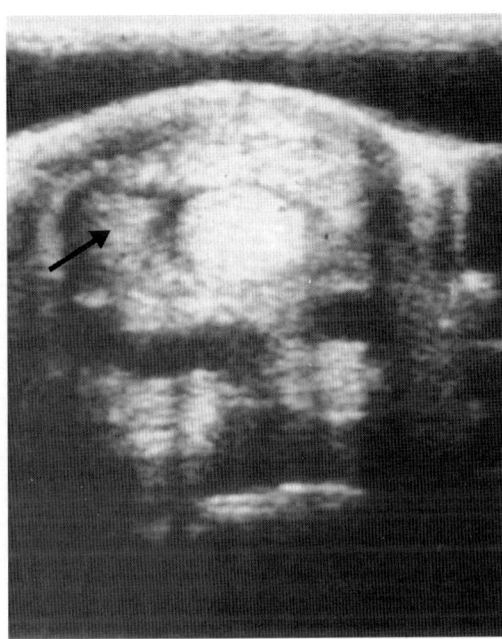

Fig. 74-2 • Stage 3 tenosynovitis of the digital flexor tendon sheath with adhesions and synovial mass formation *(arrow).*

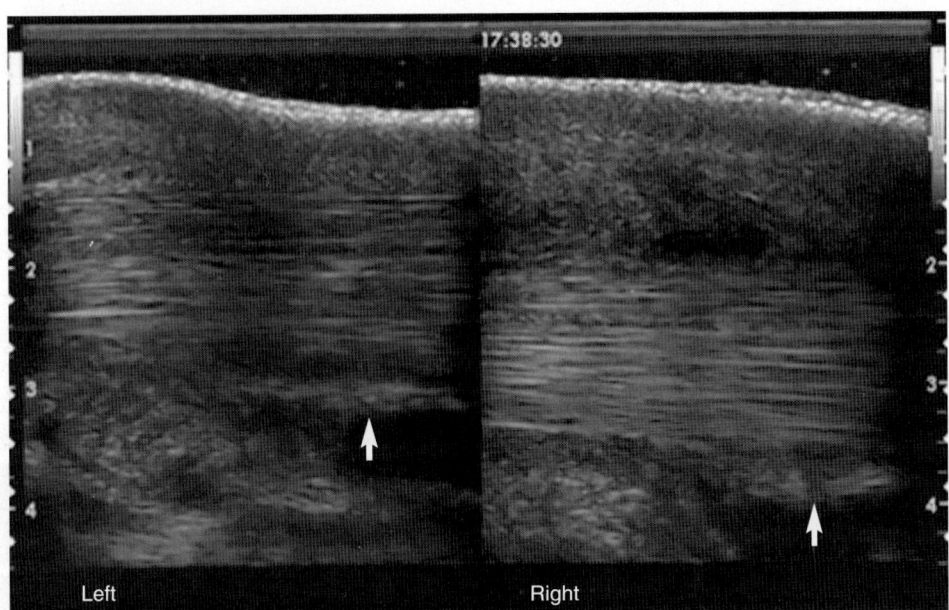

Fig. 74-3 • Longitudinal ultrasonographic images from the midline immediately proximal to the metatarsophalangeal joint *(distal to the left).* The left limb has a normal manica flexoria *(arrow).* In the right hindlimb, the manica flexoria is displaced from the dorsal surface of the deep digital flexor tendon and is thickened *(arrow).*

evidence of synovial proliferation represents stage 1, or the effusive stage of synovitis. More pronounced, often asymmetrical distention of the proximal pouch, which feels firm on palpation and is accompanied by synovial proliferation, is stage 2. In stage 3 synovitis, extensive synovial proliferation occurs with or without adhesion formation in the sheath. Adhesions are manifest as echogenic material between the tendon and wall of the DFTS and can be more easily seen when fluid from marked distention provides negative contrast. Care must be taken to avoid undue pressure on the ultrasound transducer, which will obliterate this fluid from the field of view. However, the presence of adhesions can be easily overestimated with ultrasonography.

Treatment

An important aspect of the decision making is the differentiation of primary versus secondary tenosynovitis. Treatment of horses with acute primary tenosynovitis consists of rest with bandage immobilization, cold therapy, and systemic antiinflammatory medication. The latter can be commenced with a single systemic dose of a short-acting corticosteroid (dexamethasone phosphate [0.06 mg/kg intravenously] or betamethasone phosphate [0.04 mg/kg intravenously]), followed by a 5-day systemic course of flunixin meglumine (1.1 mg/kg daily) or phenylbutazone (4.4 mg/kg daily). After the initial 7 to 14 days, in-hand-walking can be resumed for 2 weeks, before returning the horse to riding. If the clinical signs have not resolved after 7 to 14 days, intrathecal injection of hyaluronan and a corticosteroid (40 to 80 mg of methylprednisolone acetate or 10 mg of triamcinolone acetonide) can be considered provided that no primary cause, such as tendon injury, of the tenosynovitis is suspected. A potential adverse effect of this treatment is that the intrathecal injection of a corticosteroid will interfere in the healing of an injured tendon and may enable a horse with a complicating digital flexor tendon injury to return to soundness temporarily, thereby potentially allowing it to exacerbate the underlying cause for continued irritation of the DFTS. Therefore the clinician should attempt to ensure, with the aid of ultrasonographic evaluation, that no injuries to the digital flexor tendons in the DFTS exist before intrathecal corticosteroids are administered. However, one should remember that many marginal tears of the SDFT or the DDFT within the DFTS may not be identifiable with ultrasonography, especially if they are located at the level of the ultrasonographic blind spot beneath the ergot. Evaluating specific images (see above), measuring the cross-sectional area of each digital flexor tendon (see Chapter 16), and comparing the same measurements in the contralateral limb may help veterinarians recognize subtle digital flexor tendon injuries, without obvious changes in echogenicity. One of the Editors (SJD) treats suspected primary DFTS tenosynovitis by intrathecal administration of corticosteroids immediately after recognition of lameness; persistence of lameness or recurrence of lameness within 2 to 3 weeks is a good indicator that there may be a more complicated injury.

However, in horses that are unresponsive to this treatment or in horses with suspected primary causes (such as those characterized by thickening and fibrosis of the PAL, adhesions, synovial masses, or tears to the digital flexor tendons), tenoscopic exploration of the DFTS is warranted. Tenoscopy provides both diagnostic and therapeutic capabilities. In forelimb injuries, the majority of the tendon lesions involve marginal tears of the lateral, most commonly, or medial margins of the DDFT proximal to the base of the PSBs (Figure 74-4).[14,15] These tears are most appropriately managed by debridement of the prolapsed tendonous tissue. Open suture repair of the tears is invasive, does not offer any improvement over tenoscopic debridement, and is not recommended. In contrast, in hindlimbs, the more common abnormality (with the same clinical signs) is tearing of the lateral or medial attachments of the manica flexoria to the SDFT (Figure 74-5).[15]

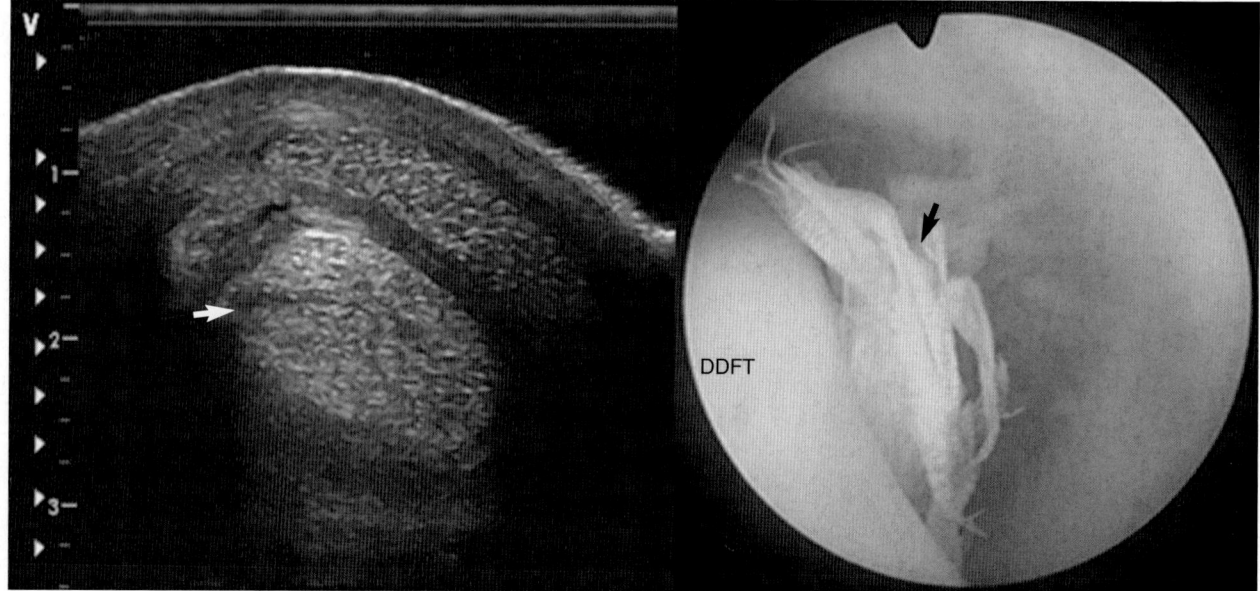

Fig. 74-4 • Oblique transverse ultrasonographic image *(left, lateral to the left)* showing a lateral border tear of the deep digital flexor tendon (DDFT) and *(right)* the tenoscopic appearance with the torn fibers prolapsing from the border of the tendon *(arrow)*.

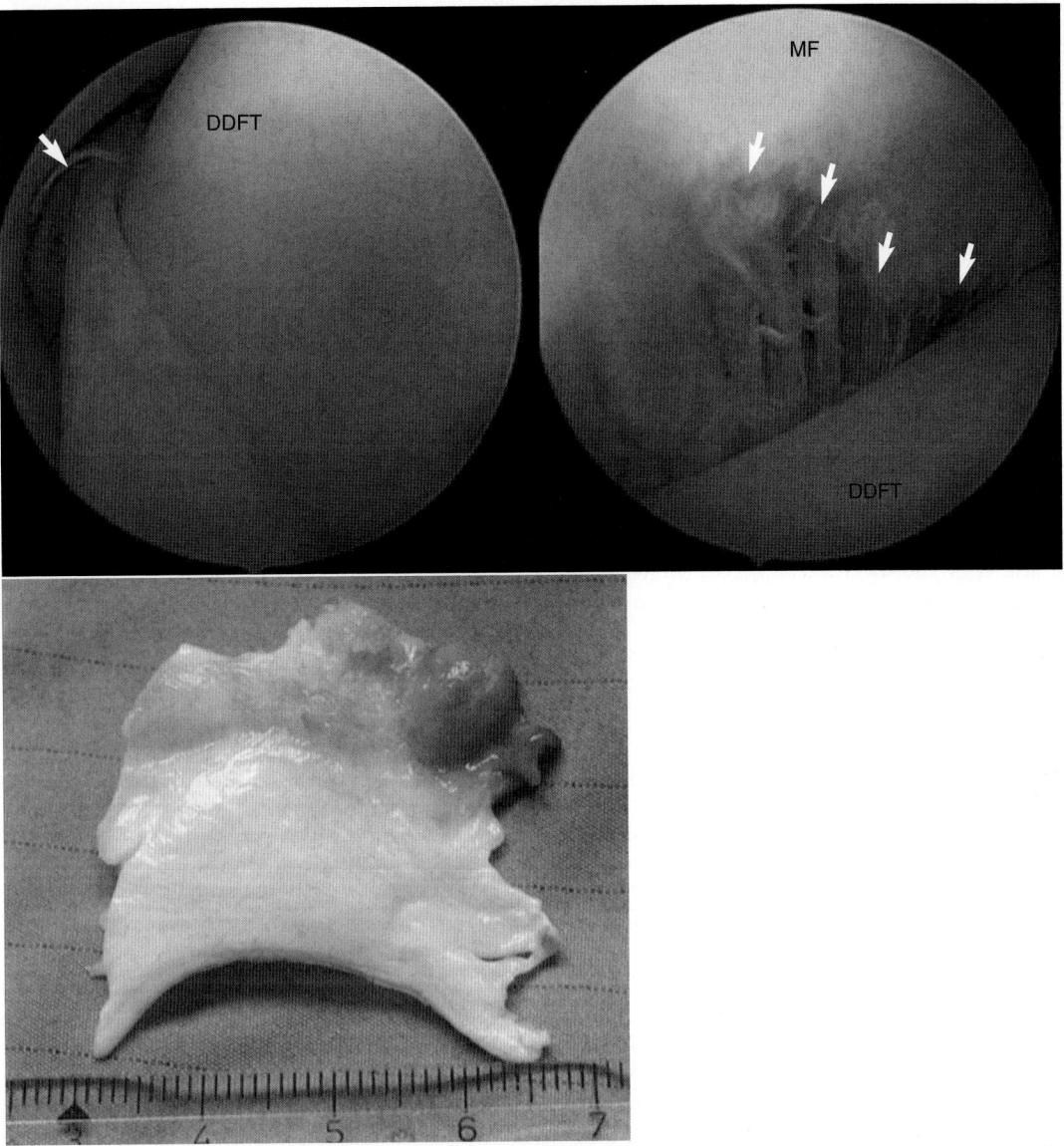

Fig. 74-5 • Tenoscopic view of a manica flexoria tear *(top images; arrows)*. The top left image shows a partial tear viewed from the abaxial part of the proximal aspect of the digital flexor tendon sheath. The top right image shows an almost complete tear taken with the endoscope positioned between the manica flexoria and the deep digital flexor tendon (DDFT). The bottom image shows the manica flexoria after resection. *MF*, Manica flexoria.

These horses are managed by removing the manica flexoria in its entirety (see Figure 74-5). This is achieved using medial and lateral endoscopic portals and medial and lateral instrument portals to introduce a hook knife that is used to transect all remaining attachments of the manica flexoria to the medial and lateral borders of the SDFT. The manica is then pulled through one of the instrument portals (where enlargement of the skin portal is usually necessary) before the proximal synovial attachment is transected to complete removal.

Prognosis

The prognosis for horses with acute, uncomplicated non-infectious tenosynovitis is favorable if treatment starts immediately. The prognosis for those with complex teno-synovitis with synovial masses and adhesions is more guarded but lameness can resolve after tenoscopic debridement and PAL desmotomy. In one report, 18 of 25 horses returned to athletic soundness.[12] Of those horses with a primary tendon injury, the prognosis depends more on this primary pathology. Only 40% of horses with longitudinal tears of the DDFT within the DFTS returned to the same level of exercise after debridement, with the prognosis being even worse (18%) if the tears were long.[15] This is similar to those horses with DDF tendonitis within the DFTS not associated with marginal defects, where seven of 24 horses (29%)[16] made a full recovery (see Chapter 70). However, one of the Editors (SJD) has recently had much better success with management of horses with core lesions by intralesional injection of cultured mesenchymal stem cells. Seventy-six percent of horses with excision of manica flexoria tears returned to the previous level of work.[15] Negative prognostic indicators in addition to the site of the tear were chronicity and marked preoperative distention of the DFTS.[15] However, conservative management of horses with acute small marginal tears of the SDFT is often successful.

Infectious Tenosynovitis

Infectious tenosynovitis is a critical condition in the horse because of the severity of lameness, the difficulty in eliminating infection from the DFTS, and the high risk of long-term sequelae such as adhesions and fibrosis, which contribute to permanent lameness even if infection is eliminated.

Etiopathogenesis

The most common cause of DFTS infection is a penetrating wound. Occasionally, small puncture wounds that readily seal over may not be recognized as the cause of acute, severe lameness associated with DFTS infection. Penetrating injuries to the DDFT in the pastern region are frequently undiagnosed at the outset.[15] Most penetrations in this region lead to infectious tenosynovitis and rarely infectious tendonitis of the DDFT. However, occasionally a traumatic penetration may enter the DDFT through its distal mesotendon and form a localized abscess that remains separate from the intrathecal space, thereby preventing infectious tenosynovitis. Infection may also occur after intrathecal injection or surgery of the PAL. Rarely, hematogenous spread of infection to the digital sheath may result from bacteremia.

Diagnosis

Heat and effusion of the DFTS and severe lameness are classic signs of DFTS infection. Typically horses are reluctant to put the heel of the affected limb to the ground. Exception to this may be seen in horses with an open wound to the DFTS that allows free drainage of infected synovial fluid. The reduction in intrathecal pressure and bacterial numbers provided by continuous flow of synovial fluid may reduce inflammation and lameness considerably. With a closed wound, however, the affected sheath is grossly distended. Generalized and painful lower limb edema caused by cellulitis associated with the entry wound may hinder specific palpation that would aid in identifying DFTS distention. Horses with penetrating injuries to the DDFT in the pastern region are characterized by moderate to severe lameness, localized swelling in the pastern, and a pronounced pain response to focal pressure on the palmar surface of the DDFT in the pastern region.

Radiography and ultrasonography are useful to recognize complicating factors such as osteitis or osteomyelitis, concurrent tendon injury, foreign bodies, and infectious tendonitis. Contrast radiography may help confirm a penetrating tract. In the absence of a penetrating tract, confirmation of the diagnosis relies on synovial fluid analysis. This should be performed as early as possible when DFTS infection is suspected. A total nucleated cell count greater than or equal to 30,000/µL, with more than 90% neutrophils, and a total protein concentration greater than or equal to 4.0 g/dL are considered pathognomonic for infection. Attempts should be made to identify bacteria by Gram stain and culture. Using broth culture bottles enhances the likelihood of obtaining a positive culture. Bacteria cultured from wounds or draining tracts are not representative of intrathecal bacterial populations. Positive cultures have been reported from 67% to 81% of horses with infectious tenosynovitis.[18] Of the positive cultures in one study, 46% were mixed cultures. *Streptococcus* and *Klebsiella* species were the most common isolates from adult horses with infectious tenosynovitis.[19] In another study, iatrogenic synovial infection was more likely to result in a pure culture of *Staphylococcus aureus*, whereas Enterobacteriaceae were most frequently cultured from synovial sepsis caused by a penetrating wound.[20]

Treatment

As for joint infections (see Chapter 65), the principles of antimicrobial therapy, synovial debridement, and drainage apply to infections of the DFTS. Treatment of infectious tenosynovitis must consist of aggressive intrasynovial and systemic broad-spectrum antimicrobial therapy with lavage of the sheath. Regional intravenous perfusion of antibiotics,[21] slow-release antibiotic-depot systems in collagen or polymethylmethacrylate,[22,23] and antibiotic infusion pumps (MILA Joint Infusion System; MILA International, Inc., Florence, Kentucky, United States)[24] all have been used to maximize the intrathecal concentration of antibiotics over a protracted period.

The ideal surgical treatment for DFTS infection consists of tenoscopic debridement of fibrin, foreign material, adhesions, and synovial masses along with simultaneous lavage.[25] Needle lavage is usually relatively less effective at achieving resolution of the infection because of the blind-ending pouches in the DFTS. Transection of the PAL can relieve pain that results from excessive fluid accumulation and fibrosis and thickening of the sheath wall in horses with chronic infectious tenosynovitis. This is best performed through a tenoscopic approach to minimize the risk of wound dehiscence that accompanies a transcutaneous approach. After tenoscopy, portals usually are closed but can be left open for continued drainage if desired with chronic infection. Indwelling fenestrated drains may be placed at surgery for continued through-and-through lavage. Fenestrated polyvinylchloride or silicone drains are preferable to Penrose drains because they allow for lavage and drainage. The drain is covered with a sterile dressing under a bulky pressure bandage, and lavage is continued twice daily for 3 to 5 days. Because adhesion formation and fibrosis are the most common causes for surviving horses' failure to return to the intended use, specific recommendations have been made to reduce the incidence of these crippling complications. After removal of the drain and healing of the skin portals, hyaluronan is injected into the sheath at 14-day intervals to reduce adhesion formation. These injections are best started between 7 and 14 days after injury during the time of fibrosis and adhesion formation.

Provided adequate debridement and lavage have been achieved tenoscopically, primary closure of an open DFTS shortly after injury is usually indicated. However, closure may be contraindicated in some horses with extensive contamination and/or inadequate debridement because closure may trap bacteria in the sheath. In such horses, cleaning the wound thoroughly and maintaining it under sterile wraps to allow for healing by second intention to occur may be preferable, or consideration may be given to delayed closure when the wound is sufficiently clean and lameness has resolved.[18]

Early passive motion and handwalking exercise were advocated to prevent restriction of range of motion.[18,19] Elevation of the heel often causes improved weight bearing and ambulation during this period. Cast immobilization of the distal limb is contraindicated during treatment for DFTS infection if the digital flexor tendons are intact. Although immobilization limits recurrent inflammation associated with continuous movement of the damaged tissues, it limits drainage and promotes the restrictive nature of any scar tissue and adhesions. However, immobilization effects more rapid soft tissue healing and therefore is indicated to decrease wound motion once infection has been resolved. A commercial or homemade splint is adequate for immobilization.

Prognosis

Horses with wounds of the DFTS have a good prognosis for return to soundness if the wound is diagnosed and treated before infectious tenosynovitis develops. If infection occurs, the prognosis is guarded. Although the prognosis for elimination of infection and survival was described as good in most studies (as high as 100% in one study[20]), another study reported a 45% failure of return to soundness and intended use for horses with infectious DFTS tenosynovitis. Even if infection can be resolved successfully, fibrosis, adhesions, and occasionally tendon rupture or osteomyelitis of the PSB may cause permanent lameness. Most authors believe that the chance of resolution is related directly to the duration of infection.[18]

PALMAR ANNULAR LIGAMENT SYNDROME

Etiopathogenesis

The PAL counteracts a tendency of the PSBs to move in a dorsal and abaxial direction during weight bearing. The medial and lateral branches and the extensor branches of the SL effect strong traction in a dorsal direction at the respective insertion sites on the abaxial surface of the PSBs during extension of the fetlock joint. This traction is balanced by the intersesamoidean ligament and the PAL.[1] The role of disease of the PAL as a cause of lameness is a subject of debate. Thickening of the PAL has been associated with lameness in a number of different diseases of the DFTS and associated structures. All these diseases have characteristic clinical manifestation of distention of the DFTS and thickening of the PAL in common and therefore as a group have been referred to as *palmar annular ligament syndrome*. Other terms that have been used to describe this clinical presentation include *stenosis of the fetlock canal*, *palmar annular ligament constriction*, *fetlock canal dysfunction*, and *stenosing palmar ligament desmitis*. The role of desmopathy in this syndrome is supported by histopathological evidence of chronic inflammation and repair tissue in PAL biopsies from horses with clinical disease.[24-28] Undoubtedly, however, the cause of PAL desmitis is multifactorial. Direct external trauma to the PAL may be caused by laceration or by direct impact (e.g., overreach). Overextension of the fetlock at high speed is likely to be associated with high tensile forces in the PAL and may lead to injury and failure of the PAL under tension. Excessive tendon swelling within the DFTS, although uncommon, may result in sustained pressure on and inflammation of the PAL (see Chapter 69, Figure 69-2). Finally, chronic inflammation of the DFTS (noninfectious or infectious tenosynovitis) leads to fibrosis and thickening of the fibrous part of the DFTS capsule, which includes the PAL. In some horses the subcutaneous connective tissue in the area of the PAL becomes greatly

thickened and fibrotic. Once an inflammatory response is initiated, the PAL becomes thickened, whatever the cause. Thickening of the PAL reduces the space within the fetlock canal and results in a relative stenosis. The continuous pressure from the tendons associated with this relative stenosis is a source of trauma and perpetuates this sequence of events, leading to further inflammation, fibrosis, and thickening of the PAL and persistent pain (Figure 74-6).

A positive relationship exists between incidence of PAL desmitis and increasing age of the horse, a predisposition in some breeds (Paso Fino and Warmbloods), and location (especially hindlimbs in the mentioned breeds).[26] Rarely, small avulsion fractures may occur at the site of insertion of the PAL to the palmar border of a PSB after overextension injury or local trauma (see page 754 and Figure 72-17).[29]

Diagnosis

Occasionally, acute lameness may be caused by PAL injury without tenosynovitis. Clinical signs include localized heat, swelling, and pain on palpation of the palmar aspect of the fetlock. The clinical signs of the more common chronic PAL syndrome are characteristic. Horses have long-term, persistent, mild to moderate lameness that improves little with rest and worsens with return to exercise. A fetlock flexion test exacerbates lameness. DFTS distention with a notch in the palmar outline of the fetlock is virtually pathognomonic for PAL syndrome (Figure 74-7). This notch is caused by the inability of the DFTS to distend at the site of intimate attachment between the SDFT and the dorsal surface of the thickened, inelastic PAL. Sometimes enlargement of the PAL or the overlying subcutaneous tissues results in a localized bulge rather than a notch over the palmar aspect of the fetlock region. Extension of the affected fetlock often is decreased during weight bearing at walk or trot, and occasionally affected horses are reluctant to put the heel of the affected foot to the ground. This splinted fetlock posture is assumed by the affected horse to decrease pressure of the digital flexor tendons on the inflamed PAL.

Lameness often is improved, but not always completely eliminated, by intrathecal analgesia. The response to a low four- or six-point nerve block is often better. Sometimes a palmar nerve block performed at the base of the PSBs improves lameness. Fibrosis of the PAL and DFTS may result in mechanical gait restriction, which cannot be abolished totally by regional analgesia.

Various imaging techniques can be used to support the clinical diagnosis of PAL desmitis. In horses with chronic lameness, entheseous new bone may be present at the PAL insertions on the palmar border of one or both PSBs. Air tenography or ultrasonography must be used to demonstrate thickening of the PAL or the overlying subcutis. The ultrasonographic appearance of a diseased PAL differs between affected horses and may be helpful in differentiating the etiopathogenic mechanisms behind each injury. An unaffected PAL can be difficult to identify because it is only 1 to 2 mm thick, and imaging the ligament in the sagittal midline is complicated by the vinculum between the PAL and the SDFT, which makes resolution of the ligament difficult. The PAL is identified most easily at its attachment to a PSB by tilting the transversely positioned

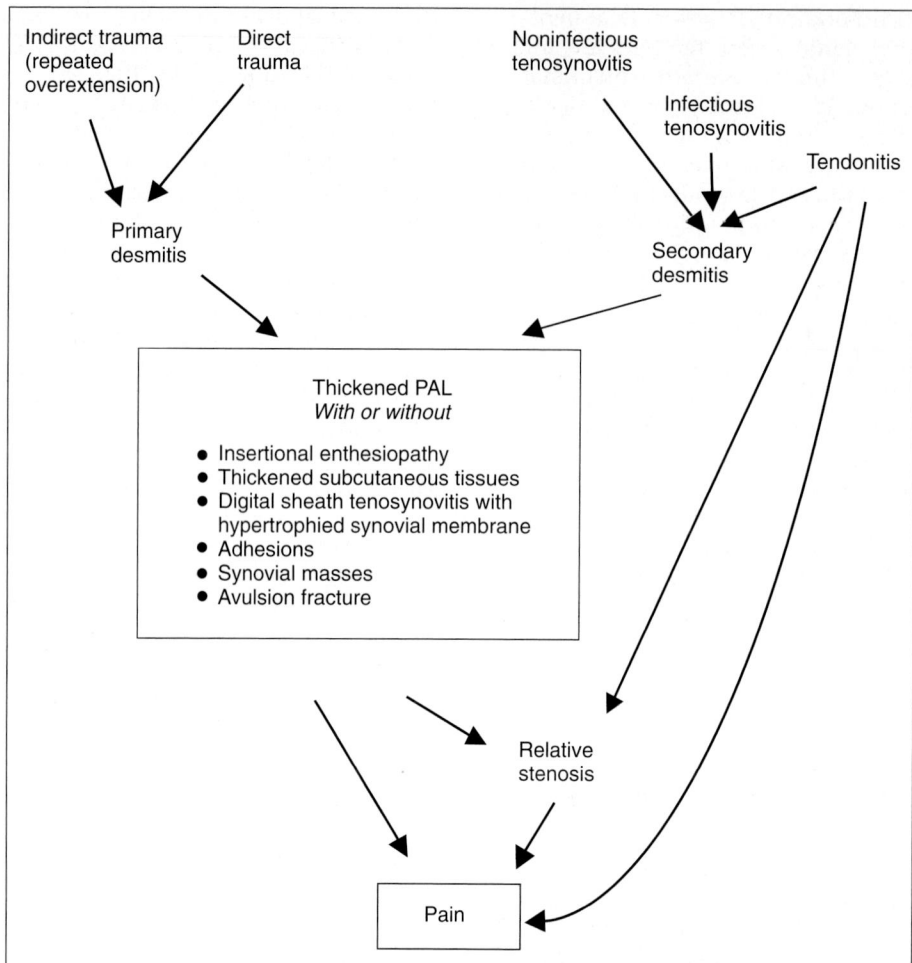

Fig. 74-6 • Etiopathogenesis of palmar annular ligament *(PAL)* syndrome.

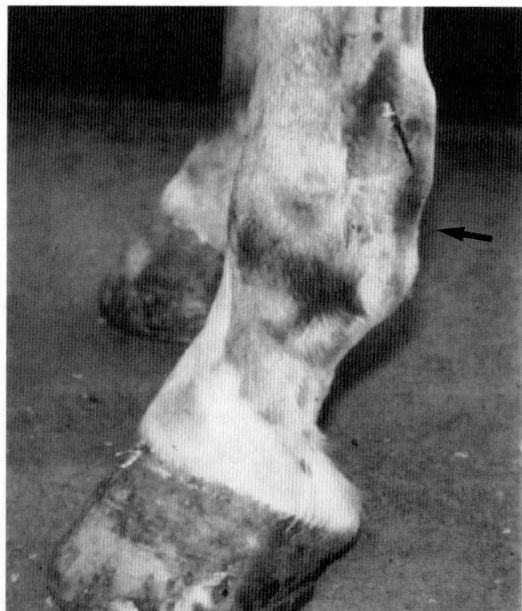

Fig. 74-7 • Digital flexor tendon sheath distention with characteristic notch in the plantar outline of the fetlock region *(arrow)* in a horse with plantar annular ligament syndrome.

transducer laterally or medially from the palmar midline. The ligament then can be followed toward the midline. Several measurements of the thickness of the PAL should be made on transverse and longitudinal images to obtain reliable data. Because of the difficulties in consistently identifying the PAL, some clinicians have proposed measuring the distance between the palmar surface of the SDFT and the skin surface.[30] Any increase in thickness more than 5 mm is considered to be abnormal. However, three different structures contribute to this measurement, each of which can be thickened to varying degrees in different pathology and in different breeds: the subcutaneous tissues, the PAL, and the parietal and visceral layers of the DFTS.

Primary Palmar Annular Ligament Thickening

Primary PAL thickening is characterized by ultrasonographic evidence of thickening of the PAL, without evidence of pathological conditions of the structures within the DFTS (Figure 74-8). Although tenosynovitis is present, the synovial lining of the sheath is not substantially thickened. With acute desmitis, the ligament is enlarged and contains focal hypoechoic areas, or it is diffusely hypoechoic. PAL thickening may be accompanied by extensive subcutaneous fibrosis. This condition occurs more

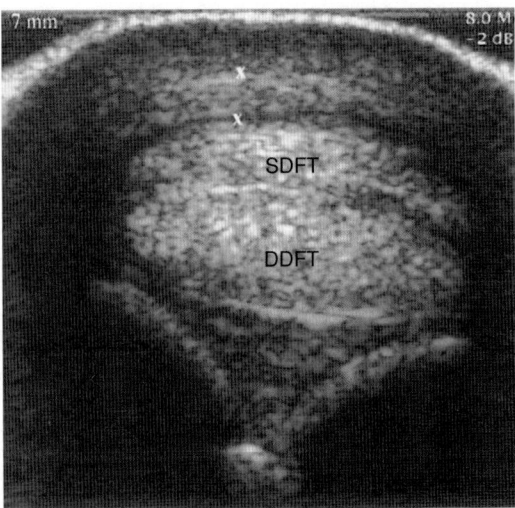

Fig. 74-8 • Transverse ultrasonographic image of the distal metacarpal region at the level of the proximal sesamoid bones. There is primary enlargement of the palmar annular ligament. The palmar annular ligament (*X* to *X*) measured 7 mm in thickness. *SDFT*, Superficial digital flexor tendon; *DDFT*, deep digital flexor tendon.

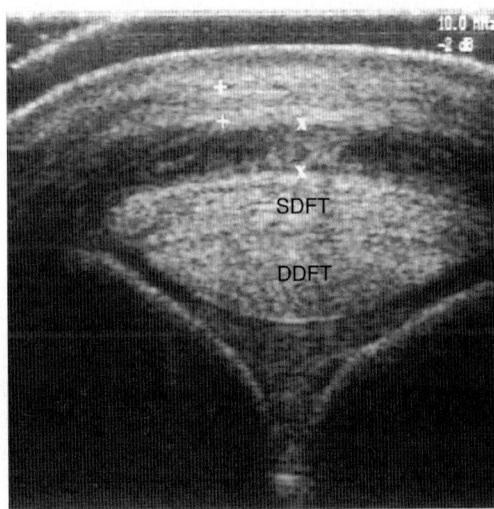

Fig. 74-9 • Transverse ultrasonographic image of the distal metacarpal region at the level of the proximal sesamoid bones. There is thickening of the palmar annular ligament (+ to +) and the synovial membrane of the digital flexor tendon sheath (*X* to *X*). *SDFT*, Superficial digital flexor tendon; *DDFT*, deep digital flexor tendon.

commonly in hindlimbs than forelimbs, and ponies and cob-type horses seem particularly prone. Thickening may be present bilaterally in a unilaterally lame horse but is always greater in the lame limb. Some horses have developed sequential lameness in more than one limb.

Primary Tenosynovitis with Secondary Palmar Annular Ligament Thickening

Ultrasonographic differentiation between secondary PAL thickening and primary desmitis is sometimes difficult, but the synovial lining of the DFTS usually is considerably thickened, including the lining at the level of the PAL

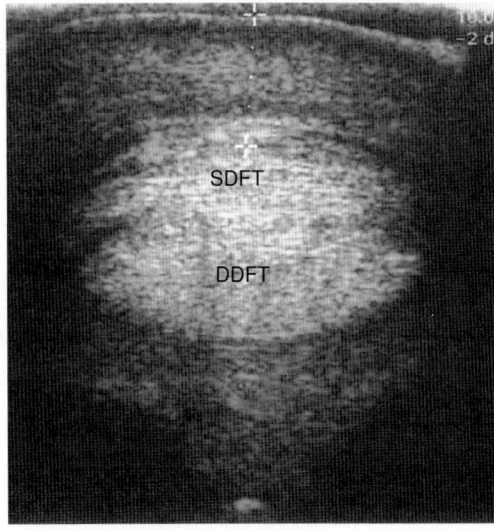

Fig. 74-10 • Transverse ultrasonographic image of the distal metacarpal region. There is subcutaneous fibrosis, with minimal thickening of the palmar annular ligament (PAL), associated with clinical signs of PAL syndrome. Although the distance from the skin to the plantar surface of the superficial digital flexor tendon amounts to 9.19 mm (+ to +), the PAL is only 1.59 mm thick. *SDFT*, Superficial digital flexor tendon; *DDFT*, deep digital flexor tendon.

(Figure 74-9). Horses with chronic, complex tenosynovitis may have adhesions and synovial masses.

Subcutaneous Fibrosis with a Normal or Minimally Enlarged Palmar Annular Ligament

Subcutaneous fibrosis in the region of the PAL can produce clinical signs similar to those of PAL thickening and often can be distinguished only by careful ultrasonographic imaging (Figure 74-10). These injuries frequently are caused by focal trauma to the PAL area and can involve portions of the PAL and the surface of the underlying SDFT.

Tendon Injuries with Secondary Palmar Annular Ligament Thickening

Injuries of the SDFT, manica flexoria, or DDFT within the fetlock canal may result in inflammatory tenosynovitis, which also can lead to PAL thickening. Although tendonitis usually can be diagnosed by ultrasonography, many focal longitudinal tears of the SDFT and DDFT remain undetected, especially if they are located at the level of the ultrasonographic blind spot beneath the ergot.

Treatment and Prognosis

Treatment of horses with acute PAL desmitis with rest and topical antiinflammatory medication often results in rapid resolution of lameness and swelling. In many horses, however, PAL desmitis becomes a chronic condition, treatment of which requires surgical release (desmotomy) of the inflamed and thickened PAL. Desmotomy resolves pain from traction on the ligament during weight bearing and eliminates pressure from structures within the stenotic fetlock canal on the PAL. This can be performed via a traditional surgical approach, using an open or a minimally invasive technique. A minimally invasive approach through a small skin incision in the proximal recess of the DFTS is simple and quick, but subcutaneous transection of the PAL is performed blind (see Chapter 69). However, confirmation of a relative stenosis within the fetlock canal in these horses is difficult preoperatively unless movement of the tendons through the canal is visibly impeded. The best evaluation is achieved tenoscopically, albeit in a non–weight-bearing limb, by assessing the ease with which a 5-mm endoscopic cannula can be passed from distal to proximal through the fetlock canal. This has an additional benefit of enabling the surgeon to simultaneously evaluate the entire DFTS and treat any concurrent pathological conditions, such as longitudinal tendon tears, adhesions, and synovial masses, which may be the primary cause of the PAL thickening. Desmotomy of the PAL can then be achieved tenoscopically either with a slotted canula used for carpal tunnel release in people (Smith & Nephew Dyonics Inc., Andover, Massachusetts, United States) or by direct tenoscopic evaluation and use of a freehand, hook knife or Metzenbaum scissors.[11] A minimally invasive approach (incisional or tenoscopic) decreases the risk of wound dehiscence and fistulation and allows for earlier, safe return to exercise. If a traditional open approach is used, particular attention should be paid to careful closure of the subcutaneous tissues in two layers, as well as of the skin, to minimize the risks of synovial fistulation and wound dehiscence. Contrary to previous reports, our opinion is that horses that have undergone an open surgical approach to the DFTS should not be returned to exercise before healing of the incision is complete. Instead the horse should be confined to a stable and the limb enclosed in a firm, padded bandage until the time of suture removal at 2 weeks. After this, a gradually increasing exercise regimen can be initiated (2 weeks walking in hand, 4 weeks lunging) before return to ridden work. Some authors report the need for 4 to 6 months of rest and controlled exercise before soundness can be expected.[29]

Specific recommendations for treating PAL syndrome can be made according to the specific ultrasonographic characteristics. Unresponsive primary desmitis requires PAL desmotomy. In horses with primary tenosynovitis with secondary PAL desmitis, therapeutic planning should be aimed at discovering and treating the primary cause of the synovitis (e.g., infection, traumatic tendon injuries, and hypertrophic synovitis), with or without the need for PAL desmotomy. Tenoscopy is indicated in these horses.

If the stenotic effect is caused by extensive subcutaneous fibrosis over the PAL, conservative management with rest and antiinflammatory medication is occasionally successful in resolving lameness. However, if this approach fails to bring resolution, surgical release of the PAL and subcutaneous ring of fibrosis may resolve lameness. Occasionally, complete resection of the PAL is performed in horses in which there is persistent focal and intense pain over the PAL. The use of a C-shaped skin incision to create a medially or laterally based flap and preservation of the subcutaneous tissues, including the fat of the ergot, followed by careful closure and short-term (2 to 4 weeks) cast immobilization can give remarkably good cosmetic and

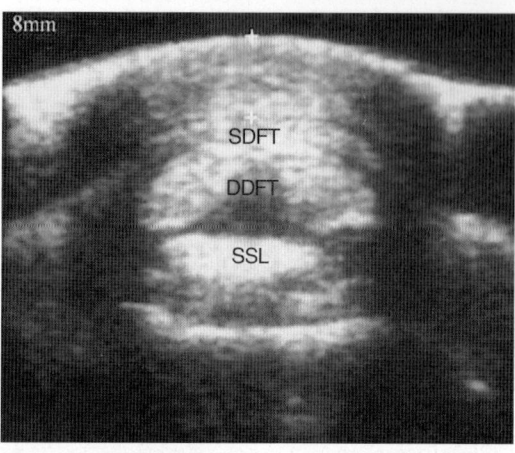

Fig. 74-11 • Transverse ultrasonographic image of the proximal pastern region of a hindlimb. The distance from the skin surface to the plantar surface of the superficial digital flexor tendon (SDFT) (+ to +) is enlarged to 8 mm in this horse with chronic desmitis of the proximal digital annular ligament. *DDFT*, deep digital flexor tendon; *SSL*, straight sesamoidean ligament.

functional end results (Figure 74-11). However, resection should only be considered for horses with primary PAL pathology unresponsive to conservative management. Lameness associated with small avulsion fractures of the palmar border of the PSB may be relieved by PAL desmotomy near its insertion site. In one study, however, three horses regained soundness without surgery after 3 to 6 months of controlled exercise.[27] Finally, the resolution of tendonitis of the SDFT or DDFT within the DFTS may be assisted by PAL desmotomy, although the benefit of surgical treatment has proved less obvious in these horses.[13,30] Despite these reports, PAL desmotomy has proved useful in managing SDF tendonitis in Standardbreds (see Chapter 69).[31] The prognosis after surgical desmotomy is generally favorable for soundness in horses with desmitis of the PAL without tendonitis and has ranged from 64% to 87%.[12,29] Factors with a negative influence on outcome are the presence of tendonitis, infection, or adhesions. Although in one study adhesions reduced the return to soundness to 44% after PAL desmotomy,[30] a different study showed that 72% of horses with complex tenosynovitis made a full recovery after tenoscopic debridement and PAL desmotomy.[12] In a study of 71 horses with chronic PAL desmopathy with or without subcutaneous fibrosis, 22 of 44 (50%) returned to full athletic function, whereas only eight of 27 (33%) horses with concurrent tendon pathology returned to full function.[27]

DISEASES OF THE INTERSESAMOIDEAN (PALMAR) LIGAMENT OF THE FETLOCK
Etiopathogenesis
When the fetlock overextends, the proximal scutum slides distally to the metacarpal condyle and its palmar surface undergoes pressure from the flexor tendons. Moreover, in this position the distal medial and lateral extensor branches of the SL induce high tension on the abaxial surface of the PSBs, thus creating high tension on the intersesamoidean ligament.[32] The effect of these forces could provide a

biomechanical explanation for injuries to the intersesamoidean ligament. Post mortem examination of 305 pairs of PSBs revealed radiological changes in 25.8% and gross abnormalities of the intersesamoidean ligament in 25.9%,[33] although premortem recognition of intersesamoidean ligament pathological conditions causing lameness has been considerably less common.[30] Diseases of the intersesamoidean ligament have been classified by the ultrasonographic and radiological appearance as rupture of the intersesamoidean ligament, avulsion fracture of the intersesamoidean ligament from the PSBs, desmitis of the intersesamoidean ligament (noninfectious and infectious), and enthesopathy of the intersesamoidean ligament.[32,35-37] Infectious desmitis and axial osteomyelitis of the PSBs usually are associated with infectious arthritis of the fetlock joint or infectious tenosynovitis of the DFTS. Which condition precedes the other is not always obvious. If infectious desmitis or osteomyelitis is the primary condition, a hematogenous route for the infection is likely.

Diagnosis

Injuries of the intersesamoidean ligament usually cause acute-onset, moderate to severe lameness. Horses with enthesopathy with thinning of the intersesamoidean ligament and erosion of the flexor surface of the corresponding PSB may have a more insidious course. Avulsion fractures of the axial border of the PSBs often are accompanied by fetlock effusion, usually involve the lateral PSB, and usually occur in conjunction with a displaced lateral condylar fracture of the third metacarpal bone[31] Lameness accompanying these conditions is improved, but not always abolished, by intrasynovial analgesia of the fetlock joint or the DFTS and is eliminated by a low four-point block. Scintigraphy may be required to find the exact site of the pathological condition. In horses with suspected infectious desmitis or osteomyelitis, cytological examination of synovial fluid of the fetlock joint or DFTS often, but not always, indicates synovial infection.

Diagnosis of injury to the intersesamoidean ligament and associated structures mainly is based on abnormal imaging features. Evidence of osseous fragmentation or radiolucency along the axial border of the PSB, predominantly centered at the proximal half of the intersesamoidean space, indicates desmitis, enthesopathy with osteitis, avulsion fracture, or osteomyelitis. Evidence of osteolysis also may be observed along the palmar surface of the PSBs in association with enthesopathy of the intersesamoidean ligament. Ultrasonographic abnormalities include enlargement of the distance between both PSBs with intersesamoidean ligament rupture (>6 mm), enlargement of the intersesamoidean ligament, and alteration of the echogenicity within the intersesamoidean ligament in horses with desmitis, and asymmetrical reduction in the thickness of the intersesamoidean ligament and irregular bony outline to the palmar surface of a PSB in association with enthesopathy.

Treatment and Prognosis

No effective treatment exists for rupture of the intersesamoidean ligament with abaxial displacement of the PSB or for enthesopathy with thinning and degeneration of the intersesamoidean ligament within the DFTS, and the prognosis for soundness in either situation is grave. We have observed complete recovery in a general purpose riding and jumping horse with intersesamoidean desmitis and a small avulsion fracture of the axial border after a prolonged confinement (6 months). Some reports also have documented favorable outcome for horses with noninfectious desmitis with or without avulsion fracture after arthroscopic removal of fracture fragments and debridement of the osteochondral defect and the associated discolored area of the intersesamoidean ligament.[35,36] Histological evaluation of the damaged intersesamoidean ligament in these horses revealed chronic inflammation and granulation tissue, with thrombosis of the microvasculature. All horses with noninfectious desmitis treated surgically in one study returned to previous level of performance, although the horses' intended uses were not mentioned.[35] Recovery time was 7 to 12 months. In the same study, similar treatment was generally unsuccessful for horses with infectious desmitis and osteomyelitis.[35]

DISEASES OF THE DIGITAL ANNULAR LIGAMENTS

Desmitis and avulsion fractures of the proximal insertion sites of the proximal digital annular ligament may occur.

Etiopathogenesis

Hyperextension of the fetlock causes differential movement between the SDFT and the proximal phalanx. The proximal digital annular ligament is adhered intimately to the palmar surface of the SDFT in this region, and the proximal digital annular ligament inserts to the proximal phalanx at two levels; thus this differential movement may result in injury of the proximal digital annular ligament or its insertions. Additionally, external trauma to the palmar aspect of the pastern may result in desmitis of the proximal digital annular ligament. Desmitis of the proximal digital annular ligament also has been described in association with injury of the SDFT or infectious tenosynovitis with thickening of the DFTS in horses with infectious desmitis and osteomyelitis.[37] It has been suggested that thickening of the proximal digital annular ligament or fibrosis of the subcutaneous tissues on the palmar aspect of the pastern may result in functional constriction of the DFTS and the digital flexor tendons, causing lameness, as is the case with the PAL syndrome.[36]

Diagnosis

Characteristic clinical findings in horses with desmitis of the proximal digital annular ligament are soft tissue thickening in the palmar pastern region, prominent palmar protrusion of the DFTS distal to the proximal digital annular ligament, and improvement in lameness score by a palmar nerve block or intrathecal analgesia of the DFTS. Ultrasonography provides a definitive diagnosis. The normal proximal digital annular ligament is not visible on ultrasonographic examination, but the palmarodorsal thickness of the combined skin–proximal digital annular ligament layer should not exceed 2 mm. In horses with proximal digital annular desmitis, this distance increased to 4 to 5 mm (see Figure 74-11).[36] It is important to rule out pathological conditions of the digital flexor tendons or

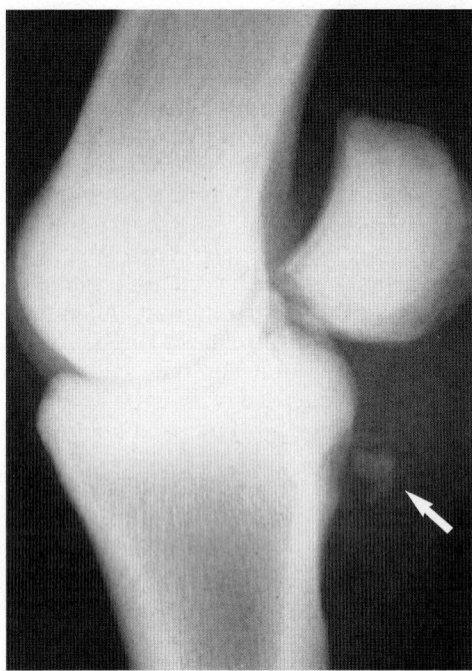

Fig. 74-12 • Lateral radiographic image of a metatarsophalangeal joint. An avulsion fracture fragment *(arrow)* involves the proximal insertion of the proximal digital annular ligament to the plantarolateral border of the proximal phalanx.

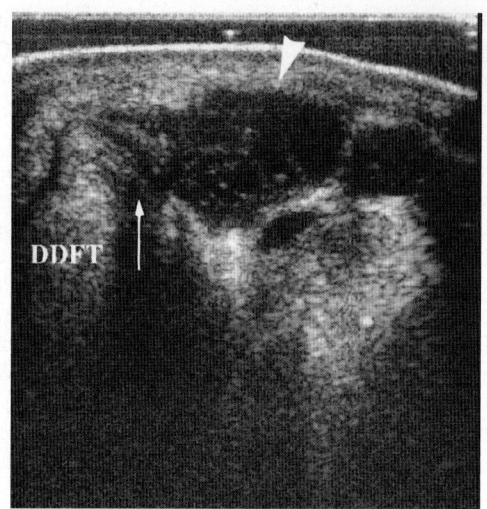

Fig. 74-13 • Transverse ultrasonographic image over the lateral aspect of the distal metatarsal region of a horse with a synovial ganglion of the digital flexor tendon sheath (DFTS). There is subcutaneous fluid collection *(arrowhead)* outside the boundary of, but in communication with, the DFTS *(arrow)*. DDFT, Deep digital flexor tendon.

distal sesamoidean ligaments as causes of soft tissue swelling in the palmar pastern region (see Chapter 82).

Avulsion fractures of the proximal insertion of the proximal digital annular ligament were seen as a cause of lameness in three horses.[37] There were few localizing signs, and diagnosis relied on response to nerve blocks and radiography. Radiographs showed an avulsion fracture fragment at the insertion site of the proximal digital annular ligament on the palmarolateral or palmaromedial border of the proximal phalanx (Figure 74-12).

Treatment

Desmitis of the proximal digital annular ligament with constriction of the DFTS was treated successfully in two horses by desmotomy of the proximal digital annular ligament.[36] Two horses with avulsion fractures of the proximal digital annular ligament were treated with 2 months of rest alone, and one horse was treated with 6 weeks of immobilization, followed by 6 weeks of rest. All three horses returned to the previous level of performance.[36]

Injury of the distal digital annular ligament has recently been recognized as a potential contributor to lameness, either as a primary injury[39] or as one of a complex of injuries.[40] Diagnosis required magnetic resonance imaging. Seven horses with pain localized to the digit had diffuse or focal thickening of the ligament associated with increased signal intensity in T1- and T2-weighted images, with or without concurrent lesions of the DDFT within the adjacent DFTS. Surgical transection of the ligament successfully resolved lameness in those horses in which the injury was considered primary.[39] However, it is difficult to conceive how transection was achieved because of the intimate

anatomical relationship between the DDFT and the distal digital annular ligament.

SYNOVIAL GANGLION OR HERNIA OF THE DIGITAL FLEXOR TENDON SHEATH

A synovial hernia or ganglion is a thin-walled cyst originating from a tendon sheath or joint capsule.[41,42] Hernias of the DFTS result from a traumatic defect in the fibrous layer of the DFTS wall, allowing the synovial lining to herniate through it. Ganglia are thought to result from trauma involving all layers of the sheath wall and are not lined by synovium. Subsequent irritation to the hernial sac causes secretion of synovium and filling of the sac. The opening in some hernial sacs or ganglions can act as a one-way valve that prevents movement of synovial fluid back to the DFTS. Injection of a radiodense contrast medium into the DFTS has resulted in flow of the contrast medium from the parent synovial cavity into the ganglion (Figure 74-13), but not vice versa. We have encountered such a ganglion at the level of the proximolateral recess of the DFTS in five horses, associated with lameness, which was abolished by intrathecal analgesia of the DFTS.[43] Diagnostic imaging and surgical exploration revealed a cystic structure, connected to a small slitlike opening in the DFTS wall. Resection and closure of the DFTS wall defect resulted in resolution of lameness. However, such structures can often be seen incidentally unassociated with lameness.

TENDONITIS OF THE SUPERFICIAL AND DEEP DIGITAL FLEXOR TENDONS WITHIN THE DIGITAL FLEXOR TENDON SHEATH

Tendonitis of the SDFT and DDFT within the digital sheath is discussed in Chapters 69 and 70.

The Carpal Canal and Carpal Synovial Sheath

Sue J. Dyson

ANATOMY

The carpal canal encloses the carpal synovial sheath, which contains the superficial (SDFT) and deep (DDFT) digital flexor tendons. The dorsal wall of the carpal canal is formed by the common palmar ligament of the carpus, which is a thickened part of the fibrous joint capsule that extends distally as the accessory ligament of the DDFT (ALDDFT). Proximally the accessory ligament of the SDFT (ALSDFT) forms the medial wall of the canal. Laterally the carpal canal is formed by the accessory carpal bone and the accessorioquartale and accessoriometacarpeum ligaments extending distally. The caudal antebrachial fascia, flexor retinaculum, and palmar metacarpal fascia form the palmar aspect of the canal.

The carpal synovial sheath extends from 7 to 10 cm proximal to the antebrachiocarpal joint to the midmetacarpal region. The proximal recess is wide and extends between the ulnaris lateralis and lateral digital extensor muscles laterally, but it is firmly supported on the medial aspect by the antebrachial fascia. The distal recess extends between the DDFT and its accessory ligament. If the carpal sheath is distended, swelling can be seen on the lateral aspect of the distal antebrachium and between the DDFT and its accessory ligament, medially or laterally in the metacarpal region.

The ALSDFT arises from the caudomedial aspect of the radius about 10 cm proximal to the antebrachiocarpal joint. The ALSDFT is a fibrous fan-shaped band that merges with the SDFT at the level of the antebrachiocarpal joint and prevents overload of the SDFT muscle during overextension of the metacarpophalangeal joint. After desmotomy of the ALSDFT in cadaver specimens, strain on the SDFT is increased.[1] At the level of the distal aspect of the radius is an extension from the lateral aspect of the sheath wall between the SDFT and DDFT. At the level of the accessory carpal bone is a mesotendon extending from the lateral aspect of the DDFT to the sheath wall. In clinically normal horses, the amount of fluid within the carpal sheath varies, but it is usually the same bilaterally in each horse.

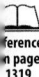
References on page 1319

Fluid within the sheath may be seen readily by ultrasonography between the DDFT and its accessory ligament in normal horses, with no palpable distention of the sheath wall.[2] Within the proximal part of the carpal sheath, the SDFT and DDFT contain muscular tissue and therefore have hypoechoic regions within them on ultrasonographic examination.[3-5] However, the ALSDFT is uniform in its echogenicity.[4,5] The position of the accessory carpal bone prohibits ultrasonographic examination from the caudal aspect of the carpus. The carpal sheath and its contents are evaluated most easily from the distal caudomedial aspect of the antebrachium and carpus and the palmar aspect of the proximal metacarpal region. The heterogeneous echogenicity of the digital flexor tendons proximally can make definitive diagnosis of a tendon lesion difficult, but comparison with the contralateral limb may be helpful. Endoscopic evaluation may yield further information and permit surgical debridement of torn fibers (see Chapter 24).

The transverse ridge of the distal aspect of the radius is at about the same level as the distal physis. Irregular roughening of this ridge may be seen radiologically in normal horses and should not be confused with entheseous new bone associated with tearing of the attachment of the ALSDFT further proximally.

Occasionally abnormalities cannot be detected using conventional imaging techniques and magnetic resonance imaging (MRI) is required (see Figure 75-1, *B*). Normal MRI anatomy of the carpal region has recently been described.[6]

CLINICAL SIGNS

Lameness associated with the carpal synovial sheath is usually accompanied with some distention of the sheath. There may be generalized thickening in the region of the flexor retinaculum. The horse may have restricted flexibility of the carpus, with pain on passive flexion. Alternatively, the horse may resent full extension of the carpus. Rarely, increased pressure within the carpal sheath may result in compromised blood flow within the median artery and reduction in arterial pulse amplitudes in the more distal part of the limb.[7] Palpation of the structures within the proximal part of the carpal sheath is not possible, but the SDFT, DDFT, and ALDDFT should be assessed carefully in the metacarpal region. Lameness varies from mild to severe and usually is improved by intrathecal analgesia. Clinical investigation should include radiographic and ultrasonographic examinations. In the absence of effusion of the carpal sheath, intrathecal analgesia should be performed to verify the source of pain and the clinical significance of any postulated lesion.

Carpal sheath effusion is not always associated with a primary lesion within the sheath per se but can be seen in association with injuries of the ALDDFT, the proximal aspect of the suspensory ligament, trauma or fractures involving the antebrachiocarpal joint, and cellulitis in the distal aspect of the antebrachium, carpus, or proximal metacarpal region (see Chapters 14 and 37).

IDIOPATHIC SYNOVITIS

Synovitis of the carpal sheath usually results in acute-onset, moderate to severe unilateral lameness associated with distention of the carpal sheath. No palpable abnormalities of the digital flexor tendons are apparent. Ultrasonographic examination reveals an abnormal amount of fluid within the sheath but no other structural abnormality. Horses usually respond well to box rest and controlled walking exercise for 4 to 6 weeks, combined with intrathecal administration of corticosteroids and hyaluronan. If lameness is recurrent, synovectomy may be required.

INTRATHECAL HEMORRHAGE

Hemorrhage within the carpal sheath may be idiopathic, result from trauma (e.g., a fall), or occur secondary to either a tear of the SDFT or DDFT, a tear of the ALSDFT, or a fracture of the accessory carpal bone (see pages 446 and 780). The horse may be very lame. Diagnosis is confirmed by synoviocentesis. The fluid within the sheath may appear more echogenic than synovial fluid. Careful ultrasonographic examination of the digital flexor tendons and the retinaculum should be performed to identify any primary lesion. In the absence of a primary tendon lesion and fracture, some relief of pain may be gained by draining blood from the sheath. This should be followed by administration of hyaluronan to reduce the risks of subsequent adhesion formation. The horse should be rested for 4 to 6 weeks with administration of nonsteroidal antiinflammatory medication. The prognosis is usually good unless there is underlying primary pathology.

TRAUMA RESULTING IN CHRONIC ENLARGEMENT OF THE CARPAL SHEATH

A horse may have acute distention of the carpal sheath and moderate to severe lameness after a fall. In the acute stage, ultrasonographic examination may reveal only an abnormal amount of fluid within the sheath, but over the next several weeks thickening of the sheath wall and the palmar retinaculum may become apparent, with echogenic fibrous material within the sheath (Figure 75-1). The margin of the SDFT or DDFT may be poorly demarcated, and either structure may be enlarged. Some horses respond satisfactorily to rest and controlled exercise combined with repeated medication of the sheath with hyaluronan. Early aggressive treatment seems to yield the best results. Passive flexion of the carpus also may be beneficial. If lameness persists for more than 6 weeks, endoscopic evaluation of the sheath and its contents should be considered (see Chapter 24).

DESMITIS OF THE ACCESSORY LIGAMENT OF THE SUPERFICIAL DIGITAL FLEXOR TENDON

Desmitis of the ALSDFT is an unusual injury in show jumpers, event horses, dressage horses, and Thoroughbred racehorses, but it seems to occur more commonly in European Standardbred trotters.[8] The condition is rarely recognized in North American trotters.[9] Lameness is usually sudden in onset and associated with localized swelling.

Diagnosis is based on ultrasonographic examination. Abnormalities of the ALSDFT include enlargement, abnormal fiber pattern, and reduced echogenicity. Enlargement of the ALSDFT results in increased distance between the caudal aspect of the radius and the median artery. Injuries to the ALSDFT are often seen with other injuries either in the carpal canal, including superficial digital flexor (SDF) tendonitis or thickening of the flexor retinaculum, or elsewhere.[10,11] These injuries include tenosynovitis of the flexor carpi radialis tendon sheath and suspensory desmitis.

Treatment consists of box rest and controlled exercise for up to 6 months, combined with intrathecal administration of hyaluronan and corticosteroids. The prognosis for horses with simple injuries is fair. Six of eight horses with

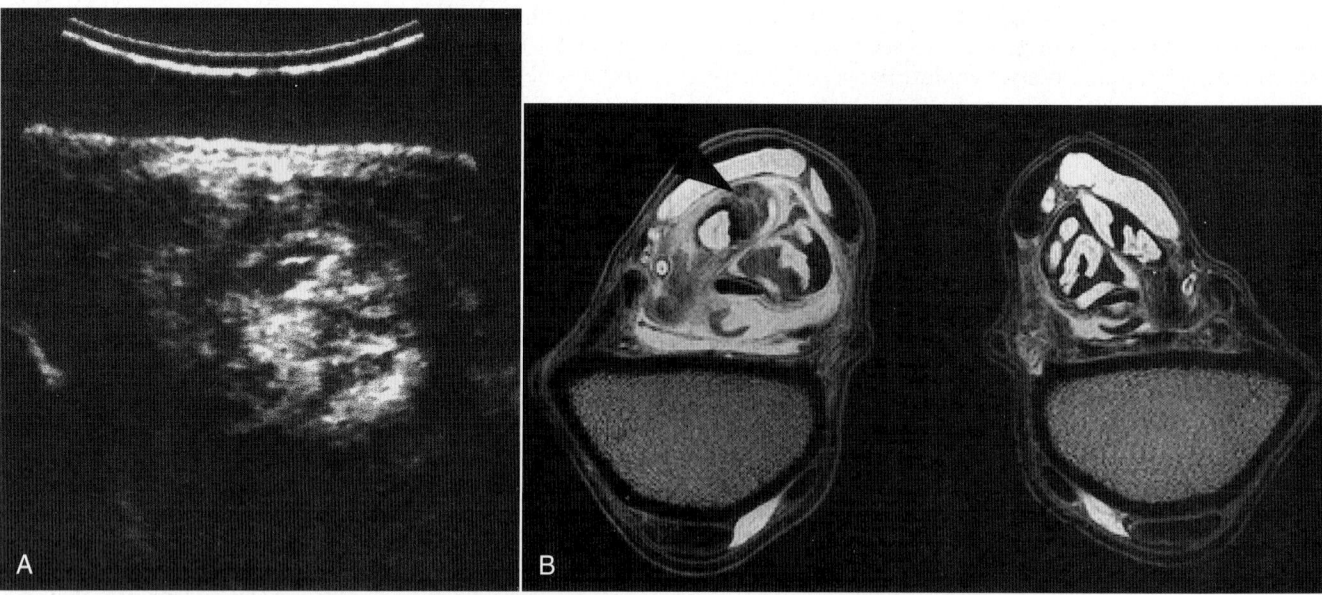

Fig. 75-1 • A, Transverse ultrasonographic image of the carpal sheath of a 9-year-old dressage horse with chronic left forelimb lameness of 3 months' duration. Medial is to the left. There is thickening of the sheath wall and enlargement of the superficial digital flexor tendon (SDFT), but no internal structural abnormality could be defined because of the normal heterogeneous echogenicity of the tendon at this level from muscle tissue. The horse failed to respond to intrathecal medication or endoscopic debridement of the proliferative synovial membrane. **B,** Transverse T2* gradient echo magnetic resonance image of the carpus at the level of the musculotendonous junction of the SDFT of the left *(shown on the left)* and right forelimbs of a horse with chronic left forelimb lameness. There is enlargement of the left fore SDFT. Normal muscle tissue is replaced by an area of low signal intensity consistent with fibrosis *(arrow)*.

uncomplicated desmitis of the ALSDFT returned to the former athletic function.[10] However, horses with concurrent injuries were more likely to suffer recurrent lameness. Debridement of the torn ALSDFT using a tenoscopic approach combined with rest and intrathecal medication was successful in a trotter.[9]

SUPERFICIAL DIGITAL FLEXOR TENDONITIS

Older horses (>15 years of age) and occasionally Standardbred racehorses may show acute SDF tendonitis within the carpal canal (see Chapter 69).[2] In the acute stage, the carpal sheath is distended, but the horse may show no palpable abnormality of the SDFT in the metacarpal region or only slight peritendonous edema proximally. Diagnosis is based on ultrasonographic identification of lesions of the SDFT. In some horses, lesions may not be detectable acutely but may become apparent over the next several weeks. Some older horses initially show SDF tendonitis, which progresses proximally to involve the SDFT within the carpal sheath. These horses have a poor prognosis regardless of the method of management.

Younger horses may develop SDF tendonitis in the proximal metacarpal region. Such lesions may extend proximally into the carpal region, with only slight distention of the carpal sheath. A high proportion of these lesions result in recurrent lameness if treated conservatively. In horses with chronic tendonitis, surgical treatment by desmotomy of the ALSDFT combined with transection of the carpal retinaculum and proximal metacarpal fasciotomy should be considered (see Chapter 69). Moderate results have been achieved in a small number of racehorses and ponies.[9]

INJURY OF THE SUPERFICIAL DIGITAL FLEXOR TENDON AT THE MUSCULOTENDONOUS JUNCTION

Rupture of the SDFT at the musculotendonous junction is usually the result of a fall and is a catastrophic injury meriting humane destruction of the horse. There is rapid development of soft tissue swelling in the antebrachium. The horse is severely distressed and is unable to fully load the limb, and if it tries to do so there is abnormal sinking of the fetlock. Diagnosis is usually made based on the results of clinical examination.

Focal tears of the SDFT at the musculotendonous junction occur rarely and result in moderate to severe lameness associated with distention of the carpal sheath. Diagnosis is based on ultrasonographic examination,[5] which may not be straightforward because the normal muscle tissue is anechogenic. Hematoma formation may be seen as a region of increased echogenicity. Careful comparison with the contralateral limb reveals that the tendon is enlarged, and there may be echogenic material extending from the tendon margins, reflecting tearing. Horses with low-grade lesions within the musculotendonous junction may respond favorably to conservative management but those with large tears warrant a more guarded prognosis. Surgical debridement, performed tenoscopically, has yielded disappointing results, with most horses remaining lame despite prolonged rest.

INJURY OF THE FLEXOR RETINACULUM

Primary injury of the flexor retinaculum is rare but does occasionally occur. More commonly, thickening and loss of echogenicity are seen ultrasonographically in association with other injuries, such as desmitis of the ALSDFT, carpal sheath tenosynovitis, or SDF tendonitis.

DEEP DIGITAL FLEXOR TENDONITIS

Primary deep digital flexor (DDF) tendonitis within the carpal sheath is unusual, but marginal tears have been identified endoscopically in a small number of horses with persistent lameness associated with carpal sheath distention. Surgical debridement has resulted in clinical improvement. Secondary tears on the cranial aspect of the DDFT may occur with a solitary osteochondroma or a distal radial physeal exostosis (see the following sections). Carpal sheath distention with incomplete rupture of the cranial head of the DDFT has been reported.[12] Hemorrhagic fluid was aspirated from the sheath, and disruption of the DDF muscle was identified by ultrasonography.

Occasionally DDF muscle injuries occur proximal to the carpal sheath, resulting in localized swelling and lameness. Ultrasonography is required for definitive diagnosis.[5] Acute injuries result in a region of reduced echogenicity reflecting muscle tearing and hemorrhage, whereas a more chronic injury may be hyperechogenic reflecting hematoma formation or fibrosis. Off-incidence artifact can be used to differentiate between a hematoma and fibrosis.

SOLITARY OSTEOCHONDROMA

An osteochondroma is an exostosis continuous with the cortex of the bone and is covered by cartilage. The distal caudal radius is a common site, immediately proximal to the distal radial physis. An osteochondroma is readily identifiable radiologically and by ultrasonography. Almost invariably an impingement lesion is found on the cranial aspect of the DDFT. Treatment is by surgical removal of the osteochondroma and debridement of any torn fibers of the DDFT. Treatment usually produces an excellent functional and cosmetic result.[2]

DISTAL RADIAL PHYSEAL EXOSTOSES

Small spikes or exostoses may develop on the distal caudal aspect of the radius at the level of the physis.[11] These vary in size and have the potential to create tears in the cranial aspect of the DDFT (Figure 75-2). Importantly, it is the exostoses that occur on midline and not those that can be seen peripherally on oblique radiographic images that irritate and injure the DDFT. Careful examination of a dorsopalmar radiographic image of the carpus is required. Although some can be identified radiologically, others are only identified using ultrasonography. A typical history is of sporadic severe lameness that frequently resolves very rapidly (within hours). The carpal sheath may be mildly to moderately distended at the time of lameness, but in some horses there are no detectable localizing clinical signs, creating a diagnostic challenge. Surgical removal of the spike and debridement of torn tendon fibers usually yield an excellent prognosis.

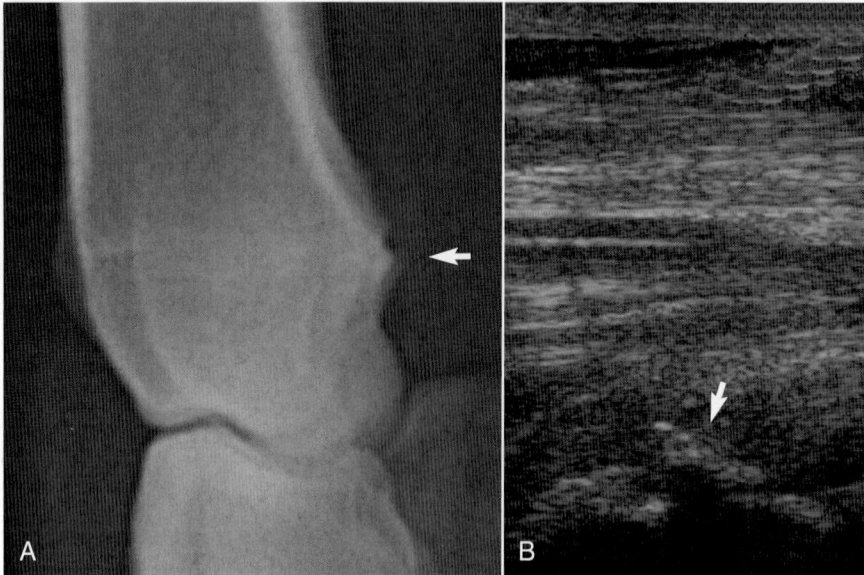

Fig. 75-2 • A, Lateromedial radiographic image of the distal radius of a 7-year-old Warmblood dressage horse with sporadic severe lameness, associated with distention of the carpal sheath. There is a physeal exostosis *(arrow)* on the caudodistal aspect of the radius that was impinging on the deep digital flexor tendon (DDFT). **B,** Longitudinal ultrasonographic image of the carpal sheath obtained from the caudomedial aspect. Proximal is to the right. There is an exostosis *(arrow)* impinging on the DDFT.

FRACTURES OF THE ACCESSORY CARPAL BONE

Fractures of the accessory carpal bone are often the result of a fall and result in acute-onset, moderate to severe lameness (see Chapter 38). The majority have a vertical configuration.[14,15] Reports are conflicting about the incidence of carpal canal syndrome secondary to a fibrous union or nonunion of the accessory carpal bone.[14-16] Seven of 11 horses returned to full athletic function without complications after a vertical (frontal) fracture of the accessory carpal bone, despite healing by fibrous union in the six horses reexamined radiographically.[15] The four remaining horses were sound: two were retired for breeding, and two were used for pleasure riding. I have had similar experience. However, if lameness associated with thickening of the carpal sheath wall persists, resection of a piece of the carpal retinaculum may be successful.[14] Radiographs should be inspected carefully because occasionally chip fractures of the articular margin of the accessory carpal bone occur alone or concurrently with a more typical vertical fracture. Horses with such fractures warrant a more guarded prognosis. Small chip fractures may be removed surgically, but osteoarthritis of the antebrachiocarpal joint may rapidly ensue. Horses with severely comminuted fractures warrant a guarded prognosis.

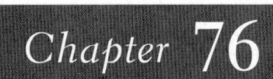

Chapter 76

The Tarsal Sheath

Eddy R.J. Cauvin

References on page 1319

The tarsal sheath corresponds to the synovial sheath of the lateral digital flexor tendon at the level of the hock. Tenosynovitis of this sheath is a well-recognized condition[1-6] and can be caused by a wide range of lesions. Nonpainful, chronic distention in the absence of obvious pathological lesions, often called *idiopathic thoroughpin*, is common and should be distinguished from other debilitating causes of tenosynovitis, many of which can cause persistent, severe lameness.[7,8] Specific lesions within the sheath can be difficult to confirm clinically.[8,9]

FUNCTIONAL ANATOMY

The deep digital flexor tendon (DDFT) in horses is formed by the fusion in the proximal metatarsal region of the thin medial digital flexor tendon and the larger lateral digital flexor tendon.[10-13] The two tendons pass within separate sheaths. The lateral digital flexor muscle covers the caudal aspect of the tibia and is joined by the tibialis caudalis muscle in the distal aspect of the crus. The tendon starts 2 to 4 cm proximal to the tarsocrural joint and passes medial to the tuber calcanei over a fibrocartilage-covered groove on the plantar aspect of the sustentaculum tali of the calcaneus. The lateral digital flexor tendon passes over the thick plantar ligament on the distal, medial aspect of the tarsus, medial to the superficial digital flexor tendon (SDFT), before being joined by the medial digital flexor tendon 1 to 3 cm distal to the tarsometatarsal joint.

The tarsal sheath is 16 to 20 cm long and starts near the musculotendonous junction of the lateral digital flexor

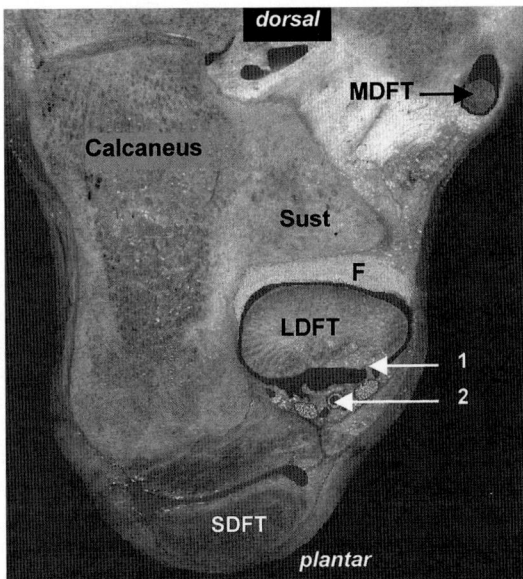

Fig. 76-1 • Transverse section of the proximal tarsus, showing the lateral digital flexor tendon (LDFT) in the fibrocartilaginous groove (F) on the plantar aspect of the sustentaculum tali (Sust). Lateral is to the left. Vessels and nerves course within the retinaculum (2), lateral to the attachment of the mesotendon (1). MDFT, Medial digital flexor tendon; SDFT, superficial digital flexor tendon.

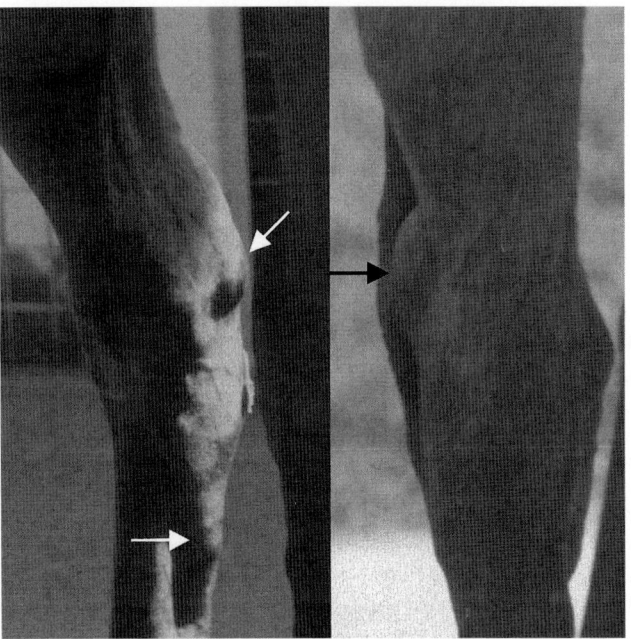

Fig. 76-2 • Distention of the tarsal sheath, giving the typical thoroughpin swelling, medially in the distal caudal aspect of the crus and proximal metatarsal region (white arrows) and laterally, caudal to the tibia (black arrow).

tendon in the distal caudal aspect of the crus. At this level the tarsal sheath forms a large pouch between the lateral digital flexor muscle and the common calcanean tendon. The distended pouch is largest over the lateral aspect of the crus. At the level of the tarsocrural joint the sheath extends laterally to surround the lateral digital flexor tendon. Cranially a rigid groove is formed by fibrocartilaginous thickening of the tarsocrural joint capsule. The sheath terminates as a recess dorsomedial to the DDFT in the proximal third of the metatarsal region.

The tarsal sheath is enclosed at the level of the sustentaculum tali by a thick, transversely oriented ligament, the plantar retinaculum (Figure 76-1), and in the distal tarsus by a superficial fascia. The plantar nerves and vessels run within the retinaculum, in the plantar two thirds of its width, that is, plantar and plantaromedial to the lateral digital flexor tendon. The sheath is lined by a parietal synovial membrane with few villi, except distally. This membrane reflects plantarly to wrap around the tendon, leaving a thin but continuous membrane, or mesotendon, along the plantaromedial aspect of the lateral digital flexor tendon. This membrane carries vessels to the tendon and therefore should be preserved during surgery.

CAUSES OF TARSAL TENOSYNOVITIS

Distention of the tarsal sheath (Figure 76-2) is commonly termed *thoroughpin*, or *true thoroughpin*,[14] but the condition may have distinct causes (see Figure 6-30).

Idiopathic Thoroughpin
Slight to moderate distention of the tarsal sheath is often seen in young horses.[8,9] It also occurs in adults, particularly in Warmbloods and Western performance horses and horses with a straight hock conformation, after extended box rest

or transport. Effusion also may result from acute inflammation in nearby tissues, congestion, and edema in the distal limb (sympathetic effusion). The distention usually is not associated with signs of inflammation or lameness and tends to resolve spontaneously.[8] However, the distention can become recurrent or persistent in some horses.

Traumatic Thoroughpin
Tenosynovitis may be induced by trauma, leading to acute inflammation and hemorrhage in the sheath. In my experience, direct trauma to the medial plantar aspect of the sheath is common and most often results from a kick by another horse. Tenosynovitis also may result from hitting hard objects during jumping or occasionally from interference from the contralateral hind foot. These traumatic injuries may be associated with a chip fracture or fragmentation of the medial edge of the sustentaculum tali at the insertion of the plantar retinaculum.[3,13] Transverse fracture of the calcaneus involving the sustentaculum tali also was described.[3] In most horses no signs of direct trauma are apparent, and overstretching, or sprain, which may or may not involve the lateral digital flexor tendon, is suspected of causing acute tenosynovitis.[8,9] Intrathecal hemorrhage always causes substantial inflammation and pain and can induce the formation of fibrinous adhesions. The inflammation often leads to chronic distention, with synovial thickening, fibrosis, and fibrous adhesion formation between the lateral digital flexor tendon and parietal sheath lining, which occasionally can cause persistent pain and mechanical lameness. Acute tenosynovitis without overt lameness also has been described.[9]

Primary Lateral Digital Flexor Tendon Injuries
Sprain injuries to the lateral digital flexor tendon do occur in the tarsal sheath region and are characterized

ultrasonographically by longitudinal fraying and irregular hypoechoic lesions at the level of the sustentaculum tali. These lesions may be caused by overstretching and compression of the tendon over the bone.

Infectious Tenosynovitis

Direct trauma to the medial aspect of the hock can result in breach and contamination of the tarsal sheath.[3,9,13,15] The medial edge of the sustentaculum tali is the most prominent relief on the medial aspect of the tarsus, and a wound at this level often disrupts the retinaculum, thus opening the sheath.[6,13] Puncture wounds are rare in my experience, but they may occur, especially in the distal caudal aspect of the crus. Iatrogenic contamination induced by intrathecal injection is also common and should be suspected in horses with worsening of the lameness and signs of inflammation after such injections.[9] If untreated, suppurative tenosynovitis may lead to infectious tendonitis, destruction of the fibrocartilage, and eventually osteitis or osteomyelitis of the calcaneus.[3,4,6,13] Infection also may result from extension of abscesses in adjacent tissues.

Other Causes

One horse with hemangiosarcoma involving the tarsal sheath has been described.[7] Chondrosarcomata, extending from the tarsocrural joint, and systemic lupus–like synovitis have been reported as rare causes of thoroughpin.[9]

DIAGNOSIS OF TARSAL SHEATH INJURIES

Clinical Signs

Distention of the tarsal sheath is visible in the distal aspect of the crus, particularly laterally between the common calcanean tendon and the tibia and, to a lesser extent, on the medial caudal aspect of the crus (see Figures 6-30 and 76-2). Such distention should not be confused with swellings associated with the plantar pouch of the tarsocrural joint (see Chapter 44), situated farther distally between the tuber calcanei and distal aspect of the tibia (bog spavin) or with distention of other bursae, for example, the deep calcanean bursa and calcanean bursa of the SDFT (see Chapter 79).[8,10] False thoroughpin may result from soft tissue masses such as hematomata, tarsal sheath herniation, granulation tissue,[8,9] or abscesses (see Chapter 79). Distention of the tarsal sheath also may be detected in the proximal metatarsal region on the medial aspect of the DDFT.

In horses with idiopathic tenosynovitis, the swelling is soft and nonpainful and unassociated with lameness.[9,16] In inflammatory conditions, swelling is soft, warm, and painful in the acute stage and nearly hard and rarely painful in chronic injuries. The degree of lameness varies.[3,7] The level of pain is not always correlated with the severity of the condition. Prominent pain usually is induced by hock flexion in acute and chronic injuries, and the degree of hock flexion may be greatly decreased. Confirming that the lameness is associated with the sheath may be necessary by using intrathecal injection of 5 to 10 mL of local anesthetic solution and by elimination of other sources of pain. Synoviocentesis may be difficult in horses with acute injuries because of edematous, hypertrophic, and congested synovial membrane.

Confirming infection is not always easy in all horses in the absence of a wound. Wounds over the sustentaculum tali always should be considered suspicious and warrant a contrast tenovaginogram or tenovaginocentesis.

Radiography

Radiographic examination is paramount in all horses with severe tarsal tenosynovitis to rule out fractures or osteitis of the sustentaculum tali and tuber calcanei (see Chapter 44).[2-4,13] Lesions are most visible on dorsoplantar and dorsomedial-plantarolateral oblique images to highlight the medial and plantaromedial aspects of the calcaneus (Figure 76-3). A flexed skyline image of the plantar aspect of the sustentaculum tali (flexed proximocaudal-distoplantar image) is essential to demonstrate some lesions[17] (Figure 76-4). Contrast radiography is also useful to highlight the surface of the fibrocartilage and the outline of the lateral digital flexor tendon[18] but has been replaced largely by ultrasonography.[12] However, contrast radiography remains a useful technique to confirm puncture wounds into the sheath. After collecting synovial fluid, 5 mL of an iodinated contrast medium mixed with 5 mL of Hartman's solution is injected in the proximal pouch of the sheath, and lateromedial, dorsomedial-plantarolateral oblique, and dorsoplantar radiographic images are obtained to highlight a communication with the skin.

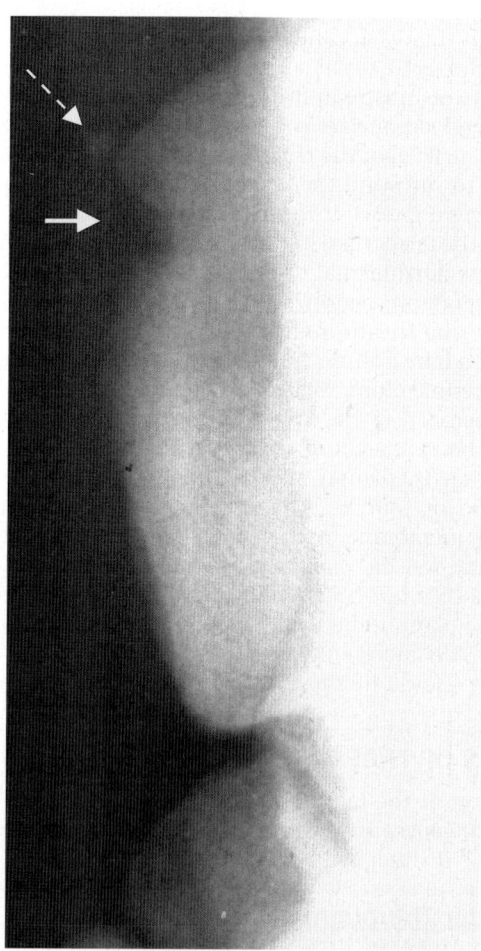

Fig. 76-3 • Dorsomedial-plantarolateral oblique radiographic image of the calcaneus, showing erosion *(plain arrow)* and fragmentation *(dotted arrow)* of the edge of the sustentaculum tali.

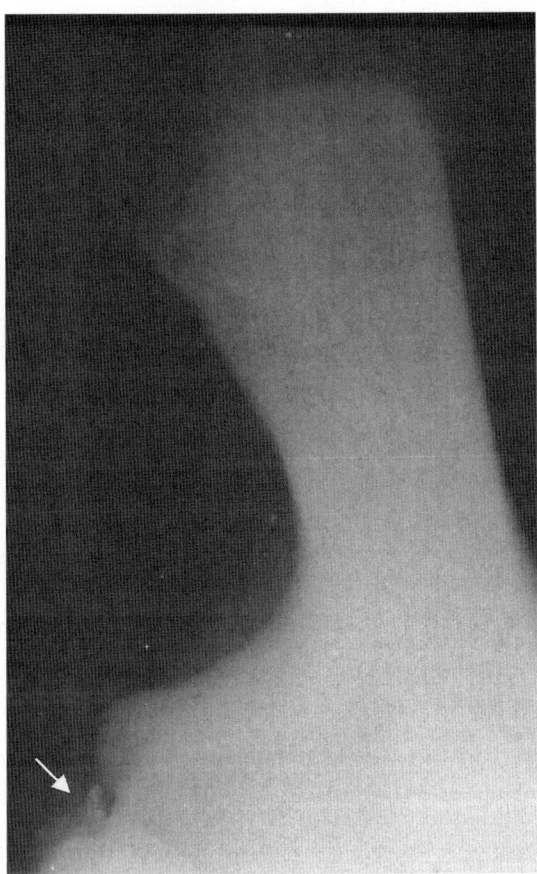

Fig. 76-4 • Skyline radiographic image of the calcaneus, highlighting fragmentation of the edge of the sustentaculum tali *(arrow)*, medial to the groove.

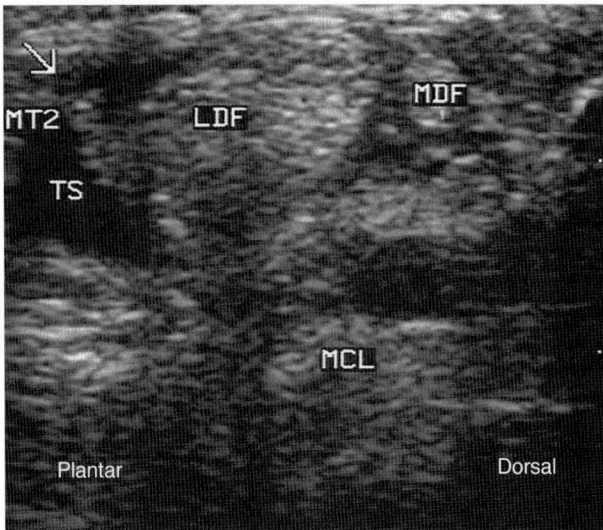

Fig. 76-5 • Transverse ultrasonographic image of the tarsal sheath at the level of the tarsometatarsal joint obtained from the plantaromedial aspect. Plantar is to the left. There is hyperplasia of the synovial membrane around the lateral digital flexor tendon *(LDF)* and a well-organized adhesion between the tendon and parietal sheath wall *(arrow)*. The tarsal sheath *(TS)* is distended. *MCL,* Medial collateral ligament; *MT2,* plantar border of the second metatarsal bone; *MDF,* medial digital flexor tendon.

Ultrasonography

Ultrasonographic examination of the tarsal sheath is best performed with a linear 7.5-MHz or higher-frequency transducer. The lateral digital flexor tendon is best imaged from the medial aspect of the limb.[12,13,19] Accurate imaging requires high-definition equipment and experience. The chestnut can be trimmed and soaked with warm water to improve imaging. In idiopathic distention, the sheath is filled with anechogenic fluid, and no evidence of synovial membrane hyperplasia is apparent. In acute tenosynovitis, the sheath is distended, and substantial thickening of the synovial membrane occurs. Hemorrhage is seen frequently as a hypoechogenic, whorl-like structure in the proximal pouch. Lesions may be seen in the lateral digital flexor tendon, but they are relatively rare. Longitudinal tears and superficial fraying are the most common types of lesions, but they should not be confused with hyperplasia of the visceral synovium covering the tendon. Early fibrinous adhesions may be visible. The integrity of the fibrocartilage groove and retinaculum can be assessed, and fragmentation of the edge of the sustentaculum tali may be detected.[8,13] In chronic injuries, substantial fibrosis may be seen around the sheath, and often there are large adhesions between the lateral digital flexor tendon and parietal sheath, especially in the proximal pouch (Figure 76-5). The visceral lining is usually thick (several millimeters) and has increased echogenicity. Horses with chronic lameness and those that have received numerous injections of

corticosteroids may have large, nodular fibrocartilaginous or partially mineralized masses, termed *ossicles.*[2,9] Differentiating these from chip fractures or mineralization of the tendon or sheath lining without the use of tenoscopy may be difficult. Ultrasonography can help to differentiate true from false thoroughpin (see Chapter 79). Infection is characterized by severe inflammation of the synovial lining, and the fluid is often echogenic and heterogeneous because of the fibrin clots and debris.[6,13] This may not be obvious early in the condition.

Tenovaginocentesis

Tenovaginocentesis (collecting fluid from the tendon sheath) is useful to rule out infection and confirm inflammation.[9,15] The fluid may be normal in appearance, but it is usually contaminated by blood. A moderate increase of cellularity (<8000/mcL) may be evident, except in horses with acute traumatic injuries where the nucleated cell count can exceed 10,000/mcL. Generally infection is associated with a thin, cloudy to purulent fluid and cell counts well in excess of 10,000/mcL. Note that centesis should be carried out after ultrasonography to avoid bleeding and gas artifacts.

Tenoscopy

Tenoscopy (see Chapter 24) is rarely necessary as a purely diagnostic method because the tarsal sheath is evaluated adequately with ultrasonography in most horses. A major exception is in infectious conditions, where it may be useful to assess potential damage to the fibrocartilages, which may not be visible with other diagnostic imaging methods.[13,20]

MANAGEMENT OF TARSAL TENOSYNOVITIS

Idiopathic and Traumatic Tenosynovitis

Treatment is of little value in horses with idiopathic tenosynovitis, which generally resolves spontaneously.[8,9,16]

Reduced (but not interrupted) exercise, sweats, and systemic antiinflammatory therapy can be helpful.[9] It is not advisable to place a needle in the sheath because this may cause bleeding and subsequent inflammation.

Treatment of acute tenosynovitis is controversial. In the absence of tendon or bony lesions, rest, systemic or local nonsteroidal antiinflammatory drugs (NSAIDs), local dimethylsulfoxide creams, and cryotherapy (ice packs or cold hosing) are often effective.[9] The horse should be rested in a box for 24 to 48 hours and then walked out in hand to reduce sheath fibrosis. Hyaluronan may be useful for horses with more severe tenosynovitis or in horses in which lateral digital flexor tendon lesions are present. Intrathecal corticosteroids may be useful in horses with acute tenosynovitis, but they certainly are contraindicated if tendon lesions exist. The latter carry a poor prognosis, except for superficial fraying.[8,9] Bone fragments should be removed by tenoscopy because they can cause chronic inflammation and interference with the tendon.

In horses with more chronic tenosynovitis with associated lameness, corticosteroids such as methylprednisolone acetate (40 mg), triamcinolone acetonide (10 mg), or betamethasone have been used with varying success.[8,9] Fluid retrieval to decrease the volume of the sheath, followed by rest and the application of pressure bandages may produce temporary relief of the distention,[9] but recurrence is common, probably because of chronic proliferative synovitis. Recurrent swelling is often worse than originally seen. Repeated injections have been associated with mineralization of the tendon and synovial lining, and rupture of the lateral digital flexor tendon was reported[9]; therefore repeated injections are not recommended. If possible, the cause of the chronic inflammation should be ascertained. With bony fragments, ossicles, or adhesions, conservative treatment and medical therapy are often disappointing, and surgical debridement appears to be the most effective treatment.[9,13] Debridement is best achieved by tenoscopy (see Chapter 24) (Figure 76-6). NSAIDs are administered for 1 to 2 weeks postoperatively, and the horse is restricted

to box rest for 10 days, after which handwalking starts several times daily. The horse may be turned out in a small paddock or ridden gently after 2 to 3 weeks. Hyaluronan may be injected intrathecally at least 10 days after surgery.

Infectious Tenosynovitis

Horses with acute infectious tenosynovitis may be treated by thorough lavage of the tarsal sheath, with 5 L of sterile, polyionic isotonic fluids, through large-bore catheters or needles placed in the proximal pouch and distal recess of the sheath.[9,15] Lavage may be carried out in the standing horse, but it is best performed with the horse under general anesthesia for accurate needle placement and use of a high-velocity, high-pressure lavage system. This technique is less useful if purulent material, adhesions, or bony lesions are present. These horses are best treated by tenoscopic lavage and debridement.[13] All debris and hypertrophic synovium, frayed areas on the lateral digital flexor tendon, and lesions on the sustentaculum tali (Figure 76-7) are debrided, preferably using motorized equipment, and bone fragments are removed. Drains are rarely necessary, except with recurrent infectious tenosynovitis, but in horses with chronic lameness, leaving a 2- to 4-cm incision (the endoscopic portal) open for drainage is advisable. If a wound is present at the level of the sustentaculum tali, this may be used as an endoscopic portal and then enlarged and left to heal by second intention. Drainage can be prolonged, and primary closure and use of a closed suction drain may be preferable. Fragmentation and osteitis of the sustentaculum tali outside the sheath are best approached through a separate incision. Curettage to the level of healthy bone is performed. Damage to the long medial collateral ligament of the tarsus should be assessed. Aminoglycoside antimicrobial drugs may be inserted into the tarsal sheath at the end of surgery. The horse is treated with systemic broad-spectrum antibiotics (see Chapter 65) for at least 2 weeks postoperatively. NSAIDs are used for at least 5 days and may be continued as necessary. A pressure bandage is applied from foot to midcrus

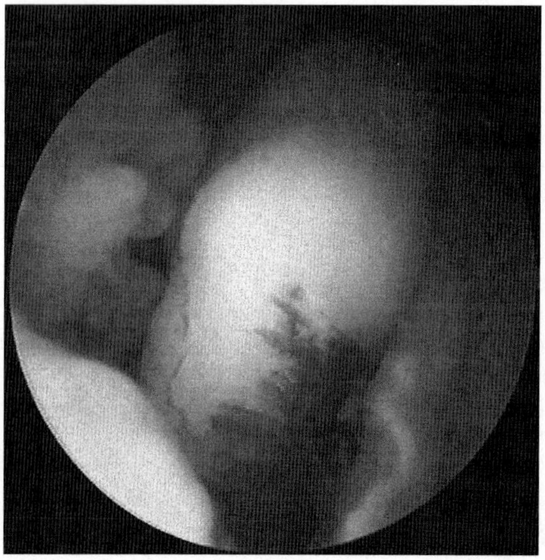

Fig. 76-6 • Tenoscopic view of the tarsal sheath at the level of the sustentaculum tali. A large ossicle is seen lateral to the lateral digital flexor tendon.

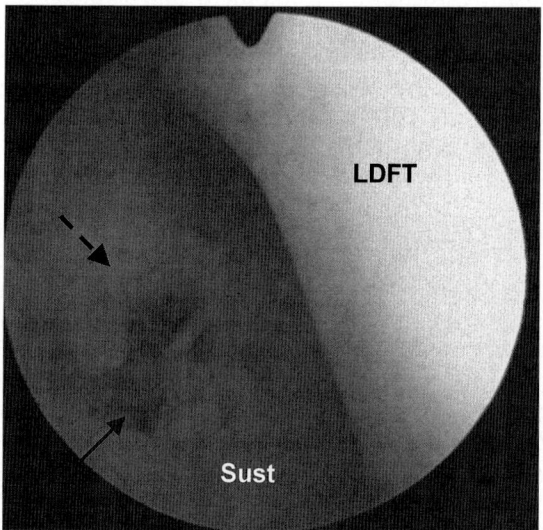

Fig. 76-7 • Tenoscopic view of the tarsal sheath at the level of the sustentaculum tali *(Sust)*. A small erosion in the fibrocartilage *(plain arrow)*, surrounded by fibrinous pannus *(dotted arrow)*, is secondary to subacute infectious tenosynovitis. *LDFT,* Lateral digital flexor tendon.

and changed every 1 to 3 days, depending on the amount of exudate produced. The horse should be rested in a box until the wound has healed and then walked out in hand for 2 to 3 weeks before being turned out in a small paddock.

In horses with chronic infectious tenosynovitis with substantial damage to the fibrocartilaginous groove on the sustentaculum tali or to the lateral digital flexor tendon, open surgery was advocated.[6,8] The tarsal sheath is approached through a desmotomy (longitudinal transection) of the flexor retinaculum to debride all the lesions, followed by the application of a fenestrated drain and repeated lavages for several days. The retinaculum is left unsutured to relieve pressure, and the skin is closed over it.[6] A tenectomy of the damaged lateral digital flexor tendon within the sheath was performed in one horse unresponsive to this approach. However, this was associated with clinically significant complications from poor healing of the wound. In another horse, midmetatarsal tenotomy of the DDFT was carried out, with a heel extension shoe applied to prevent digital hyperextension. This decreased the lameness, presumably by decreasing shearing of the lateral digital flexor tendon on the roughened sustentaculum tali. In my opinion, most horses respond to tenoscopic treatment. More aggressive techniques should be reserved for horses that are unresponsive or those with severe damage to the tendon.

Prognosis

The prognosis is good in horses with idiopathic thoroughpin,[8,9,16] although some horses may have persistent, nonpainful distention of the tarsal sheath. In these horses surgery to imbricate the stretched synovial sheath has been advocated,[9] but recurrence is common. The prognosis is fair in horses with acute tenosynovitis treated medically[8,9] and in horses with chip fractures of the sustentaculum tali treated by tenoscopy.[13] In chronic traumatic tenosynovitis, some horses may respond to a single injection of corticosteroids,[3] but most have recurrent distention and lameness caused by adhesion formation and peritenovaginal fibrosis. These may respond well to tenoscopic treatment,[13] but a guarded prognosis should be given if lameness is a prominent feature. In horses with infection the prognosis is fair with prompt drainage and curettage, but poor in horses with severe tendon lesions or extensive damage to the sustentaculum tali.[2,4,9] A fair prognosis was reported with aggressive surgical debridement in horses with osteitis/osteomyelitis of the sustentaculum tali, even if chronic.[20]

Chapter 77

Extensor Tendon Injury

Jane C. Boswell and Michael C. Schramme

The extensor tendons of the carpus and digit and the respective synovial sheaths are vulnerable to injury because they lie relatively unprotected in the subcutaneous fascia on the dorsal surface of the limb. This chapter discusses lameness caused by injuries and disorders of the extensor tendons of the carpus and digit. Injuries of the extensor tendons of the hock (gastrocnemius and calcaneal tendons) are discussed elsewhere (see Chapter 80).

ANATOMY

The extensor carpi radialis (ECR) muscle is the largest extensor muscle of the forelimb and has a prominent muscle belly on the cranial aspect of the antebrachium. The ECR muscle extends the carpus, smoothes carpal joint movement by dampening oscillations as the hoof strikes the ground, and flexes the elbow.[1,2] The extensor carpi radialis tendon (ECRT) extends through most of the muscle belly and appears on the surface of the muscle in the middle of the antebrachium. The tendon passes through the middle groove at the distal end of the radius, over the dorsal aspect of the carpus, and inserts on the metacarpal tuberosity on the dorsal proximal aspect of the third metacarpal bone.[1] As the tendon passes over the carpus, it is bound by the extensor retinaculum and enveloped by a synovial sheath, which extends from 8 to 10 cm proximal to the carpus, to the level of the middle carpal joint. Distal to the sheath the ECRT is attached to the carpometacarpal joint capsule. There is usually a small bursa beneath the tendon at the level of the third carpal bone.[1,3]

The common digital extensor (CDE) muscle is a compound muscle with three heads (humeral, radial, and ulnar) that lies lateral to the ECR muscle on the craniolateral aspect of the radius and acts to extend the digit and carpal joints and to flex the elbow. The main common digital extensor tendon (CDET) appears on the surface of the muscle in the middle of the antebrachium and passes distally through the lateral groove on the cranial distal aspect of the radius and over the capsule of the carpal joints. As the tendon passes distally over the dorsal aspect of the metacarpal region, it courses medially and reaches the dorsal midline just proximal to the fetlock. At the level of the distal aspect of the proximal phalanx the tendon becomes wider as it is joined by extensor branches of the interosseous tendon (suspensory ligament). The CDET inserts on the extensor process of the distal phalanx and the dorsal surface of the proximal extremities of the proximal and middle phalanges.

The CDET is enveloped by a synovial sheath as it passes over the carpus. The sheath extends from about 8 cm proximal to the carpus to the proximal end of the metacarpal region.[1,3] A bursa is present between the tendon and the dorsal pouch of the fetlock joint capsule.[1,3,4]

A small tendon also arises from the smaller head (the radial head) of the CDE muscle. This tendon runs through the synovial sheath of the principal tendon and then passes laterally to fuse with the lateral digital extensor tendon (LDET) or may continue separately between the CDET and LDET to the fetlock. A small tendon may also arise from the ulnar head of the CDE muscle, which either fuses with the principal tendon or inserts on the joint capsule dorsal to the fetlock joint.

eferences on page 1320

The lateral digital extensor (LDE) muscle is smaller than the other extensor muscles and is situated caudal to the CDE muscle. The action of the LDE muscle is to extend the digit and carpus. The LDET arises at the level of the distal third of the antebrachium and passes distally through the groove on the lateral styloid process of the radius and over the lateral aspect of the carpus. The tendon becomes larger and flattens distal to the carpus as it joins the tendon of the radial head of the CDE muscle and a strong band from the accessory carpal bone. The LDET runs lateral to the CDET and gradually inclines toward the dorsal aspect of the metacarpal region and inserts on the eminence on the dorsal proximal aspect of the proximal phalanx.[1]

A synovial sheath envelops the LDET as it passes over the carpus. It begins 6 to 8 cm proximal to the carpus and extends to the proximal end of the metacarpal region.[1,3] At the fetlock a small bursa lies between the tendon and the joint capsule.[1]

The extensor carpi obliquus is a small muscle that extends the carpus. The tendon of the extensor carpi obliquus arises at the distal end of the radius and courses distally, cranially, and medially over the ECRT and then passes through the oblique groove at the distal end of the radius to insert on the base (head) of the second metacarpal bone. The tendon is enveloped by a synovial sheath.[1]

In the hindlimb, the long digital extensor (LoDE) muscle is situated superficially on the craniolateral aspect of the limb and acts to extend the digit and flex the hock. The tendon of the muscle begins in the middle of the muscle belly and passes distally over the dorsal aspect of the hock, where the tendon is bound by the extensor retinacula and enveloped by a synovial sheath. The sheath extends from slightly proximal to the level of the lateral malleolus of the tibia to the proximal third of the metatarsal region. The long digital extensor tendon (LoDET) is joined by the LDET about 10 cm distal to the tarsus. In the angle of this union the extensor digitorum brevis also joins the principal tendon of the LoDE.[1] Distal to this point the arrangement of tendons is the same as in the forelimb.

The LDE muscle lies on the lateral surface of the crus caudal to the LoDE muscle. The LDET runs through the entire length of the muscle belly and emerges at the level of the distal third of the tibia. The tendon descends through the groove on the lateral malleolus of the tibia, where it is bound by the extensor retinacula, and usually blends with the LoDET. In some horses the tendon does not insert on the LoDET but passes separately lateral to the LoDET and inserts on the eminence on the dorsal proximal aspect of the proximal phalanx, like the corresponding tendon in the forelimb.[1] The tendon is surrounded by a synovial sheath that extends from 4 to 6 cm above the lateral malleolus of the tibia to the proximal third of the metatarsal region.[1,3]

DIAGNOSTIC TECHNIQUES

Many disorders of the extensor tendons, particularly acute injuries, may be diagnosed by careful clinical examination, gait analysis, and palpation. Diagnostic perineural or intrathecal analgesia may be useful in horses with chronic injuries to the extensor tendons to determine the importance of clinical findings. Synoviocentesis of distended tendon sheaths or bursae also may be helpful to distinguish between tenosynovitis caused by injury or infection.

Plain radiography is of little value in identifying soft tissue injuries of the extensor tendons unless radiodense foreign material or bone fragments are present. Radiology may be useful to evaluate mineralization within the tendons or the synovial sheaths, enthesopathy, and associated osseous abnormalities. Contrast radiography may demonstrate a penetrating tract, intrathecal adhesions, or synovial fistulae between the extensor tendon sheaths and carpal joints.[5,6]

Ultrasonography is a safe, noninvasive method of evaluating the extensor tendons, the synovial sheaths, and the bursae. A 7.5- or 10-MHz transducer and standoff pad are used to image the extensor tendons and the respective tendon sheaths. Careful evaluation of transverse and longitudinal images allows the clinician to determine the extent of tendon damage, the presence of foreign bodies within the tendon or tendon sheaths, synovial membrane hyperplasia, and intrathecal adhesions.[7]

CONDITIONS AFFECTING THE EXTENSOR TENDONS

Laceration of the Digital Extensor Tendons

Lacerations of the extensor tendons commonly occur in the metacarpal or metatarsal regions of the limbs because of their superficial location at these sites (see Chapter 81). Extensor tendon lacerations are more common in the hindlimb[8-11] and are frequently associated with considerable soft tissue damage and opening of the extensor tendon sheaths.

Transection of an extensor tendon below the carpus or tarsus leads to reduced ability to extend the digit, which results in an exaggerated, rapid flip of the hoof at the end of the swing phase of the stride, intermittent knuckling over at the fetlock, or tripping at the walk. The horse, however, will bear weight in a normal posture if the foot is placed flat on the ground. This gait abnormality is more obvious in horses with hindlimb injuries and when the laceration is near the fetlock because remaining peritendonous fascial attachments provide some support to the distal part of the tendon in more proximal injuries.

Lacerations with transection of the extensor tendons proximal to the carpus, and at or just proximal to the tarsus, are also common. Transection of the CDET and ECRT commonly occurs proximal to the carpus and often results in pain on flexion of the carpus. Transection of the LoDET proximal to or at the tarsus results in greater tarsal flexion during the swing phase of the stride and intermittent knuckling of the digit. Within a few days of transection of an extensor tendon the horse learns to adapt its gait, and tripping and knuckling of the fetlock become less frequent.

The diagnosis of extensor tendon laceration is often apparent from the gait deficit. If necessary, the diagnosis may be confirmed by exploration of the wound with a sterile, gloved finger after aseptic preparation and wound lavage. Plain and contrast radiography should be used to evaluate concomitant joint or bone damage and to help to identify foreign bodies.

After aseptic preparation, wounds over the extensor tendons should be debrided and lavaged. It is important to debride any exposed or obviously devitalized bone and, where possible, to cover bone with skin to reduce the risk of sequestrum formation. Primary apposition of the lacerated tendon is unnecessary even if a large gap has formed between the distracted tendon ends. Progressive ultrasonographic evaluations show that fibrous tissue develops between the transected tendon ends; this tissue gradually becomes more organized and regains the linear arrangement of collagen along the line of the original tendon. This fibrous tissue provides an adequate mechanical link between the tendon ends, allowing extensor function of the digit to return.[12]

Although lacerations of extensor tendons may heal without external coaptation, wound healing is facilitated and exuberant granulation tissue formation is controlled if limb immobilization is used during the first 3 to 6 weeks after injury. Immobilization may be achieved using a polyvinylchloride (PVC) splint or cast. Full-limb PVC splints may be applied to the dorsal or palmar aspect of the forelimb to prevent knuckling of the fetlock and carpal flexion. In the hindlimb, a distal limb splint applied to the dorsal or plantar aspect of the limb can be used. Application of a shoe with a toe extension may help facilitate flat foot placement and prevent tripping or knuckling over of the fetlock in the early postinjury period. Casts provide an inexpensive and efficient means of immobilizing the limb and tendon ends and are especially useful when extensor tendon lacerations occur with extensive, contaminated wounds, in which primary wound closure cannot be achieved.

After removal of the cast or splint, the horse should remain confined to a box stall for another 4 to 6 weeks. During this period the toe should be trimmed short so that it does not catch to cause knuckling and disruption of the organizing fibrous tissue. A controlled exercise program of in-hand walking exercise may be initiated at this time to strengthen the tendon and improve gliding function. Passive range of movement exercises may also be beneficial. If no signs of knuckling are present after 10 to 12 weeks of controlled exercise, a gradual return to athletic use may begin.

The prognosis for return to athletic function after extensor laceration is good.[8-11] In a retrospective study of 156 horses with extensor tendon lacerations, 74% returned to soundness and 60% of sports horses returned to previous activity at the same, or higher, level.[10] In this study there was a significant influence on positive outcome if primary closure of the wound was performed, with horses 2.6 times more likely to return to soundness compared with those horses in which wound closure was not performed. Complications in that study included wound infection and dehiscence, exuberant granulation tissue, and sequestrum formation. Stringhalt may also occur as a complication of lacerations or injury to the extensor tendons in the dorsoproximal aspect of the metatarsal region. It is speculated that stringhalt may result from adhesion formation, which decreases the ability of the long or LDETs to stretch during hock flexion, or from abnormalities in the myotatic reflex, which governs extensor muscle tone and relaxation.[13]

Rupture of the Common Digital Extensor Tendon

Rupture of the CDET occurs in foals and may be present at birth or may develop within the first few weeks of life. This

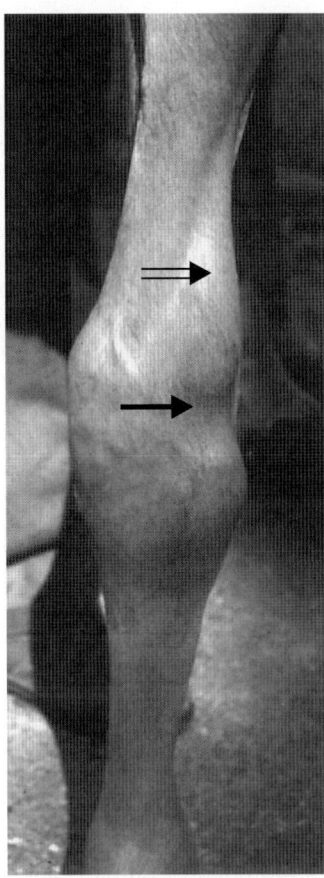

Fig. 77-1 • Fluctuant swelling over the dorsolateral aspect of the carpus in a foal with rupture of the common digital extensor tendon (CDET). The injury shows the typical transverse depression in the sheath where the CDET has ruptured *(solid arrow)* and the bulge in the sheath where the transected distal part of the tendon is situated *(open arrow).*

condition may be primary or secondary to flexural deformities of the carpus or metacarpophalangeal joint that result in increased tension in the CDET.[14] Rupture of the CDET may be an inherited condition because Arabians and Quarter Horses were overrepresented in one retrospective study.[15]

As rupture of the CDET always occurs within the synovial sheath,[14] affected foals have a characteristic fluctuant swelling over the dorsolateral aspect of the carpus at the level of the distal carpal joints (Figure 77-1). Palpation reveals fluid distention of the tendon sheath, and the ruptured ends of the CDET can usually be identified. Affected foals may have a normal stance but often stand with the carpus slightly flexed (over-at-the-knee appearance) and frequently knuckle forward on the fetlock. Most affected foals, however, quickly accommodate the gait and learn to flip the distal aspect of the limb during the swing phase of the stride.

Diagnosis of rupture of the CDET is based on careful palpation and is confirmed by ultrasonography. Radiography of the carpus should be performed to rule out cuboidal bone malformation.

In foals with primary injuries without associated flexural deformities, treatment usually involves box rest and the application of well-padded bandages to support the carpus and prevent abrasion of the dorsum of the fetlock.

In foals that exhibit frequent knuckling over on the fetlock, or foals with concurrent flexural deformities of the carpus, a PVC splint should be applied to the palmar aspect of the limb, extending from the elbow to the fetlock. For foals with concurrent cuboidal bone malformation, tube casts from the elbow to the fetlock should be used to provide carpal support. Foals with splints usually walk comfortably, and sufficient fibrosis has usually developed after 2 to 4 weeks to allow removal of the splints. However, the foal should be maintained in padded bandages for several more weeks to maintain pressure on the area of tendon rupture to minimize the resultant blemish.

It has been suggested that the ruptured ends of the CDET are unlikely to reunite but adhere to the tendon sheath and that the LDET assumes the function of the CDET.[15] However, anecdotal evidence indicates that the tendon ends may rejoin in some horses.[16] Consequently, foals with primary rupture of the CDET, without concurrent cuboidal bone malformation, usually have an excellent prognosis for athletic performance with minimal blemish. Foals with concurrent cuboidal bone malformation or flexural deformities have a more guarded prognosis for athletic performance.[17,18]

RUPTURE OF THE EXTENSOR CARPI RADIALIS TENDON

Rupture of the ECRT is a rare condition of adult horses.[15] Partial rupture may also occur rarely, particularly in horses that are used for jumping.[19] Complete and partial rupture of the ECRT usually occurs within the synovial sheath on the dorsal aspect of the carpus. The injury is believed to result from trauma associated with repeated overflexion of the carpus.[15] Partial rupture of the ECRT was reported to be a consequence of tendon damage caused by exostoses on the distal aspect of the radius.[19]

Acute rupture of the ECRT is characterized by pain and distention of the tendon sheath. Extension and flexion of the carpus are limited, which may result in dragging of the toe.[20] In horses with chronic injuries of the ECRT, distention of the tendon sheath persists but is usually painless unless an associated inflammatory tenosynovitis occurs.

Complete rupture of the ECRT results in excessive carpal flexion during limb protraction and consequently a higher arc of foot flight in the affected limb. Limb extension may be characterized by a double movement as the carpus suddenly snaps into extension.[21,22] Atrophy of the ECR muscle may be evident in horses with chronic injuries. Partial rupture of the ECRT may be associated with mild lameness and restricted carpal flexion.[19]

Diagnosis of rupture of the ECRT may be confirmed by careful palpation, ultrasonography, and contrast radiography.[6,7] Plain radiography should be used to evaluate associated osseous lesions.

Horses with acute, complete rupture of the ECRT may be treated surgically. Tenosynovectomy with primary suturing of the tendon ends, or substitution of the extensor carpi obliquus tendon by tendon anastomosis, has been described.[15] Other authors, however, believe that surgical apposition of the tendon ends is unnecessary and advocate tenoscopy, which allows characterization of the extent of the injury, debridement of the damaged tendon ends, and lavage of the sheath. After surgery the limb should be

immobilized in a tube cast or splint for 2 to 4 weeks. Once the cast and sutures have been removed, passive range-of-movement exercises should be instituted to prevent the formation of intrathecal adhesions and to reduce carpal joint capsule fibrosis, which result in a limited range of carpal flexion. The prognosis for return to athletic performance for horses with complete rupture of the ECRT is unfavorable. The prognosis for return to athletic performance for horses with partial rupture of the ECRT is guarded to fair, but tenolysis and partial tenosynovectomy may benefit some horses.[15,20]

Trauma to the Extensor Carpi Radialis Tendon

Single episode trauma, such as a kick injury, or repetitive trauma from hitting fixed cross-country fences or pawing at a door, may result in a primary injury of the ECRT, often accompanied by tenosynovitis, with or without adhesion formation between the tendon and tendon sheath. Such injuries may be accompanied by new bone formation on the distal aspect of the radius. The ECRT is usually palpably enlarged, with associated distention of the tendon sheath. Ultrasonographic examination confirms enlargement of the tendon and determines the extent of injury to the tendon and the presence of adhesion formation. Although horses with mild injuries often respond well to medical management, those with severe injuries may require en bloc surgical removal of the injured tendon and the synovial lining of the tendon sheath. Cosmetic results are often poor, but the prognosis for athletic function is reasonable.

Enthesopathy of the Insertion of the Extensor Carpi Radialis Tendon

In the racing Standardbred, tearing of the ECRT attachment at its insertion on the proximodorsal aspect of the third metacarpal bone can cause lameness, and these tears may play a role in the cause of fractures of the dorsomedial aspect of the proximal end of the third metacarpal bone (see Chapter 37).[23]

CONDITIONS AFFECTING THE EXTENSOR TENDON SHEATHS

Tenosynovitis

Idiopathic Tenosynovitis

Idiopathic tenosynovitis may be defined as swelling with synovial effusion but without active inflammation, pain, or lameness.[15] Idiopathic tenosynovitis of the extensor tendon sheaths has been reported in foals at birth.[24] In adults the condition tends to develop insidiously. The pathogenesis in newborn foals is unknown, but in adult horses the pathogenesis is presumed to be caused by chronic trauma.[15] However, distention of the LoDE sheath in hindlimbs often occurs bilaterally, is unassociated with any history of trauma, and is of unknown cause.

Ultrasonographic examination usually reveals anechogenic fluid within the sheath. Occasionally, hypoechoic lesions are identified within the enclosed tendon, the clinical significance of which is unknown because lameness is rarely present.

As idiopathic tenosynovitis usually is not associated with pain or lameness, treatment is unnecessary unless the owner is concerned about cosmesis. Treatment by injection of corticosteroids (10 to 20 mg triamcinolone acetonide or 40 to 80 mg methylprednisolone acetate) and pressure bandaging often only provides a temporary resolution of tendon sheath effusion.[15] Anecdotal reports suggest that intrathecal injection of 4 to 15 mg of atropine sulfate, alone or with corticosteroids and hyaluronan, may cause permanent resolution of the effusion. Atropine sulfate is purported to reduce the production of synovial fluid from synoviocytes; however, its anticholinergic effects mean that its use has been associated with transient signs of mild colic and depression. The Editors have never recognized any side effects of intrathecal injection of atropine.

Acute Traumatic Tenosynovitis

Acute tenosynovitis is characterized by a rapidly developing effusion of a tendon sheath, accompanied by heat, pain, and variable lameness. Acute tenosynovitis of the extensor tendon sheaths is often caused by trauma, such as a fall or hitting a jump with the carpus.[19] This injury is common in event horses, in which it often is not associated with lameness.[16]

Diagnosis of acute tenosynovitis is based on clinical signs and ultrasonography. Ultrasonography is useful to evaluate concurrent tendonitis of the extensor tendons and to differentiate acute tenosynovitis from other conditions that are associated with soft tissue swelling over the dorsal aspect of the carpus, including hygroma, cellulitis, synovial hernia, and effusion of the carpal joints (see Chapter 38).

Horses with acute tenosynovitis of an extensor tendon sheath are treated by rest, cold hydrotherapy, and nonsteroidal antiinflammatory drugs (NSAIDs). Aspiration of fluid and injection of corticosteroids are reserved for horses that do not respond to more than 1 week of conservative treatment.[25]

Infectious Tenosynovitis

Infectious tenosynovitis is characterized by dramatic synovial effusion, heat, pain, swelling, and severe lameness. Contamination from a penetrating wound is the most common cause of infectious tenosynovitis, but infection also may arise from hematogenous spread of bacteria and iatrogenic infection.[26] Infection of the CDET sheath has been reported as a complication of hemicircumferential periosteal transection.[27] After penetration of a tendon sheath, severe lameness does not become evident unless infection becomes established. If the tendon sheath is open and draining, then the lameness may be less severe.[28]

Once infection is established, rapid and aggressive treatment is necessary to prevent synovial hyperplasia, fibrosis of the tendon sheath, intrathecal adhesion formation, and damage to the extensor tendons. Prompt recognition of infectious tenosynovitis is essential for a successful outcome. Diagnosis of infectious tenosynovitis is based on clinical signs and must be confirmed by synovial fluid aspiration and analysis. Infected synovial fluid is typically turbid and has a low viscosity, an elevated total nucleated cell count ($>30 \times 10^9$/L, with more than 90% neutrophils), and a total protein concentration of more than 40 g/L. Contrast radiography (Figure 77-2) or ultrasonography may be useful to confirm a communication between a penetrating wound and the tendon sheath, especially if horses are examined soon after injury.

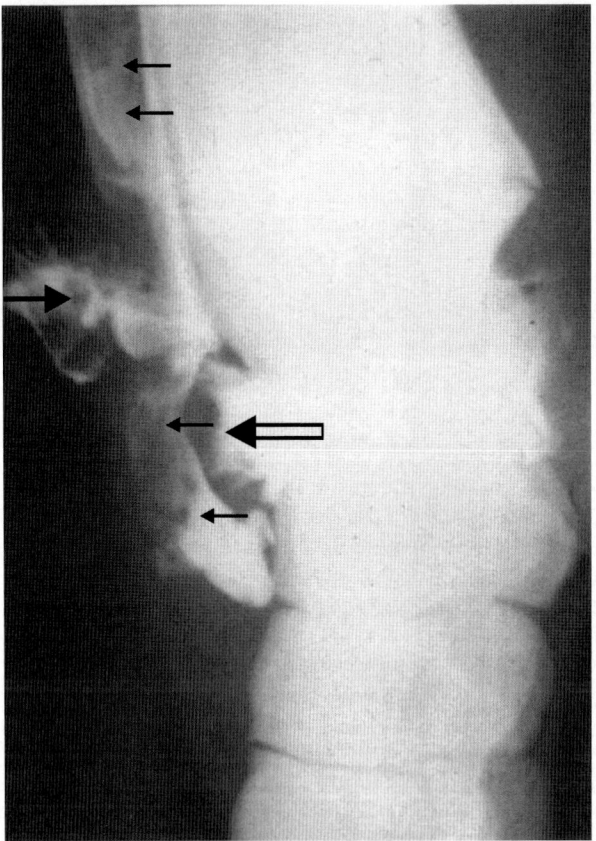

Fig. 77-2 • Lateromedial radiographic image of a carpus. Dorsal is to the left. Positive-contrast medium has been injected into the extensor carpi radialis tendon sheath and antebrachiocarpal joint in a horse that had sustained a deep puncture wound over the dorsal aspect of the carpus. Radiopaque contrast agent is present near the skin surface *(solid arrow)*, outside the tendon sheath *(small arrows)*, confirming penetration of the extensor carpi radialis sheath. The antebrachiocarpal joint *(open arrow)* was not involved.

The primary aim of treatment of horses with infectious tenosynovitis is the rapid elimination of bacteria and rapid return of the normal synovial environment. This is best achieved by wound debridement, lavage of the tendon sheath with copious amounts of sterile isotonic fluids, and the provision of bactericidal levels of appropriate antibiotics within the sheath.

Appropriate systemic and intrathecal antibiotic therapy should be initiated immediately. The presence of *Enterobacteriaceae* most commonly is associated with tendon sheath infection caused by a penetrating wound, whereas staphylococci are most commonly identified as the cause of iatrogenic infections of a tendon sheath.[26] The most effective combination of antibiotics for the treatment of infectious tenosynovitis is amikacin and cephalosporin (>85% effective).[29] However, the cost of these drugs may be prohibitive, and other drug combinations, such as penicillin and gentamicin, may be considered. The initial selection of antibiotic should be altered according to bacterial susceptibility if a positive culture is obtained from the synovial fluid.

Wound debridement and lavage of the affected tendon sheath with copious amounts of sterile isotonic fluids are important to reduce concentrations of bacteria and inflammatory mediators. Early in the infection, effective lavage may be achieved by through-and-through lavage using large-bore needles or arthroscopic egress cannulas. In more established infectious tenosynovitis, leukocytes and fibrin accumulate within the sheath, necessitating tenoscopic debridement. If satisfactory debridement and lavage have been achieved, primary closure of the sheath may be performed. The horse should be monitored closely for lameness, and repeated synovial fluid samples should be taken at 2- to 3-day intervals to monitor for return of infection. Alternatively the sheath may be left open, or a closed suction drain system may be inserted into the sheath for further elimination of inflammatory mediators and fibrin. The drain should be left in place for 3 to 5 days, but careful management is important to prevent ascending suprainfection.

Systemic antibiotic therapy should be continued for at least 2 weeks after the resolution of clinical signs. Once the infection has been eliminated, intrathecal injection of corticosteroids or hyaluronan may be used, with physiotherapy, to reduce adhesion formation and restore the normal gliding movement of the tendon within its sheath. However, both drugs may cause immunosuppression within the sheath and may potentiate dormant infection. Early return to controlled exercise is also important to reduce intrathecal adhesion formation.

If chronic infectious tenosynovitis becomes established, exploration of the tendon sheath and radical synovectomy may be required (see the following discussion). Successful outcomes have been reported after complete resection of the intrasynovial part of the CDET in horses with chronic infectious tenosynovitis and tendonitis.[30,31]

The prognosis for return to soundness after infectious extensor tenosynovitis is more favorable than for infectious flexor tenosynovitis,[26,28] possibly because extensor tendons are non–weight bearing compared with flexor tendons. The prognosis for return to soundness is generally good after early surgical intervention and appropriate antibiotic therapy for horses with infectious extensor tenosynovitis.

Chronic Tenosynovitis

Chronic tenosynovitis of the extensor tendon sheaths is characterized by persistent synovial effusion, fibrous thickening of the sheath, and subcutaneous edema.[32,33] Chronic tenosynovitis results in variable, sometimes severe, lameness, restricted carpal flexion, and a gait characterized by circumduction of the affected limb during protraction.[33] However, in some horses there is no gait abnormality.

Chronic tenosynovitis commonly arises after penetrating injuries to the carpal extensor sheaths, which may result in the inoculation of foreign material or bacteria into the synovial cavity and establishment of an infectious or noninfectious chronic tenosynovitis. The condition commonly occurs in horses jumping natural fences because of penetration of the sheath by thorns.[33] Chronic tenosynovitis also may occur after acute tenosynovitis and may be associated with partial tendon rupture.[22,32] Chronic inflammation of the tendon sheath causes granulomatous proliferation of the synovium, connective tissue deposition in the fibrous capsule, and fibrous adhesion formation between the tendon and its sheath, resulting in restriction of movement and pain on carpal flexion.[32,33]

Diagnosis of chronic tenosynovitis is based on clinical signs of effusion and thickening of the affected sheath (Figure 77-3) and restricted carpal flexion. Radiography of the carpus often reveals palisading new bone formation on

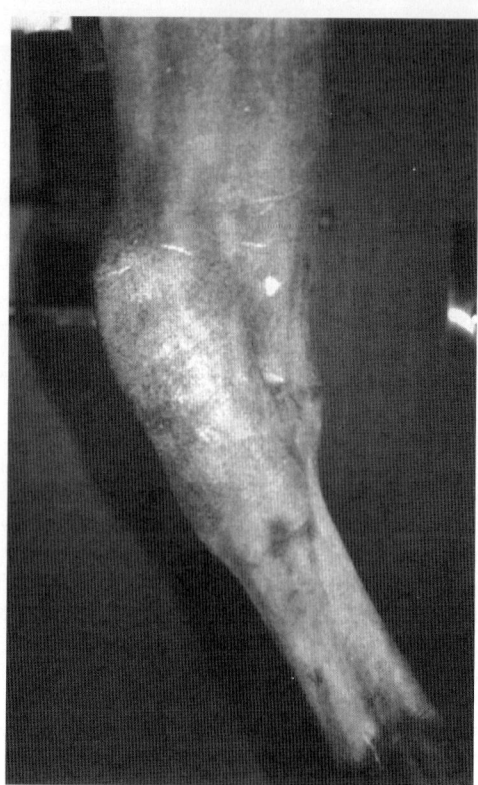

Fig. 77-3 • Chronic distention of the tendon sheath of the extensor carpi radialis in a horse with chronic tenosynovitis.

the craniodistal ridges of the radius adjacent to the affected sheaths (Figure 77-4) and entheseous new bone formation on the dorsal aspect of the carpal bones.[33] Synovial fluid aspirates vary from serosanguineous to turbid, with an increased nucleated cell count and total protein concentration. Ultrasonography may demonstrate tendon damage, synovial hypertrophy, foreign bodies, and intrathecal adhesions.

Conservative treatment with antibiotics, analgesics, intrathecal corticosteroids, and symptomatic physiotherapeutic procedures such as bandaging, cold hosing, massage, and forced exercise is usually unrewarding.[19,22,32,33] Good results, however, have been reported after both tenoscopic and open surgical intervention.[19,33,34] Tenoscopic examination of the sheaths of the ECRT, CDET, and LDET allows radical synovectomy of the hyperplastic synovium, removal of intrathecal adhesions, and debridement of damaged tendon and is associated with a good prognosis for resolution of lameness. The cosmetic appearance of most distended extensor tendon sheaths after tenoscopic surgery can be substantially improved, although most have some residual fibrosis.[34] The prognosis for soundness after open surgical exploration and radical synovectomy has been reported to be good,[33] although the resultant scar may cause a substantial blemish. After surgery, an intensive program of physiotherapy involving manual flexion and extension of the carpus and an ascending program of in-hand walking exercise should be initiated. Early passive motion to stimulate cavitation and reformation of the synovial lining and prevent adhesion formation is considered an essential part of the treatment.[33] Initially, carpal flexion is resented, and administration of NSAIDs and sedatives may be required.

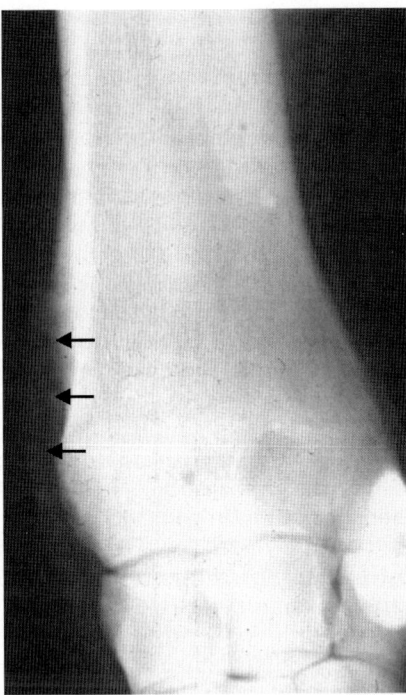

Fig. 77-4 • A craniolateral-caudomedial oblique radiographic image of the distal aspect of the radius in a horse with chronic tenosynovitis of the extensor carpi radialis tendon sheath. There is palisading new bone formation (arrows) on the craniomediodistal ridge of the radius adjacent to the tendon sheath.

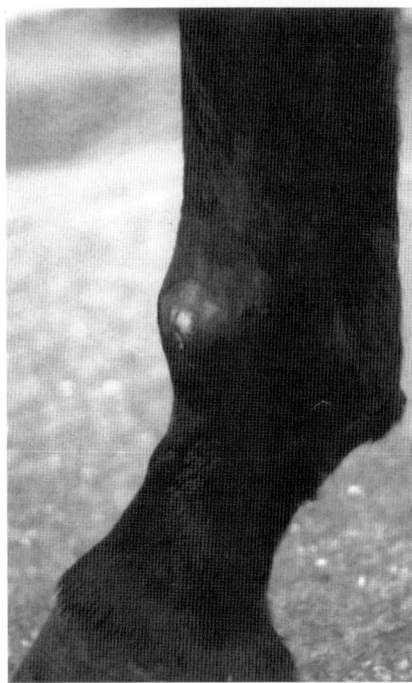

Fig. 77-5 • Prominent soft tissue swelling over the dorsal aspect of the fetlock region in the hindlimb of a horse with severe lameness. This is a supratendonous infectious bursitis and should not be confused with infectious arthritis of the metatarsophalangeal joint. Arthrocentesis of the metatarsophalangeal joint through a dorsal approach may result in iatrogenic infectious arthritis.

Full flexion of the carpus should be achieved by 30 days after surgery.

Osteochondromatosis

Synovial osteochondromatosis of the ECRT sheath has been reported.[35] Synovial osteochondromatosis is characterized by the formation of multiple small osseous bodies within a synovial-lined structure. The cause is unclear but it may be associated with trauma. Clinical signs include swelling on the dorsal surface of the carpus characterized by multiple, firm subcutaneous nodules and crepitus during joint movement, and lameness is usually evident. Diagnosis is confirmed by radiography and ultrasonography.[35] No information is available for the surgical treatment of osteochondromatosis of the extensor tendon sheaths in horses, but partial synovectomy and endoscopic removal of the osteochondral bodies was successful in other synovial cavities in horses and other species.[36]

Intersynovial Fistulae

Intersynovial fistulae are uncommon, but they have been documented between the CDET sheath and antebrachiocarpal joint,[37] the CDET sheath and middle carpal joint,[15] and the ECRT sheath and middle carpal joint.[5] The cause of these fistulae is unclear, but they are considered to be traumatic in origin and may occur in horses with carpitis or carpal fractures.[5,37] Typically, horses with intersynovial fistulae have chronic lameness and distention of the affected tendon sheath. Synovial fluid can be massaged from the joint to the tendon sheath. Diagnosis may be confirmed by contrast radiography[6] and intrasynovial analgesia. Surgical treatment is advocated in the management of intersynovial fistulae,[15] but little information concerning

the prognosis of affected horses is available because reports of this condition are rare. Use of tenoscopic approaches to close fistulae between the carpal joints and extensor tendon sheaths has been largely unsuccessful.[34] Surgical treatment involving a combination of endoscopically assisted synovectomy and limited open exposure of the fistula, and closure of the fibrous layers of the joint and tendon sheath are generally recommended.[34]

Infectious Bursitis

Infectious bursitis may occur in any of the bursae associated with the extensor tendons over the dorsal aspect of the fetlock. The condition is seen most commonly in horses that jump natural obstacles (e.g., event and National Hunt horses). Typically these horses have swelling over the dorsal aspect of the fetlock (Figure 77-5) and mild-to-severe lameness. Infectious bursitis may affect the subtendonous bursae or more commonly affects an acquired subcutaneous (supratendonous) bursa on the dorsal aspect of the LoDET in the fetlock region.[38] Occasionally both bursae may communicate around the lateral or medial aspect of the LoDET. Some horses have a severe, non–weight-bearing lameness. This condition frequently is confused with infectious arthritis of the metacarpophalangeal or metatarsophalangeal joints. Diagnosis is confirmed by ultrasonographic examination or contrast radiography[6] and synoviocentesis. Synoviocentesis from the palmar or plantar pouch of the adjacent metacarpophalangeal or metatarsophalangeal joint should be used to rule out joint infection. Treatment consists of surgical drainage and debridement and appropriate antimicrobial therapy. The prognosis for return to soundness is good.

Chapter 78

Curb

Mike W. Ross and Ronald L. Genovese

References on page 1320

The historical definition of *curb* is enlargement on the plantar aspect of the fibular tarsal bone (calcaneus) caused by inflammation and thickening of the (long) plantar ligament.[1] There is confusion regarding the cause of curb; a seminal publication uses this historical definition in the text but describes curb as superficial digital flexor (SDF) tendonitis in a figure legend.[2] By ultrasonographic evaluation curb was redefined as a complex of soft tissue injuries that occurs on the distal plantar aspect of the tarsus.[3,4] Long plantar (LP) desmitis is only one of many injuries that causes curb. However, the indelible term *curb* has been used for hundreds of years[5] and is still useful to describe swelling of the distal, plantar aspect of the tarsus (excluding the calcaneal bursa and proximal aspect of the calcaneus). In the rest of this chapter, *curb* is used specifically to mean the clinically apparent soft tissue swelling of the plantar aspect of the tarsus seen best from the side. Conformational abnormalities or bony exostoses can mimic or contribute eventually to formation of curb.

CLINICAL APPEARANCE OF CURB

The convex profile typical of curb is best seen from the side (Figure 78-1). Careful evaluation of swelling from all perspectives, palpation, and thorough lameness examination are critical. Curb must be differentiated from other swellings of the hock, including capped hock, effusion, edema and fibrosis of the calcaneal bursa (see Chapter 79), tarsal tenosynovitis (see Chapter 76), thoroughpin (with or without involvement of the tarsal sheath), and bony enlargements of the distal hock region (see Chapter 44). Injuries of the deep digital flexor tendon (DDFT) as it courses along the plantaromedial aspect of the hock within the tarsal sheath can produce typical signs of curb, but they account for only a small percentage of injuries in horses with curb.

Horses with sickle-hocked conformation are said to be *curby* (see Chapter 4). Sickle-hocked and in-at-the-hock conformation lead directly to curb, a finding most common in Standardbred (STB) and Thoroughbred (TB) racehorses. Prognosis for STB racehorses with sickle-hocked conformation and curb is worse in a trotter than in a pacer. Trotters with sickle-hocked conformation are usually fast early in training and racing, but this conformation is often career limiting. Sickle-hocked conformation is also undesirable in TB racehorses. Horses with sickle-hocked conformation often develop curb first, but they then independently or concomitantly develop other lameness associated with the distal hock joints. Tarsal region lameness begins with curb in 2- and 3-year-olds and progresses to osteoarthritis of the centrodistal and tarsometatarsal joints or slab fractures of the central tarsal bone, or more commonly the third tarsal bone.

Horses can have curby conformation without developing curb, and horses with normal hindlimb conformation can develop curb. The proximal aspect of the fourth metatarsal bone (MtIV) is often prominent in horses with sickle-hocked conformation. The most dramatic example of altered joint morphology occurs in young foals with tarsal crush syndrome, the result of delayed or incomplete ossification of the tarsal cuboidal bones (see Chapter 44).

Firm, fibrous soft tissue swelling can develop just proximal to the MtIV as a sequela to injection or local analgesia of the tarsometatarsal joint, presumably from local trauma, hemorrhage, or leakage into the subcutaneous tissues. Mild bony proliferation or fragmentation of the proximal aspect of the MtIV, or of the fourth tarsal bone, can cause focal swelling easily mistaken for curb.

Considerable variation in clinical signs occurs, and the injury cannot be categorized, or a management program and prognosis established, without thorough clinical and ultrasonographic examinations. Historically, owners and trainers consider curb to be an annoying, self-limiting problem that rarely causes lameness or poor performance, that responds to a single treatment that is uniformly effective, and that is cured by treatment. Most racehorse trainers are opposed to resting a horse with curb unless lameness is performance limiting, so veterinarians often are faced with management decisions without an option for even short-term rest or a reduction in training intensity. Many traditional therapies have no data to support efficacy. Thus, progress in understanding and management of this complex soft tissue injury has been limited.

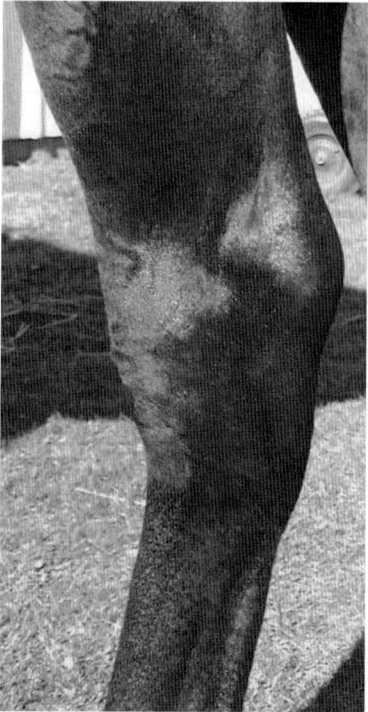

Fig. 78-1 • A Standardbred racehorse with typically appearing curb. Swelling associated with the distal, plantar aspect of the tarsus is centered over the centrodistal and tarsometatarsal joints. In this horse swelling was caused by superficial digital flexor tendonitis.

Lameness ranges from none, mild, or severe depending on the structure involved and extent of injury. Lameness tends to be worse if the soft tissue structure involved is located dorsal to the superficial digital flexor tendon (SDFT) in the plantar aspect of the tarsus (i.e., the DDFT and/or the long plantar ligament [LPL]), if SDFT injury is diffuse, or if a mixed injury involves more than one structure. Diagnosis is straightforward in horses with obvious lameness seen at a trot in hand and painful swelling, but lameness may be evident only as a slight loss of performance or unlevelness when the horse is performing maximally and may be perceived only by trainers, drivers, or riders. A horse with chronic curb may not exhibit signs of pain during palpation, or lameness at a trot in hand, but can show lameness at speed, and convincing a trainer that the long-term swelling is a source of pain may be difficult. The area should be palpated carefully with the limb bearing weight and flexed. Swelling may be firm and fibrous, with few signs of active inflammation, or may be warm, painful, and edematous. Acute, compliant, or mushy swelling is associated with hemorrhage or other subcutaneous fluid accumulation and sometimes deeper soft tissue injury. Horses with this form of curb usually have acute, moderate-to-severe lameness. Horses with distal hock joint pain often exhibit a painful response when direct pressure is placed on plantar hock structures, including the SDFT, proximal aspect of the MtIV, second metatarsal bone, and proximal aspect of the suspensory ligament. Often swelling is not detected in these horses. Response to upper limb flexion varies and is nonspecific. Direct digital palpation followed by trotting is useful, because horses with active inflammation show increased lameness.

Because horses with curb can have concomitant osteoarthritis or other problems of the distal hock joints, differentiation of the source of pain is important but difficult. Diagnostic analgesia is useful but not foolproof. If horses are lame at a trot in hand, local infiltration of local anesthetic solution subcutaneously over the curb is effective. A minimum of 20 to 30 mL of local anesthetic solution should be infiltrated along the lateral, plantar, and medial aspects of the curb. Small-gauge needles should be avoided (to avoid needle breakage), and the injection should be performed with the limb in flexion, because horses may object to several injections. If horses are not visibly lame at a trot in hand, examination at the track or under saddle should be performed. Selective intraarticular analgesia of the distal hock joints and sequential perineural analgesia to rule out the lower limb are essential. A tibial nerve block alleviates pain with curb, but it is seldom done because other common sources of pain are abolished similarly.

Radiography and scintigraphy help differentiate other sources of pain, but ultrasonography is the imaging method of choice to determine which structures are involved and the extent of damage.

APPLIED ANATOMY AND NORMAL ULTRASONOGRAPHIC EXAMINATION OF THE PLANTAR ASPECT OF THE TARSUS

Plantar to the calcaneus are skin, subcutaneous tissues, a thin fibrous tissue layer, the SDFT, and the LPL (Figure 78-2). Medially the DDFT courses distally over the sustentaculum tali, within the tarsal sheath. Normally the tarsal sheath has a small amount of fluid that can be seen during ultrasonographic examination, but it is not felt. The LPL originates from the calcaneus, closely adheres to this bone, and inserts distally on the plantar surface of the fourth tarsal bone and the MtIV. The plantar aspect of the tarsus can be divided into zones to classify findings (Figure 78-3) or the distance measured from the proximal aspect of the

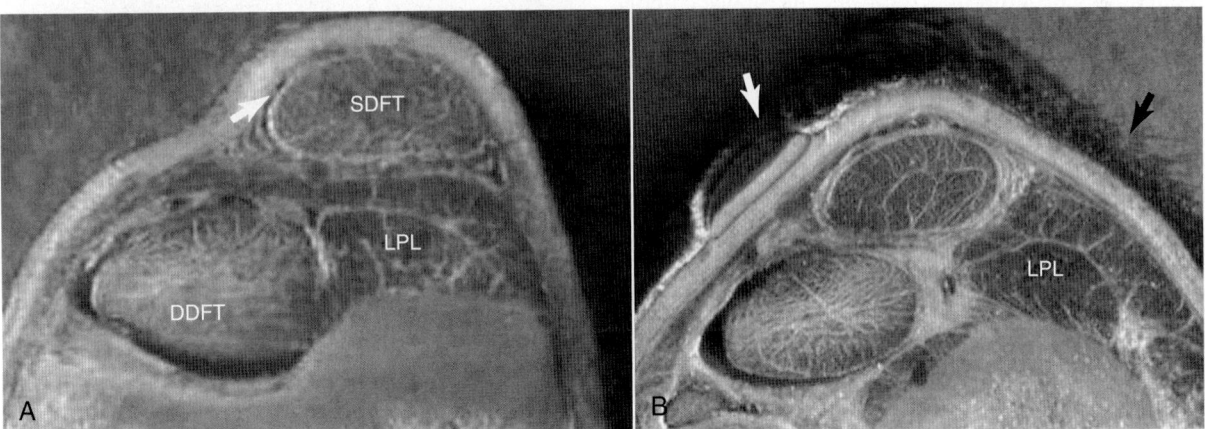

Fig. 78-2 • **A,** Cross-section of the left tarsus at the level of zone 1A (lateral is to the right and plantar is uppermost). At this level the superficial digital flexor tendon *(SDFT)* and long plantar ligament *(LPL)* are located on the plantar aspect of the calcaneus, and ultrasonographic examination of these structures is completed with the transducer on the plantar midline. For imaging of the deep digital flexor tendon *(DDFT)*, the transducer must be positioned plantaromedially. In this specimen from a normal horse the thin peritendonous and periligamentous tissue *(arrow)* layer can be seen. **B,** Cross-section of the left tarsus distal to the section shown in **A** at the level of zone 1B2 (same orientation as **A**). Note that the LPL is now located plantarolaterally; for accurate anatomical and cross-sectional data information regarding the LPL to be obtained, an ultrasound transducer must be placed along the plantarolateral aspect of the limb *(black arrow)*. At this level the DDFT is located plantaromedially, and for accurate depiction of this structure ultrasonographically the transducer must be placed on the plantaromedial aspect of the limb *(arrow)*.

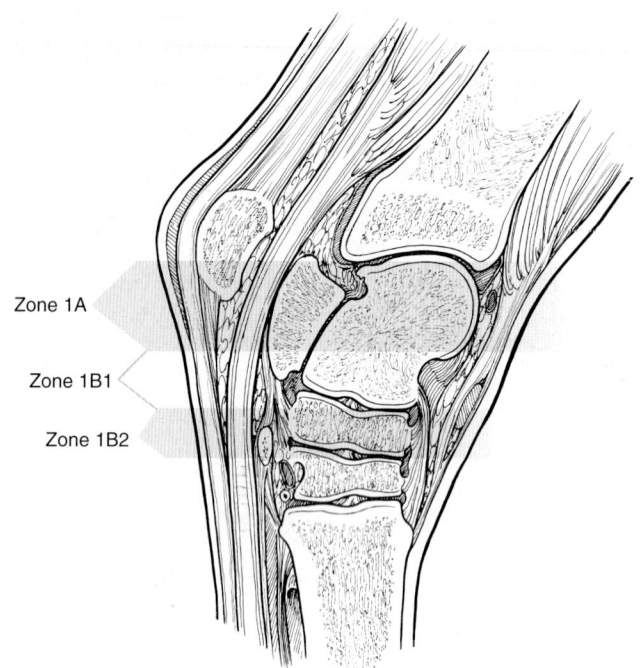

Fig. 78-3 • The plantar aspect of the tarsus is divided into zones 1A and 1B. Because zone 1B is rather large and important, the zone is sometimes subdivided into 1B1 and 1B2. An alternative technique for recording level of injury is to measure distally from the proximal aspect of the calcaneus.

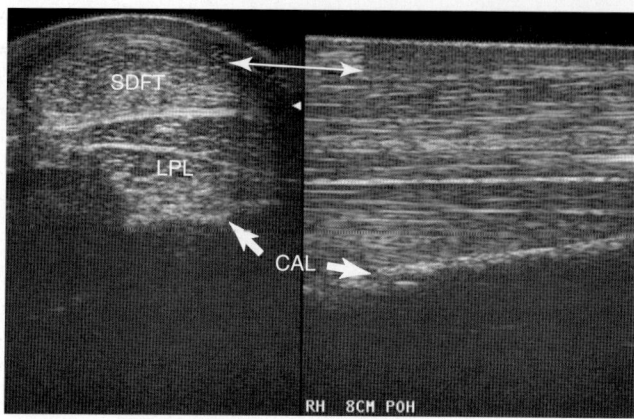

Fig. 78-4 • Transverse (left) and longitudinal (right) midline ultrasonographic images at 8 cm distal to the point of the hock. A thin subcutaneous fibrous tissue layer runs along the plantar surface of the superficial digital flexor tendon (SDFT) (double-headed arrow). The SDFT (crescent-shaped) is narrower in a medial-to-lateral direction and somewhat thickened compared with further proximally. In the longitudinal scan the normal SDFT has a dense parallel fiber pattern. Deep to the SDFT the long plantar ligament (LPL) is at full thickness (plantar-to-dorsal direction), is rectangular, and is attached firmly to the calcaneus (CAL). At this level the deep digital flexor tendon is out of view medially and must be evaluated by placing the transducer plantaromedially.

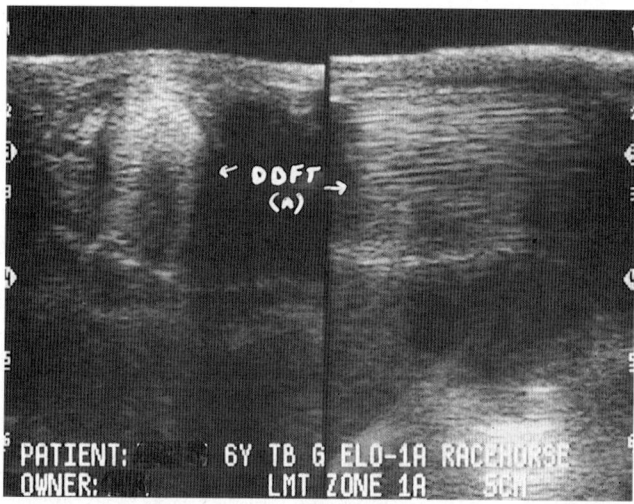

Fig. 78-5 • Transverse (left) and longitudinal (right) ultrasonographic images from the plantaromedial aspect of the left hock 5 cm distal to the point of the hock. In the transverse image the tarsal sheath surrounds the deep digital flexor tendon (DDFT). The tendon is oval and has a large eccentric hypoechoic region composed of residual muscle tissue, but this defect could be caused by incident angle artifact.

calcaneus (point of hock). Swelling comprising curb occurs in zone 1 of the tarsal and metatarsal regions but can extend into zone 2 if SDF tendonitis occurs. Transverse and longitudinal images of both limbs should be obtained from the plantar midline, plantaromedial (to evaluate the DDFT), and slightly plantarolateral (to evaluate the distal aspect of the LPL). Measurement of cross-sectional area (CSA) is important to confirm lesions in which enlargement has occurred but with no overt fiber damage. Precise placement of the ultrasound transducer is important because the LPL changes size and shape as it courses distally. Knowledge of normal ultrasonographic anatomy is crucial (Figures 78-4 to 78-7).[3,4]

CURB: A COLLECTION OF SOFT TISSUE INJURIES[3]

One hundred and ten horses with curb were examined using ultrasonography, including 87 (79%) racehorses (72 STB and 15 TB) and 23 nonracehorse sports horses (six field or show hunters, six Western performance horses, four show jumpers, two event horses, two gaited horses, two horses of unknown use, and one dressage horse).[3] Mean and median ages (range 1 to 13 years) were 3.4 and 3.0, respectively. There were 32 late yearlings or 2-year-old horses, of which all were STBs; 24 of these STBs were examined before or near the time of a qualifying race. There were 24 intact males, 35 females, and 51 geldings. No sex predilection was found. Curb occurred in the left hindlimb (LH) in 60 horses, right hindlimb (RH) in 37 horses, and bilaterally in 13 horses. Of the 13 horses with bilateral curb, 11 were STBs. Within STBs there were 61 pacers and 11 trotters, compared with an expected population (ratio of pacers:trotters is 3:1 in North America) of 54 pacers:18

trotters. Curb was thought to result from excessive stress or strain from race training (80 horses), direct trauma (11 horses), previous injection (three horses), associated injuries (three horses), and an apparent "bad step" or unknown cause (13 horses). The most common reported form of direct trauma was stall or wall kicking. Curb was the primary reason for examination in 94 horses, was a compensatory lameness in 10 horses, and was seen in association with other tarsal injury or ipsilateral hindlimb lameness in six horses. Sixty-three horses were lame, and although lameness score was not uniformly recorded in the

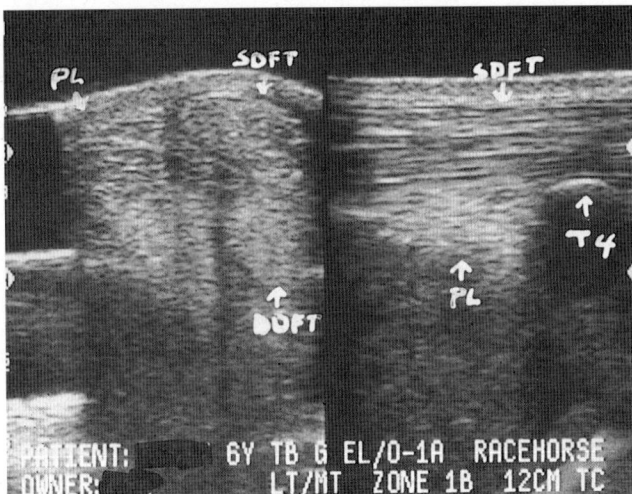

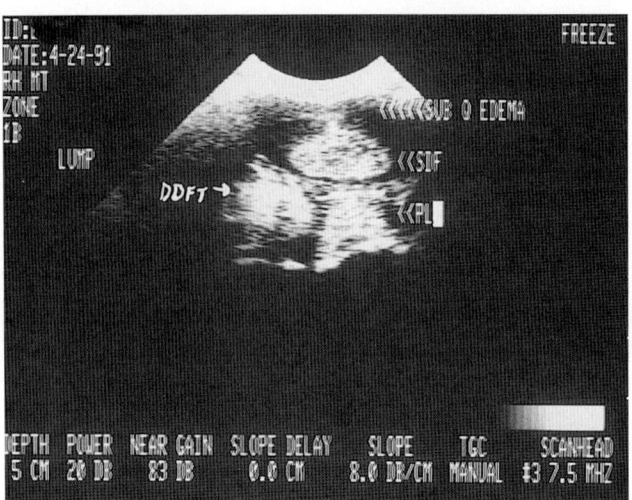

Fig. 78-6 • Transverse *(left)* (medial is to the right) and longitudinal (proximal is to the left) *(right)* plantarolateral ultrasonographic images 9 cm distal to the point of the hock at the level of the fourth tarsal bone *(T4)*. The long plantar ligament *(PL)* is a multiseptated structure, and large plantar fiber bundles are not normally perfectly aligned with dorsal bundles. In transverse images the PL normally may appear to lack echogenicity, and the size and shape change at the insertion on the fourth tarsal bone. The PL is wide at the insertion on the fourth tarsal bone (longitudinal scan).

Fig. 78-8 • Transverse midline ultrasonographic image (medial is to the left) of the plantar aspect of the hock of 2-year-old Standardbred gelding obtained in zone 1B. There is subcutaneous edema *(arrows)* and thickening. The superficial digital flexor tendon *(SDFT)*, deep digital flexor tendon *(DDFT)*, and long plantar ligament *(PL)* were normal. This horse was managed using a peritendonous injection of corticosteroids.

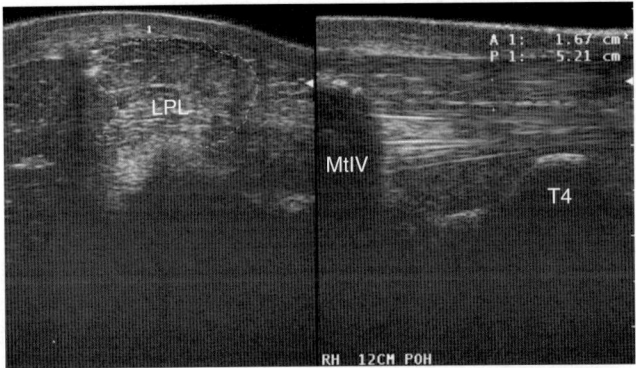

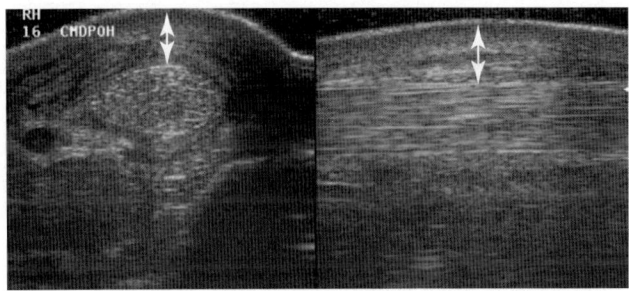

Fig. 78-9 • Transverse *(left)* (medial is to the left) and longitudinal ultrasonographic images of zone 1B2 of the right hock in a 2-year-old trotter with curb. Thickening and mild fluid accumulation in the peritendonous and periligamentous tissues *(double-headed arrow)* are present, but the underlying soft tissue structures are normal. In the longitudinal image the plantar swelling giving the clinical profile associated with curb can distinctly be seen.

Fig. 78-7 • Transverse *(left)* (medial is to the left) and longitudinal *(right)* (proximal is to the right) plantarolateral ultrasonographic images 12 cm distal to the point of the hock, just distal to the insertion of the long plantar ligament *(LPL)* on the fourth tarsal bone *(T4)*. The LPL is thick in the plantar-to-dorsal direction. A midline image would show the superficial digital flexor tendon and deep digital flexor tendon, but at this level a plantarolateral transducer placement is needed to assess the LPL. In the transverse image the normal heterogeneous fiber pattern of the LPL and cross-sectional area measurement can be seen. In the longitudinal image the LPL is seen attaching to the fourth metatarsal bone *(MtIV)* distally.

medical record, recorded lameness scores ranged from 1 to 2 out of 5. Horses with LP desmitis, those with SDF tendonitis extending distally from zone 1 into zone 2 of the proximal metatarsal region, those with deep digital flexor (DDF) tendonitis, and those with combined soft tissue injuries exhibited most pronounced lameness. Swelling (prominence of curb) was pronounced in horses with recent or combined soft tissue injury and in those with hematoma or abscess formation in the peritendonous and periligamentous (PT-PL) tissue. Swelling was described as fibrous in nature in many horses, particularly in STBs in which curb was chronic and in horses in which previous management

included cryotherapy, topical counterirritation, or thermocautery. However, in acute injuries the swelling was often edematous, warm, and painful on palpation.

Ultrasonographic diagnosis included peritendonous-periligamentous (PT-PL) swelling without injury of the SDFT, DDFT, and LPL (29 [26%] horses) (Figures 78-8 to 78-10), PT-PL swelling primarily consisting of hematoma (six horses), and PT-PL swelling primarily consisting of abscess formation (five horses). Overall, 40 (36%) horses had swelling confined to the PT-PL tissues without other underlying soft tissue injury. There were 32 (29%) horses with PT-PL swelling and SDF tendonitis (Figure 78-11); 25 horses with PT-PL and LP desmitis (Figure 78-12); five horses with LP desmitis alone; five horses with DDF tendonitis; complex tarsal soft tissue injury of the LPL, PT-PL tissues, and gastrocnemius tendon in two horses; and tarsocrural collateral desmitis in one horse. Overall, only 32 (29%) horses had involvement of the LPL.

Management and outcome in these 110 horses with curb were difficult to assess, and information in medical

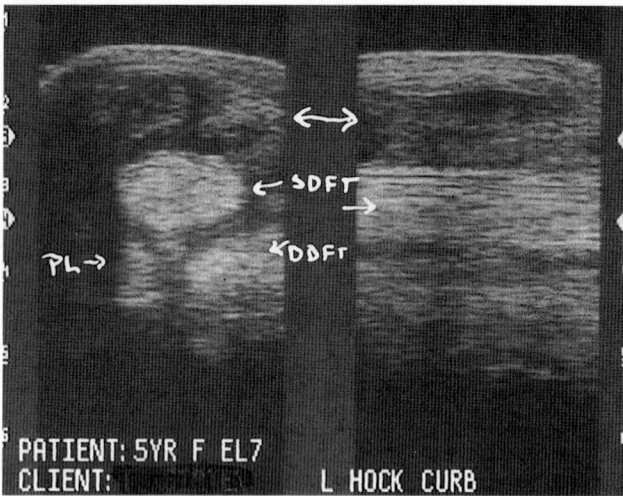

Fig. 78-10 • Transverse *(left)* (medial is to the right) and longitudinal midline ultrasonographic images of the hock in zone 1B in a 5-year-old Thoroughbred racehorse. There is soft tissue swelling of heterogeneous echogenicity of the peritendonous and periligamentous tissues and fibrous adhesion *(double-headed arrow)* plantaromedial to the superficial digital flexor tendon *(SDFT)*. The SDFT, deep digital flexor tendon *(DDFT)*, and long plantar ligament *(PL)* are normal.

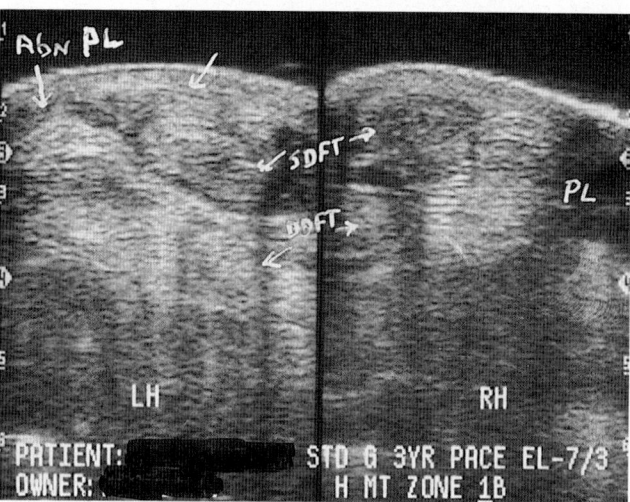

Fig. 78-12 • Transverse plantarolateral ultrasonographic images of the left hindlimb *(LH)* (abnormal) and right hindlimb *(RH)* (normal) plantar tarsi in zone 1B of 3-year-old Standardbred pacer. The left long plantar ligament *(PL)* is enlarged, with an indistinct central hypoechoic lesion. *DDFT,* Deep digital flexor tendon; *SDFT,* superficial digital flexor tendon.

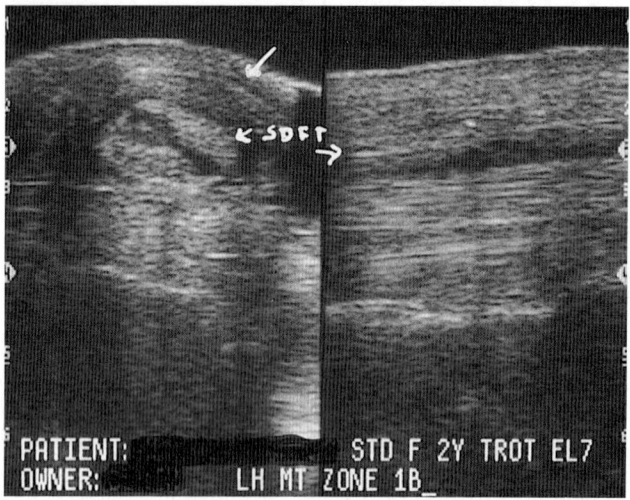

Fig. 78-11 • Transverse *(left)* and longitudinal midline ultrasonographic images of the plantar aspect of the hock of 2-year-old Standardbred racehorse with curb resulting from peritendonous and periligamentous tissue injury and superficial digital flexor tendonitis. Subcutaneous fibrous tissue accumulation *(top arrow)* plantar to the superficial digital flexor tendon *(SDFT)* and a central anechoic lesion of the SDFT can be seen, findings verified in the longitudinal view. Cross-sectional area of the affected superficial digital flexor tendon was 33% greater than that of the contralateral normal tendon.

records was lacking. There was a tendency for clinicians to manage horses with curb that were not lame or those in which curb was a compensatory issue with subcutaneous injections of a corticosteroid-containing preparation in combination with a reduction in exercise intensity or a short period of rest. Most of these horses had PT-PL swelling. Horses in which curb caused actual lameness were generally managed with rest and nonsteroidal antiinflammatory drug (NSAID) administration, but cryotherapy and

topical counterirritation were often performed as well. Horses with severe SDF tendonitis extending into zone 2, LP desmitis, DDF tendonitis, or combination soft tissue injury were given long-term rest (>3 months) and controlled return to exercise, but they were the group most likely to do poorly or to remain lame. Horses (five) with PT-PL swelling and abscessation had surgical drainage and appropriate antimicrobial therapy and successfully returned to exercise. Associated ipsilateral lameness conditions included osteoarthritis of the centrodistal and tarsometatarsal joints and metatarsophalangeal joint pain.

Curb was previously described as simply LP desmitis,[1,2,5] but is a collection of plantar tarsal soft tissue injuries. In fact, in 68% of horses with curb in this study, the LPL was normal ultrasonographically, and horses with curb were more likely to have injury of the PT-PL tissue alone or in combination with SDF tendonitis than injury of the LPL.[3] Curb should not be used synonymously with LP desmitis. Although not directly studied, CSA measurement (see Figure 78-7) of all soft tissue structures should routinely be performed and compared with measurements from the contralateral limb (some horses are bilaterally affected), because common forms of SDF tendonitis and LP desmitis are often associated with increased CSAs rather than frank fiber tearing.

Curb is primarily an injury of racehorses, especially STBs. Gait, speed, and training methods differ between racing breeds, and STB racehorses have a higher prevalence of conformational abnormalities, such as sickle-hocked and in-at-the-hock conformation. These conformational abnormalities have not been directly studied, and a cause-and-effect relationship is therefore difficult to establish. However, sickle-hocked conformation may increase load on the distal plantar soft tissue structures, predisposing to curb. Weight and load distribution are considerably different in STBs and TBs. Curb develops frequently in STB racehorses that train and race on a thin, near-hard surface, contrary to many soft tissue injuries that result from work on deep surfaces. Many curbs develop in young STB racehorses early in training when they are jogging and not formally performing speed work. In some instances track surfaces are inconsistent and perhaps slippery, because early training is done in the winter months. In many horses clinical signs are recurrent and progressive, and the development of clinical signs early in training supports a theory that curb develops primarily as a result of overload of plantar soft tissue structures, in a roughly plantar-to-dorsal direction, because the most common tissue involved is the PT-PL tissues. For instance, in our study SDF tendonitis was not seen in horses without PT-PL tissue enlargement, suggesting that PT-PL injury may have preceded injury of the SDFT.[3] Pronounced lameness in horses with SDF tendonitis was seen only when injury progressed distally into zone 2 in the proximal metatarsal region; in some horses sickle-hocked conformation and alleged loss of support of the hock produced what appeared as a dropped hock. Horses with this form of curb, LP desmitis, or combination injury are most likely to be lame. Curb was more common in the LH limb, and although it is tempting to associate this finding with counterclockwise training, many horses developed curb before speed work commenced in that direction. Perhaps in STBs the conventional practice of giving horses many slow miles of jogging in a clockwise direction may place additional load on the outside LH, predisposing to curb. Curb appears more common in pacers than trotters. Nonracehorse sports horses develop curb, but only sporadically, and lameness is often moderate to severe and most commonly is associated with PT-PL tissue swelling, although other structures are sometimes involved.

Peritendonous and Periligamentous Inflammation

PT-PL tissue swelling occurs alone or with abnormalities of one or more of the SDFT, DDFT, or LPL. PT-PL tissue injury can occur secondary to direct trauma from horses kicking a wall or trailer door, or rarely from a direct kick or interference injury from another horse, resulting in acute, large, painful swelling. Ultrasonographic examination most often reveals frank hemorrhage and edema. More commonly the horse has neither a history of trauma nor clinical findings suggesting trauma. We suspect that PT-PL tissue injury reflects excess loading or strain of the plantar tarsal soft tissue structures from race training. Extensive jogging of young STBs early in training may cause dramatic increase in hock loading, and tension and overstretching of thin PT-PL tissue occurs. PT-PL tissue injury may be an accumulated overload injury and may develop secondarily to other lameness. The PT-PL tissue is most plantar in location, is thin, may be most vulnerable to injury from abnormal strain, and may be the first tissue in progression to be injured. Conformational abnormalities may predispose the horse to such injuries. The cause of such soft tissue injury in mature nonracehorses is unknown, and although swelling can develop with relatively mild lameness, more often lameness is moderate to severe.

Clinical examination reveals localized soft tissue swelling, often with heat and pain on palpation, with or without lameness. Previous application of liniments or blisters or pin firing may create sore skin and considerable soft tissue swelling. Ultrasonographic findings depend on the duration of the injury. Acute lesions have an accumulation of anechoic fluid subcutaneously; in more chronic injuries,

swelling is from subcutaneous echogenic material (see Figures 78-8 to 78-10). The SDFT, DDFT, and LPL should be inspected carefully, but they are frequently normal.

Management depends on the degree of lameness, the stage of training, the race or competition schedule, and the owner's or trainer's wishes. Blistering is used widely, but we question its value. Although not supported by scientific evidence, thermocautery (pin firing) appears to be an effective management tool, perhaps because it enforces rest. However, prolonged rest is rarely necessary in racehorses, and many horses can be managed by local injection of corticosteroids (triamcinolone acetonide, 9 mg) without substantial interruption of training. More than one treatment may be required if the swelling and lameness do not resolve. A lame horse must be rested to prevent injury to deeper structures. In nonracehorses with moderate-to-severe lameness, lameness may take several weeks to resolve. If the swelling becomes firm, fibrous, and pain free but lameness recurs, further investigation is warranted, because other causes of tarsal pain often develop in STB and TB racehorses with curb.

Infection can occur from direct trauma with skin penetration, previous injection, or severe topical counterirritation. If infection is suspected, cytological examination and culture are indicated. If a hematoma resulting from trauma is large or recurrent or if the curb is infected, establishing drainage is often necessary. A distal incision is made to provide drainage, and fibrin and debris are removed. Care must be taken to avoid penetration of the tarsal sheath when creating the incision. A drain is inserted if necessary, and the hock is bandaged. Culture usually reveals *Staphylococcus* species, and appropriate antimicrobial and NSAID therapy is instituted. Horses are rested for 2 to 3 weeks to allow the tissues to heal, even though lameness from PT-PL tissue injury was not present before infection developed. Prognosis in horses with infection of PT-PL tissues is excellent but is far worse in those with infection of the SDFT, DDFT, or tarsal sheath.

Superficial Digital Flexor Tendonitis

A common finding in horses with curb is SDF tendonitis. Sickle-hocked conformation may predispose the horse to tendonitis, which can occur alone but rarely is seen without concomitant inflammation of the PT-PL tissues. Pathogenesis likely involves progressive or accumulated overload injury of first the thin, fragile PT-PL tissues and later the SDFT.

Previous PT-PL tissue injury appears to predispose to subsequent SDF tendonitis if the training level is increased quickly. PT-PL injury may simply be an early stage of a progressive lesion that eventually involves the SDFT or LPL. Progressive injury occurs frequently if horses with PT-PL tissue injury are treated with cryotherapy, internal blisters, or corticosteroids, and training intensity is accelerated before mature fibrous tissue can form. In horses with PT-PL tissue injury and SDF tendonitis, lameness varies, but it is much more likely to be observed than in horses with only PT-PL tissue injury. Lameness may be acute in onset and often is seen at fast speeds, but it can be seen in some horses at a trot in hand. SDF tendonitis occurs commonly in young STB racehorses but usually at a later stage of training than PT-PL tissue injury. Ultrasonographic examination reveals enlargement of the CSA of the SDFT, with a variable change in echogenicity and fiber pattern, depending on the severity of the injury (see Figure 78-11). Often, subcutaneous edema or fibrosis occurs, depending on the chronicity of the injury.

In horses with SDF tendonitis, rest is an important part of management. Lesions usually are localized to the plantar aspect of the tarsus; those extending farther distally are associated with more severe lameness, and horses have a poorer prognosis. Horses with localized lesions have a fair prognosis, although the prognosis is worse in trotters than in pacers. Horses with mild acute SDF tendonitis, with enlargement of the tendon without fiber tearing, should be rested for 3 to 4 weeks. Without rest, progressive fiber damage may occur, resulting in prolonged recovery. Horses with more severe injuries may require up to 4 months of stall rest and controlled walking exercise.

In some STB racehorses actively racing, SDF tendonitis can be managed symptomatically, without giving rest, if the lesion is well localized and mild. Rest is always the best option but one often met with resistance from trainers. Mild lameness may be observed at speed or while the horse is trotting in hand, but severe lameness should not be evident. Ultrasonographic examination often reveals PT-PL tissue injury with enlargement of the SDFT, but core lesions are not present. In most horses local therapy using cold water hosing and poultice application, NSAID therapy, and subcutaneous injection of a corticosteroid preparation is successful. Subcutaneous injection of methylprednisolone acetate (200 mg) and Sarapin (25 mL) medial, plantar, and lateral to the SDFT is often done by practitioners with apparent success. Care is taken not to inject corticosteroids directly into the substance of the SDFT and LPL. Horses are given 10 to 14 days of jogging and light training before racing again. Nonracehorses with localized lesions usually respond well to rest for up to 3 months and have a favorable prognosis. Intralesional injections of fresh bone marrow, platelet-rich plasma, cultured stem cells, or other preparations may help healing and improve long-term prognosis, but we currently have no experience with intralesional therapy in this location.

Horses with severe SDF tendonitis have severe mushy swelling. If not given rest, these horses develop progressive tearing of the SDFT distal to the hock in the metatarsal region and lose support of the hock. Long-term rest (9 to 12 months) is recommended, but prognosis for return to previous race class is poor and in trotters, grave.

Deep Digital Flexor Tendonitis

DDF tendonitis is a rare cause of curb. Horses with curb resulting from DDF tendonitis are usually acutely lame and have substantial swelling. Mixed injury with DDF tendonitis accompanying SDF tendonitis and LP desmitis occurs, but it is unusual. Horses with DDF tendonitis have concomitant PT-PL tissue inflammation and effusion of the tarsal sheath (tenosynovitis). The DDFT simply can be enlarged compared with the contralateral limb or can have anechoic or hypoechoic core lesions. During ultrasonographic examination, the DDFT should be evaluated carefully from the midline and plantaromedial aspects. Lameness often is pronounced, and rest is recommended for a minimum of 4 to 6 months, but prognosis is guarded because lameness can recur. Serial ultrasonographic

examination, corrective shoeing, and controlled exercise are given.

Long Plantar Desmitis

LPL injury usually causes acute lameness, but chronic soft tissue swelling and progressive lameness can occur. Soft tissue swelling often is pronounced. Although LP desmitis can occur in racehorses, this form of curb appears to be equally common in other types of horses, such as Western performance horses. In one of the Editor's experience (SJD) LP desmitis is rare in sports horses in Europe. LP desmitis can be well localized or diffuse. Cross-sectional measurements of the LPL are critical, because desmitis often manifests as ligament enlargement rather than overt fiber tearing. Subtle thickening of the LPL may cause high-speed lameness, and evaluation of the CSA may be the only method to identify early lesions in these horses. Lesions can occur at any level within zones 1A and 1B, and injury may involve the insertion of the LPL on the MtIV (see Figure 78-12).

Conservative management is best for horses with LP desmitis, because lameness and swelling often are pronounced. Owners and trainers of nonracehorses are often open to a conservative approach involving ample rest (3 months) to rehabilitate horses with curb properly. Intervening with therapy to enforce rest is not necessary. Controlled return to exercise is straightforward in this type of horse, because walking and trotting under saddle can be given easily. Graded exercise programs are not administered as easily or desired in STB racehorses compared with nonracehorse sports horses. Lunging and walking and trotting under saddle are usually not practical, although riding trotters is popular among trainers originally from Europe. Walking and light jogging in a jog cart are the best methods for graded exercise in a STB racehorse. We do not recommend turnout exercise in any horse with soft tissue injury, because we feel strongly that this prolongs recovery and may lead to reinjury, but we realize our recommendations may not be followed. Cryotherapy, topical counterirritants, subcutaneous injections, and thermocautery are less likely to influence inflammation and healing of the LPL than more superficial causes of curb, but these treatments are sometimes requested. As experience is gained with intralesional therapy for management of soft tissue injuries in horses, it will undoubtedly be applied to injuries in the plantar aspect of the tarsus.

Curb can result from LP desmitis at its insertion on the MtIV. These horses do not have extensive swelling but focal thickening just proximal to the MtIV. Mild soft tissue swelling must be differentiated from a prominent but normal MtIV seen in yearlings with sickle-hocked conformation. Horses with curb resulting from distally located LP desmitis show lameness and mild, focal swelling and are managed with rest.

Mixed Soft Tissue Injuries

Ultrasonographic examination of curb nearly always identifies PT-PL tissue inflammation and in many horses an abnormality of the SDFT, DDFT, or the LPL. Occasionally, however, simultaneous injury of the SDFT and LPL occurs in addition to PT-PL tissue inflammation. This is most common in nonracehorse sports horses, in which lameness and swelling are severe. Long-term rest is recommended, but prognosis is guarded.

Chapter 79

Bursae and Other Soft Tissue Swellings

Sue J. Dyson

A bursa is a flattened, closed sac interposed between structures subject to friction or at points of unusual pressure, such as bony prominences and tendons. Bursae are lined with a cellular membrane resembling synovium and are classified according to position (subcutaneous, subligamentous, submuscular, and subtendonous) and according to the method of formation (congenital or acquired).

Acquired bursae develop because of pressure and friction over bony prominences. Tearing of the subcutaneous tissues results in accumulation of transudative fluid, which becomes encapsulated by fibrous tissue. In chronic injuries fibrous bands may develop within the capsule.

SUPRASPINOUS BURSA

The supraspinous bursa overlies the summits of the dorsal spinous process of the second to fifth thoracic vertebrae, under the funicular part of the nuchal ligament. Inflammation of the supraspinous bursa and surrounding soft tissues, so-called *fistulous withers,* is usually infectious in origin and may be a sequela to trauma. *Streptococcus* and *Staphylococcus* species, *Brucella abortus,* and *Onchocerca cervicalis* have been considered important causative agents.[1-3]

Clinical signs of supraspinous bursitis are generalized soft tissue swelling, heat and pain, and often draining tract(s). Osteitis or osteomyelitis of the dorsal spinous processes of the cranial thoracic vertebrae may be concurrent. Care must be taken not to misinterpret the normal granular radiopaque appearance of normal, incompletely ossified summits of the dorsal spinous processes.[4] Diagnostic ultrasonography and radiology are useful for determining the extent of the infection, for identifying a foreign body, and for evaluating signs of osteitis or osteomyelitis.

Treatment is by aggressive surgical debridement of all infected tissue and establishment of adequate drainage, taking care not to penetrate the dorsoscapular ligament. Several surgical procedures may be required to resolve the infection successfully.[1-3]

INTERTUBERCULAR (BICIPITAL) BURSA

The intertubercular (bicipital) bursa is discussed in Chapter 40.

HYGROMA

Hygroma is discussed in Chapters 38 and 67.

NAVICULAR BURSA

The navicular bursa is discussed in Chapters 24 and 30.

TROCHANTERIC BURSA

The Editors have no clinical experience of trochanteric bursitis. This condition is discussed further in Chapter 47.

CALCANEAL BURSA

The calcaneal or intertendonous bursa lies between the tendons of the gastrocnemius and the superficial digital flexor muscles, proximal to the hock, and extends distally on the plantar aspect of the calcaneus to the distal aspect of the hock (Figure 79-1). In most horses a communication exists between the calcaneal bursa and the gastrocnemius bursa. There is communication between the calcaneal bursa and the subcutaneous bursa in 37% of horses.

Injuries of the calcaneal bursa are not common and are usually the result of trauma. However, mild distention of the calcaneal bursa often is seen with gastrocnemius tendonitis (see page 803). Mild distention also may be seen unilaterally or bilaterally, as an incidental finding unassociated with lameness.[5] Primary inflammation of the bursa results in acute-onset lameness associated with distention of the bursa. Hemorrhage into the bursa also may occur. Conservative management by rest, with or without injection of short-acting corticosteroids, usually results in resolution of lameness, although enlargement of the bursa may persist.

More commonly, infection of the bursa is caused by a penetrating injury or is secondary to infectious osteitis of the calcaneus[6,7] (see Chapter 44).

Chronic distention of the calcaneal bursa also has been seen with well-circumscribed osteolytic lesions on the

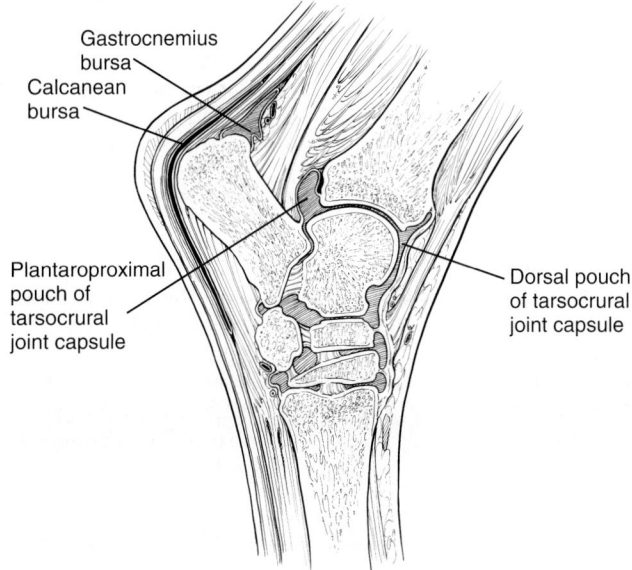

Fig. 79-1 • Diagram of a sagittal section of the hock region showing the relative positions of the calcaneal and gastrocnemius bursae.

Labels: Gastrocnemius bursa; Calcanean bursa; Plantaroproximal pouch of tarsocrural joint capsule; Dorsal pouch of tarsocrural joint capsule

eferences on page 1320

tuber calcanei, which were thought to represent enthesopathy at the insertion of the gastrocnemius tendon.[8]

Further investigation should include diagnostic ultrasonography, radiography of the calcaneus, and synoviocentesis. Radiographic examination should include a flexed skyline image of the calcaneus.[9] The internal structure of the bursa may be evaluated endoscopically,[10] but some underlying bony lesions may not be visible if the insertion of gastrocnemius is intact.[8] Endoscopy has been used diagnostically and therapeutically in horses with infectious osteitis, or bursitis, and in those with osteolytic lesions.

Horses with primary infection of the calcaneal bursa should be treated by debridement and lavage of the bursa and broad-spectrum antimicrobial therapy. Horses with infectious and noninfectious lesions of the calcaneus have been managed conservatively and surgically, with rather disappointing results.[6-8] Repeated surgeries are often required, and a substantial number of treated horses have persistent lameness.

SUBCUTANEOUS ABSCESS OVER THE TUBER CALCANEI

Puncture wounds in the region of the hock frequently result in penetration of the calcaneal bursa and infectious bursitis. Less commonly a subcutaneous abscess develops associated with firm, painful swelling on the plantar aspect of the hock and lameness. The extent of soft tissue swelling may make accurate palpation difficult, and ultrasonography is essential to determine whether or not the calcaneal bursa is involved. Radiographic examination of the calcaneus is also required. Treatment is by radical surgical debridement. The long-term functional outcome is usually satisfactory, although there is usually residual swelling (capped hock).

GASTROCNEMIUS BURSA

The subgastrocnemius bursa usually communicates with the calcaneal or intertendonous bursa. Mild distention may be present, unassociated with lameness. Primary injuries of the gastrocnemius bursa are rare. The bursa may be distended in association with gastrocnemius tendonitis, resulting in a capped hock appearance (see page 804). Occasionally, infection may occur because of a puncture wound or extension of infection from the calcaneal bursa.

CAPPED HOCK

A capped hock appearance may be caused by distention of the gastrocnemius bursa, distention of the subcutaneous bursa, or development of an acquired bursa over the tuber calcanei (see Figure 6-28). An acquired bursa develops because of repetitive trauma, such as the horse kicking the stable walls or leaning backward on its hindlimbs when traveling. Capped hock usually has no associated lameness. Protection of the hocks with hock boots may help to prevent deterioration.

CUNEAN BURSA

The cunean bursa lies underneath the cunean tendon on the medial aspect of the hock. Inadvertently penetrating the bursa is easy if one is inexperienced in injecting the centrodistal joint. Although the potential for primary bursitis exists, neither of the Editors of this text recognizes primary bursitis as a cause of lameness in racehorses or other sports horses. Gabel recognized a syndrome, "cunean tendonitis and bursitis–distal tarsitis syndrome of harness racehorses," but appreciated that horses showed substantially better improvement in gait after intraarticular analgesia of the distal hock joints than after infiltration of the cunean bursa alone.[11] Nonetheless, a component of periarticular soft tissue pain may occur in Standardbred trotters and pacers with distal hock joint pain, and treatment of the cunean bursa with corticosteroids frequently is used as part of management. Cunean tenectomy is practiced by some, but it has largely fallen from favor. Subcutaneous injection of corticosteroids and Sarapin over the proximal aspect of the second metatarsal bone may yield better results than medication of the cunean bursa.[5]

CAPPED ELBOW

A capped elbow is an acquired bursa that develops over the olecranon of the ulna. The bursa results from repeated trauma from the heel of the shoe on the ipsilateral forelimb when the horse is lying down. The condition generally is not associated with lameness and is merely a cosmetic blemish. The use of a sausage boot around the pastern prevents trauma from the shoe, and usually the swelling diminishes substantially and rapidly in size. Horses with chronic injuries have been treated by injection of corticosteroids, orgotein, or dysprosium-165, with disappointing results, or surgically, with better cosmetic results.[12]

ACQUIRED BURSA ON THE DORSAL ASPECT OF A HIND FETLOCK

Firm swelling on the dorsal aspect of the hind fetlocks of horses that jump fixed fences is common. These lesions are false bursae that overlie the extensor tendon and are usually of no consequence, except cosmetically. However, a puncture wound may result in infection, causing enlargement of the bursa and surrounding soft tissue swelling, localized heat, and pain on palpation.[5] In contrast to infection in a joint or tendon sheath, lameness is usually only mild to moderate. Ultrasonography is useful to better identify the causes of the soft tissue swelling, and diagnosis is confirmed by synoviocentesis and identification of many nucleated cells. Surgical treatment is required, and the prognosis is good.

FALSE THOROUGHPIN

A *thoroughpin* is the colloquial name for distention of the tarsal sheath, but more commonly the term is misused to describe a variety of swellings that may develop in the distal aspect of the crus cranial to the gastrocnemius tendon. These conditions are otherwise called *false thoroughpins* and should be differentiated from distention of the tarsal sheath, tarsocrural joint capsule (see Chapter 44), or calcaneal bursa (see page 799). A false thoroughpin occurs laterally more commonly than medially and may develop unilaterally or bilaterally. A false thoroughpin

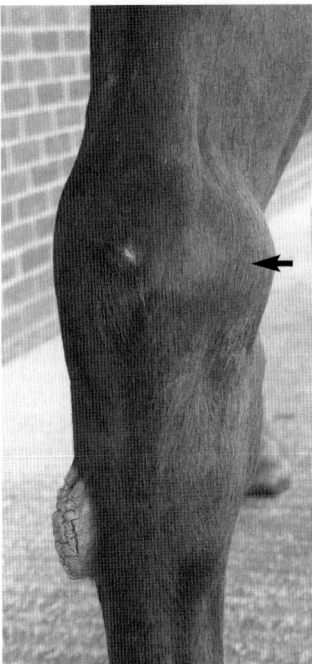

Fig. 79-2 • Plantar view of a right hock. A false thoroughpin *(arrow)*. The swelling in this horse was acute in onset, but it was unassociated with lameness. The horse was maintained in full work, and despite this the swelling reduced in size. Ultrasonographic evaluation revealed a unilocular fluid-filled cavity.

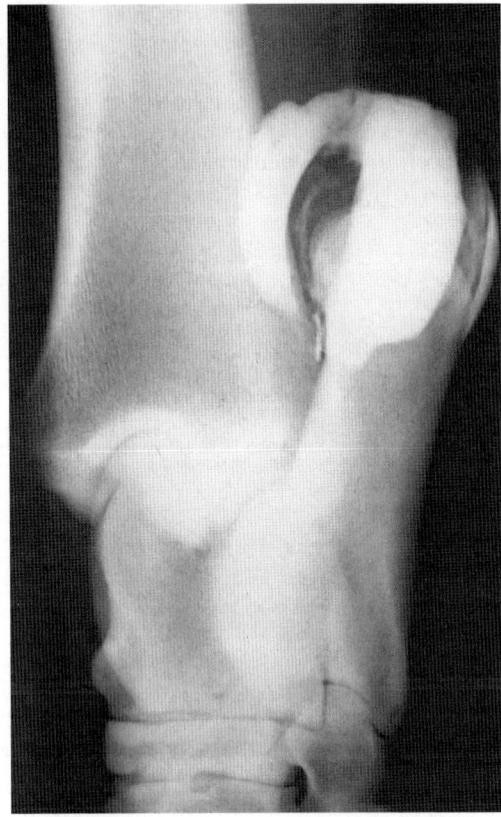

Fig. 79-3 • Dorsolateral-plantaromedial oblique radiographic image of a hock. A positive-contrast radiographic study of false thoroughpin. This fluid-filled cavity did not communicate with the tarsal sheath.

varies in size from small to large. In contrast to distention of the tarsal sheath or the plantar outpouching of the tarsocrural joint capsule, these swellings cannot be balloted from laterally to medially and do not extend distal to the hock (Figure 79-2). They may be sudden or insidious in onset and may or may not be associated with lameness.

The causes vary and are poorly understood. False thoroughpins are usually solitary, fluid-filled sacs (Figure 79-3), unilocular or multilocular, with a wall of variable thickness, with or without large echogenic fibrous bands traversing them (Figure 79-4). They may develop secondary to local hemorrhage or because of herniation of the tarsal sheath or the calcaneal or gastrocnemius bursae.[13-15]

Diagnostic ultrasonography is useful to identify the nature and extent of the swelling (see Figure 79-4). Unlike the tarsal sheath, no tendon is within the cavity. Positive-contrast radiography can be used to demonstrate whether any communication exists between adjacent structures (see Figure 79-3).

A false thoroughpin may be an incidental clinical finding unassociated with lameness. The condition is seen commonly in horses with a base-narrow hindlimb conformation.[5] Other causes should be excluded before one concludes that a false thoroughpin is the cause of lameness. Even if the swelling is acute in onset, in the absence of lameness I have maintained horses in work with no deleterious effects. Sometimes such swellings spontaneously reduce in size, but some swelling is likely to persist.

Long-term lameness associated with a false thoroughpin has been seen in a number of horses with chronic hindlimb lameness that has not responded to conservative management. Surgical excision of large multiloculated

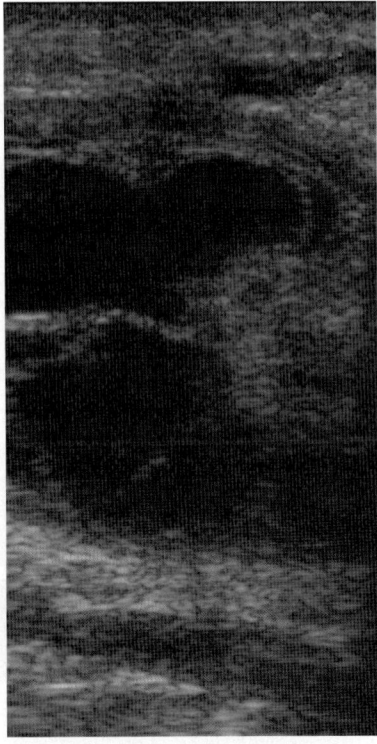

Fig. 79-4 • Longitudinal ultrasonographic image of a false thoroughpin. Proximal is to the left. There is a thick-walled fluid-filled cavity with some echogenic bands.

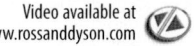

cystlike lesions has resolved lameness successfully in some horses,[5] although cosmetic results may be disappointing.

Spherical Masses Close to the Fetlock

Small, focal, hard, nonpainful spherical swellings are sometimes seen on the palmarolateral (plantarolateral) or palmaromedial (plantaromedial) aspect of the fetlock adjacent to the digital flexor tendon sheath (DFTS). These do not generally cause lameness. Ultrasonographic examination reveals a fluid-filled mass. Lameness associated with herniation of the DFTS is discussed in Chapter 74, page 776.

Chapter 80

Other Soft Tissue Injuries

Sue J. Dyson

RUPTURE OF THE FIBULARIS (PERONEUS) TERTIUS

Anatomy

The fibularis (peroneus) tertius is an entirely tendonous muscle that lies between the long digital extensor and the cranialis tibialis muscles, which cover the craniolateral aspect of the tibia. The fibularis tertius originates from the extensor fossa of the femur. Distally the fibularis tertius divides into branches that enfold the tendon of insertion of the tibialis cranialis and insert on the dorsoproximal aspect of the third metatarsal bone, the calcaneus, and the third and fourth tarsal bones. The tendon is an important part of the reciprocal apparatus of the hindlimb, which coordinates flexion of the stifle and hock.

The fibularis tertius is the most echogenic structure on the craniolateral aspect of the crus and is identified readily by ultrasonography as a well-demarcated hyperechogenic structure relative to the surrounding muscles (Figure 80-1).

History and Clinical Signs

Rupture of the fibularis tertius invariably is caused by trauma resulting in hyperextension of the limb; for example, a horse trying to jump out of a stable and getting one hindlimb caught on the top of the stable door. This usually results in rupture of the tendon in the middle of the crus but occasionally farther distally. Alternatively, rupture may be caused by a laceration on the dorsal aspect of the tarsus, resulting in transection of the tendon. Occasionally, partial tearing of the tendon occurs, usually at the level of the tarsocrural joint, with prominent swelling. Occasionally the reciprocal apparatus is partially but not totally disrupted. Avulsion injuries of the origin of the tendon rarely occur in young foals. Injury close to the origin is unusual in mature horses, occurring in two of 25 adult horses with fibularis tertius injury.[1]

The clinical signs are pathognomonic, because rupture of this tendon allows the hock to extend while the stifle is flexed. When standing at rest, the horse may appear

Reference on page 1321

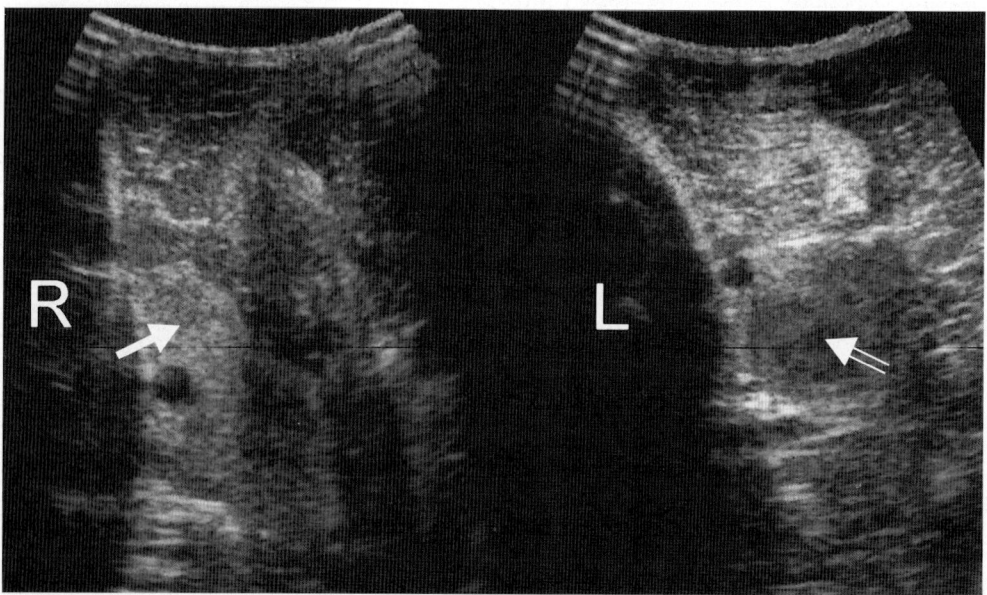

Fig. 80-1 • Transverse ultrasonographic images of the craniolateral aspect of the midcrus of 7-year-old horse with left hindlimb lameness of 2 months' duration. The fibularis tertius is the most echogenic structure in the center of the image of the right *(R)* hindlimb *(solid arrow)*. Compare this with the image of the left *(L)* hindlimb, in which the fibularis tertius is markedly hypoechoic *(open arrow)*. Note also that the overlying muscle is increased in echogenicity compared with the right hindlimb.

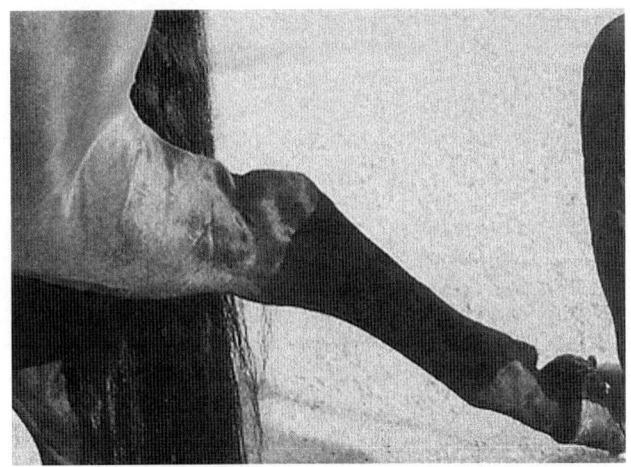

Fig. 80-2 • A horse with rupture of the fibularis tertius. The hock can be extended while the stifle is flexed. Note also the characteristic dimple in the contour of the caudodistal aspect of the crus. Clinical signs developed after the horse had attempted to jump out of its stable and had got hung up on the door. The horse made a complete recovery.

clinically normal, although with acute injury careful palpation may reveal some muscle swelling on the craniolateral aspect of the crus or farther distally. When the horse walks, it should be viewed carefully from behind and from the side. The hock may extend more than usual. The tendons of gastrocnemius and the superficial digital flexor muscles may appear unusually flaccid, and a dimple is seen on the caudal aspect of the crus about one handbreadth proximal to the tuber calcanei. At the trot the horse appears severely lame, with apparent delayed protraction of the limb because of overextension of the hock.

If the limb is picked up and pulled backward, the hock can be extended gradually and "clunks" into complete extension while the stifle remains flexed. A characteristic dimple appears in the contour of the caudal distal aspect of the crus (Figure 80-2). If rupture is only partial, or if lameness is chronic and some repair has taken place, clinical signs may be less severe and the diagnosis less obvious.

Presumably, strain of this tendon can occur, resulting in lameness, but I have no experience of this, and to my knowledge this condition has not been documented.

Diagnosis
The diagnosis of rupture of the fibularis tertius is based on the pathognomonic clinical signs. The site of rupture can be identified with ultrasonography (see Figure 80-1). The normally echogenic structure is not clearly identifiable and may be replaced by a region that is hypoechoic relative to the surrounding muscles. In horses with chronic injuries the surrounding muscles may become hypertrophied. Usually no associated radiological abnormalities are apparent in adult horses, although avulsion fracture of the origin has been described in foals.

Treatment
Confinement to box rest for 3 months, followed by a slow resumption of work, usually results in total resolution of clinical signs. Most horses are able to return to full athletic function without recurrence of clinical signs; however, injury may recur if work is resumed prematurely. Healing

should be monitored ultrasonographically. Fifteen of 21 horses (71%) retuned to full athletic function, with a mean convalescent period of 41 weeks.[1] Performance horses were less likely to return to their former activity than pleasure horses. Site and cause of injury (laceration or trauma) did not influence the outcome, but the presence of other injuries adversely influenced the prognosis. Delayed recognition of the clinical signs and failure to confine the horse may result in a chronic lesion, which fails to heal satisfactorily. However, compensatory hypertrophy and/or fibrosis of surrounding muscles may permit functional recovery.[1,2]

COMMON CALCANEAL TENDONITIS

The common calcaneal tendon consists of components from the superficial digital flexor and gastrocnemius tendons and from the biceps femoris, soleus, semimembranosus, and semitendinosus muscles. Contributions from the last two muscles are called the *axial* and *medial tarsal tendons.* So-called "common calcaneal tendonitis" has resulted from a kick in the hock region.[3] Unfortunately, the horse was not examined with ultrasonography until 5 months after injury, at which time soft tissue swelling was marked. Ultrasonographic examination revealed that the superficial digital flexor and gastrocnemius tendons appeared normal, but the axial and medial tarsal tendons were enlarged. The horse made a complete functional recovery.

GASTROCNEMIUS TENDONITIS

Tendonitis of the gastrocnemius is a relatively unusual cause of hindlimb lameness in the horse.[4-6] Disruption of the gastrocnemius in neonatal foals is discussed separately.

Anatomy
The gastrocnemius muscle arises from two heads that terminate in the midcrus in a common tendon. Proximally the tendon lies caudal to the superficial digital flexor tendon (SDFT); farther distally the tendon lies laterally and is ultimately cranial, inserting on the tuber calcanei. The SDFT and gastrocnemius tendons are separated by a bursa, the calcaneal or intertendonous bursa, that extends to the midtarsal region. A small bursa, the subgastrocnemius bursa, also lies cranial to the insertion of the gastrocnemius tendon on the tuber calcanei. A communication usually exists between these bursae. The intertendonous bursa also communicates with a subcutaneous bursa in approximately 37% of horses.

The tendon of the gastrocnemius may still contain some muscular tissue as far distally as the level at which it lies lateral to the SDFT. This results in hypoechoic regions within the tendon.

Gastrocnemius tendonitis usually occurs distally, distal to the musculotendonous junction. Rarely, damage occurs at the musculotendonous junction.[7] Occasionally, injuries occur at the origin of the gastrocnemius on the distal caudal aspect of the femur.[8]

History and Clinical Signs
Lameness may be acute or gradual in onset and varies from mild to severe. Distention of the subgastrocnemius and

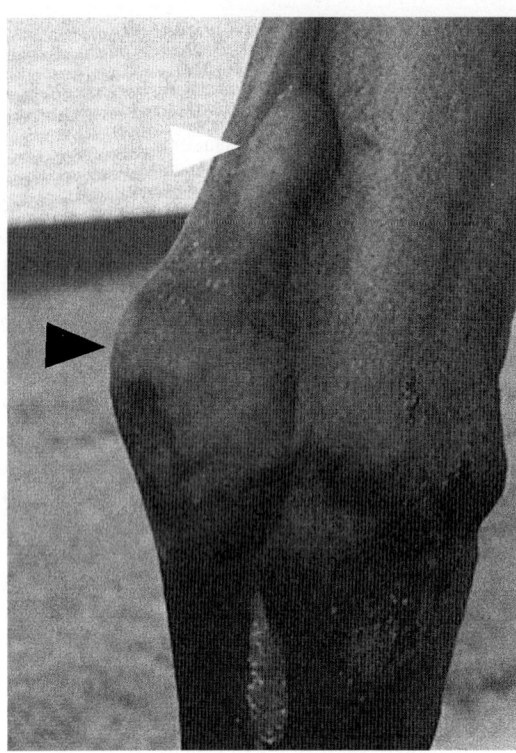

Fig. 80-3 • Medial view of the left hock of a 7-year-old Thoroughbred with acute-onset lameness associated with gastrocnemius tendonitis. Note the capped-hock appearance *(black arrowhead)* and the distention of the calcaneal bursa *(white arrowhead)*.

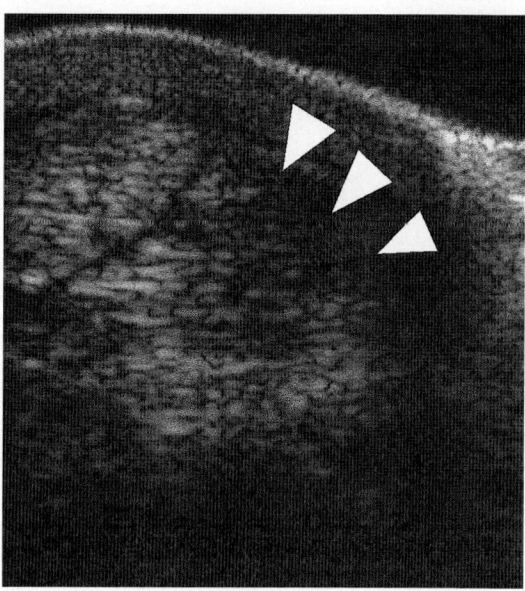

Fig. 80-4 • Transverse ultrasonographic image of the caudal distal aspect of the crus of a 6-year-old mare with left hindlimb lameness that was alleviated by perineural analgesia of the tibial nerve. Medial is to the left. The gastrocnemius tendon is enlarged, its caudal lateral aspect is poorly defined *(arrowheads)*, and there is a large hypoechoic region consistent with gastrocnemius tendonitis.

calcaneal bursae frequently is associated with gastrocnemius tendonitis, and the horse often develops a capped-hock appearance because of distention of the subcutaneous bursa (Figure 80-3). However, these swellings can occur without lameness or detectable pathological conditions of the gastrocnemius or SDFT (see page 799). Mild enlargement of the gastrocnemius tendon may occur, but this can be difficult to appreciate. Eliciting pain by palpation usually is not possible. Occasionally there are no palpable abnormalities.

Severe lameness is characterized by a reduced height of arc of foot flight, shortened cranial phase of the stride, and a tendency to hop off the caudal phase of the stride. Horses with less severe lameness have no specific gait characteristics. Lameness often is accentuated by proximal or distal limb flexion. Two of four horses with injury to the origin of the gastrocnemius muscle had an unusual gait characterized by internal rotation of the affected limb (outward movement of the calcaneus).[8] One of the Editors (MWR) has seen a horse with gastrocnemius tendonitis exhibit a similar, unusual gait in the affected limb. Care should be taken to not overinterpret this clinical finding in sound horses, because bilaterally symmetrical internal rotation of the hindlimbs can be a normal finding. A severe injury at the origin of the gastrocnemius muscle may result in an abnormal posture, with the hock of the affected limb lower than that of the contralateral limb.

Diagnosis
Lameness associated with gastrocnemius tendonitis is improved substantially by perineural analgesia of the tibial nerve, possibly because of local diffusion of the local

anesthetic solution. Diagnosis is confirmed by ultrasonographic examination. Comparison with the contralateral limb is useful. Lesions usually occur distal to the musculotendonous junction but do not involve the insertion on the tuber calcanei.

The tendon usually is damaged in the distal aspect of the crus, where it lies cranial to the SDFT. Ultrasonographic abnormalities include enlargement of the tendon, poor definition of the margins, and focal or diffuse hypoechoic or anechoic regions (Figure 80-4). Usually no detectable radiological abnormalities are apparent. In young Thoroughbred racehorses there may be increased radiopharmaceutical uptake (IRU) in the tuber calcanei, which should prompt investigation of the gastrocnemius tendon as a potential cause of lameness. Ultrasonographic assessment of the gastrocnemius tendon is also warranted if lameness is abolished by perineural analgesia of the tibial and fibular nerves, but no potential cause of lameness is identified in the hock or proximal metatarsal regions.

Injury at the origin of the gastrocnemius muscle on the caudal aspect of the femur may be associated with IRU and, if chronic, radiological evidence of proliferative new bone formation.[8]

Treatment and Prognosis
Conservative treatment with box rest and controlled exercise for up to 12 months generally has resulted in progressive improvement in lameness associated with gastrocnemius tendonitis and improvement in the ultrasonographic appearance of the tendon. Horses with mild lesions have been able to return to full athletic function without recurrent lameness, but those with more severe lesions have a more guarded prognosis.[5,6] Overall 14 of 25 horses managed conservatively have returned to full athletic function.[9] However two horses with moderate or severe lesions that

failed to respond to conservative management subsequently returned to full athletic function after intralesional treatment with β-aminopropionitrile fumarate.[9] Three of four horses with injury of the origin of the gastrocnemius returned to athletic use, but recurrent injury occurred in the fourth horse.[8]

DISRUPTION OF THE GASTROCNEMIUS IN NEONATAL FOALS

Disruption of gastrocnemius in neonatal foals is an unusual cause of hindlimb lameness or an inability to stand.[10,11] The condition has often been associated with dystocia. Partial or complete rupture usually occurs at the proximal musculotendonous junction, resulting in soft tissue swelling over the caudodistal aspect of the femur. Injury is usually unilateral, although it is occasionally bilateral. Diagnosis is based on the stance of the foal and detection of soft tissue swelling and is confirmed by ultrasonography. Foals able to bear weight are treated by stall rest alone; a sleeve cast or splints are applied to those that are unable to load the limb. Complications include severe hemorrhage associated with the injury, leading to cardiovascular compromise (three of 28 foals, 11%); concurrent disease (17 of 28, 61%); abscess formation at the site of rupture (four of 28, 14%); and cast sores (seven of 18, 39%).[11] Historically the prognosis was considered guarded,[10] but in a recent report 23 (82%) of 28 foals survived to discharge from the hospital, and 13 (81%) of 16 horses that reached 2 years of age trained or raced.[11]

SUBLUXATION AND LUXATION OF THE SUPERFICIAL DIGITAL FLEXOR TENDON FROM THE TUBER CALCANEI

Lateral (see Figure 6-29), or less commonly medial, luxation or subluxation of the SDFT from the point of the hock may occur along with damage to or rupture of the retinacular bands that insert medially and laterally on the tuber calcanei. Although usually a unilateral injury, the condition can occur bilaterally.

Lateral displacement of the SDFT occasionally occurs secondarily to hyperextension of the hind fetlock associated with progressive breakdown of the suspensory apparatus in older horses (see Figure 72-24 and page 760).

Anatomy
The SDFT lies caudally in the distal aspect of the crus and broadens to form a cap over the tuber calcanei. At this level, broad, thick retinacular bands extend medially and laterally to insert on the tuber calcanei. The calcaneal bursa is interposed between the SDFT and the tendon of gastrocnemius.

History and Clinical Signs
Partial or complete disruption of one of the retinacular bands that attach the SDFT to the tuber calcanei can result in subluxation or, more commonly, luxation of the SDFT laterally or medially. Occasionally the SDFT tendon splits sagittally, with the tendon luxating both medially and laterally. Lameness is usually sudden in onset and severe, although occasionally mild lameness precedes this, associated with soft tissue swelling in the region of the

point of the hock. Frequently no history of trauma is apparent, and the injury often occurs as the horse is being worked. The horse may suddenly stop and may become extremely distressed, especially if the tendon repeatedly moves on and off the tuber calcanei. The horse may kick out repeatedly with the limb. The tendon may return to its normal position when the horse bears weight. Soft tissue swelling rapidly ensues, resulting in a capped hock appearance, making accurate palpation difficult. If the horse is kicking repeatedly when moving, one may conclude wrongly that the soft tissue swelling developed as the result of trauma caused by kicking.

With subluxation of the SDFT, the tendon is usually positioned normally at rest. Careful observation of the tendon as the horse moves may reveal instability. With luxation it may be possible to see that the SDFT has been displaced laterally or, less commonly, medially. If the tendon remains luxated, then the horse tends to be less agitated, although obviously in pain in the acute stage. Careful palpation may reveal instability of the tendon or its displacement to an abnormal position.

In horses in which lateral displacement occurs secondary to hyperextension of the fetlock, the condition may be insidious in onset and slowly progressive and unassociated with acute lameness.

Diagnosis
Ultrasonographic examination is helpful if the tendon is displaced by confirming its abnormal position, but such examination can add to confusion if the tendon is in the normal position when the horse stands still. It may be possible to identify a partial tear in the medial, or less commonly the lateral, retinacular band. The calcaneal bursa may be distended, and if the condition is chronic there may be synovial proliferation. Occasionally there is a longitudinal split in the SDFT, which adversely affects prognosis.

Treatment
In the acute stage pain relief is essential, and tranquilization may be necessary to calm the horse. If the SDFT is unstable and is moving constantly on and off the tuber calcanei, management in the acute and chronic phases may be difficult. If the tendon is permanently dislocated laterally or medially, the distress usually resolves rapidly. Antiinflammatory drugs are best avoided, because the surrounding soft tissue swelling helps stabilize the tendon. If the tendon has luxated laterally, prolonged rest (6 months) usually results in resolution of pain, although a mechanical lameness may persist. This limits the horse's function for dressage, but these horses may be able to race or show jump at a high level. The prognosis associated with medial luxation is more guarded and tends to be associated with a greater degree of mechanical lameness.

If the SDFT is unstable initially, the tendon may with time and progressive further disruption of the attaching retinacular bands become more stable in a luxated position. Peritendonous injection of a sclerosing agent, P2G (Martindale Pharmaceuticals, Romford, Essex, England), has been helpful in stabilizing the luxated tendon in a limited number of horses.[9] Surgical transection of a partially torn retinacular band has helped in chronic subluxation.[9] Attempts at surgical stabilization of the SDFT in its normal position often have been disappointing, although successful results have been reported.[12,13] Surgical stabilization is worth considering only if the horse is temperamentally suited to a full-limb cast. Prognosis is influenced by the ease of reconstruction of the torn retinaculum, which depends on the site of the tear (close to the tendon, close to the bone, or midway) and its age.

BICEPS BRACHII TENDONITIS

Biceps brachii tendonitis is discussed in Chapter 40.

INFECTION OF THE COMMON DIGITAL EXTENSOR TENDON

Infection of the common digital extensor tendon and its sheath is usually the result of a puncture wound with or without deposition of a foreign body such as a blackthorn. It results in swelling, heat, pain, and lameness (see also page 789). Successful management was described by complete resection of the infected tendon.[14]

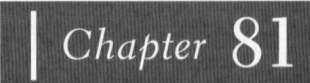

Chapter 81

Tendon Lacerations

Sue J. Dyson and Alicia L. Bertone

References
on page
1321

Tendon lacerations are serious injuries in horses because of the loss of the biomechanical function of the tendon, the slow return of tendon strength, the immediate strenuous loading demanded by a horse, and the complications of scarring. Nonetheless, early diagnosis, wound management, limb support, and long-term surgical and medical management have resulted in a good prognosis for most horses with extensor tendon lacerations and a fair prognosis for most of those with flexor tendon lacerations.[1,2] The extensor (dorsal) aspect of the limb is often damaged by

wire or a sharp object over which the horse has jumped. The flexor (palmar or plantar) aspect of the limb may be traumatized by circumferential wire injuries, landing on a sharp object, or being struck. The latter may be self-inflicted or from another horse.

DIAGNOSIS

Gross Appearance of the Wound

Any laceration over the dorsal or palmar/plantar surface of the limb distal to the stifle or elbow, especially across the dorsal aspect of the tarsus, distal dorsal aspect of the tarsus, dorsal metatarsal region, distal aspect of the radius, dorsal metacarpal region, and dorsal fetlock region may involve a tendon (Figure 81-1). Extensor tendons and the superficial digital flexor tendon (SDFT) are positioned directly under the skin; therefore minor-appearing wounds can transect these tendons completely. Direct visual inspection may reveal transected tendon fibers protruding from the

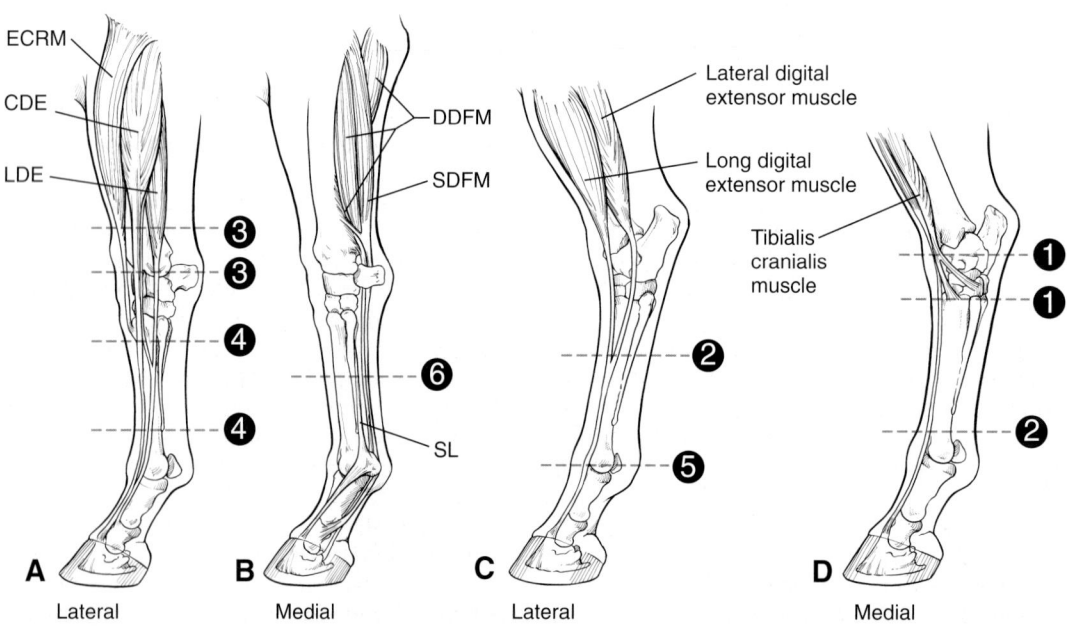

Fig. 81-1 • Diagram illustrating common sites of tendon injury. **A,** Lateral forelimb. **B,** Medial forelimb. **C,** Lateral hindlimb. **D,** Medial hindlimb. *1,* Dorsal tarsus; *2,* dorsal metatarsal region; *3,* distal radius; *4,* dorsal metacarpal region; *5,* dorsal fetlock region; *6,* palmar metacarpal region; *ECRM,* extensor carpi radialis muscle; *CDE,* common digital extensor muscle; *LDE,* lateral digital extensor muscle; *DDFM,* deep digital flexor muscle; *SDFM,* superficial digital flexor muscle; *SL,* suspensory ligament. (Adapted from Bertone AL: Tendon laceration in tendon and ligament injuries. Part II, *Vet Clin North Am Equine Pract* 11:293, 1995.)

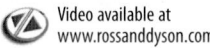
wound. However, injuries sustained at the gallop may result in a skin wound removed from the site of tendon damage because of the movement of the skin during exercise. The position of the wound relative to synovial structures should be evaluated with care because concurrent synovial contamination or infection reduces the prognosis and necessitates specific emergency treatment.

Evaluation of Gait

Each tendon serves a biomechanical function. Complete severance of a tendon results in a posture or gait change, which may be pathognomonic for disruption of the tendon integrity.

Extensor Tendons

Transection of an extensor tendon below the carpus produces a reduced ability to extend the digit, which is detected as an exaggerated, rapid (uncontrolled) dorsal flip of the hoof at the walk. This subtle change is easiest to detect if the lateral and common (or long) digital extensor tendons are transected completely. Intermittently the horse knuckles at the fetlock joint and places the digit on the dorsal surface of the pastern and fetlock joint. The gait abnormality is more obvious in a hindlimb and with lacerations in close proximity to the fetlock. Remaining peritendonous fascial attachments provide some support in horses with more proximal injuries. Horses with extensor tendon lacerations bear weight fully in a normal posture, unless other aspects of the wound create lameness and pain.

Transection of extensor tendons proximal to the carpus and at, or just proximal to, the tarsus also commonly occurs. Proximal to the carpus, transection of the extensor carpi radialis and common digital extensor tendons is most frequent. Flexion of the carpus may cause pain. The tendon sheath is often involved.

Proximal or dorsal to the tarsus, transection of the long digital extensor, cranialis tibialis, and fibularis (peroneus) tertius tendons is most frequent. If the fibularis tertius is disrupted, the hock can be extended while the stifle is flexed, indicating loss of the reciprocal apparatus. The gastrocnemius tendon develops a characteristic wrinkle in this extended position (see Figure 80-2 and page 802). The degree of gait abnormality may be mild. Transection of all the extensor tendons over the tarsus still allows full weight bearing with the foot flat on the ground. A greater tarsal extension during the swing phase of the stride and intermittent knuckling of the digit can be detected.

Digital Flexor Tendons

Transection of the digital flexor tendons below the carpus or tarsus produces pain on weight bearing and therefore lameness and gait abnormality. Transection of the SDFT is most common because it has the most superficial position of the two digital flexor tendons. The suspensory ligament (SL) is deep to the deep digital flexor tendon (DDFT) and is therefore least commonly injured with lacerations. A horse with complete transection of the SDFT may stand normally, or it may bear weight on the toe of the hoof to minimize movement of the tendon ends with fetlock joint extension. Complete transection of one branch of the SDFT in the pastern may not alter the stance during full load bearing. Administration of phenylbutazone for pain may eliminate lameness, and a gait abnormality may become

hard to detect. The DDFT and SL support the fetlock joint together with the SDFT. Therefore slight hyperextension of the fetlock because of disruption of the SDFT may be difficult to detect unless the contralateral limb is picked up. The greater the number of structures transected, the less support to the fetlock and other distal joints and the greater the likelihood of vessel and nerve transection. Elevation of the toe is pathognomonic for transection of the DDFT.

Digital Palpation of the Wound

Digital palpation is a simple and direct way to determine the extent of damage to structures below the skin. Integrity of the tendons is readily determined by feel. Partial tears can be distinguished from complete tears, and this affects treatment (see Partial Tendon Lacerations section). The tendon ends are often palpable beneath the skin proximal and distal to the wound, but they may be removed from the wound if the injury was sustained while the horse was galloping. The muscular attachment to the proximal end pulls the proximal tendon end farther from the wound. The wound should be clipped around the edges and cleansed thoroughly with a dilute antiseptic solution such as chlorhexidine before exploration. Gross debris can be debrided manually from the wound. Sterile gloves should be worn for the digital exploration after the wound is clean. Digital palpation may reveal involvement of a tendon sheath or joint capsule; however, small tears of these synovial structures may not be palpable. Sterile preparation of the skin and injection of a balanced electrolyte solution into the synovial structure in question at a site distant from the wound may demonstrate communication if solution exits the wound. Synovial fluid also can be obtained and submitted for cytological evaluation. Hemorrhage or inflammation is usually present in the synovial fluid if a sheath has been penetrated. Mild inflammatory changes can be seen in synovial structures adjacent to tendon injuries, even if no actual communication with the wound occurs.

Ultrasonographic Evaluation

Ultrasonographic evaluation of the tendons can quantitate the degree of tendon damage, particularly in horses with partial tears. Ultrasonographic examination is not necessary for diagnosing complete tears and therefore is performed rarely. Ultrasonography may also be technically difficult in the region of a skin wound because air in the wound impairs transmission of ultrasound waves. A partial laceration of the SDFT may be associated with the development of longitudinal splits extending proximodistally as a result of altered shear stresses. Complete transection of a branch of the SDFT in the pastern region may result in a shift of position of the branch proximal to the transection toward the side of the intact branch.

Ultrasonographic evaluation can be useful during the healing phases of horses with partial or complete tendon lacerations.[3] The amount of repair tissue should increase early in repair and then decrease as the tissue matures and gains strength. In digital flexor tendons, about 6 weeks are required for the tendon to gain the strength to support 450 kg, and the strength of the repair tissue is largely because of an increase in tissue mass. The repair tissue cross-sectional area is greater than the original tendon area, but the strength of that tissue per unit area is reduced.[4] The quality of the repair tissue can be monitored with ultrasonography. Ultrasonographic examinations should show progressively increased homogeneity of echogenicity, reduction in the hypoechoic areas of damaged tendon or early immature repair tissue, and appearance of parallel arrangements of fibers.

EMERGENCY MANAGEMENT

Treatment of Shock

Trauma is often severe in horses with lacerated tendons, particularly digital flexor tendons. Some horses may be trapped for hours in wire or entangled in equipment. Blood loss may be extensive if major arteries to the distal limbs have been transected. The loss of the function of a limb is painful and stressful. Initial management of these horses can be lifesaving. If possible, the horse should be caught and brought into a warm, clean area for examination and further treatment. If the horse has severe tachycardia (>100 beats/min) with pale mucous membranes and is reluctant to move, initial treatment should be performed on site. If the wound is still bleeding, a clean pressure bandage should be applied to stop the bleeding and provide some support to the limb. If the function of the limb is impaired mechanically, a splint should be applied over the bandage to minimize further damage with movement. Use of tranquilizers and sedatives should be kept to a minimum until the degree of blood loss and shock can be assessed and treated. Most sedatives are peripheral vasodilators and may produce substantial hypotension in a hypovolemic horse. Some horses may be in stress-induced shock from pain, with extreme catecholamine release. The effect of tranquilizers may be unpredictable and potentially can worsen the bleeding. Securing the horse in a familiar, warm, clean environment and stabilizing the injured limb may resolve the stress-related shock and allow assessment of hemorrhagic shock by evaluating peripheral pulse strength and quality, heart rate, and mucous membrane color. If hemorrhagic shock is severe, the most important treatment is intravenous fluid volume replacement, which can be in the form of high-volume isotonic fluids (20 to 60 L minimum per 450 kg of horse) or hypertonic saline (9% NaCl; 1 L per 450 kg of horse), followed by isotonic fluid replacement. Hypertonic fluid therapy can be effective for rapid expansion of the vascular space in hemorrhagic shock, but hypertonic solutions dehydrate the interstitium and induce a profound renal diuresis. Therefore it is critical that isotonic fluid therapy begins within 30 minutes to 1 hour after hypertonic fluid administration. Hypertonic fluid therapy is practical because of the convenience of the small volumes necessary and works well if the horse is referred or transported to a facility that has access for fluid administration.

Transportation

For transportation the injured limb should be placed toward the back of a trailer. The horse's weight shifts to the front of a trailer during braking, which is often less controlled than acceleration. The horse's head should not be tied tightly, so the head and neck can be used for balance. The limb should be supported with a padded pressure bandage and a splint for transport.

MEDICAL MANAGEMENT

All horses with tendon lacerations need medical therapy, whether surgery to reappose tendon ends is elected or not. If tendon laceration, partial or complete, is diagnosed, a more thorough aseptic preparation of the wound should be performed. These procedures require sedation, restraint, and local or regional analgesia.

Wound Cleansing and Debridement

The hair should be clipped circumferentially from above the wound (to the estimated top of the bandage) and the entire limb distal to the wound. Drainage of serum and exudate from the wound is often voluminous, and removal of the hair makes subsequent cleaning of the limb easier and more thorough, thereby minimizing bacterial growth and contamination. A 10-minute scrub of the wound with an antiseptic solution should be performed. If bone and tendon are exposed, care must be taken to minimize trauma to these tissues. A minor sterile instrument pack may be helpful in trimming heavily contaminated tissues and lacerated tendon ends, as well as for removing hair and debris from deep in the wound. Lacerated tendons should be trimmed at the edges to remove traumatized tissue that is expected to become necrotic. Debridement of tendon ends should be most conservative in horses with digital flexor tendon lacerations, for which apposition of tendon ends with suture is recommended.

Systemic and Local Medications

Tetanus toxoid should be administered to any horse with a tendon laceration, and tetanus antitoxin should be given if no vaccination history exists. Because all wounds are contaminated at injury and compound wounds have extensive soft tissue injury, broad-spectrum antimicrobial drugs should be administered systemically for a minimum of 3 days. Metronidazole should be considered in horses with grossly contaminated distal extremity wounds. The duration of antimicrobial therapy may be longer in horses with heavily contaminated wounds, wounds healing by second intention, infected wounds, wounds involving a tendon sheath, or wounds with delayed treatment (>24 hours). Wound lavage should be copious, usually with a minimum of 5 L of a balanced electrolyte solution.

SURGICAL TREATMENT

Surgery in the form of wound closure is performed in most horses with open wounds involving tendons. Primary closure is preferred, if possible, to provide the best success of obtaining primary wound healing, minimal scar formation, and the fewest complications associated with the transected tendon. However, wounds that are heavily contaminated, older than 24 hours, or heavily traumatized should have a delayed closure (1- to 3-day delay) performed to reduce the contamination and necrotic debris before closure. The decision to close a wound older than 24 hours must be made based on the condition of the wound and surrounding structures. Wounds in horses that have been managed appropriately from the time of injury until surgery can be closed at any time, if tissue loss is minimal and infection is not present.

Extensor Tendons

Transected extensor tendons heal well without primary suturing of the tendon, even if a large gap has formed between the tendon ends. Serial ultrasonographic evaluations show fibrosis occurring between the tendon ends that eventually becomes more organized and regains the linear arrangement of collagen along the pattern of the original tendon. This fibrous tissue seems to provide a mechanical link between the tendon ends because extensor function of the digit returns in most horses. In our experience, a palpable thinning of the new tendon and an enlargement at the old tendon ends usually remains, even after 1 year.

Horses with lacerated extensor tendons have a good prognosis, with 73% of injured horses returning to athletic soundness and 18% to pasture soundness.[2] In that study, 62% of the affected horses were treated with a three-layer cotton bandage, 23% with a splint and bandage, and 10% with fiberglass casts.

It is important that the horse is confined to box rest for at least 6 weeks so that lameness does not ensue. With lameness the hoof may be positioned on the toe, and the force of the digital flexor tendons maintains this position, particularly without the counterforce of the extensor tendon. Chronic flexor pull may result in permanent flexural deformity and lameness. If flexor dominance is noted, a splint or cast should be applied (see Chapter 86).

In our experience, the best cosmetic outcome, as well as chances of achieving primary wound closure, occurs with using a fiberglass cast for 3 to 6 weeks. The cast provides the most immobility to the limb and the lacerated tendon ends. Early fibrosis matures more quickly, without disruption of the early granulation tissue.

Digital Flexor Tendons

Horses with complete laceration of one or more digital flexor tendons are best treated with tendon suturing, wound closure, and postoperative immobilization for about 6 weeks. Digital flexor tendons support the weight of the horse on loading. Thus healing and return to full strength is a slow process, one that does not return to normal for at least 6 months. In studies investigating methods of tendon repair, immobilization of the limb in a cast without suturing produced a significantly weaker repair that resulted in the clinical sequela of a hyperextended fetlock joint.[4,5] The amount of scar tissue filling the tendon gap was significantly less in this group compared with the sutured groups and was the reason for the reduced strength. Therefore suturing of digital flexor tendon injuries is recommended. Monofilament suture (nylon or polyglyconate) produced the greatest strength of repair compared with carbon fiber suture when placed in a double-locking loop pattern (nylon) or three-loop pulley pattern (polyglyconate) for apposition of tendon ends or for spanning tendon gaps.[4-6] The limb should be cast for at least 6 weeks, with the fetlock joint in mild flexion, by building a heel support with casting tape or plaster to provide a level weight-bearing surface with the ground.

Repairs of flexor tendon lacerations above the hock (i.e., gastrocnemius tendon, DDFT, or SDFT) should follow the same principles, but the prognosis is decreased because of the greater difficulty in maintaining a full-limb cast, larger size of the tendons at this location, and greater biomechanical stresses to support the hock with weight bearing.

Partial Tendon Lacerations

Horses with partially transected tendons can be treated successfully without suturing but with wound closure and limb immobilization. Partial transection of digital flexor tendons usually involves the SDFT only or the axial margin (medial or lateral) of the SDFT and DDFT. If the limb is immobilized, the remaining fibers of tendon provide the stability for the torn tendon ends to remain in apposition and provide the strength to prevent further tendon tearing during healing. Anecdotally, if more than 75% of the SDFT is lacerated, tendon suturing may provide a reduced gap and faster healing and improve the repair. If the SDFT is completely transected along with a partial laceration of the DDFT, the SDFT should be treated with suturing as previously described and the DDFT left unsutured.

Lacerations in Tendon Sheaths

If a laceration enters a tendon sheath, then therapy is altered to include aggressive lavage of the sheath and wound, intrathecal administration of antibiotics, close monitoring of sheath fluid cytological condition, longer use of systemic antibiotics, and limb immobilization. If tissue loss is minimal, wounds entering tendon sheaths should be closed primarily. Primary closure and fiberglass cast application offer the best chance of early healing and minimize the potential for the complications of ascending infection, chronic drainage and fistulae formation, and fibrosis.

CONVALESCENT THERAPY
Shoeing

After removal of a cast or splint for horses with extensor tendon lacerations, a gradual return to full weight bearing is recommended. Shoeing recommendations are simple and include trimming or shoeing level, without toe extensions that may catch and produce knuckling. For horses with digital flexor tendon lacerations, an elevated and extended heel shoe can be applied and the heel lowered sequentially over the next 6 weeks to a flat position. For severe lacerations involving the DDFT, SDFT, or SL, an extended heel shoe may always be required for additional flexor support.[7]

Graduated Exercise

Horses with extensor tendon injuries have not been evaluated as closely during the healing process to assess tissue maturation and return of strength as those with digital flexor tendon injuries. Because the function of the extensor tendon is to extend the digit and not endure a load on weight bearing, return to full strength may occur sooner than for digital flexor tendons. Horses should remain in a box stall or a confined area during the wound healing phases and early fibroblastic repair phases of tendon healing (3 to 6 weeks). After this time, handwalking and controlled exercise such as swimming can begin to strengthen the tendon and improve gliding function. After 10 to 12 weeks of controlled exercise, and if no signs of knuckling or flexor dominance are present, gradual return to athletic use can begin.

Horses with digital flexor tendon lacerations require a more gradual convalescent period. After the first 6 weeks of immobilization, the next 6 weeks should be spent in confinement and regaining a normal foot posture and full weight bearing. Heel support shoes are applied during this time. After 12 weeks, handwalking can begin and gradually increase in frequency and duration over the next 3 to 6 weeks. Controlled exercise with walking, lunging, swimming, or ponying (leading from another horse) is preferred to turnout. Turnout can be given after the horse is sound at the walk and trot and ultrasonographic examination demonstrates extensive fibrosis and mature scar tissue. Heavy athletic use should not begin until 8 to 12 months after the injury.

PROGNOSIS

Successful outcome (soundness) occurs in about 75% of horses with extensor tendon lacerations and up to 54% of horses with digital flexor tendon lacerations.[1,2,8] The prognosis for horses with partial disruption of the SDFT, DDFT, or both is better than for those with complete lacerations.[8] Long-term failures are attributable to continued pain from extensive adhesions, joint pain, other injury at the time of laceration, tendon sheath adhesions, tendon contracture, palmar (plantar) annular ligament constriction, reinjury, and failure of the repair to regain adequate strength to support the joint, leading to breakdown. Reinjury to a damaged tendon may occur during healing, but such a tendon can heal successfully, although convalescence is prolonged. In general the prognosis is better for pleasure riding horses than for sports horses, but especially with injuries involving the digital flexor tendons of a hindlimb, complete function may be restored. An association exists between lacerations of either or both the long and lateral digital extensor tendons in the proximal part of the metatarsal region and the subsequent development of stringhalt several months later.[9]

Chapter 82

Soft Tissue Injuries of the Pastern

Virginia B. Reef and Ronald L. Genovese

References on page 1321

Injuries to the digital flexor tendons and ligaments in the pastern are a common cause of lameness in horses.[1-6] Injuries to the collateral ligaments or the palmar or plantar ligaments of the proximal interphalangeal joint are a less frequent cause of lameness.[1,7-9] Swelling, heat, and sensitivity of the affected tendon or ligament to palpation often accompany lameness. Ultrasonographic evaluation of the pastern is indicated when local swelling, heat, and sensitivity are detected, or when effusion occurs in the digital flexor tendon sheath (DFTS).[10] The cause of the swelling can be determined by ultrasonography, and the severity of the injury can be characterized. The clinician should keep in mind that peripheral longitudinal splits in the digital flexor tendons within the DFTS are difficult to detect and can be missed ultrasonographically.[10] If injury occurs to the superficial or deep digital flexor tendons (SDFT, DDFT) in the metacarpal or metatarsal region, ultrasonographic examination should include an evaluation of these structures in the pastern. Lameness associated with soft tissue injuries of the pastern also can occur without localized soft tissue swelling, and ultrasonographic examination is indicated if pain is localized to the region using diagnostic analgesia and no radiological abnormality is detected, or entheseous new bone is seen. The clinician should bear in mind that intraarticular analgesia of the metacarpophalangeal or metatarsophalangeal joints, the proximal interphalangeal joint, and the DFTS is not necessarily specific and may influence closely related structures such as the distal sesamoidean ligaments and the palmar ligaments of the proximal interphalangeal joint. It also may be important to use diagnostic analgesia to determine whether the injury causing soft tissue swelling in the pastern region is the source of the lameness. Nuclear scintigraphy may help to determine whether entheseous new bone is active, and magnetic resonance imaging (MRI) has the potential to provide additional information. This chapter focuses on lesions diagnosed using ultrasonography, but the absence of detectable ultrasonographic abnormalities does not preclude soft tissue pathology causing pain.

ANATOMY

Most of the soft tissue structures in the pastern are on the palmar or plantar aspects and are similar in the forelimbs and hindlimbs. The following describes the forelimb but applies equally to the hindlimb. The SDFT forms a thin ring around the DDFT at the ergot and in the proximal-most portion of the pastern and then bifurcates into medial and lateral branches. The origin of the branches has a teardrop shape. The cross-sectional area (CSA) of each SDFT branch gradually enlarges as the branch extends distally along the palmarolateral and palmaromedial aspects of the pastern, until the branches insert on the distal aspect of the proximal phalanx and on the proximal aspect of the middle phalanx. The DDFT lies immediately dorsal to the SDFT and extends along the midline to its insertion on the distal phalanx.[1-6,11-15] The DDFT has a bilobed shape in the pastern and is surrounded by the DFTS. The oblique (middle) sesamoidean ligaments (OSLs) originate from the base of the lateral and medial proximal sesamoid bones (PSBs) as two large, round to oval branches. These branches become smaller in CSA as they extend distally. The branches join in the proximal to mid aspect of the proximal phalanx and insert as a broad band on the palmar aspect of the middle of the proximal phalanx. The straight sesamoidean ligament (SSL) also has its origin at the base of the PSBs and the palmar ligament and extends distally in the midline, palmar to the OSL, to insert on the scutum medium of the middle phalanx.[1-6,11-13,16] The SSL lies dorsal to the DDFT and has an hourglass shape, larger proximally and distally, and narrowest in the middle.

The DFTS surrounds the SDFT and DDFT throughout the proximal aspect of the proximal phalanx to the bifurcation of the SDFT.[1-6,11-15,17] The entire length of the DDFT is included in the DFTS, except for a small area in the distal palmar aspect of the pastern, just proximal to the bulbs of the heel. The dorsal aspect of the DFTS extends farther distally than its palmar aspect. The proximal digital annular ligament is adhered closely to the palmar aspect of the SDFT in the proximal aspect of the pastern.[1,3-5,18] The distal digital annular ligament forms a sling over the distal part of the DDFT. These two structures are thin in normal horses.

The abaxial and axial palmar ligaments of the proximal interphalangeal joint originate in pairs from the medial and lateral aspects, respectively, of the middle of the proximal phalanx and dorsal to the SDFT branches. They insert on the scutum medium abaxial to the branches of the SDFT (abaxial palmar/plantar ligament) and between the SSL and the branches of the SDFT (axial palmar/plantar ligament). These are large, round to oval ligaments that extend in a diagonal direction from the origin to the insertion. The collateral ligaments of the proximal interphalangeal joint originate from a small eminence on the lateral and medial aspects of the proximal phalanx, distal to the origin of the palmar ligaments, and arc across the joint to insert on a small eminence on the lateral and medial aspects, respectively, of the proximal aspect of the middle phalanx.[1,3,7,11] The proximal interphalangeal joint has a closely adhered joint capsule.

The common digital extensor tendon is located on the dorsal aspect of the pastern.[1] The extensor branches of the suspensory ligament (SL) join the common digital extensor tendon in the distal part of the proximal phalanx. The main insertion of the common digital extensor tendon is on the extensor process of the distal phalanx, but there are also areas of insertion onto the proximal and middle phalanges. A bursa is present between the tendon and the proximal interphalangeal joint.

ULTRASONOGRAPHIC ANATOMY

The pastern has been divided into five zones: three zones for the proximal phalanx and two zones for the shorter middle phalanx[1-6,12-15] (see Chapter 16).

Superficial Digital Flexor Tendon

In the proximal aspect of the pastern (zone P1A), the SDFT is imaged from the palmar aspect and is homogeneously echogenic and has a thin, half-moon shape in the transverse plane.[1-6,12-14] In longitudinal images the SDFT has a parallel fiber pattern and a triangular shape along the midline in zone P1A because its thickness decreases distally. In normal horses, distinguishing the proximal digital annular ligament from the DFTS and the palmar border of the SDFT is difficult. The proximal digital annular ligament can be identified if thickened by following it medially and laterally to its attachment to the proximal aspect of the proximal phalanx. The body of the SDFT ranges in thickness (palmar to dorsal) from 2 to 6 mm in P1A to 1 to 4 mm over the middle of the proximal phalanx.[3] The teardrop-shaped branches in the proximal to mid pastern region (at the junction of zones P1A and P1B) are imaged from the palmaromedial and palmarolateral aspects

are followed individually to triangular-shaped insertions. The SDFT branches are similarly homogeneously echogenic, with a parallel fiber pattern throughout. The branches of the SDFT range in thickness from 4 to 7 mm in the proximal pastern to 7 to 12 mm distally.[15] The CSA of the two SDFT branches ranges from 0.3 to 0.4 cm^2 in the distal portion of zone P1A where the branch begins, increases to 0.4 to 0.6 cm^2 in zone P1B, and further enlarges to 0.6 to 0.8 cm^2 near the insertion.

Deep Digital Flexor Tendon

The DDFT has an oval to bilobed appearance in the pastern and is imaged on the palmar midline of the pastern until the DDFT is lost from view distally.[1-6,12-15] The two lobes are symmetrical. The fibers of the DDFT extend obliquely from a deeper to a more superficial position in the more distal portion of the pastern and are separated from the SSL by an anechogenic space. The dorsopalmar thickness and lateral to medial width of the DDFT decrease in the mid pastern and increase again in the distal aspect of the pastern. The DDFT measures 5 to 10 mm (palmar to dorsal) in the proximal aspect of the pastern, slightly less in the mid pastern, and 7 to 12 mm in the distal aspect of the pastern. The width of the DDFT in a lateral-to-medial direction ranges from 18 to 33 mm in the proximal aspect of the pastern, decreasing to 15 to 23 mm in the mid pastern, and increasing in the distal aspect of the pastern to 23 to 32 mm.[3] Along the dorsal aspect of the DDFT in the mid pastern region is a synovial fold of the DFTS that is imaged readily, surrounded by a small amount of anechogenic synovial fluid. In the distal pastern region, the palmar aspect of the DDFT adheres to the synovial membrane of the DFTS.

Oblique Sesamoidean Ligaments

Injury to the OSLs is often missed ultrasonographically because the origin and proximal to midportion of each OSL (where the majority of the injuries are) are not imaged from the palmaromedial and palmarolateral aspects of the limb. The origin of the medial or lateral OSL is best found by placing the ultrasound transducer over the base of the medial or lateral PSB and scanning distally over the bone to its base, angling the transducer proximally to image the origin of the respective OSL.[1-6,12,13] Alternatively, the origin of an OSL can be found by following the SL branches distally over the respective PSBs to the base. Immediately distal to the base of the PSB is the origin of an OSL, best located initially in its transverse section as a large, round to oval structure. The OSLs merge in the distal part of zone P1A into a broad, rectangular band dorsal to the DDFT. The OSLs then insert on the palmar or plantar aspect of the proximal phalanx in zone P1B. An OSL is the most difficult tendon or ligament to follow longitudinally to its insertion because the ligament extends diagonally from its origin to its insertion in two different planes. Following the medial or lateral OSL from its origin to the main body of OSL requires a transducer angle of about 45 degrees from the base of the PSBs to the palmar midline of the proximal phalanx. Properly aligning the transducer and eliminating off-normal incidence artifact is difficult. The OSLs may appear less echogenic because of an oblique orientation. The OSLs are thickest in the medial to lateral direction proximally. Each OSL measures 12 to 20 mm (lateral to medial) in the proximal aspect of P1A, decreasing to 9 to 17 mm just before their convergence, and 0 to 9 mm (one side only) at their insertion. The palmar to dorsal thickness of the OSLs is 5 to 12 mm in P1A, decreasing to 2 to 6 mm just proximal to the convergence, and decreasing again to 0 to 3 mm at the insertion. The mean CSA of an OSL determined with MRI is reported to be 0.86 cm^2 in the proximal third, 0.56 cm^2 in the middle third, and 0.40 cm^2 in the distal third.[19] However, there may be size differences between the medial and lateral OSLs.[20]

Straight Sesamoidean Ligament

The origin of the SSL is found by angling the transducer in a proximal and dorsal direction from the proximal-most aspect of the pastern, just underneath the ergot, to image the ligament and the base of the PSBs. The SSL becomes a more oval-shaped structure and is palmar to the OSLs in zone P1B. The SSL remains dorsal to the DDFT as it inserts on the scutum medium.

The dorsal-to-palmar thickness of the SSL gradually increases as the medial to lateral width decreases. The SSL measures 5 to 9 mm (palmar to dorsal) proximally, increasing slightly over the distal aspect of the proximal phalanx to 6 to 12 mm, and increasing again to 8 to 14 mm at the scutum medium. The medial-to-lateral thickness of the SSL ranges from 17 to 30 mm in zone P1A, decreases to 10 to 15 mm, and then widens over the scutum medium to 45 to 65 mm.[3] The SSL is echogenic with normal parallel fiber alignment throughout, except at the insertion. A central symmetric hypoechoic area is commonly imaged in clinically normal horses at the insertion of the SSL.[16] Care must be taken to be sure that lesions are not created at the insertion of the SSL because of the difficulty in aligning the transducer perpendicular to the ligamentous fibers owing to the horse's heel. Comparison of this area with the contralateral normal limb should aid in determining whether a suspected lesion is real.

Cruciate Sesamoidean Ligaments

The cruciate sesamoidean ligaments are imaged only in the proximal-most portion of the pastern and measure 2 to 4 mm in a palmar to dorsal direction.[3]

Collateral Ligaments

The collateral ligaments of the proximal interphalangeal joint are easiest to examine by imaging in both longitudinal and transverse planes. The collateral ligaments of the proximal interphalangeal joint are homogeneously echogenic structures, with a parallel fiber pattern at the origin on the distal aspect of the proximal phalanx to the insertion on the proximal half of the middle phalanx.[1,2]

Proximal Interphalangeal Joint

The proximal interphalangeal joint is easiest to image initially in the longitudinal plane by identifying the joint space, and then a transverse evaluation of the joint can be made.[7] Fluid normally is not imaged in the proximal interphalangeal joint.

Palmar/Plantar Ligaments of the Proximal Interphalangeal Joint

The palmar ligaments of the proximal interphalangeal joint can be imaged from the origin on the middle of the proximal phalanx to the insertion on the proximal palmar aspect of the middle phalanx. These ligaments are paired on the medial and lateral aspects of the pastern and are located by placing the transducer dorsal to the branch of the SDFT. The more abaxial branch originates first and is easier to follow than the more axial branch. Each branch has a round to oval shape, is homogeneously echogenic with a parallel fiber pattern, and must be followed individually from origin to insertion.

Digital Nerves

The digital nerves are located dorsal to the lateral and medial aspects of the SDFT, adjacent to the lateral or medial palmar digital arteries.[1] The nerves are found most easily by identifying the digital vein and artery, looking immediately adjacent (palmar) to the digital vein and the adjacent SDFT. The nerves are tiny, homogeneously echogenic circular structures. The normal thickness of the palmar or plantar digital nerves is 2 to 3 mm, with a CSA of 0.5 to 1 mm^2.[1]

TENDON AND LIGAMENT INJURIES

In the fore pastern, the SDFT is the most frequently injured tendon or ligament in all performance horses.[1-6,21] The OSLs are the second most commonly injured structures in the fore pastern, followed by injuries to the DDFT and SSL.[1-6] In the hind pastern, injuries to the DDFT are most common, with a low incidence of injuries to the other tendonous and ligamentous structures.[1-5] Injuries to the DDFT are accompanied most often by tenosynovitis of the DFTS.[1-6] Injuries to the collateral ligaments of the proximal interphalangeal joint occur infrequently and are more common in the forelimb.[1,3,7] Injuries to the palmar/plantar ligaments of the proximal interphalangeal joint are also uncommon and occur in forelimbs (most common) and hindlimbs. The tendonous and ligamentous structures in the pastern have little covering, and thus they are vulnerable to injury with puncture wounds and lacerations. Ultrasonographic evaluation of the pastern region in a horse with an acute laceration or puncture wound to the pastern should be performed aseptically and is an integral part of the evaluation of these soft tissue structures to determine whether injury occurred and the severity of the injury.

Superficial Digital Flexor Tendonitis

Injuries to the branches of the SDFT are more common in the forelimb.[1-6,21,22] Injury in the pastern may occur in isolation, without an injury to the SDFT in the metacarpal or metatarsal region, or may be an extension of a more proximal tendon injury. Extension of the SDFT injury into the proximal pastern region, and less frequently into the mid and distal pastern, is more common in the forelimb. Abnormal conformation such as a long pastern, an underrun heel, or an axially displaced heel may predispose to injury of an SDFT branch.

Lameness usually occurs at the onset of injury, is more common with SDFT injuries in the pastern than with those in the metacarpal or metatarsal region, and may persist longer, lasting for 1 to 4 weeks. Longitudinal swelling that extends in a proximal-to-distal direction along the lateral or medial aspect of the pastern throughout its length is often characteristic.[1,2,21] Focal heat and sensitivity usually

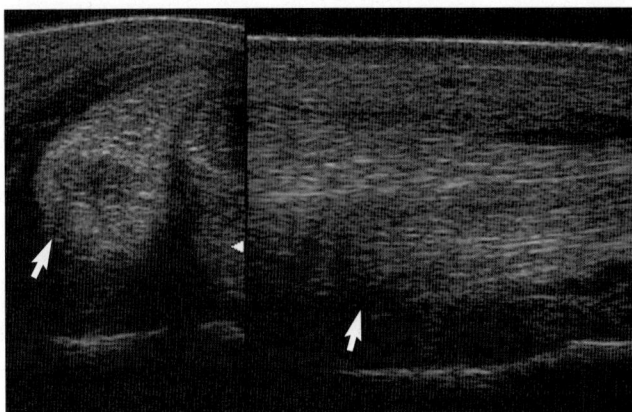

Fig. 82-1 • Ultrasonographic images of the right front medial branch of the superficial digital flexor tendon obtained in the proximal part of zone P1C in a horse with a recent injury. The anechoic to hypoechoic core lesion is apparent within the branch *(arrows)* in the transverse *(left)* and longitudinal *(right)* views. Fiber disruption and short linear fibers are imaged within the lesion in the longitudinal view, consistent with a recent injury and early healing. The horse was 1 of 5 degrees lame, with focal swelling, heat, and sensitivity to palpation.

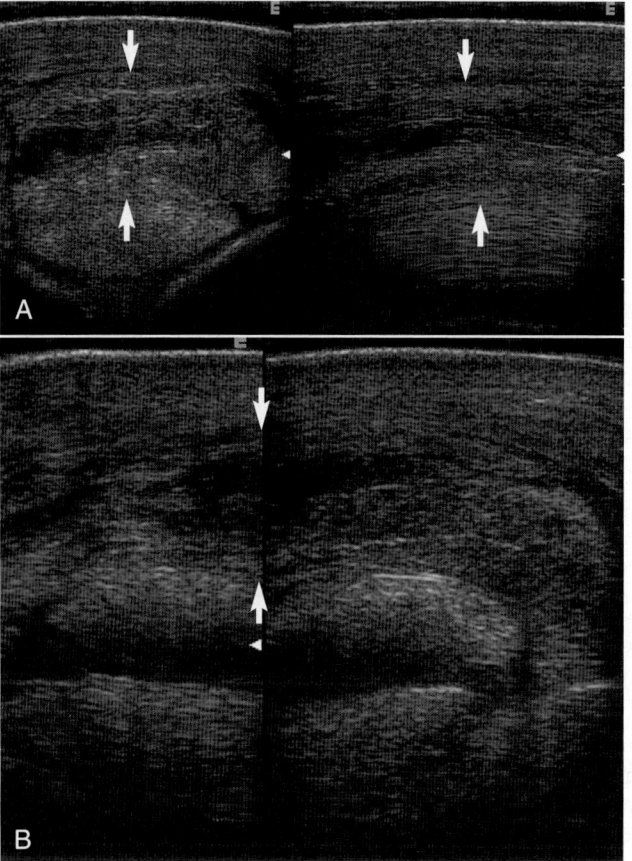

Fig. 82-2 • Ultrasonographic images of the left superficial digital flexor tendon (SDFT) in the metacarpal region **(A)** and pastern **(B)** obtained from a horse with an acute severe injury to that tendon. This horse was lame at the walk, with substantial swelling of the SDFT in the metacarpal and pastern regions and heat and sensitivity of the tendon on palpation. The metacarpophalangeal joint dropped on weight bearing. **A,** The SDFT is enlarged *(arrows)* and contains a large central anechoic lesion completely lacking in tendon fibers. The SDFT was severely injured in the metacarpal region from 7 to 32 cm distal to the accessory carpal bone. The SDFT in zone 3C is surrounded by a thickened hypoechogenic digital flexor tendon sheath (DFTS). The transverse image is on the left, and the longitudinal image is on the right. **B,** The SDFT in zone P1A is markedly enlarged *(arrows)* with a central anechoic lesion that extended distally to the insertion of the lateral branch. The surrounding DFTS and peritendonous tissues are greatly thickened and hypoechogenic, and the distinction between the palmar margin of the SDFT and the peritendonous structures is difficult to discern. The lateral branch of the SDFT has nearly complete fiber disruption that extends to its insertion. The lateral side of the proximal pastern is the right image, and the medial side of the pastern is the left image. The SDFT and the DFTS were so enlarged that they could not be imaged in their entirety in a single image. Therefore the two halves of the SDFT were displayed together in these transverse images.

accompany this swelling. However, in horses with acute injuries, no localizing clinical signs may be apparent, but lameness is alleviated by palmar (abaxial sesamoid) nerve blocks. Generally, swelling develops within 3 to 4 days. Ultrasonographic examination in the absence of swelling may result in false-negative results. Subluxation of the proximal interphalangeal joint can occur in horses with severe injury to or complete rupture of the SDFT in the pastern. Dropping of the fetlock joint with weight bearing can occur in horses with severe SDFT injury.

Core injuries are the most common detected by ultrasonography (Figure 82-1), followed by diffuse injury to the affected branch.[1,2] Complete ruptures or near complete ruptures of the branches do occur, but they are less frequent. These injuries can be unilateral or bilateral and uniaxial or biaxial, although uniaxial injuries are most common. The frequency of injury to the medial or lateral SDFT branch varies with the type of racing or sporting activity.[21,22] Peritendonous soft tissue swelling is common. Avulsion fracture of the insertion of the SDFT branch occurs infrequently. Ultrasonographic evaluation of the more proximal aspect of the SDFT in the metacarpal or metatarsal region is indicated to determine whether the injury is an extension of a more proximal injury (see Chapter 69) (Figure 82-2). Ultrasonographic evaluation of the contralateral fore or hind pastern is recommended because bilateral disease may be present, more frequently in the forelimb. Radiological examination of the pastern is indicated for all horses with subluxation of the proximal interphalangeal joint, avulsion fractures at the insertion of the SDFT branch, or a ruptured SDFT branch.

Treatment for horses with acute superficial digital flexor tendonitis in the pastern is similar to that in the metacarpal or metatarsal region.[1,2] Horses with SDFT injuries in the pastern may have a poorer prognosis for returning to racing than those with injuries in the metacarpal region, with a more frequent recurrence of injury.[1,2,22] Extension of the injury from the pastern to the metacarpal area may also occur, resulting in a shortened racing career.[21] However,

successful return to performance does occur for horses with SDFT branch injuries. Rare horses are able to continue to compete with SDFT branch injuries, without a period of rest, but these are the exceptions rather than the rule. Healing of the SDFT occurs similarly to that in the metacarpal region, with an increase in the echogenicity of the lesion and the subsequent appearance of short, usually randomly aligned linear echoes. Rehabilitation of horses with injuries to the SDFT branch is similar to that described for proximally located tendonitis and is based on the injury severity (see Chapter 69). A minimum of 6 months in a

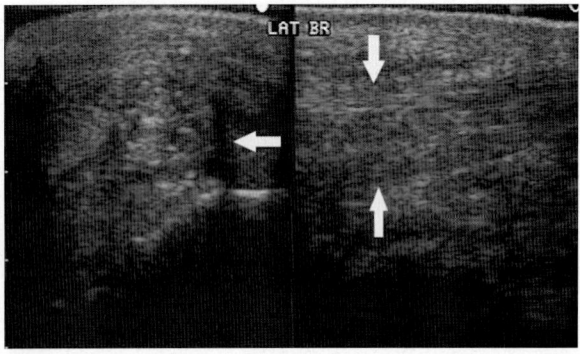

Fig. 82-3 • Ultrasonographic images of the left front lateral branch of the superficial digital flexor tendon obtained in zone P1B of a horse with a chronic healed core injury. The horse had sustained the original injury more than 5 years earlier, and after a long, controlled exercise program the horse had raced successfully several times a year, although some small areas of reinjury were detected periodically, necessitating short periods of downtime from race training. The original central core lesion is still visible in this branch as an echogenic central area, with a thin hypoechoic rim (arrow) in the transverse view (left) and longitudinal (right) views. In the longitudinal view, the central area of the tendon has a more random fiber pattern than the periphery (arrows).

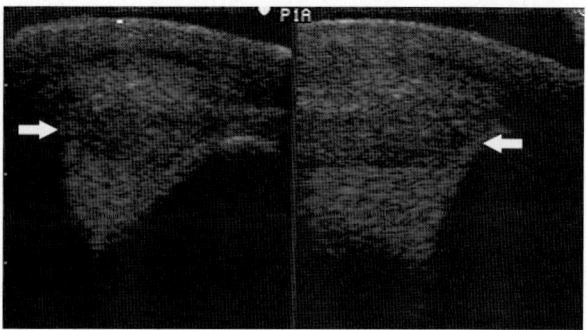

Fig. 82-4 • Ultrasonographic images of the origin of the left hind lateral oblique sesamoidean ligament (OSL) obtained in zone P1A. Most of the OSL is hypoechoic (arrow) in the transverse (left) and longitudinal (right) views (proximal is to the right). Substantial fiber disruption is visible in the longitudinal view, beginning at the base of the proximal sesamoid bone (arrow). There is no normal fiber pattern imaged at the origin of the lateral OSL. The more anechoic abaxial region represents a more recent injury, whereas the more echogenic area axially with a random fiber pattern represents a more chronic area of injury that is repairing. Some periligamentous echogenic soft tissue thickening surrounds the branch. The horse had a concurrent distal suspensory desmitis involving both suspensory branches that extended from 37 to 47 cm distal to the point of the hock. The horse was 2 of 5 degrees lame and had local heat, swelling, and mild sensitivity of the lateral OSL.

controlled exercise program is needed for horses with mild SDFT branch injury, whereas 12 months or more are indicated for those with severe injury to the SDFT branch to maximize the horse's chance of returning to its previous level of competition. Ultrasonographic monitoring of tendon healing is an important part of the rehabilitation program. A central echogenic scar surrounded by a hypoechoic halo may be detected in the SDFT branch with a healed core lesion (Figure 82-3). Peritendonous echogenic tissue representing immature and maturing fibrous tissue often is imaged adjacent to the injured SDFT branch and can result in adhesions between the branch and the surrounding tendonous and peritendonous structures. New areas of fiber disruption often occur adjacent to the previously healed area or are associated with adhesions to the surrounding tendonous or peritendonous structures.

Deep Digital Flexor Tendonitis

Deep digital flexor tendonitis is discussed in Chapter 70.

Distal Sesamoidean Desmitis

Oblique Sesamoidean Desmitis

Desmitis of an OSL is the most common distal sesamoidean ligament injury and is seen in all types of performance horses.[1-6] Horses with a valgus or varus limb conformation or a long sloping pastern may be at increased risk for OSL injuries. Swelling in the pastern region in horses with OSL injuries is characteristic because this ligament runs diagonally across the proximal to mid pastern, and swelling of the pastern usually occurs in this direction. Many horses have a boxy appearance to the fetlock joint from swelling at the origin of an OSL. Most horses have local swelling, heat, and pain detected on palpation of the affected ligament and lameness in the affected leg. However, some lesions restricted to the origin of the ligament occur without palpable abnormalities. Chronic injuries may be associated with dorsal enlargement of the dorsal articular margins of

the proximal interphalangeal joint. Subluxation of the proximal interphalangeal joint can also occur in horses with either chronic injuries or complete rupture of the OSLs. This is characterized clinically by a dorsally convex profile of the pastern. Complete biaxial rupture of the OSLs is more common in Thoroughbreds and can have catastrophic implications. Injury to the medial OSL is more common than lateral OSL injury and is more common in the forelimb than in the hindlimb.[3] Hindlimb OSL injuries are more common in nonracehorses. Horses with SL injury are also at increased risk of injuring the OSLs. Therefore ultrasonographic evaluation of the SL is recommended for all horses with oblique sesamoidean desmitis.

Discrete core lesions often are seen in both OSLs, although diffuse areas of fiber damage and splits also occur (Figure 82-4). Injuries to the insertion of an OSL are usually diffuse (Figure 82-5). Periligamentous soft tissue thickening is often seen. Comparison of the ultrasonographic findings in the affected limb with the contralateral limb is recommended to be sure that subtle or early injuries are not missed. The origin and insertion of the OSLs should be carefully evaluated for avulsion fractures.[1,2] Avulsion fractures usually occur in association with fiber tearing in the distal sesamoidean ligaments and occur from the base of the PSBs (Figure 82-6) and the insertion on the proximal phalanx. Avulsion fractures remain visible for years after the original injury, long after the associated desmitis in the distal sesamoidean ligament has resolved. Radiographs of the fetlock (particularly the PSBs) and the pastern regions should be obtained in all horses with OSL desmitis, paying careful attention to the base of the PSBs. However, it is important to recognize that entheseous new bone on the base of one or both of the PSBs or on the midpalmar aspect of the proximal phalanx can be seen as incidental radiological abnormalities, unassociated with lameness or active desmitis. Homogeneously radiodense mineralized bodies

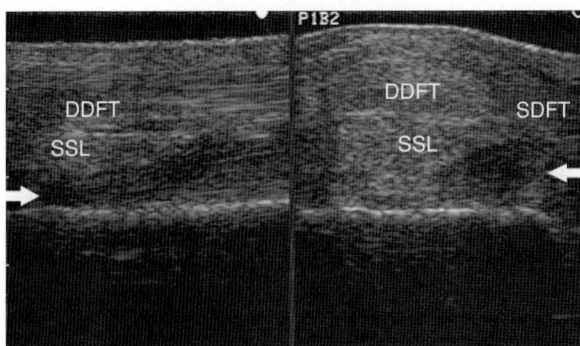

Fig. 82-5 • Transverse *(right)* and longitudinal *(left)* ultrasonographic images of the right fore lateral oblique sesamoidean ligament (OSL) obtained where the two OSLs join. The lateral aspect of the transverse view is on the right side of the image. This horse had sustained an acute injury to the lateral OSL from the base of the lateral proximal sesamoid bone to its insertion. A large anechoic to hypoechoic core lesion *(arrows)* is visible. The horse was lame at the walk, with mild subluxation of the proximal interphalangeal joint and local swelling, heat, and sensitivity along the entire lateral OSL. *DDFT,* Deep digital flexor tendon; *SSL,* straight sesamoidean ligament; *SDFT,* superficial digital flexor tendon.

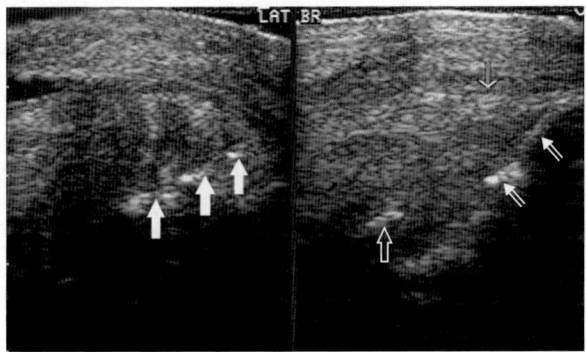

Fig. 82-6 • Transverse *(left)* and longitudinal *(right;* proximal to the right) ultrasonographic images of the medial oblique sesamoidean ligament (OSL) obtained in zone P1A of the left forelimb in a horse with chronic active desmitis of the OSL and a small basilar sesamoid fracture. The hyperechogenic bony fragment *(open arrow)* is distracted away from the base of the proximal sesamoid bone (PSB) in the longitudinal view. Hyperechoic areas are visible in the transverse view *(large arrows),* and areas of amorphous and random fiber pattern are imaged in the longitudinal view, proximal and distal to the fracture fragment. There is cortical irregularity of the base of the PSB *(small arrows)* in the longitudinal image. The horse was 1 of 5 degrees lame, with thickening of the base of the lateral PSB but no heat or local sensitivity.

are also sometimes seen distal to the PSBs as incidental findings.

Since MRI has become used more frequently in the search for a diagnosis for horses with pain causing lameness localized to the fetlock or pastern region by diagnostic analgesia, the limitations of ultrasonography for injury diagnosis in the pastern have become more apparent.[19,20,23] Injuries of the OSLs, SSL, and cruciate ligaments may be overlooked. Moreover, local analgesic techniques may be confusing. Pain associated with proximal lesions of these ligaments can be abolished by intraarticular analgesia of the fetlock or by intrathecal analgesia of the DFTS.[23] However, care should be taken in the interpretation of signal intensity alterations on magnetic resonance images of the OSLs because of the magic angle effect,[24] and the variable alignment of fibers in the proximal part of the

ligaments.[25] Lesions characterized by an increase in size of an OSL and increased signal intensity in T1- and T2-weighted images can be seen as incidental findings in association with other primary causes of lameness.[20] However, genuine primary lesions can be identified.[19,23] Thirty-nine sports horses with pain localized to the fetlock region underwent MRI because conventional imaging techniques failed to yield a diagnosis.[23] Injury of one or more of the distal sesamoidean ligaments was identified as the primary cause of lameness in 21 (54%) horses.

Horses with acute injuries to the OSLs should be managed in the same way as those with other tendon and ligament injuries, with initial antiinflammatory therapy and exercise restriction.[1,2] A controlled exercise program with incremental increases in the exercise level should be based on ultrasonographic monitoring. As the injury heals, the CSA of the ligament usually decreases, the echogenicity of the lesion increases, and linear echoes are imaged in the area of previous fiber tearing. A long recuperative period usually is indicated for horses with desmitis of an OSL to maximize the chance of return to athletic function.

Prognosis for horses with OSL injury is guarded to grave for returning successfully to racing and other competitive athletic activities and depends on the severity of the injury. Horses with coexisting suspensory desmitis, basilar fractures of the PSBs, or subchondral palmar third metacarpal or plantar third metatarsal bone disease have a poorer prognosis for return to athletic function. The incidence of recurrence of OSL injury is high. Prognosis is grave for athletic horses with subluxation of the proximal interphalangeal joint associated with distal sesamoidean desmitis.

Straight Sesamoidean Desmitis
Injuries to the SSL occur infrequently and may occur alone or with other soft tissue injuries.[1-6] These injuries usually are associated with lameness, but focal heat, swelling, and sensitivity are not always detected. Lameness is usually acute in onset and may be severe. Some horses, especially those with proximal lesions, never develop localizing soft tissue swelling, and diagnosis depends on localizing pain to the pastern region by diagnostic analgesia and subsequent ultrasonographic identification of a lesion. The ease with which the most proximal aspect of the ligament can be seen depends on the conformation of the horse and the position of the ergot. Ultrasonographic evaluation of the SSL is most difficult in horses with short pasterns and easiest in those with relatively long, upright pasterns.

Small splits or core lesions may be seen in the SSL.[1-6] Large areas of fiber disruption in the SSL are uncommon (Figure 82-7). Areas of periosteal proliferative change or avulsion fractures at the insertion of the SSL on the proximal aspect of the middle phalanx may be seen (Figure 82-8). Avulsion fractures of the origin of the SSL are less common than with OSL desmitis, but the base of the PSBs should be evaluated carefully.

Treatment for horses with SSL desmitis is similar to that recommended for horses with OSL desmitis.[1-6] Horses with mild injuries have returned successfully to racing, but the prognosis for horses with more severe lesions is guarded for any form of competitive athletic function because recurrent injury is common. Horses with multiple tendonous or ligamentous injuries in the pastern have a guarded to grave prognosis for returning to full athletic function.

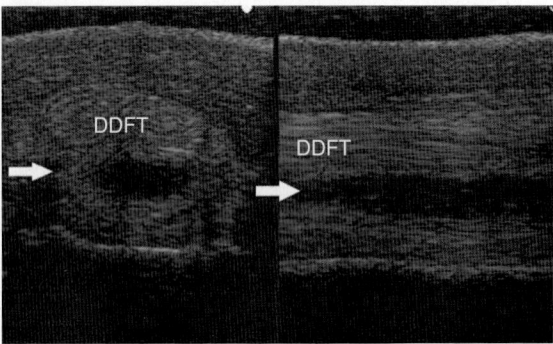

Fig. 82-7 • Ultrasonographic images of the right hind pastern obtained in zone P1A from a horse with an acute injury to the straight sesamoidean ligament (SSL). The horse was lame at the walk, with swelling of the proximal palmarolateral aspect of the pastern and local heat and sensitivity. The large anechogenic lesion *(arrows)* in the plantar aspect of the SSL is visible in the transverse view *(left)*, with complete fiber disruption in this region that is best imaged on the longitudinal view *(right)*. The SSL is mildly enlarged along the midline in the dorsal to palmar direction. Note also the markedly thickened subcutaneous tissues.

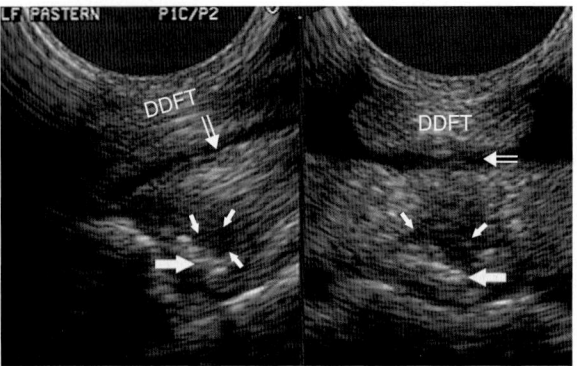

Fig. 82-8 • Ultrasonographic images of the left fore straight sesamoidean ligament (SSL) obtained in zone P1C-P2A from a horse with an acute severe injury to the SSL and an avulsion of its insertion onto the scutum medium. The horse was lame at the walk, with subluxation of the proximal interphalangeal joint and substantial soft tissue swelling of the palmar pastern, with local heat and pain on palpation of the oblique sesamoidean ligament (OSL) and SSL. The hypoechoic lesion *(small arrows)* in the distal-most portion of the SSL and the hyperechogenic fragment distracted away from the middle phalanx *(large arrows)* are visible in the transverse *(right)* and longitudinal *(left)* views. There is anechogenic effusion *(open arrows)* in the digital flexor tendon sheath. *DDFT,* Deep digital flexor tendon.

Cruciate Sesamoidean Desmitis

Desmitis of the cruciate sesamoidean ligaments is rare and difficult to diagnose by ultrasonography because of the location of these ligaments.[1,2]

Proximal Digital Annular Desmitis

Desmitis of the proximal digital annular ligament or proximal digital annular ligament constriction occurs infrequently (see Chapter 74).[1,3] Affected horses usually have chronic moderate to severe lameness. Distention of the palmar pouch of the DFTS is usually present, in addition to subtle distention proximal to the palmar annular

ligament of the fetlock. Thickening of the proximal digital annular ligament and skin usually is substantial, with a combined thickness of 4 to 5 mm (normal thickness is 1 to 2 mm) and distention of the DFTS.[21] Ultrasonographic evaluation of horses with proximal digital annular desmitis often reveals thickening of the synovium of the DFTS, in addition to the proximal digital annular ligament, and may reveal tendonitis of the SDFT or DDFT. Adhesions between the SDFT and the proximal digital annular ligament are suspected when restricted movement of the tendon relative to the proximal digital annular ligament is imaged during a dynamic examination.

Distal Digital Annular Desmitis

See Chapter 74 for a discussion of distal digital annular desmitis.

SOFT TISSUE SWELLING

Soft tissue swelling in the pastern, without tendonous or ligamentous injury, can result from skin irritation caused by liniments, blisters, local therapeutic ultrasound or cold laser treatment, local trauma from a blow, bandaging, or bell (overreach) boots, or from a skin infection. Ultrasonographic findings of thickened anechogenic to echogenic subcutaneous tissues, with normal tendonous and ligamentous structures, are typical for injury or inflammation to the skin and subcutaneous tissues. Thickening of the skin also may be seen in horses with skin irritation or infection. These horses usually respond well to local or systemic antiinflammatory therapy.

TENOSYNOVITIS OF THE DIGITAL FLEXOR TENDON SHEATH

Tenosynovitis of the DFTS is discussed in Chapter 74.

ABNORMALITIES OF THE PASTERN JOINT

Lameness and local swelling are two common findings in horses with injuries of the collateral or palmar ligaments of the proximal interphalangeal joint.[1,3-5,7-9] Swelling is usually primarily medial and lateral, although it can be circumferential. Acute desmitis of the collateral ligaments may be confirmed by ultrasonography, with decreased echogenicity and loss of fiber pattern, with or without an associated avulsion fracture (Figure 82-9).[1,3-5,7] In horses with more chronic injuries, enthesophyte formation at the origin and the insertion of the collateral ligaments usually is detected. A smoothing of these areas of insertional injury occurs as the desmitis becomes inactive. Similar ultrasonographic findings may be detected in horses with acute (Figure 82-10) and chronic injury (Figure 82-11) to the palmar ligaments of the pastern. These horses have a guarded prognosis for return to full athletic function. Bony proliferative changes associated with "high ringbone" are also easily imaged ultrasonographically.

NEURITIS/NEUROMA

Neuritis of the palmar (plantar) digital nerves results in acute lameness associated with exquisite pain on palpation of the nerves and localized heat and swelling.

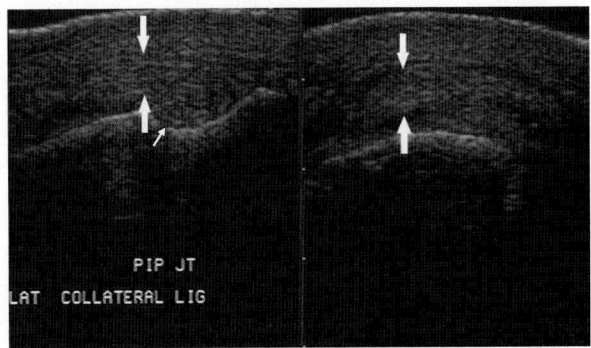

Fig. 82-9 • Longitudinal ultrasonographic images of the lateral collateral ligament of the proximal interphalangeal joint of the right hindlimb of horse with moderate lameness and localized swelling. The thickening of the lateral collateral ligament *(large arrows)*, the hypoechoic areas of fiber disruption, and the short random fiber pattern seen in the longitudinal view are consistent with desmitis. The distal portion of the proximal phalanx is on the right side of both longitudinal images, and the proximal portion of the middle phalanx is on the left side of both images. The right image is the proximal portion of the lateral collateral ligament, and the left image is the distal portion of the ligament. The small anechoic slit between the proximal and middle phalanges represents the joint space *(small arrow)*. There is marked bony proliferative change (irregular bone at the joint space), especially on the proximal aspect of the middle phalanx. Some echogenic subcutaneous thickening is present superficial to the collateral ligament.

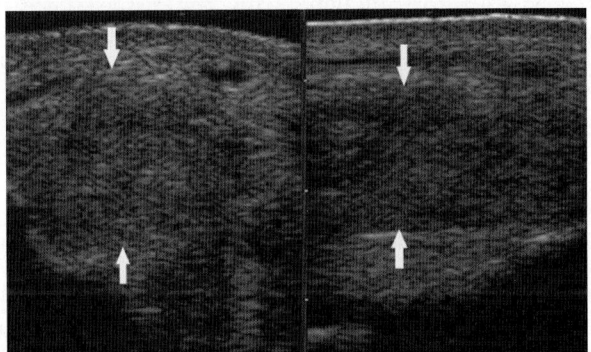

Fig. 82-10 • Ultrasonographic images of the left abaxial plantar ligament of the proximal interphalangeal joint in a horse with severe desmitis associated with mild lameness and localized swelling. There is marked enlargement of the ligament. It is hypoechoic and circular to oval in the transverse view *(left)* and has a random fiber pattern in the longitudinal view *(right)*. The arrows outline the margins of the ligament. A small amount of echogenic peritendonous subcutaneous tissue is visible.

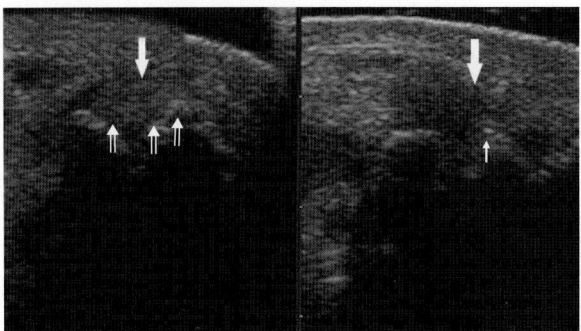

Fig. 82-11 • Ultrasonographic images of the lateral palmar ligament of the proximal interphalangeal joint *(large arrows)* in a horse with chronic severe desmitis and severe enthesopathy. The bony proliferative changes of the proximal phalanx *(small arrows)* in the transverse *(left)* and longitudinal views *(right)* make imaging the ligament in its entirety in either plane impossible at the ligament's origin. The visible portion of the ligament contains hypoechoic areas adjacent to the bony proliferative change in both views and near the ligament's origin in the longitudinal view. The gelding was 2 of 5 degrees lame, with thickening over the lateral and medial aspects of the proximal phalanx, but no heat or local sensitivity was detected.

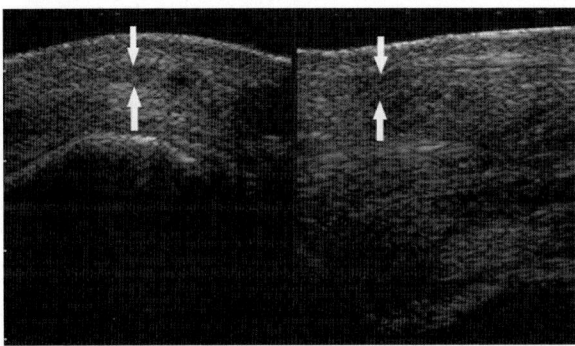

Fig. 82-12 • Transverse *(left)* and longitudinal *(right)* ultrasonographic images of the right fore medial palmar digital nerve obtained from a horse with a neuroma resulting in acute onset of moderate lameness with local swelling, heat, and exquisite sensitivity to palpation. The enlarged nerve ending *(arrows)*, oval to circular shape, is located palmar to the digital artery in the transverse view and superficial to the medial branch of the superficial digital flexor tendon in both views. The cross-sectional area of the nerve is markedly increased. Anechoic and hypoechoic areas disrupt the nerve ending *(arrows)*. Notice also the perineural soft tissue thickening.

Ultrasonography shows swelling and decreased echogenicity of the nerve (Figure 82-12). Neuromas following palmar digital neurectomy initially appear as focal painful swellings over the stump of the digital nerve. With ultrasonography, the nerve appears enlarged and hypoechoic, with perineural soft tissue swelling in horses with an acute neuroma. The neuroma becomes more echogenic and heterogeneous with increasing chronicity of injury. A large amount of perineural echogenic tissue may be present in horses with chronic neuromas.

Chapter 83

Skeletal Muscle and Lameness

Stephanie J. Valberg and Sue J. Dyson

DIAGNOSIS OF SPECIFIC MUSCLE DISORDERS IN THE HORSE

Diagnosis of a particular muscle disorder is best accomplished with a thorough neuromuscular examination. The key components of the examination include the following.

History

A history of stiffness, muscle cramping, pain, muscle fasciculations, exercise intolerance, undiagnosed lameness, weakness, or muscle atrophy may all indicate a muscle disorder. Further characterization requires a detailed account of the horse's performance level, exercise schedule, previous lameness, diet, vaccination history, signs of respiratory disease, duration, severity and frequency of muscle problem, any factors that initiate the muscle problem, and all medications with which the horse is being treated.

Physical Examination

A detailed evaluation of the muscular system includes inspection of the horse for symmetry of muscle mass while standing with forelimbs and hindlimbs exactly square. Any evidence of fine tremors or fasciculations should be noted before palpating the horse. Horses originating in the southwestern United States that have muscle pain and fasciculations should have their ears examined with an otoscope for ear ticks (*Otobius megnini*).[1] The entire muscle mass of the horse should be palpated for heat, pain, swelling, or atrophy comparing contralateral muscle groups. Firm, deep palpation of the lumbar, gluteal, and semimembranosus and semitendinosus muscles may reveal pain, cramps, or fibrosis. The triceps, pectoral, gluteal, and semitendinosus muscles should be tapped with a fist or percussion hammer and observed for a prolonged contracture suggestive of myotonia. Running a blunt instrument such as artery forceps, a needle cap, or a pen over the lumbar and gluteal muscles should illicit extension (swayback), followed by flexion (hogback) in healthy horses. Guarding against movement may reflect abnormalities in the pelvic or thoracolumbar muscles, or pain associated with the thoracolumbar spine (see Chapter 52) or sacroiliac joints (see Chapter 51). The horse should be observed at the walk and the trot for any gait abnormalities, and some horses should be ridden.

Ancillary Diagnostic Tests

Muscle Enzymes

Skeletal muscle necrosis may be identified by determining the activity in blood of serum enzymes or proteins that are normally present in high concentration within intact muscle cells but leak out into the bloodstream following cell damage. Three enzymes are used routinely to assess muscle necrosis: creatine kinase (CK), aspartate transaminase (AST), and lactate dehydrogenase (LDH). Serum myoglobin has also been used as a marker of acute muscle necrosis.[2,3] The permeability of the muscle cell membrane, rate of enzyme production, alternate tissue sources of the enzyme, and rate of enzyme excretion/degradation may also influence serum enzyme activities.

Serum Creatine Kinase

Isoforms of CK are found in skeletal muscle (MM), cardiac muscle (MB), and nervous tissue (BB). CK is a relatively low-molecular-weight protein (80,000 Da) that is intimately involved in energy production within the cell cytoplasm. It is liberated within hours of muscle damage, or increased cell membrane permeability, into the extracellular fluid and usually peaks at 4 to 6 hours after muscle injury (half-life [$t\frac{1}{2}$] is 108 min).[4] A threefold to fivefold increase in serum CK from normal values is believed to represent necrosis of approximately 20 g of muscle tissue.[5] Rhabdomyolysis results in a proportionately greater increase in the MM isoform than the MB isoform, although some investigators disagree with the tissue specificity of serum CK isoforms in the horse.[6] Limited elevations in CK (<1000 U/L; high range of normal value = 380 U/L) may accompany training or transport.[7] Extreme fatiguing exercise (e.g., endurance rides or the cross-country phase of a Three Day Event) may result in CK activities being increased to more than 1000 U/L, but usually less than 5000 U/L. Under these circumstances, serum CK activities rapidly return to baseline (i.e., <350 U/L in 24 to 48 hours). Recumbent horses also may have slightly elevated CK activities that are usually less than 3000 U/L. In contrast, more substantial elevations (from several thousand to hundreds of thousands of units per liter) in the activity of this enzyme may occur with rhabdomyolysis.[3]

Serum Aspartate Transaminase

Serum AST, previously known as serum glutamic-oxaloacetic acid and aspartate aminotransferase, is a larger-molecular-weight protein that has high activity in skeletal and cardiac muscle and also in liver, red blood cells, and other tissues. Elevations in AST are not specific for myonecrosis, and increases could be the result of hemolysis, muscle, liver, or other organ damage. AST activity increases more slowly in response to myonecrosis than does CK, often peaking between 12 and 24 hours after the insult. In addition, AST is cleared slowly by the reticuloendothelial system and may persist for 2 to 3 weeks after rhabdomyolysis ($t\frac{1}{2}$ is 7 to 10 days).[4,8]

By comparing serial activities of CK and AST, information concerning the progression of myonecrosis or muscle cell membrane permeability may be derived. Elevations in CK and AST reflect relatively recent or active myonecrosis or muscle cell stress; persistently elevated serum CK indicates that myonecrosis or muscle stress is likely ongoing. Elevated AST activity accompanied by decreasing or normal CK activity indicates that myonecrosis has ceased. The degree of elevation of CK and AST does not necessarily reflect the severity of clinical signs.

References on page 1321

Serum Lactate Dehydrogenase

LDH is a tetramer made up of combinations of the M and H subunits, with five isoenzyme forms found in various organs within the body. Electrophoretic separation suggests that the M_4 (LDH_5) and M_3H (LDH_4) isoforms are found predominantly in skeletal muscle. Elevations in LDH may be detected in horses with rhabdomyolysis, myocardial necrosis, and/or hepatic necrosis.[7] Therefore concurrent measurement of serum CK is necessary to establish that rhabdomyolysis is present.

Myoglobin

Elevation in plasma/serum myoglobin concentrations indicates acute muscle damage. Myoglobin is a low-molecular-weight protein (16,500 Da) that leaks into plasma immediately after muscle damage and is rapidly cleared in the urine by the kidney. Approximately 200 g or more of muscle must be damaged before it is detectable in the urine in people.[9] Normal serum concentrations in resting horses have been determined by nephelometry (range, 0 to 9 mcg/L), with measured concentrations with rhabdomyolysis ranging from 10,000 to 800,000 mcg/L.[2,3]

Exercise Response Test

Diagnosing chronic exertional rhabdomyolysis (ER) may be problematic in horses that do not have acute clinical signs and have normal serum AST and CK at rest. In such horses, an exercise challenge can be helpful to detect subclinical ER. In addition, quantifying the extent of rhabdomyolysis during mild exercise is helpful in deciding how rapidly to put a horse back into training. Blood samples should be taken before exercise and 4 to 6 hours after exercise to evaluate peak changes in CK. Serum CK activity measured immediately postexercise will not reflect the amount of damage occurring during the exercise test. Small fluctuations in serum CK activity may occur with exercise from enhanced muscle membrane permeability, particularly if exercise is prolonged or strenuous and the horse is untrained.[10] A submaximal exercise test is often valuable for detecting rhabdomyolysis because it provides more consistent evidence of subclinical rhabdomyolysis than maximal exercise tests.[3,11] Fifteen minutes of trotting is often sufficient to produce subclinical muscle damage in horses prone to chronic exertional myopathies.[12] If signs of stiffness develop before this, exercise should be concluded. A normal response would be less than a threefold to fourfold increase from basal CK.

Thermography

Thermography may be useful for identification of superficial abnormal temperature changes from muscle damage but has little value in horses with deeper injuries. However, there are many potentially confusing issues such as recent removal of a rug or tack. Careful comparisons of the left and right sides should be made. Muscle inflammation is seen as an area of increased temperature in the skin directly overlying the affected muscle. The most common sites of muscle strain identified thermographically include the longissimus dorsi, the origin or body of the middle gluteal, the insertion of the gluteals on the greater and third trochanters of the femur, biceps femoris, semitendinosus, semimembranosus, and adductor muscles.[13]

Nuclear Scintigraphy

Nuclear scintigraphy is useful for identification of some forms of muscle damage and may alert the clinician to an area of deep muscle damage that had not been suspected based on clinical examination. In human athletes, technetium-99m stannous pyrophosphate has been used to assess the degree of skeletal muscle damage and to delineate areas of damage.[14,15] It is thought that abnormal uptake of the radiopharmaceutical reflects an early stage of muscle damage from episodic ischemia, which is reversible in some fibers but may lead to muscle necrosis in others.[14]

Technetium-99m–methylene diphosphonate (MDP) is taken up in some damaged muscle in the horse and is best seen in the bone (delayed) phase images, that is, 3 hours after injection. Scintigraphy has been used most commonly in horses with a history of poor performance, with or without stiffness after exercise, to confirm a diagnosis of equine rhabdomyolysis.[16] The mechanism of MDP binding is unknown, but the release of large amounts of calcium from damaged muscle or the exposure of calcium binding sites on protein macromolecules in the damaged muscle may be responsible. Diffuse linear areas of increased radiopharmaceutical uptake (IRU) are commonly seen in the caudal epaxial muscles and the muscles of the hindquarters and thigh in some but not all horses with ER (Figure 83-5). Less commonly there is IRU in the triceps and latissimus dorsi muscles.

The use of scintigraphy for the diagnosis of other muscle injuries has not been documented in the horse, but in one author's experience (SJD) it can be helpful in some horses with either proximal forelimb or hindlimb muscle injuries. Uptake of the radiopharmaceutical tends to be much more focal and much less intense than in horses with rhabdomyolysis. In some, but not all, horses the region of IRU has correlated with a region of increased echogenicity identified ultrasonographically.

Ultrasonography

Diagnostic ultrasonography is potentially useful for identification of muscle trauma and fibrosis, provided that there is physical disruption of the muscle and assuming that one knows where to look. Muscles have a rather typical striated echogenic pattern,[17,18] but this varies according to the muscle group, and careful comparisons must be made between similar sites in contralateral limbs, in both transverse and longitudinal images. The appearance of muscle is also sensitive to the way the horse is standing and whether the muscle is under tension; therefore it is important that the horse is standing squarely and bearing weight evenly. Muscle fascia appears as well-defined relatively echogenic bands. Care must be taken in identifying large vessels and artifacts created by them.

In an acute injury, muscle fiber disruption is seen as relatively hypoechoic areas within muscle, with loss of the normal muscle fiber striation. The jagged edge of the margin of the torn muscle may be increased in echogenicity. Tears in the muscle fascia may be identified. The muscle defect may be filled by a loculated hematoma that is slowly replaced by hypoechogenic granulation tissue. With muscle fiber repair there is a progressive increase in echogenicity. Relatively hyperechogenic regions may develop as a result of fibrous scarring, which may result in long-term gait abnormalities. Hyperechogenic regions causing shadowing artifacts reflect mineralization.

Muscle Biopsy

The routine examination of muscle biopsies has resulted in the identification of a number of specific equine myopathies. To fully characterize a neuromuscular disorder and its rate of progression, muscle fiber sizes, shapes, and fiber type distribution, mitochondrial distribution, polysaccharide staining pattern, neuromuscular junctions, nerve branches, connective tissue, and blood vessels should be examined in frozen sections using a battery of tinctorial and histochemical stains.[19]

A number of basic pathological responses of muscle can be identified in formalin-fixed, paraffin-embedded sections. These include inflammation, muscle fiber necrosis, muscle fiber regeneration, variations in muscle fiber sizes and shapes, alterations in the number of cell nuclei, vacuolar change, and proliferation of connective tissue. However, there are many pathological alterations that cannot be detected in formalin-fixed tissue but can readily be seen in histochemical stains of fresh-frozen biopsy samples.[20] Histochemical stains of frozen tissue allow muscle fiber types to be distinguished, differentiation between neurogenic and myogenic atrophy, characterization of vacuolar storage material, characterization of inclusion bodies, and assessment of mitochondrial density. In addition, frozen samples may be used for biochemical analysis of substrate concentrations and enzyme activities, as well as DNA isolation.

When considering collection of muscle biopsies, some general guidelines are applicable. Preferably, samples should be collected from what is considered abnormal/diseased muscle. A 6-mm outer diameter (Jorgen KRUUSE A/S, Langeskov, Denmark) percutaneous needle biopsy technique can be used to obtain small muscle samples through a 1.5-cm skin incision using a local anesthetic solution subcutaneously. If this technique is used, enough muscle should be obtained to form a 1.5-cm^2 sample at a minimum. However, these samples do not tolerate well shipment to an outside laboratory. The optimum biopsy for shipment of histopathological tissues to a laboratory is collected using surgical or open techniques and performed under local analgesia. Care must be exercised to infiltrate only the subcutaneous tissues, not the muscle, with the local anesthetic solution. The objective is to obtain approximately 2-cm^3 of tissue; hence a suitably long skin incision is required. Subsequently two parallel incisions 2 cm apart should be made longitudinal to the muscle fibers with a scalpel. The muscle should only be handled in one corner using forceps, and care should be taken not to crush the tissue. The muscle sample is then excised by transverse incisions 2 cm apart, and the tissue is fixed appropriately.

Samples submitted for routine histopathology can be placed in formalin. Samples for histochemical analysis require fixation in isopentane (methylbutane) chilled in liquid nitrogen to ensure rapid freezing and minimization of freeze artifact. In the field, where freezing is not possible, fresh samples wrapped in gauze slightly moistened with saline can be shipped in a water-tight hard container on icepacks to specialized laboratories. Samples that potentially may be used for biochemical analysis should be immediately frozen in liquid nitrogen. Samples for electron microscopy (EM) require appropriate fixation in glutaraldehyde preparations. Ideally, thin sections of muscle for EM should be clamped in vivo to maintain fibers at a resting length before they are excised. However, if pathology other than the alignment of thick and thin myofilaments is to be investigated, small muscle pieces can be excised and placed directly in appropriate EM fixative.

Responses of strips of fresh muscle to stimuli such as caffeine, halothane, and a variety of other agents can be performed on site by specialized laboratories, but these tests are largely research tools.[21,22]

Electromyography

A specific diagnosis of the cause of muscle atrophy, muscle fasciculations, or myotonic dimpling after tapping the muscle can be aided by performing electromyography (EMG). EMG of normal skeletal muscle shows a brief burst of electrical activity when the needle is inserted in muscle and then quiescence, unless motor units are recruited (motor unit action potentials), or the needle is very close to a motor endplate (miniature endplate potentials). Normal muscle shows little spontaneous electrical activity unless the muscle contracts or the horse moves. Motor unit action potentials can be evaluated to assess amplitude, duration, phase, and number of phases. Myopathic changes include a decrease in duration and amplitude of motor unit action potentials.[23,24] Horses with abnormalities in the electrical conduction system of muscle, or denervation of motor units, show abnormal spontaneous electrical activity in the form of fibrillation potentials, positive sharp waves, myotonic discharges, or complex repetitive discharges.

Based on the information obtained on neuromuscular examination and muscle biopsy, a diagnosis can usually be obtained. The following classification system may be helpful to narrow down rule-outs for muscle disease in horses:

I. Nonexercise-associated rhabdomyolysis
   A. Inflammatory myopathies
      1. Immune-mediated
         a. Infarctive hemorrhagic purpura
         b. Immune-mediated myopathy
      2. Infectious
         a. Clostridial myositis
         b. *Streptococcus equi* myositis
         c. Anaplasma myositis
         d. Viral myositis
         e. Sarcocystis myositis
   B. Nutritional myopathy
      1. Vitamin E and selenium deficiency
   C. Toxic myopathy
      1. Ionophore toxicity
      2. Pasture myopathies
         a. Rayless goldenrod/white snakeroot
         b. *Cassia occidentalis*
         c. Atypical myoglobinuria
   D. Traumatic myopathy
      1. Compressive anesthetic myopathy
      2. Trauma
   E. Metabolic myopathy
      1. Glycogen branching enzyme deficiency in Quarter Horses

2. Type 1 and type 2 polysaccharide storage myopathy
3. Malignant hyperthermia
II. Exertional rhabdomyolysis
  A. Focal muscle strain
  B. Extrinsic (sporadic) tying-up
    1. Dietary imbalances, vitamins, minerals, electrolytes
    2. Exercise in excess of training
    3. Exhaustion syndrome
  C. Intrinsic (chronic) tying-up
    1. Type 1 polysaccharide storage myopathy
    2. Type 2 polysaccharide storage myopathy
    3. Malignant hyperthermia
    4. Recurrent ER
    5. Idiopathic chronic ER
III. Exertional myopathy with normal CK
  A. Mitochondrial myopathy
IV. Muscle atrophy
  A. Myogenic atrophy
    1. Disuse
    2. Cachexia
    3. Cushing's disease
    4. Immune-mediated myositis (rapid atrophy)
    5. Type 2 polysaccharide storage myopathy
    6. Severe rhabdomyolysis
  B. Neurogenic atrophy
    1. Equine protozoal myelitis
    2. Local nerve trauma
    3. Equine motor neuron disease
V. Muscle fasciculations
  A. Pain, fear
  B. Electrolyte abnormalities
  C. Hyperkalemic periodic paralysis
  D. *O. megnini* ear tick infestation
  E. Myotonic dystrophy
  F. Stiff horse syndrome
  G. Equine motor neuron disease
  H. Focal nerve irritation

MUSCULAR PAIN, STRAIN, AND TEARS

The role of muscle pain and injury in lameness and poor performance in the horse is rather poorly recognized. In human athletes, muscle fatigue, muscle stiffness, and muscle soreness are well-recognized entities, although the pathological processes in the absence of detectable structural abnormalities are not completely understood. Increased intramuscular pressure may be associated with muscle pain after prolonged vigorous exercise in human athletes.[14]

Delayed-onset muscular stiffness or soreness (DOMS) is recognized in people as pain that develops 24 to 48 hours after unaccustomed use of certain muscles and usually resolves spontaneously, assuming the muscles are not over-worked again.[25] Continued overstress may result in structural damage to myofilaments. However, specific training involving the activity that provoked the original DOMS decreases the amount of soreness associated with that condition over time.

Muscle soreness in the pectoral region after repeated jumping efforts is commonly recognized, especially in event horses several hours after completing the cross-country phase of a Three Day Event.[26] It seems to improve with massage.

Muscle fiber tearing and hemorrhage can result in acute muscular pain in human athletes. A palpable defect or swelling can be detected in superficial muscles. For deeper muscles, ultrasonography is required for accurate diagnosis.

Muscle fibrosis and mineralization have been well documented in the horse following tearing of the semi-membranosus and semitendinosus muscles (see Fibrotic Myopathy section, page 558), but acute lesions here and elsewhere in the limbs have been poorly documented.[27-29] The use of diagnostic ultrasonography[17,18] has helped in the diagnosis of both acute and more chronic muscle lesions, but diagnosis often remains a challenge because of the deep location of some affected muscles and the lack of localizing clinical signs.

In one author's (SJD) experience, the most commonly recognized muscle injury sites in the forelimb include biceps brachii, brachiocephalicus, the pectorals, and the musculotendonous junction of the superficial digital flexor (Figures 83-1 to 83-4). In the hindlimb, semimembranosus and semitendinosus, adductor, gracilis, gluteal, and gas-trocnemius muscle injuries have been recognized most frequently. Acute muscle tearing and hemorrhage can result in severe pain and lameness and other clinical signs mimicking colic. Swelling around the damaged muscle, assuming it is superficial, may not appear until 24 to 48 hours later.

Muscle tension and spasm in the thoracolumbar region are well-documented sources of pain contributing to poor performance in association with primary hindlimb lameness, but primary muscle pain in this region has often tended to be overlooked by many veterinarians, although recognized by physiotherapists. Localized muscle soreness and the interpretation of abnormal sensitivity of acupuncture points are potentially confusing. Protective muscle spasm may also develop secondary to a primary lesion of either the thoracolumbar spine or the sacroiliac region (see Chapters 49 to 52).

Jeffcott et al[30] demonstrated that injection of lactic acid into the left longissimus dorsi muscles could significantly diminish performance of Standardbred (STB) trotters worked at speed on a treadmill, although changes in gait were subtle.

One author (SJD) has seen a number of horses that had suddenly lost performance during competition or training, either following a particularly extravagant jump or after an awkward jump. The horses had subsequently become reluctant either to jump or to gallop downhill. Clinical examination revealed intense muscle spasm in the caudal thoracic and lumbar regions, with associated pain. Manipulation to release muscle spasm resulted in relief of pain and rapid restoration of normal performance. Acute back muscle pain may also be induced by a fall.

Localized back muscle soreness is readily induced by a poorly fitting saddle. It may also be caused by a rider who either sits crookedly or is unable to ride completely in balance with the horse. This may be because of the ineptitude of the rider or the shape of the saddle and the way in which it sits on a particular horse and thus positions the rider. Such muscle pain is usually localized to the saddle area and may be associated with slight soft tissue swelling.

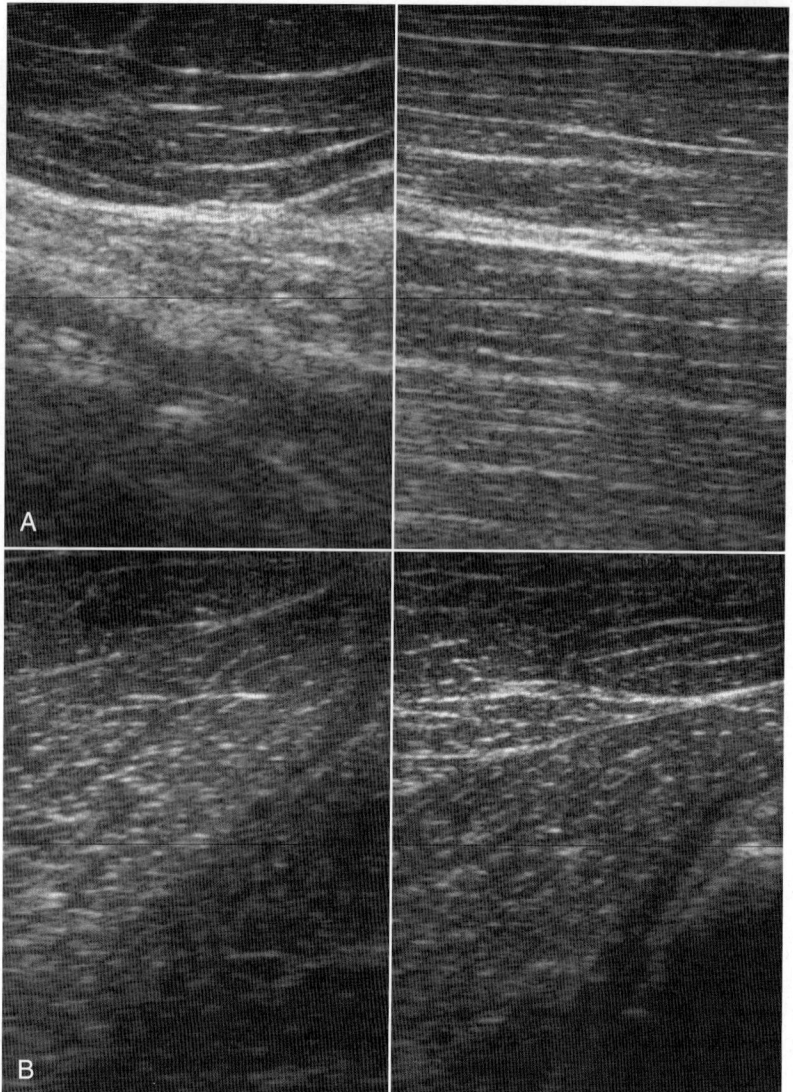

Fig. 83-1 • A and **B,** Longitudinal ultrasonographic images of the muscles at the base of the neck on the left and right sides of an advanced-level event horse with restricted forelimb gait (*left* images indicate left side; *right* images indicate right side). The horse had severe pain and tension in the strap muscles at the base of the neck on the left side and slight muscle atrophy. Note the increased echogenicity of the deeper muscle on the left side compared with the right. The horse was treated by H-wave stimulation that resulted in progressive relief of the muscle spasm and clinically significant improvement in gait and ability to jump.

Thermographic examination may be helpful to demonstrate to an owner the associated localized inflammation. Pressure measurements can also be used (see Figure 117-6), although there is some variability in the accuracy of different commercially available systems.

Diagnosis

History and Clinical Examination

It is important to establish whether there was a history of a fall or other traumatic event, the duration of clinical signs, whether swelling was noted, and whether the horse had exhibited lameness or had performed poorly.

The detection of muscle swelling from recent trauma or loss of muscle bulk as a result of fibrosis, chronic injury, or atrophy requires the horse to stand completely squarely, bearing weight evenly on all limbs and looking straight ahead. The horse should be appraised visually and by careful, systematic palpation, looking for defects in the muscle, muscle swelling, areas of abnormal muscle firmness from fibrosis, muscle tension, or spasm, and areas of pain.

In an acute injury resulting in muscle tearing or rupture, it may be possible to palpate a defect in the very early stages, but this will become filled with hemorrhage, inflammatory exudate, and edema. Careful palpation should enable detection of most acute superficial muscle injuries, but localization of deeper muscle injury may be more difficult. Identification of chronic muscle strain is more challenging because clinical signs are more subtle. The horse must be as relaxed as possible to assess properly the response to firm and deep palpation. If the muscle is sore, the horse may react by increasing tension in anticipation of pain or by pulling away. There may be "knots" within the area of damaged muscle.

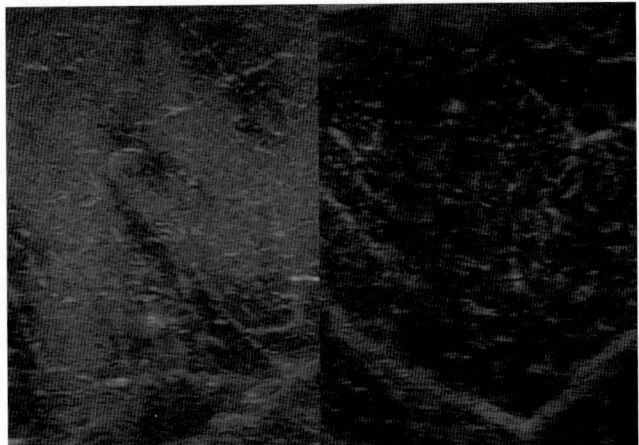

Fig. 83-2 • Transverse ultrasonographic images of the right *(left)* and left *(right)* gracilis muscles of a 12-year-old Thoroughbred cross event horse with acute-onset right hindlimb lameness of 6 days' duration, with slight swelling of the muscle, pain on palpation, and diffuse edematous swelling in the crus. At the time of lameness onset, the horse showed signs attributed to colic. A focal region of increased echogenicity in the right gracilis muscle is caused by muscle fiber tearing and hemorrhage.

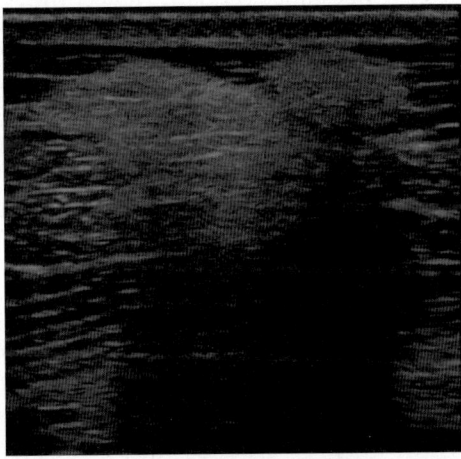

Fig. 83-3 • Transverse ultrasonographic image of the left brachiocephalicus muscle of a Grand Prix dressage horse that showed left forelimb lameness only when performing lateral movements, such as half pass. The lameness was not altered by any local analgesic technique. There is a focal area of increased echogenicity, caused by muscle fibrosis, resulting in acoustic shadowing.

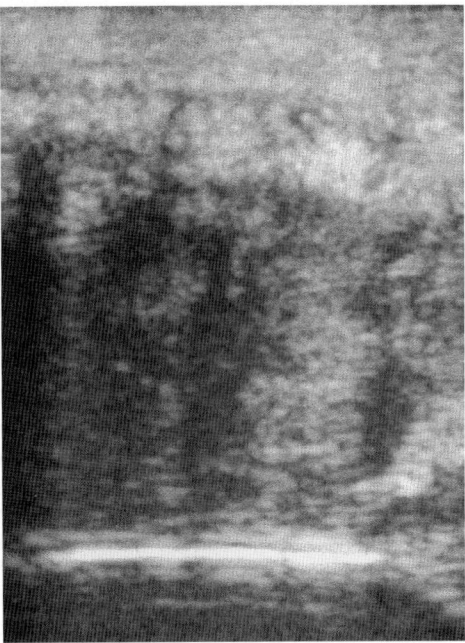

Fig. 83-4 • Longitudinal ultrasonographic image of the cranial aspect of the antebrachium of a 7-year-old hunter. The horse had developed acute-onset lameness 3 months previously, associated with substantial soft tissue swelling on the cranial aspect of the antebrachium. The extensor carpi radialis muscle is enlarged greatly and has hypoechoic and hyperechoic regions, with little normal muscle architecture.

A show jumper with sore gluteal muscles may not push off as strongly with the affected limb, resulting in the hindquarters drifting toward the ipsilateral side as the horse jumps.

Muscle Stimulation

Muscle-stimulating machines can be helpful in the identification of superficial muscle injuries. Intermittent electrical stimulation of focal areas within a muscle results in muscle contraction and relaxation. The strength of stimulus can be varied. Horses vary in sensitivity and tolerance of the procedure, so careful comparisons must be made between the left and right sides. Damaged muscle tends to respond greater to lower stimulus strength, and contraction and relaxation are less smooth and may induce pain.

Thermography, Nuclear Scintigraphy, and Ultrasonography

Thermography, nuclear scintigraphy, and ultrasonography are discussed on pages 819 and 820.

Muscle Enzymes

Determination of serum muscle enzyme concentrations is rarely of value in identification of muscle soreness or trauma but is useful for detecting horses with rhabdomyolysis (see page 813).

Treatment

The aims of treatment include repair of damaged muscle, relief of both muscle spasm and pain, restoration of normal circulation, minimization of fibrous scar formation, and remobilization of muscles. The precise mode of treatment will depend on the type of muscle injury and the stage of injury and repair. Treatment modalities include laser,[31,32]

The neck, limbs, and thoracolumbar region should be moved passively to detect any limitations in movement or pain induced by movement. The horse should be observed moving at both the walk and the trot to identify any characteristic gait abnormalities, such as an abnormal hind foot placement from fibrotic myopathy (see Chapter 48) or sinking of a front fetlock as a result of rupture at the musculotendonous junction of the superficial digital flexor (see Chapter 13). However, it must be borne in mind that muscle soreness resulting in compromise of performance may not result in overt lameness because pain may only be induced when the muscle contracts strongly or is stretched maximally. Pain associated with a brachiocephalicus muscle in a dressage horse may only be evident in particular movements such as half pass (see Figure 83-3).

therapeutic ultrasound,[31] H wave, transcutaneous electrical stimulation, electromagnetic therapy,[33] massage,[26] passive stretching combined with box rest, and a graduated, controlled exercise program. Relief of acute muscle spasm may require chiropractic manipulation. During return to work, the exercise program must be carefully moderated according to the site of the injury and to avoid overstress in the early stages of repair while encouraging a progressive increase in strength. These subjects are discussed more fully elsewhere (see Chapters 92 through 96).

Prevention

Because equine muscle injuries are poorly recognized there has been little work on prevention. However, there is evidence to document the beneficial effects of warm-up before strenuous exercise.[34-36] Warm-up enhances blood flow to active muscle and increases muscle temperature. This results in better oxygen delivery to exercising muscle, improved enzyme function, and increased range of motion. The best warm-up program for each type of exercise remains poorly defined; however, warm-up should aim to prepare the physiological systems, without contributing to excessive heat generation or fatigue.

EXERTIONAL RHABDOMYOLYSIS

ER has numerous etiologies and is a common complex cause of poor performance. About 3% of exercising horses had an episode of ER in the past 12 months.[37] It occurs in a variety of breeds, including draft breeds, Warmbloods, Thoroughbreds (TB), STBs, Arabians, Morgans, Quarter Horses, Appaloosa, American Paint horses, and many more.[37-41] In draft breeds, ER can be particularly debilitating, and terms such as *Monday morning disease, azoturia,* or *paralytic myoglobinuria* are used.[42] A milder syndrome occurs in lighter breeds, and the terms *tying-up, set fast, myositis,* and *chronic intermittent rhabdomyolysis* are used to describe muscle necrosis or muscle cell stress following any form of exercise in the lighter horse breeds.[43,44] Several specific causes have been identified for ER. Otherwise successful athletic horses may have a sporadic episode of ER from extrinsic causes such as dietary imbalances, concurrent respiratory infections, and inappropriate training regimens. In horses chronically afflicted with ER there may be an intrinsic dysfunction of muscle metabolism or muscle contraction.

Sporadic Exertional Rhabdomyolysis

The most common extrinsic cause of sporadic ER is exercise that exceeds the horse's underlying state of training.[44] Horses that are advanced too quickly in training, horses that are only ridden sporadically while being continually fed full rations, and horses performing strenuous exercise such as racing or endurance riding without sufficient conditioning commonly develop rhabdomyolysis. In addition, rhabdomyolysis may be more common in horses exercising during an outbreak of respiratory disease. Both equine herpesvirus–1 and equine influenza virus have been implicated as causative agents.[38,45]

Clinical Signs

Classically, horses lose impulsion and develop a stiff, stilted gait, particularly involving the hindquarters during exercise. There is excessive sweating and a high respiratory rate from pain. The horse may be unable to walk forward after resting because of firm painful muscle contractures involving the back and hindquarters. Signs are most commonly seen after 15 to 30 minutes of light exercise.[40,46] A horse with severe rhabdomyolysis shows signs of colic, becomes recumbent, and develops occult myoglobinuria. The urine may be discolored and has an abnormal smell. Attempts to move more severely affected animals may result in extreme pain, obvious anxiety, and exacerbation of the condition.

ER is often symmetrical, involving gluteal, biceps femoris, semitendinosus, and semimembranosus muscles. Forelimbs are less commonly overtly affected. ER may accompany the exhaustion syndrome in endurance horses with concurrent evidence of a rapid heart rate, dehydration, hyperthermia, synchronous diaphragmatic flutter, and collapse.[47] Muscle contractures are not always consistent in either endurance horses or event horses with ER.

Diagnosis is usually obvious based on the clinical signs, but measurement of serum muscle enzyme activities provides an assessment of the severity of muscle damage and confirms the diagnosis. The degree of elevation of muscle enzyme activity does not necessarily reflect the severity of clinical signs.

Treatment of Acute Rhabdomyolysis

If an attack has occurred during exercise some distance from where the horse is normally stabled, the horse should not be made to walk home. It should be transported back home or left in a nearby stable. If an attack has occurred at a competition, the horse should be treated there and should not be transported home over a long distance until at least 24 to 48 hours later.

The objectives of treatment are to relieve anxiety and muscle pain, as well as to correct fluid and acid-base deficits. Acetylpromazine (0.04 to 0.07 mg/kg), an α-adrenergic antagonist, is helpful in relieving anxiety and may increase muscle blood flow. Its use is contraindicated in dehydrated horses. Alternatively, xylazine (0.4 to 0.8 mg/kg) may provide short-term relief from anxiety. In horses with extreme pain, detomidine (0.02 to 0.04 mcg/kg) combined with butorphanol (0.01 to 0.04 mg/kg) provides excellent sedation and analgesia. Nonsteroidal antiinflammatory drugs (NSAIDs) such as ketoprofen (2.2 mg/kg), phenylbutazone (2.2 to 4.4 mg/kg), or flunixin meglumine (1.1 mg/kg) provide additional pain relief. Analgesic treatment is continued to effect, but most horses are relatively pain free within 18 to 24 hours.

Intravenous or intragastric dimethyl sulfoxide (as a <20% solution) can be used as an antioxidant, antiinflammatory, and osmotic diuretic in severely affected horses. Corticosteroid administration is advocated by some veterinarians in the acute stage. If the horse is recumbent, methyl prednisolone succinate (2 to 4 mg/kg intravenously [IV]) should be given once. Muscle relaxants such as methocarbamol (5 to 22 mg/kg, IV slowly) seem to produce variable results, possibly depending on the dosage used. The administration of dantrium sodium (2 to 4 mg/kg orally [PO]) in severely affected horses may decrease muscle contractures and possibly prevent further activation of muscle necrosis. This can be repeated in 4 to 6 hours.

Severe ER can lead to renal compromise from ischemia and the combined nephrotoxic effects of myoglobinuria, dehydration, and NSAIDs. The first priority in horses with hemoconcentration, or myoglobinuria, is to reestablish fluid balance and induce diuresis. In horses with mild rhabdomyolysis, administration of fluids via a nasogastric tube may be adequate, but generally fluids are better given intravenously. Balanced polyionic electrolyte solutions are best. If severe ER is present, then isotonic saline or 2.5% dextrose in 0.45% saline may be necessary because horses often have hyponatremia, hypochloremia, and hyperkalemia. If hypocalcemia is present, then supplementing intravenous fluids with 100 to 200 mL of 24% calcium borogluconate is recommended, but serum calcium should not exceed a low normal range. Affected horses are usually alkalotic, making bicarbonate therapy inappropriate.[48]

Ten liters of fluids may be given rapidly. The total fluid replacement is based on an estimation of the degree of dehydration and the clinical response: if the horse is mildly dehydrated (5%), give 10 L fast and then 15 L over the next 4 to 6 hours; if dehydration is severe (20%), give 10 L fast and then 50 L at 4 L/h. If the horse is recumbent, consider using at least two intravenous giving sets and infusing into both the jugular and the cephalic veins. Suture the catheters in place.

Ideally, reassessment of the packed cell volume and concentrations of total plasma protein and serum electrolytes after the initial period of therapy should provide a successful guide for the therapeutic regimen. However, in the practical situation, the clinical response to therapy is usually an adequate indicator. In severely affected horses, regular monitoring of blood urea nitrogen and/or serum creatinine is advised to assess the extent of renal damage. Diuretics are usually contraindicated unless the horse is in oliguric renal failure.

Horses should be stall rested on a hay diet for a few days. Small paddock turnout in a quiet area for a few hours twice a day is then helpful. Horses may be handwalked at this time but not for more than 5 to 10 minutes at a time. For horses with extrinsic (sporadic) ER, rest with regular access to a paddock should continue until serum muscle enzyme activities are normal. Training should be resumed gradually, and a regular exercise schedule that matches the degree of exertion to the horse's underlying state of training should be established. Avoid lunging exercise until the horse is back in normal work. If the horse has a day or several days off, the dietary energy concentrations should be reduced accordingly.

Chronic Exertional Rhabdomyolysis

Horses that have repeated episodes of ER from a young age, or from the time of purchase, or when they are put back into training after a long period of rest may have a chronic dietary imbalance or underlying intrinsic abnormality of muscle function. Chronic forms of ER are seen in many breeds of horses, including draft horses, Warmbloods, Quarter Horses, American Paint horses, Appaloosas, TBs, Arabians, STBs, Morgans, and crossbreds.[39,44,49-55] Many of the horses with intrinsic muscle defects will have repeated episodes of rhabdomyolysis with minimal exercise, even when the dietary and training recommendations for sporadic ER are followed. Three specific intrinsic causes of ER have been identified to date: recurrent exertional rhabdomyolysis (RER),[56] type 1 polysaccharide storage myopathy (PSSM),[57,58] and type 2 PSSM.[59] It is likely that there are other specific causes that have yet to be identified (idiopathic chronic ER). In all these intrinsic forms of chronic ER, it appears that there are specific environmental stimuli that are necessary to trigger muscle necrosis in genetically susceptible animals.[46,56] Horses cannot be cured of a susceptibility to this condition, but if the specific disease is identified, changes in management can be implemented to minimize episodes of rhabdomyolysis.

Chronic Dietary Imbalance

Horses consuming a high-grain diet appear to be more likely to develop ER than horses fed a low-grain or fat-supplemented diet.[46,56,60] The grain itself may not be responsible for rhabdomyolysis; however, high starch intake may trigger rhabdomyolysis in horses with particular myopathies such as RER and PSSM.

Electrolyte depletion in horses can occur from dietary deficiency and losses in sweat with strenuous exercise. Sodium, potassium, magnesium, and calcium play key roles in muscle fiber contractility. With severe acute electrolyte depletion, such as that found after endurance exercise, serum electrolytes may be below normal ranges.[47] With chronic dietary depletion, however, serum concentrations may not reflect total body electrolyte imbalances.[61,62] Work by Harris et al[61,62] established renal fractional excretions as a technique to evaluate electrolyte concentrations in horses with chronic ER. Blood and urine samples are obtained concurrently, and creatinine and electrolyte concentrations are measured in both. [Serum creatinine]/[urine creatinine] multiplied by the reciprocal for urine and serum electrolyte concentrations × 100 provides the fractional excretion of a particular electrolyte. It can be difficult to obtain consistently representative renal fractional excretions of electrolytes in horses from catheterized samples.[63] In the United Kingdom, a number of horses with chronic ER had low fractional excretions of sodium, and daily dietary supplementation of 60 g (2 oz) of NaCl resulted in abatement of clinical signs. Other horses had high phosphorus excretion, suggesting a dietary calcium/phosphorus imbalance, and decreasing bran while providing a daily calcium supplement (60 g of $CaCO_3$) was helpful in reducing clinical signs of ER.[62] Hypokalemia was suggested to play a role in chronic ER, although it is not a common finding in horses consuming adequate quantities of forage.[64,65] Supplementation with good quality forage or 30 g of KCl/day ("lite" salt) is recommended for horses with low renal fraction excretion of potassium.

Another postulated cause of ER is the increased generation of free radicals from oxidative metabolism associated with exercise. Selenium, acting via the enzyme glutathione peroxidase, and vitamin E, acting within the lipid component of cell membranes, scavenge free radicals and prevent lipid peroxidation of cell membranes. Primary selenium deficiency is common in young horses living in areas with selenium-deficient soil; however, it has rarely been demonstrated as a cause of ER.[40] In fact, many racehorses with chronic ER have higher concentrations of selenium and vitamin E from zealous dietary supplementation by the owner.[66] Riding horses, however, that are not on green pasture for 2 or more years may develop a deficiency of vitamin E, which could contribute to muscle soreness. It is not known whether horses that experience repeated episodes of ER may generate more free radicals than normal horses. A higher generation of free radicals in horses with chronic ER may explain the perceived benefit of repeated administration of selenium and vitamin E in TB horses with chronic ER.[67] Adequate values are more than 0.07 mcg/mL for blood selenium and more than 2.0 mcg/mL for serum vitamin E.

Recurrent Exertional Rhabdomyolysis

About 5% to 10% of TB racehorses develop ER during a racing season, and 75% of these horses have more than four episodes in 4 months.[55] Approximately 6% of National Hunt horses[68] and 13% of polo horses develop ER.[69] Horses with a nervous disposition, especially fillies, are highly predisposed.[56] Research studies suggest that a subset of TB horses with chronic ER have RER.[11,12,22] RER appears to be an inherited, intermittent, stress-induced defect in the regulation of muscle contraction.[12,22] A breeding trial using TB horses with RER confirmed that the characteristic abnormality in muscle contracture is inherited in an autosomal dominant fashion.[70] Recurrent episodes of rhabdomyolysis in STBs and Arabian horses may be from a similar abnormality, but this has not been confirmed. A heritable basis for RER in STBs was supported by equine lymphocyte antigen profiles in affected horses.[50]

Factors that trigger RER in susceptible horses include gender, temperament, excitement, stress, dietary starch, exercise duration/intensity, season, and lameness.[40,41,56,71] Females are most commonly afflicted with RER (67% female, 33% male), particularly those that are 2 years of age and in race training.[56,71] Nervous horses are five times more likely to develop RER, and horses with lameness are four times more likely to develop RER. Susceptible horses receiving more than 5 kg of concentrate feed (oats, corn, molasses mix) are more likely to develop RER than those receiving 2.5 kg of concentrate feed/day.[56] Dietary effects of high carbohydrate in horses with RER may in part be related to the psychogenic effects of grain on excitability. In horses with RER, glycogen storage does not increase substantially.[60,72] Inclement weather has been cited as a trigger of RER, and the condition is reported more commonly in the autumn and winter in the United Kingdom.[40]

A contribution of reproductive hormones to triggering RER was postulated because the incidence appears to be highest in mares.[41,56,71] Many owners report that episodes of RER occur most commonly during estrus, but in one study of racehorses, no direct correlation was shown between progesterone fluctuations and serum CK activity.[73] It is likely that the estrus cycle is one of many factors that combine to trigger RER in susceptible horses. Many racetrack practitioners report that the incidence of RER declines when susceptible mares are treated with testosterone. Hypothyroidism and lactic acidosis were suggested as a cause of RER but have never been substantiated.[3,60,74-76]

Clinical Signs

Horses with RER have intermittent elevations in serum CK activity.[3,11,67,68] Episodes of muscle stiffness, sweating, and firm muscle contractures often occur in horses once they become fit and are frequently associated with excitement at the time of exercise. In TBs, RER occurs most frequently during training when horses are held to a slow gallop.[56] In STBs, RER often occurs 15 to 30 minutes into jogging.[3] Obvious clinical signs are rare after racing. A history of poor performance and elevated serum AST and CK may be the only presenting complaints in some horses. Older TBs used as riding horses may have very intermittent episodes of RER associated with layup of fit horses. Event horses often develop clinical signs after the steeplechase phase or in the "10 minute box" of a long format Three Day Event, or less commonly after warm-up for the cross-country phase of a short-format Three Day Event or during the cross-country phase. Muscle stiffness, reluctance to collect, and lack of power may be present on a continual basis between episodes in some of these older horses. Arabian horses often develop clinical signs with little exertion, frequently in association with excitement.

In some riding horses, the clinical signs of a mild attack may be very subtle and are easily missed by the rider. The horse is maintained in work and may actually experience daily episodes resulting in cumulative muscle damage (Figure 83-5).

Diagnosis

A submaximal exercise test (page 819) is useful for identification of RER in a horse with a history of poor performance unrelated to signs typical of tying-up. Nuclear scintigraphy (page 819) may demonstrate IRU in the affected muscles of some, but not all, affected horses.

Muscle biopsies from horses with RER that are in training have a characteristic histological appearance (Figure 83-6). These horses have increased numbers of centrally located nuclei in mature muscle fibers. They may have evidence of varying stages of muscle degeneration and regeneration, and they have normal to slightly increased muscle glycogen staining.[11] Histopathological changes are often lacking in horses that have been laid up for a period before biopsy. In addition, RER is characterized by abnormal sensitivity of intact muscle bundles to contractures induced by the addition of caffeine or halothane to a muscle bath.[21,22] Elevated myoplasmic calcium concentration was reported in muscle of horses with acute ER[77] and

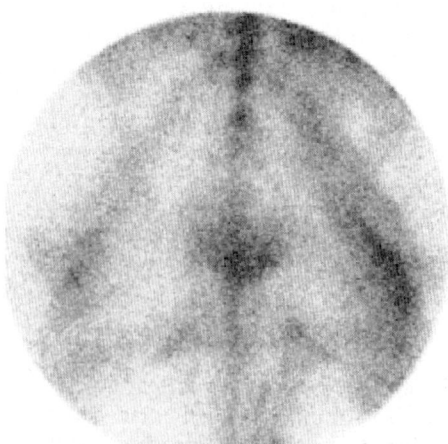

Fig. 83-5 • Dorsal scintigraphic image of the pelvic region of an 8-year-old show jumper mare with a history of poor performance and reluctance to work. Cranial is at the top. There are linear areas of moderately increased radiopharmaceutical uptake in the muscles, associated with chronic, recurrent exertional rhabdomyolysis.

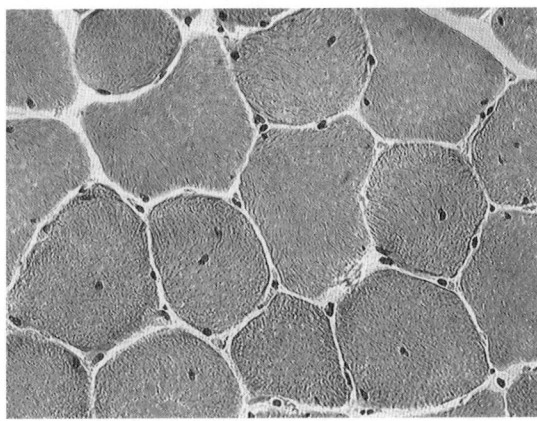

Fig. 83-6 • Cryostat-cut sections of a biopsy of the semitendinosus muscle of a Thoroughbred with recurrent exertional rhabdomyolysis (RER) stained with hematoxylin and eosin. Note the presence of centrally located nuclei in mature muscle fibers. This is a common feature of biopsies of horses with RER.

in myoblasts derived from TBs with RER.[12] There are physiological similarities between the contracture results of RER and contracture tests for malignant hyperthermia (MH). Biochemical studies of isolated muscle cell membranes[78] and linkage analysis[79] do not support an identical biochemical basis for MH and RER. The increased halothane sensitivity of the muscles in RER horses may explain why many TBs with RER develop rhabdomyolysis under halothane anesthesia.[80]

Management
In the past, horses have been box stall rested for several weeks following an episode of RER. It is our opinion that this is counterproductive and increases the likelihood that the horses will develop rhabdomyolysis when put back into training. The initial muscle pain usually subsides within 24 hours of acute RER, and daily turnout in a small paddock can be provided at this time. Subsequently, a gradual return to performance is recommended once serum CK is close to normal range.

Prevention
Prevention of further episodes of RER in susceptible horses includes standardized daily routines and providing an environment that minimizes stress. This should include desensitizing horses to stressful situations, moving to a quiet area of the barn, regular turnout, and positioning near compatible horses. Daily exercise is essential, whether in the form of turnout, walking on a horse walker, lunging, or riding. There should be a long, slow, warm-up period.

The diet should be adjusted to include a balanced vitamin and mineral supplement, high-quality hay (but not alfalfa), and a minimum of soluble carbohydrates (<3 kg of high-starch concentrate). Postexercise serum CK activity in horses with RER is influenced by the amount of energy horses are fed daily, as well as the composition of the diet. When 500-kg TBs with RER were fed 88 MJ (21 Mcal) of energy and exercised for 30 minutes a day, serum CK activity after exercise was within the normal range. There was no measurable effect of feeding a starch-based (2.5 kg of an oat, corn, molasses mix) or a fat-based (2.3 kg of rice bran; 20% digestible energy [DE] from fat) supplement with

hay on muscle necrosis.[60] However, when the energy level was increased to a level that was closer to what is normally fed to racehorses (117 MJ or 28 Mcal), the source of energy had a significant effect on postexercise CK activity. Horses fed a high proportion of energy in the form of starch (5 kg of oat, corn, molasses mix) had significantly higher CK levels after exercise than horses fed 25% of total DE as fat (Re-Leve, Hallway Feeds, Lexington, Kentucky, United States).[72] Therefore it would appear that TBs susceptible to RER that are in moderate to high intensity training should be fed concentrate feeds that are relatively low in starch (<20% DE) and high in fat (20% DE or a feed that is 10% to 12.5% fat by weight) to minimize postexercise muscle damage. Vegetable oils can be used to supplement low-starch feeds (a maximum of 600 mL/day, with 800 U of vitamin E). However, it is difficult to achieve adequate caloric intake for TBs in race training by adding vegetable oil to low-starch feeds such as hay cubes. For hard keepers, a complete low-starch, high-fat pelleted feed containing vegetable oils and/or rice bran works well and provides a balanced ration. One such feed, Re-Leve, has been shown to lower serum CK activity in exercising TBs with RER. No more than half of the total of forage should be fed as alfalfa: lower-starch hays such as grass or meadow, timothy, brome, or oat hay are preferable. Corn and barley should be avoided because they are particularly high in starch.

The use of low doses of acetylpromazine tranquilizers (0.005 to 0.01 mg/kg) 30 minutes before exercise is believed to help some nervous or excitable horses. Long-acting tranquilizers such as fluphenazine have been used successfully by some practitioners. Dantrolene (2 to 4 mg/kg PO) given 1 hour before exercise has proven to be effective in preventing RER in some horses.[81,82] Dantrolene is used to prevent MH in people and swine by decreasing the release of calcium from the calcium release channel. Phenytoin has also been advocated as a treatment for horses with RER.[83] Dosages are adjusted in horses to maintain serum levels of 8 to 10 mcg/mL. Initial doses begin at 6 to 8 mg/kg PO for 3 to 5 days. Doses can be increased by 1-mg/kg increments every 3 days until RER is prevented but should be cut back if horses appear drowsy. If possible, serum phenytoin concentrations should be assessed regularly at the initiation of treatment. Phenytoin acts on a number of ion channels within muscle and nerves, including sodium and calcium channels. Unfortunately, long-term treatment with dantrolene or phenytoin is expensive, and efficacy has not been established.

In some mares in which episodes of RER coincide with estrus, suppression of estrus using progesterone implants or injections may be helpful. This should be done in conjunction with dietary and training alterations. Anecdotal information from racehorse trainers suggests injection with testosterone cypionate decreases RER in TB mares; however, this may be a banned substance in many racing districts.

The above management is effective in reducing RER in many horses, but some remain intractable. Nervous young racing fillies and older riding horses, especially event horses, present the greatest challenge in management.

Polysaccharide Storage Myopathy
A subset of horses with chronic ER have a storage disorder characterized by the accumulation of glycogen and an abnormal polysaccharide in skeletal muscle.[58] Abnormal

polysaccharide accumulation occurs in a variety of European and North American breeds of riding and driving horses that have a history of muscle stiffness and increased serum CK activity after exercise.[51,53,84,85]

Recently an autosomal dominant gain-of-function mutation was identified in the glycogen synthase gene (*GYS1*) in Quarter Horses with PSSM.[57] This mutation is found in at least 20 different breeds of horses in Europe and North America. Affected breeds include Quarter Horses; American Paint horses; Appaloosas; draft horses, including American Cream, Belgian, Percheron, Cob Normande, Trekpard, Haflinger, Morgan, Mustang, Rocky Mountain Horse, and Tennessee Walking Horse breeds; mixed breed horse; Cobs; Hanoverians; Rheinlander; and Warmbloods of unspecified type.[53,59] Because some horses with elevated muscle glycogen content do not possess the *GYS1* mutation, PSSM is now subdivided into type 1 and type 2.[59] Type 1 PSSM refers to horses with the *GYS1* mutation. The prevalence of the PSSM from the *GYS1* mutation ranges from 8% in Quarter Horses and Paints[52] to 36% in Belgian draft horses,[54] with no reported cases in the few TBs, STBs, and Arabians tested.[53,59] Type 2 refers to horses with excessive muscle glycogen that do not have the *GYS1* mutation. Type 2 PSSM appears to account for about 25% of PSSM seen in Quarter Horse–related breeds and 80% of PSSM seen in Warmblood breeds.[59] The acronyms EPSM and EPSSM have also been used for polysaccharide storage myopathy, although they do not indicate a specific genotype.[86]

Clinical Signs

Horses with both forms of PSSM often have a calm and sedate demeanor. Clinical signs of muscle stiffness, reluctance to exercise, exercise intolerance, or overt muscle contractures and reluctance to move usually are apparent at the commencement of training.[46,51] Most horses have numerous episodes of ER or a consistent history of poor performance; however, some mildly affected horses have only one or two episodes of ER per year.[46] In Quarter Horses, type 1 PSSM has the highest frequency in halter horses, followed by pleasure horses and working cow horses. It is uncommon in racing Quarter Horses. Serum CK activities are often elevated in untreated Quarter Horses, even when horses are rested, and while clinical signs are active, CK will usually increase by 1000 U/L or more 4 hours after 15 minutes of exercise at a trot.[87] Muscle atrophy, renal failure, and severe colic-like pain are less common presenting complaints. Both type 1 and type 2 PSSM occur in Quarter Horse and Paint horse foals and weanlings without rhabdomyolysis necessarily being induced by exercise (see page 829).

Draft horses with type 1 PSSM show signs of a generalized decrease in muscle mass, overt muscle atrophy, weakness in the hindlimbs with difficulty rising, reluctance to backup, and gait abnormalities.[54,55,88-90] ER can be a debilitating feature of type 1 PSSM in draft breeds. Although shivers was suggested to be a sign of PSSM, recent studies show there is no causal relationship (see Chapter 48).[54] Draft horses with PSSM often have only a mild elevation in serum CK and AST. The prevalence of type 1 PSSM is so high in many draft breeds that many homozygous affected horses can be identified.[91] These homozygotes may have more severe clinical signs.

Warmbloods derived from draft crosses may have type 1 PSSM. Many European Warmblood breeds are more frequently affected by type 2 PSSM.[59] One of the most common presenting complaints in Warmbloods with PSSM is a gait abnormality characterized by lack of impulsion and shifting undiagnosed lameness.[51] Warmbloods with PSSM also present with sore muscles and ER.

Diagnosis

A diagnosis of type 1 PSSM can be made by testing whole blood or hair root samples for the *GYS1* mutation (http://www.vdl.umn.edu/vdl/ourservices/neuromuscular.html). Type 2 PSSM at present must still be diagnosed by muscle biopsy. The distinctive features of type 1 PSSM in muscle biopsy samples are numerous subsarcolemmal vacuoles and dense, crystalline periodic acid–Schiff (PAS)-positive, amylase-resistant inclusions in fast twitch fibers.[58] A false-negative diagnosis of type 1 PSSM by muscle biopsy may occur if biopsy samples are small or if horses are less than 1 year of age. Muscle biopsies from horses with type 2 PSSM have increased PAS staining for glycogen and aggregates of granular PAS-positive polysaccharide in the cytoplasm or under the sarcolemma.[91] The PAS-positive polysaccharide in type 2 PSSM is frequently, but not always, amylase sensitive. False-positive diagnosis is possible for type 2 PSSM in highly trained horses that normally have higher muscle glycogen concentrations or in formalin-fixed sections that show a greater deposition of subsarcolemmal glycogen in healthy horses. Other features that may be present with both forms of PSSM include muscle necrosis, macrophage infiltration of myofibers, regenerative fibers, and atrophied type 2 fibers.

Etiology

Muscle glycogen concentrations in horses with type 1 PSSM are 1.5 to 4 times normal, and glucose-6-phosphate concentrations are up to 10 times normal.[92] Increased muscle glycogen concentrations in type 1 PSSM appear to be from increased and unregulated glycogen synthase activity as a result of a gain-of-function mutation in the *GYS1* gene.[57] Horses with PSSM show increased glycogen synthase activity both in the basal state and when stimulated by glucose-6-phosphate. Elevated insulin in the bloodstream can further enhance glycogen synthase activity. Abnormal amylase-resistant polysaccharide appears to result from production of a polysaccharide with a higher ratio of straight glucose chains, which are created by glycogen synthase, relative to branched chains, which are created by the less active glycogen branching enzyme. Rhabdomyolysis in type 1 PSSM appears to result from a deficiency of energy within individual contracting muscle fibers.[93] The genetic defect combined with a high-starch diet appears to produce substrate-limited muscle oxidative metabolism by both impairing production of acetyl coenzyme A from glycogen and by preventing lipolysis and delivery of free fatty acids to skeletal muscle mediated by insulin release. Clinical signs of muscle pain in horses with the *GYS1* mutation may be exacerbated by enhanced individual insulin sensitivity,[92] as well as by meals that produce elevated blood glucose and insulin levels.[94] The etiology of type 2 PSSM is not known at present.

Management

Horses with acute rhabdomyolysis can be managed in a fashion similar to that described for sporadic rhabdomyolysis (see page 824).[87] Episodes of rhabdomyolysis can be lowered by 75% or more by feeding a diet that is low in starch, supplemented with fat and high in fiber.[46,94] The primary factor to consider in PSSM horses is their body weight and energy requirements. Overweight horses should begin with a weight-reduction program consisting of grass hay, a ration balancer, a grazing muzzle, and daily exercise following an overnight fast, which elevates plasma free fatty acid levels through lipolysis. Horses with PSSM are much less tolerant of dietary starch and sugar than horses with RER. Horses with a normal body weight should consume diets consisting of good quality grass hay and no high-starch concentrate feed. Instead, a low-starch fat-supplemented feed, such as rice bran–based feeds, complete feeds designed for PSSM, or 250 to 500 mL (1 to 2 cups) of vegetable oil soaked into a low-starch pellet should be provided.[94,95] Although 1 lb of fat per day has been recommended on some Internet websites, recent research has shown that half as much fat usually works well for many horses with type 1 PSSM.[94] The amount of digestible energy obtained through starch and sugar should be less than 10% and fat more than 13% per day. Daily exercise is absolutely essential to return PSSM horses to athletic endeavors. As much daily turnout as possible combined with a very gradual training program has a significant impact on decreasing serum CK activity within 30 days.[94] Box stall rest for more than 12 h/day appears to increase the incidence of rhabdomyolysis in these horses.

Malignant Hyperthermia

Etiology

An autosomal dominant mutation in the skeletal muscle ryanodine receptor (*RYR1*), which is altered in pigs and people with MH, was originally identified in Quarter Horses that developed severe reactions to general anesthesia.[96] The prevalence of the *RYR1* mutation is in general low; however, within a family of Quarter Horses with type 1 PSSM the prevalence is high.

Clinical Signs

Horses with both the MH mutation and the *GYS1* mutation for PSSM show intermittent but severe signs of muscle pain, stiffness, cramping, and sudden death associated with mild exertion.[97] Quarter Horses with MH that were masked with halothane and then intubated and maintained on halothane showed a marked increase in body temperature, metabolic acidosis, rigor, and death.[98]

Diagnosis

Genetic testing is recommended in Quarter Horse and Paint horses with a family history of postanesthetic complications or with difficult-to-manage forms of PSSM. Testing is available through the Veterinary Diagnostic Laboratory at the University of Minnesota (http://www.vdl. umn.edu/vdl/ourservices/neuromuscular.html).

Treatment

The most successful outcome for a horse with suspected MH would be pretreatment with oral dantrolene (4 mg/kg) 30 to 60 minutes before induction of general anesthesia. There is no cost-effective means to deliver dantrolene to horses intravenously once an episode has begun. Unfortunately, once a fulminant episode is underway it is difficult

to prevent cardiac arrest. Horses with both PSSM and MH respond to a low-starch, high-fat diet and regular daily exercise.[97]

NONEXERTIONAL RHABDOMYOLYSIS

Although exertion is the most common trigger for rhabdomyolysis in horses, many horses can suffer severe rhabdomyolysis without any preceding exertion. Nonexertional rhabdomyolysis may have metabolic, immune-mediated, infectious, nutritional, or toxic causes.

METABOLIC MYOPATHIES

Polysaccharide Storage Myopathy

Clinical Signs

The most common form of PSSM causes the development of muscle necrosis, pain, and firm muscles in adult horses with the onset of training (see section on Polysaccharide Storage Myopathy, page 828). A subset of horses with both type 1 and type 2 PSSM and a concurrent illness may develop rhabdomyolysis without any preceding exercise. Rhabdomyolysis may be so severe that horses become recumbent and unable to rise. Initial muscle swelling and firmness may give way to substantial atrophy after a few days. This form of PSSM was described in weanling and yearling Quarter Horses with concurrent bacterial pneumonia or diarrhea.[99] In addition to serum CK greater than 200,000 U/L, electrolyte abnormalities such as hyponatremia, hypochloremia, hypocalcemia, hyperphosphatemia, and hyperkalemia are common as a result of the loss of partitioning between extracellular and the large intramuscular fluid compartment and, in some horses, renal compromise.[100] Foals with type 2 PSSM may have a history of a stiff gait and difficulty producing the power required to stand successfully from a recumbent position without assistance. Serum CK activity in these foals may only be moderately elevated, and the primary clinical signs are weakness and pain. Horses with both type 1 PSSM and the mutation for MH (*RYR1*) can develop severe nonexertional rhabdomyolysis and sudden death.

Diagnosis

A diagnosis of type 1 PSSM and MH can be made by genetic testing. A diagnosis of type 2 PSSM is based on identification of abnormal polysaccharide in PAS stains of muscle biopsies (Figure 83-7). A diagnosis may be complicated by the fact that rhabdomyolysis in weanlings with PSSM may precede the later stage of accumulation of abnormal polysaccharide.[101] The diagnosis of PSSM in a weanling may be supported by the identification of PSSM in a muscle biopsy from the dam or sire.[99]

There are many other differential diagnoses for acute rhabdomyolysis in foals. Neonatal foals may have modest increases in CK at birth in conjunction with elevated creatinine and a history of placentitis or dystocia.[102] Septicemia could potentially cause an inflammatory reaction in skeletal muscle of neonatal foals. Most commonly, myodegeneration is caused by vitamin E and selenium deficiency with subsequent peroxidation of cell membranes by oxygen free radicals (see page 834).[103] Young Quarter Horses have developed acute rhabdomyolysis on infection

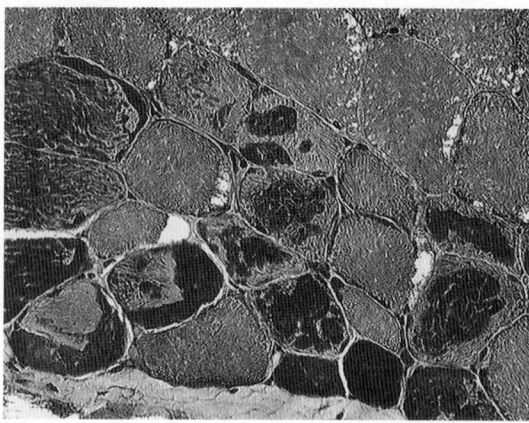

Fig. 83-7 • Cryostat-cut sections of a semitendinosus biopsy of a horse with polysaccharide storage myopathy stained with periodic acid–Schiff (PAS) and counterstained with hematoxylin. Note the presence of white subsarcolemmal vacuoles in some fibers and the dark PAS-positive granular inclusions representing abnormal polysaccharide in numerous other muscle fibers.

with *Streptococcus equi* (see page 832).[104] Mild elevations in CK also occur in Quarter Horses with glycogen branching enzyme deficiency (GBED).

Treatment

Acute treatment of rhabdomyolysis is similar to that recommended in the Sporadic Rhabdomyolysis section (pages 824 and 825). Special considerations for foals include stall confinement in those showing pronounced stiffness or weakness and assistance to rise and suckle every hour. Nutritional support in the form of mare's milk or foal pellets should be supplied if they do not suckle adequately. Either the mare should be switched to a low-starch high-fat supplement that the foal can share or the mare's grain should be kept inaccessible to the foal. In recumbent foals, in addition to intravenous fluids and nutritional support, a constant rate infusion of detomidine, lidocaine, butorphanol, or ketamine may be useful to control severe pain and struggling. Dantrolene sodium (4 mg/kg, every 4 to 6 hours, PO) may decrease muscle cell necrosis. Assistance to stand every few hours either manually or using a sling is necessary to improve muscle function and circulation. Cautious handwalking for no more than a few minutes at a time is recommended once the foal is stable and strong enough to ambulate. Whenever possible, stall confinement should be limited to less than 48 hours after the episode of rhabdomyolysis and stiffness subside because prolonged stall confinement may result in an increased incidence of rhabdomyolysis episodes as a result of PSSM. Small paddock turnout with limited ability to move around is recommended once stiffness subsides.

Dietary management of weanling foals is similar to that of adults except that foals have a higher protein requirement than adults, especially with regard to lysine. Feeding alfalfa hay rather than grass hay, combined with balanced commercial low-starch high-fat ration, is recommended to meet nutritional needs of weanlings. In some foals, this may provide excessive sugar, and grass hay may be necessary. As much turnout as possible with other horses to encourage daily exercise is recommended for long-term management of foals with PSSM.

The prognosis for weanlings with nonexertional rhabdomyolysis is guarded because of the high likelihood of recurrence.

Glycogen Branching Enzyme Deficiency (GBED)

Clinical Signs

GBED is a fatal autosomal recessive glycogen storage disorder distinct from PSSM in Quarter Horse and Paint foals.[105,106] A mutation in the glycogen branching enzyme gene *(GBE1)* causes a deficiency in the glycogen branching enzyme (GBE) responsible for producing a normally configured glycogen molecule in numerous tissues.[107] Approximately 8% of Quarter Horses and Paint horses are carriers of the mutation, and 3% of second and third trimester aborted fetuses submitted to two diagnostic laboratories were found to be homozygous for GBED.[108] Pleasure horses and working cow horses have the highest incidence of GBED carriers.[109] Many foals with GBED are undiagnosed because of the similarity of clinical signs with many neonatal diseases and the current lack of awareness of available genetic testing for stillborn foals and aborted fetuses.

Clinical signs appear to be caused by a lack of intracellular glucose stores for normal tissue metabolism. Foals may be aborted, stillborn, weak after birth, or live to up to 18 weeks of age. Death may be sudden when foals are exercised on pasture, associated with weak respiratory muscles, or the result of euthanasia from persistent recumbency. Treatable flexural deformities of all limbs and recurrent hypoglycemia occur in some affected foals. Persistent leukopenia, intermittent hypoglycemia, and moderate elevations in serum CK (1000 to 15,000 U/L), AST, and γ-glutamyl transferase activities are common laboratory findings.

Diagnosis

Routine post mortem examination usually reveals few abnormalities apart from pulmonary edema in some foals and basophilic inclusions in skeletal muscle and cardiac tissues in foals more than 1 month of age. PAS staining of muscle, heart, and sometimes liver shows notable lack of normal PAS staining for glycogen and a variable amount of abnormal PAS-positive globular or crystalline intracellular inclusions. EM and iodine spectra absorption indicated that the polysaccharide is filamentous, with a very minimally branched structure. The most accurate diagnosis of GBED can be obtained through genetic testing of the foal for homozygous status or the dam/sire for heterozygous status. Many stallion owners offer a free repeat breeding to owners that lose foals, and if a diagnosis is not established, the owner will have a 25% chance of having another GBED-affected offspring on repeat breeding. The Veterinary Genetics Laboratory at the University of California, Davis (www.vgl.ucdavis.edu) and Vet Gen in Michigan (www.vetgen.com) are licensed by the University of Minnesota to test for GBED. Mane or tail hairs with roots intact can be submitted. Diagnostic laboratories should be encouraged to screen aborted fetuses for GBED either through PAS staining of cardiac samples or via genetic testing. Testing also should be strongly advised for prepurchase evaluation of broodmares or stallions.

INFLAMMATORY MYOPATHIES

Immune-Mediated Myopathies

Infarctive Hemorrhagic Purpura

Mild elevations in serum CK activity have been observed in conjunction with purpura hemorrhagica in horses. Rarely, some horses vaccinated for, or exposed to, *S. equi* within the past month develop variable edema, extremely high serum CK activity, acute colic, firm swellings within muscle and under the skin, and unilateral lameness.[110] Infarctions of skeletal muscle, subcutaneous tissue, and focal areas of the gastrointestinal tract and lungs resulting from a severe vasculopathy are found in these horses. Infarctive purpura is characterized by leukocytosis, hyperfibrinogenemia, and hypoalbuminemia. A diagnosis is often established based on clinical signs of marked pain, inflammatory leukogram, low serum albumin concentration, leukocytoclastic vasculitis in skin and affected tissues, and very high *S. equi* M protein titer. Successful treatment requires early detection, penicillin for 14 days, and prolonged high doses of dexamethasone (0.12 to 0.2 mg/kg) for at least 10 days, followed by tapering doses of prednisolone at an initial dose of 2 mg/kg. Aggressive steroid treatment is required because horses treated with lower doses progress to intestinal infarction and death.

Immune-Mediated Myositis

Immune-mediated polymyositis (IMM) often occurs in Quarter Horses, although other breeds may be affected. Horses are usually either 8 or less or 16 or more years of age.[111,112] In approximately one third of horses with IMM, a triggering factor appears to have been exposure to *S. equi* or a respiratory disease.[111]

Clinical Signs

The most prominent clinical sign of IMM in Quarter Horses is rapid onset of muscle atrophy, particularly affecting the back and croup muscles, accompanied by stiffness and malaise. Atrophy may progress to involve 50% of the horses' muscle mass within 1 week and may lead to generalized weakness. Focal symmetrical atrophy of cervical muscles has been reported in a pony with IMM.[112]

Diagnosis

Hematological abnormalities are usually restricted to mild to moderate elevations in serum CK and AST activity. However, in some horses with chronic myositis, serum muscle enzyme activities are normal. Muscle biopsy of epaxial and gluteal muscles shows lymphocytic vasculitis, anguloid atrophy, myofiber infiltration with lymphocytes, fiber necrosis with macrophage infiltration, and regeneration in acute stages (Figure 83-8). Biopsies of semitendinosus or semimembranosus muscles may show some evidence of atrophy and vasculitis, but substantial inflammatory infiltrates may be absent in these muscles. The extent of the inflammatory infiltrates in epaxial muscles is such that a diagnosis can often be established from several formalin-fixed samples obtained using an 18-gauge disposable biopsy needle.

The lymphocytic infiltrates seen in muscle samples from horses with IMM contain a high CD4/CD8 ratio with no evidence of IgG binding to myofibers.[111] The reason

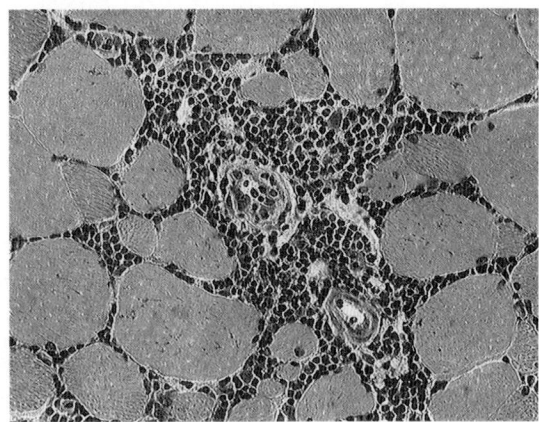

Fig. 83-8 • Immune-mediated myositis: Cryostat-cut sections of a biopsy of the longissimus dorsi from a horse with rapid muscle atrophy stained with hematoxylin and eosin. Note the prominent cuffing of the blood vessels with mononuclear cell infiltrates and the lymphocytes surrounding a number of muscle fibers that is characteristic of immune-mediated myopathy in Quarter Horses.

why specific muscle groups are affected in horses with IMM is unclear.

Treatment

Horses with concurrent evidence of streptococcal infection should be treated with antibiotics. It is prudent to avoid intramuscular injections. Administration of corticosteroids appears to immediately improve signs of malaise and inappetence and prevents further progression of muscle atrophy. Recommended dosages are dexamethasone (0.05 mg/kg) for 3 days, followed by prednisolone (1 mg/kg for 7 to 10 days) tapered by 100 mg/week over 1 month. Serum CK activity often normalizes after 7 to 10 days of treatment. Muscle mass will usually gradually recover over 2 to 3 months even without corticosteroid treatment. Recurrence of atrophy in susceptible horses is common and may require reintroduction of corticosteroid therapy.

Infectious Myopathies

Virus-Associated Myositis

Necrosis of skeletal and cardiac muscle may occur in association with viral diseases such as equine influenza and equine infectious anemia. In most situations, viral-induced muscle damage represents a component of systemic multiple organ system involvement. Equine influenza A2 has been found to cause severe rhabdomyolysis, and equine herpesvirus–1 has been reported to induce primary muscle stiffness and clinical signs resembling ER.[38,45]

Sarcocystosis Myositis

Cysts of the sporozoan parasite *Sarcocystis* are commonly seen in routine histological sections of the heart, esophageal, and skeletal muscle. More than 90% of horses more than 8 years of age have sarcocysts in esophageal muscles, and 6% of healthy horses have one or more nonreactive sarcocysts in gluteal muscle biopsies.[52] Cysts usually pose no problem, but multisystemic dysfunction occurs with heavy infestations. Horses with heavy infestation show signs of fever, anorexia, stiffness, weight loss, muscle fasciculations, atrophy, and weakness.[113] Diagnosis of sarcocystosis requires history, clinical signs, laboratory evaluation, and the demonstration of an inflammatory reaction to immature cysts in muscle biopsies. Infection occurs from contamination of feed by infected canine feces. Successful treatment of one horse with sarcocystosis using phenylbutazone, trimethoprim sulfa, and pyrimethamine was reported.[113]

Streptococcus equi Rhabdomyolysis

Severe rhabdomyolysis was reported in young Quarter Horses in association with concurrent *Streptococcus equi equi* submandibular lymphadenopathy and/or guttural pouch empyema.[104] Myonecrosis could be from toxic shock resulting from profound nonspecific T-cell stimulation by streptococcal superantigens and the release of high levels of inflammatory cytokines. An alternative explanation may be bacteremia with local multiplication and production of exotoxins or proteases within skeletal muscle. *S. equi* bacteria were identified in affected muscle using immunofluorescent stains for both Lancefield group C carbohydrate and *S. equi* M protein. There is currently no evidence that the *S. equi* involved is an atypical genetic strain of *S. equi*.

Clinical Signs

Horses develop a stiff gait that progresses rapidly to severely painful, firm, swollen, epaxial, and gluteal muscles. Horses often become recumbent, unable to rise, and unrelenting pain may necessitate euthanasia within 24 to 48 hours.

Diagnosis

Hematological abnormalities include mature neutrophilia, hyperfibrinogenemia, and marked elevations in CK (115,000 to 587,000 U/L) and AST (600 to 14,500 U/L) concentrations. Titers to the M protein of *S. equi* are low in affected horses, unless horses are recently vaccinated for strangles. Titers to another protein called *S. equi* myosin binding protein were high in a small number of horses that were tested.[104] At post mortem, large, pale areas of necrotic muscle are evident in hindlimb and lumbar muscles. The histopathological lesions are characterized by severe acute myonecrosis, with a degree of macrophage infiltration. Sublumbar muscles often show the most severe and chronic necrosis as indicated by greater macrophage infiltration of myofibers.

Treatment

A high mortality rate has been reported. Appropriate therapy includes intravenous penicillin therapy combined with an antimicrobial that inhibits protein synthesis, such as rifampin. In addition, flushing infected guttural pouches and draining abscessed lymph nodes will diminish the bacterial load. NSAIDs and possibly high doses of short-acting corticosteroids may assist in diminishing the inflammatory response. Control of unrelenting pain is a major challenge in horses with severe rhabdomyolysis. Constant-rate infusion of lidocaine, detomidine, or ketamine may provide better anxiety and pain relief than periodic injections of tranquilizers. Horses should be placed in a deeply bedded stall and moved from side to side every 4 hours if they are unable to rise. Some horses may benefit from a sling if they will bear weight on their hindlimbs when assisted to stand.

Anaplasma-Associated Rhabdomyolysis

Clinical signs of acute rhabdomyolysis were reported in a horse in conjunction with *Anaplasma phagocytophilia* infection (formerly *Ehrlichia equi*).[114] Typical clinical signs of fever, malaise, and limb edema are accompanied by severe muscle stiffness. Hematological findings include anemia, thrombocytopenia, neutropenia, morula visible in granulocytes, and marked elevations in serum CK and AST concentrations. A diagnosis is confirmed by polymerase chain reaction testing of blood for *A. phagocytophilia*. A direct toxic effect of *A. phagocytophilia* on muscle cells is postulated. The horse in this report was successfully treated with supportive care and oxytetracycline.[114]

Clostridial Myositis

Clostridium septicum, Clostridium chauvoei, Clostridium sporogenes, and mixed infections cause acute myonecrosis in horses with a high fatality rate. *Clostridium perfringens* type A is another cause of myonecrosis; however, with early and aggressive treatment mortality rates for infection with this bacterium are about 20%.[115] There is usually only one primary site of infection that is associated with an injection or deep wound.[116,117] Clostridial spores may lie dormant in skeletal muscle,[118] or direct clostridial spore deposition into the tissue may occur in association with a penetrating injury. If suitable necrotic conditions exist, the spores convert to the vegetative, toxin-producing form of the organism. Powerful exotoxins responsible for the local necrotizing myositis and systemic toxemia are released by proliferating clostridia. Myocardial damage occurs in some horses.

Clinical Signs

Horses often have a history of colic, vaccination, exertional myopathy, penetrating wound, and/or intramuscular injections in the preceding 48 hours. Affected horses usually rapidly develop depression, swelling, and crepitus at the injection site, as well as a fever, toxemia, and tachypnea.[116] Crepitus is not always present.[115] Tremors, ataxia, dyspnea, recumbency, coma, and death may occur within the next 12 to 24 hours. Hematology and serum biochemical analyses usually reflect a generalized state of debilitation and toxemia (e.g., hemoconcentration and a stress/toxic leukogram may be present). Moderate elevations in the activities of serum CK and serum AST usually occur; however, they often do not reflect the toxicity of clostridial myonecrosis.

Diagnosis

Ultrasonographic evaluation of swollen areas may reveal fluid and characteristic hyperechogenic gas accumulation. A specific diagnosis is best made from aspirates of affected tissues examined via direct smears, fluorescent antibody staining, and anaerobic bacterial culture. Cut tissue from the affected area may reveal abundant serosanguineous fluid with an odor of rancid butter. At post mortem, swelling, crepitus, and autolysis are rapid, and blood-stained fluid is often observed discharging from body orifices.

Treatment

Aggressive antibiotic therapy, wound fenestration, aggressive surgical debridement over the entire affected area, and supportive care are the hallmarks of successful treatment.[115]

High doses of intravenous potassium penicillin are recommended every 2 to 4 hours until the horse is stable (1 to 5 days), combined or followed by oral metronidazole. Supportive fluid therapy and antiinflammatory agents for control of pain and swelling are recommended. Short-acting corticosteroids such as prednisolone or hydrocortisone may be used for initial therapy of systemic/toxic shock, but continued use is contraindicated in the face of overwhelming infection. Extensive skin sloughing over the affected area is common in surviving horses.

Postinjection Muscle Soreness and Abscessation

Intramuscular injection of a variety of drugs and vaccines may be followed by severe localized muscle soreness, with or without swelling. Injections in the neck may result in neck stiffness and a bilaterally shortened forelimb stride. Injections in the gluteal muscle mass or thigh region can cause unilateral hindlimb stiffness and lameness. These reactions are usually transitory, but occasionally muscle abscessation is a sequel.

A muscle abscess results in localized swelling, heat, and pain. The extent of the abscess, its depth, and the thickness of the walls may be determined ultrasonographically. Surgical drainage or complete abscess excision is required.

Other Muscle Abscesses

Suppurative myositis may arise through penetrating injuries, hematogenous spread of infection, or via local spread of infection. Initially there is an ill-defined cellulitis, which may heal or progress to a well-defined abscess (Figure 83-9). An abscess may heal, expand, or fistulate, usually

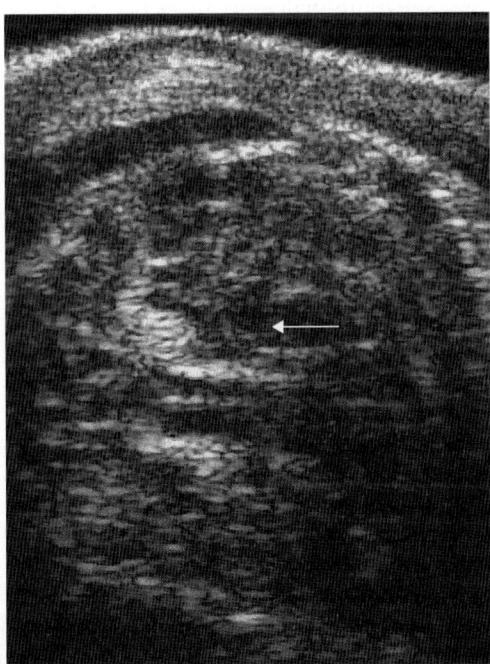

Fig. 83-9 • Transverse ultrasonographic image of the lateral aspect of the antebrachium of a pony with cellulitis previously unresponsive to antimicrobial treatment. There was extensive soft tissue swelling throughout the antebrachium and carpal regions, with effusion in the carpal sheath and the tendon sheaths of extensor carpi radialis and the long and lateral digital extensor tendons. The pony was severely lame. There is a loculated, partly fluid-filled developing abscess *(arrow)*.

to the skin surface. Once fistulated, the abscess may collapse and heal or result in a chronic granuloma with intermittent discharge. *Staphylococcus aureus*, *S. equi*, and *Corynebacterium pseudotuberculosis* are commonly isolated from skeletal muscle abscessation.

The effect of an abscess on the horse's gait depends on its location and can vary from mild stiffness to severe lameness.

Diagnosis is confirmed by ultrasonography or by culture of aspirated fluid. Abscesses lying deep within muscles can be difficult to diagnose. There may be an elevated fibrinogen level and nucleated white blood cell count. The synergistic hemolysin inhibition test, detecting antibodies to *C. pseudotuberculosis*, can be helpful for detection of internal abscesses.[99]

Treatment consists of poulticing, lancing, flushing, and draining. Occasionally surgical excision may be required for complete removal. The use of antimicrobial drugs is controversial but may be recommended for corynebacterial abscesses. Commonly recommended drugs include procaine penicillin (20,000 U/kg IM twice daily) and crystalline penicillin (20,000 to 40,000 U/kg IV four times daily) alone or in combination with rifampin (5 mg/kg PO twice daily). If antimicrobial therapy is used, it should be continued for several weeks.

Prognosis is usually good for horses with superficial abscesses. Horses with deep abscesses are more difficult to manage successfully. Prolonged resolution or recrudescence often occurs with corynebacterial abscesses.

Traumatic Myopathies

Postanesthetic Myopathy

Postanesthetic myopathy occurs as a unilateral problem, such as triceps myopathy, a bilateral problem, such as hindlimb adductor myopathies, or as a generalized condition.[102] In horses anesthetized in lateral recumbency, the dependent triceps muscle is most commonly affected, whereas the longissimus dorsi and gluteal muscles are usually affected in horses positioned in dorsal recumbency.

Hypoperfusion of muscle groups is the most important causative factor, often the result of increased intracompartmental pressure. Positioning of the horse on the operating table is critical. Compressing muscles against a hard, unyielding surface, venous drainage obstruction, and hypotension may all be contributory factors. Generalized myopathies may occur independent of positioning, and hypotension may play a greater role in these horses. The longer the duration of general anesthesia, the higher the risk.

Clinical Signs

Clinical signs are usually evident as soon as the horse tries to stand but may be delayed for up to 2 hours. Horses with severe myopathy may be unable to stand. Triceps myopathy is often characterized by a dropped elbow stance similar to that seen in horses with radial nerve paralysis. Involvement of the gluteal muscles may result in unwillingness to bear weight on the hindlimbs. Horses may appear distressed, with profuse sweating, tachycardia, and tachypnea. The degree of distress depends on the severity of the muscle damage. Affected muscles may feel very firm to near hard. There may be localized swelling.

Diagnosis

Diagnosis is confirmed by measurement of serum CK concentration. The concentration is often increased after general anesthesia, but levels greater than 2000 U/L indicate the presence of myositis. The CK concentration may be normal immediately after the horse stands, but as blood flow returns to the affected muscles, the concentration will increase and peak 4 hours after initiation of the event.

Treatment and Prognosis

Treatment aims to relieve distress and pain, to encourage perfusion of muscles, and to keep the horse standing if at all possible. Pain relief is provided by NSAIDs, such as phenylbutazone (4.4 mg/kg) or flunixin meglumine (1 mg/kg), combined with opiate analgesics (e.g., butorphanol, 0.1 mg/kg) if necessary. Sedation with detomidine in horses with severe pain or acepromazine (0.05 mg/kg) in those with mild pain may be required. Constant-rate infusions of detomidine or butorphanol may be beneficial for pain control. Fluid therapy is important to maintain renal perfusion and urine output and to ensure adequate muscle perfusion. A balanced polyionic electrolyte solution should be infused at up to 20 mL/kg/h for the first several hours.

The prognosis for horses with unilateral myopathy is usually good, although with severe damage there may be residual muscle fibrosis, which may compromise function. With persistent clinical signs, ultrasonographic examination may be useful to determine the extent and severity of muscle damage.[119] The prognosis for generalized myopathy is more guarded.

Prevention

Prevention requires careful preoperative planning to minimize the time under general anesthesia, careful positioning of the horse on the operating table, and maintenance of arterial blood pressure greater than 60 mm Hg using fluid therapy and inotropic agents such as dobutamine (1 to 5 mcg/kg/min). The position of the horse on the operating table is in part dictated by the surgical procedure. With horses in lateral recumbency, the dependent forelimb should be pulled forward, and the upper limb should be supported at least parallel to the table. The hindlimbs should be supported parallel to, or above parallel, and adequately separated to permit venous drainage. With horses in dorsal recumbency, support of the forelimbs or hindlimbs in a semiflexed position using an overhead hoist or side bars can be helpful.

Gastrocnemius Muscle Injury

Gastrocnemius muscle injury in foals and adult horses is discussed in Chapter 80.

Fibrotic Myopathy

Fibrotic myopathy is discussed in Chapters 47 and 48.

Compartment-like Syndrome in the Antebrachium

Compartment syndrome is a condition in which high pressure within a closed fascial space reduces capillary blood perfusion below a level necessary for tissue viability. The syndrome develops in skeletal muscle enclosed by relatively noncompliant osseofascial boundaries.[122] Elevated intracompartmental pressure may result from increased intracompartmental fluid or from decreased compartment size. Increased pressure from fluid accumulation may be the result of muscle trauma and hemorrhage or a sequel to prolonged ischemia and subsequent reperfusion and edema. Prolonged elevated pressure greater than 30 mm Hg resulted in myonecrosis in the dog.[123]

A compartment-like syndrome was described in the horse involving the caudolateral muscle compartment of the antebrachium.[124] This encloses the lateral digital extensor, ulnaris lateralis, superficial and deep digital flexor and flexor carpi ulnaris muscles, and also the median artery, vein, and nerve.

Lameness is a sequel to trauma and is acute and severe in onset, with reluctance to bear weight on the limb associated with firm swelling on the caudolateral aspect of the antebrachium. Digital pulse amplitudes in the more distal part of the limb may be reduced if the limb is flexed or extended. With time, the affected muscle mass may become cold.

Treatment is by fasciotomy. Incising the superficial fascia over ulnaris lateralis resulted in immediate separation of the fascia by 3 to 4 cm and rapid relief of clinical signs.[124]

▣ NUTRITIONAL MYOPATHIES
John Maas and Stephanie J. Valberg

NUTRITIONAL MYODEGENERATION

Etiology

Nutritional myodegeneration (NMD) (white muscle disease, nutritional muscular dystrophy) is an acute degenerative disease of cardiac and skeletal muscle caused by a dietary deficiency of selenium and/or vitamin E.[103,125] Marginally to severely selenium-deficient areas occur in regions of numerous countries throughout the world.[125,126] This syndrome occurs in young, rapidly growing foals born to dams that consumed selenium-deficient diets during gestation. The disease has also been implicated in masseter muscle myopathy and occasionally nonexertional rhabdomyolysis in adult horses. Selenium and vitamin E appear to be synergistic in preventing NMD. However, based on prophylaxis and response to treatment, selenium deficiency appears to be the most important contributor.

Clinical Signs

Foals with primary necrosis of myocardium and respiratory muscles have dyspnea, a rapid irregular heartbeat, profound weakness, recumbency, and sudden death.[100,103] The skeletal muscle form of NMD frequently has a slower onset of muscular weakness, trembling, stiffness, or inability to stand. Most affected foals are able to stand only for short periods. Supporting muscle groups may appear swollen and may be hard and painful on palpation. Commonly affected muscle groups include the gastrocnemius, semitendinosus, semimembranosus, and biceps femoris and muscles of the lumbar, gluteal, and neck regions. If the diaphragm and intercostal muscles are affected, the foal may show respiratory distress and evidence of increased abdominal effort when breathing. Myocardial damage and signs consistent with cardiac dysfunction may be apparent. Dysphagia from necrosis in the tongue may be the only sign in some affected foals and is frequently accompanied by aspiration pneumonia. Foals with primary muscular NMD often show improvement after a few days of rest and treatment with selenium and can often stand and walk within 3 to 5 days. In the western United States, selenium-responsive NMD is seen in adult horses that were extremely deficient in selenium during the winter (snow on the ground), and the only clinical signs have been myoglobinuria (red snow) and mild stiffness in the morning.

Clinical Pathology

Substantially elevated serum CK concentration in the thousands to hundreds of thousands of units per liter along with high AST and LDH activities occur during myodegeneration. Progressively decreasing CK activity can be used as a prognostic indicator of cessation of myodegeneration. Hyperkalemia, hyperphosphatemia, hyponatremia, hypochloremia, and hypocalcemia can occur with severe rhabdomyolysis when the normal distinction between extracellular and intracellular compartments is destroyed by massive tissue necrosis.[100] Myoglobinuria is common. Elevated serum protein concentrations and hemoconcentration commonly reflect dehydration in foals unable to nurse or drink water, as well as fluid shifts into damaged tissues. Neutrophilia is common because of the high incidence of aspiration pneumonia.

Diagnosis

Whole blood selenium and plasma vitamin E samples can be used to assess intermediate to long-term nutritional status. Whole blood selenium analysis is preferred over plasma and serum.[127] Whole blood selenium concentrations ranging from 0.07 to more than 0.1 ppm are considered normal. Short-term oral or intramuscular supplementation of selenium can confuse interpretation of circulating selenium concentration. Selenium-dependent glutathione peroxidase (GSH-Px) formed in the red cells during erythropoiesis also provides an index of body selenium status. Adequate GSH-Px activities are greater than 20 to 50 U/mg of hemoglobin/min in horses. However, GSH-Px reference values are only specific to the laboratory where the analysis is performed and must be validated by comparison with blood selenium concentration. The activity of GSH-Px in red blood cells of domestic species remains constant for 4 to 6 days when maintained at 39° F (4° C); after this time, significant decreases occur. The critical concentration of vitamin E (α-tocopherol) in plasma is 1.1 to 2 ppm. Vitamin E deteriorates rapidly in plasma samples. Therefore plasma samples for α-tocopherol analysis need to be put on ice immediately, protected from the light by wrapping in tin foil, and stored frozen (−21° F, −70° C) if analysis is to be delayed.

Pathology

Bilaterally symmetrical myodegeneration is a consistent finding in NMD.[103] Skeletal muscle degeneration is characterized by pale discoloration and a dry appearance of affected muscle, white streaks in muscle bundles, calcification, and intramuscular edema. The white streaks seen in muscle bundles represent bands of coagulation necrosis or, in horses with chronic disease where insults may have occurred weeks before, may represent fibrosis and calcification. Affected muscle bundles are often adjacent to apparently normal or minimally affected muscle. Histologically, affected muscle fibers may be hypercontracted and fragmented, with some mineralization of muscle fibers and macrophage infiltration.[128] Tissue biopsies and tissue specimens obtained at necropsy can be assayed for selenium content. Normal liver concentrations of selenium are 1.05 to 3.5 ppm on a dry matter (DM) basis. Fresh liver is approximately 30% DM in adult horses.

Pathophysiology

During normal cellular metabolism, highly reactive forms of oxygen (free radicals) are produced. These include hydrogen peroxide, hydroperoxides, lipoperoxides, superoxide, various hydroxy radicals, and singlet oxygen. Vitamin E is active within the cell membrane as a lipid-soluble antioxidant that scavenges free radicals that otherwise might react with unsaturated fatty acids to form lipid hydroperoxides. In contrast, GSH-Px destroys hydrogen peroxide and lipoperoxides that have already been formed and converts them to water or relatively harmless alcohols. Other enzymes such as catalase and superoxide dismutase are also involved in this protective process. It is believed that a deficiency of selenium results in rhabdomyolysis through oxidant damage to muscle cell membranes. The precise interrelationships between selenium, vitamin E, other metabolic factors, and triggering mechanisms in NMD are not fully understood because many horses deficient in selenium and/or vitamin E have no evidence of muscle disease. In certain situations, deficiencies of both selenium and vitamin E are necessary for disease to occur. In other horses, NMD can occur when a deficiency of only one of the nutrients is present and the other is normal in blood and tissues.

Treatment and Prognosis

Myocardial damage is often extensive and incompatible with life with the cardiac form of NMD. Only rarely is treatment successful. In contrast, the skeletal form of NMD is more generally amenable to treatment, although the prognosis for clinical recovery from the skeletal form of NMD is guarded and depends often on whether secondary complications such as respiratory disease develop. In all horses with NMD, therapy should involve specific supplementation with selenium and vitamin E and general supportive care.

Alleviation of selenium-responsive NMD requires the use of injectable selenium products. These are available with selenium concentrations varying from 1 mg/mL of selenium to 5 mg/mL, with all products containing 50 mg/mL (68 U) of vitamin E as DL-α-tocopherol acetate. The label dose for selenium is 0.055 to 0.067 mg/kg (2.5 to 3 mg/45 kg) body weight given intramuscularly or subcutaneously. Dosage of these injectable products should not be greatly increased above the label dose to prevent an inadvertent selenium toxicosis. Absorption and distribution of injectable selenium occur rapidly and may account for the rapid improvement in clinical signs seen in reversible cases.

The amount of vitamin E in vitamin E/selenium combinations is insufficient for vitamin E supplementation. Injectable vitamin E products are now available that contain 300 U vitamin E/mL as D-α-tocopherol (Vital E, Schering-Plough Animal Health, Boxmeer, The Netherlands). Administration of these products increases the tissue and/or plasma level of vitamin E activity for approximately 3 weeks. The bioavailability of vitamin E from injectable products depends on the form of vitamin E (the alcohol form, D-α-tocopherol, being the most active) and the amount and quality of the solution emulsifier used. Oral vitamin E supplementation is a good approach to supplement dietary levels with natural vitamin E providing the highest bioavailability. Daily recommended levels of supplementation for horses range from 600 to 1800 mg of DL-α-tocopheryl acetate.[129] Oral α-tocopherol is now available for all species and contains 500 U vitamin E/mL (Emcelle, Stuart Products, Inc., Bedford, Texas, United States). The recommended dosage of this product is 0.5 to 1.5 U/kg body weight.

Supportive therapy may include administration of antibiotics to help combat secondary pneumonia and infected decubital lesions that are common in recumbent horses. If dysphagic, horses should be fed via nasogastric tube, and provision of adequate energy intake and attention to the fluid and electrolyte balance are of critical importance if recovery is to be successful. Hyperkalemia may be life threatening in affected foals. Mineralocorticoids, alkalinizing fluids, and dextrose and insulin may be used to reduce circulating potassium concentrations.[100]

Prevention and Control

NMD is prevented and controlled through supplementation of selenium and vitamin E. Oral supplementation for horses at 1 mg/day of selenium increases blood selenium concentrations above levels known to be associated with NMD.[130,131] Supplementation of pregnant mares is advised in areas known to be selenium deficient; however, only limited selenium may cross the placenta.[107] Supplementation during lactation increases the levels of selenium in milk and thus provides a potential means of selenium supplementation in foals; however, evidence in cattle indicates that this increased level of selenium in milk may not meet the foal's nutrient requirements.[132] Supplementation of selenium by use of injectable selenium products alone would require treatment every 30 to 45 days and would provide only partial amounts of the recommended level of selenium.[133]

Regardless of the method of supplementation, periodic blood (or tissue) sampling of horses at risk is necessary to ensure maintenance of desired levels of selenium. In high-risk areas, samples should be taken every 60 to 90 days to determine selenium status in susceptible horses and every 6 to 12 months to monitor supplementation. Based on these assessments, adjustments to the rate or extent of selenium supplementation may be made. Feeding horses properly prepared and stored hay and grain or allowing them access to high-quality green forage should ensure adequate vitamin E intake.

TOXIC MYOPATHIES

Ingestion of a number of toxic substances in feed or forage may cause rhabdomyolysis in horses.

Ionophores

Ionophores are commonly added to ruminant feeds to promote growth and to control coccidia. However, horses are 10 times more sensitive to the toxic effects of ionophores in feed than cattle. When equine feeds are inadvertently contaminated with ionophores or horses eat cattle feed, cardiomyopathy is the most common chronic sequela, although some horses may die acutely with colic-like signs, myoglobinuria, hypokalemia, cardiac arrhythmia, and tachypnea.[134]

Pasture Myopathies

Tremetone

Horses ingesting 0.5% to 2% body weight of tremetone-containing plants are likely to die from skeletal muscle and cardiac muscle necrosis. Horses show marked depression, weakness, low head posture, and increased cardiac and respiratory rate. Serum AST and CK concentrations are often markedly elevated, and serum electrolyte abnormalities such as hypocalcemia, hyponatremia, hypochloremia, hyperkalemia, and hyperphosphatemia may be present. Treatment is generally supportive as described in the section on acute ER. Tremetone was identified in white snakeroot (*Eupatorium rugosum*) and rayless goldenrod (*Isocoma wrightii*). White snakeroot grows in shaded areas of the eastern and central United States.[135-137] Rayless goldenrod is common in the southwestern United States on open pastures. Tremetone remains active in the hay and in the stalks of the dead plants on pasture, so both the fresh and the dried form of the plants should be kept from horses.[136]

Cassia occidentalis

Muscle necrosis may also occur in horses ingesting *Cassia occidentalis* seeds prevalent in the southeastern United States.[138] Horses develop incoordination, recumbency, and death. Gross skeletal muscle lesions are not present, but histopathological lesions include segmental myonecrosis.

Blister Beetles

One of 70 horses poisoned with blister beetles developed muscle necrosis.[139]

Atypical Myoglobinuria

Atypical myoglobinuria occurs sporadically in horses kept at pasture, usually with no supplemental feeding.[140,141] It has been recognized most commonly in the United Kingdom and Europe, but a similar syndrome has been seen in the midwestern United States.[142] The cause is unknown but appears to involve disruption in lipid metabolism from exposure to a toxin in well-grazed, cool wet pastures.[143,144] It occurs most often in spring and autumn and is often associated with a sudden deterioration in weather conditions.[141,145] The clinical signs are sudden in onset and rapidly progressive, frequently resulting in death. Several horses in a group may be affected, although some may remain without symptoms. Affected horses are reluctant to move, have muscle weakness, fasciculations, and may become recumbent. Choke may be present, and gut sounds may be reduced, with a reduction in fecal production, although appetite may be unaffected. Heart rates may be markedly elevated, and pulmonary edema may be present. The horses do not show signs of pain, despite post mortem evidence of widespread myopathy. Metabolic and respiratory acidosis, elevated cardiac troponin I concentration, substantial increases in serum CK and AST levels, and myoglobinuria are common.

Post mortem examination reveals widespread myodegeneration in skeletal muscles and the myocardium. Special stains for lipid reveal excessive lipid storage in the heart, diaphragm, and other oxidative postural muscles.[142,143] Multiple chain lengths of acylcarnitines are elevated in urine or plasma.[144] Supportive therapy including antioxidants such as vitamin C, vitamin E, riboflavin, and intravenous fluids containing dextrose is recommended. Mortality is high in affected horses.

Disorders Associated with Muscle Fasciculations or Myotonia

A variety of muscle disorders exist in the horse that can cause muscle fasciculations, muscle cramping, and, in some, recumbency. These include metabolic alkalosis combined with hypocalcemia, hypomagnesemia, infestation with ear ticks, myotonia congenita and dystrophic myotonia, and hyperkalemic periodic paralysis. With the exception of ear ticks, these disorders are not associated with a marked elevation in serum CK activity.

Hypocalcemia in Horses

Hypocalcemia (lactation tetany, transport tetany, idiopathic hypocalcemia, and eclampsia) is a relatively rare disorder in horses. Clinical signs of increased muscle tone may resemble tetanus. Horses may show a stiff, stilted gait, rear limb ataxia, muscle fasciculations (especially temporal, masseter, and triceps muscles), trismus, dysphagia, salivation, anxiety, profuse sweating, tachycardia, elevated body temperature, cardiac dysrhythmias, synchronous diaphragmatic flutter, convulsions, coma, and death.[146] Clinical signs of excitability are usually seen when serum calcium values are less than normal but more than 8 mg/dL. Values of 5 to 8 mg/dL usually produce tetanic spasms and incoordination. Concentrations less than 5 mg/dL usually result in recumbency and stupor. This disorder often progresses and may cause death within 48 hours, particularly in lactating mares. A metabolic alkalosis, hypomagnesemia/hypermagnesemia, and hyperphosphatemia/hypophosphatemia have all been found in association with hypocalcemia in horses.[147,148]

Treatment involves the intravenous administration of calcium solutions such as 20% calcium borogluconate or those recommended for the treatment of parturient paresis in cattle. Administration of these solutions at the rate of 250 to 500 mL/500 kg diluted 1:4 with saline or dextrose will often result in full recovery, although in some horses it may take several days.[146] Relapses do occur. If no response to an initial infusion occurs, a second dose may be given 15 to 30 minutes later. Cardiac rate and rhythm should be closely monitored when calcium-containing solutions are infused intravenously.

Ear Tick–Associated Muscle Cramping

Intermittent painful muscle cramps not associated with exercise were described in horses with severe *Otobius. megnini* infestations.[1] These horses show intermittent signs of severe muscle cramping of pectoral, triceps, abdominal, or semitendinosus/semimembranosus muscles lasting from minutes to a few hours, with severe pain that often resembles colic. Horses may fall over when stimulated. Between muscle cramps, horses appear to be normal. Percussion of triceps, pectoral, or semitendinosus muscles results in a typical myotonic cramp. Horses have serum CK activities ranging from 4000 to 170,000 U/L. Numerous ear ticks, *O. megnini*, can be identified in the external ear canal of affected horses. Without treatment for ear ticks, the spasms continue; however, local treatment of the ear ticks using pyrethrins and piperonyl butoxide results in recovery within 12 to 36 hours later. Acepromazine is helpful to relieve painful cramping.

Myotonia

Myotonic muscle disorders represent a heterogeneous group of clinically similar diseases that share the feature of delayed relaxation of muscle after mechanical stimulation or voluntary contraction. Skeletal muscle ion channel dysfunction producing abnormal muscle membrane excitability or abnormalities in mRNA processing[149,150] appear to be the shared abnormality among myotonias in many species.

Clinical Signs

Foals with myotonia congenita usually have conspicuously well-developed musculature and mild hindlimb stiffness.[151-153] Gait abnormalities are usually most pronounced when exercise begins and frequently diminish as exercise continues. Bilateral bulging (dimpling) of the thigh and rump muscles is often obvious and exacerbated by stimulation of affected muscles by percussion. Affected muscles may remain contracted for up to 1 minute or more with subsequent slow relaxation. A variety of breeds of horses have been described with this disorder, but an inherited basis for myotonia has not been established.

A more severe progressive form of myotonia that eventually results in debilitating muscle atrophy, fibrosis, and stiffness has been observed in Quarter Horse foals.[154-157] At birth, foals with myotonia dystrophica appear well-muscled, and slight stiffness disappears with exercise. As the condition progresses, muscle hypertrophy is less obvious, atrophy may occur, and exercise may produce debilitating muscle contractures. Foals may become so stiff they are unable to stand. This condition resembles myotonia dystrophica in people in that numerous organ systems may be involved. Retinal dysplasia, lenticular opacities, and gonadal hypoplasia have been reported in one such Quarter Horse foal.[155]

Diagnosis

A diagnosis of both forms of myotonia is best made by EMG. High-frequency crescendo-decrescendo action potentials with a classic "dive-bomber" pattern are characteristic for myotonia. Muscle biopsies may be normal or show fiber hypertrophy and an increased proportion of type 1 fibers with myotonia congenita. Muscle biopsies from horses with myotonia dystrophica show fiber-type grouping, increased numbers of cells with centrally located nuclei, sarcoplasmic bodies, ring fibers, and fibrosis.[154,156]

Treatment

Foals with myotonia congenita do not usually demonstrate progression of clinical signs beyond 6 to 12 months of age. Phenytoin may diminish clinical signs, but no long-term treatment is available.[83] The prognosis for foals with myotonia dystrophica is extremely poor, and most foals are euthanized by 1 year of age.

Stiff-Horse Syndrome

A condition called stiff-horse syndrome has been described in Belgium and is characterized by stiffness and muscle spasms, associated with an abnormally straddled posture.[158] The muscle spasms were typically triggered by voluntary movements, such as going to eat from the manger or being led from the stable. EMG showed persistent motor unit activity in the axial and gluteal muscles. The clinical signs were responsive to oral prednisolone therapy but recurred after treatment stopped. Several similar cases have been seen in the United Kingdom.[159,160] The etiology of the condition is currently unknown. Similar conditions have been recognized in people, some of which are thought to be autoimmune.

Muscle Fasciculation of Unknown Cause

One horse had a history of sudden onset severe hyperesthesia and intense muscle fasciculations of the longissimus dorsi muscles in the thoracolumbar region, stimulated by light touch.[159] No underlying cause was identified. It was speculated that pain may be neuropathic in origin, and the horse responded to treatment with gabapentin (4 mg/kg PO BID), with complete resolution of clinical signs.

Muscle Fasciculation Associated with Osteoarthritis of the Caudal Cervical Synovial Articulations

Several horses have shown an episodic transient forelimb lameness, unresponsive to local analgesic techniques in association with ipsilateral or bilateral fasciculation of the pectoral and shoulder muscles after exercise, and neck stiffness.[159] All have had massive enlargement of the synovial articulations between the sixth and seventh cervical vertebrae, with ventral buttressing. Episodic nerve root impingement is thought to be the underlying cause of the muscle fasciculation and lameness. Intraarticular medication with corticosteroids has resulted in short term (months) resolution of clinical signs.

◼ HYPERKALEMIC PERIODIC PARALYSIS

Sharon J. Spier

Hyperkalemic periodic paralysis (HyPP) is an autosomal dominant trait affecting Quarter Horses, American Paint horses, Appaloosas, and Quarter Horse crossbreds worldwide.[161-163] The genetic disease has been linked to a prolific Quarter Horse sire named Impressive. Current estimates indicate that 4% of the Quarter Horse breed may be affected.[162,164,165] Affected horses may have been preferentially selected as breeding stock for pronounced muscle development, and there is evidence of selection of HyPP-affected horses as superior halter horses by show judges.[164]

Clinical Signs

Clinical signs among horses carrying the same mutation range from asymptomatic to daily muscle fasciculations and weakness. In the majority of horses, intermittent clinical signs begin by 2 to 3 years of age, with no apparent abnormalities between episodes. Ingestion of diets high in potassium (>1.1%), such as those containing alfalfa hay, molasses, electrolyte supplements, and kelp-based

supplements, or sudden dietary changes commonly trigger episodes.[161,162,166-168] Fasting, general anesthesia or heavy sedation, trailer rides, and stress may also precipitate clinical signs; however, the onset of signs is often unpredictable without a definable cause. Other possible precipitating factors that have been noted in people and horses are exposure to cold, fasting, pregnancy, and concurrent disease and rest following exercise. Exercise per se does not appear to stimulate clinical signs, and serum CK shows no change to very modest increases during episodic fasciculations and weakness.

In most horses, clinical episodes begin with a brief period of myotonia, with some horses showing prolapse of the third eyelid. Sweating and muscular fasciculations are observed commonly in the flanks, neck, and shoulders. The muscle fasciculations become more generalized as additional muscle groups are involved. Stimulation and attempts to move may exacerbate muscular fasciculations. Some horses may develop severe muscle cramping. Muscular weakness during episodes is a common characteristic of HyPP. Horses remain standing during mild attacks. In more severe attacks, clinical signs may progress to apparent weakness with swaying, staggering, dog sitting, or recumbency within a few minutes. Heart and respiratory rates may be elevated, and horses may show manifestations of stress yet remain relatively bright and alert during episodes. Affected horses usually respond adversely to noise and painful stimuli during attacks. Episodes last for variable periods, usually from 15 to 60 minutes. Several horses have died during acute episodes. Respiratory distress occurs in some horses as a result of paralysis of upper respiratory muscles, and a tracheostomy may be necessary. In addition, young horses that are homozygous for the HyPP trait have been observed to manifest a respiratory stridor and periodically may develop obstruction of the upper respiratory tract.[169,170] Horses homozygous for HyPP may have dysphagia or respiratory distress, and endoscopic findings include pharyngeal collapse and edema, laryngopalatal dislocation, and laryngeal paralysis. Once the episode subsides, horses appear normal with no apparent or minimal gait abnormalities. Although HyPP horses appear normal between attacks, examination using EMG reveals abnormal fibrillation potentials, complex repetitive discharges with occasional myotonic potentials, and trains of doublets between episodes.[162,171]

Etiology

HyPP is caused by a point mutation that results in a phenylalanine/leucine substitution in a key part of the voltage-dependent skeletal muscle sodium channel α-subunit.[163] In horses with HyPP, the resting membrane potential is closer to firing than in normal horses. Sodium channels are normally briefly activated during the initial phase of the muscle action potential. The HyPP mutation results in a failure of a subpopulation of sodium channels to inactivate when serum potassium concentrations are increased. As a result, an excessive inward flux of sodium and outward flux of potassium ensues, resulting in persistent depolarization of muscle cells and temporary weakness.

Diagnosis

In most affected horses, hyperkalemia (6 to 9 mEq/L), hemoconcentration, and hyponatremia occur during episodes, but acid-base balance is normal.[161,162] Serum potassium concentrations return to normal following cessation of clinical signs. Some affected horses may have normal serum potassium concentrations during minor episodes of muscle fasciculations. Differential diagnoses for hyperkalemia include delay before serum centrifugation, hemolysis, acidosis, renal failure, severe rhabdomyolysis, and high-intensity exercise.

Because veterinarians may not be present during acute episodes, the definitive test for identifying HyPP is the demonstration of the base-pair sequence substitution in the abnormal segment of the DNA encoding for the α-subunit of the sodium channel. Submission of mane or tail hair should be made to appropriate genetic laboratories.

Descent from the stallion Impressive on the sire's or dam's side in a horse with episodic muscle tremors is strongly suggestive of HyPP. To increase public awareness of this genetic defect, mandatory testing for HyPP with results designated on the Registration Certificate began for foals descending from Impressive born after January 1, 1998. In response to requests from the membership, in 2004 the American Quarter Horse Association Stud Book and Registration Committee ruled that foals born in 2007 and later testing homozygously affected for HyPP (H/H) will not be eligible for registration.

Treatment

Low-grade exercise can sometimes abort a mild episode, or if horses are just beginning to exhibit clinical signs. Feeding grain or corn syrup to stimulate insulin-mediated movement of potassium across cell membranes may also be helpful. Other treatment options that may abort an episode include intramuscular administration of epinephrine (3 mL of 1:1000/500 kg) and administration of acetazolamide (3 mg/kg PO every 8 to 12 hours). Many horses experience spontaneous recovery from episodes of paralysis and appear normal by the time a veterinarian arrives.

During severe episodes, administration of calcium gluconate (0.2 to 0.4 mL/kg of a 23% solution diluted in 1 L of 5% dextrose) will often provide immediate improvement. An increase in extracellular calcium concentration raises the muscle membrane threshold potential, which decreases membrane hyperexcitability. To reduce the serum potassium, intravenous dextrose (6 mL/kg of a 5% solution) alone or combined with sodium bicarbonate (1 to 2 mEq/kg) can be used to enhance intracellular

movement of potassium. With severe respiratory obstruction, a tracheostomy may be necessary.

Control

Decreasing dietary potassium and increasing renal losses of potassium are the primary steps taken to prevent HyPP episodes.[167,168] Avoid feeding high-potassium feeds such as many electrolyte and kelp supplements, alfalfa hay, canary grass hay, orchard grass hay, brome hay, soybean meal, and molasses. Optimally, later cuts of timothy or Bermuda grass hay; grains such as oats, corn, wheat, and barley; and beet pulp should be fed in small meals several times a day. Regular exercise and/or frequent access to a large paddock or yard are also beneficial. Pasture works well for horses with HyPP because the high water content of pasture grass makes it unlikely that horses will consume large amounts of potassium in a short period. Ideally, horses with recurrent episodes of HyPP should be fed a diet containing between 0.6% and 1.1% total potassium concentration. Because there is a wide variation in potassium concentration of forages depending on maturity and soils, it is advisable to have feeds analyzed for potassium concentrations and other nutrient requirements. Commercially available complete feeds with a guaranteed K^+ content may be more convenient for some HyPP horses, especially for owners with few horses.

For horses with recurrent episodes of muscle fasciculations even with dietary alterations, acetazolamide (2 to 4 mg/kg PO every 8 to 12 hours) or hydrochlorothiazide (0.5 to 1 mg/kg PO every 12 hours) may be helpful. These agents work through different mechanisms; however, both cause increased renal potassium ATPase activity. In addition, acetazolamide stabilizes blood glucose and potassium by stimulating insulin secretion. Breed registries and other associations may have restrictions on the use of these drugs during competitions because diuretics mask prohibited substances.

Prognosis

In most horses, HyPP is a manageable disorder, although recurrent episodes may occur and severe episodes may be fatal. Owners of affected horses should be strongly discouraged from breeding these horses for the long-term health of the Quarter Horse and other breeds. Breeding of an affected horse to a normal horse has a 50% chance of producing a foal with HyPP. Owners of affected horses should advise veterinarians of HyPP status before general anesthesia or procedures requiring heavy sedation.

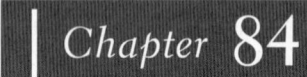

Principles and Practices of Joint Disease Treatment

C. Wayne McIlwraith

References on page 1325

The joint is an organ, and there are a number of ways in which traumatic damage occurs to it, ultimately resulting in degradation of articular cartilage. In 1966, the concurrent damage to joint capsule and ligament attachments that accompanied osteochondral fragmentation and cartilage damage was described.[1] However, the fact that synovitis and capsulitis could cause degradation of articular cartilage was not known until later. Experimentally, cartilage morphological damage and loss of glycosaminoglycan (GAG) staining occurred in the absence of instability or traumatic disruption of joint soft tissues.[2] Surveys estimate that approximately 60% of lameness is related to osteoarthritis (OA).[3,4] Rapid resolution of synovitis and capsulitis is critical in management of OA because synovitis induces cartilage matrix degradation. The goals of treatment of traumatic joint injuries are twofold: to return the joint to normal as quickly as possible and to prevent occurrence or to reduce the severity of OA, thus to minimize lameness and joint deterioration. Medical management is largely used to minimize OA, but timely surgery to remove osteochondral fragments, to reduce and repair large intraarticular fractures in an appropriate fashion, to diagnose accurately ligamentous and meniscal injuries using arthroscopy, and to manage manifestations of osteochondrosis can be critical to prevent OA. This chapter addresses both medical and surgical management.

MEDICAL TREATMENT

The goal to manage acute synovitis, with or without capsulitis, is to return the joint to normal as quickly as possible. In addition to reducing lameness and returning the horse to work, suppression of synovitis and capsulitis is important to prevent the byproducts of inflammation from compromising articular cartilage and causing OA. Pain relief and minimizing the potential microinstability associated with excessive synovial effusion are both also critical. As information increases regarding potential targets for therapeutic intervention, the range of treatment options has increased. Medications that provide pain relief, but for which any therapeutic action at the level of cartilage matrix has not been defined, are termed symptom-modifying osteoarthritic drugs (SMOADs). Disease-modifying osteoarthritic drugs (DMOADs) are those agents that can positively influence either the articular cartilage or the synovial environment. DMOADs were previously called chondroprotective drugs.

Nonsteroidal Antiinflammatory Drugs

Nonsteroidal antiinflammatory drugs (NSAIDs) are antiinflammatory agents that inhibit some components of the enzyme system that converts arachidonic acid into prostaglandins and thromboxane. Prostaglandin (PG) E_2 (PGE_2) is the product associated with synovial inflammation and cartilage matrix depletion and was demonstrated in the synovial fluid of horses with OA.[5,6] Phenylbutazone is the most commonly used NSAID in the horse, given at a dose of 2.2 mg/kg, once or twice daily. However, results are variable both in horses with naturally occurring OA[7] and in experimental trials using an equine OA model developed at Colorado State University (CSU), which has been used to assess a number of commonly used medications.[8] Lameness scores were lowest after administration of the combination of phenylbutazone with flunixin meglumine compared with phenylbutazone alone, but concerns with secondary side effects (including acute necrotizing colitis) were raised.[8]

All NSAIDs inhibit cyclooxygenase (COX) activity to some degree,[5,6] but more recently two different isoenzymes called COX-1 and COX-2 were reported with potential importance in the horse. COX-1 maintains the "good" or "housekeeping" portion (constitutive part) of the COX pathway.[9] COX-1 is important in the balance of normal physiology of the gastrointestinal and renal systems but plays a lesser role in the inflammatory COX cascade. COX-2 is associated with inflammatory events, especially those driven by macrophages and synovial cells, plays a minor role in normal physiology, and is considered the "bad" or "inducible" portion of the COX pathway. Drugs that preferentially inhibit COX-2 have been developed. Although it is logical that inhibition should minimize side effects,

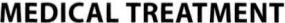

there is some suggestion that complete inhibition of COX-2 may not be optimal for either the joint or the horse.[9-11] Whereas COX-1 is mainly responsible for the protective functioning of prostaglandins, COX-2 may play an accessory constitutive role in the COX pathway.

The mainstream view is still that the beneficial effects of selective COX-2 inhibition in OA are ideal. Anecdotally, carprofen (Rimadyl, Pfizer, New York, New York, United States) was used at CSU in horses that developed high serum creatinine levels and diarrhea in association with phenylbutazone use. These side effects disappeared when horses were given carprofen; a protective effect was seen, implying there may be more preferential COX-2 inhibition than with phenylbutazone therapy. Firocoxib, a member of the class of drugs that selectively inhibits the COX-2 isoenzyme, is now approved for use in horses to control pain and inflammation associated with OA in general, and its pharmacokinetics during prolonged use have been determined.[12]

Although prostaglandin inhibition provides effective symptomatic relief, there may be long-term deleterious effects of some NSAIDs on cartilage metabolism.[11] In vitro work in the horse had initially shown no evidence of deleterious effects on cartilage metabolism.[13] However, in a more recent study, phenylbutazone was given to horses for 14 days, and serum was tested on articular cartilage explants in vitro. There was decreased proteoglycan synthesis to a degree similar to that with recombinant human interleukin–1β.[14] However, in the absence of any clinical associations between phenylbutazone use and articular cartilage degeneration, continued appropriate use of NSAIDs is justified.

A new, licensed topical NSAID preparation, 1% diclofenac sodium cream (Surpass, IDEXX Laboratories, Greensboro, North Carolina, United States), is now available in the United States but not in Europe. Previous research in people indicated topical NSAID could be clinically beneficial while reducing systemic side effects. Antiinflammatory effects were demonstrated experimentally using an induced subcutaneous inflammation model.[15] A clinical field trial of the topically applied diclofenac liposomal cream for the relief of joint inflammation showed promising results,[16] and more recently its value was demonstrated in equine OA using an osteochondral fragment–exercise model (see the section on Intraarticular Corticosteroids).[8]

Intraarticular Corticosteroids

The use of intraarticular corticosteroids for treatment of equine OA was extensively reviewed in 1996, and the benefits and deleterious side effects were more recently clarified.[17] Based on my observation of an apparent lack of correlation between the previous use of betamethasone esters (Betavet Soluspan, Schering-Plough Animal Health Corp., Union, New Jersey, United States) and articular cartilage degradation during arthroscopic surgery for osteochondral chip removal, experimental studies were initiated for the three most commonly used intraarticular corticosteroids. Methylprednisolone acetate (MPA) (Depo-Medrol, Pharmacia and Upjohn Co., Kalamazoo, Michigan, United States), triamcinolone acetonide (TA) (Vetalog, Bristol Myers Squibb for Fort Dodge, Fort Dodge, Iowa, United States), and betamethasone esters (Betavet Soluspan) were evaluated using an osteochondral fragment–exercise model.[18-20] Betamethasone (Betavet Soluspan, now available as Celestone Soluspan) was tested first. Osteochondral fragments were created arthroscopically on the distal dorsal aspect of the radial carpal bone in both middle carpal joints in 12 horses, and one joint was treated with 15 mg of betamethasone at 14 and 35 days after surgery.[18] The contralateral control middle carpal joint was injected with saline. No deleterious side effects on articular cartilage were demonstrated. Exercise produced no harmful effects in the presence of betamethasone.[18]

In subsequent studies with intraarticular corticosteroids (as well as other treatments), the research model was modified so that the contralateral joint was not used as a control. The chip fragment model was also modified to more effectively produce early osteoarthritic change. Eighteen horses were randomly assigned to three groups: MPA or TA was injected 14 and 28 days after surgery, and horses were exercised on a high-speed treadmill for 6 weeks, beginning on day 15 after surgery. Results were compared with control joints treated with corticosteroids but which had no osteochondral fragment, as well as with a second control osteochondral fragment group treated with polyionic fluid (Figure 84-1).[19,20] In joints containing an osteochondral fragment and treated with MPA, there was a trend (not statistically significant) for lower lameness scores. However, there were significantly lower synovial fluid PGE[2]

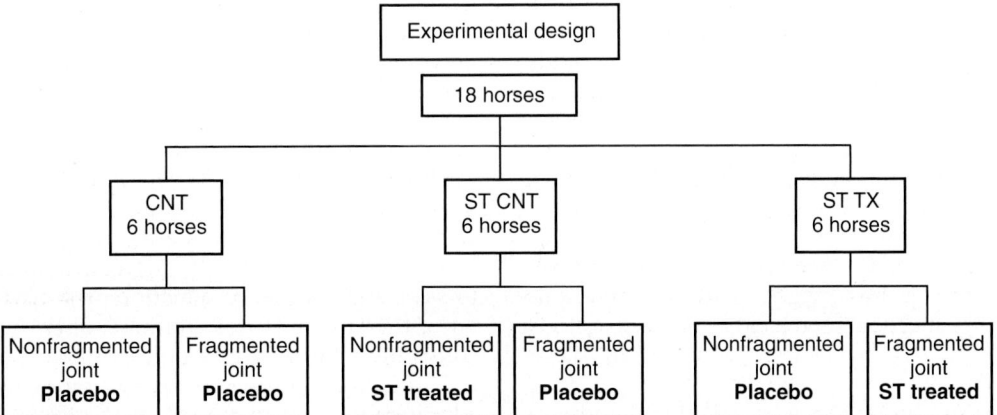

Fig. 84-1 • Design of experiments to assess the value of direct intraarticular injection of a corticosteroid into an osteoarthritic joint (ST TX), as well as injection of intraarticular corticosteroid in a remote joint (ST CNT) compared with a saline-injected control (CNT). (Reproduced with permission. McIlwraith CW: From arthroscopy to gene therapy—30 years of looking in joints, *Proc Am Assoc Equine Pract* 51:65, 2005.)

concentrations and lower scores for intimal hyperplasia and vascularity (no effect on cellular infiltration in the synovium compared with placebo-treated joints) in MPA-treated joints compared with control joints. Of more importance, modified Mankin scores (a score of histopathological change in articular cartilage) were significantly increased in MPA-treated joints compared with control joints, suggesting deleterious effects of intraarticular administration of MPA.[19] This is in contrast to the results with TA (Vetalog).[20] Horses that were given 12 mg of TA in a joint containing a fragment (TA TX) were less lame than horses in the two control groups (see Figure 84-1). Horses treated with TA had lower protein and higher hyaluronan (HA) and GAG concentrations in synovial fluid. Synovium from treated groups had less inflammatory cell infiltration, intimal hyperplasia, and subintimal fibrosis. Analysis of articular cartilage morphological parameters evaluated using a standardized scoring system was significantly better from TA control (no fragment) and TA treatment groups compared with the control placebo-treated fragment group. The results supported favorable effects of TA on lameness scores, synovial fluid, synovium, and articular cartilage morphological parameters, both with direct intraarticular administration and remote site administration compared with placebo injections.[20] Evaluation of intraarticular TA on subchondral bone showed no deleterious effects.[21] In other work, repetitive intraarticular administration of MPA to exercising horses altered mechanical integrity of articular cartilage but had no effect on subchondral or cancellous bone.[23]

Based on these and recent in vitro results demonstrating a protective effect of TA,[24] I recommend TA be used especially in high motion joints. Some have recommended low doses of MPA to alleviate potential negative effects. However, based on in vitro titration studies, commonly used "low doses" are unlikely to have the same clinical effects because a greater concentration of corticosteroid is needed to inhibit the catabolic compared with the anabolic effects on articular cartilage.[25] On the other hand, clinical improvement is seen in horses administered low doses, an observation that is more important to a clinician than are experimental data.

Despite scientific studies demonstrating the efficacy and chondroprotective properties of TA, some practitioners fear the potential of TA to cause laminitis. Laminitis did not occur in 1200 horses treated with TA when the total dose did not exceed 18 mg.[26] From this study, 18 mg was established as a maximum dose. A more recent study reported no association between the occurrence of laminitis and the intraarticular use of TA.[27] There was a recent legal case in the United Kingdom in which a horse developed catastrophic laminitis after receiving 8 mg of TA in each tarsus and 20 mg of dexamethasone into its back.[28] This led to a review of the literature, which revealed that there was a lack of good evidence linking laminitis to corticosteroid injection; it was suggested that a large-scale multicenter trial was needed.[29] A related retrospective study from one clinician[29,30] revealed that laminitis associated with intraarticular injection of corticosteroids had occurred in 3 of 2000 (0.15%) horses. TA was used the majority of the time, and the upper total dose ranged from 20 to 45 mg.[30] The relationship between corticosteroid use and laminitis is discussed further in Chapter 34.

Another traditional cliché is that although it is better not to use MPA in high-motion joints, using it in low-motion joints (such as the distal tarsal joints) is appropriate. This implies that we do not care about the state of the articular cartilage in these joints, and perhaps corticosteroids may promote ankylosis. There is currently no evidence that ankylosis can be promoted in this fashion. The other side of this argument is that we should preserve articular cartilage whenever we can. Intraarticular injection of MPA or TA (with or without hyaluronan [HA]) in horses with OA of the distal hock joints led to a positive outcome in only 38% of horses (suggesting to the authors that surgical treatment may lead to better long-term prognosis).[31] There was no significant difference between treatment with either MPA or TA, thus questioning any clinical advantages of the use of MPA.[31] However, this was a relatively small study performed on a referral population of horses, and these results may not be representative of the overall response of horses with distal hock OA to intraarticular medication.

Intraarticular corticosteroids are commonly combined with HA, and there is a perception that the HA might be protective against any deleterious effects of corticosteroids (MPA). This perception is based on tradition rather than scientific proof but has become common thinking among equine practitioners.[3] Some support can be gained from a 1-year, single-blind, randomized study in which 24 human patients were treated with intraarticular HA once weekly for 3 weeks and then again at 6 months (total of six injections).[32] Sixteen of these patients also had TA before the first and fourth HA injections, and using the Western Ontario and McMaster Universities Index of OA (WOMAC) scores, the results were better with the combination of these two products. There was no progression of OA as evaluated using magnetic resonance imaging in either group.[32] Two in vitro equine studies evaluated whether HA might have a mitigating effect against the deleterious effects of MPA. In the first study, HA addition had little effect on MPA-induced cartilage matrix proteoglycan catabolism in cartilage explants.[33] In the second study, MPA combined with HA had beneficial effects on proteoglycan metabolism in interleukin-1 (IL-1)–treated equine chondrocytes (but there were no comparisons between HA alone and MPA plus HA).[34] The combination of MPA and HA increased PG synthesis compared with IL-1–treated controls.[34]

Hyaluronan (Sodium Hyaluronate)

HA is a nonsulfated GAG, and the biological characteristics and therapeutic use of HA in equine OA were reviewed previously.[35,36] HA has modest analgesic effects,[37] but more emphasis is placed on its antiinflammatory effects that may be physical (steric hindrance) or pharmacological (inhibition of inflammatory cells and mediators).[36] Various in vitro studies have shown HA protects against IL-1–driven prostaglandin synthesis and inhibits free radicals, but the ability of HA to inhibit matrix metalloproteinase (MMP) activity is questionable.[38,39] Several inflammatory mediators can augment HA production by synovial fibroblasts in vitro; therefore elevated synthesis of HA in early OA may constitute a protective response by the synovium to joint inflammation.[36] While providing a rationale for exogenous administration, it may explain the elevated levels of HA in response to intraarticular injection of a number of medications.[19,20]

In my opinion, HA alone is useful in horses with mild to moderate synovitis, but the adjunctive use of corticosteroids is necessary in most horses with OA. However, based on clinical evidence in people, although the immediate effects may not be dramatic, the evidence for long-term disease-modifying activity of HA is accumulating.[40] Claims that HA preparations of molecular weight exceeding 1×10^6 Da may provide superior clinical results and chondroprotection than lesser-molecular-weight products remain controversial.[36,41,42]

In a randomized, double-blind, and placebo-controlled clinical study, 77 Standardbred trotters with moderate to severe lameness were treated with HA, polysulfated glycosaminoglycan (PSGAG), or placebo for 3 weeks. Mean initial lameness score was significantly reduced during treatment and at the last examination in all three groups ($P < 0.01$).[43] Additionally, the prevalence of sound horses increased significantly from 1 to 3 weeks of treatment into the last examination in all three groups. Both drugs (250 mg of PSGAG intraarticularly four times or 20 mg of HA intraarticularly twice) were superior to placebo for reduction of lameness score during treatment and the total study period, time until soundness occurred, and the number of sound horses at the last examination. Thus placebo and drug therapy were effective in the treatment of naturally occurring traumatic arthritis in horses, but HA and PSGAG gave better results than placebo. In a second study, the researchers compared intraarticular saline with rest alone in 38 Standardbreds with traumatic arthritis.[44] The mean lameness was significantly lower when 2.0 mL of 0.9% NaCl solution was injected compared with control horses.[44] This raises the question: is this effect the result of withdrawing fluid and/or placing a needle in the joint?

Most recently, intraarticular HA was tested in the CSU equine OA model.[45] OA was induced by the osteochondral fragment–exercise model in one middle carpal joint of 24 horses. Eight horses received HA (20 mg) (Hyvisc, Boehringer Ingelheim GmbH, Ingelheim am Rhein, Germany) and amikacin (125 mg) intraarticularly on study days 14, 21, and 28. A second group of eight horses received PSGAG (250 mg) and amikacin (125 mg) intraarticularly on study days 14, 21, and 28. The remaining eight horses were control horses. There were no adverse treatment-related problems. Synovial effusion was reduced with PSGAG compared with controls. No changes in other clinical signs (lameness, response to flexion, joint effusion, and radiological findings) were seen with PSGAG or HA compared with controls. Histologically, however, there was significantly less articular cartilage fibrillation seen with HA treatment compared with controls (despite no significant reduction in vascularity and subintimal fibrosis of the synovium). The conclusion was that HA had beneficial disease-modifying effects and was a viable therapeutic option in equine OA.[45] The result of a questionnaire survey of 20 members of the American Association of Equine Practitioners (14 responses) showed that it was uncommon for the respondents to administer intraarticular HA initially or alone, particularly in horses with established OA.[3] Twelve of 14 supplemented HA injections with other forms of treatment (usually intraarticular corticosteroids).[3]

The use of intravenous HA (Legend [or Hyonate], Bayer HealthCare LLC, Animal Health Division, Shawnee Mission, Kansas, United States) in the treatment of OA is now common. Using intravenous HA in the experimental osteochondral fragment–exercise model, there was significant improvement in clinical lameness, decreased PGE_2, and total protein levels in the synovial fluid, as well as decreased hyperemia and cellular infiltration of the synovium.[46] However, in a survey, most clinicians were not impressed by the efficacy of intravenous HA and its short duration of action in the treatment of OA, particularly when used alone.[3]

Based on the reports from the manufacturing company, the majority of intravenous HA is used "prophylactically" in athletic horses with the attributed benefits being subjective. The prophylactic value of intravenous HA was studied in both Quarter Horse and Thoroughbred racehorses. One hundred and forty horses participated in the Quarter Horse study and received either intravenous saline or HA every 2 weeks for the duration of the 9-month study.[47] Trends for HA-treated horses to race longer, require an intraarticular injection of corticosteroid earlier, have a better speed index, have a higher average number of starts, and earn more money were observed when compared with placebo-treated horses. The Editors note that the better performance results could be due to earlier corticosteroid treatment in the HA-treated compared with placebo-treated horses. A second unpublished study was conducted in Thoroughbred racehorses using synovial fluid markers and starting with horses without musculoskeletal problems. No significant differences were found between HA- and placebo-treated horses. However, there are anecdotal positive reports regarding the prophylactic use of intravenous HA from trainers in various equine disciplines.

Polysulfated Glycosaminoglycan

PSGAG belongs to a group of polysulfated polysaccharides and includes, in addition to PSGAG (Adequan, Luitpold Pharmaceuticals Inc., Animal Health Division, Shirley, New York, United States), pentosan polysulfate. These drugs are DMOADs, and therefore PSGAG has been traditionally used when cartilage damage is presumed present rather than in the treatment of acute synovitis.[48] However, recent work questions this traditional approach (see below). Use of DMOADs is meant to prevent, retard, or reverse the morphological cartilaginous lesions of OA, with the major criterion for inclusion being prevention of cartilage degeneration. The principal GAG in PSGAG is chondroitin sulfate (CS), and the product is made from an extract of bovine lung and trachea modified by sulfate esterification.

Adequan was reviewed extensively in 1996.[48] One in vitro study demonstrated that PSGAG was the only drug tested (others included phenylbutazone, flunixin meglumine, betamethasone, and HA) that inhibited stromelysin.[49] There have been three other in vitro studies on the effect of PSGAG on equine cartilage that had contradictory results. PSGAG caused increased collagen and GAG synthesis in both articular cartilage explants and cell cultures from normal and osteoarthritic equine articular cartilage.[50] However, other work found a dose-dependent inhibition of proteoglycan synthesis, little effect on proteoglycan degradation, and no effect on proteoglycan monomer size.[51] Various studies have supported the value of intraarticular PSGAG (250 mg) in equine OA, including a clinical study,[52] a study using a Freund's adjuvant-induced OA model,[53] and a carpal synovitis model using sodium monoiodoacetate.[54] In the latter study, there was significant reduction of articular cartilage fibrillation erosion, less chondrocyte death, and markedly improved GAG staining.[54] However, PSGAG had no benefit in healing preexisting articular cartilage lesions in the latter study[54] or in a different study in ponies.[55]

I have traditionally recommended the use of intraarticular PSGAG after arthroscopic surgery when there is substantial loss of articular cartilage (most commonly in the carpus). I observed rapid resolution of synovitis and hemarthrosis after PSGAG administration that otherwise tended to be persistent after arthroscopy when there was secondary loss of articular cartilage. A recent study using the CSU equine osteochondral fragment–exercise model compared intraarticular PSGAG with either intraarticular HA or saline and revealed that synovial fluid effusion was significantly reduced with PSGAG compared with both saline and HA. The degree of vascularity and subintimal fibrosis of the synovium was significantly reduced with PSGAG treatment compared with controls.[45] The main value of intraarticular PSGAG appears to be for severe (and acute) synovitis (most commonly seen after arthroscopic surgery when there is considerable debridement of bone). However, the U.K. data sheet expressly states, "Do not inject into actively inflamed joints. In the presence of active joint inflammation, therapy with a suitable antiinflammatory drug should be given prior to intraarticular treatment with Adequan."

Administration of PSGAG intramuscularly has become popular. However, intramuscular PSGAG (500 mg every 4 days for seven treatments) produced relatively insignificant effects in horses with sodium monoiodoacetate–induced synovitis (limited to slightly improved GAG staining).[56] In a more recent study using the osteochondral fragment–exercise model in which intramuscular PSGAG was used as a positive control (administered every 4th day for 28 days starting 14 days post-OA induction), decreased GAG levels in the serum 14 days posttreatment was the only significant beneficial effect.[57] In this study, better improvement was seen in horses given extracorporeal shock wave therapy.

In a 1996 survey, PSGAG was considered more effective than HA for the treatment of subacute OA and less effective for idiopathic joint effusion and acute synovitis[58]; however, there is currently only weak evidence to justify intramuscular administration. It was reported that articular cartilage concentrations of PSGAG after intramuscular administration are capable of inhibiting some cartilage degrading enzymes,[59] but the duration of effective concentration is unclear. A number of articular degradative enzymes were reduced in an in vitro study in other animals, but direct evidence of effectiveness in the horse is lacking.[59,60]

In the questionnaire survey of veterinarians cited previously, indications for use of intramuscular PSGAG varied widely, including acute and/or chronic OA.[3] PSGAG was also used as a preventative measure, and information from the manufacturer reports that 90% of sales are for such "prophylactic" use. There have been no scientific studies on prophylactic use, and efficacy is difficult to prove or disprove.

A principal driving force for the persistent use of intramuscular PSGAG in preference to intraarticular administration is the work demonstrating a slightly increased risk of infection following intraarticular injection compared with corticosteroids and HA.[61] However, a companion study found that all risks could be obviated with concurrent intraarticular injection of amikacin sulfate, 125 mg (0.5 mL).[62] In a survey of 20 practitioners, it was reported that six of seven racehorse veterinarians used intraarticularly administered PSGAG, at least occasionally, whereas a similar number of nonracehorse veterinarians avoided the practice.[3] Intraarticular use of PSGAG is still common in Europe. A recent multivariable analysis of factors influencing the outcome of two treatment protocols in 128 horses responding positively to intraarticular analgesia of the distal interphalangeal joint showed significant positive effects with an intraarticular PSGAG therapy protocol of three intraarticular injections approximately 8 days apart.[63] Antimicrobial drugs were not administered, and no adverse results were reported.

Pentosan Polysulfate

The use of pentosan polysulfate (PPS) was reviewed in 1996, but at that time reports of its efficacy were only anecdotal.[64] PPS is a heparinoid compound but is unique because it is derived from beechwood hemicellulose instead of animal sources. Commercial products available include Cartrophen Vet (Biopharm, Australia Pty Ltd, Bondi Junction, NSW, Australia) (licensed for use in small animals in Australasia and Europe, but not in horses) and more recently Pentosan Equine Injection (Nature Vet Pty Ltd., Glenorie, NSW, Australia; 250 mg/mL PPS sodium), which is licensed in Australasia. In experimental studies in sheep, weekly intraarticular injections of PPS for 4 weeks improved joint function and reduced mean radiological scores and Mankin histological scores of articular cartilage damage in femoral condyles.[65]

Recently, we found favorable results using PPS given at a dose of 3 mg/kg body weight once weekly for 4 weeks (Pentosan Equine Injection). Using the carpal osteochondral fragment–exercise model, there was a significant decrease in articular cartilage fibrillation ($P < 0.05$) and a strong trend ($P = 0.06$) for improvement in overall cartilage histological appearance (modified Mankin score). Furthermore, although there was improvement in most other parameters (lameness, joint flexion, synovial fluid total protein concentration, synovial fluid collagen degradation products, and aggrecan synthesis), results were not statistically significant.

Combination Intraarticular Therapy

HA and corticosteroids are commonly combined. Without corticosteroids, the efficacy of intraarticular HA (based on short-term clinical response) is limited to horses with mild to moderate synovitis but is markedly enhanced with corticosteroids. Some veterinarians have used HA in conjunction with MPA, thinking that the former would mitigate the effects of the latter, but this is questionable (see page 842). In human medicine, localized, severe, acute inflammatory reactions (SAIRs) were associated with the use of highly cross-linked HA products.[66] Although no adverse reactions were reported using Hylan G-F 20 (Synvisc, Genzyme, Cambridge, Massachusetts, United States) in people with knee OA,[67] others have reported SAIRs and reduction of the risk with concurrent intraarticular corticosteroid administration.[68] The risk of adverse reactions after Hylan G-F 20 administration may increase with the second or third injection.[69] This may be because of an immunogenic mechanism associated with fermented HA products; the problem was not seen with naturally extracted HA.[69] Anecdotally, there have been more adverse reactions in horses following synthetic HA injections compared with naturally extracted HA. The combination of TA and insulin-like growth factor-I (IGF-I) has been evaluated in vitro with positive results.[70]

The Editors add that various other combinations of intraarticular products have been used by practitioners to manage horses with OA. A combination of hyaluronan and PSGAG (and amikacin sulfate) has been used, apparently quite safely, to manage chronic OA in Standardbred racehorses and anecdotal reports suggest this combination gives better results than injection of either product alone. Studies evaluating efficacy and safety of combination therapy have not been done. A new product, Polyglycan (Arthrodynamic Technologies, Versailles, Kentucky, United States), is a combination of HA, glucosamine, and CS and is marketed as a postsurgical lavage solution. This product is currently being used to manage OA in horses as an intraarticular or intramuscular injection and anecdotal reports suggest the efficacy of this combination approach is similar to that seen with PSGAG alone. Preliminary studies are underway.

Oral Joint Supplements

Oral joint supplements are loosely classified as nutraceuticals. The term "nutraceutical" combines the word "nutrient" (nourishing food or food component) with "pharmaceutical" (a medical drug)[71] and describes a broad list of products sold under the premise of being a dietary supplement (i.e., a food) but for the expressed intent of treatment or prevention of disease. The claims (usually made by manufacturers) to aid in equine joint health are often very weak. Unlike a feed, a nutraceutical is unlikely to have an established nutritive value. Feeds are required to have nutritive value, and labels must be accountable. Joint supplements fall between food and drugs, and there is no requirement for labels to list ingredients or nutrient profiles as required for feeds. They are sold with the intent to treat or prevent disease without first undergoing proper drug approval.[71] Joint supplements are fed to horses to heal the lame or make chronically unsound horses sound or to prevent joint problems from occurring. However, when an owner or trainer first uses oral supplements, the source of pain is rarely diagnosed. A role in prevention of OA is hard to disprove but serves as a rationale to use nutraceuticals and many licensed drugs. In 2005, nutraceutical sales in the United States reached more than 1 billion U.S. dollars for companion animals, and that figure was expected to double in the next 3 years. To equine practitioners, this is disturbing because this industry is, for the most part, unregulated by the Food and Drug Administration, and there is only weak in vivo scientific evidence to support use of the their products.[72]

None of the oral supplements or nutraceuticals are licensed, and proof of efficacy is generally lacking. Most products include variable amounts of glucosamine and/or CS along with other ingredients. The first oral GAG products available for equine use included a CS product extracted from bovine trachea (Flex-Free) and a complex of GAGs and other nutrients from the sea mussel *Perna canaliculus* (Syno-Flex)(Vita Flex Nutrition, Council Bluffs, Iowa, United States). More recently, glucosamine hydrochloride, CS, manganese, and vitamin C have been marketed as a nutraceutical (Cosequin) (Nutramax Laboratories, Inc., Edgewood, Maryland, United States), and a number of other products have simulated Cosequin. There are now many other commercially available products containing

various concentrations of glucosamine, chondroitin sulfate, manganese, vitamin C, methylsulfonylmethane (MSM), fish oils, and other constituents. The different labeling methods make it extraordinarily difficult to compare objectively the relative amounts of the different constituents between products. Glucosamine sulfate is a precursor of the disaccharide subunits of cartilage proteoglycans. Glucosamine salts are well absorbed orally in people[73]; however, in the horse oral bioavailability of glucosamine hydrochloride was only 2.5%, interpreted as poor absorption, but with extensive tissue uptake thereafter.[74] In dogs, glucosamine is poorly absorbed when given orally (12%), probably because of extensive first-pass metabolism in the gastrointestinal tract and/or liver.[75]

In a more recent study, eight adult female horses with no evidence of joint disease were randomly assigned to two groups (n = 4) in a crossover study.[76] Glucosamine hydrochloride (20 mg/kg) was administered by nasogastric intubation or intravenous injection. The maximum serum and synovial fluid glucosamine concentrations were substantially higher after intravenous administration (288 ± 53 µM and 250 µM, respectively) than by the oral route (5.8 ± 1.7 µM and 0.3 to 0.7 µM). The levels of glucosamine found in synovial fluid after oral administration were lower than those that have been used in vitro to study glucosamine action in tissue culture.[76]

CS consists of alternating disaccharide subunits of glucuronic acid and sulfated *N*-acetylgalactosamine molecules and is a principal GAG of aggregating proteoglycan (aggrecan). CS is less sulfated but resembles PSGAG in structure and mechanism of action. Oral absorption of CS was tested in horses. A low-molecular-weight CS (0.80 kDa) was evaluated by quantifying the disaccharide content using a validated method that combined enzymatic digestion of plasma followed by fluorescence high-performance liquid chromatography.[77] Low-molecular-weight CS was absorbed better than glucosamine; its absorption may be influenced by the molecular weight of the polymer.[77]

In vitro studies can potentially help to determine at what concentrations glucosamine or CS may inhibit a catabolic response in equine cartilage explants. A study of cartilage disks incubated with lipopolysaccharide (LPS) in varying concentrations of glucosamine, CS, or both revealed that glucosamine concentrations as low as 1 mg/mL decreased nitrogen oxide production, but that CS at either 0.25 or 0.5 mg/mL had no effect. Glucosamine concentrations as low as 0.5 mg/mL decreased PGE_2 production, whereas CS did not affect PGE_2 production. A combination of CS and glucosamine decreased MMP-9 activity but had no effect on MMP-2; there was a trend for decreasing MMP-13 protein concentrations.[78]

In vitro dose titration studies of glucosamine hydrochloride and CS alone and in combination were performed in our laboratory. There were no detrimental effects of either glucosamine hydrochloride, CS, or a combination of both on normal cartilage metabolism. High doses of either glucosamine or CS or the combination limited total GAG release, whereas intermediate doses enhanced GAG synthesis and total cartilage content.[79] The same dosages tested on IL-1–conditioned articular cartilage explants revealed no treatment effects for either glucosamine or CS alone, but a protective effect of high doses of the two combined for total GAG release. This study suggested that a combination of CS and glucosamine might be beneficial to cartilage metabolism by preventing GAG degradation. However, the question of effective concentration of glucosamine after oral administration remains an issue.[76]

An oral HA product showed no efficacy in our osteochondral fragment–exercise model. However, a clinical study evaluating the use of an oral HA product after arthroscopic surgery for tarsocrural joint osteochondritis dissecans (OCD) revealed a significant reduction in postoperative synovial fluid effusion in treated horses compared with controls.[80]

The osteochondral fragment–exercise model was used to test avocado and soybean unsaponifiable (ASU) extracts.[81] The placebo control group (n = 8) received molasses orally once daily, whereas the ASU-treated horses (n = 8) received 6 g of ASU plus a similar volume of molasses orally. At the termination of the study, horses treated with ASU had significantly improved total gross examination score (articular cartilage erosion plus synovial hemorrhage score) in the OA joint compared with placebo control horses.[81] There were significant decreases in synovial intimal hyperplasia and the cartilage disease score and a trend for decrease in lameness scores. Although improvement was modest, it was greater than that seen with other parenteral (intramuscular PSGAG and intravenous HA) and oral (HA) products tested using the same model.

Platinum Performance (Platinum Performance Inc., Buellton, California, United States) is a combination of rare earth minerals and omega-3 fatty acids that is used postoperatively, but all information is anecdotal. There is potential value of using omega-3 polyunsaturated fatty acids (PUFAs) in the management of OA. PUFA administration reduces inflammatory mediators in equine monocytes, corresponding to an increase in the ratio of omega-3 to omega-6 fatty acids in cell membrane phospholipids.[77,78] In an in vitro study, the role of α-linolenic acid and omega-3 PUFA, as well as its antiinflammatory potential for the reduction of equine synovial inflammation, was evaluated in an established LPS model.[79] Whereas LPS significantly increased production of PGE_2 and decreased production of HA, treatment with α-linolenic acid at the highest dose inhibited prostaglandin production.[79]

Summary of Use of Conventional Medications

Conventional medications still form a large part of the equine veterinarians' armamentarium. Increased attention is being paid to physical therapy regimens and positive results demonstrated with shock wave therapy (see Polysulfated Glycosaminoglycan, page 843); these could possibly decrease the need for medication for equine joint disease. COX-2 inhibitors may be useful when a horse does not tolerate phenylbutazone well. Intraarticular corticosteroids continue to be the principal intraarticular therapy. The use of MPA has decreased appropriately, and the value of betamethasone esters and TA is recognized, but there is still an overuse of MPA, and I consider its use in high-motion joints to be below the standard of care. (One of the Editors [MWR] respectfully disagrees. Given the short-lived effect of TA, limited dosages [20 to 40 mg/joint] of MPA are still used in high-motion joints if a sustained effect of antiinflammatory therapy is needed.) Continued availability of licensed medication is a challenge. Intraarticular HA continues to be used in conjunction with corticosteroids. Recent research challenges the value gained from

intramuscular PSGAG, but results have been positive with intraarticular use of the drug. It is predicted that PPS will become a licensed medication, and its value has been documented scientifically. Oral nutraceuticals continue to be somewhat of a "black box" as far as efficacy is concerned, but positive results in a controlled study with avocado and soybean extracts are exciting.

The Editors respectfully point out that the osteochondral fragment–exercise model of OA is not necessarily representative of naturally occurring OA in sports horses. Although it is a reliably reproducible model of OA, drugs may have a different effect in naturally occurring OA compared with this experimental model. Comparisons between the efficacy of various drugs and other treatment modalities using the experimental model are also not easily made because in most of the studies significant results are achieved with the tested drug compared with control horses for one or more of the many measured parameters. The studies are relatively short term compared with the career of many equine athletes and only assess short-term outcomes. The studies using this model have unquestionably enhanced knowledge about the potential efficacy of a variety of drugs, but these results are not necessarily transferable to all high- and low-motion joints with naturally occurring OA.

NEWER BIOLOGICALLY BASED THERAPIES

Biological therapy specifically modulates key mediators, and our improved understanding of critical mediators in equine traumatic arthritis and OA has led to the identification of new targets for therapy. Two obvious targets identified include MMPs and IL-1.

Inhibition of Metalloproteinases as a Therapeutic Approach

MMP inhibitors include peptide-based (including hydroxamic acids), non–peptide-based (including chemically modified tetracyclines such as doxycycline), and naturally occurring inhibitors (such as omega-3 fatty acids, i.e., fish oils; see the section on Oral Joint Supplements).

In vitro studies assessed the MMP inhibitor BAY 12-9566 using an IL-1 degradation model (tenfold concentration [1 nM : 10 µM] increases) in equine and canine articular cartilage explants.[85] There was a significant dose-dependent reduction in the catabolic effect of IL-1α on the release of proteoglycans and type II collagen. In vivo assessment of MMP inhibition has not been performed in the horse. However, a canine study of experimentally induced OA (cranial cruciate ligament transection) failed to demonstrate efficacy with an MMP inhibitor,[86] and the prospect for these being valuable therapeutically in the horse seems low.

Inhibiting Interleukin–1

The most commonly accepted mediator at the top of the cascade for cartilage degradation in OA is IL-1. However, tumor necrosis factor (TNF) has received most attention in rheumatoid arthritis in people, leading to the novel therapy of using an anti-TNF monoclonal antibody adalimumab (Humira, Abbott Laboratories, Abbott Park, Illinois, United States) and recombinant human TNF receptor etanercept (Enbrel, Wyeth Pharmaceuticals, Madison, New Jersey, United States).[87]

IL-1 activates MMP, aggrecanase, and PGE_2 release by acting through IL-1 receptors on the cell membrane (Figure

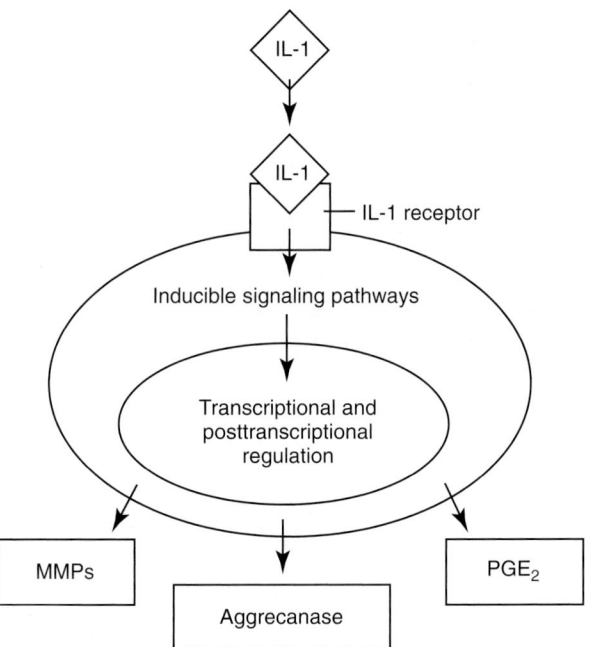

Fig. 84-2 • Diagram of interleukin-1 (IL-1) activation of metalloproteinase, aggrecanase, and prostaglandin E₂ release acting through IL-1 receptors on the cell membrane. (Reproduced with permission. McIlwraith CW: From arthroscopy to gene therapy—30 years of looking in joints, *Proc Am Assoc Equine Pract* 51:65, 2005.)

84-2). IL-1 can be inhibited through the natural antagonist, IL-1 receptor antagonist (IL-1ra), which binds to the cell membrane IL-1 receptor to block IL-1. IL-1 can also be inhibited by using soluble receptors, where IL-1 receptors are released from the cell membrane and bind IL-1.[87] Soluble receptors are used to inhibit TNF, but there are no current techniques for using IL-1–soluble receptors therapeutically. Cell membrane IL-1 receptors can be inhibited by using recombinant proteins or gene therapy (see Chapter 63). The first therapeutic application of IL-1ra for equine use involved the direct transfer of the equine IL-1ra gene sequence to synoviocytes using an adenoviral vector.[88,89] Complete inhibition of carpal OA confirmed the critical role of IL-1 in the osteoarthritic process.[89] Although both symptom- and disease-modifying effects were demonstrated and the magnitude of therapeutic value was greater than any other medication tested to date, repeated delivery of IL-1ra using gene transfer necessitates a better vector, which is currently being researched.

The limitations with gene transfer therapy have led to the development of alternative methods of delivering IL-1ra to joints. The concept of IL-1ra, IRAP (Arthrex Vet Systems, Naples, Florida, United States) was developed in Europe as a product named Orthokine (Orthogen AG, Dusseldorf, Germany). To make IRAP, peripheral blood is collected in a syringe containing glass beads soaked in chromium sulfate and is incubated for 24 hours and is then centrifuged. The autologous modified serum (autologous conditioned serum [ACS]) is then used for one or more intraarticular injections. Marked elevation of IL-1ra without elevated expression of IL-1 or TNF, that is, preferential up-regulation of "good" cytokines without concurrent up-regulation of "bad" cytokines, was documented.[90] In 2004, Arthrex Biosystems began marketing IRAP in the United States, and their unpublished data confirmed up-regulation

of IL-1ra but not to the same extent as previously reported.[90] Up-regulation of proteins is probably through stimulation of monocytes by the beads and syringe, and it is likely that more than IL-1ra is up-regulated, a concept currently being studied at CSU using mass spectroscopy.

IRAP was tested in a double-blinded, placebo-controlled, experimental study using the osteochondral fragment–exercise model and was shown to have both symptom and disease-modifying effects in horses.[91] In eight placebo and eight ACS-treated horses, 6 mL of phosphate-buffered saline (PBS) solution or ACS, respectively, was injected into the OA-affected joint on days 14, 21, 28, and 35. No adverse treatment-related events were detected. Horses that were treated with ACS had significant improvement in lameness scores, significantly decreased synovial hyperplasia, and less gross cartilage fibrillation and synovial hemorrhage than PBS-injected horses. Synovial fluid concentration of IL-1ra (assessed using a mouse anti-IL-1ra antibody) was increased after treatment with ACS.[91] All reports concerning clinical efficacy of ACS are anecdotal; there have been no controlled clinical trials.

Mesenchymal Stem Cells

Mesenchymal stem cells (MSCs) have been used intraarticularly in the horse for a number of "indications." Both clinical experience and research studies are limited to adult-derived MSCs, and bone marrow remains the gold standard as a source of MSCs. However, other sources such as muscle, cartilage, and adipose tissue contain multipotent MSCs. MSCs from bone marrow or digestive tissue are isolated by simple adhesion and proliferation of MSCs to tissue culture surfaces, a technique that yields a near-homogenous MSC population and is called culture expansion.[92] Work is proceeding on establishing cell surface antigens that characterize MSCs. There are distinct differences between cultured-expanded MSCs and those available through non–culture-expanded sources, such as the Vet-Stem technique (Vet-Stem Regenerative Veterinary Medicine, Poway, California, United States), in which harvested fat undergoes tissue digestion, producing a nucleated cell population called stromal vascular fraction. Stromal vascular fraction is believed to contain approximately 2% to 4% MSCs. Much of the other literature regarding culture-expanded adipose-derived MSCs cannot necessarily be compared with the Vet-Stem technique.

Intraarticular use of MSCs was investigated in a study comparing adipose-derived stromal cells, bone marrow–derived cultured MSCs, and placebo in the equine osteochondral fragment–exercise model. There were no significant treatment effects in any group, with the exception of improvement in synovial fluid PGE₂ levels in horses treated with bone marrow–derived MSCs compared with the placebo group.[93] Based on this study, we cannot recommend the use of MSCs for the treatment of OA. However, the results of an ovine OA model using medial meniscectomy and cranial cruciate ligament transection, evaluating intraarticular autogenous bone marrow–derived MSCs, were encouraging.[94] There was regeneration of the medial meniscus and decreased progression of OA. Meniscal regeneration could be critical in decreasing OA in this model, whereas OA in the equine osteochondral fragment–exercise model has a different pathogenic pathway. Based on the ovine study, considerable interest was generated at CSU in using intraarticular MSCs to treat soft tissue injuries in the femorotibial joints after arthroscopy, apparently with good clinical results.

Calcitonin

There is some evidence to suggest a direct chondroprotective effect of calcitonin, which, together with its well-established effects on bone resorption, makes it a potential biological therapy for OA.[95,96] Calcitonin is used to treat osteoporosis.[97] In some in vitro work, calcitonin was shown to attenuate collagenase activity, targeting type II collagen.[98] Dogs with OA induced using the cranial cruciate ligament transection model given 400 U/day of calcitonin had significantly reduced histological changes in the articular cartilage of unstable knees. Calcitonin enhanced HA content, as well as the size distribution and relative abundance of aggrecan aggregates in cartilage in both operated and nonoperated knees. In the calcitonin group, the cartilage content of keratin sulfate increased in the operated joints.[96]

Radiation Synovectomy

Synovectomy is hardly a specific biological therapy but is included so its potential use can be recognized. Synovectomy is a well-developed technique for removal of synovial-based inflammation in people with rheumatoid arthritis, but surgical synovectomy is technically difficult, time consuming, and requires general anesthesia.[99] Samarium-153 ([153]Sm) bound to hydroxyapatite microspheres ([153]SmM) effectively ablated normal equine synovium, with minimum radiation hazards to the horse or medical personnel.[99] Radiation emissions from [153]SmM are primarily absorbed by synovium; thus the clinician can target this intraarticular tissue specifically. [153]Sm-hydroxyapatite complex minimizes exposure to other organs or support personnel. In another study, the effects of [153]SmM on reactive synovium in a surgically induced model of synovitis were investigated.[100] Although there was a transient flare causing lameness, effusion, and edema for 48 to 72 hours, [153]SmM destroyed inflamed synovium. There may be potential (with further testing) for radiation synovectomy in horses with persistent synovitis unresponsive to conventional therapy.[100]

SURGICAL TREATMENT

Arthroscopy has revolutionized management of joint disease (see Chapter 23).[101-103] Readers are referred to *Diagnostic and surgical arthroscopy in the horse*[104] for details including advantages and disadvantages of the technique. Arthroscopic surgery remains the gold standard for diagnosis and assessment of pathological joints. Diagnostic arthroscopy is especially valuable when response to medical treatment of a joint is suboptimal. In many instances, cartilage lesions are more extensive than suggested from radiographs but are consistent with the degree of clinical signs.

By 1990, equine arthroscopy had gone from being a diagnostic technique used by a few veterinarians to the accepted way of performing joint surgery.[101] Prospective and retrospective data substantiated the value of arthroscopy in management of carpal chip fractures,[105] fragmentation of the dorsal margin of the proximal phalanx,[106] carpal slab fractures,[107] OCD of the femoropatellar[108,109] and scapulohumeral[110] joints, subchondral cystic lesions of the femur,[111] and various manifestations of osteochondrosis of the tarsocrural joint.[112] Diagnostic arthroscopy led to the

recognition of previously undescribed articular lesions, many of which are treated using arthroscopic techniques.

Since 1990, there have been further advances in diagnosis and management of joint disease based on new pathobiological knowledge gained from arthroscopy.[102,113-118] Previously thought of as inaccessible, the palmar aspects of the carpal and distal interphalangeal joints are now routinely evaluated arthroscopically.[119-121] Arthroscopy led to the discovery of soft tissue injuries, previously undiagnosed, such as tearing of the medial palmar intercarpal ligament.[122-126] In the fetlock joint, we now know success rates after arthroscopy for horses with osteochondral fragments of the palmar/plantar aspect of the proximal phalanx,[127,128] treatment of OCD of the distal dorsal aspect of the third metacarpal/metatarsal bones,[129] and apical, abaxial, and basilar fragments of the proximal sesamoid bones.[130-134] The arthroscopic approach to the plantar pouch of the tarsocrural joint first documented in 1990[101] was more recently reviewed.[135]

Considerable advances have been made in arthroscopic surgery of the stifle joint. Results for the management of OCD of the femoropatellar joint and a syndrome of fragmentation of the distal aspect of the patella occurring after medial patellar desmotomy and success when treating certain patellar fractures were documented.[101,136-138] The use of arthroscopic surgery to treat subchondral cystic lesions of the medial condyle of the femur[139] and proximal tibia[140] has been reported. In fact, pathogenesis of cystic lesions in the medial femoral condyle, once thought to only be a manifestation of osteochondrosis, was recently redefined. Subchondral cystic lesions were traumatically induced by surgically creating a defect, 3 mm deep and 5 mm wide, in the subchondral bone plate.[141] Arthroscopic curettage and drilling into the cyst wall of naturally occurring subchondral cysts sometimes caused cyst enlargement and recurrent lameness; alternative methods for management have developed. Examination of the fibrous tissue of medial femoral subchondral cystic lesions demonstrated the production of local mediators and neutral MMPs, which caused bone resorption in vitro.[142] Production of nitric oxide, PGE_2, and MMPs in media of explant cultures of equine synovium and articular cartilage has also been demonstrated in normal and osteoarthritic joints.[143] Therefore injection of corticosteroids into the lining membrane of subchondral cysts has been performed clinically with favorable results (Figure 84-3).[144]

Cartilage lesions of the medial femoral condyle occur, but surgical manipulation is limited.[145] Adjunctive therapy using IRAP or MSCs has become popular, but results are anecdotal. Arthroscopy has allowed great advances in the recognition and treatment of meniscal tears and cruciate ligament injuries.[146-148] Horses with grade I and grade II meniscal tears can be managed successfully, but those with lesions that are not completely accessible do not respond well (Figure 84-4). Arthroscopy has been used to facilitate removal and repair of fragments from the intercondylar eminence of the tibia.[149,150] Techniques to manage disease of the caudal pouches of the femorotibial joints are now published.[147,151-154] Limited diagnostic and surgical arthroscopy of the coxofemoral joint can be performed.[155,156] Arthroscopy is no longer confined to the limbs, and the arthroscopic anatomy of the temporomandibular joint was described recently.[157]

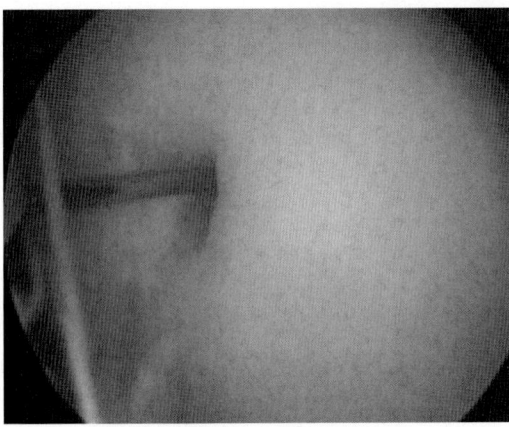

Fig. 84-3 • Arthroscopic view of an 18-gauge spinal needle being used to inject triamcinolone acetonide into the lining of a subchondral cystic lesion. (Reproduced with permission. McIlwraith CW: From arthroscopy to gene therapy—30 years of looking in joints, *Proc Am Assoc Equine Pract* 51:65, 2005.)

Arthroscopic-assisted repair with internal fixation of both nondisplaced and displaced articular fractures has become routine and includes fractures of the metacarpal/metatarsal condyles and carpal slab fractures (Figure 84-5).[158-160] Techniques for evaluation and treatment of diseases of smaller joints[161-164] and in large joints in which lameness is seldom encountered are well developed.[165] Results of arthroscopic surgery are often limited by extensive cartilage damage, an observation that has led us back to scientific research as discussed below.

Recent Progress at Healing Articular Cartilage Lesions and Resurfacing Joints

Progressive loss of articular cartilage is the real challenge in horses with OA, and failure of osteochondral defects to heal is a major limiting factor in the prognosis after treatment of articular fractures. Arthroscopic techniques that enhance both the quantity and quality of cartilage repair tissue, while using the well-documented advantages of arthroscopic surgery, have been attempted.[166-169] Repair, as

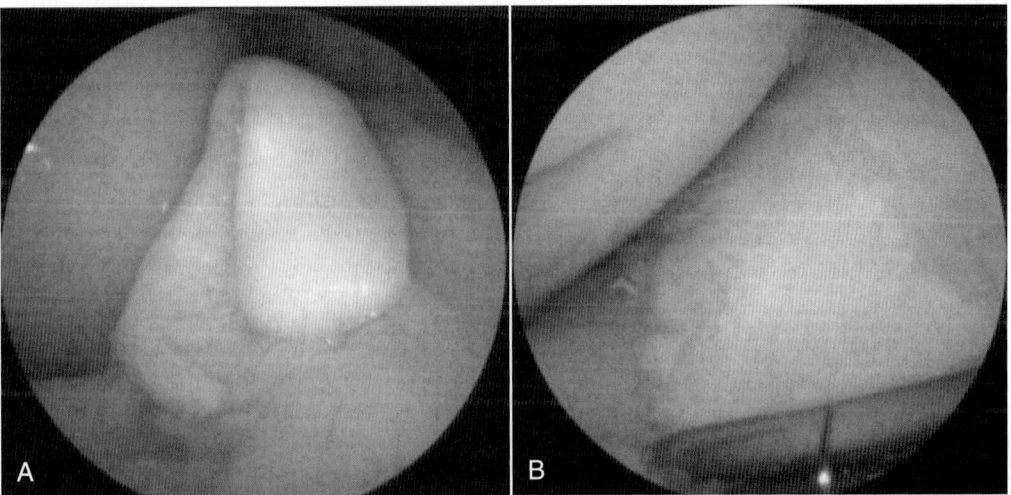

Fig. 84-4 • A grade II tear of the medial meniscus before **(A)** and after removal and debridement of the torn portion **(B)**. (Reproduced with permission. McIlwraith CW: From arthroscopy to gene therapy—30 years of looking in joints, *Proc Am Assoc Equine Pract* 51:65, 2005.)

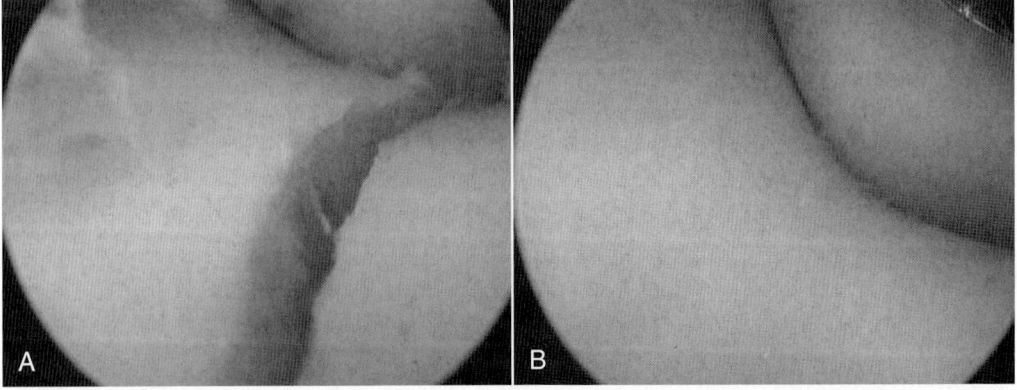

Fig. 84-5 • Arthroscopic view of a displaced fracture of the lateral condyle of the distal aspect of the third metacarpal bone before **(A)** and after **(B)** reduction: under arthroscopic guidance and internal fixation. (Reproduced with permission. McIlwraith CW: From arthroscopy to gene therapy—30 years of looking in joints, *Proc Am Assoc Equine Pract* 51:65, 2005.)

occurs in full-thickness cartilage defects, is defined as replacement of damaged or lost cells and matrix with new cells and matrix, but the original structure and function may not be restored. Regeneration is a special form of repair, in which cells replace lost or damaged tissue with a tissue identical to the original, the aim of continuing investigations in resurfacing. Overall, attempts at improving the repair of articular defects can be divided into stimulation of endogenous repair and articular grafting.

Stimulation of Endogenous Repair

Stimulating endogenous repair involves techniques to provide access for marrow elements to populate the cartilage defect. The simplest method, debridement of the defect, provides fibrocartilaginous repair with high concentrations of type II collagen but low levels of proteoglycan (GAG).[170,171] In addition to simple debridement, other methods of endogenous repair include partial-thickness chondrectomy, spongialization, subchondral bone drilling, abrasion arthroplasty, and most recently, micropicking or microfracture.

Debridement and the Need for Removal of Calcified Cartilage

The time-honored surgical principle of debridement to the level of subchondral bone is well known, but recent work at CSU revealed that if the calcified cartilage layer is left, healing is markedly restricted.[169,172] If the calcified cartilage was removed, there was a significant increase in the amount of repair tissue in defects compared with controls at 4 and 12 months.[173] There was also significant enhancement of repair tissue attachment and calcified cartilage reformation in defects from which the calcified cartilage had been removed (Figure 84-6).

Partial-Thickness Chondrectomy

Partial-thickness chondrectomy down to relatively healthy chondral tissue (cartilage shaving) for partial-thickness defects and fibrillation smoothes the cartilaginous area and may decrease further tissue exfoliation, producing (in conjunction with joint lavage) an early remission of synovitis. However, controlled work in the horse is still necessary. In rabbits in which articular cartilage was shaved on the underside of the patella, there was no evidence of repair.[174] Ultrastructural studies after arthroscopic cartilage debridement questioned any regeneration and suggested deleterious effects.[175]

Spongialization, Abrasion Arthroplasty, and Subchondral Bone Drilling

Spongialization is removal of sclerotic subchondral bone from the base of a full-thickness defect, a procedure sometimes done in horses. However, subchondral bone cysts can form, and I believe that an intact subchondral bone plate is essential for maintaining a foundation for repair.

Abrasion arthroplasty, also called superficial intracortical debridement, as opposed to deep cancellous debridement, is used on sclerotic degenerative lesions in people.[176] The concept is controversial because it is necessary to expose cancellous bone to reach both blood supply and primitive MSCs. Critics have pointed to variables such as patient selection, arthroscopic debridement, and joint irrigation, as well as variation in the degree of pathological change in the joint.[177] In an in vitro study, low oxygen tension was demonstrated to be chondrotrophic and led to the corollary that excessive oxygen tension is not conducive to cartilage formation. Deep debridement to cancellous bone exposes the defect to blood and MSCs, but also to higher oxygen tensions; some people have questioned whether increasing oxygen tension to the defect is beneficial or not.[178] Follow-up biopsies after abrasion arthroplasty showed type I and type III collagen and only limited amounts of the much wanted type II collagen.[176]

Subchondral drilling had similar rationale in providing access through the cancellous bone plate, while still preserving most of the subchondral bone plate. In a study on full-thickness defects of the third carpal bone of horses, satisfactory functional healing was not achieved.[179]

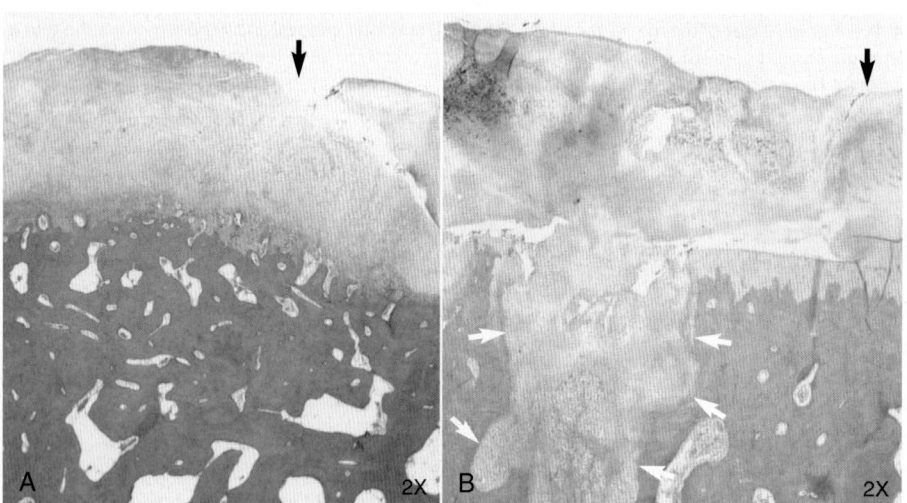

Fig. 84-6 • Histology 12 months after articular cartilage defects in the medial femoral condyle were treated with microfracture and with the calcified cartilage removed **(A)** and retained **(B).** In addition to improved repair tissue, there is partial restoration of the calcified cartilage layer and better attachment of the repair tissue to the underlying bone in the section shown in **A.** Black arrows show the junction of repair tissue *(left)* and retained cartilage. White arrows in **B** show a micropick hole in subchondral bone. (Reproduced with permission. McIlwraith CW: From arthroscopy to gene therapy—30 years of looking in joints, *Proc Am Assoc Equine Pract* 51:65, 2005.)

Subchondral Micropicking (Microfracture)

Subchondral microfracture, or micropicking, was a technique developed by Dr. Richard Steadman and is extensively used in people.[180,181] The technique was shown to provide equivalent repair to the commercially available autologous chondrocyte implantation process of Carticel (Genzyme, Cambridge, Massachusetts, United States).[182] Micropicking is a simple and atraumatic way to provide pluripotential cells and growth factors while minimizing heat (associated with drilling with other techniques) and providing a rim of bone around the pick holes that may provide a foundation to enhance repair tissue attachment. Studies in the horse showed that the amount of repair tissue significantly increased when cartilage defects debrided down to subchondral bone were micropicked compared with debridement alone. A short-term study revealed that there was a significant increase in type II collagen mRNA production 8 weeks after microfracture.[172] Although aggrecan production gradually increased between 2 and 8 weeks, this expression was not influenced by microfracture.[172]

Further Manipulation of Endogenous Healing Using Growth Factors (Protein Administration or Gene Therapy)

We may be able to manipulate cells to produce improved repair tissue matrix. Several naturally occurring polypeptide growth factors play an important role in cartilage homeostasis.[183,184] However, endogenous manipulation not only involves the use of growth factors to promote synthesis of matrix components (anabolism) but also should inhibit proteinases and inflammatory factors that can cause ongoing degradation after surgery (catabolism) (Figure 84-7). IGF-I and transforming growth factor–β (TGF-β) have matrix anabolic activity and are also considered important in counteracting the degradatory and catabolic activities of cytokines and MMPs. Three-dimensional cultures of equine chondrocytes in fibrin gels were evaluated with either IGF-I or TGF-β and cultured without serum supplements; these two growth factors stimulated matrix component elaboration in a dose-dependent manner, with the most profound effects occurring at the highest concentration of IGF-I and TGF-β.[185,186] In other cartilage explant studies using normal and IL-1–depleted cartilage, IGF-I had a positive effect on equine cartilage homeostasis.[187] Because of these results, IGF-I was selected as a candidate growth

factor for evaluation in the horse. Elution studies showed that IGF-I–laden equine fibrin had maximal stimulatory levels of IGF-I (>50 ng/mL) remaining for a minimum of 3 weeks.[188] In vivo evaluation after placement of 25 μg of IGF-I in fibrin into cartilage defects in the femoropatellar joint showed improved cell populations, with more cartilage-like architecture after 6 months.[189] However, type II collagen levels only increased to 47%, half of that found in normal articular cartilage, compared with a type II collagen content of 39% in the control defects, comparable with the levels seen in empty full-thickness defects.[190]

Other work in the same laboratory suggested IGF-I worked better in combination with a chondrocyte or a MSC graft, resulting in more complete cartilage repair.[191] At 8 months after implantation of a mixture of chondrocytes in 25 mcg of IGF-I in femoropatellar defects in horses, there was improved joint surface, 58% type II collagen, and better neocartilage integration at the defect edges. Resurfacing of articular defects using autogenous fibrin laden with 50 mcg of IGF-I in 30 million chondrocytes/mL of fibrin was used in horses with OCD and subchondral cystic lesion of the fetlock and stifle joints. The chondrocytes were mixed with fibrinogen and IGF-I with activated thrombin to provide a two-component system for immediate injection. This polymerization process developed immediately on injection into the articular defect.[167]

Using gene therapy techniques (previously discussed with IL-1ra), transplanted chondrocytes were transfected with IGF-I.[192,193] Transfecting transplanted chondrocytes with bone morphogenetic protein–7 accelerated cartilage repair.[194]

In a collaborative effort between CSU, Cornell University, University of Pittsburgh, and Harvard University, the usefulness of a combined gene therapy protocol using IL-1ra to decrease the effects of IL-1 on cartilage repair in combination with IGF-I (previously shown to enhance cartilage healing in an equine model, as well as to also reduce the deleterious effects of IL-1) was investigated.[195-197] Using an osteoarthritic IL-1 coculture (synovium and articular cartilage) system, gene transduction of IGF-I and IL-1ra proteins was demonstrated using an adenoviral vector with protection of proteoglycan loss in the cartilage.[195] There was also restoration of cartilage matrix without IL-1 present using the same in vitro system.[196] The combination gene therapy protocol was then evaluated using full-thickness articular

Homeostasis of articular cartilage

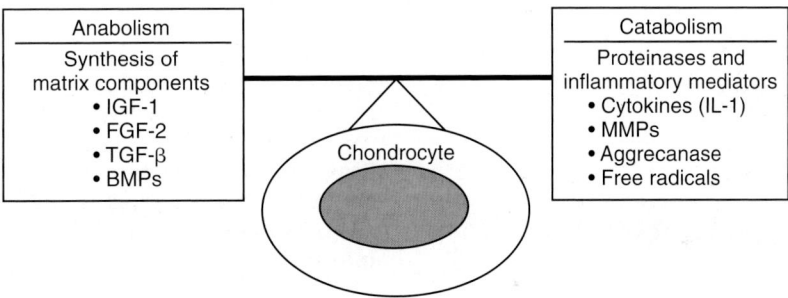

Fig. 84-7 • Diagram of homeostatic pathways that can represent potential ways of endogenously manipulating articular cartilage. *IGF*, Insulin-like growth factor; *FGF-2*, fibroblast growth factor-2; *TGF-β*, transformin growth factor-β; *BMPs*, bone morphogenetic proteins; *MMPs*, matrix metalloproteinases; *IL-1*, interleukin-1. (Reproduced with permission. McIlwraith CW: From arthroscopy to gene therapy—30 years of looking in joints, *Proc Am Assoc Equine Pract* 51:65, 2005.)

chondral defects treated with microfracture in the horse.[197] This protocol enhanced the quality of the repair tissue in full-thickness equine chondral defects compared with microfracture alone, and there was increased type II collagen and aggrecan content in the defects.[197]

Articular Grafting

Reattachment of Cartilage Flaps and Periosteal and Sternal Grafts

Direct repair of large OCD defects by replacing the flap and providing fixation with polydioxanone (PDS) pins was done successfully in horses.[198] However, attempts with direct grafting of periosteum or sternal cartilage met with disappointing results.[170,171,199]

Implantation of Autologous Chondrocytes

Early attempts at grafts of cultured chondrocytes or cartilage regenerative cells in a matrix were also relatively unsuccessful.[200-202] Currently there is one commercially available technique of autologous chondrocyte implantation into human knees, and it is used principally for focal erosive defects[203,204] and OCD.[205] This is a two-stage procedure. After collection of cartilage, it is cultured; 3 weeks later, a piece of autogenous periosteum is sutured into the defect, and the cultured chondrocytes are injected beneath it. Despite reports implying excellent results, failures, particularly with detachment of the graft, can occur, and recently a clinical study with a 2-year follow-up period showed no superiority over microfracture alone.[182] Grafting in this manner was used experimentally in 10-mm–diameter defects on the lateral trochlear ridge of talus and resulted in significantly improved defect filling with a well-integrated neocartilage and comparable expression of cartilage-specific markers.[206]

I have conducted experiments at CSU using a solid form of autologous chondrocyte culturing. Cartilage (300 mg) was harvested from the lateral trochlear ridge of the femur, and chondrocytes were cultured on a collagen membrane and reimplanted at 4 weeks. The results were significantly superior to empty defects and defects implanted with matrix alone. However, it is still a two-stage technique, and this remains a caveat.[207]

A one-stage technique for treatment of 15-mm defects in the trochlear ridge of the femur in the horse was evaluated.[208] An articular cartilage biopsy was taken from the lateral trochlear ridge of the femur (follow-up evaluation at 12 months revealed no apparent morbidity associated with the cartilage biopsy). The cartilage was morselized into approximately 1 mm^3 and suspended in fibrin on a membrane (a PDS-reinforced foam). This morselized cartilage-fibrin-PDS membrane combination was then placed into the defect with the membrane uppermost and fixed with three specially developed PDS-polyglycolic acid (PGA) staples. The follow-up results at 12 months were excellent. The technique is now being tested in people.

What about Stem Cells?

The use of MSCs in medical management of OA was previously discussed (see Mesenchymal Stem Cells, page 847). The relative chondrogenic potential of bone marrow–derived or adipose-derived MSCs was evaluated after expansion in monolayer culture and implantation into agarose or peptide gels.[209] GAG accumulation in hydrogels seeded with culture-expanded MSCs and containing TGF-β after 21 days of culture was significantly enhanced with bone marrow–derived MSCs compared with adipose-derived MSCs, and there was also superior type II collagen expression. Implantation of MSCs (using fibrin as a vehicle) into femoral trochlear defects in the horse showed early benefit at 30 days, but there were no significant differences between treated and control joints at 8 months.[210] Direct intraarticular injection of MSCs is currently being tested at CSU. We contend that MSCs act as trophic mediators; in addition to dividing and differentiating, MSCs secrete a variety of cytokines and growth factors, and these bioactive factors suppress local immune reactions, inhibit fibrosis and apoptosis, enhance angiogenesis, and stimulate mitosis and differentiation of tissue-intrinsic reparative or stem cells.[211] These effects, which are referred to as trophic effects, are distinct from the direct differentiation of MSCs into repair tissue.

Osteochondral Grafts

The use of osteochondral plugs to repair experimentally created defects in the medial condyle of the femur was initially investigated using sternal osteochondral grafts.[212,213] Techniques of autogenous and allogeneic osteochondral plug grafting using mosiacplasty were reported with some success, but the technique is challenging.[214,215]

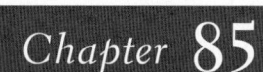

Analgesia and Hindlimb Lameness

Rose M. McMurphy

The benefits to providing analgesia for both acute and chronic pain are well established in many species. Inadequate treatment of pain can result in inappetence and weight loss, increases in serum cortisol and catecholamines, tachycardia, hypertension, and compromise of the immune system.[1] Increases in serum cortisol and catecholamines can cause derangements in serum glucose, protein metabolism, and immune function. In addition, horses with a painful limb may remain recumbent for prolonged periods, with resultant decubital ulcer formation and secondary infection.

References on page 1329

EPIDURAL ANALGESIA

Designing an appropriate plan for analgesia in a horse, particularly for those with severe, chronic pain, can be challenging. Parenterally administered opioids and α₂-adrenergic agonists may be associated with side effects such as ataxia, excitement, and adverse effects on the gastrointestinal and cardiovascular systems. Nonsteroidal antiinflammatory drugs (NSAIDs) can cause gastrointestinal ulceration or renal disease, and they may be inadequate for horses with acute, intense pain. Epidural administration of drugs provides more localized analgesia and fewer systemic effects than parenteral administration.

Epidural drug administration places a drug in close proximity to its site of action within the spinal cord or the spinal nerves as they exit the spinal cord. A greater analgesic effect may be achieved with a smaller total dose of a drug. The duration of analgesia is usually longer than with parenteral administration. Pain that is related to a disease process of a hindlimb is particularly amenable to treatment with epidural analgesia. The site of injection for epidural drug administration in horses is usually the first coccygeal (caudal) interspace. When deposited into the epidural space, the drug diffuses across the meninges, into the cerebrospinal fluid (CSF), and then into the spinal cord. The degree of cephalad diffusion of the drug within the CSF depends on several factors, including the volume of the drug injected, concentration of the drug, and lipid solubility.[2] Although studies in dogs and people have reported analgesic effects with epidural morphine or α₂-agonists that extend to the midthoracic area or farther cranially,[3,4] this is generally not the case in horses.[5-8] This limits the use of epidural analgesia in horses to the treatment of hindlimb pain.

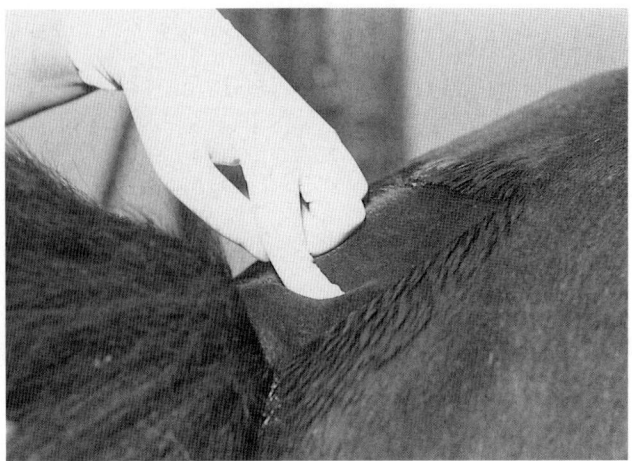

Fig. 85-1 • The first coccygeal interspace between the first and second coccygeal vertebrae is identified while the clinician raises and lowers the tail and palpates for the articulation between these two vertebrae. This space is just caudal to the most angular portion of the bend of the tail.

TECHNIQUE FOR EPIDURAL ADMINISTRATION

Caudal epidural drug administration can be done by single injection at the first coccygeal interspace or by placement of an epidural catheter at this same site for repeated drug administration. The lumbosacral space is also a potential site of injection, and its use may result in a more rapid onset of hindlimb analgesia. However, positioning the tip of the needle within the epidural space rather than the subarachnoid space can be difficult. Subarachnoid administration of drugs in the horse is certainly acceptable, but the dose should be reduced by 40% to 50%.

The first coccygeal interspace (between the first and second coccygeal vertebrae) is identified while raising and lowering the tail and palpating for the articulation between these two vertebrae. This space is just caudal to the most angular portion of the bend of the tail, about 5 cm cranial to the first long tail hairs (Figure 85-1). The site should be prepared aseptically. Administration of 2 to 3 mL of 2% lidocaine subcutaneously using a 25-gauge needle helps decrease the response of the horse to placement of the needle for epidural injection. An 18- or 20-gauge, 6.35-cm spinal needle with stylet is recommended for epidural injection in horses, although many clinicians use a standard 18-gauge needle. The bevel of a spinal needle is not as sharp as that of a standard needle and the bevel angle is less acute. This design makes it easier to identify penetration through the interarcuate ligament and the subsequent loss of resistance as the epidural space is entered. The needle is inserted at a 30- to 60-degree angle to horizontal, with the tip pointed cranioventrally, and is advanced until it contacts the floor of the vertebral canal (Figure 85-2). The depth of insertion is 3 to 6 cm,

depending on the size of the horse and the angle of the needle. The needle placement can be tested by attempting to inject 2 to 3 mL of air or solution in a 3-mL syringe. Resistance to injection should be little or absent. Appropriate epidural injection of local anesthetic solution and xylazine often is confirmed when anal tone decreases and the tail relaxes, but because the drugs most commonly used for epidural analgesia of the hindlimb (morphine, detomidine) have little or no effect on motor nerves, these responses will be absent.

EPIDURAL CATHETER PLACEMENT

The site for insertion of an epidural catheter is the same as for a single epidural injection. Placement of the catheter requires the use of a needle with a curved point (Tuohy, Becton, Dickinson, Franklin Lakes, New Jersey, United States) that will direct the catheter cranially, along the floor of the vertebral canal (Figure 85-3). The epidural catheter is made of polyamide (nylon) or Teflon, with a closed or open end, and it can be purchased with a wire stylet if desired. I use an 18-gauge, 8.89-cm Tuohy needle and a 20-gauge, 100-cm radiodense, polyamide catheter with a closed tip (bullet tip) without a stylet (Figure 85-4). Epidural catheters have marks every centimeter and multiple marks at 10, 15, and 20 cm from the end. Before needle and catheter placement, slide the catheter inside the needle and note the distance from the tip of the needle to the hub on the catheter. The clinician then should determine which mark on the catheter will be at the hub of the needle once the catheter has been advanced to the desired position.

As with the single epidural injections, strict attention should be paid to aseptic technique, and sterile gloves must be worn. Lidocaine is injected into the subcutaneous tissues at the desired site. A small incision is made through the skin with a No. 11 scalpel, because the Tuohy needle has a blunt tip. Once the needle has been positioned, the bevel should be directed cranially (the notch on the hub of the needle should face cranially). The catheter is threaded

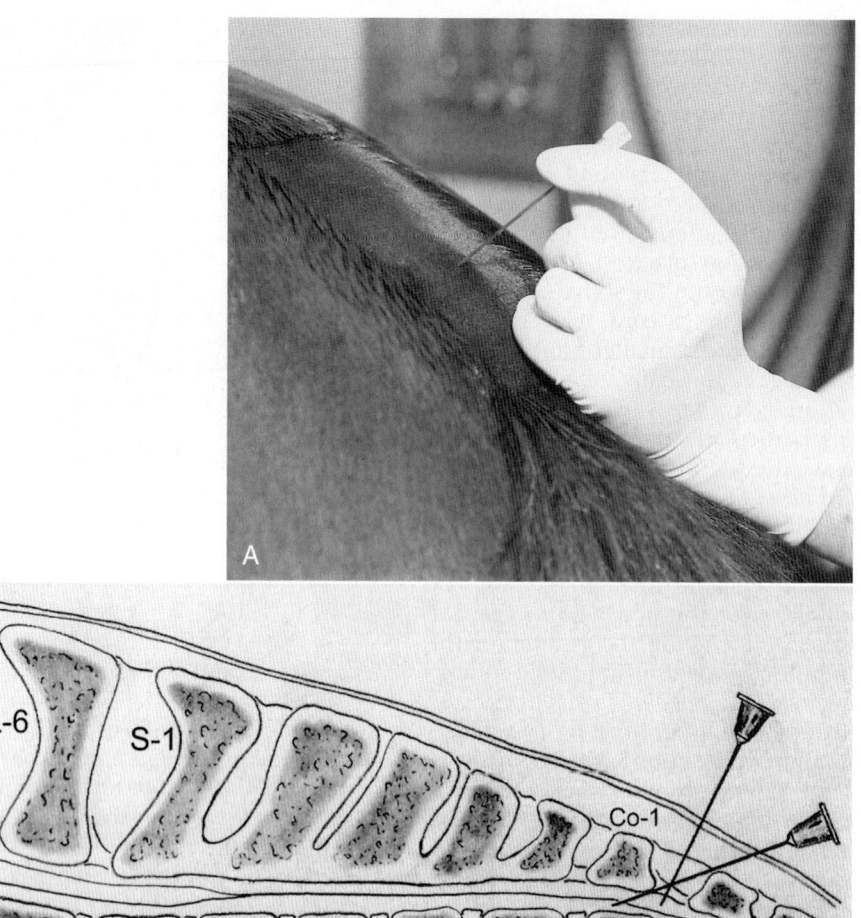

Fig. 85-2 • **A,** The needle is inserted at a 30- to 60-degree angle to horizontal and is advanced until it contacts the floor of the vertebral canal. **B,** Sagittal view of the sacral vertebrae and placement of the needle within the epidural space. *Co-1,* First coccygeal vertebra; *L-6,* sixth lumbar vertebra; *S-1,* first sacral vertebra.

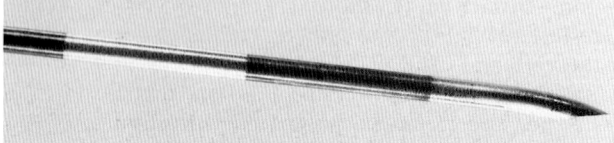

Fig. 85-3 • Curved point of a Tuohy needle.

through the needle and along the floor of the vertebral canal (Figure 85-5). Provided the needle is positioned in the epidural space, the advancing catheter receives little resistance. If the tip of the needle is angled incorrectly, the catheter tends to bump up against the vertebrae and will not advance. If this occurs, the needle is withdrawn 1 to 2 mm and the catheter is rotated slightly as it is advanced. It is critical that once the catheter has advanced any distance outside of the needle, it never be withdrawn back into the needle. This may result in cutting or shearing off of the catheter. The catheter is advanced 5 to 10 cm past the tip of the needle, and the tip is positioned in the mid-sacral region. Once the catheter has been positioned, the needle is carefully withdrawn over the catheter and

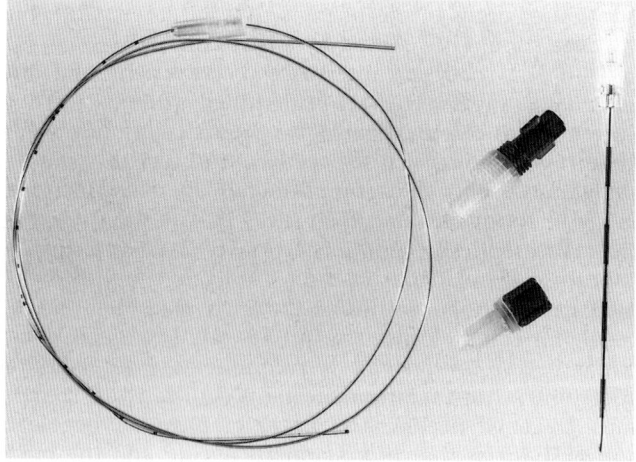

Fig. 85-4 • Tuohy needle and epidural catheter.

removed (Figure 85-6). Most epidural catheters intended for human use are very long to facilitate positioning of the injection port in a convenient place on the body. I usually cut the catheter with a scalpel (scissors tend to crush the catheter), leaving about 10 cm of the catheter to secure to

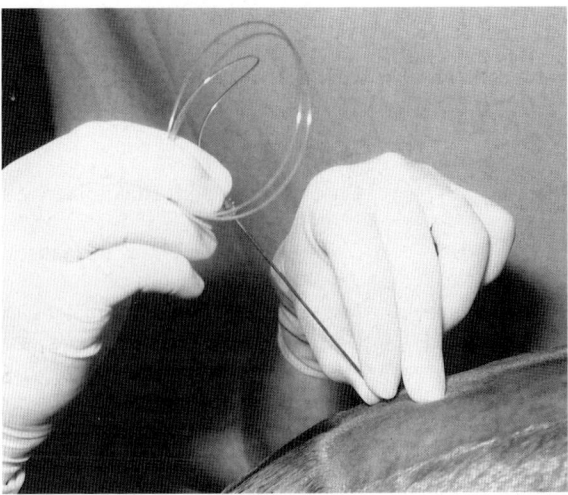

Fig. 85-5 • The epidural catheter is threaded through the needle and along the floor of the vertebral canal. If the catheter will not advance, the needle is withdrawn 1 to 2 mm, and the tip of the needle is angled up slightly.

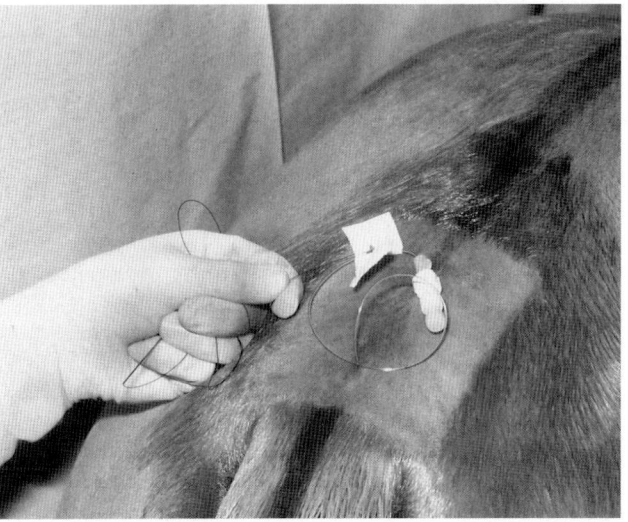

Fig. 85-7 • The catheter or syringe adapter is attached, and an injection cap is secured to the adapter. A portion of tape is secured to the catheter at the point of insertion and then sutured to the skin.

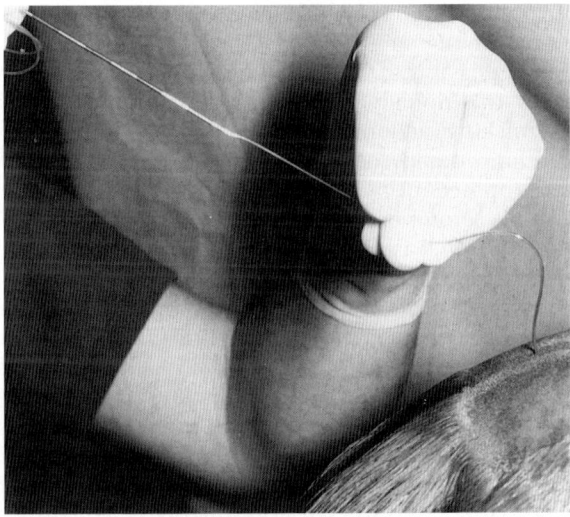

Fig. 85-6 • Once the catheter is in place, the needle is carefully withdrawn over the catheter and removed.

the horse. The catheter or syringe adapter is attached, and an injection cap is secured to the adapter. A portion of tape is secured to the catheter at the point of insertion and then sutured to the skin (Figure 85-7). The syringe adapter also should be sutured to the skin, making sure tension will be minimal on the catheter during any movement of the horse. The catheter and injection cap then are covered with a sheer, adhesive dressing. Each injection into the catheter is made through the catheter cap after thoroughly cleaning it with alcohol, while wearing sterile gloves. It is critical that the catheter system remains sterile. A bacterial filter can be inserted between the syringe adapter and the catheter cap as an added precaution. The catheter site should be examined daily for signs of inflammation or infection, which would necessitate removing the catheter and submitting the tip for culture. With diligent aseptic

technique and catheter care, I have kept catheters in place for 2 weeks in horses, and some researchers have reported epidural catheters being maintained for 5 weeks in research horses.[9]

DRUG SELECTION

Epidural Opioids

The primary advantage of epidural administration of an opioid is the intense and prolonged, segmental (localized) analgesia achieved without either sedation or the possible excitement that may accompany the parenteral administration of an opioid. Unlike epidural local anesthetic solutions or xylazine, epidural opioids do not affect neuromuscular function or the sympathetic nerves.

The analgesia obtained with epidural opioids is primarily from the effect of the opioid within the spinal cord rather than from a supraspinal location. Opioids bind to presynaptic receptors of the afferent nerve terminals in the dorsal horn and inhibit the release of excitatory neurotransmitters such as glutamate and substance P. Opioids also act postsynaptically to inhibit transmission of impulses in ascending tracts. Evidence also shows that opioids enhance the effects of descending inhibitory pathways on the processing of pain within the dorsal horn.[10]

The onset and duration of action of epidural opioids vary greatly among drugs. The time to onset of analgesia reflects the time required for a drug to diffuse from the epidural space, across the meninges, into the spinal fluid, and ultimately into the spinal cord. Physicochemical properties of the drug, such as molecular weight, molecular shape, degree of ionization, and particularly lipid solubility influence the diffusion across the meninges.[3,11] The more lipid-soluble drugs, such as fentanyl and butorphanol, have a rapid onset but a shorter duration of action, whereas the more water-soluble drug, morphine, has a delayed onset and a very long duration of action (Table 85-1).[3] This delay in onset of analgesia with morphine can be particularly long in horses, and the drug may not reach peak effect

TABLE 85-1

		ANALGESIA				
DRUG	DOSE (mg/kg)	ONSET (min)	DURATION	SEDATION	ATAXIA	COMMENTS
Morphine	0.1	150-180	12-18 hr	Minimal	No	Onset time for peak analgesia may be up to 6 hours
Butorphanol	0.04	?	2.5-3 hr	No	No	Degree of analgesia may be inadequate
Tramadol	1.0	30	6-12	No	No	
Xylazine	—	—	—	—	Marked	Not suitable for hindlimb analgesia
Detomidine	0.05	10-25	2-3 hr	Moderate	Mild	Decreased heart rate, blood pressure, and respiratory rate
Ketamine	1-2	5-10	30-75 min	Mild	Mild	Ataxia only at higher doses
Detomidine and morphine	0.03 and 0.1-0.2	10-25	12-18 hr	Moderate	Mild	Decreased heart rate, blood pressure, and respiratory rate

Characteristics of Analgesia and Side-Effects after Epidural Administration of Various Drugs

for several hours.[12] The more water-soluble opioids also tend to have greater degree of cranial diffusion within the CSF.[2]

Morphine remains the opioid of choice even though numerous other opioids have been evaluated for epidural analgesia in horses (see Table 85-1).[5-7,13-15] Fentanyl has a faster onset of action but a considerably shorter duration of action (4 to 6 hours). Butorphanol provides inadequate analgesia. Analgesia after epidural administration of hydromorphone and methadone has been described in research horses.[15] The onset of analgesia is more rapid than with morphine, and the duration of analgesia in the lumbar and sacral regions is approximately 4 hours. There may be benefit to using a drug with a more rapid onset, particularly in horses with an epidural catheter, which can facilitate more frequent administration. The utility of these drugs in horses with hindlimb pain remains to be evaluated.

I use preservative-free morphine (Abbott Laboratories, North Chicago, Illinois, United States) that is intended for epidural use at a dose of 0.1 mg/kg. The disadvantage of this preparation is the volume required. There are parenteral preparations of morphine that have been used for epidural administration in horses in an attempt to lower the cost, but some of these may contain substances such as phenol or formaldehyde, which may be neurotoxic. A preparation of morphine (25 mg/mL) with sodium bisulfite as an antioxidant (morphine sulfate, Hospira, Lake Forest, Illinois, United States) has been used in the horse epidurally, but the dose to be administered should be diluted in 20 mL of sterile saline solution. Epidural morphine has been used at a dose of up to 0.2 mg/kg combined with epidural detomidine.[16,17] The higher dose may potentially speed the onset of action and extend the drug's duration, but it may increase the incidence of side effects.

Potential side effects include respiratory depression, pruritus,[18] and urinary retention. These are rarely seen in horses and can be treated with naloxone (0.005 to 0.01 mg/kg). I have experience with a horse that developed substantial central nervous system effects after administration of morphine (0.2 mg/kg in 50 mL of saline solution), resulting in collapse, tachypnea, muscle rigidity, and hypoxemia. The horse was treated with naloxone (0.01 mg/kg), furosemide (2 mg/kg), diazepam (0.01 mg/kg), and a neuromuscular blocker to facilitate positive-pressure ventilation

after intubation and anesthesia with isoflurane. The horse recovered.

Epidural α₂-Adrenergic Agonists

Epidural administration of an α_2-adrenergic agonist can induce profound analgesia mediated by α_2-adrenergic receptors in the spinal cord.[19] The exact mechanism for the analgesia is not known. However, the α_2-adrenergic agonists traditionally were thought to induce analgesia by mimicking action of norepinephrine released from descending noradrenergic inhibitory pathways.[20] Additional proposed mechanisms of action include modulation of pain via serotonergic and adenosinergic pathways, inhibition of the release of substance P, and effects on opiate receptors.[21,22]

Xylazine, an α_1- and α_2-receptor agonist, is commonly used to induce analgesia of the perineal area of horses.[23] However, xylazine is not suitable for severe hindlimb lameness because of its effects on somatic motor innervation.[8] Doses that exceed 0.25 mg/kg can cause substantial ataxia and have the potential to cause temporary hindlimb paralysis. Detomidine is a more selective α_2-adrenergic agonist that primarily affects nerve fibers involved in pain transmission (C fibers and A delta fibers) and appears to have limited effect on somatic motor function at clinically used doses. Detomidine is therefore less likely to cause motor dysfunction and hindlimb paralysis, making it more appropriate for the treatment of horses with hindlimb pain. However, detomidine has a relatively short duration of action (see Table 85-1) and also has systemic effects, such as decreased blood pressure and heart and respiratory rates. Detomidine is best used with morphine and can provide additional analgesia. I use a combination of morphine (0.1 mg/kg) and detomidine (30 mcg/kg).

Other Drugs for Epidural Analgesia

Ketamine is an *N*-methyl-D-aspartate (NMDA) receptor antagonist that can be effective for pain resulting from central sensitization in the spinal cord and hyperalgesia caused by continuous nociceptive input from damaged tissue. Epidural ketamine has been administered to people and animals for treatment of acute and neuropathic pain with mixed results. Research horses given 1 mg of ketamine per kilogram epidurally had reduced postincisional pain (flank incision) for several hours and demonstrated no signs of ataxia or sedation.[24] Epidural ketamine may be a suitable adjunct to other forms of analgesia, particularly in horses with inadequate analgesia from epidural morphine.

Tramadol is a centrally acting analgesic with effect on opiate, adrenergic, and serotonergic receptor systems. Tramadol (1.0 mg/kg) administered as a caudal epidural analgesic to horses induces analgesia, beginning at 20 minutes, that lasts approximately 6 hours in the sacral region and 5 hours in the lumbar and thoracic regions, with the analgesia in the more cranial regions being less intense.[12] The duration of this analgesia is slightly shorter than that of epidurally administered morphine, with a faster onset of action.

CLINICAL APPLICATIONS

Epidural analgesia can make a profound difference in the comfort and convalescence of horses and is frequently used in conjunction with other forms of analgesia, such as NSAIDs. Epidural analgesia is often used during the first stages of recovery from various disease processes, when the pain may be more intense, or immediately before or after surgical treatment of hindlimb injuries or disease. Procedures such as fracture repair and arthrodesis can cause pain intraoperatively and postoperatively. Preoperative administration of epidural opioids can decrease the concentration of inhalation anesthetic required, and some evidence shows that preoperative administration of epidural opioids is effective preemptive analgesia. Evidence also shows that effective preemptive analgesia can make postoperative pain management more successful. Because the onset of action of epidural morphine is prolonged in horses, administration of the drug 1 to 3 hours before induction of general anesthesia may be necessary to achieve the greatest effect postoperatively. A clinical impression exists that horses treated with epidural morphine have longer recovery times. My own impression is that recovery might be slightly prolonged, but not dangerously so, and that the horses are far more comfortable in the immediate postoperative period. Epidural administration of morphine provides analgesia that is far superior to what can be achieved with NSAIDs and parenterally administered opioid agonist-antagonists, such as butorphanol, without substantial systemic effects.

Horses with trauma to a hindlimb that require long-term therapy may benefit from the placement of an epidural catheter. I have left catheters in place for 1 to 2 weeks in some horses and as of yet have seen no complications attributable to the catheter. In some horses, however, the analgesia seems gradually to become less effective, despite increases in the dose and frequency of administration of epidural morphine. The addition of 30 mcg of epidural detomidine per kilogram every 6 to 8 hours has been beneficial in such horses. Ketamine,[9] tramadol, or other α_2-agonists, such as medetomidine, may have a role in treating horses with pain that is refractory to epidural morphine.

CONTRAINDICATIONS AND COMPLICATIONS

Complications associated with epidural analgesia can be grouped according to those caused by the drugs administered, those caused by the actual insertion of the needle or the catheter, and those secondary to the maintenance of

an epidural catheter. Complications reported with epidural morphine are rare in horses. Detomidine may cause cardiopulmonary depression, sedation, and ataxia. Careful assessment of the horse's cardiovascular status and appropriate dosage of the drug can minimize the risks associated with epidural detomidine.

Introduction of the needle or catheter into the epidural space potentially can cause trauma to the spinal nerve roots or the epidural venous sinus. Substantial bleeding in horses with normal clotting times and platelet numbers is unlikely. The possibility exists that if the tip of the needle is in the venous sinus, the drug administration will be intravenous as opposed to epidural and will not have the desired effect of prolonged, segmental analgesia. I have also, on one occasion, inadvertently catheterized the epidural venous sinus. If blood is obtained after aspiration of the catheter, the catheter (and needle if still in place) should be removed and a new catheter placed.

Potential complications secondary to the maintenance of an epidural catheter include localized soft tissue inflammation and, rarely, epidural abscess, vertebral osteomyelitis, and meningitis. The catheter site should be inspected daily for signs of infection or inflammation. Technical problems with the epidural catheter (dislodgement, kinking) are more likely to result in early removal of the catheter than other complications.[25]

Possibly the most serious potential complication would be the inadvertent injection of an inappropriate substance or an overdose of the drug into the epidural catheter. The epidural catheter should be clearly marked as such, and all personnel working with that horse should be instructed in the care of the catheter and the amount and type of drugs that are administered through the catheter.

NOVEL ANALGESIC DRUGS AND ADJUNCTIVE THERAPIES

The transdermal route of drug administration can be used for opioid administration in horses. The transdermal therapeutic system for fentanyl administration is used in horses by applying patches to either the neck or the lateral aspect of the antebrachium.[26,27] Two 10-mg patches (Duragesic 100 mcg/hr, Janssen Pharmaceutical, Titusville, New Jersey, United States) are generally used for adult horses. A pharmacokinetic study of transdermal fentanyl found that serum levels of fentanyl considered to be analgesic were present within 8 to 15 hours and were maintained for up to 32 hours. The application of fentanyl patches in conjunction with NSAIDs in horses with pain from soft tissue and orthopedic disease resulted in decreased overall pain scores, but improvement in the horses with orthopedic disease was minimal and lameness scores did not change.[27] My experience with transdermal fentanyl in horses is similar. Clinical signs in horses with soft tissue injuries and abdominal pain may improve, but the analgesic benefit in horses with acute or substantial orthopedic pain is questionable.

Subanesthetic doses of intravenous ketamine have been used to provide analgesia in small animals and people. A constant rate infusion of as low as 0.4 mg/kg/hr in horses results in plasma levels of ketamine above those needed to provide analgesia in people, and doses of 1.2 mg/kg/hr were analgesic in research horses with minimal changes in behavior.[28,29] The efficacy of low-dose constant infusions of ketamine in painful horses is yet to be determined. I have used low-dose ketamine (0.3 mg/kg bolus and 1 mg/kg/hr) in a limited number of horses that were in pain despite opioid therapy, and horses appeared to show modest to marked improvement.

Other adjunctive analgesic agents used in veterinary medicine include the anticonvulsant gabapentin (Neurontin, Pfizer, New York, United States). The proposed analgesic mechanism is mediated by binding to a presynaptic voltage-gated calcium channel in the dorsal root ganglia and spinal cord, which inhibits calcium influx and subsequent release of excitatory neurotransmitters.[30] Gabapentin has become an established therapy in some types of neuropathic pain, and its use for acute, perioperative pain is being investigated. Limited pharmacokinetic data in horses have revealed maximal plasma levels that were lower than those in people and dogs given a similar dose.[31] There is a single case report of a mare with femoral neuropathy that was given 2.5 mg/kg of gabapentin every 8 hours. The authors concluded that gabapentin appeared to be an effective treatment for neuropathic pain in that horse.[32] My only experience with gabapentin is in dogs with severe neuropathic or chronic pain, with responses varying from excellent to poor. One of the Editors (SJD) has treated several horses with suspected neuropathic pain with complete remission of clinical signs; however, horses with severe, chronic pain associated with laminitis have shown only limited improvement.

Chapter 86

Bandaging, Splinting, and Casting

Alan J. Ruggles and Sue J. Dyson

Indications for bandaging and cast application include protection of limbs during transport and performance, reduction of soft tissue swelling, protection of surgical wounds, management of skin defects and granulation tissue, protection of surgical implants, management of fractures, and first aid before transport of injured horses. This chapter discusses methods of bandage, splint, and cast application and the acute management of a horse with a suspected fracture or soft tissue injury.

STABLE AND TRAVELING BANDAGES

Bandages used routinely as stable bandages or for transport consist of a padded, quilted, fleece, or an interwoven sheet of cotton as a protective layer, held in place by a flannel wrap or commercially available bandage material. Horses that continually wear stable bandages tend to develop ridges in the hair coat, and this should be noted at a prepurchase examination. Proper bandaging prevents limbs from filling in a stabled horse and helps to prevent injury during transport. The coronary band region is particularly vulnerable during transport, loading, and unloading, and the bandage ideally should extend to cover this area. Alternatively, overreach (bell) boots should be used. Improper bandage application or management can cause the development of white hairs, transient edema, and structural damage to soft tissue structures and, under severe circumstances, pressure necrosis. An excessively tight bandage can result in severe tissue necrosis within 24 hours, resulting in full-thickness skin loss and damage to the underlying soft tissues. The midmetacarpal region seems to be particularly vulnerable. Alternatively, commercially available boots can be used for transport, the best of which extend from proximal to the dorsal aspect of the carpus, or the plantar aspect of the tarsus, to cover the coronary band. The use of exercise bandages and boots for protection and support is discussed in Chapter 37.

BANDAGING WOUNDS

The principles of bandages used to protect wounds are to absorb exudate, reduce soft tissue swelling, and provide an environment conducive to wound healing. Each wound has its own characteristics that make a specific type of bandage, or even the absence of a bandage, ideal. All bandages prevent or reduce edema by providing pressure. A bandage can immobilize a region to a certain extent; the degree of immobilization depends on the type of material used and the manner of its application.

Surgical wounds are generally created under ideal conditions, and proper apposition of the skin edges occurs during suturing. Protection is provided by a nonadherent, porous dressing (Telfa, Kendall Co., Mansfield, Massachusetts, United States) over the wound. The dressing is held in place with a sterile gauze roll (Conform, Kendall Co.), and then a cotton combine roll 45 cm wide (for the lower limb only), or alternatively a soft conforming bandage (Soffban, Smith and Nephew, Hull, North Humberside, United Kingdom). The gauze is held in place with an elastic conforming bandage (Vet-Wrap, 3M Animal Care Products, St Paul, Minnesota, United States; Elastikon, Johnson and Johnson, Arlington, Texas, United States). These dressings are changed every 2 to 3 days, or earlier as needed, until suture removal. In some circumstances bandaging may be prolonged to reduce postoperative swelling and improve cosmetic results. If a full-limb bandage is placed to extend above the carpus or tarsus, an additional bandage 40 cm wide is applied above the first bandage. A layer of gauze is used over the combine and cotton, and an elastic conforming bandage (Elastikon) is then applied. Finally, additional elastic tape is used to secure the top of the bandage to the skin. These types of bandages are used postoperatively for most horses undergoing orthopedic procedures, such as arthroscopy or splint removal, and for most horses with limb wounds, assuming the limb is stable.

In a forelimb the area of the bandage over the accessory carpal bone is incised with a scalpel blade to prevent rub sores from developing. In a hindlimb the point of the hock can be covered by the bandage if duration of bandaging is anticipated to be less than 1 week. If prolonged bandaging is required, the point of the hock should not be covered, to prevent rub sores and potential development of white hairs.

Roll cotton (cotton wool) rather than combine roll may be used for the proximal portion of carpal bandages, because it stays in position best. Roll cotton is particularly useful for reducing soft tissue swelling after desmotomy of the accessory ligament of the superficial digital flexor tendon. A nonadherent layer and conforming gauze are covered by elastic adhesive bandaging tape before application of a full-limb padded bandage. This provides protection of the wound from the environment and prevents hematoma and seroma formation. Care must be taken to avoid excessive tension being applied to the elastic adhesive tape to prevent pressure necrosis.

Pressage Bandages

Pressage bandages (S.C. Meades, Cardiff, Wales) are commercially produced elasticized bandages designed specifically for the carpus and hock and available in three sizes. They provide an excellent method of securing a light bandage in place and providing pressure, with a minimal risk of pressure sores, and are used routinely by one author (SJD). Two turns of an elastic conforming bandage over the proximal extent of the Pressage bandage and application of a stable bandage in the more distal part of the limb help to keep the Pressage bandage from slipping.

Ether Bandages

Ether bandages are used to cover surgical incisions, but they do not provide any compression to the incision. For the ether bandage to stay, the area to which it is applied must be clipped or preferably shaved. Cleansing of the skin with surgical scrub, followed by alcohol rinsing, provides the best environment on which to apply this bandage. Strips of adhesive elastic tape approximately 15 cm in length are cut, and ether is applied to the adhesive side of the bandage tape. The ether-soaked bandage is then applied over gauze sponges and held in place while the ether evaporates and the adhesive dries to the skin and elastic tape. Three or four strips of elastic tape typically are used. Ether bandages are extremely adherent and very useful to protect surgical wounds made for stifle arthroscopy, bone grafts from the tuber coxae, and plate fixation of the olecranon (Figure 86-1). Because of the explosive nature of ether, proper precautions should be followed in its use and storage. Commercially available Primapore (Smith and Nephew) or Coverderm (DeRoyal, Powell, Tennessee, United States) dressings provide a simpler alternative but are less adherent.

Stent Bandages

Stent bandages are towels or gauze rolls that are sutured over wounds to protect the wound from the environment or to relieve tension at the sutured site. A sterile hand towel or gauze sponges, rolled like a cigar to the proper width of

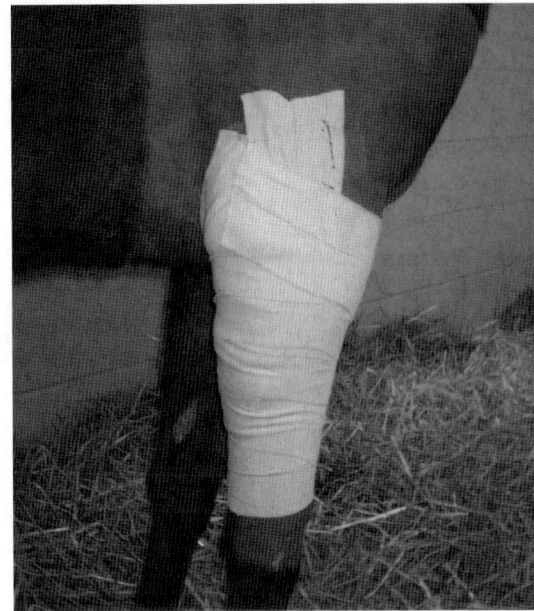

Fig. 86-1 • Application of an ether bandage over an incision for repair of a fractured olecranon in a yearling.

the wound, are sutured over the wound with No. 2 or larger suture. A cruciate pattern is usually used. Stent bandages are used after shoulder arthrotomy, after olecranon or femur fracture repair, to cover wounds over the point of the hock, and for other incision sites unsuitable for bandaging. If the stent is to be changed routinely, then loop sutures are placed on both sides of the incision, and umbilical tape can be used as suture to hold the bandage in place between changes.

Wet-to-Dry Bandages

Wet-to-dry bandages are used to absorb exudates and to provide an environment conducive to wound healing, particularly in the proliferative phase of wound healing. After cleansing of the wound, sterile sponges moistened with saline solution are applied to the wound and held in place with normal bandaging techniques. The bandage is changed daily, or as needed, and the process can be repeated as often as necessary until a granulation bed has formed.

With any wound there is a combination of dressings, bandaging, immobilization, and systemic therapy that is appropriate. The management changes as the wound heals, and sometimes alternative strategies need to be adapted. Careful attention to the progress of the wound and understanding of wound healing principles optimize outcome.

Foot Poultice

If a subsolar abscess is suspected, applying a poultice may be necessary, along with foot soaks, to soften the sole to permit drainage and to draw the abscess. A commercial poultice such as Animalintex (3M Animal Care Products; Robinson Animal Healthcare, Chesterfield, United Kingdom) is the simplest to use. A half piece is usually adequate. It should be thoroughly soaked in hot water and partially squeezed out before being applied to the sole of the foot. The poultice is covered by a thick layer of cotton wool, and then conforming bandage is wrapped around the foot to hold the poultice in position. To keep the moisture in, the foot can be placed in a used intravenous fluid bag, which is then covered by duct tape to provide a durable bandage.

Robert Jones Bandage

A Robert Jones bandage is used when additional support or compression is required. The bandage is particularly useful for immobilizing the limb of a horse with a suspected fracture for transport or for recovery from general anesthesia after fracture or wound repair—for example, after lag screw repair of a simple proximal phalangeal fracture or a condylar fracture of the third metacarpal bone. The Robert Jones bandage also can provide limb support if the suspensory apparatus is disrupted, can control severe posttraumatic limb edema, and can provide substantial pain relief to a horse with a severely injured superficial digital flexor tendon. This bandage has a multilayered construction. Compared with a single-layered bandage, a Robert Jones bandage compresses air-filled cotton wool layers to increase rigidity and spread pressure evenly. A half-limb bandage requires four to five rolls of cotton wool, eight to 10 conforming bandages, and three to four rolls of elastic adhesive tape. A full-limb bandage needs twice as much. For a half-limb bandage for a forelimb, the cotton wool should be applied snugly from the foot to the distal aspect of the carpus, incorporating the foot. The first layer, using one and a half to two rolls of cotton wool, should be 2 to 3 cm thick. This layer is then compressed using several conforming bandages at least 15 cm wide. Each bandage is applied using fairly firm, constant pressure to compress the cotton wool evenly. Filler layers of cotton wool usually are needed at the top and bottom of the bandage to create a uniform cylinder. A length of cotton wool is folded in half and placed around the top and bottom of the bandage as a filler layer. Another 2- to 3-cm layer of cotton wool is then applied and is compressed using a conforming bandage. At least three layers are constructed to create a thickness of 6 to 8 cm. The entire length of the bandage is then covered with elasticized tape, which should extend the entire length of the bandage and above and below it, to prevent dirt and bedding material from getting into the bandage. The end of one roll of elasticized bandage and the beginning of the next should overlap to prevent unraveling of the bandage. The end of the last roll is covered by zinc oxide tape. A full-limb bandage is applied similarly. In a forelimb the bandage should extend the entire length of the limb, incorporating the elbow; in a hindlimb the bandage should extend to the proximal aspect of the tibia.

Splinting

Splints should be used to support unstable fractures, when disruption of the suspensory apparatus is suspected, and when a full-limb Robert Jones bandage is used to provide additional support. Proper splinting helps protect bone from further trauma, prevents further soft tissue damage, and may also increase the horse's comfort. Wood or plastic guttering (diameter about 112 mm), cut in half to give a U shape, can be used. Polyvinyl chloride (PVC) piping is lightweight, inexpensive, and strong, but wood is generally more suitable for lateral splints. The length of the splint

depends on the size of the horse and the position of the injury. It is critical that the splints be adequately padded, especially at the top and bottom, to avoid rub sores. A gutter splint can be padded throughout its entire length with cotton wool. Wooden splints should be padded at the top and bottom. The splint should be covered with elastic adhesive tape proximally and distally to prevent it from becoming damaged and developing rough, sharp edges. A splint generally is applied over the dorsum to immobilize the distal aspect of the limb. If a transverse or oblique fracture is suspected, or if support of the suspensory apparatus is lost, the limb should be splinted to align the dorsal cortices of the third metacarpal bone and phalanges to eliminate the bending forces of the metacarpophalangeal joint. An assistant is needed to hold the limb off the ground, supporting it under the antebrachium. One layer of the Robert Jones bandage is applied, and then the splint is strapped to the dorsum of the limb before application of the second layer of the Robert Jones bandage. The splint should be well reinforced at the toe. If a sagittal plane fracture or subluxation or luxation of a joint is suspected, supporting the limb in its normal position is preferable. The splint then can be applied over the full thickness of the Robert Jones bandage. To immobilize the carpal region, or if a fracture in the midmetacarpal region is suspected, caudal and lateral splints are used, extending to the elbow (Figure 86-2). With a fracture of the midradius or proximal aspect of the radius, abduction of the limb is prevented by placement of a lateral splint extending from the ground to the middle of the scapula. The top of the splint must be well padded to prevent rub sores. With a fracture of the

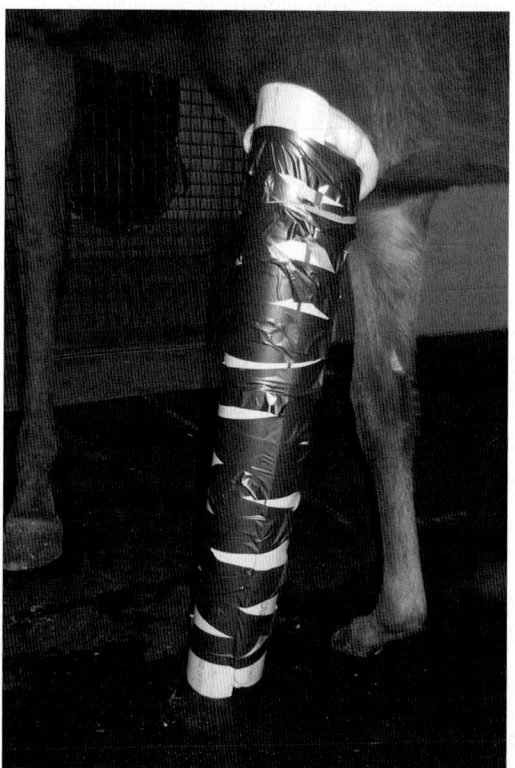

Fig. 86-2 • Full-limb forelimb bandage with lateral and caudal polyvinyl-chloride splints for an unstable diaphyseal third metacarpal bone fracture in a foal.

ulna and loss of triceps function, it is best to fix the carpus in extension by using a caudal splint extending from the ground to the proximal aspect of the olecranon. In some horses with olecranon fracture this type of splinting makes it more difficult to ambulate, and in those horses this splinting is not used initially. Similar principles apply in a hindlimb. Not all horses tolerate immobilization of a hindlimb, and the clinician must be prepared for the horse to react adversely when it first moves. For horses with fractures of the distal metatarsal region and distally, the limb is held above the hock by an assistant while the Robert Jones bandage and dorsal splint are applied. With a suspected fracture of the midmetatarsal and proximal metatarsal regions, the Robert Jones bandage should be applied with the limb bearing weight, and plantar and lateral splints are applied. The plantar splint should extend up to the proximal aspect of the calcaneus, to fix the tarsus to the distal limb fracture. Wood splints are stronger than gutter splints. Splinting of the hock and distal tibial regions aims to counteract the destabilizing effect of flexion of the stifle through the reciprocal apparatus. To immobilize the hock, a lateral splint is contoured to the angle of the hock by heating PVC gutter pipe over a flame, or by using a 12-mm steel rod that can be shaped by hand but is strong enough to provide support. The splint should extend to the proximal aspect of the tibia. An additional contoured splint can also be placed distal to the stifle and proximal to the fetlock on the plantar (caudal) side.

Several commercial splints are available that are particularly useful in an emergency situation, being easy to apply and rapidly providing pain relief by immobilization of the limb. These include the Kimzey Leg Saver Splint (Figure 86-3) (Kimzey, Woodland, California, United States) and the Monkey Splint (Kruuse, North Yorks, United Kingdom). They are all designed to align the dorsal cortices of the distal limb bones and are appropriate for fractures

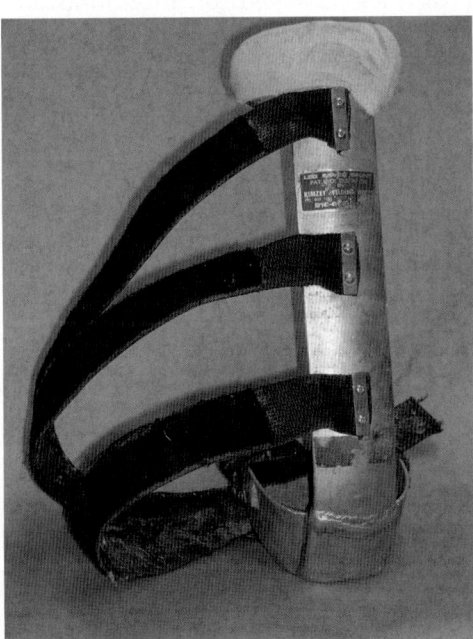

Fig. 86-3 • Kimzey Leg Saver Splint used for first aid treatment of traumatic disruption of the suspensory apparatus.

and luxations distal to the distal third of the metacarpal or metatarsal regions or suspensory apparatus breakdown. The Kimzey Splint also has an extension that reaches to the proximal aspect of the antebrachium and is suitable for use in horses with fractures up to the carpus.

TRANSPORT OF AN INJURED HORSE

With appropriate immobilization of a limb, a horse with a suspected fracture or major soft tissue injury can be safely transported long distances to a clinic with suitable diagnostic and surgical facilities and a skilled surgeon. Ideally the horse should be transported in a low-loading vehicle. Alternatively the horse should be loaded via a loading ramp, or with the ramp of the vehicle placed on a slope, so that the incline up the ramp into the vehicle is shallow. Ideally a horse with a forelimb injury should travel facing backward so that major load is placed on the hindlimbs when the vehicle decelerates. A horse with a hindlimb injury should travel facing forward. Appropriate but not excessive sedation may be required for transport of a fractious horse. A clinic expecting to receive such horses also should have a loading ramp to minimize the incline down which the horse has to walk when unloaded.

CAST BANDAGE

Cast bandages are a combination of a standard bandage, casting tape, and splint material (typically PVC). Clinical indications for this technique include management of wounds over the carpus, including transverse lacerations or hygroma resection. After placement of a standard bandage, two layers of cast material are placed over the bandage in the area to be splinted. The splint is then applied and held in place while at least two additional layers of casting tape are applied. In 2 to 3 days the cast material is split to create a bivalve to allow access to the surgical site. The cast can then be reapplied to provide immobilization.

CAST APPLICATION

Indications for cast application include after fracture repair or suturing of lacerated tendons or for wound management. Commonly used materials include plaster of Paris, resin-augmented plaster, and fiberglass. Fiberglass casting tape consists of knitted fiberglass fabric impregnated with polyurethane resin and is preferred and used most commonly because of its greater strength, lighter weight, and quicker setting times, despite increased cost. Full-limb (up to elbow or stifle) and half-limb (up to carpus or tarsus) casts can be applied. Full-limb casts are not well tolerated by all horses, and the horse's temperament should be assessed carefully, particularly before application of a full hindlimb cast. Casts are changed as needed because of rub sores, suture removal, inspection of the limb, and/or breaking or buckling of the cast, usually within 4 weeks after placement. In some circumstances a cast can be left on for up to 6 to 8 weeks; however, the risks of cast rubs increase the longer the cast is left on the horse The use of hydrocolloidal dressings (Tegaderm, 3M Health Care, St Paul, Minnesota, United States) directly over pressure points is useful

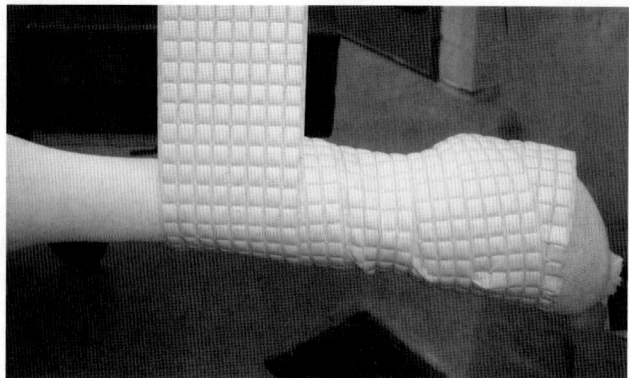

Fig. 86-4 • Procel Cast Liner being applied before fiberglass casting tape.

to prevent and/or treat cast rubs. The placement of a cast effectively lengthens the injured limb. Placement of a shoe equalizes the limb lengths and helps to prevent excessive weight bearing in the unaffected limb. Support of the contralateral foot with a wedge cuff shoe (Nanric Ultimate, Nanric, Lawrenceburg, Kentucky, United States) and sole support (Advanced Cushion Support, Nanric) is recommended if a horse is to be maintained in a cast for a long time.

Casts can be applied in a conscious, sedated horse but are commonly applied with the horse under general anesthesia, after internal fixation or wound repair. The limb should be clean and dry before cast application. Sterile dressings are applied over the surgical site, and a thin layer of nonbinding material such as cotton cast padding should be used to secure the wound dressings. A double layer of sterile stockinette is applied over the limb and extends above the proximal extent of the cast. Four to 5 cm of orthopedic felt is placed at the proximal extent of the cast. Wider felt is used for full-limb casts. In addition, orthopedic felt with the centers cut out can be placed over bony prominences, such as the styloid processes or accessory carpal bone in full-limb casts, to avoid rubs. The felt is secured with adhesive tape. Wire can be placed through holes made in the hoof wall near the toe and secured to a twitch handle to provide a means for an assistant to hold the limb and maintain the proper angle of the digit. In general, the hoof is placed at or near a weight-bearing position. Alternatively, the hoof can be extended to a lesser extent by manual pressure at the toe. Cast padding is applied and overlapped about 50%. The use of 3M Custom Support Foam (3M Healthcare), which has a polyurethane resin–impregnated cast padding, is helpful in reducing cast rubs. Another cast padding product is Procel Cast Liner (W.L. Gore and Associates, Flagstaff, Arizona, United States), which remains dry and allows the skin to remain dry through evaporation (Figure 86-4). It is important not to use too much cast padding, because the cast will compress it and the cast will become loose, predisposing

the horse to rub sores. Casting tape (3M Scotchcast, 3M Healthcare; 10 to 12 cm wide) is applied, beginning on the orthopedic felt at the top of the cast. The material is spiraled down the limb, taking care not to apply it too tightly, while avoiding wrinkles. Because the limb is not a perfect cylinder, wrinkles tend to develop in areas where contouring is necessary. Tension across the width of the casting tape eliminates potential folds or wrinkles. The next roll of casting tape begins where the first leaves off. At least five rolls of casting tape are used on the limb to construct a half-limb cast, and sometimes one or two additional rolls. When this is complete, more casting tape should be applied at the fetlock and distally, because this is the most common site of breakage. If the distal limb is extended using wires through the hoof wall, the toe region is not cast until the rest of the limb is finished and the twitch handle is no longer necessary. The wire and twitch handle are removed and the foot is covered with one to two rolls of casting tape. If a heel wedge is required, folded casting tape or a wood wedge can be incorporated in the casting tape applied to the hoof. Polymethylmethacrylate (Technovit, Jorgenson Laboratories, Loveland, Colorado, United States) is applied to the bottom of the cast, especially if the cast is to remain more than 2 weeks, to prevent wearing through of the casting tape.

For application of a cast in a standing horse the same protocol is followed, except a 2.5- to 5-cm block is placed under the horse's hoof, so that the heel is left hanging slightly over the edge of the block, and the cast is applied. After the limb has been cast, the limb is lifted and casting tape and polymethylmethacrylate are applied to the hoof. When standing casts are applied for first aid treatment of unstable fractures, a dorsal splint can be incorporated to maintain the bony column in a straight line. Foot casts are useful in managing heel bulb lacerations and in the prevention of support limb laminitis.

Potential cast complications include rub sores and cast breakage. Rub sores can occur over any bony prominence or any area where cast folds or fingerprints are present. Common sites for cast rubs include the proximal dorsal metacarpal and metatarsal regions, proximal sesamoid bones, and heel bulbs in half-limb casts; and the elbow, distal aspect of the radius, accessory carpal bone, stifle, and point of the hock in full-limb casts. Increased lameness, fever, drainage, heat, foul odor, and swelling proximal to the cast are signs of cast rubs. Rub sores are common complications of cast application and usually are managed easily by cast change or removal. Failure to recognize rub sores can lead to serious problems, such as large wound defects, infections of synovial structures, or laminitis in the supporting limb. Proper application and careful monitoring of cast is essential to prevent serious rub sores.

Transfixation Pin Casts
The use of transfixation pin casts is discussed in Chapter 87.

Chapter 87

External Skeletal Fixation

David M. Nunamaker

HISTORY AND DEVELOPMENT

Using external skeletal fixation to treat fractures in the horse has only recently received some enthusiasm from equine surgeons. Although external skeletal fixation of fractures works well in small animals and has undergone periods of enthusiastic use, these same devices do not withstand the loads of weight bearing in an adult horse and therefore are not versatile enough to meet the needs of equine surgeons. Using transfixation pins in plaster, transfixation pins in fiberglass casts, or an external skeletal fixation device, has allowed salvage of some horses with difficult fractures that could not have been saved using internal fixation (Figure 87-1).

The incorporation of a walking bar cast, with transfixation pins placed in the bone above the fracture, was described in 1991 to manage fractures in horses and ponies.[1] An overall success rate of 57% was reported for a variety of fractures in 35 horses and 21 ponies. The authors suggested that using transfixation pins incorporated into the cast material may help prevent fracture through these pin sites. Major complications of the technique included infection in nine horses or ponies, fracture through the bone or pin sites in six horses or ponies, and loss of circulation to the distal phalanx in two horses or ponies. Complications in the remaining seven nonsurvivors were not reported.[1] Using in vitro tests, McClure and colleagues[2,3] suggested that a walking bar was not necessary when using fiberglass casts and that divergent transfixation pins may be helpful in preventing fracture through the pin tract sites.

Although transfixation pins have been used successfully in fiberglass casts, this technique represents a compromise compared with classical external skeletal fixation. In horses managed with transfixation pin casts, wounds, skin, and pin sites must be covered in the cast, and at the time of every cast change, fractures are remobilized, allowing fracture collapse or shortening of the limb segment. In addition, pin loosening, pin breakage, and local infection at pin sites are common sequelae of this form of transfixation pinning, often necessitating pin replacement through new pinholes. The use of tapered-sleeve pins (TSPs) in a fiberglass cast has been reported.[4] This technique increases the strength and durability of the pin and appears superior to use of unprotected pins alone, and fewer pins may be needed in the pin cast.[4] This technique is used as an intermediate step after removal of the newly designed TSP external skeletal fixation device (ESFD) (see later).

The development of an equine ESFD in our laboratory had its origins before the first horse was treated in 1981, and we described the design and development of that device in the first 15 horses in 1986.[5] The ESFD was designed to allow immediate full weight bearing in an adult horse

and was used in horses with severely comminuted fractures of the distal aspect of the limb, in which internal fixation was not indicated or was impossible to carry out. A follow-up study including five additional horses along with further development of the device was published in 1992.[6]

Although the previous models of the ESFD proved the feasibility of using external skeletal pin transfixation in a frame device for immediate full weight bearing in an adult horse, there were substantial problems associated with the treatment itself. The original device used three unprotected 9.6-mm–diameter centrally threaded stainless steel pins loaded in bending within the intact bone (the third metacarpal bone [McIII]) above the fracture site, with two sidebars that connected the pins to a ground support through a base plate that was nailed to the horse's hoof, much like a shoe. This allowed the forces of weight bearing to bypass a comminuted fracture with support through the pins, sidebars, and base. Six (22%) of 27 horses in which the original device was used developed fractures of the McIII through one of the pin holes (usually the proximal pin hole while wearing the device) either when wearing the device or shortly after removal of the device. Problems associated with catastrophic failure of the McIII through a pin hole after device removal were controlled by removing the device while the horse was standing rather than subjecting horses to the rigors of recovery from general anesthesia. After this modification there were no further incidents of McIII fracture after device removal (used in 12 horses without incident).

In 2001 we described a radical change of design of the transfixation pins that was aimed at reducing the incidence of these McIII failures through the pin holes.[7] Several horses treated with this new design as well as horses treated with the old design were among a larger group of 64 horses with comminuted proximal phalangeal fractures reported in 2004.[8]

Mechanics of External Skeletal Fixation

The normal loading regimen for a transfixation pin is in bending. This is similar to hanging a weight in the middle of a clothesline stretched between two poles. The weight of the object causes the clothesline to sag, which can be compared with bending of the transfixation pin when the horse's weight is transmitted down the bone through the pins to the sidebars. The amount of deflection in the pin is related to the load, the pin diameter, the pin material, the distance from the bone to the sidebar, and the cortex thickness. Pin stiffness is a function of the fourth power of its diameter, whereas pin deflection is proportional to the cube of the distance between the bone and the sidebars. These power relationships show that very small changes in pin diameter or distance to the sidebars make a large difference in the performance parameters of the device. Theoretically to prevent bending of the pin one should reduce the bone-sidebar distance to zero, and the pin diameter should approach infinity. Obviously these parameters are unacceptable in a clinical situation, in which skin and soft tissues represent a barrier to the zero distance, and large holes drilled into bone will decrease bone strength leading to failure, especially if the diameter of the hole is greater than 30% of the smallest cross-sectional diameter of the bone.[4]

References on page 1330

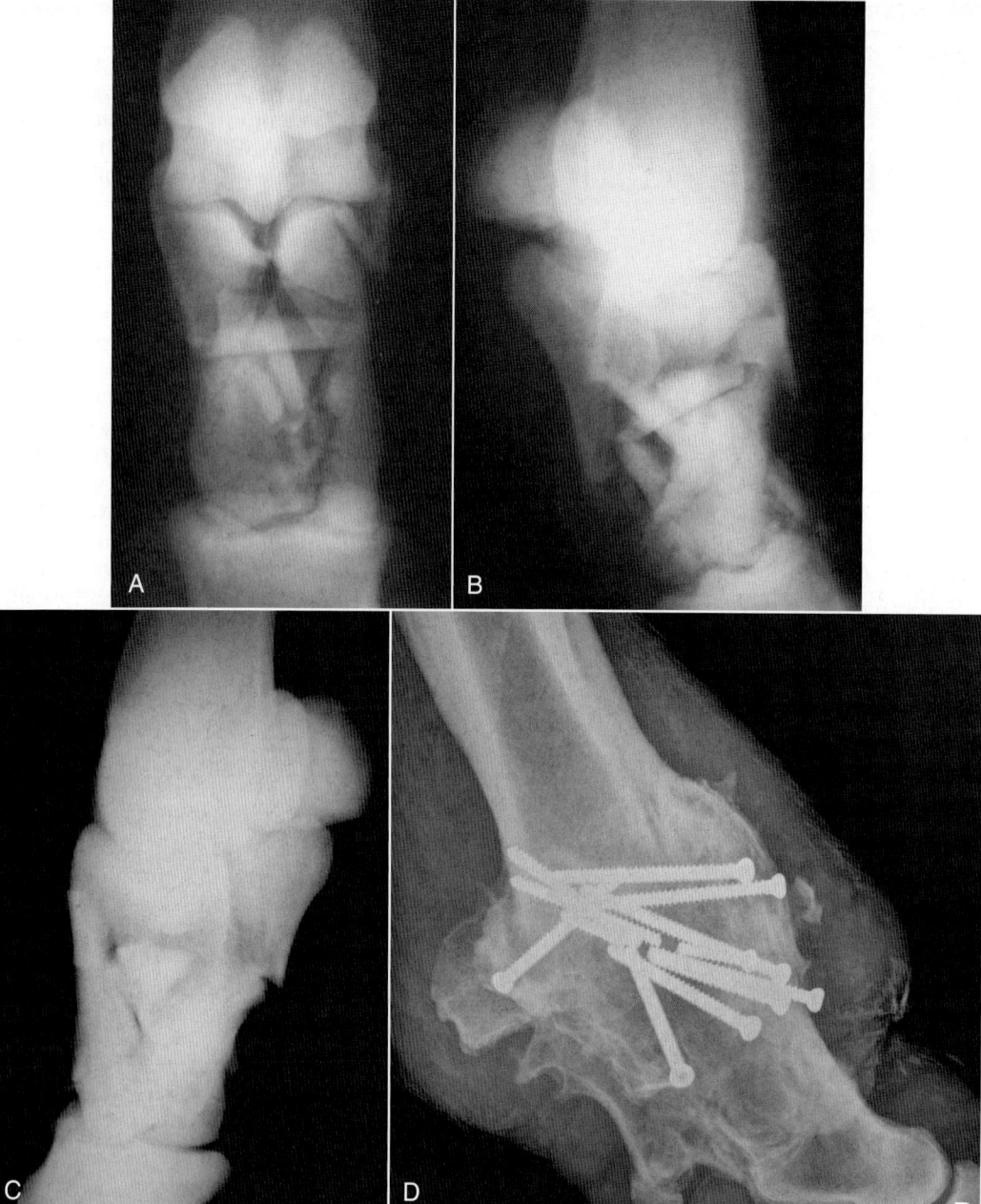

Fig. 87-1 • Dorsopalmar **(A)**, dorsolateral-palmaromedial oblique **(B)**, and dorsomedial-palmarolateral oblique **(C)** preoperative radiographic images show a severely comminuted fracture of the proximal phalanx. The fracture was open and the horse was managed using a tapered sleeve pin external skeletal fixation device. **D,** Five years after fracture there is radiological evidence of healing of the proximal phalanx and fusion of the metacarpophalangeal joint, but healing was delayed by motion (see broken screws). The proximal interphalangeal joint fused spontaneously, as usually occurs when the original fracture enters this joint. To date this mare has successfully foaled five offspring.

Up to 90% of the magnitude of the total stress at the bone-pin interface is attributed to stresses generated by the bending moment.[7] The highest stresses are seen on the surface of the bone at the pin junction, and because bone fails (breaks) at about 2% strain regardless of load, lowering the bone-pin stress should allow an increased load before failure. The solution for this problem was to load the pin uniformly in shear instead of bending to get a uniform load all along the pin as it passed through the bone.[7] To accomplish this goal we used transcortical pins that slid into a tapered sleeve. The TSP ends are threaded and compress the tapered sleeves against the bone when fasteners (nuts and lock washers) are used to provide tension in the pins. The pins are then biaxially loaded in tension via the nuts and in shear via the axial load on the bone (Figure 87-2).[7]

Although the device could be made in many sizes, it was sized for light horses, ranging from an adult Arabian to larger Warmblood crosses. It ideally fits Thoroughbred (TB) and Standardbred (STB) horses, in which the device has been used most frequently. Two 7.94-mm pins are incorporated into the tapered sleeve and attached through a welded collar steel tube system to the aluminum-magnesium

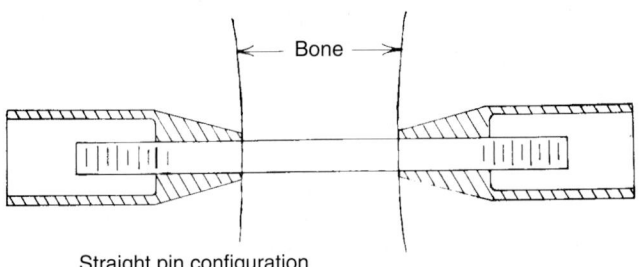

New Transcortical Pin
with Tapered Supports

Bone

Straight pin configuration

Fig. 87-2 • This drawing shows the concept of sleeves that slide over the transfixation pins to give protection from bending in the external skeletal fixation device. The large diameter of the sleeves and the proximity to the bone eliminate bending as a loading mode and ensure a more uniform loading on the pin in shear. This protects the outer bone cortex from the loads of a bending pin and allows the device to be loaded to about 10 times body weight before bone failure.

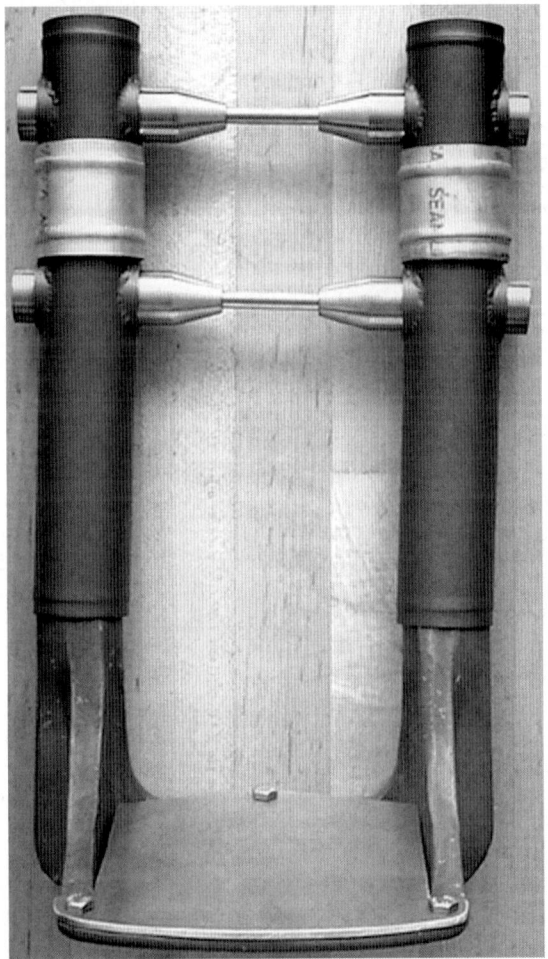

Fig. 87-3 • The present tapered sleeve pin external skeletal fixation device is shown. The device is assembled easily over the tapered sleeves using the footplate attached to the base.

base through an aluminum foot plate. The device is always applied with the horse under general anesthesia (Figure 87-3).

The TSP ESFD with all the tools to apply and remove it is commercially available (rane@magnolia-net.com,

Ron Nash Engineering, 977 Stephens Highway, Magnolia, Arkansas, United States).

PREOPERATIVE PLANNING, INDICATIONS, TIPS, AND LIMITATIONS

The TSP ESFD was designed to treat horses with catastrophic injuries of the distal limb. Indications include comminuted fractures of the proximal phalanx when no strut (intact piece of bone from the proximal to the distal articular surface) is available for use with internal fixation (see Chapter 35), comminuted fractures of the middle phalanx, fracture dislocations, or traumatic disruptions of the suspensory apparatus with massive soft tissue injury (see Chapters 36 and 104). Expanded use of the ESFD could be considered in horses with severe laminitis. In its present form the TSP ESFD is designed for use when the McIII or the third metatarsal bone (MtIII) is intact. The only other requirement is that the blood supply to the distal limb must be intact. In addition to applying the ESFD, it is sometimes helpful to insert bone screws, used in lag fashion through stab incisions, to hold large fragments together. This can be done under radiographic guidance, and these fixations do not need to resist weight-bearing forces, because the ESFD supports the entire weight of the horse. It is necessary that the hoof fits on the base plate of the device, and, if large, the hoof needs to be trimmed. This must be accomplished to allow the aluminum base plate to attach to the magnesium-alloy base using the three cap screws. A compression bandage (elastic bandage) is wrapped around the fractured bone before and during surgery to bring the bone fragments closer together and reduce swelling, which helps with reduction of badly comminuted fractures.

Abbreviated instructions for application of the TSP ESFD are included to show the simplicity of the system. The procedure is completed with the horse under general anesthesia. The only surgical requirement for application of the device is to drill two holes in the McIII, although additional internal fixation may be used when appropriate. The footplate is attached using a glue-on system (www.soundhorse. com). The limb is prepared for aseptic surgery. With the drill guide supplied, two 7.94-mm holes are drilled, one at the junction of the proximal and middle thirds and the other at the junction of the middle and distal thirds of the McIII from the lateral aspect. Holes are placed in the center of the bone and marrow cavity and perpendicular to the long axis of the bone. This is facilitated using the dual drill guide, which places the holes parallel and properly spaced. Next the 7.94-mm pins are inserted using the threaded cap to protect the threads. The sleeves over the pins are assembled on the medial and lateral sides and secured with nuts. The sleeve-skin junction is wrapped with a sterile bandage, and the rest of the assembly is performed using nonsterile technique. The side tubes are then assembled using ring connectors over the tapered sleeves on both sides of the limb. The base is slid into the distal ends of the tubes, and the base is fastened to the footplate using cap screws supplied. The reinforcing rods are then inserted into tubes on the medial and lateral sides, and electrical tape is placed around all the tubular junctions to prevent leakage. The fracture is reduced and stabilized by placing traction on the limb in a position that allows the tubes to be filled. The polymer (Conathane UC41, Cytec Industries, Olean, New

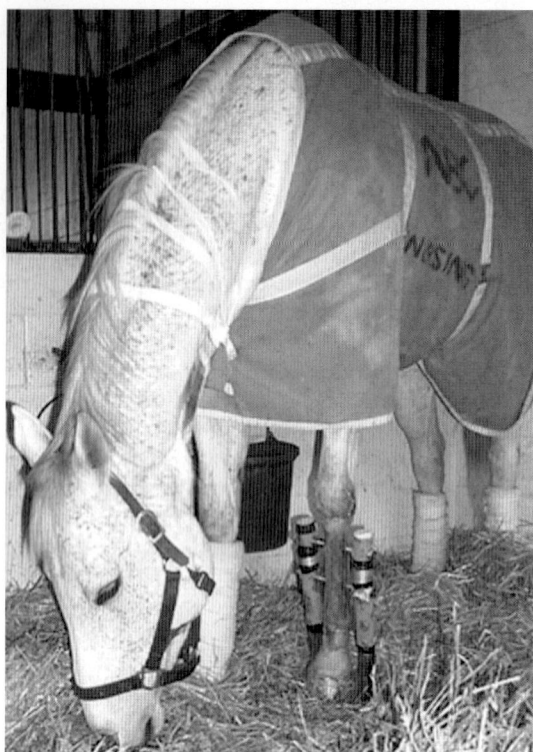

Fig. 87-4 • A tapered sleeve pin external skeletal fixation device is used to manage a horse with a comminuted fracture of the middle phalanx.

York, United States) is then mixed (2:1 by volume) and poured into the sidebars. The tubing is cooled, using cold saline solution if necessary, to prevent heating of the pins. Last, the now wet sterile wrap around the tapered sleeves is removed, and the ESFD is covered with a bandage. The horse is then recovered from general anesthesia. The current ESFD is shown being worn in Figure 87-4.

The contralateral foot often has a shoe applied that elevates the limb so that the horse stands squarely. Without this elevated shoe the horse has a tendency to point the foot in the TSP ESFD while standing. It is important to keep the horse standing squarely on both limbs to help prevent laminitis from occurring in the supporting, non-injured limb.

POSTOPERATIVE CARE

After recovery from general anesthesia the horse is immediately fully weight bearing and usually comfortable on the limb. In fact, this is a major advantage of this type of fracture management. Skin care around the pin sites is important during the initial postoperative period and is done easily using antiseptic-soaked sponges. The TSP ESFD is checked for tightness using an appropriate deep socket wrench every few days. Pin loosening does not occur, because one has the ability to tighten the pins with the fastener nuts already in place, which is easily done and does not require sedation of the horse. Reducing pin loosening helps to diminish pin tract infections and allows the horse to remain fully weight bearing. Local antiseptic application at the pin sites may decrease severity of pin site infections. Some horses may be discharged from the hospital with the TSP ESFD in place. If the owner or trainer

can provide pin care, discharging the horse as soon as possible decreases the cost of hospitalization. The horse is returned to the hospital for removal of the TSP ESFD after 8 to 10 weeks. Although the device can be left on longer, substantial osteoporosis of the McIII or the MtIII below the lowest pin may be detrimental to the end result. Radiologically the fracture site may not appear healed (based on the observation of mature callus) at this time, because osteoid will have formed, but calcification of this soft callus will not yet have occurred without the stimulus of weight bearing. The TSP ESFD is removed in the standing, sedated horse, and a fiberglass cast is applied. Serial radiographic examinations are then performed until radiological evidence of fracture healing is visible. Spontaneous fusion of the proximal interphalangeal joint will occur in horses with comminuted fractures of the proximal phalanx. If arthrodesis of the metacarpophalangeal or metatarsophalangeal joint is necessary, additional internal fixation, usually screws alone, will be needed because spontaneous fusion rarely occurs (see Figure 87-1). Most horses with fractures of the proximal phalanx managed with the TSP ESFD need arthrodesis of the metacarpophalangeal or metatarsophalangeal joint to maintain comfort.

REMOVING THE EXTERNAL SKELETAL FIXATION DEVICE

Removal of the ESFD is accomplished with the horse standing, with use of light sedation and a special pin removal device supplied by the manufacturer. The foot plate is removed using a sharp box knife, cutting the material at the junction of the hoof and plate.

An electric Sawzall or hacksaw can be used to cut the lateral sidebar tube just below the lower tapered sleeve on one side of the frame very quickly.

The nuts are removed from the threaded pins on the tapered sleeves. The pin extractor is placed over the distal tapered sleeve and the pin engaged and removed by turning the extractor with an end wrench. This is repeated as necessary on the proximal tapered sleeve. Once the pins have been removed, the frame can be lifted away. A standing cast is usually applied to preserve the structure and function of the extremity for an additional time until healing is sufficient for unrestricted weight bearing. It is at this juncture that the TSPs can be incorporated into the cast if desired. Radiographic examination is helpful in making these decisions.

RESULTS OF TREATMENT (2008)

Of 27 horses managed with the original ESFD (three 9.6-mm unprotected pins through the McIII or the MtIII) over a period of 14 years, nine survived (33%). The complication of the McIII or the MtIII fracture through pin sites in six horses led us to abandon this device and introduce the two-pin TSP ESFD in 1996. Early experience with the TSP ESFD has been favorable, and five (71%) of seven horses survived; only one horse developed a fracture through the pin site. Both nonsurvivors had chronic infections of the original fracture site and laminitis on the contralateral forelimb. Four fractures were open, six were comminuted fractures of the proximal phalanx (see Figure 87-1), and one was a comminuted fracture of the middle phalanx.

ferences
on page
1330

Chapter 88

Counterirritation

David R. Ellis and Stephen P. Dey III

BRIEF HISTORY AND OUTLINE OF TECHNIQUES

Counterirritation techniques have long been a part of veterinary therapy, particularly in horses. Major veterinary texts, such as those by Percivall,[1] Wooldridge,[2] and even Stashak[3] as late as 1987, devoted considerable attention to indications and techniques. To some this now seems misguided and even cruel, but one has to read only a few of the older texts to admire the authors' inquiring minds and their thorough observations on matters medical and particularly orthopedic. They were not far from the truth, but they did not have the benefit of modern anesthetics or imaging equipment to learn and apply more direct and rational therapies. Techniques currently used include hot or cold firing and blisters, but use of those therapies is much reduced because of changes in horse ownership and veterinary attitudes. This chapter considers both British (DRE) and North American (SPD) perspectives.

BLISTERING

Limited availability of ingredients and ignorance of preparation and safe use has restricted blistering of horses in the United Kingdom. Although veterinary surgeons or equine wholesalers are the source, the horse owner is usually the user. More severe blisters, such as those containing cantharides or croton oil, are used less commonly than the working blisters that are iodine or mercuric iodide based and mainly used on splints, sore shins, or curbs. The technique involves rubbing or brushing the liquid preparation onto the clipped skin once daily until a scale forms. The horse is kept in light exercise, such as walking, trotting, or hack cantering, and this phase usually is undertaken after the initial rest and antiinflammatory treatment have removed heat, swelling, and pain (i.e., 7 to 10 days after initial clinical signs). When the heat and soreness from counterirritation has settled, which takes 2 to 3 weeks, the horse resumes work.

Irritation from working blisters is minimal, and protective measures such as antiinflammatory treatment, keeping the horse crosstied, or fitting a bib or cradle are not necessary.

Strong blister was made mostly from cantharides (Spanish fly) or croton oil, but nowadays these ingredients are difficult to obtain and, because they are not licensed drugs in the United Kingdom, are probably illegal for a veterinary surgeon to import without a permit. As a consequence the strong blister that is used most commonly is made as a cream using red mercuric iodide. The skin is clipped and the blister rubbed into the area for 5 minutes. Excess is removed and petroleum jelly is applied to flexor surfaces distal to the blistered areas. The horse is kept shod

for blistering, in case it paws the ground, and a neck cradle is applied until the initial inflammatory phase has subsided. It is essential that the horse continues walking exercise, usually 30 minutes twice daily. A substantial risk of laminitis or lymphangitis exists if blistered horses do not have this regular exercise. When blisters form and burst, they are left alone and sprayed with antibiotic powder. Rarely is the reaction severe enough to warrant antiinflammatory treatment. After 10 days the blistered areas of the legs are smeared with petroleum jelly, which is left on overnight and then washed off with warm water and soft soap. This softens and lifts the scabs free, without causing bleeding or further irritation. Any blistered areas that are still moist are dressed with antibiotic wound powder, and walking is continued. Scabs that persist after 7 to 10 days are removed by repeating this procedure. After 6 weeks the horse can be turned out to pasture or start light ridden exercise. The program for a return to training depends on the nature and progress of the original injury.

Areas treated most commonly with strong blister are the digital flexor tendon region of forelimbs and the fetlock joints. Indications are tendonitis, tenosynovitis, suspensory desmitis, and chronic effusion of fetlock joints.

In North America, curbs frequently are treated by blistering (see Chapter 78), and both hindlimbs are usually treated. The area is clipped and rubbed aggressively for 3 minutes with medical-grade turpentine and then with kosher salt for 3 minutes, alternating for a total of 15 minutes. This is repeated once daily for 3 days. The horse is exercised immediately after each treatment for at least 20 minutes. The skin excoriates and remains thickened and inflamed for some time, but therapeutic effects are almost immediate.

Blistering also is used to manage suspensory desmitis, tendonitis, sesamoiditis, and other fetlock problems. The severity of the injury determines which blister is used and the degree of exercise modification. If horses with suspensory desmitis or tendonitis are being treated, the metacarpal or metatarsal region usually is wrapped (bandaged) with a gauze layer, a leg quilt, and a bandage to control swelling. Moving areas such as the carpus or tarsus are not wrapped.

The blistering process is allowed to continue for 5 days, and then a firing paint is applied to the area for another 7 days, with the bandages reset every day if the blistering process involves the metacarpal (metatarsal) or fetlock region. After the firing paint application period ends, usually an iodine glycerin-based product is applied every day to soften the blister scabs and help lift the outer skin layers that have separated. Once a horse begins to be painted with the firing paint, it can be exercised on a walker or in a small paddock. This reduces inflammation and begins to reestablish normal venous and lymphatic flow.

Internal blisters have more widespread use in North America compared with Europe. A 2% iodine mixture, in almond oil or a lighter base, can be injected into tissues. One author (SPD) treats muscle soreness by injection of 1 mL of internal blister per site using an 18-gauge needle of variable length, depending on the depth of the injection. The mechanism of action is unknown, but trainers usually report that the gait improves (see Chapter 47).

Internal blisters also are used to treat horses with suspensory desmitis, curbs, and splints. Varied results may reflect the inconsistency of the available products.

CAUTERY OR FIRING

Cautery or firing is performed less frequently in the United Kingdom since the Royal College of Veterinary Surgeons deplored the practice in 1991. Cautery or firing is used for horses with injuries to soft and hard tissues, and some clinicians and clients are still enthusiastic about its value. Pin or needle firing is the most common technique.

Cold firing is used mainly for horses with persistent sore shins or splints, and the thermal injury is made with liquid nitrogen (see Chapter 89). The procedure is done soon after the initial inflammatory phase has subsided and is preferred for horses with intractable injuries that have not responded to antiinflammatory measures or blisters. The area is clipped, the horse is sedated, and local anesthesia is administered. An ordinary firing iron can be cooled by leaving it in the liquid nitrogen, or a special "gun" point freezes a small area of skin. Spots of lubricant gel on the areas to be fired improve the contact. The pattern should not allow the frozen spots to be closer than 3 cm apart. No systemic or local treatment is needed, and the horse is kept in walking exercise for 6 weeks. Ultimately the skin develops persistent white point scars. Results have been good enough to ensure its continuing use, but the rationale is difficult to ascertain. Cold firing probably causes local analgesia of some duration within periosteal nerves and may necrose small areas of the periosteum and underlying cortical bone.

Acid firing enjoyed a vogue several years ago but has deservedly fallen from use. Concentrated nitric acid was soaked into a small cork, which was then pressed onto the clipped and desensitized skin. The inflammatory reaction was substantial, but, like line firing, acid firing appeared to affect only the skin and not the underlying tendon.

Line or bar firing was used for horses with tendonitis or curbs. For the lines to be made evenly, the area was clipped the day before firing and covered with a mustard plaster overnight, which caused subcutaneous edema to smooth out the grooves between the structures before firing. Curved, blade-shaped irons were used, and management was the same as for pin firing. One author (SPD) has minimal experience with this technique but agrees with Silver and colleagues[4] that it would not be "a useful therapeutic exercise."

Horses are still pin fired regularly in the United Kingdom. The procedure is used for horses with superficial digital flexor tendonitis, suspensory desmitis, and sesamoiditis and has value for those with persistently painful splints. Pin firing is no longer used for distal hock joint pain or carpitis. The horse is fired after the initial inflammatory response has subsided and when the area is no longer warm or painful, 4 to 6 weeks after the injury. The area is clipped and anesthetized before being dressed with surgical spirit. Firing is started 10 to 15 minutes later and patterned no closer than 3 cm apart over the structure being treated. It is important to use a fine point so that minimal burning of the adjacent skin occurs. The point penetrates the underlying tendon or periosteum. An iodine-based ointment is then applied, and petroleum jelly is smeared distally, particularly in the flexural regions of joints. The horse is crosstied, or fitted with a cradle, and walked in hand twice daily for 30 minutes. As for blistered horses, walking is essential. It is wise to keep front shoes on, and only rarely is analgesia indicated. The area is powdered with antibiotic daily and after 10 days is smeared with petroleum jelly, which is left on overnight and washed off the following morning, as previously described. Walking exercise continues for at least 6 weeks, and then the horse can start to spend increasing periods of time turned out in a paddock. The horse should not return to training for about 1 year after a soft tissue injury. Those horses that have had bony tissue fired, such as with splints, can return gradually to training after 6 weeks of walking.

In North America, pin firing is used mostly to treat horses with splints, curbs, tendon and ligament injuries, and fetlock and surrounding soft tissue injuries. A similar pattern is used for pin firing curbs and splints (SPD). Marks are made down the center of the lesion, 1 cm apart. Alternating rows, medially and laterally, 0.5 cm between the original marks, are then made. When firing tendons or ligaments, a similar pattern is used, but the point never goes through the deep layer of epidermis. However, areas of maximum damage are refired to ensure deeper penetration to focus the healing process. The horse may require sedation and analgesia for 24 hours after treatment to control pain. The area is painted with firing paint for 10 days; it is covered with gauze, a quilt, and bandage. Another 30 days of rest are required before reevaluation of the horse. The total convalescent period depends on the initial injury. In sports horses, use of cryotherapy to treat splints and some soft tissue injuries is more common. Although cryotherapy is less invasive, the procedure is often less effective (see Chapter 89).

Current thoughts on thermal injury to tissues still emphasize the gulf between veterinary science and veterinary practice. Although much excellent science has illuminated the injury and healing of strained tendons, such injuries are still the most substantial injuries a flat racehorse can sustain and are a long-term threat to the horse's continuing career. Horses that race over fences (steeplechasers) or hurdles seem to manage better than those that race at a faster pace on the flat. The expectation that counterirritation would produce a fiber pattern with crimp and better-quality collagen may have been ill-founded, but the successful results that veterinarians have experienced over the years need to be explained. Perhaps the mechanical side effect of pin fire scars, evening out the differing strength and elasticity along the length of the injured tendon and in the contralateral limb, has kept pin firing in equine orthopedics. Beyond enforced rest and low-grade exercise, seeing benefit accruing from blisters used in horses with tendon strain is difficult.

Aggressive antiinflammatory treatment in the early postinjury phase is important, but one author (DRE) is uncertain if subcutaneous corticosteroids are essential for a good long-term result.

Treatment regimens such as intralesional glycosaminoglycans or β-aminopropionitrile fumarate have disappointed, and the results of surgical splitting or desmotomy of the accessory ligament of the superficial digital flexor tendon have not always justified the expense in the United Kingdom. Prolonged rest and controlled exercise regimens seem as successful as any treatments.

The choice of treatment still emerges from consensus among the experiences of the veterinary surgeon, the trainer, and the owner. All equine veterinary surgeons share the fervent hope that successful and rational therapy for horses with strained flexor tendons will emerge soon.

Restrictions on using firing by the Royal College of Veterinary Surgeons were initiated by a question in the Houses of Parliament about the firing of horses. The Horserace Betting Levy Board then funded a research program by the Bristol group, led by Professor Ian Silver. This work was published in a supplement to the *Equine Veterinary Journal*.[4] Extensive discussion followed, but in 1991 the Royal College of Veterinary Surgeons tried to outlaw the technique of firing tendons by declaring that they deplored it and would bring disciplinary action against any member performing it. This was not well received by a substantial number of respected equine veterinary surgeons, and the policy was one that had been poorly thought through, did not recognize hard tissue firing, and proved to be unenforceable. A compromise was later reached, whereby veterinary surgeons had to show that other treatments had failed and to justify their choice of firing a particular horse. The technique continues to be used, but since the introduction of ultrasonography and the retirement of veterinarians who preferred it, the use of firing has diminished considerably. One author (DRE) believes that firing would have gradually disappeared without legislation.

Techniques currently used in equine orthopedics have become more conservative since the introduction of ultrasonography and the development of finer sensitivity among horse owners. The regular monitoring of these horses has enabled more rational advice to be given regarding healing of the lesions and programming of exercise. Thus the implementation of direct therapy has taken second place among certain groups of clinicians. They remain cynical about therapy while maintaining client confidence through regular observation of the horse. Splitting or needle decompression of a tendon core lesion soon after injury is a rational first step, followed by regular monitoring and controlled, graded exercise throughout a long convalescence. The old adage of "the longer the rest, the better" still seems valid.

ferences n page 1330

Chapter 89

Cryotherapy

Kjerstin M. Jacobs and Thomas P.S. Oliver

Cryotherapy has been used widely in veterinary medicine since the 1970s, primarily for tumor ablation. Percutaneous cryotherapy, called *freeze firing* or *freezing*, is a useful palliative technique for various musculoskeletal disorders in the horse, but little research has been published on specific techniques or results.[1-4] Most of the information in this chapter comes from our clinical experience using cryotherapy to manage selected lameness conditions. Cryotherapy generally is used for pain management, and our recommendations are made assuming the horse will continue or resume athletic performance. The term *cryotherapy* (cold therapy) is sometimes used to refer to intentional cooling of a body part to reduce inflammation or the effects of inflammatory mediators. For instance, cryotherapy is used to prevent laminitis by inducing digital vasoconstriction (see Chapter 34).

MECHANISMS OF CRYONECROSIS

Freezing mammalian tissue results in direct and indirect cell destruction. Direct cell injury occurs by formation of intracellular and extracellular ice crystals, which destroy cell walls and cause intracellular dehydration, respectively. Intracellular dehydration causes severe electrolyte concentration and pH shifts, which damage lipoprotein membranes and organelles. Loss of cellular homeostasis results in cell death. Indirect cell injury occurs by damage to the endothelium of arterioles and venules, causing increased vascular permeability, edema, and hemoconcentration. Local tissue damage occurs from thrombosis and infarction of small vessels. Two rapid-freeze, slow-thaw cycles are used. Rapid freezing maximizes intracellular crystal formation and crystal size. Slow thawing causes additional cell damage by a process of recrystallization, during which time crystals increase in size before melting. Precooled tissue freezes faster than normal tissue; therefore a second freeze-thaw cycle optimizes the processes of tissue destruction.

Because cryotherapy causes tissue destruction in situ, fibrous structures such as epineurium remain intact. This allows for regeneration of large myelinated nerves. Experimental percutaneous cryotherapy of equine palmar and plantar digital nerves resulted in neuropraxia (temporary ablation of nerve function, with the axons remaining intact) or axonotmesis (wallerian degeneration of axonal tissue, with the fibrous supportive tissue remaining intact). All nerves regenerated.[5] The degree of nerve damage is temperature dependent, with lower temperatures resulting in longer duration of analgesia.[6]

Presumably, percutaneous cryotherapy causes destruction of local type C nerve fibers. Type C fibers are small, unmyelinated, nociceptive nerve fibers that contribute to chronic pain. The inflammatory response to cryotherapy appears to cause thickening and fibrosis of certain soft tissues, such as the suspensory ligament and subcutaneous tissues, and although this effect has not been studied, the clinical result is a stronger ligament and one less likely to be reinjured in the same location. Cryogens must be used judiciously on the distal aspect of the limb to avoid cryonecrosis of tendon, ligament, joint tissues, or cortical bone.

BASIC TECHNIQUE

Cryotherapy instruments and cryogens are described elsewhere, and only basic principles are discussed here.[7-9] Instruments used to apply cryogens vary from simple cryoprobes to cryounits with continuous closed-system flow of cryogen liquid. We use liquid nitrogen that is stored in a commercial 10- to 20-L tank. For all techniques we use individual brass probes, 1.5 cm in diameter (Figure 89-1), precooled in liquid nitrogen and positioned on the lesions for a double freeze-thaw cycle consisting of freezing (60 seconds), thawing (60 seconds), and freezing (60 seconds). Local edema formation is minimal and has no effect on the second freezing cycle. Earlier work suggested that a thaw duration of 15 seconds was optimal, but our modified cycle appears effective.[4] We prefer to use solid metal probes, because consistent freezing to a specific depth is easy to control (Figure 89-2). The cooling ability of solid metal probes has been questioned, but in one study solid metal probes were most effective in freezing to specific depths.[7]

Cryotherapy is well tolerated by most horses, but sedation and a twitch are used. Local analgesia (a ring block proximal to the freeze site) may be necessary for highly

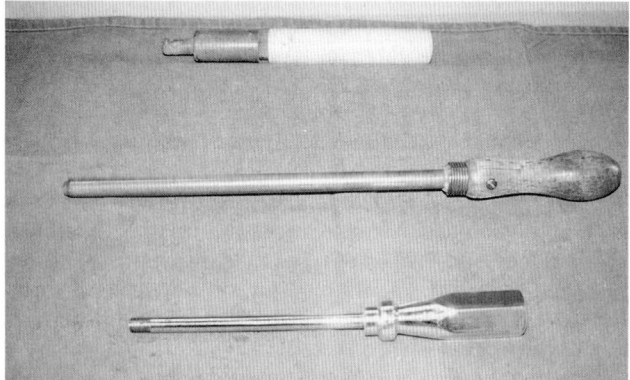

Fig. 89-1 • Solid brass cryoprobes commonly used for cryotherapy in the horse.

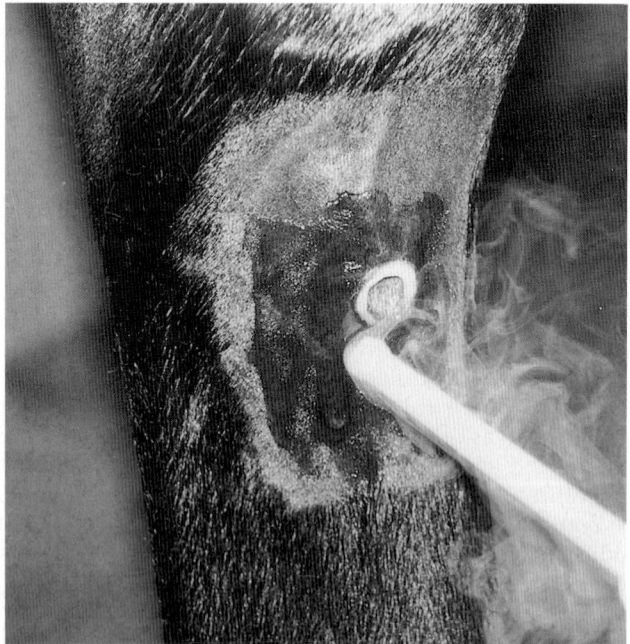

Fig. 89-2 • Cryotherapy is being used to manage pain associated with an exostosis of the fourth metatarsal bone in a Standardbred racehorse. A double freeze-thaw cycle has been used in one site, and the probe is being applied at a distal site.

strung or fractious horses. The area over the lesion is clipped with a No. 40 blade and cleaned of gross contamination with iodophor or chlorhexidine solution. The limb is dried, and a 0.5-cm–thick layer of water-soluble gel is applied generously over the site. This layer provides a template to ensure accurate positioning for the second freeze cycle.

The metal probe tip is applied to the skin for 60 seconds, then removed to allow thawing, and reapplied (see Figure 89-2). No benefit accrues from a third freeze-thaw cycle, and in fact a third cycle may lead to underlying bone necrosis. Freeze sites should be located 1 cm apart in staggered, parallel rows that cover the lesion site and extend 1.5 cm beyond the margins of the lesion. If freezing sites are closer than 1 cm, the areas of skin necrosis will coalesce and later slough.

After completion of the procedure, the leg is cleaned of lubricant and the sites are covered with an antibacterial spray. The leg should be left unbandaged, but it is kept dry, and antibacterial spray is applied daily until skin healing is complete. Local soft tissue swelling and edema develop and persist for 7 to 10 days and then gradually resolve. The administration of antiinflammatory agents should be avoided, because this medication limits the intended effect of cryotherapy. Percutaneous cryotherapy destroys melanocytes in skin cells, so hair regrowth will be white. This negative cosmetic effect should be considered when discussing complications of cryotherapy.

TREATMENT OF SPECIFIC LESIONS

Diagnosis always should be confirmed using diagnostic analgesia, because results obviously are improved if the painful area is identified correctly. Most horses return to full function and race performance within several days to weeks, but some (e.g., those treated for severe suspensory desmitis) require up to 120 days of rest after treatment. When managing horses with suspensory desmitis, rest is paramount but is a source of frustration for trainers and owners, who often want to rush a horse back to the races.

Splint Exostoses (Splints)

Horses with exostoses of the second, third, and fourth metacarpal and metatarsal bones should not be treated until acute inflammation has subsided, because cryotherapy may exacerbate periosteal reaction. Horses are given 2 weeks of rest during which a poultice is applied for 5 days, followed by the application of a cedar oil blister for 5 to 7 days. Scurf from the blister is removed by sweating before cryotherapy is performed. Horses with chronic splints can be managed with cryotherapy without this 2-week preparation period. After cryotherapy in any horse, stall rest is recommended for 3 to 5 days. The horse then may be jogged or galloped lightly and brought back into full training within 7 to 10 days after treatment. Prognosis is good for return to racing. The procedure may be repeated at the same site, or at additional sites, if pain recurs or new sites develop.

Second and Fourth Metacarpal or Metatarsal Bone Fractures

Ostectomy of distal fragments of the second or fourth metacarpal or metatarsal bones is ideal, but in some horses surgery is not an option and cryotherapy can provide analgesia. Acute inflammation must be resolved before treatment. A single freeze site is placed directly over the fracture site, and four more sites are frozen in a circular pattern around the fracture site. Prognosis and rest depend mostly on extent of associated suspensory desmitis, if present, because horses with simple splint bone fractures can return to work immediately. Horses with mild suspensory desmitis have a good prognosis for return to racing and usually receive 60 days of rest after cryotherapy. Horses with severe suspensory desmitis require a minimum of 120 days of rest and have a guarded prognosis.

Periostitis of the Third Metacarpal Bone (Bucked Shins)

Cryotherapy can be used to manage pain associated with bucked shins (see Chapter 102) once acute inflammation has subsided. A dorsal cortical fracture of the third metacarpal bone must be ruled out, because cryotherapy in horses with fracture is contraindicated. Once swelling and palpable pain resolve, cryotherapy is performed using three vertical rows of eight or nine freeze sites per row. After cryotherapy, 2 weeks of stall rest with handwalking followed by 4 weeks of turnout exercise is given. Prognosis is excellent, and few horses require additional treatments.

Suspensory Desmitis

Ultrasonography must be performed first to determine the severity and extent of desmitis (see Chapters 16 and 72). Before cryotherapy, acute inflammation is managed using rest, antiinflammatory medication, and local therapy, such as cold-water hosing and poultice application. Cryotherapy is then performed using a vertically oriented row of freeze sites, beginning 3 cm proximal and extending 3 cm distal to the lesion. It is crucial that freeze sites be 1 cm apart and that each site be located directly over the body of the suspensory ligament and not over the deep and superficial digital flexor tendons. Cryotherapy is performed over each affected branch. If suspensory body desmitis is present, the procedure is performed on the medial and lateral aspects. Horses are given a minimum of 2 weeks of stall rest with handwalking, followed by 2 weeks of turnout or swimming physiotherapy. The suspensory ligament and overlying tissue become fibrotic and rigid after treatment, and, although tissue may appear strong to laypersons and the horse may be sound at the walk and trot, it is essential to recommend a conservative return to training and racing. Prognosis always is guarded, but most Standardbred racehorses return to racing. Suspensory desmitis is often a compensatory condition caused by contralateral limb lameness, or lameness in a diagonal or ipsilateral limb, and management of the primary problem is critical in decreasing recurrence of suspensory desmitis. Cryotherapy is seldom effective for long-term management of suspensory desmitis if primary lameness continues. After developing suspensory desmitis, horses may drop in race class and value, but cryotherapy has been a useful adjunct in managing pain and allowing continued racing. The Editors believe that cryotherapy should not be performed for suspensory branch and body lesions in Thoroughbred racehorses because of the risk of catastrophic failure of the suspensory ligament (see Chapter 104).

Distal Hock Joint Pain (Bone or Jack Spavin, Cunean Tendonitis)

Cryotherapy is useful in managing horses with distal hock joint pain. A double horizontal row of freeze sites over the proximal and distal borders of the cunean tendon is used. The horse is given stall rest with handwalking for 2 weeks. Prognosis is excellent for return to racing in the Standardbred racehorse.

Osteoarthritis of the Proximal Interphalangeal Joint

Chronic pain from osteoarthritis of the proximal interphalangeal joint (see Chapter 35) may be alleviated partially by cryotherapy. Cryotherapy is most useful in horses in which palmar digital neurectomy fails to abolish all pain originating from the proximal interphalangeal joint, especially in those with severe bone lysis and proliferation and in which arthrodesis is not an option. Pain relief sometimes can be achieved by placing cryotherapy sites 1 cm apart, encircling the proximal interphalangeal joint proximal to the lesion, and directly over the sites of bony proliferation. It is important to avoid the superficial digital flexor and deep digital flexor tendons. After treatment, horses are given stall rest with handwalking for a minimum of 3 weeks. Prognosis is guarded.

Curb

Curb, a collection of injuries located along the distal, plantar aspect of the tarsus, can be managed successfully using cryotherapy (see Chapter 78). Acute inflammation must be resolved, a process that may take as long as 7 to 10 days. The number of cryotherapy sites depends on the size of the curb, but 8 to 12 sites are usually required. Horses are given stall rest with handwalking for 2 to 3 weeks, but further rest depends on the structure involved and severity of initial lameness. The technique works best on horses with curb as a result of inflammation of the peritendonous tissue or mild superficial digital flexor tendonitis (see Chapter 78). Prognosis is usually good, but some horses require additional treatment within 6 to 12 months.

Cryoneurectomy

Cryotherapy can be useful to provide analgesia to the palmar or plantar aspect of the digits, but the degree of cryoanalgesia depends on the technique used. Percutaneous cryoneurectomy has limited clinical use, because only temporary pain relief (3 to 4 weeks) is achieved.[5] Cryoneurectomy has been found to be more effective in producing neuroanalgesia than simple transection, but the former procedure requires a surgical approach.[10] The nerves are exposed and transected, and the proximal ends are frozen.

A modified approach can be used.[5] The palmar or plantar digital nerves are exposed, and a double freeze-thaw technique is used to freeze the nerve within the perineurium, but the nerve is not transected. Analgesia is longer than with percutaneous cryotherapy, but having to expose the nerves limits the practical application of this technique.

Tendonitis

We feel that management of superficial digital flexor or deep digital flexor tendonitis with cryotherapy is contraindicated. After cryotherapy, fibrous tissue formation along the tendon fibers and possible scarring and adhesions of the digital flexor tendon sheath can occur and limit prognosis. Although we are aware of horses that have raced after cryotherapy for tendonitis, we suggest that other management options be explored (see Chapters 69 and 70).

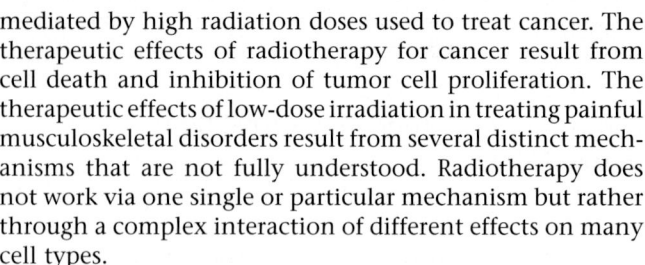

Chapter 90

Radiation Therapy

Alain P. Théon

References
on page
1330

Radiation therapy is the use of ionizing radiation to treat people and animals with malignant tumors and, occasionally, selected benign diseases. These diseases can be classified as inflammatory, degenerative, and hyperproliferative. The analgesic action of ionizing radiation for chronic orthopedic conditions has long been recognized and was first reported soon after the discovery of x-rays.[1] The effectiveness of radiotherapy has been demonstrated in people with painful, degenerative joint diseases that were refractory to first-line conservative treatment—for example, nonsteroidal antiinflammatory drugs (NSAIDs) and physiotherapy.[2] In horses radiation therapy was found to be effective for painful degenerative and inflammatory musculoskeletal conditions early in the development of veterinary radiation therapy.[3] However, limited access to treatment facilities for horses, fear of the long-term hazards of ionizing radiation, and the availability of potent antiinflammatory drugs have decreased the impact of radiation therapy in the overall management of equine lameness. Although most clinical studies on using radiation therapy for equine chronic orthopedic conditions were reported in the 1960s and the 1970s, interest is currently renewed because of a better understanding of the mechanisms of action of radiation and identification of specific indications for treatment. The emergence of the specialty of veterinary radiation oncology will provide the expertise and personnel for expanding the applications of radiation therapy for treatment of noncancerous conditions at veterinary schools and private referral practices. Controlled studies are required to validate the experience-based indications, compare radiation therapy with other treatment options, and improve radiation parameters (single and total dose and fractionation). Several clinical trials have been undertaken at our institution, but adequate long-term observations and reliable assessment of clinical data according to objective orthopedic criteria are difficult to document.

RADIOBIOLOGICAL ASPECTS

Radiotherapy of nonmalignant conditions requires low doses of radiation, usually one fifth to one tenth the dose used in cancer treatment. The radiobiological mechanisms involved in the therapeutic effects of low-dose radiation used for benign conditions are different from those mediated by high radiation doses used to treat cancer. The therapeutic effects of radiotherapy for cancer result from cell death and inhibition of tumor cell proliferation. The therapeutic effects of low-dose irradiation in treating painful musculoskeletal disorders result from several distinct mechanisms that are not fully understood. Radiotherapy does not work via one single or particular mechanism but rather through a complex interaction of different effects on many cell types.

Early data indicating an increase in dermal blood flow and cutaneous temperature after treatment[4] led to the misconception that radiation therapy produces a deep counterirritation that promotes increased blood flow and cell recruitment to the treated area to expedite healing.[5] This theory, however, is not supported by any current data. The previously observed effects merely reflect inaccurate dosimetry that resulted in high radiation doses to the skin. In addition, evidence shows that counterirritation during the chronic stage of inflammation prolongs healing time and results in further damage.[6]

Modern theories on mechanisms of low- to medium-dose radiation for treatment of noncancerous conditions are based on new experimental data. The mechanisms are grouped into antiinflammatory effects, analgesic effects, and antiproliferative effects.

Antiinflammatory Effects

Whereas good evidence exists that high radiation doses induce strong inflammation in normal tissues, equally good evidence exists that low radiation doses have the opposite effect in inflamed tissues. Low-dose radiation therapy has a pronounced antiinflammatory effect on acute and chronic inflammatory processes in joints and periarticular tissues. In experimental animal models of osteoarthritis (OA), low-dose irradiation reduced bone loss, synovial proliferation, cartilage degradation, joint swelling and pain.[7]

The antiinflammatory effects of irradiation are not caused by cytotoxic effects, because the low doses used are not lethal to cells, and activated inflammatory cells, including lymphocytes,[8] monocytes, and macrophages,[9] have lost the clonogenic potential and are therefore radioresistant.

Clinically observed antiinflammatory effects of low-dose radiation do not result from elimination of inflammatory cells but appear to be caused by functional alteration and regulation of cells involved in the inflammatory response including endothelium, macrophages, and granulocytes.[10] Adhesion of white blood cells to activated endothelial cells and induction of nitric oxide synthetase in activated macrophages are reduced. Radiation decreases leukocyte adhesion, thereby reducing recruitment of granulocytes to inflamed tissue, which results in decreased proteolytic enzyme release and reduced tissue necrosis.

Radiation-induced inhibition of nitric oxide production results in reduced inflammatory reaction.[9,11] Good evidence also exists that radiation-induced reduction of monocyte and macrophage cytokines prevents excessive fibrosis.[12] This may explain subjective reduction in joint capsule fibrosis and the functional improvement after treatment of OA.[13]

Analgesic Effects

The analgesic effects of ionizing radiation on degenerative and inflammatory disorders are manifested by early effects of short duration, followed by long-term, delayed effects. The delayed effects, characterized by long-lasting pain relief that develops several weeks after treatment, result from the antiinflammatory effects of radiation. Early effects, characterized by fast pain mitigation, result from radiation-induced modulation of the afferent nociceptive pathways. Analgesia involves non–opioid- and opioid-mediated mechanisms. Although the opioid-mediated analgesia is poorly understood,[14] the nonopioid mechanisms (which include modification of pain transmission and perception) appear to be mediated in part by nitric oxide.[15-17] Radiation-induced decrease in local nitric oxide production results in desensitization of the nociceptors[18] and prevention of neuropathic pain development.[19]

Antiproliferative Effects

Ionizing radiation inhibits cell proliferation and temporarily reduces the production of new cells. This mechanism is assumed for prevention of new bone growth and treatment of chronic synovitis. Low-dose radiation does not interfere with normal bone healing, because native osteoblasts are not irreversibly inactivated by radiation. However, irradiation can inhibit excessive new bone formation from existing bone and within muscle after trauma or surgery. Radiation target cells are pluripotent mesenchymal stem cells that are stimulated to proliferate and differentiate into osteoblasts after trauma (e.g., injury or surgery) as a result of the healing process.[20]

Surgical trauma initiates a sequence of events during which cell proliferation takes place within a specific time. Radiation administered during this period induces a delay in cell production that results in a full and permanent therapeutic effect. In people the ability of irradiation treatment to interfere with the formation of heterotopic bone is limited to 4 hours before surgery to 48 hours after surgery.[21] In horses the timing of radiotherapy to prevent new bone growth is also important, and irradiation usually is performed immediately after surgery. In ponies with experimental osteochondral defects in the antebrachiocarpal and middle carpal joints, radiation therapy was not effective in preventing periostitis and periarticular osteophytes when given 6 weeks after surgical trauma.[21] For mature ossification, irradiation alone has no value beyond pain control.

In treating chronic synovitis the antiproliferative effects of irradiation only delay progression of the disease process, because no critical period exists during which cell proliferation is required for the expression of damage. The goal of radiation-induced synovectomy is to ablate inflamed, proliferative synovium, with the expectation that after treatment the regenerated synovium will be free of disease.

Treatment Side Effects

Much of the concern surrounding using irradiation to manage benign conditions is the presumed risk of radiation-induced malignancy. The low doses used, however, are below the threshold associated with an identifiable risk of malignant transformation. In horses, development of in-field sarcoma secondary to radiation therapy to manage benign conditions has not been reported. Reported skin and bone damage likely reflect inadequate treatment techniques according to modern standards.

Skin Damage

Skin damage including epilation, dry desquamation, and regrowth of depigmented hair was often seen when low-energy orthovoltage radiation or insufficiently filtered radioisotope sources were used. The use of modern irradiation techniques and high-energy megavoltage radiation has eliminated the risk of skin overdose, and skin reactions are no longer observed.

Osteopenia

Similar to findings in people, experimental[22,23] and clinical[24] studies in mature horses have shown that low doses of radiation (<10 gray [Gy]) do not affect bone density measured radiologically and do not increase risk of fracture. Although irradiation inhibits excessive bone remodeling and periosteal reactions after surgery, it does not appear to interfere with bone healing. In immature horses, the use of radiation therapy to treat periostitis and OA is discouraged because radiation interferes with bone growth.[25]

IRRADIATION TECHNIQUES

The administration of ionizing radiation is analogous to the prescription of medications based on pharmacological principles. Irradiation of nonmalignant diseases should be carried out by a veterinary radiation therapist familiar with all technical and clinical aspects of modern radiation therapy. Long-term follow-up has to be assured because of the responsibility for radiogenic late effects.

Radiation doses are expressed in Gy, the Système International unit, which has replaced the roentgen (R) and the rad (radiation absorbed dose; 1 Gy = 100 rad).

Before treatment, areas to be irradiated must be identified radiologically to ensure delivery of the radiation dose to the appropriate target volume. Radiotherapy techniques vary considerably based on tissue involved, location, and equipment available. Two methods of irradiation available for treatment of benign lesions in horses are teletherapy (external beam therapy) and brachytherapy.

External Beam Irradiation

Teletherapy involves the external administration of radiation therapy (at a distance of 50 to 100 cm from the area to be treated) by machines that emit x-rays or γ-rays, which can be collimated and directed precisely at the lesion. No difference exists in the mechanism of action between x-rays and γ-rays. In the past, treatments were done with low-energy orthovoltage x-ray units[26-28] producing low-energy x-rays (60 to 90 keV), and the radiation dose was given in a series of three to five exposures. Dosimetry was inaccurate because of the poor penetration of radiation and movement of the standing horse, which was physically restrained during treatment. Currently, teletherapy is done exclusively with megavoltage (4 to 6 megavolts [MV]) radiation delivered by linear accelerators that produce high-energy x-rays or telecobalt units that produce high-energy γ-rays.[29] The advantages of megavoltage radiation include skin sparing, deep penetration into tissue, and precise dosimetry. A distinct disadvantage of this technique is the need for general anesthesia to ensure accurate positioning and immobilization of the horse during treatment. Delivering a single radiation dose ranging from 8 to 12 Gy takes 6 to 8 minutes, so complete immobilization is crucial. Accurate radiological definition of the area to be treated is essential for efficacy and sparing of the surrounding normal tissues.

This treatment method requires high investment in equipment and involves the registration of the radiation therapy unit with government agencies. As a result, such treatments for horses are usually provided at veterinary schools.

Brachytherapy

Brachytherapy is a treatment in which radioactive sources are applied directly to the area to be treated. The short distance between the radiation source and the lesion allows delivery of the radiation dose with minimal exposure to surrounding, uninvolved normal tissues. The disadvantage is radiation exposure to the radiotherapist during positioning and removal of the sources and to personnel responsible for the care of horses during treatment.

Treatment involves using sealed radioactive sources implanted directly into tissues (interstitial brachytherapy) or arranged into an applicator positioned on the skin above the area to be treated (surface brachytherapy). An alternative approach consists of injecting unsealed radioisotopes into a joint space (intracavitary brachytherapy) to deliver the radiation dose directly to the synovium.

This treatment method requires minimum facility and equipment investment, but obtaining a license for laboratory and industrial use of radioactive materials is necessary. This type of license is issued only to an individual who can document extensive training and experience in the safe use of radioisotopes for medical and veterinary purposes.

Interstitial Brachytherapy

Radon gas (^{222}Rn) in beads and radioactive gold (^{198}Au) pellets that emit γ-rays have been used for interstitial brachytherapy. Radioactive sources are inserted permanently and slowly deliver the radiation dose to the surrounding tissue, until complete decay occurs. To minimize personnel exposure, the implantation procedure is done in two steps: first, the insertion of unloaded needles in tissues according to specific radiation planning rules; and second, the loading of the needles with radioactive sources using a special implantation instrument. Achieving consistently satisfactory implants requires a good deal of practice. Treatment is expensive, because radioactive sources can be used only once. This technique is now used rarely and is not allowed in most areas of the United States (the reader may inquire at the local department of social and health services for state regulations, or with the appropriate government agency in other countries). The major drawback is the potential radiation hazard, because the implant is still radioactive when the horse is discharged from the hospital.

Surface Brachytherapy

Surface brachytherapy (plesiotherapy) involves using a surface applicator containing an array of linear radioactive sources. The most common brachytherapy technique involves inserting radioactive sources in the form of rigid needles applied on the skin overlying the lesion. Radioactive cobalt (^{60}Co) and cesium (^{137}Cs) emit a useful beam of γ-rays and are the most common radioisotopes used. Rigid (cast)[30] or flexible (pack)[31] applicators must be light, immobile, well fitted, and comfortable because they are left in position for an extended period to deliver the radiation dose. Dose distribution in tissues depends on arrangement and number of radioactive sources. Treatment doses range from 5 to 15 Gy, given at a low dosage rate over 48 to 72 hours (Table 90-1). Horses must be confined to an isolation facility during treatment to manage the radiation safety hazard posed by large ambient exposure rates around the applicator. Once the dose has been delivered and the pack has been removed and stored in a shielded container, a radiation hazard no longer exists. The horse then can be discharged safely from the hospital.

Surface application has a distinct disadvantage over a therapeutic x-ray machine, because movement of the pack above the skin affects the radiation dose distribution on the area to be irradiated. The potential for source damage, release of radioactive material, and contamination of the facility for several years are other disadvantages.

Intracavitary Brachytherapy

Intracavitary brachytherapy is a new approach developed to concentrate the radiation dose in the target tissue and is used primarily to treat synovitis. Radiation is delivered by intraarticular administration of unsealed β-emitting radioisotopes. The short emission range of the β particles (electrons) provides a high radiation dose to the synovium in contact with the radioisotope without causing damage to articular cartilage or surrounding skin. Diseased synovium is ablated, but the effects on the periarticular tissues and underlying cartilage are minimal.

Several formulations have been developed to prevent leakage of radioisotope from the site of injection. Radiocolloids labeled with radioactive gold (^{198}Au), yttrium (^{90}Y), phosphorus (^{32}P), and rhenium (^{186}Re), and particulate radiopharmaceuticals labeled with radioactive dysprosium (^{165}Dy), holmium (^{166}Ho), and samarium (^{153}Sm) have been used successfully in people. The radioisotope used is based on the energy of the β radiation emitted and the expected thickness of the synovium.[32] In a large joint with a thick synovium, deep penetration with high-energy β radiation is desirable for sufficient treatment of inflamed tissue.[33] Ferric hydroxide macroaggregate labeled with high-energy ^{166}Ho β radiation emitter (penetration depth of 3 mm in tissue) deeply ablated synovium but injured normal intraarticular and periarticular structures, resulting in edema and effusion in the treated joint. The use of lower-energy β radiation with shallower penetration may be limited to mild synovial hyperplasia but results in less periarticular soft tissue injury.[34] Hydroxyapatite microspheres labeled with ^{153}Sm β radiation emitter (penetration depth of 1 mm in tissue) were safe and effective for intraarticular administration in horses.

TABLE 90-1

			NUMBER	RETURN TO	
CONDITION	TREATMENT TECHNIQUE	RADIATION DOSE	OF CASES	RACING (%)	REFERENCES

Radiation Therapy for Painful Degenerative and Inflammatory Musculoskeletal Conditions in Horses

CONDITION	TREATMENT TECHNIQUE	RADIATION DOSE	NUMBER OF CASES	RETURN TO RACING (%)	REFERENCES
Osteoarthritis					
Carpus	Plesiotherapy with γ-radiation (^{222}Rn, ^{60}Co)	5-10 Gy	39	80	13, 26, 41, 42
	Plesiotherapy with γ-radiation (^{137}Cs)	12 Gy	51	84	39
	Teletherapy with orthovoltage x-rays (HVL: 0.5-1.3 mm Cu)	5-15 Gy given in 3 to 7 dose fractions	38	71	26-28
PIP joint	Plesiotherapy with γ-radiation (^{60}Co)	8 Gy	1	100	26
	Plesiotherapy with γ-radiation (^{137}Cs)	12 Gy	22	77	39
	Teletherapy with orthovoltage x-rays (HVL: 0.5 mm Cu)	4-10 Gy given in 3 to 7 dose fractions	21	62	27
MCP joint	Plesiotherapy with γ-radiation (^{222}Rn, ^{60}Co)	5-9 Gy	19	74	13, 26, 42
	Plesiotherapy with γ-radiation (^{137}Cs)	12 Gy	25	60	39
	Teletherapy with orthovoltage x-rays (HVL: 1.3 mm Cu)	12-15 Gy given in 3 dose fractions	5	40	26
Sesamoiditis	Plesiotherapy with γ-radiation (^{222}Rn, ^{60}Co)	5-9 Gy	10	80	13, 26, 41, 42
	Plesiotherapy with γ-radiation (^{137}Cs)	12 Gy	12	80	39
	Teletherapy with orthovoltage x-rays (HVL: 1.3 mm Cu)	10-12 Gy given in 3 dose fractions	4	75	26
Navicular osteitis	Plesiotherapy with γ-radiation (^{222}Rn)	4.5-9 Gy	4	50	41
	Teletherapy with orthovoltage x-rays (HVL: 1.3 mm Cu)	12-15 Gy given in 3 dose fractions	2	100	26
Villonodular synovitis	Postoperative teletherapy with orthovoltage x-rays	12 Gy given in 4 dose fractions	14	90	36
Tendonitis or Desmitis					
Suspensory ligament	Plesiotherapy with γ-radiation (^{222}Rn)	4.5-7 Gy	4	50	41
	Plesiotherapy with γ-radiation (^{137}Cs)	12 Gy	17	64	39
Digital flexor tendon	Plesiotherapy with γ-radiation (^{222}Rn, ^{60}Co, ^{182}Ta)	7-15 Gy	4	25	30, 42
	Plesiotherapy with γ-radiation (^{137}Cs)	12 Gy	7	71	39
	Teletherapy with orthovoltage x-rays (HVL: 0.5-1.3 mm Cu)	4.5-15 Gy given in 3 to 7 dose fractions	5	80	26, 28
New Bone Growth					
Splints	Plesiotherapy with γ-radiation (^{222}Rn)	4.5-9 Gy	4	50	41
	Plesiotherapy with γ-radiation (^{137}Cs)	12 Gy	20	55	39
	Postoperative plesiotherapy with γ-radiation (^{60}Co)	5 Gy	5	100	13
McIII periostitis	Plesiotherapy with γ-radiation (^{222}Rn)	9 Gy	2	100	40
	Teletherapy with orthovoltage x-rays (HVL: 0.5 mm Cu)	4-10 Gy given in 3 to 7 dose fractions	8	37	28

HVL, Half-value layer; *McIII,* third metacarpal bone; *MCP,* metacarpophalangeal; *PIP,* proximal interphalangeal.

CLINICAL APPLICATIONS

Irradiation was efficacious for treatment of painful degenerative and inflammatory musculoskeletal conditions in horses. The treatment goal is long-term pain relief and return to racing or performance. Although modern standards of clinical research cannot be applied to these clinical studies, the general message is a remarkable consistency in the response pattern.

Although radiation therapy should not be used indiscriminately, it should not be viewed as a last resort. Radiation therapy is effective in managing refractory, chronic stages of various degenerative disorders and should be used for conditions that do not respond within a few months to conservative treatments, including administration of NSAIDs, local injections (corticosteroids or other antiinflammatory products), physical therapy, and physiotherapy. Strenuous exercise should be avoided, and the horse should be given state-of-the-art physiotherapy after radiation therapy is used. General recommendations include stall rest with handwalking for 30 to 90 days and a gradual return to regular training over 60 to 90 days.

A summary of clinical results of radiotherapy for painful refractory orthopedic conditions is found in Table 90-1. Overall success rate was 60% to 70%, although data are not contemporary and techniques are different from those practiced today. Onset and duration of analgesia were often difficult to measure. Low success rates were found in horses with chronic conditions or in those in which many unsuccessful treatments had previously been performed.

Chronic Synovitis

When synovitis plays a major role in the arthritic process, radiation therapy may be advantageous. Treatment is directed at reducing synovial inflammation and proliferation to prevent progressive joint deterioration and control of joint effusion, fibrosis, and pain. Inflamed synovium induces damage to the articular surfaces by causing effusion, up-regulation of endothelial adhesion molecules, liberation of inflammatory mediators and destructive enzymes, and alterations in the synovial fluid constituents.[35]

Chemical, surgical, or radiation-induced synovectomy can be performed. Similar to surgical synovectomy, radiation synovectomy destroys diseased synovium, and the intent is to allow regeneration of normal synovium and amelioration of clinical signs. In people the duration of response after radiation synovectomy is related inversely to the amount of cartilage and bone destruction. These findings emphasize the importance of screening horses for radiological evidence of cartilage and bone destruction before considering radiation synovectomy. It is imperative to discriminate pain arising from inflamed synovium from that originating from cartilage or bone damage, so that horses with pain from the latter, which is likely to be unaffected by radiation synovectomy, do not undergo unnecessary treatment.

Irradiation is recommended in horses with chronic OA, after osteochondral fragment removal if synovium is proliferative, in horses with idiopathic synovitis, and potentially as an ancillary treatment for infectious arthritis. The role of radiation therapy in treating infectious arthritis is limited to preventing chronic synovitis and treating reactive arthritis. Radiation therapy should not be used until bacteria have been eliminated, because the antiinflammatory effects of radiation can exacerbate infection. In addition, radiation therapy should be limited strictly to adult horses, because the antiproliferative effects of radiation damage growing bones and joints in young horses. External beam irradiation can be used as an adjuvant to incomplete surgical synovectomy.[36,37] Radiation doses of 7 to 10 Gy do not cause delayed wound healing or wound complications when the incision is excluded from the field of radiation. Intraarticular administration of [153]Sm may be used as a single modality when thickness of the inflamed synovium does not exceed 1 mm.[32,38] Treatment doses ranging from 7 to 34 Gy have been found to be safe in horses.[38] For thicker synovial conditions the use of higher-energy radionuclides such as holmium ([166]Ho) and rhenium ([186]Re) may be required. Treated horses may experience transient pain (lameness), pitting edema, and effusion. In people, concomitant intraarticular injection of triamcinolone acetonide prevents transient local reaction and reduces pain.

Degenerative Bone and Joint Disorders

Radiation therapy is used to treat various types of equine lameness caused by inflammatory and degenerative changes affecting bones, joints, and tendons. The most common indications for radiation therapy include chronic traumatic arthritis and OA of the carpal and fetlock joints,

sesamoiditis, active carpitis with swelling and mild mineralization, and chronic carpitis. Radiographic examination should be performed before radiation therapy is performed. This helps ensure that the cause of lameness is not an osteochondral fragment or another condition that is best handled surgically. The antiinflammatory and analgesic effects of radiation may stabilize the injury process in subacute and chronic painful disorders, when periarticular new bone proliferation is minimal and damage to cartilage is not obvious. Horses with joints with end-stage OA are unlikely to benefit from irradiation.[27] Because radiation has no inhibitory effect on the degenerative processes in OA, the treatment goal is limited to pain relief.

Radiation therapy can be used for horses with tendonitis, tenosynovitis, and desmitis. Long-term results in horses with acute and subacute conditions are better than in those with chronic conditions. In horses with chronic OA in which substantial periarticular radiological changes have occurred, radiation therapy is used to control inflammation and pain and to prevent excessive fibrosis and calcium deposition, which can result in dysfunction, reduced joint motion, and deformity. Horses with severe OA that show extensive new bone, large amounts of mineralization of soft tissues, and evidence of cartilage destruction are not treated routinely because they rarely improve enough to perform satisfactorily.

Treatment results have not been uniform because of many variables, including severity and location of the lesion, degeneration of the articular cartilage and preexisting OA, radiation dose and technique used, and duration of rest after treatment. In addition, questionable causes and pathogenesis make degenerative disorders prone to polypragmasy. Finally, the effects of enforced rest periods in the overall management are not known, which makes definitive assessment of the value of radiation therapy impossible.

The efficacy of plesiotherapy using ^{137}Cs packs was evaluated in 147 horses (46% Thoroughbreds, 27% Quarter Horses, and 12% Standardbreds) treated at the University of California, Davis, Veterinary Medical Teaching Hospital.[39] The treatment dose was 12 Gy given over 24 to 32 hours. Treatment responses were judged to be good, meaning that the horse returned to racing and was sound, or poor, meaning that the horse showed no response or the response was temporary. However, this was not a controlled study, and the results should be interpreted cautiously. Treatment was most effective for horses with carpitis, OA of the proximal interphalangeal joint, and sesamoiditis and least effective for those with OA of the metacarpophalangeal joint and splints (see Table 90-1) Results were less favorable for treatment of horses with desmitis and tendonitis.

Because of the radiation hazard associated with the use of radioactive sources, treatments are currently done at the University of California, Davis, Veterinary Medical Teaching Hospital with a linear accelerator. Depending on the volume of the lesion to be treated and the size of the joint, irradiation is done with 4 MV (Clinac 4, Varian, Lake Oswego, Oregon, United States) or 6 MV (Clinac 2100 C, Varian) x-rays. Horses were anesthetized in a recovery stall adjacent to one of the two radiation therapy suites. Interim results in 14 horses with refractory OA of the proximal interphalangeal joint or with osteophytes associated with mild OA followed for a minimum of 12 months after treatment indicate that irradiation is effective in controlling pain even after unsuccessful previous treatments including surgery, medical treatment, laser therapy, acoustic shock wave therapy, or ultrasound hyperthermia. Eighty-three percent of horses had a good clinical response, meaning that these horses returned to their previous performance level.

Preventing New Bone Growth

Posttraumatic exostosis occurs after repair of bone fractures (third carpal bone and third metacarpal or metatarsal bone condylar fractures) and after certain surgical procedures, such as arthrodesis and distal splint bone removal. Radiological changes are usually more advanced than are clinical signs and functional impairment. Risk factors that predispose horses to develop exostoses are not known. A history of previous new bone growth after surgery is the most substantial predisposing condition. Although a report described regression of excessive callus on a splint bone,[40] horses with painful mature exostosis or periarticular and soft tissue calcification usually do not benefit from radiotherapy except for pain relief. These horses require excision of calcified tissue followed by postoperative irradiation.

Radiation therapy is a powerful prophylactic treatment to prevent abnormal ossification in stress-related bone and periosteal injury in race horses. Treatments should be done with high-energy radiation, such as that produced by linear accelerators or telecobalt units. Doses of 8 to 10 Gy are given in a single treatment. The effective therapeutic window reaches from a still-undefined preoperative time to about 2 days after surgery or traumatic soft tissue injury. In an ongoing prospective study conducted at the University of California, Davis, Veterinary Medical Teaching Hospital, prophylactic irradiation was given to horses at risk for developing abnormal mineralization after surgery or horses with a previous history of periarticular calcification and exostosis. A single dose of 10 Gy (1000 rad) was given using a linear accelerator immediately after surgical curettage of the excessive bony proliferation. Depending on the surgical field and the size of the joint, irradiation was done with 4 MV (Clinac 4, Varian) or 6 MV (Clinac 2100 C, Varian) x-rays. While horses were still under general anesthesia after surgery, they were moved from the operating room to one of the two radiation therapy suites for irradiation. Close proximity of the two rooms at the hospital minimized the potential for surgical and anesthetic complications during transportation. Interim results in 34 horses with carpal chip fractures (N = 10) and exostosis after trauma or splint bone fracture (N = 24) with a minimum of 12 months' follow-up after treatment indicated that irradiation was effective in long-term prevention of abnormal postoperative mineralization. Eighty-three percent of horses had a good clinical response, meaning that horses returned to previous performance level. Although subjective evaluation criteria are insufficient to define the role of radiotherapy compared with other therapies, a third of the treated horses with heterotopic ossification after previous surgical treatments had complete radiological response lasting more than 1 year.

Chapter 91

Rest and Rehabilitation

Barrie D. Grant

The number of publications about the effects of exercise on bone, cartilage, and tendons has increased substantially. The results of these investigations have allowed not only the research community but also practicing veterinarians to gain more insight into the effects of mild, moderate, and strenuous exercise on the skeletal system, especially regarding the pathogenesis of fractures and osteoarthritis. Unfortunately, results of controlled studies of the effects of deconditioning on bone, cartilage, and tendons have not been disseminated widely. Presently each clinician recommends a rest and rehabilitation program based often on intuition, anecdotal experience, and tradition. These recommendations have withstood the test of time, however, and can serve as a guide.

The number of alternative therapies and therapists has also increased. Although some benefits to this approach are possible, many of the modalities have not been tested in a standard scientific method, and popularity often is based on the principle that alternative approaches are less expensive and have faster results.

PRINCIPLES OF REST AND REHABILITATION PROGRAMS

The following are some basic principles that should be considered when formulating a specific plan for a specific injury.

1. Is the diagnosis complete? An incomplete diagnosis and thus treatment lead to poor results. Arthroscopic removal of a carpal fracture in the apparently lame limb will have poor results if there is an osteochondral fracture in the contralateral fetlock joint. Hindlimb suspensory desmitis is unlikely to resolve satisfactorily if mild ataxia is concurrent. An expedient, complete, and accurate diagnosis affords the best chance for long-term success.
2. Horses can tolerate extensive periods of stall confinement without becoming deranged psychopaths. They do need to be in clean airy stalls, so they can see other horses, and energy intake should be reduced. Clinicians should avoid walking horses every 4 or 5 days to see how they are doing, because horses tend to find any excuse suddenly to jump or rear and may sustain reinjury.

3. The heart and muscles do not undergo any clinically significant deconditioning for at least 4 weeks after a standard anaerobic training program. Therefore many horses with minor injuries, or even a suspicion of a minor ligament or tendon problem, possibly can heal with 4 weeks of rest, with little loss in performance. The cardiac parameters actually improve 5 days after the last extensive training effort. Little will be lost and much could be gained if experienced jumping and dressage horses with lameness problems could be walked under tack for a week before major events.

4. An earlier return to training, in the form of walking under saddle, swimming, or controlled exercise on a treadmill, can reduce the chance of further injury than if a previously stall-confined horse is turned out in a paddock and allowed to run, buck, slide, and turn quickly. If paddock turnout is used, then administering sedation and gradually increasing the size of the paddock are recommended. Leaving a horse in a paddock continuously also is best once the horse has been introduced to the freedom. If a horse is stabled each evening, then it tends to buck and play again each morning when released.

REST

The basic principle of rest is to reduce the force and strain on injured tissue and allow the normal reparative processes to proceed without further insult. Muscle tissue can heal in a much shorter period than tendons or ligaments, but the repair of cartilage is accomplished by the metaplasia of replacement tissue, which takes 4 to 6 months. The quality and quantity of rest depends on the severity of the condition, the disposition of the horse, the owner, and the trainer, and their expectations.

Complete Immobilization

Although complete immobilization can be accomplished with internal fixation, external coaptation with a cast also can reduce the motion of fracture fragments and excessive strain placed on damaged ligaments or tendons. The long-term use of cast immobilization can result in osteoarthrosis (fracture disease) and osteopenia. Normal joints can tolerate at least 4 weeks of cast immobilization without significant irreversible change to the articular cartilage.[1] Well-designed splints and braces offer an alternative for conditions that do not require complete rest or can be used for intermediary support in the transition from a cast to having no external support.

References on page 1331

Stall Rest

Stall rest is the most common form of rest recommended and is highly effective as long as weekly episodes of outside activity do not interrupt it. The effects of controlled exercise on articular cartilage remain controversial. French and colleagues[2] concluded that early postoperative exercise is not detrimental to repair of experimentally created osteochondral defects of the carpus. Other investigators suggested deleterious effects of early exercise on the healing

of carpal osteochondral defects.[3] However, exercise may be beneficial in maintaining normal concentrations of glycosaminoglycan in insulted articular cartilage.[4] The administration of polysulfated glycosaminoglycans may have a protective effect against the deleterious results of early postoperative exercise on experimentally induced osteochondral defects.[3] Only a cost-benefit investigation with a sufficient number of horses will show if the expense of the medication is justified, with an earlier return to competition compared with horses restricted to stall rest.

Owners are always concerned about the effect that enforced stall rest can have on the mental status of horses, but provided that energy intake is restricted and horses have visual contact with other horses, most adapt satisfactorily. During inactivity many horses lose muscle mass and tone, which are rapidly restored, and horses that become overweight are less likely to return to athletic competition than leaner cohorts. It is important to stress good husbandry practices, because soiled wet bedding or infrequent hoof care can lead to chronic hoof problems. I have seen many horses with joint disease develop subsolar hematomas on the opposite limb, predisposing to or because of the joint disease. These hematomas can become subsolar abscesses if the husbandry is inadequate.

Experience has shown that 60 days is the minimum amount of time necessary for the repair of soft tissues after orthopedic surgery,[2] but convincing eager and aggressive owners and trainers that this time is a positive economic decision is often difficult.

Reduction of Excessive Movement

In horses with severe orthopedic and neurological problems, recent improvement in slings has helped to reduce the risk of further injury from difficulties in lying down and getting up and the risk of laminitis in the contralateral limb. I prefer the Liftex sling (Liftex, Warminster, Pennsylvania, United States) to the more complicated Anderson sling (CDA Products, Potter Valley, California, United States) for everyday use, although I recognize that the Anderson sling has some features that are helpful in lifting severely injured or neurologically compromised horses. Not all horses tolerate a sling, especially those under a year of age, and further injury can possibly occur if a horse becomes violent. Giving the horse a small amount of acepromazine reduces anxiety before a sling is applied. Having a short introductory period for the first session and rewarding acceptable behavior with food is helpful. Slings are not meant to provide vertical stability to horses that cannot stand by themselves. Slings are best used to provide a method for injured horses to reduce weight bearing for short periods. Experienced horses take full weight off the limbs and sit as a person might in a hammock for short periods, two or three times an hour.

Use of crossties or overhead chains can also prevent excessive movement and force on injured areas from horses lying down and struggling to rise. Young horses may not accept this form of restraint well, which may increase the chance of injury because they fight the system. However, most Thoroughbred flat racehorses in training adapt satisfactorily. It is important to allow horses three or four sessions a day with the head down to prevent pneumonia, which can occur with improper drainage of pulmonary secretions.

Paddock Rest

After stall confinement, tradition has stressed a period of paddock rest before a horse is returned to active training. When to give paddock rest and how it is administered are based on each individual horse. The type of injury, response to treatment, personality of the horse and owners, and the season of the year are major considerations. In my experience horses can overexercise and reinjure healing tissue or incur new injuries when turned out. The use of small paddocks (6×6 m) to inhibit running is a suitable compromise.

The initial introduction of the horse to the paddock is the time when most mishaps can occur. Sedation, protective boots (tendons and bell or overreach boots), and avoiding muddy, snowy, frozen conditions and unfamiliar horses greatly reduce injuries. Ideally the horse should be allowed to remain in the paddock at all times, instead of being turned out each morning after a night of stall confinement. It is necessary to continue to monitor the general health care of the horse, including anthelmintic prophylaxis and immunization against respiratory pathogens that are spread easily among horses communicating over adjacent fences. Foot care is still a concern. Many horses may require shoeing to prevent abnormal hoof wear, which could result in an uneven gait when they return to active training.

Ridden Walking

After stall confinement and handwalking, I prefer to ride the horse at walk, beginning with 10 minutes a day and progressing to 30 minutes a day after 30 days, rather than using paddock exercise. This increase of activity is felt to stimulate the maturation of repair tissue in cartilage and tendons.

EXERCISE

Exercise as a basic component of rehabilitation has as its most basic goal to return an injured horse to at least its previous level of performance. The owner and/or trainer need(s) to have a realistic idea of what is possible with each type of injury and the relative severity of the injury, considering the inherent risks of each form of athletic performance. For example, for an elite dressage horse with a severe hindlimb suspensory injury, attempts to return to elite competition may well be a fool's errand, especially if the horse does not have an elite rider. The selection of an alternative form of competition, such as show jumping, that is not associated with such a high incidence of suspensory problems might suit the horse better.

There are two diverging approaches regarding the intensity of exercise used in rehabilitation. The most common is a protective program that uses the minimum amount of conditioning necessary to return a horse to competition without excessive forces and overuse. For example, a racehorse with pathology on the weight-bearing joint surfaces often has exercise limited to soft rebounding surfaces, using shock absorbing shoes and being ridden by a lighter rider, at less than maximal speeds for shorter periods. This approach has been successful but takes advantage of each horse's inherent ability to perform at a higher level of activity than it has been trained for, because horses are competitive and most want to please their riders.

Although many disciplines allow horses to perform soundly repeatedly while underconditioned, there are others such as flat and hurdle racing, eventing, and endurance disciplines that do not. From personal experience, entering and starting a horse of questionable soundness or underconditioned because of an unsoundness in a 50-mile endurance race most often results in a tired, lame, and stressed companion that must be led the last 10 miles over rough trails either in the blazing sun or cold, wet darkness. As veterinarians, owners, and trainers, we should not take advantage of our noble companions by exploiting their willingness to perform at a higher level of competition than they have been prepared for.

The opposite approach is the mindset that the injured tissue needs to be stimulated to be stronger than normal. Familiar to anyone who has gone through physical therapy after knee surgery, this is the approach used by human physical therapists. They prescribe the use of weights, Cybex machines, treadmills, and verbal intimidation to attain new levels of strength and fitness before permitting a return to standard training. In order for this method to be successful and not result in reinjury, a commitment to a longer time must be made. A recent study from Australia using the thickness of the dorsal cortex of the third metacarpal bone (McIII), as measured by serial radiography as a barometer, determined that it required a mean of over 500 days to achieve a maximum thickness. This same study also showed that a higher stress load than normal is required to stimulate the McIII to model to this degree.

Passive Exercise

Passive exercise can begin immediately after joint surgery to reduce the amount of postoperative immobility. Theoretically, passive exercise improves distribution of nutrients to chondrocytes and reduces the number of synovial adhesions to any osteochondral defects on the edge of a joint. The type of reparative tissue that develops under synovial adhesions is fibrous and not the hyaline-like material that fills a full-thickness defect when no synovial tissue has adhered to the defect.[5] I routinely begin passive joint movement on the first postoperative day. The joint is flexed just to the position that produces discomfort 15 to 20 times twice a day, for 30 days. Passive exercise is not indicated in joints with any detectable instability or in which a problem with primary healing of the joint capsule exists.

Handwalking

Handwalking is the mildest form of active exercise and often is recommended along with stall rest. Although recommending handwalking early in the postoperative period is easy to appease owners, trainers, and caretakers, it is also essential to realize that early disruption of a primary clot in an osteochondral defect can result in poor healing of the defect.[5] The chances of excessive and unpredictable behavior that can result in removal of the clot are increased with removing an active horse from a stall for short periods. The benefits of complete stall rest for the first 30 days far outweigh any benefit that 5 to 10 minutes of handwalking may produce. Handwalking for 5 to 10 minutes a day beginning at day 30, and gradually increasing to 30 minutes at postoperative day 60, is common practice. Handwalking seems to be the most objectionable form of exercise to owners and caretakers, because horses act up or the potential for them to do so is anticipated and dreaded. The new form of caged horse walkers appears to be much safer and, although horses are constantly turning, this appears to be a suitable form of exercise to replace handwalking. Alternatively, ridden walking exercise can be used.

Aquatreds and Swimming

Using swimming pools and submerged treadmills (aquatreds) is still popular and at least in specific locations has withstood the test of time. Minimal controlled data are available to document the benefits of these modalities for treating horses with athletic injuries. That the cardiopulmonary system responds substantially to swimming has been documented, but only anecdotal information exists for aquatreds. Both modalities assist in increasing joint mobility and producing some physical activity in a controlled environment. The force to the axial skeleton is reduced, and this benefits horses with a nondisplaced fracture or a joint with advanced osteoarthritis. However, the reduction of the weight-bearing force in rehabilitation may not be desirable, because osteoporosis develops when training is curtailed for more than 30 days.[6] Returning the skeletal system to its previous competitive state requires a longer time than for muscles and the cardiopulmonary system. Reconditioning the muscles by swimming or aquatreds, before reconditioning the skeletal system, increases the possibility of having horses that are too eager and able to produce more force than the bones, joints, tendons, and ligaments can tolerate. The recognition that stress fractures of the humerus are more common in horses returned to training after only 30 to 60 days of rest bears testimony to the inability of the skeletal system to adapt to the stress of training as quickly as the muscle does.[7]

High-Speed Treadmills

The increase in the number of privately owned treadmills could increase the quality of healing of horses with athletic injury. High-speed treadmills have a number of benefits for reconditioning equine athletes. The speed, distance, slope, heart rate, and climatic conditions can be controlled, monitored, and, with some systems, even programmed. Work effort can be increased with a weighted saddle and raising the slope of the treadmill, without having to increase the speed. The force on the tendons can be increased slowly by increasing the slope of the treadmill slowly.

Using treadmills for exercising horses is now accepted widely because the injury rate has been low if good judgment is used, especially when introducing a new horse. It is important to realize that training on a treadmill is not the same as racing or training on a racing surface. Horses require twice as much work on a treadmill at maximum oxygen consumption (VO_2) to produce the same muscle changes as galloping on a training track with a rider.[8] Horses also require speeds of at least 14 m/sec to produce the same changes on implanted strain gauges in the McIIIs as breezing on a racetrack.[9] Some treadmills cannot achieve this speed, and lay operators often are reluctant to exercise horses at 14 m/sec because they feel the horses may become injured.

We have found little problem with long-term training on a treadmill. Horses usually trot 1000 m at 4 m/sec and then gallop for 2000 m at 10 m/sec. We have not recognized any foot problems that may result from excessive time on the treadmill,[10] although the training plates are hot to the touch after a training session. A constant fine mist applied to the treadmill belt is supposed to reduce the heat. Recently it has been shown that prolonged treadmill training can result in carpal articular cartilage changes.[11]

Active Training

The importance of periodic monitoring for any subtle clinical signs as a horse progresses through the final stages of training before competition cannot be overstated. The trainers with the most success in returning horses with athletic injuries to a successful career are those who are patient and careful observers. Horses often show signs of increased inflammation and gait abnormalities as the training intensity increases from tack walking and jogging to galloping. Reducing the amount and quality of the exercise for 30 days may be all that is necessary to reduce the inflammation, without medication.

Hill Training

It is possible to produce the same training effect by exercising horses on moderate inclines (e.g., ½ mile at 13% incline) at a 50% reduction in the speed of horses trained on a racetrack.[12] Trotting downhill is not necessary for most conditioning programs other than endurance or cross-country eventing. Trotting downhill may lead to an increase in the incidence of proximal suspensory problems and also increases the forces on the stifle joint. I used interval training in 15 2-year-old Thoroughbreds being trained for racing, using a program consisting of three intervals, with the first at an extended trot, the second at a canter, and the third at a gallop, and found the horses had minimal unsoundness and were competitive. Walking the horses downhill allowed time to recover and kept the horses relaxed and manageable.

SECTION 2
Complementary (Nontraditional) Therapy

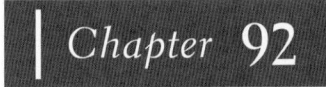

Acupuncture

■ EQUINE ACUPUNCTURE FOR LAMENESS DIAGNOSIS AND TREATMENT

Allen M. Schoen

Interest in veterinary acupuncture for lameness diagnosis and treatment has increased greatly in the public and veterinary medical communities. With this increased awareness has come an increase in veterinary acupuncture research and thus a better understanding of the physiological basis of acupuncture and its clinical applications. Acupuncture may be used as an adjunct diagnostic and therapeutic tool to our traditional lameness examination and to the treatment of lameness, but it is not meant to be a substitute.

With the increased interest in equine acupuncture, there has also been additional controversy and use and misuse of this modality. It is important to understand the scientific basis, traditional Chinese medical theories, and clinical indications and limitations if acupuncture is to be used in a professional manner as part of an integrated approach to equine lameness. Currently, equine acupuncture is practiced by veterinarians trained in the Western medical perspective of scientific acupuncture and the traditional Chinese and Japanese medical theories. The approach may vary slightly based on the practitioner's perspective.

The history of equine acupuncture dates back to 2000 to 3000 BCE during the Shang and Chow dynasties in China. Around 650 BCE Bai-le wrote *Bai-le's Canon of Veterinary Medicine,* one of the first veterinary textbooks, which described acupuncture and moxibustion in equine medicine. The first atlas of equine acupuncture points and channels, *Ma Jing Kong-xiue Tu,* was written during the Sui period, from 581 to 618 CE.[1] Equine back pain was first addressed in the ancient veterinary textbook *Yuan-Heng Liao Ma Ji (Yuan-Heng's Therapeutic Treatise of Horses).*[2] Periodically, anecdotal reports of using equine acupuncture would come to the Western world. The first substantial introduction occurred in the 1970s, when the International Veterinary Acupuncture Society was established and developed training programs in veterinary acupuncture in the United States. In 1996 the American Veterinary Medical Association stated, "Veterinary acupuncture and acutherapy are considered valid modalities, but the potential for abuse exists. These techniques should be regarded as surgical and/or medical procedures under state practice acts. It is recommended that extensive continuing education

References on page 1331

programs be undertaken before a veterinarian is considered competent to practice acupuncture."[3] Postgraduate education in veterinary acupuncture throughout the world—including Australia, Europe, Scandinavia, North and South America, and other areas—is offered by the International Veterinary Acupuncture Society, based in Fort Collins, Colorado.[4] The Chi Institute of Traditional Chinese Medicine in Reddick, Florida[5]; Colorado State University College of Veterinary Medicine continuing education program in Fort Collins, Colorado[6]; Tufts University School of Veterinary Medicine in North Grafton, Massachusetts[7]; and the Veterinary Institute for Therapeutic Alternatives in Sherman, Connecticut[8] also offer postgraduate programs. All of the programs are in the United States.

SCIENTIFIC BASIS

Acupuncture may be defined in a Western medical perspective as the stimulation of specific predetermined points on the body to achieve a therapeutic or homeostatic effect. Recent research has provided evidence for the anatomical classification of acupoints. Acupuncture points are areas on the skin of decreased electrical resistance or increased electrical conductivity. Acupuncture points correspond to four known neural structures. Type I acupoints, which make up 67% of all acupoints, are considered motor points. The motor point is the point in a muscle that, when electrical stimulation is applied, will produce a maximal contraction with minimal intensity of stimulation. Motor points are located near the point where the nerve enters the muscle. Type II acupoints are located on the superficial nerves in the sagittal plane on the midline dorsally and ventrally. Type III acupoints are located at high-density foci of superficial nerves and nerve plexuses. For instance, acupoint GB-34 is located at the point where the common fibular (peroneal) nerve divides into the deep and superficial branches. Type IV acupoints are located at the muscle-tendon junctions, where the Golgi tendon organ is located.[9] Recently, histological studies have revealed that small microtubules, consisting of free nerve endings, arterioles, and venules, penetrate through the fascia at acupuncture points (Figure 92-1).[10]

Acupuncture has many varied physiological effects on all systems throughout the body. No one mechanism can explain all the physiological effects observed. Traditional Chinese medical theories have explained these effects for 4000 years, based on empirical observations and descriptions of naturally occurring phenomena. Western medical theories include the gate and multiple gate theories, autonomic theories, humeral mechanisms, and bioelectric theories.[10] Detailed discussions of the neurophysiological basis of acupuncture are reviewed in a number of texts.[9-12] Essentially, acupuncture stimulates various sensory receptors (pain, thermal, pressure, and touch), which stimulate sensory afferent nerves, which transmit the signal through the central nervous system to the hypothalamic-pituitary

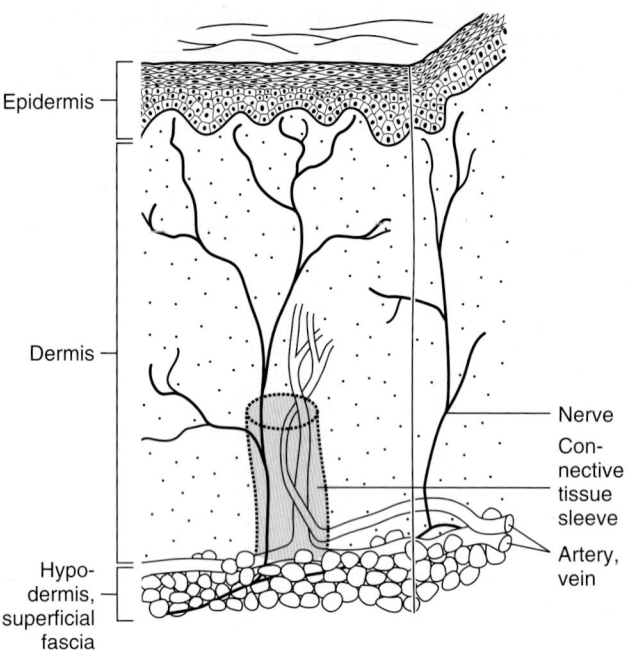

Fig. 92-1 • Schematic drawing of the skin, showing a neurovascular bundle wrapped by a sleeve of loose connective tissue deep to an acupoint. (From Schoen AM, ed: *Veterinary acupuncture: ancient art to modern medicine,* ed 2, St Louis, 2001, Mosby.)

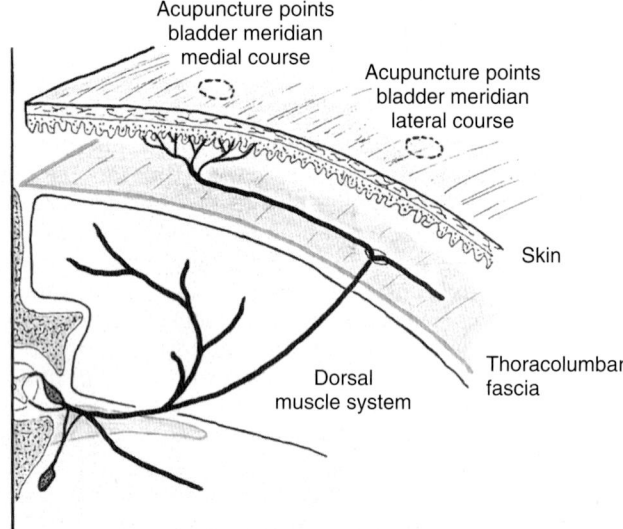

Fig. 92-2 • Cutaneous nerve entering the dermis at an acupuncture point along the bladder meridian. (From Schoen AM, ed: *Veterinary acupuncture: ancient art to modern medicine,* ed 2, St Louis, 2001, Mosby.)

system (Figure 92-2). The acupoints correlate with cutaneous areas containing higher concentrations of free sensory nerve endings, mast cells, lymphatics, capillaries, and venules. Various neurotransmitters and neurohormones are then released and have subsequent effects throughout the body. Research in rabbits using electroacupuncture-induced neural activation, detected by the use of manganese-enhanced functional magnetic resonance imaging, demonstrated a corresponding cerebral link between peripheral acupoints and central neural pathways. Research such as this is aiding in further understanding the effects

of local peripheral stimulation on specific areas in the brain.[13] Electroacupuncture has also been found to stimulate endogenous opioids, vasoactive peptides, adreno-corticotrophic hormone, cortisol, and catecholamine in cerebrospinal fluid and peripheral plasma in ponies.[14] Bossut and colleagues[15] documented changes in plasma cortisol and β-endorphin in horses subjected to electroacupuncture for cutaneous analgesia. Changes in serum protein and blood gas concentrations also have been demonstrated in donkeys after acupuncture.[16,17] Xie and colleagues[18] documented that electroacupuncture could relieve experimental pain in the horse via the release of β-endorphin. They found that acupuncture stimulation using local acupuncture points with high frequency (80 to 120 Hz) is more effective than using distal points with low frequency (20 Hz). They found that acupoints close to the painful areas require high-frequency electroacupuncture stimulation, whereas the acupoints far from the painful areas may be stimulated with low-frequency electroacupuncture. Electroacupuncture generally is considered to have stronger effects than other types of acupuncture methods.[18] The degree of stimulation appears to depend on the location of the specific acupoints.[19,20]

Through understanding the neurophysiology and neuroanatomy of acupuncture, one can appreciate that acupuncture may stimulate nerves, increase local microcirculation to joints and muscles, relieve muscle spasms, and cause a release of various neurotransmitters. Clinically, one may see the benefits of these effects in treating equine lameness caused by soft tissue injury, muscle spasms, nerve trauma, and other conditions.

TRADITIONAL CHINESE MEDICAL THEORIES

Acupuncture has been used in China to treat equine lameness for a few thousand years. Chinese acupuncture was based on the empirical use of acupoints for certain conditions. Historically, acupuncture meridians were not acknowledged in animals. Specific empirical points based on experience were identified and named for location or function. Equine acupuncture meridians, or pathways, have been transposed onto horses from human acupuncture maps only in the past 40 years.

Traditional Chinese medicine acupuncture diagnosis and treatment are based on the pattern differentiations that are developed from two main theories of traditional Chinese medicine: the Five Element theory and the Eight Principles, which require a great deal of study.[21] The traditional Chinese medicine diagnosis is defined as a specific pattern based on imbalances in the five elements (also called *five phases*), imbalances and disorders in specific meridians or organs, or specific patterns of disharmony. The diagnosis is based on a physical examination of the horse, including evaluation of the tongue and pulse. Tongue inspection includes evaluation of the color of the tongue, the moistness, and the color and thickness of any tongue coating. Palpation of the jugular pulse would be described as *weak, strong, wiry,* and so on. Tongue and pulse examination and an overall examination would lead to a traditional Chinese medicine diagnosis and treatment of appropriate acupuncture points. Xie[22] describes a traditional Chinese medicine five-step method for diagnosis and treatment. This includes the following:

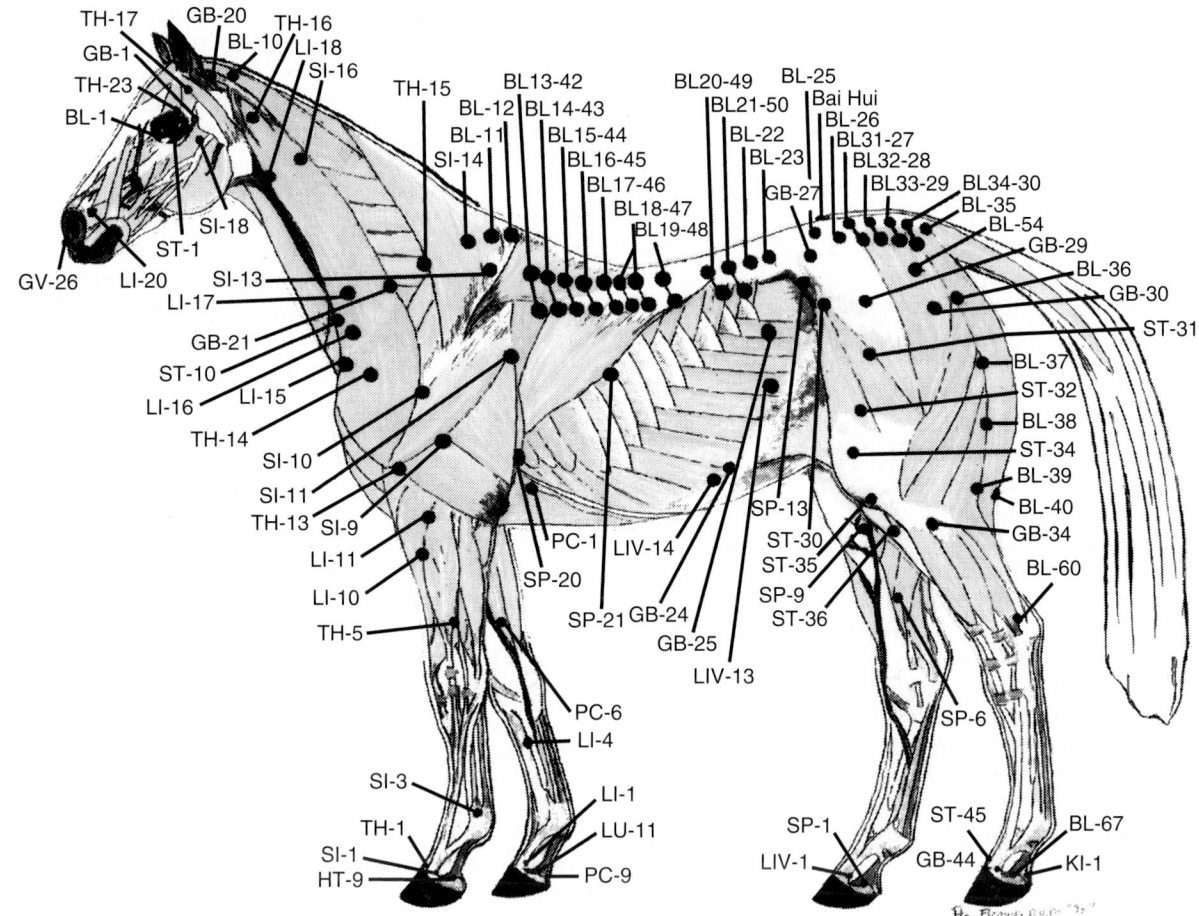

Fig. 92-3 • Acupoints of the horse: lateral view in relation to muscles. (Courtesy Peg Fleming. From Schoen AM, ed: *Veterinary acupuncture: ancient art to modern medicine,* ed 2, St Louis, 2001, Mosby.)

1. Collection of empirical data from the history, tongue, and pulse examination and diagnosis
2. A Western medical examination
3. A traditional Chinese medicine pattern differentiation
4. A treatment strategy based on traditional Chinese medicine
5. A selection of appropriate acupuncture points, Chinese herbs, or both

In contrast, the Japanese technique, frequently termed *meridian therapy,* is based more on palpation of the acupuncture points and the reaction. The anatomical location of equine acupoints is based on the traditional Chinese acupuncture atlases or a transpositional atlas based on transcribing human acupuncture points onto the equine anatomy. The location of the points is similar in each method, though anatomical variation exists, as discussed by Fleming[23] (Figure 92-3).

TECHNIQUES AND INSTRUMENTATION

Numerous techniques exist to stimulate acupuncture points. The following modes of stimulation are commonly used in equine acupuncture: dry needle stimulation, electroacupuncture, aquapuncture, moxibustion, laser stimulation, gold implants, and acupressure. Each method has its indications and limitations. Dry needle stimulation and aquapuncture are used most routinely in the West.

Aquapuncture is the injection of various solutions into the acupuncture points. The hypodermic needle is stimulating the acupuncture point as a traditional acupuncture needle would. In addition, the solution is stimulating the pressure receptors for a period, and the solution is having its specific effect as well. Solutions injected include saline, vitamins such as B_{12}, nonsteroidal analgesics, local anesthetic solutions such as lidocaine, and occasionally homeopathic and herbal solutions, depending on the veterinarian's preference. Electroacupuncture, using a portable electroacupuncture unit, normally is used for nerve stimulation to treat severe chronic cervical, thoracolumbar, or lumbosacral problems or an affected joint, tendon, or ligament. These electroacupuncture units have electrodes attached to the acupuncture needles. Positive results with electroacupuncture have been documented for treatment of lameness in horses. Electroacupuncture decreased the lameness score in horses ($P < .001$).[24] Although poorly documented, electroacupuncture without needles is sometimes applied as well. Moxibustion is a form of thermostimulation using a Chinese herb, *Artemisia vulgaris.* Low-level or cold laser therapy is also used to stimulate acupuncture points. Gold implants have been used to treat navicular disease and chronic back pain and provide long-term stimulation of acupoints. This approach is an adaptation of the Chinese technique of sutures embedded into acupoints. Acupressure often is taught to the client to administer between acupuncture treatments to potentiate the effect. Detailed descriptions of these techniques are provided by Altman.[25]

From a Western medical perspective, acupuncture point selection is based on locating points on the body where stimulation produces a beneficial change in the central nervous system by modulating ongoing physiological activity, releasing local muscular spasms, and increasing local microcirculation. From a traditional Chinese medicine perspective, acupoints are selected based on a pattern differentiation developed from the Five Element theory or Eight Principles. The choice of acupoints based on the Eight Principles depends more on tongue and pulse findings and a comprehensive history. The Japanese approach to point selection follows a diagnostic acupuncture point examination, palpating diagnostic acupoints, including association (Shu) points on the dorsal aspect of the thoracolumbar region, alarm (Mu) points on the ventral aspect of the abdomen, and other diagnostic points. Many clinicians choose their points based on a combination of Chinese, Japanese, and Western diagnostic techniques, including tongue and pulse examination and diagnosis, diagnostic acupuncture point examination, sometimes including Ting points (points around the coronary band), and a comprehensive Western medical examination and history.[26,27] The number of acupuncture points treated may vary from one to more than 20, depending on the condition treated and the approach and experience of the practitioner. The depth of needle insertion varies from 1 mm to 12 cm, depending on the location of the point, such as the coronary band versus dorsal lumbar musculature. The number of treatments required depends on the condition treated and the chronicity of the problem, usually ranging from one to eight treatments. The length of treatment varies from 5 to 30 minutes.

Manual therapies, such as chiropractic or osteopathy, are often applied along with acupuncture. They appear to work synergistically, acupuncture relieving muscle spasms and increasing circulation, chiropractic helping to correct skeletal fixations (see Chapter 93), and osteopathy affecting the fascia and skeletal structures (see Chapter 95). The combination of these therapies often leads to a more rapid response and greater efficacy, with fewer treatments required.

CLINICAL APPLICATIONS IN LAMENESS EXAMINATION AND TREATMENT

Acupuncture Diagnostic Examination

Acupuncture and manual therapies may be used diagnostically to aid in evaluating various lameness and performance problems. Acupuncture is an excellent diagnostic aid as an adjunct to a conventional lameness examination. Many of the diagnostic acupoints are located lateral to the dorsal midline, between the longissimus and iliocostalis muscles, along the acupuncture meridian known as the *bladder meridian*.[26] In addition, some diagnostic points are actually trigger points, knots or tight bands in a muscle. For instance, a triceps trigger point is often sensitive to palpation when a distal forelimb lameness is present and correlates with the acupoint Small Intestine 9. A triceps trigger point may not indicate exactly where the lameness

is or what the cause is, but it does indicate that something is reactive in that region (Figure 92-4).

Diagnostic acupoints also are located around the coronary band on the forelimb and hindlimb, known as *Ting* points (Figure 92-5).[15] Each diagnostic acupuncture point may have four or five meanings, depending on which other points show up as reactive on the examination. For instance, one point, Large Intestine 16 (located in a depression on the cranial border of the scapula, at the intersection of the cranial margin of the scapular muscles and the caudal margin of the brachiocephalicus muscle, cranioventral to the first thoracic vertebrae) may be reactive in horses with forelimb lameness, cervical conditions, or a contralateral hindlimb lameness.[26] Sensitivity on acupoints along the bladder meridian, lateral to the dorsal midline, along the back may indicate that a hindlimb lameness is related to the stifle or hock, or that a primary back problem is related to the saddle fit, the rider, or a conformational problem. Sensitivity at acupoints suggesting a problem in the hock region also may be reactive with nearby injuries, such as a proximal suspensory problem. In addition, reactivity may indicate internal organ problems via a somatovisceral reflex. The combination of reactive points often aids the clinician in localizing the cause of the problem and determining a diagnosis. Often a horse may have a localized distal limb lameness along with a back problem. Sometimes acupoint diagnosis assists the veterinarian in figuring out which may have come first, the distal limb lameness or the back problem, based on the degree of sensitivity of the various points. Acupuncture diagnosis can be an excellent adjunct to conventional lameness examination, flexion tests, diagnostic analgesia, radiography, ultrasonography, and other diagnostic approaches. Not uncommonly we use all of our diagnostic capabilities, including nuclear scintigraphy and magnetic resonance imaging, and still do not arrive at a diagnosis. Acupuncture is often an excellent adjunct technique that may assist in elucidating the problem. In people, musculoskeletal pain often is accompanied by muscle shortening in peripheral and paraspinal muscles from spasms and contractures, and secondary trigger points and autonomic manifestations of neuropathies are also present in chronic musculoskeletal pain.[28] Patterns of trigger points distant to the primary problem, compensating for the primary musculoskeletal problem, also have been found.[29] These patterns are also evident in equine acupuncture lameness examinations. For instance, the horse may have a primary hock or stifle problem and may then develop compensatory patterns of trigger points in the back and neck and contralateral forelimb. These patterns show up as standard patterns of trigger points that may assist the veterinarian in the primary diagnosis.

An integrative approach to diagnosis is incorporated along with the acupuncture diagnostic palpation examination and includes evaluation of conformation, saddle fit, shoeing, and rider and training programs and the conventional lameness examination. Chiropractic evaluation, including static and motion palpation, also is included, which allows for a more comprehensive evaluation of all potential causes of lameness.

Acupuncture Therapy for Lameness

Acupuncture has been reported to be effective for treating various musculoskeletal pain–producing conditions and

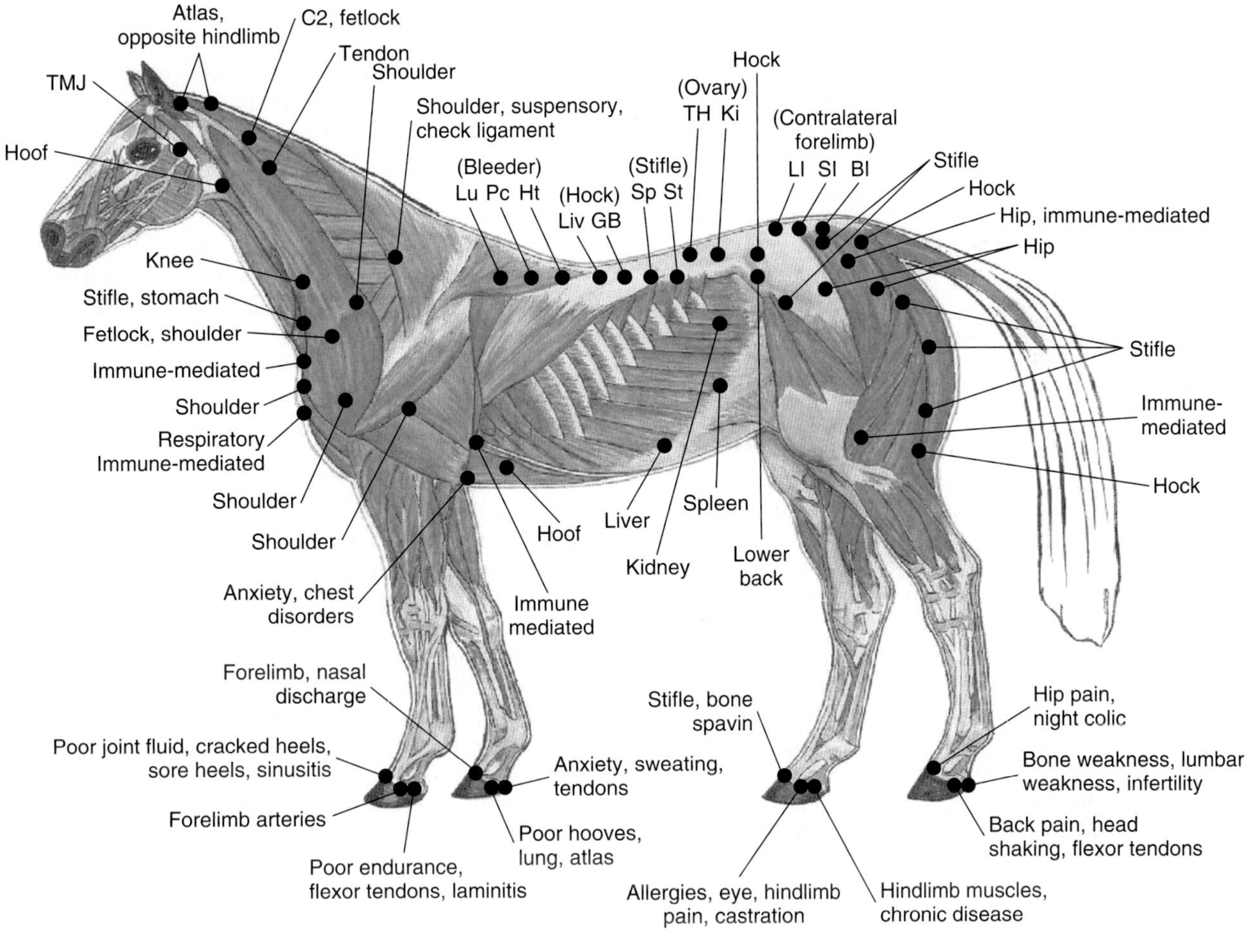

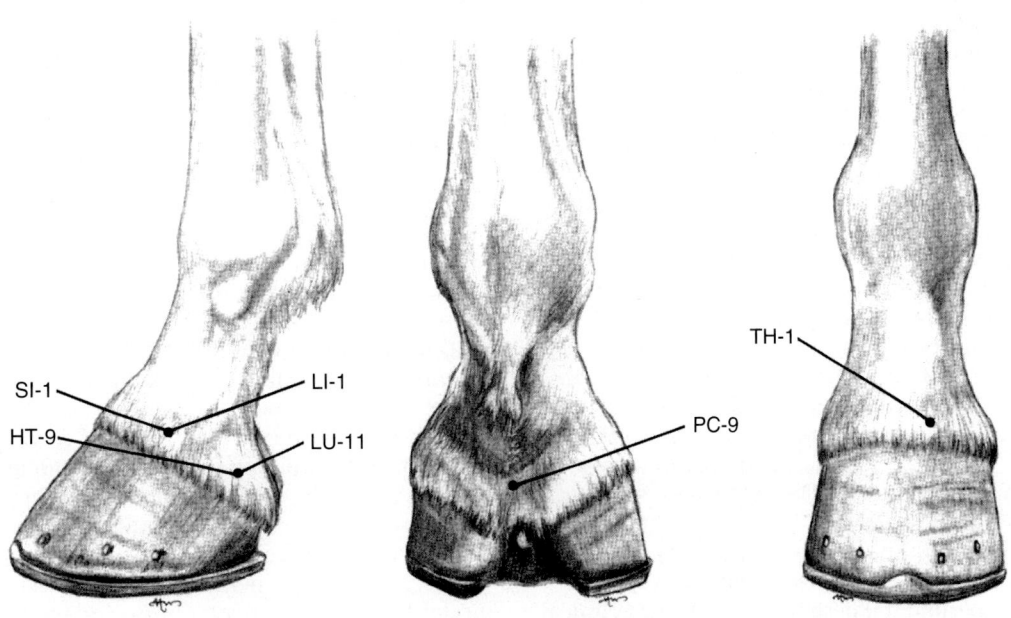

Fig. 92-4 • Diagnostic acupuncture palpation points. (Courtesy Peg Fleming. From Schoen AM, ed: *Veterinary acupuncture: ancient art to modern medicine*, ed 2, St Louis, 2001, Mosby.)

Atlas, opposite hindlimb
C2, fetlock
Tendon
Shoulder
TMJ
Shoulder, suspensory, check ligament
Hoof
Hock
(Ovary)
TH Ki
(Contralateral forelimb)
(Bleeder)
Lu Pc Ht
(Hock)
Liv GB
(Hock)
(Stifle)
Sp St
LI SI Bl
Stifle
Hock
Hip, immune-mediated
Hip
Knee
Stifle, stomach
Fetlock, shoulder
Immune-mediated
Shoulder
Respiratory
Immune-mediated
Shoulder
Shoulder
Anxiety, chest disorders
Hoof
Liver
Spleen
Kidney
Lower back
Stifle
Immune-mediated
Hock
Immune mediated
Forelimb, nasal discharge
Stifle, bone spavin
Hip pain, night colic
Poor joint fluid, cracked heels, sore heels, sinusitis
Anxiety, sweating, tendons
Bone weakness, lumbar weakness, infertility
Forelimb arteries
Poor hooves, lung, atlas
Back pain, head shaking, flexor tendons
Poor endurance, flexor tendons, laminitis
Allergies, eye, hindlimb pain, castration
Hindlimb muscles, chronic disease

Fig. 92-5 • *Ting* points of the equine front foot. In a lateral position the points are SI-1 and HT-9; in a medial position the points are LI-1 and LU-11. (From Schoen AM, ed: *Veterinary acupuncture: ancient art to modern medicine*, ed 2, St Louis, 2001, Mosby.)

SI-1
HT-9
LI-1
LU-11
PC-9
TH-1

has been found to be beneficial in treating cervical, thoracolumbar, and lumbosacral hyperpathia,[30,31] chronic back pain, chronic lameness, osteoarthritis, and colic. Hyperpathia, increased pain sensation detected as muscle spasms and increased sensitivity of acupuncture points, is often secondary to numerous causes, including work-related muscle soreness and injuries, metabolic diseases, infectious diseases, and underlying soft tissue and orthopedic problems. Wherever possible, primary underlying causes of lameness should be explored with appropriate diagnostic procedures. Conventional and complementary therapies should be considered based on what is most appropriate for the particular condition.

Back Pain

Chronic back pain can be a major cause of poor performance and may be caused by soft tissue damage or lesions to the thoracolumbar vertebrae. Numerous studies have documented the benefits of acupuncture for equine back pain.[32-42]

Xie and colleagues[24] documented the success of electroacupuncture for treating chronic back pain in performance horses in a controlled clinical trial. They found that three electroacupuncture sessions were needed for clinical improvement. Conventional medical approaches, including the administration of muscle relaxants and analgesics, usually offer only temporary and minimal improvement, decreasing the clinical signs but not addressing the specific problems. Acupuncture is able to address specific muscle spasms and trigger points. Research suggests that electroacupuncture may be stronger and more effective than dry needle techniques or aquapuncture.[24] Clinically, aquapuncture and dry needle techniques appear to be effective.

Pain Associated with Lameness of the Distal Aspect of the Limb

Acupuncture has been reported to be beneficial in horses with various distal limb lameness[43-65] and has been beneficial in treating lameness related to the shoulder, elbow, carpus, tarsus, fetlock, stifle, hip, and numerous soft tissue injuries. In one study evaluating acupuncture in the treatment of distal limb lameness, Xie and co-workers[24] found that electroacupuncture can partially relieve pain caused by the mechanical pressure induced by tightening a screw against the sole. They found that electroacupuncture significantly reduced the degree of lameness ($P < 0.001$). Electroacupuncture simultaneously increased plasma β-endorphin concentration, which suggests that endorphin release may be one of the pathways in which acupuncture relieves experimental pain. Electroacupuncture did not alter adrenocorticotrophic hormone concentrations, which indicates that the hormone may not be involved in this type of analgesia. This indicates that the mechanism of acupuncture analgesia is not merely a nerve block, as with local anesthetic solution, but that acupuncture analgesia also has central-acting effects. This correlates well with other clinical studies demonstrating the benefits of acupuncture in relieving equine lameness caused by joint contusion, muscular atrophy, rheumatic pain, and laminitis. Using a similar experimental design in a controlled clinical trial, Hackett and colleagues[65] found that acupuncture alleviated equine pain, based on heart rate measurements as an indicator of pain response. In this study acupuncture

was found to be more beneficial than nonsteroidal antiinflammatory medications.

The experience of numerous clinicians suggests that acupuncture, combining local and distant points and using various techniques, can be beneficial as a primary or secondary modality. In clinical practice, acupuncture is beneficial in resolving chronic back pain. Establishing a primary cause of back pain is critical and includes evaluating the feet, saddle fit, rider, training, and conformation. If pain primarily is caused by conformation problems, long-term resolution may include periodic electroacupuncture, traditional acupuncture, or gold bead implantation.

Acupuncture and chiropractic are used successfully in treating various equine musculoskeletal conditions as primary treatments or as adjuncts to conventional veterinary therapeutic techniques. For instance, a horse may have primary distal hock joint pain and may be treated with an intraarticular injection. However, the injection may not completely resolve hock lameness. The horse may still "not be right" or may "be off." Often secondary compensation and subsequent patterns of trigger points, muscular spasms in the longissimus, and vertebral fixations in the lumbar and cervical regions remain unresolved. Acupuncture and chiropractic therapy may then be used to treat the sequelae of the primary hock problem successfully. Hence the clinician then may resolve 100% of the lameness and increase client satisfaction.

Acupoint selection for lameness may include specific local points or ah shi (tender points) around a specific joint or region, points related to the secondary compensation for the primary lameness, and points based on traditional Chinese medicine or Japanese meridian therapy. Acupuncture may be used as primary therapy for distal limb lameness if conventional medical approaches have not demonstrated substantial improvement, or as an adjunct to conventional therapy. Horses with limb lameness that may benefit from acupuncture include those with laminitis; navicular disease; carpal, metacarpal, tarsal, fetlock, and pastern problems; soft tissue injuries; and some idiopathic problems. Horses with acute and chronic laminitis have responded favorably to acupuncture using dry needles, hemoacupuncture, or electroacupuncture. In the treatment of laminitis, local points around the coronary band are used along with distant points based on traditional Chinese medicine therapy.

SUMMARY

Acupuncture can be beneficial in diagnosing and treating various lameness conditions, including distal limb and back problems. A thorough conventional diagnostic examination should be conducted along with an acupuncture diagnostic examination. All therapeutic options appropriate for a specific lameness condition should be considered. The advantages and disadvantages of each therapy should be discussed. Acupuncture can be considered as a primary therapy or as an adjunct treatment, depending on the condition. No one form of medicine has all the answers. Clinicians should consider the most appropriate conventional and complementary diagnostic and therapeutic modalities for the particular horse and its owner to develop a comprehensive, integrative approach to equine lameness. Acupuncture is one of these complementary approaches that may be beneficial for the lame horse.

ACUPUNCTURE CHANNEL PALPATION AND EQUINE MUSCULOSKELETAL PAIN

William H. McCormick

The key to the diagnosis and treatment of equine musculoskeletal pain with acupuncture is the Oriental examination. The preferred use of acupuncture in a healthy, nonlame sports horse implies the anticipation and rectification of abnormalities before they become clinical entities. However, in the presence of overt pathology, the descriptive methodology and therapeutic protocol of acupuncture will proceed as in a presupposed normal horse. The basic principle of Traditional Oriental Medicine (TOM) as stated in Mandarin Chinese is *bien jheng lun jhi,* or in translation, "treatment is based on pattern differentiation."[1] The *si jhun,* or four examinations of (1) looking, (2) asking, (3) palpating, and (4) listening and smelling, are the criteria for determining patterns. A patient's pattern is defined by the sum total of the signs, symptoms, tongue, and pulse as determined by the *si jhun.*[2] Palpation is the most easily adapted of the four examinations for horses. In current equine practice the underpinning logic of TOM is combined with the precise palpation of the Japanese tradition and the linear analysis of Western equine lameness diagnosis.

How does the Oriental pattern-based therapy differ from the Western disease-based approach? The Western practitioner arrives at a diagnosis by physical examination supported by the available technologies such as nerve blocks, radiography, nuclear scintigraphy, and other techniques. The strict practitioner of TOM must rely on the patterns demonstrated by the horse using the *si jhun* without technical support. For example, in a horse with pain in the palmar aspect of a foot one might expect the following patterns, to name only a few: *Blood Stasis,* or fixed pain; *Qi Stagnation,* or moving, referred muscle pain; *Liver Depression,* or anger expressed in stereotypical behavior; and *Heart Qi Vacuity,* or anxiety. The total of the patterns is a description of the presentation of the disease in TOM. Most diseases exhibit a number of different patterns. Furthermore, therapy is defined by the pattern, because each pattern must be addressed in the subsequent therapeutic principles. In other words, the pattern of *Blood Stasis* (fixed pain) requires the use of a TOM therapy that will *Quicken the Blood and Resolve Stasis. Qi Stagnation* requires *Moving Qi.* The stated functions of each acupoint or herbal medicinal are used to determine which acupoints or medicinals to select. The proper use of the descriptive methodology of TOM forces a practitioner to describe each individual in terms of patterns that will then be used to determine therapy. None of this replaces Western structural diagnosis, but the scope of one's physical examination is greatly enhanced.

One must evaluate the use of acupuncture by the elimination of abnormal pattern(s). However, any other therapy, be it Western or Oriental, can also be evaluated in terms of its effect on the pattern(s). For the purpose of practical illustration, consider that a horse with pain in the palmar aspect of the foot is not lame, but the rider complains of a change in performance caused by pain—for example, stiff in the corners, late leaving the ground when jumping, sore

back. In such a horse the TOM pattern may add important information, whereas radiography, scintigraphy, and magnetic resonance imaging are technological overkill, expensive, unwieldy, and perhaps misleading. It may be less invasive and more efficient to treat the horse with available modalities such as shoeing, drugs, acupuncture, and herbs and to subsequently evaluate the change in pattern and performance. Sophisticated imaging techniques can and should be used to establish a structural anatomical diagnosis when possible. The therapeutic advantage of an integrated Western and Oriental approach is most applicable to a subclinically or functionally sore horse, as opposed to a horse with a structural lameness.

There is one examination within TOM that can be conducted in a timely manner and that can add information about every horse's response to musculoskeletal pathology. Channel Diagnosis is a technique by which individual acupoints are palpated to determine the characteristics of those sites. Most acupoints are linked in groups called *channels,* which allow for a systematic organization. The acupoints themselves are specific anatomical sites on the body that a practitioner can use for diagnosis and treatment (Figure 92-6).[3] Usually an acupoint is in a palpable depression in regions of high electrical conductance.[4] Although there are 173 acupoints described in the traditional veterinary literature,[5] less than 20 diagnostic acupoints are needed for the assessment of the response of the horse to exercise.

The qualitative acupoint description attained through palpation can be useful in a Western context. Acupoint examination should include a grading system for reactivity and a recording of those reactions over time. I use the following simple grading system for acupoints in Excess. As opposed to the characteristic of Deficiency, acupoints in Excess are the easiest to appreciate and locate, because they are actively sensitive and energetically rise to meet the examiner's palpation. The grading scheme is as follows: Grade I is a normal, supple, and nonpainful response to deep (1 to 5 cm) palpation. Grade II is a slight muscle twinge that is fatigable. Grade III is consistent pain or avoidance response to deep palpation. Palpation of an acupoint with Grade IV sensitivity will elicit a sharp avoidance response accompanied by a kick or a bite. Sensitivity of Grades III and IV are of sufficient severity to warrant therapy.

The Deficiency pattern is the mirror image of the Excess pattern. Whereas the Excess pattern reflects the superficial response of the organism to adversity, the Deficiency pattern reflects a more subtle depth of pathology.[6] Unfortunately, the determination of the presence of a Deficiency pattern requires the clinician to recognize the horse's minimal passive resistance to palpation. The Deficiency pattern can best be appreciated after the practitioner has injected intraarticular antiinflammatory medication in a degenerative joint. In such a horse the Excess pattern of muscle hyperreactivity related to the joint will be dramatically dissipated, but there will remain a low resistance that can easily be missed in superficial palpation. The sharper the Excess perceived by the examiner the greater the probability of the presence of underlying, hidden Deficiency. The difference between these two patterns in sports horses is theorized to be caused by the difference in reflex muscle tension caused by synovial receptors (Excess)

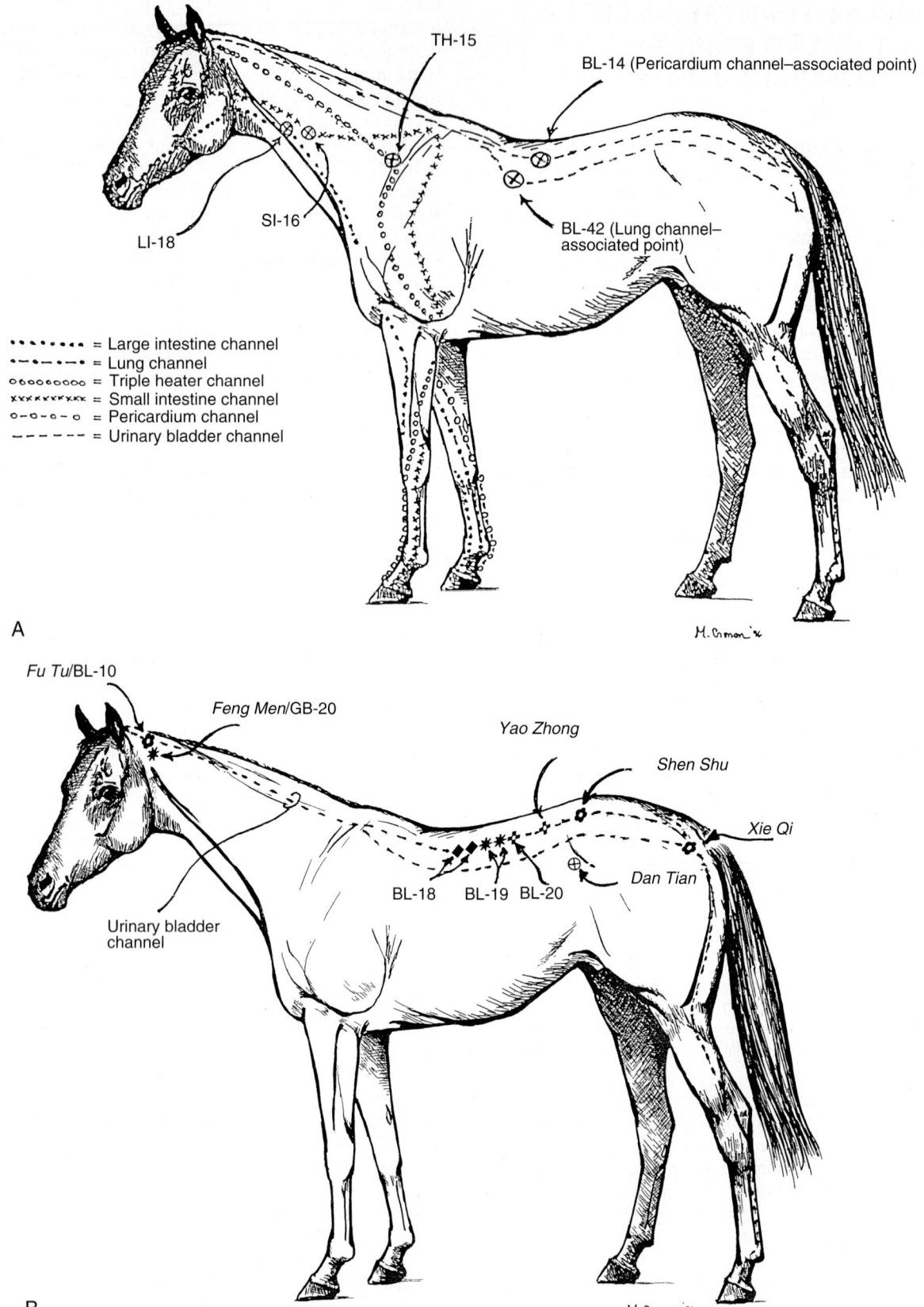

= Large intestine channel
= Lung channel
= Triple heater channel
= Small intestine channel
= Pericardium channel
= Urinary bladder channel

TH-15

BL-14 (Pericardium channel–associated point)

SI-16

LI-18

BL-42 (Lung channel–associated point)

A

Fu Tu/BL-10

Feng Men/GB-20

Yao Zhong

Shen Shu

Xie Qi

Urinary bladder channel

BL-18   BL-19   BL-20

Dan Tian

B

Fig. 92-6 • A, The principal acupoints used in the diagnosis of channel pain referable to the equine forelimb. **B,** The principal acupoints used in the diagnosis of channel pain referable to the equine hindlimb. (Courtesy William E. Jones.)

BOX 92-1

Traditional Oriental Medicine Acupoints and International Veterinary Acupuncture Transpositional Points for Best Overall Assessment of a Horse

1. Large Intestine (LI) 18: An acupoint at the level of the caudal aspect of Viborg's triangle on the ventral aspect of the sternocleidomastoid muscle at the junction of the third (C3) and the fourth (C4) cervical vertebrae. The distal course of this channel passes over the dorsomedial aspect of the distal extremity of the forelimb.[7,8]

2. Small Intestine (SI) 16: An acupoint located caudal to the angle of the mandible in a depression on the dorsal border of the sternocleidomastoid muscle, and dorsal to the transverse processes of C3 and C4 or approximately 8 to 10 cm caudal to LI 18. Distally the SI channel courses over the dorsolateral aspect of the forelimb.[7,8]

3. Triple Heater (TH) 15: An acupoint located on the cranial border of the scapula in a depression approximately one third of the distance from the cranial angle of the scapula to the shoulder joint. TH 15 is defined by the ventral borders of the cervical serratus and the cervical trapezius muscles. The course of this channel crosses the dorsal midline of the distal extremity of the forelimb.[5,7]

4. Urinary Bladder (UB) 42: An acupoint located in a depression over the seventh intercostal space just caudal to the scapular cartilage in a muscular groove between the longissimus thoracis and the iliocostalis thoracis muscles, approximately 20 cm from the dorsal midline. UB 42 is the *Shu* or associated point for the Lung (LU) channel, which runs over the distal medial aspect of the equine forelimb.[5,7]

5. Urinary Bladder (BL) 14: An acupoint that is approximately 12 cm lateral to the midline and parallel to the caudal border of the dorsal spinous process of the ninth thoracic vertebra. In the ninth intercostal space, this acupoint is situated approximately 10 cm caudal and dorsal to UB 42. UB 14 is the *Shu* point of the Pericardium (PC) channel in the IVAS (International Veterinary Acupuncture Society) transpositional system. The PC channel courses over the palmar midline of the distal aspect of the digit.[7,9]

6. Urinary Bladder (BL) 18, *Gan Shu:* An acupoint located approximately 12 cm lateral to the caudal border of the dorsal spinous processes of the thirteenth and fourteenth thoracic vertebrae, at the thirteenth and fourteenth intercostal spaces in the muscular groove between the iliocostalis and the latissimus dorsi muscles. BL 18 is associated with the Liver channel, the distal course of which passes over the distal dorsomedial aspect of the hindlimb.[7,10]

7. Urinary Bladder (BL) 19, *Dan Shu:* An acupoint located approximately 12 cm lateral to the caudal border of the dorsal spinous processes of the fifteenth and sixteenth thoracic vertebrae, at the fifteenth and sixteenth intercostal spaces in the muscular groove between the iliocostalis and the latissimus dorsi muscles. BL 19 is associated with the Gall Bladder channel, which courses over the dorsolateral distal aspect of the hindlimb.[7,10]

8. Urinary Bladder (BL) 20, *Pi Shu:* An acupoint located approximately 12 cm lateral to the caudal border of the spinous process of the seventeenth thoracic vertebra, at the last intercostal space in the muscular groove between the iliocostalis and the latissimus dorsi muscles. BL 20 is associated with the Spleen channel, which crosses the distal medial aspect of the hindlimb.[7,10]

9. *Yao Zhong:* An acupoint approximately 12 cm lateral to the dorsal midline between the third and the fourth lumbar vertebrae, midway between the caudal border of the last rib and *Shen Shu,* a traditional veterinary acupoint. *Yao Zhong* is associated with the Stomach channel, which courses over the dorsal distal aspect of the hindlimb.[5,11]

10. *Shen Shu:* An acupoint approximately 6 cm lateral to the lumbosacral space. *Shen Shu* is the traditional veterinary acupoint associated with the Kidney channel, which courses over the plantaromedial aspect of the tarsus and the plantar midline of the distal aspect of the hindlimb.[5,11]

11. *Xie Qi:* An acupoint in the muscular groove between the biceps femoris and the semimembranosus muscles and at a level horizontal to the anus. *Xie Qi* is used as the associated point of the Urinary Bladder channel, which courses over the plantarolateral distal aspect of the hindlimb.[5,11]

12. *Feng Men* (Gall Bladder [GB] 20): An acupoint in a depression cranial to the wing of the atlas, 6 cm ventral to the dorsal midline and 3 cm caudal to the ear base. *Feng Men* reflects the distal dorsolateral aspect of the hindlimb.[5,10]

13. *Fu-Tu* (BL 10): An acupoint in a depression cranial to the wing of the atlas, 6 cm caudal to the ear base and 4.5 cm ventral to the dorsal midline. *Fu-Tu* reflects the distal plantarolateral aspect of the hindlimb.[5,10]

14. *Dan Tian* (GB 28): An acupoint in a depression 4.5 cm ventral to the tuber coxae at the origin of the tensor fascia latae muscle. *Dan Tian* reflects the distal dorsolateral aspect of the hindlimb.[5,12]

and extrasynovial structures (Deficiency). A nonarticular example of extreme Excess and Deficiency patterns in the horse occurring simultaneously would be that of tying-up, in which the "boardlike" quality of the superficial muscles prevents any deep palpation of Deficiency in the underlying structurally affected tissues.

Each of the following acupoints corresponds to a TOM channel or meridian, which in turn is named after an internal organ. The twelve channels govern the flow of *Qi,* or life forces, for the whole body. I mix TOM acupoints with International Veterinary Acupuncture Society (IVAS) transpositional points to give the best overall assessment of a horse (Box 92-1).

What meaning can we attribute to reactive acupoints? I published a series of articles on the use of reactive acupoints in Excess for pain referable to the shoulder joint,[12] metacarpophalangeal joint,[13] distal interphalangeal (DIP) joint,[14] and the joints of the distal aspect of the hindlimb.[15] These articles were based on 712 lame and "sore" horses. Over 14 years, which succeeded 13 years of strictly Western lameness practice, many thousands of examinations were conducted to establish a protocol and to subsequently

confirm the principles for evaluating reactive acupoints. In another study 350 working sports horses and racehorses were represented as serviceably sound, but 37% of the horses were lame and 39% had reactive acupoints.[16] When the lame horses were compared with the sound horses with respect to reactive acupoints, 25% of the sound horses had Grade III or IV reactive acupoints, whereas 63% of lame horses had similar abnormalities.[16] Therefore, reactive acupoints in the channels were frequently observed and bore a close relationship to lameness and, by implication, a similar relationship to subclinical musculoskeletal pain.

The following is a set of guidelines for palpating acupoints in Excess:

1. Palpable reactive acupoints in musculoskeletal disease are dependent on neural control through the spinal reflex (Figure 92-7).
2. Reactive acupoints that reflect the distal aspect of the limb can be differentiated from local muscular injury, somatovisceral pain, spinal neurogenic pain, and myofascial pain by intraarticular medication. That is to say, if a pattern of reactive acupoints is

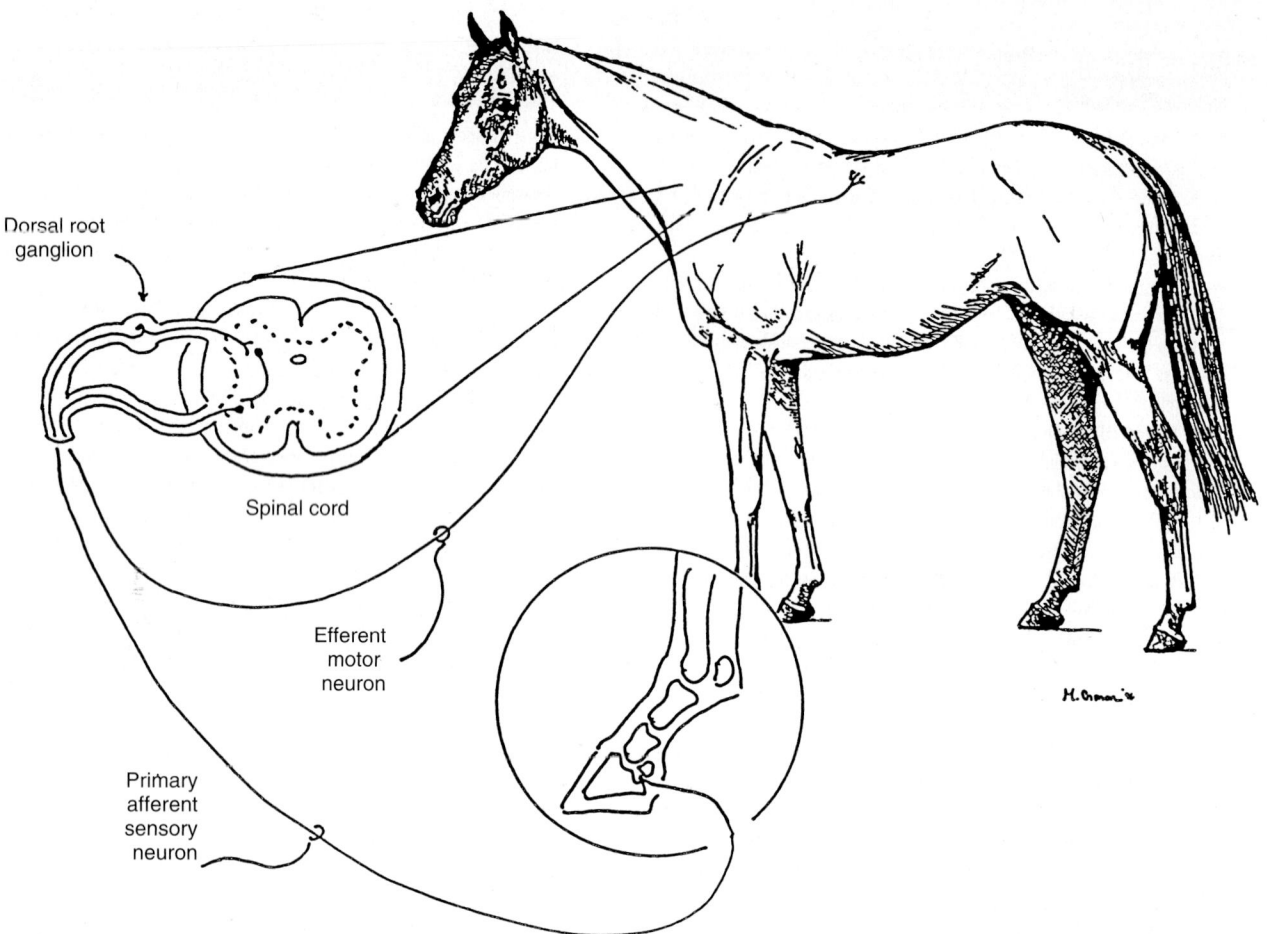

Dorsal root
ganglion

Spinal cord

Efferent
motor
neuron

Primary
afferent
sensory
neuron

Fig. 92-7 • The mediation of channel pain through the spinal reflex. (Courtesy William E. Jones.)

present and if intraarticular medication abolishes the pattern, then the treated joint(s) alone are responsible for the changed reactive acupoints regardless of what other pathology may be present. Intraarticular mepivacaine hydrochloride* will change acupoint reactivity within 10 minutes. Intraarticular triamcinolone acetonide,† methylprednisolone acetate,‡ or hyaluronan§ will change the acupoints within 24 hours.

3. In musculoskeletal extremity pain (*Bi Syndrome*), acupuncture channel reactivity in Excess reflects only synovial inflammation in the DIP, proximal interphalangeal (PIP), metacarpophalangeal, and carpal joints in the forelimbs and the DIP, PIP, metatarsophalangeal, and distal tarsal joints and the stifle in the hindlimbs. Reactive acupoints in Excess do not reflect nonsynovial pain such as subchondral bone or extraarticular structures. Reactive acupoints in Excess are frequently present as a warning or as part of a complex disease presentation, as in fetlock inflammation together with superficial digital flexor tendon pathology, or DIP joint inflammation in association with laminitis.

4. Potentially any joint can produce any pattern of reactive acupoints, but some joints have patterns that occur statistically more frequently than others, such as BL 14 reactivity in DIP joint inflammation,[14] *Yao Zhong* in metatarsophalangeal joint inflammation,[15] or *Yan Chi* in stifle joint inflammation.[3,17,18] The channel that courses across the inflammatory site and the severity of inflammation will determine the reflected acupoint and the reactivity of that acupoint. For example, pain in the palmar aspect of the foot is reflected at the acupoint BL 14, which is stimulated by pericardium channel (PC) channel reactivity (see Figure 92-6). However, BL 14 can also be stimulated by palmar inflammation in the pastern, fetlock, or carpus.

5. Complex diseases are represented by a number of different patterns occurring simultaneously. The projection of reactive acupoints by inflamed synovial structures is one clinical finding that can be easily confirmed by practical Western diagnostic tests. If a careful evaluation of the acupoints was performed before a joint injection, then the effect on the acupuncture pattern can be evaluated after the injection.

6. Somatovisceral dysfunction can be reflected in the channel palpation of sports horses. The internal organs that are frequently represented are lungs,

*Carbocaine-V, Upjohn.
†Vetalogue, Solvay.
‡Depo-Medrol, Upjohn.
§MAP 5, Vetrepharm.

stomach, liver, and ovary or testis. Because somato-visceral patterns tend to be more subdued than the Excess patterns of joint inflammation, the former can be obscured. Elimination of musculoskeletal patterns by joint medication can reveal the underlying somatovisceral patterns.

7. Neurogenic pain is reflected in acupoint projection from spinal structures such as the cervical and thoracolumbar facet joints, or the sacroiliac joint. Acupoints reflecting spinal pain are manifest in the associated segment as opposed to being proximally or distally projected. The grade of reactivity of these structures is more often Grade III and, as in somatovisceral pain, can be obscured by extremity pain of an equal or more severe grade. Neurogenic pain results in the muscular splinting of the spine and a loss of systemic flexibility. Some flexibility can be added back into the system by hyperextension of the joints of the distal extremities. The cost of the greater range of articular motion is joint inflammation, which is reflected in the acupuncture channels. Thus, neurogenic pain is commonly accompanied by extremity inflammation.

8. Myofascial pain in people has been well described,[19] and more recently myofascial pain in the horse has been described.[20] However, self-perpetuating discrete myofascial trigger points palpated within a tight band of muscle are quite rare in the horse. The cleidobrachialis muscle is one of the few muscles in the horse that is amenable to the strict definition of myofascial pain.

When a horse with subclinical pain but with a multi-pattern acupoint abnormality is examined, intraarticular medication may remove one or more patterns. If a horse has acupoint examination abnormalities reflecting the extremities of both the forelimbs and hindlimbs and the distal hock joints are injected, and if, indeed, the primary source of inflammation is the tarsus, then the whole acupuncture presentation will change. But if there is concomitant involvement of the hind fetlock, stifle, or forelimb joints, then only the pattern reflecting the distal aspect of the tarsus will change. The patterns that reflect the other joints will remain the same. Nonarticular peritarsal pathology such as painful hind splints or suspensory desmopathy will not directly cause a pattern that is reflected in reactive acupoints in Excess. Rather, the Excess pattern will reflect only the distal aspect of the tarsus. Joint infection is also not reflected in Excess acupoints.

It is good practice to routinely reexamine horses that have received joint therapy or acupuncture on both day 1 and day 7. Reexamination allows for a rider or trainer's evaluation as well as a careful reassessment by the veterinarian. If the pattern is balanced and the horse is doing well, then one's efforts should be directed toward maintaining the acupuncture balance. The remaining points of low reactivity can be managed using acupuncture or manual therapy. However, if lameness or sharply reactive acupoints remain, then the basic premise of one's diagnosis must be reevaluated.

The effect of other medications and management changes can be assessed. Shoeing changes will directly affect acupuncture balance, as will the forgiveness of track surfaces and training and management regimens. It is the responsibility of the trainer to bring the equine athlete up to the peak of fitness without going over the edge. The acupuncture examination is one of the ways that "the edge" can be defined. From the Western point of view, the presence of acupoints in Excess in musculoskeletal conditions indicates that affected joints have not been able to spontaneously recover from exercise-induced hyperflexion. Excess acupoint reactivity in joint pain is a function of highly innervated intraarticular synovial structures that are activated by the mediators of traumatic inflammation,[21] which in turn are activated by joint hyperextension. The distribution, incidence, and severity of Excess acupoint activity depend on the spatial distribution of nociceptor sites within specific joints and the quantity and characteristics of released inflammatory mediators within those joints. Lameness is a function of a much broader range of pain perception.

Joints that project reactive acupoints vary according to the horse's use. Thoroughbred racehorses have a greater incidence of synovial inflammation in the metacarpophalangeal joint, reflecting the proximal dorsal aspect of the proximal phalanx versus the DIP joint, whereas the converse is true for show hunters. In both types of horses I find a high incidence of distal hock joint pain. Steeplechase horses and show jumpers have a high incidence of hind fetlock inflammation, and numerous ipsilateral joints can be involved. It is difficult to determine multiple joint inflammation if lameness is not severe enough to abolish using diagnostic analgesia. Careful examination of horses after joint therapy and over time should reveal changes in acupoint reactivity. Horses returning to competition after a long rest tend to revert to the same acupuncture patterns that they displayed during previous training. In horses recovering from surgery, the acupuncture pattern is a sensitive early sign of a need for changes in management.

Two papers published in English define the limits of acupuncture in sports horses. Martin and Klide's work on back pain showed the efficacy of modulation of muscle tension on the performance of equine athletes.[22] Steiss showed that acupuncture in foot lameness was no better than that expected in untreated controls.[23] Martin and Klide were treating the TOM pattern of *Qi Stagnation* or abnormal muscle tension as opposed to Steiss's fixed pain pattern of *Blood Stasis*. The strength of acupuncture is its ability to restore normal physiological activity in the face of functional abnormality. Hackett, Spitzfaden, and May showed that pain modulation after digital electroacupuncture is similar to that provided by phenylbutazone therapy.[24] However, foot pain cannot be as easily reversed as abnormal back muscle tension. Acupuncture can be used effectively as an adjunctive therapy if muscle hyperactivity is part of the pattern. Careful examination of the channels should provide evidence of patterns with a good therapeutic potential.

The basis of acupuncture diagnosis and therapy in musculoskeletal disease depends on pattern differentiation. The patterns most easily determined by the Western practitioner involve the precise palpation of key acupoints in Channel Diagnosis. Acupoint reactivity of musculoskeletal dysfunction is a reflection of the body's response to intraarticular trauma. Because only highly innervated synovial structures of a small number of joints of the extremities are reflected by reactive acupoints, the primary disease may be reflected only indirectly or not at all. However, abnormal patterns are extremely common and are worth investigating regardless of the type of therapy contemplated. At the least, the abnormal pattern is a warning. The ease that one has in elimination of a pattern over time will give an idea of the persistence and severity of the underlying traumatic pathology.

The pattern projected by synovial structures is a protective mechanism, the presence of which is the teleological function of limitation of joint excursion. Therefore,

effective treatment must go beyond the elimination of acupoint imbalance and address all the underlying problems as well. Because disease in TOM consists of all of the existent abnormal patterns, treatment of multipattern abnormalities must be undertaken. In my experience the channel approach to horses with subclinical pain is effective and useful. With the exception of lameness from muscle tension, acupuncture is generally not sufficient by itself to address lameness that is obvious enough to abolish using diagnostic analgesia.

Chapter 93

Chiropractic Evaluation and Management of Musculoskeletal Disorders

Kevin K. Haussler

MANUAL THERAPY AND CHIROPRACTIC

Manual therapy involves the application of the hands directly to the body, with the goal of treating soft tissue injuries or articular dysfunction. Chiropractic, osteopathy, massage therapy, therapeutic touch, and certain physical therapy techniques are considered forms of manual therapy. Chiropractic is a health profession concerned with the diagnosis, treatment, and prevention of disorders of the musculoskeletal system and the effects of these disorders on the nervous system and general health.[1] The word *chiropractic* is derived from the Greek words *cheir,* meaning "hand," and *praktikos,* meaning "concerning action." The goal of chiropractic is to optimize health through the inherent healing ability of the body (i.e., homeostasis) as affected by and integrated through the nervous system.[2] The practice of chiropractic focuses on the relationship between structure (primarily the spinal column) and function (as coordinated by the nervous system) and how that relationship affects the preservation and restoration of health. Chiropractic uses controlled forces (i.e., adjustments), which are applied to specific joints or anatomical regions, to induce therapeutic responses through induced changes in joint structures, muscle function, and neurological reflexes. Research in people demonstrated reductions in pain and muscle hypertonicity and increased joint range of motion after chiropractic treatment.[2,3]

Joint mobilization and manipulation are two types of induced articular movements used in musculoskeletal rehabilitation to restore joint function. Mobilization is characterized as repetitive joint movements induced within the normal physiological range of joint motion (Figure 93-1). Joint manipulation (e.g., chiropractic adjustment) occurs within the paraphysiological zone, which lies outside of the active (i.e., patient induced) and passive ranges of joint

References on page 1333

motion. In people, joint mobilization and manipulation induce different physiological responses. Manipulation in people relieved adjacent spontaneous myoelectrical activity immediately, whereas mobilization did not.[2]

PRACTITIONER QUALIFICATIONS

Equine practitioners have seen a proliferation in the use of chiropractic techniques on horses, in one form or another. Veterinarians currently do not receive any formal education in chiropractic principles or techniques; therefore many equine clinicians do not have a basic understanding of chiropractic principles or clinical applications. Conversely, chiropractors (doctors of chiropractic) do not have any formal training in comparative anatomy, physiology, or pathology or clinical equine experience. Veterinary medicine, for the most part, has been forced to acknowledge the use of chiropractic and other nontraditional modalities by horse owners who have sought practitioners who use these techniques and have experienced their perceived therapeutic effects.[4] However, limited research has been done to evaluate the clinical effectiveness of chiropractic techniques in horses. If veterinarians have not taken the time or made the effort to learn more about these nontraditional techniques, objectively evaluating the use of chiropractic, discussing the indications or contraindications for a specific treatment modality, or applying these techniques clinically is difficult. Therefore owners often seek advice about alternative therapies or treatment from

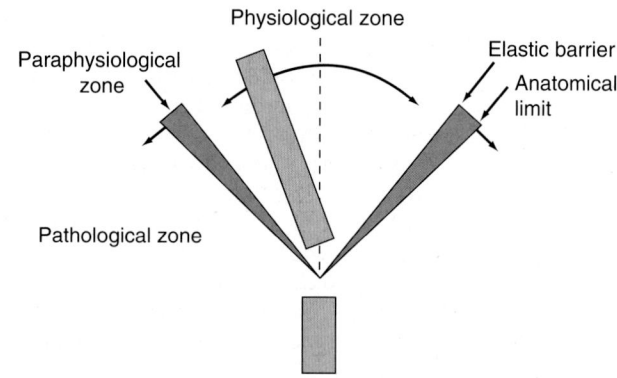

Fig. 93-1 • Schematic representation of the three articular zones of joint motion: physiological, paraphysiological, and pathological. The elastic barrier and the anatomical limit mark the transitional boundaries among the three articular zones.

someone who is not their regular veterinarian and often without his or her knowledge. To complicate matters, many laypersons claiming to be equine chiropractors are not professionally trained or licensed in chiropractic or veterinary medicine. These lay practitioners often have a limited knowledge of equine musculoskeletal anatomy, physiology, biomechanics, and pathology. Because of the potential misapplication, chiropractic evaluation and treatment should be provided only by licensed professionals (i.e., veterinarians or chiropractors working under the direct supervision of a veterinarian) who have pursued additional postgraduate training in animal chiropractic principles and techniques. The primary organizations in North America currently involved in training and certifying veterinarians and chiropractors in animal chiropractic are Options for Animals, based in Wellsville, Kansas; Parker College of Chiropractic in Dallas, Texas; and the Healing Oasis Wellness Center in Sturtevant, Wisconsin and in Canada. An additional course on equine osteopathy is offered at the Vluggen Institute in San Marcos, Texas. Equine manual therapy courses in Europe include Focus on the Equine Spine in the Netherlands; McTimoney College of Chiropractic in England; the International Academy of Veterinary Chiropractic in both Germany and England; and a Healing Oasis Wellness Center–sponsored course in Germany.

Most state chiropractic and veterinary medical boards do not allow chiropractors to treat animals unless they are working under the direct supervision of a veterinarian. This requires that the veterinarian and chiropractor work together in evaluating and treating the horse and provide appropriate follow-up care as indicated. It is strongly recommended that owners and referring veterinarians seek out licensed professionals (veterinarians or chiropractors) who have had specialized training and experience in chiropractic evaluation and treatment of horses. Veterinarians who have not pursued formal postgraduate training are not qualified to provide chiropractic care and risk producing more harm than potential benefit. It is a good idea to ask equine chiropractors about their professional and postgraduate training or certification, horse experience, and the types of techniques that they use (i.e., hands only versus more aggressive techniques, or the use of additional instruments). Chiropractic and osteopathy require a working knowledge and understanding of vertebral anatomy, physiology, biomechanics, pathology, and rehabilitation. Combining the knowledge and expertise of the veterinary and chiropractic professions provides practitioners with new insights and methods for diagnosing and managing horses with select vertebral or musculoskeletal disorders. A similar multidisciplinary approach has developed in human medicine in the last 20 years to address chronic pain syndromes and vertebral column disorders.

HISTORY OF EQUINE CHIROPRACTIC

Chiropractors often have been asked to treat the horses of clients who have experienced the benefits of chiropractic care for their own back or neck problems. Horse owners often want the opportunity to have the same type of care for their horses, without the potential adverse effects of medications or surgery. The recent increased awareness of the prevalence and management options to address back problems with which traditional veterinary medicine has

had difficulty in dealing has also stimulated horse owners' interest in complementary forms of treatment.[5] Any vertebral column disorder can have serious effects on a horse's ability to perform. Back problems can be classified into three basic types of injuries—those involving the muscles, tendons, and ligaments (soft tissue injuries); bones and joints (osseous injuries); or nervous system (neurological disorders). However, several concurrent injuries have been reported in 17% of horses with back pain.[6] Diagnosis of the underlying vertebral pathological conditions in horses with back pain is important for the appropriate treatment and management of these disorders (see Chapter 52).

Many horses in which chiropractic may be useful often have a history of a traumatic event or an injury related to overexertion.[7] Trauma may occur as a single event (i.e., macrotrauma), such as a trailer accident, flipping over backward, or substantial falls over jumps. Severe musculoskeletal injuries may improve gradually, but they never resolve totally, or debilitating arthritis or soft tissue fibrosis may subsequently develop. Chronic overuse injuries (i.e., microtrauma) usually are associated with poor saddle fit, improper riding techniques, inadequate shoeing, or faulty conformation. Long periods of confinement, inconsistent training programs, or cumulative stresses and strains related to prolonged, high-level athletic activities also may predispose horses to musculoskeletal injuries and reduced performance. Older horses, like elderly people, are susceptible to loss of vertebral column flexibility, joint degeneration, and loss of muscle strength. Aged horses also have increased healing times and increased chances of having chronic conditions or abnormal musculoskeletal compensations from prior injuries. Chiropractic techniques have helped identify and treat some of these previously undiagnosed or poorly managed problems in horses. Most veterinarians use chiropractic techniques to complement their conventional veterinary practice.

COMPLEMENTARY APPROACHES

Prevalence of back problems in horses varies greatly (from 0.9% to 94%), depending on the specialization or type of practice surveyed: general practice, 0.9%; Thoroughbred racehorse practice, 2%; veterinary school referrals, 5%; mixed equine practice including dressage, show jumpers, and eventing, 13%; spinal research clinic, 47%; and equine chiropractic clinic, 94%.[8] Clinicians often have difficulties when dealing with horses with no obvious localized pain or vague, unspecified lameness. Neck or back problems and limb injuries often are interrelated. Distal limb injuries can cause an alteration in carriage of the affected limb and altered gait, which subsequently can overwork or injure proximal limb musculature and the paraspinal musculature. Similarly, vertebral column injuries can produce gait abnormalities, increased concussive forces, and distal limb lameness. The diagnostic dilemma facing clinicians is to decide whether the limb or the vertebral column is the primary or initial cause of the horse's clinical problem. Unless the primary cause of the neck or back pain is identified and treated, most horses will have recurrent back pain when returned to work after a period of rest or a trial of antiinflammatory medications. Nonspecific back pain most likely is related to a functional impairment and not a structural disorder. Therefore many back problems may be related to muscle or joint dysfunction, with secondary soft tissue irritation and pain generation.[9]

Chiropractic provides expertise in evaluating vertebral column disorders and can provide an additional means of diagnosis and early treatment options in certain types of gait abnormalities or performance problems. Prepurchase examinations using chiropractic examination techniques can help identify horses that have chronic underlying neck or back problems.[7] Chiropractic addresses subclinical conditions or abnormal biomechanics, which may progress to future debilitating musculoskeletal injuries. Chiropractors are trained in using physiotherapy modalities, strength training exercises, massage, stretching techniques, and other forms of musculoskeletal and nerve rehabilitation. Equine chiropractic is a complementary modality that can be used in veterinary medicine for the diagnosis, treatment, and potential prevention of select musculoskeletal disorders in horses. However, although a few recent studies have investigated the short-term effectiveness of chiropractic intervention in the horse, none have addressed performance benefits, long-term efficacy, and the safety or cost-effectiveness of chiropractic procedures in equine veterinary medicine.

PATHOPHYSIOLOGY AND MECHANISMS OF ACTION

The vertebral motion segment is the functional unit of the vertebral column and includes two adjacent vertebrae and the associated soft tissues that bind them together. The basic elements of joint dysfunction include altered articular neurophysiology, biochemical alterations, pathological conditions of the joint capsule, and articular degeneration.[2,3] Vertebral segment dysfunction (i.e., chiropractically defined subluxation) is a vertebral lesion characterized by the following:

1. Asymmetrical or loss of normal joint motion (Figure 93-2)
2. Diminished pain thresholds to pressure in the adjacent paraspinal tissues or osseous structures
3. Abnormal paraspinal muscle tension
4. Visual or palpatory signs of active inflammation or chronic tissue texture abnormalities (e.g., edema, fibrosis, hyperemia, or altered temperature)[2]

Numerous theories have been proposed and tested over the years to explain the causes of vertebral segment dysfunction in people and its effects on the neuromusculoskeletal system.[2,3] The chiropractically defined vertebral subluxation complex is a theoretical model that incorporates the complex mechanical and biochemical interactions of injured nervous, muscular, articular, ligamentous, vascular, and connective tissues.[10] The theory of a "bone out of place" is outdated and not supported by current spinal research in people.

The goal of chiropractic treatment is to reduce pain and muscle hypertonicity, restore joint motion, and stimulate neurological reflexes. The exact mechanisms by which chiropractic techniques produce therapeutic effects are not certain. Chiropractic treatment may reduce musculoskeletal pain by stimulating nociceptive reflexes and release of neuropeptides (i.e., endorphins and enkephalins).[2,11,12] Concurrent muscle spasms restrict joint motion and may contribute to the further development of joint stiffness. In people, palpatory changes in osseous symmetry after manipulation often are associated with soft tissue alterations and not actual reduction of an articular misalignment.[9] Chiropractic care can improve restricted joint motion and may reduce the associated harmful effects of joint immobilization.[2,3] In response to chronic pain or stiffness, new movement patterns are learned by the nervous system and adopted in an attempt to reduce pain or discomfort. Long after the initial injury has healed, adaptive or secondary movement patterns that predispose additional joints or muscles to injury may persist.[9] Chiropractic treatment is thought to affect mechanoreceptors (i.e., Golgi tendon organ and muscle spindles) to induce reflex inhibition of pain and reflex muscle relaxation and to correct abnormal movement patterns.[10,12] Additional modalities used to address altered movement patterns in people and horses include stretching or relaxing hypertonic muscles, strengthening weak muscles, and reeducating movement patterns.[9]

Successful chiropractic treatment requires specific techniques and psychomotor skills.[3] A thorough knowledge of vertebral anatomy and joint biomechanics is required for proper chiropractic evaluation and treatment. Joint manipulation often induces a palpable release or movement of the restricted articulations. An audible cracking or popping also may be heard during chiropractic treatment as the applied force overcomes the elastic barrier of joint resistance.[13,14] The rapid articular separation produces a cavitation of the synovial fluid.[15] Radiological studies of synovial articulations after manipulation in people have shown a radiolucent cavity within the joint space (i.e., vacuum phenomenon) that contains 80% carbon dioxide and lasts for 15 to 20 minutes. A second attempt to recavitate the joint will be unsuccessful and potentially painful until the intraarticular gas is reabsorbed (i.e., refractory period).

EQUINE CHIROPRACTIC RESEARCH

The focus of recent equine manual therapy research has been on assessing the clinical effects of chiropractic techniques on relieving pain, improving flexibility, and restoring spinal motion symmetry. A veterinarian's ability to physically induce movement in a horse's back has been questioned. Pilot work in three horses that were instrumented with spinal transducers attached to Steinman pins implanted into dorsal spinous processes at adjacent vertebrae demonstrated that manually applied forces associated

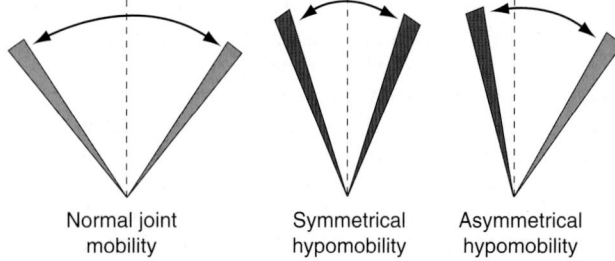

Fig. 93-2 • Diagram of patterns of normal and altered joint range of motion. Symmetrical joint hypomobility is characterized by generalized stiffness. Asymmetrical joint hypomobility is characterized by reduced joint mobility in one or more directions (e.g., left lateral bending).

with chiropractic techniques were able to produce substantial segmental spinal motion.[16] The induced spinal motions were usually beyond the normal range of segmental motion that was measured during treadmill locomotion (up to 227% larger segmental spinal range of motion induced by high-velocity, low-amplitude thrusts than measured at the walk). The next logical research question would be what, if any, are the therapeutic effects of these induced spinal movements? In two randomized, controlled clinical trials, pressure algometry was used to measure mechanical nociceptive thresholds (MNTs) in the thoracolumbar region and to evaluate whether chiropractic treatment can reduce back pain (or increase MNTs) relative to findings in a control group of horses.[17,18] The first study evaluated 24 horses in active exercise, with the treatment group receiving high-velocity, low-amplitude thrusts applied to the thirteenth thoracic vertebra (T13) to the sixth lumbar vertebra (L6) region.[17] At 2 weeks, 21 of 29 (72%) treated sites had increased MNTs, six (21%) sites had decreased MNTs, and two (7%) sites had similar MNTs. Although MNTs in all 10 treated sites within the T13 to L6 region increased, magnitude was significant in only 7 (24%) sites when compared with the control group. In the second study 38 horses without previously recognized clinical signs of back pain were randomly divided into five treatment groups with MNTs measured at seven bilateral sites at the T9 to second sacral (S2) vertebral levels.[18] Single applications of instrument-assisted (Activator) high-velocity, low-amplitude thrusts and massage therapy were given at day 0 in two groups at sites of pain, muscle hypertonicity, or stiffness. Phenylbutazone was given orally at a dose of 2 g twice a day for 7 days in the third group, and active and inactive horses were assigned to two control groups. MNTs were measured at Days 0, 1, 3, and 7. The Day 7 median MNTs had increased by 27% in the chiropractic group, 12% in the massage therapy group, and 8% in the phenylbutazone group, with less than 1% changes in both control groups.[18] Future research is recommended to evaluate long-term effects and the potential synergistic effects of combined therapies (e.g., chiropractic and massage therapy) for treating back pain.

Additional studies assessed the effects of equine chiropractic techniques on passive spinal mobility (i.e., flexibility) and longissimus muscle tone.[19,20] The first study used 10 horses to objectively measure vertical displacement, applied force, and stiffness at five thoracolumbar intervertebral sites in an experimentally induced back pain model using a randomized, crossover study design.[19] The chiropractic treatment induced a 15% increase in vertical displacement and a 20% increase in applied force, compared with control measurements, indicative of increased spinal flexibility and increased tolerance to applied pressure. The second study measured changes in muscle tone and electromyographic (EMG) activity within the longissimus muscle immediately after spinal manipulation or reflex inhibition therapy, compared with a control group.[20] Significant decreases in muscle tone and EMG activity were measured in both treatment groups, compared with no significant changes within the control group. Additional studies are needed to determine how long the increased flexibility and reduced muscle tone persist in horses treated with chiropractic techniques and whether these therapies can improve performance.

The last two studies document the potential beneficial effects of chiropractic treatment on spinal movement patterns in horses with documented back pain.[21,22] In a dressage horse with back pain and severe loss of performance, objective spinal kinematic assessment was performed before and up to 8 months after the last chiropractic treatment.[21] A right lateral bending restriction (functional scoliosis) was diagnosed, and two high-velocity, low-amplitude treatments were applied, 3 weeks apart. Symmetry of spinal movement indices improved dramatically after the first chiropractic treatment and remained improved above baseline at 8 months after the last treatment. It was concluded that manipulation had a measurable influence on kinematics of the thoracolumbar spine; however, this improvement was not judged equivalent to clinical improvement. A follow-up study assessed limb and spinal kinematics before and 1 hour and 3 weeks after chiropractic treatment in 10 horses.[22] Significant changes in spinal kinematics were noted at the walk and trot, but no changes were noted in limb kinematics. The main overall effect was more thoracic region flexion, a reduced inclination of the pelvis, and improvement of the symmetry of the pelvic motion pattern. It was concluded that chiropractic treatment elicited slight but clinically significant changes in thoracolumbar and pelvic kinematics and that changes may be beneficial.

CLINICAL EVALUATION

Chiropractic, like any medical evaluation, begins with a thorough history, discussion of the chief complaint, and observation of the horse from a distance for conformation, posture, and signs of lameness. Chiropractic evaluation and treatment are not a substitute for a thorough lameness examination and diagnostic workup, because many horses have musculoskeletal conditions that are identified readily and managed with traditional approaches. In veterinary medicine, many structural abnormalities of the vertebral column are becoming easier to diagnose with newer imaging modalities (e.g., scintigraphy and ultrasonography). Currently most clinicians are not well educated or experienced in procedures required to perform a thorough functional evaluation of the equine vertebral column. Therefore horses with conditions not diagnosed readily using traditional modalities, or with suspected concurrent neck or back problems, may require referral for chiropractic evaluation.

Horses with conditions that may be responsive to chiropractic care have a variety of nonspecific or vague problems (Box 93-1). The focus of the chiropractic examination is placed on evaluating static and dynamic characteristics of the musculoskeletal system. Initially the horse's general attitude and behavior are monitored for signs of pain or discomfort. Vertebral column conformation then is evaluated for proper alignment and symmetry, with special attention to the top line, shape and height of the withers, and osseous pelvic symmetry. A short-coupled horse is thought to have a higher incidence of osseous disorders, whereas a long-backed horse is more prone to soft tissue injuries.[23] Conformation is a structural relationship of body segments, whereas postural analysis deals more with functional relationships. The horse is made to stand on a hard, level surface and is evaluated for a preferred or shifting

BOX 93-1

Potential Clinical Indications for Chiropractic Evaluation and Treatment of Horses

Poor performance
Back or neck pain
Reduced neck or back flexibility
Not able to raise or lower head and neck
Localized muscle tightness
Vague lameness
Uneven or asymmetrical gait
Recent change in spinal conformation
Difficult or improper saddle fit
Discomfort with saddle placement
Resentment of tightening of the cinch or girth
Stiff and slow to warm up
Bucking or pinning ears when ridden
Lame only when ridden
Constantly on one rein or line
Difficulty with a lead or gait transition
Refusing jumps
Resisting collection
Difficulty with turning in one direction
Consistent stumbling or toe dragging
Muscle mass asymmetry
Pelvic asymmetry
Not standing squarely on all limbs
Difficulty standing for the farrier
Holding tail to one side
Resentment of being groomed
Behavior or avoidance problem

Modified from Willoughby SL: *Equine chiropractic care,* Port Byron, IL, United States, 1991, Options for Animals Foundation.

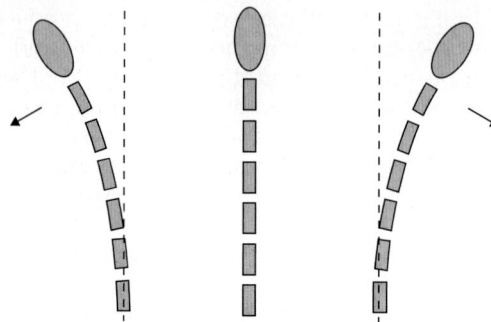

Fig. 93-3 • Diagram of normal segmental vertebral contributions to overall vertebral column mobility during active left and right lateral bending. Note the smooth vertebral curve produced by cumulative segmental joint motion.

characterized by localized pain, muscle hypertonicity, and reduced joint motion.[10] Palpation is used to localize and identify soft tissue and osseous structures for changes in texture, tissue mobility, or resistance to pressure.[23,25] Soft tissue layers are evaluated from superficial to deep in two ways: by increasing digital pressure and by shifting attention with discrete palpatory movements. Shapes of structures, transitions between structures, and attachment sites also may be palpated.[9] Soft tissue texture and mobility can be compared among the skin, subcutaneous tissue, thoracolumbar fascia, and muscle. Response to palpation is important, especially in evaluating tenderness or hypersensitivity. Osseous palpation involves evaluating osseous structures for pain, morphology, asymmetries, and alignment. Many horses with dental problems or malocclusion have localized pain during palpation of the temporomandibular joints and hypertonicity of the adjacent muscles of mastication. Osseous asymmetry of the space between the ramus of the mandible and the lateral wing of the atlas (first cervical vertebra) can be identified in horses with upper cervical congenital malformations, in horses with poll trauma caused by pulling back or falling over, or in some horses that head toss. Such asymmetry can also be seen in some otherwise clinically normal horses. The apices of the thoracic and lumbar spinous processes are readily palpable in most horses, unless they are grossly overweight. The dorsal apices of individual spinous processes are palpated with firm manual pressure, while monitoring for a localized pain response or muscle hypertonicity, indicative of local injury or impinged spinous processes. Palpable deviations of individual spinous processes are common, but usually they are not associated with spinous process fracture or vertebral malposition (i.e., bone out of place), as is commonly thought. Overlapping or malaligned dorsal spinous processes are often caused by spinous process impingement, developmental asymmetries in the neural arch, or isolated dorsal spinous process deviation of unknown cause.[5,26] During induced kyphosis, the abaxial borders of each individual thoracolumbar spinous process and the overlying supraspinous ligament are palpated for pain, thickening, or deviation from midline. The tubera sacrale are palpated for height asymmetries and evaluated for a localized pain response to manual pressure applied dorsally or during abaxial compression. The apices of the sacral spinous processes (of the second to fifth sacral vertebrae) are palpated for pain or deviation from midline.

stance, head and neck carriage, vertebral curvatures, and muscular symmetry. Chiropractic gait analysis focuses on evaluating regional vertebral mobility and pelvic motion symmetry, in addition to the typical assessment of forelimb and hindlimb lameness. Gait analysis may help to rule out distal limb disorders and to rule in vertebral dysfunction, although limb lameness has been reported in about 85% of horses with back problems.[24] Motion asymmetries, restricted vertebral or pelvic mobility, not tracking straight, and lack of propulsion are a few characteristics that are evaluated. Tape on the tubera coxae or vertebral column midline may make subtle motion asymmetries easier to see. Normal vertebral column motion consists of small cumulative amounts of segmental motion, which produce an overall smooth curve or movement of the vertebral column (Figure 93-3). Evaluation of the horse's response to having a saddle placed and being ridden is important for a complete assessment of horses with back problems. Inspection of the tack for proper use and fit is always suggested on initial examination. Saddles and restraint devices should be evaluated for proper fit, padding, and positioning on the horse.

A thorough physical examination is used to eliminate other, more common causes of lameness or neurological disorders. Chiropractic evaluation focuses on evaluating and localizing segmental vertebral dysfunction, which is

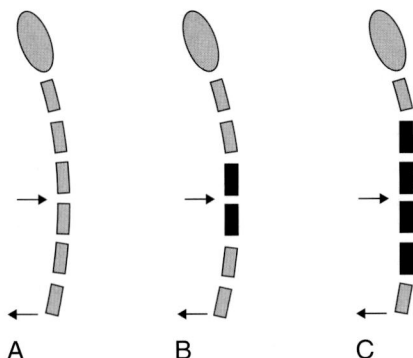

Fig. 93-4 • Diagram of segmental vertebral motion during manually induced left lateral bending of the vertebral column. Arrows indicate direction of applied forces to vertebral column. **A,** Normal segmental motion of the vertebral column. **B,** Locally restricted vertebral motion involving two vertebrae. **C,** Regionally restricted vertebral motion involving several vertebrae.

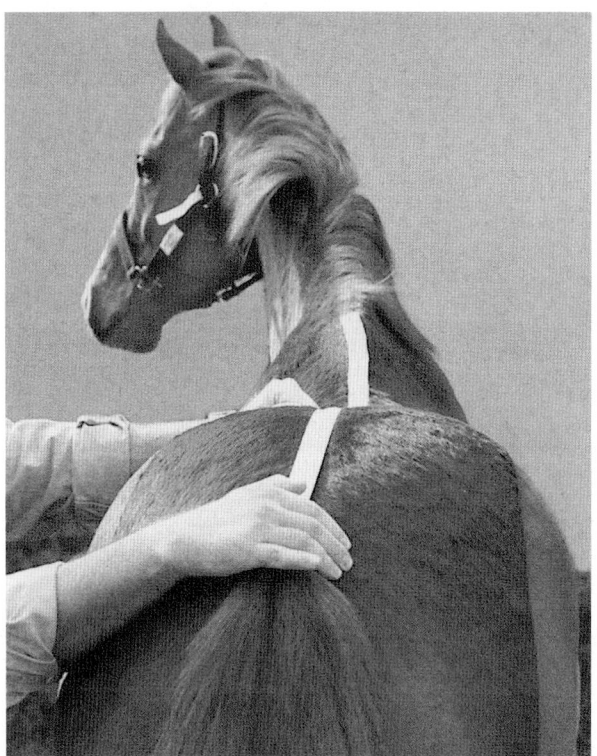

Fig. 93-5 • Demonstration of motion palpation with induced left lateral flexion of the thoracolumbar vertebral column.

A complete musculoskeletal examination includes assessment of active and passive ranges of joint motion for all axial and appendicular articulations. Active joint range of motion is evaluated during induced vertebral movements (carrot stretches) and gait analysis. Assessment of passive range of motion requires muscular relaxation as the articulations are moved passively throughout the individual joint ranges of motion (Figure 93-4). Abnormal segmental vertebral motion is detected when joint motion is asymmetrical or restricted bilaterally (see Figure 93-2). Causes of segmental vertebral motion restrictions include capsular fibrosis, effusion, and inflammation. Regional causes of vertebral movement restrictions may include periarticular soft tissue adhesions, musculotendonous contractures, or, more commonly, protective muscle spasms. Combining the evaluation of joint range of motion and the presence or absence of pain at the extremes of joint motion, diagnostic interpretations can be implied.[27] Normal joint motion is painless, suggesting that articular structures are intact and functional. Normal joint mobility that has a painful end range of movement suggests that a minor sprain of the associated articular tissues is present. Painless joint hypomobility suggests that a contracture or adhesion is present. Painful hypomobility suggests the presence of an acute strain with secondary muscle guarding. Painless hypermobility of an articulation may indicate a complete rupture, whereas painful hypermobility suggests a partial tear of the evaluated structure.

Motion palpation is used to evaluate each vertebral segment for loss of normal joint motion and overall resistance to induced motion (see Figure 93-4; Figure 93-5). Vertebral segments with altered motion palpation findings can occur with or without localized muscle hypertonicity and pain. Using palpation to evaluate the musculoskeletal system requires an understanding of how joint motion is assessed.[9] Moving an articulation from a neutral position first involves evaluating joint motion that has minimal and uniform resistance. As the articulation is moved toward the end range of motion, a gradual increase in the resistance to movement occurs (i.e., elastic barrier) (see Figure 93-1). End range of motion starts when any change in resistance to passive joint movement is palpable. The elastic barrier is evaluated by bringing the articulation to tension and applying gentle, rhythmic oscillations to qualify the resistance to movement. The normal joint end feel is initially soft and resilient and gradually becomes more restrictive as maximal joint range of motion is reached. This elastic barrier marks the end of physiological joint movement. A pathological or restrictive end range of motion is palpable earlier in passive joint movement and has an abrupt, restrictive end feel compared with normal joint end feel. The goal of palpating joint movement is to evaluate the initiation of motion resistance, the quality of joint motion and end feel, and the overall joint range of motion. Joint movement beyond its normal anatomical limits is characterized by ligamentous or articular capsule disruption and joint subluxation.

Individual vertebral segments are evaluated for altered motion palpation findings in flexion and extension (Figures 93-6 and 93-7); right and left lateral flexion (see Figures 93-4 and 93-5); and right and left rotation. In a relaxed horse the articulations of the individual second to sixth cervical vertebrae are assessed for the presence or loss of the normal elastic barrier during combined lateral flexion and rotation. The articulation between the fourth and fifth cervical vertebrae seems to be commonly affected in most performance horses, presumably because of locally altered biomechanical influences. The individual spinous processes of the third to twelfth thoracic vertebrae are deviated manually from midline, while monitoring for signs of reduced vertebral motion, localized pain, and induced muscle hypertonicity. Horses with poorly fitting saddles (e.g., tree too narrow) resent motion palpation of the affected vertebrae. The remaining thoracolumbar region is assessed in lateral bending and flexion and extension for similar signs of joint dysfunction. While the clinician stands next to the

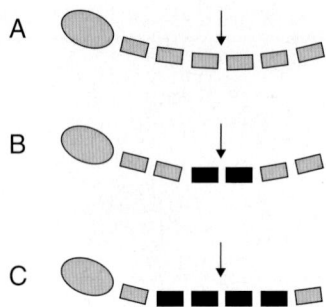

Fig. 93-6 • Diagram of segmental vertebral motion during manually induced extension of the vertebral column. Arrows indicate direction of applied forces to vertebral column. **A,** Normal segmental motion of the vertebral column. **B,** Locally restricted vertebral motion involving two vertebrae. **C,** Regionally restricted vertebral motion involving several vertebrae.

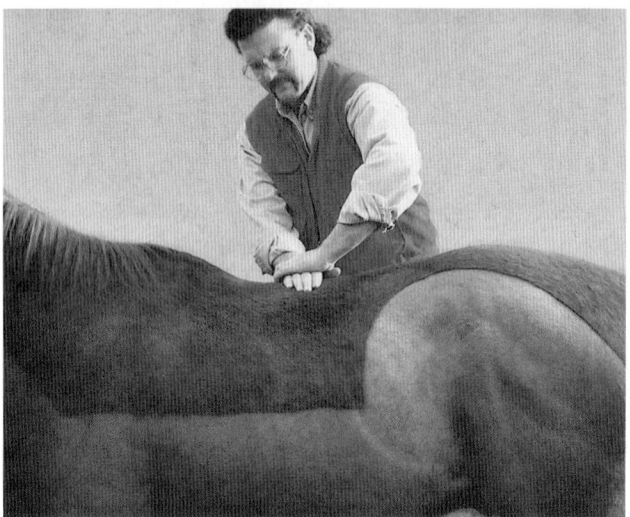

Fig. 93-7 • Demonstration of motion palpation with induced extension of the thoracolumbar vertebral column.

horse, segmental vertebral motion in lateral bending is assessed with one hand lying over the intervertebral articulation to be evaluated. The other hand is placed at the tail head and is used to induce rhythmic oscillations to the caudal vertebral column. Normal lateral bending is maximal at the midthoracic vertebral region and gradually diminishes toward the lumbosacral junction. Conversely, flexion and extension are minimal in the thoracic region and gradually increase until the lumbosacral junction, the site of maximal flexion and extension. Segmental vertebral motion in flexion and extension requires the clinician to be on an elevated surface to induce ventrally directed rhythmic oscillations to the intervertebral articulations of the thirteenth to sixteenth thoracic vertebrae. The sacroiliac joints are evaluated for motion restriction or pain during induced joint motion, with an applied force directed ventrally over the tuber coxae, or during abaxial compression of the tubera sacrale (see Chapter 51). The caudal vertebrae are assessed by manipulation of individual vertebrae or by application of axial traction. The range of motion of the individual forelimb and hindlimb articulations also are evaluated in flexion and extension, internal and external rotation, abduction and adduction, and circumduction

for signs of reduced joint motion, localized pain, and induced muscle hypertonicity. Palpation of the entire musculoskeletal system, including joint motion assessment of the axial and appendicular skeleton, can be accomplished within 15 to 20 minutes.

A neurological examination is indicated to evaluate horses with back problems to rule out traumatic, infectious, and toxic causes (see Chapter 11). Postural reactions also help to assess the proprioceptive status, which may be compromised in horses with certain vertebral column disorders. Rectal palpation is a commonly forgotten diagnostic test in horses with back problems. Osseous palpation rectally is useful for evaluating fractures, pelvic canal symmetry, and lumbosacral or sacroiliac joint osteoarthritis (OA). Externally induced pelvic motion during rectal palpation helps to assess lumbosacral joint motion internally. Palpation of the iliopsoas muscles for pain, swelling, or asymmetry is also important in evaluating horses with back pain. An orthopedic examination commonly is indicated to rule out or identify concurrent limb problems. Hematological evaluation, diagnostic analgesia, muscle biopsies, or cerebral spinal fluid analysis may be required in certain horses before chiropractic assessment and treatment. Imaging modalities that may contribute to a definitive diagnosis in horses with neck or back problems include radiography, myelography, ultrasonography, scintigraphy, computed tomography, and thermography. A thorough diagnostic workup and a definitive diagnosis, when available, are important for tailoring the appropriate chiropractic treatment and rehabilitation program. Horses with developmental osseous abnormalities, cervical vertebral fractures, thoracolumbar impinged dorsal spinous processes, equine protozoal myelitis, and sacroiliac joint luxation have been referred to me for chiropractic consultation. It was critical that these horses be properly diagnosed and that inappropriate chiropractic treatment not be applied, especially as the sole or primary therapeutic modality.

INDICATIONS FOR CHIROPRACTIC CARE

Chiropractic provides additional diagnostic and therapeutic approaches that are not currently available in veterinary medicine. The principal indications for equine chiropractic evaluation are acute or chronic neck or back pain, localized or regional joint stiffness, poor performance, and an altered gait that is not associated with overt lameness (see Box 93-1). Musculoskeletal conditions that are chronic or recurring, are not diagnosed readily, or do not respond to conventional veterinary care also may be indications for chiropractic consultation. A thorough diagnostic workup is required to identify soft tissue and osseous pathological conditions, neurological disorders, or other lameness conditions that may not be responsive to chiropractic care. Horses with a localized limb lameness or diagnosed neurological disease are better treated with conventional veterinary medicine. However, if a residual lameness continues or a secondary vertebral column disorder (e.g., stiffness or asymmetry) is identified, then concurrent chiropractic care is indicated. Horses that have concurrent hock pain (e.g., OA) and a stiff, painful thoracolumbar or lumbosacral vertebral region are best managed by using a multidisciplinary approach of concurrent medical treatment of the hock OA and chiropractic evaluation and treatment of the back problem. Most horses respond favorably to concurrent management, and owners appreciate a complete and thorough medical evaluation and treatment. Similarly, horses with chronic forelimb lameness often have compensatory pain and stiffness in the withers region, which are readily addressed with chiropractic or physical therapy techniques.

The primary clinical signs that equine chiropractors assess are areas of localized musculoskeletal pain, muscle hypertonicity, and restricted joint motion. This triad of clinical signs can be found in a variety of horses with distal limb disorders, but it is most evident in those with neck or back problems. In general, localized pain, reduced vertebral segment motion, and local muscle spasms in the vertebral column are indications of a primary spinal disorder. In contrast, regional or diffuse pain, generalized stiffness, and widespread muscle hypertonicity are indications of a chronic or secondary spinal disorder, and further diagnostics should be done to identify the primary cause of lameness or poor performance. Chiropractic care may provide symptomatic relief in horses with early vertebral OA if related to joint hypomobility and subsequent immobilization degeneration. Research suggests that spinal manipulation also may affect certain visceral disorders (e.g., cardiovascular, respiratory, and gastrointestinal) through somatovisceral reflexes in animals and people.[2,3] However, consistent and predictable long-term changes in visceral disorders rarely occur with chiropractic treatment in people or horses.

Specially trained veterinarians or chiropractors, with advanced training and experience in equine chiropractic techniques, should be able to evaluate vertebral column disorders and determine if the condition will respond to chiropractic care, if further diagnostic evaluation is required, or if the horse would be better managed with traditional veterinary care. Unfortunately, equine chiropractors often are asked to treat horses as a last resort, when all else has failed or the disease has progressed to an irreversible condition. Chiropractic care has helped some of these horses with chronic conditions when other types of conventional treatment have failed. However, chiropractic is usually much more effective in the early stages of clinical disease versus end-stage disease, where reparative processes have been exhausted. Chiropractic care and other holistic modalities often fail when used as a last resort.

CONTRAINDICATIONS

Chiropractic is not a cure-all for every back problem and is not suggested for treatment of horses with fractures, infections, neoplasia, metabolic disorders, or nonmechanically related joint disorders. Horses with serious diseases requiring immediate medical or surgical care need to be treated by conventional veterinary medicine before any chiropractic treatment is initiated. However, chiropractic care may contribute to the rehabilitation of most horses postoperatively, or those with medical conditions, by helping to restore normal musculoskeletal function. Chiropractic care usually is contraindicated in horses with acute stages of soft tissue injury. However, as the soft tissue injury heals, chiropractic has the potential to help restore normal joint motion, thus limiting the risk for future reinjury.[9] Acute episodes of pain associated with OA, impinged

dorsal spinous processes, and severe articular changes, such as joint subluxation or luxation, are often contraindications to chiropractic care. All horses with neurological diseases should be evaluated fully to assess the potential risks or benefits of chiropractic treatment. Cervical myelopathy occurs because of structural and functional disorders in the cervical vertebrae. Static compression caused by malformation and dynamic lesions caused by vertebral segment hypermobility are contraindications to cervical manipulation. However, adjacent hypomobile vertebrae may require chiropractic treatment to help restore joint motion and reduce biomechanical stresses in the affected vertebrae. Chiropractic care cannot reverse severe degenerative processes or overt pathological conditions.

CHIROPRACTIC TECHNIQUES

Most of the current knowledge about equine chiropractic was borrowed from chiropractic techniques, theories, and research used in people and adapted to horses. Therapeutic trials of chiropractic manipulations often are used because knowledge is limited about the effects of equine chiropractic. Chiropractic addresses mechanically related disorders of the musculoskeletal and nervous systems and provides a conservative means of treatment and prevention for horses with back problems. Chiropractic treatment uses an applied, controlled force to a specific anatomical region or osseous structure to produce a desired therapeutic response. Chiropractic manipulations are applied to areas of vertebral segment dysfunction. The condition of the horse is monitored closely as the neuromusculoskeletal system responds to the applied treatment. The applied treatment influences joint, muscle, and nerve function via mechanical and biological mechanisms.[2] The therapeutic dosage of the applied chiropractic manipulation is modified by the number of vertebrae treated, the amount of force applied, and the frequency of treatment. The goal of chiropractic care is to restore normal joint motion, stimulate neurological reflexes, and reduce pain and muscle hypertonicity. Comparisons of sensitivity to palpation, muscle tone, and joint motion are made before and after treatment to evaluate the response to chiropractic treatment.

Clinicians and clients often ask, how can a 500-kg horse be treated with chiropractic techniques? The answer is one vertebral segment at a time. Recent equine chiropractic research has demonstrated that forces applied to instrumented vertebral segments do induce substantial vertebral motion, usually beyond the normal range of segmental motion that occurs during locomotion.[16] Segmental vertebral motion characteristics induced during chiropractic treatment in horses are similar to those reported in people.[28] In a relaxed horse, the mass (i.e., vertebral segment) that is affected by the rapidly applied force is proportionately smaller than the mass of the clinician applying the treatment. However, if the horse does not relax the paraspinal musculature, then the mass that is affected increases dramatically from the mass of a few vertebral segments to the mass of the entire vertebral region, or potentially the entire horse. Effective joint mobilization or manipulation cannot be applied to a nervous, tense horse without risk of injury to the horse or the clinician. Chiropractic treatments in horses usually are done without any sedation or other medications, but they may occasionally be done with the horse under general anesthesia, or coupled with intraarticular injections, if indicated.[29] Typical indications for manipulation in people under anesthesia include chronic myositis or fibrosis, or acute musculoskeletal pain, where reflex muscle spasms prevent a thorough assessment or impede manipulative treatment. Untrained professionals who do not have a thorough understanding of joint physiology, vertebral anatomy, or chiropractic principles resort to overly aggressive and forceful means of applying an external force (e.g., mallets and 2 × 4s). Small, rapidly applied manual forces are easier to control and have a lower risk of soft tissue or bone injury than more forceful types of manipulation. A good rule of thumb is that if the procedure does not look like something that the practitioner would be willing to have done to himself or herself, then the procedure should not be done to a horse.

Horses are usually held by a trained handler on a loose lead during chiropractic treatment. The cervical vertebrae, sacrum, and extremities are evaluated and manipulated as needed from ground level. However, the thoracolumbar vertebrae and pelvis often require an elevated surface on which to stand for effective manipulation and proper positioning of the clinician (see Figure 93-7). Equine chiropractic is physically demanding and requires substantial mental concentration. The clinician and the horse must be relaxed and focused on each other. Environmental distractions are counterproductive to effective chiropractic care. Muscle relaxation allows evaluation of the elastic barrier of the joint. Motion palpation is used to evaluate joint motion restrictions so that the manipulative thrust can be applied correctly. Stabilization of adjacent joints or vertebral segments is required for proper joint manipulation.

Typically, an immediate reduction in pain and an increase in segmental vertebral motion are noted. Most horses also have increased muscle relaxation, but other therapies (e.g., acupuncture or stretching) often are used with chiropractic treatment to completely resolve any remaining muscle hypertonicity. In general, horses with conditions with an acute onset respond rapidly, whereas those with chronic conditions usually require longer treatment or rehabilitation. Horses with acute pain or vertebral column trauma may require initial antiinflammatory medication, physiotherapy modalities (e.g., ice), or rest before chiropractic treatment. If stiffness, local muscle hypertonicity, or pain remain, then two or three chiropractic treatments may be indicated. Horses with chronic neck or back stiffness may require monthly evaluation and treatment for several months' duration. Owners often request chiropractic evaluation at the beginning of the performance season or a few days after athletic competition or as a general assessment of the overall musculoskeletal system. Similarly, horses may benefit from chiropractic treatment several days before an event. Because of ethical considerations or possible masking of musculoskeletal dysfunction, it is not recommended that chiropractic treatment be performed immediately before or during any competition.

Posttreatment recommendations for actively training horses usually include stall rest or pasture turnout for one day, which provides an opportunity for the musculoskeletal system to respond to the applied treatment without immediate reexposure to potential inciting factors of the vertebral segment dysfunction. The horse returns to normal work the next day, unless other musculoskeletal injuries are present, for which appropriate care is recommended. If stiffness or soreness is noted after chiropractic treatment, then an additional day of rest is suggested.

COMPLICATIONS OR ADVERSE EFFECTS

Potential adverse effects from properly applied chiropractic treatments include a transient stiffness or worsening of the condition after treatment (e.g., aggravated clinical signs, worsening of preexisting state, regional soreness, or lameness).[3] Adverse reactions from properly applied vertebral manipulation are typically uncommon, but they may occur immediately after treatment or insidiously within 6 to 12 hours. The undesired effects usually last less than 1 to 2 days and resolve without concurrent medical intervention. If increased or acute musculoskeletal dysfunction or lameness is noted after chiropractic treatment, then a thorough reexamination and appropriate medical treatment or physiotherapy should be pursued. If the condition does not improve with conservative care, referral for more extensive diagnostic or therapeutic modalities is recommended. Potential harmful side effects from improperly applied manipulation from untrained individuals may include permanent articular damage or loss of function (e.g., torn ligaments, injured muscles, luxated joints, fractures, or possible paralysis if a severe underlying pathological condition is present).

ADJUNCT RECOMMENDATIONS AND PROGNOSIS

Chiropractic care often is supplemented with massage, physiotherapy modalities, and stretching or strengthening exercises to help soft tissue rehabilitation and to help restore normal vertebral joint motion (see Chapter 94). These concurrent therapies also help to encourage owner participation in the healing process and provide close monitoring of the horse's progress. Other recommendations may include changes in training schedules or activities, corrective shoeing, or tack changes. Horses with poorly fitting saddles often have localized pain and muscle hypertonicity in the caudal withers region. Saddle refitting, coupled with chiropractic treatment of the painful withers region, leads to rapid recovery and management of a common problem for many horse owners. In one instance a horse with a 6-month history of consistently resenting saddle placement and bucking the owner off was treated chiropractically and the next week won 11 ribbons at the local country fair. Many horses with repetitive-use disorders may benefit from cross-training activities. Clinicians report synergistic therapeutic effects with the combined use of chiropractic, acupuncture, and other holistic modalities in horses. In general, horses with conditions with an acute onset respond rapidly and have a good prognosis for return to function. Horses with chronic injuries may gain only short-term improvement of restricted motion, pain, or muscle hypertonicity. This corresponds to current research on joint immobilization and spinal learning.[9] Horses with chronic conditions usually require a series of treatments to effect a more lasting improvement. Musculoskeletal health depends on movement and use. Scientific evidence suggests that long-term rest and inactivity are contraindicated for back problems in people.

SUMMARY

A thorough knowledge of equine vertebral anatomy, biomechanics, and pathology is required to understand the principles and theories behind chiropractic and to apply its techniques properly. Because of its potential misuse, spinal evaluation and manipulative therapies should be provided only by specially trained veterinary clinicians or licensed manual therapists. Anecdotal evidence and clinical experience suggest that chiropractic is an effective adjunct modality for the diagnosis and conservative treatment of select musculoskeletal-related disorders in horses. Recent research including randomized, controlled clinical trials supports the efficacy of equine chiropractic techniques for reducing pain, improving flexibility, reducing muscle tone, and improving symmetry of spinal kinematics. Additional studies are needed to monitor the long-term changes and improvements in performance. Chiropractic provides additional diagnostic and therapeutic means that may help equine clinicians to identify and treat select musculoskeletal disorders. Chiropractic provides specialized evaluation and treatment of joint dysfunction and conservative treatment of neuromusculoskeletal disorders that currently lack treatments in traditional veterinary medicine.

Chapter 94

Electrophysical Agents in Physiotherapy

Amanda Sutton and Tim Watson

Electrotherapy has been a component of physiotherapy practice since the early days, but its delivery has changed remarkably and continues to do so. All electrotherapy modalities involve the introduction of some physical energy, which brings about one or more physiological changes that are used for therapeutic benefit. To appropriately select the most suitable modality, it is necessary to:
1. Determine the nature of the problem to be addressed
2. Establish the physiological changes that need to take place
3. Select the modality that is most able to bring about the changes in the tissue(s) concerned
4. Choose the appropriate dose
5. Apply the treatment

ELECTROTHERAPEUTIC WINDOWS

The effectiveness of electrotherapeutic treatment is influenced by a number of factors, including the time after the injury at which treatment is applied, the "dose" administered, the amplitude or strength applied, and the frequency. An energy delivered at a particular amplitude has a beneficial effect, whereas the same energy at lower amplitude may have no demonstrable effect. Laser therapy provides a good example—one level will produce a distinct cellular response, whereas a higher dose may be destructive. A modality applied at a specific frequency (pulsing regimen) may have a measurable benefit, whereas the same modality applied using a different pulsing profile may not achieve equivalent results.

THERAPEUTIC ULTRASOUND

Ultrasound (US) is a form of mechanical energy, not electrical energy, and therefore, strictly speaking, is not electrotherapy but falls into the group of electrophysical agents.[1] Mechanical vibration at increasing frequencies is known as sound energy. In children and young adults, the normal audible sound range is 16 Hz to 15,000 to 20,000 Hz. Higher frequencies are known as US. The frequencies used in therapy are typically between 1.0 and 3.0 MHz (1 MHz = 1 million cycles/sec).

References
on page
1333

Sound waves are longitudinal waves consisting of areas of compression and rarefaction. When exposed to a sound wave, particles of a material oscillate about a fixed point rather than move with the wave itself. Any increase in the molecular vibration in a tissue can result in heat generation; thus US can be used to produce thermal changes in the tissues, although current therapeutic usage does not focus on this phenomenon.[1,2] The vibration of the tissues may also have nonthermal effects. As the US wave passes through the tissue, the energy levels within the wave decrease as energy is transferred to the tissues.[1]

Therapeutic Ultrasound Waves

US waves are characterized by frequency, wavelength, and velocity. Frequency is the number of times a particle experiences a complete compression/rarefaction cycle in 1 second. The wavelength is the distance between two equivalent points on the waveform in the particular medium. In an "average tissue," the wavelength at 1 MHz is 1.5 mm and at 3 MHz is 0.5 mm. The velocity is the speed at which the wave (disturbance) travels through the medium. In a saline solution, the velocity of US is approximately 1500 m/sec compared with approximately 350 m/sec in air (sound waves can travel more rapidly in a denser medium). The velocity of US in most tissues is thought to be similar to that in saline.

These three factors are related but are not consistent for all types of tissue. Typical average therapeutic US frequencies are 1 and 3 MHz, although some machines produce additional frequencies (e.g., 0.75 and 1.5 MHz), and the "long wave" US devices typically operate at 40 to 50 kHz, a much lower frequency than "traditional US" but still beyond human hearing range.

Ultrasound Waveform

The US beam is not uniform and changes in its nature with distance from the transducer. The US beam nearest the treatment head is called the near field. The behavior of the US waves in the near field is not regular, and areas of interference and energy can be many times greater than the output set on the machine (up to 12 to 15 times greater).

Ultrasound Transmission through the Tissues

Tissues present impedance to the passage of sound waves. The specific impedance of a tissue is determined by its density and elasticity. For the maximal transmission of energy from one tissue to another, the impedance of the two tissues needs to be as similar as possible. An air gap between the generator and the skin will result in the majority of the US energy being reflected rather than transmitted to the underlying tissues.

Coupling media, water, various oils, creams, and gels, are used to bridge the air gap. Ideally, the coupling medium should be fluid so as to fill all available spaces, be relatively viscous so that it stays in place, have an impedance appropriate to the media it connects, and allow transmission of US with minimal absorption, attenuation, or disturbance. At present, the gel-based media appear to be preferable to the oils and creams. Water is a good medium and can be used as an alternative. The addition of active agents (e.g., antiinflammatory drugs) to the gel is widely practiced but remains incompletely researched.

Studies[3,4] have considered the effect of animal hair on the transmission of US to the underlying tissue and report that best penetration is achieved by clipping the hair. In addition to the reflection that occurs at a boundary because of differences in impedance, there will also be some refraction if the wave does not strike the boundary surface at 90 degrees. Essentially, the direction of the US beam through the second medium will not be the same as its path through the original medium; its pathway is angled. The treatment head is ideally placed perpendicular to the skin surface (i.e., at 90 degrees). If the treatment head is at an angle of 15 degrees or more from the perpendicular to the plane of the skin surface, the majority of the US beam will travel through the dermal tissues (i.e., parallel to the plane of the skin surface) rather than penetrate the tissues as would be expected.

Care of the Machine

The US treatment head should be cleaned with an alcohol-based swab between treatments to minimize the potential transmission of microbial agents between horses.[5]

Contraindications

- Do not expose either an embryo or fetus to therapeutic levels of US by treating over the uterus during pregnancy
- Malignancy (DO NOT treat over tissue that is or may possibly be malignant; however, an area from which a malignancy was removed can be treated)
- Tissues in which bleeding is occurring or could reasonably be expected (typically within hours of injury)
- Substantial vascular abnormalities
- The eye
- The cardiac area in advanced heart disease
- Active physes in young foals

Precautions

US should be used at the lowest intensity, which produces a therapeutic response, in a continuous mode, moving the applicator throughout the treatment (speed and direction are not issues). The US machine should be regularly calibrated.[6]

Treatment Record

Records should be maintained of the machine used, the machine settings (frequency, intensity, time, and pulse parameters), the area to be treated (size and location), and any immediate or untoward effects.

Absorption and Attenuation

The absorption of US energy follows an exponential pattern: more energy is absorbed in the superficial tissues than in the deep tissues.[7,8] Thus as the US beam penetrates further into the tissues, a greater proportion of the energy has been absorbed; therefore there is less energy available to achieve therapeutic effects. The half value depth represents the depth in the tissues at which half the surface energy is available and is different for each tissue and US frequency. Tissues with high protein content are greatest absorbers of US energy. Those with higher water and low protein content absorb little. This is very important when electing US as a suitable modality.[1] It is impossible to know the thickness of each tissue layer in an individual horse; therefore average half value depths are used for each frequency: 3 MHz = 2.0 cm; 1 MHz = 4.0 cm. Tissues with absorption are tendon, ligament, fascia, joint capsule, and scar tissue. In cartilage and bone, a majority of US energy striking the surface is likely to be reflected.[7-9]

Therapeutic Effects of Ultrasound

The therapeutic effects of US are influenced by the treatment parameters chosen and are commonly divided into thermal and nonthermal.

Thermal

Therapeutic US may produce heat,[10] especially in periosteum, collagenous tissues (ligament, tendon, and fascia), and fibrotic muscle. If the temperature of the damaged tissues is raised to 40 to 45° C, there is hyperemia, which may be therapeutic and help resolve chronic inflammation.[11] However, nonthermal effects are probably more important.

Nonthermal

The nonthermal effects of US are from cavitation and acoustic streaming.[7,12] Cavitation, the formation of gas-filled voids within tissues and body fluids, occurs in two types—stable and unstable—which have different effects. Stable cavitation occurs at therapeutic doses of US and is the formation and growth of dissolved gas bubble accumulation. The "cavity" acts to enhance the acoustic streaming phenomena. Unstable (transient) cavitation is the formation of bubbles at the low pressure part of the US cycle. These bubbles then collapse very quickly, releasing a large amount of energy that is detrimental to tissue viability. However, this does not occur at therapeutic levels if good technique is used.

Acoustic streaming is a small-scale eddying of fluids near a vibrating structure such as cell membranes and the surface of a stable cavitation gas bubble and affects diffusion rates and membrane permeability.[11] Sodium ion permeability is altered, resulting in changes in the cell membrane potential. Calcium ion transport is modified, which in turn leads to an alteration in the enzyme and cellular secretions.

The result of the combined effects of stable cavitation and acoustic streaming is that the cell membrane becomes "excited" (up-regulates), thus increasing the activity levels of the whole cell. The US energy acts as a trigger for this process, but it is the increased cellular activity that is in effect responsible for the therapeutic benefits of the modality.[1,2,13]

Some US machines offer variable time: typical pulse ratios are 1:1 and 1:4. In 1:1 mode, the machine offers an output for 2 ms followed by 2 ms of rest. In 1:4 mode, the 2-ms output is followed by 8-ms rest period.

Ultrasound Application in Relation to Soft Tissue Repair

The process of tissue repair is a complex series of cascaded, chemically mediated events that lead to the production of scar tissue.

Inflammatory Phase

US induces the degranulation of mast cells, causing the release of arachidonic acid and its subsequent cascade.[9,13] Thus therapeutic US is proinflammatory rather than antiinflammatory. The benefit of US may not be to "increase" inflammation, although if applied too intensely at this stage, it is a possible outcome; rather, US should act as an "inflammatory optimizer."[1] The inflammatory response is essential for effective tissue repair, and the more efficient the process, the more effectively it can advance to the next phase (proliferation). Studies have failed to demonstrate an antiinflammatory effect of US, and results suggest US is ineffective.[14] US may be effective at normalizing inflammatory events and may have therapeutic value in promoting overall repair.[1,7]

Proliferation

During the proliferative phase (scar production), US is proproliferative and stimulates (cellular up-regulation) fibroblasts, endothelial cells, and myofibroblasts.[1,9] US may maximize efficiency, producing the required scar tissue in an optimal fashion. Low-dose pulsed US increased protein synthesis and enhanced fibroplasia and collagen synthesis.[15-17] Recent work has identified the critical role of numerous growth factors in relation to tissue repair, and there is some evidence for an effect of US on growth factors and heat shock proteins.[13,17]

Remodeling

During the remodeling phase of repair, the somewhat generic scar is refined such that it adopts functional characteristics of the tissues that it is repairing. Remodeling involves reorientation of the collagen fibers[18] and a change from predominantly type III to more mature type I collagen. Therapeutic US increases tensile strength and scar mobility by enhancing collagen fiber orientation and the collagen profile change from type III to type I.[19] US enhances functional capacity scar tissue.[19]

Other Applications of Therapeutic Ultrasound

Ultrasound for Fracture Repair

The application of very low-dose US over a fracture (whether healing normally, delayed, or nonunion) can be of benefit, but the effective "dose" is lower than most therapy machines can deliver. Higher-intensity US over a fracture can initiate a strong pain response, a property that may be helpful to locate stress fractures.[1]

Ultrasound at Trigger Points

US can be used to stimulate acupuncture trigger points with measurable benefit.[20]

PULSED ELECTROMAGNETIC FIELD THERAPY

Wires carrying an electric current produce a surrounding magnetic field. The magnetic field around a long straight wire is in the form of concentric circles around the central wire. When a current flows in a circular coil, an electromagnetic field is induced. A pulsed electromagnetic field (PEMF), which is emitted from an applicator, is transmitted through the tissues and is absorbed in those of low impedance (muscle and nerve), which are highly vascular, and tissues in which there is edema, effusion, or recent hematoma.[21] PEMF therapy may have beneficial effects on damaged tissue cells, particularly at the cellular level.

Normal healthy cells have a selectively permeable membrane.[22] When membrane integrity is lost through disease, chemicals that would otherwise not enter the cell can now enter, drastically lowering the voltage potential across the cell. The application of a PEMF to affected cells may restore cell membrane potential, transport, and ionic balance by either a direct ionic transport mechanism or an activation of various pumps (sodium/potassium).[23,24] PEMF therapy is important in the inflammatory phase and reduced healing time after oral surgery in people.[25] PEMF therapy may reduce pain.

Bone is a calcified collagenous structure and can develop a piezoelectric potential on its external and internal surfaces. Most studies have failed to show PEMF therapy significantly improves bone remodeling.[26] A small but statistically significant effect of PEMF stimulation on cancellous bone graft incorporation was found in a small study (eight ponies), but missing data prohibit drawing any strong conclusions.[27]

The clinical effects of PEMF therapy, US, and laser are all similar; the key difference in clinical use relates to where the energy is absorbed rather than the effects achieved.[21] They have little or no effect on normal cells because "abnormal" cells respond to lower energy levels than normal cells.[21] US is better absorbed by dense collagen-based tissues and laser by superficial vascular tissues, whereas PEMF therapy is absorbed primarily in wet, ionic, low-resistance tissues such as muscle, nerve, areas of edema, hematomas, and effusion.

Primary Effects of Pulsed Electromagnetic Field Therapy

The primary effects of PEMF therapy include[28]:
1. Increased number of white cells, histiocytes, and fibroblasts in a wound
2. Improved rate of edema dispersion
3. Promotion of absorption of hematoma

4. Reduction (resolution) of the inflammatory process
5. Prompting a more rapid rate of fibrin fiber orientation and deposition of collagen
6. Promotion of collagen layering at an early stage
7. Stimulation of osteogenesis

PEMF therapy in the equine market consists mainly of either full-body rugs to target the tissues of the body, back, and neck, or paired coils that are strapped or bandaged to a limb.

CONTRAINDICATIONS

- Pregnancy
- Bleeding
- Severe circulatory compromise or deficit including ischemic tissue
- Physes in growing foals

LASER THERAPY

Low-level laser therapy (LLLT) is popular in people and animals. Laser is an acronym for *l*ight *a*mplification by the *s*timulated *e*mission of *r*adiation. Laser light differs from ordinary light in that it is highly amplified and nondivergent. It forms part of the electromagnetic spectrum.[29] High-power lasers (>10 W) are commonly used surgically but are not discussed here.[30] Low-power lasers (<500 mW, <35 J/cm²) are used in the management of pain, wound healing, and soft tissue injury.[31]

Biophysics of Laser

Light wavelengths between 600 and 1300 nm are typically used with laser therapy.[32] This includes both visible light and the near part of the infrared spectrum. Laser differs from other radiation in its unique properties of monochromacity (single wavelength), coherence (waves in phase), and collimation (waves in parallel).[29] However, there exists some debate as to the necessity of such expensive properties, especially coherence.[33] Superluminous diodes, lacking the property of coherence, are also used therapeutically.[31] Superluminous diodes (660 and 870 nm) are equally effective in stimulating fibroblast proliferation as coherent, laser light (820 nm).

The lasing medium determines the wavelength emitted, and media such as helium neon (HeNe, 632.8 nm), gallium arsenide (GaAs, 904 nm), and gallium–aluminum–arsenide (GaAlAs, 820 nm) are used clinically.[33] When used, the laser beam is scattered, reflected, transmitted, or absorbed.[32] The magnitude of each depends on the application technique, the nature of the tissue being treated, and the wavelength of the incident light.[30] Given the low irradiation level used, the effects are likely to be photochemical because there is no appreciable temperature increase.[32]

When applying LLLT, energy density (J/cm²) is an important recorded value, and ranges of 0.1 to 4 J/cm² and 1 to 10 J/cm² are used.[29,32] However, some advocate values as high as 30 J/cm².[31]

Because penetration is wavelength dependent, an infrared beam (wavelength, 800 to 900 nm) penetrates further than a visible red beam (wavelength, 600 to 650 nm).[31] As a result, visible red laser light is used to treat wounds and skin conditions, whereas infrared laser light is used for deeper conditions.[29,31]

Energy density (J/cm²) is measured at the skin surface, but energy density applied to deep target tissues is unknown because of the exponential tissue absorption of the energy and uncertainty about penetration depth.[29] Longer wavelengths penetrate further than shorter wavelengths.[33,34] However, actual penetration and energy density at a target site can only be speculated. Hair and skin pigmentation may adversely influence penetration.

Laser therapy is used widely in animals,[35] and 50% of UK veterinary surgeons surveyed in 1993 were aware of it.[36] Of animal physiotherapists surveyed, 64% used laser therapy, which equaled the number using US therapy.[37] Although LLLT has gained popularity during the past 20 years,[31] acceptance is hampered by a paucity of supportive studies using standard research protocols,[38-40] and there are both advocates[30] and detractors.[41] In a randomized controlled clinical trial, LLLT had a significant pain-relieving effect, reduced joint swelling, and caused an objective improvement in hand function in people with rheumatoid arthritis.[42]

LLLT in Veterinary Medicine

LLLT may be used in the treatment of nerve compression, bruising, wounds, tendon and ligament injuries, edema, and for pain relief.[35,43-46]

Clinical Applications

In cell cultures, LLLT wavelengths of 660 and 870 nm (noncoherent) and 820 nm (coherent) encouraged macrophages to release factors that stimulate fibroblast proliferation and thus promote healing.[33] LLLT reduced experimentally induced inflammation by 20% to 30%.[47,48] In vitro experiments showed an effect of laser on cells; however, the results of in vivo study results are inconsistent.[49-51]

There is general agreement on dose guidelines for LLLT,[39] but an infinite number of combinations and permutations of parameters are possible.[52] Rationale behind protocols remains unclear, although laboratory findings indicate effects are dose dependent.[53]

Human Studies

Tissue healing and pain control are the main areas for which laser therapy is used in people.[29] Wound healing, soft tissue injuries, and pain apparently respond well.

Pain

LLLT may be used for management of pain.[29] Laser significantly reduced pain and improved movement in people with rheumatoid arthritis[42] and osteoarthritis.[53]

LLLT can directly induce analgesia when locally applied and indirectly when used at acupuncture and trigger points.[32] People with cervical pain were managed with LLLT, and axonal beading by delayed nerve transmission was thought to occur.[52]

Studies in horses are lacking, but 14 horses diagnosed with chronic back pain were treated with laser (904 nm) acupuncture in an uncontrolled clinical trial.[54] Back pain was eliminated in 10 horses, nine of which continued to perform at an acceptable standard 1 year later.

Musculoskeletal Use in People

Twelve musculoskeletal conditions (excluding osteoarthritis) were included in a meta-analysis, in which there was an equal number of positive and negative outcomes.[55]

There was no evidence to support the use of LLLT for post-traumatic joint disorder, myofascial pain, and rheumatoid arthritis. A Cochrane review of the use of a 904-nm laser concluded that LLLT was effective for fast pain relief and quicker functional recovery, most specifically in the treatment of rheumatoid arthritis.[56] Using ultrasonographic assessment, there was a decrease in tendon diameter in people with de Quervain's tenosynovitis after 2 to 4 J/cm^2 LLLT (wavelength not specified).[57]

Animal Studies

Of U.K. chartered physiotherapists surveyed in 1994, 64% used laser in the treatment of horses and dogs.[58] Laser therapy in animals is used for pain relief, wound healing, and to promote hoof growth.[43]

There are mixed results in research studies of LLLT in animals.[31] In an uncontrolled clinical trial in Standardbreds, there was a successful outcome after treatment of soft tissue injuries using a 904-nm laser.[59]

Wounds

In experimental studies using LLLT, results are often inconclusive or mixed, with both positive[59] and negative outcomes.[60] Closure of chronic canine wounds was thought to be enhanced in a noncontrolled case report,[61] but this article is typical of much of the LLLT literature—anecdotal evidence lacking the necessary scientific format for appropriate analysis. Sutured teat wounds in dairy cattle were irradiated by LLLT, and histopathological examination and laser Doppler flowmetry demonstrated improved healing.[62] The effect of laser on equine wound healing was reported.[63] Surgically transected rat medial collateral ligaments exposed to laser (GaAlAs) gained a larger fibril diameter compared with controls.[64] Laser research is generally poor quality, with inadequate study design, lack of controls, and inconsistent recording of treatment parameters.[32] However, enough evidence exists to justify continued investigation.[65]

ELECTRICAL STIMULATION

Transcutaneous electrical nerve stimulation (TENS) is widely used to modify pain, whereas neuromuscular electrical stimulators (NMES) are used for muscle reeducation, prevention of muscle atrophy, and enhanced joint movement. Almost all electric stimulators are TENS units; they work transcutaneously through surface electrodes to excite nerves. TENS can stimulate muscle fiber activation in both normal and denervated muscle. NMES is used to treat a wide variety of physiological disorders and injuries in people and animals. It is the administration of an electrical current generated by a stimulator that travels through leads to electrodes placed on the skin to depolarize the motor nerve and produce a skeletal muscle contraction.

Electrical Current/Waveforms

Three types of current are commonly used:
1. Continuous direct current—unidirectional electrical current that flows for 1 second or longer
2. Continuous alternating current—changes direction of flow at least once every second (e.g., interferential)
3. Pulsed current (AC or DC)—unidirectional or bidirectional flow of charges (AC or DC) that periodically stops for a finite period. All NMES are pulsed current stimulators.

The phase duration is the time in which the current flows from the baseline in one direction and back to the baseline. The current may be monophasic, in which the pulse duration and the phase duration are the same, or biphasic, when the two phases make up one pulse. Pulsed current consisting of a bidirectional flow of charge is called biphasic pulsed current. When the duration of flow in each direction is the same, but the amplitude-dependent features differ, then the biphasic current is termed asymmetrical. Zero net DC current occurs when the total charge in one phase equals the total charge of the other phase. Both pulsed AC and DC current forms are commonly used in portable and clinical model NMES units.

Parameters Used in Neuromuscular Electrical Stimulation

Amplitude

Increasing the current intensity (milliamps) induces a stronger force of muscle contraction by recruitment of motor nerves at greater distances from the electrode. Lowering the skin's resistance decreases the driving voltage necessary for skin penetration, making stimulation more comfortable. Fortunately, horses have low skin resistance, and less current intensity is required to produce a sensory and motor effect.

Increased current amplitude is required to produce a given amount of muscular force if the pulse or phase durations are short. Symmetrical or asymmetrical biphasic pulsed currents use intermediate current amplitude levels.

Pulse Duration

Pulse duration of 200 to 400 μs produces powerful contractions while minimizing the likelihood of recruiting many pain fibers. As the pulse duration increases, smaller-diameter pain fibers are recruited.

Pulse Rate

Pulse rate (frequency and pulse per second) is the number of pulses delivered per second and is measured in hertz (Hz). Tetanic muscle contractions may be produced with frequencies as low as 20 Hz. A maximum force contraction generally occurs between 60 and 100 Hz, and fatigue will occur as frequency increases.

Duty Cycle

Duty cycle is the ratio of on time to total cycle time, expressed as a percentage. On time is the period in which a series of pulses is delivered. Off time is the time between on times. As the on time increases, muscle fatigue increases. A horse with severe atrophy may require a longer off time to recover between contractions; therefore monitoring of fatigue is required.

Ramp

Ramp refers to a gradual change in current amplitude and results in a gradual and more comfortable change in force of muscle contractions.

Recruitment

NMES recruits type II (fast-twitch) fibers before type I (slow-twitch) fibers, the reverse of the muscle recruitment pattern seen in a volitional contraction.[66] Increasing the pulse duration increases the recruitment of smaller diameter motor units at the same depth. Increasing the amplitude or pulse duration affects the strength of contractions because additional muscle fibers are recruited. Increasing the frequency results in the existing motor units firing at a faster rate and increases the strength of contractions, but it will also result in more fatigue.

Indications for NMES Treatment

NMES is commonly used for the treatment and rehabilitation of people who have had neurological or orthopedic injury. Examples include spinal cord injury, paralysis, or paresis from neurological disease and more commonly in joint disease or joint pain. NMES is used to mobilize and strengthen after edema, contractures, or surgical procedures resulting in nerve injury, to minimize atrophy, improve strength, halt the loss of volitional control, improve sensory awareness, decrease pain, and correct gait.

NMES was shown to halt muscle atrophy and improve recovery after reinnervation in rats with surgically severed peroneal nerves,[67,68] although there may be detrimental effects, including altered muscle structure[69] and muscle-generating capacity.[70] NMES of the triceps brachialis muscle in monkeys enhanced oxidative capacity and increased fiber size.[71] Capillary proliferation was seen in response to increased muscle blood flow, resulting in proliferation of endothelial cells. Microvascular perfusion is enhanced when applied at intensities that produce muscle contractions.[72]

Overall Effects of NMES

Increased muscle strength, muscle mass, and oxidative capacity plus the ability to overcome the effects of reflex inhibition on muscles are possible effects.[73,74] Care must be taken to avoid muscle fatigue, probably caused by the preferential recruitment of type II muscle fibers. If current intensity is too high, painful contractions may develop.

Transcutaneous Electrical Nerve Stimulation

TENS provides a degree of pain relief (symptomatic) by specifically exciting sensory nerves and thereby stimulating either the pain gate mechanism or the opioid system. These different physiological mechanisms dictate how TENS is applied.

TENS is noninvasive and has few side effects compared with drug therapy. The most common side effect is an allergic-type skin reaction seen in 2% to 3% of people and usually caused by the material of the electrodes, the conductive gel, or the tape used to hold electrodes in place. Most TENS applications are now made using self-adhesive, pregelled electrodes, which have several advantages, including reduced cross-infection risk, ease of application, lower allergy incidence rates, and lower overall costs.

Machine Parameters

The current intensity (strength) is in the range of 0 to 80 mA (up to 100 mA). Although small, this current is sufficient because the primary targets are the sensory nerves, and provided these nerves are depolarized, TENS can be effective. The machine delivers "pulses" of electrical energy, and pulse rate varies from about 1 or 2 pulses/sec (pps) up to 200 or 250 pps. In addition to the stimulation rate, the duration (or width) of each pulse may be varied from 40 to 250 μs.

Most modern machines have a burst mode in which the pulses are allowed out in bursts or "trains," usually at a rate of 2 to 3 bursts/sec. Modulation mode, which uses a method of making the pulse output less regular and therefore minimizing the accommodation effects, is sometimes available. Short-duration pulses can be effective because the sensory nerves have relatively low thresholds and depolarize following stimulation for less than a millisecond. The pulses delivered by the TENS stimulators vary between manufacturers but tend to be asymmetrical biphasic modified square wave pulses. Biphasic pulses have no net DC component, so skin reactions from a buildup of electrolytes under the electrodes are uncommon.

Mechanism of Action

Pain relief from TENS occurs by activating the pain gate mechanism and/or the endogenous opioid system. Pain relief from the pain gate mechanism involves excitation of the Aβ sensory fibers, and by doing so, reduces transmission of noxious stimuli from the "c" fibers through the spinal cord and hence onto the higher centers. Ideal pulse rate for Aβ fibers is high (90 to 140 Hz or pps), but it is unlikely a single frequency works well for every horse.

Alternatively, Aδ fibers respond preferentially to much lower stimulation rates (2 to 5 Hz), and when stimulated activate an opioid mechanism that causes the release of endogenous opiates (enkephalins) in the spinal cord.

Both nerve types can be stimulated simultaneously by using burst mode stimulation. High-frequency stimulation (about 100 Hz) is interrupted (or burst) at the rate of about 2 to 3 bursts/sec.[75] Pulses at 100 Hz activate Aβ fibers and the pain gate mechanism, but burst excitation of Aδ fibers activates the opioid mechanism with release of enkephalins.[75] For some horses, this is by far the most effective approach to pain relief.

Traditional TENS (Hi TENS, Normal TENS)

Traditional TENS uses stimulation at a relatively high frequency (90 to 130 Hz) and uses a relatively narrow pulse width (start at about 100 μs). Thirty minutes is the minimal effective time, but it can be delivered for as long as needed. The main pain relief is achieved during the stimulation, with a limited "carryover" effect, that is, pain relief after the machine has been switched off.

Acupuncture TENS (Lo TENS, Acu-TENS)

Acupuncture TENS uses low-frequency stimulation (2 to 5 Hz) with wider (longer) pulses (200 to 250 μs). The intensity used is usually greater than with traditional TENS, resulting in a definite strong sensation. Thirty minutes are needed to deliver a minimally effective dose. Opioid levels are slow to build up, and the onset of pain relief may be slower than with the traditional mode. Once sufficient opioid has been released, it keeps working after cessation of the stimulation. Many human patients find that the stimulation at this low frequency at intervals throughout the day is an effective strategy. The "carryover" effect may last for several hours.[75]

Brief Intense TENS

Brief intense TENS achieves rapid pain relief, but the strength of the stimulation may be too intense and intolerable. The pulse frequency (90- to 130-Hz band) and the pulse width (200-μs plus) are high. The current is delivered at, or close to, the tolerance level, and the energy delivered is high compared with the other approaches. Fifteen to 30 minutes is all that can be tolerated.

Stimulation Intensity

In human medicine, the most effective intensity management appears to be related to what the patient feels during stimulation, and this may vary from session to session. In veterinary medicine, it is not possible to determine the sensory response in the same way. Horses show a visible endorphin response demonstrated by body posture and eye dilation. Resentment is clearly displayed by a high head carriage, tail swishing, and an obvious dislike to what is being done.

Electrode Placement

For maximal benefit, target the stimulus at the appropriate spinal cord level (appropriate to the pain) by placing the electrodes on either side of the lesion (painful area). Some alternatives that are effective, most of which are based on the appropriate nerve root level: stimulation of appropriate nerve root(s), the peripheral nerve, motor point(s), trigger point(s), or acupuncture point(s),[76] or appropriate dermatome, myotome, or sclerotome.[77]

A two-channel application can be effective for treatment of vague, diffuse, or particularly extensive pain or the management of a local and a referred pain combination (one channel used for each component).

Contraindications (from Human Medicine)

- Application of the electrodes over the trunk, abdomen, or pelvis during pregnancy
- Patients who have an allergic response to the electrodes, gel, or tape[79]
- Dermatological conditions
- Patients with current or recent bleeding, hemorrhage, or with compromised circulation (e.g., ischemic tissue, thrombosis, and associated conditions)
- Application over the anterior aspect of the neck or carotid sinus

Precautions

- If there is abnormal skin sensation, the electrodes should preferably be positioned in a site other than this area to ensure effective stimulation
- Avoid active physes

TENS is a noninvasive method of giving pain relief; however, despite extensive studies in people,[66,67,72,76-80] there are few studies analyzing the therapeutic effect in veterinary medicine.

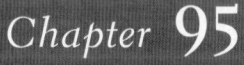

Chapter 95

Osteopathic Treatment of the Axial Skeleton of the Horse

Chris Colles* and Julia Brooks

Osteopathy originated in the United States with a Kansas physician, Andrew Taylor Still. He envisaged a system of healing that placed emphasis on the structural integrity of the body as being vital to the well-being of the organism. As knowledge of physiology and anatomy advanced, a concept evolved of the nervous system as an information network constantly changing and adapting in response to sensory information from the body and the environment. This knowledge allows a move away from the idea of pathological dysfunction as the only cause of illness to a concept of physiological (or somatic) dysfunction.[1] To use a computer analogy, the body may suffer from software failure (physiological malfunction) and hardware failure (pathological malfunction). To extend the analogy, osteopathy may be thought of as a form of reprogramming.

Chiropractic treatment evolved at around the same time as osteopathy and is similar but subtly different. The differences are largely philosophical; both forms of treatment rely on mobilization of joints. Chiropractors in equine practice tend to look primarily for positional changes associated with skeletal dysfunction. Treatment is directed principally at restoring joint mobility, with manipulation directed to the local site of dysfunction.

The osteopathic approach considers local tissue dysfunction as the direct result of trauma or the breakdown of compensatory mechanisms consequent to past trauma. The diagnostic approach is based on identifying patterns of dysfunction, with minimal reliance on positional factors and emphasis on the interactions of the entire spine. Treatment is aimed not only at restoring local function but also at identifying and removing factors that predispose to acute relapse. Therefore treatment frequently involves tissues distant to the perceived area of local dysfunction.

NEUROPHYSIOLOGICAL BASIS OF OSTEOPATHY

It is not uncommon in clinical practice to encounter horses that exhibit musculoskeletal signs for which no pathological cause can be established. The osteopathic philosophy accommodates these horses with the concept of somatic dysfunction. This concept is fundamental to osteopathy and describes a disturbance in the neurological networks that affects the function of the body (software failure). In other words, somewhere in the course of entering information from the environment and body, processing the information in the central nervous system, and then generating a motor response, something has gone wrong. Clinically this presents as a horse with signs such as stiffness, loss of performance, poor coordination, or gait abnormality for which no pathological process can be identified. Osteopathic treatment is directed at changing the signals to the

References on page 1335

*In the previous edition, this chapter was coauthored by the late Mr. A.G. Pusey, DO, FeCert. I am very grateful to Miss J. Brooks, DO, MSc, wife of the late Mr. Pusey, for assistance in updating this chapter.

neural network to modify the way sensory information is processed and thus to correct the motor response generated in the central nervous system.

To explore this concept, it is necessary to appreciate aspects of neurological activity not only under normal circumstances and as part of the protective response to injury, but also when long-term and inappropriate changes occur that adversely affect function of the body.

Normal Neurophysiology

In a normal horse, sensory and motor systems work together to achieve optimum function.

Sensory Component

The peripheral sensory system has two categories of neurons that provide information to the central nervous system. The division is made based on fiber size. The fast, low-threshold large fibers carry the sensation of touch and proprioception, and the high-threshold small fiber system (C and Aδ fibers) conveys potentially painful nociceptive and temperature modalities. In the spinal cord, these neurons synapse on interneurons where the first stage in information processing occurs. How the signals from the periphery are modified and sent onward to cortical areas for interpretation relies in part on the balance between large fiber input and small fiber nociceptor activity. This balance forms the basis of the pain gate theory where small fiber input, which may potentially be decoded as pain, can be held in check by large fiber activity. Under normal circumstances, much of the nociceptive input is screened out at the spinal cord level and never progresses to register as a painful sensation.

The sensory information will initiate and/or modify activity of the motor system.

Motor Component

The basic motor pattern is one of mutual inhibition of flexor and extensor neurons,[2] providing a balance between agonist and antagonist muscles. To refine the movements, proprioceptive information is sent constantly from muscle spindles and joint receptors back to the spinal cord. As sensory nerves enter the spinal cord, they send off sprays of ascending and descending collateral fibers, which synapse on interneurons that have connections within the spinal cord segment, with other spinal segments up and down the cord, and with tract cells up to the brainstem. The result is a network of neurons processing information from the body and environment. These generate flexible patterns of motor activity (sometimes referred to as *central pattern generators* [CPGs]). Thus a pattern of nerve activity is generated where the primary function is to move a limb, but simultaneously vital secondary functions are engendered—for example, changing the tone in the central musculature to counteract the changing load on the axial skeleton.

CPGs can cause many different routine patterns by virtue of the number and variety of interconnections, whose characteristics are determined by cellular and synaptic connections of the neurons. These patterns develop over time by a process of repetition and learning. Thus the inconsistent swing of a learner golfer becomes a confident, automatic swing after many hours of repetitive practice. This involves a process of chemical changes within a neuron and new synaptic connections with other neurons, which speed up or "fast track" a particular response and result in a consistent and reproducible pattern of motor activity.

Autonomic Component

Alongside skeletal activity, autonomic changes such as alterations in blood flow are incorporated to provide the necessary humeral environment for motor activity.

Response to Injury

In response to injury, a number of events occur, which involve not only the sensory and motor pathways but also the autonomic system. A painful stimulus is conveyed from the periphery along small caliber nociceptors to the spinal cord. If the stimulus is of sufficient intensity, it will pass on to the brain to register pain. It will stimulate motor neurons in the ventral horn, resulting in paravertebral and peripheral muscle spasm,[3] and stimulate sympathetic activity in the lateral horn, causing reduced blood flow to the skin.[4] These neurophysiological changes represent a protective response against further injury and will, in the short term, affect the function of the body.

Once these defensive measures are activated, a control mechanism exists at the level of the spinal cord to modify this activity to prevent constant discomfort. Mediated by the large fiber system input of discriminatory touch and proprioception and by descending inhibitory cortical activity, the pain gate can be closed to painful stimuli. This can be demonstrated by rubbing an injured area to ease pain. It is the balance between large and small fiber stimulation and higher center input that determines the activity of the interneurons and therefore sensory, motor, and autonomic responses.

In the short term, these responses are protective. If they persist, however, changes occur in the activity of the neuronal network that results in altered pain states and impaired function.

Altered Neurophysiology

It is tempting to consider the reactions of the neurons to injury as hard wired, with a certain level of stimulus giving a corresponding magnitude of response. In fact, these neuronal networks are plastic, and the sensitivity of neurons to stimuli can be altered at any point in the pathway. In some circumstances, this process of sensitization or facilitation, as it is sometimes called, can be useful, for example, patterns of motor neuron firing during the acquisition of a new skill. However, when pain circuits are involved, a lower firing threshold may result in neurophysiological changes that affect function of the body long after the original injury has resolved. This is the basis of the somatic dysfunction concept that encompasses distortion in sensory, motor, and autonomic activity in the absence of any obvious pathology.

Sensory Effects

A lowered threshold for firing may occur at any point in the sensory system extending from peripheral receptors through to the spinal cord and brain. In response to injury, nociceptor nerve endings produce neurochemicals such as substance P.[5] Combined with other inflammatory mediators such as prostaglandins and serotonin, the firing threshold is lowered, and the intensity at which the nociceptors will fire is increased. This local sensitization is generally responsive to treatment with antiinflammatory medication.

If nociceptor activity is intense or prolonged, changes can occur in the chemistry and structure of the interneurons of the spinal cord.[6] These can be traced 3 to 7 days after only 45 minutes of moderate nociceptive stimulation.[7] These changes lower the threshold for interneuron firing in a process called *facilitation* or *"wind-up."* They become supersensitive to afferent input and internal network activity within the spinal cord and will activate a pain circuit at an inappropriately low level of nociceptive input. This is the mechanism underlying hyperesthesia.

A further stage in this central sensitization of interneuron pools is the development of allodynia, where even an innocuous stimulus such as a light touch results in a pain response. The clinical manifestation may be a "cold-backed" horse or one with sensitivity around the poll. Furthermore, the central pain pathways may be driven without any peripheral input at all. In experiments when afferent activity was blocked by sectioning the dorsal (sensory) root, a sensation of pain accompanied by autonomic and motor responses may still be present, driven by the output of the sensitized interneurons. This means that pain persists long after the original injury has resolved. Even when pain is no longer felt, the neuronal pool remains sensitive, and relatively low levels of nociceptive activity will produce a pain response inappropriate to the magnitude of the stimulus. This may account for horses with recurrent injuries that occur with minimal physical provocation.

Another characteristic of central sensitization is the development of antidromic activity in the sensory nerves. Although under normal circumstances a sensory neuron is stimulated at the periphery and transmits a signal back toward the spinal cord, it is in fact capable of firing from the center outward to the receptor, in what is termed the dorsal root reflex.[8] On reaching the periphery, depolarization of the nerve endings has the same effect as depolarization as a result of a noxious stimulus from an injury. Proinflammatory neurochemicals are released from the nerve into the surrounding area and trigger an inflammatory cascade. This centrally driven inflammatory response may explain those cases of intermittent limb swellings and dysfunction for which no pathological cause can be identified.[6]

Alongside the deleterious effects of persistent sensory changes, there are motor and autonomic effects that will affect neuromusculoskeletal function.

Motor Effects

Part of the response to injury is contraction of muscle, which protects the area from further harm. In the short term, this is a helpful emergency measure. However, persistent muscular changes are not desirable. There are a number of biomechanical, neurophysiological, and biochemical consequences arising from a muscle that remains in a contracted state.

From a biomechanical perspective, muscle spasm causes asymmetry of and restriction in joint movement. This not only has a local effect but also causes adaptation of movement by other parts to accommodate this loss of function. These distant sites may themselves become symptomatic in the long term.

On a neurophysiological level, persistent contraction reduces joint movement and results in length changes in muscle fibers. This diminishes the amount of large fiber input from muscle spindles and joint receptors into central interneuron pools and shifts the balance in favor of small fiber nociceptor activity and stimulation of pain circuits.

The other consequence of reducing information from proprioceptors is that it impairs the ability of the central processing centers to map the position of the body in space. This is of particular importance in the cranial cervical spine, where the greatest concentration of proprioceptors is found[9] and which is a vulnerable area when a horse falls. Joint stiffness and muscle contraction in this area following an injury will alter feedback from this level. This affects the ability of motor pattern generators throughout the spinal cord to modify activity in response to alterations in body position and may produce changes ranging from subtle gait disorders to ataxia. Clinically there may be no obvious signs, but it will affect the horse's potential and leave it more susceptible to acute injury.

Biochemical effects of muscle spasm influence factors that regulate the number of sarcomeres, which are the building blocks of muscle mass. Although stimulation of muscle by motor neurons is an important ingredient in muscle development, another clinically significant factor is stretch of the muscle fibers.[10] Stretch results in the production of a substance referred to as mechano–growth factor, which stimulates development of muscle mass. Lack of movement through an area may be responsible for the loss of topline and underdeveloped quarters often seen in a stiff horse.

Autonomic Effects

Alongside the sensory and motor effects that are characteristic in somatic dysfunction, altered autonomic patterns are also generated.

Thermography can be useful to detect this aspect of somatic dysfunction. In a "normal" horse, a reproducible thermographic pattern is observed, reflecting cutaneous blood flow.[11] Where facilitated segments exist, sympathetic activity in the lateral horn reduces surface blood flow, giving distinctive segmental cooling. In addition to local segmental changes, the pattern may be disrupted throughout the length of the spine, giving a visual record of changes in autonomic nerve output.[10]

Clinical Implications for Altered Neurophysiology

These mechanisms may explain some of the nonspecific lameness and back pain that tend to be recurrent. A diagnosis based on pathological condition of tissue (demonstrated by radiographic and scintigraphic examinations or by diagnostic analgesia) is not possible because the abnormality results from physiological changes in the motor, sensory, and autonomic patterns generated by the facilitated neuronal segment. Gait disturbance may be observed, and muscle spasm, joint stiffness, and tissue texture changes may be appreciated by palpation and passive motion testing.

EFFECTS OF OSTEOPATHIC TREATMENT

The concept of somatic dysfunction means that if an injury is treated exclusively at the periphery but central sensitization has occurred, then treatment may be ineffective or the benefits may be short lived.

On a neurophysiological level, osteopathy seeks to reduce this central sensitization of the facilitated segment by increasing large fiber signaling into the central nervous system. This shifts the balance of input away from small fiber nociceptive traffic, thereby closing the pain gate and inhibiting pain circuits. This has the effect not only of reducing discomfort but also of increasing movement, improving proprioception, encouraging muscle development, and promoting nutrition to the musculoskeletal system.

In practical terms, most techniques are directed toward restoring movement to stiff joints to optimize maintenance of postural position and functioning of the body. Local musculature is relaxed and mobility improved, which is associated with an increase of mechanoreceptor activity carried by the large fiber system into the interneuron pool. The treatment may take a number of forms, including soft tissue techniques, articulatory techniques, and mobilization and functional techniques.

Soft tissue and articulatory techniques stretch the skin, fascia, and muscles to improve pliability of and nutrition to the periarticular tissues and also to allow the joints to move in a full range. These techniques include massage and repetitive flexion and extension of restricted joints.

Mobilization techniques involve taking a joint with poor mobility to the point of maximum resistance (the restrictive barrier) and pushing through this barrier with a short-amplitude, high-velocity thrust. This causes relaxation of the muscles and improved mobility resulting from a sudden increase in large fiber input from mechanoreceptor activity, which resets the balance of inputs into the spinal cord and reduces central sensitization.

A successful approach in horses with long-standing, complex injuries is the use of functional techniques. This uses the concepts of ease and bind. A normal joint reaches a point (usually at the middle of its range of movement) where tension on the capsular ligaments and the overlying muscles is minimal. This is the point of ease, where a joint tends to rest naturally. Any movement away from the point increases tension or bind. This information is used by the central nervous system to monitor joint position and to generate an appropriate pattern of motor activity. Where the normal relationships between the joint structures have been disturbed, this point of ease is offset, and afferent information from that joint is changed. New reference points become imposed on the established networks, and the joint is less able to perform appropriately or to coordinate movement with other joints.

This new abnormal point of ease may be detected clinically by testing each range of movement (flexion/extension, side bending, rotation, translocation, and traction/compression). With the joint held in the position of ease, tension is minimal, and therefore afferent input into the spinal cord is minimal. This appears to reduce conflicting information entering the network and allows the old pattern to reassert itself. The old pattern is preferred by the system because over time neuronal connections have been created that fire more readily to generate this original learned response. This form of treatment relies on the osteopath establishing and maintaining one or, more commonly, several joints at the point of ease until the original

central pattern generators can reassert influence over the newly acquired patterns. This is a learned skill on the part of the osteopath and requires considerable tactile sensitivity and skill to adjust the tissues as the neurological patterns are modified. Among injured horses is a clinically challenging subgroup of 4- to 6-year-old horses that develop clinical signs as work becomes more demanding, rather than as a response to direct trauma. In these horses, it is tempting to conjecture that some form of perinatal injury may have occurred that has prevented the normal patterns from developing. These horses frequently undergo more treatment and require more careful rehabilitation than other horses.

Details of osteopathic techniques are beyond the scope of this chapter, but the reader is referred to an excellent textbook.[11]

DIAGNOSIS AND CASE SELECTION FOR OSTEOPATHIC TREATMENT

Diagnosis should involve selection of horses with a somatic dysfunction and exclusion of horses with a pathological condition. Initially a conventional veterinary lameness examination should be performed. If the examination indicates a change in quality of movement rather than lameness, or if lameness is centered in the axial skeleton and no pathological process can be demonstrated readily (e.g., by radiological or scintigraphic evaluation), then the likelihood of a somatic dysfunction as the cause of lameness should be considered. Somatic dysfunction alters the way a horse moves and so may contribute to pathological change (e.g., synovitis in an overloaded joint). Once a primary pathological condition has been excluded, the process of making an osteopathic diagnosis can proceed. This diagnosis is based on somatic dysfunction, that is, how the component parts of the horse work together as a whole and how different areas of dysfunction or stiffness may contribute toward the problem.

An accurate case history is essential and should include the type of work the horse is expected to do and the level it is expected to attain. The history also highlights past injuries and illnesses and may reveal idiosyncrasies in behavior or movement that, although noticed by the owner, have not interfered with performance sufficiently to be a cause for concern. When considering the history, these subtle disturbances in motor function may, in retrospect, have been early signs of the coming crisis.

Examination begins by assessing muscle development and distribution of weight through all limbs in the standing horse. The horse should stand naturally with all cannon bones vertical and not shift weight constantly between limbs. Muscle development should be symmetrical, and the areas of muscle should be consistently developed throughout the horse. Areas of poor development over the top of the back, neck, or quarters should be noted. Similarly, uneven development or hypertrophy may be substantial. In particular, hypertrophy of the pectoral muscles may indicate that forward propulsion of the horse depends unduly on the forelimbs because of poor hindlimb function. Hypertrophy of the muscle over the atlas and axis frequently accompanies restricted joint movement at this level. Foot placement, shape, and shoe wear are also important for locating areas of dysfunction. When assessing feet, however, it is necessary to differentiate between change caused by altered limb movement and problems caused by poor farriery.

Movement at a walk is more revealing than at the trot, when the horse tends to fix the neck and back to guard against pain. Observation gives an impression of how the horse moves as a whole and indicates which areas are functioning poorly. Balance and fluidity of movement from head to tail are as important as stride length, foot placement, and frank lameness. How the horse copes with long and short turns indicates problems with lateral flexibility. In particular, when the horse is turned short, the head and neck should flex evenly in the direction of the turn, and the hindlimbs should be crossed as the quarters move around. All limbs should be moved with easy flowing strides, showing consistent stride length and straight limb flight. The feet should be placed easily, and in particular the hind feet should not dig into the ground when placed. Limb movement that appears heavy, stiff, inconsistent, or mechanical should alert the observer to potential problems. Excessive head and neck movement in time with the limbs is also abnormal. Substantial lateral movement of the pelvis, often associated with patches of worn hair under the back of the saddle, indicates reduced movement in the lumbosacral spine. The pelvis and tail being carried to one side also indicates uneven tone in the spinal musculature. Uneven height between the tubera coxae also should alert the clinician to potential problems.

The transition from walk to trot can be revealing, and any tendency to raise the head or skip in the transition indicates problems, probably in the region of the cervicothoracic junction. Assessing individual joint movements is useful, but it requires considerable skill and powers of observation. Running the hands down the paravertebral muscles from the occiput to the tail may reveal areas of muscle hypertrophy or spasm, and most importantly tissue texture can be felt. Moving the joints through the relevant ranges of motion identifies those that are stiff.

Diagnosis requires consideration of past injuries, the way the horse moves overall, and identification of dysfunction in specific areas. Initially, the clinician may only be able to form a working hypothesis, which will be refined once treatment begins. Where problems have been present for some time, the horse will have developed altered patterns of posture and movement to work around poorly functioning areas. These alterations may occur at several levels because of the interconnections of the neural networks. Ascertaining what is the site of the primary injury and what are secondary changes may be difficult.

INFRARED THERMOGRAPHIC IMAGING

Thermographic examination in the horse has proved to be an invaluable tool to confirm somatic dysfunction.[12] It is important to realize that areas of cooling are more important in diagnosing sympathetic dystonia than are increased temperatures. Thermography is prone to artifactual results, and interpretation can be reliable only if image acquisition is carried out in a temperature-controlled environment (between 18 and 22° C) using an absolutely consistent technique.

The horse must be clean and dry because moisture absorbs infrared radiation and causes false readings. Hair length should be consistent because hair has an insulating effect, and horses that have clipped coats or rubs from rugs present difficulties in interpretation. Different coat colors may be of different hair length or density, which causes artifacts. When moulting, areas of different colored hair may moult at different times, again giving rise to artifactual results. Before performing a thermographic examination, horses should be acclimatized to the room temperature for as long as it takes for the surface temperature to remain stable. The time required depends on the difference in ambient temperature of the environments inside and outside the thermography room. The room should be free of drafts and direct sunlight.

In a normal horse, a reproducible thermographic pattern is observed, reflecting cutaneous blood flow.[13] Where facilitated segments exist, sympathetic activity in the lateral horn reduces surface blood flow, giving distinctive segmental cooling. In addition to local changes, the pattern may be disrupted throughout the length of the spine, giving a visual record of changes in autonomic nerve output. Certain specific injuries give areas of increased blood flow and an increase in surface temperature. These injuries are usually around the head or in the lower limbs, where little or no overlying muscle is present.

In a normal horse, the surface temperature should be within 1.5° C over the neck and body of the horse and in the limbs proximal to the carpus and tarsus. The head and lower limbs are generally cooler. A useful guide when setting the thermographic factors is to assume the eye will be the hottest normal area and to set up the camera with this as the maximum temperature. Changes of 5 to 6° C are severe, so a temperature range of about 6° C is ideal. If the horse has parts of the coat clipped, then changes in the level of the window may be required to accommodate the clipped areas of the body. Particularly important is a dorsal view of the back, where a relatively warm dorsal midline stripe is seen, with the muscle on either side symmetrical and between 0.5 and 1° C cooler. When interpreting thermographs of the neck and back, changes of less than 1° C from the normal may be discounted. Changes in excess of 1° C usually indicate sympathetic dystonia, the importance of which must be interpreted in the light of information regarding clinical signs seen and the use to which the horse is put. It is likely that horses frequently suffer low-grade back pain or stiffness, which may not be of particular clinical significance if they live relatively sedentary or gymnastically undemanding existences (e.g., a racehorse or hunter performs satisfactorily with minor changes in the cranial aspect of the neck or thoracolumbar spine, which would cause unacceptable stiffness or gait modification in an event or dressage horse).

Figure 95-1, *A* to *C* (Color Plate 5), shows the thermographic appearance of a completely normal horse. One should bear in mind that few horses meet this degree of perfection, but they may still perform adequately at the required use. The most common area of the spine to show joint stiffness is the cranial aspect of the neck, with changes to the occipitoatlantal and atlantoaxial joints. This group of injuries results in a cold band running obliquely ventrally in the neck from about the level of the occiput (Figure 95-2; Color Plate 6). This band becomes narrower with time, and although a substantial temperature change is visible in the acute stage, over an initial period (probably

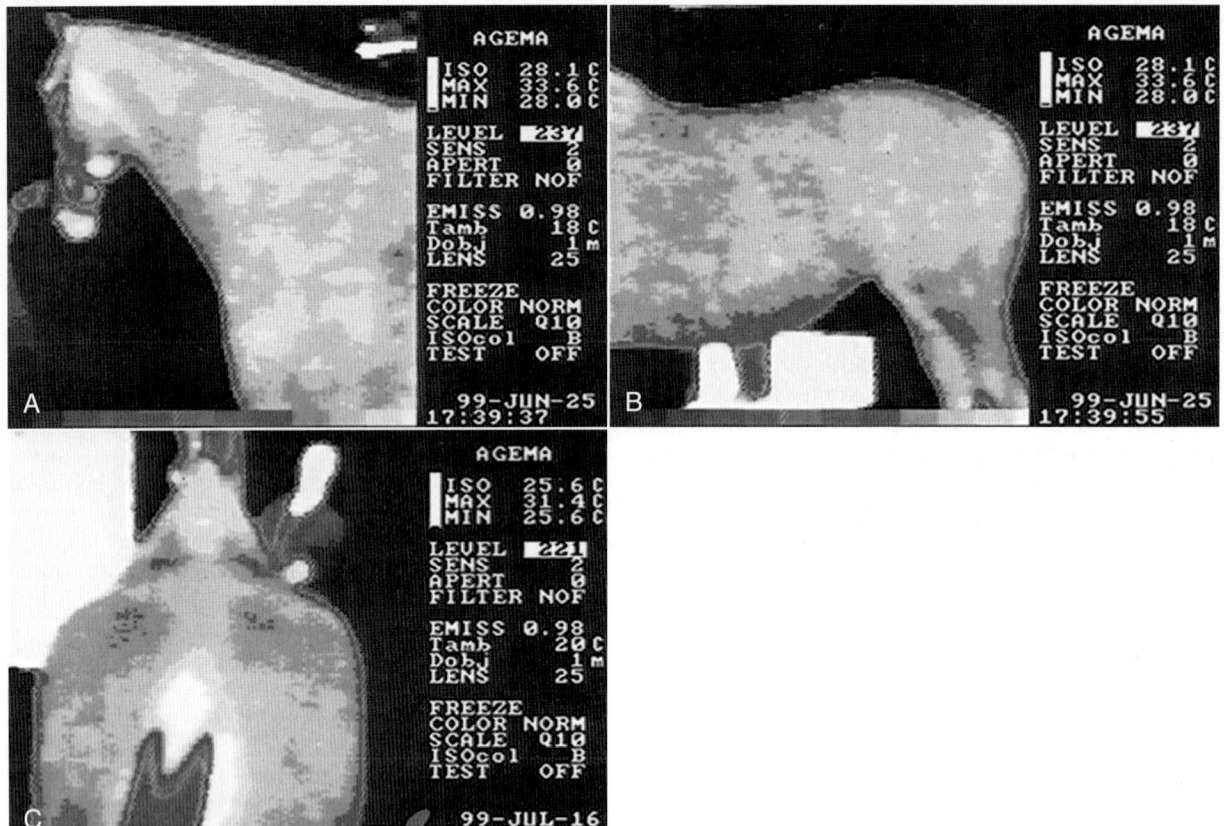

Fig. 95-1 • Thermographs show the appearance of normal horses. The color scale represents 5.6° C using 10 colors; that is, each color represents about a 0.5° C change in temperature. The color bar under the image shows the colors used; those to the right side are the hottest, and those to the left are the coldest. White is above the top of the scale, and black is below the scale. **A,** Lateral image of the head, neck, and shoulder. **B,** Lateral image of the thorax, abdomen, and hindquarters. **C,** Oblique dorsal image from behind the horse looking toward its head and neck. Temperature variation is 1° C over the neck, trunk, and hindquarters. A warm midline dorsal stripe along the back extends from the withers to the base of the tail, with symmetrical muscle temperature on either side.

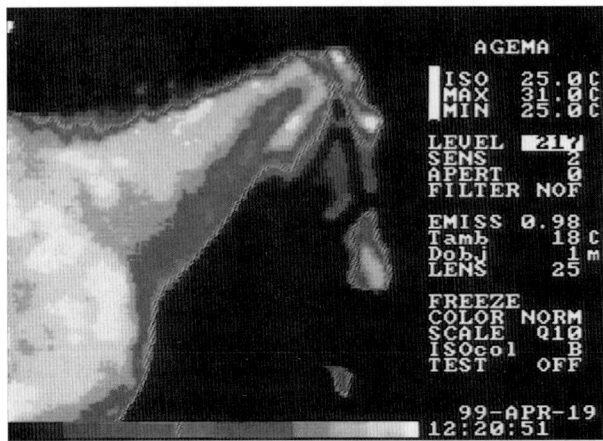

Fig. 95-2 • Lateral image of the neck of horse with reduced mobility in the occipitoatlantal and atlantoaxial joints. A cool line runs obliquely from the region of the atlantoaxial joint caudally to the base of the neck and is 1.5° C cooler than the surrounding muscle, indicating an area of sympathetic dystonia.

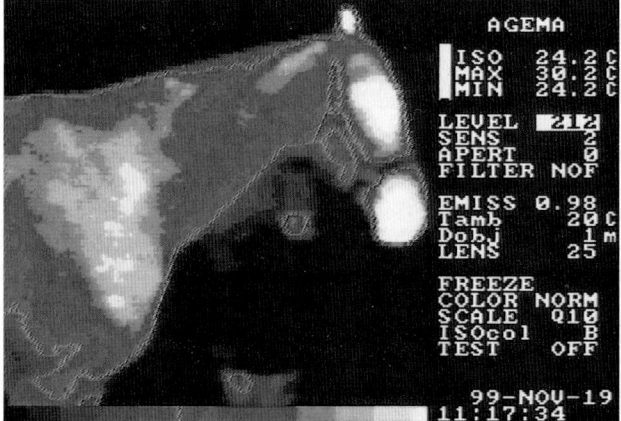

Fig. 95-3 • Lateral image of the neck of horse with reduced mobility in the neck. There is clinically significant cooling from the occiput caudally to the level of the sixth and seventh cervical vertebrae, indicating a problem involving all joints in the neck.

about 2 years), the temperature change becomes less noticeable. Stiffness or injury farther caudal in the neck is accompanied by cooling of the surface temperature overlying the affected area (Figure 95-3; Color Plate 7). Because the nerve supply to the muscles of the shoulder arises from the caudal

aspect of the neck, injuries to the spine between the shoulders are difficult to see thermographically, but a cold band running vertically down the back of the shoulder region (Figure 95-4, *A*; Color Plate 8, *A*), usually accompanied by cooling of the entire thoracic area and hindquarters, is an

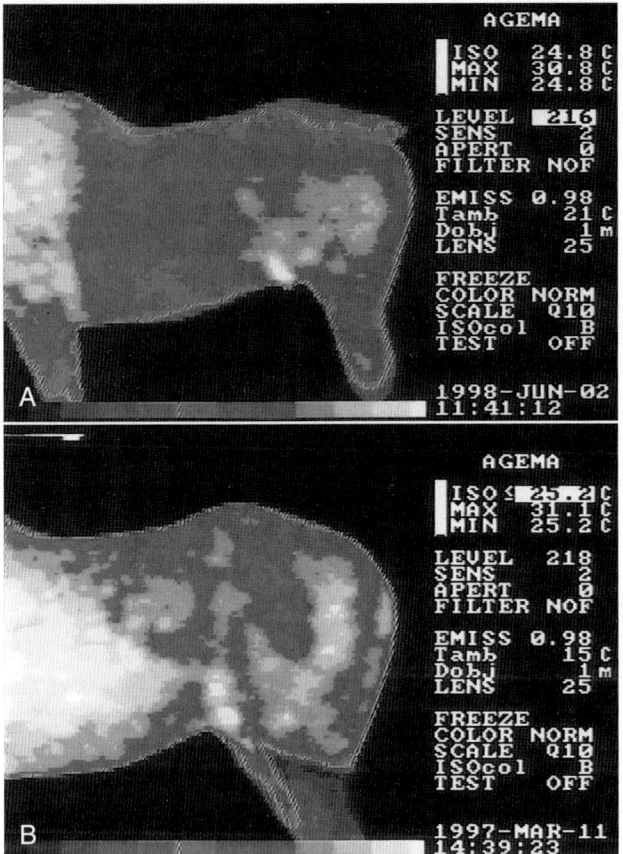

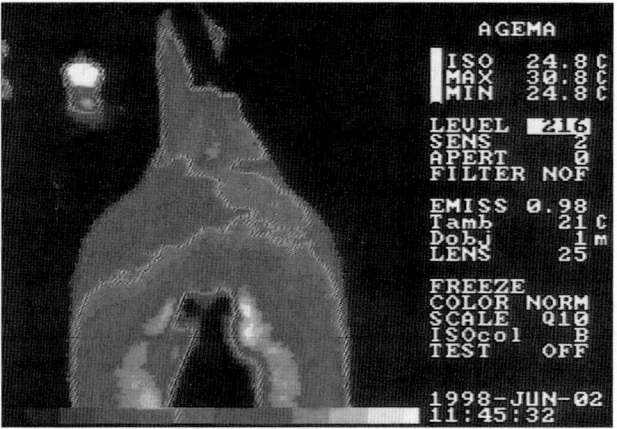

Fig. 95-5 • Dorsal image of horse showing abnormal temperature patterns of the thoracolumbar spine. Note the complete loss of the normal central stripe, with substantial cooling indicating the presence of reduced mobility of the entire thoracolumbar spine and pelvis. The asymmetrical nature of the temperature pattern indicates the horse is likely to move with an asymmetrical gait, resulting from increased muscle tone on the left side of the body.

Fig. 95-4 • Lateral images of the thoracolumbar area of two horses, both showing substantial cooling in the musculature of the dorsal spine from the saddle region caudally. **A,** The vertical cranial boundary to the zone of cooling indicates that the injured area is in the region of the cervicothoracic junction, but the shoulder muscles overlying this area receive innervation from the lower neck, partly masking the muscles supplied by the upper thoracic area. **B,** The typical appearance of cooling in the muscle resulting from an injury to the region of the twelfth thoracic vertebra, with the cranial border of the region running obliquely ventrally and caudally. This horse has been clipped, but long hair left on the hindlimb produces an area 5° C cooler than the surface temperature of the thorax of the horse.

indicator of injury to the cervicothoracic area. Cooling of the hindquarters arising caudal to a diagonal band from the level of about the twelfth thoracic vertebra generally indicates injury at this level of the thoracic spine (Figure 95-4, *B*; Color Plate 8, *B*). Two other changes are of particular clinical significance. Any break in the normal dorsal stripe running along the midline of the back or substantial cooling on either side of this stripe indicates a change in sympathetic activity in that region (Figure 95-5; Color Plate 9). Second, cooling of the distal aspect of a limb may be clinically significant. If the ambient temperature decreases below about 15° C, normal physiological changes reduce blood flow in the distal aspect of the limbs to conserve body temperature. This causes cooling of the distal aspect of the limbs (distal to the carpus or tarsus, unilaterally or bilaterally), but such limbs should still show a surface temperature 5 to 6° C cooler than the trunk temperature. If severe injury has occurred at the base of the neck or in the lumbar region, then the temperature of the distal aspect of the limb may decrease to equal the ambient temperature.

More detailed analysis of the thermographic changes seen is beyond the scope of this chapter.

TREATMENT

Because of the vast number of interneural connections and the ramification of effects on the spinal cord, the entire spine must be considered as one interrelated structure, and treatment may have to be provided at several levels. Sedating the horse is useful because treatment requires identification of specific areas of stiffness or reduced movement. If the horse is sedated adequately, then the absence of conscious movement allows the osteopath to feel underlying deficiencies more easily. Sedation is particularly helpful when using functional techniques that monitor subtle changes in joint position. Osteopaths in the United Kingdom undergo a 4-year university course that includes considerable theory and practical training. The techniques used require considerable practical experience to be successful; therefore this chapter can only begin to outline treatment.

After the osteopath performs the static and moving examinations described earlier, he or she starts a physical examination, feeling the tone and physical character of the muscles and the extent of movement of the joints, usually starting at the head and working along the neck and back to the tail. It is necessary to try to determine which joints show restricted movement, which areas show abnormalities caused by primary injury, and which changes are secondary to the primary affected areas. Experience allows the osteopath to determine which area must be treated first. The areas showing somatic dysfunction tend to be interrelated and must be treated in a specific order if treatment is to be successful. Starting treatment on an area showing restricted movement secondary to another abnormal area is doomed to failure. However, treatment of a key area often results in dramatic relaxation throughout the spine. The basic techniques of treatment have already been outlined and rely on stimulating the activity of the large caliber fibers, thereby inhibiting the interneuron pool and blocking the small fiber (pain) signals. The results are effective in most horses, and once the neural activity returns to normal, the horse tends to maintain this state.

In a small number of horses the problem may be so ingrained and widespread that general anesthesia may be needed to facilitate assessment and treatment. The plane of anesthesia is light, and the horses are in good health; thus the risks of the procedure are minimal. Assessment of individual joint complexes can be made throughout the spine with the horse under general anesthesia. It is remarkable how often gross dysfunction of these complexes can be detected with the horse anesthetized, when they had previously been effectively concealed by the capacity of the body to set up compensatory mechanisms. Treatment is still based on the principles outlined above, but the horse is positioned on its back, allowing movements such as rotation of the thoracolumbar spine, which cannot be achieved in a standing horse. Using all limbs simultaneously is also possible, allowing functional techniques (outlined previously) to produce a massive large fiber input to the interneuron pool. This is done by moving each limb to its position of ease, and then holding the position until relaxation is felt. By moving the limbs to maintain the positions of ease, the sympathetic dystonia can be unwound gradually. This technique, used with the horse under general anesthesia, allows a potent but gentle treatment to be carried out. In a standing, conscious horse, techniques are necessarily limited and are most effective with relatively short-term injuries.

RESULTS OF TREATMENT

Pusey et al[14] reported on a trial carried out over 4 years, treating horses with chronic dysfunction using osteopathic techniques. Eighty percent of treated horses returned to the previous use, performing at the same or a better level than before treatment, at least 12 months after the last treatment. As might be expected, the authors concluded that results were substantially better among the later horses because of increasing experience of treatment techniques.

Another study was made of horses that had been treated under general anesthesia, having failed to respond satisfactorily to treatment under sedation. Follow-up information was obtained at least 1 year after the treatment was finished. Thirty-five horses were treated. Twenty-four (71%) of these had maintained improvement and returned to the previous level of work: 11 at the previous level and 13 at a higher level than previously. Eight (24%) horses did not respond to treatment, and two horses deteriorated. One horse was not available for follow-up evaluation. The authors concluded that given that these horses had long-term intractable problems, this was a justifiable and useful treatment technique.

We hope this brief overview shows the potential for osteopathy in a complementary role, alongside veterinary science, in treating neuromusculoskeletal problems in the horse.

Chapter 96

Shock Wave Therapy

Scott R. McClure

References on page 1335

HISTORICAL PERSPECTIVE

Early studies in people in which shock waves (SWs) were used to disintegrate ureteral stones resulted in radiologically evident remodeling of the pelvis.[1] These findings sparked the initial studies investigating the use of SWs in orthopedic applications. These studies and anecdotal clinical use resulted in the initial five standard indications used in human medicine: (1) calcifying tendonitis of the shoulder (tendinosis calcarea), (2) tennis elbow (lateral epicondylitis), (3) golfer's elbow (medial epicondylitis), (4) heel spurs (plantar fasciitis), and (5) pseudarthrosis. Focused shock wave therapy in horses started in Germany in 1996, and applications were primarily based on those from human medicine.[2] Because of positive experiences treating people with insertional desmopathies, the first equine application was the use of shock wave therapy (SWT) in horses with proximal suspensory desmitis. Initial clinical responses were positive; therefore SWT was attempted in numerous other equine conditions, including navicular syndrome and distal hock joint pain.[3,4] Initially, the probe

was positioned behind the navicular bone from the heel, but when ultrasonographic imaging showed that the distal sesamoidean impar ligament could be seen through the frog, this location was then used to administer SWT to the navicular bone and associated structures.

The first equipment was large, requiring water cycling and degassing, and use was limited to horses under general anesthesia. The development of more affordable, portable, and durable equipment led to an initial expansion of its use and applications. However, as further knowledge was gained in equine medicine and surgery, the use of SWT has contracted somewhat, and attention is now paid to applications that consistently provide good clinical outcomes.

SHOCK WAVE GENERATORS

Two distinctly different pressure waves have been loosely described as SWT, SWs and radial pressure waves (RPWs). True SWs are pressure waves that meet specific physical parameters, including a rapid rise time (within nanoseconds), high peak pressures, and a gradual decrease in pressure over a few milliseconds, often with a negative pressure component (Figure 96-1 and Table 96-1).[5] SWs occur naturally associated with lightning, planes breaking the sound barrier, or explosions. Electricity is used as a driving energy source to generate SWs used for medical purposes. RPWs are generated by pneumatically powered sources that drive a metal rod to strike a plate in contact with the skin surface. RPWs have slower rise times and lower peak pressures than

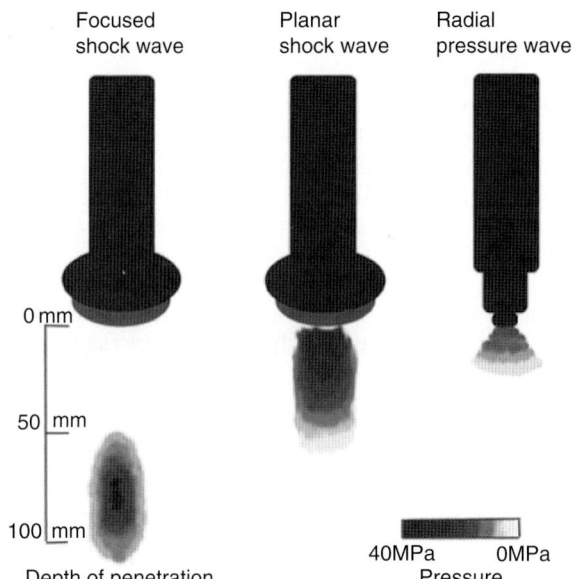

Fig. 96-1 • The schematic demonstrates the three types of pressure waves described. Focused shock waves concentrate the pressure at a focal point that can be centered up to approximately 75 mm deep. Planar shock waves are not focused and have a more diffuse pattern with less penetration. Radial pressure wave generators have a lower maximum pressure and deposit the maximum pressure on the surface. (Reprinted with permission from Robinson EN, Sprayberry KA: *Current therapy in equine medicine,* ed 6, St. Louis, 2009, Saunders.)

TABLE 96-1

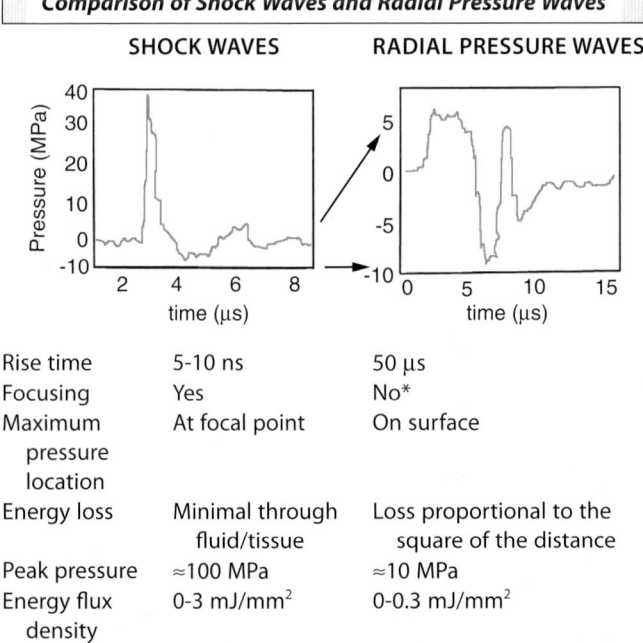

Comparison of Shock Waves and Radial Pressure Waves

	SHOCK WAVES	RADIAL PRESSURE WAVES
Rise time	5-10 ns	50 μs
Focusing	Yes	No*
Maximum pressure location	At focal point	On surface
Energy loss	Minimal through fluid/tissue	Loss proportional to the square of the distance
Peak pressure	≈100 MPa	≈10 MPa
Energy flux density	0-3 mJ/mm^2	0-0.3 mJ/mm^2

Reprinted with permission from Robinson EN, Sprayberry KA: *Current therapy in equine medicine,* ed 6, St. Louis, 2009, Saunders.
*Includes "focused" end piece.

SWs. Differences between SWs and RPWs are important because they may not affect tissue similarly; consequently, the type and equipment used are critical when evaluating the effect on tissues and efficacy of treatment. Editors' note: However, published results in the horse have to date

shown little difference in efficacy. A comprehensive review of SWs and RPWs, along with a description of equipment currently available, was recently published.[6]

DOSE DEPENDENCE

There is a dose effect of SWT that is a combination of the energy flux density (EFD) and the number of pulses. The EFD (mJ/mm^2) is the amount of energy (millijoules) in the focal area (mm^2). There is a lower limit of EFD that must be reached for SWT to be effective and an upper level over which EFD is high enough to create damage at any number of pulses. This range depends on species, tissue being treated, waveform, and generator.

It is difficult to transpose doses from other species to horses. When 1000 pulses at an EFD of 0.28 mJ/mm^2 was applied to rabbit Achilles tendons, there was a useful inflammatory reaction; but there was inflammation and tendon necrosis at 0.6 mJ/mm^2.[7] However, EFDs of 0.6 mJ/mm^2 or more are used in horses without complications. The minimal dose to achieve the desired effect is not known, and we may not need to use such high levels. There is a current trend to use low EFDs for a number of applications. One thousand pulses at 0.18 mJ/mm^2 stimulated neovascularization of the tendon-bone junction in dogs.[8] A dose of 200 pulses at 0.12 mJ/mm^2 was better than 500 pulses in an Achilles tendonitis model in rats.[9] At this time, the ideal energy levels and pulse numbers remain empirical in most equine applications.

The frequency (pulses/sec) of the pulse application appears unimportant, although SWT using lower frequencies takes longer. From a biological standpoint, frequency of all equine SWT applications is relatively slow, and tissue heating or other untoward biological effects seen at high rates do not occur, although white hair occasionally develops at treatment sites.

APPLICATIONS

Bone

Early studies of SWs on bones yielded variable results and were confusing. Very-high-energy treatment of rodent and rabbit bones resulted in physical disruption of the bone and periosteum, which led to the thought that bone remodeling in response to SWT was the result of physical damage.[10,11] In other studies using more appropriate tissue and in different species, bone remodeling occurred without physical disruption. The ability for SWT to stimulate bone healing resulted in an interest to use SWs for the management of nonunion fractures. In one study, nonunion fractures were created in 10 dogs using segmental radial osteotomies.[12] Five dogs were treated with 4000 SWs at 0.54 mJ/mm^2, and five served as untreated controls. All treated dogs had osseous union by 12 weeks compared with only one untreated control dog.[12] The first widespread musculoskeletal use of SWs in people was for management of nonunion fractures. Clinical trials have consistently demonstrated bone healing following SWT in delayed union fractures and nonunion fractures. Wang reported 80% success[13]; Schaden, 75% success[14]; and Rompe, 72% success—results that were remarkably consistent.[15]

The mechanisms of SW-induced osteogenic stimulation are currently being investigated. There were increased osteoprogenitor colony-forming units from the marrow of rat femora 24 hours after treatment with 500 SWs at 0.16 mJ/mm². [16] A dose response was seen with the highest supernatant concentrations of transforming growth factor–β1 (TGF-β1) after 500 SWs; lower numbers of pulses were ineffective, and higher numbers were inhibitory. The same treatment protocol (500 SWs at 0.16 mJ/mm²) was administered to rats with segmental bone defects and resulted in increased expression of TGF-β1 and vascular endothelial growth factor–A (VEGF-A) mRNA and increased osteoprogenitor cells. [17] In both studies, it appeared that SWT stimulated osteogenesis without physical disruption of the bone. Subsequent studies have shown that SWT increases concentrations of VEGF and bone morphogenic protein–2, as well as neovascularization and ultimately an increase in load to failure in a rabbit femoral fracture model. [18]

The application of SWT to bone was the initial musculoskeletal application in people and horses. The applications and outcomes in human medicine have grown and are positive. The applications of SWs in horses have not been pursued as aggressively as may have been expected. One initial concern was the potential for the creation of microfractures that could weaken the bone after treatment, a theory that has some support. The application of 9000 pulses of RPWs at 0.175 mJ/mm² or 9000 SWs at 0.15 mJ/mm² to cadaver third metacarpal bones (McIIIs) from racehorses that suffered catastrophic injuries of the contralateral limb caused a small but significant increase in microcrack density, and RPWs increased microcrack length. [16] In dorsal cortical bone specimens of the McIII 2000 pulses of SWs or RPWs subjected to pulse increments of either 500-SWs (0.15 mJ/mm²) or RPWs (0.16 mJ/mm²), there were no detectable changes in modulus of elasticity. [17] Histologically, there were no increases in microfractures demonstrated with either SWs or RPWs. [17] Microfractures did not develop in an in vivo study in which 1000 pulses at a high EFD (1.8 mJ/mm²) were used.

In an in vivo equine pilot study that used 2000 SWs at 0.89 mJ/mm², two treated McIIIs had 30% more activated osteons than the contralateral untreated control McIII. [18] SWs were compared with periosteal irritation (stimulated by scarifying the periosteum with a needle) in the third metatarsal bone (MtIII) of four horses. The SW-treated MtIIIs had 56% more double-labeled osteons than those with only periosteal irritation, and the osteonal response was located at both the endosteal and the periosteal surfaces. This preliminary finding demonstrated that SWs exert an effect on bone that is different from simple periosteal scarification. Scintigraphic and histological examination of the fourth metatarsal bone after 2000 pulses at 0.15 mJ/mm² showed increased radiopharmaceutical uptake in the treatment area and an increased number of osteoblasts. [19]

Twenty-two Thoroughbred (TB) racehorses with dorsal metacarpal disease (see Chapter 102) manifest as pain on palpation, a thickened dorsal cortex of the McIII, and longitudinal radiolucent lines that were unresponsive to conventional therapy were treated with RPWs. [20] Three treatments at 2-week intervals were administered, and a modified training program was instituted. The mean time to the first race was 4.5 months. Similar results are seen with focused SWT. I treat horses with periostitis with focused SWT (0.14 mJ/mm², 800 pulses), give 1 week of walking, and then resume training for 2 weeks; the cycle is repeated two more times. When horses are treated early in the disease process, most can continue in training without an extended rest period.

Horses with stress fractures of the tibia, humerus, and the McIII are candidates for management with SWT. Without controlled studies, it is difficult to compare SWT with healing in horses with nontreated fractures or in those receiving osteostixis. It is my impression that TB racehorses with dorsal cortical fractures of the McIII can return to training in a similar period as those that have received osteostixis. Six of 10 horses with McIII stress fractures were pain free and/or showed radiological evidence of healing by 90 days. [21] Two horses took more than 120 days, and two were retired for other reasons. In 20 horses with single oblique dorsal cortical McIII stress fractures treated with RPWs, the mean time from the last treatment to the first race was 5 months. [20]

Horses with fractures of the second and fourth metacarpal (metatarsal) bones and exostoses are frequently treated with SWT. Focused SWT was used in four horses with closed fractures and in three with open, infected, comminuted fractures of the proximal aspect of the splint bones. [22] Horses with infected fractures were first treated locally and systemically with antibiotics, local wound curettage, and ostectomy of small loose fragments. SWT began when signs of infection were resolved and the skin was healed. The horses were treated with three treatments at 10- to 14-day intervals. They were administered 600 to 900 pulses, depending on the size of the lesion, at an EFD of 0.15 mJ/mm². Radiographs were obtained after the third treatment and 4 weeks later. Handwalking began after the second or third treatment. In horses without an infection, training began 10 to 12 weeks after fracture, whereas in those with infected fractures, training began 13 to 16 weeks after fracture. All the horses were sound and returned to normal use. There were no horses that did not undergo SWT for comparison.

Horses with fractures of the distal phalanx that can be approached with SWT through the frog are good candidates for treatment, but efficacy is anecdotal. Because it is not possible to get the SWs to penetrate through the hoof wall or the sole, fractures must be near the center of the distal phalanx and accessible through the frog. Some horses have shown positive outcomes.

There are only limited reports of using SWT in horses with long bone fractures and arthrodesis stabilized with internal fixation. Expense is a consideration, but access to apply SWT is a major limiting factor. SWT cannot be used effectively on horses with external coaptation such as a cast. SWT improved callus formation in the immediate postoperative period in dogs with bilateral 3-mm osteotomy gaps in the midtibia stabilized with a plate and treated with 2000 pulses at 0.18 mJ/mm². [23] At 12 weeks there was more radiologically visible callus and more histologically evident cortical bone formation than in control untreated dogs. [23] Early treatment of fractures may be beneficial in the horse.

Tendons and Ligaments

In vivo studies of tendon and ligament injuries have provided support for the use of SWT. Rabbits with collagenase-induced patellar tendonopathy were treated twice with

1500 pulses at 0.29 mJ/mm^2.[24] Tendons were harvested 4 and 16 weeks after SWT. SW-treated tendons had a 7% and 10% increase in strength at 4 and 16 weeks, respectively, compared with untreated controls. There were increased hydroxyproline concentrations in treated tendons and more blastlike tenocytes after 4 weeks. When 500 SWs at 0.12 mJ/mm^2 were applied to long digital tendon grafts placed to stabilize surgically disrupted anterior cruciate ligaments in rabbits, the treated bone–tendon interface had more trabecular bone ingrowth than controls.[25] The contact between the bone and tendon was improved, and subsequently the strength of the graft was increased 24 weeks postoperatively. Growth factors known to affect tendon repair, including TGF-β1 and insulin-like growth factor I, were increased after SWT in rats.[9]

Tissue explants were used to evaluate the effect of SWs on healthy pony tendons and ligaments.[26] Six hundred pulses at 0.14 mJ/mm^2 increased glycosaminoglycan (GAG) and protein synthesis in explants harvested 3 hours after treatment. However, by 6 weeks there was a decrease in GAG and collagen synthesis.[26] In a similar study, samples harvested at 3 hours after treatment revealed histological findings of disorganization of matrix structure and increase in degraded collagen.[27] Gene expression of type I collagen and matrix metalloproteinase 1 was increased at 6 weeks after SWT.[27] In these studies the degraded collagen and disorganization of the collagen at 3 hours after treatment warrant some concern about a possible detrimental effect of SWT. However, these studies were done in normal pony tendon and ligament, and one would expect these findings to already be present in injured soft tissues.

The most common application and the greatest amount of SW research in the horse have related to tendons and ligaments.

SUSPENSORY DESMITIS

To study the effects of SWT in horses, ultrasonography was used to monitor healing in two studies of suspensory ligaments after collagenase-induced desmitis.[28,29] In both studies, ultrasonographic measurements showed the defects healed faster in the SW-treated groups. Different outcomes were evaluated histologically in each study, but a positive effect of SWT was found in both studies. In forelimbs treated with SWT, there was increased metachromasia consistent with increased production of extracellular matrix in the SWT group.[28] In hindlimbs there were more newly formed small collagen fibrils in the SWT group.[29] The exact mechanisms by which these outcomes occur are not fully understood and it is unknown if the differences between treated and controls would result in a stronger outcome or less recurrence of injury in horses with suspensory desmitis. Immunocytochemical evaluation of suspensory ligaments treated by SWT showed increased TGF-β1 after treatment.[29]

Clinical response to SWT is consistently better in forelimbs than in hindlimbs. In a retrospective clinical study of horses with forelimb proximal suspensory desmitis (PSD) managed with 2000 pulses at 0.15 mJ/mm^2, 61.8% of horses with desmitis were in full work by 6 months, and 55.9% were still working at 1 year.[30] Editors' note: However, it must be borne in mind that many horses with forelimb PSD respond well to conservative management of rest alone (see Chapter 72). Of horses with hindlimb suspensory desmitis, 40.9% were in full work at 6 months, but only 18.2% were in full work at 1 year.[30] Results using RPW therapy in horses with forelimb or hindlimb lameness of at least 3 months' duration before treatment associated with PSD were remarkably similar.[31,32] Response was related to lesion severity determined ultrasonographically. At a recent equine practitioners' meeting,* the consensus on outcome was similar to these reports. Many practitioners do not consider horses with hindlimb suspensory desmitis to be good candidates for SWT alone. A combination of SWT and plantar fasciotomy to relieve alleged pressure on the proximal aspect of the suspensory ligament and to stimulate healing of the defect may provide a better prognosis. Horses with body and branch desmitis are also commonly treated and thought to have acceptable outcomes; however, there have been no controlled clinical trials, and information is anecdotal.

SUPERFICIAL DIGITAL FLEXOR TENDONITIS

There are two studies that have evaluated the short-term effect of SWT on collagenase-induced superficial digital flexor (SDF) tendonitis in the midmetacarpal region.[33,34] Ultrasonographically, the treated and control groups were similar throughout the studies. Histologically, the treated tendons were more "mature," indicating that the healing process was occurring at a faster rate. Treated tendons had more parallel collagen fibers than controls in one study, and treated tendons had increased neovascularization in the other study. In both studies there was an initial decrease in inflammation associated with SWT, but in neither study was tendon strength evaluated. A notable finding after SWT of tendonitis is the rapid improvement in clinical appearance. The peritendonous inflammation that results in the "bowed" appearance decreases quickly after SWT. One must be careful not to interpret that as tendon healing. The echogenicity and fiber alignment of the tendon injury must be monitored with ultrasonography.

ADDITIONAL APPLICATIONS
Osteoarthritis

Osteoarthritis (OA) of the distal hock joints was one of the first applications of SWs in the United States. In an early study of 74 horses with "bone spavin" refractory to medical therapy given SWT using a single high energy (0.89 mJ/mm^2) treatment of 2000 pulses, 59 (80%) horses improved by 90 days.[4] There are horses with OA of numerous joints that anecdotally have improved after SWT.[35] However, responses are mixed. In some horses, lameness decreases for a few months after SWT, whereas in others there is no change. I cannot find a logical explanation. SWT was evaluated experimentally in an osteochondral fragment–exercise model of OA of the middle carpal joint (see Chapter 84).[36] In treated horses, there was a decrease in total protein concentration in synovial fluid and less lameness on day 28 compared with controls.[36]

---

*Applying Regenerative Therapies for Tendon and Joint Caused Lameness of Horses, Bonn, Germany, October 6-7, 2008.

Navicular Syndrome

Clinical signs in horses with navicular syndrome may improve after SWT.[37,38] In 16 horses with long-term follow-up examination treated with 1000 pulses through the frog and 1000 pulses from between the heel bulbs under general anesthesia at 0.89 mJ/mm², masked video analysis from before and 6 months after treatment showed 56% of horses improved at least 1 lameness grade.[37] Owners reported 69% of the horses returned to the previous level of activity. There was no comparative control group. In another study, all 26 horses treated under general anesthesia with 3000 pulses at 0.56 mJ/mm² were free of lameness at 6 months.[38]

Navicular syndrome is complex, and as diagnostic techniques have improved, we now know that pain can originate from the deep digital flexor tendon, navicular bursa, the collateral sesamoidean or distal sesamoidean impar ligaments, the navicular bone itself, or other structures. SWT is indicated for horses that do not adequately respond to medical therapy and corrective shoeing. However, it must be recognized that navicular syndrome is a progressive disease, and SWT is not a cure.

Collateral Ligament Injury of the Distal Interphalangeal Joint

There is a recent report of the use of SWT or RPW therapy for the treatment of horses with collateral ligament injuries of the distal interphalangeal joint. There was no significant difference in outcome for horses managed by box rest and controlled exercise alone or combined with SWT or RPW therapy.[39]

Back Pain

SWT has been used for numerous causes of back pain, including impinging dorsal spinous processes, OA of articular facet joints, and soft tissue injury. There are two approaches to therapy for back pain. First is the treatment of specific sites of bony pathology identified by radiography, scintigraphy, and ultrasonography. Both sides of the back are treated with 35- and 80-mm probes (designed to treat equine backs; Equitron, Sanuwave Inc., Marietta, Georgia, United States) at 0.15 mJ/mm². Most horses improve after one or two treatments. A dose of 50 pulses/cm of bone "sclerosis" was suggested.[23] Second, horses that have back pain without specific skeletal pathology may respond to treatment of the muscle with SWT.[2,40] The 35- and 80-mm probes are moved along the dorsum of the horse. When the horse shows a painful reaction or muscle fasciculation, 80 to 100 pulses are applied at the site. There are anecdotal reports of SWT used for treating sacroiliac disease; an 80-mm probe may reach the dorsal sacroiliac ligaments but is unlikely to reach the sacroiliac joints per se.

Some horses with OA of the cervical articular facets (see Chapter 53) respond well to SWT, and others have a limited response. It is important to identify the specific facet joint to be treated and focus the SWs on the facet similarly to an injection into the joint. Two to three treatments at 2- to 3-week intervals are performed. If response is acceptable, then the treatment is repeated as needed.

Therapy Planning

When considering the application of SWs, obviously an accurate diagnosis is imperative. Next one needs to consider whether one can and should focus SWs on the pathology. SWs will not penetrate the hoof wall. Bone can be treated; however, 70% of the energy is lost in the bone. Therefore little energy is available on the opposite side of the bone. Most focused generators have a series of standoffs that adjust the depth of penetration. Any site that can be seen ultrasonographically can be treated with SWs, and ultrasonography can be used to measure the required depth if necessary. RPWs are different from the more powerful focused SWs in that the energy of the wave decreases proportional to the square of the depth; thus the depth of penetration is limited.

A three-dimensional treatment plan should be used to apply SWs to the full width and depth of the injured area.[23] For example, to treat a horse with PSD, the entire width and depth of the proximal aspect of the suspensory ligament are treated by using two probes, one with a 20-mm and the other with a 35-mm focal distance (and a commonly used generator; Equitron, Sanuwave Inc.). From the palmar midline, both probes are used to administer SWT to the axial aspect of the suspensory ligament, and then the 20-mm probe is used from oblique angles just palmar and axial to both splint bones to treat the remaining abaxial aspects of the ligament. The probes are slowly moved around the treatment area when applying SWT. This should expose the entire proximal suspensory ligament and the palmar/plantar aspects of the third metacarpal or metatarsal bones to the SWs.

SWs will completely reflect at an air interface, and it is important to avoid air interfaces during treatments near the thorax and abdomen. The pressure wave will be reflected and can cause hemorrhage at the interface. It is important to have the generator in good contact with the skin surface. Typically, the hair is clipped with a No. 40 blade. To obliterate the air interface found between the probe and skin, ultrasound coupling gel is the best agent to use, but water, mineral oil, and petroleum jelly are all suitable. It is best to slowly move the probe in the direction of the clipped hair, and then move back up and down again, with care taken to recoat the area with the gel. The convex radial generators may get air bubbles in the concavity, making coupling difficult.[41]

Combination therapies are frequently used to treat soft tissue injuries. Platelet-rich plasma and pig's urinary bladder matrix (ACellVet, Webster Veterinary Supply, Sterling, Massachusetts, United States) injected intralesionally in combination with SWT may result in some additive effects. My personal experience is favorable when I use a combination of ACellVet in horses with SDF tendonitis at the time of the first of three SWTs. The direct effect of SWs on stem cells in vivo is unknown. For this reason, when used together, I suggest SWT should precede the injection of stem cells, and the next SWT should be delayed for 3 weeks. Editor's Note: Since the effect of SWs on stem cells is unknown and given that stem cell therapy is still unproven and rather expensive, it may be best to select either SWT or stem cell therapy rather than combine the modalities.

Potential Complications

Very few complications are seen with SWT. There are dose-related effects, and it is possible to overtreat an area. With most commonly available devices, there are general guidelines to assist the veterinarian to calculate the appropriate dose. Transient swelling at the treatment site is occasionally noted and is more commonly seen when using RPW devices. White hairs may develop at the treatment site. As noted above, air- or gas-filled structures should be avoided. What is the effect of SWs on a physis? Some say it stimulates growth, whereas others say it inhibits growth. Studies in rabbits showed SWs can lead to premature closure of a physis; however, this work has not been repeated in horses.[42]

Analgesia

Analgesia has been a welfare concern since the beginning of SWT in the horse. There are concerns that analgesia after treatment may result in worsening of an injury when a horse returns to work. In vivo evaluation of skin sensation after both focused SWT and RPW therapy showed some analgesia for 48 hours after treatment.[43] There was no analgesia of the nerve field after the application of SWs and RPWs directly to the palmar digital nerve; thus it was concluded that analgesia was a local effect. In horses with unilateral navicular syndrome and OA where analgesia was measured as a change in increase in peak vertical force after treatment, analgesia from SWT was identified that peaked at 48 hours after application.[44] In a similar study using horses with unilateral navicular syndrome and RPWs, no analgesia was found.[45] The RPWs may not reach the depth sufficient to affect pain sensation from the palmar foot structures. Many racing and horse show jurisdictions have specific rules about SWT, and they should be consulted.

SECTION 1
Poor Performance

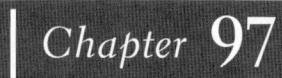

Poor Performance and Lameness

Sue J. Dyson

Horses may be presented to a veterinarian because of a change in performance or behavior or failure to live up to the expected level of performance, rather than because the rider or trainer has recognized overt lameness. Many of these horses do have musculoskeletal problems. The type of complaint often reflects the discipline in which the horse is used. For example, an event horse may be assessed because it has started stopping at drop fences, whereas a dressage horse may be evaluated because it takes uneven steps behind in passage or piaffe.

CHALLENGE OF ASSESSMENT

This type of horse presents the veterinarian with a diagnostic challenge that may involve assessment not only of the horse, but also of the horse and rider together and the rider's ability. Such an assessment requires knowledge of the sport in question and an ability to recognize when the problem is a lack of athletic ability or a mental problem rather than a pain-related musculoskeletal disorder or some other pathological condition, such as an upper airway disorder. The assessment also requires good knowledge and appreciation of how horses normally move and the variations among different breeds and types and an ability to recognize subtle changes in gait, such as a slightly reduced lift to the stride or stiffness in movement of the back. The assessment requires basic knowledge of equine locomotion and how gait may be modified by pain and also requires the ability to recognize when a rider may actually be creating the problem. Training methods and style of riding may contribute to the development of lameness.

This section sets out to discuss some of the different problems that may be encountered and the types of conditions that may be the cause of poor performance and to suggest some methods of approach to diagnosis. These may vary to some extent depending on whether the clinician is dealing with a competent professional rider or trainer or an inexperienced or even experienced amateur who lacks ability.

HISTORY

It is essential to obtain a comprehensive history to determine whether the horse has genuinely performed better previously at this level of competition, or moved better, and precisely what changes have been observed. It is important to listen carefully to the owner to properly understand the perceived problem, however small it might be. This is particularly important if the clinician does not have prior knowledge of the horse.

Determine the answer to the following questions:
1. What are the age and training history of the horse?
2. Does the horse have the musculoskeletal coordination and strength to do what is being asked?
3. Has the horse recently moved up a level of competition? Does the horse have the confidence or athletic ability to cope?
4. What is the current work program? How does this vary from day to day? Is the horse allowed turnout?
5. Has a recent change in the work pattern or intensity or some other change in management occurred?
6. Has the bit been changed?
7. Did the horse sustain a fall or any other trauma before the onset of the problem?
8. Has a recent change in the rider or trainer occurred?
9. Has an alternative rider been tried?
10. Has the horse ever exhibited clinical signs consistent with exertional rhabdomyolysis?
11. Under what circumstances is the problem apparent?

Viewing videos of the horse when it was performing normally sometimes can be helpful to compare with the findings of your own clinical evaluation. If the horse has recently changed ownership, comparing video recordings of the horse ridden by the previous rider and by the current rider can be useful to determine whether a change in riding style or training techniques may be responsible for making a previously subclinical problem become symptomatic, or to determine if the problem could be related directly to the manner in which the horse is being worked.

The types of clinical problems that may be encountered are listed in Box 97-1.

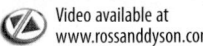
BOX 97-1

Types of Clinical Problems

References
on page
1336

- Not jumping as well: knocking down rails. This may be pain related or may be caused by the rider presenting the horse poorly to the fence.
- Not jumping as well: stopping. This may be a horse or rider confidence or ability problem, or may be pain related.
- Not making distances in combination fences. This may occur because the horse is landing too steeply, saving one or both front feet and therefore having too much ground to make up, or through lack of push from behind, reflecting a hindlimb lameness. Alternatively, if the horse is presented poorly to the first element of the fence, the subsequent elements become increasingly difficult.
- Reluctance to land leading on a specific leg. This can reflect a forelimb or less commonly a hindlimb lameness. Peak ground reaction forces at landing are significantly greater in the trailing forelimb than in the leading forelimb[1]; therefore a tendency to land with the right forelimb leading is most likely a reflection of right forelimb pain. However, stress on the suspensory apparatus is greater in the leading forelimb; therefore in association with suspensory pathology a horse may avoid landing with the affected limb leading.
- Napping (resistance) on the approach to a fence off a turn. Nappiness may be pain related or behavioral.
- Not jumping straight (e.g., jumping to the right), with a tendency for the hindlimbs to drift toward the direction in which the horse is jumping (to the right). This usually reflects pain or weakness in the ipsilateral hindlimb of the side to which the horse is jumping. Less commonly the problem may be caused by reluctance to land on the contralateral forelimb (e.g., the left).
- Loss of hindlimb power. This may be caused by back pain or hindlimb lameness. Less commonly it may be the result of low-grade hindlimb ataxia.
- Change in the shape the horse makes over a fence—for example, loss of bascule (jumping with a rounded arc over a fence). This may reflect back pain or forelimb or hindlimb lameness, or possibly gastric ulceration. It may also reflect the way in which the horse is presented to the fence.
- Rushing fences. This can be the way an excitable horse always jumps, but if the horse used to jump normally, rushing the fence usually reflects a painful problem. However, if the horse has been stopping for whatever reason and has been chased to the fences, it will inevitably rush. If a horse is overly restricted by the rider's hands it may also try to rush to escape.
- Loss of action. This can reflect the way in which the horse has been ridden and trained. Some loose, free-moving young dressage horses become much more restricted in their stride when ridden exercise is commenced. An apprehensive rider may restrict a potentially exuberant horse. A bored horse, particularly with a Warmblood mentality, may just switch off and refuse to go forward freely and loosely. Loss of action also may reflect forelimb or hindlimb lameness or back pain.
- Stiffness. Stiffness should be evaluated carefully to differentiate loss of action and back stiffness from restriction of gait caused by a bilateral forelimb or hindlimb lameness.
- Inability to perform medium or extended trot. Unless a horse is properly balanced with adequate hindlimb impulsion, it cannot perform medium or extended trot. Horses vary considerably in the ability to collect and extend. In general the Thoroughbred breed has much less natural ability than many of the Warmblood breeds. Some horses have to learn how to perform a medium and an extended trot and must first develop sufficient muscular coordination and power before they are able to do so. However, if a horse was previously able to work in medium and extended paces and now cannot do so, or if the rhythm becomes irregular, this can reflect forelimb or hindlimb lameness or back pain.
- Inadequate hindlimb impulsion in trot, with a tendency to break to canter if asked to work harder. This usually reflects hindlimb lameness.

- Difficulty in performing specific dressage movements—for example, right half pass. This often reflects a back or sacroiliac joint region problem or hindlimb lameness.
- Tendency to become disunited behind in canter. This usually reflects hindlimb lameness. However, it is important to recognize that young horses can find maintaining true canter difficult, sometimes just in one direction, or sometimes in both directions. This often can be overcome by training and development of muscular strength and coordination. Some trained horses that canter true when ridden may become disunited when cantering on the lunge. Hindlimb lameness may predispose to a horse becoming disunited. If the problem occurs to a similar extent on both reins, it often reflects a bilateral problem, but if it occurs on only one rein, the problem is more likely to be unilateral.

  Although the canter stride is initiated by the trailing hindlimb, which bears weight alone, the stance time, peak vertical ground reaction forces, and range of motion of the proximal limb joints are higher in the leading hindlimb.[2,3] Therefore if the horse consistently becomes disunited on the left rein, this is likely to reflect discomfort in the leading left hindlimb.
- Late flying changes, or difficulty in changing from right to left or from left to right. This usually results from hindlimb lameness.
- Inability to maintain a consistent rhythm in piaffe, passage, or canter pirouettes. This usually reflects a hindlimb lameness.
- Unlevelness in certain movements. Mild irregularities in rhythm may be detectable only in certain movements—for example, left half pass and right shoulder in. Such irregularities can reflect forelimb or hindlimb lameness or may be induced by the rider overrestricting with the hand and not creating sufficient hindlimb impulsion. Dressage riders often refer to *bridle lameness,* implying that lameness is not true because it cannot be detected when the horse is trotted in hand or lunged. This usually is a misnomer, because most bridle- or rein-lame horses have a genuine lameness, which may be apparent only when the horse is ridden.
- Crookedness, or reluctance to take the bit evenly on the rider's left and right hands. This can result from a training problem or can be caused by lameness or unwillingness to accept the bit because of oral pain. Less commonly it may reflect temporomandibular joint pain.
- Taking unequal-length strides behind in walk, despite appearing sound in all other gaits. This can be seen in some otherwise normal horses that show no response to systemic administration of analgesic drugs. This syndrome is generally seen only when the horse is ridden and in some horses is apparent only when the horse walks on the bit, and not when it walks on a long rein. It is characterized by a shortened cranial phase of the stride. Local analgesic techniques from the foot to the coxofemoral joint usually have no effect on this gait. Radiographic, ultrasonographic, and nuclear scintigraphic examinations are usually unrewarding. Alternatively, irregular strides may reflect hindlimb lameness also seen at other gaits.
- Lameness apparent only when the horse is working to a contact, on the bit, and not when worked on a long rein. Problems in these horses can be difficult to solve. Some reflect a forelimb lameness, upper forelimb muscular pain, or caudal cervical pain.
- Inability to engage the hindlimbs on the forehand. This usually reflects hindlimb lameness or back pain.
- Hanging, or on one line. This often reflects hindlimb lameness or forelimb lameness in a Standardbred.
- Loss of power cross-country. This may be caused by subclinical exertional rhabdomyolysis, discomfort associated with superficial digital flexor tendonitis, or other causes of lameness. Alternatively, the horse may have acute-onset back muscle pain.
- Reluctance to jump drop fences. This can be a rider or horse confidence problem, but it also may be caused by forelimb lameness or back pain.

(Continued)

BOX 97-1

Types of Clinical Problems—cont'd

- Cold-backed behavior when tacked up or first mounted. This is manifest by the horse tensing, roaching the back, sometimes freezing and refusing to walk forward, and then sometimes exploding into a series of violent bucks. Often this abnormal behavior stops within a few minutes, and the horse then works completely normally.

  Cold-backed behavior can be unrelated to pain and may be a problem initiated by pain, which then becomes a behavioral response. Such behavior may reflect fear, especially if a rider has fallen off several times, and less commonly is associated with chronic pain because of a rib fracture, fractured sternum, or nerve-related pain.

  The behavior may be precipitated by rapidly tightening the girth, especially if the girth has an elastic inset.

  Cold-backed behavior is generally manageable by an experienced rider, but such behavior is potentially dangerous to a nervous or inexperienced rider. Affected horses should be tacked up slowly and the girth tightened progressively, walking the horse forward each time. The horse should be lunged and made to go forward at the trot and the canter before being mounted. The rider should be legged up onto the horse and should not attempt to mount from the ground.

  Horses with cold-backed behavior may improve with careful management but should never be trusted completely.
- Bucking. Bucking behavior can be similar to cold-backed behavior, or it may occur only after the horse has been ridden for a period. Although the horse may appear to buck with a flexible back, primary back pain is sometimes the underlying cause. Back pain secondary to hindlimb lameness may also result in bucking. Bucking can be a behavioral problem unrelated to pain.
- Bucking and kicking out to one side is often a manifestation of sacroiliac joint region pain.
- Rearing. Rearing is often part of nappy or resistant behavior: the horse tests the rider. Relatively rarely is rearing associated with a pain-related problem such as sacroiliac region pain.
- Bolting. Bolting may result from pain of any cause (e.g., bilateral hindlimb proximal suspensory desmitis) or may be a behavioral problem.

- Tendency for the saddle to slip to one side. This may be because of the rider's inability to sit straight, a poorly fitting saddle, or unilateral hindlimb lameness. The saddle usually slips to the side of the lame hindlimb.
- Reluctance to work on the bit. Difficulties in working on the bit may be one of the first signs noted by a rider when the horse develops a minor musculoskeletal problem involving the back or limbs, or a mouth problem.
- Head-shaking behavior when ridden. There is a poorly understood syndrome in which horses head-shake generally only when ridden, although if the horse is severely affected the behavior may also be apparent on the lunge and occasionally in the stable. Such horses are usually worse in the summer months. Affected horses sneeze frequently and may strike out with a forelimb or repeatedly try to rub their nose on one or both forelimbs. The behavior may be controlled in some horses by placement of a net over the horse's nostrils. Mildly affected horses may perform normally when jumping and may show signs only when worked on the flat. Severely affected horses may be virtually impossible to ride.
- Unwillingness to work. This may be behavioral or pain related. Warmblood breeds in particular are strong-willed horses that easily recognize when their rider is not competent enough, and rapidly a vicious circle can ensue. However, reluctance to work equally may reflect lameness or back pain.
- Nappy (resistant) or evasive behavior. This may reflect pain or the dominance of the horse over the rider. Although some horses have a compliant temperament and never take advantage of an incompetent handler or rider, other horses rapidly recognize lack of ability, or apprehension of the rider, and develop resistant or awkward behavior.
- Progressive agitation with work, with or without loss of action. This may reflect the horse's temperament or pain caused by exertional rhabdomyolysis, for example.
- Episodic complete loss of rhythm and lack of synchronization of movement of all limbs. This may reflect a multilimb lameness, but it may also be an evasion or reflect tension. If the horse puts its head up and hollows its back, maintaining a regular rhythm is difficult. Working the horse in draw reins, changing the work environment, and using sedatives or analgesic drugs can help to differentiate a pain-related problem from an evasion.

Investigation of this type of horse is time-consuming and usually requires repeated clinical examinations, together with ancillary diagnostic techniques. Ideally the horse should be in full work at the time of the investigation. The horse must be assessed in its entirety, including full visual appraisal and palpation at rest, evaluation of the horse moving in hand and on the lunge on soft and hard surfaces, and assessment of the response to flexion tests. Ridden exercise is crucial.

CLINICAL ASSESSMENT

It is generally essential to see the horse ridden by the regular rider, performing the movements that are causing difficulty. If the veterinarian does not feel competent to judge the rider and the influence the rider may be having on the problem, the assistance of a professional rider or trainer may be necessary. However, it is important to recognize that not all so-called "experts" are truly experts, and the advice of a misguided professional may serve only to muddy the waters.

It is important to appreciate the profound influence that back pain arising from the thoracolumbar or sacroiliac regions can have over the horse's entire manner of moving.

Back pain not only may induce back stiffness, but also may result in the horse holding itself tensely and not accepting the bit properly, with a restriction in stride length and reduced lift to the stride in all limbs. Bilateral hindlimb proximal suspensory desmitis may have a similar effect.

Clinical assessment of back pain is not easy. A normal horse should be able to flex and extend the thoracolumbar spine repeatedly in the sagittal plane and flex from side to side with ease, without inducing tension in the epaxial muscles. Holding the back stiffly, sinking on the hindquarters to avoid extension, and showing evidence of muscle fasciculation or spasm may indicate pain. Alteration of facial expression and a tendency to bite or kick out may also reflect pain. However, some nervous, thin-skinned horses guard the back and do not flex normally unless they are relaxed completely. Some stoical cob-type horses show little response at all. Some horses respond to digital palpation, whereas in others firmer pressure must be applied, using, for example, the closed tips of a pair of artery forceps to induce flexion and extension of the back.

In a normal horse at the trot and canter appreciable up-and-down movement of the back occurs, along with swing from side to side, with an easy swinging movement of the tail. The degree of movement is to some extent determined by the horse's natural athleticism. The degree of movement often is reduced with back pain. The degree of restriction of movement reflects the temperament of the horse and hence its reaction to pain and the severity of the pain. Clinical signs of back pain may be subtle unless the horse is assessed while it is ridden. Restricted back mobility may be more obvious when the rider sits continuously in the saddle, in sitting trot and canter, compared with when the rider sits lightly, or rises up and down in the trot. Movement of the tail may be restricted. The restricted movement of the back may be much more obvious to a rider than to an observer and may induce back pain in the rider. Further investigation of thoracolumbar and sacroiliac pain is discussed elsewhere (see Chapters 50 through 52).

It is important to recognize that many horses with hindlimb lameness show signs only when the horse is ridden. The modification of stride variables because of hindlimb lameness is much less than for forelimb lameness. The diagonal on which the rider sits in rising trot often substantially influences the lameness. Lameness is usually most obvious when the rider sits on the diagonal of the lame limb and may be unapparent on the other diagonal. The horse may deliberately try to make the rider sit on the nonlame diagonal. Low-grade irregularities in gait may be most apparent when the horse changes direction when performing small figures of eight (e.g., loss of rhythm, swinging the hindquarters to the outside of the circle, crossing the inside hindlimb in underneath the body during protraction, coming slightly above the bit) or when decelerating from canter to trot or from trot to walk (e.g., failure to "sit down" behind and engage the hindlimbs), or may be manifest as hopping into trot from walk. Subtle delayed release of the patella may be apparent only as a horse decelerates.

Recurrent low-grade equine rhabdomyolysis may occur almost every time an affected horse is ridden, without any of the classical clinical signs of tying up. Measurement of serum concentrations of creatine kinase and aspartate transaminase reveals elevation of both. Some of these horses have increased radiopharmaceutical uptake in the affected muscles in bone phase images if examined using nuclear scintigraphy.

It is often necessary to compare the horse's performance when ridden by a different rider, bearing in mind that riders with varying abilities can make horses appear different, and riders of differing weights and ability to follow the rhythm can make a great difference in the horse's gait. A good rider can make a slightly nappy horse go forward freely, with a totally rhythmical stride, whereas a less competent rider may be unable to ride the horse through, and the horse may take uneven steps behind because it is not going forward enough. A heavy rider or a rider who is unable to ride properly in balance may induce hindlimb lameness. The same horse ridden by a lighter rider may be completely sound. A horse that evades the bit and runs along with its head in the air may take irregular steps in front and behind and appear stiff in the back, especially if a rider attempts to make the horse work on the bit. The same horse, when encouraged to submit and work on the bit when ridden by an expert with draw reins, may appear completely different, relaxing the back, stepping under more from behind and becoming much more rhythmical. It is often necessary to separate the owner from

the horse diplomatically to assess how the horse responds to a skilled rider over several days.

It is also important to recognize that inappropriate work patterns on the flat or over fences actually can induce musculoskeletal pain, which may progress to chronic lameness. For example, repeatedly placing the horse too close to a jump (putting the horse in deep), which also alters the bascule over the fence and the way in which the horse lands, may predispose the horse to patellar ligament soreness. This may alter the horse's way of moving and predispose to the development of pain elsewhere. In the early stages the problems potentially may be managed with a change in work program and methods of training the horse. However, long-term problems may be more difficult to resolve satisfactorily.

Paradoxically, it may be helpful to see a usually well-ridden horse with a subtle performance problem ridden by a less clever rider. The professional rider may be making subtle adjustments to the gait inadvertently and thereby masking gait irregularities reflecting low-grade lameness.

The fit of the tack and its suitability must be evaluated. The veterinarian should not assume that because the saddle was fitted by a professional saddle fitter that it necessarily does fit. The position of the bit in the mouth, the size of the bit relative to the size and shape of the mouth, and the suitability and the severity of the bit should all be assessed. The mouth should be inspected carefully to ensure that no lacerations of the tongue, gums, or corners of the horse's mouth have occurred and that the teeth have no sharp points or hooks.

In some instances the horse may appear to be clinically normal, and it is necessary to try to establish whether the complaint is indeed pain related. In my experience, phenylbutazone is the most effective analgesic drug for trying to determine whether a problem is pain related. The drug must be given at a high enough dose (minimum 4.4 mg/kg twice daily) for long enough (at least 7 days if the horse does not respond within 2 to 3 days). A comparison with records of the horse's attitude, behavior, and action before, during, and after treatment should be assessed as objectively as possible. A positive response confirms the presence of a pain-related problem, whereas a negative response does not definitively exclude a pain-induced problem. The potential exists to create a placebo effect for the rider, and in selected horses, "blinding" the rider to the treatment may be worthwhile.

If the problem seems to induce considerable anxiety and tension when the horse is worked, mild tranquilization with acepromazine or sedation with detomidine can be helpful to determine if the problem is pain induced or reflects tension. The tension actually may be induced by the rider or the environment in which the horse is worked. Working the horse in a different situation with another skilled rider can be helpful.

If the horse is fresh and exuberant, minor gait abnormalities can be difficult to assess, especially in a big moving dressage horse. In these circumstances mild sedation can be useful.

It is important to try to determine if a problem reflects pain or weakness caused by a neurological problem. Low-grade hindlimb toe drag may reflect a mild proprioceptive deficit rather than lameness. When in doubt, a comprehensive neurological examination should be performed (see

Chapter 11). This is particularly important in areas (North and South America) where equine protozoal myelitis occurs. In other countries it is important to establish whether the horse has ever been to America.

It is also important to recognize that some horses that are mild wobblers, with mild hindlimb gait abnormalities seen when moving loose or in hand, may actually move loosely and freely when ridden, with apparently good coordination, and perform rather well in low-level dressage and other competitive disciplines despite a problem. However, such horses usually lack strength and coordination to perform more advanced dressage.

Diagnostic Analgesia

In some horses, taking an educated guess about a potential source of pain and medicating the suspect joints with, for example, triamcinolone acetonide and assessing the response to medication (so-called "diagnostic medication") may be necessary. For example, in a dressage horse taking uneven-height steps behind in piaffe, or failing to maintain a regular two-time rhythm in piaffe, medicating the distal hock joints may be worthwhile. However, it is necessary to recognize that a negative response does not definitively exclude distal hock joint pain as the primary problem. Paradoxically, in some horses the response to intraarticular analgesia may be better than the response to intraarticular medication, whereas in others the response to medication is better than the response to analgesia, even in the absence of radiological abnormalities.

Frequently through careful clinical evaluation of the horse, a low-grade, bilateral, symmetrical lameness can be identified that can be investigated further through local analgesic techniques and then appropriate imaging modalities. With low-grade bilateral forelimb lameness, blocking both front feet simultaneously, for example, may be more useful than blocking one at a time and then assessing the change in the horse's overall way of moving. With poor hindlimb propulsion, blocking the region of the origin of both hindlimb suspensory ligaments may be more useful than blocking one at a time. In some horses concurrent forelimb and hindlimb lameness may be detected. This may be manifest as lack of athleticism or animation, lack of power, or merely reduced stride length. Alternatively, back stiffness may be identified, requiring further investigation by radiography, nuclear scintigraphy, and ultrasonography.

Diagnostic Imaging

Thermographic evaluation, particularly of the neck and back, is thought by some to be helpful in diagnosing low-grade performance abnormalities (see Chapters 25 and 95). However, others have found thermography much less rewarding. It is vital to recognize the normal thermographic patterns, the responses to exercise, and the many other external factors that may influence the results.

In horses in which no obvious gait abnormalities can be identified or in which subtle changes are noted that cannot be investigated further by local analgesic techniques, performing a comprehensive nuclear scintigraphic examination of the horse may be helpful (see Chapter 19). However, interpretation of the results can be notoriously difficult, because areas of IRU are not necessarily synonymous with pain, and not all musculoskeletal problems are

associated with IRU. For example, bilateral proximal suspensory desmitis may result in a slightly restricted and stiff hindlimb gait, with or without stiffness of the back, but nuclear scintigraphic examination findings may be normal. Great care must be taken not to overinterpret the results of scintigraphic examination. Results must be correlated carefully with the clinical signs, the responses (where possible) to local analgesic techniques, and the response to diagnostic medication.

Gastroscopy may be valuable to determine the presence of gastric ulceration. Alternatively the response to medication with omeprazole can be assessed.

Evaluation of gait and other aspects of performance on a high-speed treadmill are discussed in Chapter 98.

COMMON PERFORMANCE PROBLEMS

The most common causes of poor performance not related to readily recognizable overt lameness are listed in Box 97-2.

These horses are time-consuming to investigate, often requiring a multifaceted approach to diagnosis. It is important to recognize that the failure to perform optimally may be the result of several problems, and recognition of all of

---

BOX 97-2

Common Performance Problems

Possible Clinical Problems
Bilateral foot pain
Bilateral fetlock pain
Bilateral proximal suspensory desmitis, forelimb or hindlimb
Bilateral carpal pain
Thoracolumbar or sacroiliac pain
Intermittent upward fixation of the patella or delayed release of the patella
Bilateral distal hock joint pain
Tying up

Rider-Induced Problems
Handbrake on (i.e., too much restriction by the rider's hands) and no legs
Overweight; inability to follow the rhythm
Lack of confidence
Overhorsed rider being too restrictive
Misunderstanding of how to achieve "on the bit"
Poor eye for a stride; therefore repeatedly placing the horse in less than ideal positions for take off for a fence, making the jump more awkward or necessitating more effort
Sitting crookedly
Lack of rapport with the horse
Trainer-induced problem
Monotonous training program with no variation

Horse Problems
Lack of ability
Unsuitable temperament
Loss of confidence
Lack of rapport with the rider
Staleness
Lack of focus in a dual-purpose breeding stallion and competition horse
Inconsistency of a mare

these may be crucial to successful management. Determination of all the postulated sites of pain causing poor performance is based on an assessment of a detailed history of performance; the results of palpation including the response to stimulation of acupuncture points; evaluation of the horse moving in hand, on the lunge, and ridden, both when work is first initiated and later in the work program; and the response to flexion tests and chiropractic assessment of joint mobility, sometimes combined with assessment of the response to local analgesic techniques. Although it is often essential to see the regular rider riding the horse, separating the horse from the rider for several days can be helpful, particularly with horses ridden by amateurs or semiprofessionals. It is essential to have access to adequate facilities to see the horse ridden (or driven) properly on a daily basis and to be able to perform local analgesic techniques and then reevaluate the horse ridden or driven under the same circumstances.

eferences
on page
1336

Chapter 98

Experiences Using a High-Speed Treadmill to Evaluate Lameness

Benson B. Martin Jr., Sue J. Dyson, and Mike W. Ross

The advent of the high-speed treadmill has led to many advances in evaluating equine poor performance in exercise physiology, gait analysis, cardiac disease, and lameness diagnosis.[1-5] This chapter describes our experience using a high-speed treadmill for lameness evaluation in the performance horse.

Lameness has been implicated as a cause of poor performance in several studies involving a complete physical examination, lameness examination, and where possible a high-speed treadmill examination.[1-3] In one study, 74% of horses were found to have lameness as a component of poor performance.[1] In another study, in which horses with no apparent history of lameness were examined because of poor performance, clinically important lameness in 23.9% of horses precluded a high-speed treadmill investigation.[2] In a third study, 4.3% of horses sound enough to undergo a high-speed treadmill examination for poor performance were clinically significantly lame after high-speed treadmill exercise.[3]

In our experience, convincing trainers and owners that lameness is a cause for poor performance can be difficult. Several studies using a shoe model to induce lameness to assess the metabolic cost of pain related to lameness suggested a trend that pain related to lameness may not increase the metabolic cost of exercise, but it does increase the heart rate in response to pain.[6-8] However, another study suggested that a metabolic cost of pain and exercise does occur.[9] Pain may alter a horse's ability or willingness to perform up to expectations or previous performance levels.[10]

CRITERIA FOR CASE SELECTION

The most common criterion for a treadmill lameness examination is lameness that occurs at only high speeds or after an extended period of exercise. The treadmill examination is used most commonly in Standardbred (STB) racehorses or endurance horses. However, a treadmill lameness examination can be used in any breed or discipline, although a horse in which lameness is apparent only when the horse is ridden may be unsuitable.

Horses in which a complete lameness investigation, including diagnostic analgesia and appropriate imaging technologies, fails to reveal a diagnosis are potential candidates for treadmill lameness examination. Additional candidates include horses that require considerable work at low, medium, or higher speeds before the lameness becomes apparent, such as endurance horses or STB racehorses. A treadmill lameness examination also may be useful in horses that are fractious or otherwise pay little attention when jogged in hand or ridden. Horses must pay close attention when trotting on a treadmill and therefore have a more even, rhythmical, relaxed gait that is easier to evaluate.

HISTORY

Important historical facts need to be ascertained. Some questions are general, and some are use related. Some may need to be repeated in a different order to elicit an accurate answer. Questions may include those listed in Box 98-1.

EQUIPMENT

The treadmill must have a speed of at least 7 to 10 m/sec. Most horses will not canter until the speed exceeds 7 m/sec. Lameness is usually evident at lower speeds, but occasionally it is necessary to see a horse trot at up to 7 m/sec for lameness to become manifest. In addition, for further poor performance evaluation the treadmill needs a speed of at least 14 to 15 m/sec and the capability of being elevated to at least a 6-degree slope. Ideally the treadmill should be mounted in the ground, which is safer. In our experience clients and horses easily adapt to an in-the-ground treadmill. It is easier to use video equipment with a treadmill in the ground, rather than above the ground.

At least 4 to 5 m of space in front of, behind, and on either side of the treadmill is needed to allow for equipment, cameras, and personnel and to allow room for the horse to move off the front, rear, or side. The moving treadmill surface is relatively forgiving. In one study in which a horse had a strain gauge placed on the left third metacarpal bone, bone strain was measured as the horse galloped on a dirt track, on a wood chip track, and on a treadmill. Compared with the dirt track bone strain was 75% less when the

BOX 98-1

Questions to Ask When Determining History

General Questions

How long has the horse been lame?

When do you notice the lameness?

Does the lameness improve with exercise?

Does the lameness become worse during or after exercise?

Does the horse ever appear to become anxious or frantic?

Does the horse sweat?

Has the horse's performance level changed?

Has the horse changed how well it performs?

Has the horse changed the style of performance?

Has the horse had any behavioral changes?

Has the horse been treated for lameness?

Has the horse been "tapped"?

Has the horse ever had any joints treated?

Has the horse received any intramuscular treatments?

Has the horse received any other therapy or medication?

How much and for how long?

What has been the response?

Does the horse receive any special supplements (e.g., sodium bicarbonate)?

What type of shoes does the horse wear and why?

Does the horse have any special shoeing or trimming and why?

Use-Specific Questions

Standardbred Racehorses

At what speed is the horse the worst?

At which gait (trot or pace) is the lameness most easily seen?

Is the horse worse on the straight or on turns?

Is the horse worse when turned in the correct direction of the track?

Is the horse worse when jogging?

What is the horse's normal gait?

Has any change in the horse's gait occurred, and what is the change?

Is the horse on a line?

Is the horse on a shaft?

Does the horse get into his knees?

Is the horse worse when jogging free legged or in full harness?

Is the horse worse when checked up?

Does the horse use any special gaiting equipment?

Does the horse wear any head poles?

Does the horse wear any other special equipment and why?

Thoroughbred Racehorses

Does the horse bear in or out?

Does the horse break out of the starting gate as well as before?

Does the horse require any special bit or tack and why?

At what speed is the lameness best seen or felt?

Is lameness worse with or without a rider?

Endurance Horses

How far does the horse have to go before the lameness appears (time or distance)?

What does the lameness feel like or look like?

Does the horse have any bruising of the feet?

Does the horse feel or look like it is tying up?

Does the horse sweat normally?

Dressage and Show Horses

Is the horse worse when ridden?

Is the horse worse on a large turn or small turn?

Is the horse worse going up or down a hill?

Is the horse worse when collected or on a free rein?

horse galloped on the wood chip track and an additional 75% less when it galloped on the treadmill.[11]

Kinematic analyses include high-speed cinematography, videography, electrogoniometry, or accelerometry to quantify the movements of the limbs and torso during exercise. Kinetic analyses use instrumented shoes, force plates, and pressure-sensitive mats to measure forces that affect, arrest, or modify motion. The reader is referred to Chapter 22 and other references. Many of these systems are expensive, time-consuming, and cumbersome and require considerable expertise to use. The ideal gait analysis system provides considerable data, which are obtained easily, are visually and statistically analyzed, and are not too expensive. The system must be fast enough to assess correctly diagnostic analgesic techniques in a timely fashion and simple enough to not alter the gait of the horse.[12,13]

Simple systems can be assembled with a digital video camera, a tripod, and a computer, using simple video editing software to review and edit the images. If a computer is not available, video editing tape decks can be used. The camera or cameras are placed perpendicular to the side and front or rear of the treadmill. Caution must be used with the rear camera. Enough light must be available for adequate video viewing (at least two 1000-W lights or equivalent).[12,13]

The video camera should be a digital camera (some Hi-8 cameras are still functional) with a video stabilization system and should have a shutter speed of at least 1/2000 (digital) or 1/4000 (analog).[14] Most consumer-grade cameras film at 30 frames per second (fps). Therefore some video loss is apparent compared with more sophisticated (200 fps) and expensive systems. Digital and Hi-8 video create less video noise and provide a superior viewing experience. For rapid viewing the recorded tape can be placed into a digital videocassette recorder that has a jog-shuttle device for stop frame viewing or frame grabbing. Alternatively, video editing tape decks, which are more expensive than traditional videocassette recorders, can be used. Digital images also can be reviewed on a computer and thus more accurately analyzed and edited. Turnkey systems including hardware and software using universal serial bus or IEEE 1394 rapid transfer technology are available.

Using video technology allows the clinician to critically examine the baseline lameness and lameness after diagnostic analgesia, record them in real time, analyze the differences in real time slow motion, maintain a permanent record for follow-up examinations, and demonstrate to the owner or trainer the difference in gait before and after a successful block. Video analysis also can be useful in demonstrating initial footfall, footfall after trimming or shoeing, and the effects of different types and weights of shoes. The technology gives one a new appreciation for lameness, motion, conformation, and gait at a walk, trot, or higher speed. The camera is much more sensitive than the human eye and can answer many questions and create new ones.[12,15,16]

PREPARATION OF THE HORSE AND SAFETY CONSIDERATIONS

It is important that a horse be reasonably fit to perform an accurate treadmill lameness examination. STBs should be trained down to at least a 2-minute mile. Endurance horses, in which lameness may not occur for several miles, need to be at least fit enough to accomplish this task easily. Other horses should be in regular work. To do otherwise places the horse and examination at risk. Unfit horses run the risk of exertional myopathy, thus obfuscating the results of any lameness examination.

We prefer horses to wear shoes when being examined for lameness. Tremendous friction and therefore heat are generated by the contact of the horse's foot and the tread-mill belt. Whenever a foot contacts the belt, the foot slips and therefore causes friction. Many research horses that exercise daily on a high-speed treadmill have chronic foot problems secondary to the heat generated. This heat can be enough to melt the glue of glue-on shoes at higher speeds. If the horse is not shod, the toes of the hind feet can break off and bleed, leading to substantial lameness for several weeks. We do not place any type of tape on the horses' shoes. We recommend using flat shoes, with no toe grabs, stickers, borium, or turndowns. This minimizes wear to the treadmill belt, which when used daily lasts 9 to 12 months before replacement is required. We recommend that shoeing changes be made 3 to 5 days before a treadmill examination, in case foot problems related to shoeing are found that may mask the horse's actual primary lameness.

Examination for lameness on a treadmill requires at least three people. One person controls the treadmill and the horse's head, one person stands behind the horse to keep it moving forward if necessary, and one person is the clinician. The clinician is responsible for operating the video equipment and observing the horse at a walk, trot, and any other desired gait. Occasionally, two people are required at the head for fractious horses.

Schooling of the average horse usually takes about 30 minutes to 1 hour before the horse is ready to be examined for lameness. Most (>99%) horses can be schooled and examined for lameness or poor performance in the same day. This period includes acclimating the horse to the treadmill and the fan noise, standing on the treadmill with the machine off, and moving with the treadmill at the walk, the trot, or pace at medium speed, a canter at low speed (7 m/sec) for non-STBs, and then at rest. STBs then are harnessed and moved up to a speed of about 7 m/sec for 200 to 300 m. Most horses adapt easily using this method of schooling, which is safe and successful in 99% of horses examined for lameness or poor performance. Occasionally, horses are recalcitrant or scared and need to be reschooled a day later and usually adapt well. Some horses (<1%) cannot be examined because the examination would not be safe for the horses or personnel.[17]

Safety of horses and personnel is paramount. Personnel must be cautioned to be alert at all times and not to stand behind the horse when the treadmill is moving. Shoes and horses can come off the treadmill without warning. Substantial injuries (e.g., tendonitis) occur in less than 1.5% of horses. Lacerations, broken-up hind feet, and myositis occur in less than 5% of horses.[17] All horses wear protective boots on all limbs. All STBs are schooled first without equipment (tack), but with protective boots, and then they wear the normal equipment plus protective boots if they move at speeds greater than 7 m/sec.

To minimize the risk of injury to personnel and horses, it is important to have a trained team to examine each horse. Personnel should block any windows through which the horse can see out, eliminate as many noise distractions

as possible, and ensure that no doors can be opened in front of the horse during schooling or exercise. This allows the horse to concentrate on keeping up with the treadmill and minimizes fright or distraction of the horse during the examination.

LAMENESS DIAGNOSIS

Most lameness is seen best in all breeds with a minimum of equipment in place. STBs, which usually race checked up, are examined first with a minimum of equipment (i.e., no hobbles) and not checked up. Many lameness conditions in STBs can be obfuscated, changed, or eliminated when a horse wears its equipment and in particular, when checked up. Other horses are examined wearing just a halter unless some equipment change exacerbates the lameness (rare). A riding horse may need to wear side reins. Occasionally, STBs with carpal or stifle lameness are worse when wearing hobbles.

Horses are first examined at the walk and then at the trot and are recorded on video. Recording from the side is useful to evaluate stride length and frequency. Examination from the rear is helpful in evaluating the swing of the forelimbs and hindlimbs and the footfall.

Observation of lameness using a treadmill is different from the standard lameness examination because the horse is stationary relative to the observer, allowing viewing and video recording of the horse's gait from the side, front, and rear. The most useful gaits for observing lameness are the trot and pace. These are symmetrical gaits and allow for easier evaluation of lameness and gait rhythm.[13]

The horse should become comfortable at the trot, so that the lameness or gait abnormality can be established. An audible rhythmic pattern to the gait also becomes apparent. The horse is in rhythm (normal) or out of rhythm (lame). In addition to video recording for later viewing, it is important to evaluate the lameness concurrently to establish a baseline. If lameness is not readily apparent, reviewing the video immediately before performing diagnostic analgesia may be advantageous. Although detecting a difference in footfall is a standard part of any lameness examination, in our experience footfall may be exacerbated on a treadmill. Sound horses that trot have a symmetrical, diagonal, two-beat gait, and pacers have a symmetrical, lateral two-beat gait. The horse should be observed carefully for a change in how the horse swings its forelimbs or hindlimbs. In STB pacers, any change in how the horse moves from side to side at the poll or hips, when viewed from the rear after diagnostic analgesia, is important. These horses, whether pacing free-legged (no harness) or when in harness or checked up, have a tendency to swing from side to side and land more heavily or with greater excursion on the sound side. An in-depth description of these gaits is available.[13]

In addition to elimination of lameness, a change in stride characteristics may occur, including stride frequency, length, and swing plane. Some horses not accustomed to the treadmill, or not comfortable on the treadmill, may have an increased stride frequency and shortened stride length, which also may be seen in lame horses.[13] Once accustomed to the treadmill, many sound horses exercised at medium to higher speeds on a treadmill have a longer stride and thus a lower stride frequency.[18] However, lame horses may have an increased stride frequency and shortened stride length.[19] This can best be demonstrated and seen using video.

Other, more subtle changes include improvement in gait fluidity, improvement in use of the head and neck and shoulder, and change of an anxious eye expression, flexion of major joints, foot flight, width and rhythm of gait, and footfall. Occasionally, horses may become stiff or anxious and lame or lamer in front or behind during or after exercise. Exercise should be discontinued. Exertional myopathy (see Chapter 83) or aortoiliac thrombosis (see Chapter 50) should be considered likely causes.[20,21]

ADDITIONAL TESTS

It is useful to measure creatine kinase and aspartate transaminase concentrations before and after exercise to monitor horses for subclinical myopathy, overt myopathy, or previous undiagnosed myopathy.[21] If aortoiliac thrombosis is suspected, a rectal examination and an ultrasonographic examination per rectum should be performed. Horses with aortoiliac thrombosis commonly become lame behind during or shortly after commencement of exercise.[20] They have an anxious look and can sweat more profusely than their level of exercise would dictate.

The treadmill provides a smooth, even surface at a constant, controllable speed and a horse that is stationary relative to the observer. Some horses are lame in hand, but not on a treadmill, and some are lame on a treadmill, but not in hand. Horses that are lame only on turns are difficult to evaluate on a treadmill, which operates only in a straight line. Some horses will not tolerate working on a treadmill.[22-24]

SECTION 2
The Racehorse

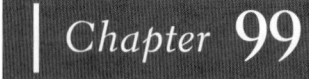

The Sales Yearling

■ PURCHASE EXAMINATION OF A THOROUGHBRED SALES YEARLING IN NORTH AMERICA

Benson B. Martin Jr., John C. Kimmel, and Mark W. Cheney

References on page 1336

Veterinary inspection of a Thoroughbred (TB) yearling at public auction requires expertise and experience.[1-13] Previously, yearlings commonly were examined after purchase, and if a problem was discovered subsequently, a lengthy, expensive, and frequently unsatisfactory arbitration for buyer and seller alike was implemented. Recently a shift has occurred toward a comprehensive examination of yearlings before purchase.

It is important that the veterinarian's role be defined in advance with all the necessary parties, such as the potential trainer, owner, and syndicate manager. Clinicians should determine whether they are prepared to offer advice concerning the pedigree or whether their advice will be strictly veterinary. It should be made clear that no guarantees of future performance can be given. Any potential conflicts of interest must be declared, including whether the veterinarian is involved as an agent, breeder, purchaser, or consignor.

Veterinarians should establish precisely for whom they are working and to whom information can be divulged. They should not give privileged, confidential information to anyone else. Provide a representative estimate of the fee for the examination. Sometimes a buyer may wish to gain access to information obtained by another. This is acceptable provided that the original client gives permission. In this way the fee may be split between two or more prospective purchasers. If clinicians work regularly with purchasers, they may be able to contribute to their buying policy, which may include consideration of pedigree information, budget, conformation type, sex, and potential resale breeding value. Excellent communication with trainers is important, because they ultimately have most control of the horse when it enters training.

It is also important to establish a good relationship with the consignor or agent. Veterinarians should be courteous and respectful, should arrange a mutually suitable time to examine the yearling, and should request permission before carrying out endoscopic or radiographic examinations.

Experience is essential to make accurate interpretations of conformational or gait abnormalities, radiological or endoscopic findings, and the results of examination of the eyes and heart. Knowledge of pedigrees also can be helpful.

CONDITIONS OF SALE

It is important to be aware of the conditions of sale for each sales company. These conditions usually differ with the age of the horse, use of the horse, and sales company. Sales are weighted in favor of the consignors and conducted with an attitude of caveat emptor. The warranty is limited, with no implied warranty for use or soundness other than those conditions published in the sales catalog. The repository is an area at the sale location set up for viewing radiographs, and videotapes of the upper airway at rest, in selected horses. If veterinarians determine this information is not adequate or satisfactory, it is their responsibility to obtain the desired information. They should examine all available information carefully. If any problem is discovered after the sale that was evident in the repository information, the consignor is not liable. The sales company makes no warranty about the accuracy or completeness of repository information and makes no interpretation of it. Repository information is for the convenience of potential buyers and as a courtesy of the consignors and also decreases the exposure of yearlings to repetitive and stressful examinations. Other information, such as previous surgery, medical problems, eye problems, current medication, vaccination status, Coggins and equine viral arteritis status, and availability of radiographs, may be available from the consignor, if the veterinarian asks.

PRESALE OR POSTSALE EXAMINATION

Currently many persons prefer presale inspection. This eliminates the process of arbitration, places the onus of disclosure on the consignor, and makes the buyer responsible for obtaining all available information before sale. If the buyer does not obtain such information (such as identification of a chip fracture), the buyer has no recourse. With examination after sale the only problems for which a horse may be returned are listed in the catalog as conditions of sale. The veterinarian is responsible for knowing these conditions and the terms under which arbitration can occur. Arbitration usually must be implemented within 24 hours after the sale of the yearling, and the yearling must still be on the sale grounds. Failure to comply with this negates any chance of arbitration.[14] Arbitration usually involves three veterinarians representing the sales company, the consignor, and the buyer respectively.

CLINICAL EXAMINATION

A yearling TB is immature, and its physical appearance may change considerably. Developing the skills to predict how each horse may develop by learning from experienced persons is worthwhile. Assess the general attitude of the horse, its eye, and its presence. Be aware that many yearlings are tranquilized for ease of inspection, so one may not get a true picture of the horse's attitude, which can be important in training and racing. Evaluate the horse's conformation (see Chapter 4). Look at the horse's feet, because the old adage "no foot, no horse" is true. Assess the horse's shoulder, hip, top line, and length of back and then the lower limbs. A good shoulder and hip can accommodate many conformational defects lower in the limb. In our opinion the following conformational abnormalities may predispose to lameness and should be avoided: back at the knee, tied in behind the knee, offset knees, and exceptionally straight hindlimbs. Carefully evaluate the shoeing and trimming of the feet, because good farriers can make a horse that toes in or out appear to be almost normal, and they are very adept at repairing an abnormal hoof appearance. After examining the horse walking in hand, perform a more detailed examination in the stall, out of sight of the general public, as a courtesy to the consignor. Assess carefully any swellings, and palpate the joints, tendons, and ligaments. Examine the eyes and auscultate the heart. Look for evidence of previous periosteal stripping or other surgery, evident as dermal thickening or white hair in areas where surgery is commonly performed.

ENDOSCOPY, ECHOCARDIOGRAPHY, AND OPHTHALMOLOGY

The veterinarian should ask the consignor or his manager for his assistance and permission to perform an endoscopic, radiographic, and echocardiographic examination of the horse, and should arrange a time to do so. A resting endoscopic examination of the horse's upper airway should include stimulating the horse to swallow and holding off the horse's airway. This allows more complete evaluation of the horse's upper airway function at rest. Echocardiographic examination is not performed routinely but can be used to assess heart size and left ventricular free-wall contractility or to detect abnormalities.[15] A brief eye examination should be conducted, looking carefully, in particular, for corneal scars.

RADIOGRAPHY AND RADIOLOGY

For many yearlings, radiographs are obtained up to 30 days before the sale and are stored in the repository at the sale. Most states allow only veterinarians licensed in the state to examine these radiographs. The examining veterinarian is responsible for ensuring that all the desired images are present, that the radiographs are properly identified, and that they are of suitable quality. The radiographs should be interpreted carefully. If the radiographs are incomplete, of poor quality, or absent completely, the veterinarian should arrange to have his or her own complete set of radiographs obtained. In our opinion a comprehensive examination consists of 46 images, plus any additional images needed on the basis of clinical examination. These images include the following:

- Front feet: lateromedial (LM) and dorsopalmar (DPa)
- Front fetlocks: DPa, LM, flexed LM, dorsolateral-palmaromedial oblique (DL-PaMO), and dorsomedial-palmarolateral oblique (DM-PaLO)
- Carpi: DPa, LM, flexed LM, DL-PaMO and DM-PaLO
- Hind fetlocks: dorsoplantar (DPl), LM, dorsolateral-plantaromedial oblique (DL-PlMO), and dorsomedial-plantarolateral oblique (DM-PlLO)
- Tarsi: DPl, LM, DL-PlMO, DM-PlLO
- Stifles: caudocranial, LM, and caudolateral-craniomedial oblique (CdL-CrMO)

However, the following 36 images are those required by the Keeneland sales repository in 2009:

- Front fetlocks: dorsal 15° proximal-palmarodistal oblique, LM, flexed LM, DL-PaMO, and DM-PaLO
- Hind fetlocks: dorsal 15° proximal-plantarodistal oblique, LM, flexed LM, DL-PlMO, and DM-PlLO
- Carpi: flexed LM, DL-PaMO, and DM-PaLO
- Tarsi: D10°L-PlMO, LM, and DM-PlLO
- Stifles: LM and Cd20°L-CrMO including the medial condyle of the femur in its entirety

This provides a comprehensive, but not all-inclusive, picture of the horse's musculoskeletal system. Other sales companies may have different requirements. The veterinarian is responsible for ascertaining the requirements.

A number of common radiological findings may eliminate a horse from further consideration.[16] Fractures of the carpus, distal phalanx, tarsus, proximal sesamoid bones, and the second or fourth metacarpal (metatarsal) bones generally are considered unacceptable, whereas small osteochondral fragments on the dorsal aspect of a fetlock joint may be acceptable. Osteoarthritis (OA) of the carpus, fetlock, or proximal interphalangeal joint is not acceptable. However, small osteophytes on the dorsoproximal aspect of the third metatarsal bone (MtIII) do not necessarily preclude a successful athletic career.

The relevance of osteochondrosis depends on the location of the lesion, its size and severity, the presence or absence of OA, and the prognosis for racing after surgical treatment. A yearling with a small fragment may be amenable to surgical treatment and should be discussed with the buyer. If a fragment has been removed previously and no evidence of OA exists, the horse may be a reasonable risk for purchase. Horses with osteochondral fragmentation of the cranial aspect of the intermediate ridge of the tibia or small lesions of the lateral trochlear ridge of the femur usually are treated successfully by surgical removal. Horses with osteochondral fragments on the proximoplantar aspect of the proximal phalanx in the hindlimbs (which may actually be traumatic in origin) represent a reasonable risk.

If an osseous cystlike lesion is identified, especially one involving the stifle or fetlock, the horse generally should be considered at high risk for developing lameness. Other radiological abnormalities that may preclude purchase include sesamoiditis, laminitis, and active splints.

Few objective studies detailing the relevance of radiological changes and race performance are available for review. In a study to determine prevalence of radiological changes in the repository radiographs of 1162 TB yearlings selling in Kentucky, fragmentation of the dorsal proximal aspect of the proximal phalanx in the forelimb (1.6%) was more common than that of the palmar aspect (0.5%), whereas in the hindlimb fragmentation of the proximal plantar aspect of the proximal phalanx (5.9%) was more common than that of the dorsal aspect (3.3%).[5] Radiolucent defects, bony fragments, and loose osseous fragments of the distal aspect of the third metacarpal bone (McIII, 2.8%) and the MtIII (3.2%) were found, and most yearlings (98%) had radiologically apparent vascular channels of the proximal sesamoid bones. Irregular channels (>2 mm wide or with nonparallel sides) were more common (79%) than were regular vascular channels (56%). The cranial aspect of the intermediate ridge of the tibia (4.4%) was the most common site of osteochondral fragmentation in the tarsus.[5] The authors concluded that although some radiological changes were common, others such as fragmentation and radiolucent defects were uncommon, and if rare, the effect of radiological changes on race performance would be difficult to study.[5] In a second study race performance of these yearlings was evaluated, and overall 81% started a race as a 2- or 3-year-old.[6] Fourteen of 24 horses (58%) with moderate or severe palmar supracondylar lysis of the McIII, 8 of 14 (57%) of those with enthesophyte formation of the proximal sesamoid bones, and 19 of 30 (63%) with radiological changes of the dorsomedial aspect of the middle carpal joint started a race.[6] The odds of starting a race with these three radiological changes were three times lower than the overall population, a result that was statistically significant.[6] Twenty-five of 36 (69%) of yearlings with

fragmentation of the dorsoproximal aspect of the proximal phalanx in a hindlimb raced, a percentage that was lower than in the overall population but not statistically significant.[6] Yearlings with enthesophyte formation of the proximal sesamoid bones in the hindlimbs placed in a significantly smaller percentage of starts and earned significantly less money per start.[6]

DRUG SCREENING FOR ANABOLIC STEROIDS AND OTHER PROHIBITED PRACTICES

In 2008, Keeneland instituted a policy stating that "a limited warranty provides that any yearling entered at the Keeneland Fall Yearling Sale shall not have been administered any exogenous anabolic steroids within 45 days of the date of the sale." A prospective purchaser may have the horse tested for the presence of exogenous anabolic steroids. If the blood is found to be positive, the buyer has the right to rescind the sale and return the horse to the seller.

The following practices are prohibited once a horse has entered the sale ground:
1. Extracorporeal shock wave therapy
2. Acupuncture and/or electrostimulation with the intent of altering laryngeal function
3. Internal blister (behind the carpus) to alter conformation

PURCHASE EXAMINATION OF A THOROUGHBRED SALES YEARLING IN EUROPE

David R. Ellis

Yearling sales occur in Europe later in the year than in the United States. The earliest, at Deauville in Normandy, is in early August, but in England and Ireland the main sales are conducted from the end of September to early December.

MONITORING AND SALE SELECTION

Most higher-class farms that offer yearlings regularly monitor the growth rates, weights, and conformation of the young stock. Such monitoring often is done with veterinary help and is conducted in close cooperation with the farrier. This should ensure that any corrective farriery is undertaken as early as possible, thus gaining maximum benefit and not leaving correction until too late in the growth of the animal. The second growth spurt, from 9 to 12 months of age, is an important window of opportunity in which to make substantial changes through corrective techniques. Regular veterinary inspections also help to detect disease, such as acquired deformities or developmental orthopedic disease, early enough to allow successful remedial measures to be undertaken. As in the United States, selection of the sale at which the yearling is to be offered is made in the spring, usually April. A few consignors conduct radiological surveys at this time to help with this selection and to deal with potential problems such as bone chips and osteochondrosis.

PREPARATION

Yearlings are brought in from pasture 6 to 8 weeks before sale for increasingly intensive preparation. This involves walking exercise with the horse led by hand, sometimes using uphill work, or using a walker. Treadmills were once used commonly, but they have fallen from favor because they tend to give a horse a goose-stepping type of action. Lunging is introduced later in preparation, particularly for the heavier or fatter yearlings, and this will be short and at a sharp trot and canter, on both reins and often twice daily. Lunging is more important to sale preparation in Europe because most yearlings, particularly the more expensive, will undergo respiratory examination at the canter by the purchaser's veterinary surgeon immediately after sale. Education and fitness are important if this post-sale test is to be conducted safely and satisfactorily. A substantial risk of injury exists during lunging if the exercise is not conducted carefully and on a suitable surface. Interference injuries, such as brushing or overreach wounds, can be prevented by using protective boots, farriery, and careful buildup of speed and fitness and particularly by using a sympathetic surface. Surfaces such as deep sand or dry wood chips may become too deep or slide away under the horse. Paddock turf can be too firm and slippery to be safe. Modern surfaces, such as Fibresand (Fibresand UK, Mansfield Sand, Nottinghamshire, United Kingdom) or Polytrack (Martin Collins Enterprises, Hungerford, United Kingdom) on a slight camber are safer. Some of the more successful vendors place more emphasis on lunging to achieve fitness and muscle condition than on walking. Excessive walking usually makes the person leading the yearling fitter and leaves the yearling bored and slovenly.

Yearlings usually come up from summer grazing in good, perhaps heavy, body condition. Converting the fat yearling into a well-muscled potential athlete by judicious feeding and exercise is an art. Overfeeding the leaner yearling may lead to physitis (see Chapter 57). As the weather starts to cool, most yearlings will be rugged (blanket applied) in the stable to ensure that they do not start changing to a winter coat. This change in management means that less energy is required in the diet.

Using medication to promote growth or body condition is much less common nowadays, partly because certain vendors became renowned for these practices and suffered in the long term. Anabolic steroids are not licensed for use in the horse, now deemed in mainland Europe to be a food animal. Several years ago Tattersalls, the important Bloodstock Auctioneers, conducted a pilot program of drug testing yearlings for steroids at their premier sale to assess for steroid use. Although the results were never published, the effect of this exercise was salutary.

During the preparation period, front shoes will be fitted, and some changes can be made to hoof trimming and balance to conceal slighter conformation faults, fill horn defects, and ensure that hoof wear during exercise is not excessive. Few yearlings will be fitted with hind shoes. It is important that the final shoeing not be too close to the sale date, so that tight nails or other shoeing problems do not cause lameness.

Orthopedic problems encountered in the yearling year can include physitis—mainly at the distal radial physis, but occasionally also the distal tibial physis—splints, sesamoiditis and strain of suspensory ligament branches, osteochondrosis, or bone cysts or osseous cystlike lesions. Horses with bone cysts often have clinical lameness when forced exercise commences, as in sale preparation, or breaking in immediately after sale. Managing orthopedic problems in the months before the sale not only requires the ideal veterinary measures according to the disease, but also requires giving consideration to the importance that potential purchasers place on the problem (little perhaps in yearlings with small settled splints) and to alternative strategy if the chosen sale has to be missed. If, for example, a yearling develops a bog spavin that requires surgical removal of osteochondral fragments 3 months before sale, having the joint back to normal, the clipped hair regrown, and the yearling adequately fit to offer for auction would be a close race to run. The ethics of offering such a yearling also have to be considered.

CONDITIONS OF SALE

Conditions of sale for yearlings at the main European auction houses do not include orthopedic conditions or surgery, with the exception of denerving at Doncaster (United Kingdom) and Goffs (Ireland). The latter auction house also deems wobblers to be returnable. Purchaser power and the example from the United States have introduced more presale radiographic examinations at premier sales. These now mostly are conducted by the vendor, and films of standard images of the carpi, the hocks, all fetlocks, and the stifle joints are available for examination by purchasers' veterinary surgeons. No official repository exists, but viewing facilities are available at the sale paddocks.

Radiographs are not essential to a profitable sale, because some of the most successful vendors at Tattersalls have not allowed presale radiography or endoscopy. They stand by their yearling on orthopedic matters and rely on the auctioneer's condition of sale regarding wind conditions. The latter is more stringent than in the United States regarding laryngeal hemiplegia but does not include other upper respiratory disorders that are considered intermittent, treatable, or so rare (e.g., rostral displacement of the palatine arch has been detected three times in 17 years) as to be dealt with on a single-case basis. Conditions of sale for English and Irish yearlings state that a horse is returnable if it is found to make a characteristic abnormal inspiratory sound when actively exercised (a roar or whistle at the canter) and to have endoscopic evidence of laryngeal hemiplegia that was not declared before sale. Horses are lunged for this examination soon after sale and before they leave the sale paddocks.

ORTHOPEDIC CONDITIONS

The most commonly found orthopedic condition to cause difficulty after sale is a subchondral bone cyst in the medial femoral condyle (see Chapter 46). Characteristically, lameness occurs soon after the horse starts lunging exercise for breaking in. Clinicians experienced with yearlings always obtain radiographs of a yearling's stifles if lameness develops in a hindlimb under these circumstances, with no obvious clinical sign of origin of pain. Vendors usually are approached with a view to taking the horse back, particularly if the money has not changed hands, but not all will

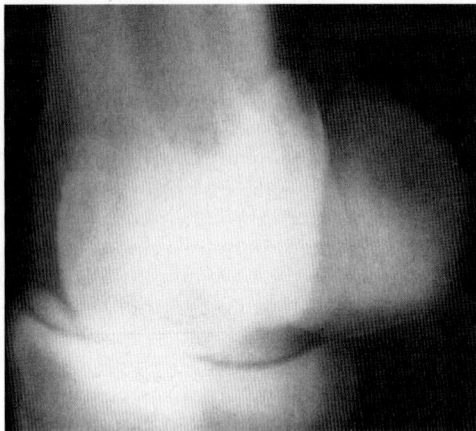

Fig. 99-1 • Dorsolateral-palmaromedial oblique radiographic image of a metacarpophalangeal joint. Irregularity and enthesophyte formation on the abaxial margin of the lateral proximal sesamoid bone reflect sesamoiditis. (Courtesy I.M. Wright, Newmarket, England.)

do so. No case has yet come to court, and it must be admitted that after conservative or surgical treatment some such horses have gone on to race satisfactorily, but not as 2-year-olds.

Conditions commonly found during prepurchase veterinary examination include the following:

- Enlargement of the proximal sesamoid bones can be the most important condition, because enlargement may result from fractures sustained as a young foal that have healed by fibrous union (see Chapter 36). Enlargement is often multiple and can involve the apex or the base of the bone. Sesamoiditis, with or without suspensory branch desmitis, also is seen in yearlings (Figure 99-1).
- Any effusion of a joint must be viewed with suspicion, particularly if forced flexion is painful. Purchase cannot be recommended, and even if good-quality radiographs reveal no abnormality, a guarded opinion is given.
- Asymmetry of front feet is common, and a slightly narrow hoof need not detract, providing the hoof is not twisted or shear heeled. Feet are sometimes overcorrected, which leaves them unlevel when viewed from the front standing on a hard, level surface or when the foot is held up and the solar surface is inspected. These conditions can cause orthopedic problems in training, and only mild imbalances are acceptable. A narrow, boxy foot is probably a lesser evil than a broad, flat foot with a collapsed heel.
- Lameness rarely is seen at sale examinations, but it can be difficult to spot because routine examination involves only inspection at the walk. Trotting can confirm or deny lameness. Ataxia can be difficult to discern because the frequently inspected yearling tires during the day and can appear weak. Also, some yearlings are given mild sedatives to control behavior, which may give a similar effect.
- Presale injuries are common. Yearlings travel by road or ferry, and knocks and abrasions often cause more distress to the vendor than the yearling. Capped hocks are particularly common but rarely important.

ULTRASONOGRAPHIC EXAMINATIONS

Ultrasonographic examinations have been introduced by some purchasers. Ultrasonography has been used mainly to measure dimensions of the cardiac chambers, but some horses that have had injuries or other soft tissue anomalies may be offered with ultrasonographic images provided by the vendor or, with the vendor's permission, may be examined by ultrasonography by a purchaser's veterinarian. Conditions that may warrant such an examination to give purchasers confidence include thickening of suspensory ligament branches or fleshy superficial digital flexor tendons (SDFTs). The former is seen distally where the suspensory ligament branch attaches to the proximal sesamoid bone and usually results from a mild strain. Whatever the fiber pattern appearance in these horses, they often need considerable patience in training as 2-year-olds but ultimately can stand racing. Fleshy tendons are a thickening or bowing of the SDFT in the forelimbs that is seen in yearlings or 2-year-olds in training. They show minimal or no soreness on digital pressure and on ultrasonographic examination have an increased cross-sectional area of the middle third of the tendon and a coarseness of fiber pattern, but no core lesion or accumulation of fluid (Figure 99-2). These horses do well if they are shown patience in training (horses with mild lesions are capable of light cantering exercise but not galloping) and are not given aggressive veterinary treatment. With regular monitoring the tendon(s) usually thins and straightens to normal during the summer months, and many horses can be raced as 2-year-olds. This condition is probably an adaptive mild inflammation, because it occurs in yearlings that have had no managed exercise and in 2-year-olds in early training. Fleshy tendons should not be considered in the same serious manner that a strain or core lesion would demand in an older horse and pose only a slightly greater risk of tendonitis later in the racing career. Local antiinflammatory medication or counterirritation is sometimes applied, but the efficacy is dubious.

◼ NORTH AMERICAN STANDARDBRED SALES YEARLING
Mike W. Ross

Veterinary inspection of the Standardbred (STB) sales yearling at the major sales is limited compared with that of the North American TB yearling. At most sales the number of veterinarians inspecting horses for their own potential purchase is similar to the number of those hired by owners and trainers to provide opinions.

LOCATION AND TIME OF MAJOR SALES

The major sales take place in the fall in Kentucky and Pennsylvania, with smaller sales elsewhere. Small consignors may sell directly through the sales company, but large breeding farms or well-known agents sell most STB sales yearlings. Separate dispersal sales of broodmares, sucklings, and weanlings occur with the yearling sales or at a later date. Horses of racing age sell at various sales across North America, but no specific sales occur for 2-year-old horses in training.

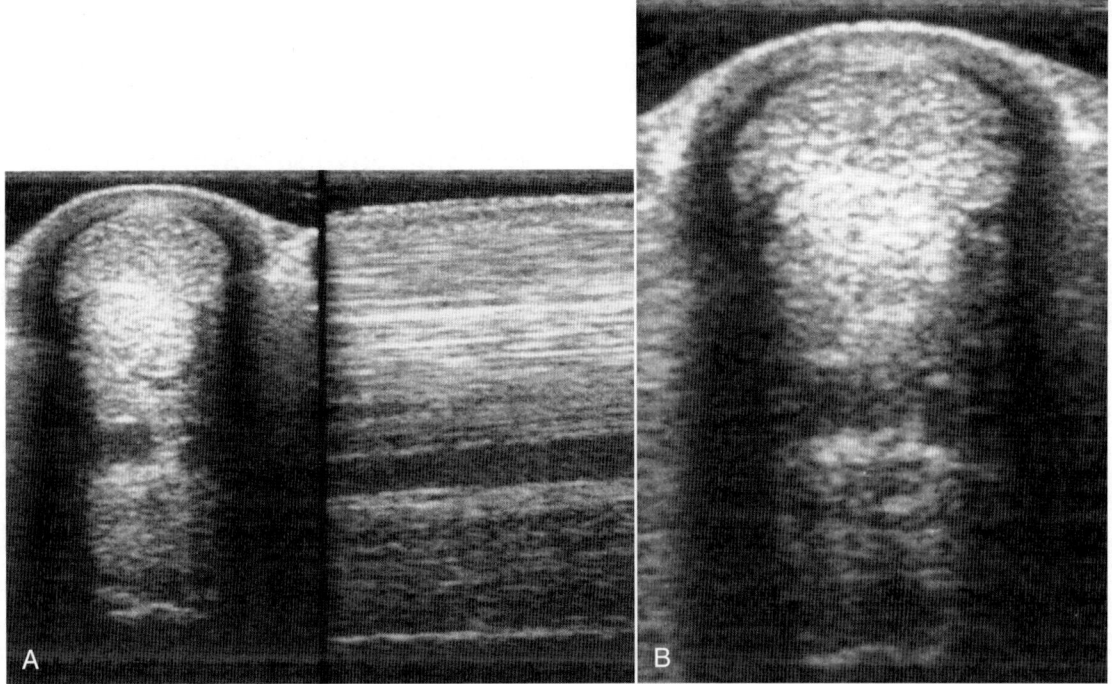

Fig. 99-2 • A, Transverse (on the left) and longitudinal ultrasonographic images of the midmetacarpal region of a 2-year-old Thoroughbred with fleshy tendons. Subcutaneous edema and enlargement of the superficial flexor tendon are present. **B,** Enlarged transverse image of horse shown in **A.** The entire cross-sectional area of the tendon has a diffuse reduction in echogenicity.

CONDITIONS OF SALE

All STB sales yearlings sell as is, meaning that when the hammer falls, the buyer owns the yearling in the condition in which it was sold and must pay according to the conditions of sale. The sales companies are not responsible for determining the suitability of the horse for racing or for unsoundness discovered after the sale. The sales company announces the yearling's sex and reproductive changes or abnormalities (gelding, spayed, ridgeling, cryptorchid), if the yearling was conceived by embryo transfer, and if the horse has been "nerved." Consignors sign a contract with the sales company that includes details about remediation if a dispute regarding soundness occurs, but the legal responsibility is with the consignor, not the sales company. Arbitration, according to the laws of the state in which the yearling was sold, is used if a suitable arrangement cannot be made.

Consignors, usually large farms acting as agents or independent sales agents, have a separate contract with individual owners to represent them at a sale. Owners are required to give information about neurological status, cribbing, fractures, neurectomy, or unsoundness of sight or wind at least 30 days before sale. The consignor determines if information regarding these conditions is announced at the sale, but no contract stipulates that known conditions, such as lameness or previous surgery, be announced at the sale. To prevent disputes and to preserve their integrity, consignors may request that surgical procedures, such as arthroscopy to remove osteochondritis dissecans (OCD) fragments, or other pertinent information be announced. Verbal announcements and the availability of presale radiographs and surgical reports may be detrimental to the sale price, despite resolution of the condition, although removal of tarsocrural OCD fragments is usually acceptable. Philosophical differences exist among consignors, and only some provide presale information. Thus little incentive exists to disclose information or to investigate problems before sale. Many owners prefer that problems not be investigated so that the yearling may be consigned without disclosure.

RESOLUTION OF DISPUTES

The consignor is primarily responsible for adjudicating conflicts about STB sales yearlings. Because sales companies stipulate yearlings are sold as is and arbitration is the final remedy for disputes, consignors often are forced to provide flexible remediation when disputes arise. If consignors are owners, they deal with problems directly with buyers. If consignors are agents for owners, they become the intermediary. In most instances consignor and buyer attempt to avoid arbitration. Problems arise when a condition is found after the sale, usually on postsale radiographs, that is judged to be detrimental to the yearling's future potential as a racehorse. The buyer refuses to pay and contacts the consignor. Influential large buyers can often stand their ground, and the consignors may refund money, give credit to the buyer for the future purchase of a yearling, pay for surgery if necessary, or lower the sale price. If agreement cannot be reached, arbitration ensues. The high prevalence of OCD fragments means that most disputes concerning these are judged in favor of the consignor. Disputes regarding carpal chip or other fractures, osseous cystlike lesions, extensive radiolucency of the proximal sesamoid bones, or unusual OCD or traumatic conditions often are resolved in favor of the buyer. Fractures are considered important, and the term should be avoided if a condition is known by most to be a manifestation of OCD. Failure to disclose a condition is most difficult to prove but often is suspected by disgruntled owners.

ROLE OF THE VETERINARIAN

Because repository radiographs are not available, the veterinary presence at major sales is minimal. Veterinarians are sometimes asked to accompany buyers to farms before sale, or to the sale itself, but are handicapped by not having the ability to review radiographs. Influential buyers may be able to convince consignors to allow radiographic and endoscopic examinations and may otherwise threaten not to bid on horses. Veterinarians often are asked to judge conformation and interpret what effect abnormalities may have on future race performance. They may be asked to review pedigrees, but in general, trainers and owners are extremely knowledgeable. Veterinarians are usually prohibited from performing radiographic and endoscopic examinations at a sale or, if they are allowed to do so, must perform the examinations after normal sale hours. However, these examinations usually are allowed for horses of racing age.

CONFORMATION

A definite relationship between conformation and the development of certain lameness conditions exists in the STB sales yearling (see Chapter 108). A difference in the relevance of abnormal conformation exists between a trotter and pacer. Sickle-hocked conformation is acceptable in a pacer, unless severe, but in a trotter this conformation leads to lameness. A sickle-hocked trotter is usually fast but lame. Mild sickle-hocked conformation is considered by some to be desirable in a pacer, but in horses of either gait, this abnormality predisposes to curb, osteoarthritis of the distal hock joints, and fracture of the central or third tarsal bones (see Chapters 44 and 78). In-at-the-hock conformation is undesirable in a trotter and a pacer. Calf-knee or back-at-the-knee conformation is prevalent in STB yearlings, and if mild and in a pacer the conformation is acceptable, but in a trotter this abnormality should be avoided. Any conformational abnormality of the carpus in a trotter should be considered carefully. Bench-knee or offset-knee conformation is undesirable in a trotter or pacer (see Chapter 38). Tied-in below the knee leads to superficial digital flexor tendonitis, especially in a pacer (see Chapter 69). I believe TB racehorses can tolerate clubfoot conformation better than STBs, and this abnormality should be avoided. Metacarpal and metatarsal exostoses are common, but usually of little concern, unless large or proximally located near the carpus or tarsus, respectively.

Videotapes of yearlings in action (loose exercise in paddocks or jogging on the track) are usually available and are thought to be much more informative in trotters than in pacers. Desirable characteristics of trotters include a wide gait behind and a narrow gait in front. An acceptable trotter can be base narrow and toed out in front, because hindlimbs often land lateral to the forelimbs (called *passing gaited*), and interference injury is minimal. Base-narrow, toed-out conformation predisposes a pacer to considerable interference injury. In pacers, base-wide forelimb conformation

is acceptable, whereas in a trotter this predisposes to interference. Toed-in conformation, if mild, is acceptable in a pacer but not in a trotter, because interference injury and lateral branch suspensory desmitis are problems.

RADIOGRAPHY AND RADIOLOGY

Because no repository for radiographs is provided and many consignors actively discourage presale radiography, radiographs are usually unavailable. However, some farms examine all STB sales yearlings radiologically before the sale, remove OCD fragments, and have radiographs available on request. Because OCD fragments of the tarsocrural joint generally cause effusion in late weanlings and early yearlings, these often are removed surgically before sale, but this may not be announced. Radiographs may be available for other types of injuries, such as lumps or bumps in the metacarpal or metatarsal region or elsewhere, to demonstrate that the injury is unlikely to affect future race performance.

Radiographs commonly are obtained after sale and may lead to questions about future soundness and, in some horses, arbitration. In general, radiological changes that affect racing performance are radiolucent defects of the proximal sesamoid bones (sesamoiditis and osseous cyst-like lesions), large conglomerate OCD fragments involving the plantar processes of the proximal phalanges (intraarticular and extraarticular fragments) in trotters, osseous cystlike lesions of the distal aspect of the proximal phalanx and middle and distal phalanges, large OCD lesions of the lateral trochlear ridge of the femur and subchondral bone cysts in the medial femoral condyle, single or multiple fragments located in the distal sesamoidean ligaments (rare form of fragmentation seen in the forelimb, thought to be a manifestation of OCD), carpal chip fractures, and various forms of osteoarthritis. The mere presence of OCD fragments does not necessarily affect sale price if the condition is known before the sale, and certainly in most yearlings does not preclude future soundness and successful racing. The most common sites of OCD involve the tarsocrural joint and the metatarsophalangeal and metacarpophalangeal joints. Once discovered, these fragments are often removed prophylactically before training begins. Management of STBs with fragments in the metatarsophalangeal joint is discussed elsewhere (see Chapter 42).

FUTURE DIRECTION

Many disputes occur between buyers and consignors concerning abnormalities in postsale radiographs, lameness, or neurological disease. Determination of when a lesion developed, if a true fracture exists, real or perceived effects on prognosis, and chain of custody (in whose care the yearling was when the problem was noticed) complicate final payment. These issues generally are resolved between the consignor and buyer (see the previous discussion), but occasionally arbitration is necessary and usually favors the consignor. Availability of presale radiographs in a repository would be preferable and a strong forward step for the STB industry, and although this change is not yet well accepted, mandatory radiographic examination is gaining support from some of the most influential owners and agents.

Chapter 100

Pathophysiology and Clinical Diagnosis of Cortical and Subchondral Bone Injury

Elizabeth J. Davidson

PATHOPHYSIOLOGY

Bone is an amazing living tissue that is able to conform and adapt to its environment. When bone is exposed to a load, it deforms. This deformation is elastic and within certain limits; bone returns to its original state once the load is removed. If the degree of deformation is beyond bone's upper limit, complete failure occurs. Under other conditions, bone may be subject to loads that are persistently different. Alterations in bone strain patterns develop, and the bone responds accordingly. Bone will then counteract the variation in load by changing its inertial properties via the processes of modeling and remodeling. In time, bone will modify its shape and structure, effectively adapting to the load under which it is placed (Wolff's law).

The term *modeling* refers to the geometric sculpting of bone by formation or resorption.[1] With modeling, osteoblasts and osteoclasts work independently, resulting in increased or decreased bone density. Resorption occurs when strain patterns are below the minimum threshold, and bone formation occurs when bone strain is above the maximum strain threshold.[1] In cortical bone, modeling adaption results in periosteal thickening (bone formation) or thinning (bone resorption). In trabecular bone, subchondral sclerosis or osteoporosis ensues. Eventually, modeling alters the size, shape, and density of bone. *Remodeling* refers to the coordinated action of osteoclasts and osteoblasts resulting in the removal of biomechanically inferior bone and replacement with new bone.[1] Osteoclasts move through bone at a much quicker rate than osteoblasts; therefore bone resorption (within weeks) is followed by bone formation (months).

Bone modeling and remodeling are active ongoing processes and can occur in the same bone at the same time. These processes are driven by site-specific bone strain patterns, although the exact mechanism by which strain induces bone change is unknown. Throughout life, bone continually adapts to its physiological loads by modeling and/or remodeling until its mechanical stimulus is normalized. These processes ensure the mechanical integrity of the skeleton. For example, when a horse undergoes athletic training, its bones are exposed to increasing and varying loads at specific locations. In turn, bone responds by adding more bone to regions of higher load. An adaptive site-specific response to race training in Thoroughbred (TB)

horses is the dramatic thickening that occurs in the dorsomedial aspect of the third metacarpal bone (McIII).

In ideal situations, a balance exists between load and the rate of bone adaptation. Repetitive cyclic loading produces an accumulation of focal microdamage at sites that are maximally stressed. Microdamage incites a bone response, followed by successful repair and remodeling. If there is imbalance between removal and replacement, the very process of bone repair may contribute to a bone's failure. Because osteoclasts act more quickly than osteoblasts, transient weakness occurs after damaged bone has been removed and before completion of bone replacement. Prolonged or rapid increases in load, such as those during high-speed workouts and racing, result in an accumulation of microdamage. The resorptive phase of remodeling may then exceed replacement capacity and transiently weaken the bone.[2,3] This focal weakness can function as a stress riser and allow initiation of a complete fracture or fragmentation under otherwise normal physiological loading.[4]

Failure of the bone to adapt in a timely fashion combined with continual and compounded microdamage results in stress-related bone injury.[5] Horses undergoing race training and racing are particularly susceptible to injury because their bones are constantly subjected to large repetitive loads. Risk for injury is high until a satisfactory adaptive bone response is completed.[3] Evaluation of postmortem specimens indicates that most musculoskeletal injuries are overuse injuries. Evidence of stress remodeling has been observed in equine long bones (the McIII, humerus, scapula, or tibia), the third carpal bone (C3), the pelvis, and vertebrae.[6-14] Site-specific pathology includes periosteal callus, sclerosis of endosteal or subchondral bone, and focal osteoporosis.

Stress-related cortical bone injury is commonly referred to as a *stress* or *fatigue fracture*. Stress fractures occur in horses undergoing intense exercise (repetitive high-strain loading) and are not correlated with a specific traumatic event.[3,8,15-17] They are associated with activities that produce repetitive loading of the involved bone. Repeated cyclic loading of cortical bone results in loss of stiffness, reduction in strength, and development of microcracks. With continued loading, microcracks propagate and coalesce into macrocracks (i.e., stress fractures). Stress fractures are regularly identified, clinically and at postmortem examination, in consistent locations presumably at sites of maximal load. They are very common in racehorses and are a well-recognized cause of lameness. If the stress remodeling continues in an unbalanced fashion, trauma to an already fatigued bone can lead to catastrophic fracture. Periosteal callus, indicative of preexisting reparative response, at equine cortical fracture interfaces[6,13] is common and provides evidence of a continuum of stress-related bone injury.

Like cortical bone, subchondral bone is susceptible to stress-related bone injury. Although features of bone modeling and remodeling are similarly induced, depending on the mechanical impact periosteal callus is not seen. Normally, the compliant subchondral plate acts as a shock absorber between articular cartilage and subchondral bone, thereby dissipating the impact to the articular surface. Repeated loading results in subchondral bone mineralization and subsequent stiffening to combat the increased

ferences
n page
1337

bone strain. The progressive increased bone density of the trabecular bone adjacent to the subchondral plate of the radial fossa of the C3 and the palmar condyles of the McIII or plantar condyles of the third metatarsal bone (MtIII) are examples of a subchondral response in race-trained horses.[12,18,19] As with cortical bone, repetitive loading of the subchondral bone may result in a repair process dominated by the resorptive phase of remodeling. Associated focal subchondral osteoporosis and microcracks may result. Small cracks may develop into larger fractures, resulting in fragmentation and overt fracture along articular margins.[20] Preexisting subchondral sclerosis is commonly seen in racehorses with distal McIII condylar fractures[21] and is a proposed precursor to C3 slab fractures.[12,22] Sclerotic subchondral bone may result in articular cartilage damage. Progressive cartilaginous erosion and ulceration has been identified at areas of increased subchondral thickness.[9,23,24] Collapse of subchondral bone resulted in flattening and indentation of cartilage, osteochondral fragmentation, and ultimately osteoarthritis (OA).[7,9,20]

CLINICAL EXAMINATION

A pathological continuum of cortical and subchondral stress-related bone injury causes lameness, subchondral sclerosis, subchondral lucency, incomplete (stress or fatigue) and complete fracture, and, in horses with subchondral damage, the eventual development of OA. Clearly, early and accurate diagnosis of stress-related bone injury in racehorses is important for the well-being of the horse and the safety of the industry. However, clinical recognition of these injuries can be challenging, and, although stress fractures are a well-recognized cause of lameness in racehorses,[11,15,16,25-34] most of these injuries occur in the absence of a specific traumatic event.[3,8,15-17,30] Characteristic history includes acute onset of lameness after racing or training that responds to rest.[25-27,30,35] Over time, lameness may worsen or linger, and some horses may have a history of weeks to months of poor performance, intermittent unilateral lameness or lameness in numerous limbs, or reports from exercise riders or drivers that horses are not "right."[27,36,37] Lameness scores at the time of diagnosis are quite variable, with some horses exhibiting no lameness and others being severely lame. Physical findings such as swelling or sensitivity to palpation are often subtle or absent. This is especially true in horses with upper limb long bone stress fractures, in which palpation may be at best difficult.

Clinical signs of cortical bone injury include periosteal thickening and local sensitivity. This is easily recognized in horses with the bucked-shin complex[38-40] (see Chapter 102). However, in the majority of long bones, overlying soft tissue and muscle prohibit clear identification. Localized signs of cortical pain in the tibia or humerus are uncommon and frequently absent.[16,25,28,31] When noted, pain during palpation and percussion of the medial diaphysis of the tibia occurs in as few as 30% of affected horses.[25] Careful palpation may reveal focal pain in horses with avulsion fracture of the proximal palmar or plantar aspect of the McIII or the MtIII, respectively.[41] Pain on palpation or profound muscle spasm of the affected side and ventral displacement of a tuber sacrale are consistent but subtle

physical abnormalities in horses with stress fractures of the wing of the ilium.[15,30] Flexion tests, time-honored clinical tools to help exacerbate and localize lameness, often have inconclusive results, and findings may even be absent in horses with cortical bone injury.[24,42]

Clinical signs of subchondral bone injury are also variable and often subtle. Injuries are frequently bilateral, and overt unilateral limb lameness is unusual. Affected horses may simply be performing at a lower level than expected. Overlying cartilage is minimally affected early in the disease process, and joint effusion is absent. Early subchondral bone injury of the distal aspects of the McIII and the MtIII rarely causes fetlock effusion,[36,43-45] and carpal effusion is often less than expected based on severity of lameness in Standardbreds (STBs) with subchondral lucency of the C3.[46,47] Diagnostic analgesia is essential for accurate diagnosis, but perineural techniques are consistently more effective than intraarticular analgesia, presumably because pain is associated with subchondral bone and not synovitis, capsulitis, and overt cartilage damage (see Chapter 42). Veterinarians and trainers are often incredulous when a diagnosis of subchondral bone injury is made by use of diagnostic analgesia and scintigraphic examination when clinical signs are lacking. As with cortical bone injury, flexion test results are inconsistent and often negative in horses with subchondral bone injury.[36,46] Subchondral increased radiopacity may be radiologically apparent, but it is often difficult to determine whether this is successful adaptive change or a maladaptive or nonadaptive response. In those horses with severe or chronic subchondral bone injury, clinical signs are often more obvious. Synovitis, lameness, and OA may be noted.

DIAGNOSTIC ANALGESIA

Although diagnostic analgesia is one of the most valuable tools used to localize the authentic source of pain, there are several considerations in horses with stress fractures and subchondral bone injury. At the time of evaluation, horses must be lame enough to visually assess response to diagnostic analgesia. Horses with stress fractures are notorious for being lame immediately after intense exercise but subtly lame or sound at the time of lameness examination. Neither perineural nor intraarticular analgesia can be used to diagnose upper limb stress fractures; however, such fractures should be suspected when lameness cannot be improved by routine distal limb diagnostic analgesia.* In addition, response to diagnostic analgesia is often variable. Lameness associated with cortical or subchondral injury of the proximal palmar aspect of the McIII may improve with high palmar analgesia or intraarticular analgesia of the middle carpal joint.[27,41,42,50] Pain associated with nonadaptive subchondral remodeling of the distal aspect of the McIII or the MtIII may be alleviated by using a low palmar or plantar or the lateral palmar metacarpal or plantar metatarsal block.[51] Often these horses will not improve with intraarticular analgesia and are similarly unresponsive to intraarticular medications.[36,43,44] Diagnostic analgesia is a good starting point but must not be used alone.

---

*References 25, 26, 28, 34, 48, 49.

DIAGNOSTIC IMAGING

Radiography and Radiology

Radiography remains hugely important in the diagnosis of bone injury in racehorses; however, it is insensitive during early phases of stress-related bone injury and often inadequate for subtle subchondral changes. Radiology provides structural information, much of which must be several weeks old before it can be seen. Lag time for enough structural change to occur to be seen radiologically is an obviously serious limitation of radiography, especially when one is attempting to localize and identify early or subtle bone injury. It takes 2 to 3 weeks or more before radiological changes of periostitis are apparent (see Chapter 15).[52-55] Even frank fracture lines or compression injury of subchondral bone can take days to weeks to be recognized. Supplementary radiographic images of site-specific regions may enhance detection of injury. For example, the dorsal 30° proximal 45° lateral-palmar (or plantar) distal medial oblique and dorsal 30° proximal medial-palmar or plantar distal lateral oblique ("down-angled") images (Figure 100-1) are useful for evaluation of subchondral injury of the condyles of the McIII or the MtIII.[51,55] A dorsal 60° proximal 45° lateral-palmar distal medial oblique image or dorsal 60° proximal 45° medial-palmar distal lateral oblique image of the distal phalanx is necessary for identification of palmar process fractures.[56-58] Even with additional images, subtle subchondral radiolucency and increased radiopacity are often difficult to recognize because density differences must be at least 30% to 50% and lesions 1 to 1.5 cm in diameter before recognition is possible.[52] Another obvious limitation of radiography is the inability to distinguish whether the radiologically apparent lesion is an active process or simply the result of an adaptive bone response.

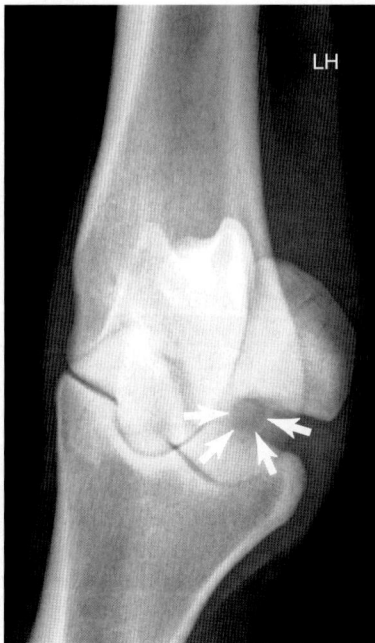

Fig. 100-1 • A dorsal 30° proximal 45° lateral-plantar distal medial oblique ("down-angled") radiographic image of 3-year-old Standardbred with subchondral lucency *(arrows)* of the distal plantarolateral aspect of the third metatarsal bone.

Nuclear Scintigraphy

Increased awareness of location and prevalence of stress-related bone injuries and scintigraphic examination of affected racehorses enhance early detection of bone pathology before catastrophic fracture. Nuclear scintigraphy is an extremely sensitive method of detecting exercise-induced bone remodeling (see Chapter 19). Normal bone response in the dorsal aspect of the McIII, the proximal sesamoid bones (PSBs), and the metacarpal condyles is easily identified and has typical patterns of increased radiopharmaceutical uptake (IRU) in horses undergoing high-speed exercise.[59,60] Scintigraphy is useful to detect abnormal alterations in local bone metabolism such as increased activity from cyclic loading and provides a foundation for the diagnosis of stress fractures, stress remodeling, and subchondral trauma.* A focal, moderate-to-intense area of IRU is the scintigraphic hallmark of stress fracture.

Several circumstances exist in which scintigraphy is invaluable for the diagnosis of cortical or subchondral bone injury. Racehorses with stress fractures often have a history of acute severe lameness that abates with rest. These horses have few localizing clinical signs and are diagnostic challenges. Scintigraphy can be used as a screening tool and obviates the need for numerous radiographic images. In addition, a negative bone scan is invaluable because it rules out active bone disease and virtually eliminates the possibility of a stress fracture.[52,54] Another scenario is when a racehorse fails to respond to diagnostic analgesia. This is especially true in horses with upper limb stress fractures. Scintigraphy is also helpful for horses with bone injury in numerous areas or multiple limbs. Racehorses with stress remodeling of the distal aspects of the McIII or the MtIII are often in this category.

Scintigraphy is more sensitive than radiography for the identification of stress-related bone injury, and a positive bone scan may precede conclusive radiological change by at least 2 to 3 weeks.[52-54] In reports of scintigraphic examinations of racehorses, nearly half of areas of IRU were not associated with radiologically detectable abnormalities.[61,63,64] A positive bone scan may also enhance the recognition of subtle radiological changes[41] and assist in determination of a structural abnormality as an active process or a reflection of past change. For example, radiographs of a 3-year-old TB racehorse reveal extensive thickening of the dorsal cortex of the McIII, but the bone scan is negative. Gradual resolution of IRU of the dorsal cortex of the McIII can be interpreted as evidence of satisfactory healing of a previously identified dorsal cortical fracture. On the other hand, a persistent fracture line without concurrent moderate-to-intense IRU may indicate the development of a nonunion, because the amount of radiopharmaceutical uptake reflects the rate of bony repair.[29] Carpal pain is not likely in a STB with radiological evidence of extensive sclerosis of the C3 but with only mild or no IRU seen scintigraphically.

Ultrasonography

Ilial wing fractures can be detected ultrasonographically.[15,17,30,66,67] Hematoma formation, irregular bone contour (indicative of callus formation), and breaks in the

---

*References 25, 27, 31, 32, 35, 41, 52-54, 56, 60-65.

normal hyperechogenic contour of bone may be seen if the fracture involves the dorsal surface of the bone (see Figure 49-3, page 566). A displaced fracture is seen as hyperechogenic bony structure distracted from adjacent bone ("stair-step" sign). Ultrasonographic abnormalities are usually most severe at the caudal margins of the fracture.[66,67] These findings are supported by postmortem studies in horses with ilial wing fractures.[11,13] Serial ultrasonographic examinations can be used to determine if the fracture has healed but should not be the single means of diagnosis. Because of variability in conformation of the ilium and other factors, ultrasonographic findings should be combined with a thorough clinical examination and, if necessary, scintigraphic and occasionally radiographic examinations.[15,66]

Magnetic Resonance Imaging and Computed Tomography

Slice-by-slice high-resolution images obtained during magnetic resonance imaging (MRI) detect alterations within bone early in a disease process before they are detectable by most other imaging modalities. In people, MRI is frequently used when conventional radiological findings are unremarkable, because MRI has better spatial resolution and specificity. Low signal intensity on T1- and T2-weighted gradient echo (GRE) or proton density (PD) images is the classic appearance of stress-related bone injury. Increased signal intensity in the trabecular and/or cortical bone on short tau inversion recovery (STIR) sequences or fat-suppressed T2-weighted fast spin echo sequences may reflect a bone contusion or fracture, depending on the distribution of altered signal intensity. Computed tomography (CT) may identify linear alteration in signal intensity in the cortex and endosteal and periosteal callus and is more sensitive than plain radiography. As with conventional radiography, false-negative findings are not uncommon. Obvious limitations of MRI and CT acquisition include costly equipment, often the need for general anesthesia, and the inability to image equine upper limbs and pelvis.

SPECIFIC LOCATIONS OF CORTICAL AND SUBCHONDRAL BONE INJURY

Knowledge of the prevalence of stress-related bone injuries provides insight into the likelihood of an area causing clinically important problems, especially when diagnostic analgesia fails to localize the lameness, or radiological and ultrasonographic examination findings are unremarkable. The type of training and racing largely determines the location of injury and whether the injury involves cortical or subchondral bone (Tables 100-1 and 100-2). In lame STBs, IRU is most commonly associated with exercise-induced subchondral bone remodeling, and prevalent sites include the PSBs followed by the C3 and the tarsus.[63] The distal palmar or plantar aspect of the McIII or the MtIII is also a frequent location of IRU and, when combined with IRU of the PSB, is the most common location of stress remodeling.[55,63] In TBs, IRU of the distal palmar or plantar aspects of the McIII or the MtIII is the most common abnormal scintigraphic finding.[62] In the forelimbs, sites of prevalence are the distal palmar aspect of the McIII, followed by the carpus and the dorsal cortex of the McIII.[62] In the hindlimbs, the distal plantar aspect of the MtIII is the most common abnormal area, followed by the tarsus and tibia.[62]

TABLE 100-1

Prevalences of Sites of Increased Radiopharmaceutical Uptake in the Forelimbs of Racehorses

SITE	STANDARDBRED (%)	THOROUGHBRED (%)
Phalanges	14	10
Proximal phalanx	7	—
Middle phalanx	0	—
Distal phalanx	7	—
Proximal sesamoid bone	32	6
Third metacarpal bone		
Distal palmar	21	50
Dorsal	0	15
Proximal palmar	3	4.5
Carpus (C3)	43	17
Radius	2	4
Humerus	0	10
Scapula	0	2

From Arthur RM, Constantinide D: Results of 428 nuclear scintigraphic examinations of the musculoskeletal system at a Thoroughbred racetrack, *Proc Am Assoc Equine Pract* 41:84, 1995; and Ehrlich PJ, Dohoo IR, O'Callaghan MW: Results of bone scintigraphy in racing Standardbred horses: 64 cases (1992-1994), *J Am Vet Med Assoc* 215:982, 1999.
C3, Third carpal bone.

TABLE 100-2

Prevalences of Sites of Increased Radiopharmaceutical Uptake in the Hindlimbs of Racehorses

SITE	STANDARDBRED (%)	THOROUGHBRED (%)
Phalanges	—	3
Proximal phalanx	11	—
Middle phalanx	0	—
Distal phalanx	1	—
Proximal sesamoid bone	35	6
Third metatarsal bone		
Distal plantar	19	28
Dorsal	2	3
Proximal plantar	4.5	<1
Tarsus	33	19
Tibia	0	11
Femur	4.5	2
Pelvis	—	6

From Arthur RM, Constantinide D: Results of 428 nuclear scintigraphic examinations of the musculoskeletal system at a Thoroughbred racetrack, *Proc Am Assoc Equine Pract* 41:84, 1995; and Ehrlich PJ, Dohoo IR, O'Callaghan MW: Results of bone scintigraphy in racing Standardbred horses: 64 cases (1992-1994), *J Am Vet Med Assoc* 215:982, 1999.

Distal Phalanx

IRU associated with the distal phalanx in the absence of radiological abnormalities in racehorses that subsequently developed distal phalanx fractures suggests that these fractures are not single-event injuries, but rather the result of repetitive stress.[56,57] Clinical examination findings include unilateral lameness localized to the digit using palmar digital analgesia. A fracture usually results in acute, severe lameness. If the fracture is articular, distal interphalangeal joint distention may be noted, and lameness is often alleviated by intraarticular analgesia.[58] Response to hoof tester application is variable and often unreliable. Distal phalangeal fractures occur more often in the forelimbs than the hindlimbs, and STBs may be overrepresented.[56,57] The lateral aspect of the left front and the medial aspect of the right front distal phalanges are most commonly affected, a finding that may reflect compression of these sides of the distal phalanx during counterclockwise racing in the United States.[56-58] The distribution of distal phalangeal fractures in racehorses from the United Kingdom or continental Europe is unknown.

Numerous scintigraphic images including lateral, dorsal, and solar images are recommended for complete and accurate diagnosis.[59] Oblique radiographic images of the palmar processes of the distal phalanx should be obtained to assist in identification of subtle radiolucent lines, particularly in horses with IRU identified scintigraphically.[59,61]

Palmar or Plantar Aspects of the Metacarpophalangeal/Metatarsophalangeal Joints

The true incidence of distal palmar or plantar subchondral injury of the McIII or the MtIII is unknown (see Chapters 36 and 42). Scintigraphic studies have indicated as many as 50% of TBs[62] and 20% of lame STBs may be affected.[63] Subchondral bone injury of the MtIII was identified as a major cause of hindlimb lameness in STB racehorses.[55] The proposed pathogenesis of subchondral injury to the distal palmar or plantar aspects of the McIII or the MtIII includes a progression of subchondral remodeling in response to repetitive stress including trabecular thickening (sclerosis). Under normal circumstances, this functional adaptation attenuates the load and spares stress on the articular cartilage. Under pathological conditions, this adaptation fails to protect the joint. Microcracking of the subchondral bone and cartilage[68-70] and/or focal necrosis[7,9] ensue, promoting the development of OA.

Subchondral bone changes in the distal aspect of the McIII or the MtIII may precede and predispose to condylar fractures.[71] The adapted and thicker subchondral bone of the condyles is significantly stiffer than adjacent bone, which results in a gradient between the relatively less dense sagittal ridge and the condylar bone. Strain accumulation at this interface may lead to an increase of localized fatigue damage, predisposing it to catastrophic failure.[71] Alternatively, larger cracks may be a manifestation of smaller microcracks, which originate in the sclerotic zone as part of the resorption phase of the remodeling response.[20] Regardless of the underlying chain of events, preexisting pathology such as focal regions of osteoporosis and microdamage in the surrounding bone have been identified in bones of horses with lateral condylar fracture of the McIII/MtIII.[21,70,71] Fracture lines pass through areas of localized porosity.[21,71]

Early in the disease process, when lameness is thought to be related to subchondral bone pain, abnormal physical examination findings are often lacking and clinical signs can be easily overlooked. Lameness is mild or apparent only at high speeds, joint effusion is uncommon, and most horses do not manifest a positive response to flexion tests.[36,55] When the hindlimbs are affected a bunny-hopping type of gait or lack of impulsion may be noted

when horses canter.[45] In horses affected bilaterally, a short, choppy, uncomfortable gait or an intermittent, shifting hindlimb lameness may be present. Perineural analgesia is more effective than intraarticular analgesia in abolishing pain at this stage of the disease process. Either a low palmar or plantar or lateral (medial) palmar metacarpal or plantar metatarsal nerve block is recommended,[51] because intraarticular analgesia of the fetlock joint inconsistently abolishes subchondral pain.[36,43] Perineural analgesia in one limb will often result in horses then exhibiting contralateral limb lameness. Radiological evaluation is frequently unremarkable; however, IRU in the distal palmar or plantar aspects of the McIII or the MtIII is diagnostic if lameness has been localized using diagnostic analgesia. As the disease progresses, lameness worsens, and horses are more likely to have a positive response to a lower limb flexion test. Both a positive bone scan and abnormal radiological findings (increased subchondral radiopacity and radiolucency) are apparent. Later, joint effusion, more prominent lameness, and a positive response to intraarticular analgesia may be noted.

Scintigraphy is the method of choice for diagnosis as radiographs are often negative or equivocal, especially in the early stages of disease. Standing lateral, plantar, and flexed lateral scintigraphic images are recommended (Figure 100-2). The most common scintigraphic abnormality is focal IRU of the distal palmar or plantar aspects of the McIII or the MtIII, but the PSBs may be involved. Flexed lateral images are especially helpful to differentiate IRU of the distal aspect of the McIII or the MtIII from that involving the PSBs.[55] In a retrospective study of lame STBs undergoing scintigraphic evaluation, 20% of images had IRU associated with the palmar or plantar aspect of the fetlock joints.[63] It is not uncommon for more than one limb to be affected[62] or for IRU to be identified in all four fetlock joints.[61] Front and hind fetlock joints are commonly concomitantly affected.[61,63] Metatarsophalangeal joint lameness may be more common in STBs because

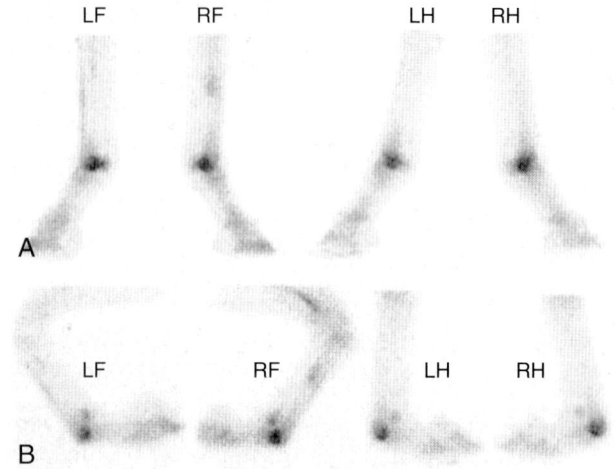

Fig. 100-2 · A, Delayed phase lateral scintigraphic images of the distal aspect of the limbs of a 4-year-old Thoroughbred with focal, intense increased radiopharmaceutical uptake (IRU) in the palmar and plantar aspects of the metacarpophalangeal and metacarpophalangeal joints. **B,** The flexed lateral images confirm that IRU is confined to the distal palmar or plantar aspect of the third metacarpal and metatarsal bones, not the proximal sesamoid bones or the proximal phalanx.

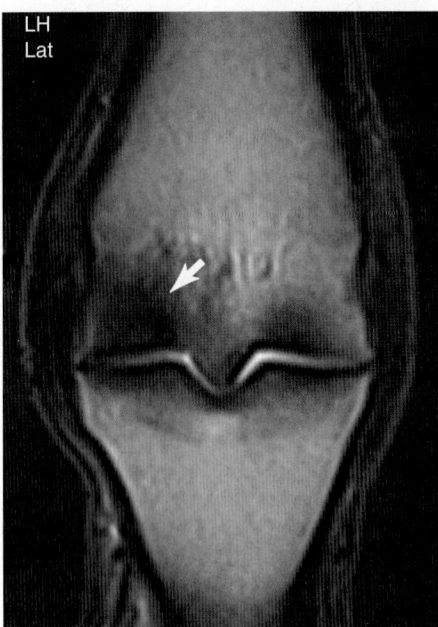

Fig. 100-3 • Dorsal T2-weighted gradient echo magnetic resonance image of the right metatarsophalangeal joint of a 3-year-old Standardbred racehorse with moderate right hindlimb lameness, which subsequently improved with lateral plantar metatarsal analgesia. There is a hypointense signal *(arrow)* within the lateral condyle of the distal aspect of the third metatarsal bone, consistent with increased bone density.

of gait and load distribution, and IRU of the distal plantarolateral aspect of the MtIII predominates.[55] In TBs, IRU in the distal palmar aspect of the McIII is more common than IRU in the distal plantar aspect of the MtIII, and bilateral IRU is prevalent.[61,62]

In addition to routine radiographic images of the metacarpophalangeal and metatarsophalangeal joints, "down-angled" oblique images are recommended for complete evaluation of the distal palmar or plantar aspects of the McIII or the MtIII.[51,55] Less than half of horses with IRU will have radiological abnormalities.[55,61,63] When apparent, bony changes include subchondral lucency and increased radiopacity (see Figure 100-1).[45,55] Radiological evidence of lucency may represent a later stage of the remodeling process and may be indicative of necrotic subchondral bone.[7,55]

Advanced imaging (MRI and CT) has improved our understanding of subchondral bone damage in fetlock joints and has great potential for early detection and implementation of management techniques directed toward injury prevention. Bony changes identified during MRI include small areas of high signal intensity within dense, sclerotic subchondral bone on STIR and T2-weighted images consistent with fluid, fibrosis, or bone necrosis within the subchondral bone and hypointense regions within the condyle on PD images consistent with increased bone density (Figure 100-3).[72] Through the use of CT, subchondral increased radiopacity in the condyles[59,69,71] and bone porosity at the site of condylar fracture[69,71] have been identified in cadaver specimens.

Dorsal Cortex of the Third Metacarpal Bone

Stress-related bone injury of the dorsal cortex of the McIII (bucked-shin complex) is a well-recognized disease of racehorses, particularly young TBs, in which incidence has been reported to be as high as 70%.[38] There are two clinical syndromes, diffuse periostitis (bucked shins) and dorsal cortical fracture (saucer, fatigue, stress fracture), thought to be closely related and representing a continuum of stress-related bone injury (see Chapter 102).

Race training in TBs results in repetitive loading on the McIII. The McIII then responds by modeling and remodeling, adding to and increasing the density of the dorsal cortex. Under balanced conditions, the dorsal cortex thickens, the minimum moment of inertia changes significantly, and the bone is then adapted.[3] Histological examination of classically trained TBs shows that bone remodeling is confined to the dorsomedial surface of the bone.[73] If the modeling process is unable to keep up with bone strain, more bone stiffness is lost, and more periosteal new bone is formed. This resulting microdamage manifests itself clinically as "bucked shin."[73] The relatively thinner dorsolateral cortex is subject to lower strains during race training, never responding with clinically significant modeling and remodeling. As the speed of training increases and the high-strain cycles accumulate, this thinner poorly adapted dorsolateral cortex may sustain incomplete cortical stress fractures.[73]

Classically, TBs develop bucked shins early in training, at or about the time of high-speed work, usually in the 2-year-old year. Clinical signs are usually sufficient for diagnosis. The condition is characterized by pain, heat, and swelling on palpation of the dorsal aspect of the McIII.[29,38,44,60] Frank lameness may be present, but subtle signs such as unwillingness to train at high speeds may be apparent.[29,60] In North American TBs the left forelimb may be more commonly affected than the right, although the disease occurs bilaterally. This injury is rarely seen in older horses, especially those that have raced successfully. Racehorses trained and raced in Europe may develop bucked shins when they relocate to North American dirt tracks.[40] Once the condition is recognized and the horse recovers, it rarely recurs. Clinical signs of dorsal cortical fractures include firm protuberance on the dorsal aspect of the McIII, usually in the middle third of the diaphysis. Application of firm digital pressure often elicits pain. Dorsal cortical fractures usually develop some months after the acute phase of bucked shins and most commonly in 3-year-old TB racehorses. About 10% to 12% of horses with bucked shins will also have dorsal cortical stress fracture.[38,40] Dorsal cortical fractures can occur along the proximal, middle, or distal dorsal aspects of the McIII but are most common in the middle third of the bone.

Although signs of dorsal McIII pain are common in TBs, STBs seldom exhibit it. In fact, TBs are 8.6 times more likely to develop dorsal metacarpal disease than STBs.[60] Bucked shins occasionally occur in pacers in June or July of the 2-year-old year and are unusual in trotters. Dorsal cortical fractures occur rarely, usually in 3-year-old pacers in the midportion of the racing year. Because mechanical properties of the McIII are not significantly different between STBs and TBs,[39] the disparity in prevalence is most likely the result of differences in training regimens between the breeds. STBs race at slower speeds than do TBs and in a different gait. In addition, STBs typically train long, slow jogging miles before introduction to speed work, unlike TBs, which typically have an earlier introduction of speed

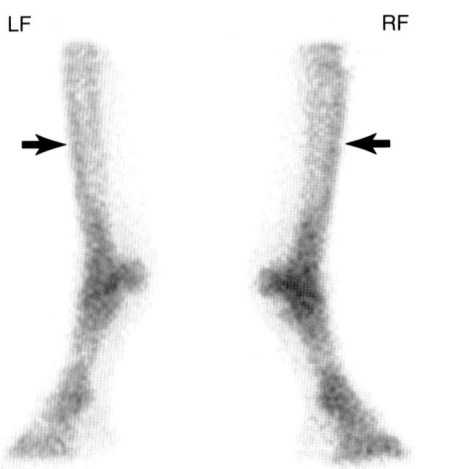

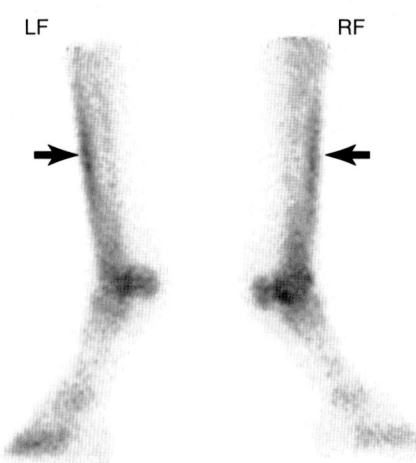

Fig. 100-4 • Delayed phase standing lateral scintigraphic images of the distal forelimbs of a young Thoroughbred in active race training with normal, adaptive uniform and diffuse radiopharmaceutical uptake in the dorsal cortex of the third metacarpal bones *(arrows)*.

Fig. 100-5 • Delayed phase lateral scintigraphic images of the distal fore-limbs of a 3-year-old Thoroughbred with diffuse moderate increased radio-pharmaceutical uptake (IRU) in the dorsal cortex of the third metacarpal bones *(arrows)*. This pattern of uptake is consistent with a diagnosis of bilateral periostitis (bucked shins). The distal palmar aspects of both third metacarpal bones exhibit mild IRU as well.

work during training. When compared with the TB McIII, STB McIIIs are significantly more developed before onset of racing,[39] a finding that would explain an apparent resistance to the development of bucked shins in young STBs.

Radiological diagnosis of stress-related bone injury of the dorsal aspect of the McIII is often delayed after clinical diagnosis. When apparent, periostitis is identified by the presence of periosteal new bone (bony thickening or roughening) over the dorsal or dorsomedial aspect of the McIII. A diagnosis of dorsal cortical stress fracture is confirmed by the presence of a short, oblique, linear radiolucency at 30- to 45-degree angle to the dorsal cortex and is often noted in conjunction with periostitis. Well-exposed and well-positioned plain, digital, or computed radiographic views are required.

Mild, diffuse IRU in the dorsal cortex of the McIII is common in young TBs in training and is attributed to the rate of accelerated modeling that occurs in the McIII during training. Patterns of uptake considered a normal finding in these horses include mild, uniform, and diffuse IRU in the dorsal cortex of the McIII relative to the palmar cortex, but activity should be less than in the metaphyses (Figure 100-4).[29] Scintigraphic studies of racehorses evaluated for lameness indicated that 45% to 68% of TBs[29,60] and 95% to 97% of STBs[60] have some IRU in the dorsal aspect of the McIII, but most of these horses do not have clinical signs of metacarpal pain. Periostitis (bucked shins) is evident by uniform and diffuse IRU in the dorsal cortex of the McIII relative to the palmar cortex and metaphyses (Figure 100-5).[29] IRU consistent with periostitis may be noted in as many as 12% to 34% of TBs[29,60,62] and 1% to 3% of STBs.[60] Clinical signs of periostitis correlate well with scintigraphy; most horses with abnormal IRU also have metacarpal pain. Dorsal cortical fractures are evident as focal moderate-to-intense IRU in the dorsal cortex of the McIII[29,60] (Figure 100-6) and are occasionally identified in combination with periostitis.[29] Focal IRU is a much more important finding in establishing the diagnosis of fracture than is intensity of IRU. In STBs, dorsal cortical stress fractures are exceedingly

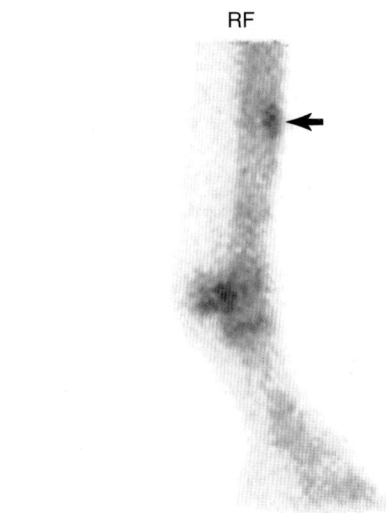

Fig. 100-6 • Delayed phase lateral scintigraphic image of the distal right forelimb of a 3-year-old Thoroughbred with focal, intense increased radio-pharmaceutical uptake in the dorsal cortex of the right third metacarpal bone. This pattern of uptake is consistent with a diagnosis of a dorsal cortical fracture.

uncommon, reported in only 1% of the population of lame horses undergoing scintigraphic examination.[60]

Proximal Palmar Aspect of the Metacarpal Region

Proximal palmar metacarpal region pain is a common cause of forelimb lameness in athletic horses (see Chapter 37).[27,35,41,42,50] Many pathological bony processes have been described, including avulsion fracture of the McIII at the origin of the suspensory ligament, palmar proximal cortical incomplete fracture of the McIII, and stress reaction or stress fracture of the McIII.[27,35,41,42] The differential diagnosis is based on clinical findings, perineural analgesia, and diagnostic imaging. Scintigraphic, ultrasonographic, radiographic, and/or MRI examinations are often required to confirm and categorize a diagnosis. Making a clear distinction between primary bony injury and secondary bone modeling that occurs in some horses with proximal suspensory desmitis can be challenging without MRI. Physical examination findings are often lacking.[27,35,42,50,74] Moderate-to-severe lameness is the most consistently observed clinical sign* and typically occurs at or near racing speeds.[27,42,50] Some horses respond to focal digital pressure on the proximal palmar aspect of the McIII,[27,41,42,50,74] and few have evidence of heat or swelling.[74] Proximal palmar metacarpal region pain is confirmed by improvement in lameness severity after diagnostic analgesia. Multiple techniques for analgesia of this region include lateral palmar, high palmar, and subcarpal analgesia, local infiltration of the proximal palmar aspect of the McIII, and middle carpal analgesia.†

Radiological evaluation may reveal a plethora of bony abnormalities. The classic appearance of an avulsion fracture of the suspensory origin consists of a crescent-shaped radiolucent defect of the proximal aspect of the McIII seen on a dorsopalmar image. Incomplete longitudinal fracture is seen as a linear or slightly oblique radiolucency in the proximal aspect of the McIII, medial to the midline.[35,42] Increased radiopacity of the subchondral bone is best identified on a dorsopalmar image and may be seen alone, in conjunction with fracture, or in association with bony modeling secondary to proximal suspensory desmitis. More subtle radiological findings such as periosteal reaction, enthesophyte formation, and small radiolucent defects in combination with positive scintigraphic findings are also diagnostic.

Focal moderate or intense IRU in the proximal palmar aspect of the McIII confirms the presence of stress-induced bone injury and may represent avulsion fracture,[41] incomplete fracture,[35] stress reaction, or stress fracture of the McIII[27] but can also be seen in association with acute, severe proximal suspensory desmitis. Radiological abnormalities are inconsistently identifiable in horses with IRU,[27,35,41] and the clinical importance of subtle or questionable radiological abnormalities is enhanced with positive bone scan findings.[41] Scintigraphy is quite useful for differentiation of middle carpal and carpometacarpal joint lesions, particularly in horses with lameness abolished by middle carpal analgesia.

Ultrasonographic examination is recommended for identification of confounding and/or contributing suspensory desmitis. Individual variation in size and shape of the proximal aspect of the suspensory ligament, artifacts, and variable amounts of muscular tissue complicate ultrasonographic interpretation. Ultrasonographic images underestimate ligament size because the medial and lateral margins are difficult to evaluate; they are less anatomically detailed than MRI images,[75] and low-grade lesions may be missed.

Recent experience with MRI has demonstrated superior ability to assess both soft tissue and bone injury in the proximal palmar aspect of the McIII.[74,75] High signal intensity on STIR sequences is indicative of fluid or edema (bone contusion), fibrosis, or necrosis and may be caused by the bone's response to tearing of the origin of the proximal aspect of the suspensory ligament, but may also reflect primary osseous injury.[74] Low signal intensity on PD and T2-weighted GRE images is indicative of increased bone density and may be a sign of chronic injury.[74]

Subchondral Injury of the Third Carpal Bone

The C3 adapts to high-intensity exercise by increasing its subchondral density by bone modeling.[22,76-80] The radial facet of the C3 is particularly vulnerable to repetitive loads encountered during race training (see Chapter 38).[76,77,79] Histological changes include progressive thickening of the subchondral bone plate at the expense of medullary space that ultimately produces a bony bridge between the proximal and distal cortices.[12,22] Although some degree of sclerosis is a normal adaptive response,[22] continued modeling in response to loading may cause excessive increase in bone density. In horses with extreme sclerosis, cancellous bone appears to have been almost entirely converted into compact cortical bone, and abnormal dissipation of forces between articular cartilage and subchondral bone may ensue. With subchondral bone density increases, the shock-absorptive capacity decreases, predisposing to cartilage damage[81] and OA. Cartilaginous lesions[18,79] and reduced cartilage stiffness[79] have been noted in sites of maximal subchondral density; however, the interactive mechanism by which bone changes may affect cartilage, and vice versa, is disputed and the subject of intense study.

Modeling of the subchondral bone at the expense of the marrow and vascular spaces may also lead to ischemia of the subchondral bone,[9,12,22] although the role of ischemia has not been clearly delineated and remains controversial. Further mechanical abuse to ischemic regions may cause progression to focal osteolysis and gross subchondral loss, predisposing to chip or slab fracture.[9,12,22] Histological and/or gross sections of C3 slab fractures indicate that these injuries are pathological fractures, occurring in chronically damaged necrotic bony tissue.[9]

The localized increase in bone density is evident radiologically as increased radiopacity and loss of trabecular structure (sclerosis) on a dorsoproximal-dorsodistal oblique (skyline) image of the distal row of carpal bones. Histological evidence of increased subchondral bone density corresponds to increased radiopacity noted radiologically[22,77,82] and is usually localized to the radial fossa of the C3.[82,83] C3 sclerosis and associated subchondral bone pain were implicated as an important cause of carpal lameness in STB and TB racehorses.[46,63,83-85] In addition, increased radiopacity is seen in most horses with fractures of the C3.[83,86] However, some degree of increased radiopacity represents a normal physiological adaptation to exercise, and not all horses with severe increased radiopacity are lame.[22,84,85] Therefore the value of radiology and the clinical significance of increased radiopacity of the C3 can be questioned. The presence of IRU supports the clinical significance of radiologically apparent increased radiopacity of the C3.

Subchondral lucency of the C3, commonly in combination with increased radiopacity of the radial fossa, causes lameness in STBs.[46,47,63,85] The pathogenesis is not clearly understood, but it may result from osteochondral collapse and cartilage damage because of chronic degenerative subchondral bone.[46,82] Subchondral lucency is not a disease of racehorses in early training and may be the end result of a continuum of compression injury of the sclerotic C3.[46]

The amount of sclerosis that can be considered physiological and how the transition to pathology can be

---

*References 27, 35, 41, 42, 50, 74.
†References 27, 35, 41, 42, 50, 74.

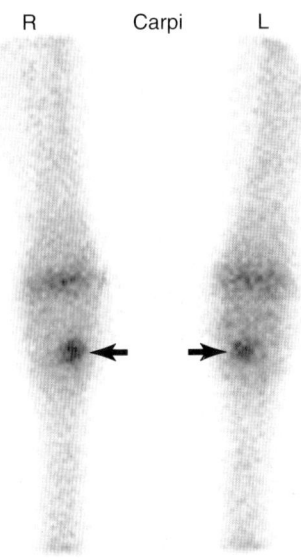

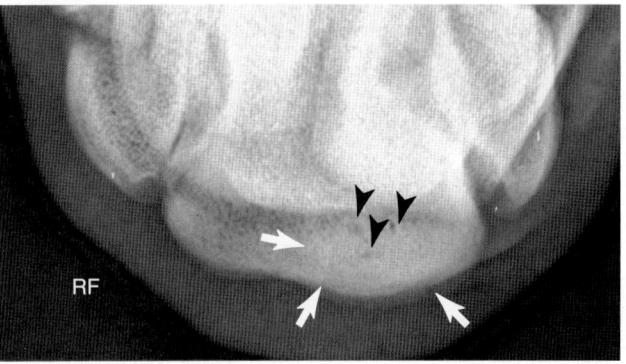

Fig. 100-8 • Dorsoproximal-,dorsodistal (skyline) radiographic image of the distal row of carpal bones of the right carpus of the horse in Figure 100-7 showing increased radiopacity (sclerosis) *(white arrows)* and small radiolucent defects *(black arrows)* of the radial fossa of the third carpal bone.

Fig. 100-7 • Dorsal delayed phase scintigraphic image of the carpal region in a 2-year-old Standardbred with focal intense increased radio-pharmaceutical uptake in the third carpal bones *(arrows)*.

detected or prevented remain a major diagnostic dilemma. Therefore the clinical diagnosis of C3 subchondral bone injury can be challenging. The majority of horses with authentic subchondral C3 pain are lame, and often the degree of lameness is more pronounced than other clinical signs. As with other subchondral bone injuries, joint effusion, positive response to a carpal flexion test, and pain on palpation are often lacking.[44,46,47,85] Horses with carpal pain tend to place the limb more widely than expected during protraction and may abduct the limb during advancement.[44,46] Diagnostic analgesia in combination with well-exposed, well-positioned radiographic images and positive bone scan findings are recommended for diagnosis.

Scintigraphic examination reveals focal IRU of the C3 or the medial aspect of the subchondral bone of the middle carpal joint (Figure 100-7). Flexed dorsal images of the carpus help to differentiate IRU of the C3 from the radial carpal bone. In retrospective studies IRU of the C3 is common in lame STBs and frequently bilateral.[63] IRU in the C3 is also noted in TBs, and about one third of horses are bilaterally affected.[62] Radiological evidence of increased radiopacity accompanies IRU in about half of injured horses.[63] Horses with focal, moderate-to-intense IRU are more likely to have radiological abnormalities (Figure 100-8).[63]

Radius

Stress fractures of the radius are uncommon.[26,62,63] They are usually unilateral and midshaft,[26] although bilateral fractures are seen occasionally.[26,62] Enostosis-like lesions can mimic stress fractures and are seen more commonly in the radius than are stress fractures during scintigraphic evaluation (see Chapter 39).[87] Enostosis-like lesions are characterized by focal areas of IRU often close to the nutrient foramen and not involving the cortex.[87] Correct and careful positioning and/or additional images assist in differentiation.[87] Radiological abnormalities are typical for stress remodeling; periosteal bone reaction and fracture lines are identified infrequently. Enostosis-like lesions appear as

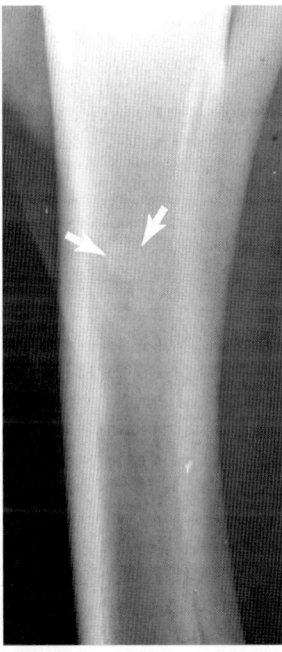

Fig. 100-9 • Lateromedial radiographic image of the left radius reveals multiple rounded intramedullary radiopaque lesions typical of enostosis-like lesions.

focal intramedullary radiopacities corresponding to areas of IRU (Figure 100-9).[87]

Humerus

Complete, catastrophic humeral fractures in TB racehorses are now known to be associated with preexisting pathology (periosteal callus and incomplete fracture).[6] Increased awareness of incomplete humeral stress fractures and scintigraphic examination of horses with undiagnosed forelimb lameness have enhanced early detection.

Stress fractures of the humerus are relatively common in young TB racehorses in early or mid training,[2,6,25,26] and half of affected horses are unraced before diagnosis.[25] Race training after a lay-up period may be a predisposing factor, because return from lay-up has been strongly associated with increased risk of complete humeral facture.[2] Initially, stress fractures of the humerus were reported

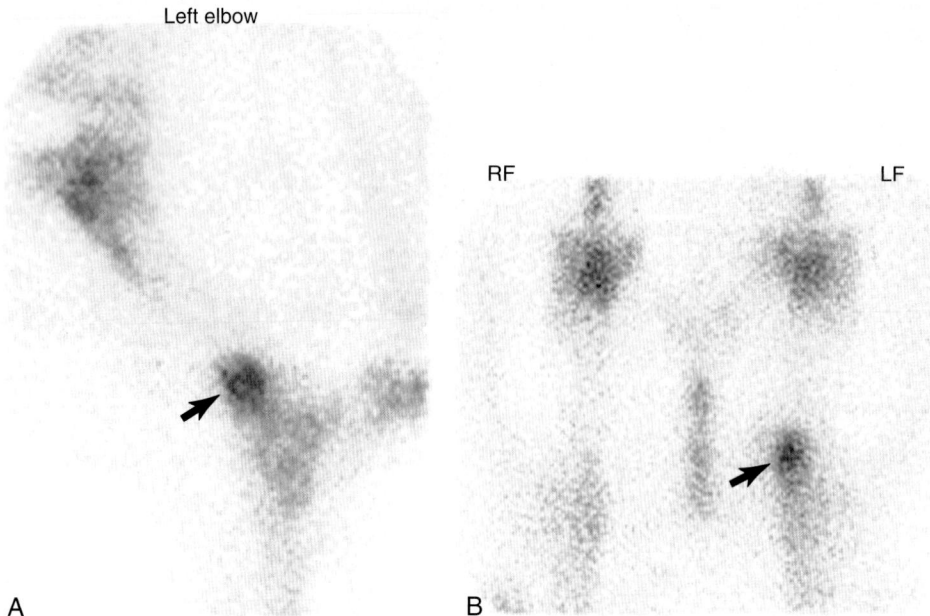

Left elbow

RF   LF

A   B

Fig. 100-10 • **A,** Lateral delayed phase scintigraphic image of the left elbow region of a 3-year-old Thoroughbred with focal, intense increased radiopharmaceutical uptake in the distal cranial aspect of the humerus *(arrow)*. **B,** In merged cranial delayed phase scintigraphic images of the right and left shoulder regions, the increased radiopharmaceutical uptake is more prominent on the distal medial aspect of the left humerus *(arrow)*.

more commonly in the left forelimb,[26] but more recent studies showed no difference between left and right forelimbs.[6,25] Bilateral humeral stress fractures and recurrence are uncommon.[25,26] The prevalence of humeral stress fractures in STBs is low and the location and conformation of stress-related bone injury of the humerus in STBs may be different than that of the TB.[34,63] Differences in training and racing regimens may be responsible for the low prevalence of humeral stress fractures in STBs.

Most affected horses are unilaterally lame.[25,26,34] Typical of horses with stress fractures, lameness is often severe immediately after exercise and improves quickly with box rest.[25,26] Lameness may be more severe than with stress fractures elsewhere in the forelimbs. Physical examination findings are generally unremarkable, and few affected horses show pain during upper limb manipulation.[25,34] Lameness is not abolished with distal limb analgesia[25,26,34] and may become worse.[25] Intrathecal analgesia of the bicipital bursa may partially improve lameness severity in horses with stress fractures of the proximal aspect of the humerus because of diffusion of local anesthetic solution.[34]

Nuclear scintigraphy is the most sensitive method to diagnose humeral stress fractures; there is focal IRU in the humeral cortex.[25,26,34] The caudoproximal[25,26] and the craniodistal[25,34] aspects of the humerus and usually the medial cortex are the most common sites (Figure 100-10). Rarely, areas of IRU that are seen extending from the proximal caudal cortex to the distal cranial cortex of the humerus are highly suggestive of an incomplete spiral fracture. The scintigraphic pattern generally follows the same pattern as complete humeral fractures.[6] Radiological examination is less sensitive, positive in only half of horses with focal IRU associated with the humerus, but is more specific than scintigraphy.[25] Callus formation and less commonly a distinct fracture line may be noted (Figure 100-11).

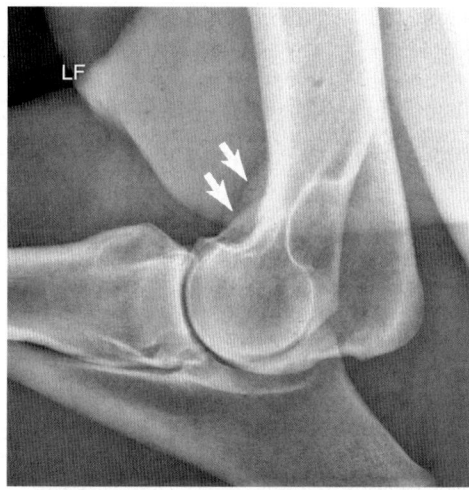

LF

Fig. 100-11 • Lateromedial radiographic image of the left elbow region showing callus formation *(arrows)* along the distal cranial aspect of the humerus consistent with a healing stress fracture.

Scapula

Postmortem examination has identified scapular stress fractures as singular and focal and occurring along the distolateral aspect of the scapular spine.[13] Periosteal callus, indicative of preexisting bone stress, is also found in association with complete fractures.[13] Although rare, stress fractures of the scapula should be considered when an upper forelimb stress fracture is suspected clinically.[48,49] Affected TB racehorses have a history typical of other stress-related bone injuries—acute unilateral forelimb lameness after racing or speed work.[48,49] To date, scapular stress fractures remain unreported in STBs. Few localizing clinical examination findings are apparent. Injured horses have a negative response to diagnostic analgesia of the distal limb and infrequently a positive response to upper limb manipulation.[48,49] Diagnosis is confirmed scintigraphically with focal, intense IRU in the scapula along the caudal ventral aspect,[48] the middistal spine of the scapula, or the supraspinous fossa.[49] Radiological abnormalities are difficult to detect in horses with proximally located stress fracture but may be apparent in those with distal fractures. Ultrasonographic examination may reveal bony irregularity and/or a "stair-step" appearance of the site of injury.

Tibia

Tibial stress fractures occur predominately in TBs and are one of the more common causes of acute hindlimb lameness in the racehorse.[25,26,88] Tibial stress fractures occur infrequently in STBs and Quarter Horses.[16,26,28,31,89] Most tibial stress fractures occur during race training, and in one study, more than half of affected horses had had at least one 60-day lay-off period within the last three starts before injury.[32,33] Most affected horses are 2- or 3-year-olds,[25,28,32,33] but fractures occur in older TBs and STBs as well.[26,28,89] Fractures may occur unilaterally and are seen equally in the right and left hindlimbs. However, unilateral lameness may be associated with bilateral fractures. Fractures occur in a variety of locations, including proximocaudal, middiaphyseal, and distomedial.* Bilateral lameness and bilateral fractures may occur,[25,31,32,88] and fractures can occur in the contralateral tibia at a later date.[25] Tibial stress fracture can propagate to a complete fracture even with enforced stall confinement.[32]

Typically, horses have moderate-to-severe acute lameness after racing or training.† Affected horses may be more lame than horses with stress fractures in other locations and should be suspected of having a tibial stress or spiral fracture if acute non–weight-bearing hindlimb lameness is present. There are few localizing signs on physical examination. Some affected horses have a positive response to firm pressure and percussion of the medial diaphysis of the tibia.[25] Horses may have a positive response to upper limb flexion[16,25,26,31] and pain when torsion is placed on the tibia.[45] History and a negative response to diagnostic analgesia in the remainder of the limb are important.[25,26,28]

Tibial stress fractures are identified as focal areas of IRU, and numerous sites of injury have been described.§ The thickness of the soft tissue overlying the lateral aspect of the midcrus may impede detection in all affected horses in lateral images; therefore additional caudal or oblique images are recommended for horses with subtle areas of IRU in the tibia and in those in which there is a high index of suspicion but no convincing area of IRU is seen in standard images. The most common site of IRU is in the caudolateral aspect of the middiaphysis (Figure 100-12) or the proximocaudal aspect of the tibia.ǀ Stress fractures of the caudomedial cortex may occur but are uncommon. Occasionally, diffuse areas of IRU in the distal aspect of the tibia are seen with spiral tibial stress fractures (Figure 100-13). Postmortem studies correlate with scintigraphic findings and have identified periosteal callus in a variety

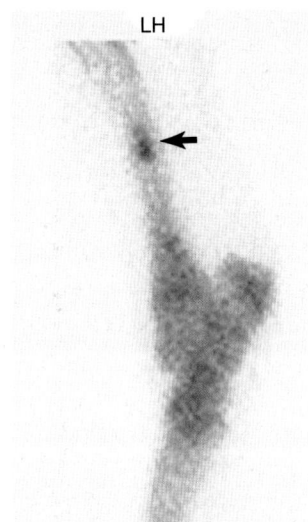

Fig. 100-12 • Lateral delayed phase scintigraphic image of the left tibia of a Thoroughbred racehorse with left hindlimb lameness. There is focal moderate-intense increased radiopharmaceutical uptake *(arrow)* in the caudal, lateral aspect of the tibial diaphysis consistent with a tibial stress fracture.

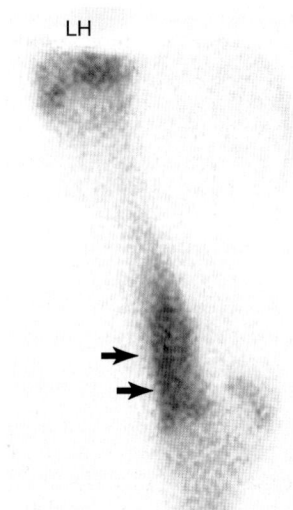

Fig. 100-13 • Lateral delayed phase scintigraphic image of the left tibia of a Thoroughbred racehorse with severe left hindlimb lameness. There is diffuse intense increased radiopharmaceutical uptake *(arrows)* in the distal aspect of the tibial diaphysis consistent with a spiral tibial stress fracture. Despite enforced stall confinement, the horse sustained a catastrophic fracture 30 days after diagnosis.

of locations.[13] Radiological examination can confirm diagnosis in the majority of but not in all horses.[25,28,31,32] Radiological abnormalities include cortical thickening, periosteal or endosteal bony reaction, and an oblique cortical fracture line.*

Ilium

The ilium is the most common site of stress-related bone injury in the pelvis (see Chapter 49).[11,13,15,17,67] Within the ilium the most frequent site is 10 to 15 cm lateral to the

*References 13, 25, 26, 28, 32, 88, 90.
†References 25, 26, 28, 32, 89, 90.
§References 25, 26, 28, 31, 32, 62.
ǀReferences 25, 28, 31, 32, 89, 90.

*References 25, 26, 28, 31, 32, 88.

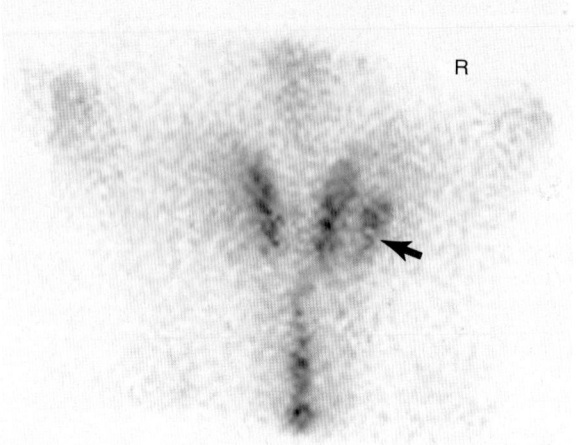

Fig. 100-14 • Dorsal delayed phase scintigraphic image of a 3-year-old Thoroughbred with moderate, focal increased radiopharmaceutical uptake *(arrow)* in the right ilium. This is a common area of uptake seen in racehorses with stress fractures of the ilium. Cranial is to the top of the image.

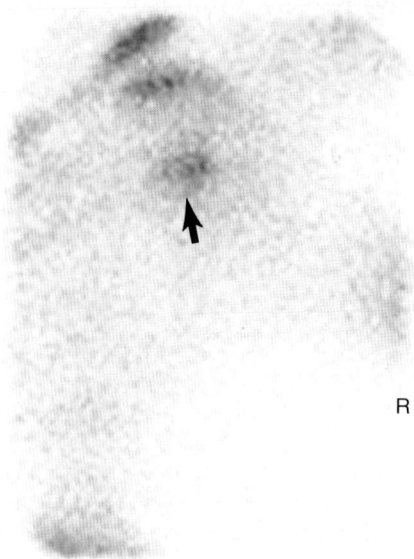

Fig. 100-15 • Right oblique delayed phase scintigraphic image (cranial is to the right) of the same horse as shown in Figure 100-14. Increased radiopharmaceutical uptake consistant with an ilial stress fracture *(arrow)* can readily be seen.

tuber sacrale.[15] Fractures usually originate at the caudal border of the ilium near the sacroiliac joint and course in a craniodorsal or craniolateral direction.[11] They may be unilateral and incomplete; however, bilateral injury is frequently seen.[11,15,67] Horses usually sustain an ilial stress fracture during race training,[2,33] and female and older racehorses are more likely to be affected, although this prevalence is derived from postmortem specimen data.[2,11] Fractures extending into the ilial shaft are occasionally seen, especially in National Hunt racehorses in Europe, and horses with this type of ilial stress fracture have a more guarded prognosis than those with fractures limited to the ilial wing.

Initially, most affected horses are lame, although lameness severity varies and lameness often resolves rapidly within 24 to 48 hours.[15,30,67] Shortened stride, hunched up back, and plaiting may be apparent.[15,67] Mildly affected horses may lack propulsion and exhibit poor action behind without overt lameness.[15] Horses may exhibit pain on palpation of the tuber sacrale on the affected side.[15,30,67] Subtle, ventral displacement of the ipsilateral tuber sacrale may be noted when fracture is complete, but this clinical finding is easily missed.[15,30,67] Muscle atrophy and resultant asymmetry of the sacral region may also be noted in horses with chronic fractures. Rectal palpation is useful if the fracture involves the ilial shaft and is complete. Gentle rocking of the pelvis while palpating may reveal the presence of crepitus or hematoma with complete fractures.[67]

Scintigraphic evaluation reveals marked, focal IRU associated with the ilial wing, just lateral to midline (Figure 100-14). Right and left dorsal oblique images of the pelvis enhance the diagnosis by decreasing superimposition and improving image geometry of surrounding structures (Figure 100-15).[12,91] Less commonly there is linear IRU extending from the tuber coxae axially along the caudal cortex of the ilial wing. Fractures of the ilial shaft may be more difficult to detect because of the greater overlying muscle mass resulting in shielding; subtle IRU consistent with a fracture is easily overlooked.

Ultrasonographic examination has been discussed previously (see page 937). Pelvic radiography is useful only for diagnosis of complete ilial stress fractures and requires general anesthesia in most horses. However, diagnostic images of the tuber coxae, the ilial shaft, the acetabulum of the pelvis, and the ischium can be obtained in a standing, sedated horse.

Lumbar Vertebrae

A postmortem study of Californian TBs identified lumbar vertebral stress fractures in 50% of specimens.[11] Lesions were characterized by incomplete fracture and focal periosteal proliferation. Vertebral laminar stress fractures were mostly unilateral, and affected specimens tended to be from older horses. All vertebral stress fractures were continuous with vertical articular clefts of the cranial articular facets, near the junction of the dorsal spinous process in most. They were positively associated with the severity of both impingement of dorsal spinous processes and OA of synovial articulations. Although they were a common postmortem finding, the clinical prevalence is less in a normal racing population. Antemortem physical examination findings of affected horses are vague at best. Nonspecific signs of back pain such as poor performance, hunched-up lumbar spine, and poor hindlimb propulsion may be noted. Scintigraphic abnormalities of the lumbar vertebrae are not common.[92] There is focal intense IRU in the affected vertebra; a dorsal image can help to determine if the lesion is on the left or the right. Radiological examination may reveal marked enlargement of the affected synovial articulation and a generalized increase in radiopacity.

Chapter 101

Bone Biomarkers

Joanna Price

References on page 1338

Bone is a complex tissue that undergoes change throughout life by the processes of bone formation by osteoblasts and bone resorption by osteoclasts.[1] Modeling and subsequent remodeling of bone are required for bone health and allow the skeleton to respond rapidly to changes in its internal and external environment. Bone formation and resorption of bone are "coupled"[2]; the cycle of remodeling begins with the recruitment of osteoclasts, which attach to the bone surface and resorb the subjacent bone matrix. After osteoclasts evacuate a resorption pit, osteoblasts differentiate from mesenchymal precursors and fill in the lacuna with new bone matrix.[3] In a healthy adult skeleton, formation and resorption are balanced. However, the balance is changed during growth, in response to altered exercise, by hormonal changes, during ageing, after therapeutic intervention, in metabolic bone disease, in neoplasia, and in response to injuries such as stress fractures.[4-6] Changes in subchondral bone metabolism are also potentially important in the pathogenesis of osteoarthritis (OA).[7,8] A challenge is to develop sensitive and specific noninvasive methods to detect changes in bone turnover in vivo. Abbreviations used in this chapter are summarized in Box 101-1.

Changes in bone mass and structure are assessed using techniques such as quantitative ultrasound (QUS), dual energy x-ray absorbiometry (DEXA), and quantitative computed tomography (QCT).[9-11] However, it may take several months for changes in bone mass and architecture to be of a sufficient magnitude to be detected with these methods. Furthermore, QCT and DEXA are not straightforward to use in a conscious horse, and use is restricted to ex vivo or in vivo research studies. Magnetic resonance imaging (MRI) is being used increasingly to study bone pathology in people,[12] but in a standing horse it can be used only for the distal aspect of the limb. It is expensive and not appropriate for screening potentially at-risk populations. In contrast, bone biomarkers measure dynamic changes in bone cell activity and can be measured in body fluids using relatively inexpensive straightforward methods. Biomarker measurements can be repeated at frequent intervals and so are convenient to use in the field. Although bone biomarkers remain predominantly research tools, considerable investigation has been undertaken on potential clinical applications. Soon it is highly likely that selected biomarkers will be used in conjunction with other tools to identify at-risk horses.[13,14]

Ideally, a biomarker should be measurable in body fluids by a sensitive and specific technique and be specific to its tissue of origin. Detailed molecular characterization of bone has led to the development of biomarkers with increased specificity. Progress in equine bone biomarker research has been led by work in people—in particular, use of biomarkers to detect osteoporosis.[15-17] There are a number of equine-specific assays, but most assays in use were originally developed for people.

Bone biomarkers are generally classified as markers of bone formation or markers of bone resorption or degradation, although some reflect changes in both processes (Tables 101-1 and 101-2). In general, bone biomarkers are enzymes expressed by osteoblasts or osteoclasts or organic components released during the synthesis and resorption of bone matrix.[15-17] However, many bone biomarkers are present in tissues other than bone and may therefore be influenced by other physiological processes. Because each biomarker may reflect a different physiological process, it is preferable to assay for a combination of markers, as this will provide more information on bone (re)modeling. However, human studies have shown that in certain diseases individual markers give more useful information than others,[15] and the same may be true in horses. Other criteria that determine the value of any biochemical marker are whether the factors that control its synthesis and metabolic pathway are understood and what factors influence its biological variability. For many biomarkers used in human clinical studies, surprisingly little is known about the regulation of synthesis and metabolism, and in horses even less is understood about these variables.

BOX 101-1
Abbreviations

ALP	Alkaline phosphatase
BALP	Bone-specific alkaline phosphatase
BGP	Bone gla-protein
BMD	Bone mineral density
CTX	Type I collagen C-terminal telopeptide
DEXA	Dual-energy x-ray absorbiometry
DMD	Dorsal metacarpal disease
DPD	Deoxypyridinoline
GGHyl	Glucosylgalactosylhydroxylysine
Ghyl	Galactosylhydroxylysine
HPLC	High-performance liquid chromatography
Hyp	Hydroxyproline
ICTP/CTX-MMP	Carboxy-terminal cross-linked telopeptide of type I collagen
IGF-1	Insulin-like growth factor 1
IRMA	Immunoradiometric assay
MRI	Magnetic resonance imaging
NTX	Type I collagen N-terminal telopeptide
OA	Osteoarthritis
OCa	Osteocalcin
PICP	Carboxy-terminal propeptide of type I collagen
PINP	Amino-terminal propeptide of type I collagen
PYR	Pyridinoline
QCT	Quantitative computed tomography
QUS	Quantitative ultrasound
RIA	Radioimmunoassay
WGL	Wheat germ lectin

TABLE 101-1

Bone Formation Biomarkers				
BIOMARKER	METHODS USED	BODY FLUID	SOURCE	COMMENTS
Bone-specific alkaline phosphatase (BALP)	ELISA	Serum SF	Bone	Some cross-reactivity with liver ALP?
Osteocalcin	RIA ELISA	Serum SF	Bone	Specific osteoblast product
Type I collagen propeptide (PICP)	RIA ELISA	Serum SF	Type I collagen	May be contribution from tissues other than bone

ALP, Alkaline phosphatase; *ELISA*, enzyme-linked immunosorbent assay; *RIA*, radioimmunoassay; *SF*, synovial fluid.

TABLE 101-2

Bone Resorption Biomarkers				
MARKER	METHODS USED	BODY FLUID	SOURCE	COMMENTS
Deoxypyridinoline (DPD)	HPLC ELISA	Urine Serum	Mature collagen in bone and dentin	Good specificity
Carboxy-terminal cross-linked telopeptide of type I collagen (ICTP, CTX-MMP)	RIA	Serum	Type I collagen	May be contribution from tissues other than bone
Carboxy-terminal cross-linking telopeptide of type I collagen (CTX-I)	ELISA ECLA	Urine Serum SF	Type I collagen	May be contribution from tissues other than bone
Collagen I (Col 1)	Indirect determination by subtracting Col CEQ from C1, 2C (both measured by ELISA)	Serum SF	Type I collagen	May be contribution from tissues other than bone

ECLA, Electrochemiluminescence assay; *ELISA*, enzyme-linked immunosorbent assay; *HPLC*, high-performance liquid chromatography; *RIA*, radioimmunoassay; *SF*, synovial fluid.

BIOMARKERS THAT REFLECT CHANGES IN BONE FORMATION

Bone formation biomarkers are synthesized by osteoblasts and reflect different aspects of osteoblast activity. They are all measured in serum or plasma (see Table 101-1).

Bone-Specific Alkaline Phosphatase

Alkaline phosphatase (ALP) is associated with the plasma membrane of osteoblasts and is required for osteoid formation and matrix mineralization.[18] Total serum ALP is derived from numerous sources and is not a specific marker of bone formation. However, because posttranslational modifications of tissue-specific ALP (which encodes bone, liver, and kidney isoforms of ALP) occur, different methods have been developed that enable separation and quantification of these isoforms. Although numerous techniques exist to characterize equine ALP isoenzymes, electrophoresis and precipitation of bone-specific ALP (BALP) with wheat germ lectin (WGL) are used most commonly.[19,20] The WGL assay is more specific than a human immunoradiometric (IRMA) assay, which shows some cross-reactivity with liver ALP in horses.[19] However, other, more user-friendly human immunoassays have now been validated for use in horses.[21] BALP predominates in serum during growth, and this is reflected in the high concentrations of BALP measured in young horses, although the proportion of the bone isoform decreases to approximately 50% in adults.[22] The observation that ALP activity in subchondral bone is increased in equine osteochondrosis[23] provided the first indication that BALP may be a useful marker for analyzing changes in subchondral bone associated with equine joint disease (BALP as a potential biomarker for joint disease is discussed in a later section).

Osteocalcin

Osteocalcin (OCa), which is otherwise known as *bone gla-protein* (BGP) is the most abundant noncollagenous protein in bone matrix, and a small fraction is released into the circulation after synthesis by osteoblasts. The only other cells to express OCa protein are odontoblasts and hypertrophic chondrocytes, so OCa has tissue specificity, and it has been widely used as a sensitive and specific marker of osteoblast function in human clinical studies. Numerous studies have described the measurement of OCa in horses and the factors that influence OCa levels.[24-27] Several methods have been used to measure OCa in horses, and a number of equine-specific assays have been developed; recently I used a competitive human immunoassay that has been validated for equine use.[28] OCa is highly labile; therefore samples should be processed rapidly (within 90 minutes). For OCa assays, equine serum can be stored at −20° C for up to 26 weeks, although long-term storage should be below −25° C.[29] OCa levels are affected by general anesthesia; therefore sampling during surgery may give misleading results.[30]

The Carboxy-Terminal Propeptide of Type I Collagen

Type I collagen is the most abundant collagen in bone, and the procollagen molecule contains both amino (PINP) and carboxy-terminal (PICP) extension domains, which are split off before fibril formation and released into the circulation. These propeptides provide quantitative measures of newly synthesized type I collagen, and in people serum levels reflect the rate of bone formation. PICP can be measured in horses by human radioimmunoassay (RIA).[31] However, type I collagen is not bone specific, and synthesis in other soft tissues may contribute to PICP concentrations in serum. For example, increased levels have been observed after tendon injury,[32] and there is a peak in PICP levels during rapid weight gain in growing Thoroughbreds (TBs).[33] Unfortunately, the human PINP assays that I have tested to date do not appear to show species cross-reactivity.

BIOMARKERS THAT MEASURE CHANGES IN BONE RESORPTION

The majority of bone biomarkers that reflect osteoclastic resorption of bone matrix are degradation products of type I collagen (see Table 101-2). Originally, collagen-related resorption biomarkers were measured in urine samples collected over a 24-hour period, but in practice this is difficult in the horse. More recently developed resorption markers can be measured in serum and synovial fluid.

Cross-Linked Collagen Telopeptides

Cross-links are located at the amino (N-) and carboxy (C-) termini in the type I collagen molecule, and a number of peptide assays have been developed for measuring telopeptides generated during osteoclastic resorption. The first of these was a RIA for the carboxy-terminal telopeptide of type I collagen (ICTP), which works well for serum of the horse. Because the enzyme cathepsin K cleaves the telopeptide, the assay is now abbreviated to CTX-MMP.[16] I and others used ICTP quite extensively in early bone biomarker studies in horses.[31,33-35]

More recently an immunoassay (CTX) was developed that recognizes ICTP containing an isoaspartyl peptide bond[36] and has been used increasingly in equine studies.[37,38] In people, CTX has been widely used to monitor changes in bone remodeling in osteoporosis and in joint disease,[15,37] although concentrations are affected by diet.

Other Biomarkers of Bone Resorption

A number of other biomarkers have been used to monitor bone resorption in the horse, including hydroxyproline (Hyp), hydroxylysine glycosides, and the pyridinium cross-links of collagen.[39-42] Pyridinoline (PYD) or hydroxylysyl pyridinoline (HP) is found in cartilage, bone, ligaments, and vessels, whereas deoxypyridinoline (DPD) or lysyl pyridinoline (LP) is found almost exclusively in bone and dentin.[43] During osteoclastic resorption the cross-links are cleaved and the components released into the circulation. Pyridinium cross-link concentrations measured in serum and urine are mainly derived from bone, and for many years urinary DPD, measured by high-performance liquid chromatography (HPLC), was considered the gold standard of resorption markers in human clinical research. HPLC

also provides a reliable method for measuring total urinary DPD and PYD concentrations in the horse. There are age-related decreases in PYD and DPD levels and a significant diurnal pattern in excretion.[44] In a study of acute tendon injury, urine PYD and DPD concentrations were increased, which probably reflects increased bone resorption associated with disuse.[40] I have used HPLC to measure DPD and PYD in horse serum, but this assay can be used reliably only in horses younger than 2 years of age, because serum concentrations in skeletally mature horses are below the limit of detection.[41] A human immunoassay was used to measure the free fraction of equine urinary DPD, and this assay can be adapted for the measurement of serum DPD.[45,46] Type I collagen degradation can also be determined indirectly by subtracting concentrations of a specific type II collagen degradation biomarker, Co1 234CEQ,[47] from concentrations of a biomarker that measures degradation of both type II and type I collagen (originally called COL2-3/4C$_{short}$, now referred to ascC1,2C).[48]

FACTORS THAT INFLUENCE BIOCHEMICAL MARKERS OF BONE CELL ACTIVITY IN HORSES

Because bone markers reflect instantaneous changes in bone cell activity, a large number of factors can be a source of preanalytical variability—controllable factors (e.g., food intake, circadian changes, or exercise) and uncontrollable factors (e.g., gender, age, or intercurrent disease).[49] A failure to define and appropriately manipulate controllable sources of variability and to account for uncontrollable variability limits interpretation of the results of bone marker measurements in clinical studies. Fortunately, the analytical variability of the assays is low if carried out by a specialist laboratory.

Circadian Variability

Human studies have shown that circadian variability may have a significant effect on markers of bone turnover, particularly urinary markers of bone resorption.[49] These circadian rhythms can be affected by age, disease, fasting, and drugs. Circadian rhythms in urinary PYD and DPD excretion have been described in adult geldings with peak levels occurring between 02.00 and 08.00—a pattern of change similar to that described in people.[40] In a study of six 2-year-old TB mares, changes in three bone biomarkers (OCa, ICTP, and PICP) and insulin-like growth factor 1 (IGF-1) were measured over a 24-hour period. There was a significant circadian rhythm for OCa (estimated peak at 09:00) and IGF-1 (estimated peak at 17:30) but no significant circadian rhythm for PICP or ICTP.[50] Others had previously described circadian rhythmicity in OCa levels in horses of different ages, although this remains somewhat controversial.[25,40,51] Light may also influence OCa concentrations.[25] No circadian variability in CTX concentrations was found.[51] I recommend collecting samples at a similar time of day, preferably first thing in the morning before exercise.

Diet

Human studies have shown that fasting significantly reduces the circadian variation in serum levels of CTX.[52] To date, no effect of feeding on bone biomarkers has been described. Little is known about the influence of diet on bone turnover markers in horses; no short-term effect on

OCa concentrations was found after feeding.[25] Calcium supplementation has been found to suppress bone turnover in women.[53] Dietary mineral supplements, widely used in horses, may influence bone markers.

Seasonal Changes

Time of year may influence bone turnover in horses, and this may be particularly important during growth. Monthly variability in ALP and OCa concentrations has been found in Finnhorse foals[54]; bone turnover markers in TB yearlings have been found to increase between midwinter and early summer.[33] A similar seasonal pattern of change in OCa was seen in a longitudinal study of 30 Ardenner horses from approximately 1 to 2 years of age.[37] CTX-I concentrations are also affected by season, with levels reaching a nadir in November before rising from November to April. In TBs the influence of season on bone biomarkers declines with age. Bone biomarkers were measured every month in more than 100 2-year-old TBs, and season did not have a significant effect on OCa, PICP, or ICTP concentrations.[34]

Age

In horses, as in people, bone biomarkers are higher during skeletal growth than in adults. I do not know if bone turnover increases in old horses as it does in people. An inverse relationship with age was described for several bone biomarkers in different horse breeds including OCa,* BALP,[19,22,31] PICP, ICTP,[33,34,56] PYD, and DPD.[44] The decrease in bone turnover markers is most substantial during the first year of life, but levels do not plateau until 3 to 4 years of age. Comparison of ICTP, PICP, and OCa changes with age in early- and late-born foals showed that age-related decreases in these biomarkers were more distinct in late-born foals,[56] indicating a difference in the rate of skeletal development in foals born at different times of year. This may reflect increased activity in late-born foals that were turned out to pasture immediately after birth, whereas early-born foals were initially kept confined. Generally, biomarkers of bone formation and bone resorption have a similar pattern of change, because bone remodeling involves resorption of bone at some sites (e.g., the endosteum) and formation at others (e.g., periosteal surfaces and the metaphyses). However, an age-related decrease in CTX-I concentrations is not observed. There was no effect of age on CTX-I concentrations in 30 Ardenner horses 1 to 2 years of age[37]; however, levels increased at 2 to 52 weeks of age.[38,57] These results call into question the bone specificity and thus the value of this biomarker in the horse.

Any study of bone biomarkers must control for the effects of age, especially in young horses. Serial marker measurements (i.e., use of the horse as its own control) are likely to be most informative in young horses. Ideally each laboratory should establish its own reference ranges for each marker in horses of different ages. Published reference ranges are of questionable value because absolute levels of these biomarkers vary significantly among laboratories.

Gender

In people there are gender differences in bone biomarkers, and these vary with age.[49] In horses this may depend on the specific biomarker and/or the horse's age. There were higher OCa levels in TB fillies of 24 to 36 months of age, but no gender difference was observed in younger horses.[55] There was no effect of gender on OCa and CTX-I concentrations,[37] on OCa concentration in Standardbreds of different ages,[24] or on OCa or ICTP concentrations in Warmblood or draft horses older than 4 years of age.[26] However, in a longitudinal study of 2-year-old TBs in race training in the United Kingdom (84 colts and 63 fillies), ICTP and OCa concentrations were higher in colts than in fillies, but there was no gender difference in PICP concentrations.[34] Lower biomarker concentrations in fillies may reflect smaller bone size and/or earlier sexual maturation.

Pregnancy, Lactation, and the Estrous Cycle

The calcium requirements during pregnancy and lactation are met, at least in part, by changes in maternal bone turnover, and in people an increase in markers of bone resorption precedes an increase in markers of bone formation.[58] Although not extensively studied in horses, OCa levels were unchanged in Selle Francais mares during the first 5 months after birth.[59] Bone cell activity in people is regulated by sex hormones.[60] In horses both OCa and ICTP concentrations were higher during the luteal phase of estrus,[61] which is consistent with lower estrogen concentrations being associated with increased bone turnover. The stage of estrus must be considered as a potential source of uncontrollable variability in bone biomarker concentrations in horses as in people.[49]

Breed

Ethnic differences in bone turnover have been described in people,[49] and horse type must also be considered as a potential effect on bone markers. The concentrations of OCa were lower and ICTP levels higher in draft horses compared with Warmbloods[26], which may relate to different rates of bone remodeling. This is not surprising considering the wide variation in skeletal size between different types of horse.

Intercurrent Disease

Little is known about the effect of different diseases on equine bone biomarkers. Any condition that affects bone metabolism (e.g., nutritional hyperparathyroidism) or marker clearance (e.g., kidney disease) will influence marker concentration. Liver disease may lead to increased cross-reactivity of BALP assays with the liver isoform of ALP. Fortunately these diseases are not common in equine athletes. However, an unrelated undiagnosed disease could contribute to circulating levels of a biomarker and misinterpretation of results.

CLINICAL APPLICATIONS FOR BONE BIOMARKERS

Bone biomarkers have been used in human medicine to study metabolic bone disease, particularly postmenopausal osteoporosis,[16,17] for prediction of fracture risk and bone loss, and for monitoring the effects of therapy.[62-64] The most valuable clinical applications for bone biomarkers in the horse, particularly if measured serially in the same horse, will be for identification of horses at risk of injury or for monitoring the effects of treatment. An important research application is to monitor the effects of exercise on

---

*References 24, 26, 37, 38, 55, 56.

the equine skeleton. However, because bone biomarkers reflect turnover in the *whole* skeleton and are affected by numerous variables there will always be an overlap between marker levels in normal and affected horses. Thus, in my opinion, it is unlikely that any bone biomarker measured as a "one off" will be able to function as a diagnostic test with a high level of discriminatory power.

Bone Biomarkers and Fracture

In order to assess bone biomarkers as predictors of risk of fracture (or any other condition), prospective studies are required that relate baseline bone biomarker levels to subsequent risk of injury. Bone biomarkers can be used to predict osteoporotic fracture in people.[62,63] In a prospective study bone biomarkers (ICTP, PICP, CTX-I, and OCa) were measured at the start of the training season in more than 500 2-year-old and more than 300 3-year-old flat racehorses to determine if fracture could be predicted in the subsequent training season.[65] The incidence of fracture was 11.6% (60 horses) but the bone biomarkers measured were unable to identify horses that sustained a fracture. Measurement of bone biomarkers longitudinally (monthly) in flat racehorses in training also failed to demonstrate a relationship between biomarkers and fracture.[66] However, a field study of horses in training undertaken in the United States showed a relationship between biomarkers and injury risk.[67] Whether bone biomarkers have better predictive value in older horses when the biological variability associated with skeletal growth is reduced remains to be determined.

Bone Biomarkers and Dorsal Metacarpal Disease

Dorsal metacarpal disease (DMD) is a common problem in young racehorses associated with accumulated distance trained at canter and high speed.[68] In a study of 165 2-year-old TBs in training it was demonstrated that bone biomarkers measured at the start of training may have value for identifying horses at risk of developing DMD in the subsequent training and racing season.[69] OCa, PICP, and ICTP were measured in November to early December, and training and veterinary records monitored for the next 10 months. OCa and ICTP were significantly higher in horses that subsequently developed DMD (horses with DMD were defined as having an episode where clinical signs of DMD were sufficiently severe for a horse to miss 5 consecutive days of training). A multivariable logistic regression model indicated that horses with ICTP concentrations above 12,365 mcg/L and older than 20.5 months are 2.6 times more likely to develop DMD.

Bone Biomarkers and Osteochondrosis

Several studies have used biomarkers to identify young growing horses which have, or are at risk of, developing developmental orthopedic disease (DOD), osteochondrosis in particular. Osteochondrosis is associated with changes in bone as well as cartilage[70] and so it is appropriate to study both bone and cartilage biomarkers in the context of this condition. A small cross-sectional study demonstrated that ICTP concentrations were elevated in DOD, indicating that this disease is associated with increased bone resorption.[71] However, in a study of Hanoverian foals there was no relationship between bone biomarker concentrations (OCa, ICTP, and PICP) and predisposition

to develop osteochondrosis,[56] although this study did not grade the severity of osteochondrosis. In contrast, there was a relationship between OCa concentrations and severity of osteochondrosis at 5 months in Dutch Warmblood foals.[72] There was also a significant correlation between OCa concentrations at 2 weeks of age and the number of osteochondrosis lesions detected radiologically at 5.5 and 11 months,[38] although there was no significant relationship between CTX-I and radiological status. OCa concentration at 2 weeks of age was also significantly related to necropsy score in hindlimb joints. Further studies in larger populations are required to confirm whether OCa, together with specific cartilage biomarkers, provide a reliable clinical tool for identifying young horses at risk of developing osteochondrosis.

Bone Biomarkers and Osteoarthritis

A substantial amount of research has been directed at the value of biomarkers for assessing cartilage and bone anabolism and catabolism in equine OA.[73] The relationship between biomarkers of bone degradation and synthesis is reviewed because subchondral bone plays an important role in the pathogenesis of traumatic joint disease.[74]

BALP is a potentially useful marker for analyzing changes in subchondral bone in equine OA. ALP activity in subchondral bone is increased in equine osteochondrosis.[23] In a cross-sectional study of OA, synovial fluid concentrations of BALP were significantly correlated with levels of two cartilage biomarkers and the degree of joint damage identified by arthroscopy.[75] In TB racehorses with osteochondral injuries in the fetlock joints, BALP concentrations in serum were significantly lower than in unaffected controls.[21] BALP concentrations were significantly higher in synovial fluid from affected carpal joints compared with normal joints. Concentrations of BALP in serum with less than 30 U/L and more than 22 U/L and a ratio of synovial fluid to serum BALP greater than 0.5 were predictive of osteochondral injury. OCa also reflects bone anabolism but was not useful in detecting early subchondral bone disease in exercised horses.[76] However, a later study by the same group used a range of serum biomarkers to differentiate joint pathology and exercise-induced changes; OCa concentrations did correlate with measures of pain and modified Mankin score.[77] More recently a large number of bone and cartilage biomarkers were measured in treadmill-exercised 2-year-olds with or without an experimentally induced OA lesion.[78] OCa and type I collagen degradation were increased in the synovial fluid of OA joints compared with exercise-alone joints. Serum OCa and type I collagen concentrations were also significantly higher in OA-affected horses. CTX-I was not useful for separating early experimentally induced OA from exercise alone. In contrast, in human OA, CTX-I had value as a marker of bone resorption.[15]

EFFECTS OF EXERCISE ON BONE BIOMARKERS

The responsiveness of bones to changes in mechanical load ensures that skeletal mass and architecture are sufficiently robust to prevent injury.[79] Bone biomarkers provide a potentially valuable tool for studying the effect of exercise on bone and thus could possibly be used to help identify those training regimens that are osteogenic compared with those that may be harmful, if the effects of exercise and disease can be distinguished.[78] There are conflicting results on the effects of exercise on bone biomarkers in horses. It was suggested that a higher OCa:ICTP ratio in Warmblood horses compared with draft horses may reflect a positive modeling response in horses having regular daily work.[26] Increased PICP, ICTP, and BALP concentrations have been found in treadmill-exercised 2-year-old female TBs compared with unexercised controls,[80] perhaps reflecting increased remodeling from accumulated fatigue damage associated with 18 months of training on a hard surface. In contrast, a follow-up study showed that a much shorter period of training, which increased bone mineral density in the exercised group, was associated with decreased ICTP and OCa concentrations.[81] A decrease in OCa was also observed when Quarter Horses commenced race training,[82] and two other studies showed lower OCa concentrations at the end of a training period.[83,84] In TBs in commercial race training there were decreased OCa concentrations as the intensity of work increased.[66] However, OCa levels increased in young Standardbreds after 6 months of race training.[85] In an experimental study designed specifically to discriminate between changes in cartilage and bone biomarkers with treadmill exercise and OA, synovial fluid and serum OCa and collagen I concentrations increased.[78] There was no clear pattern of change with CTX-I, whereas a previous study in Warmblood foals found higher CTX-I levels in foals trained for the first 5 months of life compared with those raised at pasture or in a box stall.[57]

Changes in bone turnover may not be revealed using bone biomarkers because a training regimen is not sufficiently osteogenic. For example, lunging yearling Quarter Horses had no effect on OCa levels[86]; no change on DPD or OCa concentrations was observed when previously stabled Arabian horses returned to training.[45]

Although increased loading has anabolic effects on bone, disuse is catabolic and leads to increased resorption. Bone biomarkers have shown that a period of immobility may predispose horses to injury. When Arabian yearlings were confined to a stable, serum concentrations of the resorption marker DPD increased, whereas levels of the formation marker OCa decreased compared with levels in controls kept at pasture. There was a decrease in bone mineral content.[45] A decrease in OCa levels after transfer of foals from pasture to winter stabling has been described.[54] However, age and/or a horse's previous exercise history may influence the effect of immobility on bone turnover because OCa and Hyp levels were unchanged during a 12-week period of stall confinement in older Arabian horses despite a decrease in bone mineral content.[42]

MONITORING RESPONSES TO THERAPY

To date, monitoring responses to therapy has proved to be one of the most valuable applications of bone biomarkers in human medicine.[16] The newer bone resorption markers in particular provide a very sensitive measure of the effects of antiresorptive agents on bone turnover. In osteoporotic women, type I collagen N-terminal telopeptide (NTX) and CTX decrease within months of bisphosphonate treatment.[64] There is already some evidence that in horses bone biomarkers may be useful for monitoring responses to therapy and also for assessing the potentially harmful

effects of drugs on the equine skeleton. For example, bone biomarkers have showed that corticosteroids have a negative effect on osteoblast activity, and in the long term this could lead to osteoporotic changes in bone.[87,88] OCa levels have been found to be significantly decreased after intravenous, intramuscular, and oral administration of dexamethasone and triamcinolone acetonide.[87,88] In contrast, levels did not decrease after intraarticular injection of methylprednisolone acetate, which suggests that this route of corticosteroid administration may not have long-term adverse effects on bone.[89] Serum BALP did not reflect decreased mineral apposition rate associated with phenylbutazone administration[20]; however, this was a relatively short-term study, and in people changes in bone formation biomarkers may not occur for several months after treatment.[54] Bone marker levels were increased after growth hormone administration in horses and thus could be useful as indirect measures for detecting its abuse in racehorses.[90] More recently, CTX-I and BALP were measured in a study designed to test the effect of the bisphosphonate tiludronate on disuse osteoporosis induced by the application of a cast to the left forelimb.[91] There was a transient, rapid decrease in CTX-I after tiludronate administration.

In my opinion the use of bone and cartilage markers to monitor the effects of treatment may be one of the most important applications for the markers in equine orthopedics, to provide an objective reflection of how treatment regimens influence catabolic and anabolic processes in bone.

In conclusion, bone biomarkers provide a relatively inexpensive, straightforward, and noninvasive method for studying changes in the activity of cells responsible for forming and resorbing bone. To the basic scientist bone biomarkers can contribute to understanding the cellular mechanisms that underlie normal and abnormal bone development and (re)modeling. To the clinical researcher bone biomarkers provide insight into disease pathogenesis and assist in developing prevention and treatment strategies for equine musculoskeletal diseases. The inherent biological variability of bone biomarkers means that they are unlikely to be appropriate for diagnosing bone disease with absolute certainty when measured on a single occasion. This notwithstanding, there is accumulating evidence that bone biomarkers are potentially useful in the clinical setting, particularly when measured longitudinally with other biomarkers and used alongside diagnostic imaging modalities. Future research needs to be directed at replicating results obtained from experimental and relatively small clinical studies in large multicenter studies. There needs to be greater understanding of how variables such as exercise, growth and intercurrent disease may influence bone biomarkers, and administrators of laboratories need to start developing cost-effective, reliable biomarker panels appropriate for different clinical scenarios. If work in this area continues to progress, in 10 to 15 years bone biomarkers will likely be part of an established repertoire of tools that equine clinicians will have at their disposal for identifying horses at risk for developing disease, for achieving early diagnosis of bone and/or joint diseases, and for monitoring disease and repair progression. Inevitably this will lead to a reduction in the prevalence of lameness and wastage in equine athletes, racehorses in particular, an outcome which remains a priority and a major challenge.

Chapter 102

The Bucked-Shin Complex

▣ ETIOLOGY, PATHOGENESIS, AND CONSERVATIVE MANAGEMENT

David M. Nunamaker

Conditions of fatigue failure of bone and inadequacy of bone modeling and remodeling of the third metacarpal bone (McIII) in the racehorse are part of a condition known as *bucked shins* or *dorsal metacarpal disease*.[1,2] Bucked shins start in young healthy racehorses, usually Thoroughbreds (TBs) and Quarter Horses, but occasionally Standardbreds (STBs), that undergo intense training for racing, usually as 2-year-olds, while the skeleton is still immature and in the growth phase (Figure 102-1, *A*). The true incidence of

References on page 1340

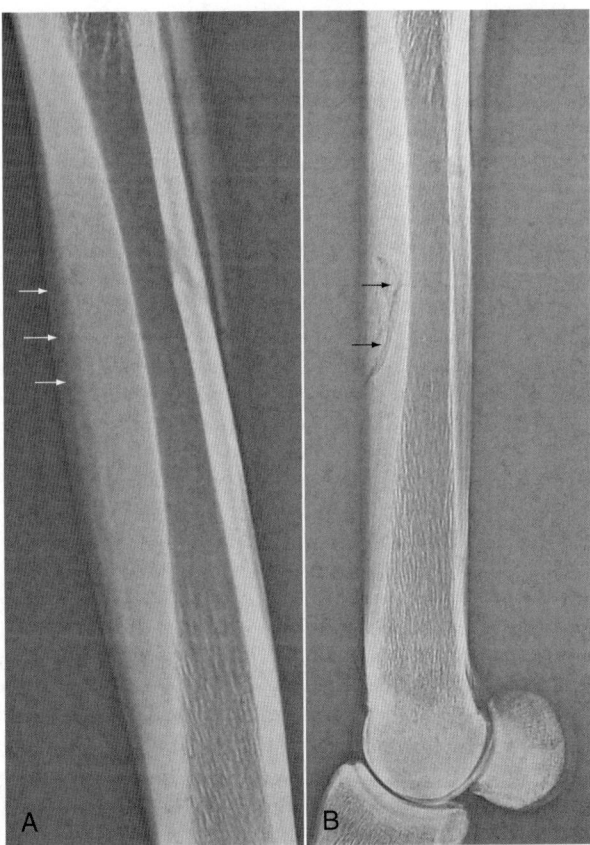

Fig. 102-1 • A, Dorsolateral-palmaromedial oblique radiographic image of a third metacarpal bone (McIII). Periosteal new bone formation *(arrows)* over the dorsomedial aspect of the McIII is evidence of bucked shins. **B,** Lateromedial radiographic image of the metacarpal region. This dorsal cortical fracture of the dorsolateral aspect of the McIII represents a common type of fatigue (stress) fracture *(arrows)* that usually occurs months after an episode of bucked shins.

bucked shins is unknown and may vary geographically, but reports range from 30% to 90%. A North American questionnaire cited an incidence of 70%.[1] Stress fractures (dorsal cortical or saucer fractures) usually occur some months after initial signs of bucked shins and may be a potentially life-threatening injury if a horse is raced or exercised at speed (see Figure 102-1, *B*). The diagnosis of bucked shins is easy and often made by the trainer or owner. The history of sudden tenderness or soreness of the left McIII (in North America) or both the McIIIs after high-speed work or the first race, or soreness developing the day after, are cardinal signs of early bucked shins. Horses with severe disease manifest acute lameness and extreme sensitivity to palpation of the dorsal cortex of the McIII and are unwilling to train or race. All gradations of pain or disability may be seen. Swelling and tenderness may suggest new bone proliferation. Radiology is helpful to determine the amount of periosteal new bone formation, which determines prognosis. Large accumulations of periosteal new bone on the dorsal or dorsomedial surface of the McIII suggest a serious imbalance between exercise and bone fatigue and may portend actual stress fractures that will be seen on the dorsolateral aspect of the McIII some months later.

RESEARCH FINDINGS

An understanding of the etiology, pathomechanics, and pathogenesis of bucked shins in the TB is helpful in determining prevention and/or treatment modalities and training regimens. It was formerly suggested that bucked shins resulted from microfractures on the dorsal aspect of the McIII, caused by high-speed exercise. However, microfractures should heal without periosteal callus, which does not fit with the clinical observation of extensive periosteal new bone on the dorsomedial aspect of the McIII. Work in our laboratory led us to propose a different cause of bucked shins[3] and an exercise program that significantly reduces the incidence of bucked shins and may help to eliminate catastrophic stress fractures. The following summarizes our investigations.

Geometric Properties of the Third Metacarpal Bone: Comparison of Thoroughbreds and Standardbreds

The McIIIs of TBs and STBs of known age were examined, and comparisons were made between breeds of a particular age group and among the age groups of a particular breed. The second moments of area relate to bending stiffness in dorsopalmar and mediolateral directions and were used to determine the minimum and maximum principal moments of inertia (I_{min} and I_{max}). The most significant changes in the bone occurred at the midsections between the ages of 1 and 2 years, but continued change occurred until age 3 or 4 years. I_{min} was smaller in the yearling TBs but larger in the adult TBs compared with STBs. During the first 2 to 4 years of life, I_{min} changed to a greater extent in TBs.[4]

In Vitro Comparison of Local Fatigue Failure of the Third Metacarpal Bone

Dumbbell-shaped specimens machined from adult McIIIs from TBs and STBs were tested in fully reversed cyclic bending experiments using a constant-strain rotating

Thoroughbred and Standardbred McIII Fatigue Data

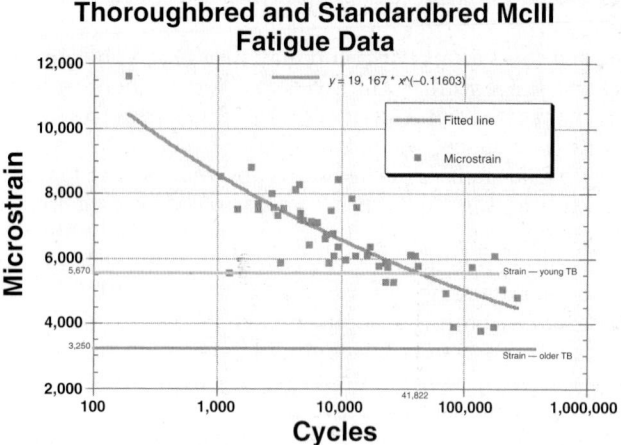

Fig. 102-2 • In vitro fatigue data are plotted for the adult Thoroughbred (TB) and Standardbred. The regression line shows where the third metacarpal bone *(McIII)* will fail from repeated cycles. Superimposition of the strain levels of young TBs shows that 41,822 cycles would result in fatigue failure. The superimposition of an older TB shows that more than a million cycles would be needed before bone failure.

cantilever model that measured load decrement. All tests were performed at 40 Hz and continued until the specimen broke or had a 30% loss of stiffness. Three different offsets were used to establish nominal strains of 7500, 6000, or 4500 microstrain in the specimens.

Data were analyzed using a power regression model for each horse and for each breed. Statistical differences were not found among the curves for individual horses of the same breed or for the curves between breeds. Pooled data then were used to describe fatigue characteristics of cortical specimens of the McIIIs from TBs and STBs of various ages, subjected fully to reversed cyclic loading (Figure 102-2).[5] The bone from young horses was much more susceptible to fatigue failure.

Because the in vitro fatigue was similar in TBs and STBs, other factors appeared to be important in the pathogenesis of fatigue failure of bone in the TB. This, together with the different inertial properties noted in STBs and TBs, led to the hypothesis that differences in training regimens or racing speeds between breeds might influence the incidence of disease.

Third Metacarpal Bone Stiffness Measurements

Whole bone stiffness measurements were made from horses of 2 months to 28 years of age using an Instron testing machine (Instron, Canton, Massachusetts, United States) and a nondestructive three-point dorsopalmar bending test. The bones showed general increases in stiffness until they reached a plateau at about 6 years of age.

The material included the McIIIs from 12 2-year-old TBs, three of which had bucked shins. These three horses had differences in stiffness between the left and right McIIIs of 16% to 27%, respectively, whereas other trained or control 2-year-olds had considerably smaller left-right differences.[6]

In Vivo Strain Measurements: Relationship to Exercise

Bone strain in the McIII was measured in horses of varying ages, training at or near racing speed, by placing a rosette strain gauge on the dorsolateral aspect of the McIII and recording using telemetry.[7] The mean peak compressive strain in four horses 2 years of age was −4841 ± 572 microstrain, compared with −3317 in a horse 12 years of age. One 2-year-old developed bucked shins, and its strain measurements were about 6 standard deviations greater than in the other three.

After acquiring in vivo strain data, we correlated these data with in vitro fatigue data previously generated by determining the average number of cycles that a young TB would gallop in training before the onset of bucked shins. The training records of six 2-year-old TBs that developed bucked shins were analyzed to determine the total distance worked before the onset of bucked shins. Stride length at canter, gallop, and racing speed was measured in a group of TBs to determine the number of strides (cycles) per mile. The total number of gait cycles was estimated based on the distances covered at a canter, at a gallop, and at work. The six horses were trained in these gaits for 10,000 to 12,000 cycles per month and developed bucked shins at 35,284 to 53,299 training cycles. These data were compared with the in vitro data described previously and showed good correlation (see Figure 102-2).

Changing from the trot to the gallop changed the principal strain direction by more than 40 degrees on the dorsolateral surface of the McIII. Although trotting horses showed tensile strains in the long axis of the bone on the dorsal or dorsolateral surface, at racing speeds this same surface of the bone showed compressive strains.[8]

Relationship of Exercise to Bone Fatigue

With the understanding that slow-speed gaits produced tensile strains on the dorsal surface of the McIII, whereas high-speed exercise induced compressive strains, a study was undertaken to determine the effects of different training regimens and track surfaces on the modeling and remodeling of the McIII in TBs.

Eight untrained 2-year-old TBs were divided into four groups of two horses each. Classical training methods were used for the horses in groups I and II. Group I horses trained on a dirt track. Group II horses trained on a wood chip track. Group III horses (control group) were not trained, but they were allowed free exercise in a large pasture. Group IV horses were trained using a modified classical training program on a dirt track.

The classical training program consisted of daily gallops (approximately 18-second furlongs or 11.2 m/sec) of 1 to 2 miles per day (1.6 to 3.2 km), followed by shorter workouts or breezes at racing speed (approximately 14-second furlongs or 14.4 m/sec) once every 7 to 10 days that increased in distance from 2 to 6 furlongs (0.4 to 1.2 km) progressively over the course of the study. The modified classical training method used similar daily gallops, but the frequency of the high-speed workouts increased to three per week, and distances increased progressively from 1 to 4 furlongs (0.2 to 0.8 km). After 5 months the McIIIs were harvested from all horses. Microradiographs of bone sections were made to determine the extent of the remodeling activity (Figure 102-3). Bone modeling on the periosteal and endosteal surfaces of the McIII changed the cross-sectional geometry differently among the experimental groups. Classically trained horses (groups I and II) responded with appositional new bone formation on the

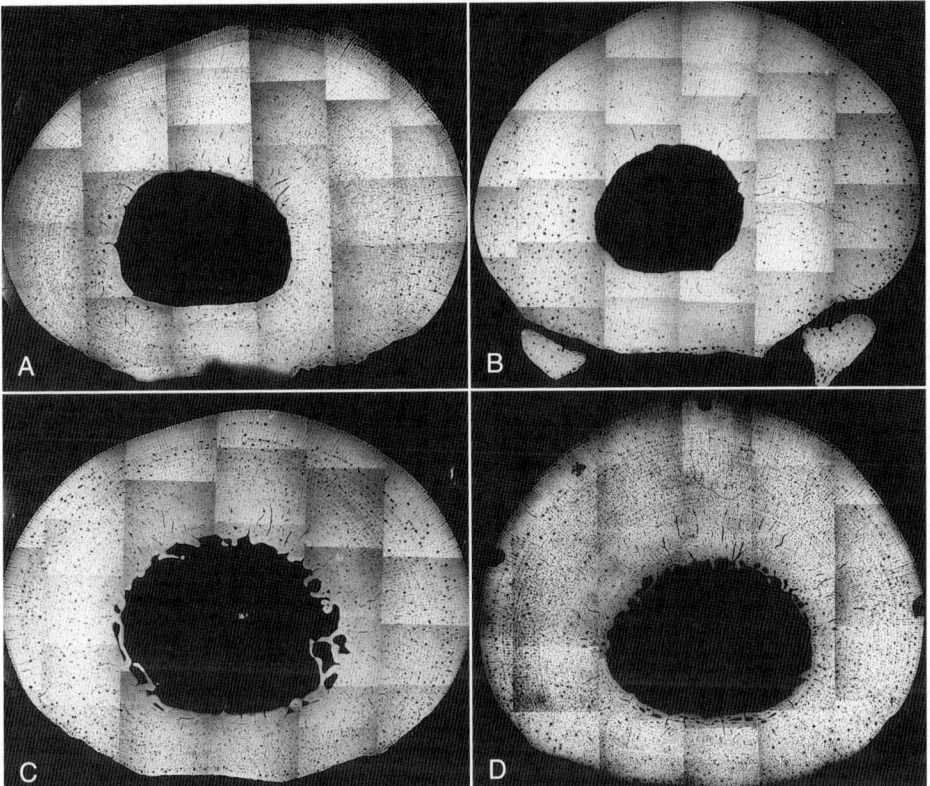

Fig. 102-3 • Fifty-percent length cross-sections of the third metacarpal bone were used to make these microradiographs. Individual photographs were taken with cross-sections magnified four times, and giant montages (approximately 50 × 70 cm) were constructed to be able to evaluate individual haversian systems of each individual bone of each horse. Lateral is to the left. **A,** Group I horses: classically trained on a dirt track. **B,** Group II horses: classically trained on a wood chip track. **C,** Group III horses: controls. **D,** Group IV horses: modified training on a dirt track. Changes in modeling, remodeling, and shape can be seen easily by comparing different groups. Group II horses appear to be earlier in the remodeling cycle than are group I horses, which already have remodeled in the medial and lateral cortices. All specimens are from the left forelimb, and increased new bone formation is seen on the medial surface of the classically trained horses (groups I and II). Modified training (group IV) and the control horses (group III) do not show this change. The lack of haversian remodeling in the dorsal-dorsolateral cortex of the classically trained horses in groups I and II is notable. In this area catastrophic stress fractures occur in racehorses.

dorsomedial periosteal surface, giving the impression that the medullary cavity, although reduced in diameter, was displaced laterally. Horses in the modified training group (group IV) had bone deposition dorsally and a slightly larger medullary cavity that was not displaced laterally. Control horses (group III) had new bone formation on the medial, lateral, and dorsal surfaces. The medullary cavity remained large and centrally placed. Examination of the McIII inertial properties showed that I_{min} in groups I, II, and III was similar, but the I_{min} of group IV horses was greater and was similar to the I_{min} previously reported for mature racehorses.

Microradiographic sections from the middiaphysis of the McIII showed that bone remodeling occurred only medially and laterally in groups I and II. Filling of secondary haversian systems with new bone was most complete in group I specimens, indicating that the remodeling process was advanced further in horses exercised on a harder surface. A distinct lack of remodeling activity was apparent in the dorsal and dorsolateral regions in groups I and II. Horses in groups III and IV showed extensive remodeling throughout the cortex, including remodeling in the dorsal and dorsolateral aspects.

These data suggested that in horses training on a hard surface, bone remodeling occurred at a faster rate than in horses training on a compliant (wood chip) surface. Previous studies showed that classically trained horses on a hard surface have a higher incidence of bucked shins than do horses trained on a more compliant surface. One horse in group I developed bucked shins during the training period. Inertial properties (I_{min}) of the McIII in the dorsopalmar direction were no different in horses trained on a hard or soft track. Horses in group IV had a significant change in I_{min} of the dorsal cortex of the McIII, similar to that seen in adult racehorses evaluated previously that were no longer at risk for developing bucked shins.[3] This supported the concept that exercise could be designed to optimize the shape and modeling or remodeling status of the McIII and thus reduce the incidence of bucked shins.[9]

Exercise Programs Designed to Decrease the Incidence of Fatigue Failure

To determine the efficacy of an adapted training program in decreasing the incidence of bucked shins, a prospective and retrospective study was performed using work training data from five commercial training stables. Two of the stables (2 and 5) were already using our modified classical training program, and the others (1, 3, and 4) were training in a classical manner. Horses in stables 1, 2, and 4 were trained on a commercial racetrack, whereas those in stables 3 and 5 were trained on private farm training tracks. All horses in the study were TBs, 2 years of age, and starting training for the first time and were followed for 1 year. Data collection stopped if horses developed bucked shins, were sold, or stopped training because of another event not related to bucked shins. The study included 11 years of training data from 226 2-year-olds. Fifty-six of the 226 horses developed bucked shins, and 170 horses completed the observation period or were sold.

Regression analysis and survival analysis techniques were used to explore the data. Horses in stable 2 had the best survival, and those in stables 1 and 4 the worst, and evaluation of data suggested that relationships between galloping and breezing were important. Horses in stable 2 had the highest breezing rate and the lowest incidence of bucked shins, whereas those in stables 1 and 4 had the highest galloping rates and the highest incidence of bucked shins.

Galloping increased the likelihood of bucked shins by 36.4%, whereas breezing short distances was protective, reducing the likelihood of bucked shins by 98.6%.[10] It is important to note that long-distance breeze rates are detrimental.[11] The winter of 1994 brought severe ice storms to the northeast. Horses in stable 2 could not be trained using the modified program and instead were trained using the standard classical program. An unintentional crossover design was created, and 62% of the horses trained that year developed bucked shins. When 1994 data are not used, only 9.3% of horses developed bucked shins.

In Vitro Bone Testing

In vitro compression testing of cylindrical specimens obtained from the McIIIs of 16 horses (139 specimens) in four different training regimens that included no training were tested to failure to determine differences in modulus and strength. These specimens included three horses that developed bucked shins. Because these in vitro studies showed no statistical differences in the material properties of bones with different training regimens, a change in material properties of bone is not a factor in the etiology or pathogenesis of bucked shins. From this study and previous ones carried out in our laboratory, it can be hypothesized that early in a TB's racing career the McIII experiences extreme strain conditions. These strains cause bone apposition on the dorsal periosteal surface of the McIII in an attempt to lessen the strains. This causes a change in the geometric properties (section properties) but not the material properties of the existing bone.

DISCUSSION

Two decades of evolutionary experiments and clinical observations based on an initial observation of a significant difference in the incidence of fatigue fractures between TB and STB racehorses have led to a natural model for fatigue failure of bone.[11,12] We can now compare in vitro and in vivo fatigue behavior and observe bone adaptation with different exercise regimens. Adaptive exercise was shown

to change the geometric properties of the McIII without changing the material properties, to influence bone modeling and remodeling, and to reduce the incidence of bucked shins and catastrophic fatigue failure of the McIII in the TB.[13]

Comparisons of TBs and STBs show major changes in inertial properties of the McIII resulting from growth and superimposed training. Comparisons of young TBs that are susceptible to fatigue failure, with older, resistant horses suggest that changes in bone inertial properties are an important factor affecting the incidence of bucked shins. Large McIII I_{min} values reflect probable increases in the McIII stiffness in the dorsopalmar direction and thus reduced peak strain during high-speed exercise. The inertial properties of the proximal aspect of the tibia were shown to predict development of fatigue fractures in military recruits,[14,15] just as the inertial property measurement of the McIIIs of 5-year-old TBs shows that these horses are no longer at risk for bucked shins.[4]

In vivo strain measurements of the McIII demonstrated higher peak strains under physiological loading than ever had been reported previously in any species. Although in vitro test conditions differed from the in vivo loading, both involved significant bending components that can be expected to produce accumulated fatigue failure in bone. Superimposition of the in vivo strains reported for the young and older horses at racing speed produced a striking predictive relationship for risk of developing bucked shins (see Figure 102-2).

Large surface strains, measured in vivo at high speeds on the dorsolateral aspect of the McIII in young TBs in training, contrast dramatically with the smaller strains measured in adults that have raced successfully. Strains, under a given load regimen, measured on the surface of bone relate to the modulus and inertial properties (section modulus) of the bone. Because inertial properties were shown to increase with age, and bone strains during high-speed exercise were shown to decrease in older horses, the hypothesis was that changes in bone inertial properties and modulus serve to lower the peak bone strains as a young racehorse matures. However, training regimens possibly can outpace adaptive response. In fact, we observed that a certain percentage of young horses actually increased the McIII surface strains after several months of training. Whole bone stiffness measurements showed right-to-left differences of up to 27% in horses in training, whereas no right-to-left difference was found in the nontrained control horses. Because bucked shins occur bilaterally but sequentially in TBs, usually on the left side before the right, the developmental stiffness changes in limbs possibly are not synchronized but may respond to the predominance of the left lead used by the horse in its racing gait as the horse works in a counterclockwise direction. Maximal strains at exercise and bone stiffness parameters probably change with time and may be declining on one side, while increasing on the other. Increasing bone strain measured at high speed during training, as seen in four of seven TBs, suggested rapid bone stiffness changes in vivo from exercise. Because we now believe that material properties of the bone do not change dramatically during this phase of training, this means that the horses must be providing larger forces on the bone (running faster or applying increased muscular input into the bones).

If Wolff's law is applied strictly, it follows that a bone that adapts to a particular peak tensile strain may not be prepared adequately to resist far larger peak compressive strains in the same location. Hence training adapts bone to training, and training that mimics racing adapts bone to racing.

An in vitro fatigue study of equine McIIIs showed a difference in fatigue resistance to bending loads in different anatomical quadrants. Bone that was loaded in bending around the physiological bending axis had greater fatigue resistance than bone bent at 90 degrees to this axis.[16]

We hypothesized that to adapt adequately for racing, the McIII should be exposed during training to strains of the actual magnitude and direction experienced during racing. Furthermore, the high incidence of bucked shins in TBs suggested that loading to produce such peak strains and concomitant adaptive remodeling did not occur in a large number of TBs in classical training programs before racing.

Previous in vivo studies using a functionally isolated rooster ulna, have shown that low numbers of loading cycles (four per day) were adequate to maintain bone mass. Thirty-six cycles were enough to stimulate bone formation.[17] The resulting periosteal new bone formation is the same type of bone reaction observed in the TB McIII with fatigue injury.

With these observations taken into account, an exercise (training) regimen was developed that modestly increased the small numbers of high-load cycles using peak load magnitudes and directions that were seen during racing. Increasing the number of short-distance workouts (breezes) from once every 7 to 10 days, as occurs with classical training programs, to three per week produced large changes in modeling, remodeling, and inertial property measurements of the McIII. Classical training produced little progressive change in the inertial properties of the McIII, whereas the new modified training program showed inertial property development that equaled or surpassed that observed in established older successful TBs, those horses apparently no longer susceptible to bucked shins.[3]

The idea of using exercise to produce adaptive bony remodeling is not new. Woo and colleagues[18] showed that 12 months of exercise in young pigs produced dramatic changes in the femur, increasing cross-sectional area by 23% and inertial properties (I_{min}) by 27%, without intrinsic bone property changes.[18] Milgrom and co-workers[19] looked for exercise that can adapt bone and showed that playing basketball for 2 years or more was protective in reducing the incidence of bone fatigue failure in military recruits.

In the 11-year longitudinal study, we proved that adaptive exercise could be used to reduce the incidence of bucked shins. The relative incidence of bucked shins in classically trained TBs is probably higher than we found. The mean time taken for horses to develop bucked shins was about 25 days shorter than the mean time to loss for other reasons. Bucked shins developed in most horses by 200 days in training. We would not expect horses in the modified training program to experience additional fatigue fractures after the observation period, because the McIII should resemble more closely that of adult, nonsusceptible racehorses.

Adaptive exercise changed the geometric parameters of a specific bone in a way that would be expected to reduce

fatigue damage while significantly reducing the incidence of bucked shins. This correlation, although not explicit proof of the interrelationship between the factors measured, is convincing.

In addition, approximately 10% of the catastrophic breakdown injuries involving the skeleton of TB racehorses are complete fractures of the McIII. These injuries are direct sequelae to fatigue fractures of the dorsolateral aspect of the McIII that are often seen several months after horses develop bucked shins. Theoretically, if bucked shins could be prevented there would be an immediate 10% decrease in the incidence of these catastrophic fractures and thereby a decrease in racing fatalities.

TRAINING TO PREVENT BUCKED SHINS

A training program was developed to limit the incidence of bucked shins and can be modified by trainers to suit their situations.[12,20]

The principles of this training program are the following:

1. Bone changes its shape and structure based on its use (Wolff's law). It therefore follows that training adapts bone to training, racing adapts bone to racing, and training that mimics racing adapts bone to racing.
2. Short, high-speed workouts are introduced into the training program early and often (two per week) to introduce bone to the forces it will experience during racing.
3. Galloping is done in moderation (1 mile/day, 6 days/week). Long gallops result in high mileage that may induce high-strain cyclic fatigue of bone.
4. Jogging is used for warm-up only and is not used to increase a horse's level of fitness, because jogging induces tension on the dorsal surface of the McIII. Once bone adapts to racing (6 to 8 months), this training program is no longer needed, because bone will not regress into its previous shape and architecture. Any successful program can then be instituted.

These principles were developed based on experimental studies that showed that at slow gaits the dorsal surface of the McIII is under tension and at high speed is bending to produce compression. Structurally, materials are designed differently to support tension or compression. Think how strong a rope is in tension and how useless it is in supporting loads in compression. Short, high-speed exercise exposes the bone to compression on its dorsal surface and introduces the bone to the loads expected during a race. Experimental studies showed that this sort of training regimen changed the cross-section of the McIII to the adult racing shape within 6 months.

Long, low-speed jogging adapts the bone only to jogging, creating tension on the dorsal surface of the McIII. In stable 2 in the icy winter of 1994 the horses were jogged for 30 days, without any high-speed exercise, and then resumed the exercise program. The incidence of bucked shins increased fivefold compared with previous years and returned to normal the following year. Although training is not a cookbook recipe for success, the fundamentals of the program are described here with an actual schedule.[12]

The schedule assumes that the young horse is broken to ride in the fall and is able to gallop 1 mile (18- to

20-second furlongs) by the end of December. The training program starts in January and can be broken into three stages. The principle involved is that the horse's bones need to see the strain environment of racing as soon as possible so that bone modeling and remodeling can begin in a timely manner. The training program is 6 days a week with Sundays off. The horses walk to and from the racetrack. On the track the horse walks ½ mile and jogs ½ mile to warm up. The horse then gallops 1 mile.

> **Stage 1**—Using the strategy just described, the horse will finish the gallops two times a week with a ⅛-mile open gallop in 15 seconds. This speed work is done on Tuesdays and Saturdays. This speed and distance of the open gallop is repeated 10 times (5 weeks).
>
> **Stage 2**—After 5 weeks of stage 1 gallops, the horse moves up in distance so that two times a week (Tuesday and Saturday) the horse will finish its gallop with ¼ mile in 30 seconds (15-second furlongs). This speed work is repeated 10 times, which takes up the next 5 weeks. All open gallops in stage 1 and stage 2 are at the end of the gallop and are included in the 1-mile gallop.
>
> **Stage 3**—After the completion of stage 2, the horse continues its training using speed work once a week (Saturday), breezing ¼ mile in approximately 26 seconds (13-second furlongs). This is repeated four times (4 weeks). In stage 3 the daily gallops are extended to 1¼ miles twice a week. After the fourth week the ¼-mile breeze is continued with a strong "gallop out" for an additional furlong. This makes the 3-furlong total about 40 seconds. This is done for an additional 3 weeks, giving stage 3 a total time of 7 weeks.

After stage 3, the McIII shape and architecture are effectively established for the longer high-speed workouts necessary for racing. The horse can now go on to 4- to 6-furlong workouts as needed to further develop other body systems to complete fitness for racing. The total time of this initial training program is 119 to 147 days, depending on the availability of a race for the horse. This does not include any downtime for sickness or injury. Gate work is started early and often in this program. The horses are introduced to the gate in January as the program starts. All young horses are turned out in a small paddock for 1 to 1½ hours of exercise before daily training. This training program has shown no increase in the injury rate of young horses. An excellent byproduct of this training program is the mental development of these 2-year-olds. Because of the very relaxed atmosphere of walking to and from the racetrack, these horses exhibit no anxiety about work. For this training program to work, the rider cannot be in a hurry to get back to the barn and on the next horse. The 2-year-olds are not anxious about speed work because it has been in the weekly schedule since the beginning of training. All the horses walk back to the barn. Walking is a great exercise that does not seem to negatively influence bone modeling or remodeling. The schedule described here for training to negate bucked shins is just that—a schedule. An understanding of the principles behind this training regimen is important. Training programs that take advantage of this information can be developed that will meet an individual horse's needs.

Horses that develop respiratory disease during training and are off for 10 days or more are backed up about 10 days in the training program. Shin sore horses are treated for soreness with phenylbutazone and ice water and are walked until soreness is gone. These horses then get put in an abbreviated program in which the breezing distances and galloping distances are cut in half. These horses are usually coming from a classical training program, in which bucked shins is a common occurrence. When presented with these horses (often from a 2-year-old in training sale), one is far better off putting them into this bone-conditioning program initially rather than going on with them and hoping that they do not develop bucked shins, as they invariably do. These horses take far longer to get to the first race. Sore horses should be individually evaluated based on clinical and radiological signs. In most horses that develop early shin soreness the training program can be modified and the horse can continue training. A short rest period with handwalking, the administration of phenylbutazone, and the application of ice water can get most horses back into training rather quickly.

Although bucked shins are commonly accepted by veterinarians, trainers, and owners as a normal training event in young TB racehorses, with estimated losses to the industry of $10,000,000 per year in lost training and racing days, they are far more important than that! Horses with bucked shins are at increased risk to develop dorsal cortical fractures of the McIII and then may have catastrophic failure of the McIII during racing. Horses without bucked shins are at very low risk to develop these fractures.

Horses with bucked shins can be trained using this program, provided that the horse is sound and periosteal new bone formation is not substantial. The secret is to decrease the horse's galloping distance (cut it in half) and add short high-speed workouts. For example, if a horse usually gallops 1½ miles/day, reduce the distance to ¾ mile/day and introduce short workouts twice weekly. We usually back the horse up about 1 month in its exercise program and get the high-speed workouts started over short distances. If horses are sore or lame, training is stopped and cold therapy and administration of nonsteroidal antiinflammatory drugs (NSAIDs) are begun. Once sound, horses are returned to training. In some horses NSAIDs may need to be administered for chronic soreness, but horses with frank lameness should be allowed to rest until sound.

If a horse's training schedule is interrupted by an unrelated lameness or upper respiratory tract disease, remodeling that starts with bone resorption is sudden. When the primary problem resolves, if horses are returned to training at a level similar to that before rest but the McIII porosity is increased, the horse is at risk for bucked shins. Therefore if a horse is out of the exercise program for 10 days or more, the horse should be backed up in its training schedule to minimize the risk of bucked shins when it restarts training.

With proper training the incidence of bucked shins can be reduced dramatically (almost eliminated). This can be accomplished without increasing the training time or risking added injury. The added benefit of this program is the concurrent absence of dorsal cortical fractures of the McIII in horses without previous bucked shins.

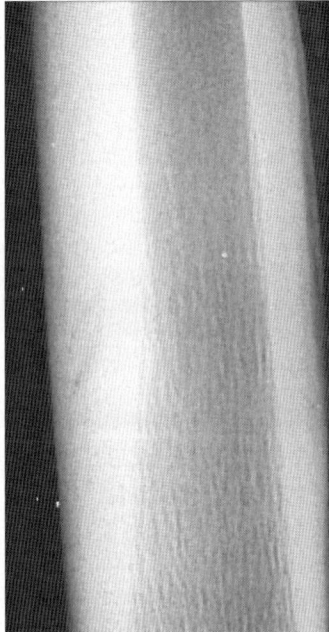

Fig. 102-4 • Lateromedial radiographic image of a third metacarpal bone (McIII) of a 4-year-old Thoroughbred. Dorsal is to the left. Typical dorsal cortical stress fracture of the third metacarpal bone, cortical thickening of the McIII, and numerous oblique fracture lines are present. This horse is a candidate for drilling or screw placement.

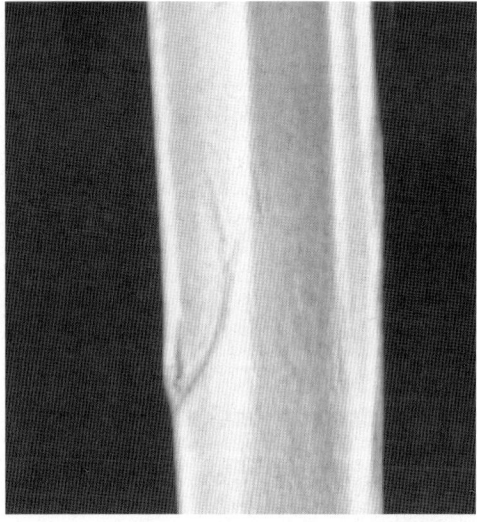

Fig. 102-5 • Lateromedial radiographic image of the third metacarpal bone (McIII) of a 2-year-old Thoroughbred. Dorsal is to the left. There is a severe, dorsal cortical fracture of the McIII. Conservative management in horses with severe fractures is recommended. This fracture is saucer-shaped in appearance and could propagate during recovery from general anesthesia.

◼ STRESS FRACTURES OF THE THIRD METACARPAL BONE: SURGICAL MANAGEMENT

Alan J. Ruggles

Most stress fractures of the McIII occur on the dorsolateral aspect of the left forelimb but may be bilateral (Figure 102-4). Treatment options include controlled exercise (see page 958), screw placement in the dorsal cortex, and cortical drilling around the fracture line. Recently extracorporeal shock wave therapy has been used with apparent early success (Editors, see Chapter 96). The placement of a screw does not result in interfragmentary compression, but it may have a local effect on bone modeling and remodeling. Cortical drilling is thought to improve vascularization and new bone formation at the fracture line.[1] Advantages of cortical drilling alone are that a second surgery is not necessary to remove the screw, and in some horses this procedure can be performed with the horse in a standing position, obviating the need for general anesthesia. However, drill breakage in a standing horse is a risk and, if the bit piece is not retrieved, may lead to chronic lameness. Clinical reports indicate that the use of cortical drilling and screw placement has a lower rate of fracture recurrence than cortical drilling alone. Success rates were 97% and 85%, respectively.[2,3] I use the combination technique.

Horses with radiological evidence of substantial endosteal or periosteal healing often heal satisfactorily without surgical intervention. Horses with severe fractures that are in multiple locations, or spiral around the bone, have a risk of catastrophic failure on recovery from general anesthesia and usually are treated conservatively (Figure 102-5). To my knowledge no objective reports of conservative management of dorsal cortical stress fractures exist. In my experience conservative management is less reliable than surgical treatment and does not result in a reduction in training days missed. In addition, I have experienced a higher rate of recurrent fracture, or failure of fracture to heal, with conservative compared with surgical management.

SURGICAL PROCEDURE

The horse is positioned in lateral recumbency under general anesthesia with the affected limb uppermost. Both limbs can be operated on from this position. The periosteal new bone usually can be felt through the skin, and a 6- to 8-cm vertical incision is made over the fracture, usually between the common and lateral digital extensor tendons. Radiographic examination is used if necessary. The periosteum should not be elevated. A sharp 2.5-mm drill bit is used to drill a thread hole for a 3.5-mm screw perpendicular to the fracture line. Screws are placed as positional screws rather than in lag fashion. Only the dorsal cortex is drilled. Overdrilling may result in impact on the palmar cortex and instrument breakage. During or after screw placement, radiological examination is necessary to determine proper screw placement. The screw is placed after countersinking, tapping, and measuring to determine appropriate screw length. Usually a single screw is used, but occasionally several screws are used for a long fracture. Five or six unicortical drill holes approximately 1 cm apart are made using a 2.5-mm drill bit in the region of the fracture, before routine closure and bandaging of the limb.

If dorsal cortical drilling alone is performed with a horse in the standing position, under sedation and perineural analgesia, a 3.2-mm drill bit is used to decrease the risk of drill breakage if the horse moves during the procedure.

POSTOPERATIVE TREATMENT

Four weeks of stall rest with handwalking followed by 4 weeks of small paddock turnout, continued handwalking, or swimming are recommended. Screw removal is performed with the horse standing at 8 weeks, based on fracture healing. Return to light jogging can occur 2 weeks after screw removal, but more intense training should not start until at least 16

weeks after surgery and should be based on lack of clinical signs of lameness and radiological signs of healing.

PROGNOSIS

Prognosis is considered good, with 85% to 97% of horses returning to racing.[2,3] Recurrence of fracture is more common after cortical drilling alone, compared with the combination of cortical drilling and screw placement. Catastrophic failure has occurred after cortical drilling alone but not with the combined technique.

Chapter 103

On-the-Track Catastrophes in the Thoroughbred Racehorse

W. Theodore Hill

References on page 1341

Horses in racing and high-intensity training are subject to a variety of musculoskeletal injuries. For North American racing the overall incidence of musculoskeletal injuries ranges from 3.3 to 7.3 per 1000 starts, depending on variables such as reporting criteria and degree of follow-up. A much closer range of 1.1 to 1.8 injuries per 1000 starts is reported for horses with catastrophic injuries resulting in euthanasia.[1] Catastrophic or fatal injuries are documented more reliably and are considerably less subject to bias or misinterpretation by the reporter. The rates for training injuries may be somewhat higher, although accurate acquisition and evaluation of these data is more difficult. To date, limited information is available regarding training injuries.[1,2] Several factors cannot be controlled during training, making information obtained inaccurate and incomplete. The absence of a veterinary observer during most training sessions allows many lameness incidents to go unreported. Often only injuries requiring an ambulance come to the attention of a track veterinarian. During training, no standard exists for soundness, medication use, and exercise rider skill. Differences between training injuries and racing injuries are documented when they exist. In July 2008, the Jockey Club launched the Equine Injury Database (EID) to provide the racing industry with a national database for racing and training injuries. The purpose of the EID is to collect comprehensive data to serve as a resource for epidemiological study to improve safety and prevent injuries. Additional information on the EID can be found at www.incompasssolutions.com.

Information about racing injuries presented in this chapter applies to racing worldwide. However, discussions of the regulatory veterinarian primarily refer to racing in the United States.

REGULATORY VETERINARIAN

The official veterinarian and staff members at a U.S. Thoroughbred racetrack have many duties. The primary responsibility is monitoring the soundness of horses during racing and, to some degree, training. This task is accomplished by an efficient prerace inspection and observation of all horses before, during, and after a race. After the horse has been identified, a visual assessment is made of the overall condition and attitude, and vital parameters are assessed. Ideally the temperature, pulse, and respiratory rates are recorded, and the eyes and mouth are examined closely. The mouth should be free of any inflammation or lacerations, which the bit would aggravate, possibly causing control difficulties for the rider. The forelimbs and hindlimbs are palpated, and attention is paid to the type of shoes worn and the condition of the feet. When bar shoes, aluminum pads, or quarter crack patches are noted, closer inspection of the foot is indicated. A palmar digital neurectomy is permitted in most jurisdictions. The clinician must always check for a neurectomy to ensure compliance with the rules. Usually a horse that has undergone neurectomy must be reported to the track veterinarian and its name conspicuously displayed for claiming races.

Any horse determined to be sick or unsound for racing is reported to the track stewards and withdrawn from the day's racing card. Only the stewards have the authority to officially scratch a horse, although in practice a track official rarely questions the veterinarian's recommendation. The veterinary department must function as an independent authority, and neither management nor anyone connected to a horse should interfere with the veterinarian's decisions.

Once withdrawn for a veterinary reason, a horse is usually placed on an ineligible list and requires further evaluation before being permitted to race again. Depending on the nature of the illness or lameness, the evaluation may involve only a quick check; if the condition is more serious, a monitored workout and thorough examination may be required. The importance of the prerace inspection and follow-up examinations of identified horses cannot be overstated. Evidence exists that horses with prior pathological conditions are at increased risk for recurrent or more severe injury, possibly career-ending or catastrophic.[3,4]

A veterinarian is present in the paddock, where horses are saddled, and at the starting gate. An injury or lameness requires prompt evaluation and contact with the stewards for a late withdrawal. The track veterinarian is the ultimate authority over all horses in the paddock and on the racetrack during racing and training.

Racing officials rely on the veterinarian for information and guidance. Objective data on injuries may assist the track superintendent to address concerns about the track surface and dispel rumor and exaggeration among horsemen. The stewards and judges need the veterinarian's input regarding the use, safety, and validity of new equipment such as shoes, bandages, protective eye covering, bridles, and therapy modalities. The official veterinarian also can be an invaluable source of information on medication for private practitioners, horsemen, and racing officials.

A brief comment on managing spills is appropriate. A *spill* is defined as a sudden fall of horse and rider that usually causes other horses and riders to fall. Ideally, one may call for immediate assistance from other veterinarians and experienced track personnel to assess and attend promptly to more than one horse injured in the incident. Horses may rise after a spill, although seriously injured, and move to other areas on the racetrack, thus further complicating the situation. A prompt overall assessment of the number of horses involved, the location on the track, and the major injuries is essential to prevent misallocation of resources. Triage and communication, with preferably one experienced veterinarian coordinating the activities, are key to an efficient professional outcome.

MANAGEMENT CONSIDERATIONS

Efficient management of an on-the-track catastrophe while maintaining the horse's best interests is the primary objective. The key elements required include trained personnel, equipment, and communication.

Communication is critical to make the best use of available resources. The track veterinarian must be prepared to respond to the injured horse and direct support personnel and equipment at the scene. The injured horse is under the care and direction of the track veterinarians until it is moved to a clinic or stable to be attended by a veterinarian employed by the owner or trainer. A stable veterinarian may be called to the scene for severe injuries and if time permits. The track veterinarian acts promptly to attend to the injured horse on the track, thus facilitating an efficient transfer for further evaluation and treatment. Efficiency is important for the care of the injured horse and to allow the official veterinarian to be in position for subsequent races without undue delay. Ideally a communication network of two-way radios and mobile telephones works well to keep an orderly process in motion. Radio communication with track departments such as security is used to relay information as required.

The operator of the horse ambulance should have sufficient training to fully understand the ambulance features and how to use them. Knowing how to back up and position the loading doors properly is essential. Failure to accomplish these basic skills could cause further injury or delay proper treatment.

In most situations, track personnel are the first on the scene of the injured horse, but in some countries, such as those of the United Kingdom and Ireland, a veterinarian follows the race and would be on the scene immediately. Track personnel routinely are equipped with radios and are

crucial for initiating communication with veterinarians and providing the immediate care. Knowing who and how to call for assistance can save valuable time and distress for all involved.

Those individuals should be instructed in the basics of emergency care. The track veterinary department should provide such instruction to ensure a defined, reliable standard, without confusion and delay. Topics such as restraint, controlling hemorrhage, support of an injured limb, and when to apply a splint are well worth the time. Most if not all persons are willing to do whatever may be required to assist an injured horse, but they are often reluctant for fear of making a mistake. These first-line providers of emergency care should be encouraged and recognized for their valuable assistance. Splint selection and application should be kept as simple as possible to avoid potential legal complications, which fortunately are uncommon. An overzealous and poorly trained person may assume too much responsibility, however, placing the horse at risk of further injury and subjecting track management to extensive liability. Outriders, who monitor training in the mornings, may be instructed in using a commercially available support, such as a Kimzey splint (Kimzey, Woodland, California, United States). The splint may be applied safely whenever loss of support in the fetlock joint is obvious, because the splint is simple, quick to apply, and generally well tolerated. Restraint is often a critical issue for horse and handlers' safety. Usually keeping the horse quiet and still while supporting a distal limb injury is adequate until a veterinarian arrives to provide professional care. However, in some situations the horse is best kept recumbent (e.g., a horse with such a severe injury that it is unable to remain standing, even with assistance). Such horses may lunge repeatedly and fall, risking further injury and endangering all present. A fallen rider near the horse may be incapable of movement for several minutes while being attended, making control and restraint of the horse all the more imperative.

EQUIPMENT

Substantial improvements in equine ambulance design have contributed to minimizing secondary injury and complications, increasing the chances of saving seriously injured horses. The ambulance should be partitioned, be well ventilated, allow ample daylight, and be equipped with interior lights. Sturdy, rubber floor matting and padded sidewalls, all easily washed, are required. A partition separating the horse holding area and a forward compartment provides a storage area and some protection for handlers. Ideally the ambulance trailer can be lowered hydraulically to facilitate loading of a severely injured horse and eliminating the need for a rear ramp. Side access doors with ramps provide convenient and safe off-loading, without having to back the horse up or turn it around. An extremely valuable feature is a movable middle partition, which serves as a squeeze chute to help support the horse during transport. A seriously injured horse will make excellent use of this feature by leaning on it or the wall when turning, thus drastically reducing lateral movement and unnecessary weight bearing. The Kimzey Equine Ambulance is an excellent example of such a fully equipped vehicle.

The ambulance should be well equipped with splints and bandaging materials. Splints to support the metacarpophalangeal (fetlock) joint are essential, as are compression boots in two or three sizes. Bandage material should include sterile pads, gauze and cotton bandages, and elastic and adhesive wraps. Sufficient material to make a modified Robert Jones bandage always should be available. Duct tape is an excellent means to secure a heavy support bandage or splint, preventing shifting and providing axial stability. Inflatable compression splints are sometimes helpful to stabilize carpal fractures, but application of a cotton-and-elastic bandage is often faster and more effective.

Some of this material can be kept in the equine ambulance, but space and security considerations require that most of the splints and medications are kept in a track vehicle that transports the veterinarians. Emergency supply bags can be equipped and organized to facilitate quick access at the location of the injured horse.

Containers of ice should be kept on board the ambulance during racing for prompt application to horses with acute injuries. Rubbing alcohol is also useful for cooling horses in warm climates.

Although it is not frequently required, a portable oxygen supply with a simple flow delivery system and two endotracheal tubes should be readily available. A sling of suitable design to support a horse for extended periods is recommended (Liftex, Warminster, Pennsylvania, United States).

MEDICATION

Security concerns may preclude keeping medications in the ambulance in some jurisdictions. An emergency bag with selected drugs is an efficient means to attend to an injured horse on the track and in the ambulance. A suggested inventory includes butorphanol, xylazine, flunixin meglumine, ketamine hydrochloride, detomidine, hydrocortisone sodium succinate, epinephrine, phenylbutazone, and euthanasia products. It should be noted that the American Association of Equine Practitioners Euthanasia Guidelines (2007) state that the sole use of skeletal muscle relaxants is unprofessional and inhumane; however, the guidelines do not preclude the use of these drugs as an adjunct to a barbiturate or other acceptable drugs to facilitate a humane procedure. These can be a valuable aid to safely manage an uncontrollable horse that cannot be removed from the racetrack for euthanasia. An assortment of syringes, needles, tourniquet, scalpels, scissors, hemostats, and blood collection tubes complete the emergency kit.

TRAINING INJURIES

Humeral Fractures

During morning workouts and gallops, horses are subject to the same injuries as those that occur in racing. A few injuries, such as humeral fractures, are not encountered commonly in racing, but they are often seen while horses are only galloping. For the reporting period of 1993 to 2000, 12 of the 15 humeral fractures observed occurred during morning training.[5] Horses with spiral humeral fractures, with or without displacement, almost always are considered candidates for immediate euthanasia. The injuries usually involve the horse falling suddenly and

remaining down, although some do rise. The rider may have no warning before the fall, but some horses may change leads and bobble or shorten the stride.

The diagnosis is straightforward if the horse is standing. The horse bears little or no weight, and the limb is in a hanging position, with the horse unable to advance the leg if encouraged to move. There may be obvious swelling of the area, and palpation or manipulation with auscultation often reveals crepitus. Horses that are down on the track when the veterinarian arrives are diagnostic challenges. They may make some attempt to rise, particularly with encouragement, but with the fractured humerus on the down side they are rarely successful. Rolling the horse over can be accomplished with at least two people and the use of shanks or similar equipment to avoid being kicked in the process. Once the horse is turned over, the fracture is often apparent and the horse may rise with the good forelimb down. These horses often fall dramatically when the fracture occurs and may be slow to recover because of the shock of both the fall and the fracture.

Although some injured horses may be loaded and transported to the stable, no treatment is recommended other than analgesia and physical support. These horses are extremely difficult to load without the assistance of capable and readily available personnel. Loading becomes substantially more difficult with time, and the increased swelling and pain make the horse reluctant to move at all after several minutes. A horse is best left supported on the equine ambulance until the stable veterinarian arrives to confirm the diagnosis before euthanasia. At the request of an owner, or to satisfy insurance requirements, radiography may be attempted to document the diagnosis, particularly for horses with minimally displaced fractures. For most horses with this severe injury, radiographs are obtained more humanely post mortem. Humeral and scapular fractures do occasionally occur during racing, and horses should be managed in the same manner.

Collision Injuries

Collision injuries usually are associated with training, because many horses are often on the track, exercising at various speeds, distances, and directions. Maintenance equipment and personnel moving on and near the training surface, open gaps permitting access to the track, and insufficient outriders to monitor and control the congestion all predispose to collision injuries with other horses and inanimate objects. Injuries may be of any type but include trauma to the head, axial skeleton, shoulder, and pelvis. Bruising and lacerations from impact are not uncommon. The severity can range from minor abrasions and contusion to severe, life-threatening fracture and hemorrhage.

Location of Injuries on the Racetrack

Considerable anecdotal and published information exists regarding the location of injury occurrences on the track surface.[5,6] Any injury type can be encountered at any point in a race, and trained personnel should be prepared to respond to any location. From experience, it is safe to conclude that most catastrophic injuries occur in turns and in the stretch run to the finish. Most racing operations position the equine ambulance in the area of the $\frac{1}{2}$- to the $\frac{1}{4}$-mile pole to be available for a prompt response.

Many injuries are evident immediately after a race and when horses are pulling up and begin galloping back to be unsaddled. Horses with carpal chip or proximal sesamoid bone (PSB) fractures and new or recurrent tendonitis or suspensory desmitis usually show lameness after they are pulled up. The jockeys should alert an outrider for assistance. Some riders may be hesitant to pull up and dismount because of inexperience and uncertainty, but the track veterinarian should make this policy clear to the jockeys and encourage conservative, prudent decisions. Any horse suspected of being lame, by a jockey or outrider, should be held at that location until evaluated by an official veterinarian.

Horsemen, riders, and officials often express concern about unsafe track conditions. Extreme conditions, such as freezing, washouts, and gross discrepancies in uniformity, may be potentially hazardous. However, muddy or sloppy conditions are not a significant risk factor for serious injury, but they may contribute to rundown injuries, the bruising and abrading of soft tissue at the palmar or plantar aspect of the fetlock from contact with the track surface. Random injuries can cause poor performance. Most catastrophic injuries occur on a fast racetrack.[3,5-7] Muddy and sloppy tracks usually produce numerous late withdrawals and smaller fields, especially if a race was originally scheduled for the turf. Thus some degree of selection of horses occurs in these races. In addition, horses that are not in contention and showing response entering the stretch on a poor track usually are not encouraged persistently by the riders. They are allowed to ease themselves, a situation that may not occur on a fast track with the rider more optimistic of a good finish.

PUBLIC RELATIONS AND MEDIA ISSUES

The track veterinarian must be keenly aware of humane considerations and prepared to respond to questions from the media, patrons, horsemen, and track personnel.

In situations that expose the public to catastrophic injuries in the racehorse, the track veterinarian also must be cognizant of esthetic considerations, such as using screens and covers to eliminate unnecessary viewing of horses and the process of euthanasia. During racing, time constraints may become critical to management. Most seriously injured horses can be supported, loaded, and transported for further evaluation off the track. On-track euthanasia should be reserved for those few horses for which no other alternatives exist.

During the 1990 Breeders Cup at Belmont Park, catastrophic injuries resulted in the euthanasia of three horses and considerable media attention. The need for more efficient liaison with the media was demonstrated clearly. In response, the American Association of Equine Practitioners initiated the "On Call" program at the 1991 Kentucky Derby and has continued this program to date. The program consists of veterinarians with media training who donate their time to respond to questions from the media regarding equine health care concerns. The "On Call" veterinarian is available to provide accurate and expert commentary, answering vital questions during a busy event, thus releasing the event veterinarians to attend the injured horse. More than 100 equestrian events are supported by an "On Call" veterinarian each year.

RACING INJURIES
Fractures of the Forelimb

Fractures range in severity from relatively minor chip and nondisplaced incomplete fractures to open, comminuted fractures of long bones, which are considered the most severe on-the-track catastrophes. Fortunately the latter are rare. Available data support the clinical findings that most fatal fractures involve the forelimb and that most of these fractures are of the carpus or more distal part of the limb.[1] This section provides an overview of the most common types of fractures that are encountered on the racetrack, beginning with the foot and working proximally in the forelimb and hindlimb.

Foot and Pastern

Fractures of the distal phalanx are often articular, but they may be nonarticular and involve only a palmar process. An affected horse usually completes the race or begins easing in the later stages, rather than pulling up abruptly. Distal phalanx fractures commonly are diagnosed after the race while the horse is on the track or is cooling out. Lameness may vary in intensity, but it usually increases to non–weight-bearing status within 30 to 60 minutes. Moderate-to-severe lameness is present, without palpable swelling. Nondisplaced third metacarpal bone (McIII) or proximal phalangeal fractures should be considered as a differential diagnosis. If the lameness is apparent at a walk, a compression boot to stabilize the limb distal to the carpus may be useful until other fractures are ruled out. Distal phalangeal fractures are not as commonly diagnosed on the track as fractures of the proximal phalanx, and some may be missed initially, only to be diagnosed later and go unreported.

Middle phalangeal fractures are rare as a primary injury and usually are seen as part of a multiple injury breakdown of the fetlock and pastern.

Fractures of the proximal phalanx usually occur suddenly during a race or while the horse is pulling up. Such fractures range from an incomplete fracture to varying degrees of fragmentation and severe comminution. Most horses with these fractures are lame and require prompt analgesia and application of a supportive splint or bandage. These horses do not tolerate a heavy compression boot well. Displaced fractures are diagnosed readily on the track. These require considerable attention to provide adequate support for transport to prevent further bone and soft tissue damage, thus optimizing the chances of repair and recovery. Proximal phalangeal fractures are the most commonly diagnosed injury of the pastern and occur equally in the left and right forelimbs.

Metacarpophalangeal Joint

The metacarpophalangeal joint is involved in most catastrophic injuries. Horses with simple, nondisplaced condylar fractures of the McIII usually develop acute lameness at the end of a race or after the race. Lameness is noticeable at a walk by the time the horse is loaded. With minimal swelling, diagnosis is presumptive initially, and appropriate supportive measures are required. Although the lameness may be substantial, localizing the injury is often difficult when displacement and swelling are minimal. However, some condylar fractures of the McIII are diagnosed after the horse has returned to the stable to cool out, without the assistance of an ambulance. An open, comminuted McIII condylar fracture causes severe lameness. The horse is pulled up during a race or immediately after the race. The proximal aspect of the displaced fragment penetrates the skin with some mild hemorrhage, making the diagnosis readily apparent.

Because the potential for further displacement and contamination is great, considerable care must be exercised to support the fracture site. Preferably a sterile bandage should be applied to the area and then the limb supported with a heavy bandage or compression boot. Excessive movement of the horse should be avoided while the horse is loaded and transported on the ambulance. Newer ambulances are equipped with a sliding partition to support the horse firmly. The prognosis is guarded because of the compound (open) nature of this injury, and extreme care in managing these horses on the track is essential to a successful outcome.

Proximal Sesamoid Bones

The PSBs are a frequent site of racing and training injury. The PSBs of the forelimbs are primarily involved. Classically, a simple fracture of a PSB results in a progressive lameness while the horse is cooling out after successfully completing a race or workout. The official veterinarian may not see many of these horses and may learn of their injuries only after receiving information from the test barn personnel, trainers, or attending veterinarians.

A more severe sagittal or midbody fracture of one or both of the PSBs causes severe, acute lameness during a race or immediately after a race. If only one PSB is involved, the loss of support of the metacarpophalangeal joint is minimal. The limb should be held by the first attendant on the scene, to prevent weight bearing and further movement, before application of a Kimzey splint. Once supported, these horses are relatively cooperative and confident to move for loading and transport.

In horses with biaxial PSB fractures, loss of metacarpophalangeal joint support is immediate. A dramatic drop of the metacarpophalangeal joint occurs whenever the horse attempts to bear weight. The limb must be supported immediately and the horse controlled to allow prompt application of a splint. These horses may attempt to move on the injured limb and, if they are not restrained, may cause substantial secondary damage to the soft tissues of the fetlock joint (see Chapters 36 and 104).

Fractures involving the metacarpophalangeal joint frequently are complex and involve some combination of condylar fractures of the McIII and PSB fractures, thus compromising the suspensory apparatus. Horses running at race speeds that sustain a McIII condylar or PSB fracture continue to gallop several strides on the injured limb before pulling up. Often they may unseat the rider and gallop considerable distances before being stopped. Additional fractures and disruption of the suspensory ligament (SL) and distal sesamoidean ligaments may result, and the injury may become open, with subluxation and disarticulation of the metacarpophalangeal joint. Depending on the severity of the injury, some of these horses may be manageable for ambulance transport. However, many require immediate euthanasia because of the extensive damage. The metacarpophalangeal joint is involved in two thirds of all catastrophic racing injuries at the New York Racing Association tracks.[5]

Third Metacarpal Bone

Condylar fractures of the McIII were discussed previously. Horses with minimal displacement of the fracture have a good prognosis for return to racing after surgery. Those with substantial displacement of the fracture or skin penetration have a less favorable prognosis, but with proper on-track management, many can have a reasonable outcome in an alternative career.

The McIII diaphysis is the site of a common racing and training injury referred to as *bucked shins* (see Chapter 102). If not properly managed, horses with bucked shins may not stride out well, move with a choppy action, and trail the field during a race. These horses may be pulled up by the jockey, but they require little on-track care.

Dorsal cortical fracture of the McIII may result from the bucked-shin complex and is an injury that is seen most frequently in late 2-year-olds or in 3-year-olds. Lameness may be intermittent, and palpation of the affected area often provides inconsistent findings. Dorsal cortical fracture of the McIII poses a serious risk to horse and rider if not detected and properly treated. If a horse with a fracture is returned to training and racing prematurely or the fracture is undiagnosed, a complete diaphyseal fracture may develop. This catastrophic injury causes a horse to fall without warning during morning workouts or a race, risking serious injury to the rider and others in close proximity. The track veterinarian is faced with an essentially unmanageable horse. The fracture usually is comminuted and open. The limb distal to the fracture site is often attached by only tendons and remaining skin. The horse may attempt to rise or manage to rise, but it is extremely unstable and usually falls again. For the safety of all assisting at the scene and for the riders who may still be down on the track, the horse should physically be kept down by capable track personnel. Immediate euthanasia is indicated. If the trainer or owner is present and requests another opinion, the attending veterinarian can sedate or anesthetize the horse long enough for another veterinarian to be summoned. Attempts to develop an anesthetic protocol to facilitate transport of these horses for potential surgical intervention have been unsuccessful. Historically, this catastrophic injury has been the cause of spectacular horse spills in racing, causing considerable loss to the horse industry, serious jockey injury, and negative media attention. Because essentially no treatment alternatives are available, all effort must be directed toward prevention. Accurate diagnosis and the removal of horses from high-intensity training and racing are essential.

Carpus

Although the carpus is a frequent site for lameness, it is seldom an area associated with catastrophic injury (see Chapter 38). Carpal chip and slab fractures cause a range of clinical signs. Small chip fractures may be difficult to detect and, without obvious effusion or pain on palpation, are difficult to differentiate from McIII condylar fractures. A horse with a carpal slab fracture, especially if displaced, is usually severely lame. If a slab fracture is suspected, the carpus should be supported with a cotton wrap and elastic bandage or an inflatable compression splint. Comminuted carpal fractures occur and cause collapse of the proximal and distal rows of carpal bones and obvious instability. Although a horse with numerous carpal fractures may fall, most horses pull up abruptly, stopping in just a few strides. The horse is in acute distress and non–weight bearing and usually is difficult to load and transport. If possible, a horse with a comminuted carpal fracture should be examined by consulting veterinarians, because euthanasia may be highly likely. Such examination avoids unnecessary movement and distress for the horse. Some horses may be salvaged for breeding purposes with surgery and extensive nursing care.

Radius

Radial fractures are rare. For an 8-year period, four horses were destroyed because of comminuted radial fractures. It is interesting to note that all four horses sustained a fracture of the left radius.[5]

Shoulder

Fractures of the shoulder, though rare, are always catastrophic. Those of the humerus most often occur during training and were discussed previously (see page 962). The scapula may fracture during a race, and in my experience the injury always involves the joint. The horse may fall suddenly, but some horses manage to pull up in the race without going down. Horses are severely lame and have rapid, severe swelling from hemorrhage, great difficulty in advancing the limb, and a dropped shoulder appearance. This is an excellent example of the benefit of viewing the entire horse from a short distance before commencing a close-up examination.

Inexperience with this injury often leads the clinician to an early misdiagnosis of a lower limb problem, only to be frustrated and embarrassed when enlightened by lay assistants. Swelling over the area may become extensive in a few moments but may be overlooked if one remains focused on assessing the distal aspect of the limb. On numerous occasions, support splints have been applied to the limb distal to the carpus, with the shoulder recognized as the primary injury only when attempting to load the horse onto the ambulance.

Nevertheless, once the diagnosis is made, the horse may be difficult to load, even with abundant help. As a rule, horses are more willing to attempt to move shortly after the injury occurs. Once loaded, the use of a movable partition for support is a tremendous aid. Euthanasia is best performed while the horse is still in the ambulance.

Fractures of the Hindlimb

Pastern

Fractures of the hind phalanges occur considerably less frequently than in the forelimb. Similar injuries occur, but fractures of the proximal phalanx predominate. Only 10 proximal phalangeal fractures of a hindlimb were diagnosed for the period 1993-2000 at the New York Racing Association tracks, compared with 28 for the forelimbs.[5] Horses appear considerably more able to support on only one hindlimb, and to protect the injured site from further weight bearing, than to support on only one forelimb. Open fractures are much less common than in forelimbs, and the prognosis for horses with hindlimb fractures is better than for those with forelimb fractures. A lightweight splint and bulky bandage are recommended, because horses do not tolerate a heavy splint or boot well. Complex fractures involving the proximal and middle phalanges and the third metatarsal bone (MtIII) may be seen, although these are rare.

Third Metatarsal Bone

MtIII condylar fractures occur less commonly than those seen in the McIII. Horses do not tolerate the weight of a compression boot on a hindlimb and often do better with a thick support bandage. It is important to obtain good-quality radiographs, because many of these fractures are located medially and have a tendency to spiral, making surgical repair a challenge.

Tarsus and Tibia

Fractures of the tarsus are an uncommon cause of acute training and racing injuries. Osteoarthritis of the distal tarsal joints commonly results in reluctance to break from the gate and overall poor performance, but it rarely causes an acute on-track incident.

Catastrophic tibial fractures are rare and generally result from preexisting stress fractures (see Chapter 45). Complete fracture may occur hours after a race or training, when the horse is moving about and resting in the stall. In horses with obscure hindlimb lameness, scintigraphic examination is a valuable diagnostic aid for preventing catastrophic injury.

Stifle and Femur

Femoral fractures are rare in the racing Thoroughbred. Osteochondrosis lesions of the distal aspect of the femur are not uncommon and cause subtle hindlimb lameness that is often difficult to diagnose (see Chapter 46). Stifle lameness, including that caused by osteochondrosis lesions, often leads to compensatory lameness conditions. Tarsal or stifle problems may not cause catastrophic injury primarily but rather lead to a compensatory forelimb lameness and secondary breakdown, often involving the PSBs and metacarpophalangeal joint. Accurate diagnosis and treatment of many mild-to-moderate lameness conditions often helps prevent more serious injury.

Acute hindlimb lameness, other than that caused by complete tibial or femoral fracture, is generally difficult to assess on the track. The horse may pull up abruptly or be lame at the completion of a race and often is reluctant to bear weight. Unlike those with forelimb lameness, horses with acute severe hindlimb lameness are often relatively easy to load into an ambulance and transport with minimal effort. The clinician must keep in mind that a horse may have an incomplete fracture, such as of the MtIII. Thus maximizing support while the horse is in the ambulance and walking the horse minimally should be standard care for these horses.

Pelvis

Pelvic fractures can cause acute hindlimb lameness and occur predominantly in fillies while racing or training (see Chapter 49). From 1993 to 2000 at the three New York Racing Association tracks, a diagnosis of pelvic fracture was made in 20 horses, 17 of which were fillies.[5] A horse with a pelvic fracture is in obvious distress and reluctant to move, but with proper analgesia and physical assistance, most horses can be loaded and relocated carefully to a stall. Extreme care must be taken, because displacement of the fracture is a potential risk, specifically in horses with iliac wing or shaft fractures. Severe hemorrhage and death can occur even when a horse is in an ambulance or stall. This potential for fracture displacement and hemorrhagic shock keeps survival numbers discouragingly low. Of the 20 horses with pelvic fractures, six horses died within 1 hour, and 11 were euthanized at the scene or less than 1 week after injury.[5] With increased use of scintigraphy and early diagnosis of stress-related bone injury, the hope is that catastrophic injuries such as displaced pelvic fractures can be avoided.

Head and Axial Skeleton

Horses involved in collisions or spills may sustain any number of head or spinal injuries. Loose horses attempting to jump railings and run through gaps frequently fall, but they seldom sustain serious injury. Young horses not uncommonly become fractious while being saddled, rearing, lunging, and occasionally falling. Horses with obvious injury, regardless of the severity, should be withdrawn from the race immediately. The track veterinarian must take responsibility for withdrawing a horse after a fall, often consulting with the trainer or owner. The most serious head injuries usually result from flipping in the saddling paddock and striking the hard ground or a wall partition. Sinus hemorrhage, although dramatic and at times copious, is generally not a serious concern. Horses that sustain a hard blow to the head may become disoriented and show ataxia initially. Prompt treatment with corticosteroids and dimethyl sulfoxide may be indicated while the horse is kept quiet in a reasonably safe area. Horses should be led to and held in a grass paddock away from trees and fences. If ataxia subsides, the horse may be moved to a stall by ambulance or by walking with attendants.

I find it interesting that some horses may appear normal immediately after a hard fall and head trauma, only to become dull and ataxic or reluctant to move after a short time. Initial conservative management is recommended for any horse after a hard fall. The horse should be monitored closely while moving to the stable, and track personnel should communicate their concerns personally to the attending veterinarian whenever possible. A horse that sustains a serious fall resulting in fractures at the base of the skull is often recumbent, has aural hemorrhage, and unfortunately dies quickly. Fractures or other injuries of the axial skeleton may occasionally result from falling, but a definitive diagnosis may be difficult to make. A horse may be stunned or winded, may remain recumbent after falling, and may make no attempt to rise. Vital signs are usually normal. After it is ensured that the airway is unobstructed and after the saddle has been removed, the horse is given time to rise. Oxygen from a continuous-flow mask and an intravenous corticosteroid (hydrocortisone sodium succinate, 100 to 500 mg) are recommended. It may be 30 minutes or longer before a winded horse is ready to get up. When ready, and with a mild prompt of a slap on the neck or rump, many horses then stand unassisted. Some may be slower and assume a sternal position briefly before rising. Those that are unstable and appear weak behind will need assistance, by helping lift on the tail.

If a horse attempts to rise unsuccessfully several times even with assistance, rolling it on its other side may be best. Injury to the down limb may have occurred. A horse

with fractures of the cervical or thoracic vertebrae makes little or no attempt to move, depending on the level of injury.

Horses that are down on the track with normal vital signs and no apparent limb injury must be presumed to have injury of the axial skeleton. The horse can be positioned on a mat while still recumbent and carefully pulled onto the ambulance for transport to the stable or emergency clinic. An anatomical diagnosis may be established, but the prognosis is poor for horses that have not stood successfully by 12 to 24 hours.

Soft Tissue Injuries

Injuries sustained at the speeds of racing and training workouts are often complex, with soft tissue and bone injury. Fracture of a PSB or the McIII causes abrupt loss of action and compensation by the horse and concomitant reaction by the rider. Several strides may follow with some weight bearing on the affected limb. What began as a simple fracture may progress to a catastrophic, life-threatening injury in only seconds because of progressive soft tissue and bony disruption.

The soft tissues supporting the metacarpophalangeal joint are particularly prone to injury. Disruption of the digital flexor tendons or SL can cause gross hyperextension of the metacarpophalangeal joint and potential damage to the digital vessels and nerves. Inadequate perfusion of the injury site may limit or prevent a successful surgical repair or other attempts at recovery.

The metacarpophalangeal joint may subluxate with a primary soft tissue injury. This usually results from a traumatic disruption of the suspensory apparatus, although complete disruption of the digital flexor tendons also may be involved secondarily. If the luxation is closed, the joint may become locked in hyperextension, requiring manual reduction before a splint can be applied. If open luxation occurs, the distal aspect of the McIII can be seen. Complete luxation usually results from a complete disruption of the SL or the distal sesamoidean ligaments. Immediate support of the limb and splint application are essential for a closed injury. A horse with an exposed, open fetlock injury must be euthanized on the track.

Digital Flexor Tendon Injuries

Digital flexor tendon injury (tendonitis) primarily involving the superficial digital flexor tendon (SDFT) is a substantial cause of economic loss in the Thoroughbred industry. Tendonitis varies in severity, but horses with even the most minor tear require time to recover and return to training. Racing data from the three New York Racing Association tracks support a recurrence rate approaching 25% for horses with tendonitis.[3] The overall rate is clearly higher when one considers horses lost to follow-up or reinjured before reaching racing fitness.

Acute tendonitis is usually not apparent on the racetrack and usually is diagnosed by the attending veterinarian several hours later. Severe or total disruption of a SDFT causes obvious lameness at the completion of training or a race. Lameness usually increases rapidly, and hyperextension (dropping) of the metacarpophalangeal joint is apparent.

Recurrent tendonitis is usually more severe than the initial injury. A horse may pull up before completing training or a race. Swelling is often substantial, the mid-metacarpal region lacks definition, and the metacarpophalangeal joint drops moderately. The degree of swelling may preclude accurate diagnosis of what soft tissue structure is involved. The prerace inspection is particularly important in horses with a history of tendonitis, because this may be the determining factor in preventing reinjury. Careful palpation for sensitivity and swelling can reveal subtle changes that may have gone undetected by the trainer and exercise rider, because these horses usually continue to train without obvious lameness. The track veterinarian may require an ultrasonographic evaluation before permitting the horse to race. Comparison with previous examination findings may demonstrate a clinically significant lesion, although the horse is sound at the trot and gallop. Despite all efforts, tendon reinjury occurs to some horses during racing or in workouts. When reinjury does occur, the application of a compression boot or splint is required. Horses with severe tendonitis, even with loss of metacarpophalangeal joint support, can heal with time to become pasture sound.

Digital flexor tendonitis in a hindlimb is unusual, but tendons are vulnerable to severe laceration and blunt trauma by being cut down during a race. Injury may occur when the foot of a following horse strikes the tendons of the hindlimb. The shoe, particularly one with a toe grab, may lacerate and completely sever the SDFT and less commonly the deep digital flexor tendon. Wounds often are badly contaminated, and prognosis is guarded because of complications from infection. A clean support bandage is applied initially, and light sedation and analgesia are given. Further splinting is usually unnecessary and is not well tolerated. Immediate transport to an emergency hospital is strongly advised.

Suspensory Ligament Injuries

Injuries of the SL and digital flexor tendons have many similarities, are relatively common, vary considerably in severity, and predominantly involve a forelimb. Branch or body desmitis often is detected after the morning exercise when the horse is cooling out. Moderate or severe desmitis causes acute lameness, possibly with some degree of metacarpophalangeal joint drop, but swelling may initially be minimal. A presumptive diagnosis is made while the horse is still on the track, but differentiating between a SL and digital flexor tendon injury may be difficult. An important principle in emergency management is providing immediate support. A splint that supports the metacarpophalangeal joint is always indicated whenever suspensory disruption is suspected. Obvious dropping of the metacarpophalangeal joint during weight bearing reinforces the decision to use a standard Kimzey splint. PSB fractures often may occur concomitantly, but they may not always be readily apparent. Progressive loss of metacarpophalangeal joint support occurs as the severity of suspensory tearing increases. If the injury is closed, the on-track management remains the same. Complete SL disruption and disarticulation of the metacarpophalangeal joint was discussed previously (see page 966).

The distal sesamoidean ligaments are a vital component of the suspensory apparatus, and even mild desmitis should be considered a serious injury in Thoroughbred racehorses. Horses with mild desmitis look similar to those with digital flexor tendon or SL injuries. These injuries may

appear to heal, but recurrence is common and problematic. My strong clinical impression is that horses with previous distal sesamoidean desmitis are at risk to develop catastrophic injury, and close monitoring of the status of these injuries is imperative when horses return to training. Any indication of recurrence of desmitis is sufficient cause for retirement or at least additional time off for reevaluation. Reinjury is often catastrophic, with complete rupture of the ligaments, proximal displacement of the PSBs, and disarticulation of the metacarpophalangeal joint with multiple secondary injuries. Euthanasia usually is required for these horses.

REGULATORY CONSIDERATIONS

Attending veterinarians must be aware of their responsibility to the regulatory body, that is, the state racing commission or its equivalent. Some jurisdictions require a written report to be filed for any horse euthanized on official racetrack grounds. In lieu of a formal report, a good policy is to contact the track stewards and state or association veterinarian to inform them of catastrophic injuries that occur during training or racing. A necropsy and samples for pathological examination may be commission requirements and are vital for statistical evaluation of injuries at the racetrack. Important information can be obtained relative to the nature of the injury, track condition, age and sex of the horse, and other possible risk factors. The official track veterinarian, whether state or association, is fully knowledgeable of commission requirements and appropriate procedures and so is a valuable source of information for the veterinary practitioner on the backstretch. Free exchange among professionals is mutually beneficial. The official veterinarian frequently requires the prompt assistance of the stable veterinarian to continue the management and treatment of a seriously injured horse.

EUTHANASIA AND INSURANCE

When attending to a horse with a catastrophic injury, the veterinarian should instruct the owner to notify the insurance carrier, if applicable, as soon as possible. In the event that euthanasia is not immediately essential but is later considered, most insurance companies require a second opinion. Horses with catastrophic injuries may require immediate euthanasia at the scene on the racetrack when supporting and loading the horse onto the ambulance is not possible. Regardless of the circumstances, thorough documentation with photographs of the injury and specifics of the incident should be maintained. If possible, radiographs should be obtained to document the nature of the injury. It is always advisable to have a representative of the stable present to provide consent for euthanasia, but this is rarely the owner. When consent cannot be obtained, the veterinarian on the scene must do whatever is indicated to alleviate distress and protect the horse from further injury until a consulting veterinarian arrives.

On rare occasions the veterinarian may be confronted with an uncontrollable horse or a situation in which euthanasia is the only course of action remaining, consent and consulting opinion being unavailable. After exhausting reasonable attempts to stabilize the horse and obtain assistance, the professional decision for euthanasia can be exercised without excessive concern. Documentation in these horses should include necropsy examination. Although the situation is extremely unlikely to result in a legal challenge, thorough communication and documentation are always advisable. Euthanasia is the final option available to the clinician and is justified to prevent further pain and distress. Although the technical aspects of the procedure are simple, resulting in a fast and humane death for the horse, veterinarians must exercise discretion and sensitivity. As disturbing as the situation may be for the attending veterinarian, there is no way to gauge the emotional and esthetic impact on others who might be present. Persons with direct connections to the injured horse, track workers, media representatives, and patrons may all be within viewing range. An effort to screen the horse from onlookers during euthanasia and while removing the body is recommended. Those immediately connected with the horse should be afforded the opportunity to leave, although some will wish to remain. Finally, the veterinarian must remain in control of the scene, being cognizant of not only the needs of the horse, but also the concerns and safety of all others present.

Chapter 104

Catastrophic Injuries

Dean W. Richardson

Surprisingly, it is difficult to define exactly what comprises a catastrophic injury, but one definition might be any injury that will unquestionably end athletic function and will require extensive treatment to save the horse's life. Comminuted fractures, severe limb lacerations with major vascular damage and extensive tissue loss, and ligamentous injuries leading to overt joint instability are straightforward examples and are easily categorized as "catastrophic." Problems arise when the gross appearance of an injury is initially not representative of its severity or when the severity of the injury is overestimated because of its gross appearance. The attending veterinarian often has to calm the client long enough to allow proper decision making. Most horses with catastrophic injuries can be stabilized well enough to be transported to a referral facility, or at least long enough to permit a complete investigation of therapeutic options and probable outcomes. A quick decision to euthanize might be the easiest and best option, but in some instances it may not be correct, and it most certainly is not revocable.

General principles for emergency first aid of severe distal limb injuries are as follows:

1. Immobilize with a dorsal splint that aligns the phalanges with the third metacarpal bone (McIII). This can be either with a prefabricated splint (e.g., Kimzey Leg Saver, Kimzey, Woodland, California, United States; Figure 104-1), or with a stave of split polyvinylchloride (PVC) pipe or something similar over a lightly padded bandage. The dorsal splint should extend from the proximal aspect of the McIII to the ground, covering the entire dorsal aspect of the hoof wall. The heel must be pulled upward toward the dorsal aspect of the splint to align the phalanges with the McIII. If a prefabricated splint is not available, a lightly padded bandage with a splint applied to the dorsal aspect of the metacarpal region, phalanges, and hoof serves the same purpose if the heel is kept elevated. This can be done by taping the heel and a heel wedge with nonelastic tape (e.g., duct tape) to the dorsally applied splint. Excessive padding should be avoided because it allows dorsal flexion within the bandage and shifting of the splint. A prefabricated splint is not ideal for all injuries because it may not provide medial-to-lateral stability, but it is usually adequate for first-aid stabilization. For injuries involving the upper limb a Robert Jones Bandage

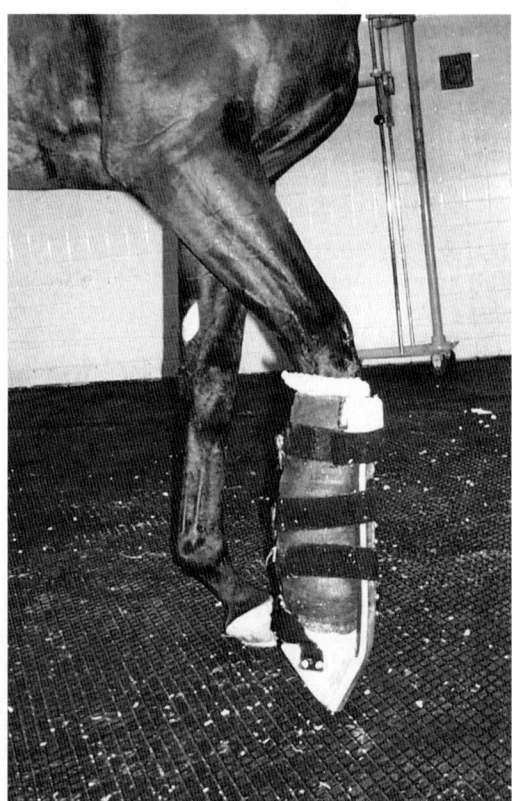

Fig. 104-1 • A Kimzey Leg Saver has been applied to the right forelimb of a racehorse with traumatic disruption of the suspensory apparatus. Note that the distal aspect of the limb is held in position with a dorsal splint attached to a footplate that keeps the phalanges in alignment with the third metacarpal bone. When splinted horses usually comfortably bear weight when walking, they stand with the splinted limb forward in a flexed non–weight-bearing position (as shown). Excessive load is placed on the contralateral limb. Limb length disparity occurs as a result of the added length of the splint, making it necessary to elevate and pad the contralateral foot (not shown).

with splinting material incorporated within the bandage should be applied (see Chapter 86).

2. Tranquilize or sedate adequately to minimize further injury and allow examination. Xylazine or detomidine is usually adequate.

3. It is often difficult to know the exact nature of an injury without using diagnostic imagining, so *do not* make assumptions. If possible, immobilize the area of injury and transport the horse to a referral center for evaluation.

4. Do not hesitate to use parenteral antiinflammatory agents and analgesics. Many attending clinicians worry that antiinflammatory therapy may prompt an injured horse to use a limb, causing further damage; unless perineural analgesia is used, a horse with an injured limb will be unlikely to sustain further injury under the influence of parenteral medication.

5. If there is any skin damage, the horse should immediately be given broad-spectrum antimicrobial drugs intravenously.

6. Transport an injured horse in a *tight* stall, as tight as it can be, so that the horse can easily lean against side walls for support. Do not tie the head tightly. In general, horses with forelimb injuries should be transported facing backward, and those with hindlimb injuries facing forward.

7. Most important, do not make rash decisions concerning treatment and prognosis.

The reader is referred to Chapter 86, and there are two excellent recent reviews that detail emergency stabilization of equine fractures.[1,2]

erences
n page
1341

TYPES OF CATASTROPHIC INJURIES

Traumatic Disruption of the Suspensory Apparatus

Traumatic disruption of the suspensory apparatus is almost exclusively an injury that occurs in the forelimbs of Thoroughbred (TB) racehorses, but it can occur in the hindlimbs and in Standardbred (STB) and Arabian racehorses. It may occur more often in North America than in Europe, although any horse running at high speed may sustain this injury, including young foals that are chasing the dams in a pasture. Speed alone does not account for the injury, and it is likely that fatigue of the flexor muscles supporting the fetlock joint and digit leads to higher stresses in each component of the suspensory apparatus. There also may be a history of the horse being bumped or making a misstep.

The history and clinical presentation of adult horses with traumatic disruption of the suspensory apparatus are straightforward, because the horses are either breezing or racing and pull up acutely and severely lame. The fetlock joint drops as the horse attempts to bear weight. Many horses become anxious or even frantic as they attempt to control the injured limb. Obvious swelling and pain are present over the site of the injury. In foals the diagnosis is often not made as quickly.[2,3] The typical history of a foal with traumatic disruption of the suspensory apparatus (or lesser injuries of the suspensory apparatus) is of being turned out in a large field with its dam and other mares and foals shortly after birth, or after confinement to a box stall for an extended period. As the mare runs with the other horses, the foal attempts to keep up, running at speed and to the point of exhaustion. This results in the same

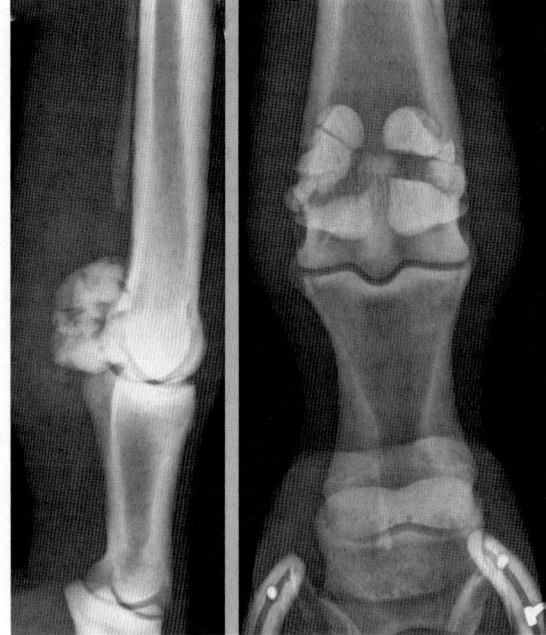

Fig. 104-2 • Lateromedial *(left)* and dorsopalmar radiographic images of a Thoroughbred racehorse with traumatic disruption of the suspensory apparatus as a result of comminuted fractures of both proximal sesamoid bones. The radiographs were obtained with the horse in a non–weight-bearing position. This horse later underwent successful surgical management using fetlock arthrodesis.

combination of speed and fatigue that leads to this injury in racehorses. The clinical signs of complete disruption of the suspensory apparatus in foals are similar to those in adult horses but less dramatic.

The hallmark clinical signs, fetlock drop and severe lameness, are seen in horses with complete disruption of any portion of the suspensory apparatus. The most common injury in both adult horses and foals is fracture of both proximal sesamoid bones (PSBs) (Figure 104-2). The fractures are often comminuted, especially in the basilar portions. The second most common type of traumatic disruption of the suspensory apparatus is complete avulsion of the distal sesamoidean ligaments. This is easily recognized radiologically by the proximal displacement of the intact PSBs (Figure 104-3). The least frequently recognized type of traumatic disruption of the suspensory apparatus is a complete tear of the body or both branches of the suspensory ligament (SL) (Figure 104-4). The Paso Fino, Peruvian Paso, and some other older horses have a degenerative condition of the SL that leads to suspensory apparatus failure that is particularly problematic in the hindlimbs. However, these horses do not have acute, severe lameness, which is typically seen in racehorses (see Chapter 72). In horses with traumatic disruption of the suspensory apparatus, excessive extension of the fetlock may result in stretching and damage to the digital vessels, which may cause avascularity or hypovascularity of the digit. Simultaneous damage to the superficial and deep digital flexor tendons is also common and should be assessed ultrasonographically if there is a suspicion of severe injury. Although PSB fractures and suspensory injuries are both common hindlimb injuries, the most severe breakdown injuries usually involve the forelimbs.

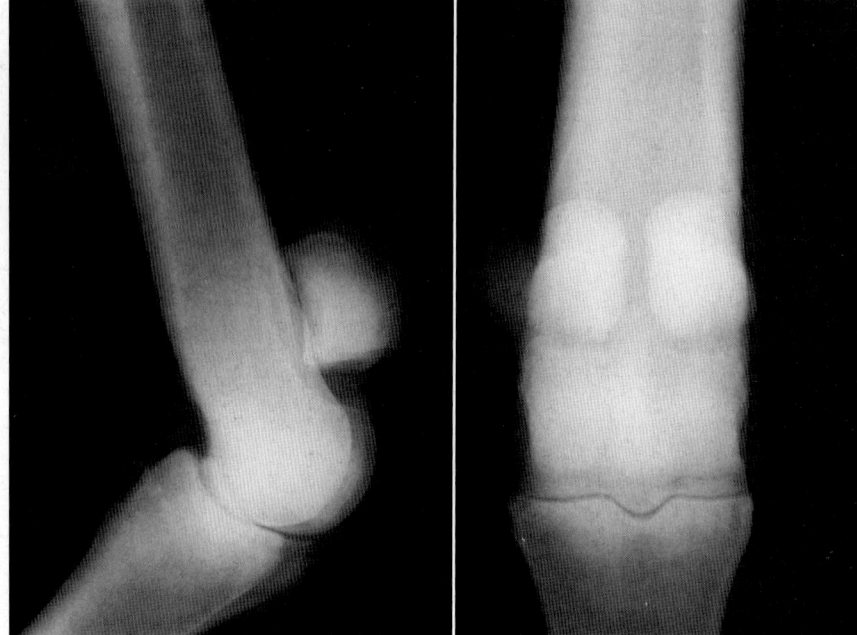

Fig. 104-3 • Lateromedial *(left)* and dorsopalmar radiographic images of a Thoroughbred racehorse with traumatic disruption of the suspensory apparatus as a result of complete rupture of the distal sesamoidean ligaments. Proximal displacement of the proximal sesamoid bones and hyperextension (drop) of the fetlock joint can be seen in these weight-bearing radiographic images.

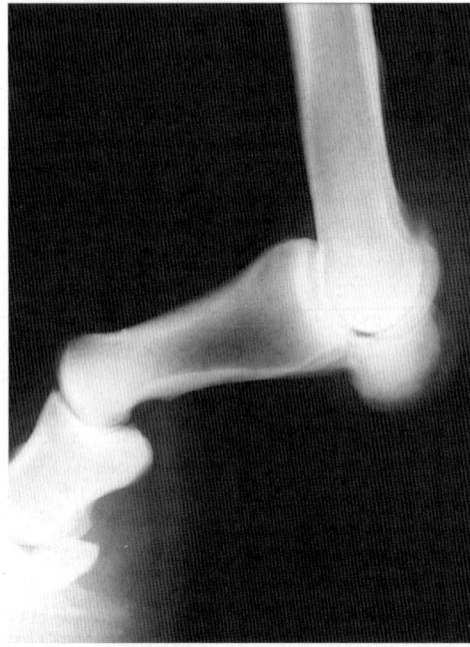

Fig. 104-4 • Lateromedial radiographic image of a horse with traumatic disruption of the suspensory apparatus as a result of a nearly complete tear of the body of the suspensory ligament. A similar appearance is observed in horses with severe injury of both branches of the suspensory ligament. Dorsal subluxation (hyperflexion) of the proximal interphalangeal joint occurs as a result of suspensory ligament disruption. Surgical or nonsurgical management can be chosen in horses with this injury.

Traumatic disruption of the suspensory apparatus is virtually always a career-ending injury. The only exceptions are horses with simple, displaced midbody fractures of both PSBs that can be individually repaired and suspensory body or branch injuries in some STBs. It is important to recognize the severity of the injury so that an informed decision can be made concerning treatment. Most horses can be saved as pasture sound or breeding horses, but treatment often is prolonged and expensive regardless of the therapeutic approach selected.

First Aid

As outlined previously, an important principle is to align the McIII and the phalanges using a homemade splint or a commercially available splint (see Figure 104-1). I much prefer the commercially available splint. Most horses are less anxious and are able to move comfortably immediately after the splint is applied. Other first aid measures include the administration of nonsteroidal antiinflammatory drugs (NSAIDs), intravenous fluids to replace water and electrolytes lost through sweating, and broad-spectrum antibiotics. Antibiotics should be given even if the fracture is ostensibly closed. High concentrations of antibiotics in the fracture hematoma are desirable, because skin abrasions and lacerations over hypovascular tissue are common. The vascularity of the foot should be assessed by palpation of the digital vessels and assessment of hoof temperature. Aspirin may be of some value in limiting the vascular injury. Horses that are extremely anxious and difficult to calm should be given xylazine or detomidine, with or without butorphanol, as needed for restraint and to prevent further self-injury.

Nonsurgical Management

Nonsurgical management involves long-term splinting with a goal of achieving sufficient fibrosis of the injured tissues that satisfactory support of the fetlock returns. The primary advantage of this approach is avoiding the risks associated with operating in a hypovascular and possibly contaminated surgical site. The surgical and technical expertise and equipment required are modest, and the expense of *initial* treatment is relatively small. There are serious disadvantages of nonsurgical management. Developing fibrosis may not be adequate to support the fetlock joint in a horse exercising at pasture; this is more problematic in horses with distal sesamoidean ligament avulsions than fractured PSBs. Scar tissue may slowly fail when stallions enter a breeding shed or a mare carries a foal. Most horses are uncomfortable on the splinted limb and cannot use it normally because of an abnormal posture (see Figure 104-1), and they are at risk for supporting limb breakdown and laminitis. Long-term splinting also demands meticulous daily bandage changes to prevent rub sores at the proximal dorsal metacarpal region and suppurative dermatitis of the palmar aspect of the pastern and heel bulbs. In my opinion, nonsurgical management is not the best choice in most horses with traumatic disruption of the suspensory apparatus, especially those with comminuted fractures of the PSBs, or rupture of the distal sesamoidean ligaments.

Successful long-term splinting of horses with traumatic disruption of the suspensory apparatus involves meticulous nursing care. Most clinicians use a prefabricated splint because of the ease of its removal and application. The Kimzey splint can be improved for long-term use by welding on a heel extension to increase the load-bearing surface area. This helps minimize the tendency to develop rub sores at the proximal, dorsal edge of the splint. The prefabricated splints are not perfectly fitted for every horse. Therefore some modifications in padding may be required to avoid excessive pressure at the proximal, dorsal metacarpal region. Regardless of which type of splint is used, the limb should be checked daily for developing sores or dermatitis, particularly in the palmar aspect of the pastern. If the leg is washed, it should be dried before a bandage is applied. Skin infection can be very difficult to manage. Both systemic and local antibiotics are usually necessary. A shoe with a thick pad and heel elevation should be applied to the contralateral foot. A thick shoe is necessary to mitigate the limb-length discrepancy that exists when the contralateral limb is splinted, but it is difficult to give an exact degree of heel elevation.

The most critical decisions when using nonsurgical management of a horse with traumatic disruption of the suspensory apparatus with splints are when to remove the splints and how to gradually return the horse to more normal fetlock and digit joint angles. Upright splinting is used in most horses for approximately 6 weeks, but many, particularly those with distal sesamoidean ligament avulsions, may require much longer. The process of dropping the fetlock should be gradual. This can be done by splinting at decreasing angles (a difficult task when using a prefabricated splint) or using a fetlock support shoe incorporating an adjustable sling. Horses should be confined to a stall for a prolonged period (4 to 6 months), because a single misstep can lead to tearing of the still-maturing scar tissue. Although external coaptation has worked well in individual horses and in some clinicians' hands, long-term results do not appear to be as good as surgical arthrodesis (fusion). Surgical fusion has considerable potential complications, but solid fusion of the fetlock joint is unlikely to slowly fail and cause progressive discomfort in horses used for breeding. Horses in which nonsurgical management was used appear to have more long-term lameness problems when compared

with those in which surgical management was used. The more serious the injury, the less likely it is that a nonsurgical approach will prove satisfactory. Although a splint will definitely allow adequate early management, both laminitis at 6 to 8 weeks postinjury and chronic pain or instability when the splint is removed occur commonly.

Surgical Management

Surgical management of horses with traumatic disruption of the suspensory apparatus generally involves fetlock arthrodesis, although repair of simple, displaced midbody fractures of the PSBs can be performed to preserve some degree of fetlock joint function. The major advantage of arthrodesis is that the procedure usually affords the horse immediate, comfortable use of the limb and, barring surgical infection or failure, avoids the problems associated with prolonged overload of the contralateral limb. Because the fixation is usually very stable, postoperative immobilization is minimal, and the various complications of casts and splints can be avoided. The primary disadvantage of surgical arthrodesis is an increased risk of infection when compared with nonsurgical management. In addition, successful arthrodesis requires both surgical expertise and investment in equipment and facilities.

The most widely used technique for fetlock arthrodesis is the application of a dorsal plate and the creation of a tension band on the palmar aspect of the fetlock joint.[3] Dorsal plating without a tension band on the palmar aspect of the fetlock is ill-advised because the plate is cycled in bending and the fixation may fail. Cyclic fatigue of even a large bone plate consistently results in plate failure unless a tension band technique of some sort is used. There are small variations in the techniques preferred by experienced surgeons with this procedure, but all have the same primary mechanical goals. I currently use a 10-hole, broad locking compression plate with a combination of 5.0-mm locking head screws and 5.5-mm cortex screws, and two 1.25-mm wires placed in figure-eight fashion along the palmar aspect of the fetlock joint.

The major complication of internal fixation for fetlock arthrodesis is infection. However, because this repair is very strong and stable, healing can occur even in the face of infection. The combination of instability and infection, however, rarely results in success, and reoperation on horses with unstable, infected sites is usually necessary to achieve fusion. Implant failure also is a concern, but proper technique and the use of large screws make this complication uncommon.

A common long-term complication associated with traumatic disruption of the suspensory apparatus is osteoarthritis of the proximal or distal interphalangeal joints. The joints are stressed by the fusion of the fetlock joint and often by the presence of serious injury to the digital flexor tendons and distal sesamoidean ligaments that insert on the phalanges.

Many horses with traumatic disruption of the suspensory apparatus sustain open, contaminated fractures or such extensive soft tissue damage that internal fixation may carry an unacceptable risk of infection. External skeletal fixation is an alternative means of managing horses with such injuries (see Chapter 87).

The prognosis for any horse with traumatic disruption of the suspensory apparatus depends on the specific nature and severity of the injury. Horses with distal sesamoidean ligament avulsions have a poorer prognosis than those with displaced fractures of the PSBs, because the latter tend to form fibrous scar tissue more quickly. Horses with the relatively uncommon suspensory body or bilateral branch tears have the best prognosis, because they seem to heal more quickly and have less fetlock joint instability. At least 60% to 75% of horses with closed disruptions of the suspensory apparatus and an intact blood supply should be saved with proper treatment. Horses with open injuries have a much poorer prognosis regardless of the therapy chosen, and those with open injuries with vascular compromise have a very poor prognosis.

Additional complications of traumatic disruption of the suspensory apparatus, regardless of treatment, include laminitis or breakdown of the contralateral limb. The primary complications of long-term splinting are rub sores and inadequate fibrosis, which lead to instability and chronic pain.

Other Catastrophic Distal Limb Fractures

Horses with other distal limb fractures have highly variable prognoses, but most horses with catastrophic fractures of the distal extremity can be successfully treated (for life if not function) if proper first aid and technically competent surgical treatment are performed. It is critical to prevent skin penetration of bone fragments, vascular injury, and prolonged delays in treatment. Because distal limb injuries can nearly always be temporarily immobilized relatively easily, decisions to euthanize should be made only after having informed discussions with the owner.

Severely comminuted fractures of the proximal and middle phalanges can be managed with the relatively simple technique of transfixation pin casting (Figure 104-5).[4,5] The important advantages of transfixation techniques are that they are technically easy to perform and provide consistent early comfort. Without an open approach to the fracture site the surgeon can avoid causing further damage to already severely compromised tissues. The major disadvantages of transfixation techniques are

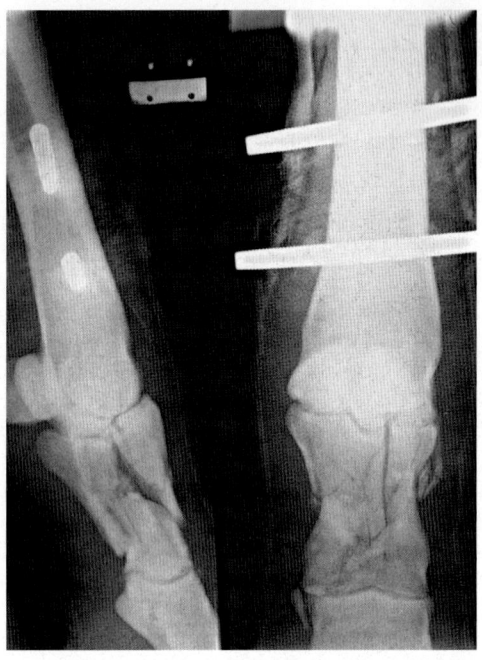

Fig. 104-5 • Lateromedial and dorsopalmar radiographic images of a horse with a comminuted fracture of the proximal phalanx stabilized using transfixation pin casting. This type of fixation allows immediate weight bearing and obviates the need to invade the fracture site and further compromise injured soft tissues. Eventually both the metacarpophalangeal and the proximal interphalangeal joints will fuse, but horses with catastrophic phalangeal fractures can be salvaged using this technique.

catastrophic fractures through the pin holes and early loss of acceptable comfort from pin loosening or infection.

Horses with major fractures above the carpus and tarsus are not as easy to deal with humanely on an emergency basis. It is certain that any overtly unstable fracture in the proximal limb will be an extremely expensive proposition to address surgically and that the prognosis is always guarded to poor at best. The only common exception might be horses with humeral fractures that may successfully heal with just stall confinement.

Chapter 105

Track Surfaces and Lameness: Epidemiological Aspects of Racehorse Injury

Tim D.H. Parkin

The racing surface is often regarded as the most important factor likely to influence the risk of injury. The effect that different course designs and surface types have on injury

has been discussed for many years,[1,2] and the surface and its management are obvious targets for immediate scrutiny after a racing injury. Certainly there are significant differences in the risk of injury among races held on turf, all-weather, and dirt tracks. On turf tracks there is also a significant effect of the firmness of the ground on injury risk. However, there are many other potentially less obvious factors that may also be related to the type and quality of the racing surface that influence the risk of injury during racing. In this chapter, the strength of evidence provided by a range of epidemiological studies is examined. Associations between injury and surface characteristics during both racing and training are described. The risk of injury on different surfaces and evidence from multivariable epidemiological studies that include surface characteristics are summarized. Comparisons of the same racecourse where changes have been made are discussed, and priorities for future research are identified.

 References on page 1341

RACING SURFACES

The Risk of Injury on Different Racing Surfaces

Musculoskeletal injuries are the most common reason for time lost in training, retirement from racing, and euthanasia in racehorses worldwide.[3-7] In the majority of locations, nonturf surfaces appear to be associated with an approximately twofold greater risk of injury. From 1999 to 2003 in the United Kingdom, the overall incidence of catastrophic distal limb fractures (including fractures of the carpus and tarsus) in all-weather flat races was 0.74 per 1000 starts compared with 0.37 per 1000 starts in turf flat races.[8] The risk of catastrophic musculoskeletal injury on dirt has been reported to be 1.12 per 1000 starts compared with 0.58 per 1000 starts on turf on two racecourses in Ontario, Canada,[9] The risk of fracture injury for horses racing on three New York Racing Association tracks from February 1, 1983 to mid October 1985 was 2.1 per 1000 starts on dirt compared with 1.1 per 1000 starts on turf.[10]

Results in a study from Florida did not concur.[11] In this study the incidence of injury was significantly higher in turf races (2.3 per 1000 starts) than in dirt races (0.9 per 1000 starts).[11] This may be a particular characteristic of racing in Florida because the turf races were more likely to involve larger fields and be longer races than those reported in other studies. Both of these factors were associated with the risk of injury in previous studies,[12-17] indicating that turf racing may be a proxy marker for these other risk factors.

Fractures predominate as a major type of injury, and the bones distal to the carpus or tarsus are most often affected.[3,4] Postmortem investigations conducted in the United Kingdom have enabled estimates of the risk of different types of fracture on different racing surfaces (Figure 105-1).[8] The overall incidence of catastrophic distal limb fractures in all-weather flat races was 0.74 per 1000 starts compared with 0.37 per 1000 starts in turf flat races. In other words, the relative risk (RR) of catastrophic distal limb fracture on all-weather surfaces compared with turf was 2.0 (95% confidence interval [95% CI] 1.3 to 3.1). There were also significant differences in the risk of certain types of fracture on these surfaces. In particular, fractures of the lateral condyle of the third metacarpal bone (McIII) were 3.2 times (95% CI 1.6 to 6.6) more likely to occur on all-weather surfaces than turf racecourses, and biaxial proximal sesamoid bone (PSB) fractures were 4.6 times (95% CI 1.8 to 11.6) more likely to occur on all-weather surfaces than turf racecourses.[8] Some fracture types were more common on the turf. For example, catastrophic fractures of the proximal phalanx were twice as common (RR 2.0; 95% CI 0.6 to 6.7) on turf than on all-weather surfaces.[8]

Similar postmortem studies have been conducted in other racing jurisdictions. In California[3,18] and Kentucky[14,19] the PSBs followed by the McIII were the most common sites of fracture. These were catastrophic fractures included in the California Horse Racing Board postmortem program from dirt tracks[3,18] and all injuries recorded at four tracks in Kentucky.[14,19] In contrast, injuries on three New York Racing Association dirt and turf tracks from 1986 to 1988 were more similar to those in the United Kingdom, with fractures of the McIII being most common.[20] Information on fatal musculoskeletal injuries from a number of racing jurisdictions within the United States (33 racetracks in 15 different states) revealed that McIII fractures were slightly more common than those of the PSBs.[21] However, an unknown number of "ankle breakdowns" in these data would have been caused by a PSB fracture and suspensory apparatus disruption. PSB fractures were also reported as the most common "serious accident" on eight racecourses in Japan.[22] In Australia, the situation is more similar to that in the United Kingdom, with fractures of the McIII and then of the PSBs predominating.[23] Clarification of differences in the risk of individual fracture types on different surfaces and further international comparisons will aid in the understanding of the pathogenesis of different fractures and ultimately may result in novel preventative measures being developed.

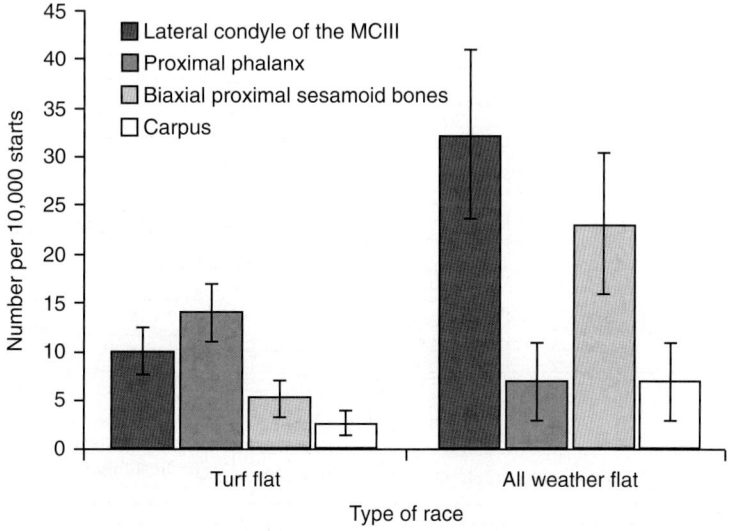

Fig. 105-1 • The distribution of catastrophic forelimb distal limb fractures on UK racecourses, by flat race surface type, from January 1999 to December 2003 (showing standard error bars). *MCIII*, Third metacarpal bone.

Simple comparisons of injury rates are useful in establishing priorities for future work at the local or regional levels. However, when establishing causal relationships, raw comparisons should be interpreted with caution. To state that the differences in injury rates on different surfaces in different racehorse populations are directly caused by surface characteristics is dangerous. There are many differences in the Thoroughbred populations racing in different locations. For example, at the time of the following study, different shoe types such as toe grabs were permitted in the United States.[24] There were strong associations between the use of toe grabs and the risk of both suspensory apparatus failure and condylar fracture of the McIII. In particular, the risk of suspensory apparatus failure was substantially increased in horses using regular-height toe grabs compared with those using no toe grabs.[24] In many other racing jurisdictions, toe grabs are not permitted, so meaningful international comparisons need to account for differences in shoe types as well as many other important contributory factors.

Even within a racing jurisdiction, direct comparisons between turf and all-weather tracks should not be made without consideration of all potential explanatory factors. For example, in the United Kingdom the prize money available and class of flat race held on the all-weather racecourses are generally lower than for flat races held on turf. This is obviously potentially an important confounding factor, as one of the reasons for poor performance may be subclinical or previous injury. It is therefore possible that horses in all-weather flat races are inherently more likely to sustain an injury, regardless of the surface on which they are racing. The type of surface may be important, but it is imperative to consider all potential factors in the same analysis. In order to deal with confounding variables, epidemiologists build multivariable or multiple regression models. These models adjust the size of effect and significance of risk factors by accounting for the effect of other confounding variables that are associated with both the outcome and other explanatory variables (Figure 105-2).

Further examples of potential confounding variables include track configuration,[25] training regimens of the local trainers who most often use the tracks,[26-28] and weather conditions and experience of the jockeys.[29] All of these variables and many more should be considered and accounted for when interpreting differences in injury risk on different racing surfaces. A causal web can be built to account for all potential confounders. A simplified version of the causal web designed for investigations of fatality during racing in Victoria, Australia[30,31] is shown in Figure 105-3. It is particularly useful with such complex diagrams to divide variables into the different horse, race, track, and jockey factors and then to identify which of these factors

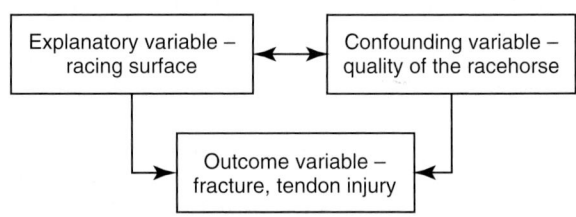

Fig. 105-2 • An example of the relationship among explanatory, confounding, and outcome variables that should be accounted for when determining the true size and significance of associations between important risk factors and the outcome of interest.

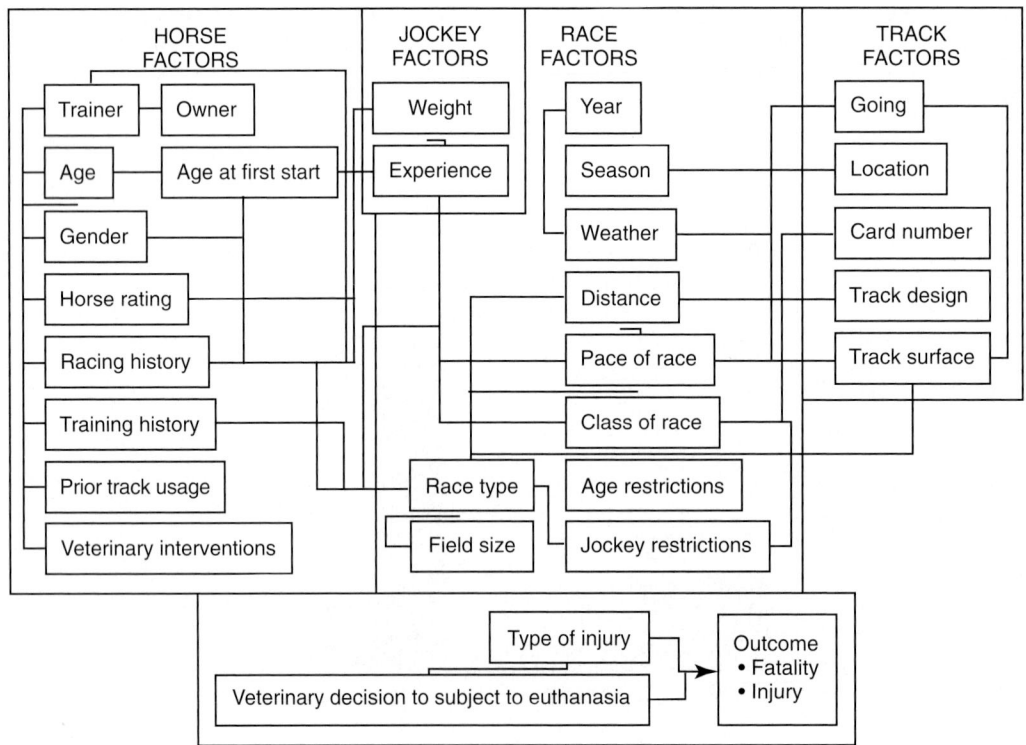

Fig. 105-3 • Causal web for consideration of risk factors and interactions among them for fatality during racing in Victoria, Australia.[30,31]

are likely to influence others as well as affecting the likelihood of the outcome of interest.

Evidence from Multivariable Epidemiological Studies

There are relatively few multivariable epidemiological studies that have included surface type in models while also accounting for the effect of many other factors. The likely reason for this is that when performing case-control studies it is common to select control (unaffected) horses from the same race in which the case horse was running. This obviously means that race-matched case-control sets are also matched on surface type, making comparison of this factor impossible. The rationale behind this study design is that in order to identify horse-level factors it is easiest to exclude (by matching) the potentially strong influence that race-level factors may have on the outcome. Even among studies that have specifically investigated race-level factors, control races, in which no horses were injured, are often matched on race and surface type.[17] This is done to account for the strong effect of race type and surface on injury risk so that other, more subtle race-level risk factors can be identified. Given the fact that until recently the majority of courses were not in a position to change their track type, the priority was to identify modifiable risk factors to reduce the likelihood of injury on the surfaces already in use.

Results from the few multivariable studies that did include surface type have not been consistent. In New York, racetrack location (one particular track) and dirt surfaces were significantly associated with an increased risk of injury.[20,32] However, in Florida, horses racing on turf tracks were more likely to be injured than those racing on dirt.[11] This association remained significant even when field size and race distance (both associated with surface type) were accounted for.

Therefore, to date complex multivariable models have not fully addressed the effect of surface type on injury risk. Ideally, large-scale collaborations among racing jurisdictions with different racing surfaces, using multivariable analysis to account for other potential risk factors, are needed if firm conclusions are to be drawn. Although expensive and time-consuming, such an initiative would also help to avoid repetition of studies and duplication of investment in different jurisdictions investigating the same problems. Large-scale collaborations can dramatically improve statistical power, ensuring that small effects of different risk factors can be identified.

Studies within the Same Racecourse

The goal of most multivariable epidemiological studies is to identify modifiable risk factors to enable the design and implementation of appropriate and effective interventions. In the field of racetrack epidemiology, monitoring the effect of a change is as close as the industry will get to a randomized controlled trial. If all other factors remain the same and sufficient time is given for interventions to have a statistically significant effect, a change in one variable (e.g., surface type) may be interpreted as causing a change in the outcome variable (e.g., risk of injury). Although there has been a change from dirt to synthetic surfaces at a number of tracks around the world, to date few have reported how these new surfaces have affected injury rates.

It is likely too early to see statistically significant differences in changes of surfaces on racetracks in the United States. However, in Japan, changes were made to Hanshin Racetrack after it was found to have a higher rate of racing injuries than other racetracks.[25] Changes included slowing the pace of races, widening the third and fourth corners, and including an upgrade slope in the finishing stretch. A better cushion was installed in both the turf and dirt tracks. In the following year there were significant reductions in the incidence of severe racing injuries (both fracture and nonfracture).[25]

In 2000 the British Horseracing Authority established an Equine Welfare database that provides all race, horse, course, trainer, jockey, and racecourse details for every race on all 60 racecourses in the United Kingdom. Comparison of the risk of fatality and long-term injury on the different courses before and after the introduction of new surfaces provides some of the most convincing evidence available to assess the effect of surface type on injury risk. These data were provided by members of the Equine Science and Welfare department at the British Horseracing Authority.[33] The synthetic surfaces at three all-weather racecourses were replaced or relayed from 2001 to 2007. At two of these tracks the surface was changed to Polytrack from either Equitrack or Fibresand. At a third track an old Fibresand surface was replaced by a new Fibresand surface that was subsequently relayed 2 years later.

The change from Fibresand to Polytrack on one course resulted in a statistically significant reduction (50%) in the risk of fatality (RR 0.48 [95% CI 0.3 to 0.78]; $P = 0.002$). However, there was no significant reduction in the risk of long-term injury on this track ($P = .026$). In contrast, a change from Equitrack to Polytrack on a second course resulted in a significant drop in the risk of long-term injury (RR 0.37 [95% CI 0.2 to 0.7]; $P = 0.002$) but no significant change in the risk of fatality ($P = 0.73$).

These studies demonstrate that all aspects of course design must be considered to enable the provision of the safest racing conditions. On some courses with certain climatic conditions, turf may be the only appropriate surface. However, in other situations, synthetic surfaces (especially the more recent designs) may present a similar level of risk as turf. All racing jurisdictions should endeavor to provide the best racing conditions and seek the most robust current evidence when deciding which surface to introduce. In addition, comparisons and subsequent judgments on success or failure should be made only once sufficient time has passed for statistically significant differences in risk to be identified.

Quality of the Racing Surface

Turf Tracks

The firmness of the turf racing surface was reported as a risk factor for musculoskeletal injury.[6,17,34] In all studies there was an approximately linear increase in risk of injury from heavy and soft going (footing) through to firm or hard. The firmer the surface, the greater the risk of injury. Racing on firm or hard ground increased the risk of catastrophic lateral condylar fracture of the McIII fivefold, compared with racing on anything between good-firm and heavy.[29] Harder tracks, with less moisture content, may have less cushion, causing greater forces to be exerted and increasing the risk of injury.[35-37] This may be the case for most fracture types, but when lateral condylar fractures of the McIII were investigated, there was a threshold of good-firm going, above which the risk was greatly increased. Observations such as these could help elucidate the true pathogenesis underlying what is believed to be a stress-related fracture.[38] Further studies to identify methods to both effectively measure and modify the track firmness, specifically in jump racing, in which lateral condylar fractures of the McIII are most common, are warranted.

All-Weather Tracks

Recently there has been considerable interest in the replacement of dirt surfaces with new synthetic surfaces, particularly in the United States. Anecdotally the effect on injury rates has been variable. There remains much to learn about track maintenance with newer surfaces, and a particular type of synthetic surface may be more suitable than others in certain locations with particular climatic conditions. It may be years before statistical analysis of injury rates can be performed; therefore it is essential that accurate records of the number of starts and injuries be maintained for all tracks to enable effective future comparison.

Synthetic surfaces may lose the properties that make them safer than dirt surfaces, and inappropriate maintenance may well result in significant deterioration of the surface. Based on race data from the United Kingdom from 1987 to 1993, the overall fatality rate in all-weather flat races was determined to be 0.6 per 1000 starts compared with 0.8 per 1000 starts in turf flat races.[4] At the time there were only two all-weather racecourses in use, both of which were still relatively new, having started racing toward the end of 1989. In contrast, today starts at all-weather tracks in the United Kingdom are significantly more likely to result in injury or fatality than starts at turf tracks.[6,8] All-weather surfaces must be installed to customize maintenance regimens and surface characteristics with prevailing local weather conditions.

TRAINING SURFACES

It is understandable that the focus of epidemiological studies be race day fatalities and injuries, because they attract much media attention and have a substantial impact on the public perception of racing. In addition, epidemiological race day data are much more readily available than training data, simplifying study design and logistics. Training injuries are extremely important, and given the amount of time at risk there are many more nonfatal injuries during training than racing. One study in the United Kingdom followed a population of approximately 1200 horses for 2 years and reported that 78% of nontraumatic fractures occurred during training.[39] It is important to consider the effect of the training surface on lameness incurred during training and also during racing. The quality, type, and maintenance of training surfaces are at least as important as the same aspects of the racing surface. However, to date there are relatively few studies that have investigated the effect of different training surfaces on injury or lameness.

In some racing jurisdictions where the majority of training occurs at the same location as racing and sometimes on the main racetrack itself, it is difficult to compare the effects

of different surfaces. However, in other jurisdictions, such as the United Kingdom, the vast majority of training occurs on private or public gallops located away from racecourses, and in this scenario there are many other factors that may contribute to differences in injury rates on different surfaces (e.g., training regimen, topography, and population demographics). Therefore identifying definitive associations with surface type has proved difficult. Nevertheless, there are differences. There is a higher incidence of dorsal metacarpal disease on dirt than on wood fiber training surfaces in the United States.[40] Horses in the United Kingdom that spent a majority of time training on Equitrack were less likely to develop a fracture than those training on other surfaces.[41] During a study investigating racecourse catastrophic fracture a marginal association with the use of sand gallops during training was identified.[26]

Recent work from Ontario, Canada indicated that catastrophic musculoskeletal injuries were more likely to occur on turf (0.64 per 1000 workouts) than on dirt (0.39 per 1000 workouts).[9] Although not statistically significant, these differences are in contrast to the findings of previous studies and defy the common perception that turf is the safer surface. There is limited detailed discussion in the report, and results may be an example of an unavoidable limitation of observational epidemiological studies. Such studies identify associations, but often it is impossible to determine cause or effect. Horses may have been trained on turf, a more forgiving surface, because they were not as sound as those training on dirt. Turf-trained horses may have been inherently more likely to sustain a catastrophic musculoskeletal injury, regardless of the surface on which they were being trained. A further example of this potential effect was seen in a study in the United Kingdom,[26,29] in which horses doing no fast work during training were found to be significantly more likely to sustain a catastrophic distal limb fracture during racing. Bones of these horses may not have been adapted and may have been at risk to fail when racing, or the horses may have had subclinical injury or preexisting pathology that prevented them from training at full speed but increased the likelihood that they would sustain a fracture during racing.

Horses training in the United Kingdom on an unnamed all-weather surface were eight times more likely to have sustained a pelvic or tibial stress fracture.[28] Horses were included if they had been trained on this surface 70% of the time during the exposure period (30 or 60 days before fracture date). Horses that had trained less than 70% of the time on one surface were defined as the reference group (mixed surfaces), with which other surfaces were compared. The 70% cutoff was arbitrary. Incline and maintenance of the training surface were not taken into consideration, and there was a significant degree of unexplained trainer-level variability.[28] Further investigations measuring other trainer- or training yard–level variables are required before definitive statements about the effect of training surfaces on injury and lameness can be made.

FUTURE DIRECTIONS

Physical properties of racing surfaces and injury rates were studied. As early as the 1970s a dynamic testing machine was developed to simulate the peak impact force of a horse's hoof on a racing surface.[35] There was a decreased risk of lameness on surfaces with a loose cushion and soft base in a survey of racecourses in California conducted at the same time as the testing machine was being used.[35] Significant differences in surface moisture content at six different locations around Canterbury Downs racecourse, Shakopee, Minnesota, were identified, even though the subbase moisture did not change significantly.[13] Several areas of abnormal compaction were identified at starting chutes and areas of the course exposed to high traffic density.[13,42] During the study six horses broke down in the compacted areas. More recently, moisture content of the track cushion was shown to alter the energy return and impact resistance.[43] It is interesting to note that these authors also suggest that these properties may be optimal for horses traveling at relatively narrow ranges of speeds. Given the potential differences in the way individual horses interact with the racing surface[43] and the fact that tracks are not uniform,[13,42] there is a requirement for large-scale population level studies using accelerometers (in conjunction with Global Positioning Systems [GPSs] and heart rate monitors) to monitor hoof-surface interactions during normal training.

Accelerometers placed on different anatomical locations are now being used more frequently. In the early 1980s, accelerometers placed on the dorsal aspect of the hoof showed typical decelerations on a sand track of 85 g

(g = acceleration of gravity, 9.8 meters/sec^2) on impact.[36] This author also cited Fujisawa (personal communication), who reported that the typical deceleration on impact on turf was 175 g compared with 84 g to 125 g on dirt. Promising recent developments in wireless data acquisition systems (WDASs) suggest that population-wide studies are not far off. A WDAS was used to identify significant differences in impact accelerations in horses using toe grabs compared with flat racing plates[44] and on different surfaces.[45]

The potential to use the horse as the device to measure hoof-surface interactions is being pursued by a number of groups around the world. Technological advances have reduced the cost and weight of GPSs and accelerometers. Assuming jockey and horse safety are not compromised, WDASs will enable population studies to be conducted during normal training. The volume of data acquired will require specialist analytical techniques so that these data can be combined with routinely collected training, medical, and racing data to enable new risk factors for injury and lameness to be identified. These risk factors will be at the level of hoof-surface interaction and will provide novel insights into the pathogenesis of many different injuries. Only then will the true extent of the role the surface plays in the development of injury in the Thoroughbred be realized.

Chapter 106

The North American Thoroughbred

Rick M. Arthur, Jeff A. Blea, Mike W. Ross,
Patrick J. Moloney, and Mark W. Cheney

DESCRIPTION OF THE SPORT

King James I of England established horse racing as the Sport of Kings in the early seventeenth century, and the earliest English immigrants brought the sport to the American colonies. Colonials imported fine-blooded horses and staged informal race meets almost as soon as they hit land. Richard Nicolls took command of New Amsterdam, renamed New York, became the first governor of the colony in 1664, and established a racecourse.

Many of the founding fathers of the new country, including George Washington and Thomas Jefferson, raced horses. John Wickham, Aaron Burr's attorney at his treason trial, lost one of the top American stallions of the emerging Thoroughbred (TB) breed, named Boston, in a card game in 1835. Nathaniel Rives won the difficult 2-year-old colt and ignored advice to geld him. Boston not only won 40 of 45 starts, but he also sired Lexington. A foal of 1850, Lexington became the top racehorse in the country by winning from New York to New Orleans.

Lexington was named for the Kentucky town that became the center of TB breeding. Horsemen quickly realized that healthy horses could be raised on the limestone base of Central Kentucky, and the horse Lexington helped establish the area by becoming the top sire in the United States for 16 years.

Racetracks sprang up in many cities, and although the industry suffered during the Civil War, Saratoga was the exception. The New York social elite took in the waters at the Spa to escape the heat and humidity of the city, attended the races during the day, and partied through the summer evenings in spite of the war. A few years after the conflict, Col. M. Lewis Clark founded the Louisville Jockey Club to conduct race meets in Kentucky. In 1875 the Louisville Jockey Club opened a new racetrack, later called Churchill Downs, and that year Aristides won the first edition of the Kentucky Derby (the Derby).

The Derby did not begin as America's most famous race. Col. Matt Winn's genius at marketing in the early twentieth century was required to create the legend the Derby has become. When the filly Regret won the race in 1915, the Derby rose to prominence quickly as a premier American sporting event and a major stop for 3-year-old TBs.

Fans were disappointed when owner Sam Riddle and trainer Louis Feustel deemed the Derby too early in the year for their strapping colt Man o' War, the horse that had broken many records the previous year, winning 9 of 10 races. However, Man o' War added to his reputation without the Derby, going through a perfect season of 11 wins in as many races. To many he remains the finest TB racehorse the United States has ever produced.

A new moral climate was sweeping the nation after the turn of the century. Gambling, including on horse racing, was banned in many states as a precursor to Prohibition, which began in 1919. Kentucky was the exception, and horsemen and racing fans found many ingenious ways to skirt the law. The need for more state revenue from the Great Depression in the 1930s prompted the ban on racehorse wagering to be lifted in many states. Until the 1970s horse racing was often the only legalized form of gambling in most states. From the 1930s to the 1960s horse racing, boxing, and baseball were the most popular sports in the United States.

War Admiral, sired by Man o' War, gained such a following in the 1930s that the whole country listened to the Seabiscuit–War Admiral match race. Because the older Seabiscuit had lost his first 17 races as a 2-year-old, everyone expected War Admiral to win. Yet Seabiscuit, "the people's horse," beat War Admiral that day, and in 1938 Seabiscuit was said to have had more newspaper space than Hitler.

As a 3-year-old, War Admiral won the Derby, the Preakness, and the Belmont Stakes, races that became known as the Triple Crown. Only 11 horses have ever won all three races. In 1948 Citation so impressively captured the series that some thought the horse replaced Man o' War as the greatest racehorse. That argument persisted for the next 25 years, despite the achievements of horses such as Native Dancer, Swaps, Kelso, and Dr. Fager, none of which won the Triple Crown. However, in 1973 a bright chestnut colt, Secretariat, so captured the public imagination when he won the Triple Crown that *Time, Newsweek,* and *Sports Illustrated* all put him on the cover. He won the 1½-mile Belmont Stakes by a spectacular 31 lengths.

Although the Triple Crown increased in stature, California developed a strong racing circuit. Santa Anita, east of Los Angeles, opened in 1934 and gained immediate attention by offering the then unheard-of sum of $100,000 (U.S.) for the inaugural Santa Anita Handicap. Across town, Hollywood Park began attracting movie stars and established its own fixture, the Hollywood Gold Cup. Bing Crosby and friends built Del Mar about 100 miles south.

As transportation by air became more popular in the last half of the 20th century, horses from the East and West began meeting regularly. In fact, Affirmed, the latest horse to win the Triple Crown, in 1978, prepared for racing at Santa Anita and Hollywood Park.

Regional rivalries became popular, which added to the success of the Breeders' Cup series, inaugurated at Hollywood Park in 1984. Unlike the Triple Crown, which is solely for 3-year-olds, Breeders' Cup Day offers races for various divisions. Two-year-olds show what might emerge at the next year's Kentucky Derby. European horses often invade for the grass events and more recently have achieved notable success on synthetic surfaces. The Breeders' Cup Classic attracts elite runners on the dirt from coast to coast and from abroad.

The Breeders' Cup epitomizes the tenacity of the racing TB. Spectacular victories—including the triumph of Sunday Silence over archrival Easy Goer in the 1989 Classic, the victory of Personal Ensign over the Kentucky Derby–winning filly Winning Colors in the 1988 Distaff, and the devastating move Arazi made to capture the 1991 Juvenile after shipping to the United States from France—are legendary. American TBs regularly compete in Europe, Japan, Australia, and Dubai. Not even King James I could have envisioned the Sport of Kings developing into the international phenomenon it is today.

TB racing always has been an expensive sport. Since the introduction of pari-mutuel gambling, financial support and revenue have been derived from two groups: racehorse owners and the gambling public. The third leg of the horse racing industry is the racetrack operator. Racetracks are generally for-profit corporations, with the exception of Del Mar, Keeneland, Oak Tree at Santa Anita, and a few others. Racehorse ownership was once the domain of the wealthy, but now opportunities and partnership options are available for many. In the past, most owners maintained breeding operations to supply horses for their personal racing stables; commercial breeders were few. The focus of breeding was for successful racehorses, and rigorous selection for soundness was as important as racing ability. Commercial breeders have now become a major source of racehorses and have a different goal. They produce horses to satisfy the commercial market, an entirely different objective, often unrelated to producing a racehorse.

Commercial breeders offer horses at public auction, primarily as yearlings but also as weanlings and 2-year-olds in training. The auction market is fashionable and in many ways fickle and trendy. Buyers favor precocious yearlings, relatively more mature than others. Yearlings with sprinting bloodlines and well-muscled yearlings sell better than those with a classic distance pedigree and conformation for all but the most expensive horses. Little is known of soundness of the sire and dam. Although these trends are worrisome, one positive consequence has been the ever-improving quality of horse offered at public auctions. Now some of the best-pedigreed horses in the world are sold at public auction, a fact not true 30 years ago, and even traditional owners and breeders have entered the lucrative commercial market.

The commercial market is a straightforward avenue for owners to buy a high-quality racehorse without maintaining broodmares. The September Keeneland yearling sale offers nearly 5000 yearlings over a 10-day period. Numerous other sales are conducted throughout the year. Presale examination is an important part of veterinary practice at racetracks (see Chapter 99). The auction environment can be an extremely high-pressure setting for the veterinarian because the knockdown price may reach millions of dollars.

Owners can also buy horses in claiming races. In claiming races the prospective owner buys the horse for a predetermined price *before* the race, and the horse is considered sold once the starting gate opens, regardless of whether the horse wins or even finishes the race. Purses and monies from purchase (claim) go to the previous owner. Potential buyers of claiming horses cannot examine the horse, but they can watch it walk into the saddling paddock. Buying a horse by claiming gives an owner a ready-made racehorse, whereas owners and breeders have to wait at least 3 years before racing a homebred horse, and yearling buyers have to wait at least a year. Unfortunately, the risks in claiming are considerable, because the claiming game has no honor and the new horse may already be at the end of its career.

Racetrack operators have changed to meet demands of the racing fans. The state, racetrack operator, and horsemen, through purse distributions, obtain income from a percentage of the moneys wagered, called *handle*. Revenue from simulcasting races across the United States and internationally is now an important source of handle, and Internet and at-home wagering are already realities. There was a time in the 1970s when Santa Anita and Hollywood Park had a higher daily average attendance than the Los Angeles Dodgers baseball stadium. On-the-track attendance has dwindled and contributes only a fraction to purses and commissions compared with what it did 40 years ago, when a fan had to come to the track to place a wager. Unfortunately, for reasons the racing industry is now regretting, the revenue sharing from off-track sites is much less than when the same amount of money is wagered on-track. The amount of revenue generated for purses and racetrack operators has not kept up with inflation, thereby placing greater economic stress on all industry participants. The importance of simulcasting to the future of horse racing has led to consolidation of racetrack ownership.

Because track operators emphasize handle, races are run in a manner to encourage betting. Races must be competitive, and the more horses the better. An anathema to the nongambling race fan and many horsemen is that gamblers bet more money on a large field of poor-quality horses than on a small field of high-quality horses. In the United States, field size rarely exceeds 12 horses, because dirt racetracks are relatively narrow and have tight turns, and turf courses, usually inside of the main dirt track, are even narrower with tighter turns.

Races are made to be competitive by restricting which horses are eligible to run in a particular race. Most important are age, gender, distance, and surface (turf or dirt). Sex and age restrictions limit which horses are allowed to compete in a race. Age is a major factor, and 2-year-olds are never raced against older horses, because they would not be competitive. Distaff races are those restricted to fillies and mares, and although the distaff side is not excluded from open races, such races are seldom competitive, except early in the 2-year-old year.

Distance and surface are conditions selected to suit the horse. Another set of conditions, handicaps and allowances, can be confusing but works well. Handicap and allowance races are set up to even the race by varying the weight carried by the horse. Weight variation is a subjective value, determined by racing officials for handicap races. In allowance races, weight variation is determined by a set of published criteria. For example, 3-year-olds carry less weight than older horses, fillies less than colts, and nonwinners may get additional weight off.

Most races in the United States are claiming races. In claiming races, horses of similar ability are pitted together. Because of the risk of losing a horse by claim, owners and trainers are discouraged from running more valuable horses to steal a purse. The claiming aspect of American racing is popular, but it has several negative effects on racing.

Stakes races are for the best horses. Stakes races require an entry fee and some require an additional starting fee. Stakes races are raced according to sex, age, distance, and surface. Stakes races are graded, listed, or restricted. Restricted stakes races, popular in recent years, restrict eligibility to the state of foaling or to conditions similar to allowance races. Stakes races are run even if only one horse is entered, but this is rare and is called a *walkover*. Stakes can be handicaps, allowances, or weight-for-age races. In weight-for-age races all horses carry the same weight, except for the well-established allowances for age and gender. The Kentucky Derby is a weight-for-age race for 3-year-olds. All horses are assigned the same weight (126 lb [57.3 kg]), but a filly receives a weight allowance and carries 123 lb (55.9 kg). The best stakes races are graded by a national committee and classified as Grade 1, Grade 2, or Grade 3; Grade 1 races are the top races. The Kentucky Derby and Breeders' Cup Classic are examples of Grade 1 races. The North American graded stakes races are analogous to the European group or pattern races.

Nonstakes races fall into several categories. Maiden races are for horses that have never won a race and can be allowance or claiming races. Races can be restricted to horses that have not won a certain number of lifetime starts. Other specific conditions for races can include eligibility for horses that have not won a race in a certain time period or over a certain distance. Claiming races also are restricted by age, gender, distance, and surface. Although races are devised to maximize competitiveness, the uncertain offering of races for nonstakes horses greatly complicates training and veterinary care, because timing for future races can be difficult to judge.

Stakes races are predominantly for horses 2 and 3 years of age, whereas horses may continue to race in claiming races up to 10 to 12 years of age. Claiming horses may drop progressively in class and value, and the lowest level of TB racing in the United States is considerably below that of the United Kingdom. Much of the following discussion reflects our dealings with high-quality, younger horses. These situations are easier for the veterinarian to be in control and to dictate the diagnostic approach and therapeutic plan, working with the trainer. With low-value claiming horses the trainer is more likely to dictate what is treated and with what. Frequently joints are treated with corticosteroids alone, rather than in combination with hyaluronan. Regardless of level of competition, it is important to establish and maintain a good owner-trainer-veterinarian relationship. This helps ensure the health of the racehorse and the success of the racing venture (JAB).

CONFORMATION

Many mild conformational defects appear to be well tolerated by TB racehorses (MWC, PJM). Mild toe-out and toe-in conformation causes few problems, but horses with moderate or severe toe-out conformation develop interference injuries. Toe-out conformation may predispose the horse to subsolar bruising of the medial heel. The most severe conformational defect is calf-knee or back-at-the-knee conformation. This defect leads directly to carpal lameness. Short, straight pasterns increase concussion, and long, sloping pasterns are undesirable because they may lead to soft tissue injuries or fractures of the proximal sesamoid bones (PSBs). Offset (bench) knee conformation leads to splint disease, injury of the antebrachiocarpal joint, and proximal suspensory desmitis (PSD). Horses that are tied in behind the knee develop tendonitis. Sickle-hocked conformation leads directly to lameness of the distal tarsal region. Horses with straight hindlimbs develop lameness of the stifle region and are prone to upward fixation of the patella.

TRACK SURFACE AND LAMENESS

Track surface is an important factor in the development of lameness and frequently is overlooked or neglected in lameness discussions (PJM, MWC) (see Chapter 105). Track surface dictates frequency and type of lameness. Injuries are often blamed on track surfaces, but musculoskeletal injuries are multifactorial. Shoeing, medication, training patterns, commercial breeding, and many other factors have all been implicated in the high injury rates in racehorses, and as often as not injuries cannot be fairly blamed on track surface (RMA, JAB). The most important factor in fatal racing injuries is not the track surface, but the horse (RMA). Almost all horses that develop fatal musculoskeletal racing and training injuries have evidence of preexisting pathology at the site of the fatal injury. They are repetitive stress injuries. Regardless, track surfaces play an important part in injury development, and the veterinarian needs to appreciate the types of injuries that are likely to develop in the track surfaces in his or her practice area.

Surfaces that favor speed also predispose horses to catastrophic breakdowns. Quality of racing surface is much more important than whether the surface is dirt or turf. Hard racetracks with little cushion are the worst surfaces. One of us (MWC) observed 38 horses with bone injury in a 4-week period when horses were training and racing on a hard racetrack. When sand was added to the track and the cushion increased from 6 to 11 cm, over the ensuing 4-week period only four horses developed bone injury. However, race times increased substantially. Horses need not train on hard surfaces to be able to race on them. Training on a forgiving surface then racing on a fast surface is safer than the opposite approach or working on a hard surface constantly. Consistent and uniform surfaces are the safest, allowing horses to remain sound and reducing incidence of injury (JAB). Track surfaces can change dramatically, especially in inclement weather.

Banking around turns can influence how horses negotiate turns and lameness distribution and expression. The hindlimbs of horses negotiating flat turns appear to slip out from under them, and in some instances horses nearly go down.

Track surface can make a difference in how horses with injuries are managed or rehabilitated. Horses rehabilitating after fractures or other bone injuries should not train on hard tracks. Likewise, horses coming back after soft tissue injuries or racing with minor infirmities should not be trained on deep or muddy tracks.

Many European horses that previously trained on grass now race in North America. Most race and continue to train on grass, but some make the switch to training and racing on dirt successfully (see Chapter 107). Our impression is that European horses appear to have fewer forelimb and more hindlimb lameness problems than North American TBs. European horses often train on long straightaways, and this, combined with a forgiving surface (grass), is a situation different from training on dirt in North America. Horses bred to race on the turf appear to have an inherent conformational difference that allows superior performance on grass. Synthetic racing surfaces fall somewhere between dirt and turf relative to horse surface preferences. Turf horses are much more likely to be competitive on synthetic surface, even if they do not handle dirt tracks.

Just as there are horses that do well or poorly on dirt or turf, there are horses that handle synthetic surfaces well and horses that do not.

In recent years more attention has been placed on track surfaces than ever before. The major change has been the introduction of synthetic surfaces in North America. The first Breeders' Cup events run over a synthetic surface were at Oak Tree at Santa Anita in 2008 and 2009. Synthetic surfaces are primarily sand, some fiber material, and a wax or polymer used to coat the sand and bind the material together. Unlike dirt tracks, which are usually cambered to drain horizontally, synthetic tracks are designed to drain vertically and require a drainage system built into the track. The racing results from synthetic surfaces have been mixed. In California, where the racing commission mandated synthetic surfaces by the beginning of 2008, racing fatalities dropped 40% when main track racing fatalities were compared with the same main tracks when they were dirt from 2004 to 2007. The training fatalities at the same tracks have not significantly improved with the synthetic surfaces. The distribution of racing and training injuries resulting in fatalities has changed. There are many more hindlimb injuries with synthetic surfaces compared with dirt (RMA). There are also numerous reports of increases in soft tissue injuries, primarily involving the proximal aspect of the suspensory ligament (SL). Although synthetic surfaces appear promising, the technology is relatively new, and the synthetic surfaces have had installation and maintenance problems.

A better understanding of the relationship between track surfaces and injury has been woefully neglected in the past. A number of research efforts have begun to better characterize the important relationship between track surfaces, biomechanics, and ultimately injuries. A safe racing surface has become of paramount importance to racing as the highly public injuries to Barbaro in the 2006 Preakness and Eight Belles in the 2008 Kentucky Derby have made equine welfare concerns a public debate. Marketing surveys by the racing industry have shown racing fatalities are of major concern to the general public. There can only be increasing emphasis on equine safety in the future.

MEDICATION AND DRUG TESTING CONSIDERATIONS

Horse racing has always regulated the use of medications, but more recently the relatively permissive North American medication regulatory scheme has come under greater scrutiny. Outside North America most racing jurisdictions operate under International Federation of Horseracing Authorities (IFHA) rules. IFHA rules prohibit the use of nonsteroidal antiinflammatory drugs (NSAIDs) within several days of racing, whereas all North American racing jurisdictions allow some use of at least one NSAID the day before racing. Whether the permissive NSAID regulations and other medication policies contribute to the higher racing fatality rates in North America than most other racing jurisdictions using IFHA rules is debatable. Further complicating the issue, racing regulatory veterinarians, the veterinarians responsible for the prerace examinations have begun to question whether North American NSAID regulations are compromising their examinations by masking clinical signs of inflammation. Currently, an approximate

4-mg/kg dose of phenylbutazone about 24 hours before racing is permitted in North America and conforms to the blood level of lower than 5 mcg/mL on raceday.

The policies and regulations governing the use of corticosteroids, particularly intraarticular corticosteroids, are also under scrutiny. Most racetrack veterinarians believe intraarticular corticosteroids are most effective if used 5 to 10 days before racing (RMA, JAB). Unfortunately, changes in the way races are carded today have made planning for races problematic except for stakes races. Trainers cannot confidently plan for races on a certain date and feel forced to wait until the horse is in a race to perform intraarticular injections, sometimes as little as 2 days before the a race. The American Association of Equine Practitioners is recommending that racehorses should not receive intraarticular corticosteroid injection within 5 days of racing. Racing regulatory veterinarians have called for an outright prohibition within 5 to 7 days of racing (RMA). Most corticosteroids are Association of Racing Commissioners International (ARCI) Class 4 drugs, and recent research efforts have been directed toward increasing the sensitivity of drug screening for corticosteroids. Research suggests triamcinolone acetonide and betamethasone have chondroprotective properties when used prudently. On the other hand, one of the most commonly used intraarticular corticosteroids, methylprednisolone acetate, does not fare as well in laboratory studies but is still a preferred intraarticular corticosteroid of many racetrack practitioners because of potency and consistency of clinical response. The pharmacodynamics of intraarticular corticosteroids is just now being studied in horses. With a better understanding of the clinical response to these drugs, combined with advances in laboratory detectability, the way corticosteroids are used may change dramatically within a few years.

Withdrawal time information is not readily available in all jurisdictions for many common therapeutic drugs used for equine lameness. The state-by-state regulation of racing in the United States and the large number of drug-testing laboratories complicates racetrack veterinary practice. Prudence dictates that all veterinarians treating horses intended to race at state-sanctioned racetracks be familiar with the drug testing and medication regulations in that jurisdiction. Resources that may be of use to racetrack veterinarians are the ARCI and the Racing Medication and Testing Consortium (RMTC). Both organizations have websites with information on medication and veterinary practice regulations as well as drug testing.

LAMENESS EXAMINATION

A racetrack clinician has distinct advantages over other practitioners. A racetrack veterinarian is involved intimately in the day-to-day operation of a racing stable and becomes familiar with the normal gait, disposition, and general health care factors of each horse, such as appetite, coat condition, weight, training and racing status, and performance. Numerous examinations can be performed easily if needed. Horses can be examined before and after training to see if lameness worsens or improves.

History

The most important piece of information is the training history. What did the horse do today, yesterday, and the day before? How far is the horse from racing? When was the last fast work or race? Did any problems occur? Did the horse want to train? Did the horse lug in or out? Did the horse cool out normally? When did the trainer or exercise rider notice a problem? When was the last time the horse was shod? Is the horse receiving any medication? NSAIDs and corticosteroids can easily compromise the veterinarian's ability to properly evaluate lameness (RMA, JAB). The entire veterinary medical history is important for the veterinarian to know, but the past medical history of claiming horses is usually unavailable.

Most fractures occur in horses with a history of a recent hard workout or race. Sometimes lameness may not become apparent until the horse returns to the track several days later, but the injury occurred in the previous workout or race. Humeral stress fractures are the exception, because they usually occur in horses returning to work after not having worked for 45 to 90 days. Horses that lug in (drift toward the inside rail) or lug out (drift toward the outside rail) usually are moving away from the source of pain, but not always. The gallop is a complicated gait, and some horses may drift toward the side of pain while galloping at high speed, perhaps reflecting the lack of power on the affected side (MWR). Most horses in North America finish a race on the right lead. Finishing a race on the left lead may be normal for a horse, but in some horses finishing on the left lead may be a sign of high-speed lameness. A left-lead finish should prompt careful investigation of the left forelimb and right hindlimb as potential sites of lameness (MWR). Many lameness conditions are insidious in onset. Subtle signs, such as a horse that is unusually nervous and prefers to break into the gallop instead of jogging, are easy to overlook. Lameness the day after a shoeing change may implicate a close nail or a drastic change in hoof angle.

The age of the horse is important. Dorsal third metacarpal bone (McIII) disease and other stress-related bone injuries are unusual to diagnose in older horses if they do not have problems at 2 or 3 years of age. Older claiming horses are much more likely to have chronic osteoarthritis (OA), osteochondral fragmentation, or tendon injuries.

Palpation

The physical examination should be routine and complete. Horses are first examined in the stall, where they are comfortable and are more willing to tolerate manipulation. One of us (PJM) feels strongly enough about thorough examination that if trainers want to start with a visual examination while horses are tacked up and proceed directly to injection, they should find another veterinarian. Many lameness conditions are acute, and signs of inflammation are clearly useful. Horses with chronic lameness can be challenging, but long-term association with a horse is of great benefit. Regardless, the examination is the same. Palpation is critically important in evaluating racehorses, possibly the single most important clinical skill a racetrack veterinarian can develop. Very subtle abnormalities or changes from previous examinations can often be the key to developing the most effective diagnostic plan (JAB). With the horse standing squarely, all limbs are palpated for heat, pain, and swelling. During individual flexion of the front fetlock joints and carpi, pain response is important. Pain during carpal flexion almost always indicates a problem in that region. The clinician should remember that during lower limb flexion tests, joints other than the fetlock are being stressed. If concerned, we flex joints independently if possible. Whenever a pain response is elicited, the same palpation technique should be used to compare the response with that of the contralateral limb. There is considerable individual variation from one horse to another, particularly with more subtle responses. All aspects of the PSBs should be examined with the limb in flexion. SL branches, body, and origin and digital flexor tendons are carefully palpated along the entire length. The dorsal aspect of the McIII is palpated by placing the palm of the hand around the tendons and applying firm finger pressure. The forelimb is then brought forward while elevated, and the dorsal cortex of the McIII is palpated with firm thumb pressure. Careful palpation of the dorsal and palmar aspects of the McIII is important in detecting fracture of this bone (MWC).With the palm of the hand on the dorsal aspect of the McIII, the fingers can be used to palpate the proximal aspect of the SL and each splint bone. Care must be taken when examining the dorsal and palmar metacarpal regions, because the clinician may inadvertently cause pain on the dorsal cortex by examining the palmar aspect of the metacarpal region and vice versa (PJM). Proximal palmar metacarpal pain is important to detect, but false-positive results can occur (MWC). Any suspicious response should be evaluated further with ultrasonography (PJM). The carpus is flexed and the dorsal surfaces of the antebrachiocarpal and middle carpal joints are palpated with thumb pressure. An effort should be made to stretch the joint capsule around the borders of each carpal bone, because stretching often elicits pain if a lesion is present. To evaluate the elbow and shoulder regions, the limb is pulled backward and forward. With the limb extended, a jerking, upward motion sometimes causes pain in horses with humeral stress fractures. The shoulder joint and intertubercular (bicipital) bursa should be palpated with firm digital pressure.

The hands should be run lightly over the back to assess for sore or tense muscles. The lumbar and sacroiliac regions, gluteal muscles, and greater trochanter of the femur should be palpated from each side. Although the process appears hazardous, the gluteal muscles and greater trochanter also should be palpated from behind. If necessary a forelimb can be elevated. Firm pressure should be used to detect gluteal myositis or trochanteric bursitis. Standing behind the horse is the best way to compare effusion of the femoropatellar joints. Each hindlimb should be examined in the standing and flexed positions. The Churchill test should be performed bilaterally (see Chapter 6). A positive response suggests distal hock joint pain. Negative findings on palpation and manipulation do not eliminate a joint from consideration, but positive findings often point to the source of pain causing lameness.

Movement

It is mandatory to observe the horse during the first few steps out of the stall. Then the horse is usually walked down the shed row and back. Occasionally the horse is trotted immediately. If a horse appears "stiff" initially, it is useful to walk the horse a couple of times around the shed row to help discern if the lameness is real or if mild stiffness is a normal characteristic of that horse. This is important

with older horses that may have chronic problems. Horses with painful conditions do not generally warm out of lameness (JAB). It is important to trot the horse at a comfortable speed for the *horse,* not the handler, and the horse must be trotted far enough to reach an even speed. The head must be free, without allowing the horse to throw the head. Surface is important, and the harder, the better; soft surfaces may hide lameness. The horse is trotted in a straight line and while circling. Trotting the horse in a circle is the best way to differentiate diagonal or ipsilateral lameness (i.e., left forelimb from right or left hindlimb) and exacerbates many lameness conditions. Horses with tibial stress fractures are much worse while circling. Horses with third carpal bone pain and medial foot lameness are worse with the affected limb on the outside of a circle. Horses with lameness of the fetlock joint are usually worse with the affected limb innermost. Although characteristics of lameness while trotting are important, they are subjective.

At times, observing a horse under tack is useful. Often horses with hindlimb lameness are best examined on the racetrack, because many horses do not use themselves behind. Only when horses are absolutely sound in hand is examination at speed warranted, and even then, with the exception of understanding the complaint of the rider, obtaining useful diagnostic information is rare. However, one of us (PJM) likes to examine horses with obscure lameness on the track, under tack at the trot.

The usefulness of flexion or other manipulative tests is debatable. Lameness may be exacerbated, but disagreement exists over what a positive response means. For instance, when performing fetlock flexion, a positive response is common even in horses with lameness unrelated to the fetlock joint (RMA). One of us (PJM) finds fetlock and lower limb flexion tests worthwhile, but not carpal flexion, and finds hindlimb flexion tests nonspecific. One of us (MWC) finds forelimb flexion tests useful but finds all but the lower limb flexion test in the hindlimbs questionable. Finally, one of us finds the carpal flexion test the most specific and accurate flexion test; horses with a positive response generally have carpal region pain, and there are few false-positive results (MWR; see Chapter 8). Hindlimb flexion tests lack specificity (MWR). Each clinician needs to develop a protocol and be consistent.

Diagnostic Analgesia

Diagnostic analgesia is important to localize sources of pain, and sequential, distal-to-proximal, intraarticular, and perineural blocks should be performed. One of us (PJM) feels strongly that shortcuts, such as skipping immediately to a low palmar or plantar block rather than performing a palmar or plantar digital block first, lead only to misdiagnoses. Another (MWC) feels confident in clinical examination and blocks only when unsure of his diagnosis but admits that when a trainer or owner wants a definitive answer, this approach is unacceptable. However, to diagnose proximal plantar metatarsal pain definitively, a block must be performed. Blocking horses with long winter coats can be difficult. For distal McIII or third metatarsal bone (MtIII) bone disease, one of us (MWC) uses specific palmar or plantar metacarpal or metatarsal analgesia. A novel approach is taken to desensitize the distal 50% to 75% of the McIII. Five milliliters of local anesthetic solution are injected into the nutrient foramen. This block is not specific for bony disease, because the nearby accessory ligament of the deep digital flexor tendon can be affected; however, injury of this ligament is rare.

Whether to clip for intraarticular injections or analgesia is personal preference, but two of us do not clip (MWC, PJM). Although medicating and performing intraarticular analgesia simultaneously is acceptable, one of us (MWC) prefers to wait at least 1 day after blocking to medicate.

Horses may be difficult to handle during analgesic procedures or during intraarticular injections, but usually a lip chain or twitch provides adequate restraint. A good handler must be in control of the horse during the procedure. Gentle, confident, sure hands with painless technique are best (PJM). If sedation is necessary, a combination of 5 mg butorphanol and 200 mg xylazine or 2.5 mg (0.25 mL) detomidine is useful (MWC). However, sedation for diagnostic analgesia should be kept to a minimum. Acepromazine (5 to 10 mg intravenously [IV]) is useful, because the lameness may be exacerbated as a horse trots more quietly. This amount is usually adequate during the analgesic procedure (JAB).

Diagnostic analgesia is often necessary to identify the exact location of pain causing lameness. It is quite useful when two or more limbs or areas are affected. In the forelimb, intraarticular analgesia of the fetlock joint is an excellent and preferred starting point. Palmar disease of the fetlock joint (subchondral bone pain) is common, and if there is a positive response, this block identifies pain in this region. However, if degree of lameness does not change, low palmar or low plantar and palmar metacarpal or plantar metatarsal perineural analgesia (four-point block) should be performed, because subchondral bone pain of the distal aspect of the McIII or the MtIII may not be eliminated using intraarticular analgesia (MWR). Intraarticular analgesia of the fetlock joint will abolish pain associated with an articular fracture of the PSB, pain from which may be abolished using palmar digital analgesia. When the carpus is being blocked, intraarticular analgesia of each joint is useful to determine location of the pain causing lameness. A dorsal approach to the carpus is beneficial to prevent diffusion of local anesthetic solution to the proximal aspect of the SL. It is possible to abolish pain from a fracture of the third carpal bone with subcarpal analgesia. Time of response to intraarticular analgesia is important. A positive response may be seen with an intraarticular problem within minutes. When a positive response to intraarticular analgesia of the middle carpal joint is seen only after 30 minutes, it is important to evaluate the SL. In the hindlimb, a plantar digital nerve block is the preferred starting point.

Approaches and techniques have been well published. A sterile preparation should be performed for intraarticular injection. Gloves are not required but are a personal preference. After injection the limb is bandaged with "foam air" or Vetrap; alcohol and clean cotton bandages are used for the next 12 hours. Concurrent intraarticular medication is often administered but may be more beneficial to the joint if administered 24 hours later.

Diagnostic analgesia is a critical piece of the lameness puzzle. Proper allotment of time is necessary. Consistent interpretation of lameness is essential during the procedure (JAB).

IMAGING CONSIDERATIONS

Routine radiographic images often are supplemented with views looking specifically at problem areas of the TB racehorse. For instance, for the metacarpophalangeal and metatarsophalangeal joints, flexed dorsopalmar or dorsoplantar (DPa, DPl), dorsal 35° distal-palmaro(plantaro) proximal oblique, standard horizontal DPa or DPl, lateromedial (LM), flexed LM, and dorsolateral-palmaro(plantaro) medial oblique and dorsomedial-palmaro(plantaro)lateral oblique images should be considered routine. Additional images of the PSBs may be useful in evaluating fractures of the PSBs or palmar erosions of the McIII or the MtIII. The cassette is placed on the ground and a 45° (or 60°) oblique skyline image of each PSB is obtained (JAB). For the carpus the four standard images and a skyline image of each of the proximal and distal rows of carpal bones are routine. A flexed dorsal 45-degree lateral–palmaromedial oblique image should be considered when evaluating a distal radial carpal bone fracture (JAB).

Scintigraphic examination is important, because TB racehorses frequently develop cortical and subchondral stress-related bone injuries. Horses with obscure or undiagnosed lameness and those suspected of having stress-related bone injuries are candidates for scintigraphic examination. Because complete fracture often results from preexisting stress-related bone injuries in cortical and cancellous bone, horses with signs consistent with pelvic, tibial, humeral, and McIII or MtIII stress fractures should undergo scintigraphic examination before continuing in work. However, interpretation is not always straightforward. False-negative results have been found in horses with preexisting tibial stress fractures (PJM) and false-positive results in those with modeling reflecting changes in work intensity. Therefore experienced interpretation is essential, and follow-up examinations are required if findings do not concur with clinical observations.

For ultrasonographic examination, horses are routinely clipped. Ultrasonographic examination is valuable in diagnosing and staging tendonitis, suspensory desmitis, carpal tenosynovitis, lateral branch superficial digital flexor tendonitis, and other swellings of the pastern, swellings of the medial stifle region, and distal sesamoidean desmitis. Digital ultrasonography is the gold standard (JAB).

SHOEING

Trimming and shoeing of the TB racehorse are extremely important. In many practices, veterinarians are not involved in trimming and shoeing, and decisions often are made exclusively by trainers and farriers. The veterinarian should make every effort to work with the farrier regarding shoeing changes when a musculoskeletal problem renders them necessary (JAB). Because recent evidence has linked catastrophic injury to toe grabs on shoes, now a general trend is to see horses shod with low grabs, or none at all. Toe grabs are thought by many to cause forelimb lameness. Hindlimb toe grabs are often associated with hindlimb injuries on synthetic surfaces. There is virtually no slide of the foot on synthetic surfaces, and toe grabs can be a contributor to lameness (JAB). The rationale for using grabs is questionable, because the forelimbs are propelled by the hindlimbs, and traction on the front feet makes little sense.

Toe grabs may shorten the cranial phase of the stride, prevent forward sliding of the forelimbs, and cause lameness. One of us (MWC) has observed many horses that are stiff and short in front, and by simply removing the grabs and applying Queens plates (aluminum shoes with a low toe grab; Victory Racing Plate Company, Baltimore, Maryland, United States), lameness abates in 2 to 3 days. Steel shoes are a good alternative when horses resume training after a lay off. Training barefoot is often beneficial for horses that continue to develop sole bruises as a result of track surfaces. Training and racing without shoes may be beneficial for horses with distal hindlimb pain such as that caused by subchondral bone injury of the distal aspect of the MtIII (MWR). Lameness associated with toe grabs appears most commonly on dirt tracks with hard bases and cushions of less than 7.5 cm. For racing on dirt the Queens plates or variations are popular, and for turf the Queens plates and Queens XT shoes are required. Turndown shoes have received negative press, but they may be advantageous in horses with low heels. Slight turndowns without toe grabs on hind feet may actually benefit horses with hock and stifle pain. Many lameness problems may be created or exacerbated by poor shoeing, including PSD, tendonitis, and fractures of the PSBs. One of the major problems is shoeing horses with small shoes. Overzealous use of acrylic can cause severe foot lameness. Horses with thin walls are predisposed to nail bind, and those with sheared heels sustain repeated heel bruising. Glue-on shoes may be beneficial in the short term but can be detrimental if used long term. Using a three-quarter shoe is an alternative for bruised quarters. Cut-out or half aluminum plates are useful for a bruised or sore heel. Accurate diagnosis is essential (JAB).

Shoeing for synthetic racing surfaces is a hotly debated issue. In California many trainers are using Queens plates or Queens XT shoes all around for the synthetic surfaces. Rarely are traction devices used behind because of the concern that the natural slide for hindlimbs on dirt is lost on synthetic surfaces when shod with toe grabs, calks, or other traction devices. Many trainers and farriers keep flat or low toes on the hind feet when horses are training and racing on synthetic surfaces. California changed regulations permitting horses to race barefoot on synthetic surfaces. Although this is still fairly unusual, horses perform quite well without shoes on synthetic tracks. More commonly, horses are trained barefoot, especially the hind feet.

INABILITY TO MAKE A DIAGNOSIS

In many horses, despite a methodical and time-consuming approach to diagnostic analgesia, the source of pain cannot be identified (MWC). These horses are referred for additional clinical and scintigraphic examinations (MWC, PJM). Horses with stress-related bone injuries may show few clinical signs, and scintigraphy is the imaging modality of choice. Lameness in young horses in training may be more difficult to diagnose than that in horses that are racing (MWC). Many horses with undiagnosed lameness are confined to at least 6 weeks of walking. The advances of ultrasonography, digital radiography, computed tomography, and magnetic resonance imaging (MRI) have made the inability to make a diagnosis a rarity (JAB).

TEN MOST COMMON LAMENESS CONDITIONS

1. Lameness of the foot
2. Lameness of the metacarpophalangeal or metatarsophalangeal (fetlock) joints
3. Suspensory desmitis
4. Lameness of the carpus
5. Superficial digital flexor tendonitis
6. Tibial stress fractures
7. Distal hock joint pain
8. Myositis
9. Dorsal third metacarpal bone disease
10. Other stress fractures

SPECIFIC LAMENESS CONDITIONS

Lameness of the Foot

The most common cause of lameness in the TB racehorse is foot pain. Horses may be observed in the stall to pile bedding under the feet, presumably to cushion the feet or to change angles. Lameness is often worse with the affected limb on the inside of a circle. Heat at the coronary band and increase in digital pulse amplitude are frequent signs. TB racehorses have little hoof. Many are shod at least monthly, but most are shod more frequently, with thin, lightweight shoes. When shoes are changed frequently, little natural hoof is available with which to work if adjustments are necessary. The tendency is for the farriers to remove too much foot, particularly toward the heel, resulting in low heels. Thin feet have prompted the use of acrylics to augment the hoof wall, but overzealous use may itself result in foot soreness (MWC). Soreness and bruising are common, particularly on the medial quarter, just forward of or at the bar. The center of load distribution for a TB racehorse is medial and palmar to the anatomic center of the foot, close to the medial bar.

Most racehorses react positively to the application of hoof testers because only a thin covering of horn protects the sensitive structures of the foot. Degree of sensitivity to hoof testers is important and is learned through experience. Hoof tester examination is best done when an assistant holds the foot (RMA). Hoof testers can be placed carefully on front and hind feet, and slight differences in positioning make a substantial difference. Left and right feet should be compared at least twice before conclusions are reached. The diagnosis of palmar foot pain can be confirmed readily by selective medial or lateral palmar digital analgesia. Horses with a naturally wide gait, or with carpal pain, bruise the medial quarters and can have concomitant foot pain. Acquired bruises of this nature are difficult to treat in horses with wide gaits without lameness and without managing primary lameness in those with carpal pain. In most horses with foot lameness, diagnosis is made with clinical findings and diagnostic analgesia. If abnormalities of the sole or hoof wall cannot be found, radiographic examination is occasionally necessary (PJM). In most horses without fracture, lameness resolves in 2 to 3 weeks with specific therapy and the administration of NSAIDs.

Bruised Heels or Quarters

Lameness caused by bruised heels or quarters is often mild, and horses usually are kept in training. More often than not, little heat is associated with a bruised quarter. Mild dilation of one or both digital arteries and hoof tester sensitivity are the most common signs. The best treatment is rest, however. The foot should be examined for any conformational or shoeing faults; sheared heel or unbalanced feet are common causes of bruised quarters. Horses with toed-out conformation often bruise the medial aspect of the heel (MWC). Corrective shoeing is really the only treatment option. Steel shoes distribute force along the hoof wall evenly and can be applied to horses in training but not racing. Bonded shoes can be applied to horses that are racing. If the foot is warm, the horse should stand in ice water, but if the foot is normal in temperature, the horse should stand in a foot tub of hot water with Epsom salts. A poultice of warm, cooked flaxseed or commercially available products such as Animalintex (3M Animal Care Products, St Paul, Minnesota, United States) should be applied. A common practice of applying hoof-hardening agents such as iodine and turpentine should be avoided, because hard hooves bruise easily.

Abscesses

Foot abscesses are a common problem, particularly during the wet seasons. A foot abscess is the most common eventual diagnosis when a horse is found three-legged in the stall in the morning without a recent history of hard work or racing. TBs are prone to foot abscesses because of the manner and frequency of shoeing. Foot abscesses occur most commonly in the medial quarter, where bruising is also most common. Sole abscesses not involving the quarter are uncommon, take more time to resolve, and cause different clinical signs than do abscessed quarters. Although abscesses in the heel or quarter usually are located easily and precisely with hoof testers, a sole abscess can produce a large area of soreness. Identifying the specific area of pain is often difficult.

Horses with foot abscesses are best managed with hot water baths with Epsom salts and poulticing. The longer the horse stands in hot water with Epsom salts, the better. Ideally, the shoe should be removed, and the abscess should be allowed to open naturally. Usually more damage is done to the hoof wall by attempting to open the abscess manually than by allowing it to open naturally. Probing the white line to identify an abscessed area can be worthwhile. Sole abscesses are more likely to require manual opening and debridement than are abscessed quarters. The integrity of the hoof wall needs to be evaluated and preserved, if possible, but wet, infected areas need to be exposed, opened, and dried. Foot abscesses or infections also can originate from grabbed quarters, which occur frequently in horses that stumble out of the starting gate. When grabbed, the hoof wall of the quarter may separate at the heel bulb or quarter, well down the foot. The opened area becomes contaminated with track dirt, and infection can occur several days to weeks after the original injury. Fortunately a pathway for drainage is already present.

Quarter Cracks

Quarter cracks are common for the same reasons as bruising and abscessation. The quarters and heels take continual pounding, particularly in a TB racehorse with poor hoof wall support. Quarter cracks may be caused by poor hoof balance but most commonly result from innate hoof weakness. Farrier-incurred hoof imbalance can contribute to the development of quarter cracks, but most commonly a single horse in a stable has numerous cracks. Horses with an initial crack are prone to develop subsequent cracks in the same hoof or other hooves. A horse ran successfully with seven quarter crack patches at one time (RMA). If identified early, quarter cracks can be patched readily with acrylic or epoxy resin. The goal is to stabilize the hoof wall and eliminate uneven movement. Mild cracks should be patched if any movement occurs at all. As little patching material as possible should be used to stabilize the hoof wall. If a quarter crack is infected, a drainage path needs to be established. If the quarter crack is infected systemic antibiotics are warranted. An acrylic patch should never be applied until the infection has resolved (JAB). Some epoxy resins are much harder than the natural hoof wall, and trapped infection eventually drains through natural tissues rather than the patch. The incidence of quarter cracks is markedly reduced on synthetic surfaces (JAB).

Osteoarthritis of the Distal Interphalangeal Joint

Most lameness conditions of the foot seen in other sports horses also occur in racing TBs. Considerable controversy exists regarding the frequency of osteoarthritis (OA) of the distal interphalangeal (DIP) joint. Some veterinarians diagnose the problem regularly, whereas others never recognize it. In our experience, OA of the DIP joint is uncommon. Effusion is the most common clinical sign. Osteophytes may be seen on the extensor process of the distal phalanx. Frequently, horses with bilateral OA of the DIP joint have poor performance rather than overt lameness, and lameness is worse at the end of a race (MWC).

Navicular Syndrome

Navicular disease and navicular bursitis are unusual or rare conditions in the TB racehorse (PJM). Lameness can be localized using palmar digital analgesia, but most often horses have bruises, cracks, and abscesses, and those with navicular syndrome are unusual. One of us (MWC) diagnoses navicular bursitis commonly. Rarely, fractures of the navicular bone, bipartite formation, or other anomalous conditions of the navicular bone can occur in young TBs, either in the forelimbs or hindlimbs. Successful management of this type of palmar foot pain has been achieved by injecting the digital cushion with orgotein (Palosein) and Sarapin and methylprednisolone acetate, applying a bar shoe, increasing heel angle, and giving NSAIDs. Intraarticular injection of the DIP joint with hyaluronan and corticosteroids affects numerous structures in the foot and improves the condition of horses with navicular syndrome or OA of the DIP joint.

Distal Phalanx Fractures

Fractures of the distal phalanx occur occasionally. Most fractures are nonarticular palmar process (wing) fractures, and horses do well with the application of a bar shoe. Articular wing fractures are more serious. Extensor process fragments are rare and can be removed arthroscopically.

Palmar digital neurectomy is permitted in most racing jurisdictions, but it must be reported to the race office. Indications for neurectomy are few, but occasionally a horse with a distal phalangeal fracture and chronic pain is a candidate. Occasionally, palmar digital neurectomy is performed in horses with recurrent quarter cracks to eliminate pain, but the procedure does nothing to solve the original problem. Surgical neurectomy should be performed because percutaneous techniques are often ineffective.

Lameness of the Fetlock Joint

The metacarpophalangeal or metatarsophalangeal (fetlock) joint, carpus, and tarsus are the most important joints associated with lameness in racing TBs, especially the fetlock joints. Clinical findings of fetlock joint lameness usually include effusion, heat, a positive response to flexion, and elimination of lameness using intraarticular analgesia. However, in some horses with subchondral bone pain, clinical signs such as effusion are often lacking, and perineural blocks are most effective. The most common lameness conditions of the fetlock can be divided into four categories: synovitis, distal palmar McIII or MtIII disease, fractures, and OA.

Synovitis

Fetlock joint pain associated with effusion, pain on joint manipulation, a positive response to a distal limb flexion test, and moderate lameness is common, but horses generally respond well to intraarticular treatment with hyaluronan and corticosteroids (repeated if necessary), combined with systemic treatment with polysulfated glycosaminoglycans (PSGAGs). Intravenous hyaluronan may be useful in these horses. However, recurrence of clinical signs indicates that the horse should be removed from training, because continued training may result in chronic OA (MWC). The use of autologous conditioned serum (interleukin-1 receptor antagonist, IRAP) has gained popularity for management of synovitis (JAB).

An increase in forelimb tenosynovitis of the digital flexor tendon sheaths (DFTSs) has been noted in horses trained and raced on synthetic surfaces. Lameness is acute. The DFTS is distended and warm to palpation, and there is a marked response to lower limb flexion. Ultrasonographic and radiographic examinations are often normal and unrewarding. These horses typically become sound in 7 to 10 days with the administration of NSAIDs, walking, and the application of a topical poultice (JAB). Firing and blistering may be useful.

Distal Third Metacarpal or Metatarsal Bone Disease

Stress and maladaptive or nonadaptive remodeling, a form of stress-related bone injury, of the distal aspects of the McIII and the MtIII is a common cause of lameness. During training and racing, these areas undergo considerable modeling and remodeling, change shape, and are at risk to develop fracture and cartilage damage. Scintigraphic examination reveals focal areas of increased radiopharmaceutical uptake (IRU) and is the imaging modality of choice for diagnosis, because radiographs are often negative. Ultimately, damage to the distal aspect of the McIII and the MtIII leads to OA and fracture. Early in the course of the disease pain originates from subchondral bone, without effusion or heat. However, intraarticular analgesia is usually effective in partially eliminating pain. Perineural analgesia of the palmar or plantar and palmar metacarpal or plantar metatarsal nerves (low four-point block) or a modification

of the diagnostic technique is usually quite successful in abolishing pain. In a hindlimb the lateral plantar metatarsal nerve can be blocked independently of the other three nerves in the conventional low four-point block; in most horses improvement is noted, or a horse will then show contralateral hindlimb lameness. Often contralateral limb lameness is quite prominent and lameness grade can be 1 or 2 degrees higher than in the original limb (MWR). If lateral plantar analgesia produces only partial improvement or if no improvement is noted, the conventional low four-point technique should then be completed. In some horses all fetlock joints are affected simultaneously, and the horse appears sore all over. This disease is often referred to as "bone bruising" but is a form of chronic, stress-related bone injury characterized by the development of dense, painful sclerotic bone, rather than acute, subchondral bone injury from a single-event form of trauma. Distal McIII or MtIII disease is so prevalent that some veterinarians first perform intraarticular analgesia of the fetlock joint rather than beginning with palmar or plantar digital analgesia. As the disease progresses, radiological changes can include flattening of the distal palmar aspect of the McIII or the MtIII, increased radiopacity and radiolucency, and, when severe, large areas of subchondral lucency of the McIII or the MtIII. A form of severe flattening of the distal palmar aspect of the McIII has been recognized and may result in severe OA by the end of the 3-year-old year (MWC). Negative radiological findings do not eliminate this disease as a source of pain, and scintigraphy is more sensitive for its detection. Areas of IRU can represent subchondral bone damage from nonadaptive remodeling or fracture, and a combination of imaging modalities is necessary to differentiate these conditions. Increased radiopacity representing sclerosis of the distal palmar or plantar aspects of the McIII and the MtIII may be visible. Interpretation of sclerosis is subjective and should correlate to scintigraphic findings and clinical signs. Subtle fracture lines do occur in the subchondral bone plate of the distal condyle of the McIII and the MtIII. These become evident on successive radiographs. Surgical fixation of a visible fracture in the subchondral bone plate is the preferred treatment (JAB). Rest, a minimum of 4 months, to allow healing of sclerotic subchondral bone is recommended in horses without fracture, the most common situation. Bisphosphonate therapy has become popular, but there is little evidence to date to support the use of bisphosphonates unless administered in horses that are resting or in a reduced training program (see Chapter 42, page 490). One author (MWR) has used subchondral forage in two TBs with unilateral hindlimb lameness as a result of subchondral bone injury, and although both horses returned to racing, one developed recurrent lameness as a result of the same condition. Recurrence of lameness is a common problem in 40% to 50% of horses with conservative management.

Osteochondral Fragmentation

Osteochondral fragments (chip fractures) of the proximal, dorsal aspect of the proximal phalanx are common in TB racehorses. Fragments are more often medial than lateral, but they can occur biaxially and bilaterally. Fragments are more common in forelimbs but do occur in hindlimbs as well. Often disease of the fetlock joint occurs before fragments are recognized. Subtle radiological changes in the silhouette of the dorsal rim of the proximal phalanx are important and indicate that this area is experiencing stress. The distal dorsal aspect of the McIII at the joint capsule attachment can be injured at the same time that chip fractures are seen.

Once fractures are recognized, arthroscopic surgery should be performed. After surgery the horse can be back in training in as little as 6 weeks if cartilage damage is minimal. Horses with small fragments can be managed conservatively using local ice therapy, NSAIDs, and a reduction in exercise intensity. Inflammation (effusion) subsides within 7 to 10 days, and training can be resumed. Small osteochondral fragments appear to demineralize and no longer irritate the joint. If inflammation and lameness recur, the horse should be taken out of training, and surgery is recommended. Intraarticular injection of corticosteroids and hyaluronan is one option and is effective at reducing inflammation, but if training and racing continue, deep scoring of the articular cartilage of the distal aspect of the McIII occurs and leads to OA. If the goal is long-term racing, surgery should always be recommended.

Osteoarthritis

OA is a common problem and usually is associated with fractures of the proximal phalanx or palmar or plantar McIII or MtIII disease, but it can develop as a primary condition. Arthroscopic examination often reveals considerable articular cartilage scoring and thinning, or complete erosions through the articular cartilage, without any evidence of an associated fracture. Because OA is chronic and cartilage cannot regenerate, the disease must be identified early so preventative measures can be taken. Judicious use of NSAIDs and intramuscular PSGAGs is the best long-term treatment for OA of the fetlock joint. If present, fractures need to be repaired or fragments removed. Young horses should be taken out of training and allowed to mature. Immature horses are particularly prone to overextension injury of the fetlock joint. Some horses may require PSGAGs throughout the racing career. Oral supplements may be beneficial, but intramuscular administration is best. Repeated use of intraarticular corticosteroids exacerbates chronic OA, but whether this is a direct result of the medication or simply allowing a horse to continue in training and racing is unknown. Unfortunately, heat, effusion, positive response to flexion, and lameness resulting from OA need to be treated, because horses are expected to perform. Intraarticular injections are unavoidable, and a combination of hyaluronan and corticosteroids is preferred (RMA). Horses with recurrent synovitis may need additional injections in combination with 2 to 3 weeks of rest (MWC). In spite of information to the contrary, methylprednisolone acetate is the drug of choice, because if used prudently at well spaced intervals, the drug is preferable to repeated injections of shorter-acting corticosteroids (RMA). Intraarticular injections of PSGAGs every 2 weeks are beneficial in horses with chronic OA (PJM). IRAP therapy is gaining popularity for treatment of OA in the fetlock joint. It should be used in conjunction with rest or as a postoperative treatment for better efficacy (JAB).

Other Conditions

Distal McIII or MtIII condylar fractures, PSB fractures, sesamoiditis, and proximal phalangeal fractures are discussed in Chapters 35, 36, and 42. Distal McIII or MtIII condylar fractures often result from maladaptive or nonadaptive remodeling and may be more common in certain racetrack practices than others. One of us (PJM) includes these fractures as a top 10 lameness condition. Prognosis is much better in horses with incomplete fractures, with or without surgery. One author (PJM) recommends surgery in horses with fractures longer than 4 to 5 cm above the joint surface. Surgical fixation may yield a better long-term prognosis than conservative management in horses with short condylar fractures of the McIII and the MtIII since quality of healing may be better and recurrence of the injury less (MWR).

Lameness of the Carpus

The carpus is similar to the fetlock joint in several ways. The third carpal bone undergoes considerable modeling and remodeling with associated subchondral bone pain, similar to the distal palmar or plantar aspect of the McIII or MtIII. Fractures and OA are often the end-stage result of this process of stress-related bone injury. The response of the third carpal bone to stress-related bone injury is similar to that of cortical bone.

Nonadaptive Remodeling of the Third Carpal and Radial Carpal Bones

The third carpal bone and other carpal bones such as the radial carpal bone become sclerotic (model) to withstand the stress of training and racing. The change in the third carpal bone is seen on a skyline radiograph as increased radiopacity of the radial fossa. The mere presence of increased radiopacity does not establish a diagnosis because a certain amount of increased radiopacity reflects a normal, adaptive response. At what point the sclerotic process becomes pathological is not known. Diagnostic analgesia should be used to establish the authentic source of pain. Sclerotic bone eventually becomes painful if the condition of stress remodeling becomes pathological, called *maladaptive or nonadaptive remodeling*. If training and racing continue, bone loss, lysis, or fracture occurs. Third carpal bone subchondral bone pain is common, particularly in young horses, but because pain involves bone, no treatment other than reducing training and racing intensity is available.

Diagnosis of third carpal bone subchondral bone pain can be challenging, because many young horses do not develop effusion. Heat may be present over the dorsal aspect of the carpus, and horses move wide and tend to abduct the limb during advancement (MWC). Response to flexion varies, but in horses with subchondral bone pain, response is often negative. Diagnostic analgesia is essential for diagnosis. Careful interpretation of the results of diagnostic analgesia is necessary because inadvertently blocking the proximal palmar metacarpal region with middle carpal analgesia and vice versa is easy (MWC). The middle carpal and antebrachiocarpal joints always should be blocked separately. Radiological changes of increased radiopacity and later radiolucency can be seen with good-quality skyline images, but they are missed easily with poorly positioned and exposed images. To assess radiographic exposure, the veterinarian should evaluate the second and fourth carpal bones. These bones rarely have alterations in trabecular pattern, and both bones should be clearly visible on the skyline image. Scintigraphy is an excellent tool with which to diagnose stress-related bone injuries of the third carpal bone and other carpal bones, and although not needed in many horses, scintigraphy assists in early diagnosis and helps convince skeptical trainers and owners. Sclerosis of the third carpal bone changes the mechanical properties of bone, and sclerotic bone is brittle and at risk of fracturing. Few osteochondral fragments or small (chip) or large (slab) fractures of the third carpal bone occur in normal bone. At the time of arthroscopic surgery to repair a third carpal bone frontal slab fracture, a wedge-shaped piece of sclerotic and often necrotic bone often can be found between the fracture fragment and parent third carpal bone.

Once painful sclerosis of the third carpal bone develops, treatment is difficult. Rest may not help remodel dense bone, so prevention is important. The training programs of young TBs with evidence of third carpal bone sclerosis should be modified, but trainers are often unwilling. Although little evidence supports using isoxsuprine or aspirin to improve blood flow, some veterinarians prescribe these medications. Bisphosphonate therapy has become popular but there is little conclusive evidence regarding efficacy. Extracorporeal shock wave therapy (ESWT) is useful in treating horses with third carpal bone remodeling and pain. The benefits of therapy will be achieved only in conjunction with rest or a substantial reduction in training. There will be no radiological changes; however, there will be a reduction in pain when full training resumes (JAB).

Carpal Fractures

Osteochondral fragmentation of the carpus is a common problem. Clinical signs are unique for each fracture type, and radiographic examination is most important. Horses with distal radial carpal bone fractures exhibit pain on direct palpation of the fracture site and often have effusion of the middle carpal joint. Horses with third carpal bone pain and fractures are unwilling to rock on the limb, evaluated by picking up the contralateral limb and forcing the horse to rock on the affected limb by putting side-to-side pressure against the horse's body. Horses with distal, lateral radius fractures generally have pain on direct palpation. Horses with proximal intermediate carpal and radial carpal bone fractures may be surprisingly lame, without obvious palpable abnormalities.

A rare fracture, but one to keep in mind, is a sagittal fracture of the proximal aspect of the intermediate carpal bone (MWC). Horses train and race but come back to the barn obviously lame (grade 3 of 5). When walking and jogging, they exhibit a stiff-legged gait and obvious abduction during advancement. Horses respond positively to carpal flexion, and lameness is abolished using antebrachiocarpal analgesia. Intraarticular treatment does not improve lameness. The skyline image of the proximal row of carpal bones is mandatory for diagnosis, because fractures will be missed on other views. Early arthroscopic surgery is recommended, because OA can develop if horses are continued in work with a fracture.

Arthroscopic surgery has improved the management of horses with carpal joint lameness greatly. Removal of small osteochondral fragments and repair of large fragments substantially reduces the severity of OA. PSGAGs can be useful in limiting the development of OA, particularly if pain is originating from the third carpal bone. After surgery in horses with carpal osteochondral fragmentation, one of us (MWC) recommends hyaluronan injection 2 to 3 weeks later. Horses with fractures of the middle carpal joint need additional rest compared with horses with antebrachiocarpal joint fractures (MWC). One of us (PJM) prefers to manage horses with incomplete or nondisplaced third carpal bone slab fractures conservatively by giving 60 days of rest and reevaluating the horse. The prognosis for TB racehorses with displaced third carpal bone slab fractures even with surgery is only guarded. Horses with fractures extending into the weight-bearing surface of carpal bones more than 0.5 cm have a poor prognosis. Horses with recurrent and chronic OA appear to benefit from topical blisters and 3 or more months of rest.

Osteoarthritis

In young horses with early signs of OA, rest is recommended. In horses with chronic OA that are able to race, intraarticular injection of a combination of hyaluronan and PSGAG produces better results than does injection of either product alone (MWC). In horses with mild or moderate lameness, intraarticular injection of hyaluronan and triamcinolone acetonide a minimum of 5 to 7 days before racing (depending on racing commission rules) decreases clinical signs for 6 to 8 weeks. Most horses exhibiting carpal lameness appear to benefit from the intramuscular administration of PSGAG once every 4 days for seven or eight treatments, and intravenous injection of hyaluronan appears beneficial before racing.

Rest should be recommended for young horses with early OA even though recurrence of signs is common. NSAIDs are useful in managing pain in horses with OA of the carpus.

Intercarpal Ligament Damage

Because the complex carpal joint is highly dynamic and moveable, fractures and soft tissue damage can lead to OA. Although fractures are more common, injury of the medial palmar intercarpal ligament has been recognized (see Chapter 38).

Another rarely seen lameness of the carpus is related to an osteochondroma of the distal aspect of the radius (see Chapter 75). Rarely, exostoses of the caudal perimeter of the distal radial physes are seen. These horses are acutely lame after exercise and sound within a few hours. Marked carpal sheath swelling and resistance to carpal flexion are usually obvious. Radiologically, there is an osteochondroma proximal and medial to the distal radial physis. There is usually marked carpal sheath effusion seen on ultrasonographic examination. The osteochondroma structure and a lesion in the DDFT are often evident. Surgery to remove the osteochondroma or exostoses is the treatment of choice. Prognosis depends on the degree of damage to the DDFT and the tendency for the osteochondroma to reappear (JAB).

Suspensory Desmitis

Proximal Suspensory Desmitis

Suspensory desmitis is a very important cause of lameness in the TB racehorse and previously has been underestimated. Suspensory desmitis is much more common in forelimbs than in hindlimbs (PJM). Hindlimb PSD is difficult to diagnose because horses have a stiff, hopping-type gait similar to that in horses with tibial stress fractures, and heat and swelling are unusual (MWC). Lameness in horses with forelimb PSD is similar to that in horses with carpal disease. Horses travel wide, with a shortened cranial phase of the stride, and are worse with the limb on the outside of a circle. Conformational faults such as offset knees and upright pasterns and fetlock joints predispose horses to PSD. PSD is most commonly a 2-year-old lameness condition, perhaps caused by immaturity, and can be diagnosed by manual palpation in some horses, but that is the exception rather than the rule (MWC). An increase in occurrence of PSD has been noted in horses that race and train on synthetic surfaces. This may be related to the inability of the foot to slide, causing increased stress on the SL (JAB). More often, horses with PSD require diagnostic analgesia, and one author (RMA) uses the lateral palmar block, the site for which is just below the accessory carpal bone. With the lateral palmar block it is unlikely to inadvertently cause analgesia of the carpometacarpal and middle carpal joints. In many horses, lameness thought to originate from PSD, after a positive response to high palmar analgesia, was later found to originate from the carpus (MWC).

Considerable variation occurs in the ultrasonographic appearance of the proximal aspect of normal and diseased SLs. Overt tears are easy to diagnose. Chronic tears have an abnormal ultrasonographic appearance despite absence of clinical signs (JAB). Hypoechoic areas can be identified in sound horses. Furthermore, bony pathological conditions of the proximal, palmar aspect of the McIII can be seen in horses without obvious tearing of the SL. Avulsion fractures of the McIII are diagnosed in horses that develop acute, severe lameness abolished by lateral palmar analgesia. Scintigraphy is the best way to diagnose bony injury of the proximal aspect of the McIII in horses without ultrasonographic evidence of PSD and negative radiological findings. Avulsion fracture of the McIII is associated with focal, intense IRU, but many horses have diffuse IRU of the proximal aspect of the McIII. Whether these horses have chronic avulsion injury or whether this represents stress reaction or other injury of the proximal aspect of the McIII is unknown. Regardless, horses with bony injury of the proximal, palmar aspect of the McIII have a good prognosis if given a minimum of 120 days of rest. Horses with PSD often can be managed and allowed to continue racing. Local infiltration with corticosteroids or other products is of questionable benefit, and systemic therapy is more effective and rewarding (RMA). Others disagree and recommend local injection with triamcinolone acetonide in horses with mild PSD (PJM). The combination of Sarapin, methylprednisolone acetate, and in some horses Palosein has been successful, and 2-year-old horses may never take another lame step (MWC). Systemic corticosteroids and NSAIDs reduce inflammation enough to relieve the lameness. Where regulations permit, phenylbutazone and triamcinolone acetonide (12 to 18 mg intramuscularly) can be administered 3 to 5 days before racing. A good alternative is two Naquasone (a combination of the diuretic trichlormethiazide [200 mg] and dexamethasone [5 mg]) 48 hours before racing, if permitted by the rules of racing. Triamcinolone acetonide lasts longer, but Naquasone contains a diuretic that is also useful for reducing swelling. An ice boot or an ice tub is beneficial. Platelet-rich plasma (PRP) may be beneficial for treating horses with lesions of the SL. A single treatment or treatment in combination with autogenous stem cells appears promising, when combined with removal from training for 4 to 6 months. Prognosis is good. ESWT is also useful in horses with PSD. Repeated treatments every 10 days for 6 weeks is ideal. The horse should be jogging during the treatment (JAB).

Horses in which lameness is mild when trotted in hand or even under tack but that refuse to give a full effort toward the end of a race should be given rest.

Corrective shoeing can make a difference in horses with PSD. In fact, PSD may be secondary to lameness of the foot (MWC). The toe should be shortened, and the shoe should have only minimal toe grabs. Horses with PSD do not develop catastrophic disruption of the suspensory apparatus but return from a race sore.

Suspensory Branch Desmitis

Suspensory branch desmitis is a different situation and can easily lead to catastrophic breakdown if horses are managed improperly. Early detection is critical because suspensory branch desmitis is a predisposing factor for condylar fractures of the McIII. If there is any detectable change or swelling of a suspensory branch, an ultrasonographic examination should be performed. Subtle clinical changes can predispose the horse to catastrophic breakdown and must be identified early (JAB). Management of suspensory branch desmitis with infiltration of corticosteroids in a TB racehorse is a high-risk treatment, with no therapeutic benefit to the horse. Systemic antiinflammatory therapy similar to the approach described for PSD is useful for horses with suspensory branch desmitis, but the horse should not be raced if the SL remains hot and painful. Suspensory branch desmitis is a dangerous injury.

In horses with suspensory branch desmitis the splint bones should be evaluated carefully. Radiographs should be obtained to check for fracture, flaring, or thickening of the second and fourth metacarpal bones. A clear relationship exists between suspensory branch desmitis and pathological conditions of the splint bone. Splint ostectomy is recommended in horses with fractured, flared, or thickened splint bones, not just in those with fracture.

Midbody Desmitis

Horses with midbody desmitis can be managed similarly to those with PSD, but if desmitis extends distally into the branches, the risk of catastrophic breakdown exists. Horses with suspensory desmitis may benefit from rest (45 to 120 days) and blistering (PJM).

Bucked Shins: Dorsal Metacarpal Disease

Bucked shins or dorsal metacarpal disease (periostitis) is common but readily manageable (see Chapter 102). This condition is simply the mismatching of exercise with modeling and remodeling of the McIII necessary for the bone to withstand the rigors of training and racing. Bucked shins are most commonly seen in young horses early in training. The simplest and best treatment is to modify the training program to match the horse. With bucked shins, horses are usually only mildly lame after exercise, unilaterally or bilaterally (PJM). Bucked shins are common in young horses with other primary lameness conditions, particularly of the hindlimbs (MWC). Heat and pain over the dorsal cortex of the McIII are commonly found, but care must be taken not to place pressure on the palmar metacarpal structures while palpating the dorsal cortex (PJM). One of us (MWC) feels that careful palpation of the palmar cortex is useful in identifying McIII disease. Clinical signs are usually sufficient for diagnosis, but low or high palmar nerve blocks, infiltration of the nutrient foramen of the McIII, or local infiltration of local anesthetic solution occasionally is required (MWC). Radiographs reveal a typical modeling response, but in some horses with fracture, computed or digital radiographs should be obtained, because fractures may be missed on conventional films (PJM). Scintigraphic examination can be useful, mostly in horses with dorsal cortical fracture (MWC).

Great strides have been made in changing training techniques to manage TB racehorses with bucked shins (see Chapter 102). This requires close monitoring of the dorsal cortex of the McIII. Overall, the incidence of authentic dorsal cortical fractures has decreased greatly. Although all trainers have horses with bucked shins, those that still have major problems train in the old-fashioned style. There is a noticeable reduction of bucked shins in horses racing and training on synthetic surfaces (JAB).

Once inflammation is noticed, ice, NSAIDs, and topical cooling muds, such as Uptite poultice (Uptite, Lawrence, Massachusetts, United States), are often all that is necessary if training intensity is reduced and modified. Once the periosteum becomes hot, thickened, and sore over a large portion of the dorsal cortex of the McIII, modifying training is usually too late. Training should be stopped, and when necessary thermocautery may still be the best treatment, once inflammation has subsided (RMA, PJM, MWC). When done properly thermocautery is humane and effective. An old-time racetrack practitioner was asked a few years ago if he still fires horses, and if so, why? His response was simple: "I can tell you in two words: It works." The real problem with thermocautery is perception. Most persons who adamantly are opposed to thermocautery generally have no experience with the procedure. Regardless, alternative treatments are available, but none in one author's opinion work as well as thermocautery (RMA). All treatments require extended periods of rest or light training. Others prefer a relatively new technique called *periosteal scratching*. A 16-gauge needle is used to create linear incisions of the periosteum using aseptic technique. This procedure, as with thermocautery, is combined with rest and is done after the inflammation has subsided (PJM). Prognosis after periosteal scratching is estimated to be 70% (MWC). ESWT is an effective therapy for bucked shins. The success of treatment relies on training modification. Treatment is performed every 10 days for 3 to 5 treatments. During that time the horse should only walk and jog (JAB).

Bucked shins can progress to dorsal cortical (stress) fracture if horses with periostitis are forced to continue training. Stress fractures occur most commonly on the dorsolateral aspect of the McIII, but those located in the distal third to distal fourth of the McIII are most problematic. Fractures in this location under the extensor tendons can be difficult to palpate, but they may be extensive.

Horses with bucked shins should not be lame at the jog 1 to 2 days after the last workout, but if lameness persists, a dorsal cortical fracture should be suspected. Radiographs should be obtained. Success in treating horses with dorsal cortical fracture relates directly to the duration of fracture. Horses with acute fractures are treated more easily than those with chronic fractures. In horses with acute fractures, rest, with or without thermocautery, is successful. Chronic dorsal cortical fractures are essentially nonunions and heal slowly or not at all and require surgery. Cortical drilling (forage, osteostixis) using numerous small-diameter holes drilled across the fracture line is effective and in one author's opinion is the treatment of choice (RMA). Rarely a cortex bone screw placed in lag fashion or as a positional screw is needed. The question of whether compression using lag screw technique is necessary or if screws are best placed as set or positional screws remains unanswered. Implants must be removed before training begins. ESWT in combination with rest appears promising for the management of dorsal cortical fractures of the McIII (MWR).

Superficial Digital Flexor Tendonitis

Superficial digital flexor tendonitis usually is advanced before lameness is observed and diagnosis is made. Lameness is one of the last clinical signs observed. Prognosis for racing is poor when lameness is present (JAB). Superficial digital flexor tendonitis is usually a career-threatening or career-ending injury, and estimates indicate that superficial digital flexor tendonitis is the single most common injury ending a TB racehorse's career. However, many horses with superficial digital flexor tendonitis return to racing or, on occasion, race through the injury. One author (RMA) feels strongly that local infiltration of corticosteroids and continued racing are contraindicated. Intralesional injection of corticosteroids can cause tendon necrosis and result in complete rupture of the superficial digital flexor tendon (SDFT). Some horses may be able to race after treatment with systemic corticosteroids, NSAIDs, and ice therapy. The SDFT will set up on occasion, but that is certainly an exception, and horses fall in value.

Recognizing superficial digital flexor tendonitis before overt fiber tearing occurs has distinct advantages. To recognize tendonitis early, horses must be monitored closely, and ultrasonographic examination must be performed at the earliest indication of inflammation. Heat and swelling are early clinical signs but may not indicate necessarily that the tendon is involved, because peritendonous injury can cause similar signs. *The key is pain on palpation of the suspect tendon.* Pain, even without obvious heat or swelling, is an important clinical finding. Ultrasonographic examination must include cross-sectional area measurements, because subtle enlargement of the SDFT precedes fiber tearing. Once early superficial digital flexor tendonitis has been recognized, horses should be given rest, or at least the training intensity should be reduced.

One author (RMA) prefers to manage horses with core lesions of the SDFT with tenoplasty (tendon splitting). The surgery can be done with the horse standing and is inexpensive, and aftercare is minimal. To perform tendon splitting, a core lesion must be present, and the earlier the procedure is done, the better. A double-edged tenotome is used. The tendon fibers are split longitudinally with five rows of about 15 percutaneous stab incisions each. After surgery horses are surprisingly sound. Horses with superficial tearing along the edge of a SDFT have a poor prognosis with any treatment and may be the only candidates for peritendonous injection of corticosteroids, provided the horse is removed from training and rested. PRP and stem cell therapy appear promising in treating SDFT core and peripheral lesions. Ongoing research is needed to determine long-term efficacy. Lesions are typically resolved ultrasonographically at 60 days. Rehabilitation is critical to success, and the horse should not have a saddle on its back for 8 to 10 months. ESWT has been unrewarding in getting horses back to racing after an acute tendon injury. It does, however, have some merit in treating horses with chronic tendonitis (JAB). One author prefers the use of surgical management (MWR; see Chapter 69). A combination of desmotomy of the accessory ligament of the superficial flexor muscle (superior check ligament) and tenoplasty is recommended. Prognosis in the TB racehorse, however, is no higher than 50% to 60%, and recurrence of tendonitis is common.

Horses with superficial digital flexor tendonitis should have as much time off as possible. However, if owners and trainers are unwilling to give 6 to 8 months of rest before the horse returns to training, any treatment is a waste of time. One of us (PJM) has stopped recommending any form of surgery or injections and simply recommends walking rest for 4 to 16 weeks. A blister is applied at least twice, and tendon healing is monitored with ultrasonography. Even with this approach, recurrence rate is 60% to 80%. The trainer plays a major role in rehabilitating horses with superficial digital flexor tendonitis. Those that are successful give the horse the most time off and are patient getting the horse fit before starting hard work.

Tibial Stress Fractures

Tibial stress fractures are the most common cause of acute, pronounced, unilateral hindlimb lameness in the TB racehorse. Lameness from tibial stress fractures usually is recognized after a hard workout or after breaking from the gate. Lameness can be severe, and the horse may not bear weight on the limb. Tibial stress fractures are usually unilateral, but bilateral fractures can cause unusual hindlimb lameness (PJM). Similar to humeral stress fractures, tibial stress fractures can occur after a horse has had 60 to 90 days of training, often after a period of rest for an unrelated cause. Tibial stress fractures can occur anytime during training and racing, and the association between a layup period and the early development of a tibial stress fracture is not as well established as for horses with humeral stress fractures (MWR). Two of us (RMA, PJM) do not find manual palpation of the tibia useful diagnostically, but one of us (MWC) finds deep palpation and tibial percussion helpful. Scintigraphy is the diagnostic modality of choice. Less than 50% of horses diagnosed with tibial stress fractures using scintigraphy have radiologically apparent fractures, even if follow-up examination is performed after 2 weeks. If scintigraphy is unavailable, even small areas of periosteal, endosteal, or cortical change should be considered important, if clinical signs suggest tibial stress fracture. Tibial stress fractures are located most commonly on the caudolateral cortex, proximally or midshaft, but can occur caudolaterally and caudomedially distally. Bilateral tibial stress fractures are occasionally seen, even in horses with unilateral hindlimb lameness. One of us (PJM) has examined a number of horses with clinical signs consistent with tibial stress fracture but in which scintigraphic examination findings were negative. Horses returned to the track and developed complete tibial fractures. Now this author (PJM) recommends reexamination in 3 weeks. False-negative

results are unusual in horses with stress-related bone injuries unless fractures are located medially and only lateral scintigraphic images are obtained (MWR). Horses that are trained on synthetic surfaces with hindlimb toe grabs appear to have an increased incidence of tibial stress fractures. Whether synthetic surfaces increase the incidence of tibial stress fracture as compared with dirt surfaces is unclear and will not be answered without clinical research (JAB). A recent trend is for practitioners to take digital radiographic images of a tibia in a TB racehorse suspected of having a tibial stress fracture in lieu of obtaining a scintigraphic examination. There are many normal irregularities of the cranial tibial cortex and care must be taken not to make an erroneous diagnosis; the practitioner should keep in mind the common distribution of tibial stress fractures (see above). One of the authors (MWR) has never recognized an authentic tibial stress fracture involving the cranial cortex.

Horses with tibial stress fractures are given 90 to 120 days of rest. The prognosis is excellent. The crus is well muscled and has a good blood supply, and callus formation of the tibia does not interfere with nearby structures. Complications develop when horses have spiral fractures and severe lameness or when horses with unrecognized tibial stress fractures are trained or raced. Catastrophic failure can result. Tibial stress fractures can recur if horses are given inadequate time for healing, but this is otherwise unusual.

Some horses with only mild lameness at the time of initial diagnosis and in which lameness rapidly resolved can be kept in light work. In these horses scintigraphic examination reveals mild IRU, and radiographs are negative. Horses are given a minimum of 60 days without hard work, but if lameness recurs, additional rest for 90 to 120 days is recommended. Aspirin at 60 grains orally (PO) sid is thought to be of benefit during rest (JAB). When the horse becomes sound, light training may begin (JAB).

Tibial stress fractures were misdiagnosed as stifle lameness for years at some racetracks, and the same error is still made today. Even with the introduction of high-quality nonportable radiography equipment at referral centers, the diagnosis of a tibial stress fracture has been difficult to make because radiographs are often negative and clinicians have to isolate pain, a difficult task in many TB racehorses. Scintigraphy has taught us that tibial stress fracture is an important and frequent cause of hindlimb lameness in TB racehorses.

Distal Hock Joint Pain

Distal hock joint pain, or distal tarsitis, is a common cause of hindlimb lameness. One of us (MWC) feels strongly that the hock joint is the most important articular structure in equine locomotion. Compensatory lameness caused by primary distal hock joint pain is important. The skeleton of the TB foundation sire Eclipse at the Racing Museum in Newmarket and the skeleton from an extinct breed from the La Brea Tar Pits in Southern California reveal extensive osteoarthritic changes. Radiological changes in the tarsometatarsal joint of young horses are common and can be found in yearlings before training begins. The importance of osteophyte formation involving the dorsal proximal aspect of the MtIII, often called *juvenile spavin*, is difficult to evaluate without signs of lameness.

Horses with distal hock joint pain have a typical gait. The hindlimbs travel close together and may even cross midline. Horses with bilateral lameness may not show overt lameness, but they are observed to be not right behind (PJM). This has been described as a "bicycling" gait because the hindlimbs appear to mimic the action of peddling a bicycle (JAB). However, this gait is not pathognomonic for distal hock joint pain, and diagnostic analgesia should always be used to confirm the source of pain causing lameness. Some horses may break from the gait slowly, may not switch leads properly behind, or may crossfire and develop abrasions on the medial aspect of the tarsus (MWC). Horses often wear the lateral aspect of the toe of the shoe. Horses that have a positive Churchill test response likely have distal hock joint pain involving the tarsometatarsal joint (RMA). Some clinicians place emphasis on upper limb flexion, and certainly the response rate is high, but this test lacks specificity. Diagnostic analgesia should be performed to localize pain causing lameness to the distal hock joints. Distal hock joint pain can cause lameness without radiological changes, particularly in young horses, but radiological changes can be present in horses with pain originating elsewhere. Involvement of the centrodistal (distal intertarsal) joint is difficult to assess without radiological and scintigraphic examinations. Nuclear scintigraphy is useful to identify slab fractures of the third and central tarsal bones. Oddly, horses with radiologically evident periarticular osteophyte formation may show little IRU.

The simplest and best treatment is intraarticular injection of methylprednisolone acetate (100 mg) into each affected joint. The centrodistal and tarsometatarsal joints are small, and injecting more than 3 mL of medication without encountering resistance is often difficult. Using hyaluronan gives little advantage, because the joints are low-motion joints (RMA). However, two of us (PJM, MWC) use hyaluronan (20 mg) and methylprednisolone acetate (40 mg), and one of us (MWC) feels strongly that the combination of hyaluronan and corticosteroids prolongs the racing careers of affected horses by delaying progression of OA. Rarely the cunean bursa is injected. There appear to be few complications following repeated injections of corticosteroids into low-motion joints, such as the centrodistal and tarsometatarsal joints. If the diagnosis is correct, the response to therapy is rewarding. However, lameness recurring rapidly after one or two injections may indicate that the primary source of pain is elsewhere or that subchondral pain is a substantial component of lameness. Corrective shoeing may help horses with distal hock joint pain. A high hoof angle (≥54 degrees) and the application of slight turndown shoes may help horses push off and may prevent sliding. In horses with primary, chronic distal hock joint pain, turnout or complete rest actually may worsen lameness, and better results are achieved in these horses by maintaining a low level of training (MWC).

The tarsocrural joint usually is not involved, but if effusion exists, one author (RMA) injects the joint with hyaluronan and corticosteroids, because the joint is a high-motion joint. If dark synovial fluid is obtained during arthrocentesis of the tarsocrural joint, cartilage damage should be suspected (MWC). Repeated injections of corticosteroids into the tarsocrural joint should be avoided.

Myositis

Exertional rhabdomyolysis (ER) and nonspecific localized myositis frequently are overlooked sources of lameness in TB racehorses. ER is a common problem, especially in young horses, and primarily is seen in fillies. Male horses can be affected, but much less frequently. Diagnosis usually is not a challenge if a veterinarian observes a hot, sweaty horse with obvious muscle cramps. Lameness is mostly bilateral, is transient after exercise, and resolves within a few hours. A horse with ER should be sound at the trot even when lameness is present at the walk. If ER is suspected and the horse jogs lame, a lameness examination should be performed (JAB). Some horses have unilateral lameness with ER. Colts often develop unilateral forelimb ER, resembling other causes of upper limb pain. Horses may have generalized whole body stiffness if ER is unrecognized and untreated. Elevated serum levels of creatine kinase and aspartate transaminase are necessary to diagnose ER definitively. Horses at risk are given acetylpromazine (5 to 15 mg IV) before exercise to prevent ER. Dantrolene (500 mg PO) given 4 hours before exercise is used in horses that have had serious episodes of ER and have missed training.

Interestingly, some horses are found to have IRU during bone (delayed) phase scintigraphic imaging, and serum muscle enzyme levels may be normal or only mildly elevated. In some horses a history of previous ER is known, but others have no known history of ER. Large muscles or individual muscle bellies within muscles can be affected. Lameness associated with IRU in skeletal muscles may or may not be seen, depending on the muscles involved. These horses typically require rest for a period of 6 weeks (JAB). Muscles of the hindlimb most commonly are affected, such as the gluteal, biceps femoris, and semitendinosus muscles, but forelimb or trunk muscles can be involved, rarely.

Gluteal myositis occurs in TB racehorses. Lameness is characterized by a reluctance to reach forward during the cranial phase of the stride and to push off to extend the hindlimbs at the end of the stride. Lameness may result from a loose, cuppy racetrack that breaks away from the horse. Whether the trochanteric bursa is involved is unclear. Pain is best identified by using direct digital pressure over the greater trochanter of the femur. Local pain is eliminated with injection of corticosteroids (methylprednisolone acetate, 100 mg/site) with an 8-cm, 18-gauge spinal needle into the middle gluteal muscle. The needle is directed horizontally at a 45-degree angle to the sagittal plane toward the opposite tuber coxae. One author (RMA) does not make any effort to inject the trochanteric bursa.

The lumbar region is prone to myositis. Diagnosis is made by palpation of pain and recognition of hindlimb stiffness. An effective treatment is methocarbamol (10 g PO tid). This high dose is effective with no substantial side effects. The withdrawal time for methocarbamol can be long in some racing jurisdictions. Alternatively the affected muscles can be injected with corticosteroids diluted with Sarapin (2.5 mL of a mixture of 50 mL Sarapin and 200 mg methylprednisolone acetate per site).

Other Stress Fractures

TB racehorses are prone to stress-related bone injuries of several sites other than the tibia, including the humerus, pelvis, and scapula. Humeral stress fractures account for an estimated 5% to 8% of the fatal musculoskeletal injuries in any given year in California. Horses typically develop lameness 45 to 90 days after returning to training, following rest for an unrelated cause. Acute lameness quickly abates within 1 to 2 days, typical of many horses with stress fractures. The cranial phase of the stride is shortened, and the horse may drag the forelimb. This fracture is dangerous. When humeral stress fractures displace, they spiral and invariably cause the destruction of the horse on humane grounds. However, when identified before displacement, fractures heal well without complications. Fractures are nonarticular and rarely recur. Horses are given 90 to 120 days of rest. Scintigraphic examination is the best method to diagnose humeral stress fractures, because location precludes adequate radiographic examination in many horses. Humeral stress fractures occur medially and involve the proximal caudal cortex immediately below the humeral head; the caudal distal cortex (rare); and the cranial, distal medial cortex. Distal-medial humeral stress fractures may be more common in horses training on synthetic surfaces (JAB). Radiographs may show proliferative changes and fracture lines in horses with fractures of the distal, craniomedial aspect of the humorus, but often in other sites neither the fracture line nor proliferative changes can be seen. Proximally, any loss of distinction in the proximal caudal aspect of the humerus should be considered diagnostic for a humeral stress fracture until proved otherwise.

Stress fractures of the scapula are rare but do occur in the TB, and clinical signs are similar to those caused by humeral stress fractures. Nuclear scintigraphy is the only way to diagnose this fracture. Most scapular fractures occur where the spine of the scapula meets the neck, in the same location as scapular fractures that necessitate destruction on humane grounds.

Pelvic stress fractures are underestimated grossly, overlooked, and misdiagnosed as a source of lameness in racehorses. Pelvic stress fractures most commonly involve the ilium, anywhere from the tuber sacrale to the tuber coxae. Stress fractures at the base of the tuber sacrale frequently are misdiagnosed as strains of the sacroiliac ligament. Fractures involving the base of the tuber coxae can be incomplete or complete (knocked-down hip).

Pelvic stress fractures can be catastrophic injuries, if a fracture becomes complete and displaced and results in laceration of the iliac artery. All horses with stress fractures usually have a history of transient recent lameness. Considerable evidence indicates that catastrophic pelvic fractures develop from preexisting stress-related bone injuries in horses that were continued in training. The incidence is markedly higher in fillies. Nuclear scintigraphy is useful for identifying pelvic stress fractures, but several factors decrease sensitivity, including the overlying muscle mass. Even a minor area of IRU should be considered important. Motion-correction software improves accuracy and image quality. Ultrasonographic examination can be used to identify fracture if displacement exists but is less sensitive than scintigraphy. Ultrasonography is most useful in horses that cannot be moved. Pelvic stress fractures should be included in the differential diagnosis of any TB with hindlimb lameness. Horses returning from training with severe, undiagnosed hindlimb lameness should be tied and not allowed to become recumbent until a pelvic fracture

can be eliminated as a source of pain. Horses with a pelvic stress fracture may not exhibit severe lameness and may be confused with those suspected of having sacroiliac pain or pelvic muscle pain.

Sacroiliac strain is diagnosed in horses when lameness results from slipping while the horse is coming out of the starting gate (MWC). Horses with sacroiliac pain resent pressure applied between the tubera sacrale. Certainly, sacroiliac strain needs to be differentiated from pelvic fracture, because management may include local, deep injections of corticosteroids and Sarapin. Injecting the back or hip muscles in a horse with a pelvic fracture gives no benefit and incurs considerable risk.

The prognosis for horses with pelvic stress fractures is good, unless displacement exists. Even horses with complete, displaced fractures of the tuber coxae can return to racing if the displacement is not severe.

Other Lameness Conditions

Stifle

Stifle lameness causes unilateral and occasionally bilateral lameness in TB racehorses (MWC, PJM). Horses have mild or moderate lameness and appear to swing the limb. Other characteristics include a stiff hindlimb gait, not using the hindlimbs or weak behind, getting out in the straightaway, slipping behind, and locking up behind. The most common clinical finding is effusion of the medial femorotibial joint. Lameness is exacerbated by upper limb flexion. Pain on palpation of the medial collateral ligament is found occasionally.

Diagnostic analgesia is important, but eliminating the lameness totally in most horses is difficult. Radiological findings are generally negative, unless osteochondritis dissecans or subchondral bone cysts are present. Horses with osteochondrosis usually are treated surgically as young horses before arriving at the racetrack. Ultrasonographic examination is useful in identifying soft tissue lesions such as collateral desmitis, and when identified, affected horses are given 7 to 10 days or more of handwalking.

Most horses with stifle lameness appear to have synovitis or early OA. Differences of opinions exist regarding the type of intraarticular injections to use in the stifle. One of us (MWC) uses hyaluronan and betamethasone but avoids using methylprednisolone acetate, because synovitis may worsen. On the other hand, one of us (PJM) uses hyaluronan (50 to 200 mg) and methylprednisolone acetate (160 to 200 mg) in the medial and lateral femorotibial joints.

Secondary Shoulder Region Pain

Horses with forelimb lameness characterized by a shortened cranial phase of the stride may have some degree of secondary muscle soreness in the shoulder region or mild intertubercular (bicipital) bursitis (MWC). Horses often have primary lameness in the foot or fetlock joint, but management of the primary lameness conditions does not alleviate all clinical signs. Injection of a combination of methylprednisolone acetate, isoflupredone acetate, and hyaluronan into the bicipital (intertubercular) bursa and 2 days of handwalking resolves remaining clinical signs in some horses.

Chapter 107

The European Thoroughbred

Robert C. Pilsworth

HISTORY OF HORSE RACING IN THE UNITED KINGDOM

As long as people have ridden horses, matches of speed have been held informally between proud owner-riders. Racing horses under saddle was certainly established in England by the time of the Roman occupation. Chester boasts the longest running unbroken series of race meetings in the United Kingdom on the original site, the strangely named Roodeye. This area of land (translated, island of the cross) has been used for horse racing continuously since 1539. Interestingly, racing was introduced to replace football (soccer), which had been banned a few years earlier because of the number of severe injuries and fatalities it produced. The original prize money was substantial for the time, being "in the XXXI yere (31st year) of King Henry Theght (VIII), a bell of sylver, to the value of three shillings and three pence, is ordayned to be the reward of that horse which shall runne before all others."

Since the time of James I (1603 to 1625), a link has existed between royalty and the town of Newmarket in Suffolk, leading to its reputation as the headquarters of racing in the United Kingdom. Charles I, the successor of James I, established regular spring and autumn race meetings in Newmarket and built a palace and stables, some of which have survived. Racing at that time consisted of matches between pairs of horses, over long distances by modern standards, usually accompanied by hefty personal wagers between their aristocratic owners. Distances as long as 4 to 6 miles were not unusual. During the succeeding two centuries the race distances declined, as did the age at which horses were allowed to race. Initially horses had to be older than 5 years of age, but this was reduced gradually until in 1859 even yearlings were allowed to race. This practice soon ceased, but 2-year-old racing had become established and became, unfortunately in the opinions of many, part of the Thoroughbred (TB) spectrum. During this time the breed itself changed considerably.

Arab horses had been imported sporadically to Britain from the time of the Crusades (twelfth century AD). Usually seized in battle, these Arab horses would have been relatively slow and sturdy horses, used for carrying warriors into battle. In the seventeenth century, a marriage alliance between Charles I and the Portuguese Royal Household allowed Charles access to the Arab horses of the Barbary Coast, and several stallions made the long journey, mainly over land, back to the United Kingdom. Three horses alone—the Byerley Turk, the Darley Arabian, and the Godolphin Barb—founded the entire breed of the TB we know today, producing profound changes in size and conformation from the native English stock. Eighty percent of the TB racehorses alive today are descended from just one of these stallions, the Darley Arabian, through his great-great-grandson Eclipse.

As the distance of races decreased, speed became an increasing factor, and the fields of competitors increased in size. Eventually the handicap system was introduced in an attempt to avoid the dominance of the sport by a few exceptionally gifted individual horses. All this led to an increase in interest in racing as a spectator sport and a vehicle for gambling. From the nineteenth century onward, racing was more or less recognizable as the sport we enjoy today.

PATTERN OF RACING

The most prestigious races in Europe belong to a worldwide system of accreditation, which groups together races of similar standing. The best horses competing at top level meet each other in a group of internationally acknowledged races known as Group 1. This group includes all the classics in the United Kingdom and the most prestigious races throughout Europe and North America. Beneath Group 1 are two other groupings (Group 2 and Group 3) for horses that have excellent ability but are not up to the extreme rigors of Group 1 racing. Competitors in these races face a weight for performance penalty system. For example, a Group 1 winner running in a Group 2 race carries a weight penalty in an attempt to equalize the competition.

The next tier down from Group races includes the Listed races. Again, the International Pattern Committee decides which races are of sufficient stature to belong to this list. Usually horses enter a Listed race when they have already won a maiden and possibly another race with specific conditions. Such horses have few other realistic options because after two wins a horse carries a lot of weight in an open handicap. Often success in a Listed race increases potential breeding value far more than winning such a handicap. These limited opportunities are often the reason why horses that are good, but not good enough to be top class, are sold out of Europe to continue racing in North America, where races are more suitable. Horses racing in North America are also often able to recoup in prize money the owner's investment, a situation that is often impossible racing in Europe, with its relatively lower prize money.

Beneath the upper echelon of horses racing in Listed and Group company is an open handicap system in which horses are allocated weight according to speed rating. These speed ratings are assessed by professional handicappers, who monitor the performance of the horses when they run in the first three maiden races or less if they win. The horse's rating rises and falls during its racing career, depending on its most recent form. Although this system is obviously open to abuse by trainers running horses at inappropriate distances or on unsuitable ground to lower their racing weight, the system does allow horses of moderate or differing ability to compete against one another on near equal footing and produce an exciting finish. The handicappers' dream is of all horses finishing within a length or so of each other.

Until recently all flat racing in the United Kingdom took place on turf. This led to a certain divergence in bloodlines and ability patterns of racehorses in North America and Europe. About 20 years ago, all-weather racing on a synthetic surface was developed at two tracks, Lingfield and Southwell. Although initially introduced for hurdle racing as a way of keeping the betting public satisfied when the National Hunt cards had to be abandoned through bad weather, both tracks rapidly discontinued hurdle racing on all-weather surfaces because of the high injury rate. This left the way open for flat racing on the all-weather tracks to become established. Since that time, new synthetic tracks have also opened at Wolverhampton, Kempton, and Great Leighs.

The synthetic all-weather track surface is not the same as the dirt commonly used in North America. The depth of the cushion is greater, and the material is a composite of oil, plastics, fibers, and sand. Few races with large prize money are run on the synthetic surfaces, and the racing has tended to be of a more humble grade, but that is slowly beginning to change. These tracks give horses of limited ability somewhere to race and also allow trainers with small stables to compete with each other in the absence of both top-level horses and the larger yards, although this too is beginning to change. Several successful all-weather horses have made a transition to racing in North America to end up running in Group (graded stakes) races on dirt, and the all-weather surface can act to some extent as a screening academy to pick out horses that seem particularly adept at performing on these artificial surfaces, although not all horses make a successful transition from synthetic surfaces to dirt racing.

Flat racing is popular in the United Kingdom, Ireland, and France but less so in the rest of Europe. Although training centers exist in Germany along with a substantial number of high-grade races, flat racing has not really caught the imagination of the public in the same way as in Britain and Ireland and receives little media attention. Ireland always has had a strong tradition of horsemanship, and racing, centered around the Curragh, is buoyant and popular. Standardbred racing is equally popular in France, Germany, and Scandinavia, where flat racing opportunities are limited. Many European countries enjoy racing in the absence of a substantial breeding industry, and this creates a market for the surplus racehorses produced and raced in the United Kingdom, Ireland, and France. Horses in these countries are raced at 2 years of age and, ability permitting, 3 years of age, and at the end of the 3-year-old career many are submitted for sale if they have not shown sufficient ability to be retained for racing as older horses. This makes room in the yards for the incoming yearlings. These large dispersal sales at the end of the 3-year-old career supply the horses for National Hunt racing in the United Kingdom and for flat racing areas of the world lacking breeding programs. The need for yards to clear out the less gifted 3-year-olds to make room for the influx of yearlings also produces enormous pressure on trainers and consequently their veterinary surgeons to have a racehorse fit and able to race at 2 and 3 years of age, often without consideration for the long-term consequences of any treatments.

The small window of opportunity available to these horses impinges directly on many of the surgical and medical management decisions that need to be made when problems arise. The economics and practicality of any advice given have to be considered from the owner's viewpoint and the welfare of the horse.

COMPARISONS WITH RACING IN NORTH AMERICA

One of the major differences between training and racing in North America and Europe is in the geographical location and logistics of stabling and training of the horses. In the United States, almost all horses train at the racetrack and are stabled there continuously. In Europe, the horses live and train in yards often well away from the racetrack. These yards tend to be clustered around a training area, with gallops and conditioning canters available for use by local trainers. The horses travel daily to race at racecourses that may be up to 200 miles away.

In the United States, the horses, trainers, jockeys, and veterinary surgeons tend to move from one racecourse to another, but they stay at each track for long periods. Racing at each location takes place for many days or even weeks before horses and trainers move on to another track. Although some horses stay behind at one track, racing does not occur at that track when the primary focus is elsewhere.

In Europe, racing seldom occurs at any one racecourse for more than 3 consecutive days. Horses are trained in traditional stables, some of which date back many centuries. Horses travel to racecourses the day before racing, if the journey is particularly long, or even on the day of the race. Some horses make extremely long round trips. For example, it is not unusual for a trainer in Arundel on the south coast to send horses as far north as Ayr in Scotland, a round trip of 936 miles. Obviously the cost of transport has to be weighed against the potential gains, but the traditional system of training and traveling to the races in the United Kingdom seems to be holding up for now.

In 2000, two of the all-weather racetracks opened training barns adjacent to the track with a view to introducing American-style training, track side. How popular and successful this system is going to be and whether it will spread to other racecourses remain to be seen.

In North America, almost all training and racing takes place on a left circle (counterclockwise), and this might be expected to have influences on the incidence rates of injury to the left and right limbs for many lesions, such as proximal sesamoid bone (PSB) fractures, third metacarpal (McIII)/metatarsal (MtIII) bone condylar fractures, and tendonitis (see Chapter 106). In the United Kingdom, much conditioning work and even race speed training take place in straight lines (Figure 107-1). Racing itself can be on straight tracks (e.g., 1000 and 2000 Guineas at Newmarket), predominantly to the left (Epsom Derby), or to the right (Doncaster St. Ledger). The tracks themselves divide into about one third right-handed and two thirds left-handed throughout the country. This has an important impact on the lack of specific incidence of injury to the left or right limbs. One large fracture survey in Newmarket showed few instances of left or right dominance for any injury.[1]

Making categorical comments about the impact the new synthetic tracks have made on specific lameness and injury in the United Kingdom is difficult for several reasons:

References on page 1342

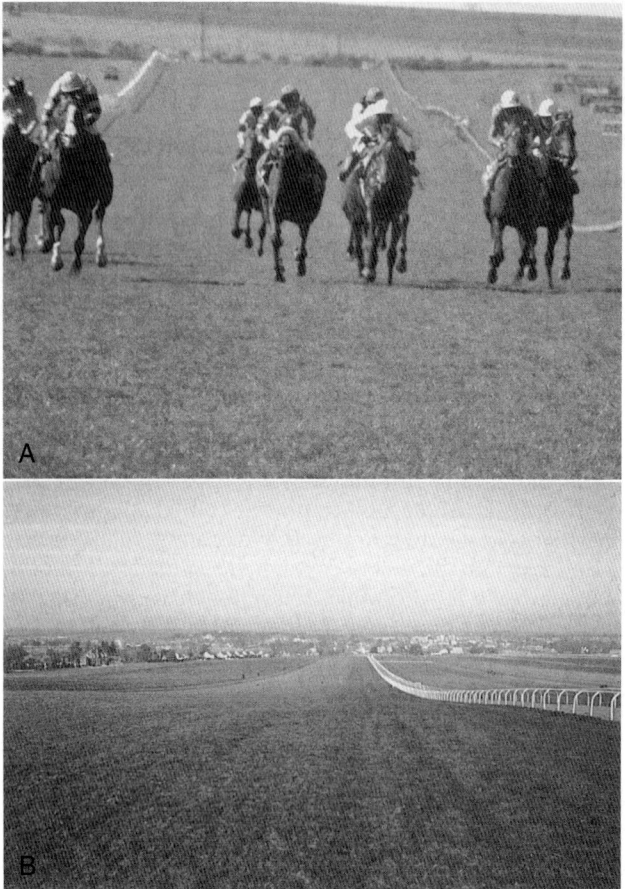

Fig. 107-1 • A, Horses approach the finish of the long and lonely Rowley mile racetrack at Newmarket. This photograph illustrates the undulating nature of the straight 1-mile track over which both 3-year-old Group 1 classics are run. **B,** The long straight of the training track gallops up Warren Hill just outside Newmarket. Two different all-weather synthetic surfaces are also available (between the white railings). The rest of the heath is used in strips, which are changed daily using movable markers. Each strip of grass is used only once every 3 years.

1. Although the racing is on a specific surface, because of the way British horses travel long distances to race, the horses in any race have trained on a variety of surfaces at home. Because it is believed that the accumulation of the daily work sets up stress-related injuries, the actual failure that may take place in a race often can have little to do with the track surface on which the horses are racing that day.
2. Tendonitis is relatively rare in the populations of 2- and 3-year-olds in a large flat training yard, and one might expect to see one bowed tendon in a yard of 100 horses in any one season. Horses that race on all-weather tracks have a far higher incidence, but they often include many older horses (3 to 9 years of age) and a higher number of horses with chronic, low-grade gait abnormalities, both of which could help to increase the incidence of tendon injuries.
3. The incidence of fractures in horses racing on all-weather surfaces seems to be higher than on good grass, but turf described as firm or hard is just as testing. Generalizations about turf versus artificial surfaces in terms of impact on injury have to be more specific because turf

can vary from bottomless mud to baked clay in midsummer. The older population of horses that race on the all-weather tracks, many of which carry a legacy of subchondral bone change from the previous training at 2 and 3 years of age for turf racing, could influence the higher incidence of fractures.

TRAINING REGIMENS IN EUROPE

Yearlings arrive in the yards for breaking from the sales in September and October and, unlike the situation in North America, often go straight to the trainer for breaking rather than to a specialist pretraining center.

After breaking, the yearlings usually start steady cantering exercise until Christmas. As the racing season approaches, horses showing precocity and ability to withstand faster exercise step up in pace throughout February and March. The first 2-year-old races occur in April, encouraging hard training of skeletally immature horses. However, until the racing calendar changes and while these races are open and available, trainers will train horses for them.

All-weather racing has altered the seasonal impact of flat racing in the United Kingdom forever, and some flat race horses now train throughout the year. However, most of the high-quality flat race horses do not compete on the all-weather circuit and are put into a slow-speed maintenance program from November until January, involving light cantering and trotting. Fillies may be turned out for a period.

All this is substantially different from the position in North America, where the horses often do not arrive at the racetrack until they are fully broken, in cantering exercise, and ready to do fast work. The breaking and pretraining often takes place in specialized pretraining centers, away from the city center tracks. This has important effects on the perception of racetrack veterinarians in North America concerning the incidence of developmental orthopedic disease linked to lameness. In North America, developmental orthopedic disease often causes lameness leading to diagnosis and removal from training *before* a horse reaches the racetrack; therefore horses with developmental orthopedic disease are not commonly seen by track veterinarians. An example is a subchondral bone cyst in the medial femoral condyle. Subchondral bone cysts are a regular occurrence in the annual intake of yearlings in the United Kingdom, diagnosed by the trainers' veterinarians. Discussion with colleagues working at California racetracks reveals that they rarely see horses with subchondral bone cysts, presumably because of the effect of the earlier screening at the pretraining centers.

Once on the track in North America the racing is often less seasonal and less age specific, removing a lot of the pressure for success at 2 or 3 years of age within a short season. Whether a horse races on turf or dirt does not matter: historically, all training took place on dirt, and this should be borne in mind by veterinarians assessing horses for potential purchase to move from Europe to America. Asking potential purchasers whether the horse is intended for turf or dirt racing is largely irrelevant because the daily training almost certainly will be on dirt. The dirt surface is more testing in many ways than anything these horses have seen before, and horses able to train and perform well on grass sometimes fail to make the transition to dirt. In the past couple years, a few training tracks and racetracks in North America have moved to synthetic surfaces. It will be interesting to see whether this makes for an easier transition for horses moving from Europe to race in North America, and what impact it has on the types and frequency of training and racing injuries.

CLINICAL HISTORY

Taking a detailed history is a prerequisite for a medical examination in any species. In racehorse practice one often sees a succession of lame horses during any morning in several different yards, and the detailed information may be limited. The trainer may not be present to supply it. However, one should always try to ascertain the following information before examining a TB racehorse for lameness:

1. How old is the horse? This is probably the single biggest determinant for different types of lameness. The chronological age is important, but far more important is the skeletal naivete of the horse. An unbroken horse of 3 or 4 years of age behaves in essentially the same way as an unbroken yearling, regardless of the difference in age, and may suffer similar problems when confronted with an inappropriate training program.

2. What stage of training has the horse reached? Has a horse reached race-speed exercise yet; is it simply trotting; or has it entered normal conditioning cantering exercise? For a yearling that is lame while being broken or in early cantering exercise, one has to consider subchondral bone cysts and other osseous cystlike lesions, osteochondritis dissecans (OCD), and associated osteoarthritis (OA). Problems may be bilateral, resulting in a peculiar gait. Bilateral iliac wing stress-related bone injury or sacroiliac joint pain considerably affects the freedom of movement of the hindlimbs and may mimic the clinical signs of exertional rhabdomyolysis, but plasma creatinine kinase (CK) levels often will be normal or only slightly raised (500 to 1500 IU/L).

   Stress-induced bone injuries are more likely to become apparent as work intensity increases. Stress-induced bone injuries include all of the long bone stress fractures of the humerus, tibia, the McIII, and the MtIII, and the iliac wing and shaft of the pelvis. Similarly, in a 2-year-old that has reached advanced training speed, the carpus and metacarpophalangeal joint are common sources of forelimb lameness, and lateral condylar stress injuries of the MtIII are common causes of hindlimb lameness. A 2-year-old in advanced training is less likely to have lameness associated with a subchondral bone cyst, osseous cystlike lesion, or OCD because these lesions usually cause lameness when the horse is younger and beginning its conditioning exercise. However, occasionally subchondral bone cysts and osseous cystlike lesions may arise or result in clinical signs for the first time at 3 years of age or even older.

3. Has the horse raced yet? If a horse has raced successfully at 2 years of age, the horse is unlikely to have hidden osseous cystlike lesions or OCD. Also, the skeleton has probably been conditioned adequately, and the incidence of stress fractures can be expected to be lower. However, in countries where racing is seasonal, 3-year-olds can "detrain" through the closed season if they are not maintained in cantering exercise. Stress fractures then may occur in the following season if speed training starts too quickly. A Californian study showed an associative link between the occurrence of stress fracture of the humerus and previous long-term removal from training.[2]

   If a horse did not race at 2 years of age, then all the differential diagnostic criteria used in the recently broken 2-year-old should be applied to the 3-year-old.

4. Has the horse had any previous orthopedic problems? Often in practice one knows each horse individually, and one is able to recall the problems that affected the horse in its early years. The history of a horse with previous problems may guide the use of diagnostic analgesia in an unorthodox, but timesaving, manner to establish whether the current lameness is a recurrence of a previous problem.

5. What is the pattern of the lameness? One should ascertain whether the lameness is constant from day to day and for how many days the horse has shown a gait abnormality. The veterinarian should ask whether the lameness gets better or worse within an exercise period. In some conditions, such as proximal suspensory desmitis (PSD), the lameness tends to get worse as the horse exercises, only to resolve with 24 to 48 hours of rest. Horses with lameness from other causes, such as OA, often warm out of clinical signs considerably from the start of exercise.

   In horses with acute-onset, severe lameness, questions of clinical history become less important because the horse is often not bearing weight, and a suspicion of skeletal failure is raised. Knowing whether this horse has been a good mover before onset of severe lameness is often helpful because some injuries (McIII/MtIII bone condylar fractures, PSB fractures) often are associated with poor gait before the actual fracture takes place. The same is true of horses with slab fractures of the third carpal bone, which often are preceded by a long period of subchondral bone sclerosis associated with bilateral third carpal bone pain (Figure 107-2). One of the most useful questions to ask about a horse with severe lameness is what stage of training the horse has reached because only advanced training to fast canter or gallop speeds usually results in bone failure. However, bacterial infection subcutaneously or within the hoof also can produce severe lameness.

6. Has the horse had a prolonged layoff for any reason? Horses brought back from a long period of box rest after illness or injury, without adequate previous bone conditioning, can get bizarre injuries from unusually low-speed exercise. These include complete, displaced scapular and humeral fractures, bilateral fractures of the PSBs and tibias, or displaced fractures of the proximal phalanx or condyles of the McIII. This is a reminder of the vital need for time to allow adequate skeletal conditioning necessary to avoid injury.

Clinical Examination

The veterinarian always should get the horse out and see it walk and trot to determine which limb is lame. Riders are notoriously unreliable at detecting the correct lame limb. The veterinarian should determine whether the lameness is unilateral or bilateral by the way the horse

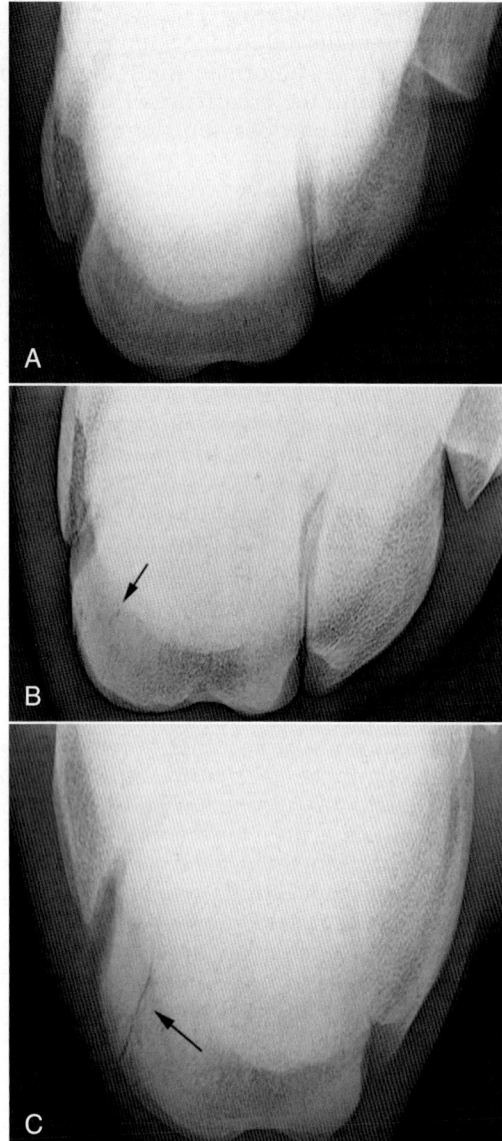

Fig. 107-2 • Flexed dorsal 60° proximal-dorsodistal oblique radiographic images of the left third carpal bone (C3) of three Thoroughbreds (TBs). Lateral is to the right. **A,** Normal. However, this complete lack of increased radiopacity is rare in a TB in advanced training, most of which show some degree of radiopacity of the radial fossa of C3. **B,** Dense increased radiopacity of the radial fossa of C3. Normal trabecular pattern is lost, and the bone has a "ground glass" appearance. There is increased osteolysis at the site of a normal nutrient foramen (*arrow* in the center of increased radiopacity). This stiffening of the bone predisposes it to injury or fracture. **C,** A nondisplaced sagittal fracture of C3 that propagates through the center of an area of severe increased radiopacity representing mineralization of bone (*arrows*).

moves. Many racehorses are slightly lame in all limbs and have a typical crouching, shuffling trot or may try repeatedly to break into a canter because trotting is so uncomfortable. New lameness may be superimposed on a chronic level of unsoundness.

Increasing experience usually leads one away from the belief that any one injury is linked to a particular gait. Lameness typical of a shoulder or a stifle tends to become a more remote belief because so-called typical lamenesses so often are linked eventually to the most unexpected site. However, a few types of lameness do remain that seem to

be linked to one particular pathological syndrome. Young TBs often show bilateral forelimb lameness related to carpal pain. These horses often trot with the limbs abducted from the midline and not fully flexed during forward motion. This gives a rolling, stiff-legged forelimb gait. The horse's attempt to get the contralateral limb down quickly to get off the sore limb as soon as possible shortens the forward phase of the stride, leading to a choppy, stilted action. However, horses affected with bilateral front fetlock pain or PSD trot in a very similar way if the pain level is the same in both limbs, and it may simply be that because carpal lameness is a common manifestation of this gait, we have come to link the two more firmly than we should.

Pain associated with the metatarsophalangeal joint is often bilateral and leads to a fairly characteristic gait typified by low limb flight, often with dragging of the toe during protraction, and an exaggerated rocking pelvic excursion dorsoventrally on both sides (sometimes termed the *Marilyn Monroe trot*) because the horse dips off each painful limb. Horses with a humeral stress fracture often abduct the limb, with shortened cranial protraction at the walk. One Newmarket trainer described this gait recently as "trotting like a pig in a tight skirt," which, although not a likely scenario, is in fact just how they look..

Having ascertained which limb is the lamest, the limb should be examined in detail using basic examination protocols (see Chapters 4 through 8 and 10). The following specific points apply to the TB racehorse.

1. Many racehorses show a pain response to squeezing of the foot with hoof testers, which is not related to a current lameness. The TB has a thin-soled foot, which often is shod incorrectly, causing soft-tissue bruising on the palmar aspect of the foot. If the horse responds to hoof testers in the lame limb, I normally test the contralateral foot to see whether the response is different. If the response to hoof testers is the same in both limbs, the foot may not be the primary source of pain causing lameness.

2. Suspensory branches are best appraised by centering each branch between opposing thumbs and following the branch from the most proximal portion that is palpable distally to the PSB. Subtle thickening in the suspensory branch not palpable with fingertips may be detected as the thumbs separate running toward the PSB.

3. The metacarpophalangeal joint should be checked for distention of the palmar pouch of the joint capsule. Thumb pressure is applied to the dorsoproximal aspect of the proximal phalanx and the dorsodistal aspect of the McIII, common sites for fragmentation and impingement lesions producing soreness. The limb then should be flexed partially and the response to flexion of the metacarpophalangeal joint monitored. Many young horses show a mild pain response to flexion, and the contralateral limb should be compared to gauge whether a difference exists. However, in a 2-year-old a bilateral pain response may reflect true problems in both limbs. In a normal horse the metacarpophalangeal joint should not be painful to flex.

4. The proximal aspect of the suspensory ligament (SL) should be examined with the limb raised by squeezing the ligament between the thumb or fingertips and the palmar surface of the McIII, first medially and then laterally. Normal untrained horses show no pain

response. However, many young racehorses show a variable degree of discomfort on SL palpation. Differentiating pathological and normal response to palpation associated with increased training can be difficult.

5. The dorsal surface of the McIII should be squeezed using the fingertips with the limb raised and the pain response noted as an indication of sore shins. The surface of the shin should be palpated for periosteal thickening or even focal callus formation associated with a stress fracture.

   Running a finger distally on the shin with a horse bearing weight often causes a horse to buckle the limb even if it has been months or even years after shin soreness has subsided and is not a reliable diagnostic test.

6. To detect distention of the antebrachiocarpal or middle carpal joint capsules, pushing on the dorsal surface of the joint with the finger and thumb of one hand while observing the palmar pouches of the joints is useful. Mild effusion then may be detected.

7. Many young racehorses resent extension of the shoulder joint in the absence of a lesion.

8. Many racehorses mildly object to forced tarsal flexion equally in both hindlimbs unrelated to a lesion. A profound response to flexion of the tarsus of the lame limb, which is not matched in the contralateral limb, usually signifies a tarsal bone fracture or a stress fracture of the distal aspect of the tibia. If pain is noted on flexion, thumb pressure should be applied to the proximodorsal aspect of the MtIII and the dorsolateral surface of the tarsal bones to determine a pain response. Pain response is often marked if there is a slab fracture of the third tarsal bone.

9. The tibia is a common site for stress fractures and is examined by curling the fingers around the caudal surface of the tibia from the medial aspect and squeezing on a common predilection site for stress fracture, the caudal surface of the distal third of the tibia. Torsion of the tibia also is attempted by flexing the limb, applying lateral traction to the os calcis with one hand while maintaining firm contact on the stifle with one's shoulder, and medially twisting the distal aspect of the MtIII with the other hand (Figure 107-3). A horse with an incomplete linear stress fracture will show a profound pain response to torsion and may try to kick. It may also not want to take weight on the limb for a few seconds after its release, which is a sign characteristic of marked cortical involvement. The other limb should be examined, bearing in mind that these fractures can be bilateral, although pain and degree of lameness are often asymmetrical.

10. The pelvis is another frequent site of stress fractures and is examined by monitoring the position of the bony landmarks—the tubera sacrale, tubera coxae, third trochanter of the femurs, and tubera ischia—looking for displacement (see Chapter 49). Response to deep palpation of the muscles that lie between these sites is also noted. The most common clinical sign in horses with a nondisplaced pelvic fracture is guarding of the musculature as a response to deep palpation. Guarding gives a hard, boardlike texture to the muscle and often is accompanied by fasciculation of the gluteal mass and an avoidance response. Similar clinical signs can be seen in horses suffering from exertional

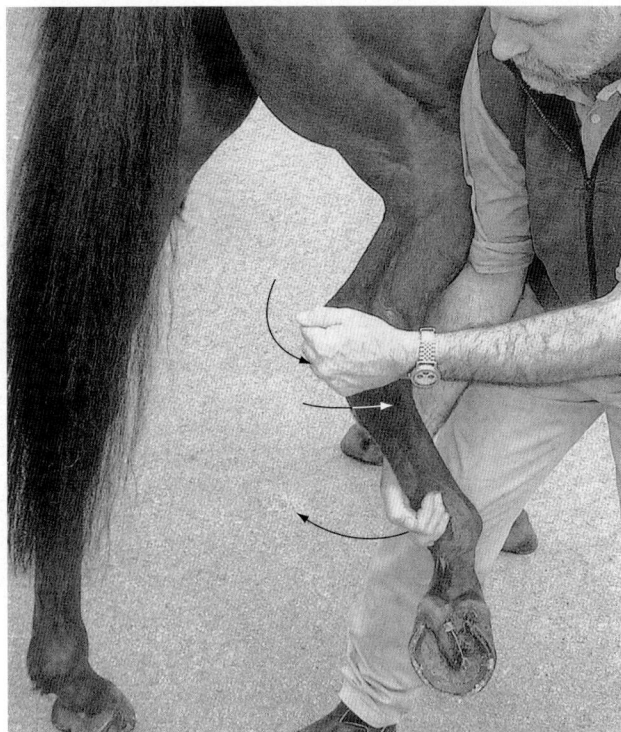

Fig. 107-3 • Application of torsion to the tibia. The metatarsophalangeal joint is rotated medially, the os calcis laterally, and firm shoulder pressure maintained with the stifle. Horses with a stress fracture of the tibia often show a sharp pain response to this test and will often be unwilling to bear weight on the limb for some seconds subsequently.

rhabdomyolysis, and this may be a difficult differential diagnosis to establish. Muscle enzyme concentrations may be elevated (CK, 500 to 1500 IU/L) in horses with a pelvic fracture. The tail should be raised and lowered, and tail tone should be monitored. A flaccid tail often indicates a sacral or coccygeal fracture.

Imaging Considerations
Radiography and Radiology
Many lesions in the TB racehorse are associated with subtle changes in bone density and structure rather than overt fragmentation of bone. These variations result in subtle changes in radiopacity (increased radiolucency or radiopacity), which often are seen best on high-quality radiographs using single-screen film and excellent radiographic technique or more recently by using digital radiography. However, we should be aware when using digital radiography that the "standard" appearance of bone is lost. By altering the algorithms and scaling, we can alter contrast and obliterate the signs of increased radiopacity of bone at will. This is particularly true in appraisal of the "skyline" projection of the third carpal bone, where assessment of increased radiopacity is critical in advising on future workload of young horses and can be made MORE difficult by the ease of image manipulation now available to us digitally.

Radiography is notoriously unreliable in detecting early fracture lines and subchondral bone collapse. For this reason, if lameness is linked to a particular site by diagnostic analgesia and nothing is visible radiologically, repeating the radiography 2 weeks later is often advisable. Any horse with subtle changes in bone density can be rested long

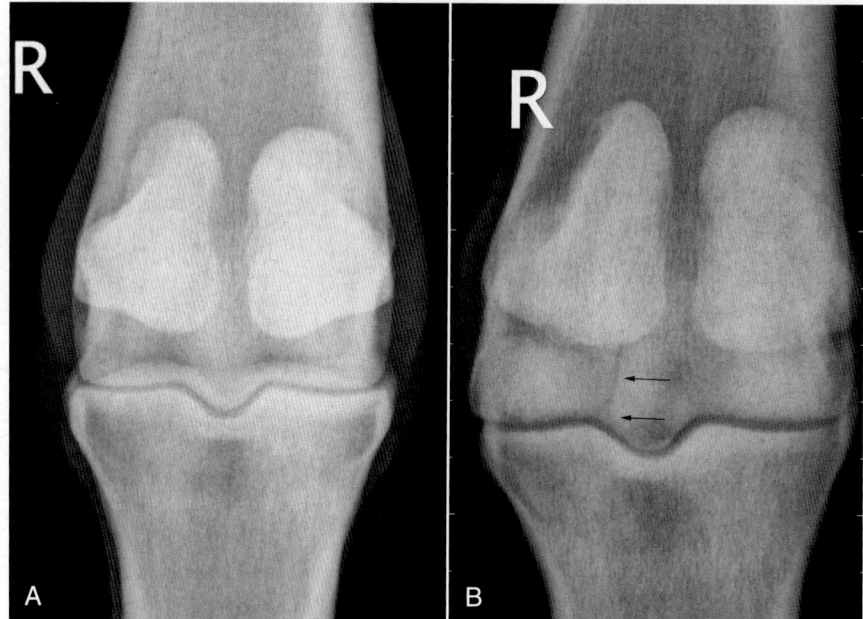

Fig. 107-4 • A, Weight-bearing dorsal 20° proximal-palmarodistal oblique radiographic image of a right meta-carpophalangeal (MCP) joint. Lateral is to the left. No gross abnormality is seen. **B,** Flexed dorsal 125° distal-palmaroproximal oblique radiographic image of the same MCP joint. There is an incomplete linear fracture *(arrow)* in the lateral condyle that was not visible on any other image.

enough where additional damage can be seen. During investigation of individual joints, special projections are often most useful (Figure 107-4). Radiographic examination of the metacarpophalangeal and metatarsophalangeal joints always should include the flexed dorsopalmar image, which is extremely useful for evaluating the palmar and plantar aspect of the condyles (see Figures 107-4 and 107-5).[3,4] In a hindlimb this view often is achieved best as a plantarodorsal image. The limb is cupped loosely by a hand underneath the tarsus and allowed to hang in a semi-flexed position. The cassette is placed in a cassette holder and positioned on the dorsal aspect of the metatarsopha-langeal joint, and the x-ray machine is positioned above and behind to achieve the orthodox 125-degrees image.

The lateral condyle of the MtIII bone is a predilection site for subchondral bone injury, represented by sclerosis in the early stages and subchondral bone loss and radiolu-cency as the condition advances. This can be highlighted by a dorsal 30° proximal 45° lateral–plantarodistal medial oblique image (down angled oblique) developed by Ross[5] (see Figure 107-5, *C*).

Another unorthodox image that can be helpful in trying to evaluate subchondral bone radiopacity and fissur-ing in the distal palmar/plantar aspect of the McIII/MtIII is a steeply angled (60°) dorsopalmar/plantar image (i.e., dorsal 60° proximal-palmarodistal oblique view), centered on the palmar/plantar aspect of the condyles, projecting the PSBs proximally. Areas of fissuring and radiolucency adjacent to the sagittal ridge of the McIII/MtIII or promi-nent increased radiopacity of the subchondral bone can sometimes only be seen on this image (see Figure 107-5, *A*). This image was developed in response to frustration in being unable to see marked changes in this site seen on magnetic resonance imaging (MRI) examination using conventional radiographic images (Figure 107-6).

Radiographic examination of the carpus always should include a flexed dorsal 55° proximal-dorsodistal oblique (skyline) image of the third carpal bone, which is some-times the only image in which lesions in this bone can be seen clearly. The image is easy to do well but is still often done poorly. Small changes in the angle of projection make a substantial difference to the amount of the third carpal bone visible in the resultant image.[6] One should not be satisfied unless the entire radial fossa is seen clearly (see Figure 107-2).

The relevance of changes in bone density should not be underestimated. Many stress fractures of the long bones are seen only by the occurrence of endosteal or periosteal callus. Periosteal callus may only be visible with the aid of a bright light or more extreme digitally produced "window-ing." Fracture lines are relatively rare. Despite the difficulty in imaging incomplete fracture lines sometimes, some horses may go on to develop complete, displaced fractures during periods of box rest, reminding us that the evidence must have been there if only we could have seen it.

Scintigraphy

Scintigraphy has allowed enormous advances to be made in the detection and understanding of stress fractures in the racehorse.[7-9] Scintigraphy should not be used as a first line of investigation in horses with obvious single-limb lameness, unless a strong clinical suspicion exists that the humerus, pelvis, or tibia is involved and radiography has been unrewarding. Examination of an entire TB race-horse that cannot trot and has multilimb lameness is often useful. These horses are difficult to assess using diag-nostic analgesia because one is often racing against time, moving from one limb to another with the predominant lameness constantly changing. Scintigraphy in these horses often results in a list of lesions that can be investigated

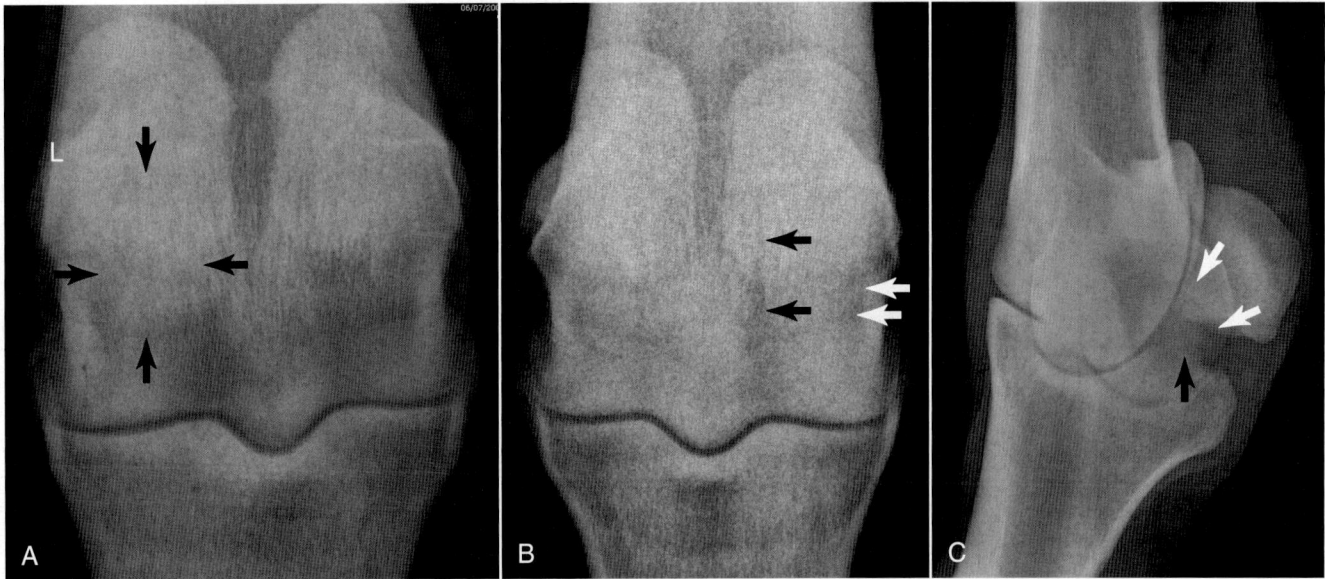

Fig. 107-5 • A, Dorsal 60° proximal-palmarodistal oblique image of the left metacarpophalangeal (MCP) joint; lateral is to the right. This steeply angled dorsopalmar image was developed in an attempt to see subchondral bone change diagnosed by magnetic resonance imaging examination, but not seen on conventional radiographs. There is a zone of severe bone mineralization (increased radiopacity, *arrows*) associated with an advanced subchondral bone injury in the medial condyle. Normal trabecular pattern of the condyle is lost (cf., lateral condyle). **B,** Dorsal 60° proximal-palmarodistal oblique image of a right fore MCP joint; lateral is to the left. There is less marked mineralization of the medial condyle *(white arrows)* than in **A,** but there is radiolucency/fissuring in the most palmar portion of the parasagittal aspect of the medial condyle *(black arrows)*. This horse was lame at the walk, and pain was localized to the MCP joint by local analgesia. This fissuring was not visible on orthodox radiographic images. **C,** Dorsal 30° proximal 45° lateral-plantarodistal medial oblique image. This image highlights the region of the lateral condyle in contact with the lateral proximal sesamoid bone when the joint is at full weight bearing, a common site of focal stress injury. Focal bone mineralization (increased radiopacity) is evident *(white arrows)* with a central area of radiolucency *(black arrow)*, which probably represents bone necrosis and resorption. This degree of change is usually irreversible and associated with chronic lameness. These changes cannot be seen on any other radiographic image.

radiologically and by judicious use of diagnostic analgesia. The other roles of scintigraphy include examining a site identified by diagnostic analgesia but in which no abnormality can be found radiologically and safety screening of an initially severely lame horse that has become sound before a diagnosis has been reached. Thus making a diagnosis in these horses at post mortem is avoided. Clients should be educated to not request the scintigraphic "fishing trip" as a first line of enquiry.

Ultrasonography

Ultrasonography is the imaging modality of choice for investigating soft tissue injuries in the metacarpal and metatarsal regions (see Chapter 16). In the young TB affected with PSD, lesions are often subtle, with enlargement and bulging of the palmar border with consequent loss of the neat rectangular shape of the normal SL as the only finding.[1] Large anechogenic defects and obvious fiber tearing are not common.

The clinical relevance of bilateral enlargement of the superficial digital flexor tendons along with intratendonous edema in a 2-year-old may be difficult to interpret because normal tendons increase in size in response to training[10] (see Figure 99-2). If obvious distortion of the contour of the tendons exists, I advise that the horse not gallop or race at 2 years of age. The horse is maintained in alternate-day trotting and cantering for 3 months. This treatment

has not led to true tendonitis at 3 years of age in any horse. I refer to these horses as having juvenile tendonitis but have never been comfortable that this degree of caution is mandatory. Perhaps these horses could do more work without further injury.

Ultrasonography is also useful for detecting and monitoring some fractures of the ilial wing and shaft and ischium of the pelvis (see Chapter 49).

Diagnostic Analgesia

Having carried out the clinical examination described, one structure causing lameness may be obvious. For example, the horse may show a sharp pain response on palpation of the SL or distention of the middle carpal joint capsules with pain on flexion. Diagnostic analgesia may not be necessary in these horses, and diagnostic imaging of the site may be the next step. Many horses have a list of diagnostic possibilities: the horse may have shown a pain response to hoof testers and some tenderness to palpation of the SL and have some distention of the middle carpal joint capsule. To tease apart these findings, diagnostic analgesia is mandatory. Diagnostic analgesia is done most efficiently at a clinic rather than a training yard because the procedure is time consuming. If a horse is fresh when admitted for diagnostic analgesia, the increase in muscle tone and general excitement can obscure a mild lameness, and acetylpromazine (2 to 5 mg/horse

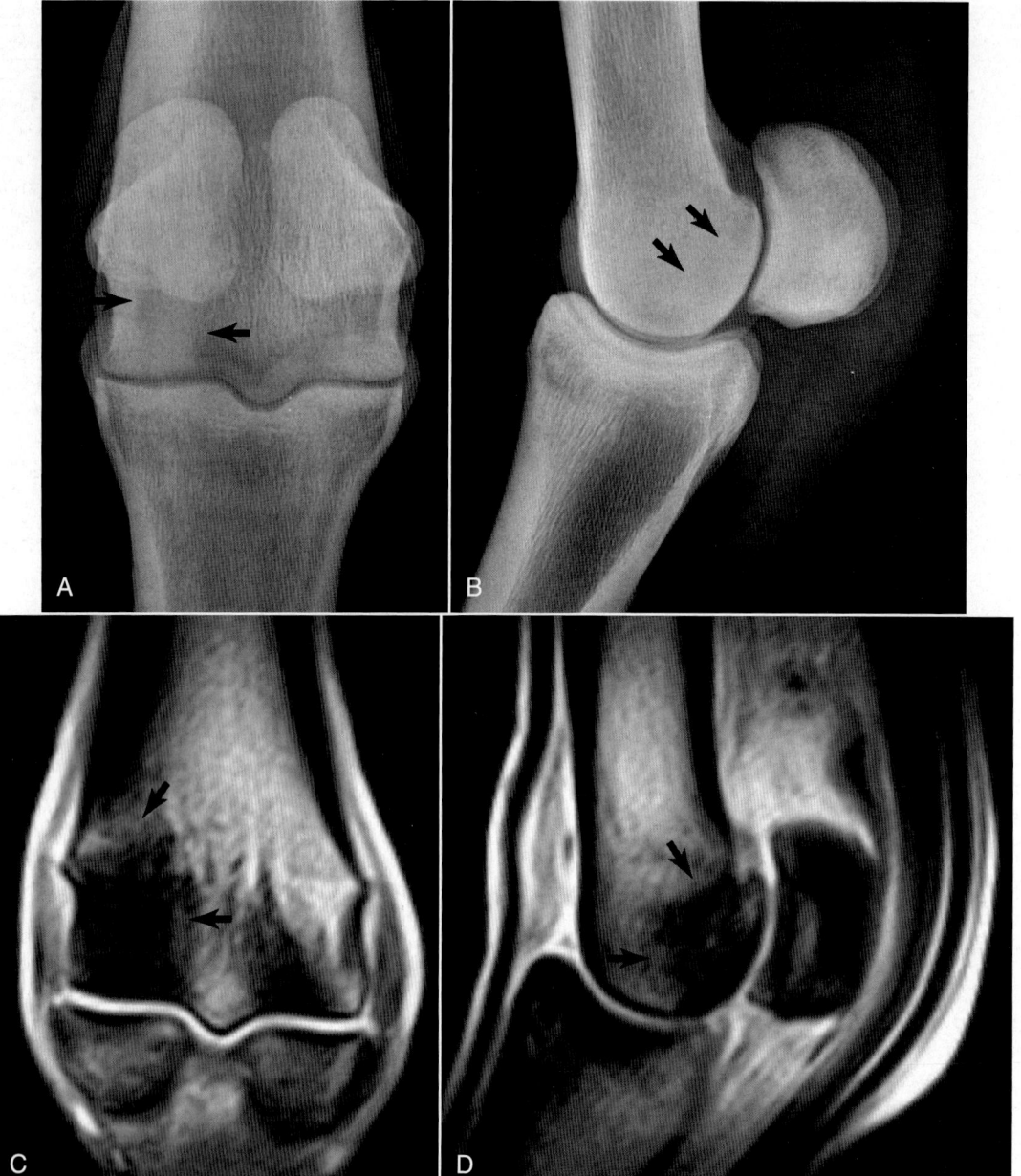

Fig. 107-6 • Dorsal 15° proximal-palmarodistal oblique **(A)** and lateromedial **(B)** images of the left fore fetlock of a 2-year-old TB, with lameness localized to the metacarpophalangeal (MCP) joint by regional and intraarticular analgesia. There is mild increased radiopacity of the palmar aspect of the medial condyle *(arrows)*, but within the range one might encounter in sound horses. T1-weighted gradient echo motion-corrected low-field magnetic resonance images, dorsal **(C)** and parasagittal **(D)** plane, of the same MCP joint. There is diffuse marked decreased signal intensity within the palmar aspect of the medial condyle *(arrows)* and to a lesser extent in the lateral condyle. This is consistent with mineralization (bone sclerosis) underestimated in the radiograph. (Courtesy Sarah Powell, Rossdale and Partners, Newmarket, England.)

intravenously) can help settle the horse without affecting its ability to trot.

If the horse is admitted to a clinic for a day, a positive block can be allowed to wear off, so that more localized blocks can be carried out. For this reason, my own first block in a forelimb is usually biaxial palmar digital nerve blocks so that the foot can be eliminated or investigated in greater detail later. Many horses with mild lameness exhibit a detectable worsening of the degree of lameness if the foot is desensitized and is not the source

of pain, which can be useful when investigating intermittent or low-grade lameness. I used to first perform palmar (abaxial sesamoid) blocks, but I increasingly found that this often abolished pain from the fetlock or the distal metacarpal or metatarsal regions and thus was not reliable as an indicator of primary foot pain.

If lameness is abolished using palmar digital analgesia, a more detailed investigation of the foot and distal extremity is carried out, perhaps with the shoe removed. If effusion of the distal interphalangeal joint is present, an intraarticular block is performed. In rare instances, palmar digital nerve blocks will abolish pain later proven to originate from the distal condyle of the McIII or the MtIII; therefore this should also be checked by intraarticular analgesia of the fetlock joint if the subsequent block results do not make logical sense.

If the horse is unchanged after palmar digital analgesia, a low palmar and palmar metacarpal (four-point) block is used. This may alleviate lameness; not improve lameness, indicating the problem is much higher; or give a 30% to 50% improvement in lameness, which is observed commonly in horses with PSD. However, recently I have become aware that horses with severe, advanced subchondral bone sclerosis and injury of the distal aspect of the McIII/MtIII seen on MRI may not be rendered completely sound by either a low four-point block or intraarticular analgesia of the fetlock joint, although the lameness may be substantially improved by both. There is a danger if one assumes that a 50% improvement in lameness following a low four-point block, followed by total soundness after a subcarpal block indicates that the origin of pain is in the proximal aspect of the SL or the McIII. This block response may divert attention away from the actual site of pathology in the fetlock.

The next logical step is the subcarpal block, which I perform using 1.6-cm needles and 2.5 mL of mepivacaine in the recess immediately palmar to the top of the second and fourth metacarpal bones. Short needles and small volumes of local anesthetic solution are used in an attempt to reduce the frequency of false-positive analgesia of the middle carpal joint. False-positive responses can occur by inadvertent direct penetration of the distopalmar outpouchings of the carpometacarpal joint[11,12] or by diffusion of local anesthetic solution up the fascial planes to a site proximal to the middle carpal joint.

A positive subcarpal block is always allowed to wear off, and the middle carpal joint is blocked subsequently to ascertain which site is responsible for the pain causing lameness. Unfortunately, in some horses complete soundness follows both the middle carpal joint and subcarpal blocks. When this occurs, ultrasonographic examination of the proximal aspect of the SL and a radiographic examination of the carpus are performed before an informed guess is made about the most likely source of lameness. If no lesions are found after imaging both sites, defining the source of pain categorically may not be possible, and the horse is a candidate for nuclear scintigraphy. MRI is also proving extremely useful in unpicking the complexity of lameness in this site.[13] I avoid using the lateral palmar nerve block because in my hands it is too nonspecific and has abolished lameness that originates from the SL, proximal aspect of the McIII, and both joints of the carpus on occasions. In an experimental study, no penetration of the antebrachiocarpal and middle carpal joints occurred as a result of lateral palmar analgesia, although commonly the carpal synovial sheath was penetrated (Editors).[12]

Negative subcarpal and middle carpal analgesia are followed by median and ulnar nerve blocks. Although these blocks leap-frog the antebrachiocarpal joint, median and ulnar nerve blocks usually abolish lameness associated with lesions of this joint. Intraarticular analgesia of the antebrachiocarpal joint may fail to abolish pain associated with chip fractures of the distal aspect of the radius in some

horses.[14] The jump directly to median and ulnar blocks avoids the possibility of false-negative responses misleading the lameness diagnosis.

Negative median and ulnar blocks usually are followed by advice to carry out scintigraphy because scapulohumeral joint lameness is relatively rare and intraarticular analgesia does not alleviate lameness associated with humeral stress fractures, which are common. Although OCD and osseous cystlike lesions of the scapulohumeral joint are found in late yearlings and early 2-year-olds, these often show scintigraphically and can be confirmed later by radiological examination and diagnostic analgesia if necessary. Intraarticular analgesia of the elbow and scapulohumeral joints is performed if the median and ulnar blocks and scintigraphy fail to establish the seat of pain causing lameness. However, it has been my experience that intraarticular analgesia of the elbow joint can on occasion abolish lameness later proven to have originated from a site more distal in the limb, presumably by diffusion of local anesthetic solution from the joint in proximity to the median nerve; therefore a positive elbow block may need to be interpreted with caution.

Hindlimb investigation follows a slightly less rigorous approach for three reasons:

1. Some young TBs become difficult with repeated needle entry of the hindlimbs, resulting in a serious risk to the veterinary surgeon, the member of staff holding the horse, and the horse itself.

2. The common occurrence of stress fractures in the more proximal sites in the hindlimb, particularly in the tibia and the pelvis, means that many horses potentially would be blocked in detail from toe to stifle, without producing any improvement in lameness. For this reason a six-point (low plantar) block above the metatarsophalangeal joint is performed first in a hindlimb. A positive response to a six-point block is allowed to wear off, and the response to intraarticular analgesia of the fetlock joint is assessed. If these blocks produce negative results, a subtarsal block is performed, followed by tarsometatarsal (TMT) joint analgesia. If the horse behaves satisfactorily, tibial and fibular (peroneal) nerve blocks are performed. It is common for pain originating from stress fractures of the distal aspect of the tibia to be abolished by tibial and fibular nerve blocks, and postblock radiographic screening after a positive result to this block should include the distal aspect of the tibia. If lameness is still present, the horse may be allowed to rest, undiagnosed, or the stifle is examined radiographically, or scintigraphy is performed, depending on the wishes of the trainer and owner. Only if lameness recurs after a period of rest and the absence of a scintigraphic diagnosis are the stifle joints blocked.

3. Bilateral lameness associated with subchondral injury to the lateral condyle of the MtIII is common in TBs and often can be abolished by blocking the lateral plantar metatarsal nerve only, just dorsal to the button of the splint, using 2 mL of local anesthetic solution.[15] This often produces an overt lameness in the contralateral limb. This block is easy to perform, and the problem is common; therefore it is tempting to use this block first in horses showing the typical bilateral tight, choppy gait abnormality often seen in this condition.

Shoeing Considerations

TB racehorses have notoriously bad horn quality and hoof conformation. They appear to have uniformly thin soles and a tendency to develop long toes and low heels. Medial to lateral hoof balance is vital to the TB racehorse remaining sound, but it is sometimes not pursued adequately. All horses should be shod wide at the heel to allow full weight bearing by the horn structures. However, in racehorses this tends to produce an abundance of pulled shoes by the trapping of the metal of one shoe underneath the other foot in the stable, particularly on rubber floors, which do not allow the trapped shoe to slip out. This encourages farriers to tuck the shoes out of reach under the foot, which leads to progressive collapse of the heel and long-toe, low-heel conformation. Farriers have to be reassured that they will not be held responsible for pulled shoes within the stable and that the health of the horse's foot is more important than the management problems sometimes associated with correct shoeing.

Interference injuries are not as common in the TB as in Standardbreds and are more common when horses are on a reduced exercise plane or in 2-year-olds in early training. Interference injuries seem to become less common as the horse strengthens and becomes more fit. In every horse such injuries should be approached as a joint exercise, with the full involvement of the farrier. Interference injuries, such as scalping, that suddenly begin to occur regularly in a horse previously unaffected can be an early sign of gait alteration reflecting pain, and the horse's action at the walk and trot should be carefully evaluated.

The following approaches may be helpful.

Brushing Injuries of the Hindlimbs

Hindlimb brushing injuries are caused by the contralateral foot in flight and produce cuts on the medial aspect of the fetlock or the proximal aspect of the pastern. Most of these horses toe out and are base narrow, and some swing the foot inward during protraction at walk and trot. Traditionally three-quarter round shoes have been used, with the medial branch missing. Over time, however, this shoeing results in progressive collapse of the medial hoof wall, pushing the limb even further out of line, and brushing may actually increase. An alternative is to use light steel or alloy plates behind. This lowers the weight of the foot and often stops the problem. If this fails, we use a 2-cm lateral trailer on the shoe. Half-round shoes are always a help because they remove the cutting edge if interference does take place.

Brushing Interference in the Forelimbs

Brushing in forelimbs is difficult to treat. Affected horses usually toe out considerably from distal to the metacarpophalangeal joint and are base narrow. Horses often first show interference when galloping at speed, and injury causes substantial hemorrhage and swelling over the medial PSB. This swelling then makes future interference even more likely, and a downward spiral begins. The steps I usually take involve careful correction of medial to lateral hoof imbalance by the farrier, rest and antiinflammatory treatment to reduce swelling, and application of closely fitted half-round section shoes. Topical application of dimethyl sulfoxide containing flumethasone is indicated unless there is an open wound. If a full-thickness skin wound is present, topical antisepsis and systemic antibiotic treatment may be indicated to prevent undue swelling at the site. Ultrasonographic examination sometimes reveals a subcutaneous seroma, which responds well to needle drainage and injection of a small amount of corticosteroids (dexamethasone, 2 to 4 mg).

Protection of the site of injury on return to training with a thin layer of cohesive exercise bandage can help, but great care should be taken in applying this type of bandage because the lack of padding can all too easily produce a bandage bow (bind). Even with all these measures, it is not uncommon for affected horses to suffer repeated intermittent problems throughout their careers.

Scalping, Forging, and Overreaching

Scalping, forging, and overreaching are produced by the hind foot arriving in the site occupied by the front foot too soon in the gait cycle.

Scalping produces cuts on the dorsal aspect of a hindlimb pastern, too dorsal to have been caused by the contralateral limb. Scalping is caused by the tip of the front shoe striking the front of the advancing hind pastern, as the horse just misses forging. Such injuries often are avoided by a four-point trim or shortening the toe and using a rolled-toe shoe in front to speed breakover fractionally, thus getting the front foot out of the way by the time the hind foot arrives. If this alone fails, then using a light steel or alloy plate with a square toe in front and heavy steel shoes behind often eliminates the problem. The same measures are used to reduce true forging, when the hind shoe strikes the tip of the front shoe, producing the characteristic steel-on-steel noise from which the name is derived. Forging can be more common when horses jog on a soft synthetic or sand surface, which "holds" the front foot and prevents its early clearance, and rolling and damping these track surfaces before use can help. Overreaching, when the hind toe strikes the bulb of the front heel, can be approached in the same way. Overreach boots can help but can only be used in slow work. Overreaching is most common when the horse is fresh and being restrained hard in its exercise or is being exercised in deep sand, preventing easy limb clearance. For this reason these horses can be helped by judicious use of mild sedation before exercise (10 to 25 mg of acetylpromazine orally, 30 minutes before exercise) and by exercising on a nonimpeding surface. In many horses all these measures can cease as the horses become fully fit.

TEN MOST COMMON LAMENESS CONDITIONS

The following are the 10 most common lameness conditions; these are discussed in detail in this section.
1. Foot-related lameness
2. Suspensory desmitis
3. Fetlock lameness and subchondral bone injuries to the distal aspect of the third metacarpal/metatarsal bone
4. Lameness associated with the middle carpal joint
5. Lameness subsequent to bacterial infection
6. Stress fractures of the long bones (third metacarpal bone, tibia, and humerus) and pelvis
7. Exostoses of the second and fourth metacarpal/metatarsal bones (splints)
8. Undiagnosed hindlimb lameness

9. Fractures of the proximal phalanx and condyles of the distal aspect of the third metacarpal/metatarsal bone
10. Lameness associated with the tarsometatarsal joint

Foot-Related Lameness

TB feet are usually thin soled, and most racing TBs have a pain response to hoof testers, even in the absence of genuine lameness. To minimize laminar bruising, good shoeing technique is essential, and horses should not be exercised on a surface that is too firm. Medial-to-lateral foot balance is also vital but often neglected. Farriers often are expected to shoe in the dark of the early morning, with the horse loose in the stable on deep bedding. This often leads to poor visual assessment of foot–pastern axis and balance. Clinicians should help farriers to change this attitude in favor of a system that allows these skilled professionals to achieve their potential. Such a change involves providing staff members to lead out and hold the horses for the farrier to inspect.

Bruising usually is diagnosed when the horse shows an exquisite pain response to hoof testers in a fairly localized area, but no obvious tract leading to the deeper structures. Careful paring with a hoof knife often reveals pink discoloration in the horn layers immediately above the area of the bruise. Removing the shoe and applying a poultice to the foot for a day is usually successful in managing this condition. If the horse is close to a race and time is of the essence, the foot is iced morning and night in an attempt to decrease the pain associated with the bruise. Once the pain is clearly found to be only from the bruising and no pus pocket has formed under the sole, poulticing is stopped to dry up the sole again before shoeing. If foot lameness is associated with infection, then draining the subsolar abscess is mandatory. Although traditional textbooks talk about radical curettage and establishing sufficient drainage, in the racing TB removal of too much horn is associated with an extended period of lameness because of laminar damage and pain from exposed soft horn. Initially the hole to the pus pocket should be as small as possible. Once drainage has been established, hoof testers can be used to expel pus and to pull in soaking agents or hydrogen peroxide. The hole often can be enlarged using a bent 16-gauge needle. The foot usually is soaked then in warm salt water for 10 minutes morning and night and in between is wrapped in saline-soaked cotton wool dressing contained within polyethylene. Walking these horses twice a day if the degree of lameness permits is a good idea to encourage extrusion of the pus, which leads to quicker return to full work and decreases the risk of rhabdomyolysis on return to training. Some infections within the foot are infuriating because although an exquisite pain response occurs and a clear penetration tract leads into the foot, blood in the sensitive laminae is reached before the infected focus is found. The horse then usually resents further digging in the sensitive laminae. Radiological examination is justified in these horses to rule out infectious osteitis of the distal phalanx, usually evident as a radiolucent area. This condition, if confirmed, is treated by radical curettage after sedation, local nerve blocks, and application of a tourniquet. A treatment (hospital) plate is then applied.

Traumatic corns can be one of the most frustrating conditions with which to deal. Affected horses usually have a long-toe, low-heel conformation and inwardly collapsing heel bulbs. Intense pain occurs when hoof testers are applied across the seat of the corn, and yet exploration simply reveals subsolar blood pockets or bleeding tissue. When these are exposed, localized prolapse of the sole may occur at the seat of the corn. These horses take a long time to regain soundness and normally are shod with a bar shoe to bridge the weight bearing from the nonaffected heel to the wall of the other quarter. The horse should be kept in walking exercise only for at least 2 weeks to allow some horn growth before an attempt at retraining. Training and racing on hard surfaces is contraindicated, which can be realistic advice in the United Kingdom. These horses may be more difficult to manage if sold to train on the tracks in North America. The farrier should be involved in attempting to bring up the heel angle in these flat-footed horses, and the four-point trim is often helpful in achieving this quickly. Medial-to-lateral balance should be checked because traumatic corns often occur on the lower aspect of a heel of a horse that has been allowed to become unbalanced. This seems to occur because of second contact concussion as the foot strikes the ground in a biphasic manner, which is corrected by lowering the longer side of the heel to make sure that the foot strikes the ground evenly.

Sometimes a breach in the horn at the seat of the corn allows infection to enter, producing an infected corn. The condition often is linked to swelling and pain or even discharge of pus at the bulb of the heel above the corn. Drainage, poulticing, and remedial shoeing are the standard treatments.

For lameness associated with the horse being pricked by the farrier, with or without development of infection, use of a glue-on shoe when the horse is reshod after the problem has been resolved is sometimes a good idea. Most farriers shoeing racehorses are extremely skilled, and if they have managed to puncture the sensitive laminae during a routine shoeing, the cause is usually because the horse has extremely little wall outside the white line. The direct glue-on technique, using a normal alloy racing plate stuck directly to the sole without nails, allows the horse 3 to 4 weeks of extra horn growth before further nailing is done. The more traditional tab-glue shoes are less satisfactory because the shoes tend to become loose and the horse's foot shape may change. This is not the case with direct glue-on shoes. Horses that repeatedly lose shoes and have increasing wall avulsion and damage are treated best using direct glue-on shoes to allow time for wall recovery. More recently another type of glue-on shoe has been developed by farrier Rob Sigafoos (the Sigafoos shoe). This is constructed incorporating a collar of strong synthetic fabric into the structure of the shoe, which is glued directly to the dorsal wall of the hoof. The advantages with this shoe are that the heel bulbs are not bound in and can expand over the shoe, and that the shoe can be set properly under the foot in a normal position. Horses have trained and raced with success in these shoes.

Suspensory Desmitis

The forelimb SL can be injured at any location, but PSD is most common in a young racehorse. PSD is often bilateral, although the lameness observed is almost always unilateral. PSD is characterized by weight-bearing lameness of grade of 1 to 3 of 5, which seems to disappear rapidly after periods of rest. Even 24 hours of box rest often renders these horses sound. However, within an exercise period, the lameness is typified by becoming worse the more the horse does (warms into the lameness). Horses with PSD often show pain when the SL is squeezed between the thumb and the back of the McIII with the limb flexed. The veterinarian should start at the apex of the PSB and work along the SL, squeezing it against the bony structures of the limb. The response should be compared with the contralateral limb. Most normal young TBs show some degree of tenderness to palpation of the SL, although unbroken and untrained horses of the same age usually do not. This may indicate that many racehorses suffer a degree of PSD during early training in the absence of observable clinical signs. Lesions of the origin of the SL can be present without pain on palpation because it is difficult to apply accurate digital pressure in the proximal metacarpal region.

Local analgesia is discussed on page 1001. When performing subcarpal analgesia, the needles should be applied to the syringe before injection to prevent the introduction of air into the fascial planes, which can preclude later ultrasonographic examination. This air appears as a hyperechogenic band between the SL and the accessory ligament of the deep digital flexor tendon, obscuring evaluation of the SL.

The other common predilection site for injury of the SL is the interface of the distal aspect of a branch and the ipsilateral PSB. These lesions usually occur when the horse starts fast exercise. In horses with conformational defects, the same site can be affected in both forelimbs. For example, in a horse with offset carpi and toed-in conformation, the lateral branch of the SL and the lateral PSB are affected. Typical radiological changes of sesamoiditis are seen with clear disruption of the SL/PSB interface. Central hypoechoic lesions are identified by use of ultrasonography, along with irregularity of the PSB surface and even fragment avulsion. The SL branches often are enlarged palpably, but ultrasonographic imaging often reveals this to be a zone of periligamentous fibrosis, rather than true swelling of the branch itself.

Horses with PSD are confined to box rest for 2 to 4 weeks until clinically sound and then walk on a horse walker for 4 to 6 weeks, followed by 1 month of walking and trotting exercise. Ultrasonographic reassessment is recommended to determine whether the horse should start alternate-day cantering exercise or continue trotting for another month. Horses with distal branch lesions may have a guarded prognosis if substantial sesamoiditis exists. Most of these horses are taken out of training altogether as 2-year-olds and given the same rest program as horses with PSD. At the end of the period of controlled exercise, the horse usually is turned out and brought back in at the end of the year for further education, before resuming training as a 3-year-old. This distal branch/proximal sesamoid bone surface interface lesion is one of the few clinical situations in which I have been convinced that extracorporeal shock wave therapy (ESWT) has improved prognosis and reduced reinjury rate. I use weekly treatments of 3000 to 4000 shocks using a dual lithotripsy machine in ballistic mode at 4 Bar for 6 weeks in conjunction with controlled exercise.

Most young racehorses with PSD have an increase in the dorsopalmar thickness of the proximal aspect of the SL to greater than 1 cm, and irregularity of contour, with bulging of the normally flat palmar border (palmar bowing),

detectable by ultrasonography. The fiber pattern may be heterogeneous. Ultrasonographic monitoring of these lesions may reveal a decrease in size of the SL, with more linear borders as healing progresses. However, in many horses, the SL never returns to normal. Exercise level is increased when the ligament shows good echogenicity, although it still may be enlarged. Some horses seem to have long-term hypoechoic lesions within the SL that do not change with further rest.

Less commonly, a unilateral, acute, focal core lesion occurs in the SL after a race or gallop associated with lameness, swelling in the subcarpal region, and an exquisite pain response to palpation. Occasionally the SL seems to split, with the most dorsal surface being linearly avulsed, presumably by fluid or hemorrhage. This results in considerable thickening and striation of the SL.

The prognosis for mild to moderate PSD in 2-year-old TBs is good, but the prognosis is more guarded in horses with acute core injuries. Some of these horses take 4 to 5 months before they are able to withstand training and have a risk of reinjury. The prognosis in older horses is also guarded to poor.

In a 3-year-old horse that had PSD at 2 years of age, mild lameness may recur as training speed increases, in the absence of any real changes that can be identified using ultrasonography, radiography, or scintigraphy. This lameness always can be abolished by subcarpal analgesia. These horses with subcarpal "ache" often can be managed by administration of 5 to 10 mg of triamcinolone acetonide in 3 mL of local anesthetic solution, injected in the same site as a subcarpal block. Lameness often is abolished for long periods after this treatment, without apparent degeneration of the SL, even with continued training. It is vital to complete a full diagnostic evaluation before treatment in these horses to eliminate the possibility of training horses tolerating incipient catastrophic lesions under the influence of corticosteroids. For those working under jurisdictions that do not allow the presence of drugs at race time, such as in the United Kingdom, clinicians should be aware that the detection period for triamcinolone acetonide at this site can approach 30 days, and shorter-acting agents such as dexamethasone may be preferred.

Fetlock Lameness and Subchondral Bone Injuries to the Distal Aspect of the Third Metacarpal/Metatarsal Bone

All racehorses begin training when they are skeletally immature and relatively weak, and this leads to frequent damage to the pressure points on either side of high motion joints. Lameness can result from impingement lesions at the site of contact between the distal extremity of the McIII and the proximal eminence of the proximal phalanx as the fetlock sinks in hyperextension. Lesions include damage to the cartilage, synovitis, osteochondral fragmentation, or very often a combination of all three. The typical early sign is of a distended fetlock with pain on flexion and a mild degree of lameness. Radiological examination often reveals new bone at the proximal extremity of the sagittal ridge of the McIII and remodeling or minor fragmentation of the proximal eminence of the proximal phalanx. We should resist the temptation to "fix" these joints in a 2-year-old by intraarticular medication because heat and inflammation tell us that the joint is having problems. These horses need some time. External application of ice, in conjunction with reduction of exercise to jogging for a couple of weeks, with or without the use of oral NSAIDs, gives these horses some chance to recover. The treatment may need to be repeated two or three times before the horse can train without trouble. There is often substantial pressure to keep such horses in training, with a request for intraarticular corticosteroid treatment. We all succumb to this pressure on occasion, but we should always point out to the trainer and owner that after corticosteroid administration, any healing processes will cease for a considerable time. The pain response, which is protecting the joint from overuse, will also be abolished or diminished, allowing more damage to occur. There will be a price to be paid later in the horse's career. In an older horse, ongoing OA can often be traced back to an early interventional therapy, followed by a cycle of continued intraarticular treatment. There is often an ever-diminishing response to treatment until there is an end-stage joint with cartilage wear, fibrillation, or collapse, along with severe pathological change in the subchondral bone.

Subchondral bone injury is an extremely common cause of lameness in young TBs and is vastly underacknowledged. Subchondral bone pain seems to be increasingly implicated in much joint-related lameness in other classes of horses (e.g., navicular syndrome, tarsal pain, and third carpal bone pain). In the young TB, subchondral bone injuries in the distal aspect of the MtIII and the McIII often are linked to bilateral or quadrilateral lameness, which limits performance. Horses with bilateral subchondral bone injuries of the distal aspect of the MtIII fail to push from behind at exercise. Often these horses appear to bunny hop for the first section of canter. The rider reports that the horse feels wrong behind and does not perform as well as it previously did. The clinical history (see page 997) and response to diagnostic analgesia (see page 1001) have been described. With American-bred horses, equine protozoal myelitis (EPM) is an important differential diagnosis because the clinical appearance can be similar. Onset of clinical signs can be delayed, so that a yearling bred in America and sold in Europe could have EPM.

Subchondral bone injuries are extremely difficult or impossible to identify radiologically. If lesions are visible radiologically, these are usually end stage, and horses warrant a guarded prognosis (see Figure 107-5). These lesions usually represent necrosis and collapse of subchondral bone and are visible as a crescent-shaped radiolucency in the middle of the lateral condyle of the MtIII, seen on flexed plantarodorsal or flexed dorsoplantar images (see Figure 107-4, *B*). Increased radiopacity of the lateral condyle also occurs and is most visible on a lateromedial image. Deliberate overexposure may be necessary to demonstrate a triangular region of increased radiopacity just palmar/plantar to the midpoint of the articular surface (Figure 107-7). All racing TBs seem to develop some degree of sclerosis in this site as a normal physiological response to loading from the PSB as the limb assumes full extension. MRI examination reveals changes associated with dense mineralized subchondral bone and sometimes focal areas of increased signal intensity in fat-suppressed images, which may reflect microfracture, fibrosis, or bone necrosis (see Figure 107-6).

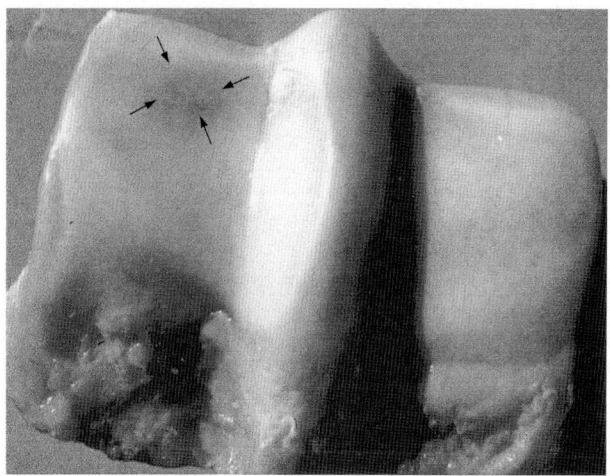

Fig. 107-7 • Post mortem specimen of the distal aspect of a third metatarsal bone from a horse with plantarolateral focal increased radiopharmaceutical uptake seen on a bone scan. Lateral is to the left. The specimen was collected when the horse was euthanized for unrelated reasons. The area in the center of the plantarolateral aspect of the condyle is dark, and the cartilage surface is irregular *(arrows)*. Histopathological sections cut through the site revealed abnormal irregular and necrotic subchondral bone. Compare with the lesion in Figure 107-5, *C*.

On scintigraphic examination, these stress injuries are remarkable because increased radiopharmaceutical uptake (IRU) is focal in nature and markedly increased. On a plantar image, IRU in the MtIII is mistaken easily for IRU in a PSB because the shape of the lesion is similar to that bone. However, on a lateral image, the PSBs can be seen clearly plantar to the region of the IRU, localized within the condyle itself (Figure 107-8). In the forelimb, subchondral bone injuries in the metacarpophalangeal joint seem to occur most commonly in the medial condyle, but can also be present in the lateral condyle or both. Horses usually have bilateral lameness and trot with the head held low with a short, stumbling gait as they try to get off each weight-bearing limb as fast as possible. If all fetlock joints are injured, a horse may refuse to trot and attempt to break into a slow, rolling canter as speed increases. Lameness often becomes apparent in the contralateral limb after local analgesia of one metacarpophalangeal/metatarsophalangeal joint. Radiological examination is often unremarkable, but scintigraphy confirms focal IRU in an active early lesion. Use of flexed dorsal and flexed lateral scintigraphic images is helpful in pinpointing the exact location of the lesion, particularly in the front limb (see Figure 107-8). In the more chronic stage, there may be only mild IRU, yet the pain and lameness can be more intense. We should not forget that the mere presence of mild IRU does not necessarily mean painful and vice versa.

Treatment is difficult, and we have no protocol that results in uniform resolution of lameness. Many different treatment regimens have been used, including intraarticular injection with hyaluronan or corticosteroids; systemic medication with isoxsuprine, aspirin, polysulfated glycosaminoglycans, or tiludronate; and rest alone.[16] Often the lameness disappears rapidly after the instigation of rest but returns when the horse resumes fast galloping speed. Although some horses have been able to perform without further problems, predicting which horses may respond

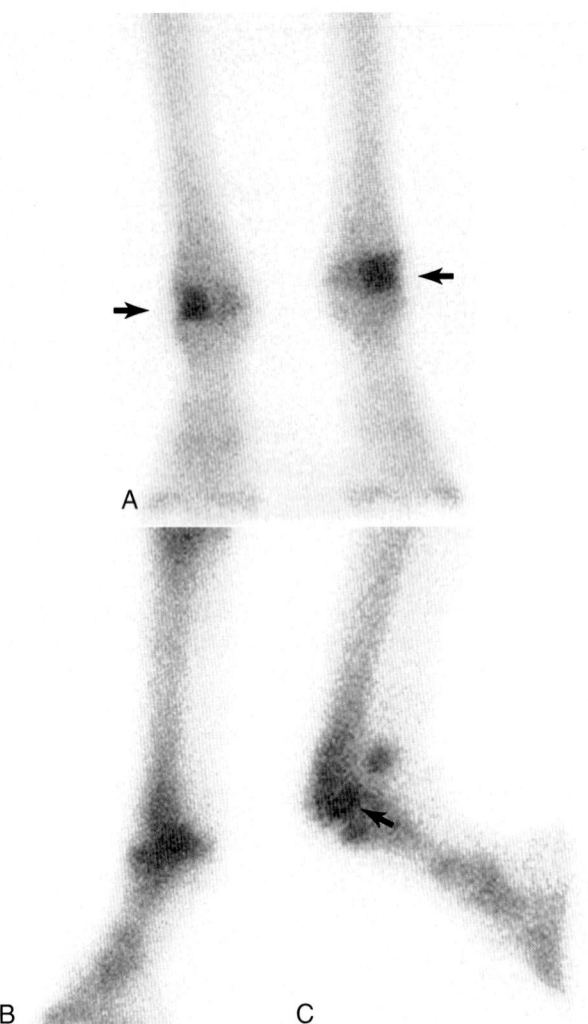

Fig. 107-8 • **A,** Plantar delayed (bone) phase scintigraphic image of horse with bilateral stress injuries to the lateral condyle of the third metatarsal bone. The shape and distribution of the increased radiopharmaceutical uptake (IRU; *arrows*) easily can be mistaken for that associated with the lateral proximal sesamoid bone (PSB). **B,** Lateral delayed (bone) phase scintigraphic image of the same horse. If there is doubt as to the exact location of the IRU, a flexed lateral image (**C**) is useful in moving apart the PSB and the plantar aspect of the lateral condyle. This clearly shows the IRU to be situated in the plantar aspect of the condyle *(arrow)* rather than the PSBs, which are moved away from the joint in this image. (Courtesy Sue Dyson, Animal Health Trust, Newmarket, England.)

favorably is not possible. However, those with subchondral lucency and sclerosis rarely remain sound. This does not mean that these horses cannot perform, and many racehorses seem to withstand training despite lameness. However, this may be a performance-limiting problem that directly interferes with racing ability and determines the level at which the horse can compete.

Because horses with advanced lesions rarely return to sustained soundness, it is advisable to stop hard training as soon as the condition is noted in a 2-year-old and allow 3 months of rest. This is not a guarantee that the problem will not recur at 3 years of age, but going on with training these young horses in the face of this lameness seems illogical. Many horses can be trained at 3 years of age without problems. When the clinical syndrome appears in a horse

aged 3 or more for the first time, the prognosis is much worse than when subchondral bone lesions occur in a 2-year-old and the horse is allowed to rest. In an older horse, end-stage pathological damage in the affected condyle is more common. These horses may well have been trained through the problem at 2 years of age, with a low-grade bilateral lameness that was not recognized.

Some horses first show hindlimb lameness associated with the lesions in the lateral condyles of the MtIII after a race on unsuitably firm ground. They are described as "jarred up." Although the clinical appearance of a jarred-up horse has long been recognized, no precise definition of the syndrome has ever been made. The syndrome may well represent multifocal subchondral bone pain. Affected horses may never regain normal action. The reasons why some horses become progressively lamer whereas others can race with success and maintain a steady-state lameness are not understood.

A few horses with subchondral bone injury have been examined at post mortem (see Figure 107-7). The degree of damage to the subchondral bone at the injury site easily explains why some horses are untrainable. We need to understand why some horses develop these lesions whereas others do not, whether the type of training surface may be a predisposing factor, what pathological mechanisms are involved, and why these lesions produce pain. Ideally, we also need to track some young TB horses using repeat MRI scans from the time they are broken right through training to see when these lesions develop and what impact they have on gait and race performance.

Lameness Associated with the Middle Carpal Joint

Several distinct syndromes are associated with the middle carpal joint. One of the most common syndromes is exemplified by a 2-year-old in early training that develops an increasingly short, choppy gait at the trot. The limbs are held abducted during the protraction phase, and the carpi are barely flexed. This gives a stiff, rolling action. Often the horse has bilateral middle carpal joint effusion and pain on carpal flexion. Injection of local anesthetic solution into one middle carpal joint produces lameness (grade 1 to 2 of 5) in the contralateral limb. The gait changes so that the desensitized limb is often brought back toward the midline. Some of these horses have mild increased radiopacity of the third carpal bone, seen on a skyline image, but others have no detectable radiological abnormality. These horses probably are suffering from pain produced by concussion of immature cartilage and excessive torsion on untrained ligaments within the carpus, and should be given rest. If excessive effusion occurs, the joint may be drained and medicated with triamcinolone acetonide (5 mg) and hyaluronan, but only if rest is to follow. Nonsteroidal antiinflammatory drugs (NSAIDs) may be administered for the first 4 or 5 days of rest. Most horses are restricted to box rest for 1 month, followed by walking exercise for 2 weeks, followed by 1 month of trotting before resuming full training. Many horses never show lameness again during the second introduction to exercise loading.

The second syndrome, which may include some horses in the first category if training has continued, involves development of more severe sclerosis in the third carpal bone and remodeling of the distal aspect of the radial carpal bone. Focal overloading of the third carpal bone results from a conformational defect (offset carpi with toe in is the worst) or from a mismatch between loading of the limb and time allowed for adaptation. These horses are usually bilaterally lame; often one lame limb dominates, and contralateral limb lameness is only recognized when the lamest limb is blocked. Radiological signs include increased radiopacity in the radial fossa of the third carpal bone seen on the skyline image, associated with local areas of rarefaction around the nutrient foramina or with small comma-shaped fissure fractures extending from the dorsal aspect of the third carpal bone. Further training of these horses risks development of a full sagittal fracture (see Figure 107-2).

Despite statements to the contrary in the literature, I believe that the early sclerotic changes in the third carpal bone are reversible after a period of box rest. However, there seems to be a certain degree of pathological damage from which there is no return. Once the radial fossa becomes completely devoid of trabecular detail and has a "ground glass" appearance radiologically, the changes are often permanent. These lesions often are associated with recurrent lameness each time the horse reaches racing speed. Therefore identifying increased radiopacity of the third carpal bone at an early stage is vital. Screening radiographic examinations of the third carpal bone in a 2-year-old may be useful before starting full race-speed galloping. Without radiological information, lameness may be the first indicator of sclerosis, which may already be advanced.

Lame horses with third carpal bone sclerosis are confined to box rest for 2 months, followed by 1 month of walking exercise. Radiographic examination is then repeated. I advise that these horses are not trained with a view to racing at 2 years of age, although they may reenter the training environment so that they acclimatize to respiratory disease and other management problems that might influence the 3-year-old career.

Problems related to the distal aspect of the radial carpal bone are also common, associated with lameness and distention of the middle carpal joint capsule. Radiological abnormalities include spur formation on the distal aspect of the radial carpal bone and radiolucent changes in the same site leading to modeling of the dorsal margin. This usually leads to or is associated with coexistent secondary sclerosis of the opposing third carpal bone because the load becomes borne by the medullary bone, instead of the weight-bearing pillar of the dorsal cortex. These radiological abnormalities result from overloading the carpus, leading to bone stiffening, cartilage damage, and secondary OA. Debate exists over whether spurs should be removed surgically. OA of the middle carpal joint is already established. Although removing the spur is logical, it is not curative, and the horse will still require treatment the following season. With cheap horses and in yards where money is tight, many horses with mild carpal OA can be treated once by intraarticular medication with hyaluronan and triamcinolone acetonide, followed by 4 to 6 weeks of rest and a graded return to exercise.

If a chip fracture occurs, then removal of the fragments is probably still mandatory. One should explain to the owner and trainer, however, that the horse has preexisting OA that will persist after surgery and that further problems should be anticipated the following season.

The antebrachiocarpal joint is more forgiving than the middle carpal joint in the amount of pathological change

that can be seen radiologically in the absence of clinical signs. Large fragments can be removed surgically with a favorable prognosis for horses the following season. Some horses can continue to train and race without obvious impairment even with chip fractures left in situ in this joint.

A small group of horses with middle carpal joint pain remains in which lameness recurs after periods of rest, despite absence of radiological changes. These horses often have unilateral lameness associated with middle carpal joint effusion. Some of these horses have tears of the palmar intercarpal ligaments. Response to conservative treatment often is disappointing, and even after prolonged periods of rest, lameness recurs as soon as work intensity increases. I normally medicate these horses with hyaluronan and corticosteroids, but in the absence of a firm diagnosis, this empirical treatment is illogical and usually unrewarding. Diagnostic arthroscopy probably is always indicated in these horses but is also often unhelpful in producing a permanent cure. We should also always be aware that local anesthetic solution in the middle carpal joint can abolish pain arising from the SL, carpal ligaments, and many other structures, and it may be very simplistic to assume a positive middle carpal joint block means we have problems only in the middle carpal joint. MRI examinations of some of these horses have been carried out recently and reveal a catalog of abnormalities in structures all around the site of the block.[13]

Lameness Subsequent to Bacterial Infection

Bacterial infection in a limb of a horse can cause a degree of pain greater than almost any other injury, including a displaced fracture. Although wounds in any part of a limb can become infected, leading to an obvious swelling and lymphangitis, some discrete syndromes in the racehorse deserve mention.

Staphylococcal Abscesses on the Palmar Aspect of the Metacarpophalangeal Joint

Horses exercising on sand, synthetic, or wood chip surfaces seem to be prone to bacterial infections around the ergot that produce small, focal abscesses, which can be difficult to find if the horse has a winter coat. The horse often initially points the limb, is severely lame (grade 4 of 5), with swelling on the palmar aspect of the metacarpophalangeal joint. Manipulation of the joint is resented. The abscess can mimic the appearance of an infected joint and must be differentiated because synoviocentesis inadvertently may introduce infection into the joint. Careful evaluation shows that the metacarpophalangeal joint capsule is not distended. By working through the hair coat with the fingernails, localizing the point of a small abscess is often possible. The horse shows a severe pain response, and a pink porelike hole may be observed discharging serosanguineous pus. Bacteriological culture almost invariably results in the growth of a hemolytic *Staphylococcus aureus*.

Treatment is by external application of kaolin paste or a similar open poultice, combined with systemic antibiotic therapy along with NSAIDs and forced walking exercise. Horses are normally sound after 12 to 24 hours, and if this is not the case, then the diagnosis should be reestablished. Bandaging should be avoided because the limb often continues to swell and the bandage may become constricting, which can lead to ischemic necrosis and sloughing of the skin.

Focal Peritarsal Cellulitis

Focal peritarsal cellulitis is a syndrome that appears to be related to the architecture of lymphatic drainage and is characterized by acute-onset severe lameness (grade 4 or 5 of 5), often with a shocklike state, hyperventilation, and sweating.[16] Rectal temperature is elevated (39 to 40° C). Clinical examination of the limb reveals an exquisitely painful area on the dorsomedial aspect of the hock with focal swelling (Figure 107-9). Brushing this area lightly with the fingertips usually causes the horse to stagger sideways and abduct the limb sharply to get away from the pain. Almost always a small skin lesion of some sort is evident in the distal part of the limb, through which the initial infection may have entered.

Although the horse is severely lame in the stable, if forced to walk, the lameness usually improves after a few steps, and the horse bears weight reasonably well. The focal swelling on the medial aspect of the tarsus appears to be linked to a nidus of lymphatic drainage because the swelling is so consistently positioned. The pain is so great because of involvement of the retinaculum and fascia immediately above and beneath the site, causing a compartment-like syndrome. Some North American clinicians describe emergency surgical drainage of these abscesses, with or without fasciotomy. However, conservative treatment using antibiotics (oxytetracyclines or ceftiofur), along with NSAIDs

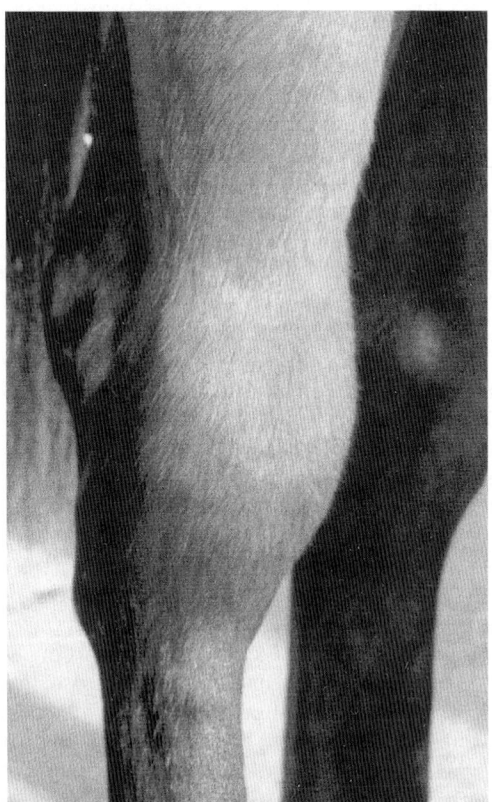

Fig. 107-9 • A horse with focal peritarsal cellulitis. There is tight focal distention caused by swelling associated with infection in the deep fascia beneath the skin, retained at either extremity of the tarsus by the retinacular ligaments. This produces a profound degree of pain for the horse.

administered morning and night, and forced exercise several times daily is usually adequate.

Often within 24 hours the swelling changes from a small egg-sized swelling on the medial aspect of the hock to involve the entire distal part of the limb. Swelling gradually resolves with exercise over the next month.

A great risk of laminitis in the contralateral limb exists in the early stages because of the combination of severe lameness in the affected limb and toxin production from the abscess. Therefore it is vital that the horse is stabled on deep bedding during its initial treatment and that regular exercise is encouraged despite obvious lameness in the affected limb.

Axillary and Scrotal Intertrigo Infections

Horses are affected by skinfold infections, particularly in the axilla and groin. The infection begins in the fold of skin and causes an exudative, purulent dermatitis. The swelling of the affected region results in more occlusion and development of anaerobic infections deep in the skin folds. Affected horses often stand with the limb abducted and appear as if they have a proximal long bone fracture. Because the swollen skin folds close themselves off, these lesions can be missed unless the limb is pulled away from the body to expose the raw pink exudative dermatitis. Treatment is by systemic administration of antibiotics and analgesics and topical cleansing of the affected area with a debriding agent, followed by application of an antibiotic ointment. Fusidic acid creams are often effective because most of these infections involve staphylococci. Topical treatment often requires profound sedation of the horse so as to be carried out safely because of the pain involved. Exercise should be limited to a short period of handwalking, until the edema of the skin folds of the axilla subsides, because walking produces friction that makes the condition worse. Less commonly the area between the scrotum and the medial aspect of the thigh can be involved, especially in horses exercising on dirt or sand. Affected horses walk in a crouching gait, with abduction of each hindlimb during protraction. Once the acute infection has resolved, daily use of a talcum powder designed for use in babies is helpful in avoiding recurrent chaffing of the edematous skin during exercise for the first couple of weeks.

Stress Fractures of the Long Bones and Pelvis

Post mortem studies carried out on racehorse fatalities in California have revealed that many horses have evidence of previously undetected stress fractures of the long bones. We have been aware clinically of these fractures for some time, particularly when they became complete and displaced in horses in training. With the advent of scintigraphy, the early diagnosis of these stress fractures increased.

Certain rules apply to all stress fractures in the TB. Fractures usually occur after repeated cyclical loading of bone over time rather than as an acute incident. Lameness itself may be *acute* in onset, as the bone reaches the stage where it can no longer bear weight and the cortex begins to collapse. However, because the lesions are chronic in nature, radiological signs that we tend to link to bone healing and remodeling, such as periosteal new bone formation, irregular ill-defined lucencies in the cortex, and occasionally cortical displacement, may be detectable at the onset of lameness. Because stress fractures result from repeated focal overloading, they tend to occur in predilection sites in the bone, reflecting the architecture of that bone and the manner in which weight is borne during locomotion. The repeatability of these sites makes looking for these injuries on radiographs more straightforward.

Skeletal bone seems to detrain almost as effectively as it can be trained. For this reason, any horse that has been removed from training for longer than 3 weeks should be given sufficient time to allow reconditioning of the skeleton on return to training. Stress fractures may occur in horses of any age if they have been removed from training for a period of more than 1 month and have been returned to cantering exercise too rapidly.

Periostitis of the Dorsal Cortex of the Third Metacarpal Bone (Sore or Bucked Shins)

Sore shins are a common problem in 2-year-old racehorses or in older horses that have not reached race speed previously or have had a long layoff. Most of these horses are not shown to a veterinary surgeon. The stable staff and trainers know how to recognize sore shins and treat them in a variety of traditional methods. It is advisable to restrict the horse to trotting until the area is no longer painful to light fingertip pressure with the limb flexed. The horse is then reintroduced to the exercise level one step beneath the level that produced the soreness. This speed is maintained for 1 month before increasing. If the shin soreness returns as speed increases, the cycle is repeated.

Rarely, more invasive therapy is required for horses that have three serial episodes and for which normal management strategies have failed. The shin is pin fired under local analgesia, and the horse is walked for 2 weeks and then trotted for 2 weeks before gradually increasing speed work. Freeze-firing is a local temporary neurectomy only and confers no long-term benefit. The shin is a barometer of what is going on in the rest of the skeleton, and when sore the shin indicates that the skeleton needs more time to adapt. Freeze-firing simply lets us ignore this and allows the horse to develop real damage elsewhere. This subject is controversial, and the views expressed here are not shared by all veterinarians.

Fracture of the Dorsal Aspect of the Third Metacarpal Bone

Fracture of the dorsal aspect of the McIII presents as an extension of the sore shin complex. When a true stress fracture (dorsal cortical fracture) is present, the pain to palpation usually is localized to one area rather than being distributed across the entire surface of the shin. Normally a periosteal callus is present at the site of the fracture, causing a bump on the surface of the McIII. Radiographic examination should include unorthodox lesion-oriented oblique images because the fracture lines are often extremely difficult to see, particularly in the acute phase of the injury. Horses are usually slightly lame, but continued training results in an increase in lameness after each exercise period, which reduces rapidly. A lame horse with focal periostitis that is painful to palpation should be considered to have a stress fracture at that site, even if the fracture is not visible radiologically. Treatment is by rest, which can include walking exercise. These injuries normally take about 1 month to heal, after which light training may begin, but 3 months should elapse before full training speeds are achieved. If the injury has progressed to a clear tangential fracture line in the cortex, some veterinarians recommend surgical drilling (osteostixis), or even screw insertion across the fracture line, to encourage healing. This has never been necessary in my experience. ESWT is also used to treat horses with this type of fracture, but its clinical efficacy remains to be proved. Normally early diagnosis allows full healing with conservative treatment alone.

Tibia

Stress fractures of the tibia are one of the most common causes of hindlimb lameness in 2-year-old racehorses in race training. In the seasonal racing calendar, when yearlings enter training in October or November, peak incidence of tibial stress fractures is in April or May as speed work increases. The tibia has three main predilection sites. The most common in naive horses entering training for the first time is the proximolateral cortex, 7 to 8 cm distal to the proximal articular surface of the tibia. Stress fractures in this site are visible radiologically as poorly defined callus, often associated with an oblique fracture line in the cortex itself. The second common predilection site, often seen in a 3-year-old or in a 2-year-old in more advanced training, is in the caudal distal cortex, 10 cm proximal to the tarsocrural joint. On radiological examination endosteal callus can be seen as a subtle sunburst of increased radiopacity extending forward from the caudal cortex on a lateromedial image. On a caudocranial image, a lucent line is usually visible, surrounded by an area of increased radiopacity in the middle of the distal aspect of the tibia. The third common site is the middle of the medial cortex. In this site, the injuries usually are seen as periosteal and endosteal new bone formation only, and fracture lines are visible only rarely.

Occasionally a complete, comminuted displaced fracture of the tibia can occur during racing or training. The prognosis in these horses usually is hopeless. In Newmarket complete tibial fractures occurring at exercise have almost disappeared following the advent of scintigraphy, suggesting that in the past some complete fractures were the end stage of chronic stress fractures, which are now detected early.

Diagnosis of tibial stress fracture is difficult because these injuries may not be affected by diagnostic analgesia. The typical history is of a 2-year-old being brought into faster speed exercise or of a 3-year-old that did not race at 2 years of age being prepared in the same way. The lameness is usually acute in onset and can be severe (grade 3 or 4 of 5) but usually diminishes rapidly with rest. Forced flexion of the hock and torsion of the tibia produce pain in horses with severe lameness (see Figure 107-3). Scintigraphy is ideal to confirm these lesions, but the degree of IRU seen in the middiaphyseal and distal metaphyseal sites is often mild, particularly if the horse is imaged early.

Treatment is by rest and a gradual return to training. The horse is restricted to box rest initially for 2 to 6 weeks depending on the severity of the radiological signs. Occasionally stress fractures of the tibia become complete and displaced during periods of convalescence after normal recumbency. The horse should be tied up by the head for the first 3 to 4 weeks if the weight-bearing ability of the tibia is severely compromised (for precautions, see Chapter 49). Less severely affected horses are exercised as soon as it is practical. If a treadmill or horse walker is available, horses can be walked as soon as clinically sound, allowing a total healing period of between 2 and 3 months. Trotting exercise can be included in the second and third months.

Humerus

A horse with a humeral stress fracture has acute-onset forelimb lameness with features of proximal forelimb pain. The horse walks with a short cranial phase to the stride and circumducts the limb in protraction. Substantial weight-bearing lameness is evident at the trot. Horses often drag the toe of the affected limb in the bedding during protraction in the stable. The lameness rapidly diminishes, and in 2 days horses may be sound, only to go severely lame again after return to exercise.

Two main predilection sites exist for humeral stress fractures. Scintigraphic examination is ideal for diagnosis. One site is on the caudal cortex just distal to the humeral head, about 5 cm distal to the weight-bearing surface. Loose periosteal callus usually is visible, with increased radiopacity of adjacent bone and occasionally incomplete tangential fracture lines. The other site is the cranial or, less frequently, caudal cortex of the distal aspect of the humerus about 5 cm proximal to the elbow joint surface. A focal sunburst of callus usually is visible on a mediolateral radiographic image, and a linear fracture line is sometimes seen. Treatment is as described for tibial stress fractures. Complete, displaced humeral fractures can occur in exercise, and horses have a hopeless prognosis.

Pelvis and Axial Skeleton

Fractures of the sacral wing of the ilium are often stress fractures and are described in detail elsewhere (see Chapter 49). Laminar stress fractures of the vertebrae immediately adjacent to the pelvis have been described.[17] A full review of the scintigraphic appearance of stress fractures in the TB has been published.[9] There is usually a unilateral lameness for which no other reason can be ascribed after routine diagnostic analgesia and survey radiography. Scintigraphic examination of these horses reveals focal IRU associated with the lumbar vertebrae on the same side as the lameness. Some horses simply show bilateral poor hindlimb propulsion, short stepping at the walk, and a hunched-up lumbar spine, coupled with poor performance without obvious lameness. Being certain that the laminar stress fracture is the cause of the reduced performance is difficult. However, if scintigraphy reveals an active bone injury in the spine, continuing full training cannot make sense, and these horses subsequently are allowed to rest. Although this lesion is described as widespread in the Californian pathological survey, the clinical presentation is uncommon. I have examined the lateral lumbar spine routinely in all bone scan images over a 2-year period and have not encountered the lesion as a common incidental finding.

Exostosis of the Second and Fourth Metacarpal/Metatarsal Bones (Splints)

Splints are more of a nuisance in a racehorse than a major problem. They are clinically obvious, and a sharp pain response can be elicited by squeezing the area. Splints normally are associated with lameness in the initial stages, although this can subside rapidly. Splint lameness is one of the few conditions with which lameness is often more obvious with the affected limb on the outside of a circle. Splints are common in horses of 2 years of age but can occur in horses of any age, particularly if they experience a change in loading because of a different type of training surface or, paradoxically, a reduction in training workload, or a different angle of camber in the surface on which they are training. In many horses a fracture line is not detectable radiologically, but most horses with obvious exostosis formation associated with lameness probably do have fractures within the body of the bone, which often can be identified scintigraphically. Many of these "splints" will continue to show marked IRU for months or even years after clinical signs have settled. A period of stable rest with walking exercise is probably indicated until the horse is clinically sound. The horse then can recommence trotting for 2 to 4 weeks to allow the injury to heal fully. If pain on palpation and lameness immediately recur when the horse returns to exercise, then pin firing may be considered to encourage more aggressive callus formation. This is one of the few orthopedic indications in which firing achieves a good clinical result in most horses. Horses with displaced fractures of the distal aspect of the second and fourth metacarpal/metatarsal bones are treated by surgical removal of the distal portion of the bone.

Numerous comminuted fractures of the second and fourth metacarpal/metatarsal bones sometimes result from external trauma and heal surprisingly well. Many fragments may be identified by digital palpation with a gloved finger through an open wound and confirmed radiologically. Most horses with fractures heal satisfactorily with antibiotic treatment, bandaging of the wound, and stable rest. If infectious osteitis does occur with sequestrum formation and recurrent fistulation, then affected bone should be removed surgically. Open comminuted fractures of the fourth metatarsal bone can lead to infection ascending into the TMT joint and should be closely monitored.

Undiagnosed Hindlimb Lameness

Despite all our modern diagnostic aids, the cause of hindlimb lameness in a large number of horses remains elusive. Given the huge muscle mass involved in the hindquarters of the horse, some must have muscular origin and insertion pathological conditions, as well as pain from muscular overexertion. In human athletes, lameness is commonly linked to strains, tears, and cramps in the semimembranosus and semitendinosus muscle groups and in the adductor and gluteal muscles. Horses are presumably no different. As yet, no definitive test appears to be available to confirm genuine muscle injury. Thermography is helpful in some horses but is disappointing in others, and only reflects changes in skin temperature. Increases in CK and aspartate transaminase levels, although pathognomonic for exertional rhabdomyolysis, do not seem to occur following genuine tears of muscle tissue. Presumably these tears result in little cellular disruption, the damage being more in the fascial planes and connective tissue.

If a horse remains undiagnosed after all available diagnostic analgesia and imaging modalities have been used, then the horse is confined to box rest with walking exercise only for 1 month. Most horses become sound in this period. The horse then returns to walking and trotting exercise for 1 month before resuming a normal ascending exercise program. Although admitting defeat and being unable to give a definitive diagnosis is frustrating, one should try to avoid attributing a definite cause for the lameness if no evidence exists to support it. Trainers and clients should be educated to accept the fact that ascribing lameness to injury of a specific structure in every horse is not possible.

Fractures of the Proximal Phalanx and Distal Condyles of the Third Metacarpal/Metatarsal Bone

The most dramatic example of a proximal phalanx fracture is a split pastern that is a frequent injury, particularly in a 2-year-old racehorse as it enters fast work. The length and configuration of these fractures include complete sagittal fractures involving both articular surfaces, multiple comminuted displaced fractures, and incomplete fractures extending short distances from the proximal articular surface. Diagnosis is usually straightforward in horses with a complete fracture or an extensive incomplete fracture. With extreme injury, a horse pulls up severely lame during or at the end of exercise. With less severe injuries, horses may finish exercise apparently sound but become increasingly lame on return to the stable. The horse is usually not bearing weight by the time of examination. Pain always occurs on flexion of the metacarpophalangeal or metatarsophalangeal joint and on pressure applied with the fingertips to the proximal phalanx along its sagittal dorsal midline. Radiological examination is usually confirmatory.

Short incomplete sagittal fractures of the proximal phalanx can be notoriously difficult to see radiologically, when the fracture line only extends 1 or 2 cm into the bone. Clinical signs are of a severe lameness (grade 3 of 5) that rapidly improves so that the horse may be sound within 2 days. Flexion of the fetlock joint is usually not painful. Firm squeezing of the proximal dorsal surface of the proximal phalanx usually is resented, particularly approaching the proximal articular surface, and this is a reliable clinical sign. A horse with this type of fracture should be given box rest for at least 2 weeks before further radiography. Short, incomplete fractures easily become complete comminuted fractures if a horse is exercised after 2 weeks of rest because the fracture weakens by normal osteoclastic activity. Therefore although the horse may be sound, a premature return to work may result in a catastrophic fracture. See Chapter 35 for a discussion of management of horses with fractures of the proximal phalanx.

Fractures of the condyles of the McIII or the MtIII are a frequent injury, but they occur more often in 3- and 4-year-olds than in 2-year-olds. The lateral or medial condyle can be affected, and fractures of the medial condyle of the MtIII often spiral proximally. The whole fracture may not be seen on one radiographic image, and several oblique images should be obtained to determine the extent of the fracture before contemplating general anesthesia for surgical fixation. Spiral fractures present a risk during recovery from general anesthesia.

A complete, displaced condylar fracture presents little diagnostic challenge. The horse is extremely lame and resents palpation of the lateral or medial condyle. Flexion of the metacarpophalangeal/metatarsophalangeal joint invariably is associated with sharp pain, and joint capsule distention and effusion usually occur because of hemorrhage. Short, incomplete condylar fractures are more difficult to diagnose. Lameness is usually severe (grade 2 or 3 of 5) and diminishes rapidly with rest. Horses often become lame again as soon as they are returned to cantering exercise. Diagnostic analgesia localizes lameness to the metacarpophalangeal/metatarsophalangeal joint, but nothing may be seen radiologically. A flexed dorsopalmar image is vital if these lesions are to be seen adequately.[3] If radiography is performed in the field, using portable equipment, then an upright flexed image that moves the PSBs proximally is useful to identify the fracture[4] (see Figure 107-4).

If a condylar fissure is suspected, the horse should be restricted to walking and trotting exercise for 2 weeks before follow-up radiography is performed. Many horses that eventually develop full, displaced condylar fractures are described as having been bad movers before injury, and almost certainly prodromal pathological damage contributes to the cause of these fractures. See Chapter 36 for a discussion of management of horses with fractures of the McIII and the MtIII.

Pain Associated with the Tarsometatarsal Joint

Sore hocks are probably much more common in the United States than they are in the United Kingdom. TMT joint lameness can be bilateral or unilateral and often does not resolve with rest, and the response to intraarticular administration of corticosteroids varies extremely. I treat horses with triamcinolone acetonide (10 mg) at the time of intraarticular analgesia to avoid having to reenter the joint. After this therapy, many horses are sound, and lameness never returns. However, other horses require intermittent repeated medication, and others will not respond at all. The withdrawal period for racing free of medication is probably longer for triamcinolone acetonide than many other corticosteroids and can be in excess of 20 days after injections of the distal hock joints in the United Kingdom.

Horses with bilateral lameness are more difficult to diagnose. Bilateral plantar stress injuries in the distal aspect of the MtIII should be eliminated first by diagnostic analgesia because the gait of affected horses is similar. If diagnostic analgesia is negative, local analgesia of one TMT joint should be performed in the hope that an obvious lameness will become visible in the contralateral limb. Care should be taken if medicating both TMT joints to avoid a laminitis-inducing dose of corticosteroid (i.e., no more than 20 mg of triamcinolone acetonide per horse). The very prolonged detection period of depot preparations of drugs such as methylprednisolone acetate virtually rules out the use of this drug in horses racing under European medication rules.

| *Chapter* **108**

The North American Standardbred

James B. Mitchell, John S. Mitchell,
Paul M. Nolan, and Mike W. Ross

DESCRIPTION OF THE SPORT

The Standardbred (STB) was developed as a racing breed by registering any horse that could trot or pace 1 mile in a set time, called the standard. An early standard was 2:30 (2 minutes, 30 seconds, 0 fifths). Early STBs were diverse because they were different types with a large genetic pool. Crossing many types resulted in a strong, rugged breed that lacked refinement of the head, ears, and bone structure. Trotters were large and coarse, whereas pacers were smaller and more refined. The breed has progressed rapidly by selective breeding in the past 4 decades. Although trotters and pacers now are bred separately, the physical appearance has become more alike, and both lines have a racy appearance similar to Thoroughbreds (TBs). Early trotters were farm or buggy horses, selected for good disposition and durability, traits that are still characteristic. Early STBs were raced several 1-mile races in the same day, called heats, a part of the sport demanding stamina and gameness.

A TB stallion, Messenger, imported from England in 1788, was prominent in the formative period of the STB. Many of his offspring had a natural inclination to trot. In 1849, a descendent of Messenger sired Hambletonian 10, the foundation sire of the STB breed. The breed developed in the northeastern United States, where it was influenced by the Hackney and Morgan breeds and local mixed-breed horses.

The STB races at two different gaits: the trot, a diagonal two-beat gait in which the left forelimb (LF) and right hindlimb (RH) move together, and the pace, a lateral two-beat gait in which the LF and left hindlimb (LH) move together. High knee action and a lateral (left to right) nodding of the head are typical of a trotter (Figure 108-1, *A*). A trotter travels straight ahead (see Figure 108-1, *A*) (Figures 108-2, *A*, and 108-3), but a pacer sways from side to side while moving forward (see Figure 108-1, *B*).

Fifty years ago trainers had to spend several months determining at which gait a STB was more talented; some could not handle speed at either gait. As late as the 1970s and 1980s, it was not unusual for a horse to race one season at one gait and the next season at the other. A few horses raced at different gaits weekly, but today most STBs race at only one gait. Many foals pace or trot naturally. Although trotters trot while racing, they occasionally break into a pace when they are lame. Pacers often jog—the term used for trotters and pacers when trotting the slow or wrong way (clockwise) of the track at the trot—but train and race at the pace. The pace is faster than the trot. The current (2009) world record for the pace during a parimutuel race is 1:46.4 (all-age, any size track) and that for the trot is 1:49.3 on a track longer than 1 mile and 1:50.1 on a 1-mile or smaller racetrack. Many purists in the sport do not consider a world record on a racetrack longer than 1 mile to be equivalent to that obtained on a smaller racetrack because there is only one turn compared with two or more on smaller racetracks. Many pacers race near record time, but trotters do not. Trotters and pacers do not race against each other in parimutuel races. A STB racehorse must qualify for racing, meaning the horse must better or match a minimal speed before being entered into a parimutuel race. Another form of speed test is called a time

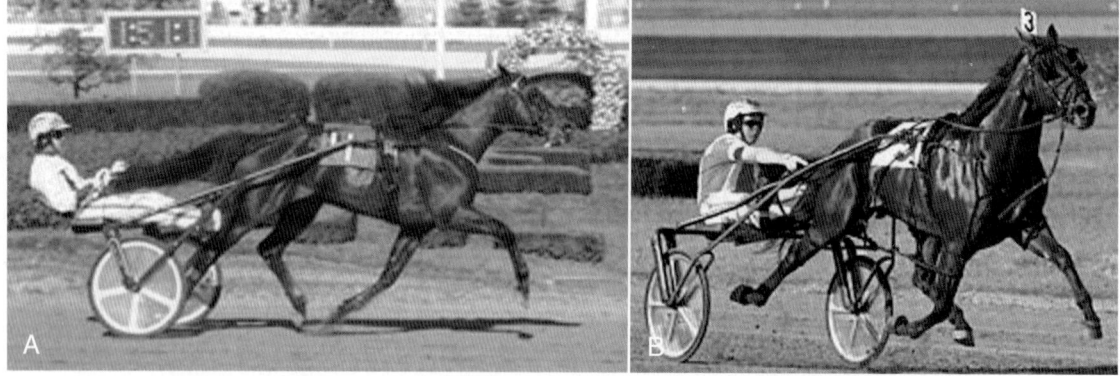

Fig. 108-1 • A, Muscle Hill, a champion 3-year-old trotting colt of 2009, is seen here with driver Brian Sears. This talented young trotter equaled the all-age trotting world record of 150.1 in his overwhelming victory in the Hambletonian, raced at the Meadowlands racetrack outside of New York City. **B,** Paul MacDonell guides Somebeachsomewhere, a champion 3-year-old pacing colt in 2008. Somebeachsomewhere equaled the all-age pacing world record with his 146.4 performance at the Red Mile in Lexington, KY. (Courtesy United States Trotting Association, Columbus, Ohio, United States.)

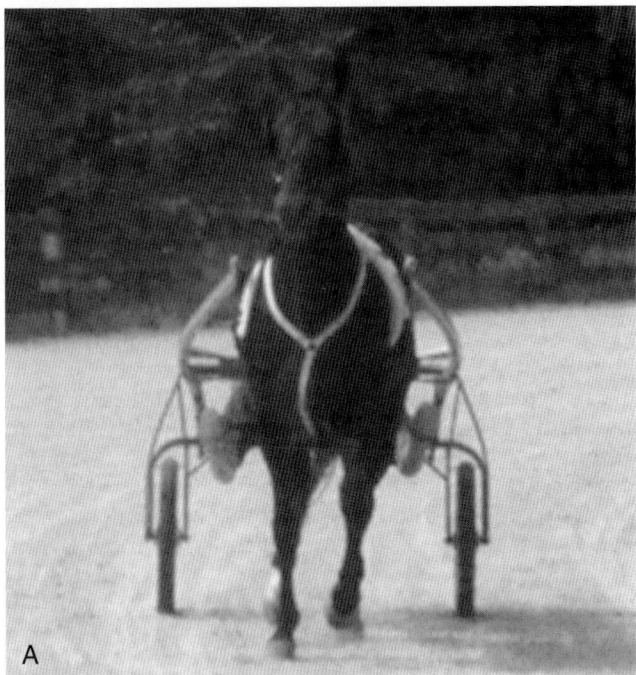

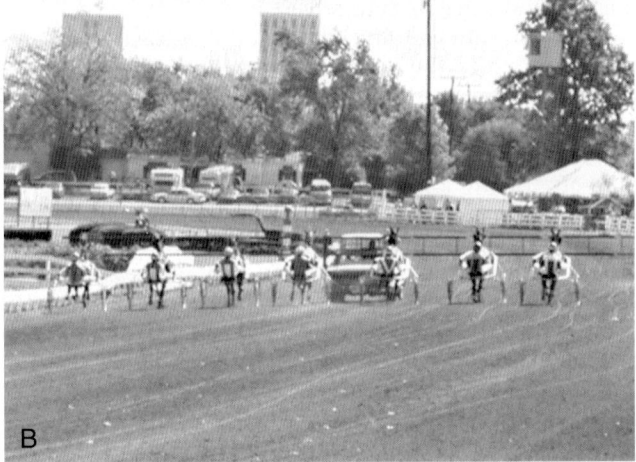

Fig. 108-2 • A, A young trotter is on the left shaft coming out of a turn on a small farm track. On this track a horse has to negotiate four turns to train 1 mile. **B,** Horses approach the start of a race at the Red Mile, Lexington, Kentucky, a track that is 1 mile long. Compared with the turn in **A**, the turn on this track is substantially larger, and horses must negotiate only two turns for a 1-mile race.

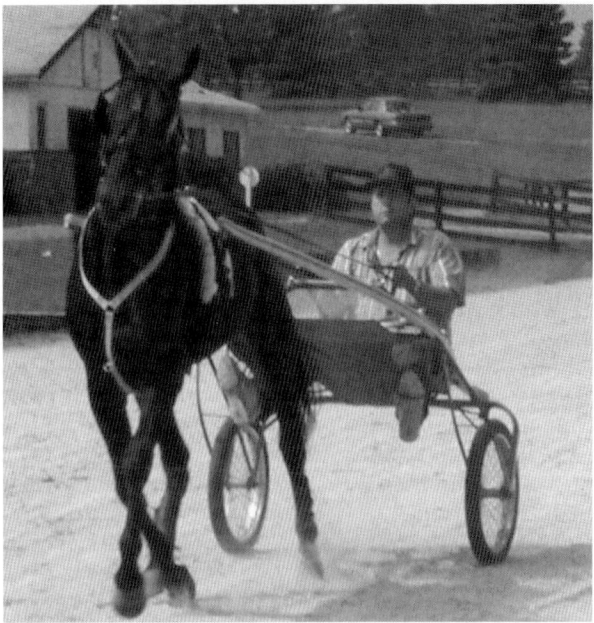

Fig. 108-3 • This trotter is on the left line and the right shaft in the straightaway. The horse's head is turned to the left because the driver (Rich Ringler) has to pull harder on the left rein to keep the horse going straight. The horse's hindquarters are closer to the right shaft. This combination of left line and right shaft would be consistent with left hindlimb lameness.

trial. At certain 1-mile-long racetracks, horses compete against a prompter, usually a TB in harness, and go as fast as possible, but the prompter cannot pass the STB. The world record for the time trial is 1:46.1 set by a pacer. Mean race times of STBs are decreasing constantly (the horses are becoming faster) because of selective breeding, changes in track surfaces and banking, popularity of 1-mile racetracks (racing is faster because horses only negotiate two turns), refinement in race bikes (sulky), and advances in veterinary care.

Early trotters were raced under saddle and then with carts and wagons, with a time under 3 minutes being noteworthy. Sulkies appeared regularly in races in the 1840s, and the 2:30 barrier fell in 1845, becoming a time standard for the era. Race times fell steadily, and in 1897 a stallion named Star Pointer paced a mile in under 2 minutes.

The first horse to trot the 2-minute mile was Lou Dillon in 1903.

North American STBs start a race behind a moveable starting gate, a vehicle carrying a barrier to keep the horses in line until the gate pulls away, at which time the horses accelerate to start the race evenly. In some countries, horses start from a standing start, a staggered standing start, or a moving start without a gait. In Europe, races are only for trotters, and top 3-year-old and older North American trotters often are sold to European buyers.

STBs in North America are divided into four classes. The first is the International trotter that races in the top competitions in North America and Europe. The second is the Grand Circuit or stakes horse that travels from track to track, racing against the top 2- and 3-year-old horses. These horses may earn more than 1 million dollars a year. The third class includes the greatest number of horses stabled at or near a parimutuel track. These horses race repeatedly at one or two different tracks and are referred to as overnight horses. Overnight horses are raced in condition races, grouping similar quality horses by earnings, age, or sex, or in claiming races, where horses are grouped by price. The fourth class, county fair racehorses, popular mostly in the northeast and midwest United States, race for small purses at county fairgrounds, often under adverse track conditions, but they provide thrills for fans and owners beyond those of races with richer purses.

Amateur STB driving and racing under saddle are hobby-type events that are increasing in popularity. STBs compete at horse shows in the roadster classes, hitched to a bike or wagon, and also as road horses under saddle. Former STB racehorses are not only popular in the Amish community, but they also can be found performing diverse sporting activities such as low-level dressage and jumping. The Standardbred Retirement Foundation (http://www.adoptahorse.org) helps to find homes for former racehorses; the Harness Racing Museum and Hall of Fame (http://www.harnessmuseum.com) and the United States Trotting Association (http://www.ustrotting.com) are worthy causes and valuable sources of information about the North American STB.

TRAINING

A classically trained STB has about 9 months of schooling and training before its first race. Most horses start training in the fall at 1½ years of age and begin racing the next summer. Many states have racing programs for 2-, 3-, and 4-year-old horses and require a horse to be nominated early in life. Eligibility then is maintained by periodic payments, called stake payments, creating a large pool of money divided among the winners of elimination and final events. Although some stake races receive track or corporate purse assistance, owners who put up their own money support most races. Stake races are limited by age and sex. For example, 2-year-old trotting fillies race together. Stake payments must be made early in the spring, before talent and speed of individual horses can be confirmed, and owners, trainers, and veterinarians must decide which horses to stake. Emphasis on racing young STBs and the money necessary to maintain stakes eligibility place extreme pressure on trainers to race horses at 2 and 3 years of age. Horses often are pushed farther and faster than is reasonable, placing them at risk of stress-related bone injury, usually of subchondral bone. Many owners do not realize the difficulty of having a horse compete based on a calendar of scheduled events, expecting the horse to peak for the biggest purses, rather than on the horse's training and fitness level. The process of nominating and planning for stakes races is an art and science, and often a staking service is hired to organize periodic stake payments. Stake payments are a considerable expense, and some owners spend several hundred thousand dollars a year. Horses not nominated, those dropped from stakes programs because of injury or lack of talent, or those in which payments were missed are still eligible for overnight racing. More and more late closer and entry-only stakes are becoming available for nonstaked horses.

A STB is trained in a jog cart that is stronger, longer, and about three times as heavy as the 14-kg sulky or race bike. A young pacer is soon equipped with hobbles, which are leather or plastic straps encircling the ipsilateral forelimbs and hindlimbs, to keep legs moving in unison (see Figure 108-1, B). A horse capable of sustaining a pace without hobbles is called a free-legged pacer, but few race without hobbles. Hobbles can cause areas of hair loss on the cranial aspect of the forearm and the caudal aspect of the crus called hobble burns, which are typical marks of a pacer. Trotting hobbles, which are straps encircling both forelimbs that run through a pulley underneath the horse, have become popular and are being used on more and more trotters in recent years, even those competing in top stakes races. Trotting hobbles may stabilize the trotting gait at speed. Some in the industry frown on the use of these equipment additives, claiming they may give an unfair advantage and historically have not been used.

Equipment is important in understanding gait and lameness. Head poles, boots, brace bandages, gaiting straps, and gaiting poles are used to improve gait and performance, as well as to assist in steering the horse at racing speed. A head pole keeps the horse from turning the head and neck to the opposite side. A horse with right forelimb (RF) lameness usually bears left, called bearing in or on the right line, because the driver pulls on the right line, causing the horse to turn the head to the right. This horse would wear a left head pole. Gaiting straps and poles run alongside the horse and attach to the cart beside the driver's seat and are used to keep the horse straight. Horses with unilateral hindlimb lameness often carry the hindquarters near the contralateral shaft, called being on the shaft. A horse with RH lameness goes on the left shaft and requires a left gaiting pole or strap. Boots are applied to minimize interference injury. Some horses chronically interfere, whereas interference in others is accidental. Soft brace bandages are used for protection and to widen the hindlimb gait.

Training the Young Standardbred
Yearling STBs are introduced to the harness and bridle in the stall and then are line driven at a walk for several days before being hitched and jogged on the track. Once the horses can go to the track with a single driver, trainer, or groom, they are jogged 1 to 2 miles each morning, usually in a clockwise direction (wrong way) first. Young STBs are encouraged to jog at the intended gait as soon as possible. STBs are usually jogged 6 days a week at slow speed. This is usually natural for trotters, but many pacers need hobbles or special shoeing. Weight usually is added to hind shoes of pacers, especially to the outside web, whereas the front feet may be left unshod. In trotters, weight is added to the front shoes. Shoeing and equipment changes begin early to produce the best gait possible.

Jogging is increased 1 mile every few weeks, up to 4 to 5 miles daily. Horses are taught to jog both ways of the track. Most young horses are jogged in groups, so horses overcome fear of traveling in close proximity. In large stables, horses are trained in sets of three to five to teach passing and racing in tight quarters and to simulate racing. In addition to jogging, horses are trained fast every 3 to 4 days initially, but later twice weekly, going counterclockwise (the race or right way on the track). Horses are trained 2 and sometimes 3 fast miles on training days but usually go back to the barn for a breather (to blow out) between fast miles (trips). STBs develop tremendous stamina compared with TBs, but fatigue and strain cycles predispose them to stress-related injury of the subchondral bone, not commonly of cortical bone unlike TBs. When the fastest miles approach racing speed, young horses are ready for baby or schooling races to learn how to leave the starting gait. It is interesting that most STBs are trained, schooled, and qualified in the morning daylight and then make the first parimutuel start at night under the lights.

Retraining a Racehorse
The classic retraining approach involves jogging 2 to 5 miles a day and additional training one to two times a week. A fast workout usually consists of two to three fast trips, which are simulated race miles taken at increasing speed. Horses usually are allowed to blow out between

trips. Some are given double headers, which are two 1-mile workouts without returning to the barn, but they walk or jog slowly between trips. A break is when a horse leaves the expected gait and breaks into a gallop. Many training miles are given to obtain maximum physical fitness and to condition the horse to travel at speed without breaking. Many training miles are considered necessary to evaluate and adjust equipment and shoeing. Diagnostic analgesia can be performed between trips.

Alternative training methods produce good results and are customized to the disposition and physical condition of the horse. Trainers now use interval training, straight tracks, inclines and hills, swimming, towing behind a vehicle, and mechanical walkers or joggers. With relocation of European trainers to North America, more alternative techniques have been introduced, including riding trotters between races.

Once racing, work is customized to each horse's needs. Hard training using the classic training method consists of one race and two training trips per week, but in this system horses are under considerable stress. Now that the breed is refined and heat races are fewer, racing horses are given much less training between races, and fast work may not be given at all. Reducing exercise intensity between races is important in managing STBs with chronic lameness.

LAMENESS AND POOR RACING PERFORMANCE

Lameness is the leading cause of poor performance and a major cause of STBs making breaks. Some overnight and stakes horses are chronically lame but race weekly, although lame horses race slower, and horses drop in class as lameness progresses. The major effect of lameness is seen during the last quarter of the race, called the last quarter time. Lower-class horses usually have a fast opening quarter but slow last quarter time, whereas open and stakes horses have fast quarter times anytime during the race. Evaluation of last quarter time is useful to determine cause and severity of poor race performance. Lameness often costs a horse 1 to 2 seconds in last quarter race time, equating to 5 to 10 horse lengths. For example, a horse that normally paces the last quarter in 27.1 seconds but for the last few starts has been coming home in 28.4 to 29.2 seconds is probably lame, although concomitant respiratory and metabolic problems cannot be overlooked.

TRACK SURFACE AND LAMENESS

STBs usually race around an oval track, ½ to 1 mile in circumference; a 1-mile track is most common. Races are usually 1 mile, but a few are ⅝-mile sprints to 2-mile races. The track surface is a crushed rock base, covered with a packed, sandy soil and a thin sand or stone dust surface. STB racing requires a much firmer track surface than galloping horses. Sulky tires are more efficient if rolling over a firm smooth surface, and the STB gaits require a firmer and smoother surface than does the gallop. Track surfaces have become firmer because year-round racing requires a surface suitable for racing in rain and subfreezing temperatures. Hard tracks with loose surfaces require horses to wear shoes with added grabs and welded-on spots of borium to avoid slipping. Excessive slipping or overzealous use of shoes with additives predisposes horses to lameness. A soft or deep surface can predispose horses to tendonitis and suspensory desmitis. Hard tracks with a covering of loose stone dust are slippery and may predispose horses to carpal synovitis, bruised soles, and muscle soreness. Racetracks get soft and sticky with small amounts of rain and hard and unyielding with heavy rainfall that may wash the top surface into the infield. Recently, a three-dimensional dynamometric horseshoe was used to measure acceleration and other forces on the front hoof of French trotters performing at high speed on two different track surfaces, all-weather waxed and crushed sand track surfaces.[1,2] Hoof deceleration was significantly less, and there was a 50% attenuation of shock when horses performed on the waxed surface, suggesting this surface had better shock-absorbing qualities compared with a crushed sand surface.[1] The amplitude of the maximal longitudinal braking force was significantly lower and occurred 6% later in the stance phase. The magnitude of the ground reaction force at impact was lower on the waxed track compared with the crushed sand track surface.[2] The attenuation of loading rate, amplitude of horizontal braking, and shock at impact on waxed surfaces suggested that there is likely a reduction in stress in the distal aspect of the forelimb, results that may be important in training normal horses or rehabilitating STBs with infirmities.[2]

References on page 1342

TRACK SIZE AND LAMENESS

Track size has substantial implications in the development and expression of lameness. Tracks are 1 mile, ⅞ mile, ⅝ mile, and ½ mile, and in general race times are lower (faster) on large tracks. Because most STB races are 1 mile, track size determines the number of turns during the race. During a race on a ½-mile track, a STB must negotiate four turns. Turns on smaller racetracks are much tighter than those on larger tracks (see Figure 108-2). There is a single racetrack larger than a 1-mile oval, Colonial Downs in Virginia, at which a short race meet is held each year; on this track, races involve negotiating a single turn. Horses racing with mild chronic lameness are less likely to sustain speeds necessary to be competitive on larger tracks, so they may race on smaller tracks; however, if lameness is worse in the turns, the horse may be less competitive on small tracks and better suited for a 1-mile track. If lameness is worse in the straightaway, the horse may be best suited for a small track. This is particularly important when lameness worsens as the race goes on because large tracks have a long straightaway at the end.

During counterclockwise racing, right-sided lameness conditions exert more influence, even though the LF and LH are on the inside. Horses with left-sided lameness can race successfully on small tracks and apparently negotiate turns well. However, those with right-sided lameness cannot trot or pace the turns well, most likely from the effect of centripetal and compressive forces. Ideally, all racehorses should be sound, but many horses can race successfully with mild infirmity. Horses with substantial lameness should be treated or rested until the condition improves.

CONFORMATION

Forelimb and hindlimb faults lead to lameness and interference. Severity often depends on gait. A trotter should be as long from front to back as it is tall. Trotters are passing gaited if hind feet land outside the front feet, and in-line gaited if hind feet land in plane with the front feet. Wide hindlimb gait is advantageous because it allows a passing gait. Trotters can be mildly to moderately toed out in front without substantial interference problems, but they should not be toed in because winging out leads to interference and lateral suspensory branch desmitis. Pacers can be wide and mildly toed in but not toed out because this fault predisposes the horse to hitting the knees. A club foot is less well tolerated by a STB than a TB and usually results in foot lameness. Low, underslung heels and long toes are acquired by attempts to increase stride length or to decrease interference. Back at the knee is undesirable and leads directly to carpal lameness in a trotter, but it is better tolerated by a pacer. Offset (bench) knee is a major fault, and although horses may race successfully, lameness of the carpus and metacarpal region often develops. Mild carpus valgus is tolerated by pacers but can lead to lameness of the carpus and metacarpal region. Pacers that are tied in behind the knee are at risk of developing superficial digital flexor tendonitis, but surprisingly trotters are not. Short, straight pasterns and short backs are undesirable.

A serious hindlimb fault leading directly to moderate to severe lameness is sickle-hocked conformation (see Chapters 4 and 78). Mild sickle-hocked conformation typified many early pacers and is desired by some trainers. Sickle-hocked trotters are fast but develop curb and osteoarthritis (OA) of the distal hock joints, particularly severe in the dorsal aspect, and are chronically unsound. Sickle-hocked conformation predisposes all STBs to the development of slab fractures of the third and central tarsal bones. Straight hindlimb conformation is unusual but is a severe fault, leading to metatarsophalangeal and stifle joint lameness and suspensory desmitis. In horses with straight hindlimb conformation, excessive extension of the metatarsophalangeal joint occurs. Long, sloping pasterns also predispose horses to fetlock hyperextension, but a primary metatarsophalangeal joint weakness is seen in some trotters with normal pastern lengths, in which the base of the proximal sesamoid bones (PSBs) is level with the middle of the proximal phalanx. Abnormal elasticity or loss of support from the suspensory apparatus predisposes horses to run-down injury and suspensory desmitis. Run-down injury is more commonly seen in the hindlimbs. Cow-hocked conformation is prevalent in trotters but is not problematic unless severe. In-at-the-hock conformation predisposes horses to OA of the distal hock joints, curb, and medial splint bone disease. Base-wide and base-narrow conformational faults, if severe, can lead directly to interference and lameness.

DISTRIBUTION OF LAMENESS

STB racehorses have a higher percentage of hindlimb lameness than TBs. The STB trains and races using a two-beat gait: two limbs bear weight simultaneously. Load is shared almost equally between forelimbs and hindlimbs. The caudal location of the cart and driver (load) and the addition of the overcheck apparatus shift the center of balance caudally, increasing hindlimb lameness (see Figures 2-2 and 2-3). The distribution of forelimb to hindlimb lameness is approximately 55% to 45%.

LAMENESS IN THE YOUNG STANDARDBRED

The top 10 list (see page 1024) contains those conditions seen in STB racehorses of all ages when grouped together, but unraced 2- and early 3-year-olds develop a subset of lameness conditions. Osteochondrosis (see Chapters 54 and 56), splint exostoses (splints), and curbs are common. Forelimb splints are usually medial but can occur laterally. Hindlimb splints are almost always medial and are more common in trotters. Splints can cause primary lameness or be secondary to carpal lameness, especially if the exostosis is proximal. Forelimb splints develop when the limb is carried or lands abnormally. Young horses develop splints from difficulty learning the racing gait and by making breaks. While breaking, pacers often hit themselves because galloping in hobbles is difficult. Curb is common in young pacers and may be recognized while horses are jogging, before training begins (see Chapter 78).

Carpal lameness is common in young horses. The middle carpal joint is the most common site, but synovitis can occur in the antebrachiocarpal joint. Carpal lameness is caused by early subchondral stress-related bone injury of the third carpal bone and is particularly common in trotters. Paddock turn out for 30 days is recommended. Middle carpal joint lameness must be differentiated from proximal suspensory desmitis (PSD). The thought once was that the distal radial physis was a source of occult carpal region lameness, but diagnosis was never confirmed. Physeal pain is a rare diagnosis today, but some veterinarians believe such pain is a possible source of so-called colt soreness.

Bucked shins are rare but do occur in 2-year-old pacers in July and August. Most bucked shins occur in the forelimbs. Genuine bucked shins rarely occur in trotters, but interference trauma of the dorsal cortex of the third metatarsal bone (MtIII) is common.

Distal hock joint pain is a common cause of acute unilateral lameness, but if pain is bilateral, overt lameness may not be present. Horses appear stiff and sore when starting out and warm out of lameness. Gait abnormalities and repeated breaking may cause distal hock joint pain. Lameness may be difficult to abolish completely with intraarticular analgesia because pain is multifactorial, arising from periarticular soft tissues and secondary gluteal myositis and trochanteric bursitis. Horses should be rested for 1 week and given nonsteroidal antiinflammatory drugs (NSAIDs) such as phenylbutazone (2.2 to 4.4 mg/kg orally [PO] twice daily). Intraarticular injections are avoided if possible, but treatment of the tarsometatarsal (TMT) joint with hyaluronan alone, or in combination with corticosteroids, often resolves residual lameness. Using a less aggressive training schedule for 20 to 30 days is recommended. Shoeing should be evaluated, and grabs and calks should be removed or minimized.

Interference injuries are common and plague many STBs throughout the racing career. Trotters interfere primarily by striking the toe of the ipsilateral front foot to the shin, pastern, or coronary band regions of the hindlimb (see Chapter 7 and Figure 7-2). Interference from a front foot striking the medial aspect of the contralateral forelimb (cross-firing) occurs occasionally in trotters but is a major form of interference injury in pacers. Injury to second (McII) and third metacarpal (McIII) bones, PSBs, carpus, heel, and hoof wall causes bruising and hematoma formation. Contusions can lead to soreness or frank lameness and can cause an altered gait. A trotter attempting to avoid striking the LH shin shortens the cranial phase of the stride, causing what appears to be a pelvic hike, mimicking LH lameness. Deliberate hiking can alter load distribution, causing compensatory lameness in the RH and RF. Local trauma is treated, and changes in equipment and shoeing, such as applying brace bandages and boots, are performed. A brief (5 to 7 days) reduction in exercise intensity is useful to allow a young horse to gain confidence in the corrected gait.

Young horses with poor gait should be examined carefully for neurological disease. Equine protozoal myelitis (EPM) is endemic in STBs and can be a real cause of gait deficits or a catchall diagnosis (see Chapter 11).

CLINICAL HISTORY

Clinical history is critical for lameness diagnosis and to put lameness into context with other causes of poor racing performance. The attending veterinarian with an established relationship with the horse may know the horse's history. A trainer often refers to mild lameness by saying, "The horse is just sore, Doc," or "The horse is off when jogging, but throws it away when going the right way." STBs have unusual resiliency and race rather well with chronic lameness, but lameness does not resolve with speed. Owners do not understand this concept. Signs of lameness become less visually apparent when horses go fast. Because STBs often race with numerous compensatory lameness problems, one must be open to the possibility that current lameness is not worsening of an existing problem but is an entirely new one.

A good starting place is to determine the chief complaint from the person(s) closest to the horse, usually the groom and trainer. What differs now from the horse's normal activity, gait, or performance? Has a change in training or racing schedule occurred? Has there been a change in track surface? A horse noticed to be stiff and sore up front when walking to the track may be foot sore the day after the horse raced on a hard track. Have any equipment or shoeing changes been made? Additions of head poles, gaiting straps, and boots point to high-speed lameness and gait abnormalities. Shoeing changes, such as adding or removing bar shoes, are important because horses used to wearing bar shoes may have sore feet if bars are removed. Metacarpophalangeal joint lameness may be worse if bars are added. Stress-related bone injury of the metatarsophalangeal joint is seen soon after aluminum shoes with toe grabs are applied. Is the horse receiving any current medication, and when was the horse last examined? What treatments, if any, were given? Although an acute injury or worsening of chronic OA can cause acute synovitis, inflammatory and infectious arthritis can develop days to weeks after intraarticular injections, particularly if corticosteroids were used, because these drugs can suppress signs of inflammation and infection for weeks. Infectious arthritis is common 14 to 21 days after intraarticular injection, but often owners and trainers are incredulous because recent injections were not performed. What have the trainer and groom done recently to solve or treat the problem? Topical therapy may reduce or worsen inflammation and mask or augment clinical signs. Skin soreness after application of paints and blisters can cause a false-positive response to deep palpation.

Is the horse a trotter or a pacer? This information is critical. The usual distribution of pacers to trotters is about 3:1. Interference problems are different between gaits. Trotters often develop contralateral or diagonal compensatory lameness, whereas pacers most often develop ipsilateral compensatory lameness. A pacer with a left carpal lameness often develops LH compensatory lameness, but a trotter is more likely to develop compensatory lameness in the RH. Although this distribution of compensatory lameness is common when examining horses trotting in hand, load distribution and interference issues may complicate and change visual appearance of where primary lameness originates when a STB is pulling a cart on the track and on which gait the horse is performing. The distribution of lameness differs between gaits. Fractures of the proximal phalanx and the McIII and the MtIII and superficial digital flexor tendonitis are less common in trotters. Trotters with stifle lameness, specifically OA of the medial femorotibial joint, can cope better than pacers. Race times are different. Prognosis for certain problems such as osteochondral fragments of third carpal and radial carpal bones is worse in trotters. Pacers are more likely than trotters to start a race and to have five starts before and after surgical removal of osteochondral fragments of the carpus.[3] Osteochondrosis is common in certain bloodlines of trotters and pacers.

Is the condition worse at the trot or pace? Trotters and many pacers trot while jogging the wrong way but assume the intended gait when turned the right way. Most forelimb lameness conditions are less obvious at the pace, but hindlimb lameness differs. In general, STBs with stifle lameness are worse at the pace than the trot. If trainers comment that the horse is worse at the pace than at the trot, the veterinarian should suspect stifle lameness until proved otherwise. Pacers wear hobbles, but trotting hobbles are often used in trotters making breaks.

Is lameness different depending on what direction the horse moves? Problems on the right side are worse going the right way of the track (counterclockwise). Horses with medial foot and carpal lameness may show signs in the turns, especially entering the turning radius going the right way, but not when jogging.

What is the horse's last quarter time? Although high-speed lameness can cause a 1- to 2-second decrease in last quarter time, horses with mechanical upper airway disease and rhabdomyolysis have a 2- to 4-second reduction, and those with severe lameness or atrial fibrillation have a 5- to 10-second reduction in last quarter time.

Is the horse on a line? This is one of the most important pieces of information to obtain. Trainers sometimes dismiss young horses being mildly on the line because nervous and inexperienced horses may change directions suddenly, but in reality most of these abnormal movements are caused by lameness. During counterclockwise racing of a horse on the right line, the driver has to increase the tension (pull harder) on the right rein to keep the horse straight and prevent it from bearing toward the infield. Just the opposite occurs when horses are on the left line (see Figure 108-3). Because of bit pressure, when a horse is on the left line, it turns or cocks the head to the left, toward the inside rail, and vice versa. If history is unclear, the veterinarian should watch the horse on the track and observe head position. Because most horses bear away from pain, a horse on the right line is most often lame on the right side, but exceptions occur. A common finding is metacarpophalangeal effusion and a positive response to lower limb flexion. The trainer states, "The horse was on the left line when finishing the mile, but is usually on the right line especially in the turns." Primary lameness may be in the right carpus, but chronic RF lameness has caused compensatory overloading and lameness of the left metacarpophalangeal joint, and both areas should be evaluated and potentially treated. Most horses on a line from forelimb lameness have foot or carpal lameness. However, problems located medially, such as medial sole bruising, quarter cracks, or carpal lameness, paradoxically can cause a horse to be on the contralateral line. Horses may lose power in the affected limbs and drift at speed toward the lame side. Therefore a horse with a medial LF quarter crack could be on the right line, whereas those with a right carpal lameness could be on the left line. All limbs should be examined because not all horses read the book. "If a horse is on the left line, think right hind," one old saying goes, and rarely a horse with RH bruised or cracked heels will be on the left line.[4]

Horses on a line without overt signs of lameness are among the most difficult lameness mysteries to solve. Because compensatory lameness problems may be numerous in a horse in which primary lameness cannot be ascribed, deciding on which limb to begin diagnostic analgesia is a dilemma. Most horses need to be examined at speed after blocking, a time-consuming and frustrating process. In many horses on a line, obscure sources of pain such as subchondral bone can be difficult to identify, and horses often are referred for scintigraphic examination. Most horses chronically on a line have had many intraarticular or other injections, and trainers will state, "We've done his knees, hocks, stifles, and feet and nothing helped." Often forgotten are the metatarsophalangeal joints. In many horses numerous sites of pain must be managed simultaneously rather than sequentially. Recommending numerous intraarticular and regional injections, a shoeing change, and a change in exercise intensity in a horse that is on a line is not unusual.

Is the horse on a shaft? A horse with RH lameness drifts to the left (see Figure 108-2) and positions the hindquarters closer to the left shaft of the sulky and is thus on the left shaft; the reverse is true with LH lameness (see Figure 108-3). Not all hindlimb lameness problems cause horses to be on a shaft. Horses with OA of the medial femorotibial joint may not be on a shaft, but those with distal hock joint pain will be. A horse may be falsely on a shaft if it is hard on a line and the driver pulls hard to keep the horse straight, compelling the horse to twist its entire body, positioning the hindquarters close to one shaft to maintain balance.

Is the horse worse in the turns or on the straightaway? Although nothing is pathognomonic, a few findings are consistent. Horses with front foot lameness, splints, and curbs get worse as the mile progresses and so appear worse on the final straightaway. Horses with distal hock joint pain appear to be worse when going into or coming out of a turn but usually can pace and trot the turns successfully. Horses with carpal, metatarsophalangeal, and stifle joint lameness are worse in the turns. If a horse gets rough in the first turn just after leaving the gate, a medial

RF problem such as a splint or carpal lameness should be suspected.

On what size track does the horse race? The relationship of track size to expression of lameness and the differences between left- and right-sided lameness problems were discussed (see page 1017).

Is the horse making breaks? Unsound trotters often break stride and gallop but occasionally break into a pace. Lame trotters may pace when trotted in hand. Because high-speed lameness often causes pacers to gallop and trotters to pace or gallop, it seems that the gallop may be the easiest gait that a lame horse can maintain at speed. The most difficult gait to maintain at speed is the trot, followed by the pace, and lastly the gallop (MWR). Interference injury causes breaks, and current shoeing or recent changes should be evaluated. A different way to hang up a horse, meaning how to shoe and equip it, may be all that is needed.

The veterinarian must be current on all medication rules in the racing jurisdiction because changes, such as recent (2009) modifications of allowable blood levels of corticosteroids, may impact management strategy.

LAMENESS EXAMINATION

The lameness examination can be divided into three stages: palpation, observation while moving on a lead shank, and observation under harness. The veterinarian should avoid narrowing the examination to the area suspected by the groom and trainer but should first stand back and observe the horse and watch the horse moving around and coming out of the stall. Subtle neurological signs may be apparent. Asymmetry, such as muscle atrophy, may point toward chronic lameness or neurological disease.

Palpation

Careful palpation is the art of diagnosis in the racehorse but often is sacrificed because palpation is time consuming. Palpation is critical in STBs because of numerous compensatory lameness problems. The veterinarian needs to be able to "read" the horse to make a diagnosis. A successful lameness detective respects what the horse is trying to say. The veterinarian should move over the entire horse with a light touch to see whether a withdrawal response is elicited. A light touch along the neck and gluteal regions may elicit pain from secondary muscle soreness or painful previous intramuscular injection sites. Horses often exhibit a withdrawal response when a limb is first picked up, indicating a problem even before the specific region is manipulated. Horses may exhibit false-positive responses in areas that have been recently painted, blistered, or freeze fired. Once horses have been freeze fired for splints and curbs, many trainers assume the problem has been solved and are incredulous if the veterinarian suggests the area is still the source of pain. Cryotherapy is not a panacea and may have to be repeated, or another form of management may be needed (see Chapters 78 and 89).

Palpation should be done in a quiet place, before the horse is trotted in hand, so that all potential lameness problems are detected. Careful and detailed examination of the front feet should be performed. Hoof tester examination is critical, but most horses show a painful response for 1 to 2 days after racing, particularly if the track was hard.

Effusion of the distal interphalangeal (DIP) joint capsule often accompanies early OA and sore feet. Shoes on the front and back feet should be evaluated critically for wear, type, weight, and the presence of additives. The proximal, dorsal aspect of the proximal phalanx should be palpated for pain associated with midsagittal fractures of the proximal phalanx. Palpation findings in the metacarpophalangeal and metatarsophalangeal joints often do not correlate well with degree of lameness, response to diagnostic analgesia, and results of scintigraphic examination. The presence of mild warmth (heat) on palpation, a subtle clinical finding, is an important observation for detection of subchondral bone pain in the distal aspect of the McIII or the MtIII. Pain on palpation of the PSBs may indicate sesamoiditis. Normally a horse responds little to compression of the suspensory ligament (SL), deep digital flexor tendon (DDFT), and superficial digital flexor tendon (SDFT). Pain is often the first sign of desmitis or tendonitis. Chronic enlargement of the SL and SDFT is common in lower-class horses, and although a horse may not react to palpation, it may have associated high-speed lameness. Splint exostoses are most painful after training or racing but may be nonpainful several days later. Standing and flexed subcarpal palpation may reveal pain associated with PSD, longitudinal and avulsion fractures of the McIII, proximal superficial digital flexor tendonitis, and a dorsal medial articular fracture of the McIII.

No palpable abnormalities may be associated with carpal lameness. The veterinarian should carefully assess for warmth and compare the limb with the contralateral limb. If the horse has been clipped for the application of a paint or blister, the affected area will feel warm compared with the surrounding unclipped skin. Effusion occurs in 2-year-old horses early in training, but it often is minimal in horses with subchondral bone pain. The antebrachiocarpal joint is rarely a site of carpal lameness in older racehorses, but in young horses, especially trotters, effusion may occur. The medial aspect of the carpus and the distal aspect of the antebrachium are common sites for interference injury. Carpal tenosynovitis is unusual to rare, but occasionally hyperextension injury and hemorrhage occur. Rarely, almost always in trotters, desmitis of the accessory ligament of the SDFT occurs, associated with carpal tenosynovitis. Pacers develop hobble burns and cellulitis in the proximal aspect of the antebrachium. Elbow and shoulder joint lameness is rare, but horses may exhibit pain when the biceps brachii, intertubercular bursa, and other muscles are palpated or the shoulder joint is flexed, from muscle soreness secondary to primary carpal lameness. The neck, back, and rump regions should be palpated for symmetry and muscle soreness. Young horses will occasionally manifest sore withers from an improperly fitted harness. Because intramuscular injections of counterirritant and antiinflammatory solutions are common in STBs, careful palpation is necessary to discover deep abscesses causing pain, lameness, and fever. Disease of the thoracic dorsal spinous processes is rare. In a 16-year period, only one of nearly 2400 STBs undergoing scintigraphic examination had increased radiopharmaceutical uptake (IRU) in the dorsal spinous processes or the intervertebral synovial joints, and no bony abnormalities were found in the pelvis.[5]

Secondary muscle soreness of the gluteal region is a common problem, and the diagnosis of trochanteric bursitis often is made based on a painful response to compression. Trochanteric bursitis (whorl bone disease) may be overdiagnosed and difficult to authenticate, but injections often improve hindlimb gait and performance (see Chapter 47). Rhabdomyolysis also can cause pain on palpation of the rump region. Young horses with loose stifles often knuckle behind, but palpation is often negative. Pain associated with the medial aspect of the stifle may be present, but abnormalities when manipulating the patella are absent. Femoropatellar effusion in young horses can signal osteochondrosis. The medial femorotibial joint capsule should be palpated because OA is the most important cause of lameness of the stifle. The crus is a rare site of pain. Hobble burns on the caudal aspect can cause soreness in young pacers.

The tarsocrural joint is the most common site for osteochondrosis, and effusion in young horses should prompt radiographic examination. Periarticular pain in the distal aspect of the tarsus and proximal metatarsal region often accompanies distal hock joint pain. The Churchill test is done routinely, but in addition to those with distal hock joint pain, STBs often respond positively with other common distal limb lameness. Bony enlargement (bone spavin) is rare. Plantar soft tissue swelling and pain associated with curb is a common cause of lameness (see Chapter 78). The plantar metatarsal region commonly is overlooked, but it should be palpated carefully for the presence of suspensory desmitis. Signs of inflammation may be difficult to detect because the SL is enclosed within the bony confines of the metatarsal bones. The first evidence of suspensory desmitis is mild enlargement and pain of the suspensory body in the midmetatarsal region. Compression of the splint bones puts indirect pressure on the SL and explains why the Churchill test is nonspecific. The dorsal aspect of the MtIII is a common site for interference injury in trotters. Palpation of the fetlock region is critical because the region is an important source of lameness, but often no localizing clinical signs are apparent. Mild warmth may signal the presence of subchondral bone injury. Pain from interference injury should be differentiated from that associated with midsagittal and dorsal plane fracture of the proximal phalanx. The hind foot is an unusual source of lameness, but fractures of the distal phalanx, bruising, navicular disease, and OA of the DIP joint are diagnosed occasionally. STBs normally respond positively to hoof testers placed across the heel.

Movement

The horse should be examined at a walk and trot in hand. The pace is a forgiving gait, and head and neck nod and pelvic hike can be difficult to see. Evaluating lameness in pacers is easier while they are trotting, but correlation between lameness seen in hand and during pacing at high speed is questionable. Forelimb lameness is less obvious at the pace. Degree of pelvic hike is comparable at the pace and trot. Baseline lameness should be determined before the harness is applied because horses that are fracture lame should not be taken to the track, and a good correlation exists between lameness seen in hand and in harness in horses with obvious lameness. The ability to trot horses in hand at the racetrack may be limited because of too much activity, lack of room, and often poor or slippery surfaces. Flexion tests are performed but lack specificity. The carpal flexion test is the most reliable and specific of all flexion tests. Direct compression of a painful splint, the proximal aspect of a SL, and a curb followed by trotting is useful. Subtle hindlimb lameness is best evaluated in harness because little correlation may exist with lameness seen in hand. Pulling a cart and different surface likely explain this observation. Subtle (less than grade 1 of 5) hindlimb lameness at the trot in hand should be taken with a grain of salt. Observation on the track puts lameness into perspective and allows evaluation of compensatory lameness. Although there may be a lack of correlation between lameness seen in hand and that observed on the track or at speed, any lameness condition may be an important contributor to poor performance. Lameness is most pronounced when horses are jogged slowly and is much less obvious with speed. High-speed lameness is evaluated by communication with the trainer and by resolving signs such as being on a line by using diagnostic analgesia.

DIAGNOSTIC ANALGESIA

Diagnostic analgesia is essential to pinpoint lameness, but trainers and owners often prefer treatment of a suspected area rather than lengthy investigation. With weekly racing, no time may be available for blocking because levels of local anesthetic solution will be detectable. Diagnosis often is made based on response to treatment. Many common lameness conditions involve subchondral stress-related bone injury, and often horses can be blocked sound but do not improve with intraarticular treatment. Perineural analgesia is more effective than intraarticular analgesia for diagnosing subchondral bone pain.

Controlling as many variables as possible is important when observing STBs in harness. The same gait, equipment, driver, approximate speed, and track direction should be used. Sometimes horses exhibit lameness when driven by the groom but not the trainer because trainers expect a higher level of performance and often carry a whip. A false-positive response occurs when a horse exhibits lameness at the pace but after diagnostic analgesia returns to the track without hobbles equipment and trots soundly. The diagnostic analgesia procedure should be the only variable. STBs often warm out of lameness and should be evaluated immediately when starting out after each block. Overzealous use of a twitch and rough handling may compromise evaluation, and administration of drugs can add another variable. If horses are observed in harness after diagnostic analgesia, the person driving the horse should be instructed to return the horse to the stable as soon as improvement is recognized because training a horse after blocking risks further injury.

Complete description of blocking techniques is found in Chapter 10. A few points about diagnostic analgesia in the STB must be kept in mind. Palmar or plantar digital analgesia desensitizes most of the foot. Horses with metacarpophalangeal or metatarsophalangeal joint lameness can be sound after palmar or plantar digital analgesia, particularly those with midsagittal fracture of the proximal phalanx.[6] Palmar nerve blocks at the level of the PSBs are avoided because inadvertent analgesia of fetlock pain can be misinterpreted as lameness of the foot or pastern. Individual carpal joints should be blocked separately, and differentiation between carpal and proximal metacarpal region lameness is necessary. The median and ulnar nerve block is underused.

A low plantar block must be done routinely, or many lameness conditions will be diagnosed erroneously as high up. The fetlock region is a major source of hindlimb lameness. Although subchondral bone pain of the distal aspect of the MtIII (McIII) can be abolished using intraarticular analgesia of the fetlock joint, most consistently pain is abolished using perineural analgesia. A modification of the low plantar technique, blocking only the lateral plantar metatarsal nerve, can be completed and the horse evaluated. If lameness abates, then pain associated with the lateral aspect of the fetlock joint is diagnosed; however, if no response is seen sequentially, the medial plantar metatarsal nerve, then the medial and lateral plantar nerves must be blocked. The high plantar block is often overlooked, but PSD cannot be substantiated without it. The centrodistal (CD) joint is difficult to enter but should be blocked separately from the tarsometatarsal (TMT) joint because communication occurs in only 8% to 39% of horses. The medial femorotibial joint should be blocked separately from the femoropatellar joint, even though they communicate in a high percentage of horses.

IMAGING CONSIDERATIONS
Radiography
Routine radiographic examination of STBs does not differ from that of other sports horses. However, a few specific images should be kept in mind. Down-angled oblique (dorsal 60° proximal 45° lateral-palmarodistal medial oblique and dorsal 60° proximal 45° medial-palmarodistal lateral oblique) and horizontal oblique (dorsolateral-palmaromedial oblique [DL-PaMO] and dorsomedial-palmarolateral oblique) images should be obtained to evaluate the DIP joint and palmar processes of the distal phalanx. The tangential (palmaroproximal-palmarodistal oblique) image of the navicular bone is less valuable in the STB than in other older sports horses. To evaluate the distal aspect of the McIII (or MtIII) for subchondral stress-related bone injury and the space between the proximal palmar (or plantar) aspect of the proximal phalanx and the base of the PSBs for the presence of fragments, down-angled oblique (dorsal 30° proximal 45° lateral-palmarodistal medial oblique and dorsal 30° proximal 45° medial-palmarodistal lateral oblique) images should be obtained (see Chapter 42). The most important images of the carpus are the DL-PaMO image and the tangential (skyline) image of the distal row of carpal bones. In STBs it is essential to have a well-exposed and well-positioned skyline image to evaluate the third carpal bone for increased radiopacity, radiolucency, and osteochondral fragments (see Chapter 38). Radiological changes of OA of the CD and TMT joints and slab fractures of the third tarsal bone are seen best on the lateromedial and dorsomedial-plantarolateral oblique (DM-PlLO) images. A common misconception is that changes associated with bone spavin occur medially but not in young STBs. The DM-PlLO image is essential in evaluating the tarsocrural joint for osteochondrosis fragments because two common locations—the cranial aspect of the intermediate ridge of the tibia and the lateral trochlear ridge of the talus—are evaluated best using this image. The caudocranial image is essential when evaluating the

medial femorotibial joint for narrowing, osteophytes, and subchondral bone cysts. Inadequate exposure and positioning often result in images that cannot be interpreted.

Digital and computed radiography are useful in evaluating stress-related bone injury of subchondral bone and incomplete fractures. Computed tomography is useful to evaluate subchondral bone and fracture configuration. Magnetic resonance imaging is useful to evaluate subchondral bone and soft tissues of the distal aspect of the limb, but scintigraphic examination is still used routinely for investigation of high-speed lameness and poor performance and continues to have great value in lameness diagnosis in STBs.

Ultrasonographic Examination

Suspensory desmitis, superficial digital flexor tendonitis, curb, and desmitis of the distal sesamoidean ligaments are common in the STB, and ultrasonographic examination is essential for diagnosis and assessing prognosis (see Chapter 16).

Scintigraphic Examination

Referral for scintigraphic examination is common, and horses with poor performance often have numerous areas of IRU, indicating high-speed lameness is a part of the problem. Common areas of IRU include the distal phalanx, metacarpophalangeal joint (medial condyle of the McIII and PSBs), proximal aspect of the McIII, carpus, especially the third and radial carpal bones, metatarsophalangeal joint (proximal aspect of the proximal phalanx and distal plantarolateral aspect of the MtIII and PSBs), the proximal plantar aspect of the MtIII, subchondral bone of the TMT and CD joints and the medial femorotibial joint (see Chapter 19).

PROCEEDING WITHOUT A DIAGNOSIS

Proper identification of lameness as the cause of poor performance and localizing the site(s) of pain can be challenging and relies heavily on experience. It is particularly important to differentiate lameness from interference because interference can cause signs that mimic lameness, lameness can result from interference, and lameness can cause interference. Horses on a line without obvious lameness and a negative response to diagnostic analgesia can be frustrating. Horses can become stubborn and react to equipment and twist and bend the head and neck, causing signs similar to being on a line. Occasionally, horses with tooth-related pain get on a line. An ocular problem is a rare cause of a horse being on a line. Trainers may use bridles with partial blinds or vision-restricting cups to control a horse on a line.

Simultaneous RF and RH or LF and LH lameness, or even primary hindlimb lameness, can be difficult because hindlimb lameness can cause a head nod mimicking ipsilateral forelimb lameness. Diagnostic analgesia should start in the hindlimb. In trotters with foot and carpal lameness the caudal phase of the lame forelimb is longer, and to avoid interference, the cranial phase of the ipsilateral hindlimb is shortened (hiking), mimicking hindlimb lameness. Pelvic hike abates when the source of forelimb lameness is localized. If the lameness problem is complex and frustrating, it is possible that a fresh perspective from a colleague or advanced imaging may help.

To differentiate lameness from interference gait abnormalities, phenylbutazone (4.4 mg/kg twice daily for 5 to 10 days) is administered (the bute test). Horses with pain should improve, whereas those with pure interference gait abnormalities should not. However, not all horses with musculoskeletal pain respond to NSAIDs, particularly those with chronic lameness or numerous compensatory problems. Alternatively, the veterinarian should medicate the suspected area and see whether performance improves because mimicking the maximal exertion of racing is difficult. A trotter on a line only going into the first turn may be helped by injection of corticosteroids around a mildly painful medial splint or into the middle carpal joint. Sometimes treating a different area between several races may allow a fortuitous discovery, but this requires good record keeping, and it may be expensive. Occasionally, horses with subtle or nondescript lameness or a rough gait are managed using a shotgun approach, and numerous intraarticular treatments are given simultaneously. This approach should be reserved for horses in which normal management procedures have failed and an important race is rapidly approaching. Sometimes a positive response to intraarticular corticosteroid injections results from systemic absorption and effect on a distant, rather than the intended, site.

A brief turnout period of 7 to 10 days is sometimes useful. In 2-year-olds, a decision often is made to stop training and give 3 to 4 months of turnout rather than risk compensatory lameness or fracture. The decision to stop training a horse should not be taken lightly. Getting an older horse back to the same level of racing is often difficult, even with a planned turnout period, and jogging the horse three to four times a week to maintain condition and range of joint motion may be best. The older the horse is, the more difficult it is to return the horse to racing. Older horses with chronic lameness do not thrive with rigorous training and often come out of a solo training mile lamer than after schooling or qualifying races. Older horses often are raced into fitness rather than trained rigorously. A common mistake is to train or race these horses too often.

A complete neurological examination should be performed in any horse with gait deficits and even some with overt lameness, if neurological signs are noticed concomitantly. EPM is frequently diagnosed, but positive identification of the source of neurological signs is difficult to make because serum and cerebrospinal fluid analyses are not accurate (see Chapter 11). The immunofluorescent antibody test (University of California, Davis, California, United States) ascribes a numerical value (titer) to the levels of antibodies to the organisms causing EPM and appears to be more accurate than the Western blot technique, and results of this test have correlated better with clinical signs in STBs suspected of having EPM. A common method to manage horses when all else fails is to treat for EPM and observe the results. Some horses improve despite having no overt neurological signs.

SHOEING AND LAMENESS

Shoeing to obtain ideal high-speed gait is an art, especially in trotters that are difficult to balance. The farrier must be a part of the lameness team. Veterinarians have to take a back seat to the trainer and farrier and cannot be overtly critical of the shoeing approach. Sore front feet are common, and many approaches are used. Sometimes a simple shoeing change redistributes load away from a sore area, and a common approach in trotters is a switch from a half-round to a flip-flop shoe (see Figure 109-5). Classically, trotters are shod with more weight up front, whereas pacers are shod with more weight behind. Recently the tendency has been to lighten shoe weight in trotters and pacers in front and behind. The typical hind shoe of a pacer (a half-round, half-swedge) has been replaced by an aluminum shoe with a low toe grab. Aluminum shoes are used commonly in front in pacers. In trotters, heavy front shoes may predispose to interference injury and carpal lameness, and now aluminum shoes often are used behind, allowing a lighter shoe to be used in front. Light aluminum shoes with grabs allow maximal track purchase and increase speed, but they may worsen existing OA of many distal joints behind and in front. A STB can jog and train abnormally with a sprung shoe or a broken bar shoe. Special attention should be given to the medial half of the front feet because interference bruising is substantial.

A low-heel, underslung foot is not common in modern day STBs, although low-heel, long-toe conformation was previously favored in the erroneous assumption that it would increase stride length. When combined with heavy shoes, long toes prolong breakover, increase stress on the dorsal aspect of the forelimb, and predispose the horse to lameness. Using a shorter toe and more upright front foot is a major improvement in trimming trotters.

Quarter cracks and other hoof wall defects are common. Acrylic and composite repair of hoof defects have aided many sore-footed STBs. Acrylic often is applied to augment the hoof wall. In horses with thin walls, shoes are difficult to maintain, especially when shoes may be changed every 2 to 3 weeks. Overzealous application of acrylic can weaken a normal hoof wall.

TEN MOST COMMON LAMENESS CONDITIONS IN THE NORTH AMERICAN STANDARDBRED RACEHORSE

1. Front foot lameness
2. Carpal lameness
3. Metatarsophalangeal joint lameness
4. Distal hock joint pain and other tarsal lameness
5. Suspensory desmitis: forelimb and hindlimb
6. Metacarpophalangeal joint lameness
7. Splint bone disease
8. Stifle joint lameness
9. Rhabdomyolysis and muscle soreness
10. Other soft tissue lameness: curb and superficial digital flexor tendonitis

SPECIFIC LAMENESS CONDITIONS OF THE STANDARDBRED RACEHORSE

Front Foot Lameness

Front foot lameness is the most common lameness condition. Palmar foot pain abolished using palmar digital analgesia is a common finding, but the veterinarian should keep in mind that palmar digital analgesia also abolishes most of the pain associated with the DIP joint and toe and lower pastern regions. Occasionally, palmar digital analgesia can abolish pain associated with the fetlock joint. Palmar foot pain can be caused by a bruised heel, corns, sheared heel, hoof cracks, contracted heel, wall separations and gravel, stress remodeling and stress fractures, traumatic fractures, OA, or various combinations of these conditions.

Bruises, Corns, and Abscesses

Bruised feet can be caused by faulty conformation such as that seen in a large, flat-footed horse that develops bruising of the heel and bars. Small, narrow-footed horses are prone to quarter and heel cracks and a sore heel. Young STB feet are trimmed and pared and subjected to daily concussion on a firm and unforgiving surface. Aggressive paring can predispose to palmar sole bruising. Overt lameness may not be seen. Horses are often sore when starting from the barn and warm out of lameness after jogging a short distance. Because early carpal lameness can produce similar signs, careful hoof tester examination is necessary and often reveals profound sensitivity across the heel.

Base-wide, toed-out conformation causes overload of the medial heel bulb and quarter, and long, sloping pasterns cause overload of the palmar aspect of the foot. Shoes that are too narrow or those with short branches can cause sole bruising and corns. Horses that interfere (cross-firing or forging) are often shod with the inside branch of the shoe turned in to prevent grabbing and pulling of the shoe, and this can cause corns. Shoeing to correct interference is important but so is management of lameness that may lead to interference. Tubbing and soaking may compound the problem, creating a softer, more easily bruised sole. Poulticing may reduce inflammation initially, but continuous poulticing has the same undesirable result. The sole should be hardened with daily applications of an iodine-based paint, such as Rites paint, an iodine-ether preparation. Attention should be given to the stall bedding because an overly dry stall may lead to dry, cracking hoof walls. Digging out a bruise prolongs lameness and predisposes the hoof to abscessation. A wide web, concave inner surface steel bar shoe is applied if the horse can tolerate this much weight. A trainer may prefer a lighter aluminum bar or egg bar shoe. Full pads may afford protection for an upcoming race, but bruises cannot be reassessed, and sole paint cannot be applied. In trotters the flip-flop shoe is advantageous because the pad can be lifted and the sole painted, and without shoe branches the heel can spread. Deep-seated bruises can become corns; corns can fissure and crack; and bacterial invasion can cause infection. With abscessation, judicious paring to establish drainage is necessary, but the more sole that is removed, the longer it takes to heal. Soaking in warm water with Epsom salts (magnesium sulfate) and then wrapping with ichthammol (an iodine-based drawing salve) promotes drainage.

Sheared Heel

Quarter and heel cracks, wall separations, and a contracted heel can result from a sheared heel. Improper and asymmetrical rasping over time results initially in lowering of one heel bulb and later to vertical heel walls, a contracted heel, and flaring of the wall on the side of the lower heel bulb. With medial-to-lateral hoof imbalance, the vertical heel strikes the ground first, and uneven impact causes structural breakdown between the bulbs of the heel. The heel bulbs are painful, and little resistance is offered to digital displacement of the bulbs in opposite directions. Corrective shoeing involves shoeing the steep side full and floating the quarter. The flared wall is shod tight and rasped off over several trimmings. For a horse with a long-toe and underrun heel predisposed to sheared heel, the toe should be shortened and the heel maintained. Recurrent quarter and heel cracks are common sequelae.

Hoof Cracks

Hoof cracks, depending on location, are known as heel or quarter cracks. Cracks may begin at the coronary band or at the bearing edge of the hoof wall. If the quarter crack extends to the sensitive laminae, local tenderness and variable lameness result. Horses with dry, shelly feet or vertical walls are predisposed to quarter cracks. Untreated chronic inflammation, inappropriate rasping of the periople, and application of excessive acrylic predispose horses to dry feet because exposure of horn tubules results in loss of moisture. Indiscriminate cutting of bars predisposes horses to a contracted heel and results in vertical walls. A vertical wall is more likely to crack than a normal one. Quarter cracks can develop if horses are shod with the web of the shoe set in. To manage quarter cracks, weight bearing is prevented by floating, and artificial support to the weakened and cracked wall is applied using a full or egg bar shoe. Extensive, deep, or painful cracks are repaired and stabilized. Acrylic patches are now preferred, but the crack must be prepared by paring and drying with iodine paint or gentian violet; otherwise, infection may develop.

Contracted Heel

A contracted heel can result from palmar foot pain rather than cause it. Dry, brittle feet cannot expand normally and may contract, as does a foot that has a long toe and low heel. When faced with a choice, farriers too often pick a shoe that fits tight (narrow), rather than full (wide), when the horse really needs a size in between. The wall inevitably grows to the small shoe and contracts. The indiscriminate use of acrylic results in heel contraction because the material restricts expansion. Acrylic should be placed on the weight-bearing wall surface only to repair broken or brittle walls for nail placement or for rebuilding low heels. The last shoe nail should be placed at the bend in the foot quarter, rather than in a more palmar location, to prevent restriction of heel movement. Other causes of palmar foot pain reduce weight bearing at the heel, leading to contraction. To manage a contracted heel, the quarter is softened, the toe is shortened, and an extended bar shoe that fits full (wide) is applied. Lowering the heel to achieve frog pressure is contraindicated.

Wall Separation and Gravel

Gravel is caused by separation of the white line at the quarter and heel and bacterial invasion. Lameness, insidious at first, progresses to nearly non–weight bearing. Digital pulse amplitude is increased, and the horse responds intensely to hoof tester pressure over the affected area. The coronary band or heel bulb becomes sensitive just before infection breaks out. Local therapy such as soaking and poulticing may hasten coalescence and proximal migration of exudate. If pastern cellulitis occurs, broad-spectrum antimicrobial agents should be given. The horse is generally sound within 24 hours after drainage, but a full pad may be necessary to avoid repeat infection during wall healing. Wall separations and gravel are common complications to sheared heels and dry, brittle feet. Seedy toe is an infected wall separation at the toe.

Sidebone

Ossification of the cartilages of the foot (sidebone) is a rare cause of lameness. Ossification may be hastened in horses with poor hoof conformation, particularly in those with chronic medial to lateral hoof imbalance or in those in which interference injury occurs. Sidebone is found more often radiologically in aged horses with large, round, flat feet, but it may be seen incidentally in yearlings. If sidebone is painful to digital palpation, a bar shoe with heel clips and local subcutaneous injection of corticosteroids and Sarapin (High Chemical Company, Levittown, Pennsylvania, United States) may provide temporary relief. Interference injury may cause fracture and infection of a cartilage of the foot.

Fractures of the Distal Phalanx

Fractures of the distal phalanx occur most commonly in the LF lateral and RF medial palmar processes and are usually articular (Figure 108-4).[7] Clockwise training and racing may account for asymmetrical location of fractures. Nonarticular palmar process and midsagittal fractures are rare. Predisposing factors include hard racing surfaces (most fractures occur during a race, more often in winter months), foot imbalance, impact on an uneven surface, and overloading. Fractures of the distal phalanx are unlikely single-event injuries and are the sequelae to maladaptive or nonadaptive remodeling of the distal phalanx that results from stress-related bone injury. IRU often is seen in the lateral aspect of the LF and medial aspect of the RF

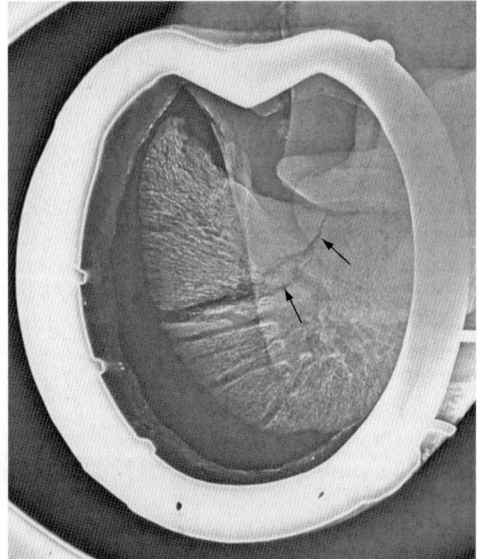

Fig. 108-4 • Dorsomedial proximal-palmarolateral distal oblique xeroradiographic image of the right front foot of a Standardbred racehorse. There is a typical articular fracture of the medial palmar process *(arrows)* of the distal phalanx. The horse is shod with a bar shoe with clips.

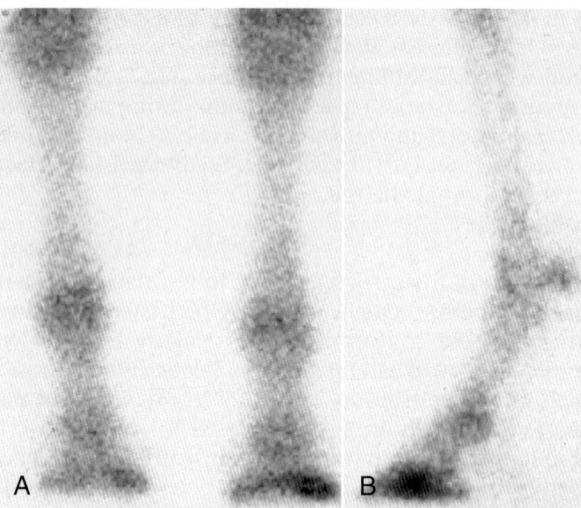

Fig. 108-5 • A, Dorsal delayed (bone phase) scintigraphic image showing a typical distribution of increased radiopharmaceutical uptake of the Standardbred front feet. The left forelimb is on the right. **B,** Lateral delayed (bone) phase scintigraphic image of the left forelimb. This Standardbred was lame in the left forelimb, and lameness was localized to the lateral aspect of the distal phalanx. In the left forelimb, stress remodeling of subchondral bone of the distal phalanx was diagnosed. Increased radiopharmaceutical uptake involving the lateral aspect of the left forelimb and medial aspect of the right forelimb distal phalanx is thought to be caused by counterclockwise training and racing, and stress-related bone injury can lead to fracture in these locations.

distal phalanx in horses with lameness abolished by palmar digital analgesia but in which radiographs are negative (Figure 108-5).[8] Most fractures of the distal phalanx occur in aged horses. Treatment includes application of a wide web, concave inner surface steel straight or egg bar shoe with two side clips on each side. Horses are given 3 months of stall rest and then 3 months of turnout in a small paddock. Most fractures are complete but nondisplaced; mild displacement results in a step in the articular surface. Fractures take months to heal, and some appear to develop chronic nonunions, although many horses return to racing soundness even with a radiologically apparent nonunion. Distal phalangeal fractures in the hind feet are unusual to rare but generally involve the medial plantar process and are articular in location.[5] OA of the DIP joint often occurs, particularly in horses with displacement or nonunion, but unless severe, prognosis for racing is good. Osteochondral fragments of the extensor process of the distal phalanx are unusual, but arthroscopic removal of small fragments and repair of large ones are indicated. Prognosis is fair, but OA of the DIP joint can affect prognosis negatively.

Osteoarthritis of the Distal Interphalangeal Joint

The earliest sign of primary OA of the DIP joint is effusion. Effusion is also common in horses with nondescript foot soreness. Intraarticular injections of hyaluronan and corticosteroids are often performed into the DIP joint. Progressive OA can cause severe lameness, chronic fibrosis, and thickening of the DIP joint capsule, radiological evidence of proliferative changes on the dorsal aspect of the middle phalanx and extensor process of the distal phalanx, and narrowing of the DIP joint space.

Other Foot Lameness

Navicular disease is a rare cause of palmar foot pain. In 2-year-olds and early 3-year-olds, IRU in the navicular bone is seen in delayed (bone) phase scintigraphic images, indicating abnormal bone modeling, but rarely do radiographs show substantial changes, except for mild medullary increased radiopacity. Navicular bone fracture, cysts, and acute separation of bipartite navicular bone are diagnosed rarely in forelimbs and hindlimbs. Horses with bipartite bones or fractures have a poor prognosis, and palmar digital neurectomy is recommended. Keratomas in young racehorses are not seen, but they can occur rarely in broodmares or older STBs being used for alternative sporting activities.

Undiagnosed foot lameness—sore feet—is common. Horses have sensitivity to hoof testers and likely have soft tissue trauma, but a definitive diagnosis cannot be made. Treatment of the DIP joint with corticosteroids and hyaluronan, perineural injection of antiinflammatory agents, and shoeing changes are recommended.

Carpal Lameness

The carpus is the most common articular location for lameness and conformational faults. In 2-year-olds, carpal synovitis is common. High prevalence of carpal lameness is caused in part by racing young, immature STBs around tight turns on firm surfaces. The medial aspect of the middle carpal joint and the right carpus are predisposed to injury. Lateral injury of the carpus is unusual. Heat, effusion, and pain on careful palpation of the dorsal surfaces are common. Heat (the perception of warmth) on the dorsal aspect of the carpus is the earliest clinical sign of subchondral bone injury of the dorsomedial aspect of the middle carpal joint. Lameness varies with severity of injury, and horses carry the limb in an abducted position during advancement (see Chapter 38). Response to flexion varies, and diagnosis should be confirmed using intraarticular or median and ulnar analgesia. Secondary shoulder muscle soreness often develops. Horses warm out of lameness, and weeks to months may pass before consistent lameness is seen. Radiographs are usually negative or equivocal initially, but increased radiopacity of the third carpal bone and mild marginal osteophyte production can predispose the horse to small osteochondral fragments or slab fractures of the third carpal bone. The mere presence of increased radiopacity of the third carpal bone, however, is not diagnostic for subchondral bone pain because mild sclerosis is an adaptive response to race training (Figure 108-6). Diagnosis of subchondral bone pain as a result of maladaptive or nonadaptive remodeling is made using a combination of abnormal clinical and imaging findings. In a radiological study evaluating degree of increased radiopacity of the third carpal bone, exercised horses had significantly more increased radiopacity than nonexercised control horses, and lameness referrable to the middle carpal joint developed more commonly in STBs with higher degrees of third carpal bone increased radiopacity.[9] Thirty percent of STBs in the study developed lameness of the middle carpal joint.[9] In a separate study the same investigators determined the importance of middle carpal joint pain in STBs and found carpal lameness to be present in 28% of STBs overall and in 56% of those with forelimb lameness.[10] Carpal lameness was the most common reason for more

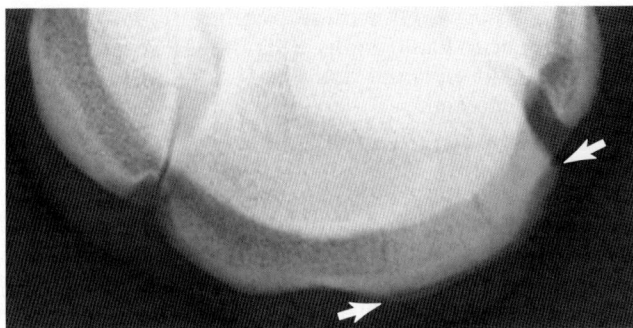

Fig. 108-6 • Dorsoproximal-dorsodistal digital radiographic image of the right distal row of carpal bones in a 2-year-old Standardbred filly that was sound and racing successfully at the time of this radiological study conducted as part of an examination before purchase (medial is to the right). Mild-to-moderate increased radiopacity of the radial fossa (between *arrows*) is seen as an adaptive response to training and racing. This filly continued to race successfully for the remainder of the 2- and 3-year-old racing years.

than 1 month of rest in STBs in race training. Few clinical signs such as effusion were present. Risk factors were faulty conformation and intense speed training.[10] Diagnostic analgesia remains a most important aspect of clinical diagnosis, given the lack of early clinical signs associated with subchondral bone injury. Scintigraphic examination often reveals focal areas of IRU, usually involving the third carpal bone or the subchondral bone of the dorsomedial aspect of the middle carpal joint collectively; bilateral lesions are common (see Figure 19-16). Stress-related bone injury results in a continuum of subchondral and overlying cartilage damage, eventually leading to OA or osteochondral fragments. Rest is the best form of management but is usually unacceptable to trainers and owners. Topical counterirritation with iodine paints is still popular and is used with apparent success because blistering usually is accompanied by a reduction in exercise intensity. The administration of NSAIDs for 3 to 5 days and a brief period of reduced exercise (2 weeks) may be an acceptable compromise between the veterinarian and the trainer, but keep in mind that although a reduction in training intensity is helpful, bone cannot heal in 2 weeks, and pain may not subside. Intraarticular injections of hyaluronan or polysulfated glycosaminoglycans (PSGAGs) may reduce inflammation and theoretically may be useful in cartilage healing, but these often are used in a palliative rather than therapeutic manner, given a lack of synovitis in most horses. Injections may be of little benefit when pain originates from subchondral bone. Ten 2-year-old STBs with mild carpitis were treated with three to five weekly intraarticular injections with PSGAGs (Adequan, Luitpold Pharmaceuticals, Inc., Shirley, New York, United States) and were compared with a control group receiving NSAIDs and topical counterirritation.[11] The treated group had substantially less carpal lameness during the ensuing racing season. All horses raced, but horses in the control group required intraarticular injections to maintain soundness. Early aggressive intraarticular therapy may forestall development of progressive OA in young STBs. Extracorporeal shock wave therapy has gained popularity as an adjunctive therapy in the management of STBs with subchondral bone injury and OA. With the exception of a palliative analgesic effect, the role of this

modality in potentiating healing remains unknown. The possibility exists that as a result of the analgesic effect horses could be continued in training well past the ability of injured bone to adapt.

Palmar foot pain may play a role in the development of carpal lameness in young STBs. Early carpal lameness is easier to treat if palmar foot pain is recognized early and managed aggressively. In horses with bruised bars and poor medial-to-lateral hoof balance, the application of wide web bar shoes reduces inflammation and signs of carpal lameness. In all ages of trotters, the flip-flop shoe appears to be effective in reducing clinical signs of carpal lameness. Small osteochondral fragments of the carpus are the most common fractures and involve the third and radial carpal bones and rarely other bones in the middle carpal and antebrachiocarpal joints. Arthroscopic surgical removal and PSGAG therapy after surgery are recommended. Frontal (dorsal) and sagittal slab fractures occur commonly, and repair using screws placed in lag fashion is recommended. Small, frontal slab fracture fragments can be removed. Although rest is an option in horses with nondisplaced fractures, internal fixation may shorten recovery period and reduce risk of recurrence (see Chapter 38).

Metatarsophalangeal Joint Lameness
The metatarsophalangeal joint is a common source of pain causing lameness in STBs, and diagnostic analgesia is usually essential for diagnosis.

Stress and Maladaptive or Nonadaptive Remodeling
Stress and maladaptive or nonadaptive remodeling of the metatarsophalangeal joint most often involves the distal, plantarolateral aspect of the MtIII, PSBs, and the proximal aspect of the proximal phalanx (see Chapters 19 and 42).[6,12] Initially the horse has a variable, subtle, high-speed lameness, most commonly manifested around turns or by the horse making breaks. Later, grade 1 to 2 of 5 hindlimb lameness is seen at the trot in hand. Lameness can be localized to the metatarsophalangeal joint, but it does not improve with intraarticular treatment. Palpation findings are negative or equivocal. Horses show variable responses to flexion and have negative radiological findings but positive responses to diagnostic analgesia. The low plantar or lateral plantar metatarsal block is most effective, but horses may respond partially to intraarticular analgesia (and may require 12 mL of local anesthetic solution). Later, increased radiopacity and radiolucent changes of the plantarolateral aspect of the MtIII are seen on down-angled radiographic images. Ultrasonographic evaluation may reveal a defect in articular cartilage late in the disease process. Scintigraphic examination is the best way to establish a diagnosis and shows focal IRU involving the distal aspect of the MtIII (see Figures 19-6, 19-20, 42-1 through 42-3, and 42-6 through 42-9). The disease can affect both hindlimbs. The distal aspect of the MtIII appears at risk to develop stress-related bone injury before other sites in the metatarsophalangeal joint, possibly from anatomical variations or uneven loading during the full extension and landing phases of the stride. Shoe additives such as calks or grabs may play an adverse mechanical role. The metatarsophalangeal joint is a high-motion joint and subject to high-strain cyclic fatigue (repetitive loading) that is encountered during intense exercise around turns and on hard surfaces. This

continuum of stress-related bone injury can lead to OA and fracture (see Chapter 42).

Exercise intensity is reduced for 1 to 3 weeks. If lameness is prominent, a 3- to 4-month rest period is necessary. Exercise reduction allows the modeling and remodeling processes to equilibrate and microdamage to heal. A flat shoe is applied or the horse is left bare footed. Cold water therapy and the administration of NSAIDs (phenylbutazone or acetylsalicylic acid) appear helpful initially. Intraarticular injections of hyaluronan and PSGAGs may help, but early in disease, overlying cartilage damage and synovitis are not prominent, and response to intraarticular injections is minimal. When radiolucent changes and synovitis develop, response to intraarticular injections is better, but prognosis is worsened. Extracorporeal shock wave and radial pressure wave therapy may be useful in providing partial analgesia and may prolong training and racing. Bisphosphonate therapy is currently used for many conditions, including subchondral bone pain, OA, and other bone-related problems, but efficacy is unknown (see Chapter 42, page 490). In TBs there is a higher risk of catastrophic breakdown than in STBs, although the wisdom of training and racing a STB with chronic pain is certainly debatable. Whenever possible, frank advice must be given to trainers and owners about the long-term sequelae of continued training and racing a STB with a condition that may lead to OA.

Fractures

Acute, severe lameness is seen most commonly in STBs with fractures of the metatarsophalangeal joint, but some horses can race with incomplete fractures. Horses shorten the cranial phase of the stride, land on the toe, and rapidly compensate with other limbs. Often no effusion or pain on flexion is apparent unless a fracture is displaced. Diagnostic analgesia and examination in harness are avoided if a fracture is suspected because comminution or displacement can occur. Radiographs, including flexed dorsoplantar or 125° dorsoplantar and flexed lateromedial images, should be obtained.

Midsagittal fractures of the proximal phalanx are most common, causing severe intermittent or severe unrelenting lameness, depending on fracture length and configuration. Fractures can be short, incomplete with mild periosteal proliferation on the dorsal aspect of the proximal phalanx (Figure 108-7) or long, incomplete or complete midsagittal fractures, fractures that break out of the lateral cortex, and comminuted fractures (see Figure 36-10). Horses with short, midsagittal fractures often race or train because lameness is intermittent and often abates after several days. Clinical signs precede radiological evidence of fracture for 7 to 21 days, and scintigraphic examination reveals focal IRU in the proximal aspect of the proximal phalanx (see Figure 19-20, *C*). Horses with short, midsagittal fractures can be rested or have internal fixation and have a good prognosis with either treatment.[13] Long incomplete, complete, displaced, or comminuted fractures should be repaired. Prognosis depends on degree of comminution and displacement and whether a strut of bone is intact to which to attach fragments. Horses with comminuted fractures rarely race again and are at risk of infection, fracture displacement, and OA of the metatarsophalangeal and proximal interphalangeal joints and contralateral limb laminitis (see Chapter 35).

Dorsal plane (frontal) fractures of the proximal phalanx can be unilateral or bilateral, are most common in the RH, and occur in trotters and pacers (see Figure 42-11 and accompanying text). Fractures of the PSBs are common and most often involve the lateral PSB. Small medial abaxial fragments can be difficult to identify. Apical PSB fractures are most common, but abaxial, midbody, and rarely basilar fractures occur, and the combination of suspensory

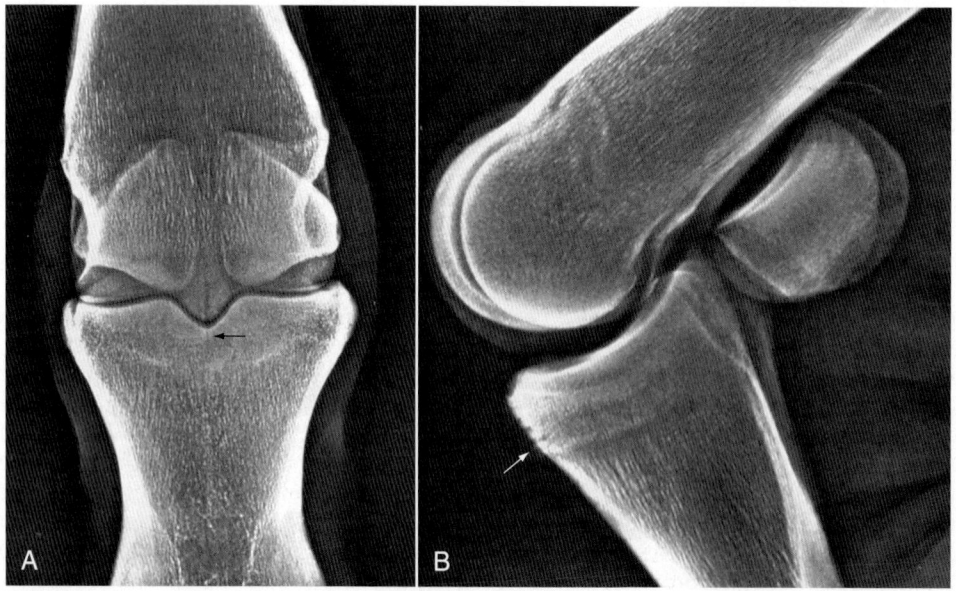

Fig. 108-7 • Dorsoplantar (**A**) and flexed lateromedial (**B**) xeroradiographic images showing a short, incomplete, midsagittal fracture of the proximal phalanx *(arrow)*. There is slight periosteal new bone on the proximodorsal aspect of the proximal phalanx seen in the flexed lateromedial image *(white arrow)*. Radiological changes often lag behind clinical signs, and follow-up radiological and scintigraphic examinations often are needed to establish a diagnosis.

desmitis, and splint bone and PSB fractures is not uncommon. Horses show acute lameness after training or racing, with grade 3 to 4 of 5 lameness, and prefer to bear weight only on the toe. Effusion and a positive response to flexion are usually present, and the diagnosis is confirmed radiologically. Ultrasonographic examination of the SL should be performed to establish baseline information and assess prognosis. Surgical removal of apical, abaxial, and basilar fragments and surgical repair of displaced midbody fractures using bone screws or wiring techniques are recommended. Prognosis is guarded in trotters and fair in pacers that have raced before fracture. Horses in which fractures occur early in training appear to have a poor prognosis. Of 43 STBs with apical PSB fractures no difference in prognosis was found between pacers and trotters; 86% of fractures involved the hindlimbs. Prognosis was better in STBs with hindlimb PSB fractures than with forelimb injuries. Eighty-eight percent of horses that raced before injury raced after injury, whereas only 56% of those previously unraced raced after injury. Neither fracture fragment dimensions nor associated suspensory desmitis negatively affected outcome.[14] These latter two findings are surprising given our experience.

Condylar fractures of the McIII or the MtIII occur, and fractures of the lateral condyles are more common than those of the medial condyles. Medial condylar fractures of the MtIII outnumber those occurring in the McIII. Clinical signs are similar to those caused by midsagittal fracture of the proximal phalanx, but diagnosis can be difficult unless good-quality radiographs with appropriate views are obtained. A flexed dorsoplantar or 125° dorsoplantar image should be obtained. Medial condylar fractures often spiral proximally and should be repaired, although even with repair there is a risk of catastrophic failure of the bone. In general, lateral condylar fractures of the McIII or the MtIII are best managed using surgical fixation, although STBs with short, incomplete fractures can be successfully managed conservatively. Regardless of management method, prognosis is favorable; 12 of 13 STBs with incomplete condylar fractures of the MtIII and 7 of 9 with incomplete condylar fractures of the McIII raced after injury.[15] Four of six surviving horses with medial spiral fractures of the MtIII raced after injury.[15] In that study, TBs were overrepresented and STBs were underrepresented when compared with the hospital population; TBs had significantly more lateral condylar fractures and forelimb condylar fractures than did STBs.[15]

Osteochondrosis

The metatarsophalangeal joint is a major site for osteochondrosis, and the most common manifestation is plantar fragmentation. A complete discussion of axial, articular fragments and abaxial, nonarticular fragments and other forms of osteochondrosis can be found in Chapter 42. Some debate exists over the management of STBs with axial, articular fragments and abaxial, nonarticular fragments and other fragments. Horses with axial, articular fragments and dorsal fragments respond well to arthroscopic removal and postoperative intraarticular injections of PSGAGs or hyaluronan. We believe that surgical removal prolongs racing careers and decreases metatarsophalangeal joint lameness. Some horses, particularly pacers, race successfully without surgery.

Proliferative synovitis, radiolucent defects of the PSBs, traumatic small osteochondral fragments of the proximal phalanx, and OA are discussed in Chapter 42.

Distal Hock Joint Pain and Other Tarsal Lameness

The hock joint is under considerable stress and strain, especially going into turns and with quick acceleration. Distal hock joint pain and progressive OA of the TMT and CD joints are common. However, distal hock joint pain should not be a default diagnosis, and careful lameness examination, including diagnostic analgesia, should always be performed. Injection of the "knees and hocks" is commonplace in the STB sport, despite our experience highlighting the importance of the metatarsophalangeal joint as a cause of hindlimb pain. Horses with distal hock joint pain warm out of lameness, often dramatically, because they may come out of the barn or paddock on the toe and eventually be able to train or race successfully. Horses show a mildly shortened cranial phase of the stride and a stabbing type of gait, with medial deviation of the limb during protraction and landing first on the outside toe (stabbing laterally), but this gait is not pathognomonic for distal hock joint pain. Palpation in a flexed position often reveals pain of periarticular soft tissue structures, and the Churchill test is often positive. Upper limb flexion is positive, but diagnostic analgesia is essential for diagnosis. Radiographs may show evidence of OA in older horses, but radiographs are negative or equivocal in most 2- and 3-year-olds. Changes are seen most often in the DM-PlIO image, but dorsoplantar, lateromedial, and slightly off dorsoplantar images can be helpful. Scintigraphic examination confirms that OA of the TMT joint is most common, and changes are lateral and dorsolateral (Figure 108-8). Focal IRU is sometimes seen involving only the CD joint in horses that failed to respond to intraarticular analgesia of the TMT joint, emphasizing the need to block and treat each joint separately.

Treatment comprises intraarticular injections, NSAIDs, shoeing changes, and rest. Early, intraarticular hyaluronan is useful to decrease inflammation, and concomitant use of NSAIDs such as phenylbutazone (4.4 mg/kg PO daily for 5 days and 2.2 mg/kg PO daily for 5 days) is recommended initially. Later, as OA progresses, methylprednisolone acetate (80 mg/joint every 6 to 8 weeks) is most effective to manage inflammation. A series of intraarticular and intramuscular injections of PSGAGs also can be given. In horses with severe OA, 4 to 6 months of rest is successful, but recurrent lameness often mandates a limited racing schedule (10 to 15 starts/year). The toe is shortened, and a flat aluminum or steel squared-toe shoe is applied to allow easy breakover. All shoe additives are removed to decrease shear stress.[11]

Slab fractures of the third tarsal bone and fractures of the proximal, dorsomedial aspect of the MtIII result from stress-related bone injury or from pathological fractures in horses with OA (see Chapter 44). Third tarsal bone fractures are the most common and are best seen on a DM-PlIO image. Fractures of the central tarsal bone are usually oblique, involve the dorsal aspect of the bone, occur without concomitant OA, and are best seen in lateromedial images. Conservative management is recommended in horses with nondisplaced fractures, but displaced fractures should be repaired. Ninety-two percent of horses with slab fractures of

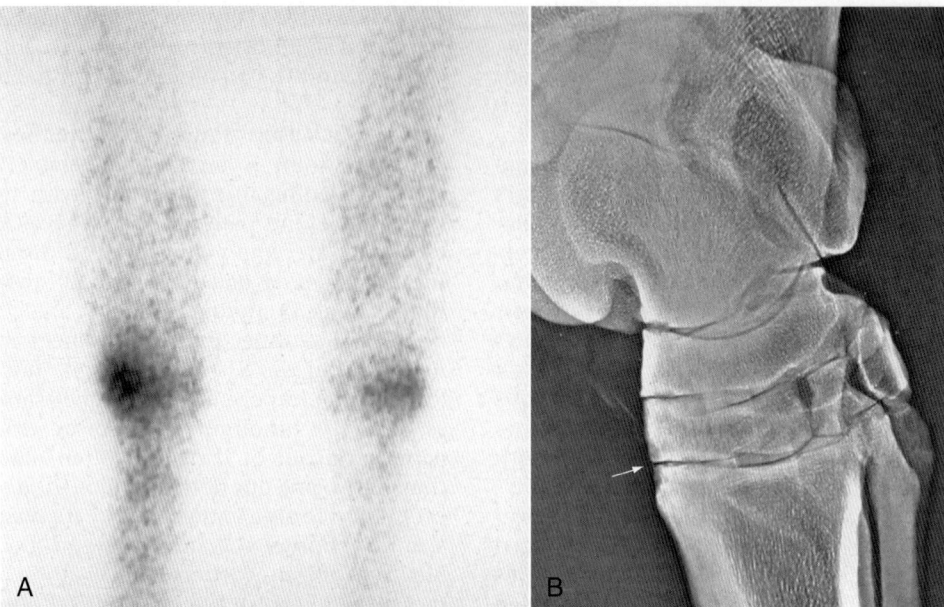

Fig. 108-8 • A, Plantar delayed (bone) phase scintigraphic image of the hocks. There is focal, nucleate *(right)* and intense *(left)* increased radiopharmaceutical uptake in the dorsolateral aspect of both tarsometatarsal joints (left hindlimb is on the left) in this 2-year-old Standardbred filly. **B,** Dorsomedial-plantarolateral oblique xeroradiographic image of the left hindlimb showing minimal changes *(arrow)*. Lameness and scintigraphic evidence of distal tarsitis precede radiological changes by many months.

the third tarsal bone and 88% with slab fractures of the central tarsal bone raced after conservative management.[16]

The tarsocrural joint is often injected, but tarsocrural joint lameness is uncommon, except in young horses with osteochondrosis. Trainers often request injection of the upper and lower hock joints (tarsocrural and TMT joints), but lameness most likely is caused by pain associated with the distal hock joints. Bog spavin occurs most commonly in weanlings and yearlings, and radiological identification of osteochondrosis fragments prompts surgical removal. Most yearlings begin training without fragments. Although debate exists about the importance of tarsocrural osteochondrosis and lameness, we recommend surgical removal to resolve current inflammation, if present, and to prevent future lameness. However, osteochondrosis fragments are seen in some older racehorses in which neither lameness nor effusion is present. Tarsocrural lameness may occur without effusion, and diagnostic analgesia is necessary to differentiate the site of hock pain. Good-quality radiographs are essential to discover occult osteochondrosis fragments and fractures. The DM-PlLO image is best for evaluating the cranial aspect of the intermediate ridge of the tibia and a slightly oblique dorsoplantar image (dorsal 5° to 7° lateral-plantaromedial oblique) is best to evaluate the medial malleolus. The most common sites for osteochondrosis are the cranial aspect of the intermediate ridge of the tibia, lateral trochlear ridge of the talus, medial malleolus of the tibia, medial trochlear ridge of the talus, and lateral malleolus of the tibia. Medial malleolar fragments appear to be increasing in importance, particularly in trotters, although a heightened awareness and improved imaging may be uncovering fragments in this location that may have previously been missed. Osteochondrosis fragments can be large, numerous, loose, and free floating, and cartilage damage can be prominent even in yearlings;

however, prognosis is good with removal. If distention of the tarsocrural joint is unexplained, osteochondrosis of the medial malleolus of the tibia should be suspected, and diagnostic arthroscopy is recommended. Small osteochondrosis fragments (dewdrop lesions) of the distal aspect of the medial trochlear ridge of the talus may be incidental but can cause lameness if displaced or if impinging on the central tarsal bone. Surgical removal is recommended.

Tarsocrural OA occurs in older horses (usually >5 years) and may be associated with osteochondrosis because fragments often are seen concomitantly. OA causes progressive lameness and effusion, but intraarticular analgesia should be performed to validate the source of pain. Large volumes of local anesthetic solution (30 to 50 mL) are necessary because pain is severe; false-negative responses occur if 10 to 15 mL is used. Radiographs may reveal prominent increased radiopacity and narrowing of the tarsocrural joint space, but end-stage OA can be present with only subtle radiological abnormalities (Figure 108-9, *A*). Scintigraphic evaluation reveals diffuse IRU on both sides of the tarsocrural joint and is useful to differentiate OA from sagittal fracture of the talus (Figure 108-9, *B*) or subchondral injury of the distal aspect of the tibia. Prognosis is grave.

Sagittal fracture of the talus is unusual. Acute, grade 3 to 4 of 5 lameness is localized to the tarsocrural joint by diagnostic analgesia, but often subtle tarsal lameness precedes fracture. Focal IRU is seen involving the talus (see Figure 108-9, *B*), and slightly oblique dorsoplantar images reveal subchondral lucency or fracture. Eight of 11 horses with sagittal fracture of the talus were STBs, and 7 raced after being managed conservatively.[17]

Enthesitis of the long, lateral collateral ligament of the tarsocrural joint, on the lateral aspect of the calcaneus, results in mild to moderate lameness and mild tarsocrural

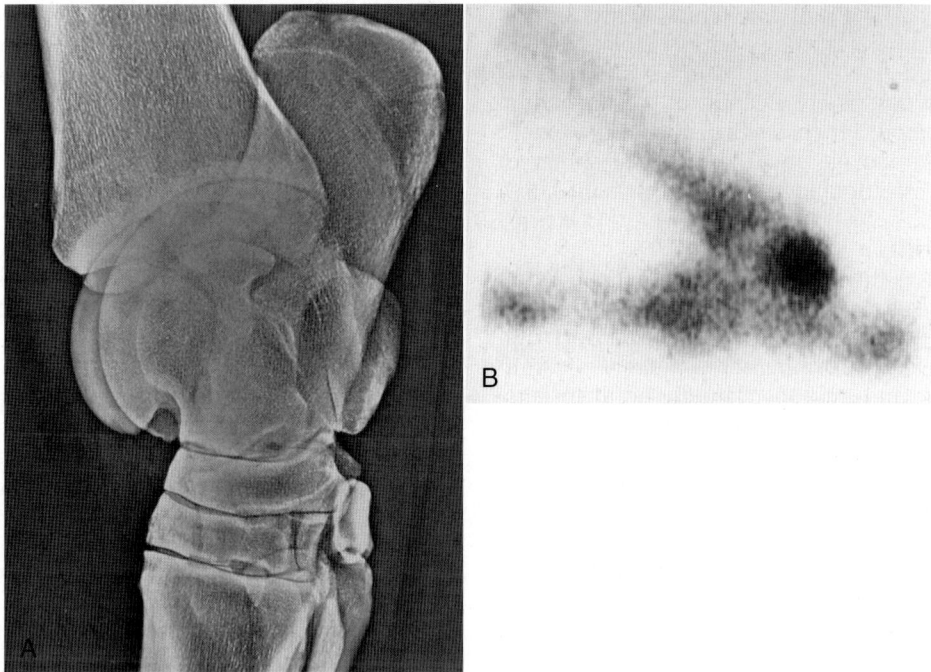

Fig. 108-9 • A, In this dorsomedial-plantarolateral oblique xeroradiographic image, the tarsocrural joint space is narrow, indicating end-stage OA of the tarsocrural joint, but this radiological sign is difficult to recognize because proliferative changes are minimal. **B,** Flexed lateral delayed (bone) phase scintigraphic image of a different Standardbred with a sagittal fracture of the talus. With flexion, the area of moderate to intense increased radiopharmaceutical uptake moves with the talus and can be differentiated clearly from end-stage osteoarthritis (OA) or distal tibial subchondral trauma.

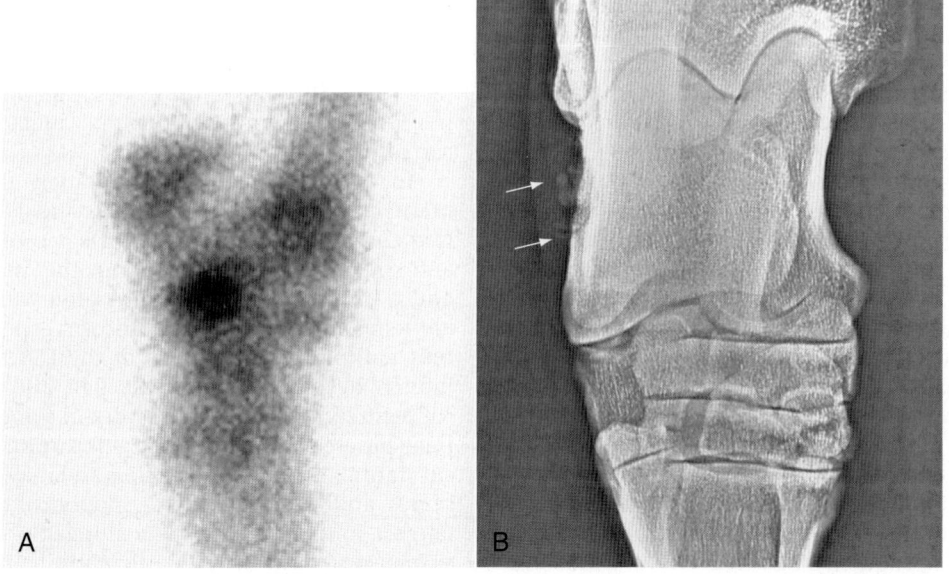

Fig. 108-10 • A, Lateral delayed (bone) phase scintigraphic image of a hock showing focal, moderate to intense increased radiopharmaceutical uptake in the calcaneus. **B,** Dorsoplantar xeroradiographic image showing proliferative changes associated with the collateral ligament attachment on the lateral aspect of the calcaneus *(arrows).*

effusion (Figure 108-10). Soft tissue swelling is easy to miss initially, and radiological changes lag behind clinical signs for at least 14 to 21 days; however, lameness abates or is improved considerably with tarsocrural analgesia. Scintigraphic examination reveals focal IRU in the lateral aspect of the calcaneus. Local injections and radiation therapy may allow continued racing, but rest to allow enthesitis to subside is often necessary.

Injury of the fibularis tertius tendon anywhere from the midcrus to the distal tarsus can occur but is rare, and injury usually occurs at the insertion on the MtIII and the third tarsal bone. Soft tissue swelling is present, and the hock can be pushed forward without concomitant extension of the stifle with the limb in standing position. Horses require 4 to 6 months of rest.

Inflammatory synovitis or infection of the tarsocrural joint is not uncommon. Prognosis depends on the extent of existing cartilage damage and the financial ability of owners to manage infection aggressively (see Chapter 65).

Suspensory Desmitis

Suspensory desmitis is the most common soft tissue injury and can be classified as unilateral branch desmitis, bilateral branch desmitis, body desmitis, and PSD. Suspensory desmitis is often an overload compensatory lameness condition because fatigue and improper landing occur in lame horses. Suspensory desmitis is seldom a single-event injury but is caused by accumulated damage over weeks to months (see Chapter 72). Diagnosis is made by careful palpation from the origin to the insertion of the SL with the limb in standing and flexed positions. The splint bones and PSBs are examined for associated injuries. One of us (JBM) has found that horses with core lesions are lamer, but exhibit fewer outward signs of inflammation, than those with peripheral lesions. Horses with suspensory branch desmitis are common and heal quicker (6 to 8 weeks) with lower recurrence than do those with body desmitis and PSD (4 to 6 months). Core lesions recur frequently. Because suspensory desmitis is often a compensatory injury, the primary lameness needs to be resolved. For example, OA and osteochondral fragments of the left carpus frequently cause suspensory desmitis of the RF in horses of both gaits, RH suspensory desmitis in trotters, and LH suspensory desmitis in pacers.

Ultrasonographic examination is critical in assessing the SL, and its entire length should be examined systematically. In hindlimbs, enlargement of the origin and body is more common than core lesions, and cross-sectional area measurements of the affected and contralateral limb are mandatory. Branches are evaluated for change in shape, loss of margin definition, central or marginal hypoechoic lesions, subcutaneous hemorrhage and edema, fibrosis and calcification, irregular contour (step line defects), and avulsion fragments of the PSBs. The intersesamoidean ligament rarely is involved.

Forelimb unilateral branch desmitis results from toed-in or toed-out conformation, hoof imbalance, and uneven landing. To correct interference injury with knee knocking resulting from toed-out conformation, the hoof is commonly lowered on the inside, causing uneven loading and medial unilateral branch desmitis, whereas in horses with toed-in conformation, lateral unilateral branch desmitis occurs. Improper impact can occur from fatigue or if a horse is stopped suddenly. Lameness varies with severity of injury and presence of associated splint and PSB disorders.

Forelimb bilateral branch desmitis is caused by acute or chronic hyperextension of the metacarpophalangeal joint. Prognosis depends on the degree of fetlock drop seen when the contralateral limb is held in flexion. Concomitant PSB fractures can occur. Dorsal subluxation (flexion) of the proximal interphalangeal joint is seen in horses with bilateral branch desmitis and body desmitis, whereas palmar subluxation (extension) is seen in horses with distal sesamoidean desmitis and loss of palmar support. If the axis of the proximal interphalangeal joint is altered, the prognosis for racing is poor.

Forelimb body desmitis often begins just proximal to the bifurcation of the SL, and careful palpation reveals pain and mild enlargement. The first sign may be mild swelling, without lameness, and training and racing are often continued, leading to further suspensory desmitis. Horses often race successfully with chronic suspensory branch desmitis, but if desmitis progresses into the body, lameness becomes pronounced. There is a considerable difference in the potential for catastrophic breakdown injury with branch desmitis between TBs and STBs. Rarely, a STB develops catastrophic injury of the suspensory apparatus as a result of chronic suspensory desmitis, whereas continued racing with any suspensory branch desmitis is dangerous in TBs. Chronic enlargement and thickening of the SL often cause bowing of the splint bones, and concussion leads to fracture. Horses with recalcitrant swelling of the SL should be examined with ultrasonography because exuberant exostosis from fractures may encroach on the SL and cause swelling and pain.

Proximal palmar metacarpal pain is common and often called a check ligament problem, although genuine desmitis of the accessory ligament of the DDFT is rare. Palmar metacarpal pain can be caused by avulsion or longitudinal fracture of the McIII and stress reaction/stress fracture of the McIII, but PSD is most common. STBs often have pain on palpation of the proximal palmar metacarpal region and may have compensatory PSD, with primary lameness elsewhere. Lameness is noticed in the first half of the support phase of stride. An exaggerated head nod is often noted (JSM). A carpal type of gait may be seen. Lameness is most prominent when the affected limb is on the outside of a circle. Local analgesia and ultrasonographic examination should be performed. Radiographs are necessary to identify bone injury. Scintigraphic examination is useful to differentiate proximal metacarpal pain from carpal pain.

In hindlimbs, unilateral branch desmitis, bilateral branch desmitis, body desmitis, and PSD occur but less frequently than in forelimbs. Degree of lameness varies, and similar concerns exist about the MtIII, a splint bone, and a PSB involvement. Horses often land on the toe and are reluctant to put the heel down, especially if a concurrent pathological condition of the PSB exists. Suspensory branch desmitis often occurs first and can be managed successfully with continued work in some horses, but proximal progression toward the bifurcation and body causes substantial increase in lameness and may involve the splint bones, and often horses lose support of the metatarsophalangeal joint. Racing can no longer continue. Hindlimb suspensory desmitis is particularly important in young trotters. Many top 2- and 3-year-old trotters have been retired because of hindlimb suspensory desmitis. Second to carpal lameness, hindlimb suspensory desmitis is the most dangerous, career-limiting cause of lameness in trotters.

Early PSD can go unrecognized because of lack of obvious swelling. Local analgesia is critical for diagnosis. Once desmitis involves the body, swelling may be recognized, but damage is now extensive.

Inflammation can be suppressed, but rest is essential for healing. Rest is not well received by owners and trainers, who often exert pressure to keep a horse in work.

Cryotherapy is used to manage horses with suspensory branch desmitis and distal body desmitis. Horses with marginal lesions respond well but not those with core lesions. Cryotherapy decreases pain and seems to promote more or better-organized scar tissue. Periligamentous injections of sclerosing agents such as sodium oleate promote fibrosis and can be used to cause a swollen SL to "set up." Periligamentous injections of corticosteroid mixtures reduce inflammation and lameness, but if training and racing continue, further damage occurs. Many naive owners lack understanding that the latest popular injection does not promote healing but simply masks inflammatory signs. Although horses may continue to race a few more starts, further damage inevitably occurs. Horses with PSD often can be managed using injections of corticosteroids, internal blisters, and, if available, radiation therapy, and if lameness is mild and support is not lost, racing may continue. Shock wave therapy has gained prominence and shows promise.

Rest is the best approach, and there is no substitute. Between 3 to 6 months of rest may be necessary to allow healing. A combination of stall rest, handwalking, walking in the jog cart, and swimming is recommended. We do not recommend turnout, but many horses are blistered and turned out, although this has been shown to be detrimental to healing. Healing progress is assessed by ultrasonography. Surgical management using a modified Asheim approach (ligament splitting, or desmoplasty) and ostectomy of fractured splint bones and PSB fragments is recommended. Desmoplasty and injection of fresh liquid bone marrow have been used successfully (MWR). Other intraligamentous injections with products such as platelet-rich plasma and stem cells have shown modest success. One of us (MWR) has performed bone marrow injection and fasciotomy on a limited number of top trotters with hindlimb PSD and body desmitis with modest success.

Prognosis depends on level of injury, gait (trotters worse than pacers), severity of injury (poor prognosis with fetlock drop), and associated bony pathological conditions. Unless the SL is totally disrupted, prognosis for racing is good, but racing class is an important consideration because few STBs return to the same or improved race class after sustaining suspensory desmitis (Figure 108-11).

Metacarpophalangeal Joint Lameness

Fatigue from underconditioning and other factors causing overload may lead to hyperextension of the metacarpophalangeal joint. Hyperextension leads to injury of the dorsal aspect of the joint, such as small osteochondral fragments of the proximal phalanx and proliferative synovitis, and to injury of the palmar aspect of the joint, such as fractures of the PSBs and suspensory branch insertional injury. Traumatic disruption of the suspensory apparatus is rare but usually involves rupture of the SL. Stress-related bone injury of subchondral bone leading to OA and fracture occurs in the metacarpophalangeal joint, as described for the metatarsophalangeal joint. In a STB with normal conformation, metacarpophalangeal effusion should be a red flag (a barometer), often a sign of compensatory lameness. Young horses often have bilateral metacarpophalangeal synovitis secondary to palmar foot pain because toe-first landing overloads the joint. Corrective trimming and shoeing often helps. In older horses unilateral carpal lameness

often causes contralateral metacarpophalangeal synovitis. Primary lameness of the metacarpophalangeal can begin when horses break stride, stumble, or stop quickly.

OA and stress-related bone injury are the most common problems of the metacarpophalangeal joint. Early radiographs are usually negative, but radiolucency and increased radiopacity of the distal medial aspect of the McIII develop later. Scintigraphic evidence of IRU is more prominent medially, unlike in the metatarsophalangeal joint, in which IRU is more common laterally. In older horses (about 4 years of age) with progressive severe OA, narrowing of the medial joint space indicates severe cartilage damage. Owners are incredulous that the horse has end-stage OA because lameness can be acute and severe, and fracture often is suspected.

Early OA is treated using intraarticular injection of hyaluronan alone or a combination of hyaluronan and PSGAGs. The latter is preferred, and three to four weekly injections are combined with a reduction in exercise. Horses that do not respond may have proliferative synovitis, usually seen in older horses with chronic OA. Injecting the joint in the dorsal pouch may be difficult, and little synovial fluid may be present. Surgical resection of synovial pads and postoperative intraarticular injections of PSGAGs are recommended.

Fractures and osteochondritis dissecans occur, but palmar fragments are rare (see Chapter 36).

Splint Bone Disease

Exostoses and Fractures of the Second and Fourth Metacarpal Bones (Splints)

Splints are a common problem in 2- and 3-year-olds (see page 1018). Poor conformation and hard track surfaces predispose horses to splints. Whether tearing of the interosseous ligaments occurs is unknown. Medial splints are most common. Yearlings can begin training with dormant, so-called field splints that become active as training advances. Splints rarely cause severe head nodding lameness, but put a horse on a line and signs become worse as work progresses. Splints on the abaxial surfaces of the McII and McIV are visible and can be palpated readily, but those on the axial surfaces require the limb to be lifted to relax the SL. Axially-located splints cause more obvious lameness than do abaxially-located splints.

Management includes reducing inflammation and limiting callus. Cold-water therapy and poultice should be applied, and horses are given NSAIDs. Blistering and external heat therapy may be contraindicated if reduction in the size of the callus is desirable. Ionophoresis with corticosteroids is successful. Perilesional injection of corticosteroids and cryotherapy are used successfully. Cryotherapy is a common therapeutic option often performed in STBs, but after the procedure local pain and inflammation persist, complicating palpation during reexamination. In these STBs, resolution of signs of lameness or other horse-related factors, such as a reduction or cessation of being on a line, is often used as evidence of clinical improvement. Cryotherapy may need to be repeated, and if necessary additional local therapy can be given once cutaneous sores from the procedure heal. If signs fail to abate, a fracture may be present. Improper toe-heel impact and medial-to-lateral hoof imbalance predispose horses to splints. Chronic

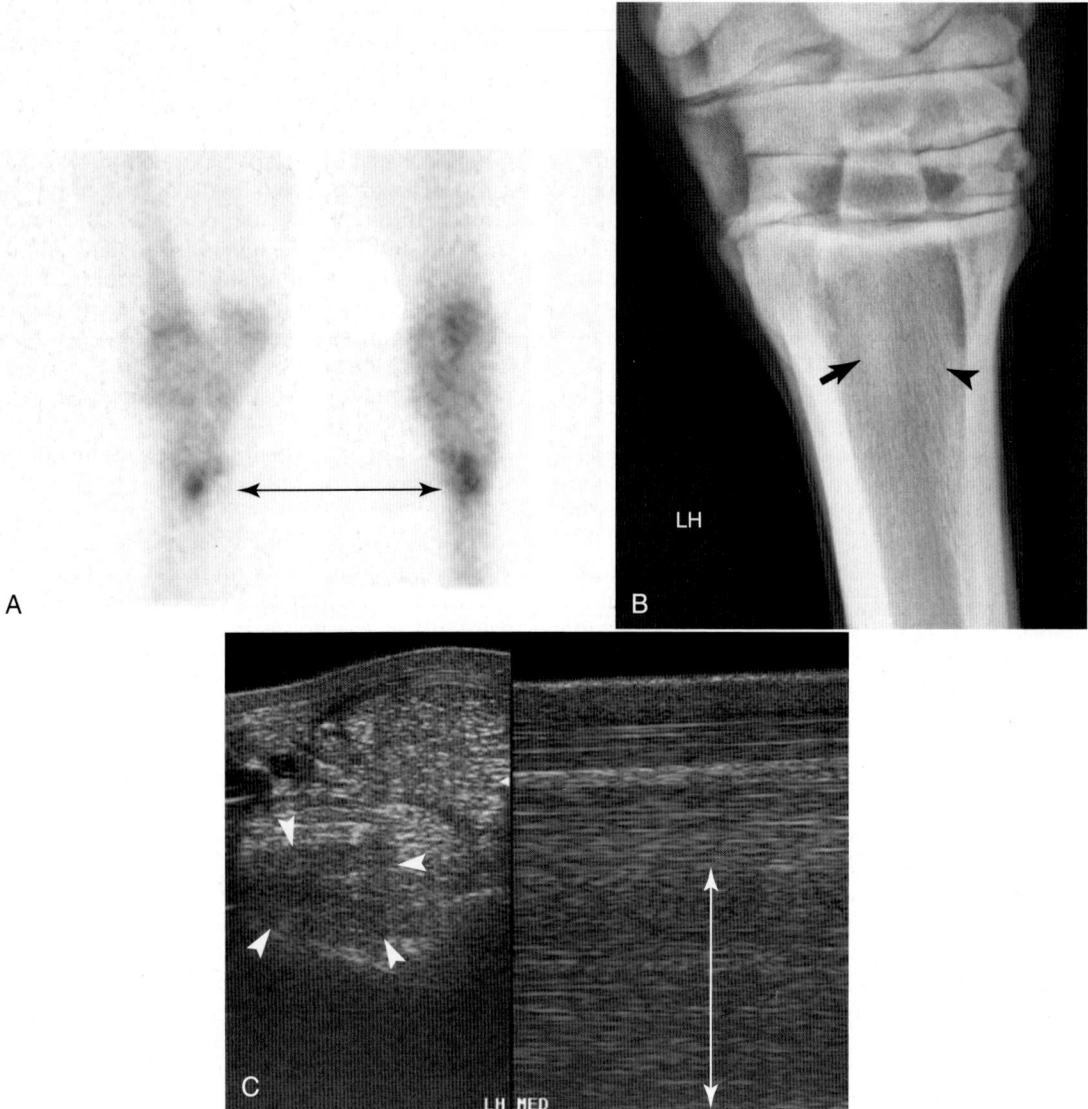

Fig. 108-11 • Images of a 3-year-old Standardbred colt pacer in May after being trained and qualified for racing; the colt had won divisional honors the previous year but developed substantial (3 of 5) left hindlimb lameness as a result of complex injury in the proximal plantar metatarsal region. **A,** Delayed phase lateral *(left)* and plantar scintigraphic images showing focal, intense increased radiopharmaceutical uptake in the proximal, plantar aspect of the third metatarsal bone (MtIII) indicative of bony injury at the origin of the suspensory ligament *(double-headed arrow)*. **B,** Dorsoplantar digital radiograph (lateral is to the left) of the left proximal metatarsal region showing increased radiopacity *(arrow)* and mild radiolucency *(arrowhead)* of the MtIII; neither avulsion nor longitudinal fracture was seen, but changes of this magnitude in bone indicate the lesion is chronic. **C,** Transverse *(left)* and longitudinal ultrasonographic images acquired with the transducer medial to the plantar midline showing enlargement *(double-headed arrow)* of the proximal aspect of the suspensory ligament (cross-section area measured 2.4 cm²) and a large hypoechogenic region *(arrowheads)*. This colt was retired from racing.

splint disease in older horses is almost always related to palmar foot pain. Aggressive therapy for palmar foot pain and restoring normal hoof strike is critical. Direct trauma from interference and breaking must be prevented.

Fractures of the McII and the McIV can be caused by direct trauma. Interference injury can cause fracture of the McII, and accidents involving carts and other equipment predispose horses to fractures of the McIV. If fractures are located proximally and displacement exists, surgical fixation using small plates and screws is best. McIV fractures can heal functionally without fixation. Most distal splint

bone fractures are secondary to suspensory desmitis. Exuberant callus can impinge on the SL. Fracture callus and fragments should be removed.

Exostoses and Fractures of the Second and Fourth Metatarsal Bones

Exostoses most commonly involve the MtII, but chronic painful splint exostoses are not as common as in the forelimb. Perilesional corticosteroid therapy is recommended (80 mg of methylprednisolone and 8 mL of Sarapin, (High

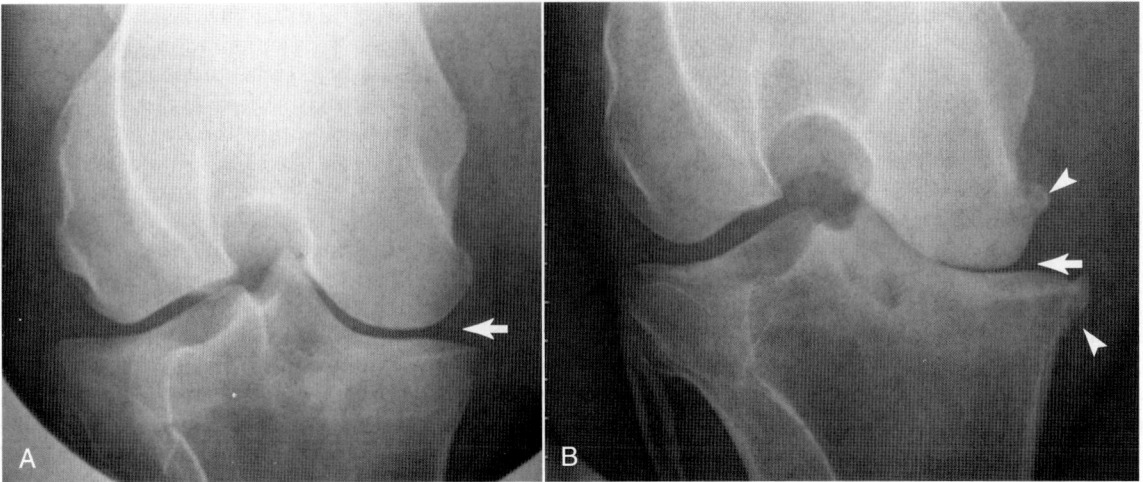

Fig. 108-12 • A, Caudocranial digital radiographic image of the left stifle of a 4-year-old Standardbred (STB) trotter with marked narrowing of the medial femorotibial joint (MFTJ, *arrow*). Radiological evidence of narrowing on a well-positioned caudocranial image is the earliest sign of osteoarthritis (OA) of the MFTJ. **B,** Advanced OA of the MFTJ is seen in this caudocranial image of a 9-year-old STB pacer. Absence of an obvious MFTJ space *(arrow)*, marginal osteophyte formation *(arrowheads)* of the distal, medial aspect of the femur and proximal medial aspect of the tibia, and radiolucency of the distal aspect of the medial femoral condyle can be seen. This horse was 4 of 5 lame in the left hindlimb, and the prognosis for racing is grave.

Chemical Company). Fractures of the MtII and the MtIV occur occasionally and usually result from direct trauma, but distal splint fractures can be secondary to suspensory branch desmitis. Fracture fragments should be removed.

Stifle Joint Lameness

The stifle joint often is incriminated as a source of pain, but diagnostic analgesia identifies a problem in the more distal part of the limb. OA of the medial femorotibial joint is the most important stifle lameness, but osteochondrosis should be considered in young horses. OA is a progressive disease beginning in late 2-year-olds, and degree of lameness varies from grade 1 to 4 of 5. Distention of the medial femorotibial joint capsule is an important finding, but in some STBs this is a subtle finding. The limb may be carried forward slightly lateral or outward during the cranial phase of the stride. The cranial phase is shortened, and lameness is worse in the turns. Radiographs are usually negative or equivocal in 2-year-olds, and arthroscopic evaluation reveals generalized cartilage thinning and fissure formation. Later, in caudocranial radiographic images, narrowing of the medial femorotibial joint space and mild osteophyte formation on the proximal medial aspect of the tibia and distal medial aspect of the femur are visible (Figure 108-12, A). Scintigraphic examination can confirm extensive OA. Diffuse IRU involves both sides of the medial femorotibial joint and is best seen in a caudal image, although if extensive IRU can be seen in a lateral image as well. Arthroscopic evaluation at this time reveals exposed subchondral bone and severe synovitis, but therapeutic value of arthroscopy is negligible. If the diagnosis of OA is made in a 2-year-old, a period of 3 to 4 months of rest is recommended. The stifle joint often is injected in horses without stifle lameness, and few untoward effects are seen. Treatment of STBs with OA of the medial femorotibial joint with methylprednisolone acetate is contraindicated early in the course of the disease. Although the drug is effective and allows continued

racing, OA can progress rapidly, resulting in severe lameness. Hyaluronan (40 mg) and isoflupredone acetate (4 to 6 mg) or triamcinolone acetonide (4 mg), interleukin-1 receptor antagonist protein, or PSGAGs (750 to 1000 mg) are preferred, and although they are less effective than methylprednisolone acetate, they decrease inflammation and prolong the racing career. Systemic administration of PSGAGs or hyaluronan is helpful. Methylprednisolone acetate is necessary for older horses with advanced OA, but if no improvement is seen, the racing career is usually over (see Figure 108-12, B). Once severe lameness occurs, rest may improve comfort slightly, but horses will not tolerate training again. Trotters can tolerate racing with more advanced OA than can pacers.

In young horses osteochondrosis can cause lameness and effusion in early training, prompting radiographic examination, but signs of osteochondrosis often are seen in weanlings and yearlings, and surgery is performed before training begins. Osteochondritis dissecans of the lateral trochlear ridge of the femur is most common; it causes considerable effusion of the femoropatellar joint and if bilateral may cause a bunny-hopping gait. Surgical treatment, 4 to 6 months of rest, and intraarticular therapy are recommended. Prognosis for racing is good unless lesions are severe or cartilage damage of the patella is advanced. Subchondral bone cysts most commonly involve the medial femoral condyle but can occur in the proximal aspect of the tibia. Lameness is often progressive, with horses first being on a line. Surgical debridement of the cyst is recommended, although injection of corticosteroids beneath the lining of the cyst and into the cyst cavity under arthroscopic guidance can be used. After debridement, lameness persists for several months, but this approach may be a better long-term solution. Horses need a minimum of 6 to 8 months of rest to allow healing and for lameness to abate. Prognosis is fair (70%) for successful racing.

Rhabdomyolysis and Muscle Soreness

We divide muscle lameness into metabolic disease (recurrent exertional rhabdomyolysis [RER]) and nonmetabolic disease (muscle soreness). Signs vary, but horses appear stiff and hindlimbs are not fully engaged in the stride unilaterally or bilaterally. Palpation often reveals muscle pain but must be done carefully because aggressive, sudden, and deep palpation elicits false-positive responses.

RER occurs more commonly in females and can cause swollen muscles. Overt clinical signs of tying up after racing and training can be seen, but subclinical RER can be a cause of poor performance. Myoglobinuria and elevation of serum creatine kinase (CK) and aspartate transaminase (AST) levels are diagnostic. Horses are managed initially with intravenous fluids, NSAIDs, tranquilization, and methocarbamol (22 mg/kg intravenously [IV] or 33 mg/kg PO twice daily). Care must be taken when using acetylpromazine and methocarbamol simultaneously because effects may be additive, and horses may act severely tranquilized (JSM). Walking is recommended in horses with mild RER but is contraindicated in those with severe RER. Dantrolene sodium (2 mg/kg IV or via nasogastric tube) and intravenous dimethyl sulfoxide solution are recommended in horses with severe RER. Large quantities of intravenous or oral fluids should be administered. After an acute episode, signs may recur or subclinical myositis may persist, reflected by elevations in CK and AST concentrations. Enzyme levels should return to baseline before intense training or racing resumes.

In horses with subclinical RER or those with recurrent acute episodes, we recommend a management protocol that includes a reduction in carbohydrate intake, especially before exercise, a high-fat diet, vitamin E and selenium supplementation, supplementation with oral potassium, and a regular 7-day exercise program combining jogging, brief periods of intensive training, and paddock exercise, if feasible. Chronic administration of dantrolene sodium (2 mg/kg) or phenytoin (8 to 10 mg/kg PO twice daily) is recommended, but racing jurisdiction rules must be followed.

Nonmetabolic myositis is common, and gait is similar to that described for stifle lameness. Signs are similar to RER, but serum CK and AST levels are usually within or just above normal limits. The middle gluteal muscle and associated tendons commonly are affected unilaterally or bilaterally. Myositis may be a secondary problem or a primary source of pain after traumatic injuries such as accidents during transport, paddock injuries, slipping while racing on muddy or other undesirable surfaces, or by making a break. Horses are managed initially with muscle relaxants, NSAIDs, and rest (5 to 7 days). Horses with chronic soreness are treated with an internal counterirritant or corticosteroids injected strategically in the sore areas (see Chapter 88).

Curb and Superficial Digital Flexor Tendonitis

Other soft tissue injuries such as curb and superficial digital flexor tendonitis occur commonly. Curb in the STB is discussed in detail in Chapter 78. Superficial digital flexor tendonitis is discussed in detail in Chapter 69. Surgical management using desmotomy of the accessory ligament of the superficial digital flexor muscle (superior check desmotomy) and annular desmotomy if tendonitis involves the distal metacarpal region are recommended.

Chapter 109

The European and Australasian Standardbreds

■ THE EUROPEAN STANDARDBRED
Fabio Torre

DIMENSIONS AND CHARACTERISTICS

The European Standardbred (STB) is historically the result of different crosses between the classic American bloodlines and European families. The French STB is known for its stamina and aptitude for long distances. The American-derived families, however, have been selected for speed and racing at a fixed distance of 1 mile and are represented more widely in Italy and Sweden. Several countries (especially France, Italy, Germany, and the Scandinavian countries) have developed individual bloodlines and today are able to produce good-quality STB trotters. In Europe no races are available for pacers. In Table 109-1 the STB population and racing activity of different European countries are listed.

Europe has a large number of racetracks for STBs, and they are characterized by different circuit lengths, surfaces, and designs. Half-mile tracks have been replaced progressively by 1-km (⅝-mile) tracks, and no 1-mile racetracks (with the exception of training centers) are present in Europe. The most characteristic and popular racetrack is the Plateau de Gravelle in Vincennes, Paris, where the Prix d'Amerique is held. The track surface is made of pressed charcoal powder; slopes and descents are present; and the circuit is egg-shaped, which is unique in Europe, where other racetracks have a regular design. Another famous French racetrack, Cagnes-sur-Mer in Nice, is well known for being 1200 m in length and for hosting the Criterium de Vitesse, one of the main European free-for-all races. In Sweden, Solvalla racetrack in Stockholm represents the heart of the Swedish STB racing, and in late May the multiple-heat race Elitlopp is held. In Norway, in addition to well-developed STB racing (the main racetrack being Bjerke near Oslo), races for Warmblood horses (a breed historically devoted to hard work but now genetically selected for speed) are still popular and meet the special interest of the local public.

TABLE 109-1

Distribution of Standardbreds Born in Different European Countries, Summary of the Racing Activity, Earnings, and Betting						
COUNTRY	NEWBORNS PER YEAR (NO.)	RACING DAYS (NO.)	RACES (NO.)	RACING STANDARDBREDS (NO.)	TOTAL EARNINGS (EURO)	MONEY FOR BETTING (EURO)
Denmark	870	404	3,702	3,367	5,963,019	52,414,070
Finland	1,750	585	3,716	5,159	8,230,345	174,133,572
France	12,062	1,773	9,980	13,188	133,880,408	2,851,925,331
Germany	2,049	811	9,609	7,242	26,137,229	168,811,395
The Netherlands	548	170	1,506	1,508	3,422,242	38,163,810
Italy	4,700	1,606	13,823	10,158	73,504,710	1,336,481,000
Norway	890	502	2,281	2,753	18,724,000	253,123,200
Sweden	5,040	937	8,529	12,942	63,781,182	1,045,013,432
Austria	310	124	1,206	1,144	3,060,177	9,748,299
Belgium	706	190	1,628	1,836	2,414,831	37,602,040
Spain	372	289	1,918	970	686,334	1,187,325

Data from UET (European Trotting Union), update December 1999.

TABLE 109-2

Racetrack Distribution in Different European Countries				
COUNTRY	RACETRACKS (NO.)*	HALF-MILE RACETRACKS (NO.)	1-KM RACETRACKS (NO.)	>1-KM RACETRACKS (NO.)
Denmark	9	1	7	1
Finland	43	0	43	0
France	240	0	0	4
Germany	16	3	0	5
The Netherlands	7	1	3	1
Italy	25	11	13	0
Norway	9	1	7	0
Sweden	26	1	25	0

Data from UET (European Trotting Union), update December 2000.

*The total number includes all racetracks in which at least 1 day of racing is held, but less important, occasional, and fairlike tracks (which are especially popular in France) are not considered in the subsequent columns.

A variety of track designs and purposes are present in Europe. For example, a large number of small country tracks are found in France, and local races are organized in a fairlike fashion, whereas the main racing activity is concentrated in Paris. In Italy, however, important races have a more even distribution among racetracks, Milan and Rome being the main places. In Table 109-2 the distribution of racing tracks in the main European countries is summarized.

Differences exist in availability of prize money among different countries, and this makes France and Italy the most attractive countries for trainers and owners. A number of well-known trainers started to move in the early 1980s toward France and Italy, especially from northern Europe, and this has enhanced the exchange of experiences between trainers and veterinarians.

Prize money distribution among horses of different ages has strongly influenced racing, especially in Italy, where 2- and 3-year-olds have the richest races. Higher purses for younger horses have also affected breeding programs and have stimulated an interest in many of the orthopedic problems affecting young horses, especially osteochondrosis, which has been studied widely in northern Europe.

APPROACHING LAMENESS PROBLEMS

Only STB trotters are allowed to race in Europe, and this makes the trainer's work more challenging. Any possibility to switch gaits or to move an unnaturally fast gaited trotter to a potentially good pacer is precluded. When the fast gait is compromised by biomechanical problems and substantial interference between limbs (unlike in the pacer), corrections aimed at avoiding interference are attempted. Finding a solution for mechanical problems is not always possible, and corrective shoeing that alters the natural gait may cause compensatory lameness in different locations.

A series of mechanical limitations may be present at the beginning of training, and relatively soon they are followed by pain-related problems, usually affecting joints and less frequently digital flexor tendons and the suspensory ligament (SL). A less than 100% natural trotting athlete is more likely than a natural trotter to have its gait totally compromised, even by a mild subclinical lameness problem, and consequently gait limitations increase. However, anything that is attempted by the trainer to improve gait (corrective shoeing, special equipment that prevents turning the head and neck toward one side, or shifting the hindlimbs toward one shaft) forces the horse to a nonnatural fast gait and often results in lameness. In fact, when a nonnatural gait is forced, the end result is usually that a single limb (or a biped) is overloaded, and the uneven loading is exacerbated by the progression of training.

When young horses start training, they frequently have been subjected to basic lameness and radiological evaluations. This allows trainers the opportunity to treat conditions such as osteochondrosis or to be aware of other abnormalities. Prepurchase radiographic examinations and, when needed, preventative arthroscopic surgery (mostly for osteochondrosis of the tarsocrural joint and osteochondral fragments in the fetlock joints) are now practices that have received general acceptance. The reason to operate early is to have the horse rested before any training program is started. In yearlings eligible for autumn sales, it is important to perform surgery early to have presale radiographs without evidence of osteochondral fragments and to decrease effusion before the sale.

When moderate gait anomalies are present, experienced trainers usually give the horse time and keep going with a light exercise program instead of making radical changes. This allows, in many horses, a complete maturation of the equine athlete, and when the growth is complete and the muscular function well conditioned, the gait in many horses automatically improves without injuring the immature skeleton. Shoeing is also central in early training. Light plastic shoes are ideal to allow foot growth and expansion and to minimize trauma in the early phases of fast training.

LAMENESS EXAMINATION

Horses with acute, severe lameness should be allowed to rest. Radiographs are frequently diagnostic, revealing the most common severe musculoskeletal injuries affecting trained STBs, such as incomplete sagittal fractures of the proximal phalanx, fractures of the proximal sesamoid bones (PSBs), splint bone fractures, fractures of the third or radial carpal bones, fractures of a palmar process of the distal phalanx, fractures of the lateral condyle of the third metacarpal bone (McIII), slab fractures of the third tarsal bone, and stress fractures of the palmar aspect of the McIII or the plantar aspect of the third metatarsal bone (MtIII). Apical fractures of the PSBs are a common injury in young STBs, and the lateral PSB in the hindlimbs is the most common location.[1]

References on page 1343

The conditions mentioned previously represent injuries of the racing STB requiring rest or surgical repair. More commonly the veterinarian is consulted for mild or obscure lameness, gait disturbances, or poor performance. In any case, a thorough history is mandatory before the lameness examination is initiated.

A basic lameness history must include the following:
- What is the trainer's complaint?
- What is the horse's gait (naturally born vs. artificial trotter)?
- Describe the shoeing management: recent changes, difficulties in combining appropriate shoeing and fast gait, ideal shoeing for the horse, and attempts at correcting the problem.
- What is the horse's recent performance?
- When was the onset of the problem and correlation with previous lameness, if any?

- When does the problem arise during the race? Does the horse worsen in the turns or on the straight? Is the horse better at the beginning of the race and does it worsen at the end?
- Is the horse lame after the race?
- What about the day after the race?
- How is the horse during daily jogging (a question best addressed to the groom or assistant trainer)?
- How does the horse behave when trained clockwise (although races are counterclockwise)?
- Is the horse better when trained on a straight track, when available?
- Does the problem worsen on a particular racetrack and specifically on hard tracks?
- Is the horse on a line or on a shaft?
- Does the horse break stride? If so, when? At the start, approaching turns, in turns, coming out of turns, or in the straightaway?
- Does the horse deviate left in the turns and right on the straight lines? Does the tendency worsen at the end of the race?
- Has the horse been submitted to any previous lameness examination?
- Was the horse subjected to any previous treatment with paints, ointments, or local injections, and did the horse improve with therapy?
- Was any other problem diagnosed or suspected (exercise-induced pulmonary hemorrhage, rhabdomyolysis)?

Concerning conformation, the clinician should check the following:
- Foot conformation (club foot or low heel, toed in, toed out, hoof wall angle, correction of the lateral-to-medial balance, quality of the horn, characteristics of the sole and quarters, type of shoeing). Club feet may indicate osteoarthritis (OA) of the distal interphalangeal (DIP) joint. Toed-out horses have the most frequent gait disturbances because they tend to hit the contralateral carpus or the ipsilateral metatarsal region. Toed-in horses have less important gait problems, but the uneven distribution of the weight is likely to produce lameness associated with the middle carpal joint or suspensory desmitis.
- Potentially clinically significant conformational abnormalities include torsional defects proximal to the hoof (fetlock and carpus and, more rarely, the tarsus), uncorrected angular limb deformities, offset (bench) knees, tied in behind the knees, straight conformation of the hindlimbs. Any of these abnormalities invariably produces secondary injuries such as suspensory desmitis, superficial digital flexor (SDF) tendonitis, and middle carpal joint lameness.
- Conformation of the foot is important. Asymmetrical foot size is often a consequence of reduced weight bearing and lameness on one side, and the smallest foot is generally on the lame side.

Palpation

Many clinicians spend little time palpating a lame horse, a practice that I believe is a mistake. Areas of warmth (heat), especially in the hoof wall, must be detected, and regions of special interest include the fetlock joints, the metacarpal and metatarsal regions, carpus, hock, stifle, and back.

In the forelimb, the DIP joint capsule just above the coronary band is palpated to detect effusion. The character of the digital pulse is evaluated and compared between limbs.

Hoof tester examination can be considered part of palpation. When possible, feet are first tested without removing the shoes, and ideally the horse should be kept shod until any examination in movement is completed. When diagnostic analgesia is needed, hoof testing must precede palmar digital analgesia, and shoes may be removed temporarily if bar shoes or pads prevent accurate testing. These six points are tested in each horse: lateral and medial quarters, lateral and medial middle sole, and lateral and medial toe. Testing the frog rarely produces useful information, and squeezing the quarters from lateral to medial with hoof testers may cause pain unrelated to the primary lameness.[2] Pain arising from the quarters, especially mild pain medially, should not be overrated because this region is frequently sensitive to hoof testers in normal horses. The contralateral foot may serve as a reference. In my experience the right medial quarter is the most common region to find pain elicited by hoof tester examination in STBs, and this is probably secondary to the counterclockwise direction of racing. This may be a clinically significant finding, but generally a painful response is considered more important when it arises from the toe or from the lateral side of the sole. When shoes are removed, a further evaluation of the lateral-to-medial balance is performed. The sole itself is observed, and when it appears flat and painful, this may correlate with type of shoes and padding that are used. Overzealous padding may add to, rather than relieve, pressure on the sole. A leather or rubber layer may allow sand to pack quickly under the pad and create pressure and secondary bruises. These horses are better managed with shoes in which the contact is limited to the hoof wall and no contact is made with the sole.

In the forelimb the fetlock joint is examined for effusion, alteration of the dorsal outline, and enlargement of the suspensory branches. The latter are palpated carefully with the joint flexed. Each branch is pressed gently axially, and alterations in consistency and pain response are noted. Range of motion of the fetlock joint is assessed. In a normal STB, the fetlock joint can be flexed up to 90 degrees (angle between the McIII and the proximal phalanx) without eliciting a painful response. With one hand holding the dorsal pastern region, the dorsal aspect of the fetlock joint can be palpated further by using the other hand to compress the dorsal joint capsule against the bony prominences of the sagittal ridge and condyles of the McIII. Horses with osteochondritis dissecans (OCD) or a hypertrophic synovial pad exhibit a painful response. The bony profile of the McIII must be followed with fingers to detect painful areas in the dorsal, lateral, and medial aspects. Palmar soft tissues are evaluated with the limb in a weight-bearing position and while being held off the ground. Each structure is palpated accurately to detect heat, pain, and edema in horses with acute lesions or fibrotic consistency and adhesions in those with chronic conditions. Fingers must be pressed firmly, deep in the proximal palmar metacarpal region, where pain originating from the proximal aspect of the SL is hard to detect. The carpus is better evaluated by

holding the limb in a moderate degree of flexion. Careful digital palpation along the dorsal aspect should be performed. Of particular importance is the dorsomedial aspect where a thickened joint capsule and painful response correspond to the common finding of OA of the middle carpal joint. Palpation of the forelimb proximal to the carpus is rarely helpful. Elbow and shoulder lameness are rare, and bicipital bursitis has seldom been reported.

In the distal aspect of the hindlimb, palpation is similar to that described for the forelimb with the exception that foot lameness is less important. The metatarsophalangeal joint region is best evaluated while holding the limb in a semiflexed position. When the proximal metatarsal and distal tarsus regions are palpated, some false-positive painful reactions frequently are elicited, especially on the medial aspect. This pain frequently is overemphasized in horses with back pain, especially when the trainer thinks the horse has primary lameness in the tarsus. Effusion of the tarsocrural joint often indicates the likely presence of osteochondrosis (OC). The stifle must be palpated deeply and carefully because the joint is complex, but the structures that can be assessed are limited. The femorotibial joints seldom appear distended, but effusion of the medial femorotibial joint is an important abnormal clinical sign. More frequently, joint effusion is limited to the femoropatellar joint, but because the femoropatellar and medial femorotibial joints communicate, inflammation in one may result in effusion of both. With the exception of acute trauma, painful responses to palpation are rare in this area, even from the patellar ligaments that are identified easily. On the medial side, scar tissue and irregularities or enlargement of the medial patellar ligament may suggest previous desmotomy. When associated with femoropatellar effusion, the latter sign may suggest apical patellar fragmentation, and radiographic examination is indicated. The stifle can be flexed only in unison with most other hindlimb joints, so a painful response is not specific. With moderate flexion the medial collateral ligament can be stressed by the veterinarian pulling the tibia in a lateral direction with both hands and pressing the shoulder against the femur.

Palpation of the back is aimed at evaluating pain arising from joints (intervertebral, lumbosacral, sacroiliac, and sacrococcygeal), nerve roots, and muscles. The latter are the most likely origin of pain elicited by palpation, but other problems must be ruled out if associated clinical signs (atrophy, asymmetry) are present. Pain in the gluteal area may be secondary to many problems, including straight hindlimb conformation, hock or stifle pain, sore feet, gait imbalance, and stiff corrective harness equipment. Therefore pain in this area should not be treated as a primary problem unless a thorough clinical examination has ruled out other sources of pain.

Movement

After palpation, the horse is examined during movement. I commonly tranquilize each horse I examine for lameness. Tranquilization (10 mg of acetylpromazine maleate intravenously) improves the possibilities of handling the horse and lowers the risk of injuries to the veterinarian. Furthermore, the horse appears less stiff; mild lameness becomes somewhat more obvious; and the horse stands better for radiographic or ultrasonographic examination. The trainer must be consulted before injecting a tranquilizer because this practice may preclude racing because of doping regulations (the term used in Europe for a blood or urine drug test for a prohibited substance). Lameness is rarely detectable at the walk, but it is important to observe the way the horse lands with each foot to identify lateral-to-medial hoof imbalance. The horse is then trotted in a straight line on a firm surface, and the character of movements is observed. Abduction or circumduction of forelimbs is considered characteristic of carpal lameness because the horse appears to attempt to avoid flexion. In the hindlimb, stiffness has been related anecdotally to distal hock joint pain but in fact is not a specific sign. In horses with pain arising from the distal part of a hindlimb (frequently the metatarsophalangeal joint), the horse tends to moderately overflex the hock and stifle to shorten the weight-bearing phase of the stride.[3] In horses with more severe lameness, drifting forward of the sound limb is observed, and a drop of the fetlock joint is easily seen. Abduction of the hindlimb is thought to be related to stifle lameness.

Flexion tests are used to supplement findings during movement and are similar to those used in other sports horses. Flexion of the carpus is accomplished by pulling the metacarpal region laterally, and the clinician's elbow may act as a lever against the horse's radius to stress the medial aspect. In young horses affected by carpitis, this maneuver frequently elicits pain.

DIAGNOSTIC ANALGESIA

Diagnostic analgesia can be performed in sequence from distal to proximal, or, to save time, selective analgesic techniques can be used. For example, European trotters with a positive response to forelimb lower limb flexion inconsistently respond to palmar digital analgesia; therefore analgesia of the metacarpophalangeal or DIP joints may be the first option. Perineural analgesia is preferred, however, to avoid minor risks of joint infections or to save the opportunity to provide intraarticular therapy immediately (when working in stables, trainers frequently are interested more in treatment than in diagnosis). I frequently start with low plantar analgesia in the hindlimbs because lameness of the digit is rare. In young STBs with forelimb lameness and a positive response to carpal flexion, I block the middle carpal joint first.

In horses with obscure lameness or when lameness is only apparent during fast exercise, examining the horse on the track may be useful. The horse is rigged in full harness and first examined trotting in a clockwise direction. Speed then is increased, and the horse is turned to train in a counterclockwise direction, the same as racing. Clinicians can drive the horse themselves, sit in a two-seat wagon, or observe the horse from a car or from a distance. In my opinion, watching the horse during exercise is important, especially when routine training and racing can be simulated, and I prefer the horse to be driven by its usual trainer. Having the horse fully equipped, mimicking the stress of racing, and observing the horse in turns are important advantages to this form of lameness examination.

Diagnostic analgesia is useful, but the clinician must be aware of related risks and make the trainer and owner aware as well. Diagnostic blocks should be avoided in horses suspected of having incomplete fractures. Radiographic examination should precede diagnostic analgesia

in these horses. When examining a horse on the track after local analgesia, the trainer should be told to limit the speed as much as possible, avoiding any sudden stop or sharp turn. An experienced trainer normally is able to appreciate the benefits of a block quickly and without stressing the horse. Examination at speed is needed to make a diagnosis in horses with plantar process osteochondrosis fragmentation of the proximal phalanx and fragmentation of the distal border of the distal phalanx.

DIAGNOSTIC IMAGING

Sophisticated equipment for diagnostic imaging is now available in most European equine clinics. Scintigraphy is available in Europe but is limited to large referral hospitals. Radiography remains the mainstay of equine diagnostic imaging, and the availability of excellent portable units has improved the radiographic examination under field conditions. Digital radiography offers advantages in terms of imaging processing, time saving, radiation protection, and easier image storage. Ultrasonographic examination is commonly performed.

Common pathological findings in the distal limb of European trotters include osteophyte formation on the distal aspect of the middle phalanx, sometimes associated with modeling of the extensor process of the distal phalanx, as seen on a lateromedial image of the foot (Figure 109-1). This radiological pattern often is associated with heel growth proceeding faster than toe growth (club foot). When associated with a positive lower limb flexion test and lameness abolished using analgesia of the DIP joint, this radiological finding is important and indicates the presence of OA. Fragmentation of the extensor process of the distal phalanx has controversial clinical significance, but in my experience these fragments cause synovitis of the DIP joint and should be removed using arthroscopy.

The dorsoproximal-palmarodistal oblique radiographic image of the distal phalanx, unlike scintigraphy, rarely helps in diagnosing pain arising from stress remodeling of the distal phalanx; thus the diagnosis of pedal osteitis is

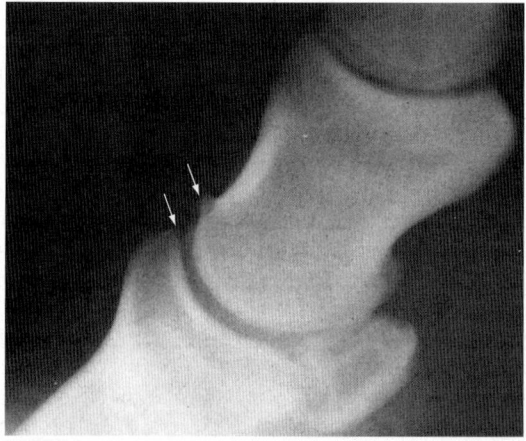

Fig. 109-1 • Lateromedial radiographic image of the distal interphalangeal joint of a Standardbred trotter. Osteophyte formation on the distal border of the middle phalanx associated with moderate remodeling of the extensor process of the distal phalanx (*arrows*) is a common pathological finding in European trotters.

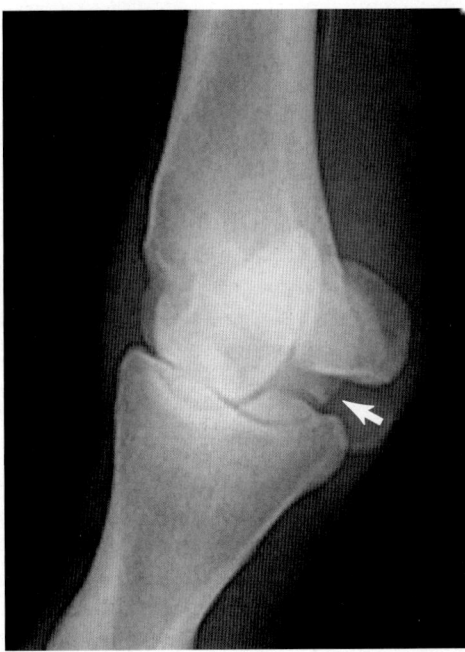

Fig. 109-2 • Dorsoproximal 45-degrees medial-plantarodistolateral obli-que radiographic image of a hind fetlock of a 2-year-old Standardbred. There is plantar fragmentation *(arrow)* of the proximal medial aspect of the proximal phalanx.

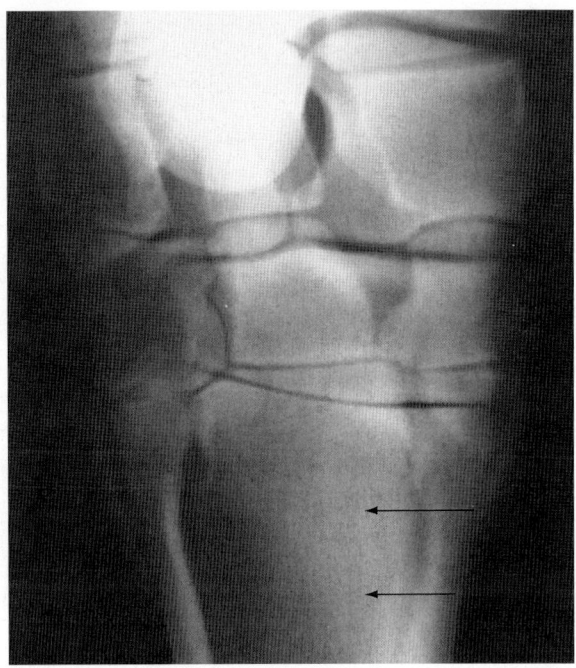

Fig. 109-3 • Dorsopalmar radiographic image of the proximal metacarpal region of a Standardbred trotter (lateral is to the left). Increased radio-pacity of the palmar cortex of the proximal aspect of the third metacarpal bone *(arrows)* is a common finding in trotters with chronic proximal sus-pensory desmitis.

limited to horses with chronic lameness characterized by substantial radiolucency.[4] Fragmentation of the lateral and medial palmar processes of the distal phalanx, although controversial as a cause of acute lameness, may be an important source of pain best managed by shoeing.

The flexed lateromedial image of the metacarpophalan-geal or metatarsophalangeal joints is useful in evaluating lesions of the distal aspect of the McIII or the MtIII. In the hindlimb, the oblique images must be acquired in a proxi-mal to distal direction (down-angled) to see better the area between the proximal phalanx and the base of the PSBs. Fragmentation of the proximal plantar aspect of the proxi-mal phalanx represents a major cause of subtle hindlimb lameness (Figure 109-2).

A dorsopalmar image of the carpus helps to evaluate the proximal suspensory origin from the McIII, and focal or diffuse increased radiopacity of the McIII may be found (Figure 109-3). In yearlings and young horses, this image allows examination of the distal radius, and pathological modifications of the growth plate on the medial side (phy-sitis) are a frequent cause of early lameness. The most common lesions of the carpus are seen with the dorsolateral-palmaromedial oblique image and the dorsal 35° proximal-dorsal distal oblique (skyline) image of the flexed carpus to highlight the distal row of carpal bones. The radiographs must be of excellent quality, and the appropriate projec-tion must be obtained because false-negative radiographic images are frequent. Abnormal findings include areas of radiolucency in the dorsoproximal articular border of the radial fossa of the third carpal bone, radiolucent lines sug-gestive of fractures, and increased radiopacity of the third carpal bone.[5] A moderate degree of increased radiopacity in the radial fossa of the third carpal bone is considered normal in racing horses, but more severe increased

radiopacity associated with radiolucent areas represents a pathological finding.[6,7]

In the hindlimb the centrodistal and tarsometatarsal joints frequently appear normal radiologically even when distal hock joint pain is diagnosed clinically as the source of pain. Scintigraphy is an excellent tool for diagnosing OA of these joints.[8] The tarsocrural joint is a predilection site for OC in STBs, and the presence of fragments associated with effusion may represent an indication for arthroscopic surgery. Lesions affecting the lateral trochlear ridge of the talus and medial malleolus of the tibia more frequently cause lameness and effusion than do those of the cranial aspect of the intermediate ridge of the tibia. In horses with effusion but without obvious fragmentation, a specific dorsal 10° to 15° lateral-plantaromedial oblique image is required to evaluate the axial aspect of the medial malleo-lus. Subtle osteochondral fragmentation or radiolucency easily can be overlooked (Figure 109-4).

Curb is not seen frequently but can develop in the early stages of training in young horses. Curbs represent thicken-ing of the plantar aspect of the hock and must be differenti-ated from the soft swelling caused by distention of a tarsal sheath. Abnormal stress to the plantar soft tissue structures can be predisposed by sickle-hocked or cow-hocked con-formation. Accurate palpation differentiates curb from tarsal tenosynovitis. Ultrasonographic evaluation helps characterize the soft tissue structures involved in curb and assess severity (see Chapter 78). In the European STB, curb nearly invariably represents inflammation and thickening of the long plantar ligament, but ultrasonographic evalua-tion is necessary to differentiate long plantar desmitis from other soft tissue injury.

Trainers frequently ask for radiography or ultrasonog-raphy of the stifle because they seem to incriminate this

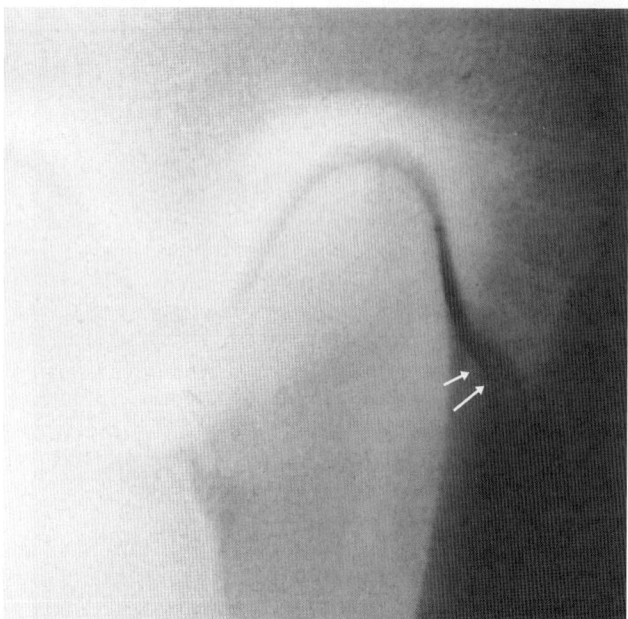

Fig. 109-4 • Dorsal 15° lateral-plantaromedial oblique radiographic image of the hock of a 2-year-old Standardbred colt. There is axial fragmentation of the medial malleolus of the tibia *(arrows)*, which is difficult to detect unless oblique images are obtained. The condition can cause effusion of the tarsocrural joint and lameness.

joint as the source of pain causing lameness in horses with obscure hindlimb lameness. Radiography of the stifle is important in foals and yearlings with femoropatellar effusion. Lateromedial and caudocranial images must be obtained. OCD of the lateral trochlear ridge and, less frequently, subchondral bone cysts of the medial femoral condyle can cause effusion and lameness in young STBs. Ultrasonographic evaluation of the stifle is useful in detecting soft tissue injuries, but these lesions are rare in STBs. Mild dimples or cartilaginous defects on the articular surface of the medial femoral condyle can be detected using ultrasonographic examination by holding the stifle in a semiflexed (90 degrees) position.

FINAL DIAGNOSIS, PROGNOSIS, AND TREATMENT OPTIONS

A final diagnosis is made easily when the horse has obvious severe lameness, as is the case in horses with the more common fractures and tendon or ligament injuries (incomplete sagittal fracture of the proximal phalanx, PSB fracture, carpal chip or slab fractures, SDF tendonitis, and acute suspensory desmitis). Surgery or rest most often is recommended for these horses. In some horses, rest is the best option, and accurate monitoring of the healing process must follow (fracture of the distal phalanx, stress fractures of the proximal aspect of the McIII, and proximal suspensory desmitis [PSD]).

OA of the DIP joint, the metacarpophalangeal or meta-tarsophalangeal joints, or the middle carpal joint (particularly in young horses) can cause chronic lameness. Racetrack clinicians frequently inject the tarsometatarsal (TMT), centrodistal, and tarsocrural joints, but the true prevalence of problems arising from these joints has not been substantiated using diagnostic analgesia. Problems affecting the proximal aspect of the hindlimb, in the absence of visible lameness, frequently are diagnosed, but definitive diagnosis is difficult to substantiate.

Intraarticular therapy includes corticosteroids or nonsteroidal antiinflammatory drugs (NSAIDs) and, more recently, interleukin-1 receptor antagonist protein (IRAP). A series of four intraarticular injections of polysulfated glycosaminoglycans (PSGAGs), 250 mg every fourth day and then at weekly intervals, is helpful to treat juvenile OA, especially in the carpus. PSGAGs also have been useful parenterally (500 mg every 4 days for seven treatments).[9] High-molecular-weight hyaluronan (20 to 40 mg) may be used alone or with corticosteroids. Hyaluronan (20 to 40 mg) may be used intravenously.[10] The most popular corticosteroids for intraarticular therapy in horses include methylprednisolone acetate (40 to 60 mg), betamethasone disodium phosphate or betamethasone acetate (3 to 9 mg), and triamcinolone acetonide (6 mg). A basic treatment includes three intraarticular injections using 60 mg of methylprednisolone acetate for the first injection, followed by two injections of 40 mg at 2-week intervals. A similar protocol may be applied to betamethasone disodium phosphate and betamethasone acetate (6 to 9 mg the first time followed by two injections of 6 mg each). This treatment is usually helpful in horses with chronic OA of the DIP joint, the metacarpophalangeal or metatarsophalangeal joints, and the distal tarsal joints and sometimes resolves acute synovitis in young horses. When using triamcinolone acetonide (6 mg), clinicians must be aware of systemic effects and problems (laminitis and rhabdomyolysis) if several joints are injected at the same time. Although the cause is unsubstantiated, these complications may develop because of iatrogenic hyperadrenocorticism. Corticosteroids must be used in compliance with doping regulations.

Liniments, paints, and blisters are still popular, and despite lack of scientific support, they appear strongly tested by time. Iodide-based light paints diluted in dimethyl sulfoxide may be helpful in improving circulation to the distal aspect of the limbs and help to remove edema. Stronger blisters (with iodide mercury, cantharis, cedar oil, or turpentine) may play a role in improving circulation in some areas, but trainers must be made aware of possible secondary effects of the chemical-induced inflammation (scars, adhesions, cellulitis, and excessive joint inflammation) and that using most irritant blisters is no longer justified. Thermocautery (pin firing) is now less popular in Europe but is still used to treat STBs with curbs and proximal splint exostoses. Paints and blisters are used more frequently in France and Italy than in northern Europe.

CORRECTIVE SHOEING

Corrective shoeing is important for many STBs with forelimb lameness conditions. Generally speaking, a good lateral-to-medial balance and an ideal dorsal hoof wall angle must be provided before any shoe is applied. Then a large-based (wide-web) shoe is ideal but not always possible because of gait characteristics. Many trainers prefer thinner and lighter shoes because they are associated with increased speed. In horses with a flat sole the shoe must be in contact only with the wall border, and any rubber, leather, or silicon pad must be avoided. In these horses a rigid (aluminum) sole may prove helpful, but frequent cleaning is required to avoid sand accumulation under the sole. In horses with OA of the metacarpophalangeal or metatarsophalangeal joints, bar shoes must be avoided because the bar prevents the natural slipping of the foot when landing and increases stress on these joints. A bar shoe may prove helpful in horses with SDF tendonitis, but I prefer to leave this shoe on only during the recovery phase and during light training, whereas an open shoe is preferred for fast training and racing.

TRAINING PROGRAMS

Alternative training programs can be a valuable adjunct therapy, especially when dealing with unnatural fast-gaited trotters. Clockwise jogging and training, training on straight tracks (using interval training schedules), and swimming are preferred. Training programs aimed at reducing speed and stress on the large upper limb muscles, such as fast trotting in a circle in deep sand and use of heavy wagons or wagons with preselected brake sets (power carts), have been used, but scientific studies and objective data to support use of these alternatives are lacking.

PROCEEDING WITHOUT A DIAGNOSIS

Progress in diagnostic imaging has made the situation rare in which a clinician cannot determine a diagnosis. When available, whole body scintigraphic examination in horses with occult lameness is useful. Results of scintigraphy must not be overinterpreted, and clinicians must be aware that conditions may be subtle or difficult to detect. Bone remodeling around OCD or osseous cystlike lesions may be subtle. When detailed clinical examination has failed to reveal a diagnosis, I suggest the following options:
1. The horse should be reassessed 10 to 15 days later. This may help in horses with acute lesions without initial radiological abnormalities and when scintigraphy is not available.
2. A second opinion can be considered, especially if the horse can be referred to a center that is equipped with advanced imaging equipment.
3. The horse should be treated with NSAIDs (phenylbutazone 2.2 mg/kg/day orally [PO] for 5 days and then every second day for 10 days) and then reevaluated.
4. The clinician should treat the most likely site or sites of pain with short-acting corticosteroids. Some trainers prefer this approach because they believe the horse does not lose time and often believe something has been done. In some horses, experienced horsemen may help the clinician effectively by asking for a specific therapy that may help the situation.
5. The clinician should give the horse a period of controlled exercise or rest. This decision is particularly helpful when dealing with young horses, in which early training may have promoted bone and soft tissue maladaptation and remodeling that requires time to heal. Before resting the horse, a complete radiographic examination is a good idea because horses with advanced disease may have a poor prognosis or may require additional rest.

TEN MOST COMMON LAMENESS CONDITIONS

The following are the 10 most common lameness conditions:
1. Hoof or foot pain
2. Osteoarthritis of the distal interphalangeal joint
3. Osteoarthritis of the metacarpophalangeal joint
4. Lameness associated with middle carpal joint pain
5. Proximal palmar metacarpal pain including proximal suspensory desmitis
6. Sesamoiditis
7. Suspensory branch desmitis
8. Lameness of the metatarsophalangeal joint
9. Superficial digital flexor tendonitis
10. Osteochondrosis of the tarsocrural joint

LAMENESS IN THE EUROPEAN TROTTER
Hoof Pain

This nonspecific definition refers to a number of conditions, including what most clinicians and trainers call foot pain. Lameness varies, and the response to flexion may be equivocal. Negative flexion tests in a lame horse may suggest nonarticular hoof pain, and the same applies to horses in which the trainer's complaint is pain (with compromised gait) at the end of the race. Horses may break stride on the last turn or may get on a line in the straightaway.

A thorough examination of the feet, including hoof tester examination, is performed as previously described. A series of selective diagnostic analgesic procedures follows. Palmar digital analgesia commonly improves lameness by 75% to 90%. If a less than 50% response is obtained, palmar blocks at the base of the PSBs are performed. I avoid analgesia of the DIP joint because I may choose to medicate the joint. Recent evidence suggests analgesia of the DIP joint is not specific, and pain originating from the sole may be abolished.[11]

Diagnostic imaging includes radiography and scintigraphy. Stress remodeling of the distal phalanx is a common finding in trained STBs. Radiographs are usually negative, although occasionally marginal changes of the distal phalanx are seen.

Management includes corrective shoeing, controlled exercise, DIP joint injections, and local application of iodide ointments or blisters. Temporary pain relief has been reported anecdotally after perineural injection of cobratoxin, alcohol, or other preparations and after percutaneous cryotherapy. There can be complications such as substantial local inflammation and abscess formation with perineural injections. Horses with mild lameness respond to corrective shoeing: rubber or leather soles may be added to wide-web shoes, or different types of rubber flaps may be used temporarily. Light training for 2 to 3 weeks is suggested, and the horse is best trained on a soft track or on a straight track if available. Swimming is a good alternative method of training.

Osteoarthritis of the Distal Interphalangeal Joint

History, character of the lameness, response to flexion tests, and shape of the hoof are points to consider when OA of the DIP joint is suspected. Horses can be lame or reported to be intermittently lame. The tendency is for horses to develop OA of the DIP joint and club foot because the hoof growth in the heel region is faster than in the toe region. Evaluation and trimming of the hoof wall to lower the dorsal angle may help prevent this conformational change. Palpation of the area over the coronary band may elicit pain, especially medially where the condition must be distinguished from chronic collateral ligament strain of the DIP joint. Mild pain also may be detected by palpation of the proximal aspect of the SL in the forelimb and muscles of the back, two common compensatory lameness conditions. Diagnosis can be frustrating because horses are not always improved with DIP analgesia (this may suggest pain originating in the subchondral bone), and the gait may be abnormal because of other problems frequently secondary to pain originating from the DIP joint. An 80% to 90% positive response to perineural analgesia must be considered clinically relevant.

Lateromedial radiographs of the distal aspect of the limb frequently show a prominent osteophyte on the distal aspect of the middle phalanx, sometimes associated with secondary remodeling of the proximal aspect of the distal phalanx (see Figure 109-1). Fragmentation of the extensor process of the distal phalanx may also be observed, in which case the hoof wall frequently has a grossly triangular shape. OA of the DIP joint may be bilateral but is most commonly unilateral.

Suggested therapy includes intraarticular therapy with corticosteroids, PSGAGs, high-molecular-weight hyaluronan, or a combination of these drugs three times at 7-day intervals (14 days when using corticosteroids); IRAP therapy represents a new promising alternative. Corrective trimming to decrease excessive heel growth and maintaining the hoof angle at about 50 degrees appear important. Wide-web shoes distribute load on a large surface area, and when possible, a rubber or leather pad is needed. The shoe should have a rolled toe to ease breakover. A thick rubber pad (flap or flip-flop) is used sometimes to replace the classic shoe (Figure 109-5).

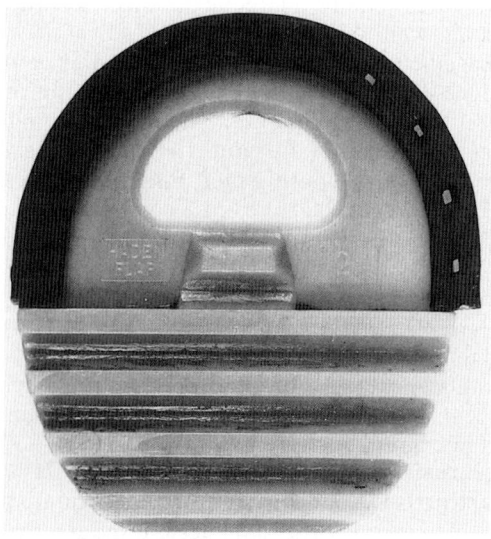

Fig. 109-5 • A flap or flip-flop shoe can be useful in trotters with foot pain.

Osteoarthritis of the Metacarpophalangeal Joint

OA of the metacarpophalangeal joint may be acute or chronic. Acute synovitis is seen in young horses when training is intensified or when the track surface changes. Clinical signs include mild to moderate lameness, pain on palpation, and lameness after flexion. Radiographs are usually negative in young horses, but flattening or more severe changes of the sagittal ridge of the McIII in older horses with chronic OA often are seen. Contrast radiology reveals a filling defect corresponding to a hypertrophic synovial pad of the distal, dorsal aspect of the McIII. Ultrasonographic examination reveals various degrees of dorsal joint capsule thickening and increase in echogenicity of the synovial pad. Intraarticular analgesia abolishes the lameness in most horses.

In horses with acute synovitis, training program modulation (2 to 3 weeks of light jogging), corrective shoeing (wide-based shoes and pads), and intraarticular corticosteroids (a series of three injections at 2-week intervals) may resolve the problem. In these horses, concurrent pathological conditions of the articular cartilage, subchondral bone, and the synovial pad usually are lacking or mild. Horses with hypertrophic synovial pads benefit from arthroscopic surgery to remove the thickened tissues because response to medical management is poor. This is frequently the case in older horses, in which advanced OA is often present. Prognosis after surgery is only fair to guarded, however.

Middle Carpal Joint

The middle carpal joint is the most common site of lameness in young STBs. Typically, affected horses tend to trot with a wide gait, abducting the affected limb or limbs in an attempt to minimize carpal flexion.[12] Visual inspection from a dorsolateral perspective reveals abnormal contour of the dorsomedial aspect of the carpus. Palpation often elicits a painful response over the dorsal aspect of the radial and third carpal bones. Usually the response to carpal flexion is positive, and intraarticular analgesia abolishes lameness in most horses. A negative result from intraarticular analgesia does not rule out the middle carpal joint as the source of pain causing lameness because subchondral bone damage under a relatively normal cartilage layer may cause pain that may not be desensitized completely. Radiographs are usually diagnostic, especially the skyline image of the distal row of carpal bones. Abnormal radiological findings range from complete slab fracture of the third carpal bone to more subtle signs of radiolucency of the radial fossa of the third carpal bone. Scintigraphy is a sensitive and excellent tool in the early diagnosis of middle carpal joint injury.[8]

Training program modulation and intraarticular injections of PSGAGs, hyaluronan, or small amounts of corticosteroids are the first steps in the treatment program. Arthroscopy is suggested when evidence of more severe bone damage exists. Chip fractures in STBs most frequently involve the third and radial carpal bones. Counterclockwise racing, especially in the turns, concentrates forces along the medial aspect of the right forelimb, and this makes the right middle carpal joint more predisposed to injuries.[13-15] The proximal border of the third carpal bone is involved more frequently than the distal border of the radial carpal bone in the STB trotter, unlike in the Thoroughbred (TB) and in the pacer.[13,15,16] Arthroscopic surgery and rest generally yield a fair to good prognosis.[15] STBs with incomplete slab fractures of the third carpal bone may heal with rest, possibly preceded by diagnostic arthroscopy and curettage of the lesion. Horses with complete slab fractures are best treated by internal fixation. Thin fragments are removed. When arthroscopy shows substantial loss of articular cartilage, the micropick technique may increase the possibilities of cartilage repair.[17] Arthroscopic findings in young STBs have been shown to correlate poorly with radiological findings, and lesions appear frequently more severe than expected.[16] In horses without radiological changes, I frequently find depressions and discoloration of articular cartilage (especially in the radial fossa of the third carpal bone), loss of articular cartilage in focal areas of the third and radial carpal bones, and partial or complete tearing of the medial palmar intercarpal ligament. Ligament injuries, especially affecting the medial palmar intercarpal ligament, must be suspected in the absence of radiological abnormalities.[18] However, medial palmar intercarpal ligament injuries are rare. These horses are treated using arthroscopic trimming and are given 4 to 6 weeks of stall rest followed by 4 weeks of stall rest with handwalking exercise, and joints are injected with short-acting corticosteroids.

Proximal Palmar Metacarpal Pain Including Proximal Suspensory Desmitis

Proximal palmar metacarpal pain affects many more horses than we once thought. Mild pain in the proximal palmar aspect of the metacarpal region may be secondary to other gait disturbances and may reflect attempts to maintain balance when trotting fast. In these horses the lesion rarely is substantiated by ultrasonography, but pain may be detected with accurate palpation (racetrack clinicians used to diagnose and treat "blind splints" in this area).

PSD is usually acute in onset, and direct palpation of the SL elicits pain. A carpal flexion test is often positive. Intraarticular analgesia of the middle carpal joint produces a variable amount of improvement, but some degree of lameness still is elicited by flexion. Subcarpal analgesia (4 mg of local anesthetic solution placed axial to each of the second and fourth metacarpal bones or direct infiltration of 2% mepivacaine over the proximal aspect of the SL) usually abolishes lameness.

Diagnostic imaging includes radiography, scintigraphy, and ultrasonography. Scintigraphy is useful in identifying horses with bony injury, including horses with an avulsion fracture of the McIII at the origin of the SL, those with enthesopathy, or those with a longitudinal fracture of the McIII. Horses with PSD without bony involvement may have positive pool phase images, but delayed images are usually negative. Radiography (dorsopalmar and flexed lateromedial images) may reveal associated longitudinal or avulsion fractures of the proximal, palmar aspect of the McIII or, in horses with chronic lameness, increased radiopacity of the McIII at the SL origin (see Figure 109-3). Ultrasonography is useful in identifying patterns of ligamentous injury, palmar cortical bone damage, and monitoring the healing process.

The prognosis is fair to good, provided the affected horse is subjected to walking exercise and controlled training with concurrent monitoring of the healing process. STBs may tolerate an acceptable level of training with

chronic injuries of the SL compared with TBs, possibly because of the increased percentage of muscle fibers present in the SL.[19] The prognosis in horses with PSD is better than those affected with lesions in the suspensory body.

Therapy includes 6 to 8 weeks of rest followed by 4 to 6 weeks of 20 to 60 minutes of walking exercise or swimming. Local application of blisters and injections of corticosteroids or PSGAGs may help but rarely shorten the healing period. Cryotherapy has gained some popularity in treating STBs with PSD in racetrack practice, but its usefulness has not been substantiated scientifically. Several biological therapies have gained recent acceptance: intralesional injection of bone marrow,[20] isolated or cultured stem cells, and platelet-rich plasma (PRP). However, more research and clinical work are required to substantiate their value. Shock wave therapy also has been used to treat horses with PSD in recent years (see Chapter 96).

Sesamoiditis

Sesamoiditis may be defined as enthesopathy at the insertion of the branches of the SL to the abaxial surface of the PSBs. The condition also may affect the base of PSBs, but this form is rare and is best defined as distal sesamoidean desmitis. Two types of sesamoiditis are recognized. Type 1, or juvenile sesamoiditis, is characterized by radiolucent lines (vascular channels) in the proximal third of a PSB, radially oriented as seen in lateromedial or oblique radiographic images, and is a frequent feature in young (2- and 3-year-old) STBs (Figure 109-6). This radiological pattern is not always associated with lameness, and no link has been observed between the presence of these lines and PSB fractures.[21] Affected horses tend to be lame after training, but pain subsides with rest. Intraarticular analgesia does not abolish lameness. Lameness disappears after perineural analgesia of the medial and lateral plantar (palmar) nerves. The condition usually involves one or both hindlimbs, and the lateral PSB is affected more frequently. Scintigraphic examination reveals increased radiopharmaceutical uptake (IRU), but radiological changes are seen in only 50% of STBs with scintigraphic abnormalities.[8] The lateral PSB

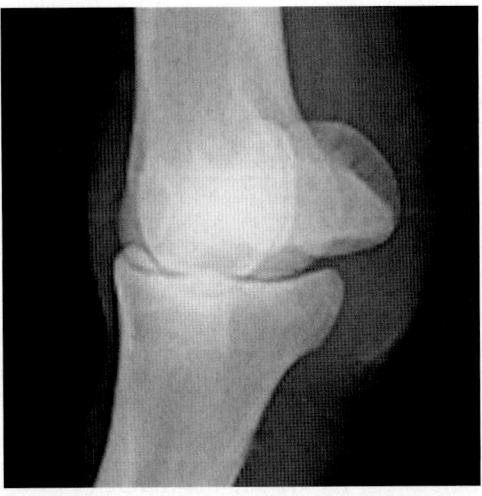

Fig. 109-6 • Dorsolateral-plantaromedial oblique radiographic image of a metatarsophalangeal joint of a lame 2-year-old Standardbred colt with juvenile sesamoiditis. Note the radiolucent lines in the lateral proximal sesamoid bone.

represents one of the most frequent locations for IRU in racing STBs.[8,22]

Type 2 sesamoiditis is chronic, frequently affects a single PSB, and is found more commonly in the forelimbs of older horses. Radiological signs of type 2 sesamoiditis (evidence of radiolucent lines in the proximal half of the bone, irregular palmar/plantar and abaxial outline of the bone, enthesophytes, and mineralization of the adjacent intersesamoidean ligament) are associated with ultrasonographic evidence of suspensory insertion desmitis. One or both suspensory branches often are involved. Focal loss of echogenicity in horses with acute disease and increased echogenicity in horses with chronic lameness are common abnormal ultrasonographic findings. The insertion on the PSB (enthesis) becomes grossly irregular.

In horses with type 1 sesamoiditis, treatment involves rest, slow training, or turnout for 30 to 90 days, depending on the degree of lameness present. Radiological monitoring of the lesion is probably not helpful because lameness may improve substantially despite the persistence of radiolucent lines. More information is provided by scintigraphy initially and during follow-up examination. Medical treatment includes local application of paints or mild blisters and corrective shoeing (bars must be avoided; the quarters must be lowered moderately; and shoes must provide a wide base in the hindlimbs). Medical treatment is aimed at improving local blood flow, and isoxsuprine hydrochloride (0.6 to 1.2 mg/kg PO twice daily) and sodium acetylsalicylate (10 mg/kg PO twice daily) are recommended for 45 to 60 days. The efficacy of this therapy, however, is questionable. The prognosis is fair if lameness is not severe and if the horse tends to warm out of lameness. If severe lameness is observed and associated radiological changes are pronounced, the prognosis is guarded. These horses are best given long periods of rest and paddock turnout (6 to 8 months). Treatment of horses with type 2 sesamoiditis includes rest, corrective shoeing (wide-web aluminum shoes, leather pad, with particular attention to lateral-to-medial hoof balance), local application of dimethyl sulfoxide, and paints and blisters. Pin firing is no longer justified. Cryotherapy has become popular in recent years, but in my opinion its clinical efficacy is poor. The prognosis is fair, but hoof balance must be monitored to prevent recurrence. Low-level or alternative (swimming) training is indicated.

Suspensory Branch Desmitis

Suspensory branch desmitis can be acute or chronic and is caused by lateral-to-medial hoof imbalance, exercise over uneven track surfaces, strains, and chronic fractures of the second and fourth metacarpal/metatarsal (splint) bones. Acute desmitis can be associated with metacarpophalangeal/metatarsophalangeal joint effusion. Shoeing changes, particularly when the hoof angle is modified (usually increased), frequently precede the condition, and when treating the condition, hoof imbalances must be identified and corrected. Ideally the dorsal hoof angle in the forelimb should be kept between 48 and 52 degrees, with a shoe providing good support to the heel. The routine training regimen, track conditions, and the counterclockwise direction of racing may affect the distribution of suspensory branch desmitis. In my experience the right forelimb and right hindlimb are most commonly affected, and lesions of the medial branch are twice as common as those of the

lateral branch. Radiography and ultrasonography are performed to assess ligament damage and bone involvement. Enlargement and loss of definition of the margins of the branch, focal hypoechogenic areas, or diffuse loss of echogenicity and hyperechogenic foci in horses with chronic desmitis are the most frequent ultrasonographic findings.[23] Radiologically the ipsilateral splint bone may appear deviated abaxially, and in horses with chronic lameness, adhesions may develop between the splint bone and suspensory branch, causing fracture during fast exercise. For the latter reason, radiological monitoring of the splint bones is suggested in horses with chronic desmitis. The insertion of the branch on the PSB must be assessed by ultrasonography for the presence of insertional desmitis.

The treatment in horses with acute desmitis includes rest, antiinflammatory drugs (phenylbutazone 2.2 mg/kg), or local application of dimethyl sulfoxide and poultices. Intraarticular injection of corticosteroids may be beneficial when the condition is associated with metacarpophalangeal/metatarsophalangeal joint effusion. In horses with chronic or severe desmitis, rest and local application of mild blisters may help. Fast training must be avoided when possible, and corrective shoeing must be provided. Alternative training programs, especially swimming physiotherapy, are indicated and can allow an acceptable level of exercise without worsening the lesion.

Metatarsophalangeal Joint

The metatarsophalangeal joint represents a major source of hindlimb lameness in STBs.[24] Lameness of the metatarsophalangeal joint and specifically the plantar aspect is frequently subtle, and diagnosis can be challenging. Malor nonadaptive modeling of the plantar aspect of the metatarsophalangeal joint, proximal plantar fragmentation of the proximal phalanx, and nonunion of the lateral eminence of the proximal phalanx represent the most common conditions. Traumatic OC of the distal plantar aspect of the condyles of the MtIII and mineralization of the distal sesamoidean ligaments are observed rarely.

Subchondral nonadaptive remodeling of the MtIII has been described and represents a scintigraphic finding, with a corresponding radiological pattern not easily identifiable (Figure 109-7).[22] Proximal plantar fragmentation of the proximal phalanx has been reported by several authors in radiological surveys of young STBs and is commonly seen (see Figure 109-2).[25,26] Plantar fragments from the proximal phalanx rarely are associated with lameness at a trot in hand. Trainers' complaints include gait disturbances during fast exercise, especially in turns, and the tendency for the horse to be on one shaft. Intraarticular analgesia of the metatarsophalangeal joint can alleviate lameness, but a fast exercise test is required, and owners must be aware of the potential consequences of this procedure. For this reason, when the clinical pattern indicates pain arising from the metatarsophalangeal joint, a radiographic examination including the oblique images (dorsoproximolateral-plantarodistomedial oblique and dorsoproximomedial-plantarodistolateral oblique) is required. In horses with plantar process OC fragments, arthroscopic surgical removal of fragments is indicated. The prognosis after surgical treatment is good. In horses with nonadaptive remodeling of the distal aspect of the MtIII, rest or reduced training, intraarticular injections of PSGAGs, or low doses of corticosteroids and hyaluronan are recommended.

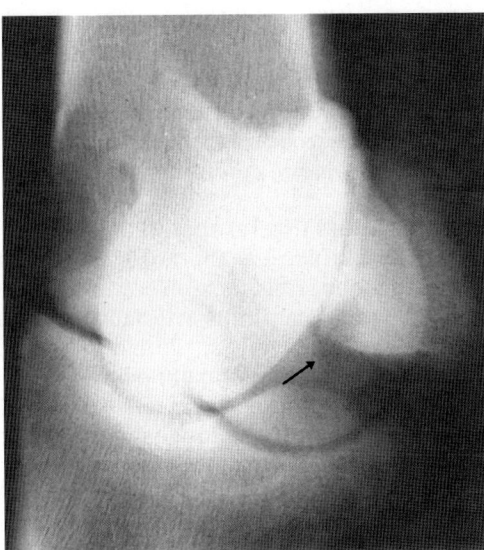

Fig. 109-7 • A radiolucent defect *(arrow)* in the distal, plantarolateral aspect of the third metatarsal bone is visible on the dorsal 45° lateral 30° proximal-palmarodistal oblique radiographic image, the result of stress or nonadaptive remodeling.

Superficial Digital Flexor Tendonitis

The incidence and morbidity of STBs with SDF tendonitis are lower compared with TBs, but tendonitis of the superficial digital flexor tendon (SDFT) and suspensory desmitis represent the main indications for ultrasonographic examination of the distal aspect of the forelimbs in STB racehorses in Europe.

In my experience, most of the lesions are located in the middle and distal thirds of the SDFT. A core lesion located in the palmarolateral border of the tendon characterizes more than 30% of the lesions identified using ultrasonography. More rarely central core lesions are seen. Horses with chronic lesions have the typical pattern of diffuse tendonitis. Therapy includes rest; corrective shoeing; local application of antiinflammatory ointments, poultices, dimethyl sulfoxide, paints, or blisters; tendon splitting; desmotomy of the accessory ligament of the SDFT; and desmotomy of the palmar annular ligament. Intralesional injections of hyaluronan or PSGAGs have been reported. Promising results after bone marrow, cultured stem cell, and PRP therapy have been reported anecdotally. My treatment of choice in horses with acute lameness includes corrective shoeing (moderate lowering of the heels, correcting lateral-to-medial balance, and using wide-based shoes without pads, especially rubber pads), local application of dimethyl sulfoxide, cold water therapy twice a day, poultice application, and walking exercise for 2 to 4 weeks. The initial treatment is followed by the local application of an iodide blister, and the horse is given an additional 4 to 8 weeks of walking exercise. The horse usually is able then to resume jogging unless lameness is present. Ultrasonographic examination is performed 12 weeks later.

In horses with recurrent tendonitis, my treatment of choice includes desmotomy of the accessory ligament of the SDFT (superior check desmotomy). Desmotomy of the palmar annular ligament also is performed when substantial tendonitis involving the distal aspect of the tendon or digital flexor tendon sheath effusion is present. After

surgery, horses are given 2 weeks of box stall rest, followed by 8 weeks of walking exercise.

Tendonitis of the SDFT within the pastern region is less common but more difficult to manage than tendonitis in the metacarpal region. Lameness is more pronounced, and recurrence of clinical signs is common. With ultrasonography, lesions can be detected at the tendon insertion over the lateral or medial aspect of the middle phalanx. Treatment includes rest, local and systemic antiinflammatory drugs, blisters, corrective shoeing, and alternative training, particularly swimming. Monitoring of the healing process is important to prevent recurrence.

Osteochondrosis of the Tarsocrural Joint

Joint effusion represents the most common feature of tarsocrural OC, a condition with a reported prevalence ranging between 4% and 20%.[25-33] Tarsocrural OC frequently is diagnosed in yearlings, and breeders are particularly concerned because the condition may lower the yearling's price at the autumn sales. For this reason, tarsocrural effusion in yearlings now represents a frequent indication for radiographic examination and preventative arthroscopy.

Lameness associated with OC is rare, but selected lesions may cause gait disturbances. In horses with effusion and osteochondral fragmentation, it is important to rule out other causes of lameness. Lesions affecting the lateral trochlear ridge of the talus and medial malleolus of the tibia are more likely to cause lameness and synovial effusion than are lesions of the cranial aspect of the intermediate ridge of the tibia. Focal areas of radiolucency or loss of radiopacity on the medial malleolus may be associated with osteochondral fragmentation and may represent an indication for diagnostic arthroscopy.[34] In young horses with effusion, arthroscopic removal of fragment(s) represents the best option. Prognosis after arthroscopic treatment of tarsocrural OC is good, but synovial effusion may persist especially when OC involves the lateral trochlear ridge of the talus and the medial malleolus.[35,36] Studies performed in Europe found no significant differences in the racing performance and longevity of STB trotters with or without tarsocrural OC.[1,32,37]

◼ THE AUSTRALASIAN STANDARDBRED

R. Chris Whitton

DESCRIPTION OF THE SPORT

Standardbred (STB) horses have been racing in Australia and New Zealand for more than 140 years. In both countries the sport does not enjoy the same high profile as Thoroughbred (TB) racing, and prize money is generally lower, which attracts fewer professional trainers than TB racing. Owner/trainers are common, with many stables having fewer than 10 horses. Horses can begin racing at 2 years of age and generally race until 8 or 9 years of age.

Most races are for pacers, with trotting races being much less common. In Australia, races range in distance from 1600 to 2600 m, and most pacing races are from a mobile start, with an occasional standing start. All trotting races are from a standing start. In New Zealand, races tend to be longer, up to 3200 m, and standing starts are more common.

Regional meetings carry prize money of $A2000 (Australian dollars) to $A5000 per race, whereas metropolitan meetings offer $15,000 per race. The 15 most valuable pacing races in Australia and New Zealand make up what is called the Grand Circuit. Prize money for Grand Circuit races ranges from $A125,000 to $A1,000,000 for the Interdominion Pacing Championship Final and the New Zealand Cup. Prize money for trotting races is substantially less than that for pacers. The Interdominion trotter's Championship Final carries a $A250,000 prize, and New Zealand's Row Cup has a prize of $NZ300,000.

An increased number of stakes programs for young horses have become available in recent years. The Australasian Breeders Crown is held over all states of Australia and both islands of New Zealand for 2-, 3-, and 4-year-old pacers and trotters. Australian Pacing Gold is a program for yearlings sold at the sales of the same name and also has feature races for 2-, 3-, and 4-year-olds. The value of these programs puts great pressure on trainers and clinicians to persist with young horses that may benefit from rest.

Race speeds generally are expressed as mile rates, which is the time taken to travel 1 mile averaged over the whole race. Tight tracks result in slightly slower rates than large tracks. Typical mile rates for pacers in 1600-m races are 1:56 to 1:58. For 2400-m races, mile rates of 2 minutes are typical.

TRACK SURFACE OR TRAINING SURFACE AND LAMENESS

Most of the racetracks are 700 to 1000 m in circumference, and races are run in a counterclockwise direction, except for the north island of New Zealand, where races are run clockwise. Track surfaces vary but usually consist of sand or fine gravel. Banking of turns tends to be modest, although a trend to greater degrees of banking and resulting reduced injury rates has been demonstrated. Many trainers have their own homemade training track that is often just graded dirt or sand and not always well maintained, and recurrent subsolar bruising can be a major problem. Banking on these tracks tends to be minimal. In coastal areas, training on the beach is popular and considered beneficial for horses with injuries.

TRAINING METHODS

A typical training program involves a period of jogging exercise, generally of about 6 weeks, and these sessions generally last 35 to 40 minutes. Higher-speed work in hobbles (pace work) is introduced two to three times a week. A typical workout is two intervals of half to three-quarter pace over 1½ miles. The speed of these workouts is steadily increased over 4 to 6 weeks until speeds approaching those of race speed are achieved. A horse that is racing generally is hobbled twice a week and jogged on the other days. Training in New Zealand is similar, with the major difference being the tendency to house horses in paddocks rather than in stables.

LAMENESS EXAMINATION

Experience in examining STBs for lameness is essential because of their awkward gait, even when trotting. A high incidence of lameness occurs in horses in full work, and numerous sites of pain are common.

Examination at Rest (Preferably in a Stable)

The clinician should observe the horse standing for any obvious swelling, abnormal weight bearing, and areas of hair loss on the proximal limbs associated with the position of the hobbles. The clinician should palpate the neck and back to detect any areas of pain; palpate the supraspinous ligament, dorsal spinous processes, and dorsal sacro-iliac ligament, along with the longissimus dorsi muscles; and then examine each limb in turn. Palpation is performed with the limb bearing weight and not bearing weight. The veterinarian should palpate the digital pulse amplitude in the distal aspect of the pastern or over the abaxial surface of the proximal sesamoid bones (PSBs). Observe each joint and palpate for swelling or effusion. Palpate the tendons and ligaments for heat, pain, and swelling. Particular attention should be paid to all levels of the suspensory ligaments (SLs) of the forelimbs and hindlimbs. The clinician should take time to examine the hind fetlock joints for effusion. Flex the joints firmly to detect pain, and apply hoof testers to each foot.

Trotting in a Straight Line

The horse should be trotted on a firm flat surface. Many horses pace initially, which makes the diagnosis of subtle lameness difficult. Persistence is important because most horses will trot after two or three runs up and down. The horse should be observed trotting away from and toward the observer and should be observed from the side.

Flexion Tests

Flexion tests have limitations but are a useful addition to the lameness examination. It is important to perform hindlimb fetlock flexion tests separately from proximal limb flexion tests because hindlimb fetlock problems are common.[1]

DIAGNOSTIC ANALGESIA

Nerve blocks generally are required where no cause of lameness is obvious or the importance of a clinical finding is not clear. Where no localizing clinical signs are apparent, I use a standard approach: in the forelimb a pastern ring block is performed. The veterinarian should avoid nerve blocks at the level of the PSBs because distinguishing between PSB pain and foot pain is difficult. This is followed by a low four-point block and then a subcarpal block and intraarticular blocks of the middle carpal joint and then the antebrachiocarpal joint. Should the horse fail to respond to these blocks, median and ulnar nerve blocks are performed to rule out the lower limb as a source of pain. Rarely are blocks of the elbow joint, intertubercular (bicipital) bursa, or shoulder joint required.

A similar sequence of blocks is used in the hindlimb. A single lateral plantar metatarsal nerve block may be performed if plantar condylar subchondral bone pain is suspected. A subtarsal block is followed by an intraarticular block of the tarsometatarsal joint and then the centrodistal joint. The tarsocrural joint is seldom blocked because there is generally swelling associated with intraarticular pathological conditions. Tibial and fibular blocks are performed to rule out the lower limb as the source of pain. Occasionally an intraarticular stifle block is required, in which case all compartments should be blocked at one time.

IMAGING CONSIDERATIONS

Radiography remains an important imaging technique. Oblique images of the distal phalanx are important when a fracture is suspected because some may be missed on dorsopalmar images. A flexed lateromedial image of the metacarpophalangeal joint should be obtained to highlight the sagittal ridge of the distal aspect of the third metacarpal bone (McIII) and the dorsal surfaces of the PSBs. Proximodistal oblique images of the hind fetlocks are obtained to demonstrate fragments of the proximal plantar aspect of the proximal phalanx and the lateral condyle of the third metatarsal bone (MtIII). Carpal images should always include a skyline image of the third carpal bone.

Ultrasonographic examination of the digital flexor tendons and SLs commonly is required. Superficial digital flexor tendon (SDFT) lesions are often peripheral rather than core lesions. Lesions also may involve the distal third of the metacarpal region or the proximal metatarsal region, areas that are examined less commonly by ultrasonography and may be more difficult to assess. Cross-sectional area measurements comparing affected and nonaffected limbs are essential when assessing subtle lesions. When examining the SLs, it is important to assess the full length because lesions can affect the origin, body, and branches.

Scintigraphy is useful for assessing STBs with complex lameness, STBs that fail to improve with diagnostic analgesia, and when pain is localized but no abnormalities are detected with radiography or ultrasonography. Stress fractures are common and can be insidious in onset. Typical sites include the third tarsal bone, lateral cortex of the tibial shaft, and the distal phalanges. Subchondral bone injuries may not be observed on radiographs yet are well documented with bone phase scintigraphic images.

PROCEEDING WITHOUT A DIAGNOSIS

Intraarticular corticosteroids often are used to assist in diagnosing subtle hindlimb lameness. Bilateral intraarticular injection of the tarsometatarsal and centrodistal joints may be used in horses in which hindlimb lameness is too subtle for accurate assessment by nerve blocks. Triamcinolone acetonide is the most commonly used intraarticular corticosteroid because of its relatively short and predictable detection time. Treatment of metatarsophalangeal joints also is often performed because lameness can be subtle. The clinical relevance of fragments of the plantar aspect of the proximal phalanx is often questionable, and intraarticular therapy may be the only method of confirming that metatarsophalangeal joint pain exists.

SHOEING CONSIDERATIONS

Most horses are shod and trimmed by the trainer or owner. Therefore the quality varies extremely. Steel rim shoes generally are used, with trailers on the hind feet being universal. These shoes are thin and provide little protection for the sole. An occasional horse is trained and raced barefoot. Wider web aluminum shoes, similar to those used on TB racehorses, are available, but the use of these shoes is less common. These shoes generally have steel inserts to improve grip. Glue-on shoes rarely are used. In an attempt to promote increased length of stride, toes are often left overlong but there is no evidence to support this traditional approach. The combination of overlong toes and the lack of sole protection predisposes horses to subsolar bruising. Manipulation of shoeing methods is used for horses that hit the carpi during the swing phase. Generally this is trial and error. Heavier shoes tend to exaggerate any abnormal movement in the swing phase and result in higher hoof flight.

TEN MOST COMMON LAMENESS CONDITIONS

1. Subsolar bruising
2. Foot abscess
3. Osteoarthritis of the metacarpophalangeal or metatarsophalangeal joint and other conditions
4. Carpal joint disease
5. Suspensory desmitis
6. Superficial digital flexor tendonitis
7. Osteoarthritis of the distal tarsal joints
8. Fracture of the distal phalanx
9. Sagittal fracture of the proximal phalanx
10. Osteochondrosis of the tarsocrural joint

DIAGNOSIS AND MANAGEMENT OF LAMENESS

Subsolar Bruising and Abscessation

The diagnosis of subsolar bruising is based on pain with the application of hoof testers over the sole, either localized or generalized, and increased lameness after concussion of the foot. Lameness is localized to the foot with a pastern ring block, and radiography is performed to rule out a fracture of the distal phalanx. Chronic bruising may result in radiolucency and modeling of the margins of the distal phalanx, but these changes do not necessarily mean that the bruising is active. Scintigraphy will allow assessment of active inflammation and bone metabolism. Hemorrhage within the horn of the sole may or may not be evident. Horses with acute lameness are treated with rest and nonsteroidal antiinflammatory drugs. Careful attention should be paid to foot balance, and wide-web aluminum shoes should be fitted.

Osteoarthritis of the Fetlock Joint

Osteoarthritis (OA) of the metacarpophalangeal or metatarsophalangeal (fetlock) joint may or may not be associated with joint effusion and swelling. Usually the horse shows pain on passive flexion and a positive response to a fetlock flexion test. Lameness should be improved with a low four-point block or intraarticular analgesia. If lameness is recent, no radiological abnormalities will be apparent, but more chronic lameness is associated with modeling changes on the dorsal aspects of the proximal phalanx and the McIII or the MtIII. Modeling also may be observed on the articular margins of the PSBs and the palmar or plantar aspect of the proximal phalanx. In advanced OA, subchondral radiolucent or cystic lesions may be observed in the palmar or plantar aspect of the condyles of the McIII or the MtIII. This is most common in the lateral condyle of the MtIII and is best observed on a proximodistal oblique radiographic image. Scintigraphy may be required for horses with few radiological changes and demonstrates increased radiopharmaceutical uptake in the subchondral bone.

Proliferative Synovitis

Proliferative synovitis occasionally causes lameness in STBs. Lameness generally is localized to the metacarpophalangeal joint by either perineural or intraarticular analgesia. Abnormal concavity proximal to the dorsal and occasionally the palmar aspects of the sagittal ridge of the McIII is observed on lateromedial radiographic images. Ultrasonography demonstrates enlargement of the synovial pad medial or lateral to the sagittal ridge of the McIII on the dorsal aspect, which must be differentiated from the joint capsule. Intraarticular corticosteroids may be used, but the results often are disappointing. Surgical excision of the synovial pad using arthroscopy is usually effective in resolving the lameness. The prognosis is poorer in horses with modeling of the palmar aspect of the McIII because this usually reflects the presence of more advanced chronic OA.

Axial, Articular (Type 1) Osteochondral Fragments of the Proximal Plantar Aspect of the Proximal Phalanx

Fragments of the proximal plantar aspect of the proximal phalanx are best observed on proximodistal oblique radiographic images of the metatarsophalangeal joints. These views should be included in the workup of horses with low-grade hindlimb lameness or a history of not running straight. Lameness is generally mild or not present at low speeds. Most horses have a positive flexion test of the affected fetlock, and about half have joint effusion.[3] Osteochondral fragments of the proximal plantar aspect of the proximal phalanx are most commonly found medially but can occur laterally or biaxially. These fragments are present by 1 year of age and are thought by some to be traumatic in origin. Treatment involves arthroscopic removal, and treated horses can be returned to training within 6 weeks. Intraarticularly administered corticosteroids are sometimes used to determine the relevance of these lesions because not all are associated with poor performance.

Carpal Joint Disease

Lameness caused by carpal pain is common in Australasian STBs, affecting up to 30% of horses in training. In the absence of intraarticular fractures, lameness is often bilateral, and effusion is mild or absent. Because of the lack of localizing signs, intraarticular analgesia must be used to localize the pain causing lameness to the carpus. Radiographs should always include a skyline image of the third carpal bone. Often only increased radiopacity with or without focal radiolucent defects of the third carpal bone is observed.

Intraarticular fractures of the carpal bones generally involve the middle carpal joint. Fractures involving the antebrachiocarpal joint are less common and lameness is generally mild. More severe lameness is seen in horses

with slab fractures or severe joint injury. Joint swelling and pain on flexion are common. Treatment options include arthroscopic surgery to remove diseased bone and cartilage, intraarticularly administered corticosteroids, and rest.

Suspensory Desmitis

In most horses with suspensory desmitis, swelling and pain on palpation of the affected area of the SL are obvious, but lesions confined to the origin may be more difficult to diagnose, and subcarpal or subtarsal nerve blocks are required for diagnosis. Ultrasonographic examination confirms desmitis based on increased cross-sectional area and areas of decreased echogenicity. Radiological examination is used to assess the palmar or plantar aspect of the McIII or the MtIII and the PSBs at the proximal and distal attachments of the SL. The ideal treatment involves an initial period of rest and antiinflammatory treatment to allow the inflammation to resolve, followed by a period of controlled exercise. Horses should not return to full work for 12 months. In practice this is not always possible, and many horses can be managed by reducing the workload for shorter periods, treating with antiinflammatory drugs, and monitoring the response with ultrasonography.

Superficial Digital Flexor Tendonitis

Tendon injuries are easy to diagnose when the midmetacarpal or midmetatarsal area is involved. Swelling and pain on palpation are indications for ultrasonographic examination to confirm the diagnosis and differentiate from peritendonous inflammation. Horses with moderate to severe injuries are treated with rest and antiinflammatory therapy until the swelling is reduced, followed by a controlled exercise program. Intralesional injection of bone marrow or bone marrow–derived stem cells has been used, but long-term follow-up data on efficacy are currently lacking. Full work should not be reintroduced until 12 months after injury. Less severely injured horses may be kept in work, provided the exercise level is reduced and the tendon is monitored by ultrasonography. Such management is more successful in horses with hindlimb injuries. Tendon injuries at the level of the digital flexor tendon sheath (DFTS) may result in secondary palmar annular ligament (PAL) constriction and tenosynovitis. Lameness and effusion of the DFTS are observed when the horse is returned to training. Provided healing of the tendon injury is adequate, the PAL can be sectioned tenoscopically and the horse rapidly returned to training to prevent the formation of adhesions.

Osteoarthritis of the Distal Tarsal Joints

Confirmation of the distal tarsal joints as the source of pain causing lameness involves using intraarticular analgesia or intraarticular medication in horses with more subtle lameness. Although radiographs are useful for determining the extent of bony changes, they are not always diagnostic. Scintigraphy is more sensitive and may also reveal stress fractures of the third tarsal bone or the proximal dorsal aspect of the MtIII. Treatment involves intraarticular injection of long-acting corticosteroids. Triamcinolone acetonide is the most commonly used because of its reliable excretion times and reliable duration of action.

Fracture of the Distal Phalanx

STBs with a sudden onset of forelimb lameness after racing or fast work but with no localizing signs should be suspected of having a fracture of the distal phalanx. Application of hoof testers usually elicits pain, but this is not always consistent. Oblique radiographic images of the foot often are required to assess the fracture properly. It is important to determine whether the fracture enters the DIP joint. Most fractures are intraarticular. In horses that race counterclockwise, left forelimb fractures are generally of the lateral palmar process, and right forelimb fractures are generally of the medial palmar process. Occult fractures are occasionally identified with scintigraphy. Horses with nonarticular fractures are treated with a bar shoe with quarter clips or a rim shoe, and 12 months of rest. Horses with articular fractures may be treated in the same manner or by internal fixation with a single 4.5-mm screw placed in lag fashion along with a bar shoe with quarter clips. Evidence of the relative success of these treatments is limited, with the choice depending on individual preference. Reports indicate that 50% to 75% of Australian STBs with fracture of the distal phalanx are able to race following treatment with a bar shoe.[2] It is recommended that a bar shoe be maintained when horses return to racing to reduce the risk of refracture.

Sagittal Fracture of the Proximal Phalanx

The clinical presentation of horses with sagittal fractures of the proximal phalanx depends on fracture configuration. Horses with short, incomplete fractures may have chronic lameness that is localized to the fetlock joint with nerve blocks. Longer fractures often cause acute onset of lameness. Swelling may be present, and the horse often has pain on palpation of the dorsal aspect of the proximal phalanx. Nerve blocks are contraindicated because of the risk of progression of the fracture. Radiological examination confirms the diagnosis. Horses with nondisplaced fractures may be treated with external coaptation. Internal fixation with screws placed in lag fashion is recommended for horses with complete and displaced fractures. Horses with short, incomplete fractures may heal with rest. Internal fixation has been recommended for horses with fractures that fail to heal.

Tarsocrural Osteochondrosis

The most common osteochondrosis lesion affecting the tarsocrural joint of STB horses involves the cranial aspect of the intermediate ridge of the tibia. Most horses have effusion of the tarsocrural joint, and lameness is absent or subtle. Radiographs demonstrate fragmentation of the cranial aspect of the intermediate ridge of the tibia. The fragments are removed arthroscopically.

Stifle Disease

Lameness localized to the stifle is rare in the STB racehorse. These horses appear to be able to race successfully with radiological evidence of OA of the femorotibial joints. Direct trauma to the stifle may result in soft tissue and bony injuries as in other types of horses. Trainers often are concerned that a horse may be locking its stifles, but this generally resolves with increased fitness, and sectioning of the medial patellar ligament is rarely necessary.

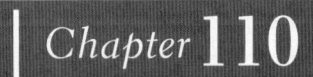

The Racing Quarter Horse

Nancy L. Goodman

HISTORY AND DESCRIPTION OF THE SPORT

Racing Quarter Horses (QHs) are the sprinters of the racing world, competing at distances of 220 yards (one furlong, 201 meters) to 870 yards (795 meters). The explosive power exerted while leaving the starting gate and the ability to attain speeds of more than 50 mph (80 km/h) to run 440 yards (402 meters) in less than 21 seconds distinguishes the QH from other racing breeds. The American QH originates from colonial Virginia in the 1600s where imported English Thoroughbreds (TBs) were crossed with "native" breeds of Spanish descent to produce a compact, heavily muscled horse that excelled at running short distances. They were known as Quarter Pathers or Quarter Milers, named after the quarter-mile distance at which they excelled. The first race records came from Enrico County, Virginia, in 1674, where match races were run down village streets and in small level fields. Gambling on races was popular at the time, with plantations changing hands over lost bets.[1]

References on page 1343

When settlers moved west with their horses, racing grew along with the popularity of the breed recognized for its versatility for ranch work and innate "cow sense." The first official QH racetrack was Rillito Park in Tucson, Arizona, opening in 1943. The American Quarter Horse Association (AQHA) was formed in 1940 to register and preserve the breed that presently represents the largest breed association in the world with more than 3 million members. QH racing is now nationwide and spans over five countries on three different continents. In North America alone, $123 million in purse money was paid out in 2007.[1] Many racing QH owners, trainers, and jockeys raise horses or participate in Western performance events (roping, cutting, reining, showing, and rodeo events), and they take deep pride in the accomplishments of their horses. Winning the All American Futurity, held each year on Labor Day at Ruidoso Downs, Ruidoso, New Mexico and featuring a $2 million purse ($1 million going to the winner), has been the dream of most everyone in the industry. Los Alamitos Racetrack, a predominantly QH track in southern California, offers at least five races during the year with high dollar purses, with the Los Alamitos Two Million Futurity being the richest. The Champion of Champions race held at the end of the racing year is the most prestigious race for older horses, representing winners of the top races during the year.

Emphasis in the sport is on 2-year-old racing (Futurities), requiring qualifying heats where horses with the 10 fastest times compete in a final 2 weeks later. Horses must be nominated to Futurities with periodic payments to maintain eligibility. The same applies to Derbies held for 3-year-olds, but the purse money is less than for 2-year-olds. Yearling sale prices are driven by precocious, nicely conformed, and well-bred individuals to compete in these lucrative Futurities at 2 years of age and then Derbies the following year.

The AQHA Racing Challenge is a program that was designed to provide more racing opportunities for older American QHs. At this time, 59 races take place in 11 regions across the United States, Canada, Mexico, and South America throughout the year. The horses compete in one of six different types of races, depending on age and ability. The series culminates with a championship night held in different locations.[1]

The AQHA stud book has remained open to the breeding of TBs ever since the QH breed was formally established. Breeding to TBs is a useful outcross to expand an otherwise small gene pool and maintain the classic quarter-mile distance of 440 yards because some QHs run best at even shorter distances of 300 to 350 yards. Unlike the Jockey Club, artificial insemination is the norm for breeding, and embryo transfer is popular.

TRAINING THE RACING QUARTER HORSE

Horses are usually broken in the latter part of the yearling year to prepare for racing as 2-year-olds. They are not allowed to race before March of the 2-year-old year, and they are restricted from racing 440 yards until later in the year.[2] The early races are very short (220 to 300 yards), and the training schedule is light compared with the racing TB. Most of the 2-year-old QHs are very precocious, big bodied, and naturally fast. They can perform well with a low level of fitness, possibly a risk factor for injury. Once they are fit, they gallop fewer days than does a TB, and fitness in many older racehorses is maintained using a mechanical horse walker at the barn. To race for the first time, the horse must have two satisfactory morning works (qualifying). They generally work from the gate in "sets" of two horses at a time for a specific distance.

LAMENESS RELATED TO TRACK SURFACE

QHs race on varying track surfaces around the country, but trainers prefer a firmer surface when possible because a loose or sandy surface poses problems with breaking at speed from the starting gate and getting enough traction for sprinting at high speeds. A new set of injuries is seen when racing on a sandier type of track, especially superficial digital flexor (SDF) tendonitis. Hindlimb lameness, muscle strains, back soreness, and suspensory injuries are also increased. The firmer track is favored, but it may lead to the high incidence of joint and bone injury seen as a result of greater concussive forces. No statistics are available at this time for QH injuries racing on the newer synthetic tracks.

CONFORMATION RELATING TO LAMENESS

Conformational factors that may contribute to lameness in the forelimb are relative large body mass, poor carpal conformation (back at the knee and bench kneed), upright pasterns, and small feet. Major hindlimb conformational defects (sickle hocks, cow hocks, too straight in the stifles) are undesirable in the QH racehorse because breaking sharply from the starting gate is necessary to be competitive. Any serious hindlimb lameness may limit the horse's usefulness.

LAMENESS EXAMINATION

There is no set procedure for lameness examination, but a systematic approach is essential for completeness. An efficient approach is required, however, because many trainers like to examine every horse before it is entered to race. Soundness is imperative for optimum racing performance in the QH breed because races are so short and therefore won or lost by photo finishes on a regular basis. Horses with lameness may be fractious in the starting gate, and those with hindlimb lameness may be slow to break from the gate. Close lameness monitoring is required to maintain QHs in peak condition, and intraarticular therapy is frequently used because of the high level of joint trauma associated with the speed and concussion in these elite athletes.

Watching the horse walk out of the stall and down the shed row is useful and a good time to obtain a history from the trainer or barn foreman. A QH with a sore carpus may be noted immediately by a characteristic wide placement of the limb while walking. History is very useful, such as "the horse was getting hotter than usual at the track this morning," or "he is digging a hole in the stall and standing in it." Large barns often keep records of lameness work on each horse, and it is always useful to quickly review past radiographs and joint injections. Observing the horse walk and jog on a hard level surface may accentuate the lameness and aid in diagnosis. Hoof testers should always be used to define foot pain. Joint flexion and palpation are particularly useful owing to the high prevalence of joint problems.

When flexing the carpus, if the limb is raised forward and upward so that the radius is in the horizontal position, the veterinarian may observe an immediate tell-tale withdrawal response of the neck and shoulder muscles as a response to pain. Relaxing the limb, the joints are palpated by placing the thumbs along the individual dorsal borders of the carpal bones while the fingers apply pressure behind the joint to further localize the pain causing lameness. Moving in a distal direction, the dorsal aspect of the metacarpal region, suspensory ligament (SL), digital flexor tendons, and any splints should be palpated for a painful response. The fetlock is flexed, and the suspensory branches are palpated. The distal interphalangeal (DIP) joint is palpated for heat and excessive joint effusion. The digital pulse amplitudes should always be checked because they frequently will be elevated in horses with acute problems of the foot. Excessive synovial effusion, tenderness to palpation, and heat or filling in a specific area of the limb should be noted. The horse's back, loin, and gluteal muscles are briefly palpated and observed for asymmetry, and then the separate compartments of the stifle are palpated. The medial femorotibial joint is the most common area of soreness in the stifle and may or may not have effusion. A positive Churchill test may be indicative of hock soreness and is quickly performed before palpating the distal aspect of the limb. The history of a poor performance (especially leaving the gate) or recognition of hindlimb lameness at the initial jog usually prompts a more complete examination, with proximal and distal limb flexion tests.

Diagnostic blocks are used when necessary to localize the lameness (see Chapter 10).

IMAGING CONSIDERATIONS

Because of the high incidence of joint injury, digital radiography is the most frequently used modality. The carpus and fetlock are the joints most commonly examined radiologically. Ultrasonographic examination is used for definition of suspensory, tendon, and joint injuries. Ultrasonographic examination is generally unrewarding for detection of proximal suspensory injuries in the QH. SDF tendonitis occurs with varying frequency, depending on the characteristics of the racing surface, and lesions vary widely in severity. Nuclear scintigraphy is used less than in the TB, but it is especially helpful in the diagnosis of tibial stress fractures.

SHOEING

The most serious shoeing problems in the QH are the same as in the TB: long toe, low excessively sloping heel, and medial-to-lateral hoof imbalance. Most racehorses are shod close to or on race day. Therefore corrective shoeing is not used as often as needed in many horses because of the risk of sore feet on race day. Horses race in aluminum shoes, and various kinds of pads are used for foot sore horses, including rim pads, wedge pads, full plastic pads, and even full aluminum pads with an assortment of different hoof packings. The most controversial topic at the moment is the use of toe grabs. Toe grabs have been associated with catastrophic injury in the racing TB, and use of these shoe additives is restricted in some states. Historically, many QH racehorses have raced with high toe grabs (>6 mm) to prevent stumbling and slipping from the starting gate and to maintain traction at high speeds. Now many QHs race without a toe grab or a 2-mm toe grab in front. Some leading trainers of QHs believe that the injury rate has been greater with the recent change to smaller toe grabs at the shorter sprinting distances.

A racetrack study including TBs, QHs, and other breeds showed that the prevalence of underrun heels was a significant risk factor for suspensory apparatus failure. The length of toe grabs was not shown to be significant in this study.[3] Further investigation of toe grabs in relation to racing surfaces is necessary.

TEN MOST COMMON LAMENESS CONDITIONS OF THE RACING QUARTER HORSE

1. Synovitis of the carpal and metacarpophalangeal joints
2. Arthrosis of the distal interphalangeal joint and problems associated with the foot
3. Dorsal metacarpal disease
4. Osteochondral fragmentation of the carpus
5. Osteochondral fragmentation of the metacarpophalangeal joint
6. Distal hock joint pain
7. Stifle lameness
8. Proximal suspensory desmitis
9. Tibial stress fractures
10. Miscellaneous fractures of importance

SPECIFIC LAMENESS CONDITIONS

The following lameness conditions are the most relevant for the QH racing breed. Most of the topics are covered extensively in other chapters, and therefore this section is meant as a review of QH injuries and differences from those of the TB.

Synovitis of the Carpal and Metacarpophalangeal Joints

Synovitis of the carpus is the most frequent condition seen in the young racing QH. Back-at-the-knee conformation is common, and this predisposes to carpal injury during hyperextension of the joint while running. Many 2-year-olds have a large body mass and are inherently fast sprinters, reaching very fast speeds without much conditioning. Synovitis is characterized by heat and synovial effusion of the affected joints, with the absence of radiological changes. Lameness may be present but is generally not severe. Carpal flexion and palpation are used to localize the affected joints. Symptomatic treatment includes the use of ice, leg sweats or poultice, and nonsteroidal antiinflammatory drugs (NSAIDs). Intravenous hyaluronan (Legend, Bayer HealthCare, Animal Health Division, Shawnee Mission, Kansas, United States) or intramuscular polysulfated glycosaminoglycans (PSGAGs) (Adequan, Luitpold Pharmaceuticals Inc., Animal Health Division, Shirley, New York, United States) are often used as systemic treatment. Intraarticular therapy is very effective, with a good response from corticosteroids with or without hyaluronan.

The metacarpophalangeal joint of the forelimb is another frequent site of pain causing lameness in QHs. Heat and synovial effusion are the first signs of synovitis, along with a varying degree of lameness. The condition is often bilateral, and radiological examination is negative. In my opinion, capsulitis does not occur with the same frequency as in the TB because QHs in training do far less galloping than TBs; therefore much less stress is placed on the soft tissue structures of the metacarpophalangeal joint. The treatment is the same as for carpal synovitis. If the condition does not resolve with intraarticular therapy, or if it recurs rapidly, the training program should be altered, or the risk of further joint damage is likely, with osteoarthritis (OA) the end result. Many 2-year-olds are entered in numerous Futurities, so training revolves around these races. Trainers try to keep horses on schedule for these race dates, without sustaining injuries that jeopardize the racing careers or require extended layup periods.

Arthrosis of the Distal Interphalangeal Joint and Problems Associated with the Foot

DIP joint synovitis is a clinically significant cause of lameness in the QH.[4] The breed is well known for having undersized feet in relation to the body size, and this, coupled with the tendency for racehorses to develop a long toe and an excessively sloping heel, probably leads to greater stresses to the foot than in other breeds. QHs also have short upright pasterns, and they race at higher speeds on a harder track surface. Bilateral forelimb lameness is seen that can be accentuated by jogging on a hard surface. The stride is shortened with a transfer of weight to the hindlimbs. Horses typically respond to the application of hoof testers over the central third of the frog (as in navicular syndrome). Increased digital pulse amplitude is usually evident, and DIP effusion may be palpated above the coronet in many horses. Younger horses (2- and 3-year-olds) with synovitis show a greater degree of localizing inflammatory signs than older horses with chronic OA.[5]

Intraarticular analgesia may be used to localize the pain causing lameness, and I use intraarticular analgesia in combination with intraarticular medication when necessary to confirm the diagnosis. Radiographs are frequently normal but may show some degree of radiolucent changes along the margin of the distal phalanx and, rarely, radiological changes associated with navicular syndrome. OA of the DIP joint occasionally will be evidenced by the presence of osteophytes involving the distal aspect of the middle phalanx or the extensor process of the distal phalanx. A generalized suspensory soreness, as well as soreness in the area of the bicipital bursa, is often palpated secondary to inflammation of the DIP joint. Back pain may also be associated with the presence of sore feet and can be detrimental to racing performance because of the horse's reluctance to break sharply and extend its stride.[4] These secondary clinical signs usually disappear after resolution of the foot soreness.

Antiinflammatory medications and corrective shoeing are used to treat DIP joint synovitis. The shoeing is in accordance to individual needs, most commonly backing up the shoe as much as possible and protecting the sole. A wide variety of pads are used, including rim pads, full pads, and aluminum pads with various sole packings. Wedge pads or shoes may be used to correct the low heel conformation, but care must be taken because often the heel pain is exacerbated. Some horses are trained in bar shoes until they are ready to race. NSAIDs (usually phenylbutazone) are used, and the feet are iced twice daily during the acute stage.

Intraarticular corticosteroids are effective in relieving pain. Betamethasone esters or triamcinolone acetonide, with or without hyaluronan, is preferred especially if frequent joint injection is necessary. In my experience, frequent use of methylprednisolone acetate (Depo-Medrol, Pharmacia and Upjohn Co., Kalamazoo, Michigan, United States) in the DIP joint will produce severe OA over time.

Other important common problems of the foot include bruises, abscesses, grabbed quarters, and quarter cracks, which are discussed in Chapter 28.

Dorsal Metacarpal Disease

Bucked shins and stress fractures of the dorsal aspect of the third metacarpal bone (McIII) are mainly problems of the 2-year-old QH racehorse but are occasionally seen in a 3-year-old. Dorsal metacarpal disease is basically a bone remodeling phenomenon of the dorsal aspect of the McIII

along the lines of stress, resulting in various degrees of periostitis and osteoporosis.[6] The incidence is less now that trainers understand this bone remodeling process as it relates to exercise. There are four categories of this syndrome in QHs[5]:

1. The acute stage is seen when the horse's shin is hot and extremely sensitive to touch and the gait is "peggy" but radiographs are normal. This would be after a race or qualifying work.
2. "Shin splint" is used to describe a pea-sized bump seen directly below the carpus in association with considerable lameness. It is detected by manual palpation while sensitivity in the remainder of the shin is absent. Radiologically, a small area of periostitis is present.
3. The chronic shin stage is seen with horses that have not responded to treatment, and there is thickening over the dorsal aspect of the metacarpal region. Horses show little pain to palpation but are sore to jog and usually suffer from poor racing performance. Signs of periostitis and remodeling of the dorsal aspect of the McIII are seen radiologically.
4. Stress fractures are most often seen in 2-year-old QHs in contrast to TBs, which often sustain stress fractures from 3 to 5 years of age.[6] Many of the fractures are longitudinal and cannot be seen to exit the cortex. The stress fractures may be present bilaterally, and the dorsolateral cortex of the McIII is the most common location, as in the TB. Longitudinal fractures heal well with rest, and surgery is not indicated.

The treatments are variable, depending on the owner, trainer, and the horse's racing schedule. Extracorporeal shock wave therapy is a popular treatment, but some of the older methods such as electrical hyfercation, pin firing, and periosteal scraping are still used. They are all used with varying periods of rest depending on disease severity.

Osteochondral Fragmentation of the Carpus

The incidence of osteochondral fragmentation (chip fractures) of the carpus is very high in the racing QH. Numerous chip fractures are often seen, and many times they are bilateral. The distal aspect of the radial carpal bone is the most common site for a chip fracture, followed by the proximal aspect of the intermediate carpal bone. It is not uncommon to have distal radial carpal chip fractures in both middle carpal joints and proximal intermediate carpal bone chip fractures in both antebrachiocarpal joints in the same horse.[7] Most are the result of cyclic trauma leading to alteration in bone structure.[8]

The diagnosis is generally made by physical examination and radiological assessment to confirm the location of the fragments. The lameness is fairly obvious; most horses have a characteristic wide placement or circumduction of the involved limb at the walk. Most horses are sensitive to flexion of the carpus and palpation of the dorsal aspect of the carpal bones. Heat and synovial effusion are often present. Arthroscopic surgery is the treatment of choice, although some less valuable claiming horses are injected with corticosteroids and raced. Distal radial carpal fractures in particular are associated with progressive cartilage damage and OA if the horse continues to race with a chip fracture. Preoperative radiographs of the contralateral carpus often reveal chip fractures. Many QHs have numerous surgeries because of the high incidence of osteochondral chip fragmentation.

Occasionally tearing of the medial palmar intercarpal ligament is seen with or without a chip fracture. The condition is suspected when intraarticular analgesia eliminates lameness, but there are no obvious radiological abnormalities, or only a small fragment can be seen. The horse shows a disproportionate degree of lameness compared with the radiological findings. The diagnosis of tearing of the medial palmar intercarpal ligament can only be confirmed by arthroscopic surgery.[9]

Osteochondral Fragmentation of the Metacarpophalangeal Joint

Intraarticular chip fractures of the dorsal, proximal aspect of the proximal phalanx are commonly seen in the forelimb of racing QHs (but less commonly than carpal chip fractures). These fractures are considered to be traumatic hyperextension injuries. They occur primarily on the medial aspect but may also occur laterally.[10] Horses usually exhibit lameness and synovial effusion and are positive to flexion of the fetlock joint. In some horses there are large fragments (especially compared with those fragments occurring in TBs), with a long frontal component. It may be necessary to use a flat blade knife to surgically remove the fragment from the joint capsule during arthroscopic surgery (Figure 110-1).

OA may be seen in association with chip fractures of the proximal aspect of the proximal phalanx especially in older horses, manifested as wear lines and erosions on the distal articular surface of the McIII.[10] Defects on the palmar distal aspect of the McIII are far less common than in the TB, but they do occur in older QHs, and the prognosis is similarly poor.

Fragments of the palmar and plantar aspects of the proximal phalanx are seen less frequently than are dorsal fragments and are not always a source of lameness.[11] They are removed arthroscopically when clinically relevant.

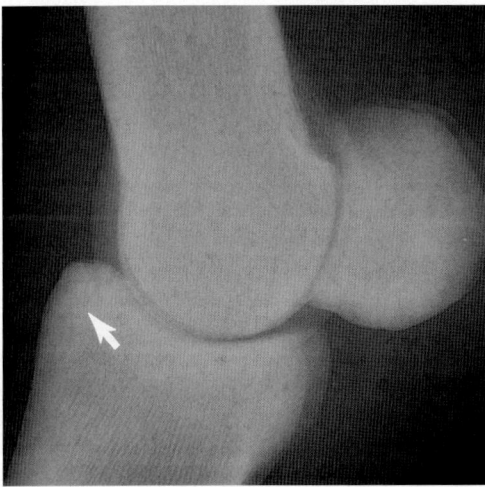

Fig. 110-1 • Lateromedial digital radiographic image of a metacarpophalangeal joint in a racing Quarter Horse with a large osteochondral fracture *(arrow)* of the dorsal, proximal aspect of the proximal phalanx. Large dorsal plane fractures are common in the racing Quarter Horse. (Courtesy Dr. C.W. McIlwraith, Ft. Collins, CO, United States.)

Fractures of the proximal sesamoid bones (PSBs)—apical, abaxial, and basilar—are relatively common in the QH, despite such fractures being considered fatigue-related injuries.

Distal Hock Joint Pain

Lameness associated with the pain arising from the distal hock joints, as well as other hindlimb lameness, is associated with a failure to break sharply from the starting gate. Proximal limb flexion tests may be equivocal, but a positive Churchill test (see page 60) along with a history of poor performance may be indicative of distal hock joint pain, although a negative test does not rule this out. The condition is usually bilateral, and the horse may track closely behind or a hindlimb may cross axially during protraction when observed from behind. Horses that wear patches behind to protect from scalping or horses with laceration marks seen on the medial aspect of the hock are highly suspect for distal hock joint pain. Radiographs are negative in many instances, or subtle abnormalities may be seen. Intraarticular corticosteroids are effective at relieving pain and/or improving performance. Even though the tarsometatarsal and centrodistal joints are low motion joints, maintaining articular cartilage is important because these joints rarely fuse spontaneously. Betamethasone esters and triamcinolone acetonide have been shown to have fewer deleterious effects on cartilage than methylprednisolone acetate.[12,13] If methylprednisolone acetate is used, low doses should be considered (20 to 40 mg).

Stifle Lameness

The most common site of stifle pain is the medial femorotibial joint, and this is the same as in the racing TB. Stifle pain can cause poor performance. The horse may be positive to proximal limb flexion or palpation, but usually intraarticular analgesia is required to localize the pain causing lameness. It is not always clear whether the condition is synovitis or early OA. Radiological examination is useful to assess the joint and rule out certain conditions. Ultrasonographic examination is useful to identify soft tissue lesions.[14] Most horses with stifle pain respond well to intraarticular therapy, but if lameness persists diagnostic arthroscopy is necessary to make a definitive diagnosis. Lameness associated with the femoropatellar joint is often accompanied by joint effusion. In recent years most osteochondritis dissecans lesions are removed surgically before a horse starts racing. Upward fixation of the patella may be a problem in immature horses in early training.

Subchondral bone cysts of the medial femoral condyle can be an important problem. Arthroscopic surgery with injection of triamcinolone acetonide into numerous areas of the cyst lining has been recently reported as successful and is now the preferred treatment.[15]

Proximal Suspensory Desmitis

Forelimb proximal suspensory desmitis (PSD) is usually seen as an acute, profound lameness (grade 4 of 5) the day after a race and often affects the fastest horse in the trainer's barn. The horse may walk on the toe, without dropping the heel to contact the ground. Such severe lameness associated with PSD rapidly subsides, similar to that seen in QHs with a stress fracture of the third carpal bone. If digital palpation is unrewarding, perineural analgesia of the lateral palmar nerve may be necessary to localize the pain causing lameness without blocking the middle carpal joint. Radiography and ultrasonography should be performed. Nuclear scintigraphy may be used but is not usually necessary for the diagnosis. QHs with acute PSD usually respond well to shock wave treatment and altering the training schedule as necessary.

Tibial Stress Fractures

Stress fractures of the tibia are seen in young horses about the time of their second qualifying work or first race. Diagnosis has become more common with access to nuclear scintigraphy. The lameness is unilateral and severe; the left hindlimb is affected most commonly. This may be because horses are pulling up quickly from a high rate of speed before entering a left-hand turn on the racetrack. Unlike in the TB, in which tibial stress fractures occur most frequently in the caudolateral cortex, the most common location of tibial stress fractures in the QH is the distal medial aspect of the tibia.[16] Nuclear scintigraphy is the most accurate means of diagnosis; digital radiography performed 7 to 10 days after injury may identify a lesion. Rest is required for at least 90 days before resuming training.

Miscellaneous Fractures of Importance

The three most common fractures resulting in catastrophic injury in the racing QH and TB are those of the PSB, the McIII, and the humerus.[17] Although most often associated with racing and fatigue in TBs, biaxial and comminuted PSB fractures occur in the QH with resulting disruption of the suspensory apparatus and the integrity of the MCP joint. Fractures of the McIII and the humerus are a cause of catastrophic injury in the QH. Horses generally are able to walk after shoulder injury, but the definitive diagnosis is usually made the next day when the pain and swelling are localized.

Another important injury is severe carpal bone fractures (slab fractures and comminuted fractures), many of which are amenable to surgery. Whenever pain causing severe lameness is localized to the carpus, a thorough radiographic examination, including skyline images, is necessary to ensure that degenerative lesions, incomplete sagittal fractures, and any nondisplaced fractures may be seen before a catastrophic injury occurs. All the recognized third carpal bone fractures can be seen in the QH, but a higher percentage of large dorsal plane slab fractures involve both the radial and intermediate facets than in the TB (Figure 110-2). The slab fracture is often displaced, with the distal margin of the radial carpal bone collapsing into the proximal aspect of the third carpal bone fracture site (Figure 110-3). Internal fixation using screws placed in lag fashion is necessary for proper healing and to prevent further collapse of the joint.

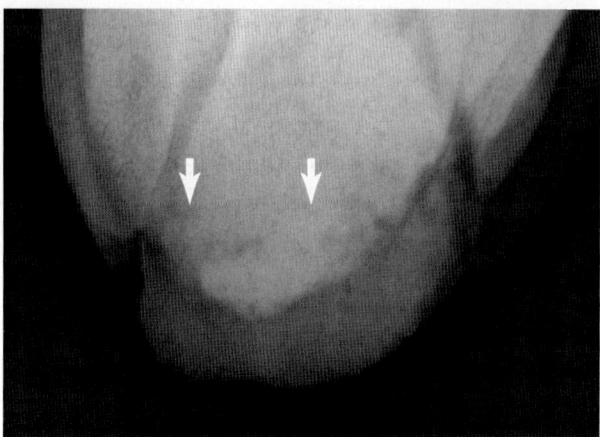

Fig. 110-2 • Dorsoproximal-dorsodistal (skyline) digital radiographic image of the distal row of carpal bones in a racing Quarter Horse with a large dorsal plane slab fracture *(arrows)* of the third carpal that spans the entire radial and intermediate fossae. (Courtesy Dr. C.W. McIlwraith, Ft. Collins, CO, United States.)

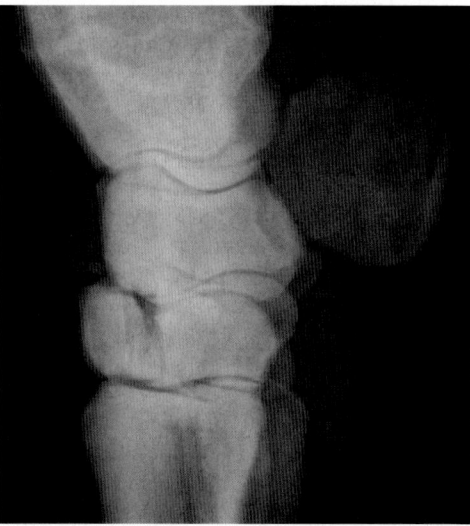

Fig. 110-3 • Lateromedial digital radiographic image of a racing Quarter Horse with a large, displaced dorsal plane slab fracture of the third carpal bone (C3). With dorsal displacement of C3 there is distal movement of the overlying radial carpal bone causing carpal instability. Prognosis for future racing is guarded, and surgical repair is necessary. (Courtesy Dr. C.W. McIlwraith, Ft. Collins, CO, United States.)

Comminuted carpal fractures caused by slab fractures involving both rows of carpal bones are catastrophic injuries seen in QHs. Challenging, salvage surgical procedures, such as partial arthrodesis or panarthrodesis using numerous bone plates, are necessary.

Although less frequent, fractures of the lumbosacral vertebrae are particularly devastating because they not only result in the death of the horse but as a result of the horse falling on the jockey, they often also result in severe injury to the rider.

Chapter 111

Lameness in the Arabian Racehorse: Middle East and North America

Robert Andrew Dalglish and Mark C. Rick

HISTORY OF RACING

The Arabian racehorse originates directly from the Thoroughbred (TB) foundation sires of all light or hot-blooded horses. In the seventeenth century, these TB sires—the Darley Arabian, Godolphin Barb, and Byerly Turk—were imported to England and bred to the Queen's mares. The Arabian was used originally as a war horse, and although the true beginnings of the Arabian horse are under a shroud of mystery and legend, the consensus is that the Middle Eastern desert Bedouin tribes played a large role in the breeding and early development of the breed.

Throughout the Middle East and Europe, Arabian racing and performance are more deeply rooted than in North America. The popularity of Arabian racing has grown enormously in the United Kingdom in the last 15 to 20 years, with a growing number of professional trainers and jockeys and a progressive increase in prize money, in part because of the high Middle Eastern sponsorship. Arabian racing in North America and around the globe is less popular, and the number of races is fewer and the amount of prize money is less compared with TB, Standardbred, and Quarter Horse racing.

The Arabian Horse Registry of America, founded in 1908, includes many types and uses. Known for stamina, speed, and elegance, Arabian horses often were bred and raised for showing in halter and performance classes. In the latter part of the twentieth century, Arabian horse popularity and breeding selection shifted to criteria based more on aesthetics than athleticism.

The Arabian racehorse lineage reflects more athleticism than is found in Arabian show horses. Consistent winners often are more heavily muscled and have stronger hindquarters with a more sloping croup and a lower head and neck carriage than a typical Arabian show horse. Recent influx of new breeding lines has given rise to concern and controversy over the purity of the lineage and the possible infusion of impure Arabian blood. Certain new stallions appear to be much taller and longer, with a body type similar to the modern day TB racehorse. Constant vigilance and careful documentation of lineage is required to preserve the pure Arabian racehorse breed.

Arabian racehorses race on the same surfaces as TB racehorses. In North America selected meets are held from California to Delaware, from Florida to Michigan, in Colorado, Texas, and Washington, and at a few other tracks. Arabian racehorses perform in fair meets, allowance races, claiming races, and futurity nominated stakes races. Racing

Arabian horses also compete in the United Kingdom, Poland, France, Russia, and South America and in many Middle Eastern countries. In North America, racing begins on March 1 of the 3-year-old year. Race distances are similar to those for TB races, but the length and configuration of the racecourses vary. Shorter sprint distances, $4\frac{1}{2}$ to 6 furlongs, often are run on the small tracks, whereas the longest race (2 miles [3.2 km]) is usually run on a large track. Typically, races are $4\frac{1}{2}$ furlongs to $1\frac{3}{4}$ miles (881 m to 2.8 km). In the United Arab Emirates (UAE) races are 5 to 12 furlongs (1 km to 2.4 km), and horses race on both dirt and turf. A sound Arabian racehorse may compete as often as every 7 to 10 days, but most are given 2 weeks between races. Because relatively few Arabians are raced, lack of entries may mandate racing whenever enough horses are entered to meet race conditions rather than when trainers and owners prefer. Racing in the United Kingdom starts in late April. Until 2001, horses did not race until 4 years of age, but in 2001 a restricted number of races for horses 3 years of age were introduced. These are high-value races and also attract horses trained in France and other European countries. Races range from 5 furlongs to 3 miles (1 km to 4.8 km). In the UAE, Arabian races average 9.5 runners.

In 1999 the International Federation of Arabian Horse Racing Authorities (IFAHR) was formed for the purpose of cooperation among all national and international Arabian horse racing associations throughout the world. The IFAHR is registered in France. Founding member countries were France, Germany, Belgium, the UAE, Qatar, Switzerland, the United Kingdom, Austria, Holland, Russia, Saudi Arabia, the United States, Turkey, Egypt, Spain, Sweden, Morocco, and Poland. In the UAE, Arabian horseracing has taken place for over two decades. Abu Dhabi, where Arabian horse racing takes place almost every week during the racing season from November to March, is the largest of the seven emirates and has also become the leader in international sponsorship of Arabian racing since 1996, supporting major races in countries such as England, the United States, France, Russia, Holland, and Belgium. The Gulf State of Qatar is also an important sponsor of international Arabian racing. Several UAE breeders maintain operations throughout Europe and the United States and are a constant force at international auctions, where stock is acquired to race in their domestic market and eventually to support breeding programs. The majority of Arabians racing in the UAE are from North American and French bloodlines. Breeding of purebred Arabian racehorses is now very popular; over 60% of the Arabian racehorses competing in the UAE today are bred in the UAE.

TEN MOST COMMON RACING-RELATED LAMENESS CONDITIONS IN THE MIDDLE EAST ARABIAN RACEHORSE

1. Metacarpophalangeal joint lameness
2. Superficial digital flexor tendonitis
3. Suspensory desmitis including proximal suspensory desmitis and avulsion fractures of the third metacarpal bone
4. Distal hock joint pain and osteoarthritis

5. Lameness of the foot
6. Myopathies
7. Stifle and carpal lameness
8. Back pain
9. Dorsal third metacarpal bone disease
10. Fractures of various bones, including stress fractures

TEN MOST COMMON RACING-RELATED LAMENESS CONDITIONS IN THE NORTH AMERICAN ARABIAN RACEHORSE

1. Dorsal third metacarpal bone disease
2. Superficial digital flexor tendonitis
3. Suspensory desmitis
4. Stifle lameness
5. Tarsocrural osteochondrosis and distal hock joint pain
6. Back pain
7. Proximal sesamoid bone fractures
8. Metacarpophalangeal joint lameness
9. Carpal osteochondral fragmentation
10. Lameness of the foot

METACARPOPHALANGEAL JOINT LAMENESS AND CARPAL OSTEOCHONDRAL FRAGMENTATION

In North America, osteochondral fragmentation or chip fractures of the carpal and metacarpophalangeal joints occur in Arabian racehorses but less frequently than in TBs and Quarter Horses. Smaller body size, a more gradual training regimen, and older age of horses racing likely account for the difference in incidence. However, in Middle East Arabian racehorses, lameness associated with the metacarpophalangeal joint is the most common problem encountered; carpal pain associated with osteochondral fragmentation is unusual. Early signs of arthrosis without chip fracture resolve quickly, with minor interruption in race training. The diagnosis of fetlock or carpal osteochondral fragments is straightforward. Arthroscopic surgery to remove osteochondral fragments is well accepted and successful. The prognosis depends on location, size, duration, previous treatment, and amount of associated cartilage damage. Horses with acute osteochondral fragments with only mild cartilage damage have a good prognosis. The decision for surgery often is based on economic factors.

Proliferative synovitis (villonodular synovitis) and associated fragmentation of the dorsal proximal aspect of the proximal phalanx occurs in the young Arabian racehorse. Horses have characteristic signs of effusion and a noticeable dorsal swelling. Dorsal swelling can be insidious and go unrecognized early in the disease process. Plain radiographs often reveal soft tissue swelling on the dorsal distal aspect of the third metacarpal bone (McIII) and osteochondral fragments of the proximal phalanx. Radiolucent changes in the McIII are seen in horses with severe proliferation. Ultrasonographic examination usually reveals enlargement of the dorsal synovial pad. One of us (MCR) recommends arthroscopic evaluation, removal of osteochondral fragments, and debridement of the synovial pad with a 5.2- or 3.4-mm suction punch (Dyonics, Andover, Massachusetts, United States).

In older Arabian racehorses, chronic osteoarthritis (OA) of the metacarpophalangeal joint is recognized. The trainer complains of poor performance or racing below previous levels. The metacarpophalangeal joint is enlarged from effusion or fibrosis and is warm. Horses usually respond positively to lower limb or fetlock flexion tests. Comprehensive radiographic examination should be performed. Radiological evidence of OA, such as marginal osteophytes of the proximal sesamoid bones (PSBs) and joint space narrowing, enthesophytes at capsular attachments, and soft tissue thickening, often is seen. OA of the metacarpophalangeal joint is seen frequently without osteochondral fragments and appears to be related to chronic wear and tear. In some horses OA can be managed by judicious use of intraarticular medication, but the prognosis for return to previous racing levels is guarded. In Middle East Arabian racehorses OA of the metacarpophalangeal joint and associated lameness are a major problem. Clinical signs include fetlock effusion, a positive response to lower limb and fetlock flexion tests, and a positive response to intraarticular analgesia and medication. Horses have typical radiological changes. The prognosis for continued racing is generally good, but numerous intraarticular injections of hyaluronan and corticosteroids are often needed to maintain adequate clinical comfort. Subchondral bone pain is suspected to be a factor in horses with few radiological changes or in those with increased radiopacity of the distal aspect of the McIII.

SUPERFICIAL DIGITAL FLEXOR TENDONITIS

Superficial digital flexor (SDF) tendonitis (bowed tendon) is common and occurs from a combination of training overload and fatigue. Faulty forelimb conformation appears to be a factor, and the heavier Arabian racehorses from French bloodlines are more prone to injury of the superficial digital flexor tendon (SDFT) than those of North American origin. Lesions are found in the body and/or in the medial and lateral margins of the SDFT.

Occasionally horses run uphill at the end of a race, and SDF tendonitis occurs commonly under this condition. Sudden changes in track surfaces or training conditions are associated with an increased incidence of tendonitis. Injuries are often cumulative, and an initial injury that is overlooked or badly managed develops into a severe, career-threatening injury. Severe SDF tendonitis usually is recognized by the trainer because swelling, heat, and pain are present during palpation. More subtle swelling and pain are detected during careful palpation by a veterinarian. Thorough ultrasonographic examination is imperative to confirm the diagnosis. Careful assessment requires proper horse preparation, sedation, clipping and cleaning of the leg, and use of a high-quality ultrasound machine and a 7.5- to 10-MHz (or greater) linear transducer. Cross-sectional area (CSA) of the tendon and lesion, fiber alignment, and echogenicity of the lesion are evaluated, and any associated pathological conditions such as palmar annular ligament constriction, carpal tenosynovitis, or other soft tissue damage are assessed. Swelling is often mild if horses have been given local and systemic antiinflammatory therapy and rest. A slight increase in CSA measurement may be the only indication of SDF tendonitis, and comparison with the contralateral SDFT is mandatory. Initial management includes rest, local ice and bandage application, and administration of systemic nonsteroidal antiinflammatory drugs (NSAIDs). Horses with mild or moderate SDF tendonitis often are sent to a layup or rehabilitation farm for 3 to 6 months, where a monitoring and controlled exercise program should be initiated. Follow-up examinations are performed at 2-month intervals to determine quality of the healing and the appropriate time to return the horse to race training. A slow return to training includes progressive walking, jogging, cantering, speed work (breeze), and then racing. Time span and progression depend on maintaining an acceptable ultrasonographic appearance during each incremental increase in stress or exercise level. Tendon splitting and desmotomy of the accessory ligament of the SDFT used separately or concomitantly are successful in horses with moderate or severe tendonitis. Intralesional injections of β-aminopropionitrile fumarate (Bapten; no longer commercially available) have been used successfully. More recently, intralesional injection of autologous stem cells derived from either bone marrow or fat and platelet-rich plasma (PRP) have been used with success. One of us (AD) has successfully used intralesional injection of the porcine urinary bladder matrix product A-Cell (A Cell Vet, Columbia, MD, United States) for Arabian racehorses with SDF tendonitis and suspensory desmitis.

Prognosis varies with the severity of the injury and the stage of racing when the injury occurred. Because many Arabian horses race as older horses, even stallions and mares, providing up to a year or more of rest is not uncommon, assuming the lesion heals, before returning the horse to race training. Horses with substantial SDF tendonitis often reinjure the same area of the tendon, develop a new injury of the previously damaged tendon, or develop tendonitis of the contralateral SDFT. SDF tendonitis does occur in the hindlimb, but less often than forelimb injury, and Arabian racehorses with hindlimb SDF tendonitis have a better prognosis than those with forelimb injuries.

SUSPENSORY DESMITIS

Forelimb suspensory desmitis is an intermittent problem of many Arabian racehorses early in training. Suspensory desmitis is not considered to be as debilitating or career limiting as it is for TB racehorses. A trainer often complains that the horse is sore, but overt lameness is not present. The differential diagnosis includes bucked shins, SDF tendonitis, and metacarpophalangeal joint and carpal joint lameness. Careful palpation reveals pain and enlargement of the suspensory ligament. Although ultrasonographic examination should be performed to confirm and grade desmitis, a pattern of subtle inflammation and soreness often precedes lesions detectable by ultrasonography. Scintigraphy may be useful but is seldom recommended. Suspensory desmitis is not severe, and most often the finding of body soreness in response to increased training intensity is the only apparent clinical sign. Traumatic disruption of the suspensory apparatus is rare. Horses with suspensory desmitis usually are kept at the track because they do not require or benefit from extensive time off. We recommend 1 to 2 weeks of rest or simply a decrease in training intensity to allow for tissue adaptation. The prognosis for horses with suspensory desmitis is good if the condition is

recognized early and horses are given a period of much-reduced work intensity and slow rehabilitation.

Proximal suspensory desmitis (PSD) is a clinically significant and often underdiagnosed cause of lameness in Arabian racehorses in the Middle East. One of us (AD) feels strongly that PSD and related injuries, such as avulsion fracture at the origin of the suspensory ligament on the McIII, are some of the most underrecognized sources of pain causing lameness in the Arabian racehorse. Pain associated with forelimb PSD and associated injuries can be abolished by performing lateral palmar analgesia at the level of the distal aspect of the accessory carpal bone after first performing low palmar (low four-point) analgesia. Infiltration of local anesthetic solution at the proximal aspect of the suspensory ligament can be used, but the combined carpometacarpal and middle carpal joints may be inadvertently desensitized; however, in Middle East Arabian racehorses these articular structures are rarely a source of pain. Once one forelimb is blocked, the horse often demonstrates contralateral forelimb lameness because PSD is often bilateral. Although changes associated with PSD can be identified ultrasonographically, often in Arabian racehorses ultrasonographic evidence of PSD is mild, but scintigraphically, focal areas of increased radiopharmaceutical uptake (IRU) of the proximal palmar aspect of the McIII are found, a finding that corroborates that bone injury is present. Although a diagnosis of PSD is often made in these horses, early stress fracture of the McIII may more appropriately describe this clinical syndrome, because in most horses PSD exists without concomitant McIII injury (Editors).

Treatment of Arabian racehorses with PSD and associated injuries includes an immediate removal from training, rest, and a controlled exercise program. Intralesional therapy with PRP and A-Cell and extracorporeal shock wave therapy have been used with some success. Generally, a good prognosis for return to athletic function is given. Avulsion fracture of the McIII at the suspensory ligament origin occurs less commonly and may cause sudden, severe lameness during exercise.

Proximal suspensory ligament injuries of the hindlimbs are less common than those involving the forelimbs and are more difficult to diagnose, but they are an important cause of pain causing lameness; they should be considered when investigating hindlimb lameness and carefully differentiated from distal hock joint pain.

TARSOCRURAL OSTEOCHONDROSIS AND DISTAL HOCK JOINT PAIN

Tarsocrural osteochondrosis is an occasional cause of hindlimb lameness. If bog spavin is recognized when the horse is a weanling or yearling, arthroscopic surgical removal of osteochondritis dissecans (OCD) fragments usually is performed then. However, horses may arrive at the racetrack or training stable with mild tarsocrural effusion. Moderate tarsocrural effusion is commonly observed in many Middle East Arabian racehorses without evidence of osteochondrosis. Although horses are usually not lame, trainers request that the joints be drained and injected with hyaluronan and corticosteroids. If lameness is observed, if a horse has a positive response to upper limb flexion, or if moderate effusion is persistent, then radiographs should be obtained. If OCD fragments are found, we recommend arthroscopic surgery and a short (2- to 3-month) period of rest before training resumes.

Distal hock joint pain occurs in the Arabian racehorse and is seen most commonly after changes in track surfaces. These horses often do not push off or propel themselves well behind, may refuse to grab the bit or bow the neck, and use the front end to pull ahead, a gait that may lead to secondary forelimb lameness. Clinical signs often are lacking, and an upper limb flexion test may be only mildly positive. Radiological findings are often negative, but scintigraphic examination reveals IRU in the distal hock bones. OA of the centrodistal and tarsometatarsal joints is common in Middle East Arabian racehorses, and distal hock joint pain is the most common cause of hindlimb lameness. Intraarticular injection of corticosteroids produces a good response, and repeated injection is not deleterious to the future function of the hock (AD). Recently, adjunctive use of tiludronate has proved beneficial. Distal hock joint pain should be differentiated from pain originating from PSD.

LAMENESS OF THE FOOT

Although Arabian horses are alleged to have solid foot structure, they do get sore feet. Long-toe, low-heel conformation is not common. Arabian horses are protected from some of the lameness conditions of the feet simply because of small body size and weight. Sore feet develop after a fast workout or race on a hard, packed racetrack. Trainers often recognize signs, and the condition is managed using ice baths, NSAIDs, and 3 to 4 days of rest.

In the Middle East, lameness attributable to the distal interphalangeal (DIP) joint is characterized by effusion, a positive response to intraarticular analgesia, and a positive response to medication with hyaluronan and corticosteroids. The DIP joint is a relatively common source of pain causing lameness in the Middle East Arabian racehorse. Although marked radiological changes may not be apparent, a response to intraarticular therapy can be dramatic, but injections may have to be repeated to maintain comfort. Less commonly, in older Arabian racehorses, "navicular syndrome" is diagnosed as the cause of foot lameness. Horses may improve for a short time with intraarticular injections into the DIP joint. In horses with pain originating from the navicular bone without concomitant deep digital flexor tendonitis tiludronate is given adjunctively. Other common causes of foot-related lameness are abscesses, bruised heels and quarters, and poor foot balance.

MYOPATHY

In the Middle East one of us (AD) has managed many Arabian racehorses, especially those from certain bloodlines, with recurrent exertional rhabdomyolysis (RER). This condition can manifest as acute "tying-up"(usually following a change in management such as a return to training after a period of rest) or as a cause of poor performance in horses with subclinical, chronic elevations in the serum muscle enzyme concentrations of creatine kinase (CK) and aspartate transaminase (AST). RER appears to be caused by an inherited, intermittent, stress-induced defect in regulation of muscle contraction (see Chapter 83). RER can be successfully managed with exercise and dietary changes. Starch in the diet is replaced by rice bran (which can be fed in specialized feeds). Ensuring that the horse has regular exercise including short periods of fast exercise is an essential component of the management of horses with RER. Acute RER invariably occurs during periods of submaximal exercise. The condition is monitored by regularly following blood CK and AST levels. CK is quickly excreted through the kidney, and therefore a chronic elevation in serum levels of CK is indicative of ongoing muscle damage. Because AST is metabolized in the liver, serum levels are slower to rise and fall during acute, initial muscle damage.

STIFLE AND CARPAL LAMENESS

In North America the most common source of hindlimb soreness is the stifle region. In the Middle East Arabian racehorse, stifle region pain is uncommon, as is lameness associated with the carpus, and these conditions are grouped together. Early in training a horse may become sore and stiff, usually bilaterally. Intermittent upward fixation of the patella is common as in other young sports horses. Stifle soreness is common in young horses shod with flat shoes and training on a soft track. Soft tissues around the stifle become inflamed. Clinical signs include a shortened stride and an unwillingness to extend the stride behind, or actual upward fixation of the patella, with characteristic stifle and hock extension and toe drag. With early detection, horses with stifle region lameness are assumed to have a soft tissue problem and are managed by decreasing training intensity and the administration of NSAIDs. Occasionally an internal blister is injected around the patellar ligaments, especially if evidence of upward fixation of the patella exists. If effusion of the femoropatellar joint accompanies the upward fixation of the patella, radiographs should be obtained. Results are usually negative, but some horses have underlying OCD of the lateral trochlear ridge of the femur. Surgical debridement is recommended, especially if a flaplike lesion exists. OCD lesions usually are detected early in race training if they are clinically important. In Middle East Arabian racehorses the most common source of stifle region pain is lameness related to osteochondrosis lesions, OCD, and subchondral bone cysts. In North America, subchondral bone cysts of the medial femoral condyle are rarely seen. Horses with subchondral bone cysts are treated by rest, injection with corticosteroids, or surgery. If radiographs reveal evidence of OA, such as enlargement of the medial tibial plateau, or if ultrasonographic examination reveals flattening, wrinkling, or other change of the medial meniscus, then the prognosis for racing is diminished. If subchondral bone cysts are discovered early in training, horses are best managed with arthroscopic surgery. The prognosis for a horse with a sore stifle, ligament laxity, and intermittent upward fixation of the patella is good, assuming a favorable response to alterations in training regimen. Lameness in Arabian racehorses with sore stifles appears similar to that seen in young TBs with tibial stress fractures, but the origin of pain is different. The prognosis for horses with osteochondrosis varies but is poorer if evidence of OA exists.

BACK PAIN

Primary hindlimb lameness causes secondary back pain in most Arabian horses, particularly those with primary lameness of the stifle and hock joints. Often back pain resolves after management of the primary hindlimb lameness. However, treatment of back pain concomitantly allows earlier resolution of both problems. Exercise riders or jockeys may suspect back pain and often report a sensitivity or soreness over the top line. Horses usually show pain on palpation or when pressure is applied along the back. The back is palpated carefully, and pressure should be applied uniformly and gently. Thermography has been of some value in horses with back pain resulting from a poorly fitting saddle. The saddle can be evaluated thermographically and compared with any warm spots on the horse's back. Nuclear scintigraphy may reveal IRU in the summits of the dorsal spinous processes. Radiological examination may confirm overriding of the dorsal spinous processes. However, radiological and scintigraphic findings are often negative, and back pain is assumed to originate from soft tissues. Nonetheless, if back pain is severe, we suspect a bony source of pain. The back can be evaluated by ultrasonography, dorsally or rectally, for myositis, nerve root impingement or enlargement, and osteophytes associated with the vertebral articulations. Lumbosacral and sacroiliac pain is often detected in Middle East Arabian racehorses, and a positive response to pressure over the tubera sacrale may indicate that sacroiliac region pain is contributing to an abnormal gait, if present. IRU in the sacroiliac region can help establish a diagnosis, and one of us (AD) often injects corticosteroids in horses with this finding, not only to manage pain in these horses, but also to help establish a diagnosis.

DORSAL THIRD METACARPAL BONE DISEASE

Many racehorses trained intensely at speed at a young age experience the sore-shin or bucked-shin complex. Although intense training may not begin until the 3-year-old year and the Arabian racehorse is smaller in stature and weight than its TB counterpart, bucked shins remain a major cause of lameness requiring reduction in training intensity. Trainers are well aware of this problem and often can diagnose it accurately based on clinical findings and the observation of a sore horse, traveling short. A veterinarian usually confirms the diagnosis clinically, but in some horses radiography and occasionally scintigraphy are necessary. With advanced dorsal McIII cortical pain, typical dorsal cortical periostitis or a dorsal cortical fracture is seen radiologically (see Chapter 102). With periostitis comes intense, diffuse IRU, whereas focal IRU is seen in horses with a dorsal cortical fracture (see Chapter 19). However, scintigraphy is used more commonly to diagnose stress-related bone injury and stress fracture of other long bones in Arabian racehorses. Conservative management is preferred with rest, reduction in strenuous training, or return to the layup farm. Pin firing and blistering are not used routinely. Dorsal cortical fractures are rare, but if present, one of us (MCR) prefers surgical management using osteostixis (dorsal cortical drilling) or insertion of a bone screw placed in lag fashion in the dorsal cortex of the McIII. The prognosis is good.

Although this condition is recognized in Middle East Arabian racing, it does not appear to be as common as in North America, and horses are usually successfully managed conservatively.

FRACTURES OF VARIOUS BONES, INCLUDING STRESS FRACTURES

PSB fractures do occur in Arabian racehorses but are less common than in TBs. Clinical signs, management, and prognosis are similar to those in the TB racehorse (see Chapter 36). Other fractures, such as midsagittal fractures of the proximal phalanx and condylar fractures of the distal aspect of the McIII, are rare in North America. However, in the Middle East both medial and lateral condylar fractures of the McIII occur quite commonly. Lateral condylar fractures predominate. Horses with fractures of the proximal phalanx and condyles of the McIII are managed surgically. Less commonly, humeral and tibial fractures occur. Complete fractures are easily diagnosed and necessitate immediate euthanasia. Horses with humeral and tibial stress fractures often require scintigraphic examination for diagnosis but have a good prognosis if fractures are recognized early when incomplete and the horses are properly given complete box rest. Pelvic stress fractures are being recognized more frequently in Middle East Arabian racehorses; one of us (AD) believes that these fractures have been underdiagnosed. Scintigraphy usually produces a conclusive diagnosis. Avulsion fractures of the origin of the suspensory ligament from the McIII with or without associated PSD occur in the forelimbs and hindlimbs, cause acute-onset lameness, and are commonly diagnosed in the Middle East Arabian racehorse. Conservative management is successful, but prognosis is adversely affected by concomitant PSD.

PROCEEDING WITHOUT A DIAGNOSIS

Lameness in Arabian racehorse should be investigated in a logical manner as with all lameness examinations, taking into account the usual wishes of the owner and trainer to retain the horse in training if possible. In some horses in which joint pain is suspected but clinical signs are vague, a concurrent intraarticular injection of hyaluronan, corticosteroids, and local anesthetic solution can be used as a diagnostic and therapeutic approach. Occasionally, lameness is suspected but a diagnosis cannot be made. Horses with such lameness are characterized by a drop in performance, an increase in race times, a subtle gait change, a refusal to switch leads, a drop in class, or soreness, but no clinical signs of overt lameness are observable. In this situation, we usually recommend a whole-body scintigraphic examination, but correlating findings with clinical signs is often difficult. Comprehensive evaluation for poor performance considers not only a musculoskeletal problem but also cardiovascular and muscle abnormalities. Sometimes, Arabian horses may be thought to be more fragile and highly strung than other racehorses, and some trainers attribute poor performance to this portion of the horse's personality. However, Arabians are used for endurance riding (see Chapter 118), in which average speeds of more than 25 km/hr are often sustained over a course of 120 km, a fact that confirms the breed's strong metabolic endurance characteristics. One of us believes strongly that if an Arabian cannot endure race training, there is invariably a musculoskeletal defect or injury (AD).

Chapter 112

National Hunt Racehorse, Point to Point Horse, and Timber Racing Horse

Sue J. Dyson, Robert Joseph Van Pelt,
Kevin P. Keane, James Wood, and Anthony Stirk

DESCRIPTION OF THE SPORT

For as long as horses have been domesticated and ridden, they have been raced. The oldest record of racing in Britain shows that the Romans used to race their horses in Chester. Subsequently, little is known about any organized horse racing during the Middle Ages, but by about 1150 racing had become established at Smithfield, a horse market, where horses were tried and sometimes raced before sale. By the early part of the sixteenth century, racing had returned to Chester, where the prize for the winner in 1511 was a silver bell.

All of these races were on turf with no obstacles to negotiate. At about the same time that horses were competing for the Chester bell, fox hunting (rather than hunting deer or wild boar) started to become established and rapidly increased in popularity. One reason for this may have been the changing agricultural landscape as more and more land was enclosed, providing natural obstacles for those following the hunt to jump. Inevitably, rivalry developed among those who regularly followed fox hunts across country regarding who had the fastest horse, and a new sport was born, known as steeplechasing. The origin of the name is simple. Because no courses were defined over which the races could take place, the participants had to race from one church to another, using the high church steeple toward which they were heading as a landmark. The riders could choose their own route and had to jump a variety of fences such as hedges, banks, walls, timber fences, and brooks during the course of the race. The first steeplechase of this type was held in Buttevant in Ireland in 1752, when two neighbors raced between Buttevant church and the St Leger church, a distance of 4½ miles (7.2 km).

Eventually this new sport was formalized, with specially constructed courses that allowed more participants to take part and more spectators to watch. The first such organized race meeting in Britain was held at St Albans in 1830. The Grand National was first staged in 1839, the National Hunt Steeplechase followed at Market Harborough in 1859, and the first meeting at Cheltenham (Prestbury Park), arguably the best known modern jump racing venue, was in 1898.

As the sport developed, regulating it became important, but the Jockey Club, which had been regulating flat racing since the mid-eighteenth century, regarded the new sport with suspicion. Accordingly, a separate National Hunt Committee was established in 1866 and continued to run

jump racing until 1969, when it and the Jockey Club merged to bring all racing, on the flat and over jumps, in Britain under one governing body. The National Steeplechase Association oversees racing over fences in the United States.

Modern National Hunt racing now consists of several categories, all run on turf on clockwise and counterclockwise courses. Horses run under similar rules in the United Kingdom, Ireland, and France. Elsewhere in Europe, racing over fences takes place but on a much lower scale. Most races are hurdle races or steeplechases, but some races run over more natural obstacles remain—some that are run over exclusively timber fences, and some, called *National Hunt flat races,* that are run without obstacles.

Apart from the fences, three major differences exist between National Hunt and flat racing, which are important in the epidemiology of the injuries that may occur in the different sports. These differences are the race distance, the age of the horses, and the weights of the riders. All National Hunt races are more than a minimum of 2 miles (3.2 km) compared with the minimum distance of 5 furlongs (1 km) on the flat, and the horses are at least 3 years of age. Forty percent of National Hunt Flat races involve horses of 4 years of age, a slightly higher percentage are 5 years of age, and less than 20% are 6 years of age or older. Most horses competing in flat races are 2 or 3 years old, but it is not unusual for horses over the age of 10 to race in National Hunt races, especially in steeplechases. Finally, National Hunt horses carry 10 stone (63.5 kg) to 11 stone 12 lb (75.3 kg), considerably more weight than flat horses.

Hurdle races are held over fences smaller than those encountered in steeplechasing. In Britain, most hurdles are derived from the simple portable fences used to create temporary pens for sheep, although small brush hurdles are being trialed. They are usually 72 inches (1.83 m) wide and must be not less than 42 inches (107 cm) from top to bottom bar and constructed of ash or occasionally oak. Several hurdle sections are placed end to end to produce an obstacle that must be at least 30 feet (9 m) wide. Each hurdle section consists of two uprights with pointed legs that are driven into the ground and five horizontal rails, between which is interwoven birch or another suitable material. Gorse, which is durable but has sharp thorns, is not permitted. The hurdles must be driven into the ground at an angle of 62 degrees so that the top bar is set back 20 inches (51 cm) from the vertical, and the effective height of the hurdle is 37 inches (94 cm). All of the exposed timber parts must be padded with a minimum of ½ inch (1.3 cm) of high-density polyethylene or closed cell foam rubber (Figure 112-1).

Timber hurdles have the advantage that if a horse misjudges the fence and does not jump it cleanly, the hurdle gives way on impact. Old style hurdles were not padded as well as the modern versions and occasionally led to lacerations on the dorsal aspects of the hindlimbs, which could be extensive with degloving injuries of much of the metatarsal region. These injuries have been virtually abolished by the new padding.

In countries other than Britain and Ireland, timber hurdles are replaced by fences that look like small versions of steeplechase fences. Such fences also are seen on a small

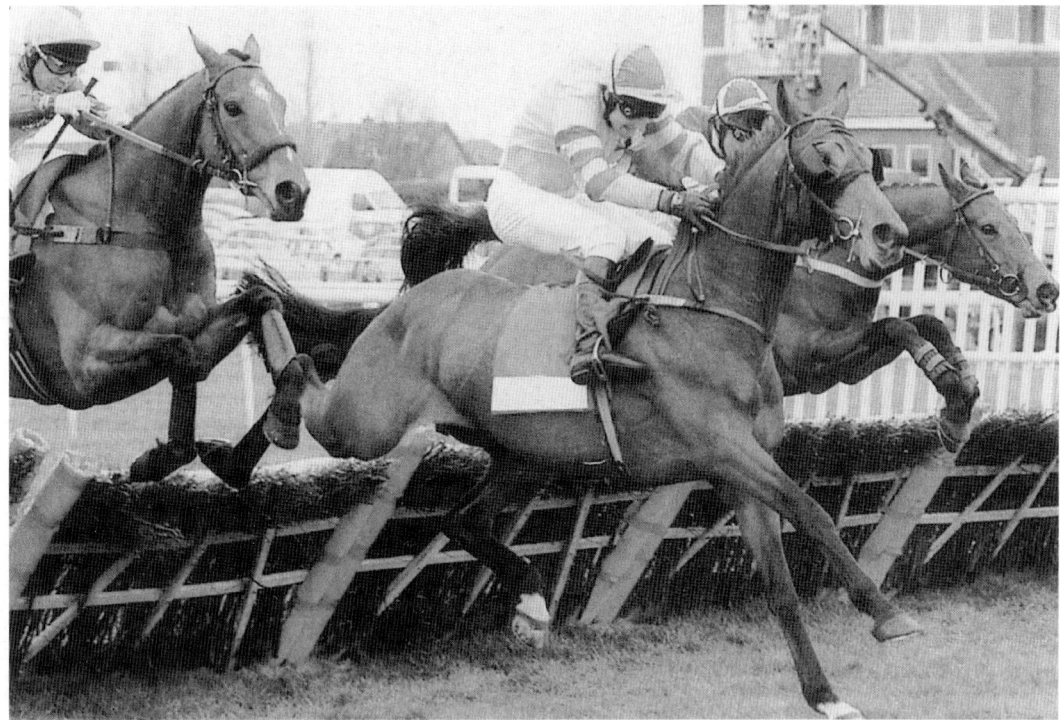

Fig. 112-1 • A hurdle race. The jump of the leading horse, which has almost run through the hurdle, is awkward, the hindlimbs are positioned asymmetrically, and the horse's back is hollow.

number of racecourses in Britain, and proponents of these types of fences argue that they provide a better introduction to racing over obstacles for horses that ultimately are intended to be steeplechasers. This may be true, but only 35% of horses that run over hurdles convert to steeplechasing, indicating that hurdle racing has become a specialty sport that draws many of its participants from horses that have raced previously on the flat.

Steeplechases are run from 2 to 4½ miles (3 to 7 km) over fences that, with the exception of those at Aintree, over which the Grand National is held, have a standard construction. The course must have at least six fences per mile, one of which must be an open ditch, with the other plain fences. The plain fences must be a minimum of 54 inches high (1.37 m) and constructed of birch, or birch and spruce, in a frame. The use of gorse is not permitted. The base of the fence must be 72 inches (1.83 m) from front to back, with the thickness of the fence at its top not less than 18 inches (46 cm) (Figure 112-2, *A*). Plain fences usually have a guard rail on the face of the fence that usually is padded with the same material as the hurdles. An open ditch has similar overall dimensions, but the ditch in front of the fence, which may or may not be dug out, must be at least 72 inches (183 cm) from front to back and be delineated by a takeoff board that is up to 24 inches high (146 cm). Designers of racecourses also, if they wish, may include a water jump in steeplechases. These consist of a smaller fence, up to 36 inches (91 cm) high, with a 108-inch (2.74-m)–wide water ditch, which must be 3 inches (7.6 cm) deep, on the landing side of the fence.

Point to point races (see Figure 112-2, *B*), named because originally they were run from one point to another, represent the amateur branch of steeplechasing and are restricted to horses that have qualified to race by hunting with a registered pack of hounds. Races for such horses also take place on licensed racecourses and are known as *Hunters' Steeplechases* (or Hunter chases).

Some races, notably in France, at Punchestown in Ireland, and at Cheltenham in Britain, are run over more natural obstacles, including banks and growing hedges. Timber races are held over upright (United States) or sloping (Britain) post and rail fences (Figure 112-3). To make the obstacles less dangerous, the top rails may be sawn through so that they will knock down if they are hit hard.

Finally, National Hunt flat races are staged for horses that have not run previously on the flat and are at least 3 years old. The races are intended to teach horses to acclimatize to the environment of a racecourse and the rigors of a race, without the additional hazard of obstacles. They also provide a way of demonstrating a horse's ability so that it can be sold. Colloquially, National Hunt flat races are known as "bumpers," because originally they were restricted to amateur riders, and the combination of inexperienced riders and horses led to their pejorative nickname.

NATIONAL HUNT HORSES

British and Irish National Hunt horses may be Thoroughbreds, which are registered in the General Stud Book, or non-Thoroughbreds, which are in the Non-Thoroughbred register. Many top-quality French jumping horses are of the Selle Français breed. Horses are started in jump racing by one of two routes. They are raced on the flat at 2 or 3 years of age before moving on to hurdling and possibly to steeplechasing, or they are bred specifically for National Hunt racing. Red Rum, who won the Grand National on three occasions, is an example of a horse that started racing

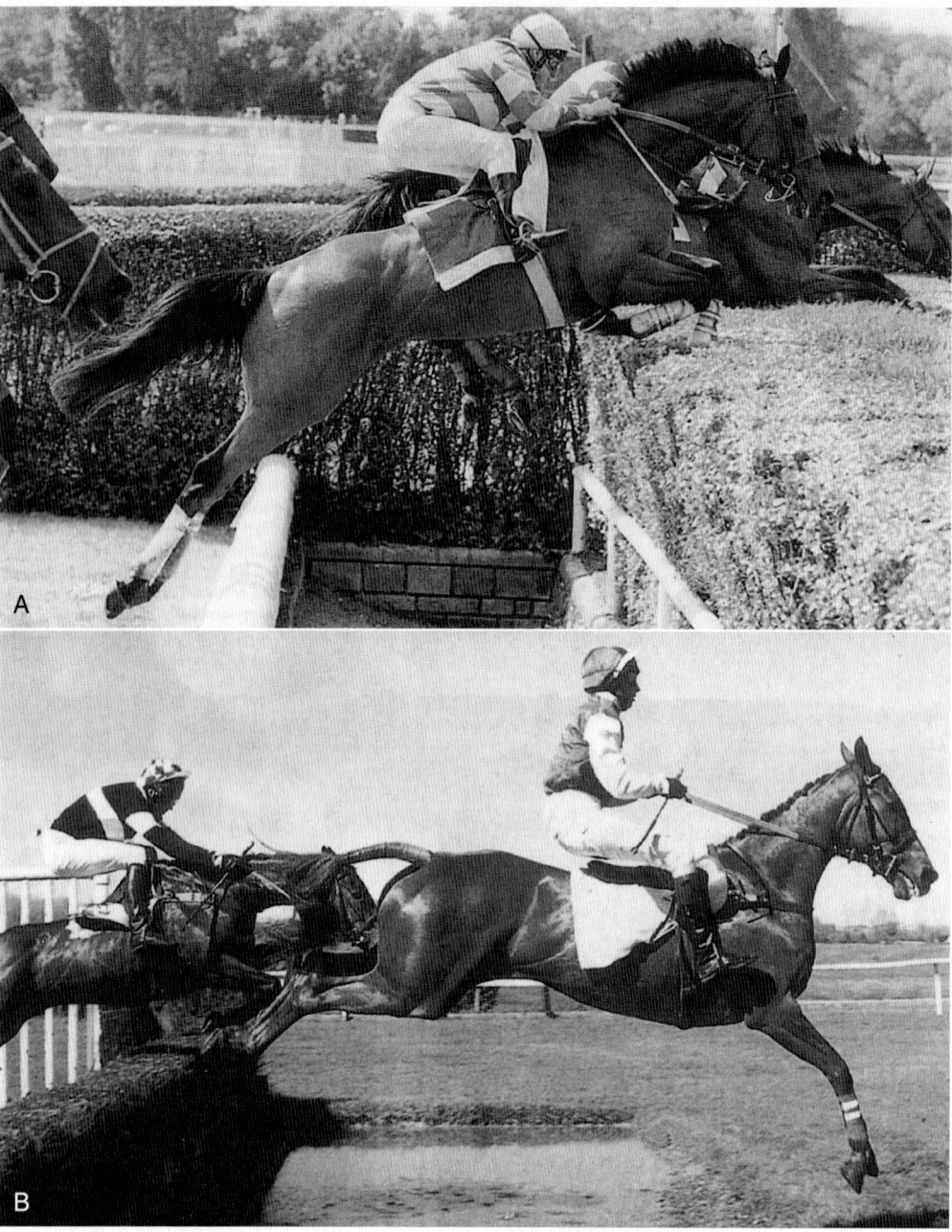

Fig. 112-2 • A, A steeplechase race in France. **B,** A point to point race. The fences are smaller than in steeplechase races, and the amateur jockeys tend to be less well positioned.

in flat races as a 2-year-old. In general, however, horses that graduate from the flat tend to stay in hurdle races, and only 35% of horses that race over hurdles go on to race in steeplechases. Geldings tend to predominate in both types of race.

Steeplechasers tend to be bred for that particular type of racing and are usually bigger-framed Thoroughbreds compared with flat racehorses. Breeding steeplechasers is less straightforward than breeding for flat races, because most steeplechasers are geldings, meaning that it is unlikely that males can be chosen based on racecourse performance. Finding performance-tested mares also is difficult, because the average age of steeplechasers is the highest of all racing categories, and by the time a mare has proved her ability, she may be past her breeding prime. Therefore most

stallions that are popular as sires of steeplechasers are horses that have shown stamina on the flat and then prove to sire successful progeny. Many mares that are used to breed steeplechasers are chosen because of pedigree rather than performance.

Once foaled, many horses destined for steeplechasing are left unbroken until 3 or 4 years of age, when they are often sold as National Hunt *stores* (horses bred specifically for National Hunt racing) intended to start a racing career at 4 or 5 years of age. This traditional system has been used for many years and could be said to have stood the test of time. Recently, National Hunt breeze-up sales have been introduced and are gaining in popularity. However, some research suggests that horses benefit from an early introduction to regular exercise and from early racecourse

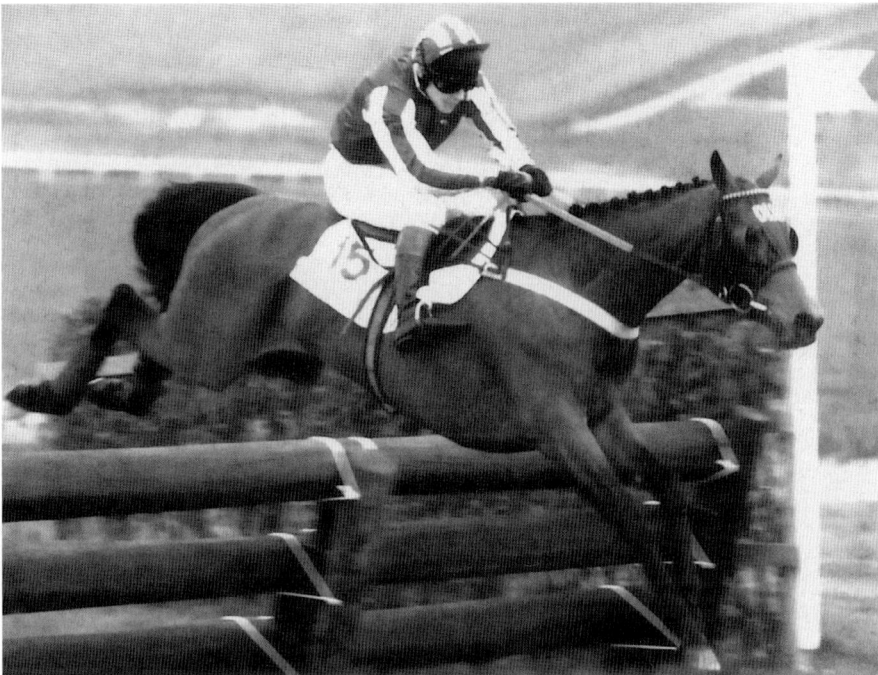

Fig. 112-3 • A timber race. The horse is jumping well, and the rider is in good balance.

References on page 1344

experience, and this may reduce the risks of injury.[1] Moreover, the later that horses enter training, the higher the risk of fatal injury.

TRAINING NATIONAL HUNT HORSES

At its simplest, training involves conditioning the cardiovascular, respiratory, and musculoskeletal systems of horses to tolerate maximal exercise. The skill of the trainer is to exert the horse sufficiently to achieve this while avoiding physical injury and without inducing an aversion to hard work. Human athletes, being motivated to succeed, tolerate extreme discomfort during training to achieve their goals. Horses have to be encouraged to exercise and never to anticipate that the result of exercise will be discomfort or pain.

Horses that move to National Hunt racing from flat racing receive the basic conditioning as yearlings and young 2-year-olds. Store horses, however, may do little regular exercise until they are virtually skeletally mature at 4 years. Because they are older, thinking that they require less time to adapt to exercise is tempting, whereas the reverse may be true. It is therefore essential that early preparation is graduated gently and that early signs of failure to adapt, such as sore shins or joint effusions, are noted and training intensity adjusted. If clinical signs go unrecognized or ignored, more serious skeletal defects may develop, such as stress fractures of the tibia, humerus, or pelvis, which may precede catastrophic fractures on the gallops or racecourse. Traditionally, store horses spent at least 6 weeks walking and trotting on quiet roads and tracks before they commenced any faster work. This initial slow preparation has now been abandoned by many trainers, partly because of the difficulty of finding a suitable safe, quiet environment and partly because of the economic pressure to see the horse on the racecourse.

Most trainers of National Hunt horses now use a simple adaptation of interval training over distances of about 1000 m, almost invariably up an incline that may be steep. An average morning workout would be an initial slow warm-up, followed by two brisk canters up the incline on an easy morning, alternating with three faster ascents on a work morning.

One of the most important aspects of training National Hunt horses is teaching them to jump appropriately. Hurdle races are conducted at a fast pace, and some trainers believe that horses that jump the obstacles without touching them, and with the same action as a show jumper, use energy unnecessarily and concede ground to rivals who jump low and flat. This is possible because the timber hurdles give way if the horse hits them, although the ease with which they do this depends on the ground into which the legs of the hurdles have been driven. Once horses have acquired this style of jumping, some trainers argue that the horse finds it difficult to jump the larger, more solid, steeplechase fences. This accounts for the relatively low number of horses that make the transition from hurdling to steeplechasing and the demand in Britain by some trainers for a brush hurdle that, although relatively small, has to be jumped with care. Specialist steeplechasers are encouraged to jump much as horses intended for other disciplines that involve jumping, and they jump low poles and logs, with and without a rider, before progressing to larger obstacles. However, the amount of training carried out over fences by steeplechasers is proportionately much less in the United Kingdom and Ireland than for event horses or show jumpers.

RACING NATIONAL HUNT HORSES

Jump racing developed as a winter sport, probably originally because of the connection with fox hunting, which

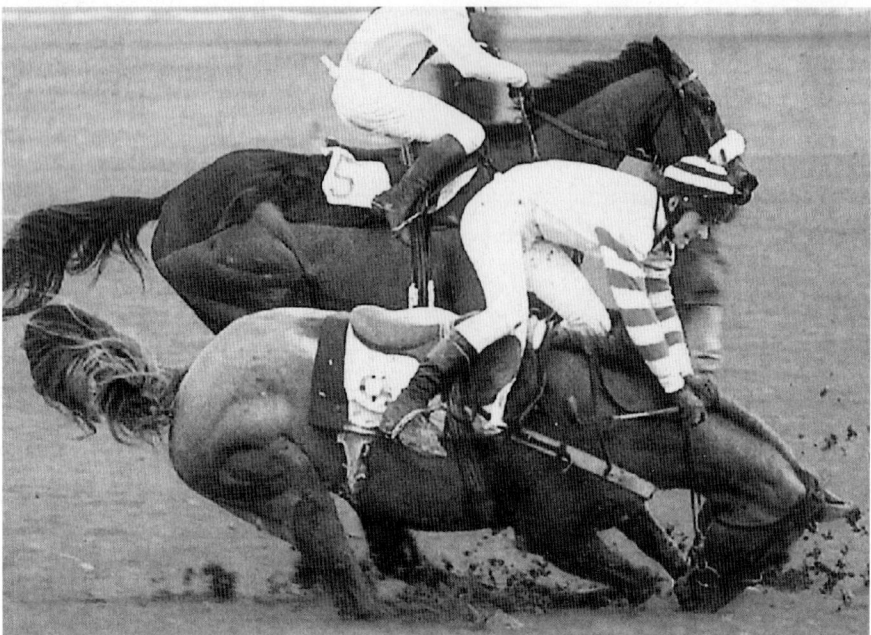

Fig. 112-4 • A faller at a point to point race. Note the extreme position of the hindlimbs.

also is conducted during the winter months. However, jump racing is now held in Britain throughout the year, although those courses that hold summer jump meetings are required to ensure by artificial irrigation that the ground conditions are kept no worse than good to firm. This is because epidemiological studies have shown that firm ground conditions are more likely to be associated with serious injuries. The reason for such a relationship is complex. It is probably related to the speed at which the horses travel, but other complex factors influence the interaction of the horse's foot with the ground under various conditions, some of which are related to ground hardness, and these require further research and elucidation. Jump racing remains seasonal, however, because the major races take place from November to March, and many horses spend a few weeks turned out during the summer. Seasonal racing influences injury management, because if a horse sustains a clinically significant injury in, for example, late February, the owner or trainer applies pressure for the horse to be ready for the next season—that is, to resume training by October of the same year.

Horses are trained by individual trainers spread throughout the United Kingdom, Ireland, and France and may travel long distances to compete. Therefore any single veterinary surgeon usually does not deal with more than four or five trainers and their horses. At race meetings the horses are subjected to prerace veterinary inspections, and each race is monitored carefully by veterinary surgeons driving on the outside of the track alongside the race and a veterinarian observing the entire race from an appropriate vantage point.

Point to point races are held from January to June. Point to point racing is an amateur sport, raced over obstacles that are smaller and softer versions of the steeplechase fences on licensed racecourses. Some horses that perform well in point to points successfully graduate to steeplechasing, and this route to steeplechasing is chosen by some owners in preference to hurdle racing, possibly after one

or more National Hunt flat races. While National Hunt horses run on average between four and five times per year, point to point horses may run more frequently during the season, because the race meetings are usually held at weekends. However, the average number of starts per point to point horse in 2000 was only three.

Because of the two distinct sources of horses that enter National Hunt racing, a wide variety of injuries is seen, ranging from injuries related to beginning training to degenerative injuries associated with overuse. In addition to the injuries sustained while the horse is in training, a National Hunt horse is more prone to injury after a fall than is a flat racehorse (Figure 112-4). It is also important to be aware that horses that are skeletally mature when they begin training (4- to 5-year-old store horses) still undergo the same pathophysiological processes that lead to stress fractures, albeit in different sites from the 2- or 3-year-old Thoroughbred. Because National Hunt racing continues throughout the year, the going under foot (footing) can vary, and extremes of both soft and firm going place the National Hunt horse under extra stress from injury.

A substantially higher death rate occurs in National Hunt racing compared with flat racing.[1-7] In a retrospective analysis of data from all starts from January 1990 to December 1999, 2015 deaths were recorded on racecourses from 719,099 starts.[1] The death rate per 1000 starts was substantially higher in steeplechasers (6.7; 34.5% of the total) and hurdlers (4.0; 43.4% of the total) compared with flat racehorses (0.9; 18.8% of the total). Spinal injuries occur much more frequently in hurdlers (19% of all hurdler deaths) and steeplechasers (23% of steeplechaser deaths) compared with flat racehorses (1% of flat racehorse deaths). Tendon breakdown injuries resulting in humane destruction at the racecourse were also substantially higher in hurdlers (20% of hurdler deaths) and steeplechasers (14% of all steeplechaser deaths) compared with flat racehorses (8% of flat racehorse deaths). Risk of mortality was associated with a number of variables. With steeplechase horses a higher risk occurred in horses that started steeplechase racing at 8 years of age or older. The weight carried was also influential, with horses carrying more than 70 kg minimum weight being at greater risk. Races longer than 4 miles were associated with a higher risk than shorter races. Heavy going, resulting generally in slower speeds, reduced the risk. Good to firm or hard going increased the risk of mortality in hurdlers and steeplechasers.

TIMBER RACING

Timber racing is considerably more popular in the United States than in the United Kingdom and is more structured. Novice or stakes horses compete only against one another, with greater prize money for stakes races, the most valuable being the Maryland Hunt Cup. The most prestigious race in the United Kingdom is the Marlborough Hunt Cup. Historically the stakes races with the largest amounts of prize money have been open only to amateur jockeys; however, recent rule changes have allowed for professionals to ride in these races in the United States. Timber racing horses often have raced previously on the flat or over hurdles, are usually 6 to 12 years of age, and may have injuries from earlier racing, particularly osteoarthritis (OA) of numerous joints and stable superficial digital flexor tendon (SDFT) injuries.

TRACK SURFACE OR TRAINING SURFACE AND LAMENESS

The surfaces and terrain over which horses train vary extremely because the trainers are dispersed widely geographically. Much of the work is done on grass, but fast work often is done on all-weather purpose-built gallops.

Many horses hack up to a mile to and from the gallops, ensuring good warm-up and cool-down. However, the standard of maintenance of the gallops varies. Poor gallops with an inconsistent surface varying from soft to deep may increase the risk of tendon injuries or predispose horses to stumbling and accidents such as third carpal bone fractures. Many trainers are based in areas of chalk downland (natural rolling hills with a chalk subsoil), which drains well, but the large number of flints (sharp stones) in the soil may result in a high incidence of bruised soles or sole punctures unless the horses have well-conformed feet. The steepness of the terrain over which the horses do fast work may influence injury. An increased number of pelvic fractures was noted after a new gallop was laid, the last section of which was up a steep incline (RvP). In a yard of 40 horses, one or two horses per year sustained pelvic or tibial stress fractures, but after the new gallop there were seven iliac wing fractures (three right, four left), two sacroiliac subluxations (one bilateral, one right), and two tibial stress fractures. These injuries may have been caused by hind foot slippage. After the gallop was recontoured, the problem resolved.

The influence of falls on the nature of injuries is substantial.[2-7] Most falls occur on landing over a fence. Falls may result from the horse or jockey making a jumping error, from interference by another horse still in the race, or from a loose horse that had previously unseated its rider. The fall of one horse may result in the fall of one or more other horses (Figure 112-5). Thus injuries may result from the fall and impact with other horses. Falls may result in fatal fractures of the cervical or thoracolumbar vertebrae. Rib fractures usually result from a fall and may cause severe lameness and/or respiratory signs. Other fractures seen commonly, usually resulting from a fall, include scapular, radial, and humeral fractures; fractures of the accessory

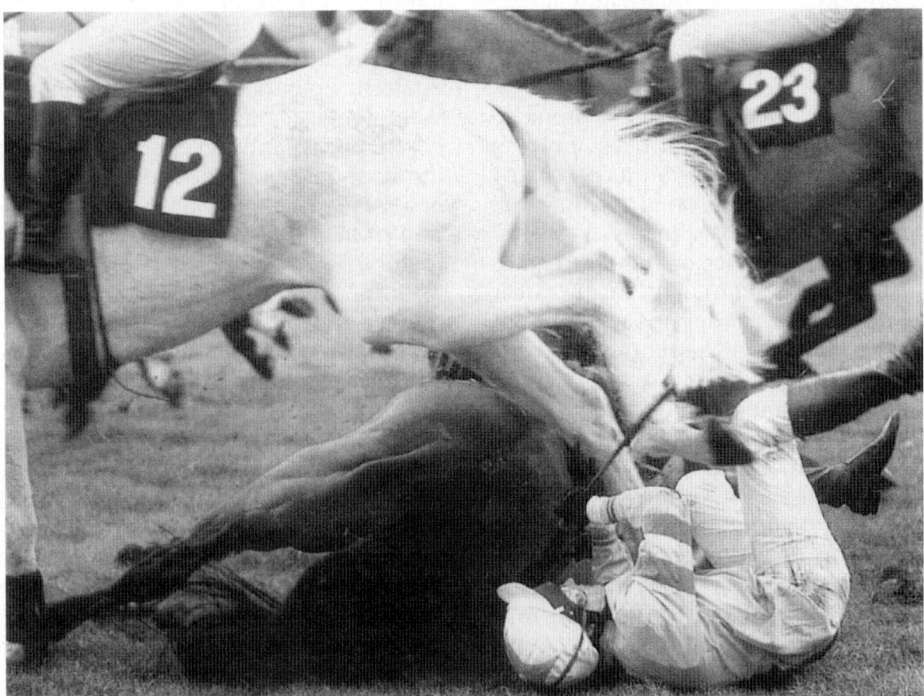

Fig. 112-5 • Horse no. 12 is about to be brought down by a fallen horse and jockey.

carpal bone; and fractures of the lateral malleolus of the tibia. Major muscle ruptures, especially in the hindlimbs (e.g., semimembranosus, quadriceps, or adductor) also usually result from a fall. Rupture of the fibularis tertius may occur if the horse falls with forced hyperextension of the hock.

A significant statistical correlation exists between certain factors and the incidence of injury on racetracks:

- Increased firmness of the going results in an increased injury rate in all forms of National Hunt racing.
- Increased incidence of injury on firm ground is further increased by increasing the length of the race.
- In hurdle races run over more than 2½ miles with only a few obstacles (six to eight), the casualty rate increases compared with the same distance with nine or more fences.
- Races ridden by amateur riders carry a higher risk of serious injuries.

Digital flexor tendon lacerations frequently are sustained as horses race over fences and generally occur on the palmar aspect of the metacarpal region, proximal to the proximal sesamoid bones (PSBs). It is important to recognize that the site of a skin laceration may not coincide with the site of a tendon laceration.

Some important injuries occur more commonly during racing than training. Luxation of the SDFT from the tuber calcanei sometimes occurs. Rupture of the musculotendonous junction of the superficial digital flexor (SDF) muscle is an unusual injury, but is an important injury in steeplechasers. SDF tendonitis is common in National Hunt horses,[5-7] and recurrent injuries may result in complete rupture of the tendon.

CONFORMATION AND LAMENESS

With an increasing proportion of National Hunt horses starting training earlier and running first on the flat at 3 years of age and then over hurdles at 4 years of age, the trend has been toward using smaller, lighter-framed horses. Although such horses are not necessarily more prone to injury, they seem less able to cope with deep, holding going often encountered in the winter months compared with the more traditionally bred rangy National Hunt store horses, which are often rather late maturing.

For a National Hunt steeplechaser or hurdler to race until 10 years of age is not uncommon, so the racing career is considerably longer than for a European flat racehorse. Horses should be well balanced and proportioned, with good feet and adequate bone for body size and weight. Horses with back-at-the-knee conformation, carpus valgus, offset knees, or substantial toed-in or toed-out conformation particularly may be predisposed to forelimb problems. A long back may be associated with an increased risk of back problems. A horse with straight hocks or long, sloping hind pasterns may have an increased risk of hindlimb lameness.

In a study evaluating variation in conformation in a cohort of National Hunt horses, Thoroughbreds were found to be different from other breeds in lengths, joint angles, and deviations, but variation was small.[8] In a group of 108 National Hunt horses an increase in intermandibular width, flexor angle of the shoulder joint, and coxal angle (angle between the ilium and ischium) had a positive effect on race performance.[9] Performance decreased with increases in girth width and hind digit length and with valgus conformation of the metacarpophalangeal joint, and the risk of superficial digital flexor tendonitis increased with increased metacarpophalangeal joint angle and carpus valgus limb deformity.[9] The risk of pelvic fracture decreased with an increase in coxal angle, but risk increased with greater tarsus valgus limb deformity.[9]

LAMENESS EXAMINATION

Diagnosis of lameness starts with a full history, which should include stage of training, because, for example, a 6-year-old store horse starting training is as susceptible to stress fractures as an immature athlete. The clinician should establish whether the horse has run recently. Is the lameness of recent onset, or is it a chronic problem that has been getting progressively worse? Some trainers request advice as soon as lameness is recognized, whereas others may restrict the horse to light work and seek veterinary advice only if lameness persists. Some trainers treat a lame horse with phenylbutazone. Many trainers are happy for horses to come out rather short, shuffly, and stiff and warm up to move more freely; however, more overt lameness usually supervenes, or a back problem develops secondarily.

It is important to determine if the horse has had any time off recently with the present trainer or a previous trainer that may suggest a previous injury. There may be a history of warmth associated with the palmar metacarpal region that, if the horse has been subsequently rested, may not be obvious on clinical examination. Does the horse have any history of trauma? Jumping history is also important: did the injury occur while the horse was schooling over fences or in a race? Did the horse fall or collide with another horse (Figure 112-6)? Does the lameness resolve with rest or does the horse warm out of lameness?

If the horse had a history of a fall, it is important to establish how the horse fell. It may be possible to review video footage. Did the horse turn a full somersault, land on its pelvis, and develop lameness thereafter? A pelvic injury should be suspected. Did the horse fall at the end of a 3-mile race on heavy going and lay winded? Information from the racecourse veterinarian may be particularly useful.

If a horse has a history of poor jumping performance, trying to establish if the horse has ever been a good jumper over hurdles or fences is worthwhile. Many of these horses are lame. The veterinarian needs to find out how the horse is jumping. Does the horse stand off the fences or jump flat? If a horse does not want to take off, it may have a hindlimb problem. If the horse jumps flat, it may have a back problem. If the horse is reluctant to land, it may have a forelimb problem.

If a horse is presented for evaluation for poor performance, it is important to try to assess the orthopedic component. About 50% of horses with poor performance are lame. When did the horse last race, and over what ground conditions? Did the jockey make any comments when he dismounted? Has the horse coughed? Is rectal temperature routinely monitored? Routine hematological

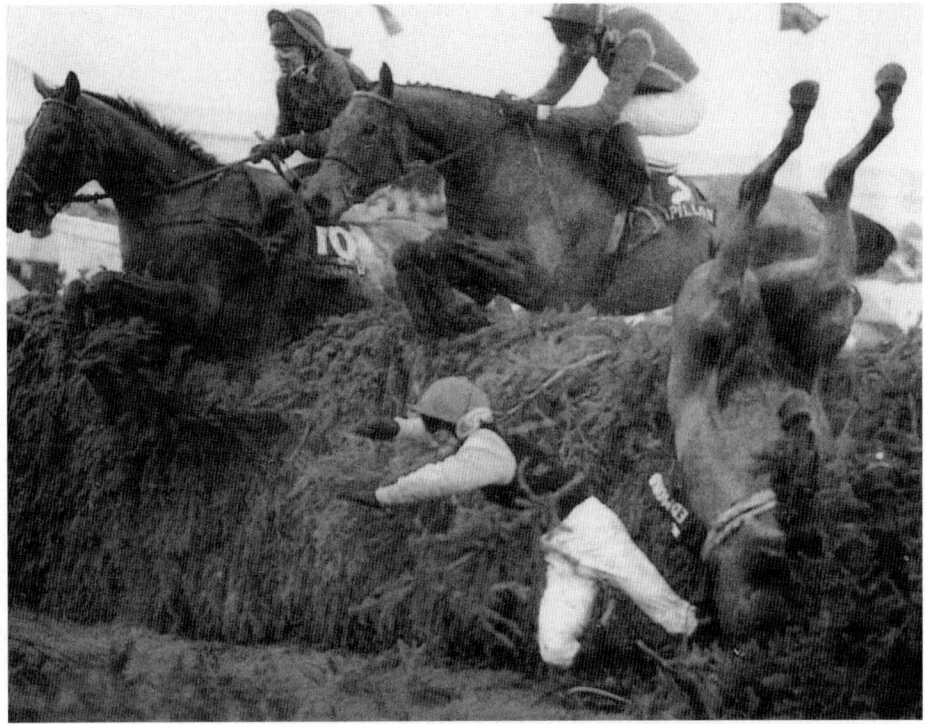

Fig. 112-6 • A fall at the Chair at the Grand National. The horse pitches steeply and lands on its neck.

examination and measurement of fibrinogen, comparing results with a baseline for that horse, are useful for detecting systemic abnormalities. Endoscopic examination of the upper airways and trachea, combined with a tracheal wash, are useful screening tools to eliminate a respiratory component to the problem.

The clinical examination does not differ from a routine lameness evaluation of any other type of horse, but because many horses have chronic problems with which they have been living until more obvious lameness supervened, the entire horse should be assessed, not just the postulated lame limb. In view of the high incidence of SDF tendonitis and suspensory desmitis, particular attention should be paid to the palmar metacarpal soft tissues. If the horse has a history of a fall while jumping, particular attention should be paid to the neck, back, and pelvic regions.

A thorough clinical examination may reveal palpable abnormalities in the palmar metacarpal region, evidence of effusion, or pain on flexion of a particular joint. Skeletal pelvic asymmetry or muscle wastage over the quarters also may be evident. Back and pelvic reflexes and the tone of the back and pelvic muscles should be assessed. Is any evidence of guarding apparent? Abnormal shoe wear may give clues about which limb or limbs are lame, which is otherwise not always easy to determine in a horse moving short because of pain in several limbs.

Dynamic examination at the walk and trot in a straight line, followed by flexion tests, should be followed by examination on firm and soft going on the lunge at the trot and canter. The horse should be turned tightly to the left and to the right. If a history of a fall exists, a complete neurological examination should be performed.

If a horse is lame after a recent fall, the investigative approach depends on the degree of lameness and the rate of improvement. A horse with a pelvic injury is usually very lame initially, although lameness associated with an ilial wing fracture usually improves substantially within 24 hours. Lameness associated with an ilial shaft fracture is usually persistent, and the horse remains extremely lame. These horses should be crosstied, assuming the horse's temperament is suitable. Some ilial wing fractures can be detected with ultrasonography, but the diagnosis of others requires nuclear scintigraphy. Nuclear scintigraphy may give false-negative results if done before 5 to 7 days after injury. If a horse shows only mild to moderate lameness after a recent fall, the horse generally is allowed rest for 7 to 10 days and is then reassessed, and only if lameness persists is further investigation carried out.

DIAGNOSTIC ANALGESIA

If no obvious cause of lameness is apparent, then diagnostic analgesia is performed, but no particular differences in approach exist for this type of horse. However, if clinical signs suggest an intraarticular problem, such as synovial effusion and pain on passive manipulation of a joint, then intraarticular analgesia of the suspect joint may be performed first. If intraarticular analgesia is carried out, clipping a small area is preferred, but some trainers are reluctant to allow this, and provided that the hair coat is not excessively long, a timed 5-minute surgical scrub is performed before injection.

If a fracture is suspected based on the history or clinical signs, diagnostic analgesia is not performed. A horse that pulled up lame on the gallops or finished work and then became severely lame while walking home may have a stress fracture. Stress fractures of the third metacarpal bone (McIII), the third metatarsal bone (MtIII), and the tibia are common. If a stress fracture is suspected, the horse is examined radiographically or scintigraphically.

If soft tissue swelling is identified clinically, then ultrasonography is performed routinely as the next diagnostic step.

IMAGING CONSIDERATIONS

Radiography is performed routinely using standard radiographic images. Special images at different angles may be required for demonstrating specific lesions, based on the preliminary examination. Some stress fractures are difficult to identify radiologically, and if a fracture is suspected on clinical grounds, radiographic examination is repeated 10 to 14 days later.

If the clinician suspects an abnormality of the palmar metacarpal soft tissues, an ultrasonographic examination should be performed. In view of the high incidence of bilateral lesions, both limbs should be examined routinely. A systematic approach is essential, focusing on the SDFT, deep digital flexor tendon, and suspensory ligament (SL) in turn. It is almost invariably necessary to clip the metacarpal and metatarsal regions to achieve satisfactory image quality, because most National Hunt horses have thick guard hairs. However, satisfactory images of the pelvis usually can be obtained after washing with chlorhexidine for about 10 minutes, soaking with alcohol, washing off (to avoid alcohol-induced damage to the transducer), and liberally applying coupling gel.

Transverse and longitudinal images of the metacarpal and metatarsal regions are required to gain a full appreciation of the severity of injury. An injury index giving a quantitative assessment of damage can help in communication with trainers and may help to convince them of the clinical significance of an injury associated with only mild clinical signs. Each structure should be evaluated sequentially from proximally to distally at predetermined measured intervals (4 or 5 cm) distal to the accessory carpal bone or each zone should be examined (see Chapter 16). Cross-sectional area (CSA) or circumferential measurements are made at comparable sites in each limb. Measurement of the size of damaged fibers is also useful. One author (RvP) describes the severity of a core lesion by multiplying the percentage of CSA of the tendon damaged by the length of the lesion and by the percentage of the fibers damaged within the injury (assessed visually). For example, a core lesion that occupies 10% of the CSA of the tendon, extends 10 cm proximodistally, and is assessed visually as having 75% of the fibers within the core lesion damaged has an index of $10 \times 10 \times 0.75 = 75$. A similar lesion occupying 30% of the CSA has an injury index of $30 \times 10 \times 0.75 = 225$. All images should be recorded routinely for future comparisons.

Nuclear scintigraphy is indicated as a screening tool when a lame horse is presented after a bad fall, particularly when a moderate-to-severe lameness has persisted for more than 3 or 4 days. Scintigraphy also may be indicated if severe, sudden-onset lameness occurs with no localizing clinical signs to rule out fracture before a dynamic workup is contemplated. Scintigraphy often is more rewarding in horses with acute injuries than those with chronic lameness. Scintigraphy usually can be targeted to specific areas such as the pelvis or both hindlimbs unless the horse has lameness involving several limbs. During evaluation of the pelvis, radioactive urine in the bladder can confound

interpretation. The use of furosemide may help, but this drug may make the horse fidgety, and catheterization of the bladder, followed by flushing with warm water, may be preferable.

PROCEEDING WITHOUT A DIAGNOSIS

National Hunt horses have a longer career than flat racehorses, and less prize money is available to be won. Therefore the pressure to get a horse sound quickly often is less, and many trainers accept resting the horse if a diagnosis cannot be achieved by the techniques described previously. However, an attempt to reach a diagnosis always should be made.

SHOEING CONSIDERATIONS AND LAMENESS

Most National Hunt horses train and run in light steel shoes with one toe clip in front and two side clips on hind shoes. Some trainers change to a hind shoe with a single toe clip for racing. Good shoeing is essential. Given the high incidence of foot problems causing lameness, a good relationship with a skilled farrier is invaluable. Poor foot conformation, especially low collapsed heels, may predispose the horse to SDF tendonitis. Bar shoes combined with a rolled toe often are used for horses with collapsed heels. If a foot is conformed poorly, the risk exists of shoes being pulled off repeatedly in training, particularly if the branches of the shoe are set too far medially or laterally.

THE TEN MOST COMMON CAUSES OF LAMENESS IN STEEPLECHASERS, HURDLERS, AND POINT TO POINT HORSES

1. Superficial digital flexor tendon injuries
2. Suspensory ligament injuries
3. Lameness associated with the carpus
4. Lameness associated with the hocks
5. Lameness associated with the pelvis
6. Lameness localized to the feet
7. Fractures of the third metacarpal bone; pelvic and tibial fractures
8. Lameness localized to the metacarpophalangeal joints
9. Traumatic injuries, particularly of the back and neck, after falls
10. Back problems

DIAGNOSIS AND MANAGEMENT OF LAMENESS IN STEEPLECHASERS, HURDLERS, AND POINT TO POINT HORSES

Superficial Digital Flexor Tendonitis

Epidemiological studies have demonstrated a 16% to 43% incidence of SDFT injuries in National Hunt horses, with some reports but not all studies documenting variations among trainers (10% to 40%).[7,10,11] Although most of the injuries occur in the forelimbs, hindlimb injuries also occur. Horses 5 years old or younger were less at risk, whereas the maximum injury rate was seen in horses 12 to 14 years of age.[9] Many trainers routinely assess forelimb

SDFTs daily, and some are adept at detecting relatively subtle lesions. Veterinary involvement may enhance these skills. Many, but not all, trainers are keen to have ultrasonographic assessment of suspected tendon injuries. Some trainers tend to ignore suspicious injuries at the end of a season, contrary to veterinary advice. This may be one reason why a peak incidence of tendon injury tends to occur at the beginning of the season when horses start galloping after a short summer break. Other horses may have been kept in training late in the season to get an extra race and may have sustained injury, which may or may not have been manifested clinically. A second peak incidence of injuries tends to occur at the end of the season, perhaps related to races run on faster going. SDF tendonitis is more common in steeplechasers than in hurdlers, but this may reflect the older population of the horses rather than the type of racing itself. The degree of lameness at the time of acute injury may reflect the severity of tendon damage.

Horses with acute lesions are managed with aggressive antiinflammatory treatment for 5 days, including systemic nonsteroidal antiinflammatory drugs (e.g., phenylbutazone and eltenac), with or without a single dose of corticosteroids (e.g., dexamethasone), and cold hosing several times daily. Cold water bandages or cold kaolin is applied to the limbs. Some thin-skinned horses are prone to blistering, so any bandaging must be done with care. Other popular proprietary poultices, such as Animalintex (Robinson Animal Health Care, Chesterfield, United Kingdom) and a variety of clay-based preparations, may irritate small unnoticed wounds and are therefore avoided.

An initial ultrasonographic examination is performed about 7 days after the injury is first recognized. Horses with central core lesions may be treated by decompression, using needle fenestration or a fixed blade. This is performed with the horse sedated and with use of regional analgesia. Follow-up ultrasonographic examinations frequently are performed 3 to 4 weeks after injury, because the preliminary examination may underestimate the degree of damage because of ongoing enzymatic degradation. This gives a baseline scan for the injury.

Many differing views are given on the best management of SDF tendonitis in National Hunt horses. Adequately rehabilitating a tendon that was injured late in a season so that the horse can race the following season without a disproportionately high risk of reinjury is difficult. Firing remains a popular treatment, and because many owners and trainers are prepared to rest a horse for 12 months after firing when they would not give such a long convalescent period if rest alone was recommended, this treatment still is carried out widely. Nonetheless, the reinjury rate remains high, so many alternatives have been tried with various success. These alternatives range from at least 9 months of field rest, intralesional injection of hyaluronan, polysulfated glycosaminoglycan, a phenol derivative, β-aminopropionitrile fumarate, platelet-rich plasma, or growth factors, combined with a variety of exercise regimens. Intralesional β-aminopropionitrile fumarate combined with a strictly controlled exercise program has produced good results in selected horses (RvP, SJD) but is no longer commercially available; however, the time for return to racing often is prolonged, in part dictated by the time of injury and the seasonal nature of racing.

The average time to return to racing was 17 months. Preliminary results with cultured mesenchymal stem cell injections indicate that recurrent injury rate after treatment may be reduced compared with other treatments.[12] The reinjury rate in the injured or contralateral limb 2 years after returning to full work was approximately 33% in 83 horses treated with mesenchymal stem cells[12] compared with 55% of 28 horses managed conservatively or with β-aminopropionitrile fumarate.[13] Forty-two percent of horses treated with mesenchymal stem cells were still racing 2 years after returning to full work.[12] The owner or trainer must be committed to at least 3 to 4 months of walking exercise after treatment, and some horses are unsuited to this temperamentally, unless a horse walker is available. Regardless of the methods of management, a slow, gradual rehabilitation before resumption of ridden work seems beneficial. Ideally the horse should be walking on a horse walker daily for 3 months before resuming ridden exercise. The horse can be turned out during this 3-month period. A cage horse walker in which the horse is free and in which the speed can be set manually to encourage the horse to walk briskly is best.

Serial ultrasonographic examinations are particularly useful as exercise is resumed—about 1 month after walking begins, then again before cantering commences, and a third time before fast work commences. Commonly as work intensity increases, small hypoechogenic areas develop, especially in areas in which the fiber pattern is not parallel. In some horses these lesions disappear, provided the horse is maintained at the same exercise level, whereas in others a core lesion redevelops, and the trainer should be warned accordingly.

The prognosis is related partly to the severity of injury.[14] In a follow-up study of 73 National Hunt and point to point racehorses, lesions were graded by ultrasonography as mild (<50% CSA or <100 mm in length), moderate (50% to 75% CSA or 110 to 160 mm in length), or severe (>75% CSA or >160 mm in length). All mildly affected horses returned to training, and 63% raced. Fifty percent of horses with a moderate lesion resumed training, and 23% raced. However, only 30% of horses with severe lesions resumed training, despite up to 6 months longer convalescence, and 23% raced. The mean reinjury rate of those resuming work was 40% in the period of follow-up (9 to 30 months).

The type of racing in which the horse is involved may influence the prognosis for return to racing after SDF tendonitis. Fifty-one (73%) of 70 hurdlers raced five or more times after desmotomy of the accessory ligament of the SDFT for treatment of tendonitis compared with 39 (58%) of 67 steeplechasers.[15]

Cellulitis, skin necrosis, and necrosis of the underlying SDFT are poorly understood conditions that have been recognized in National Hunt horses (SJD) and flat race horses that have run over long distances (>1½ miles) (RvP). Many horses run in boots or exercise bandages, which are removed after racing. Whether exercise bandages would be on long enough to cause pressure necrosis is debatable. The typical history is that a proprietary claylike substance (Kaolin, Ice-Tite) or commercial poultice (e.g., Animalintex) is applied to the metacarpal regions after racing, with or without overlying bandages. The applied substance is removed the following day. Clinical signs may be apparent within 24 to 72 hours, with the development of peritendonous edema and serum ooze, progressing to skin slough and slough of deeper tissues, which may take several weeks. The degree of damage varies among horses, and one or both limbs may be affected. One author (SJD) has seen this unassociated with SDF tendonitis, whereas another (RvP) often has seen concurrent SDF tendonitis. The prognosis depends on the depth of the lesions. One author (RvP) recommends that horses be thoroughly cooled after racing before anything is applied topically to the limbs, to minimize the risks of these complications. If a SDFT injury is suspected, then the advice of the course veterinarian should be sought.

Suspensory Desmitis

Suspensory desmitis is a major problem in National Hunt horses, especially steeplechasers and point to point racehorses.[3,10,11] However, in a study of 1119 horses in training followed over two seasons, SDFT lesions were more common (1.71/100 horse months in training) than SL injuries (0.23/100 horse months).[11] Injuries of the body or branches occur in forelimbs and hindlimbs, sometimes with a fracture of the distal third of the second metacarpal bone (McII) or second metatarsal bone (MtII), fourth metacarpal bone (McIV) or fourth metatarsal bone (MtIV), apical or abaxial proximal sesamoid fractures, or sesamoiditis. Proximal suspensory desmitis does occur in forelimbs and hindlimbs and is recognized more commonly in hindlimbs, but the true incidence may be underestimated.

Body and branch injuries of the SL often go unrecognized until the ligament is grossly enlarged; possibly some of these are cumulative injuries rather than single-event injuries. More careful monitoring of the SLs by regular palpation with the limb not bearing weight may lead to earlier detection of important lesions. The degree of swelling sometimes makes it difficult to palpate accurately the distal end of the McII and the McIV.

Assessment of structural damage is done by ultrasonography in a way similar to that described for SDFT lesions. Lesions are assessed acutely (up to 7 days after injury and 4 to 6 weeks later) to determine the baseline degree of injury. Some of the swelling contributing to the apparent swelling of a SL branch is often a periligamentous reaction. Radiographic examination is necessary to evaluate the McII or the MtII, the McIV or the MtIV, and the PSBs.

Body and branch injuries are associated with a prolonged convalescence irrespective of the way in which they are managed, and returning to racing often takes longer than for a horse with SDF tendonitis. The rate of recurrent injury is high. Surgical removal of fractures of the McII or the McIV (or the MtII or the MtIV) has little bearing on the horse's final outcome.

Conservative management of rest alone, splitting the SL, intralesional injections of β-aminopropionitrile fumarate, and pin firing have been used with no clinically significant differences in outcome. There is anecdotal evidence that mesenchymal stem cell treatment or platelet-rich plasma may improve healing and reduce reinjury rate.

Lameness Associated with the Carpus

Synovitis and OA of the middle carpal joint are common and are treated by intraarticular injection with hyaluronan, with or without triamcinolone acetonide. A horse with synovitis may be treated more conservatively than a flat racehorse when the pressure is great to maintain the horse in training if at all possible. With a young National Hunt horse with a career of several years ahead, restricting the horse to walking exercise until clinical signs have resolved fully often is more prudent.

Chip fractures of the dorsal border of any of the carpal bones are common and often are associated with preexisting OA. Treatment is by surgical removal of the fragment(s), and prognosis depends on the degree of OA; most horses are able to return successfully to racing. Slab fractures of the third carpal bone are also common but are not always associated with obvious clinical signs. Lameness is often mild and associated with only slight effusion of the middle carpal joint.

Accessory carpal bone fractures usually result from a fall and are common in National Hunt horses. Most fractures are longitudinal (vertical) and occur midway between the dorsal and palmar borders of the bone, but less commonly articular chip fractures occur on the proximal or distal dorsal articular margin. The latter must be removed surgically; otherwise, severe OA ensues. Horses with the more common longitudinal fractures do not require treatment other than prolonged rest. Some fractures heal only by fibrous union, but the prognosis for return to racing is good. Some horses have effusion in the carpal sheath when work is resumed, which responds well to the intrathecal administration of triamcinolone acetonide and for which retinacular release is seldom necessary.

Lameness Associated with the Hock

The degree of lameness caused by hock pain varies, and lameness is more commonly unilateral, unlike the bilateral lameness usually seen in the flat racehorse. The most common cause is osteoarthritis (OA) of the distal hock joints, although traumatic injuries also occur. The horse may adduct the lower limb as the leg is brought forward at the walk and trot. The lameness often worsens after flexion and when the lame limb is on the inside on the lunge. More subtle signs of poor jumping or back pain may herald a problem originating in the hocks.

Lameness most often is alleviated by intraarticular analgesia of the tarsometatarsal joint. It is rare to have to inject the centrodistal joint as well, despite the variable communication between the joints and the fact that osteoarthritic changes seen radiologically often affect both joints. Radiography of the hocks should include four standard views, because radiological changes may be visible only on one projection. Abnormalities range from mild periarticular osteophyte formation to osteolysis, with narrowing of the joint spaces, with or without periarticular new bone. Occasionally, young horses in the first year in training have clinically significant radiological changes in one limb. The damage was probably present before onset of training and may be associated with collapse of the distal tarsal bones or a traumatic incident earlier in the horse's life.

Care should be taken when interpreting scintigraphic images of the hocks in National Hunt horses. Often areas of increased radiopharmaceutical uptake (IRU) are seen but do not appear to correlate with clinical signs of lameness. Treatment of horses with OA of the distal tarsal joints usually consists of intraarticular medication of the tarsometatarsal joint with combinations of hyaluronan and corticosteroids. Consideration should be given to chemical fusion of painful distal hock joints in young National Hunt horses.

Traumatic injuries involving the hock are common. Injuries frequently sustained after a fall include fracture of the lateral malleolus of the distal aspect of the tibia and tearing of the attachments of the collateral ligaments. The lameness in horses with lateral malleolar fractures can be mild, and lesions may be missed if radiography is not carried out. Ultrasonography may be more useful than radiology for the early diagnosis of collateral ligament injury. Follow-up radiology some weeks later may reveal some entheseous new bone formation. Horses with these injuries have a good prognosis for a return to racing, although improvement in lameness may be slow. Some debate exists about the optimal management of horses with lateral malleolar fractures: conservative or surgical. Both treatments carry favorable prognoses. Surgical removal is usually easiest by making an incision directly over the fracture fragment(s) rather than by attempting arthroscopic removal. Arthroscopic surgical techniques can be used successfully, particularly if motorized equipment such as a synovial resector is available to improve visibility and help with dissection of ligamentous attachments (Editors).

Lameness Associated with the Pelvis

Lameness associated with the pelvis in the National Hunt horse is more likely to result from a traumatic incident than a stress fracture. Falls or poor landings while jumping (see Figure 112-4) may lead to subluxation of the sacroiliac joint or pelvic fractures. However, iliac stress fractures also occur, especially in horses entering training at 5 years of age or older. A strong correlation between pelvic lameness and working horses on loose all-weather surfaces, especially on unmanaged wood chip surfaces and particularly uphill, has been noted (AS, RvP). In a study of 1119 horses in training followed over two seasons there were 111 fractures, 17% of which were pelvic fractures.[11]

Clinical signs can vary from severe lameness with obvious crepitus to mild stiffness. It is important to examine the pelvis per rectum when pelvic damage is suspected. A horse with an iliac fracture sustained during a fall may be lame initially and improve rapidly within 48 hours. If an iliac wing fracture is nondisplaced, the horse could return to cantering exercise before lameness recurs. Muscle spasm may result in substantial asymmetry of the tubera coxae in the acute stage, but this usually also resolves within 24 hours. Severe lameness associated with an iliac shaft or acetabular fracture is invariably persistent. Iliac stress fractures may cause only mild clinical signs, and sometimes the most important abnormality is shortening of the contralateral forelimb stride as the horse moves off from standing still. This gait abnormality rapidly resolves.

Fractures of the iliac wing involving the dorsal surface often can be diagnosed by ultrasonography, but incomplete stress fractures involving the ventral aspect cannot be seen.

Nuclear scintigraphy is invaluable for assessing pelvic pain. Assessment of pelvic fractures should be delayed for at least 5 to 7 days after injury to avoid false-negative results. If scintigraphy indicates IRU in the region of the coxofemoral joint, obtaining numerous oblique scintigraphic images is worthwhile to try to assess whether the fracture involves the joint. Other scintigraphic changes seen include IRU at the greater and third trochanters of the femur associated with damage to the insertions of the deep and middle gluteal tendons and the superficial gluteal insertion, respectively.

Horses with nondisplaced iliac wing fractures have a good prognosis, whereas the prognosis for those with fractures of the iliac shaft[16] or iliac fractures involving the acetabulum is poor.

Lameness Associated with the Front Feet

Lameness associated with the front feet may vary from a shortened gait to obvious lameness. The most common causes of foot lameness include solar bruising, corns, and subsolar abscesses. Other commonly recognized causes of foot lameness in the National Hunt horse include pedal osteitis, palmar foot pain, and fractures of the distal phalanx. Palmar foot pain may be caused by bruising of the heel bulbs or may be caused by deeper pain associated with the deep digital flexor tendon or navicular bone, with a much poorer prognosis. Horses that train on downland are particularly at risk for bruising of the feet or penetrating injuries of the sole caused by flints. The latter may result in infectious osteitis of the distal phalanx. Protective aluminum pads may prevent solar penetrations but do not prevent bruising, because the pad is distorted and puts pressure on the sole if a horse stands on a flint.

In horses with chronic lameness associated with foot pain, local analgesia, radiography, and ultrasonography sometimes can be unrewarding or give equivocal results. Nuclear scintigraphy using soft tissue and bone phase images is sometimes helpful. Magnetic resonance imaging is increasingly useful.

Fractures of the Third Metacarpal and Metatarsal Bones

The most common long bone fractures in National Hunt horses are condylar fractures of the McIII (or the MtIII) and pelvic and tibial fractures. In a study of 1119 horses followed in training over two seasons, there was a total of 111 fractures, 17% of which involved the McIII or the MtIII.[11] Former store horses were more at risk of fracture than former flat racehorses, although this difference was not significant. Fractures of the MtIII frequently involve the medial condyle and may spiral proximally. Full evaluation of the fracture may require numerous oblique radiographic images of the MtIII. Such fractures are more common in hurdlers than in steeplechasers. With prompt surgical treatment by internal fixation, the prognosis is good. Compound, comminuted fractures of the distal aspect of the McIII and the MtIII may occur during racing and may be associated with luxation of the fetlock. These horses have a guarded prognosis for return to racing.

Incomplete proximal palmar cortical fatigue fractures of the McIII occur commonly, especially in horses older than 4 years of age entering National Hunt or point to point training for the first time. Preexisting increased radiopacity in the proximomedial aspect of the McIII detected when lameness is first recognized in some horses suggests that abnormal bone modeling has existed for some time, subclinically or without clinical signs being recognized. Lesions are often bilateral. Lameness is characterized by the horse becoming lamer the farther it trots and then improving if walked a few steps. Usually no localizing clinical signs are apparent, and diagnosis depends on localizing pain to the proximal palmar metacarpal region and identifying radiological lesions or scintigraphic evidence of increased bone turnover, in the absence of ultrasonographic abnormalities of the proximal aspect of the SL. Treatment of 3 months of rest with a graduated return to work is usually successful, and recurrent injury is unusual.

Less commonly, transverse stress fractures of the distal metaphyseal region of the McIII cause acute-onset lameness. No localizing signs may be apparent, but lameness is alleviated by a four-point nerve block of the palmar and palmar metacarpal nerves. Usually preexisting callus formation is evident on the distal metaphyseal region of the McIII on the dorsal or palmar aspects.

Lameness Associated with the Metacarpophalangeal Joint

Most lameness associated with the metacarpophalangeal (fetlock) joint is degenerative. Fetlock lameness is often present bilaterally with a shortened forelimb gait, warmth around the joint, and reduction of range of motion. Flexion often exacerbates lameness. Lameness often is improved by intraarticular analgesia of the metacarpophalangeal joint. Radiography may reveal periarticular osteophytes or a small fragment on the dorsoproximal border of the proximal phalanx. If the PSBs and SL attachments are involved in sesamoiditis, a low palmar or four-point nerve block is required to alleviate lameness. New bone formation and osteolysis may occur on the abaxial surface of the PSBs at the attachments of the SL. This form of sesamoiditis more commonly is associated with damage to the attachments of the SL onto the PSB rather than a primary PSB disease and is seen much more frequently in National Hunt horses than other types of horses. The condition is related to the stress to which the palmar metacarpal soft tissues are subjected during jumping and galloping.

Treatment options include the following:
1. Injection of the fetlock joint with hyaluronan, with or without corticosteroids
2. Arthroscopy and removal of any free fragments
3. Blistering of the palmar aspect of the fetlock to treat sesamoiditis

The prognosis for lameness affecting the fetlock is more guarded in the National Hunt horse than in the flat racing horse but such lameness occurs much less frequently.

Neck Lesions

Neck trauma usually results from a fall (see Figure 112-6) and is more common in steeplechasers and point to point racehorses than in hurdlers.[2-7] Neck trauma may result in ataxia or a stiff neck, with or without forelimb lameness, and can cause death. Ataxia may be transient or persistent. Radiographic examination should be performed if ataxia or neck pain and stiffness persist for more than a few days. Fractures in the cranial or midneck regions are most common, but occasionally fractures occur caudally, which may be difficult to assess without a fixed, high-output x-ray machine. Nuclear scintigraphy can be helpful in localizing

such fractures, but false-negative results in the caudal cervical spine are possible. Horses with persistent ataxia have a guarded prognosis. Most horses with a fracture unassociated with ataxia can return to racing despite residual neck stiffness.

Back Pain

Back pain in the National Hunt horse may be primary or may develop secondary to chronic lameness in one or more limbs and is being recognized with increasing frequency. Nuisance problems include the development of seromas underneath the saddle, which are probably attributable to an ill-fitting saddle and poor riding. Most trainers regularly use a physiotherapist, who may be the first person asked to look at a horse that is not right. Only if the horse fails to respond to one or two treatments, or if the physiotherapist recognizes obvious lameness, is veterinary advice sought. A good working relationship with the physiotherapist is valuable, because without a doubt the rehabilitation and long-term management of horses with chronic back pain can be helped by regular physiotherapy treatment. Moreover, certain findings on palpation have been shown to predict the occurrence of some pelvic and hindlimb fractures.[17] However, the veterinarian should have responsibility for both the diagnosis and the development of the treatment program.

Knowledge of back problems in National Hunt horses has increased greatly with more routine use of nuclear scintigraphy. Thorough investigation of the back is warranted in horses with chronic back pain, with a history of jumping awkwardly (see Figure 112-1), or after bad falls. Physical examination of the back often can be unrewarding concerning specific diagnosis, because the examination may reveal only stiffness and pain on palpation. Underlying problems such as active kissing spines (impinging, overriding, or overlapping dorsal spinous processes) or OA of the synovial intervertebral articulations (facet joints) are common in National Hunt horses and can be ruled in or out using scintigraphy and radiography. In a horse with an acutely sore back after a fall, scintigraphy can be used to determine if any bony damage occurred. The clinician should bear in mind that falls may involve more than one horse, and a fallen horse may get shunted (pushed) by one behind. Serious vertebral fractures can produce nothing more than severe stiffness and guarding in some horses after a fall, if the spinal cord itself is not compromised. For example, scintigraphy may reveal intense focal IRU suggesting a fracture in the region of the second or third lumbar vertebra. Radiology may demonstrate an obvious change in orientation of the spinous processes at this level, without being able to demonstrate a fracture. Lateral and dorsal scintigraphic images are useful to identify fractures of the transverse processes of the lumbar vertebrae.

Ultrasonographic examination is also useful for identifying some soft tissue injuries such as desmitis of the supraspinous or dorsal sacroiliac ligaments.

Horses with traumatic injuries often respond well to prolonged rest combined with physiotherapy. Horses with kissing spines often improve after local infiltration with corticosteroids.

Successful management of chronic back pain needs a broad approach. Many National Hunt horses have an inadequate jumping education and poor technique (see

Figure 112-1). Traditionally in the United Kingdom and Ireland, horses learn to jump by loose schooling over small fences; horses are schooled ridden over two or three small fences, once or twice when they are fresh. In France horses often are trained to jump out of deep going, when they are tired, providing a better grounding for racing conditions. The standard of riding of the work riders is often only moderate, and employing some staff with a background of working with event horses or show jumpers may be beneficial. Time should be spent teaching the horse to jump properly. Often more time is available in the summer break period to devote to such problems.

Additional work from the field, or keeping the horse in work, or bringing the horse in early should be advised. The horse should be encouraged to work in a round outline by exercising in draw reins to improve the development of the epaxial muscles. The horse can be given a warm-up period on a horse walker before being ridden. Use of a well-fitting hunting saddle rather than a racing saddle should be encouraged. After exercise the horse may benefit from being led home from the gallops rather than ridden.

Other Injuries

National Hunt horses seem particularly vulnerable to lacerations involving the distal palmar (plantar) aspect of the metacarpal (metatarsal) region, which may involve the SDFT or the digital flexor tendon sheath (DFTS), usually resulting from the horse being struck or from penetration by a sharp stone. Such horses with these injuries should be treated early and aggressively, especially if the DFTS is involved. With early lavage of the DFTS using an arthroscope, combined with intravenous broad-spectrum antimicrobial treatment for 5 to 7 days, the prognosis is usually excellent unless substantial damage of the SDFT has occurred.

A high number of complex injuries to the palmar (plantar) soft tissues of the pastern have been seen in National Hunt horses as sequelae to previous SDF tendonitis in the metacarpal region or as primary injuries. Although injury to one or both branches of the SDFT may occur alone, simultaneous injuries of the oblique and straight sesamoidean ligaments are not uncommon. The prognosis for horses with such injuries is generally guarded.

THE TEN MOST COMMON CAUSES OF LAMENESS IN TIMBER RACING HORSES

1. Superficial digital flexor tendonitis
2. Suspensory desmitis
3. Osteoarthritis of the distal hock joints
4. Thoracolumbar or pelvic pain
5. Distal sesamoidean desmitis
6. Osteoarthritis of the metacarpophalangeal joint
7. Soft tissue trauma of the stifle
8. Interference injuries during racing
9. Timber shins
10. Fracture of the patella

DIAGNOSIS AND MANAGEMENT OF LAMENESS IN TIMBER RACING HORSES

Lameness falls into three groups: acute injury or breakdown after racing, chronic wear injury caused by the horse's age and length of competitive career, and traumatic injuries caused by interference from another horse or hitting a fence.

Eighty-five percent of acute injuries after racing are caused by SDF tendonitis and SL desmitis. Many timber horses have had previous SDFT injuries from earlier flat racing. The long courses (up to 4 miles), variable turf quality and terrain, fatigue, and poor weather conditions predispose horses to injury. Injuries range from small tears to catastrophic breakdowns that may necessitate humane destruction. Regular clinical and ultrasonographic monitoring is useful for detecting subtle changes and for making recommendations about running on specific footing (ground) conditions (KK).

Once recognized, horses with OA of the metacarpophalangeal and the distal hock joints require management, because increased lameness may be induced by the increased work leading up to a race. Keeping horses as comfortable as possible throughout training is preferable, which may necessitate intraarticular medication two or three times during a season, using hyaluronan for the metacarpophalangeal joints and hyaluronan and corticosteroids for the distal hock joints (KK). Orally administered glucosamine and chondroitin sulfate are used commonly. It is important to keep the horse well shod and to use cold hydrotherapy after strenuous exercise.

Traumatic injuries sustained during racing are common, with the hindlimbs particularly vulnerable because of the horse hitting fences at speed. Damage to the quadriceps muscles, periarticular soft tissues of the stifle, and stifle joint is common, although determination of the severity of injury is usually easiest several hours after a race rather than immediately. Radiological examination is indicated to rule out a patellar fracture, which requires surgical management. Bruising of the patellar ligaments is common, with or without effusion of the femoropatellar joint, and is treated by drainage of excess synovial fluid and injection of hyaluronan (4 to 6 mL) combined with controlled exercise and nonsteroidal antiinflammatory drugs.

Timber shin describes firm enlargement of the dorsal aspect of the metatarsal region because of chronic bruising of the long digital extensor tendon, with fibrosis of the tendon and peritendonous soft tissues. Timber shin is unsightly and is not associated with long-term lameness, but recent trauma results in lameness from severe swelling of the leg, with pain on protraction.

Injuries sustained by interference from another horse, for example, traumatic heel bulb laceration or strike injuries on the palmar or plantar aspect of the fetlock, are common (see other injuries on this page). Injuries also can result from falls—for example, fracture of the accessory carpal bone—or from a galloping horse treading on a faller.

Chapter 113

The Finnish Horse and Other Scandinavian Cold-Blooded Trotters

Kristiina Ertola and Jukka Houttu

HISTORY OF THE BREEDS

The Finnhorse is the only original horse breed in Finland. Sweden and Norway also have similar cold-blooded breeds. The Finnhorse has been known for about 1000 years and originally was used for farm and forest work and in the army. The Stud Book of the Finnhorse was founded in 1907 for draft and carriage horses but is now divided into four parts for racing trotters, riding horses, draft horses, and small pony-type horses. Seventy-five percent of the registered Finnhorses are trotters. The Finnhorse is heavy and well muscled, with a short neck and usually a heavy head. The average height is 155 to 160 cm, but pony-sized Finnhorses exist. Swedish and Norwegian cold-blooded horses are slightly lighter and smaller than Finnhorses, with an average height of 150 to 160 cm.

Trotting competitions are the main use of Finnhorses. In Scandinavia all harness races are for trotters; there are no pacing races. The first records of trotting races are from 1817, when races were arranged on the ice of the river Aura in Turku. The first races with official timing took place in 1862 in Viipuri. In the early years the trotting races were arranged by the state to support and develop horse breeding in Finland. In the first races the distance was 2138 m, and they were on a straight track. The horses raced individually, and prizes were given according to the times. The first official Finnish record was from 1865 by the mare Brita. The average time for 1000 m was 1.51.3 (1 minute 51.3 seconds, equivalent to a mile in 2 minutes 59 seconds). Today the record is held by Viesker and is 1.19.9 (2:08.5). Betting was first introduced in 1928 but developed slowly until the 1960s, after which rapid growth followed.

In Sweden, racing also was started in the early nineteenth century on roads and icetracks. The first permanent tracks were built in the early twentieth century. The first official record in Sweden was in 1829, 1.37.6 (2:37), held by a Norwegian horse, Sleipner Varg. Today the record is 1.17.9 (2:05) by a Swedish stallion, Jarvsofaks. When racing became more popular, Swedish and Norwegian horsemen started trading horses across the border, and the Swedish and Norwegian breeds began to merge together. Today the breeds are genetically alike, and they now are considered to be the same breed. Sweden and Norway have a close collaboration in breeding and racing, and their horses race in the same races.

Today the races are held at modern dirt tracks, and in the same events there are separate races for Finnhorses and

Standardbreds (STBs). The Finnhorses are allowed to race first at the age of 3 years, but not uncommonly they start racing as late as 5 or 6 years of age. They are allowed to race until 16 years of age, and a Finnhorse usually is considered to be best from 7 to 10 years of age. Some stakes races are held for 4- and 5-year-olds, but the main events are for older horses. The biggest event for Finnhorses is the Kuninkuusravit, the Royal Trot, which is held annually in July or August at a different track in Finland each year. The race is one of the major sporting events in Finland, attracting about 50,000 people. Separate races are held for mares and stallions; geldings are excluded. To be allowed to race in the Kuninkuusravit, the horse has to be approved for public breeding and has to be entered in the Stud Book, which requires inspection and approval by a special board. The horses race three times in 2 days over distances of 1609 m, 2100 m, and 3100 m, and the final result is based on the total time for all three races. To win the royal title is the greatest honor a Finnhorse can ever achieve; the best stallions have won the title five times (Vieteri, Vekseli, and Viesker), and the best mares, four times (Suhina and Valomerkki). This is good proof of stamina and endurance, which are typical for the Finnhorse at its best.

In Sweden and Norway horses usually start racing at 3 years of age and are allowed to race until the age of 15. Stakes races are open to Swedish and Norwegian horses, and big races are held for 3- and 4-year-olds and for older horses. Finnish horses are not allowed in these races, and only a few races are held in which all Scandinavian horses race together.

TRAINING A COLD-BLOODED TROTTER

Traditionally the horses have been bred and trained by farmers, and many remain home bred and trained. There are no sales for Finnhorses, Swedish, or Norwegian trotters. Most horses are broken at 2 years of age, spend the next summer at pasture, and then start more serious training in the winter at 3 years of age, often with a summer break. Farm and forest work has historically been part of the training to build up strength. Speed work is not done at all at this stage, and traditionally some trainers have never used speed work. Horses started racing at 5 to 6 years of age and raced themselves to condition. However, many professional trainers now train cold-blooded horses, and the horses are better prepared for the races and start racing younger. The race times for the beginners are faster, which has caused problems for many old-school trainers. Many Finnhorses are not natural trotters, and building them up to speed takes time and training. If fast speeds are demanded too early, gait abnormalities develop at higher speeds, and horses lose complete control of the trotting action while appearing sound at a slower trot.

Training cold-blooded trotters takes much more time than for STBs, making training more expensive and leading to problems in getting new owners and trainers. In all Scandinavian countries, fewer cold-blood races are held than STB races, and they are concentrated in the north. Nonetheless, cold-blood racing is supported by the central racing organizations of each country and continues to thrive.

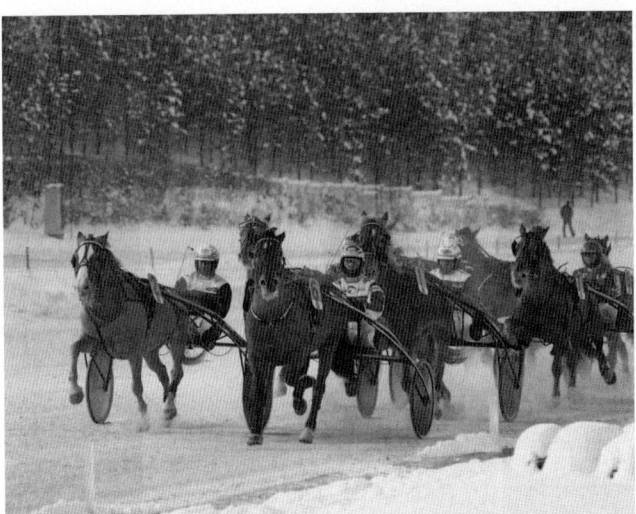

Fig. 113-1 • Winter racing. (Courtesy Olavi Ilmonen, Lahti, Finland.)

RACETRACKS AND WEATHER CONDITIONS

The racetracks in Scandinavia are 1000-m oval dirt tracks, and the horses race counterclockwise. The climate is cold in the winter, and the tracks freeze and get covered by snow (Figure 113-1). In winter temporary tracks also are made on ice for smaller races with no betting. The variable climate causes track problems. In late autumn when the track is frozen but not yet covered by snow, the surface can be treacherous. Snowfall makes the tracks smooth but not hard, and provided the horse is shod properly, the track is not slippery. In the springtime, when the snow begins to melt, the track conditions vary throughout the day, being hard in the morning after a night frost, becoming good for a few hours when the frost melts, and then becoming wet and soft the rest of the day. Keeping the track in good condition requires much skill.

Because of the long winter, much of the training has to be done on snowy or icy surfaces. Snow is a good surface on which to train a horse, but special shoeing with studs is essential so that the horses do not slip. In the winter many trainers do much of the speed work in snow, which can be deep. The training speeds can be lower because of the resistance, but the training effect is equal or even better than when the training is done on the track. Snow provides a soft and smooth surface, acting as a shock absorber. Many horses with lameness problems race better in winter because of the training in snow. Horses also are trained on the ice of lakes, which is also a good surface. The surface of the ice gives slightly, and shoes with studs can get a good grip. The worst training surface is ground that is frozen hard like asphalt; this type of surface causes many lameness problems.

SHOEING CONSIDERATIONS

In the winter (November to April) special requirements for shoeing are needed to prevent the horses from slipping on ice. Studs, 5 to 15 mm in length with sharp tips that offer a good grip on the ice or snow, are screwed into the shoes. Four to 15 studs are used per shoe; more studs usually are used in the hind shoes. It is important to have enough studs for the horse to avoid slipping slightly at every step, causing joint and muscle soreness. A risk of interference injuries exists, and some horses with poor action cannot race in the winter. Forelimb heel injuries are common if a horse breaks stride. Elbow boots may be necessary to protect the elbows from stud-induced trauma. Some lameness problems get worse during the winter, because traction from the studs stops the feet abruptly. Hock-related lameness is often worse during the winter, and tendon and suspensory ligament (SL) problems increase.

The shoeing of racing Finnhorses is otherwise much like that of STBs, but many Finnhorses are not natural trotters and tend to gallop or pace, so many trainers use special shoeing to help the horse to balance. Young horses often need heavy front shoes with toe weights and bell (overreach) boots when they are learning to trot. The total weight per foot can be up to 500 to 800 g, and this predisposes the horses to lameness, particularly tendon and SL injuries. Improvements in breeding have decreased the number of horses with severe balancing problems. On the hind feet Finnhorses usually wear normal STB shoes. The lateral branch of the shoe is often longer and bent slightly outward (trailer) to make the hind action wider and therefore avoid interference between the forelimbs and hindlimbs. Although many STBs race unshod, this is rare in Finnhorses.

CONFORMATION AND LAMENESS

The Finnhorse is a heavy, draft-type horse compared with other racehorses. The forehand is heavier than the rear of the horse and is combined with a heavy head and a thick and short neck, causing much stress to the forelimbs. Finnhorses often stand back at the knee, and this sometimes is combined with lateral deviation of the carpus (offset knees). Forelimb tendon, SL, and carpal injuries are not uncommon. The hindlimbs are usually conformed better in Finnhorses than the forelimbs. The most common faults are sickle hocks and cow hocks, which can cause curbs or other lameness problems in the tarsal area. Fetlock conformation is often good, and most Finnhorses have big hooves with good-quality horn.

LAMENESS EXAMINATION

Many Finnhorses complete a racing career without serious lameness problems and require substantially less veterinary treatment than STBs, perhaps because of slower racing speeds. The lameness examination for a Finnish horse is similar to that for a STB racehorse, and similar problems occur. Clinical history is particularly important, and the following questions should be asked:

1. How long has the horse been in training, and how has it been trained? What is the duration of lameness, and has the horse ever trotted sound at high speed? A Finnhorse often develops slowly and has to be taught to trot. Therefore many action problems in young horses are not caused by lameness but by lack of coordination. Lack of strength or condition may predispose horses to lameness.
2. Does the horse trot straight? Is the horse hanging on a line? Is the horse hanging on a shaft? Does the

horse need sidepoles or headpoles? A great many lameness problems show only at higher speeds, especially in the early stages of the problem. This is particularly true with hindlimb lameness. With right hindlimb lameness the horse's rear end usually turns to the left shaft, and the horse hangs on the right line. Correspondingly, problems in the left hindlimb cause hanging on the left line and turning the rear end to the right shaft. A horse with bilateral lameness may move straight. With forelimb lameness this tendency to be on a line is less obvious.

3. Does the horse trot better in turns or on straightaways? In which direction are the turns better? In a counterclockwise direction, horses with right hindlimb lameness are usually worse in the turns. Horses with left hindlimb lameness are worse in the straightaways and usually are worst in the turns in a clockwise direction.
4. Is the horse better on soft or hard surfaces? Sidebones often cause lameness on hard surfaces, as do many other foot problems.
5. Is the horse worst when it starts to trot? Does the horse warm into or out of the lameness problem? In young horses (4- to 5-year-olds), bilateral hind fetlock pain is a common cause of lameness, resulting in a short hindlimb stride when first trotting. The lameness usually improves if the horse is jogged for about 1000 to 3000 m.
6. Do the studs in the shoes affect the lameness in the winter? Many horses with carpal or tarsal lameness are worse with studs.

The veterinarian should assess the type and use of the horse and its conformation, muscular development, and general condition and should systematically palpate all the limbs, because concurrent lameness in several limbs often occurs.

Many horses are trained with sleighs in the winter and are harnessed with collars. If the collar is not fitted properly, it can cause shoulder musculature soreness. Soreness of the shoulder or scapular musculature also can point to other problems in the forelimbs, especially when the lameness is bilateral. Inflammation of the carpal sheath is common because of the heavy front of Finnhorses and the conformation of the carpi and invariably is associated with palpable distention. Proximal suspensory desmitis (PSD) sometimes occurs, and pain may be induced by palpation of the proximal metacarpal region.

The second (McII) and fourth (McIV) metacarpal bones in Finnhorses are sometimes thick and prominent, but this is not usually relevant (Figure 113-2), although thick metacarpal bones are sometimes seen in horses with PSD or tenosynovitis of the carpal sheath. Ossification of the cartilages of the foot usually can be felt by thickening and loss of elasticity in the region of the coronet, but pain is seldom evident on palpation.

In the hindlimbs special emphasis needs to be given to palpation of the tarsus. Tarsal pain is common in Finnhorses with poor conformation. Curbs are common in younger horses (3 to 6 years of age), and distal hock joint pain is common in older horses. The Churchill test works well in Finnhorses. Stifle lameness is not common in Finnhorses, and upward fixation of the patella is rare. Osteochondrosis of the lateral trochlear ridge of the femur occurs

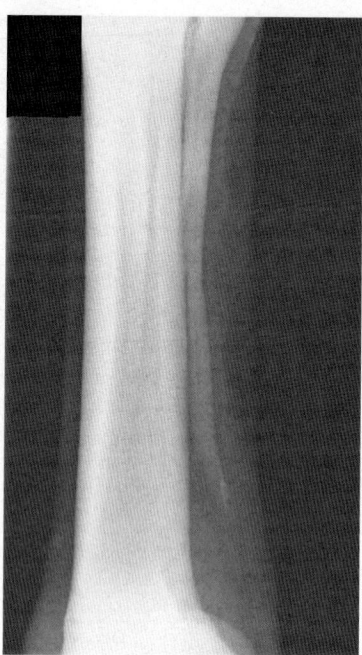

Fig. 113-2 • Dorsomedial-plantarolateral oblique radiographic image of the metacarpal region. The second metacarpal bone is enlarged, which usually has no clinical significance.

occasionally in foals and young horses, sometimes with large defects that respond poorly to arthroscopic debridement.

The gait and response to flexion tests can be evaluated properly only when the horse is calm and well controlled by the handler. It is essential that the horse trots straight and not too fast. Many horses are too eager and excited and need to be sedated or tranquilized mildly for flexion tests. Acepromazine (0.01 to 0.025 mg/kg) or romifidine (0.01 to 0.03 mg/kg) is suitable. Sedation is especially important for Finnhorse stallions, which are often difficult to handle, and sometimes two leaders are necessary to control the horse and keep it trotting straight. Horses used for riding can be examined in a circle on the lunge, but trotters are seldom taught to lunge.

When flexion tests are performed, it is essential for the veterinarian always to examine all limbs and not only those that are suspected to be lame. The tests always should be done in a similar manner and order. When doing flexion tests, the clinician should note all reactions. We do not think false-positive reactions exist, only reactions of different grades. The clinician needs to collect all the information and decide which reactions are clinically significant. Proximal and distal limb flexion tests are done separately in the forelimbs and hindlimbs, using a force of approximately 40 kPa for 60 seconds.

In general, all the trotting Finnhorses also are examined at the track at high speeds. Many action problems, especially in the young horses, show only at high speeds. The horse is harnessed in a higher sulky than normal, so the driver of the vehicle does not obscure the horse. The veterinarian drives a car behind or beside the horse at the racetrack. Examining the horse from the car is more helpful than driving the horse, because the clinician can be some distance away from the horse to see the action more clearly, and abnormalities can be assessed more easily.

Diagnostic analgesia is used as in STBs. The clinician must keep in mind that high-speed lameness seldom can be resolved totally by analgesic techniques. Every block changes the horse's action, and when the veterinarian does several blocks on the same horse, assessing the meaning of each block is difficult. When examining a horse with high-speed lameness, the clinician must believe what vision, touch, and experience indicate.

IMAGING CONSIDERATIONS

In Finnhorse trotters, radiological changes are found much less commonly than in STBs. Carpal chip fractures are rare in Finnhorses, and sclerosis of the third carpal bone is unusual. Osteochondrosis is also rare in the Finnhorse, though the prevalence has been increasing slightly in the past decade. Because osteochondrosis is unusual, radiographic examination of young Finnhorses is not performed routinely if clinical signs are absent. Controlling osteochondrosis in Finnhorses is attempted by obtaining radiographs of all stallions that are proposed for public breeding. Stallions with osteochondrosis generally are not accepted. Ossification of the cartilages of the foot is a common radiological finding in Finnhorses. Navicular disease is a rare diagnosis. Enlargement of the McII and the McIV is common and often does not cause clinical signs. Flakelike fragments adjacent to the McII usually result from interference.

Ultrasonography is invaluable for assessing soft tissue injuries and may be more useful than radiography in examining the splint bones, because splint bone problems often are associated with carpal canal syndrome or PSD.

UNDIAGNOSED LAMENESS

Some young trotting Finnhorses trot soundly at slow speeds and show no signs of lameness during a lameness examination, but when asked for speed, the horses lose the action completely. Loss of rhythm causes this; the horse simply cannot trot at higher speeds. This often happens to talented horses that have early speed with little training but do not have the strength to maintain it. The training regimen must be aimed at building strength, especially in the hindlimbs. Horses are trotted in 1- to 3-minute intervals with resistance from a special resistance cart, in deep snow, or uphill. Training takes a long time, sometimes up to a year, until these horses learn to trot again, and some horses never recover. Because the main racing events are for aged horses, time is not as big a factor for Finnhorses as for STBs. It is quite possible for a horse to recover completely and become a top-class racehorse at an older age.

TEN MOST COMMON CAUSES OF LAMENESS

1. Carpal conditions
2. Tarsal conditions
3. Superficial digital flexor tendonitis
4. Suspensory desmitis
5. Curb
6. Ossification of the cartilages of the foot
7. Splints
8. Metatarsophalangeal joint pain
9. Tenosynovitis of the digital flexor tendon sheath
10. Loss of rhythm

LAMENESS CONDITIONS TYPICAL OF FINNHORSES

Carpal synovitis is common in Finnhorses, and signs are similar to those seen in STBs. In the early stages a horse warms out of lameness quickly. Often horses with carpal problems begin to roll over and may try to pace or gallop instead of trotting. The horse may trot if the shoes are weighted more, but this may accentuate the primary problem. Without treatment the lameness worsens, and the horse begins to hang on a line and gradually becomes overtly lame. Radiological changes rarely are seen, probably because of the slower racing speeds compared with those of Thoroughbreds and STBs. Treatment consists of intraarticular medication with hyaluronan, polysulfated glycosaminoglycans (PSGAGs), or corticosteroids, alone or in combination, together with rest for several weeks. Recently the use of autologous conditioned serum (ACS) has been increasing in treating joint lameness with good results.

Carpal canal syndrome is also common in Finnhorses, sometimes simultaneously with carpitis, sometimes on its own. Ultrasonography is useful for confirming the diagnosis. The treatment is usually rest combined with intrathecal administration of hyaluronan or corticosteroids. Some horses do not respond to conservative therapy, and surgical treatment using tenoscopy may be necessary. Osteochondromas of the distal caudal aspect of the radius are seen tenoscopically, often accompanied by lesions of the deep digital flexor tendon (DDFT). The severity of these osteochondromas is difficult to assess radiologically, and often the diagnosis is made by tenoscopy. Surgical removal of the osteochondroma and debridement of torn fibers of the DDFT result in a good prognosis for racing.

Tarsal lameness is common in Finnhorses and is the most frequent cause of hindlimb lameness, usually because of distal hock joint pain. Mild lameness in horses is not noticed easily at slow speeds, but with increasing speed the horse begins to drag the affected limb, and the rear end moves to the opposite shaft. The horse usually hangs on the line on the side of the affected limb. Radiological evidence of osteoarthritis may or may not be apparent. Radiological changes are seen less frequently than in STBs. Intraarticular treatments with corticosteroids, hyaluronan, or PSGAGs are used widely. Treatment with intravenous (IV) tiludronate is often beneficial. In some horses cunean tenectomy can be useful.

Superficial digital flexor (SDF) tendonitis and suspensory desmitis are common. SDF tendonitis usually occurs in forelimbs, and poor conformation or overweighting the shoes may be predisposing factors. In the hindlimb, tendon injuries are usually traumatic. Suspensory desmitis occurs more frequently in forelimbs than hindlimbs, probably because of the heavy front conformation. Suspensory branch injuries are most common.

Finnhorses cope better with chronic suspensory desmitis than do STBs because of the lower racing speeds, longer rest periods, ability of the horses to race at an older age, and thus better opportunities to heal. Suspensory desmitis is sometimes associated with splint bone fractures or exostoses.

Treatment of Finnhorses with SDF tendonitis and suspensory desmitis is most often conservative, with long rest

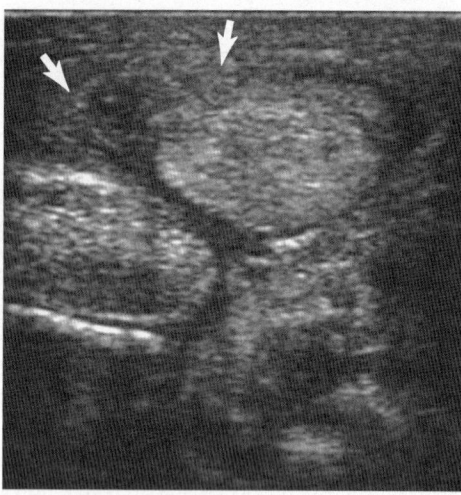

Fig. 113-3 • Transverse ultrasonographic image of the plantar distal aspect of the hock. Medial is to the left. There is extensive subcutaneous heterogeneous echogenic material *(arrows)* plantar to the superficial digital flexor tendon in a horse with curb.

periods. Tendon splitting or desmotomy of the accessory ligament of the SDF tendon (SDFT) sometimes is used for tendonitis. Hot firing has been a traditional treatment for Finnhorses with tendonitis and desmitis for many decades, and some veterinarians still use it in some horses, though with mixed success. Stem cell treatments are used as in other breeds.

Curbs (soft tissue enlargement in the plantar tarsal and proximal plantar metatarsal regions) often are seen in young horses (3 to 5 years old) in early training, especially those with sickle hocks (see Chapter 78). Curbs seldom cause spontaneous lameness. Usually the signs show first at higher speeds, when the cranial phase of the stride in the affected limb is shortened, and the horse begins to drag the limb. Ultrasonographically, peritendonous and peri-ligamentous inflammation is the most common finding (Figure 113-3). Injuries of the SDFT or the DDFT are rarely seen. Most veterinarians treat horses with curbs symptomatically, without ultrasonographic examination to determine the structure involved. Treatments include rest, corticosteroid or dimethyl sulfoxide injections, or pin firing. Cryotherapy is not used as widely as pin firing. The prognosis with all treatments is very good.

Ossification of the cartilages of the foot (sidebones) is a common finding in the front feet of heavy horses, occurring in 80% of Finnhorses. The condition is more common in females than in males and positively correlates with the size of the horse. The grade of the ossification is usually mild, but extensive ossification sometimes occurs. The cause is unclear, but a heritable component exists. In a recent study evaluating ossification of the cartilages of the foot in 964 Finnhorses, females had more ossification than males, and this difference increased with age.[1] The ossification in the medial cartilages progressed significantly with age in females but not in males, and in lateral cartilages the increase in ossification with age was evident in both sexes.[1] Estimates of heritability for the ossification parameters varied slightly between the cartilages as well as between the front feet.[1] For total ossification, the estimates of heritability varied from 0.31 (right lateral) to 0.50 (left

medial) and were slightly higher for ossification at the base of the cartilages.[1] High genetic correlations were found for total ossification between the medial and lateral cartilages in the foot and for parallel ossification parameters between the right and left feet.[1] The authors concluded that the estimates of heritability were relatively high, and both cartilages and front feet have a similar genetic tendency to ossify.[1] The cartilages start ossifying at an early age, unassociated with training of the horse. Other contributory factors may include hoof conformation, shoeing, and concussion.

The clinical relevance of sidebones is questionable. Most horses with mild or moderate ossification show no clinical signs. Ossification is detected only by radiology. With extensive ossification the cartilages are palpable proximal to the coronary band. Palpation does not induce pain. In general, horses with large sidebones show some clinical signs, especially on hard ground. Lameness at slow speeds is rare, but at high speeds with increased concussion the forelimb stride is shortened and the horse breaks to pace or gallop. In a study of 21 Finnhorses with ossification of the cartilages of the front feet, there was no significant relationship between height of the ossifications measured radiologically and increased radiopharmaceutical uptake (IRU) in the cartilages of the foot. Separate centers of ossification were not associated with IRU.[2] Intense IRU was seen unilaterally in four horses, medially in one horse, and laterally in three. In two of these horses a unilateral palmar digital nerve block relieved the mild lameness.[2] In the other two horses no obvious lameness was seen, but both had a history of being stiff or having locomotion problems during high-speed trot.[2] In two horses with IRU in the lateral cartilage of the foot, an incomplete fusion line was found radiologically between a large separate center of ossification and the base. The third horse had extensive ossification with bony protrusions, suggestive of chronic enthesopathy in a narrow foot.[2] In all cartilages of the foot with intense IRU and/or lameness, the ossified part of the cartilage was wider and more irregular compared with other ossifications.[2] The authors concluded that IRU and a different radiological appearance of affected cartilages from that of unaffected cartilages within the same horse were definite signs of clinical relevance. Obscure locomotion problems were more commonly associated with ossification of the cartilages than true lameness.[2]

The diagnosis is confirmed radiologically, using dorso-palmar images. Osteoarthritis of the distal interphalangeal joint and navicular disease may cause similar clinical signs and may be present concurrently with sidebones.

The treatment options are limited, because the condition persists. Shoeing with egg bar shoes, often combined with thick pads, is helpful in some horses. Most horses with sidebones can race with moderate-to-good success when shod properly and raced only on good surfaces. Because of the hereditary background, all Finnhorse stallions that are used for public breeding have to be free of sidebones, radiologically, before being accepted.

Splints are fairly common in the forelimbs of young, growing horses, and affected horses are usually treated conservatively with rest. Most splints resolve spontaneously, but local corticosteroid injections or cryotherapy sometimes is used. Interference injury may result in a

References
on page
1344

flake of bone detached from the McII. These fragments do not heal with rest and horses respond poorly to corticosteroid injections or cryotherapy. Surgical removal is usually necessary.

Chronic tenosynovitis of the digital flexor tendon sheath (DFTS) is a common cause of lameness in aged cold-blooded trotters and usually develops gradually, with mild or moderate swelling and no lameness for long periods. In time the DFTS becomes fibrotic, and masses and adhesions develop. At this stage constriction by the palmar annular ligament (PAL) may occur. Many horses can perform well despite chronic tenosynovitis, especially in hindlimbs. Intrathecal administration of hyaluronan, with or without corticosteroids, is used for horses with acute tenosynovitis. Frequent corticosteroid injections often seem to increase tenosynovial masses. Physiotherapy and especially shock-wave therapy are often beneficial in treating Finnhorses with chronic tenosynovitis, not only for controlling pain but also for helping to keep the DFTS as elastic as possible. Tenoscopy and transection of the PAL is used if the condition is advanced. Cold-blooded horses with chronic tenosynovitis seem to respond more poorly to treatment than do STBs with similar lesions. This may be because Finnhorses are often older and of greater weight.

In young Finnhorses, bilateral hindlimb fetlock pain is fairly common and causes a short and stiff hindlimb stride when they start to trot, which improves with exercise early in the condition. When both hind fetlocks are blocked simultaneously, the action changes completely. Pain is considered to be associated with subchondral bone remodeling of the distal aspect of the MtIII. A variety of treatments have been used, including shockwave therapy, joint lavage, and intraarticular treatment with PSGAGs, hyaluronan, or corticosteroids, often combined with parenteral administration of NSAIDs. In some Finnhorses IV tiludronate infusion is more beneficial than intraarticular treatments. If lameness is severe, surgical drilling of the subchondral bone is performed. Horses remain lame for several months, but the long-term prognosis is reasonable.

Osteochondrosis is rare in Finnhorses, but when it does occur, osteochondrosis most often is seen in the cranial aspect of the intermediate ridge of the tibia and causes effusion of the tarsocrural joint. Treatment is removal of the fragment(s) by arthroscopy. The femoropatellar joint is another typical predilection site for osteochondrosis in Finnhorses, and osteochondrosis of this joint causes clinical signs in young horses. Finnhorses with large defects of the lateral trochlear ridge of the femur have a guarded or poor prognosis.

SECTION 3
Nonracing Sports Horses

Chapter 114

Prepurchase Examination of the Performance Horse

Richard D. Mitchell and Sue J. Dyson

The purchase or prepurchase examination is a much discussed and sometimes feared subject for equine practitioners. Careless conduct and poor documentation can leave veterinarians wishing they had not agreed to perform the examination, whereas forethought and good planning can lead to a rewarding experience for the practitioner and the client. In the United States the examination is referred to as the *purchase examination,* because in many cases the deal already has been completed, whereas in Europe the examination usually is referred to as the *prepurchase examination,* because generally the purchaser has agreed to buy the horse subject to a satisfactory veterinary examination. In some countries (e.g., Holland), where many horses are sold through professional dealers, a horse may be purchased by the dealer and then examined by a veterinarian on behalf of the dealer before resale within a few days. In Europe young competition horses may be sold at auction and are subjected to a prepurchase examination before the sale.

The terms of sale usually permit a purchaser to have an additional independent examination performed within a predetermined time after the sale.

GOALS OF THE EXAMINATION

When requested to evaluate a horse for purchase, the veterinarian should keep several goals in mind. First, the examination should be an objective assessment of the horse's physical condition. Second, the examination should be a fact-finding mission to aid the purchaser in his or her decision to make a purchase. This may involve the veterinarian in making some predictions based on experience and probability, but care must be taken to be factual and objective. Last, the examination can serve as a formal introduction to a horse for which the practitioner may provide long-term care. Such relationships may affect the veterinarian's decision-making process relative to a client's needs.

It is helpful to have knowledge of the disciplines for which the horse has been and is to be used. Various equine sports place differing demands on the horse, and the clinician should be aware of sometimes subtle, yet important, differences. Some physical characteristics or conditions may be acceptable for certain levels of performance but not acceptable for others. For example, a previous strain of a superficial digital flexor tendon (SDFT) may be an acceptable risk for a show hunter but may carry a high risk for an event horse. Veterinarians should avoid performing prepurchase examinations on horses that will be involved in disciplines with which they are not familiar.

The veterinarian needs to discuss the goals of the examination and horse ownership with the prospective purchaser. Understanding the client, the trainer, and what is expected of the horse will help the veterinarian in assessing the horse's potential suitability. Passing or failing the horse is not the veterinarian's job, but it is his or her role to advise on how existing conditions may affect the future use of the horse. It is therefore self-evident that prepurchase examinations should not be performed by recent graduates, who may be fully competent in performing clinical examinations but generally do not have the experience of how to interpret the findings of the examinations and are not in a position to evaluate risk. The prospective purchaser requires advice about the risks of proceeding with the purchase. Prior knowledge of clients, their expectations of the horse, and their attitude toward risk make offering such advice easier, compared with clients about whom clinicians know little.

A veterinarian must be open-minded and should consider himself or herself to be a facilitator for the sales contract: the vendor wishes to sell the horse, the purchaser may have searched for a long time to find a suitable horse, and the veterinarian's role is to enable the transaction to take place if such is reasonable. Nonetheless, the veterinarian must be streetwise and recognize that a minority of unscrupulous vendors may try to misrepresent a horse. *Caveat emptor.* Veterinarians also should be aware that prospective purchasers often are keen to buy horses and in their enthusiasm may wish to overlook any problems that are identified during the examination. A veterinarian who believes that the risks of buying a horse are too high is responsible for trying to dissuade the purchaser from proceeding further. If the purchaser ignores the advice, it is essential that the veterinarian documents adequately his or her observations and advice. Purchasers can have remarkably selective memories when things start to go wrong.

The scope of the examination can range from a comprehensive clinical examination of the horse, using basic powers of observation, to a complex investigation using advanced techniques such as radiography, ultrasonography, endoscopy, thermography, scintigraphy, and magnetic resonance imaging (MRI). The wishes of the buyer are important in determining the extent and depth of the examination, which also must be dictated to some extent by the value of the horse and its future athletic expectations. Some consideration to cost should be given, but not at the cost of the quality of the examination. The veterinarian should allow some latitude for deciding what is needed to answer questions posed by the clinical examination.

CONTRACT

A veterinarian enters a business arrangement with a purchaser when he or she agrees to perform a prepurchase examination. It is imperative for the veterinarian to understand the buyer's intentions for the horse and the expectations of the proposed examination. The terms, details, and costs of the examination should be discussed at the time of the initial request. The extent and depth of the examination and its limitations should be emphasized.

This is straightforward when the veterinarian is dealing directly with the purchaser, assuming that the purchaser has knowledge of horses. The terms of agreement become more difficult when a veterinarian is speaking to an agent for the potential owner or to the prospective rider of the horse, when the actual purchaser has no knowledge of horses. Such persons may have expectations of the horse as if it were a mechanical object like a car.

Purchaser's Reservations
The veterinarian is responsible for the following:
1. Establishing whether the purchaser has any reservations about the horse.
2. Determining whether the horse has been in regular work until the examination.
3. Warning the client of the hazards of performing an examination on a horse that has not been in regular work; previous lameness or back problems may be inapparent until the horse is in regular work. It may be helpful to suggest that the purchaser check the horse's official competition record to determine whether any unexpected breaks from competition have occurred.

Purchase for Resale
If the horse is to be purchased for resale, this should be noted. The purchaser should be warned that the clinician's interpretation of the findings may not be identical to that of another veterinary surgeon. The examining veterinarian may regard the horse as a reasonable risk for purchase, but this is not a guarantee that others have the same opinion. All observations should be well documented so that comparisons can be made should questions arise at a subsequent resale examination. Such notes may well help save a sale in the future and save face for the initial veterinarian.

Insuring the Horse
It is important to establish if the horse will be insured for loss of use for a specific athletic activity or for veterinary fees. The purchaser should be advised that the examining veterinarian may consider the horse a reasonable risk for purchase but that does not necessarily equate with the horse being a normal insurance risk. The veterinarian may consider that a small, well-rounded osseous opacity on the dorsal aspect of the distal interphalangeal joint is unlikely to be of clinical significance, but for an insurance company to place an exclusion on problems related to the joint would not be unreasonable. The veterinarian should advise the purchaser that if such problems arise, the purchaser should communicate with the insurance company before completing the purchase transaction.

Blood Tests and Limitations
The client should be informed clearly that the results presented are good for the day of examination, but predictions about future soundness and suitability are impossible. The limitations of analysis of blood for drugs must be detailed, bearing in mind the difficulties of detection of many drugs administered by the intraarticular route. The client should be warned that several days may elapse before the results of blood tests are known and that the purchase transaction should not be completed until the results are known. The

veterinarian should discuss with the client how the findings will be transmitted and what kind of report will be issued.

Conflicts of Interest

Any potential conflicts of interest for the veterinarian must be disclosed to the buyer. Previous dealings with the vendor, although the vendor may not be a current client, could be perceived as a conflict of interest. In the horse world today, not to have such conflicts arise is difficult, but such conflicts should be acknowledged, and the buyer should be given the option of having someone else perform the examination.

COMMUNICATION WITH THE VENDOR

The vendor must understand clearly what facilities are required for the examination and should be advised that the horse should be stabled before the examination and not worked earlier in the day. If the vendor is unable to be present at the examination, the veterinarian should establish the answers to a number of important questions in advance:

1. How long has the horse been in the owner's possession?
2. Is the horse in regular work?
3. Has the horse had any previous lameness?
4. Has the horse had any previous medical problem?
5. Is the horse receiving any medication, or has it done so in the last 8 weeks?
6. Does the horse have any vices (crib-biting, wind sucking, box walking), or does it bite or kick?
7. Has the horse been seen to shake its head?
8. Has the horse had previous surgery?
9. Does the horse normally live in or out?
10. Does the horse have dry or soaked hay or a haylage preparation?
11. When was the horse last trimmed or shod?

Ideally vendors should sign a copy of their responses to these questions (Figure 114-1).

When the examination actually is performed, ideally all involved parties or their agents should be present. This provides an environment in which the veterinarian can ask pertinent questions of the buyer and seller regarding the horse's history and future use and can assure the buyer that a complete examination has been performed. Problems that arise during the examination can be discussed with the purchaser.

The veterinarian should not compromise the standard of the examination because of physical conditions. If modifying the procedure of the usual examination technique is necessary, such should be noted in the subsequent report, and the purchaser should be advised accordingly. The limitations of the conclusions drawn from the examination should be documented. If an uncooperative vendor or agent makes conducting the usual examination difficult, the veterinarian may choose not to continue the examination to protect the interests of the buyer and personal interests.

EXAMINATION AT A DISTANCE

A client may request the veterinarian to examine a valuable competition horse that is a long distance away or possibly in a foreign country. A number of alternative strategies can be applied. It may be prudent to first have the horse undergo radiographic examination and proceed with visiting the horse only if these radiographs are considered acceptable. The veterinarian is of course relying on the honesty of everyone concerned that the radiographic images provided are current images of the horse in question. It is critical that the veterinarian provide clear guidelines of the views required and be prepared not to compromise on quality. Alternatively, the veterinarian can travel and examine the horse and be present for the radiographic assessment. However, this may mean that the clinical examination is compromised by inadequate riding facilities at a veterinary clinic or that substantial time is spent traveling between the site where the horse is examined and the veterinary clinic where ancillary tests are performed. However, clinic facilities may be required anyway for additional examinations such as ultrasonography or endoscopy.

A client may inform the veterinarian of an intended purchase of a horse from a foreign country and that it has been recommended that he or she employ a specific clinician from that country to carry out the prepurchase examination. The client should be warned that the method of carrying out and reporting the examination may differ from what he or she is used to seeing and may have limitations of which he or she is unaware. For example, in some countries in Europe the examination is much more limited and does not encompass assessment of conformation. It is not usual practice to examine the horse being ridden. It is worthwhile developing a group of professional colleagues whose clinical expertise and trustworthiness the veterinarian respects, one of whom can be recommended to the purchaser. The veterinary surgeon performing the examination should be requested to communicate with the client's own veterinarian and to send radiographs for assessment. Discussion between two colleagues—one who has examined the horse and the other who knows the client—can result in a highly satisfactory outcome.

CLINICAL EXAMINATION AT REST

Various national bodies have established guidelines for the way in which a prepurchase examination should be carried out and reported, to which the veterinarian obviously should adhere. The legal responsibilities for the veterinary surgeon and the vendor may vary in different countries. For example, in Holland the expectations of the veterinary examination performed on behalf of an amateur purchaser are higher than for a professional purchaser. In Denmark, if clinically significant radiological abnormalities that obviously predate the purchase are discovered soon after purchase, the vendor is liable.

The clinical examination should evaluate all organ systems as comprehensively as possible. The examination should be methodical and repeatable. Using a checklist may help. The principal aims of this chapter are to focus on the examination of the musculoskeletal and neurological systems[1,2] and to discuss the interpretation of abnormal findings.

The veterinarian should identify the horse, including name, breed, sex, age, markings, tattoos, freeze marks, brands, and height. In Europe a freeze brand L signifies that

References on page 1344

Text continued on p. 1088

BEVA Prepurchase Examination Worksheet

Purchaser's name and address   ....

....

Telephone no.   ....

Agent's name and address   ....

....

Telephone no.   ....

Vendor's name and address   ....

....

Telephone no.   ....

Intended use of horse   .... Stated age .... Stated height ....
Purchaser's reservations   ....

Is horse to be insured?   ☐ YES *Permanent incapacity/All risks of mortality* ☐ NO

Name   .... Breed   ....

Sex   ☐ *Gelding*   ☐ *Mare*   ☐ *Entire*

Colour   ....

Size   .... *Estimate app./Measurement/By documentation*

Duration of current ownership?   ....

In current work?   ☐ YES   ☐ NO   ....

Was horse stabled prior to examination?   ☐ YES   ☐ NO   ....

Receiving medication or received medication in last 4 weeks?

☐ YES   ☐ NO   ....

Previous lameness?   ☐ YES   ☐ NO   ....

Previous medical problems?   ☐ YES   ☐ NO   ....

Previous surgery?   ☐ YES   ☐ NO   ....

Vices?   ☐ YES   ☐ NO   ☐ *Cribbing*   ☐ *Windsucking*   ☐ *Weaving* ....

Behavioural abnormalities?   ☐ *Head shaking*   ☐ *Box walking*   ☐ *Biting*   ☐ *Other*   ....

Bedding?   ☐ *Straw*   ☐ *Shavings*   ☐ *Paper*   ☐ *Other*   ☐ *Lives out*   ....

Food?   ☐ *Dry hay*   ☐ *Soaked hay*   ☐ *Haylage/silage* ....

Husbandry?   ☐ *Stabled*   ☐ *At grass*   ☐ *In & out*   ....

When was horse last shod?   ....

Vendor's declaration: To the best of my knowledge the answers to the above questions are correct.

Signature of vendor/vendor's agent: ....

Fig. 114-1 • British Equine Veterinary Association prepurchase examination worksheet. *D*, Dorsal; *Di*, distal; *L*, lateral; *LF*, left forelimb; *LH*, left hindlimb; *M*, medial; *O*, oblique; *P*, proximal; *Pa*, palmar; *Pl*, plantar; *RF*, right forelimb; *RH*, right hindlimb; *URT*, upper respiratory tract. (Courtesy British Equine Veterinary Association.)   *Continued*

Examined at ....

....

On ....

At ....AM/PM

Present ....

....

....

....

Weather ....

....

....

....

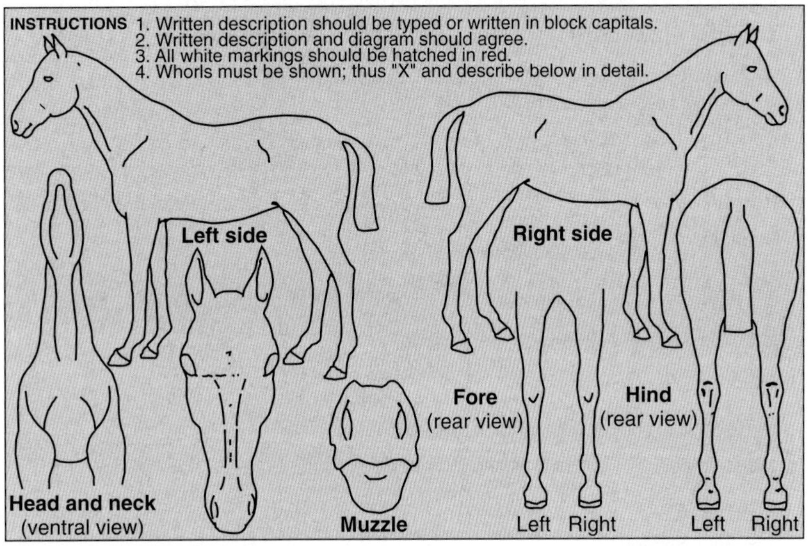

Identification

Head ....

....

Neck ....

....

Limbs: LF ....

RF ....

LH ....

RH ....

Body ....

....

Acquired marks/Brands/Freeze brands ref loss of use ....

Microchip scanned ☐   Not scanned ☐   Present? Yes/No   No. ....

Stage 1–Preliminary Examination (tick if normal/note abnormalities)

Bodily condition: Overweight ☐   Good ☐   Lean ☐   Poor ☐

Stance, attitude, and demeanour ....

Head   Ears ....

Eyes (including ophthalmoscopic examination) ....

Nose ....

Gums ....

Mandible ....

Other ....

Age and teeth   Wolf teeth   Yes/No   Location ....

Incisor	Permanent	Infundibulum	Dental Star	Enamel Spot	Shape
1					
2					
3					

Fig. 114-1 • cont'd

Hook incisor 3–Left .... Hook incisor 3–Right ....

Galvayne's groove Left.. Galvayne's groove Right ....

Angle ....

Abnormal wear ....

Molars ....

Approximate age .... Range .... Documented age ....

Integument

Surgical scar   Laryngoplasty ☐   Ventriculectomy ☐   Laparotomy ☐   Medial patellar desmotomy ☐   Neurectomy ☐

                Other   ☐

Other acquired scars ....

Sarcoids   Yes/No (note location) ....

Melanomata   Yes/No (note location) ....

Other ....

Faeces, urination ....

Respiratory system   Spontaneous cough   Yes/No   Cough reflex   Yes/No

                            Auscultation of thorax ....

Cardiovascular system ....

Urogenital system ....

Nervous system ....

Conformation

LF ....

RF ....

LH ....

RH ....

Body ....

Hindquarters

       Symmetrically muscled Yes/No   Tubera sacrale symmetrical   Yes/No

Musculoskeletal system

LF ....

RF ....

LH ....

RH ....

Back ....

Bulb of heel sensation ....

Feet   Horn quality   Good ☐   Poor   ☐

        Foot pastern axis   Straight ☐   Broken back ☐   Broken forward   ☐

        Hoof testers ....

        Trimming & shoeing ....

        Symmetry ....

Fig. 114-1 • cont'd

Stage 2–Trotting up (tick if normal/note abnormalities)

Walk ....

Trot ....

Circle ....

Reverse ....

Flexion test   Yes/No

LF   ☐ –   ☐ + ...

RF   ☐ –   ☐ + ...

LH   ☐ –   ☐ + ...

RH   ☐ –   ☐ + ...

Lunged on soft   Yes/No   Left rein ....

Right rein ....

Lunged on hard   Yes/No   Left rein ....

Right rein ....

Stage 3–Strenuous Exercise (tick if normal/note abnormalities)

Ridden/lunged   Inside/outside   State going ....

Trot ....

Canter ....

Gallop ....

Respiratory noise   No/Yes   < Inspiratory   Nasal discharge   Yes/No

Expiratory   Cough   Yes/No

Auscultation ....

Recovery ....

Stage 4–Rest

Observations ....

Crib biting   Yes/No

Stage 5–Second Trot and Foot Examination (tick if normal/note abnormalities)

Walk ....

Trot ....

Circle ....

Reverse ....

Flexion test   Yes/No   Lunged on firm surface   Yes/No

LF ....

RF ....

LH ....

RH ....

Shoes removed   Yes/No

Fig. 114-1 • cont'd

General observations ....

Blood collected   Yes/No   Analysed/stored

☐ NSAID only   ☐ Full screen   ☐ Health profile

Specialised Techniques
Radiography

Area Examined	**Views (circle which used)**	**Comments**
LF Foot	LM, DPr-PaDiO, PaPr-PaDiO	....
RF Foot	LM, DPr-PaDiO, PaPr-PaDiO	....
L Mc/P Joint	LM, DL-PaMO, DM-PaLO, DPa	....
R Mc/P Joint	LM, DL-PaMO, DM-PaLO, DPa	....
L Carpus	LM, DL-PaMO, DM-PaLO, DPa	
R Carpus	LM, DL-PaMO, DM-PaLO, DPa	....
L Hock	LM, DL-PIMO, PIL-DMO, DPL	....
R Hock	LM, DL-PIMO, PIL-DMO, DPL	
Other		....

Ultrasonography

Yes/No   Area examined & comments ....
....

Endoscopic examination of URT   ☐ Yes   ☐ No ....
....

Other special techniques
....
....

Signed .... Date .... Time ....

Record of discussion   ☐ In person   ☐ Telephone   Date .... Time ....
....
....
....

Suitable for purchase   ☐ Yes   ☐ No   ☐ Deferred: reason ....
Certificate issued (Date)   ....
Signed   ....

Fig. 114-1 • cont'd

the horse has previously been a loss of use insurance case. The horse's identity should be compared with its passport or vaccination certificate.

The horse first should be examined in the stable, with assessment of demeanor, attitude, stance, and conformation and thorough observation and palpation of the head, neck, back, and limbs as described in Chapters 4 to 6. Collection of blood samples may be performed at this stage or when the examination is completed and the veterinarian deems that purchase will probably be recommended. More

comprehensive evaluation of the feet, overall conformation, and evaluation of muscle symmetry is best performed outside, where the horse can be viewed better from all angles.

If the horse will be used for show purposes, in which the cosmetic appearance of the horse is important, the veterinarian should draw the purchaser's attention to all possible abnormalities, such as a prominent base (head) of the fourth metatarsal bone that a lay judge may misconstrue as a curb. If the purchaser has expressed reservations about a swelling such as a splint, the veterinarian should be sure to document its size and possible importance. If the purchaser is concerned about the horse's hock conformation, recommending radiographic examination of the hocks is worthwhile, even if the veterinarian considers the conformation to be acceptable and the horse appears sound.

Conformation

Although assessment of conformation as far as it may influence future lameness is considered an important part of the examination in the United States and United Kingdom, this is not usual practice, and in Holland, for example, is not included. It is important to recognize that breed differences in conformation exist and that what might be acceptable in one breed does not necessarily apply to others. The relevance of conformational abnormalities in part is dictated by the discipline in which the horse is involved.[1]

Most Arabian horses have a short-coupled and slightly lordotic back; thus they are likely to have some degree of impingement of dorsal spinous processes. This is unlikely to compromise the horse's show performance. However, a dressage horse with a short back may well develop a clinical problem associated with impinging dorsal spinous processes when working at an advanced level. In such a horse the flexibility of the back at rest and when the horse is moving in hand and ridden must be assessed with great care, paying great attention to the freedom and elasticity of the gaits. Even if the horse is currently free of clinical signs, the purchaser should be advised that problems may occur in the future.

Young Warmblood breeds have a relatively high propensity for intermittent upward fixation or delayed release of the patella, especially those with a straight hindlimb conformation. Although the condition may be manageable in some, in others it can become a chronic problem, albeit a subtle one, resulting in low-grade discomfort and unwillingness to work. The veterinarian should observe the horse carefully as it moves over in the stable, to assess smooth or jerky movement of the patella on the left and right sides, and should check carefully for a surgical scar and the size of the medial patellar ligament, which if enlarged is likely to reflect a previous desmotomy or desmoplasty.

Very straight conformation of the hocks and abnormal extension of the hind fetlock joints are predisposing factors for and may be indicative of proximal suspensory desmitis and suspensory branch injury. The client should be advised of the potential importance of such findings and asked whether he or she wishes the examination to be continued. It may be preferable that the examination be terminated at this stage rather than the veterinarian running up a large bill and antagonizing the vendor by wasting more time.

The clinician should pay particular attention to the conformation of the feet and relate this to the type of ground surface on which the horse will have to work. A horse with flat feet and thin soles is not a good candidate for endurance riding. A horse with crumbly hoof walls is predisposed to losing shoes, and this can be disastrous for Three Day Event horses. Although changing the horse's nutrition and foot management may result in some improvement, accurate prediction of the degree of improvement that may be achieved is difficult. Sheared heels and

underrun heels in the forelimbs or hindlimbs may be primary problems or predispose horses to altered ways of moving, causing soreness in the more proximal parts of the limbs. These findings are particularly important in jumping and dressage horses and those used for cutting and reining.

The veterinarian should assess the forelimb conformation carefully from the front and ensure that the foot is positioned symmetrically under the central limb axis of the more proximal parts of the limb. A disproportionately high incidence of distal limb joint problems occurs in horses in which the pastern and foot are set more to the outside, with a tendency for the medial wall to become more upright and the lateral wall to be flared (Figure 114-2).

Many Warmblood breeds naturally have much narrower and upright foot conformation than other breeds. This predisposes the horses to develop thrush, and careful stable hygiene and foot cleanliness are necessary to control this problem. Asymmetry of front foot shape and size always should be documented and may reflect previous lameness in the limb with the more contracted foot, but it also may reflect development of a mild flexural deformity of the distal interphalangeal joint when the horse was a foal, which may be of no long-term relevance. The veterinarian should beware if the feet are long and misshapen; this finding may mask underlying conformational problems or asymmetry in foot shape and size. Postponing

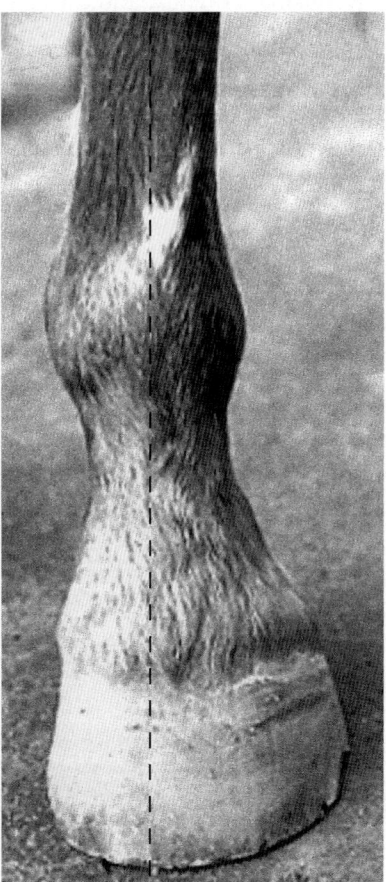

Fig. 114-2 • Dorsal view of a forelimb with clinically significant conformational abnormalities. Medial is to the left. Note the position of the foot and pastern relative to the central axis of the metacarpal region *(dotted line)*. The hoof capsule is distorted, and the foot shape is asymmetrical.

further assessment of the horse until the feet have been trimmed and shod properly may be preferable.

Some conformational abnormalities, such as over at the knee, do not appear to influence a horse's future soundness greatly but must be described. Failure to document observations leaves the veterinarian open to litigation if future problems arise.

Muscle Symmetry

Muscle asymmetry of the hindquarters may reflect previous or current hindlimb lameness, although it is not necessarily associated with future chronic lameness. Muscle asymmetry should alert the veterinarian to pay particular attention to the hindlimb gait in hand, on the lunge, and ridden and to the response to flexion tests. Asymmetry is an indication for flexion tests before and after ridden exercise. The potential clinical significance of muscle asymmetry must be discussed with the purchaser. Slight asymmetry of the tubera sacrale is a common finding and frequently is not of clinical significance. Nonetheless, the purchaser should be informed of its potential clinical significance.

Tendons and Ligaments

Particular attention should be paid to the size, shape, and stiffness of the tendonous and ligamentous structures of the metacarpal and pastern regions, bearing in mind that if the horse has sustained a bilateral tendon injury, both tendons may be enlarged slightly, and the clue to previous damage may be rounding of the margins of the tendons or abnormal stiffness. The clinical significance of a previous injury to the SDFT or suspensory ligament must be assessed in light of the horse's previous and future career. These injuries carry a high risk of recurrence in racehorses, event horses, high-level show jumpers, and endurance horses. However, the horse may perform satisfactorily as a hunter, a dressage horse, or a pleasure horse or at a low level in more demanding sports. The purchaser should be advised that further information about the repair of the injury may be obtained by ultrasonographic examination. Further information about when the injury was sustained and what the horse has done since then may be helpful. Decision making must be based on the athletic expectations of the horse, all other aspects of the horse's suitability, and whether the horse is being bought for resale. If the horse is a perfect schoolmaster for a junior rider and the price is reasonable, the risk/benefit ratio may be acceptable.

Assessment of Joints

Many horses have mild fetlock joint capsule distention or thickening. The relevance of distention must be assessed based on the environmental temperature: if it is cold, joint capsules are more likely to be tight than if it is warm. Asymmetry between left and right is of greater clinical significance than bilateral symmetry. The joints should be assessed carefully for any evidence of restricted range of motion or pain on manipulation. The range of motion varies among horses and is in part a reflection of age and work history, but asymmetry between left and right should be viewed with caution. The response to distal limb flexion and the horse's action on the lunge on a hard surface must be assessed carefully. Distention of the antebrachiocarpal or middle carpal joint capsules is rarely an insignificant

finding and even if unassociated with detectable lameness should prompt radiographic examination.

During hindlimb assessment, care should be taken to differentiate between pain on flexion of the proximal limb joints and reluctance to stand on the contralateral hindlimb, perhaps associated with sacroiliac pain. Abnormal limb flexion may be present if the horse is a shiverer. A high incidence of this condition occurs among high-performance Warmblood breeds, and it does not appear to compromise performance. However, an intending purchaser must be warned that the condition may be progressive and may make the horse difficult to trim and shoe.

Flexibility of the neck and back should be assessed, and the presence of any abnormal muscle tension or abnormal reaction to palpation of acupuncture trigger points should be noted. The veterinarian also should pay attention to the presence of sarcoids in a position where they may be abraded by tack. If a sarcoid is identified, the client always must be warned that such lesions may increase in number, but assuming that the client is aware of the risks, a small number of lesions at sites removed from the tack should not mitigate against purchase. The mouth should be examined carefully. Large hooks on the rostral aspect of the first upper cheek teeth are usually an indicator that large hooks also may be present on the caudal aspect of the lower caudal cheek teeth, which may be difficult to manage.

Sensation in the heel region of the forelimbs and the reaction to vigorous application of hoof testers should be assessed carefully to determine if a previous neurectomy may have been performed. The absence of a visible or palpable scar does not preclude previous surgery.

ASSESSMENT OF GAIT

The horse should be examined moving freely at a walk and trot on a firm surface, with particular attention directed to the stride length and lift to the stride relative to the horse's type. The veterinarian should bear in mind that a horse with a bilateral forelimb or hindlimb lameness may not appear overtly lame, but merely may have a slightly restricted gait. The veterinarian should beware of the situation encountered particularly in a professional's yard when the horse is encouraged by an assistant to trot excessively quickly, is unduly restrained, or is excessively fresh and trots crookedly. The horse must trot in a regular, relaxed rhythm with freedom of the head and neck; otherwise, lameness may be missed. The veterinarian should pay particular attention to how easily the horse turns when changing direction and the flexibility of the neck and back. If the horse trots in a particularly loose and extravagant way, the veterinarian should bear in mind that the horse may be mildly ataxic. Ataxia may not jeopardize a dressage horse when competing at lower levels, but when finer degrees of muscular strength and coordination are required in advanced dressage, performance may be compromised. The safety of a mildly ataxic horse jumping must be questioned. The veterinarian should watch the horse carefully as it decelerates, when signs of mild ataxia or jerky movement of the patella associated with its delayed release may be apparent. Watch the horse turning in small circles and moving backward, assessing flexibility of the neck and back, limb coordination and placement, and any quivering movement of the tail suggestive of shivering.

Flexion Tests

The interpretation of flexion and extension tests is controversial.[3,4] The force applied, the duration of flexion, the way in which the joints are flexed, and the work history of the horse may all influence the response. Positive results of flexion tests in a horse that does not demonstrate lameness before flexion may not be a cause for termination of the examination, unless other suspicious clinical signs have been identified already. The horse should be evaluated on the lunge and ridden for evidence of lameness. Many positive results on flexion tests are found to change during the course of the exercise examination (perhaps as the horse warms up or loosens up), and these may not have clinical significance. A difference in response between distal limb flexion of the left and right forelimbs may be more important than a symmetrical response. A positive response to carpal flexion or to proximal limb flexion of a hindlimb must be viewed with caution. Veterinarians should aim to perform flexion tests as consistently as possible so that they know the ranges of response anticipated in clinically normal horses.

Lunging and Ridden Exercise

The requirements for lunging and ridden or driven exercise vary among the guidelines for prepurchase examinations in different countries and also are dictated by the type of horse under examination. The methods used for a 3-year-old Thoroughbred racehorse differ from those for a 6-year-old destined for eventing. Seeing the horse lunged on soft and hard surfaces and ridden is helpful to gain maximum information about any potential lameness problems. The vendor should be encouraged to use any protective boots or bandages that might be used normally. Subtle lameness or restriction in gait because of thoracolumbar or sacroiliac discomfort may not be evident until the horse performs specific movements when it is ridden.[5,6] Small figure eights and upward and downward transitions may be particularly revealing. Watching the horse do what it specifically is intended to do is good practice. The veterinarian should watch the horse being tacked up and mounted to learn about any cold back behavior or evidence of back pain or other behavioral abnormalities. The horse should be worked reasonably hard relative to its fitness. In many European countries, evaluating a ridden horse is not standard practice, and if an examination is being performed on behalf of the client by a foreign veterinarian, the client should be advised accordingly.

Clinicians who have the prerequisite skill and experience may wish to evaluate horses further by riding or driving them themselves. Feeling the horse in this fashion may answer questions regarding a peculiar gait or way of going and may aid the evaluation of subtle lameness or respiratory noises. Such practice should be done with caution, because legal problems could arise from an unfortunate accident. A signed disclaimer may be helpful in this situation.

After strenuous exercise the horse should be allowed to stand for 15 to 20 minutes before being reevaluated in hand at the walk and the trot. This is a mandatory part of the examination in the United Kingdom but is not practiced widely in the rest of Europe. Previously inapparent lameness now may become evident. Any previously questionable response to flexion tests may be reassessed.

EVALUATION OF IDENTIFIED PROBLEMS

The veterinarian should now have gained enough information either to discontinue the examination after consultation with the purchaser or to make recommendations for further special examinations. If the horse is lame and a potential cause that may resolve is obvious (e.g., nail bind), reevaluating the horse on a subsequent occasion may be worthwhile, but the veterinarian should try to ensure that the horse has been worked properly for several days before the reexamination.

The veterinarian should always bear in mind that in a mature competition horse, it is relatively unusual not to identify some problems. Taking no risks and advising against purchasing the horse is easy, but that actually may be doing the purchaser, the vendor, and the veterinary profession a disservice. It is important to weigh the risks and describe them to the purchaser as objectively as possible, based on previous experience. At this point having in-depth knowledge of the purchaser, his or her aspirations for the horse, and the attitude to risk and financial ability to take the consequences of risk is most valuable. Further information obtained from radiographic and ultrasonographic examinations may help provide further objective information on which decisions can be based. Decisions also must be related to the horse's recent competition record, its age, and the future expectations for athletic performance. Low-grade hindlimb lameness associated with mild radiological changes of the distal hock joints might be an acceptable risk for a horse as a schoolmaster for a young rider, but similar abnormalities identified in a 6-year-old about to step up a level in competition must be regarded as potentially more serious. A veterinarian always must bear in mind that minor problems may become major problems with a change of rider, work pattern, and environment.

RECTAL EXAMINATION

Rectal examination is not a routine part of a prepurchase examination and should be performed only with the vendor's consent if indicated clinically or if a mare is to be used later for breeding or has a recent history of breeding.

RADIOGRAPHIC EXAMINATION

Radiographic examination is not a standard part of a prepurchase examination. The extent of routine radiographic examination in the United States and some European countries is probably higher than elsewhere. In Holland and Germany a strict grading system for evaluation of radiographs is used. The purchaser must be made aware that the presence of some radiological abnormalities is not necessarily synonymous with future lameness and the absence of radiological changes does not preclude future lameness.[7] If radiographs are to be obtained for a specific area, then a comprehensive set of radiographs should be ordered to avoid missing lesions apparent on only one images. In many European countries, obtaining only three images in evaluation of the hocks and omitting a dorsomedial-plantarolateral oblique image are common. This practice may risk the veterinarian missing lesions such

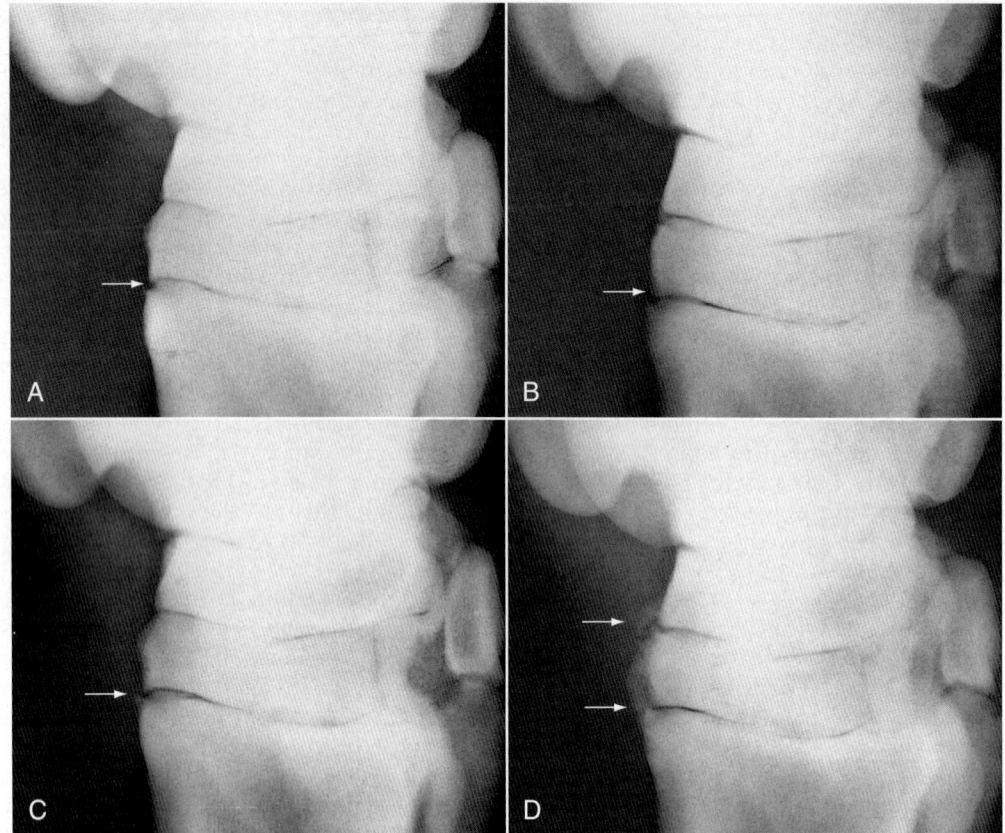

Fig. 114-3 • Dorsomedial-plantarolateral oblique radiographic images of the left **(A)** and right **(B)** hocks of a 9-year-old Grand Prix show jumper. There is a small osteophyte on the proximal aspect of the third metatarsal bone (MtIII) *(arrow)*, and subtle modeling of the articular margins of the centrodistal joint is present in each hock. The horse was clinically sound. **C** and **D,** The same horse 24 months later. At this stage the horse showed right hindlimb lameness that was alleviated by intraarticular analgesia of the tarsometatarsal joint. Considerable periarticular osteophyte formation (arrows in **D**) involves the centrodistal and tarsometatarsal joints of the right hock **(D).** The spur on the dorsoproximal aspect of the left MtIII was little changed *(arrow).*

as periarticular osteophytes, which are present only on the dorsolateral aspect of the joints (Figure 114-3).

The regions to be examined and the interpretation of findings are dictated by the previous and intended career of the horse and the results of the clinical examination. Examination of the front feet, fetlock, and hock joints is considered routine in many countries. Evaluation of the carpi, hind fetlock and pastern joints, stifles, and dorsal spinous processes of the thoracic region may be considered. It is, however, important not to overinterpret the clinical significance of some radiological abnormalities, bearing in mind the variability among breeds and the knowledge that even some obvious changes may be clinically insignificant. For example, Warmblood breeds have a tendency to have a greater number of radiolucent zones along the distal border of the navicular bone than do Thoroughbreds (Figure 114-4). A relatively high incidence of spur formation on the dorsoproximal aspect of the middle phalanx occurs in Warmbloods (Figure 114-5), but this rarely is associated with lameness. However, one of the authors (RDM) recognizes a higher incidence of clinically significant osteoarthritis (OA) of the proximal interphalangeal joint in Warmblood horses compared with other breeds.

Evidence of abnormal radiolucent zones in the proximal sesamoid bones (sesamoiditis) (Figure 114-6) should

alert the veterinarian to reevaluate the branches of the suspensory ligament. An ex-racehorse may have periosteal new bone on the dorsal aspect of one or more carpal bones, but this is unlikely to influence the horse's career as an event horse. A horse with a small osteochondral fragment on the dorsal aspect of the distal interphalangeal or metacarpophalangeal joint is often asymptomatic.

A small spur on the dorsoproximal aspect of the third metatarsal bone (MtIII) is a frequent incidental finding.[8] However, such findings also must be described to the purchaser, and the potential future clinical significance must be discussed. Small spurs on the dorsoproximal aspect of the MtIII do not necessarily reflect OA but may reflect entheseous new bone at the attachment of the fibularis (peroneus) tertius or cranialis tibialis. Despite the fact that these spurs are a common finding, accurately predicting the future behavior is impossible. Some spurs may reflect OA and may be progressive (see Figure 114-3). A 3-year-old that has done little work and has small osteochondral fragments at the cranial aspect of the intermediate ridge of the tibia may be asymptomatic, but if fragments became unstable with increased work, it might result in distention of the tarsocrural joint capsule, and surgical removal may be indicated. Such a finding in a mature competition horse is usually of no consequence. Complete fusion of the

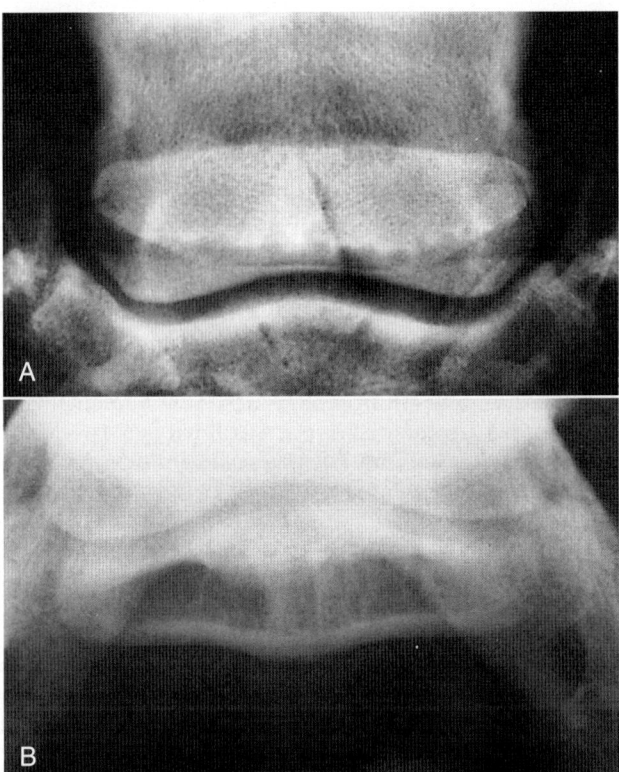

Fig. 114-4 • A, Dorsoproximal-palmarodistal oblique image of the right front foot of a clinically normal 6-year-old Dutch Warmblood horse with good foot conformation. Note the large size and number of the radiolucent zones along the distal border of the navicular bone. The horse competed successfully for many years with no evidence of foot pain. **B,** Palmaroproximal-palmarodistal oblique image of the same foot. Note the large, oval-shaped lucent zones in the medulla of the navicular bone.

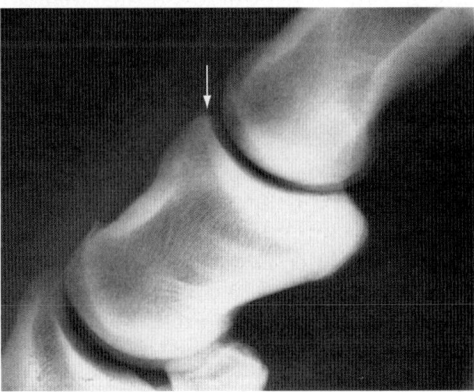

Fig. 114-5 • Lateromedial radiographic image of the left front pastern of a clinically normal 7-year-old Belgian Warmblood show jumper. Note the modeling of the dorsoproximal aspect of the middle phalanx *(arrow)*. Such spurs are a common finding in Warmblood breeds and usually are not associated with lameness.

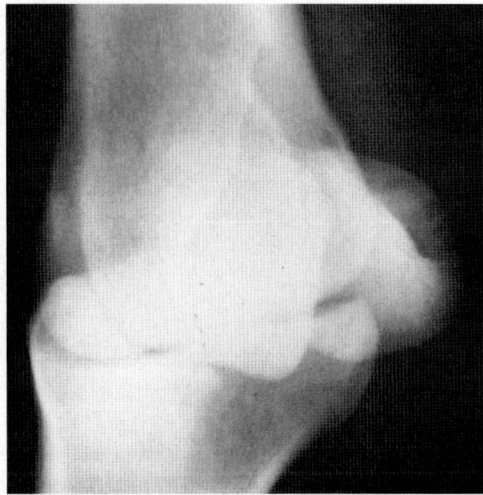

Fig. 114-6 • Dorsolateral-palmaromedial oblique image of a 6-year-old Thoroughbred that had raced previously on the flat and was used now for eventing. Note the large lucent zones in the lateral proximal sesamoid bone. The horse had no history of lameness.

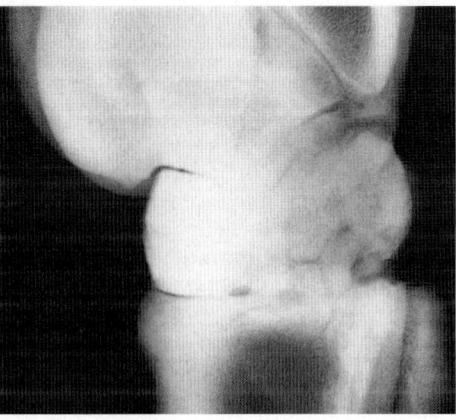

Fig. 114-7 • Lateromedial radiographic image of the left hock of a 9-year-old clinically normal Thoroughbred advanced event horse. The centrodistal joint is fused completely. The horse competed successfully for another 8 years before being retired because of a tendon injury.

centrodistal (distal intertarsal) joint may be identified unassociated with any other radiological change of the hock (Figure 114-7). Some horses may compete successfully with such changes for many years, but occasionally lameness subsequently develops because of pain associated with the talocalcaneal-centroquartal (proximal intertarsal) or tarsometatarsal joints. Well-rounded osseous opacities frequently are identified distal to a proximal sesamoid bone (Figure 114-8). These are often innocuous, but ultrasonographic evaluation of the distal sesamoidean ligaments may be indicated. Evidence of osteochondrosis of the trochleas of the femur is of concern in a 3-year-old, even if the horse is asymptomatic, whereas mild flattening of the lateral trochlear ridge of the femur in a 10-year-old jumper free from lameness would be of no concern.

NUCLEAR SCINTIGRAPHIC EXAMINATION

Nuclear scintigraphic examination is not a routine part of a prepurchase examination. If the horse is clinically normal, the interpretation of results of whole body screening is difficult. This practice should be discouraged. In selected horses when interpretation of the clinical significance of specific radiological abnormalities may be in dispute, focused nuclear scintigraphic examination may be helpful.

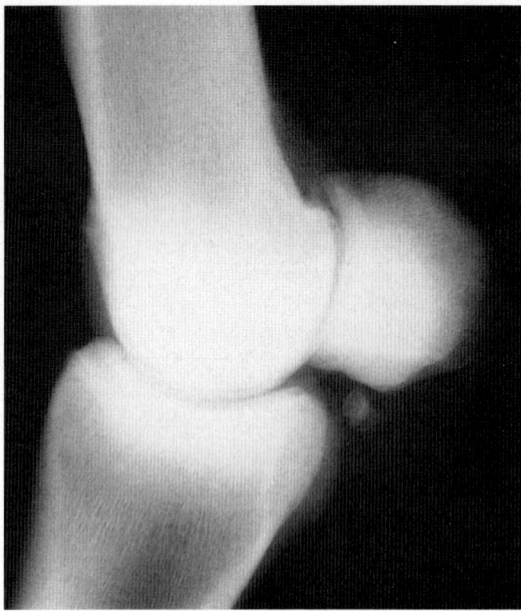

Fig. 114-8 • Lateromedial radiographic image of the left forelimb of a clinically normal 7-year-old Thoroughbred. There are two well-rounded osseous opacities distal to the proximal sesamoid bones. Such opacities are usually clinically innocuous.

ULTRASONOGRAPHIC EXAMINATION

Ultrasonographic examination of the limbs requires three important prerequisites: high-class image quality, experience of interpretation (knowledge of normal anatomy and its variations and the ability to detect abnormality and to interpret its potential clinical significance), and client compliance. A number of clinical situations occur in a prepurchase examination in which ultrasonographic examination provides invaluable clinical information not otherwise available. These situations include the following:

- An event horse that has competed in a Three Day Event within the last 6 months but has not competed since or a racehorse that has run recently but has not done fast work since. Strain of the SDFT, unilateral or bilateral, is a common injury in event horses and racehorses. Clinical signs of localized heat and swelling may resolve quickly or even pass unnoticed by the vendor (see Chapter 69). Clinical signs of tendonitis may be inapparent at the prepurchase examination but may become evident when fast work is resumed. If the left and right SDFTs are slightly enlarged with rounded margins but are symmetrical, this may pass unnoticed during the clinical evaluation.
- An event or racehorse that has not competed or raced in the last several months during the season. The purchaser may have given a plausible explanation for this, but the clinician should be suspicious that the absence from competition may reflect injury.
- Known previous tendon or ligament injury. Ultrasonographic examination gives more objective information than can be obtained from palpation alone but does not give information about strength of the structure.

- Suspected enlargement of one or more tendonous or ligamentous structures, detection of localized heat, or pain on palpation.
- Moderate enlargement of a digital flexor tendon sheath, especially if unilateral, particularly in a forelimb.
- Enlargement on the palmar (plantar) aspect of the pastern. It can be difficult to determine by palpation alone if thickening reflects localized fibrosis or swelling of a tendon or ligament.

Interpretation of findings in a horse with no identifiable clinical abnormality may not be straightforward, but enlargement of a tendon or ligament usually does reflect previous injury, the future relevance of which depends on the intended use of the horse, chronicity of the lesion, severity of the lesion, and degree of healing.

If ultrasonographic examination is recommended but is refused by the vendor or the purchaser, this should be noted on the prepurchase examination certificate.

THERMOGRAPHIC EXAMINATION

Thermography also may provide a useful indicator of low-grade inflammation and help to identify signs of early tendonitis, suspensory desmitis, and splint development. However, a normal thermographic appearance does not preclude the presence of a subclinical tendon lesion.

MAGNETIC RESONANCE IMAGING

The availability of MRI (especially the standing application) may lead to requests for more "thorough" examinations. MRI should be discouraged as a routine procedure because of the high probability of finding lesions in otherwise sound mature performance horses. It may be appropriate in situations where unusual radiological or ultrasonographic lesions are found, to further assess the possible clinical significance.

BLOOD TESTS

The use of blood tests is controversial, and limitations should be discussed with the prospective purchaser. Screening for nonsteroidal antiinflammatory drugs, mood-altering drugs, sedatives, and possibly also corticosteroids is advisable, but the purchaser must be aware that blood tests are less sensitive for these drugs and metabolites than is urine analysis. If the vendor knows in advance that the horse will be tested, this knowledge may provide a deterrent to the unscrupulous. Alternatively, blood may be collected and stored suitably and be analyzed only if a problem arises within the first few weeks of purchase. In the United Kingdom the Veterinary Defence Society and the Horse Race Forensic Laboratory run a scheme jointly. The vendor signs a form to permit collection of the sample in a specialized container provided by the Horse Race Forensic Laboratory, to which is applied a bar-coded label. The purchaser can elect to have the sample analyzed immediately for a fee or it can be stored at the Horse Race Forensic Laboratory at no charge with the potential for analysis at a later date. This system has proved to be legally robust.

The purchaser must be aware that drugs administered intraarticularly may not be detectable, depending on the nature of the drug and the time of administration relative to the time of examination. In professional dealers' yards in Europe, a high incidence of joint medication to mask lameness occurs.

If the horse is being purchased in one country for export to another, testing for evidence of specific diseases may be necessary. For example, horses entering the United States should be tested for equine infectious anemia, dourine, glanders, and piroplasmosis. A horse from an area where African horse sickness has occurred should be tested. Testing stallions going to the United States for equine viral arteritis is advised. Positive horses may not be permitted back into the European Union and other regions without extensive testing and potential limitations.

Screening for contagious equine metritis may be indicated. Use of hematological and serum biochemical screening and other assays, such as measurement of cortisol and insulin, as an aid to detect equine Cushing's syndrome in older horses is controversial. Routine hematology and serum biochemistry may be useful to ensure that the horse is healthy at the time of the examination. Serum testing for equine protozoal myelitis potentially is misleading and should be actively discouraged.

NERVE BLOCKS

In some circumstances, nerve blocks may aid interpretation of clinical findings. A horse may appear completely sound under all circumstances but have an unusually short forelimb stride. Does this reflect bilateral foot pain, or is this gait completely normal and natural for this horse? With the vendor's permission this question could be answered by bilateral perineural analgesia of the palmar nerves at the level of the proximal sesamoid bones. However, nerve blocks are not without complications and only establish the region of the pain causing lameness at best. Pursuing this course may prove frustrating and not elucidate the cause of the lameness

If a horse is lame but the vendor claims that the horse has never been lame previously, the situation should be discussed with the purchaser. Reexamining the horse on a subsequent occasion may be best, but the vendor should be advised that after resolution of the lameness the horse must be worked for at least a week before reassessment. The veterinarian should ask the vendor to sign a form declaring that the horse has been worked properly and has not received medication, and the veterinarian should collect blood for medication testing when the horse is reexamined.

The examining veterinarian's role is not to perform a lameness investigation; this would be unethical. A lameness investigation is a job for the vendor's own veterinarian.

SUMMARY OF OBSERVATIONS

The veterinarian should summarize the basic assessment of the horse's physical condition for the buyer. Abnormalities of conformation, clinically insignificant swellings, and any clinical abnormality should be discussed and documented. The initial report should be made verbally to the client or the client's agent. When dealing with an agent,

informing the agent that the client also will be receiving a complete written report is wise. Comments should be as factual as possible, with minimal personal bias, but findings must be interpreted and the risk assessed and documented.

Although the veterinarian is working for the buyer, the veterinarian does have an obligation to the seller. The findings should not be discussed with anyone other than those involved in the sale. With permission of the buyer, the veterinarian can divulge any and all information to the seller.

A written report reviewing the findings of the examination should be provided to the buyer. The American Association of Equine Practitioners has an excellent set of guidelines for reporting the prepurchase examination (www.aaep.org/purchase_exams.htm). This report can serve as documentation of clinically significant findings for future reference.

The veterinarian should advise the buyer about the risks of purchase, without making the decision for the buyer. The veterinarian is not responsible for assessment of the suitability of the horse for a rider or for determining an appropriate value for the horse. However, if the horse is clearly likely to be unsuitable for the purchaser because of temperament or ease of management or riding, the purchaser should be advised accordingly.

GUIDELINES FOR REPORTING PREPURCHASE EXAMINATIONS

The American Association of Equine Practitioners has approved the following guidelines for reporting equine prepurchase examinations. The spirit of these guidelines is to provide a framework that aids the veterinarian in reporting a purchase examination and to define that the buyer is responsible for determining if the horse is suitable. These guidelines are neither designed for nor intended to cover any examinations other than prepurchase examinations (e.g., limited examinations at auction sales and other special purpose examinations such as lameness, endoscopic, ophthalmic, radiographic, and reproductive examinations). Although compliance with all of the following guidelines helps to ensure a properly reported prepurchase examination, the veterinarian has the sole responsibility for determining the extent and depth of each examination. The American Association of Equine Practitioners recognizes that for practical reasons not all examinations permit or require veterinarians to adhere to each of the following guidelines.

1. All reports should be included in the medical record.
2. The report should contain the following:
   a. A description of the horse with sufficient specificity to identify it fully
   b. The time, date, and place of the examination
3. The veterinarian should list abnormal or undesirable findings discovered during the examination and give his or her qualified opinions as to the functional effect of these findings.
4. The veterinarian should make no determination and express no opinion as to the suitability of the horse for the purpose intended. This issue is a business judgment that is solely the responsibility of the

buyer that he or she should make on the basis of a variety of factors, only one of which is the report provided by the veterinarian.

5. The veterinarian should record and retain in the medical record a description of all the procedures performed in connection with the examination, but the examination procedures need not be listed in detail in the report.

6. The veterinarian should qualify any finding and opinions expressed to the buyer with specific references to tests that were recommended but not performed on the horse (e.g., radiography, endoscopy, blood and drug tests, electrocardiography [ECG],

rectal examination, nerve blocks, laboratory studies) at the request of the person for whom the examination was performed.

7. The veterinarian should record and retain the name and address of parties involved with the examination (e.g., buyer, seller, agent, witness).

8. A copy of the report and copies of all documents relevant to the examination should be retained by the veterinarian for a period of years not less than the statute of limitations applicable for the state in which the service was rendered. Local legal counsel can provide advice as to the appropriate period of retention.

Chapter 115

Lameness in the Show Hunter and Show Jumper

Robert P. Boswell, Richard D. Mitchell, Timothy R. Ober, Philippe H. Benoit, Christopher (Kit) B. Miller, and Sue J. Dyson

HISTORICAL PERSPECTIVE

Show jumping and related competitions have origins in hunting sport and military tradition. The show hunter, most popular in North America, has evolved from the traditions of fox and stag hunting. These horses were expected to provide fast, safe, and athletic passage for the rider, and considerable pride was taken in being well mounted and having the horse admired. Today in the show ring these horses are judged for beauty, athletic ability, manners, and way of going. Jumping style is important and must be coupled with consistent performance.

Some competitions encourage the development of a young horse to a higher level of training, others award a mature horse for outstanding performance, and others separate amateur and professional riders. Horses often are selected based on suitability for a particular division of competition.

The modern show jumper has many of its origins with military traditions. Many cavalry officers were by necessity highly skilled and accomplished horsemen. Thus when the era of the modern Olympics began, the equestrian competitors were military men. With the mechanization of the military and the replacement of the cavalry with motorized transport, the private sector became more involved in Olympic show jumping. Many of the early civilian competitors were retired military men. Show jumping has become increasingly more popular, and many talented riders have emerged on the national and international scenes. Since the 1960s many women have entered this sport, once dominated by men.

STRUCTURE OF THE SPORT

Show jumping combines athletic effort of the horse and rider. The scoring process is objective, with the winner jumping the course with the fewest rails knocked down and, in the jump off, in the fastest time. Heights of fences range from 1 m at novice level to 1.7 m for advanced competitions. The course should be completed within an allowed time, and some competitions are considered as speed classes in which jumping and time faults are combined. As the jumps get bigger, the potential for injury increases, and many conditions develop from repetitive strain. Many of the fences are set at distances to each other so that the horse must adjust stride length to fit in the appropriate number of strides. A good horse must have explosive power and great athleticism, combined with carefulness—a desire not to hit fences. Contrary to many equine sports, similar numbers of mares and geldings or stallions compete (Figure 115-1).

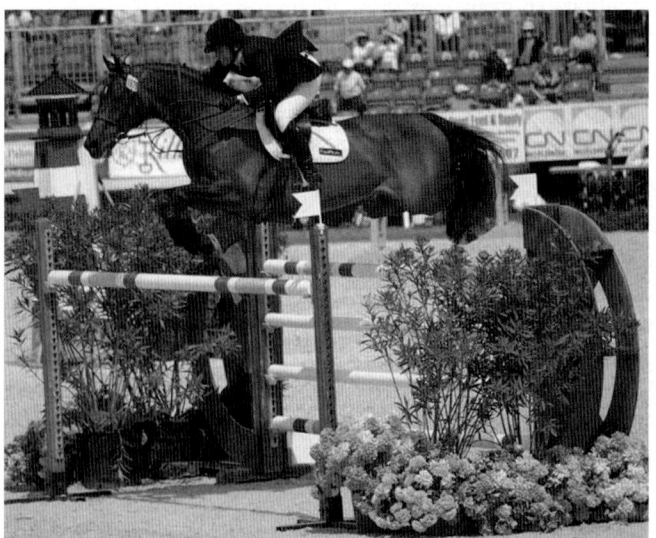

Fig. 115-1 • A Grand Prix show jumper jumping a large oxer at Spruce Meadows, Calgary, Canada, a venue with one of the most lucrative prize structures worldwide. Note the symmetrical position of each of the forelimbs and hindlimbs. Asymmetry may reflect an underlying pain-related problem. The horse is jumping squarely across the fence; jumping obliquely may reflect hindlimb pain and uneven propulsion.

Some older horses compete at levels of competition lower than they have reached to be schoolmasters for less experienced riders. These older horses may experience unique problems related to age and use. Today show jumping is a highly diverse and competitive sport enjoyed all over the world from beginner level to the level of the Olympic Games. At the top level the sport is entirely professional, with horses changing hands for huge prices and with large amounts of prize money available, putting pressure on the veterinarian to keep horses sound. Competition continues throughout the year, with outdoor shows during the summer months and indoor shows during the winter, so horses potentially get few breaks.

CHARACTERISTICS OF THE JUMPING SPORTS HORSE

Many breeds are capable of show jumping and related activities and include Thoroughbreds (TBs), European Warmbloods, TB-Warmblood crosses, and American Quarter Horses and related crosses. The European Warmbloods most often are represented by the Hanoverian, Holsteiner, Trakehner, Dutch Warmblood, Selle Français, Swedish Warmblood, and Irish crossbred breeds. Breeding in continental Europe has become highly specialized and has developed in part through financial support from state governments. Most modern day top-level show jumpers are naturally well-balanced, good-moving athletes. Various pony breeds, such as the Welsh crosses, are used for children (see Chapter 126).

Current preferences are for lighter and taller horses, with moderate muscling. This body type is associated with greater speed and agility, which are assets to a modern show jumper. This body type also benefits hunters because these horses have graceful movement, with good extension and natural balance. Larger horses, if not excessively heavy, are at an advantage for show jumping because of greater stride length and overall strength and power. The TB long has been preferred by American trainers for the hunter ring; however, in recent years Warmblood breeds have gained favor because of a calmer nature and better manners.

Horses often start competing at 4 years of age, reach peak ability at 9 to 12 years of age, and may continue to compete until 18 to 20 years of age.

TRAINING

Training of the hunter and jumper emphasizes using the hindquarters for engagement and collection, which places more weight and stress on the hindlimbs as they are brought forward and under the rider during locomotion. Such a posture is somewhat unnatural for the horse, whose normal inclination is to distribute weight over the forehand. These stresses may contribute to or accelerate the development of problems of the thoracolumbar and pelvic regions, and ligaments and joints of the hindlimbs. Early in the training of a young horse, lameness often reflects musculotendonous problems and relates to lack of adaptation to work.

When training over fences begins, new loads on the hindlimbs occur that place more stress on soft tissues and joints. Stresses on the forelimbs also are increased because they are involved in takeoff and landing. The forelimbs are involved in setting up the jump and aiding in the directional change from horizontal to vertical. On landing the forelimbs receive considerable impact loads and absorb the entire weight of the horse. Increased load places more stress on the foot, distal limb joints, and the soft tissues of the forelimbs.

Horses must learn to adjust stride length by shortening or lengthening the stride, to jump from a line perpendicular to a fence or at an angle, to turn quickly, to change leading legs in canter, and to jump from variable speeds of approach. Unwillingness to change leads or always favoring one lead when landing after a fence may indicate a problem (see Chapter 97). Much of the basic flat work training is similar to dressage.

Many lameness conditions encountered early in a horse's training begin as subtle performance-limiting problems, progress relatively slowly, and may disappear with further conditioning. However, excessive training leads to the development of important problems such as chronic muscle soreness, fatigue, joint inflammation, and behavioral changes. Slow, steady work with a gradual buildup in exercise intensity and duration results in fewer joint and soft tissue problems later.

TRAINING AND COMPETITION SURFACES

Training, warm-up, and competition surfaces play a substantial role in the development of lameness in a jumper. Soft, deep footing requires much more effort by the horse and is responsible for early fatigue of muscles, tendons, and ligaments. Injuries include gluteal muscle strain and spasm, suspensory desmitis, desmitis of the accessory ligament of the deep digital flexor tendon (ALDDFT), and superficial digital flexor (SDF) tendonitis as well as inflammation of or trauma to any of the soft tissue structures in the hoof, pastern, and metacarpal and metatarsal regions. Sandy soils contribute to the development of hoof wall problems. Hard surfaces may result in bone- and joint-related injuries, as well as distal limb and foot problems such as subsolar bruising, distal interphalangeal (DIP) joint synovitis, and osteoarthritis (OA) of the proximal interphalangeal (PIP) and DIP joints.

Formerly most high level outdoor competitions in Europe took place on grass, but there is an increasing trend for some of the higher-level competitions to take place on all-weather surfaces. The nature of the footing depends highly on the weather and can vary extremely. To enhance traction, screw-in studs often are used in the front and hind shoes. Studs may be used in the medial and lateral branches of the shoe or just the lateral branch to reduce risk of interference injuries. If studs are used in only one branch of the shoe, this immediately creates mediolateral imbalance and the potential for abnormal torque. Studs also alter the dorsopalmar balance, especially if the ground is firm. Horses that flex the carpi excessively during jumping may have to wear a girth guard to protect the sternal region from self-inflicted injuries. If a horse is jumping on firm going, studs concentrate the forces of impact and can predispose the horse to deep-seated bruising of the foot. There is a tendency in horses with poor-quality horn for the hoof wall to break in the region where studs are placed. In some circumstances studs may halt the normal slide of a foot on landing and thereby predispose to injury.

Excessive work, such as long period of lunging a hunter to calm it down, prolonged competitive efforts, and long show schedules of repeated competitions play a role in the development of many injuries in hunters and jumpers.

CONFORMATION AND LAMENESS

Conformational abnormalities of the foot predispose horses to lameness. An underrun heel, long toe, and a broken hoof-pastern axis frequently contribute to palmar foot pain and DIP joint synovitis. Horses with improper medial-to-lateral hoof balance may develop a sheared heel, crushed bar, and chronic foot pain. Base-wide or base-narrow forelimb conformation may contribute to injuries to the suspensory ligament (SL), its branches, and the distal sesamoidean ligaments.

Toe-in or toe-out forelimb conformation may predispose horses to PIP and metacarpophalangeal joint problems. Short, more upright pasterns predispose horses to navicular disease and DIP joint and PIP joint synovitis or OA. These horses are often straight through the shoulder as well and lack the stride and extension necessary for jumping. Long, more sloping pasterns sometimes are associated with sesamoiditis and soft tissue injuries to the distal aspect of the limb.

Over-at-the-knee conformation may predispose horses to SL strain and should be avoided in selecting a jumper. Offset-knee conformation predisposes a jumper to medial splint problems. However, attention always should be paid to subclinical contralateral hindlimb lameness in a mature horse that develops an acutely painful medial splint bone. Subtle angular limb deformities are rarely a problem, provided proper attention is paid to shoeing and hoof balance.

Extremely sickle-hocked conformation is associated with weak hindlimbs and places more stress on the plantar tarsal soft tissues and the centrodistal and tarsometatarsal joints. A straighter hock is actually more desirable, but an overly straight hock may predispose to SL strain and distal hock joint pain, especially in association with an extended fetlock and long pastern conformation.

Horses that are extremely straight through the stifle are poor jumping prospects and have a high incidence of instability and upward fixation of the patella. A more angular stifle gives the horse a longer, more powerful stride and is thought to provide more strength for jumping.

A long, sloping hip and croup are desirable characteristics in a jumping horse, providing strength and power. Horses with a flat croup often suffer from thoracolumbar and sacroiliac pain. Asymmetry of the tubera sacrale and tubera coxae can be seen in the absence of lameness and may reflect previous trauma. An experienced rider usually can manage these horses.

Horses with excessively base-wide or base-narrow hindlimb conformation place abnormal stress on the feet and joints. Base-wide horses may have an increased incidence of hock problems, whereas base-narrow horses may have more stifle problems.

SHOEING CONSIDERATIONS

Many lameness problems are a direct result of improper trimming and shoeing. Neglected feet are frequently a source of lameness, and a poorly shod foot also may contribute to lameness by forcing the horse to transfer abnormal and excessive stresses to other parts of the limb or to other limbs. Many of the Warmblood breeds have relatively tall, narrow upright feet, which are predisposed to the development of thrush and sheared heels. Others have wide flat feet that can be carelessly shod into a broken back hoof-pastern axis with an underrun heel and abnormal orientation of the distal phalanx. Studs in the shoes may create foot imbalance and may increase the severity of interference injuries. A good cooperative relationship with an experienced farrier is an essential element in lameness prevention and management. This can be a problem for top-level competition horses that are constantly moving from show to show and are being trimmed and reshod by different people with varying ability. The time of shoeing relative to the day of competition is important because trimming may alter biomechanical forces. To avoid increased stresses on the soft tissue structures within the hoof capsule, it is suggested that the horse be shod within a maximum of 4 weeks from competition. In Europe we consider 7 to 15 days to be the optimum interval between shoeing and competition (PHB, SJD).

LAMENESS EXAMINATION

Before a horse is examined because of a suspected lameness problem, several factors should be considered. If the horse is currently competing, will any diagnostic tests or treatment have an effect on the horse's ability to continue competition? Knowledge of the competition rules and drug use guidelines are essential. Has the horse recently competed? Has a change in exercise intensity or duration been made? Does the horse have a new trainer? When was the horse last shod? If the horse has been competing away from home, it is important to determine if another veterinary surgeon already has examined and treated the horse, and if so with what.

The lameness examination should begin as the horse is walked from the stall or paddock to the examination room or area, because movements such as a small circle to reverse its direction may offer clues as to which limb or limbs may be affected. It is not uncommon for there to be concurrent lameness in more than one limb. Careful observation and palpation of the joints of each limb as well as the neck and back are performed while the horse is held quietly. Passive flexion tests and evaluation of the lateral movements of the head, neck, and back are performed.

A dynamic examination should be performed beginning with an observation of the horse at the walk in a straight line, in small circles, and in a figure eight. The horse should next be examined at the trot in hand on a firm, level surface. Lunging on firm footing in small circles in both directions should be performed, as this often exacerbates subtle lameness, especially if involving the foot.

It is sometimes necessary to see the horse ridden to determine which limb is lame. The rider may also be asked to change the diagonal at the trot and figure eight to increase the load on a specific limb when it is on either the inside or the outside of the circle.

Examinations performed after strenuous exercise or after competition may be useful; more subtle lameness may then be more obvious. It should also be noted and recommended that the veterinarian observe the "way" or "style" the horse trains and jumps. Defects in the horse's position and way of jumping that would have otherwise gone unnoticed may be observed during a routine physical or lameness examination. Watching videos of the horse may also allow the practitioner to see abnormalities of the horse's balance or gaits when in motion. Knowing what is "normal" may also help the practitioner detect early or subtle changes in movement before an obvious lameness is manifest.

Proximal and distal limb flexion tests should be performed on all limbs. The method and duration of flexion are a matter of personal preference but should be consistent and interpreted with care, bearing in mind that joints and soft tissue structures may be stressed simultaneously. It has become common practice for top-level competition horses to be examined periodically throughout the year to try to detect early warning signs of impending problems. A positive response to flexion is often followed by treating the stressed joint(s). The true value of this practice is difficult to determine objectively.

Once the lame limb(s) has been identified, the limb is carefully reexamined. Hoof tester response should also be assessed. An obvious source of pain may be identified, but perineural or intraarticular analgesia often is required to localize the source(s) of pain. Results are sometimes confusing and always should be related to the clinical examination.

Aseptic preparation is essential for intrasynovial injections to minimize the risk of infection. Two authors (RPB, CBM) also administer gentamicin intravenously before entering any synovial space. The conditions of the work area and the temperament of the horse being examined influence which analgesic technique to use. Intrasynovial analgesia may be delayed or not performed if no clean, dry place is available for safe injection. Although intraarticular analgesia is considered to be more specific than perineural analgesia, it may influence periarticular pain. In some instances regional or intraarticular analgesia may not be safely performed without first tranquilizing the horse. This may interfere with the lameness examination, especially if the lameness is low grade. Lameness is reassessed after the effects of sedation have worn off. Alternatively the horse is sedated, the suspected joint is treated with the appropriate drug(s), and the horse is reevaluated in a few days. The treatment is therefore substituted for intraarticular analgesia. In situations in which subtle lameness makes interpretation of nerve blocks difficult, in those horses with multiple-limb lameness, in horses that are difficult or dangerous, or when comprehensive blocking fails to localize the lameness, other techniques such as nuclear scintigraphy should be considered.

When horses are competing regularly, especially away from home, owners, riders, trainers, and peers often put pressure on the veterinarian to treat the horse based on an index of clinical suspicion rather than on a complete lameness evaluation including local analgesia. Although this can be successful and a positive response to treatment clearly indicates a correct diagnosis, one must bear in mind that some injuries do require rest for the best long-term outcome. A merely transient response to treatment or a lack of response warrants further investigation of the lameness, and this routinely should include local analgesic techniques.

IMAGING CONSIDERATIONS

Only after successfully localizing the source of pain causing lameness or after an extensive physical examination has provided the veterinarian with a reasonable indication of the problem should the examination progress to diagnostic imaging, including radiography, ultrasonography, and, if indicated, nuclear scintigraphy, computed tomography, or magnetic resonance imaging (MRI). Routine techniques are used, with no special images. High-quality diagnostic imaging is related directly to the veterinarian's success as a diagnostician. The routine use of both ultrasonography and radiography is strongly encouraged, as soft tissue structures are commonly involved in injuries of the bone and joints. The complete extent of the injury may be identified; the presence of a soft tissue component may influence both the treatment options and the prognosis. Frequent ultrasonographic examinations make a practitioner more confident in correctly recognizing an abnormality.

FAILURE TO MAKE A DIAGNOSIS

Every veterinarian, no matter how astute as a lameness diagnostician, eventually will be confused or unsure or simply have no idea as to why a particular horse is lame, and consultation with associates or referral to other experts should be considered. Just as a good relationship with a farrier is paramount to the successful management of many foot-related problems, good relationships with other veterinarians are necessary and may be helpful when one is faced with a difficult or confusing lameness. The veterinarian must be honest and open about the horse with the owners and trainers; inclusion of other professionals in the case or referral for advanced imaging may ultimately lead to both an accurate diagnosis and enhancement of the veterinarian's relationship with the client if handled well. Reexamination at a later date also may be beneficial. Some bone lesions may take a few weeks to become visible radiologically, so the veterinarian should consider reimaging if the pain causing lameness has been localized to a specific area.

The use of many medications for a "shotgun" approach to treatment may be a veterinarian's only hope when all diagnostic methods are either unrewarding or not available and if previously attempted "trial therapies" have failed. Such medications include but are not limited to nonsteroidal antiinflammatory drugs (NSAIDs), doxycycline, tiludronate, intramuscular polysulfated glycosaminoglycans (PSGAGs), intravenous hyaluronan, and oral nutraceuticals.

TREATMENT

In recent years the trend has been toward much more aggressive treatment, with many different treatment modalities often being combined to manage a single condition. Although in some circumstances this can be justified, it does mean that the veterinarian is often not sure which treatment really is effective. More targeted treatment based on a precise diagnosis actually may be equally effective. A thorough understanding of the overall "pain map" of the horse can lead to a confident approach to treatments even in the absence of objective data from the lameness examination. The pain map essentially represents the postulated sites of pain causing poor performance based on an assessment of a detailed history of performance; the results of palpation including the response to stimulation of acupuncture points; evaluation of the horse moving in hand, on the lunge, and ridden, both when work is first initiated and later in the work program; and the response to flexion tests and chiropractic assessment of joint mobility, sometimes combined with assessment of the response to local analgesic techniques (TRO).

TEN MOST COMMON LAMENESS PROBLEMS OF SHOW HUNTERS AND SHOW JUMPERS

1. Foot pain
2. Distal hock joint pain
3. Suspensory desmitis
4. Thoracolumbar region pain
5. Fetlock region pain
6. Stifle pain
7. Osteoarthritis or trauma of the proximal interphalangeal joint
8. Croup and hip region pain
9. Superficial digital flexor tendonitis and desmitis of the accessory ligament of the deep digital flexor tendon
10. Cervical osteoarthritis and pain

Many of these problems are interrelated, and more than one problem may occur simultaneously. We have attempted to list these in relative order of frequency; however, this is not intended to imply that one is more serious than another.

DIAGNOSIS AND MANAGEMENT OF COMMON CAUSES OF LAMENESS

Foot Pain

Foot Soreness

The most common site of forelimb lameness and overall lameness in a hunter or jumper is the foot. The horse naturally supports 60% to 65% of its body weight over the forelimbs, and impact forces during jumping dramatically increase load and structural stresses in tissues within the hoof capsule. This may be exacerbated by training regimens that do not focus on improving strength from behind and therefore the overall balance of the horse.

The manner in which a horse is shod has tremendous importance in the development of hoof- and foot-related problems. A long toe and underrun heel are common hoof conformational defects and frequently contribute to heel pain because of hoof wall separation or bruising in the heel, quarter, and bar areas. The heel itself may be excessively long and collapsed inward, and the horse actually may be bearing weight on the outer wall. This often results in sensitivity to hoof tester pressure applied to each heel bulb and when the heel bulbs are squeezed together. A flattened and chronically bruised heel and bar area (corns) may be seen after removal of the shoe.

Lameness is often improved by analgesia of the palmar digital nerves. Lateromedial radiographic images of the foot may reveal that the distal phalanx is abnormally oriented, in extreme situations so that the palmarmost aspect of the bone is lower (more distal) than the toe (so-called

"negative palmar angle"). The so-called "negative palmar angle" appears to occur more commonly in the United States than in Europe. The solar margins of the distal phalanges may be irregular. In horses with chronic lameness, deep digital flexor (DDF) tendonitis and distal sesamoidean impar desmitis may contribute to pain associated with an underrun heel. However, these soft tissue injuries have been documented using MRI in show jumpers with both poor and good foot conformation (SJD).

Some horses with underrun heels and poor angulation of the distal phalanges do not respond well to shoeing. Removing the shoes, trimming back the abnormal heel wall, and placing the foot in a support bandage are recommended. One author's (RPB) preference is to fashion a cushion support for the palmar aspect of the hoof using a two-part putty elastomer material (EDSS, Equine Distal Support System, Penrose, Colorado, United States). Using the sulci of the frog for support is believed to suspend the heel and promote the new growth to be more vertical in its orientation. This process, however, requires a long-term commitment by the owner and trainer, because new heel growth may take up to 6 months to be sufficient for the reapplication of shoes. One author floats the heel using a ¾ rim pad and either a heart bar shoe or a pour-in pad in an effort to keep the horses in work and competition (CBM).

Attention should be paid to the role of training and overall management of the horse, specifically as it relates to hindlimb strength and comfort.

Subsolar Bruising

Horses with subsolar bruising often respond well initially to Epsom salt poultices or cooked linseed hoof packs and NSAIDs (e.g., phenylbutazone) followed by corrective shoeing. Rasping excessive toe from the solar surface proximally up the dorsal wall to create a 45-degree angle with the ground surface and application of a shoe fitted full at the heel may be of benefit by removing resistance to breakover. Ideal breakover is located between two points; the first is located by extending a line distally along the dorsal surface of the distal phalanx to the bearing surface, and the other by drawing a perpendicular line from the dorsal distal aspect of the distal phalanx to the bearing surface. Egg bar shoes may be required to gain adequate heel support. Shoes such as the EDSS natural balance shoe (Equine Digital Support System), with the web behind and squared off at the toe, also improve breakover and reduce stress in the palmar portion of the foot. We do not recommend the long-term application of plastic wedge pads or egg bar shoes because they actually may contribute to further crushing of the heel and promote the heel bulbs to slide forward and grow horizontally. Leather pads may be helpful in some horses if sole pain is present and sole protection is desired. In horses with a chronic problem, long-term use of aspirin (60 g once daily or 20 g bid for 5 days) may be helpful. Hoof growth supplements containing biotin and methionine also may be of benefit, and we recommend feeding of biotin (100 mg to 1 g for 3 to 12 months, either alone or combined with zinc, cysteine, and DL-methionine daily) to promote hoof wall growth. Careful attention should be paid to the condition of the gastric mucosa with long-term NSAID use in show horses, because gastric ulceration may occur or worsen. Concurrent administration of acid pump inhibitors such as omeprazole should be considered.

Extreme sensitivity to hoof testers may be evident along the periphery of the sole at the level of the distal phalanx. Such pain may be associated with bruising, solar margin fractures, laminar inflammation or inflammation of the distal phalanx caused by chronic concussion from hard ground, or excessive sole pressure from the shoe. These conditions may be more common in North America (with its harder and dryer footing) than in Europe. Radiology is necessary for diagnosis of solar margin fractures of the distal phalanx. Shoeing should be directed at reducing local pressure on the affected areas and improving the overall hoof balance. Egg bar shoes and rim pads are often effective, but soft sole pours that provide extra cushion and shock absorption also help. Two-part putty elastomer is thought to benefit by providing support and lift from the sulci of the frog. Care should be taken with a pour or putty elastomer to avoid overfilling, causing excessive sole pressure.

Subsolar Abscess

Subsolar abscesses occur commonly and result from shoe nails improperly applied, poor environmental conditions, a shoe moving slightly, and poor hoof structure. Onset of clinical signs may be rapid, such as immediately after a show, or may occur within the first several days after shoeing. The additional trauma of jumping exacerbates the condition, leading the rider or trainer to suspect trauma or serious injury. Warmth in the hoof wall, increased digital pulse amplitudes, and focal, extreme sensitivity to hoof tester application are usually diagnostic, provided that the hoof horn is not excessively hard. Perineural analgesia is rarely necessary to confirm the suspected diagnosis and also may be confusing, because not all horses respond positively. After blocking and trotting the horse to reassess lameness, reexamination of the solar surface of the foot may reveal purulent drainage from the area of suspicion. Treatment is directed toward liberal opening of the solar surface of the foot at the point of maximum sensitivity to establish adequate drainage. If drainage is not established, bandaging the foot with hyperosmotic agents such as products containing magnesium sulfate (Epsom salts) is recommended. Twice daily soaking of the foot with a hot, supersaturated solution of Epsom salts with the bandage left on is also recommended for 3 to 5 days. Once drainage has been established, the foot is bandaged in a similar fashion, and NSAIDs also may be administered to reduce the inflammation. Antibiotics rarely are indicated but are sometimes used if soft tissue swelling occurs above the coronary band.

Navicular Disease

Navicular disease may initially be misdiagnosed as inflammation of the DIP joint. It is also likely that navicular disease is overdiagnosed in horses with simple heel pain. The diagnosis of navicular disease carries the stigma of a permanent and disabling lameness and is upsetting to the horse owner and trainer. Therefore the veterinarian should make an exhaustive effort to rule out all other possible sources for the pain causing lameness before making the diagnosis.

Lameness in horses with navicular disease usually is characterized by a slow, insidious onset. Early signs include shortening of the stride length, tripping, toe stabbing, and an intermittent unilateral lameness, although the lameness is almost always bilateral. Show horses are often more lame the day after a competition. Some horses with no previous lameness history become suddenly lame and are often refractory to standard therapies. Recent experience using MRI suggests that a proportion of horses that were previously thought to have navicular disease have primary lesions of the deep digital flexor tendon (DDFT) within the hoof capsule (SJD). Some horses with navicular disease also have an acute-onset unilateral lameness. The response to hoof testers varies, and often the horse shows only resentment when the heel bulbs are squeezed together. The wedge test may accentuate lameness; however, a positive response is not pathognomonic for the disease. Lameness may be increased after distal limb flexion, but the response is nonspecific. Lameness is almost always eliminated by palmar digital nerve blocks, and a previously undetected lameness often appears in the contralateral limb. Analgesia of the DIP joint or the navicular bursa often improves or abolishes the lameness.

Interpretation of the radiological appearance of the navicular bone is not easy; many horses with navicular bone pain have no detectable radiological abnormality. Radiolucent cystlike lesions in the body of the bone, large lollypop-shaped radiolucent areas on the distal border of the bone, increased thickness of the flexor cortex, and enthesophyte formation on the proximal and distal borders of the bone should be considered clinically significant.

Nuclear scintigraphy may be useful in horses that appear normal radiologically. The solar image is most useful and may reveal increased radiopharmaceutical uptake (IRU) in the navicular bone, reflecting abnormal bone metabolism. Lateral pool phase images may also be useful for highlighting horses that may have DDF tendonitis within the hoof capsule.

Ultrasonographic examination of the navicular bone and its associated soft tissue structures through the window of the frog may be useful, especially if MRI is not an option. It potentially allows assessment of the palmar aspect of the navicular bone, and the DDFT and the distal sesamoidean impar ligament and the insertions on the distal phalanx. MRI is useful for the diagnosis of various forms of navicular disease, identifying bone abnormalities not visible radiologically (Figure 115-2) and associated soft tissue injuries.

Therapy for navicular disease includes pain management and corrective shoeing. Clients should be advised that this disease rarely is cured and requires a long-term commitment to its management. Horses with chronic, refractory lameness may require neurectomy.

Trimming and shoeing should be directed toward facilitating breakover, providing support to the palmar aspect of the foot, and in some horses elevating the heel to reduce tension in the DDFT. A full fitted egg bar shoe with a rockered toe or the EDSS natural balance shoe may be useful. The forward edge of the shoe should be set back from the toe and the branches fitted full at the heel. Leather wedge pads have been used to elevate the heel; however, the foot should be monitored closely to prevent crushing of the heel. A commercially available aluminum wedge-shaped shoe also may be used to provide heel elevation. It should also be noted that horses with palmar foot pain associated

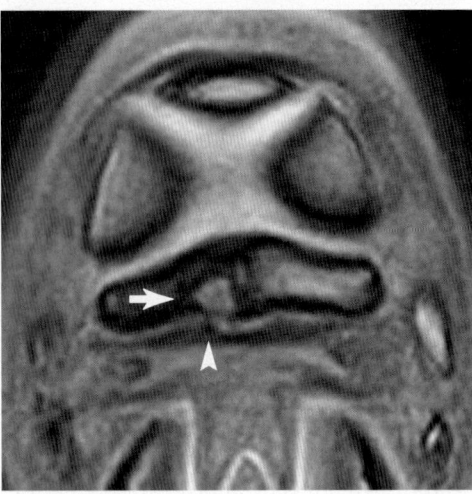

Fig. 115-2 • Transverse T1-weighted gradient echo magnetic resonance image of a foot. Medial is to the left. There is increased signal intensity in the flexor cortex of the navicular bone medial to the sagittal ridge *(arrow)*, dorsal to which signal intensity in the spongiosa is also increased, bounded dorsally by a rim of reduced signal intensity. There is dorsal irregularity of the deep digital flexor tendon in the same sagittal plane as the navicular bone defect *(arrowhead).*

with injury to the DDFT often demonstrate improvement in lameness when shoes are removed.

Medical management includes the use of NSAIDs, isoxsuprine, pentoxifylline, tiludronate, and aspirin; intraarticular injection of the DIP joint and intrathecal injection of the navicular bursa with corticosteroids and hyaluronan; and rest. Many of these therapies, usually in combination, have proved successful in short-term management of this condition, and we generally would recommend the least-invasive therapies first. The degenerative nature of this disease, however, ultimately usually results in the failure of any treatment, and palmar digital neurectomy may be considered. Surgical case selection is important, and consideration should be given to the overall condition of the horse and its level of performance. This procedure is not allowed for horses competing under Fédération Equestre Internationale (FEI) rules. Horses with evidence of DDF tendonitis and PIP or DIP joint OA are not considered good candidates because of the possibility of rupture of the DDFT or exacerbation of OA. Some horses may experience temporary pain relief from the application of a chemical nerve block using a mixture of corticosteroids, ammonium sulfate, and Sarapin locally injected at the level of the palmar digital nerves. This procedure may work well initially, only to gradually lose its effectiveness.

Shock wave therapy recently has been introduced as a noninvasive therapeutic option for pain management in horses with navicular disease. Several investigators have reported good results, but differences in equipment and protocols require further investigation. Positive results may be short-lived.

Sheared Heel
Sheared heel can be a serious problem in hunters and jumpers. Lameness is often insidious in onset, or a critical point of instability may be reached, producing a more acute lameness. Subtle conformational abnormalities and

poor hoof balance likely contribute to this condition. The medial heel bulb often is displaced proximally, with the remainder of the foot splayed laterally. When viewed from the solar surface of the foot, the lateral half of the foot is larger and flared compared with the medial half. The medial heel bulb may be painful to hoof testers, and the heel bulbs may be manipulated independently. Analgesia of the medial palmar digital nerve frequently improves lameness, but usually it is necessary to desensitize both heel bulbs before the horse appears sound. Many horses demonstrate radiological abnormalities of the medial palmar process of the distal phalanx, such as roughening or demineralization of the margin of the bone, presumably because of chronic trauma and inflammation. The therapeutic goal is to stabilize the heel bulbs and reduce pressure on the driven up or proximally displaced bulb. Stabilization most often is accomplished best by improving balance and breakover so that the foot lands flatly and relieving the affected heel from excessive loading during weight bearing. In a jumper an egg bar shoe with or without a pour-in pad to stabilize the heel is usually satisfactory. Horses with more severely affected feet may benefit from a heart bar, diagonal bar, or G-bar shoe. A rim pad with the portion to lie beneath the affected heel cut away may float the heel enough to allow that side to descend into a more normal position. Six to 9 months of persistent treatment are required before a more stable heel structure is established.

Distal Interphalangeal Joint Synovitis and Osteoarthritis
Inflammation of the DIP joint is common in jumping horses and usually results in subtle lameness that is frequently bilateral. Palpable joint effusion may or may not be present. Many horses, but not all, respond positively to a distal limb flexion test. Forelimbs are most commonly affected, but the hindlimbs also may be involved. The horse may have a reduction in stride length, and lameness is most obvious when the horse circles on firm footing. The rider or trainer may complain of a reduction in jumping performance, such as a reluctance to leave the ground and landing in a heap. Very hard surfaces for training or competition and surfaces that are too soft, irregular, and unstable may be predisposing factors. Soft footing, although not seemingly likely to contribute to excessive concussion, produces torsional forces on the DIP joint that strain the periarticular soft tissues. An underrun heel, long-toe conformation is probably the single most important contributing factor. The horse often shows a painful response to hoof testers with pressure applied from either heel to the opposite side of the frog and from the center of the frog to the dorsal hoof wall. Lameness usually is improved with analgesia of the palmar digital nerves and eliminated with palmar (abaxial sesamoid) nerve blocks or intraarticular analgesia of the DIP joint.

Radiological changes may be absent or subtle; however, in horses with more chronic or severe disease, active periosteal bone may be present on the dorsal aspect of the middle phalanx, and modeling of the extensor process of the distal phalanx may occur. With chronic, severe OA of the DIP joint there may be subchondral radiolucent areas in the distal phalanx consistent with collapse of the joint. Prominent radiolucent areas representing synovial invaginations may be present on the distal border of the

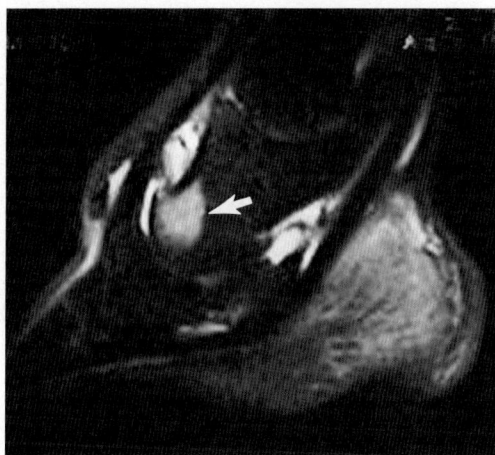

Fig. 115-3 • Parasagittal fat suppressed short tau inversion recovery (STIR) magnetic resonance image of the phalanges. There is a well-demarcated region of increased signal intensity on the distal dorsal aspect of the middle phalanx *(arrow)*, reflecting bone trauma. This was associated with reduced signal intensity in T1-weighted images.

navicular bone. Ultrasonographic examination of the collateral ligaments should be performed.

Nuclear scintigraphy is useful to rule out bone involvement. An area of IRU in the synovial structures of the joint may be visible in pool phase studies. Differentiating the palmar pouch of the DIP joint from the navicular bursa is difficult, and both structures may be involved in horses with severe lameness.

MRI has proven extremely useful in identifying abnormalities in and around the DIP joint including osseous trauma of the distal aspect of the middle phalanx (Figure 115-3). However, osseous trauma of the middle phalanx can occur alone, without DIP joint pain.

Therapy for horses with DIP joint synovitis depends on the severity of the lameness and the horse's competition schedule. Proper trimming and shoeing as for palmar foot pain with attention to the medial-to-lateral hoof balance is essential. The use of NSAIDs is common. Peripheral vasodilating agents such as isoxsuprine are of questionable value, although higher-than-standard doses appear to be clinically effective.

Intraarticular injection of high-molecular-weight hyaluronan and corticosteroids (triamcinolone acetonide or betamethasone) with proper shoeing and an appropriate amount of rest usually yields the best results. Occasionally, repeated injections are necessary after 4 to 6 weeks; however, injections repeated more frequently than once every 3 months should be avoided and should prompt a thorough review of the shoeing and hoof balance. Nutraceuticals and parenterally administered chondroprotective agents (PSGAGs) may be beneficial. Interleukin-1 receptor antagonist protein (IRAP) is helpful in managing recurrent inflammation in the DIP joint. A series of three or four injections given 7 to 10 days apart often is effective at relieving lameness associated with chronic synovitis.

Other primary sources of pain causing forelimb overload should be investigated.

Collateral Ligament Injury of the Distal Interphalangeal Joint

Some horses with synovitis of the DIP joint that are unresponsive to therapy should be evaluated for possible collateral ligament injury of the DIP and other anatomically related injuries. In a few horses, we (RDM, SJD) have identified enlargement and disruption of the infrastructure of the collateral ligament ultrasonographically, sometimes with focal IRU at the site of insertion on the distal phalanx, occasionally extending into the ipsilateral palmar process (SJD, RPB). MRI must be considered the gold standard for imaging structures in this area. Horses with collateral ligament injury should be managed with corrective shoeing and rest. Work level is reduced substantially. Extracorporeal shock wave or therapeutic ultrasound therapy combined with prolonged rest (at least 6 to 9 months) may be effective. Palmar digital neurectomy has been an effective management tool in horses failing to respond to conservative management (SJD).

Distal Hock Joint Pain

Distal hock joint pain is the second most common reason for lameness in a hunter or jumper and is the most common hindlimb lameness. Conformational defects, developmental abnormalities, and the incredible torsional stresses placed on the distal hock joints during jumping are thought to contribute to lameness. A variety of subtle signs becomes manifest before the onset of clinical lameness. Often the trainer or rider complains of a loss in the horse's stride length, poor impulsion, and a change in the horse's jumping style. Many horses may develop a tendency to switch leads in front of a jump or may have difficulty jumping from a particular lead. The horse consistently may develop the tendency to jump to one corner of the obstacle, and wider jumps appear to require more effort than usual or even necessary.

Clinical examination often reveals sensitivity to palpation of the muscles of the lumbar area and shortened cranial phase of the stride. The upper limb flexion test may reveal resentment of flexion and may or may not have a positive result. Some horses are reluctant to move forward immediately into a trot after flexion and may canter away from the veterinarian. Other horses may demonstrate an overall loss of balance after proximal limb flexion, manifesting as an induced forelimb lameness (TRO). The Churchill test often has a positive result in horses with tarsometatarsal (TMT) joint pain, but the result may be negative with centrodistal (CD) joint pain. Some horses with proximal suspensory desmitis (PSD) also respond positively to both proximal limb flexion and the Churchill test (RPB, RDM). Tarsocrural effusion may or may not be present. We (RPB, RDM) rarely perform regional perineural analgesia of the fibular and tibial nerves, because we consider the procedure difficult to interpret and somewhat dangerous to perform. Intraarticular analgesia of the CD and the TMT joints is preferred. However, a negative response to intraarticular analgesia does not preclude CD and TMT joint pain, and using fibular and tibial nerve blocks to identify some horses with distal hock joint pain may be essential. With practice this is a highly reliable and safe technique (SJD). With subtle hindlimb lameness or complaints of poor performance and no apparent lameness, it may be necessary for the horse to be ridden and for the rider to interpret the results of the block. The veterinarian should allow this with only the most experienced and talented riders.

Radiological changes vary from none to severe, with what may appear as total radiological evidence of joint fusion. Radiological changes do not necessarily correlate to the degree of lameness, but extensive radiolucent regions are often associated with moderate lameness. Osteochondral fragments on the cranial aspect of the intermediate ridge of the tibia, or at the distal aspect of the medial trochlea of the talus in a mature athlete in the absence of lameness, are usually an incidental finding of little if any clinical significance. However, fragments on the cranial aspect of the intermediate ridge of the tibia are occasionally associated with OA of the tarsocrural joint. The severity of the degenerative changes may be similar in the CD and the TMT joints; however, the TMT joint often has less severe abnormalities. The reason for this is unclear.

Nuclear scintigraphy can be helpful and reveals IRU in the distal aspect of the tarsus. Occasionally, small, focal, moderate-to-intense areas of IRU may reflect focal areas of loss of joint space, bone trauma, or tearing of interosseous ligamentous attachments.

It has been generally accepted that radiological evidence of distal joint(s) fusion is desirable, because the suggestion is that once joint fusion has occurred, the inflammation and therefore the pain should disappear. This is an unfortunate myth. Surgical arthrodesis is a currently accepted treatment for horses with OA of the CD or TMT joints that have become refractory to routine therapies. We challenge this belief and have observed evidence to the contrary. Once arthrodesis has occurred, the normal function of the joint is lost. The distal joints are responsible for the dissipation of the twisting or torsional forces and shear stress in that area. With this capability gone, these forces are concentrated, and stress fracture of the central or the third tarsal bones may occur or OA of the talocalcaneal-centroquartal (proximal intertarsal) joint may develop (RPB, SJD).

Treatment of horses with distal hock joint pain varies. Intraarticular injections of corticosteroids (20 to 40 mg methylprednisolone acetate, up to 10 mg triamcinolone acetonide, or 5 to 7.5 mg betamethasone in each joint) and hyaluronan (2 mL per joint) is usually the first treatment, combined with NSAIDs, and is usually the best and most expeditious means of treatment. With radiological evidence of severe OA we use a long-acting corticosteroid alone. Treating horses with more mildly affected joints with a low corticosteroid dose in combination with hyaluronan may be chondroprotective and extend the useful life span of the joint. Combined therapies have grown popular because of the perception that they work better and the effects last longer. Most horses respond favorably, and the riders comment on how much better the horse performs. Many horses, especially those with demanding show schedules, have the hocks (and perhaps other joints also) routinely injected at intervals predetermined by the history of when the horse previously became unsound after previous injections. Maintenance treatment is performed about 1 month earlier. This reduces the risks of loss of performance, recurrent lameness, or development of a secondary problem. However, we strongly advocate that horses should undergo periodic clinical reappraisal to determine the current cause or causes of suboptimal performance or lameness. Recurrent apparent hock pain should lead to investigation of other causes of lameness such as caudal back pain and PSD.

Many horses also are treated with oral nutraceuticals, parenterally administered PSGAGs, and intravenously administered hyaluronan. These products are incorporated into a maintenance program designed to keep the horse comfortable and prolong the interval between intraarticular joint injections. Frequently the large size of these horses means that they are treated with twice the normal dose of PSGAGs. Horses often are treated with intramuscularly administered PSGAGs and intravenously administered hyaluronan the evening before competition. Occasionally, horses with joints unresponsive to corticosteroids and hyaluronan do respond to intraarticularly administered PSGAGs, with or without corticosteroids. Once the horse has been made more comfortable, an exercise program consistent in intensity and duration, emphasizing strengthening the hindquarters and abdominal muscles, improves performance. Shock wave therapy has been effective in controlling the pain associated with severe OA of the distal tarsal joints. In addition, intravenous tiludronate has proven beneficial in some horses. Shoeing is aimed at encouraging breakover in the center of the hoof by squaring the toe. Alternative therapies such as muscle massage and acupuncture are used commonly with traditional therapies.

Suspensory Desmitis

Injury to the SL is the most common soft tissue injury and certainly one of the most serious injuries of jumping horses. Early lesions may go unnoticed by even the most skilled horseman, because the rider or trainer is aware of only a vague problem that the horse warms out of fairly quickly. With bilateral hindlimb injury the rider may complain of loss of power. Exercise continues, and the injury eventually worsens to the point of causing enough damage to produce obvious lameness. With forelimb injury the lameness usually is more pronounced when the horse is trotted in a circle with the affected limb on the outside and also may be exacerbated in soft footing. With hindlimb injury lameness may be worse with the lame(r) limb on either the inside or the outside of a circle. Midbody and branch lesions are diagnosed easily by palpation; however, diagnosis of PSD is more challenging. The distal limb flexion test may be resented and substantially increase the lameness in horses with midbody and branch lesions, whereas carpal flexion and upper hindlimb flexion frequently accentuate lameness associated with PSD, which can cause confusion with hock pain. Perhaps injuries to the distal aspect of the branches and at the insertion onto the proximal sesamoid bones (PSBs) may lead to fetlock joint instability. Careful examination of the distal aspect of the ipsilateral splint bone should be performed in horses with chronic desmitis of the branches or distal aspect of the body. A high palmar metacarpal nerve block, direct infiltration of the SL origin, or analgesia of the lateral palmar nerve eliminates lameness in the forelimb. Analgesia of the proximal aspect of the hindlimb SL requires caution, because injury to both the veterinarian and the horse can occur. Analgesia is best performed with the horse restrained with a twitch and the leg positioned in the veterinarian's lap as if the horse's foot were being examined. Displacing the digital flexor tendons medially and isolating the SL for injection is thus easier. The SL is infiltrated with local anesthetic solution from the axial aspect of the lateral splint bone, fanning across the SL from lateral to medial. During injection, the local anesthetic solution should go in with considerable resistance if it is being deposited within the SL itself. Another technique involves having an assistant hold the limb in a similar fashion and making an injection medially 1.5 cm distal to the chestnut along the axial margin of the DDFT in a dorsolateral direction. Depositing 3 to 6 mL of local anesthetic solution within the SL can then be accomplished, usually with little objection by the horse. Alternatively, perineural analgesia of the deep branch of the lateral plantar nerve can easily and safely be performed with the limb bearing weight (SJD). With direct infiltration of the ligament, soundness should be almost immediate. Some risk exists of entering the distal palmar outpouchings of the carpometacarpal joint capsule using direct infiltration in the forelimb, causing potential diagnostic confusion; however, infiltration in the hindlimb inadvertently entering the tarsometatarsal joint is less likely. With hindlimb injury there may be associated pain in the sacroiliac joint region.

Ultrasonographic examination of the SL may reveal obvious lesions; however, finding minimal evidence of damage in horses with acute injuries is not uncommon. Recent nerve blocks may confuse interpretation, so ultrasonographic examination is best delayed for 1 to 2 days. Alternatively, ultrasonographic examination may precede nerve blocks. In our opinion, ultrasonographic imaging of the proximal SL in the hindlimb is difficult. The transducer should be placed on the plantaromedial aspect of the limb to get the best-quality images A cross-sectional area of greater than 1.5 cm^2 suggests PSD, even in the absence of a focal or diffuse loss of echogenicity. Comparison with the contralateral hindlimb is essential.

Radiographic examination of the proximal aspect of the third metacarpal bone (McIII) or third metatarsal bone (MtIII) may demonstrate increased radiopacity with or without radiolucent defects in a dorsopalmar (dorsoplantar) image or subcortical increased radiopacity in lateromedial images. Incidental radiological changes can be seen in hindlimbs, especially in older horses.

Nuclear scintigraphy has proved useful in characterization and prognosis of some horses with PSD. The pool phase occasionally reveals pooling of radiopharmaceutical in the ligament. A characteristic pattern of IRU is present in the forelimbs and hindlimbs in the bone phase. The lateral image is most important in the forelimb because focal IRU is present on the proximopalmar aspect of the McIII if bone injury accompanies PSD. PSD occurs often without chronic changes in the palmar or plantar cortex of the McIII or the MtIII. Dorsal images of the forelimb are less sensitive than lateral images because the limb is farther away from the gamma camera. In hindlimbs lateral and plantar images have similar sensitivity. The veterinarian should not mistake for a lesion IRU in the proximolateral aspect of the metatarsal region in plantar images, which is a normal finding. Ultrasonographic abnormalities of the SL and abnormal scintigraphic images confirm injury to the bone at the origin of the SL, indicating a complex injury involving two tissue types and adversely affecting the prognosis. IRU in the proximal aspect of the McIII or the MtIII in the absence of detectable ultrasonographic abnormalities may reflect primary osseous injury, which can be confirmed using MRI. MRI has also been useful in the diagnosis of PSD

when the condition is not evident ultrasonographically and for identification of concurrent osseous pathology.

Medical therapy for horses with suspensory desmitis varies. NSAIDs combined with rest and physical therapy have historically been considered the only option, and clients were advised that treatment could take 6 to 12 months. We recommend stall rest for 10 to 14 days after the injury, with twice daily handwalks in an effort to cool the ligament down. Recently, new therapies (adult bone marrow–derived stem cells, growth factors, platelet-rich plasma [PRP], pigs' urinary bladder matrix [A-Cell]) have become available and show early promise; however, long-term follow-up on a large number of horses is required. After the injection the limb is kept bandaged for at least 2 weeks. Phenylbutazone is administered (2 g bid for 4 days and then 1 g bid for 10 days) after the injection. Walking under saddle then is commenced for 20 to 30 minutes once or twice daily for the next 30 days. Follow-up ultrasonographic examinations are performed after 30 days and every 30 to 60 days thereafter. The duration and intensity of exercise gradually are increased based on the ultrasonographic appearance of the SL and the clinical appearance of the horse. Trotting begins once the horse is sound. Some veterinarians in North America recommend an internal blister, using 2% iodine in almond oil infiltrated into the SL. Light exercise is continued immediately after this therapy, with a gradual return to full work. Shoeing should be improved if necessary. In horses with acute PSD with no substantial ultrasonographic changes, local injection of corticosteroids may decrease inflammation and eliminate pain. We use triamcinolone acetonide (12 to 18 mg), betamethasone (30 mg), or isoflupredone acetate. Sarapin (4 mL) also may be added. If there is IRU in the McIII or the MtIII, there is anecdotal evidence that tiludronate may be effective.

Recently a surgical procedure has been reported in which the tight fascia overlying the proximal aspect of a hindlimb SL is transected in order to reduce pressure or in this apparent compartment syndrome. Bone marrow aspirate collected from the sternum then is injected into the area of the injury in an effort to stimulate healing. Early results from this technique appear promising; however, further investigation and long-term follow-up information are needed. Neurectomy of the deep branch of the lateral plantar nerve together with fasciotomy have been used successfully for management of horses with hindlimb PSD, with approximately 70% of horses returning to long-term full athletic function (SJD). Osteostixis of the proximal plantar aspect of the MtIII may also help with some horses with chronic injuries with radiological abnormalities but is invasive and has yet to be shown effective in a large number of horses.

Shock wave therapy has been used successfully to treat suspensory desmitis of the origin, body, and branches, especially in horses with bone involvement at the origin. This technique provides profound analgesia and therefore may decrease or even eliminate the lameness.

Horses with larger lesions within the body of the SL or its branches may benefit from splitting alone. This appears to allow a more complete healing of core lesions, which otherwise may be slow to resolve.

Therapeutic ultrasound or infrared laser therapy may aid and reportedly speed healing, although evidence is mainly anecdotal.

Shoeing should be directed at supporting the toe and preventing it from sinking deeper into the ground surface than the heel on weight bearing. If this happens, the heel is elevated, the fetlock drops, and strain is applied to the suspensory apparatus. A shoe with a wide toe is commercially available and helps to prevent the toe from sinking.

Selection of the footing during the convalescent period and when work is resumed is vital, together with careful modification of the training program.

Back Pain

Back pain is common in jumpers, and although signs are recognized easily, the etiological diagnosis may be elusive and complex. The trainer or owner may perceive that a horse has back pain from many clinical signs including sensitivity to grooming and saddling, resistance to rider weight, overall body stiffness, poor performance, and pain on palpation of the muscles over the back. Careful examination of the horse under saddle and over fences and a good working relationship with professional riders can be of great help in interpreting and localizing the type of back pain. Many clinical signs are also common to other diseases or injuries and may be secondary to clinical or subclinical hindlimb lameness resulting in or from an altered gait. Primary back pain may be caused by muscle strain, impingement or overriding of the spinous processes, diskospondylosis, sacroiliac desmitis, supraspinous desmitis, OA of the synovial intervertebral articulations (facet joints), and sacroiliac joint pain.

The veterinarian should first attempt to rule out any lameness. Horses with distal hock joint, stifle, or gluteal muscle pain may swing the hindlimb outward away from the body or inward toward the midline in an attempt to reduce the degree of joint flexion required to advance the limb. Hindlimb lameness should be suspected in horses with simultaneous gluteal and back pain. Horses with bilateral hindlimb PSD may hold the back stiffly and mimic a horse with primary back pain. Chronic forelimb soreness, particularly involving the foot, also may contribute to cervical and/or thoracic pain because of an inverted way of jumping that somewhat protects the foot on landing. Teeth problems or neck pain also should be considered.

Severe back pain suggests a primary back problem. The horse may move with a shortened, stiff gait and appear to be flat or hollowed out in the back when ridden but appear much more comfortable when moving free in a paddock or on the lunge. Injection of local anesthetic solution into the painful areas of the back may change the horse's movement.

Impinging Spinous Processes

Radiology of the thoracolumbar spinous processes may reveal impingement with increased radiopacity, bone proliferation, and radiolucent defects. Nuclear scintigraphy can be used to diagnose and support the diagnosis of spinous process impingement and osteitis, although false-negative results are sometimes obtained. Occasionally, areas of IRU are visible in the spinous processes without any radiological changes, and supraspinous ligament desmitis should be considered.

The treatment for impingement of the spinous processes or supraspinous desmitis is similar. NSAIDs and methocarbamol are prescribed routinely for a prolonged period. Sarapin and corticosteroids frequently are injected between and around the impinging spinous processes. The locations for injection are determined best by placing a radiodense marker on the top of the back during radiography and then identifying the affected vertebrae by clipping the hair. Mesotherapy may be useful: small doses of flumethasone, lignocaine, Traumeel (a homeopathic remedy), and normal saline are delivered intradermally with 0.4- to 0.6-cm 27-gauge needles on a multiport injection rack. Numerous rows of skin blebs are formed after the injections, and pain relief is almost immediate. Shock wave therapy is also helpful.

Muscle Injury and Pain

Acute muscle strain may be accompanied by spasm, which is evident as a firm, painful swelling. Palpation of the psoas and lumbar muscles can also be performed transrectally, and pressure may also be applied to the caudal and ventral sciatic nerve roots as well. Immediate application of ice and administration of NSAIDs such as phenylbutazone or naproxen are beneficial One author (RPB) also administers 20 to 40 mg of dexamethasone once daily for 2 days in horses with acute pain. Later, moist heat and therapeutic ultrasound reduce pain and inflammation. Local treatment with mesotherapy is useful when treating back muscle pain. Acupuncture has proved useful in managing horses with back pain no matter what the cause. Chiropractic manipulation may be of some benefit in relieving pain and muscle spasm. Pulsating magnetic field therapy is used routinely in show jumpers for the long-term management of back pain. Shock wave therapy has also been used successfully to treat and manage jumpers with back muscle pain.

Saddle fit always should be evaluated critically in a horse with chronic or recurrent back pain, and thermography may be helpful, together with advice available through most good saddle manufacturers.

Fracture of the Withers

Fracture of the withers is not uncommon if a horse flips over backward. The withers area may appear flat and is extremely painful to palpation. The horse plaits in front and holds the neck stiffly. Radiographs are diagnostic. Treatment is directed toward reducing pain and inflammation by applying ice and administering NSAIDs immediately after the injury. Bone sequestrae occasionally develop, and purulent drainage may appear weeks after the injury. However, most fractures are uncomplicated, and horses usually may be able to return to work after 6 to 12 months.

Sacroiliac Joint Pain

Sacroiliac strain is common in show jumpers. Many horses have chronic low-grade pain that never seems adversely to affect the ability to perform. With severe pain a horse may stand parked out (the hindlimbs are extended unusually) and rest one hindlimb. Unilateral lameness may develop, and the horse's performance then is affected severely. The horse may experience pain on palpation around the lumbosacral region and directly over the tubera sacrale, but this is not specific. Exerting pressure on one of the tubera sacrale may reveal slight motion and even may be resented by the horse. The horse may offer considerable resistance when one of the hind feet is picked up and the limb is flexed high. Rocking the pelvis may cause the horse to grunt. Injection of local anesthetic solution deep into the muscles directed toward the sacroiliac articulations should be performed with caution because the horse may lose its ability to stand. Transrectal ultrasonographic examination may reveal irregular margins of the caudal aspect of the sacroiliac joint and may be useful to support a clinical diagnosis. Evaluation of the ventral sacral nerve roots and the lumbosacral joints may be useful. Nuclear scintigraphy may reveal little if any IRU in this region and is therefore unreliable, but with modern motion-correction software and improved image quality, useful information is acquired in some horses (SJD).

Rest and time are the most important factors influencing the outcome. Horses lame from acute sacroiliac strain may require at least 6 months to heal. Severely affected horses should be given stall rest for 30 days, followed by 2 to 3 months of controlled paddock rest. Light exercise then may begin, gradually increasing the intensity and duration of the work. In our experience, acupuncture has been extremely useful for pain management and the treatment of muscle spasm.

Horses with less severe injuries may be managed successfully by local injections of corticosteroids and Sarapin deep into the painful areas. These horses are able to continue to exercise and compete successfully. The procedure involves directing a 15- to 25-cm needle from a point just medial to one of the tubera sacrale along the inner surface of the ilium deep toward the sacroiliac articulation or using ultrasound guidance and approaching the sacroiliac joint from a cranial dorsal ipsilateral aspect and a caudal dorsal route to treat both sides of the horse. One author (RPB) prefers to use all three approaches on each side. A combination of corticosteroids and Sarapin is injected; however, some practitioners have reported good results with IRAP and bone marrow aspirate as well. Deep injections from either side of midline to the transverse processes of the caudal lumbar vertebrae also help. For 2 weeks after treatment, the rider is cautioned not to collect the horse or perform aggressive lateral movements. Proper and careful rehabilitation is paramount to avoiding recurrence of the problem. Horses with sacroiliac disease are more predisposed to injury when competing at indoor shows, performing high jumps with tight turns.

Injection of the acupuncture points on either side of or parallel to the sacrum with the same solution also may be performed. Chiropractic manipulation often is attempted in horses with sacroiliac injury. Although chiropractic has proved useful as a diagnostic tool and may be of benefit with mild sacroiliac strain, manipulation of the sacrum in horses with more severe injuries never replaces the need for prolonged rest. Pulsating magnetic field therapy, cold laser, and therapeutic ultrasound may be used for the long-term management of chronic sacroiliac problems.

Osteoarthritis of the Thoracolumbar Synovial Intervertebral (Facet) Joints

OA of the synovial intervertebral (facet) joints may be contributing to thoracolumbar region pain, and diagnosis is by radiography and ultrasonography. Ultrasound-guided periarticular injections through the fascia of the multifidus muscle may be of benefit. Careful and progressive warm-up exercises are important.

Fetlock Joint

Synovitis and Osteoarthritis

Metacarpophalangeal or metatarsophalangeal joint synovitis and OA are common in older horses with lengthy careers. Chronic capsulitis results in a thickened, prominent joint capsule with a dramatic decrease in the flexibility of the joint. At least a moderate amount of joint effusion occurs, but many sound horses may have chronic effusion, thickening of the joint capsule, and reduced range of motion. The source of pain is confirmed by a low four-point palmar or plantar nerve block or intraarticular analgesia.

Radiological examination may reveal osteophyte formation on the proximal aspects of the proximal phalanx and the PSBs and flattening of the sagittal ridge of the McIII or the MtIII. The McIII or the MtIII may have a scalloped appearance on the dorsal or palmar/plantar aspect in horses with advanced OA. Subchondral radiolucent areas may develop in the McIII or the MtIII or the proximal phalanx and may result from severe, focal trauma or end-stage OA. The prognosis for horses to return to athletic competition after the development of these lesions is considered poor. Acute fractures and small chips are uncommon in hunters and show jumpers. Small, round, smooth fragments on the proximodorsal aspect of the proximal phalanx are seen in forelimbs and hindlimbs. These fragments represent osteochondrosis and are rarely associated with lameness but occasionally may become unstable and require removal.

Nuclear scintigraphy may reveal mild-to-moderate IRU in the distal, dorsal aspect of the McIII or the MtIII, the proximodorsal aspect of the proximal phalanx, or both. In some horses flexed lateral images are required to separate the bones, especially if IRU in one area is so intense that identifying the adjacent structures is impossible.

In the absence of substantial radiological abnormalities, medical therapy should include NSAIDs, intraarticularly administered corticosteroids and hyaluronan, and orally and parenterally administered PSGAGs. Horses with chronic OA or those difficult to manage may benefit from regular treatment with IRAP. Physical therapies such as icing, cool water therapy, poultices, sweats, cold laser, therapeutic ultrasound, support wraps, and rest are also beneficial. Arthroscopic exploration of the metacarpophalangeal joint is indicated if the response to medical treatment is transient or poor. Clients should be advised that although the causal problem may be revealed, treatment may not be possible. Debridement of damaged cartilage and subsequent replacement with fibrocartilage may be curative; however, excessive erosion of the articular cartilage warrants a poor prognosis for continued jumping.

Therapeutic shoeing targeted at providing support to the palmar aspect of the foot, such as a wide-web shoe, may be of benefit (RDM, RPB). One author prefers an aluminum shoe with short branches, which decreases extension of the fetlock, especially when the horse is landing (PHB). Proper medial-to-lateral hoof balance is also important in reducing torque on the metacarpophalangeal joint.

Sesamoiditis

Sesamoiditis frequently is associated with chronic suspensory branch desmitis. Horses are variably lame and may warm out of the lameness. The distal limb flexion test usually is resented and results in increased lameness. The suspensory branches may be palpably thickened and painful. Intraarticular analgesia of the metacarpophalangeal or metatarsophalangeal joint may improve lameness but does not alleviate it. Lameness is abolished by a low four-point palmar/plantar nerve block.

Abnormal radiological findings include linear lucent zones or lytic areas within the body of the PSB. A generalized loss of bone opacity or proliferative, reactive bone also may be present on the abaxial margins in association with suspensory branch desmitis and insertional lesions of the SL and palmar/plantar annular ligament. We find proximodistal oblique images of the PSBs useful.

Nuclear scintigraphy is sensitive to inflammation in the PSBs, and IRU in the PSBs often is intense. A flexed lateral image helps to separate the PSBs from the McIII or the MtIII. Dorsal or plantar images are required to distinguish between the medial and lateral PSBs.

Treatment for horses with sesamoiditis includes rest, NSAIDs, and supportive shoeing similar to that prescribed for fetlock joint problems. Shock wave therapy may be helpful.

Stifle Joint Pain

Problems involving the stifle joint are common in show jumpers and frequently accompany problems in the tarsus. Joint effusion is present variably. Stifle pain may be primary and related to trauma, mechanical problems, developmental diseases, and OA, or it may be secondary to other lameness. Primary problems include OA, osteochondrosis, meniscal and cruciate ligament trauma, upward fixation or delayed release of the patella, and patellar desmitis. Signs may be subtle at first, with mild shortening of the stride or switching leads at the canter or gallop. Caudal back pain also may be present. The proximal or upper limb flexion test may or may not have a positive result, and the veterinarian should look closely for subtle gait changes such as a shortening of the cranial phase of the stride. Separation of stifle and tarsal pain may be accomplished by flexing the stifle with the hock slightly extended so that the metatarsal region is held behind the tail and perpendicular to the ground, with the tibia held parallel to the ground. The Churchill test also may help to separate hock from stifle pain. Cranial to caudal motion of the tibia relative to the femur during weight bearing (cruciate test) may produce a change in stride; however, it is not routinely performed and has been replaced by abducting and adducting the limb in an attempt to stress the stifle (RDM). However, intraarticular analgesia always is required to confirm the source of pain.

Horses with straight stifle conformation are predisposed to upward fixation and instability of the patella. Pain results from subsequent patellar ligament strain and synovitis. Although the limb may be observed to lock in extension, more frequently a slight hesitation in the advancement of the limb is noted. Femoropatellar effusion may be present. Ultrasonographic examination of the patellar ligaments may reveal desmitis characterized by enlargement and a focal or diffuse hypoechogenic region. Horses with transient upward fixation of the patella benefit from NSAIDs and an increased exercise program designed to increase muscle tone in the quadriceps group, which stabilizes the patella. Failure to respond to these measures may justify a more aggressive procedure, such as local injection of 2% iodine in almond oil at the proximal aspect, middle portion, and insertions of all three patellar ligaments and into the muscle just proximal to the stifle. This procedure has proved effective in treating transient upward fixation of the patella and subtle soreness in the adjacent muscles. A "splitting" (desmoplasty) of the medial patellar ligament may be performed in horses with more severe upward fixation of the patella. This induces desmitis of the ligament and subsequent thickening. Anecdotal reports describe benefit from estrone sulfate, estradiol, and calcium channel blockers. Jumpers with primary patellar ligament injuries require rest.

Cranial Cruciate Ligament and Meniscal Injury

Trauma to the cranial cruciate ligament produces profound lameness. Intraarticular analgesia of the femorotibial joints may or may not abolish the lameness, and radiographs of the stifle may be normal in horses with an acute injury. With chronic injury new bone may be seen cranial to the intercondylar eminences, most obvious in a flexed lateromedial image. Injury to the medial meniscus is most common. Intraarticular analgesia of the femorotibial joint on the affected side usually produces improvement in the lameness. Radiographs may reveal osteophyte formation on the proximomedial aspect of the tibial plateau indicative of OA and a subjective decrease in the joint space width on the affected side.

Ultrasonographic examination of the stifle is routinely performed and enables assessment of parts of the medial and lateral menisci, the cranial meniscal ligaments, the articular surfaces of the medial and lateral condyles and trochlear ridges, the medial and lateral collateral ligaments, the patellar ligaments, and the tendons originating from the femur and tibia. The presence of joint effusion can also be assessed. Evaluation of the cranial cruciate ligament is challenging.

Osteochondrosis and Subchondral Bone Cysts

Osteochondrosis and subchondral bone cysts should be considered in a young Warmblood that has recently started training or increased its training intensity and has developed lameness localized to the stifle. Intraarticular analgesia usually at least partially eliminates the lameness. We recommend blocking all three joint spaces.

Radiographs are usually diagnostic. Arthroscopy may be indicated. Horses with subchondral bone cysts and other lesions in the medial femoral condyle usually have a poorer prognosis than those with osteochondrosis of the lateral trochlear ridge of the femur. We recommend radiography of the stifles as part of the routine radiographic study when a young Warmblood is examined for purchase.

Nuclear scintigraphy of the stifle in horses with osteochondrosis may reveal little if any IRU. Both caudal and lateral images should be obtained. IRU (to any degree) in the medial femoral condyle in a caudal image almost always is associated with a pathological condition (RPB).

Synovitis and Osteoarthritis

Mature horses may develop synovitis and OA of any one or a combination of the stifle joints. Often the femoropatellar and medial femorotibial joints are involved; however, lateral femorotibial OA may occur alone. Intraarticular analgesia of all three joints should be performed.

The diagnosis may or may not be confirmed radiologically. Osteophyte formation on the proximal medial aspect of the tibia is not uncommon. Nuclear scintigraphy may reveal mild-to-moderate IRU in the femoral condyle and the opposing surface of the tibia on the affected side in a caudal image. Ultrasonographic examination often reveals mild soft tissue inflammation and may be more sensitive than radiography for identification of periarticular osteophytes.

Intraarticular injection of corticosteroids and hyaluronan usually has favorable results. Each joint should be injected separately with double doses of a high-molecular-weight hyaluronan combined with methylprednisolone acetate (40 to 80 mg) or betamethasone (5 to 10 mg). In many horses treatment of the medial femorotibial joint alone is successful (RDM, SJD). NSAIDs, parenterally administered PSGAGs, and intravenously administered hyaluronan are also beneficial and may be used routinely with nutraceuticals as part of a maintenance program. Adequate rest also should be prescribed; however, strict stall confinement is usually not appropriate. Walking these horses under saddle for 30 minutes once or twice daily is preferred. Alternative therapies such as those described for distal tarsitis are also beneficial. Acupuncture commonly is used for managing horses with stifle pain. Recurrent synovitis of a stifle that has been injected repeatedly is suggestive of a more serious injury such as meniscal damage causing some degree of joint instability; therefore, prolonged rest or exploratory arthroscopy should be considered.

Pastern

The pastern region is subject to considerable stress in the jumping horse. OA of the PIP joint is not uncommon and often is associated with OA of the DIP joint. Horses with base-narrow or toe-in conformational defects are affected most frequently. Distal sesamoidean desmitis is also a common problem. Trainers complain that many horses with OA of the PIP joint start out stiff when training and feel much better after warming up, but eventually the lameness becomes persistent. With chronic injury comes obvious thickening in the distal aspect of the pastern. Palmar (abaxial sesamoid) nerve blocks normally eliminate the lameness, although a low palmar (four-point) block sometimes is required. Intraarticular analgesia of the PIP joint also usually produces soundness. The veterinarian must beware that a palmar digital nerve block may alleviate lameness associated with OA of the PIP joint because of proximal diffusion of the local anesthetic solution and the distal palmar extension of the joint capsule.

There is usually greater RU in the subchondral bone of the PIP joints of sound jumping horses relative to other joints. With OA the intensity of the IRU usually increases. We (RPB, RDM) therefore believe that subclinical OA of the PIP joint is common. Radiological changes in horses with OA of the PIP joint include osteophyte formation on the proximodorsal aspect of the middle phalanx. Subchondral osseous cystlike lesions in the proximal aspect of the middle phalanx may be associated with severe trauma or end-stage OA. Acquired osseous cystlike lesions usually are associated with focal, intense IRU.

Management of horses with OA of the PIP joint includes using NSAIDs, intraarticularly administered corticosteroids and hyaluronan, and orally and parenterally administered PSGAGs. The horse should be trimmed and shod to reduce resistance to breakover at the toe and to balance the foot to land as flatly as possible. Occasionally, wedge pads provide comfort by opening up the dorsal aspect of the joint space. Shock wave therapy has been of benefit to horses with advanced ringbone and may be combined with intraarticular injection. Horses with severe OA of the PIP joint may respond poorly to medical management, and arthrodesis may be required. Arthrodesis is often successful in the hindlimbs of jumping horses, but results are often unsatisfactory in forelimbs. Tibial neurectomy also has been used successfully.

Soft Tissue Injury

Injury to the distal sesamoidean ligaments may or may not be accompanied by obvious swelling or pain on palpation. The oblique sesamoidean ligaments are most commonly affected, but jumpers with this injury have a better prognosis than those with injuries to the straight sesamoidean ligament. Analgesia of the palmar (abaxial sesamoid) nerves usually eliminates the lameness. Ultrasonographic examination reveals focal or diffuse hypoechogenic regions in the affected ligament. Palmar or plantar displacement of the DDFT medially or laterally may be secondary to distal sesamoidean ligament injury. The veterinarian should image all structures carefully in the pastern, because several structures may be injured simultaneously. DDFT injuries are more common in the pastern than in the metacarpal region (Figure 115-4). Chronic strain at the insertion of the oblique sesamoidean ligaments may be evident radiologically as enthesophyte formation on the palmar or plantar lateral and medial borders of the proximal phalanx.

Horses with strains and tears of the distal sesamoidean ligaments usually respond to supportive shoeing, NSAIDs, and rest. Horses with acutely torn ligaments may benefit from cast or splint application for about 1 month. Physical therapy such as therapeutic ultrasound may speed recovery. Shock wave therapy is routinely used to treat horses with injuries to the soft tissue structures in the palmar or plantar aspect of the pastern. Regenerative therapies such as those previously mentioned for the treatment of suspensory desmitis may also be of benefit. Injury to these ligaments usually requires 6 to 12 months for convalescence. Returning the horse to work too soon results in thickening and fibrosis of the pastern and prolonged lameness.

Croup and Hip Region Pain

Strain and inflammation of the gluteal muscles are common in jumping horses and sometimes result from an altered gait secondary to lameness elsewhere in the ipsilateral or contralateral hindlimb. Primary strain may occur in a horse during jumping, when a horse refuses a jump, or after a fall. Palpation of the gluteal muscles at the insertion on the greater trochanter and third trochanter of the femur and over the middle gluteal region reveals milder reactivity in horses with secondary strains and a much more severe response or resentment after a primary muscle injury. Upper limb flexion tests may be positive, especially if the gluteal soreness is secondary to lameness involving the hock or stifle. Ultrasonographic examination of the

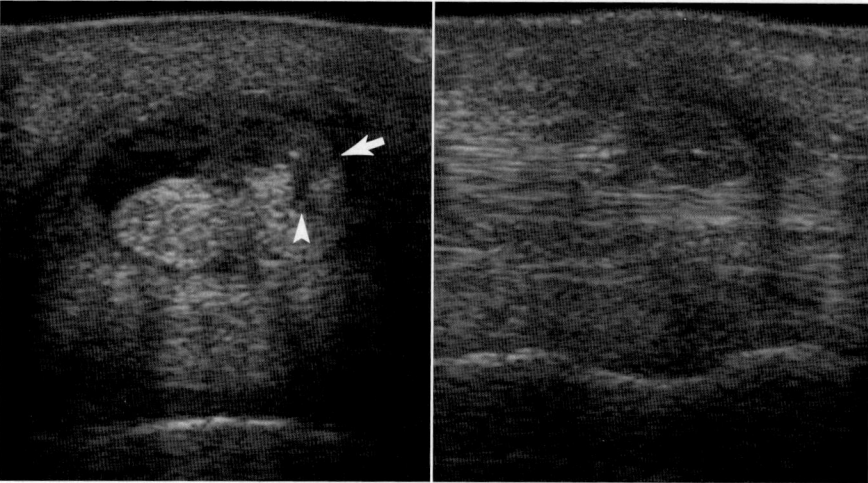

Fig. 115-4 • Transverse (left) and longitudinal (right) ultrasonographic images of the palmar aspect of the pastern. Lateral is to the right and distal is to the right. There is an abnormal amount of fluid in the digital flexor tendon sheath. The lateral lobe of the deep digital flexor tendon (DDFT) is enlarged (arrow) with disruption of the palmar border and echogenic material palmar to this. There is a vertically orientated hypoechogenic defect extending across the lateral lobe of the DDFT seen in the transverse image (arrowhead).

coxofemoral joint may rarely reveal increased fluid indicative of effusion, the result of synovitis or OA. Nuclear scintigraphy may support that diagnosis with IRU in dorsal or oblique images of the coxofemoral joint.

Treatment depends on the severity of the muscle injury or inflammation. Identification and appropriate treatment of the primary lower limb lameness, if present, may do much to reduce mild soreness in just a few days. Most horses with mild injury also respond well to NSAIDs, local application of moist heat, dimethyl sulfoxide, and therapeutic ultrasound. Methocarbamol (20 mg/kg orally bid) may be of benefit. Acupuncture treatments, and in horses with severe injuries local injection of corticosteroids mixed with Sarapin (mix Sarapin, prednisolone, and betamethasone in equal parts in a 12-mL syringe and inject 3 mL per site), provide pain relief. Injections are performed on either side of the spine into the sorest portions of the muscle at 5- to 8-cm intervals or at specific acupuncture sites. Injections may also be made around the region of the greater trochanter of the femur. Ultrasound-guided injection into the coxofemoral joint when synovitis or OA is suspected is recommended. Rest and a reduction in the intensity and duration of exercise also may help. Some horses may require total rest, with exercise limited to handwalking, for several weeks.

Superficial Digital Flexor Tendonitis, Tenosynovitis of the Digital Flexor Tendon Sheath, and Desmitis of the Accessory Ligament of the Deep Digital Flexor Tendon

Superficial Digital Flexor Tendonitis

Injury to the superficial digital flexor tendon (SDFT) in a hunter or jumper is far less common and severe than in a racehorse, probably because the horse is not trained at high speeds. Injuries are more likely to result from a misstep in deep footing rather than from muscle or tendon fatigue proceeding to failure, but low-grade injuries occur frequently in top-level horses from about 10 years of age.

Recurrent injuries to the SDFT and ALDDFT may occur in association with foot pain, which changes the biomechanical stress on the digital flexor tendons (PHB). Spontaneous rupture of the SDFT also is seen in old (midteens) jumpers. Often no indication of any tendonitis is apparent before rupture. We also have seen several aged horses no longer in competition with spontaneous SDFT rupture. Geldings are overrepresented, and there may be an association between this severe trauma and hormonal imbalance.

The diagnosis of SDF tendonitis is normally not difficult, and unlike injury to the DDFT usually is not accompanied by substantial lameness, unless an acute injury occurs in the proximal metacarpal region. Lesions in the proximal metacarpal region may be a diagnostic challenge because of lack of swelling. Ultrasonographic evaluation is recommended to assess the severity, location, and extent of the injury. Several reexaminations are important to determine the rate of healing and predict the time to return the horse safely to competition.

The therapeutic goals for management of a hunter or jumper with an acutely injured digital flexor tendon are rapid reduction of the inflammatory response and elimination of edema. This is achieved with the administration of NSAIDs, low doses of corticosteroids, and diuretics. Ice, hydrotherapy, and support bandages also are used and applied as soon as possible, and often the trainer applies them before the veterinary examination. For horses with strains or injury without actual fiber tearing (type 1 or 2 lesions), peritendonous injection of corticosteroids or intralesional injection of hyaluronan may dramatically decrease the size of the tendon and produce favorable cosmetic results. The trainer must be advised not to exercise the horse and that total healing actually may be delayed slightly. After the injection the limb should be supported with a firm, modified Robert Jones bandage to prevent the return of any swelling. Tendon splitting has been indicated in horses with substantial core lesions (type 3 or 4 with a diameter greater than 0.5 cm). Ultrasound-guided intralesional injections of IRAP, PRP, or A-Cell may be of benefit for lesions of this type and severity. The benefit of a splitting is obtained with the multiple injections required to deliver an adequate volume of product. During the procedure the material is seen going into and coming out of the tendon and causing peritendonous or subcutaneous swelling. Perhaps this produces a "lavaging" effect and removes some of the blood, serum, and inflammatory mediators from the core lesion. It is one author's opinion that this lavaging effect is actually beneficial and that larger volumes of fluid should be used when possible (RPB). Therapeutic ultrasound after the initial phase of healing (3 to 4 weeks after injury) encourages resolution of inflammation and promotes healing. Shock wave therapy is also sometimes recommended after the injection; there is debate about frequency and intensity of treatment.

Overall, the time required for digital flexor tendons to heal sufficiently so the horse may return to jumping depends on the severity of the injury and to some degree the location of the injury. Routine SDF tendonitis takes less time to heal than an injury to the SL at the same location. A mild injury takes 3 to 4 months and a severe injury takes about 12 months to heal. Monthly ultrasonographic examinations are used to determine the physical therapy schedule and the optimum time for the horse to return to jumping. Horses often can continue to compete despite active SDFT injuries, although the lesions may slowly get worse.

Tenosynovitis of the Digital Flexor Tendon Sheath
SDFT or DDFT injury within the digital flexor tendon sheath (DFTS) frequently is seen in jumpers at any age or level of competition (Figure 115-4). Tenosynovitis also occurs without tendon injury. SDF tendonitis may result in chronic tenosynovitis and often plagues older horses. Tenosynovitis is slightly more prevalent in hindlimbs, presumably because of the strain caused by the push-off in jumping. The DFTS may be warm and swollen. Digital pressure at the proximal and distal aspects of the DFTS usually is resented. Pressure applied directly over the palmar or plantar aspect of the fetlock also may cause pain. Results of a distal limb flexion test are usually positive. Moderate effusion is usually present in horses with an acute injury, but those with chronic injuries may have a thickened, fibrotic DFTS and much less fluid. The proximal aspect of the DFTS may show effusion, yet none may occur distally in the pastern. Lack of effusion likely results from a compartment syndrome with thickening of the DFTS synovium, the SDFT, and possibly the palmar/plantar annular ligament, thus preventing the flow of fluid distally past the PSBs. However, DDFT lesions in the pastern may be associated with distention of the DFTS localized to the pastern. DDFT lesions may be core injuries readily identified using ultrasonography or marginal tears more reliably diagnosed using tenoscopy (see Figure 115-4). Lameness may vary and may be evident only after flexion of the distal aspect of the limb. Intrathecal analgesia of the DFTS usually improves lameness. Ultrasonographic examination should include the fetlock and pastern regions and reveals increased fluid, allowing the tendons and a thickened synovium to be evaluated easily. The digital flexor tendons may appear to be normal.

Therapy for horses with tenosynovitis of the DFTS varies depending on the severity of the problem and the structures involved. Antiinflammatory therapy consisting of ice, cool water therapy, poultices, NSAIDs, and corticosteroids is effective in horses with mild primary injuries of the DFTS. In horses with more severe injuries, intrathecal injection of corticosteroids and hyaluronan is beneficial. Rest is essential. Horses with mild injuries may return to work in 1 to 2 weeks, but those with more severe injuries require more time. Good trimming and shoeing are beneficial. Transient response to treatment usually implies associated tendon injury. Horses with chronic, unresponsive tenosynovitis may require tenoscopic examination and possibly desmotomy of the palmar or plantar annular ligament.

Desmitis of the Accessory Ligament of the Deep Digital Flexor Tendons
Desmitis of the ALDDFT is a common problem, especially in older show jumpers, and often results in sudden onset of lameness after landing over a fence, with rapid development of localized swelling. In some horses there is only mild-to-moderate swelling below the carpus on the day after jumping, with minimal to no lameness. Ultrasonography is required to determine the location, severity, and extent of the injury and subsequently to monitor healing. Treatment is similar to that for SDF tendonitis, and rapid and aggressive use of systemic NSAIDS as well as local injection of corticosteroids to control early inflammation is important. A premature return to work may result in recurrent injury and ultimately adhesion formation between the ALDDFT and the SDFT. However, many horses with mild-to-moderate strains can be managed with shortened rest periods and aggressive antiinflammatory therapy. Once inflammation has been controlled, the horse can return to work and may handle a normal workload even without meaningful healing of the injury. This depends on the severity of the injury, in particular the proportion of the cross-sectional area of the ligament affected. As long as pain and swelling are controlled, lameness is controlled and the horse can perform in many instances even without a completely healed ligament (TRO). Shock wave therapy may be useful.

Cervical Osteoarthritis and Pain
Soreness in the cervical region can seriously affect a jumper's performance. OA of the cervical facet joints is common but may not always cause clinical signs. Muscle strain in the cervical region can also occur. Neck pain may be evidenced by an unwillingness to flex the neck laterally or dorsoventrally, by being "hard" on one side of the mouth, or by an overt forelimb lameness, which first may appear as a reluctance to advance the limb. Enticing the horse with a carrot to stretch and flex from side to side may reveal an unwillingness or limited range of motion. There may be pain on palpation. Lameness related to neck pain may appear similar to primary forelimb pain, but it is not abolished using diagnostic analgesia of the lame limb. Shoulder pain may mimic cervical pain, but analgesia of the shoulder joint or bicipital bursa may improve the lameness.

Nuclear scintigraphy is a potential screening method (RPB), but greater radiopharmaceutical uptake is frequently normally seen in the caudal cervical facet joints compared with further cranially (SJD). Comparison of left and right lateral images is crucial (SJD). Lateral and oblique radiographic images are useful for identification of OA, bearing in mind that many horses with radiologically apparent lesions do not have clinical signs (SJD). Ultrasonography may yield additional information about joint effusion and joint capsule thickening.

Ultrasound-guided intraarticular injections of the facet joints can be used both diagnostically and therapeutically.

One author (RPB) routinely injects the affected facet joints and those immediately cranial to and caudal to the suspected joint; however, it is also his experience that regional injection also produces a positive response. Methylprednisolone acetate, 20 mg, is injected as a 3-mL solution in sterile saline at each site.

Chapter 116

Lameness in the Dressage Horse

Svend E. Kold and Sue J. Dyson

THE SPORT

Dressage is the ultimate athletic challenge in equestrian sports because it combines balance, suppleness, and power in a unique gravity-defying manner. A good horse gives the impression of athletic elegance and expressive animation. The gaits are described using terms such as *balance, suppleness,* and *hindlimb activity.* The first demand is that the horse be completely obedient, going wherever the rider wants and carrying out movements at his or her request. In doing so the horse has to rely on its rider, trust the rider, and accept the rider as its superior. The key to the training and development of a dressage horse from the lowest levels to International Grand Prix is gymnastic exercises, with the aim of strengthening the muscles and thereby avoiding injury to joints and tendons associated with an increased workload.

The Fédération Equestre Internationale (FEI) dressage rules state that the object of dressage is the harmonious development of the physique and ability of the horse. Through the levels of dressage training, the center of gravity of the horse and rider is placed further caudally, achieved by increasing the degree of flexion and loading of the hindlimbs, while at the same time freeing the front end of the horse to create a more airborne, uphill set of movements. This can be obtained only by increasing the power of the hindlimbs, by synchrony in movement between the forelimbs and the hindlimbs, and through the freedom of movement of the back.

In the German equestrian literature the following terms describe the aims of the correctly trained dressage horse:
- *Takt* (rhythm)
- *Lossgelassenheit* (looseness and suppleness)
- *Anlehnung* (contact with the bit)
- *Schwung* (energy and swing)
- *Geraderichten* (straightness)
- *Versammlung* (collection)

Dressage is an international sport, although it always has had its main center of excellence in Northern Europe, most particularly Germany, but in later years also in Holland, Denmark, and Sweden. More recently, teams from Spain, the United Kingdom, and the United States have started to challenge for medal positions in international competitions. Dressage developed from the military institutes and only in the twentieth century became a truly civilian sport. Even up to the time of the Second World War, military officers participated at all the major dressage games.

In Europe the competitive sport has been divided into three levels: L, M, and S. L covers novice level (novice and elementary); M covers medium and advanced medium; and S covers Prix St Georges, Intermediare I and II, Grand Prix, and Grand Prix Special. The movements required at each of these levels reflect the horse's degree of collection, with the L classes expressing balance and freedom of movement, M classes requiring more collection and lateral movements, and S classes demanding ultimate collection to enable movements of maximum collection and suspension, such as piaffe, passage (Figure 116-1), and canter pirouettes (Figure 116-2). However, even the most skilled rider or trainer has difficulty selecting the right horses, because many promising young horses with excellent gaits fail to learn passage and piaffe, probably because of our insufficient knowledge of the biokinematics of collection.[1]

Lateral movements apply specific, unique strains to different structures within the skeleton. In shoulder-in, half-pass, renvers, and travers the horse is bent evenly in its neck and body but moves on more than two tracks. In shoulder-in, the horse moves on three tracks (1, outside hindlimb; 2, inside hindlimb and outside forelimb; and 3, inside forelimb) with the body at an ideal angle of 30 degrees to the direction of movement. In travers (quarters-in) and renvers (head to the wall) the horse moves on four tracks. These movements create an unusual strain on the horse's back and pelvis and an additional twisting movement on the appendicular joints.

The increased engagement of the hindlimbs developed through collected work allows for greater storage of elastic strain energy in the hock joints and pelvis, which, via the increased lifting of the forehand, allows for high-energy movements such as medium and extended trot. The term *cadence* is associated closely with working through the back and self-carriage and requires complete freedom without which movements will be inferior. Self-carriage reflects a level of training in which the horse has learned to balance itself and its rider and additionally has developed its musculature to allow movement with greater range of freedom. This process takes time, and it is not unusual to see a degree of hindlimb gait irregularity in 4-year-old horses in the early part of training; normally this is a reflection of lack of balance and will improve with training and time.

Anlehnung (contact with the bit) is an important concept to understand, requiring the horse to move freely forward

Reference on page 1344

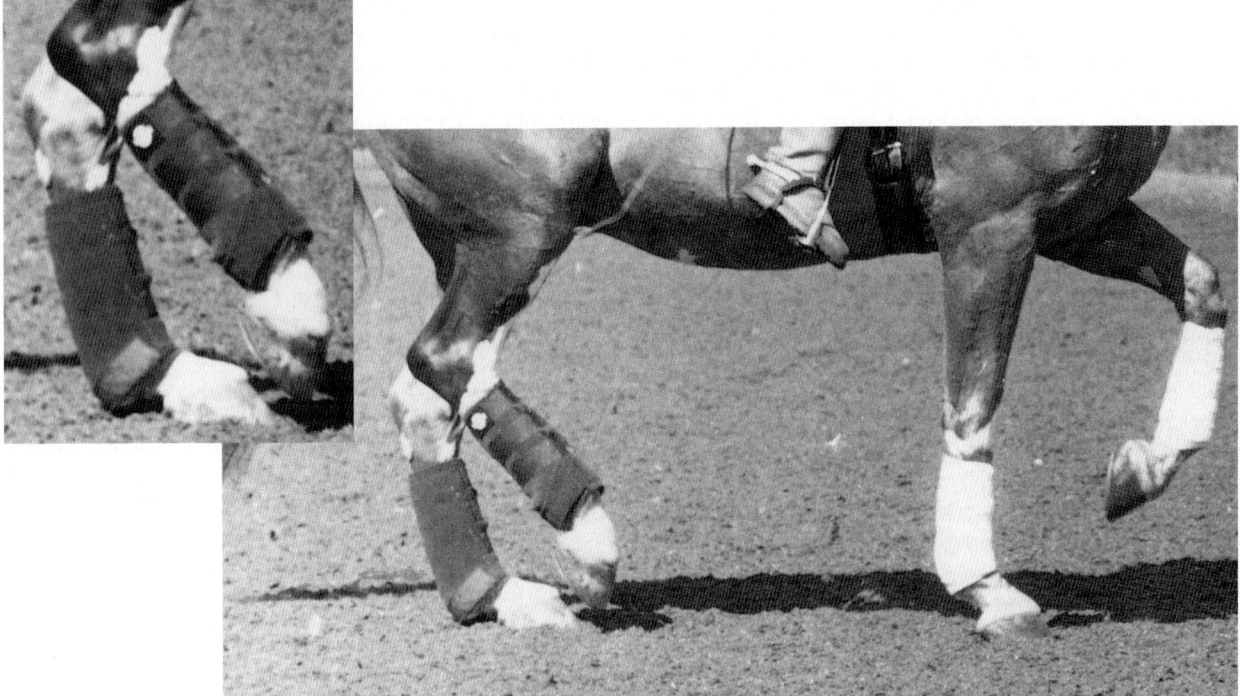

Fig. 116-1 • Passage. Note the severe extension of the left metatarsophalangeal joint *(inset)*.

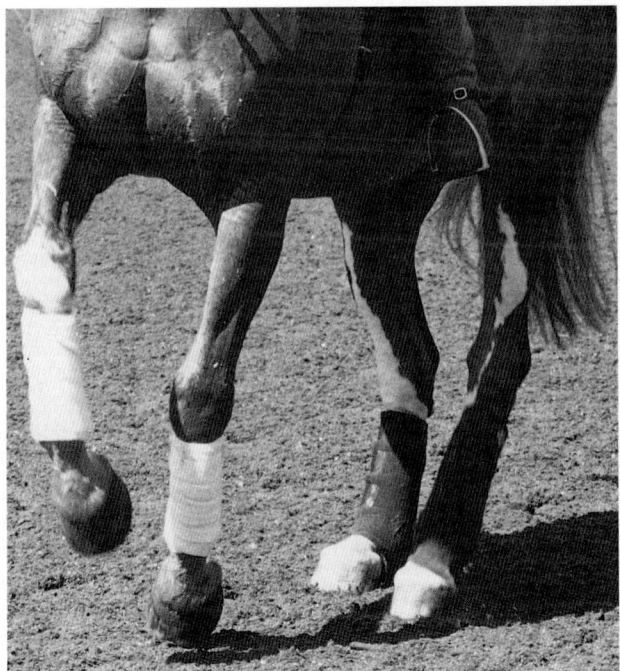

Fig. 116-2 • Canter pirouette to the left. The horse intermittently takes all weight on the hindlimbs, resulting in extension of the metatarsophalangeal joints and great strain on the suspensory apparatus.

with impulsion, to take and accept the bit, and to react to it without resistance. The FEI rules require the horse to work on the bit—that is, with the front of the head positioned in, or slightly in front of, the vertical plane. In recent years the tendency has been toward training dressage horses in an over-bent fashion, with the horse's forehead behind the vertical plane, in its extreme form referred to as *rollkur*. This is said to be a requirement for developing the trapezius and rhomboidius as well as other muscles of the shoulder and withers region and thus enabling a greater lift of the forehand via the shoulder girdle. Although this method of training contradicts the FEI requirement for the horse's forehead to be in a vertical plane, top riders are able to place the horse's head in virtually any position according to what is required. There has been considerable debate about rollkur being a forced and unnatural position; however, to date there is no scientific evidence to suggest that it is in any way detrimental to physical well-being, assuming that it is performed well. Moreover, some of the most successful dressage horses are trained using rollkur as part of the regular work program. However, as with any method of training, it is important that the horse be allowed regular stretching and rest periods to avoid muscular fatigue, which may predispose to injury.

"Contact with the bit" and "working on the bit" are terms that are frequently misunderstood. The horse must move with energy and impulsion and work through the back to enable correct contact with the bit. Stiffness in the back often results in poor and incorrect bit contact. Increased bit lathering as an indication of improved bit function is frequently seen after successful treatment of back pain. Misinterpretation of the role of the bit leads to restriction of the horse by the hands, which inevitably results in loss of action and gait irregularities. Thus inappropriate riding and training can potentially produce clinical problems.

THE DRESSAGE HORSE

Most dressage horses competing internationally are Warmbloods (WBLs) with a high proportion of Thoroughbred (TB) breeding. Dressage horses today combine the elegance and athleticism of the TBs with the power and trainable mind of the WBLs, which have been selected for many generations for these traits. Few pure TBs reach international standard dressage. The TB has been bred to run fast or show courage jumping obstacles cross-country, which are not of great value when the rider requires complete obedience to perform movements that go as much upward and sideways as forward. Most TBs also lack the strength and quality in all three paces compared with the WBLs, in particular the walk and the trot. Most TBs do not show the same degree of natural engagement of the hindlimbs typical of many WBLs. Many of the greatest TB sires in postwar European dressage breeding (Der Löwe, Velten, and Pik As) have been neither particularly physically impressive nor equipped with more than an average trot. Previously TB stallions in WBL breeding were required to have a minimum general handicap to ensure that they had been physically and mentally strong enough to stand up to training and race consistently and reasonably successfully. Spanish horses have increased in popularity, often being easier to train than WBLs, readily learning and executing piaffe and passage, but lacking the expression and animation of the gaits of the most successful WBLs. Lipizzaner horses are rather similar and are used by the Spanish Riding School in Vienna, but are rarely used as competition horses. Mares, geldings, and stallions are used; stallions may combine competition work with breeding (usually by artificial insemination).

A dressage horse must be naturally well balanced. The head and neck must be set sufficiently high to facilitate working uphill and for easy contact with the bit to be made. The shape of the withers region is important, so that the saddle sits easily in the correct position. The dressage rider spends a lot of time sitting in the saddle in sitting trot; therefore correct weight distribution is critical.

Most dressage horses are broken at 3 or 4 years of age and begin competing in young horse classes at 5 years of age. Medium classes are reached by the age of 7 and many future Grand Prix dressage horses do a small tour at the age of 8 and 9. Once a dressage horse has reached Grand Prix level, the training predominantly involves repetition of movements, maintaining suppleness, and increasing physical power. Thus dressage horses rarely succumb to acute stress-induced traumatic injuries but are more likely to succumb to repetitive, accumulative subclinical injuries that may surface at irregular intervals. This means that with correct training and management, dressage horses can continue to compete at the highest level at an advanced age, often as old as 15 to 20 years. Many of the Lipizzaner stallions at the Spanish Riding School in Vienna are touring and performing adequately after 20 years of age.

A true link between conformation and soundness is difficult to establish, because what creates an outstanding dressage horse in terms of conformation does not necessarily create a particularly sound dressage horse, and vice versa. However, in a study of 4-year-old Swedish WBL horses, highly significant correlations were found between conformation and movement and between conformation and orthopedic health, whereas no correlation was found between the overall conformation score and competition performance.[2] A series of elite dressage horses had larger hock joint angles and more sloping shoulders than more average horses, whereas good forelimb movements were

characterized by a large range of flexion of the elbow and carpal joints during the second half of the swing phase. This is what previously has been referred to incorrectly as shoulder freedom. It is important that a young horse naturally places the hindlimbs well underneath itself, because the approach angle does not seem to be influenced by training.[1]

Wear-and-tear lesions frequently occur because of a less-than-ideal joint and limb angulation, but many other factors influence the durability of the horse, including genetic predisposition and management conditions before skeletal maturity. The main requirement must be the ability of the horse to balance itself at all paces, because imbalance and asynchrony in movement apply unusual strains on many structures. Holmström found that a large positive diagonal advanced placement (the time difference between the hindlimb and contralateral forelimb contacting the ground) correlates with high trot scores and suggests this as being an important indicator of the horse's natural balance.[1] The positive diagonal advanced placement does not change with more collection and therefore may become a useful selection criterion. Holmström also found that a group of selected elite horses with high gait scores had significantly larger stride duration, increased hind stance phase duration, and greater diagonal advanced placement than a group of horses with low gait scores.[1] It should be noted, however, that advanced diagonal placement results in a single hindlimb bearing all the horse's weight, with increased extension of the metatarsophalangeal joint and thus increased strain on the suspensory apparatus. Medium and extended trots result in greater extension of the fetlock joints compared with working and collected trots, thus stressing the suspensory apparatus. Many talented young horses that are professionally produced for sale by auction are worked in a much bigger trot than a true working trot, which also results in high loads on the suspensory apparatus, predisposing to injury in all four limbs.

TRAINING SURFACES

Dressage horses are trained predominantly on artificial surfaces with a high degree of cushion, providing a consistency in the training surface not paralleled in other equestrian sports. All dressage competitions in mainland Europe take place on artificial surfaces, and only in England does dressage at the lower levels (L) still take place on grass. A multitude of artificial surfaces have been developed over the last 20 years. Most are based on silica sand mixed with a variety of rubber and polyvinyl chloride material, together with a binding and dust-limiting agent such as Vaseline, which ensures that such surfaces remain dust- and frost-free down to at least −5° C. This standardization of working and competition surfaces unquestionably plays a huge role in the low occurrence of many acute orthopedic problems in the dressage horse. Some trainers, however, consider constant working of repetitive movements on ideal surfaces likely to soften the limb structures and therefore recommend that the horses occasionally be jumped or hacked on less ideal surfaces to provide a stimulus for joint, tendon, and ligament adaptation and generally improve proprioception. We believe that working on a variety of surfaces and "cross training" are helpful for maintaining both musculoskeletal soundness and a correct mental attitude.

Arena maintenance is paramount for a good surface. An effective drainage system through central and perimeter drains is also absolutely essential. Dead corners of deep sand predispose horses to momentary loss of balance and may predispose to the development of lameness. Any sudden change of surface integrity also predisposes horses to lameness. Young horses in particular work more easily and confidently on firmer modern artificial surfaces, where they can obtain a more confident grip and are less likely to fatigue. In a recent questionnaire-based study of British dressage horses the effect of arena surfaces on both lameness and undesirable gait traits such as tripping or slipping was investigated.[3] The results indicated that wax-coated and sand and rubber surfaces were associated with less detrimental surface properties than sand, sand and PVC, woodchip, or grass. Woodchip was most strongly associated with the detrimental characteristic of slipping, and sand with tripping. Findings indicated that any arena surface should have a base, and limestone was recommended, with crushed concrete best avoided. In a related study, work on sand-based arena surfaces resulted in a 1.36 times greater likelihood of having lameness in the previous 2 years compared with other surfaces.[4] However, very regular work on sand appeared to have a protective effect. Regular work on an outside arena resulted in a 0.61 times reduced risk of lameness compared with horses worked in indoor arenas. Deep, patchy, or uneven going under normal conditions and patchy, boggy, or deep surfaces in wet conditions increased the risk of lameness.

TACK

The horse must be comfortable in its tack if it is going to work optimally. Dressage saddles are designed to position the rider with a deep seat and with an extended leg position. The surface area over which the weight is distributed must be as large as possible, to avoid focal pressure points. The use of gel pads and layers of numnahs (saddle pads) is not a substitute for good saddle fit. The saddle must fit the horse and the rider and must position the rider in appropriate balance. The fit must be assessed with and without a rider. The shape of the horse's back musculature may change as the horse develops muscular strength and power; therefore a previously well-fitting saddle may become constricting. It should also be remembered that the withers and back may expand during a training session, sometimes effectively rendering the saddle too small.

Acceptance of the bit is crucial in a dressage horse. Horses vary considerably in the shape of the mouth and the sensitivity of the corners of the lips, bars, and tongue. Great variation also exists in the thickness of the tongue among horses. A slight crack in the corner of the mouth, caused by an inappropriate bit, can cause major problems with proper acceptance of the bit and the horse's willingness to work straight. At S level, horses have to compete wearing a double bridle—that is, the mouth has to accommodate both bradoon (snaffle) and curb bits. These vary greatly in shape and design, and selection of the most appropriate can be critical.

LAMENESS EXAMINATION

Examining a lame dressage horse does not differ in any great detail from examining any other equine athlete. However, examination frequently requires spending more time observing the horse being ridden, because many dressage horses reproduce the perceived problem, often no more than a resistance, only when ridden and sometimes only during certain movements. This, however, does not mean that the horse should not be examined in hand, including walking and trotting on a straight line and lunging on hard, nonslip surfaces (such as gravel) and on softer artificial surfaces. Not only does lunging on tarmac or concrete carry the risk of the horse slipping, with potentially disastrous consequences, but also in most horses such lunging alters the gait so much that it has little value in a lameness examination of an extravagantly moving dressage horse. Leading the horse on a circle at a trot also tends to alter the horse's stride. The horse does not have the freedom to move its neck and instead will set its head on the leader's hand. Many big moving exuberant dressage horses are a safety hazard either to trot in hand or to lunge and lameness is easily masked, especially if low grade. The use of sedatives such as romifidine or detomidine can be helpful, although it is an art to select the most appropriate dose. Repeated sedation may be required to permit accurate interpretation of the response to nerve blocks.

In many horses the usual rider has to be available to reproduce the described problem, if lameness is not overt. However, one should remember that just as bad riders create lameness, so good riders may hide lameness. The latter may take place completely unintentionally and may involve no more than a corrective change of point of balance of the rider through a corner, but enough that for a long time the problem may not be observable from the ground. Most veterinarians who are not competent riders are not experienced fully to appreciate the subtle differences in high-quality dressage horses, and attempting to ride the horse to better appreciate the problem may create an embarrassing situation. They are better advised to spend more time observing the horse from the ground. However, one of the authors (SJD) who is an experienced rider often finds it hugely valuable to ride a horse to be able to better understand the feel of subtle problems.

The veterinarian should not just focus on the limbs when watching the horse ridden. It is important to observe changes such as a change in lathering of the mouth, audible change in the rhythm of the stride, or even absence of teeth grinding or grunting after a particular diagnostic test. The position of the head and neck, the suppleness of movement through the back, the balance of the horse, and its ability to engage the hindlimbs in downward transitions are all important features.

For many horses the veterinarian relies heavily on the perceived observations of the rider during the lameness examination; this may involve the appreciation of subtle changes of gait, or even just an impression of a stronger rhythm or less heavy contact on the bit after a peripheral nerve block. Many riders feel through their own body if the horse is working crookedly, that is, not straight and not in complete balance, and will be able to tell the clinician if this feeling has been altered by any of the diagnostic tests.

In many horses, alternating between lunging and ridden work is useful, often going back to lunging with full tack after the horse has been ridden to see a possible difference in the gait from being ridden. Generally, horses with back pain appear worse while ridden than when lunged, with a loss of freedom and athleticism.

A useful test is to ask the rider to deliberately ride on the wrong diagonal, that is, to sit to the trot in the saddle when the inside forelimb is bearing weight. Horses with forelimb or hindlimb lameness and horses with back pain may alter the gait when the weight-bearing diagonal (of the horse) is changed. The difference in the horse's outline and attitude when changing between sitting and rising trot also may add valuable information.

It can be helpful to see the horse ridden in two 10-m–diameter circles in a figure eight. A low-grade hindlimb lameness may be highlighted as the horse changes direction, characterized by loss of rhythm and fluidity of movement, swinging the hindquarters outward, and a tendency for the inside hindlimb to cross in under the body during protraction. Careful observation of downward transitions from trot to walk may reveal that the horse does not "sit down" properly behind but stays somewhat croup high and takes slightly shortened steps behind. Low-grade unilateral hindlimb lameness may manifest only in certain movements, such as canter pirouette to the side of the lame limb. The horse may be unable to maintain the three-time canter rhythm and may try to jump out of the movement. The horse may find flying changes in canter difficult in the change toward the side of the lame limb—that is, a horse with right hindlimb lameness may perform flying changes from right to left without difficulty but perform less well from left to right, becoming croup high and/or changing late behind. Half-pass away from the lame limb may be less good—that is, a horse with right hindlimb lameness may find half-pass to the left more difficult than to the right.

In some horses lameness is created by the rider. This most commonly occurs with amateur riders who misunderstand the principles of obtaining an outline and riding the horse forward into a contact with the bit. Overrestriction by the hands, with inadequate impulsion, can create gait irregularities. Lower-level trainers are sometimes unable to appreciate these problems and may themselves be unable to work the horse better. Using a good professional rider who is not the horse's trainer to work the horse during the examination is therefore preferable. Determining definitively whether the problem is one of riding or of training or a reflection of a genuine lameness may require observing the horse over several days. A rider who sits consistently crookedly can create back pain and loss of hindlimb rhythm and symmetry. Some dressage horses are exuberant and expressive movers and also strong-willed characters that may refuse to go forward properly if ridden by an enthusiastic but less competent amateur rider, especially if the rider is somewhat apprehensive and inclined to be overrestrictive. Nappy (resistant) behavior and unwillingness to work may reflect a pain-related problem, but not necessarily so.

One should remember that not all horses are athletes. Many owners tend to think that all horses can learn to do dressage. Veterinarians must in certain situations be prepared to offer the opinion that the particular horse has too many shortcomings physically or psychologically to be able to perform advanced dressage. A veterinarian may be able to help a horse overcome a specific problem but cannot provide missing athleticism.

The veterinarian should not forget to check the obvious. The horse may be apprehensive about taking the bit, may take irregular steps, or may be reluctant to bend properly. Wolf teeth frequently are blamed for reluctance to accept the bit properly and for irregularities in gait. Provided that a wolf tooth is immediately in front of the first upper cheek tooth and is not mobile, the tooth rarely is associated with pain.

Horses with a short poll and a relatively large mandible have difficulty in acquiring the correct degree of neck flexion. In these horses it is also important to check that airflow is not impaired. Restricted airflow is not necessarily accompanied by an audibly abnormal inspiratory and/or expiratory noise.

If a diagnosis cannot be made because clinical signs are too subtle, or if it is difficult to determine whether the clinical problem is pain related, working the horse while treating it with antiinflammatory medication (2 to 4 g phenylbutazone per day orally [PO]) for 2 to 3 weeks may be useful. If lameness returns once the medication has been withdrawn, the performance problem can be attributed to pain. The lameness also may be worse, making further investigation easier. If the horse appears to have a low-grade bilateral problem, starting by blocking one limb (forelimb or hindlimb) to see if a contralateral limb lameness immediately becomes obvious can be useful. Blocking both limbs simultaneously and then reassessing the overall freedom of movement and balance may also be of enormous value.

DIAGNOSTIC ANALGESIA

In principle, no differences exist between dressage horses and other equine athletes with regard to diagnostic analgesia. However, the horse's response should be assessed both when ridden and when trotted in hand. Because only minor irregularities in gait are often the point of investigation in lame dressage horses, it is particularly important that the conditions, including the surface, the person handling the horse, and the tempo with which the horse is lunged remain consistent throughout the lameness investigation. Starting the investigation on one surface only to change surface halfway through the nerve blocks should therefore be avoided. Indoor arenas obviously are of great assistance in terms of providing a consistent working surface in severe weather conditions.

Although the sequence of the nerve blocks in theory should be the same in all equine athletes, known common lameness sites in dressage horses often make focusing on these areas possible in order to save time and to avoid an unnecessary number of injection sites and undesirable number of clipped sites. If clipping is essential, many riders prefer that the entire limb (and contralateral limb) be clipped symmetrically rather than producing many small clipped sites in one limb.

IMAGING CONSIDERATIONS

Imaging of a lame dressage horse is no different from imaging any other equine athlete. However, the frequent lack of overt lameness in a submaximally performing dressage horse often necessitates the use of every possible diagnostic modality available. This is particularly true for evaluation of the neck and the back, both of which are important structures for balance and coordination. These are areas in which diagnostic analgesia is less easy than in the limbs but is nonetheless important.

Radiographic evaluation of the thoracolumbar region requires fixed or semimobile radiographic equipment. Use of a Dodger-T aluminum wedge to attenuate the primary x-ray beam facilitates acquisition of high-quality images of the dorsal spinous processes.[5]

Diagnostic ultrasonography of the thoracolumbar and pelvic regions is also useful, used transcutaneously or per rectum to image the supraspinous ligament and epaxial musculature, the synovial articulations (facet joints), and the ventral aspects of the lumbosacral and sacroiliac joints.[6] An ability to obtain high-quality images of the suspensory ligament is crucial, but according to the shape of the proximal aspect of the hindlimbs this may or may not be possible. In some horses magnetic resonance imaging (MRI) may be required for accurate diagnosis.

Nuclear scintigraphic evaluation can be particularly helpful in evaluating the thoracolumbar and pelvic regions. However, a study in clinically normal WBL riding horses showed that mild increased radiopharmaceutical uptake (IRU) in the summits of the dorsal spinous processes may be seen. Thus, as with all imaging techniques, great scientific integrity is demanded to distinguish between normal variations and pathological lesions, and results must be correlated carefully with clinical observations and with other imaging modalities.

Computerized thermographic image analysis has been reported as being helpful but in our experience is often misleading, and it is no longer used routinely.

TEN MOST COMMON LAMENESS CONDITIONS IN DRESSAGE HORSES

The conditions are listed not necessarily in strictly decreasing order of importance or frequency.
1. Proximal suspensory desmitis
   a. Hindlimbs
   b. Forelimbs
2. Suspensory branch lesions
3. Synovitis or osteoarthritis of the forelimb distal interphalangeal joints
4. Desmitis of the forelimb accessory ligament of the deep digital flexor tendon
5. Osteoarthritis of the centrodistal and/or tarsometatarsal joints
6. Synovitis of the middle carpal joint (possibly with palmar intercarpal desmitis)
7. Synovitis or osteoarthritis of the metacarpophalangeal and metatarsophalangeal joints
8. a. Palmar or plantar annular desmitis
   b. Tenosynovitis of the digital flexor tendon sheath: forelimbs and hindlimbs
9. Palmar cortical stress fracture of the third metacarpal bone
10. Thoracolumbar and sacroiliac pain

In our experience many of these conditions can cause overt unilateral lameness. However, bilateral conditions may be less easily recognized and the horse may be presented for investigation because of an insidious onset of progressive unwillingness to work or loss of quality of paces. In-depth investigation of such horses often reveals the presence of lameness in three or four limbs, with or without thoracolumbar or sacroiliac joint region pain.

PROXIMAL SUSPENSORY DESMITIS: HINDLIMBS

Probably the most important cause of lameness in dressage horses working at medium and advanced levels is proximal suspensory desmitis (PSD), although a recent study showed that nonelite dressage horses were also at high risk.[7] The carrying capacity of the hindlimbs is increased with increased collection required for more advanced work, and movements such as piaffe, passage, and canter pirouettes (see Figure 116-2) place great strain on the hindlimb suspensory apparatus. Advanced diagonal placement, a gait characteristic of some excellent moving horses, increases stance duration and also results in the horse bearing weight on a single hindlimb, both of which may contribute to repetitive overload. Suspensory desmitis is believed to be caused by an accumulation of repetitive strains within the suspensory ligament (SL) and its proximal origin. The observation that some horses develop PSD in all four limbs suggests that some horses may have some genetic predisposition to injury.

Detection of PSD is often delayed because of its bilateral nature, which often means that overt hindlimb lameness is not present or immediately noticed by the rider. The condition may be manifested as a loss of performance, increased stiffness, change in contact with the bit, or resistances, if bilateral. If unilateral, problems may arise with specific movements such as canter pirouette or flying changes. In our experience dressage horses tolerate hindlimb PSD less well than show jumpers or event horses, probably because the temperament of the horses is different and the enjoyment of jumping can override low-grade pain.

Accurate diagnostic nerve blocks therefore are required to reveal lameness. When no obvious lameness is present, lameness may be created subsequently in the contralateral hindlimb by diagnostic analgesia of either of the hindlimbs. A negative response can be misleading, and it is often necessary to block both hindlimbs simultaneously, after which there may be a substantial improvement in gait. Direct palpation of the region often fails to indicate a problem because of the deep location of the proximal aspect of the SL. The clinical diagnosis is confirmed by positive subtarsal analgesia (of the deep branch of the lateral plantar nerve), together with negative intraarticular analgesia of the tarsometatarsal (TMT) joint. In some horses PSD and distal hock joint pain occur together and additional intraarticular analgesia of the TMT joint is required for complete resolution of lameness. In other horses, especially those with lesions involving the most proximal aspect of the SL, a tibial nerve block is required to abolish lameness. In some horses, usually those with bilateral PSD, there is coexistent sacroiliac region pain. There may be substantial clinical improvement after bilateral subtarsal nerve blocks, but the quality of the paces, especially canter, and the balance of the horse may not be normal. Further improvement is seen after infiltration of local anesthetic solution around the sacroiliac joint regions. In some young horses, often those that have been professionally produced and sold through public auction in continental Europe, that have developed problems within the first few months of purchase, resolution of hindlimb lameness may reveal a forelimb lameness, often bilateral, also the result of PSD.

Extensive ultrasonographic and radiological changes often reflect a chronic and long-standing problem. Ultrasonographic images may reveal enlargement of the proximal aspect of the SL in both transverse and longitudinal planes, with areas of reduced echogenicity, most often involving one or both of the dorsal quadrants of the ligament. However, in other horses ultrasonographic abnormalities may be much more subtle; areas of increased echogenicity may reflect chronic fibrosis. Radiological diagnosis requires high-quality radiographs of the proximal metatarsal region; dorsoplantar and lateromedial images are the most useful. Irregularity of the proximal plantar cortex of the third metatarsal bone (MtIII) may occur in the region of the origin of the SL, with a varying degree of endosteal new bone resulting in increased radiopacity of the trabecular bone over a distance of up to 5 cm. On dorsoplantar images this may be seen as a centrally or laterally positioned area of increased radiopacity within the trabecular metaphysis of the MtIII. One should remember, however, that such radiological changes may be present in an asymptomatic horse because of previous problems (either subclinically or clinically manifested), leading to the risk of a false-positive diagnosis. Diagnosis should never be based only on radiological evaluation.

Occasionally, nuclear scintigraphy can be useful in horses with early desmitis in which no radiological changes are present and subtle, equivocal abnormalities are detected with ultrasonography. IRU may occur in the proximoplantar aspect of the MtIII in bone phase (delayed) images. Pool phase (soft tissue) images are rather insensitive, and not all horses have associated IRU in the proximal plantar metatarsal region. Thus a negative bone scan does not preclude PSD. Moderate-to-intense IRU usually reflects entheseous reaction. MRI may be required for definitive diagnosis.

Treatment of this condition is often frustrating because of the chronic nature of the problem at the time of its detection. However, in well-conformed young horses with recent onset of clinical signs, rest may be all that is required, with a careful progressive resumption of work after approximately 3 months. Corrective trimming to restore foot balance is important; shoeing using egg bar shoes provides some support in horses with hyperextension of the fetlock joint. In horses with chronic injuries prolonged rest (3 to 6 months) often provides a disappointing response, and a controlled exercise program may be more successful. Periligamentous, subfascial injection of hyaluronan plus a corticosteroid (e.g., 40 mg of methylprednisolone acetate or 10 mg of triamcinolone acetonide) is now used frequently and is believed to provide an initial reduction in inflammation to enable a reasonably pain-free walking program to be initiated. This frequently is continued for as long as 12 weeks before slow, balanced trotting on a good surface is initiated.

The ultrasonographic appearance of the SL often changes little, even in horses that are returned successfully to full training. Egg bar shoes are often removed when normal training is initiated, because many riders believe that they provide too much breaking action on ground impact of the hindlimbs. The likelihood of recurrence of

PSD is high, and special care should be taken not to overwork the horse on deep or holding surfaces or to change suddenly to a different surface. Modification of the training program is often required, particularly in terms of avoiding a fatiguing training session in deep or loose surfaces. Medium and extended paces should be avoided as far as possible during training.

Some horses have chronic lameness that fails to respond to therapy. Some horses with mild or moderate ultrasonographic lesions respond to serial shock wave therapy or radial pressure wave therapy, initially using three treatments at 2-week intervals. There is often substantial improvement in lameness and ultrasonographic appearance of the ligament. Further treatments can be given if required.

Ultrasound-guided injection of core lesions with platelet-rich plasma (PRP) has recently shown encouraging results. Neurectomy of the deep branch of the lateral plantar nerve, with or without fasciotomy, has a role in horses that fail to respond to medical management or in horses with a long-term history of suboptimal performance. Concurrent medication of the tarsometatarsal joint is required for complete resolution of lameness in some horses. The presence of a straight hock conformation or hyperextension of the hind fetlock is a poor prognostic indicator.

In view of the relatively common occurrence of PSD becoming apparent in young horses soon after purchase after preparation for sale by auction, one of the authors (SJD) recommends a 3-month period of rest after purchase and then introduction of a graduated work program to try to prevent PSD becoming clinically apparent.

PROXIMAL SUSPENSORY DESMITIS: FORELIMBS

Forelimb PSD is seen more often than hindlimb PSD in younger horses and may result from hyperextension of the carpus in extravagantly moving horses, in particular horses volunteering extended trot. PSD often results from the horse working on less than ideal surfaces. Lameness is often unilateral and acute in onset but is sometimes bilateral. Most sound horses resent firm manual squeezing of the body of the SL but the proximal region of the SL is difficult to access by palpation; therefore local analgesic techniques are required to verify the source of pain.

In horses with peracute PSD, slight swelling in the proximal metacarpal region may occur, but this often resolves within 24 hours. The horse may react to firm pressure applied over the proximal aspect of the SL. Lameness may be transient unless the horse is worked again. In these horses, the veterinarian relies on a history of acute-onset lameness that is usually worse with the affected limb on the outside of a circle. However this is not pathognomonic for PSD. Lameness is often easier to feel (by a rider) than to see from the ground. In some horses lameness is never apparent either in hand or on the lunge but is only seen ridden, incongruously with the lame limb on the inside of a circle. The appearance of lameness may be influenced by the diagonal on which the rider sits.

Lameness may be worse after palmar (abaxial sesamoid) nerve blocks, probably because the horse loses some proprioceptive information from the foot and therefore is less able to protect the loading of the suspensory apparatus.

Some improvement is often seen after perineural analgesia of the palmar and palmar metacarpal nerves at the junction of the proximal two thirds and distal one third of the metacarpal region, either because of proximal diffusion of local anesthetic solution or the presence of pain in the more distal aspects of the suspensory apparatus. Lameness is usually substantially improved or resolved by blocking the lateral palmar nerve or the palmar metacarpal nerves at subcarpal level. However, in some horses an ulnar nerve block is required. Because of the close proximity of the middle carpal joint capsule, horses with a positive response to subcarpal analgesia should later be evaluated with intraarticular analgesia of the middle carpal joint to exclude articular pain from the carpus.

Radiography is frequently of little or no value in dressage horses with forelimb PSD. Ultrasonography is required to confirm the diagnosis. Use of a virtual convex array transducer and/or acquisition of images obtained while the limb is flexed may be required to identify abaxial lesions. Because subtle lesions may be present and may be a reflection of a previous pathological condition (possibly subclinical), high-quality ultrasonographic images of both limbs are required for comparison, together with knowledge of normal variations. Lesions vary from subtle enlargement of the proximal aspect of the SL with normal echogenicity to large areas of reduced echogenicity. In some young horses no ultrasonographic abnormalities have been detected, but MRI has confirmed the presence of PSD.

Rest, often for 12 to 16 weeks, together with a controlled, ascending walking program (in hand, using a horse walker, or ridden) is the treatment of choice. Careful trimming to restore foot balance is crucial. Intralesional injection using 2 mL of a polysulfated glycosaminoglycan (PSGAG) or PRP may also be tried.

The prognosis is good in horses with early PSD, provided that the horse is managed carefully subsequently, avoiding the medium or extended trot in training. In horses with chronic PSD the risk of recurrence is moderately high. Shock wave therapy has been useful in treating some of these horses. In others injection of mesenchymal stem cells or desmoplasty has produced a successful outcome. In some horses the ultrasonographic appearance may not change substantially, despite a favorable clinical response to treatment, leading to later risk of a false-positive diagnosis in an asymptomatic horse.

DESMITIS OF THE SUSPENSORY LIGAMENT BRANCHES: FORELIMBS AND HINDLIMBS

Desmitis of a branch of the SL is often acute in onset and results in palpable enlargement of the suspensory branch and often moderate lameness. Occasionally, both medial and lateral branches are involved in a hindlimb. The branch is painful to palpation. Diagnosis is confirmed by ultrasonography. Enlargement of the branch is often accompanied by periligamentous fibrosis characterized by subcutaneous echogenic material. There is often a central (sometimes eccentric) hypoechogenic or anechogenic core lesion. The interface between the ligament branch and the proximal sesamoid bone (PSB) may be disrupted. This is best seen on longitudinal images and merits a more guarded prognosis. If both branches in a hindlimb are involved, echogenic material may be visible between the branches.

The PSBs may or may not show radiological evidence of enthesopathy, with parallel linear opacities extending from the palmar or abaxial margin. Dystrophic mineralization within the SL branch is occasionally seen on ultrasonographic and radiographic images.

Treatment is prolonged rest (4 to 6 months) with a slow return to exercise. Intralesional injections using 1 mL of a PSGAG may be tried but generally have met with disappointing results. Counterirritation (pin firing) has been tried on horses with old, indurated lesions associated with chronic lameness, but again generally with disappointing results. Some horses have responded to intralesional treatment with β-aminopropionitrile fumarate. Encouraging results also have been obtained recently with shock wave therapy (three treatments at 2-week intervals), combined with a controlled walking exercise program for 3 to 4 months. However, the presence of extensive periligamentous fibrosis is a poor prognostic indicator.

The risk of recurrence is high. Any predisposing causes such as limb deviations or lateromedial imbalance of the feet should be corrected or at least adjusted.

SYNOVITIS OR OSTEOARTHRITIS OF THE DISTAL INTERPHALANGEAL JOINT

Pain arising from the distal interphalangeal (DIP) joint is a frequent diagnosis in all sports horses. The unique anatomical position of the DIP joint, with the forces distributed on it through the rigidity of the hoof capsule and the forward thrust of the deep digital flexor tendon (DDFT) and the navicular bone during weight bearing and limb protraction, are likely to be contributory factors. Lateral-to-medial imbalance of the foot also contributes to the joint trauma in many horses.

The diagnosis is made by comparing the response to intraarticular analgesia with that of (minimal volume, 0.5 mL per branch) perineural analgesia of the palmar digital and palmar (abaxial sesamoid) nerves as well as intrasynovial analgesia of the navicular bursa. The interpretation of the response to intraarticular analgesia is not black and white, and the clinician must learn to build up a picture of a composite, often complicated distal forelimb lameness. Recent studies have confirmed that intraarticular analgesia of the DIP joint is not specific and can influence pain associated with the navicular bone, distal phalanx, DDFT, and even subsolar tissues. A rapid (within 5 minutes) positive response to a small volume (maximum of 6 mL) of local anesthetic solution may be a good indicator of the possible response to subsequent intraarticular medication. A good response to subsequent treatment requires at least 75% clinical improvement after intraarticular analgesia, together with absence of relevant radiological changes involving the DIP joint or the navicular bone.

Radiological changes usually involve the extensor process of the distal phalanx and the dorsoproximal margin of the navicular bone. One should remember that considerable variation exists in the shape and size of the extensor process between limbs and within sound horses. Minor modeling changes may not be of clinical significance. Small, mineralized fragments proximal to the extensor process may be seen incidentally. Large fragments may require surgical removal to prevent secondary osteoarthritis (OA).

Intraarticular medication using a number of individual drugs or a combination of drugs has given encouraging results, although results vary among clinicians and populations of horses. Horses with recent onset of usually unilateral lameness with palpable distention of the DIP joint capsule may respond favorably to 10 mg of triamcinolone acetonide or up to 40 mg of methylprednisolone acetate, combined with a short period of controlled walking exercise (e.g., 2 weeks on a horse walker) followed by 2 weeks of ridden walking. Injection with hyaluronan probably will provide a similar response in such horses. However, in horses with more chronic lameness, the response to corticosteroids is less favorable, and the most successful long-term results have been seen after a triple series of intraarticular injections of a PSGAG.[8] PSGAGs received some negative press after a research study in North America in 1989 suggested that PSGAGs have a potentiating effect on a subinfectious dose of *Staphylococcus aureus* in a joint. Subsequently, this preparation has been used sparingly intraarticularly and in many horses only in combination with intraarticular amikacin. We have not seen any negative reaction (inflammatory or infectious) to numerous intraarticular injections of PSGAGs and do not use systemic or intraarticular antibiotics. Strict asepsis and a skillful technique are essential. Because of its distal location in the limb, we recommend that DIP joints always be bandaged for at least 24 hours after injection. Eighty-two percent of dressage horses returned to soundness after PSGAG medication of the DIP joint, compared with 65% in a similar-sized group of horses competing in cross-country jumping.[8] In most horses the initial triple injection proved adequate, and additional injections in horses successfully treated using this technique were rarely needed.

Autologous conditioned serum containing interleukin-1 receptor antagonist protein (IRAP) has proved beneficial for management of horses with DIP joint or navicular bursa pain.

Corrective shoeing by improving the foot-pastern axis and reestablishment of correct hoof balance should always be combined with intraarticular medication, but changes should be performed slowly. Heart bar shoes often are used for an initial 3- to 6-month period.

DESMITIS OF THE ACCESSORY LIGAMENT OF THE DEEP DIGITAL FLEXOR TENDON: FORELIMBS

Desmitis of the accessory ligament of the DDFT (ALDDFT) frequently occurs as an acute injury associated with sudden onset of lameness and palpable inflammation (heat and swelling) in the proximal one third or one half of the metacarpal region. Overextension of the carpus caused by imbalance in young horses or resulting from imperfect working surfaces is often believed to be a contributory cause.

The diagnosis is confirmed by ultrasonography in both transverse and longitudinal planes. There is often substantial enlargement of the ALDDFT, together with loss of definition of the margins and areas of reduced echogenicity. A definite, hypoechogenic core lesion is recognized infrequently.

Horses with desmitis of the ALDDFT respond better to a controlled ascending walking exercise program than to complete box rest. Controlled walking for 3 to 6 months often is required in horses with severe desmitis, despite the initial lameness often resolving considerably sooner. The

risk of recurrence is moderately high. Local invasive treatment of desmitis of the ALDDFT seldom has been rewarding, although some horses have responded favorably to treatment with β-aminopropionitrile fumarate and more recently with PRP.

DESMITIS OF THE ACCESSORY LIGAMENT OF THE DEEP DIGITAL FLEXOR TENDON: HINDLIMBS

Desmitis of the proximal aspect of the ALDDFT of hindlimbs results in acute-onset lameness usually associated with soft tissue swelling in the proximoplantar aspect of the metatarsal region. Diagnosis is confirmed by ultrasonographic examination; it is important to examine the limb from the plantaromedial aspect; otherwise, lesions may be missed (see Figure 71-3).

OSTEOARTHRITIS OF THE CENTRODISTAL AND TARSOMETATARSAL JOINTS

Lameness or poor performance (e.g., inability to collect in order to perform piaffe or passage) associated with pain arising from the centrodistal (CD) or TMT joints occurs frequently in dressage horses. Likewise, a horse with an outstanding freedom of movement in the trot may have an unexplainably poor canter associated with distal hock joint pain. In collected paces there is increased tarsal loading and joint compression,[9] which may predispose to tarsal injury in dressage horses. The pattern of subchondral bone thickness in the distal tarsal bones reflecting loading pathways is different in elite performance horses compared with general-purpose horses.[10] This may be related to circling and other specific movements, and potentially predisposes to pathological change.

A poor correlation exists between the clinical signs, including response to intraarticular analgesia of the TMT and CD joints, and the radiological appearance of these joints. Many dressage horses have confirmed pain from the joints but have fairly equivocal, if any, radiological changes. One should remember that the degree of joint collapse and osseous ankylosis always is underestimated from radiographs because of the curvilinear nature of the joints and the low radiodensity of immature bone bridging the joint centrally. Nuclear scintigraphy may be a sensitive indicator of increased bone modeling in the absence of radiological abnormalities or in horses with equivocal changes and also can be helpful in horses with subtle lameness, when the response to local analgesic techniques is difficult to interpret. Alternatively, diagnostic medication with intraarticular corticosteroids may be helpful.

Pain is often bilateral, and the presenting problem is often shortening of the hindlimb stride and an inability to collect, rather than overt lameness. An advanced horse may show irregularities of rhythm in piaffe and passage. Clinical signs mimicking back pain, rather than overt lameness, may be present.

Most horses respond to intraarticular analgesia of the TMT and CD joints, although occasionally a better response is seen after fibular and tibial nerve blocks or after treatment of the joints. Intraarticular analgesia of the TMT joint and the response to subtarsal analgesia should be compared. In horses with advanced radiological changes, false-negative responses to intraarticular analgesia may occur.

Horses with few or no radiological changes may respond satisfactorily to intraarticular medication with a corticosteroid (e.g., up to 40 mg of methylprednisolone acetate or 10 mg of triamcinolone acetonide), IRAP, or 1 mL of a PSGAG if lameness is of longer duration. Medical treatment often is combined with a program of controlled walking exercise for 2 to 4 weeks (pending response to treatment), together with alterations of the shoeing. Horses that tend to plait or swing the affected limb axially during protraction may benefit from a lateral extension shoe, which may help to normalize posture and hindlimb gait pattern with an additional effect on secondary back pain.

Repeated medication of the joint(s) may be required at monthly or quarterly intervals. A longer response may be achieved by combined use of corticosteroids and hyaluronan.

Additional PSGAG medication given intramuscularly on a weekly basis (500 mg/mL, 7 times 5 mL) may be beneficial. Tiludronate infusion has given poor results. Glucosamines and chondroitin sulfate given orally on a daily basis are often administered, but clinical efficacy remains largely unproven.

If substantial radiological changes are present, the joint is changed irreversibly, and the horse fails to respond to repeated intraarticular medication, fusion of the joints by surgery or by intraarticular injection of sodium monoiodoacetate or ethyl alcohol can be considered, but the prognosis for high-level dressage is guarded.

SYNOVITIS OF THE MIDDLE CARPAL JOINT

Lameness associated with pain in the middle carpal joint has been seen in many dressage horses, in particular young horses that still may be struggling to establish balance and synchronicity in all paces with the additional weight of the rider. Lameness is often mild and most frequently unilateral, being most noticeable when the limb is on the outside of a 10-m diameter circle. Intermittent hyperextension of the carpus, often on a tight circle, is believed to be involved.

If the response to analgesia of the middle carpal joint is positive, the proximal SL should be examined by ultrasonography to preclude injury.

Usually, no radiological or ultrasonographic changes are present involving the middle carpal joint. Arthroscopy of the middle carpal joint sometimes reveals damage to one (most frequently the medial) or both of the palmar intercarpal ligaments, which show edema, petechial hemorrhage, and fraying of superficial fibers.

Most horses respond well to intraarticular medication using a triple series of 1 to 2 mL of a PSGAG given 8 days apart, or treatment with short-acting corticosteroids combined with hyaluronan. Six to 8 weeks of ridden walk or on a horse walker should be followed by a modified training program for at least another 3 months.

SYNOVITIS OR OSTEOARTHRITIS OF THE METATARSOPHALANGEAL AND METACARPOPHALANGEAL (FETLOCK) JOINTS

Fetlock joint disease is not a common problem in dressage horses and certainly does not seem to be as common in this type of equestrian sport as in others. The absence of

galloping across often firm and irregular surfaces associated with cross-country jumping is a likely explanation.

The diagnosis is confirmed by palpation and intraarticular analgesia. In the absence of radiological changes, intraarticular medication using a corticosteroid (e.g., 10 mg of triamcinolone acetonide), together with 2 mL hyaluronan in horses with synovitis, or 1 mL of PSGAG in horses with more long-standing OA, frequently has proved successful. IRAP treatment has also proven successful. Generally the response to medication is good and the likelihood of recurrence is low in the forelimbs. The response is poorer in hindlimbs. Horses with radiological abnormalities consistent with OA warrant a more guarded prognosis.

PALMAR OR PLANTAR ANNULAR LIGAMENT DESMITIS

Desmitis of the palmar (plantar) annular ligament (PAL) occurs more commonly in forelimbs than in hindlimbs and usually results in acute-onset lameness. The PAL has localized heat and is palpably enlarged, with pain elicited by firm pressure. Mild distention of the digital flexor tendon sheath (DFTS) may occur. Diagnosis is confirmed by ultrasonography. The PAL is thickened, with a diffuse reduction in echogenicity or focal hypoechogenic areas. Horses with acute desmitis usually respond well to box rest and controlled walking exercise for 3 months. In the acute phase, nonsteroidal antiinflammatory drugs (e.g., phenylbutazone 2 g bid PO for 5 days) are beneficial. If associated with a degree of synovitis of the DFTS, intrasynovial treatment of the DFTS with a corticosteroid may assist in resolution of lameness.

Radial pressure wave treatment has also proven a useful alternative to surgery. Tenoscopic resection of the ligament is reserved for horses not responding to conservative management.

TENOSYNOVITIS OF THE DIGITAL FLEXOR TENDON SHEATH

Tenosynovitis of the DFTS often results in sudden-onset lameness associated with distention. Some horses have long-standing distention of the DFTS without lameness (windgalls), especially in the hindlimbs, but subsequently develop clinically important tenosynovitis. Constriction of the DFTS by the PAL may be apparent. Lameness may vary from mild to severe and usually is accentuated by distal limb flexion. If distention of the DFTS is acute in onset, then local analgesia is usually unnecessary. However, if distention of the DFTS has been present for some time, then the source of pain should be confirmed by local analgesia. Intrathecal analgesia of the DFTS usually results in substantial improvement in lameness but often does not alleviate it fully. Perineural analgesia of the palmar or plantar (midcannon) and palmar metacarpal or plantar metatarsal nerves usually eliminates lameness. Improvement sometimes is seen after perineural analgesia of the palmar nerves at the level of the PSBs. Excluding the metacarpophalangeal joint as a potential source of pain by intraarticular analgesia may be necessary.

Ultrasonographic examination should be performed in the metacarpal and pastern regions. Usually an abnormal amount of fluid within the DFTS allows better visibility of the normal synovial plicae extending from the medial and lateral margins of the DDFT in the distal metacarpal region and the synovial fold on the palmar aspect of the DDFT in the pastern region. These should not be mistaken for adhesions or tears of the DDFT. In horses with chronic tenosynovitis, the DFTS wall may be thickened, with echogenic bands within the DFTS representing adhesions. Ultrasonography frequently underestimates adhesion formation. The superficial digital flexor tendon (SDFT) and DDFT should be inspected carefully, because tenosynovitis may be secondary to a primary pathological tendon condition. Lesions of the DDFT occur more commonly, either as ill-defined core lesions or marginal tears, most frequently of the lateral margin. The latter can be difficult to detect by ultrasonography. Enlargement of the cross-sectional area of the tendon compared with the contralateral limb suggests a lesion, which may be confirmed only by tenoscopic evaluation of the sheath. Mineralization within the DDFT warrants a guarded prognosis. Horses with early tenosynovitis without adhesions or detectable lesion of the DDFT respond well to intrasynovial administration of a corticosteroid (e.g., 10 mg of triamcinolone acetonide) or 2 mL of hyaluronan, together with a pressure bandage and box rest with handwalking for 4 to 6 weeks. Horses with small core lesions of the DDFT may respond satisfactorily to conservative management, but those with large core lesions have a more guarded prognosis. However, ultrasound-guided injection of cultured mesenchymal stem cells has yielded encouraging results in a small number of horses.

If the horse fails to respond adequately to medical therapy, then surgical exploration is warranted. Tenoscopic evaluation should be performed to evaluate the extent of adhesion formation and to detect longitudinal tears in the medial or lateral margins of the DDFT, which may extend proximally under the manica flexoria. Resection of intrasynovial adhesions and lavage, with or without resection of the PAL, may resolve the problem. Horses with lesions of the DDFT that may be debrided warrant a more guarded prognosis. Surgery is frequently followed by intrasynovial injection of 2 mL of hyaluronan, repeated 4 to 6 weeks later to reduce inflammation and to try to prevent adhesions from reforming.

The response to surgery depends on the chronicity of the problem, the amount of intrasynovial adhesions, and the presence of lesions of the DDFT. Horses with lesions involving the forelimbs appear to have a better prognosis than those involving the hindlimbs. Surgery is accompanied by 8 to 12 weeks of absence from training, although controlled walking in hand or on a horse walker is essential to try to stretch any adhesions that reform.

PROXIMAL PALMAR CORTICAL STRESS FRACTURE OF THE THIRD METACARPAL BONE

Proximal palmar cortical stress fracture of the third metacarpal bone (McIII) occasionally is seen in dressage horses, especially young horses, with an acute onset of moderate-to-severe lameness. Hyperextension of the carpus, imbalance, and limb asynchrony in immature horses are believed to be contributing factors.

The diagnosis is sometimes suspected when pain is induced by digital pressure on the palmaroproximal aspect

of the McIII. When the horse trots on a firm surface, the lameness tends to increase the farther the horse trots. If the horse turns and then trots again, lameness appears to be improved and then increases again. Lameness usually is improved substantially by perineural analgesia of the palmar metacarpal nerves in the subcarpal region. If the fracture extends into the carpometacarpal joint, improvement also may be seen after intraarticular analgesia of the middle carpal joint.

On radiographs a fracture may be recognized on a dorsopalmar image as a linear radiolucent line, usually in the medial aspect of the McIII and extending up to 8 cm, possibly with surrounding increased radiopacity. In some horses a fracture line cannot be seen, although increased radiopacity is present. In some horses no radiological abnormality is identified. In these horses, the diagnosis is confirmed by nuclear scintigraphy, with focal intense IRU in the proximal palmar aspect of the McIII. Alternatively, MRI can be used but is generally unnecessary.

Treatment is complete box rest for 6 weeks, followed by 6 weeks of controlled walking exercise. The prognosis is good, and the likelihood of recurrence low.

THORACOLUMBAR AND SACROILIAC PAIN

Thoracolumbar and sacroiliac region pain are frequent causes of reduced performance in dressage horses. In a questionnaire survey concerning British dressage horses, so-called back pain occurred in 25% of horses in a 2-year period.[4] However, in a high proportion of horses lameness was subsequently identified. It is therefore important to appreciate that the appearance of back stiffness and recognition of back pain may reflect an underlying lameness, which is sometimes subclinical. Although caudal thoracic back muscle soreness may be secondary to primary hindlimb lameness, primary back pain does occur commonly and is usually not associated with overt lameness, although poor hindlimb impulsion or intermittent hindlimb gait irregularity can be seen. Sacroiliac joint region pain often develops secondarily to hindlimb PSD. The horse may have a history of unwillingness to perform certain movements, stiffness, loss of impulsion and cadence, loss of action, or being less easy to work in a correct outline. Sometimes bucking or other nappy (resistant) behavior remain the only clinical observations. The horse usually moves better on the lunge than when being ridden. The most common causes of back pain include the following:
1. An ill-fitting saddle
2. The rider sitting crookedly
3. Primary muscle spasm
4. Impingement of dorsal spinous processes in the mid-thoracic to cranial lumbar regions
5. OA of the synovial articulations (facet joints) in the region of the thoracolumbar junction
6. Sacroiliac disease
7. A combination of lesions in the thoracolumbar and sacroiliac regions

Definitive diagnosis of the cause of back pain can be a diagnostic challenge. It may be helpful to work in conjunction with a skilled physiotherapist or chiropractor. Liaison with an experienced high-quality saddle fitter may also be valuable. Obvious causes such as ill-fitting saddle or the position of the rider should be eliminated first before proceeding with more sophisticated diagnostic tests such as radiography, ultrasonography, nuclear scintigraphy, and thermography. If back muscle tension or spasm is obvious, assessing the response to treatment using physiotherapy (e.g., manipulation and therapeutic ultrasound) or antiinflammatory medication may be worthwhile before further investigation.

Thermography provides pictorial images of the surface temperature of the body, which gives a physiological identification of changes in tissue perfusion or sympathetic neuromuscular dysfunction. Thermography is a useful tool to demonstrate to an owner the effect of a poorly fitting saddle or the rider sitting crookedly and also may be useful in identifying acute superficial ligament or muscle injuries.

Nuclear scintigraphy may be more sensitive than radiology for detecting lesions in the thoracolumbar or sacroiliac regions, but radiology potentially gives more structural information, such as the proximity of the dorsal spinous processes. It is important to verify the clinical significance of any lesions identified by infiltration of local anesthetic solution whenever possible. If dorsal spinous processes are extremely crowded, injecting between them may not be possible, but injecting around them (20 to 50 mL of mepivacaine) usually results in substantial improvement within 15 minutes of injection, although this may confirm "back pain" rather than pain specifically arising from impinging dorsal spinous processes.

Ultrasound guidance is necessary for infiltration around synovial articulations.

Treatment is aimed at removing any predisposing factor and control of pain. Local infiltration with corticosteroids (e.g., methylprednisolone acetate combined with mepivacaine) or Sarapin is successful in some horses. If pain associated with impinging dorsal spinous processes fails to be controlled by medical management, surgical treatment should be considered. Infiltration of corticosteroids, Sarapin, or a sclerosing agent, P2G (Martindale Pharmaceuticals, Romford, Essex, United Kingdom), around the sacroiliac joints produces clinical improvement in some horses with pain associated with these joints. Acupuncture can be a useful adjunctive therapy for pain management. The daily work pattern and training methods used by the rider and trainer should also be reviewed for successful long-term management. Regular lunge work in a Pessoa may be of benefit. Exercises to increase core muscle strength are important. Slow warm-up in a pace that the horse finds easy is also valuable.

Chapter 117

Lameness in the Three Day Event Horse

Andrew P. Bathe

SPORT OF EVENTING

The sport of eventing generally is considered the most all-around test of a horse's athletic ability, and therefore the horses tend to be jacks-of-all-trades rather than excelling in any one particular area. The competition consists of three disciplines, namely dressage, show jumping, and cross-country, with the latter being the most influential phase. The Three Day Event or Concours Complet International (CCI) is the pinnacle of the sport (Figure 117-1) and is run over 4 days: 2 days of dressage, followed by a day for the speed and endurance phases and a day of show jumping. In the traditional long-format event the speed and endurance test consists of roads and tracks at trotting speed, a steeplechase, and the actual cross-country phase over fixed obstacles. This is a severe athletic test, and horses normally compete in only two or maximally three such competitions in a year. Since 2004 a "short format" Three Day Event has been introduced, which excludes the steeplechase and endurance phases but leaves the cross-country phase. This is cheaper to stage and potentially requires a smaller site on which to run the competition. At CCI**** level the course must be 6720 to 6840 m in length, with up to 45 jumping efforts at an optimum speed of 570 mpm, to therefore be completed within 11 to 12 minutes. It has resulted in some horses competing in three or occasionally four such competitions in one year.

CICs (international One Day Events), One Day Events or Horse Trials, compress the same disciplines into a shorter time frame but without the roads and tracks and steeplechase phases. The distance and thus time for the cross-country phase are also much shorter, and there are fewer jumping efforts, so that many such competitions may be completed in a season. For most advanced horses, One Day Events are used as training for the Three Day Events, although a large number of recreational competitors aspire to compete in only One Day Events. There are an increasing number of relatively high–prize money CICs, encouraging international level horses to compete more frequently. The emphasis of this chapter is the Three Day Event horse, because the extreme demands placed on this horse give characteristic patterns of lameness, whereas the novice One Day Event horse can be considered a standard riding club or recreational horse from a veterinary point of view.

Eventing is an established Olympic sport and a substantial equine industry. The highest grade of competition is the four-star event (CCI****). Traditionally these have been the English events of Badminton and Burghley, although there are now more elite level competitions around the world including Lexington, Kentucky, United States and Lumhulen, Germany. The sport has a high-risk element for rider and horse, and a noticeable recent trend has been to try to make courses safer, with the introduction of fences with frangible pins to try to minimize the frequency of rotational falls.

The sport includes substantial veterinary involvement. During a Three Day Event, the horse is examined by the

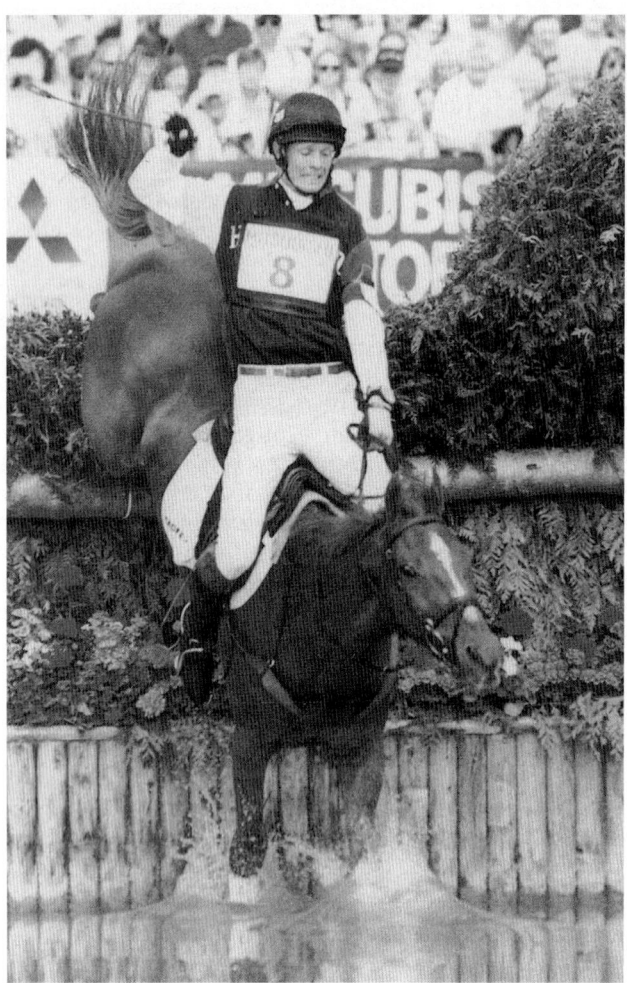

Fig. 117-1 • Example of a cross-country fence at CCI**** level. (Courtesy Kit Houghton Photography, Bridgewater, Somerset, United Kingdom.)

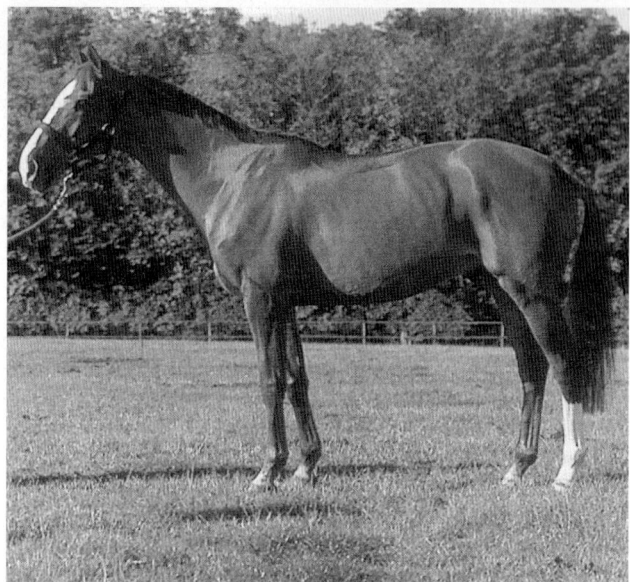

Fig. 117-2 • An ideal modern eventing stamp. This 16.1-hand–high New Zealand Thoroughbred gelding was an individual Olympic and World Championship gold medalist. (Courtesy Badminton Speciality Feeds, Oakham, Rutland, United Kingdom.)

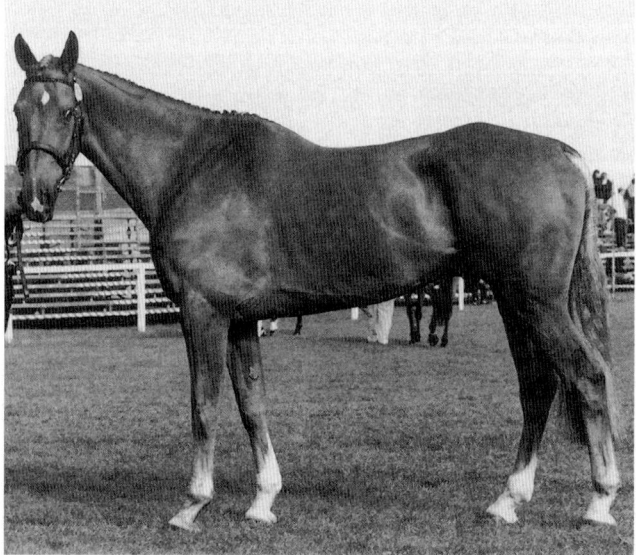

Fig. 117-3 • Example of a successful but tall and hunter-bred horse. This 17-hand–high gelding Thoroughbred-cross Irish draft horse was a Badminton CCI**** winner and Open European Championship Team gold medalist. (Courtesy Kit Houghton Photography, Bridgewater, Somerset, United Kingdom.)

official veterinarians on arrival, the day before commencing the dressage, before and after the cross-country, and the morning before show jumping. The horse must be deemed fit to compete—that is, the horse must be sound—throughout the competition, and thus any orthopedic disorders are of great clinical significance. A mild degree of hindlimb gait asymmetry may be acceptable to the Inspection Panel, but any noticeable forelimb lameness normally is not permitted.

HORSE TYPES

Because the Three Day Event places great emphasis on the horse's speed and stamina, there is a preference toward the Thoroughbred (TB) or predominantly TB crossbreeds. A substantial proportion of horses are of uncertain or unknown breeding. Exceptions have been notable, but Warmbloods and classic Irish hunter types normally do not have the endurance required at the top level. Such horses often may do extremely well at the lower levels, however, because they move and jump better than the pure TB. Figure 117-2 demonstrates what could be considered the ideal modern eventing stamp, a highly successful New Zealand TB. A horse's ability and mental aptitude are the most important determinants, and other body types are

successful (Figure 117-3). An average ideal size would be 16.2 hands, but the rules are not hard and fast. The short-format Three Day Event has perhaps slightly reduced the emphasis on pure galloping ability, and because the courses usually have the same number of jumping efforts, sometimes in a shorter course, there is a need for the horses to be quick and nimble.

The financial value of event horses is considerably lower than that of racehorses, show jumpers, or dressage horses, so any horse with outstanding ability in one of these phases is likely to be used in that sport first. If the horses do not succeed, then they may be tried as potential event horses. These horses bring with them any injuries they may have accumulated, but because of the different stresses imposed during eventing, this may not be a problem. For example, event horses tolerate low-grade carpal pathological conditions from previous race training. A small number of horses are bred specifically for eventing. Stallions generally are considered to lack the courage required to compete at the top level, and because the horse takes a number of years to reach its peak, choosing proven sires is a problem. The predominantly TB Irish sports horse and the relatively larger-boned New Zealand and Australian TBs are sought after.

Event horses normally commence dressage and show jumping training at 4 years of age and start competing in prenovice and novice One Day Events from the age of 5. Depending on the horse's ability and rider's skill and patience, a horse usually competes in its first (graded as a CCI* or CCI**) Three Day Event at 6 to 7 years of age. A substantial proportion of horses do not have the ability, courage, or physical durability to proceed beyond the CCI** or CCI*** level to the top grade of CCI****.

INFLUENCE OF THE SPORT ON LAMENESS

Event horses are generally skeletally mature when they commence training and are not trained at the same speed or intensity as racehorses. They therefore have different patterns of injury, although most of the problems are still related to training. Primary long bone pathological conditions are rare. Soft tissue injuries such as tendonitis are common and often career limiting. The amount of endurance training necessary produces repeated cyclic loading, and problems such as osteoarthritis (OA) are common. The other subset of event horse injuries is acute traumatic injuries sustained during competition. Because the horses are jumping large fixed obstacles at speed, they are prone to falls and to direct traumatic fractures. The short format does not seem to have led to a dramatic difference in the type or incidence of injuries. Horses may tolerate low-grade soft injuries better than with the long format, and in the long run there might be a decrease in the incidence of injuries.

Fence design has changed in recent years. Square-shaped fences are avoided, and rounded top contours are now more common. These fences give horses more leeway to correct mistakes and cause less severe direct impact trauma. The fences may be 1.2 to 1.4 m high, with a 2-m spread and a 2-m drop, so substantial strain can be placed on the supporting structures of the limbs on landing. The quality of the terrain also appears to have an important impact on the incidence of lameness problems. The competitions are run predominantly on turf, the nature of which depends on the soil type, local weather, and management factors. At the lower level, financial constraints generally preclude much improvement on the quality of the ground, but some of the top events try to maintain a permanent track that is tended carefully.

The prolonged period and intensity of training required for horses to reach an elite level means that those horses not metabolically or physically suited to the sport are selected out. For instance, few elite horses have recurrent exertional rhabdomyolysis or navicular syndrome. Three Day Events are regulated by the Fédération Équestre Internationale. A strict medication control program is enforced and permits only emergency medication at the competition after official veterinary approval or the use of a small number of permitted forms of medication, including antibiotics, rehydration fluids, and preparations for treating gastric ulcers.

TRAINING METHODS

References on page 1344

Event horses train in all three disciplines, with the actual methods varying greatly among riders. A complete description of training methods is available elsewhere.[1] Most competing horses have natural cross-country ability, so little time generally is spent on training for this, because the progression of competitions provides sufficient experience. Event horses normally are selected for natural jumping action, but jumping technique during the cross-country phase is different from that needed for show jumping. Therefore event horses may not be as careful when show jumping and can have a tendency to touch poles. Most event horses are show jumped regularly, especially during the off season. The event horse's weakest link is usually the dressage phase. The movements required are no more than a medium level of pure dressage, but the different breeding and level of fitness of these horses means that the major challenge can be to control the horse's temperament. Most of the skills training revolves around dressage, and a high standard now is required to be competitive at the top level.

Fitness training is a major component of the preparation for a Three Day Event and is where most orthopedic damage is incurred. The horse is likely to undergo a 3- to 4-month training period for the target Three Day Event. Training methods vary greatly among riders and often depend on local factors such as the availability of hills for trotting or all-weather gallops. Restricting the horse to training solely on an artificial surface is not advisable, because this seems to predispose the horse to injury when the horse actually competes on a natural surface.

Event horses normally receive a 6-week initial period of walking and trotting on the roads, and then commence cantering exercise. Different riders vary in their use of conventional or interval training but usually peak the quantity of work at around three canters of 8 minutes, or shorter if a hill is available. The quality of the work usually is increased closer to the Three Day Event to include faster work. One Day Events are used to monitor the horse's fitness and as additional training. The dressage and jumping training also substantially contributes to the fitness regimen. Older, experienced horses can get to major competitions with relatively few preparatory runs in comparison with less experienced horses, making it easier to manage low-grade injuries.

The majority of riders have not substantially reduced the intensity of their training for short-format competitions. The initial impression was that horses were finishing short-format competitions more tired than at a long-format competition. This was unexpected because of the lower overall effort of the shorter format. It may have been a result of the more intense nature of jumping the same number of fences in a shorter course. There may also have been an element of riders not preparing their horses as intensively for what was thought to be a less demanding competition. A study comparing cross-country recovery rates at a CCI** in long and short formats showed no significant difference between the two groups.[2]

CONFORMATION AND LAMENESS

Although the horse's stamp may vary the basic conformation must be correct. Eventing is unforgiving to conformational defects compared with show jumping and dressage. The general principles are the same as for any equine athlete. Serious conformational defects include being back at the knee, having upright pasterns and hocks, and having a moderate or severe toed-out conformation. Of slightly lesser importance are having a long or short back, being over at the knee, or having long, sloping pasterns. Defects such as offset knees and a slight-to-moderate toed-in conformation seem to be less important. A good foot conformation is always desirable, but many event horses have the TB trait of weak feet with collapsed heels.

The prepurchase examination for a young event prospect with hopes of a Three Day Eventing career is likely to be strict. The conformation should be assessed critically at this stage. Although the horse may have sufficient talent, defects in conformation may not allow it to stand up to the 5 or so years of training necessary to reach the top level of the sport. Conversely, it is possible to be more lenient in the interpretation of subtle problems when performing a prepurchase examination on an older, experienced horse. The horse's competitive record should be assessed carefully, because advanced horses are likely to have accumulated wear-and-tear changes during an extended career. Any conformational or subtle soundness queries can be addressed in light of the horse's proven ability to perform its task.

CLINICAL HISTORY

A routine lameness history should be obtained, emphasizing and obtaining the following information:
- Horse's competitive level
- Competition targets and timing, ahead or behind in its fitness schedule
- Previous problems
- Recent competitive or training program
- Current medications
- Prodromal signs
- Onset acute or insidious
- Exact nature of problem (limb swelling, lameness, or poor performance)
- Progression of problem
- Response to treatment

LAMENESS EXAMINATION

My standard approach is described, and the regions requiring particular attention and the most rewarding procedures are outlined for horses with subacute or chronic lameness problems. Care should be taken to palpate all limbs and the back thoroughly, because many concurrent or compensatory injuries can be found that way. Because many problems are subtle, the horse should be examined on a variety of surfaces and at different gaits.

Particular attention should be paid to the feet. The size, shape, and conformation should be assessed in relation to the size and breed of horse. The suitability of the shoe type for that horse should be determined, because farrier preference may have been influenced by fashion. The fit of the shoe should be correlated with stage in the shoeing cycle. Fortunately, the trend is to move away from the traditional problem of shoeing the horse short and tight at the heel. The hoof should be palpated for heat and any cracks or defects. The sole should be pared and hoof testers carefully applied over the entire solar surface, assessing the solar compliance and any pain response. Horses with recurrent bruising associated with soft soles may not have demonstrable pain on examination, but the lack of solar rigidity is clearly evident. Percussion may be helpful in a small proportion of horses. An increased digital pulse amplitude can be helpful in determining the presence of any inflammation in the foot and is especially important if the amplitude is asymmetrical in a limb or between feet. A subtle increase in digital pulse amplitude is best evaluated after trotting the horse in hand on a hard surface.

The horse should be palpated carefully for distention of the distal interphalangeal (DIP) and metacarpophalangeal or metatarsophalangeal (fetlock) joint capsules. The range of joint flexion and any resentment to flexion should be assessed carefully. Particular attention should be paid to the palmar metacarpal structures for presence of subtle, diffuse filling and any discrete swelling, heat, or pain in the tendonous or ligamentous structures. Owners and riders of event horses tend to be thorough in their own palpation of this region and often know the normal contours of their horse well. However, they often are misled by distention of the medial palmar vein or diffuse swelling from a more distal inflammatory lesion.

In the hindlimbs, pain on palpation over the cunean bursa and in response to the Churchill test should be determined. The medial femorotibial and femoropatellar joint capsules should be palpated to detect distention. The muscle tension in the back and hindquarters should be assessed carefully. Trigger points and painful foci should be determined, and the range of spinal flexibility in response to running a blunt object along the back should be assessed.

During the static examination the horse should be assessed for symmetry. The horse's condition and degree of muscling should be assessed in relation to its level of fitness. The freeness of stride, dynamic foot placement, and foot flight arcs should be assessed at the walk. At the trot any head nod and the range of gluteal excursion should be assessed to determine any lameness. Lunging in a circle on a hard surface frequently is used to exacerbate subtle lameness. However, it is also critical to see the horse lunged on a soft surface, a portion of the lameness examination that often is omitted. Different lameness conditions may be evident on different surfaces, and this comparison is valuable. For instance, a horse may have a low-grade concussive distal limb lameness evident when lunged on the hard surface. However, the primary problem may be proximal suspensory desmitis (PSD), pain from which is evident only when the horse is lunged on a soft surface. Notwithstanding the value of evaluating all the lameness problems present, many of these horses have numerous, low-grade sites of pathological conditions to which they have adapted. Evaluating these can be a frustrating business, and it is important to determine the current problem noticed by a knowledgeable owner or rider. Event horses are often remarkably tolerant of low-grade pain to which they become accommodated compared with dressage horses. Evaluation of the horse while the horse is being ridden can be more difficult, but this form of movement can exacerbate low-grade lameness. Riding may be the only way of observing problems evident during certain movements, such as lack of hindlimb impulsion during a change of gait or when jumping. Seeing the horse ridden by a different, preferably more experienced rider can be helpful in some horses suspected of having back pain or when schooling or behavioral problems are present.

Determining the normal range of soundness is a difficult and contentious issue. Because of age and level of work, most top-level event horses have some degree of orthopedic pathological condition. I prefer to score lameness on a scale of 0 to 10, with 0 being sound and 10 being non–weight bearing. An advanced horse should be sound in the forelimbs when trotted in a straight line, but a large proportion demonstrate a 1 of 10 bilateral forelimb lameness when trotted in a circle on a hard surface. Some horses that are competing satisfactorily may show a greater degree of symmetrical lameness, but asymmetry in lameness may indicate that an important problem exists. Advanced horses can demonstrate up to a 2 of 10 hindlimb lameness when trotted in a straight line, without being penalized for this in a trot-up at a Three Day Event. Many have a 2 to 3 of 10 bilateral hindlimb lameness while circling on a hard surface. Hindlimb lameness evident on soft surfaces is likely to produce lower dressage scores, because the horse will exhibit poor and asymmetrical action.

Flexion tests are useful to exacerbate any subtle lameness problems, but these tests are not specific. Flexion tests can be particularly helpful in evaluating horses with lameness evident only immediately after they have completed an event. These horses can be frustrating, because they are often clinically sound when evaluated subsequently. A persistent positive response to flexion that can be alleviated by diagnostic analgesic techniques is important. Limb protraction, retraction, adduction, and abduction can be helpful in exacerbating upper-limb pain. Turning the horse in a tight circle can be used to assess coordination and flexibility. The range of cervical movement is assessed by observing the horse reach for food (voluntary movement) and by manual manipulation (forced movement). Many horses can cheat and reach the flank by rotation of the upper cervical region, rather than by full lateral flexion of the entire neck.

Different considerations apply when examining the horse with a history of an acute, severe lameness, usually after the cross-country phase of a competition. A comprehensive evaluation of an acutely lame horse must be performed (see Chapter 13) and is described in detail elsewhere.[3] Unfortunately, localizing signs may be minimal, the horse may be in cardiovascular shock, and initial efforts must be directed at providing support to the horse and the suspected region of injury. Fractures are caused most commonly by external trauma. Particular attention should be paid to the shoulder region for signs of fracture of the supraglenoid tubercle of the scapula and to the stifle for effusion or periarticular swelling associated with patellar or other fractures. Soft tissue injuries such as severe suspensory desmitis or superficial digital flexor (SDF) tendonitis may cause acute, severe lameness.

DIAGNOSTIC ANALGESIA

Diagnostic analgesia is an important tool in lameness diagnosis in event horses. Because the horse may have many palpable abnormalities, differential diagnosis is important. However, no localizing clinical signs may be apparent, and diagnostic analgesia is critical to identifying the painful region. Specific treatment can be given if a problem is identified accurately. A positive response to intraarticular analgesia usually means a horse is likely to respond to intraarticular medication, leading to a quicker return to work. In horses with lameness problems too subtle for accurate interpretation of diagnostic blocks, intraarticular administration of corticosteroids may be useful to assess the long-term response to treatment. Even with experienced riders this method of management can have a placebo effect, because the rider may desire for the problem to be veterinary rather than from schooling.

Perineural and intrasynovial analgesic techniques are used commonly. Intraarticular analgesia is particularly helpful because many problems are joint related, and a quick and definitive diagnosis can be achieved. Owners greatly resist clipping of the hair during the competition season, and clipping is not necessary in fine-coated animals if a thorough scrub is performed. The preferred techniques for the most commonly performed blocks are described subsequently.

The palmar digital nerve block should be performed as far distal as possible, angling the needle axially and distally to the cartilages of the foot. Separate medial and lateral blocks may be helpful to localize the pain to a specific heel. Blocking the palmar nerves at the level of the fetlock is less likely to desensitize the fetlock joint with a block performed just below the base of the proximal sesamoid bones (PSBs), rather than at the level of the PSBs. The palmar portion of a low four-point block should be performed just proximal to the digital flexor tendon sheath (DFTS) to decrease the risk of proximal migration of local anesthetic solution, taking care to go above or below the communicating branch of the palmar nerves. The lateral palmar nerve block is a satisfactory method of achieving proximal palmar metacarpal analgesia. Because the middle carpal joint is not a likely source of pain in event horses, the risk of confusing pain from this site with that from the origin of the suspensory ligament is minimal.

The DIP joint is injected most easily at a site on the dorsal midline, using a vertically directed needle. Six milliliters or less of local anesthetic solution should be used to decrease the risk of diffusion from the joint. For the fetlock joints I prefer the lateral sesamoidean ligament approach because most horses do not have gross joint distention and the fixed anatomy of this approach is reliable.

In the hindlimbs the DIP, proximal interphalangeal, and metatarsophalangeal joints often are overlooked sources of pain. Perineural analgesia normally starts with plantar blocks performed at the base of the PSBs, followed by a low six-point block if necessary. Analgesia of the proximal plantar metatarsal region can be performed most easily by blocking the lateral plantar nerve 1 cm distal to the tarsometatarsal (TMT) joint. This blocks the nerve before it branches into the plantar metatarsal nerves and carries a minimal risk of inadvertent penetration of the distoplantar outpouchings of the TMT joint capsule.

IMAGING CONSIDERATIONS
Radiography
Radiography is the mainstay of imaging, but a few special considerations are necessary in event horses. Lateromedial and dorsopalmar radiographs of the digit can be helpful in assessing foot balance. The palmaroproximal-palmarodistal oblique image often is underused in assessing subtle pathological conditions of the navicular bone and the palmar processes of the distal phalanx. Some fractures of the distal phalanx are only detectable in this radiographic image. The flexed cranioproximal-craniodistal image of the stifle is especially valuable for assessing the medial aspect of the patella for fractures. It is important to angle the x-ray beam so that the trochlear ridges are not superimposed over the patella, because some fractures or evidence of comminution may otherwise be obscured. A relatively underexposed and undercollimated lateromedial image is also beneficial to detect small, displaced fragments, which otherwise may be missed.

Ultrasonography
Ultrasonographic evaluation of the palmar metacarpal structures is a vital part of the lameness evaluation of an event horse. SDF tendonitis is a common and career-threatening injury, and if the veterinarian has any doubt about even a subtle problem, an ultrasonographic examination should be performed. Even when primary forelimb lameness is located at a distal site, the most important lesion may be a compensatory tendonitis in the contralateral limb.

It is usually not necessary to clip the coat, particularly if the hair is fine, and diagnostic images can be obtained after thorough scrubbing and the liberal application of alcohol and gel. The coat may be clipped to obtain maximal detail if subtle tendonitis needs to be investigated. Clients are often reluctant to have the coat clipped for a precautionary scan during the competitive season, because they perceive that the horse will be flagged as having a problem when it next competes. In my experience, sufficient detail is visible in fine-coated horses without clipping, although the clients are warned that greater image quality can be obtained with clipping, and if the image quality is nondiagnostic, the coat needs to be clipped. Often the difficulty is not in identifying abnormalities within the tendon but in determining the relevance of any changes that are present. Many advanced horses have changes in fiber pattern of the superficial digital flexor tendon (SDFT). Transverse and longitudinal views should be obtained in a systematic fashion. Different focus, gain, and frequency settings optimize evaluation of different structures. The cross-sectional area (CSA) of the SDFT should be obtained routinely, because sequential monitoring of this may allow the early detection of tendonitis. Determining the CSA also assists in assessing the current importance of chronic lesions, which is an important and helpful part of the ultrasonographic examination and should not be omitted.

Ultrasonography also can be helpful in assessing articular and periarticular pathological conditions in structures such as the patellar ligaments. Examination of the ventral sacroiliac ligaments per rectum also can be valuable when pain in this region is suspected.

Scintigraphy
Nuclear scintigraphy is a useful technique for evaluating some lame event horses. Scintigraphy commonly is used in horses with hindlimb lameness, back problems, multiple limb lameness, and forelimb lameness with an equivocal or negative response to diagnostic analgesia. Image quality can be a concern, because event horses are skeletally mature and the degree of pathological bone conditions is low. Normal bone uptake can be limited, except in horses with acute trauma. Good technique is therefore essential to obtain diagnostic images, and postprocessing techniques, such as using motion-correction software, can be helpful. Case selection is also important, because the more chronic and low-grade the problem, the lower the likelihood of finding an obvious focal region of increased radiopharmaceutical uptake (IRU). Examples of conditions for which scintigraphy can be rewarding include nonlocalized foot pain (pedal osteitis and insertional injury of the deep digital flexor tendon [DDFT] attachment), stress fractures (although these are rare overall), and OA of the thoracolumbar synovial articulations (facet joints).

Normal scintigraphic patterns are described elsewhere.[4] Regions that commonly have greater radiopharmaceutical (RU) than elsewhere in event horses, but without associated pathological conditions, include the distal phalanx, the subchondral bone of the proximal interphalangeal joint, the subchondral bone of the fifth and sixth cervical and sixth and seventh cervical articulations, and the distal tarsal bones. The distal aspect of the tarsus appears to have active bone remodeling when evaluated scintigraphically, but many event horses do not show lameness or a positive response to either flexion tests or local analgesia. In a study evaluating the accuracy of scintigraphy in horses with confirmed distal hock joint pain, we found a positive predictive value of 0.70 and a negative predictive value of 0.91 for focal IRU.[5] Because of this high false-positive rate, scintigraphy should be used with thorough clinical examination. Although relying on scintigraphy in fractious horses may be tempting, authenticating the diagnosis using diagnostic analgesia is important.

Thermography
Thermography has been used for more than 30 years but is still a developing diagnostic modality. The technology has improved recently, and thermography units are now affordable. The handheld infrared imaging cameras are particularly attractive. Thermographic imaging provides a sensitive representation of skin surface temperature, but many confounding variables make interpretation of these images difficult. To develop expertise involves a steep learning curve, and considerable amounts of time and experience are necessary to make consistently useful interpretations. Major advantages include that the technique is noninvasive and is performed quickly. Thermography is similar to scintigraphy because it is a physiological rather than an anatomical imaging technique. Given the high prevalence and importance of soft tissue injuries in event horses, thermography has applications in detection and in monitoring response to therapy. Because of low specificity,

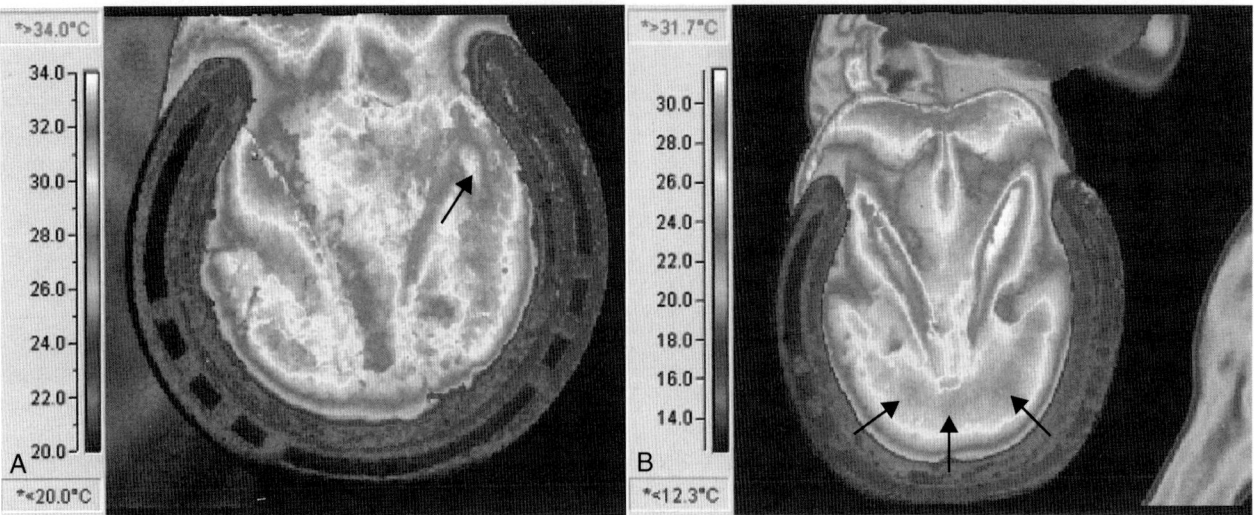

Fig. 117-4 • Examples of different thermographic foot patterns (solar images). **A,** This horse has a medial corn, manifested as a focal hot spot *(white) (arrow)* within an area of increased temperature. **B,** This horse has subacute laminitis, with a pattern of increased heat in the region of the tip of the distal phalanx *(arrows)*.

however, thermography should be used with other imaging techniques.

Thermographic imaging is useful in evaluating foot balance and in differentiating various types of inflammation of the foot (Figure 117-4; Color Plate 10). Examinations before and after exercise are particularly useful for this purpose. Similarly, preexercise and postexercise thermograms are helpful in identifying specific superficial muscle injuries. Accurate identification of local muscle strain permits treatment to be focused on the affected area, with a consequently shortened convalescent period. Thermography is also a useful tool in evaluating neck and back problems, although interpretation is more complex in these regions.

Thermography can be particularly useful in monitoring SDF tendonitis and can be used as part of a routine screening procedure, with regular examinations in the run up to a Three Day Event. Thermography can detect small lesions before clinical signs are evident, or it can be helpful in determining if a chronic lesion is active (Figure 117-5; Color Plate 11). If thermography suggests a lesion is present, then ultrasonographic examination is indicated. During the convalescent phase after injury, regular thermographic screening allows detection of any signs of inflammation in the affected region, as the plane of exercise is increased. Care must be taken to avoid artifacts from bandaging, previous clipping, and topical medication.

Magnetic Resonance Imaging

The increased availability and use of magnetic resonance imaging (MRI) have revolutionized the diagnosis and management of foot lameness in recent years. Diagnostic images can now be obtained in a standing horse, without the risk and expense of general anesthesia. This imaging modality is thus much more likely to be used early in the investigation of a lameness problem (see Chapter 21). In horses with foot lameness with no clinically significant radiological signs nor obvious superficial inflammation or pain, MRI can be helpful. Even if there are no relevant findings, the horse can be managed with corrective farriery

and a relatively early return to exercise once the lameness has subsided, with a greater degree of confidence that there is not an underlying soft tissue injury that will be adversely affected. It can also be helpful in assessing the degree of activity of ultrasonographic findings in more proximal soft tissues, and indeed in detecting lesions that are not evident ultrasonographically. Evidence of bone trauma may be detected that is not radiologically apparent.

SADDLE PRESSURE ANALYSIS

Computerized saddle pressure analysis using a force-sensing array system allows an objective assessment of pressure distribution beneath the saddle (Figure 117-6; Color Plate 12). Poor saddle fit is an important problem in event horses and is discussed elsewhere in greater detail (see page 1132). Computerized saddle pressure analysis is straightforward to perform and is complementary to conventional saddle fitting. By allowing an objective assessment, computerized saddle pressure analysis can be useful to confirm a problem to a rider, owner, or saddler. The better systems allow dynamic assessment of saddle fit at exercise, which is not otherwise possible.

PROCEEDING WITHOUT A DIAGNOSIS

Although a diagnosis can be made in most lame event horses, factors such as the experience level of the veterinarian, the thoroughness of the lameness workup, the number of imaging modalities available, and the nature, severity, and stage of the disease process affect diagnostic ability. If a horse is seen repeatedly on a first-opinion basis, stepping back and reassessing the horse as if from the start is sometimes necessary. It may be necessary to refer the horse for a second opinion or for advanced imaging techniques, such as scintigraphy, if these have not been performed. In some horses the precise diagnosis continues to remain elusive. In horses with obscure forelimb lameness, I routinely perform an ultrasonographic examination of the palmar metacarpal soft tissue structures, because tendonitis

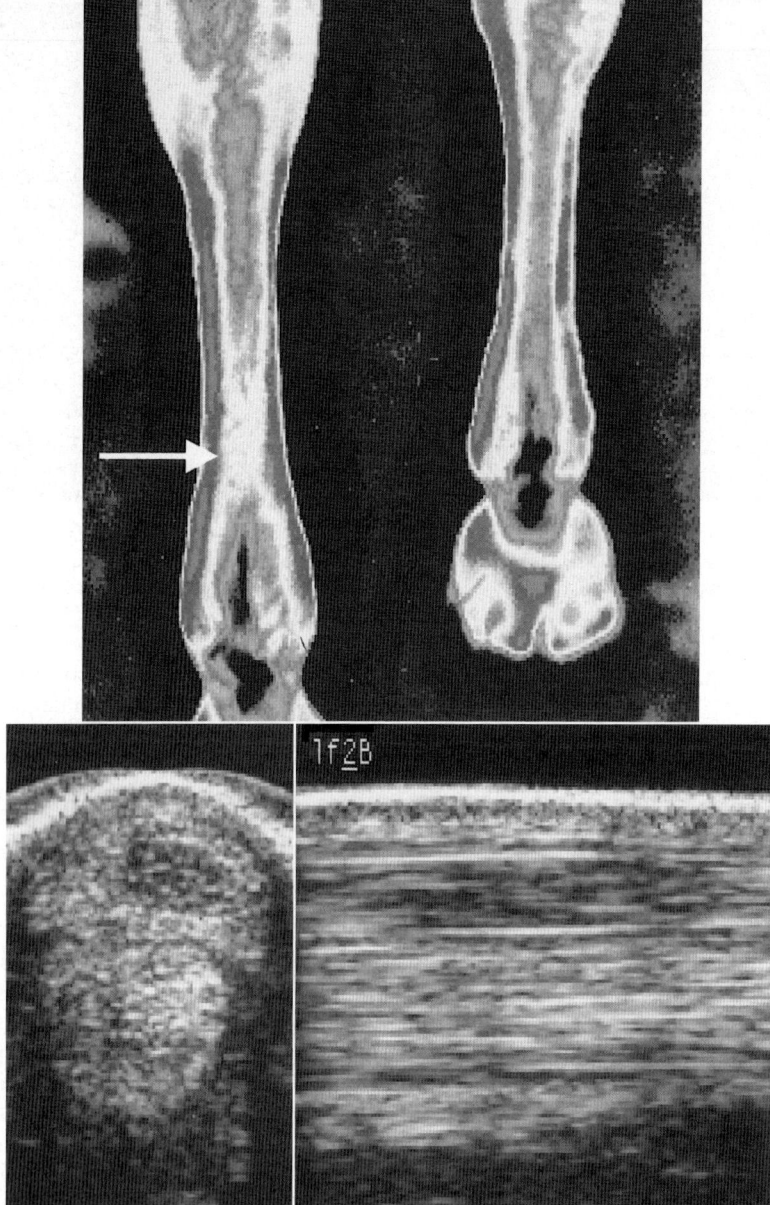

Fig. 117-5 • Palmar thermographic image and subsequent transverse (on the left) and longitudinal ultrasono-graphic images of the metacarpal region of an advanced event horse 10 days after successfully completing a Three Day Event. The horse was having a routine examination, and no clinical localizing signs were evident in the tendon. The thermogram (top) demonstrates a focal hot spot over the distal aspect of the left superficial digital flexor tendon (arrow), and the ultrasonographic images reveal a hypoechogenic core lesion in the same region.

and desmitis are important and highly prevalent. Serial CSA measurements of the SDFTs should be obtained, because the most relevant problem with an undiagnosed low-grade lameness may be a compensatory tendonitis in another limb. Any evidence of tendonitis indicates that exercise level should be decreased. Similarly, any persistent clinical signs of swelling in the palmar metacarpal structures should prompt a cautious approach. Even in the absence of ultrasonographic changes, mild swelling should alert the veterinarian to the possibility of a subclinical problem with tendonitis or desmitis. It is important not to rely too much on ultrasonography for diagnosis of soft tissue injuries, because early lesions may not be apparent.

Generally in horses with low-grade, undiagnosed lameness the response to a period (a few days to weeks) of rest should be assessed. If the response is poor, then most horses with an undiagnosed, low-grade hindlimb lameness can be continued in work, with or without the use of a systemic nonsteroidal antiinflammatory drug (NSAID) such as phenylbutazone. Greater caution normally is advised in horses with undiagnosed forelimb lameness, because the risk of developing a career-limiting injury with continued exercise is greater compared with similar injuries in the hindlimbs. If a subtle problem persists, then it may be necessary to increase exercise intensity to exacerbate the problem to a point at which diagnostic local analgesia can be performed. If a competition is imminent,

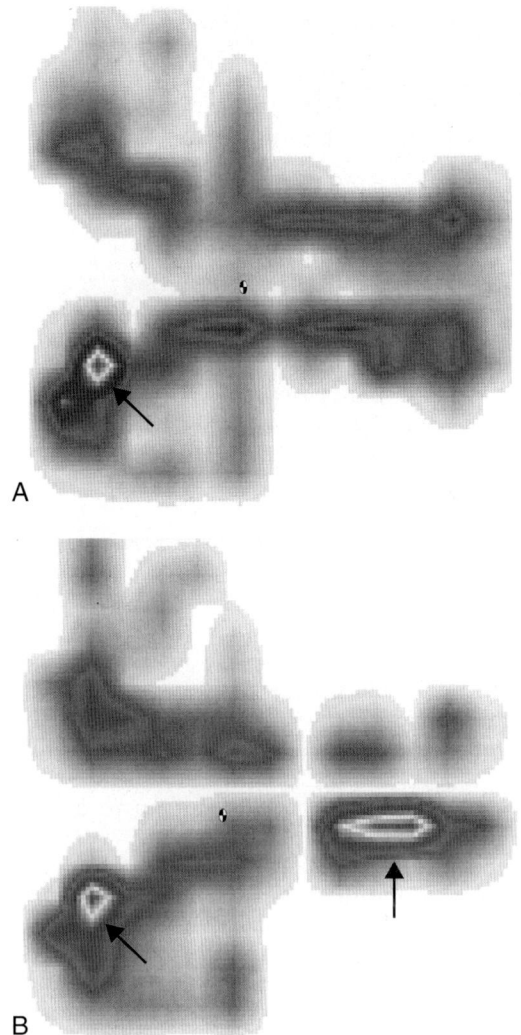

Fig. 117-6 • Computerized saddle pressure analysis images. Cranial is to the left, and left is to the bottom. **A,** This image shows a poorly fitting saddle, with a focal pressure point in the left wither region *(arrow)*. **B,** This image demonstrates failure of a gel pad to alleviate the pressure point and the development of an additional pressure point caudally *(arrows)*.

the owner or rider may apply considerable pressure to treat the most likely problem in the hope of rendering the horse sufficiently sound to compete.

If lameness is severe without initial diagnosis, then the horse should be given box rest, and the workup should be repeated until a diagnosis is achieved. If an upper limb soft tissue problem or a back problem is suspected, then a physiotherapeutic, chiropractic, or osteopathic opinion can be helpful. Although veterinary opinion is divided on the validity and value of these techniques, an owner frustrated by the lack of a veterinary diagnosis is likely to turn to these. Horses with poor performance may have schooling or behavioral problems. Assessment by an experienced and different rider can be helpful.

SHOEING CONSIDERATIONS

Foot problems are a major problem in event horses, and the importance of high-quality farriery in minimizing the incidence of lameness cannot be overemphasized. Regular and good farriery is critical in maintaining good medial-to-lateral and dorsal-to-palmar (plantar) hoof balance. Types of shoes vary among the traditional fullered hunter-type shoes, continental flat shoes, four-point style shoes, and various types of bar shoes. For routine shoeing the conventional fullered shoe offers the advantage of superior grip. Many farriers prefer the extra width of the flat section shoe, because this shoe is easier to fit, has sufficient width at the heel, and gives extra sole cover. If not applied correctly, flat-section shoes may cause excessive sole pressure in horses with flat feet. Traction devices are necessary if flat section shoes are put on horses working on tarmac. Natural balance shoeing has become popular recently in event horses, but although the technique suits some horses, others may actually develop lameness because of improper shoeing technique. However, the natural balance concept of a more palmar location for the breakover point has been well accepted. Seeing horses shod with the shoe set well back is now common, and quarter clips rather than toe clips are most common. This is helpful in horses with long-toe conformation, OA of the DIP joint, or navicular syndrome. A rolled-toe shoe may give a similar effect, although bringing the breakover point back to the same degree is difficult, and care must be taken to set the shoe back sufficiently.

The most common therapeutic shoe used in event horses is the bar shoe. The egg bar shoe is used commonly to manage horses with navicular syndrome and other causes of palmar foot pain and to provide support in horses with a collapsed heel. Egg bar shoes are heavy if they protrude beyond the heel bulbs and may be pulled off. Shoe loss is an important issue in event horses, more so than in other sports horses. As a compromise the straight bar shoe may provide additional foot stability while reducing the risk of shoe loss. In horses that require egg bar shoes, overreach boots can be used to reduce the risk of shoe loss, and by using a more palmar point of breakover, the front feet may leave the ground more quickly compared with horses with conventional shoes. In horses with a weak heel or quarter, laminar separation, or focal osteitis of the distal phalanx, an egg bar shoe may provide inadequate support and a heart bar shoe can be beneficial. This shoe is heavy, does not project as far beyond the heel as does the egg bar shoe, and transfers some portion of weight-bearing load to the frog. In horses with pain localized to one heel bulb or quarter, a half bar shoe can provide sufficient support and is lighter than a full heart bar shoe.

Pads are used relatively infrequently in event horses. Although pads may provide short-term benefit in horses with sole pain, they promote excess movement of the clenches and premature shoe loosening. Full pads cause a poor microenvironment of the foot. Packing the soles of the hoof has become popular in recent years because it is thought to protect the soles and to have anticoncussive effects, but without the risk of premature shoe loosening. Modern synthetic hoof repair materials can be beneficial in horses that have lost portions of the hoof wall, because the defect can be filled and shoe nails can be placed subsequently. However, routine use of hoof repair materials to augment hoof wall in horses with poor-quality, cracking, and flaking feet should be discouraged and may even cause the problem to persist. If used, repair material should be removed at the end of the season, and the horse should be turned out without shoes. The foot may break up initially but will grow back stronger without the repair materials.

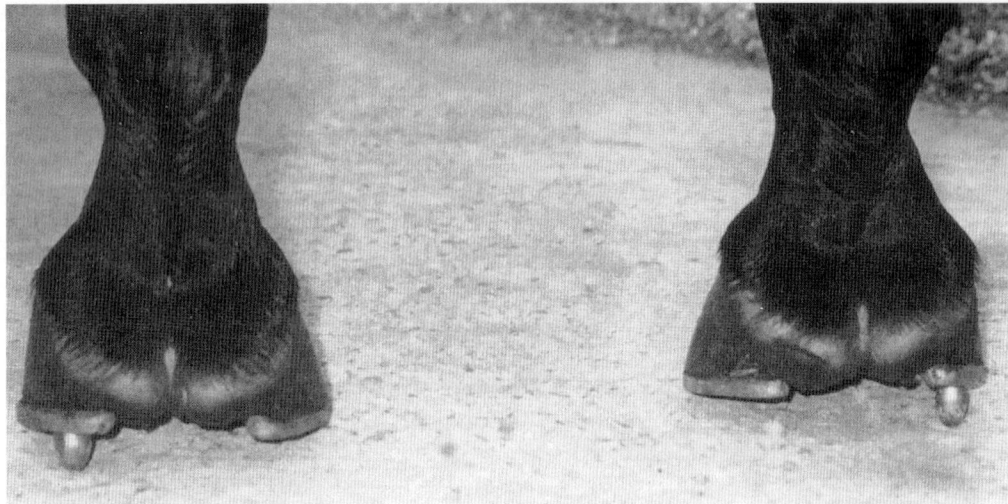

Fig. 117-7 • Palmar view of horse with single studs, showing the degree of medial-to-lateral imbalance induced when the horse is on a hard surface.

Steel shoes are used routinely, but some riders switch to aluminum shoes at a Three Day Event. The foot must be of sufficient quality to cope with the lower degree of support offered by the more flexible aluminum shoe, and switching is not recommended if the horse has any history of foot-related lameness. Any speed and recovery benefits of the lighter shoes do not appear to be obvious in event horses. Synthetic shoes rarely are used.

Road nails or studs often are used, especially in broad section shoes, to decrease the risk of slipping on the roads during walking and trotting exercise. Improper use of road nails or studs may cause hoof imbalance. If the grip point is positioned near the middle of the foot (rather than near the heel), the foot may rock over this point during weight bearing. Event horses commonly wear studs for competition. Some advocate that a single stud be worn simply on the basis that if the stud is on the outside, the risk of the horse treading on itself is less. With a single stud, the foot can still twist, causing less jarring to the limb overall. Conversely, a single stud severely imbalances the foot, and because the roads and tracks phase of a long-format Three Day Event often includes sections of metaled road or tracks, this could induce excessive strain on the joints (Figure 117-7). Studs should be avoided for the roads and tracks phase if logistically possible. However, some horses will jump with confidence only if two or more studs per foot are applied. The studs always should be chosen based on ground conditions, and a blunt inside stud decreases problems from tread injury. Care should be taken to avoid positioning a stud hole over an area of defective hoof wall. Horses are normally reshod 1 week before a Three Day Event, because if a horse is pricked or any foot soreness occurs after shoeing, the horse has time for recovery.

TACK CONSIDERATIONS

Saddle fit is of great importance in event horses. Injuries to the withers and back may manifest as poor performance in the dressage or show jumping phases of competition. Different saddles are required for the different disciplines of eventing, predisposing the horse to fitting problems. The fit of the saddle to the horse is sometimes a secondary consideration to riders, who may have a particular saddle in which they feel secure. Event horses often have high withers, and fitting a saddle is often difficult. Saddle fit can be affected adversely by the tendency of event horses to lose weight dramatically in the run up to a Three Day Event. Therefore a saddle that is fitted 2 weeks before an event can sit too low by competition time. Unfortunately, the use of pads and numnahs to correct poor saddle fit is not effective. Computerized saddle pressure analysis has shown that even gel pads are ineffective in alleviating focal pressure points, and that numnahs and pads placed beneath well-fitting saddles can be detrimental (see Figure 117-6).[6] Thick or numerous pads elevate the saddle and put pressure on the midline and over the dorsal spinous processes, a situation that impedes spinal flexibility.

Opinions vary on the benefits of protective leg wear. Tendon boots are used almost universally for the cross-country phase, because the risk of direct traumatic injury to the distal aspect of the limb is high. However, the additional insulation increases the temperature of the distal aspect of the limb. There are theoretical concerns that elevation in temperature could damage tenocytes and predispose the horse to tendonitis, although no clinical evidence indicates that this occurs. Some boots have reinforced sections to give additional protection against speedy cut injuries to the palmar aspect of the tendons, but the large rigid section may rub against the tendons at exercise and cause abrasions. Conversely, some of the flimsy boots do not give sufficient protection against this kind of laceration. Bandages give a greater degree of conformity, but they are more difficult to apply correctly and require inclusion of a reinforcing layer if they are to provide substantial protection. Neither bandages nor boots reduce risk of tendon strain but simply protect against direct trauma.

TEN MOST COMMON LAMENESS CONDITIONS

Some conditions are more common during training, and others are more common at competitions. The overall prevalence is as follows:

1. Thoracolumbar and cervical soreness and restriction
2. Foot soreness (bruising, imbalance, and nail bind)
3. Traumatic osteoarthritis
   a. Distal interphalangeal joint
   b. Metacarpophalangeal and metatarsophalangeal joints
   c. Tarsometatarsal and centrodistal joints
   d. Proximal interphalangeal joint
4. Superficial digital flexor tendonitis
5. Suspensory desmitis
   a. Branch desmitis
   b. Proximal suspensory desmitis
6. External trauma
   a. Lacerations including overreaching injury
   b. Penetrations
   c. Stifle bruising
7. Pain in the sacroiliac region
8. Fractures of the stifle region
9. Other fractures
10. Rhabdomyolysis

DIAGNOSIS AND MANAGEMENT OF LAMENESS

Thoracolumbar and Cervical Soreness and Restriction

Neck and back soreness are common clinical findings in event horses, although they do not always limit performance. Soreness may be secondary to lameness as occurs, for example, when pain on palpation of the brachiocephalicus muscle is found in horses with distally located forelimb lameness. Primary problems may be subtle, and determining the importance of clinical findings can be difficult. To know an individual horse's normal degree of sensitivity and flexibility can be extremely helpful, because any changes can be correlated with the onset of a performance problem. Questioning a knowledgeable owner, groom, or physiotherapist can be helpful. Sometimes the clinical significance of any soreness can be assessed only by the horse's response to treatment.

Event horses are particularly prone to muscle soreness when exercise intensity is varied or increased. Intense dressage training initially causes a transient period of lumbar muscle soreness, especially during the sitting trot. Areas of focal pain and muscle spasm may be easily palpable, but assessing flexibility and range of movement is also important. Radiographs are not helpful in diagnosing the relevance of dorsal spinous process impingement, and clinical signs, scintigraphic examination, and a positive response to local analgesia or treatment are necessary to confirm if a lesion is active and/or causing pain. Ultrasonographic examination can be helpful in diagnosing supraspinous ligament injury. Thermography is helpful in detecting acute soft tissue injuries in the thoracolumbar region (see Chapter 25).

Many horses with neck and back pain respond well to physiotherapy. If range of movement is decreased, then mobilization of the affected region is beneficial (see Chapters 93 to 95), which then can be followed by continued stretching exercises, performed by the owner or rider. Massage is beneficial but yields only temporary improvement. Various modalities such as laser, therapeutic ultrasound, and neuromuscular stimulation can be helpful. Results with extracorporeal shock wave therapy have been encouraging in some horses. In some horses, chiropractic manipulation is beneficial. Acupuncture also can be effective if performed by an experienced practitioner. Given the range of physiotherapeutic treatment options available, the degree of experience necessary for optimal treatment results, and the nature of these therapeutic modalities, I suggest that veterinarians work with an experienced and qualified therapist. It behooves the veterinarian to be familiar with these techniques, because case selection and palpation skills can improve.

Horses with caudal cervical restriction caused by OA of the synovial articulations (articular facet joints) may show a positive response to intraarticular medication with triamcinolone acetonide (5 mg) injected under ultrasonographic guidance. Each affected facet joint is injected, and the horse is rested for 2 weeks, after which time improvement is normally dramatic. Horses with mild to moderate impingement of the thoracic dorsal spinous processes can be treated successfully using local injection of methylprednisolone acetate (40 mg) and Sarapin (6 mL). The horse is lunged or long reined for 2 weeks and then returned to exercise. The duration of effect can be as short as 6 weeks, but in a large proportion of horses, the problem resolves without repeat medication. Marks provides a review of the various veterinary options in treating back pain.[7] The importance of management and riding factors in treating these conditions cannot be overemphasized. Rehabilitation and reschooling of horses with moderate-to-severe pain are necessary to build up the local musculature and to develop flexibility.

Foot Soreness (Bruising, Imbalance, and Nail Bind)

Foot soreness is a common clinical problem in event horses. Transient sole bruising is frequent, especially in flat- and thin-soled horses. Foot imbalance predisposes horses to soreness, and medial-to-lateral hoof imbalance is commonly present. In horses with a collapsed heel, pain to hoof testers and corns are commonly found. Horses with persistent foot lameness may have laminar separation or focal osteitis of the distal phalanx, and scintigraphy is helpful in differential diagnosis. Poor foot conformation in many horses can predispose them to nail bind or pricking when shod. Shoes often are pulled off, which can lead to breakup of the wall and further problems with shoe security. Regular, high-quality farriery is more important in maintaining good hoof quality than is the feeding of supplements or use of topical applications. Good stable hygiene is also important. Shoeing aspects have been discussed (see page 1131).

Osteoarthritis

Distal limb joints are especially prone to traumatic joint disease, especially in the forelimb. OA of the DIP joint is most common, followed by that of the metacarpophalangeal joint. OA of the proximal interphalangeal joint is rare. Diagnosis is confirmed by observing a positive response to intraarticular analgesia, effusion or fibrosis, a positive response to flexion, and low-viscosity synovial fluid. Radiographs are often unremarkable in horses with early or low-grade OA. Response to intraarticular medication is normally excellent. Combining hyaluronan with a low dose of corticosteroid such as triamcinolone acetonide (5 mg) produces the greatest therapeutic effect. Hyaluronan alone produces an inconsistent response, and low doses of triam-cinolone acetonide have been shown to be chondroprotective. Medium-viscosity hyaluronan usually is used initially based on economic factors, but high-molecular-weight products may give a greater effect in some horses. Systemic administration of hyaluronan (intravenously) or polysulfated glycosaminoglycan (intramuscularly) is not nearly as effective as is specific intraarticular medication. Systemic medication does not carry the same risk of iatrogenic infection and is easier to administer and so is used frequently as an adjunct therapy. Prophylactic use of systemic therapy frequently is used in horses in the run up to a Three Day Event or to manage those with pathological conditions of numerous joints or generalized stiffness. Feeding of nutraceuticals such as chondroitin sulfate and glucosamine is also common practice. Although in vitro evidence of efficacy is substantial, no convincing clinical studies demonstrate efficacy in vivo. In fact, studies have demonstrated a lack of oral absorption of chondroitin sulfate[8-10] and glucosamine[10] in horses.

In horses with OA of the DIP and metacarpophalangeal joints that has been unresponsive to medication, and especially with radiological evidence of osteochondral fragmentation, arthroscopic evaluation can be beneficial. Focal areas of cartilage and subchondral bone damage may be identified, and the horse often responds positively to debridement. Access is limited in the DIP joint, but lesions often are found on the extensor process of the distal phalanx.

OA of the TMT and centrodistal joints is not infrequent, but the distal tarsal joints show scintigraphic evidence of remodeling even in normal event horses. Horses with authentic OA of these joints usually respond well to medication with low doses of long-acting corticosteroids (40 mg of methylprednisolone acetate). The condition rarely seems to progress sufficiently to necessitate chemical or surgical arthrodesis.

Superficial Digital Flexor Tendonitis

Although not the commonest lameness problem in event horses, tendonitis is the most substantial cause of wastage[11] because of prolonged convalescence and high recurrence rates. Although tendonitis can occur as a single-event injury, especially if the horse falls,[12] stumbles, or trips badly, the condition most commonly results from repetitive cyclic loading. Unlike the suspensory ligament, tendons in adult horses do not strengthen in response to exercise and therefore are prone to develop accumulated microdamage during intense training. This damage can give the prodromal signs of slight filling or heat in the palmar metacarpal structures. The clinical signs of a SDFT strain then may develop acutely after a training canter or competition. For horses to develop subclinical tendonitis after a Three Day Event is not uncommon. The condition may not be apparent during the rest period after the competition but develops into clinical tendonitis when the horse resumes training or competitive work, even after 3 to 6 months. Close monitoring is thus essential, and I recommend routine ultrasonography after each Three Day Event. Ultrasonographic evaluation is important to assess the severity of injury and to determine a prognosis and an appropriate treatment plan. Lesion length and percentage of CSA involvement should be determined. Tendons may increase in CSA up to

10% normally with intense training, but this tends to return to baseline at the end of the season. If ultrasonographic examination is performed soon after injury, the extent of the lesion may not be apparent and severity may be underestimated. Severity of tendon damage is assessed most accurately 1 to 4 weeks after injury.

Initial treatment of event horses with SDF tendonitis is aimed at limiting inflammation and preventing any further tendon damage. The horse should be given box rest for 2 to 4 weeks, and antiinflammatory therapy should be commenced. Systemic NSAIDs appear to decrease swelling and pain, and no evidence indicates that they impede healing. Conversely, prolonged corticosteroid administration may interfere with fibroplasia, although a single systemic dose helps decrease inflammation without any apparent detrimental effects.

Support bandages or firm stable bandages should be applied for the first few weeks to reduce swelling. Topical dimethyl sulfoxide can be useful to decrease inflammation early after injury but should not be used for more than 5 days, because it can weaken collagen fibers and blister the skin. Local treatment with cold water hosing and ice application is beneficial while the signs of acute inflammation persist. For horses with mild-to-moderate injuries, the benefits of being able to perform local therapy seem to outweigh the greater external support that can be provided by application of a Robert Jones bandage.

In horses with severe SDF tendonitis in which loss of support (sinking) of the metacarpophalangeal joint has occurred, external support using a Robert Jones bandage is recommended. A heel wedge should be applied if the horse is severely lame. Heel elevation theoretically does not decrease load on the SDFT but appears to provide analgesia to horses that stand with the heel off the ground. In horses with severe breakdown injury, support with a proprietary splint, such as a Kimzey Leg Saver (Kimzey, Woodland, California, United States) is recommended.

Controlled exercise, to encourage development of a longitudinal fiber pattern but without placing excessive load on the tendon to damage the healing fibers, is the mainstay of recuperation. Serial ultrasonographic examinations are helpful to determine the appropriate rate of progress and the response to increasing exercise. After the period of box rest, walking in hand normally is commenced. Mechanical horse walkers appear detrimental in the early stages of healing, because constant turning places excessive load on a weak tendon. However, such walkers are extremely helpful after the initial 4 to 6 weeks of walking in hand, when duration of walking is increased. A major problem during this stage is degree of tolerance shown by the horse to this restricted level of exercise. Many horses are too excitable to be walked safely in hand, but they behave appropriately on a horse walker or if ridden under saddle. Exercise programs must be tailored to account for rider competence and the horse's behavior. Once trotting has been commenced, the horse normally settles down into the exercise regimen.

A large number of treatment options exist for managing event horses with tendonitis. Tendon splitting, usually performed percutaneously in the standing horse, appears beneficial in horses with acute core lesions. Tendon splitting may decompress the core lesion and allow neovascularization but is most effective when performed in the first 10 days after injury. Intralesional injection of hyaluronan or a polysulfated glycosaminoglycan has not proved beneficial. Initial clinical studies investigating intralesionally administered β-aminopropionitrile fumarate unfortunately lacked representative control groups, and a licensed product is no longer available.

Intralesional injections of growth factors have been tried. Insulin-like growth factor-1 (IGF-1) and equine growth hormone, which induces the production of IGF-1, have been studied. I have had success in a small number of horses using transforming growth factor–β (TGF-β) in horses with tendonitis. The drug appears to promote fibroplasia. Although this gives a quicker healing rate and horses have returned to work successfully, whether the expected increase in strength and decrease in elasticity are desirable is theoretically debatable. I have had rewarding results using TGF-β in horses with chronic tendonitis. When ultrasonographic evidence of poor infilling exists, intralesional injection of TGF-β improves fiber pattern, and horses are able to withstand increased exercise intensity. After treatment, some horses have returned to CCI**** level and have completed successfully in up to three events. Platelet-rich plasma (PRP) has been used more for ligamentous than tendonous injuries.

Desmotomy of the accessory ligament of the superficial digital flexor tendon (superior check desmotomy) also can be beneficial in selected horses, and performing the technique tenoscopically carries a much lower risk of postoperative incisional problems. Because of the risk of general anesthesia, I reserve its use for horses with recurrent tendonitis when there are very high owner expectations and for horses in which the ultrasonographic appearance of the SDFT deteriorates inappropriately during the controlled exercise regimen. In a small number of horses in trotting exercise after tendonitis, increased CSA and decreased echogenicity are observed. Even after the plane of exercise is reduced to walking for another 6 to 8 weeks or even longer, the ultrasonographic appearance of the SDFT does not change. After desmotomy, however, these horses tolerate an increased plane of exercise without ultrasonographic deterioration or subsequent recurrence of tendonitis. Because the procedure may increase the risk of suspensory desmitis after surgery, desmotomy should not be used in horses with a concurrent pathological condition of the suspensory apparatus. In a comparative discussion of outcomes for National Hunt horses with tendon injuries treated with different methodologies, superior check ligament desmotomy was the only one to show a significant improvement in outcome in comparison with conservative management, with shock wave therapy, IGF-1, and firing showing only trends toward improved outcomes.[13]

Stem cell therapy has become popular in some quarters (see Chapter 73), but I have not yet seen any clinically significant improvement in outcome and await the results of long-term studies. The expense and the delay in instigating treatment are off-putting. I currently use intralesional injections of bone marrow concentrate, made by processing bone marrow in a commercial system usually used for preparing PRP. This should yield some stem cells as well as growth factors and can be done on an outpatient basis.

Extracorporeal shock wave therapy (ESWT) can be beneficial. Subjectively I have felt that there is an improvement in the longitudinal fiber pattern. It is particularly useful in horses with mild or chronic tendonitis when there is no clear core lesion for injection.

Systemic medication with a polysulfated glycosaminoglycan is used as an adjunct treatment in horses with tendonitis. Ease of administration and lack of potential complications make such treatment popular, but no evidence indicates that any systemic medication, or feed supplement for that matter, has beneficial effects in tendon healing.

My current approach tends toward combined therapies, as none of the treatments individually have been shown to make any dramatic difference in outcome. Horses with core lesions would be treated with intralesional medication, followed by a course of ESWT and superior check ligament desmotomy if finances and the severity of the lesion justified it.

The total convalescent period depends on severity of initial injury, how well the injury appears to heal determined by ultrasonography, and the degree of compliance with the controlled exercise regimen. In horses with mild tendonitis (subtle loss of fiber pattern and <10% increase in CSA) as few as 6 weeks of walking exercise is sufficient. Horses with loss of fibers and frank tendonitis require a convalescent period of 9 to 15 months. Recurrence rate is less in horses that are given at least a year to recuperate before commencing full work. After tendonitis, many horses can be managed successfully to complete one Three Day Event, but sustaining the horse through a number of Three Day Events without recurrence is more difficult. A small number of horses seem to suffer recurrent clinical signs regardless of management protocol, and these are best restricted to One Day Events, in which they will often then compete successfully for many years.

Suspensory Desmitis
The two main levels of suspensory injury in the Three Day Event horse are branch desmitis and PSD. Midbody desmitis is rare. Suspensory branch desmitis can be considered an occupational disease of event horses. Advanced horses commonly develop inflammation and enlargement of the branches after a Three Day Event, and the condition is often transient with no associated lameness. Viewed by ultrasonography, the branches have periligamentous fibrosis with no areas of obvious hypoechogenicity, although some loss of longitudinal fiber pattern may occur. In many horses this pathological condition is missed or ignored, and the horse is just turned out. Even a short period of controlled exercise often decreases the risk of recurrence, however. Some degree of synovitis of the metacarpophalangeal joint commonly occurs and usually responds favorably to intraarticular medication.

PSD is a common cause of forelimb lameness.[11] Lameness may be acute in onset, with inflammation obvious after exercise, or the disease can be insidious without any localizing signs. Diagnostic analgesia is mandatory, and ultrasonographic examination is valuable. Radiographic and scintigraphic examinations are useful adjunct tools. Most horses have true desmitis, although a small number have enthesopathy and associated bone remodeling, with clinically significant IRU and minimal ultrasonographic abnormalities. Most horses respond well to 4 to

9 months of controlled exercise, and no convincing evidence exists that any intralesional medications are beneficial. ESWT is commonly used to treat horses with suspensory desmitis. The analgesic effect may encourage a premature return to full exercise, thus increasing the risk of recurrence, and patience is still required in the rehabilitation of horses with acute injuries. ESWT is useful in horses with chronic, active desmitis, especially those with bone involvement that does not respond appropriately to controlled exercise.

I feel that PSD in hindlimbs is a most important but underdiagnosed condition. Similar to that seen in forelimbs, hindlimb PSD may cause acute or chronic lameness. The prognosis is generally much poorer for horses with hindlimb PSD, however, because of the development of a local compartment syndrome and associated pressure on the plantar metatarsal nerves. Thus most horses remain chronically lame, even after the ligament appears healed on ultrasonographic images. I have had success in treating event horses with persistent, chronic lameness with static or healed ligaments resulting from hindlimb PSD using local infiltration of triamcinolone acetonide (10 mg). Although lameness abates, treatment needs to be repeated at 6-month intervals and may be detrimental to the ligament in the long term. Thus a surgical technique has been developed for use in horses with chronic desmitis that has yielded extremely good results.[14]

The surgical technique involves the resection of a 4-cm segment of the common (deep) branch of the plantar metatarsal nerve, distal to its origin from the lateral plantar nerve. This is combined with incision of the fascia (fasciotomy) overlying the origin of the suspensory ligament. This technique combines decompression with analgesia and has allowed horses to return to a normal level of work within 3 months. The horses are restricted to walking only for the first month, after which time turnout and ascending exercise are permitted. I have operated on hundreds of horses, with a long-term success rate of around 75% and a low risk of more extensive suspensory ligament damage developing.

External Trauma
Event horses are prone to traumatic lacerations during competition, the most common being overreach injuries to the heel bulbs and skin abrasions and lacerations, particularly to the carpus and stifles.[11] Standard principles of treatment apply, although owners often apply pressure to minimize healing time during the competition season. Aggressive early treatment is advised, and horses with deep foot or pastern wounds should be managed with a fiberglass cast for 10 to 14 days, a treatment that may shorten the convalescent period. Wounds should be assessed carefully for synovial penetrations. Thorn penetrations from brush or hedge fences can lead to infectious arthritis of the carpal or stifle joints, with only minimal clinical signs evident initially.

Direct trauma from jumping solid fences is common. Trauma directly over bone can lead to a severe, transient lameness. Acute lameness from this type of bone bruising can be difficult to differentiate from a fracture on an initial clinical examination. Trauma over the soft tissues may lead to the development of a considerable hematoma or edema, so local cold and pressure are indicated in the early stages.

Pain in the Sacroiliac Region
A low-grade form of sacroiliac disease is common in event horses and is manifest as a loss of impulsion and scope when jumping, with a reduced hindfoot flight arc. Most advanced event horses have bony pelvic asymmetry when critically assessed. Clinical signs include pain on palpation around the tubera sacrale and resentment of gentle lateral rocking action when the horse is in a weight-bearing position, with the opposite hindlimb held up. Often, associated muscle soreness and spasm are present in the surrounding musculature, notably the middle gluteal muscle. Most of these horses appear to have sacroiliac joint instability, but minimal evidence of IRU is seen on scintigraphic examination. Clinical signs can be localized by assessing the response to infiltration of local anesthetic solution around the dorsal aspect of the sacroiliac joint, using a spinal needle angled ventrocraniolaterally from just caudal to the opposite tuber sacrale. Ultrasonographic evaluation of the ventral sacroiliac ligaments per rectum also can be helpful to localize any pathological abnormality. The condition usually occurs when the horse is unfit and being brought into work or when the plane of exercise is increased. Sacroiliac pain often is self-limiting because the musculature increases as the plane of exercise increases and stabilizes the sacroiliac joint. Administering a systemic NSAID such as phenylbutazone helps the horse work through the period of lameness. Physiotherapy can assist in treating the local muscle spasm, and some horses improve with chiropractic or osteopathic manipulation. Horses with refractory pain sometimes improve after the local infiltration of methylprednisolone acetate (120 mg) or a sclerosing agent (e.g., P2G Solution [50 mL], Martindale Pharmaceuticals, Romford, United Kingdom), using the same approach as for local analgesia. Horses are continued in the same plane of work, and improvement normally is reported within a week. The duration of response varies, and some horses do not require repeat treatments.

Fractures in the Stifle Region
Fractures of the patella are common in event horses,[15] and the imaging aspects have already been discussed. For medial fractures, surgical removal offers the best prognosis. The original surgical description is for an incision 15 to 25 cm in length, but I prefer to use arthroscopic guidance, enabling me to create a minimal surgical incision (5 to 7 cm) centered directly over the fragment. This is satisfactory for small fragments and also allows for thorough evaluation of the femoropatellar joint and easy removal of any loose fragments.

Other Fractures
Fractures caused by direct trauma of the distal phalanx and second and fourth metacarpal bones are not uncommon. Occasionally, condylar fractures of the third metacarpal or metatarsal bones or sagittal fractures of the proximal phalanx occur during training or competition, although they are rare. The standard considerations apply for evaluation and treatment. Vertebral or upper limb fractures can occur after a fall, and the initial evaluation can be complicated by adrenaline dominance.

Rhabdomyolysis

Recurrent rhabdomyolysis is relatively rare in advanced-level horses, because horses prone to this disease are selected out at the lower levels. Sporadic episodes are common at Three Day Events, however. Many potential trigger factors exist, including the stress of travel, stabling away from home, the competition itself, dehydration, climate changes, electrolyte imbalance, and dietary changes. I have noted a particularly high incidence in horses that were switched to haylage products immediately before a competition. This practice is done frequently because of the greater convenience of the small, packaged bales. A period of at least 4 to 6 weeks is recommended to allow adaptation to the new diet. The clinical manifestations at a Three Day Event can vary from collapse and recumbency on the roads and tracks phase in long-format competition to slight stiffness developing many hours after the completion of the cross-country phase of either short- or long-format competition.

To reduce the risk of rhabdomyolysis, attention should be paid to avoiding the trigger factors. Vitamin E levels are frequently low in event horse diets. Many commercial electrolyte preparations do not contain sufficient quantities of salt, and horses may be at risk if owners follow manufacturers' recommendations. Routine blood sampling to monitor the muscle-derived enzymes aspartate transaminase and creatine kinase is performed frequently, but considerable fluctuation in asymptomatic event horses can occur,[16] making interpretation difficult. This variation tends to decrease as horses become fitter, as the muscle cells appear less leaky. With the recognition of polysaccharide storage myopathy as a cause of rhabdomyolysis, some event horses have been successfully managed on a diet high in fat and low in soluble carbohydrates, although actual diagnosis is difficult to confirm.

PREVENTION OF LAMENESS

When considering the time involved to train a horse to the top level and the potential for a long athletic career, preventing lameness is especially desirable in event horses. However, many important factors are beyond the veterinarian's influence. The number and frequency of competitions, having the opportunity to choose events with good going and an appropriate riding surface, and a high standard of riding ability are factors difficult to control. The veterinarian may be able to assist with other factors such as a high standard of farriery and optimizing training programs. Regular veterinary monitoring can be valuable by allowing the early detection and treatment of any lameness problems. Monitoring for incipient SDF tendonitis by performing periodic clinical examinations, using thermographic and ultrasonographic examinations, and monitoring serum markers of tendonitis can be useful. Serial determination of markers such as cartilage oligomeric matrix protein (COMP) holds promise. Initial studies have shown that COMP increases as training intensity increases, and higher COMP levels are found in horses that subsequently developed SDF tendonitis.[17] The concurrent use of all of these maximizes the veterinarian's ability to detect subclinical tendonitis.

Many medications and supplements are sold with the aim of decreasing the risk of orthopedic disease. In racehorses, intramuscularly administered polysulfated glycosaminoglycan and intravenously administered hyaluronan have been shown to decrease the number of races missed, although the incidence of injuries was not decreased. Thus these drugs seem to be acting as antiinflammatory rather than as disease-modifying agents. Many commercial feed supplements are available but have unproven efficacy and variable and uncertain composition.

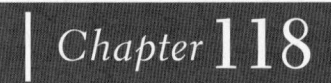

Lameness in Endurance Horses

Martha M. Misheff

EVOLUTION OF ENDURANCE

Modern endurance is the most rapidly evolving equine sport. It has its roots in the long distance races of the ancient Bedouin across the desert. Later British and American cavalry used endurance tests as part of their military training, and nineteenth century Austrians had a Vienna to Budapest ride. Despite this long history, organized endurance riding is a young sport. The first modern endurance ride, the 100-mile (160-km) Tevis Cup from Nevada to California, has been run every year since 1955. The Tom Quilty Gold Cup, a prestigious 100-mile endurance race named for its founder, was established in 1966 and is held every year in a different part of Australia. The oldest endurance organization, the American Endurance Ride Conference, has been in existence only since 1972. Since 1984, all international endurance competitions have been held under the auspices of the Fédération Équestre Internationale (FEI). The Endurance World Championships are held every 2 years in a different host country, and endurance is now the fastest growing FEI sport. More countries participate in international endurance championships than in the international championships of any other FEI discipline.

DESCRIPTION OF THE SPORT

The FEI Rules for Endurance describe the sport as a test of "the competitor's ability to safely manage the stamina and fitness of the horse over an endurance course in a competition against the track, the distance, the climate, the terrain and the clock." It is the clock, however, that determines the winner because the winner is the competitor who completes the course in the shortest time and passes the final veterinary inspection and forensic testing. As the sport of endurance has grown, it has come under intense scrutiny with regard to equine welfare. In addition, there is a great deal of debate within the endurance community as to whether the more media- and spectator-friendly events favoring increasing speeds over shorter distances (120 km) are preferable to the more traditional sport of slower speeds over longer distances and more challenging terrain. In March 2008, an Endurance World Forum was held in Paris to discuss these and other concerns, and a task force was appointed to revamp current rules governing the sport. The new rules went into effect in 2009; the current championship distance remains unchanged at 160 km (100 miles). The 2008 Endurance World Championships in Malaysia marked the first time that this event was internationally televised.

Each country has its own National Federation, and national competitions may be run under national rules. All international and championship competitions are run under FEI rules, and there are rigorous qualification requirements that must be met to participate. Concours de Raid d'Endurance International (CEI) competitions are divided into 4-star (championship level) through 1-star (low-level) events, depending on the distance covered and age requirements of the horse. Horses must be at least 5 years of age to compete in qualifying events, with age requirements increasing through the star rating. Horses must be at least 8 years of age to compete in championships and CEI 4-star competitions.

VETERINARY CONTROLS

Veterinary controls are an integral part of endurance events, and horses must undergo and pass an initial veterinary inspection and subsequent inspections after each phase of the competition. The total distance of the ride is divided into segments of 20 to 40 km, usually laid out in a cloverleaf pattern with a central Vet Gate area. After riding each section, the competitor must pass the Vet Gate or veterinary checkpoint, where panels of veterinarians evaluate horses for lameness and metabolic criteria. The heart rate must be at or less than 64 beats per minute (bpm) within 20 minutes of arrival from the course to each Vet Gate and within 30 minutes of arrival to the final inspection after crossing the finish line. FEI rules allow the Veterinary Commission the latitude to lower the heart rate criterion if extreme weather conditions are deemed severe enough to warrant it.

The time is taken when the competitor comes in off the course into the crewing area. The competitor has 20 minutes in which to "clock in" to the Vet Gate, or the horse will be eliminated on a time penalty. Heart rate decreases to less than 64 bpm within 1 to 3 minutes of arrival in most elite endurance horses. The time is recorded again when the horse enters the Vet Gate. There is a mandatory hold time after each phase of the competition, which begins from the time of entry into the Vet Gate. Therefore speed of entry into the Vet Gate is a critical opportunity to gain time. If the horse's heart rate is higher than 64 bpm on initial inspection he is "spun" or required to go out of the Vet Gate and return for a reinspection when the heart rate meets the 64-bpm criterion. A horse is permitted one reinspection within the 20-minute time limit at the Vet Gates, but no second chance to meet the heart rate requirement is permitted at the finish. Intensive crewing (rapid cooling with copious amounts of ice water) is common at high-level competitions, and top-level horses generally come in off the course, have saddles removed, are cooled, have the heart rates checked, and go directly into the Vet Gate. Most championship venues have instituted digital heart rate monitors on which the heart rate for each horse is publically displayed at the end of the trotting lane. A second heart rate is measured by direct auscultation 1 minute after the commencement of a 40-meter trot, and the difference between the first and second heart rates is calculated. This is known as the cardiac recovery index (CRI) or Ridgway Test, after Dr. Kerry Ridgway. Although not a criterion for elimination in and of itself, a positive CRI, in which the second heart rate is elevated more than several beats above the first one, is an indication that the horse merits further evaluation. Other metabolic parameters, such as mucous membrane color, capillary refill time, skin turgor, and auscultable intestinal borborygmi, are checked and recorded. The presence of any saddle sores, girth rubs, or bitting lesions is also noted. A heart rate above the maximum allowed, injury, or "consistently apparent" lameness are grounds for elimination. Synchronous diaphragmatic flutter is a common condition in endurance horses and may be grounds for elimination if other metabolic abnormalities are concurrently present. Time-keeping systems for arrival from and departure to the course are automated at high-level events, with riders presenting a digitized "slash card" at timing checkpoints. After passing the veterinary examination, the horse is returned to the crewing area, where it is fed, groomed, and watered before called to return to the course. The horse is not permitted to leave the exit gate until the hold time for each phase is completed. A computerized record of the competitor position, exit time, time taken for the horse to present, and average speed is available at each Vet Gate and at the finish. Endurance horses are not permitted to compete on performance-enhancing medication, and medication control programs are in place to test for substances that are not permitted, in accordance with FEI rules for all equestrian disciplines.

Although national competitions may use the same veterinarians for control and treatment, FEI competitions require separate veterinarians dedicated to each. There are specific requirements regarding the number of commission and treatment veterinarians per number of competitors according to the star rating of the competition. Typically, a horse that is eliminated by a control (Commission) veterinarian for a lameness or metabolic problem is referred to the treatment veterinarian for further evaluation. If the treatment veterinarian deems that treatment is prudent, it is provided at a field clinic at the ride site, or in some cases the horse is transported to a local referral veterinary clinic or to its home stable for treatment. Team veterinarians are usually so busy with other competitors that have not been eliminated that they are happy to have the assistance of the treatment veterinarian. However, it is important that treatment and team veterinarians closely liaise with one another to provide the best possible care. Ride site clinics at large venues or championships offer sophisticated treatment (e.g., blood analysis, fluid therapy, digital radiography, ultrasonography, electrocardiography, endoscopy), and only those horses that require continued care, further diagnostics, or surgical treatment are referred.

Top-level international modern endurance is an extreme sport. Competitors and experienced endurance veterinarians recognize that proactive provision of post-competition fluid therapy is beneficial in rapidly returning the horse to normal hydration and homeostasis. In my opinion, fluid therapy should not be withheld in an effort to reduce "treatment rates," and competitors whose horses receive fluid therapy to optimize recovery should not be penalized.

TYPE OF HORSE

Most endurance rides are open to horses of any breed, but horses of Arabian extraction are most popularly used for endurance riding because they have light build and stamina for long distance rides. Larger, heavier framed horses are less able to sustain the speed required over the distances traveled. Endurance horses, compared with other athletic horses, tend to be small and light, although in the past 10 years there has been a trend toward taller more robust Anglo-Arab types. Like human marathon runners, good endurance horses tend to be ectomorphs, but speed, cardiac recovery capacity (the ability to rapidly decrease the heart rate after a fast gallop over long distances), and conformation that is likely to withstand the pressure of the demands to which endurance horses are subjected are currently the most sought-after qualities.

TRAINING METHODS AND COMPETITION SPEEDS

Training methods differ considerably among trainers, but most would agree that it takes 2 to 3 years of training to make a good endurance horse. Training distance and frequency depend largely on individual circumstances (terrain, weather, availability of pasture, or turn-out paddocks), but most regularly competing endurance horses are ridden 6 days a week. A typical program might include daily rides of 10 to 20 km, with weekly or 10-day interval 30- to 80-km rides. Horses are ridden at a walk, trot, and canter, with the proportion of the time spent at each gait varying considerably. Horses being prepared for a 100- to 160-km ride will usually perform a 60- to 80-km training ride on at least two occasions before competition. New qualification requirements mandate that horses complete successive rides at lesser distances before being permitted to compete at the next increased distance level. Overtraining of endurance horses tends to be more of a problem than undertraining, particularly by novice trainers.

Endurance competition has rapidly evolved from amateur operations where the same person owned, trained, and rode the same horse for many years, competing for pleasure, with small prizes in kind, to large stables with numerous horses run by professional trainers competing for international recognition, luxury automobiles, and hundreds of thousands of dollars in prize money. The value of a horse winning or running successfully in a prestigious international competition increases exponentially. Speeds at high-profile rides over mountainous terrain have not substantially changed, but as the sport has continued to develop, speeds of competition over flat terrain have increased dramatically. Essentially, at the highest levels the sport has changed from endurance riding to endurance racing. The winner of the 2008 World Championship in Malaysia averaged 18 km/h (5 m/sec) for 160 km, at night,

in a torrential downpour, and with high humidity. A world record time for 160 km of 6 hours, 28 minutes, 28 seconds riding time was set in January 2008. Although the total average speed for all phases was 24.71 km/h (6.86 m/sec), the final 19-km loop was covered at an average speed of 30.29 km/h (8.41 m/sec). It must be borne in mind that as an average over 19 km, actual speeds for short bursts can be substantially higher. As winning speeds at the classic 160-km distance have increased, speeds at the shorter 120-km and 100-km distance have increased even more. In these races, average speeds for some phases reach more than 36 km/h (10 m/sec), which is the equivalent of an "open gallop." It is not unusual to have flying finishes with fractions of seconds separating finishing places. Ten years ago this would have been unheard of. Opinions differ as to whether this is desirable progress, but from a veterinary standpoint, at rides where speeds are increasing, it means that we are beginning to see more flat-racing types of musculoskeletal injuries, as well as serious metabolic abnormalities. Although water is available on the course every 5 to 8 km, riders competing at distances less than 160 km rarely stop on the course to water their horses. The horses are watered when they come into the crewing area.

COURSE TERRAIN

Endurance horses compete and train over some of the most highly variable terrain of any sports horses, including rocky mountains, through creeks, across sandy deserts, along tarmac, gravel, or dirt roads, and across grassy fields, depending on where the ride is held. Course terrain clearly has a bearing on the type of injury, generally in a straightforward way. Stone-bruised feet and painful joints are more common when horses are worked on hard, rocky ground, whereas ligament and tendon injuries are more often observed in horses worked on soft or sandy ground. Downhill grades, if slippery or taken at speed, tend to produce a plethora of dorsal carpal injuries as a result of falls. A relatively recent innovation is the grading and harrowing of long stretches of the course, much like a racetrack without the cushion. Many large endurance stables now train horses on racetracks. This has resulted in an increase in racing-type fractures and superficial digital flexor tendon (SDFT) injuries.

LAMENESS AND CONFORMATION

Lameness in endurance horses can be divided into three categories involving (1) ligaments or tendons, (2) muscle, or (3) joints, bones, or feet. Lameness affecting endurance horses can also be separated into transient problems that may be cause for elimination on the day of competition but then resolve and more persistent problems that are likely to be recurrent. In the relatively recent past, many endurance horses competed over an 8- to 10-year period, and horses with the most glaring conformation defects tended to weed themselves out by attrition. Developments in the sport, most notably increases in speeds of competition, have paralleled the shortening of the competitive life of top-level endurance horses by several years. Astute veterinary advisors make a concerted effort to avoid young horses with flat, asymmetrical, or contracted feet, major angular limb deformities, offset cannon bones, and long, slack, or

References on page 1345

short, upright pasterns because these may contribute to later unsoundness problems.[1] Although poorly conformed horses may be successful in the short term or at less-demanding levels of competition, it is an exceptional poorly conformed horse that stays sound and is successful over the time that it takes to reach championship level.[2] Flaws that are not extreme may be present without compromising the overall function of the horse but are preferentially avoided when possible. Horses with toe-in conformation appear to be more likely to develop splint exostoses that may impinge on the suspensory ligament (SL), causing desmitis, and horses with recurrent suspensory desmitis are ultimately unsuitable for endurance.

THE LAMENESS EXAMINATION AND PROCEEDING WITHOUT A DIAGNOSIS

A lameness examination in any horse is most easily and efficiently performed when the lameness is visible, and the endurance horse is no exception. It is usually not possible to make a specific diagnosis if a horse is not lame at the time of examination. Endurance horses are problematic because often a mild transient lameness that resulted in elimination from competition may not be visible the next day or even later the same day, although many horses have painful superficial digital flexor tendons (SDFTs) and SLs after a race. Low-grade, inconsistent, nonspecific lameness that cannot be localized is a frustratingly common scenario faced by veterinarians charged with keeping endurance horses sound. When possible, watching the horse trot while lame, application of hoof testers, noting the presence of any palpable abnormalities, and response to flexion or other manipulative tests help to narrow the possible causes. Diagnostic analgesia, adhering to the principle of starting at the bottom and working upward, is the standard most useful means of localizing the source of pain causing lameness when no palpable abnormalities are present. Sometimes, despite a careful and complete lameness examination, diagnostic analgesia, and ancillary diagnostic aids such as radiography, ultrasonography, scintigraphy, and even magnetic resonance imaging (MRI), a specific diagnosis cannot be reached. Some horses never "block out." A careful neurological examination should then be performed because subtle neurological deficits may mimic or produce lameness. In other horses, pain causing lameness can be isolated to a specific region, but no lesion can be found. Like other athletic horses, endurance horses may have subtle gait abnormalities emanating from numerous areas, all contributing to suboptimal performance but difficult to identify individually. The advent of MRI has elucidated some previously elusive conditions of the distal aspect of the limb, especially in the proximal palmar metacarpal region and the foot.

Horses with pain causing lameness localized using diagnostic analgesia or clinical examination to a specific region in which there are no detectable radiological or ultrasonographic lesions should be reexamined by the most appropriate conventional imaging modality after 2 to 4 weeks or should undergo scintigraphic or MRI examination if warranted by the degree of lameness present. Stress fractures are particularly notorious for not being detectable on the first radiological examination and being readily apparent later. However, stress fractures are usually detectable using scintigraphy or MRI. If the lameness has resolved and no lesion is detected on a recheck examination, it is reasonable to return the horse to light training. If lameness recurs, the lameness examination should be repeated.

Although "full-body" scintigraphy is ideally avoided, it is sometimes beneficial in horses that have an acute lameness that cannot be specifically localized. We have recognized the propensity for stress fractures to turn into catastrophic fractures; therefore obtaining a specific diagnosis is increasingly important. It should be borne in mind that the percentage of positive scintigraphic findings is higher for horses with acute, severe lameness than in those with chronic, low-grade lameness. Sometimes, despite every attempt at imaging and reimaging, the clinician is still left with a lame horse and no diagnosis. When this point is reached, a prolonged rest period (8 to 12 months) may be helpful.

COMMON CAUSES OF LAMENESS IN ENDURANCE HORSES

The principal cause of lameness is proximal palmar metacarpal pain,[1-4] but the other top 10 causes of lameness in endurance horses tend to vary somewhat in ranking from season to season. Although the problems listed here are the most frequently encountered, not only is the ranking variable, but also pathology in the proximal palmar metacarpal region and in the fetlock can be divided into subcategories that may overlap and are difficult to separate. The advent of the availability of sophisticated imaging techniques, especially MRI, has made it more difficult to write a list of the 10 most common causes of lameness in endurance horses because of the ability to recognize to a greater degree the interrelatedness of the anatomical structures involved. In addition, some injuries appear to be part of a spectrum or continuum that progresses through phases with time. Bearing this in mind, the following are the lameness problems seen most commonly:

1. Proximal palmar metacarpal pain
   Proximal suspensory desmitis
   Proximal palmar metacarpal stress pathology
   Pathology associated with the second and fourth metacarpal bones
2. Foot problems
3. Metacarpophalangeal and metatarsophalangeal osteoarthritis, synovitis, and periarticular pathology
4. Stress-related injury of the distal aspect of the third metacarpal bone
5. Superficial digital flexor tendonitis
6. Myalgia of the paravertebral and gluteal muscles
7. Osteoarthritis of the centrodistal and tarsometatarsal joints
8. Desmitis of the suspensory ligament body and branches
9. Other bone injury
10. Exertional rhabdomyolysis

PROXIMAL PALMAR METACARPAL PAIN

The leading cause of chronic or recurrent lameness in endurance horses, regardless of terrain, is pain in the proximal palmar metacarpal region. Proximal suspensory desmitis (PSD) is often the primary problem. Pain associated with the lesions of the palmar aspect of the third metacarpal bone (McIII) or less commonly pain associated with the second (McII) or the fourth (McIV) metacarpal bones, or the interosseous ligaments between the McII and McIII and the McIV and McIII may contribute to lameness. Injury to the proximal metatarsal region of the hindlimb also occurs but is less common.

Proximal Suspensory Desmitis

Desmitis of the SL typically develops in the later stages of a race when the horse becomes fatigued but may occur in the earlier stages of a race in an unfit horse or a horse that has had previous SL injury. It is also a common training injury. Lameness caused by PSD may be sudden in onset and severe or be more insidious in onset. Often, there is little or no detectable swelling, but careful palpation may elicit a painful response. However, many horses resent palpation of the proximal aspect of the SL and will give a false-positive response to even the most gentle and careful palpation. Horses with forelimb PSD are usually positive to distal limb flexion. Diagnostic analgesia is critical to definitively localize pain to the proximal palmar metacarpal region. The proximal palmar metacarpal region may be desensitized by (1) blocking the deep branch of the lateral palmar nerve laterally at the edge of the accessoriometacarpal ligament distal to the accessory carpal bone and the medial palmar nerve (high two-point or Wheat block, after Dr. John D. Wheat), (2) direct infiltration, (3) performing a high palmar and palmar metacarpal nerve block ("high four-point"), or (4) blocking the lateral palmar nerve in the longitudinal groove on the medial aspect of the accessory carpal bone.[5] The first and last techniques have the advantage of avoiding inadvertent penetration of the distal palmar outpouchings of the carpometacarpal joint and the last technique avoids penetration of the carpal canal. Although lameness in endurance horses is seldom localized to the carpus, carpometacarpal joint pathology is increasingly recognized. When a high index of suspicion of proximal palmar metacarpal pain exists but the horse does not improve with one of the blocks, the block should be repeated, or one of the others should be tried because there may be some variability in response. Ultrasonographic examination of the SL is generally performed if diagnostic analgesia has localized the source of the pain causing lameness to this area. Ultrasonography is a less precise imaging modality than MRI, but it is more accessible and readily available to a general practitioner and remains a highly useful technique. PSD is characterized by loss of echogenicity of the dorsal-most fibers immediately distal to the carpometacarpal joint. Symmetry is important in determining whether acute SL injury has occurred, and the further distally the fiber loss extends (from zone 1 into zone 2), the worse the injury.[6] Both forelimbs should be compared. Often, bilateral change is present, but the clinically affected side appears less echogenic (Figure 118-1). Examination of the limb in flexion with the digital flexor tendons and accessory ligament of the deep digital flexor tendon (DDFT) pushed aside can allow more complete evaluation of the medial and lateral lobes of the suspensory origin. If the pain causing lameness has been localized to the proximal palmar metacarpal region but the ultrasonographic appearance of the SL is within normal limits, there are several possible explanations: (1) inflammation of the ligament may exist without accompanying structural change; (2) abnormalities may be present in the ligament that are

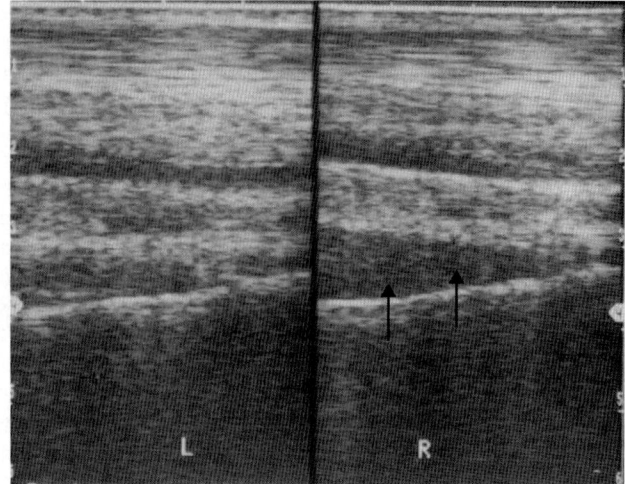

Fig. 118-1 • Longitudinal ultrasonographic images of the palmar metacarpal soft tissues. The left forelimb is on the left. There is marked loss of echogenicity and disruption of the fiber pattern in the proximal aspect of the right suspensory ligament *(arrows)*. Some loss of echogenicity is also seen in the proximal aspect of the nonlame left forelimb.

not detectable with ultrasonography[7]; and (3) there is pathology of other structures. It should be noted that most horses that have undergone any strenuous work will have some degree of ultrasonographic change (e.g., loss of echogenicity, fiber malalignment) in the proximal aspect of the SL[6]; the challenge is determining its clinical significance. Therefore combining the use of diagnostic analgesia and ultrasonographic comparison between limbs can be helpful in determining the relevance of a lesion. However, it is frustrating that there appears to be little correlation between ultrasonographic appearance of the SL, response to analgesia, ability to return to training, and incidence of recurrent lameness. MRI has revealed that this may be either because of SL damage that is present but undetectable using ultrasonography or injury of other structures.

Initial management of horses with PSD regardless of whether ultrasonographic changes are present is aimed at reducing inflammation. Combination therapy using systemic corticosteroids (a single injection of intramuscular [IM] triamcinolone acetate, 0.03 mg/kg), rest, a 7- to 14-day course of nonsteroidal antiinflammatory drugs (NSAIDs), and local therapy (e.g., ice, cold hydrotherapy, poulticing, and bandaging) is beneficial. Lameness in some horses with transient soreness and pain on palpation resolves without further problems. Infiltration along the axial borders of the McII and the McIV with corticosteroids is sometimes helpful to reduce acute proximal SL inflammation in the short term and may enable a horse to compete successfully if no structural abnormalities are present. The short-term benefit must be weighed against the risk of enabling the horse to compete and sustain further damage. It is critical to rule out stress fractures in the proximal aspect of the McIII before infiltrating corticosteroids to minimize the risk of complete fracture. Correct foot balance is critical because a poorly balanced foot may contribute to SL strain. Weekly extracorporeal shock wave therapy (ESWT) for 3 to 5 weeks is used to reduce pain after the initial inflammatory period. Newer treatment modalities used with increasing frequency are intraligamentous injection of platelet-rich plasma, autologous stem cells derived from fat or bone marrow, and matrix derived from the urinary bladder of pigs (ACell Vet, ACell, Inc., Columbia, Maryland, United States). Although healing time is not shortened, these treatments may increase the quality of healing and decrease reinjury rate.[8] Surgical splitting of the proximal aspect of the SL and osteostixis of the proximal aspect of the McIII or the third metatarsal bone (MtIII) was described in three dressage horses in which conservative management had failed and in which there was entheseous new bone on the McIII or the MtIII.[9] This was reportedly successful. Fasciotomy is a technique used by some clinicians who treat other types of sports horses. I do not have enough experience with either technique to comment on their potential value in endurance horses. To accurately evaluate efficacy of various treatments, we must continue to define more precisely which structures have been injured. In general, I have had the most consistent success in endurance horses using initial antiinflammatory treatment, ESWT, rest, ensuring good foot balance, and a controlled rehabilitation and exercise program.

The horse should be restricted to handwalking until no lameness is apparent at a trot in hand on a hard surface without the benefit of systemic NSAIDs. The horse may then be gradually reintroduced to work if no structural abnormalities in the SL were identified. However, ultrasonographic examination should be repeated to confirm that no clinically significant structural change is present because the appearance of fiber damage observed ultrasonographically can lag behind the clinical perception of pain. Training may progress gradually if the lameness does not recur. If substantial structural change is present in the SL, if other ligamentous or osseous pathology has been identified, or if the lameness is persistent or recurrent, strenuous work should be avoided for at least 8 to 12 months. Although other sports horses may be able to return to training sooner, elite endurance horses are not able to quickly recover and require a considerably longer period. PSD is particularly treacherous to a horse's career because, initially, a horse often responds to a short period of rest, but the horse then becomes lame again when increased exercise is attempted. This scenario may happen repeatedly after short rest periods.

Much of the recommended rehabilitation program for horses with tendon or ligament injury depends on the horse's temperament and the amount of help and facilities available, but the best success is achieved with a controlled and gradual increase in exercise over 8 to 12 months. This may include turnout in a single-horse small paddock not much bigger than a stall; treadmill, handwalking, or walking machine exercise; and walking under tack. The bottom line has never changed: horses working in high-speed, strenuous athletic disciplines that sustain substantial damage to the SL (or SDFT) need 8 to 12 months of rest. The reason conventional wisdom becomes conventional is that it has withstood the test of time. Horses that sustain severe PSD may take 18 months to return to full training and will always be at increased risk of reinjury.

Stress Pathology of the Proximal Palmar Aspect of the Third Metacarpal Bone

Stress pathology of the proximal palmar aspect of the McIII includes avulsion and stress fractures, as well as more subtle bone and ligamentous change. Some avulsion fractures associated with the origin of the SL can be identified

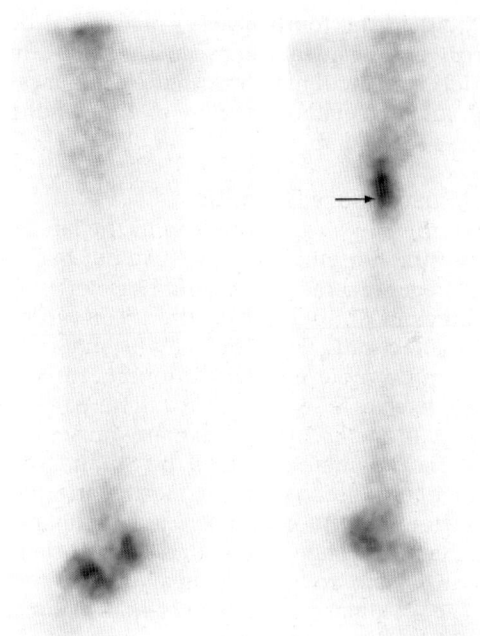

Fig. 118-2 • Lateral bone phase scintigraphic images of the left and right forelimbs. There is intense focal increased radiopharmaceutical uptake (IRU) in the proximopalmar aspect of the right third metacarpal bone (McIII) (arrow) at the origin of the suspensory ligament. Note also IRU in the proximal aspect of the proximal phalanx of the left forelimb and IRU of the distal aspects of the McIII in both forelimbs.

using radiology or ultrasonography; others not identifiable using these imaging modalities are apparent using scintigraphy (Figure 118-2). MRI has enabled the recognition of fractures, prefracture pathology, and other changes occurring in the proximal palmar metacarpal and metatarsal regions unapparent using other imaging techniques. Avulsion fractures are part of an array of proximal palmar metacarpal pathology that includes palmar cortical and endosteal abnormalities, enthesophyte formation at the origin of the SL, severe palmar McIII so-called "bone bruising" characterized by increased signal intensity in fat-suppressed MR images, and stress fractures or linear defects within the cortex consistent with linear incomplete cortical fractures.[3,7] Some proximal metacarpal fractures originate at the carpometacarpal joint surface; others originate from avulsion fractures that propagate distally.[10] Incomplete fractures can be difficult to diagnose; one horse with bilateral proximal palmar McIII cortical fractures that extended into the diaphysis displayed a crouching stance, giving the appearance of a primary hindlimb lameness.[10] The crouched stance in this horse and unusual gait occurs in horses with other bilateral forelimb fractures and is often confused with hindlimb pain (Editors). Horses with incomplete fractures should be box-rested for 30 to 60 days and confined alone in a small paddock or handwalked for an additional 60 days before resuming exercise. If unrecognized, there is a substantial risk that incomplete cortical fractures may propagate to become complete, with disastrous consequences (Figure 118-3).

Pathology Associated with the Second and Fourth Metacarpal Bones

Periostitis or exostosis of the McII and the McIV (splints) is much less common than other injuries in the proximal

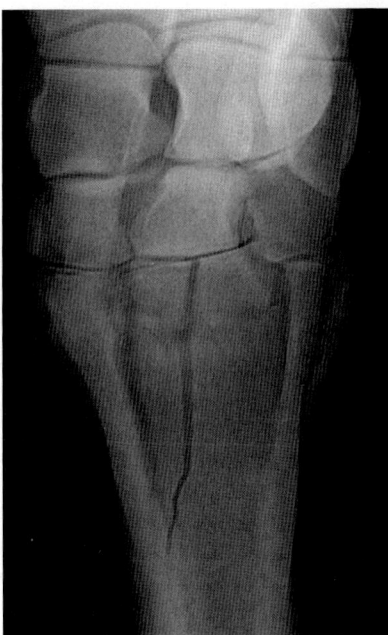

Fig. 118-3 • Dorsopalmar radiographic image of the metacarpal region. Lateral is to the right. There is a wide intraarticular fracture of the proximal aspect of the third metacarpal bone, extending from the carpometacarpal joint distally and medially.

palmar metacarpal region and is included because of the close anatomical relationship to other structures in the region. It may be a minor problem necessitating a 2- to 4-week break from training, but abnormalities of the McII and the McIV may be associated with pathology of adjoining structures. Abnormalities identified with MRI include interosseous ligament pathology and reactive synostoses between the McII or the McIV and the McIII. This may be seen in association with injuries of the palmar cortex of the McIII and/or the SL, and the clinical significance of some of these findings is still undetermined. Loss of separation between either the McII or the McIV and the medial and lateral lobes of the SL with subsequent soft tissue apposition and adhesion formation may also occur and be of clinical significance. Radiological examination of an enlargement of the McII or the McIV should be performed to rule out a fracture. Ice, cold hydrotherapy, dimethyl sulfoxide (DMSO) gel, NSAIDs, and bandaging are used to reduce inflammation during the inflammatory period. Cryotherapy can also be used to reduce inflammation and will sometimes enable horses with reactive splint exostoses to continue in training and competition. Most uncomplicated splints resolve with time and treatment, although a nonpainful enlargement remains. If the exostosis continues to enlarge or if the area remains painful, training should be discontinued to avoid impingement on and damage to the SL. Sometimes SL damage occurs before recognition of the problem, and affected horses require a longer rest period. Fractures of the distal aspect of the McII or the McIV should be surgically removed, and horses should be given rest. Horses with splint exostoses that appear reactive or large enough to impinge on the SL may also be surgical candidates, although opinions differ. Horses undergoing distal splint ostectomy because of a fracture have a better prognosis than those receiving ostectomy because of

exostosis.[1] It may be that once SL damage has occurred, the window of opportunity for surgical intervention without adhesion formation is past. Any associated injury to the SL is the limiting factor in how quickly and how successfully horses with splint exostoses can be returned to work.

FOOT PROBLEMS

Problems with the feet are a frequent cause of elimination from endurance competitions, as well as being a common cause of chronic or recurrent pain. Foot problems occur in both forelimbs and hindlimbs but are more regularly seen in the forelimb. Many lameness eliminations related to the feet are transient in nature: bruising or a dislodged shoe. The importance of a properly trimmed, well-balanced, well-shod foot cannot be overemphasized, and a good farrier is an integral part of a successful endurance team. Because endurance horses train and compete over very long distances, foot balance has a huge impact on the support structures of the limb. Trimming and shoeing with a long toe and low heel can lead to direct heel trauma, as well as increased strain on the SL and digital flexor tendons. Good medial-to-lateral balance is vital to avoid problems with collateral ligaments of the distal limb joints and the collateral sesamoidean and distal sesamoidean impar ligaments. Farriers who are accustomed to working with horses that wear keg shoes may be impatient with the requirements of endurance horses, which can sometimes require a more innovative and time-consuming approach aimed at providing the foot with increased protection and support. Many, if not most, endurance horses are shod with full pads for the day of a race, which are later removed. Silicon gel is often used for this purpose.

Sole bruises occur frequently in horses traveling over hard ground. Horses show a bilateral lameness manifest as a shortened, choppy gait. Application of hoof testers around the solar margins of the foot elicits a painful response. Lameness is often more pronounced in one limb. Diagnostic analgesia of the foot in which the lameness is most noticeable may then result in contralateral limb lameness. Sole bruising may be accompanied by increased radiopharmaceutical uptake (IRU) in the distal phalanx and changes indicative of distal laminar and bone inflammation on MRI ("pedal osteitis").[11] Radiological abnormalities include loss of bone opacity at the margins of the distal phalanx and increased size and number of vascular channels, resulting in a ragged appearance. Lateromedial radiographic images may reveal modeling at the distal aspect of the distal phalanx, sometimes described as a "ski jump" appearance. Management is aimed at protecting the solar margins and reducing concussion. Wide-webbed, seated-out shoes, full pads, or rim pads can be used to accomplish these goals. Distal interphalangeal (DIP) joint synovitis may occur concurrently and is treated by intraarticular medication (hyaluronan and corticosteroid combinations). Sore feet often occur in conjunction with distal hock joint and back pain and may be the inciting cause. Each area must be addressed individually, as well as the horse as a whole, for treatment to be successful.

Palmar foot pain is less common in Arabian and Arabian crossbreeds than in larger breeds, but it does occur and can be an important cause of lameness. As more MRI examinations are performed, abnormalities in the navicular region are identified with increasing frequency. Injuries identified in endurance horses with lameness abolished using palmar digital analgesia have included so-called "edema" of the navicular bone (i.e., increased signal intensity in the spongiosa in fat-suppressed images); distal border irregularities of the navicular bone; lesions of the DDFT from the level of the navicular bone to its insertion, with increased signal intensity in the palmar aspect of the navicular bone in fat-suppressed images; adhesions between the DDFT and the navicular bone; and disruption of the collateral sesamoidean ligament and its attachment to the dorsolateral aspects of the middle phalanx.

Endurance horses frequently exhibit inflammation of the coronary band ("coronitis") in the first 24 hours after competition. It may be focal (usually dorsal) or all the way around and is usually painful on palpation. Separation of the hoof wall from the coronary band may occur, and there may be oozing of serum from the coronary band. This is sometimes, but not always, accompanied by a bounding digital pulse. Interestingly, as alarming as this is, these horses do not usually progress to typical laminitis. The outer layer of hoof wall may peel away from the coronary band, but the horse is not lame, and there is no rotation or sinking of the distal phalanx. The episode is marked by bruising and a distinct defect in the hoof wall that usually grows out without further incident.[1,3]

Endurance horses are also subject to laminitis that may be traumatic or metabolic in origin. Clinical signs become apparent 24 to 72 hours after competition. The severity may range from frightening, but mild, to disastrous. Horses without rotation or sinking are generally able to return to endurance competition. Horses with the worst outcomes often show few prodromal clinical signs. Proactive measures aimed at preventing laminitis should be considered in all high-risk horses after competition (those that are severely hemoconcentrated, exhausted, or have rhabdomyolysis, ileus, or diarrhea) because it is not possible to predict which horses will or will not have a satisfactory outcome. Continuously standing all four feet of the horse in an ice water slurry or water at 1° C up to the level of the carpus has proved to prevent onset of laminar damage[12,13] but will not halt laminitis that is already occurring.[13] Any horse that begins to shift weight or show any signs of discomfort after competition should certainly be treated, but by the time these signs are apparent, progression of the disease may be well underway. Flunixin meglumine (0.25 mg/kg intravenous [IV], thrice daily), phenylbutazone (2.2 to 4.4 mg/kg twice daily), acepromazine (0.0 25 mg/kg IM four times daily), pentoxifylline (7.5 mg/kg orally [PO] thrice daily) (Editors Note: Also see comments on page 373), and DMSO (1 g/kg IV diluted to 10% solution once or twice daily) are routinely used in various combinations, with the caveat that the horse should receive fluid therapy before administration of NSAIDs or acepromazine. Sole and frog pressure are also provided.

METACARPOPHALANGEAL AND METATARSOPHALANGEAL OSTEOARTHRITIS, CAPSULITIS, SYNOVITIS, AND PERIARTICULAR PATHOLOGY

Osteoarthritis (OA) of the metacarpophalangeal (MCP) and metatarsophalangeal (MTP) joints and periarticular

pathology is related to the ongoing nature of degenerative processes, chronic wear and tear associated with training and competing, and the fact that endurance horses may compete for several years. OA of the MCP or the MTP joints may occur with or without joint effusion and may be unilateral or bilateral, but is most often bilateral. OA is far more common in the MCP joints but also occurs in the hindlimbs. There is usually pain on flexion, and the joint often has a decreased range of motion and thickening of the joint capsule; acute or chronic synovitis may be present. Radiological changes may be subtle, such as narrowing of the joint space, or may consist of more obvious periarticular osteophyte or enthesophyte formation and joint modeling. Hypertrophy of the dorsal synovial pads with associated bone lysis at the proximal aspect of the sagittal ridge of the McIII is common, and osteochondral fractures may occur. Radiological changes do not always correlate with clinical significance; therefore diagnostic intraarticular or perineural (low palmar and palmar metacarpal) analgesia is used to confirm the site of pain. MRI findings may include effusion of the MCP joint with dorsal soft tissue accumulation and chronic, fibrotic synovial tissue and associated dorsal proximal plica formation. Lesions of the distal sesamoidean ligaments may contribute to periarticular pain. Using MRI a diagnosis of medial oblique sesamoidean desmitis is more common than lateral oblique desmitis. Acute, traumatic synovitis or capsulitis of the MCP joints may occur occasionally, but in general long-term management of chronic OA is the more common scenario, and management is similar to that in any other athletic horse. Local therapy (e.g., ice, cold hydrotherapy, poultice, and sweats), intramuscular glycosaminoglycans, intravenous hyaluronan, and judicious use of intraarticular hyaluronan and corticosteroids are beneficial. Repeated intraarticular corticosteroid injections may lead to a reduced response. Interleukin-1 receptor antagonist protein therapy may have long-term benefit, but most team and stable veterinarians preparing for a big race tend to continue to use intraarticular corticosteroid–hyaluronan combinations because the effects are more predictable. Withdrawal periods must be borne in mind. Horses with markedly hypertrophied dorsal synovial pads and osteochondral fragments usually require surgery.

STRESS PATHOLOGY OF THE DISTAL ASPECT OF THE THIRD METACARPAL OR THIRD METATARSAL BONE

Repetitive overloading injury of bone can lead to athletically induced fractures. Most fractures in endurance horses propagate from the MCP or the MTP joints, and lateral condylar fractures of the McIII are the most common type.[14] This is consistent with reported common fracture locations in Thoroughbred racehorses.[15,16] MRI has proved to be a valuable tool in early identification of stress pathology that is not visible radiologically. Identified abnormalities include asymmetry in trabecular architecture between the medial and lateral condyles of the McIII and the MtIII, and superficial palmar or plantar fissure lines at the articular surface. Alteration in structure of the articular surface and osteochondral and some subchondral irregularities associated with the medial and lateral condyles of the McIII and the MtIII are likely to be a reflection of traumatic or degenerative cartilage and underlying bone damage, increasing potential for fracture at these sites.[16-21] Bone trauma (so-called "bruising") and, more commonly, chronic subchondral bone modeling of the distal aspect of the McIII or the MtIII of mature horses are recognized causes of pain, but may not increase risk of fracture formation.[11,20,21] When pathological changes thought to increase the risk of fracture formation are identified, it is clearly prudent that the horse not continue training. However, it is not always clear what changes are pathological and increase fracture risk and what changes may reflect adaptive response to training. There is increasing evidence to support that many fractures in athletic horses occur not as isolated instances of a "bad step" but as a progression of pathological changes and stress remodeling over time, ultimately resulting in bone failure.[15-19]

Condylar fractures of the McIII or the MtIII may be complete or incomplete, displaced or nondisplaced, and may or may not be associated with joint effusion. Nondisplaced fractures are not always readily diagnosed but should be considered high on the list of differential diagnoses in an acutely lame endurance horse. The importance of careful physical examination and diagnostic imaging cannot be overemphasized because nondisplaced fractures risk becoming displaced if undiagnosed and sufficient confinement, support, and repair or stabilization are not provided. Many nondisplaced fractures are not diagnosed until several days after the occurrence of the injury and may require special imaging techniques. The presence of "moderate injury of the suspensory apparatus" increased the risk of condylar fracture in Thoroughbred racehorses.[22] Given the high prevalence of PSD in endurance horses and the increasing numbers of condylar fractures identified, it is tempting to think that there may also be an association in endurance horses, and evaluation of risk factors for fracture in endurance horses is in progress.[3]

An unusual fracture type seen with increasing frequency in mature endurance horses is a transverse compression fracture of the distal metaphysis of the McIII at the residual physis (Figure 118-4). Horses with compression fractures of the distal aspect of the McIII have pain on palpation in the lateral condylar region and are usually suspected to have lateral condylar fractures, although no joint effusion is present. I have observed one horse with bilateral nondisplaced compression fractures, which had unilateral forelimb lameness. Horses with unilateral or bilateral nondisplaced fractures respond well to conservative management. One 7-year-old horse with no previous history of lameness pulled up grade 4 of 5 lame after a 40-km qualifying ride and had a transverse compression fracture with displacement of the distal epiphysis of the McIII.

Diagnosis in horses with bilateral fractures of the McIII or MtIII is challenging. Two horses with bilateral forelimb condylar fractures were reluctant to move and had a stance similar to horses with acute laminitis, rocked back onto the hindlimbs. Another horse with bilateral hindlimb lateral condylar fractures and a concurrent hindlimb sagittal fracture of the proximal phalanx appeared to have unilateral hindlimb lameness (on the side with the proximal phalangeal fracture) and was reluctant to move. On initial examination at the ride venue there was a palpable condylar fracture. After the limb with the obvious fracture was splinted and analgesics had been administered, the horse

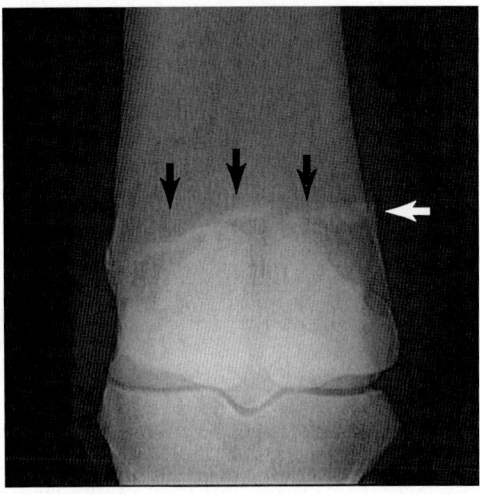

Fig. 118-4 • Dorsopalmar radiographic image of a metacarpophalangeal joint, obtained with a horizontal x-ray beam so that the proximal sesamoid bones are superimposed over the epiphysis of the third metacarpal bone, distal to the physis. Lateral is to the right. There is a transverse compression fracture of the distal aspect of the third metacarpal bone at the residual physeal scar characterized by increased radiopacity of the physis *(black arrows)* and a small step incongruity laterally *(white arrow).*

walked reasonably comfortably. Subsequently swelling developed over the lateral condyle of the MtIII of the contralateral limb, and radiography revealed bilateral fractures, with a complete, displaced, comminuted lateral condylar fracture in the less lame contralateral limb.[10] It must be recognized that bilateral fractures do occur but may not be obvious. However, if a horse has an unusual stance or is reluctant or unable to move, radiographs of both limbs should be obtained to rule out fractures of the proximal phalanx and the distal and proximal aspects of the McIII or the MtIII. It should be standard practice to obtain radiographs of the contralateral limb before placing a horse under general anesthesia for surgery.

SUPERFICIAL DIGITAL FLEXOR TENDONITIS

Superficial digital flexor (SDF) tendonitis may be acute or chronic, low grade or severe. Acute ruptures or partial ruptures occur occasionally during competition. Although more common in forelimbs, SDFT injury also occurs in hindlimbs. Initial management is directed at trying to reduce swelling and inflammation and to relieve pain. Ice, bandaging, and NSAIDs are used to this effect. Dehydrated horses should not be treated with NSAIDs until they are rehydrated. Horses that sustain a rupture or partial rupture of the SDFT have a poor prognosis for return to endurance competition.

Horses with less severe damage to the SDFT can be more challenging to diagnose and manage. Training injuries, wherein the SDFT may be warm and tender on palpation, occur relatively frequently. Lameness is often not apparent. The initial unremarkable ultrasonographic appearance may belie underlying structural damage, which is not yet visible. A second examination should be performed 7 to 10 days later because the ultrasonographic appearance is often worse at that time than it is initially. Horses with transient heat and tenderness but no swelling or fiber damage can usually be safely returned to training within 2 to 4 weeks after the resolution of clinical signs. If the tendon is enlarged or if fiber separation has occurred, a substantially longer absence from training and competition is required.

Endurance horses that sustain tendon injuries in training or competition are managed similarly to any athletic horse. A one-time dose of intramuscular triamcinolone acetonide (0.03 mg/kg), local application of ice for the first few days, cold hydrotherapy, bandaging, poulticing, and NSAIDs for 2 to 3 weeks are beneficial in reducing initial inflammation. Surgical splitting of those tendons with central core lesions, autogenous liquid bone marrow injection of split SDFTs, and intralesional stem cell, platelet-rich plasma, or ACell injection may be beneficial, but whether these therapies are more beneficial than rest alone is uncertain. Endurance horses with SDF tendonitis have traditionally had a better prognosis for return to competition than horses that race over short distances at higher speeds. Prognosis may be less encouraging in the future as speeds of endurance competitions increase.

PARAVERTEBRAL AND GLUTEAL MYALGIA

Paravertebral myalgia is related to repetitive stress over long distances and is exacerbated by a fatigued, unbalanced rider. Unbalanced movement of the horse contributes to muscle fatigue and often occurs as a result of the horse altering his gait to protect weaknesses. Unfortunately, concomitant diminished rider capability occurs in horses experiencing muscle fatigue. Horses ridden by fit, experienced riders are less subject to battering of the paravertebral muscles than those ridden by novices or poorly balanced riders. FEI rides require that a minimum weight of 75 kg be carried. A fit, competent rider is able to adjust his or her weight distribution to help a tiring horse, but a horse ridden by a less capable rider may be better off with the dead weight of a lead pad.

A horse that has strained or injured the paravertebral muscles appears stiff or rigid rather than lame, and instead of flexing and extending the spine normally when palpated, the horse tends to stiffen, squat, or crouch. It may be difficult or impossible to differentiate muscle pain from pain emanating from vertebral articular facets or dorsal spinous processes. Paravertebral myalgia can occur from a gait change induced by sore feet or sore hocks. Treatment consists of removing the inciting cause when possible and reducing inflammation. Most horses respond to 2 weeks of reduced exercise in conjunction with NSAIDs and pulsed muscle massage. Injection of the paravertebral muscles with an antiinflammatory agent can also be beneficial. The longissimus dorsi muscles are injected bilaterally, approximately 3 cm lateral to the dorsal midline, at five to six sites approximately 5 cm apart using a 22-gauge 1.5-inch needle, from the midthoracic area moving caudally, with 2 mL/injection site of an aqueous solution of soluble salts of the volatile bases from Sarraceniaceae (Sarapin, High Chemical Company, Levittown, Pennsylvania, United States) alone or mixed equally with estrone sulfate (50 mg).

Inflammation of the gluteal muscles also occurs with relative frequency in horses subjected to strenuous work over long distances. The horse exhibits stiffening and shortening of stride; pressure on the superficial and middle gluteal muscles produces a painful response; and the horse may crouch down or move away during palpation.

Swelling or asymmetry may be apparent in the acute stages, with elevation of serum muscle enzyme concentrations. Severe inflammation of the gluteal muscles and accompanying rhabdomyolysis are serious problems that are discussed in the metabolic abnormalities section (see page 1147). NSAIDs must never be administered to a horse with acute gluteal muscle inflammation unless it can be ascertained that hydration and renal function are not compromised. Endurance horses with mild gluteal muscle inflammation usually respond to NSAID therapy, pulsed muscle massage to alleviate muscle pain and spasm, and a short (2 to 3 weeks) rest period. Gluteal soreness may occur in conjunction with forelimb lameness because horses may alter the hindlimb gait to avoid interference. The primary lameness must be managed to hasten resolution of gluteal muscle inflammation.

OSTEOARTHRITIS OF THE DISTAL HOCK JOINTS

OA of the distal tarsal joints usually affects both the tarsometatarsal (TMT) and centrodistal joints and is often bilateral, with one limb usually more affected than the other. Joint effusion is not palpable, but occasionally during joint injection of the TMT joints one gets the impression that there is increased pressure and volume of synovial fluid. Affected horses are positive to hindlimb flexion and show variable sensitivity to the Churchill test. Radiological abnormalities include joint space narrowing and osteophyte formation but do not always correlate with clinical signs. If the clinical picture is one of distal hock joint pain, intraarticular medication is usually administered; a positive response is empirical evidence of a correct diagnosis. This approach obviates the need to go back after a positive response to intraarticular anesthesia to administer intraarticular medication. Distal hock joint pain frequently occurs concurrently with paravertebral muscle pain and sore front feet: the "terrible triad." This is likely to be a result of a horse with sore front feet altering his gait in such a way as to cause strain in the paravertebral muscles and hocks. The best results are obtained when all three problems are treated simultaneously; otherwise, the pain in one area and gait alteration and soreness in another become a never-ending and ever-enlarging cycle.

If pain is localized to the tarsus but radiological findings are negative, consideration should be given to the possibility of less common causes. I have evaluated two endurance horses with nondisplaced parasagittal fractures of the talus. Pain was localized to the tarsocrural joint using diagnostic analgesia. In both horses there was IRU, and a clear fracture line was visible with MRI (Figure 118-5). MRI examination has been useful to diagnose incomplete fracture of the third tarsal bone and evidence of bone repetitive overloading injury in the talus, central, and third tarsal bones. Curb, inflammation of the long plantar ligament, or SDFT distal to the calcaneus may also be a cause of pain in the tarsal area but is usually identified by local pain and swelling.

DESMITIS OF THE SUSPENSORY BODY AND BRANCHES

Desmitis of the suspensory body and branches is more obvious than PSD because there is usually palpable swelling. It most frequently occurs as acute, often severe, traumatic

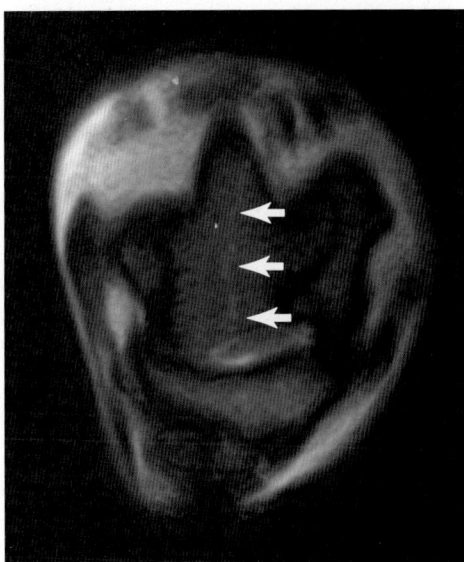

Fig. 118-5 • Transverse magnetic resonance image of a hock at the level of the talus. There is linear increased signal intensity from dorsal to plantar consistent with a sagittal fracture *(arrows)* of the talus.

injury during training or competition. Low-grade, chronic desmitis often precedes acute onset of lameness. Ultrasonographic examination of the SL body and branches is easier to interpret than ultrasonography of the proximal aspect of the SL. Initial and long-term management is essentially the same as for horses with PSD. Suspensory desmitis often occurs in conjunction with pathology of the fetlock joint, which must be managed simultaneously.

OTHER BONE INJURY

It is clear that most common fractures result from accumulated microdamage,[15-20] but inconsistent, unpredictable surfaces may cause increased and uneven loads on the structural integrity of bone.[23] Horses that get loose or run off over uneven ground or variable surfaces (sand to tarmac) may sustain unusual fractures. The presence of preexisting stress pathology increases this risk. Veterinarians working at endurance rides should be prepared to deal with emergency fracture management. A Kimzey splint over a suitable bandage is the most convenient and effective means of stabilizing a lower limb fracture or disruption of the suspensory apparatus. "Ski-boot" splints are equally effective but are more difficult to fit and apply correctly. Additional splint materials for stabilization of upper limb fractures, such as polyvinylchloride pipe cut into circumferential thirds and to appropriate lengths or a Kimzey splint with a proximal extension, should also be available.

While fractures of the distal aspect of the McIII or the MtIII are most common, the second most common fracture in endurance horses involves the proximal phalanx, and, importantly, horses often have acute lameness with limb instability from displaced fractures.[14] Sagittal fractures are the most common followed by those that are comminuted. Proximal phalangeal fractures also occur in the dorsal plane and the dorsal and sagittal planes combined. Numerous radiographic views are essential to elucidate fracture configuration.

Less common fractures include radial, humeral, and scapular stress fractures diagnosed scintigraphically. A horse with a complete humeral fracture had no initial swelling or crepitus, but the limb could be abducted to an abnormal degree, and the presence of a fracture was confirmed radiologically. Other less common fractures of the distal phalanx (type V), proximal sesamoid bone (apical), middle phalanx (abaxial palmar eminence fracture), third trochanter of the femur, and pelvis (ilium and ischium) are occasionally seen.

EXERTIONAL MYOPATHY

Exertional myopathy, rhabdomyolysis, or myositis in endurance horses is not so much a lameness problem, but it is part of a larger picture of fatigue and metabolic abnormalities. It manifests as stiffening and shortening of the stride in all four limbs and may be accompanied by trembling and profuse sweating. It usually occurs either in the very early or very late stages of a ride. Severely affected horses often have pronounced swelling, hardening, or asymmetry of the gluteal muscles. Fluid therapy (0.9% sodium chloride) is the mainstay of treatment, and horses with severe myopathy may require large volumes (40 to 80 L) of fluids. Horses with myoglobinuria ideally should urinate normal-colored urine before administration of flunixin meglumine (0.55 to 1.1 mg/kg or 250 to 500 mg/450-kg horse). When in doubt as to the status of renal function, it is better to give the lower dose and repeat if necessary. Blood urea nitrogen and creatinine concentrations should be monitored, if possible. Portable, relatively inexpensive, user-friendly blood analyzers now make it possible to monitor renal function indicators and muscle enzymes, as well as electrolytes and packed cell volume. Methocarbamol (5 to 25 mg/kg IV) is helpful in many horses. DMSO (1 g/kg IV in a 10% to 20% solution) may also be beneficial. Dantrolene is not generally used because it is not available in an intravenous form, is expensive and not well absorbed when administered orally at recommended dosages, and is ideally given before exercise to be most effective. Horses that have suffered a clinical episode of exertional myopathy or myositis should not be returned to training until muscle enzyme concentrations return to normal values, bearing in mind that what is normal for a particular endurance horse may be higher than published ranges for other types of horses. Some endurance horses in regular training that show no clinical signs of myositis may have resting aspartate transaminase (AST) and creatine kinase (CK) values that commonly reach the range of 1000 U/L to 40,000 U/L or higher after a race or long training ride.[3] Resting CK and AST values, as well as those after races or long rides, for individual horses must be known to determine whether elevated muscle enzyme concentrations are a result of new muscle damage causing lameness or the reason for subclinical poor performance.

METABOLIC PROBLEMS

Avoidance, diagnosis, and management of metabolic problems are some of the many controversial topics currently faced by the sport of endurance. Veterinarians experienced in the sport of endurance racing believe that fatigued, metabolically compromised horses are at increased risk of developing musculoskeletal injury. The highly competitive nature of the sport has led to a large number of horses with metabolic abnormalities. Although veterinarians are now more adept at recognizing subtle signs of exhaustion and often treat horses proactively, a substantial number of horses still have serious problems. The "exhausted horse syndrome" described many years ago[24] is still very much in evidence today. Exhausted horses undergo massive but poorly understood fluid and electrolyte shifts that lead to multiple organ system compromise. Initially, there is persistent elevation of the heart rate, a prolonged capillary refill time, and profound ileus that do not respond as anticipated to fluid therapy, electrolyte supplementation, or analgesics. Synchronous diaphragmatic flutter may be present. Horses with ileus and signs of abdominal pain should be checked for the presence of gastric distention by passing a nasogastric tube. Small intestinal volvulus after endurance competition is a recognized phenomenon,[2,25] and horses with gastric reflux that do not respond to analgesics should be referred. A number of horses with small intestinal volvulus have experienced intractable pain and required intravenous general anesthesia for transport. Although dangerous, use of this technique has resulted in successful outcomes in horses that otherwise would not have survived.[2] Two horses transported under intravenous general anesthesia that subsequently underwent small intestinal resection and anastomosis successfully returned to race the following season.

It cannot be overemphasized that exhausted, hypovolemic, or dehydrated horses or those with severe myositis must not be treated with NSAIDs until they are adequately reperfused. To do so risks renal failure, and these horses are already at high risk for renal failure as a result of hemodynamically mediated vasoconstriction. Vasoconstriction may contribute to subsequent renal ischemia that is exacerbated by NSAID-mediated inhibition of prostaglandin synthesis. If severe lameness or myositis is present, many veterinarians are lured into treating immediately with phenylbutazone or flunixin meglumine. This temptation must be resisted. Lame horses, even those with fractures and without overt evidence of metabolic compromise, should receive fluid therapy before NSAID administration. Horses with acute tendon or ligament injuries should have the affected limb placed in ice, and those with fractures should have appropriate external coaptation applied. Endurance horses should receive at least 10 L, and preferably 15 to 20 L, of intravenous 0.9% sodium chloride (or other available isotonic fluid) to restore renal perfusion before NSAID administration. This volume represents approximately half of the required fluid replacement volume for a moderately hypovolemic horse. Treatment of moderate hypovolemia, the decrease in circulating plasma volume responsible for clinical signs of tachycardia and prolonged capillary refill time, and dehydration (excessive loss of water from the body tissues) generally requires a *minimum* of 50 mL/kg of crystalloid fluids to replace deficits (20 L in a 400-kg horse). Horses with severe hypovolemia require large-volume replacement (60 to 90 mL/kg). The endpoint for fluid therapy is based on the response to treatment, which is closely monitored.

High-volume fluid replacement is by far the most effective treatment for horses suffering from severe hypovolemia that have collapsed or are on the verge of collapse. Two intravenous catheters should be placed; 14- or 12-gauge catheters are adequate if fluids can be delivered under pressure, and 10-gauge catheters are more difficult to place and usually require a cutdown. It is important that catheters are 140 mm (5.5 inches) long and are sutured in place to prevent dislodgement and extravasation of fluid. Aseptic technique is imperative to avoid the unwelcome complication of infectious thrombophlebitis. Horses with profound hypoglycemia may collapse, be reluctant to move, or exhibit a "sawhorse" stance and respond well to administration of 50 to 100 mL of 50% dextrose diluted in 3- or 5-L bags of saline, repeated as needed. Prednisolone sodium succinate (2.2 mg/kg IV or 1 g/450-kg horse; Solu-Delta-Cortef, Pfizer Inc., New York, New York, United States) can be helpful in stabilizing horses that have collapsed or are showing neurological signs, but it should be borne in mind that exhausted, hypovolemic, or dehydrated horses are also at risk for subsequent pleuropneumonia and laminitis, and large doses of corticosteroids may increase this risk. Profound leukopenia may precede the onset of pleuropneumonia, and appropriate antibiotic therapy should be instituted in leukopenic horses. It is wise to recheck the white blood cell count and creatinine levels of distressed horses the day after the race, even if they have been previously treated because endurance horses may be immunosuppressed or azotemic following competition. Laminitis may strike several days following postrace exhaustion. Prophylaxis for laminitis should be instituted in horses that are depressed, inappetent, leukopenic, or febrile.

Synchronous Diaphragmatic Flutter

Synchronous diaphragmatic flutter, or "thumps," a condition in which the phrenic nerve is stimulated by atrial depolarization, causing contraction of the diaphragm and consequent "thumping" of the flank in time with the heartbeat, has traditionally been considered a sign of serious electrolyte imbalance, most commonly hypocalcemic, hypochloremic metabolic alkalosis.[25] In my experience, blood levels of total or ionized calcium are often normal, and the presence and degree of alkalosis are variable. Measured electrolyte values may not reflect total body stores, and there is no convenient way to simultaneously measure chloride and ionized calcium. Many horses with thumps have no other identifiable abnormalities, and rest, food, and water may be all the treatment required. Before 2009, FEI rules dictated that horses be eliminated for thumps, but now disqualification is left to the discretion of the Commission Veterinarians. Most Commission Veterinarians require that horses with thumps be reexamined; if the condition is still present after the horse has been rested, fed, and watered, the horse is usually eliminated. Unfortunately, most horses with thumps take longer to resolve the condition than the limited time period given in which to represent, even if other metabolic abnormalities are not present. Horses eliminated from competition may be completely normal, and Commission Veterinarians may be in a bit of a conundrum: they do not wish to send a potentially compromised horse back out onto the course, nor do they wish to eliminate a competitor that is capable of safely completing. One must not lose sight of the forest for the trees, and it is essential to look at the overall picture.

Horses with thumps accompanied by serious metabolic abnormalities usually respond to intravenous calcium supplementation (100 to 300 mL of 20% to 23% calcium borogluconate diluted in 3 or 5 L of saline given over 15 to 20 minutes, to effect). It has been proposed that horses prone to thumps be fed a low-calcium diet before competition to enable more efficient mobilization of calcium from bone reserves during periods of stress.[26] Although making physiological sense, this strategy has not been successful. Unfortunately, some horses appear to have a low threshold for development of thumps and are likely unsuitable for endurance use.

Prevention of Metabolic Problems

Many, if not most, metabolic problems could be avoided by the use of common sense, but in the heat of competition common sense is one of the first things lost. Although both horse and rider get tired, an astute rider is able to determine when the horse has had enough. The horse should be stopped if it is not eating and drinking at rest stops, is reluctant to move forward, or is stumbling.

Misuse of electrolyte replacement preparations is common, and concentrated electrolyte preparations that are force-fed may be detrimental if the horse does not drink. They increase the tonicity of the gastrointestinal lumen, cause fluid influx, and contribute to dehydration. Poorly formulated electrolyte preparations full of sugar cause hyperglycemia and a subsequent insulin-mediated hypoglycemic crash. Hay fed to a well-hydrated horse acts like a sponge, or water reservoir, in the large intestine. Whereas in flat racehorses hay and water are often withheld before racing, endurance horses should be encouraged to eat hay and should have free access to water before competition so that they will have a fluid reserve available for absorption from the large intestine.

Now one compulsory recheck examination is required at one or more Vet Gates at all FEI rides. This recheck examination has been exceedingly useful in identifying horses that pass the initial veterinary examination but then deteriorate during the mandatory hold period. Without a "second look," horses may return to the course and further worsen. Focusing on the overall safety of the horse by early identification of metabolic and lameness problems is paramount and is in the best interests of the horse. It is incumbent on those of us entrusted with the stewardship of these horses to ensure that we do our utmost to manage them wisely.

Chapter 119

Lameness in the Polo Pony

Paul Wollenman, P. J. McMahon, Simon Knapp, and Mike W. Ross

HISTORY OF THE SPORT

Polo was the first equestrian sport in recorded history. With strong ties to military traditions, the game originated in China in AD 272 and was often substituted for war games in preparation for military battle. Polo evolved into an organized sport and spread into Greece, India, and China, where the British colonies adopted the game. During the nineteenth century, the game became more refined in Great Britain and eventually found its way into the northeastern United States in 1876. Today polo continues to be one of the fastest and most dangerous equine sports in the world. Polo is no longer a sport only for the wealthy; an increasing number of small clubs start up each year that attract people of moderate incomes to take lessons, buy horses, and begin to play. The sport has become more complex, with international professional players competing year-round on different teams. Thus professional polo coaches, umpires, trainers, and breeders have emerged, solidifying polo as a genuine equine sport industry. Playing seasons in the northern and southern hemispheres are followed by nomadic players, grooms, horses, and spectators. During the winter months in the United States, thousands of horses enter Florida and California, where the tropical climate is conducive to world-class polo tournaments. During the spring, summer, and fall seasons these horses travel across the Midwest, up the northeast coast and into Canada. The high-goal season begins in the summer in England and Spain, but in the southern hemisphere, the season in Argentina commences in the fall.

POLO AS AN INDUSTRY

Today three types of polo are played: outdoor, indoor (arena), and snow polo. Outdoor polo is by far the most popular and is played on a large, finely manicured grass field measuring 274 m (300 yards) by 137 m (150 yards) (Figure 119-1). Injuries are related to fatigue (because of the distances covered), stopping, turning, speed, and surface consistency, depending whether the soil beneath the grass is compact or soft. Arena polo is played in much smaller arenas and is more common in collegiate settings. Injuries tend to be less frequent and are usually impact related. Snow polo is regarded as a novel exhibition sport played on the surface of a frozen lake and produces surprisingly few injuries. Obviously, footing and surface conditions often can be responsible for the type of lameness seen. Heavy, soft, grass polo fields and deep, sandy, uneven exercise tracks are frequently responsible for proximal suspensory desmitis (PSD), suspensory branch desmitis, and metacarpophalangeal joint sprains. Hard fields, exercise tracks, and polo field sideboards may cause hoof and pastern region injuries, and hard, fast ground predisposes horses to superficial digital flexor (SDF) tendonitis.

In outdoor polo each team is composed of four players, and each member brings an average of seven to eight horses to the field. A game normally runs for six chukkers (a chukker is 7 minutes), and a different horse is used for

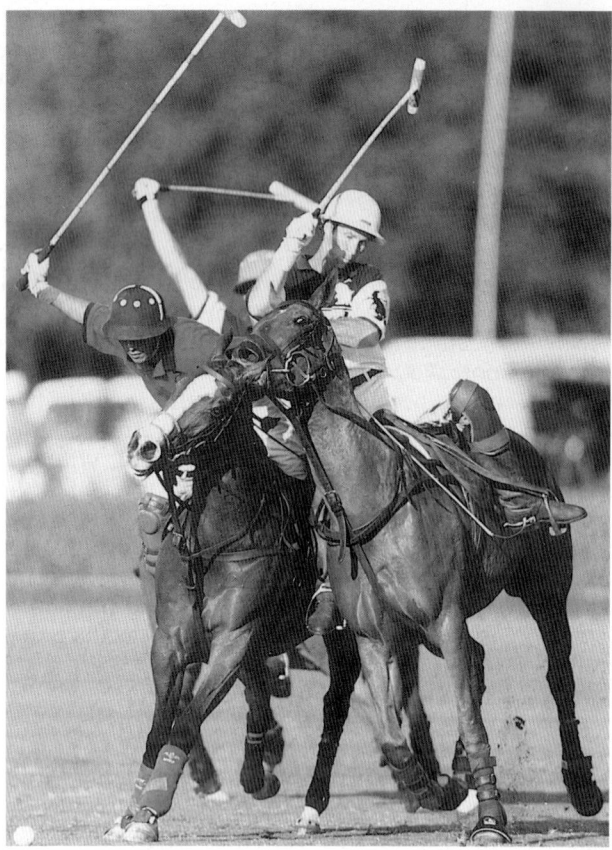

Fig. 119-1 • Outdoor polo is the most popular format for the game today. Close proximity of horses and riders explains why polo ponies often develop injuries related to direct trauma. Polo is only played right-handed.

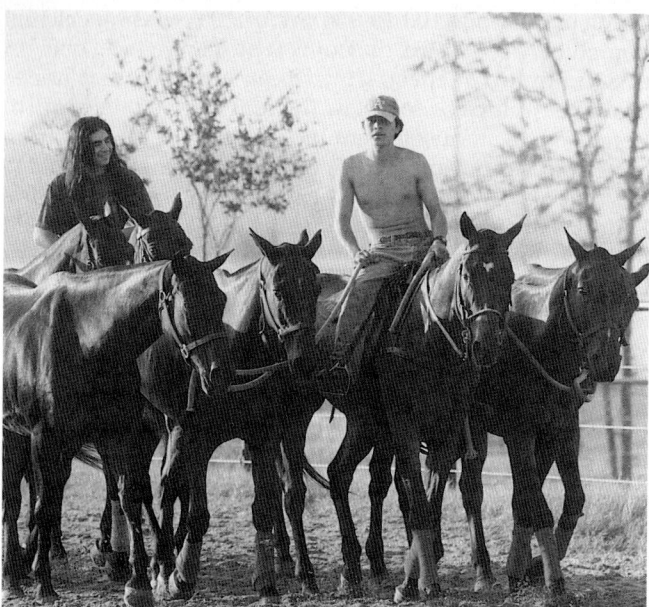

Fig. 119-2 • Daily legging up is an important part of training polo ponies. Ponies often are tied together in sets of four to five, and although this practice saves time, horses in close contact are at risk of traumatic injury.

each chukker. In higher goal polo, numerous mounts are used in single chukkers. Therefore in a single match there may be 50 to 55 horses playing over 1.5 hours. The number of horses that are required to mount a polo team makes each owner's total investment much larger than that for other equine disciplines.

Polo requires the speed and stamina of a Thoroughbred (TB) or a TB-cross horse, the ability to stop and turn quickly, and the boldness to meet and collide with other horses at high speed. Although called ponies, polo horses stand 15 to 16 hands tall, and mares are preferred to geldings at a ratio of 10:1. Most trainers look for a fine neck and throat-latch, a good strong shoulder, powerful hip, quiet disposition, and a responsive, light mouth. Many horses have not raced, so few racetrack-related injuries are found in polo ponies. Argentina, New Zealand, and Australia are the only countries that specifically breed large numbers of horses for polo competition. Horses indigenous to these countries tend to have more bone than those in the United States and Europe, rendering them slightly more durable. Argentina has historically produced the most horses used solely for polo. Since 1970, thousands of Argentine horses have been imported into the United States and Europe, primarily because such a large selection was available at low cost. During the 1970s, inexpensive American former racehorses were sold as polo prospects, but many had numerous orthopedic problems. Today the price of high-goal Argentinian polo ponies continues to increase, and as the cost of importing horses into the United States increases,

economic demands necessitate a greater influx of American TBs into polo. Recently, embryo transfer has been used by players from the United States. Embryos are collected from top playing mares during the off-season and from retired superior mares to produce numerous foals each year. Argentina and, to a lesser extent, Australia have led the movement toward embryo transfer.

Most horses are 3 to 4 years old when introduced to the game, and 2 years of training and playing generally are required before a pony becomes seasoned. Exceptionally talented horses are playing high-goal polo at 6 years of age. By the age of 12 to 14 years, speed usually has begun to diminish, and horses are sold to less demanding players. By the age of 15 to 16 years, depending on temperament, polo ponies may be sold to beginners before being retired.

Neck reining is paramount in training a polo prospect because the rider uses only one hand for control. Wide range of movement, the ability to stop and turn quickly, and the ability to exhibit rapid bursts of speed are required. How well and smoothly the horse performs these maneuvers often determines the number of years the horse stays sound and competes successfully. In addition to schooling, fitness training consists of daily galloping (legging up). Ponies often are tied together in sets of four to five. This time-saving practice teaches the horses to travel more calmly together in close contact but can result in traumatic injuries to the lower limbs (Figure 119-2).

Polo ponies are shod with special rim shoes in front that allow for traction and pivoting without applying excessive torque to the lower limb. Medial and lateral heel calks on the hind shoes are helpful for stopping abruptly but often result in coronary band and pastern region lacerations to other horses during competition. For safety reasons, the Great Britain Polo Association only permits a lateral calk on each hind shoe, whereas the United States Polo Association allows medial and lateral heel calks. The size limit for calks is regulated but seldom enforced.

Therapeutic corrective shoeing is problematic in playing horses (those actively being used in polo competition) because they may lose traction and maneuverability. Some common shoeing modifications include squared, rolled, and rocker toes; elevated and full-shod heels; and padded soles. The standard support and protection afforded the horse during exercise are leg wraps and coronet boots. All legs are wrapped with double-layer rolled cotton bandages. Impact-resistant European racing boots may be added to cover the metacarpal regions to protect against mallet and hoof trauma. More recently, especially on previously injured limbs, cotton leg bandages have been replaced with neoprene fabric wraps that extend below the fetlock joint and provide additional support. Despite these additional protective barriers, horses may still injure tendons and receive skin lacerations during a game or practice.

Drug testing of polo ponies is not yet compulsory in the United States, and no mention of prohibitive medication is addressed in the United States Polo Association rulebook; however, limited testing is done in Great Britain and France. Attending veterinarians often work for many competing teams within the same tournament, and prompt assessment of injuries is important. Low doses of nonsteroidal antiinflammatory drugs (NSAIDs) are commonly used, especially in horses with wounds and solar bruising. The general aim is to have as many sound horses as possible sharing the workload during a match to avoid the practice of double-chukkering (using the same horse for two chukkers).

Minor conformation abnormalities in polo ponies often can be overlooked, but some faults predispose ponies to specific injuries. Long toes and underrun heels may result in tendonitis of the deep digital flexor tendon (DDFT) and palmar foot pain. Toed-in horses are prone to develop lateral suspensory branch desmitis, whereas toed-out horses are more likely to injure the medial branch. Horses with long pasterns and long third metacarpal bones (McIII) are at increased risk of tendonitis of the superficial digital flexor tendon (SDFT).

The most common sources of lameness in polo ponies are similar to those seen in most other equine sports. Polo ponies are at higher risk for traumatic injury because of the high-impact play and the practice of tethering of horses in close proximity to other horses during shipping, exercise, and polo tournaments. Causes of lameness often seen concurrently include palmar foot pain and PSD and osteoarthritis (OA) of the fetlock joint with chronic suspensory branch desmitis.

LAMENESS EXAMINATION

Horses should be stabled overnight so that they cannot warm out of subtle lameness. The horse is first examined in the stall and then as it walks from the stall. The horse is observed at a trot in a straight line on a hard surface and is circled in both directions. Most polo ponies are reluctant to lunge. If necessary, the horse may be observed under saddle, but Argentine ponies generally resist trotting when ridden.

A systematic examination at rest is begun with the hoof and hoof tester evaluation and then continued proximally in the limb, noting evidence of pain, swelling, or obvious injury. Findings always should be compared with the contralateral limb, especially when palpating the body of the suspensory ligament (SL). Joints are assessed for range of motion and a painful response to flexion. Lower limb flexion is followed by carpal or upper hindlimb flexion. Walking the horse briefly between flexion tests to allow an aggravated response to wear off is wise.

One of us (PJM) attends to many older polo ponies that have effusion of the metacarpophalangeal joints, manifest a positive response to flexion, and even may have visible and radiological evidence of OA, but lameness often is abolished using low palmar digital analgesia. Palpation may reveal one or more fractured splint bones with callus, but the rest of the limb should be examined because the cause of lameness may be elsewhere.

If a definitive diagnosis cannot be made, diagnostic analgesia is performed. Because drug tests are not performed, local anesthetic solutions can be used for diagnostic purposes in actively competing horses. When performing a nerve block, it is important to remember that the block may affect a larger area than intended, primarily related to diffusion of local anesthetic solution to surrounding tissue. High palmar analgesia can mask middle carpal joint pain, and palmar nerve blocks performed at the base of the proximal sesamoid bones (PSBs) can eliminate pain associated with the fetlock joint. For this reason, the horse should be observed at the trot shortly after injection of local anesthetic solution and then again after an appropriate wait.

To reduce time and money spent on lameness diagnosis, one author (PW) prefers to block large areas during the initial examination. Specific blocks then are performed, if necessary, the following day. For example, a horse that shows neither a sensitivity to hoof tester examination nor an increased digital pulse amplitude may go sound after palmar nerve blocks performed at the base of the PSBs. The following day the same horse may show slight improvement after palmar digital analgesia and a 100% improvement with intraarticular analgesia of the distal interphalangeal (DIP) joint. However, two authors (PJM and MWR) prefer to start distally and work proximally in a systematic fashion.

Intraarticular analgesia is used extensively in polo ponies because it is more specific than perineural analgesia. Although intraarticular analgesia requires aseptic preparation and carries a small risk of infection, clients are generally receptive. If lameness is localized to a specific joint on clinical examination, therapeutic agents such as corticosteroids and hyaluronan can be added to local anesthetic solution to confirm diagnosis and initiate treatment simultaneously. One author (PW) uses combination diagnostic and therapeutic arthrocentesis typically in the DIP and proximal interphalangeal (PIP) joints. The horse's immediate response to local analgesia is noted, and response to therapy is usually evident 2 to 3 days later. Another author (PJM) frequently uses combination diagnostic and therapeutic injections in the DIP and distal hock joints. Combination injections can also be used simultaneously to diagnose and treat back pain. The dorsal aspect of the dorsal spinous process and the interspinous space can be infiltrated with a combination of local anesthetic solution, Sarapin (High Chemical Company, Levittown, Pennsylvania, United States), and a corticosteroid. Response to infiltration is evaluated immediately by riding the horse after injection, and response to medication is evaluated over the next several days.

Because metacarpophalangeal joint disease and splint bone injury are common sources of pain in the polo pony, one author (PJM) prefers specifically to differentiate these sources of pain by first performing intraarticular analgesia of the metacarpophalangeal joint and then later performing a low palmar block. If low palmar analgesia is performed first, both potential sources of pain are eliminated. If pain is detected on palpation of bony exostoses of the splint bones, these areas can be blocked first, before a systematic blocking strategy is followed. One author (PJM) refers to this as the splint block. This block is performed by first blocking the palmar metacarpal nerve distal to the exostoses. If improvement is not seen, the palmar metacarpal nerve just proximal to the exostoses is then blocked (2 mL of local anesthetic solution). A biaxial splint block can be performed if exostoses are found medially and laterally. This block should be done well below the origin of the SL to clearly differentiate PSD from splint bone disease. Splint disease, mainly from direct trauma from mallets and calk trauma, is common in hindlimbs. Diagnostic analgesia is performed as described in the forelimb.

Hindlimb PSD has become a common diagnosis because we are now more aware of it. In the United Kingdom, a variation of the high plantar nerve block, analgesia of the deep branch of the lateral plantar nerve (see Chapter 10), is commonly used to diagnose PSD. Three milliliters of local anesthetic solution is injected deep to the proximal aspect of the lateral splint bone, and 2 mL each is placed over the medial and lateral plantar nerves. If this block is unsuccessful in abolishing pain, each hock joint compartment is blocked subsequently. This procedure then is followed by fibular and tibial nerve blocks. In Argentina, chemical neurolysis (long-term nerve block) of the fibular and tibial nerves frequently is performed for horses with distal hock joint pain or PSD (PJM).

UNDIAGNOSED LAMENESS

In some horses the lameness is inconsistent and/or subtle, and diagnostic analgesia cannot be performed. Nerve trauma on the abaxial aspect of a PSB may cause episodic, transient severe lameness. An option in a horse with mild inconsistent lameness is to treat with phenylbutazone (2 g orally [PO] twice daily) for 5 days and then reassess the horse. If lameness resolves and does not return after treatment is discontinued, the horse gradually is put back into work. In horses with inconsistent lameness that fail to respond to rest or therapy, we recommend nuclear scintigraphic examination. Exercise intensity can be increased in horses with subtle lameness but is done so with caution. Lameness may become more apparent to the point at which diagnostic analgesia can then be performed. In a horse with recurrent episodes of hindlimb lameness, the veterinarian should be aware of the possibility of an iliac stress fracture (SK).

Occasionally, a polo pony becomes acutely non–weight bearing, with lameness lasting only a few minutes and resolving before examination is possible. If this sort of episode becomes recurrent in the same limb and physical examination reveals no clinically significant findings, we refer the pony for nuclear scintigraphic examination.

Consultation with colleagues and second opinions are always options. It is also important to consider the option of extended turnout. Because the career of a polo pony can last 12 to 15 years, owners are often willing to give the horse 6 to 12 months of turnout to avoid any further injury. If subtle lameness resolves with phenylbutazone therapy, the polo pony can compete because there is no drug testing in polo competition. However, this option must be elected with caution.

Several lameness problems may exist simultaneously in a polo pony, a fact that makes observing the primary or baseline lameness difficult. Subtle signs such as the failure of a horse to stop appropriately, a horse that jumps on after stopping, or a horse that turns one way or the other when stopping (which is probably from outside hindlimb pain; horses turn away from lameness) may reflect low-grade lameness. If these observations have been made, having the horse ridden to witness the problems first hand is useful. In one author's experience (PJM), the most common source of pain in this type of situation is from the distal hock joints.

IMAGING CONSIDERATIONS

Conventional, computed, and digital radiography are the mainstays of imaging, with the front feet and front fetlock joints and hock joints being examined most frequently. The introduction of computed and digital radiography has provided great advantages because, with the exception of faulty positioning or movement, obtaining nondiagnostic radiographs is almost impossible. Exposure can be adjusted at the time of processing, and subtle details that would have been difficult to see on conventional radiographs can now readily be detected and scrutinized easily with computed and digital radiography. Images can be enlarged, and the contrast and brightness can be improved, which are important factors in the diagnosis of incomplete fractures.

Scintigraphic examination is particularly useful in polo ponies with undiagnosed lameness and in those with palmar foot pain, but it is not always helpful in horses with chronic lameness (SK). Motion-correction software has been an important innovation.

Ultrasonography is extremely important in evaluating the damage and healing processes in tendons and the SL in forelimbs and hindlimbs. Transverse images are used more frequently in identifying lesions, whereas longitudinal images aid in assessing healing. Ultrasonographic evaluation of the supraspinous ligament is often useful in horses with obscure hindlimb lameness. We have not found thermography particularly useful in our practices.

Magnetic resonance imaging (MRI) has become available in university settings and in some private equine practices. Despite a long learning curve in the interpretation of magnetic resonance images, many differential diagnoses and prognoses have emerged. Nowhere is this more evident than in obscure foot and pastern lameness with no detectable radiological abnormalities.

Diagnostic arthroscopy in horses with OA of the metacarpophalangeal or carpal joints can be valuable in evaluating the condition of joint surfaces. Palmar intercarpal ligament injury has been diagnosed in ponies with lameness localized to the middle carpal joint but lacking radiological and scintigraphic abnormalities. Tenoscopy and bursoscopy also can be useful diagnostically and therapeutically.

TEN MOST COMMON LAMENESS PROBLEMS IN POLO PONIES

1. Superficial digital flexor tendonitis
2. Metacarpophalangeal osteoarthritis
3. Proximal palmar metacarpal pain and suspensory desmitis
    a. Proximal suspensory desmitis and third metacarpal bone disease
    b. Body suspensory desmitis and splint bone disease
    c. Suspensory branch desmitis and sesamoiditis
4. Injury to the hoof and distal phalanx
5. Palmar foot pain including navicular disease and deep digital flexor tendonitis
6. Distal interphalangeal joint osteoarthritis
7. Desmitis of the accessory ligament of the deep digital flexor tendon
8. Splint bone disease
9. Distal hock joint pain
10. Gluteal myositis and back pain

SUPERFICIAL DIGITAL FLEXOR TENDONITIS

SDF tendonitis is the most common soft tissue injury seen in polo ponies and is by far the most common reason for early retirement. SDF tendonitis can be divided into three categories by location on the limb—high (proximal), midmetacarpal, and low (distal)—or by cause: trauma, speed, and fatigue.

We believe that most peripheral injuries of the SDFT result from tendon trauma while the limb is bearing weight. However, the Editors note that peripheral injuries commonly are seen in other sports horses, such as Standardbred racehorses and reining horses, in which direct trauma is usually not a factor. These injuries occur much more frequently at the midmetacarpal region on the lateral aspect and to a lesser extent on the palmar surface of the tendon (Figure 119-3). Proximal SDF tendonitis also can be caused by trauma (PJM). These areas have a high degree of exposure to swinging mallets and flying hooves. Despite new protective boots, the SDFT is still traumatized with surprising frequency. Traumatic tendon injuries are generally noticed 1 to 2 days after the incident and are characterized by a slight widening of the tendon (not a banana-shaped profile). Lameness is usually not present, but the area is warm and tender to palpation. Some horses have recurrent heat and swelling that resolves quickly with topical and systemic antiinflammatory therapy. Peripheral tendon fiber lesions may involve 20% or less of the cross-sectional area (CSA) of the tendon. However, careful ultrasonographic examination of the medial and lateral borders of the SDFT and critical evaluation of longitudinal images are necessary. Recurrent tendonitis leads to typical swelling and later lameness commonly found with moderate or severe SDF tendonitis.

Core lesions and lesions of the SDFT adjacent to the DDFT are thought to be injuries related to speed and fatigue. Hard, fast ground may be a predisposing factor. SDF tendonitis may result in a banana-shaped profile of the

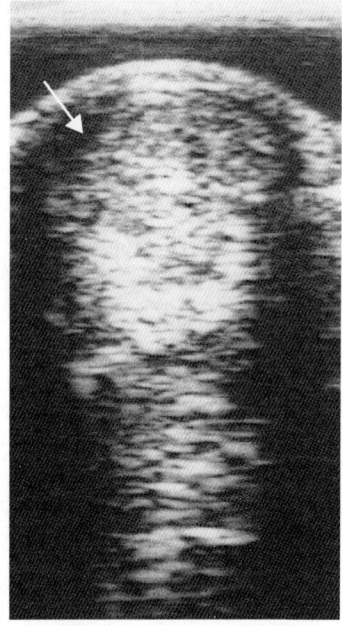

Fig. 119-3 • Transverse ultrasonographic image of the palmar metacarpal region of a polo pony with traumatic tendonitis of the lateral aspect of the superficial digital flexor tendon *(arrow)*. Lateral is to the left. After initial diagnosis, the horse continued to play, and the lesion progressed.

metacarpal region. Core lesions compromising between 20% and 25% of the CSA of the SDFT are serious, and the risk of recurrence is high (Figure 119-4). Horses with small CSA tears that extend more than 2.5 cm in length or those with distally located tendonitis involving SDFT impingement by the palmar annular ligament (PAL) are at high risk of recurrence. Despite appropriate therapy, these horses often have chronic and recurrent lameness, and ultrasonographic evaluation reveals a lesion that often fails to heal.

Initial therapy for any polo pony with tendonitis regardless of location or cause includes the application of ice boots and cold-water hosing, sweats, and compression wraps, as well as the administration of NSAIDs. A combination of injection and rest or surgical management has been successful (MWR).

Medical Management

Peritendonous injections over lesions and intralesional injections have become the mainstay of today's preferred therapy for SDF tendonitis. The aim of this therapy is to return the injured segment of tendon to its elastic state and maintain tensile strength. Peritendonous injections of short-acting corticosteroids and hyaluronan may help to reduce inflammation and improve the cosmetic appearance of the tendon profile, but it is important that corticosteroids are not injected directly into a tendon. Peritendonous corticosteroid injection is frowned on in the United Kingdom (PJM). Autologous adult mesenchymal stem cells, platelet-rich plasma (PRP), and porcine bladder matrix (PBM) have emerged as the biological-based therapies of choice and have markedly increased the success of medical management. One author (PW) prefers an ultrasonographic guided injection of PRP directly into lesions and prefers to use only small volumes of the prepared serum into the

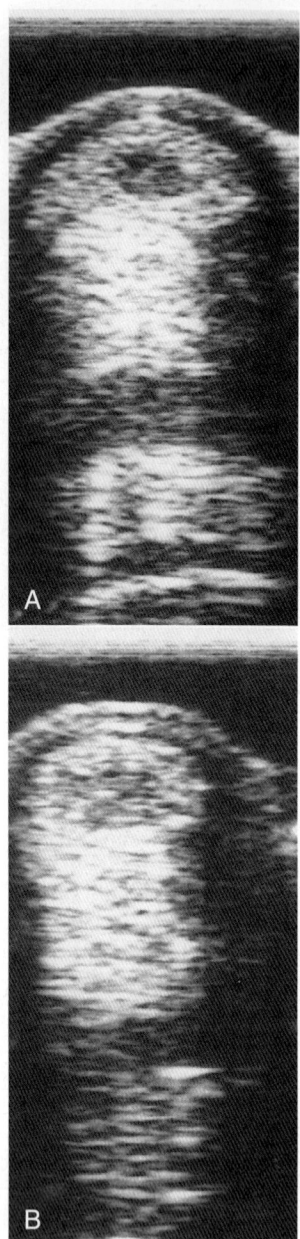

Fig. 119-4 • Initial **(A)** and 40-day follow-up **(B)** transverse ultrasonographic images of the palmar metacarpal region of a polo pony with a typical core lesion of the superficial digital flexor tendon. Tendon splitting was done immediately after the initial image was obtained. The core lesion is more echogenic in the follow-up image but can still be seen.

lesion. Results using adult fat-derived stem cells are equally satisfactory, but this technique requires preinjection surgical collection, as well as transit time, and is substantially more expensive than using in-house processed PRP. PBM is commercially available (ACellVet, ACell Inc., Columbia, Maryland, United States), requires no surgical harvesting or transit time, and is comparable in price to PRP processing, although it occasionally causes postinjection flares. These flares can be reduced by using a small volume of PBM rather than using the entire reconstituted vial. Daily topical icing and rebandaging, along with NSAIDs, are good precautionary therapies to reduce reactions.

Ultrasonographic assessment of tendons 2 months after injection with one of these biologically based products has revealed remarkable filling within hypoechogenic lesions on transverse images. At 6 months after treatment there is good fiber alignment seen on longitudinal images. The real endorsement of success is that approximately 80% of horses with first-time bowed tendons treated with these products have returned to the same level of polo without recurrence of injury within 8 to 12 months.

Surgical Management

Tendon splitting is now seldom used as a standalone therapy to manage polo ponies with SDF tendonitis. If used, tendon splitting within 1 week after injury appears to be beneficial in decompressing the lesion. Tendon splitting must be done early because granulation tissue forms quickly and cannot be decompressed. After appropriate sedation, perineural analgesia, and aseptic preparation, 30 to 40 incisions with a No. 11 scalpel blade in a stabbing manner (a fan-shaped pattern is avoided) are used to decompress only the affected tendon segment. One author prefers using a double-edged tenotome in a fan-shaped pattern (MWR). The procedure can be performed with the limb in a weight-bearing or flexed position, but a weight-bearing position is preferred. With experience, the texture of diseased tendon can be differentiated from surrounding normal tendon structure. Bandages are applied, and horses are confined to a box stall and given controlled, increasing handwalking over the next 8 to 10 weeks. Controlled exercise is recommended for a minimum of 4 to 6 months before any form of turnout exercise is given, but client compliance with this timetable is poor unless a horse walker is available. Unfortunately, most horses are turned out to pasture after blistering within 1 month of injury, a conventional practice we believe is harmful to tendon healing. Total time of turnout exercise (after controlled exercise) is 8 to 12 months. Follow-up ultrasonographic evaluation is important to monitor healing and to determine when exercise level can be stepped up. Desmotomy of the accessory ligament of the SDFT (superior check desmotomy) has been useful in horses with large core lesions (CSA >25%) and in those with small tears (CSA <15%) that are more than 2.5 cm in length. Combining the surgical procedures of desmotomy and tendon splitting early after injury has been successful in returning horses with tendonitis of the SDFT to polo. After surgery, horses are given stall rest and handwalking for 4 to 6 weeks, with a total of 4 to 6 months of controlled exercise, before being turned out or conditioned for polo. Desmotomy of the PAL occasionally is performed when the SDFT is injured and enlarged just above the ligament. This surgery interrupts a self-perpetuating cycle of injury that develops between the enlarged tendon and the thickened PAL. One author (PW) believes that horses with distal tendonitis of the SDFT involving the PAL should initially be treated with peritendonous injection of short-acting corticosteroids followed by compression wraps, not only to reduce the size and improve cosmetic appearance of the SDFT but also to prevent the need for desmotomy of the PAL.

The most common reasons for therapeutic failure in horses with SDF tendonitis are lack of ultrasonographic follow-up evaluation after tendon splitting to determine whether additional therapy is needed, poor owner compliance concerning walking the horse and stretching the injured tendon in the early stages of healing, not allowing for adequate rest before the horse is returned to work, and failure to perform ultrasonographic examination at the time of initial injury, resulting in an inability to evaluate maximal medical improvement before returning the horse to unsupervised work.

METACARPOPHALANGEAL (FETLOCK) OSTEOARTHRITIS

OA of the fetlock joint is the most common articular problem in polo ponies and the most common articular problem necessitating early retirement. Former racehorses with mild OA, osteochondrosis, chip fractures, and chronic capsulitis may be sold for use as polo ponies and have a high risk of redeveloping lameness. The fetlock region of any polo pony with forelimb lameness should be examined carefully. Lameness apparently originating from the fetlock joint based on the clinical observations of pain on palpation, decreased range of motion, and a positive response to distal limb flexion must be differentiated from suspensory branch desmitis and splint bone disease. Intraarticular analgesia is important for differentiation. A full set of radiographs should be obtained. One author (PJM) recommends using large cassettes to assess the fetlock joint and distal aspect of the splint bones. Common radiological findings include fragmentation of the dorsoproximal aspect of the proximal phalanx (Figure 119-5), radiolucent areas in the distal aspect of the McIII, proliferative new bone formation on the palmar aspect of the PSBs, and mineralization of the proximal and distal fetlock joint capsule attachments (Figure 119-6).

Intraarticular injections are the mainstay of treatment. One author (PW) injects both short-acting corticosteroids and hyaluronan. Another author (PJM) prefers polysulfated glycosaminoglycan (PSGAG; Adequan, Luitpold Animal Health, Shirley, New York, United States) therapy or short-acting corticosteroids and hyaluronan or a combination of atropine, short-acting corticosteroid, and hyaluronan. Intramuscular injections of PSGAGs at biweekly intervals for 1 month and then possibly weekly for the entire season

are recommended. Horses that do not respond well to intraarticular injections of corticosteroids may be candidates for serial interleukin-1 receptor antagonist protein (IRAP) injections or arthroscopic evaluation because many of these horses have considerable cartilage damage. IRAP is now commercially available for in-hospital collection, incubation, and administration and is generally administered at bimonthly intervals for a series of three to five doses. IRAP was initially used by one author (PW) in polo ponies that were unresponsive to corticosteroid therapy and was used in conjunction with hyaluronan. Unless the IRAP is prepared with strict asepsis and processed preferably in a sterile hood, it is well advised to use a 2-μm filter to ensure sterility during the injection process. If using hyaluronan in conjunction with the IRAP, be sure to inject the hyaluronan either first or after the filter is removed from the needle hub because the viscosity of the hyaluronan is too thick to pass through the filter. Now many veterinarians, including one auther (PW), are using IRAP as their first line of therapy to treat both acute and chronic joint disease, and its good success tends to appear later rather than earlier in the life of an osteoarthritic joint. Daily icing, poulticing, and NSAID administration can help reduce inflammation in horses with chronic OA. In horses with chronic OA, radiological abnormalities may be extensive, but many horses are serviceably sound (Figure 119-7).

Fetlock joint capsulitis is often a concurrent problem with fetlock OA and can be an additional source of pain and a cause of restricted motion. On rare occasions it can be the only cause of pain and resentment of joint flexion. One author (PW) has seen substantial benefit from mesotherapy applied to the dorsal aspect of the fetlock joint. After aseptic preparation and performing a "ring block" of the fetlock joint, the author uses a 3-tipped mesotherapy injector with 27-gauge × 4-mm needles to inject the area with corticosteroid (triamcinolone acetonide, 9 mg), Sarapin (4 mL), and mepivacaine (4 mL) dorsomedially and dorsolaterally. A compression wrap/sweat is applied for 24 hours after the injection. This treatment usually results in greater range of pain-free motion of the joint and may also be used in conjunction with intraarticular therapy.

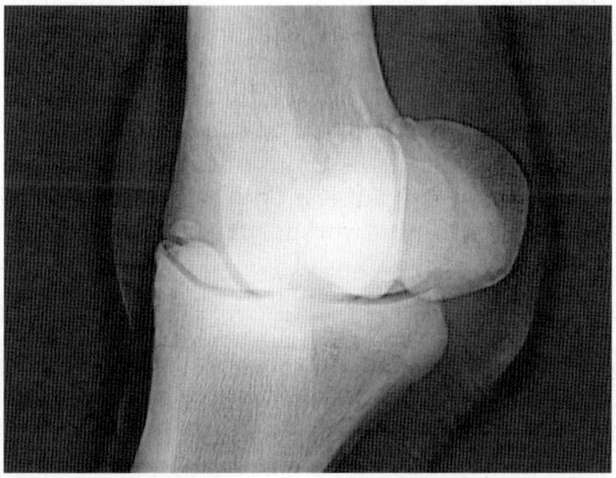

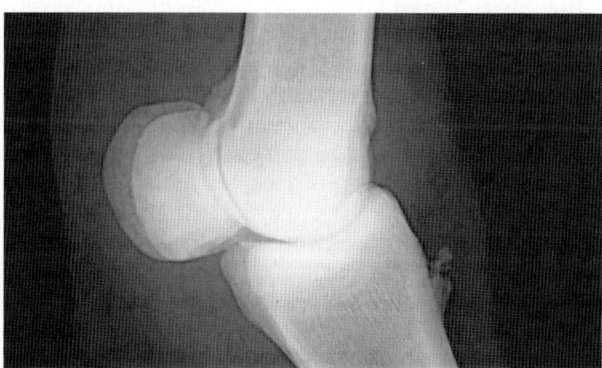

Fig. 119-5 • Dorsolateral-palmaromedial oblique radiographic image of a metacarpophalangeal joint of a polo pony with osteoarthritis. Soft tissue swelling is apparent; a rounded osteochondral fragment is on the proximal dorsomedial aspect of the proximal phalanx; and proliferative changes involve the proximal aspect of the proximal phalanx and proximal sesamoid bones.

Fig. 119-6 • Slightly oblique lateromedial radiographic image of a metacarpophalangeal joint. Mineralization at the insertion of the lateral digital extensor tendon and metacarpophalangeal joint capsule on the proximal aspect of the Lroximal phalanx is a common radiological finding in polo ponies with osteoarthritis of the fetlock joint. Although the finding is important, it does not preclude successful playing.

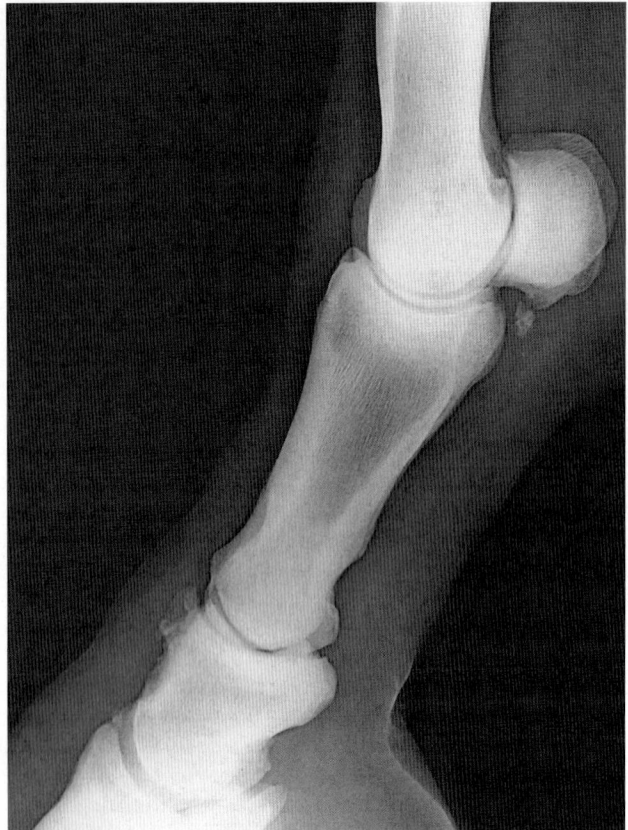

Fig. 119-7 • Lateromedial radiographic image of the distal aspect of a forelimb of a serviceably sound polo pony. There is modeling of one of the proximal sesamoid bones (and a mineralized radiopacity distally) and the dorsoproximal aspect of the proximal phalanx, as well as osteoarthritis and osteochondral fragmentation of the proximal and distal interphalangeal joints.

Chronic proliferative synovitis (villonodular synovitis) is common in polo ponies with chronic OA of the fetlock joint and may be associated with capsular tearing (SK). The dorsal aspect of the fetlock joint develops an apple-shaped appearance, with only mild or moderate effusion. Chronic proliferative synovitis is most common in horses previously used as racehorses and becomes evident after several years of polo. Radiographs may reveal an abnormal contour of the distal dorsal aspect of the McIII, and positive contrast radiographs may be diagnostic. We prefer ultrasonographic examination because ultrasonography helps differentiate between horses that are surgical and nonsurgical candidates. Chronic proliferative synovitis masses of 1.5 cm or larger should be removed arthroscopically to maximize long-term prognosis, whereas horses with smaller masses respond well to rest and intraarticular corticosteroid injections. Intraarticular atropine sulfate also has been used successfully (SK) to reduce effusion.

SUSPENSORY DESMITIS

Suspensory desmitis is seen at three levels: PSD, suspensory body desmitis, and suspensory branch desmitis.

Proximal Suspensory Desmitis

PSD occurs frequently, and diagnosis is confirmed using high palmar or lateral palmar analgesia. PSD results from polo ponies exercising on soft, uneven footing and is not necessarily related directly to playing polo. Lameness is usually only visible at a trot and varies in degree. The cranial phase of the stride is shortened, and lameness is usually most prominent with the affected limb on the outside of a circle. Palpation of the proximal palmar metacarpal region often reveals neither pain nor clinically appreciable enlargement of the SL. Polo ponies with PSD often fail to improve with rest and NSAID administration. Longitudinal ultrasonographic images are most useful in the diagnosis of PSD, but negative ultrasonographic findings do not necessarily eliminate the possibility of injury. MRI is useful to evaluate the bone–ligament interface, particularly in horses in which PSD is difficult to diagnose because there are no detectable changes on radiographs or on ultrasonographic images. CSA measurements on transverse images are occasionally helpful if the same area is measured in the affected and contralateral limbs. One author (PW) has found that variation in CSA measurements leads to misdiagnosis because even in normal polo ponies obtaining reliable repeat measurements is difficult. Hypoechogenic muscle tissue should not be confused as a lesion (SK).

PSD causes more subtle lameness and clinical signs in polo ponies than in other sports horses. Subtle injury and enlargement may cause the ligament to be pinched or compressed by overlying dense fascia, especially in hindlimbs. Horses with long-standing PSD often have increased radiopacity of the proximal aspect of the McIII visible in lateromedial or dorsopalmar radiographic images. Absence of increased radiopacity does not rule out PSD because horses with soft tissue injuries often lack bony involvement. Avulsion fractures of the McIII at the origin of the SL, incomplete longitudinal fractures of the McIII, and stress reaction can occur independently or concomitantly to PSD. Radiological and ultrasonographic examinations may reveal small or large fragments or proliferative changes and radiolucency associated with the palmar cortex of the McIII. Computed and digital radiography, nuclear scintigraphy, and MRI are beneficial in diagnosing bony injury and differentiating it from PSD. Follow-up radiographs may be necessary because avulsion or longitudinal fractures may not show up on initial radiographs.

Even without treatment, almost all polo ponies with PSD and bony causes of proximal palmar metacarpal pain recover within a 3-month rest period. However, horses that are notably lame at a walk, stand somewhat unstably, and occasionally buckle at the carpus of the affected limb may require up to 6 months of rest. In polo ponies with PSD in which a quick return to work is mandated, local injection into and around the origin of the SL with a combination of short-acting corticosteroids and PSGAGs hastens resolution of clinical signs. Ponies are walked for 1 week and then put in light work the second week. By the third week they may be galloped and are able to play shortly thereafter. Owners tend to keep polo ponies with PSD in work if the end of the season is near because ponies are turned out routinely for 3 to 6 months after the season. Owners may gamble successfully by continuing to play the horse through the end of the season without permanently damaging the ligament. Polo ponies rarely get hindlimb PSD, but when they do, prognosis is guarded, and treatment by neurectomy often is required.

In horses with chronic PSD, once bony involvement has been ruled out, local injections of corticosteroids and Sarapin or internal blister may be warranted. In the United Kingdom and Europe, injection of corticosteroids into the proximal aspect of the SL is frowned on because this medication may slow healing and may mask the presence of fractures (SK and PJM). This is especially true in horses with acute injuries. Numerous applications of shock wave therapy are popular and may prove beneficial. Horses with known bony injury should be given rest. One author (PW) prefers the use of concentrated bone marrow–derived stem cells to infiltrate the origin of the SL in combination with fasciotomy.

Body Suspensory Desmitis

Body suspensory desmitis is a serious and often career-ending injury. Diagnosis is straightforward if the SL is thickened and painful. Ultrasonographic examination is crucial in assessing SL damage, but radiology is important to evaluate the medial and lateral splint bones because splint bone disease often is associated with suspensory desmitis in a polo pony. Radiographs should be obtained even if obvious areas of pain or bony and soft tissue swelling associated with the splint bones are absent. Treatment of polo ponies with acute body suspensory desmitis includes immediate application of cold or ice therapy, alternating with topical sweats, and administration of NSAIDs. Periligamentous infiltration of short-acting corticosteroids early after injury improves cosmetic appearance and may minimize adhesion formation between the SL and splint bones. Injections are performed in polo ponies only if the owner agrees the horse is in need of long-term rest. The horse gradually is returned to handwalking in 5 to 7 days and can be turned out after 3 weeks. Intralesional injections of concentrated bone marrow into SL body tears have proven beneficial and successful, and one author (PW) prefers this over PBM and fat-derived adult stem cells. Sclerosing agents (e.g., ethanolamine) injected into the SL may be helpful (SK). Two authors (PW and PJM) believe that long-term box stall rest may increase the chance of adhesion formation. One author (MWR) prefers controlled exercise rather than turnout exercise and believes strongly that turnout exercise is the "antithesis of healing." Ultrasonographic evaluation of ligament healing is important. One author (PJM) has observed many polo ponies with distal body suspensory desmitis that involves the bifurcation and invariably at least one branch. If desmitis at the suspensory bifurcation is severe, the polo pony may never fully recover. The best results are seen with a combination of periligamentous injections of dimethyl sulfoxide (DMSO) and corticosteroids and long-term rest. Performance level may need to be dropped to junior polo, and even at this level lameness may be persistent or recurrent.

Suspensory Branch Desmitis

Suspensory branch desmitis is common in polo ponies. The lateral branch is injured more frequently than the medial branch, and occasionally both branches are injured simultaneously. Pivoting of the distal limb at high speeds is likely the cause of suspensory branch desmitis. Faulty conformation is another important predisposing factor. Horses that are toed in tend to develop lateral suspensory branch desmitis, whereas those that are toed out tend to develop

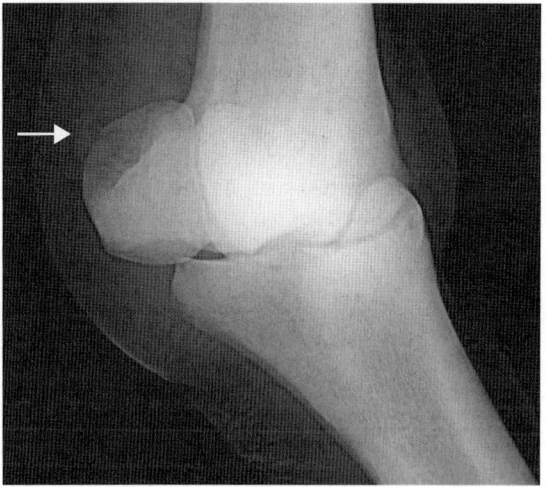

Fig. 119-8 • Dorsolateral-palmaromedial oblique radiographic image of a metacarpophalangeal joint, with mineralization in the lateral branch of the suspensory ligament at the attachment to the proximal sesamoid bone *(arrow)*. Note also the soft tissue swelling.

medial suspensory branch desmitis. Palpation of the branches while the fetlock joint is in partial flexion is a preferred technique of one author (PW). Firm palpation and lower limb flexion followed by trotting exacerbates the degree of lameness. Ultrasonographic examination of the branches is accomplished easily and allows assessment of the degree of suspensory branch desmitis. Radiography should be performed to evaluate the distal aspects of the splint bones because fracture and fracture displacement are common in ponies with suspensory branch desmitis. Mineralization in a branch close to attachment on a PSB may occur in horses with chronic injury (Figure 119-8). Horses with acute injuries are treated identically to those with suspensory body desmitis. The appearance of the branch can be restored cosmetically to near normal over time with periligamentous injection of short-acting corticosteroids. The branch can be split 2 to 3 weeks after injury, although results in the United Kingdom have been disappointing (SK). In the United States, one author (PW) believes that branch splitting in conjunction with shock wave therapy has had superior results compared with adult stem cell or PRP injections. Horses with suspensory branch desmitis need about 6 months of layup time before returning to polo training. One author (PJM) believes that adhesions between the inflamed branch and surrounding tissue or the ipsilateral splint bone negatively influence prognosis, and corticosteroid injections may limit adhesion formation. Surgical adhesiolysis and distal ostectomy of the fractured splint bone may be useful in horses with chronic suspensory branch desmitis and splint bone fracture, but the cosmetic appearance is usually less than desirable. Counterirritants still are used in Europe with variable results. We believe that pin firing (hot firing) is not successful for horses with suspensory body desmitis, but it can be useful for horses with suspensory branch desmitis as a last resort.

INJURY TO THE HOOF AND DISTAL PHALANX

Polo more than other types of equine sporting activity predisposes horses to direct hoof trauma. Direct trauma results from swinging mallets, horses stepping directly on the hard polo balls used during playing, interference or direct impact from hooves of nearby horses, and from horses stepping on wooden sideboards at great speed. Calk or stud injuries to the hoof wall and pastern region are most common. Careful evaluation of wounds for involvement of deeper structures, such as the PIP and DIP joints, is necessary. A common lameness that occurs during polo competition is called *getting stung*, referring to a sudden crippling lameness, lasting only a few minutes, generally resulting from a blow to the hoof or pastern by a mallet or hoof of another horse. The horse is usually sound within minutes of the incident with no clinical evidence of injury. Occasionally, a fracture occurs that may not be evident radiologically for up to 14 days.

Fractures of the Distal Phalanx

Acute fractures of the palmar processes of the distal phalanx often occur from mallet blows, and because polo is played right-handed, fractures usually are seen in the medial aspect of the left forelimb and lateral aspect of the right forelimb. Oblique fractures are sometimes difficult to see in conventional radiographic images, and several dorsoproximal-palmarodistal oblique images may be necessary. Rarely, fractures of the solar margin or of the extensor process of the distal phalanx are seen. Management of polo ponies with distal phalangeal fractures is similar to that in other sports horses.

PALMAR FOOT PAIN INCLUDING NAVICULAR DISEASE

Palmar foot pain in polo ponies with TB and TB-cross ancestry appears to be decreasing, primarily because of the successful efforts of farriers and owners. The problem may be worse in American TBs than in TBs originating from the United Kingdom, Argentina, Australia, and New Zealand (PJM). The long-toe and underrun heel complex and the tendency to shoe front feet with shoes with short branches that sit tight at the heel (to prevent front plates from being pulled off by hind feet) gradually have been corrected. Squared or rolled toe shoes, with or without an elevated heel (world plates and natural balance plates), have reduced the number of polo ponies with broken pastern foot axes and have reduced DDFT tension caused by prolonged breakover. Owners have allowed farriers to reset polo plates more frequently during the playing season and to perform more frequent four-point trims during the off-season than in previous years. The causes of palmar foot pain are often difficult to differentiate from navicular disease because the horse may show a painful response to hoof testers, and lameness is abolished using palmar digital analgesia. Differentiation may be possible using intraarticular analgesia of the DIP joint, radiography, and scintigraphy. Many polo ponies with palmar foot pain have secondary pain at the origin of the SL, which is thought to be caused by alteration of gait.

A common source of palmar foot pain is laminar tearing at the heel. Sudden stops force the horse to use the heels of the front feet as brakes. Corns or heel bruising can cause poor performance and lameness. Corns are diagnosed easily using hoof testers and by carefully inspecting the seat of the corn for hemorrhage or discoloration. One author (PJM) has seen many polo ponies toward the end of the polo season with bilateral, biaxial horn staining resembling chronic corns that apparently did not result in overt lameness. Management of polo ponies with palmar foot pain resulting from corns is similar to that used for undiagnosed palmar foot pain, including the application of wedge pads to relieve heel pain for a few games, or by using the four-point trimming method with natural balance or straight bar shoes and acrylic rubber frog and heel support. One author (SK) has found that four-point shoeing provides poor grip and traction and considers it unsuitable for polo ponies. However, most feel these shoeing techniques appear to decrease stress on the heel and the DDFT and navicular region. Hoof growth stimulants and NSAID administration may help horses with palmar foot pain.

Osteitis of the Distal Phalanx (Pedal Osteitis)

Although definition and accurate diagnosis of osteitis of the distal phalanx remain obscure, many polo ponies with palmar foot pain have evidence of disease in the margins of the distal phalanx on scintigraphic and radiographic images. There may be new bone projecting distally from the palmar aspect of the distal phalanx seen on a lateromedial radiographic image. This finding should be interpreted carefully on radiographs obtained during purchase examinations.

Navicular Disease

Navicular disease in a polo pony is characterized by chronic forelimb lameness, which is abolished using palmar digital analgesia, intraarticular analgesia of the DIP joint, or analgesia of the navicular bursa, often with little radiological abnormality. Nuclear scintigraphy may be helpful to differentiate navicular disease from other causes of palmar foot pain. Most horses with early navicular disease respond positively to intraarticular administration of hyaluronan and corticosteroids into the DIP joint. The administration of NSAIDs and isoxsuprine and the application of corrective shoeing techniques (see Palmar Foot Pain section) are valuable. Those ponies unresponsive to intraarticular injections of the DIP joint may improve after injection of the navicular bursa, best performed under radiographic guidance. MRI has become extremely valuable in differentiating between navicular bone pathology and soft tissue pathology. Therapy, length of rest, and prognosis differ for horses with deep digital flexor (DDF) tendonitis versus those with acute navicular bone pain. Horses with acute navicular bone injury that fail to respond to treatment of the DIP joint or navicular bursa are rested for 3 to 6 weeks and treated with NSAIDs; work is then resumed for the rest of the season with continued treatment with NSAIDs. Horses with advanced navicular disease or those unresponsive to therapy may be dropped from medium- or high-goal polo. Horses with DDF tendon (DDFT) injury have a much more guarded prognosis and are treated by 6 to 12 months of rest. Initially a frog support is applied and the heel is elevated, combined with stall rest, handwalking for 4 weeks, and NSAIDs. This is followed by 3 months of shoeing with full heel support and then turnout unshod, with monthly trimming for the remainder of the convalescent period. Palmar digital neurectomy is considered undesirable and is not routinely performed. Chemical neurolysis (long-term foot block) is of limited value. Cryoneurectomy can give limited relief, but the palmar digital nerves regrow and lameness recurs. Concomitant or solitary injury of the DDFT does not appear to be as common in polo ponies as in other sports horses (PJM). Shock wave therapy may offer a viable solution for these horses.

DISTAL INTERPHALANGEAL OSTEOARTHRITIS

Early (synovitis) and chronic OA of the DIP joint can cause lameness in the polo pony, but diagnosis can be challenging because of the lack of specificity of analgesic techniques in the foot. For example, if more than 6 mL of local anesthetic solution is injected into the DIP joint and lameness is evaluated after 3 to 5 minutes (SK) or 10 minutes (PW), pain from other areas of the foot, including the sole, can be blocked inadvertently. This effect can be avoided by using smaller amounts of local anesthetic solution. Horses with synovitis have DIP joint effusion and manifest only a mildly painful response to lower limb flexion. However, this test may be positive in horses with many sources of pain, including either the navicular bone or the fetlock joint. Management of horses with OA of the DIP joint usually includes intraarticular medication. Short- or long-acting corticosteroids are preferred to injection with hyaluronan. One author (PJM) combines corticosteroids and DMSO because DMSO may improve distribution of corticosteroids to all parts of the joint and the navicular bursa. The DIP joint is the only joint in which one author (PW) uses PSGAGs, combined with short-acting corticosteroids. Another author (PJM) favors using PSGAGs in horses unresponsive to injections with corticosteroids. Most of these horses have clinical and radiological evidence of advanced OA. In some polo ponies, lameness does not improve directly after intraarticular analgesia but inexplicably resolves 24 to 36 hours later, when presumably the effects of the corticosteroid begin. After intraarticular injection, horses are given 3 weeks of limited exercise and a tapered dose of NSAIDs. Weekly intramuscular administration of PSGAGs for a minimum of 30 days and the application of corrective shoes to ease breakover are recommended.

DESMITIS OF THE ACCESSORY LIGAMENT OF THE DEEP DIGITAL FLEXOR TENDON

Trainers and owners commonly confuse chronic desmitis or acute tears of the accessory ligament of the deep digital flexor tendon (ALDDFT) with bowed tendons. Desmitis of the ALDDFT occurs in polo ponies, especially older ponies (SK), but is less frequent than SDF tendonitis. Mild desmitis is characterized by a meaty, nontender swelling of the proximal palmar metacarpal region between the SL and DDFT. Horses with severe or complete tears can have prominent swelling at or near the junction of the ALDDFT with the DDFT, but neither lameness nor the response to palpation is commensurate with the degree of damage. Diagnosis must be confirmed and healing monitored using ultrasonographic examination. Initially, horses are managed with rest, cold therapy including ice, application of sweats, and administration of NSAIDs. Local infiltration of short-acting corticosteroids around (but not in) the ALDDFT can help cosmetic appearance. Stall rest for 2 weeks is recommended, and thereafter horses can be turned out for 4 to 6 months. Follow-up ultrasonographic examination reveals

an enlarged, hyperechogenic ALDDFT. Prognosis for future soundness and return to polo is usually excellent in horses with small (<30% mass) tears, but swelling persists. Chance of recurrence is slim. In horses with large tears (>30% mass) or near ruptures, the chance to return to competitive polo is slim, even with 1 year off work.

SPLINT BONE DISEASE

Traumatic exostoses (Figure 119-9) caused by swinging mallets and fractures of the splint bones are common in polo ponies and are sometimes referred to as *bamboo fever*. Although trauma is usually the inciting cause of exostoses, injury of the SL may play a role (PJM). Horses with splint exostoses resent direct palpation, but many do not manifest overt signs of lameness. If lameness is present but the exostosis is only mildly painful, a splint block (see page 1152) should be performed to confirm the diagnosis. Splint disease can make a veterinarian look foolish because an acute injury may be confused with PSD, but subsequent development of a large golf ball-size swelling reveals the true diagnosis. Oblique radiographic images are most helpful for evaluating the splint bones.

Local infiltration of corticosteroids and Sarapin is used to treat polo ponies with acute splint exostoses. Other injections include a combination of corticosteroids, Sarapin, calcitonin, and medroxyprogesterone acetate. Calcitonin (400 IU) and medroxyprogesterone acetate (200 mg) are used commonly in Europe (PJM). Rest, compression wraps, sweats, and the administration of NSAIDs are useful. Polo ponies with chronic exostoses seem to benefit from pin freezing (cryotherapy), and this is the treatment of choice, with a quick return to work in 14 days. Cryotherapy appears to stimulate remodeling of chronic proliferative splint exostoses, and often a cosmetically acceptable limb profile is seen within 6 months. Despite the resulting white spots, clients seem to accept this form of therapy because of a high success rate. Thermocautery (hot firing) has merit, and early results of shock wave therapy appear promising (PJM).

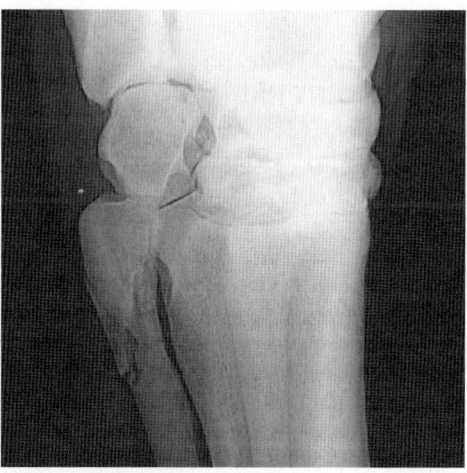

Fig. 119-9 • Dorsolateral-plantaromedial oblique radiographic image of the metatarsal region. There is a comminuted fracture of the proximal aspect of the fourth metatarsal bone caused by mallet injury (called bamboo fever). This fracture usually does not require internal fixation, and prognosis for future soundness is good.

Proximal splint bone fractures may require surgical fixation, and certainly horses need prolonged stall rest and a slow return to work. If fractures are nonarticular and fragments are not displaced or are displaced minimally, prognosis is favorable.

Polo ponies with nondisplaced diaphyseal splint bone fractures respond well to cryotherapy. Cryotherapy not only produces local analgesia but also induces deep fibrous tissue formation that stabilizes fracture fragments. Cryoprobes (No. 17 pointed probes, Veterinary Ophthalmic Specialties, Inc., Moscow, Idaho, United States) are applied two at a time in firm contact with the skin covering the abnormal splint for 1 minute at each site, at sites 1.5 cm apart. Applying two probes at different sites simultaneously decreases treatment time. Preselected aim point patterns for pin freezing are marked by commercially available office white correction fluid. Because each site is to be frozen only once to minimize surface skin necrosis, technicians often draw the pattern on a piece of paper before freezing and check off the appropriate sites once the probes have been applied. A major reason for failure of pin freezing splints is the use of cryospray units to apply nitrogen, rather than using prefrozen probes. Pointed probes pressed firmly into the skin form better ice balls on the surface of the bone, creating a much better bone response, remodeling, and flattening of the exostosis. Maintaining a 1-minute freeze with no movement of the subzero probes is also useful. Failure to pattern the pin freeze outward to slightly beyond the perimeter of the preexisting splint exostosis often results in continued growth of the exostosis above and below the therapy area. After cryotherapy, the limb is kept wrapped for up to 3 weeks, but ponies return to exercise within 4 to 7 days. Ponies with nondisplaced splint bone fractures are given rest for 4 to 6 weeks. Distal splint bone fractures can be diagnosed easily using longitudinal ultrasonographic images or radiography. These fractures usually are associated with chronic suspensory branch desmitis, which is thought to cause bowing of the distal aspect of the splint bone and subsequent displacement and proliferative changes (Figure 119-10). Distal fracture fragments generally are removed surgically, and concomitant splitting of the involved SL branch(s) is often performed.

DISTAL HOCK JOINT PAIN

Polo ponies can play successfully with moderate to severe radiological changes in the distal hock joints (Figure 119-11). Most of the distal hock joint pain appears to be subclinical, meaning lameness is not the most noticeable clinical sign. Most polo ponies with distal hock joint pain are noticed by owners or riders to lack quick jump-out speed and the ability to stop abruptly and are noticed to be running through the bridle. These ponies generally improve if they are given ample warm-up time before playing. Distal hock joint pain appears to be one source of pain with which a polo pony can live, but such pain is a major cause of poor performance and may induce compensatory lameness such as PSD in the forelimbs as a result of overload. Proximal limb flexion tests may elicit little response, and detecting pain or effusion using careful palpation is difficult in some horses. Because lameness is not necessarily proportional to radiological changes, scintigraphic examination is helpful,

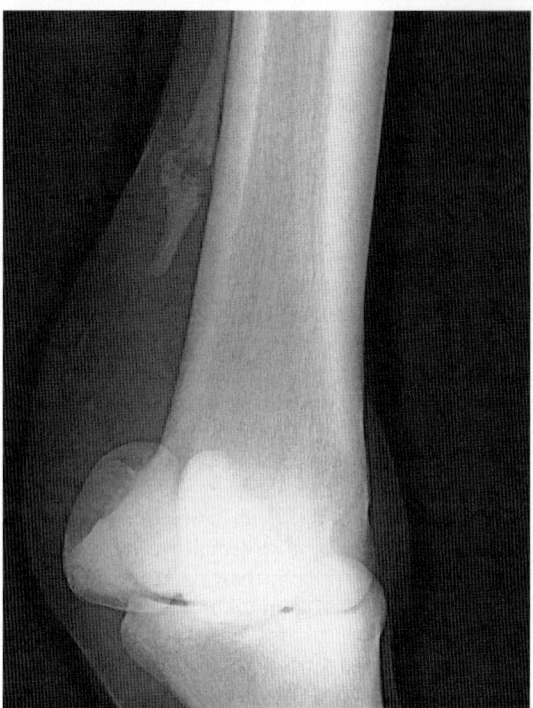

Fig. 119-10 • Dorsolateral-palmaromedial oblique radiographic image of the metacarpal region. A chronic displaced fracture of the fourth metacarpal bone is associated with suspensory branch desmitis. The second metacarpal bone is bowed away from the third metacarpal bone; chronic proliferation has resulted from instability; sesamoiditis is apparent; and the suspensory branch has mineralization.

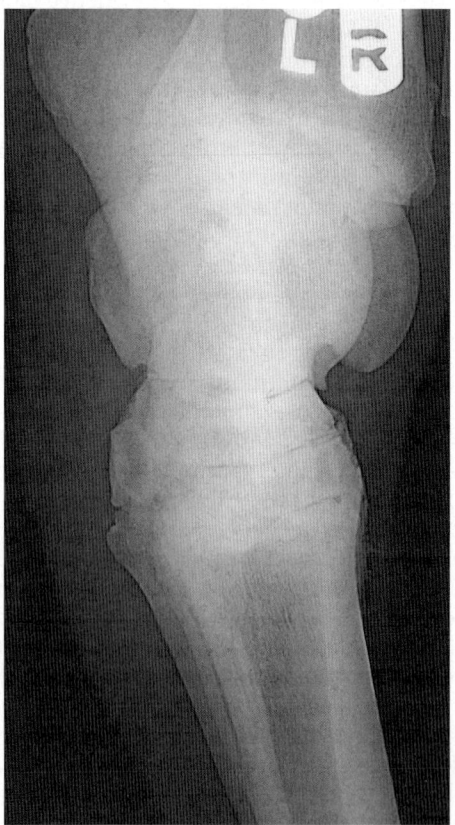

Fig. 119-11 • Dorsomedial-plantarolateral oblique radiographic image of a left hock with radiological evidence of advanced osteoarthritis. This polo pony was not lame.

especially in polo ponies with subtle hindlimb lameness. Diagnostic analgesia is an important tool if lameness is perceptible, and in horses with bilaterally symmetrical lameness, analgesia of one hindlimb may induce obvious contralateral lameness. Combining diagnostic and therapeutic injections is commonplace because the practice saves time and money. The tarsometatarsal and centrodistal (distal intertarsal) joints are injected most commonly with methylprednisolone acetate, but in some ponies the tarsocrural joint also is injected. Intramuscular administration of PSGAGs and intravenous injection of hyaluronan throughout the playing season appear to be helpful in allowing horses to play up to potential. Horses are kept in work and placed on low doses of NSAIDs throughout the season, and training is limited.

GLUTEAL MYOSITIS AND BACK PAIN

Gluteal myositis often accompanies subclinical hindlimb lameness and is often a compensatory problem. One or both hindlimbs have a shortened cranial phase of the stride. Deep palpation of the gluteal muscles elicits pain, although the muscles never feel as hard as they do in ponies with rhabdomyolysis. If possible, it is important to determine whether gluteal myositis is a primary or secondary problem. Gluteal myositis can be differentiated easily from rhabdomyolysis because serum creatine kinase and aspartate transaminase levels are invariably normal. Polo ponies with gluteal myositis can be treated with local injections directly into the gluteal muscles and between the biceps femoris and semitendinosus muscles. The horse is allowed light work and is placed on NSAIDs. One author (PW) has had modest success using a 5-day series of rubeola virus immunomodulator. If gluteal myositis is secondary, the primary source of pain must be identified and managed successfully.

Back pain in polo ponies is often secondary to lameness or results from mismanagement, including use of ill-fitting saddles, overweight amateur riders, and mouth problems. Poor dentition from lack of, or inappropriate, tooth floating procedures causes sharp molars to come in contact with gag bits. Horses carry the head and neck high to avoid pain and tend to hollow the back. Back pain can become a permanent or chronic problem if horses are mismanaged continually. Back pain generally is characterized by a painful response to palpation along the lateral edges of the longissimus dorsi muscles. The horse exhibits a crouching gait when mounted and during initial walking under saddle.

Intramuscular injections of corticosteroids combined with Sarapin (2:1 ratio) are performed along the length of the longissimus dorsi muscle, from the caudal border of the trapezius muscle to the level of the tuber coxae, 15 cm lateral to the dorsal midline. Injection sites are placed every 15 cm, and 5 mL of the mixture is administered at each site. Mesotherapy is also extremely beneficial and is often used in conjunction with deep muscle injections. After preparation of the lumbar region, mesotherapy is performed using a 5-tipped mesohead with 27-gauge × 4-mm needles. A volume of 35 mL of flumethasone, Sarapin, mepivacaine, and Traumeel is used to inject two passes down each side of the dorsal midline. Generally horses are ponied (led from another horse) for 5 days before being ridden. Relief from

pain is quick and predictable with this treatment. Because back pain may be compensatory to primary distal hock joint pain or other lameness, it is important to evaluate the hindlimbs and pelvis carefully. Primary management of the distal hock joint pain and local treatment of acupuncture points in the back are common.

Dorsal spinous process impingement can be a source of back pain, and one author (PJM) believes this is a major cause of back pain in the polo pony. Diagnosis should be confirmed by assessing the effect of local analgesia and/or performing scintigraphy (SK). Treatment involves injection of the spaces between the dorsal spinous processes with corticosteroids and Sarapin. Shock wave therapy may be beneficial (PJM and PW). Horses with back pain are given NSAIDs and are kept fit during a 4- to 6-week period using ponying (being led from another horse) exercise. In Europe, a common management regimen includes paddock exercise as much as possible, lunging exercise with the horse's head down, and little warm-up before polo games. Internal blisters have been used with some success, but care must be taken when injecting these compounds because deep muscle abscesses can develop. Faradism is useful for longissimus dorsi and gluteal muscle strain (SK).

OTHER CONDITIONS
Dislocation (Luxation) of the Superficial Digital Flexor Tendon
Although rare, avulsion injury and dislocation of the SDFT from the tuber calcanei is seen nearly once each year in a busy polo pony practice, resulting in extreme panic by the pony, necessitating sedation. The SDFT usually dislocates laterally, but diagnosis may be difficult before swelling develops. In our experience, surgical techniques, including primary repair, mesh augmentation, and laterally located screws combined with full-limb cast application, are neither successful nor necessary. Most horses respond well to confinement in a small pen and subsequent turnout for 6 to 12 months. Turnout exercise is recommended as soon as possible. Despite the fact that the SDFT remains displaced, causing a slight mechanical lameness and enlargement of the calcaneal and gastrocnemius bursae, horses tend to perform well at the canter and gallop, with a fair to good prognosis for medium- and low-goal polo. Some polo ponies with lateral dislocation of the SDFT in one limb develop the same condition in the opposite limb 1 or 2 years later (PJM).

Fractures of the Cranial Thoracic Dorsal Spinous Processes (Fracture of the Withers)
Fracture of the withers is fairly common. Polo ponies are often tied next to each other for long periods, and a frightened horse occasionally rears up and flips over (Figure 119-12), resulting in fractures of the longest dorsal spinous processes at the withers. Often up to four dorsal spinous processes are fractured, with ventral displacement of the fragments resulting in a flattened appearance of the withers. Ponies are usually only mildly painful to palpation but are generally reluctant to lower the head when grazing. The affected horse may travel with a painful, stiff, extended head and neck carriage, and some horses grunt with every

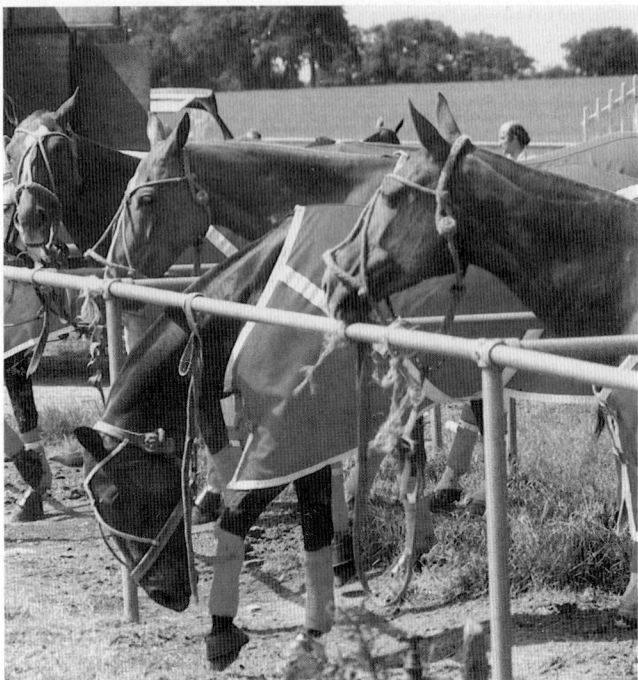

Fig. 119-12 • Polo ponies commonly are tied to rigid bars and in close proximity to each other. Occasionally a polo pony flips over and fractures the thoracic dorsal spinous processes at the withers.

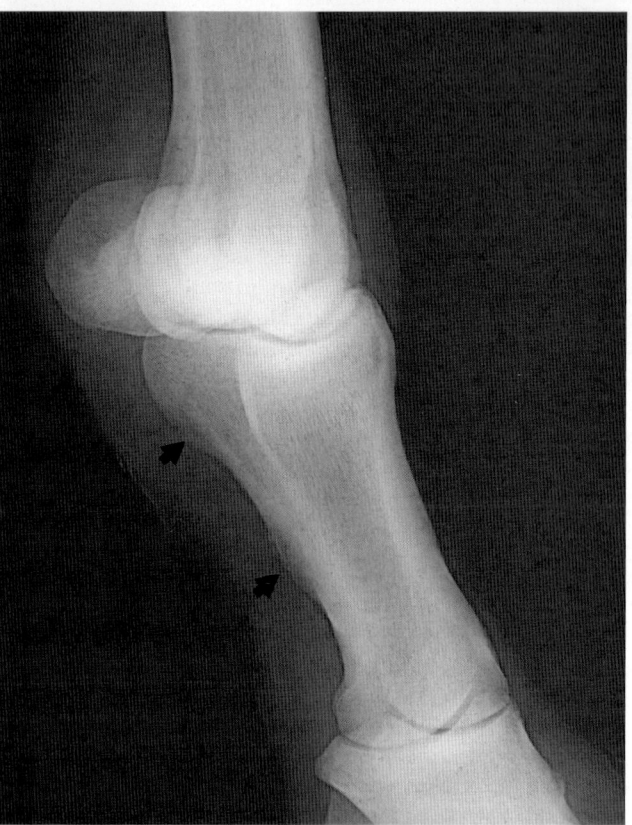

Fig. 119-13 • Dorsomedial-palmarolateral oblique radiographic image of the distal aspect of a left forelimb. Proliferative new bone (arrows) along the palmar medial aspect of the proximal phalanx is typical of a mallet injury. Polo is played right-handed, and trauma usually involves the medial aspect of the left forelimb and the lateral aspect of the right forelimb proximal phalanges.

stride. The prognosis for return to polo is excellent after rest for 4 to 6 months, as long as secondary infection does not develop. Special consideration should be given to saddle fit; a croup strap may be necessary to keep the saddle from sliding forward.

Proximal Interphalangeal Osteoarthritis and Other Pastern Region Injuries

OA of the PIP joint (high ringbone) occurs occasionally in polo ponies and is seen most frequently in green horses (generally Quarter Horses or Quarter Horse/TB crosses) playing on rough terrain in the western United States and generally results from irregular footing. Pain originating from the PIP joint is difficult to diagnose in horses with acute disease without radiological changes, but it can be identified scintigraphically. OA of the PIP joint is often difficult to manage, and although motion of this joint is limited, lameness can be inappropriately severe. Rest (60 to 90 days), NSAID therapy, and intraarticular long-acting corticosteroid therapy are recommended.

A common finding in oblique radiographic images of the pastern region is periosteal new bone on the medial aspect of the left forelimb and the lateral aspect of the right forelimb proximal phalanges (Figure 119-13). Because polo always is played right-handed, powerful neck shots always hit the right side of each forelimb. Lameness is usually insignificant and short lived. These radiological changes should not be confused with those resulting from enthesitis at the attachment sites of the distal sesamoidean ligaments. To differentiate OA of the PIP joint from these proliferative changes, intraarticular analgesia or pinpoint perineural or local analgesic techniques should be performed.

Sesamoiditis

Inflammation (sesamoiditis) of the PSBs can be caused by direct mallet or hoof trauma and by stress-related injury at the suspensory branch insertions. Traumatic sesamoiditis occurs in the medial PSB in the forelimbs from interference injury and in the lateral PSB in the forelimb and hindlimb from mallet trauma. Diagnosis of sesamoiditis is straightforward using radiography and scintigraphy, but ultrasonographic evaluation provides information about the suspensory attachment as well. One author (PJM) believes that shock wave therapy is a promising treatment modality for sesamoiditis.

Fractures of the PSBs are rare, and response to surgery is similar to that of other sports horses. Ponies with fractures of the base of the PSBs rarely return to athletic soundness with or without surgery. Polo ponies with basilar fractures and desmitis of the oblique sesamoidean ligament often can be helped by using shock wave therapy (PJM). An apical fracture of the PSB may be mistaken for mineralization of the suspensory branch. Polo ponies with apical fractures of the PSBs have a good prognosis, provided that SL injury is not concurrent. Horses with apical fractures associated with sesamoiditis and insertional suspensory branch desmitis often have recurrent lameness. It is important to differentiate true fractures from sesamoiditis or a commonly seen radiological abnormality in older polo ponies, one to three stress lines in the PSBs, which most often are considered incidental changes.

Digital Flexor Tenosynovitis and Desmitis of the Palmar Annular Ligament

Tenosynovitis of the digital flexor tendon sheath (DFTS) is common in polo ponies. Debate exists as to whether this syndrome is caused by desmitis of the PAL or whether the PAL is a passive structure causing only constriction of the inflamed DFTS. The terms *tenosynovitis* and *desmitis of the PAL* are sometimes used synonymously, but tenosynovitis with mild thickening of the PAL is more common than primary desmitis. A normal or slightly thickened PAL can restrict SDFT movement in horses with tendonitis, but this is a separate entity (see page 1153). In polo ponies, desmitis of the PAL can be solitary and diagnosed in horses with healthy digital flexor tendons. It can lead to tenosynovitis or can accompany tenosynovitis. Primary desmitis of the PAL occurs most frequently from interference injury, when a hind foot strikes a forelimb PAL, or from direct mallet trauma. Initial trauma may be minor, but continued trauma can lead to substantial injury (Figure 119-14). Whether primary or secondary, tenosynovitis with thickening and compartmentalization of the DFTS can occur proximal and distal to the PAL. Diagnosis can be made by combining the results of clinical examination and intrathecal analgesia. Ultrasonographic evaluation is crucial and should include dynamic studies in which the digital flexor tendons and DFTS are evaluated for possible adhesions between tendons, DFTS, and the PAL. Concomitant

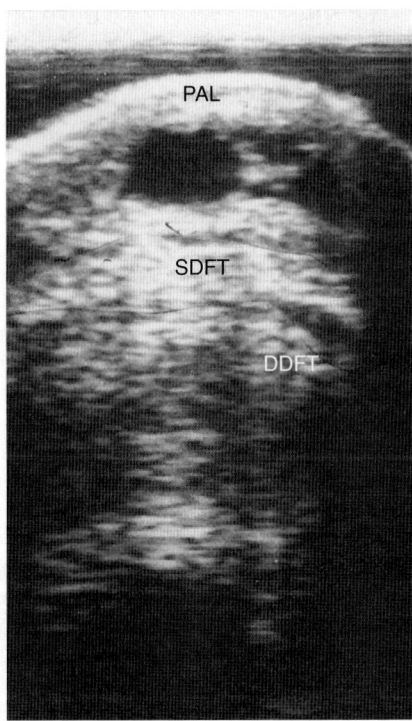

Fig. 119-14 • Transverse ultrasonographic image of the distal palmar metacarpal region. An acute injury caused by direct trauma resulted in a chronically thickened palmar annular ligament and huge anechogenic areas within it. *PAL,* Palmar annular ligament; *SDFT,* superficial digital flexor tendon; *DDFT,* deep digital flexor tendon.

conditions, such as OA of the fetlock joint, sesamoiditis, and demineralization of the PSBs at the medial and lateral attachments of the PAL, should be assessed radiologically. Initial management is to apply cold therapy and sweats and to administer NSAIDs. Decompression of the DFTS and injection of hyaluronan and corticosteriods then is followed by 3 weeks of stall rest. Tenoscopy is valuable in identifying horses with tendon tears and to perform adhesiolysis. Palmar annular desmotomy in horses with chronic desmitis or in those with chronic tenosynovitis may be helpful. Definitive therapy should be instituted early and aggressively to minimize adhesion formation.

Desmitis of the Distal Sesamoidean Ligaments

Desmitis of the distal sesamoidean ligaments (bowed pastern) is seen occasionally in polo ponies and usually involves the straight sesamoidean ligament. Diagnosis is made by detecting pain and swelling, performing perineural analgesia (palmar nerve blocks at the base of the PSBs), and using ultrasonographic examination.

Polo ponies with recurrent injury may not resent palpation, and ultrasonographic examination is necessary to differentiate this from other injuries. Proliferative changes along the base of the PSBs and abaxial surface of the proximal phalanx (at the insertion of the oblique sesamoidean ligaments) are often seen. These injuries may be career ending and at best are performance limiting. Long-term rest for 6 months is often necessary. Numerous applications of shock wave therapy have shown promise, and some owners request pin firing as a last resort.

Carpal Region Lameness

The carpus is an uncommon source of lameness in the polo pony. Preexisting chronic radiological changes are often incidental findings, even in horses with reduced range of carpal flexion and mild effusion. Carpal chip fractures can occur, but they are unusual. Tearing of the medial palmar intercarpal ligaments can cause lameness. Transient traumatic carpitis occasionally is seen after direct trauma from a mallet or ball. Rupture of the carpal sheath is a rare cause of lameness in the polo pony; one author (PJM) has seen two horses with massive swelling in the distal aspect of the antebrachium, and ultrasonographic evaluation revealed rupture of the carpal sheath. Prognosis is not known.

Fractures of the proximal aspect of the splint bones can lead to OA of the carpometacarpal joint. Fracture of the medial splint bone is most serious, but polo ponies usually respond well to conservative management.

Horizontal and vertical fracture of the accessory carpal bone may occur after collapse or a fall. Ponies are occasionally hit on the forehead by a hard-struck polo ball, rendering them unconscious and causing the hind hoof to hit the back of the carpal region. Fracture can also occur if a horse trips inadvertently on a loose polo wrap. Prognosis appears to be indirectly proportional to fracture displacement. Treatment is conservative. Physiotherapy, forcing full carpal flexion, is helpful to restore normal mobility (SK). Tenosynovitis of the carpal sheath can occur primarily or after fracture of the accessory carpal bone and in ponies with tendonitis of the SDFT and DDFT, as well as in horses with desmitis of the accessory ligament of the SDFT, but this condition is rare.

Desmitis of the Accessory Ligament of the Superficial Digital Flexor Tendon

In the United Kingdom, between 10 and 15 polo ponies each year are diagnosed with desmitis of the accessory ligament of the SDFT, which may occur because of the fast and aggressive play of modern polo (PJM). Awareness of the condition and use of ultrasonography may have resulted in increased recognition.

One high-goal player had five horses with this problem in a single year. Diagnosis is made by eliminating the distal aspect of the limb as a source of pain, by palpating pain and swelling in the distal aspect of the antebrachium and in the carpal sheath, and by ultrasonographic assessment. Conservative management is usually successful, including the periligamentous injection of hyaluronan and corticosteroids. Surgical resection of the accessory ligament of the SDFT may be indicated, particularly in polo ponies with considerable fibrosis and bony proliferation on the caudal distal aspect of the radius or in those that stand over at the knee.

Upper Forelimb Lameness

Lameness associated with the antebrachium, elbow, and shoulder regions is uncommon in polo ponies. Occasionally, fractures of the radius or olecranon and wounds with bony sequestration occur from kick trauma. Repair of fractures of the olecranon has been successful. Shoulder region soft tissue trauma, fracture of the supraglenoid tubercle of the scapula, and suprascapular nerve injury occur occasionally from falls, dangerous play, or wrecks.

Other Hindlimb Lameness

The distal aspect of the hindlimb is subject to the same type of bony injuries as seen in the forelimb, with the exception of navicular disease. Fractures of the distal and proximal phalanges and PSBs occur with the same frequency as in the forelimb, but prognosis is better in the hindlimb. In the hindlimb, OA of the fetlock joint, SDF tendonitis, suspensory desmitis, and desmitis of the ALDDFT are not nearly as common as in the forelimb.

Two soft tissue problems occur specifically in the hindlimbs. A form of severe suspensory desmitis occurs in older polo ponies with exceedingly straight hock conformation. The hind fetlock joint drops, and the pastern region is parallel to the ground. However, lameness is often minimal, and despite the abnormal angle of the fetlock joint, these horses can continue to play for years with the help of support wraps. The second specific soft tissue injury of the hindlimb is spontaneous rupture of the common digital extensor tendon above the fetlock joint. This injury results in lameness and hyperflexion of the fetlock joint at the trot. These horses respond well to conservative management, with support wraps and rest, and prognosis is excellent.

Lameness from stifle injuries is uncommon. Osteochondrosis occasionally causes effusion and lameness or poor performance if present bilaterally. Collateral ligament injury may occur from severe bumps. Kick wounds to the tibial crest can cause pronounced lameness and may result in a fracture. Polo ponies with a history of poor stopping or turning ability respond favorably to injection of counterirritants (blisters) around the patellar ligaments and the insertion of the vastus lateralis and rectus femoris muscles. Horses are kept in a working schedule following these injections and typically may be played successfully several days later.

Pelvic injury in polo ponies is infrequent but may result from dangerous play, such as a high-angle ride off behind the saddle (SK), and is best diagnosed using scintigraphy. Stress fractures of the ilium and traumatic fracture of the acetabulum occur but are rare. Disparity in height of the tubera sacrale often is seen, but with no effect on performance.

Rhabdomyolysis

Rhabdomyolysis, or tying up, is fairly common, especially in mares. Two types of horses are predisposed to this syndrome. Unfit horses placed into work too rapidly often develop a stiff gait at the trot and tenderness to palpation over the dorsal musculature. Muscle enzyme levels are only moderately elevated, and horses respond well to rest and NSAIDs. The most common form of rhabdomyolysis is seen in fit polo mares after an extended layup period for illness, unrelated lameness, or foul weather that prevents horses from being played regularly. Rhabdomyolysis can also occur on cold, clear mornings or blustery days during which a decrease in barometric pressure occurs. Horses generally become affected after exercise (when they return to the barn or trailer), are reluctant to move, and have firm, tight gluteal regions. Epaxial muscles rarely are involved. Clinical signs may be confused with colic because horses with rhabdomyolysis often paw, stretch out, and sweat profusely. Muscle enzyme levels are elevated greatly. Management is similar to that described for other sports horses (see Chapter 83). Nutritional management appears to be important in Europe, where bran, which is high in phosphorus (reduces calcium), is fed to reduce recurrence.

Gracilis Muscle Tear

Gracilis muscle tears are seen in several polo ponies each year and are characterized by lameness at the trot and dramatic swelling in the medial thigh region. Abduction of the flexed hindlimb elicits a painful response, and a large hematoma generally develops soon after the injury. The administration of NSAIDs and DMSO intravenously, and the topical application of cold water are beneficial. If necessary, seroma fluid can be drained surgically 5 to 7 days after injury, and exercise is limited for a minimum of 2 weeks.

Equine Protozoal Myelitis

Mild neurological signs typical of equine protozoal myelitis (EPM) or lameness associated with the disease can be confused with other causes of musculoskeletal pain, in particular hindlimb lameness. EPM is prevalent in the United States but is rare in England (PJM). Occasionally, a polo pony in the United Kingdom that was imported from the United States develops clinical signs consistent with EPM under the stress of the latter half of the season.

Chapter 120

The Western Performance Horse

■ THE CUTTING HORSE

Jerry B. Black and Robin M. Dabareiner

DESCRIPTION AND HISTORY OF THE SPORT

The cutting horse was born of necessity long ago on the open grass plains of West Texas. This was the era of Western history that included big cattle drives from the open ranges of ranches such as Burnett and the 6666 Ranch, Waggoner Ranch, the Pitchfork Ranch, and the Matador Ranch to Dodge City, Kansas. Cutting horses enabled big country ranches, where no barbed-wire fences existed, the only means of working vast herds of cattle. In those days the task of the horse was simple, at least by definition. Guided by the rider, the cutting horse entered a herd of cattle quietly and deliberately. A single cow was cut, or separated, from the herd. The natural instinct of the cow is to return to the safety of the rest of the herd. The cutting horse, through breeding and training, controlled the cow with a series of moves and countermoves. The speed, agility, balance, and quickness of the cutting horse kept the cow from the herd, where other cowboys would hold the cut. The horse and rider would reenter the herd again and again, cutting cattle out until the work was done. Only the top hands earned the right to ride the best horses of the remuda (herd), the cutting horses.

The unique skills of the cutting horse were a great source of pride to the frontier cowboy. This often led to impromptu or jackpot cuttings on the open range or, from about 1900, in outdoor pens of the large ranches. From this love of the cutting horse, as well as the subsequent competition to determine who had the best horse, came the roots of cutting as we know it today. The first cutting horse contest for money was held at the 1898 Cowboy Reunion in Haskell, Texas. Twelve cutting horses competed for a purse of $150. From this start, regular events occurred on ranches of the Southwest and at the Fort Worth Stockyards. Rules and prizes varied greatly, but the ability of the cutting horse to separate a single cow from the herd always was and continues to be the goal of the competition. From these roots the National Cutting Horse Association was formed in 1946 during the Fort Worth Exposition and Fat Stock Show. The stated purpose of the organization was to standardize the rules and judging of competition and to preserve the tradition and history of the cutting horse with the ranching and livestock industry.

Today competitions approved by the National Cutting Horse Association occur throughout the United States and Canada. In addition, many association members from other countries, such as Australia, are conducting competitions outside North America. The format of these competitions and other Western performance horse disciplines, such as reining, presents a unique challenge to the equine veterinarian.

TRAINING

Training of the cutting horse begins at 2 years of age. Usually 60 to 90 days are spent in basic training before the horse is introduced to cattle. This generally is accomplished by turning one cow into a round pen that is 38 to 54 m in diameter. The horse is taught to mirror the movements of the cow as the cow moves around the perimeter of the arena. This process of training a cutting horse is repetitive and is done several days a week for months. The object of training is for the horse to develop an ability to perform identical movements with the cow. Simply put, when the cow stops or stops and turns, the horse does the same maneuver. This type of training is accomplished by asking the horse to stop with the aid of a bridle and turning the horse to move with the cow. The key to training is a complete and balanced stop. With time, a stop ultimately is followed by the instinctive ability of the horse to "read" the movement of the cow and to turn in the direction the cow is going. Because this ability to watch a cow and respond to its movement is instinctive to the working stock horse, breeding is of the utmost importance. Without this genetic instinct a horse simply does not respond to the movement of a cow and does not initiate a stop or turn as necessary to continue to track the cow. A good cutting horse trainer knows in a relatively short period if a young horse has the instinct and athletic ability to be a successful cutting horse. A finished cutting horse must perform the necessary moves to keep a cow in proper position away from the herd, without any hand cues from the rider, relying on instinct alone to read the movement of the cow. Reining the horse is permitted only to make the cut of a single cow out of the herd. After the cut is successfully made, the reins are placed in a relaxed position on the horse's neck, and only leg cues are permitted from the rider during the actual working time. The ability of a horse to contain an individual cow provides the excitement of competition in cutting.

Training of a cutting horse prospect that has shown good potential continues when it is a 3-year-old, preparing it for the first major competitions, the futurities. The futurity is the first of the horse's aged event competitions that continue for 4 years. No horse can compete in aged events beyond 6 years of age. Aged events consist of two elimination go-rounds, followed by the semifinal and the final competition. Substantial musculoskeletal stress is placed on these athletic performance horses, with multiday competitions over a short period. In addition, the horses usually are practiced with cattle daily, including the day of competition, to sharpen performance skills. Competition in these aged events is heavy, with the major shows having more than 500 entries in a single age division. Purses in this type of event can exceed a total of $1 million. The nature of this aged event competition, with large purses in numerous events over a 4-year period, has caused the cutting horse economy to grow rapidly during the past several years. Select yearling and training sales are conducted annually that are beginning to parallel the racing industry in financial return on sales. This has contributed to the current popularity and resurgence of breeding of cutting and Western stock horses, which in turn will ensure the preservation of the tradition and heritage that this horse played in the history of the great Old West.

LAMENESS EXAMINATION

The increasing popularity of the cutting and reining horse for show and performance is occurring nationally and internationally. Sales of this type of horse have increased to Europe, South America, and other countries. In North America, the revival of interest stems primarily from excellent programs instituted by associations such as the National Cutting Horse Association and the National Reining Horse Association. These associations encourage owner participation at an amateur level in cutting and reining events. This type of performance horse creates a new diagnostic and treatment challenge for attending veterinarians, partially because of the rigid training schedules necessary for 3- to 6-year-old horses to compete in futurities and aged events.

Hindlimb lameness presents one of the more interesting diagnostic challenges to an equine clinician. The lameness is often difficult to diagnose and even more difficult to manage. A systematic approach must be developed to achieve an accurate diagnosis consistently. The veterinarian must use a routine that is repeated with each horse and must allow sufficient time to complete a thorough examination. Western stock horses may be difficult to evaluate while being led. These horses usually are not taught to lunge and are often difficult to trot in hand. A 10- to 15-m round pen with firm footing has proved to be beneficial for evaluating lameness.

DIAGNOSIS AND MANAGEMENT OF SPECIFIC LAMENESS

Hindlimb lameness is more common than forelimb lameness in cutting horses. Mixed lameness with swinging and supporting components is common in hindlimbs, especially in upper limb lamenesses such as those involving the hock, stifle, and hip or sacroiliac region. Hindlimb lameness may be associated with two sources of pain: for example, chronic hock lameness and secondary lumbar and gluteal myositis. This section focuses on selected hindlimb lamenesses of the hock, stifle, and thoracolumbar regions.

Selected Lameness of the Tarsus

Osteoarthritis of the Distal Tarsal Joints (Distal Hock Joint Pain)
Osteoarthritis (OA) of the distal tarsal joints is seen most commonly in horses that have repeated, excessive compression and rotation of the hocks at high speed, and a high incidence occurs in young working cow horses and in cutting and reining futurity prospects, reflecting the demanding training schedules of 5 to 6 days a week at 2 and 3 years of age. Sickle hocks, cow hocks, and narrow hocks also may predispose horses to lameness. OA also may develop secondary to partial collapse of the central and third tarsal bones, and affected horses often develop

lameness within the first year after birth. In one author's practice (JBB), routine survey radiology of the tarsus in 20, 2-year-old cutting horse prospects before training began revealed evidence of OA in 11 (55%).

Clinical signs include reduced height of the foot flight arc, resulting in abnormal toe wear, and a shortened cranial phase of stride. Hard work increases the degree of lameness, although most horses are lame and stiff when first taken out of the box stall and improve to some degree during the initial warm-up. Trotting in a circle increases the degree of lameness. Gait alteration or lameness may be observed with the affected limb on the inside or outside of a circle. Cutting, reining, and stock horses are reluctant to stop properly. Upper limb flexion often increases the degree of lameness. Palpation of the distal medial aspect of the hock may reveal an exostosis and soft tissue thickening. Deep palpation of the area can cause a painful withdrawal response. Thoracolumbar pain is present in about 50% of horses.

Diagnosis is based on a positive response to intraarticular analgesia and radiology. Radiological abnormalities are often only seen in a dorsolateral-plantaromedial image in 2- to 4-year-old cutting horses, findings that differ from those seen in other young sports horses.

Therapy varies depending on the degree of lameness. Rest is generally not helpful in horses with advanced OA, and obtaining trainer compliance if the lameness is subtle is difficult. Training usually is continued with the help of nonsteroidal antiinflammatory drugs (NSAIDs), such as phenylbutazone (2 g daily or 1.5 g twice daily) and intraarticularly administered antiinflammatory drugs. Shoeing changes include removing excessive toe, squaring the toe of the shoe, and extending both branches of the shoe for more heel support. Half-round shoes help aid breakover in some horses with cow-hocked or sickle-hocked conformation. Changes in training schedules include more paddock or free-choice exercise and longer warm-up periods before training. Training in deep surfaces, overtraining, or conditioning in circles should be avoided. Varying the gait frequently during training and conditioning helps the horse to stay more comfortable.

Intraarticular medication is used to keep chronically lame horses in competition. A combination of methylprednisolone acetate (40 mg) and hyaluronan (10 to 20 mg) is injected separately into the centrodistal (distal intertarsal) and tarsometatarsal joints in horses with advanced OA. The veterinarian should not rely on communication between the two joints. If good results are achieved, these injections are repeated as necessary every 12 to 16 weeks. Horses with early OA respond favorably to intraarticular treatment with hyaluronan (20 mg of Hylartin-V, Pfizer Inc., New York, New York, United States) and triamcinolone acetonide (3 to 6 mg). Intravenous injections of hyaluronan (Legend [Bayer HealthCare LLC, Animal Health Division, Shawnee Mission, Kansas, United States]; 40 mg in 7-day intervals, series of three) or intramuscular injections of polysulfated glycosaminoglycan (PSGAG; 500 mg of Adequan [Luitpold Animal Health, Shirley, New York, United States] intramuscularly [IM] in 5-day intervals, series of four to eight) are used frequently as concurrent therapy. Combinations of intermediate-acting corticosteroids and hyaluronan administered intraarticularly have been used in horses that are lame immediately before leaving for circuit shows or important multiday competitions, such as cutting horse, snaffle bit, and reining horse futurities.

Therapeutic levels of NSAIDs may be necessary during competition if allowed by the breed, performance, or state drug regulations governing the event. Phenylbutazone (2 g daily or 1.5 g twice daily) is usually effective. However, many stock horse trainers believe that this drug tends to dull the mouth and sides of the horse, thus limiting bit and spur response. Other NSAIDs that are effective include flunixin meglumine (Banamine [Intervet/Schering-Plough Animal Health, Roseland, New Jersey, United States]; 1 mg/kg daily) or ketoprofen (Ketofen [Pfizer Inc.]; 2 mg/kg daily). Horses vary in response to the therapeutic effects of each NSAID. If one drug is not effective, a different one should be assessed. Tiludronate and interleukin-1 receptor antagonist protein (IRAP) have recently been introduced, but long-term follow-up results are not known. Tiludronate is administered as a single intravenous infusion. IRAP is injected three to five times at 1- to 2-week intervals. Focused extracorporeal shock wave therapy is used in horses refractory to intraarticular medication.

Surgery has been an important adjunct to OA therapy in horses requiring repeated intraarticular injections or continual therapy with NSAIDs. Horses with mild to moderate radiological changes but normal joint spaces respond favorably to cunean tenectomy. Horses with substantial intraarticular changes and joint space collapse are treated best surgically with a combination of cunean tenectomy and arthrodesis (fenestration) of the affected joint or joints using a 3.2-mm drill bit and creating three to four tracts. The horse is returned to work as soon as possible after surgery to encourage ankylosis. Handwalking is begun the day after surgery, and light riding at a walk may begin 2 to 3 weeks later. Light riding exercise continues for another 3 weeks, and full training begins 45 to 60 days postoperatively if the horse is reasonably comfortable. Phenylbutazone, 2 g once daily as needed, is used initially if obvious lameness persists. Most horses show almost immediate improvement after surgery. This improvement may be caused partially by the release of intraosseous pressure after the fenestration procedure, plus cessation of the rotational effect of the cunean tendon on the distal aspect of the tarsus. Radiological evidence of ankylosis occurs over a prolonged period, even up to 1 year postsurgery. Soundness does not seem to be related to radiological evidence of ankylosis.

Prognosis varies depending on the degree of OA, the number of joints involved, and the type of competition in which the horse is engaged. Surgery offers the best prognosis for horses with chronic lameness. It is possible that chemical fusion with ethyl alcohol may offer a shorter convalescent time.

Arthrosis of the Tarsocrural Joint
Distention of the tarsocrural joint capsule is usually the result of osteochondrosis or trauma. Osteochondrosis lesions occur on the cranial aspect of the intermediate ridge of the tibia, the trochlear ridges of the talus, and the lateral or medial malleoli of the tibia. Trauma is related to quick turns, hard stops, loss of balance, and poor footing. Faulty conformation, such as overly straight angulation of hock and stifle joints, may be a predisposing factor.

Distention of the tarsocrural joint capsule is observed most easily on the dorsomedial aspect of the hock, but swelling also occurs in the plantar pouches, laterally or medially. The horse may have pain on palpation. A proximal limb (hock) flexion test may or may not be positive, depending on the degree of joint capsule distention and synovitis. Radiographic examination is essential to determine the cause and should be repeated after 10 to 14 days if initial radiographs are normal.

Horses with osteochondrosis are treated surgically. Horses with traumatic distention of the tarsocrural joint are treated by intraarticular injection of intermediate-acting corticosteroids and hyaluronan, two or three times, 14 to 21 days apart. Intraarticular injections often are followed by hyaluronan (40 mg) administered intravenously weekly for 3 weeks. All injected hocks are bandaged concurrently to help reduce joint effusion. Pressage elastic contour bandages (Jupiter Veterinary Products, Harrisburg, Pennsylvania, United States) provide adequate pressure and are easy to maintain. The horse is given rest for 3 to 6 weeks.

Exploratory or diagnostic arthroscopy is justified in any horse that does not respond to conservative therapy, permitting identification of subtle osteochondrosis lesions not detectable radiologically and soft tissue injuries, as well as providing joint lavage.

The prognosis is good if treatment is initiated early and if all fragments and debris are removed soon after the synovitis is recognized in horses with osteochondrosis lesions or severe trauma. If conformation is the predisposing cause, the prognosis is poor.

Selected Lameness of the Stifle
The stifle is a large, complex joint composed of two articulations: the femorotibial and femoropatellar joints. One author's experience (JBB) has been that during arthroscopy of the femorotibial joint, despite high intraarticular fluid pressure, obvious distention of the femoropatellar joint capsule does not occur. Thus little or no distention of the femoropatellar joint capsule occurs in association with disease of the femorotibial joint. When performing intraarticular analgesia of the stifle, all three compartments should be injected separately.

Osteochondrosis
Osteochondrosis of the trochlear ridges of the femur is seen commonly in young horses. Clinical signs include distention of the femoropatellar joint capsule and varying degrees of lameness, depending on the amount of joint surface involved. Diagnosis is confirmed radiologically. Arthroscopic surgery is the treatment of choice to debride all diseased cartilage and bone and to remove all free-floating bone and cartilage. Aftercare consists of 45 to 60 days of stall rest, followed by an equal amount of stall and paddock confinement. Training generally resumes 3 to 6 months postoperatively. Intraarticularly administered hyaluronan (20 mg) followed by intramuscularly administered PSGAGs (500 mg in 5-day intervals, series of four to eight) 2 to 3 weeks after surgery has helped to reduce postoperative synovitis.

Subchondral Bone Cysts
Subchondral bone cysts of the medial condyle of the femur are the most frequently recognized bony lesions of the stifle

in one author's (JBB) practice. Affected horses are lame at the walk or trot in one or both hindlimbs. The degree of lameness varies greatly among horses. Some horses are subtly lame, requiring riding or repeated flexion to produce a recognizable lameness. Others have acute, severe lameness and are unwilling to trot. Moderately lame horses tend to swing the toe medially during protraction. This contrasts with horses with painful conditions of the femoropatellar joint or patellar ligaments, with which the horse often carries the stifle out or abducts the limb. Lameness may be more obvious with the affected limb on the inside of a circle.

Subtle distention of the femorotibial joint capsule may be palpated between the medial patellar and medial collateral ligaments. Some horses resent deep digital pressure over the medial femoral condylar region.

Diagnosis of subchondral bone cysts is based on clinical signs and response to intraarticular analgesia using 30 mL of mepivacaine and radiology. Conservative treatment for the most part yields only temporary improvement in the lameness and is used only when a performance horse needs to compete for the remainder of the season or when finances prohibit surgical intervention. Conservative treatment consists of intraarticular injections of hyaluronan, with or without corticosteroids such as betamethasone or triamcinolone acetonide. Intramuscularly administered PSGAGs, given in a series of four to eight injections at 5-day intervals, are also used. Many trainers report a pronounced effect about 24 hours after administration of PSGAGs. Therapeutic levels of systemic NSAIDs may be also necessary during multiday competitions. Owners should be informed that continued training and competition over an extended period might lead to secondary OA.

There are several treatment options, but the treatment of choice in our experience is curettage and fenestration of the subchondral bone cyst. Before 1988, this procedure was done through an arthrotomy incision. Although the surgery was successful in most horses, wound dehiscence and prolonged hospitalization were of great concern. Currently the surgery is performed by arthroscopy, with the horse placed in dorsal recumbency and the limb in flexion. This position provides adequate visibility and good access to the cystic lesion via an instrument portal. Postoperative hospitalization is minimal, and to date no postoperative complications have been seen. The horse is confined for 60 days after surgery. Handwalking for 10 minutes daily is allowed during confinement. Free-choice exercise for an additional 2 to 4 months is allowed. Training usually resumes 6 months postoperatively or earlier, if the horse is sound. Surgical success is about 50% to 60%. Most of these horses return to a competitive level of performance, if given adequate rest. Recently arthroscopic injection of corticosteroids into the fibrous tissue of subchondral cystic lesions has been described.[1] A retrospective study examined 52 horses with subchondral cystic lesions in the medial femoral condyle that were injected with arthroscopic guidance with a reported success rate of 77%. Preexisting osteophytes had a negative impact on outcome. This seems like a viable first option for treatment, and if unsuccessful then surgical debridement and fenestration can be performed.

References on page 1345

Upward Fixation of the Patella

Partial or complete upward fixation of the patella is a common cause of stifle pain, which can eventually produce articular changes of the patella. Upward fixation of the patella can occur in any type of body conformation and hindlimb angulation and may be related to the anatomical formation and depth of the notch on the proximal aspect of the medial trochlea of the distal aspect of the femur. Lack of condition and loss of condition are contributory factors. Poor coordination between extensor and flexor groups of the stifle and lack of quadriceps development may explain why upward fixation is seen in young horses at the beginning of training. One of us (JBB) examined two horses in which upward fixation of the patella was secondary to a subchondral bone cyst in the medial femoral condyle. Upward fixation may have been caused by alteration of gait and foot placement because of pain in the medial femorotibial joint. Upward fixation resolved after arthroscopic treatment of the subchondral bone cyst. The duration of locking varies from an almost instantaneous release, with only slight backward jerk evident, to a complete locking that can last for hours and may require surgical release.

Diagnosis is based on clinical signs. Often, although no obvious upward fixation occurs in extension, the limb snaps with an audible click while in an extended position. Occasionally, pushing the patella over the top of the trochlear ridge when the limb is in extension can produce the locking. Clinical signs often are exacerbated if the horse is walked down a steep slope. The diagnosis is sometimes based almost entirely on the owner's or trainer's description of the condition.

Treatment should remain conservative when possible. If complete upward fixation has occurred for any period, the femoropatellar joint usually has effusion. Treatment should be aimed initially toward reducing inflammation and resting the tissues involved. The usual treatment schedule includes administration of systemic corticosteroids (20 mg of dexamethasone [Azium, Intervet/Schering-Plough Animal Health] IM daily) for 1 to 3 days, followed by 3 to 5 days of NSAIDs (2 g of phenylbutazone twice daily). Handwalking for 5 to 10 minutes is allowed if no further upward fixation occurs, but no free-choice exercise is allowed. Excessive toe is removed, and wedged shoes or wedge pad and flat shoes are used if the heel is low. Half-round shoes allow the horse to break over in its most comfortable and natural position.

Once the initial inflammation has subsided, a conditioning program is started. Long warm-up periods are essential. Thirty minutes of walking and trotting, followed by an increasing amount of extended trotting on the straightaway are recommended. Once the horse becomes conditioned, trotting in the hills is prescribed, where possible. The concept of conditioning is to improve quadriceps development and tone and to improve overall coordination. Horses that are underweight should be fed to gain weight and to improve the overall body condition and the condition of the muscles involved in movement of the stifle.

Horses that do not respond to conservative treatment may require an internal blister, medial patellar desmotomy, or medial patellar desmoplasty. Internal blister is accomplished by local infiltration of 2% iodine in peanut or almond oil injected directly into the body of the medial patellar ligament. Care must be taken to avoid the accidental penetration and injection of the femoropatellar joint with the counterirritant solution. If this is unsuccessful, splitting the medial patellar ligament is a viable option. This can be performed in either a standing sedated horse or under intravenous anesthesia. The area over the medial patellar ligament is clipped and scrubbed, and a number 15-scalpel blade or 14-gauge needle is inserted at 1-cm intervals and used to scarify the ligament perpendicular to the longitudinal axis of the limb. The thought is that by creating inflammation and scar tissue, the ligament will tighten, thereby preventing upward fixation of the patella. This treatment has been very successful in one of our hands (RMD). Medial patellar desmotomy should be reserved as a last form of therapy because the postoperative complications include fragmentation of the distal aspect of the patella, soft tissue fibrosis, and mechanical alteration of gait.

Femorotibial Joint Pain

Subtle soft tissue injuries may occur in the femorotibial joint, resulting in low-grade lameness that is most evident when the horse trots in circles. Such injuries often occur as training is increased. A typical example is a young cutting horse that is being worked hard on cattle before a futurity. The horse has a shortened cranial phase of stride and lowered foot flight, causing toe drag. Results of hindlimb flexion tests are generally negative. Mild distention of the medial femorotibial joint capsule may be palpable. Diagnosis is based on clinical signs, response to intraarticular analgesia of the femorotibial joint, and the absence of radiological abnormalities.

Treatment comprises intraarticular medication with hyaluronan and corticosteroids such as triamcinolone acetonide (6 mg), plus intramuscularly administered PSGAGs. Systemic NSAIDs are given in decreasing doses over 10 to 14 days. All trailers and calks are removed from shoes. A wedge pad may be added with an egg bar shoe or extended branch shoe, depending on the amount of heel support needed.

Training is resumed after 14 to 21 days of rest. Long warm-up periods and extended straightaway trotting are recommended to condition the muscles of the upper hindlimb.

Prognosis is good if a consistent training schedule is maintained. Horses with irregular training schedules and frequent periods of several days off between exercise sessions tend to have recurrent problems.

Thoracolumbar Injuries

Thoracolumbar Myositis

Soft tissue injuries of the thoracolumbar region produce back soreness and are common injuries in a working stock horse. Thoracolumbar myositis may coexist with hindlimb lameness, such as distal hock OA, or may be a primary traumatic lesion, frequently caused by the extraordinary forces of rotation and propulsion placed on the hindlimbs. Other factors include rigid training and competition schedules such as the fall futurities for 3-year-olds that result in an overworked young horse.

Local myositis involving the muscles of the thoracolumbar and pelvic region can have a profound effect on the performance of a stock horse. A cutting horse has three basic components to work: the stop, turn, and ability to track a cow in mirror image across the arena at high speed. Localized back pain results in decreased performance in all of these, without obvious lameness. The trainer perceives that the horse is simply not trying. Consequently, a horse with back pain is forced to try even harder and soon falls into the overworked category.

Clinical signs of thoracolumbar myositis include pain to palpation of the affected muscle groups and associated spinous processes, obvious discomfort during saddling or mounting, subtle bilateral or unilateral hindlimb lameness, unwillingness to stop in form, and overall lack of performance. Flexion tests are seldom positive, unless the back problem coexists with distal hock joint pain. One may reasonably believe that arthrosis of vertebral articulations in the lumbar and lumbosacral region exists in some horses. However, because of the depth and mass of the muscles involved, distinguishing the exact pathological condition or even the exact site of the injury is impossible.

Therapy is aimed at reducing inflammation and controlling the associated muscle pain and spasms. Prolonged rest periods from training always are indicated but in reality are difficult to achieve because of the rigid schedule of preparation for competition. For example, an average futurity horse being prepared for the National Cutting Horse Association futurity in December of its 3-year-old year accumulates a $20,000 to $24,000 debt in training and entry fees alone before competition. Convincing an owner and trainer that a horse should be allowed to rest immediately before the futurity is difficult, if appropriate therapy has even a remote chance of being effective.

The systemic use of skeletal muscle relaxants such as methocarbamol (10 mg/kg orally [PO] twice daily for 5 to 10 days) has been effective in treating cutting horses with generalized back pain. Dexamethasone (10 mg PO twice daily for 3 to 4 days) is indicated in horses with acute pain. Horses with chronic back pain may be treated successfully during competition with a single dose of triamcinolone acetonide (12 to 16 mg IM) and methocarbamol administered orally. NSAIDs generally have not been effective unless the back pain is secondary or coexists with distal hock joint pain. Care must be taken to comply with any medication rules.

Specific localized pain may be treated successfully by local injection of methylprednisolone acetate (200 to 400 mg) and Sarapin (50 mL; High Chemical Company, Levittown, Pennsylvania, United States). Treatment is repeated every 10 to 14 days until pain subsides.

Other management considerations are important for recovery. Horses with low, underslung heels of the hind feet should be shod using raised heels. Evaluation of the fit of the saddle, type of pad, and specific pressure points when ridden should be considered. Other modalities of therapy, such as pulsed electromagnetic field and therapeutic ultrasound, have been useful in keeping a horse in competition. Long warm-up periods without the rider for 30 to 45 minutes by ponying (leading from another horse) at a walk and trot always are indicated. The trainer must be cautioned that overwork and severe fatigue must be avoided at all times.

Sacroiliac Region Pain

Strain and subluxation of the sacroiliac joint are not uncommon in working stock horses because of twisting and rotation of the back and pelvis during work. This rotation is complicated by the weight of tack and the rider, who is attempting to maintain balance and remain stationary on top of the horse during sudden hard stops, turns, and bursts of speed.

Many of the clinical signs observed in horses with thoracolumbar myositis are also common in those with sacroiliac region pain because the epaxial muscles go into spasm to provide stability to the traumatized sacroiliac joint. However, bilateral or unilateral lameness with stiffness and alteration of gait usually are associated with sacroiliac region pain. Protrusion of the tubera sacrale may be evident when the horse is walking away from the observer. Flexion of the contralateral limb for 2 minutes may result in elevation of the tuber sacrale, hip hike, and stiffness of the affected limb. Digital palpation adjacent to the tuber sacrale and over the gluteal regions usually elicits pain. Local infiltration of local anesthetic solution may result in improvement, but rarely are clinical signs fully alleviated.

Deep intramuscular injections of methylprednisolone acetate (400 mg) and Sarapin (50 mL) into the region of the sacroiliac joint have been effective in treatment. Disposable needles at least 10 cm long are necessary to reach the affected area. Strict aseptic technique must be followed. Injections usually are repeated after 2 to 3 weeks. Concurrent systemic therapy with NSAIDs is beneficial. Horses must have rest, and 2 to 6 months out of training is often necessary, with strict stall confinement for the first 30 to 45 days.

Proper therapy and management of injuries to the thoracolumbar and sacroiliac regions generally are rewarding if initiated early in the course of the disease. Horses with chronic recurrent problems usually can be managed to allow some level of competition.

Forelimb Lameness in the Cutting Horse
Forelimb lameness in the cutting horse is similar to that described in the roping horse (see the following section).

◼ THE ROPING HORSE
Robin M. Dabareiner

TEAM ROPING HORSE
Description of the Sport
A unique handicapping system implemented in the early 1990s has contributed to team roping becoming a rapidly growing equestrian sport. Team roping began as a rodeo event many years ago, evolving from the everyday work of cowboys on ranches. If a cow needed to be treated on the open range, the only method of restraint was to secure the head and heel of the animal, or to team rope it. The cowboys soon began wagering among themselves to see which team of a header and heeler could accomplish this feat in the shortest time. Currently nearly 1 million people compete in team roping competitions in North America.

Because of the large number of participants, team roping has become of great economic importance. Many team roping organizations exist nationally, but the most prestigious is the United States Team Roping Championships. The numbering or handicapping system of the team ropers was begun by the United States Team Roping

Championships and has become standard. A number, from 1 to 9, with 9 being the highest level of ability, is assigned to each of the team ropers. This number is based on various factors, including ability, previous prize earnings, experience, age, and physical handicaps.

The roping categories also are assigned a numerical value that cannot be exceeded by the total handicap numbers of the two participating ropers. The highest level of roping is the open roping, which is open to any roper but usually is entered by professional ropers (numbered 9), allowing the world champions to compete together. The lowest number is a true beginner, who would be a number 1 or 2. This handicap system allows the lower-level ropers to compete as a team with the world champions and to level the playing field of competition at all levels. The entry fees of the participants usually generate the purse money in a jackpot fashion. A portion of the entry fee is held out by the producer of the roping to pay for the arena, the cattle, and advertising, and the rest of the fee is placed in the purse money to be divided among the winners.

Dally team roping is a timed event involving five basic elements: the header, the heading horse, the heeler, the heeling horse, and the steer. The steers that are used for the team roping event are usually horned cattle called Corriente cattle, often from Mexico. Other types of cattle used are longhorns or other native homed breeds ranging in weight from 170 to 320 kg.

A typical run in dally team roping begins with a steer contained in a chute at the end of an arena. The heading box is to the left of the chute, and the heeling box is to the right of the chute. When the header calls for the steer, or asks that the steer be released from the chute, the chute gate is opened and the steer is allowed a head start called the score. If the header leaves the heading box before the steer crosses the score line, or reaches the predetermined head start, then the team is issued a penalty of 10 seconds. The timing of the run is begun when the steer crosses the score line.

When cued by the riders, the horses leave the roping box much as a racehorse leaves the starting gate to attain maximum speed as quickly as possible. As the header approaches the steer with the heading horse running at full speed, the horse is trained to rate off, or to slow up slightly, once the horse reaches the hip of the steer, to position the steer properly so that the header may rope the steer. Team roping has three legal head catches: both horns (a clean horn catch), a half head (one horn and the nose of the steer), or a neck. All other catches are considered illegal, and the team is given a no time.

After the header successfully catches the head of the steer and dallies (wraps in a full circle) the rope around the saddle horn, the heading horse drops its hindquarters and slows somewhat as it sets the steer and brings the steer's head around to the left. As the steer's body progresses to the left, the heading horse also is turned to the left and is moved out in front of the steer to allow the header to pull it across the arena at about a 90-degree angle to the original direction of travel, maintaining a constant slower speed, thus allowing the heeler to get into position to rope the hindlegs of the steer.

As the header sets and turns the steer, the heeler turns left following the steer and positions just behind and slightly to the left of the steer as it is taken across the arena.

As the heeling horse follows the steer in this position, maintaining a constant speed equal to that of the header and steer, the heeler properly times his swing and then releases the heel rope, placing the loop under the steer and ropes the hindlegs of the steer. If only one hindleg is caught, then the team is issued a 5-second penalty. As the slack is taken out of the heel loop and as the dally is made on the saddle horn, the heeling horse is signaled to drop its hindquarters and come to an abrupt stop.

As the heading horse progresses away from the heeler with the steer still in tow, the ropes come tight, and when tight, the heading horse is cued to spin around to the right while maintaining a tight rope to face the steer. When the facing is complete, the rope is tight and in a straight line from the saddle horn of the header to the head of the steer and is tight from the hind feet of the steer to the saddle horn of the heeler, and then the flagman signals the end of the run and the time is taken.

The roping can be accomplished by experts in 6 to 7 seconds but requires thousands of hours of practice to achieve this and to minimize the danger to all the participants. Runs recorded in the range of 3.4 to 3.6 seconds have been made by the World Champion–caliber team ropers.

Conformation

The horses, predominately geldings, used in team roping are usually American Quarter Horses (QHs), preferred because of exceptional athletic ability, quick acceleration over short distances, and a good mind. Other breeds are rarely used. The head horse must be larger and faster than the heel horse. Head horses typically weigh 545 to 590 kg and are heavily muscled to tow the steer across the arena. The heel horse is smaller and quicker with more cow sense than the head horse. Horses that are trained for cutting but no longer are competing often make good heel horses because of size and cow sense. Team ropers prefer a mature,

experienced horse, and so horses are usually over the age of 10 years, and many top ropers have horses in the mid to late teens. Therefore repetitive injuries are common, but because horses often have had several owners, a complete medical history is rarely available. In a recent retrospective study looking at lameness and poor performance in horses used solely for team roping, horses used for heading were significantly heavier (median weight, 545 kg; range, 473 to 603 kg) and older (median age, 12 years) than heeling horses (median weight, 490 kg; range, 441 to 545 kg; median age, 9.5 years).[1]

Training

The training of heading and heeling horses involves thousands of team roping runs and many thousands of miles of hauling. The horse must anticipate every variable of a team roping run, so that rider intervention is unnecessary. This allows the roper to focus on nothing but the speed of the run, which is an important factor contributing to injury. The current high demand for a finished team roping horse has greatly increased the value of these horses, and because replacement is difficult, veterinary advice is now sought more often.

Historical Data and Decreased Performance

It is imperative for a clinician to know whether a team roping horse is used primarily as a heading or heeling horse. In addition, a thorough description of the owner's complaint of a change in or decreased performance provides valuable insight into the underlying problem, bearing in mind that often in the early stages little or no lameness may be present. Eighty-nine of 118 (75%) team roping horses had a history of lameness, and 29 (25%) had an owner complaint of decreased or altered performance.[1] The type of performance change differed between horses used for heading or heeling (Figures 120-1 and 120-2).

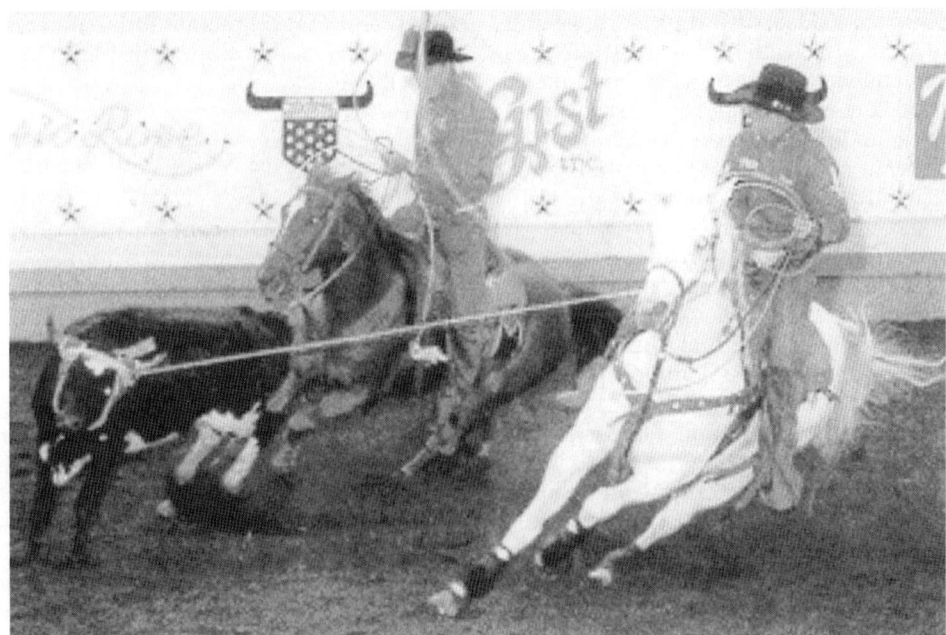

Fig. 120-1 • A header roping the steer and making a 90-degree turn to set the steer for the heeler. The weight of horse and rider results in excessive loading of the right forelimb of the head horse (gray horse).

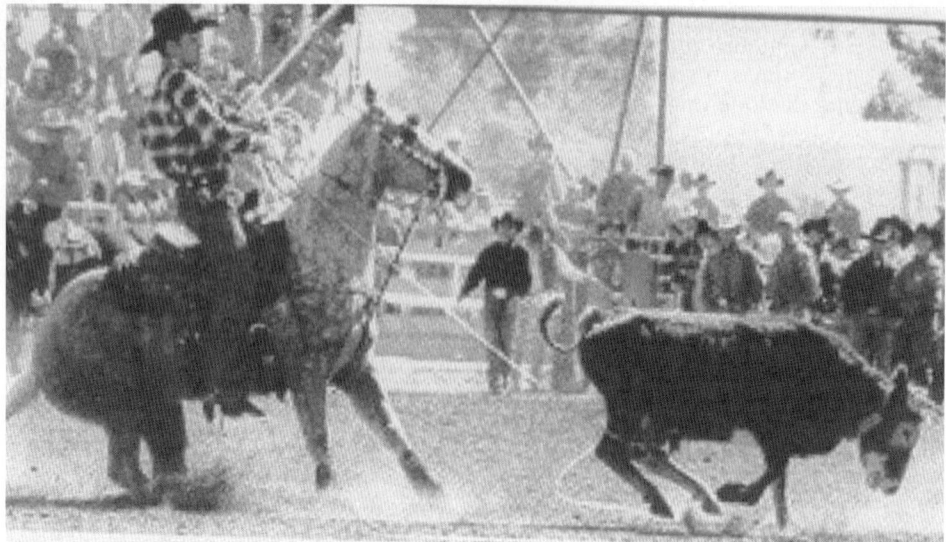

Fig. 120-2 • A heel horse stopping after the heeler throws his rope. Note the flexion of the hock joints during the stop and the extreme forward placement of both hindlimbs.

Lameness Examination

Team roping horses experience many of the same problems as any of the Western performance horses. In the heading horse, the right forelimb is placed under tremendous force after the steer is roped and just before turning 90 degrees. The right forelimb is placed cranially and laterally to decelerate and brace against its forward motion and the weight of the steer, thus placing tremendous strain on this limb (see Figure 120-1). A study reported that horses used for heading had significantly more right forelimb lameness (72%) than heeling horses (43%).[1] The heading horse also had significantly more bilateral forelimb lameness (25%) compared with the heeling horse (9%).[1] Heeling horses that did not turn properly into the steer after it switched directions often had left forelimb lameness.[1] The distal tarsal joints are loaded with the rider's weight, the horse's weight, the deceleration of the full-speed forward motion, and the weight of the steer as primarily rotational forces. This occurs as the horse is asked to set and get under the steer and pull the steer's weight forward across the arena. After a successful catch by the heeler, the heading horse must face or spin around to the right while the hocks and distal hindlimbs are loaded as described, and do so with the addition of a backward motion to maintain tightness of the rope. Although more forelimb versus hindlimb musculoskeletal problems were observed in horses used for heading, distal hock joint pain and osteoarthritis (OA) were the most common problems observed in the hindlimbs.

The heeling horse often has a similar history, with problems in the heeling box, not making the corner properly as the steer is set and turned, or nickering and bouncing out of the stop at the completion of a run while maximal tension is on the ropes. Clinical examination often reveals pain on palpation of the caudal lumbar area, the gluteal muscles, and over the point of both hips. This pain often is accompanied by the owner complaint that the horse is sore in the kidneys. If only the distal tarsal joints are involved, effusion usually is not detectable, but the horse may be reluctant to allow palpation of the medial aspect of the tarsus, as if anticipating pain. The dorsomedial distal aspect of the tarsus may be enlarged. High-quality radiographic examination of the hocks is essential. Intraarticular analgesia is often ineffective because the horse has developed performance problems in response to the pain experienced during every run, and the pain is anticipated, even though the area has been blocked. Thus horses become intractable in the roping box because they dread the pain that they will experience during the run. However, horses often respond well to intraarticular therapy when they realize, after several runs, that the pain has been lessened or stopped. The most common musculoskeletal problems causing lameness in horses used for heeling were (1) left forelimb palmar foot pain, (2) distal tarsal joint OA, (3) palmar foot pain and distal tarsal joint pain, (4) left forelimb pastern joint OA, and (5) hindlimb fetlock OA.

Diagnosis and Management of Specific Lameness

Palmar Foot Pain

Given the usual QH conformation of large body size and small feet or short, upright pastern conformation, navicular disease and injuries to structures within the palmar aspect of the foot are common. Right forelimb or bilateral palmar foot pain and left forelimb palmar foot pain were the most common problems identified in heading and heeling horses, respectively. Palmar foot pain results in a slowly progressive lameness, often bilateral, and horses may initially respond to intraarticular medication of the distal interphalangeal (DIP) joint, NSAIDs, and corrective shoeing. Soft tissue injuries of the palmar aspect of the foot (e.g., injury of the distal sesamoidean impar ligament [DSIL], a collateral ligament of the DIP joint, or the deep digital flexor tendon [DDFT] in the region of the navicular bone) are also common in heading horses and usually are acute, occurring during a roping event. Lameness is improved by perineural analgesia of the palmar digital nerves or intraarticular analgesia of the DIP joint. Often no radiological abnormality is apparent. Diagnosis of the specific structure injured can usually only be determined by magnetic resonance imaging (MRI).

The diagnosis of palmar foot pain is not complicated, but determining which structure is damaged can be challenging. Diagnosis is based on a combination of historical data and the response to perineural and intraarticular analgesia, high-quality radiographs, and possibly advanced diagnostic techniques such as nuclear scintigraphy, computed tomography, or MRI. Severity and duration of the lameness, the horse's activity, potential owner compliance, and the experience of the owner's farrier should be considered when determining therapy. The horse's hoof wall quality, conformation, environment, and occupation all affect treatment.

A thorough musculoskeletal examination should include palpation of the digital pulse amplitudes and assessing the hoof capsule for increased heat. In 97% of 23 horses with palmar foot pain there was increased digital pulse amplitude in the most severely affected limb. Hoof tester evaluation can be beneficial in determining pain location. Pain involving the navicular area is identified by application of intermittent hoof tester pressure over the middle third of the frog, which results in persistent non-fatigable reflex withdrawal of the hoof from the examiner. However, false-negative results may occur, especially during periods of dry weather when the horse's feet are excessively hard or in horses with thick soles and hard frogs. It is important to assess whether the withdrawal reflex is resulting from real pain and not a whimsical reaction by the horse. The results from both front feet should be compared. Horses with an injury of the DSIL or the insertion of the DDFT seem particularly sore with hoof tester pressure near the junction of the middle and dorsal thirds of the frog. Horses with underrun heels, bruised heels, or damaged laminae in the heel area often have more pain over the affected heel. It is important, if possible, to differentiate peripheral versus central hoof pain with a thorough hoof tester examination.

Many of the middle-aged roping horses diagnosed with palmar foot pain have moderate to severe radiological lesions of the navicular bone. My initial treatment involves correcting any existing hoof imbalance. I apply a 2-degree wedge pad or wedge shoe, which decreases the pressure on the navicular area by about 25%. If the horse's foot was imbalanced and/or poorly shod, then correcting these problems combined with systemic NSAID therapy (phenylbutazone 1 g twice daily for 10 days) and rest may temporarily resolve the lameness. If the owner cannot rest the horse or the feet are properly shod, then I medicate the DIP joint using a combination of 9 mg of triamcinolone acetonide, 10 to 20 mg of hyaluronan, and 125 mg of amikacin.[2] Postinjection care involves 4 to 5 days of no roping and NSAID therapy (phenylbutazone 2 g daily for 5 days). Approximately 60% of horses respond to DIP joint medication and, depending on severity of disease and level of work, will remain sound for 4 to 6 months. If the horse does not respond to DIP joint medication, then I medicate the navicular bursa with 10 mg of hyaluronan and 9 mg of triamcinolone acetonide, or if a severe bony lesion exists, I use 20 mg of methylprednisolone acetate plus 125 mg of amikacin. I reserve navicular bursa medication only for those not responding to DIP medication and known not to have an acute soft tissue injury (e.g., a DDFT lesion). Horses with chronic collateral sesamoidean ligament pathology, identified by the presence of a spur on the proximomedial or proximolateral aspects of the navicular bone, usually do not respond to DIP joint medication but do respond to treatment of the navicular bursa. I caution the owner that navicular bursa injections are invasive and may lead to subsequent DDFT pathology and/or rupture. Palmar digital neurectomy is the last resort in treating horses with palmar foot pain because of its short-lived results (average 2 years of soundness) and numerous complications, such as severe infection, DDFT rupture, and DIP joint subluxation.

Soft Tissue Injuries

Ligament or tendon injury occurred in about 15% of heading horses, especially in the right forelimb, and in about 10% of heeling horses, usually in the left forelimb.[1] The structure affected varied, but the suspensory apparatus, the accessory ligament of the DDFT, DDFT, superficial digital flexor tendon (SDFT), and the distal sesamoidean ligaments were all involved. These injuries usually cause lameness of varying degrees, and diagnosis by clinical examination is straightforward. Ultrasonography should be used to confirm the diagnosis. Distal sesamoidean ligament injury may be more difficult to diagnose but often results in acute, moderate to severe lameness (grade 2 to 3 of 5) after a run, associated with pain on palpation of the palmar aspect of the pastern. Perineural analgesia of the palmar digital nerves may improve the lameness, but analgesia of the palmar nerves at the base of the proximal sesamoid bones is needed for complete soundness. Fractures of the middle phalanx are also common; therefore the horse should be examined by radiography and ultrasonography. Ultrasonographic evidence of enlargement or reduction in echogenicity in the straight (SSL) or oblique sesamoidean ligaments (OSL) is diagnostic (Figure 120-3). Radiological examination is usually negative if lameness is acute; however, chronic injury is often associated with entheseous new bone on the palmar aspect of the proximal phalanx or on the proximopalmar aspect of the middle phalanx associated with OSL or SSL injury, respectively.

In hindlimbs, deep digital flexor tendonitis, tenosynovitis of the digital flexor tendon sheath, and proximal suspensory desmitis (PSD) are common, especially in the left hindlimb of head horses. When turning to face the steer, the head horse turns 180 degrees at fast speeds, putting a rotational torque on the distal aspect of the left hindlimb (Figure 120-4).

The management of roping horses with these soft tissue injuries varies with which structure is affected and severity of the lesion, although the initial treatment is similar. The first 2 weeks consist of daily ice therapy for 20 minutes two to three times per day, NSAIDS (phenylbutazone 1 g twice daily for 7 days), stall rest with 10 minutes of handwalking, and a support bandage. This is followed by a variable period of stall rest with 15 to 20 minutes of daily handwalking. When the horse is sound and there is 80% resolution of any lesion seen using ultrasonography, a controlled exercise program is initiated to strengthen the affected structure (Box 120-1).

The horse remains confined until the controlled exercise program is completed. Lameness and ultrasonographic

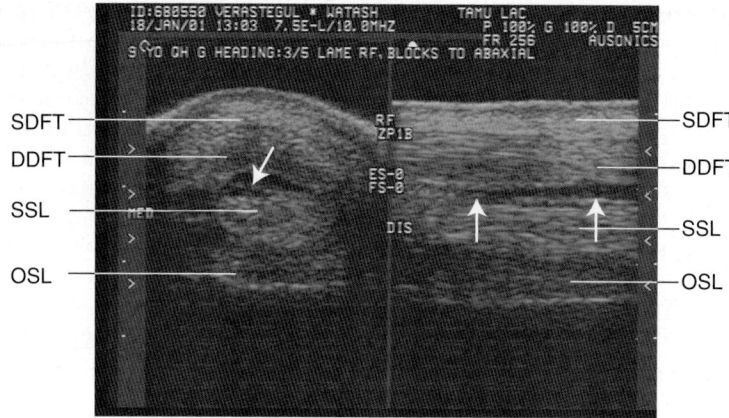

Fig. 120-3 • Transverse *(left)* and longitudinal *(right)* ultrasonographic images of the midpastern region of the right forelimb of a head horse. There is a hypoechogenic lesion in the straight sesamoidean ligament *(arrows) (SSL)*. *SDFT,* Superficial digital flexor tendon; *DDFT,* deep digital flexor tendon; *OSL,* oblique sesamoidean ligament.

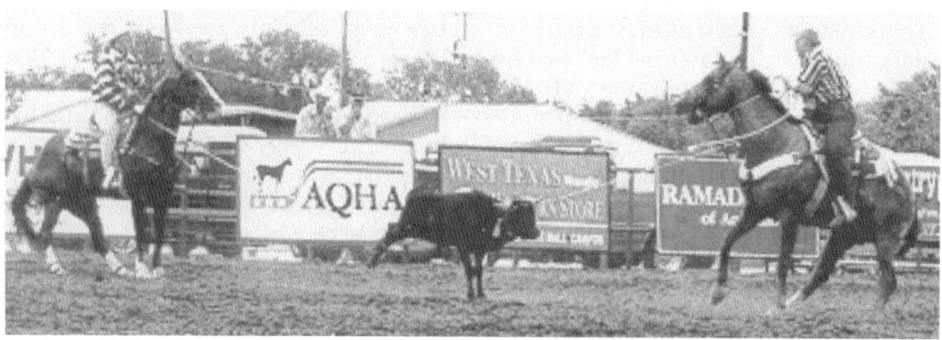

Fig. 120-4 • A head horse *(right)* turns to face the heeler at the end of the run. Note the strain placed on the left hindlimb.

BOX 120-1

Exercise Regimen after Mild Injuries to Forelimb Suspensory Ligament or Accessory Ligament of the Deep Digital Flexor Tendon

Weeks 1-2	The horse is given stall rest or a small run (6 × 10 m) with support bandage on the limb, ice therapy, and nonsteroidal antiinflammatory drugs.
Weeks 2-6	Length of time depends on severity of the lesion and structure affected. Horses are rechecked and ultrasonographic examination is performed at 3-month intervals until the horse is sound and the lesion is 75% to 80% healed. The horse is handwalked 10 minutes daily.
Weeks 6-8	Confinement is continued with 15 minutes of handwalking twice daily.
Weeks 9-12	Confinement is continued with 30 minutes of handwalking daily.
Weeks 13-16	If horse is sound at the trot, then confinement is continued, but the horse is walked under saddle or is ponied 15 minutes a day plus 5 minutes of trotting. Five minutes of walking and trotting are added every third day. The horse is reexamined by ultrasonography before returning to roping activity.

examinations are repeated before the horse returns to roping activity or turnout.

Distal Hock Joint Pain

OA of the distal hock joints is common, and heeling horses seem especially at risk. Most respond well to intraarticular medication of the centrodistal and tarsometatarsal joints. Middle-aged horses with moderate or severe OA are treated with 40 mg of methylprednisolone acetate and 125 mg of amikacin per joint. Younger horses or horses with mild to no radiological lesions are treated as above except 10 mg of hyaluronan is added to each joint. Postinjection care is 7 to 10 days off before returning to roping. The toes are squared on the hindlimbs to ease breakover and decrease torque on these joints.

Back and Pelvic Region Pain

Injury to the back and pelvic area is seen, especially in heading horses. Strain or tearing of the sacroiliac ligaments or epaxial musculature can occur. Radiographic evaluation is difficult and often unrewarding, but ultrasonographic examination may reveal longissimus lumborum and gluteal muscle tearing and can be used to evaluate the sacroiliac area. Lameness predisposing to back pain must be eliminated. Rest combined with topical heat (hot towels) and dimethyl sulfoxide or diclofenac (Surpass, IDEXX

Pharmaceuticals, Inc., Greensboro, North Carolina, United States) helps many horses, but often months of rest are needed before the pain is eliminated. Treating the painful areas with local injections hastens the recovery time. I prefer a combination of 5 mL of methylprednisolone acetate, 5 mL of Sarapin, and 5 mL of prednisolone diluted with 30 mL of mepivacaine and then depositing 3 to 5 mL in several sites around the painful muscle or ligament. The horse is given 2 to 3 weeks of light riding, with no roping activity, and then is reevaluated by ultrasonography. Most horses return to roping activity within 4 weeks from the time of injury.

Obviously all team roping horses are also susceptible to any of the same injury problems that other equine athletes experience. Most of these injuries produce overt lameness, and diagnosis is usually straightforward.

Shoeing Considerations

Because roping horses are often middle-aged, are used frequently, and commonly have palmar foot pain, maintenance of proper hoof balance is critical in keeping these horses sound. Long toes and collapsed heels are common. The heels grow too far forward and are left unsupported and thus are at risk of abnormal concussion. We recommend trimming the heel back to the widest part of the frog and setting the shoe further back on the foot; thus the heels of the shoe end at the widest aspect of the frog. Care must be taken to fit the front shoes properly so that little of the medial side of the shoe is exposed because head horses have a tendency to grab this portion of the shoe and pull off a shoe, especially the left front shoe. Easing the breakover of the limb can be accomplished by rockering the shoe. A rim shoe or steel natural balance shoe provides good traction and allows an easier breakover by the rounded and rockered toe region of the shoe construction. The natural balance shoe has a wider web than a normal shoe and is beneficial for horses with sore feet acquired from performing on harder ground. If trimming alone cannot establish a correct hoof-pastern angle, a 1- to 2-degree wedge pad is recommended. We prefer a cutout pad because a full pad often traps moisture and can lead to thrush. Care must be taken to avoid pad pressure over the central region of the frog in horses with navicular pain.

In horses with deep digital flexor tendonitis, we recommend applying a 2- to 3-degree wedge pad for the initial 4 to 5 months of rest to decrease tension on the DDFT. The wedge is reduced gradually over three shoe resets, once the horse is sound. In horses with distal hock joint pain, we try to ease breakover of the hind feet by squaring the toes or by setting the shoe back under the toe 0.3 cm. Avoiding any type of trailer or extension on the rear shoes is also preferable, especially for a heading horse, because this can aggravate pain associated with distal hock OA.

CALF ROPING AND BREAKAWAY ROPING HORSES

Description of the Sport

Calf roping originated on ranches of the Old West when sick calves were roped and tied down for medical treatment. Success in calf roping depends on the teamwork between a cowboy and a horse. After the calf is given a head start (like a scoreline in team roping), horse and rider chase the calf, and as the rider ropes the calf, the rider dismounts and runs to the calf. As the rider dismounts, the horse must sit back on its hind end and come to a sudden stop, which takes the slack out of the rope and stops the running calf. This allows the cowboy to catch the calf and throw the calf to the ground, termed *flanking the calf*. Once on the ground, the cowboy ties three of the calf's legs together with a pigging string. The horse is trained to "work the rope" as the cowboy ties the calf, meaning to back up if needed to keep the rope tight, thus keeping the calf still for the rider to tie. When the cowboy completes his tie, he throws his hands up in the air as a signal to the judge that his run is complete. The calf must stay tied for 6 seconds. A 10-second penalty is added if the calf roper breaks the barrier at the beginning of the run. An 8- to 9-second run is considered good, and Jeff Chapman of Athens, Texas set the arena record in 1997 when he roped and tied a calf in 6.8 seconds.

Breakaway roping is similar to calf roping except the participants are women and children and the rider does not dismount and tie the calf. Instead, the calf is given a similar score or head start, and the horse and rider chase the calf and rope it around the neck. The rope used for breakaway roping has a quick-release device on it so that when the rope becomes tight, it snaps open and the calf runs free. After the calf is roped, the horse stops abruptly, the rope tightens and breaks away, and time is called. The rider remains on horseback. A typical breakaway time is 3.0 to 4.0 seconds.

Conformation

QHs are used for calf roping and must be athletic and well trained. Because the rider must dismount during calf roping, calf horses are usually not tall, often 14.2 or 14.3 hands high. Calf horses also have wide-base and muscular frontquarters and hindquarters. Many ropers believe that the performance demands on a calf horse are greater than those of a team roping horse.

Historical Data and Poor Performance

Calf roping and breakaway roping horses often show an alteration in performance before an observable lameness. There are no scientific studies specifically evaluating calf and breakaway roping horses. However, anecdotally the most common owner complaint is that a calf horse quits "working the rope," that is, after the calf is roped, the horse does not want to back up and keep tension on the rope for the rider to catch and tie the calf. This is usually associated with hindlimb lameness. Another common complaint is that the horse ducks to the right or left after the calf is roped instead of stopping in a straight line. If the horse ducks to the right, this is usually because of left-sided pain that the horse is trying to avoid. A horse that will not run hard to the calf usually has front foot pain.

Diagnosis and Management of Specific Lameness

Calf horses have lameness similar to that of team roping horses with a few exceptions. Hindlimb lameness is more common in horses used for calf roping. OA of the distal hock joints is the most common problem, but stifle lameness also occurs frequently, such as collateral ligament or meniscal injury. However, diagnosis is usually not possible until after bony changes are seen radiologically, months after the initial injury. Bony reaction at the proximal medial aspect of the tibia is diagnostic. With rest, NSAIDs, and intraarticular medications, these horses often can return to roping, but at a lower level, perhaps as a calf roping horse for a child or beginner. Hindlimb proximal suspensory desmitis, traumatic fetlock OA, and fractures of the proximal sesamoid bones and middle phalanx are common. The most common forelimb lameness is palmar foot pain, often resulting from improper shoeing.

Shoeing Considerations

The same shoeing considerations are used for balance and protection of the navicular region in the forelimbs as described for team roping horses. Rim shoes or half round shoes are commonly worn on the front feet. In the hindlimbs if the toes of the feet are too short, so that the horse has a broken forward hoof-pastern axis, then the hind toe digs deep into the ground and the limb stops abruptly, causing sudden torque on the distal aspect of the limb. Having more toe length and a shoe that fits full with the heel branches of the shoe extending to the heel bulbs is preferable, so that the horse slides as it stops. This not only protects the heel bulbs from the ground surface, but it also puts less strain on the distal aspect of the limb. Horses used for calf roping often wear skid boots, protective leg gear aimed at minimizing friction between the ground surface and the plantar aspect of the hindlimb fetlock joints, because the horse skids to a stop.

◼ THE REINED COW HORSE

Van E. Snow*

The National Reined Cow Horse Association was initiated in 1949 as the California Reined Cow Horse Association and changed its name in 1970. The purpose of the association is to preserve the training traditions of the vaqueros, the horsemen of early California, who trained their horses for ranch work. As a result of selective breeding and refined training techniques, reined cow horses today are able to achieve more with livestock than was ever thought possible.

The National Reined Cow Horse Association held its first Snaffle Bit Futurity in 1970 in Sacramento, California. Bobby Ingersoll, a renowned cow horse trainer, had the idea to showcase the best all-around cow horses in the world. The competition involves showing the horse in three different disciplines: herd work (cutting), rein work, and cow work (working a cow down a fence). In the Snaffle Bit Futurity, the top 20 horses from the first round of competition come back and do another round over 2 days, starting again with even scores. The sport of reined cow horse has evolved from 1970, when 27 horses competed for $3900, to now when hundreds of horses compete at their annual futurity for nearly $1 million.

The professionals compete on numerous horses in four divisions: snaffle bit, hackamore, two rein, and bridle. Competition consists of numerous levels, including professional, nonprofessional, amateur, and limited open. An auction is held each year at the reined cow horse futurity

at which horses that range from 1 to 12 years of age and breeding stock horses are available for sale.

Affiliate groups of the National Reined Cow Horse Association are organized in Canada, Germany, Belgium, and Australia, and a strong interest in the group exists in most of Europe and in South and Central America. No restrictions exist as to the breeds allowed to compete in the futurities. Numerically the American Quarter Horse dominates, but Paint horses often compete successfully, and an Appaloosa has won.

The competition requires that a horse be accomplished in its ability to run, stop, turn, and "read" and control a cow. These horses also must have a high level of endurance. These qualifications do not necessarily dictate a particular body type, but a reined cow horse tends to be a taller, leaner horse than a cutting horse. Stallions, mares, and geldings compete equally, as do all genders and age groups of riders.

Reined cow horses typically begin training when they are less than 2 years old and start to compete at 3 years of age. They have about 20 months to learn all of the events and to become conditioned well enough to withstand the rigors of competition. This requires that the training surface, shoeing, and judgment of the trainer be optimal throughout the 20-month period.

Most trainers have become knowledgeable in the prevention and the early detection of lameness. Musculoskeletal evaluations are done quarterly on the futurity prospects, beginning in the fall of the 2-year-old year. These evaluations include a complete lameness evaluation, including flexion tests. At this time, good baseline information on each horse is established, and future insidious problems can be detected before they become unmanageable. In the past, it was commonplace for a trainer to blame himself or herself or the horse's attitude for not being able to accomplish a certain task, when in fact low-grade lameness was developing. The trainer would continue to train the horse, and often a serious lameness would develop. For a trainer to suspect a subtle lameness and to have the horse evaluated is much more common now. Lameness detected at this point is usually manageable.

A reined cow horse continues to compete beyond 3 years of age. As 4-year-olds, they can continue in the snaffle bit or begin in the hackamore or bridle class. The 5-year-olds are shown in the hackamore or bridle class, and the 6-year-olds compete in the bridle class. Hackamore and bridle horses compete in the reining and cow work divisions, but they do not do herd work. The intention is to finish a horse's education by the time the horse is 6 years old.

TRAINING SURFACES

The training surface has a strong influence on lameness in terms of incidence, degree of severity, and type of injury. In general, an arena or round pen is best constructed as follows: the original ground is graded to a 1.5% grade from one corner to the other and is compacted to 95%. A 15-cm thickness of base material such as limestone rock dust is then added, watered, and compacted to 95%. The type of base used is dictated by what is available in the area, but it should be smaller-sized particles (not small rocks) that have interlocking edges. A 1.5% grade should be maintained. Sand is then added to the top of the base to a thickness of at least 5 cm and not more than 12 cm in the arena, and from 10 to 15 cm in a round pen. Adding the sand at the minimum levels first and then adding more later if necessary is recommended. In general, less injury occurs with thinner layers of sand, but performance may be enhanced with thicker layers of sand. Fine beach sand is the best because it has low abrasive characteristics and is light. These qualities are important because the sand gets between the skin and protective boots and also comes in direct contact with the back of the pasterns and fetlocks. If the sand is coarse and abrasive, it damages the skin and causes lameness. The density of the sand is important because a horse has to push the sand during sliding stops, and if the sand is too heavy, it causes injury and destroys the horse's confidence.

Water content of the training surface is also an important consideration. In general, applying water a few hours before use is a good idea, so that the water is distributed evenly. If the training surface is too deep with sand or if the base is not consistent, I see more soft tissue injuries such as tendonitis, suspensory injuries, curbs, and sprained backs. If the training surface is too hard, I tend to see bone injuries such as osteitis of the distal phalanx, navicular syndrome, sesamoiditis, or fractured proximal sesamoid bones.

THE RELATIONSHIP OF TRAINING TO LAMENESS

The types of injuries commonly seen tend to vary as the training progresses. The young 2-year-olds have hoof and sole problems during the initial breaking process, before they are shod, associated with an increased digital pulse amplitude and sensitivity to hoof testers. Subchondral bone cysts in the medial femoral condyle and osteochondrosis of the fetlock may manifest at this time. Chip fractures, present but unnoticed when the horse was a foal or yearling, may become clinically apparent when ridden work starts.

The work during the latter half of training for a 2-year-old involves more speed and collection, and low-grade lamenesses may develop that later become persistent problems. These lamenesses include suspensory desmitis, navicular syndrome, and hock and stifle pain. The 3-year-old year involves even more collection, cow work at speed, and harder stops. We generally see a continuation of the 2-year-old problems, if they are not managed well, and also more acute injuries to soft tissue and chip fractures of the fetlock and carpus.

CONFORMATION AND LAMENESS

Conformation has an effect on the development of lameness, but I believe that conformation often is overemphasized. The component of conformation that has the biggest effect on soundness is body conformation and the degree of balance in motion. I have seen many horses whose conformation was not impressive when viewed at a standstill but were impressive when evaluated in motion. Balance in motion is that somewhat immeasurable quality that gives one the impression that the horse could jump, stop, turn, or do almost anything on any given stride without effort. In my experience, these horses remain sound while performing to an exceptional level, whereas horses that

have less balance suffer more frequent injury. Although static conformation related to lameness is important and should be evaluated, in my opinion, conformation in motion is equally important.

The most common conformation problems that I see are toed in and toed out. These problems predispose the horse to lameness but are present to some degree in nearly all horses. Most often these conformational abnormalities are associated with injury to the suspensory ligament (SL) and also can be associated with injury to the collateral ligaments of the digit. I try to manage these conformation faults before they cause injury to the horse by trimming and shoeing. A horse that toes out initially contacts the ground with the outside toe quarter with improper trimming. The hoof then slides along the ground and begins to rotate the toe out. The inside heel bulb then makes contact with the ground, and the hoof rotation stops. However, this rotational force continues up the limb and places unnatural strain on the soft tissues below the carpus and eventually causes damage. I recommend removing more wall from the hoof at the point of contact and beveling the toe so that breakover is accomplished easily over a wide area. My goal is to get the entire hoof to contact the ground evenly and eliminate the rotational force. Horses that toe in generally contact the ground at the inside toe quarter. Horses with this problem need more hoof removed from the inside toe, the goal being to cause the foot to land flat.

LAMENESS EVALUATION

I begin the lameness examination by obtaining as complete a history as possible. I establish the duration of lameness; any change in lameness, if the horse has been rested or kept in work; any response to treatment; alteration in lameness with work; when the horse was last trimmed and shod; any changes in footing, type of work, or shoeing; if lameness was associated with turnout or work; if the horse has received any intramuscular injections; if the horse kicks the paddock or stall; if the horse is turned out with others; if the horse stumbles; any known trauma; whether the lameness occurred insidiously or suddenly; and if the horse stands normally. Generally, the best history is obtained from the grooms and trainer, although some owners can provide information.

I watch the horse at the walk, trot, and canter, loose in a 9-m round pen, and on firm footing on a 2% slope. The degree of lameness often is amplified when the horse is loose, on hard ground, and allowed to work on a slight slope. Some lameness characteristics are best seen at a slow trot and some at an extended trot. The round pen enables one to evaluate the horse's ability to hold leads. Detecting low-grade ataxia is also easier when the horse works free, especially during downward transitions.

Lameness may be manifest in how a horse does a sliding stop; lameness may be accentuated after several sliding stops from a canter. A horse may slide stronger on one hindlimb than the other. The complaint is often made that a horse is not stopping as well as previously, although lameness is not noticed. A horse may begin a sliding stop normally but then pick up the painful limb halfway through the stop and replace it. The stop is not held evenly. The stop becomes normal if pain is removed by local analgesia.

Another common situation occurs when a horse is cutting a cow; the horse runs off at one end or does not come back with the cow as strongly at one end. The hindlimb farthest from the cow before the weak turn is generally the lame limb. If this horse is asked to do rollbacks in a round pen, the horse is much weaker when it reverses direction one way. Generally, the hindlimb on the outside of the circle after the weak rollback is the lame limb.

Competition is now so great that the difference between winning and losing is sometimes a matter of which horse feels the best. Performance diminishes before outright lameness is noted. Hindlimb lameness is particularly common in reined cow horses because of hock or stifle pain or proximal suspensory desmitis.

Flexion tests include flexion of the digit in all limbs and carpal, hock, and stifle flexions. Notes are made on the results and whether the horse resented flexion. The digit is flexed in an oblique plane (applying medial and lateral torque), and any resentment or decreased elasticity is noted.

All the soft tissue structures are palpated, and any enlargements and sensitivity are noted. Hoof testers always are applied to the front feet, as well as to the hind feet of horses with hindlimb lameness. Any lameness or weakness is classified in degrees (grade 1 to 5); by the limb involved; by weight bearing or non–weight bearing or mixed status; by the effect of walking in a circle or on a straight line, on an incline or decline; by flexion tests; and by the effects of prolonged digital pressure over sensitive areas.

If lameness is serious enough possibly to be caused by fracture, radiography is performed first; otherwise, diagnostic analgesia is used to establish the source of pain. Intraarticular analgesia is more specific than regional analgesia, which can be done at a later time if necessary; therefore I often start with intraarticular blocks, especially in forelimbs. I rely on the flexion tests to direct the start point. If flexion of the distal limb is normal but carpal flexion is positive, I usually use perineural analgesia of the proximal palmar metacarpal and palmar nerves (high four-point). If lameness persists, I perform intraarticular analgesia of the carpus. If flexion of the distal limb is positive, I perform intraarticular analgesia of the distal interphalangeal (DIP) joint first and then proceed to the pastern and fetlock joints if necessary to eliminate the pain causing lameness. If intraarticular analgesia is not helpful and the flexion test is still positive, I perform perineural analgesia of the palmar digital nerves, followed by the digital nerves at the base of the proximal sesamoid bones (PSBs) and later a "low four-point block." Knowing whether the problem is articular is useful because horses with articular problems are often more amenable to treatment.

For intraarticular analgesia I do a three-step povidone-iodine (Betadine, Purdue Products L.P., Stamford, Connecticut, United States) and alcohol skin preparation and use sterile gloves. I place a subcutaneous bleb of local anesthetic solution before injection and combine local anesthetic solution with gentamicin sulfate (40 mg).

In a hindlimb I usually use perineural analgesia proximal to the fetlock, local infiltration around the region of the origin of the SL, intraarticular analgesia of the centrodistal and tarsometatarsal joints separately, and intraarticular analgesia of the femoropatellar and medial femorotibial joints. The lateral femorotibial compartment

rarely is involved. If the response to a low four-point block is positive but the response to plantar nerve blocks at the base of the PSBs is negative, intraarticular analgesia of the metatarsophalangeal joint is performed the following day.

IMAGING CONSIDERATIONS

Once the region of pain is localized, the area is examined using radiography and ultrasonography to identify the exact structure that has been damaged and to assess the degree of damage. The more specific I can be at this point, the more reliable the prognosis and treatment are. If the diagnosis is not specific, scintigraphy often is used. Generally, a differential diagnosis list is generated based on the physical examination. Developing a therapeutic plan based on a tentative or vague diagnosis is a mistake. Nearly all diagnoses are tentative until the pain has been localized as specifically as possible through the use of diagnostic analgesia and appropriate imaging.

PROCEEDING WITHOUT A DIAGNOSIS

Sometimes the site of pain causing lameness cannot be discovered, even after all the joints and nerves have been blocked and a complete scintigraphic examination has been performed. I then treat the horse for myofascial pain with drugs or chiropractic therapy. If the horse responds to these therapies, then this is indirect evidence of the cause. Another possible cause is equine protozoal myelitis (EPM). Horses with EPM may show chronic lameness without other neurological signs.

LAMENESS AND SHOEING CONSIDERATIONS

Proper foot balance is critical to resolving all lameness problems successfully. The foot should be trimmed to land evenly. Any medial-to-lateral imbalance should be removed by trimming. If the point of contact is the lateral toe quarter, then enough of the lateral wall should be removed so the foot lands flat. The foot should be trimmed or a wedge used to achieve a hoof angle that is the same as the pastern angle (about 55 degrees in forelimbs and 57 degrees in hindlimbs). A square-toed shoe that has a wide bevel, which extends from the medial to lateral toe nail holes, commonly is recommended and is useful. The shoe should be set back so the dorsopalmar axis is shortened. The heels are trimmed so the shoe comes in contact with the wall at the widest section of the frog. These specifications are designed to remove rotational forces up the limb that occur in horses with medial-to-lateral imbalances, to provide mechanical advantage to the palmar/plantar aspect of the limb that occurs in horses with a long toe and low heel, and to reduce concussion to the digit that occurs in horses with the two-phase foot impact associated with foot imbalance.

An egg bar shoe is used for horses with moderate to severe tendonitis, suspensory desmitis, or an apical PSB fracture. A reverse shoe is used sometimes for horses with navicular syndrome, ringbone, sesamoiditis, suspensory desmitis, tendonitis, constricted palmar/plantar annular ligament, carpitis, and tarsitis. Horses with bruising in the sole are shod with soft dental acrylic pads. Horses with heel and quarter cracks are managed with egg bar shoes.

TEN MOST COMMON LAMENESS CONDITIONS IN THE REINED COW HORSE

1. Suspensory desmitis
2. Osteoarthritis of the centrodistal and tarsometatarsal joints
3. Navicular syndrome
4. Hoof-related problems such as bruises, abscesses, and cracks
5. Superficial digital flexor tendonitis
6. Subchondral bone cysts, osteochondrosis, and traumatic injuries of the stifle
7. Fetlock arthrosis
8. Sesamoiditis
9. Distal interphalangeal joint synovitis or osteoarthritis
10. Osteitis of the distal phalanx

TREATMENT OF LAMENESS

Suspensory Desmitis

For horses with suspensory desmitis, it is important to optimize foot balance as previously described. Corrective shoeing is designed to minimize any further physical damage and therefore prevent further pain and inflammation. Other treatments provide short-term results and are aimed at reducing the existing inflammation.

Horses with minor to moderate fiber disruption are treated with perilesional injections of Sarapin and corticosteroids. If the lesion is proximal, a sterile skin preparation is recommended, with the addition of gentamicin sulfate (40 mg) in case the carpometacarpal joint is entered inadvertently. The drugs are injected under the loose tissue between the SL and the accessory ligament of the deep digital flexor tendon. Middle carpal joint pain may occur concurrently and is treated using intraarticularly administered corticosteroids, provided that no radiological abnormalities are apparent. Physical therapy in the form of electrical stimulus modalities or low-level light laser therapy is started 3 days after injection and continued as needed through the intended competition. Magnets of 600 to 1200 G placed over the site have been used successfully and are kept in place for 60 days and then as needed for soundness.

The lesion is monitored monthly using ultrasonography. If conservative treatment fails, extracorporeal shock wave therapy (ESWT) is used and administered with the horse under general anesthesia. Up to four treatments have been used, combined with rest for 60 to 90 days.

Centrodistal and Tarsometatarsal Joint Pain

Intraarticular injection of corticosteroids is effective at relieving pain and inflammation in the centrodistal and tarsometatarsal joints. Horses are allowed to rest for at least 10 days after injection, and then work gradually is increased as soundness dictates. The systemic use of hyaluronan and acetylglucosamine is helpful for maintenance. Orally administered chondroitin sulfate and glucosamine products also have been useful. If medication is ineffective, joint drilling or forage to induce joint ankylosis, or periarticular ESWT can be used effectively.

Navicular Syndrome

Navicular syndrome is diagnosed based on a positive response to palmar digital analgesia and analgesia of the DIP joint, radiography, and scintigraphy. Radiology can be misleading, and in my opinion scintigraphy is the most reliable method of diagnosis. Corrective shoeing is essential. Isoxsuprine hydrochloride (600 mg) is given orally once daily for 60 days. Aspirin (15 g) also is given orally once daily for 60 days. If this combination provides relief, it is continued for another 60 days or until the horse finishes the futurity season. Injection of the DIP joint with corticosteroids, or a combination of corticosteroid and hyaluronan, often provides temporary relief (about 30 days).

If a horse fails to respond to corrective shoeing and medications, ESWT is indicated and has been effective, except in horses with entheseous new bone at the attachment of the collateral sesamoidean ligaments. Palmar digital neurectomy is used as a last resort.

Traumatic Hoof Injuries

Horses with bruises and cracks in the hooves respond well to egg bar shoes with soft dental acrylic pads or metal pads. A horse with a quarter crack is treated by trimming the wall palmar/plantar to the defect, so that no contact is made with the shoe, that is, floating the heel. The air gap is up to 6 mm deep and is reopened daily using a hacksaw blade to relieve pressure between the hoof wall and the shoe until the defect has grown out. If the crack is moving and bleeding, a copper patch is attached to the wall with screws to span the defect and therefore stabilize it.

Superficial Digital Flexor Tendonitis

Ultrasonography is used to characterize size and position of the lesion in horses with superficial digital flexor tendonitis. If a lesion is small, the owner or trainer usually decides to continue preparing for the futurity. It is important to try to determine the circumstances that caused the lesion to develop to eliminate further damage. Possible causes for tendonitis include poor hoof balance, deep footing, fatigue, speed, overexertion from working a difficult cow, uncontrolled exercise (turnout), interference from hindlimbs, tight bandages, poorly fitting support boots, and hanging a leg on a hot walker, tie rope, or fence.

Therapy for tendonitis involves depositing corticosteroids in the loose subcutaneous tissue in the proximity of the lesion. The leg is wrapped in a gelocast for 3 days and then is treated with ice and laser or electrical stimulus therapy. The horse is walked in hand or under saddle for 15 minutes twice daily for 7 days. Training then is resumed. The leg is maintained in a support wrap continuously. Shoeing, good footing, and conservative training are critical to the healing process.

Stifle Pain

If no abnormalities are detected in the stifle radiologically, the affected joints are treated with intraarticularly administered corticosteroids and hyaluronan. The horse is prescribed weekly injections of systemic acetylglucosamine, which continue through the futurity. Subsequent intraarticular injections are not performed sooner than 6 months and preferably not at all.

If radiological evidence of osteochondrosis of the trochlear ridges of the femur exists, the same therapy is effective.

The prognosis for horses with subchondral bone cysts of the medial femoral condyle is dismal, and I do not recommend that these horses continue training to be futurity horses.

Metatarsophalangeal Joint Pain

Metatarsophalangeal joint pain may be caused by traumatic osteoarthritis, fracture of a PSB, sesamoiditis, fragments detached from the proximoplantar aspect of the proximal phalanx, or periarticular soft tissue injury. If no radiological lesions are present, the horse is treated with intraarticularly administered betamethasone and hyaluronan, followed by 10 days of rest. Systemic glucosamine is given every 2 weeks as maintenance therapy. Orally administered glucosamine and chondroitin sulfate also seem to be useful in managing metatarsophalangeal joint pain. Shoeing imbalances must be corrected concurrently.

Sesamoiditis

The foot must be properly balanced to treat sesamoiditis. Egg bar shoes with a square toe and a wide roll or bevel are used. The shoe is set back to minimize the leverage on the palmar/plantar aspects of the fetlock. The hoof angle is optimal when it matches the pastern angle. Isoxsuprine hydrochloride (600 mg) and aspirin (15 g) are given orally once daily for 60 to 90 days. Electromagnetic energy is applied to the affected region every other day for 3 months and thereafter as needed for soundness. The amount of training is dictated by the degree of soundness.

Distal Interphalangeal Joint Pain

The foot must be properly balanced to treat reined cow horses with DIP joint pain. Soft dental acrylic pour-in–type pads and shock-absorbing rim pads can be helpful. Intraarticular injection of a corticosteroid and hyaluronan is followed by the systemic use of acetylglucosamine and hyaluronan. It is imperative that training is continued on a soft surface.

Osteitis of the Distal Phalanx

Soft dental acrylic pour-in–type pads and shock-absorbing rim pads are used to treat horses with osteitis of the distal phalanx. The horse is treated with isoxsuprine hydrochloride (600 mg), aspirin (15 g), and phenylbutazone (2 g) given orally once daily for 60 days and then as needed for soundness. Training must be done in soft footing to reduce concussion to the foot. ESWT has recently been introduced to manage horses with osteitis of the distal phalanx. The Editors question whether shock waves can penetrate the hoof capsule, or whether they have adequate depth of penetration if administered via the heel bulbs.

■ BARREL-RACING HORSES

Robin M. Dabareiner

Barrel racing began in 1948 when a group of Texas ranch women started riding horses around a cloverleaf pattern of barrels and the fastest horse around the course was the winner. Barrel racing has evolved into a multimillion-dollar industry called the Women's Professional Rodeo Association (WPRA). From this original organization many

other barrel racing associations, which host numerous futurities for horses 4 or 5 years of age or younger and derbies for older horses, have arisen.[1-5] Now (from the WPRA website) "WPRA barrel racers compete for millions of dollars each year, culminating in twelve circuit finals rodeos held throughout the country, the Dodge National Circuit Finals Rodeo held in Pocatello, Idaho in April, and the Wrangler National Finals Rodeo held in Las Vegas each December." The major competitions are divided into rodeo, futurities, derbies, open jackpots, and professional levels. Futurities and derbies are classified by age of the horse. Open competitions are open to any horse or rider and are highly competitive. Within the open jackpots, a new classification of barrel racing has developed, termed a *3D* or *4D competition*, which includes a handicapping system that allows less experienced horses or riders to compete with seasoned horses and riders.

Barrel racing is a timed event with the clock beginning when a predetermined line is crossed. Three barrels (55-gallon steel drums) are positioned in a triangle or cloverleaf (Figure 120-5). The contestant must turn the left or right barrel first (most choose to turn the right-hand barrel first) in a manner that the path always crosses. The distance covered for the pattern varies with the size of the arena, but generally the distance from the starting line to the first

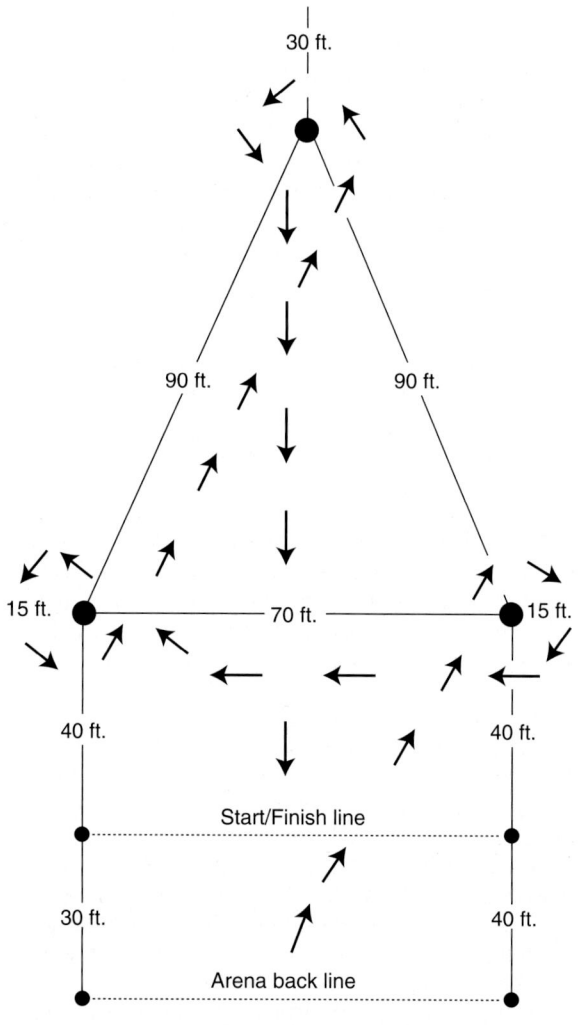

Fig. 120-5 • Diagram of barrel racing cloverleaf.

barrel is 14 to 18 m. The distance between the first and second barrel is 21 to 27 m and between the second and third barrel is 27 to 32 m. The horses must start at the alleyway or entrance to the arena, run at full speed to the first barrel, slow down and complete a 360-degree turn around the barrel, speed up and run to the second barrel, turn 360 degrees, head to the third barrel, turn 360 degrees, and then sprint to the finish line. The fastest time to complete the pattern varies with distance of the pattern and arena size, but a good run for a large arena pattern is 15 to 16 seconds. An electric eye timing system usually is used, and times are recorded in hundredths of a second. If a rider hits a barrel and tips it over, a 5-second penalty is imposed. If the horse and rider fail to negotiate the pattern correctly, they are disqualified. The arena is often leveled after each horse.

CONFORMATION

Horses are predominately American Quarter Horses (QHs) and Appendix horses (QH and Thoroughbred [TB] crosses), but occasionally TB, Paint, or Arabian horses are seen. Speed, quick acceleration, and agility to slow down quickly to turn the barrel are essential. Many barrel horses have QH racehorse pedigrees. Some prefer stockbred horses, which usually have a calmer personality. Geldings are preferred. Horses usually range from 14.3 to 15.1 hands. Barrel horses are not usually as muscular and wide based as calf roping horses. They usually have long, leaner muscle mass that provides the speed and flexibility needed to perform the 360-degree turns. In a recent retrospective study evaluating musculoskeletal problems in 118 horses used solely for barrel racing, the median age was 9 years (range, 3 to 19 years), median weight was 509 kg (range, 409 to 611 kg), and 73% were geldings and 27% were mares.[6]

TRAINING

Futurity competitions are popular because of the amount of prize money, and training usually starts at 2 years of age. Futurity horses often have short careers because of the pressure to perform at a high level of competition at only 4 to 5 years of age, resulting in advanced osteoarthritis (OA), often in the distal tarsal joints. Successful futurity horses seldom have long-term careers because of behavioral problems or performance-limiting injuries.

Horses that are 5 years of age or older, started slowly, and are allowed to mature before performing in serious competition may compete professionally for 5 years.[2] The average age of a professional barrel horse is 10 to 15 years. Horses may compete in 50 to 100 rodeos per year and spend much time traveling. An experienced barrel horse is trained by practicing turns but rarely uses the barrels because the horse learns to anticipate the pattern and tires of it. Many professional horses are ponied (led from another horse) or are ridden just enough to keep them fit for competition, but they are never really worked unless competing.

Older, semiretired horses that are well trained to the barrel pattern, but not fast enough for upper-level competition, may be used for a child or beginner. These horses do make repetitive barrel pattern runs in a practice pen for the rider to learn and often have use-related injuries, requiring much maintenance therapy to withstand the number of practice runs needed to teach a beginner.

HISTORICAL DATA AND POOR PERFORMANCE

Barrel racing is the one equine discipline that most riders train and ride their own horses. Unlike roping events where many variables exist (e.g., cow selection and partners), there are few variations in the barrel horse pattern or run. Size of arena and ground surface may affect the speed of the run, but the barrel pattern is constant, and most riders know what time to expect from their horse for a given arena size. Therefore more barrel horses are examined because of a change or decrease in performance (40%) compared with roping horses (about 25%), rather than overt lameness. In a recent study, 45% of barrel horses that had an owner complaint of running past or wide around the first (right) barrel had a right forelimb musculoskeletal problem.[6] Unilateral or bilateral forelimb foot pain or subclinical epistaxis was observed in horses that had a recent decrease in speed. Horses that were reluctant to turn to the left had either a left forelimb or hindlimb musculoskeletal problem.

Other musculoskeletal problems depend on the horse's age and level of competition. A young futurity barrel horse may run up the fence, that is, the horse does not turn around the barrel but runs past it up the arena, or it may refuse to enter the arena. No lameness may be detectable, and the veterinarian has to determine whether the young horse is mentally stressed and showing behavioral problems or is responding to pain. Several options are presented to the owner to help determine whether the horse is responding to pain or it is a result of overtraining. One option is to administer phenylbutazone (2.2 mg/kg daily for 2 weeks and then 1.1 mg/kg daily for 2 weeks) for 30 days and to keep the horse in barrel race training. If the horse returns to normal performance, then it is concluded that the horse is most likely experiencing pain. If the problem does not resolve, then I try to address any behavioral problems. If problems persist, I often suggest giving the horse a 3- to 6-month break from barrel racing and have the horse work cattle or perform other less intense activities. A second option is to increase the workload and try to establish whether lameness can be identified and then located with diagnostic analgesia, but few owners select this option. Older, experienced horses usually have pain-related problems.

Most barrel racers train their own horses, and the quality of training is inconsistent, and performance changes may be induced by the rider. Determining which barrel is the problem barrel is helpful. An owner may complain that the horse will not stay in the ground for the first barrel but works fine for the second and third barrels. The horse may perform well for the first barrel but does not make a good turn around the second barrel. The first barrel (usually going to the right) is the hardest barrel and most often a problem because the horse is running at full speed when it reaches the barrel and must slow quickly to make the 360-degree turn. When the horse is turning the barrel, the inside forelimb and hindlimb appear to be under the greatest pressure (Figure 120-6). If the owner complains that the horse is swinging wide or pulling away from the first barrel, the horse does not want to turn to the right and is probably trying to avoid right hindlimb or right forelimb pain.

The teeth are always evaluated to eliminate bitting problems as a cause of performance changes.

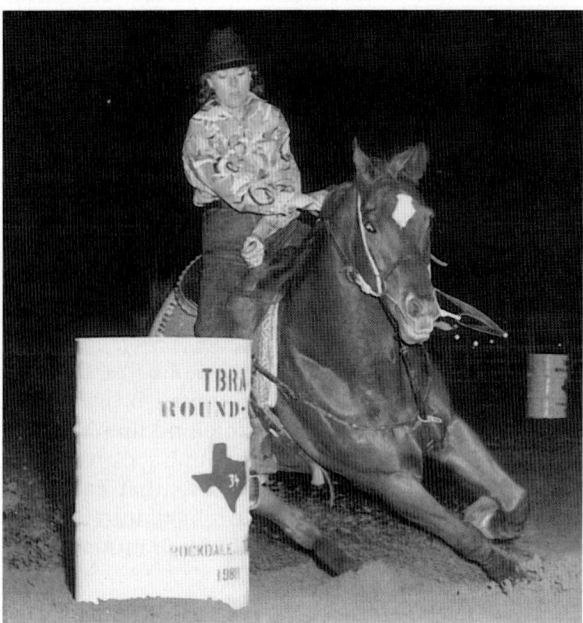

Fig. 120-6 • A barrel horse turning a barrel. Note the pressure on the inside hindlimb. This horse is on the backside of the barrel coming out of the turn and is in correct position. At this point in the barrel turn, a horse with hindlimb pain becomes uncollected and swings wide around the barrel.

LAMENESS EXAMINATION

A barrel horse does not run at top speed over long distances like flat racehorses; therefore fatigue-type injuries like superficial digital flexor tendonitis or fetlock and carpal chip fractures are seen less commonly than in racehorses. Some of the common injuries seen in barrel horses are attributed to the twisting and turning motion of the horse at high speeds (see Figure 120-6).

In a recent study, the most common musculoskeletal problem observed in horses used solely for barrel racing was (1) forelimb foot pain (33%), with the right front more often affected; (2) OA of the distal tarsal joints (15%); (3) suspensory branch desmitis or tendon injury (14%); (4) a combination of foot pain and distal tarsal pain (12%); and (5) medial femorotibial joint pain (10%).[6]

If an obvious lameness is not detected when trotting the horse in a straight line or large circle, the horse is trotted in hand in a small circle (1.5- to 3-m radius), mimicking the barrel turn, which will exacerbate the lameness. This may be the only time the horse shows lameness.

DIAGNOSIS AND MANAGEMENT OF SPECIFIC LAMENESS

QHs and Appendix QHs make up most of the barrel horses. Sore feet, navicular area pain, and palmar foot pain are the most frequent causes of forelimb lameness, with poor hoof conformation and farriery and hard arena surfaces being predisposing factors. Diagnosis and management are similar to those described for the team roping horse.

Distal hock OA is the second most common musculoskeletal problem and most common hindlimb problem most resulting in reduced performance or lameness. Diagnosis

is based on intraarticular analgesia, radiology, response to treatment, and sometimes nuclear scintigraphy. The centrodistal and tarsometatarsal joints are treated using methylprednisolone acetate (40 to 60 mg/joint) or triamcinolone acetonide (6 mg/joint) alone or in combination with hyaluronan (10 mg/joint) plus 125 mg of amikacin. Ideally the horse should have 7 to 10 days of turnout or light exercise before returning to barrel racing, but often the competition schedule does not allow this. Response to treatment may take up to 3 weeks. If the horse does not respond to treatment, we reevaluate the horse for lameness.

Hindlimb proximal suspensory desmitis (PSD) and suspensory branch desmitis are common in older, seasoned horses and can be career-ending injuries. Deep sand in arenas may contribute to the high incidence. Moderate lameness (grade 2 to 3 of 5) often is exacerbated by upper limb flexion. The horse usually has no swelling or minimal swelling and no heat and pain for proximal suspensory body lesions, but these will be seen in horses with suspensory branch desmitis. Local analgesia is essential to verify the source of pain. Radiology of the proximal metatarsal area is often negative, although if the condition is chronic, endosteal reaction or entheseous new bone may be present, seen as increased radiopacity. Ultrasonographic examination may reveal an enlarged and hypoechogenic SL, but some horses have no detectable structural abnormalities. The latter are treated by local infiltration of triamcinolone acetonide (9 to 12 mg) and reduced work. With acute, mild PSD, horses often return to work in 2 to 4 weeks. I also recommend confining the horse to a small area to avoid further damage from excessive uncontrolled exercise. If ultrasonographic abnormalities are detected, the horse is confined to a small area (12- × 30-foot [3.7 × 9.1 m] run) with no riding for 60 to 90 days before reexamination. Complete healing often takes 6 to 12 months, and some horses never return to full athletic function. After the initial 2 weeks of ice therapy, rest, nonsteroidal antiinflammatory drugs, and support bandages, the horse is reevaluated. If the lesion is extensive or severe (type 2 or greater on a scale of 0 to 4), then novel tissue healing therapies such as platelet-rich plasma (PRP) or stem cells are injected into the lesion under ultrasonographic guidance to enhance quality of ligament fiber repair. I have had more experience with PRP and prefer it to stem cell therapy, but both may be beneficial in ligament healing. Hindlimb PSD can be difficult to treat because of the constricting thick fascia surrounding it. If the horse is not sound after 4 to 6 months (depending on severity of lesion) of confinement, then I have had good success performing a fasciotomy and neurectomy of the deep branch of the lateral plantar nerve. Postsurgery care consists of 60 days of stall rest with 20 minutes of daily handwalking and 60 days of controlled exercise program before returning to barrel racing or turnout activity.

PSD is also common in forelimbs. Deep arenas and long toes and low heels are predisposing factors. The prognosis for barrel racing horses with forelimb PSD is good, with most horses responding well to rest and controlled exercise for 3 to 4 months. Tendon protection boots are recommended.

Medial femorotibial joint pain also frequently occurs and is treated in a similar manner as described above for cutting horses (see page 1167). If the lameness is recurrent after several intraarticular injections, diagnostic arthroscopy is recommended. Metacarpophalangeal joint synovitis results in mild lameness (grade 1 to 2 of 5) that is exacerbated by fetlock flexion. The horse often strongly resists fetlock flexion. Lameness and response to fetlock flexion are eliminated by intraarticular analgesia. Radiology is usually negative. The horse is treated with intraarticularly administered triamcinolone acetonide (6 mg) and hyaluronan (20 mg). The problem may or may not recur. If recurrence is frequent, diagnostic arthroscopy is recommended.

Many times horses have undergone several types of alternative therapies (e.g., equipment changes, acupuncture, chiropractic, and herbal therapy) in an attempt to correct the perceived problems before being checked by a veterinarian. Often, for some inexplicable reason, an accurate diagnosis and conventional medical therapy are sought only after failure of these other treatments. Many owners rely on diagnosis from a fellow competitor and request treatment that was successful in another horse. This makes client communication difficult.

SHOEING CONSIDERATIONS

Traction, especially in the deep and often muddy arenas in which horses compete, is critical. A rim shoe is used most commonly on all feet, with one rim higher than the other to provide added traction. A rounded toe provides easier breakover than a normal flat steel shoe. Hind shoes may have square toes.

Recently the natural balance shoe has gained popularity as owners are becoming more aware of good farriery principles and are trying to correct long-toe, low-heel problems. The natural balance shoe is available in steel or aluminum. Steel construction is preferred because of the added weight, which provides better traction than an aluminum shoe. The natural balance shoe has a rockered toe that eases breakover of the forelimb and is built with a wider web than a normal shoe, which benefits a sore-footed horse competing on hard surfaces.

OTHER CONSIDERATIONS

Exercise-induced pulmonary hemorrhage is common in barrel horses. The owner may complain that the horse has lost a step or has become slower. If a musculoskeletal reason for the performance change cannot be determined, a respiratory evaluation is indicated. Obvious bleeding from the nostrils rarely is seen, but endoscopic examination within 30 minutes of the barrel race often reveals tracheal hemorrhage. Presently no drug testing or rules prevent drug administration for competition. Most horses receive phenylbutazone or flunixin meglumine 4 to 6 hours before competition and furosemide (4 to 8 mL/horse).

◼ THE EUROPEAN WESTERN PERFORMANCE HORSE

Franco Ferrero

The Western performance horse sports have developed in Europe, especially in Germany and Italy, since the mid-1980s, with reining and cutting the most popular sports. Most horses are American Quarter Horses (QHs) and are traditionally broken at 18 months of age. The intense training needed to show 3-year-olds in the futurity competitions results in many horses not competing at 4 years of age because of behavioral or lameness problems. In an attempt to reduce injuries, there has been a move to shift bigger purses to 4-year-olds. In addition, the Fédération Équestre Internationale (FEI) has recently acknowledged reining as an official discipline, and only horses 6 years of age or older can compete under FEI rules. This is slowly changing the European approach to training of reining QHs.

There is zero tolerance of any drugs in competing horses, and antidoping testing takes place at most official shows in Europe for both professional and nonprofessional classes. This influences the treatment strategies that can be used for lameness. The strict medication rules also influence advice given concerning purchase of horses with pre-existing lameness problems. Increasing attention is being paid to welfare, and strict rules govern which bits and harness are acceptable. Excessive use of spurs or whips may result in suspension of the rider. Common procedures like hair clipping around a horse's nose and ears are not recommended when competing in Germany.

TEN MOST COMMON LAMENESS CONDITIONS IN 2- TO 8-YEAR-OLD EUROPEAN WESTERN PERFORMANCE HORSES

1. Lameness of the foot
2. Lameness of the hock
3. Superficial digital flexor tendonitis
4. Lameness of the stifle
5. Suspensory desmitis
6. Lameness of the metacarpophalangeal/metatarsophalangeal (fetlock) joint
7. Lameness of the carpus
8. Exostoses of the second metacarpal bones (splints)
9. Curb
10. Fracture of the medial plantar process of the middle phalanx

LAMENESS OF THE FOOT

Common causes of foot pain include subsolar abscessation, solar bruising, osteoarthritis (OA) of the distal interphalangeal (DIP) joint, osteitis or fracture of a palmar process of the distal phalanx, and navicular syndrome. Oblique radiographic images of the palmar (plantar) processes of the distal phalanx and a palmaroproximal-palmarodistal oblique image of the navicular bone are particularly valuable.

Poor foot conformation is often an important predisposing factor for the development of foot pain. The foot is often upright with overgrown angles of the wall and heel, flattening of the sole at the toe, and an underdeveloped frog. Bar shoes exacerbate high heel conformation because they prevent the heel bulbs from sinking into the ground; the bar of the shoe concentrates loading and reaction forces from the ground in the bars and underlying structures inducing palmar foot pain.

In such horses trimming of the bars and wall at the heel increases the length of the loading plane, thus distributing ground reaction forces over a wider area. If the horse works on soft ground, reaction forces on the palmar aspect of the foot can be reduced by applying aluminum shoes with

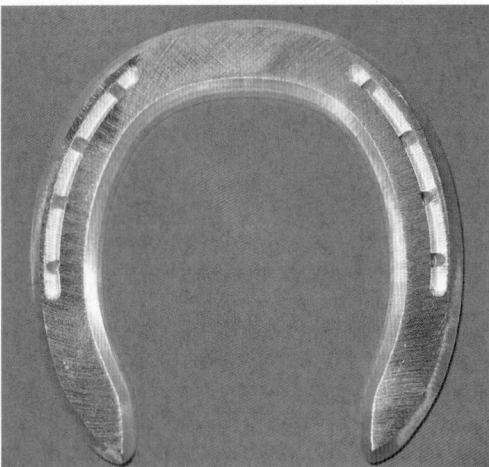

Fig. 120-7 • A typical shoe used in reining horses is made of aluminum and is beveled along the entire outer surface to reduce torsional forces associated with sudden turns and spins.

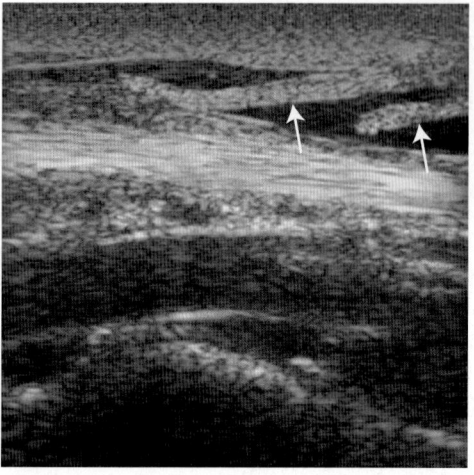

Fig. 120-8 • Longitudinal ultrasonographic image of the long digital extensor tendon sheath on the dorsolateral aspect of the hock. Proximal is to the left. There is extensive echogenic material covering the extensor tendon and echogenic bands (arrows) extending between the tendon and the synovium.

thinned and beveled heels; if the horse works on harder ground, a complete pad must be inserted between the shoe and the foot, and the shoe must be well concaved on the inner surface to prevent direct pressure to the sole through the pad itself. Shearing forces at the toe can be decreased by moving the breakover point back with a rolled-toe shoe.

Most of the top-level reining QHs are now shod with premade aluminum shoes beveled along the entire outer surface (Figure 120-7; Colleoni/Zaffi design, Farrier Product Distribution, Shelbyville, Kentucky, United States). These are available in either an open or bar type. The beveled outer surface helps the foot to breakover in most of the demanding figures (like spins or roll backs) that produce marked oblique and twisting forces on the distal aspect of the limb. A rocker toe shoe or squared toe is used less frequently because it can restrict the length of the stride.

Treatment of reining horses with navicular syndrome during the show season is challenging because of the long detection times of most commonly used drugs either for local injection or for oral use. Horses with navicular syndrome often have long toe and underrun heel conformation. Treatment involves restoration of a more correct hoof-pastern axis and use of an egg bar or bar shoe to increase the loading area of the foot. A bar shoe also prevents the heel from sinking into the ground and reduces tension on the deep digital flexor tendon. Tendon lesions usually occur toward the insertion. Some are detectable ultrasonographically, but magnetic resonance imaging (MRI) is superior for diagnosis.

The hind feet are subject to enormous loading and twisting forces when horses perform quick stops or when spinning or doing a roll back. Reining horses are shod behind with sliding plates (sliders), which are usually kept long at the heels. A long-heeled shoe concentrates load at the angle of the heel and can create resistance to turning.

LAMENESS OF THE HOCK

Lameness associated with tarsocrural joint is infrequent; however, many veterinarians still inject all three compartments of the hock routinely, thus increasing chances of articular reaction and infection.

OA of the distal hock joints is common. In 2-year-olds there is a high prevalence of partial collapse of the central and third tarsal bones with secondary OA. This is usually accompanied by a camped-under, sickle-hocked, or cow-hocked conformation of one or both hindlimbs.

I use a hock torsion test to try to differentiate pain arising from the centrodistal or tarsometatarsal joints. With the hock in a semiflexed position, I apply a medial to lateral rotational force on the longitudinal axis of proximal aspect of the third metatarsal bone. If the horse reacts quickly or tries to kick, this indicates centrodistal joint pain, whereas if the reaction is slower and the horse gradually lifts and abducts the limb, the test suggests tarsometatarsal joint pain. The hock torsion test is not the "Churchill test." When performing the torsion test there must be neither direct compression on the medial aspect of the hock nor any compression of the suspensory ligament (SL).

Treatment of horses with OA of the distal hock joints is by intraarticular administration of corticosteroids and sodium hyaluronan. Care must be taken with withdrawal times for horses competing under FEI rules. Horses refractory to intraarticular medication are treated by surgical (drilling) or chemical (sodium monoiodoacetate or ethyl alcohol) arthrodesis. Arthrodesis is most effective in 2-year-olds.

Tenosynovitis of the long digital extensor tendon sheath on the dorsolateral aspect of the tarsus may result in a shortened cranial phase of the hindlimb stride. Ultrasonographic examination of the sheath may reveal tendon lesions and extensive tenosynovial adhesions (Figure 120-8). Treatment involves intrathecal injection of corticosteroids. If chronic, tenoscopic debridement of adhesions and partial retinacular release are indicated.

SUPERFICIAL DIGITAL FLEXOR TENDONITIS

Acute superficial digital flexor tendonitis is a common cause of lameness in 2-year-old reining and cutting horses. Chronic injuries are seen in older horses that have not received proper treatment of acute lesions. Two groups of

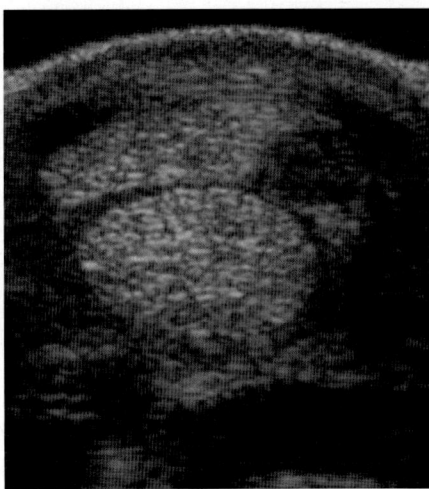

Fig. 120-9 • Transverse ultrasonographic image of the distal metacarpal region of a 3-year-old Quarter Horse filly in full training. Medial is to the left. There is an acute anechogenic lesion of the lateral aspect of the superficial digital flexor tendon, which is swollen.

horses are predisposed to superficial digital flexor tendon (SDFT) injury: (1) young thin-legged Appaloosas, Paints, and QHs with conformation defects such as tied in below the knee, offset knees, and calf knees; and (2) well-built 3-year-old QHs intensely trained, especially working on spins in preparation for the futurity.

Lesions almost invariably affect the most lateral or medial border of the SDFT, usually extending for 3 to 5 cm in the middle or distal third of the metacarpal region, and are seen as diffuse areas of reduced echogenicity (Figure 120-9). Extreme uneven loading of the medial or lateral side of SDFT occurs while the horse is spinning or performing rapid turn backs. To reduce leverage and shearing forces acting on a hoof's quarters in the breakover phase of the spin, top-level reining QHs are currently shod with aluminum shoes beveled along the entire outer surface (see Figure 120-7).

Treatment of horses with acute tendon lesions is aimed at reducing inflammation and edema with rest, cold packs, poultice, stall bandage, oral nonsteroidal antiinflammatory drugs followed by peritendonous injection of low doses of short-acting corticosteroids mixed with antiedema drugs. Intralesional, ultrasound-guided injection of platelet rich plasma (PRP) is performed 10 to 14 days after injury. For acute SDFT lesions in reining or cutting QHs, it is recommended that the horse should not return to full athletic function until at least 8 months after injury.

LAMENESS OF THE STIFLE

Stifle pain is caused by subchondral bone cysts in the medial femoral condyle, traumatic OA, medial collateral ligament injury, osteochondrosis of the femoral trochleas, and fragmentation of the distal aspect of the patella in horses that underwent previous medial patellar desmotomy.

Digital radiography has enhanced the ability to detect subtle alteration in shape of the joint surface of the medial femoral condyle and early changes of subchondral bone opacity in early stages of the disease.

Intraarticular therapy should avoid use of the depot form of corticosteroids because it has been associated with rapid progression of OA and persistent lameness associated with the medial femorotibial joint in reining and cutting QHs. Surgical management of horses with medial femoral condyle cysts using arthroscopically guided injections of methylprednisolone acetate into the cyst lining or curettage results in a 50% to 60% chance for return of the horse to previous level of competition. Rest for 6 to 8 months is mandatory.

SUSPENSORY DESMITIS

Proximal suspensory desmitis (PSD) and desmitis of the branches of the SL are common. PSD affects young reining and cutting QHs in early or advanced training. Lameness is usually intermittent and can vary in intensity from grade 1 to 3 of 5, depending on workload; the horse is lamer with the affected limb on the outside of the circle. Lameness is abolished with analgesia of the lateral palmar nerve. Subtle ultrasonographic changes can be difficult to identify, and comparison with the contralateral limb is useful. Radiology is useful for identification of increased opacity in the proximal aspect of the third metacarpal/metatarsal bone.

Treatment of horses with PSD is based on rest, intralesional injection of PRP, shock wave therapy, radiotherapy/hyperthermia (INDIBA, Sant Cugat del Vallés, Barcelona, Spain). Corrective shoeing comprises an open aluminum shoe wide at the toe and thinned and beveled at the heels. A horse with an uncomplicated PSD lesion requires 90 days of convalescence. The presence of increased bone opacity at the origin of the SL is a poor prognostic indicator, with many horses remaining chronically lame.

Desmitis of a branch of the SL is frequently induced by medial-to-lateral foot imbalance; the wall is lower on the lateral side, and this induces more tensile stress on the lateral branch of the SL. Affected horses often have an offset knee or carpus valgus/fetlock varus and toe-in conformation.

Ultrasonographic examination often reveals hypoechogenic lesions of the most axial part of the branch. Therapy consists of periligamentous injection of corticosteroids and antiedema drugs and intraarticular treatment of the fetlock joint. Horses with chronic branch desmitis are treated with shock wave therapy, hyperthermia, controlled exercise, and repeated local application of working blisters. Shoeing correction involves the use of an open aluminum shoe with wider web on the side of the injured SL branch and balancing the foot.

LAMENESS OF THE FETLOCK JOINT

Osteochondrosis is frequent in front and hind fetlock joints. Most lesions in the dorsal aspect of the joint involve the sagittal ridge of the third metacarpal (McIII) or metatarsal (MtIII) bones, whereas lesions of the palmar (plantar) aspect originate from palmar (plantar) processes of the proximal phalanx.

OA of the fetlock joint is frequently accompanied by insertional desmitis of the SL branches or desmitis of the SL body at the level of its bifurcation. Both the fetlock joint and the SL must be treated for a successful outcome.

Chronic synovitis may result in supracondylar lysis in 2-year-old QHs. Scintigraphy can be useful for identification of increased radiopharmaceutical uptake in the palmar aspect of the condyles of the third metacarpal bone, reflecting bone trauma in horses with no detectable radiological abnormality.

Western performance horses with early fetlock joint OA are managed using serial intraarticular injections with sodium hyaluronan, polysulfated glycosaminoglycans or interleukin-1 receptor antagonist protein (autologous conditioned serum). The prognosis is good. However, if there is thinning of articular cartilage and subchondral bone sclerosis or the presence of cystic lesions in the distal aspect of the condyles of the third metacarpal or metatarsal bones, the prognosis is poor, irrespective of medical or surgical treatment.

LAMENESS OF THE CARPUS

Faulty conformation of the carpi is often present, especially offset knees. Lesions of the carpus include OA of the antebrachiocarpal and middle carpal joints, self-induced trauma of either the accessory carpal bone or the dorsal aspect of the carpus incurred during hard spinning, tenosynovitis of the carpal sheath, chip fractures of the radial or third carpal bones, increased radiopacity (sclerosis) of the radial facet of the third carpal bone, or sagittal fracture.

Sclerosis and sagittal fracture of the third carpal bone are the result of shearing forces caused by uneven loading of the medial aspect of the third carpal bone produced by repeated spinning and galloping in small circles.

EXOSTOSIS OF THE SECOND OR FOURTH METACARPAL/METATARSAL BONES (SPLINTS)

Medial splints are common in 2-year-old reining and cutting QHs, frequently associated with a carpus valgus or offset knee conformation; lateral splints are less common but are occasionally seen in horses with an offset third metacarpal bone and base-narrow conformation.

Splints usually produce transient lameness, but horses with chronic lameness can be managed by freeze firing to reduce local pain and lameness. Shin splints—bony swelling on the proximal dorsomedial aspect of the McIII—are occasionally seen in very hard-stopping horses. The swelling is caused by periosteal and endosteal reaction to microfractures produced by repeated compression cycles of the dorsal cortex of the MtIII. Treatment is rest and handwalking for 30 to 45 days and freeze firing to reduce swelling and pain.

CURB

Curb is seen in 2-year-old QHs that have a sickle-hocked/cow-hocked conformation as a result of partial collapse of cuboidal hock bones. Ultrasonographic examination helps to determine which tendonous or ligamentous structure is involved and to decide the appropriate treatment.

FRACTURE OF THE PLANTAR PROCESS OF THE MIDDLE PHALANX

A fracture of the medial plantar process of the middle phalanx is the result of an avulsion caused by extreme pulling of the distal enthesis of the insertion of the SDFT during a stop. The tension in the medial branch of the SDFT may be the result of the wide stance of the hindlimbs that some horses adopt during the last phase of a sliding stop.

Shoeing should aim to correct horses that stop too wide by an inward rotation of the shoe or by applying medial heel extensions (trailers). Surgical management of horses with this middle phalangeal fracture by internal fixation with compression screws has had disappointing results. Prognosis is also poor following digital neurectomy and prolonged rest. Arthrodesis of the proximal interphalangeal joint might be a better choice.

◼ THE RACING QUARTER HORSE

See Chapter 110.

Chapter 121

Walking Horses

James T. Blackford and James C. Sternberg

DESCRIPTION OF THE SPORT

The Tennessee Walking Horse, commonly called the *Walking Horse,* is a light horse breed developed in middle Tennessee for use on southern plantations during the eighteenth century. The average Walking Horse is 15 to 16 hands tall and weighs 500 to 600 kg. The Tennessee Walking Horse is a composite breed, created by crossbreeding Canadian and Narragansett Pacers and Morgan,

Standardbred, and Thoroughbred horses. The Tennessee Walking Horse Breeders' and Exhibitors' Association was formed in 1935. Because of the versatility of the Walking Horse, along with a characteristic racking gait within the breed, a second breed association was recognized in 1971, the Racking Horse Breeders' Association. Members of this group of horses are commonly referred to as *Racking Horses.*

A Walking Horse performs three gaits: the flat-foot walk, running walk, and canter. Both walks are four-beat gaits, with one foot up and three feet in various phases of striking the ground. The footfall sequence is left hind, left front, right hind, and right front. High-stepping forelimbs with an extended reach characterize the flat-foot walk. The hind foot overreaches the imprint of the front foot by 15 to 55 cm in a straight, smooth, gliding motion. This overstride is unique to the breed and is referred to as the *big lick.* The horse's head and neck nod, and the ears flick forward and backward in rhythmical fashion with the rise and fall of the front feet. The appearance is that of pulling with the forelimbs and driving or pushing with the hindlimbs. The speed of the flat-foot walk is from 4 to 8 miles per hour (6.4 to 12.8 km per hour). At the running walk, the gait is basically the same but faster (10 to 20 mph [16 to 32 km/h]). The canter is a three-beat gait, with a left or right lead. In the canter the horse lifts the forehand, giving an easy rise and fall, in a rolling motion. The gait is referred to commonly as the *rocking-chair canter* because of the high, rolling movement of the horse's body.

The Racking Horse gait is a bilateral four-beat gait, with one foot striking the ground with the other three limbs in various phases of elevation. The gait often is referred to as the *single-foot gait*. When shown, a Racking Horse performs the show walk, slow rack, and fast rack. The show walk is a smooth, collected, slow and easy four-beat gait. At the slow rack the horse's head is held with the neck arched and ears erect. The fast rack is similar in form to the slow rack, but the horse displays speed and leg action. The natural head nod must not be exaggerated at the slow or fast rack.

In both breeds the collected gaits of a show horse (a gaited horse in performance shoes and tack) shift the center of gravity caudally, compared with most other light breeds, with increased loads on the hindlimbs resulting in a high incidence of hindlimb lameness.

Both breeds are used for show, trail, and pleasure riding. Horses are shown at halter, in harness, and under tack, with English or Western saddles. Horses that are shown wear a light shoe similar to a standard keg shoe, a plantation shoe, or a performance shoe, depending on the class. The plantation shoe cannot exceed 3.8 cm in width and 1.3 cm in thickness, and the heel calk cannot exceed 2.5 cm in height. The performance shoe, or stack, is a shoeing technique used to accentuate the show horse gaits. The shoe is constructed of several layers of flat or wedge pads, stacked one on top of another, placed between a nail pad at the solar margin and a metal shoe on the contact surface. Pads are made of leather, plastic, or hard rubber. The amount of height or extension the shoe provides must not exceed 50% of the natural hoof wall length, measured from the coronary band to the tip of the toe. Pleasure horses are commonly flat shod.

Although the highest population of Walking and Racking Horses is presently in the southeast United States, they are becoming more popular across North America, especially for trail and pleasure riding, because of the physical endurance and gentle disposition of the breeds. The show season generally is considered to be year-round, picking up in the spring and peaking in the fall with the national championships. The Tennessee Walking Horse National Celebration is held in Shelbyville, Tennessee, each year and is an 11-day event ending with the crowning of the national champions on the Saturday before Labor Day. The Racking Horse Celebration is held each year in Decatur, Alabama, during the last 2 weeks in September.

LAMENESS EXAMINATION

Lameness evaluation of a gaited horse is best performed with the horse under complete tack with a rider. It is impossible to duplicate the head set, balance, and shifting of the horse's center of gravity caudally without a rider. The horses generally exercise in a large, oval arena, and to perform a good evaluation, one needs to provide a place where the horse has room to work in all gaits. The ground surface in this area should be firm. A veterinarian's impression when evaluating a show horse for the first time will be that the horse's problem must be in the forelimb and more specifically the foot. In light of the negative publicity the stacked shoe receives, focusing one's attention on this area is easy. Even as the horse is walked at halter, this impression may not change, because of the awkward nature of the horse handling the bulky shoe. In our experience, few problems are associated directly with the shoe, except hoof wall avulsions, when the shoe is accidentally pulled off in the show ring. Measures to control bleeding must be taken immediately, followed by good wound care. Hoof wall composites then can be used to restore hoof wall function. If an elevated shoe is removed completely and suddenly from an immature, developing horse early in training, removal causes a dynamic mechanical flexural deformity. The horse knuckles over at the fetlock joint because of the pain associated with pulling of the deep and superficial digital flexor tendons.

Unfamiliarity with the standard gaits of Walking and Racking Horses, especially when shod with a stacked shoe, may result in confusion with ataxia, particularly at faster speeds. However, anecdotally, our impression is that a high incidence of cervical vertebral malformation does indeed occur in Tennessee Walking Horses, so this should be kept in mind.

Tennessee Walking Horses are stoic and seem to have a high pain tolerance. Problems encountered in flat-shod Walkers or Rackers mirror the lameness problems seen in other light breeds; therefore the following discussion focuses on show horses in stacked shoes. The hoof tester evaluation is of limited value on the front feet of performance-shod horses. Careful palpation and manipulation of the limbs are performed routinely. Careful evaluation of the foot and shoe should not be overlooked. Use of pressure-shoeing techniques by unscrupulous owners and trainers causes soreness and increases the big lick, conditions that occasionally arise in a performance-shod horse and should not be overlooked. The technique is performed by overtrimming the hoof wall and thus increasing sole pressure. A carefully placed nail in the nail pad encroaching on the sole or the sensitive laminae may be noted. A foreign object, such as a stone inserted between the pad and the sole, inflicts discomfort. Assessment of digital pulse amplitudes, tapping on the hoof wall with hoof testers or a shoeing hammer, and response to nerve blocks may determine the problem.

Problems seen in the forelimbs commonly are associated with imbalances in the shoeing, leading to an uneven height of the forelimb carriage. To evaluate the forelimb carriage, the observer should draw an imaginary line at the chest level, watching the carpal action to determine which leg is carried lower to the imaginary line as the limb advances, indicating the problem limb. When this problem is detected, careful evaluation of the shoeing technique and comparison between limbs are indicated. Correction of foot imbalance may resolve the problem. Osteoarthritis of the distal interphalangeal joint (low ringbone) frequently is seen in older horses but is not always correlated with lameness. Proximal suspensory desmitis usually is caused by slipping while shod with an elevated shoe and may be associated with localized pain on palpation. Bicipital bursitis is seen occasionally. The horse may have asymmetry in shoulder motion and pain on palpation of the area, especially when the limb is raised. Abduction or adduction of the shoulder is performed. As in most breeds, sole abscesses are common in flat- or performance-shod horses, as is laminitis.

The highest percentage of lameness seen in our practice with Walking and Racking Horses is associated with the hindlimbs, because of loading of the hindlimbs during exercise. As each hindlimb strikes the ground and the horse's weight is carried through the stride, a rotational, twisting motion also is seen throughout the entire limb before the leg is advanced. This is especially noticeable in the Walking Horse at the faster gaits. The shifting weight and the twisting motion increase stress on the joints and surrounding support structures. Osteoarthritis of the distal hock joints and stifle is common. A positive response to the Churchill test is helpful in isolating pain to the distal hock joints. Careful palpation of the medial patellar ligament is particularly important in this type of sports horse, because at one time almost all of the show horses were subjected to medial patellar desmotomy with hopes of

improving the overreaching stride of the rear legs. Although the medial patellar desmotomy site only occasionally is found to be the origin of the lameness in these horses, the possibility should not be overlooked. The practice is not as common today as in the past; however, many trainers from the old school feel that having the desmotomy performed is important. Upper- and lower-limb flexion tests are performed. Local analgesia is used to define the source of pain. Trochanteric bursitis occurs in Walking and Racking Horses and is related to the rotational, twisting motion of the hindlimbs. The horse has pain on deep palpation over the greater trochanter of the femur, during upper limb flexion tests, and when the hip is stretched forward or backward, abducted or adducted, and rotated.

Other conditions are encountered in these horses. Some have muscular weakness in the hindlimbs, especially young unconditioned horses. When weakness is combined with straight hindlimbs, instability of the patella is common. Chronic hip and stifle soreness caused by a trailer on the outside of the shoe may be an underlying cause of lameness. Osteochondrosis occurs in the forelimbs and hindlimbs. We see a substantial number of horses that are thought to be lame but have equine protozoal myelitis.

Chapter 122

Lameness in the American Saddlebred and Other Trotting Breeds with Collection

Scott D. Bennett

DESCRIPTION OF THE SPORT

The American Saddlebred, Morgan, Hackney Pony, National Show Horse, and Arabian (see Chapter 123) show horses are described as *trotting breeds with collection*. Lameness in disciplines such as dressage, road horses, and road ponies is similar. The American Saddlebred and National Show Horse have five gaits: walk, trot, canter, slow gait, and rack. The slow gait and rack are manmade gaits. These horses also perform in three gaited classes (walk, trot, and canter), fine harness classes, pleasure driving, pleasure-gaited classes, and equitation. Morgan and Arabian horses are shown similarly, but without the slow gait or rack. Hackney ponies are shown in harness, pleasure driving, and road pony classes. Show classes are further divided for professional, amateur, and juvenile riders. Equitation, hunt seat, Western, and numerous young horse and in-hand halter classes are available.

In road horse classes, Standardbreds, Morgans, American Saddlebreds, or Standardbred-cross horses are shown

at the walk, trot, and road gait pulling a bike similar to a sulky used for Standardbred racehorses. These horses usually are more animated in gait than Standardbred racehorses and go both ways around the ring when performing. The road gait is a high-speed performance gait.

To understand lameness in a gaited show horse, the veterinarian must first understand the difference in locomotion between running and gaited horse disciplines. Concussion (impact) is a part of every gait. How a horse distributes concussion is related directly to athletic ability and the longevity of the horse's career. Better equine athletes are more efficient in the distribution of concussion through the limbs and body. A superior equine athlete appears capable of using energy of concussion efficiently and distributing it for dispersion and recovery. Normally kinetic or stored energy from proper distribution of concussion causes recoil of the tissues receiving the energy of concussion. Tissue injury results in an inability to disperse concussive energy properly. Maintaining healthy hoof wall, bone, cartilage, tendons, ligaments, and muscles in a good conditioning and gait management program is essential. A veterinarian must be familiar with the gaits, because gait analysis is an important part of evaluating poor performance and subtle lameness. Many times a veterinarian may be dealing with a gait abnormality caused by the bit, saddle fit, or faulty shoeing rather than lameness.

Gaits of show horses are complex and must be synchronous to maintain distribution of concussion. Synchrony must be achieved in up to five gaits and is altered by the different gait specifications. Unlike most other horses the normal load distribution between forelimbs and hindlimbs in a show horse is about 35% and 65%, respectively (see Chapter 2). A show horse does not have to perform at racing speed. Synchrony of concussion and weight distribution are totally different compared with many sports horses, and because much concussion is dispersed through the hindlimbs, hindlimb lameness is more prevalent. In some other sports horses the head and neck are raised and lowered with the stride, a movement that assists in balance, energy distribution, and propulsion. A show horse, like a dressage horse, maintains a fixed and flexed head and neck carriage. This further shifts the balance and energy of concussion to the hindlimbs.

Show horses carry more body weight for a fleshier look than the greyhound-like racing counterparts. Riders of show horses, as a rule, also are heavier than racing jockeys.

Longevity of show horses compared with racehorses is related directly to speed of performance, which is dramatically less. Racehorses must change energy distribution at high speed quickly, potentially leading to catastrophic breakdown, but such actions and injuries in show horses are rare. A show horse often can remain competitive into the late teens and early twenties, but chronic wear and tear may result in lameness.

Although show horses do not perform at speed, high head carriage and high limb action and motion are strenuous. Show horses perform numerous gait changes and transitions going in both directions of the ring, and for a high-level (stake class) five-gaited class to last from 30 to 40 minutes is not unusual.

Because five-gaited movements and transitions are complex and arduous, compensatory lameness is common. A methodical approach to lameness diagnosis must be used to differentiate primary and compensatory lameness. A superior show horse distinctly separates its different gait movements, raising each carpus above the horizontal, with a high hock action. The horse drives off its hindlimbs with a flexed high head and neck carriage. Responsiveness to the bit, with an alert expression and attitude, and forward placement of the ears are desirable. Just as racehorses are bred for speed, show horses are bred for animated motion.

AMERICAN SADDLEBRED

The American Saddlebred has a long history and aptitude for different gaits and is derived from many different lineages. The breed was developed in a young country where the best horses could be bred to the best. The American Saddlebred was developed as a horse of usefulness and beauty that could work in the field, pull a buggy or carriage, and have gaits that were smooth for travel under saddle.

The ability of the American Saddlebred to perform lateral gaits (slow gait and rack) came from the Narragansett pacers, which were among the earliest known easy-riding pacers. The Narragansett pacers were derived from French Canadian pacers of Arabian and Andalusian descent that were bred 100 to 200 years before the American Revolutionary War and had a comfortable saddle gait. Early settlers brought these horses, known as *saddlers*, to Kentucky. During the late 1830s and 1840s, many of these easy-riding saddlers were bred to the Thoroughbred foundation sires Denmark and Montrose. These crossbreeds were then bred to horses of trotting blood, from which the Standardbred breed was developed. Offspring of these crosses became favorite mounts of cavalry during the Civil War because they had an easy gait, versatility, and an ability to withstand the pressures of war. On April 7, 1891,

the American Saddlebred Breeders Association was founded in Louisville, Kentucky, and became the first all-American breed registry. In recent years the American Saddlebred has gained popularity in South Africa and has been crossed with European Warmblood and carriage bloodlines (e.g., Dutch Carriage Horse). During the 1980s, the National Show Horse was derived from American Saddlebred and Arabian lineage.

The American Saddlebred ranges in height from 152 to 178 cm (15 to 17.2 hands; average 160 cm [15.3 hands]) and varies in weight from 455 to 545 kg. Colors include chestnut, bay, black, gray, golden (palomino), and spotted (chestnut, black, or bay mixed with white). As described in *Modern Breeds of Livestock*[1]:

References on page 1345

> [The] American Saddlebred has a strikingly long neck and considerable arch to the neck. The American Saddlebred is refined in appearance; has long, sloping pasterns that give spring to the stride; has a long, level croup; is strong and short-coupled; and has a back with high, well-defined withers above the level of the hips. The American Saddlebred is famous for refinement, smoothness, proportion, and a beautiful and handsome presentation and projects an alert, curious, expressive personality.

There are shows for American Saddlebreds throughout the United States and South Africa. The World Championship Horse Show is held each year in Louisville, Kentucky. Shows are run under the guidelines of USA Equestrian, which establishes rules, regulations, and drug-testing procedures. A veterinarian must be aware of current drug and medication rules, and failure to do so may result in fines and penalties to the horse, owner, and trainer.

SADDLEBRED GAITS

The five gaits of the American Saddlebred and other gaited horses are as follows[2]:

1. *Walk and flat walk*—The flat walk is a relaxed, elastic, ground-covering, and collected four-beat gait, maintaining proper form and consistency in stride. The gait is required in pleasure classes. The animated walk is a highly collected gait, exhibiting much primp at a slow, regulated speed, with good action and animation. The gait can be a two- or four-beat gait and is performed with great style, elegance, and airiness of motion.

2. *Trot*—The trot is a natural, diagonal two-beat gait. A balanced trot features coordinated motion with straight, true shoulder motion of forelimbs, with flexing hocks carried close together. The gait is executed in a highly collected manner and should display the horse's athletic ability.

3. *Slow gait*—The slow gait was developed from the pace to be a four-beat gait with each of the feet striking the ground separately. In the takeoff the ipsilateral front foot and hind foot start almost together, but the hind foot contacts the ground first. The slow gait is a highly collected gait, with most of the propulsion coming from the hindquarters, whereas the forequarters assist in the pull of the final beats. The slow gait is not a medium rack. The slow gait is a restrained gait, executed slowly, but with true and distinct precision, and speed is penalized. The gait is

high, lofty, brilliant, and restrained, denoting the style, grace, and polish of the horse.

4. *Rack*—The rack is a four-beat gait in which each foot meets the ground at equal, separate intervals. The gait is smooth and highly animated, performed with great action and speed in a slightly unrestrained manner. Desired speed and collection are determined by the maximum rate at which a horse can rack in form. Racking in form should include the horse remaining with a good set head and should be performed by the horse in an effortless manner from the slow gait, at which point all strides become equally rapid and regular. Any tendency to become trotty, pacey, or hitchy-gaited is penalized.

5. *Canter*—The canter is slow, lofty, and fluid, with a definite three-beat cadence. High action, a good way of going, and proper collection are paramount. The propulsion is in the hindquarters, with the leading forelimb sustaining the concussion of the final third beat. A brief interval occurs when all feet are off the ground. The gait is an ambidextrous gait, executed on the lead that is toward the center of the ring to relieve stress and aid in balance.

LAMENESS EXAMINATION

The history of lameness and poor performance must be discussed with the trainer and rider to seek their perception. This should include noting any problems with the bridle and the way a horse pulls on the bit and bridle. Show horses with hindlimb lameness often fight the bit and try to lower the head, an observation known as *diving in the bit*. Horses that become one-sided in the bit may have contralateral hindlimb or ipsilateral forelimb lameness. Faulty bit and bridle placement may cause gait abnormalities, particularly of the hindlimbs. Keeping the head up and fixed in position in a horse that dives in the bit is difficult. A horse with forelimb lameness is more likely to raise up out of the bridle. A horse cannot produce a gait properly or do proper gait transitions when being pushed into an uncomfortable bridle or if the rider is using the bit improperly. It is important to determine if the rider is using the bit to balance the horse or himself or herself. A rider using the bit poorly can induce a gait abnormality. Bit and bridle responsiveness is often a wild card that must be played during examination of a show horse for gait abnormalities and lameness.

Problems with a particular gait may indicate the source of lameness. Back pain is seen in horses that have difficulty in the canter, a condition known as *being broke in the middle*. This occurs with asynchronous movement of the forelimbs and hindlimbs. Broke in the middle also can be caused by stifle pain that causes a reduction in the cranial phase of the stride. Most commonly, however, broke in the middle is caused by stringhalt. Stringhalt prevents the limb from moving forward at a time when the forelimbs are required to go faster, causing a mismatch in synchronization between the forelimbs and hindlimbs. Distal hock joint pain and back pain can cause a hitching motion of the hindlimbs, jerking the lame limb caudally and leaving the hocks behind the motion.

Examination first begins in a stall before the horse is worked. Careful palpation with emphasis on the tendons,

ligaments, joint capsules, and bulbs of the heels should be performed. Palpation of the back and gluteal muscles before working is important, because the horse can warm out of soreness in these areas. Digital pulse amplitudes should be assessed.

The horse should be evaluated during movement under tack. Harness horses, road horses, and ponies should be examined while working with and without the overcheck (checked up and without the check). Five- and three-gaited horses should be examined performing each gait going in both directions. Often horses are lame only while going in one direction or only in the turns. Horses with lameness from the hock distally are often worse with the lame limb on the inside, whereas those with pain located more proximally are lame with the lame limb on the outside of the turn. Forelimb lameness is usually worse with the affected limb on the inside.

In most show horses flexion tests can be performed with a rider or in harness. The horse's temperament may make this difficult, but I find that the horse being ridden or jogged in a cart after flexion is helpful.

DIAGNOSTIC ANALGESIA

Diagnostic analgesia in show horses is similar to that described for other sports horses. I start distally and work proximally.

IMAGING CONSIDERATIONS

Conventional and computed or digital radiography are used extensively. Scintigraphy is most useful in horses with complex lameness, because primary and compensatory issues are difficult to differentiate. The solar scintigraphic image is mandatory to evaluate horses with palmar foot pain in which radiographs are negative, and may reveal evidence of abnormal modeling of either the navicular bone or the distal phalanx. Areas of increased radiopharmaceutical uptake in the distal phalanx may indicate excessive pressure that can be relieved by corrective shoeing. Thermography is of value in diagnosing tendonitis, sole pressure, muscle inflammation, and suspensory desmitis. Ultrasonographic examination is useful to confirm and assess damaged soft tissues and healing. Diagnostic arthroscopy is used occasionally.

Magnetic resonance imaging (MRI) has added hugely to the ability to diagnose and differentiate difficult lameness problems. Evaluation of the soft tissues, ligaments, and tendons of the feet, fetlocks, hocks, carpus, and stifles has created a quantum leap in the ability to diagnose bone, cartilage, and soft tissue injury.

SHOEING GAITED HORSES

Shoeing gaited horses to assist with motion and gait transitions is an art form in itself. In general a long toe and high heel in front help to delay breakover and cause high knee action. In the past, weighted shoes and lead weights screwed into the bottom of shoe pads were used to induce animation. In recent years a transition to "lighter is better" has occurred, and now the focus is on fitness and training techniques to teach a horse to elevate its limbs to achieve animation. Shoeing depends to a great extent on a horse's ability, conformation, and desired gait performance (e.g., five-gaited, three-gaited, or harness). For example, a three-gaited horse may have a long foot with long toe and heel length to delay breakover in the forefeet and hindfeet. This gives the extreme highly animated knee and hock action expected from a top three-gaited horse. In contrast, in a five-gaited horse a lower hind heel angle is used to assist with a longer hindlimb stride needed for the slow gait and rack. Compared with three-gaited horses, lighter and shorter front feet are maintained in five-gaited horses to promote speed at the trot and rack.

Shoeing with high heels and long toes, with or without pads, predisposes the American Saddlebred to a contracted heel, sheared heel, and quarter cracks. The recent use of cushion polymer compounds to maintain frog pressure is helpful, because frog pressure is lost with high heels and pads. Cushioned polymers placed in the collateral sulci (grooves) of the heel and over an atrophied frog have dramatically reduced hoof problems. Medial-to-lateral hoof balance is paramount.

TEN MOST COMMON LAMENESS CONDITIONS

The 10 most common lameness conditions in show horses are the following:
1. Distal hock joint pain (tarsitis)
2. Gluteal myositis and back pain
3. Palmar foot pain, including contracted heel, sheared heel, quarter cracks, navicular syndrome, tears of the deep digital flexor tendon, and injury of the distal sesamoidean impar ligament
4. Osteitis of the distal phalanx (pedal osteitis)
5. Osteoarthritis and osteochondrosis of the tarsocrural joint
6. Osteoarthritis and osteochondrosis of the fetlock joint
7. Osteoarthritis and osteochondrosis of the stifle joint
8. Suspensory desmitis
9. Tendonitis and desmitis, including deep digital flexor tendonitis, superficial digital flexor tendonitis, and desmitis of the accessory ligament of the deep digital flexor tendon
10. Splint exostosis

SPECIFIC LAMENESS CONDITIONS

Distal Hock Joint Pain and Distal Tarsitis

There are two types of show horses: those that have distal hock joint pain and those that are getting it. Show horses with distal hock joint pain typically jerk the hindlimb caudally (hitching) and leave the hocks behind in motion. Many horses stab the toe, rather than landing normally with the heel first.

Distal hock joint pain without radiological abnormality is common in 2- and early 3-year-olds just starting to rack. As training and showing proceed, radiological evidence of osteoarthritis (OA), such as loss of joint space and periarticular osteophytes, can become apparent as early as 5 years of age and may be severe by 12 years of age.

The tarsometatarsal joint is by far the most valuable point of intraarticular injection in show horses. Occasionally, injection of the centrodistal (distal intertarsal) joint also is required. I prefer to use hyaluronan and a low-dose

corticosteroid combination and recommend oral supplementation with glucosamine and chondroitin sulfate–containing products. Magnetic therapy appears beneficial in horses with early onset of pathology. Horses with lameness that does not improve are considered candidates for shock wave therapy and/or treatment with interleukin-1 receptor antagonist protein (IRAP). Arthrodesis of the distal hock joints, using a drilling technique combined with laser ablation, is recommended in horses with severe pain or evidence of osteonecrosis of the distal tarsal bones detected radiologically or possibly earlier using MRI.

Although cunean tenectomy was once widely used, effects of the procedure are short-lived, and I do not recommend it. If a horse is hitching through the turns of a show ring, a 45° flat outside trailer is used on the hind shoe for support. The shoe is set back, and the toe is squared or rolled to improve breakover.

Gluteal Myositis and Back Pain

Show horses are prone to gluteal myositis and back pain, which are often secondary to primary distal hock joint pain. A willing horse hyperflexes its back to compensate for lower hindlimb pain. The middle gluteal muscle passes over the greater trochanter of the femur and the trochanteric bursa. Gluteal myositis and tendonitis are common sequelae to distal limb pain, but they can cause primary lameness. Trochanteric bursitis (whorl bone disease) can accompany gluteal myositis.

In horses with subacute gluteal myositis, upper limb flexion may stretch the gluteal muscles and produce a transient improvement in gait. Transient improvement may be seen by gently massaging the greater trochanter and gluteal muscles. However, in horses with chronic myositis with involvement of the trochanteric bursa, deep massage and pressure may make lameness worse. Horses with subacute primary gluteal myositis commonly have a tightrope trot (plaiting). Plaiting is associated with distraction and rotation of the hindlimb, with subsequent lateral movement of the hip, motion that may cause gluteal muscle strain. Horses that plait usually have base-narrow conformation, and corrective trimming in the form of spreading the stance (lowering the outside hoof walls) may help.

Back pain is identified easily using digital pressure along the thoracolumbar region, abaxial to the spinous processes. Many horses are in so much pain that one can almost put them on the ground with digital pressure. Diagnostic analgesia usually is not necessary. However, small amounts of local anesthetic solution injected at numerous sites along the affected muscles may give enough relief to allow evaluation for lameness that has been hidden by back or gluteal pain.

Management of horses with gluteal myositis and back pain requires a multifaceted approach, including local injection of Sarapin and corticosteroids. In most horses nonsteroidal antiinflammatory drugs (NSAIDs), methocarbamol, electrical stimulation, magnetic therapy, therapeutic ultrasound, and anticoncussion saddle pads are used in various combinations. Exercise regimens using stretching and flexing during the warm-up period are also beneficial. Acupuncture and chiropractic modalities often are used and can be of benefit if performed by skilled practitioners. Extracorporeal shock wave therapy (ESWT), with or without intramuscular injection of a combination of

Sarapin, dimethyl sulfoxide (DMSO), and a low dose corticosteroid, is effective for immediate relief. Diagnosis and treatment of primary lameness problems, if present, are of utmost importance.

Palmar Foot Pain

Because show horses are shod intentionally with a high heel and long toe to produce high motion, they are prone to a contracted and/or sheared heel. Full or wedge pads are often applied to achieve the desired motion, and the lack of frog pressure can cause atrophy of the soft tissues of the heel. Without proper frog support, the bulbs of the heel contract and a sheared heel often develops. As the heel contracts or a sheared heel develops, more stress is applied to the quarters, predisposing the hooves to quarter cracks. Differentiation of causes of palmar foot pain is critical but difficult, because palmar digital analgesia affects these conditions and navicular syndrome similarly.

Recently more concern has arisen about maintaining frog pressure. Soft, acrylic polymers are now used for frog support in horses with frog atrophy. Turnout for several months, during which the horse is barefoot, may help. Expansion springs can be used to assist in reestablishing proper heel conformation. Severe quarter cracks are repaired using a lacing technique, applying screw compression plates, or nailing. Floating the heel bulb and quarter located under the crack is important to reduce weight bearing, allowing showing to continue.

Navicular disease is not uncommon, but in horses without abnormal radiological findings the diagnosis should be confirmed using scintigraphy. The aforementioned conditions of the hoof capsule and supporting soft tissues are much more common.

Treatment of soft tissue causes of palmar foot pain involves maintaining comfort while proper anatomy is reestablished. Corrective shoeing, NSAIDs, and long-term foot blocks often are used. If navicular disease is confirmed, intraarticular treatment of the distal interphalangeal (DIP) joint using hyaluronan and corticosteroids is recommended. Drugs aimed at improving peripheral perfusion or decreasing intraosseous pressure such as isoxsuprine may be useful with NSAIDs, long-term foot blocks, and corrective shoeing. ESWT appears promising in managing palmar foot pain.

MRI has been particularly beneficial for differentiating navicular disease, navicular bone cystic disease, deep digital flexor (DDF) tendonitis (see Chapter 32), adhesions of the DDF tendon (DDFT), distal sesamoidean impar desmitis, cartilage defects of the DIP joint, disruptions of the laminae and hoof capsule, and hemorrhage or abscessation of the structures of the foot. Blood flow studies using MRI contrast techniques are invaluable for evaluation of circulatory disturbances of the foot.

Osteitis of the Distal Phalanx

In horses with high stepping gaits the distal phalanx is prone to injury. Trauma to the solar margin such as bruising and fracture occurs. A careful evaluation for improper sole pressure or medial-to-lateral hoof imbalance should be performed. Well-exposed and well-positioned radiographs are essential. Digital venography may reveal compression of blood vessels within the hoof capsule and is useful to pinpoint a location of trauma.

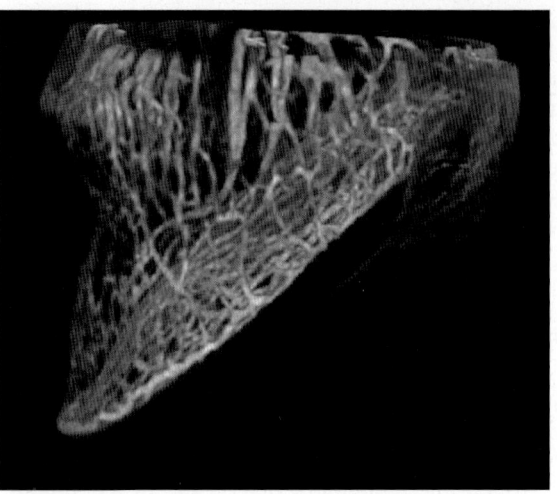

Fig. 122-1 • Sagittal T1-weighted magnetic resonance contrast venogram in a normal horse, produced using three-dimensional reconstruction after soft tissue and bone subtraction techniques were applied.

Fractures of the distal phalanx are rare. Solar scintigraphic images are useful to diagnose fractures and other areas of distal phalangeal trauma and can help to formulate a corrective shoeing plan. Thermography may be useful for diagnosis of distal phalanx trauma.

For horses without distal phalangeal fracture, management includes corrective balancing and shoeing to relieve improper sole pressure and to provide support, NSAIDs, and isoxsuprine. If effusion of the DIP joint is present, intraarticular treatment with hyaluronan and corticosteroids, or IRAP is beneficial.

MRI of the distal phalanx may identify evidence of bone contusions. MRI blood flow contrast studies are more accurate than standing venograms and a computerized three-dimensional rotation can be accomplished with soft tissue and bone subtraction (Figure 122-1).

Osteoarthritis and Osteochondrosis of the Tarsocrural Joint

Lameness of the tarsocrural joint is not as common as distal hock joint pain. Osteochondrosis of the tarsocrural joint in show horses is similar to that described for other sports horses. The most common location is the cranial aspect of the intermediate ridge of the tibia. Although show horses with osteochondrosis lesions may compete successfully without surgical intervention, effusion and capsulitis are indications that surgery should be performed. Prognosis after arthroscopic surgery is favorable. However, prognosis for show horses with osteochondrosis lesions of the trochlear ridges of the talus is guarded. Osteophytes and small fragments of the distal aspect of the medial trochlear ridge are not a major source of lameness.

The diagnosis of OA of the tarsocrural joint is derived from the results of physical examination, flexion tests, diagnostic analgesia, radiography, nuclear scintigraphy, and MRI. Horses with early OA of the tarsocrural joint are managed with intraarticular injections of hyaluronan, with or without corticosteroids. Oral supplementation with glucosamine and chondroitin sulfate–containing compounds appears beneficial. Intramuscular and intravenous administration of polysulfated glycosaminoglycans and hyaluronan, respectively, are helpful. NSAIDs may be necessary. Horses with chronically distended tarsocrural joints (so-called boggy hocks) usually respond well to routine intraarticular medications, but if they are refractory, I add 0.5 mL atropine sulfate. IRAP appears effective for management of horses with chronic capsulitis and OA of the tarsocrural joint.

MRI of the tarsocrural joint and distal aspect of the tibia has permitted identification of soft tissue damage, tibial stress fractures, and bone cysts communicating with the tarsocrural joint, which may be associated with damage to the opposing cartilage and subchondral bone.

Osteoarthritis and Osteochondrosis of the Fetlock Joint

Conditions of the fetlock joint in show horses are essentially the same as seen in other sports horses. The most common conditions are osteochondral fragments of the proximal dorsal aspect of the proximal phalanx and sesamoiditis. Plantar process osteochondrosis fragments are uncommon but are recognized. During prepurchase examinations, I obtain lateromedial radiographic images of each metatarsophalangeal joint specifically to evaluate for plantar process fragments. Fractures of the proximal sesamoid bones occur infrequently. Osseous cystlike lesions of the distal aspect of the third metacarpal bone (McIII) and osteochondritis dissecans (OCD) lesions of the sagittal ridge of the McIII occur infrequently and are less devastating than in racing breeds. Mineralized proliferative synovitis lesions are often confused with osteochondral fragments, but show horses with this condition have a favorable prognosis. Primary OA of the fetlock joint is seen commonly in show horses that wing the lower limb while moving, but radiographs are often negative.

Diagnosis of lameness of the fetlock joint is routine, using radiography, nuclear scintigraphy, ultrasonography, and, when necessary, MRI. Nuclear scintigraphy is most useful in diagnosing sesamoiditis.

Arthroscopic removal of osteochondral fragments of the proximal phalanx is not always necessary, because many show horses compete well and require little maintenance therapy when fragments involve the front fetlock joints. When fragments involve the hind fetlock joints, arthroscopic removal is recommended, because these horses have gait abnormalities characterized by a skipping motion that are accentuated at the rack and slow gait. This is particularly evident in horses with plantar process fragments of the proximal phalanx.

Horses with sesamoiditis respond well to corrective shoeing (lowering the heel), NSAIDs, isoxsuprine, and injection of hyaluronan and corticosteroids into the fetlock joint. Shock wave therapy appears to be effective in managing horses with chronic sesamoiditis, collateral ligament damage, and severe arthritic changes. Treatment with IRAP with or without ESWT is beneficial in horses with severe OA.

MRI may be helpful for evaluation of the articular cartilage and subchondral bone and for identification of injuries of the intersesamoidean ligament (Figure 122-2), oblique sesamoidean ligaments, straight sesamoidean ligament, palmar annular ligament, and digital flexor tendons.

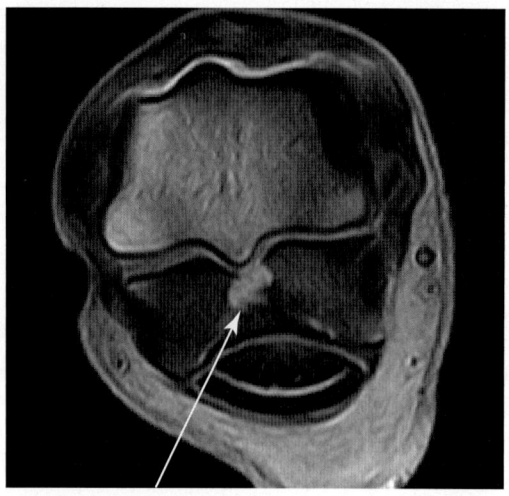

Fig. 122-2 • Transverse high-resolution spin echo magnetic resonance image of a metacarpophalangeal joint (dorsal is to the top and lateral to the left) showing an area of increased signal intensity *(arrow)* in the intersesamoidean ligament. This lesion was debrided arthroscopically.

Osteoarthritis and Osteochondrosis of the Stifle Joint

OA of the stifle joints is a common lameness in show horses, particularly in horses being pushed to perform at a young age. Normal weight distribution favoring the hindlimbs, coupled with learning the slow gait and rack at a young age, predispose the horses to stifle pain. Horses with stifle lameness usually have a shortened cranial phase of the stride and are said to be "humping up in the hip" at the beginning of the caudal phase of the stride. Lameness often is pronounced with the limb on the outside of the ring and is worse in the turns. Diagnosis is made using assessment of gait, diagnostic analgesia, radiography, nuclear scintigraphy, and MRI if needed. Subchondral bone cysts of the medial femoral condyle and OCD of the trochlear ridges of the femur are commonly diagnosed in young show horses with stifle effusion. Arthroscopic surgery, debridement, and fragment removal are recommended in those horses with effusion and lameness. Prognosis for a five-gaited horse with OCD of the stifle is guarded, even with surgery. Many of these horses can compete successfully in other divisions such as harness, pleasure driving, and equitation.

Distal patellar fragmentation and cartilage damage are seen in older horses, and horses respond well to intraarticular injections of hyaluronan and corticosteroids. Arthroscopic surgery is recommended in horses refractory to this therapy.

Lateral luxation of the patella occasionally is diagnosed in foals, which have a guarded prognosis. Atrophy of the trochlear groove of the femur usually occurs with this condition, which may be genetic and familial.

Upward fixation of the patella is seen in young horses with underdeveloped quadriceps muscles. Most improve with training in a jog cart to build up the hindlimb musculature in lieu of intense riding and training. Trainers must be advised to be patient. Medial patellar desmotomy should be used as a last resort and should be done only if radiographs of the stifle are negative. Horses with early OA

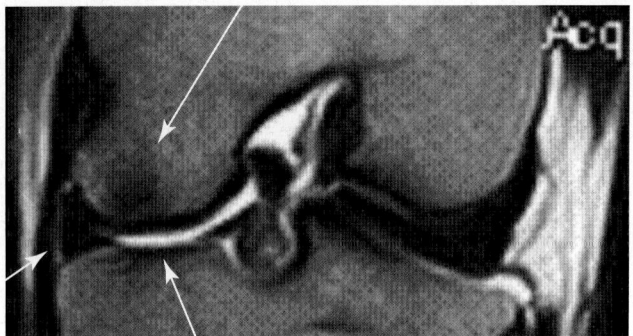

Fig. 122-3 • Dorsal turbo spin echo magnetic resonance image of a stifle joint (proximal is to the top and medial is to the left) in a show horse showing an area of low signal intensity consistent with bone injury of the distal aspect of the medial femoral condyle *(upper arrow)* and corresponding mild injury of the proximal medial aspect of the tibia *(lower arrow)*. The medial meniscus *(left arrow)* is shaped abnormally.

and negative radiographs are managed by decreasing training intensity and implementing a jogging program to develop the hindlimb musculature. A weighted drag behind the cart is added later, before the normal riding program resumes. Internal blisters are used commonly. Intraarticular injection of hyaluronan and corticosteroids alleviates clinical signs, but without modification of exercise the results are short-lived.

Horses with chronic OA are maintained using intraarticular injections, oral supplements, intramuscularly and intravenously administered polysulfated glycosaminoglycans, and NSAIDs.

MRI may reveal degeneration of the meniscal cartilages in areas of contact with osseous cystlike lesions of the proximal aspect of the tibia or subchondral bone cysts in the medial femoral condyle. Identification of injury of the meniscal cartilages, meniscotibial ligaments, and cruciate ligaments is important for establishing a prognosis and formulating a management plan in show horses with stifle joint disease (Figure 122-3).

Suspensory Desmitis
Show horses with long pasterns and high heels are prone to suspensory desmitis because the fetlock drops excessively and stretches the suspensory ligament. Show horses trained in deep footing (sand or mud) are at increased risk for suspensory desmitis. Avulsion fracture of the McIII at the origin of the suspensory ligament may occur in association with suspensory desmitis. Suspensory desmitis is more common in forelimbs than in hindlimbs. Treatment of show horses with suspensory desmitis involves rest, NSAIDs, periligamentous injection of corticosteroids, leg sweating, magnetic therapy, and support wraps. Rest includes handwalking, because horses with suspensory desmitis appear to respond better to limited, controlled exercise than to stall rest alone. The heel should be lowered and a palmar or plantar extension applied.

ESWT has been extremely beneficial in show horses with suspensory body or suspensory branch injuries, and particularly those with proximal suspensory desmitis. Intralesional injection with IRAP or stem cells, combined with ESWT, has been most effective.

MRI may give additional information about suspensory pathology compared with ultrasonography, permitting identification of adhesions to the second or fourth metacarpal (metatarsal) bones.

Tendonitis
Performing in deep, muddy, outdoor show rings and a long-toe, high-heel hoof conformation predispose horses to tendonitis of the superficial digital flexor tendon (SDFT) and DDFT and desmitis of the accessory ligament of the DDFT. As a rule tendonitis is not nearly as devastating in show horses as in racehorses.

Horses with tendonitis respond well to sweats, peritendonous injection of corticosteroids, NSAIDs, magnetic therapy, and ESWT. Rarely, show horses require tendon splitting and desmotomy of the accessory ligament of the DDFT or the accessory ligament of the SDFT. Serial ultrasonographic examinations are important to monitor healing.

Splint Exostoses
Splint exostoses are caused by lunging young horses in tight circles too fast and too long. Direct trauma from interference can cause splint exostosis or fracture. Once splints become inactive, they rarely cause lameness, unless the mineralization impinges on the suspensory ligament or if the exostosis is so large that it repeatedly becomes traumatized. Diagnosis is made by palpation and radiological assessment for fracture. Treatment consists of leg sweats, subcutaneous injections of corticosteroids over the exostosis, and ESWT in horses refractory to sweating and injections. Surgical removal of distal splint bone fracture fragments, large exostoses, or nonunions that impinge on the suspensory ligament should be performed.

OTHER LAMENESS CONDITIONS
Stringhalt
Stringhalt is common in the show horse and needs to be differentiated from other hindlimb lameness conditions. Local anesthetic solution (5 mL at each of three sites) is injected into the lateral digital extensor muscle, and the horse is observed while ridden 10 minutes later. If gait is improved, I recommend lateral digital myotenectomy. Previous trauma to the lateral or common digital extensor tendons can predispose horses to stringhalt (see Chapter 48).

Semimembranosus or Semitendinosus Myositis
Myositis of the semimembranosus or semitendinosus sometimes can mimic stringhalt and cause bizarre gait abnormalities similar to fibrotic myopathy. Horses and ponies (particularly road ponies) show restriction of the cranial phase of the stride. The hindlimb appears to hang up in a flexed position, or the horse is short-strided. Typically a trainer says the horse cannot get underneath itself. This occurs particularly in gaited horses that cannot perform the slow gait or rack. This condition may be an early form of fibrotic myopathy.

Diagnosis involves injecting 5 mL of local anesthetic solution in three or four sites each in the semimembranosus and semitendinosus muscles. The horse is evaluated ridden in 10 minutes, and often the change is dramatic.

Short-lived benefit is seen by injecting the involved muscles with Sarapin and a corticosteroid and using electrotherapy. The best solution appears to be tenotomy of the medial branch of the semitendinosus muscle, the same procedure described for surgical management of horses with fibrotic myopathy.

Tibial Stress Fractures

Young show horses, particularly young, talented five-gaited prospects, can become suddenly difficult to gait. Typically the trainer says, "The horse was one of the best young prospects I ever had, and then suddenly I lost him," or "Everything came undone." Tibial stress fractures are the show horse counterpart to bucked shins in the Thoroughbred. Diagnosis is difficult and usually involves ruling out everything else first and proceeding to nuclear scintigraphy, the most consistent and best method of diagnosis. Horses are given 60 days of jogging and are reassessed.

Hindlimb Extensor Tenosynovitis

The long digital extensor tendon sheath at the level of the hock can become inflamed and distended, a condition that is particularly prevalent in talented gaited horses. There is usually an indentation of the distended sheath just below the hock, caused by constriction by the retinaculum.

Although lameness is unusual, severe distention of the sheath may cause a stiff gait, because the horse cannot flex the hock normally. Tenosynovitis may be confused with bog spavin. If left untreated, the synovium becomes hypertrophic, and movement of synovium under constricting retinaculum causes a hitch in hindlimb gait. Treatment consists of draining synovial fluid and injecting a combination of hyaluronan, corticosteroids, and 0.5 mL of atropine sulfate. Massaging with DMSO and a corticosteroid is also beneficial.

Cervical Myositis

The degree of neck flexion required in show horses often causes pain, particularly in young horses. Older horses may develop OA of the facet joints, especially of the fifth to seventh cervical vertebrae. Diagnosis is based on radiological examination and nuclear scintigraphy. Myelography may be necessary if there is evidence of hindlimb incoordination. Horses with cervical myositis and pain often are observed to be fighting the bit. Diagnosis is made by palpation. Injection of Sarapin and corticosteroids in the affected muscles, methocarbamol, electrical stimulation, and NSAIDs are used. Acupuncture and chiropractic procedures also may be beneficial. ESWT may be beneficial in horses with OA of the facet joints. Ultrasound-guided intraarticular injection may also be of benefit.

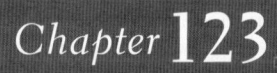

Lameness in the Arabian and Half-Arabian Show Horse

Jeffrey A. Williams and Bradley S. Root

HISTORY OF THE ARABIAN

The Arabian is one of the oldest breeds in the world. The horse originated in the deserts of the Middle East and was used by the Bedouins for transportation and in battle. The Arabian breed was noted for its speed and endurance. Three Arabian stallions (the Godolphin Barb, Byerley Turk, and Darley Arabian) imported to Europe during the late 1600s and early 1700s became the foundation of a new breed of horse, the Thoroughbred. Today, 93% of all modern Thoroughbreds can be traced to these three sires. In the 1800s many royal families of Europe established Arabian stud farms. Two of the most notable were the Polish National Arabian Stud in Poland and the Crabbet Arabian Stud in England. The Arabian is thought to have an influence on many of the light horse breeds that have developed throughout history. A typical Arabian ranges from 14.1 to 15.1 hands in height. The American Horse Show Association breed standards describe the Arabian as having a

small, slightly dished face with large eyes set well apart, small ears, deep and wide jowls, a small muzzle, and large nostrils. The horse should have a long, arched neck; a long, sloping shoulder; well-sprung ribs; a short back with a relatively horizontal croup; and natural, high tail carriage. The limbs should have large, well-defined joints, short cannon bones, sloping pasterns of good length, and round feet of proportionate size.[1]

The Half-Arabian studbook originated with the United States Army Remount Service after World War II and was acquired by the International Arabian Horse Association in 1951. Half-Arabians must have a registered purebred Arabian sire or dam. The Anglo-Arabian is a cross between an Arabian and a Thoroughbred, whereas the more recently developed National Show Horse is a cross between an Arabian and a Saddlebred. Many Half-Arabians are double registered.

References on page 1345

HISTORY OF THE SPORTING EVENT

The International Arabian Horse Association was created in 1950 to join the local and regional clubs across America into one united association. The International Arabian Horse Association promotes and coordinates all Arabian and Half-Arabian horse show activities and develops horse show rules. The International Arabian Horse Association also maintains the Half-Arabian and Anglo-Arabian registries, whereas the Arabian Horse Registry of America maintains the registry and pedigree records for purebred Arabian horses in the United States and Mexico.

The first United States National Arabian and Half-Arabian Show was held in 1966. The United States National

Show is held in October in Tulsa, Oklahoma. A separate Youth National show for riders under 18 years old is held in July of each year in Albuquerque. The Canadian National Horse Show is held in August in Regina, Saskatchewan. The Sport Horse Nations, an event for Arabians and Half-Arabians competing in dressage, working hunter-jumper, and carriage-driving categories, is held at a different time and location each year. The United States and Canada are separated into 18 regions, each of which holds an annual show. Horses can qualify for the national show by placing in the top five at a regional show or by accumulating points at Class A shows. Some of the major shows in the United States other than the regionals and nationals are the Scottsdale Show (Arizona), the Buckeye Show (Ohio), the Pacific Slopes Show (California), the East Coast Championship (Pennsylvania), and the Pro-Am Challenge (Texas). Major international shows are held in England, France, South America, and Australia.

Performance classes for Arabian and Half-Arabian horses cover a broad spectrum and are listed in Box 123-1. Each of these classes is held separately for Arabians and Half-Arabians. They may be divided further into sections for junior owner, adult amateur owner, amateur owner, junior exhibitor, and amateur. The Park horse has a strong animated trot, with the forearm horizontal and the limb extending fully forward. The hock has a well-raised driving action. The walk and canter are animated and collected. The English Pleasure horse is shown at a walk, trot, strong trot (faster and more animated than the normal trot), canter, and hand gallop. Its gaits are less animated than those of the Park horse, although the forearm, at the trot, is horizontal. The same gaits are used in the Country English Pleasure class, but horses have lower limb action,

and high action is penalized. The Country English Pleasure horse must also halt, stand quietly, back, and walk off on a loose rein. With all pleasure classes the horse must give the appearance of being a pleasure to ride. Park horses and English Pleasure horses are shown with the head carried high and considerable flexion at the poll. Saddle seat attire is required.

In the English Show Hack class a horse must perform each gait (walk, trot, and canter) in a normal, collected, and extended manner. A transition between gaits should be noticeable, and high knee action is not expected. Horses in the Hunter Pleasure division are shown under saddle at the walk, trot, canter, and hand gallop. The neck should be carried lower, the head should be carried with less bend at the poll, and the horse should be in a generally longer frame than the English Pleasure or Show Hack horse. Working Hunters are shown over a course of fences set at levels of 0.6 to 1 m and are judged on performance, manners, and soundness. Jumpers are shown over courses of jumps that vary in height from 0.9 to 1.05 m. The maximum width (spread) is 1.5 m.

Horses in driving classes are shown pulling a four-wheeled (Formal and Pleasure) or two-wheeled (Pleasure and Country Pleasure) vehicle. The gaits judged in the Formal, Pleasure, and Country Pleasure driving classes correspond to the Park, English Pleasure, and Country English Pleasure classes under saddle. The Roadster is a driving class that focuses on the trot at three different speeds.

The Western Pleasure horse is shown at the walk, jog (trot), lope (slow canter), and hand gallop. Ideally, contact with the reins is light, the head is carried low (approximately at the level of the withers), and the jog and lope are slow, easy gaits. The Working Western horse classes include reining, working cow horse, trail, cutting, and Western riding.

BOX 123-1

Performance Classes for Arabian and Half-Arabian Horses

Park horse
English Pleasure
Country English Pleasure
Hunter Pleasure
English Show Hack
Hunter
Jumper
Dressage
Formal Driving
Pleasure Driving
Country Pleasure Driving
Roadster
Combination (Driving and Riding)
Mounted Nature Costume
Ladies Side Saddle
Western Pleasure
Reining
Working Cow horse
Trail
Cutting
Equitation (Hunter Seat, Saddle Seat, and Stock Seat): youth classes only
Western Horsemanship (youth only)

TRAINING: IMPACT OF INDUSTRY

The Arabian and Half-Arabian are versatile breeds, as shown by the many sports in which they compete. These include halter, endurance (see Chapter 118), pleasure, jumping, dressage, reining, cutting, and racing (see Chapter 111). Young performance horses are not shown under saddle until they are 3 years old. They then compete in futurity classes for horses 3 years of age or junior horse classes for horses 5 years of age or younger. Because these horses do not compete in performance classes until 3 years of age, this allows more time for adequate skeletal development compared with racehorses and Quarter Horses that start training before 2 years of age. The reason that training of Arabian show horses is started later than some other breeds may be partly smaller size and late maturation, but it is also related to the fact that no performance classes are available for 2-year-olds, and therefore no economic incentives exist to start intensive training early.

Early training and conditioning typically involve a substantial amount of work in a round pen or by lunging. Excessive training in small circles causes increased torque on the joints and support structures of the distal aspect of the limbs. Young horses trained in this manner commonly develop bilateral distal forelimb lameness involving numerous structures. These problems tend to be exacerbated by uneven and excessively hard or deep footing.

Rules govern the shoeing of Arabian and Half-Arabian show horses. The rules vary with age, breed, discipline, and the country of the competition. Foot length, shoe weight and shape, and pad usage are individualized for each horse to optimize the height and arc of flight of the forelimbs and hindlimbs. In English Pleasure horses, a common shoe is the toe-weighted shoe, constructed by forging more steel in the toe of the shoe. The long foot and weighted shoes are used to enhance forelimb motion. Unfortunately this can contribute to strain on the suspensory ligament (SL) and joints of the distal aspect of the limb.

In all performance divisions horses are shown in a collected frame. In each division the type of work performed, the body position required, and the conformational defects of an individual horse contribute to the common lameness conditions. Differences are apparent in gaits, degrees of collection, and head and neck position in the various divisions. In the English Pleasure division, for example, the degree of collection, neck elevation, and poll flexion required shift weight to the hindlimbs and increase the work of the back and abdominal muscles. These positional factors can cause hindlimb lameness (especially involving the stifle and SL) and back pain. In the Western Pleasure and Reining divisions, similar problems are seen because of the amount of collection required. These horses also incur a variety of lameness conditions because they commonly are worked for longer periods than English Pleasure horses. In the Western Pleasure and Reining classes, because any departure from a quiet, steady position is penalized, fatigue can be part of the class preparation.

CONFORMATION AND LAMENESS

Mild-to-moderate carpus valgus and toed-out conformation commonly are seen and do not appear to have a major impact on soundness (Figure 123-1). One reason is that the carpus is not a common location for lameness. If these conformational faults are severe, horses are at risk of suspensory desmitis. Horses with long sloping pasterns, back-at-the-knee conformation, or offset knees are also predisposed to suspensory desmitis. These conformational faults are more common in the Half-Arabian and National Show Horse than in purebred Arabians and are more common in certain pedigrees.

Horses with low, underrun heels certainly are prone to lameness from palmar foot pain. This fault can be difficult to correct, even with careful attention to shoeing and trimming. A small, upright, contracted foot (club foot) can be a source of lameness and appears to be increasing in incidence. Inflammation of the soft tissues such as the SL, accessory ligament of the deep digital flexor tendon (ALDDFT), palmar foot structures, and distal sesamoidean ligaments tend to be more common in horses with club foot conformation.

A long, weak (sway) back and a short croup may predispose horses to soreness in the thoracolumbar, sacroiliac, and gluteal areas. Because problems in these areas are a common cause of poor performance, this type of conformation is a serious fault. Horses with cow-hocked conformation are the rule rather than the exception, but this conformation seems to have little effect on soundness.

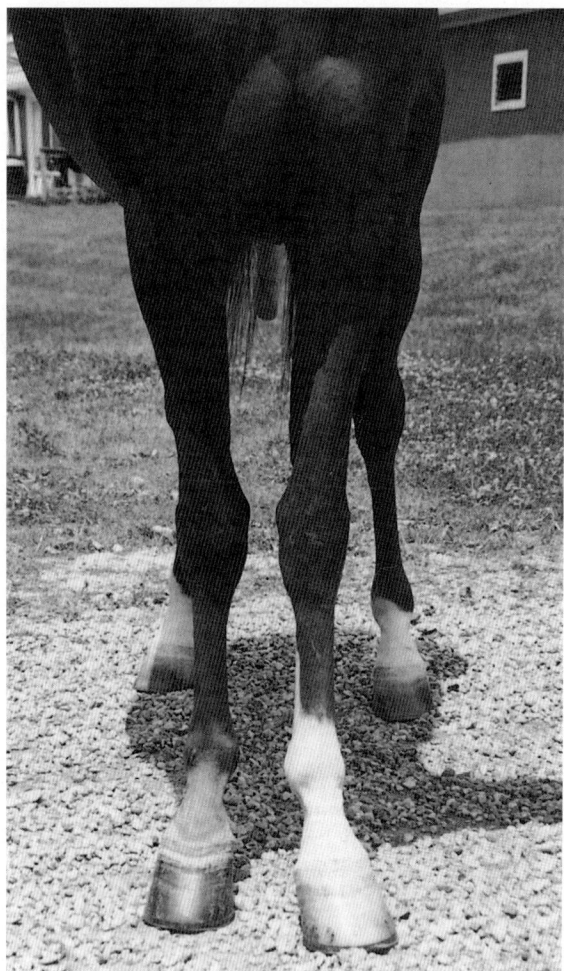

Fig. 123-1 • A 4-year-old Half-Arabian with toed-out, carpus valgus, back-at-the-knee conformation. These are common conformation faults in the Arabian and Half-Arabian breeds and may predispose the horses to suspensory desmitis.

LAMENESS EXAMINATION

History

When describing lameness, trainers often comment that problems occur or are more noticeable during the first direction or the second direction of the show ring. This refers to the directional order in which rail classes are run. In the first direction horses enter the ring and travel counterclockwise (on the left rein), and in the second direction horses travel clockwise (on the right rein). Important questions regarding history include the division in which the horse competes; onset, degree, and progression of the lameness; previous or current treatment; and response to therapy. Additional information that can be helpful includes knowing which direction is harder for the horse at the trot (jog) and canter (lope), whether the horse pulls unevenly on the reins, whether the horse tracks straight in each direction, whether the horse falls out of leads behind (in the hindlimbs) in corners (i.e., becomes disunited in canter or breaks from canter to trot), and whether the rider rides the correct or incorrect diagonal in each direction (the horse may throw the rider up on one diagonal preferentially).

The age of the horse is important, because osteochondrosis is more likely to affect young horses recently started into training than older horses, but in older horses osteoarthritis (OA) is common. It is important to find out when the horse was last shod, and if any recent shoeing changes have been made. Altering medial-to-lateral hoof balance or hoof angle may increase pressure in certain areas and lead to bruising of the heel or sole. Increasing the hoof angle by raising the heel may increase load on the SL, which may lead to suspensory desmitis. The type and condition of the footing the horse has been working on is important to consider. Often footing at shows is less than ideal and in many cases is too hard, leading to the development of bruised feet. Conversely, if footing is too deep, it may lead to tendon and ligament injuries.

STATIC EXAMINATION

Visual Examination

Stepping back to visually examine the horse for overall symmetry of the limbs and upper body is helpful. Asymmetry of upper limb muscle groups may be a sign of atrophy from denervation, chronic lameness, or neurological disease. Asymmetry in the height and position of the points of the shoulders, the tubera sacrale, the tubera coxae, or the tubera ischii can indicate subluxations or fractures. The size, shape, and symmetry of the feet are important to note. Abnormalities such as club feet, an underrun or sheared heel, growth rings, dished dorsal hoof walls, and a contracted heel are some of the more common problems. Joint swelling, soft tissue swellings, poor conformation, scars, and abnormal structures such as splints are recognized quickly.

Palpation

Thorough palpation of the distal aspect of the limbs is performed with the horse in weight-bearing and non–weight-bearing positions. Degree of joint and tendon sheath filling; abnormal contours of bones, tendons, and ligaments; and intensity of the digital pulse amplitudes are best evaluated while the horse is bearing weight. With the limb elevated, painful response to palpation of tendons, ligaments (origins and insertions), and splints; pain on joint flexion; and range of motion of joints are assessed. Effusion of the distal interphalangeal (DIP) and stifle joints (especially the medial femorotibial joint) is common. To evaluate filling in the medial femorotibial joint, it is helpful to have the horse bearing weight with the limb being palpated slightly cranial to the opposite limb and perpendicular to the ground.

Response of an Arabian or Half-Arabian to palpation of the SL varies greatly, depending on the horse. Differences between limbs should be considered important, and change in the response over time is noteworthy. Many horses have a pain response to palpation of the SL but have primary lameness localized to the foot. Possibly the SL is painful because of a compensatory gait caused by a primary foot problem. In contrast, absence of inducible pain, especially in the proximal suspensory region, does not rule out this area as a source of pain causing lameness.

Careful palpation of the cervical, thoracic, and lumbosacral regions is useful in diagnosing the reason for poor performance and lameness. Asymmetry, abnormal contours, and painful response to palpation are important to assess. Particular attention should be paid to the thoracolumbar musculature, the spinous processes, and the sacral tuberosities, because these areas commonly are involved in horses that perform poorly.

Hoof Tester Examination

Many Arabian and Half-Arabian show horses wear full pads in front during training and showing. Although sometimes inconvenient, especially at a competition, removing the shoe and pad for a complete hoof tester examination is helpful if the veterinarian suspects a foot problem. Some indication of painful areas may be obtained with the shoe and pad on, but many areas can be missed. Bruised heels and soles are common, especially at shows where footing may be too hard and horses are being worked longer than normal. Bruised heels and soles are two of the most common sources of lameness. Improvement in lameness can be dramatic if areas of bruising can be trimmed to reduce pressure or if the shoe is modified to eliminate weight bearing on a bruised area. Many horses show pain when hoof testers are applied across the heel but no pain with an individual heel bulb, the sole, or the bars of the hoof. These horses are in as much pain with the shoe and pad on, and therefore this situation may relate to structures deeper in the heel of the foot, rather than simply bruising of the sole.

Medial-to-lateral hoof imbalances may contribute to lameness and should be addressed whenever lameness exists and sore feet have been identified with hoof testers. In general, pain is associated with the high side of the foot or that area making ground contact first.

Pain in the toe region occurs less commonly than in the heel, especially for horses in the English and Park divisions, and likely is related to the way the foot is trimmed. These horses usually have a long toe and thick sole that may protect sensitive structures from bruising and exaggerate heel-first landing in the forelimbs. When pain over the middle of the frog is detected, bruising, palmar foot pain, or navicular-related pain should be considered. Diagnostic analgesia should be performed to confirm the relevance of hoof tester examination, because false-positive reactions occur.

DYNAMIC EXAMINATION

Flexion Tests

Flexion tests are important, but responses should be interpreted carefully. A painful response to flexion of joints and the degree of lameness should be assessed. Many false-positive distal limb flexion tests occur in Arabian and Half-Arabian show horses. Many horses without lameness show pain to static flexion and a positive response when trotted. In a lame horse a distal limb flexion test is not specific. For example, in a lame horse with a positive response to a distal limb flexion test, lameness may be localized anywhere from the foot to the distal metacarpal region. Carpal flexion usually is performed only in a static situation because we do not feel that substantial additional information is gained by trotting the horse. Horses that resent carpal flexion may have proximal suspensory desmitis (PSD), superficial digital flexor tendonitis, or carpal tenosynovitis, because bony injury of the carpus itself is unusual in Arabian and Half-Arabian show horses.

Initially the entire hindlimb is held in flexion and then individual distal limb flexion and proximal limb flexion tests are performed. We attempt to stress the stifle independently of the tarsus by holding the distal tibia upward and behind the horse for 60 seconds. This test can also elicit pain from the lumbosacral and sacroiliac joint regions. These flexion tests are not specific, but they may increase the index of suspicion in a certain area. For example, horses with hindlimb PSD or distal hock joint pain respond positively to proximal limb flexion and must be differentiated based on the results of other tests. Mildly positive hindlimb flexion test results can be seen in sound horses that are actively training and showing. These mildly positive flexion test results may be related to subtle lameness or subclinical pain, or could be a normal response. For horses that have been competing successfully to have a moderate-to-severe positive response to a distal limb flexion test after a lengthy show is not unusual. This fact needs to be taken into account when prepurchase examinations are performed directly after horses have competed.

Examination in Hand and under Saddle

Horses should be examined at the walk and at the trot on the straight in hand. It is also helpful to examine horses at the walk in a figure-eight pattern. Examination on both hard and soft surfaces can be helpful. If possible, examining the horse at all appropriate gaits on the lunge line (or long line) and under saddle or in a cart is helpful. Multiple-limb lameness, especially contralateral forelimb and hindlimb lameness and bilateral front foot lameness, is common, which is important to keep in mind. The possibility of subtle neurological deficits should be considered during all phases of the lameness examination. In some horses lameness may not be apparent unless the horse is under tack and working near the higher end of its performance capabilities. This type of lameness is more difficult to diagnose, and diagnostic analgesia is usually required. Subtle lameness can be masked by a rider restricting free head movement or by controlling body position. The diagonal on which the rider sits can alter the appearance of lameness. When riding the *left* diagonal, the rider sits when the left forelimb and right hindlimb bear weight, and on the *right* diagonal the rider sits when the right forelimb and left hindlimb bear weight. The correct diagonal is the *left* when trotting clockwise and the *right* when trotting counterclockwise. In general a horse appears more lame behind when the rider sits when the lame limb is bearing weight, and the horse may try to throw the rider to the opposite diagonal. A horse with right hindlimb lameness appears more lame when the rider sits on the left diagonal. In Park, English, or Country English Pleasure classes, where riders are not penalized for riding the incorrect diagonal, horses often are ridden on the diagonal that minimizes lameness. Often a lameness is involved when a horse is seen being ridden on the incorrect diagonal when traveling in one direction and on the correct diagonal going the other way. These horses are referred to as *right* or *left diagonal horses*. An inconsistent relationship exists between the degree of forelimb lameness and the diagonal on which the rider sits, but lameness may be modified by switching diagonals.

It is important to note whether the observed lameness is constant regardless of direction or pattern. It is important to note if lameness varies, whether the involved limb is on the inside or outside of a circle, whether the horse is on the straight or in a turn, and whether lameness is worse when the horse is on hard or soft ground. The only gait deficit visible in horses with subtle forelimb lameness may be a slight difference in the height or arc of flight of the involved limb. Often a head nod is absent, but the horse appears unsteady in the face (movement of the nose from a fixed position) because of the discomfort of the limb from landing or from pushing off the ground.

DIAGNOSTIC ANALGESIA

If possible, it is important to perform diagnostic analgesia to confirm the source of pain. For example, many horses that appear to have foot pain because of sensitivity to hoof testers or pain on palpation of the SL actually have pain elsewhere. Under United States Equestrian Federation (USEF) rules, with a properly filed medication report, local anesthetic solution such as mepivacaine can be administered up to 24 hours before a class.

If lameness is to be reassessed with the horse under saddle or in a cart, intraarticular rather than perineural nerve blocks are preferred, because of possible loss of proprioception, which may lead to tripping or stumbling. After perineural blocks, horses may pull shoes or show an altered or awkward gait regardless of the lameness. If perineural blocks are performed in horses under saddle or in a cart, the rider or driver should be cautioned. Hindlimb nerve blocks can be difficult in uncooperative horses, and a tranquilizer (10 to 15 mg acepromazine intravenously) may be administered to fractious horses. Lameness may be more obvious after a tranquilizer is administered, but the risk of permanent penile prolapse with the use of acepromazine in stallions or geldings should be considered. In some horses, diagnostic analgesia of the hindlimbs may be impossible. On occasion the response to intraarticular medication, administered under heavy sedation, may be assessed as a diagnostic aid. Other diagnostic procedures such as nuclear scintigraphy, radiographic and ultrasonographic examinations, and magnetic resonance imaging (MRI) may be employed.

NEUROLOGICAL EXAMINATION

An Arabian or Half-Arabian show horse with neurological disease may show subtle to overt clinical signs of lameness, weakness, or ataxia, which may be mistaken easily for signs of musculoskeletal pain. Watching the horse turn in tight circles, back up, and walk a figure eight can be performed quickly and may pinpoint subtle deficits that were not noted or were less noticeable earlier in the examination.

Traumatic injuries caused by fractious horses falling during handling and training and equine protozoal myelitis are common causes of neurological disease and dysfunction in Arabian and Half-Arabian show horses in North America. OA of the caudal cervical facets is common, but is not necessarily of clinical significance. Clinical signs can include focal muscle atrophy, reduced lateral flexion of the neck, and subtle or overt forelimb lameness and ataxia. Radiographic examination and nuclear scintigraphy may be helpful in diagnosis. Ultrasound-guided injections of the cervical facet joints are commonly performed. Two rare neurological conditions that may be confused with lameness and are much more common in Arabians than in any other breed are cerebellar abiotrophy and occipito-atlantoaxial malformation. Cerebellar abiotrophy is a congenital neurological abnormality that may have an inherited susceptibility and has been reported only in the Arabian horse and Gotland pony. Typical signs occur around 2 to 4 months of age and include head tremor, incoordination, hypermetria, and proprioceptive deficits. Horses may live into adulthood, and anecdotal evidence suggests that the condition may stabilize or improve, although for these horses to improve sufficiently to be useful performance horses is unlikely. Occipito-atlantoaxial malformation is an inherited congenital malformation that has been reported most frequently in Arabians. The severity of clinical signs varies greatly, from splinting of the neck to progressive ataxia and weakness to congenital tetraparesis. Reduced atlantooccipital movement and abnormal head carriage with the neck extended are common findings.[2] Diagnosis is confirmed radiologically (see Figure 53-4, B). Developmental cervical vertebral anomalies also may cause ataxia.

UNDIAGNOSED LAMENESS

When a diagnosis of the cause of lameness cannot be made after all available diagnostic procedures have been performed, a veterinarian should consider the following:

1. Tack problems: A poorly fitting saddle may create abnormal pressure on the withers or lumbar region and cause poor performance or lameness. A poorly fitted bit or bridle that causes the horse to flip its head or lean into or away from the bit also can affect performance greatly.
2. Dental problems (causing behavior that may lead to poor performance): Sharp enamel points, wolf teeth, and fractured or infected tooth roots may all cause abnormal head carriage and poor performance.
3. Painful skin lesions in the area of the girth, saddle, or bridle may affect performance.
4. A poorly skilled rider pulling on the horse while posting or with poor balance or timing may affect the horse's performance.
5. Recurrent exertional rhabdomyolysis affects performance.
6. Subtle neurological deficits may affect performance.

If these problems are ruled out and a diagnosis still cannot be made, the veterinarian could try empirical treatment including a period of rest, a course of nonsteroidal antiinflammatory drugs (NSAIDs), systemic corticosteroids, intravenously administered hyaluronan, oral or systemic polysulfated glycosaminoglycans (PSGAGs), acupuncture, or chiropractic manipulation.

TEN MOST COMMON LAMENESS CONDITIONS OF THE ARABIAN AND HALF-ARABIAN SHOW HORSE

1. Bruised and inflamed feet
2. Osteoarthritis of the distal interphalangeal joint and palmar foot pain
3. Suspensory desmitis
4. Osteoarthritis of the stifle joints
5. Thoracolumbar, sacroiliac, and gluteal pain
6. Osteoarthritis of the metacarpophalangeal and metatarsophalangeal joints
7. Distal hock joint pain
8. Splint bone injuries
9. Osteoarthritis of the proximal interphalangeal joint
10. Desmitis of the accessory ligament of the deep digital flexor tendon

DIAGNOSIS AND MANAGEMENT OF LAMENESS

Bruised and Inflamed Feet

Differential diagnosis for lameness in the foot of an Arabian or Half-Arabian show horse includes sole bruising, osteitis of the distal phalanx, foot abscess, penetrating wounds, fractures, laminitis, navicular syndrome, OA of the DIP joint, collateral desmitis of the DIP joint, and palmar foot pain. The most common foot problems are bruising, OA of the DIP joint, and palmar foot pain.

Bruising is diagnosed by finding localized or generalized pain in the sole and by ruling out other lameness conditions. Digital pulse amplitudes are usually normal at rest unless bruising is severe and commonly increase abnormally with exercise. Discoloration of the sole by hemorrhage usually occurs later and may not be seen with acute sole bruising. The most common causes of bruising are hard footing or poor medial-to-lateral hoof balance. The high side (longer when viewed from the palmar aspect) is usually the bruised side, and treatment may be as simple as balancing the hoof. If hoof balance is judged to be adequate, then a pad can be cut out or the shoe can be beveled to reduce pressure on the bruised area. A common problem is a low, underslung heel. One foot may be affected, whereas the other tends to be upright or club footed. Horses with low, underslung hoof conformation commonly develop a bruised heel. Although raising the heel angle with a degree pad may appear desirable, this correction actually may cause further heel bruising by concentrating the force on the heel. We recommend the use of both a bar shoe and frog pads or a pad cut out over a heel bulb. The shoe may also be gently rockered into the pad (by grinding the heel portion of the pad) to reduce impact at the heel.

Horses with club foot conformation also may develop a contracted heel. Treatment involves identification and medical treatment of any existing palmar foot pain and shoeing fully in the quarters. Some horses with a low, underslung heel or with club foot conformation may not be lame, and therefore attempts at correction should be tempered.

In a flat-footed horse, sole bruising may occur in areas underlying the shoe, where the sole is not concave enough to prevent contact with the shoe or pad. In these horses a concave inner surface shoe should be used. Pads and packing material are important in treating and preventing bruised feet, but bruising can still be a problem. Silicone, tar, and oakum and newer products such as advanced cushion support are commonly used packing materials. However, if the packing is too firm, it may create rather than prevent sole bruising. Radiographs should be obtained to measure sole depth. A minimum of 15 to 20 mm of sole at the toe region of the distal phalanx is required. Venograms are useful for identifying areas and severity of vascular compression to aid in shoeing and in deciding aftercare. Osteitis of the distal phalanx refers to a noninfectious inflammation of the distal phalanx, which in many horses appears to occur secondary to chronic sole bruising. The diagnosis is made radiologically by observing radiolucent changes and modeling along the solar margins and proliferative new bone along the dorsal aspect of the distal phalanx. Horses that have these radiological changes in the toe region also may have chronic bruising, laminitis, solar margin fractures, or club-footed conformation. In the heel the margins of the distal phalanx are normally irregular and less well defined radiologically, and a distinction between bruising and osteitis is harder, if not impossible, to make. In most horses, however, the treatment is similar.

Treatment of horses with acutely bruised feet also includes the administration of NSAIDs and physical therapy. If treatment is necessary during or close to a show in North America, NSAIDs must be given according to the USEF rules for therapeutic medication under which the Arabian and Half-Arabian divisions operate. The 2008 guidelines state that horses can receive phenylbutazone at a dose of 4.4 mg/kg once daily for 5 days in a row no closer than 12 hours before a class. If 2.2 mg of phenylbutazone per kilogram is given by mouth every 12 hours, then the drug can be administered at any time before a class. Under USEF rules, two NSAIDs from a list of seven (flunixin meglumine, ketoprofen, naproxen, meclofenamic acid, firocoxib, diclofenac, and phenylbutazone) are allowed to be given at the same time, except that phenylbutazone and flunixin meglumine may not be given to the same horse within 7 days of a class. If bruising is severe and a second NSAID is required, intravenously administered ketoprofen (2.2 mg/kg sid) is helpful. This should be given no closer than 6 hours before a class. Specifics of NSAID use at USEF competitions are listed in the USEF handbook and can be viewed online. Isoxsuprine (400 mg orally [PO] bid) can be used to increase blood flow to the foot and, although controversial, appears to be helpful in many horses.

Physical therapy includes standing the horse in ice (15 minutes in and 15 minutes out for three repetitions, repeated several times a day) for the first 24 hours, followed by soaks in hot water and Epsom salts (15 to 20 minutes, three times daily). After soaking, the bottom of the foot can be packed with a poultice and wrapped. An effective poultice is a slurry of dimethyl sulfoxide (DMSO) and Epsom salts. If areas of the sole are particularly soft, painting on a mixture of formaldehyde hardens the sole. Feet with weak or damaged walls should not be soaked.

Osteoarthritis of the Distal Interphalangeal Joint and Palmar Foot Pain

Synovitis or acute inflammation of the DIP joint is common and likely represents an early form of OA. Lameness is usually mild to moderate and frequently is bilateral. Lameness tends to be more obvious in circles or tight turns, frequently with the affected limb on the *outside* of a circle. When horses are affected bilaterally, the only signs may be a shortened cranial phase of the stride and reluctance to go forward. Effusion of the DIP joint can be palpated just proximal to the coronary band on the dorsal aspect of the limb. Horses may show pain when hoof testers are applied across the heel, but examination of the sole of the foot is unremarkable, unless other problems such as bruising or navicular syndrome are present. Many young horses develop DIP synovitis early in training and lameness improves with a short period (14 to 28 days) of rest and the administration of NSAIDs. DIP synovitis is also common in older show horses, in which it may be associated with poor foot conformation or a heavy show schedule.

No radiological abnormalities are detected unless the condition is chronic and advanced OA develops. Lameness is abolished by analgesia of the DIP joint or palmar nerve blocks at the base of the proximal sesamoid bones (PSBs). Mepivacaine (3 mL) deposited over the medial and lateral palmar digital nerves just above the bulbs of the heel also substantially alleviates pain originating from the DIP joint.[3] Analgesia of the DIP joint is not specific, but use of a small volume (6 mL) of local anesthetic solution and evaluation of the response within 6 to 8 minutes may minimize the effects of diffusion into the digital nerves and inadvertent misdiagnosis.

It is important to remember that several problems may coexist in the foot, and sorting out a single specific diagnosis can be difficult. Horses with a low, underrun heel often have bruising, osteitis of the distal phalanx, and OA of the DIP joint. Horses with navicular syndrome may have bruising in the toe area related to decreased weight bearing on the heel. Scintigraphic examination may be useful in differentiating these potential causes of lameness.

Horses with early, acute OA of the DIP joint should be evaluated clinically for abnormalities of hoof balance and hoof angle. Shortening and rolling the toe of the shoe or rockering the shoe into the pad to ease breakover can be helpful. Shortening the toe in English show horses may not be well accepted by trainers because they think it decreases the desired forelimb action. If the lameness is moderate or severe, the horse should be allowed to rest for 30 days or the workload should be reduced drastically. Intraarticular medication with hyaluronan (20 mg) and a corticosteroid (40 mg methylprednisolone acetate or 6 to 10 mg triamcinolone acetonide) and systemic phenylbutazone (2.2 mg/kg PO bid for 5 days) are recommended. Intraarticular medication with interleukin-1 receptor antagonist protein (IRAP), usually as a three-dose series, is a useful alternative treatment. If lameness is mild, training can resume 2 to 3 days after the injections. Treatment with hyaluronan (40 mg intravenously once a week for 3 weeks) or PSGAGs (500 mg intramuscularly once every 5 days for four to seven treatments) sometimes is used also, but it should not be a substitute for intraarticular therapy. These products frequently are used as "maintenance" medications (one dose every 2 to 4 weeks) and for preshow medication (one dose 24 to 72 hours before a class) for joint-related lameness.

Palmar foot pain is a frequent cause of lameness. Horses may or may not show pain on hoof tester examination, but lameness is eliminated by palmar digital analgesia. Causes include navicular syndrome, deep digital flexor tendonitis, distal sesamoidean impar desmitis, collateral sesamoidean ligament injury, inflammation of the navicular bone, fragmentation of the distal border of the navicular bone, and congenital bipartite or tripartite navicular bones. Reaching a specific diagnosis in some horses may be difficult. Radiology, ultrasonography, and MRI may be used to determine the specific cause(s) of lameness.

Although it is important to identify the source of lameness as specifically as possible, the treatment options in horses with palmar foot pain are somewhat limited and similar regardless of the cause. Rest, systemic corticosteroid and NSAID administration, therapeutic shoeing, extracorporeal shock wave therapy (ESWT), medication of the DIP joint or navicular bursa and the administration of tiludronate in horses with navicular involvement, and palmar digital neurectomy are the most common treatments. Mesenchymal stem cell or platelet-rich plasma (PRP) injections may be used to treat horses with distal deep digital flexor tendon (DDFT) lesions. Natural balance shoes are not used routinely for English and Park horses because they decrease forelimb motion.

Suspensory Desmitis

PSD is one of the most common lameness conditions of the metacarpal and metatarsal regions. Although more prevalent in the forelimb, PSD is a common hindlimb problem and typically is an insidious lameness but may have an acute onset. Lameness is more obvious when the affected limb is on the outside of a circle and is worse on turns than in straight lines. Usually no swelling is detectable, and the response to palpation is unreliable. Definitive diagnosis is based on the response to diagnostic analgesia, combined with radiological and ultrasonographic examinations. Many treatments are available, including the use of systemic antiinflammatory agents; local injections of antiinflammatory agents or counterirritants; intralesional injections of mesenchymal stem cells or PRP; topical agents with support wraps; ESWT, magnetic, laser, and ultrasound therapies; and various surgical procedures.

A decision must be made whether the horse is sound enough to remain in work, as in horses with a chronic low-grade PSD, or whether the horse should be allowed to rest. If the horse is to remain in work and local injections are to be part of the treatment regimen, a veterinarian has two options. An antiinflammatory agent such as a short-acting corticosteroid, possibly mixed with hyaluronan or a PSGAG, may be used, followed by a few days of handwalking, before the horse resumes work. Alternatively, a counterirritant such as 1 to 2 mL of 2% iodine in almond oil is injected, followed by continued work. In both instances the work is limited to graduated periods of walking and low-speed trotting for several weeks. The walking and trotting generally are performed in escalating timed intervals. The canter or lope is not recommended initially, because the affected limb is the only limb on the ground for a portion of the gait sequence. The weight of the shoes and pads may be reduced during the initial portion of the recovery period. If the injury is too severe for the horse to remain in work, the horse is confined and handwalked until recovery is sufficient to begin a regimen of low-impact, controlled exercise. These horses are not turned out, because they tend to reinjure themselves with free exercise.

PSD tends to recur with prolonged intense exercise. Horses with bilateral club feet, low underrun heels, one club foot and one foot with a low heel, or substantial rotational and angular deformities are predisposed to PSD. Horses with a chronic lameness in the contralateral limb or the diagonal limb also are predisposed to lameness because of compensatory loading. It is important to identify other problems, because resolution of lameness in another limb may be crucial to the long-term resolution of PSD.

Suspensory branch desmitis also occurs frequently. An acute injury causes pain, heat, and swelling over the affected branch and a positive response to distal limb flexion. Usually some distention of the fetlock joint capsule occurs. Diagnosis is confirmed by ultrasonography, and the PSBs should be evaluated radiologically. Horses with acute injuries are treated symptomatically with ice, poulticing, NSAIDs, and systemic corticosteroids. If sesamoiditis is present, isoxsuprine or pentoxifylline treatment may be helpful. The shoeing should be evaluated, and imbalance (frequently a low heel bulb on the affected side) corrected. If possible, the toe should be shortened, or a rolled toe shoe should be used to ease breakover. Horses with chronic active suspensory branch desmitis may benefit from injection of corticosteroids (methylprednisolone acetate and isoflupredone acetate) subcutaneously in the affected area. Most horses are managed similarly to horses with PSD. Suspensory branch desmitis tends to recur, can be difficult to manage successfully, and may be a career-ending injury.

Suspensory desmitis in the hindlimbs also occurs frequently. Horses with camped-out conformation may be predisposed. Diagnosis and treatment are similar to those described for forelimb desmitis. In hindlimb PSD compartment syndrome may be identified. Transection of the proximal metatarsal retinaculum (fasciotomy) can be helpful. Hindlimb PSD is often chronic, and horses require periodic therapy to remain sound.

Osteoarthritis of the Stifle Joints

The stifle is a common source of lameness, and apart from occasional acute injuries most often horses have chronic, low-grade lameness that may not be evident when examined in hand. Riders may complain that horses are hard on one side of the mouth, tracking with a shoulder or hip in or out, falling out of a hind lead in the corners (becoming disunited in canter or breaking to trot), and bending poorly. Horses with stifle pain also have difficulties in downward transitions, because they cannot maintain a collected frame and tend to fall out behind. If a horse is forced to maintain collection, the head may be raised. Horses exhibit increased discomfort going downhill. If the work area has even a slight grade, an affected horse appears more comfortable going up the grade than down. Horses also fatigue easily in deep footing, with loss of collection, diving forward in the bridle (English divisions), raising out of the bridle (Western and Hunter divisions), and loss of hindlimb cadence at the trot. Lameness is worse in turns and improves in the straight portions of the arena.

The medial femorotibial and femoropatellar joint capsules may be distended, and fibrous thickening from a previous medial patellar desmotomy or desmoplasty (splitting) and other abnormalities from previous injuries may be apparent. Various flexion tests, such as pulling the limb caudally, may exacerbate lameness, but these tests are not reliable and may be dangerous to perform. Intraarticular analgesia usually is required. The medial femorotibial joint, the femoropatellar joint, and the lateral femorotibial joint are affected with decreasing frequency and generally are blocked individually in that order. Radiographic examination should include caudocranial, lateromedial, and oblique images. Ultrasonographic examination, nuclear scintigraphy, and diagnostic arthroscopy are sometimes required.

Most commonly lameness is improved by intraarticular analgesia of the medial femorotibial joint, but radiological findings are negative or equivocal. Affected horses are thought to have chronic inflammation of the soft tissues of the joint and synovitis. Some of these horses eventually develop an enthesophyte on the proximal medial aspect of the tibia. Lameness often recurs, because lameness reflects the type of work the horse performs, the collected frame required, and conformational weaknesses, such as lack of angulation in the hip, stifle, and hock, camped-out conformation, and weak hindquarters in general. The condition is managed by adapting the work level between shows and the show schedule of the horse to accommodate for lameness, by corrective shoeing, and by using systemic antiinflammatory agents and intraarticular medication. Corrective shoeing is individualized but involves trimming the foot short and using a light shoe that assists breakover. Increasing the hoof angle in a long-toed low-heeled foot can be helpful. Many horses break over the dorsomedial aspect of the toe, and that portion of the shoe can be rolled or shaped to ease breakover. A worn shoe can be examined for breakover location (Figure 123-2). Some horses are more sound barefooted behind and compete that way. To maintain soundness at shows, horses are maintained at a work level between shows that does not require intraarticular treatment. Systemic administration of hyaluronan and a PSGAG may help. Systemic and intraarticular antiinflammatory therapy is begun before competition to minimize lameness during the competition. If a horse requires frequent therapy between shows, it has a poor chance of enduring a competition in good form.

Counterirritant therapy in the form of 2% iodine in oil commonly is injected in various patterns along the patellar and collateral ligaments of young horses, in horses with loose stifles, and in horses that have been rested as the intensity of training increases and that exhibit nonspecific pain or weakness in the stifle area. Counterirritants are not used as a replacement for intraarticular therapy but may be used concurrently. Injections usually are limited to 1 to 5 mL to reduce postinjection inflammation and to decrease scarring from numerous injections. Work is continued, but the intensity is reduced for a short time as the horse recovers.

Osteochondrosis is the second most common problem seen in the stifle. Osteochondral fragments from the femoral trochleas can be removed arthroscopically; usually horses have a favorable prognosis. Horses with lameness caused by subchondral bone cysts in the medial femoral condyle have a poorer prognosis. Some horses respond to intraarticular or intralesional corticosteroids. Surgical treatment may fail to resolve the lameness.

Thoracolumbar (Back), Sacroiliac, and Gluteal (Croup) Pain

Work-related back and croup pain is common in horses because of working in a collected frame frequently or for extended periods, compensatory altered carriage caused by injuries to the distal aspect of the limb, poor saddle fit, poor balance and timing of a rider, injuries from falling and weakness from immaturity, lack of conditioning, or poor conformation (long, weak back).

Back pain should be suspected when behavioral changes such as kicking out during lead changes in canter and uncharacteristic bucking occur. The horse is observed for muscle asymmetry while it stands with the body straight and the limbs squared on a level surface. The back and croup are palpated for areas of pain, using gradual pressure with the flat surface of the digits. Flexion, extension, and lateral flexion of each area of the back should be induced, and ease of mobility evaluated. Unilateral abnormalities may indicate concurrent injuries to the distal aspect of the limb. Unilateral lumbar pain often results from compensatory carriage of the hindlimbs to that side. Unilateral sacroiliac inflammation or dorsal ligamentous thickening often results from overbearing on that side from a chronic contralateral or diagonal limb injury. For example, horses with a chronic left front or left hind lameness may have swelling and pain in the area of the right tuber sacrale. Rectal examination is used to evaluate pelvic symmetry and ventral lumbar muscular pain. Other diagnostic modalities include radiography, ultrasonography, nuclear scintigraphy, and thermography, but physical examination remains the most important and reliable method of diagnosis. Myositis also occurs commonly and is diagnosed by history, observation of altered gait, palpation, and serum enzyme assay.

A variety of treatments is used, and these are discussed thoroughly elsewhere. Usually a period of rest is indicated, along with resolution of any associated lameness, followed by a period of reduced exercise. Systemic and local antiinflammatory agents are administered. Other therapies include cold and heat therapy, acupuncture, chiropractic therapy, massage therapy, and magnetic, electromagnetic, laser, and ultrasound therapy.

Successful treatment of horses with back and croup injuries depends on identifying initiating causes and making appropriate changes to alleviate these causes if possible. Educating the rider is also helpful, because changes

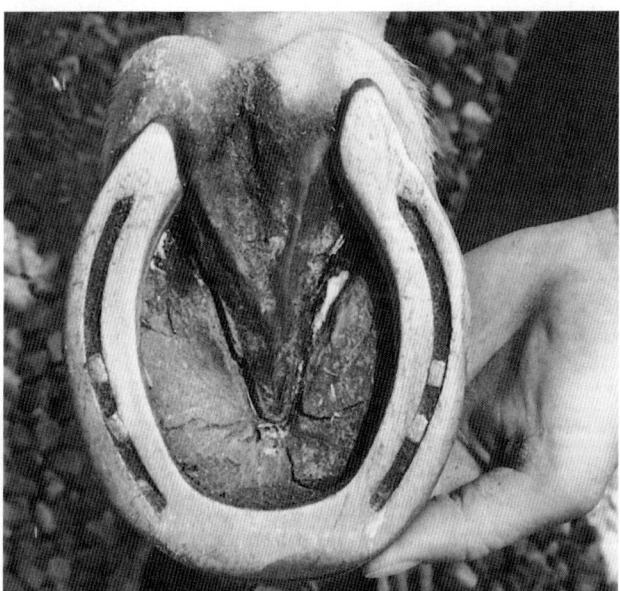

Fig. 123-2 • A left hind shoe indicating natural breakover medial to the toe area (medial is right). Future shoes will be formed to allow breakover in this area rather than directly at the center of the toe.

in training routines or tack may be helpful in preventing recurrence.

Osteoarthritis of the Metacarpophalangeal and Metatarsophalangeal Joints

Synovitis of the metacarpophalangeal and metatarsophalangeal joints, an early form of OA, causes effusion, pain on static fetlock flexion, and a positive response to a distal limb flexion test. The condition is frequently bilateral. Because mild effusion in sound Arabian and Half-Arabian show horses is seen commonly, it is important to perform intraarticular or perineural analgesia to confirm the source of pain when OA of the metacarpophalangeal or metatarsophalangeal joint is suspected. Radiological assessment is performed to determine the extent of osteoarthritic abnormalities. Many Arabian and Half-Arabian show horses perform well in spite of mild OA of the fetlock (Figure 123-3). Treatment is similar to that recommended for OA of the DIP joint, except that a shorter-acting corticosteroid such as triamcinolone acetonide or betamethasone is used for intraarticular medication.

Distal Hock Joint Pain

OA of the centrodistal and tarsometatarsal joints, called distal tarsitis, is common. Tarsal lameness is often bilateral, although one limb usually is affected more severely. Affected horses have reduced hock flexion at the trot and tend to travel with a hip off to one side, especially in the corners (drift away from the lame limb). Rider complaints

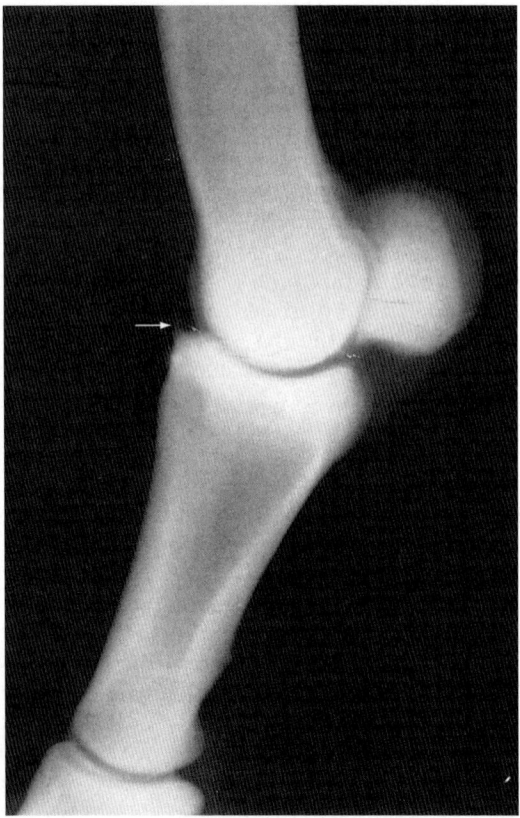

Fig. 123-3 • Lateromedial radiographic image of a metacarpophalangeal joint of a sound Half-Arabian show horse. There is a moderately sized osteophyte *(arrow)* on the proximal dorsal aspect of the proximal phalanx, reflecting osteoarthritis.

are similar to those regarding horses with stifle lameness. Western horses may tend to rate poorly and lope (canter) with a four-beat rather than a three-beat action. Reining horses tend to raise up in spins to the affected direction, bend poorly, stop unevenly or on the forehand, and change leads late behind in flying changes. Diagnosis is based on palpation, including the Churchill test, flexion tests, diagnostic analgesia, radiography, and occasionally ultrasonography and nuclear scintigraphy. Treatment consists of systemic administration of antiinflammatory agents and intraarticular medication with corticosteroids, possibly with hyaluronan (60 to 80 mg of methylprednisolone acetate and 10 mg of hyaluronan per joint), repeated as necessary, often two or three times during a show season. If medical therapy fails, chemical, laser, and surgical fusion techniques are available. ESWT and intravenous tiludronate administration have both been used successfully. Cunean tenectomy usually is not performed because the procedure commonly does not resolve lameness. Corrective shoeing involves inspecting the old shoe and squaring the new shoe to accommodate the breakover, setting the shoe back, shortening the toe, reducing the weight of the hind shoe, and occasionally using asymmetrical trailers.

Splint Bone Injuries

Proliferative periostitis, referred to as *splints,* and fractures of the second and fourth metacarpal bones and to a lesser extent fractures of the second and fourth metatarsal bones are common, especially in young horses. Diagnosis of splint-induced lameness is made using palpation, diagnostic analgesia, and radiography. Associated suspensory desmitis should be considered and assessed by ultrasonographic examination. Predisposing causes include conformational defects such as offset knees or base narrow and toed out. Heavy shoes and pads can exacerbate a tendency to wing in and cause interference. Poor footing that is excessively deep or hard can contribute to the development of splints. Immature horses in excessive work, or wearing shoes and pads that are too heavy for their level of fitness, are predisposed to splints. Shoeing with improper medial-to-lateral balance, obesity, and dietary imbalances can be contributory causes.

Proliferative periostitis originates from injury to the interosseous ligament, resulting in the development of proliferative fibrous connective tissue that subsequently mineralizes. Radiology is used to assess the injury and to determine the presence of fractures. Osteolysis of the third metacarpal or metatarsal bone and of the splint bone at the site of the injury is a sign of substantial inflammation and can indicate a prolonged recovery. Treatment includes rest (2 to 4 weeks), cold therapy, systemic and local administration of antiinflammatory agents, topical agents with support wraps, ESWT, and magnetic therapy. Large exostoses that interfere with surrounding soft tissue structures can be excised surgically.

Work-related fractures are predominantly distal, closed fractures and are thought to result from overexcursion of the SL during fetlock hyperextension. These fractures frequently are displaced, heal by nonunion, and tend to irritate surrounding soft tissues. For these reasons they commonly are removed surgically. Lameness in horses with mid–splint bone nondisplaced fractures often resolves with conservative therapy. Initial therapy is similar to the treatment of a true splint, except that local administration of corticosteroids is not performed. If conservative therapy fails, surgical excision of the exostosis and distal portion of the splint bone may be performed. Horses with fractures of the proximal aspect of a splint bone are evaluated on an individual basis, because some respond to conservative therapy, whereas others require surgical intervention.

Osteoarthritis of the Proximal Interphalangeal Joint

Incidental radiological changes (lipping and spurring) indicating mild OA of the proximal interphalangeal (PIP) joint in Arabian and Half-Arabian show horses are not uncommon. Moderate-to- severe OA, however, would be expected to cause chronic lameness. In most horses OA of the PIP joint is caused by chronic repetitive trauma, although OA secondary to a single severe injury is possible. In young horses osteochondrosis in the form of osseous cystlike lesions and fragmentation may be involved. The importance of any radiological abnormalities should be validated using diagnostic analgesia. Distal limb flexion is usually positive, and lameness should improve with palmar nerve blocks at the base of or at the level of the PSBs or intraarticular analgesia of the PIP joint. Treatment is similar to that recommended for horses with OA of the DIP joint.

Desmitis of the Accessory Ligament of the Deep Digital Flexor Tendon

Desmitis of the ALDDFT occurs less frequently than does PSD and is usually diagnosed in horses with club feet or low, underrun heels. Footing that accumulates under the shoe, creating a rocking motion of the foot during the weight-bearing phase of the stride, may predispose horses to desmitis. Lameness is usually acute in onset, and palpation often reveals a painful thickening along the length of the ligament that can be confused with the DDFT. If the condition is chronic and low grade, diagnostic analgesia may be required. Diagnosis is confirmed with ultrasonography. Treatment involves prolonged rest and systemic and local administration of antiinflammatory agents, PRP, or mesenchymal stem cells. Adjuncts include cold therapy, topical agents with support wraps, and magnetic, laser, ESWT, and ultrasound therapy. Because the predisposing conformational defect remains, the condition tends to recur.

Chapter 124

Lameness in the Driving Horse

Kevin P. Keane and Graham Munroe

DESCRIPTION OF THE SPORT

This chapter deals with horses used for competitive driving purposes, those driven privately for pleasure, and those used as beasts of burden as a mode of transportation. The sport of driving horses in competition is relatively new and has many variations, requiring different types of horses performing different tasks. Certain breeds or breed types are perfectly suitable for one form of driving sport but not another, and variation in the size, type, and breed of horse used is considerable. Horses and ponies are used, and the term *horse* is used in this chapter to refer to both, except when specific reference to a pony is required.

In the United Kingdom and Europe there is a much greater availability of a variety of driving competitions than currently exists in North America. The sport is growing in Australia, South Africa, and South America. Pleasure driving includes presentation classes in the show ring and general driving on roads and tracks. Presentation classes are grouped broadly into hackney and nonhackney types, the difference being based on the phenotype of the horse as opposed to a breed registry. A competitor pays close attention to the harness, the attire of the driver, and an appropriate carriage to suit the horse, because judging is subjective and relies on strict adherence to tradition, based on a suitable match of horses and carriage. The horses perform movements requested by the judges, and style and quality of the gaits are scored subjectively. These horses compete at the walk and trot (a park pace being roughly equal to a slow working trot). Pleasure driving events also can include drives at the walk or trot on roads and tracks of up to 5 to 10 miles.

Competitive driving includes combined driving or horse driving trials and scurry driving. Scurry driving is seldom seen in North America but has a strong following in the United Kingdom and other parts of Europe. Scurry driving consists of a single horse (mainly ponies) or more commonly pairs of horses competing over a tight, coned course in a show ring against the clock. The horses and carriages are often small to allow the narrow gates (the gap between a pair of cones) and corners to be negotiated at speed. Horse driving trials are a driven form of horse trials, or eventing, and like its ridden counterpart, driving is a highly athletic, physically demanding sport for the horse and driver.

Driving trials as an international equestrian sport started in 1968, when the Fédération Équestre Internationale (FEI) international rules were drawn up under the instigation of HRH Prince Philip, who was then the President of the Federation. The first international horse driving trials event took place in 1971 in Hungary. Initially the competition was only for horse teams (four-in-hand). A team is composed of four horses, two before two; those in front are called *leaders,* and those closer to the coach, *wheelers.* As the sport developed and individuals of more modest means entered the fray, competitions for singles (one horse), tandems (two horses harnessed one behind the other), and pairs (two horses harnessed side by side) rapidly blossomed. These classes were further divided into those for ponies (less than 148 cm or 14.2 hands high) and horses. The sport is now structured at various levels depending on the ability of the driver and horse(s). Disabled driving has recently been introduced. The FEI is responsible for the international rules that cover the World and European championships and selected international events such as the Royal Windsor International Driving Grand Prix. The national associations liaise with the FEI and are responsible for running the national events and championships and producing national rules. Local driving clubs (found in Europe, the United Kingdom, and the United States) also run local events that may differ substantially in standards and requirements of competitors, but they essentially mimic FEI rules. Important events include the Royal Windsor (United Kingdom), Aachen and Riesenbeck (Germany), Breda (Holland), Saumur (France), Waregem (Belgium), St Gallen (Switzerland), and Fair Hill (United States). World championships are held every 2 years for singles, pairs, and teams for horses, and a European championship is held for pony teams. The World Equestrian Games, held every 4 years, which also host World Championships, allow four-in-hands only to compete. The first World Pony Championships (singles, pairs, and teams) were held in Saumur in 2003. Competitions in Europe run from April to September, with championships held toward the end of this period. However, in the last 5 years there has been a growth in indoor driving events, culminating in the FEI World Cup, which is a series of events within Europe. Indoor driving competitions often consist of three phases: precision and paces, cone driving, and time driving through marathon obstacles.

Horse driving trials consist of three phases—dressage, marathon, and cones—usually spread over 3 days, but in lower standard competition all three may take place over 1 to 2 days. The first phase is a driven dressage test, which consists of a set sequence of movements that are judged by a number of officials against a standard of absolute perfection. The test is designed to highlight the obedience, paces, and suppleness of the horse(s), and the skill of the driver in handling of the reins. The second stage is the marathon, which tests the fitness and stamina of the horse(s) and the judgment of pace and horsemanship of the driver. The cross-country marathon can be divided into three or five sections (depending on the level of competition); for each section a maximum and minimum time are allowed (Table 124-1).

The speeds and time allowances are adjusted for different classes, especially ponies. At the end of sections B and D are mandatory 10-minute halts. During the second of

these, the horses are subjected to veterinary checks for lameness, injuries, and fitness (respiratory rate, pulse rate, dehydration, temperature, and speed of recovery). Section E has eight obstacles. Each obstacle is made up of a number (up to six) of lettered gates. The aim is to drive through these gates (between white and red markers) within each obstacle in the correct alphabetical sequence in the shortest possible time. Most injuries occur on the marathon, although lameness may not become apparent until later, just before the third phase, the cone competition. The object of the cone phase is to test the fitness and suppleness of the horse after the marathon phase by driving through a course of narrowly spaced pairs of cones (up to a maximum of 20) within an allotted time. Each cone has a ball balanced on top of it that is dislodged easily if the horse or carriage strikes the cone. The winner of the competition is the competitor with the fewest penalty points.

Veterinary inspections of horses taking part in an event also occur before the dressage day, at the end of the marathon, and at the beginning of the cone competition. Lameness at any of these inspections usually leads to elimination from the event, although considerable variation exists in the definition of working soundness among veterinarians, particularly regarding hindlimb problems.

Horses used by Amish and Mennonite sects (United States) as beasts of burden are nearly always Standardbreds or American Saddlebred horses and are driven as singles. The horses are driven when needed, with no structured fitness training, and lameness is common.

TYPES OF HORSES USED

The type of horses used for driving varies considerably with the particular form of the sport or use to be undertaken. For pleasure and presentation driving, the type of horse used is related mainly to the size and type of the carriage and the overall effect the driver is trying to convey to the judges (e.g., country or town turnout, meaning an informal or formal appearance of the coach, harness, and driver's attire). Horses used include Shires, Clydesdales, and Percherons in heavy horse turnouts such as drays; Hackneys (including crosses), Thoroughbreds, and Warmbloods in smart town turnouts; Cobs, larger pony types such as Welsh Cobs, Welsh Section C, Dales, Fells, Fiordlanders, and Friesians in country turnouts; and smaller pony types such as Welsh Mountain Section A, Shetlands, New Forest, and Dartmoor in small carriage turnouts. The aforementioned breeds primarily cover the variety seen in the United Kingdom and Europe. In the United States Warmblood, Warmblood crosses, Welsh, Hackney, Morgan, and Friesians are used most often for pleasure and driving trials. Most presentation and pleasure driving is undertaken with a single horse turnout. The horses range from 4 to 20 years of age, and many have been or are used for other equestrian disciplines. Scurry driving usually involves single or pairs of small ponies or pony-type horses such as Shetlands, Welsh Mountain, New Forest, and Dartmoor. These ponies are often younger than pleasure-driving horses and are less likely to be used for other equestrian sports, except perhaps combined driving trials.

Horses used for driving trials must be older than 4 years of age before they can compete, and records show 19-year-old horses competing at world championship level. Many

TABLE 124-1

| | | | AVERAGE |
| *Basic Format of the Five-Stage Marathon* | | | |
	LENGTH	GAIT	SPEED (KPH)
Section A	≈10 km	Any type, usually trot	15
Section B	1 km	Walk	7
Section C	4 km	Fast trot	19
Section D	1 km	Walk	7
Section E	10 km	Trot, canter	14

of the best driving trial horses are 12 to 19 years of age and have been used earlier for other purposes. This long working life and slow introduction to work at a young age, together with little high-speed and more slow-speed conditioning work and regular winter breaks, has a considerable effect on the type of lameness seen in these horses. The types of horses and ponies used vary greatly. In continental Europe, Warmblood breeds are particularly popular; for example, Gelderlanders, Swedish Warmbloods, Dutch Warmbloods, Hanoverians, and Holsteiners, with a modern trait being ever-increasing size. In the United Kingdom less uniformity occurs in the horses used; for example, Hackney crosses, Cobs, Welsh Cobs, Lipizzaners, Lusitanians, Orlovs, and some Warmbloods and Thoroughbred crosses. The most popular ponies used for driving trials in Europe are Welsh Sections A, B, and C, Haflingers, and New Forest crosses.

In the practice radius of one of the authors (KK) is a unique opportunity to observe, evaluate, and diagnose lameness conditions in driving horses used by members of the Amish and Mennonite religious sects as a mode of transportation. Several regions throughout North America have populations large enough to provide a reasonable number of horse owners for which to provide veterinary services. The incidence of lameness is influenced by the necessity of driving reasonably long distances on asphalt surfaces (up to 30 miles [48 km] in one day), with sometimes a single horse pulling a Meadowbrook cart containing up to seven family members. Electricity is not used by the Amish sect and is consequently not available, so a veterinarian must be guided by the ability to palpate precisely and interpret the findings often without the adjunct diagnostic procedures relied on daily, such as radiography and ultrasonography. The veterinarian also faces great pressure because a lame horse may strand an Amish owner.

TRAINING

The training regimen for driving horses varies considerably depending on the type of driving to be undertaken and the level of competition to be attempted. Top-class horse driving trial horses require a regimented fitness program of up to several hours daily, with techniques for such fitness varying from trainer to trainer. In addition some time is spent practicing cone driving, and hazard training through schooling obstacles set up to mimic what is seen in competition. In pleasure or presentation driving, horses normally are worked intermittently, mainly on roads and tracks at the walk and trot, usually in the summer months, with a rest or turnout to grass in the winter. With the introduction of indoor winter competition, winter breaks may be reducing. In scurry driving the training required is more intense, with a combination of regular road work at the walk and trot to increase overall fitness, alongside school and field work concentrating on bending, suppleness, and turning at speed with accuracy. The scurry driving season can extend over longer periods of the year, when competition comes indoors. Amish horses attain a less quantitative level of fitness through irregular use and essentially no training.

Conditioning exercise tends to start in February, aiming for the first events in late April. Competitions are then available almost every weekend (Thursday to Sunday)

throughout the summer, culminating in the national and international championships in August to October.

The type or breed of horse used in driving and the way the horse is trained have an important effect on the type and incidence of lameness. Differences in conformation, gait, and size have an influence. Generally, ponies are less likely to develop lameness, are easier to train to fitness, and are more agile. When compared with horses, pony conformation and foot shape are better and they carry less weight. Unfortunately, alongside this general toughness is all too frequently allied a "cussed" temperament. Cob-types are similar to ponies in temperament and hardiness but are heavier and more powerful, often leading to low-grade osteoarthritis (OA) in later life. They often require considerable training to allow the necessary control and obedience to be obtained. Welsh Cobs and hackney-types and crosses have particularly exaggerated natural forelimb actions, which over long periods of use may increase wear-and-tear injuries in the forelimbs such as metacarpophalangeal joint problems. Some of the larger breeds, such as the Warmbloods, have poor conformation, especially in the hindlimbs, such as straight in the stifle and hock, which has a major effect on the incidence of lameness. Most driving horses are not broken to harness until they are 3 to 4 years old and are not worked until they are 5 to 6 years old. Therefore conditions prominent at an earlier age, such as osteochondrosis of the tarsus and stifle, are uncommon.

The incidence of lameness in driving horses is much influenced by a long working life; the training, which is mainly flat work at the walk and trot; the different stresses and strains placed on them by the carriage (increased pressure on the hindlimbs, especially distally); the regular rest periods during the driving career; slow start in life; and whether they have been used for other purposes, previously or concurrently. All of these factors contribute to a low incidence of lameness, especially from fractures or acute soft tissue injuries seen in racehorses, but an increased incidence of low-grade wear-and-tear injuries, particularly of the hindlimb joints. In recent years the increasing competition and prestige at the top end of the sport, particularly internationally, have led to increased demands on horses, less patience to wait for horses to mature or to become seasoned, and consequently more lameness.

GROUND CONDITIONS

Training is usually carried out on roads or tracks of varying surfaces, depending on the region and country involved. In the United Kingdom this is mainly tarmacadam roads and firm tracks, whereas in the eastern United States, tarmacadam, dirt, and gravel roads and precut paths through agricultural fields predominate. Training for dressage and cones is usually in grass paddocks, although some drivers have access to all-weather areas. The variable, often hilly terrain in the United Kingdom and United States helps develop fitness. In Europe some of the competitions and areas for training are flat and have a sandy soil, which gives an even, absorbent, good surface for exercise. The firm surfaces on which many driving horses train and work tend to increase concussion to the feet and joints; recent evidence has shown bone density is increased (strengthened) by driving on such surfaces, but firm surfaces are unlikely to prevent injury to tendons and ligaments as was once thought. Repeated concussion over many years may contribute to low-grade joint disease and means that good foot conformation and shoeing are imperative to help offset some of this constant trauma. The variable and unpredictable ground conditions present on marathon courses contribute to injuries to joints, such as the fetlock, and to ligaments and the digital flexor tendon sheath (DFTS).

CONFORMATION

The huge variety of breeds and types of horses used in driving means that no particular traits of conformation have been established as representative of this type of work. Many of the Warmbloods, which are the most common breeds on the continent of Europe and are now becoming so popular elsewhere in the world for riding and driving, have a conformation that appears to predispose them to OA of the distal hock joints. The hindlimbs are often straight through the hock and stifle, but some horses are sickle hocked and cow hocked. There is a high prevalence of osteochondrosis in Warmbloods, especially of the tarsocrural and stifle joints, which may manifest itself later in the working life of the horse. The headlong dash in recent years for bigger and stronger Warmblood driving horses has in our opinion led to a heavier, less agile horse, often with small feet and limited bone, which cannot help the horse cope with work over the many years that the horse is driven. Foot conformation in some of the carriage breeds, such as the Hackney, Orlov, Gelderlander, and Lipizzaner, can be upright and boxy, which may decrease concussion protection by the foot and increase trauma reflected up the limb. Many of the native breeds or crosses have good conformation and inherent limb soundness, which is reflected in their low level of lameness. The exception to this statement is the pleasure or presentation pony that is worked irregularly and kept at grass in the summer. The overweight (show condition) nature of these ponies and the access to large amounts of grass predispose them to laminitis, which more reflects owner management than suggests inherent unsoundness.

LAMENESS EXAMINATION

Examination of lameness in the driving horse differs little from the standard approach. The major objectives are to decide if the horse is lame, to determine which limb or limbs and which portion or portions of the limb(s) are affected, and to determine a pathological process. This process is complicated in a driving horse, particularly as the horse ages, because of the possibility of old or unimportant lesions and the low-grade and often bilateral nature of some causes of lameness. Further problems are related to intermittent or variable lameness. Identification of lameness is more difficult in a driving horse when being driven, especially lameness in a hindlimb, than in a ridden horse.

The history should consist of typical questions asked before any standard lameness evaluation—for example, how the lameness was first recognized, what the duration of the lameness has been, whether the lameness is worse on hard or soft ground, and whether the horse has responded to any treatments used. In addition, because driving horses are exercising between two poles that are parallel to the ground, straightness is generally fairly easy

for the driver to observe. Is the horse resting one hip on the right or left shaft? Is the horse leaning more on one rein than the other? With pairs and four-in-hand, is one horse taking more of the workload, indicating unwillingness of the other horse to pull an equal load? Have any changes in tack or harness been made? The veterinarian should observe the stance and attitude of the horse, areas of muscle atrophy, limb and foot conformation, and the presence of swellings before assessing the horse moving in hand at the walk and trot on a hard, flat surface. Examination in harness and carriage is rarely useful, because lameness is sometimes less evident while the horse is pulling, rather than moving freely and without restriction on a lunge line. When a driver or trainer feels that the lameness for which the horse is being presented is observed only when in work, that is, driven, seeing the horse in harness then may be necessary. Standard flexion tests of the forelimbs and hindlimbs are useful, but as a horse ages the likelihood of a positive result in an otherwise working, sound horse increases. Exercise on the lunge or in hand on a circle is helpful in horses with bilateral or mild lameness. Exercise on different surfaces (hard and soft) and when possible on a slight incline uphill and downhill can be useful.

Identification of the affected lame limb(s) should be followed by detailed palpation and manipulation of the limb(s), with the limb bearing weight and in a flexed position. Assessment of any swelling by digital palpation and manipulation of the limb(s) to determine whether pain can be elicited can help to differentiate old, clinically insignificant lesions. In older horses distention of fetlock and tarsocrural joint capsules and DFTSs is a common, clinically insignificant finding. Skin scars and areas of fibrosis from previous trauma may further complicate the localization of the site of pain causing lameness. Careful examination of the foot with hoof testers is important. The use of diagnostic analgesia is considered vital to rule out incidental lesions or previously managed chronic problems.

DIAGNOSTIC ANALGESIA

Many of the causes of lameness in driving horses are related to chronic wear-and-tear injuries in one or more joints. Distention of a joint capsule or DFTS can be an incidental finding. Localization of pain by a logical system of regional analgesia is central to our approach to lameness diagnosis and is particularly useful in horses with bilateral or multiple limb lameness, because such an approach allows the effect on the gait of one or more of the lame limbs to be removed, allowing identification of additional lame limb(s). In most horses localization of pain is initially undertaken by a sequence of perineural analgesic techniques beginning distally and moving proximally in a logical manner. In the forelimbs the sequence is palmar digital; palmar (abaxial sesamoid); low palmar and palmar metacarpal (four point); high palmar (subcarpal); and median, ulnar, and musculocutaneous. In the hindlimb the sequence is plantar (abaxial sesamoid); low six point; analgesia of the proximal aspect of the suspensory ligament (SL) (see Chapter 10 for numerous described techniques); intraarticular blocks of either specific joints of the tarsus or suspected stifle joints; and then tibial and fibular (peroneal) nerve blocks. Nerve blocks of the antebrachium or crus are useful when the veterinarian is uncertain if the lesion is above or below midlimb. Once that has been determined, more specific blocks may be planned proximally or distally as needed. If the veterinarian suspects a particular site, performing an intraarticular block at that site first may be more efficient. It may be necessary to perform intraarticular blocks after perineural analgesia. Sites for intrasynovial analgesia are prepared aseptically (with or with out clipping, at the discretion of the veterinarian), and fresh bottles of mepivacaine or bupivacaine, needles, and syringes are used. Gloves are mandatory for intrasynovial techniques. Assessment of response can be difficult in horses with mild or intermittent lameness or when several painful sites exist. The veterinarian should be as certain as possible of the degree of improvement in the lameness, but unfortunately this is sometimes equivocal. In a driving horse the most common intrasynovial structures injected are, in the forelimb, the distal interphalangeal (DIP), proximal interphalangeal (PIP), and metacarpophalangeal joints and the DFTS; and, in the hindlimb, the PIP, metatarsophalangeal, tarsometatarsal (TMT), centrodistal, and tarsocrural joints and the DFTS. Local infiltration of local anesthetic solution around areas of possible damage, such as periosteal reactions and ligament insertions, may be helpful in horses with specific injuries.

IMAGING CONSIDERATIONS

Many causes of lameness in a driving horse, especially in older horses, are related to problems in the distal aspect of the limb and the hock joints. Considerable variation in the radiological appearance of these structures can occur, representing normal anatomical variability, old injuries, incidental findings, or wear and tear. Only by localizing the site of pain to a particular joint by intraarticular analgesia is interpreting these findings possible. Standard radiographic images are obtained. Upper limb injuries are often induced by trauma, are not localized easily by diagnostic analgesia, and are difficult to examine with small x-ray machines. Ultrasonography is particularly useful in examining some of these injuries, not only to differentiate the soft tissue components (e.g., hematoma, muscle injury, edema, and wounds), but also to examine the cortical outline of the bones in the proximal aspect of the limb (shoulder and stifle regions) for evidence of fractures or other damage. Comparison with the opposite limb is helpful in determining what is normal in these areas.

Ultrasonography is essential for examining the DFTS and associated structures and for definitive diagnosis and monitoring of desmitis of the SL or the accessory ligament of the deep digital flexor tendon (ALDDFT). It may also be useful for evaluation of joints for detection of collateral ligament or joint capsule injury and identification of periarticular modeling or articular cartilage damage.

DIFFICULTIES IN DIAGNOSIS

The most difficult problem in diagnosing pain causing lameness in a driving horse is an intermittent, often low-grade lameness that may flare up with increased exercise or competition. Many lame driving horses have bilateral hindlimb problems, often with several sites of pain contributing to lameness. If making progress in these horses

by standard examination techniques is impossible, scintigraphic examination may be useful. The advantages of scintigraphy include the ability to cover many areas of the body (forelimbs and hindlimbs, back and pelvis) at one session, the noninvasive nature of the technique, and its use to monitor healing. The disadvantages include cost, lack of local availability, and lower sensitivity of the technique in localizing chronic sites of inflammation compared with acute injuries. Several sites may be detected as having increased radiopharmaceutical uptake, and other techniques, such as local analgesia, are necessary to assess clinical significance. Making a definitive diagnosis is not always possible, but it is important to treat what is diagnosable or visible and to monitor the horse's progress carefully during convalescence. A reassessment of the horse at regular stages may cast further light on the problem. We frequently tell clients that the best option is to treat what we are able to identify and monitor the progress of such treatment through periodic reassessment. Rest may be easy to accomplish in driving horses because they have a long working life, and in pairs and teams a spare horse may be available to take the lame horse's place, allowing competition to be continued.

A problem occasionally encountered in lameness from harness and carriage use is an abnormal gait, often intermittent, seen only while the horse is working in harness, usually with the carriage. Lameness often is manifested at the collected trot in the forelimb, and an extra lift in the shoulder movement during protraction is apparent. Usually only one forelimb is affected. The horse appears normal at the walk and extended trot, and the problem is not exacerbated by exercise. The actual diagnosis of this condition remains obscure, but one possible theory revolves around the effect of a neck collar on the action of the scapula while the horse is in harness: a mechanical interference. In some horses, changing from a neck collar to a breast band harness appears to stop the problem.

SHOEING

Most driving horses are shod conventionally, with few special techniques or shoes. Many are shod with flat, fullered shoes set rather short and tight at the heels to minimize interference injuries to the horse and the other member(s) of the pair or team. Other reasons for such shoeing given by farriers and owners include minimizing shoe loss in the varying surfaces of the competition and preventing inadvertent removal by the wearer or another horse by standing on the shoe. Short-shoeing a horse, with a tight fit in the heel, exacerbates poor foot conformation, whether the horse has upright, boxy feet or long-toed and low, weak-heeled feet.

The use of studs and occasionally calks, especially in the hind feet, is common in an attempt to increase grip in the marathon phase of competition. In the teams, the wheelers, where the power is mainly delivered, often have studs or calks. If studs have to be used, we prefer to see them put in only for the marathon and, if possible, only for the obstacles. The extra grip studs can give may lead to ligament or joint damage, particularly in the lower limb. The use of studs or calks all the time, especially on hard tracks and roads, increases heel trauma and changes the forces transmitted up the limbs. Unilateral studs and calks are not acceptable, and their use should be actively discouraged.

TEN MOST COMMON LAMENESS CONDITIONS

A 15-year retrospective study of the clinical practice of one of the authors (KK) led to the formation of the following list of common lameness conditions, in order of incidence. Some variation in incidence occurs from leaders to wheelers in four-in-hand teams and in other countries, such as the United Kingdom.

1. Suspensory desmitis
2. Foot lameness: heel pain, corns, and navicular region pain
3. Distal hock joint pain
4. Exertional rhabdomyolysis
5. Tenosynovitis of the digital flexor tendon sheath
6. Osteoarthritis of the proximal and distal interphalangeal and fetlock joints
7. Stifle lameness
8. Lesions associated with turnout: solar abscesses and bruising, mud fever, rain scald, cracked heels, and kick wounds
9. Interference and traumatic injuries of forelimbs and hindlimbs
10. Desmitis of the accessory ligament of the deep digital flexor tendon and superficial digital flexor tendonitis

DIAGNOSIS AND MANAGEMENT OF LAMENESS

Suspensory Desmitis

Desmitis of the SL, both body and branches, is common, particularly in Amish and Mennonite carriage horses. Seventy percent of the Amish carriage horses are Standardbreds, nearly all of which have raced previously and have preexisting chronic, healed, or healing suspensory desmitis. Forelimbs (80%) and hindlimbs (20%) are affected. Body and branch lesions occur with similar prevalence in forelimbs, but branch injuries predominate in hindlimbs.

Suspensory desmitis may cause an acute-onset, moderate lameness, but often a low-grade insidious lameness is reported by the owner or driver. There is often considerable swelling and inflammation associated with the SL. Horses with branch lesions especially have a positive response to a lower limb flexion test. Diagnosis usually is based on clinical examination and is confirmed by ultrasonography, but in some horses diagnostic analgesia is required to confirm that the SL is the source of pain.

With branch lesions radiological examination of the proximal sesamoid bones (PSBs) and splint bones is required to identify concurrent fractures or sesamoiditis, which influence prognosis. PSB fractures usually are seen in Standardbred horses that have raced previously and were retired with a fracture, pain from which becomes apparent after a second career as an Amish driving horse. Amish and Mennonite horses with a less-than-good prognosis may be culled.

Rest is essential. The duration is determined by improvement in lameness, reduced sensitivity on palpation, and improvement in fiber pattern assessed by ultrasonography. In the initial, acute stages, cold hosing, icing for a few days, and support wrapping are recommended. The combined oral use of dexamethasone and a diuretic is helpful in decreasing inflammation and filling without masking pain. It is important to provide appropriate palmar or plantar support, and if necessary an egg bar shoe is used to increase the weight-bearing surface.

In horses with the most severe injuries, and in situations in which economics does not play a role in selection of treatment, a more aggressive approach may be considered. Very good results have been obtained with surgical treatment of horses with large core lesions in the body of the SL. After perineural analgesia and localization of the core lesion by ultrasonography, we use a sharpened teat bistoury to enter the core lesion with the limb bearing weight. A rigid 18-week slow progressive exercise schedule is then employed. Alternatively, intralesional injections of autologous platelet-rich plasma (PRP) or stem cells can be performed. Several different commercial kits are available for retrieval and harvesting of biological material. We are encouraged by the results to date, but the number of driving horses managed using these techniques is insufficient to report the level of success.

Some clients prefer to turn out a horse with suspensory desmitis rather than adhere to a structured rehabilitation. Our impression is that lesions heal more slowly, often with less acceptable cosmetic results, compared with horses in which controlled exercise is used. Horses with branch injuries are treated conservatively with a long, slow progressive exercise schedule, with periodic ultrasonographic monitoring. Therapeutic ultrasound treatment also is recommended.

Prevention of suspensory desmitis is achieved primarily by selecting well-conformed horses with a good hoof-pastern axis and good feet and continually reassessing hoof balance, the adequacy of heel support, and the angle of the pastern relative to the limb conformation.

Foot Lameness

Foot lameness is common in driving horses and is traumatic, degenerative, or inflammatory. Lameness varies from simple trauma (puncture wounds and bruises) to infectious conditions such as thrush, degenerative conditions such as navicular syndrome, and a host of lesions caused or affected by quality of shoeing.

Carriage horses receive a moderate amount of direct trauma resulting in wounds to the digit. The lack of available prepared and manicured training surfaces often necessitates fitness work on gravel roads and through streams and wooded areas, and solar punctures by stumps or sharp objects are not uncommon. Injuries to the coronary region of horses in pairs and four-in-hand occur when driving conditions are difficult, as in the hazards, when one or more horses may be stepped on by an adjacent horse.

Although wounds of the coronary band are generally obvious, a puncture of the sole may not be readily apparent. A horse with a puncture may or may not be lame at the time of injury. The excitement of competition allows horses to continue without overt signs of discomfort, even with frank injury to the sole. Once back in the stable or sometimes the following day, lameness becomes apparent. Many wounds of the sole and frog are difficult to see, and they can be missed easily. Frog and sole tissue tends to close over the entry site, particularly if the offending object was sharp. If foreign material remains in the foot, severe lameness is usually present. We recommend being very aggressive with "unroofing" sole or frog puncture sites in horses with severe lameness, because it may be the only way to tell if vital structures are contaminated, and removal of organic material is imperative. Most horses respond well to curettage and soaking in antiseptic solutions, but protracted lameness is usually a sign of infection. Contrast radiology is useful to detect direction and depth of a tract. When a veterinarian cannot determine if vital structures are involved, surgical exploration or magnetic resonance imaging (MRI) examination may be indicated.

Bruises and corns are diagnosed by localizing pain to the sole or heel, evaluating the history, ruling out other causes of foot lameness, and identifying areas of solar discoloration. Treatment for bruising is directed at protecting the sole. In susceptible horses with a chronic tendency toward bruising, use of foot soaks or preferably packing gel with dimethyl sulfoxide with an overwrap frequently is indicated for flare-ups. Horses with corns require changes in shoeing to relieve pressure on the heel and constant monitoring of the heel growth to discourage an underrun, rolled in heel.

Synovitis of the DIP joint occurs as an acute or, less commonly, as a recurrent condition. Effusion of the DIP joint and lameness generally are exacerbated by distal limb flexion. Diagnosis is confirmed by intraarticular analgesia. Treatment consists of phenylbutazone (2 g sid) or flunixin meglumine (500 mg sid) for several days, icing of the digit, and intramuscular administration of a polysulfated glycosaminoglycan (PSGAG), with or without intraarticular administration of hyaluronan or corticosteroids.

Navicular syndrome may be more prevalent in carriage horses of certain breeds. The European Warmbloods, particularly the heavier horses, appear to be at risk. Navicular syndrome is nearly nonexistent in driving ponies. Horses with navicular syndrome have an insidious lameness that usually resolves with palmar digital analgesia. Occasionally a horse has sudden onset of moderate-to-severe lameness without any history of a chronic problem. These horses may have dramatic lesions apparent radiologically without a reasonable explanation for why the lameness occurred suddenly rather than gradually. A critical evaluation of hoof balance is important, and we recommend using bar or egg bar shoes. Very good results have been obtained by intrathecal injection of the navicular bursa with hyaluronan and triamcinolone acetonide (4 to 6 mg) along with improved shoeing. Horses with more pronounced lameness may also be treated with phenylbutazone (1 to 2 g orally [PO] sid).

The greatest number of carriage horses with foot pain fit into a broad category of palmar foot pain (also see Chapter 30). Lengthy drives on hard surfaces result in chronic contusions to the hoof capsule and subsequent lameness. Palmar foot pain often is correlated with the degree of work the horse is undertaking currently and may occur seasonally in susceptible horses. Lameness varies from slight to moderate and is exacerbated by circling on hard ground with the affected limb on the inside of a circle. Hoof tester examination may reveal pain from the medial or lateral sulcus across to that quarter, but a large number of horses have no reaction. Lameness is eliminated by perineural analgesia of the palmar digital nerves. Intraarticular analgesia of the DIP joint and intrathecal analgesia of the navicular bursa ideally should be performed to rule out these structures as sources of pain. Radiological examination usually is unrewarding.

Assessment of hoof balance and shoeing is necessary, and until any imbalance has been corrected, recommending other therapies is pointless. We have had good results from increasing the length of support or ground surface in the dorsal or palmar direction of the hoof, without any other therapy. Many horse owners do not understand when instructed to move the weight-bearing surface farther palmarly, and they simply raise the heel. Talking directly with the farrier and providing explanatory diagrams to the client are worthwhile. If the heels are too weak or inadequate to allow for corrective trimming, using egg bar shoes until heel growth is adequate may be necessary.

Distal Hock Joint Pain

OA of the distal hock joints is common, particularly in older and larger horses (>10 years old). Many of these horses are not presented by the owner or driver as overtly lame but with a history referring to lack of performance or action, stiffness, back problems, or poor bending. Some horses with OA, especially from teams, are not identified until veterinary inspections at events. Many older driving horses, particularly those in horse driving trials at a high level, have an uneven hindlimb gait, especially when trotted in hand, and have a positive response to upper limb flexion tests. The horse often is said to warm or work into its work (warm out of lameness), and owners do not request investigation. A high percentage of these horses have low-grade OA of the distal hock joints. In some horses acute lameness or gradual worsening of lameness (often described as unilateral lameness by the driver) leads to lameness investigation. In the Warmblood breeds an earlier incidence of this problem has become apparent in recent years, with horses of 5 to 8 years old showing severe OA and even ankylosis of affected joints. Many have poorly conformed and small hocks, and in some OA appears to be a sequela to developmental orthopedic disease in a young, growing horse.

Diagnosis is based on clinical examination, intraarticular analgesia, and radiology. Many horses have bilateral lameness, with one limb worse than the other, and evidence of gluteal muscle atrophy. Poor hock conformation (sickle hocked, straight, or cow hocked) predisposes some horses to OA. Shoe and hoof wear may indicate toe dragging or abnormal lateral breakover. Swelling may be palpable or visible at the seat of spavin. Tarsocrural joint distention is a common incidental finding, but it may indicate proximal intertarsal (talocalcaneal-centroquartal) joint involvement. The gait often is characterized by reduced foot flight arc and hock flexion, leading to toe dragging, and adduction of the limb medially underneath the body to land and then breakover laterally. On the lunge, lameness of the inside hindlimb may be worse, with shortening of the cranial phase of the stride and a tendency to fall toward the handler. Bilateral lameness is common, although one limb is often worse, leading to a choppy or stilted gait.

Flexion tests of the upper hindlimb are often positive bilaterally, but the response varies enormously depending on the stage and extent of the disease and the individual horse. Positive flexion test results in the hindlimbs of older driving horses are common, even in the absence of lameness.

Initially, lameness can be localized to the hock region using perineural analgesia, although intraarticular analgesia is more specific. Previously the centrodistal and TMT joints were blocked separately, but more recently only the TMT is blocked, on the basis of recent research confirming the high rate of diffusion of mepivacaine between the two joints.

A poor correlation exists between the degree of lameness and the extent of radiological abnormalities. Scintigraphic examination may be indicated in the absence of radiological abnormalities.

Treatment depends on a variety of factors including the degree of lameness, other concurrent causes of lameness (e.g., back problems), the type and extent of radiological abnormalities, the age of the horse, the level of work, the competition undertaken, the time and cost constraints, and the response to previous treatment. Conservative treatments often are used when financial constraints exist, when lameness is mild, or when radiologically the disease is advanced, or simply to assess the effects of treatment before more radical therapy is considered. Surgical treatments involve the willingness of the owner to make the financial investment and subject the horse to the risk of general anesthesia. We usually assess all aspects on an individual basis before embarking on a standard treatment plan, involving three monthly clinical and radiological examinations.

In general, because of the low-grade and chronic nature of the complaint in driving horses, a horse initially may be treated conservatively with corrective shoeing (graduated toe heel shoe, rolled at the toe, with or without lateral extension), a controlled graduated exercise program (up to 90 minutes) placing an emphasis on walking and trotting in a straight line (ridden or driven), and oral medication with variable levels of nonsteroidal antiinflammatory drugs (NSAIDs) (usually phenylbutazone) to control pain and encourage a more normal action. Many driving horses make considerable clinical progress with this regimen, but few high-level driving trial horses are able to return to competition quickly. Resolution of lameness may take up to 18 months and in some horses never happens if conservative treatments are used. Predicting the course of the disease and ultimate result in any one horse is difficult early and requires consideration of all the clinical and radiological findings. Many horses improve, but they do not become sound and have minimal progression of radiological abnormalities over 6 to 12 months. Horses with more obvious lameness, or those that are unable to cope with exercise with orally administered phenylbutazone, may be candidates for intraarticular injections with long-acting corticosteroid preparations (10 mg triamcinolone acetonide or 40 mg methylprednisolone acetate per joint). This may result in improvement for 3 to 6 months, and repeated injection usually is required. The use of NSAIDs or corticosteroids is not allowed in official competitions, and drugs must be withdrawn according to the manufacturers' recommendations before any competition. The use of tiludronate has increased with mixed results. Pentosan polysulfate (Cartrophen) is used by some clinicians, but there is controversy over its efficacy, and the drug is not licensed for use in the horse in Europe.

Arthrodesis is used in horses that fail to respond to conservative or intraarticular treatment or are in too much pain to achieve ankylosis by exercise, and when time to return to performance soundness is important. In horses with minimal radiological changes, intraarticular injection of sodium monoiodoacetate is performed using general anesthesia. In horses with more advanced radiological abnormalities or those in which monoiodoacetate has failed to achieve ankylosis, surgical treatment using three drill holes is used in each joint. Controlled exercise postoperatively is essential for success with either treatment. Although many driving horses with OA of the distal tarsal joints are useable with treatment, complete resolution of lameness is unusual.

Exertional Rhabdomyolysis

Carriage horses have isolated episodes of tying up during competition or strenuous exercise, and this is a true exertional rhabdomyolysis. Competition horses may develop mild signs of muscle stiffness affecting the hindquarters, during or at the conclusion of an exertional session, such as the marathon. The condition may become apparent in the 10-minute box, during the formal veterinary examination section, or before the marathon course. Clinical signs are invariably subtle and may be interpreted as fatigue by an inexperienced competitor. Affected horses should be withdrawn from the competition to avoid further skeletal muscle damage. Treatment should include administering antiinflammatory drugs and low doses of acepromazine (5 to 25 mg total dose) and ensuring adequate hydration. Horses should not be walked out of the stiffness and should be moved by trailer from the 10-minute box to a treatment stall.

To prevent further episodes, the feeding up to and including a competition and a horse's fitness program should be evaluated and amended as necessary. Teaching drivers how to assess a horse's fitness by measurement of temperature and pulse and respiratory rates on the stress days of training sessions is particularly valuable.

Acute, severe rhabdomyolysis (tying up) also occurs in horses driven by the Amish and Mennonites. These are frequently emergency situations. Horses have true, severe exertional rhabdomyolysis and are often in recumbency when examined. The clinical signs in nonrecumbent horses are extreme muscle stiffness and swelling over the topline and gluteal muscle groups, increased heart rate, sweating, and coliclike symptoms. The history is consistent: the horse became stiff while being driven, but the driver needed to continue to a destination and may have been driven another 1 to 15 miles [1.6 to 24 Km]. The condition in colloquial Amish terminology is referred to as *kidney shot*.

Rehydration and controlling pain and shock are imperative. Tranquilizers are particularly helpful, and measurement of packed cell volume and total protein concentration is useful for monitoring hydration. Measurement of creatine kinase may be useful prognostically in recumbent horses, although the initial response to treatment and the ability to get the horse on its feet are primary factors in determining whether the horse can be saved. Creatine kinase concentrations are often 400,000 to 800,000 IU/L (normal 130 to 400 IU/L), and we have treated horses successfully with levels up to 600,000 IU/L. Without prompt emergency attention, nearly all of the more severely affected horses die or are ultimately humanely destroyed. Most horses that remain recumbent after 24 hours are lost.

Horses are viewed by Amish farmers as utilitarian and necessary for transportation, and prevention of fatal exertional rhabdomyolysis is not necessarily easy. Owners should be advised of the need to match exercise with the intake of concentrates. If possible, the horse's entire body can be clipped if the onset of summer or warm weather is sudden or the winter coat is still present. Clipping can be done using a gas-powered generator for the clippers. Clipped horses have less risk of severe dehydration, and a clipped horse apparently is less prone to rhabdomyolysis than a hirsute horse.

Tenosynovitis of the Digital Flexor Tendon Sheath

Tenosynovitis of the DFTS is a common cause of acute hindlimb lameness. Often extreme swelling of the DFTS occurs and is turgid and firm, which contrasts to chronic, benign distention of the DFTS in which fluid in an overly stretched sheath can be balloted from side to side.

With horses with acute tenosynovitis there is a substantial response to lower limb flexion, and in some horses (5%) a non–weight-bearing lameness develops. Using perineural analgesia is unnecessary, but intrathecal analgesia using 6 to 10 mL of mepivacaine can be used to confirm the source of pain. Synoviocentesis is best performed distal to the fetlock and is facilitated by applying a disposable elastic bandage around the distal metatarsal region to push the fluid into the distal outpouching of the sheath on the plantar aspect of the pastern (Figure 124-1). Once

the sheath has been entered, an assistant cuts off the bandage, and local anesthetic solution is injected.

Radiological examination is usually negative, but is necessary to be certain that no unexpected lesion is missed. Ultrasonographic examination is essential to determine if tenosynovitis is associated with a lesion of the deep digital flexor tendon (DDFT), which requires a longer convalescence, and horses have a more guarded prognosis than those with primary tenosynovitis.

Treatment is based on reducing inflammation and controlling exercise. Uncontrolled turnout results in prolonged healing, and stall rest followed by walking in hand is preferable. A horse with an acute injury is treated with icing for 40 minutes twice a day, for 2 to 3 days, and orally administered NSAIDs. Intrathecally administered hyaluronan is beneficial. Caution should be exercised in the use of corticosteroids, which may provide temporary relief and often give the client a false sense of security regarding the rate of healing. Isoflupredone acetate is recommended, is short acting, and may control the acute flare-up without having any long-term effect that makes monitoring progress difficult. Methylprednisolone acetate lasts at least twice as long and may predispose the horse to develop dystrophic mineralization in the sheath. We have had better long-term results with conservative medical management than with surgical treatment by desmotomy of the plantar annular ligament.

Prevention of tenosynovitis and tears of the DDFT is difficult, because most injuries are acute and unforeseeable,

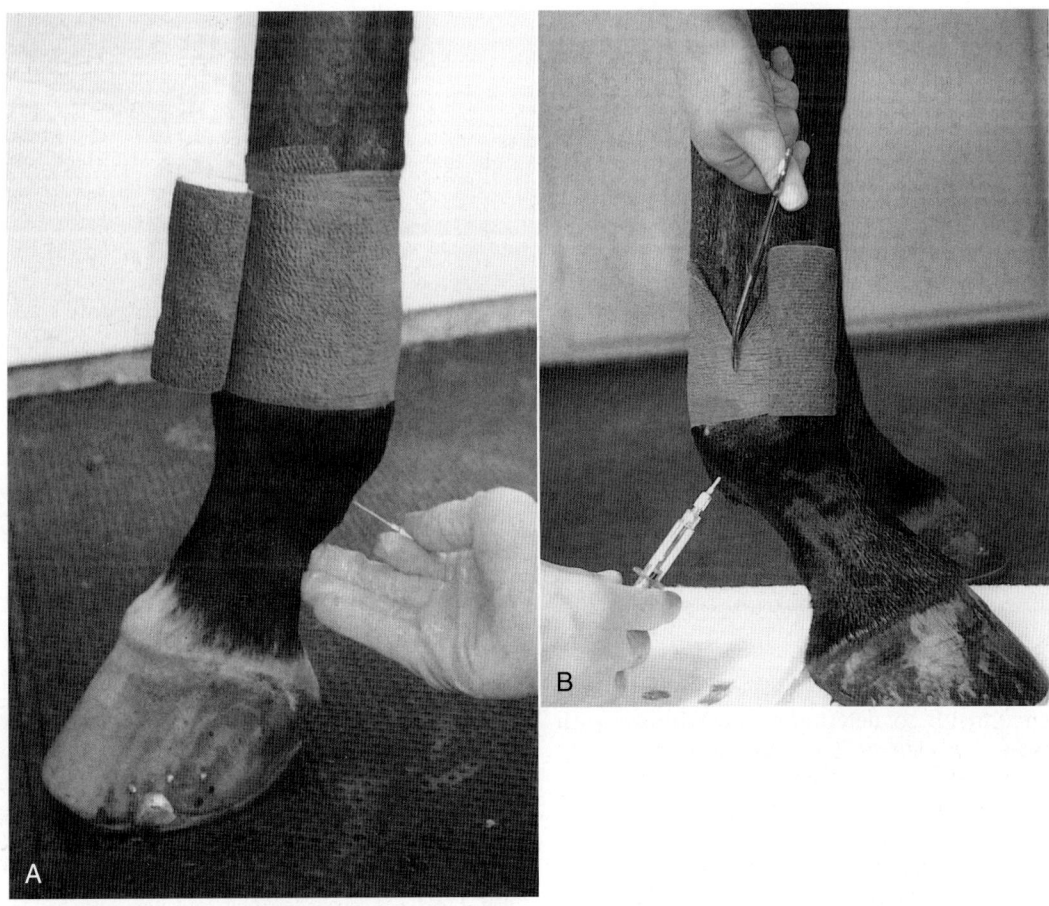

Fig. 124-1 • A, Application of a pressure bandage isolates fluid in the distal, plantar outpouching of the digital flexor tendon sheath, facilitating synoviocentesis. **B,** An assistant cuts the compression bandage during injection.

occurring during strenuous exercise. A team horse previously used as a wheeler may be better placed as a leader. The foot should be kept well balanced, with a full-fitting shoe providing adequate plantar support.

Chronic Osteoarthritis of the Lower Limb Joints

Many driving horses develop chronic OA of the DIP, PIP, and metacarpophalangeal joints as a result of wear and tear because of the work they undertake, the length of time they are used, and other factors such as conformation, foot shape, and shoeing. Radiological examination of these joints, especially in the hindlimbs and in larger horses, often reveals a variety of intraarticular and periarticular abnormalities that may be associated with lameness. Older driving horses often live with low-grade hindlimb gait abnormalities associated with low-grade joint pain. This low-grade, chronic, and often multiple leg or multiple joint pain can be exacerbated by excessive or different exercise regimens, leading to acute flare-ups, increased lameness (often unilateral), joint flexion pain, periarticular heat, and joint swelling. Radiographs obtained at this time reveal little more than the preexisting abnormalities. Intraarticular analgesia may be essential to localize the pain causing lameness, but multiple limb and joint involvement can make localization difficult. Nuclear scintigraphy may be helpful, but it is expensive, and often it is used only after early treatment has proved unsuccessful.

Treatment of horses with acute flare-ups of OA involves cold therapy such as cold hosing or ice packs, compression bandaging, systemic NSAIDs, topical applications of various antiinflammatory substances, and intraarticular or systemic medications such as corticosteroids, hyaluronan, interleukin-1 receptor antagonist protein (IRAP), and PSGAGs. Rest and a controlled, graduated return to exercise are important. Management of horses with chronic OA involves a careful review and possible modification of the horse's work program, judicious use of NSAIDs, physiotherapy techniques such as laser or ultrasound treatment, and systemic medication with hyaluronan or PSGAGs. The prognosis varies enormously depending on the severity and extent of the problem, the way in which the individual horse responds to pain, and the level of work required to keep the horse sound and competing. In many horses, if the hindlimbs are affected and especially if the condition is bilateral and the horse is part of a pair or team, then the chronic low-level lameness is not observed, is undiagnosed, or is ignored. An acute flare-up may lead to recognition of the problem and diagnosis. Prognosis for horses with the first acute flare-up is reasonable, but those with further occurrences warrant more aggressive management, which if unsuccessful worsens the overall prognosis.

Stifle Lameness

A definitive diagnosis of the cause of stifle pain in driving horses is often difficult to determine. Most horses with stifle lameness are wheelers of a four-in-hand or one of a pair. It is generally accepted that wheelers supply 60% of the workload in pulling, which may affect the incidence of stifle lameness. Lameness is usually acute in onset and unilateral, with no stifle effusion or other localizing clinical signs. Stifle flexion may cause more obvious accentuation of lameness than other hindlimb flexion tests. Lameness is improved by intraarticular analgesia.

Radiographs uniformly are negative. Ultrasonographic examination may sometimes reveal a lesion, but in more than 80% of horses no cause of pain can be identified. However, with digital ultrasonographic imaging and improved operator skill the likelihood of establishing a diagnosis may improve. Arthroscopic exploration may be warranted, but this is expensive, and only a limited part of the stifle can be assessed. The prognosis generally is guarded for horses with a known meniscal or cruciate ligament injury and for those without a specific diagnosis. The best results have been achieved after intraarticular treatment with hyaluronan, combined with systemic administration of PSGAG and rest or rigidly controlled exercise, walking in hand.

We recommend that horses not resume work until 60 days after complete resolution of lameness *and* when they no longer manifest a positive response to stifle flexion.

Direct Trauma

Traumatic injuries to the limbs and body of a driving horse are common.

Interference Injuries

Distal limb lacerations of varying severity are common, especially in horses that are part of a team, particularly in combined driving, and are caused by overreaching (forelimbs) or by interference from other horses. The most common lesions involve the heel and coronary band (Figure 124-2), although wounds to the midpastern and distal palmar (plantar) aspect of the metacarpal (metatarsal)

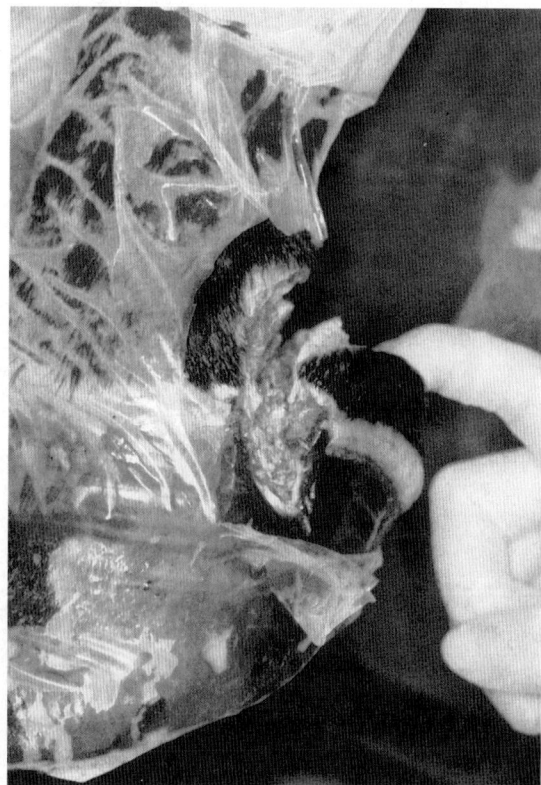

Fig. 124-2 • A severe heel bulb laceration sustained by a driving horse during a team competition, probably caused by interference from another horse.

region occur frequently. Many wounds are superficial and consist only of contaminated skin, but it is essential to check for injury to the digital flexor tendons and the DFTSs, joint integrity, and damage to the coronary band. The horse should be restrained properly, the affected area clipped and vigorously cleaned, and the damage assessed before medical or surgical treatment is initiated. In some horses detailed examination using digital palpation with sterile gloves, radiography, ultrasonography, and even surgical exploration may be necessary. Early and aggressive treatment may improve the prognosis considerably in the short and long term.

Injuries to the Brisket, Lower Neck, Antebrachium, Stifle, and Crus

Injuries usually occur during the marathon phase of driving trials, especially in the obstacles, or after runaways and accidents in any driven horse. The tendency of some drivers in combined driving in recent years to drive the carriage as a battering ram through the obstacles has increased the incidence of these injuries. Skin lesions occur, especially in the brisket and caudal aspect of the neck and upper forearm regions, and can range from full-thickness lacerations to mild hair loss and deeper bruising (Figure 124-3). In some horses little is visible externally except

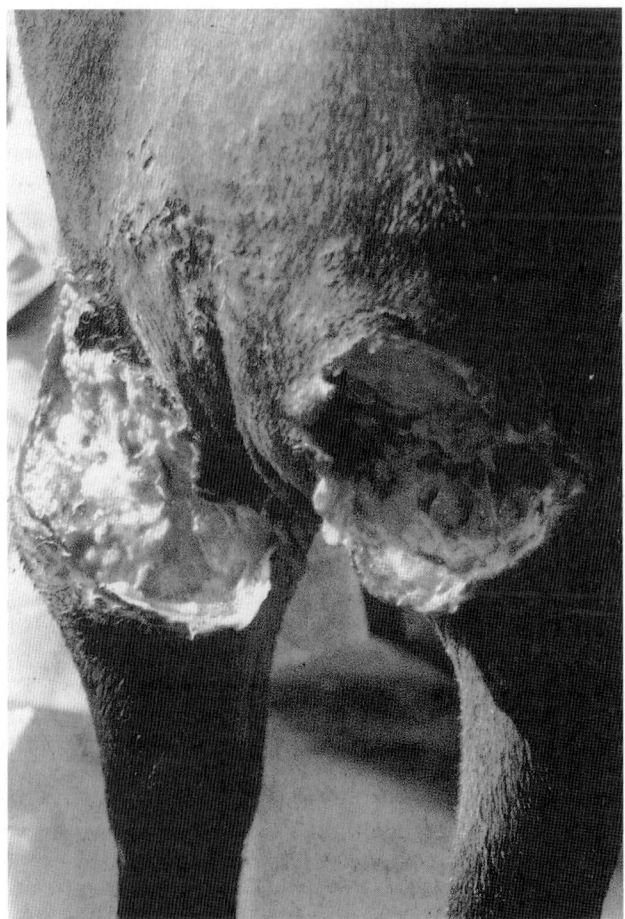

Fig. 124-3 • A severe traumatic injury to the upper forelimb and brisket regions caused by a collision with an obstacle in the marathon.

mild swelling to suggest the site of impact. Stiffness or lameness often develops several hours later. Severe trauma, particularly involving broken shafts or obstacles, can lead to life-threatening injuries to the chest, abdomen, or vital vascular structures.

The injured area should be examined carefully, particularly when lacerations are present. In these, thorough lavage and cleaning, followed by digital exploration using sterile gloves to assess for additional deeper damage, are essential. Surgical repair may be necessary. Horses with blunt soft tissue damage and bruising benefit from light walking in hand, cold therapy, topical and systemic antiinflammatory medication, and physiotherapy techniques.

Desmitis of the Accessory Ligament of the Deep Digital Flexor Tendon

Desmitis of the ALDDFT is a common cause of forelimb lameness. Older horses, including ponies, are more likely to be affected, and injury can occur at exercise or during turnout. Onset is usually acute, with unilateral forelimb lameness occurring during or immediately after exercise. Swelling of the ALDDFT occurs with edematous swelling of the surrounding soft tissues. In horses with severe desmitis, periligamentous hemorrhage can occur. Palpable pain is rare, but heat usually is apparent.

Ultrasonographic examination is used to determine the extent of injury. Diffuse lesions are more common than focal core lesions. Damage to other tendon structures is uncommon, but adhesions to the superficial digital flexor tendon (SDFT) or DDFT do occur, particularly in horses with chronic recurrent injuries.

Treatment of horses with acute injuries includes cold therapy, compression bandaging, box rest, and topical or systemic antiinflammatory medications. We regularly recommend the use of systemic PSGAG therapy and therapeutic ultrasound physiotherapy from 7 days after injury. Graduated walking in hand is encouraged from 7 days after injury, increasing in duration up until 12 weeks, when limited free exercise is allowed. Ultrasonography is essential to determine when healing is sufficient to allow exercise to begin. A total convalescent period of 6 to 15 months may be required. Some injuries, particularly in older horses, do not heal satisfactorily. Occasionally horses with chronic injuries with adhesions have been treated by desmotomy of the ALDDFT, but the prognosis for return to full soundness is guarded. Recently a small number of horses with severe injuries have been treated with PRP, but it is too early to evaluate success.

Superficial Digital Flexor Tendonitis

Superficial digital flexor tendonitis is not common in a driving horse, although the condition is seen occasionally as a flare-up of a lesion sustained previously in another discipline, or in wheelers when the going during the marathon phase has been soft and deep. Most lesions are in the distal half of the metacarpal region and are generally mild. Diagnosis is based on clinical and ultrasonographic examinations. The prognosis for return to full work as a driving horse is generally good, because most of the injuries are mild and the type of work to be undertaken is usually slow.

Chapter 125

Lameness in Draft Horses

Dallas O. Goble

The draft horse today enjoys a position in the world far different from when it was considered primarily a work animal. Draft horses supplied power for farming, transportation of commodities, lumbering, road building, and all such tasks until the 1930s, when the gasoline engine essentially replaced the horse. Isolated areas still continued to use the draft horse for farming and some lumbering activities until the early 1940s. After this period, draft horses were used primarily for specialty areas such as movie production, theme parks, parades, and frontier celebrations. But in some communities, religion and family tradition mandated the continual use of draft horses as a power source for farming. During the 1950s and 1960s, draft horses decreased in numbers in the United States, and subsequently the genetic pool was decreased. Draft horses started gaining popularity in the late 1970s and early 1980s and have once again become a popular member of the horse industry.

Draft horses today are different from those of the early 1900s. They perform different functions and are owned for a different purpose. Owning a draft horse is far more likely to be simply a hobby than an economic part of the family income. Many horses are used strictly for show purposes in classes such as halter, fine harness, and equitation, or for parades and advertising. Draft horses are used for trail riding, pleasure riding, fox hunting (often crossbred with Thoroughbreds), and other pleasure uses. In some mountain areas where selective lumbering of individual trees is undertaken, draft horses are still used today. With a resurgence of interest in mules, draft horse mares often are used in the breeding programs. Draft horses frequently are crossed with Thoroughbreds to change the genetic pool for the breeding of large hunter, jumper, and Three Day Event horses. Pulling contests are popular in certain areas and represent an additional use of the modern-day draft horse.

MODERN-DAY DRAFT HORSES

The most important physical change of the modern-day draft horse is its size. In many modern breeding operations, size is the main criterion used for selection. When draft horses were used predominantly as working horses, the average weight was 680 to 775 kg (1500 to 1700 lb) and the average height was 1.6 to 1.7 m (15.5 to 17 hands). This size was optimal for the multipurpose activities these horses performed on most farms and ranches. They pulled the plow, mowed and racked hay, helped round up cattle, and often took the family to church on Sunday. Draft horses today are more frequently in the range of 820 to 1000 kg (1800 to 2200 lb) and measure 1.8 to 2 m (17.5 to 19.5 hands) in height. As a result of selection based on size as the dominant characteristic, conformation and quality

have suffered in some respects. Distribution of lameness also has changed. Foot size and quality have not increased proportionately with body size and weight. Osteoarthritis (OA) is common in draft horses and likely is related to body size rather than the use of the horse. Hybrid vigor, once thought to be advantageous, has decreased by using the practice of line breeding for selected traits. The large size of a draft horse sometimes misleads one to think the horse can withstand greater stress and disease than can light horses, but I have not found this to be true. Draft horses may not recover as well as light horses with the same injury or disease. Because draft horses have a tendency to be stoic, recognizing a severe problem early in the disease process may be difficult. This tendency may cause a costly delay in diagnosis and management. The physical size of draft horses today has hindered veterinary care and treatment. Veterinarians tend to be unsure of drug dosage and appropriate treatment schedules because of the large body size. Many hobby horse owners do not have facilities adequate to handle a 1000-kg horse and may not be knowledgeable in draft horse care. Draft horses are not always well trained or easy to handle, and owners are sometimes unable to lend assistance when needed. These facts have curtailed the interest of many practicing veterinarians who have difficulty rationalizing being stepped on by a 1000-kg draft horse as fun. In addition, finding high-quality foot care for a draft horse is sometimes difficult, because most farriers are experienced with light horses. Farriers feel similar to veterinarians: "Why hold up a 1000-kg horse twice as long as needed to hold up a 500-kg horse?" In addition, farriers who shoe draft horses have to stock nails, shoes, and bar stock often on special order or low-volume items, a fact that dramatically increases overhead expenses. Thankfully, some veterinarians and farriers are willing to treat and specialize in draft horse care.

The following discussion related to draft horse lameness reflects my personal clinical experiences and not necessarily what may be in the equine literature. Lameness distribution may vary from my observations depending on the use, location, individual draft breed studied, or other factors associated with different populations of horses.

LAMENESS EXAMINATION

Diagnosis and management of lameness in a draft horse may seem more intimidating simply because of the large size of the horse and the infrequency with which requests are made for examination compared with light horses. In reality, draft horses experience the same problems as do light horses, although the distribution is different, and the principles of diagnosis and management are the same. The lameness examination is the same as in light horses, and any deficiency of hands-on experience can be overcome by a systematic and thorough examination. Palpation of peripheral nerves (palmar and plantar digital nerves, in particular) can be difficult because of thick skin and hair, and veterinarians are sometimes reluctant to attempt perineural or intraarticular blocks. The anatomy is the same, but the ability to palpate the nerves is diminished by these factors and also by subcutaneous thickening that some draft horses develop in the lower part of the limb.

Draft horse lameness diagnosis and management lagged behind those of light horses for many years. First, as long as the horse could still accomplish farm work, less concern was shown for a horse that limped slightly. Possibly the person behind the plow or cultivator also limped and accepted it as part of doing the job. Second, economic considerations were a major factor in the farming operation. This does not reflect necessarily a lack of care, but it was simply an accepted part of working in that day and time. But today, draft horses are afforded the same concerns and care given to the light horse, and only modification of most treatment protocols needs to be made.

Detailed description of the lameness examination can be found in earlier chapters. Special attention should be paid to several critical points, however. Draft horses are more stoic than light horses, and as a result lameness may be advanced when first recognized. For example, draft horses with OA of the proximal interphalangeal (PIP) or distal interphalangeal (DIP) joints may have severe radiological changes, but the owner may report that the horse only recently showed signs of lameness. Granted, many owners are inexperienced, but even the experienced owner may not recognize a problem until it is well advanced. This can be explained partially by the fact that a draft horse often is used at a gait (walk) that makes lameness less obvious, and the horse frequently is hitched with one to seven additional horses, and an individual horse's problems are less discernible in a group.

When possible, observing the horse at a walk and trot on soft and hard surfaces is useful. Hoof tester examination, in my experience, is less reliable in draft horses than in light horses. Small hoof testers are of questionable value. Even with long-handled hoof testers, it is difficult to apply enough pressure to produce a positive response. Foot lameness should be suspected if a horse shows grade 1 of 5 lameness on soft footing but grade 3 of 5 lameness on a hard surface. The examination always should include backing the horse at least two or three times and observing the horse at the walk and trot in a circle and in tight turns. Sometimes conditions such as shivers, stringhalt, or intermittent upward fixation of the patella are seen only during these maneuvers.

Lower limb flexion tests are less rewarding in draft horses than in light horses. It is difficult to apply sufficient pressure during the flexion test to accentuate pain in this region. A draft horse may be less willing to trot after a flexion test, making it difficult to determine a true positive response. Most light horses will trot after flexion, even when the reaction is highly positive, but a draft horse will not trot off as readily without strong urging. In addition, draft horses often are not accustomed to being trotted in hand routinely. Hindlimb upper limb flexion tests in a draft horse are a more reliable indicator of hindlimb lameness than in a light horse.

I prefer to perform diagnostic analgesia with the horse in a standing position, rather than having an assistant elevate the limb. This is especially true when attempting palmar digital nerve blocks or palmar nerve blocks at the base of the PSBs. Palpating anatomical landmarks in this area when a draft horse is bearing weight is easier than when the limb is elevated. To maintain the limb in an elevated position or to restrain the limb in this position can be difficult. Adequate restraint usually can be achieved by the application of a nose twitch.

TEN MOST COMMON LAMENESS PROBLEMS

Over several years I evaluated 745 draft horses admitted with a chief complaint of lameness. The following list shows the top 10 lameness conditions that I observed in order of decreasing frequency (33 horses had other problems):

1. Foot lameness (abscess, hoof cracks, laminitis, and sidebone) — 260
2. Tarsal lameness (osteoarthritis, bog spavin, and osteochondrosis) — 207
3. Splints — 84
4. Tendonitis and suspensory desmitis — 45
5. Osteoarthritis of the distal interphalangeal or proximal interphalangeal joints — 44
6. Fetlock lameness (sesamoiditis, osteoarthritis, and osteochondrosis) — 23
7. Thoroughpin — 18
8. Carpal lameness (traumatic or infectious carpitis) — 13
9. Stifle lameness (traumatic, upper fixation of the patella; osteochondrosis) — 10
10. Myopathy — 8

LAMENESS COMMON TO THE FORELIMB AND HINDLIMB

Foot

The foot is the most common source of pain causing lameness in draft horses. A thorough and complete examination of the foot is paramount to diagnosis and management of lameness. Hoof quality and conformation have suffered in modern-day breeding selection, and as a result we tend to have large horses that are supported on feet that lack hoof size and quality. I suggest that breeders of draft horses give strong consideration to hoof conformation when making critical selections for breeding programs.

Subsolar Abscess

The most common cause of foot lameness in a draft horse is a subsolar abscess, a problem most frequently encountered in a forelimb. The high incidence of subsolar abscess formation in draft horses can be related to several factors. First, obtaining consistent farrier care may be difficult in many locations, and foot care may be neglected. Second, draft horses often have poor hoof quality and easily develop hoof cracks or severely chipped and broken hoof walls. Clydesdales have particularly poor hoof quality. Many draft horses have dropped soles, predisposing them to bruising and subsolar abscess formation.

A pair of large, good-quality hoof testers provides the simplest method of determining the location of the abscess. Tapping the hoof wall or sole with a hammer (or the hoof testers) can help locate the abscessed area. In horses that recently have been shod or reset, each nail should be examined. An abscess associated with a nail usually develops 5 to 11 days after shoeing. Hoof cracks causing instability of the hoof capsule can cause lameness even though the area of abscessation may have resolved. If a foreign body is lodged in the hoof (nail, glass, or other penetrating object), a fistulogram (contrast radiograph) should be performed. A subsolar abscess can become a life-threatening problem if osteitis of the distal phalanx develops or penetration of the DIP joint, deep digital flexor tendon (DDFT), or navicular bursa occurs. Proper diagnosis is mandatory; otherwise, the long-term prognosis becomes worse.

Once the abscess is located, the sole should be pared with caution, especially if the horse has a dropped sole or has a concomitant full-thickness hoof wall crack. Overzealous sole paring may result in extensive mechanical damage to laminae and loss of hoof wall strength. Adequate drainage is paramount, but removing a large amount of sole is not necessary, even when substantial undermining has occurred. In draft horses, it is important to err toward a conservative approach, at least initially. Thorough flushing of the foot with povidone-iodine or chlorhexidine diacetate solution should be done at least once a day for 3 days or until the drainage has stopped. The foot can be soaked in a saturated solution of magnesium sulfate for 3 to 5 days to reduce inflammation and to aid in drainage. Finding a soak boot large enough for draft horse feet at a reasonable cost is difficult, and I have found an easy solution by using a 1 m length of truck tire inner tubing. The tubing is slipped half its length over the foot, and then up the leg, with the remaining half doubled back up the leg and secured in place by a wrap of choice (Figure 125-1). The tube then can be filled with the soak solution. Draft horses with an uncomplicated subsolar abscess do not need to be treated with systemic antibiotics. However, if cellulitis of the coronary band and pastern region is present, the administration of antibiotics is indicated. Trimethoprim-sulfadiazine (15 mg/kg orally [PO] bid) or ceftiofur sodium (1 mg/kg intravenously [IV] bid or intramuscularly [IM]) is my usual choice. Judicious use of nonsteroidal antiinflammatory drugs (NSAIDs) is indicated, but these drugs should

not be used for extended periods of time or at levels that may mask a more serious problem. Phenylbutazone, 4 g PO or 2 g IV, on the first day is sufficient. Thereafter, 3 g and then 1 g are given orally on the second and third days, respectively. A tetanus booster should be administered if the horse's vaccination status is not current or is unknown.

If the horse's condition is not improved in 3 days, the horse should be reexamined. Radiography and positive contrast fistulography should be performed. A fistulogram is performed using contrast material administered through a Foley catheter. The foot should be held off the ground when contrast medium is infused and should be held up for 2 minutes thereafter. The foot is then placed in a weight-bearing position, and radiographs are obtained immediately. During weight bearing, a fistulous tract often is closed by soft tissue compression. If deeper structures are involved (DIP joint, DDFT, distal phalanx, or navicular bursa), an extensive treatment program is initiated, including bacterial cultures, surgical drainage or curettage, lavage of the affected area, and the administration of broad-spectrum intravenous antibiotics. The initial antibiotic treatment usually includes 20,000 IU of potassium penicillin per kilogram four times a day and 6.6 mg of gentamicin per kilogram once a day. Bacterial culture and susceptibility testing results may require changing the antibiotic regimen.

Hoof Wall Cracks

Forelimb hoof wall cracks were found in 67% of the 260 draft horses examined for lameness of the foot, although not all were the primary cause of the horse's current problem. Full-thickness hoof wall cracks need to be stabilized when they cause lameness. The crack should be cleaned carefully and curetted, and normal hoof wall should be present on each side of the defect. The technique of dovetailing may provide additional support if hoof repair material is used. Dovetailing is accomplished most easily using a 1-cm (⅜-inch) round burr on an electric drill and undermining the hoof wall at about a 45-degree angle, leaving a shelf of hoof wall down to the white line on each side of the defect for the full length of the crack. This provides additional surface area for a stronger repair and reduces the likelihood that the repair material will come out. Care must be exercised to avoid damage to the sensitive laminae or to create bleeding during this procedure because these may predispose to abscess formation beneath the repair material. If the horse is initially unshod, a shoe with clips may be sufficient to provide support and to immobilize the defect. Radiator hose clamps and 1-cm long, No. 8 metal screws can be used to stabilize the crack. Because infection is often a problem, the radiator clamp method can be used initially, when filling the defect with repair material is contraindicated. Antibiotic-impregnated repair material has been used, but my success with this material in draft horses has been limited, and my preferred method is a shoe and the radiator clamp and screw combination. It is important to have at least two screws through each piece of clamp and on each side of the defect to add stability. The top clamp should be placed at the proximal limit of the crack. I generally space the clamps 1.9 cm (¾ inch) apart, and the number of clamps needed depends on the length, depth, and amount of instability in the crack and on the size of radiator clamp used. The clamps are removed as the defect grows and are replaced if broken. The clamps must

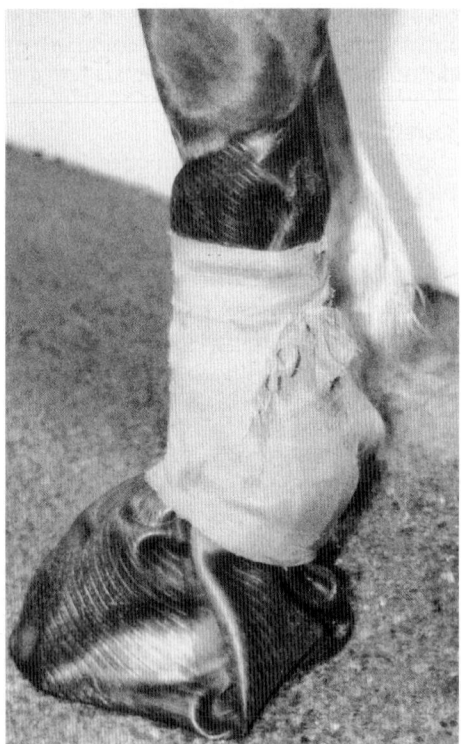

Fig. 125-1 • Draft horse with rubber inner tube in place and used as a soak boot for a foot abscess.

be tightened carefully, because lameness from laminar pain will be worse if the clamps are too tight. This problem is corrected by adjusting the clamp with a screwdriver.

Laminitis

Laminitis in draft horses is a serious lameness condition, and prognosis for complete resolution often is guarded to unfavorable. Regardless of the cause (e.g., grain overload, colitis, metritis, retained placenta, toxemia), once the pathophysiological process of laminitis is in motion, the end results are similar. The solution to the primary cause often is solved more easily than the secondary problem of laminitis. This is especially true in mares with retained placenta, in which the retained placenta and metritis are solved easily, but secondary complications may be devastating. Many of these mares develop severe laminitis with distal displacement (sinking) of the distal phalanx.

I would like to contrast my observations of draft horses with laminitis to similar conditions in light horses. Laminitis carries a more guarded or unfavorable prognosis in draft horses for many reasons. Our ability to manage secondary problems is less satisfactory in draft horses. Size, when we consider a 1000-kg as opposed to a 400- to 500-kg horse, is the most important factor. Slings are seldom big enough, and hoists or hoist support systems may not be available to lift a draft horse safely. Locating a farrier who will work on a chronically lame draft horse and forge therapeutic shoes on a consistent basis is often difficult. Management of draft horses with myositis, decubital ulcers, infections, pneumonia, and other secondary complications is more difficult and costly. The owner must be informed clearly of cost, and a dedicated team (owner, farrier, and veterinarian) must be assembled to manage these complications. I generally tell clients that at least 1 year will pass before the horse's level of function can be assessed reasonably.

Classification of laminitis is confusing, and I make little attempt to classify laminitis based on chronicity or by using the Obel grading system (see Chapter 34). Regardless of classification used, prognosis for return to function is poor if lameness is severe and persists for longer than 10 days with intensive treatment. In my experience, two major differences exist between draft horses and light horses. First, draft horses develop laminitis more frequently and severely in the hindlimbs. Second, draft horses are more likely to develop distal displacement (sinking) of the distal phalanx once laminitis occurs (Figure 125-2). This latter difference may be related to hoof quality or hoof care in general and the important role that body weight plays in causing distal displacement. In addition, shoeing methods that flair the hoof wall simply to give the impression of a large foot weaken laminar support. Distal displacement can occur in horses with traumatic laminitis without a traditional laminitic episode. Traumatic laminitis and sinking can occur unilaterally, only to then occur weeks to months later in the opposite foot. Traumatic laminitis caused by incorrect shoeing can be reduced greatly or eliminated when proper shoeing is provided on a regular basis.

Diagnosis of laminitis is not difficult except in draft horses with traumatic laminitis that is slowly progressive, without an acute episode typically seen with laminitis in a light horse. These horses often have a dropped sole (including the frog in many horses), with the entire sole at a level below the hoof wall. Increased digital pulse amplitudes may be missed easily in a draft horse, but hoof tester sensitivity and abnormal stance are important clinical signs. Initial and follow-up radiographs should always be obtained.

Management of draft horses with laminitis is similar to that of light horses, but some precautions need to be taken.

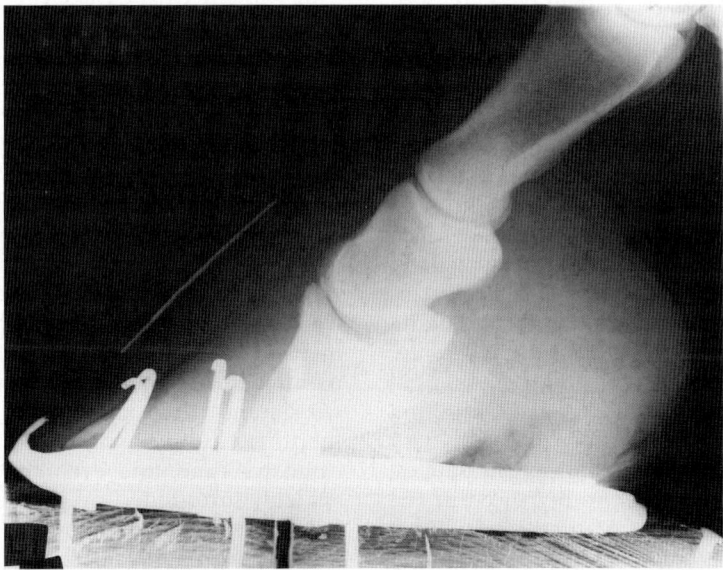

Fig. 125-2 • Lateromedial radiographic image of the front foot of a draft horse mare that had developed laminitis in all four limbs within 24 hours of foaling and retention of the placenta. The radiographic image was obtained 10 days after foaling. The proximal end of the radiodense marker on the dorsal hoof wall is at the level of the coronary band. Both extensive sinking and rotation of the distal phalanx have occurred. Note also the broad radiolucent line in the dorsal hoof wall, the result of laminar necrosis. The mare was managed until the foal was weaned, but humane destruction was ultimately necessary.

Pain amelioration is important but often difficult to achieve. Clydesdales, for instance, are susceptible to gastric and colonic ulcers when treated with phenylbutazone. The Belgian horses that I have treated with phenylbutazone seem less susceptible to ulcers than do Clydesdales. In Clydesdales I seldom if ever administer more than 4 g phenylbutazone PO daily or 3 g IV daily, unless no other alternative is available. The dose should be lowered as quickly as possible, and the high dose should be maintained for a maximum of 5 to 7 days. Although this dose is low based on milligrams per kilogram, Clydesdales have many gastrointestinal complications with higher doses. Flunixin meglumine, meclofenamic acid, and other NSAIDs can be used, but phenylbutazone is the most frequently used and cost-effective drug. Butorphanol tartrate (0.01 to 0.02 mg/kg) can be used with phenylbutazone to lower the necessary dose of NSAIDs. Butorphanol tartrate alone is not a satisfactory analgesic for draft horses with laminitis, but it is useful with NSAIDs, and can be administered three or four times each day.

To provide frog support initially, I use pieces of rubber stall matting, 1.9 cm (¾ inch) thick. The matting is cut to fit the foot and frog and then secured with fiberglass cast material. To increase thickness, two rubber pads can be glued together. To raise the heel in draft horses with acute laminitis, a hand grinder can be used to make a wedge pad from the rubber mat. I believe raising the heel helps to reduce pain and rotation of the distal phalanx. The heel should be elevated 10 to 14 degrees. The single most important factor in draft horses with laminitis is to avoid excessive paring of the sole. Paring the sole away to make it look like a normal sole is putting the curse of death on draft horses with laminitis. This practice removes natural protection from rotation or sinking, and the sole supports the foot better than anything we can apply externally.

Radical hoof wall resection should be avoided. I recall two horses that were referred after complete dorsal hoof wall resection. In both horses the remaining hoof wall lacked strength, and although one horse was shod and the other was unshod, the distal phalanx rotated and sank through the remaining hoof wall in both horses, which were euthanized. If hoof wall resection is indicated, a shoe with side or quarter clips is applied *before* the procedure is performed. The entire hoof wall should not be removed at one time, but resection should be staged over 2 to 3 weeks. If the hoof wall spreads and crowding of the side clips occurs or if further rotation or sinking of the distal phalanx is observed, any further resection is delayed. The coronary band should be assessed each day for signs of sinking (depression at the top of the coronary band). Radiography is helpful but does not replace careful physical examination. Horses with subsolar abscesses are treated by drilling small holes (3 to 5 mm) through the hoof rather than by resection of large portions of hoof wall and sole (see Figure 129-1). Two or more holes may need to be placed in the hoof wall or sole to provide adequate drainage and to flush the site. Drilling small holes does not reduce hoof wall strength compared with paring or removing large portions using conventional methods.

Sidebone

Mineralization of the cartilages of the foot (sidebone) is a common radiological finding in draft horses, particularly in the forelimbs, but is an infrequent cause of lameness. Of 113 draft horses with sidebones, 80 had the condition bilaterally in the forelimbs, and 28 horses had it bilaterally in the hindlimbs. Five horses had unilateral involvement. Draft horses with angular limb deformities are more likely to develop sidebone than are horses with normal bone structure. Sidebone is more common in draft horses with poor hoof quality than in horses with normal hooves. Trauma to the heel and quarters and reduced palmar support are contributing factors. If sidebone is the cause of lameness, lameness grade is usually mild (1 to 2 of 5). Lameness is most common in horses 4 to 7 years of age. Sidebone fractures, occurring in older horses, can cause acute lameness. Lameness is usually most apparent when the horse is working on pavement or other hard surfaces. On soft surfaces the hoof can tip or angle, whereas on hard surfaces the bony column cannot move. Lameness is most obvious when horses are working in circles or tight turns.

Lameness associated with sidebone can be difficult to confirm. Palmar or plantar digital nerve blocks usually greatly improve clinical signs, and palmar nerve blocks at the base of the PSBs abolish lameness. Both nerve blocks provide analgesia to numerous other structures that are more frequent causes of lameness, however. Physical examination is more helpful than is diagnostic analgesia. Tapping on the upper one fourth of the hoof wall (while avoiding hitting the coronary band) with hoof testers or a hammer may elicit pain. A lateral or medial wedge test often causes lameness (see Chapter 8). Thermography is valuable in some horses, showing increased temperature in the area of the sidebone. Radiography is of limited value, because the mere presence of mineralization is not conclusive evidence for lameness diagnosis. Nuclear scintigraphy and magnetic resonance imaging have the potential to help to obtain a definitive diagnosis.

Treatment includes rest and hoof care. The hoof should be trimmed level. Hoof strike should be evaluated dynamically (how it strikes the ground during movement) rather than by just viewing the hoof in a static position. Vertical and parallel grooving may allow the hoof wall to expand and may reduce pressure, but I have not found grooving highly rewarding. The horse should have stall rest or small paddock confinement for 4 to 8 weeks and NSAID therapy. The foot must be balanced properly before the horse resumes a normal exercise program. Fractures associated with large sidebones may be accompanied by OA of the DIP joint. Rarely the PIP joint is involved. Surgical management of draft horses with sidebone fractures often is unrewarding, and I do not recommend it unless conservative management efforts have failed. Conservative management includes an extended period of stall rest (8 to 12 weeks) and then small, level paddock exercise for 6 to 8 months. Healing as shown on radiographs may require extensive time, and even then the fracture still may be evident, surrounded by proliferative exostosis. Unilateral palmar digital neurectomy also can be performed. This will provide relief in most horses unless there is concurrent OA of the DIP or PIP joints.

Quittor

Quittor is defined as a chronic infectious condition associated with one of the cartilages of the foot. A mixed bacterial infection causing chronic or recurrent drainage at or

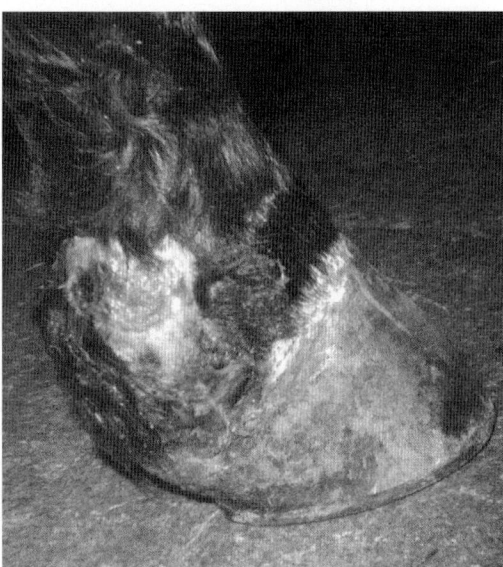

Fig. 125-3 • Draft horse foot showing chronic scar and granulation tissue associated with quittor.

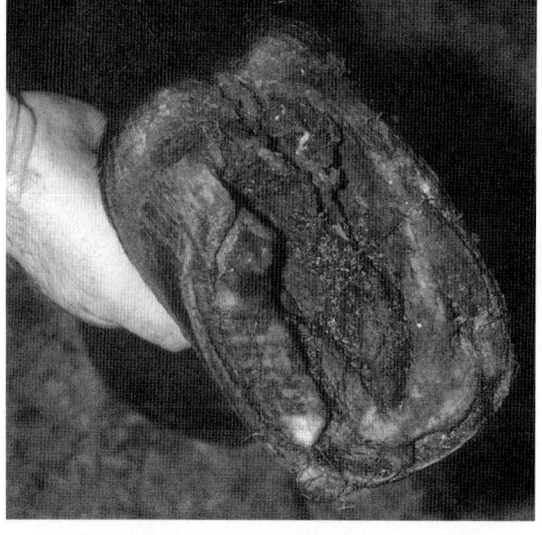

Fig. 125-4 • Draft horse foot showing the typical appearance of thrush complicated by canker beneath the superficial layer of the frog.

near the coronary band is most common (Figure 125-3). Trauma is the most common cause of the condition referred to as *necrosis of the cartilage*. Wire cuts and wounds incurred from large calks on the shoes when horses are working in harness or being transported are common histories. Quittor is considerably less common today than it once was.

Surgical management is the only option, because scar tissue and limited circulation preclude successful conservative management with local or systemic antibiotics. Excision of necrotic cartilage and scar tissue is best. Samples should be submitted for aerobic and anaerobic bacterial culture and susceptibility testing. Standing surgery can be performed, but I prefer to use general anesthesia, which reduces the chance of the DIP joint being penetrated, improves the ability to provide hemostasis, and provides maximal restraint during surgery. A tourniquet at the level of the fetlock joint provides excellent surgical hemostasis, and as a precaution I always administer prophylactic broad-spectrum antibiotics before surgery. The DIP joint occasionally is opened, and although penetration does not necessarily indicate surgical failure, an open joint alters the postoperative management protocol. If necrotic material (cartilage or scar tissue) extends distal to the coronary band, adequate distal drainage and flushing require drilling a hole in the hoof wall.[1]

References on page 1346

Osteitis of the Distal Phalanx

Many draft horses have flat soles and bear substantial weight on the sole and thus are prone to sole bruising and osteitis of the distal phalanx. The condition is most prevalent in the forelimbs and often is associated with improper shoeing or lack of proper hoof care. Draft horses with osteitis of the distal phalanx may assume a stance similar to that seen with traumatic laminitis. Hoof tester examination may be helpful to differentiate these conditions. A laminitic horse is most sensitive immediately dorsal to the apex of the frog in line with the dorsal third of the toe. With osteitis of the distal phalanx, hoof tester pain response usually is less severe and more likely involves the sole in

general. Soles may be pink or red, showing indications of bruising, and lameness is worse on hard surfaces or gravel. Mildly affected horses warm out of the lameness, but in horses with severe pain, lameness increases as exercise continues. Radiographs can be difficult to interpret, and a definitive diagnosis is best reached using nuclear scintigraphy, observing increased radiopharmaceutical uptake in the distal phalanx. Management includes the judicious administration of NSAIDs and corrective shoeing. The sole should be protected and minimally pared. Pads frequently are used initially but may be counterproductive in the long run, because the sole has a tendency to become soft and lose thickness. Pads are needed for the first few shoe changes but then should be removed, and the sole should be hardened. To harden the sole, a common mixture referred to as *sole paint* (composed of equal parts of 7% iodine, buffered formalin, and liquid phenol) is applied. This solution is applied to the sole once each day for 3 to 5 days or until the sole becomes hard. Overzealous application can cause the sole to become too hard. Paddock rest for 45 to 60 days is given. If shorter rest periods are given, recurrence is common. Hard, frozen, or rough surfaces should be avoided.

Canker

Canker is not common but is a difficult problem to solve. Canker is proliferative pododermatitis of the frog that may extend to undermine the sole and heel bulbs. The condition can occur in one or all feet and has no predilection for forelimbs or hindlimbs. Often horses are thought to have nonresponsive thrush, but later when the problem persists, canker is diagnosed (Figure 125-4). Canker is seen more commonly in draft horses than in light horses, a fact that may reflect differences in hoof care and environment or simply may represent a breed predisposition. Two clinical signs that differentiate canker from thrush are a foul odor (necrotic) and the presence of granulation-like tissue that bleeds easily when manipulated (Figure 125-5). Lameness is highly variable depending on the severity and

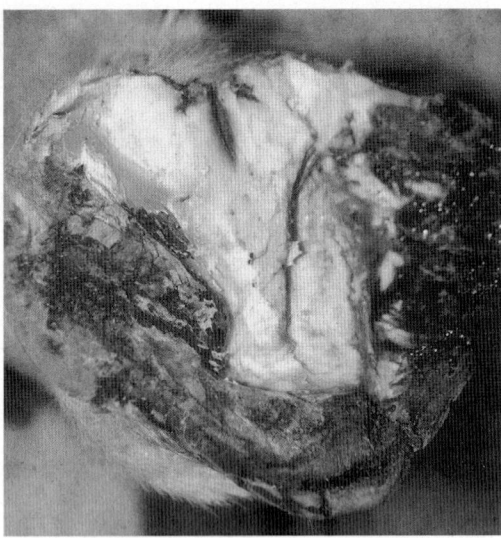

Fig. 125-5 • Chronic canker with proliferative granulation tissue. Infected granulation tissue has undermined the sole and heel.

number of feet involved. Once the superficial layer of tissue is removed, bleeding is often profuse. Creamy exudate is typical initially, especially if the owner has initiated treatment with caustic preparations.

Successful treatment of canker requires patience on the part of the owner and the veterinarian because recurrence is common. The application of a hospital plate shoe is critical, because this shoe allows for long-term treatment and protects the sole. It is important to note that pressure on the sole appears beneficial to healing, similar to that seen with granulation tissue at any site. Hospital plate shoes reduce the cost associated with daily care and management of a bandage. The shoe allows the horse to be exercised. The hospital plate shoe is made and fitted to the foot, and then the foot is blocked. A tourniquet is placed at the level of the fetlock joint, because bleeding during debridement is often profuse. Complete debridement of all abnormal proliferative tissue is often not possible and in fact may be counterproductive, because aggressive debridement may expose uninvolved deep tissue. Dry gauze sponges are packed to apply pressure on the frog and sole when the plate is replaced. Metronidazole appears to be the best topical agent, but I have used tetracycline and sulfapyridine powder successfully. The dressing should be changed daily for the first 10 to 14 days and then as needed. Debridement often needs to be repeated several times. Long-term treatment is necessary, and the owner needs to be prepared to provide it. Caustic compounds are not effective and in fact may worsen the condition. In the final stages of healing, when cornification of the frog is complete, caustic agents may be applied. Sole paint is applied to the sole for 8 to 10 days before the hospital plate shoe is removed. Horses are administered trimethoprim-sulfamethoxazole (15 mg/kg) for 3 weeks starting the day before initial debridement. Penicillin (20,000 IU/kg IM) is also effective, but oral antimicrobial agents are administered more easily.

Osteoarthritis of the Proximal and Distal Interphalangeal Joints, Ringbone

OA of the PIP or DIP joint was diagnosed in 26 draft horses in my series.

Ringbone has been described classically as being periarticular or articular in nature. The prognosis for draft horses with articular ringbone is worse than for those with the periarticular form. Pulling horses (heavy loads) are affected most commonly, especially in the hindlimbs. OA of the PIP and DIP joints appears to occur with similar frequency, because in 26 horses, 11 had PIP, 10 had DIP, and 5 had PIP and DIP joint involvement. Horses with OA of the PIP joint remained serviceably sound for 2.6 years, whereas horses with OA of the DIP joint or of both joints were serviceably sound for only 11 months. Early diagnosis appears to be an important criterion for an improved prognosis, and reducing workload, instituting corrective shoeing, and providing medical management can make a substantial difference in delaying the progression of OA.

Draft horses with short, upright pasterns are predisposed to OA of the PIP and DIP joints, and other factors such as angular limb deformities, toed-in or toed-out conformation, hoof imbalance, and trauma may play a substantial role. Horses required to work on pavement are predisposed to OA of the PIP and DIP joints. Proliferative periarticular changes often result from lacerations or wire cuts. Horses with moderate-to-severe lameness have obvious enlargement of the pastern or coronary band area and heat. The degree of lameness varies from grade 1 to 5, and it worsens with lower limb flexion or after rotation of the digit. Rotation causes a substantial positive response if collateral ligaments are involved in horses with the periarticular form. In horses with OA of the DIP joint, palmar digital nerve blocks generally result in substantial improvement in lameness score. Thorough examination of the foot must be done to eliminate other potential causes of lameness. If the diagnosis is unclear after radiological examination, intraarticular analgesia should be performed. In horses with OA of the PIP joint, palmar digital nerve blocks may provide some improvement in lameness score, but palmar nerve blocks at the level of the PSBs are needed to improve lameness substantially. Intraarticular analgesia can also be used.

Management depends on when the diagnosis is first made. Draft horses with OA and mild lameness should be given rest in a small level paddock for 4 months. I do not use stall rest unless horses are very active, because I have had greater success allowing the horse to walk in a confined area. Hoof imbalance should be corrected, and the horse should be shod with flat shoes without calks, toe grabs, or borium. I recommend oral glucosamine or chondroitin sulfate supplementation or intramuscular injection of a polysulfated glycosaminoglycan (PSGAG). I also inject the joints with a corticosteroid and hyaluronan. Initial and follow-up radiographic examinations are recommended. If the horse is sound and radiological changes do not progress, the horse is put back into a light exercise program, whereas if radiological changes worsen, additional rest and injections are given. Many horses with OA perform for extended periods of time without recurrence of lameness. Horses with severe OA of the PIP or DIP joints have an unfavorable prognosis for athletic use. Medical management is of little benefit, and although spontaneous fusion of the PIP joint may occur, giving an accurate time estimate of when this may occur is difficult. Spontaneous fusion of the DIP joint seldom occurs. Surgical arthrodesis of the PIP joint can be performed by using bone plates or the three-screw technique with 5.5-mm bone screws (see Chapter 35). A half-limb cast is placed for at least 4 to 6 weeks after surgery. In draft horses the surgical procedure is more difficult than in light horses because the joints are large, removing articular cartilage is difficult, and horses may have difficulty with recovery from general anesthesia. Draft horses in general do not recover well from extended periods (>2 hours) of general anesthesia. The surgical procedure can be long, in particular if there is substantial periarticular new bone formation and fibrosis. Implants can break because of the large size of a draft horse. Because of this, I have used an alternative technique of drilling across the joint with a 4.5- or 5.5-mm drill bit and then applying a half-limb cast without using implants. In horses with substantial periarticular bone proliferation or fibrosis, this technique is my method of choice. Intraoperative radiographs are mandatory to ensure proper placement of the drill bit within the joint. I drill at three to five sites in a fan-shaped pattern from each side of the joint to destroy as much articular cartilage as possible. Breaking a drill bit in the joint is possible, and if this happens, removing the bit generally is not worth the extra time required. The palmar digital artery, vein, and nerve must be avoided during this procedure. A half-limb cast encompassing the foot is applied and maintained for 12 to 16 weeks. Advantages of this technique over those involving implants are that this technique is faster, requires shorter anesthesia periods, and requires no major skin incisions, and implant failure is not a concern. Pain control must be used to maintain reasonable comfort to avoid contralateral laminitis, which is always a concern.

Metacarpophalangeal (Fetlock) Joint Lameness

Problems associated with the fetlock joint are less frequent in draft horses than in other breeds, and most result from direct trauma. Fetlock joint problems plague horses that perform at speed, and therefore draft horses seldom have lameness in this region. Sesamoiditis does occur in draft horses and usually results from suspensory desmitis and insertional injury at the level of the PSB. Sesamoiditis is more common in the hindlimbs than in the forelimbs. An unusual problem of the fetlock joint in young draft horses is osteochondritis dissecans (OCD).

Splints

Exostoses of the second and fourth metacarpal or metatarsal bones (splints) most commonly affect the second metacarpal bone, as in light horses. In 84 draft horses diagnosed with splints, 71 horses had forelimb involvement. Lameness associated with true splint (tearing of the interosseous ligament) is not common in draft horses. Lameness caused by splints is most prominent in the first 2 to 3 weeks after the condition is first recognized and usually resolves with 6 to 8 weeks of rest. Because draft horses do not perform at speed or change direction quickly, splints do not cause long-term lameness. Splints can result from interference injury from the contralateral limb, a problem that usually is corrected by proper shoeing and trimming. Local infiltration of local anesthetic solution in the region of the splint may be performed if the diagnosis is in question. Although a splint may be painful during palpation, missing a problem in the more distal aspect of a limb is easy; therefore diagnostic analgesia should be performed distal to the splint

before local infiltration. Radiographs should be obtained to check for a fracture.

To manage a draft horse with lameness resulting from a splint, I administer NSAIDs for 5 to 7 days and recommend stall rest. If the condition is acute, I use cold water therapy or ice boots for 20 to 30 minutes twice daily and apply support wraps. The horse should be handwalked for 10 minutes twice daily. In horses with chronic splints, I recommend a sweat (50/50 mixture of glycerin and alcohol) for 7 to 10 days. Paddock exercise can be given for 12 hours each day. A total rest period of 60 to 90 days is usually adequate. I avoid overzealous treatment with topical or internal blisters.

Fractures of the splint bones are rare but usually involve the fourth metatarsal bone (MtIV), and they often occur from kick wounds. These fractures often are comminuted and usually infected, because owners do not seek veterinary attention until 2 to 3 weeks after injury. Severe lameness often is not seen or is short lived, so the owner usually is not concerned until drainage starts. If the tarsometatarsal (TMT) joint is involved and infected, the prognosis for return to original use is unfavorable. Many of these fractures heal if horses are given rest and treated with antibiotics. If the articular surface of the TMT joint is not involved, displacement of fragments is minimal, and if the horse is not an athlete, horses with this injury can be treated conservatively. Standing curettage of a draining tract and removal of sequestra can be accomplished in many horses with use of sedation and local analgesia. A culture and antimicrobial sensitivity testing are performed, and the horse is placed on appropriate antibiotics for 3 to 4 weeks; the outcome is often satisfactory. For economic reasons this method also is chosen by some owners for horses intended for athletic use. However, I believe the problem is best treated surgically in those horses that are expected to be athletes. Surgical removal of the distal fractured segment of the MtIV is recommended occasionally, and horses usually have a good prognosis. If greater than 80% of the total length of the MtIV is removed, I use a screw to stabilize the proximal fragment. I do not like placing a screw into an area of known infection if I can avoid doing so. In horses with substantial displacement or a fracture involving the articular surface, internal fixation to realign the fracture is indicated, if the injury is less than 3 weeks old. Fractures older than 3 weeks old can be difficult to realign because callus formation occurs quickly.

Tendonitis and Suspensory Desmitis

Digital flexor tendonitis and suspensory desmitis are not as common in the draft horse as one might expect. Of 45 horses examined for these soft tissue problems, the distribution of these combined soft tissue injuries between the forelimbs and hindlimbs was similar, in contrast to most sports horses. Suspensory desmitis is more common in hindlimbs and often is seen with sesamoiditis. Tendonitis and suspensory desmitis are more common in draft horses that pull heavy loads or weighted sleds. Clinical signs include heat, pain, swelling, and lameness, and diagnosis is usually straightforward. Horses with hindlimb proximal suspensory desmitis may have more subtle clinical signs, and diagnostic analgesia is usually necessary. In horses with early forelimb superficial digital flexor tendonitis, the anastomosing branch of the palmar nerves may be enlarged and sensitive to palpation before the tendon itself shows clinical abnormalities. Ultrasonographic examination should be performed.

Management of draft horses with tendonitis and suspensory desmitis is similar to that in light horses. Ultrasonographic examination, rest, and a staged return to work are important. I am an advocate of percutaneous tendon or suspensory ligament splitting under ultrasonographic guidance in draft horses. The surgery can be accomplished in a standing horse, using local analgesia and sedation, thus avoiding the need for general anesthesia. Prognosis is guarded to favorable in draft horses with forelimb tendonitis and suspensory desmitis. Draft horses with hindlimb injury, however, have a guarded to unfavorable prognosis, especially if horses are used for pulling heavy loads. Broodmares with chronic, severe suspensory desmitis must be given special attention during late pregnancy because of weight gain. These mares should be housed on level surfaces and alone. Situations that require the mare to move quickly to avoid an aggressive pasture mate or cause the mare to slip while going over rough terrain should be avoided. Muddy or slick footing also should be avoided. Stall rest, although advantageous for healing of the suspensory ligament, is avoided, because these broodmares usually develop substantial ventral edema.

Other Forelimb Lameness

Other causes of forelimb lameness are unusual. Upper limb lameness usually is caused by direct trauma and is not the result of athletic use. Carpal, elbow, or shoulder joint lameness is not common. I have examined only 13 draft horses with carpal lameness. Various manifestations of osteochondrosis are seen in the elbow and shoulder joints.

Sweeny, a neuromuscular disorder thought to be associated with injury of the suprascapular nerve, does occur with some frequency in draft horses. Muscle atrophy may not be obvious for weeks to months, depending on the extent of the injury. Sweeny may result from acute direct trauma, but in draft horses insidious trauma from a collar is the most common cause. This is especially true of poorly fitting collars, or old and worn collars in which the padding is no longer adequate. Collars of inadequate size often are used on today's large-sized draft horses. Some draft horses with Sweeny continue to perform adequately despite muscle atrophy. Diagnosis is made by observing muscle atrophy over the scapula, especially affecting the supraspinatus muscle. Lameness is most likely functional and not related to pain, because horses cannot extend the shoulder joint normally. In some horses, however, the shoulder joint actually may subluxate when the horse is walking or especially turning in a circle. Subluxation results more frequently from external trauma from being kicked or from running into a solid object rather than from collar injury and may involve additional nerve injury.

Management of horses with acute trauma of the shoulder area includes the administration of NSAIDs, corticosteroids, and dimethyl sulfoxide and performance of physical therapy. A water hose with a hard stream of water can be useful for physical therapy. Liniments, massage, handheld muscle stimulators, and heating pads can be useful physical therapeutic modalities as well. The administration of dimethyl sulfoxide (0.3 g/kg sid IV for 3 to 5 days) is recommended in the acute phase. Prognosis is difficult to assess, but if improvement is not seen in the first 6 to 8 weeks after diagnosis, prognosis becomes less favorable. I have not attempted scapular notch resection in draft horses, but knowing the complications associated with the procedure in light horses leads me to hesitate recommending it.

Unusual Signs Consistent with Lameness Caused by Mange Mites

In the United Kingdom a clinically significant incidence of mange occurs in draft breed horses.[2] Draft horses often are presented for evaluation of presumed lameness because of a stiff, stilted gait and with abnormal stamping of the limbs to the ground. In these horses careful clinical evaluation reveals areas of dermatitis, but this condition can be confused easily with musculoskeletal pain. I have not seen this to be a problem in draft horses in the United States.

Hindlimb Lameness

Hindlimb lameness occurs frequently in draft horses, and the most common cause is lameness associated with the tarsus (hock joint). Draft horses in general have a predisposition to develop tarsitis, and lameness does not seem to be related to use. The custom of lowering the inside wall of the hoof and attempting to turn the hocks, a shoeing change thought to improve the horse's pulling ability, may predispose a draft horse to tarsitis. To my knowledge, however, this has never been proved in a controlled study. Draft horse shoes often have a large calk on the heel of the lateral branch of the shoe, increasing torque and shear stress on the entire limb. Heel calks are especially detrimental in horses that work on hard surfaces, because the calk does not sink into the surface, thus putting even greater stress on the limb. This method of shoeing causes a flaring of the lateral hoof wall and predisposes the hooves to separation and breakdown of laminae. Even if this method of shoeing is abandoned, at least 12 to 18 months are required for the foot to return to normal.

Tarsus

Draft horses with hock lameness show a variety of clinical signs. The perceived problems by the owner also vary considerably. The horse may stop pulling or may rest its butt on the stall wall when in the barn. Breeding stallions may be reluctant to mount a mare, and when mounted, they may be unable to maintain erection. Horses may be reluctant to back up, back up in crooked fashion, and have difficulty going up and down inclines. The horse may take short strides in harness or may have a change in attitude, sometimes biting other horses. Because the prevalence of hock joint lameness is high, carefully considering this region when evaluating a draft horse with hindlimb lameness is always wise.

Diagnosis may be straightforward, based on clinical signs, or may require diagnostic analgesia to pinpoint the problem. Upper limb flexion tests in draft horses appear to be slightly more accurate as an indicator of hock lameness than the same tests are in light horses, but false-negative results do occur. Pulling the medial splint bone with the fingers (Churchill test) with the limb in flexion also may be of value. The horse may show a positive response while standing, or lameness may be exacerbated after this

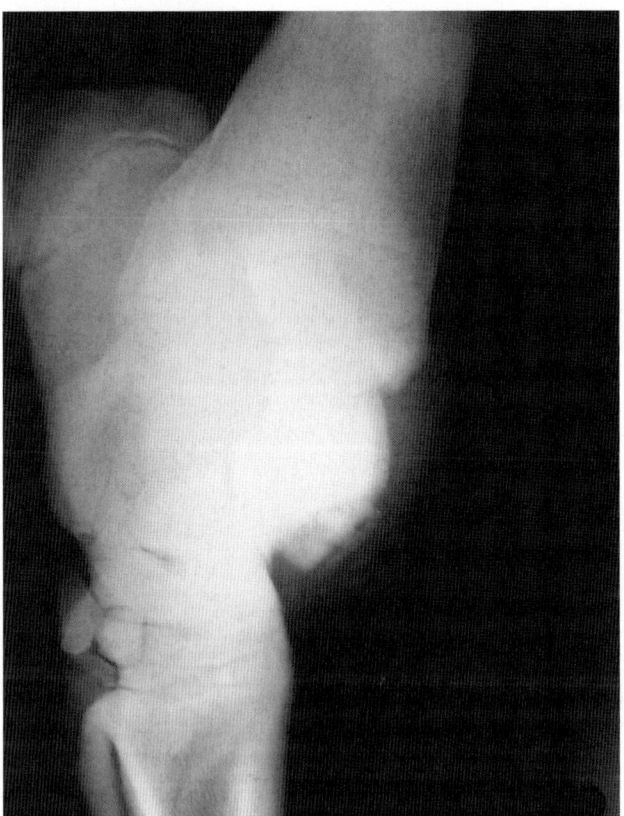

Fig. 125-6 • Dorsomedial-plantarolateral oblique radiographic image of a hock of a yearling draft horse. The radiograph was deliberately underexposed to highlight the extensive osteochondrosis lesion involving the distal half of the lateral trochlear ridge of the talus.

maneuver is performed. When the horse is trotting, careful attention is given to the vertical movement of the wings of the ilium (hip or pelvic hike), but if the problem is bilateral, a pelvic hike may not be obvious. Stride length may be shortened when the horse is viewed from the side, and when evaluated from behind or in front, horses have a tendency to swing the limb toward the midline and then place the limb laterally as it strikes the ground. Horses may scuff the toes because of the low arc of limb flight. Bony exostosis on the dorsal medial aspect of the hock joint may be obvious or absent.

Tarsocrural effusion, or bog spavin, is observed commonly in draft horses. This clinical observation often does not correlate with the source of pain. Even if osteochondrosis is suspected or confirmed, intraarticular analgesia always should be performed (Figure 125-6). Although present, OCD fragments may not be the major source of pain, and surgical removal of these fragments may not resolve lameness. Often in draft horses with OCD there is severe tarsocrural effusion, which may improve but is unlikely to resolve even after arthroscopic removal of the offending fragments (Editors). Arthroscopic removal of OCD fragments is often less rewarding in adult horses. In draft horses younger than 2 years of age, arthroscopic removal of OCD fragments is more likely to resolve lameness, however. The decision to perform surgery is based on the level of performance, cosmetic considerations related to joint distention, location of the lesion, and, most important, whether lameness resolves with tarsocrural analgesia.

Horses with OCD lesions located more distally on the trochlear ridges of the talus have a more favorable prognosis than those with lesions located on the proximal aspect. Horses with OCD lesions associated with the cranial aspect of the intermediate ridge of the tibia have a favorable prognosis if lesions are removed early before chronic synovitis or capsulitis occurs. With only a limited number of horses from which to draw experience, lesions seemingly occur more frequently on the lateral trochlear ridge of the talus (tibial tarsal bone) than in any other location in a draft horse. OCD lesions associated with the cranial aspect of the intermediate ridge of the tibia are also quite common in draft horses (Editors).

Lameness associated with OA of the centrodistal and TMT joints is common. Intraarticular analgesia is often necessary, although some veterinarians medicate these joints and assess the clinical response to this treatment. I prefer to perform intraarticular analgesia and consider management options once a definitive diagnosis has been made, however. In my opinion, conservative management should be attempted before corticosteroids are used. I block the TMT and the centrodistal joints first with the horse standing squarely on each limb. In draft horses with exostoses on the medial aspect of the tarsus (bone spavin), confidently blocking the centrodistal joint may be difficult. Two-percent mepivacaine hydrochloride (7 to 12 mL) is injected into each joint using a 20- to 22-gauge, 2.5- to 4-cm needle in the standard locations (see Chapter 10). In most draft horses a twitch is adequate for restraint. Radiographs should be obtained, but unfortunately they are unreliable in confirming the diagnosis of OA. In some draft horses with substantial radiological changes, lameness may originate elsewhere, whereas in some horses with minor or equivocal radiological changes, severe lameness from early OA of these joints is diagnosed. Radiological examination helps to select management options and to determine prognosis, however.

Management of a draft horse with OA of the distal hock joints includes physical and medical and surgical options. Correction of any shoeing or trimming problems should be performed before any other treatment. The foot is balanced in a medial-to-lateral direction according to conformation to achieve a level foot strike. My definition of a level foot strike is that the foot lands evenly when contacting the ground during movement. I remove the large calks and trailers that often are placed on the lateral branch of the shoes. If the horse is not going to be worked for a period, I prefer to shoe the horse without any special trim (calks, toe grabs, or inside rims). The dorsal aspect of the shoe is placed at the white line, and the toe is rasped back to the level of the shoe. Squared-toe shoes also can be used. The heels of the shoe should extend far enough behind to support the plantar aspect of the heel completely. In some horses slight heel elevation improves breakover and comfort. If the lateral hoof wall is flared, it must be rasped at each shoeing, and the lateral branch of the shoe gradually must be adjusted to conform properly to a more normal hoof shape. If borium is needed for traction on hard surfaces, it should be placed so that it provides a level surface on the bottom of the shoe. Uneven stress from borium points may cause hoof wall cracks. Usually, using six to 10 spots of borium on the shoe adequately supports the foot and also provides adequate traction.

Medical management may include oral supplementation, intramuscular administration of PSGAGs, and intravenous administration of hyaluronan. NSAIDs are recommended at the time of shoeing changes, but long-term use of NSAIDs is usually not a solution in the management of chronic distal hock joint pain. Chronic administration often results in gastrointestinal ulceration and additional problems such as colic or colitis. Horses with distal hock joint pain can be given 2 to 3 g of phenylbutazone daily. Intraarticular injection with hyaluronan alone has limited value in draft horses with OA of the distal hock joints, and I prefer to use hyaluronan with methylprednisolone acetate. If there are economic restrictions, the corticosteroid is most important and can be injected alone. The dose of these compounds is similar to that used in the light horse and is not based necessarily on body weight. I increase the corticosteroid dose by about 25% using methylprednisolone acetate (100 mg) in each of the centrodistal and the TMT joints. If treating bog spavin, I use methylprednisolone acetate (120 mg) and hyaluronan (40 mg). I seldom if ever use triamcinolone acetonide in draft horses, because of a concern about laminitis induction and the fact that I often am injecting several joints simultaneously.

Cunean tenectomy is used in some horses, especially those that have obvious enlargement on the medial aspect of the hock (Figure 125-7). Cunean tenectomy is accomplished in a standing horse using local analgesia and sedation. Horses often are put back into work once the skin sutures are removed, 12 to 14 days after surgery.

Stifle Joint

Draft horses have long been thought to have more stifle joint lameness than do light horses, but when reviewing the records of 745 draft horse lameness examinations, only 10 horses had primary lameness of the stifle joint. Perhaps long ago, when draft horses were used daily to pull heavy loads, the frequency of stifle lameness may have been far greater than it is today. Of these 10 horses, three had bilateral idiopathic effusion of the femoropatellar joint. One horse had bilateral subchondral bone cysts of the medial femoral condyles, one had upward fixation of the patella, and five had trauma from kick injuries. Poor conformation and extended stall confinement predispose some draft horses to upward fixation of the patella. Emaciated horses or those with substantial weight loss also are predisposed to the condition. I make every attempt to correct upward fixation of the patella by using conservative management including foot care, improving muscle tone or conditioning, and improving nutritional intake. Raising the heel often alleviates the problem, and block wedges to raise the angle of the hind feet 6 to 10 degrees are needed. Heel elevation is reduced gradually as the problem is rectified. Improved muscle tone and exercise are beneficial, as is avoiding prolonged periods of stall confinement. Backing exercise strengthens the quadriceps muscles and is a useful form of physical therapy. Internal blisters, injected at the origin and insertion of the patellar ligaments, may cause mild fibrosis and thus tighten the joint. This treatment is used less frequently now than in the past because the preparations need to be special ordered. I seldom if ever elect medial patellar desmotomy as my initial treatment. If conservative management is unsuccessful, desmotomy needs to be performed. The procedure should be done in

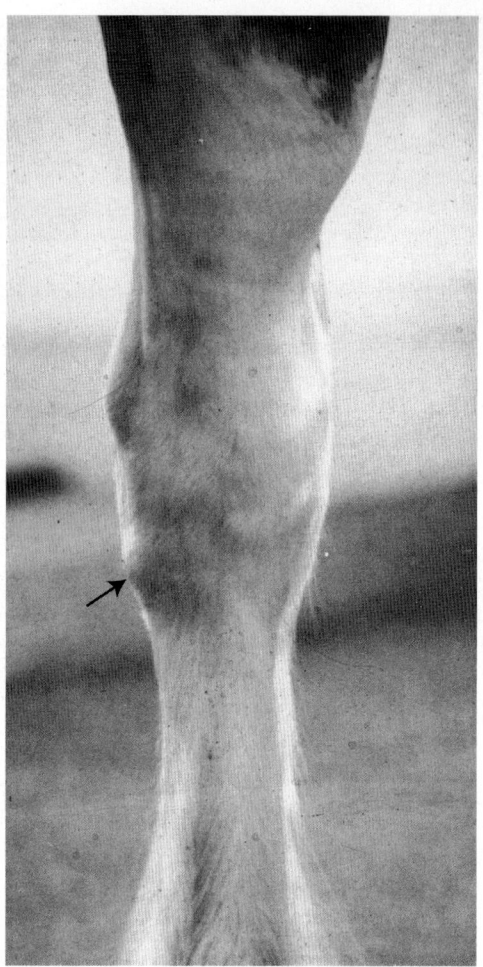

Fig. 125-7 • The dorsal aspect of the left hock of a draft horse showing bony exostosis of the dorsal medial aspect *(arrow)*. If lameness was confirmed to originate from the lower hock joint region, this horse would be a candidate for cunean tenectomy.

the standing horse and not under general anesthesia and should be done with a sharp, strong-backed bistoury. This procedure should not be attempted in a draft horse with an ordinary scalpel handle and blade, because the risk of the blade breaking during the surgery is real. Medial patellar desmoplasty (splitting) would be a suitable alternative to desmotomy in draft horses (see Chapter 48 [Editors]).

Shivers

Shivers is considered a progressive, degenerative neuromuscular disease predominantly affecting draft horses or other large-breed horses (see Chapter 48). Various causes have been suggested, including immune-mediated disease following viral infection or strangles and exposure to organophosphates. Polysaccharide storage myopathy has been put forth as a possible cause, but like previous proposed causes, this one may go by the wayside. Clinical signs include an involuntary jerking or twitching most frequently affecting the hindlimbs and the tail. A reflex-like maximum degree of flexion can be seen. Clinical signs often are noticed first by the farrier, because manually picking up the hindlimb frequently stimulates the jerking movements. Signs may be most obvious when the horse first starts to walk, or is backed up or is turned sharply.

On occasion, twitching of the muzzle, lips, and ears and forelimb involvement occur. The condition may improve with rest but usually returns when the horse is put back into work.

Currently, no effective treatment is available. Shivers has been confused with stringhalt in some horses, and the surgical procedure, lateral digital flexor tenectomy, has been performed erroneously. Muscle biopsy to check for polysaccharide storage myopathy and treatment with high-fat, low-carbohydrate diets may be warranted, but definitive proof that polysaccharide storage myopathy is the cause of shivers may be difficult to substantiate. Horses still can be worked, but often owners elect to use them sparingly.

LAMENESS OF FOALS, WEANLINGS, AND YEARLINGS

Young draft horses require careful monitoring and early attention to lameness conditions. Lameness is often multifactorial and is related to nutrition, genetics, and environment. Early diagnosis and management of lameness appear more critical in draft horse foals than in light horse foals. Often the size and strength of draft horse foals gives the erroneous impression that they can overcome many problems.

Infectious Arthritis

Infectious arthritis is common in draft horse foals and may be related to a high frequency of umbilical problems. Umbilical hernia, umbilical infection, and patent urachus are more common in draft horse foals than in light horses. Careful examination and treatment of the umbilicus at birth is mandatory, and the umbilicus should be monitored closely for a minimum of 3 weeks. Compared with light horse foals, draft horse foals are often slower to stand and nurse after birth, leading to many infectious processes. Owner education is important, not only in assisting slow foals up to nurse but also in careful, daily evaluation of joints. Early and aggressive management of infectious arthritis and umbilical remnant infections should be performed (see Chapters 65 and 128).

Developmental Orthopedic Disease

Draft horses are affected by all of the various manifestations of developmental orthopedic disease (DOD), including flexural deformities, epiphysitis and physitis, osteochondrosis, angular limb deformities, and vertebral malformations (wobbler syndrome). A multifactorial cause is suspected, including nutrition (calcium/phosphorus ratios and trace mineral levels) and hereditary factors (certain bloodlines have a high prevalence). Hereditary factors are complex and include high growth rate, feed deficiency conversion, milk production, and individual horse size.

Physitis and Epiphysitis and Flexural Deformities

Physitis and epiphysitis and flexural deformities are closely related and seldom if ever a single problem. These conditions are seen over a wide age range from 6 weeks to 24 months, but peak occurrence is in foals 4 to 12 months of age. When raising large horses, owners have a tendency to overfeed, resulting in high-energy rations, fast growth, and nutritional stress, all of which include the possibility of DOD. My experience with some 300 draft horse foals suggests a distinct correlation between the frequency of DOD and nutritional management. Foals having the highest frequency of DOD were fed free-choice high-quality alfalfa hay, approximately 0.015 kg of feed per kilogram of body weight per day of a 16% protein grain ration, and two vitamin-mineral supplements. Foals were fed in groups of six to 10 in 5- to 6-acre paddocks. Group feeding allowed the aggressive eater to consume far more than the prescribed amount of grain, and of course hay was fed free choice. None of the foals was thin or malnourished, but numerous foals were obese. Overweight foals, yearlings, and 2-year-olds do not exercise properly, a fact that exacerbates problems associated with excess ration. Under these conditions, two to four foals per group were affected with DOD each year.

To correct this problem, the nutritional program was revamped. The owner accepted the fact that yearling size would be slightly less than previously attained, but that DOD would occur less frequently. Anecdotally, buyers of yearlings from this group had complained in previous years that 2-year-olds had become lame when training had started. The nutrition was changed as follows. The hay ration was given at a 50/50 mixture of alfalfa to timothy. Hay was fed at a rate of 0.015 kg per kilogram of body weight per day, or the amount the foals could consume in about 16 hours. The grain ration was reduced to approximately 0.01 kg per kilogram of body weight per day of a 14% protein ration. Only one vitamin-mineral supplement was given. Foals were grouped according to size, age, and disposition and were monitored closely and checked every 2 weeks by the farm veterinarian. Changes in conformation (becoming upright in the pastern and fetlock) or enlargement (heat and pain) of the growth plates were noted.

Any foal with a change in the pastern or fetlock angle (developing more upright conformation), joint effusion, or physitis was treated immediately. Stall rest was given for 7 to 10 days, the feed intake was reduced, and the foal subsequently was given controlled exercise in a small paddock. Foals were fed only timothy hay, and the grain ration was reduced to 0.002 kg per kilogram of body weight per day. They were placed on phenylbutazone (2.2 mg/kg bid for 3 consecutive days and then every other day for 3 more days). They were maintained in this environment until the problem resolved. Any hoof imbalance or growth abnormality was treated. A 60% decrease in DOD was noted the first year, and now that farm management has become more attentive to noticing early signs of DOD, the frequency of this complex of diseases is now less than 10%.

Osteochondritis Dissecans and Osteochondrosis

In my experience, osteochondrosis is observed more commonly in draft horse foals than in light horse foals. In draft horse foals the tarsocrural and femoropatellar joints are affected most commonly. Any joint can be affected, including the cervical vertebrae. Horses with osteochondrosis show varying degrees of lameness from 1 to 4 of 5 degrees. Lameness is less frequent with osteochondrosis lesions of the tarsocrural joint than with osteochondrosis of the stifle. Loose OCD fragments in the femoropatellar joint should be removed as soon as possible. Arthroscopic surgery does not guarantee success but improves the prognosis for athletic use. In my experience, draft horses have a more guarded prognosis for future soundness with osteochondrosis of the stifle than do light horses. I am unsure if this is related simply to the size of the horse or the amount of pulling many of these draft horses are expected to do, but only about 50% of draft horses are sound after surgery. Early diagnosis and surgical management improve prognosis considerably. In some foals without loose OCD fragments, conservative management has resulted in a favorable outcome. Large OCD defects involving the lateral trochlear ridge of the femur have healed based on radiological examination, but this process may take up to 6 months to occur.

Chapter 126

Lameness in the Pony

Andrew M. McDiarmid

Horses under the height of 14 hands 2 inches (148 cm) at the withers generally are recognized as ponies. Despite this classification, ponies of some breeds are referred to as *horses:* for example, Icelandic (toelter) horses. Many native pony breeds are found throughout the world—for example, Asturian (Spain), Connemara (Ireland), Fell (England), Gerrano (Portugal), Highland (Scotland), M'Bayar (Senegal), Merens (Pyrenees), Ob (Russia), Pindos (Greece), and Welsh ponies. Several small island breeds also exist—for example, Balearic, Eriskay, Faroe Island *horse,* and Chincoteague ponies. The size and conformation of most pony breeds have evolved over centuries because of specific work requirements and geographical isolation. Several breeds are endangered, including the Yonaguni and Noma in Japan and Sorraia in Spain, and some have become extinct— for example, the Fen, Galloway, and Tarpan. Attempts are actively being made to prevent extinction of several breeds—for example, the Kerry bog pony in Ireland and the Taishuh in Japan. In recent times new breeds of pony have evolved, including the Welara and Pony of the Americas. Despite this, most ponies are crossbred.

Ponies have a considerable range of height, weight, and conformation and are involved in most spheres of equine work, including show jumping, eventing, dressage, driving, and general pleasure activities. Many ponies show great athletic ability, and when used for show jumping, they often jump heights similar to their own height at the withers. Ponies have a long life expectancy and can remain in athletic work well into their twenties. Although a small number of ponies are used for high-level competition work such as eventing and show jumping, most are used for general purpose work, when they may be ridden only in the summer months. General purpose ponies tend to be much less valuable than horses and are ridden predominantly by children, which may create emotional and financial conflicts for owners (parents) when deciding the appropriate treatment of a seriously injured pony. Many general purpose ponies remain at grass all year round and do not have access to a stable. Successful competition ponies often change ownership, at high prices, every 2 or 3 years as children outgrow them.

Few reports in the literature describe orthopedic conditions specifically affecting the pony. In this chapter I hope to give an overview of some of the conditions that are recognized in the pony.

LAMENESS AFFECTING THE PONY

Ponies develop orthopedic problems similar to those in horses, but the overall prevalence of lameness in the pony is less than in the horse. This may be because of differences in temperament and body weight. With a relatively older population the incidence of some specific orthopedic conditions affecting older ponies may appear higher than in horses, but the prevalence is often unclear and may, for some conditions, be similar (e.g., laminitis as a result of Cushing's disease).

LAMENESS EXAMINATION

Gait assessment in ponies can be challenging because they can have a higher limb speed than horses, and the larger, heavier pony breeds (e.g., Highland) often have a base-wide gait behind, which may make assessment of hindlimb lameness difficult. Several breeds also have gaits additional to walk, trot, and canter; these include the South African, Basotho pony, and Icelandic horse. For small ponies the handler may have to walk when leading a trotting pony, rather than run, to keep the limb speed to a rate at which the observer can detect low-grade lameness.

The low height of some ponies compared with most veterinary surgeons may create difficulties with assessment of the lower limb, and excessive force or torsion can easily be applied to the distal joints when a flexion test is performed.

In small ponies, care should be taken not to apply excessive pressure with hoof testers and, if the veterinary surgeon is tall, not to flex or twist the lower limb excessively in an effort to raise the foot to a convenient height to use the testers. Paradoxically, in comparison with horses many ponies have harder hoof horn, making eliciting foot pain difficult, so care always should be taken when assessing the response to hoof testers. The use of small or adjustable hoof testers is advisable for ponies.

Ponies can have a positive response to lower limb flexion tests despite being sound and performing to the owner's expectations.

DIAGNOSTIC ANALGESIA

Some ponies are strong-willed, which can limit a conventional lameness evaluation using perineural or intrasynovial analgesia. Using a nose twitch or a low dose of an α_2-sedative may aid this (e.g., 40 to 60 mcg of romifidine per kilogram or 0.6 to 0.9 mg of xylazine per kilogram

References on page 1346

intravenously). In some ponies the lower limbs may have thick skin and be very hairy, making accurate palpation of the structures difficult, particularly finding the site for a palmar digital nerve block. I am conscious that because of the relatively shorter limbs in ponies, local anesthetic solution may diffuse further than in the horse, and a reduced amount of local anesthetic solution is used for perineural analgesia (e.g., 1 mL of mepivacaine hydrochloride for each nerve for palmar digital or palmar [abaxial sesamoid] analgesia).

IMAGING CONSIDERATIONS

For most clinical situations a similar number of radiographic images are required to examine the lower limb of a pony as for a horse. Although obtaining good-quality radiographs of the lower limb is generally easier, some important lesions may be more subtle than in the horse, particularly those involving the distal interphalangeal (DIP) joint and navicular bone. Conversely, one should note that a substantial amount of joint degeneration can be present in some sound ponies. It is therefore important in the pony to undertake intrasynovial analgesia to confirm that any periarticular and intraarticular abnormalities are associated with joint pain.

In some ponies, particularly those kept at grass, a substantially increased thickness of skin in the distal limbs, pelvis, and thoracolumbar areas can be present and reduces skin penetration by ultrasound waves, resulting in poor ultrasonographic images. I have found that shaving the hair and hosing the area to be scanned with warm water for 15 minutes often substantially improves the quality of the image.

TEN MOST COMMON CONDITIONS AFFECTING COMPETITION PONIES

Competition ponies appear to have a reduced prevalence of lameness in comparison with horses; however, the common conditions they develop mimic those found in competition horses. The following list contains the 10 most common lameness conditions in the ponies treated in my practice:
1. Laminitis and other foot-related injuries
2. Distal hock joint pain, osteoarthritis of the distal tarsal joints (bone spavin)
3. Desmitis of the accessory ligament of the deep digital flexor tendon
4. Conditions of the digital flexor tendon sheath
5. Osteoarthritis of the metacarpophalangeal joint
6. Superficial digital flexor tendonitis
7. Exertional rhabdomyolysis
8. Osteoarthritis of the carpus
9. Osteoarthritis of the femorotibial joint
10. Injuries of the palmar or plantar annular ligament

LIMB DEFORMITIES

Mild angular limb deformities in ponies are common, but few affect performance or require medical or surgical correction. In many native breeds in the United Kingdom a small degree of carpal and fetlock valgus deviation is common. The persistence of a full-length ulna and fibula

has been associated with the development of severe angular limb deformities in Shetland ponies.[1] This may be a form of atavism, the inheritance of a characteristic from remote, rather than recent, ancestors.

Congenital laxity of the digital flexor tendons in the hindlimb of Shetland ponies is not uncommon and can be associated with hyperextension of the DIP joint. Treatment is similar to that in the horse.

Adactyly (absence of all or part of a normal digit) and polydactyly (duplication of all or part of a digit beyond the normal number) and other congenital musculoskeletal defects have been recorded in ponies.[2]

JOINT DISEASE
Osteochondrosis

Rarely do ponies have lameness associated with osteochondritis dissecans (OCD). Histopathological evidence of osteochondrosis specifically in ponies has been reported only in the lateral trochlear ridge of the femur.[3] Based on a limited number of ponies, in my opinion the most commonly affected joints are the tarsocrural and femoropatellar joints, and lesions are found at the same recognized sites as in the horse—namely, the cranial aspect of the intermediate ridge of the tibia, trochlear ridges of the talus, the medial and lateral malleoli of the tibia, and the lateral trochlear ridge of the femur. Osteochondrosis has been seen particularly in ponies bred for showing,[4] perhaps because these ponies were receiving high feed intakes in an effort to improve show ring appearance.

Lameness associated with a subchondral bone cyst in the medial femoral condyle in the stifle is not uncommon in the pony.

Osteoarthritis

Ponies develop osteoarthritis (OA) in similar joints as horses. However, many ponies have mild-to-moderate joint degeneration, are clinically sound, and perform to the level of the owner's expectation (Figure 126-1). OA in ponies tends to be primary rather than secondary to a previous intraarticular condition, such as intraarticular chip fractures, OCD, osseous cystlike lesions, or ligamentous damage.

Scapulohumeral Joint

Shetland and Miniature Horses have a higher prevalence of OA of the scapulohumeral joint than do other equine breeds.[5-7] This typically occurs in young ponies; the mean age in one survey was 5.2 years. The lameness is usually unilateral but can be bilateral and is sudden in onset and severe (grade 4 to 5 of 5) in degree. Lameness is characterized by a reduction in the cranial phase of the stride and a low arc of foot flight. Radiological abnormalities may not be present in the acute stage.[5] Ultrasonography may be used to assist in the diagnosis.[8] No reported treatment has resulted in successful resolution of the lameness. Some Shetland ponies have a flatter and more shallow glenoid cavity of the scapula than other equine breeds, and this may be caused by a primary joint dysplasia that could predispose Shetland ponies to OA of the scapulohumeral joint.[6] In Miniature Horses scapulohumeral joint OA can be associated with an inability of the owner or veterinarian to pick up either forelimb.[7] Ponies with severe bilateral OA of the scapulohumeral joint may exhibit an unusual,

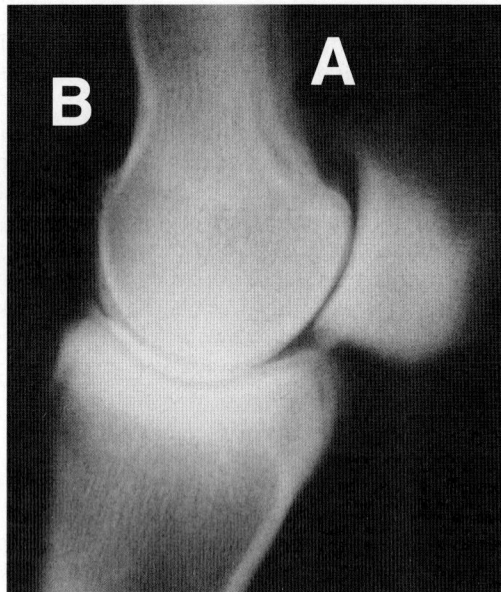

Fig. 126-1 • Lateromedial radiographic image of the metacarpophalangeal joint of a 12-year-old jumping pony. Periarticular osteophytes on the articular margins of the proximal and distal aspect of the proximal sesamoid bones reflect osteoarthritis. There is also evidence of supracondylar lysis (*A*) on the palmar aspect of the third metacarpal bone and villonodular (proliferative) synovitis (*B*) on the dorsal border. This pony had met the owners' expectation until 5 weeks before this examination.

compensatory hindlimb gait deficit in an attempt to redistribute weight to the hindlimbs (Editors).

Carpus

When compared to horses older ponies appear to have an increased incidence of OA of the carpometacarpal joint, often referred to as *carpal spavin*. The radiological abnormalities found within the carpometacarpal joint are similar to those of OA of the distal tarsal joints, and periosteal new bone and enthesophyte formation on the abaxial margins of the second and fourth metacarpal bones may also be present.[9]

I have observed several lame ponies with restricted flexion of the carpus and radiological evidence of carpal joint degeneration, but the lameness was abolished by perineural or intrasynovial analgesia in the more distal aspect of the limb. Restricted carpal flexion without overt lameness may result in a pony being presented because of a history of tripping and concern for the safety of a child rider.

Stifle

In a retrospective study of stifle lameness, a higher incidence of OA of the femorotibial joints was noted in Highland ponies compared with the normal referral horse population at the University of Edinburgh.[10] The ponies have sudden-onset, severe (grade 4 to 5 out of 5) lameness associated with damage to the menisci and collateral or cruciate ligaments. Ultrasonography and arthroscopy are useful to assess the extent of the soft tissue damage. In some of these ponies concurrent abnormalities in the articular surface of the medial femoral condyle, as described in horses, were present.[11] The extent of the meniscal and ligament damage was such that treatment was generally unsuccessful. OA

of the femoropatellar joint can occur in Shetland Ponies and Miniature Horses secondary to chronic lateral luxation of the patella[12] (see following discussion).

Hock

OA of the distal tarsal joints (bone spavin) is a common cause of hindlimb lameness in ponies, but as in other joints, intrasynovial or perineural analgesia is advisable to confirm the relevance of any radiological changes. Icelandic horses appear to be predisposed to OA of the distal hock joints.[13] An epidemiological study showed that 23% of Icelandic horses in Sweden had radiological signs of bone spavin.[14] A causal relationship has been found between hindlimb lameness and radiological evidence of bone spavin and the Icelandic horses' ages and hock angles. No relationship was found with environmental factors such as training and showing.[15] The lameness found in Icelandic horses is often mild, despite moderate-to-severe radiological changes.[13] OA of the talocalcaneal joint has been seen in ponies,[16] and in my opinion the incidence is higher in ponies than horses. Surgical arthrodesis is the preferred treatment for functional soundness, but the prognosis is guarded.[16]

Other Specific Joint Conditions

Luxation of the Coxofemoral Joint

Rupture of the coxofemoral ligaments and secondary luxation of the coxofemoral (hip) joint have a higher prevalence in the pony than in the horse (Figure 126-2).[17] This may be because in horses, unlike in ponies, the ilium tends to fracture before luxation of the hip occurs,[18] although marginal fractures of the acetabulum have been seen with luxation.[19] In the pony, ligament rupture usually occurs after trauma, and the head of the femur is often displaced in a craniodorsal direction. Affected ponies adopt a characteristic posture with outward rotation of the foot and stifle, inward rotation of the tarsus, and a pronounced shortening of the affected limb. Open or closed reduction has been used to treat the luxation, but the prognosis for long-term soundness is poor.[17] Successful closed reduction has been noted in two ponies that were seen within 12 hours of the initial injury.[19] Successful surgical management of a Miniature Horse with coxofemoral luxation using open reduction and a novel toggle suture, synthetic capsulorrhaphy, and trochanteric transposition has been reported.[20] Ponies with unsuccessful reduction or irreducible luxation can be salvaged for breeding or companion purposes by excision arthroplasty.[21] Coxofemoral luxation is often complicated by upward fixation of the patella.[18,21] Ligament rupture may occur without luxation of the coxofemoral joint, and the clinical signs are similar to those of luxation except for the absence of limb shortening.[18]

Dysplasia of the Coxofemoral Joint

Hip dysplasia has been reported in the Norwegian Dole and a Shetland pony colt.[22] In the latter, hip dysplasia was associated with the development of OA in the coxofemoral joint.

Luxation of the Patella

Lateral (sub)luxation of the patella in Shetland ponies is common.[23] The condition is usually congenital but can be

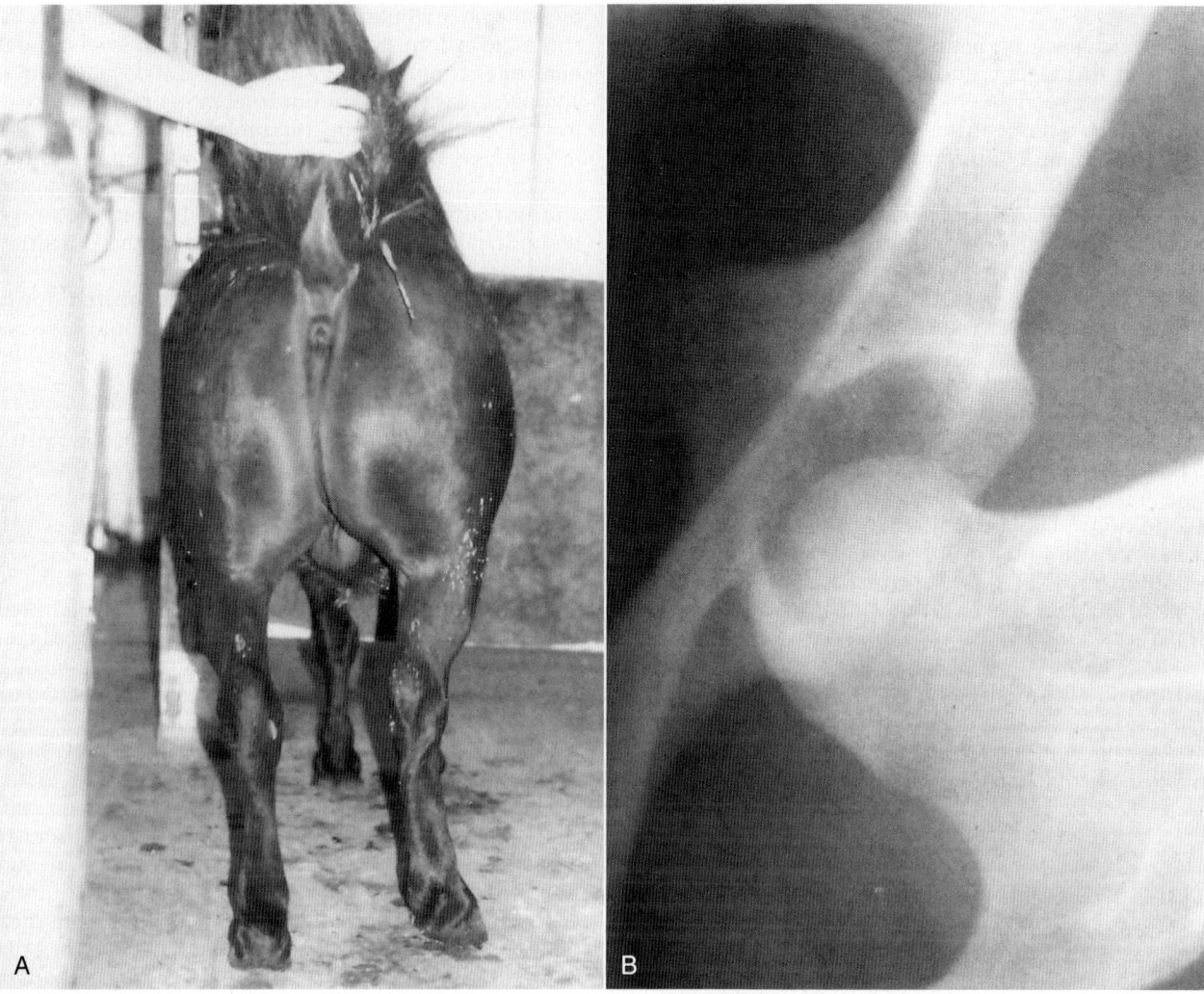

Fig. 126-2 • A, Typical appearance of luxation of the coxofemoral joint in a pony. Note the outward rotation of the stifle and foot, inward rotation of the tarsus, and shortening of the right hindlimb. **B,** Ventrodorsal radiographic image of the right coxofemoral joint demonstrating the caudodorsal luxation of the head of the femur.

acquired and affects one or both hindlimbs. A distinction should be made between (sub)luxation and congenital permanent lateral luxation (see the following discussion). The cause of the condition is thought to be malformation of the trochlear ridges and groove, but rupture of the medial femoropatellar ligament has been reported in one pony.[24] Postmortem examination usually reveals that (sub)luxation is associated with a broadening and flattening of the medial and lateral trochlear ridges of the femur, particularly the distal aspect of the medial trochlear ridge. Whether these changes are congenital or are caused by bone modeling is unknown. The clinical signs vary, but in most ponies the patella can be easily manipulated laterally and then replaced in the trochlear groove, and in some ponies the (sub)luxation can be observed during motion. The degree of (sub)luxation varies among ponies and can vary during an individual pony's life. Patellar luxation can be observed in lateromedial and caudocranial radiographic images, but to confirm (sub)luxation a cranioproximal-craniodistal oblique (skyline) image of the patella is required. In ponies with (sub)luxation the patella may appear an abnormal shape on the skyline projection, but this is caused by

rotation and abnormal positioning and not by bone modeling.[23] Ponies with lateral luxation of the patella have been treated successfully by medial imbrication and lateral release incision[12] or imbrication and recession sulcoplasty.[24] Hermans and colleagues,[23] using a limited breeding experiment with a group of Shetland ponies, found evidence to suggest monogenic autosomal recessive hereditary transmission of this defect.

Congenital permanent lateral luxation of the patella is also seen in Shetland ponies. Affected newborn foals are unable to extend the stifle fully and therefore have a crouched, squatting position when standing. The lateral trochlear ridge of the femur in affected foals is often flat rather than convex.[23] The prognosis for successful treatment is poor.

Upward Fixation of the Patella

Intermittent upward fixation of the patella is a not uncommon condition in ponies, affecting young ponies (typically 2 to 3 years old), and older ponies secondary to an orthopedic problem in the limb. The clinical presentation is similar to that in the horse.

Hemarthrosis

A higher incidence of hemarthrosis has been noted in ponies than in horses,[25] and this is often secondary to a systemic disease such as a blood clotting disorder or hepatopathy. Affected ponies have acute-onset lameness with a severely painful joint effusion(s).

Subluxation of the Proximal Interphalangeal Joint

Nontraumatic dorsal subluxation of the proximal interphalangeal (PIP) (pastern) joint has been recorded in the hindlimbs of ponies.[26] The condition usually occurs bilaterally in young ponies (Figure 126-3). Dorsal subluxation of the PIP joint is observed when the affected limb is not bearing weight. The subluxation is reduced as weight is borne on the affected limb, and an audible clunk often accompanies joint reduction. Tenotomy of the medial head of the deep digital flexor tendon (DDFT) in the proximal metatarsal region has produced good results in treating this condition.[26] Unilateral dorsal subluxation of the PIP joint has been observed in a 3-year-old pony secondary to infectious arthritis of the tarsocrural joint.[27] The subluxation resolved after successful treatment of the infectious arthritis.

Treatment of Joint Disease

Nonsteroidal antiinflammatory drugs should be used with care in lightweight ponies because they may be more susceptible to phenylbutazone toxicity.[28] (Recommendations

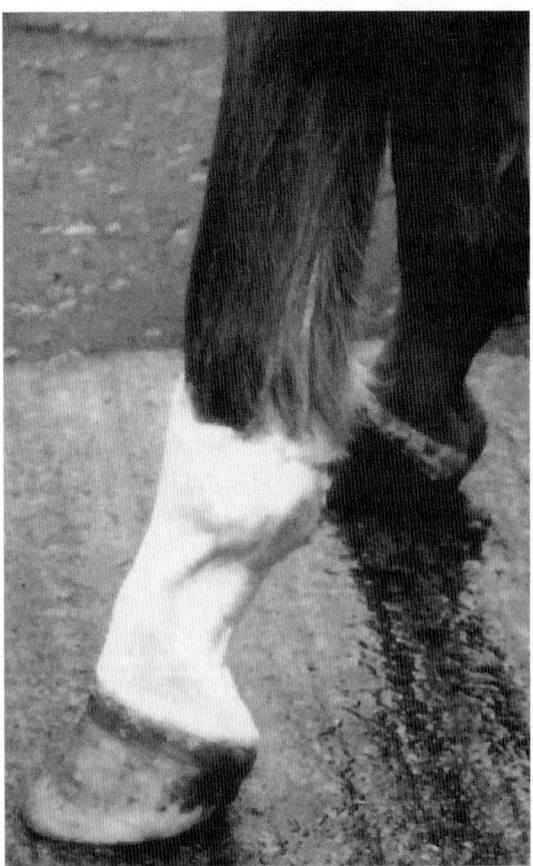

Fig. 126-3 • Bilateral nontraumatic dorsal subluxation of the proximal interphalangeal joints in a 3-year-old Welsh pony. The condition resolved after tenotomy of the medial head of the deep digital flexor tendon.

by some phenylbutazone-supplying drug companies in the United Kingdom state that the maximum level of phenylbutazone in ponies is 4.4 mg/kg orally on alternate days compared with a maximum level of 4.4 mg/kg twice daily for horses.) The ulcerogenic properties of orally administered phenylbutazone are possibly more pronounced in ponies because of less efficient gut absorption. Systemic and intraarticular corticosteroid use in ponies also has to be undertaken with caution because of the potential for development of laminitis.[29]

If arthroscopy or arthrotomy is undertaken in the diagnosis or treatment of joint disease, one should note before giving a prognosis that ponies appear to accommodate greater cartilage degeneration than horses.

A Fell pony foal with infectious arthritis should be checked for immunodeficiency syndrome before treatment is initiated.[30]

FRACTURES

Common fractures seen in horses (i.e., proximal phalangeal fractures, third carpal bone slab fractures, and condylar fractures of the third metacarpal or the third metatarsal bones) are rare in ponies. Most fractures are secondary to trauma. Hindlimb fractures, particularly involving the lateral splint bone (fourth metatarsal bone [MtIV]), often result from kicks from other horses.

In some ponies, closed fracture reduction and using a cast alone may result in successful bony union in fractures that would require internal fixation in a horse. The lighter weight of most ponies also means that the use of internal or external fixation of long bone fractures is more successful than in a horse. Repair of complete fractures of the humerus, tibia, and radius that would require euthanasia in a horse can be attempted in lightweight ponies (<300 kg).[31] Treatment may involve using intramedullary implants such as a single Steinmann pin, stacked pin fixation, or intramedullary interlocking nails. External fixation for comminuted lower limb fractures (e.g., proximal phalanx) is also more successful in the pony.[32] External fixation using a transfixation cast, with or without a U-bar,[33] or an equine modified type II external skeletal device may be successful.[34]

Many fractures of the splint bones (second and fourth metacarpal bones, and the MtIV), including proximal fractures, heal satisfactorily with conservative management in the pony. I also have found in the pony that complete excision of the MtIV as previously described[35] is successful in treating fractures of the proximal third of the MtIV; however, this occasionally leads to instability of the tarsus.

In ponies with severe or multiple fractures of the carpus, pancarpal or partial carpal arthrodesis can also be considered.[36] Arthrodesis of the scapulohumeral joint of a Miniature Horse also has been described.[37]

It may be important when undertaking internal (or external) fixation in older ponies to assess whether the pony may be compromised systemically by Cushing's disease, because this potentially could result in delayed fracture healing and problems with implant failure.

Stress fractures in ponies are rare but have been recorded.[38]

FOOT-RELATED PROBLEMS

Ponies generally tend to have better foot conformation than do horses, and the prevalence of long-toe, low-heel foot conformation appears to be lower than in the Thoroughbred. Navicular disease does occur in ponies, but the incidence is considerably lower than in the horse.[39] Intrasynovial analgesia of the DIP joint or navicular bursa should be undertaken to confirm any suspected radiological changes in the flexor surface of the navicular bone. Lesions within the DDFT and collateral ligaments of the DIP joint have been detected in ponies with the use of magnetic resonance imaging. The incidence of collateral desmitis of the DIP joint and DDFT injuries in competition ponies appears similar to that found in competition horses.[40]

Some degree of ossification of the cartilages of the foot (sidebone) is a common radiological finding in ponies,[41] especially in native pony breeds. As in horses, this is rarely associated with lameness.

LAMINITIS

The incidence of laminitis in ponies is high, and this may be the result of an innate insulin insensitivity.[42] Many of the affected ponies are obese, and a considerable amount of research has recently been carried out comparing human peripheral vascular disease and equine laminitis.[43] The term *equine metabolic syndrome* has been introduced to describe laminitis in obese mature ponies.[44] It has been proposed that hyperglycemia results from insulin insensitivity and causes impaired endothelial function and increased vascular tone. This may involve decreased nitric oxide production, increased release of endothelin-1, increased expression of matrix metalloproteinases, increased lipid oxidation, and increased vasoconstrictor eicosanoids. Dexamethasone suppression tests or adrenocorticotropic hormone (ACTH) stimulation tests give results within normal reference ranges for these ponies, ruling out underlying pars intermedia dysfunction.[44] It is now common to screen for insulin insensitivity in ponies using a variety of factors.[43] Exercise appears to improve insulin sensitivity in ponies.[45]

In the United Kingdom many ponies used for showing are obese and have a high incidence of equine metabolic syndrome. These ponies often have repetitive annual bouts of laminitis, particularly in the spring, and many respond quickly to acute therapy within a matter of days. Metformin (dimethylbiguanide) at a dose of 15 mg/kg bid orally has recently been shown to improve insulin sensitivity and is rapidly gaining considerable support in the United Kingdom for the treatment of equine metabolic syndrome.[43] Chromium has also been used to improve insulin sensitivity in ponies.[46] Trilostane, a 3-hydroxysteroid dehydrogenase inhibitor that acts to inhibit adrenal steroidogenesis, was found in one study to reduce the quantity of phenylbutazone therapy required in the treatment of horses with severe laminitis as a result of Cushing's disease.[47] It has also been used to assist conventional therapies for ponies with laminitis.[44]

If ponies with chronic laminitis do not receive corrective farriery, then many secondary complications can occur in the subsequent months, including recurrent

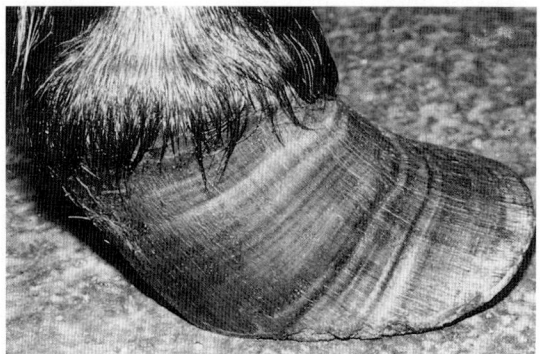

Fig. 126-4 • Foot of a pony with chronic laminitis that has not received any corrective farriery. Note the extremely long toe and laminitic rings.

subsolar hemorrhage, onychomycosis-induced white line disease,[48] and abscess formation within the dorsal wall (Figure 126-4). Dorsal wall resection is indicated in treating some ponies with laminitis, and this can reduce the incidence of chronic problems.[49] Repetitive bouts of laminitis also can lead to hoof and distal phalangeal deformation, resulting in the need for the construction of modified shoes for each foot.[50] The deformation also can result in substantial gait alterations.

In a survey of horses and ponies with laminitis, the prognosis for horses was found to be no different than that for ponies.[51] Restricted access to grass may need to be enforced to prevent laminitis in general purpose ponies that are never stabled. This can involve mowing the field, strip grazing, or muzzling the pony for part of the day. Care should be taken, however, not to undernourish ponies to prevent laminitis because of the potential development of hyperlipemia.[52]

The incidence of Cushing's disease is higher in ponies than in horses,[53] and the diagnosis of Cushing's disease should always be considered in an older pony with laminitis.

SOFT TISSUE INJURIES

Superficial Digital Flexor Tendonitis

Superficial digital flexor (SDF) tendonitis has a lower incidence in ponies than in horses. Tendonitis does occur in older ponies[54]; however, it is often associated with desmitis of the accessory ligament of the DDFT (ALDDFT).[55] Tendonitis may not necessarily occur after strenuous exercise, and the site of the superficial digital flexor tendon (SDFT) damage can be in the proximal metacarpal region or within the carpal canal.[56]

Desmitis of the Accessory Ligament of the Deep Digital Flexor Tendon

Desmitis of the ALDDFT (inferior or distal check ligament), in both the forelimbs and hindlimbs, has a higher incidence in ponies than in horses.[57-59] In an in vitro study the forelimb ALDDFT ruptured at lower forces in older horses and ponies, which suggested that an age-related degeneration occurs within the ligament.[60] Because of the relatively older pony population, the prevalence of ALDDFT desmitis therefore may be similar to that in the horse. Clinically in the forelimb, desmopathy causes an acute-onset lameness and swelling in the proximal, palmar aspect of the metacarpal region. In the hindlimb a similar situation occurs, but desmopathy can also develop as either an insidious or a sudden onset of postural changes.[59] Ultrasonography may show a focal area of reduced echogenicity or disruption of the entire cross-sectional area of the ligament. The damage may occur for part or the entire length of the ALDDFT. Prompt aggressive antiinflammatory therapy is required in the acute stage to prevent adhesion formation linking the ALDDFT to the SDFT around the parietal layer of the carpal (or tarsal) sheath.[58,59] Treatment recommended for ponies with desmitis of the ALDDFT is similar to that recommended for SDF tendonitis in the horse.[61] If extensive adhesion formation occurs in the forelimb, an acquired flexural deformity of the metacarpophalangeal joint may develop, which is difficult to treat.[58] Ponies with hindlimb ALDDFT desmitis and postural changes have a very poor prognosis for a return to full soundness.[59] I have used extracorporeal shock wave therapy in a limited number of ponies with excessive adhesion formation associated with forelimb ALDDFT desmitis. After treatment, the adhesions reduced extensively in size, but I am unsure if this altered the long-term prognosis.

Digital Flexor Tendon Sheath

Tendonitis of the DDFT within the digital flexor tendon sheath (DFTS) is not an uncommon injury in ponies,[62,63] but primary DDF tendonitis further proximally in the metacarpal or metatarsal region is rare. It is my opinion that DDFT injuries within the DFTS are more common in the heavier cob types than in lighter ponies. Ponies with tendonitis have an acute-onset lameness with a painful DFTS effusion.[63] There are two forms of injury: a focal tear within the central core area of the DDFT[62] and a marginal longitudinal tear.[63] Focal lesions within the core of the tendon can be detected by ultrasonography as areas of reduced echogenicity, occasionally with areas of dystrophic mineralization.[64] The associated lameness is abolished by intrasynovial analgesia of the DFTS. The lameness is often slow to resolve (8 to 12 months), treatment is prolonged (often 15 months), and the rate of reinjury is high after return to normal work.[62] Marginal tears of the DDFT are not always detected by ultrasonography, and tenoscopic evaluation of the DFTS is needed to determine the true extent of the damage.[63] The incidence is higher in the forelimbs than in the hindlimbs, and the tears occur more commonly on the lateral margin of the tendon.[63] After tenoscopic debridement or repair, the prognosis for ponies with marginal tears is considerably better than for those with focal core lesions.

Marginal tears of the SDFT and tears of the manica flexoria can also occur in ponies.[63] As in ponies with marginal tears to the DDFT, they are best diagnosed and treated tenoscopically.

Secondary mild thickening of the palmar (or plantar) annular ligament (PAL or PlAL) of the DFTS may accompany tears to the DDFT, SDFT, or manica flexoria. After tenoscopy and tendon debridement, it has been found that PAL desmotomy is not always necessary for a return to full soundness in ponies with such thickening.[63]

Primary desmitis of the PAL is not uncommon in ponies, may be associated with tenosynovitis of the DFTS,

and can cause secondary stenosis of the fetlock canal.[65,66] Desmopathy of the PAL or PlAL occurs more often in ponies and cob types than horses, especially in teenage ponies, and may be in part a degenerative condition. It occurs in hindlimbs more than forelimbs and results in a convex swelling on the palmar or plantar aspect of the fetlock, with localized heat and pain on palpation.[66] I have noted a higher incidence of plantar annular desmitis in ponies with chronic or repetitive laminitis. The condition may develop because of the postural and gait changes occurring with laminitis that put greater strain on the plantar structures of the fetlock joint. In such a situation, plantar annular desmitis could be described as a repetitive strain injury. Treatment initially should include antiinflammatory therapy and treatment of the laminitis. In ponies that are unresponsive to treatment or have chronic PAL desmitis, desmotomy may be required to relieve fetlock canal stenosis. Chronic enlargement of the PAL can occur without signs of lameness.[65] However, ponies with lameness associated with PAL (or PlAL) desmopathy and asymptomatic enlargement of the PAL (or PlAL) of the contralateral limb may subsequently develop lameness in the second limb.

WOUNDS

Ponies undergoing second intention (contraction and epithelialization) wound healing are less likely to have excessive granulation tissue (*proud flesh*) than are horses, and wound contraction is generally faster.[67] In ponies, leukocytes produce more inflammatory mediators, resulting in better local defenses, faster cellular debridement, and a faster transition to the repair phase of wound healing. They also appear to have better myofibroblast organization.[68] An in vitro study has also found that horse limb fibroblasts have significantly less growth than those found in ponies.[69]

OTHER CONDITIONS

The results of nuclear scintigraphic examinations of a limited number of athletic jumping ponies I have treated are similar to those described in horses[70] (i.e., increased technetium-99m [^{99m}Tc] uptake in the proximal and distal aspects of the proximal phalanx, dorsal spinous processes, and distal hock joints). As in the study in horses, not all of these lesions were associated with lameness and may represent bone adaptation to the act of jumping. In all ponies, the results of scintigraphy should be confirmed by diagnostic analgesia.

Back Pain

Back injuries in ponies, particularly involving the sacroiliac joint, appear to have a lower prevalence than in horses.[71] Ponies, however, often demonstrate abnormal behavioral problems such as bucking, secondary to hindlimb and occasionally forelimb lameness, that can be perceived by the owner as signs of primary back pain.

Muscular Disorders

Recurrent exertional rhabdomyolysis (*azoturia* or *tying up*) does affect ponies, especially excitable types and ponies used for eventing. In general purpose ponies, recurrent exertional rhabdomyolysis usually develops when the owner exercises an unfit pony. In one survey in the United Kingdom, ponies were the third most commonly affected group of horses affected by recurrent exertional rhabdomyolysis.[72] Raised blood levels of creatine kinase and aspartate transaminase confirm the diagnosis, and treatment is similar to that for the horse. Polysaccharide storage myopathy also has been reported in Welsh-cross ponies and in larger breeds of horses.[73]

Cerebellar Abiotrophy

Cerebellar abiotrophy has been recorded in Gotland[74] and Eriskay ponies.[75] The disease is inherited in the Gotland pony as an autosomal recessive gene.[74]

Chapter 127

Lameness in Breeding Stallions and Broodmares

Benson B. Martin Jr. and Sue M. McDonnell

Although maximal athletic fitness is typically not the goal for breeding stock, maintenance of musculoskeletal soundness is an important concern for breeding stallions and broodmares, especially because longevity is the usual expectation and a high percentage of these horses have existing musculoskeletal disease related to previous training and performance.

THE STALLION

Musculoskeletal fitness is critical to breeding efficiency of a stallion. The principal management goals are to maintain adequate fitness for normal breeding behavior and to avoid conditions or treatments that may adversely affect spermatogenesis or sperm viability. Libido, mounting, thrusting, and ejaculatory dysfunction represent major causes of poor breeding performance in stallions.[1] Musculoskeletal and neurological disease have been estimated to account for as much as 50% of these problems.[1,2] The goal of managing a lame breeding stallion includes maintaining comfort and fitness to sustain libido and adequate copulatory agility.

Examination

Breeding stallions require skillful handling and are most efficiently examined in an area away from other stallions and mares, in a secluded area if possible. An experienced breeding stallion handler with appropriate restraint aids is ideal. Sedation can be used, but care must be taken not to confound the examination or jeopardize fertility. Phenothiazine tranquilizers, although useful for lameness examinations, have been associated with an increased risk of paralysis of the retractor penis muscle. If acepromazine is used, we recommend a small dose (5 to 10 mg intravenously 30 minutes before the examination) well before the horse gets excited, as well as diligent observation of the stallion for several hours to monitor its ability to retract the penis normally. Should the penis not retract with tactile stimulation once the horse is again otherwise normally alert and reactive, steps can be taken immediately for physical support and management to minimize loss of erectile function.[3] For further diagnostic procedures (e.g., radiography), xylazine or detomidine and butorphanol may be necessary.

History should include signalment, information about the performance career, duration and details of breeding experience, current problem and associated details, medical history, medication, nutrition, and environment, including housing, breeding facilities (e.g., flooring and dummy), and breeding protocol (semen collection technique and stallion handling). Knowledge of old performance-related problems is useful. During the breeding season, the veterinarian should determine the breeding schedule because this will influence the diagnostic and therapeutic strategy.

Complete musculoskeletal evaluation in a breeding stallion ideally begins with a routine breeding soundness examination, including a general physical examination, examination of the internal and external genitalia, evaluation of at least two ejaculates collected 1 hour apart, and evaluation of penile microflora, as outlined by the Society of Theriogenology.[4]

The veterinarian should observe the stallion at a walk and trot in hand, preferably on an even, hard, flat surface or on grass; perform upper and lower limb flexion tests of the forelimbs and hindlimbs because osteoarthritis (OA) is common; examine the feet with hoof testers; and palpate the back. Manifestations of back pain include abnormal sinking, prolonged muscle fasciculation or guarding, and contraction of the epaxial muscles without touching the back. Back pain is common during the breeding season because of the work or secondary to lameness.

A simple neurological examination should include observation of the horse moving in small circles to the left and right, walking in a serpentine pattern with the head elevated, and assessment of hindlimb strength by pulling the tail as the horse walks. The veterinarian should look carefully for unusual patterns of muscle asymmetry, possibly indicative of equine protozoal myelitis (EPM) if the horse is in, or from, North America.

A stallion often is examined because of difficulty in breeding and should be observed during teasing, mounting, thrusting, and dismounting. Specific findings suggestive of a musculoskeletal or neurological problem include failure to couple squarely and to thrust with smooth, rhythmic pelvic action; asymmetric hindlimb weight bearing, particularly one hindlimb dangling while thrusting with the other; failure to properly flex or use the neck or back; abnormal tail posture (spiked high) and anal tone (relaxed, voiding gas or feces) during thrusting; an anxious look in the eye or atypical ear postures suggesting discomfort or

References on page 1347

distraction; failure to grasp securely with the forelimbs; lateral instability; falling during thrusting or dismount; weak, thready, or irregular ejaculatory pulses (often variable from day to day); and lameness after breeding.[1] Common manifestations of musculoskeletal pain are reluctance to mount or dismount, early dismount, squealing during dismount, or savaging the mare or handler during or immediately after mounting. Frame-by-frame videotape analysis may help to determine when discomfort occurs, as well as to identify handling factors that enhance or impair performance. Diagnostic analgesia can be difficult to perform and is often unnecessary because of the obvious signs of OA. Further investigation in selected stallions may include ultrasonography, nuclear scintigraphy, and measurement of creatine kinase before and 1 hour after breeding.

Specific Diagnostic Considerations and Therapy

Sore Back

A sore back is associated with inadequate coupling and thrusting during breeding. A stallion may fail to wrap the pelvis or neck around the mare or dummy and may tend to hold its head off the neck of the mare and paddle with the forelimbs. Thrusting is often of irregular depth and rhythm, that is, choppy and interrupted. An acutely sore back may become a chronic condition, exacerbated by breeding and an increased number of unsuccessful mounts, unless treated aggressively.

It is important to determine the primary cause of lameness and initiate the appropriate treatment. Pain can be secondary to another musculoskeletal cause such as OA, a heavy breeding schedule, poor footing, poor shoeing, poor fitting of the breeding dummy to the stallion, or allowing the stallion to advance up the side of a dummy mount so that it is thrusting with a curved back. Chronic back pain may be treated using acupuncture once weekly for 8 weeks and repeated every 3 to 4 weeks or as needed.[5] Acupuncture therapy may be combined with nonsteroidal antiinflammatory drug (NSAID) therapy, or NSAIDs may be used alone.[5,6]

Prognosis for normal breeding performance is guarded to good and varies with management factors. One key factor is ejaculatory efficiency. Once a stallion needs more than one or two mounts per breeding, expected performance diminishes rapidly.

Osteoarthritis

A stallion with OA appears stiff and painful during breeding; stiffness is often worse after rest and improves with exercise. The carpus, front fetlocks, and hocks are affected most commonly. Diagnosis may be obvious on physical examination and is confirmed radiologically.

Pain control is essential to maintain adequate breeding performance. We recommend phenylbutazone (1.5 to 2 g orally [PO] twice daily for 4 to 5 days and then 1 g twice daily for 5 to 7 days)[7] combined with a period of sexual and general rest if possible. Clinically significant improvement may not be evident for up to 5 to 10 days. Long-term, low-dose phenylbutazone treatment has no measurable effect on sperm production or testicular size,[8] but horses should be monitored for signs of toxicity, including colic, loss of appetite, diarrhea, dependent edema, and mucosal ulceration or renal disease.[9] Other NSAIDs, such as flunixin

meglumine and ketoprofen, and intraarticular or systemic medication with corticosteroids, polysulfated glycosaminoglycans, and hyaluronan may be useful in selected horses.

Arthrodesis may be warranted for severe OA of the fetlock joint, but postoperative pain may persist, requiring long-term management. Pancarpal arthrodesis may be considered for stallions with severe carpal OA or after acute, severe carpal injury. With any lameness, pain management must be used to prevent increased recumbency, which can compromise thermal regulation of the testes, especially in hot conditions, and reduce sperm viability and fertility.

Neurological Disease

Neurological disease (see also Chapter 11) is usually evident during mounting, intromission, and thrusting, with a stallion stepping on its hind feet, bearing weight on a toe rather than the sole, and sometimes knuckling over. The stallion may bear weight unevenly during thrusting, sometimes becoming high sided on the mare or dummy mount, or falling. The stallion may have reduced proprioceptive control of the penis in seeking and intromission and may have poor anal tone during thrusting. The horse may require extraordinary effort to ejaculate.

Treatment of cervical vertebral malformation (CVM) in adult horses is challenging, and management methods are important, including good footing, proper shoeing, proper positioning of the mare or dummy mount, ground collection of semen, and pharmacological aids to ejaculation when necessary (Box 127-1).[1,10] Special precautions must be taken during collection of semen or breeding to protect the stallion, the mare, and the personnel working around the stallion. The mare or dummy mount should be positioned to minimize the risk of a stallion with poor lateral stability falling. Lateral support can be provided at the hips. For semen collection, a mare that does not wiggle from side to side should be used. A dummy mount may be better but usually elicits less vigorous thrusting than a live mount and cannot be moved forward to assist the stallion with dismounting. Surgery occasionally is performed, with recovery taking many months.[11]

The management of horses with EPM (see Chapter 11) is similar to that for horses with CVM, together with daily pyrimethamine and sulfadiazine or sulfamethoxazole for at least 60 to 90 days (Table 127-1). To prevent anemia, supplementation with folate and vitamin E is advised.[12] This treatment does not affect sperm production adversely.[13]

Sore Feet

Signs of sore hind feet include shallow thrusting, failure to plant the feet securely during thrusting, thrusting on one leg, and early dismount. Signs of sore front feet or other forelimb pain include hesitancy to mount and dismount. If not resolved quickly, sore feet can lead to long-lasting psychogenic sexual behavior dysfunction.

Many breeding stallions that come from the racetrack have poor hoof quality, underrun heels, long toes, and thin soles, predisposing them to sore feet. The feet should be observed daily and trimmed every 4 to 6 weeks. Leaving stallions barefoot is best, but some may require front shoes to remain comfortable. Rarely, bilateral hind foot pain can cause similar clinical signs, and hind shoes with corrective

BOX 127-1

Management and Pharmacological Aids to Enhance Libido and Facilitate Ejaculation

Management Aids

To enhance sexual arousal

Prolonged teasing under conditions that yield the highest safe level of arousal

Breeding schedule for maximum arousal

Natural estrus stimulus and mount mare

Stable (no side-to-side movement) mount mare or dummy is necessary

Minimal distractions in the breeding area

Established breeding routine rich with conditioned stimuli for maximum arousal

Encouragement and positive reinforcement

To reduce back and hindlimb pain and accommodate musculoskeletal deficiencies

Mount mare or dummy of appropriate height and conformation

Mare or dummy down grade from stallion to reduce weight on hindlimbs

Semen collection on the ground (artificial vagina or manual stimulation)

Weight loss to reduce work of hindlimbs, particularly during breeding

Pain treatment

Lateral support at the hips during mount

Good footing (grass or dry nonslip, synthetic surface)

To increase positive stimulation of the penis

Pressure and temperature of the artificial vagina that yields best response

Hot compresses applied to the base of the penis

Pharmacological Aids

To enhance sexual arousal

Gonadotropin-releasing hormone: 50 µg of Cystorelin SC 1 and 2 hours before breeding[23]

Diazepam: 0.05 mg/kg slow IV administration[24,25]

To lower ejaculatory threshold (in copula)

Imipramine: 500 to 1000 mg PO in grain[31,32]

To induce ejaculation (ex copula)

Imipramine: 2.2 mg/kg PO followed 2 hours later by xylazine: 0.4 to 0.6 mg/kg IV[33,34]

SC, Subcutaneously; *IV,* intravenous; *PO,* orally.

TABLE 127-1

Medications			
DRUG	DOSE	ROUTE	FREQUENCY
Phenylbutazone	2.2 mg/kg	PO, IV	BID
Flunixin meglumine	1.1 mg/kg	IV, IM	BID
Ketoprofen	1.1 mg/kg	IV	SID
Aspirin	15-100 mg/kg	PO	SID
Isoxsuprine	1.2 mg/kg	PO	BID
Methocarbamol	40 mg/kg	PO	BID
Sulfamethoxazole	12.5 mg/kg	PO	BID
Sulfadiazine	12.5 mg/kg	PO	BID
Pyrimethamine	1 mg/kg	PO	SID
Folate	0.5 mg/kg	PO	SID
Vitamin E	5000 IU	PO	SID
Xylazine	150 mg	IV	AN
Detomidine	5-10 mg	IV	AN
Butorphanol	10-25 mg	IV	AN
Acepromazine	10-25 mg	IV	AN

PO, Orally; *IV,* intravenously; *IM,* intramuscularly; *BID,* twice daily; *SID,* once a day; *AN,* as needed.

trimming may be necessary (Editors). These horses may be left barefoot during the off season to allow the feet to grow more normally. Provision of soft footing in the breeding shed and weight control are important. Pain control using NSAIDs may be necessary.

Fractures of the Distal Phalanx

Fractures of the distal phalanx can be acute or chronic injuries. Most are palmar process fractures, and horses can be managed with a bar shoe with side clips reset every 6 weeks, stall rest, and NSAIDs. Sagittal fractures of the distal phalanx are more serious, but horses may be managed in the same way.

Laminitis

Common primary causes of laminitis include contralateral orthopedic injuries, colitis, Potomac horse fever, *Salmonella,* and other infectious diseases that predispose to the release of endotoxins. The treatment of horses with acute laminitis includes treating the primary disease, supporting the distal phalanx, decreasing blood pressure, treating inflammation, and managing pain (see Chapter 34).[14-16]

Chronic laminitis, with rotation of the distal phalanx, can be an important problem in breeding stallions, manifested as a stiff gait or more overt lameness in one or both front feet. Trimming, shoeing, and providing analgesia are important (see Chapter 34).

Muscle Disease

Rhabdomyolysis and other muscle diseases are usually evident during or after thrusting. Inefficient thrusting on early mounts is followed by increasing discomfort, leading to rapid mounting and dismounting. The horse may sweat profusely and have an increased respiratory rate and obvious pain. Treatment during an acute episode includes administering acepromazine (10 to 20 mg intravenously) to control anxiety and 10 to 20 L of balanced electrolyte solution intravenously, keeping the horse confined to a stall, monitoring progress, and evaluating the stallion closely for paraphimosis. In horses with chronic rhabdomyolysis, the diet should be altered to primarily hay and high-quality, low-protein, low-carbohydrate feed.[17] Methocarbamol (see Table 127-1) is useful in some horses.

Injuries

Injuries in stallions, including lacerations, punctures, abrasions, and fractures or dislocations, are managed similarly as in other horses. A common injury is abrasion or contusion of the carpus during mounting, especially with dummy mounts. A stallion with a painful carpus may fail to grasp a mare with the forelimb and may stand up on the mare or dummy. Sexual rest until the wound heals is usually best. If continued breeding is necessary, emollient topical analgesic ointment and skillful bandaging from the coronet to several centimeters above the carpus can relieve apparent discomfort, with the administration of NSAIDs if required.

Hyperextension injuries of a forelimb may occur at dismount but are usually not serious and resolve with NSAID treatment.

Aortoiliac Thrombosis

Signs suggesting aortoiliac disease include delayed ejaculation despite good libido (numerous mounts and more than 12 thrusts); progressive hindlimb weakness or pain during thrusting resulting in camping under the mare or dummy; and difficulty backing up to dismount.[18] Erection aberrations are not as common as ejaculatory dysfunction, but they can include delayed or rapid tumescence or detumescence, or loss of erection during thrusting.

Comprehensive Management

The useful breeding career of a stallion with lameness problems often can be prolonged substantially with coordinated veterinary care and breeding management. Particular concerns and challenges include the following:

1. Controlling pain without adversely affecting libido or fertility
2. Maintaining a level of fitness adequate for the breeding work without exacerbating lameness
3. Using available management and veterinary techniques to enhance libido and ejaculatory function, to reduce the work of each breeding, and to reduce the total number of breedings required over the season
4. Managing the breeding book to maximize breeding value while not exacerbating the lameness

Pain Management

Phenylbutazone is the most common NSAID used for breeding stallions. A 4-week oral treatment course (2.2 mg/kg twice daily) has no adverse effects on semen quality at the time of ejaculation or after 24 and 48 hours stored at 4° C.[8] Although fertility trials have not been done, clinical experience suggests no adverse effects of chronic treatment with phenylbutazone at levels tolerated well by a stallion. We recommend orally administered phenylbutazone daily throughout the breeding season to keep the stallion comfortable and functioning with as little effort and pain as possible to avoid a potential downward spiral of delayed ejaculation, additional effort, and exacerbated lameness.

Firocoxib is now available for horses. Although not specifically tested in breeding stallions, efficacy for lameness has been reported to be similar to that of phenylbutazone.[19]

We have used gabapentin clinically in combination with phenylbutazone in an attempt to help breeding stallions with possible neurogenic and musculoskeletal discomfort.[20] Early studies indicate that oral bioavailability of gabapentin is low compared with intravenous administration but is well tolerated at 20 mg/kg.[21]

Complementary pain management, including acupuncture,[5,6] electrostimulation, and massage therapy, may provide additional comfort, with no adverse effects, on semen quality or fertility.

Fitness and Weight Management

Routine exercise is one of the most important management factors for maintaining cardiovascular and musculoskeletal physical and mental fitness of any breeding stallion. A general recommendation for exercise for a sound breeding stallion is daily paddock exercise for a minimum of 8 hours or a minimum of 30 minutes of supervised exercise or light work. Although the common tendency is to rest a lame horse, controlled exercise is probably even more important for breeding efficiency of a lame stallion. A daily exercise program, including turnout or supervised light work, appears to clinically significantly improve the breeding efficiency of a lame stallion. The type of exercise is influenced by the degree of lameness and the temperament of the stallion. Controlled exercise may include daily riding, lunging, jogging, swimming, or exercise on a treadmill or mechanical walker.

Libido and breeding efficiency almost always improve with a stallion carrying less rather than more body weight, particularly for hindlimb lameness or incoordination. We have seen remarkable improvement in breeding efficiency and stamina after reduction in body weight in Quarter Horses with small sore feet or in stallions with aortoiliac thrombosis.

Breeding Management and Handling
Breeding Schedule

For any hand-bred stallion, and particularly for a stallion with lameness, an important goal of breeding management is to minimize the work of each breeding and the cumulative work of the season. For heavily booked stallions, total seasonal work can be reduced and efficiency of each breeding often can be improved by limiting services to one per mare cycle. This forces upgraded mare management so that she is close to ovulation when covered. This type of mare tends to be more stimulating to the stallion and to stand more solidly for breeding. For certain stallions with smaller books, availability for service often can be limited to one mare, 3 or 4 days weekly. In our experience, by shifting effort toward mare management and effectively increasing the sperm numbers per service, seasonal pregnancy rates are often as good as or better than with more frequent services.

For stallions that are breeding by artificial insemination, with good to excellent longevity of sperm motility, a reasonable book of mares can be served with collection of semen limited to two or three times weekly. For stallions in registries permitting frozen semen, it is helpful to bank frozen semen for consideration for use during busy periods or to reduce pressure for obtaining fresh ejaculates when problems arise.

Maintaining Ideal Levels of Libido

It is important to maintain good to high libido to help a stallion to ejaculate more efficiently in the face of pain, neurological dysfunction, or musculoskeletal disability. Well-tested management schemes and pharmacological aids are available to enhance libido (see Box 127-1). The most useful management tools in a stabled stallion are housing near mares and away from stallions and ample daily teasing exposure to mares.[22] Treatment with gonadotropin-releasing hormone can be useful to boost libido via increased circulating testicular steroids.[23] Diazepam, by inhibiting the memory of pain associated with breeding, may be helpful.[24,25]

Occasionally, rowdy or overenthusiastic breeding behavior complicates management and breeding of a lame stallion. The stallion handler should use judicious correction and guidance to establish and maintain organized control, without overcorrection that will diminish libido.[26] Medication is not recommended because tranquilization at a level effective to control behavior makes the stallion unstable for breeding, and using progesterone or other endocrine-mediated treatments adversely affects spermatogenesis.

Breeding Shed Handling Considerations

Most disabled stallions benefit from having the mare or dummy mount slightly down grade. This can reduce the work of the hindlimbs in supporting the body weight. For a live mount mare, a down grade is achieved best with a sloping ramp extending at least 3 m behind, in front, and to each side of the mare (Figure 127-1). A height differential between the stallion and the mare can be built with mats or by placing the mare in a pit. These work well if the mare remains stationary, but if the mare moves back, the grade may be reversed for the stallion. If the mare moves forward, the stallion can become trapped between the mare and the front edge of mats, or in the pit with the mare. When breeding a stallion with the mare downhill, it is important to avoid the peak of a knoll that slopes off to the sides,

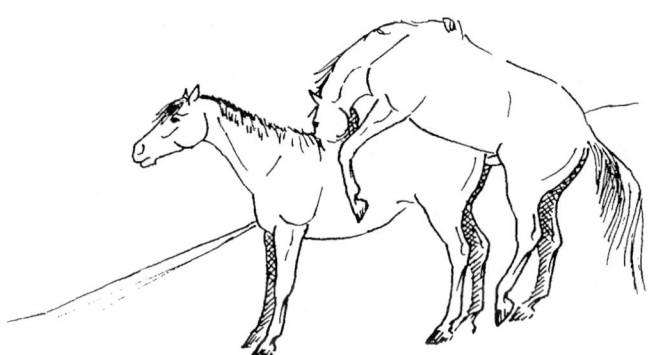

Fig. 127-1 • Mare positioned down grade for breeding.

behind the stallion, or in front of the stallion. This sets the stallion up to fall sideways should the mare move sideways or to be at further disadvantage if the mare moves backward. Once the stallion mounts, restraint of the mare should be optimized to reduce movement in any direction. Disabled stallions that are tentative to mount also can be deterred by low ceilings, cornered mares, or dummy mounts.

When using a dummy mount for stallions with hindlimb, back, or neck problems, we find that greater heights are better. Most disabled stallions do better when guided to remain mounted squarely from the rear, as opposed to across the dummy, or traveling up the side. This is best accomplished by securing the artificial vagina at a physiological angle against the dummy for the stallion to serve, rather than taking the artificial vagina to the horse.

Excellent footing in the breeding area, which is customized to a stallion's particular needs, can improve breeding efficiency greatly (Table 127-2). The surface should be nonslip even when wet, seamless and even to avoid stumbling, and provide moderate cushion. Stallions with hindlimb weakness or incoordination tend to camp under the mare. For these stallions the footing behind the mare is critical to maximize the ability to correct the stance. Although some cushion is good, it should not be so spongy or deep that the stallion gets caught up or buried in the substrate. Stallions with sore feet, especially front feet, benefit from a softer footing, particularly a soft landing during dismount. Heavy sod on well-drained soil is often the simplest and best outdoor footing. Composite rubber athletic surfaces, particularly if poured and seamless, make ideal breeding surfaces.

A stallion should be given ample freedom about the head, particularly during mounting and thrusting, to allow

TABLE 127-2

MATERIAL	FOOTING (NONSLIP)	CUSHION	CLEAN (NO DUST OR KICK-UP)	EASE OF CARE AND CLEANING	COST	COMMENTS
*Flooring Materials for Breeding Sheds**						
Rubber composite bricks or mats	+ + +	+ + +	+ + +	+ + +	$$$$	Stable, highly durable
Shredded rubber	+ Shallow − If deep	+ + +	−	+ +	$$$$	Highly durable
Poured rubber composite	− If dry − − − If wet	+ +	+ + +	+ + +	$$$$	Durable
Hard rubber mats	− If dry − − − If wet	+	+ + +	+ +	$$$	Shift, wrinkle
Fiber	+ + +	+ + +	− −	−	$$$$	Erodes
Cocoa mats	+ + +	+ +	+ +	−	$$	Shift
Wood chips	+ +	+	− − −	Replace	$	Erodes
Sawdust	+	+	− − −	Replace	$	Erodes
Wood shavings	+	+	− − −	Replace	$	Erodes
Brick pavers	− − −	− − −	+	+ + +	$$$$	
Concrete	− − −	− − −	+ + +	+ + +	$$	
Asphalt	−	− − −	+ + +	+ +	$$	
Dirt	+ At best − − − If wet	+ At best − − − If hard	− −	Replace	$	Erodes
Sand	+	+ +	− − −	Replace	$$	Erodes
Gravel fines	− − −	− −	− −	Replace	$$	Erodes

$, Inexpensive; $$, moderately inexpensive; $$$, moderately expensive; $$$$, expensive; +, positive; −, negative.
*Data reflect our opinion.

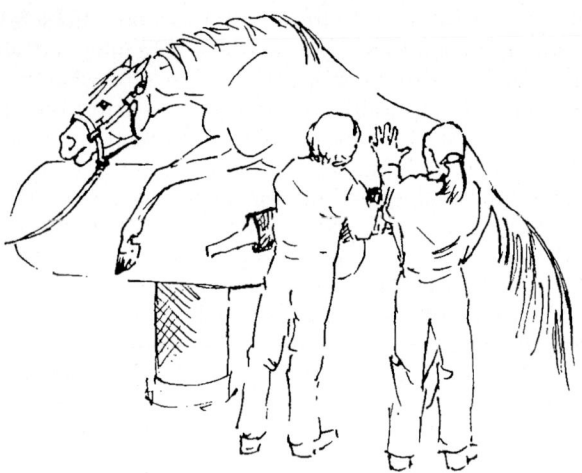

Fig. 127-2 • Spotting a stallion on the left side during breeding.

postural adjustments. Enforcing routines that work well for sound stallions, such as always keeping the head on the left side of the mare or dummy mount, may discourage a disabled horse. For severely ataxic, weak, or uncomfortable stallions, thrusting and ejaculation can be facilitated with gentle stabilizing assistance or spotting during breeding. We recommend an assistant apply gentle pressure with the hands on one or both hips to support the stallion from falling (Figure 127-2). Some stallions tolerate support from the rear, for example, with a wide strap held from either side behind the buttocks. Some resent this type of support, appearing to become trapped on the mare.

Gentle, guiding handling during dismount is important for all stallions but particularly for a disabled horse. For stallions with hindlimb weakness, pain, or incoordination, special consideration should be given to allowing the stallion as much recovery time as possible before dismount and to moving the mare slowly out from under the stallion rather than forcing the stallion to back off. Ataxic stallions that tend to step on themselves and the mare while breeding can benefit from simple, well-secured protective boots or wraps for themselves and the mare.

Monitoring Breeding Performance

Stallions with chronic musculoskeletal discomfort or disability usually deteriorate, and breeding performance should be monitored systematically so that adjustments can be made to maximize performance. A sensitive measure of improved comfort is the number, rhythmic pattern, and strength of pelvic thrusts from insertion to ejaculation. Normal, sound stallions typically require seven to nine thrusts at about 1-second intervals, with even sweep and strength, to ejaculate. The normal range of mount duration is 20 to 30 seconds, with insertion time 12 to 20 seconds. With discomfort, horses tend to require more thrusts, the sweeping pattern of the thrusts becomes less organized (irregular depth, rhythm, and strength), and the hindlimbs become more dancy as opposed to being planted with equal weight bearing on each. The head and ear positions of an uncomfortable stallion also suggest distraction (as if about to quit, fall, or dismount) as opposed to commitment. Horses with sore backs or necks tend to fail to couple closely. Thrusts may be jerky and shallow. Stallions with

hindlimb neurological deficits may bear weight unevenly, become camped under, or become tipped toward the stronger side, with the weaker hindlimb dangling. They seem particularly unable to maintain lateral stability. We recommend developing a customized record sheet for daily grading of each abnormality. Videotaping each breeding from a direct lateral view that spans the entire mount and stallion and from the rear provides the most complete record.

One Mount Rule

For longevity of a disabled stallion through a season or through a breeding career, we recommend that ejaculation should be achieved with one mount. If a horse does not ejaculate in one or at most two mounts, the horse should be taken back to the stall or paddock to rest and return fresh. This strategy often effectively yields a greater number of successful mounts, provided that conditions are optimized for the first mount. The horse should be at the highest level of arousal possible for safe handling, the mount well positioned and optimally restrained if it is a live mare, the artificial vagina at optimum pressure and temperature for semen collection, and the handling team in top form and focused. If particular procedures or medications (see Box 127-1) are known to make the horse more comfortable, enhance libido, or reduce the ejaculatory threshold, we recommend using these from the start.

Ground Semen Collections

For stallions that breed by semen collection, a valuable alternative to mounting is ground semen collection. Most stallions with good to excellent libido are excellent candidates for semen collection while standing on the ground or even while supported in a sling. This technique is particularly useful in horses with aortoiliac thrombosis, cervical vertebral malformation, EPM, and other conditions with hindlimb instability or weakness.

Pharmacologically Induced Ex Copula Ejaculation

For stallions that breed by artificial insemination, pharmacologically induced (or chemical) ejaculation can be used with the stallion at rest in his stall. Currently the generally most effective treatment (50% to 70% of attempts) is a combination of imipramine hydrochloride administered orally about 2 hours before intravenously administered xylazine hydrochloride (see Box 127-1). For a particular stallion, best results can be achieved by titrating through a range of doses for each component drug.

BROODMARE

Soundness of a broodmare is important for the demands of pregnancy and lactation and for ongoing comfort for normal expression of estrus behavior, willingness to stand for natural service when necessary, conception, and normal interactive maternal behavior.[27] Diagnosis and treatment should not adversely affect fertility or the safety of the developing fetus, or nursing foal. As a population, broodmares tend to have a high rate of husbandry-related feet and limb problems. They may have old training or racing injuries. Broodmares coming and going tend to have herd social aggression and related injuries. Broodmares also suffer lameness secondary to foaling.

Specific Diagnostic Considerations and Therapy

Sore Feet

It is recommended that maiden mares should arrive on a breeding farm at least 8 to 10 weeks before the beginning of the breeding season. This allows time to assess and monitor condition of the feet and time for trimming as needed. Early arrival also affords time to acclimate the horse to the farm routine and social environment and for advanced photoperiod manipulation (under lights). Simple sore feet are a common problem in a maiden mare coming from the racetrack. The mare may have thin-walled feet and soles, underrun heels, long toes, bruised feet, quarter cracks, or corns. The mare may have been shod for a long time and not be accustomed to being barefoot. If sore feet are suspected as a cause of lameness, the feet should be examined with hoof testers. Baseline radiography may be indicated. Soaking, poulticing, sole painting, and the administration of phenylbutazone or flunixin meglumine (see Table 127-1) may be required for effective management of mares with foot soreness. Feet of broodmares should be trimmed every 6 to 8 weeks and ideally mares should be barefoot on all limbs and certainly for the hindlimbs.

A subsolar abscess is the most common cause of acute foot pain (see Chapter 28). Other causes include a sequestrum, laminitis, or a fracture of a palmar process of the distal phalanx. A sequestrum of the distal phalanx may be removed in a standing horse,[28] eliminating the risks of general anesthesia for a developing fetus.

Laminitis

Acute or chronic laminitis can be a management problem in mares and may be secondary to pleuritis, diarrhea, severe lameness, or most commonly after foaling followed by a retained placenta (more common in draft breeds; see Chapter 125) or infectious metritis. Chronic laminitis also occurs in overweight mares, mares with a previous history of laminitis, or those that have ingested large amounts of feed or fresh pasture. Acute or chronic laminitis can have a negative effect on fertility secondary to pain.[27]

The treatment goals in broodmares with acute laminitis and chronic laminitis are similar to those described for the stallion. In our experience, some mares with chronic laminitis can be salvaged as successful broodmares with careful foot care, pain medication, good footing, separation from other broodmares and associated competition, and management similar to that described for the breeding stallion. In addition, some can conceive and deliver a normal foal, if these management techniques are successful. However, reproductive lives are often limited by laminitis.

Osteoarthritis

A broodmare with OA may need confinement to a stall or small paddock and analgesic medication (see Table 127-1). With severe OA of the fetlock or carpus, arthrodesis may be considered as a last resort in a broodmare that can no longer conceive or maintain a foal because of chronic pain.

Enlarged or Swollen Limbs

Palmar or plantar dermatitis of the pastern (scratches or mud fever) secondary to wet or muddy footing may cause lameness, particularly in hindlimbs. The mare should be removed from the wet area. Local therapy may be necessary, including washing, drying, and clipping the affected area and local application of a steroid/triple antibiotic topical ointment.

Lymphangitis is seen most commonly in the hindlimbs, is worse in later pregnancy, and causes reluctance to move, painful and pitting edema, and fever. Treatment includes stall rest, antibiotic therapy, and phenylbutazone.

A puncture wound and secondary cellulitis may cause lameness. Locating the original wound is often difficult. Aggressive antibiotic and antiinflammatory therapy is necessary. Additional treatment may include surgical drainage, hot packs, warm water hosing, and bandaging.

Hindlimb lameness may be associated with mastitis. The udder is painful to touch; the mare may not allow the foal to nurse; her appetite may decrease; and she may be febrile. Lameness resolves with symptomatic treatment of the mastitis.

Rhabdomyolysis

Acute rhabdomyolysis occurs occasionally in late gestation after particularly vigorous exercise. The mare may not come in for normal feeding or night stables and is often anxious, has a stiff walk, and may have dark-colored urine. Diagnosis is confirmed by measurement of serum creatine kinase levels. Treatment includes stall rest and NSAIDs. A mare with a foal at foot can be treated with the foal present.

Foaling-Related Injuries

Obturator nerve paralysis secondary to dystocia can result in mild to severe lameness. The mare may show difficulty in abducting the hindlimb and standing immediately after foaling. Femoral nerve paralysis secondary to dystocia results in inability to fix the patella and therefore the hindlimb. This is seen immediately after foaling. Symptomatic therapy for either condition includes NSAIDs, supportive therapy, nursing care, such as slinging if necessary, and adequate bedding and footing. The prognosis for full recovery is guarded, and a nurse mare may be needed for the foal.

Prepubic tendon rupture or ventral body wall hernias may occur during late gestation, apparently without reason. Ventral edema cranial to the udder is severe, unilaterally or bilaterally. An affected mare may have difficulty rising. It is difficult to obtain an accurate diagnosis until edema resolves after foaling. The body wall enlarges in the ventral flank. Diagnostic tests include palpation per rectum and ultrasonography. Occasionally, a tear in the ventral body wall can be palpated per rectum. Supportive treatment consists of NSAIDs, physical support of the enlarged area using large bandages, restricted exercise, close monitoring before and during foaling, a laxative diet, and assisted early induction of foaling. Successful surgical repair of ruptured prepubic tendons and large ventral body wall hernias is often unrewarding, but smaller defects can be repaired successfully. The prognosis for mares with large tears of a ruptured prepubic tendon and future use as broodmares is guarded to poor.[29] Embryo transfer may be a reasonable alternative in breeds that allow this form of management (the Editors).

Neurological Disease

The most common neurological disease of adult broodmares in the United States is EPM. Cervical vertebral malformation also occurs and should be distinguished because treatment is different. Treatment for EPM is as for a stallion, but folate supplementation is not recommended in broodmares receiving pyrimethamine because of the potential alteration in organogenesis.[30]

Old Injuries

Many broodmares have old superficial digital flexor tendon or suspensory ligament injuries that may deteriorate, or mares may sustain acute reinjury. Aged broodmares may have gradual thickening and lengthening of the hindlimb suspensory ligaments. Broodmares with acute reinjuries are treated by restricted exercise, analgesia if needed, local therapy, and ultrasonographic monitoring. Stall confinement with daily handwalking may be needed for 3 to 4 months, depending on ultrasonographic evidence of healing. Treatment of mares with hindlimb suspensory desmitis with a dropped fetlock consists of strict stall confinement, pain medication if needed, and application of an extended heel, egg bar shoe. This shoe should be removed just before foaling for safety.

Occasionally, older broodmares develop extensive new bone, especially around the carpus, causing lameness. The mare should be separated from the normal herd to reduce competition for food and water, with restricted exercise and analgesia provided.

General Husbandry and Breeding Management Considerations

Simple management and handling may improve the comfort of an acutely lame broodmare and prolong the useful life of a chronically unsound broodmare. Attention to social groupings can reduce the chance of new injury and provide greater comfort for an older or lame broodmare. Many farms separate broodmares into compatible groups, including maidens, seasoned broodmares, barren mares, and older broodmares. The goals should be to limit competition for food and water and to minimize risk of encountering manufactured obstacles during aggressive interactions. Some farms follow a buddy system, in which compatible pairs are kept together as much as possible. Convalescent broodmares often do well grouped together for rehabilitation or special medical attention. Good footing, including breeding areas, pastures, alleyways, areas around hay bunks, loading ramps, and in stalls, can prevent injury and provide comfort for a lame broodmare. Broodmares benefit from as much exercise as possible to maintain overall good musculoskeletal fitness, and obesity should be avoided.

Phenylbutazone is the most commonly used drug for the effective pain management and has limited or no effect on organogenesis. Its use may be associated with gastric ulceration and concurrent treatment with omeprazole (4 mg/kg curative or 2 mg/kg preventative) may be of value, although any effects on organogenesis have not been reported.

Emergency surgery to repair a fracture may be necessary to save the life of the mare and fetus. Ideally a preformed plan should be in place, especially close to gestation. Is the decision to save the mare and the foal or to consider a nonsurvival cesarean section to deliver the foal? If the decision is made to proceed to save the mare and fetus, administration of synthetic progesterone (30 mg/kg PO twice daily) may be helpful, especially in the first trimester of pregnancy. Elective surgery should be delayed until the mare has foaled whenever possible.

For lame or otherwise disabled mares, artificial insemination should be considered whenever possible. For natural cover, we recommend excellent footing, a gentle approach, reduced restraint, and acute pain control. To reduce the stress in broodmares with pain, maiden mares, or broodmares with a known volatile live cover breeding history, the use of 25 mg of acepromazine and 10 to 25 mg of butorphanol given together intravenously 15 to 20 minutes before breeding may increase safety without the ataxia or sudden outbursts seen with xylazine administered alone. When possible, medication, including nutritional supplements, should be avoided during gestation and early lactation, including detomidine and xylazine used alone.

Chapter 128

Lameness in Foals

Robert J. Hunt

Like all horses, foals are prone to injury and lameness; however, considering the immature and fragile musculoskeletal system, the incidence of serious injury is surprisingly low. Exposure of a foal's naive immune system to the array of pathogens places the foal at high risk of infectious causes of lameness. Degree of lameness in foals ranges from subtle and nearly imperceptible to non–weight bearing. Although no published studies document the incidence of lameness in foals, the economic impact on the horse industry is substantial when factors such as cost of diagnosis and treatment, long-term morbidity and mortality, and the effect on athletic potential are considered. Economic and emotional losses may be substantial for horse owners and breeders, enough so that they may abandon the horse industry. Most lameness is self-limiting, however, and in many instances early recognition and prompt treatment makes a difference in costly medical bills and improves the long-term soundness or survival. It is imperative that veterinarians learn to recognize the early clinical signs of these serious disorders and to initiate prompt treatment. Clients should be made aware of the potential danger of a wait-and-see approach and a delay in treatment.

EVALUATION OF A LAME FOAL

Foals often resist handling and limb manipulation, making assessing responses difficult and potentially confusing. It is imperative that the veterinarian is patient when evaluating foals. The basics of lameness localization are the same as in adult horses. The stance and any obvious swelling or sensitive areas on palpation should be noted. It is important to palpate the contralateral limb to gauge the foal's response to manipulation of that limb. Hoof and limb temperature (hot or cold) and digital pulse amplitude should be evaluated. Detailed assessment with hoof testers is invaluable in differentiating causes of hoof lameness. Any aberration in hoof development (e.g., club foot, deformed foot, unbalanced feet, or mismatched sizes of feet) should be noted. Postural or conformational changes, including sudden angular limb deviation, limb laxity, or contraction, may result from altered load bearing associated with lameness or from structural changes from injury. Careful palpation of all structures of the skeletal system, including all palpable surfaces of joints, bones, digital flexor tendons, and ligaments, with the foal in a standing position and with each limb flexed is important. Swelling should be differentiated as intraarticular, periarticular, or both.

Gait deficits in foals manifest like those in adult horses in that lameness is expressed as reduced time or weight on the lame limb.[1] The phase of the stride in which the gait is altered is the result of reducing loading of the limb during the painful portion of locomotion. Foals are more likely to show lameness in dramatic fashion by carrying a limb (i.e., not bearing weight) or exaggerating efforts to reduce load on the limb. It is important to observe the foal at a walk to discern subtle differences in stride and foot placement that may be missed at a trot.

Routine ancillary diagnostic tests used in foal lameness evaluation include diagnostic analgesia; radiographic, ultrasonographic, and nuclear scintigraphic examinations; and arthrocentesis and aspiration of other fluid pockets.[1-4] Diagnostic analgesia should be a routine component of lameness localization in foals just as in mature horses, unless a fracture is suspected. Any areas of suspect pathological bone conditions should be evaluated radiologically. Weekly follow-up radiological evaluation may be required to recognize bony changes. Soft tissue evaluation is aided by ultrasonography, especially when the veterinarian is looking for fluid pockets or alterations in soft tissue architecture. Nuclear scintigraphy has limited applications for skeletal evaluation in foals because normal radiopharmaceutical uptake in the physes can confuse or mask subtle abnormalities.

References on page 1348

NONINFECTIOUS CAUSES OF LAMENESS

Noninfectious causes of lameness include external and internal traumatic injuries and developmental or metabolic musculoskeletal diseases. Lameness also may result as a sequela to vascular disorders or may be immune-mediated secondary to an infectious problem.

Lameness resulting from external trauma varies with the area involved and the severity of the injury. Essentially any portion of the skeletal system is prone to injury. Traumatic injuries resulting in lameness are common but fortunately self-limiting in most instances. Boisterous activity, coupled with a hazardous environment, places a foal at an increased risk of sustaining injury compared with an adult horse. Trauma from other horses (a mare kicking a foal or collision injuries with other foals) is a common cause of lameness. Impact with stationary objects while a foal is being chased may result in serious injury. Internal trauma

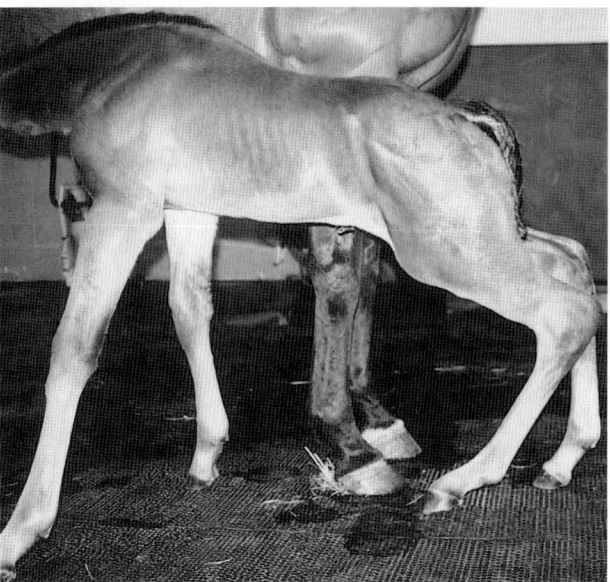

Fig. 128-1 • Typical crouched stance of a foal with rupture of the left gastrocnemius muscle subsequent to overextension while chasing a mare. The foal is unable to extend the limb or support full weight on it. Note the excessive flexion of the hock.

includes overexertion injuries, such as a foal running excessively with a mare or being chased, resulting in fracture of the proximal sesamoid bones (PSBs), or rupture of the suspensory apparatus or other soft tissue structures (Figure 128-1). Common fractures in foals include those involving the long bones, physes, PSBs, carpal and tarsal cuboidal bones, and the distal phalanx.[1,2,5,6]

Fractures of Long Bones

Clinical evaluation may be diagnostic in foals with lameness of traumatic origin. Unstable fractures or severe soft tissue injuries cause obvious, immediate clinical signs. If a fracture is suspected, radiographs are necessary to confirm the diagnosis and determine the severity of the injury (Figure 128-2).

Fractures of long bones most often result from external trauma such as a kick or having the limb pinned beneath an object while rolling. A limb misloaded while rearing may result in fracture of the tibia, femur, or pelvis. If a limb is unstable distal to the femur or humerus because of a fracture, the limb should be immobilized before transport. Surgical approaches and repair techniques for individual fracture types are described elsewhere.

Prognosis for a foal after fracture depends on anatomical location of the fracture; the complexity, orientation, and degree of soft tissue injury around the fracture; and whether the fracture is open. Secondary problems associated with prolonged lameness or confinement and immobilization often dictate the degree of long-term soundness. These problems include excessive laxity of the metacarpophalangeal or metatarsophalangeal joint, varus deviation, or deformity of the foot, such as an underslung or crushed heel and overgrowth of the toe. Mechanical laminitis is not as common as in adult horses, but it does occur. Contracture or excessive laxity of the fractured limb associated with disuse may prevent future soundness.

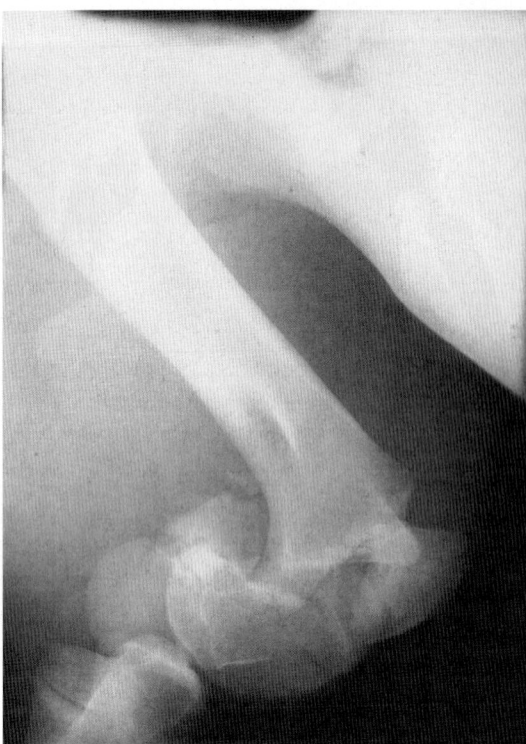

Fig. 128-2 • Slightly oblique lateromedial radiographic image of the femur of a foal. There is an unstable, displaced fracture of the distal aspect of the femur, the result of trauma. This is a Salter-Harris type II fracture.

Fractures of the radius, ulna, and tibia are generally more amenable to surgical repair than are femoral and humeral fractures. If economics do not allow surgery, conservative management of foals with femoral and humeral fractures by stall confinement is a feasible alternative to surgical intervention. Teaching the foal to support its weight on a straw bale or butt bar may alleviate load on the contralateral limb for hindlimb fractures. Complications encountered after surgical repair of femoral or humeral fractures, such as implant failure or infection, are usually fatal. Without postoperative complications, however, a foal has a greater chance of soundness for light athletic use with surgical management. Fractures of the radius and tibia require surgical stabilization if any displacement of the fracture is present. Most foals have a fair to good prognosis for light to medium athletic use or for breeding purposes. Foals with fractures of the ulna that have any displacement should undergo surgery, but those with nondisplaced fissure fractures do not require surgical fixation. Foals with nondisplaced fractures of the ulna should have stall confinement for a minimum of 8 to 10 weeks and undergo radiological monitoring every other day for the first 2 weeks and then weekly to ensure displacement does not occur. Foals with displaced, unstable fractures of the metacarpal and metatarsal bones generally have a guarded to poor prognosis for future athletic use, with or without surgery. Foals with simple, stable fractures of the metacarpal and metatarsal bones not requiring surgery have a good prognosis.

Fractures of the Pelvis

Pelvic fractures in foals are common and usually results from a foal misloading a hindlimb when rearing or from flipping over and landing on one side. Gait and degree of lameness depend on the portion of the pelvis involved and the amount of trauma to the surrounding tissue. Common sites of injury include the tuber coxae, tuber ischium, acetabulum, and the shaft of the ilium. Deep palpation of the area may elicit pain.

The characteristics of the lameness may reflect the site of injury. A foal with a fracture of a tuber ischium is reluctant to advance the ipsilateral hindlimb and has a shortened cranial phase and prolonged caudal phase of the stride. As with many pelvic injuries, the tail often is elevated and held to the opposite side, and the foal may carry the limb when running but bear full weight while walking. Conversely, foals with fractures of a tuber coxae have a shortened caudal phase of the stride, and the injured tuber coxae is often lower than the contralateral side.

Treatment for foals with pelvic fractures includes confinement for 8 to 12 weeks followed by a gradual return to controlled exercise. Improvement in the degree of lameness should be seen within 2 to 3 weeks, depending on the region of the pelvis injured. Foals with acetabular injuries may require a longer duration of confinement before improvement is seen. If the foal is fully weight bearing, controlled walking for short periods after 3 weeks can be started if the foal is tractable.

Prognosis for foals with pelvic fracture not involving the acetabulum is fair to good for light use but guarded for competitive athletics. Some horses are able to race following healing of pelvic fractures. Most foals with pelvic fractures involving the acetabulum have a poor prognosis for an athletic future; however, they generally survive to make breeding animals. In the Editors' experience, the prognosis for athletic function is not invariably poor because, in contrast to adult horses, foals have a remarkable capacity for bone remodeling, and even some severe articular fractures can heal satisfactorily, allowing normal athletic function.

Fractures of the Physes

Physeal fractures have been categorized and defined using the Salter-Harris classification scheme.[2-7] A type I fracture occurs through the physis and involves only the zone of hypertrophied chondrocytes; the adjacent epiphysis and the metaphysis are not involved. A type II fracture occurs across the physis and extends into a portion of the metaphysis. A type III fracture involves the physis and epiphysis and extends into the joint. A type IV fracture includes involvement of the physis, epiphysis, and metaphysis. A compression injury to the physis is referred to as a type V fracture. This classification scheme is applicable to pressure physes that contribute to the longitudinal growth of bone and are subject to compressive forces. Traction physes, such as the olecranon growth plate, are subject to tensile forces and are not included in this classification scheme.

Physeal fractures are common because physeal bone is weak compared with diaphyseal bone. Diagnosis of physeal injuries is made on clinical and radiological findings (Figure 128-3). Clinical signs include varying degree of lameness, pain on palpation of the injured area, swelling, and possibly instability of the limb or angular deviation of the limb

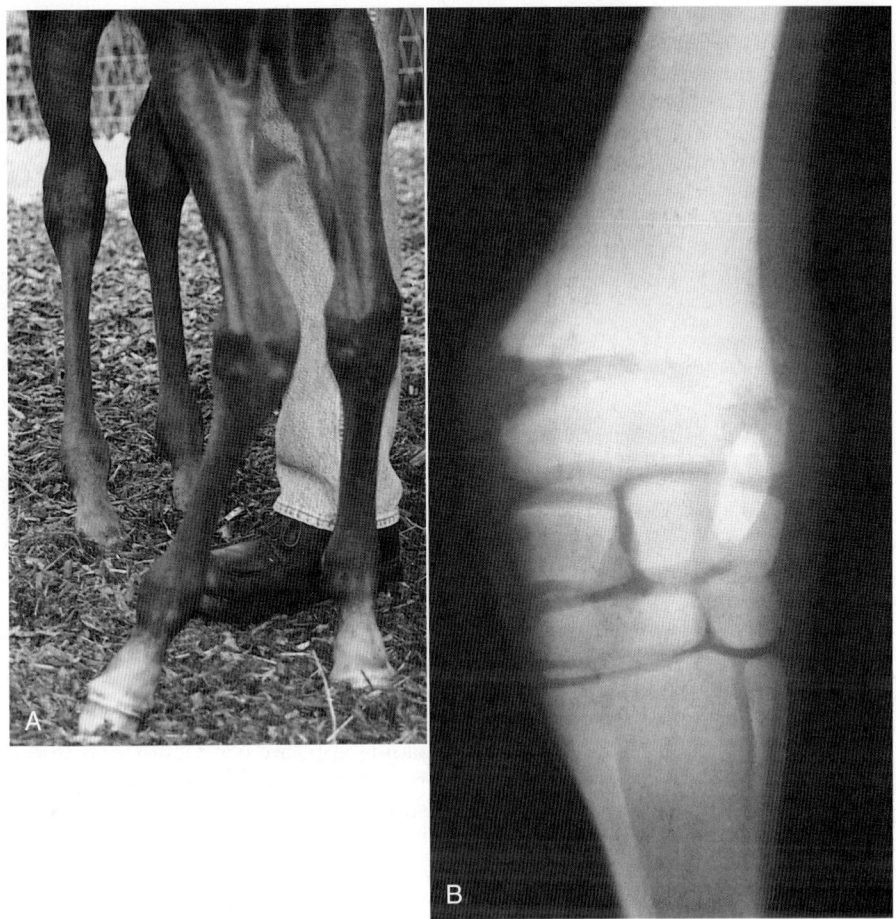

Fig. 128-3 • **A,** Marked carpus valgus deformity of the right forelimb as a result of a distal, radial physeal fracture. Note also the slight varus deformity of the left carpus. **B,** Dorsopalmar radiographic image of the right carpus. Lateral is to the right. There is a displaced Salter-Harris type III fracture of the distal radial physis. Note the widening of the physis medially, resulting in the valgus deformity.

distal to the fracture. The primary differential diagnosis for a stable physeal fracture is infectious physitis.

Surgical repair is necessary in foals with displaced, unstable physeal fractures. The major difficulty in surgical stabilization is the short section of epiphysis available for purchase. This shortcoming generally is overcome with the use of a form of T-plate, cross pins, transfixation pins, or tension-band wiring. If adequate reduction and stability are achieved, the prognosis for future soundness is good.

Cuboidal Bone Injury

Injury to the cuboidal bones of the tarsus or carpus often is associated with failure or delay of endochondral ossification in premature or dysmature neonates.[5,6] Crushing and malformation of the soft cartilaginous precursors of the cuboidal bones result in osteoarthritis and varying degrees of lameness (Figure 128-4). Outwardly the limb may appear normal or have an angular deviation, or, if a hindlimb is involved, it may be sickle hocked or curbed. Attempts at prevention of this condition are more effective than treatment after its onset, although these are limited in effectiveness. Prolonged stall confinement of premature neonates is recommended until radiological signs of ossification of the cuboidal bones occur. Ossification generally requires 4 to 8 weeks but may vary. Foals affected with crushing of

cuboidal bones rarely make competitive athletes, although most are suitable for light use, breeding, or as comfortable pasture animals. Those with milder forms of compression and modeling or tapering of the third and central tarsal bones may make competitive athletes.

Fractures of the Distal Phalanx

Nonarticular fractures of the palmar processes of the distal phalanx occur with high frequency in Thoroughbred foals (Figure 128-5). Other types of fractures of the distal phalanx occur but are less common. The forelimbs frequently are involved, and the lateral palmar process is more commonly fractured; bilateral and biaxial fractures occur occasionally. In the hindlimb, medial and lateral plantar process fractures occur evenly. Palmar/plantar process fractures may be detected radiologically as incidental findings and may not necessarily cause lameness.

Salient clinical findings associated with a fracture of a palmar/plantar process of the distal phalanx include acute onset of lameness, which may be intermittent in nature, and lameness that is almost always more noticeable on sharp turns. Foals consistently have pain when hoof testers are applied across the heel. Atypically a response may be noticed with pressure at the toe. When diffuse pain is noted during hoof tester evaluation, along with an

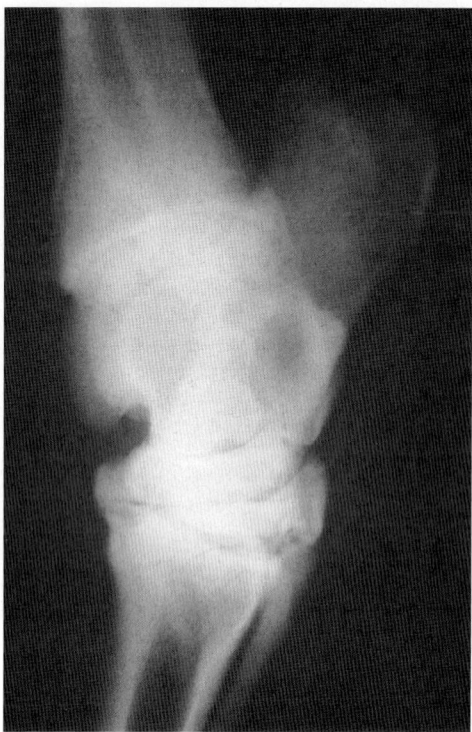

Fig. 128-4 • Slightly oblique lateromedial radiographic image of a hock of a mature horse with crushing of the third tarsal bone and secondary osteoarthritis of the centrodistal and tarsometatarsal joints, the result of incomplete ossification of the third tarsal bone as a neonate. Note the wedge shape of the third tarsal bone and the abnormal dorsal contour.

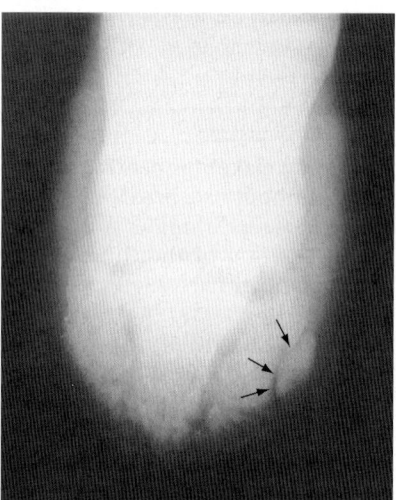

Fig. 128-5 • Dorsoproximal-palmarodistal oblique radiographic image of a foot of a foal. Lateral is to the right. There is a nonarticular fracture of the lateral palmar process of the distal phalanx (arrows).

increased temperature of the foot, subsolar abscessation should be considered.

Treatment includes confinement to a small area with soft, uniform footing for 4 to 6 weeks. Lameness should improve in the first week. External coaptation, such as a foot cast or glue-on shoe, is contraindicated and may potentiate development of club foot conformation. Follow-up

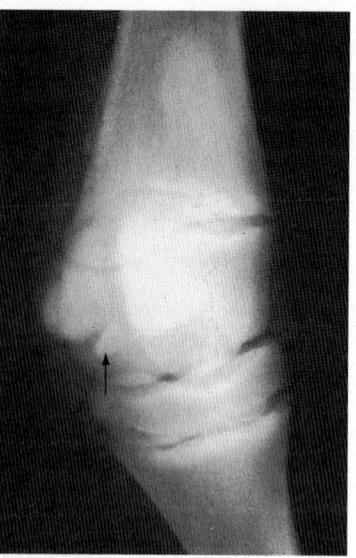

Fig. 128-6 • Dorsolateral-palmaromedial oblique radiographic image of a metacarpophalangeal joint of a foal. There is a wedge-shaped basilar fracture (arrow) of the lateral proximal sesamoid bone.

radiographs are not mandatory unless lameness persists or recurs. The prognosis is good. Differential diagnosis in foals suspect of fracture of the distal phalanx includes subsolar bruising, subsolar abscessation, infectious osteitis of the distal phalanx, and infectious arthritis of the distal interphalangeal (DIP) joint.

Fractures of the Proximal Sesamoid Bones

Fractures of the PSBs are common in young foals. Fractures usually are confined to one limb, but several limbs may be involved. Uniaxial (one) or biaxial (both PSBs) fractures in a single limb can be found. PSB fractures occur most commonly in foals between 2 weeks and 2 months of age. Fractures most often involve the base or apex of the PSB (Figure 128-6). Midbody PSB fractures occur less commonly. Hindlimb PSB fractures are less common, but they generally occur in conjunction with PSB fractures in a forelimb.

Lameness varies from moderate to severe and is exaggerated on turns. Often increased digital pulse amplitude is apparent, and palpation of the involved bone elicits a painful response. Depending on the fracture type and location, the fetlock joint capsule may be distended or regional swelling may occur over the fractured PSB. Diagnosis is confirmed radiologically.

Conservative management is recommended and involves confinement to a small area for 6 to 8 weeks. If swelling is noticed, a distal limb bandage should be applied. Surgical repair is not beneficial in foals because of the lack of substance of the PSBs. Prognosis depends on the type of fracture, number of PSBs involved, and the number of limbs involved. Most PSBs have an elongated appearance (megasesamoid) after fractures heal, but foals may be suitable for athletic use if healing is complete (Figure 128-7). The prognosis for athletic use is worse if both PSBs in one limb are affected, or if fractures occur in more than one limb, compared with a uniaxial fracture in a single limb.

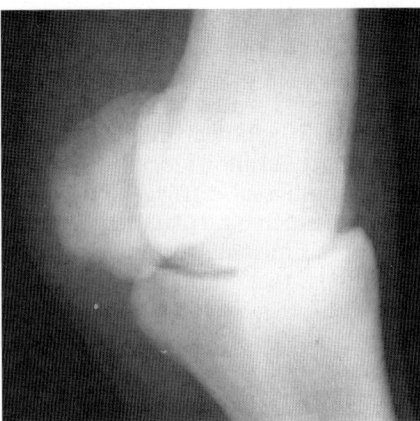

Fig. 128-7 • Dorsolateral-palmaromedial oblique radiographic image of the metacarpophalangeal joint seen in Figure 128-6, obtained when the horse was a yearling. The basilar fracture of the lateral proximal sesamoid bone has healed, resulting in an elongated, distorted appearance of the bone.

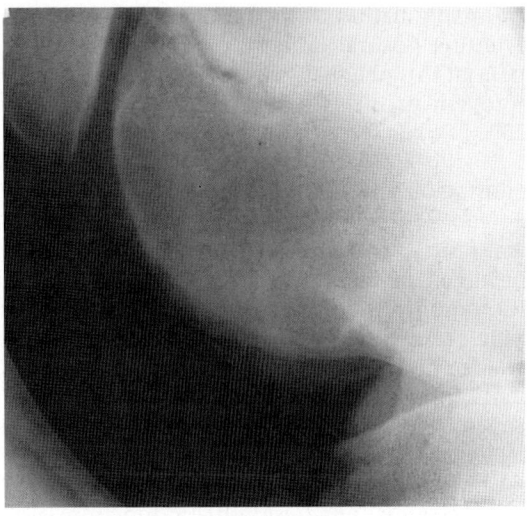

Fig. 128-8 • Lateromedial radiographic image of a stifle. There is irregularity in the outline of the cortex of the lateral trochlear ridge of the femur with subtle alteration of the subchondral bone opacity. This is the result of osteochondrosis. There are no displaced fragments; therefore surgery as a weanling is not required, although the foal should be monitored both clinically and radiologically.

Developmental Orthopedic Disease

Developmental orthopedic disease (DOD) is an uncommon cause of lameness in foals less than 2 to 4 months old.[3,8] However, DOD is a common skeletal disease in weanlings and yearlings and generally is considered self-limiting. DOD is complex and includes acquired flexural deformity, osteochondrosis, physeal dysplasia (physitis) and resulting angular limb deformity, and cervical vertebral malformation. The pathogenesis, clinical manifestations, and management are discussed in Chapters 54, 57, 59, and 60.

Diagnosis of osteochondrosis is based on clinical evaluation and radiological findings.[3,8] Clinical findings include synovial distention and varying degrees of lameness in the acute stage. Most young foals (<2 months old) afflicted with osteochondrosis have several joints or bones involved. These foals are subsequently lamer than older foals and usually have severe osteochondrosis. The cause often is not found because individual foals usually are involved, although heredity likely plays a primary role. Radiological findings may initially include osteochondral fragmentation or erosive changes in subchondral bone, or may be normal. Therefore it is important to plan on serial radiological studies to monitor the progression of changes.

Conservative management for young foals with osteochondrosis almost always is recommended and includes rest, antiinflammatory drugs, systemic chondroprotective drugs, and occasionally joint lavage and injection with hyaluronan. If a free fragment is evident, surgical retrieval may be beneficial; however, one should keep in mind that surgery for osteochondrosis is an elective procedure that should be performed at a time optimal for the foal. If a nondisplaced fragment occurs in a weanling or younger age foal, surgery may be delayed until the yearling period and monitored radiologically (Figure 128-8). Time will allow maturation of the underlying bone so minimal debridement and curettage will be necessary. In many instances the extra time allows these fragments to remineralize, and surgical removal is not necessary. In a longitudinal study of 43 Dutch Warmblood foals, osteochondrosis lesions were found at the cranial aspect of the intermediate ridge of the tibia in 68% at 1 month of age, but at 11 months of age abnormalities were detected in only 18%.[9]

Lesions in the lateral trochlear ridge of the femur developed later, with an incidence of 20% at 5 months of age, but by 11 months of age abnormalities were detected in only 3%.

Vascular Thrombosis

Vascular thrombosis is an unusual cause of lameness in foals. Usually a central focus provides emboli, the most common being a vegetative lesion on a heart valve. Clinical signs include a variable degree of lameness involving one or more limbs. The limb may feel cold during periods of lameness but normal at other times. Response to diagnostic analgesia is inconsistent. Ultrasonographic examination of the heart usually reveals a lesion on a heart valve. Although any valve may be involved, most commonly the aortic or mitral valves are affected. Bacterial blood cultures should be obtained, especially during febrile episodes, if present.

Treatment consists of long-term antimicrobial drugs, based on bacterial cultures if available, and optionally rheological agents such as pentoxifylline. Follow-up ultrasonographic examination is important to determine the effectiveness and duration of treatment. The prognosis is guarded and depends on the degree of ischemia in the distal extremity.

Traumatic Nerve Injury

Collision injuries involving the proximal aspect of the forelimb of foals may result in injury to the radial nerve or components of the brachial plexus. Most commonly a foal has a dropped elbow, is unable to advance the limb, and drags the limb during ambulation. Differential diagnosis includes fracture of the humerus, the scapula, or a cranially located rib, and radiological evaluation should be performed to differentiate these conditions. The condition may be transient, lasting only a few hours if attributable to neuropraxia, or may be permanent.

Treatment for nerve injury consists of antiinflammatory drugs, including corticosteroids and nonsteroidal drugs, and dimethyl sulfoxide. Supportive care, such as physical manipulation of the limb and splinting, may aid in preventing flexural limb deformity. Acupuncture may be beneficial in some foals with nerve injury. In general, if no improvement is seen within 3 to 5 days of treatment, only 25% of foals recover.

Miscellaneous Soft Tissue Injury

Muscle tears are common in young Thoroughbreds. Longitudinal rents, 3 to 5 cm in length, in the biceps femoris, superficial gluteal muscles, or vastus lateralis are most often seen. Commonly there is a fluctuant fluid pocket in the tear, which resolves over several weeks as the edges of the tear undergo fibrosis. Lameness is usually mild to moderate and transient in nature, lasting for several days. Less common soft tissue injuries include traumatic rupture of the suspensory apparatus or rupture of the gastrocnemius muscle, and foals with these injuries have generally had a poor prognosis for long-term athletic function. However, in a recent report 23 (82%) of 28 foals with rupture of the gastrocnemius muscle survived to discharge from the hospital, and 13 (81%) of 16 horses that reached 2 years of age trained or raced.[10]

INFECTIOUS CAUSES OF LAMENESS

Determining the location and cause of lameness in foals attributable to infection is crucial in deciding a course of therapy and assessing prognosis. As a general rule, assuming that all foal lameness is infectious in origin until proved otherwise is safest. In this instance, prompt appropriate treatment uniformly results in a more favorable outcome than if treatment is delayed.[11]

The clinical complex of infectious arthritis, tenosynovitis, infectious osteitis, or osteomyelitis occurs in foals commonly,[11-16] especially in foals less than 4 months of age but occasionally in older foals. The different forms of infection can be discussed together because the pathogenesis is common. Bacteria may gain entry through the umbilicus, respiratory tract, or gastrointestinal tract, although direct penetration of a synovial structure from external trauma may result in synovial infection. Hematogenous dissemination of bacteria allows localization into metaphyseal, physeal, or epiphyseal cartilage and is believed to be associated with the rich vascular network composed of metaphyseal loops, sinusoidal veins, and epiphyseal and transphyseal vessels that supply the end of the long bones and synovium (Figure 128-9).[2,13] The sluggish blood flow and vascular stasis of nutrient vessels approaching a cartilage interface allows bacteria to proliferate and colonize. Bacterial colonization incites an acute inflammatory response associated with kinin, complement, and coagulation system activation, eventually leading to cartilage destruction. Vasoactive amines and prostaglandins acting as chemotactic agents result in rapid accumulation of inflammatory cells. Inflammatory products released from synoviocytes, fibroblasts, chondrocytes, neutrophils, and monocytes result in the degradation of articular cartilage proteoglycan, collagen, and hyaluronan. Mediators involved include collagenases, elastases, lysosomal enzymes, plasmin, prostaglandins, metalloproteinases, monokines, and free radicals. Extrinsic mediators include interleukins, bacterial lipopolysaccharides, and physical forces placed on the damaged cartilage, all of which further compound collagen degradation. Further compromise of cartilage occurs because of poor nutrition of the chondrocytes, caused primarily by fibrin clot formation over the articular surface, and by thrombosis in the synovial vasculature. The primary mediators of infectious arthritis and eventual cartilage destruction are toxic metabolites released from chondrocytes. Cartilage matrix degradation and proteoglycan loss may occur within 2 days and collagen loss by 9 days after bacterial inoculation.[2,17,18]

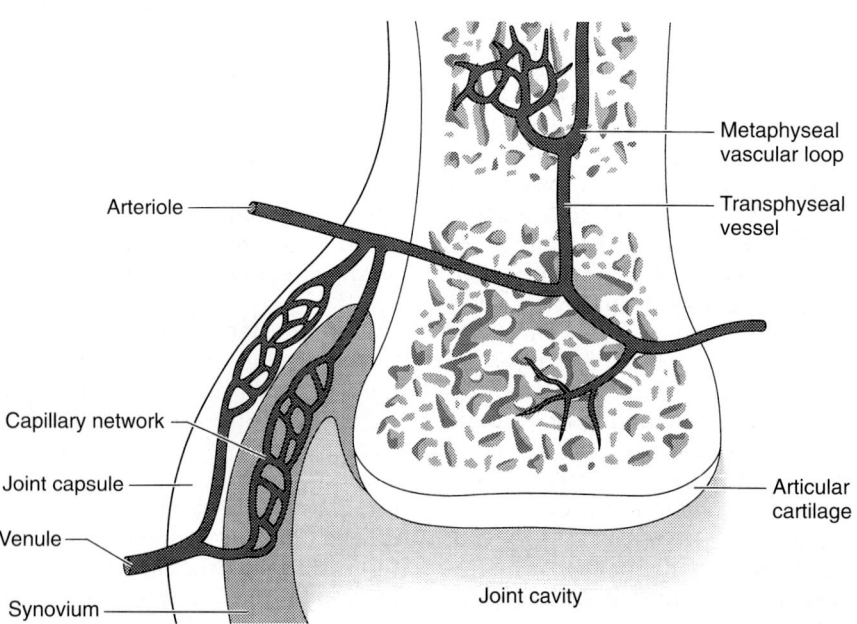

Fig. 128-9 • Vascular supply to long bone and articular soft tissue. Blood-borne bacteria may colonize at the metaphyseal vascular loop and disseminate to the physis, epiphysis, or synovial membrane. (Modified from Kobluk CN, Ames TR, Geor RJ, editors: *The horse: diseases & clinical management*, Philadelphia, 1995, Saunders.)

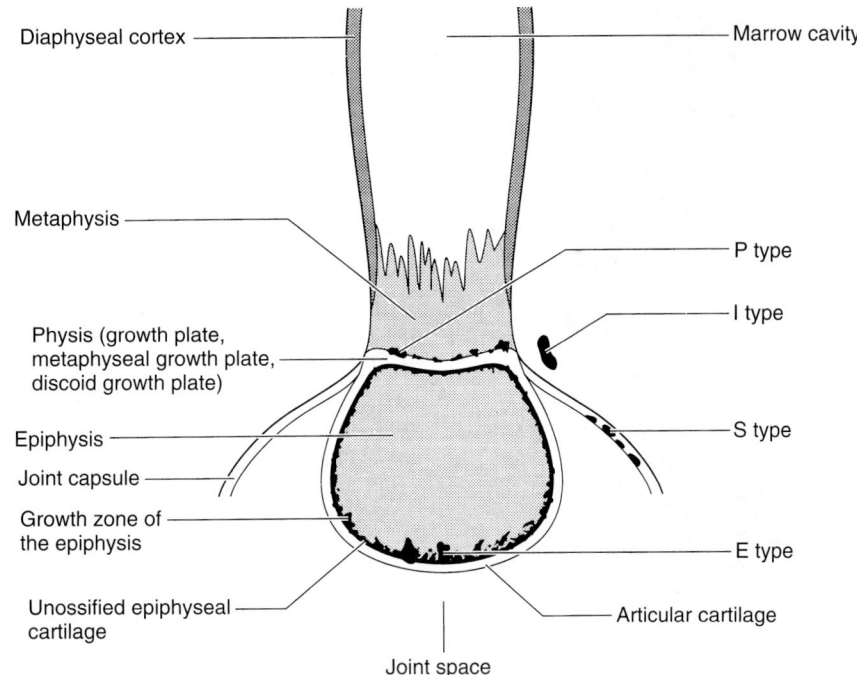

Diaphyseal cortex — Marrow cavity

Metaphysis —

— P type

— I type

Physis (growth plate, metaphyseal growth plate, discoid growth plate) —

Epiphysis —

— S type

Joint capsule —

Growth zone of the epiphysis —

— E type

Unossified epiphyseal cartilage —

— Articular cartilage

Joint space

Fig. 128-10 • Morphology of the long bone and types of S, E, P, and I infections. *P type*, Physeal-type infectious arthritis; *I type*, bacterial invasion into a physis or joint from a periarticular abscess; *S type*, infectious synovitis; *E type*, epiphyseal-type infectious arthritis. (Modified from Kobluk CN, Ames TR, Geor RJ, editors: *The horse: diseases & clinical management*, Philadelphia, 1995, Saunders.)

No explanation is apparent for disease localization in the epiphysis, metaphysis, physis, or joint. However, certain joints do appear to be affected more frequently than others. For example, the stifle, hock, metacarpophalangeal, and metatarsophalangeal joints are involved more often than the carpus or pastern. Infectious arthritis and osteomyelitis of hematogenous origin have been classified into five types based on location of the structure involved (Figure 128-10).[13,19]

Infectious synovitis (S type) affects foals usually within the first 10 days of life. Several joints are usually involved, and few, if any, radiological changes are seen. Predominant clinical signs include periarticular soft tissue swelling, effusion, and lameness. Arthrocentesis reveals an elevation in nucleated cell count (usually >50,000/mcL), and degenerate neutrophils predominate.

Epiphyseal-type (E type) infectious arthritis involves the joint and adjacent epiphysis. Foals are generally several weeks of age or older. One or more joints may be infected, and other systemic illnesses may occur concomitantly. Radiological evidence of epiphyseal involvement commonly is seen.

Physeal type (P type) may occur in foals from 1 week to 4 months of age. Degree of soft tissue swelling and lameness may vary, and generally only one site is involved. Sympathetic effusion eventually may occur in a nearby joint (articular structure in close proximity). Lesions may be seen radiologically in the metaphysis, physis, or epiphysis (Figure 128-11). Pathological fracture may result because of weakening of the involved structure.

Small tarsal or carpal cuboidal bone (T type) osteomyelitis may result in collapse of the central or third tarsal bones (Figure 128-12). Several joints commonly are affected.

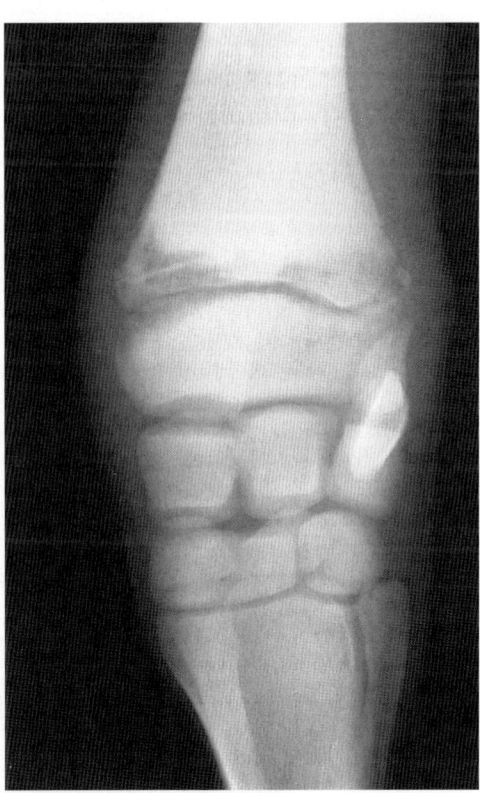

Fig. 128-11 • Dorsopalmar radiographic image of a carpus of a foal with P-type osteomyelitis of the distal radial physis. Lateral is to the right. Note the soft tissue swelling and the extensive radiolucent areas in the physis, metaphysis, and epiphysis. Infection has caused fragmentation of the lateral aspect of the metaphysis.

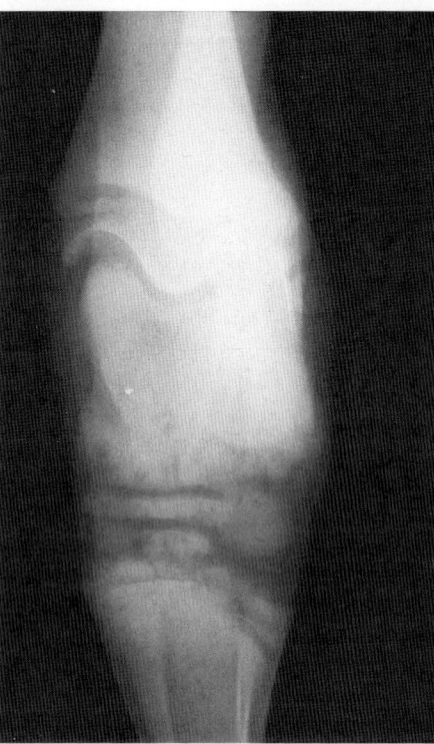

Fig. 128-12 • Dorsoplantar radiographic image of a hock of a young foal with type T osteomyelitis involving the cuboidal bones of the tarsus. Lateral is to the right. Note the mottled opacity of the central and third tarsal bones and the proximolateral aspect of the third and fourth metatarsal bones. These extensive lesions warrant a grave prognosis.

Invasion into a physis or joint from a periarticular soft tissue abscess is called I-type infection. Most commonly joints of the upper part of the limb, such as the hip or stifle, are involved. If soft tissue abscessation is detected early, infectious arthritis often can be avoided.

Most commonly foals with osteomyelitis have acute-onset lameness, diffuse regional swelling, heat, and detectable pain of the involved area. Fever is generally present before and at the onset of lameness but may go undetected. Degree of lameness depends on what bone is involved, the time frame, and stage of detection. Owners often erroneously assume lameness results from trauma because signs occur acutely. A common assumption is that the mare stepped on the foal (the Editors).

Diagnosis of complex infection is based on physical examination findings and the results of arthrocentesis (if intrasynovial involvement occurs) and radiographic examination.[2,11,13,15,16] Foals with infectious osteitis or early osteomyelitis may have no or subtle radiological changes, but within 1 to 2 weeks radiological changes consist of erosive, radiolucent changes surrounded by increased radiopacity and eventual proliferation of new bone. Therefore it is important to perform follow-up radiology to monitor the progression of the disease.

Other imaging modalities are of limited value. Sensitivity of nuclear scintigraphy alone is questionable in young foals because of the high metabolic activity of developing bone.[10] Labeled white cell imaging using nuclear medicine techniques is useful but adds expense and radiation exposure and has not gained widespread acceptance in private practice.

Ultrasonographic examination is most helpful in identifying soft tissue injury or inflammatory processes in the upper limb. Abscessation of the soft tissue adjacent to the infected bone is a common finding in foals with physeal infection. Using ultrasonographic guidance, abscesses can be aspirated for culture and antimicrobial susceptibility testing and opened, drained, and lavaged.

Arthrocentesis is the key in diagnosing infectious arthritis, but a negative culture does not rule out infection.[4,11-15,20] Joint fluid should be obtained in ethylenediaminetetraacetic acid tubes to evaluate the differential and total nucleated white blood cell count and protein concentration and for cytological evaluation. Anaerobic and aerobic culture and antimicrobial susceptibility tests should be performed. Using an antimicrobial-removal device may be of benefit to potentiate a positive culture if the foal is receiving antimicrobial drugs. Blood cultures should be collected.

In foals and horses suspected of having infectious arthritis, synovial fluid cultures are positive 64% of the time.[12,14,17,18,20] In my practice, of 158 synovial samples submitted in 1 year, there were only 64 (40%) positive isolates. Reasons for low positive culture results include previous administration of antimicrobial agents, partial success of the immune system, the intrinsic bacteriocidal properties of infected synovial fluid, poor storage, or no bacteria present in the synovial fluid.

If there is radiological evidence of osteomyelitis well away from a joint, a sample of bone and debris may be obtained using a Michelle trephine. An alternative technique is to use a 2.5- or 3.2-mm drill bit and collect the shavings for culture and antimicrobial susceptibility testing.[11] This tract then may be used for intraosseous infusion of an antimicrobial agent.

The results of hematological testing can be confusing. Complete blood count and fibrinogen level should be assessed, but results are often within normal limits initially because infection is localized. Serial hemograms should be performed in this instance. Any elevation in the white blood cell count or fibrinogen level in a lame foal with fever should be assumed to reflect bone or joint infection until proved otherwise. A normal hemogram does not rule out infectious arthritis or osteomyelitis. Foals less than 1 month of age should have immunoglobulin G levels checked to evaluate for failure of passive transfer.

Treatment of foals with infectious arthritis consists of joint lavage with sterile polyionic fluids through large-bore needles or by using an arthroscope. If a large amount of fibrin and cellular debris is in the synovial fluid, arthrotomy and lavage with or without primary closure of the joint may be indicated. Joint lavage may be repeated every 1 to 3 days depending on the clinical response. A long-term closed suction drainage system may be used as well.[11] Broad-spectrum systemic antimicrobial drugs should be started immediately and adjusted accordingly based on the clinical progression and culture and antimicrobial susceptibility testing.

Other treatments for joint and bone infection include local intraosseous injection or regional hyperperfusion with antimicrobial agents. To perform intraosseous injection, an 18- or 20-gauge needle is inserted into the physis or adjacent bone. An aminoglycoside such as amikacin (250 to 500 mg) may be used. Alternatively, a cannulated

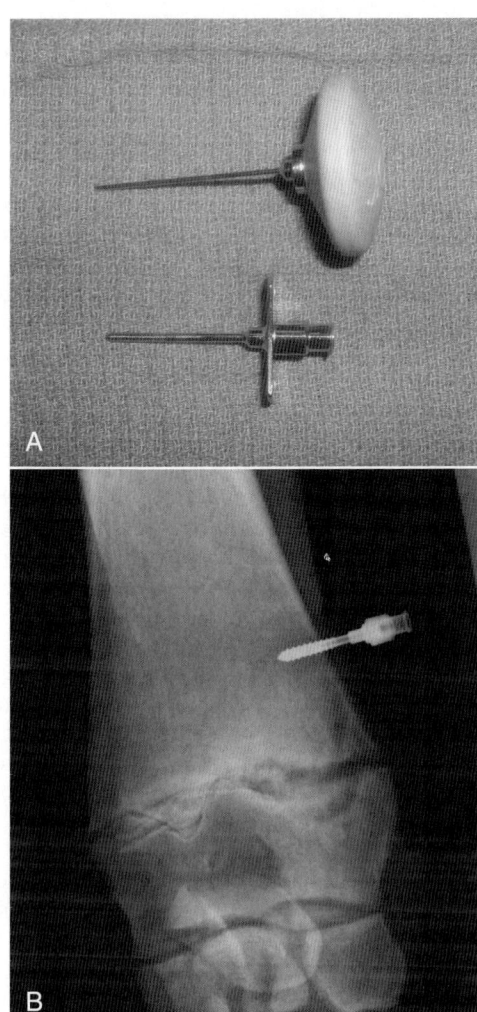

Fig. 128-13 • A, Sussmane-Raszynski intraosseous infusion needle (Cook Incorporated, Bloomington, Indiana, United States). **B,** Dorsopalmar radiographic image showing an intraosseous infusion needle inserted in the distal radius of a weanling to manage P-type osteomyelitis of the distal medial radial physis.

intraosseous infusion needle (Sussmane-Raszynski intraosseous infusion needle, Cook Incorporated, Bloomington, Indiana, United States) may be inserted and maintained for repeat use (Figure 128-13). To perform regional hyperperfusion, a site over the lateral digital neurovascular bundle is prepared aseptically, and a rubber Esmarch tourniquet is placed in the proximal metacarpal region. A 23-gauge butterfly catheter is inserted in the digital vein. An antimicrobial solution (500 mg of amikacin diluted in 10 mL of sterile water) is infused into the digital vein. The tourniquet is removed after 15 minutes, and a lower-limb bandage is applied. The procedure may be repeated as necessary. Regional digital hyperperfusion is especially useful in treating foals with infectious osteitis of the distal phalanx and infectious arthritis or osteomyelitis of the distal aspect of a limb. I have not encountered complications, such as distal limb ischemia, from tourniquet application.

Foals with infectious arthritis should be allowed to rest for a minimum of 3 to 4 weeks to prevent further traumatic cartilage damage.[2] Systemic administration of chondroprotective agents or intraarticular administration of hyaluronan may be of benefit.

Severe erosive lesions of the physis and metaphysis may result in pathological fracture and collapse of the bony column, resulting in an unstable fracture or severe angular deviation. Surgery may be indicated, but prognosis is poor for soundness if this occurs.

The prognosis for foals with infectious arthritis and osteomyelitis depends on the antimicrobial susceptibility of the organism and how early effective treatment is instituted.[12-20] In general, foals treated early for articular infections have a good prognosis for full recovery. Foals with articular infection with subchondral bone involvement have a poor prognosis, and the clinical course of disease and treatment are prolonged. Foals with focal bony lesions, involving only the physis without bone instability, have a good prognosis. Those with a pathological fracture or severe angular limb deformities have a poor prognosis and may be candidates for humane destruction.

Immune-Mediated Synovitis

Immune-mediated synovitis is a sequela to a primary inflammatory focus such as pneumonia, umbilical remnant infection, or a peripheral abscess.[11,21] *Rhodococcus equi* pneumonia is the most common primary focus of infection. The syndrome results from the deposition of immune complexes in the synovial lining and complement activation, resulting in synovitis. The condition usually involves more than one synovial structure. Foals usually have a stiff gait resulting from the synovial distention, and severe lameness is unusual.

The primary rule out for immune-mediated synovitis is early infectious polyarthritis, causing only moderate lameness and mild synovial fluid distention. Cytological evaluation of joint fluid in foals with immune-mediated synovitis commonly reveals nucleated cell counts of less than 20,000 nucleated cells/mcL. The cells are well-preserved neutrophils and large mononuclear cells. Foals with infectious arthritis generally have nucleated cell counts greater than 50,000 nucleated cells/mcL, and neutrophils are degenerate.

Therapy for foals with immune-mediated synovitis is based on identifying and resolving the underlying disease. Synovitis is self-limiting once the offending cause is removed. Systemic chondroprotective agents may be of benefit to the health of the joint because prolonged inflammation may cause cartilage damage.

Infection of the Digit

Infection of the digit is a frequent cause of severe lameness in foals. Infection may be contained to the subsolar or hoof wall regions, or it may involve the distal phalanx or the DIP joint. It is critical to differentiate between these sites as soon as possible. Infection at all sites causes increased intensity of the digital pulse amplitudes and, at some stage, increased temperature of the hoof capsule. With subsolar or wall abscessation, pressure applied with hoof testers usually produces a painful response along the toe and sole, unless overlying horn is separated from the sensitive tissue caused by accumulation of purulent material. Radiology in these foals reveals gas accumulation in the involved area. If the distal phalanx is infected, radiolucency or sequestration may be evident. Diffuse swelling at the coronary band usually means involvement of the DIP joint, and arthrocentesis should be performed in an area remote from the swelling.

Subsolar abscesses should be drained early to prevent involvement of deeper tissues. To facilitate drainage, the foot can be soaked in hot water and bandaged with an Animalintex pack (3M Animal Care Products, St. Paul, Minnesota, United States). Both procedures soften the horn. Surgical curettage of the distal phalanx and lavage of the infected bone should be performed in foals with sequestration. A sterile, antiseptic bandage should be maintained after surgery for a minimum of 3 to 4 weeks or until a healthy keratin covering has grown over the exposed bone. Ancillary treatment includes regional digital hyperinfusion using a dilute antimicrobial solution. A good prognosis is warranted in foals with infection of the distal phalanx if the disease is detected and treated early. If more than 25% of the distal phalanx is involved, prognosis for future soundness worsens. Recurrence of infection after initial curettage requires additional surgery. Because of the limited surface area and porous nature of the distal phalanx in the foal, recurrence worsens the prognosis considerably.

Chapter 129

Pleasure Riding Horse

Herbert J. Burns

Pleasure riding horses are a vital part of the equine industry, and many owners devote great amounts of time, money, and emotion to them. Although pleasure riding horses are of far less monetary value than competition horses, the overall importance to the owner should never be underestimated.

Pleasure riding horses often tend to be used seasonally and somewhat episodically. Uses include trail riding, hunting, gymkhana-type activities, showing, lesson horses (teaching horses), the pasture pet, and eating grass. Pleasure riding horses can be divided loosely into two categories: former professionals and others. The *former professionals* are horses that formerly were used for a specific athletic use, such as racing, but are no longer able to perform in the sport and have been demoted. The *others* include potential athletes that were unable to be used for the intended purpose because of lack of ability, poor conformation, or temperament, as well as horses and ponies that were bred casually as pets. The common causes of lameness in these two groups differ to some extent.

It is vital to be able to relate to the owners of pleasure riding horses, who often are inexperienced with horses, have little veterinary knowledge, but have tremendous emotional involvement with the horse and are often anxious. It is critical to first establish communication with the owner and try to relieve any anxieties. The veterinarian should explain the intended examination and treatment in straightforward, nontechnical language. Facilities for examination may be far from ideal and may complicate the examination. The veterinarian should not overinterpret a short striding gait shown by a horse trotting on an uneven paddock or a rocky driveway. The clinician should start from the basics and evaluate left-right symmetry, with the horse standing on a flat, level surface, if available, and then assess the horse moving in straight lines and circles. The veterinarian should be aware that the horse may have been living with a low-grade lameness, unrecognized by the owner, for a considerable time. If the owner is concerned about severe left forelimb lameness, the veterinarian would be prudent to avoid mentioning low-grade left hindlimb lameness observed concurrently because the lameness is probably not of material relevance and will only further worry the owner.

Interpretation of findings is in part dictated by the age and previous occupation of the horse. Many former professional horses have previous soft tissue injuries or show lameness after flexion of a variety of joints, and it is important to try to establish which is the current active disease process causing lameness. Many clinical observations reflect previous injuries and are unrelated to the current lameness.

Local analgesic techniques are useful in some situations, but the temperament of the horse, difficulties in adequate restraint, or examination facilities available may mitigate against them. Owners of pleasure riding horses may resist techniques that are invasive or potentially painful to the horse, whereas they may be fully prepared to pay large sums for advanced diagnostic techniques. The clinician should bear in mind that a twitch in the inexperienced hands of an owner may be dangerous and should consider using tranquilization (e.g., 20 mg of acepromazine) in the horse to facilitate local analgesic techniques.

In some situations an owner prefers a step-by-step diagnosis reached by assessing the response to treatment, even without a definitive diagnosis. This can provide the slow acquisition of useful information. For example, assessment of the response to nonsteroidal antiinflammatory drug treatment can be helpful. Lameness associated with a subsolar abscess is likely to deteriorate, whereas lameness from navicular disease or osteoarthritis (OA) of the proximal interphalangeal joint is likely to improve.

In former professional horses, OA and previous tendon and ligament injuries are common. Minor trauma to a joint in a horse with preexisting OA may result in severe, persistent lameness, whereas similar trauma to a normal joint probably would not result in chronic lameness. Commonly injured joints include the carpus, fetlock, hock, and stifle. Superficial digital flexor tendonitis, suspensory desmitis, and distal sesamoidean ligament injuries are common chronic injuries in former professional horses, but reinjury is comparatively unusual unless the horse is subjected to a sudden and substantial increase in exercise intensity; for example, a horse is ridden hard for 2 hours after 3 months of little or no exercise. Previous sites of chronic inflammation may become a long-term problem. For example, a horse may lose a shoe and then gallop about on hard ground, resulting in solar bruising. However, lameness may persist, and radiographs may reveal osteitis of the palmar processes of the distal phalanx. A horse with toed-out conformation may traumatize the medial proximal sesamoid bone, resulting in acute lameness, but radiology may only reveal preexisting abnormalities.

Many causes of lameness in pleasure riding horses relate to the lifestyle of pampered pets and the environment in which they are kept. Subsolar abscesses are common and often result in a severe lameness, creating panic for an owner, who assumes the horse must have sustained a fracture. Managing the owner is equally as important as treating the horse. Subsolar abscesses also may be sequelae to previous laminitis.

Creation of effective drainage is essential for successful management of subsolar abscesses. Without drainage, the use of systemic antimicrobial drugs is contraindicated in my experience because such drugs may prolong the course of the infection. In some pleasure riding horses with a hard hoof capsule, determining accurately the site of abscess may not be possible initially. I recommend intensive soaking with Epsom salts and warm water and poultice at night. Periodic survey radiographs can be useful. In horses with long-standing abscessation the appearance of a radiolucent defect associated with gas accumulation deep to the hoof capsule may allow direct drainage of the abscess through the hoof wall, rather than through the sole (Figure 129-1). Up to 30 days may pass before the abscess can be located accurately and drainage can be established. Once the abscess has opened or been opened, systemic antimicrobial drugs may be useful, especially if a large area of the foot is damaged.

Pleasure riding horses are at high risk for sustaining lacerations or puncture wounds, often resulting from impact with less than ideal fencing, such as barbed wire or a jagged post. Injuries vary from minor to severe, resulting in long-term lameness. Injuries may go unrecognized for several days because not all pleasure riding horses are inspected carefully and regularly. Many pleasure riding horses are kept in groups at pasture, and the introduction of a new horse can result in disruption of the hierarchy and the risk of horse-induced injury.

The veterinarian also should recognize that many pleasure riding horses have major conformational abnormalities that predispose them to the early development of OA. Many pleasure riding horses live to an old age, and age-related OA is not uncommon. Farrier care may be less than ideal and may predispose the horses to chronic foot pain and OA of the distal limb joints. Nail bind and excessive shortening of the toe are common farriery-related causes of lameness. It is important to establish the time of onset of lameness relative to when the horse was last shod. These problems are usually apparent within 48 hours. If a nail was driven inside the white line and immediately removed, this may predispose the horse to a subsolar abscess, which usually causes lameness within 7 to 10 days. If foot lameness develops more than 2 weeks after trimming and shoeing, the lameness is unlikely to be related to the farrier. Other primary foot problems include solar bruising, sheared heel, puncture injuries, and thrush. The relative incidence of these problems may be related to the ground conditions if the horse lives outside. Early, wet springs increase the incidence of thrush. Long, dry summers resulting in hard ground are associated with an increased incidence of bruising and sore feet.

Laminitis is a problem seen most commonly in two types of pleasure riding horses: obese ponies and older horses and ponies with a pituitary adenoma (pituitary pars intermedia dysfunction, equine Cushing's disease). Laminitis is often seasonal, occurring most in the spring and early summer and also in the autumn, if a flush of grass occurs late. Navicular disease is not uncommon, and an irregular exercise history may be a predisposing factor. Navicular disease is less common in horses that have never been shod.

Cellulitis can create an acute-onset, non–weight-bearing lameness associated with pyrexia and inappetence. In some horses minor skin abrasions can be identified through which infection was initiated, but in others the primary cause may not be identified.

The incidence of tendon and ligament injuries is low and may be related to the weather and environmental conditions or to the age of the horse. Excessively deep, muddy pastures and extremely icy conditions may predispose horses to tendonitis or desmitis. Age-related degenerative changes take place in some tendons and ligaments, and in older pleasure riding horses, even those receiving no ridden exercise, sudden onset of a severe, progressive tendonitis of the forelimb superficial digital flexor tendons may develop. Progressive stretching of the hindlimb suspensory apparatus, resulting in dropping of the fetlocks, also occurs in older horses.

Neurological problems such as radial nerve paralysis may result from trauma induced by a kick from another horse in the same field or from a collision with another horse or a static object such as a gate post. In older horses, neoplastic lesions may result in secondary lameness. For example, a large melanoma in the gluteal region of a horse I examined created pressure on the sciatic nerve and thus lameness.

Pleasure riding horses are often kept at pasture in a group, with access to field shelters of variable design. Long bone fractures, the result of a kick from a companion horse, are not uncommon, especially during the winter months. Splint bone fractures are also common.

Treatment of many of these conditions is no different than in other athletic sports horses; however, certain

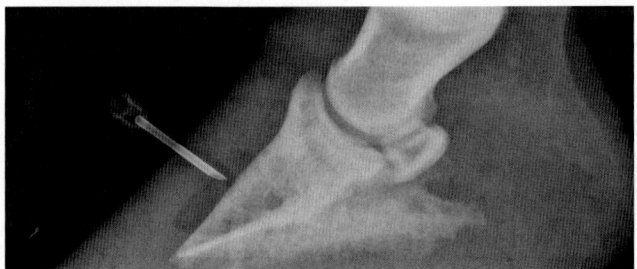

Fig. 129-1 • Lateromedial radiographic image of a foot in a pleasure riding horse with a long-standing subsolar abscess. Once a radiolucent defect is identified, a small hole can be drilled and the abscess cavity drained and medicated without opening the abscess from the sole. Lameness in this horse resolved soon after the abscess was drained.

constraints may apply that must be considered. No facilities may be available to restrict the horse's exercise or to keep it on its own. Even if surgery is contemplated, box stall rest—mandatory after most procedures—may not be possible because there may not be a stall. Some facilities are completely inadequate for performing clean procedures, such as intraarticular medication, in a safe manner. However, owners often are prepared to spend a disproportionate amount of their income on treating a condition in their much loved horse, despite a guarded prognosis; therefore it is important to describe all available treatment options. It is also critically important to explain carefully the treatment protocol, and writing it down can be useful to ensure owner compliance. The veterinarian can create a chart that the owner should complete as medication is administered.

In managing OA, the fact that a pleasure riding horse lives outside and is constantly exercising may be of benefit. I prefer to start with the least invasive therapy first and only use alternative methods if that does not work. Some oral nutraceutical agents may be of benefit, as may be intramuscular administration of polysulfated glycosaminoglycans.

Management of wounds can be difficult because client compliance is often poor. I treat pleasure horses with wounds in anticipation of a worst-case scenario, using nonsteroidal antiinflammatory drugs, broad-spectrum antimicrobial drugs, and confinement. Complete stall rest is often impossible, and restricted area turnout is a frequent compromise. If a penetrating injury possibly may have entered a joint or tendon sheath, I recommend referral for intensive therapy, stressing to the owner that this injury is potentially life threatening.

References

References can also be found on PubMed, linked to available original abstracts. http://www.ncbi.nlm.nih.gov/pubmed/

CHAPTER 1 Lameness Examination: Historical Perspective

1. Liautard A: *Lameness of horses*, New York, 1888, William R Jenkins Press.
2. Barnhart CL, ed: *The American college dictionary*, New York, 1970, Random House.
3. Ross MW, Dyson SJ. *Diagnosis and management of lameness in the horse*, Philadelphia, Saunders, 2003.
4. Adams OR: *Veterinary notes on lameness and shoeing of horses*, Denver, 1957, Colorado State University.
5. Dollar JAW: *A handbook of horseshoeing*, New York, 1898, William R Jenkins.
6. Lacroix JV: Lameness in the horse, *Am J Vet Med*, 1916.
7. Peters JE: Lameness incident to training and racing of the Thoroughbred, *J Am Vet Med Assoc* Feb:200, 1940.
8. Churchill EA: Surgical removal of fracture fragments of the proximal sesamoid bone, *J Am Vet Med Assoc* 128:581, 1956.
9. Wheat JD, Rhode EA: The surgical treatment of fractures of the proximal sesamoid bones in the horse, *J Am Vet Med Assoc* 132:378, 1958.
10. Forsell G: The operative treatment of traumatic inflammation of the navicular bursae with preservation of the deep flexor tendon, *North Am Vet* 11, 1930.
11. Lundvall RL: Fracture of the fibula in the horse, *J Am Vet Med Assoc* 129:16, 1956.
12. Delahanty DD: Defects—not fractures—of the fibulae in horses, *J Am Vet Med Assoc* 133:258, 1958.
13. Frank ER: *Veterinary surgery*, ed 7, Minneapolis, 1964, Burgess.
14. Percivall W: *Lameness in the horse*, London, 1852, Longmans, Brown, Green and Longmans.
15. Gamgee J: *A treatise on horse-shoeing and lameness*, London, 1871, Longmans, Green.
16. Bach FW: *How to judge a horse*, New York, 1893, William R Jenkins.
17. Dunlop RH, Williams DJ: *Veterinary medicine: an illustrated history*, St Louis, 1996, Mosby.
18. Stewart J: *The stable book—a treatise on the management of horses*, New York, 1858, AO Moore.

CHAPTER 2 Lameness in Horses: Basic Facts Before Starting

1. Liautard A: *Lameness of horses*, New York, 1888, William R Jenkins Press.
2. Barnhart CL, ed: *The American college dictionary*, New York, 1970, Random House.
3. *Dorland's medical dictionary*, Philadelphia, 1974, Saunders.
4. Adams OR: *Veterinary notes on lameness and shoeing of horses*, dissertation, Fort Collins, Colo, 1957, Colorado State University.
5. Ross MW, Nolan PM, Palmer JA, et al: The importance of the metatarsophalangeal joint in Standardbred lameness, *Proc Am Assoc Equine Pract* 37:155, 1992.

6. Ross MW, Nolan PM, Palmer JA, et al: The importance of the metatarsophalangeal joint in Standardbred lameness, *Vet Surg* 21:404, 1992.
7. Ross MW: Scintigraphic and clinical findings in the Standardbred metatarsophalangeal joint: 114 cases (1993-1995), *Equine Vet J* 30:131, 1998.
8. Kaneene JB, Ross WA, Miller R: The Michigan equine monitoring system. II. Frequencies and impact of selected health problems, *Prev Vet Med* 29:277, 1997.
9. United States Department of Agriculture: Equine '98 needs assessment survey results. USDA:APHIS:VS, CEAH, National Animal Health Monitoring System Pub No N236.597, Fort Collins, Colo, USDA, 1997.
10. Kane AJ, Traub-Dargatz J, Losinger WC, et al: The occurrence and causes of lameness and laminitis in the US horse population, *Proc Am Assoc Equine Pract* 46:277, 2000.
11. Ross WA, Kaneene JB, Gardiner JC: Survival analysis of risk factors associated with the occurrence of lameness in a Michigan horse population, *Am J Vet Res* 59:23, 1998.
12. Seeherman HJ, Morris E, O'Callaghan MW: Comprehensive clinical evaluation of performance. In Auer JA, ed: *Equine surgery*, Philadelphia, 1992, Saunders.
13. Morris E, Seeherman HJ: Clinical evaluation of poor racing performance in the racehorse: the results of 275 evaluations, *Equine Vet J* 23:169, 1991.
14. Kobluk CN, Robinson RA, Clayton CJ, et al: A comparison of the exercise level and problem rate of 95 Thoroughbred horses in a cohort study, *Proc Am Assoc Equine Pract* 36:47, 1990.
15. Jeffcott LB, Rossdale PD, Freestone J, et al: An assessment of wastage in Thoroughbred racing from conception to 4 years of age, *Equine Vet J* 14:185, 1982.
16. Dyson PK, Jackson BF, Pfeiffer DU, et al: Days lost from training by two- and three-year-old Thoroughbred horses: a survey of seven UK training yards, *Equine Vet J* 40:650, 2008.
17. Lucas JM, Ross MW, Richardson DW: Postoperative performance of racing Standardbreds treated arthroscopically for carpal chip fractures: 176 cases (1986-1993), *Equine Vet J* 31:48, 1999.
18. Martinelli MJ, Freeman DE, Reid SWJ: Analysis of performance parameters in the population of Standardbred racehorses in the US (1984-1993), *Proc Am Assoc Equine Pract* 42:174, 1996.
19. Martin GS, Strand E, Kearney MT: Use of statistical models to evaluate racing performance in Thoroughbreds, *J Am Vet Med Assoc* 209:1900, 1996.
20. Martin GS, Strand E, Kearney MT: Validation of a regression model for standardizing lifetime racing performances of Thoroughbreds, *J Am Vet Med Assoc* 210:1641, 1997.

21. Strand E, Martin GS, Haynes PF, et al: Career racing performance in Thoroughbreds treated with prosthetic laryngoplasty for laryngeal neuropathy: 52 cases (1981-1989), *J Am Vet Med Assoc* 217:1689, 2000.

CHAPTER 3 Anamnesis (History)

1. Liautard A: *Lameness of horses*, New York, 1888, William R Jenkins Press.
2. Young JH: Degenerative suspensory ligament desmitis. *Hoofcare Lameness* 6, 1993.
3. Mero JL, Pool RR: Twenty cases of degenerative suspensory ligament desmitis in Peruvian Paso horses, *Proc Am Assoc Equine Pract* 48:329, 2002.
4. Halper J, Kim B, Khan A, et al: Degenerative suspensory ligament desmitis as a systemic disorder characterized by proteoglycan accumulation. *BMC Vet Res* 2:1, 2006.
5. Schenkman D, Armien A, Pool R, et al: Systemic proteoglycan deposition is not a characteristic of equine degenerative suspensory ligament desmitis, *J Equine Vet Sci* 29:748, 2009.
6. Olsen K, Nann L: *Unpublished data*, Kennett Square, Pa, 1995, University of Pennsylvania.
7. Wagner PC, Grant BD, Kaneps AJ, et al: Long-term results of desmotomy of the accessory ligament of the deep digital flexor tendon (distal check ligament) in horses, *J Am Vet Med Assoc* 187:1351, 1985.
8. Steel CM, Hunt AR, Adams PL, et al: Factors associated with prognosis for survival and athletic use in foals with septic arthritis: 93 cases (1987-1994), *J Am Vet Med Assoc* 215:973, 1999.
9. Bousum P: Personal communication, 1995.
10. MacLeay JM, Sorum SA, Valberg SJ, et al: Epidemiologic analysis of factors influencing exertional rhabdomyolysis in Thoroughbreds, *Am J Vet Res* 60:1562, 1999.
11. Dyson S: Personal communication, 2000.

CHAPTER 4 Conformation and Lameness

1. Liautard A: *Lameness of horses*, New York, 1888, William R Jenkins Press.
2. Adams OR: *Veterinary notes on lameness and shoeing of horses*, Fort Collins, Colo, 1957, Colorado State University.
3. Belloy E, Bathe AP: The importance of standardising the evaluation of conformation in the horse, *Equine Vet J* 28:429, 1996.
4. Santschi EM, Leibsle SR, Morehead JP, et al: Carpal and fetlock conformation of the juvenile Thoroughbred from birth to yearling auction age, *Equine Vet J* 38:604, 2006.
5. Mawdsley A, Kelly EP, Smith FH, et al: Linear assessment of the Thoroughbred horse: an approach to conformation evaluation, *Equine Vet J* 28:461, 1996.

6. Delahunty D, Webb S, Kelly EP, et al: Intermandibular width and cannon bone length in "winners" versus "others," *J Equine Vet Sci* 11:258, 1991.
7. Hunt WF, Thomas VG, Stiefel W: Analysis of video-recorded images to determine linear and angular dimensions in the growing horse, *Equine Vet J* 31:402, 1999.
8. Clayton HM: Advances in motion analysis, *Vet Clin North Am* 7:365, 1991.
9. Leach DH, Dyson S: Instant centres of rotation of equine limb joints and their relationship to standard skin marker locations, *Equine Vet J Suppl* 6:113, 1988.
10. Holmström M, Magnusson L-E, Philipsson J: Variation in conformation of Swedish Warmblood horses and conformational characteristics of elite sport horses, *Equine Vet J* 22:186, 1990.
11. Magnusson L-E: *Studies on the conformation and related traits of Standardbred trotters in Sweden. I. An objective method for measuring the equine conformation, master's thesis*, Skara, Sweden, 1985, Sveriges Lantbruks Universitet.
12. Magnusson L-E, Thafvelin B: *Studies on the conformation and related traits of Standardbred trotters in Sweden. II. The variation in conformation of the Standardbred trotter, master's thesis*, Skara, Sweden, 1985, Sveriges Lantbruks Universitet.
13. Magnusson L-E, Thafvelin B: *Studies on the conformation and related traits of Standardbred trotters in Sweden. IV. Relationship between the conformation and soundness of four-year-old Standardbred trotter, master's thesis*, Skara, Sweden, 1985, Sveriges Lantbruks Universitet.
14. Barr ARS: Carpal conformation in relation to carpal chip fracture, *Vet Rec* 134:646, 1994.
15. Anderson TM, McIlwraith CW: Longitudinal development of equine conformation from weanling to age 3 years in the Thoroughbred, *Equine Vet J* 36:563, 2004.
16. Anderson TM, McIlwraith CW, Douay P: The role of conformation in musculoskeletal problems in the racing Thoroughbred, *Equine Vet J* 36:571, 2004.
17. McIlwraith CW, Anderson TM, Santschi BN: Conformation and musculoskeletal problems in the racehorse, *Clin Tech Equine Pract* 2:329, 2003.
18. Weller R, Pfau T, May SA, et al; Variation in conformation in a cohort of National Hunt racehorses, *Equine Vet J* 38:616, 2006.
19. Gill HE: Personal communication, 1987.
20. Gnagey L, Clayton HM, Lanovaz JL: Effect of standing tarsal angle on joint kinematics and kinetics, *Equine Vet J* 38:628, 2006.

CHAPTER 5 Observation: Symmetry and Posture

1. Valentine BA, Rousselle SD, Sams AE, et al: Denervation atrophy in three horses with fibrotic myopathy, *J Am Vet Med Assoc* 205:332, 1994.
2. Pilsworth RC, Sheperd MC, Herinckx BMB, et al: A review of 10 cases of fracture of the wing of the ilium, *Equine Vet J* 26:94, 1994.
3. Swor TM, Schneider RK, Ross MW, et al: Injury of the gastrocnemius muscle as a cause of lameness in 4 horses, *J Am Vet Med Assoc* 219:215, 2001.
4. Sack WO, Habel RE: *Rooney's guide to the dissection of the horse*, Ithaca, NY, 1977, Veterinary Textbooks.
5. Taylor SM: Disorders of the spinal cord. In Nelson RW, Couto CG, editors: *Small animal internal medicine*, St Louis, 1998, Mosby.
6. Seim HB, Prata RG: Ventral decompression for the treatment of cervical disc disease in the dog: a review of 54 cases, *J Am Anim Hosp Assoc* 18:233, 1982.
7. Ricardi G, Dyson SJ: Forelimb lameness associated with radiographic abnormalities of the cervical vertebrae, *Equine Vet J* 25:422, 1993.
8. Shoemaker RS, Martin GS, Hillmann DJ, et al: Disruption of the caudal component of the reciprocal apparatus in two horses, *J Am Vet Med Assoc* 198:120, 1991.
9. Reeves MJ, Trotter GW: Reciprocal apparatus dysfunction as a cause of severe hindlimb lameness in a horse, *J Am Vet Med Assoc* 199:1047, 1991.
10. Hanche-Olsen S, Teige J, Skaar I, et al: Polyneuropathy associated with forage sources in Norwegian horses, *J Vet Intern Med* 22:178, 2008.
11. Kraus J: Personal communication, March 2009.
12. Resnick D, Niwayama G: Osteomyelitis, septic arthritis, and soft tissue infection: mechanisms and situations. In Resnick D, editor: *Diagnosis of bone and joint disorders*, ed 3, Philadelphia, 1995, WB Saunders.

CHAPTER 6 Palpation

1. Strand E, Martin G, Crawford M, et al: Intra-articular pressure, elastance and range of motion in healthy and injured racehorse metacarpophalangeal joints, *Equine Vet J* 30:520, 1998.
2. Dyson SJ: Personal communication, 2001.
3. Kane AJ, Stover SM, Gardner IA, et al: Horseshoe characteristics as possible risk factors for fatal musculoskeletal injury of Thoroughbred racehorses, *Am J Vet Res* 57:1147, 1996.
4. Kobluk CN, Robinson RA, Gordon BJ, et al: The effect of conformation and shoeing: a cohort study of 95 Thoroughbred racehorses, *Proc Am Assoc Equine Pract* 36:259, 1990.
5. Maddren L: Personal communication, 1984.
6. Turner TA: Predictive value of diagnostic tests for navicular pain, *Proc Am Assoc Equine Pract* 42:201, 1996.
7. Castelijns HH: How to use a digital extension device in lameness examinations, *Proc Am Assoc Equine Pract* 54:228, 2008.
8. Delahanty DD: Manipulative procedures in detecting horse lameness, *Cornell Vet* 64:443, 1974.
9. Jeffcott LB, Dalin G, Drevemo S, et al: Effect of induced back pain on gait and performance of trotting horses, *Equine Vet J* 14:129, 1982.
10. Stashak TS: *Adams' lameness in horses*, Philadelphia, 1987, Lea & Febiger.
11. Barnhart CL: *The American college dictionary*, New York, 1970, Random House.

CHAPTER 7 Movement

1. Liautard A: *Lameness of horses*, New York, 1888, William R Jenkins Press.
2. Dorland WAN, ed: *Dorland's illustrated medical dictionary*, Philadelphia, 1974, Saunders.
3. Barnhart CL, ed: *The American college dictionary*, New York, 1970, Random House.
4. Adams OR: Natural and artificial gaits. In Stashak TS, ed: *Adams' lameness in horses*, Philadelphia, 1987, Lea & Febiger.
5. Dyson S: Personal communication, 2000.
6. Biewener AA, Thomason J, Goodship A, et al: Bone stress in the horse forelimb during locomotion at different gaits: a comparison of two experimental methods, *J Biomech* 16:565, 1983.
7. Leach DH, Sprigings E: Gait fatigue in the racing Thoroughbred, *J Equine Med Surg* 3:436, 1979.
8. Uhlir C, Licka T, Kübber P, et al: Compensatory movements of horses with a stance phase lameness, *Equine Vet J Suppl* 23:102, 1997.
9. Ross MW: Observations in horses with lameness abolished by palmar digital analgesia, *Proc Am Assoc Equine Pract* 44:230, 1998.
10. Evans LH: Personal communication, 1982.
11. Clayton HM: Cinematographic analysis of the gait of lame horses, *J Equine Vet Sci* 6:70, 1986.
12. Clayton HM: Cinematographic analysis of the gait of lame horses. V. Fibrotic myopathy, *J Equine Vet Sci* 8:297, 1986.
13. Wyman WEA: *Lameness in the horse*, New York, 1989, William R Jenkins Press.
14. Peloso JG, Stick JA, Soutas-Little RW, et al: Computer-assisted three-dimensional gait analysis of amphotericin-induced carpal lameness in horses, *Am J Vet Res* 54:1535, 1993.
15. Peham C, Licka T, Girtler D, et al: Supporting forelimb lameness: clinical judgment vs computerized symmetry measurement, *Equine Vet J* 31:417, 1999.
16. Ishihara A, Bertone AL, Rajala-Schultz PJ: Association between subjective lameness grade and kinetic gait parameters in horses with experimentally induced forelimb lameness, *Am J Vet Res* 66:1805, 2005.
17. Buchner HHF, Savelberg HHCM, Schamhardt HC, et al: Head and trunk movement adaptations in horses with experimentally induced fore- or hindlimb lameness, *Equine Vet J* 28:71, 1996.
18. Vorstenbosch MATM, Buchner HHF, Savelberg HHCM, et al: Modeling study of compensatory head movements in lame horses, *Am J Vet Res* 58:713, 1997.
19. Ratzlaff M, Hyde ML, Grant BD: Measurement of vertical forces and temporal components of the strides of horses using instrumented shoes, *J Equine Vet Sci* 10:23, 1990.
20. Judy CE, Galuppo LD, Snyder JR, et al: Evaluation of an in-shoe pressure measurement system in horses, *Am J Vet Res* 62:23, 2001.
21. Perino VV, Kawcak CE, Frisbie DD: The accuracy and precision of an equine in-shoe pressure measurement system as a tool for gait analysis, *J Equine Vet Sci* 27:161, 2007.

22. Keegan KG, Yonezawa Y, Pai F, et al: Evaluation of a sensor-based system of motion analysis for detection and quantification of forelimb and hind limb lameness, *Am J Vet Res* 65:665, 2004.

23. May SA, Wyn-Jones G: Identification of hindleg lameness, *Equine Vet J* 19:185, 1987.

24. Buchner HHF, Kastner J, Girtler D, et al: Quantification of hindlimb lameness in the horse, *Acta Anat* 146:196, 1993.

25. Kramer J, Keegan KG, Kelmer G, et al: Objective determination of pelvic movement during hind limb lameness by use of a signal decomposition method and pelvic height differences, *Am J Vet Res* 65:741, 2004.

26. Pfau T, Robilliard JJ, Weller R, et al: Assessment of mild hindlimb lameness during over ground locomotion using linear discriminant analysis of inertial sensor data, *Equine Vet J* 39:407, 2007.

27. Gingerich DA, Newcomb DM: Biomechanics in lameness, *J Equine Med Surg* 3:251, 1979.

28. Gingerich DA, Auer JA, Fackelman GE: Force plate studies on the effect of exogenous hyaluronic acid on joint function in equine arthritis, *J Vet Pharmacol Ther* 2:291, 1979.

29. Gingerich DA, Auer JA, Fackelman GE: Effect of exogenous hyaluronic acid on joint function in experimentally induced equine osteoarthritis: dosage titration studies, *Res Vet Sci* 30:192, 1981.

30. Schamhardt HC, Merkens HW: Quantification of equine ground reaction force patterns, *J Biomech* 20:443, 1987.

31. Merkens HW, Schamhardt HC: Evaluation of equine locomotion during different degrees of experimentally induced lameness. II. Distribution of ground reaction force patterns of the concurrently loaded limbs, *Equine Vet J Suppl* 6:107, 1988.

32. Ishihara A, Reed SM, Rajala-Schultz PJ, et al: Use of kinetic gait analysis for detection, quantification, and differentiation of hind limb lameness and spinal ataxia in horses, *J Am Vet Med Assoc* 234:644, 2009.

33. *Guide to veterinary services for horse shows*, ed 7, Lexington, Ky, 1999, American Association of Equine Practitioners.

34. Fredricson I, Drevemo S, Dalin G, et al: Treadmill for equine locomotion analysis, *Equine Vet J* 15:111, 1983.

35. Buchner HHF, Savelberg HCM, Schamhardt HC, et al: Habituation of horses to treadmill locomotion, *Equine Vet J Suppl* 17:13, 1994.

36. Kai M, Hiraga A, Kubo K, et al: Comparison of stride characteristics in a cantering horse on a flat and inclined treadmill, *Equine Vet J Suppl* 23:76, 1997.

CHAPTER 8   Manipulation

1. Nilsson G, Fredricson I, Drevemo S: Some procedures and tools in the diagnostics of distal equine lameness, *Acta Vet Scand Suppl* 44:63, 1973.

2. Ramey DW: Prospective evaluation of forelimb flexion tests in practice: clinical response, radiographic correlation, and predictive value for future lameness, *Proc Am Assoc Equine Pract* 43:116, 1997.

3. Verschooten F, Verbeeck J: Flexion test of the metacarpophalangeal and interphalangeal joints and flexion angle of the metacarpophalangeal joint in sound horses, *Equine Vet J* 29:50, 1997.

4. Dyson SJ: Evaluation of the musculoskeletal system. Part 4. The use of flexion tests and small diameter lunging. In Mair T, ed: *British Equine Veterinary Association manual: the pre-purchase examination*, Newmarket, 1998, Equine Veterinary Journal.

5. Busschers E, Van Weeren PR: Use of the flexion test of the distal forelimb in the sound horse: repeatability and effect of age, gender, weight, height and fetlock joint range of motion, *J Vet Med A Physiol Pathol Clin Med* 48:413, 2001.

6. Keg P, van Weeren PR, Back W, et al: Variations in the force applied to flexion tests of the distal limb of horses, *Vet Rec* 141:435, 1997.

7. Nilsson G: Lameness and pathologic changes in the distal joints and the phalanges of the Standardbred horse, *Acta Vet Scand (Suppl)* 43:83, 1973.

8. Strand E, Martin GS, Crawford MP, et al: Intra-articular pressure, elastance and range of motion in flexion of the equine metacarpophalangeal joint, *Am J Vet Res* 56:1362, 1995.

9. Meijer M, Busschers E, Van Weeren P: Which joint is most important for the positive outcome of a flexion test of the distal forelimb of a sound horse? *Equine Vet Educ* 13:319, 2001.

10. Dyson SJ: Personal communication, 2001.

11. Ducharme ND: Personal communication, 1981.

CHAPTER 9   Applied Anatomy of the Musculoskeletal System

1. Ashdown R, Done S: *Colour atlas of veterinary anatomy, vol 2, The horse*, London, 1987, Baillière Tindall.

2. Back W, Clayton H: *Equine locomotion*, London, 2001, Saunders.

3. Budras K, Sack WO, Rock S: *Anatomy of the horse*, ed 2, London, 1994, Mosby.

4. Denoix JM: *The equine distal limb: an atlas of clinical anatomy and comparative imaging*, London, 2000, Manson.

5. Freweined J, Habel RE, Sack WO, eds: *Nomina anatomica veterinaria*, ed 4, Ithaca, NY, 1994, World Association of Veterinary Anatomists.

6. Getty R: *Sisson and Grossman's the anatomy of domestic animals*, ed 5, vol 1, Philadelphia, 1975, Saunders.

7. Weaver J, Stover S, O'Brien T: Radiographic anatomy of soft tissue attachments in the equine metacarpophalangeal and proximal interphalangeal region, *Equine Vet J* 24:310, 1992.

CHAPTER 10   Diagnostic Analgesia

1. Melzak R, Wall PO: Pain mechanisms: a new theory, *Science* 150:971, 1965.

2. Butterworth JF IV, Strichartz GR: Molecular mechanisms of local anesthesia: a review, *Anesthesiology* 72:711, 1990.

3. Day TK, Skarda RT: The pharmacology of local anesthetics, *Vet Clin North Am Equine Pract* 7:489, 1991.

4. Jones EW: *Veterinary anesthesia*, ed 2, Philadelphia, 1987, Lea & Febiger.

5. Dyson S: Personal communication, 2001.

6. Zotterman Y: Studies in peripheral mechanisms of pain, *Acta Med Scand* 80:185, 1933.

7. Ross MW: Observations in horses with lameness abolished by palmar digital analgesia. *Proc Am Assoc Equine Pract* 44:230, 1998

8. Nagy A, Bodo G, Dyson S, et al: Diffusion of contrast medium after perineural injection of the palmar nerves: an in vivo and in vitro study, *Equine Vet J* 41:379, 2009.

9. Jones E, Vinuela-Fernandez I, Eager R, et al: Neuropathic changes in equine laminitis pain, *Pain* 132:321, 2007

10. Dyson SJ: Problems associated with the interpretation of the results of regional and intra-articular anaesthesia in the horse, *Vet Rec* 118:419, 1986.

11. Todhunter RJ: Anatomy and physiology of synovial joints. In McIlwraith CW, Trotter GW, eds: *Joint disease in the horse*, Philadelphia, 1996, Saunders.

12. Caron JP: Neurogenic factors in joint pain and disease pathogenesis. In McIlwraith CW, Trotter GW, eds: *Joint disease in the horse*, Philadelphia, 1996, Saunders.

13. Wyke B: The neurology of joints: a review of general principles, *Clin Rheum Dis* 7:223, 1981.

14. Dee R: The innervation of joints. In Sokoloff L, ed: *The joints and synovial fluid*, New York, 1978, Academic Press.

15. Fessler JF: The musculoskeletal system—functional anatomy and physiology of diarthrodial joints. In Jennings PB, ed: *The practice of large animal surgery*, vol 2, Philadelphia, 1984, Saunders.

16. Wojtys EM, Beaman DN, Glover RA, et al: Innervation of the human knee joint by substance-P fibers, *Arthroscopy* 6:254, 1990.

17. Beaman D, Graziano G, Glover R, et al: Substance P innervation of the lumbar facet joints, *Spine* 18:1044, 1993.

18. Herskovits MS, Singh IJ, Sandhu HS: Innervation of bone. In Hall BK, ed: *Bone, vol 3, Bone matrix and bone specific products*, Boca Raton, 1991, CRC Press.

19. Reimann I, Christensen SB: A histological demonstration of nerves in subchondral bone, *Acta Orthop Scand* 48:345, 1977.

20. Hague BA, Honnas CM, Simpson RB, et al: Evaluation of skin bacterial flora before and after aseptic preparation of clipped and nonclipped arthrocentesis sites in horses, *Vet Surg* 26:121, 1997.

21. Stashak TS: Diagnosis of lameness. In Stashak TS, ed: *Adams' lameness in horses*, ed 4, Philadelphia, 1987, Lea & Febiger.

22. Schumacher J, Steiger R, Schumacher J, et al: Effects of analgesia of the distal interphalangeal joint or palmar digital nerves on lameness caused by solar pain in horses, *Vet Surg* 29:54, 2000.

23. Schumacher J, Livesey L, DeGraves FJ, et al: Effect of anaesthesia of the palmar digital nerves on proximal interphalangeal joint pain in the horse, *Equine Vet J* 36:409, 2004.

24. Cornelissen BPM, Burma P, Rijkenhuizen ABM, et al: Innervation of the equine mature and immature proximal sesamoid bone by calcitonin gene-related peptide

and substance P-containing nerve fibers, *Am J Vet Res* 59:1378, 1998.

25. Ford TS, Ross MW, Orsini PG: A comparison of methods for proximal palmar metacarpal analgesia in horses, *Vet Surg* 18:146, 1989.

26. Wheat JD, Jones KJ: Selected techniques of regional anesthesia, *Vet Clin North Am Large Anim Pract* 3:223, 1981.

27. Dyce KM, Sack WO, Wensing CJG: The forelimb of the horse. In Dyce KM, Sack WO, Wensing CJG, eds: *Textbook of veterinary anatomy*, Philadelphia, 1987, Saunders.

28. Castro FA, Schumacher JS, Pauwels F, et al: A new approach for perineural injection of the lateral palmar nerve in the horse, *Vet Surg* 34:539, 2005.

29. Schumacher J, Schumacher J, de Graves F, et al: A comparison of the effects of local analgesic solution in the navicular bursa of horses with lameness caused by solar toe or solar heel pain, *Equine Vet J* 33:386, 2001.

30. Schumacher J, Schumacher J, Gillette R, et al: The effects of local anesthetic solution in the navicular bursa of horses with lameness caused by distal interphalangeal joint pain, *Equine Vet J*, 35:502, 2003.

31. Dyson SJ, Kidd L: A comparison of responses to analgesia of the navicular bursa and intra-articular analgesia of the distal interphalangeal joint in 59 horses, *Equine Vet J* 25:93, 1993.

32. Pleasant RS, Moll HD, Ley WB, et al: Intra-articular anesthesia of the distal interphalangeal joint alleviates lameness associated with the navicular bursa in horses, *Vet Surg* 26:137, 1997.

33. Keegan KG, Wilson DA, Kreeger JM, et al: Local distribution of mepivacaine after distal interphalangeal joint injection in horses, *Am J Vet Res* 57:422, 1996.

34. Gough MR, Mayhew IG, Munroe GA: Diffusion of mepivacaine between adjacent synovial structures in the horse. Part 1: forelimb foot and carpus, *Equine Vet J*, 34:80, 2002.

35. Bowker RM, Rockerhouser SJ, Vex KB, et al: Immunocytochemical and dye distribution studies of nerves potentially desensitized by injections into the distal interphalangeal joint or the navicular bursa of horses, *J Am Vet Med Assoc* 203:1708, 1993.

36. Bowker RM, Linder K, Van Wulfen KK, et al: Anatomy of the distal interphalangeal joint of the mature horse: relationships with navicular suspensory ligaments, sensory nerves and neurovascular bundle, *Equine Vet J* 29:126, 1997.

37. Schumacher J, Schumacher J, de Graves F, et al: A comparison of the effects of two volumes of local analgesic solution in the distal interphalangeal joint of horses with lameness caused by solar to or solar heel pain, *Equine Vet J* 33:265, 2001.

38. Vasquez de Mercado R, Stover SM, Taylor KT, et al: Lateral approach for arthrocentesis of the distal interphalangeal joint in horses, *J Am Vet Med Assoc* 212:1413, 1998.

39. Miller SM, Stover SM, Taylor KT, et al: Palmaroproximal approach for arthrocentesis of the proximal interphalangeal joint in horses, *Equine Vet J* 28:376, 1996.

40. Misheff MA, Stover SM: A comparison of two techniques for arthrocentesis of the equine metacarpophalangeal joint, *Equine Vet J* 23:273, 1991.

41. Ford TS, Ross MW, Orsini PG: Communications and boundaries of the middle carpal and carpometacarpal joints in horses, *Am J Vet Res* 49:2161, 1988.

42. Keily RG, McMullan W: Lateral arthrocentesis of the equine carpus, *Equine Pract* 9:22, 1987.

43. Lewis RD: Techniques for arthrocentesis of equine shoulder, elbow, stifle, and hip joints, *Proc Am Assoc Equine Pract* 42:55, 1996.

44. Sams AE, Honnas CM, Sack WO, et al: Communication of the ulnaris lateralis bursa with the equine elbow joint and evaluation of caudal arthrocentesis, *Equine Vet J* 25:130, 1993.

45. Moyer W: *A guide to equine joint injections*, Trenton, NJ, 1983, Veterinary Learning Systems.

46. Grant BG: Bursal injections, *Proc Am Assoc Equine Pract* 42:64, 1996.

47. Scrutchfield W: Injection of the navicular bursa, *Southwest Vet* 30:161, 1977.

48. Turner TA: Diagnosis and treatment of navicular syndrome in horses, *Vet Clin North Am Equine Pract* 5:131, 1989.

49. Verschooten F, Desmet P, Peremens K, et al: Navicular disease in the horse: the effect of controlled intrabursal corticoid injection, *J Equine Vet Sci* 11:8, 1991.

50. Butler JA, Colles CM, Dyson SJ, et al: *Clinical radiology of the horse*, Oxford, 2008, Wiley-Blackwell.

51. Bishop HW: A clinical review: navicular disease, *J Royal Army Vet Corps* 31:61, 1960.

52. Dietz O, Wiesner E: *Diseases of the horse*, part 1, New York, 1984, Karger.

53. Schramme MC, Boswell JC, Hamhougias KT, et al: An in vitro study to compare 5 different techniques for injection of the navicular bursa in the horse, *Equine Vet J* 32:263, 2000.

54. Harper J, Schumacher J, DeGraves F, et al: Effects of analgesia of the digital flexor tendon sheath on pain originating in the sole, distal interphalangeal joint or navicular bursa of horses, *Equine Vet J*, 39:535, 2007.

55. Sampson S, Schneider R, Tucker R, et al: Magnetic resonance imaging features of oblique and straight distal sesamoidean desmitis in 27 horses, *Vet Radiol Ultrasound* 48:303, 2007.

56. Hassell DM, Stover SM, Yarbrough TB, et al: Palmar-plantar axial sesamoidean approach to the digital flexor tendon sheath in horses, *J Am Vet Med Assoc* 217:1343, 2000.

57. Schumacher J, Livesey L, Brawner W, et al: Comparison of 2 methods of centesis of the bursa of the biceps brachii tendon of horses, *Equine Vet J* 39:356, 2007.

58. Dyson S: Lesions of the proximal aspect of the humerus and the tendon of biceps brachii, *Equine Vet Educ* 21:67, 2009.

59. Dyson SJ, Romero JM: An investigation of injection techniques for local analgesia of the equine distal tarsus and proximal metatarsus, *Equine Vet J* 25:30, 1993.

60. Dyce KM, Sack WO, Wensing CJG: The hindlimb of the horse. In Dyce KM, Sack WO, Wensing CJG, eds: *Textbook of veterinary anatomy*, Philadelphia, 1987, Saunders.

61. Sack WO, Orsini PG: Distal intertarsal and tarsometatarsal joints in the horse: communication and injection sites, *J Am Vet Med Assoc* 179:355, 1981.

62. Bell BTL, Baker GJ, Foreman JH, et al: In vivo investigation of communication between the distal intertarsal and tarsometatarsal joints in horses and ponies, *Vet Surg* 22:289, 1993.

63. Gough MR, Munroe GA, Mayhew IG: Diffusion of mepivacaine between adjacent synovial structures in the horse. Part 2: tarsus and stifle, *Equine Vet J*, 34:85, 2002.

64. Just EM, Patan B, Licka TF: Dorsolateral approach for arthrocentesis of the centrodistal joint in horses, *Am J Vet Res*, 68:946, 2007.

65. Reeves MJ, Trotter GW, Kainer RA: Anatomical and functional communications between the synovial sacs of the equine stifle joint, *Equine Vet J* 23:215, 1991.

66. Vacek JR, Ford TS, Honnas CM: Communication between the femoropatellar and medial and lateral femorotibial joints in horses, *Am J Vet Res* 53:1431, 1992.

67. Hendrickson DA, Nixon AJ: A lateral approach for synovial fluid aspiration and joint injection of the femoropatellar joint of the horse, *Equine Vet J* 24:397, 1992.

68. Hendrickson DA, Nixon AJ: Comparison of the cranial and a new lateral approach to the femoropatellar joint for aspiration and injection in horses, *J Am Vet Med Assoc* 205:1177, 1994.

69. David F, Rougier M, Alexander K, et al: Ultrasound guided coxofemoral arthrocentesis in horses, *Equine Vet J* 38:79, 2007.

70. Hughes TK, Eliashar E, Smith RK: In vitro evaluation of a single injection technique for diagnostic analgesia of the proximal suspensory ligament of the equine pelvic limb, *Vet Surg* 36:760, 2007.

71. Marks D: Medical management of back pain, *Vet Clin North Am Equine Pract* 15:179, 1999.

CHAPTER 11 Neurological Examination and Neurological Conditions Causing Gait Deficits

1. Mayhew IG: The equine spinal cord in health and disease (Milne lecture), *Proc Am Assoc Equine Pract* 45:56, 1999.

2. Divers TJ, Mohammed HO, Cummings JF, et al: Equine motor neuron disease: findings in twenty-eight horses and proposal of a pathophysiological mechanism for the disease, *Equine Vet J* 26:409, 1994.

3. Maylin GA, Rubin DS, Lein DH: Selenium and vitamin E in horses, *Cornell Vet* 70:272, 1980.

4. Craig AM, Blythe LL, Lassen ED, et al: Variations of serum vitamin E, cholesterol and total serum lipid concentrations in horses during a 72-hour period, *Am J Vet Res* 50:1527, 1989.

5. Beech J: Equine degenerative myeloencephalopathy, *Vet Clin North Am Equine Pract* 3:379, 1987.

6. Mayhew IG, Brown CM, Stowe HD, et al: Equine degenerative myeloencephalopathy: a vitamin E deficiency that may be familial, *J Vet Intern Med* 1:45, 1987.

7. Steiss JE, Traber MG, Williams MA, et al: Alpha tocopherol concentrations in clinically normal adult horses, *Equine Vet J* 26:417, 1994.

8. Traber MG, Steiss JE, Williams MA, et al: Vitamin E deficiency in horses, *FASEB J* 9:A473, 1995.

9. Marcus LC, Patterson MM, Gilfillan RE, et al: Antibodies to *Borrelia burgdorferi* in New England horses: serologic survey, *Am J Vet Res* 46:2570, 1985.

10. Cohen ND, Bosler EM, Bernard W, et al: Epidemiologic studies of Lyme disease in horses and their public health significance, *Ann N Y Acad Sci* 539:244, 1988.

11. Lindenmayer J, Weber M, Onderdonk A: *Borrelia burgdorferi* infection in horses, *J Am Vet Med Assoc* 194:1384, 1989.

12. Hahn CN, Mayhew IG, Whitwell KE, et al: A possible case of Lyme borreliosis in a horse in the UK, *Equine Vet J* 28:84, 1996.

13. Browning A, Carter SD, Barnes A, et al: Lameness associated with *Borrelia burgdorferi* infection in the horse, *Vet Rec* 132:610, 1993.

14. Granstrom DE: Equine protozoal myeloencephalitis: parasite biology, experimental disease, and laboratory diagnosis. Proceedings of the International Equine Neurology Conference, Ithaca, NY, March 1997.

15. Saville WJA, Reed SM, Granstrom DE, et al: Response of horses exposed to *Sarcocystis neurona* when monitored biweekly, *Proc Am Assoc Equine Pract* 43:8, 1997.

16. Moore RM, Trims CM: Effect of xylazine on cerebrospinal fluid pressure in conscious horses, *Am J Vet Res* 53:1558, 1992.

17. Patten B: How much blood makes the cerebrospinal fluid bloody? *J Am Med Assoc* 206:378, 1968 (letter).

18. Miller MM, Sweeney CR, Russell GE, et al: Effects of blood contamination of cerebrospinal fluid on Western blot analysis for detection of antibodies against *Sarcocystis neurona* and on albumin quotient and immunoglobulin G index in horses, *J Am Vet Med Assoc* 215:67, 1999.

19. Calabrese VP: The interpretation of routine CSF tests, *Vir Med Month* 103:207, 1976.

20. Mayhew IG, Whitlock RH, Tasker JB: Equine cerebrospinal fluid: reference values of normal horses, *Am J Vet Res* 38:1271, 1977.

21. Beech J: Cytology of equine cerebrospinal fluid, *Vet Pathol* 20:553, 1983.

22. Behrens H: Cerebrospinal liquor of horses, its withdrawal, examination, and diagnostic importance. Proceedings of the Fifteenth Annual International Veterinary Congress, Stockholm, Sweden, 1953.

23. Green EM, Constantinescu GM, Kroll RA: Equine cerebrospinal fluid: analysis, *Compend Contin Educ Pract Vet* 15:288, 1993.

24. Furr M, Chicoring WR, Robertson J: High resolution protein electrophoresis of equine cerebrospinal fluid, *Am J Vet Res* 58:939, 1997.

25. Furr MO, Tyler RD: Cerebrospinal fluid creatine kinase activity in horses with central nervous system disease: 69 cases, *J Am Vet Med Assoc* 197:245, 1990.

26. Jackson C, de Lahunta A, Divers T, et al: The diagnostic utility of cerebrospinal fluid creatine kinase activity in the horse, *J Vet Intern Med* 10:246, 1996.

27. Andrews FM, Maddux JM, Faulk D: Total protein, albumin quotient, IgG and IgG index determinations for horse cerebrospinal fluid, *Prog Vet Neurol* 1:197, 1990.

28. Cohen ND, McKay RJ: Interpreting immunoblot testing of cerebrospinal fluid for equine protozoal myeloencephalitis, *Compend Contin Educ Pract Vet (Equine)* 19:1176, 1997.

29. Saville WJA, Dubey JP, Oglesbee MJ, et al: Experimental infection of ponies with *Sarcocystis fayeri* and differentiation from *Sarcocystis neurona* infections in horses, *J Parasitol* 90:1487, 2004.

30. Howe DK, Rajshekhar YG, Marsh AE, et al: Strains of *S. neurona* exhibit differences in their surface antigens, including the absence of the major surface antigen SnSAG1, *Int J Parasitol* 38:623, 2008.

31. Mayhew IG, Donawick WJ, Green SL, et al: Diagnosis and prediction of cervical vertebral malformation in Thoroughbred foals based on semiquantitative radiographic indicators, *Equine Vet J* 25:435, 1993.

32. Moore BR, Reed SM, Biller DS, et al: Assessment of vertebral canal diameter and bony malformations of the cervical part of the spine in horses with cervical stenotic myelopathy, *Am J Vet Res* 55:5, 1994.

33. Beech J: Metrizamide myelography in the horse, *J Am Vet Radiol Soc* 20:22, 1979.

34. Papageorges M, Gavin P, Sande RD, et al: Radiographic and myelographic examination of the cervical vertebral column in 306 ataxic horses, *Vet Radiol* 28:53, 1987.

35. Maclean AA, Jeffcott LB, Lavelle RB, et al: Use of iohexol for myelography in the horse, *Equine Vet J* 20:286, 1988.

36. Henry RW, Diesem CD, Wiechers DO: Evaluation of equine radial and median nerve conduction velocities, *Am J Vet Res* 40:1406, 1979.

37. Henry RW, Diesem CD: Proximal equine radial and median motor nerve conduction velocity, *Am J Vet Res* 42:1819, 1981.

38. Blythe LL, Kitchell RL, Holliday TA, et al: Sensory nerve conduction velocities in forelimb of ponies, *Am J Vet Res* 44:1419, 1983.

39. Blythe LL, Engel HN, Rose KE: Comparison of sensory nerve conduction velocities in horses versus ponies, *Am J Vet Res* 49:2138, 1988.

40. Beech J, Dodd DC: *Toxoplasma*-like encephalomyelitis in the horse, *Vet Pathol* 11:87, 1974.

41. Beech J: Equine protozoan encephalomyelitis, *Vet Med Small Anim Clin* 69:1562, 1974.

42. Cusick PK, Sells DM, Hamilton DP, et al: Toxoplasmosis in two horses, *J Am Vet Med Assoc* 164:77, 1974.

43. Dubey JP, Davis GW, Koestner A, et al: Equine encephalomyelitis due to a protozoan parasite resembling *Toxoplasma gondii*, *J Am Vet Med Assoc* 154:249, 1974.

44. Rooney JR, Prickett ME, Delaney FM, et al: Focal myelitis-encephalitis in horses, *Cornell Vet* 50:494, 1970.

45. Saville WJA, Reed SM, Granstrom DE, et al: Seroprevalence of antibodies to *Sarcocystis neurona* in horses residing in Ohio, *J Am Vet Med Assoc* 210:519, 1997.

46. Dubey JP, Lindsay DS, Saville WJA, et al: A review of *Sarcocystis neurona* and equine protozoal myeloencephalitis (EPM), *Vet Parasitol* 95:89, 2001.

47. Daft BM, Barr BC, Collins N, et al: *Neospora* encephalomyelitis and polyradiculoneuritis in an aged mare with Cushing's disease, *Equine Vet J* 28:240, 1996.

48. Marsh AE, Barr BC, Madigan J, et al: Neosporosis as a cause of equine protozoal myeloencephalitis, *J Am Vet Med Assoc* 209:1907, 1996.

49. Marsh AE, Barr BC, Packham AE, et al: Description of a new *Neospora* species (Protozoa: Apicomplexa: Sarcocystidae), *J Parasitol* 84:983, 1998.

50. Hamir AN, Tornquist SJ, Gerros TC, et al: *Neospora caninum* associated equine protozoal myeloencephalitis, *Vet Parasitol* 79:269, 1998.

51. Reed SM: Diagnosing equine protozoal myeloencephalitis, *Compend Contin Educ Pract Vet* 22(Suppl 7A):1, 2000.

52. Toribio RE, Bain FT, Mrad DR, et al: Congenital defects in newborn foals of mares treated for equine protozoal myeloencephalitis during pregnancy, *J Am Vet Med Assoc* 212:697, 1998.

53. Lindsay DS, Dubey JP: Determination of the activity of diclazuril against *Sarcocystis neurona* and *Sarcocystis falcatula* in cell cultures, *J Parasitol* 86:164, 2000.

54. Granstrom DE, McCrillis S, Wulff-Strobel C, et al: Diclazuril and equine protozoal myeloencephalitis, *Proc Am Assoc Equine Pract* 43:13, 1997.

55. Furr M, Kennedy T: Cerebrospinal fluid and blood levels of toltrazuril 5% suspension (Baycox) in the horse following oral dosing, *Vet Ther* 1:125, 1999.

56. Lindsay DS, Dubey JP, Kennedy TJ: Determination of the activity of ponazuril against *Sarcocystis neurona* in cell cultures, *Vet Parasitol* 92:165, 2000.

57. Vatistas N, Fenger C, Palma K, et al: Initial experiences with the use of nitazoxanide in the treatment of equine protozoal encephalitis in northern California, *Vet Clin North Am Equine Pract* 21:18, 1999.

58. McClure SR, Palma KG: Treatment of equine protozoal myeloencephalitis with nitazoxanide, *J Equine Vet Sci* 19:639, 1999.

59. Cutler TJ, MacKay RJ, Ginn PE, et al: Immunoconversion against *Sarcocystis neurona* in normal and dexamethasone-treated horses challenged with *S. neurona* sporocysts, *Vet Parasitol* 95:197, 2001.

60. Saville WJA, Stich RW, Reed SM, et al: Utilization of stress in the development of an equine model for equine protozoal myeloencephalitis, *Vet Parasitol* 95:211, 2001.

61. Rooney JR: *Clinical neurology of the horse*, Kennett Square, Pa, 1971, KNA Press.

62. Nixon AJ: Cervical vertebral malformation and malarticulation. In Colahan PT, Mayhew IG, Merritt AM, et al, eds: *Equine*

medicine and surgery, ed 5, St Louis, 1999, Mosby.

63. Donawick WJ, Mayhew IG, Galligan DT, et al: Early diagnosis of cervical vertebral malformation in young Thoroughbred horses and successful treatment with restricted paced diet and confinement, *Proc Am Assoc Equine Pract* 35:525, 1989.

64. Moore BR, Reed SM, Robertson JT: Surgical treatment of cervical stenotic myelopathy in horses: 73 cases (1983-1992), *J Am Vet Med Assoc* 203:108, 1993.

65. Wagner PC, Grant BD, Bagby GW, et al: Evaluation of cervical spinal fusion as a treatment in the equine "wobbler syndrome," *Vet Surg* 8:84, 1979.

66. Mayhew IG, Grown CM, Stowe HD, et al: Equine degenerative myeloencephalopathy: a vitamin E deficiency that may be familial, *J Vet Intern Med* 1:45, 1987.

67. Blythe LL, Craig AM: Equine degenerative myeloencephalopathy. I. Clinical signs and pathogenesis, *Compend Contin Educ Pract Vet* 13:1215, 1922.

68. Beech J, Haskins M: Genetic studies of neuroaxonal dystrophy in the Morgan, *Am J Vet Res* 48:109, 1987.

69. Blythe LL: Equine degenerative myeloencephalopathy: genetics and treatment. Proceedings of the International Equine Neurology Conference, Ithaca, NY, 1997.

70. Divers TJ, Mohammed HO, Cummings JF: Equine motor neuron disease, *Vet Clin North Am Equine Pract* 13:97, 1997.

71. Divers TJ, Mohammed HO, Cummings JF, et al: Equine motor neuron disease: findings in 28 horses and proposal of a pathophysiological mechanism for the disease, *Equine Vet J* 26:409, 1994.

72. Riis RC, Jackson C, Rebhun W: Ocular manifestations of equine motor neuron disease, *Equine Vet J* 31:99, 1999.

73. De la Rùa-Doménech R, Mohammed HO, Cummings JF, et al: Association between plasma vitamin E concentration and the risk of equine motor neuron disease, *Vet J* 154:203, 1997.

74. Divers TJ, Valentine BA, Jackson CA, et al: Simple and practical muscle biopsy test for equine motor neuron disease, *Proc Am Assoc Equine Pract* 42:180, 1996.

75. Hillyer MH, Innes JF, Patteson MW, et al: Diskospondylitis in an adult horse, *Vet Rec* 139:519, 1996.

76. Dyson S: *The differential diagnosis of shoulder lameness in the horse, RCVS Fellowship Thesis*, London, 1986, Royal College of Veterinary Surgeons.

77. Henry RW: *Gait alteration in the equine pectoral limb produced by neurectomies, master's thesis*, Stillwater, Okla, 1976, Oklahoma State University.

78. Dyson S: Personal communication, 2001.

79. Hahn CN, Mayhew IG, Mackay RJ: Diseases of the peripheral (spinal) nerves. In Colahan PT, Mayhew IG, Merritt AM, et al, eds: *Equine medicine and surgery*, ed 5, St Louis, 1999, Mosby.

80. Cauvin E, Munroe GA, Mitsopoulos A: Peripheral neuropathy involving brachial plexus nerves in 2 horses, *Equine Vet Educ* 5:90, 1993.

81. Mayhew IG: *Large animal neurology: a handbook for veterinary clinicians*, Philadelphia, 1989, Lea & Febiger.

82. Ross MW: Personal communication, 2001.

83. Cahill JI, Goulden BE, Pearce HG: A review and some observations on stringhalt, *N Z Vet J* 33:101, 1985.

84. Pemberton DH, Caple IW: Australian stringhalt in horses, *Vet Annu* 20:167, 1980.

85. Slocombe RF, Huntington PJ, Friend SCE: Pathological aspects of Australian stringhalt, *Equine Vet J* 24:174, 1992.

86. Cahill JI, Goulden BE, Jolly RD: Stringhalt in horses: a distal axonopathy, *Neuropathol Appl Neurobiol* 12:459, 1986.

87. Huntington PJ, Seneque S, Slocombe RF, et al: Use of phenytoin to treat horses with Australian stringhalt, *Aust Vet J* 68:221, 1991.

88. Kannegieter NJ, Malik R: The use of baclofen in the treatment of stringhalt, *Aust Vet J* 10:90, 1992.

CHAPTER 12   Unexplained Lameness

1. Pilsworth R: Personal communication 2007.

2. Dyson S: Problems associated with the interpretation of the results of regional and intra-articular anaesthesia in the horse, *Vet Rec* 118:419, 1986.

3. Ricardi G, Dyson S: Forelimb lameness associated with radiographic abnormalities of the cervical vertebrae, *Equine Vet J* 25:422, 1993.

4. Weller R, Cauvin E, Bowen I, et al: Comparison of radiography, scintigraphy and ultrasonography in the diagnosis of a case of temporomandibular joint arthropathy in a horse, *Vet Rec* 144:377, 1999.

5. Weller R, Taylor S, Maierl J, et al: Ultrasonographic anatomy of the equine temporomandibular joint, *Equine Vet J* 31:529, 1999.

6. Ramzan P, Marr C, Meehan J, et al: A novel oblique radiographic projection of the equine temporomandibular joint, *Vet Rec* 162:714, 2008.

7. Nollet H, Vanderstraeten G, Sustronck B, et al: Suspected case of stiff-horse syndrome, *Vet Rec* 146:282, 2000.

8. Mayhew I: Personal communication, 2000.

9. Dyson S: Unpublished data, 1988-2002.

10. Divers T, Mohammed H, Cummings J, et al: Equine motor neuron disease: findings in twenty-eight horses and proposal of a pathophysiological mechanism for the disease, *Equine Vet J* 26:409, 1994.

11. Clegg P: Lyme disease, *Proc Br Equine Vet Assoc Congr* 39:155, 2000.

12. Lindenmayer J, Weber M, Onderdonk A: *Borrelia burgdorferi* infection in horses, *J Am Vet Med Assoc* 194:1384, 1989.

13. McDonnell SM: Estrous cycle–related performance problems. In Robinson NE, ed: *Current therapy in equine medicine*, ed 6, St Louis, 2009, Elsevier.

14. Cox JH, DeBowes RM: Colic-like discomfort associated with ovulation in two mares, *J Am Vet Med Assoc* 191:1451, 1987.

15. Mansmann RA: Hormonal influence on performance in the mare. In *Santa Barbara Equine Practice Newsletter*, Santa Barbara, Calif, 1991.

16. Marien T: Standing laparoscopic herniorrhaphy in stallions using cylindrical polypropylene mesh prosthesis, *Equine Vet J* 33:91, 2001.

17. Coome R, Edwards G, Rijkenhuizen A, et al: Brachial thrombosis in a mare, *Pferdeheilkunde* 23:65, 2007.

18. Anderson J, Galuppo L, Barr B, et al: Clinical and scintigraphic findings in horses with a bone fragility disorder: 16 cases (1980-2006), *J Am Vet Med Assoc* 232:1694, 2008.

CHAPTER 13   Assessment of Acute-Onset, Severe Lameness

1. Campbell N: Application of a Robert Jones bandage. In Dyson S, ed: *A guide to the management of emergencies at equine competitions*, Newmarket, UK, 1996, Equine Veterinary Journal.

2. Walmsley J: Management of a suspected fracture. In Dyson S, ed: *A guide to the management of emergencies at equine competitions*, Newmarket, UK, 1996, Equine Veterinary Journal.

3. Ellis D: Transporting an injured horse. In Dyson S, ed: *A guide to the management of emergencies at equine competitions*, Newmarket, UK, 1996, Equine Veterinary Journal.

CHAPTER 14   The Swollen Limb

1. Adam E, Southwodd L: Primary and secondary limb cellulitis in horses: 44 cases (2000-2006), *J Am Vet Med Assoc* 231:1696, 2007.

2. Fjordbakk L, Arroyo L, Hewson J: Retrospective study of the clinical features of limb cellulitis in 63 horses, *Vet Rec* 162:233, 2008.

3. Markel M, Wheat J, Jang S: Cellulitis associated with coagulase-positive staphylococci in racehorses: nine cases (1975-1984), *J Am Vet Med Assoc* 189:1600, 1986.

CHAPTER 15   Radiography and Radiology

1. Weaver J, Stover S, O'Brien Y: Radiographic anatomy of soft tissue attachments in the equine metacarpophalangeal and proximal phalangeal region, *Equine Vet J* 24:310, 1992.

2. Maulet B, Mayhew I, Jones E, et al: Radiographic anatomy of the soft tissue attachments of the stifle, *Equine Vet J* 37:530, 2005.

3. Butler J, Colles C, Dyson S, et al: *Clinical radiology of the horse*, ed 3, Oxford, 2008, Wiley-Blackwell.

4. Smallwood J, Shiveley M, Rendano V, et al: A standard nomenclature for radiographic projections used in veterinary medicine, *Vet Radiol* 26:2, 1985.

CHAPTER 16   Ultrasonographic Evaluation of the Equine Limb: Technique

1. Rantanen NW: The use of diagnostic ultrasound in limb disorders of the horse: a preliminary report, *J Equine Vet Sci* 12:62, 1982.

2. Genovese RL, Rantanen NW, Hauser ML, et al: Diagnostic ultrasonography of equine limbs, *Vet Clin North Am Equine Pract* 2:145, 1986.

3. Genovese RL, Rantanen NW, Simpson BS: The use of ultrasonography in the diagnosis and management of injuries to the equine limb, *Compend Contin Educ Vet Pract* 9:945, 1987.

4. Hausen ML: Ultrasonographic appearance and correlative anatomy of the soft tissues of the distal extremities in the horse, *Vet Clin North Am Equine Pract* 2:127, 1986.

5. Sande RD, Tucker RL, Johnsten GR: Diagnostic ultrasound: applications in the equine limb. In Rantanen NW, McKinnon AO, eds: *Equine diagnostic ultrasonography*, Baltimore, 1998, Williams & Wilkins.

6. Genovese RL, Rantanen NW: The superficial digital flexor tendon and the deep digital flexor tendon, carpal sheath, accessory ligament of the deep digital flexor tendon (inferior check ligament). In Rantanen NW, McKinnon AO, eds: *Equine diagnostic ultrasonography*, Baltimore, 1998, Williams & Wilkins.

7. Reef VB: Musculoskeletal ultrasonography. In *Equine diagnostic ultrasound*, Philadelphia, 1998, Saunders.

8. Denoix JM: Ultrasonographic examination in the diagnosis of joint disease. In McIlwraith CW, Trotter GW, eds: *Joint disease in the horse*, Philadelphia, 1996, Saunders.

9. Powis RL: *Ultrasound physics for the fun of it*, Denver, 1978, Technicare.

10. Powis RL, Powis WJ: *A thinker's guide to ultrasonic imaging*, Baltimore, 1984, Urban and Schwarzenberg.

11. Reef VB: Musculoskeletal ultrasonography. In *Equine diagnostic ultrasound*, Philadelphia, 1998, Saunders.

12. Wrigley R: Ultrasound artifacts. In Rantanen NW, McKinnon AO, eds: *Equine diagnostic ultrasonography*, Baltimore, 1998, Williams & Wilkins.

13. Pennick DG: Imaging artifacts. In Nyland TG, Mattoon JS, eds: *Veterinary diagnostic ultrasound*, Philadelphia, 1995, Saunders.

14. Kirberger RM: Imaging artifacts in diagnostic ultrasound: a review, *Vet Radiol Ultrasound* 36:297, 1995.

15. Craychee TJ: Ultrasonographic evaluation of equine musculoskeletal injury. In Nyland TG, Mattoon JS, eds: *Veterinary diagnostic ultrasound*, Philadelphia, 1995, Saunders.

16. Reef VB, Genovese RL, Davis WM: Initial long-term results of horses with superficial digital flexor tendonitis treated with intralesional β-aminoproprionitrile fumarate, *Proc Am Assoc Equine Pract* 43:301, 1997.

17. Genovese RL, Jorgensen JS: Unpublished data, 2002.

18. Hills AC: Comparative ultrasonic study of normal tendinous and ligamentous structures of the palmar metacarpus of Standardbred and Thoroughbred horses, *Proc Am Assoc Equine Pract* 42:272, 1996.

19. Wright I, McMahon PJ: Tenosynovitis associated with longitudinal tears in the digital flexor tendons in horses: a report of 20 cases, *Equine Vet J* 31:12, 1999.

20. Denoix JM: *The equine distal limb: atlas of clinical anatomy and comparative imaging*, London, 2000, Manson.

21. Genovese RL, Longo KL, Berthold B, et al: Quantitative sonographic assessment in the clinical management of superficial digital flexor injuries in thoroughbred racehorses, *Proc Am Assoc Equine Pract* 43:285, 1997.

22. Redding WR: Use of ultrasonography in the evaluation of joint disease in horses. Part 1. Indications, technique and examination of the soft tissues, *Equine Vet Educ* 3:250, 2001.

23. Genovese RL, Jorgensen JS: Clinical use of β-aminopropionitrile-fumarate (Bapten) in superficial digital flexor tendon injuries in racehorses (Session 358), *Proc Ohio Vet Med Assoc* 1998.

CHAPTER 17   Ultrasonographic Examination of Joints

1. Denoix J-M: Ultrasonographic examination in the diagnosis of joint disease. In McIlwraith W, Trotter G, eds: *Joint disease in the horse*, Philadelphia, 1996, Saunders.

2. Denoix J-M, Busoni V: Ultrasonography of joints and synovia. In White NA, Moore JN, eds: *Current techniques in equine surgery and lameness*, ed 2, Philadelphia, 1998, Saunders.

3. Denoix J-M: Ultrasound examination of joints and miscellaneous tendons. In Rantanen N, McKinnon A, eds: *Equine diagnostic ultrasound*, Baltimore, 1998, Williams & Wilkins.

4. Denoix J-M: *The equine distal limb: an atlas of clinical anatomy and comparative imaging*, London, 2000, Manson.

5. Denoix J-M, Jacot S, Perrot P, et al: Ultrasonographic anatomy of the dorsal and abaxial aspect of the equine fetlock, *Equine Vet J* 28:54, 1996.

6. Reef VB: Joint ultrasonography. *Clin Tech Equine Pract* 3:256, 2004.

7. Vanderperren K, Martens A, Declerq J, et al: Comparison of ultrasonography versus radiography for the diagnosis of dorsal fragmentation of the metacarpophalangeal or metatarsophalangeal joint in horses, *J Am Vet Med Assoc* 235:70, 2009.

8. Dyson SJ: Normal ultrasonographic anatomy and injury of the patellar ligaments in the horse, *Equine Vet J* 34:258, 2002.

9. Bourzac, C, Alexander K, Rossier Y, et al: Comparison of radiography and ultrasonography for the diagnosis of osteochondritis dissecans in the equine femoropatellar joint, *Equine Vet J* 41:686, 2009.

10. Koneberg D, Edinger J: Three-dimensional ultrasonographic in vitro imaging of lesions of the meniscus and femoral trochlea in the equine stifle, *Vet Radiol Ultrasound* 48:350, 2007.

11. Cauvin EJR, Munroe GA, Boyd JS, et al: Ultrasonographic examination of the femorotibial articulation in horses: imaging of the cranial and caudal aspects, *Equine Vet J* 28:285, 1996.

12. Coudry V, Denoix J-M: Ultrasonography of the femorotibial collateral ligaments of the horse, *Equine Vet Educ* 17:275, 2005.

13. Hoegaerts M, Nicaise M, van Bree H, et al: Cross-sectional anatomy and comparative ultrasonography of the equine medial femorotibial joint and its related structures, *Equine Vet J* 37:520, 2005.

14. Whitcomb M: Ultrasonography of the equine tarsus, *Proc Am Assoc Equine Pract* 52:13, 2006.

CHAPTER 18   Ultrasonography and Orthopedic (Nonarticular) Disease

1. Reef VB: Musculoskeletal ultrasonography. In Reef VB, ed: *Equine diagnostic ultrasound*, Philadelphia, 1998, Saunders.

2. Smith RK, Dyson SJ, Head MJ, Butson RJ: Ultrasonography of the equine triceps muscle before and after general anaesthesia and in post anaesthetic myopathy, *Equine Vet J* 28:311, 1996.

3. Jesty SA, Palmer JE, Parente EJ, et al: Rupture of the gastrocnemius muscle in six foals, *J Am Vet Med Assoc* 227:1965, 2005.

4. Dik KJ: Ultrasonography of the equine crus, *Vet Radiol Ultrasound* 34:28, 1993.

5. Dabareiner RM, Schmitz DG, Honnas CM, Carter GK: Gracilis muscle injury as a cause of lameness in two horses, *J Am Vet Med Assoc* 224:1630, 2004.

6. Swor TM, Schneider RK, Ross MW, et al: Injury to the origin of the gastrocnemius muscle as a possible cause of lameness in four horses, *J Am Vet Med Assoc* 219:215, 2001.

7. Pickersgill CH, Kriz N, Malikides N: Surgical treatment of semitendinosus fibrotic myopathy in an endurance horse—management, complications and outcome, *Equine Vet Educ* 12:320, 2000.

8. Clegg PD, Coumbe A: Alveolar rhabdomyosarcoma: an unusual cause of lameness in a pony, *Equine Vet J* 25:547, 1993.

9. Alexander K, Dobson H: Ultrasonography of peripheral nerves in the normal adult horse, *Vet Radiol Ultrasound* 44:456, 2003.

10. Reef VB: Ultrasonography of small parts. In Reef VB, ed: *Equine diagnostic ultrasound*, Philadelphia, 1998, Saunders.

11. Reef VB: Sonography. In White NA, Moore J, eds: *Current techniques in equine surgery and lameness*, Philadelphia, 1998, Lippincott.

12. Vatistas NJ, Meagher DM, Gillis CL, Neves JW: Gunshot injuries in horses: 22 cases (1971-1993), *J Am Vet Med Assoc* 207:1198, 1995.

13. Engelbert TA, Tate LP Jr: Penetrating lingual foreign bodies in three horses, *Cornell Vet* 83:31, 1993.

14. Adams R, Nixon A, Hager D: Use of intraoperative ultrasonography to identify a cervical foreign body. A case report, *Vet Surg* 16:384, 1987.

15. French DA, Pharr JW, Fretz PB: Removal of a retropharyngeal foreign body in a horse, with the aid of ultrasonography during surgery, *J Am Vet Med Assoc* 194:1315, 1989.

16. Kiper ML, Wrigley R, Traub-Dargatz J, Bennett D: Metallic foreign bodies in the mouth or pharynx of horses: seven cases (1983-1989), *J Am Vet Med Assoc* 200:91, 1992.

17. Solano M, Penninck D: Ultrasonography of the canine, feline and equine tongue: normal findings and case history reports, *Vet Radiol Ultrasound* 37:206, 1996.

18. Reef VB, Reimer J, Reid CF: Ultrasonographic findings in horses with osteomyelitis, *Proc Am Assoc Equine Pract* 37:381, 1991.

19. Shah ZD, Crass JR, Oravec DC, Bellon EM: Ultrasonographic detection of foreign bodies in soft tissues using turkey muscle

as a model, *Vet Radiol Ultrasound* 33:94, 1992.

20. Cartee RE, Rumph PF: Ultrasonographic detection of fistulous tracts and foreign objects in muscles of horses, *J Am Vet Med Assoc* 184:1127, 1984.
21. Rose PL, Penninck D: Use of intraoperative ultrasonography in six horses, *Vet Surg* 24:396, 1995.
22. Pusterla N, Latson KM, Wilson WD, Whitcomb MB: Metallic foreign bodies in the tongues of 16 horses, *Vet Rec* 159:485, 2006.
23. Dik KJ: Ultrasonography in the diagnosis of equine lameness, *Vet Annu* 30:162, 1990.
24. Pilsworth RC, Shepherd MC, Herinckx BM, Holmes MA: Fracture of the wing of the ilium, adjacent to the sacroiliac joint, in thoroughbred racehorses, *Equine Vet J* 26:94, 1994.
25. Shepherd MC, Pilsworth RC: The use of ultrasound in the diagnosis of pelvic fractures, *Equine Vet Educ* 6:223, 1994.
26. Dik KJ: Ultrasonography of the equine tarsus, *Vet Radiol Ultrasound* 34:36, 1993.
27. Dik KJ: Ultrasonography of the equine stifle, *Equine Vet Educ* 7:154, 1995.
28. Denoix J: Ultrasonography of equine joints, *Proc Am Assoc Equine Pract* 47:366, 2001.
29. Enzerink E, Dik KJ: Palmar/plantar annular ligament insertion injury: a report of four cases, *Equine Vet Educ* 13:75, 2001.
30. Santschi EM, Adams SB, Fessler JF, Widmer WR: Treatment of bacterial tarsal tenosynovitis and osteitis of the sustentaculum tali of the calcaneus in five horses, *Equine Vet J* 29:244, 1997.
31. Bassage LH 2nd, Garcia-Lopez J, Currid EM: Osteolytic lesions of the tuber calcanei in two horses, *J Am Vet Med Assoc* 217:710, 2000.

CHAPTER 19   Nuclear Medicine

1. Ueltschi G: Bone and joint imaging with 99mTc labeled phosphates as a new diagnostic aid in veterinary orthopedics, *J Am Vet Radiol Soc* 21:86, 1977.
2. Twardock AR: A personal history of veterinary nuclear medicine, *Semin Vet Med Surg (Small Anim)* 6:103, 1991.
3. Devous MD, Twardock AR: Techniques and applications of nuclear medicine in the diagnosis of equine lameness, *J Am Vet Med Assoc* 184:318, 1984.
4. Seeherman HJ, Morris E, O'Callaghan MW: Comprehensive clinical evaluation of performance. In Auer JA, ed: *Equine surgery*, Philadelphia, 1992, Saunders.
5. Lamb CR, Koblik P: Scintigraphic evaluation of skeletal disease and its application to the horse, *Vet Radiol* 29:16, 1988.
6. Dyson SJ, Pilsworth RC, Twardock AR, Martinelli MJ, eds: *Equine scintigraphy*, Newmarket, 2003, Equine Veterinary Journal.
7. Scheidegger E, Geissbühlerl U, Doherr MG, Lang J: Technetium-99m-HDP uptake characteristics in equine fractures: a retrospective study, *Schweiz Arch Tierheilkd* 148:569, 2006.
8. Dyson S, Murray R: Verification of scintigraphic imaging for injury diagnosis in 264 horses with foot pain, *Equine Vet J* 39:350, 2007.

9. Dyson S, Murray R: Use of concurrent scintigraphic and magnetic resonance imaging evaluation to improve understanding of the pathogenesis of injury of the podotrochlear apparatus, *Equine Vet J* 39:365, 2007.
10. Chambers MD, Martinelli MJ, Baker GJ, et al: Nuclear medicine for diagnosis of lameness in horses, *J Am Vet Med Assoc* 206:792, 1995.
11. Sela J, Shani J, Kohavi D, et al: Uptake and biodistribution of 99mTechnetium methylene-[32P] diphosphonate during endosteal healing around titanium, stainless steel and hydroxyapatite implants in rat tibial bone, *Biomaterials* 16:1373, 1995.
12. Kanishi D: 99mTc-MDP accumulation mechanisms in bone, *Oral Surg Oral Med Oral Pathol* 75:239, 1993.
13. Shani J, Amir D, Soskolne WA, et al: Correlations between uptake of technetium, calcium, phosphate, and mineralization in rat tibial bone repair, *J Nucl Med* 31:2011, 1990.
14. Castronovo FP, Strauss HW: Dual tracer resorption and opposition in a rat fracture model, *Nucl Med Biol* 15:181, 1988.
15. Schwartz Z, Shani J, Soskolne WA, et al: Uptake and biodistribution of technetium-99m-MD32P during rat tibial bone repair, *J Nucl Med* 34:104, 1993.
16. Okamoto Y: Accumulation of technetium-99m methylene diphosphonate: conditions affecting adsorption to hydroxyapatite, *Oral Surg Oral Med Oral Pathol* 80:115, 1995.
17. Kawano M, Taki J, Tsuchiya H, et al: Predicting the outcome of distraction osteogenesis by 3-phase bone scintigraphy, *J Nuc Med* 44:369, 2003.
18. Dore F, Filippi L, Biasotto M, et al: Bone scintigraphy and SPECT/CT of bisphosphonate-induced osteonecrosis of the jaw, *J Nuc Med* 50:30, 2009.
19. Chisin R, Gazit D, Ulmansky M, et al: 99mTc-MDP uptake and histological changes during rate bone marrow regeneration, *Nucl Med Biol* 15:469, 1988.
20. Savelkoul TJF, Visser WJ, Oldenburg SJ, Duursma SA: A micro-autoradiographical study of the localization of 99mTc(Sn)-MDP and 99mTc-MDP in undecalcified bone sections, *Eur J Nucl Med* 11:459, 1986.
21. Stokkel MP, Valdés-Olmos RA, Hoefnagel CA, et al: Tumor and therapy associated abnormal changes on bone scintigraphy: old and new phenomena, *Clin Nucl Med* 18:821, 1993.
22. Cheng KT, Shaw SM, Pinkerton TC, et al: A Walker 256 tumor-induced osteogenic small animal model for the evaluation of [99mTc] diphosphonate radiopharmaceuticals, *Int J Nucl Med Biol* 12:197, 1985.
23. Stover SM, Johnson BJ, Daft BM, et al: An association between complete and incomplete stress fractures of the humerus in racehorses, *Equine Vet J* 24:260, 1992.
24. Johnson B, Ardans A, Stover SM, et al: California racehorse postmortem program: a 4-year overview, *Proc Am Assoc Equine Pract* 40:167, 1994.
25. Stover SM, Read DH, Johnson BJ, et al: Lateral condylar fracture histomorphology in racehorses, *Proc Am Assoc Equine Pract* 40:173, 1994.

26. Mattson SE, Pearce SG, Bouré LP, et al: Comparison of intraosseous and intravenous infusion of technetium 99mTc pertechnetate in the distal portion of forelimbs in standing horses by use of scintigraphic imaging, *Am J Vet Res* 66:1267, 2005.
27. de Cock HE, Affolter VK, Wisner ER, et al: Lymphoscintigraphy of draught horses with chronic progressive lymphoedema, *Equine Vet J* 38:148, 2006.
28. Kleine LG, Solano M, Rusckowski M, et al: Evaluation of technetium Tc99m-labeled biotin for scintigraphic detection of soft tissue inflammation in horses, *Am J Vet Res* 69:639, 2008.
29. Long CD, Galuppo LD, Waters NK, Hornof WJ: Scintigraphic detection of equine orthopedic infection using Tc-HMPAO labeled leukocytes in 14 horses, *Vet Radiol Ultrasound* 41:354, 2000.
30. Alexander K, Drost WT, Mattoon JS, et al: Binding of ciprofloxacin labelled with technetium Tc 99m versus 99mTc-pertechnetate to a live and killed equine isolate of *Escherichia coli*, *Can J Vet Res* 69:272, 2005.
31. Attenburrow DP, Bowring CS, Vennart W: Radioisotope bone scanning in horses, *Equine Vet J* 16:121, 1984.
32. Pilsworth RC: Establishing a probe point counting scintigraphy system in practice, *Equine Vet Educ* 8:41, 1996.
33. Ross MW, Maxson AD, Stacy VS, Buchanan KB: First-pass radionuclide angiography in the diagnosis of aortoiliac thromboembolism in a horse, *Vet Radiol Ultrasound* 38:226, 1997.
34. Bramlage LR: Personal communication, 1998.
35. Boswell R: Personal communication, 1996.
36. Seeherman HJ: Personal communication, 1992.
37. Dyson SJ, Lakhani K, Wood J: Factors influencing blood flow in the equine digit and their effect on uptake of 99mtechnetium methylene diphosphonate into bone, *Equine Vet J* 33:591, 2001.
38. Solano M, Welcome J, Johnson K: Effects of acepromazine on three-phase 99mTc-MDP bone imaging in 11 horses, *Vet Radiol Ultrasound* 46:437, 2005.
39. Gatherer ME, Faulkner J, Voûte LC: Exposure of veterinary personnel to ionising radiation during bone scanning of horses by nuclear scintigraphy with 99mtechnetium methylene diphosphonate, *Vet Rec* 16:160, 2007.
40. Steyn PF, Uhrig J: The role of protective lead clothing in reducing radiation exposure rates to personnel during equine bone scintigraphy, *Vet Radiol Ultrasound* 46:529, 2005.
41. Dyson SJ, Weekes JS, Murray RC: Scintigraphic evaluation of the proximal metacarpal and metatarsal regions of horses with proximal suspensory desmitis, *Vet Radiol Ultrasound* 48:78, 2007.
42. Dyson S, Murray R, Branch M, et al: The sacroiliac joints: evaluation using nuclear scintigraphy. Part 1: The normal horse, *Equine Vet J* 35:226, 2003.
43. Dyson S, Murray R, Branch M, et al: The sacroiliac joints: evaluation using nuclear scintigraphy. Part 2: Lame horses, *Equine Vet J* 35:233, 2003.

44. Gorgas D, Luder P, Lang J, et al: Scintigraphic and radiographic appearance of the sacroiliac region in horses with gait abnormalities or poor performance, *Vet Radiol Ultrasound* 50:208, 2009.

45. Weekes JS, Murray RC, Dyson SJ: Scintigraphic evaluation of metacarpophalangeal and metatarsophalangeal joints in clinically sound horses, *Vet Radiol Ultrasound* 45:85, 2004.

46. White J, Busschers E, Ross MW: Clinical and scintigraphic findings in the fetlock joint of Thoroughbred racehorses, *Equine Vet J* (in preparation for submission).

47. Levine DG, Ross BM, Ross MW, et al: Decreased radiopharmaceutical uptake (photopenia) in delayed phase scintigraphic images in three horses, *Vet Radiol Ultrasound* 48:467, 2007.

48. Uhlhorn H, Eksell P, Carlsten J: Scintigraphic characterization of distal radial physeal closure in young Standardbred racehorses, *Vet Radiol Ultrasound* 41:181, 2000.

49. Metcalf MR, Forrest LJ, Sellett LC: Scintigraphic pattern of ^{99m}Tc-MDP uptake in exercise induced proximal phalangeal trauma in horses, *Vet Radiol* 31:17, 1990.

50. Ehrich PJ, Seeherman HJ, O'Callaghan MW, et al: Results of bone scintigraphy in horses used for show jumping, hunting, or eventing: 141 cases (1988-1994), *J Am Vet Med Assoc* 213:1460, 1998.

51. Bailey RE, Dyson SJ, Parkin TD: Focal increased radiopharmaceutical uptake in the dorsoproximal diaphyseal region of the equine proximal phalanx, *Vet Radiol Ultrasound* 48:460, 2007.

52. Walsh DM, Royal HD: Evaluation of a single injection of 99m-labeled diethylenetriaminepentaacetic acid for measuring glomerular filtration rate in horses, *Am J Vet Res* 53:776, 1992.

53. Campeau RJ, Bellah RD, Varma DGK: Pathologic fractures in a patient with renal osteodystrophy: failure of early detection on bone scans, *Clin Nucl Med* 12:510, 1987.

54. Trout DR, Hornof WJ, Liskey CC, Fisher PE: The effects of regional perineural anesthesia on soft tissue and bone phase scintigraphy in the horse, *Vet Radiol* 32:140, 1991.

55. Ruohoniemi M, Mäkelä O, Eskonen T: Clinical significance of ossification of the cartilages of the front feet based on nuclear bone scintigraphy, radiography and lameness examinations in 21 Finnhorses, *Equine Vet J* 36:143, 2004.

56. Nagy A, Dyson S, Murray R: Scintigraphic examination of the cartilages of the foot, *Equine Vet J* 39:250, 2007.

57. Nagy A, Dyson S, Murray R: Radiographic, scintigraphic and magnetic resonance imaging findings in the palmar processes of the distal phalanx, *Equine Vet J* 40:57, 2008.

58. Pool RR, Meagher DM: Pathologic findings and pathogenesis of racetrack injuries, *Vet Clin North Am Equine Pract* 6:1, 1990.

59. Ross MW: Scintigraphic and clinical findings in the Standardbred metatarsophalangeal joint: 114 cases (1993-1995), *Equine Vet J* 30:131, 1998.

60. Ross MW: Observations in horses with lameness abolished by palmar digital analgesia, *Proc Am Assoc Equine Pract* 44:230, 1998.

61. Rabuffo T, Ross MW: Unpublished data, 2001.

62. Lanyon LE: Functional strain as a determinate for bone remodeling, *Calcif Tissue Int* 36:S56, 1984.

63. Lanyon LE: Functional strain in bone tissue as an objective and controlling stimulus for adaptive bone remodeling, *J Biomech* 20:1083, 1987.

64. Biewener AA: Biomechanics of mammalian terrestrial locomotion, *Science* 250:1097, 1990.

65. Erlich PJ, Dohoo IR, O'Callaghan MW: Results of bone scintigraphy in racing Standardbred horses: 64 cases (1992-1994), *J Am Vet Med Assoc* 215:982, 1999.

66. Erichsen C, Eksell P, Holm KR, et al: Relationship between scintigraphic and radiographic evaluations of spinous processes in the thoracolumbar spine in riding horses without clinical signs of back problems, *Equine Vet J* 36:458, 2004.

67. Gillen A, Dyson S, Murray R: Nuclear scintigraphic assessment of the thoracolumbar synovial intervertebral articulations, *Equine Vet J* 41:534, 2009.

68. Meehan L, Dyson S, Murray R: Radiographic and scintigraphic evaluation of spondylosis in the equine thoracolumbar spine, *Equine Vet J* 41:800, 2009.

69. Dahlberg J, Ross MW: Clinical relevance of abnormal scintigraphic findings in adult equine ribs: 20 horses (1996-2008), *Vet Radiol Ultrasound* (submitted for publication).

70. Anderson JDC, Galuppo LD, Barr BC, et al: Clinical and scintigraphic findings in horses with a bone fragility disorder: 16 cases (1980-2006), *J Am Vet Med Assoc* 232:1694, 2008.

71. Durham MG, Armstrong CM: Fractures and bone deformities in 18 horses with silicosis, *Proc Am Assoc Equine Pract* 52:1, 2006.

72. Davenport CLM, Ross MW: Scintigraphic abnormalities of the pelvic region in horses examined because of lameness or poor performance, *J Am Vet Med Assoc* 224:88, 2004.

73. Morris E, Seeherman HJ, O'Callaghan MW, et al: Scintigraphic identification of skeletal muscle damage in horses 24 hours after strenuous exercise, *Equine Vet J* 23:347, 1991.

CHAPTER 20   Computed Tomography

1. Bushberg JT, Seibert JA, Leidholdt EM, Boone JM: *Computed tomography: the essential physics of medical imaging*, ed 2, Philadelphia, 2002, Lippincott Williams & Wilkins.

2. Lo WY, Puchalski SM: Digital image processing, *Vet Radiol Ultrasound* 49:S42, 2008.

3. Puchalski SM, Snyder JR, Hornof WJ, et al: Contrast enhanced computed tomography of the equine distal extremity, *Proc Am Assoc Equine Pract* 51:389, 2005.

4. Puchalski SM, Galuppo LD, Hornof WJ, Wisner ER: Intraarterial contrast-enhanced computed tomography of the equine distal extremity, *Vet Radiol Ultrasound* 48:21, 2007.

5. Sharma P, Maffulli N: Tendon injury and tendinopathy: healing and repair, *J Bone Joint Surg* 87:187, 2005.

6. Dyson S, Murray R: Magnetic resonance imaging evaluation of 264 horses with foot pain: the podotrochlear apparatus, deep digital flexor tendon and collateral ligaments of the distal interphalangeal joint, *Equine Vet J* 39:340, 2007.

7. Puchalski SM, Schultz RM, Wisner ER: Unpublished data, University of California, Davis, 2008.

8. Widmer WR, Buckwalter KA, Fessler JF, et al: Use of radiography, computed tomography and magnetic resonance imaging for evaluation of navicular syndrome in the horse, *Vet Radiol Ultrasound* 41:108, 2000.

9. Whitton RC, Buckley C, Donovan T, et al: The diagnosis of lameness associated with distal limb pathology in a horse: a comparison of radiography, computed tomography and magnetic resonance imaging, *Vet J* 155:223, 1998.

10. Puchalski SM, Galuppo LD, Drew CP, et al: Angiogenesis in equine deep digital flexor tendonopathy identified by contrast enhanced computed tomography, *Vet Radiol Ultrasound* 50:292, 2009.

11. van Hamel S, Puchalski SM, Bergman HJ, et al: *Contrast enhanced computed tomographic evaluation of deep digital flexor tendon compared to macroscopic and histologic findings in 29 limbs*, Utrecht, the Netherlands, 2008, Department of Equine Sciences, Department of Pathobiology, Utrecht University.

12. Bergman HJ, Puchalski SM, van der Veen H, et al: Computed tomography and CT arthrography of the equine stifle: technique and preliminary results in 16 clinical cases, *Proc Am Assoc Equine Pract* 53:46, 2007.

13. Kruger E, Puchalski S, Pollard RE, et al: Measurement of equine laminar blood flow and permeability by dynamic contrast enhanced computed tomography, *Am J Vet Res* 69:371, 2008.

CHAPTER 21   Magnetic Resonance Imaging

1. Murray R, Mair T: Use of magnetic resonance imaging in lameness diagnosis in the horse, *In Practice* 27:138, 2005.

2. Dyson S, Murray R: Magnetic resonance imaging of the equine foot, *Clin Tech Equine Pract* 6:46, 2007.

3. Dyson S, Murray R: Magnetic resonance imaging of the equine fetlock, *Clin Tech Equine Pract* 6:62, 2007.

4. Murray R: The equine carpus, *Clin Tech Equine Pract* 20:390, 2007.

5. Branch M, Murray R, Dyson S, et al: Magnetic resonance imaging of the equine tarsus, *Clin Tech Equine Pract* 6:96, 2007.

6. Judy C, Saveraid T, Rick M, et al: Magnetic resonance imaging of the equine stifle in a clinical setting. Proceedings of the American College of Veterinary Surgeons Surgical Summit, Washington, September 2007.

7. Murray R, Dyson S: Image interpretation and artifacts, *Clin Tech Equine Pract* 6:16, 2007.

8. Busoni V, Snaps F, Trenteseaux J, et al: Magnetic resonance imaging of the

palmar aspect of the equine podotrochlear apparatus: normal appearance, *Vet Radiol Ultrasound* 45:198, 2004.

9. Smith M, Dyson S, Murray R: Is a magic angle effect observed in the collateral ligaments of the distal interphalangeal joint or the oblique sesamoidean ligaments during standing low field magnetic resonance imaging? *Vet Radiol Ultrasound* 49:509, 2008.

CHAPTER 22   Gait Analysis for the Quantification of Lameness

1. Keegan KG, Wilson DA, Wilson DJ, et al: Evaluation of mild lameness in horses trotting on a treadmill by clinicians and interns or residents and correlation of their assessments with kinematic gait analysis, *Am J Vet Res* 59:1370, 1998.
2. Hewetson M, Christley RM, Hunt ID, et al: Investigations of the reliability of observational gait analysis for the assessment of lameness in horses, *Vet Rec* 158:852, 2006.
3. Fuller CJ, Bladon BM, Driver AJ, et al: The intra- and inter-assessor reliability of measurement of functional outcome by lameness scoring in horses, *Vet J* 171:281, 2006.
4. Arkell M, Archer RM, Guitian FJ, et al: Evidence of bias affecting the interpretation of the results of local anesthetic nerve blocks when assessing lameness in horses, *Vet Rec* 159:346, 2006.
5. Sweet AL: Temporal discrimination by the human eye, *Am J Psychol* 66:185, 1953.
6. Näsänen R, Ojanpää H, Tanskanen T, et al: Estimation of temporal resolution of object identification in human vision, *Exp Brain Res* 172:464, 2006.
7. Keegan KG, Pai PF, Wilson DA, et al: Signal decomposition method of evaluating head movement to measure induced forelimb lameness in horses trotting on a treadmill, *Equine Vet J* 33:446, 2001.
8. Winter DA: Camera speeds for normal and pathological gait analyses, *Med Biol Eng Comput* 20:4, 1982.
9. Judy CE, Galuppo LD, Snyder JR, et al: Evaluation of an in-shoe pressure measurement system in horses, *Am J Vet Res* 62:23; 2001.
10. Perino VV, Kawcak CE, Frisbie DD, et al: The accuracy and precision of an equine in-shoe pressure measurement system as a tool for gait analysis, *J Equine Vet Sci* 27:161, 2007.
11. Roepstorff L, Drevemo S: Concept of a force-measuring horseshoe, *Acta Anat* 146:114, 1993.
12. Roepstroff L, Johnston C, Drevemo S: The influences of different treadmill constructions on ground reaction forces as determined by the use of a force-measuring horseshoe, *Equine Vet J Suppl* 17:71, 1994.
13. Ratzlaff MH, Wilson PD, Hyde ML, et al: Relationships between locomotor forces, hoof position and joint motion during the support phase of the stride of galloping horses, *Acta Anat* 146:200, 1993.
14. Makoto K, Aoki O, Hiraga A, et al: Use of an instrument sandwiched between the hoof and shoe to measure vertical ground reaction forces and three-dimensional acceleration at the walk, trot, and canter in horses, *Am J Vet Res* 61:979, 2000.
15. Weishaupt MA, Hogg HP, Wiestner, et al: Instrumented treadmill for measuring vertical ground reaction forces in horses, *Am J Vet Res* 63:520, 2002.
16. Weishaupt MA, Wiestner T, Hogg HP, et al: Vertical ground reaction force-time histories of sound Warmblood horses trotting on a treadmill, *Vet J* 168:304-311, 2004.
17. Weishaupt MA, Wiestner T, Hogg HP, et al: Compensatory load redistribution of horses with induced weightbearing hindlimb lameness trotting on a treadmill, *Equine Vet J* 36:727, 2004.
18. Merkens HW, Schamhardt HC: Evaluation of equine locomotion during different degrees of experimentally induced lameness. I: Lameness model and quantification of ground reaction force patterns of the limbs, *Equine Vet J Suppl* 6:99, 1988.
19. Keg PR, Barneveld A, Schamhardt HC, et al: Clinical and force plate evaluation of the effect of a high plantar nerve block in lameness caused by induced mid-metatarsal tendinitis, *Vet Q Suppl* 16:S70, 1994.
20. Hu HH, MacAllister CG, Payton ME, et al: Evaluation of the analgesic effects of phenylbutazone administered at a high and low dosage in horses with chronic lameness, *Am J Vet Res* 226:414, 2005.
21. Symonds KD, MacAllister CG, Erkert RS, et al: Use of force plate analysis to assess the analgesic effects of etodolac in horses with navicular syndrome, *Am J Vet Res* 67:557, 2006.
22. Back W, MacAllister CG, van Heel MCV, et al: Vertical frontlimb ground reaction forces of sound and lame warmbloods differ from those in quarter horses, *J Equine Vet Sci* 27:123, 2007.
23. Dow SM, Leendertz JA, Silver IA, et al: Identification of subclinical tendon injury from ground reaction force analysis, *Equine Vet J* 23:266, 1991.
24. Ishihara A, Bertone AL, Rajaala-Schultz PJ: Association between subjective lameness grade and kinetic gait parameters in horses with experimentally induced forelimb lameness, *Am J Vet Res* 66:1815, 2005.
25. Keegan KG, Wilson DJ, Wilson DA, et al: Effects of anesthesia of the palmar digital nerves on kinematic gait analysis in horses with and without navicular disease, *Am J Vet Res* 58:218, 1997.
26. Keegan KG, Wilson DJ, Wilson DA, et al: Effects of balancing and shoeing of the forelimb feet on kinematic gait analysis in 5 horses with navicular disease, *J Equine Vet Sci* 18:522, 1998.
27. Keegan KG, Wilson DA, Smith BK, et al: Changes in kinematic variables seen with lameness induced by applying pressure to the frog and to the toe in adult horses trotting on a treadmill, *Am J Vet Res* 61:612, 2000.
28. Kramer J, Keegan KG, Wilson DA, et al: Kinematics of the equine hindlimb in trotting horses after induced distal tarsal lameness and distal tarsal anesthesia, *Am J Vet Res* 61:1031, 2000.
29. Keegan KG, Pai PF, Wilson DA, et al: A curve-fitting technique for evaluating head movement to measure forelimb lameness in horses, *Biomed Sci Instrum* 36:239, 2000.
30. Keegan KG, Yonezawa Y, Pai PF, et al: Telemeterized accelerometer-based system for the detection of lameness in horses, *Biomed Sci Instrum* 38:112, 2002.
31. Keegan KG, Arafat S, Skubic M, et al: Determination and differentiation (right vs left) of equine forelimb lameness using continuous wavelet transformation and neural network classification of kinematic data, *Am J Vet Res* 64:1376, 2003.
32. Keegan KG, Yonezawa Y, Pai PF, et al: Sensor based system of equine motion analysis for the detection and quantification of forelimb and hindlimb lameness in horses, *Am J Vet Res* 65:665, 2004.
33. Kramer J, Keegan KG, Kelmer G, et al: Objective determination of pelvic movement during hindlimb lameness using a signal decomposition method and pelvic height differences, *Am J Vet Res* 65:741, 2004.
34. Kramer J, Keegan KG: Kinematics of lameness. In *Equine sports medicine and surgery: basic and clinical sciences of the equine athlete*, St. Louis, 2004, Saunders, pp. 231-246, 55.
35. Kelmer G, Keegan KG, Kramer J, et al: Computer-assisted kinematic evaluation of induced compensatory lameness in horses trotting on a treadmill, *Am J Vet Res* 66:646, 2005.
36. DePuy T, Howard R, Keegan KG, et al: Effects of intra-articular botulinum toxin type A in an equine model of acute synovitis: a pilot study, *Am J Phys Med Rehab* 86:777, 2007.
37. Keegan KG: Evidence-based lameness detection and quantification, *Vet Clin North Am Equine Pract* 23:403, 2007.
38. Keegan KG, Messer NT, Reed SK, et al: Effectiveness of combined phenylbutazone (PBZ) and flunixin meglumine (FM) administration to alleviate lameness in horses, *Am J Vet Res* 69:167, 2008.
39. May SA, Wyn-Jones G: Identification of hindleg lameness, *Equine Vet J* 19:185, 1987.
40. Kobluk CN, Schnurr D, Horney FD, et al: Use of high speed cinematography and computer generated gait diagrams for the study of equine hindlimb kinematics, *Equine Vet J* 21:48, 1989.
41. Back W: Kinematic gait analysis in equine carpal lameness, *Acta Anat* 146:86, 1993.
42. Buchner F, Kastner J, Girtler D, et al: Quantification of hind limb lameness in the horse, *Acta Anat* 146:196, 1993.
43. Peloso JG, Stick JA, Soutas Little RW, et al: Computer-assisted three-dimensional gait analysis of amphotericin-induced carpal lameness in equids, *Am J Vet Res* 54:535, 1993.
44. Clayton HM, Bradbury JW: Temporal characteristics of the foxtrot: a symmetrical equine gait, *Appl Anim Behav Sci* 42:153, 1995.
45. Kasper CA, Clayton HM, Wright AK, et al: The effect of high doses of oxytetracycline on metacarpophalangeal joint kinematics in neonatal foals, *J Am Vet Med Assoc* 207:71, 1995.
46. Peham C, Scheidl M, Licka T: A method of signal processing in motion analysis of the trotting horse, *J Biomech* 29:111, 1995.

47. Bucher HHF, Savelberg HCCM, Schamhardt HC, et al: Head and trunk movement adaptations in horses with experimentally induced for or hind limb lameness, *Equine Vet J* 28:71, 1996.

48. Buchner HHF, Salvelberg HHCM, Schamhardt HC, et al: Limb movement adaptations in horses with experimentally induced fore- or hindlimb lameness, *Equine Vet J* 28:63, 1996.

49. Degueurce C, Pourcelot P, Audigié F, et al: Variability of the limb joint patterns of sound horses at trot, *Equine Vet J Suppl* 23:89, 1997.

50. Galisteo AM, Cano MR, Morales JL, et al: Kinematics in horses at the trot before and after an induced forelimb supporting lameness, *Equine Vet J Suppl* 23:97, 1997.

51. Pourcelot P, Degueurce C, Audigié F, et al: Kinematic analysis of the locomotion symmetry of sound horses at a slow trot, *Equine Vet J Suppl* 23:93, 1997.

52. Pourcelot P, Audigie F, Degueurce C, et al: Kinematic Symmetry Index: a method for quantifying the horse locomotion symmetry using kinematic data, *Vet Res* 28:525, 1997.

53. Uhlir C, Licka T, Kübber P, et al: Compensatory movements of horses with a stance phase lameness, *Equine Vet J Suppl* 23:102, 1997.

54. Clayton HM, Lanovaz JL, Schamhardt HC, et al: Net joint moments and powers in the equine forelimb in the stance phase of the trot, *Equine Vet J* 30:384, 1998.

55. Clayton HM, Theoret CL, Barber SM, et al: Effects of carpal synovectomy on stride kinematics of trotting horses, *Vet Comp Orthop Traumatol* 11:80, 1998.

56. Clayton HM, Lanovaz JL, Schamhardt HC, et al: Rider mass effects on ground reaction forces and fetlock kinematics at the trot, *Equine Vet J Suppl* 30:218, 1999.

57. Lanovaz JL, Clayton HM, Colborne GR, et al: Forelimb kinematics and net joint moments during the swing phase of the trot, *Equine Vet J Suppl* 30:235, 1999.

58. Clayton HM, Scharmhardt HC, Willemen MA, et al: Kinematics and ground reaction forces in horses with superficial digital flexor tendonitis, *Am J Vet Res* 61:191, 2000.

59. Clayton HM, Schamhardt HC, Willemen MA, et al: Net joint moments and joint powers in horses with superficial digital flexor tendinitis, *Am J Vet Res* 61:197, 2000.

60. Audigié F, Pourcelot P, Degueurce C, et al: Kinematic analysis of the symmetry of limb movements in lame trotting horses, *Equine Vet J Suppl*, 33:128, 2001.

61. Clayton HM, Hodson EF, Lanovaz JL, et al: The hind limb in walking horses: 2. Net joint moments and joint powers, *Equine Vet J* 33:44, 2001.

62. Peham C, Licka T, Girtler D, et al: Hindlimb lameness: clinical judgement versus computerized symmetry measurement, *Vet Rec* 148:750, 2001.

63. Audigie F, Pourcelot P, Degueurce C, et al: Fourier analysis of trunk displacements: a method to identify the lame limb in trotting horses, *J Biomech* 35:1173, 2002.

64. Clayton HM, Hoyt DF, Wickler SJ, et al: Hindlimb net joint energies during swing phase as a function of trotting velocity, *Equine Vet J Suppl* 34:363, 2002.

65. Clayton HM, Singleton WH, Lanovaz JL, et al: Sagittal plane kinematics and kinetics of the pastern joint during the stance phase of the trot, *Vet Comp Orthop Traumatol* 15:15, 2002.

66. Khumsap S, Clayton HM, Lanovaz JL, et al: Effect of walking velocity on forelimb kinematics and kinetics, *Equine Vet J Suppl* 34:325, 2002.

67. Lanovaz JL, Khumsap S, Clayton HM, et al: Three dimensional kinematics of the tarsal joint at the trot, *Equine Vet J Suppl* 34:308, 2002.

68. Meershoek LS, Lanovaz JL, Schamhardt HC, et al: Calculated forelimb flexor tendon forces in horses with experimentally induced superficial flexor tendinitis and the influence of heel wedges, *Am J Vet Res* 63:432, 2002.

69. Khumsap S, Lanovaz JL, Rosenstein DS, et al: Effect of induced unilateral synovitis of distal intertarsal and tarsometatarsal joints on sagittal plane kinematics and kinetics of trotting horses, *Am J Vet Res* 64:1491, 2003.

70. Nicodemus MC, Clayton HM: Temporal variables of four-beat, stepping gaits of gaited horses, *Appl Anim Behav Sci* 80:133, 2003.

71. Singleton WH, Clayton HM, Lanovaz JL, et al: Effects of shoeing on forelimb swing phase kinetics of trotting horses, *Vet Comp Orthop Traumatol* 16:16, 2003.

72. Clayton HM, Sha D, Stick JA, et al: Three-dimensional carpal kinematics of trotting horses, *Equine Vet J* 36:671, 2004.

73. Khumsap S, Lanovaz JL, Clayton HM: Three-dimensional kinematic analysis of horses with induced tarsal synovitis, *Equine Vet J* 36:659, 2004.

74. Ramón T, Prades M, Armengou L, et al: Effects of athletic taping of the fetlock on distal limb mechanics, *Equine Vet J* 36:764, 2004.

75. Wickler SJ, Hoyt DF, Clayton HM: The energetic and kinematic consequences of weighting the distal limb, *Equine Vet J* 36:772, 2004.

76. Buchner H: Limb movement pattern in forelimb and hindlimb lameness, *Proc Am Assoc Equine Pract* 51:128, 2005.

77. Bidwell LA, Brown KE, Cordier A, et al: Mepivacaine local anesthetic duration in equine palmar digital nerve blocks, *Equine Vet J* 36:723, 2004.

78. Clayton HM, Sha DH: Body center of mass movement in horses travelling on a circular path, *Equine Vet J Suppl* 36:462, 2006.

79. Dutto DJ, Hoyt DF, Clayton HM, et al: Joint work and power for both the forelimb and hind limb during trotting in the horse, *J Exp Biol* 209:3990, 2004.

80. Gnagey L, Clayton HM, Lanovaz JL: Effect of standing tarsal angle on joint kinematics and kinetics, *Equine Vet J* 38:628, 2006.

81. Christovão FG, Barros RML, Martins CB, et al: Three-dimensional kinematic analysis of head and limb movements of lame and non-lame colts, *Equine Comp Exer Physiol* 4:31, 2007.

82. Buchner HHF, Obermüller S, Scheidl M: Body centre of mass movement in the sound horse, *Vet J* 160:225, 2000.

83. Buchner HHF, Obermüller S, Scheidl M: Load distribution in equine lameness: a centre of mass analysis at the walk and the trot, *Pferdeheilkunde* 19:491, 2003.

84. Pfau T, Robilliard JJ, Weller R, et al: Assessment of mild hindlimb lameness during over ground locomotion using linear discriminant analysis of inertial sensor data, *Equine Vet J* 39:407, 2007.

CHAPTER 23 Arthroscopic Examination

1. McIlwraith CW, Nixon AJ, Wright IM, et al, eds: *Diagnostic and surgical arthroscopy in the horse*, ed 3, Philadelphia, 2005, Mosby Elsevier.

2. Price J, Catriona S, Welsh EM, et al: Preliminary evaluation of a behaviour-based system for assessment of post-operative pain in horses following arthroscopic surgery, *Vet Anaesth Analg* 30:124, 2003.

3. Jenner F, Ross MW, Martin BB, et al: Scapulohumeral osteochondrosis. A retrospective study of 32 horses, *Vet Comp Orthop Traumatol* 21:406, 2008.

4. Watts AE, Nixon AJ: Comparison of arthroscopic approaches and accessible anatomic structures during arthroscopy of the caudal pouches of equine femorotibial joints, *Vet Surg* 35:219, 2006.

5. Kraus BM, Ross MW: Surgical or conservative management of racehorses with sagittal slab fracture of the third carpal bone: 32 racehorses, *J Am Vet Med Assoc* 226:945, 2005.

6. Boening KJ: Instrumentation. In McIlwraith CW, Nixon AJ, Wright IM, et al, eds: *Diagnostic and surgical arthroscopy in the horse*, ed 3, Philadelphia, 2005, Mosby Elsevier.

7. Jansson N: Gas arthroscopy for removal of osteochondral fragments of the palmar/plantar aspect of the metacarpo/metatarsophalangeal joint in horses, *Vet Surg* 34:128, 2005.

8. Edwards RB, Lu Y, Cole BJ, et al: Comparison of radiofrequency treatment and mechanical debridement of fibrillated cartilage in an equine model, *Vet Comp Orthop Traumatol* 21:41, 2008.

9. Walmsley JR, Phillips TJ, Townsend HG: Meniscal tears in horses: an evaluation of clinical signs and arthroscopic treatment of 80 cases, *Equine Vet J* 35:402, 2003.

10. McIlwraith CW: Tearing of the medial palmar intercarpal ligament in the equine midcarpal joint, *Equine Vet J* 24:367, 1992.

11. Phillips TJ, Wright IM: Observations on the anatomy and pathology of the palmar intercarpal ligaments in the middle carpal joints of thoroughbred racehorses, *Equine Vet J* 26:486, 1994.

12. Story MR, Bramlage LR: Arthroscopic debridement of subchondral bone cysts in the distal phalanx of 11 horses (1994-2000), *Equine Vet J* 36:356, 2004.

13. McIlwraith CW, Yovich JV, Martin GS: Arthroscopic surgery for the treatment of osteochondral chip fractures in the equine carpus, *J Am Vet Med Assoc* 191:531, 1987.

14. Elce YA, Richardson DW: Arthroscopic removal of dorsoproximal chip fractures of the proximal phalanx in standing horses, *Vet Surg* 31:195, 2002.

15. Richardson DW: Technique for arthroscopic repair of third carpal bone slab fractures in horses, *J Am Vet Med Assoc* 188:288, 1986.

16. Wallis TW, Goodrich LR, McIlwraith CW, et al: Arthroscopic injection of corticosteroids into the fibrous tissue of subchondral cystic lesions of the medial femoral condyle in horses: a retrospective study of 52 cases (2001-2006), *Equine Vet J* 40:461, 2008.

17. McIlwraith CW, Nixon AJ: Joint resurfacing: attempts at repairing articular cartilage defects. In McIlwraith CW, Trotter GW, eds: *Joint disease in the horse*, New York, 1997, Saunders.

18. Frisbie DD, Trotter GW, Powers BE, et al: Arthroscopic subchondral bone plate microfracture technique augments healing of large chondral defects in the radial carpal bone and medial femoral condyle of horses, *Vet Surg* 28:242, 1999.

19. Frisbie DD, Morisset S, Ho CP, et al: Effects of calcified cartilage on healing of chondral defects treated with microfracture in horses, *Am J Sports Med* 34:1824, 2006.

20. Nixon AJ: Advances in cell-based grafting. Proceedings of the Twenty-Ninth Annual Surgery Forum of the American College of Veterinary Surgeons, Chicago, October 2001.

21. Wilke MM, Nydam DV, Nixon AJ: Enhanced early chondrogenesis in articular defects following arthroscopic mesenchymal stem cell implantation in an equine model, *J Orthop Res* 25:913, 2007.

22. Frisbie DD, Kawcak CE, Werpy NM, et al: Evaluation of bone marrow derived stem cells and adipose derived stromal vascular fraction for treatment of osteoarthritis using an equine experimental model, *Proc Am Assoc Equine Pract* 52:420, 2006.

23. Bodó G, Hangody L, Szabó Z, et al: Arthroscopic autologous osteochondral mosaicplasty for the treatment of a subchondral cystic lesion in the medial femoral condyle in a horse, *Acta Vet Hung* 48:343, 2000.

24. Hurtig MB, Pearce SG, Warren S, et al: Mosaic arthroplasty for resurfacing the equine third carpal bone, *Vet Surg* 30:228, 2001.

25. Hurtig MB, Pearce SG, Radcliffe R, et al: Advances in mosaic arthroplasty. Proceedings of the Twenty-Ninth Annual Surgery Forum of the American College of Veterinary Surgeons, Chicago, October 2001.

26. Bodó G, Hangody L, Modis L, et al: Autologous osteochondral grafting (mosaic arthroplasty) for treatment of subchondral cystic lesions in the equine stifle and fetlock joints, *Vet Surg* 33:588, 2004.

27. Nixon AJ, Fortier LA, Goodrich LR, et al: Arthroscopic reattachment of osteochondritis dissecans lesions using resorbable polydioxanone pins, *Equine Vet J* 36:376, 2004.

CHAPTER 24   Tenoscopy and Bursoscopy

1. McIlwraith CW, Nixon AJ, Wright IM, et al, eds: *Diagnostic and surgical arthroscopy in the horse*, ed 3, Philadelphia, 2005, Mosby Elsevier.

2. Nixon AJ: Endoscopy of the digital flexor tendon sheath in horses, *Vet Surg* 19:266, 1990.

3. Santschi MS, Adams SB, Fessler JF, et al: Treatment of bacterial tarsal tenosynovitis and osteitis of the sustentaculum tali of the calcaneus in five horses, *Equine Vet J* 29:244, 1997.

4. Menon J: Endoscopic carpal tunnel release: preliminary report, *Arthroscopy* 10:31, 1994.

5. Chow JCY: Endoscopic release of the carpal ligament: a new technique for carpal canal syndrome, *Arthroscopy* 5:19, 1989.

6. Chow JCY: The Chow technique for endoscopic release of the carpal ligament for carpal tunnel syndrome: four years of clinical results, *Arthroscopy* 9:301, 1993.

7. Southwood LL, Stashak TS, Fehr JE, et al: Lateral approach for endoscopic removal of solitary osteochondromas from the distal radial metaphysis in three horses, *J Am Vet Med Assoc* 210:1166, 1997.

8. Squire KRE, Adams SB, Widmer WR, et al: Arthroscopic removal of a palmar radial osteochondroma causing carpal canal syndrome in a horse, *J Am Vet Med Assoc* 201:1216, 1992.

9. Cauvin ERJ, Munroe GA, Boyd JS: Endoscopic examination of the carpal flexor tendon sheath in horses, *Equine Vet J* 29:459, 1997.

10. Cauvin ERJ, Tapprest J, Munroe GA, et al: Endoscopic examination of the tarsal sheath of the lateral digital flexor tendon in horses, *Equine Vet J* 31:219, 1999.

11. Booth TM: Lameness associated with the bicipital bursa in an Arab stallion, *Vet Rec* 145:194, 1999.

12. Hago BED: *An anatomical, clinical and experimental study of some synovial tendon sheaths and bursae in the horse, PhD thesis*, London, 1984, Royal Veterinary College.

13. Hay Kraus BL, Kirker-Head CA, Kraus K, et al: Vascular supply of the tendon of the equine deep digital flexor muscle within the digital sheath, *Vet Surg* 24:102, 1995.

14. Leach D, Harland R, Burko B: The anatomy of the carpal tendon sheath of the horse, *J Anat* 133:301, 1981.

15. Redding WR: Ultrasonographic imaging of the structures of the digital flexor tendon sheath, *Comp Cont Educ Pract Vet* 13:1824, 1991.

16. Edinger J, Möbius G, Ferguson J: Comparison of tenoscopic and ultrasonographic methods of examination of the digital flexor tendon sheath in horses, *Vet Comp Orthop Traumatol* 18:209, 2005.

17. Smith MR, Wright IM: Noninfected tenosynovitis of the digital flexor tendon sheath: a retrospective analysis of 76 cases, *Equine Vet J* 38:134, 2006.

18. Wilderjans H, Boussauw B, Madder K, et al: Tenosynovitis of the digital flexor tendon sheath and annular ligament constriction syndrome caused by longitudinal tears in the deep digital flexor tendon: a clinical and surgical report of 17 cases in warmblood horses, *Equine Vet J* 35:270, 2003.

19. Wright IM, McMahon PJ: Tenosynovitis associated with longitudinal tears in the digital flexor tendon in horses: a report of 20 cases, *Equine Vet J* 31:12, 1999.

20. Bertone AL: Infectious tenosynovitis, *Vet Clin North Am Equine Pract* 11:163, 1995.

21. Nixon AJ, Sams AE, Ducharme NG: Endoscopically assisted annular ligament release in horses, *Vet Surg* 22:501, 1993.

22. Barone R: *Anatomie Comparee des Mammiferes domestiques*, ed 3, vol 2, Paris, 1989, Editions Vigot.

23. Nixon AJ: Endoscopic surgery of tendon sheaths (tenoscopy). Proceedings of the Twenty-Eighth Annual Scientific Meeting of the American College of Veterinary Surgeons, San Francisco, 1993.

24. Edwards GB: Changes in the sustentaculum tali associated with distension of the tarsal sheath (thoroughpin), *Equine Vet J* 10:97, 1978.

25. Mettenleiter E, Meier HP, Ueltschi G, et al: Typical presentation of the common tendon sheath of the M. flexor hallucis longus and the M. tibialis caudalis in the horse, *Anat Histol Embryol* 21:246, 1992.

26. Nixon AJ, Schachter BL, Pool RR: Exostoses of the caudal perimeter of the radial physis as a cause of carpal synovial sheath tenosynovitis and lameness in horses: 10 cases (1999-2003), *J Am Vet Med Assoc* 224:264, 2004.

27. Richardson DW: Carpal canal syndrome. In Colahan PT, Mayhew IG, Merrit AM, et al, eds: *Equine medicine and surgery*, Goleta, Calif, 1992, American Veterinary Publications.

28. Dyson SJ, Dik KJ: Miscellaneous conditions of tendons, tendon sheaths, and ligaments, *Vet Clin North Am Equine Pract* 11:315, 1995.

29. Brokken TD: Acute carpal canal injuries in the Thoroughbred, *Proc Am Assoc Equine Pract* 34:389, 1988.

30. Cauvin ERJ, Munroe GA, Boswell J, et al: Gross and ultrasonographic anatomy of the carpal flexor tendon sheath in horses, *Vet Rec* 141:489, 1997.

31. Radue P: Carpal tunnel syndrome due to fracture of the accessory carpal bone, *Vet Clin North Am Equine Pract* 3:8, 1981.

32. Southwood LL, Stashak TS, Kainer RA, et al: Desmotomy of the accessory ligament of the superficial digital flexor tendon in the horse with use of a tenoscopic approach to the carpal sheath, *Vet Surg* 28:99, 1999.

33. Southwood LL, Stashak TS, Kainer RA: Tenoscopic anatomy of the equine carpal flexor synovial sheath, *Vet Surg* 27:150, 1998.

34. Kretzschmar BH, Desjardins MR: Clinical evaluation of 49 tenoscopically assisted superior check ligament desmotomies in 27 horses, *Proc Am Assoc Equine Pract* 47:484, 2001.

35. Textor JA, Nixon AJ, Fortier LA: Tenoscopic release of the equine carpal canal, *Vet Surg* 32:278, 2003.

36. Platt D, Wright IM: Chronic tenosynovitis of the carpal extensor tendon sheaths in 15 horses, *Equine Vet J* 29:11, 1997.

37. Ingle-Fehr J, Baxter GM: Endoscopy of the calcaneal bursa in horses, *Vet Surg* 27:561, 1998.

38. Cauvin E: Unpublished data, 2001.

39. Riggs C, Rice Y, Patteson M, et al: Infection of the intertuberal (bicipital) bursa in seven horses. Proceedings of the

Thirty-Fourth British Equine Veterinary Association Congress, Harrogate, 1995.

40. Adams MN, Turner TA: Endoscopy of the intertubercular bursa in horses, *J Am Vet Med Assoc* 214:221, 1999.

41. Wright IM, Phillips TJ, Walmsley JP: Endoscopy of the navicular bursa: a new technique for the treatment of contaminated and septic bursae, *Equine Vet J* 31:5, 1999.

42. McIlwraith CW, Turner AS: *Equine surgery advanced techniques*, Philadelphia, 1987, Lea & Febiger.

43. Richardson GL, O'Brien TR, Pascoe JR, et al: Puncture wounds of the navicular bursa in 38 horses: a retrospective study, *Vet Surg* 15:156, 1986.

44. Smith MRW, Wright IM, Smith RKW: Endoscopic assessment and treatment of lesions of the deep digital flexor tendon in the navicular bursae of 20 lame horses, *Equine Vet J* 39:18, 2007.

45. Rossignol F, Perrin R: Tenoscopy of the navicular bursa: endoscopic approach and anatomy, *J Equine Vet Sci* 23:258, 2003.

46. Cruz AM, Pharr JW, Bailey JV, et al: Podotrochlear bursa endoscopy in the horse: a cadaver study, *Vet Surg* 30:539, 2001.

CHAPTER 25   Thermography: Use in Equine Lameness

1. Stromberg B: The use of thermography in equine orthopaedics, *J Vet Radiol* 15:94, 1974.

2. Turner TA: Thermography: use in equine lameness. In Ross MW, Dyson SJ, eds: *Diagnosis and management of lameness in the horse*, St Louis, 2003, Elsevier.

3. Eddy AL, Van Hoogmoed LM, Snyder JR: The role of thermography in the management of equine lameness, *Vet J* 162:172, 2001.

4. Turner TA, Purohit RC, Fessler JF: Thermography: a review in equine medicine, *Compend Contin Educ Pract Vet* 8:855, 1986.

5. Mogg KC, Pollitt CC: Hoof and distal limb surface temperature in the normal pony under constant and changing ambient temperatures, *Equine Vet J* 24:134, 1992.

6. Tunley BV, Henson FMD: Reliability and repeatability of thermographic examination and the normal thermographic image of the thoracolumbar region in the horse, *Equine Vet J* 36:306, 2004.

7. Pollitt CC, Davies CT: Equine laminitis: its development coincides with increased sublamellar blood flow, *Equine Vet J Suppl* 26:125, 1998.

8. Bathe AP: Thermography. In Floyd AE, Mansmann RA, eds: *Equine podiatry*, St Louis, 2007, Elsevier.

9. Vaden MF, Purohit RC, McCoy MD, Vaughan JT: Thermography: a technique for subclinical diagnosis of osteoarthritis, *Am J Vet Res* 41:1175, 1980.

10. Turner TA: Hindlimb muscle strain as a cause of lameness in horses, *Proc Am Assoc Equine Pract* 34:281, 1989.

11. Graf von Schweinitz D: Thermographic diagnostics in equine back pain, *Vet Clin North Am Equine Pract* 15:161, 1999.

12. Van Hoogmoed LM, Snyder JR, Allen KA, Waldsmith JD: Use of thermography to detect performance enhancing techniques in horses, *Equine Vet Educ* 12:132, 2000.

CHAPTER 26   The Biomechanics of the Equine Limb and Its Effect on Lameness

1. Biewener A: *Oxford animal biology series*, Oxford, UK, 2003, Oxford University Press.

2. Wainwright SA, Biggs WD, Currey JD, Gosline JM: *Mechanical design in organisms*, Princeton, 1982, Princeton University Press.

3. Wilson AM, van den Bogert AJ, McGuigan MP: Optimisation of the muscle-tendon unit for economical locomotion in cursorial animals. In Herzog W, ed: *Muscle mechanics: from mechanisms to function*, 2002, John Wiley & Sons.

4. Wilson AM, Goodship AE: Exercise-induced hyperthermia as a possible mechanism for tendon degeneration, *J Biomech* 27:899, 1994.

5. Birch HL, Wilson AM, Goodship AE: The effect of exercise-induced localised hyperthermia on tendon cell survival, *J Exp Biol* 200:1703, 1997.

6. McGuigan MP, Wilson AM: The effect of gait and digital flexor muscle activation on limb compliance in the forelimb of the horse (*Equus caballus*), *J Exp Biol* 206:1325, 2003.

7. Ferris DP, Louie M, Farley CT: Running in the real world: adjusting leg stiffness for different surfaces, *Proc Biol Sci* 265:989, 1998.

8. Wilson AM, McGuigan MP, Su A, van Den Bogert AJ: Horses damp the spring in their step, *Nature* 414:895, 2001.

9. Vaughan, LC, Mason, BJE: *A clinico-pathological study of racing accidents in horses. A report of a study on equine fatal accidents on racecourses financed by the Horserace Betting Levy Board*, Dorking, 1975, Adlard and Sons, Bartholomew Press.

10. Douglas JE, Biddick TL, Thomason JJ, Jofriet JC: Stress/strain behaviour of the equine laminar junction, *J Exp Biol* 201:2287, 1998.

11. Riemersma DJ, Schamhardt HC: In vitro mechanical properties of equine tendons in relation to cross-sectional area and collagen content, *Res Vet Sci* 39:263, 1985.

12. Willemen MA, Savelberg HH, Barneveld A: The effect of orthopaedic shoeing on the force exerted by the deep digital flexor tendon on the navicular bone in horses, *Equine Vet J* 31:25, 1999.

13. Eliashar E, McGuigan MP, Wilson AM: Relationship of foot conformation and force applied to the navicular bone of sound horses at the trot, *Equine Vet J* 36:431, 2004.

14. Gustås P, Johnston C, Roepstorff L, Drevemo S: In vivo transmission of impact shock waves in the distal forelimb of the horse, *Equine Vet J Suppl* 33:11, 2001.

15. Benoit P, Barrey E, Regnault JC, Brochet JL: Comparison of the damping effect of different shoeing by the measurement of hoof acceleration, *Acta Anat (Basel)* 146:109, 1993.

16. Gustås P, Johnston C, Roepstorff L, et al: Relationships between fore- and hindlimb ground reaction force and hoof deceleration patterns in trotting horses, *Equine Vet J* 36:737, 2004.

17. Ratzlaff MH, Wilson PD, Hutton DV, Slinker BK: Relationships between hoof-acceleration patterns of galloping horses and dynamic properties of the track, *Am J Vet Res* 66:589, 2005.

18. Chateau H, Robine D, Falala S, et al: Effects of a synthetic all-weather waxed track versus a crushed sand track on 3D accelerations of the front hoof in three horses trotting at high speed. *Equine Vet J* 41:247, 2009.

19. Back W, Schamhardt HC, Hartman W, Barneveld A: Kinematic differences between the distal portions of the fore-limbs and hind limbs of horses at the trot, *Am J Vet Res* 56:1522, 1995.

20. Hjertén G, Drevemo S: Semi-quantitative analysis of hoof-strike in the horse, *J Biomech* 27:997, 1994.

21. Usherwood JR, Wilson AM: Biomechanics: no force limit on greyhound sprint speed, *Nature* 8:438, 2005.

22. Ferrari M: *Dynamic conformation: the influence of conformation on equine locomotion*, PhD thesis, 2009, University of London.

23. Witte TH, Hirst CV, Wilson AM: Effect of speed on stride parameters in racehorses at gallop in field conditions, *J Exp Biol* 209:4389, 2006.

24. Wilson AM, Seelig TJ, Shield RA, Silverman BW: The effect of foot imbalance on point of force application in the horse, *Equine Vet J* 30:540, 1998.

25. Roepstorff L, Johnston C, Drevemo S: In vivo and in vitro heel expansion in relation to shoeing and frog pressure, *Equine Vet J Suppl* 33:54, 2001.

26. Hinterhofer C, Stanek C, Haider H: Finite element analysis (FEA) as a model to predict effects of farriery on the equine hoof, *Equine Vet J Suppl* 33:58, 2001.

27. Hobbs SJ, Mather J, Rolph C, et al: In vitro measurement of internal hoof strain, *Equine Vet J* 36:683, 2004.

28. Jansen MO, van den Bogert AJ, Riemersma DJ, Schamhardt HC: In vivo tendon forces in the forelimb of ponies at the walk, validated by ground reaction force measurements, *Acta Anat (Basel)* 146:162,1993.

29. Platt D, Wilson AM, Timbs A, et al: Novel force transducer for the measurement of tendon force in vivo, *J Biomech* 27:1489, 1994.

30. Riemersma DJ, van den Bogert AJ, Jansen MO, Schamhardt HC: Influence of shoeing on ground reaction forces and tendon strains in the forelimbs of ponies, *Equine Vet J* 28:126, 1996.

31. Riemersma DJ, van den Bogert AJ, Jansen MO, Schamhardt HC: Tendon strain in the forelimbs as a function of gait and ground characteristics and in vitro limb loading in ponies, *Equine Vet J* 28:133, 1996.

32. Meershoek LS, Lanovaz JL, Schamhardt HC, Clayton HM: Calculated forelimb flexor tendon forces in horses with experimentally induced superficial digital flexor tendinitis and the effects of application of heel wedges, *Am J Vet Res* 63:432, 2002.

33. Stephens PR, Nunamaker DM, Butterweck DM: Application of a Hall-effect

transducer for measurement of tendon strains in horses, *Am J Vet Res* 50:1089, 1989.

34. Meershoek LS, Schamhardt HC, Roepstorff L, Johnston C: Forelimb tendon loading during jump landings and the influence of fence height, *Equine Vet J Suppl* 33:6, 2001.

35. Bailey CJ, Reid SW, Hodgson DR, et al: Flat, hurdle and steeple racing: risk factors for musculoskeletal injury, *Equine Vet J* 30:498, 1998.

36. Williams RB, Harkins LS, Hammond CJ, Wood JL: Racehorse injuries, clinical problems and fatalities recorded on British racecourses from flat racing and National Hunt racing during 1996, 1997 and 1998, *Equine Vet J* 33:478, 2001.

37. Crevier-Denoix N, Pourcelot P, Ravary B, et al: Influence of track surface on the equine superficial digital flexor tendon loading in two horses at high speed trot, *Equine Vet J Suppl* 41:257, 2009.

38. Davies HM, McCarthy RN, Jeffcott LB: Surface strain on the dorsal metacarpus of thoroughbreds at different speeds and gaits, *Acta Anat (Basel)* 146:148, 1993.

39. Davies HM: Estimating peak strains associated with fast exercise in thoroughbred racehorses, *Equine Vet J Suppl* 36:383, 2006.

40. Nunamaker DM, Butterweck DM, Provost MT: Fatigue fractures in thoroughbred racehorses: relationships with age, peak bone strain, and training, *J Orthop Res* 8:604, 1990.

41. Pratt GW: Model for injury to the foreleg of the Thoroughbred racehorse, *Equine Vet J Suppl* 23:30, 1997.

42. Schryver HF: Bending properties of cortical bone of the horse, *Am J Vet Res* 39:25, 1978.

43. Cheney JA, Shen CK, Wheat JD: Relationship of racetrack surface to lameness in the thoroughbred racehorse, *Am J Vet Res* 34:1285, 1973.

44. Currey J: *The mechanical adaptations of bone*, Princeton, New Jersey, 1984, Princeton University Press.

45. Den Hartog SM, Back, W, Brommer H, van Weeren PR: In vitro evaluation of metacarpophalangeal joint loading during simulated walk, *Equine Vet J Suppl* 41:214, 2009.

46. Brommer H, Brama PA, Barneveld A, van Weeren PR: Differences in the topographical distribution of articular cartilage degeneration between equine metacarpo- and metatarsophalangeal joints, *Equine Vet J* 36:506, 2004.

47. Van Heel MC, Moleman M, Barneveld A, et al: Changes in location of centre of pressure and hoof-unrollment pattern in relation to an 8-week shoeing interval in the horse, *Equine Vet J* 37:536, 2005.

48. Moleman M, van Heel MC, van Weeren PR, Back W: Hoof growth between two shoeing sessions leads to a substantial increase of the moment about the distal, but not the proximal, interphalangeal joint, *Equine Vet J* 38:170, 2006.

49. Van Heel MC, van Weeren PR, Back W: Compensation for changes in hoof conformation between shoeing sessions through the adaptation of angular kinematics of the distal segments of the limbs of horses, *Am J Vet Res* 67:1199, 2006.

50. Eliashar E, McGuigan MP, Rogers KA, Wilson AM: A comparison of three horse-shoeing styles on the kinetics of breakover in sound horses, *Equine Vet J* 34:184, 2002.

51. Viitanen MJ, Wilson AM, McGuigan HR, et al: Effect of foot balance on the intra-articular pressure in the distal interphalangeal joint in vitro, *Equine Vet J* 35:184, 2003.

52. Day P, McGuigan M, Weller R, et al: *A structural approach to treating collapsed heels*, Proceedings of the British Equine Veterinary Association Annual Congress, Birmingham, UK, 2003, p 304.

53. Willemen MA, Savelberg HH, Bruin G, Barneveld A: The effect of toe weights on linear and temporal stride characteristics of standardbred trotters, *Vet Q* 16(Suppl 2):S97, 1994.

54. Roepstorff L, Johnston C, Drevemo S: The effect of shoeing on kinetics and kinematics during the stance phase, *Equine Vet J Suppl* 30:279, 1999.

55. Hood DM, Taylor D, Wagner IP: Effects of ground surface deformability, trimming, and shoeing on quasistatic hoof loading patterns in horses, *Am J Vet Res* 62:895, 2001.

56. Benoit P, Barrey E, Regnault JC, Brochet JL: Comparison of the damping effect of different shoeing by the measurement of hoof acceleration, *Acta Anat (Basel)* 146:109, 1993.

57. Dyhre-Poulsen P, Smedegaard HH, Roed J, Korsgaard E: Equine hoof function investigated by pressure transducers inside the hoof and accelerometers mounted on the first phalanx, *Equine Vet J* 26:362, 1994.

58. Pardoe CH, McGuigan MP, Rogers KM, et al: The effect of shoe material on the kinetics and kinematics of foot slip at impact on concrete, *Equine Vet J Suppl* 33:70, 2001.

59. Wilson AM, McGuigan MP, Fouracre L, MacMahon L: The force and contact stress on the navicular bone during trot locomotion in sound horses and horses with navicular disease, *Equine Vet J* 33:159, 2001.

60. McGuigan MP, Wilson AM: The effect of bilateral palmar digital nerve analgesia on the compressive force experienced by the navicular bone in horses with navicular disease, *Equine Vet J* 33:166, 2001.

61. McGuigan MP, Walsh TC, Pardoe CH, et al: Deep digital flexor tendon force and digital mechanics in normal ponies and ponies with rotation of the distal phalanx as a sequel to laminitis, *Equine Vet J* 37:161, 2005.

62. Wilson AM: Unpublished data.

CHAPTER 27   The Foot and Shoeing

Foot Balance, Conformation, and Lameness

1. Hickman J, Humphrey M: *Hickman's farriery*, ed 2, London, 1988, JA Allen.

2. Hertch B, Hoppner S, Dallmer H: *The hoof and how to protect it without nails*, Salzhausen-Putensen, 1996, Hellmuth Kallmer.

3. Curtis S: *Farriery: foal to racehorse*, Newmarket, 1999, R & W Publications.

4. Butler D: *The principles of horse shoeing II*, ed 2, Maryville, Mo, 1985, Doug Butler Publisher.

5. Ritmeester AM, Blevins WE, Ferguson DW, Adams SB: Digital perfusion, evaluated scintigraphically, and hoof wall growth in horses with chronic laminitis treated with egg bar–heart bar shoeing and coronary grooving, *Equine Vet J Suppl* 26:111, 1998.

6. Kainer RA: Clinical anatomy of the equine foot, *Vet Clin North Am Equine Pract* 5:1, 1989.

7. Douglas JE, Mittal C, Thomason JJ, Jofriet JC: The modulus of elasticity of equine hoof wall: implications for the mechanical function of the hoof, *J Exp Biol* 199:1829, 1996.

8. Thomason JJ, Biewener AA, Bertram JEA: Surface strain on the equine hoof wall in vivo: implications for the material design and functional morphology of the wall, *J Exp Biol* 166:145, 1992.

9. Kasapi MA, Gosline JM: Strain-rate–dependent mechanical properties of the equine hoof wall, *J Exp Biol* 199:1133, 1996.

10. Landeau LJ, Barrett DJ, Batterman SC: Mechanical properties of equine hooves, *Am J Vet Res* 44:100, 1983.

11. Bertram JE, Gosline JM: Fracture toughness design in horse hoof keratin, *J Exp Biol* 125:29, 1986.

12. Douglas JE, Biddick TL, Thomason JJ: Stress/strain behaviour of the equine laminar junction, *J Exp Biol* 201:2287, 1998.

13. Douglas JE, Thomason JJ: Shape, orientation and spacing of the primary epidermal laminae in the hooves of neonatal and adult horses (*Equus caballus*), *Cells Tissues Organs* 166:304, 2000.

14. Ovnicek G, Erfle JB, Peters DF: Wild horse hoof patterns offer a formula for preventing and treating lameness, *Proc Am Assoc Equine Pract* 41:258, 1995.

15. Hood DM: Effects of ground surface on solar load distribution, *Proc Am Assoc Equine Pract* 43:360, 1997.

16. Clayton HM: Effects of hoof angle on locomotion and limb loading. In White NA, Moore JN, eds: *Current techniques in equine surgery and lameness*, Philadelphia, 1998, Saunders.

17. Ratzlaff MH, Wilson P, Hyde M, et al: Relationship between locomotor forces, hoof position and joint motion during the support phase of the stride of galloping horses, *Acta Anat (Basel)* 143:200, 1993.

18. Merkens HW, Schamhardt HC: Relationships between ground reaction force patterns and kinematics in the walking and trotting horse, *Equine Vet J Suppl* 17:67, 1994.

19. Balch OK: *The effects of changes in hoof angle, mediolateral balance, and toe length on kinetic and temporal parameters of horses walking, trotting and cantering on a high-speed treadmill*, PhD dissertation, Washington State University, 1993.

20. van Heel MC, Barneveld A, van Weeren PR, Back W: Dynamic pressure measurements for the detailed study of hoof balance: the effect of trimming, *Equine Vet J* 36:778, 2004.

21. Back W, Schamhardt HC, Harman W, Barneveld A: Kinematic differences between the distal portions of the

forelimbs and hind limbs of horses at the trot, *Am J Vet Res* 56:1522, 1995.

22. Clayton HM: The effect of an acute hoof wall angulation on the stride kinematics of trotting horses, *Equine Vet J Suppl* 9:86, 1990.

23. Lanovaz JL, Clayton HM, Watson LG: In vitro attenuation of impact shock in equine digits, *Equine Vet J Suppl* 26:96, 1998.

24. Willemen MA, Jacobs MW, Schamhardt HC: In vitro transmission and attenuation of impact vibrations in the distal forelimb, *Equine Vet J Suppl* 30:245, 1999.

25. Dyhre-Poulsen P, Smedegaard HH, Roed J, Korsgaard E: Equine hoof function investigated by pressure transducers inside the hoof and accelerometers mounted on the first phalanx, *Equine Vet J* 26:362, 1994.

26. Merkens, HW, Schamhardt HC, Hartman W, Kersjes AW: Ground reaction force patterns of Dutch Warmblood horses at normal walk, *Equine Vet J* 18:207, 1986.

27. Merkens HW, Schamhardt HC, Van Osch GJ, Van den Bogert AJ: Ground reaction force patterns of Dutch warmblood horses at normal trot, *Equine Vet J* 25:134, 1993.

28. Barrey E: Investigation of the vertical hoof force distribution in the equine forelimb with an instrumented horseboot, *Equine Vet J Suppl* 9:35, 1990.

29. Clayton HM, Lanovaz JL, Schamhardt HC, et al: Net joint moments and powers in the equine forelimb during the stance phase of the trot, *Equine Vet J* 30:384, 1998.

30. Schryver HF, Bartel DL, Langrana N, Lowe JE: Locomotion in the horse: kinematics and external and internal forces in the normal equine digit in the walk and trot, *Am J Vet Res* 39:1728, 1978.

31. Jansen MO, van den Bogert AJ, Riemersma DJ, Schamhardt HC: In vivo tendon forces in the forelimb of ponies at the walk, validated by ground reaction force measurements, *Acta Anat (Basel)* 146:162, 1993.

32. Riemersma DJ, van den Bogert AJ, Jansen MO, Schamhardt HC: Influence of shoeing on ground reaction forces and tendon strains in the forelimbs of ponies, *Equine Vet J* 28:126, 1996.

33. Johnston C, Roepstorff L, Drevemo S, Ronéus N: Kinematics of the distal forelimb during the stance phase in the fast trotting Standardbred, *Equine Vet J Suppl* 18:170, 1995.

34. Johnston C, Roepstorff L, Devemo S, Kallings P: Kinematics of the distal hindlimb during stance phase in the fast trotting standardbred, *Equine Vet J* 28:263, 1996.

35. Riemersma DJ, van den Bogert AJ, Janson MO, Schamhardt HC: Tendon strain in the forelimbs as a function of gait and ground characteristics and in vitro limb loading in ponies, *Equine Vet J* 28:133, 1996.

36. Dejardin LM, Arnoczky SP, Cloud GL: A method for determination of equine hoof strain patterns using photoelasticity: an in vitro study, *Equine Vet J* 31:232, 1999.

37. (Fischerleitner TF cited by) Kainer RA: Clinical anatomy of the equine foot, *Vet Clin North Am Equine Pract* 5:1, 1989.

38. Thomason JJ: The hoof as a smart structure: is it smarter than us? In Floyd AE, Mansmann RA, eds: *Equine podiatry*, Philadelphia, 2007, Saunders.

39. Colles CM: The relationship of frog pressure to heel expansion, *Equine Vet J* 21:13, 1989.

40. Roepstroff L, Johnston C, Drevemo S: In vivo and in vitro heel expansion in relation to shoeing and frog pressure, *Equine Vet J Suppl* 33:54, 2001.

41. Ratzlaff MH, Shindell RM, DeBowes RM: Changes in digital venous pressures of horses moving at the walk and trot, *Am J Vet Res* 46:1545, 1985.

42. Bowker RM, van Wulfen KK, Springer SE, Linder KE: Functional anatomy of the cartilage of the distal phalanx and digital cushion in the equine foot and a hemodynamic flow hypothesis of energy dissipation, *Am J Vet Res* 59:961, 1998.

43. Denoix JM: Functional anatomy of the equine interphalangeal joints, *Proc Am Assoc Equine Pract* 9:174, 1999.

44. Willemen MA, Savelberg HH, Barneveld A: The effect of orthopaedic shoeing on the force exerted by the deep digital flexor tendon on the navicular bone in horses, *Equine Vet J* 31:25, 1999.

45. Back W, Schamhardt HC, Savelberg HH, et al: How the horse moves. I. Significance of graphical representations of equine forelimb kinematics, *Equine Vet J* 27:31, 1995.

46. Leach DH, Drevemo S: Velocity-dependent changes in stride frequency and length of trotters on a treadmill, *Equine Exerc Physiol* 3:136, 1991.

47. Holmstrom M, Fredricson I, Drevemo S: Biokinematic differences between horses judged as good and poor at the trot, *Equine Vet J Suppl* 17:51, 1994.

48. Barrey E, Auvinet B, Courouce A: Gait evaluation of race trotters using an accelerometric device, *Equine Vet J Suppl* 18:156, 1995.

49. Barrey E, Landjerit B, Wolter R: Shock and vibration during the hoof impact on different track surfaces, *Equine Exerc Physiol* 3:97, 1991.

50. Drevemo S, Hjerten G: Evaluation of a shock absorbing woodchip layer on a harness racetrack, *Equine Exerc Physiol* 3:107, 1991.

51. Cheney JA, Shen CK, Wheat JD: Relationship of racetrack surface to lameness in the Thoroughbred racehorse, *Am J Vet Res* 34:1285, 1973.

52. Buchner HH, Savelberg HH, Schamhardt HC et al: Kinematics of treadmill versus overground locomotion in horses, *Vet Q* 16(Suppl 2):S87, 1994.

53. Balch O, White K, Butler D: Factors involved in the balancing of equine hooves, *J Am Vet Med Assoc* 198:1980, 1991.

54. Jackson J: *The natural horse*, Flagstaff, Ariz, 1992, Northland Publishing.

55. Turner TA: The use of hoof measurements for the objective assessment of hoof balance, *Proc Am Assoc Equine Pract* 38:389, 1992.

56. Russel W: *Scientific horseshoeing*, Cincinnati, 1901, Robert Clarke.

57. Williams G, Deacon M: *No foot, no horse*, Buckingham, 1999, Kenilworth.

58. Cripps PJ, Eustace RA: Radiological measurements from the feet of normal horses with relevance to laminitis, *Equine Vet J* 31:427, 1999.

59. O'Brien TR, Baker TW: Distal extremity examination: how to perform the radiographic examination and interpret the radiographs, *Proc Am Assoc Equine Pract* 32:553, 1986.

60. Linford RL, O'Brien TR, Trout DR: Qualitative and morphometric radiographic findings in the distal phalanx and digital soft tissues of sound Thoroughbred racehorses, *Am J Vet Res* 54:38, 1993.

61. Butler JA, Colles CM, Dyson SJ: *Clinical radiology of the horse*, ed 3, Oxford, 2008, Wiley-Blackwell.

62. Kane AJ, Stover SM, Gardner IA, et al: Hoof size, shape, and balance as possible risk factors for catastrophic musculoskeletal injury of Thoroughbred racehorses, *Am J Vet Res* 59:1545, 1998.

63. Stashak TS: *Adams' lameness in horses*, ed 4, Philadelphia, 1987, Lea & Febiger.

64. Young J: Hoof balance: methods and assessment. In White NA, Moore JN, eds: *Current techniques in equine surgery and lameness*, Philadelphia, 1998, Saunders.

65. Page B: How to mark the foot for radiography, *Proc Am Assoc Equine Pract* 45:148, 1999.

66. Moyer W, Anderson JP: Lameness caused by improper shoeing, *J Am Vet Med Assoc* 166:47, 1975.

67. Colahan P, Leach D, Muir G: Center of pressure location of the hoof with and without hoof wedges, *Equine Exerc Physiol* 3:113, 1991.

68. Firth EC, Schamhardt HC, Hartman W: Measurements of bone strain in foals with altered foot balance, *Am J Vet Res* 49:261, 1988.

69. Caudron I, Grulke S, Farnir F, et al: In-shoe foot force sensor to assess hoof balance determined by radiographic method in ponies trotting on a treadmill, *Vet Q* 20:131, 1998.

70. Wilson AM, Seelig TJ, Shield RA, Silverman BW: The effect of foot imbalance on point of force application in the horse, *Equine Vet J* 30:540, 1998.

71. Allen N, Butler D: Effect of hoof balance on hoof capsule and coffin bone, *Am Farriers J* 22:28, 1996.

72. van Heel MC, Moleman M, Barneveld A, et al: Changes in location of centre of pressure and hoof-unrollment pattern in relation to an 8-week shoeing interval in the horse, *Equine Vet J*, 37:536, 2005.

73. Peel JA, Peel MB, Davies HM: The effect of gallop training on hoof angle in Thoroughbred racehorses, *Equine Vet J Suppl* 36:431, 2006

74. Bushe T, Turner TA, Poulos P, et al: The effect of hoof angle on coffin, pastern and fetlock joint angles, *Proc Am Assoc Equine Pract* 33:729, 1987.

75. Crevier-Denoix N, Roosen C, Dardillat C, et al: Effects of heel and toe elevation upon the digital joint angles in the standing horse, *Equine Vet J Suppl* 33:74, 2001.

76. Vitanen MJ, Wilson AM, McGuigan HR, et al: Effect of foot balance on the intraarticular pressure in the distal interphalangeal joint in vitro, *Equine Vet J* 35:184, 2003.

77. Thompson KN, Cheung TK, Silverman M: The effect of toe angle on tendon, ligament and hoof wall strains in vitro, *J Equine Vet Sci* 13:651, 1993.
78. Lochner FK, Milne DW, Mills EJ, Groom JJ: In vivo and in vitro measurement of tendon strain in the horse, *Am J Vet Res* 41:1929, 1980.
79. Chateau H, Degueurce C, Denoix JM: Three-dimensional kinematics of the distal forelimb in horses trotting on a treadmill and effects of elevation of heel and toe, *Equine Vet J* 38:164, 2006.
80. Clayton HM: The effect of an acute angulation of the hind hooves on diagonal synchrony of trotting horses, *Equine Vet J Suppl* 9:91, 1990.
81. Balch O, Clayton HM, Lanovaz JL: Weight and length induced changes in limb kinematics in trotting horses, *Proc Am Assoc Equine Pract* 42:218, 1996.
82. Balch O, Clayton HM, Lanovaz JL: Effects of increasing hoof length on limb kinematics of trotting horses, *Proc Am Assoc Equine Pract* 40:43, 1994.
83. Page BT, Hagan TL: Breakover of the hoof and its effect on structures and forces within the foot, *J Equine Vet Sci* 22:258, 2002.
84. Thomason JJ: Variation in surface strain on the equine hoof wall at the midstep with shoeing, gait, substrate, direction of travel, and hoof shape, *Equine Vet J Suppl* 26:86, 1998.
85. Glade MJ, Solzman RA: Effects of toe angle on hoof growth and contraction in the horse, *J Equine Vet Sci* 5:45, 1985.
86. Moyer W, Anderson JP: Sheared heels: diagnosis and treatment, *J Am Vet Med Assoc* 166:53, 1975.
87. Page B, Anderson GF: Diagonal imbalance of the equine foot: a cause of lameness, *Proc Am Assoc Equine Pract* 38:413, 1992.
88. Snow VE, Birdsall DP: Specific parameters used to evaluate hoof balance and support, *Proc Am Assoc Equine Pract* 36: 299, 1990.
89. Caudron I, Grulke S, Farnir F, et al: Radiographic assessment of equine interphalangeal joints asymmetry: articular impact of phalangeal rotations. Part I, *Zentralbl Veterinarmed A* 45:319, 1998.
90. Caudron I, Grulke S, Farnir F, et al: Radiographic assessment of equine interphalangeal joints asymmetry: articular impact of asymmetric bearings. Part II, *Zentralbl Veterinarmed A* 45:327, 1998.
91. Caudron I, Miesson M, Grulke S, et al: Clinical and radiological assessment of corrective trimming in horses, *J Equine Vet Sci* 17:375, 1997.
92. Eliashar E, McGuigan MP, Wilson AM: Relationship of foot conformation and force applied to the navicular bone of sound horses at the trot, *Equine Vet J* 36:431, 2004.
93. O'Grady SO, Watson E: How to glue on therapeutic shoes, *Proc Am Assoc Equine Pract* 45:115, 1999.
94. Sigafoos R: Composite reconstruction of equine underrun heels, *Proc Am Assoc Equine Pract* 37:673, 1991.

Horseshoes and Shoeing
1. Willemen MA, Savelberg HH, Bruin G, Barneveld A: The effect of toe weights on linear and temporal stride characteristics of standardbred trotters, *Vet Q* 16(Suppl 2):S97, 1994.
2. Chateau C, Deguerce C, Denoix JM: Effects of egg-bar shoes on the 3-dimensional kinematics of the distal forelimb in horses walking on a sand track, *Equine Vet J Suppl* 36:377, 2006
3. Willemen MA, Savelberg HH, Barneveld A: The effect of orthopaedic shoeing on the force exerted by the deep digital flexor tendon on the navicular bone in horses, *Equine Vet J* 31:25, 1999.
4. Benoit P, Barrey E, Regnault JC, Brochet JL: Comparison of the damping effect of different shoeing by the measurement of hoof acceleration, *Acta Anat (Basel)* 146:109, 1993.
5. Gustås P, Johnston C, Roepstorff L, Drevemo S: In vivo transmission of impact shock waves in the distal forelimb of the horse, *Equine Vet J Suppl* 33:11, 2001.
6. Pardoe CH, McGuigan MP, Rogers KM, et al: The effect of shoe material on the kinetics and kinematics of shoe slip at impact on concrete, *Equine Vet J Suppl* 33:70, 2001.
7. Balch O, Clayton HM, Lanovaz JL: Weight and length induced changes in limb kinematics in trotting horses, *Proc Am Assoc Equine Pract* 42:218, 1996.
8. Clayton HM: The effect of an acute hoof wall angulation on the stride kinematics of trotting horses, *Equine Vet J Suppl* 9:86, 1990.
9. Clayton HM, Sigafoos R, Curle RD: Effect of three shoe types on the duration of breakover in sound trotting horses, *J Equine Vet Sci* 11:129, 1991.
10. Willemen MA, Savelberg HH, Jacobs MW, Barneveld A: Biomechanical effects of rocker-toed shoes in sound horses, *Vet Q* 18:S75, 1996.
11. van Heel MC, van Weeren PR, Back W: Shoeing sound Warmblood horses with a rolled toe optimizes hoof-unrollment and lowers peak loading during breakover, *Equine Vet J* 38:258, 2006.
12. Willemen MA, Savelberg HH, Barneveld A: The improvements of the gait quality of sound trotting Warmblood horses by normal shoeing and its effect on the load on the lower forelimb, *Livestock Prod Sci* 52:145, 1997.
13. Clayton HM: The effect of an acute angulation of the hind hooves on diagonal synchrony of trotting horses, *Equine Vet J Suppl* 9:91, 1990.
14. Roepstorff L, Johnston C, Drevemo S: The effect of shoeing on kinetics and kinematics during the stance phase, *Equine Vet J Suppl* 30:279, 1999.
15. Colles CM: A technique for assessing hoof function in the horse, *Equine Vet J* 21:17, 1989.
16. Dyhre-Poulsen P, Smedegaard HH, Roed J, Korsgaard E: Equine hoof function investigated by pressure transducers inside the hoof and accelerometers mounted on the first phalanx, *Equine Vet J* 26:362, 1994.
17. Willemen MA, Jacobs MW, Schamhardt HC: In vitro transmission and attenuation of impact vibrations in the distal forelimb, *Equine Vet J Suppl* 30:245, 1999.
18. Thomason JJ: Variation in surface strain on the equine hoof wall at the midstep with shoeing, gait, substrate, direction of travel, and hoof shape, *Equine Vet J Suppl* 26:86, 1998.
19. Wilson AM, Seelig TJ, Shield RA, Silverman BW: The effect of foot imbalance on point of force application in the horse, *Equine Vet J* 30:540, 1998.
20. Hertch B, Hoppner S, Dallmer H: *The hoof and how to protect it without nails*, Salzhausen-Putensen, 1996, Hellmuth Kallmer.
21. van Heel MC, Moleman M, Barneveld A, et al: Changes in location of centre of pressure and hoof-unrollment pattern in relation to an 8-week shoeing interval in the horse, *Equine Vet J* 37:536, 2005.
22. Allen N, Butler D: Effect of hoof balance on hoof capsule and coffin bone, *Am Farriers J* 22:28, 1996.
23. Moyer W, Anderson JP: Lameness caused by improper shoeing, *J Am Vet Med Assoc* 166:47, 1975.

Additional Reading
1. Butler D, Butler J: *The principles of horseshoeing III*, Crawford, Nebr, 2004, Doug Butler Enterprises.
2. Curtis S: *Farriery: foal to racehorse*, Newmarket, 1999, R & W Publications.
3. Hickman J, Humphrey M: *Hickman's farriery*, ed 2, London, 1988, JA Allen.

Natural Balance Trimming and Shoeing
1. Ovnicek G: Measurements of the sole thickness relative to the third phalanx after the dissection of nine balanced and un-balanced hooves, unpublished data, 1999.
2. Duckett D: External reference points of the equine hoof, self-published paper, 1988.

Hoof Reconstruction Materials and Glue-On Shoes
1. Reilly PT, Reilly DA, Orsini JA: The long-term results of glue-on shoes on dorsal hoof wall distortion, *J Equine Vet Sci* 29:115, 2009.

CHAPTER 28   Trauma to the Sole and Wall

1. Emery L, Miller J, Vanhoosen NV: Guidelines for shoeing and hoof care. In Emery L, ed: *Horseshoeing theory and hoof care*, Philadelphia, 1977, Lea & Febiger.
2. Moyer W: Role of corrective shoeing in prevention and correction of musculoskeletal disorders in the horse, *Calif Vet* 18:18, 1982.
3. Moyer W: Corrective shoeing, *Vet Clin North Am Large Anim Pract* 2:3, 1980.
4. Moyer W, Anderson JP: Lameness caused by improper shoeing, *J Am Vet Med Assoc* 47:166, 1975.
5. Bergman GA: Foot bruising-pads or not, *Am Farrier J* 10:341, 1984.
6. Stashak TS: *Adams' lameness in horses*, ed 4, Philadelphia, 1984, Lea & Febiger.
7. Moyer W: Examination of the musculoskeletal system. In Colahan PT, Merritt AM, Mayhew IG, Moore JN, eds: *Equine medicine and surgery*, ed 5, Philadelphia, 1999, Mosby.
8. DeBowes RM, Yovich JV: Penetrating wounds, abscesses, gravel, and bruising of the equine foot, *Vet Clin North Am Equine Pract* 5:179, 1989.
9. Kinns J, Mair T: Use of magnetic resonance imaging to assess soft tissue

damage in the foot following penetrating injury in 3 horses, *Equine Vet Educ* 17:69, 2005.

10. Boado A, Kristoffersen M, Dyson S, Murray R: Use of nuclear scintigraphy and magnetic resonance imaging to diagnose chronic penetrating wounds in the equine foot, *Equine Vet Educ* 17:62, 2005.

11. Kristoffersen M, Dyson S, Murray R, et al: Magnetic resonance imaging and scintigraphic findings in 5 horses with obscure foot lameness associated with penetrating injuries, *Proc Am Assoc Equine Pract* 50:320, 2005.

12. Honnas CM, Peloso JG, Carter GK, et al: Diagnosing and treating septic conditions of the equine foot, *Vet Med* 10:1060, 1994.

13. Honnas CM: Standing surgical procedures of the foot, *Vet Clin North Am Equine Pract* 7:695, 1991.

14. Richardson GL, O'Brien TR, Pascoe JR, Meagher DM: Puncture wounds of the navicular bursa in 38 horses: a retrospective study, *Vet Surg* 15:156, 1986.

15. Gaughan EM: Surgical treatment of septic pedal osteitis in horses: nine cases (1980-1987), *J Am Vet Med Assoc* 195:1131, 1989.

16. Steckel RR, Fessler JF, Huston LC: Deep puncture wounds of the equine hoof: a review of 50 cases, *Proc Am Assoc Equine Pract* 35:167, 1989.

17. McIlwraith CW, Turner AS: *Equine surgery: advanced techniques*, Philadelphia, 1987, Lea & Febiger.

18. Wright IM, Phillips TJ, Walmsley JP: Endoscopy of the navicular bursa: a new technique for the treatment of contaminated and septic bursae, *Equine Vet J* 31:5, 1999.

19. Moyer W: Diseases of the hoof, distal phalanx, and associated structures. In Colahan PT, Myhew IG, Merritt AM, Moore JN, eds: *Equine medicine and surgery*, ed 5, Philadelphia, 1999, Mosby.

20. Honnas CM: Standing surgical procedures of the foot, *Vet Clin North Am Equine Pract* 7:695, 1991.

21. Janicek J, Dabareiner RM, Honnas CM, Crabill MA: Heel bulb lacerations in horses: 101 cases (1988-1994), *J Am Vet Med Assoc* 226:418, 2005.

22. Stashak TS: Wound management and reconstructive surgery of problems associated with the distal limb. In TS Stashak, ed: *Equine wound management*, Philadelphia, 1991, Lea & Febiger.

23. O'Grady SE, Madison JB: How to treat equine canker, *Proc Am Assoc Equine Pract* 50:202, 2004.

CHAPTER 29 Functional Anatomy of the Palmar Aspect of the Foot

1. Sack WO: *Rooney's guide to the dissection of the horse*, Ithaca, NY, 1977, Veterinary Textbooks.

2. Kainer RA: Functional anatomy of equine locomotor organs. In Stashak TS: *Adams' lameness in horses*, ed 4, Philadelphia, 1987, Lea & Febiger.

3. Getty R: Equine osteology. In Getty R, ed: *Sisson and Grossman's the anatomy of the domestic animals*, ed 5, Philadelphia, 1975, Saunders.

4. Nickel R, Schummer A, Seiferle E, et al, eds: *The locomotor system of the domestic mammals*, Berlin, 1986, Verlag Paul Parey.

5. Bowker RM, Van Wulfen KK, Springer SE, Linder KE: Functional anatomy of the cartilage of the distal phalanx and digital cushion in the equine foot and a hemodynamic flow hypothesis of energy dissipation, *Am J Vet Res* 59:961,1998.

6. Schummer A, Wilkens H, Vollmerhaus B, et al: Blood vessels of the digital organ of the horse. In Perry P, ed: *The circulatory system, the skin and the cutaneous organs of the domestic mammals*, Berlin, 1981, Springer-Verlag.

7. Schummer A: Blutgefabe und zirkulationsverhaltnisse im zehenendorgan des pferdes, *Morph Jb* 91:568, 1951.

8. Ghoshal NG: Equine heart and arteries. In Getty R, editor: *Sisson and Grossman's the anatomy of the domestic animals*, ed 5, Philadelphia, 1975, Saunders.

9. Dyhre-Poulsen P, Smedgaard HH, Roed J, Korsgaard E: Equine hoof function investigated by pressure transducers inside the hoof and accelerometers mounted on the first phalanx, *Equine Vet J* 26:362, 1994.

10. Van Wulfen KK, Bowker RM: Microanatomic characteristics of the insertion of the distal sesamoidean impar ligament and deep digital flexor tendon on the distal phalanx in healthy feet obtained from horses, *Am J Vet Res* 63:215, 2002.

11. Bowker RM, Atkinson PJ, Atkinson TS, Haut RC: Effect of contact stress in bones of the distal interphalangeal joint on microscopic changes in articular cartilage and ligaments, *Am J Vet Res* 62:414, 2001.

12. Van Wulfen KK, Bowker RM: Evaluation of tachykinins and their receptors to determine sensory innervation in the dorsal hoof wall and insertion of the distal sesamoidean impar ligament and deep digital flexor tendon on the distal phalanx in healthy feet of horses, *Am J Vet Res* 63:222, 2002.

13. Bowker RM, Linder K, Van Wulfen KK, Sonea IM: Anatomy of the distal interphalangeal joint of the mature horse: relationships with the navicular suspensory ligaments, sensory nerves and neurovascular bundle, *Equine Vet J* 29:126, 1997.

14. Bowker RM, Dobson H: A contrast computed tomographic study of the distal interphalangeal joint and the navicular bursa in the horse. Unpublished data, 2002.

15. Molyneux GS, Haller CJ, Mogg K, Pollitt CC: The structure, innervation and location of arteriovenous anastomoses in the equine foot, *Equine Vet J* 26:305, 1994.

16. Edvinsson L, Uddman R: *Vascular innervation and receptor mechanisms*, San Diego, 1993, Academic Press.

17. Busse R, Mulsch A: Endothelium-derived relaxing factor: nitric oxide. In Sies H, ed: *Molecular aspects of inflammation*, Berlin, 1991, Springer-Verlag.

18. Moncada S, Palmer RMJ, Higgs EA: Nitric oxide: physiology, pathophysiology and pharmacology, *Pharm Rev* 43:109, 1991.

19. Kimball ES: Substance P, cytokines and arthritis, *Ann N Y Acad Sci* 594:293, 1990.

20. Bowker RM, Linder K, Sonea IM, Guida LA: Sensory nerve fibres and receptors in equine distal forelimbs and the potential roles in locomotion, *Equine Vet J Suppl* 18:141, 1995.

21. Bowker RM, Brewer AM, Vex KB, et al: Sensory receptors in the equine foot, *Am J Vet Res* 54:1840, 1993.

22. Palmieri G, Sanna L, Asole A, et al: On the collateral sesamoidean (suspensory navicular) ligament of equines: topographic relations and sensitive innervation, *Anat Histol Embryol* 73:47, 1990.

CHAPTER 30 Navicular Disease

1. Dyson S, Murray R, Schramme M: Lameness associated with foot pain: results of 199 horses (January 2001-December 2003) and response to treatment, *Equine Vet J* 37:113, 2005.

2. Blunden A, Dyson S, Murray R, et al: Histological findings in horses with chronic palmar foot pain and age-matched control horses. Part 1: the navicular bone and related structures, *Equine Vet J* 38:15, 2006.

3. Blunden A, Dyson S, Murray R, et al: Histological findings in horses with chronic palmar foot pain and age-matched control horses. Part 2: the deep digital flexor tendon, *Equine Vet J* 38:23, 2006.

4. Dyson S, Murray R, Schramme M, et al: Lameness in 46 horses associated with deep digital flexor tendonitis in the digit: diagnosis confirmed with magnetic resonance imaging, *Equine Vet J* 35:681, 2003.

5. Dik K, van den Broek J: Role of navicular bone shape in the pathogenesis of navicular disease: a radiological study, *Equine Vet J* 27:390, 1995.

6. Dik K, van den Belt A, Van den Broek J: Relationships of age and shape of the navicular bone to the development of navicular disease: a radiological study, *Equine Vet J* 33:172, 2001.

7. Stock K, Hamann H, Distl O: Variance component estimation on the frequency of pathologic changes in the navicular bones of Hanoverian Warmblood horses, *J Anim Breed Genet* 121:289, 2004.

8. Dyson S, Murray R, Blunden T, et al: Current concepts of navicular disease, *Equine Vet Educ* 18:45, 2006.

9. Ackerman N, Johnson J, Dorn C: Navicular disease in the horse: risk factors, radiographic changes and response to therapy, *J Am Vet Med Assoc* 170:183, 1997.

10. Mey G, Kleyn E, Watering C: Een onderzoek naar de eifalljke aanleg voor podotrochlitis, *Tijdschrift Dieergeneesk* 92:1261, 1967.

11. Colles C: *The pathogenesis and treatment of navicular disease in the horse, PhD thesis*, London, 1987, University of London.

12. Turner T: Role of hoof balance on navicular disease. *International Symposium on Podotrochlosis*, Dortmund, 1993.

13. Denoix JM: Les origines du syndrome podotrochleaire en relation avec la biomechanique. *Proceedings of the Sixth Geneva Congress on Equine Medicine and Surgery*, 1999.

14. Bowker R, Atkinson P, Atkinson T, et al: Effect of contact stress in bones of the distal interphalangeal joint on microscopic changes in articular cartilage and ligaments, *Am J Vet Res* 62:414, 2001.

15. Denoix JM: Functional anatomy of the equine interphalangeal joints, *Proc Am Assoc Equine Pract* 45:174, 1999.

16. Wilson A, McGuigan M, Fouracre L, et al: The force and contact stress on the navicular bone during trot locomotion in sound horses and horses with navicular disease, *Equine Vet J* 33:159, 2001.

17. McGuigan M, Wilson A: The effect of bilateral palmar digital nerve analgesia on the compressive force experienced by the navicular bone in horses with navicular disease, *Equine Vet J* 33:166, 2001.

18. Eliashar E, McGuigan M, Wilson A: Relationship of foot conformation and force applied to the navicular bone of sound horses at the trot, *Equine Vet J* 36:431, 2004.

19. Dik K, van den Belt A, Enzerink E, et al: The radiographic development of the distal and proximal double contours of the equine navicular bone on dorsoproximal-palmarodistal oblique (upright pedal) radiographs from age 1 to 11 months, *Equine Vet J* 33:70, 2001.

20. Rijkenhuizen A, Nemeth F, Dik K, et al: The arterial supply of the navicular bone in adult horses with navicular disease, *Equine Vet J* 21:418, 1989.

21. Colles C, Hickman J: The arterial supply of the navicular bone and its variations in navicular disease, *Equine Vet J* 9:150, 1977.

22. MacGregor C: *Studies on the pathology and treatment of navicular disease, PhD thesis*, Edinburgh, UK, 1984, University of Edinburgh.

23. Ostblom L, Lund C, Melsen F: Histological study of navicular bone disease, *Equine Vet J* 14:199, 1982.

24. Pool R, Meagher D, Stover S: Pathophysiology of navicular syndrome, *Vet Clin North Am Equine Pract* 5:109, 1989.

25. Wright I, Kidd L, Thorp B: Gross, histological and histomorphometric features of the navicular bone and related structures in the horse, *Equine Vet J* 30:220, 1998.

26. Wright I, Douglas J: Biomechanical considerations in the treatment of navicular disease, *Vet Rec* 133:109, 1993.

27. Dyson S, Murray R: Verification of scintigraphic imaging for injury diagnosis in 264 horses with foot pain, *Equine Vet J* 39:350, 2007.

28. Dyson S, Murray R: Use of concurrent scintigraphic and magnetic resonance imaging evaluation to improve understanding of the pathogenesis of injury of the podotrochlear apparatus, *Equine Vet J* 39:365, 2007.

29. Bowker R: Contrasting structural morphologies of "good" and "bad" footed horses, *Proc Am Assoc Equine Pract* 49:186, 2003.

30. Keegan K, Wilson D, Lattimer J, et al: Scintigraphic evaluation of 99mTc-methylene diphosphonate uptake in the navicular area of horses with lameness isolated to the foot by anaesthesia of the palmar digital nerves, *Am J Vet Res* 57:415, 1996.

31. Dyson S, Weekes J: Orthopaedic imaging. In Dyson S, Pilsworth R, Twardock R, et al, eds: *Equine scintigraphy*, ed 1, Newmarket, UK, 2003, Equine Veterinary Journal.

32. Dyson S: Subjective and quantitative scintigraphic assessment of the equine foot and its relationship with foot pain, *Equine Vet J* 34:164, 2002.

33. Murray R, Schramme M, Dyson S, et al: MRI characteristics of the foot in horses with palmar foot pain and control horses, *Vet Radiol Ultrasound* 47:1, 2006.

34. Murray R, Blunden A, Schramme M, et al: How does magnetic resonance imaging represent histological findings in the equine digit? *Vet Radiol Ultrasound* 47:17, 2006.

35. Schneider R, Gavin P, Tucker R: What MRI is teaching us about navicular disease, *Proc Am Assoc Equine Pract* 49:210, 2003.

36. Busoni V, Heimann M, Trenteseaux J, et al: Abnormal MRI findings in the deep digital flexor tendon and distal sesamoid bone in radiographically defined navicular disease—an in vitro study, *Vet Radiol Ultrasound* 46:279, 2005.

37. Verschooten F, Roels J, Lampu P, et al: Radiographic measurements from the lateromedial projection of the equine foot with navicular disease, *Res Vet Sci* 46:15, 1989.

38. Wright I: A study of 118 cases of navicular disease: radiological features, *Equine Vet J* 25:493, 1993.

39. Dyson S: Radiological interpretation of the navicular bone, *Equine Vet Educ* 268:280, 2008.

40. Kaser-Hotz B, Ueltschi G: Radiographic appearance of the navicular bone in sound horses, *Vet Radiol Ultrasound* 33:9, 1992.

41. van Wulfen K, Bowker R: Intersection of the DSIL and the DDFT and its relationship to navicular syndrome, *Proc Am Assoc Equine Pract* 43:405, 1997.

42. van Wulfen K: *Normal anatomy of navicular bone suspensory ligaments and its relationship to navicular syndrome, master's thesis*, East Lansing, Mich, 1999, Michigan State University.

43. Svalastoga E, Neilsen K: Navicular disease in the horse: the synovial membrane of bursa podotrochlearis, *Nord Vet Med* 35:28, 1983.

44. Svalastoga E, Smith M: Navicular disease in the horse: the subchondral bone pressure, *Nord Vet Med* 35:31, 1983.

45. Pleasant S, Baker G, Foreman J, et al: Intraosseous pressure and pathologic changes in horses with navicular disease, *Am J Vet Res* 54:7, 1993.

46. Bowker R, Rockerhouser S, Vex K, et al: Immunocytochemical and dye distribution studies of nerves potentially desensitised by injections into the distal interphalangeal joint or the navicular bursa of horses, *J Am Vet Med Assoc* 203:1708, 1993.

47. Bowker R, Linder K, Van Wulfen K: Anatomy of the distal interphalangeal joint of the mature horse: relationships with the navicular suspensory ligaments, sensory nerves and neurovascular bundle, *Equine Vet J* 29:126, 1997.

48. Valdez H, Adams O, Peyton L: Navicular disease in the hindlimb of the horse, *J Am Vet Med Assoc* 172:291, 1978.

49. Dyson S: Navicular disease and other soft tissue causes of palmar foot pain. In Ross M, Dyson S, eds: *Diagnosis and management of lameness in the horse*, ed 1, St. Louis, 2003, Saunders.

50. Wright I: A study of 118 cases of navicular disease: clinical features, *Equine Vet J* 25:488, 1983.

51. Beeman M: The diagnosis of navicular disease (navicular syndrome), *Proc Am Assoc Equine Pract* 31:477, 1985.

52. Hertsch von B: Untersuchung des strahlbeines. Proceedings of Sixth Geneva Congress on Equine Medicine and Surgery, 1999.

53. Dyson S, Kidd L: A comparison of responses to analgesia of the navicular bursa and intra-articular analgesia of the distal interphalangeal joint in 59 horses, *Equine Vet J* 25:93, 1993.

54. Turner T: Predictive value of diagnostic tests for navicular pain, *Proc Am Assoc Equine Pract* 42:201, 1996.

55. Schumacher J, Steiger R, Schumacher J, et al: Effects of analgesia of the distal interphalangeal joint or palmar digital nerves on lameness caused by solar pain in horses, *Vet Surg* 29:54, 2000.

56. Schumacher J, Schumacher J, De Graves F, et al: A comparison of the effects of 2 volumes of local anaesthetic solution in the distal interphalangeal joint of horses with lameness caused by solar toe or solar heel pain, *Equine Vet J* 32:43, 2000.

57. Butler J, Colles C, Dyson S, et al: Foot, pastern and fetlock. In Butler JA, Colles JM, Dyson SJ, et al, eds: *Clinical radiology of the horse*, ed 3, Oxford, 2008, Wiley-Blackwell.

58. Dik K: Radiographic examination. In Wagenaar G, ed: *The pre-purchase examination of the horse*, ed 2, Utrecht, 1992, Bunge.

59. Dik K: Personal communication, 2003.

60. Poulos P: Correlation of radiographic signs and histological changes in the navicular bone, *Proc Am Assoc Equine Pract* 29:241, 1983.

61. Poulos P: The nature of enlarged "vascular channels" in the navicular bone of the horse, *Vet Radiol* 29:60, 1988.

62. Schramme M, Murray R, Blunden A, et al: A comparison between MRI, pathology and radiology in 34 limbs with navicular syndrome and 25 control limbs, *Proc Am Assoc Equine Pract* 51:348, 2005.

63. Berry C, Pool R, Stover S, et al: Radiographic/morphologic investigation of a radiolucent crescent within the flexor central eminence of the navicular bone in Thoroughbreds, *Am J Vet Res* 53:1604, 1992.

64. Turner T: Use of navicular bursography in 97 horses, *Proc Am Assoc Equine Pract* 44:227, 1998.

65. Trout D, Hornhof W, O'Brien T: Soft tissue- and bone-phase scintigraphy for diagnosis of navicular disease in horses, *J Am Vet Med Assoc* 198:73, 1991.

66. Tiejte S: Die computertomographie im strahlbeinbereich des pferdes: ein vergleich mit der konventionellen rontgendastellung, *Pferdheilkunde* 11:51, 1995.

67. Whitton C, Buckley C, Donovan T, et al: The diagnosis of lameness associated with distal limb pathology in a horse: a comparison of radiography, computed tomography and magnetic resonance imaging, *Vet J* 155:223, 1998.

68. Widmer W, Buckwalter K, Fessler J, et al: Use of radiography, computed tomography and magnetic resonance imaging for

evaluation of navicular syndrome in the horse, *Vet Radiol Ultrasound* 41:108, 1999.

69. Dyson S, Murray R: Magnetic resonance imaging of 264 horses with foot pain: the podotrochlear apparatus, the deep digital flexor tendon and the collateral ligaments of the distal interphalangeal joint, *Equine Vet J* 39:340, 2007.

70. Dyson S, Murray R: Magnetic resonance imaging of the equine foot, *Clin Tech Equine Pract* 6:46, 2007.

71. Sampson S, Schneider R, Gavin P: Magnetic resonance imaging findings in horses with recent and chronic bilateral forelimb lameness diagnosed as navicular syndrome, *Proc Am Assoc Equine Pract* 54:419, 2008.

72. Smith M, Wright I, Smith R: Endoscopic assessment and treatment of lesions of the deep digital flexor tendon in the navicular bursae of 20 lame horses, *Equine Vet J* 38:18, 2007.

73. Bowker R, Van Wulfen K, Springer S, et al: Functional anatomy of the cartilage of the distal phalanx and digital cushion in the equine foot and a hemodynamic flow hypothesis of energy dissipation, *Am J Vet Res* 59:961, 1998.

74. Dyson S: The puzzle of distal interphalangeal joint pain, *Equine Vet Educ* 10:119, 1998.

75. Schoonover M, Jann H, Blaik M: Quantitative comparison of 3 commonly used treatments for navicular syndrome in horses, *Am J Vet Res* 66:1247, 2005.

76. Dejardin L, Arnoczky S, Cloud G, et al: Photoelastic stress analysis of strain patterns in equine hooves after four-point trimming, *Am J Vet Res* 62:467, 2001.

77. Willemen M, Savelberg H, Barneveld A: The effect of orthopaedic shoeing on the force exerted by the deep digital flexor tendon on the navicular bone in horses, *Equine Vet J* 31:25, 1999.

78. Ostblom L, Lund C, Melsen F: Navicular bone disease: results of treatment using egg-bar shoeing technique, *Equine Vet J* 16:203, 1984.

79. Ostblom L, Lund C, Melsen F: Navicular bone disease: a comparative histomorphometric study, *Equine Vet J* 21:431, 1989.

80. Rohde C, Andersen D, Bertone A, et al: Effects of phenylbutazone on bone activity and formation in horses, *Am J Vet Res* 61:537, 2000.

81. Symonds K, MacAllister C, Erkert R, et al: Use of force plate analysis to assess the analgesic effects of etodolac in horses with navicular syndrome, *Am J Vet Res* 67:557, 2006.

82. Matthews N, Gleed RD, Short CE, et al: Cardiovascular and pharmacokinetic effects of isoxsuprine in the horse, *Am J Vet Res* 47:2130, 1986.

83. Ingle-Fehr J, Baxter G: Effect of oral isoxsuprine and pentoxifylline on digital and laminar blood flow in healthy horses, *Proc Am Assoc Equine Pract* 42:214, 1996.

84. Deumer J, de Haan F, Tulp M, et al: Effect of an isoxsuprine-resin preparation on blood flow in the equine thoracic limb, *Vet Rec* 129:427, 1991.

85. Belloli C, Carcano R, Arioli F, et al: Affinity of isoxsuprine for adrenoreceptors in equine digital artery and implications for vasodilatory action, *Equine Vet J* 32:119, 2000.

86. Turner A, Tucker C: The evaluation of isoxsuprine hydrochloride for the treatment of navicular disease: a double blind study, *Equine Vet J* 21:338, 1989.

87. Pauwels F, Schumacher J, Castro F, et al: Evaluation of the diffusion of corticosteroids between the distal interphalangeal joint and navicular bursa in horses, *Am J Vet Res* 69:611, 2008.

88. Kristiansen K, Kold S: Multivariable analysis of factors influencing outcome of 2 treatment protocols in 128 cases of horses responding positively to intra-articular analgesia of the distal interphalangeal joint, *Equine Vet J* 39:150, 2007.

89. Verschooten F, Desmet P, Peremans K, et al: Navicular disease in the horse: the effect of controlled intrabursal corticoid injection, *J Equine Vet Sci* 10:316, 1990.

90. Dabareiner R, Carter K, Honnas C: Injection of corticosteroids, hyaluronate and amikacin into the navicular bursa in horses with signs of navicular area pain unresponsive to other treatments: 25 cases (1999-2002), *J Am Vet Med Assoc* 223:1469, 2003.

91. Dyson S: Unpublished data, 2008.

92. Bell C, Howard R, Taylor D, et al: Outcome of navicular bursa injections in horses with MRI-diagnosed foot pain: 23 cases (2005-2007), *Proc Am Assoc Equine Pract* 54:245, 2008.

93. Colles C: Anticoagulant therapy for navicular disease, *Vet Rec* 108:107, 1982.

94. Kirker-Head K: Use of propentofylline for the treatment of equine navicular disease, *Proc Eur Coll Vet Surg* 2:10, 1993.

95. Verschooten F, Ooms L, Desmet P, et al: Metrenperone treatment of navicular disease in horses compared with isoxsuprine: a clinical study, *J Equine Vet Sci* 10:230, 1990.

96. Crisman M: Evaluation of polysulfated glycosaminoglycan for the treatment of navicular disease: a double blind study, *Proc Am Assoc Equine Pract* 39:219, 1993.

97. Denoix J-M: Tiludronate as a new therapeutic agent in the treatment of navicular disease: a double-blind placebo-controlled trial, *Equine Vet J* 35:407, 2003.

98. Blum N: The use of extracorporeal shock-wave therapy in horses with navicular disease, *Pferdheilkunde* 21:21, 2005.

99. Wright I: Navicular suspensory desmotomy in the treatment of navicular disease: technique and preliminary results, *Equine Vet J* 18:443, 1986.

100. Diehl M: Desmotomy of the navicular collateral ligaments in horses with navicular disease, *Proc Eur Soc Vet Surg* 16:53, 1986.

101. Wright I: A study of 118 cases of navicular disease: treatment by navicular suspensory desmotomy, *Equine Vet J* 25:501, 1993.

102. Bell B, Bridge I, Sullivan S: Surgical treatment of navicular syndrome in the horse using navicular suspensory desmotomy, *N Z Vet J* 44:26, 1996.

103. Turner T: Inferior check desmotomy as a treatment for navicular disease. Proceedings of the International Symposium on Podotroclosis, Dortmund, 1993.

104. Litzke LF, Dietz O, Nagel E: Angiographie als diagnostisches hilfsmittel und periaterielle sympathektomie mit oder ohne neurektomie in der lahmheitstherapie beim pferd, *Pferdheilkunde* 3:3, 1987.

105. Jaugstetter H, Jacobi R, Litzke L, et al: Pericaskulare sympathektomie, eine therapiemoglichkeit beim podtrochlose-sesamoidose-syndrom, *Tierarztl Prax* 31:46, 2003.

106. Taylor T, Vaughan J: Effects of denervation of the digit in the horse, *J Am Vet Med Assoc* 177:1033, 1980.

107. Dabareiner R, White N, Sullins K: Comparison of techniques for palmar digital neurectomy in horses, *Proc Am Assoc Equine Pract* 43:231, 1997.

108. Jackman B, Baxter G, Doran R, et al: Palmar digital neurectomy in horses 57 cases (1984-1990), *Vet Surg* 22:285, 1993.

109. Marcoux M, Deschamps I: Nevrectomie digitale posterieure chez le cheval: etude retrospective a partir de 54 cas, *Prat Vet Equine* 25:265, 1993.

110. Mehery O: Pull through technique for palmar digital neurectomy: 41 horses (1998-2004), *Vet Surg* 37:87, 2007.

111. Zierz J, Schad D, Heeb D, et al: Chirurgische moglichkeiten zur versorgung von strahlbeinzysten sowie strukturdefekten im strahlbein, *Pferdheilkunde* 16:171, 2000.

112. Jenner F: Navicular disease with core decompression—a new approach. Proceeding of the Sixteenth Annual Convention of the European College of Veterinary Surgeons, Dublin, 2007.

CHAPTER 31 Fracture of the Navicular Bone and Congenital Bipartite Navicular Bone

1. Colles C: Repair of navicular bone fractures in the horse, *Proc Am Assoc Equine Pract* 47:270, 2001.

2. Reeves M, Yovich J, Turner S: Miscellaneous conditions of the equine foot, *Vet Clin North Am Equine Pract* 5:210, 1989.

3. Baxter G, Ingle J, Trotter G: Complete navicular bone fractures in horses, *Proc Am Assoc Equine Pract* 41:243, 1995.

4. Butler J, Colles C, Dyson S, et al: Foot, pastern and fetlock. In Butler JA, Colles CM, Dyson SJ, et al, eds: *Clinical radiology of the horse*, ed 3, Oxford, 2008, Wiley-Blackwell.

5. Murray R: Personal communication, 2001.

6. Heitzmann A, Denoix J-M: Rupture of the distal sesamoidean impar ligament with proximal displacement of the distal sesamoid bone in a steeplechaser, *Equine Vet Educ* 19:117, 2007.

7. Dyson S: Unpublished data, 1981.

8. Turner T, Malone E: How to treat navicular bone fractures, *Proc Am Assoc Equine Pract* 43:370, 1997.

9. Nemeth F, Dik K: Lag screw fixation of sagittal navicular bone fractures in 5 horses, *Equine Vet J* 17:137, 1985.

CHAPTER 32 Primary Lesions of the Deep Digital Flexor Tendon within the Hoof Capsule

1. Bowker R, Rockershouser S, Linder K, et al: A silver impregnation and immunocytochemical study of innervation of the distal sesamoid bone and its suspensory ligaments in the horse, *Equine Vet J* 26:212, 1994.

2. Bowker R, Atkinson P, Atkinson T, et al: Effect of contact stress in bones of the distal interphalangeal joint on microscopic changes in articular cartilage and ligaments, *Am J Vet Res* 62:414, 2001.

3. Denoix JM: Functional anatomy of tendons and ligaments in the distal limbs (manus and pes), *Vet Clin North Am Equine Pract* 10:273, 1994.

4. Webbon P: A post mortem study of equine digital flexor tendons, *Equine Vet J* 9:61, 1977.

5. Wright I, Kidd L, Thorp B: Gross, histological and histomorphometric features of the navicular bone and related structures in the horse, *Equine Vet J* 30:220, 1998.

6. Pool R, Meagher D, Stover S: Pathophysiology of navicular syndrome, *Vet Clin North Am Equine Pract* 5:109, 1989.

7. Van Wulfen K, Bowker R: Intersection of the DSIL and the DDFT and its relationship to navicular syndrome, *Proc Am Assoc Equine Pract* 43:405, 1997.

8. Murray R, Schramme M, Dyson S, et al: MRI characteristics of the foot in horses with palmar foot pain and control horses, *Vet Radiol Ultrasound* 47:1, 2006.

9. Blunden A, Dyson S, Murray R, et al: Histological findings in horses with chronic palmar foot pain and age-matched control horses. Part 2: the deep digital flexor tendon, *Equine Vet J* 38:23, 2006.

10. Murray R, Blunden T, Schramme M, et al: How does magnetic resonance imaging represent histological findings in the equine digit? *Vet Radiol Ultrasound* 47:17, 2006.

11. Blunden T, Murray R, Dyson S: Lesions of the deep digital flexor tendon in the digit: a correlative magnetic resonance imaging and post mortem study in control and lame horses, *Equine Vet J* 41:25, 2009.

12. Dyson S, Murray R, Schramme M, et al: Lameness in 46 horses associated with deep digital flexor tendonitis in the digit: diagnosis confirmed with magnetic resonance imaging, *Equine Vet J* 35:681, 2003.

13. Mair T, Kinns J: Deep digital flexor tendonitis in the equine foot diagnosed by low-field magnetic resonance imaging in the standing patient: 18 cases, *Vet Radiol Ultrasound* 46:458, 2005.

14. Dyson S, Murray R: Magnetic resonance imaging of 264 horses with foot pain: the podotrochlear apparatus, the deep digital flexor tendon and the collateral ligaments of the distal interphalangeal joint, *Equine Vet J* 39:340, 2007.

15. Butler J, Colles C, Dyson S, et al: Foot, pastern and fetlock. In Butler J, Colles C, Dyson S, et al, eds: *Clinical radiology of the horse*, ed 2, Oxford, 2000, Blackwell Science.

16. Ueltschi G: Radiographie und szintigraphie beim podotrochlosesyndrom, *Proc Geneva Congress Equine Med Surg* 6:119, 1999.

17. Dyson S: Subjective and quantitative scintigraphic assessment of the equine foot and its relationship with foot pain, *Equine Vet J* 34:164, 2002.

18. Dyson S, Murray R: Verification of scintigraphic imaging for injury diagnosis in 264 horses with foot pain, *Equine Vet J* 39:350, 2007.

19. Dyson S, Murray R: Magnetic resonance imaging of the equine foot, *Clin Techn Equine Pract* 6:46, 2007.

20. Busoni V, Denoix J-M: Ultrasonography of the podotrochlear apparatus in the horse using a transcuneal approach: technique and reference images, *Vet Radiol Ultrasound* 42:534, 2001.

21. Tietje S, Nowak M, Petzoldt S, et al: Die computertomographische darstellung des distalen abschnitts der tiefen beugesehne (TBS) des pferdes, *Pferdheilkunde* 17:21, 2001.

22. Puchalski S, Snyder J, Hornof W, et al: Contrast-enhanced computed tomography of the equine distal extremity, *Proc Am Assoc Equine Pract* 51:389, 2005.

23. Murray R, Roberts B, Schramme M, et al: Quantitative evaluation of equine deep digital flexor tendon morphology using magnetic resonance imaging, *Vet Radiol Ultrasound* 45:103, 2004.

24. Dyson S: Magnetic resonance imaging of the equine foot, *Clin Tech Equine Pract* 6:46, 2007.

25. Boswell J: *Proceedings of the British Equine Veterinary Association Congress*, Birmingham, UK, 2009.

26. Dyson S: Unpublished data, 2009.

27. Mair T: Personal communication, 2008.

28. Smith M, Wright I, Smith R: Endoscopic assessment and treatment of lesions of the deep digital flexor tendon in the navicular bursae of 20 lame horses, *Equine Vet J* 38:18, 2007.

29. Smith M: *Proceedings of the European College of Veterinary Surgeons Congress*, Lyons, France, 2009.

CHAPTER 33 The Distal Phalanx and Distal Interphalangeal Joint

Primary Pain Associated with the Distal Interphalangeal Joint

1. Denoix J-M: Functional anatomy of tendons and ligaments in the distal limbs, *Vet Clin North Am Equine Pract* 10:273, 1994.

2. Denoix J-M: Functional anatomy of the equine interphalangeal joints, *Proc Am Assoc Equine Pract* 45:174, 1999.

3. Chateau H, Deugueurce C, Jerbi H, et al: Normal three-dimensional behaviour of the metacarpophalangeal joint and the effect of uneven foot bearing, *Equine Vet J Suppl* 33:84, 2001.

4. Dyson S: The puzzle of distal interphalangeal joint pain, *Equine Vet Educ* 10:119, 1998.

5. Schumacher J, Steiger R, Schumacher J, et al: Effects of analgesia of the distal interphalangeal joint or palmar digital nerves on lameness caused by solar pain in horses, *Vet Surg* 29:54, 2000.

6. Schumacher J, Schramme M, Schumacher J, et al: The effect of volumes of local anaesthetic administered into the coffin joint on solar toe or heel pain, *Proc Am Assoc Equine Pract* 46:27, 2000.

7. Dyson S: Lameness due to pain associated with the distal interphalangeal joint: 45 cases, *Equine Vet J* 23:128, 1991.

8. Dyson S, Kidd L: A comparison of responses to analgesia of the navicular bursa and intra-articular analgesia of the distal interphalangeal joint in 59 horses, *Equine Vet J* 25:93, 1993.

9. Turner T: Predictive value of diagnostic tests for navicular pain, *Proc Am Assoc Equine Pract* 42:201, 1996.

10. Butler J, Colles C, Dyson S, et al: The foot, pastern and fetlock. In Butler JA, Colles CM, Dyson SJ, et al, eds: *Clinical radiology of the horse*, ed 3, Oxford, 2008, Wiley-Blackwell.

11. Denoix J-M: Ligament injuries of the distal interphalangeal joint in horses, *Proceedings of the Sixth World Equine Veterinary Association Congress*, Paris, September 1999.

12. Sage A, Turner T: Ultrasonography in the horse with palmar foot pain: 13 cases, *Proc Am Assoc Equine Pract* 46:380, 2000.

13. Denoix J-M: *The equine distal limb: an atlas of clinical anatomy and comparative imaging*, London, 2000, Manson Publishing.

14. Ross M: Observations in horses with lameness abolished by palmar digital analgesia, *Proc Am Assoc Equine Pract* 44:230, 1998.

15. Kristensen K, Kold S: Multivariable analysis of factors influencing outcome of 2 treatment protocols in 128 cases of horses responding positively to intra-articular analgesia of the distal interphalangeal joint, *Equine Vet J* 39:150, 2007.

16. Dyson S: Unpublished data, 1980-2002.

17. Verschooten F, DeMoor A: Subchondral cystic and related lesions affecting the pedal bone and stifle, *Equine Vet J* 14:114, 1982.

18. Haack D, Hertsch B, Baez C: Zystoide defekte im huftein des pferdes, *Pferdheilkunde* 14:143, 1998.

19. Wagner P, Modransky P, Gavin P, et al: Surgical management of subchondral bone cysts of the third phalanx in the horse, *Equine Pract* 4:9, 1982.

20. Honnas C, Trotter G: The distal interphalangeal joint. In White N, Moore J, eds: *Current techniques in equine surgery and lameness*, ed 2, Philadelphia, 1998, Saunders.

21. Wright I: Personal communication, 1996.

22. Heitzmann A, Denoix J-M: Rupture of the distal sesamoidean impar ligament with proximal displacement of the distal sesamoid bone in a steeplechaser, *Equine Vet Educ* 19:117, 2007.

23. Dyson S, Murray R: Magnetic resonance imaging of the equine foot, *Clin Tech Equine Pract* 6:46, 2007.

24. Dyson S, Murray R: Magnetic resonance imaging of 264 horses with foot pain: the podotrochlear apparatus, the deep digital flexor tendon and the collateral ligaments of the distal interphalangeal joint, *Equine Vet J* 39:340, 2007.

25. Blunden A, Dyson S, Murray R, et al: Histological findings in horses with chronic palmar foot pain and age-matched control horses. Part 1: the navicular bone and related structures, *Equine Vet J* 38:15, 2006.

26. Dyson S, Pool R, Blunden T, et al: The distal sesamoidean impar ligament: comparison between magnetic resonance imaging and histology, *Equine Vet J* 42:332, 2010.

27. Biggi M, Dyson S: High-field magnetic resonance imaging investigation of distal border fragments of the navicular bone

in horses with foot pain, *Equine Vet J* (In press.)

28. Biggi M, Dyson S: Comparison between radiological and magnetic resonance imaging lesions in the distal border of the navicular bone with particular reference to distal border fragments and osseous cyst-like lesions, *Equine Vet J* (In press.)

Fractures and Fragmentation of the Extensor Process of the Distal Phalanx

1. Dechant JE, Trotter GW, Stashak TS, et al: Removal of large fragments of the extensor process of the distal phalanx via arthrotomy in horses: 14 cases (1992-1998), *J Am Vet Med Assoc* 217:1351, 2000.
2. Honnas C, Trotter GW: The distal interphalangeal joint. In White N, Moore J, eds: *Current techniques in equine lameness and surgery*, ed 2, Philadelphia, 1998, Saunders.
3. Boening KJ, von Saldern F, Leendertse IP, et al: Diagnostic and surgical arthroscopy of the equine coffin joint, *Proc Am Assoc Equine Pract* 35:311, 1989.
4. Kaneps A, O'Brein T, Redden RF, et al: Characterization of osseous bodies of the distal phalanx of foals, *Equine Vet J* 25:285, 1993.
5. ter Braake F: Arthroscopic removal of large fragments of the extensor process of the distal phalanx in 4 horses, *Equine Vet Educ* 17:101, 2005.
6. MacLellan K, MacDonald DG, Crawford WH, et al: Lag screw fixation of an extensor process fracture in a foal with flexural deformity, *Can Vet J* 38:226, 1997.

Injuries of the Collateral Ligaments of the Distal Interphalangeal Joint

1. McDiarmid A: Distal interphalangeal joint lameness in horses associated with damage to the insertion of the lateral collateral ligament, *Equine Vet Educ* 10:114, 1998.
2. Denoix J-M: Ligament injuries of the distal interphalangeal joint in horses, *Proceedings of the Sixth World Equine Veterinary Association Congress*, Paris, September 1999.
3. Sage A, Turner T: Ultrasonography in the horse with palmar foot pain: 13 cases, *Proc Am Assoc Equine Pract* 46:380, 2000.
4. Dyson S, Murray R: Collateral desmitis of the distal interphalangeal joint in 62 horses (January 2001-December 2003), *Proc Am Assoc Equine Pract* 50:248, 2004.
5. Zubrod C, Farnsworth K, Tucker R, et al: Injury of the collateral ligaments of the distal interphalangeal joint diagnosed by magnetic resonance imaging, *Vet Radiol Ultrasound* 46:11, 2005.
6. Gutierrez S, White N, Werpy N, et al: Desmopathy of the collateral ligaments of the distal interphalangeal joint detected with a low-field magnetic resonance imaging system: 20 cases, *Vet Radiol Ultrasound* 50:21, 2009.
7. Dyson S, Blunden T, Murray R: The collateral ligaments of the distal interphalangeal joint: magnetic resonance imaging and post mortem observations in 25 lame and 12 control horses, *Equine Vet J* 40:538, 2008.
8. Denoix J-M: Functional anatomy of the equine interphalangeal joints, *Proc Am Assoc Equine Pract* 45:174, 1999.
9. Dyson S, Brown V, Collins S, Murray R: Is there an association between ossification of the cartilages of the foot and collateral desmopathy of the distal interphalangeal joint or distal phalanx injury? *Equine Vet J* (In press.)
10. Dyson S, Murray R: Verification of scintigraphic imaging for injury diagnosis in 264 horses with foot pain, *Equine Vet J* 39:350, 2007.
11. Spriet M, Mai W, McKnight A: Asymmetric signal intensity in normal collateral ligaments of the distal interphalangeal joint in horses with a low field MRI system: a manifestation of the magic angle effect, *Vet Radiol Ultrasound* 48:95, 2007.
12. Smith M, Dyson S, Murray R: Is a magic angle effect observed in the collateral ligaments of the distal interphalangeal joint or the oblique sesamoidean ligaments during standing low field magnetic resonance imaging? *Vet Radiol Ultrasound* 49:509, 2008.
13. Werpy N, Ho C, Kawcak C: Magic angle effect in normal collateral ligaments of the distal interphalangeal joint in horses imaged with a high-field magnetic resonance imaging system, *Vet Radiol Ultrasound* 51:2, 2010.
14. Dakin S, Dyson S, Murray R, et al: Osseous abnormalities associated with collateral desmopathy of the distal interphalangeal joint: Part 1, *Equine Vet J* 41:786, 2009.
15. Dyson S, Murray R: Magnetic resonance imaging of the equine foot, *Clin Tech Equine Pract* 6:46, 2007.
16. Dakin S, Dyson S, Murray R, et al: Osseous abnormalities associated with collateral desmopathy of the distal interphalangeal joint: Part 2. Treatment and outcome, *Equine Vet J* 41:794, 2009.
17. Smith M, Crowe O, Ellson C, et al: Surgical treatment of osseous cyst-like lesions in the distal phalanx arising from collateral ligament insertional injury, *Equine Vet Educ* 17:195, 2005.

Osseous Cystlike Lesions in the Distal Phalanx

1. Verschooten F, De Moor A: Subchondral cystic and related lesions affecting the equine pedal bone and stifle, *Equine Vet J* 14:47, 1982.
2. Bramlage L: Osteochondrosis related bone cysts, *Proc Am Assoc Equine Pract* 39:83, 1993.
3. Honnas C, Trotter GW: The distal interphalangeal joint. In White N, Moore J, eds: *Current techniques in equine surgery and lameness*, ed 2, Philadelphia, 1998, Saunders.
4. Scott E, Snyder S, Schmotzer W, et al: Subchondral bone cysts with fractures of the extensor processes in a horse, *J Am Vet Med Assoc* 199:595, 1991.
5. McIlwraith CW: Personal communication, 2001.
6. Wagner P, Modransky P, Gavin P, et al: Surgical management of subchondral bone cysts of the third phalanx in the horse, *Equine Pract* 4:9, 1982.
7. Wright I: Personal communication, 2001.
8. Story M, Bramlage L: Arthroscopic debridement of subchondral bone cysts in the distal phalanx of 11 horses (1994-2000), *Equine Vet J* 36:356, 2004.

Osseous Trauma of the Distal and Middle Phalanges

1. Dyson S, Murray R: Magnetic resonance imaging of the equine foot, *Clin Tech Equine Pract* 6:46, 2007.
2. Zubrod C, Schneider R, Tucker R, et al: Diagnosis of subchondral bone damage using magnetic resonance imaging in 11 horses, *J Am Vet Med Assoc* 24:411, 2004.
3. Olive J, Mair T, Charles B: Use of standing low-field magnetic resonance imaging to diagnose middle phalanx bone marrow lesions in horses. *Equine Vet Educ* 21:125, 2009.
4. Dyson S, Murray R: Lameness and diagnostic imaging in the sports horse: recent advances related to the digit, *Proc Am Assoc Equine Pract* 53:262, 2007.
5. Dyson S, Brown V, Collins S, Murray R: Is there an association between ossification of the cartilages of the foot and collateral desmopathy of the distal interphalangeal joint or distal phalanx injury? *Equine vet J* (In press.)
6. Dyson S, Murray R: Injuries associated with ossification of the cartilages of the foot, *Proc Am Assoc Equine Pract* (In press.)

Keratomas and Neoplastic and Nonneoplastic Space-Occupying Lesions in the Hoof

1. Hamir A, Kunz C, Evans L: Equine keratoma, *J Vet Diagn Invest* 4:99, 1990.
2. Reeves M, Yovich J, Turner A: Miscellaneous conditions of the equine foot, *Vet Clin North Am Equine Pract* 5:221, 1989.
3. Lloyd K, Peterson P, Wheat J, et al: Keratomas in horses: seven cases (1975-1986), *J Am Vet Med Assoc* 193:967, 1998.
4. Berry C, O'Brien T, Pool R: Squamous cell carcinoma of the hoof wall in a stallion, *J Am Vet Med Assoc* 199:90, 1991.
5. Gelatt K, Neuwirth L, Hawkins D, et al: Haemangioma of the distal phalanx in a colt, *Vet Radiol Ultrasound* 37:323, 1996.
6. Honnas C, Liskey C, Meagher D, et al: Malignant melanoma in the foot of a horse, *J Am Vet Med Assoc* 197:756, 1990.
7. Kunze D, Monticello T, Jakob T, et al: Malignant melanoma of the coronary band in a horse, *J Am Vet Med Assoc* 188:297, 1986.
8. Butler J, Colles C, Dyson S, et al: Foot, pastern and fetlock. In Butler JA, Colles CM, Dyson SJ, et al, eds: *Clinical radiology of the horse*, ed 3, Oxford, 2008, Wiley-Blackwell.
9. Dyson S: Unpublished data, 2001.
10. Moyer W: Keratoma. In Colahan P, Mayhew I, Merritt A, et al, eds: *Equine medicine and surgery*, ed 5, St. Louis, 1999, Mosby.
11. Chan C, Munroe G: Treatment of a keratoma in a Clydesdale horse, *Vet Rec* 140:453, 1997.
12. Pickersgill C: Recurrent white line abscessation associated with a keratoma in a riding pony, *Equine Vet Educ* 12:286, 2000.
13. Seahorn T, Sams A, Honnas C, et al: Ultrasonographic imaging of a keratoma in a horse, *J Am Vet Med Assoc* 200:1973, 1992.
14. Mair T: Personal communication, 2007.
15. Frisbie D, Trotter G: Keratomas. In White N, Moore J, eds: *Current techniques in equine surgery and lameness*, ed 2, Philadelphia, 1998, Saunders.

16. Boys Smith S, Clegg P, Hughes I, et al: Complete and partial hoof wall resection for keratoma removal: postoperative complications and final outcome in 26 horses (1994-2004), *Equine Vet J* 38:127, 2006.

Fractures of the Distal Phalanx

1. Scott E, McDole M, Shires M: A review of third phalanx fractures in the horse: sixty-five cases, *J Am Vet Med Assoc* 174:1337, 1979.
2. Honnas C, O'Brien T, Linford R: Distal phalanx fractures in horses: a survey of 274 horses with radiographic assessment of healing in 36 horses, *Vet Radiol* 29:98, 1988.
3. Yovich J, Stashak T, DeBowes R, et al: Fractures of the distal phalanx of the forelimb in eight foals, *J Am Vet Med Assoc* 189:550, 1986.
4. Kaneps A, O'Brien T, Redden R, et al: Characterisation of osseous bodies of the distal phalanx of foals, *Equine Vet J* 25:285, 1993.
5. Kaneps A, O'Brien T, Willits N, et al: Effect of hoof trimming on the occurrence of distal phalangeal fractures in foals, *Proc Am Assoc Equine Pract* 41:251, 1995.
6. Honnas C, O'Brien T, Linford R: Solar margin fractures of the distal phalanx, *Proc Am Assoc Equine Pract* 33:399, 1987.
7. Petterrson H: Fractures of the pedal bone in the horse, *Equine Vet J* 8:104, 1976.
8. Yovich J, Hilbert B, McGill C: Fracture of the distal phalanx in horses, *Austr Vet J* 59:180, 1982.
9. Honnas C, Trotter G: Articular fractures of the distal phalanx. In White N, Moore J, eds: *Current techniques in equine surgery and lameness*, ed 2, Philadelphia, 1998, Saunders.
10. Hertsch B, Neuberth M: Die isolierte ossifakation am hufbeinast des pferdes: eine differentialdiagnostische abgrenzung zu hufbeinastfraktur und hufknorpelverknocherung, *Pferdeheilkunde* 7:169, 1991.
11. Yovich J: Fractures of the distal phalanx in the horse, *Vet Clin North Am Equine Pract* 5:145, 1989.
12. Rabuffo TS, Ross MW: Fractures of the distal phalanx in 72 racehorses: 1990-2001, *Proc Am Assoc Equine Pract* 48:375, 2002.
13. Robson K, Kristoffersen M, Dyson S: Palmar or plantar process fractures of the distal phalanx in riding horses: 22 cases (1994-2003), *Equine Vet Educ* 20:40, 2008.
14. Keegan K, Twardock R, Losonsky J, et al: Scintigraphic evaluation of fractures of the distal phalanx in horses: 27 cases (1979-1988), *J Am Vet Med Assoc* 202:1993, 1993.
15. Dyson S, Murray R: Injuries associated with ossification of the cartilages of the foot, *Proc Am Assoc Equine Pract* (In press.)
16. Herthel D, Rick M, Lauper L, et al: Repair of distal phalanx fractures with articular involvement by using the titanium Herbert cannulated bone screw, *Proc Am Assoc Equine Pract* 42:170, 1996.
17. Ross M: Observations in horses with lameness abolished by palmar digital analgesia, *Proceedings of the Seventh World Equine Veterinary Association*, WEVA-SIVE 197, Sorrento, September 2001.

Pedal Osteitis: Does It Exist?

1. Rendano V: Radiographic interpretation: pedal osteitis, *Calif Vet* 33:27, 1979.
2. Linford R, O'Brien T, Trout D: Qualitative and morphometric radiographic findings in the distal phalanx and distal soft tissues of sound Thoroughbred racehorses, *Am J Vet Res* 54:38, 1993.
3. Butler J, Colles C, Dyson S, et al: Foot, pastern and fetlock. In Butler JA, Colles CM, Dyson SJ, et al, eds: *Clinical radiology of the horse*, ed 3, Oxford, 2008, Wiley-Blackwell.
4. Dyson S, Ross M: Unpublished data, 2001.
5. Moyer W, O'Brien T, Walker M: Nonseptic pedal osteitis: a cause of lameness and a diagnosis? *Proc Am Assoc Equine Pract* 45:178, 1999.
6. Nagy A, Dyson S, Murray R: Radiographic, scintigraphic and magnetic resonance imaging findings in the palmar processes of the distal phalanx, *Equine Vet J* 40:57, 2008.
7. Dyson S: Non-septic osteitis of the distal phalanx and its palmar processes, *Equine Vet Educ* (In press.)
8. Dyson S, Brown V, Collins S, Murray R: Is there an association between ossification of the cartilages of the foot and collateral desmopathy of the distal interphalangeal joint or distal phalanx injury? *Equine Vet J* (In press.)
9. Dyson S, Murray R: Injuries associated with ossification of the cartilages of the foot, *Proc Am Assoc Equine Pract* (In press.)

Osteitis of the Palmar Processes of the Distal Phalanx

1. Butler J, Colles C, Dyson S, et al: The foot, pastern and fetlock. In Butler JA, Colles CM, Dyson SJ, et al, eds: *Clinical radiology of the horse*, ed 3, Oxford, 2008, Wiley-Blackwell.
2. Trotter G: Personal communication, 2001.
3. Dyson S: Unpublished data, 2001.
4. Nagy A, Dyson S, Murray R: Radiographic, scintigraphic and magnetic resonance imaging findings in the palmar processes of the distal phalanx, *Equine Vet J* 40:57, 2008.
5. Dyson S: Non-septic osteitis of the distal phalanx and its palmar processes, *Equine Vet Educ* (In press.)
6. Dyson S, Brown V, Collins S, Murray R: Is there an association between ossification of the cartilages of the foot and collateral desmopathy of the distal interphalangeal joint or distal phalanx injury? *Equine vet J* (In press.)
7. Dyson S, Murray R: Injuries associated with ossification of the cartilages of the foot, *Proc Am Assoc Equine Pract* (In press.)

Disease of the Cartilages of the Foot

1. Nickel R, Schummer A, Bewegungsapparat S: Zehegelenke des Pferdes. In Nickel R, Schummer A, eds: *Lehrbuch der Anatomie der Haustiere*, Band 1, ed 2, Berlin, 1961, Paul Parey.
2. Bowker R, Van Wulfen K, Springer S, et al: Functional anatomy of the cartilage of the distal phalanx and digital cushion in the equine foot and a hemodynamic flow hypothesis of energy dissipation, *Am J Vet Res* 59:961, 1998.
3. Ruohoniemi M: *Ossification of the collateral cartilages of the distal phalanx in the front feet of Finnhorses, doctoral thesis*, Helsinki, Finland, 1997, University of Helsinki.
4. Butler J, Colles C, Dyson S, et al: The foot, pastern and fetlock. In Butler JA, Colles CM, Dyson SJ, et al, eds: *Clinical radiology of the horse*, ed 3, Oxford, 2008, Wiley-Blackwell.
5. Down S, Dyson S, Murray R: Ossification of the cartilages of the foot, *Equine Vet Educ* 19:51, 2007.
6. Dyson S, Murray R: Lameness and diagnostic imaging in the sports horse: recent advances related to the digit, *Proc Am Assoc Equine Pract* 53:262, 2007.
7. Nagy A, Dyson S, Murray R: Scintigraphic examination of the cartilages of the foot, *Equine Vet J* 39:250256, 2007.
8. Dyson S, Nagy A: Injuries associated with the cartilages of the foot, *Equine Vet Educ* (In press.)
9. Dyson S, Murray R: Injuries associated with ossification of the cartilages of the foot, *Proc Am Assoc Equine Pract* (In press.)
10. Dakin S, Robson K, Dyson S: Fractures of ossified cartilages of the foot: 10 cases, *Equine Vet Educ* 18:130, 2006.
11. Mair T, Sherlock C: Collateral desmitis of the distal interphalangeal joint in conjunction with concurrent ossification of the cartilages of the foot in nine horses, *Equine Vet Educ* 20:485, 2008.
12. Dyson S, Brown V, Collins S, Murray R: Is there an association between ossification of the cartilages of the foot and collateral desmopathy of the distal interphalangeal joint or distal phalanx injury? *Equine Vet J* (In press.)
13. Denoix J-M: Personal communication, 2000.

CHAPTER 34 Laminitis

Pathophysiology of Laminitis

1. Pollitt CC: Basement membrane pathology: a feature of acute equine laminitis, *Equine Vet J* 28:38, 1996.
2. Pollitt CC, Daradka M: Equine laminitis basement membrane pathology: loss of type IV collagen, type VII collagen and laminin immunostaining, *Equine Vet J Suppl* 26:139, 1998.
3. Obel N: Studies on the histopathology of acute laminitis, Almgvist and Wilcsells Bottrykeri Ab Uppsala (PhD Thesis), 1948.
4. Kyaw-Tanner M, Pollitt CC: Equine laminitis: increased transcription of matrix metalloproteinase-2 (MMP-2) occurs during the developmental phase, *Equine Vet J* 36:221, 2004.
5. Kyaw-Tanner MT, Wattlet O, van Eps AW, et al: Equine laminitis: membrane type matrix metal loproteinase-1 (MMP-14) is involved in acute phase onset, *Equine Vet J* 40:482, 2008.
6. Daradka M, Pollitt CC: Epidermal cell proliferation in the equine hoof wall, *Equine Vet J* 36:236, 2004.
7. Loftus JP, Belknap JK, Black SJ: Matrix metalloproteinase-9 in laminae of black walnut extract treated horses correlates with neutrophil abundance, *Vet Immunol Immunopathol* 113:267, 2006.
8. Loftus JP, Johnson P, Yin C, et al: Matrix metalloproteinases and structural tissue damage in equine laminitis, *J Vet Intern Med* 22:378, 2008.

9. Coyne MJ, Cousin H, Loftus JP, et al: Cloning and expression of ADAM-related metalloproteases in equine laminitis, *J vet Immunol* 129:231, 2009.

10. Budak MT, Orsini JA, Pollitt CC, et al: Gene expression in the lamellar dermis-epidermis during the developmental phase of carbohydrate overload-induced laminitis in the horse, *Vet Immunol Immunopathol* doi: 101016/jvetimm200903019, 2009.

11. Asplin K, Sillence M, Pollitt C, et al: Induction of laminitis by prolonged hyperinsulinaemia in clinically normal ponies, *Vet J* 174:530, 2007.

12. deLaat MA, McGowan CM, Sillence MN, et al: Equine laminitis: induced by 40 hours of hyperinsulinaemia in Standardbred horses, *Equine Vet J* 42:129, 2010.

13. Nourian AR, Asplin KE, McGowan CM, et al: Equine laminitis: ultrastructural lesions detected in ponies after prolonged hyperinsulinaemia, *Equine Vet J* 41:671, 2009.

14. Faleiros RR, Nuovo GJ, Belknap JK: Calprotectin in myeloid and epithelial cells of laminae from horses with black walnut extract-induced laminitis, *J Vet Intern Med* 23:174, 2009.

15. Belknap J: Pathophysiology of equine laminitis, *Proc Am Coll Vet Intern Med* 148, 2007.

16. van Eps AW, Pollitt CC: Equine laminitis induced with oligofructose, *Equine Vet J* 38:203, 2006.

17. Morgan SJ, Hood DM, Wagner IP, et al: Submural histopathologic changes attributable to peracute laminitis in horses, *Am J Vet Res* 7:829, 2003.

18. Croser EL, Pollitt CC: Acute laminitis: descriptive evaluation of serial hoof biopsies, *Proc Am Assoc Equine Pract* 52:542, 2006.

19. Nourian AR, Baldwin GI, van Eps AW, et al: Equine laminitis: ultrastructural lesions detected 24-30 hours after induction with oligofructose, *Equine Vet J* 39:360, 2007.

20. Van Eps AW, Pollitt CC: Equine laminitis model: lamellar histopathology 7 days after induction with oligofructose, *Equine Vet J* doi: 10.2746/042516409X042434116, 2009.

21. Pollitt CC, Molyneux GS: A scanning electromicroscopical study of the dermal microcirculation of the equine foot, *Equine Vet J* 22:79, 1990.

22. Black SJ, Lunn DP, Yin C, et al: Leukocyte emigration in the early stages of laminitis, *Vet Immunol Immunopathol* 109:161, 2006.

23. Loftus J, Black S, Pettigrew A, et al: Early laminar events involving endothelial activation in horses with black walnut-induced laminitis, *Am J Vet Res* 68:1205, 2007.

24. Belknap JK, Giguere S, Pettigrew A, et al: Lamellar pro-inflammatory cytokine expression patterns in laminitis at the developmental stage and at the onset of lameness: innate vs. adaptive immune response, *Equine Vet J* 39:42, 2007.

25. Visser MB: Investigation of proteolysis of the basement membrane during the development of equine laminitis, School of Veterinary Science, Brisbane, 2009, The University of Queensland. PhD thesis.

26. Kyaw Tanner M, Pollitt CC: Equine laminitis: increased transcription of matrix metalloproteinase-2 (MMP-2) occurs during the developmental phase, *Equine Vet J* 36:221, 2004.

27. Kyaw-Tanner MT, Wattle O, van Eps AW, et al: Equine laminitis: membrane type matrix metalloproteinase-1 (MMP-14) is involved in acute phase onset, *Equine Vet J* 40:482, 2008.

28. Hood DM, Grosenbaugh DA, Mostafa BM, et al: The role of vascular mechanisms in the development of acute equine laminitis, *J Vet Intern Med* 7:228, 1993.

29. Loftus JP, Belknap JK, Stankiewicz KM, et al: Laminar xanthine oxidase, superoxide dismutase and catalase activities in the prodromal stage of black-walnut induced equine laminitis, *Equine Vet J* 39:48, 2007.

30. Pollitt CC, Davies CT: Equine laminitis: its development coincides with increased sublamellar blood flow, *Equine Vet J Suppl* 26:125, 1998.

31. Robinson NE, Scott JB, Dabney JM, et al: Digital vascular responses and permeability in equine alimentary laminitis, *Am J Vet Res* 37:1171, 1976.

32. Trout DR, Hornof WJ, Linford RL, et al: Scintigraphic evaluation of digital circulation during the developmental and acute phases of equine laminitis, *Equine Vet J* 22:416, 1990.

33. deLaat MA, McGowan CM, Sillence MN, et al: Equine laminitis: induced by 48 hours of hyperinsulinaemia in Standardbred horses, *Equine Vet J* 42:129, 2010

34. Sprouse RF, Garner HE, Green EM: Plasma endotoxin levels in horses subjected to carbohydrate induced laminitis, *Equine Vet J* 19:25, 1987.

35. Parsons CS, Orsini JA, Krafty R, et al: Risk factors for development of acute laminitis in horses during hospitalization: 73 cases (1997-2004), *J Am Vet Med Assoc* 230:885, 2007.

36. MacKay RJ, Clark CK, Logdberg L, et al: Effect of a conjugate of polymyxin B-dextran 70 in horses with experimentally induced endotoxemia, *Am J Vet Res* 60:68, 1999.

37. Menzies Gow NJ, Bailey SR, Katz LM, et al: Endotoxin-induced digital vasoconstriction in horses: associated changes in plasma concentrations of vasoconstrictor mediators, *Equine Vet J* 36:273, 2004.

38. Barton MH, Collatos C, Moore JN: Endotoxin induced expression of tumour necrosis factor, tissue factor and plasminogen activator inhibitor activity by peritoneal macrophages, *Equine Vet J* 28:382, 1996.

39. Ingle-Fehr JE, Baxter GM: Evaluation of digital and laminar blood flow in horses given a low dose of endotoxin, *Am J Vet Res* 59:192, 1998.

40. Stephens KA: Studies on sublethal endotoxemia in the horse, *Southwest Vet* 36:27, 1984.

41. Milinovich GJ, Burrell PC, Pollitt CC, et al: Microbial ecology of the equine hindgut during oligofructose-induced laminitis, *ISME J* 2:1089, 2008.

42. Coyne MJ, Cousin H, Loftus JP, et al: Cloning and expression of ADAM related metalloproteases in equine laminitis, *J Vet Immunol* 129:231, 2009.

43. Rasmussen HS, McCann PP: Matrix metalloproteinase inhibition as a novel anticancer strategy: a review with special focus on batimastat and marimastat, *Pharmacol Ther* 75:69, 1997.

44. Asplin KE, Sillence MN, Pollitt CC, et al: Induction of laminitis by prolonged hyperinsulinaemia in clinically normal ponies, *Vet J* 174:530, 2007.

45. Baron AD: Insulin resistance and vascular function, *J Diabetes Complications* 16:92, 2002.

46. Bailey SR, Marr CM, Elliott J: Current research and theories on the pathogenesis of acute laminitis in the horse, *Vet J* 167:129, 2004.

47. Uemura S, Matsushita H, Li W, et al: Diabetes mellitus enhances vascular matrix metalloproteinase activity: role of oxidative stress, *Circ Res* 88:1291, 2001.

48. Mungall BA, Kyaw-Tanner M, Pollitt CC: In vitro evidence for a bacterial pathogenesis of equine laminitis, *Vet Microbiol* 79:209, 2001.

49. Milinovich GJ, Trott DJ, Burrell PC, et al: Fluorescence in situ hybridization analysis of hindgut bacteria associated with the development of equine laminitis, *Environ Microbiol* 9:2090, 2007.

50. Milinovich GJ, Trott DJ, Burrell PC, et al: Changes in equine hindgut bacterial populations during oligofructose induced laminitis, *Environ Microbiol* 8:885, 2006.

51. Johnson PJ: The equine metabolic syndrome peripheral Cushing's syndrome, *Vet Clin North Am Equine Pract* 18:271, 2002.

52. Treiber KH, Kronfeld DS, Geor RJ: Insulin resistance in equids: possible role in laminitis, *J Nutr* 136:2094S, 2006.

53. Treiber KH, Kronfeld DS, Hess TM, et al: Evaluation of genetic and metabolic predispositions and nutritional risk factors for pasture-associated laminitis in ponies, *J Am Vet Med Assoc* 228:1538, 2006.

54. Bailey SR, Habershon-Butcher JL, Ransom KJ, et al: Hypertension and insulin resistance in a mixed-breed population of ponies predisposed to laminitis, *Am J Vet Res* 69:122, 2006.

55. Bailey SR, Menzies-Gow NJ, Harris PA, et al: Effect of dietary fructans and dexamethasone administration on the insulin response of ponies predisposed to laminitis, *J Am Vet Med Assoc* 231:1365, 2007.

56. McGowan C, Frost R, Pfeiffer D, et al: Serum insulin concentrations in horses with equine Cushing's syndrome: response to a cortisol inhibitor and prognostic value, *Equine Vet J* 36:194, 2004.

57. Reeves HJ, Lees R, McGowan CM: Measurement of basal serum insulin concentration in the diagnosis of Cushing's disease in ponies, *Vet Rec* 149:449, 2001.

58. Walsh D, McGowan C, McGowan T, et al: Correlation of plasma insulin concentration with laminitis score in a field study of equine Cushing's disease and equine metabolic syndrome, *J Equine Vet Sci* 29:87, 2009.

59. Pratt SE, Geor RJ, McCutcheon LJ: Effects of dietary energy source and physical conditioning on insulin sensitivity and glucose tolerance in Standardbred horses, *Equine Exerc Physiol* 36:579, 2006

60. Durham AE, Rendle DI, Newton JR: The effect of metformin on measurements of

insulin sensitivity and β cell response in 18 horses and ponies with insulin resistance, *Equine Vet J* doi: 10.2746/042516408X042273648, 2008.

61. Bailey SR, Elliott J: The corticosteroid laminitis story: 2. Science of if, when and how, *Equine Vet J* 39:7-11, 2007.
62. French K, Pollitt CC, Pass MA: Pharmacokinetics and metabolic effects of triamcinolone acetonide and their possible relationships to glucocorticoid-induced laminitis in horses, *J Vet Pharm Ther* 23:287, 2000.
63. McCluskey MJ, Kavenagh PB: Clinical use of triamcinolone acetonide in the horse (205 cases) and the incidence of glucocorticoid-induced laminitis associated with its use, *Equine Vet Educ* 16:86, 2004.
64. Bramlage L: Personal communication, 2008.

Diagnosis of Laminitis

1. Treiber K, Kronfeld D, Hess T, et al: Evaluation of genetic and metabolic predispositions and nutritional risk factors for pasture-associated laminitis in ponies, *J Am Vet Med Assoc* 228:1538, 2006.
2. Dyson S: Unpublished data, 2006.

Medical Therapy of Laminitis

1. Baxter GM: Acute laminitis, *Vet Clin North Am Equine Pract* 10:627, 1994.
2. Pollitt CC, Pass MA, Pollitt S: Batimastat (BB-94) inhibits matrix metalloproteinases of equine laminitis, *Equine Vet J Suppl* 26:119, 1998.
3. Kyaw Tanner M, Pollitt CC: Equine laminitis: increased transcription of matrix metalloproteinase-2 (MMP-2) occurs during the developmental phase, *Equine Vet J* 36:221, 2004.
4. Kyaw-Tanner MT, Wattle O, van Eps AW, et al: Equine laminitis: membrane type matrix metalloproteinase-1 (MMP-14) is involved in acute phase onset, *Equine Vet J* 40:482, 2008.
5. Coyne MJ, Cousin H, Loftus JP, et al: Cloning and expression of ADAM related metalloproteases in equine laminitis, *J Vet Immunol* 129:231, 2009.
6. Pollitt CC, Davies CT: Equine laminitis: its development coincides with increased sublamellar blood flow, *Equine Vet J Suppl* 26:125, 1998.
7. Mungall BA, Kyaw-Tanner M, Pollitt CC: In vitro evidence for a bacterial pathogenesis of equine laminitis, *Vet Microbiol* 79:209, 2001.
8. Semrad SD, Hardee GE, Hardee MM, et al: Low-dose flunixin meglumine—effects on eicosanoid production and clinical signs induced by experimental endotoxemia in horses, *Equine Vet J* 19:201, 1987.
9. Ingle-Fehr JE, Baxter GM: Evaluation of digital and laminar blood flow in horses given a low dose of endotoxin, *Am J Vet Res* 59:192, 1998.
10. van Eps AW, Pollitt CC: Equine laminitis induced with oligofructose, *Equine Vet J* 38:203, 2006.
11. Worster AA, Gaughan EM, Hoskinson JJ, et al: Effects of external thermal manipulation on laminar temperature and perfusion scintigraphy of the equine digit, *New Zealand Vet J* 48:111, 2000.
12. Mealey RH, Carter GK, Roussel AJ, et al: Indwelling cecal catheters for fluid

administration in ponies, *J Vet Intern Med* 9:347, 1995.

13. van Eps AW, Pollitt CC: Equine laminitis: cryotherapy reduces the severity of the acute lesion, *Equine Vet J* 36:255, 2004.
14. van Eps AW, Pollitt CC: Equine laminitis model: cryotherapy reduces the severity of lesions evaluated seven days after induction with oligofructose, *Equine Vet J* 41:741, 2009.
15. Ingle Fehr JE, Baxter GM: The effect of oral isoxsuprine and pentoxifylline on digital and laminar blood flow in healthy horses, *Vet Surg* 28:154, 1999.
16. Adair HS 3rd, Goble DO, Schmidhammer JL, et al: Laminar microvascular flow, measured by means of laser Doppler flowmetry, during the prodromal stages of black walnut-induced laminitis in horses, *Am J Vet Res* 61:862, 2000.
17. Adair HS, Schmidhammer JL, Goble DO, et al: Effects of acepromazine maleate, isoxsuprine hydrochloride and prazosin hydrochloride on laminar blood flow in healthy horses, *J Equine Vet Sci* 17:599, 1997.
18. Loftus JP, Belknap JK, Stankiewicz KM, et al: Laminar xanthine oxidase, superoxide dismutase and catalase activities in the prodromal stage of black-walnut induced equine laminitis, *Equine Vet J* 39:48, 2007.
19. van Eps AW, Walters LJ, Baldwin GI, et al: Distal limb cryotherapy for the prevention of acute laminitis, *Clin Tech Equine Pract* 3:64, 2004.
20. Goetz TE: The treatment of laminitis in horses, *Vet Clin North Am Equine Pract* 5:73, 1989.
21. Peters D, Erfle J, Slobojan G: Low-dose pergolide mesylate treatment for equine hypophyseal adenomas (Cushing's syndrome), *Proc Am Assoc Equine Pract* 41:154, 1995.
22. Walsh DM, McGowan CM, McGowan T, et al: Correlation of plasma insulin concentration with laminitis score in a field study of equine Cushing's disease and equine metabolic syndrome, *J Equine Vet Sci* 29:87, 2009.
23. Durham AE, Rendle DI, Newton JR: The effect of metformin on measurements of insulin sensitivity and β cell response in 18 horses and ponies with insulin resistance, *Equine Vet J* 40:493, 2008.

Chronic Laminitis

1. Hood DM, Stevens KA: Pathophysiology of equine laminitis, *Compend Contin Educ Pract Vet* 3:s454, 1981.
2. Hood DM: The mechanisms and consequences of structural failure of the foot, *Vet Clin North Am Equine Pract* 15:437, 1999.
3. Pellmann R: *Struktur und Funktion des Hufbeinträgers beim Pferd, dissertation*, Berlin, 1995, Freie Universität.
4. Budras KD, Schiel C, Mulling C: Horn tubules of the white line: an insufficient barrier against ascending bacterial invasion, *Equine Vet Educ* 10:81, 1998.
5. Marks G: *Makroskopische, licht- und elektronenmikroskopische Untersuchungen zur Morphologie des Hyponichiums bei der Hufrehe des Pferdes, dissertation*, Berlin, 1984, Freie Universität.
6. Marks G, Budras KD: Zusammenhangstennung im corium und der epidermis

bei der chronischen hufrehe des pferdes, *Anat Histol Embryol J Vet Med Ser C* 14:187, 1985.

7. Pollitt CC: *Equine laminitis: current concepts*, Canberra, Australia, 2008, Rural Industries Research and Development Corporation.
8. Johnson P, Kreeger J, Keeler M, et al: Serum markers of lamellar basement degradation and lamellar histopathological changes in horses affected with laminitis, *Equine Vet J* 32:462, 2000.
9. Hinckley K, Henderson I: The epidemiology of equine laminitis in the UK. *Proceedings of the 35th Congress of the British Equine Veterinary Association*, Warwick, UK, 1996.
10. Morgan SJ, Grosenbaugh DA, Hood DM: The pathophysiology of chronic laminitis, *Vet Clin North Am Equine Pract* 15:395, 1999.
11. Kameya T: Clinical studies on laminitis in the racehorse, *Exp Rep Equine Health Lab* 10:19, 1973.
12. Kuwano A, Katayama Y, Kasashima Y, et al: A gross and histopathological study of an ectopic white line development in equine laminitis, *J Vet Med Sci* 64:893, 2002.
13. Stick JA, Lann HW, Scott EA, et al: Pedal bone rotation as a prognostic sign in laminitis of horses, *J Am Vet Med Assoc* 180:251, 1982.
14. Baxter GM: Equine laminitis caused by distal displacement of the distal phalanx: 12 cases (1976-1985), *J Am Vet Med Assoc* 189:326, 1986.
15. Cripps PJ, Eustace RA: Factors involved in the prognosis of equine laminitis in the UK, *Equine Vet J* 31:433, 1999.
16. Parks AH, Mair TS: Laminitis: a call for unified terminology, *Equine Vet Educ* 21:102, 2009.
17. O'Brien TR, Baker BS: Distal extremity examination: how to perform the radiographic examination and interpret the radiographs, *Proc Am Assoc Equine Pract* 32:553, 1986.
18. Linford RL: *A radiographic, morphometric, histological and ultrastructural investigation of lamellar function, abnormality and the associated radiographic findings for sound and footsore thoroughbreds and horses with experimentally induced traumatic and alimentary laminitis, PhD dissertation*, Davis, Calif, 1987, University of California, Davis.
19. Cripps PJ, Eustace RA: Radiological measurements from the feet of normal horses with relevance to laminitis, *Equine Vet J* 31:427, 1999.
20. Jones E, Vinuela-Fernandez I, Eager R, et al: Neuropathic changes in equine laminitis pain, *Pain* 132:321, 2007.
21. Wagner IP, Hood DM: Cause of airlines associated with acute and chronic laminitis, *Proc Am Assoc Equine Pract* 43:363, 1997.
22. Kameya T, Kiryu K, Kaneko M, et al: Histopathogenesis of thickening of the hoof wall laminae in equine laminitis, *Japan J Vet Sci* 42:361, 1980.
23. Mostafa MB: *Studies on experimental laminitis in the horse, PhD dissertation*, Giza, Egypt, 1986, Cairo University.
24. Budras KD, Hullinger RL, Sack WO: Light and electron microscopy of

keratinization in the laminar epidermis of the equine hoof with reference to laminitis, *Am J Vet Res* 50:150, 1989.

25. Goetz TE: Anatomic, hoof, and shoeing considerations for the treatment of laminitis in horses, *J Am Vet Med Assoc* 190:1323, 1987.

Venography

1. Redden RR: A technique for performing digital venography in the standing horse, *Equine Vet Educ* 13:128, 2001.
2. Mishra PC, Leach DH: Extrinsic and intrinsic veins of the equine hoof wall, *J Anat* 136:543, 1983.
3. Baldwin GI, Pollitt CC: Retrograde venous angiography (venography) of the equine digit during experimentally induced acute and chronic laminitis. *Proceeding of the 47th Congress of the British Equine Veterinary Association*, Liverpool, UK, 2008.
4. Eustace RA, Emery S: Partial coronary epidermectomy (coronary peel), dorsodistal wall fenestration and deep digital flexor tenotomy to treat severe acute founder in a Connemara pony, *Equine Vet Educ* 21:91, 2009.

Hoof Care of a Laminitic Horse

1. Allen DA, White NA, Fernier J, et al: Surgical management of chronic laminitis in horses: 13 cases (1983-1985), *J Am Vet Med Assoc* 189:1604, 1986.
2. O'Grady SE, Steward ML, Parks AH: How to construct and apply the wooden shoe for treating three manifestations of laminitis, *Proc Am Assoc Equine Pract* 53:423, 2007.
3. Hunt RJ, Allen DA, Baxter GM, et al: Midmetacarpal deep digital flexor tenotomy in the management of refractory laminitis in the horse, *Vet Surg* 20:15, 1991.
4. Eastman TG, Honnas CM, Hague BA, et al: Deep digital flexor tenotomy as a treatment for chronic laminitis in horses: 37 cases, *Proc Am Assoc Equine Pract* 44:265, 1998.

Deep Digital Flexor Tenotomy for Managing Laminitis

1. Allen D, White NA, Foerner JF, et al: Surgical management of chronic laminitis in horses: 13 cases (1983-1985), *J Am Vet Med Assoc* 189:1604, 1986.
2. Eastman TG, Honnas CM, Hague BA, et al: Deep digital flexor tenotomy as a treatment for chronic laminitis in horses: 35 cases (1988-1997), *J Am Vet Med Assoc* 214:517, 1999.
3. Jann HW, Williams JA, Whitfield CC, et al: Surgical treatment of chronic refractory laminitis: deep digital flexor tenotomy, *Equine Pract* 19:26, 1997.
4. Hunt RJ, Allen DA, Baxter GM, et al: Midmetacarpal deep digital flexor tenotomy in the management of refractory laminitis in horses, *Vet Surg* 20:15, 1991.
5. Burba DJ, Hubert JD, Beadle R: How to perform a mid-metacarpal deep digital flexor tenotomy on a standing horse, *Proc Am Assoc Equine Pract* 52:547, 2006.

Other Management Aspects of Laminitis

1. Sigafoos R: Personal communication, 2001.
2. Ellis J, Hollands T: Use of height-specific weigh tapes to estimate the bodyweight of horses, *Vet Rec* 150:632, 2002.
3. Tinworth K, Edwards S, Harris P, et al: Pharmacokinetics of oral metformin in insulin-resistant ponies, *Am J Vet Res* (In press.)
4. Jones E, Vinuela-Fernandez I, Eager R, et al: Neuropathic changes in equine laminitis, *Pain* 132:321, 2007.
5. Dutton D, Lashnits K, Wegner K: Managing severe hoof pain in a horse using multimodal analgesia and a modified composite pain score, *Equine Vet Educ* 21:37, 2009.
6. Love E: Assessment and management of pain in horses, *Equine Vet Educ* 21:46, 2009.

CHAPTER 35 The Proximal and Middle Phalanges and Proximal Interphalangeal Joint

1. Sack WO, Habel RE: *Rooney's guide to the dissection of the horse*, ed 1, Ithaca, NY, 1967, Veterinary Textbooks.
2. Delahunta A, Habel RE: *Applied veterinary anatomy*, ed 1, Philadelphia, 1986, Saunders.
3. Butler J, Colles C, Dyson S, et al: The foot, pastern and fetlock. In Butler J, Colles C, Dyson S, et al, eds: *Clinical radiology of the horse*, ed 3, Oxford, 2008, Wiley-Blackwell.
4. Reimer JM: *Atlas of equine ultrasonography*, ed 1, St. Louis, 1988, Mosby.
5. Dyson S, Murray R, Schramme M, et al: Lameness in 46 horses with deep digital flexor tendonitis in the digit confirmed with magnetic resonance imaging, *Equine Vet J* 35:681, 2003.
6. Gillis JP, Zardiackas LD, Gilbert JA, et al: Holding power of cortical screws after power tapping and hand tapping, *Vet Surg* 21:362, 1992.
7. Holcombe SJ, Schneider RK, Bramlage LR, et al: Lag screw fixation of noncomminuted sagittal fractures of the proximal phalanx in racehorses: 59 cases (1973-1991), *J Am Vet Med Assoc* 206:1195, 1995.
8. Tetens J, Ross MW, Lloyd JW: Comparison of racing performance before and after treatment of incomplete, midsagittal fractures of the proximal phalanx in Standardbreds: 49 cases (1986-1992), *J Am Vet Med Assoc* 210:82, 1997.
9. Markel MD, Richardson D: Noncomminuted fractures of the proximal phalanx in 69 horses, *J Am Vet Med Assoc* 186:573, 1985.
10. Markel MD, Martin BB, Richardson DW: Dorsal frontal fractures of the first phalanx in the horse, *Vet Surg* 14:36, 1985.
11. Dechant JE, MacDonald DG, Crawford WH: Repair of complete dorsal fracture of the proximal phalanx in two horses, *Vet Surg* 27:445, 1998.
12. Kraus BM, Richardson DW, Nunamaker DM, et al: Management of comminuted fractures of the proximal phalanx in horses: 64 cases (1983-2001), *J Am Vet Med Assoc* 224:254, 2004.
13. Parente EJ, Nunamaker DM: Stress protection afforded by a cast on plate fixation of the distal forelimb in the horse in vitro, *Vet Surg* 24:49, 1995.
14. Schneider RK, Ratzlaff MC, White KK, et al: Effect of three types of half-limb casts on in vitro bone strain recorded from the third metacarpal bone and proximal phalanx in equine cadaver limbs, *Am J Vet Res* 59:1188, 1998.
15. Joyce J, Baxter GM, Sarrafian TL, et al: Use of transfixation pin casts to treat adult horses with comminuted phalangeal fractures: 20 cases (1993-2003), *J Am Vet Med Assoc* 229:725, 2006.
16. Markel MD, Richardson DW, Nunamaker DM: Comminuted first phalanx fractures in 30 horses: surgical and nonsurgical treatments, *Vet Surg* 14:135, 1985.
17. McClure SR, Watkins JP, Bronson DG, et al: In vitro comparison of the standard short limb cast and three configurations of shortlimb transfixation casts in equine forelimbs, *Am J Vet Res* 55:1331, 1994.
18. Nunamaker DM: External fixation. In White NA, Moore JN, eds: *Current techniques in equine surgery and lameness*, ed 2, Philadelphia, 1998, Saunders.
19. Radcliffe RM, Cheetham J, Bezuidenhout AJ, et al: Arthroscopic removal of palmar/plantar osteochondral fragments from the proximal interphalangeal joint in four horses, *Vet Surg* 37:733, 2008.
20. Welch RD, Watkins JP: Osteochondral fracture of the proximal palmar middle phalanx in a Thoroughbred, *Equine Vet J* 23:67, 1991.
21. Dyson S: Personal communication, 2001.
22. Watkins JP, Eastman TG, Easter JL: In vitro cyclic fatigue properties of parallel screw and dorsal plate arthrodesis of the proximal interphalangeal joint, *Proc Am Assoc Equine Pract* 46:102, 2000.
23. Caron JP, Fretz PB, Bailey JV, et al: Proximal interphalangeal arthrodesis in the horse: a retrospective study and a modified screw technique, *Vet Surg* 19:196, 1990.
24. Martin GS, McIlwraith CW, Turner AS, et al: Long-term results and complications of proximal interphalangeal arthrodesis in horses, *J Am Med Vet Assoc* 184:1139, 1984.
25. MacLellan KN, Crawfrod WH, MacDonald DG: Proximal interphalangeal joint arthrodesis in 34 horses using two parallel 5.5 mm cortical bone screws, *Vet Surg* 30:454, 2001.
26. Knox PM, Watkins JP: Proximal interphalangeal joint arthrodesis using a combination plate-screw technique in 53 horses (1994-2003), *Equine Vet J* 38:538, 2006.
27. Galuppo LD, Stover SM, Willits NH: A biomechanical comparison of double-plate and Y-plate fixation for comminuted equine second phalangeal fractures, *Vet Surg* 29:152, 2000.
28. Crabill MR, Watkins JP, Schneider RK, et al: Double-plate fixation of comminuted fractures of the second phalanx in horses: 10 cases (1985-1993), *J Am Vet Med Assoc* 207:1458, 1995.
29. Dyson S: Personal communication, 2009.
30. Olive J, Mair T, Charles B: Use of standing low-field magnetic resonance imaging to diagnose middle phalanx bone marrow lesions in horses, *Equine Vet Educ* 21:116, 2009.
31. Werpy N: Diagnosis of middle phalanx bone marrow lesions in horses using magnetic resonance imaging and identification of phase effect cancellation for proper image interpretation, *Equine Vet Educ* 21:125, 2009.
32. Shiroma JT, Engel HN, Wagner PC, et al: Dorsal subluxation of the proximal

interphalangeal joint in the pelvic limb of three horses, *J Am Vet Med Assoc* 195:777, 1989.

33. Errico JA, Trumble TN, Bueno AC, et al: Comparison of two indirect techniques for local delivery of a high dose of an antimicrobial in the distal portion of forelimbs of horses, *Am J Vet Res* 69:334, 2008.

CHAPTER 36   The Metacarpophalangeal Joint

1. Brama PA, Karssenberg D, Barneveld A, et al: Contact areas and pressure distribution on the proximal articular surface of the proximal phalanx under sagittal plane loading, *Equine Vet J* 33:26, 2001.
2. Clayton HM, Sha D, Stick J, et al: 3D kinematics of the equine metacarpophalangeal joint at walk and trot, *Vet Comp Orthop Traumatol* 20:86, 2007.
3. Gray BW, Engel HN Jr, Rumph PF, et al: Clinical approach to determine the contribution of the palmar and palmar metacarpal nerves to the innervation of the equine fetlock joint, *Am J Vet Res* 41:940, 1980.
4. O'Brien TR, Hornof WJ, Meagher DM: Radiographic detection and characterization of palmar lesions in the equine fetlock joint, *J Am Vet Med Assoc* 178:231, 1981.
5. Pilsworth RC, Hopes R, Greet TRC: A flexed dorso-palmar projection of the equine fetlock in demonstrating lesions of the distal third metacarpus, *Vet Rec* 122:332, 1988.
6. Weaver J, Stover S, O'Brien T: Radiographic anatomy of soft tissue attachments in the equine metacarpophalangeal and proximal phalangeal region, *Equine Vet J* 24:310, 1992.
7. Ross MW: Scintigraphic and clinical findings in the Standardbred metatarsophalangeal joint: 114 cases (1993-1995), *Equine Vet J* 30:131, 1998.
8. Dyson S, Murray R: Osseous trauma in the fetlock region of mature sports horses, *Proc Am Assoc Equine Pract* 52:443, 2006.
9. Biggi M, Dyson S, Murray R: Scintigraphic assessment of the metacarpophalangeal and metatarsophalangeal joints with joint pain, *Vet Radiol Ultrasound* 50:536, 2009.
10. Reef VB: Joint ultrasonography, *Clin Tech Equine Pract* 3:256, 2004.
11. Denoix JM, Thill E, Houliez D, et al: Ultrasonographic examination of the metacarpophalangeal joint. Correlation between ultrasonographic and postmortem findings, *Prat Vet Equine* 29:179, 1997.
12. Vanderperren K, Martens A, Declerq J, et al: Comparison of ultrasonography versus radiography for the diagnosis of dorsal fragmentation of the metacarpophalangeal or metatarsophalangeal joint in horses, *J Am Vet Med Assoc* 235:70, 2009.
13. Hanson JA, Seeherman HJ, Kirker-Head CA, et al: The role of computed tomography in evaluation of subchondral osseous lesions in seven horses with chronic synovitis, *Equine Vet J* 28:480, 1996.
14. Schoenborn WC, Rick MC, Hornof WJ: Computed tomographic appearance of osteochondritis dissecans-like lesions of the proximal articular surface of the proximal phalanx in a horse, *Vet Radiol Ultrasound* 43:541, 2002.
15. Vanderperren K, Ghaye B, Snaps FR, et al: Evaluation of computed tomographic anatomy of the equine metacarpophalangeal joint, *Am J Vet Res* 69:631, 2008.
16. Sherlock CE, Mair TS, Braake FT: Osseous lesions in the metacarpo(tarso)phalangeal joint diagnosed using low-field magnetic resonance imaging in standing horses, *Vet Radiol Ultrasound* 50:13, 2009.
17. Zubrod C, Schneider R, Tucker R, et al: Diagnosis of subchondral bone damage using magnetic resonance imaging in eleven horses, *J Am Vet Med Assoc* 24:411, 2004.
18. Dyson S, Murray R: Magnetic resonance imaging of the equine fetlock, *Clin Tech Equine Pract* 6:62, 2007.
19. Murray R, Tranquille C, Parkin T: Using MRI for recognition/ monitoring of fetlock pathology and detection of fracture warning signs, *Proc Brit Equine Vet Assoc Congress* 48:131, 2009.
20. Dabareiner RM, White NA, Sullins KE: Metacarpophalangeal joint synovial pad fibrotic proliferation in 63 horses, *Vet Surg* 25:199, 1996.
21. Kannegieter NJ: Chronic proliferative synovitis of the equine metacarpophalangeal joint, *Vet Rec* 127:8, 1990.
22. Declercq J, Martens A, Bogaert L, et al: Osteochondral fragmentation in the synovial pad of the fetlock in Warmblood horses, *Vet Surg* 37:613, 2008.
23. Brommer H, Brama P, Barnveld A, et al: Differences in the topographical distribution of articular cartilage degeneration between equine metacarpophalangeal and metatarsophalangeal joints, *Equine Vet J* 36:506, 2004.
24. Strand E, Martin G, Crawford M, et al: Intraarticular pressure, elastance and range of motion in healthy and injured racehorse metacarpophalangeal joints, *Equine Vet J* 30:527, 1998.
25. Dyson S: Personal communication, 2009.
26. Norrdin RW, Kawcak CE, Capwell BA, et al: Subchondral bone failure in an equine model of overload arthrosis, *Bone* 22:133, 1998.
27. Riggs CM, Whitehouse GH, Boyde A: Pathology of the distal condyles of the third metacarpal and third metatarsal bones of the horse, *Equine Vet J* 31:140, 1999.
28. Parkin T, Tranquille C, Kawcak C, et al: Can condylar subchondral bone thickness predict the risk of lateral condylar fracture in the Thoroughbred? *Proc Brit Equine Vet Assoc Congress* 48:129, 2009.
29. Colon JL, Bramlage LR, Hance SR, et al: Qualitative and quantitative documentation of the racing performance of 461 Thoroughbred racehorses after arthroscopic removal of dorsoproximal first phalanx osteochondral fractures (1986-1995), *Equine Vet J* 32:475, 2000.
30. Elce YA, Richardson DW: Arthroscopic removal of dorsoproximal chip fractures of the proximal phalanx in standing horses, *Vet Surg* 31:195, 2002.
31. Kawcak CE, McIlwraith CW: Proximodorsal first phalanx osteochondral chip fragmentation in 336 horses, *Equine Vet J* 26:392, 1994.
32. Dalin G, Sandgren B, Carlsten J: Plantar osteochondral fragments in the metatarsophalangeal joints in Standardbred trotters; result of osteochondrosis or trauma, *Equine Vet J* 16:62, 1993.
33. Nixon AJ, Pool RR: Histologic appearance of axial osteochondral fragments from the proximoplantar/proximopalmar aspect of the proximal phalanx in horses, *J Am Vet Med Assoc* 207:1076, 1995.
34. Fortier LA, Foerner JJ, Nixon AJ: Arthroscopic removal of axial osteochondral fragments of the plantar/palmar proximal aspect of the proximal phalanx in horses: 119 cases (1988-1992), *J Am Vet Med Assoc* 206:71, 1995.
35. Boys-Smith S, Singer E, Clegg P: A retrospective study of 52 non-racehorses presented with a fracture of the proximal phalanx. Proceedings of the Thirteenth European College of Veterinary Surgeons Annual Congress, 2005, Lyon, France.
36. Kummerle J, Auer J, Rademacher N, et al: Short incomplete sagittal fractures of the proximal phalanx in 10 horses not used for racing, *Vet Surg* 37:193, 2008.
37. Kane AJ, Park RD, McIlwraith CW, et al: Radiographic changes in Thoroughbred yearlings. Part 1: Prevalence at the time of the yearling sales, *Equine Vet J* 35:354, 2003.
38. Kane AJ, McIlwraith CW, Park RD, et al: Radiographic changes in Thoroughbred yearlings. Part 2: Associations with racing performance, *Equine Vet J* 35:366, 2003.
39. Spike-Pierce D, Bramlage L: Correlation of racing performance with radiographic changes in the proximal sesamoid bones of 487 Thoroughbred yearlings, *Equine Vet J* 35:350, 2003.
40. Hardy J, Marcoux M, Breton L: Clinical relevance of radiographic findings in proximal sesamoid bones of two-year-old Standardbreds in their first year of training, *J Am Vet Med Assoc* 198:2089, 1991.
41. Grøndahl A, Gaustad G, Engeland A: Progression and association with lameness and racing performance of radiographic changes in the proximal sesamoid bones of young Standardbred trotters, *Equine Vet J* 26:152, 1994.
42. Barr E, Clegg P, Senior M, et al: Destructive lesions of the proximal sesamoid bones as a complication of dorsal metatarsal artery catheterisation in three horses, *Vet Surg* 34:159, 2005.
43. Anthenill L, Stover S, Gardner G, et al: Risk factor for proximal sesamoid bone fractures associated with exercise history and horseshoe characteristics in Thoroughbred racehorses, *Am J Vet Res* 68:760, 2007.
44. Schnabel L, Bramlage L, Mohammed H, et al: Racing performance after arthroscopic removal of apical sesamoid fractures in Thoroughbred horses age ≥2 years: 84 cases (1998-2002), *Equine Vet J* 38:446, 2006.
45. Schnabel L, Bramlage L, Mohammed H, et al: Racing performance after arthroscopic removal of apical sesamoid fractures in Thoroughbred horses age < 2 years: 151 cases (1998-2002), *Equine Vet J* 39:64, 2007.

46. Woodie J, Ruggles A, Bertone A, et al: Apical fracture of the proximal sesamoid bone in Standardbred horses: 43 cases (1990-1996), *J Am Vet Med Assoc* 214:1653, 1999.

47. Southwood L, Trotter G, McIlwraith C: Arthroscopic removal of abaxial fracture fragments of the proximal sesamoid bone in horses: 47 cases (1989–1997), *J Am Vet Med Assoc* 213:1016, 1998.

48. Parente EJ, Richardson DW, Spencer P: Basal sesamoidean fractures in horses: 57 cases (1980-1991), *J Am Vet Med Assoc* 202:1293, 1993.

49. Southwood LL, McIlwraith CW: Arthroscopic removal of fracture fragments involving a portion of the base of the proximal sesamoid bone in horses: 26 cases (1984-1997), *J Am Vet Med Assoc* 217:236, 2000.

50. Brokken M, Schneider R, Tucker R: Surgical approach for removal of non-articular base sesamoid fragments of the proximal sesamoid bones in horses, *Vet Surg* 17:619, 2008.

51. Henninger R, Bramlage L, Schneider R, et al: Lag screw and cancellous bone graft fixation of transverse proximal sesamoid bone fractures in horses: 25 cases (1983-1989), *J Am Vet Med Assoc* 199:606, 1991.

52. Martin B, Nunamaker D, Evans L, et al: Circumferential wiring of mid-body and large basilar fractures of the proximal sesamoid bone in 15 horses, *Vet Surg* 20:9, 1991.

53. Barclay WP, Foerner JJ, Phillips TN: Axial sesamoid injuries associated with lateral condylar fractures in horses, *J Am Vet Med Assoc* 186:278, 1985.

54. Wisner ER, O'Brien TR, Pool RR, et al: Osteomyelitis of the axial border of the proximal sesamoid bones in seven horses, *Equine Vet J* 23:383, 1991.

55. Dabareiner R, Watkins J, Carter G, et al: Osteitis of the axial border of the proximal sesamoid bones in horses: 8 cases (1993-1999), *J Am Vet Med Assoc* 219:82, 2001.

56. Radtke CL, Danova NA, Scollay MC, et al: Macroscopic changes in the distal ends of the third metacarpal and metatarsal bones of Thoroughbred racehorses with condylar fractures, *Am J Vet Res* 64:1110, 2003.

57. Yovich JV, McIlwraith CW, Stashak TS: Osteochondritis dissecans of the sagittal ridge of the third metacarpal and metatarsal bones in horses, *J Am Vet Med Assoc* 186:1186, 1985.

58. Hogan PM, McIlwraith CW, Honnas CM, et al: Surgical treatment of subchondral cystic lesions of the third metacarpal bone: results in 15 horses (1986-1994), *Equine Vet J* 29:477, 1997.

59. Tenny A, Whitcomb MB: Rupture of collateral ligaments in metacarpophalangeal and metatarsophalangeal joints in horses: 17 cases (1999-2005), *J Am Vet Med Assoc* 233:456, 2008.

CHAPTER 37   The Metacarpal Region

1. Muylle S, Desmet P, Simoens P, et al: Histological study of the innervation of the suspensory ligament of the forelimb in the horse, *Vet Rec* 142:606, 1998.

2. Keg P, van den Belt A, Merkens H: The effect of regional nerve blocks on the lameness caused by collagenase induced tendonitis in the mid metacarpal region of the horse: a study using gait analysis and ultrasonography to determine tendon healing, *J Vet Med A* 39:349, 1992.

3. Cornelissen B, Rijkenhuizen A, Barnveld A: The diagnostic nerve block of the sesamoidean nerve: desensitized structures and possible clinical applications, *Vet Q* 18(Suppl 2):S97, 1996.

4. Ford T, Ross M, Orsini P: A comparison of methods for proximal metacarpal anaesthesia in horses, *Vet Surg* 18:146, 1988.

5. Castro F, Schumacher J, Pauwels F, et al: A new approach for perineural injection of the lateral palmar nerve in the horse, *Vet Surg* 34:359, 2005.

6. Butler JA, Colles CM, Dyson SJ, et al: The metacarpal and metatarsal regions. In *Clinical radiology of the horse*, ed 3, Oxford, 2008, Wiley-Blackwell.

7. Sampson S, Tucker R: Magnetic resonance imaging of the proximal metacarpal and metatarsal regions, *Clin Techn Equine Pract* 6:78, 2007.

8. Zubrod C, Schneider R, Tucker R, et al: Use of MRI to identify suspensory desmitis and adhesions between exostoses of the second metacarpal bone and the suspensory ligament in 4 horses, *J Am Vet Med Assoc* 224:1815, 2004.

9. Brokken T, Schneider R, Sampson S, et al: Magnetic resonance imaging features of proximal metacarpal and metatarsal injuries in the horse, *Vet Radiol Ultrasound* 48:507, 2007.

10. Dyson S, Murray R: Unpublished data, 2004-2009.

11. Dyson S: Some observations on lameness associated with pain in the proximal metacarpal region, *Equine Vet J Suppl* 6:43, 1988.

12. Ross M, Ford T, Orsini P: Incomplete longitudinal fracture of the proximal palmar cortex of the third metacarpal bone in horses, *Vet Surg* 17:82, 1988.

13. Lloyd K, Kobluk P, Ragle C, et al: Incomplete palmar fracture of the proximal extremity of the third metacarpal bone in horses: ten cases (1981-1986), *J Am Vet Med Assoc* 192:798, 1988.

14. Pleasant R, Baker G, Muhlbauer M, et al: Stress reactions and stress fractures of the proximal palmar aspect of the third metacarpal bone in horses: 58 cases (1980-1990), *J Am Vet Med Assoc* 201:1918, 1992.

15. Powell S, Ramzan P, Head M, et al: Standing magnetic resonance imaging detection of bone marrow oedema-type signal pattern associated with subcarpal pain in 8 racehorses: a prospective study, *Equine Vet J* 42:10, 2010.

16. Sullivan C, Lumsden J: Distal third metacarpal bone palmar cortical stress fractures in 4 Thoroughbred racehorses, *Equine Vet Educ* 14:70, 2002.

17. Ross M, Martin B: Dorsomedial articular fracture of the proximal aspect of the third metacarpal bone in Standardbred racehorses: seven cases (1978-1990), *J Am Vet Med Assoc* 201:332, 1992.

18. Zubrod C, Schneider R, Tucker R, et al: Use of magnetic resonance imaging for identifying subchondral bone damage in horses: 11 cases, *J Am Vet Med Assoc* 224:411, 2004.

19. Dyson S, Murray R: Osseous trauma in the fetlock region of mature horses, *Proc Am Assoc Equine Pract* 52:443, 2006.

20. Bramlage L, Gabel A, Hackett R: Avulsion fractures of the origin of the suspensory ligament in the horse, *J Am Vet Med Assoc* 176:1004, 1980.

21. Dyson S, Arthur R, Palmer S, et al: Suspensory ligament desmitis, *Vet Clin North Am Equine Pract* 11:177, 1995.

22. Dyson S: *Problems encountered in equine lameness diagnosis with special reference to local analgesic techniques, radiology and ultrasonography*, Newmarket, UK, 1995, R and W Publications.

23. Dyson S: The suspensory apparatus. In Rantanen N, McKinnon A, eds: *Equine diagnostic ultrasonography*, Baltimore, 1998, Williams & Wilkins.

24. Dyson S: Proximal metacarpal and metatarsal pain: a diagnostic challenge, *Equine Vet Educ* 15:134, 2006.

25. Edwards R, Ducharme N, Fubini S, et al: Scintigraphy for diagnosis of avulsions of the origin of the suspensory ligament in horses: 51 cases (1980-1993), *J Am Vet Med Assoc* 207:608, 1995.

26. Launois T, Desbrosse F, Perrin R: Percutaneous osteostixis as treatment of the palmar/plantar third metacarpal/metatarsal cortex at the origin of the suspensory ligament in 29 cases, *Equine Vet Educ* 15:126, 2006.

27. Malone E, Les C, Turner T: Severe carpometacarpal osteoarthritis in older Arabian horses, *Vet Surg* 32:191, 2003.

28. Panizzi L, Barber S, Lang H, Carmalt J: Carpometacarpal osteoarthritis in thirty-three horses, *Vet Surg* 38:998, 2009.

29. Lang H, Panizzi L, Allen A, et al: Comparison of three drilling techniques for carpometacarpal joint arthrodesis in horses, *Vet Surg* 38:990, 2009.

30. Barber S, Panizzi L, Lang H: Treatment of carpometacarpal osteoarthritis by arthrodesis in 12 horses, *Vet Surg* 38:1006, 2009.

31. Coudry V, Denoix J-M, Didierlaurent D, et al: Use of magnetic resonance imaging to diagnose the cause of proximal metacarpal pain in a standardbred trotter, *Vet Rec* 162:790, 2008.

32. Boening J, Weiler I: New technique in splint bone surgery. Proceedings of the Forty-Fourth British Equine Veterinary Association Congress, Harrogate, 2007.

33. Bowman K, Evans L, Herring M: Evaluation of surgical removal of fractured distal splint bones in the horse, *Vet Surg* 11:116, 1982.

34. Verschooten F, Gasthuys F, De Moor A: Distal splint bone fractures in the horse: an experimental and clinical study, *Equine Vet J* 16:532, 1984.

35. Allen D, White N: Management of fractures and exostoses of the metacarpals and metatarsals II and IV in 25 horses, *Equine Vet J* 19:326, 1987.

36. Harrison L, May S, Edwards G: Surgical treatment of open splint bone fractures in 26 horses, *Vet Rec* 128:606, 1991.

37. Jackson M: Splint bone fractures in the horse: a retrospective study 1992-2000, *Equine Vet Educ* 19:329, 2007.

38. Kidd J, Dyson S, Barr A: Septic flexor tendon core lesions in five horses, *Equine Vet J* 34:213, 2002.
39. Dyson S: The metacarpal region. In Ross M, Dyson S, eds: *Diagnosis and management of lameness in the horse*, ed 1, St. Louis, 2003, Saunders.
40. Mair T, Dyson S, Fraser J, et al: Hypertrophic osteopathy (Marie's disease) in Equidae: a review of twenty-four cases, *Equine Vet J* 28:256, 1996.
41. Crawford W, Vanderby R, Neirby D, et al: The energy absorption capacity of equine support bandages. I. Comparison between bandages placed in various configurations and tensions, *Vet Comp Orthop Trauma* 1:2, 1990.
42. Crawford W, Vanderby R, Neirby D, et al: The energy absorption capacity of equine support bandages. II. Comparisons between bandages from different materials, *Vet Comp Orthop Trauma* 1:10, 1990.
43. Keegan K, Baker G, Boero M, et al: Evaluation of support bandaging during measurement of proximal sesamoidean ligament strain in horses by use of a mercury strain gauge, *Am J Vet Res* 53:1203, 1992.
44. Kobluk C, Martinez del Campo M, Harvey-Fulton K, et al: A kinematic investigation of the effect of a cohesive elastic bandage on the gait of the exercising thoroughbred racehorse, *Proc Am Assoc Equine Pract* 34:135, 1988.
45. Luhmann L, Wickler S, Hoyt D, et al: Evaluation of shock attenuation in the forelimb of horses wearing boots and wraps, *J Equine Vet Sci* 20:503, 2000.
46. Ramon T, Pades M, Armengou L, et al: Effects of athletic taping of the fetlock on distal limb mechanics, *Equine Vet J* 36:764, 2004.
47. Smith R, McGuigan M, Hyde J, et al: In vitro evaluation of nonrigid support systems for the equine metacarpophalangeal joint, *Equine Vet J* 34:726, 2002.
48. Kicker C, Peham C, Girtler D, et al: Influence of support boots on the fetlock joint angle of the forelimb of the horse at walk and trot, *Equine Vet J* 36:769, 2004.

CHAPTER 38   The Carpus

1. Getty R, ed: *Sisson and Grossman's the anatomy of the domestic animals*, Philadelphia, 1975, Saunders.
2. Whitton RC, Rose RJ: The intercarpal ligaments of the equine midcarpal joint. II. The role of the palmar intercarpal ligaments in the restraint of dorsal displacement of the proximal row of carpal bones, *Vet Surg* 26:367, 1997.
3. Whitton RC, McCarthy RH, Rose RJ: The intercarpal ligaments of the equine midcarpal joint. I. The anatomy of the palmar and dorsomedial intercarpal ligaments of the midcarpal joint, *Vet Surg* 26:359, 1997.
4. Selway SJ: Intercarpal ligament impingement: a primary cause of joint pathology, *Proc Am Assoc Equine Pract* 37:779, 1991.
5. Whitton RC, Kannegieter NJ, Rose RJ: The intercarpal ligaments of the equine midcarpal joint. III. Clinical observations in 32 racing horses with midcarpal joint disease, *Vet Surg* 26:374, 1997.
6. Bramlage LR, Schneider RK, Gabel AA: A clinical perspective on lameness originating in the carpus, *Equine Vet J Suppl* 6:12, 1988.
7. Young DR, Delaney CL, Richardson DW: Role of intercarpal ligaments in distribution and attenuation of articular contact stress in horses, *Vet Surg* 23:428, 1994 (abstract).
8. Phillips TJ, Wright IM: Observations on the anatomy and pathology of the palmar intercarpal ligaments in the middle carpal joints of thoroughbred racehorses, *Equine Vet J* 26:486, 1994.
9. McIlwraith CW: Tearing of the medial intercarpal ligament in the equine midcarpal joint, *Equine Vet J* 24:367, 1992.
10. Ford TS, Ross MW, Orsini PG: Communications and boundaries of the middle carpal and carpometacarpal joints in horses, *Am J Vet Res* 49:2161, 1988.
11. Ford TS, Ross MW, Orsini PG: A comparison of methods for proximal palmar metacarpal analgesia in horses, *Vet Surg* 18:146, 1989.
12. Dyson SJ: Problems associated with the interpretation of the results of regional and intra-articular anaesthesia in the horse, *Vet Rec* 118:419, 1986.
13. Schaer T, Ross MW: Unpublished data, 1995.
14. Waselau M, Bertone AL, Green EM: Computed tomographic documentation of a comminuted fourth carpal bone fracture associated with carpal instability treated by partial carpal arthrodesis in an Arabian filly, *Vet Surg* 35:618, 2006.
15. Anastasiou A, Skioldebrand E, Ekman S, Hall LD: Ex vivo magnetic resonance imaging of the distal row of equine carpal bones: assessment of bone sclerosis and cartilage damage, *Vet Radiol Ultrasound* 44:501, 2003.
16. Getman LM, McKnight AL, Richardson DW: Comparison of magnetic resonance contrast arthrography and arthroscopic anatomy of the equine palmar lateral outpouching of the middle carpal joint, *Vet Radiol Ultrasound* 48:493, 2007.
17. Driver AJ, Barr FJ, Fuller CJ, Barr AR: Ultrasonography of the medial palmar intercarpal ligament in the Thoroughbred: technique and normal appearance, *Equine Vet J* 36:402, 2004.
18. Foreman JH, Kneller SK, Twardock AR, et al: Forelimb skeletal scintigraphy responses in previously untrained Thoroughbreds undergoing initial treadmill training, *Equine Vet J Suppl* 34:230, 2002.
19. Kawcak CE, McIlwraith CW, Norrdin RW, et al: Clinical effects of exercise on subchondral bone of carpal and metacarpophalangeal joints in horses, *Am J Vet Res* 61:1252, 2000.
20. Kawcak CE, Frisbie DD, Werpy NM, et al: Effects of exercise vs experimental osteoarthritis on imaging outcomes, *Osteoarthritis Cartilage* 16:1519, 2008.
21. Cheetham J, Nixon AJ: Arthroscopic approaches to the palmar aspect of the equine carpus, *Vet Surg* 35:227, 2006.
22. Getman LM, Southwood LL, Richardson DW: Palmar carpal osteochondral fragments in racehorses: 31 cases (1994-2004), *J Am Vet Med Assoc* 228:1551, 2006.
23. Pool RR, Meagher DM: Pathologic findings and pathogenesis of racetrack injuries, *Vet Clin North Am Equine Pract* 6:1, 1990.
24. Young A, O'Brien TR, Pool RR, et al: Histologic and microradiographic changes in the third carpal bone of the racing thoroughbred, *Vet Surg* 7:27, 1988 (abstract).
25. Radin EL, Parker HG, Pugh JW: Response to joints to impact loading. III. Relationship between trabecular microfractures and cartilage degeneration, *J Biomech* 6:51, 1973.
26. Radin EL, Rose RM: Role of subchondral bone in the initiation and progression of cartilage damage, *Clin Orthop Relat Res* 213:34, 1986.
27. DeHaan CD, O'Brien TR, Koblik PD: A radiographic investigation of third carpal bone injury in 42 racing thoroughbreds, *Vet Radiol* 28:88, 1987.
28. Schneider RK, Bramlage LR, Gabel AA, et al: Incidence, location and classification of 371 third carpal bone fractures in 313 horses, *Equine Vet J Suppl* 6:33, 1988.
29. Tidswell HK, Innes JF, Avery NC, et al: High-intensity exercise induces structural, compositional and metabolic changes in cuboidal bones—findings from an equine athlete model, *Bone* 43:724, 2008.
30. Magnusson LE, Ekman S: Osteoarthrosis of the antebrachiocarpal joint of 7 riding horses, *Acta Vet Scand* 42:429, 2001.
31. Steel CM, Hopper BJ, Richardson JL, et al: Clinical findings, diagnosis, prevalence and predisposing factors for lameness localised to the middle carpal joint in young Standardbred racehorses, *Equine Vet J* 38:152, 2006.
32. Malone ED, Les CM, Turner TA: Severe carpometacarpal osteoarthritis in older Arabian horses, *Vet Surg* 32:191, 2003.
33. Barr ARS: Carpal conformation in relation to carpal chip fracture, *Vet Rec* 134:646, 1994.
34. Anderson TM, McIlwraith CW, Douay P: The role of conformation in musculoskeletal problems in the racing Thoroughbred, *Equine Vet J* 36:571, 2004.
35. McIlwraith CW, Anderson TM, Santschi BN: Conformation and musculoskeletal problems in the racehorse, *Clin Tech Equine Pract* 2:329, 2003.
36. Lucas JM, Ross MW, Richardson DW: Postoperative performance of racing Standardbreds treated arthroscopically for carpal chip fracture: 176 cases, *Equine Vet J* 31:48, 1999.
37. Palmer SE: Prevalence of carpal fractures in Thoroughbred and Standardbred racehorses, *J Am Vet Med Assoc* 10:1171, 1986.
38. Park RD, Morgan JP, O'Brien T: Chip fractures in the carpus of the horse: a radiographic study of their incidence and location, *J Am Vet Med Assoc* 157:1305, 1970.
39. McIlwraith CW, Yovich JV, Martin GS: Arthroscopic surgery for the treatment of osteochondral chip fractures in the equine carpus, *J Am Vet Med Assoc* 191:531, 1987.
40. Uhlhorn H, Carlsten J: Retrospective study of subchondral sclerosis and lucency in the third carpal bone of Standardbred trotters, *Equine Vet J* 31:500, 1999.

41. Uhlhorn H, Eksell P, Sandgren B, Carlsten J: Sclerosis of the third carpal bone. A prospective study of its significance in a group of young Standardbred trotters, *Acta Vet Scand* 41:51, 2000.

42. Hopper BJ, Steel C, Richardson JL, et al: Radiographic evaluation of sclerosis of the third carpal bone associated with exercise and the development of lameness in Standardbred racehorses, *Equine Vet J* 36:441, 2004.

43. Wilson BD, Neal RJ, Howard A, Groenendyk S: The gait of pacers. I. Kinematics of the racing stride, *Equine Vet J* 20:341, 1988.

44. Dabareiner RM, Sullins KE, Bradley W: Removal of a fracture fragment from the palmar aspect of the intermediate carpal bone in a horse, *J Am Vet Med Assoc* 203:553, 1993.

45. Martin GS, Haynes PF, McClure JR: Effect of third carpal slab fracture and repair on racing performance in Thoroughbred horses: 31 cases (1977-1984), *J Am Vet Med Assoc* 193:107, 1988.

46. Stephens PR, Richardson DW, Spencer PA: Slab fractures of the third carpal bone in Standardbreds and Thoroughbreds: 155 cases (1977-1984), *J Am Vet Med Assoc* 193:353, 1988.

47. Richardson DW: Technique for arthroscopic repair of third carpal bone slab fractures in horses, *J Am Vet Med Assoc* 188:288, 1986.

48. Rutherford DJ, Bladon B, Rogers CW: Outcome of lag-screw treatment of incomplete fractures of the frontal plane of the radial facet of the third carpal bone in horses, *N Z Vet J*, 55:94, 2007.

49. Kraus B, Ross MW, Boston RC: Surgical and nonsurgical management of sagittal slab fractures of the third carpal bone in racehorses: 32 cases (1991-2001), *J Am Vet Med Assoc* 226:945, 2005.

50. Fischer AT, Stover SM: Sagittal fractures of the third carpal bone in horses: 12 cases (1977-1985), *J Am Vet Med Assoc* 191:106, 1987.

51. Auer JA, Watkins JP, White NA, et al: Slab fractures of the fourth and intermediate carpal bones in five horses, *J Am Vet Med Assoc* 188:595, 1986.

52. Ross MW, Richardson DW, Beroza GA: Subchondral lucency of the third carpal bone in Standardbred racehorses: 13 cases (1982-1988), *J Am Vet Med Assoc* 195:789, 1989.

53. Levine DG, Richardson DW: Clinical use of the locking compression plate (LCP) in horses: a retrospective study of 31 cases (2004-2006), *Equine Vet J* 39:401, 2007.

54. Carpenter RS, Goodrich LR, Baxter GM, et al: Locking compression plates for pancarpal arthrodesis in a Thoroughbred filly, *Vet Surg* 37:508, 2008.

55. Lewis RD: Carpal arthrodesis: technique and prognosis, *Proc Am College Vet Surg* 64, 2004.

56. Bertone AL, Schneiter HL, Turner AS, Shoemaker RS: Pancarpal arthrodesis for treatment of carpal collapse in the adult horse: a report of two cases, *Vet Surg* 18:353, 1989.

57. Kane AJ, Park RD, McIlwraith CW, et al: Radiographic changes in Thoroughbred yearlings. Part 1: Prevalence at the time of the yearling sales, *Equine Vet J* 35:354, 2003.

58. Kane AJ, McIlwraith CW, Park RD, et al: Radiographic changes in Thoroughbred yearlings. Part 2: Associations with racing performance, *Equine Vet J* 35:366, 2003.

59. McIlwraith CW: Subchondral cystic lesions (osteochondrosis) in the horse, *Compend Contin Educ Pract Vet* 4:S396, 1982.

60. Richardson DW: Personal communication, 2000.

61. Martin BB, Reef VB: The treatment of a minimally displaced fracture of the distal radius of an adult horse, *J Am Vet Med Assoc* 191:847, 1987.

62. Dyson S: Personal communication, 2001.

63. Beinlich CP, Nixon AJ: Radiographic and pathologic characterization of lateral palmar intercarpal ligament avulsion fractures in the horse, *Vet Radiol Ultrasound* 45:532, 2004.

64. Beinlich CP, Nixon AJ: Prevalence and response to surgical treatment of lateral palmar intercarpal ligament avulsion in horses: 37 cases (1990-2001), *J Am Vet Med Assoc* 226:760, 2005.

65. Desmaizières LM, Cauvin ER: Carpal collateral ligament desmopathy in three horses, *Vet Rec* 157:197, 2005.

66. Nixon AJ, Schachter BL, Pool RR: Exostoses of the caudal perimeter of the radial physis as a cause of carpal synovial sheath tenosynovitis and lameness in horses: 10 cases (1999-2003), *J Am Vet Med Assoc* 224:264, 2004.

67. Bertone AL, Powers BE, Turner AS: Chondrosarcoma in the radius of a horse, *J Am Vet Med Assoc* 185:534, 1984.

CHAPTER 39 The Antebrachium

1. Vulcano LC, Mamprim MJ, Muniz LMR, et al: Radiographic study of distal radial physeal closure in Thoroughbred horses, *Vet Radiol Ultrasound* 38:352, 1997.

2. Butler JA, Colles CM, Dyson SJ, et al: Fusion times of physes and suture lines. In *Clinical radiology of the horse*, ed 2, Oxford, 2000, Blackwell Science. p 585.

3. Uhlhorn H, Eksell P, Carlsten J: Scintigraphic characterization of distal radial physeal closure in young Standardbred racehorses, *Vet Radiol Ultrasound* 41:181, 2000.

4. Gabel AA, Spencer CP, Pipers FS: A study of correlation of closure of the distal radial physes with performance and injury in the Standardbred, *J Am Vet Med Assoc* 170:188, 1977.

5. Pilsworth R, Shepard M: Stress fractures. In Robinson NE, ed: *Current therapy in equine medicine*, ed 4, Philadelphia, 1997, Saunders.

6. Mackey VS, Trout DS, Meagher DM, et al: Stress fractures of the humerus, radius, and tibia in horses, *Vet Radiol Ultrasound* 28:26, 1987.

7. Bramlage LR: Emergency first aid treatment and transportation of equine fracture patients. In Auer JA, Stick JA, eds: *Equine surgery*, ed 2, Philadelphia, 1999, Saunders.

8. Watkins JP: The radius and ulna. In Auer JA, Stick JA, eds: *Equine surgery*, ed 2, Philadelphia, 1999, Saunders.

9. Auer JA: Fractures of the radius. In Nixon AJ, ed: *Equine fracture repair*, Philadelphia, 1996, Saunders.

10. Bassage LH, Ross MW: Enostosis-like lesions in the long bones of 10 horses: scintigraphic and radiographic features, *Equine Vet J* 30:35, 1998.

11. Bassage LH: Unpublished data, 2000.

12. Ross MW, Boswell R, Pool RR: Unpublished data, 2000.

13. Ahern BJ, Ross MW: Clinical, scintigraphic and radiographic findings of horses with enostosis-like lesions. Unpublished observations, 2009.

14. Specht TE, Nixon AJ, Colahan PT, et al: Subchondral cyst-like lesions in the distal portion of the radius of four horses, *J Am Vet Med Assoc* 193:949, 1988.

15. Kold S, Hickman J: Three cases of subchondral cysts in the distal limb of the horse treated by bone grafting via an extra-articular approach, *Equine Vet Educ* 2:70, 1990.

16. Swinebroad EL, Dabareiner RM, Swor TM, et al: Osteomyelitis secondary to trauma involving the proximal end of the radius in horses: five cases (1987-2001), *J Am Vet Med Assoc* 223:486, 2003.

17. Mair TS, Dyson SJ, Fraser JA, et al: Hypertrophic osteopathy (Marie's disease) in Equidae: a review of twenty-four cases, *Equine Vet J* 28:256, 1996.

18. Lavoie JP, Carlson GP, George L: Hypertrophic osteopathy in three horses and a pony, *J Am Vet Med Assoc* 201:1900, 1992.

19. Susaneck SJ, Macy DW: Hypertrophic osteopathy, *Compend Contin Educ Pract Vet* 4:689, 1982.

20. Chaffin MK, Ruoff WW, Schmitz DG, et al: Regression of hypertrophic osteopathy in a filly following successful management of an intrathoracic abscess, *Equine Vet J* 22:62, 1990.

CHAPTER 40 The Elbow, Brachium, and Shoulder

1. Dyson S: The elbow, brachium and shoulder. In Ross M, Dyson S, eds: *Diagnosis and management of lameness in the horse*, St Louis, 2003, Elsevier.

2. Dyson S: The differential diagnosis of shoulder lameness in the horse, Fellowship Thesis Royal College of Veterinary Surgeons, Newmarket, UK, 1986.

3. Devine D, Jann H, Payton M: Gait abnormalities caused by selective anaesthesia of the suprascapular nerve in horses, *Am J Vet Res* 67:834, 2006.

4. Schumacher J, Livesey L, Brawner W, et al: Comparison of 2 methods of centesis of the bursa of the biceps brachii tendon of horses. *Equine Vet J* 39:356, 2007.

5. Butler J, Colles C, Dyson S, et al: The shoulder, humerus and elbow. In Butler J, Colles C, Dyson S, et al, eds: *Clinical radiology of the horse*, ed 3, Oxford, 2008, Wiley-Blackwell.

6. Bohn A, Papageores M, Grant B: Ultrasonographic evaluation and surgical treatment of humeral osteitis and bicipital tenosynovitis in a horse, *J Am Vet Med Assoc* 201:305, 1992.

7. Pugh C, Johnson P, Crawley G, Finn S: Ultrasonography of the equine bicipital tendon region: a case history report and review of the anatomy, *Vet Radiol Ultrasound* 35:183, 1994.

8. Crabhill M, Chaffin K, Schmitz D: Ultrasonographic morphology of the bicipital tendon and bursa in clinically normal Quarter Horses, *Am J Vet Res* 56:5, 1995.
9. Tnibar M, Auer J, Bakkali S: Ultrasonography of the equine shoulder: technique and normal appearance, *Vet Radiol Ultrasound* 40:44, 1999.
10. Pasquet H, Coudry V, Denoix J-M: Ultrasonographic examination of the proximal tendon of the biceps brachii. Technique and reference images, *Equine Vet Educ* 20:331, 2008.
11. Hopen L, Colahan P, Turner T, Nixon A: Nonsurgical treatment of cubital cyst-like lesions in horses: seven cases (1983-1987), *J Am Vet Med Assoc* 200:527, 1992.
12. Bertone A, McIlwraith C, Powers P, et al: Subchondral osseous cystic lesions in the elbow of horses: conservative versus surgical treatment, *J Am Vet Med Assoc* 189:440, 1986.
13. Barr A, Hillyer M, Day M: Subchondral bone cyst in the proximal radius of a horse, *Equine Vet Educ* 7:179, 1995.
14. Hardy J, Marcoux M, Eisenberg H: Osteochondrosis-like lesion of the anconeal process in two horses, *J Am Vet Med Assoc* 189:802, 1986.
15. Brown M, MacCallum F: Anconeal process of ulna: separate centre of ossification in the horse, *Br Vet J* 130:434, 1974.
16. Chopin J, Wright J, Melville L, Robinson W: Lateral collateral ligament avulsion of the humeroradial joint in a horse, *Vet Radiol Ultrasound* 38:50, 1997.
17. Oikawa M, Narama I: Enthesopathy of the radial tuberosity in two thoroughbred racehorses, *J Comp Pathol* 118:135, 1998.
18. Smith R: Personal communication, 2005.
19. Donecker J, Bramlage L, Gabel A: Retrospective analysis of 29 fractures of the olecranon process of the equine ulna, *J Am Vet Med Assoc* 185:183, 1984.
20. Anderson D, Allen D, DeBowes R: Comminuted articular fractures of the olecranon process in horses: 17 cases (1980-1990), *Vet Comp Orthop Traumatol* 8:141, 1995.
21. Richardson D: Olecranon fractures. In White N, Moore J, eds: *Current techniques in equine surgery and lameness*, ed 2, Philadelphia, 1998, Saunders.
22. Swor T, Watkins J, Bahr I, Honnas C: Results of plate fixation of type 1b olecranon fractures in 24 horses, *Equine Vet J* 35:670, 2003.
23. Swor T, Watkins J, Bahr I, et al: Results of plate fixation of type 5 olecranon fractures in 20 horses, *Equine Vet J* 37:30, 2006.
24. Wilson D, Riedesel E: Non-surgical management of ulnar fractures in the horse: a retrospective study of 43 cases, *Vet Surg* 14:283, 1985.
25. Dyson S, Greet T: Repair of a fracture of the deltoid tuberosity in a horse, *Equine Vet J* 18:230, 1986.
26. Mackay V, Trout D, Meagher D, Hornof W: Stress fractures of the humerus, radius and tibia in horses, *Vet Radiol* 28:26, 1987.
27. Stover S, Johnson B, Daft B, et al: An association between complete and incomplete stress fractures of the humerus in racehorses, *Equine Vet J* 24:260, 1992.
28. O'Sullivan C, Lumsden J: Stress fractures of the tibia and humerus in Thoroughbred racehorses, *J Am Vet Med Assoc* 222:491, 2003.
29. Adams M, Turner T: Endoscopy of the intertubercular bursa in horses, *J Am Vet Med Assoc* 214:221, 1999.
30. Yovich J, Aanes W: Fracture of the greater tubercle of the humerus in a filly, *J Am Vet Med Assoc* 187:74, 1985.
31. Grant B, Peterson P, Bohn A, et al: Diagnosis and surgical management of traumatic bicipital bursitis in the horse, *Proc Am Assoc Equine Pract* 38:349, 1992.
32. van Furst A: Retrospective study of fractures of the greater tubercle in 8 horses, *Tierarztl Umsch* 62:115, 2007.
33. Mez J, Dabareiner R, Cole R, Watkins J: Fracture of the greater tubercle of the humerus in horses: 15 cases (1986-2004), *J Am Vet Med Assoc* 230:1350, 2007.
34. Honnas C: Surgical treatment of selected musculoskeletal disorders of the forelimb. In Auer J, ed: *Equine surgery*, Philadelphia, 1992, Saunders.
35. Zamos D, Parks A: Comparison of surgical and non-surgical treatment of humeral fractures in horses: 22 cases (1980-1989), *J Am Vet Med Assoc* 201:114, 1992.
36. Dyson S: Shoulder lameness in the horse: an analysis of 58 suspected cases, *Equine Vet J* 18:29, 1986.
37. McIlwraith CW: Arthroscopy of the shoulder and elbow joint. *Proceedings of the Third Maastricht International Congress on Equine Medicine*, Maastricht, the Netherlands, 1999.
38. Jenner F, Ross M, Martin B, Richardson D: Scapulohumeral osteochondrosis: a retrospective study of 32 horses, *Vet Comp Orthop Traumatol* 21:406, 2008.
39. Doyle P, White N: Diagnostic findings and prognosis following arthroscopic treatment of subtle osteochondral lesions in the shoulder joint of horses: 15 cases (1996-1999), *J Am Vet Med Assoc* 217:1878, 2000.
40. Clegg P, Dyson S, Summerhays G, Schramme M: Scapulohumeral osteoarthritis in 20 Shetland ponies, Miniature horses and Falabella ponies (20 cases), *Vet Rec* 148:175, 2001.
41. Boswell J, Schramme M, Wilson A, May S: Radiological study to evaluate suspected scapulohumeral joint dysplasia in Shetland ponies, *Equine Vet J* 31:510, 1999.
42. Semevolos S: Scapulohumeral arthrodesis in miniature horses, *Vet Surg* 32:416, 2003.
43. Dyson S: Sixteen fractures of the shoulder region in the horse, *Equine Vet J* 17:104, 1985.
44. Dyson S: Lesions of the proximal aspect of the humerus and of the tendon of biceps brachii, *Equine Vet Educ* 21:67, 2009.
45. Coudry V, Allen K, Denoix J-M: Congenital abnormalities of the bicipital apparatus in 4 mature horses, *Equine Vet J* 37:272, 2005.
46. Seco Diaz O, Reef V, Martin B, et al. Rupture of the biceps tendon in a Thoroughbred steeplechase horse, *Equine Vet J* 35:110, 2003.
47. Gillis C, Vatistas N: Biceps brachii tendinitis and bicipital (intertubercular) bursitis. In Robinson NE, ed: *Current therapy in equine medicine 4*, Philadelphia, 1997, Saunders.
48. Fugaro M, Adams S: Biceps brachii tenotomy or tenectomy for the treatment of bicipital bursitis, tendonitis and humeral osteitis in 3 horses, *J Am Vet Med Ass* 220:1508, 2002.
49. Vatistas N, Pascoe J, Wright I, et al: Infection of the intertubercular bursa in horses: four cases (1978-1991), *J Am Vet Med Assoc* 208:1434, 1996.
50. Tudor R, Bowman K, Redding R, Tomlinson J: Endoscopic treatment of suspected infectious intertubercular bursitis in a horse, *J Am Vet Med Assoc* 213:1584, 1998.
51. Gough M, McDiarmid A: Septic intertubercular (bicipital) bursitis in a horse, *Equine Vet Educ* 10:66, 1998.
52. Booth T: Lameness associated with the bicipital bursa in an Arab stallion, *Vet Rec* 145:194, 1999.
53. Boys-Smith S, Singer E: Mineralisation of the biceps brachii tendon in a 6-year-old Cob mare, *Equine Vet Educ* 19:74-79, 2007.
54. Ramzan P: Osseous cyst-like lesion of the intermediate tubercle of a horse, *Vet Rec* 154:534, 2004.
55. Arnold C, Chaffin M, Honnas C, et al: Diagnosis and surgical management of a subchondral bone cyst within the intermediate tubercle of the humerus in a horse, *Equine Vet Educ* 20:310, 2008.
56. Little D, Redding R, Gerard M: Osseous cyst-like lesions of the intertubercular groove of the proximal humerus: a report of 5 cases, *Equine Vet Educ* 21:60, 2009.
57. Bleyaert H, Madison J: Complete biceps brachii tenotomy to facilitate internal fixation of supraglenoid tubercle fractures in three horses, *Vet Surg* 28:48, 1999.
58. Davidson E, Martin B: Stress fracture of the scapula in 2 horses, *Vet Radiol Ultrasound* 45:407, 2004.
59. Vallance S, Lumsden J, O'Sullivan C: Scapular stress fractures in eight Thoroughbred racehorses, *Proc Am Assoc Equine Pract* 53:56, 2007.
60. Whitcomb M, le Jeune S, MacDonald M, et al: Disorders of the infraspinatus tendon and bursa in three horses, *J Am Vet Med Assoc* 229:549, 2006.
61. Schneider J, Adams O, Easley J, et al: Scapular notch resection for suprascapular nerve decompression in 12 horses, *J Am Vet Med Assoc* 187:1019, 1985.
62. Dutton D, Honnas C, Watkins J: Nonsurgical treatment of suprascapular nerve injury in horses: 8 cases (1988-1998), *J Am Vet Med Assoc* 214:1657, 1999.
63. Rooney J: Radial paralysis in the horse, *Cornell Vet* 53:328, 1963.
64. Mayhew I: Paresis or paralysis of one limb. In *Large animal neurology*, Philadelphia, 1989, Lea & Febiger.

CHAPTER 41   The Hind Foot and Pastern

1. Neil KM, Axon JE, Todhunter PG, et al: Septic osteitis of the distal phalanx in foals: 22 cases (1995-2002), *J Am Vet Med Assoc* 230:1683, 2007.

2. Steel CM, Hunt AR, Adams PL, et al: Factors associated with prognosis for survival and athletic use in foals with septic arthritis, *J Am Vet Med Assoc* 215:973, 1999.

3. Getty RG, ed: *Sisson and Grossman's the anatomy of the domestic animals*, ed 5, Philadelphia, 1975, Saunders.

4. Sack WO, Habel RE, eds: *Rooney's guide to the dissection of the horse*, Ithaca, NY, 1977, Veterinary Textbooks.

5. Ross MW, Nolan PM, Palmar JA, et al: The importance of the metatarsophalangeal joint in Standardbred lameness, *Proc Am Assoc Equine Pract* 37:741, 1991.

6. Butler J, Colles C, Dyson S, et al: *Clinical radiology of the horse*, ed 3, Oxford, 2008, Wiley-Blackwell.

7. Rabuffo TS, Ross MW: Fractures of the distal phalanx in 72 racehorses, *Proc Am Assoc Equine Pract* 48:375, 2002.

8. Dyson S: Personal communication, 2001.

9. Ross MW: The hind foot and pastern. In Ross MW, Dyson SJ, editors: *Diagnosis and management of lameness in the horse*, ed 1, St. Louis, 2003, Saunders, p 418.

CHAPTER 42   The Metatarsophalangeal Joint

1. Stashak TS: *Adams' lameness in horses*, ed 4, Philadelphia, 1987, Lea & Febiger.

2. Ross MW, Nolan PM, Palmar JA, et al: The importance of the metatarsophalangeal joint in Standardbred lameness, *Proc Am Assoc Equine Pract* 37:741, 1991.

3. Dabareiner RM, Cohen ND, Carter GK, et al: Musculoskeletal problems associated with lameness and poor performance among horses used for barrel racing: 118 cases (2000-2003), *J Am Vet Med Assoc* 227:1646, 2005.

4. Dabareiner RM, Cohen NC, Carter GK, et al: Lameness and poor performance in horses used for team roping: 118 cases (2000-2003), *J Am Vet Med Assoc* 226:1694, 2005.

5. Shepherd MC, Pilsworth RC: Stress reactions to the plantarolateral condyles of MtIII in UK Thoroughbreds: 26 cases, *Proc Am Assoc Equine Pract* 43:128, 1997.

6. Specht TE, Poulos PW, Metcalf MR, Robertson ID: Vacuum phenomenon in the metatarsophalangeal joint of the horse, *J Am Vet Med Assoc* 197:749, 1990.

7. Ross MW: Scintigraphic and clinical findings in the Standardbred metatarsophalangeal joint: 114 cases (1993-1995), *Equine Vet J* 30:131, 1998.

8. Weekes JS, Murray RC, Dyson SJ: Scintigraphic evaluation of metacarpophalangeal and metatarsophalangeal joints in clinically sound horses, *Vet Radiol Ultrasound* 45:85, 2004.

9. Dyson SJ: Personal communication, 2008.

10. Sherlock CE, Mair TS, Ter Braake F: Osseous lesions in the metacarpo(tarso) phalangeal joint diagnosed using low-field magnetic resonance imaging in standing horses, *Vet Radiol Ultrasound* 50:13, 2009.

11. Dyson SJ, Murray R: Osseous trauma in the fetlock region of mature sports horses, *Proc Am Assoc Equine Pract* 52:443, 2006.

12. Zubrod CJ, Schneider RK, Tucker RL, et al: Use of magnetic resonance imaging for identifying subchondral bone damage in horses, *J Am Vet Med Assoc* 224:411, 2004.

13. Sampson SN, Schneider RK, Tucker RL, et al: Magnetic resonance imaging features of oblique and straight distal sesamoidean desmitis in 27 horses, *Vet Radiol Ultrasound* 48:303, 2007.

14. Barr A, Dyson S, Barr F, O'Brien JK: Tendonitis of the deep digital flexor tendon associated with tenosynovitis of the digital sheath in the horse, *Equine Vet J* 27:348, 1995.

15. Morgan JW, Santschi EM, Zekas LJ, et al: Comparison of radiography and computed tomography to evaluate metacarpo/metatarsophalangeal joint pathology of paired limbs of Thoroughbred racehorses with severe condylar fracture, *Vet Surg* 35:611, 2006.

16. MacKinnon M, Ross MW, VanWinkle W: Unpublished data, 2008.

17. Denoix JM, Thibaud D, Riccio B: Tiludronate as a therapeutic agent in the treatment of navicular disease: a double-blind placebo-controlled clinical trial, *Equine Vet J* 35:407, 2003.

18. Coudry V, Thibaud D, Riccio B, et al: Efficacy of tiludronate in the treatment of horses with signs of pain associated with osteoarthritic lesions of the thoracolumbar vertebral column, *Am J Vet Res* 68:329, 2007.

19. Muir P, McCarthy J, Radtke CL, et al: Role of endochondral ossification of articular cartilage and functional adaptation of the subchondral plate in the development of fatigue microcracking of joints, *Bone* 38:342, 2006.

20. Muir P, Peterson AL, Sample SJ, et al: Exercise-induced metacarpophalangeal joint adaptation in the Thoroughbred racehorse, *J Anat* 213:706, 2008.

21. Norrdin RW, Stover SM: Subchondral bone failure in overload arthrosis: a scanning electron microscopic study in horses, *J Musculoskelet Neuronal Interact* 6:251, 2006.

22. Messent EA, Ward RJ, Tonkin CJ, Buckland-Wright C: Tibial cancellous bone changes in patients with knee osteoarthritis. A short-term longitudinal study using fractal signature analysis, *Osteoarthritis Cartilage* 13:463, 2005.

23. Messent EA, Ward RJ, Tonkin CJ, Buckland-Wright C: Cancellous bone differences between knees with early, definite and advanced joint space loss: a comparative quantitative macroradiographic study, *Osteoarthritis Cartilage* 13:39, 2005.

24. MacNeil JA, Doshak MR, Sernicke RF, Boyd SK: Preservation of periarticular cancellous morphology and mechanical stiffness in post-traumatic experimental osteoarthritis by antiresorptive therapy, *Clin Biomech* 23:365, 2008.

25. Carbone LD, Nevitt MC, Wildy K, et al: The relationship of antiresorptive drug use to structural findings and symptoms of knee osteoarthritis, *Arthritis Rheum* 50:3516, 2004.

26. Delguste C, Amory H, Guyonnet J, et al: Comparative pharmacokinetics of two intravenous administration regimens of tiludronate in healthy adult horses and

effects on the bone resorption marker CTX-1, *J Vet Pharmacol Ther* 31:108, 2008.

27. Dore F, Filippi L, Biasotto M, et al: Bone scintigraphy and SPECT/CT of bisphosphonate-induced osteonecrosis of the jaw, *J Nucl Med* 50:30, 2009.

28. Foerner JJ, Barclay WP, Phillips TN, et al: Osteochondral fragments of the palmar/plantar aspect of the fetlock joint, *Proc Am Assoc Equine Pract* 33:739, 1987.

29. Fortier LA, Foerner JJ, Nixon AJ: Arthroscopic removal of axial osteochondral fragments of the plantar/palmar proximal aspect of the proximal phalanx in horses: 119 cases (1988-1992), *J Am Vet Med Assoc* 206:71, 1995.

30. Nixon AJ, Pool RR: Histologic appearance of axial osteochondral fragments from the proximoplantar/proximopalmar aspect of the proximal phalanx in horses, *J Am Vet Med Assoc* 207:1076, 1995.

31. Grøndahl AM, Dolvik NI: Heritability estimations of osteochondrosis in the tibiotarsal joint and of bony fragments in the palmar/plantar portion of the metacarpo- and metatarsophalangeal joints of horses, *J Am Vet Med Assoc* 203:101, 1993.

32. Nixon AJ: Osteochondrosis and osteochondritis dissecans of the equine fetlock, *Compend Contin Educ Pract Vet* 12:1463, 1990.

33. Nixon AJ: Fetlock plantar osteochondral fragmentation: clinical and histologic features, *Proc Vet Orthop Soc* 18:42, 1991.

34. Ross MW: Osteochondral fragmentation of the proximopalmar/proximoplantar aspect of the proximal phalanx. In White NA, Moore JN, eds: *Current techniques in equine surgery and lameness*, ed 2, Philadelphia, 1998, Saunders.

35. Grøndahl AM: Incidence and development of ununited proximoplantar tuberosity of the proximal phalanx in Standardbred trotters, *Vet Radiol Ultrasound* 33:18, 1992.

36. Jørgensen HS, Proschowsky H, Falk-Rønne J, et al: The significance of routine radiographic findings with respect to subsequent racing performance and longevity in Standardbred trotters, *Equine Vet J* 29:55, 1997.

37. Declercq J, Martens A, Maes D, et al: Dorsoproximal proximal phalanx osteochondral fragmentation in 117 Warmblood horses, *Vet Comp Orthop Traumatol* 22:1, 2009.

38. Kraus BM, Richardson DW, Nunamaker DM, Ross MW: Management of comminuted fractures of the proximal phalanx in horses: 64 cases (1983-2001), *J Am Vet Med Assoc* 224:254, 2004.

39. Markel MD, Martin BB, Richardson DW: Dorsal frontal fractures of the first phalanx in the horse, *Vet Surg* 14:36, 1985.

40. Schnabel LV, Bramlage LR, Mohammed HO, et al: Racing performance after arthroscopic removal of apical sesamoid fracture fragments in Thoroughbred horses age <2 years: 151 cases (1989-2002), *Equine Vet J* 39:64, 2007.

41. Schnabel LV, Bramlage LR, Mohammed HO, et al: Racing performance after arthroscopic removal of apical sesamoid fracture fragments in Thoroughbred horses age > or = 2 years: 84 cases (1989-2002), *Equine Vet J* 38:446, 2006.

42. Zekas LJ, Bramlage LR, Embertson RM, Hance SR: Characterisation of the type and location of fractures of the third metacarpal/metatarsal condyles in 135 horses in central Kentucky (1986-1994), *Equine Vet J* 31:304, 1999.

43. Bassage LH, Richardson DW: Longitudinal fractures of the condyles of the third metacarpal and metatarsal bones in racehorses: 224 cases (1986-1995), *J Am Vet Med Assoc* 212:1757, 1998.

44. Richardson DW: Medial condylar fractures of the third metatarsal bone in horses, *J Am Vet Med Assoc* 185:761, 1984.

45. Bramlage LR: The effect of training on the suspensory apparatus (Association for the Study of Internal Fixation course notes), Columbus, 2001, Ohio State College of Veterinary Medicine.

46. Hardy J, Marcoux M, Breton L: Clinical relevance of radiographic findings in proximal sesamoid bones of two-year-old Standardbreds in their first year of race training, *J Am Vet Med Assoc* 198:2089, 1991.

47. Grøndahl AM, Gaustad G, Engeland A: Progression and association with lameness and racing performance of radiographic changes in the proximal sesamoid bones of young Standardbreds, *Equine Vet J* 26:152, 1994.

48. Tenney WA, Whitcomb MB: Rupture of the collateral ligaments in metacarpophalangeal and metatarsophalangeal joints in horses: 17 cases (1999-2005), *J Am Vet Med Assoc* 233:456, 2008.

CHAPTER 43   The Metatarsal Region

1. Getty RG, ed: *Sisson and Grossman's the anatomy of the domestic animals*, ed 5, Philadelphia, 1975, Saunders.

2. Dyson SJ: Proximal suspensory desmitis in the hindlimb, *Equine Vet Educ* 7:275, 1995.

3. Wilson DA, Baker GJ, Pijanowski GJ, et al: Composition and morphologic features of the interosseous muscle in Standardbreds and Thoroughbreds, *Am J Vet Res* 52:133, 1991.

4. Muylle S, Vanderperren K, Saunders J, Simoens: Morphometric data on the accessory ligament of the deep digital flexor tendon in the equine hindlimb, *Vet J* Jun 27, 2009 (Epub ahead of print).

5. Bathe AP: Plantar metatarsal neurectomy and fasciotomy for treatment of hindlimb proximal suspensory desmitis, *Vet Surg* 32:480, 2003 (abstract).

6. Tóth F, Schumacher J, Schramme M, et al: Compressive damage to the deep branch of the lateral plantar nerve associated with lameness caused by proximal suspensory desmitis, *Vet Surg* 37:328, 2008.

7. Hughes TK, Lliashar E, Smith RK: In vitro evaluation of a single injection technique for diagnostic analgesia of the proximal suspensory ligament of the equine pelvic limb, *Vet Surg* 36:760, 2007.

8. Hewes CA, White NA: Outcome of desmoplasty and fasciotomy for desmitis involving the origin of the suspensory ligament in horses: 27 cases (1995-2004), *J Am Vet Med Assoc* 229:407, 2006.

9. Bischofberger AS, Konar M, Ohlerth S, et al: Magnetic resonance imaging, ultrasonography and histology of the suspensory ligament origin: a comparative study of normal anatomy of warm-blood horses, *Equine Vet J* 38:508, 2006.

10. Dyson SJ, Romero JM: An investigation of injection techniques for local analgesia of the equine distal tarsus and proximal metatarsus, *Equine Vet J* 25:30, 1993.

11. Koblik PD, Hornof WJ, Seeherman HJ: Scintigraphic appearance of stress-induced trauma of the dorsal cortex of the third metacarpal bone in racing Thoroughbred horses: 121 cases (1978-1986), *J Am Vet Med Assoc* 192:390, 1988.

12. Schallberger SP, Doherr MG, Ueltschi G: Scintigraphic appearance of the dorsal cortex of the third metacarpus and third metatarsus in the horse, *Vet Radiol Ultrasound* 45:352, 2004.

13. Weekes JS, Mruray RC, Dyson SJ: Scintigraphic evaluation of the proximal metacarpal and metatarsal regions in clinically sound horses, *Vet Radiol Ultrasound* 47:409, 2006.

14. Dyson SJ, Weekes JS, Murray RC: Scintigraphic evaluation of the proximal metacarpal and metatarsal regions of horses with proximal suspensory desmitis, *Vet Radiol Ultrasound* 48:78, 2007.

15. Launois MT, Vandeweerd JM, Perrin RA, et al: Use of computed tomography to diagnose new bone formation associated with desmitis of the proximal aspect of the suspensory ligament in third metacarpal or third metatarsal bones of three horses, *J Am Vet Med Assoc* 234:514, 2009.

16. Brokken MT, Schneider RK, Sampson SN, et al: Magnetic resonance imaging features of proximal metacarpal and metatarsal injuries in the horses, *Vet Radiol Ultrasound* 48:507, 2007.

17. Levine DG, Richardson DW: Clinical use of the locking compression plate (LCP) in horses: a retrospective study of 31 cases (2004-2006), *Equine Vet J* 39:401, 2007.

18. McClure SR, Watkins JP, Glickman NW, et al: Complete fractures of the third metacarpal or metatarsal bone in horses: 25 cases (1980-1996), *J Am Vet Med Assoc* 213:847, 1998.

19. Lescun TB, McClure SR, Ward MP, et al: Evaluation of transfixation casting for treatment of third metacarpal, third metatarsal, and phalangeal fractures in horses: 37 cases (1994-2004), *J Am Vet Med Assoc* 230:1340, 2007.

20. Ross MW, Sponseller ML, Gill HE, Moyer W: Articular fracture of the dorsoproximomolateral aspect of the third metatarsal bone in five Standardbred racehorses, *J Am Vet Med Assoc* 203:698, 1993.

21. Pilsworth RC: Incomplete fracture of the dorsal aspect of the proximal cortex of the third metatarsal bone as a cause of hind limb lameness in the racing Thoroughbred: a review of three cases, *Equine Vet J* 24:147, 1992.

22. Peterson PR, Pascoe JR, Wheat JD: Surgical management of proximal splint bone fractures in the horse, *Vet Surg* 16:367, 1987.

23. Baxter GM, Doran RE, Allen DA: Complete excision of a fractured fourth metatarsal bone in eight horses, *Vet Surg* 21:273, 1992.

24. Jenson PW, Gaughan EM, Lillich JD, et al: Segmental ostectomy of the second and fourth metacarpal and metatarsal bones in horses: 17 cases (1993-2002), *J Am Vet Med Assoc*, 224:271, 2004.

25. Bassage LH, Ross MW: Enostosis-like lesions in the long bones of 10 horses: scintigraphic and radiographic features, *Equine Vet J* 30:35, 1998.

26. Dyson SJ: Proximal suspensory desmitis in the forelimb and hindlimb, *Proc Am Assoc Equine Pract* 46:137, 2000.

27. Herthel DJ: Personal communication, 1998.

28. Smith JJ, Ross MW, Smith RK: Anabolic effects of acellular bone marrow, platelet rich plasma and serum on suspensory ligament fibroblasts in vitro, *Vet Comp Orthop Traumatol* 19:43, 2006.

29. Crowe OM, Dyson SJ, Wright IM, et al: Treatment of chronic or recurrent proximal suspensory desmitis using radial pressure wave therapy, *Equine Vet J* 36: 313, 2004.

30. Mero JL, Pool RR: Twenty cases of degenerative suspensory ligament desmitis in Peruvian Paso horses, *Proc Am Assoc Equine Pract* 48:329, 2002.

31. Halper J, Kim B, Khan A, et al: Degenerative suspensory ligament desmitis as a systemic disorder characterized by proteoglycan accumulation, *BMC Vet Res* 2:2, 2006.

32. Crabill MR, Honnas CM, Taylor DS, et al: Stringhalt secondary to trauma to the dorsoproximal region of the metatarsus in horses: 10 cases (1986-1991), *J Am Vet Med Assoc* 205:867, 1994.

CHAPTER 44   The Tarsus

1. Getty RG, ed: *Sisson and Grossman's the anatomy of domestic animals*, ed 4, Philadelphia, 1953, Saunders.

2. Lanova, J, Khumsap S, Clayton H, et al: Three dimensional kinematics of the tarsal joint at the trot, *Equine Vet J* 34:308, 2002.

3. Khumsap S, Lanovaz J, Rosenstein D, et al: Effect of induced unilateral synovitis of distal intertarsal and tarsometatarsal joints on sagittal plane kinematics and kinetics of trotting horses, *Am J Vet Res* 64:1491, 2003.

4. Badoux D: Some biomechanical aspects of the structure of the equine tarsus, *Anat Anz* 164:53, 1987.

5. Murray R, Dyson S, Weekes J, et al: Nuclear scintigraphic evaluation of the distal tarsal region in normal horses, *Vet Radiol Ultrasound* 45:345, 2004.

6. Branch M, Murray R, Dyson S, Goodship AE: Is there a characteristic distal tarsal subchondral bone plate thickness pattern in horses with no history of hindlimb lameness? *Equine Vet J* 37:450, 2005.

7. Murray R, Branch M, Dyson S, et al: How does exercise intensity and type affect equine distal tarsal subchondral bone thickness? *J Appl Phys* 102:2194, 2007.

8. Gnagey L, Clayton H, Lanovaz J: Effect of standing tarsal angle on joint kinematics and kinetics, *Equine Vet J* 38:628, 2006.

9. Sack W, Orsini P: Distal intertarsal and tarsometatarsal joints in the horse: communication and injection sites, *J Am Vet Med Assoc* 179:355, 1981.

10. Dyson S, Romero J: An investigation of injection techniques for local analgesia of the equine distal tarsus and proximal metatarsus, *Equine Vet J* 25:30, 1993.

11. Bell B, Baker G, Foreman J, Abbott LC: In vivo investigation of communication between the distal intertarsal and tarsometatarsal joints in horses and ponies, *Vet Surg* 22:289, 1993.

12. Gough M, Munroe G, Mayhew I: Diffusion of mepivacaine between adjacent synovial structures in the horse. Part 2: tarsus and stifle, *Equine Vet J* 34:85, 2002.

13. Serena A, Schumacher J, Schramme M, et al: Concentration of methylprednisolone acetate in the centrodistal joint after administration into the tarsometatarsal joint, *Equine Vet J* 37:172, 2005.

14. Updike S: Functional anatomy of the equine tarsocrural collateral ligaments, *Am J Vet Res* 45:867, 1984.

15. Deegan E, Rocken M: Zur klinisch-funktionellen anatomie des M. Interosseous medius deer hintergliedmasse Im hinblick die Insertiondesmopathies des pferdes, *Pferdeheilkunde* 24:343, 2008.

16. Kramer J, Keegan K, Wilson D, et al: Kinematics of the hind limb in trotting horses after induced lameness of the distal intertarsal and tarsometatarsal joints and intra-articular administration of anesthetic, *Am J Vet Res* 61:1031, 2000.

17. Khumsap S, Lanovaz J, Clayton H: Three-dimensional kinematic analysis of horses with induced tarsal synovitis, *Equine Vet J* 36:659, 2004.

18. Butler J, Colles C, Dyson S, et al: The tarsus. In Butler J, Colles C, Dyson S, et al, eds: *Clinical radiology of the horse*, ed 3 Oxford, 2008, Wiley-Blackwell.

19. Dyson S, Pilsworth R, Twardock R, Martinelli MJ, eds: *Equine scintigraphy*, Newmarket, 2003, Equine Veterinary Journal.

20. Weekes J, Murray R, Dyson S: Scintigraphic evaluation of the proximal metacarpal and metatarsal regions in clinically sound horses, *Vet Radiol Ultrasound* 47:408, 2006.

21. Ross M, Dyson S: Unpublished data 2009.

22. Whitcomb M: Ultrasonography of the equine tarsus, *Proc Am Assoc Equine Pract* 52:13, 2006.

23. Branch M, Dyson S, Murray R: Magnetic resonance imaging of the equine tarsus, *Clin Tech Equine Pract* 6:96, 2007.

24. Latarre R, Arcencibia A, Gil F, et al: Correlation of magnetic resonance images with anatomic features of the equine tarsus, *Am J Vet Res* 67:756, 2006.

25. Tomlinson J, Redding W, Berry C, Smallwood J: Computed tomographic anatomy of the equine tarsus, *Vet Radiol Ultrasound* 44:174, 2003.

26. Watrous B, Hultgren B, Wagner P: Osteochondrosis and juvenile spavin in equids, *Am J Vet Res* 52:607, 1991.

27. Axelsson M, Björnsdottir S, Eskell P, et al: Risk factors associated with hindlimb lameness and degenerative joint disease in the distal tarsus of Icelandic horses, *Equine Vet J* 33:84, 2001.

28. Tranquille C, Dyson S, Blunden A, et al: Effect of exercise on thickness of mature hyaline cartilage, calcified cartilage and subchondral bone thickness of equine tarsi, *Am J Vet Res* 70:1477, 2009.

29. White N, Turner T: Hock lameness associated with degeneration of the talocalcaneal articulation, *Vet Med Small Anim Clin* 75:678, 1980.

30. Pauwels F: Arthrodesis of the talocalcaneal joint for treatment of 2 horses with talocalcaneal osteoarthritis, *Vet Orthop Traumatol* 18:7, 2005.

31. Smith R, Dyson S, Schramme M, et al: Osteoarthritis of the talocalcaneal joint in 18 horses, *Equine Vet J* 37:166, 2005.

32. Dabareiner R, Carter K, Dyson S: The tarsus. In Ross M, Dyson S, eds: *Diagnosis and management of lameness in the horse*, St Louis, 2003, Elsevier.

33. Rooney J: *Biomechanics of lameness in horses*, Baltimore, 1969, Williams & Wilkins.

34. Gough M, Munroe G: Decision making in the diagnosis and management of bone spavin in horses, *Equine Pract* 20:252, 1998.

35. Fairburn A, Dyson S, Murray R: Clinical significance of osseous spurs on the dorsoproximal aspect of the third metatarsal bone, *Equine Vet J* DOI: 10:111/;2042-3306.2010.00097.x.

36. Murray R, Dyson S, Weekes J, et al: Scintigraphic evaluation of the distal tarsal region in horses with distal tarsal pain, *Vet Radiol Ultrasound* 46:171, 2005.

37. Branch M: *How is adaptive change related to pathology in the equine distal tarsal osteochondral unit?* PhD thesis, London, 2005, University of London.

38. Moyer W: Bone spavin: a clinical review, *J Equine Med Surg* 2:362, 1978.

39. McCarroll D, McClure S: Extracorporeal shock wave therapy for treatment of osteoarthritis of the tarsometatarsal and distal intertarsal joints of the horse, *Proc Am Assoc Equine Pract* 46:200, 2000.

40. Gough M: Personal communication 2008.

41. Sonnichsen H, Svalastoga E: Surgical treatment of bone spavin, *Equine Pract* 7:6, 1985.

42. McIllwraith CW, Robertson JT: *McIllwraith and Turner's equine surgery advanced techniques*, Baltimore, 1998, Williams & Wilkins.

43. Bohanon T: Pain associated with the distal tarsal joints. In Robinson E, ed: *Current therapy in equine medicine*, vol 4, Philadelphia, 1997, Saunders.

44. Sammut E, Kannegieter N: Use of sodium monoiodoacetate to fuse the distal hock joints in horses, *Aust Vet J* 72:25, 1995.

45. Dowling B, Dart A, Matthews S: Chemical arthrodesis of the distal tarsal joints using sodium moniodoacetate in 104 horses, *Austr Vet J* 82:38, 2004.

46. Shoemaker R: Use of intra-articular administration of ethyl alcohol for arthrodesis of the tarsometatarsal joint in healthy horses, *Am J Vet Res* 67:850, 2006.

47. Steenhaut M, Imschoot J, Verschooten F, et al: Partial neurectomy of the tibial nerve and neurectomy of the deep peroneal nerve as a treatment of bone spavin in the horse, *Vet Surg* 23:214, 1994.

48. Labens R, Mellor D, Voute L: Retrospective study of the effect of intra-articular treatment of osteoarthritis of the distal tarsal joints in 51 horses, *Vet Rec* 161:611, 2007.

49. Byam-Cook K, Singer E: Is there a relationship between clinical presentation, diagnostic and radiographic findings and outcome in horses with osteoarthritis of the small tarsal joints? *Equine Vet J* 41:118, 2009.

50. Rodgers M: Effects of oral glucosamine and chondroitin sulfate supplementation on frequency of intra-articular therapy of the horse tarsus, *Int J Appl Res Vet Med* 4, 2006.

51. Dechant J: Use of a 3 drill tract technique for arthrodesis of the distal tarsal joints in horses with distal tarsal osteoarthritis: 54 cases (1990-1999), *J Am Vet Med Assoc* 223:1800, 2003.

52. Edwards G: Surgical arthrodesis for the treatment of bone spavin in 20 horses, *Equine Vet J* 14:117, 1982.

53. Hague B, Guccione A: Clinical impressions of a new technique utilizing a Nd:YAG laser to arthrodese the distal hock joints, *Vet Surg* 29:404, 2000.

54. Hague B, Guccione A: Laser-facilitated arthrodesis of the distal tarsal joints, *Clin Tech Equine Pract* 1:32, 2002.

55. Zubrod C, Schneider R, Hague B, et al: Comparison of three methods for arthrodesis of the distal intertarsal and tarsometatarsal joints in horses, *Vet Surg* 14:372, 2005.

56. Miller S: Personal communication, 2009.

57. Eastman T, Bohanon T, Beeman M, et al: Owner survey on cunean tenectomy as a treatment for bone spavin in performance horses, *Proc Am Assoc Equine Pract* 43:121, 1997.

58. Ross M, Garcia-Lopez J: Personal communication, 2001.

59. Climent F, Carmona J, Cuenca R, Prades M: Eosinophilic synovitis of the tarsocrural joint in a horse, *Vet Comp Orthop Traumatol* 20:142, 2007.

60. Carstanjen B, Couturier L, Cauvin E: Ectopic cartilage formation of unknown origin in the plantar pouch of the tarsocrural joint in a yearling, *Vet Rec* 157:630, 2005.

61. Relave E, Meulyzer M, Alexander G, et al: Comparison of radiography and ultrasonography to detect osteochondrosis lesions in the tarsocrural joint: a prospective study, *Equine Vet J* 41:34, 2009.

62. Zubrod C, Schneider RK, Tucker RL, et al: Use of MRI for identifying subchondral bone damage in horses: 11 cases (1999-2003), *J Am Vet Med Assoc* 224:411, 2004.

63. Garcia Lopez J, Kirker Head C: Occult subchondral osseous cyst-like lesions of the equine tarsocrural joint, *Vet Surg* 33:557, 2004.

64. Dyson SJ, Ross MW: Unpublished data and personal observations, 2009.

65. Stephens P, Richardson D, Ross M, Ford TS: Osteochondral fragments within the dorsal pouch or dorsal joint capsule of the proximal intertarsal joint of the horse, *Vet Surg* 18:151, 1989.

66. Lindsay W, McMartin R, McClure J: Management of slab fracture of the third tarsal bone in 5 horses, *Equine Vet J* 14:55, 1982.

67. Tulamo R, Bramlage L, Coakel A: Fractures of the central and third tarsal bones in horses, *J Am Vet Med Assoc* 182:1234, 1983.

68. Martin F, Herthel D: Central tarsal bone fractures in 5 horses: report on the use of a cannulated compression bone screw, *Equine Pract* 14:23, 1992.

69. Bathe A: Distal tarsal bone fractures in Thoroughbred racehorses, Thesis for Royal College of Veterinary Surgeons Diploma in Equine Orthopaedics, 2005.

70. Elce Y, Ross MW, Woodford A, et al: A review of central and third tarsal bone fractures in 57 horses, *Proc Am Assoc Equine Pract* 47:488, 2001.

71. Baird D, Pilsworth R: Wedge-shaped conformation of the dorsolateral aspect of the third tarsal bone in the Thoroughbred racehorse is associated with the development of slab fractures in this site, *Equine Vet J* 33:617, 2001.

72. Murphy E, Schneider R, Adams A, et al: Long-term outcome of horses with a slab fracture of the central or third tarsal bone treated conservatively: 25 cases (1976-1993), *J Am Vet Med Assoc* 216:1949, 2000.

73. Santschi E: Tarsal injuries. In White SA, Moore JM, eds: *Current techniques in equine surgery and lameness*, ed 2, Philadelphia, 1998, Saunders.

74. Davidson E, Ross M, Parente E: Incomplete sagittal fractures of the talus in 11 racehorses: outcome, *Equine Vet J* 37:457, 2005.

75. Meagher D, Mackey V: Lag screw fixations of a sagittal fracture of the talus in the horse, *Equine Vet Sci* 10:108, 1990.

76. Wright I: Fractures of the lateral malleolus of the tibia in 16 horses, *Equine Vet J* 24:424, 1992.

77. Jakovljevic S, Gibbs C, Yeats JJ: Traumatic fractures of the equine hock: a report of 13 cases, *Equine Vet J* 14:62,1982.

78. Watson E, Selcer B, Allen D: What is your diagnosis? A 1- to 1.5-cm osteochondral fragment along the distal margin of the medial malleolus of the right tibia, *J Am Vet Med Assoc* 199:773,1991.

79. Moll H, Stone D, Humborg J, Jagar: Traumatic tarsal luxation repaired without internal fixation in three horses and three ponies, *J Am Vet Med Assoc* 190:297, 1987.

80. Reeves M, Trotter G: Tarsocrural joint luxation in a horse, *J Am Vet Med Assoc* 199:1051, 1991.

81. Rose P, Moore I: Imaging diagnosis-avulsion of the medial collateral ligament of the tarsus in a horse, *Vet Radiol Ultrasound* 44:657, 2003.

82. Phillips T: Unusual hock problems, *Proc Am Assoc Equine Pract* 32:663, 1986.

83. Boero M, Kneller S, Baker G, et al: Clinical, radiographic and scintigraphic findings associated with enthesitis of the lateral collateral ligaments of the tarsocrural joint in Standardbred racehorses, *Equine Vet J Suppl* 6:53, 1988.

84. Bassage L, Lopez J, Currid E: Osteolytic lesions of the tuber calcanei in two horses, *J Am Vet Med Assoc* 217:710, 2000.

85. MacDonald M, Honnas C, Meagher D: Osteomyelitis of the calcaneus in horses: 28 cases (1972-1987), *J Am Vet Med Assoc* 194:1317, 1989.

86. Post E, Singer E, Clegg P, et al: Retrospective study of 24 cases of septic calcaneal bursitis in the horse, *Equine Vet J* 35:662, 2003.

87. Hand R, Watkins J, Honnas C, et al: Treatment of osteomyelitis of the sustentaculum tali and associated tenosynovitis in horses: 10 cases (1992-1998), *Proc Am Assoc Equine Pract* 45:158, 1999.

88. Edwards G: Changes in the sustentaculum tali associated with distension of the tarsal sheath (thoroughpin), *Equine Vet J* 10:97, 1978.

89. LePage OM, Léveillé R, Breton L, Marcoux M: Congenital dislocation of the deep digital flexor tendon associated with hypoplasia of the sustentaculum tali in a Thoroughbred colt, *Vet Radiol Ultrasound* 36:384, 1995.

90. Speed J: A cause of malformation of the limbs of Shetland ponies with a note on its phylogenic significance, *Br Vet J* 114:18, 1958.

91. Hermans W: Een hereditaire anomalie bij Shetland ponies, *Tijdschr Diergeneeskd* 16:989, 1969.

92. Pilsworth R, Head R: A study of 10 cases of peritarsal infection as a cause of severe lameness in the Thoroughbred racehorse: clinical signs, differential diagnosis, treatment and outcome, *Equine Vet J* 33:366, 2001.

CHAPTER 45   The Crus

1. Lundvall RL: Fracture of the fibula in the horse, *J Am Vet Med Assoc* 129:16, 1956.

2. Delahanty DD: Defects—not fracture of the fibula in the horse, *J Am Vet Med Assoc* 133:258, 1958.

3. Ross M: Unpublished data, 2001.

4. Ruggles AJ, Moore RM, Bertone AL, et al: Tibial stress fractures in racing Standardbreds: 13 cases (1989-1993), *J Am Vet Med Assoc* 209:634, 1996.

5. Schneider RK, Milne DW, Gabel AA, et al: Multidirectional in vivo strain analysis of the equine radius and tibia during dynamic loading with and without a cast, *Am J Vet Res* 43:1541, 1982.

6. Turner AS, Mills EJ, Gabel AA: In vivo measurement of bone strain in the horse, *Am J Vet Res* 36:1573, 1975.

7. O'Sullivan CB, Lumsden JM: Stress fractures of the tibia and humerus in Thoroughbred racehorses: 99 cases (1992-2000), *J Am Vet Med Assoc* 222:491, 2003.

8. Dyson S: Personal communication, 2001.

9. Ramzan PH, Newton JR, Shepherd MC, Head MJ: The application of a scintigraphic grading system to equine tibial stress fractures: 42 cases, *Equine Vet J* 35:382, 2003.

10. Bramlage LR, Hanes GE: Internal fixation of a tibial fracture in an adult horse, *J Am Vet Med Assoc* 180:1090, 1982.

11. Young DR, Richardson DW, Nunamaker DM, et al: Use of dynamic compression plates for treatment of tibial diaphyseal fractures in foals: nine cases (1980-1987), *J Am Vet Med Assoc* 194:1755, 1989.

12. Wright IM, Montesso F, Kidd LJ: Surgical treatment of fractures of the tibial tuberosity in 6 adult horses, *Equine Vet J* 27:96, 1995.

13. Smith BL, Auer JA, Watkins JP: Surgical repair of tibial tuberosity avulsion fractures in four horses, *Vet Surg* 19:117, 1990.

14. Arnold CE, Schaer TP, Baird DL, Martin BB: Conservative management of tibial tuberosity fractures in 15 horses, *Vet Surg* 30:487, 2001.

15. Secombe CJ, Anderson BH: Diagnosis and treatment of an osteochondroma of the distal tibia in a 3-year-old horse, *Aust Vet J* 78:16, 2000.

16. Textor JA, Nixon AJ, Lumsden J, Ducharme NG: Subchondral cystic lesions of the proximal extremity of the tibia in horses: 12 cases (1983-2000), *J Am Vet Med Assoc* 218:408, 2001.

17. Engiles JB, Orsini JA, Ross MW: What's your diagnosis? Fracture of the fibula, *J Am Vet Med Assoc* 224:1429, 2004.

18. Kidd JA, Bradshaw J: Bilateral nonossifying fibromas in the proximal tibiae of a yearling Thoroughbred filly, *Equine Vet J* 34:317, 2002.

19. Story MR, Gaughan EM, Andrews GA, Balch S: Fibrosarcoma over the tarsal groove of a 14-month-old Quarter Horse, *Vet Comp Orthop Traumatol* 18:115, 2005.

CHAPTER 46   The Stifle

1. Butler JA, Colles CM, Dyson SJ, et al: The stifle and tibia. In *Clinical radiology of the horse*, ed 3, Oxford, 2008, Wiley-Blackwell.

2. Sisson S: Equine myology. In Getty R, ed: *Sisson and Grossman's the anatomy of the domestic animals*, ed 5, Philadelphia, 1975, Saunders.

3. Vacek JR, Ford TS, Honnas CM: Communication between the femoropatellar and medial and lateral femorotibial joints in horses, *Am J Vet Res* 53:1431, 1992.

4. Gough M, Munroe G, Mayhew I: Diffusion of mepivacaine between adjacent synovial structures in the horse. Part 2. Tarsus and stifle, *Equine Vet J* 34:85, 2002.

5. Walmsley JP: Unpublished data, 2008.

6. Sisson S: Equine syndesmology. In Getty R, ed: *Sisson and Grossman's the anatomy of the domestic animals*, ed 5, Philadelphia, 1975, Saunders.

7. Arnoczky SP, Marshall JL: Pathomechanics of cruciate and meniscal injuries. In Bojrab MJ, ed: *Pathophysiology in small animal surgery*, Philadelphia, 1981, Lea & Febiger.

8. Gabel AA: Diagnosis, relative incidence, and probable cause of cunean bursitis-tarsitis of standardbred horses, *J Am Vet Med Assoc* 175:1079, 1979.

9. Hendrickson DA, Nixon AJ: A lateral approach for synovial aspiration and joint injection of the femoropatellar joint in the horse, *Equine Vet J* 24:399, 1992.

10. Maulet BEB, Mayhew IG, Jones E, et al: Radiographic anatomy of the soft tissue attachments of the equine stifle, *Equine Vet J* 37:530, 2005.

11. Adams WM, Thilsted JP: Radiographic appearance of the equine stifle from birth to 6 months, *Vet Radiol* 26:126, 1985.

12. Penninck DG, Nyland TG, O'Brien TR, et al: Ultrasonography of the equine stifle, *Vet Radiol* 31:293, 1990.

13. Cauvin EJR, Munroe GA, Boyd JS, et al: Ultrasonographic examination of the femorotibial articulation in horses: imaging of the cranial and caudal aspects, *Equine Vet J* 28:285, 1996.

14. Dik KJ: Ultrasonography of the equine stifle, *Equine Vet Educ* 7:154, 1995.

15. Hoegaerts M, Nicaise M, van Bree H, et al: Cross-sectional anatomy and comparative ultrasonography of the equine medial femorotibial joint and its related structures, *Equine Vet J* 37:520, 2005.

16. Holcombe SJ, Bertone AL, Biller DS, et al: Magnetic resonance imaging of the equine stifle, *Vet Radiol Ultrasound* 36:119, 1995.

17. Bergman E: Computed tomography and computed tomography arthrography of the equine stifle: technique and preliminary results in 16 clinical cases, *Proc Am Assoc Equine Pract* 53:46, 2007.

18. Coudry V, Denoix J-M: Ultrasonography of the femorotibial collateral ligaments of the horse, *Equine Vet Educ* 17:275, 2005.

19. Jacquet S, Audigie F, Denoix J-M: Ultrasonographic diagnosis of subchondral bone cysts in the medial femoral condyle of horses, *Equine Vet Educ* 19:47, 2007.

20. Barr E, Pinchbeck G, Clegg P, et al: Accuracy of diagnostic techniques used in investigation of stifle lameness in horses: 40 cases, *Equine Vet Educ* 18:326, 2006.

21. Dyson S, McKnie K, Weekes J, et al: Scintigraphic evaluation of the stifle in normal horses and horses with forelimb lameness, *Vet Radiol Ultrasound* 48:378, 2007.

22. Steckel RR: The role of scintigraphy in the lameness evaluation, *Vet Clin North Am Large Anim Pract* 7:207, 1991.

23. Dyson S, Pilsworth R, Twardock R, et al: *Equine scintigraphy*, Newmarket, 2003, Equine Vet J Ltd.

24. Ray CS, Baxter GM, McIlwraith CW, et al: Development of subchondral cystic lesions after articular cartilage and subchondral bone damage in young horses, *Equine Vet J* 28:225, 1996.

25. Squire KR, Fessler JF, Cantwell HD, et al: Enlarging bilateral femoral condylar bone cysts without scintigraphic uptake in a yearling foal, *Vet Radiol* 33:109, 1992.

26. McCullough RW, Gandsman EJ, Litchman HE, et al: Dynamic bone scintigraphy in osteochondritis dissecans, *Int Orthop* 12:317, 1988.

27. Cymbaluk NF, Smart ME: A review of possible metabolic relationships of copper to equine bone disease, *Equine Vet J Suppl* 16:19, 1993.

28. Savage CJ, McCarthy RN, Jeffcott LB: Effects of dietary energy and protein on induction of dyschondroplasia in foals, *Equine Vet J Suppl* 16:74, 1993.

29. Phillipsson J, Andreasson B, Sandgren B, et al: Osteochondrosis in the tarsocrural joint and osteochondral fragments in the fetlock joint in standardbred trotters. II. Heritability, *Equine Vet J Suppl* 16:38, 1993.

30. Carlson CS, Cullins LD, Meuten DJ: Osteochondrosis of the articular-epiphyseal cartilage complex in young horses: evidence for a defect in cartilage canal blood supply, *Vet Pathol* 32:641, 1995.

31. Foland JW, McIlwraith CW, Trotter GW: Arthroscopic surgery for osteochondritis dissecans of the femoropatellar joint of the horse, *Equine Vet J* 24:419, 1992.

32. McIntosh SC, McIlwraith CW: Natural history of femoropatellar osteochondrosis in three young colts of thoroughbreds, *Equine Vet J Suppl* 16:54, 1993.

33. Dik K, Enzerink E: The radiographic development of osteochondral abnormalities in the hock and stifle of Dutch Warmblood foals from 1 to 11 months of age, *Equine Vet J* 31:9, 1998.

34. Dabereiner RM, Sullins KE, White NA: Progression of femoropatellar osteochondrosis in nine young horses: clinical, radiographic and arthroscopic findings, *Vet Surg* 22:515, 1993.

35. McIlwraith CW, Trotter GW: Clinical aspects of osteochondritis dissecans. In McIlwraith CW, Trotter GW, eds: *Joint disease in the horse*, Philadelphia, 1996, Saunders.

36. Nixon AJ, Fortier LA, Goodrich LR, et al: Arthroscopic reattachment of osteochondritis dissecans lesions using resorbable polydioxanone pins, *Equine Vet J* 36:376, 2004.

37. Nixon AJ: Advances in promoting cartilage healing. Proceedings of the Thirty-Fourth Annual Scientific Meeting of the American College of Veterinary Surgeons, San Francisco, Calif, 1999.

38. Rooney JR: Upward fixation—patella. In Rooney JR, ed: *The lame horse*, Cranbury, NJ, 1973, AS Barnes.

39. Stashak TS: Upward fixation of the patella. In *Adams' lameness in horses*, ed 4, Philadelphia, 1987, Lea & Febiger.

40. Brown MP, Moon PD, Buergelt CD: The effects of injection of an iodine counter-irritant into the patellar ligaments of ponies: application to stifle lameness, *J Equine Vet Sci* 4:82, 1984.

41. Turner AS, McIlwraith CW: Medial patellar desmotomy. In Turner AS, McIlwraith CW, eds: *Techniques in large animal surgery*, ed 2, Philadelphia, 1989, Lea & Febiger.

42. Tnibar MA: Medial patellar ligament splitting for the treatment of upward fixation of the patella in 7 equids, *Vet Surg* 31:462, 2002.

43. McIlwraith CW: Osteochondral fragmentation of the distal aspect of the patella in horses, *Equine Vet J* 22:157, 1990.

44. Riley CB, Yovich JV: Fracture of the apex of the patella after medial patellar desmotomy in a horse, *Aust Vet J* 68:37, 1991.

45. Walmsley JP: Medial patellar desmotomy for upward fixation of the patella, *Equine Vet Educ* 6:148, 1994.

46. Gibson KE, McIlwraith CW, Park RD, et al: Production of patellar lesions by medial patellar desmotomy in horses, *Vet Surg* 18:466, 1989.

47. Labens M, Busoni V, Peters F, et al: Ultrasonographic and radiographic diagnosis of patellar fragmentation secondary to bilateral medial patellar desmotomy, *Equine Vet Educ* 17:201, 2005.

48. McIlwraith CW: Patellar fragmentation secondary to bilateral medial patellar desmotomy, *Equine Vet Educ* 17:205, 2005.

49. Dyson SJ: Normal ultrasonographic anatomy and injury of the patellar ligaments in the horse, *Equine Vet J* 34:258, 2002.

50. Dumoulin M, Pille F, Desmet P, et al: Upward fixation of the patella in the horse: a retrospective study, *Vet Comp Orthop Traumatol* 20:119, 2007.

51. Hermans WA, Kersjes AW, van der Mey GJW, et al: Investigation into the heredity of congenital lateral patellar (sub) luxation in the Shetland pony, *Vet Q* 9:1, 1987.

52. Leitch M, Kotlikoff M: Surgical repair of congenital lateral luxation of the patella in the foal and calf, *Vet Surg* 9:1, 1980.

53. Engelbert TA, Tate LP, Richardson DC, et al: Lateral patellar luxation in miniature horses, *Vet Surg* 22:293, 1993.

54. Kobluk CN: Correction of patellar luxation by recession sulcoplasty in three foals, *Vet Surg* 22:298, 1993.

55. McIlwraith CW, Warren RC: Distal luxation of the patella in a horse, *J Am Vet Med Assoc* 181:67, 1982.

56. Howard RD, McIlwraith CW, Trotter GW: Arthroscopic surgery for subchondral cystic lesions of the medial femoral condyle in horses: 41 cases (1988-1991), *J Am Vet Med Assoc* 206:842, 1995.

57. Hance SR, Schneider RK, Embertson RM, et al: Lesions of the caudal aspect of the femoral condyles in foals: 20 cases (1980-1990), *J Am Vet Med Assoc* 202:637, 1993.

58. Textor JA, Nixon AJ, Lumsden J, et al: Subchondral cystic lesions of the proximal extremity of the tibia in horses: 12 cases (1983-2000), *J Am Vet Med Assoc* 218:408, 2001.

59. Bramlage LR: Osteochondrosis related bone cysts, *Proc Am Assoc Equine Pract* 39:83, 1993.

60. Von Rechenberg B, McIlwraith CW, Luetenegger C, et al: Fibrous tissue of subchondral bone cyst lesions (SCL) in horses produce inflammatory mediators and neutral metalloproteinases and caused bone resorption in vitro, *Vet Surg* 27:520, 1998.

61. Scott G, Crawford W, Colahan P: Arthroscopic findings in horses with subtle radiographic evidence of osteochondral lesions of the medial femoral condyle: 15 cases, *J Am Vet Med Assoc* 224:1821, 2004.

62. Stewart B, Reid CF: Osseous cyst-like lesions of the medial femoral condyle in the horse, *J Am Vet Med Assoc* 180:254, 1982.

63. Rose JA, Sande RL, Rose EM: Results of conservative management of osteochondrosis in the horse, *Proc Am Assoc Equine Pract* 31:617, 1986.

64. Greet T: The management of subchondral cysts associated with the medial femoral condyle by arthroscopic surgery in horses. Proceedings of the Seventh Annual Scientific Meeting of the European College of Veterinary Surgeons, Pörtschach, Austria, 1998.

65. Jackson WA, Stick JA, Arnoczky SP, et al: The effect of compacted cancellous bone grafting on the healing of subchondral bone defects of the medial femoral condyle in horses, *Vet Surg* 29:8, 2000.

66. Smith MA, Walmsley JP, Phillips TJ, et al: Effect of age at presentation on outcome following arthroscopic debridement of subchondral cystic lesions of the medial femoral condyle: 85 cases (1993-2003), *Equine Vet J* 37:175, 2005.

67. Wallis TW, Goodrich LR, McIlwraith CW, et al: Arthroscopic injection of corticosteroids into the fibrous tissue of subchondral cystic lesions of the medial femoral condyle in horses: a retrospective study of 52 cases (2001-2006), *Equine Vet J* 40:461, 2008.

68. Walmsley JP: Vertical tears of the cranial horn of the meniscus and its cranial ligament in the equine femorotibial joint: 7 cases and their treatment by arthroscopic surgery, *Equine Vet J* 27:20, 1995.

69. Bertone AL, Holcombe SL: Soft tissue injuries of the equine stifle, *Vet Surg* 21:383, 1992.

70. Lewis RL: A retrospective study of diagnostic and surgical arthroscopy of the equine femorotibial joint, *Proc Am Assoc Equine Pract* 23:887, 1987.

71. Walmsley JP, Phillips TJ, Townsend HGG: Meniscal tears in horses: an evaluation of clinical signs and arthroscopic treatment of 80 cases, *Equine Vet J* 35:402, 2003.

72. Walmsley JP, Phillips TJ: Unpublished data, 2001.

73. Cauvin EJ, Munroe GA, Boyd JS, et al: Ultrasonographic examination of the femorotibial articulation in horses: imaging of the cranial and caudal aspects, *Equine Vet J* 28:285, 1996.

74. De Busscher V, Verwilghen D, Bolen G, et al: Meniscal damage diagnosed by ultrasonography in horses: a retrospective study of 74 femorotibial joint ultrasonographic examinations, *J Equine Vet Science* 26:453, 2006.

75. Prades M, Grant BD, Turner TA, et al: Injuries of the cranial cruciate ligament and associated structures: summary of clinical, radiographic arthroscopic and pathological findings from 10 horses, *Equine Vet J* 21:354, 1989.

76. Rich RF, Glisson RR: In vitro mechanical properties and failure mode of the equine (pony) cranial cruciate ligament, *Vet Surg* 23:257, 1994.

77. Mueller POE, Allen D, Watson E, et al: Arthroscopic removal of a fragment from an intercondylar eminence fracture of the tibia in a two-year-old horse, *J Am Vet Med Assoc* 204:1793, 1994.

78. Baker GJ, Moustafa MAI, Boero MJ: Caudal cruciate ligament function and injury in the horse, *Vet Rec* 121:319, 1987.

79. Sanders-Shamis M, Bukowiecki CF, Biller DS: Cruciate and collateral ligament failure in the equine stifle: seven cases (1975-1985), *J Am Vet Med Assoc* 193:573, 1988.

80. Muurlink T, Walmsley J, Young D: A cranial intercondylar arthroscopic approach to the caudal medial femorotibial joint of the horse, *Equine Vet J* 41:5, 2009.

81. Watts AE, Nixon AJ: Comparison of arthroscopic approaches and accessible anatomic structures during arthroscopy of the caudal pouches of the equine femorotibial joints, *Vet Surg* 35:219, 2006.

82. Edwards RB, Nixon AJ: Avulsion of the cranial cruciate ligament insertion in a horse, *Equine Vet J* 28:334, 1996.

83. Bukowiecki CF, Sanders-Shamis M, Bramlage LR: Treatment of a ruptured medial collateral ligament of the stifle in a horse, *J Am Vet Med Assoc* 193:687, 1988.

84. Schneider RK, Jenson P, Moore RM: Evaluation of cartilage lesions on the medial femoral condyle as a cause of lameness in horses: 11 cases 1988-1994, *J Am Vet Med Assoc* 210:1649, 1997.

85. Winberg FG: Occult cartilage lesions in the stifle of young Warmblood horses: preliminary results. Proceedings of the Eighth Annual Scientific Meeting of the European College of Veterinary Surgeons, Brugge, Belgium, 1999.

86. McIlwraith CW: Surgical strategies for cartilage injury. Proceedings of the Thirty-Fourth Annual Scientific Meeting of the American College of Veterinary Surgeons, San Francisco, Calif, 1999.

87. Frisbie DD, Trotter GW, Powers BE, et al: Arthroscopic subchondral bone plate microfracture technique augments healing of large chondral defects in the radial carpal bone and medial femoral condyle of horses, *Vet Surg* 28:242, 1999.

88. Dyson SJ, Wright I, Kold S, et al: Clinical and radiographic features, treatment and outcome in 15 horses with fracture of the medial aspect of the patella, *Equine Vet J* 24:264, 1992.

89. Pankowski RL, White KK: Fracture of the patella in horses, *Comp Cont Educ Pract Vet* 7:566, 1985.

90. Dik KJ, Nemeth F: Traumatic patellar fractures in the horse, *Equine Vet J* 15:244, 1983.

91. Dyson SJ: Stifle trauma in the event horse, *Equine Vet Educ* 6:234, 1994.

92. Hunt RJ, Baxter GM, Zamos DTM: Tension-band wiring and lag screw fixation of a transverse, comminuted fracture of the patella in a horse, *J Am Vet Med Assoc* 200:819, 1992.

93. DeBowes RM, Grant BD, Chalman JA, et al: Fractured patella in a horse, *Equine Pract* 2:49, 1980.

94. Aldrete AV, Meagher DM: Lag screw fixation of a patellar fracture in a horse, *Vet Surg* 10:143, 1981.

95. Mueller POE, Allen D, Watson E, et al: Arthroscopic removal of a fragment from an intercondylar eminence fracture of the tibia in a two-year-old horse, *J Am Vet Med Assoc* 204:1793, 1994.

96. Wisner AB: Surgical removal of an avulsion fracture of the stifle joint, *Equine Vet Med Surg* 3:337, 1979.

97. Walmsley JP: Fracture of the intercondylar eminence of the tibia treated by arthroscopic internal fixation, *Equine Vet J* 29:148, 1997.

98. Montesso F, Wright IM: Removal of chip fractures of the femoral trochlear ridges of three horses, *Vet Rec* 137:94, 1995.

99. Dabareiner RM, Sullins KE: Fracture of the caudal medial femoral condyle in a horse, *Equine Vet J* 25:75, 1993.

100. Hance SR, Bramlage LR, Schneider RK, et al: Retrospective study of 38 cases of femur fractures in horses less than one year of age, *Equine Vet J* 24:357, 1992.

101. DeBowes RM, Grant BD, Modransky PD: Lag screw stabilization of Salter type IV femoral fracture in a young horse, *J Am Vet Med Assoc* 182:1123, 1983.

102. Walmsley JP, Summerhays GES: Repair of a Salter-Harris type IV fracture of the distal femur of a yearling thoroughbred by internal fixation, *Equine Vet Educ* 2:177, 1990.

103. Kirkerhead CA, Fackelman GE: Use of the cobra head bone plate distal long bone fractures in large animals: a report of four cases, *Vet Surg* 18:227, 1989.

104. Wright IM, Montesso F, Kidd LJ: Surgical treatment of fractures of the tibial tuberosity in 6 horses, *Equine Vet J* 27:96, 1995.

105. Kold SE: Traction apophysitis in a yearling colt resembling Osgood-Schlatter disease in man, *Equine Vet J* 22:60, 1990.

106. Getty R: Equine osteology. In Getty R, ed: *The anatomy of domestic animals*, ed 5, Philadelphia, 1975, Saunders.

107. Gerring EL, Davies JV: Fracture of the tibial tuberosity in a polo pony, *Equine Vet J* 14:158, 1982.

108. Smith BL, Auer JA, Watkins JP: Surgical repair of tibial tuberosity avulsion fractures in four horses, *Vet Surg* 19:117, 1990.

109. Eliasher E, Smith RKW, Schramme MC, et al: Preoperative bending and twisting of a dynamic compression plate for the repair of tibial tuberosity fracture in the horse, *Equine Vet J* 32:447, 2000.

110. Arnold CE, Schaer TP, Baird DL, et al: Conservative management of 17 horses with nonarticular fractures of the tibial tuberosity, *Equine Vet J* 35:202, 2003.

111. Blikslager AT, Bristol DG: Avulsion of the origin of the peroneus tertius tendon in a foal, *J Am Vet Med Assoc* 204:1483, 1994.

112. Holcombe SJ, Bertone AL: Avulsion fracture of the origin of the extensor digitorum longus in a foal, *J Am Vet Med Assoc* 204:1652, 1994.

113. Szabuniewicz M, Titus RS: Rupture of the peroneus tertius in the horse, *Vet Med Small Anim Clin* 62:993, 1967.

114. Dodd DC, Raker CW: Tumoral calcinosis (calcinosis circumscripta) in the horse, *J Am Vet Med Assoc* 57:968, 1970.

115. Goulden BE, O'Callaghan MW: Tumoral calcinosis in the horse, *N Z Vet J* 28:217, 1980.

116. O'Connor JP, Lucey MP: Tumoral calcinosis (calcinosis circumscripta) in the horse, *Irish Vet J* 31:173, 1977.

CHAPTER 47   The Thigh

1. Churchill EA: The methodology of diagnosis of hind leg lameness, *Proc Am Assoc Equine Pract* 25:297, 1979.

2. Churchill EA: Lameness associated with the lower back and pelvis, *Proc Am Assoc Equine Pract* 28:277, 1982.

3. Churchill EA: The diagnosis and treatment of lameness of the pelvic limb, *Proc Am Assoc Equine Pract* 33:849, 1987.

4. Hawkins DL: Diagnosis of lameness in the hind leg, *Norden News* 62:15, 1987.

5. Hawkins D, Churchill E: Unpublished data, 2001.

6. Getty R: *The anatomy of the domestic animals*, ed 5, vol 1, Philadelphia, 1975, Saunders.

7. Stashak TS: Trochanteric bursitis. In Stashak TS, eds: *Adams' lameness in horses*, ed 4, Philadelphia, 1987, Lea & Febiger.

8. Mueller POE, Hay WP: Ancillary diagnostic aids. In Colahan PT, Merritt AM, Moore JN, et al, eds: *Equine medicine and surgery*, ed 5, St. Louis, 1999, Mosby.

9. Richardson DW: The femur and pelvis. In Auer JA, Stick JA, eds: *Equine surgery*, ed 2, Philadelphia, 1999, Saunders.

10. Orsini JA, Buonanno AM, Richardson DW, et al: Condylar buttress plate fixation of femoral fracture in a colt, *J Am Vet Med Assoc* 197:1184, 1990.

11. DeBowes RM, Grant BD, Modransky PD: Lag screw stabilization of Salter type IV femoral fracture in a young horse, *J Am Vet Med Assoc* 182:1123, 1983.

12. Watkins JP: Diseases of the thigh with physical causes. In Colahan PT, Merritt

AM, Moore JN, et al, eds: *Equine medicine and surgery*, ed 5, St. Louis, 1999, Mosby.

13. Rose PL, Watkins JP, Auer JA: Femoral fracture repair complicated by vascular injury in a foal, *J Am Vet Med Assoc* 185:795, 1984.

14. Hance SR, Bramlage LR: Fractures of the femur and patella. In Nixon AJ, ed: *Equine fracture repair*, Philadelphia, 1996, Saunders.

15. Hance SR, Bramlage LR, Schneider RK, et al: Retrospective study of 38 cases of femur fractures in horses less than one year of age, *Equine Vet J* 24:357, 1992.

16. Levine DG, Richardson DW: Clinical use of the locking compression plate (LCP) in horses: a retrospective study of 31 cases (2004-2006), *Equine Vet J* 39:401, 2007.

17. Byron CR, Stick JA, Brown JA, et al: Use of a condylar screw plate for repair of a Salter-Harris type-III fracture of the femur in a 2-year-old horse, *J Am Vet Med Assoc* 221:1292, 2002.

18. Embertson RM, Bramlage LR, Herring DS, et al: Physeal fractures in the horse: I. Classification and incidence, *Vet Surg* 15:223, 1986.

19. Jesty SA, Palmer JE, Parente EJ, et al: Rupture of the gastrocnemius muscle in six foals, *J Am Vet Med Assoc* 227:1965, 2005.

20. Lescun TB, Hawkins JF, Siems JJ: Management of rupture of the gastrocnemius and superficial digital flexor muscles with a modified Thomas splint-cast combination in a horse, *J Am Vet Med Assoc* 213:1457, 1998.

21. Swor TM, Schneider RK, Ross MW, et al: Injury to the origin of the gastrocnemius muscle as a possible cause of lameness in four horses, *J Am Vet Med Assoc* 219:215, 2001.

22. Dabareiner RM, Schmitz DG, Honnas CM, et al: Gracilis muscle injury as a cause of lameness in two horses, *J Am Vet Med Assoc* 224:1630, 2004.

23. Shirai W, Momotani E, Sato T, et al: Dissecting aortic aneurysm in a horse, *J Comp Pathol* 120:307, 1999.

CHAPTER 48   Mechanical and Neurological Lameness in the Forelimbs and Hindlimbs

1. Valentine BA, de Lahunta A, Divers TJ, et al: Clinical and pathologic findings in two draft horses with progressive muscle atrophy, neuromuscular weakness, and abnormal gait characteristic of shivers syndrome, *J Am Vet Med Assoc* 215:1661, 1999.

2. Valentine BA: Polysaccharide storage myopathy in draft and draft-related horses and ponies, *Equine Pract* 21:16, 1999.

3. Slocombe RF, Huntington PJ, Friend SCE, et al: Pathological aspects of Australian stringhalt, *Equine Vet J* 24:174, 1992.

4. Huntington PJ, Seneque S, Slocombe RF, et al: Use of phenytoin to treat horses with Australian stringhalt, *Aust Vet J* 68:221, 1991.

5. Valentine BA, Rousselle SD, Sams AE, et al: Denervation atrophy in three horses with fibrotic myopathy, *J Am Vet Med Assoc* 205:332, 1994.

6. Toniato M, Torre F: Persistent acquired upward fixation of the patella in a Standardbred foal, *Equine Vet Educ* 15:233, 2003.

7. Dumoulin M, Pille F, Desmet P, et al: Upward fixation of the patella in the horse: a retrospective study, *Vet Comp Orthop Traumatol* 20:119, 2007.

8. Rooney JR: *Biomechanics of lameness in horses*, Baltimore, 1969, Williams & Wilkins.

9. Valentine BA, Hintz HF, Freels KM, et al: Dietary control of exertional rhabdomyolysis in horses, *J Am Vet Med Assoc* 212:1588, 1998.

10. Brown M, Moon P, Buergelt C: The effects of injection of an iodine counter-irritant into the patellar ligaments of ponies: application to stifle lameness, *J Equine Vet Sci* 4:482, 1984.

11. Van Hoogmoed L, Agnew D, Whitcomb M, et al: Ultrasonographic and histological evaluation of medial and middle patellar ligaments after injection with ethanolamine oleate and 2% iodine in almond oil, *Am J Vet Res* 63:738, 2002.

12. Gibson K, McIlwraith C, Park R, et al: Production of patellar lesions by medial patellar desmotomy in normal horses, *Vet Surg* 18:466, 1989.

13. Dyson S: Normal ultrasonographic anatomy and injury of the patellar ligaments in the horse, *Equine Vet J* 34:258, 2002.

14. Tnibar M: Medial patellar ligament splitting for the treatment of upward fixation of the patella in 7 equids, *Vet Surg* 31:462, 2002.

15. Tnibar M: Experiences with medial patellar ligament splitting for the treatment of upward fixation of the patella in the horse. Proceeding of the Fourteenth Annual Meeting of the European College of Veterinary Surgeons, Lyon, France, 2005.

16. Reiners SR, May K, DiGrassie W, et al: How to perform a standing medial patellar ligament splitting, *Proc Am Assoc Equine Pract* 51:481, 2005.

17. Bonder D: Personal communication, 2008.

18. Pickersgill CH, Kriz N, Malikides N: Surgical treatment of semitendinosus fibrotic myopathy in an endurance horse—management, complications and outcome, *Equine Vet Educ* 12:320, 2000.

19. Turner AS, Trotter GW: Fibrotic myopathy in the horse, *J Am Vet Med Assoc* 184:335, 1984.

20. Bramlage LR, Reed SM, Embertson RM: Semitendinosus tenotomy for treatment of fibrotic myopathy in the horse, *J Am Vet Med Assoc* 186:565, 1985.

21. Stashak TS: *Adams' lameness in horses*, Philadelphia, 1987, Lea & Febiger.

22. Magee AA, Vatistas NJ: Standing semitendinosus myotomy for the treatment of fibrotic myopathy in 39 horses (1989-1997), *Proc Am Assoc Equine Pract* 44:263, 1998.

23. Dyson S: Unpublished data, 2009.

24. Valentine B: Mechanical lameness in the hindlimb. In Ross M, Dyson S, eds: *Diagnosis and management of lameness in the horse*, ed 1, St. Louis, 2003, Saunders.

25. Crabill MR, Honnas CM, Taylor DS, et al: Stringhalt secondary to trauma to the dorsoproximal region of the metatarsus in horses: 10 cases (1986-1991), *J Am Vet Med Assoc* 205:867, 1994.

26. Torre F: Clinical diagnosis and results of surgical treatment of 13 cases of acquired stringhalt (1991–2003), *Equine Vet J* 37:181, 2005.

27. Araújo JA, Curcio B, Alda J, et al: Stringhalt in Brazilian horses caused by Hypochoeris radicata, *Toxicology* 52:190, 2008.

28. Domange C, Canlet C, Traore A, et al: Orthologous metagonomic qualification of a rodent model combined with magnetic resonance imaging for an integrated evaluation of the toxicity of Hypochoeris radicata, *Chem Res Toxicol* 21:2082, 2008.

29. Adam-Castrillo D, White NA, Donaldson LL, et al: Effects of injection of botulinum toxin type B into the external anal sphincter on anal pressure in horses, *Am J Vet Res* 65:26, 2004.

30. Wijnberg ID, Schrama SE, Elgersma AE, et al: Quantification of surface EMG signals to monitor the effect of a Botox treatment in six healthy ponies and two horses with stringhalt: preliminary study, *Equine Vet J* 41:313, 2009.

31. Nollet H, Vanderstraeten G, Sustronck B, et al: Suspected case of stiff-horse syndrome, *Vet Rec* 146:282, 2000.

32. Firshman A, Baird J, Valberg S: Prevalence and clinical signs of polysaccharide storage myopathy and shivers in Belgian Draft Horses, *J Am Vet Med Assoc* 227:1958, 2005.

33. Hanche-Olsen S, Teige J, Skaar I, et al: Polyneuropathy associated with forage sources in Norwegian horses, *J Vet Intern Med* 22:178, 2008.

34. Dyson S, Taylor P, Whitwell K: Femoral nerve paralysis after general anaesthesia in the horse, *Equine Vet J* 20:376, 1988.

35. Eliashar E, Dyson S, Archer R, et al: Two clinical manifestations of desmopathy of the accessory ligament of the deep digital flexor tendon in the hindlimb of 23 horses, *Equine Vet J* 37:495, 2005.

36. Mayhew IG: Personal communication, 2008.

37. Barrey E: Inter-limb coordination. In Back W, Clayton H, eds: *Equine locomotion*, ed 1, London, 2001, Saunders.

CHAPTER 49   Diagnosis and Management of Pelvic Fractures in the Thoroughbred Racehorse

1. Little C, Hilbert B: Pelvic fractures in horses: 19 cases, *J Am Vet Med Assoc* 190:1203, 1987.

2. Rutkowski JA, Richardson DW: A retrospective study of 100 pelvic fractures in horses, *Equine Vet J* 21:256, 1989.

3. Steckel RR: The role of scintigraphy in lameness evaluation, *Vet Clin North Am Equine Pract* 7:207, 1991.

4. Stashak TS: *Adams' lameness in horses*, ed 4, Philadelphia, 1987, Lea & Febiger.

5. Stover SM, Adams M, Reed DH, et al: Patterns of stress fractures associated with complete bone fractures in racehorses, *Proc Am Assoc Equine Pract* 39:131, 1993.

6. Shepherd MC, Pilsworth RC, Hopes R, et al: Clinical signs, diagnosis, management and outcome of complete and incomplete fracture to the ilium: a review of 20

cases, *Proc Am Assoc Equine Pract* 40:179, 1994.

7. Bathe AP: 245 fractures in thoroughbred racehorses: results of a 2 year prospective study, *Proc Am Assoc Equine Pract* 40:175, 1994.

8. Shepherd MC, Pilsworth RC: The use of ultrasound in the diagnosis of pelvic fractures, *Equine Vet Educ* 6:223, 1994.

9. May SA, Patterson LJ, Peacock PJ, et al: Radiographic technique for the pelvis in the standing horse, *Equine Vet J* 23:312, 1991.

10. Barrett E, Talbot A, Driver A, et al: A technique for pelvic radiography in the standing horse, *Equine Vet J* 38:266, 2006.

11. Dabareiner RM, Cole RC: Fractures of the tuber coxa of the ilium in horses, *J Am Vet Med Assoc* 234:1303, 2009.

12. Baum JL, Devous MD: Scintigraphic evaluation of equine lameness, *Proc Am Assoc Equine Pract* 25:307, 1980.

13. Devous MD, Twardock AR: Techniques and applications of nuclear medicine in the diagnosis of equine lameness, *J Am Vet Med Assoc* 184:318, 1984.

14. Lamb CR, Koblick PD: Scintigraphic evaluation of skeletal disease and its applications in the horse, *Vet Radiol* 29:16, 1988.

15. Berry CR, Daniel GB: *Handbook of veterinary nuclear medicine*, Raleigh, NC, 1996, North Carolina State University Press.

16. Hornof WJ, Stover SM, Koblick PD, et al: Oblique views of the ilium and the scintigraphic appearance of stress fractures of the ilium, *Equine Vet J* 28:356, 1996.

17. Dyson SJ, Martinelli MJ, Pilsworth RC, et al: *Equine scintigraphy*, Newmarket, UK, 2003, Equine Vet J Publications.

18. Pilsworth RC, Holmes MA: A low cost computer based scintigraphy system for use in lameness investigation in general practice, *Proc Am Assoc Equine Pract* 37:327, 1992.

19. Pilsworth RC, Shepherd M, Herinckx BM, et al: A review of 10 horses with fracture of the wing of the ilium, *Equine Vet J* 26:94, 1994.

20. Pilsworth RC, Shepherd MC: Scintigraphic probe point counting. II. Interpretation of scan results, *Equine Vet Educ* 8:103, 1996.

21. Raidal SL, Love D, Bailey GD, et al: Inflammation and increased numbers of bacteria in the lower respiratory tract of horses within 6-12 hours of confinement with the head elevated, *Aust Vet J* 72:45, 1995.

CHAPTER 50   Lumbosacral and Pelvic Injuries in Sports and Pleasure Horses

1. Denoix J-M: Spinal biomechanics and functional anatomy, *Vet Clin North Am Equine Pract* 15:27, 1999.

2. Dyson S, Murray R: Pain associated with the sacroiliac joint region: a clinical study of 74 horses, *Equine Vet J* 35:240, 2003.

3. Denoix J-M, Audigié F, Coudry V: Review of diagnosis and treatment of lumbosacral pain in sport and racehorses, *Proc Am Assoc Equine Pract* 51:366, 2005.

4. David F, Rougier M, Alexander K, et al: Ultrasound guided coxofemoral arthrocentesis in horses, *Equine Vet J* 39:79, 2007.

5. Dyson S: Étude de la doluer sacroiliaque chez le cheval, *Prat Vét Équine* 40:123, 2008.

6. Butler J, Colles C, Dyson S, et al: The pelvis and femur. In *Clinical radiology of the horse*, ed 3, Oxford, 2008, Wiley-Blackwell.

7. Dabareiner R, Cole R: Fractures of the tuber coxae of the ilium in horses: 29 cases (1996-2007), *J Am Vet Med Assoc* 234:1303, 2009.

8. Goodrich L, Werpy N, Armentrat A: How to ultrasound scan the normal pelvis for aiding diagnosis of pelvic fractures and transcutaneous ultrasound examination, *Proc Am Assoc Equine Pract* 52:609, 2006.

9. David F, Vinardell T, Cousty M, et al: Examen échographique de la région pelvienne chez le cheval, *Prat Vét Équine* 40:85, 2008.

10. Dyson S, Pilsworth R, Twardock R, et al: *Equine scintigraphy*, 1st ed, Newmarket, UK, 2003, Equine Vet J.

11. Dyson S, Murray R, Branch M, et al: The sacroiliac joints: evaluation using nuclear scintigraphy. Part I. The normal horse, *Equine Vet J* 35:226, 2003.

12. Erichsen C, Eksell P, Widstrom C, et al: Scintigraphy of the sacroiliac joint region in asymptomatic riding horses: scintigraphic appearance and evaluation of method, *Vet Radiol Ultrasound* 44:699, 2003.

13. Erichsen C, Berger M: Pitfalls in interpretation of pelvic scintigrams caused by soft tissue attenuation, *Vet Radiol Ultrasound* 42:179, 2001.

14. Erichsen C, Berger M, Eksell P: The scintigraphic anatomy of the equine sacroiliac joint, *Vet Radiol Ultrasound* 43:287, 2002.

15. Gorgas D, Luder P, Lang J, et al: Scintigraphic and radiographic appearance of the sacroiliac region in horses with gait abnormalities or poor performance, *Vet Radiol Ultrasound* 50:208, 2009.

16. Geissbuhler U, Busato A, Ueltschi G: Abnormal bone scan findings of the equine ischial tuberosity and third trochanter, *Vet Radiol Ultrasound* 39:572, 1998.

17. Little C, Hilbert B: Pelvic fractures in horses: 19 cases (1974-1984), *J Am Vet Med Assoc* 190:1203, 1987.

18. Rutkowski J, Richardson D: A retrospective study of 100 pelvic fractures in horses, *Equine Vet J* 21:256, 1989.

19. Dyson S: Unpublished data, 2002-2008.

20. MacLeay J, Valberg S, Sorum S, et al: Heritability of recurrent exertional rhabdomyolysis in thoroughbred horses, *Am J Vet Res* 60:250, 1999.

21. Morris E, Seeherman H, O'Callaghan M, et al: Scintigraphic identification of skeletal muscle damage in horses 24 hours after strenuous exercise, *Equine Vet J* 23:347, 1991.

22. Ross M, Maxson A, Stacy V, et al: First-pass radionuclide angiography in the diagnosis of aortoiliac thromboembolism in a horse, *Vet Radiol Ultrasound* 38:226, 1997.

23. Valentine B, Hintz H, Freels K, et al: Dietary control of exertional rhabdomyolysis in horses, *J Am Vet Med Assoc* 2:1588, 1998.

24. Harris P, Gray J: The use of the urinary fractional electrolyte excretion test to assess electrolyte status in the horse, *Equine Vet J* 4:162, 1992.

25. Harris P: Equine rhabdomyolysis syndrome in horses. In Robinson N, Wilson MR, eds: *Current therapy in equine medicine*, ed 4, Philadelphia, 1997, Saunders.

26. Haussler K, Stover S, Willits N: Pathologic changes in the lumbosacral vertebrae and pelvis in thoroughbred racehorses, *Am J Vet Res* 60:143, 1999.

27. Dalin G, Jeffcott L: Sacroiliac joint of the horse. I. Gross morphology, *Anat Histol Embryol* 15:80, 1986.

28. Jeffcott L, Dalin G, Ekman S, et al: Sacroiliac lesions as a cause of poor performance in competitive horses, *Equine Vet J* 17:111, 1985.

29. Haussler K: Osseous spinal pathology, *Vet Clin North Am Equine Pract* 15:103, 1999.

30. Rooney J: Sacroiliac luxation, *Mod Vet Pract* 60:45, 1979.

31. Tucker R, Schneider R, Sondhof A, et al: Bone scintigraphy in the diagnosis of sacroiliac injury in twelve horses, *Equine Vet J* 30:390, 1998.

32. Dyson S, Murray R, Brach M, et al: The sacroiliac joints: evaluation using nuclear scintigraphy. Part II. Lame horses, *Equine Vet J* 35:233, 2003.

33. Gorgas D, Kircher P, Doher M, et al: Radiographic technique and anatomy of the equine sacroiliac joint, *Vet Radiol Ultrasound* 48:501, 2007.

34. Reef V: Musculoskeletal ultrasonography. In *Equine diagnostic ultrasound*, Philadelphia, 1998, Saunders.

35. Denoix J-M: Ultrasonographic evaluation of back lesions, *Vet Clin North Am Equine Pract* 15:131, 1999.

36. Nagy A, Dyson S, Barr A: Ultrasonographic findings in the lumbosacral joint of 43 horses with no clinical signs of back pain or hindlimb lameness, *Vet Radiol Ultrasound* (In press.)

37. Cousty M, David F, Rossier Y, et al: Réalisation des injections échoguidées de la région sacroilaiaque, *Prat Vét Équine* 40:151, 2008.

38. Seignour M, Jacquet S, Denoix J-M: Infiltrations échoguidées des articulations synoviales intervertébrales épaxiales thoraciques et lombaires, *Prat Vét Équine* 40:149, 2008.

39. Dyson S, Worth L: Aortoiliacofemoral thrombosis. In Robinson N, Wilson MR, eds: *Current therapy in equine medicine*, ed 4, Philadelphia, 1997, Saunders.

40. Reef V, Roby K, Richardson D, et al: Use of ultrasonography for the detection of aortic-iliac thrombosis in horses, *J Am Vet Med Assoc* 190:286, 1987.

41. Warmerdam E: Ultrasonography of the femoral artery in six normal horses and three horses with thrombosis, *Vet Radiol Ultrasound* 39:137, 1998.

42. Raisis A: Personal communication, 2000.

43. Boswell J, Marr C, Cauvin E, et al: The use of scintigraphy in the diagnosis of aorto-iliac thrombosis in a horse, *Equine Vet J* 31:537, 1999.

44. Brama P, Rijkenhuizen A, Swieten H, et al: Thrombosis of the aorta and the caudal arteries in the horse: additional diagnostics and a new surgical treatment, *Vet Q* 18(Suppl 2):S85, 1996.

45. Rijkenhuizen A, Sinclair D, Jahn W: Surgical thrombectomy in horses with aortoiliac thrombosis: 17 cases, *Equine Vet J* 41:74, 2009.
46. Nixon A, Adams R, Teigland M: Subchondral cystic lesions (osteochondrosis) of the femoral heads in a horse, *J Am Vet Med Assoc* 192:360, 1988.
47. Brenner S, Whitcomb M: How to diagnose equine coxofemoral joint subluxation with diagnostic ultrasonography, *Proc Am Assoc Equine Pract* 53:433, 2007.

CHAPTER 51   Diagnosis and Management of Sacroiliac Joint Injuries

1. Jeffcott LB: Back problems in the horse—a method of clinical examination, *In Practice* 1:4, 1979.
2. Getty R: Equine osteology. In Getty R, ed: *Sisson and Grossman's the anatomy of the domestic animals*, ed 5, Philadelphia, 1975, Saunders.
3. Dalin G, Jeffcott LB: Sacroiliac joint of the horse. 2. Morphometric features, *Anat Histol Embryol* 15:97, 1986.
4. Jeffcott LB, Dalin G, Ekman S, et al: Sacroiliac lesions as a cause of chronic poor performance in competitive horses, *Equine Vet J* 17:111, 1985.
5. Ekman S, Dalin G, Olsson SE, et al: Sacroiliac joint of the horse. 3. Histological appearance, *Anat Histol Embryol* 15:108, 1986.
6. Degueurce C, Chateau H, Denoix JM: In vitro assessment of movements of the sacroiliac joint in the horse, *Equine Vet J* 36:694, 2004.
7. Goff LM, Jasiewicz J, Jeffcott LB, et al: Movement between the equine ilium and sacrum: in vivo and in vitro studies, *Equine Vet J Suppl* 36:457, 2006.
8. Haussler KK, McGilvray KC, Ayturk UM, et al: Deformation of the equine pelvis in response to in-vitro three-dimensional sacroiliac joint loading, *Equine Vet J* 41:207, 2009.
9. Denoix J-M: Ligament injuries of the axial skeleton in the horse: supraspinal and sacroiliac desmopathies. In Rantanen NW, Hauser ML, eds: *First Annual Dubai International Equine Symposium*, Dubai, UAE, 1996, Matthew R. Rantanen Design.
10. Engeli E, Yeager AE, Erb HN, et al: Ultrasonographic technique and normal anatomic features of the sacroiliac region in horses, *Vet Radiol Ultrasound* 47:391, 2006.
11. Jeffcott LB: Disorders of the thoracolumbar spine of the horse—a survey of 443 cases, *Equine Vet J* 12:197, 1980.
12. Jeffcott LB: Pelvic lameness in the horse, *Equine Pract* 4:21, 1982.
13. Adams OR: Subluxation of the sacroiliac joint in horses, *Proc Am Assoc Equine Pract* 15:191, 1969.
14. Rooney JR: Sacroiliac arthrosis and "stifle lameness," *Mod Vet Pract* 58:138, 1977.
15. Jeffcott LB: Radiographic appearance of equine lumbosacral and pelvic abnormalities by linear tomography, *Vet Radiol* 24:201, 1983.
16. Dalin G, Magnusson L-E, Thafvelin BC: Retrospective study of hindquarter asymmetry in Standardbred trotters and its correlation with performance, *Equine Vet J* 17:292, 1985.
17. Haussler KK, Stover SM, Willits NH: Pathology of the lumbosacral spine and pelvis in Thoroughbred racehorses, *Am J Vet Res* 60:143, 1999.
18. Tucker RL, Schneider RK, Sondhof AH, et al: Bone scintigraphy in the diagnosis of sacroiliac injury in twelve horses, *Equine Vet J* 30:390, 1998.
19. Dyson SJ: Sacroiliac pain: is definitive diagnosis possible? Proceedings of the 7th Congress on Equine Medicine and Surgery, Geneva, Switzerland, 2001.
20. Stecher RM, Goss LJ: Ankylosing lesions of the spine, *J Am Vet Med Assoc* 138:248, 1961.
21. Rooney JR: The cause and prevention of sacroiliac arthrosis in the Standardbred horse: a theoretical study, *Can Vet J* 22:356, 1981.
22. Gillis C: Spinal ligament pathology, *Vet Clin North Am Equine Pract* 15:97, 1999.
23. Rooney JR: Sacroiliac luxation in the horse, *Equine Vet J* 1:287, 1969.
24. Rooney JR: Sacroiliac luxation, *Mod Vet Pract* 60:45, 1979.
25. Hendrickson DA: Subluxation of the sacroiliac joint (sacroiliac strain). In Stashak TS, eds: *Adams' lameness in horses*, ed 5, Philadelphia, 2002, Lippincott Williams & Wilkins.
26. Haussler KK: Anatomy of the thoracolumbar vertebral region, *Vet Clin North Am Equine Pract* 15:13, 1999.
27. Pilsworth RC, Shepherd MC, Herinckx BM, et al: Fracture of the wing of the ilium, adjacent to the sacroiliac joint, in thoroughbred racehorses, *Equine Vet J* 26:94, 1994.
28. Dyson S, Murray R: Pain associated with the sacroiliac joint region: a clinical study of 74 horses, *Equine Vet J* 35:240, 2003.
29. Jeffcott LB: Diseases of the lumbosacral region. In Colahan PT, Mayhew IG, Merritt AM, et al, eds: *Equine medicine and surgery*, ed 5, St. Louis, 1999, Mosby.
30. Goff LM, Jeffcott LB, Jasiewicz J, et al: Structural and biomechanical aspects of equine sacroiliac joint function and their relationship to clinical disease, *Vet J* 176:281, 2008.
31. Cassidy JD, Townsend HGG: Sacroiliac joint strain as a cause of back and leg pain in man—implications for the horse, *Proc Am Assoc Equine Pract* 31:317, 1985.
32. Marks D: Back pain. In Robinson NE, ed: *Current therapy in equine medicine*, 4th ed, Philadelphia, 1997, Saunders.
33. Varcoe-Cocks K, Sagar KN, Jeffcott LB, et al: Pressure algometry to quantify muscle pain in racehorses with suspected sacroiliac dysfunction, *Equine Vet J* 38:558, 2006.
34. Engeli E, Haussler KK, Erb HN: Development and validation of a periarticular injection technique of the sacroiliac joint in horses, *Equine Vet J* 36:324, 2004.
35. Cousty M, Rossier Y, David F: Ultrasound-guided periarticular injections of the sacroiliac region in horses: a cadaveric study, *Equine Vet J* 40:160, 2008.
36. Shepherd MC, Pilsworth RC: The use of ultrasound in the diagnosis of pelvic fractures, *Equine Vet Educ* 6:223, 1994.
37. Reef VB: Diagnosis of pelvic fractures in horses using ultrasonography, *Vet Radiol Ultrasound* 33:121, 1992.
38. Tomlinson JE, Sage AM, Turner TA: Ultrasonographic abnormalities detected in the sacroiliac area in twenty cases of upper hindlimb lameness, *Equine Vet J* 35:48, 2003.
39. Kersten AA, Edinger J: Ultrasonographic examination of the equine sacroiliac region, *Equine Vet J* 36:602, 2004.
40. Butler JA, Colles CM, Dyson SJ, et al: The pelvis and femur. In *Clinical radiology of the horse*, Oxford, 2008, Wiley-Blackwell.
41. Gorgas D, Kircher P, Doherr MG, et al: Radiographic technique and anatomy of the equine sacroiliac region, *Vet Radiol Ultrasound* 48:501, 2007.
42. Erichsen C, Eksell P, Widstrom C, et al: Scintigraphy of the sacroiliac joint region in asymptomatic riding horses: scintigraphic appearance and evaluation of method, *Vet Radiol Ultrasound* 44:699, 2003.
43. Erichsen C, Berger M, Eksell P: The scintigraphic anatomy of the equine sacroiliac joint, *Vet Radiol Ultrasound* 43:287, 2002.
44. Dyson S, Murray R, Branch M, et al: The sacroiliac joints: evaluation using nuclear scintigraphy. Part 1: The normal horse, *Equine Vet J* 35:226, 2003.
45. Hornof WJ, Stover SM, Koblik PD, et al: Oblique views of the ilium and the scintigraphic appearance of stress fractures of the ilium, *Equine Vet J* 28:355, 1996.
46. Haussler KK, Stover SM: Stress fractures of the vertebral lamina and pelvis in Thoroughbred racehorses, *Equine Vet J* 30:374, 1998.
47. Davenport-Goodall CL, Ross MW: Scintigraphic abnormalities of the pelvic region in horses examined because of lameness or poor performance: 128 cases (1993-2000), *J Am Vet Med Assoc* 224:88, 2004.
48. Turner TA: Thermography as an aid in the localization of upper hindlimb lameness, *Pferdeheilkunde* 12:632, 1996.
49. Dyson S, Murray R, Branch M, et al: The sacroiliac joints: evaluation using nuclear scintigraphy. Part 2: Lame horses, *Equine Vet J* 35:233, 2003.
50. Steckel RR, Kraus-Hansen AE, Fackelman GE, et al: Scintigraphic diagnosis of thoracolumbar spinal disease in horses: a review of 50 cases, *Proc Am Assoc Equine Pract* 37:583, 1991.

CHAPTER 52   Thoracolumbar Spine

1. Robert C, Audigié F, Valette JP, et al: Effects of treadmill speed on the mechanics of the back in the trotting saddle horse, *Equine Vet J Suppl* 33:154, 2001.
2. Denoix J-M, Audigié F: The neck and back. In Back W, Clayton H, eds: *Equine locomotion*, Philadelphia, 2001, Saunders.
3. Jeffcott LB: The diagnosis of diseases of the horse back, *Equine Vet J* 7:69, 1975.
4. Jeffcott LB: Diagnosis of back problems in the horse, *Comp Cont Educ Pract Vet* 3:S134, 1981.
5. Denoix J-M: Approche sémiologique des régions lombo-sacrale et sacro-iliaque chez le cheval, *Prat Vét Equine* 24:23, 1992.

6. Girodroux M, Dyson S, Murray R: Osteoarthritis of the thoracolumbar synovial intervertebral articulations: clinical and radiographic features in 77 horses with poor performance and back pain, *Equine Vet J* 41:131, 2009.
7. Turner T, Waldsmith J, Wilson J: How to assess saddle fit in the horse, *Proc Am Assoc Equine Pract* 50.196, 2004.
8. Haussler K, Erb H: Pressure algometry for the detection of induced back pain in horses: a preliminary study, *Equine Vet J* 37:76, 2006.
9. Haussler K, Erb H: Mechanical nociceptive thresholds in the axial skeleton of horses, *Equine Vet J* 37:70, 2006.
10. Audigié F, Pourcelot P, Degueurce C, et al: Kinematics of the equine back: flexion-extension movements in sound trotting horses, *Equine Vet J Suppl* 30:210, 1999.
11. Pourcelot P, Audigié F, Degueurce C, et al: Kinematics of the equine back: a method to study the thoracolumbar flexion-extension movements at the trot, *Vet Res* 29:519, 1998.
12. Faber MJ: Kinematic of the equine back during locomotion, PhD thesis, Utrecht, Netherlands, 2001, Utrecht University.
13. Denoix JM, Audigié F, Robert C, et al: Alteration of locomotion in horses with vertebral lesions. In Lindner A, ed: *Proceedings of the Conference on Equine Sports Medicine and Science: the elite show jumper*, Essen, 2000, Arbeitsguippe Pferd.
14. Wennerstrand J, Johnston C, Roethlisberger-Holm K, et al: Kinematic evaluation of the back in the sport horse with back pain, *Equine Vet J* 36:707, 2004.
15. Schlacher C, Peham C, Licka T, et al: Determination of stiffness of the equine spine, *Equine Vet J* 36:699, 2004.
16. Peham C, Schobesberger H: Influence of the load of a rider or of a region with increased stiffness of the equine back: a modelling study, *Equine Vet J* 36:703, 2004.
17. Denoix J-M: Lesions of the vertebral column in poor performance horses. Proceedings of the World Equine Veterinary Association Symposium, Paris, 1999.
18. Denoix J-M: Ligament injuries of the axial skeleton in the horse: supraspinal and sacroiliac desmopathies, Dubai International Equine Symposium, 1996.
19. Denoix J-M: Ultrasonographic evaluation of back lesions, *Vet Clin North Am Equine Pract* 15:131, 1999.
20. Reisinger R, Stanek C: Sonographische darstellbarkeit der intervertebralgelenke on der brust-und lendenwirbesaule des pferdes, *Pferdheilkunde* 21:219, 2005.
21. Denoix J-M, Audigié F, Coudry V: Review of diagnosis and treatment of lumbosacral pain in sport and racehorses, *Proc Am Assoc Equine Pract* 51:366, 2005.
22. Erichsen C, Eksell P, Widstrom C, et al: Scintigraphic evaluation of the thoracic spine in the asymptomatic riding horse, *Vet Radiol Ultrasound* 44:330, 2003.
23. Erichsen C, Eksell P, Holm K, et al: Relationship between scintigraphic and radiographic evaluations of spinous processes in the thoracolumbar spine in riding horses without clinical signs of back problems, *Equine Vet J* 36:458, 2004.
24. Steckel RS, Kraus-Hansen AE, Fackelman GE, et al: Scintigraphic diagnosis of thoracolumbar spinal disease in horses: a review of 50 cases, *Proc Am Assoc Equine Pract* 37:583, 1991.
25. Gillen A, Dyson S, Murray R: Nuclear scintigraphic assessment of the thoracolumbar synovial intervertebral articulations, *Equine Vet J* 41:534, 2009.
26. Meehan L, Dyson S, Murray R: Radiographic and scintigraphic evaluation of spondylosis in the equine thoracolumbar spine, *Equine Vet J* 41:800, 2009.
27. Tunley B, Henson F: Reliability and repeatability of thermographic examination and normal thermographic imaging of the thoracolumbar region in the horse, *Equine Vet J* 35:306, 2004.
28. Jeffcott LB: Disorders of the thoracolumbar spine of the horse—a survey of 443 cases, *Equine Vet J* 12:197, 1980.
29. Jeffcott LB: Conditions causing thoracolumbar pain and dysfunction in horses, *Proc Am Assoc Equine Pract* 32:285, 1986.
30. Henson F, Lamas M, Knezevic S, et al: Ultrasonographic evaluation of the supraspinous ligament in a series of ridden and unridden horses and horses with unrelated back pathology, *BMC Vet Res* 3:3, 2007.
31. Alward A, Pease A, James S: Thoracic discospondylitis with associated epaxial muscle atrophy in a Quarterhorse, *Equine Vet Educ* 19:67, 2007.
32. Denoix J-M: Discovertebral pathology in horses, *Equine Vet Educ* 19:72, 2007.
33. Haussler K, Stover S: Stress fractures of the vertebral lamina and pelvis in thoroughbred race horses, *Equine Vet J* 30:374, 1998.
34. Huisheng X, Colahan P, Ott E: Evaluation of electroacupuncture treatment of horses with signs of chronic thoracolumbar pain, *J Am Vet Med Assoc* 227:281, 2005.
35. Denoix J-M: *Physical therapy and massage for the horse*, London, 1996, Manson Publishing.
36. Denoix J-M: Kinematics of the thoracolumbar spine of the horse during dorsoventral movements: a preliminary report. In Gillespie JR, Robinson NE, eds: *Equine exercise physiology*, ed 2, Davis, Calif, 1987, ICEEP Publications.
37. Denoix JM: Spinal biomechanics and functional anatomy, *Vet Clin North Am Equine Pract* 15:27, 1999.
38. Coudry V, Thibaud D, Riccio B, et al: Efficacy of tiludronate in the treatment of horses with signs of pain associated with osteoarthritic lesions of the thoracolumbar vertebral column, *Am J Vet Res* 68:329, 2007.
39. Lauk H, Kreling I: Surgical treatment of kissing spines syndrome—50 cases. II. Results, *Pferdheilkunde* 14:123, 1998.
40. Walmsley J, Petterson A, Winberg F, et al: Impingement of the dorsal spinous processes in two hundred and fifteen horses: case selection, surgical technique and results, *Equine Vet J* 34:23, 2002.
41. Perkins J, Schumacher J, Kelly G, et al: Subtotal ostectomy of dorsal spinous processes performed in 9 standing horses, *Vet Surg* 34:625, 2005.
42. Desbrosse F, Perrin R, Launois T, et al: Endoscopic resection of dorsal spinous processes and interspinous ligament in 10 horses, *Vet Surg* 36:149, 2007.

CHAPTER 53   The Cervical Spine and Soft Tissues of the Neck

1. Panzer R: Traditional Chinese veterinary medical diagnostics. In Colahan P, Mayhew I, Merritt A, et al, eds: *Equine medicine and surgery*, ed 5, St Louis, 1999, Mosby.
2. Ricardi G, Dyson S: Forelimb lameness associated with radiographic abnormalities of the cervical vertebrae, *Equine Vet J* 25:422, 1993.
3. Butler J, Colles C, Dyson S, et al: The spine. In *Clinical radiology of the horse*, ed 3, Oxford, 2008, Wiley-Blackwell.
4. Whitwell K, Dyson S: Interpreting radiographs. VIII. Equine cervical vertebrae, *Equine Vet J* 19:8, 1987.
5. Down S, Henson F: A radiographic retrospective study of the caudal cervical articular process joints in the horse, *Equine Vet J* 41: 518, 2009.
6. Gardner S, Reef V, Spencer P: Ultrasonographic evaluation of horses with thrombophlebitis of the jugular vein: 46 cases (1985-1988), *J Am Vet Med Assoc* 199:370, 1991.
7. Berg L, Nielsen J, Thoefner M, et al: Ultrasonography of the equine cervical vertebrae: a descriptive study in eight horses, *Equine Vet J* 35:647, 2003.
8. Nielsen J, Berg L, Thoefner M, et al: Accuracy of ultrasound-guided intra-articular injection of cervical facet joints in horses: a cadaveric study, *Equine Vet J* 35:657, 2003.
9. Moore B, Holbrook T, Stefanacci J, et al: Contrast-enhanced computed tomography and myelography in six horses with cervical stenotic myelopathy, *Equine Vet J* 24:197, 1992.
10. Barnes H, Tucker R, Grant B, et al: Lag screw stabilization of a cervical vertebral fracture by use of computed tomography in a horse, *J Am Vet Med Assoc* 206:221, 1995.
11. Tietje S: The value of computed tomography in horses (243 cases). I. Diseases of the head and neck, *Prakt Tierarzt* 77:1099, 1996.
12. Wijnberg I, Back W, de Jong M, et al: The role of electromyography in clinical diagnosis of neuromuscular locomotor problems in the horse, *Equine Vet J* 36:718, 2004.
13. Mayhew I: Congenital occipitoatlantal malformation in the horse, *Equine Vet J* 10:103, 1978.
14. Wilson W, Hughes S, Ghoshal N, et al: Occipitoatlantal malformation in two non-Arabian horses, *J Am Vet Med Assoc* 187:36, 1985.
15. Watson A, Mayhew I: Familial congenital occipitoatlantal malformation (OAAM) in the Arabian horse, *Spine* 11:334, 1986.
16. Funk K, Erikson E: A case of atlanto-axial subluxation in a horse, *Can Vet J* 9:120, 1968.
17. Guffy M, Coffman J, Strafuss A: Atlantoaxial luxation in a foal, *J Am Vet Med Assoc* 155:754, 1969.
18. Owen R, Smith-Maxie L: Repair of fractured dens of the atlas in a foal, *J Am Vet Med Assoc* 173:854, 1978.
19. McCoy D, Shires P, Beadle R: Ventral approach for stabilization of atlantoaxial subluxation secondary to odontoid

fracture in a foal, *J Am Vet Med Assoc* 185:545, 1984.

20. Mayhew I, Whitlock R, de Lahunta A: Spinal cord disease in the horse, *Cornell Vet* 6(Suppl):13, 1978.

21. Slone D, Bergfeld W, Walker T: Surgical decompression for traumatic atlantoaxial subluxation in a weanling filly, *J Am Vet Med Assoc* 174:1234, 1979.

22. Vos N, Pollock P, Harty M, et al: Fractures of the cervical odontoid in four horses and one pony, *Vet Rec* 162:116, 2008.

23. Mayhew J: Vertebral and paravertebral problems. In: *Large animal neurology*, ed 2, Oxford, 2009, Wiley-Blackwell.

24. Dyson S: The cervical spine and soft tissues of the neck. In Ross M, Dyson S, eds: *Diagnosis and management of lameness in the horse*, ed 1, St Louis, 2003, Elsevier.

25. Nowak M, Huskamp B: Uber einige spezielle befunde bei erkrankungen der halswirbelsaule des pferdes, *Pferdeheilkunde* 2:95, 1989.

26. Nowak M: Die insertiondesmopathie des nackenstrangursprungs beim pferd. Diagnostik, differentialdiagnostik. Proceedings of the 7th Congress on Equine Medicine and Surgery, Geneva, 2001.

27. McClure S, Weinberger T: Extracorporeal shock wave therapy: clinical applications and regulation, *Clin Tech Equine Pract* 2:358, 2003.

28. Birmingham A, Reed S, Mattoon J, Saville W: Qualitative assessment of corticosteroid cervical articular facet injection in symptomatic horses, *Equine Vet Educ* 22:77, 2010.

29. Marks D: Cervical nerve root compression in a horse, treated by epidural injection of corticosteroid, *J Equine Vet Sci* 19:399, 1999.

30. Butler J, Colles C, Dyson S, et al: Miscellaneous techniques. In *Clinical radiology of the horse*, ed 3, Oxford, 2008, Wiley-Blackwell.

31. Bullwein A, Hanichen T: Age related changes in the intervertebral disks of the cervical vertebral column in the horse, *Tierarztl Prax* 17:73, 1989.

32. Adams S, Steckel R, Blevins W: Diskospondylitis in five horses, *J Am Vet Med Assoc* 186:270, 1985.

33. Sweers L, Carstend A: Imaging features of discospondylosis in two horses, *Vet Radiol Ultrasound* 47:159, 2006.

34. MacAllister C, Qualls C, Tyler R, et al: Multiple myeloma in a horse, *J Am Vet Med Assoc* 191:337, 1987.

35. Dyson S: Problems associated with the neck: neck pain, stiffness or abnormal posture and forelimb gait abnormalities. In Robinson N, Wilson MR, eds: *Current therapy in equine medicine*, ed 4, Philadelphia, 1997, Saunders.

36. Ahern T: Cervical vertebral mobilisation under anesthesia (CVMUA): a physical therapy for the treatment of cervicospinal pain and stiffness, *J Equine Vet Sci* 14:540, 1994.

CHAPTER 54 Pathogenesis of Osteochondrosis

1. Ytrehus B, Carlson CS, Ekman S: Etiology and pathogenesis of osteochondrosis, *Vet Pathol* 44:429, 2007.

2. Wright I, Minshall G: Diagnosis and treatment of equine osteochondrosis, *Equine Pract* 27:302, 2005.

3. Olsson S-E, Reiland S: The nature of osteochondrosis in animals, *Acta Radiol* 358(Suppl):299, 1978.

4. Poulos P: Radiologic manifestations of developmental problems. In McIlwraith CE, ed: *AQHA developmental orthopedic disease symposium*, Amarillo, Texas, 1986, American Quarter Horse Association.

5. McIlwraith CW: What is developmental orthopedic disease, osteochondrosis, osteochondritis, metabolic bone disease? *Proc Am Assoc Equine Pract* 39:35, 1993.

6. Jeffcott LB: Problems and pointers in equine osteochondrosis, *Equine Vet J Suppl* 16:1, 1993.

7. Brighton CT: Structure and function of the growth plate, *Clin Orthop* 136:22, 1978.

8. Jeffcott LB: Osteochondrosis in the horse—searching for the key to pathogenesis, *Equine Vet J* 23:331, 1991.

9. Strömberg B, Rejnö S: Osteochondrosis in the horse. I. A clinical and radiologic investigation of osteochondritis dissecans of the knee and hock joint, *Acta Radiol* 358(Suppl):139, 1978.

10. Strömberg B: A review of the salient features of osteochondrosis in the horse, *Equine Vet J* 11:211, 1979.

11. Pool R: Pathologic manifestations of osteochondrosis. In McIlwraith CE, ed: *AQHA developmental orthopedic disease symposium*, Amarillo, Texas, 1986, American Quarter Horse Association.

12. Hurtig MB, Pool RR: Pathogenesis of equine osteochondrosis. In McIlwraith CW, Trotter GW, eds: *Joint disease in the horse*, Philadelphia, 1996, Saunders.

13. Summary. In McIlwraith CE, ed: *AQHA developmental orthopedic disease symposium*, Amarillo, Texas, 1986, American Quarter Horse Association.

14. Pool RR: Difficulties in definition of equine osteochondrosis: differentiation of developmental and acquired lesions, *Equine Vet J Suppl* 16:5, 1993.

15. Olstad K, Ytrehus B, Ekman S, et al: Early lesions of osteochondrosis in the distal tibia of foals, *J Orthop Res* 25:1094, 2007.

16. Rejnö S, Strömberg B: Osteochondrosis in the horse. II. Pathology, *Acta Radiol* 358(Suppl):153, 1978.

17. Dik KJ, Enzerink EE, van Weeren PR: Radiographic development of osteochondral abnormalities in the hock and stifle of Dutch Warmblood foals, from age 1 to 11 months, *Equine Vet J Suppl* 31:9, 1999.

18. Carlson CS, Cullins LD, Meuten DJ: Osteochondrosis of the articular-epiphyseal cartilage complex in young horses: evidence for a defect in cartilage canal blood supply, *Vet Pathol* 32:641, 1995.

19. Carlsten J, Sandgren B, Dalin G: Development of osteochondrosis in the tarsocrural joint and osteochondral fragments in the fetlock joints of standardbred trotters. I. A radiological survey, *Equine Vet J Suppl* 16:42, 1993.

20. Wittwer C, Hamann H, Rosenberger E, et al: Prevalence of osteochondrosis in the limb joints of South German Coldblood horses, *J Vet Med A Physiol Pathol Clin Med* 53:531, 2006.

21. van Weeren PR, Knaap J, Firth EC: Influence of liver copper status of mare and newborn foal on the development of osteochondrotic lesions, *Equine Vet J* 35:67, 2003.

22. Arnan P: [Radiographic examination of osteochondrosis in the fetlock, hock and stifle joint in two-year-old Warmblood horses: a follow-up study], doctoral thesis, Berlin, Germany, 2005, Freie Universitat Berlin.

23. van Weeren PR, Barneveld A: The effect of exercise on the distribution and manifestation of osteochondrotic lesions in the Warmblood foal, *Equine Vet J Suppl* 31:16, 1999.

24. Henson FMD, Davies ME, Jeffcott LB: Equine dyschondroplasia (osteochondrosis)—histological findings and type VI collagen localization, *Vet J* 154:53, 1997.

25. Jeffcott LB, Henson FMD: Studies on growth cartilage in the horse and their application to aetiopathogenesis of dyschondroplasia (osteochondrosis), *Vet J* 156:177, 1998.

26. Savage CJ, McCarthy RN, Jeffcott LB: Effects of dietary energy and protein on induction of dyschondroplasia in foals, *Equine Vet J Suppl* 16:74, 1993.

27. Shingleton WD, Mackie EJ, Cawston TE, et al: Cartilage canals in equine articular/epiphyseal growth cartilage and a possible association with dyschondroplasia, *Equine Vet J* 29:360, 1997.

28. Whitton RC: Equine developmental osteochondral lesions: the role of biomechanics, *Vet J* 156:167, 1998.

29. Olstad K, Ytrehus B, Ekman S, et al: Epiphyseal cartilage canal blood supply to the tarsus of foals and relationship to osteochondrosis, *Equine Vet J* 40:30, 2008.

30. Glade MJ: The role of endocrine factors in equine developmental orthopedic disease, *Proc Am Assoc Equine Pract* 33:171, 1987.

31. Kolwaczyk DF, Gunson DE, Shoop CR, et al: The effects of natural exposure to high levels of zinc and cadmium in the immature pony as a function of age, *Environ Res* 40:285, 1986.

32. Knight DA, Weisbrode SE, Schmall LM, et al: The effects of copper supplementation on the prevalence of cartilage lesions in foals, *Equine Vet J* 22:426, 1990.

33. Philipsson J, Andréasson E, Sandgren B, et al: Osteochondrosis in the tarsocrural joint and osteochondral fragments in the fetlock joints in standardbred trotters. II. Heritability, *Equine Vet J Suppl* 16:38, 1993.

34. Bramlage LR: Identification, examination, and treatment of physitis in the foal, *Proc Am Assoc Equine Pract* 39:57, 1993.

35. Savage CJ, McCarthy RN, Jeffcott LB: Effects of dietary phosphorus and calcium on induction of dyschondroplasia in foals, *Equine Vet J Suppl* 16:80, 1993.

36. Gee EK, Firth EC, Morel PC, et al: Enlargements of the distal third metacarpus and metatarsus in Thoroughbred foals at pasture from birth to 160 days of age, *N Z Vet J* 53:438, 2005.

37. Rooney JR: Osteochondrosis in the horse, *Mod Vet Pract* 56:41, 1975.

38. Trotter GW, McIlwraith CW: Osteochondritis dissecans and subchondral cystic lesions and their relationship to osteochondrosis in the horse, *Equine Vet Sci* 1:157, 1981.

39. Bramlage LR: Osteochondrosis related bone cysts, *Proc Am Assoc Equine Pract* 39:83, 1993.

40. Jeffcott LB, Kold SE, Melsen F: Aspects of the pathology of stifle bone cysts in the horse, *Equine Vet J* 15:304, 1983.

41. Ray CS, Baxter GM, McIlwraith CW, et al: Development of subchondral cystic lesions after articular cartilage and subchondral bone damage in young horses, *Equine Vet J* 28:225, 1996.

42. Kold SE, Hickman J, Melsen F: An experimental study of the healing process of equine chondral and osteochondral defects, *Equine Vet J* 18:18, 1986.

43. McIwraith CW: Subchondral bone cysts in the horse: aetiology, diagnosis and treatment options, *Equine Vet Educ* 10:313, 1998.

44. Hurtig M, Green SLK, Dobson J, et al: Correlative study of defective cartilage and bone growth in foals fed a low-copper diet, *Equine Vet J Suppl* 16:66, 1993.

45. van Weeren PR: Etiology, diagnosis, and treatment of OC(D), *Clin Tech Equine Pract* 5:248, 2006.

46. Nguyen NH, McPhee CP: Genetic parameters and responses of performance and body composition traits in pigs selected for high and low growth rate on a fixed ration over a set time, *Genet Sel Evol* 37:199, 2005.

47. Donabédian M, Fleurance G, Perona G, et al: Effect of fast vs moderate growth rate related to nutrient intake on developmental orthopaedic disease in the horse, *Anim Res* 55:471, 2006.

48. Norton SA, Zavy MT, Maxwell CV, et al: Insulin, growth hormone, glucose, and fatty acids in gilts selected for rapid vs slow growth rate, *Am J Physiol* 257:E554, 1989.

49. Olstad K, Ytrehus B, Ekman S, et al: Epiphyseal cartilage canal blood supply to the distal femur of foals, *Equine Vet J* 40:433, 2008.

50. Fortier LA, Kornatowski MA, Mohammed HO, et al: Age-related changes in serum insulin-like growth factor–I, insulin-like growth factor–I binding protein–3 and articular cartilage structure in Thoroughbred horses, *Equine Vet J* 37:37, 2005.

51. Olstad K, Cnudde V, Masschaele B, et al: Micro-computed tomography of early lesions of osteochondrosis in the tarsus of foals, *Bone* 43:574, 2008.

52. Gee E, Davies M, Firth E, et al: Osteochondrosis and copper: histology of articular cartilage from foals out of copper supplemented and non-supplemented dams, *Vet J* 173:109, 2007.

53. Sandgren B, Dalin G, Carlsten J, et al: Development of osteochondrosis in the tarsocrural joint and osteochondral fragments in the fetlock joints of standardbred trotters. II. Body measurements and clinical findings, *Equine Vet J Suppl* 16:48, 1993.

54. Gee EK, Firth EC, Morel PC, et al: Articular/epiphyseal osteochondrosis in Thoroughbred foals at 5 months of age: influences of growth of the foal and prenatal copper supplementation of the dam, *N Z Vet J* 53:448, 2005.

55. Vervuert I, Borchers A, Granel M, et al: Estimation of growth rates in warmblood foals and the incidence of osteochondrosis, *Pferdeheilkunde* 21:129, 2005.

56. van Weeren PR, Sloet van Oldruitenborgh-Oosterbaan MM, Barneveld A: The influence of birth weight, rate of weight gain and final achieved height and sex on the development of osteochondrotic lesions in a population of genetically predisposed Warmblood foals, *Equine Vet J Suppl* 31:26, 1999.

57. Pagan JD: The relationship between glycemic response and the incidence of OCD in thoroughbred weanlings: a field study, *Advances in equine nutrition*, ed 3, Nottingham, 2005, Nottingham University Press, p 319.

58. National Research Council: *Nutrient requirements of horses*, ed 5, Washington, DC, 1989, National Academies Press.

59. National Research Council: *Nutrient requirements of horses*, ed 4, Washington, DC, 1978, National Academy of Sciences, National Research Council.

60. Glade MJ, Belling TH: Growth plate cartilage metabolism, morphology and biochemical composition in over- and underfed horses, *Growth* 48:473, 1984.

61. Glade MJ, Reimers TJ: Effects of dietary energy supply on serum thyroxine, triiodothyronine and insulin concentrations in young horses, *J Endocrinol* 104:93, 1985.

62. Quarto R, Campanile G, Cancedda R, et al: Thyroid hormone, insulin, and glucocorticoids are sufficient to support chondrocyte differentiation to hypertrophy: a serum-free analysis, *J Cell Biol* 119:989, 1992.

63. Ballock RT, Reddi AH: Thyroxine is the serum factor that regulates morphogenesis of columnar cartilage from isolated chondrocytes in chemically defined medium, *J Cell Biol* 126:1311, 1994.

64. Henson FMD, Davenport C, Butler L, et al: Effects of insulin and insulin-like growth factors I and II on the growth of equine fetal and neonatal chondrocytes, *Equine Vet J* 29:441, 1997.

65. Ralston SL: Hyperglycaemia/hyperinsulinaemia after feeding a meal of grain to young horses with osteochondritis dissecans (OCD) lesions, *Pferdeheilkunde* 12:320, 1996.

66. Staniar WB, Kronfeld DS, Akers RM, et al: Insulin-like growth factor I in growing thoroughbreds, *J Anim Physiol Anim Nutr (Berl)* 91:390, 2007.

67. Werner H, Weinstein D, Bentov I: Similarities and differences between insulin and IGF-I: structures, receptors, and signalling pathways, *Arch Physiol Biochem* 114:17, 2008.

68. Yakar S, Rosen CJ, Beamer WG, et al: Circulating levels of IGF-1 directly regulate bone growth and density, *J Clin Invest* 110:771, 2002.

69. Sloet van Oldruitenborgh-Oosterbaan MM, Mol JA, Barneveld A: Hormones, growth factors and other plasma variables in relation to osteochondrosis, *Equine Vet J Suppl* 31:45, 1999.

70. Bridges CH, Harris ED: Experimentally induced cartilaginous fractures (osteochondritis dissecans) in foals fed low-copper diets, *J Am Vet Med Assoc* 193:215, 1988.

71. Bridges CH, Womack JE, Harris ED, et al: Considerations of copper metabolism of osteochondrosis of suckling foals, *J Am Vet Med Assoc* 185:173, 1984.

72. Bridges CH, Moffitt PG: Influence of variable content of dietary zinc on copper metabolism of weanling foals, *Am J Vet Res* 51:275, 1990.

73. Pearce SG, Firth EC, Grace ND, et al: Effect of copper supplementation on the evidence of developmental orthopaedic disease in pasture-fed New Zealand Thoroughbreds, *Equine Vet J* 30:211, 1998.

74. Schougaard H, Falk Ronne J, Phillipson J: A radiographic survey of tibiotarsal osteochondrosis in a selected population of trotting horses in Denmark and its possible genetic significance, *Equine Vet J* 22:288, 1990.

75. Wittwer C, Hamann H, Rosenberger E, et al: Genetic parameters for the prevalence of osteochondrosis in the limb joints of South German Coldblood horses, *J Anim Breed Genet* 124:302, 2007.

76. Grøndahl AM, Dolvik NI: Heritability estimations of osteochondrosis in the tibiotarsal joint and of bony fragments in the palmar/plantar portion of the metacarpo- and metatarsophalangeal joints of horses, *J Am Vet Med Assoc* 203:101, 1993.

77. Pieramati C, Pepe M, Silvestrelli M, et al: Heritability estimation of osteochondrosis dissecans in Maremmano horses, *Livestock Prod Sci* 79:249, 2003.

78. Dierks C, Löhring K, Lampe V, et al: Genome-wide search for markers associated with osteochondrosis in Hanoverian warmblood horses, *Mamm Genome* 18:739, 2007.

79. Wittwer C, Löhring K, Drögemüller C, et al: Mapping quantitative trait loci for osteochondrosis in fetlock and hock joints and palmar/plantar osseous fragments in fetlock joints of South German Coldblood horses, *Anim Genet* 38:350, 2007.

80. Wittwer C, Dierks C, Hamann H, et al: Associations between candidate gene markers at a quantitative trait locus on equine chromosome 4 responsible for osteochondrosis dissecans in fetlock joints of South German Coldblood horses, *J Hered* 99:125, 2008.

81. Philipsson J: Pathogenesis of osteochondrosis—genetic implications. In McIlwraith CW, Trotter GW, eds: *Joint disease in the horse*, Philadelphia, 1996, Saunders.

82. Williams RW: Expression genetics and the phenotype revolution, *Mamm Genome* 17:496, 2006.

83. Koenen EPC, Dik KJ, Knapp JH, et al: Evaluation of selection strategies against osteochondrosis for the Dutch Warmblood riding horse population. Proceedings of the 51st Annual Meeting of EAAP, The Hague, 2000.

84. Hoppe F: OC in Swedish horses: a radiological and epidemiological study with special reference to frequency and heredity, dissertation, Uppsala, Sweden,

1984, Swedish University of Agricultural Sciences.

85. Sandgren B, Dalin G, Carlsten J: Osteochondrosis in the tarsocrural joint and osteochondral fragments in the fetlock joints of standardbred trotters. I. Epidemiology, *Equine Vet J Suppl* 16:31, 1993.

86. Valentino LW, Lillich JD, Gaughan EM, et al: Radiographic prevalence of osteochondrosis in yearling feral horses, *Vet Comp Orthop Trauma* 12:151, 1999.

87. Bruin G, Creemers JJHM, Smolders EEA: Effect of exercise on osteochondrosis in the horse. In *Equine osteochondrosis in the '90s*, Cambridge, UK, 1992.

88. van den Hoogen BM, van den Lest CH, van Weeren PR, et al: Effect of exercise on the proteoglycan metabolism of articular cartilage in growing foals, *Equine Vet J Suppl* 31:62, 1999.

89. Barneveld A, van Weeren PR: Conclusions regarding the influence of exercise on the development of the equine musculoskeletal system with special reference to osteochondrosis, *Equine Vet J Suppl* 31:112, 1999.

90. McIlwraith CW: Inferences from referred clinical cases of osteochondritis dissecans, *Equine Vet J Suppl* 16:27, 1993.

91. Hernández-Vidal G, Jeffcott LB, Davies ME: Immunolocalization of cathepsin B in equine dyschondroplastic articular cartilage, *Vet J* 156:193, 1998.

92. Gläser KE, Davies ME, Jeffcott LB: Differential distribution of cathepsins B and L in articular cartilage during skeletal development in the horse, *Equine Vet J* 35:42, 2003.

93. Hernández-Vidal G, Valdes-Martinez A, Mora-Valdez F, et al: Immunolocalization of cathepsin B in chondrocytes and osteoclasts in equine dyschondroplasia (osteochondrosis), *Vet Mex* 33:395, 2002.

94. Al-Hizab F, Clegg PD, Thompson CC, et al: Microscopic localization of active gelatinases in equine osteochondritis dissecans (OCD) cartilage, *Osteoarthritis Cartilage* 10:653, 2002.

95. Laverty S, Okouneff S, Ionescu M, et al: Excessive degradation of type II collagen in articular cartilage in equine osteochondrosis, *J Orthop Res* 20:1282, 2002.

96. Billinghurst RC, Brama PA, van Weeren PR, et al: Evaluation of serum concentrations of biomarkers of skeletal metabolism and results of radiography as indicators of severity of osteochondrosis in foals, *Am J Vet Res* 65:143, 2004.

97. van de Lest CH, Brama PA, van El B, et al: Extracellular matrix changes in early osteochondrotic defects in foals: a key role for collagen? *Biochim Biophys Acta* 1690:54, 2004.

98. Vortkamp A: Interaction of growth factors regulating chondrocyte differentiation in the developing embryo, *Osteoarthritis Cartilage* 9(Suppl A):S109, 2001.

99. Semevolos SA, Brower-Toland BD, Bent SJ, et al: Parathyroid hormone–related peptide and Indian hedgehog expression patterns in naturally acquired equine osteochondrosis, *J Orthop Res* 20:1290, 2002.

100. Semevolos SA, Strassheim ML, Haupt JL, et al: Expression patterns of hedgehog signaling peptides in naturally acquired equine osteochondrosis, *J Orthop Res* 23:1152, 2005.

101. Pelton RW, Saxena B, Jones M, et al: Immunohistochemical localization of TGF beta 1, TGF beta 2, and TGF beta 3 in the mouse embryo: expression patterns suggest multiple roles during embryonic development, *J Cell Biol* 115:1091, 1991.

102. Dodds RA, Merry K, Littlewood A, et al: Expression of mRNA for IL1 beta, IL6 and TGF beta 1 in developing human bone and cartilage, *J Histochem Cytochem* 42:733, 1994.

103. Serra R, Karaplis A, Sohn P: Parathyroid hormone–related peptide (PTHrP)–dependent and –independent effects of transforming growth factor beta (TGF-beta) on endochondral bone formation, *J Cell Biol* 145:783, 1999.

104. Pateder DB, Rosier RN, Schwarz EM, et al: PTHrP expression in chondrocytes, regulation by TGF-beta, and interactions between epiphyseal and growth plate chondrocytes, *Exp Cell Res* 256:555, 2000.

105. Henson FMD, Schofield PN, Jeffcott LB: Expression of transforming growth factor beta 1 in normal and dyschondroplastic articular growth cartilage of the young horse, *Equine Vet J* 29:434, 1997.

106. Gunson DE, Kowalczyk DF, Shoop CR, et al: Environmental zinc and cadmium pollution associated with generalized osteochondrosis, osteoporosis, and nephrocalcinosis in horses, *J Am Vet Med Assoc* 180:295, 1982.

107. Campbell-Beggs CL, Johnson PJ, Messer NT, et al: Osteochondritis dissecans in an Appaloosa foal associated with zinc toxicosis, *J Equine Vet Sci* 14:546, 1994.

108. Swerczek TW: Chronic environmental cadmium toxicosis in horses and cattle, *J Am Vet Med Assoc* 211:1229, 1997 (letter).

109. Sandstead HH: Requirements and toxicity of essential trace elements, illustrated by zinc and copper, *Am J Clin Nutr* 61(Suppl 3):621S, 1995.

CHAPTER 55 The Role of Nutrition in Developmental Orthopedic Disease: Nutritional Management

1. Cunha TJ: *Horse feeding and nutrition*, ed 2, Orlando, 2007, Academic Press.

2. National Research Council: *Nutrient requirements of horses*, ed 6, Washington, DC, 2007, National Academies Press.

3. Pagan JD, Koch A, Caddel S, et al: Size of Thoroughbred yearlings presented for auction at Keeneland sales affects selling price, *Proc Equine Sci Soc Symp* 19:234, 1998.

4. Brown-Douglas CG, Pagan JD, Koch A, et al: The relationship between size at yearling sale, sale price and future racing performance in Kentucky Thoroughbreds, *Proc Equine Sci Soc Symp* 20:153, 2007.

5. Pagan JD, Jackson SG, Caddel S: A summary of growth rates of Thoroughbreds in Kentucky, *Pferdeheilkunde* 12:285, 1996.

6. Glade MJ, Gupta S, Reimers TJ: Hormonal responses to high and low planes of nutrition in weanling thoroughbreds, *J Anim Sci* 59:658, 1984.

7. Ralston SL: Postprandial hyperglycemia/hyperinsulinemia in young horses with osteochondritis dissecans lesions, *J Anim Sci* 73:184, 1995 (abstract).

8. Pagan JD, Geor RJ, Caddel SE, et al: The relationship between glycemic response and the incidence of OCD in thoroughbred weanlings: a field study, *Proc Am Assoc Equine Pract* 47:322, 2001.

9. Henneke DR, Potter GD, Kreider JL: A condition score relationship to body fat content of mares during gestation and lactation. Proceedings of the Seventh Annual Conference of the Equine Nutrition and Physiology Symposium, Warrenton, Virginia, 1981.

10. Pagan JD: Managing growth for different commercial end points. In Pagan JD, ed: *Advances in equine nutrition III*, Nottingham, 2005, Nottingham University Press.

11. Pearce SG: Copper nutrition in pasture-fed New Zealand Thoroughbreds and its role in developmental orthopaedic disease, doctoral dissertation, Palmerston North, New Zealand, 1997, Massey University.

12. Pagan JD, Brown-Douglas CG, Caddel S: Body weight and condition of Kentucky Thoroughbred mares and their foals as influenced by month of foaling, season and gender, *Proc Ky Equine Res Nutr Conf* 15:61, 2006.

CHAPTER 56 Diagnosis and Management of Osteochondrosis and Osseous Cystlike Lesions

1. Hogan PM, McIlwraith CW, Honnas CM, et al: Surgical treatment of subchondral cystic lesions of the third metacarpal bone: results in 15 horses (1986-1994, *Equine Vet J* 29:477, 1997.

2. Caron JP, Fretz PB, Bailey JV, et al: Proximal interphalangeal arthrodesis in the horse. A retrospective study and a modified screw technique, *Vet Surg* 19:196, 1990.

3. MacLellan KN, Crawford WH, MacDonald DG: Proximal interphalangeal joint arthrodesis in 34 horses using two parallel 5.5-mm cortical bone screws, *Vet Surg* 30:454, 2001.

4. Martin GS, McIlwraith CW, Turner AS, et al: Long-term results and complications of proximal interphalangeal arthrodesis in horses, *J Am Vet Med Assoc* 184:1136, 1984.

5. Schneider JE, Carnine BL, Guffy MM: Arthrodesis of the proximal interphalangeal joint in the horse: a surgical treatment for high ringbone, *J Am Vet Med Assoc* 173:1364, 1978.

6. Knox PM, Watkins JP: Proximal interphalangeal joint arthrodesis using a combination plate-screw technique in 53 horses (1994-2003), *Equine Vet J* 38:538, 2006.

7. Levine DG, Richardson DW: Clinical use of the locking compression plate (LCP) in horses: a retrospective study of 31 cases (2004-2006), *Equine Vet J* 39:401, 2007.

8. Radcliffe RM, Cheetham J, Bezuidenhout AJ, et al: Arthroscopic removal of palmar/plantar osteochondral fragments from the proximal interphalangeal joint in four horses, *Vet Surg* 37:733, 2008.

9. Fjordbakk CT, Strand E, Milde AK, et al: Osteochondral fragments involving the dorsomedial aspect of the proximal interphalangeal joint in young horses: 6 cases (1997-2006), *J Am Vet Med Assoc* 230:1498, 2007.

10. Schneider RK, Ragle CA, Carter BG, et al: Arthroscopic removal of osteochondral fragments from the proximal interphalangeal joint of the pelvic limbs in three horses, *J Am Vet Med Assoc* 205:79, 1994.

11. Story MR, Bramlage LR: Arthroscopic debridement of subchondral bone cysts in the distal phalanx of 11 horses (1994-2000), *Equine Vet J* 36:356, 2004.

12. Jenner F, Ross MW, Martin BB, et al: Scapulohumeral osteochondrosis: a retrospective study of 32 horses, *Vet Orthop Comp Traumatol* 21:406, 2008.

13. Stephens PR, Richardson DW, Ross MW, et al: Osteochondral fragments within the dorsal pouch or dorsal joint capsule of the proximal intertarsal joint of the horse, *Vet Surg* 18:151, 1989.

14. Beard WL, Bramlage LR, Schneider RK, et al: Postoperative racing performance in standardbreds and thoroughbreds with osteochondrosis of the tarsocrural joint: 109 cases (1984-1990), *J Am Vet Med Assoc* 204:1655, 1994.

15. Laws EG, Richardson DW, Ross MW, et al: Racing performance of Standardbreds after conservative and surgical treatment for tarsocrural osteochondrosis, *Equine Vet J* 25:199, 1993.

16. McIlwraith CW, Foerner JJ, Davis DM: Osteochondritis dissecans of the tarsocrural joint: results of treatment with arthroscopic surgery, *Equine Vet J* 23:155, 1991.

CHAPTER 57   Physitis

1. Salter RS, Harris WR: Injuries involving the epiphyseal plate, *J Bone Joint Surg Am* 45A:587, 1963.

2. McIlwraith CW: What is developmental orthopaedic disease, osteochondrosis, osteochondritis, metabolic bone disease, *Proc Am Assoc Equine Pract* 39:35, 1993.

3. Jeffcott LB: Problems and pointers in equine osteochondrosis, *Equine Vet J Suppl* 16:1, 1993.

4. Bramlage LR: Identification, examination and treatment of physitis in the foal, *Proc Am Assoc Equine Pract* 39:57, 1993.

CHAPTER 58   Angular Limb Deformities

1. Auer JA, Martens RJ, Williams EH: Periosteal transection for correction of angular limb deformities in foals, *J Am Vet Med Assoc* 181:459, 1982.

2. Fretz PB, Donecker JM: Surgical correction of angular limb deformities in foals: a retrospective study, *J Am Vet Med Assoc* 183:529, 1983.

3. Bertone AL, Turner AS, Park RD: Periosteal transection and stripping for treatment of angular limb deformities in foals: clinical observations, *J Am Vet Med Assoc* 187:145, 1985.

4. Auer JA: Angular limb deformities. In Auer JA, Stick JA, eds: *Equine surgery*, ed 3, St Louis 2006, Elsevier.

5. Hunt RJ: Angular limb deviations. In White NA, Moore JN, eds: *Current techniques in equine surgery and lameness*, ed 2, Philadelphia, 1998, Saunders.

6. Adams SB, Fessler JF: Surgical treatment of angular limb deformities. In Adams SB, Fessler JF, eds: *Atlas of equine surgery*, Philadelphia, 2000, Saunders.

7. Hunt RJ: New techniques in transphyseal bridging. Proceedings of the Sixteenth Annual American College of Veterinary Surgeons Symposium, 2006, Washington, DC.

8. Brauer TS, Booth TS, Riedesel E: Physeal growth retardation leads to correction of intracarpal angular deviations as well as physeal valgus deformity, *Equine Vet J* 31:193, 1999.

9. Crilly RG: Longitudinal overgrowth of chicken radius, *J Anat* 112:11, 1972.

10. Mitten LA, Bramlage LR, Embertson RM: Racing performance after hemicircumferential periosteal transection for angular limb deformities in thoroughbreds: 199 cases (1987-1989), *J Am Vet Med Assoc* 207:746, 1995.

11. Read EK, Read MR, Clark CR, et al: An evaluation of hemicircumferential periosteal transection and elevation in an angular limb deformity model (abstract). Proceedings of the Eleventh Annual American College of Veterinary Surgeons Veterinary Symposium, 2001, Chicago, IL.

12. Slone DE, Roberts CT, Hughes FE: Restricted exercise and transphyseal bridging for correction of angular limb deformities, *Proc Am Assoc Equine Pract* 46:126, 2000 (abstract).

13. Colles CM: How to aid the correction of angular limb deformities in foals using physeal stimulation, *Proc Am Assoc Equine Pract* 54:60, 2008.

14. O'Donohue DD, Smith FH, Strickland KL: The incidence of abnormal limb development in the Irish thoroughbred from birth to 18 months, *Equine Vet J* 24:305, 1992.

15. Dutton DM, Watkins JP, Honnas CM, et al: Treatment response and athletic outcome of foals with tarsal valgus deformities: 39 cases (1988-1997), *J Am Vet Med Assoc* 215:1481, 1999.

16. Dutton DM, Watkins JP, Walker MA, et al: Incomplete ossification of the tarsal bones in foals: 22 cases (1988-1996), *J Am Vet Med Assoc* 213:1590, 1998.

Suggested Readings

1. Auer JA: Angular limb deformities. In Auer JA, Stick JA, eds: *Equine surgery*, ed 3, St Louis, 2006, Elsevier.

2. Dutton DM, Watkins JP, Honnas CM, et al: Treatment response and athletic outcome of foals with tarsal valgus deformities: 39 cases (1988-1997), *J Am Vet Med Assoc* 215:1481, 1999.

CHAPTER 59   Flexural Limb Deformities in Foals

1. Auer JA: Flexural limb deformities. In Auer JA, ed: *Equine surgery*, ed 3, Philadelphia, 2006, Saunders.

2. Bohanon TC: Developmental musculoskeletal disease. In Kobluk CN, Ames TR, Geor RJ, eds: *The horse: diseases and clinical management*, Philadelphia, 1995, Saunders.

3. McIlwraith CW: Diseases of the joints, tendons, and ligaments and related structures. In Stashak TS, ed: *Adam's lameness in horses*, Philadelphia, 1987, Lea & Febiger.

4. Wagner PC: Flexural deformity of the distal interphalangeal joint (contracture of the deep digital flexor tendon). In White NA, Moore JN, eds: *Current practice of equine surgery*, Philadelphia, 1990, Lippincott.

5. Wagner PC: Flexural deformity of the metacarpophalangeal joint (contracture of the superficial digital flexor tendon). In White NA, Moore JN, eds: *Current practice of equine surgery*, Philadelphia, 1990, Lippincott.

6. Wagner PC: Flexural deformity of the carpus. In White NA, Moore JN, eds: *Current practice of equine surgery*, Philadelphia, 1990, Lippincott.

7. McIlwraith CW, James LF: Limb deformities in foals associated with ingestion of locoweed by mares, *J Am Vet Med Assoc* 181:255, 1982.

8. Lokai MD, Meyer RJ: Preliminary observation on oxytetracycline treatment of congenital flexural deformities in foals, *Mod Vet Pract* 66:237, 1985.

9. Fackelman GE: Flexure deformity of the metacarpophalangeal joints in growing horses, *Contin Educ Small Anim Pract* 1:S1, 1979.

10. Stick JA, Nickels FA, Williams MA: Long term effects of desmotomy of the accessory ligament of the deep digital flexor muscle in standardbreds: 23 cases (1979-1989), *J Am Vet Med Assoc* 200:1131, 1992.

CHAPTER 60   Cervical Stenotic Myelopathy

1. Wagner PC, Grant BD, Reed SM: Cervical vertebral malformations, *Vet Clin North Am Equine Pract* 3:385, 1987.

2. Stewart RH, Reed SM, Weisbrode, SE: Frequency and severity of osteochondrosis in horses with cervical stenotic myelopathy, *Am J Vet Res* 52:873, 1991.

3. Levine JM, Ngheim PP, Levine GJ, et al: Associations of sex, breed, and age with cervical vertebral compressive myelopathy in horses: 811 cases (1974-2007), *J Am Vet Med Assoc* 233:1453, 2008.

4. Reed SM, Bayley W, Traub J: Ataxia and paresis in horses. I. Differential diagnosis, *Compend Contin Educ Pract Vet* 3:S88, 1981.

5. Mayhew IG: Evaluation of the large animal neurological patient. In: *Large animal neurology*, Philadelphia, 1989, Lea & Febiger.

6. Powers BE, Stashak TS, Nixon AJ, et al: Pathology of the vertebral column of horses with cervical static stenosis, *Vet Pathol* 23:392, 1986.

7. Moore BR, Holbrook TC, Stefanacci JD, et al: Contrast-enhanced computed tomography and myelography in six horses with cervical stenotic myelopathy, *Equine Vet J* 24:197, 1992.

8. Ricardi G, Dyson SJ: Forelimb lameness associated with radiographic abnormalities of the cervical vertebrae, *Equine Vet J* 25:422, 1993.

9. Levine JM, Adam E, MacKay RJ: Confirmed and presumptive cervical vertebral compressive myelopathy in older

horses: a retrospective study (1992-2004), *J Vet Intern Med* 21:812, 2007.

10. Mayhew IG, Brown CM, Stowe HD, et al: Equine degenerative myeloencephalopathy: a vitamin E deficiency that may be familial, *J Vet Intern Med* 1:45, 1987.

11. Moore BR, Reed SM, Biller DS, et al: Assessment of vertebral canal diameter and bony malformations of the cervical part of the spine in horses with cervical stenotic myelopathy, *Am J Vet Res* 55:5, 1994.

12. Rush BR: Spinal radiography and myelography. In White NA, Moore JN, eds: *Current techniques in equine surgery and lameness*, Philadelphia, 1998, Saunders.

13. Whitwell KE, Dyson S: Interpreting radiographs. 8. Equine cervical vertebrae, *Equine Vet J* 19:8, 1987.

14. Papageorges M, Gavin PR, Sande RD, et al: Radiographic and myelographic examination of the cervical vertebral column in 306 ataxic horses, *Vet Radiol* 28:53, 1987.

15. Hahn CN, Handel I, Green SL, et al: Assessment of the utility of using intra- and intervertebral minimum sagittal diameter ratios in the diagnosis of cervical vertebral malformation in horses, *Vet Radiol Ultrasound* 49:1, 2008.

16. Van Biervliet J: An evidence-based approach to clinical questions in the practice of equine neurology, *Vet Clin North Am Equine Pract* 23:317, 2007.

17. Mayhew IG, Donawick WJ, Green SL, et al: Diagnosis and prediction of cervical vertebral malformation in thoroughbred foals based on semi-quantitative radiographic indicators, *Equine Vet J* 25:435, 1993.

18. van Biervliet J, Scrivani PV, Divers TJ, et al: Evaluation of decision criteria for detection of spinal cord compression based on cervical myelography in horses: 38 cases (1981-2001), *Equine Vet J* 36:14, 2004.

19. Wijnberg ID, Back W, de Jong M, et al: The role of electromyography in clinical diagnosis of neuromuscular locomotor problems in the horse, *Equine Vet J* 36:718, 2004.

20. Nollet H, Deprez P, van Ham L, et al: Transcranial magnetic stimulation: normal values of magnetic motor evoked potentials in 84 normal horses and influence of height, weight, age and sex, *Equine Vet J* 36:51, 2004.

21. Keegan KG, Arafat S, Skubic M, et al: Detection of spinal ataxia in horses using fuzzy clustering of body position uncertainty, *Equine Vet J* 36:712, 2004.

22. Donawick WJ, Mayhew IG, Galligan DT, et al: Results of a low protein, low-energy diet and confinement in young horses with wobbles, *Proc Am Assoc Equine Pract* 39:125, 1993.

23. Mattoon JS, Drost WT, Grguric MR, et al: Technique for equine cervical articular process joint injection, *Vet Radiol Ultrasound* 45:238, 2004.

24. Grisel RG, Grant BD, Rantanen NW: Arthrocentesis of the equine cervical facets, *Proc Am Assoc Equine Pract* 42:197, 1996.

25. Wagner PC, Grant BD, Bagby G: Evaluation of cervical spinal fusion as a treatment in the equine "wobbler" syndrome, *Vet Surg* 8:84, 1979.

26. Nixon AJ, Stashak TS, Ingram J: Dorsal laminectomy in the horse. III. Results in horses with cervical vertebral malformation, *Vet Surg* 12:184, 1983.

27. Moore BR, Reed SM, Robertson JT: Surgical treatment of cervical stenotic myelopathy in horses: 73 cases (1983-1992), *J Am Vet Med Assoc* 203:108, 1993.

28. DeBowes RM, Grant BD, Bagby GW, et al: Cervical vertebral interbody fusion in the horse: a comparative study of bovine xenografts and autografts supported by stainless steel baskets, *Am J Vet Res* 45:191, 1984.

29. Grant BD, Barbee DD, Wagner PC: Long term results of surgery for equine cervical vertebral malformation, *Proc Am Assoc Equine Pract* 31:91, 1985.

30. Mayhew IG: The diseased spinal cord, *Proc Am Assoc Equine Pract* 45:67, 1999.

CHAPTER 61   Osteoarthritis

1. Mankin HJ, Radin EL: Structure and function of joints. In Koopman WJ, ed: *Arthritis and allied conditions: a textbook of rheumatology*, ed 13, vol 1, Baltimore, 1997, Williams & Wilkins.

2. Sledge CB, Hari Reddi A, Walsh DA, et al: Biology of the normal joint. In Ruddy S, Harris ED, Sledge CB, eds: *Textbook of rheumatology*, ed 6, vol 1, Philadelphia, 2001, Saunders.

3. Todhunter RJ, Lust G: Pathophysiology of synovitis: clinical signs and examination in horses, *Comp Cont Educ Pract Vet* 12:980, 1990.

4. Rossdale PD, Hopes R, Wingfield-Digby NJ, et al: Epidemiological study of wastage among racehorses, 1982 and 1983, *Vet Rec* 116:66, 1985.

5. Jeffcott LB, Rossdale PD, Freestone J, et al: An assessment of wastage in thoroughbred racing from conception to 4 years of age, *Equine Vet J* 14:185, 1982.

6. Bassleer R, Lhoest-Ganthier MP, Renard AM, et al: Histological structure and functions of synovium. In Franchimont P, ed: *Articular synovium, Basel*, Switzerland, 1982, Karger.

7. Ghadially FN, Roy S: *Ultrastructure of synovial joints in health and disease*, London, 1969, Butterworth.

8. Stevens CR, Mapp PI, Revell PA: A monoclonal antibody (Mab 67) marks type B synoviocytes, *Rheumatol Int* 10:103, 1990.

9. Krey PR, Cohen AS, Smith CB, et al: The human fetal synovium: histology, fine structure and changes in organ culture, *Arthritis Rheum* 114:319, 1971.

10. Graabaek PM: Ultrastructural evidence for two distinct types of synoviocytes in rat synovial membrane, *J Ultrastruc Res* 78:321, 1982.

11. Wilkinson LS, Pitsillides AA, Worrall JG, et al: Light microscopic characterization of the fibroblast-like synovial intimal cell (synoviocyte), *Arthritis Rheum* 35:1179, 1992.

12. Gadher SJ, Woolley DE: Comparative studies of adherent rheumatoid synovial cells in primary culture: characterisation of the dendritic (stellate) cell, *Rheumatol Int* 7:13, 1987.

13. Henderson B, Pettipher ER: The synovial lining cell: biology and pathobiology, *Semin Arthritis Rheum* 15:1, 1985.

14. Roy S, Ghadially FN, Crane WAJ: Synovial membrane in traumatic effusion: ultrastructure and autoradiography with tritiated leucine, *Ann Rheum Dis* 25:259, 1966.

15. Norton WL, Lewis DC, Ziff M: Electron-dense deposits following injection of gold sodium thiomalate and thiomalic acid, *Arthritis Rheum* 11:436, 1968.

16. Müller-Ladner U, Gay RE, Gay S: Structure and function of synoviocytes. In Koopman WJ, ed: *Arthritis and allied conditions: a textbook of rheumatology*, ed 13, vol 1, Baltimore, 1997, Williams & Wilkins.

17. Danis VA, March LM, Nelson DS, et al: Interleukin-1 secretion by peripheral blood monocytes and synovial macrophages from patients with rheumatoid arthritis, *J Rheumatol* 14:33, 1987.

18. Guerne PA, Zuraw BL, Vaughan JH, et al: Synovium as a source of interleukin 6 in vitro: contribution to local and systemic manifestations of arthritis, *J Clin Invest* 83:585, 1989.

19. Bathon JM, Chilton FH, Hubbard WC, et al: Mechanisms of prostanoid synthesis in human synovial cells: cytokine-peptide synergism, *Inflammation* 20:537, 1996.

20. Landoni MF, Foot R, Frean S, et al: Effects of flunixin, tolfenamic acid, R(–) and S(+) ketoprofen on the response of equine synoviocytes to lipopolysaccharide stimulation, *Equine Vet J* 28:468, 1996.

21. Martel-Pelletier J, Cloutier JM, Pelletier JP: Neutral proteases in human osteoarthritic synovium, *Arthritis Rheum* 29:1112, 1986.

22. Canoso J: Bursae, tendons and ligaments, *Clin Rheum Dis* 7:189, 1981.

23. Gamble JG, Edwards CC, Max SR: Enzymatic adaptation in ligaments during immobilization, *Am J Sports Med* 12:221, 1984.

24. Grana WA, Larson RL: Functional and surgical anatomy. In Larson RL, Grana WA, eds: *The knee: form, function, pathology, treatment*, Philadelphia, 1993, Saunders.

25. Hvid I: Mechanical strength of trabecular bone at the knee, *Dan Med Bull* 35:345, 1988.

26. Simkin PA, Heston TF, Downey DJ, et al: Subchondral architecture in bones of the canine shoulder, *J Anat* 175:213, 1991.

27. Oettmeier R, Arokoski J, Roth AJ, et al: Quantitative study of articular cartilage and subchondral bone remodeling in the knee joint of dogs after strenuous running training, *J Bone Miner Res* 7(Suppl 2):S419, 1992.

28. Radin EL, Rose RM: Role of subchondral bone in the initiation and progression of cartilage damage, *Clin Orthop* 213:34, 1986.

29. Dequeker J, Mokassa L, Aerssens J: Bone density and osteoarthritis, *J Rheumatol* 43(Suppl):98, 1995.

30. Redler I, Mow VC, Zimny ML, et al: The ultrastructure and biomechanical significance of the tidemark of articular cartilage, *Clin Orthop* 112:357, 1975.

31. Mankin HJ, Thrasher AZ: Water content and binding in normal and osteoarthritic human cartilage, *J Bone Joint Surg Am* 57:76, 1975.

32. Mayne R, Irwin MH: Collagen types in cartilage. In Kuettner KE, Schleyerbach R, Hascall VC, eds: *Articular cartilage biochemistry*, New York, 1986, Raven Press.

33. Eyre DR: The collagens of articular cartilage, *Semin Arthritis Rheum* 21(Suppl 2):2, 1991.

34. Bruckner P, van der Rest M: Structure and function of cartilage collagens, *Microsc Res Tech* 28:378, 1994.

35. Vachon AM, Keeley FW, McIlwraith CW, et al: Biochemical analysis of normal articular cartilage in horses, *Am J Vet Res* 51:1905, 1990.

36. Mankin HJ, Brandt KD: Pathogenesis of osteoarthritis. In Ruddy S, Harris ED, Sledge CB, eds: Textbook of rheumatology, ed 6, vol 1, Philadelphia, 2001, Saunders.

37. Todhunter RJ, Wootton JA, Lust G, et al: Structure of equine type I and type II collagens, *Am J Vet Res* 55:425, 1994.

38. Eyre DR, Paz MA, Gallop PM: Cross-linking in collagen and elastin, *Annu Rev Biochem* 53:717, 1984.

39. Schenk RK, Eggli PS, Hunziker EB: Articular cartilage morphology. In Kuettner KE, ed: *Articular cartilage biochemistry*, New York, 1986, Raven Press.

40. Repo RU, Mitchell N: Collagen synthesis in mature articular cartilage of the rabbit, *J Bone Joint Surg Br* 53:541, 1971.

41. Eyre DR, McDevitt CA, Billingham MEJ, et al: Biosynthesis of collagen and other matrix proteins by articular cartilage in experimental osteoarthrosis, *Biochem J* 188:823, 1980.

42. Li Y, Lacerda DA, Warman ML, et al: A fibrillar collagen gene, Col11a1, is essential for skeletal morphogenesis, *Cell* 80:423, 1995.

43. Stallcup WB, Dahline K, Healy P: Interaction of the NG2 chondroitin sulfate proteoglycan with type VI collagen, *J Cell Biol* 111:3177, 1990.

44. Kielty CM, Whittaker SP, Grant ME, et al: Type VI collagen microfibrils: evidence for a structural association with hyaluronan, *J Cell Biol* 118:979, 1992.

45. Wu JJ, Woods PE, Eyre DR: Identification of cross-linking sites in bovine cartilage type IX collagen reveals an antiparallel type II-type IX molecular relationship and type IX to type IX bonding, *J Biol Chem* 267:23007, 1992.

46. Sandy JD, Plaas AHK, Rosenberg L: Structure, function and metabolism of cartilage proteoglycans. In Koopman WJ, ed: Arthritis and allied conditions: a textbook of rheumatology, ed 13, vol 1, Baltimore, 1997, Williams & Wilkins.

47. Poole AR, Reiner A, Tang LH, et al: Proteoglycans from bovine nasal cartilage: immunochemical studies of link protein, *J Biol Chem* 255:9295, 1980.

48. Dudhia J, Platt D: Complete primary sequence of equine cartilage link protein deduced from complementary DNA, *Am J Vet Res* 56:959, 1995.

49. Flannery C, Stanescu V, Morgelin M, et al: Variability in the G3 domain content of bovine aggrecan from cartilage extracts and chondrocyte cultures, *Arch Biochem Biophys* 297:52, 1992.

50. Mehmet H, Scudder P, Tang PW, et al: The antigenic determinants recognized by three monoclonal antibodies to keratan sulphate involve sulphated hepta or larger oligosaccharides of the poly-(N-acetyllactosamine) series, *Eur J Biochem* 157:385, 1986.

51. Poole AR: Proteoglycans in health and disease: structures and functions, *Biochem J* 236:1, 1986.

52. Poole AR: Cartilage in health and disease. In Koopman WJ, ed: Arthritis and allied conditions: a textbook of rheumatology, ed 13, vol 1, Baltimore, 1997, Williams & Wilkins.

53. Scott JE: Proteoglycan-fibrillar collagen interactions, *Biochem J* 252:313, 1988.

54. Noyori K, Jasin HE: Inhibition of human fibroblast adhesion by cartilage surface proteoglycans, *Arthritis Rheum* 37:1656, 1994.

55. Bidanset DJ, LeBaron R, Rosenberg L, et al: Regulation of cell substrate adhesion: effects of small galactosaminoglycan-containing proteoglycans, *J Cell Biol* 118:1523, 1992.

56. Heinegard D, Lorenzo P, Sommarin Y: Articular cartilage matrix proteins. In Kuettner KE, Goldberg VM, eds: *Osteoarthritic disorders*, Rosemont, IL, 1995, American Academy of Orthopaedic Surgeons.

57. Thonar EJ-MA, Masuda K, Manicourt DH, et al: Structure and function of normal adult articular cartilage. In Reginster J-Y, Pelletier J-P, Martel-Pelletier J, eds: *Osteoarthritis: clinical and experimental aspects*, Berlin, 1999, Springer.

58. Burton-Wurster N, Lust G: Deposition of fibronectin in articular cartilage of canine osteoarthritic joints, *Am J Vet Res* 46:2542, 1985.

59. Homandberg GA, Meyers R, Xie D: Fibronectin fragments cause chondrolysis of bovine articular cartilage slices in culture, *J Biol Chem* 267:359, 1992.

60. Repo RU, Mitchell N: Collagen synthesis in mature articular cartilage of the rabbit, *J Bone Joint Surg Br* 53:541, 1971.

61. Eyre DR, McDevitt CA, Billingham MEJ, et al: Biosynthesis of collagen and other matrix proteins by articular cartilage in experimental osteoarthrosis, *Biochem J* 188:823, 1980.

62. Lohmander LS, Kimura JH: Biosynthesis of cartilage proteoglycan. In Kuettner KE, Schleyerbach R, Hascall VC, eds: *Articular cartilage biochemistry*, New York, 1986, Raven Press.

63. Palmoski MJ, Brandt KD: Effects of static loading and cyclic compressive loading on articular cartilage plugs in vitro, *Arthritis Rheum* 27:675, 1984.

64. Schneiderman R, Keret D, Maroudas A: Effect of mechanical and osmotic pressure on the rate of glycosaminoglycan synthesis in the human adult femoral head cartilage: an in vitro study, *J Orthop Res* 4:393, 1986.

65. Pita J, Howell D: Micro-biochemical studies of cartilage. In Sokoloff L, ed: *The joints and synovial fluid*, New York, 1978, Academic Press.

66. Maroudas A, Bullough P, Swanson SA, et al: The permeability of articular cartilage, *J Bone Joint Surg Br* 50:166, 1968.

67. Hadler N: The biology of the extracellular space, *Clin Rheum Dis* 7:71, 1981.

68. Setton LA, Mow VC, Muller FJ, et al: Mechanical behavior and biochemical composition of canine knee cartilage following periods of joint disuse and disuse with remobilization, *Osteoarthritis Cartilage* 5:1, 1997.

69. Swanson SAV: Lubrication. In Freeman MAR, ed: *Adult articular cartilage*, Kent, England, 1979, Pitman Medical.

70. Mow VC, Mansour JM: The nonlinear interaction between cartilage deformation and interstitial fluid flow, *J Biomech* 10:1, 1977.

71. Swann DA, Radin EL: The molecular basis of articular lubrication. I. Purification and properties of a lubricating fraction from bovine synovial fluid, *J Biochem* 274:8069, 1972.

72. Radin EL, Swann DA, Weisser PA: Separation of a hyaluronate free lubricating fraction from synovial fluid, *Nature* 228:377, 1970.

73. Linn FC, Radin EL: Lubrication of animal joints. III. The effect of certain chemical alterations of the cartilage and lubricant, *Arthritis Rheum* 11:674, 1968.

74. Roberts BJ, Unsworth A, Main N: Modes of lubrication in human hip joints, *Ann Rheum Dis* 41:217, 1982.

75. Mabuchi K, Tsukamoto Y, Obara T, et al: The effect of additive hyaluronic acid on animal joints with experimentally reduced lubricating ability, *J Biomed Mater Res* 28:865, 1994.

76. Johns RJ, Wright V: Relative importance of various tissues in joint stiffness, *J Appl Physiol* 17:824, 1962.

77. Swann DA, Radin EL, Nazimiec M, et al: Role of hyaluronic acid in joint lubrication, *Ann Rheum Dis* 33:318, 1974.

78. Schwarz N, Leixnering M, Hopf R, et al: Pressure-volume ratio in human cadaver hip joints, *Arch Orthop Trauma Surg* 107:322, 1988.

79. Pedowitz RA, Gershuni DH, Crenshaw AG, et al: Intraarticular pressure during continuous passive motion of the human knee, *J Orthop Res* 7:530, 1989.

80. O'Connor J, Shercliff T, Goodfellow J: The mechanics of the knee in sagittal planes: mechanical interactions between muscles, ligaments and articular surfaces. In Mueller W, Hackenbruck W, eds: *Surgery and arthroscopy of the knee*, New York, 1988, Springer-Verlag.

81. Funk DA, Noyes FR, Grood ES, et al: Effect of flexion angle on the pressure-volume of the human knee, *Arthroscopy* 7:86, 1991.

82. Hardy J, Bertone AL, Muir WW: Pressure-volume relationships in equine midcarpal joint, *J Appl Physiol* 78:1977, 1995.

83. Myers DE, Palmer DG: Capsular compliance and pressure-volume relationships in normal and arthritic knees, *J Bone Joint Surg Br* 54:710, 1972.

84. Levick JR: Joint pressure-volume studies: their importance, design and interpretation, *J Rheumatol* 10:353, 1983.

85. Strand E, Martin GS, Crawford MP, et al: Intra-articular pressure, elastance, and range of motion in flexion of the equine metacarpophalangeal joint, *Am J Vet Res* 56:1362, 1995.

86. Kumar VP, Balasubramaniam P: The role of atmospheric pressure in stabilising the shoulder: an experimental study, *J Bone Joint Surg Br* 67:719, 1985.

87. Huberti HH, Hayes WC: Patellofemoral contact pressures: the influence of the Q-angle and tendofemoral contact, *J Bone Joint Surg Am* 66:715, 1984.

88. Simon SR, Paul IL, Mansour J, et al: Peak dynamic force in human gait, *J Biomech* 14:817, 1981.

89. Sledge CB: Biology of the joint. In Kelley WN, Harris ED, Ruddy S, et al, eds: *Textbook of rheumatology*, ed 4, Philadelphia, 1993, Saunders.

90. Mow VC, Kuei SC, Lai WM, et al: Biphasic creep and stress relaxation of articular cartilage in compression: theory and experiments, *J Biomech Eng* 102:73, 1980.

91. Kempson GE: Mechanical properties of articular cartilage. In Freeman MAR, ed: *Adult articular cartilage*, Kent, England, 1979, Pitman Medical.

92. Schmidt MB, Mow VC, Chun LE, et al: Effects of proteoglycan extraction on the mechanical properties of adult human articular cartilage, *J Orthop Res* 8:353, 1990.

93. Harris ED, DiBona DR, Krane SM: A mechanism for cartilage destruction in rheumatoid arthritis, *Trans Assoc Am Phys* 83:267, 1970.

94. Harris ED, Parker HG, Radin EL, et al: Effects of proteolytic enzymes on structural and mechanical properties of cartilage, *Arthritis Rheum* 15:497, 1972.

95. Armstrong CG, Gardner DL: Thickness and distribution of human femoral head articular cartilage, *Ann Rheum Dis* 36:407, 1977.

96. Radin EL, All IL: Does cartilage compliance reduce skeletal impact loads? The relative force-attenuating properties of articular cartilages, synovial fluid, periarticular soft tissues in bone, *Arthritis Rheum* 13:139, 1970.

97. Ochoa JA, Heck DA, Brandt KD, et al: The effect of intertrabecular fluid on femoral head mechanics, *J Rheumatol* 18:580, 1991.

98. Pugh JW, Rose RM, Radin EL: A possible mechanism of Wolff's law: trabecular microfractures, *Arch Int Physiol Biochim* 81:27, 1973.

99. Ito H, Nagasaki H, Hashizume K, et al: Time-course of force production by fast isometric contraction of the knee extensor in young and elderly subjects, *J Hum Ergol* 19:23, 1990.

100. Hough AJ: Pathology of osteoarthritis. In Koopman WJ, ed: *Arthritis and allied conditions: a textbook of rheumatology*, ed 13, vol 2, Baltimore, 1997, Williams & Wilkins.

101. Katzenstein PL, Malemud CJ, Pathria MN, et al: Early onset primary osteoarthritis and mild chondrodysplasia: radiographic and pathologic studies with an analysis of cartilage proteoglycans, *Arthritis Rheum* 33:674, 1990.

102. Knowlton RG, Katzenstein PL, Moskowitz RW, et al: Genetic linkage of a polymorphism in the type II procollagen gene (COL2A1) to primary osteoarthritis associated with mild chondrodysplasia, *N Engl J Med* 322:526, 1990.

103. Norrdin RW, Kawcak CE, Capwell BA, et al: Subchondral bone failure in an equine model of overload arthrosis, *Bone* 22:133, 1998.

104. Benske J, Schunke M, Tillman B: Subchondral bone formation in arthrosis: polychrome labeling studies in mice, *Acta Orthop Scand* 59:536, 1988.

105. Brown TD, Radin EL, Martin RB, et al: Finite element studies of some juxtarticular stress changes due to localized subchondral bone stiffening, *J Biomech* 17:11, 1984.

106. Dedrick DK, Goldstein SA, Brandt KD, et al: A longitudinal study of subchondral plate and trabecular bone in cruciate-deficient dogs with osteoarthritis followed up for 54 months, *Arthritis Rheum* 36:1460, 1993.

107. Mow VC, Ratcliffe A, Poole AR: Cartilage and diarthrodial joints as paradigms for hierarchical materials and structures, *Biomaterials* 13:67, 1992.

108. Alaaeddine N, DiBattista JA, Pelletier JP, et al: Osteoarthritic synovial fibroblasts possess an increased level of tumor necrosis factor-receptor 55 (TNF-R55) that mediates biological activation by TNF-alpha, *J Rheumatol* 24:1985, 1997.

109. Bathon JM, Chilton FH, Hubbard WC, et al: Mechanisms of prostanoid synthesis in human synovial cells: cytokine-peptide synergism, *Inflammation* 20:537, 1996.

110. May SA, Hooke RE, Lees P: Bone fragments stimulate equine synovial lining cells to produce the inflammatory mediator prostaglandin E2, *Equine Vet J Suppl* 6:131, 1988.

111. May SA, Hooke RE, Lees P: Interleukin-1 stimulation of equine articular cells, *Res Vet Sci* 52:342, 1992.

112. Farahat MN, Yanni G, Poston R, et al: Cytokine expression in synovial membranes of patients with rheumatoid arthritis and osteoarthritis, *Ann Rheum Dis* 52:870, 1993.

113. Pelletier JP, McCollum R, Cloutier JM, et al: Synthesis of metalloproteases and interleukin-6 (IL-6) in human osteoarthritic synovial membrane is an IL-1 mediated process, *J Rheumatol* 43(Suppl):109, 1991.

114. Fujikawa Y, Shingu M, Torisu T, et al: Interleukin-1 receptor antagonist production in cultured synovial cells from patients with rheumatoid arthritis and osteoarthritis, *Ann Rheum Dis* 54:318, 1995.

115. Spiers S, May SA, Bennett D, et al: Cellular sources of proteolytic enzymes in equine joints, *Equine Vet J* 26:43, 1994.

116. Clegg PD, Burke RM, Coughlan AR, et al: Characterization of equine matrix metalloproteinase 2 and 9; and identification of the cellular sources of these enzymes in joints, *Equine Vet J* 29:335, 1997.

117. Gibson KT, Hodge H, Whittem T: Inflammatory mediators in equine synovial fluid, *Aust Vet J* 73:148, 1996.

118. Auer DE, Ng JC, Seawright AA: Free radical oxidation products in plasma and synovial fluid of horses with synovial inflammation, *Aust Vet J* 70:49, 1993.

119. Alwan WH, Carter SD, Dixon JB: Interleukin-1-like activity in synovial fluids and sera of horses with arthritis, *Res Vet Sci* 51:72, 1991.

120. Morris EA, McDonald BS, Webb AC: Identification of interleukin-1 in equine osteoarthritic joint effusions, *Am J Vet Res* 51:59, 1990.

121. Niebauer GW, Wolf B, Yarmush M, et al: Evaluation of immune complexes and collagen type-specific antibodies in sera and synovial fluids of horses with secondary osteoarthritis, *Am J Vet Res* 49:1223, 1988.

122. Caron JP, Bowker RM, Abhold RH, et al: Substance P in the synovial membrane and fluid of the equine middle carpal joint, *Equine Vet J* 24:364, 1992.

123. Owens JG, Kamerling SG, Stanton SR, et al: Effects of pretreatment with ketoprofen and phenylbutazone on experimentally induced synovitis in horses, *Am J Vet Res* 57:866, 1996.

124. Hawkins DL, Cargile JL, MacKay RJ, et al: Effect of tumor necrosis factor antibody on synovial fluid cytokine activities in equine antebrachiocarpal joints injected with endotoxin, *Am J Vet Res* 56:1292, 1995.

125. Sabiston CP, Adams ME: Production of catabolin by synovium from an experimental model of osteoarthritis, *J Orthop Res* 7:519, 1989.

126. Vankemmelbeke MN, Ilic MZ, Handley CJ, et al: Coincubation of bovine synovial or capsular tissue with cartilage generates a soluble "aggrecanase" activity, *Biochem Biophys Res Commun* 255:686, 1999.

127. Bondeson J, Wainwright SD, Lauder S, et al: The role of synovial macrophages and macrophage-produced cytokines in driving aggrecanases, matrix metalloproteinases, and other destructive and inflammatory responses in osteoarthritis, *Arthritis Res Ther* 8:R187, 2008.

128. Platt D: Articular cartilage homeostasis and the role of growth factors and cytokines in regulating matrix composition. In McIlwraith CW, Trotter GW, eds: *Joint disease in the horse*, Philadelphia, 1996, Saunders.

129. Rizkalla G, Bogoch ER, Poole AR: Studies of the articular cartilage proteoglycan aggrecan in health and osteoarthritis: evidence for molecular heterogeneity and extensive molecular changes in disease, *J Clin Invest* 90:2268, 1992.

130. Mankin HJ, Lippielo L: The glycosaminoglycans of normal and arthritic cartilage, *J Clin Invest* 50:1712, 1971.

131. Curtin WA, Reville WJ: Ultrastructural observations on fibril profiles in normal and degenerative human articular cartilage, *Clin Orthop* 313:224, 1995.

132. Altman RD, Tenenbaum J, Latta L, et al: Biomechanical and biochemical properties of dog cartilage in experimentally induced osteoarthritis, *Ann Rheum Dis* 43:83, 1984.

133. Maroudas A, Ziv I, Weisman N, et al: Studies of hydration and swelling pressure in normal and osteoarthritic cartilage, *Biorheology* 22:159, 1985.

134. Shingu M, Isayama T, Yasutake C, et al: Role of oxygen radicals and IL-6-dependent matrix degradation, *Inflammation* 18:613, 1994.

135. Katrantzis M, Baker MS, Handley CJ, et al: The oxidant hypochlorite (OCl-), a

product of the myeloperoxidase system, degrades articular cartilage proteoglycan aggregate, *Free Radic Biol Med* 10:101, 1991.

136. Henrotin Y, Deby Dupont G, Deby C, et al: Production of active oxygen species by isolated human chondrocytes, *Br J Rheumatol* 32:562, 1993.

137. Roberts CR, Roughley PJ, Mort JS: Degradation of human proteoglycan aggregate induced by hydrogen peroxide: protein fragmentation, amino acid modification and hyaluronic acid cleavage, *Biochem J* 259:805, 1989.

138. Nagase J, Woessner JF Jr: Role of endogenous proteinases in the degradation of cartilage matrix. In Woessner JF Jr, Howell DS, ed: *Joint cartilage degradation: basic and clinical aspects*, New York, 1993, Marcel Dekker.

139. Werb Z, Alexander CM: Proteinases in matrix degradation. In Elli WN, Harris ED, Ruddy S, et al, eds: *Textbook of rheumatology*, ed 4, vol 1, Philadelphia, 1993, Saunders.

140. Little CB, Flannery CR, Hughes CE, et al: Aggrecanase versus matrix metalloproteinases in the catabolism of the interglobular domain of aggrecan in vitro, *Biochem J* 344(Pt 1):161, 1999.

141. Guilak F, Fermor B, Keefe FJ, et al: The role of biomechanics and inflammation in cartilage injury and repair, *Clin Orthop Rel Res* 391(Suppl):S100, 2001.

142. Campbell IK, Golds E, Mort JS, et al: Human articular cartilage secretes characteristic metal dependent proteinases upon stimulation by mononuclear cell factor, *J Rheumatol* 21:20, 1986.

143. Nagase H, Brinckerhoff CE, Vater CA, et al: Biosynthesis and secretion of procollagenase by rabbit synovial fibroblasts: inhibition of procollagenase secretion by monensin and evidence for glycosylation of procollagenase, *Biochem J* 214:281, 1983.

144. Okada Y: Proteinases and matrix degradation. In Ruddy S, Harris ED, Sledge CB, eds: *Textbook of rheumatology*, ed 6, vol 1, Philadelphia, 2001, Saunders.

145. Dean DD: Proteinase-mediated cartilage degradation in osteoarthritis, *Semin Arthritis Rheum* 20(Suppl):2, 1991.

146. Okada Y, Shinmmei M, Tanaka O, et al: Localization of matrix metalloproteinase 3 (stromelysin) in osteoarthritic cartilage and synovium, *Lab Invest* 66:680, 1992.

147. Pelletier JP, Mineau F, Woessner JF Jr, et al: Intraarticular injection with methyl prednisolone acetate reduces osteoarthritis lesions at the same time as chondrocyte stromelysin synthesis in experimental osteoarthritis, *Arthritis Rheum* 37:414, 1994.

148. Dean DD, Martel-Pelletier J, Pelletier JP, et al: Evidence for metalloproteinase and metalloproteinase inhibitor (TIMP) imbalance in human osteoarthritic cartilage, *J Clin Invest* 84:678, 1989.

149. McKie N, Edwards T, Dallas DJ, et al: Expression of members of a novel membrane linked metalloproteinase family (ADAM) in human articular chondrocytes, *Biochem Biophys Res Commun* 230:335, 1997.

150. Flannery CR, Little CB, Caterson B, et al: Effects of culture conditions and exposure to catabolic stimulators (IL-1 and retinoic acid) on the expression of matrix metalloproteinases (MMPs) and disintegrin metalloproteinases (ADAMs) by articular cartilage chondrocytes, *Matrix Biol* 18:225, 1999.

151. Arner EC, Pratta MA, Trzaskos JM, et al: Generation and characterization of aggrecanase: a soluble, cartilage-derived aggrecan-degrading activity, *J Biol Chem* 274:6594, 1999.

152. Tortorella MD, Burn TC, Pratta MA, et al: Purification and cloning of aggrecanase-1: a member of the ADAMTS family of proteins, *Science* 284:1664, 1999.

153. Abbaszade I, Liu RQ, Yang F, et al: Cloning and characterization of ADAMTS11, an aggrecanase from the ADAMTS family, *J Biol Chem* 274:23443, 1999.

154. Tortorella M, Pratta M, Liu RQ, et al: The thrombospondin motif of aggrecanase-1 (ADAMTS-4) is critical for aggrecan substrate recognition and cleavage, *J Biol Chem* 275:25791, 2000.

155. Bondeson J, Wainwright S, Hughes C, et al: The regulation of the ADAMSTS4 and ADAMTS5 aggrecanases in osteoarthritis: a review, *Clin Exp Rheum* 26:139, 2007.

156. Yamada H, Nakagawa T, Stephens RW, et al: Proteinases and their inhibitors in normal and osteoarthritic articular cartilage, *Biomed Res* 8:289, 1987.

157. Murphy G, Willenbrock R: Tissue inhibitors of matrix metalloendopeptidases, *Methods Enzymol* 248:496, 1995.

158. McCachren SS: Expression of metalloproteinases and metalloproteinase inhibitor in human arthritic synovium, *Arthritis Rheum* 34:1085, 1991.

159. Zafarullah M, Su S, Martel-Pelletier J, et al: Tissue inhibitor of metalloproteinase-2 (TIMP-2) mRNA is constitutively expressed in bovine, human normal, and osteoarthritic articular chondrocytes, *J Cell Biochem* 60:211, 1996.

160. Su S, Grover J, Roughley PJ, et al: Expression of the tissue inhibitor of metalloproteinases (TIMP) gene family in normal and osteoarthritic joints, *Rheumatol Int* 18:183, 1999.

161. Martel-Pelletier J, McCollum R, Fujimoto N, et al: Excess of metalloproteases over tissue inhibitor of metalloprotease may contribute to cartilage degradation in osteoarthritis and rheumatoid arthritis, *Lab Invest* 70:807, 1994.

162. Towle CA, Hung HH, Bonassar LJ, et al: Detection of interleukin-1 in the cartilage of patients with osteoarthritis: a possible autocrine/paracrine role in pathogenesis, *Osteoarthritis Cartilage* 5:293, 1997.

163. Ounissi-Benkalha H, Pelletier JP, Tardif G, et al: In vitro effects of 2 antirheumatic drugs on the synthesis and expression of proinflammatory cytokines in synovial membranes from patients with rheumatoid arthritis, *J Rheumatol* 23:16, 1996.

164. Westacott CI, Atkins RM, Dieppe PA, et al: Tumor necrosis factor-α receptor expression on chondrocytes isolated from human articular cartilage, *J Rheumatol* 21:1710, 1994.

165. Martel-Pelletier J, McCollum R, DiBattista J, et al: The interleukin-1 receptor in normal and osteoarthritic human articular chondrocytes, *Arthritis Rheum* 35:530, 1992.

166. Fell HB, Jubb R: The effect of synovial tissue on the breakdown of articular cartilage in organ culture, *Arthritis Rheum* 20:1371, 1977.

167. May SA, Hooke RE, Lees P: Interleukin-1 stimulation of equine articular cells, *Res Vet Sci* 52:342, 1992.

168. Tyler JA, Benton HP: Synthesis of type II collagen is decreased in cartilage cultured with interleukin-1 while the rate of extracellular degradation remains unchanged, *Coll Relat Res* 8:393, 1988.

169. Arner EC, Pratta MA: Independent effects of interleukin-1 on proteoglycan breakdown, proteoglycan synthesis and prostaglandin E2 release from cartilage in organ culture, *Arthritis Rheum* 32:288, 1989.

170. Murphy G, Hembry RM, Reynolds JJ: Characterization of a specific antiserum to rabbit stromelysin and demonstration of the synthesis of collagenase and stromelysin by stimulated rabbit articular chondrocytes, *Coll Relat Res* 6:351, 1986.

171. Platt D, Bayliss MT: An investigation of the proteoglycan metabolism of mature equine articular cartilage and its regulation by interleukin-1, *Equine Vet J* 26:297, 1994.

172. Morris EA, Treadwell BV: Effect of interleukin 1 on articular cartilage from young and aged horses and comparison with metabolism of osteoarthritic cartilage, *Am J Vet Res* 55:138, 1994.

173. Caron JP, Tardif G, Martel-Pelletier J, et al: Modulation of matrix metalloprotease 13 (collagenase 3) gene expression in equine chondrocytes by interleukin 1 and corticosteroids, *Am J Vet Res* 57:1631, 1996.

174. MacDonald MH, Stover SM, Willits NH, et al: Regulation of matrix metabolism in equine cartilage explant cultures by interleukin 1, *Am J Vet Res* 53:2278, 1992.

175. Richardson DW, Dodge GR: Effects of interleukin-1beta and tumor necrosis factor-alpha on expression of matrix-related genes by cultured equine articular chondrocytes, *Am J Vet Res* 61:624, 2000.

176. Richardson DW, Dodge GR: Cloning of equine type II procollagen and the modulation of its expression in cultured equine articular chondrocytes, *Matrix Biol* 16:59, 1997.

177. Goldring MB, Birkhead J, Sandell LJ, et al: Interleukin-1 suppresses expression of cartilage-specific types II and IX collagens and increases types I and III collagens in human chondrocytes, *J Clin Invest* 82:2026, 1988.

178. Martel-Pelletier J, Zafarullah M, Kodama S, et al: In vitro effects of interleukin-1 on the synthesis of metalloproteases, TIMP, plasminogen activators and inhibitors in human articular cartilage, *J Rheumatol* 27(Suppl):80, 1991.

179. Bathon JM, Chilton FH, Hubbard WC, et al: Mechanisms of prostanoid synthesis in human synovial cells: cytokine-peptide synergism, *Inflammation* 20:537, 1996.

180. Bandara G, Georgescu HI, Lin CW, et al: Synovial activation of chondrocytes: evidence for complex cytokine interactions, *Agents Actions* 34:285, 1991.

181. Stefanovich-Racic M, Stadler J, Evans CH: Nitric oxide and arthritis, *Arthritis Rheum* 36:1036, 1993.

182. Evans CH, Stefanovic-Racic M, Lancaster J: Nitric oxide and its role in orthopaedic disease, *Clin Orthop* 312:275, 1995.

183. Frean SP, Bryant CE, Froling IL, et al: Nitric oxide production by equine articular cells in vitro, *Equine Vet J* 29:98, 1997.

184. Bunning RA, Richardson HJ, Crawford A, et al: The effect of interleukin-1 on connective tissue metabolism and its relevance to arthritis, *Agents Actions* 18(Suppl):131, 1986.

185. Hung GL, Galea-Lauri J, Mueller GM, et al: Suppression of intra-articular responses to interleukin-1 by transfer of the interleukin-1 receptor antagonist gene to synovium, *Gene Ther* 1:64, 1994.

186. Caron JP, Fernandez JC, Martel-Pelletier J, et al: Chondroprotective effect of intraarticular injections of interleukin-1 receptor antagonist in experimental osteoarthritis: suppression of collagenase-1 expression, *Arthritis Rheum* 39:1535, 1996.

187. Pelletier JP, Caron JP, Evans C, et al: In vivo suppression of early experimental osteoarthritis by interleukin-1 receptor antagonist using gene therapy, *Arthritis Rheum* 40:1012, 1997.

188. Hawkins DL, MacKay RJ, Gum GG, et al: Effects of intra-articularly administered endotoxin on clinical signs of disease and synovial fluid tumor necrosis factor, interleukin 6, and prostaglandin E2 values in horses, *Am J Vet Res* 54:379, 1993.

189. Todhunter PG, Kincaid SA, Todhunter RJ, et al: Immunohistochemical analysis of an equine model of synovitis-induced arthritis, *Am J Vet Res* 57:1080, 1996.

190. Cornelissen BP, Rijkenhuizen AB, van den Hoogen BM, et al: Experimental model of synovitis/capsulitis in the equine metacarpophalangeal joint, *Am J Vet Res* 59:978, 1998.

191. Billinghurst RC, Fretz PB, Gordon JR: Induction of intra-articular tumour necrosis factor during acute inflammatory responses in equine arthritis, *Equine Vet J* 27:208, 1995.

192. Yaron I, Meyer FA, Dayer J-M, et al: Some recombinant human cytokines stimulate glycosaminoglycan synthesis in human synovial fibroblasts cultures and inhibit it in human articular cartilage cultures, *Arthritis Rheum* 32:173, 1989.

193. Goldring MB, Birkhead J, Sandell LJ, et al: Synergistic regulation of collagen gene expression in human chondrocytes by tumor necrosis factor-α and interleukin-1β, *Ann N Y Acad Sci* 580:536, 1990.

194. Brennan FM, Chantry D, Jackson A, et al: Inhibitory effect of TNF alpha antibodies on synovial cell interleukin-1 production in rheumatoid arthritis, *Lancet* 2:244, 1989.

195. Amos N, Lauder S, Evans A, et al: Adenoviral gene transfer into osteoarthritis synovial cells using the endogenous inhibitor IκBα reveals that most, but not all, inflammatory and destructive mediators are NFκB dependent, *Rheumatology* 45:1201, 2006.

196. Jang D, Williams RJ, Wang MX, et al: *Staphylococcus aureus* stimulates inducible nitric oxide synthase in articular cartilage, *Arthritis Rheum* 42:2410, 1999.

197. Farrell AJ, Blake DR, Palmer RM, et al: Increased concentrations of nitrite in synovial fluid and serum samples suggest increased nitric oxide synthesis in rheumatic diseases, *Ann Rheum Dis* 51:1219, 1992.

198. Jarvinen TAH, Moilanen T, Jarvinen TLN, et al: Nitric oxide mediates interleukin-1 induced inhibition of glycosaminoglycan synthesis in rat articular cartilage, *Mediators Inflamm* 4:107, 1995.

199. Pelletier JP, Mineau F, Ranger P, et al: The increased synthesis of inducible nitric oxide inhibits IL-1Ra synthesis by human articular chondrocytes: possible role in osteoarthritis cartilage degradation, *Osteoarthritis Cartilage* 4:77, 1996.

200. Hyashi T, Abe E, Yamate T, et al: Nitric oxide production by superficial and deep articular chondrocytes, *Arthritis Rheum* 40:261, 1997.

201. Oh M, Fukuda K, Asada S, et al: Concurrent generation of nitric oxide and superoxide inhibits proteoglycan synthesis in bovine articular chondrocytes: involvement of peroxynitrite, *J Rheumatol* 25:2169, 1998.

202. Stefanovic-Racic M, Mollers MO, Miller LA, et al: Nitric oxide and proteoglycan turnover in rabbit articular cartilage, *J Orthop Res* 15:442, 1997.

203. Cao M, Westerhausen-Larsen A, Niyibizi C, et al: Nitric oxide inhibits the synthesis of type-II collagen without altering Col2A1 mRNA abundance: prolyl hydroxylase as a possible target, *Biochem J* 324:305, 1997.

204. Xie QW, Kashiwabara Y, Nathan C: Role of transcription factor NF-kappa B/Rel in induction of nitric oxide synthase, *J Biol Chem* 29:4705, 1994.

205. Sasaki K, Hattori T, Fujisawa T, et al: Nitric oxide mediates interleukin-1-induced gene expression of matrix metalloproteinases and basic fibroblast growth factor in cultured rabbit articular chondrocytes, *J Biochem (Tokyo)* 123:431, 1998.

206. Murrell GAC, Jang D, Williams RJ: Nitric oxide activated metalloprotease enzymes in articular cartilage, *Biochem Biophys Res Commun* 206:15, 1995.

207. Wu GJ, Chen TG, Chang HC, et al: Nitric oxide from both exogenous and endogenous sources activates mitochondria-dependent events and induces insults to human chondrocytes, *J Cell Biochem* 101:1520, 2007.

208. Horton WE Jr, Udo I, Precht P, et al: Cytokine inducible matrix metalloproteinase expression in immortalized rat chondrocytes is independent of nitric oxide stimulation, *In Vitro Cell Dev Biol Anim* 34:378, 1998.

209. Bird JL, Wells T, Platt D, et al: IL-1 beta induces the degradation of equine articular cartilage by a mechanism that is not mediated by nitric oxide, *Biochem Biophys Res Commun* 238:81, 1997.

210. Connor JR, Manning PT, Settle SL, et al: Suppression of adjuvant-induced arthritis by selective inhibition of inducible nitric oxide synthase, *Eur J Pharmacol* 273:15, 1995.

211. Stefanovich-Racic M, Meyers K, Meschter C, et al: N-monomethyl arginine, an inhibitor of nitric oxide synthase, suppresses the development of adjuvant arthritis in rats, *Arthritis Rheum* 37:1062, 1994.

212. Pelletier JP, Jovanovic D, Fernandes JC, et al: Reduced progression of experimental osteoarthritis in vivo by selective inhibition of inducible nitric oxide synthase, *Arthritis Rheum* 41:1275, 1998.

213. Pelletier JP, Lascau-Coman V, Jovanovic D, et al: Selective inhibition of inducible nitric oxide synthase in experimental osteoarthritis is associated with reduction in tissue levels of catabolic factors, *J Rheumatol* 26:2002, 1999.

214. May SA, Hooke RA, Lees P: Identity of the E-series prostaglandin produced by equine chondrocytes and synovial cells in response to a variety of stimuli, *Res Vet Sci* 46:54, 1989.

215. Tietz CC, Chrisman OD: The effect of salicylate and chloroquine on prostaglandin-induced articular damage in the rabbit knee, *Clin Orthop* 108:264, 1975.

216. Lippiello L, Yamamoto K, Robinson D, et al: Involvement of prostaglandin from rheumatoid synovium and inhibition of articular cartilage metabolism, *Arthritis Rheum* 21:909, 1978.

217. Robinson DR, Tashijian HJ, Levine L: Prostaglandin-stimulated bone resorption by rheumatoid synovia: a possible mechanism for bone destruction in rheumatoid arthritis, *J Clin Invest* 56:1181, 1975.

218. Steinberg JJ, Hubbard JR, Sledge CB: Chondrocyte-mediated breakdown of cartilage, *J Rheumatol* 20:325, 1993.

219. Mehindate K, al-Daccak R, Aoudjit F, et al: Interleukin-4, transforming growth factor beta 1, and dexamethasone inhibit superantigen-induced prostaglandin E2-dependent collagenase gene expression through their action on cyclooxygenase-2 and cytosolic phospholipase A2, *Lab Invest* 75:529, 1996.

220. DiBattista JA, Martel-Pelletier J, Fujimoto N, et al: Prostaglandins E2 and E1 inhibit cytokine induced metalloprotease expression in human synovial fibroblasts, *Lab Invest* 71:270, 1994.

221. Yamada H, Kikuchi T, Nemoto O, et al: Effects of indomethacin on the production of matrix metalloproteinase-3 and tissue inhibitor of metalloproteinases-1 by human articular chondrocytes, *J Rheumatol* 23:1739, 1996.

222. DiBattista JA, Dore S, Morin N, et al: Prostaglandin E2 up-regulates insulin-like growth factor binding protein-3 expression and synthesis in human articular chondrocytes by a c-AMP-independent pathway: role of calcium and protein kinase A and C, *J Cell Biochem* 63:320, 1996.

223. Dieppe PA, Harkness JAL, Higgs ER: Osteoarthritis. In Wall PD, Melzack R, eds: *Textbook of pain*, ed 3, New York, 1989, Churchill Livingstone.

224. Moskowitz RW: Osteoarthritis: symptoms and signs. In Moskowitz RW, Howell DS, Goldberg VM, et al, eds: *Osteoarthritis: diagnosis and management*, Philadelphia, 1984, Saunders.

225. Richardson DW: Degenerative joint disease. In Colahan PT, Mayhew IG, Merritt AM, et al, eds: *Equine medicine and*

surgery, ed 4, Goleta, Calif, 1991, American Veterinary Publications.

226. Wyke B: The neurology of joints: a review of general principles, *Clin Rheum Dis* 7:223, 1981.

227. Dee R: The innervation of joints. In Sokoloff L, ed: *The joints and synovial fluid*, New York, 1978, Academic Press.

228. Hepplemann B, Pfeffer A, Schaible HG, et al: Effects of acetylsalicylic acid and indomethacin on single groups III and IV sensory units from acutely inflamed joints, *Pain* 26:337, 1986.

229. Nilsson G: Lameness and pathologic changes in the distal joints and phalanges of the standardbred horse, *Acta Vet Scand* 44(Suppl):83, 1973.

230. Nilsson B, Olsson SE: Radiologic and patho-anatomic changes in the distal joints and the phalanges of the standardbred horse, *Acta Vet Scand* 44(Suppl):1, 1973.

231. Kellgren JH: Pain in osteoarthritis, *J Rheumatol* 9(Suppl):108, 1983.

232. Verschooten F, DeMoor A: Subchondral cystic and related lesions affecting the equine pedal bone and stifle, *Equine Vet J* 14:47, 1982.

233. Jeffcott LB: Osteochondrosis in the horse: searching for the key to pathogenesis, *Equine Vet J* 23:331, 1991.

234. Nixon AJ: Osteochondrosis and osteochondritis dissecans of the equine fetlock, *Comp Cont Educ Pract Vet* 12:1463, 1990.

235. Lawrence JS, Bremner JM, Bier F: Osteoarthrosis: prevalence in the population and relationship between symptoms and x-ray changes, *Ann Rheum Dis* 25:1, 1966.

236. Cobb S, Merchant WR, Rubin T: The relation of symptoms to osteoarthritis, *J Chronic Dis* 5:197, 1957.

237. Arnoldi CC, Linderholm H, Mussbichler M: Venous engorgement and intraosseous hypertension in osteoarthritis of the hip, *J Bone Joint Surg Br* 54:409, 1972.

238. Stolk PWTH, Firth EC: Intra-osseous pressure of the equine third metatarsal bone, *Cornell Vet* 78:191, 1988.

239. Felson DT, Chaisson CE, Hill CL, et al: The association of bone marrow lesions with pain in knee osteoarthritis, *Ann Intern Med* 134:541, 2001.

240. Bergman AG, Willen HK, Lindstrand AL, et al: Osteoarthritis of the knee: correlation of subchondral MR signal abnormalities with histopathologic and radiographic features, *Skeletal Radiol* 23:445, 1994.

241. Zanetti M, Bruder E, Romero J, et al: Bone marrow edema pattern in osteoarthritic knees: correlation between MR imaging and histologic findings, *Radiology* 215:835, 2000.

242. Wildy KS, Nevitt MC, Kwoh CK, et al: MRI findings associated with knee pain: analysis of discordant knee pairs in Health ABC, *Arthritis Rheum* 46(Suppl 9):S148, 2002.

243. Rodeo SA, Hannafin JA, Tom J, et al: Immunolocalization of cytokines and their receptors in adhesive capsulitis of the shoulder, *J Orthop Res* 15:427, 1997.

244. Morita Y, Kashihara N, Yamamura M, et al: Inhibition of rheumatoid synovial fibroblast proliferation by antisense oligonucleotides targeting proliferating cell

nuclear antigen messenger RNA, *Arthritis Rheum* 40:1292, 1997.

245. Katayama I, Nishioka K: Substance P augments fibrogenic cytokine-induced fibroblast proliferation: possible involvement of neuropeptide in tissue fibrosis, *J Dermatol Sci* 15:201, 1997.

246. Simpkin PA: Synovial physiology. In Koopman WJ, ed: *Arthritis and allied conditions: a textbook of rheumatology*, ed 13, vol 1, Baltimore, 1997, Williams & Wilkins.

247. Tulamo RM, Houttu J, Tupamaki A, et al: Hyaluronate and large molecular weight proteoglycans in synovial fluid from horses with various arthritides, *Am J Vet Res* 57:932, 1996.

248. Saari H, Konttinen YT, Tulamo RM, et al: Concentration and degree of polymerization of hyaluronate in equine synovial fluid, *Am J Vet Res* 50:2060, 1989.

249. Tew WP, Hotchkiss RN: Synovial fluid analysis and equine joint disorders, *Equine Vet Sci* 1:163, 1981.

250. White KK, Hodgson DR, Hancock D, et al: Changes in equine carpal joint synovial fluid in response to the injection of two local anesthetic agents, *Cornell Vet* 79:25, 1989.

251. Van Pelt RW: Interpretation of synovial fluid findings in the horse, *J Am Vet Med Assoc* 165:91, 1974.

252. Bertone AL, McIlwraith CW, Powers B, et al: Effects of four antimicrobial lavage solutions on the tarsocrural joint of horses, *Vet Surg* 5:305, 1986.

253. Muttini A, Petrizzi L, Tinti A, et al: Synovial fluid parameters in normal and osteochondritic hocks of horses with open physis, *Boll Soc Ital Biol Sper* 70:337, 1994.

254. Lloyd KC, Stover SM, Pascoe JR, et al: Effect of gentamicin sulfate and sodium bicarbonate on the synovium of clinically normal equine antebrachiocarpal joints, *Am J Vet Res* 49:650, 1988.

255. Tulamo RM, Bramlage LR, Gabel AA: Sequential clinical and synovial fluid changes associated with acute infectious arthritis in the horse, *Equine Vet J* 21:325, 1989.

256. Adair HS, Goble DO, Vanhooser S, et al: Evaluation of use of dimethyl sulfoxide for intra-articular lavage in clinically normal horses, *Am J Vet Res* 52:333, 1991.

257. McIlwraith CW: Radiographically silent injuries in joints: an overview and discussion, *Proc Am Assoc Equine Pract* 37:785, 1991.

258. Whitton RC, Kannegieter NJ, Rose RJ: The intercarpal ligaments of the equine midcarpal joint. III. Clinical observations in 32 racing horses with midcarpal joint disease, *Vet Surg* 26:374, 1997.

259. Ross MW, Nolan PM, Palmer JA, et al: The importance of the metatarsophalangeal joint in standardbred lameness, *Proc Am Assoc Equine Pract* 37:741, 1991.

260. Swanson TD: Degenerative disease of the metacarpophalangeal (fetlock) joint in performance horses, *Proc Am Assoc Equine Pract* 34:399, 1988.

261. Ross MW: Scintigraphic and clinical findings in the standardbred metatarsophalangeal joint: 114 cases (1993-1995), *Equine Vet J* 30:131, 1998.

262. Bjornsdottir S, Axelsson M, Eksell P, et al: Radiographic and clinical survey of degenerative joint disease in the distal tarsal joints in Icelandic horses, *Equine Vet J* 32:268, 2000.

263. Dyson SJ: Lameness due to pain associated with the distal interphalangeal joint: 45 cases, *Equine Vet J* 23:128, 1991.

264. Schneider RK, Jenson P, Moore RM: Evaluation of cartilage lesions on the medial femoral condyle as a cause of lameness in horses: 11 cases (1988-1994), *J Am Vet Med Assoc* 210:1649, 1997.

265. Moore RM, Schneider RK: Arthroscopic findings in the carpal joints of lame horses without radiographically visible abnormalities: 41 cases (1986-1991), *J Am Vet Med Assoc* 206:1741, 1995.

266. McIlwraith CW, Yovich JV, Martin GS: Arthroscopic surgery for the treatment of osteochondral chip fractures in the equine carpus, *J Am Vet Med Assoc* 191:531, 1987.

267. Kannegieter NJ, Burbidge HM: Correlation between radiographic and arthroscopic findings in the equine carpus, *Aust Vet J* 67:132, 1990.

268. Danielsson LG, Dymling JF, Heripret G: Coxarthrosis in man studied with external counting of 85Sr and 47Ca, *Clin Orthop* 31:151, 1963.

269. Christensen SB: Localization of bone-seeking agents in developing experimentally induced osteoarthritis in the knee joint of the rabbit, *Scand J Rheumatol* 12:343, 1983.

270. Dieppe P, Cushanghan J, Young P, et al: Prediction of the progression of joint space narrowing in osteoarthritis of the knee by bone scintigraphy, *Ann Rheum Dis* 52:557, 1993.

271. Ball MA, Allen D, Parkes A: Surgical treatment of subchondral cyst-like lesions in the tibia of an adult pony, *J Am Vet Med Assoc* 208:704, 1996.

272. Erlich PJ, Seeherman HJ, O'Callaghan MW, et al: Results of bone scintigraphy in horses used for show jumping, hunting or eventing: 141 cases (1988-1994), *J Am Vet Med Assoc* 213:1460, 1998.

273. Erlich PJ, Dohoo IR, O'Callaghan MW: Results of bone scintigraphy in racing standardbred horses: 64 cases (1992-1994), *J Am Vet Med Assoc* 215:982, 1999.

274. Ulhorn H, Eksell P, Sandgren B, et al: Sclerosis of the third carpal bone: a prospective study of its significance in a group of young standardbred trotters, *Acta Vet Scand* 41:51, 2000.

275. Link TM, Stahl R, Woertler K: Cartilage imaging: motivation, techniques, current and future significance, *Eur Radiol* 17:1135, 2007.

276. Cicuttini F, Forbes A, Asbeutah A, et al: Comparison and reproducibility of fast and conventional spoiled gradient-echo magnetic resonance sequences in the determination of knee cartilage volume, *J Orthop Res* 18:580, 2000.

277. Jones G, Ding C, Scott F, et al: Early radiographic osteoarthritis is associated with substantial changes in cartilage volume and tibial bone surface area in both males and females, *Osteoarthritis Cartilage* 12:169, 2004.

278. Choquet P, Sick H, Constantinesco A: MRI of the equine digit with a dedicated low-field magnet, *Vet Rec* 146:616, 2000.

279. McKnight AL, Manduca A, Felmlee JP, et al: Motion-correction techniques for standing equine MRI, *Vet Radiol Ultrasound* 45:513, 2004.

280. Mair TS, Kinns J: Deep digital flexor tendonitis in the equine foot diagnosed by low-field magnetic resonance imaging in the standing patient: 18 cases, *Vet Radiol Ultrasound* 46:458, 2005.

281. Martinelli MJ, Kuriashkin IV, Carragher BO, et al: Magnetic resonance imaging of the equine metacarpophalangeal joint: three-dimensional reconstruction and anatomic analysis, *Vet Radiol Ultrasound* 38:193, 1997.

282. Holcombe SJ, Bertone AL, Biller DS, et al: Magnetic resonance imaging of the equine stifle, *Vet Radiol Ultrasound* 36:119, 1995.

283. Blaik MA, Hanson RR, Kincaid SA, et al: Low-field magnetic resonance imaging of the equine tarsus: normal anatomy, *Vet Radiol Ultrasound* 41:131, 2000.

284. Murray RC, Branch MV, Tranquille C, et al: Validation of magnetic resonance imaging for measurement of equine articular cartilage and subchondral bone thickness, *Am J Vet Res* 66:1999, 2005.

285. Martinelli MJ, Baker GJ, Clarkson RB, et al: Magnetic resonance imaging of degenerative joint disease in a horse: a comparison to other diagnostic techniques, *Equine Vet J* 28:410, 1996.

286. Modransky PD, Rantanen NW: Diagnostic ultrasound examination of the dorsal aspect of the equine metacarpophalangeal joint, *J Equine Vet Sci* 3:56, 1983.

287. Steyn P, Schmitz D: The sonographic diagnosis of chronic proliferative synovitis in the metacarpophalangeal joints of a horse, *Vet Radiol* 30:125, 1989.

288. Denoix JM: Ultrasonographic examination in the diagnosis of joint disease. In McIlwraith CW, Trotter GW, eds: *Joint disease in the horse*, Philadelphia, 1996, Saunders.

CHAPTER 62   Markers of Osteoarthritis: Implications for Early Diagnosis and Monitoring of the Pathological Course and Effects of Therapy

1. Nelson F, Dahlberg L, Lavery S, et al: Evidence for altered type II collagen in patients with OA, *J Clin Invest* 102:2115, 1998.

2. Shinmei M, Ito K, Matasuyama S: Joint fluid carboxy-terminal type II procollagen peptide as a marker of cartilage collagen biosynthesis, *Osteoarthritis Cartilage* 1:121, 1993.

3. Ishiguro N, Ito T, Ito H, et al: Relationship of matrix metalloproteinases and their inhibitors to cartilage proteoglycan and collagen turnover: analyses of synovial fluid from patients with OA, *Arthritis Rheum* 42:129, 1999.

4. Nelson F, Dahlberg L, Lavery S, et al: Evidence for altered synthesis of type II collagen in patients with OA, *J Clin Invest* 102:2115, 1998.

5. Mansson B, Carey D, Alini M, et al: Cartilage and bone metabolism in rheumatoid arthritis: differences between rapid and slow progression of disease identified by serum markers of cartilage metabolism, *J Clin Invest* 95:1071, 1995.

6. Lohmander LS, Ionescu M, Jugessur H, et al: Changes in joint cartilage aggrecan after knee injury and in OA, *Arthritis Rheum* 42:534, 1999.

7. Poole AR, Dieppe P: Biological markers in rheumatoid arthritis, *Semin Arthritis Rheum* 23:17, 1994.

8. Bello AE, Garrett WE Jr, Wang H, et al: Comparison of synovial fluid cartilage marker concentrations and chondral damage assessed arthroscopically in acute knee injury, *Osteoarthritis Cartilage* 5:419, 1997.

9. Hazell PK, Dent C, Fairclough JA, et al: Changes in glycosaminoglycan epitope levels in knee joint fluid following injury, *Arthritis Rheum* 38:953, 1995.

10. Poole AR: *NIH white paper: biomarkers, the OA initiative a basis for discussion*, Bethesda, MD, 2000, National Institutes of Health.

11. Al-Sobayil F, Frisbie DD, Billinghurst RC, et al: Unpublished data, 2000.

12. Sweet MBE, Coelho A, Schnitzler CM, et al: Serum keratan sulfate levels in OA patients, *Arthritis Rheum* 31:648, 1988.

13. Caterson B, Christner JE, Baker JR: Identification of a monoclonal antibody that specifically recognizes corneal and skeletal keratan sulfate, *J Biol Chem* 258:8848, 1983.

14. Brandt KD, Thonar EJ-MA: Lack of association between serum keratan sulfate concentrations and cartilage changes of OA after transection of the anterior cruciate ligament in the dog, *Arthritis Rheum* 32:647, 1989.

15. Innes JF, Sharif M, Barr AR: Changes in concentrations of biochemical markers of OA following surgical repair of ruptured cranial cruciate ligaments in dogs, *Am J Vet Res* 60:1164, 1999.

16. Innes JF, Sharif M, Barr AR: Relations between biochemical markers of OA and other disease parameters in a population of dogs with naturally acquired OA of the genual joint, *Am J Vet Res* 59:1530, 1998.

17. Frisbie DD, Ray CS, Ionescu M, et al: Measurement of synovial fluid and serum concentrations of the 846 epitope of chondroitin sulfate and of carboxy propeptides of type II procollagen for diagnosis of osteochondral fragmentation in horses, *Am J Vet Res* 60:306, 1999.

18. Laverty S, Ionescu M, Marcoux M, et al: Alterations in cartilage type-II procollagen and aggrecan contents in synovial fluid in equine osteochondrosis, *J Orthop Res* 18:399, 2000.

19. Lohmander LS, Saxne T, Heinegard DK: Release of cartilage oligomeric matrix protein (COMP) into joint fluid after knee injury and in OA, *Ann Rheum Dis* 53:8, 1994.

20. Clark AG, Jordan JM, Vilim V, et al: Serum cartilage oligomeric matrix protein reflects OA presence and severity: the Johnston County OA Project, *Arthritis Rheum* 42:2356, 1999.

21. Conrozier T, Saxne T, Fan CS, et al: Serum concentrations of cartilage oligomeric matrix protein and bone sialoprotein in hip OA: a one year prospective study, *Ann Rheum Dis* 57:527, 1998.

22. Sharif M, George E, Dieppe PA: Correlation between synovial fluid markers of cartilage and bone turnover and scintigraphic scan abnormalities in OA of the knee, *Arthritis Rheum* 38:78, 1995.

23. Misumi K, Vilim V, Clegg PD, et al: COMP in equine synovial fluids and sera. Havemeyer Symposium Molecular Markers of Cartilage and Bone Metabolism in the Horse, Northampton, UK, 2000.

24. Arai K, Misumi D, Carter SD, et al: Analysis of cartilage oligomeric matrix protein (COMP) degradation and synthesis in equine joint disease, *Equine Vet J* 37:31, 2005.

25. Salisbury C, Sharif M: Relations between synovial fluid and serum concentrations of osteocalcin and other markers of joint tissue turnover in the knee joint compared with peripheral blood, *Ann Rheum Dis* 56:558, 1997.

26. Lepage OM: Physiological variation in bone markers in horses. Havemeyer Symposium Molecular Markers of Cartilage and Bone Metabolism in the Horse, Northampton, UK, 2000.

27. Grafenau P, Eicher R, Uebelhart B, et al: General anaesthesia decreases osteocalcin plasma concentrations in horses, *Equine Vet J* 31:533, 1999.

28. Fuller CJ, Barr AR, Sharif M, et al: Cross-sectional comparison of synovial fluid biochemical markers in equine OA and the correlation of these markers with articular cartilage damage, *Osteoarthritis Cartilage* 9:49, 2001.

29. Bonde M, Garnero P, Fledelius C, et al: Measurement of bone degradation products in serum using antibodies reactive with an isomerized form of an 8 amino acid sequence of the C-telopeptide of type I collagen, *J Bone Miner Res* 12:1028, 1997.

30. Garnero P, Jouvenne P, Buchs N, et al: Uncoupling of bone metabolism in rheumatoid arthritis patients with or without joint destruction: assessment with serum type I collagen breakdown products, *Bone* 24:381, 1999.

31. Frisbie D, Billinghurst R: Unpublished data, 2001.

32. Petersson IF, Boegard T, Dahlstrom J, et al: Bone scan and serum markers of bone and cartilage in patients with knee pain and OA, *Osteoarthritis Cartilage* 6:33, 1998.

33. Petersson IF, Boegard T, Svensson B, et al: Changes in cartilage and bone metabolism identified by serum markers in early OA of the knee joint, *Br J Rheumatol* 37:46, 1998.

34. Frisbie DD, Al-Sobayil F, Billinghurst RC, et al: Changes in synovial fluid and serum biomarkers with exercise and early OA in horses, *Osteoarthritis Cartilage* 16:1196, 2008.

35. Kawcak CE, Frisbie DD, Werpy NM, et al: Effects of exercise vs experimental OA on imaging outcomes, *Osteoarthritis Cartilage* 16:1519, 2008.

36. Misumi K, Vilim V, Hatazoe T, et al: Serum level of cartilage oligomeric matrix protein (COMP) in equine OA, *Equine Vet J* 34:602, 2002.

37. Taylor SE, Weaver MP, Pitsillides AA, et al: Cartilage oligomeric matrix protein

and hyaluronan levels in synovial fluid from horses with OA of the tarsometatarsal joint compared to a control population, *Equine Vet J* 38:502, 2006.

38. Skioldebrand E, Heinegard D, Eloranta ML, et al: Enhanced concentration of COMP (cartilage oligomeric matrix protein) in osteochondral fractures from racing Thoroughbreds, *J Orthop Res* 23:156, 2005.

39. Fuller CJ, Barr AR, Sharif M, et al: Cross-sectional comparison of synovial fluid biochemical markers in equine OA and the correlation of these markers with articular cartilage damage, *Osteoarthritis Cartilage* 9:49, 2001.

40. Frisbie DD, Duffy E, Arthur R, et al: Prospective clinical study assessing serum biomarkers for musculoskeletal disease in 2- to 3-yr-old racing Thoroughbreds, *Proc Am Assoc Equine Pract* 51:301, 2005.

CHAPTER 63   Gene Therapy

1. Anderson WF: Human gene therapy, *Nature* 392:25, 1998.
2. Martin P, Thomas S: The commercial development of gene therapy in Europe and the USA, *Hum Gene Ther* 9:87, 1998.
3. Frisbie D, McIlwraith C: Evaluation of gene therapy as a treatment for equine traumatic arthritis and osteoarthritis, *Clin Orthop* 375S:S273, 2000.
4. Frisbie D, Ghivizzani S, Robbins P: Treatment of experimental equine osteoarthritis by an in vivo delivery of the equine interleukin-1 receptor antagonist gene, *Gene Ther* 9:12, 2009.
5. Haupt J, Frisbie D, McIlwraith C, et al: Duel transduction of interleukin-like growth-factor-1 and interleukin-1 receptor antagonist protein controls cartilage degradation in an osteoarthritic culture model, *J Orthop Res* 23:118, 2005.
6. Morrissey S, Frisbie D, Robbins P, et al: IL-1ra/IGF-1 gene therapy modulates repair of microfractured chondral defects, *Clin Orthop* 462:221, 2007.
7. Southwood L, Frisbie D, Kawcak C, et al: Delivery of growth factors using gene therapy to enhance bone healing, *Vet Surg* 33:565, 2004.
8. Nixon A, Haupt J, Frisbie D, et al: Gene-mediated restoration of cartilage matrix by combination insulin-like growth factor-1/interleukin-1 receptor antagonist therapy, *Gene Ther* 12:177, 2005.
9. Southwood L, Kawcak C, McIlwraith C, et al: Evaluation of Ad-BMP-2 enhancing fracture healing in an infected nonunion fracture rabbit model, *J Orthop Res* 22:66, 2004.
10. Levick J: Blood flow and mass transport in synovial joints. In Renkin EM, Michel CC, et al, editors: *Handbook of physiology, The cardiovascular system*, Baltimore, 1984, American Physiology Society.
11. Frisbie D, McIlwraith C: Gene therapy. Future therapies in osteoarthritis, *Vet Clin North Am Equine Pract* 17:233, 2001.
12. Otani K, Nita I, Macaulay W, et al: Suppression of antigen-induced arthritis in rabbits by ex vivo gene therapy, *J Immunol* 156:3558, 1996.
13. Arend W, Dayer J: Cytokines and cytokine inhibitors or antagonists in rheumatoid arthritis, *Arthritis Rheum* 33:305, 1990.

14. Arend W, Dayer J: Inhibition of the production and effects of interleukin-1 and tumor necrosis factor alpha in rheumatoid arthritis, *Arthritis Rheum* 38:151, 1995.
15. Wood D, Ihrie E, Hamerman D: Release of interleukin-1 from human synovial tissue, *Arthritis Rheum* 28:853, 1991.
16. Caron J, Fernandes JC, Martel-Pelletier J, et al: Chondroprotective effects of intra-articular injections of interleukin-1 receptor antagonist in experimental osteoarthritis, *Arthritis Rheum* 39:1535, 1996.
17. Bandara G, Mueller G, Galea-Lauri J, et al: Intra-articular expression of biologically active interleukin-I receptor antagonist protein by ex vivo gene transfer, *Proc Natl Acad Sci U S A* 90:10764, 1991.
18. Howard R, McIlwraith C, Trotter GW, et al: Cloning of equine interleukin 1 receptor antagonist and determination of its full-length cDNA sequence, *Am J Vet Res* 59:712, 1998.
19. Frisbie D, McIlwraith C: Evaluation of gene therapy as a treatment for equine traumatic arthritis. A species with clinical disease, *Clin Orthop Rel Res* 3795:5273, 2000.
20. Frisbie D, McIlwraith C: The effects of triamcinolone acetate on an in vivo equine osteochondral fragment exercise model, *Equine Vet J* 29:349, 1997.
21. Frisbie D, Kawcak C, Trotter G, et al: The effects of 6-alpha methylprednisolone acetate on an in vivo equine osteochondral fragment exercise model, *Am J Vet Res* 12:1619, 1998.
22. Goodrich L, Choi B, DudaCarbone B, et al: High-efficiency gene targeting to mammalian joint tissue using cell-complimentary adeno-associated viral vector serotypes, *Mol Ther* 13:S191, 2006.
23. Goodrich L, Choi B, DudaCarbone B, et al: Serotype-specific transduction of equine joint tissue by self-complementary AAV vectors, *Human Gene Therapy* 20:1697, 2009.
24. Goodrich L, Brower-Toland P, Warnick L, et al: Direct adenovirus-medial IGF-1 gene transduction of synovium induces persisting synovial fluid IGF-1 ligand elevation, *Gene Ther* 13:1253, 2006.
25. Goodrich L, Hidaka C, Robbins P, et al: Genetic modification of chondrocytes with insulin-like growth factor-1 enhances cartilage healing in an equine model, *J Bone Joint Surg Br* 89:672, 2007.
26. Haupt J, Frisbie D, McIlwraith C, et al: Dual transduction of insulin-like growth factor-1 and interleukin-1 receptor antagonist protein controls cartilage degradation in an osteoarthritic culture model, *J Orthop Res* 23:118, 2005.
27. Nixon A, Haupt J, Frisbie D, et al: Gene-mediated restoration of cartilage matrix for combination insulin-like growth factor-1/interleukin-1 receptor antagonist therapy, *Gene Ther* 12:177, 2005.
28. Morrisset S, Frisbie D, Robbins P, et al: IL-1Ra.IGF-1 gene therapy modulates repair of microfractured chondral defects, *Clin Orthop* 462:221, 2007.
29. Southwood L, Frisbie D, Kawcak C, et al: Delivery of growth factors using gene therapy to enhance bone healing, *Vet Surg* 33:565, 2004.

30. Southwood L, Kawcak C, McIlwraith C, et al: Evaluation of Ad-BMP-2 enhancing fracture healing in an infected nonunion fracture rabbit model, *J Orthop Res* 22:66, 2004.

CHAPTER 64   Models of Equine Joint Disease

1. Todhunter PG, Kincaid SA, Todhunter RJ, et al: Immunohistochemical analysis of an equine model of synovitis-induced arthritis, *Am J Vet Res* 57:1080, 1996.
2. McIlwraith CW, Van Sickle DC: Experimentally induced arthritis of the equine carpus: histologic and histochemical changes in the articular cartilage, *Am J Vet Res* 42:209, 1981.
3. MacDonald MH, Stover SM, Willits NH, et al: Regulation of matrix metabolism in equine cartilage explant cultures by interleukin 1, *Am J Vet Res* 53:2278, 1992.
4. Goldring MB: The role of cytokines as inflammatory mediators in osteoarthritis: lessons from animal models, *Connect Tissue Res* 40:1, 1999.
5. Back W, Barneveld A, van Weeren PR, et al: Kinematic gait analysis in equine carpal lameness, *Acta Anat (Basel)* 146:86, 1993.
6. Peloso JG, Stick JA, Caron JP, et al: Effects of hylan on amphotericin-induced carpal lameness in equids, *Am J Vet Res* 54:1527, 1993.
7. Nakai H, Niimi A, Ueda M: The influence of compressive loading on growth of cartilage of the mandibular condyle in vitro, *Arch Oral Biol* 43:505, 1998.
8. Wu QQ, Chen Q: Mechanoregulation of chondrocyte proliferation, maturation, and hypertrophy: ion-channel dependent transduction of matrix deformation signals, *Exp Cell Res* 256:383, 2000.
9. Messner K, Fahlgren A, Ross I, et al: Simultaneous changes in bone mineral density and articular cartilage in a rabbit meniscectomy model of knee osteoarthrosis, *Osteoarthritis Cartilage* 8:197, 2000.
10. Burr DB: The importance of subchondral bone in osteoarthrosis, *Curr Opin Rheumatol* 10:256, 1998.
11. Muller-Gerbl M: The subchondral bone plate, *Adv Anat Embryol Cell Biol* 141:1, 1998.
12. Frisbie DD, Kawcak CE, Trotter GW, et al: The assessment of chondrocyte proteoglycan metabolism using molecular sieve column chromatography as compared to three commonly utilized techniques, *Osteoarthritis Cartilage* 6:137, 1998.
13. Kawcak CE, Trotter GW, Frisbie DD, et al: Maintenance of equine articular cartilage explants in serum-free and serum-supplemented media, compared with that in a commercial supplemented medium, *Am J Vet Res* 57:1261, 1996.
14. Kawcak CE: Unpublished data, 2000.
15. Frisbie DD, Morisset S: Unpublished data, 2000.
16. Fortier LA, Schnabel LV, Mohammed HO, et al: Assessment of cartilage degradation effects of matrix metalloproteinase-13 in equine cartilage cocultured with synoviocytes, *Am J Vet Res* 68:379, 2007.
17. Beluche LA, Bertone AL, Anderson DE, et al: In vitro dose-dependent effects of

enrofloxacin on equine articular cartilage, *Am J Vet Res* 60:577, 1999.

18. Dechant JE, Baxter GM, Frisbie DD, et al: Effects of dosage titration of methylprednisolone acetate and triamcinolone acetonide on interleukin-1-conditioned equine articular cartilage explants in vitro, *Equine Vet J* 35:444, 2003.

19. Dechant JE, Baxter GM, Frisbie DD, et al: Effects of glucosamine hydrochloride and chondroitin sulphate, alone and in combination, on normal and interleukin-1 conditioned equine articular cartilage explant metabolism, *Equine Vet J* 37:227, 2005.

20. Munsterman AS, Bertone AL, Zachos TA, et al: Effects of the omega-3 fatty acid, alpha-linolenic acid, on lipopolysaccharide-challenged synovial explants from horses, *Am J Vet Res* 66:1503, 2005.

21. Pearson W, Lindinger MI: Simulated digest of a glucosamine-based equine nutraceutical modifies effect of IL-1 in a cartilage explant model of inflammation, *J Vet Pharmacol Ther* 31:268, 2008.

22. Huser CA, Davies ME: Validation of an in vitro single-impact load model of the initiation of osteoarthritis-like changes in articular cartilage, *J Orthop Res* 24:725, 2006.

23. Pearson W, Orth MW, Lindinger MI: Differential anti-inflammatory and chondroprotective effects of simulated digests of indomethacin and an herbal composite (Mobility) in a cartilage explant model of articular inflammation, *J Vet Pharmacol Ther* 30:523, 2007.

24. Sandler EA, Frisbie DD, McIlwraith CW: A dose titration of triamcinolone acetonide on insulin-like growth factor-1 and interleukin-1-conditioned equine cartilage explants, *Equine Vet J* 36:58, 2004.

25. Hardy J, Bertone AL, Muir WW: Local hemodynamics, permeability, and oxygen metabolism during acute inflammation of innervated or denervated isolated equine joints, *Am J Vet Res* 59:1307, 1998.

26. Hardy J, Bertone AL, Weisbrode SE, et al: Cell trafficking, mediator release, and articular metabolism in acute inflammation of innervated or denervated isolated equine joints, *Am J Vet Res* 59:88, 1998.

27. Bragdon B, Bertone AL, Hardy J, et al: Use of an isolated joint model to detect early changes induced by intra-articular injection of paclitaxel-impregnated polymeric microspheres, *J Invest Surg* 14:169, 2001.

28. Easton KL, Kawcak CE: Evaluation of increased subchondral bone density in areas of contact in the metacarpophalangeal joint during joint loading in horses. *Am J Vet Res* 68:816, 2007.

29. Elce YA, Southwood LL, Nutt JN, et al: Ex vivo comparison of a novel tapered-sleeve and traditional full-limb transfixation pin cast for distal radial fracture stabilization in the horse, *Vet Comp Orthop Traumatol* 19:93, 2006.

30. Frisbie DD, Cross MW, McIlwraith CW: A comparative study of articular cartilage thickness in the stifle of animal species used in human pre-clinical studies compared to articular cartilage thickness in the human knee, *Vet Comp Orthop Traumatol* 19:142, 2006.

31. Palmer JL, Bertone AL, Malemud CJ, et al: Biochemical and biomechanical alterations in equine articular cartilage following an experimentally-induced synovitis, *Osteoarthritis Cartilage* 4:127, 1996.

32. Gustafson SB, Trotter GW, Norrdin RW, et al: Evaluation of intra-articularly administered sodium monoiodoacetate-induced chemical injury to articular cartilage of horses, *Am J Vet Res* 53:1193, 1992.

33. Trotter GW, Yovich JV, McIlwraith CW, et al: Effects of intramuscular polysulfated glycosaminoglycan on chemical and physical defects in equine articular cartilage, *Can J Vet Res* 53:224, 1989.

34. McIlwraith CW, Fessler JF, Blevins WE, et al: Experimentally induced arthritis of the equine carpus: clinical determinations, *Am J Vet Res* 40:11, 1979.

35. Cornelissen BP, Rijkenhuizen AB, van den Hoogen A, et al: Experimental model of synovitis/capsulitis in the equine metacarpophalangeal joint, *Am J Vet Res* 9:978, 1998.

36. Owens JG, Kamerling SG, Stanton SR, et al: Effects of pretreatment with ketoprofen and phenylbutazone on experimentally induced synovitis in horses, *Am J Vet Res* 57:866, 1996.

37. Hamm D, Turchi P, Johnson JC, et al: Determination of an effective dose of eltenac and its comparison with that of flunixin meglumine in horses after experimentally induced carpitis, *Am J Vet Res* 58:298, 1997.

38. Judy CE, Galuppo LD: Evaluation of iatrogenic hemarthrosis of the metacarpophalangeal joint as a method of induction of temporary reversible lameness in horses, *Am J Vet Res* 66:1084, 2005.

39. Simmons EJ, Bertone AL, Weisbrode SE: Instability-induced osteoarthritis in the metacarpophalangeal joint of horses, *Am J Vet Res* 60:7, 1999.

40. Trotter GW: Personal communications, 1996.

41. Bertone AL, Goin S, Kamei SJ, et al: Metacarpophalangeal collateral ligament reconstruction using small intestinal submucosa in an equine model, *J Biomed Mater Res A* 84:219, 2008.

42. DePuy T, Howard R, Keegan K, et al: Effects of intra-articular botulinum toxin type A in an equine model of acute synovitis: a pilot study, *Am J Phys Med Rehabil* 86:777, 2007.

43. Murray RC, Janicke HC, Henson FM, et al: Equine carpal articular cartilage fibronectin distribution associated with training, joint location and cartilage deterioration, *Equine Vet J* 32:47, 2000.

44. Murray RC, Whitton RC, Vedi S, et al: The effect of training on the calcified zone of equine middle carpal articular cartilage, *Equine Vet J Suppl* 32:274, 1999.

45. Murray RC, Zhu CF, Goodship AE, et al: Exercise affects the mechanical properties and histological appearance of equine articular cartilage, *J Orthop Res* 17:725, 1999.

46. Kawcak CE, McIlwraith CW, Norrdin RW, et al: Clinical effects of exercise on subchondral bone of carpal and metacarpophalangeal joints in horses, *Am J Vet Res* 61:1252, 2000.

47. Bussieres G, Jacques C, Lainay O, et al: Development of a composite orthopaedic pain scale in horses, *Res Vet Sci* 85:294, 2008.

48. Dykgraaf S, Firth EC, Rogers CW, et al: Effects of exercise on chondrocyte viability and subchondral bone sclerosis in the distal third metacarpal and metatarsal bones of young horses, *Vet J* 178:53, 2008.

49. Firth EC, Rogers CW, van Weeren PR, et al: Changes in diaphyseal and epiphyseal bone parameters in thoroughbred horses after withdrawal from training, *J Musculoskelet Neuronal Interact* 7:74, 2007.

50. Moffat PA, Firth EC, Rogers CW, et al: The influence of exercise during growth on ultrasonographic parameters of the superficial digital flexor tendon of young Thoroughbred horses, *Equine Vet J* 40:136, 2008.

51. Nugent GE, Law AW, Wong EG, et al: Site- and exercise-related variation in structure and function of cartilage from equine distal metacarpal condyle, *Osteoarthritis Cartilage* 12:826, 2004.

52. Rogers CW, Firth EC, McIlwraith CW, et al: Evaluation of a new strategy to modulate skeletal development in racehorses by imposing track-based exercise during growth: the effects on 2- and 3-year-old racing careers, *Equine Vet J* 40:119, 2008.

53. Rogers CW, Firth EC, McIlwraith CW, et al: Evaluation of a new strategy to modulate skeletal development in Thoroughbred performance horses by imposing track-based exercise during growth, *Equine Vet J* 40:111, 2008.

54. Definition and classification of lameness. Guide for veterinary service and judging of equestrian events, Lexington, Ky, 1991, American Association of Equine Practitioners.

55. Yarbrough TB, Lee MR, Hornof WJ, et al: Evaluation of samarium-153 for synovectomy in an osteochondral fragment-induced model of synovitis in horses, *Vet Surg* 29:252, 2000.

56. Foland JW, McIlwraith CW, Trotter GW, et al: Effect of betamethasone and exercise on equine carpal joints with osteochondral fragments, *Vet Surg* 23:369, 1994.

57. Kawcak CE, Frisbie DD, Trotter GW, et al: Effects of intravenous administration of sodium hyaluronate on carpal joints in exercising horses after arthroscopic surgery and osteochondral fragmentation, *Am J Vet Res* 58:1132, 1997.

58. Frisbie DD, Kawcak CE, Trotter GW, et al: Effects of triamcinolone acetonide on an in vivo equine osteochondral fragment exercise model, *Equine Vet J* 29:349, 1997.

59. Frisbie DD, Kawcak CE, Baxter GM, et al: Effects of 6alpha-ethylprednisolone acetate on an equine osteochondral fragment exercise model, *Am J Vet Res* 59:1619, 1998.

60. Frisbie DD, McIlwraith CW: Evaluation of gene therapy as a treatment for equine traumatic arthritis and osteoarthritis, *Clin Orthop* 379(Suppl):S273, 2000.

61. Frisbie DD, Al-Sobayil F, Billinghurst RC, et al: Changes in synovial fluid and serum biomarkers with exercise and early osteoarthritis in horses, *Osteoarthritis Cartilage* 16:1196, 2008.

62. Kawcak CE, Frisbie DD, Werpy NM, et al: Effects of exercise vs experimental osteoarthritis on imaging outcomes, *Osteoarthritis Cartilage* 16:1519, 2008.

63. Kawcak CE, Frisbie DD, McIlwraith CW, et al: Evaluation of avocado and soybean unsaponifiable extracts for treatment of horses with experimentally induced osteoarthritis, *Am J Vet Res* 68:598, 2007.

64. Frisbie DD, Kawcak CE, Werpy NM, et al: Clinical, biochemical, and histologic effects of intra-articular administration of autologous conditioned serum in horses with experimentally induced osteoarthritis, *Am J Vet Res* 68:290, 2007.

65. Frisbie DD, Ghivizzani SC, Robbins PD, et al: Treatment of experimental equine osteoarthritis by in vivo delivery of the equine interleukin-1 receptor antagonist gene, *Gene Ther* 9:12, 2002.

66. Haussler KK, Hill AE, Frisbie DD, et al: Determination and use of mechanical nociceptive thresholds of the thoracic limb to assess pain associated with induced osteoarthritis of the middle carpal joint in horses, *Am J Vet Res* 68:1167, 2007.

67. Richardson DW, Clark CC: Effects of short-term cast immobilization on equine articular cartilage, *Am J Vet Res* 54:449, 1993.

68. van Harreveld P, Lillich J, Kawcak C, et al: Clinical evaluation of the effects of immobilization followed by re-mobilization and exercise on the equine metacarpophalangeal joint, *Am J Vet Res* 63:282, 2002.

69. van Harreveld P, Lillich J, Kawcak C, et al: The effects of immobilization followed by remobilization on bone mineral density, bone histomorphometry, and bone formation of the equine metacarpophalangeal joint, *Am J Vet Res* 63:276, 2002.

70. Delguste C, Amory H, Doucet M, et al: Pharmacological effects of tiludronate in horses after long-term immobilization, *Bone* 41:414, 2007.

71. Hurtig MB, Fretz PB, Doige CE, et al: Effects of lesion size and location on equine articular cartilage repair, *Can J Vet Res* 52:137, 1988.

72. Kold SE, Hickman J, Melsen F: An experimental study of the healing process of equine chondral and osteochondral defects, *Equine Vet J* 18:18, 1986.

73. Ray C, Baxter G, McIlwraith C, et al: Development of subchondral cystic lesions following subchondral bone trauma in horses, *Vet Surg* 23:414, 1994.

74. Frisbie DD, Trotter GW, Powers BE, et al: Arthroscopic subchondral bone plate microfracture technique augments healing of large chondral defects in the radial carpal bone and medial femoral condyle of horses, *Vet Surg* 28:242, 1999.

75. Frisbie DD: Personal communication, 2001.

76. Vachon A, McIlwraith CW, Trotter GW, et al: Neochondrogenesis in free intra-articular, periosteal, and perichondral autografts in horses, *Am J Vet Res* 50:1787, 1989.

77. Vachon AM, McIlwraith CW, Keeley FW: Biochemical study of repair of induced osteochondral defects of the distal portion of the radial carpal bone in horses by use of periosteal autografts, *Am J Vet Res* 52:328, 1991.

78. Vachon AM, McIlwraith CW, Powers BE, et al: Morphologic and biochemical study of sternal cartilage autografts for resurfacing induced osteochondral defects in horses, *Am J Vet Res* 53:1038, 1992.

79. Howard RD, McIlwraith CW, Trotter GW, et al: Long-term fate and effects of exercise on sternal cartilage autografts used for repair of large osteochondral defects in horses, *Am J Vet Res* 55:1158, 1994.

80. Hurtig MB: Experimental use of small osteochondral grafts for resurfacing the equine third carpal bone, *Equine Vet J Suppl* 6:23, 1988.

81. Frisbie DD, Morisset S, Ho CP, et al: Effects of calcified cartilage on healing of chondral defects treated with microfracture in horses, *Am J Sports Med* 34:1824, 2006.

82. Sams AE, Minor RR, Wootton JA, et al: Local and remote matrix responses to chondrocyte-laden collagen scaffold implantation in extensive articular cartilage defects, *Osteoarthritis Cartilage* 3:61, 1995.

83. Frisbie DD, Bowman SM, Colhoun HA, et al: Evaluation of autologous chondrocyte transplantation via a collagen membrane in equine articular defects: results at 12 and 18 months, *Osteoarthritis Cartilage* 16:667, 2008.

84. Edwards RB, Lu Y, Cole BJ, et al: Comparison of radiofrequency treatment and mechanical debridement of fibrillated cartilage in an equine model, *Vet Comp Orthop Traumatol* 21:41, 2008.

85. Edwards RB 3rd, Lu Y, Uthamanthil RK, et al: Comparison of mechanical debridement and radiofrequency energy for chondroplasty in an in vivo equine model of partial thickness cartilage injury, *Osteoarthritis Cartilage* 15:169, 2007.

86. Goodrich LR, Hidaka C, Robbins PD, et al: Genetic modification of chondrocytes with insulin-like growth factor-1 enhances cartilage healing in an equine model, *J Bone Joint Surg Br* 89:672, 2007.

87. Morisset S, Frisbie DD, Robbins PD, et al: IL-1ra/IGF-1 gene therapy modulates repair of microfractured chondral defects, *Clin Orthop Relat Res* 462:221, 2007.

88. Wilke MM, Nydam DV, Nixon AJ: Enhanced early chondrogenesis in articular defects following arthroscopic mesenchymal stem cell implantation in an equine model, *J Orthop Res* 25:913, 2007.

89. Koch TG, Betts DH: Stem cell therapy for joint problems using the horse as a clinically relevant animal model, *Expert Opin Biol Ther* 7:1621, 2007.

90. Gustafson SB, McIlwraith CW, Jones RL, et al: Further investigations into the potentiation of infection by intra-articular injection of polysulfated glycosaminoglycan and the effect of filtration and intra-articular injection of amikacin, *Am J Vet Res* 50:2018, 1989.

91. Gustafson SB, McIlwraith CW, Jones RL: Comparison of the effect of polysulfated glycosaminoglycan, corticosteroids, and sodium hyaluronate in the potentiation of a subinfective dose of *Staphylococcus aureus* in the midcarpal joint of horses, *Am J Vet Res* 50:2014, 1989.

92. Bertone AL, McIlwraith CW, Jones RL, et al: Comparison of various treatments for experimentally induced equine infectious arthritis, *Am J Vet Res* 48:519, 1987.

93. Bertone AL, McIlwraith CW, Jones RL, et al: Povidone-iodine lavage treatment of experimentally induced equine infectious arthritis, *Am J Vet Res* 48:712, 1987.

94. Brown NA, Kawcak CE, McIlwraith CW, et al: Architectural properties of distal forelimb muscles in horses, *Equus caballus*, *J Morphol* 258:106, 2003.

95. Brown NA, Pandy MG, Buford WL, et al: Moment arms about the carpal and metacarpophalangeal joints for flexor and extensor muscles in equine forelimbs, *Am J Vet Res* 64:351, 2003.

96. Brown NA, Pandy MG, Kawcak CE, et al: Force- and moment-generating capacities of muscles in the distal forelimb of the horse, *J Anat* 203:101, 2003.

97. Swanstrom MD, Zarucco L, Hubbard M, et al: Musculoskeletal modeling and dynamic simulation of the thoroughbred equine forelimb during stance phase of the gallop, *J Biomech Eng* 127:318, 2005.

98. Zarucco L, Swanstrom MD, Driessen B, et al: An in vivo equine forelimb model for short-term recording of peak isometric force in the superficial and deep digital flexor muscles, *Vet Surg* 32:439, 2003.

99. Merritt JS, Davies HM, Burvill C, et al: Influence of muscle-tendon wrapping on calculations of joint reaction forces in the equine distal forelimb, *J Biomed Biotechnol* 165730, 2008.

CHAPTER 65 Infectious Arthritis and Fungal Infectious Arthritis

Infectious Arthritis

1. Steel CM, Hunt AR, Adams PL, et al: Factors associated with prognosis for survival and athletic use in foals with septic arthritis: 93 cases (1987-1994), *J Am Vet Med Assoc* 215:973, 1999.

2. Smith LJ, Marr CM, Payne RJ, et al: What is the likelihood that Thoroughbred foals treated for septic arthritis will race? *Equine Vet J* 36:452, 2004.

3. Palmer JL, Bertone AL: Joint structure, biochemistry and biochemical disequilibrium in synovitis and equine joint disease, *Equine Vet J* 26:263, 1994.

4. Bertone AL: Infectious arthritis. In McIlwraith CW, Trotter GW, eds: *Joint disease in the horse*, Philadelphia, 1996, Saunders.

5. Cohen ND: Causes of and farm management factors associated with disease and death in foals, *J Am Vet Med Assoc* 204:1644, 1994.

6. Schneider RK, Bramlage LR, Moore RM, et al: Open drainage, intraarticular and systemic antibiotics in the treatment of septic arthritis/tenosynovitis in horses, *Equine Vet J* 24:436, 1992.

7. Sanchez LC, Giguere S, Lester GD: Factors associated with survival of neonatal foals with bacteremia and racing performance of surviving Thoroughbreds: 423 cases (1982-2007), *J Am Vet Med Assoc* 233:1446, 2008.

8. Meijer MC, van Weeren PR, Rijkenhuizen AB: Clinical experiences of treating septic

arthritis in the equine by repeated joint lavage: a series of 39 cases, *J Vet Med Physiol Pathol Clin Med* 47:351, 2000.

9. Schneider RX, Bramlage LR, Moore RM, et al: A retrospective study of 192 horses affected with septic arthritis/tenosynovitis, *Equine Vet J* 24:436, 1992.

10. Olds AM, Stewart AA, Freeman DE, Schaeffer DJ: Evaluation of the rate of development of septic arthritis after elective arthroscopy in horses: 7 cases (1994-1954), *J Am Vet Med Assoc* 229:1949, 2006.

11. Moore RM, Schneider RK, Kowalski J, et al: Antimicrobial susceptibility of bacterial isolates from 233 horses with musculoskeletal infection during 1979-1989, *Equine Vet J* 24:450, 1992.

12. Kawaquchi K, Church S: *Clostridium septicum* arthritis in three foals, *Aust Vet J* 82:612, 2004.

13. Raisis AL, Hodgson JL, Hodgson DR: Equine neonatal septicaemia: 24 cases, *Aust Vet J* 73:137, 1996.

14. Madison JB, Reid BV, Raskin RE: Amphotericin B treatment of *Candida* arthritis in two horses, *J Am Vet Med Assoc* 206:338, 1995.

15. Hewes CA, Schneider RK, Baszler TV, et al: Septic arthritis and granulomatous synovitis caused by infection with *Mycobacterium avium* complex in a horse, *J Am Vet Med Assoc* 226:2035, 2005.

16. Kenney DG, Robbins SC, Prescott JF, et al: Development of reactive arthritis and resistance to erythromycin and rifampin in a foal during treatment for *Rhodococcus equi* pneumonia, *Equine Vet J* 26:246, 1994.

17. Kuemmerie JM, Uhlig H, Dofler J: Severe acute inflammatory reaction (SAIR) of the fetlock joint after intraarticular hyaluronate injection in a horse, *Vet Comp Orthop Traumatol* 19:236, 2006.

18. Bertone AL, McIlwraith CM, Jones RL: Comparison of various treatments for experimentally induced equine infectious arthritis, *Am J Vet Res* 48:519, 1987.

19. Hague BA, Honnas CM, Simpson RB, et al: Evaluation of skin bacterial flora before and after aseptic preparation of clipped and nonclipped arthrocentesis sites in horses, *Vet Surg* 26:121, 1997.

20. Wright IM, Smith MR, Humphrey DJ, et al: Endoscopic surgery in the treatment of contaminated and injected synovial cavities, *Equine Vet J* 35:613, 2003.

21. Kidd JA, Barr AR, Tarlton JF: Use of matrix metalloproteinases 2 and 9 and white blood cell counts in monitoring the treatment and predicting the survival of horses with septic arthritis, *Vet Rec* 161:329, 2007.

22. Fietz S, Bondzio A, Moschos A, et al: Measurement of equine myeloperoxidase (MPO) activity in synovial fluid by a modified MPO assay and evaluation of joint diseases—an initial case study, *Res Vet Sci* 84:347, 2008.

23. Madison JB, Sommer M, Spencer PA: Relations among synovial membrane histopathologic findings, synovial fluid cytologic findings and bacterial culture results in horses with suspected infectious arthritis: 64 cases (1979-1987), *J Am Vet Med Assoc* 198:1655, 1991.

24. Tulamo R-M, Bramlage L, Gabel A: Sequential clinical and synovial fluid changes associated with acute infectious arthritis, *Equine Vet J* 21:325, 1989.

25. Tulamo R-M, Bramlage L, Gabel A: The influence of corticosteroids on sequential clinical and synovial fluid parameters in joints with acute infectious arthritis in the horse, *Equine Vet J* 21:332, 1989.

26. Crabill MR, Cohen ND, Martin LJ, et al: Detection of bacteria in equine synovial fluid by use of the polymerase chain reaction, *Vet Surg* 25:195, 1996.

27. Stahl HD, Hubner B, Seidl B, et al: Detection of multiple viral DNA species in synovial tissue and fluid of patients with early arthritis, *Ann Rheum Dis* 59:342, 2000.

28. Spiers S, May SA, Harrison LJ, et al: Proteolytic enzymes in equine joints with infectious arthritis, *Equine Vet J* 26:48, 1994.

29. Arican M, Coughlan AR, Clegg PD, et al: Matrix metalloproteinases 2 and 9 activity in bovine synovial fluids, *J Vet Med A Physiol Pathol Clin Med* 47:449, 2000.

30. Bertone AL, Palmer JL, Jones J: Synovial fluid cytokines and eicosanoids as markers of joint disease in horses, *Vet Surg* 30:258, 2001.

31. Pilleul F, Garcia J: Septic arthritis of the spine facet joint: early positive diagnosis of magnetic resonance imaging: review of two cases, *Joint Bone Spine* 67:234, 2000.

32. Graif M, Schweitzer ME, Deely D, et al: The septic versus nonseptic inflamed joint: MRI characteristics, *Skeletal Radiol* 28:616, 1999.

33. Orsini JA, Moate PJ, Engiles J, et al: Cefotaxime kinetics in plasma and synovial fluid following intravenous administration in horses, *J Vet Pharmacol Ther* 27:293, 2004.

34. Bertone AL, Tremaine WH, Macoris DG, et al: Effect of the chronic systemic administration of an injectable enrofloxacin solution on physical, musculoskeletal, and histologic parameters in adult horses, *Am J Vet Res* 217:1514, 2000.

35. Baldessari A, Bermingham E, Bargar A, et al: Evaluation of the gross and histologic changes in articular cartilage of neonatal foals dosed with enrofloxacin, *Equine Vet J* 2001 (in review).

36. Zhanel GG: Influence of pharmacokinetic and pharmacodynamic principles on antibiotic selection, *Curr Infect Dis Rep* 3:29, 2001.

37. Godber LM, Walker RD, Stein GE, et al: Pharmacokinetics, nephrotoxicosis, and in vitro antibacterial activity associated with single versus multiple (three times) daily gentamicin treatments in horses, *Am J Vet Res* 56:613, 1995.

38. Green SL, Conlon RD: Clinical pharmacokinetics of amikacin in hypoxic premature foals, *Equine Vet J* 25:276, 1993.

39. Wichtel MG, Breuhaus BA, Aucoin D: Relation between pharmacokinetics of amikacin sulfate and sepsis score in clinically normal and hospitalized neonatal foals, *J Am Vet Med Assoc* 200:1339, 1992.

40. Raisis AL, Hodgson JL, Hodgson DR: Serum gentamicin concentration in compromised neonatal foals, *Equine Vet J* 30:324, 1998.

41. Firth EC, Klein WR, Nouws JF, et al: Effect of induced synovial inflammation on pharmacokinetics and synovial concentration of sodium ampicillin and kanamycin sulfate after systemic administration in ponies, *J Vet Pharmacol Ther* 11:56, 1988.

42. Lloyd KCK, Stover SM, Pascoe JR, et al: Synovial fluid pH, cytologic characteristics and gentamicin concentration after intra-articular administration of the drug in an experimental model of infectious arthritis in horses, *Am J Vet Res* 51:1363, 1990.

43. Wininger DA, Fass RJ: Antibiotic-impregnated cement and beads for orthopedic infections, *Antimicrob Agents Chemother* 40:2675, 1996.

44. Bertone AL, Caprile KA, Davis DM, et al: Serum and synovial fluid concentration of gentamicin administered chronically to horses with experimentally induced infectious arthritis, *Vet Surg* 19:57, 1990.

45. Lloyd KCK, Stover SM, Pascoe JR, et al: Plasma and synovial fluid concentrations of gentamicin in horses after intraarticular administration of buffered and unbuffered gentamicin, *Am J Vet Med Res* 49:644, 1988.

46. Beluche LA, Bertone AL, Anderson DE, et al: Dose-dependent effect of enrofloxacin on equine articular cartilage, *Am J Vet Res* 60:571, 1999.

47. Klohnen A, Wilson DG, Hendrickson DA, et al: Effects of potentiated chlorhexidine on bacteria and tarsocrural joints in ponies, *Am J Vet Res* 57:756, 1996.

48. Wilson DG, Cooley AJ, MacWilliams PS, et al: Effects of 0.05% chlorhexidine lavage on the tarsocrural joints of horses, *Vet Surg* 23:442, 1994.

49. Swalec Tobias KM, Schneider RK, Besser TE: Use of antimicrobial-impregnated polymethylmethacrylate, *J Am Vet Med Assoc* 208:841, 1996.

50. Ostermann PA, Seligson D, Henry SL: Local antibiotic therapy for severe open fractures: a review of 1085 consecutive cases, *J Bone Joint Surg Br* 77:93, 1995.

51. Schneider RK, Andrea R, Barnes HG: Use of antibiotic-impregnated polymethylmethacrylate for treatment of an open radial fracture in a horse, *J Am Vet Med Assoc* 207:1454, 1995.

52. Holcombe SJ, Schneider RK, Bramlage LR, et al: Use of antibiotic-impregnated polymethylmethacrylate in horses with open or infected fractures or joints: 19 cases (1987-1995), *J Am Vet Med Assoc* 211:889, 1997.

53. Butson RJ, Schramme MC, Garlick MH, et al: Treatment of intrasynovial infection with gentamicin-impregnated polymethylmethacrylate beads, *Vet Rec* 138:460, 1996.

54. Gerhart TN, Roux RD, Hanff PA, et al: Antibiotic-loaded biodegradable bone cement for prophylaxis and treatment of experimental osteomyelitis in rats, *J Orthop Res* 11:250, 1993.

55. DiMaio FR, O'Halloran JJ, Quale JM: In vitro elution of ciprofloxacin from polymethylmethacrylate cement beads, *J Orthop Res* 12:79, 1994.

56. Mehta S, Humphrey JS, Schenkman DI, et al: Gentamicin distribution from a collagen carrier, *J Orthop Res* 14:749, 1996.

57. Ivester KM, Adams SB, Moore GE et al: Gentamicin concentrations in synovial fluid obtained from the tarsocrural joints of horses after implantation of gentamicin-impregnated collagen sponges, *Am J Vet Res* 67:1519, 2006.

58. Cook VL, Bertone AL, Kowalski JJ, et al: Biodegradable drug delivery systems for gentamicin release and treatment of synovial membrane infection, *Vet Surg* 28:233, 1999.

59. Nie L, Nicolau DP, Tessier PR, et al: Use of bioabsorbable polymer for the delivery of ofloxacin during experimental osteomyelitis treatment, *J Orthop Res* 16:76, 1998.

60. Laurencin CT, Gerhart T, Witschger R, et al: Bioerodible polyanhydrides for certibiotic drug delivery: in vivo osteomyelitis treatment in a rat model system, *J Orthop Res* 11:256, 1993.

61. Nelson CL, Hickmon SG, Skinner RA: Treatment of experimental osteomyelitis by surgical debridement and implantation of bioerodable, polyanhydride-gentamicin beads, *J Orthop Res* 15:249, 1977.

62. Cook VL, Bertone AL, Kowalski JJ, et al: Gentamicin-impregnated biodegradable polymer for the treatment of equine joint infection in vivo: preliminary study, *Vet Surg* 26:411, 1997.

63. Benoit MA, Moussatt B, Delloye C, et al: Antibiotic-loaded plaster of Paris implants coated with polylactide-co-glycolide as a controlled release delivery system for the treatment of bone infections, *Int Orthop* 21:403, 1997.

64. Rubio-Martinez LM, Lopez-Sanroman J, Cruz AM, et al. Evaluation of safety and pharmacokinetics of vancomycin after intraosseous regional limb perfusion and comparison of results with those obtained after intravenous regional perfusion in horses, *Am J Vet Res* 67:1701, 2006.

65. Whitehair KJ, Blevins WE, Fessler JF, et al: Regional perfusion of the equine carpus for antibiotic delivery, *Vet Surg* 21:279, 1993.

66. Whitehair KJ, Bowersock T, Blevins WE, et al: Regional limb perfusion for antibiotic treatment of experimentally induced septic arthritis, *Vet Surg* 21:367, 1992.

67. Rubio-Martinez LM, Lopez-Sanroman J, Cruz AM, et al: Evaluation of safety and pharmacokinetics of vancomycin after intravenous regional limb perfusion in horses, *Am J Vet Res* 66:2107, 2005.

68. Parra-Sanchez A, Lugo J, Boothe DM, et al: Pharmacokinetics and pharmacodynamics of enrofloxacin and a low dose of amikacin administered via regional intravenous limb perfusion in standing horses, *Am J Vet Res* 67:1687, 2006.

69. Werner LA, Hardy J, Bertone AL: Bone gentamicin concentration after intraarticular injection or regional intravenous perfusion in the horse, *Vet Surg* 32:559, 2003.

70. Meagher DT, Latimer FG, Sutter WW, et al: Evaluation of a balloon constant rate infusion system for treatment of septic arthritis, septic tenosynovitis, and contaminated synovial wounds: 23 cases (2002-2005), *J Am Vet Med Assoc* 228:1930, 2006.

71. Bolt DM, Ishihara AK, Weisbrode SE, et al: Effects of triamcinolone acetonide, sodium hyaluronate, amikacin sulfate, and mepivacaine hydrochloride, alone and in combination, on morphology and matrix composition of lipopolysaccharide-challenged and unchallenged equine articular cartilage explants, *Am J Vet Res* 69:861, 2008.

72. Karpie JC, Chu CR: Lidocaine exhibits dose- and time-dependent cytotoxic effects on bovine articular chondrocytes in vitro, *Am J Sports Med* 35:1621, 2007.

73. Bertone AL, Davis DM, Cox HU, et al: Arthrotomy versus arthroscopy and partial synovectomy for treatment of experimentally induced infectious arthritis in horses, *Am J Vet Res* 53:585, 1992.

74. Theoret CL, Barber SM, Moyana T, et al: Repair and function of synovium after arthroscopic synovectomy of the dorsal compartment of the equine antebrachiocarpal joint, *Vet Surg* 25:142, 1996.

75. Palmer J, Bertone AL, Malemud CJ, et al: Changes in third carpal bone articular cartilage after synovectomy in normal and inflamed joints, *Vet Surg* 27:321, 1998.

76. Yarborough TB, Lee MR, Hornof WJ, et al: Evaluation of samarium-153 for synovectomy in an osteochondral fragment–induced model of synovitis in horses, *Vet Surg* 29:252, 2000.

77. Ross M, Orsisni J, Richardson D, et al: Closed suction drainage in the treatment of infectious arthritis of the equine tarsocrural joint, *Vet Surg* 30:21, 1991.

78. Groom LJ, Gaughan EM, Lillich JD, et al: Arthrodesis of the proximal interphalangeal joint affected with septic arthritis in 8 horses, *Can Vet J* 41:117, 2000.

79. Wisner ER, O'Brien TR, Pool RR, et al: Osteomyelitis of the axial border of the proximal sesamoid bones in seven horses, *Equine Vet J* 23:383, 1991.

80. Honnas CM, Welch RD, Ford TS, et al: Septic arthritis of the distal interphalangeal joint in 12 horses, *Vet Surg* 21:261, 1992.

81. Nagy AD, Simofer H: Mandibular condylectomy and meniscectomy for the treatment of septic temporomandibular joint arthritis in a horse, *Vet Surg* 35:663, 2006.

82. Smith R, Kajiyama G, Schurman DJ: Staphylococcal septic arthritis: antibiotic and nonsteroidal anti-inflammatory drug treatment in a rabbit model, *J Orthop Res* 15:919, 1997.

83. Doucet M, Bertone A, Hendrickson D, et al: Comparison of efficacy and safety of paste formulations of firocoxib and phenylbutazone in horses with naturally occurring osteoarthritis, *J Am Vet Med Assoc* 232:91, 2007.

84. Moses V, Hardy J, Bertone AL, et al: The effect of various nonsteroidal anti-inflammatory drugs on lipopolysaccharide challenged and unchallenged equine synovial membrane explants, *Am J Vet Res* 162:54, 2001.

85. Moses VS, Bertone AL: Nonsteroidal anti-inflammatory drugs, *Vet Clin North Am Equine Pract* 18:21, 2002.

86. Sysel AM, Pleasant RS, Jacobson JD, et al: Efficacy of an epidural combination of morphine and detomidine in alleviating experimentally induced hindlimb lameness in horses, *Vet Surg* 25:511, 1996.

87. Sysel AM, Pleasant RS, Jacobson JD, et al: Systemic and local effects associated with long-term epidural catheterization and morphine-detomidine administration in horses, *Vet Surg* 26:141, 1997.

88. Smith G, Bertone AL, Kaeding C, et al: Anti-inflammatory effects of topically applied dimethylsulfoxide gel on endotoxin-induced synovitis in horses, *Am J Vet Res* 59:1149, 1998.

89. Visai L, Xu Y, Casolini F, et al: Monoclonal antibodies to CNA, a collagen-binding microbial surface component recognizing adhesive matrix molecules, detach *Staphylococcus aureus* from a collagen substrate, *J Biol Chem* 275:39837, 2000.

90. Smeltzer MS, Gillaspy AF: Molecular pathogenesis of staphylococcal osteomyelitis, *Poult Sci* 79:1042, 2000.

91. Balaban N, Collins LV, Cullor JS, et al: Prevention of diseases caused by *Staphylococcus aureus* using the peptide RIP, *Peptides* 21:1301, 2000.

Fungal Infectious Arthritis

1. Leitch M: Diagnosis and treatment of septic arthritis in the horse, *J Am Vet Med Assoc* 175:701, 1979.

2. Lapointe JM, Laverty S, Lovoie JP: Septic arthritis in 15 Standardbred racehorses after intraarticular injection, *Equine Vet J* 24:430, 1992.

3. Peremans K, Verschooten F, Moor AD, et al: Monoarticular infectious arthritis in the horse: 34 cases, *J Equine Vet Sci* 11:27, 1991.

4. Schneider RK, Bramlage LR, Moore RM, et al: A retrospective study of 192 horses affected with septic arthritis/tenosynovitis, *Equine Vet J* 24:436, 1992.

5. Kohli R, Hadley S: Fungal arthritis and osteomyelitis, *Infect Dis Clin North Am* 19:831, 2005.

6. Hansen BL, Andersen K: Fungal arthritis: a review, *Scand J Rheumatol* 24:248, 1995.

7. Cuellar ML, Silveira LH, Espinoza LR: Fungal arthritis, *Ann Rheumatic Dis* 51:690, 1992.

8. Cohen JM, Ross MW, Busschers E: Diagnosis and management of *Candida utilis* infectious arthritis in a Standardbred filly, *Equine Vet Educ* 20:348, 2008.

9. Madison JB, Reid BV, Raskin RE: Amphotericin B treatment of *Candida* arthritis in two horses, *J Am Vet Med Assoc* 206:338, 1995.

10. Reilly LK, Palmer JE: Systemic candidiasis in four foals, *J Am Vet Med Assoc* 205:464, 1994.

11. Riley CB, Yovich JV, Robertson JP, et al: Fungal arthritis due to infection by *Candida famata* in a horse, *Aust Vet J* 1:69, 1992.

12. Sherman KM, Myhre GD, Heymann EI: Fungal osteomyelitis of the axial border of the proximal sesamoid bones in a horse, *J Am Vet Med Assoc* 229:1607, 2006.

13. Swerczek TW, Donahue JM, Hunt RJ: *Scedosporium prolificans* infection associated with arthritis and osteomyelitis in a horse, *J Am Vet Med Assoc* 218:800, 2001.

14. Colitz CMH, Latimer FG, Cheng H, et al: Pharmacokinetics of voriconazole following intravenous and oral administration and body fluid concentrations of

voriconazole following repeated oral administration in horses, *Am J Vet Med Res* 68:1115, 2007.

15. Ross MW: Personal communication, 2009.

16. Nouyrigat P, Baume D, Blaise D, et al: *Candida* arthritis treated with intra-articular amphotericin B, *Eur J Med* 2:124, 1993.

17. Getman LG: Personal communication, 2009.

CHAPTER 66 Noninfectious Arthritis

1. Bertone AL, Hardy J, Simmons EJ, et al: Transsynovial forces of the isolated stationary equine joint, *Am J Vet Res* 59:495, 1998.

2. Hardy J, Bertone AL, Weisbrode SE, et al: Cell trafficking, mediator release, and articular metabolism in acute inflammation of innervated or denervated isolated equine joints, *Am J Vet Res* 59:88, 1998.

3. Palmer J, Bertone AL: Joint structure, biochemistry and biochemical disequilibrium in synovitis and equine joint disease, *Equine Vet J* 26:263, 1994.

4. Bertone AL, Palmer J, Jones J: Synovial fluid cytokines and eicosanoids as markers of joint disease in horses, *Vet Surg* 30:528, 2001.

5. Levick JR: Blood flow and mass transport in synovial joints. In Handbook of physiology. II. The cardiovascular system, vol 4, Bethesda, 1984, American Physiological Society.

6. Macoris D, Bertone AL: Intra-articular pressure profiles of the cadaveric equine fetlock joint in motion, *Equine Vet J* 33:1, 2001.

7. Palmer J, Bertone AL: Joint biomechanics in the pathogenesis of traumatic arthritis. In McIlwraith CW, Trotter G, eds: *Joint disease in the horse*, Philadelphia, 1996, Saunders.

8. Bragdon B, Bertone AL, Hardy J, et al: Use of an isolated joint model to detect early changes induced by intra-articular injection of paclitaxel-impregnated microspheres, *J Invest Surg* 14:169, 2001.

9. Simmons EJ, Bertone AL, Muir WW: Receptor mechanisms of enhanced vascular responsiveness of isolated equine osteoarthritic joints, *Vet Surg* 28:405, 1999.

10. Lane Smith R, Rusk SF, Ellison BE, et al: In vitro stimulation of articular chondrocyte mRNA and extracellular matrix synthesis by hydrostatic pressure, *J Orthop Res* 14:53, 1996.

11. Edwards JCW, Winchester R, Henderson B, et al: Consensus statement, *Ann Rheum Dis* 54:389, 1995.

12. Strand E, Martin GS, Crawford MP, et al: Intra-articular pressure, elastance and range of motion in healthy and injured racehorse metacarpophalangeal joint, *Equine Vet J* 30:520, 1998.

13. Hardy J, Bertone AL, Muir WW: Pressure-volume relationships in equine midcarpal joint, *J Appl Physiol* 78:1977, 1995.

14. Hardy J, Bertone AL, Muir WW: Joint pressure influences synovial tissue blood flow as determined by colored microspheres, *J Appl Physiol* 80:1225, 1996.

15. Hardy J, Bertone AL, Muir WW: Local hemodynamics, permeability and oxygen metabolism of innervated or denervated isolated equine joints, *Am J Vet Res* 59:1307, 1998.

16. Hawkins DL, MacKay RJ, Gum GG, et al: Effects of intra-articularly administered endotoxin on clinical signs of disease and synovial fluid tumor necrosis factor, interleukin 6, and prostaglandin E_2 values in horses, *Am J Vet Res* 54:379, 1993.

17. Auer DE, Ng JC, Seawright AA: Free radical oxidation products in plasma and synovial fluid of horses with synovial inflammation, *Aust Vet J* 70:49, 1993.

18. Todhunter RJ, Fubini SL, Vernier-Singer M, et al: Acute synovitis and intra-articular methylprednisolone acetate in ponies, *Osteoarthritis Cartilage* 6:94, 1998.

19. Furst DE, Breedveld FC, Burmester GR, et al: Access to disease modifying treatments for rheumatoid arthritis patients, *Ann Rheum Dis* 58(Suppl)1:I129, 1999.

20. Hawkins DL, Cargile JL, MacKay RJ, et al: Effect of tumor necrosis factor antibody on synovial fluid cytokine activities in equine antebrachiocarpal joints injected with endotoxin, *Am J Vet Res* 56:1292, 1995.

21. Bertone A: Unpublished data, 1996.

22. Sanchis-Alfonso V, Villanueva-Garcia E: Localized pigmented villonodular synovitis as a rare cause of chronic anterolateral ankle pain in an equestrienne, *Arthroscopy* 16:E15, 2000.

23. Tulamo RM, Heiskanen T, Salonen M: Concentration and molecular weight distribution of hyaluronate in synovial fluid from clinically normal horses and horses with diseased joints, *Am J Vet Res* 55:710, 1994.

24. Vilensky JA, O'Connor BL, Brandt KD, et al: Serial kinematic analysis of the canine knee after L4-S1 dorsal root ganglionectomy: implications for the cruciate deficiency model of osteoarthritis, *J Rheumatol* 21:2113, 1994.

25. Basbaum AI, Levine JD: The contribution of the nervous system to inflammation and inflammatory disease, *Can J Physiol Pharmacol* 69:647, 1991.

26. Colpaert FC, Donnerer J, Lembeck F: Effects of capsaicin on inflammation and on the substance P content of nervous tissues in rats with adjuvant arthritis, *Life Sci* 32:1827, 1983.

27. Cambridge H, Brain SD: Calcitonin gene-related peptide increases blood flow and potentiates plasma protein extravasation in the rat knee, *Br J Pharmacol* 106:746, 1992.

28. Konttinen YT, Kemppinen P, Segerberg M, et al: Peripheral and spinal neural mechanisms in arthritis, with particular reference to treatment of inflammation and pain, *Arthritis Rheum* 37:965, 1994.

29. Geor RJ, Clark EG, Haines DM, et al: Systemic lupus erythematosus in a filly, *J Am Vet Med Assoc* 197:1489, 1990.

30. Osborne AC, Carter SD, May SA, et al: Anti-collagen antibodies and immune complexes in equine joint disease, *Vet Immunol Immunopathol* 45:19, 1995.

31. Carter SD, Osborne AC, May SA, et al: Rheumatoid factor, anti-heat shock protein (65 kDa) antibodies and antinuclear antibodies in equine joint diseases, *Equine Vet J* 27:288, 1995.

32. Madison JB, Scarratt K: Immune-mediated polysynovitis in four foals, *J Am Vet Med Assoc* 192:1581, 1988.

33. Blunden AS, Smith KC, Binns MM, et al: Replication of equid herpesvirus 4 in endothelial cells and synovia of a field case of viral pneumonia and synovitis in a foal, *J Comp Pathol* 112:133, 1995.

34. Madison JB, Ziemer EL: Eosinophilic synovitis following the intra-articular injection of bacterial antigen in horses, *Res Vet Sci* 54:256, 1993.

35. Sweeney CR, Sweeney RW, Divers TJ: *Rhodococcus equi* pneumonia in 48 foals: response to antimicrobial treatment, *Vet Microbiol* 14:329, 1987.

36. Palmer J, Bertone AL, Malemud CJ, et al: Changes in third carpal bone articular cartilage after synovectomy in normal and inflamed joints, *Vet Surg* 27:321, 1998.

37. Carter BG, Bertone AL, Weisbrode SE, et al: Influence of methylprednisolone acetate on osteochondral healing in exercised tarsocrural joints of horses, *Am J Vet Res* 57:914, 1996.

38. Ross M: Personal communication, 2001.

39. Turner AS, Gustafson SB, Zeider NS, et al: Acute eosinophilic synovitis in a horse, *Equine Vet J* 22:215, 1990.

40. Crabill MR, Watkins JP, Morris EL, et al: Lead foreign body arthropathy in a horse, *J Am Vet Med Assoc* 205:864, 1994.

41. Dabareiner RM, White NA, Sullins KE: Metacarpophalangeal joint synovial pad fibrotic proliferation in 63 horses, *Vet Surg* 25:199, 1995.

42. Vickers KL, Ross MW: Atypical villonodular synovitis in a horse, *J Am Vet Med Assoc* 209:1602, 1996.

43. Roneus B, Andersson AM, Ekman S: Racing performance in Standardbred trotters with chronic synovitis after partial arthroscopic synovectomy in the metacarpophalangeal, metatarsophalangeal and intercarpal (midcarpal) joints, *Acta Vet Scand* 38:87, 1997.

44. Kannegieter NJ: Chronic proliferative synovitis of the equine metacarpophalangeal joint, *Vet Rec* 127:8, 1990.

45. van Veenendaal JC, Moffatt RE: Soft tissue masses in the fetlock joint of horses, *Aust Vet J* 56:533, 1980.

46. van der Heijden IM, Wilbrink B, Tchetverikov I, et al: Presence of bacterial DNA and bacterial peptidoglycans in joints of patients with rheumatoid arthritis and other arthritides, *Arthritis Rheum* 43:593, 2000.

47. Stahl HD, Hubner B, Seidle B, et al: Detection of multiple viral DNA species in synovial tissue and fluid of patients with early arthritis, *Ann Rheum Dis* 59:342, 2000.

48. Dyson S: Lameness associated with recurrent hemarthrosis in a horse, *Equine Vet J* 18:224, 1986.

49. Clegg P: Lyme disease, *Proc Br Equine Vet Assoc* 39:150, 2000.

50. Lindermayer J, Weber M, Onderdonk A: *Borrelia burgdorferi* infection in horses, *J Am Vet Med Assoc* 194:1384, 1989.

51. Magnarelli L, Fikrig E: Detection of antibodies to *Borrelia burgdorferi* in naturally

infected horses in the USA by enzyme-linked immunosorbent assay using whole-cell and recombinant antigens, *Res Vet Sci* 79:99, 2005.

52. Chang YF, Ku YW, Chang CF, et al: Antibiotic treatment of experimentally *Borrelia burgdorferi*–infected ponies, *Vet Microbiol* 107:285, 2005.

CHAPTER 67　Other Joint Conditions

1. Simmons EJ, Bertone AL, Weisbrode SE: Instability-induced osteoarthritis in the metacarpophalangeal joint of horses, *Am J Vet Res* 60:7, 1999.

2. Desmaizieres LM, Cauvin ER: Carpal collateral ligament desmopathy in three horses, *Vet Rec* 157:197, 2005.

3. Pool R: Tumors and tumorlike lesions of joints and adjacent soft tissues. In Moulton JE, ed: *Tumors in domestic animals*, ed 3, Berkeley, 1990, University of California Press.

4. Stashak T: Lameness. In Stashak T, ed: *Adams' lameness in horses*, Philadelphia, 1987, Lea & Febiger.

5. van Veenendaal JC, Speirs VC, Harrison I: Treatment of hygromata in horses, *Aust Vet J* 57:513, 1981.

6. Jann H: Treatment of acquired bursitis (hygroma) by en-bloc resection, *Equine Pract* 12:8, 1990.

7. Andren L, Eiken O: Arthrographic studies of wrist ganglions, *J Bone Joint Surg Am* 53:299, 1971.

8. Adams OR: *Lameness in horses*, Philadelphia, 1974, Lea & Febiger.

9. Kawcak C, Trotter G: Other conditions affecting equine joints. In McIlwraith C, Trotter G, eds: *Joint disease in the horse*, Philadelphia, 1996, Saunders.

10. Hay WP, Baskett A: Lameness caused by a ganglion in a mare, *Compend Contin Educ Pract Vet* 18:1352, 1996.

11. Llewellyn HR: A case of carpal intersynovial fistula in a horse, *Equine Vet J* 11:90, 1979.

12. McIlwraith C: Diseases of joints, tendons, ligaments and related structures. In Stashak T, ed: *Adams' lameness in horses*, Philadelphia, 1987, Lea & Febiger.

13. Johnson JE, Ryan GD: Intersynovial fistula in the carpus of a horse, *Cornell Vet* 65:84, 1975.

14. Adams SB, Fessler JF, Thacker HL: Tendon fibromas in 2 horses, *Equine Vet J* 14:95, 1982.

15. Lillich J, Gaughan E: Personal communication, 2001.

16. Vickers KL, Ross MW: Atypical villonodular synovitis in a horse, *J Am Vet Med Assoc* 209:1602, 1996.

17. Kawcak C, Goltz K: Pigmented villonodular synovitis in a mule. Unpublished data, 1999.

18. Cheli R, Zaraga L: Synovioma della grande sesamoidea nel cavallo, *Clin Vet (Milano)* 100:280, 1977.

19. Lewis R: Personal communication, 2001.

20. Riddle WE Jr, Wheat JD: Chondrosarcoma in a horse, *J Am Vet Med Assoc* 158:1674, 1971.

21. Bertone AL, Powers BE, Turner AS: Chondrosarcoma in the radius of a horse, *J Am Vet Med Assoc* 185:534, 1984.

22. Bush JM, Fredrickson RL, Ehrhart EJ: Equine osteosarcoma: a series of 8 cases, *Vet Pathol* 44:247, 2007.

23. Jenner F, Solano M, Gliatto J, et al: Osteosarcoma of the tarsus in a horse, *Equine Vet J* 35:214, 2003.

24. Cole R, Chesen AB, Pool R, et al: Imaging diagnosis—equine mast cell tumor, *Vet Radiol Ultrasound* 48:32, 2007.

25. Grant B, Lincoln S: Melanosarcoma as a cause of lameness in a horse (a case report), *Vet Med Small Anim Clin* 67:995, 1972.

26. Van Pelt RW, Langham RF, Gill HE: Multiple hemangiosarcomas in the tarsal synovial sheath of a horse, *J Am Vet Med Assoc* 161:49, 1972.

27. Johns I, Stephen JO, Del Piero F, et al: Hemangiosarcoma in 11 young horses, *J Vet Intern Med* 19:564, 2005.

28. Dunkel BM, Del Piero E, Kraus BM, et al: Congenital cutaneous, oral, and periarticular hemangiosarcoma in a 9-day-old Rocky Mountain horse, *J Vet Intern Med* 18:252, 2004.

29. Kirk MD: Radiographic and histologic appearance of synovial osteochondromatosis of the femorotibial bursae in a horse: a case history report, *Vet Radiol* 23:168, 1982.

CHAPTER 68　Pathophysiology of Tendon Injury

1. Alexander RM: Energy-saving mechanisms in walking and running, *J Exp Biol* 160:55, 1991.

2. Wilson AM, McGuigan MP, Su A, et al: Horses damp the spring in their step, *Nature* 414:895, 2001.

3. Wilson AM, van den Bogert AJ, McGuigan MP: Optimization of the muscle-tendon unit for economical locomotion in cursorial animals. In Herzog W, ed: *Skeletal muscle mechanics: from mechanisms to function*, Chichester, England, 2000, John Wiley & Sons.

4. Screen HR, Lee DA, Bader DL, et al: An investigation into the effects of the hierarchical structure of tendon fascicles on micromechanical properties, *Proc Inst Mech Eng H* 218:109, 2004.

5. Wilson AM: The effect of exercise intensity on the biochemistry, morphology, and mechanical properties of tendon, PhD thesis, Bristol, United Kingdom, 1991, University of Bristol.

6. Woo SL: Mechanical properties of tendons and ligaments. I. Quasi-static and nonlinear viscoelastic properties, 19:385, 1982.

7. Viidik A: Tensile strength properties of Achilles tendon systems in trained and untrained rabbits, *Acta Orthop Scand* 40:261, 1969.

8. Goodship AE, Birch HL, Wilson AM: The pathobiology and repair of tendon and ligament injury, *Vet Clin North Am Equine Pract* 10:323, 1994.

9. Crevier N, Pourcelet P, Denoix J-M, et al: Segmental variations of in vitro mechanical properties in equine superficial digital flexor tendons, *Am J Vet Res* 57:1111, 1996.

10. Riemersma DJ, van der Bogert AJ, Jansen MO, et al: Tendon strain in the forelimbs as a function of gait and ground characteristics and in vitro limb loading in ponies, *Equine Vet J* 28:133, 1996.

11. Stephens PR, Nunamaker DM, Butterweck DM: Application of a Hall-effect transducer for measurement of tendon strains in horses, *Am J Vet Res* 56:1089, 1989.

12. Riemersma DJ, Schamhardt HC: In vitro mechanical properties of equine tendons in relation to cross-sectional area and collagen content, *Res Vet Sci* 39:263, 1985.

13. Wilson AM, Goodship AE: Exercise-induced hyperthermia as a possible mechanism for tendon degeneration, *J Biomech* 27:899, 1994.

14. Batson EL, Paramour RJ, Smith T, et al: Are the material properties and matrix composition of equine flexor and extensor tendons determined by their functions? *Equine Vet J* 35:314, 2003.

15. Wilmink J, Wilson AM, Goodship AE: Functional significance of the morphology and micromechanics of collagen fibres in relation to partial rupture of the superficial digital flexor tendon in racehorses, *Res Vet Sci* 53:354, 1992.

16. Patterson-Kane JC, Parry DA, Birch HL, et al: An age-related study of morphology and cross-link composition of collagen fibrils in the digital flexor tendons of young thoroughbred horses, *Connect Tissue Res* 36:253, 1997.

17. Canty EG, Kadler KE: Procollagen trafficking, processing and fibrillogenesis, *J Cell Sci* 118:1341, 2005.

18. Holmes DF, Graham HK, Trotter JA, et al: STEM/TEM studies of collagen fibril assembly, *Micron* 32:273, 2001.

19. Kadler KE, Holmes DF, Trotter JA, et al: Collagen fibril formation, *Biochem J* 316:1, 1996.

20. Kadler KE, Holmes DF, Graham H, et al: Tip-mediated fusion involving unipolar collagen fibrils accounts for rapid fibril elongation, the occurrence of fibrillar branched networks in skin and the paucity of collagen fibril ends in vertebrates, *Matrix Biol* 19:359, 2000.

21. Smith RK, Goodship AE: Tendon physiology: responses to exercise and training. In Hinchcliffe K, Kaneps A, Geor R, eds: *Equine sports medicine and surgery*, St Louis, 2004, Elsevier.

22. Kraus-Hansen AE, Fackelman GE, Becker C, et al: Preliminary studies on the vascular anatomy of the equine superficial digital flexor tendon, *Equine Vet J* 24:46, 1992.

23. Kraus BLH, Kirker-Head CA, Kraus KH, et al: Vascular supply of the tendon of the equine deep digital flexor muscle within the digital sheath, *Vet Surg* 24:102, 1995.

24. Jones AJ: Normal and diseased equine digital flexor tendon: blood flow, biochemical and serological studies, PhD thesis, London, 1993, University of London.

25. Strömberg B: The normal and diseased superficial digital flexor tendon in racehorses: a morphologic and physiologic investigation, *Acta Radiol* 305(Suppl):1, 1971.

26. Smith RK, Webbon PM: The physiology of normal tendon and ligament. Rantanen NW, Hauser ML, eds: *Proceedings of the 1996 Dubai International Equine Symposium*, Bonsall, Calif, 1996, Matthew R Rantanen Design.

27. Stanley R, Goodship AE, Edwards B, et al: Effects of exercise on tenocyte cellularity and tenocyte nuclear morphology in immature and mature equine digital tendons, *Equine Vet* 40:141, 2008.

28. Goodman SA, May SA, Heinegård D, et al: Tenocyte response to cyclical strain and transforming growth factor beta is dependent upon age and site of origin, *Biorheology* 41:613, 2004.

29. Webbon PM: A histological study of macroscopically normal equine digital flexor tendons, *Equine Vet J* 10:253, 1978.

30. Cauvin ERJ: An investigation into the roles of transforming growth factor beta (TGFβ) in the development, adaptation, and repair of equine tendon, PhD dissertation, London, 2001, University of London.

31. Bi Y, Ehirchiou D, Kilts TM, et al: Identification of tendon stem/progenitor cells and the role of the extracellular matrix in their niche, *Nat Med* 13:1219, 2007.

32. Salingcarnboriboon R, Yoshitake H, Tsuji K, et al: Establishment of tendon-derived cell lines exhibiting pluripotent mesenchymal stem cell–like property, *Exp Cell Res* 287:289, 2003.

33. Strassburg S: Adult and late foetal equine tendon contain cell populations with weak progenitor properties in comparison to bone marrow derived mesenchymal stem cells, *Proc Orthop Res Soc* 52, 2006.

34. Banes AJ, Tsuzaki M, Yamamoto J, et al: Mechanoreception at the cellular level: the detection, interpretation, and diversity of responses to mechanical stimuli, *Biochem Cell Biol* 73:349, 1995.

35. McNeilly CM, Banes AJ, Benjamin M, et al: Tendon cells in vivo form a three dimensional network of cell processes linked by gap junctions, *J Anat* 189:593, 1996.

36. Murphy DJ, Nixon AJ: Biochemical and site-specific effects of insulin-like growth factor I on intrinsic tenocyte activity in equine flexor tendons, *Am J Vet Res* 58:103, 1997.

37. Dahlgren LA, van der Meulen MC, Bertram JE, et al: Insulin-like growth factor–I improves cellular and molecular aspects of healing in a collagenase-induced model of flexor tendinitis, *J Orthop Res* 20:910, 2002.

38. Frank C, Woo S, Andriacchi T, et al: Normal ligament: structure, function, and composition. In Woo SL-Y, Buckwalter JA, eds: *Injury and repair of musculoskeletal soft tissues*, Park Ridge, Ill, 1987, American Academy of Orthopaedic Surgeons.

39. Silver IA, Brown PN, Goodship AE, et al: A clinical and experimental study of tendon injury, healing, and treatment in the horse, *Equine Vet J Suppl* 1:1, 1983.

40. Hedbom E, Antonsson P, Hjerpes A, et al: Cartilage matrix proteins: an acidic oligomeric protein (COMP) detected only in cartilage, *J Biol Chem* 267:6132, 1992.

41. Mörgelin M, Heinegård D, Engel J, et al: Electron microscopy of native cartilage oligomeric matrix protein purified from the Swarm rat chondrosarcoma reveals a five-armed structure, *J Biol Chem* 267:6137, 1992.

42. Smith RK, Zunino L, Webbon PM, et al: The distribution of cartilage oligomeric matrix protein (COMP) in tendon and its variation with tendon site, age and load, *Matrix Biol* 16:255, 1997.

43. Rosenberg K, Olsson H, Morgelin M, et al: Cartilage oligomeric matrix protein shows high affinity zinc-dependent interaction with triple helical collagen, *J Biol Chem* 273:20397, 1998.

44. Thur J, Rosenberg K, Nitsche DP, et al: Mutations in cartilage oligomeric matrix protein causing pseudoachondroplasia and multiple epiphyseal dysplasia affect binding of calcium and collagen I, II, and IX, *J Biol Chem* 276:6083, 2001.

45. Hecht JT, Nelson LD, Crowder E, et al: Mutations in exon 17B of cartilage oligomeric matrix protein (COMP) cause pseudoachondroplasia, *Nat Genet* 10:325, 1995.

46. Briggs MD, Hoffman SM, King LM, et al: Pseudoachondroplasia and multiple epiphyseal dysplasia due to mutations in the cartilage oligomeric matrix protein gene, *Nat Genet* 10:330, 1995.

47. Halasz K, Kassner A, Mörgelin M, et al: COMP acts as a catalyst in collagen fibrillogenesis, *J Biol Chem* 282:31166, 2007.

48. Smith RK, Gerard M, Dowling B, et al: Correlation of cartilage oligomeric matrix protein (COMP) levels in equine tendon with mechanical properties: a proposed role for COMP in determining function-specific mechanical characteristics of locomotor tendons, *Equine Vet J Suppl* 34:241, 2002.

49. Brown DC, Vogel KG: Characteristics of the in vitro interaction of a small proteoglycan (PG II) of bovine tendon with type I collagen, *Matrix* 9:468, 1989.

50. Danielson KG, Baribault H, Holmes DF, et al: Targeted disruption of decorin leads to abnormal collagen fibril morphology and skin fragility, *J Cell Biol* 136:729, 1997.

51. Svensson L, Aszódi A, Reinholt FP, et al: Fibromodulin-null mice have abnormal collagen fibrils, tissue organization, and altered lumican deposition in tendon, *J Biol Chem* 274:9636, 1999.

52. Avella CS, Ely ER, Verheyen KL, et al: Ultrasonographic assessment of the superficial digital flexor tendon of National Hunt racehorses in training over two racing seasons, *Equine Vet J* 41:449, 2009.

53. Pickersgill C: Epidemiological studies into orthopaedic conditions of the equine athlete, MVM thesis, Glasgow, 2000, University of Glasgow.

54. Webbon PM: Post mortem study of equine digital flexor tendons, *Equine Vet J* 9:61, 1977.

55. Patterson-Kane JC, Firth EC, Parry DAD, et al: Comparison of collagen fibril populations in the superficial digital flexor tendons of exercised and nonexercised thoroughbreds, *Equine Vet J* 29:121, 1997.

56. Patterson-Kane JC, Wilson AM, Firth EC, et al: Exercise-related alterations in crimp morphology in the central regions of the superficial digital flexor tendons from young thoroughbreds: a controlled study, *Equine Vet J* 30:61, 1998.

57. Birch HL, Wilson AM, Goodship AE: Physical activity: does long-term, high-intensity exercise in horses result in tendon degeneration? *J Appl Physiol* 105: 1927, 2008.

58. Smith RKW, Birch H, Patterson-Kane J, et al: Should equine athletes commence training during skeletal development? changes in tendon matrix associated with development, ageing, function, and exercise, *Equine Vet J Suppl* 30:201, 1999.

59. Smith RK, Birch HL, Goodman S, et al: The influence of ageing and exercise on tendon growth and degeneration—hypotheses for the initiation and prevention of strain-induced tendinopathies, *Comp Biochem Physiol A Mol Integr Physiol* 133:1039, 2002.

60. Birch HL, Bailey AJ, Goodship AE: Macroscopic "degeneration" of equine superficial digital flexor tendon is accompanied by a change in extracellular matrix composition, *Equine Vet J* 30:534, 1998.

61. Cherdchutham W, Becker C, Smith RK, et al: Age-related changes and the effect of exercise on the molecular composition of immature equine superficial digital flexor tendons, *Equine Vet J Suppl* 31:86, 1999.

62. Kasashima Y, Takahashi T, Smith RK, et al: Prevalence of superficial digital flexor tendonitis and suspensory desmitis in Japanese Thoroughbred flat racehorses in 1999, *Equine Vet J* 36:346, 2004.

63. Haglund-Akerlund Y, Eriksson E: Range of motion, muscle torque and training habits in runners with and without Achilles tendon problems, *Knee Surg Sports Traumatol Arthrosc* 1:195, 1993.

64. Neuberger A, Slack HGB: Metabolism of collagen from liver, bone, skin and tendon in normal rat, *Biochem J* 53:47, 1953.

65. Perez-Castro AV, Vogel KG: In situ expression of collagen and proteoglycan genes during development of fibrocartilage in bovine deep flexor tendon, *J Orthop Res* 17:139, 1999

66. Stanley RL, Fleck RA, Becker DL, et al: Gap junction protein expression and cellularity: comparison of immature and adult equine digital tendon, *J Anat* 211:325, 2007.

67. Parkin TD, Clegg PD, French NP, et al: Risk factors for fatal lateral condylar fracture of the third metacarpus/metatarsus in UK racing, *Equine Vet J* 37:192, 2005.

68. Raleigh SM, van der Merwe L, Ribbans WJ, et al: Variants within the MMP3 gene are associated with Achilles tendinopathy: possible interaction with the COL5A1 gene, *Br J Sports Med* 43:514, 2009.

69. Mokone GG, Schwellnus MP, Noakes TD, et al: The *COL5A1* gene and Achilles tendon pathology, *Scand J Med Sci Sports* 16:19, 2006.

70. Mokone GG, Gajjar M, September AV, et al: The guanine-thymine dinucleotide repeat polymorphism within the tenascin-C gene is associated with Achilles tendon injuries, *Am J Sports Med* 33:1016, 2005.

71. Oki H, Miyake T, Kasashima Y, et al: Estimation of heritability for superficial digital flexor tendon injury by Gibbs sampling in the Thoroughbred racehorse, *J Anim Breed Genet* 125:413, 2008.

72. Weller R, Pfau T, Verheyen K, et al: The effect of conformation on orthopaedic

health and performance in a cohort of National Hunt racehorses: preliminary results, *Equine Vet J* 38:622, 2006.

73. Birch HL, Wilson AM, Goodship AE: The effect of exercise-induced localised hyperthemia on tendon cell survival, *J Exp Biol* 200:1703, 1997.

74. Burrows S: Personal communication, 2008.

75. Birch HL, Rutter GA, Goodship AE: Oxidative energy metabolism in equine tendon cells, *Res Vet Sci* 62:93, 1997.

76. Anstrom M, Westlin N: Blood flow in chronic Achilles tendinopathy, *Clin Orthop* 308:166, 1994.

77. Józsa L, Bálint BJ, Réffy A, et al: Hypoxic alterations of tenocytes in degenerative tendinopathy, *Arch Orthop Trauma Surg* 99:243, 1982.

78. Dalton S, Cawston TE, Riley GP: Human shoulder tendon biopsy samples in organ culture produce procollagenase and tissue inhibitor of metalloproteinases, *Ann Rheum Dis* 54:571, 1995.

79. Rees SG, Flannery CR, Little CB, et al: Catabolism of aggrecan, decorin and biglycan in tendon, *Biochem J* 350:181, 2000.

80. Dudhia J, Scott CM, Draper ER, et al: Aging enhances a mechanically-induced reduction in tendon strength by an active process involving matrix metalloproteinase activity, *Aging Cell* 6:547, 2007.

81. Platt DP, Wilson AM, Timbs A, et al: An investigation of the biomechanics of equine flexor tendon using an implantable microforce leaf, *J Biomech* 24:449, 1991.

82. Meershoek L: *Calculation of forelimb tendon forces in horses*, PhD thesis, Utrecht, 2001, University of Utrecht.

83. Anderson TM, McIlwraith CW, Douay P: The role of conformation in musculoskeletal problems in the racing Thoroughbred, *Equine Vet J* 36:571, 2004.

84. Denoix J-M: Functional anatomy of tendons and ligaments in the distal limbs (manus and pes), *Vet Clin North Am Equine Pract* 10:273, 1994.

85. Riemersma DJ, van den Bogert AJ: Influence of shoeing on ground reaction forces and tendon strains in the forelimbs of ponies, *Equine Vet J* 28:126, 1996.

86. Kasashima Y, Takahashi T, Birch HL, et al: Can exercise modulate the maturation of functionally different immature tendons in the horse? *J Appl Physiol* 104:416, 2008.

87. Smith RKW, Goodship AE: The effect of early training and the adaptation and conditioning of skeletal tissues, *Vet Clin North Am Equine Pract* 2008.

88. Kasashima Y, Smith RK, Birch HL, et al: Exercise-induced tendon hypertrophy: cross-sectional area changes during growth are influenced by exercise, *Equine Vet J Suppl* 34:264, 2002.

89. Williams RB, Harkins LS, Hammond CJ, et al: Racehorse injuries, clinical problems and fatalities recorded on British racecourses from flat racing and National Hunt racing during 1996, 1997 and 1998, *Equine Vet J* 33:478, 2001.

90. Hill AE, Stover SM, Gardner IA, et al: Risk factors for and outcomes of non-catastrophic suspensory apparatus injury

in Thoroughbred racehorse, *J Am Vet Med Assoc* 218:1136, 2001.

91. Ely ER, Verheyen KL, Wood JL: Fractures and tendon injuries in National Hunt horses in training in the UK: a pilot study, *Equine Vet J* 36:365, 2004.

92. Smith RK, Heinegård D: Cartilage oligomeric matrix protein (COMP) levels in digital sheath synovial fluid and serum with tendon injury, *Equine Vet J* 32:52, 2000.

93. Fackelmann GE: The nature of tendon damage and its repair, *Equine Vet J* 5:141, 1973.

94. Dahlgren LA, Mohammed HO, Nixon AJ: Temporal expression of growth factors and matrix molecules in healing tendon lesions, *J Orthop Res* 23:84, 2005.

95. Kajikawa Y, Morihara T, Sakamoto H, et al: GFP chimeric models exhibited a biphasic pattern of mesenchymal cell invasion in tendon healing, *J Cell Physiol* 210:684, 2007.

96. Williams IF, McCullagh KG, Silver IA: The distribution of types I and III collagen and fibronectin in the healing equine tendon, *Connect Tissue Res* 12:211, 1984.

97. Dahlgren LA, Brower-Toland BD, Nixon AJ: Cloning and expression of type III collagen in normal and injured tendons of horses, *Am J Vet Res* 66:266, 2005.

98. Watkins JP, Auer JA, Morgan SJ, et al: Healing of surgically created defects in the equine superficial digital flexor tendon: collagen-type transformation and tissue morphologic reorganization, *Am J Vet Res* 46:2091, 1985.

99. Crevier-Denoix N, Collobert C, Pourcelot P, et al: Mechanical properties of pathological equine superficial digital flexor tendons, *Equine Vet J* 23:23, 1997.

100. Birch HL: Personal communication, 2001.

CHAPTER 69   Superficial Digital Flexor Tendonitis

Superficial Digital Flexor Tendonitis in Racehorses

1. Rooney J, Genovese RL: A survey and analysis of bowed tendon in Thoroughbred racehorses, *J Equine Vet Sci* 2:49, 1981.

2. Dowling BA, Dart AJ, Hodgson IR, et al: Superficial digital flexor tendonitis in the horse, *Equine Vet J* 32:369, 2000.

3. Dyson S: Personal communication, 2000.

4. Avella CS, Ely ER, Verheyen KLP, et al: Ultrasonographic assessment of the superficial digital flexor tendons of National Hunt racehorses in training over two racing seasons, *Equine Vet J* 41:449, 2009.

5. Reef V: *Equine diagnostic ultrasound*, Philadelphia, 1998, Saunders.

6. Palmer S, Genovese R, Longo K, et al: Practical management of superficial digital flexor tendonitis in the performance horse, *Vet Clin North Am Equine Practice* 10:425, 1994.

7. Genovese R: Unpublished data, 2001.

8. Chesen AB, Dabareiner RM, Chaffin MK, et al: Tendinitis of the proximal aspect of the superficial digital flexor tendon in horses: 12 cases (2000-2006), *J Am Vet Med Assoc* 234:1432, 2009.

9. James F, Ross MW: Unpublished data, 2008.

10. Genovese R, Longo K, Berthold B, et al: Quantitative sonographic assessment in the clinical management of superficial digital flexor injuries in Thoroughbred racehorses, *Proc Am Assoc Equine Pract* 43:285, 1997.

11. Pacini S, Spinabella S, Trombi L, et al: Suspension of bone marrow-derived undifferentiated mesenchymal stromal cells for repair of superficial digital flexor tendon in racehorses, *Tissue Eng* 13:2949, 2007.

12. Smith RK: Mesenchymal stem cell therapy for equine tendinopathy, *Disabil Rehabil* 30:1752, 2008.

13. Dyson SJ: Medical management of superficial digital flexor tendonitis: a comparative study in 219 horses, *Equine Vet J* 36:415, 2004.

14. Jorgensen J, Genovese R: Unpublished data, 2001.

15. Genovese R, Jorgensen J: Clinical use of β-aminopropionitrile-fumarate (Bapten) in superficial digital flexor tendon injuries in racehorses. Proceedings of the Ohio Veterinary Medical Association, Columbus, Ohio, 1999.

16. Gillis C: Rehabilitation of tendon and ligament injuries, *Proc Am Assoc Equine Pract* 43:306, 1997.

17. Silver I, Brown AE, Goodship LE, et al: A clinical and experimental study of tendon injury, healing and treatment in the horse, *Equine Vet J Suppl* 1:1, 1983.

18. Genovese R, et al: Superficial digital flexor tendonitis long term sonographic and clinical study of racehorses. Proceedings of the First Dubai International Equine Symposium, Dubai, United Arab Emirates, 1996.

19. Alves ALG, Rodrigues MAM, Aguiar AJA, et al: Effects of beta-aminopropionitrile fumarate and exercise on equine tendon healing: gross and histological aspects, *J Equine Vet Sci* 21:335, 2001.

20. Genovese R: Sonographic response to intra-lesional therapy with β-aminopropionitrile-fumarate for clinical tendon injuries in horses, *Proc Am Assoc Equine Pract* 38:265, 1992.

21. Reef V, Genovese R, Davis W: Initial long-term results of horses with superficial digital flexor tendonitis treated with intra-lesional β-aminopropionitrile-fumarate, *Proc Am Assoc Equine Pract* 43:301, 1997.

22. Spurlock SL: Treatment of acute superficial flexor tendon injuries in performance horses with high molecular weight sodium hyaluronate, *J Equine Vet Sci* 19:338, 1999.

23. Dyson S: Treatment of superficial digital flexor tendonitis: a comparison of conservative management, sodium hyaluronate and glycosaminoglycan polysulfate, *Proc Am Assoc Equine Pract* 43:297, 1997.

24. Dyson S: Medical management of superficial digital flexor tendonitis: a comparative study in 219 horses (1992-2000), *Equine Vet J* 36:415, 2004.

Surgical Management of Superficial Digital Flexor Tendonitis

1. Ross MW: Surgical management of superficial digital flexor tendinitis, *Proc Am Assoc Equine Pract* 43:291, 1997.

2. Bramlage LR: Superior check ligament desmotomy as a treatment for superficial

digital flexor tendinitis: initial report, *Proc Am Assoc Equine Pract* 32:365, 1986.

3. Bramlage LR, Rantanen NW, Genovese RL, et al: Long-term effects of surgical treatment of superficial digital flexor tendinitis by superior check desmotomy, *Proc Am Assoc Equine Pract* 34:655, 1988.

4. Bramlage LR, Hogan P: Career results of 137 Thoroughbred racehorses that have undergone superior check ligament desmotomy for treatment of tendinitis, *Proc Am Assoc Equine Pract* 42:162, 1996.

5. Hogan PM, Bramlage LR: Transection of the accessory ligament of the superficial digital flexor tendon for treatment of tendinitis: long term results in 61 Standardbred racehorses (1985-1992), *Equine Vet J* 27:221, 1995.

6. Ordidge RM: Comparison of three methods of treating superficial digital flexor tendinitis in the racing Thoroughbred by transection of its accessory ligament alone (proximal check ligament desmotomy) or in combination with either intra-lesional injections of hyaluronidase or tendon splitting, *Proc Am Assoc Equine Pract* 42:164, 1996.

7. Wheat JD: New aspects on the pathology of tendon injury, *Proc Am Assoc Equine Pract* 8:27, 1962.

8. Rooney JR, Genovese RL: A survey and analysis of bowed tendon in Thoroughbred racehorses, *J Equine Vet Sci* 2:49, 1981.

9. Gillis C: Rehabilitation of tendon and ligament injuries, *Proc Am Assoc Equine Pract* 43:306, 1997.

10. Gibson KT, Burbidge HM, Pfeiffer DU: Superficial digital flexor tendonitis in Thoroughbred race horses outcome following non-surgical treatment and superior check desmotomy, *Aust Vet J* 75:631, 1997.

11. Hawkins JF, Ross MW: Transection of the accessory ligament of the superficial digital flexor muscle for the treatment of superficial digital flexor tendinitis in Standardbreds: 40 cases (1988-1992), *J Am Vet Med Assoc* 206:674, 1995.

12. Reef VB, Martin BB, Stebbins K, et al: Comparison of ultrasonographic, gross, and histologic appearance of tendon injuries in performance horses, *Proc Am Assoc Equine Pract* 35:279, 1989.

13. Dyson SJ: Personal communication, 2001.

14. Allen AK: Experience with ultrasound-guided tendon puncture or splitting, *Proc Am Assoc Equine Pract* 38:273, 1992.

15. Southwood LL, Stashak TS, Kainer RA: Tenoscopic anatomy of the equine carpal flexor synovial sheath, *Vet Surg* 27:150, 1998.

16. Shoemaker RS, Bertone AL, Mohammad LN, et al: Desmotomy of the accessory ligament of the superficial digital flexor muscle in equine cadaver limbs, *Vet Surg* 4:245, 1991.

17. Alexander GR, Gibson KT, Day RE, et al: Effects of superior check desmotomy on flexor tendon and suspensory ligament strain in equine cadaver limbs, *Vet Surg* 30:522, 2001.

18. Nixon AJ, Sams AE, Ducharme NG: Endoscopically assisted annular ligament release in horses, *Vet Surg* 22:501, 1993.

19. Denoix J-M, Guizien I, Perrot P, et al: Ultrasonographic diagnosis of spontaneous injuries of the accessory ligament of the superficial digital flexor tendon (proximal check ligament) in 23 horses, *Proc Am Assoc Equine Pract* 41:142, 1995.

20. Chesen AB, Dabareiner RM, Chaffin MK, et al: Tendinitis of the proximal aspect of the superficial digital flexor tendon in horses: 12 cases (2000-2006), *J Am Vet Med Assoc* 234:1432, 2009.

21. James F, Ross MW: Unpublished data, 2008.

22. Asheim A: Surgical treatment of tendon injuries in the horse, *J Am Vet Med Assoc* 145:447, 1964.

23. Silver I, Brown P, Goodship A, et al: A clinical and experimental study of tendon injury, healing and treatment in the horse, *Equine Vet J Suppl* 1:1, 1983.

24. Stromberg B, Tufvesson G, Nilsson G: Effect of surgical splitting on vascular reactions in the superficial flexor tendon of the horse, *J Am Vet Med Assoc* 164:57, 1974.

25. Henninger RW, Bramlage LR, Schneider RK: Short-term effects of superior check ligament desmotomy and percutaneous tendon splitting as a treatment for acute tendonitis, *Proc Am Assoc Equine Pract* 36:539, 1990.

26. Henninger RW, Bramlage LR, Bailey M, et al: Effects of tendon splitting on experimentally induced acute equine tendinitis, *Vet Comp Orthop Traumatol* 5:1, 1992.

Superficial Digital Flexor Tendonitis in Event Horses, Show Jumpers, Dressage Horses, and Pleasure Horses

1. Murray R, Dyson S, Tranquille C, et al: Association of type of sport and performance level with anatomical site of orthopaedic injury and injury diagnosis, *Equine Vet J Suppl* 36:411, 2006.

2. Singer E, Barnes J, Saxby F, et al: Injuries in the event horse: training versus competition, *Vet J* 175:76, 2008.

3. Dyson S: Superficial digital flexor tendon injuries in teenage and older horses, *Equine Vet Educ* 19:187, 2007.

4. Dyson S: Treatment of superficial digital flexor tendonitis: a comparison of conservative management, sodium hyaluronate and glycosaminoglycan polysulfate, *Proc Am Assoc Equine Pract* 43:297, 1997.

5. Dyson S: Medical management of superficial digital flexor tendonitis: a comparative study in 219 horses (1992-2000), *Equine Vet J* 36:415, 2004.

6. Smith R: Personal communication, 2008 and 2010.

7. Gibson K, Snyder J, Spiers S: Ultrasonographic diagnosis of soft tissue injuries in horses competing at the Sydney 2000 Olympic Games, *Equine Vet Educ* 14:149, 2002.

8. Smith L, Mair T: Rupture of the superficial digital flexor tendon in a forelimb in 9 mature horses, *Equine Vet Educ* 19:183, 2007.

CHAPTER 70   The Deep Digital Flexor Tendon

1. Denoix J-M: Functional anatomy of tendons and ligaments in the distal limbs (manus and pes), *Vet Clin North Am Equine Pract* 10:273, 1994.

2. Denoix J-M, Azevedo C: Images echographiques des lesions du tendon flechisseur profund du doigt, *Pract Vet Equine* 32:15, 1994.

3. Dyson S: The deep digital flexor tendon. In Ross M, Dyson S, eds: *Diagnosis and management of lameness in the horse*, St Louis, 2003, Elsevier.

4. Genovese R, Rantanen N: The deep digital flexor tendon, carpal sheath and accessory ligament of the deep digital flexor tendon (inferior check ligament). In Rantanen N, McKinnon A, eds: *Equine diagnostic ultrasonography*, Baltimore, 1998, Williams & Wilkins.

5. Brokken M, Schneide, R, Sampson S, et al. Magnetic resonance imaging features of proximal metacarpal and metatarsal injuries in the horse, *Vet Radiol Ultrasound* 48:507, 2007.

6. Sampson S, Tucker R: Magnetic resonance imaging of the proximal metacarpal and metatarsal regions, *Clin Tech Equine Pract* 6:78, 2007.

7. Nixon A, Schachter B, Pool R: Exostoses of the caudal perimeter of the radial physis as a cause of carpal synovial sheath tenosynovitis and lameness in horses: 10 cases (1999-2003), *J Am Vet Med Assoc* 224:264, 2004.

8. Barr A, Dyson S, Barr F, et al: Tendonitis of the deep digital flexor tendon associated with tenosynovitis of the digital sheath in the horse, *Equine Vet J* 27:348, 1995.

9. Dik K, Dyson S, Vail T: Aseptic tenosynovitis of the digital flexor tendon sheath, fetlock and pastern annular ligament constriction, *Vet Clin North Am Equine Pract* 11:151, 1995.

10. Wilderjans H, Boussauw K, Madder K, et al: Tenosynovitis of the digital flexor tendon sheath and annular ligament constriction syndrome caused by longitudinal tears in the deep digital flexor tendon: a clinical and surgical report of 17 cases in Warmblood horses, *Equine Vet J* 35:270, 2003.

11. Edinger J, Mobius G, Ferguson J: Comparison of tenoscopic and ultrasonographic methods of examination of the digital flexor tendon sheath in horses, *Vet Comp Orthop Traumatol* 18:209, 2005.

12. Smith M, Wright I: Noninfected tenosynovitis of the digital flexor tendon sheath: a retrospective analysis of 76 cases, *Equine Vet J* 38:134, 2006.

13. Owen R, Dyson S, Parkin T, et al: A retrospective study of palmar/plantar annular ligament injury in 71 horses: 2001-2007, *Equine Vet J* 40:237, 2008.

14. Reef V: Musculoskeletal ultrasonography. In *Equine diagnostic ultrasound*, Philadelphia, 1998, Saunders.

15. Wright I, McMahon PJ: Tenosynovitis associated with longitudinal tears in the digital flexor tendons in horses: a report of 20 cases, *Equine Vet J* 31:12, 1999.

16. Dyson S: Unpublished data, 2004-2008.

17. Fortier L, Nixon A, Ducharme N, et al: Tenoscopic examination and proximal annular ligament desmotomy for treatment of equine "complex" digital sheath tenosynovitis, *Vet Surg* 28:429, 1999.

18. Clegg P: Personal communication, 2008.

19. Edwards G: Changes in the sustentaculum tali associated with distension of the

tarsal sheath (thoroughpin), *Equine Vet J* 10:97, 1978.

20. Lepage O, Leveilee R, Breton L, et al: Congenital dislocation of the deep digital flexor tendon associated with hypoplasia of the sustentaculum in a thoroughbred colt, *Vet Radiol Ultrasound* 36:384, 1995.

21. Butler J, Colles C, Dyson S, et al: The tarsus. In *Clinical radiology of the horse*, ed 3, Oxford, 2008, Wiley-Blackwell.

22. Foerner J: Surgical treatment of selected musculoskeletal disorders of the rear limb. In Auer J, ed: *Equine surgery*, Philadelphia, 1992, Saunders.

23. Dyson S: Unpublished data, 2008.

24. Cohen J, Schneider R, Zubrod C, et al: Desmitis of the distal digital annular ligament in seven horses: MRI diagnosis and surgical treatment, *Vet Surg* 37:336, 2008.

CHAPTER 71 Injuries of the Accessory Ligament of the Deep Digital Flexor Tendon

1. Denoix J-M: Functional anatomy of tendons and ligaments in the distal limbs (manus and pes), *Vet Clin North Am Equine Pract* 10:273, 1994.

2. Muylle S, van den Perren K, Simoens P: Morphometric data on the accessory ligament of the deep digital flexor tendon in the equine hindlimb, *Vet J* Jun 27, 2009 (Epub ahead of print).

3. Riemersma D, van den Bogert A, Jansen M, et al: Influence of shoeing on ground reaction forces and tendon strains in the forelimbs of ponies, *Equine Vet J* 28:126, 1996.

4. Dyson S: Desmitis of the accessory ligament of the deep digital flexor tendon: 27 cases, *Equine Vet J* 23:438, 1991.

5. McDiarmid A: Eighteen cases of desmitis of the accessory ligament of the deep digital flexor tendon, *Equine Vet Educ* 6:49, 1994.

6. Van den Belt A, Becker C, Dik K: Desmitis of the accessory ligament of the deep digital flexor tendon in the horse: clinical and ultrasonographic features—a report of 24 cases, *Zentralbl Veterinarmed A* 40:492, 1993.

7. Dyson S, Dik K: Miscellaneous conditions of tendons, tendon sheaths and ligaments, *Vet Clin North Am Equine Pract* 11:315, 1995.

8. Denoix J-M, Azevedo C: Images echographiques des lesions du tendon flechisseur profond du doigt, *Pract Vet Equine* 32:15, 1991.

9. McDiarmid A: Acquired flexural deformity of the metacarpophalangeal joint in five horses associated with tendonous damage in the palmar metacarpus, *Vet Rec* 144:475, 1999.

10. Boswell J, Schramme M: Desmitis of the accessory ligament of the deep digital flexor tendon in the hindlimb in a horse, *Equine Vet Educ* 12:129, 2000.

11. Eliashar E, Dyson S, Archer R, et al: Two clinical manifestations of desmopathy of the accessory ligament of the deep digital flexor tendon in the hindlimb of 23 horses, *Equine Vet J* 37:495, 2005.

12. Dyson S: Desmitis of the accessory ligament of the deep digital flexor tendon. In Ross M, Dyson S, eds: *Diagnosis and management of lameness in the horse*, St Louis, 2003, Elsevier.

13. Dyson S: Injuries of the accessory ligament of the deep digital flexor tendon in the equine hindlimb: a problem of middle age, *Vet J* Aug 22, 2009 (Epub ahead of print).

14. Becker C: Function and dysfunction of the accessory ligament of the deep digital flexor tendons in horses, PhD thesis, Holland, 1996, University of Utrecht.

15. Becker C, Savelberg H, Barnveld A: In vitro mechanical properties of the accessory ligament of the deep digital flexor tendon in horses in relation to age, *Equine Vet J* 26:454, 1994.

16. Reef V: Musculoskeletal ultrasonography. In *Equine diagnostic ultrasound*, Philadelphia, 1998, Saunders.

17. Brokken MT, Schneider RK, Sampson SN, et al: Magnetic resonance imaging features of proximal metacarpal and metatarsal injuries in the horse, *Vet Radiol Ultrasound* 48:507, 2007.

18. Dyson S, Murray R: Unpublished data, 2007-2009.

19. Nagy A, Dyson S: Magnetic resonance findings in the carpus and proximal metacarpal region of non-lame horses, *Proc Amer Assoc Equine Pract* 55:408, 2009.

20. Nagy A, Dyson S: Magnetic resonance anatomy of the proximal metacarpal region in the horse, *Vet Radiol Ultrasound* 50:595, 2009.

21. Becker C, Savelberg H, Buchner H, et al: Effects of experimental desmotomy on material properties and histomorphologic and ultrasonographic features of the accessory ligament of the deep digital flexor tendon in clinically normal horses, *Am J Vet Res* 59:352, 1998.

22. Becker C, Savelberg H, Buchner H, et al: Long-term consequences of experimental desmotomy of the accessory ligament of the deep digital flexor tendon in adult horses, *Am J Vet Res* 59:347, 1998.

CHAPTER 72 The Suspensory Apparatus

1. Dyson S: The suspensory apparatus. In Rantanen N, McKinnon A, eds: *Equine diagnostic ultrasonography*, Baltimore, 1998, Williams & Wilkins.

2. Muylle S, Desmet P, Simoens P, et al: Histological study of the innervation of the suspensory ligament of the forelimb of the horse, *Vet Rec* 142:606, 1998.

3. Ford T, Ross M, Orsini P: A comparison of methods for proximal metacarpal anaesthesia in horses, *Vet Surg* 18:146, 1988.

4. Dyson S, Romero J: An investigation of injection techniques for local analgesia of the equine distal tarsus and proximal metatarsus, *Equine Vet J* 25:30, 1993.

5. Denoix JM: Functional anatomy of tendon and ligaments in the distal limbs (manus and pes), *Vet Clin North Am Equine Pract* 10:273, 1994.

6. Bramlage L, Buckowiecki C, Gabel A: The effect of training on the suspensory apparatus of the horse, *Proc Am Assoc Equine Pract* 35:245, 1989.

7. Patterson-Kane J, Firth E, Parry D, et al: Effects of training on collagen fibril populations in the suspensory ligament and deep digital flexor tendon of young thoroughbreds, *Am J Vet Res* 59:64, 1998.

8. Marks D, Mackay-Smith M, Leslie A, et al: Lameness resulting from high suspensory disease (HSD) in the horse, *Proc Am Assoc Equine Pract* 24:493, 1981.

9. Genovese R, Rantanen N, Hauser M, et al: Diagnostic ultrasonography of equine limbs, *Vet Clin North Am Equine Pract* 2:145, 1986.

10. Huskamp B, Nowak M: Insertion desmopathies in the horse, *Pferdeheilkunde* 4:3, 1988.

11. Dyson S: Some observations on lameness associated with pain in the proximal metacarpal region, *Equine Vet J Suppl* 6:43, 1988.

12. Dyson S: Proximal suspensory desmitis: clinical, ultrasonographic and radiographic features, *Equine Vet J* 23:25, 1991.

13. Brokken T, Schneider R, Sampson S, et al: Magnetic resonance imaging features of proximal metacarpal and metatarsal injuries in the horse, *Vet Radiol Ultrasound* 48:507, 2007.

14. Dyson S: Diagnosis and management of common suspensory lesions in the forelimbs and hindlimbs of sport horses, *Clin Tech Equine Pract* 6:179, 2007.

15. Castro F, Schumacher J, Pauwels F, et al: A new approach for perineural injection of the lateral palmar nerve in the horse, *Vet Surg* 34:539, 2005.

16. Dyson S: Proximal suspensory desmitis in the forelimb and the hindlimb, *Proc Am Assoc Equine Pract* 46:137, 2000.

17. Nagy A, Bodo G, Dyson S, et al: Diffusion of contrast medium after perineural injection of the palmar and palmar metacarpal nerves (low 4-point nerve block): an in vivo and in vitro study, *Equine Vet J* (In press.)

18. Ross M, Ford T, Orsini P: Incomplete longitudinal fracture of the proximal palmar cortex of the third metacarpal bone in horses, *Vet Surg* 17:82, 1988.

19. Lloyd K, Kobluk P, Ragle C, et al: Incomplete palmar fracture of the proximal extremity of the third metacarpal bone in horses: ten cases (1981-1986), *J Am Vet Med Assoc* 192:798, 1988.

20. Pleasant R, Baker G, Muhlbauer M, et al: Stress reactions and stress fractures of the proximal palmar aspect of the third metacarpal bone in horses: 58 cases (1980-1990), *J Am Vet Med Assoc* 201:1918, 1992.

21. Bramlage L, Gabel A, Hackett R: Avulsion fractures of the origin of the suspensory ligament in the horse, *J Am Vet Med Assoc* 176:1004, 1980.

22. Dyson S: *Problems encountered in equine lameness diagnosis with special reference to local analgesic techniques, radiology and ultrasonography*, Newmarket, England, 1995, R & W Publications.

23. Butler J, Colles C, Dyson S, et al: The metacarpal and metatarsal regions. In *Clinical radiology of the horse*, ed 3, Oxford, 2008, Wiley-Blackwell.

24. Martin F, Herthel D-J, Snow V, et al: Scintigraphie osseuse et diagnostic des desmites proximales du muscle interosseux III chez le cheval: a propos de 28 cas (1990-1992), *Point Vet* 26:1061, 1995.

25. Edwards R, Ducharme N, Fubini S, et al: Scintigraphy for the diagnosis of avulsions of the origin of the suspensory

ligament in horses: 51 cases (1980-1993), *J Am Vet Med Assoc* 207:608, 1995.

26. Dyson S, Murray R, Weekes J: Scintigraphic evaluation of the proximal metacarpal and metatarsal regions in horses with proximal suspensory desmitis, *Vet Radiol Ultrasound* 48:78, 2007.

27. Bischofberger A, Konar M, Ohlerth S, et al: Magnetic resonance imaging, ultrasonography and histology of the suspensory ligament origin: a comparative study of normal anatomy of Warmbloods, *Equine Vet J* 38:508, 2006.

28. Nagy A, Dyson S: Magnetic resonance anatomy of the proximal metacarpal region in the horse, *Vet Radiol Ultrasound* 50:595, 2009.

29. Dyson S, Arthur R, Palmer S, et al: Suspensory ligament desmitis, *Vet Clin North Am Equine Pract* 11:177, 1995.

30. Dyson S, Genovese R: The suspensory apparatus. In Ross MW, Dyson SJ, eds: *Diagnosis and management of lameness in the horse*, St Louis, 2003, Elsevier.

31. Boening J, Liffeld S, Matuschek S: Radial extracorporeal shock wave therapy for chronic insertion desmopathy of the proximal suspensory ligament, *Proc Am Assoc Equine Pract* 46:203, 2000.

32. Crowe O, Dyson S, Schramme M, et al: Treatment of chronic or recurrent proximal suspensory desmitis using radial pressure wave therapy, *Equine Vet J* 36:313, 2004.

33. Hewes C, White N: Outcome of desmoplasty and fasciotomy for desmitis of the origin of the suspensory ligament in horses: 27 cases (1995-2004), *J Am Vet Med Assoc* 229:407, 2006.

34. Dyson S: Proximal suspensory desmitis in the hindlimb, *Equine Vet Educ* 7:275, 1995.

35. Toth F, Schumacher J, Schramme M, et al: Compressive damage to the deep branch of the lateral plantar nerve associated with lameness caused by proximal suspensory desmitis, *Vet Surg* 37:328, 2008.

36. Murray R, Dyson S, Tranquille C, et al: Association of type of sport and performance level with anatomical site of orthopaedic injury and injury diagnosis, *Equine Vet J Suppl* 36:411, 2006.

37. Dyson S: Proximal suspensory desmitis in the hindlimb: 42 cases, *Br Vet J* 150:279, 1994.

38. Dyson S: Proximal metacarpal and metatarsal pain: a diagnostic challenge, *Equine Vet Educ* 15:134, 2006.

39. Labens R, Schramme M, Robertson I, et al: Clinical, magnetic resonance and sonographic imaging findings in horses with proximal plantar metatarsal pain, *Vet Radiol Ultrasound* 51:11, 2010.

40. Bathe A: Plantar metatarsal neurectomy and fasciotomy for the treatment of hindlimb proximal suspensory desmitis. Proceedings of the 45th Congress of the British Equine Veterinary Association, Birmingham, UK, 198, 2006.

41. Kelly G: Results of neurectomy of the deep branch of the lateral plantar nerve for treatment of proximal suspensory desmitis. Proceedings of the 16th Annual Convention of the European College of Veterinary Surgeons, Dublin, 130, 2007.

42. Launois T, Desbrosse F, Perrin R: Percutaneous osteostixis as treatment of the palmar/plantar third metacarpal/metatarsal cortex at the origin of the suspensory ligament in 29 cases, *Equine Vet Educ* 15:126, 2006.

43. Hughes T: Personal communication, 2007.

44. Pauwels F, Schumacher J, Mayhew Jvan Sickle D: Neurectomy of the deep branch of the lateral plantar nerve can cause neurogenic atrophy of the muscle fibres in the proximal suspensory ligament (M. interosseous medius), *Equine Vet J* 41:508, 2009.

45. Colbourne C, Yovich J: Suspensory ligament injuries in racing horses: ultrasonographic diagnosis and long term follow up, *Aust Equine Vet* 12:119, 1994.

46. Schnabel L, Mohammed H, Jacobson M, et al: Effects of platelet rich plasma and acellular bone marrow on gene expression patterns and DNA content of equine suspensory ligament explant cultures, *Equine Vet J* 40:260, 2008.

47. Waselau M, Sutter W, Genovese R, et al: Intralesional injection of platelet-rich plasma followed by controlled walking exercise for treatment of midbody suspensory ligament desmitis in Standardbred racehorses, *J Am Vet Med Assoc* 232:1515, 2008.

48. Dyson S: Is degenerative change within hindlimb suspensory ligaments a prelude to all types of injury? *Equine Vet Educ* (In press).

49. Minshall G, Wright I: Arthroscopic diagnosis and treatment of intra-articular insertional injuries of the suspensory ligament branches, *Equine Vet J* 38:10, 2006.

50. Enzerink E, Dik K: Palmar/plantar annular ligament insertion injury: a report of 4 cases, *Equine Vet Educ* 13:75, 2001.

51. Denoix J-M, Busoni V, Olalla M-J: Ultrasonographic examination of the proximal scutum in the horse, *Equine Vet J* 29:136, 1997.

52. Winberg F, Petterson H: Diagnosis and treatment of lesions in the intersesamoidean ligament and its adjoining structures, *Vet Surg* 23:215, 1994.

53. Dabereiner R, Watkins J, Carterm G, et al: Osteitis/osteomyelitis of the axial border of the proximal sesamoid bone in horses, *Proc Am Assoc Equine Pract* 45:156, 1999.

54. Wisner E, O'Brien T, Pool R, et al: Osteomyelitis of the axial border of the proximal sesamoid bones in seven horses, *Equine Vet J* 23:383, 1991.

55. Dyson S, Denoix J-M: Tendon, tendon sheath and ligament injuries in the pastern, *Vet Clin North Am Equine Pract* 11:217, 1995.

56. Schneider R, Tucker R, Habegger S, et al: Desmitis of the straight sesamoidean ligament in horses: 9 cases (1995-1997), *J Am Vet Med Assoc* 222:973, 2003.

57. Sampson S, Schneider R, Tucker R, et al: Magnetic resonance imaging features of oblique and straight distal sesamoidean desmitis in 27 horses, *Vet Radiol Ultrasound* 48:303, 2007.

58. Smith S, Dyson S, Murray R: Magnetic resonance imaging of distal sesamoidean

ligament injury, *Vet Radiol Ultrasound* 49:516, 2008.

59. Mero J, Pool R: Twenty cases of degenerative suspensory desmitis in Peruvian Paso horses, *Proc Am Assoc Equine Pract* 48:329, 2002.

60. Mero J, Scarlett J: Diagnostic criteria for degenerative suspensory ligament desmitis in Peruvian Paso horses, *J Equine Vet Sci* 25:224, 2005.

61. Halper J, Kim B, Khan A, et al: Degenerative suspensory ligament desmitis as a systemic disorder characterised by proteoglycan accumulation, *BMC Vet Res* 2:12, 2006.

62. Schenkman D, Armien A, Pool R, et al: Systemic proteoglycan deposition is not a characteristic of equine degenerative suspensory ligament desmitis, *J Equine Vet Sci* 29:748, 2009.

CHAPTER 73 Clinical Use of Stem Cells, Marrow Components, and Other Growth Factors

1. Benjamin M, Kaiser E, Milz S: Structure-function relationships in tendons: a review, *J Anat* 212:211, 2008.

2. Nirmalanandhan VS, Rao M, Shearn JT, et al: Effect of scaffold material, construct length and mechanical stimulation on the in vitro stiffness of the engineered tendon construct, *J Biomech* 41:822, 2008.

3. Aspenberg P: Stimulation of tendon repair: mechanical loading, GDFs and platelets. A mini-review, *Int Orthop* 31:783, 2007.

4. Nirmalanandhan VS, Shearn JT, Juncosa-Melvin N, et al: Improving linear stiffness of the cell-seeded collagen sponge constructs by varying the components of the mechanical stimulus, *Tissue Eng Part A* 14:1883, 2008.

5. Kuo CK, Tuan RS: Mechanoactive tenogenic differentiation of human mesenchymal stem cells, *Tissue Eng Part A* 14:1615, 2008.

6. Hipp J, Atala A: Sources of stem cells for regenerative medicine, *Stem Cell Rev* 4:3, 2008.

7. Nixon AJ, Goodrich LR, Scimeca MS, et al: Gene therapy in musculoskeletal repair, *Ann N Y Acad Sci* 1117:310, 2007.

8. Tweedell KS: New paths to pluripotent stem cells, *Curr Stem Cell Res Ther* 3:151, 2008.

9. Yingling GL, Nobert KM: Regulatory considerations related to stem cell treatment in horses, *J Am Vet Med Assoc* 232:1657, 2008.

10. Kisiday JD, Kopesky PW, Evans CH, et al: Evaluation of adult equine bone marrow- and adipose-derived progenitor cell chondrogenesis in hydrogel cultures, *J Orthop Res* 26:322, 2008.

11. Vidal MA, Robinson SO, Lopez MJ, et al: Comparison of chondrogenic potential in equine mesenchymal stromal cells derived from adipose tissue and bone marrow, *Vet Surg* 37:713, 2008.

12. Vidal MA, Kilroy GE, Lopez MJ, et al: Characterization of equine adipose tissue-derived stromal cells: adipogenic and osteogenic capacity and comparison with bone marrow-derived mesenchymal stromal cells, *Vet Surg* 36:613, 2007.

13. Martin DR, Cox NR, Hathcock TL, et al: Isolation and characterization of multipotential mesenchymal stem cells from feline bone marrow, *Exp Hematol* 30:879, 2002.

14. Pittenger MF, Mackay AM, Beck SC, et al: Multilineage potential of adult human mesenchymal stem cells, *Science* 284:143, 1999.

15. Herthel DJ: Clinical use of stem cells and marrow components to stimulate suspensory ligament regeneration. In Ross MW, Dyson SJ, eds: *Diagnosis and Management of Lameness in the Horse*, ed 1, St. Louis, 2003, Saunders.

16. Kovacevic D, Rodeo SA: Biological augmentation of rotator cuff tendon repair, *Clin Orthop Relat Res* 466:622, 2008.

17. Li F, Jia H, Yu C: ACL reconstruction in a rabbit model using irradiated Achilles allograft seeded with mesenchymal stem cells or PDGF-B gene-transfected mesenchymal stem cells, *Knee Surg Sports Traumatol Arthrosc* 15:1219, 2007.

18. Butler DL, Juncosa-Melvin N, Boivin GP, et al: Functional tissue engineering for tendon repair: a multidisciplinary strategy using mesenchymal stem cells, bioscaffolds, and mechanical stimulation, *J Orthop Res* 26:1, 2008.

19. Schnabel LV, Mohammed HO, Jacobson MS, et al: Effects of platelet rich plasma and acellular bone marrow on gene expression patterns and DNA content of equine suspensory ligament explant cultures, *Equine Vet J* 40:260, 2008.

20. Schnabel LV, Mohammed HO, Miller BJ, et al: Platelet rich plasma (PRP) enhances anabolic gene expression patterns in flexor digitorum superficialis tendons, *J Orthop Res* 25:230, 2007.

21. Smith JJ, Ross MW, Smith RK: Anabolic effects of acellular bone marrow, platelet rich plasma, and serum on equine suspensory ligament fibroblasts in vitro, *Vet Comp Orthop Traumatol* 19:43, 2006.

22. Chong AK, Ang AD, Goh JC, et al: Bone marrow-derived mesenchymal stem cells influence early tendon-healing in a rabbit Achilles tendon model, *J Bone Joint Surg Am* 89:74, 2007.

23. Pacini S, Spinabella S, Trombi L, et al: Suspension of bone marrow-derived undifferentiated mesenchymal stromal cells for repair of superficial digital flexor tendon in race horses, *Tissue Eng* 13:2949, 2007.

24. Smith RK: Use of bone marrow-derived mesenchymal stem cells to enhance tendon and ligament healing, *Proc Am Coll Vet Surg Symposium* CD-ROM, 2008.

25. Nixon AJ, Dahlgren LA, Haupt JL, et al: Effect of adipose-derived nucleated cell fractions on tendon repair in horses with collagenase-induced tendinitis, *Am J Vet Res* 69:928, 2008.

26. Nixon AJ, Goodrich LR, Scimeca MS, et al: Gene therapy in musculoskeletal repair, *Ann N Y Acad Sci* 1117:310, 2007.

27. Chen CH, Cao Y, Wu YF, et al: Tendon healing in vivo: gene expression and production of multiple growth factors in early tendon healing period, *J Hand Surg Am* 33:1834, 2008.

28. Bullough R, Finnigan T, Kay A, et al: Tendon repair through stem cell intervention: cellular and molecular approaches, *Disabil Rehabil* 30:1746, 2008.

29. James R, Kesturu G, Balian G, et al: Tendon: biology, biomechanics, repair, growth factors, and evolving treatment options, *J Hand Surg Am* 33:102, 2008.

30. Molloy T, Wang Y, Murrell G: The roles of growth factors in tendon and ligament healing, *Sports Med* 33:381, 2003.

31. Yoneno K, Ohno S, Tanimoto K, et al: Multidifferentiation potential of mesenchymal stem cells in three-dimensional collagen gel cultures, *J Biomed Mater Res A* 75:733, 2005.

32. Tang JB, Xu Y, Ding F, et al: Tendon healing in vitro: promotion of collagen gene expression by bFGF with NF-kappaB gene activation, *J Hand Surg Am* 28:215, 2003.

33. Zhang F, Liu H, Stile F, et al: Effect of vascular endothelial growth factor on rat Achilles tendon healing, *Plast Reconstr Surg* 112:1613, 2003.

34. Dahlgren LA, van der Meulen MC, Bertram JE, et al: Insulin-like growth factor-I improves cellular and molecular aspects of healing in a collagenase-induced model of flexor tendinitis, *J Orthop Res* 20:910, 2002.

35. Kang HJ, Kang ES: Ideal concentration of growth factors in rabbit's flexor tendon culture, *Yonsei Med J* 40:26, 1999.

36. Nurden AT, Nurden P, Sanchez M, et al: Platelets and wound healing, *Front Biosci* 13:3532, 2008.

37. Mishra A, Woodall J Jr, Vieira A: Treatment of tendon and muscle using platelet-rich plasma, *Clin Sports Med* 28:113, 2009.

38. McCarrel T, Fortier L: Temporal growth factor release from platelet-rich plasma, trehalose lyophilized platelets, and bone marrow aspirate and their effect on tendon and ligament gene expression, *J Orthop Res* 27:1033, 2009.

39. Smith RK, Korda M, Blunn GW, et al: Isolation and implantation of autologous equine mesenchymal stem cells from bone marrow into the superficial digital flexor tendon as a potential novel treatment, *Equine Vet J* 35:99, 2003.

40. Mishra A, Pavelko T: Treatment of chronic elbow tendinosis with buffered platelet-rich plasma, *Am J Sports Med* 34:1774, 2006.

41. Waselau M, Sutter WW, Genovese RL, et al: Intralesional injection of platelet-rich plasma followed by controlled exercise for treatment of midbody suspensory ligament desmitis in Standardbred racehorses, *J Am Vet Med Assoc* 232:1515, 2008.

CHAPTER 74 Diseases of the Digital Flexor Tendon Sheath, Palmar Annular Ligament, and Digital Annular Ligaments

1. Denoix J-M: Functional anatomy of tendons and ligaments in the distal limbs (manus and pes), *Vet Clin North Am Equine Pract* 10:273, 1994.

2. Andrews DR, Smith RK: Comparison of sites of synoviocentesis of the equine digital flexor tendon sheath. Proceedings of the Thirty-Seventh Meeting of the British Equine Veterinary Association Congress, Birmingham, England, 1998.

3. Hassel DM, Stover SM, Yarbrough TB, et al: Palmar-plantar axial sesamoidean approach to the digital flexor tendon sheath in horses, *J Am Vet Med Assoc* 217:1343, 2000.

4. Malark JA, Nixon AJ, Skinner KL, et al: Characteristics of digital flexor tendon sheath fluid from clinically normal horses, *Am J Vet Res* 52:1292, 1992.

5. Sampson S, Schneider R, Tucker R, et al: Magnetic resonance imaging features of oblique and straight sesamoidean desmitis in 27 horses, *Vet Radiol Ultrasound* 48:303, 2007.

6. Smith RKW, Heinegård D: Cartilage oligomeric matrix protein levels in digital sheath synovial fluid and serum with tendon injury, *Equine Vet J* 32:52, 2000.

7. Smith RKW, Onnerfjord P, Smith MR, et al: Molecular markers of tendon injury: clinical aid or research tool? Havemeyer Meeting of Molecular Markers, Estes Park, Colorado, 2005.

8. Smith RK, Webbon PM: Diagnostic imaging in the athletic horse: musculoskeletal ultrasonography. In Hodgson DR, Rose RJ, eds: *Principles and practice of equine sports medicine: the athletic horse*, Philadelphia, 1994, Saunders.

9. Verschooten F, Picavet TM: Desmitis of the fetlock annular ligament in the horse, *Equine Vet J* 18:138, 1986.

10. Hago BE, Vaughan LC: Use of contrast radiography in the investigation of tenosynovitis and bursitis in horses, *Equine Vet J* 18:375, 1986.

11. Nixon AJ: Endoscopy of the digital flexor tendon sheath in horses, *Vet Surg* 19:266, 1990.

12. Fortier LA, Nixon AJ, Ducharme NG, et al: Tenoscopic examination and proximal annular ligament desmotomy for treatment of equine "complex" digital sheath tenosynovitis, *Vet Surg* 28:429, 1999.

13. Gillis C: Digital sheath. In White NA, Moore JN, eds: *Current techniques in equine surgery and lameness*, ed 2, Philadelphia, 1998, Saunders.

14. Wright IM, McMahon PJ: Tenosynovitis associated with longitudinal tears of the digital flexor tendons in horses: a report of 20 cases, *Equine Vet J* 31:12, 1999.

15. Smith MR, Wright IM: Noninfected tenosynovitis of the digital flexor tendon sheath: a retrospective analysis of 76 cases, *Equine Vet J* 38:134, 2006.

16. Barr AR, Dyson SJ, Barr FJ, et al: Tendonitis of the deep digital flexor tendon in the distal metacarpal/metatarsal region associated with tenosynovitis of the digital sheath in the horse, *Equine Vet J* 27:348, 1995.

17. Smith RKW, Schramme MC, Voute LC, et al: Diagnosis and management of penetrating injuries to the deep digital flexor tendon in the pastern region, *Vet Surg* 24:293, 1995.

18. Honnas CM, Schumacher J, Cohen ND, et al: Septic tenosynovitis in horses: 25 cases (1983-1989), *J Am Vet Med Assoc* 199:1616, 1991.

19. Nixon AJ: Septic tenosynovitis. In White NA, Moore JN, eds: *Current practice in equine surgery*, Philadelphia, 1990, JB Lippincott.

20. Schneider RK, Bramlage LR, Mecklenburg LM, et al: Open drainage, intra-articular and systemic antibiotics in the treatment of septic arthritis/tenosynovitis in horses, *Equine Vet J* 24:443, 1992.

21. Whitehair KJ, Adams SB, Parker JE, et al: Regional limb perfusion with antibiotics in three horses, *Vet Surg* 21:286, 1992.

22. Summerhays GE: Treatment of traumatically induced synovial sepsis in horses with gentamicin-impregnated collagen sponges, *Vet Rec* 147:184, 2000.

23. Butson RJ, Schramme MC, Garlick MH, et al: Treatment of intrasynovial infection with gentamicin-impregnated polymethylmethacrylate beads, *Vet Rec* 138:460, 1996.

24. Adams SB, Lescun TB: How to treat septic joints with constant intra-articular infusion of gentamicin or amikacin, *Proc Am Assoc Equine Pract* 46:188, 2000.

25. Wright IM, Smith MR, Humphrey DJ, et al: Endoscopic surgery in the treatment of contaminated and infected synovial cavities, *Equine Vet J* 35:613, 2003.

26. Stashak TS, Vail TB, Park RB, et al: Fetlock annular ligament syndrome: results of desmotomy and factors that affect outcome in 49 horses. Proceedings of the Fifth Annual Scientific Meeting of the European College of Veterinary Surgery, Utrecht, The Netherlands, 1996.

27. Owen R, Dyson S, Parkin T, et al: A retrospective study of palmar/plantar annular ligament desmopathy in 71 horses: 2001-2006, *Equine Vet J* 40:237, 2008.

28. Torre F, Benazzi C, Potschka R: Constriction of the fetlock annular ligament: relationship between clinical and histopathological findings, *Pferdeheilkunde* 14:461, 1998.

29. Enzerink E, Dik KJ: Palmar/plantar annular ligament insertion injury: a report of 4 cases, *Equine Vet Educ* 13:75, 2001.

30. Dik KJ, Dyson SJ, Vail TB: Aseptic tenosynovitis of the digital flexor tendon sheath, fetlock and pastern annular ligament constriction, *Vet Clin North Am Equine Pract* 11:151, 1995.

31. Ross M: Personal communication, 2001.

32. Denoix JM, Busoni V, Olalla MJ: Ultrasonographic examination of the proximal scutum in the horse, *Equine Vet J* 29:136, 1997.

33. Hertsch B, Becker C: Zum Vorkommen der aseptischen Nekrose im Ligamentum palmare bzw plantare beim Pferd: ein Betrag zur Differenzierung der Gleichbeinerkrankungen, *Dtsch Tierärztl Wochenschr* 93:263, 1986.

34. Wisner ER, O'Brien TR, Pool RR, et al: Osteomyelitis of the axial border of the proximal sesamoid bones in seven horses, *Equine Vet J* 23:383, 1991.

35. Dabareiner RM, Watkins JP, Carter GK, et al: Osteitis/osteomyelitis of the axial border of the proximal sesamoid bones in horses, *Proc Am Assoc Equine Pract* 45:156, 1999.

36. Winberg F, Petterson H: Diagnosis and treatment of lesions in the intersesamoidean ligament and its adjoining structures, *Vet Surg* 23:215, 1994.

37. Denoix JM, Crevier N, Azevedo C: Ultrasound examination of the pastern in horses, *Proc Am Assoc Equine Pract* 37:364, 1991.

38. Dik KJ, Boroffka S, Stolk P: Ultrasonographic assessment of the proximal digital annular ligament in the equine forelimb, *Equine Vet J* 26:59, 1994.

39. Cohen J, Schneider R, Zubrod C, et al: Desmitis of the distal digital annular ligament in 7 horses: MRI diagnosis and surgical treatment, *Vet Surg* 37:336, 2008.

40. Dyson S: Personal communication, 2009.

41. Schramme MC, Smith RK: Diseases of the digital flexor tendon sheath, the palmar annular ligament and digital annular ligaments. In Ross M, Dyson S, eds: *Diagnosis and management of lameness in the horse*, St. Louis, 2003, Saunders.

42. Schumacher J, Auer J: A case report of a carpal ganglion in a horse, *J Equine Med Surg* 3:391, 1979.

43. Crawford A, Eliashar E, Smith RK: Surgical treatment of digital sheath synovial ganglia. European College Veterinary Surgeons Proceedings, Nantes, France, 2009.

CHAPTER 75 The Carpal Canal and Carpal Synovial Sheath

1. Shoemaker R, Bertone A, Mohammed L, et al: Desmotomy of the accessory ligament of the superficial digital flexor muscle in equine cadaver limbs, *Vet Surg* 20:245, 1991.

2. Dyson S, Dik K: Miscellaneous conditions of tendons, tendon sheaths and ligaments, *Vet Clin North Am Equine Pract* 11:315, 1995.

3. Cauvin E, Munroe G, Boswell J, et al: Gross and ultrasonographic anatomy of the carpal sheath, *Vet Rec* 141:489, 1997.

4. Denoix J-M, Busoni V: Ultrasonographic anatomy of the accessory ligament of the superficial digital flexor tendon in horses, *Equine Vet J* 31:186, 1999.

5. Jorgensen J, Stewart A, Stewart M, Genovese R: Ultrasonographic examination of the caudal structures of the distal antebrachium in the horse, *Equine Vet Educ* 22:146, 2010.

6. Nagy A, Dyson S: Magnetic resonance findings of the carpus and proximal metacarpal region of non-lame horses, *Proc Am Assoc Equine Pract* 55, 408, 2009.

7. Radue P: Carpal tunnel syndrome due to a fracture of the accessory carpal bone, *Equine Vet J* 3:8, 1981.

8. Denoix J-M: Personal communication, 1998.

9. Ross M: Personal communication, 2001.

10. Denoix J-M, Guizien I, Perrot P, et al: Ultrasonographic diagnosis of spontaneous injuries of the accessory ligament of the superficial digital flexor tendon (proximal check ligament) in 23 horses, *Proc Am Assoc Equine Pract* 41:142, 1995.

11. Denoix J-M, Audigie F: Examen echographique du carpe du cheval: lesions identifies sur 45 cas cliniques, *Prat Vet Equine* 25:193, 1993.

12. Dik K: Radiographic and ultrasonographic imaging of soft tissue disorders of the equine carpus, *Tijdschr Diergeneeskd* 115:1168, 1990.

13. Nixon A, Schachter B, Pool R: Exostoses of the caudal perimeter of the radial physis as a cause of carpal synovial sheath tenosynovitis and lameness in horses: 10 cases (1999-2003), *J Am Vet Med Assoc* 224:264, 2004.

14. Dyson S: Fractures of the accessory carpal bone, *Equine Vet Educ* 2:188, 1990.

15. Barr A: Fractures of the accessory carpal bone in the horse, *Vet Rec* 126:432, 1990.

16. Mackay-Smith MP, Cushing L, Leslie A: "Carpal canal" syndrome in horses, *J Am Vet Med Assoc* 160:993, 1972.

CHAPTER 76 The Tarsal Sheath

1. Jones RD: The diagnosis and treatment of avulsion fracture of the sustentaculum tali in a horse, *Can Vet J* 17:287, 1976.

2. Edwards GB: Changes in the sustentaculum tali associated with distension of the tarsal sheath (thoroughpin), *Equine Vet J* 10:97, 1978.

3. Dik KJ, Merkens HW: Unilateral distension of the tarsal sheath in the horse: a report of 11 cases, *Equine Vet J* 19:307, 1987.

4. MacDonald MH, Honnas CM, Meagher DM: Osteomyelitis of the calcaneus in horses: 28 cases (1972-1987), *J Am Vet Med Assoc* 194:1317, 1989.

5. Welsh RD, Auer JA, Watkins JP, et al: Surgical treatment of tarsal sheath effusion associated with an exostosis on the calcaneus of a horse, *J Am Vet Med Assoc* 196:1992, 1993.

6. Santschi MS, Adams SB, Fessler JF, et al: Treatment of bacterial tarsal tenosynovitis and osteitis of the sustentaculum tali of the calcaneus in five horses, *Equine Vet J* 29:244, 1997.

7. Van Pelt RW: Inflammation of the tarsal synovial sheath (thoroughpin) in horses, *J Am Vet Med Assoc* 155:1481, 1996.

8. Dik KJ, Leitch M: Soft tissue injuries of the tarsus, *Vet Clin North Am Equine Pract* 11:235, 1995.

9. Blumenshine KM, Dyson SJ: Soft tissue injuries of the hock. In Robinson NE, ed: *Current therapy in equine medicine*, ed 4, Philadelphia, 1997, Saunders.

10. Barone R: *Anatomie Comparee des Mammiferes domestiques*, ed 3, vol 2, Paris, 1989, Editions Vigot.

11. World Association of Veterinary Anatomists: *Nomina anatomica veterinaria*, ed 2, Vienna, 1973, Nomina Anatomica Veterinaria.

12. Dik KJ: Ultrasonography of the equine tarsus, *Vet Radiol Ultrasound* 34:36, 1993.

13. Cauvin ERJ, Tapprest J, Munroe GA, et al: Endoscopic examination of the tarsal sheath of the lateral digital flexor tendon in horses, *Equine Vet J* 31:219, 1999.

14. Stashak TS: Lameness. In Stashak TS, ed: *Adams' lameness in horses*, ed 4, Philadelphia, 1987, Lea & Febiger.

15. Bertone AL: Infectious tenosynovitis, *Vet Clin North Am Equine Pract* 11:163, 1995.

16. McIlwraith CW: Diseases of joints, tendons, ligaments, and related structures. In Stashak TS, ed: *Adams' lameness in horses*, ed 4, Philadelphia, 1987, Lea & Febiger.

17. Butler JA, Colles CM, Dyson SJ, et al: *Clinical radiology of the horse*, Oxford, 1993, Blackwell Scientific.

18. Hago BED, Vaughan LC: Use of contrast radiography in the investigation of tenosynovitis and bursitis in horses, *Equine Vet J* 18:375, 1986.

19. Mettenleiter E, Meier HP, Ueltschi G, et al: Examination of the common tendon sheath of the M. flexor hallucis longus and the M. tibialis caudalis by ultrasound in the horse, *Anat Histol Embryol* 21:246, 1992.

20. Hand DR, Watkins JP, Honnas CM, et al: Osteomyelitis of the sustentaculum tali in horses: 10 cases (1992-1998), *J Am Vet Med Assoc* 219:341, 2001.

CHAPTER 77   Extensor Tendon Injury

1. Getty R: Equine myology. In: *Sisson and Grossman's the anatomy of the domestic animals*, ed 5, Philadelphia, 1975, Saunders.

2. Rooney JR: *Biomechanics of lameness in horses*, New York, 1977, Kreiger.

3. Hago BED, Vaughan LC: Radiographic anatomy of tendon sheaths and bursae in the horse, *Equine Vet J* 18:102, 1995.

4. Denoix J-M: The equine fetlock. In: *The equine distal limb: an atlas of clinical anatomy and comparative imaging*, London, 2000, Manson.

5. Llewellyn HR: A case of carpal intersynovial fistula in a horse, *Equine Vet J* 11:90, 1975.

6. Hago BED, Vaughan LC: Use of contrast radiography in the investigation of tenosynovitis and bursitis in horses, *Equine Vet J* 18:375, 1986.

7. Tnibar M, Kaser-Hotz B, Auer J: Ultrasonography of the dorsal and lateral equine carpus: technique and normal appearance, *Vet Radiol Ultrasound* 34:4, 1993.

8. Baxter GM: Retrospective study of lower limb wounds involving tendons, tendon sheaths or joints in horses, *Proc Am Assoc Equine Pract* 33:715, 1987.

9. Foland JW, Trotter GW, Stashak TS, et al: Traumatic injuries involving tendons of the distal limbs in horses: a retrospective study of 55 cases, *Equine Vet J* 23:422, 1995.

10. Belknap JK, Baxter GM, Nickels FA: Extensor tendon lacerations in horses (1982-1988), *J Am Vet Med Assoc* 203:428, 1993.

11. Mespoulhès-Rivière C, Martens A, Bogaert L, et al: Factors affecting outcome of extensor tendon lacerations in the distal limb of horses. A retrospective study of 156 cases (1994-2003), *Vet Comp Orthop Traumatol* 21:358, 2008.

12. Bertone AL: Tendon lacerations, *Vet Clin North Am Equine Pract* 11:293, 1995.

13. Crabill MR, Honnas CM, Taylor DS, et al: Stringhalt secondary to trauma to the dorsoproximal region of the metatarsus in horses: 10 cases (1986-1991), *J Am Vet Med Assoc* 205:867, 1994.

14. Yovich JV, Stashak TS, McIlwraith CW: Rupture of the common digital extensor tendons in foals, *Compend Contin Educ Pract Vet* 6:S373, 1984.

15. Stashak TS: Lameness. In: *Adams' lameness in horses*, ed 4, Philadelphia, 1987, Lea & Febiger.

16. Dyson SJ: Personal communication, 2001.

17. Myers VS, Gordon GW: Ruptured common digital extensor tendon associated with contracted flexor tendons on foals, *Proc Am Assoc Equine Pract* 21:67, 1975.

18. Kirker-Head C: Rupture of the common digital extensor tendon. In Colahan PT, Mayhew IG, Merritt AM, et al, eds: *Equine medicine and surgery*, vol 2, St Louis, 1999, Mosby.

19. Mason TA: Chronic tenosynovitis of the extensor tendons and tendon sheaths of the carpal region in the horse, *Equine Vet J* 9:186, 1997.

20. Kirker-Head C: Rupture of the extensor carpi radialis muscle. In Colahan PT, Mayhew IG, Merritt AM, et al, eds: *Equine medicine and surgery*, vol 2, St Louis, 1999, Mosby.

21. Catlin JE: Rupture of the tendon of the extensor carpi radialis muscle in the horse, *Vet Med Small Anim Clin* 59:1178, 1964.

22. Wallace CE: Chronic tendosynovitis of the extensor carpi radialis tendon in the horse, *Aust Vet J* 48:585, 1972.

23. Ross MW, Martin BB: Dorsomedial articular fracture of the proximal aspect of the third metacarpal bone in Standardbred racehorses: seven cases (1978-1990), *J Am Vet Med Assoc* 201:332, 1992.

24. Van Pelt RW: Idiopathic tenosynovitis in foals, *J Am Vet Med Assoc* 155:510, 1969.

25. Dyson SJ, Dik KJ: Miscellaneous conditions of tendons, tendon sheaths and ligaments, *Vet Clin North Am Equine Pract* 11:315, 1995.

26. Schneider RK, Bramlage LR, Moore RM, et al: A retrospective study of 192 horses affected with septic arthritis/tenosynovitis, *Equine Vet J* 24:436, 1992.

27. Hawkins JE, Lescun TB: Sepsis of the common digital extensor tendon sheath secondary to hemicircumferential periosteal transection in a foal, *J Am Vet Med Assoc* 211:331, 1997.

28. Honnas CM, Schumacher J, Cohen ND, et al: Septic tenosynovitis in horses: 25 cases (1983-1989), *J Am Vet Med Assoc* 199:616, 1991.

29. Moore RM, Schneider RK, Kowalski JJ, et al: Antimicrobial sensitivity of microorganisms isolated from 233 horses with musculoskeletal infection during 1979-1989, *Equine Vet J* 24:450, 1992.

30. Booth TM, Clegg PD, Singer ER, et al: Resection of the common digital extensor tendon in a gelding, *Vet Rec* 146:373, 2000.

31. Booth TM, Abbot J, Clements A, et al: Treatment of septic common digital extensor tenosynovitis by complete resection in seven horses, *Vet Surg* 33:107, 2004.

32. McIlwraith CW: Diseases of joints, tendons, ligaments and related structures. In Stashak TS, ed: *Adams' lameness in horses*, ed 4, Philadelphia, 1987, Lea & Febiger.

33. Platt D, Wright IM: Chronic tenosynovitis of the carpal extensor sheaths in 15 horses, *Equine Vet J* 29:11, 1997.

34. McIlwraith CW, Wright IM, Nixon A: *Diagnostic and surgical arthroscopy in the horse*, ed 3, Philadelphia, 2005, Elsevier.

35. Newell S, Roberts RE, Baskett A: Presumptive tenosynovial osteochondromatosis in a horse, *Vet Radiol Ultrasound* 37:112, 1996.

36. Smith RK, Coumbe A, Schramme MC: Bilateral synovial chondromatosis of the metatarsophalangeal joints in a pony, *Equine Vet J* 27:234, 1995.

37. Johnson JE, Ryan GD: Intersynovial fistula in the carpus of a horse, *Cornell Vet* 65:84, 1975.

38. Voute LC, Schramme MC, Boswell JC, et al: Subcutaneous abscessation on the dorsal aspect of the metatarsophalangeal joint in six horses. Proceedings of the 39th British Equine Veterinary Association Annual Congress, Birmingham, 207, 2000.

CHAPTER 78   Curb

1. Stashak TS: Curb. In Stashak TS, ed: *Adams' lameness in horses*, Philadelphia, 1987, Lea & Febiger.

2. Sullins KE: Curb. In Stashak TS, ed: *Adams' lameness in horses*, ed 5, Philadelphia, 2002, Lippincott Williams & Wilkins.

3. Ross MW, Genovese RL, Reef VB: Curb: a collection of plantar tarsal soft tissue injuries, *Proc Am Assoc Equine Pract* 48:337, 2002.

4. Reef VB: *Equine diagnostic ultrasound*, Philadelphia, 1998, Saunders.

5. White J: *White's farriery: a treatise on veterinary medicine*, vol III, London, 1823, C Baldwin.

CHAPTER 79   Bursae and Other Soft Tissue Swellings

1. Cohen N, Carter G, McMullan W: Fistulous withers in horses: 24 cases (1984-1990), *J Am Vet Med Assoc* 201:121, 1992.

2. Gaughan E, Fubini S, Dietze A: Fistulous withers in horses: 14 cases (1984-1990), *J Am Vet Med Assoc* 193:964, 1988.

3. Hawkins J, Fessler F: Treatment of supraspinous bursitis by use of debridement in standing horses: 10 cases (1968-1999), *J Am Vet Med Assoc* 217:74, 2000.

4. Butler J, Colles C, Dyson S, et al: The spine. In *Clinical radiology of the horse*, ed 3, Oxford, 2008, Wiley-Blackwell.

5. Dyson S: Bursae and other soft tissue swellings. In Ross MW, Dyson SJ, eds: *Diagnosis and management of lameness in the horse*, St Louis, 2003, Elsevier.

6. MacDonald M, Honnas C, Meagher D: Osteomyelitis of the calcaneus in horses: 28 cases (1972-1987), *J Am Vet Med Assoc* 194:1317, 1989.

7. Post E, Singer E, Clegg P: A retrospective study of 23 cases of septic calcaneal bursitis in the horse, *Equine Vet J* 35:662, 2003.

8. Bassage L, Garcia-Lopez J, Currid E: Osteolytic lesions of the tuber calcanei in two horses, *J Am Vet Med Assoc* 217:710, 2000.

9. Butler J, Colles C, Dyson S, et al: The tarsus. In *Clinical radiology of the horse*, ed 3, Oxford, 2008, Wiley-Blackwell.

10. Ingle-Fehr J, Baxter G: Endoscopy of the calcaneal bursa in horses, *Vet Surg* 27:561, 1998.

11. Gabel A: Lameness caused by inflammation in the distal hock, *Vet Clin North Am Large Anim Pract* 2:101, 1980.

12. Honnas C, Schumacher J, McClure S, et al: Treatment of olecranon bursitis in horses: 10 cases (1986-1993), *J Am Vet Med Assoc* 206:1022, 1995.

13. Dik K, Leitch M: Soft tissue injuries of the tarsus, *Vet Clin North Am Equine Pract* 11:235, 1995.
14. Dik K, Merkens H: Unilateral distension of the tarsal sheath in the horse: a report of 11 cases, *Equine Vet J* 19:307, 1987.
15. Whitton C, Kannegeiter N: Tarsal sheath rupture in a horse, *Aust Equine Vet* 13:50, 1995.

CHAPTER 80　Other Soft Tissue Injuries

1. Koening J, Cruz A, Genovese R, et al: Rupture of the peroneus tertius tendon in 25 horses, *Proc Am Assoc Equine Pract* 48:326, 2002.
2. Dik K: Ultrasonography of the equine crus, *Vet Radiol Ultrasound* 34:28, 1995.
3. Proudman C: Common calcaneal tendonitis in a horse, *Equine Vet Educ* 4:277, 1992.
4. Dyson S, Kidd L: Five cases of gastrocnemius tendonitis in the horse, *Equine Vet J* 23:25, 1991.
5. Dyson S: Gastrocnemius tendonitis in the horse. Proceedings of the Fifteenth Bain-Fallon Memorial Lectures, Canberra, Australia, 1993.
6. Dyson S, Dik K: Miscellaneous conditions of tendons, tendons sheaths and ligaments, *Vet Clin North Am Equine Pract* 11:315, 1995.
7. Dyson S: Other soft tissue injuries. In Ross MW, Dyson SJ, eds: *Diagnosis and management of lameness in the horse*, St Louis, 2003, Elsevier.
8. Swor TM, Schneider RK, Ross MW, et al: Injury to the origin of the gastrocnemius muscle as a possible cause of lameness in four horses, *J Am Vet Med Assoc* 219:215, 2001.
9. Dyson S: Unpublished data, 2009.
10. Jesty S, Palmer J, Parente E, et al: *J Am Vet Med Assoc* 227:1965, 2005.
11. Tull T, Woodie J, Ruggles A, et al: Management and assessment of prognosis after gastrocnemius disruption in Thoroughbred foals: 28 cases (1993-2007), *Equine Vet J* 2010 (in press).
12. Scott E, Breuhas B, Gertsen K: Surgical repair of dislocated superficial digital flexor tendon in a horse, *J Am Vet Med Assoc* 181:171, 1982.
13. Phillips T: Dislocation of the superficial digital flexor tendon from the tuber calcanei, *Proc Br Equine Vet Assoc Congress* 39:82, 2000.
14. Booth T, Abbott J, Clements A, et al: Complete resection of the common digital extensor tendon in 7 horses, *Vet Surg* 33:107, 2004.

CHAPTER 81　Tendon Lacerations

1. Foland JW, Trotter GW, Stashak TS, et al: Traumatic injuries involving tendons of the distal limbs in horses: a retrospective study of 55 cases, *Equine Vet J* 23:422, 1991.
2. Belknap JK, Baxter GM, Nickels FA: Extensor tendon lacerations in horses: 50 cases (1982-1988), *J Am Vet Med Assoc* 203:428, 1993.
3. Crass JR, Genovese RL, Render JA, et al: Magnetic resonance, ultrasound and histopathologic correlation of acute and healing equine tendon injuries, *Vet Radiol Ultrasound* 33:206, 1992.

4. Bertone AL, Stashak TS, Smith FW, et al: A comparison of repair methods for gap healing in equine flexor tendon, *Vet Surg* 19:254, 1990.
5. Jann HW, Good JK, Morgan SJ, et al: Healing of transected equine superficial digital flexor tendons with and without tenorrhaphy, *Vet Surg* 21:40, 1992.
6. Easley KJ, Stashak TS, Smith FW, et al: Mechanical properties for four suture patterns for transected equine tendon repair, *Vet Surg* 19:102, 1990.
7. Flecker RH, Wagner PC: Therapy and corrective shoeing for equine tendon disorders, *Comp Cont Educ Pract Vet* 8:970, 1986.
8. Taylor S, Pascoe J, Meagher D, et al: Digital flexor tendon lacerations in horses: 50 cases (1975-1990), *J Am Vet Med Assoc* 206:342, 1995.
9. Crabhill M, Honnas C, Taylor S, et al: Stringhalt secondary to trauma to the dorsoproximal region of the metatarsus in horses: 10 cases (1986-1991), *J Am Vet Med Assoc* 205:867, 1994.

CHAPTER 82　Soft Tissue Injuries of the Pastern

1. Reef VB: Musculoskeletal ultrasonography. In Reef VB, ed: *Equine diagnostic ultrasound*, Philadelphia, 1998, Saunders.
2. Reef VB: Ultrasonic diagnosis of tendon and ligament disease. In White NA, Moore JN, eds: *Current practice in equine surgery*, Philadelphia, 1990, JB Lippincott.
3. Denoix J, Crevier N, Azevdeo C: Ultrasound examination of the pastern in horses, *Proc Am Assoc Equine Pract* 37:363, 1991.
4. Dyson S: Ultrasonographic examination of the pastern region, *Equine Vet Educ* 4:254, 1992.
5. Dyson SJ, Denoix JM: Tendon, tendon sheath, and ligament injuries in the pastern, *Vet Clin North Am Equine Pract* 11:217, 1995.
6. Redding WR: Sonographic exam of the digital flexor tendon sheath, distal flexor tendons, and soft tissues of the palmar pastern region, *Proc Am Assoc Equine Pract* 39:11, 1993.
7. Denoix J, Audigie F: Ultrasonographic examination of joints in horses, *Proc Am Assoc Equine Pract* 47:366, 2001.
8. Wright IM: Ligaments associated with joints, *Vet Clin North Am Equine Pract* 11:249-291, 1995.
9. Wright I: Ligaments associated with joints, *Proc Dubai Int Equine Symp* 241, 1996.
10. Edinger J, Mobius G, Ferguson J: Comparison of tenoscopic and ultrasonographic methods of examination of the digital flexor tendon sheath in horses, *Vet Comp Orthop Traumatol* 18:209, 2005.
11. Denoix JM: Functional anatomy of tendons and ligaments in the distal limbs (manus and pes), *Vet Clin North Am Equine Pract* 10:273, 1994.
12. Denoix JM: Diagnostic techniques for identification and documentation of tendon and ligament injuries, *Vet Clin North Am Equine Pract* 10:365, 1994.
13. McClellan PD, Colby J: Ultrasonic structure of the pastern, *J Equine Vet Sci* 6:99, 1986.

14. Redding WR: Ultrasonic imaging of the structures of the digital sheath, *Compend Contin Educ Pract Vet* 13:1824, 1991.
15. Redding WR: Evaluation of the equine digital flexor tendon sheath using diagnostic ultrasound and contrast radiography, *Vet Radiol Ultrasound* 34:42, 1993.
16. Schneider RK, Tucker RL, Habegger SR, et al: Desmitis of the straight sesamoidean ligament in horses: 9 cases (1995-1997), *J Am Vet Med Assoc* 222:973, 2003.
17. Dik KJ, Dyson SJ, Vail TB: Aseptic tenosynovitis of the digital flexor tendon sheath, fetlock and pastern annular ligament constriction, *Vet Clin North Am Equine Pract* 11:151, 1995.
18. Dik KJ, Boroffka S, Stolk P: Ultrasonographic assessment of the proximal digital annular ligament in the equine forelimb, *Equine Vet J* 26:59, 1994.
19. Sampson SN, Schneider RK, Tucker RL, et al: Magnetic resonance imaging features of oblique and straight distal sesamoidean desmitis in 27 horses, *Vet Radiol Ultrasound* 48:303, 2007.
20. Smith S, Dyson S, Murray R: Magnetic resonance imaging of distal sesamoidean ligament injury, *Vet Radiol Ultrasound* 49:516, 2008.
21. Gibson KT, Burbidge HM, Anderson BH: Tendonitis of the branches of insertion of the superficial digital flexor tendon in horses, *Aust Vet J* 75:253, 1997.
22. Reimer J: Ultrasonography of the pastern. 1. Anatomy and pathology. 2. Outcome of selected injuries in racehorses, *Proc Am Assoc Equine Pract* 43:123, 1997.
23. Dyson S. Personal communication 2010.
24. Smith M, Dyson S, Murray R: Is a magic angle effect observed in the collateral ligaments of the distal interphalangeal joint or the oblique sesamoidean ligaments during standing magnetic resonance imaging? *Vet Radiol Ultrasound* 49:509, 2008.
25. Smith M: A comparison of a high-field and a low-field magnetic resonance imaging system for evaluation of structures of the equine distal limb. PhD Thesis, University of London, 2009.

CHAPTER 83　Skeletal Muscle and Lameness

1. Madigan JE, Valberg SJ, Ragle C, et al: Muscle spasms associated with ear tick (Otobius megnini) infestations in five horses, *J Am Vet Med Assoc* 207:74, 1995.
2. Holmgren N, Valberg S: Measurement of serum myoglobin concentrations in horses by immunodiffusion, *Am J Vet Res* 53:957, 1992.
3. Valberg S, Jonsson L, Lindholm A, et al: Muscle histopathology and plasma aspartate aminotransferase, creatine kinase and myoglobin changes with exercise in horses with recurrent exertional rhabdomyolysis, *Equine Vet J* 25:11, 1993.
4. Cardinet GH, Littrell JF, Freedland RA: Comparative investigations of serum creatine phosphokinase and glutamic-oxaloacetic transaminase activities in equine paralytic myoglobinuria, *Res Vet Sci* 8:219, 1967.
5. Volfinger L, Lassourd V, Michaux JM, et al: Kinetic evaluation of muscle damage during exercise by calculation of

amount of creatine kinase released, *Am J Physiol* 266:R434, 1994.

6. Argiroudis SA, Kent JE, Blackmore DJ: Observations on the isoenzymes of creatine kinase in equine serum and tissues, *Equine Vet J* 14:317, 1982.

7. Anderson MG: The influence of exercise on serum enzyme levels in the horse, *Equine Vet J* 7:160, 1975.

8. Cardinet GH III, Fowler ME, Tyler WS: The effects of training, exercise, and tying-up on serum transaminase activities in horses, *Am J Vet Res* 24:980, 1963.

9. Rowland LP, Penn AS: Myoglobinuria, *Med Clin North Am* 56:1233, 1972.

10. Poso AR, Soveri T, Oksanen HE: The effect of exercise on blood parameters in Standardbred and Finnish-bred horses, *Acta Vet Scand* 24:170, 1983.

11. Valberg SJ, Mickelson JR, Gallant EM, et al: Exertional rhabdomyolysis in quarter horses and thoroughbreds: one syndrome, multiple aetiologies, *Equine Vet J Suppl* 30:533, 1999.

12. Lentz LR, Valberg SJ, Herold LV, et al: Myoplasmic calcium regulation in myotubes from horses with recurrent exertional rhabdomyolysis, *Am J Vet Res* 63:1724, 2002.

13. Turner T: Use of thermography in lameness evaluation, *Proc Am Assoc Equine Pract* 44:224, 1998.

14. Matin P: Basic principles of nuclear medicine techniques for detection and evaluation of trauma and sports medicine injuries, *Semin Nucl Med* 18:90, 1988.

15. Crenshaw AG, Friden J, Hargens AR, et al: Increased technetium uptake is not equivalent to muscle necrosis: scintigraphic, morphological and intramuscular pressure analyses of sore muscles after exercise, *Acta Physiol Scand* 148:187, 1993.

16. Morris E, Seeherman HJ, O'Callaghan MW, et al: Scintigraphic identification of skeletal muscle damage in horses 24 hours after strenuous exercise, *Equine Vet J* 23:347, 1991.

17. Reef V: Musculoskeletal ultrasonography. In *Equine diagnostic ultrasonography*, Philadelphia, 1998, Saunders.

18. Levaille R, Biller D: Muscle evaluation, foreign bodies and miscellaneous swellings. In Mckinnon AO, Rantanen N, editors: *Equine diagnostic ultrasonography*, Baltimore, 1998, Williams and Wilkins.

19. Cardinet GH III, Holliday TA: Neuromuscular diseases of domestic animals: a summary of muscle biopsies from 159 cases, *Ann N Y Acad Sci* 317:290, 1979.

20. Cumming WJK, Fulthorpe JJ, Hudgson P, et al: *Color atlas of muscle pathology*, London, 1994, Mosby-Wolfe.

21. Beech J, Lindborg S, Fletcher JE, et al: Caffeine contractures, twitch characteristics and the threshold for Ca(2+)-induced Ca2+ release in skeletal muscle from horses with chronic intermittent rhabdomyolysis, *Res Vet Sci* 54:110, 1993.

22. Lentz LR, Valberg SJ, Balog EM, et al: Abnormal regulation of muscle contraction in horses with recurrent exertional rhabdomyolysis, *Am J Vet Res* 60:992, 1999.

23. Wijnberg ID, Back W, de Jong M, et al: The role of electromyography in clinical diagnosis of neuromuscular locomotor problems in the horse, *Equine Vet J* 36:718, 2004.

24. Wijnberg ID, Franssen H, Jansen GH, et al: Quantitative electromyographic examination in myogenic disorders of 6 horses, *J Vet Intern Med* 17:185, 2003.

25. Cheung K, Hume P, Maxwell L: Delayed onset muscle soreness: treatment strategies and performance factors, *Sports Med* 33:145, 2003.

26. Denoix JM, Pailloux JP: *Physical therapy and massage for the horse*, Pomfret, Vermont, 2001, Trafalgar Square Publishing.

27. Harris PA, Dyson S: Muscular disorders. In Robinson NE, ed: *Current therapy in equine medicine*, Philadelphia, 1997, Saunders.

28. Marks D: Non-metabolic factors associated with myositis, *Proc Am Assoc Equine Pract* 22:229, 1976.

29. Snow DH, Valberg SJ: Muscle-anatomy: adaptations to exercise and training. In Rose RJ, Hodgson DH, eds: *The athletic horse: principles and practice of equine sports medicine*, ed 1, Philadelphia, 1994, Saunders.

30. Jeffcott LB, Dalin G, Drevemo S, et al: Effect of induced back pain on gait and performance of trotting horses, *Equine Vet J* 14:129, 1982.

31. Porter M: Equine rehabilitation therapy for joint disease, *Vet Clin North Am Equine Pract* 21:599, 2005.

32. Porter M: *The new equine sports therapy*, 1998, The Blood Horse Inc., Eclipse Press.

33. Bromiley M: *Equine injury, therapy and rehabilitation*, Oxford, UK, 1993, Blackwell Scientific Publications.

34. Tyler CM, Hodgson DR, Rose RJ: Effect of a warm-up on energy supply during high intensity exercise in horses, *Equine Vet J* 28:117, 1996.

35. McCutcheon LJ, Geor RJ, Hinchcliff KW: Effects of prior exercise on muscle metabolism during sprint exercise in horses, *J Appl Physiol* 87:1914, 1999.

36. Lund RJ, Guthrie AJ, Mostert HJ, et al: Effect of three different warm-up regimens on heat balance and oxygen consumption of thoroughbred horses, *J Appl Physiol* 80:2190, 1996.

37. Cole FL, Mellor DJ, Hodgson DR, et al: Prevalence and demographic characteristics of exertional rhabdomyolysis in horses in Australia, *Vet Rec* 155:625, 2004.

38. Freestone JF, Carlson GR: Muscle disorders in the horse: a retrospective study, *Equine Vet J* 23:86, 1991.

39. Valentine BA, McDonough SP, Chang YF, et al: Polysaccharide storage myopathy in Morgan, Arabian, and Standardbred related horses and Welsh-cross ponies, *Vet Pathol* 37:193, 2000.

40. Harris PA: The equine rhabdomyolysis syndrome in the United Kingdom: epidemiological and clinical descriptive information, *Br Vet J* 147:373, 1991.

41. Harris PA, Snow DH, Greet TR, et al: Some factors influencing plasma AST/CK activities in thoroughbred racehorses, *Equine Vet J Suppl* 9:66, 1990.

42. McCraken RW, Steffen MR: New and successful treatments for azoturia, *Am J Vet Med* 7:429, 1912.

43. Beech J: Chronic exertional rhabdomyolysis, *Vet Clin North Am Equine Pract* 13:145, 1997.

44. Hodgson DR: Exertional rhabdomyolysis. In Robinson NE, ed: *Current therapy in equine medicine*, ed 2, Philadelphia, 1987, Saunders.

45. Harris PA: An outbreak of the equine rhabdomyolysis syndrome in a racing yard, *Vet Rec* 127:468, 1990.

46. Firshman AM, Valberg SJ, Bender JB, et al: Epidemiologic characteristics and management of polysaccharide storage myopathy in Quarter Horses, *Am J Vet Res* 64:1319, 2003.

47. Carlson GP: Medical problems associated with protracted heat and work stress in horses. Proceedings of the Fifth Annual Meeting of the Association of Equine Sports Medicine, Reno, Nevada, 1985.

48. Koterba A, Carlson GP: Acid-base and electrolyte alterations in horses with exertional rhabdomyolysis, *J Am Vet Med Assoc* 180:303, 1982.

49. Beech J: Diagnosing chronic intermittent rhabdomyolysis, *Vet Med* May:453, 1994.

50. Collinder E, Lindholm A, Rasmuson M: Genetic markers in standardbred trotters susceptible to the rhabdomyolysis syndrome, *Equine Vet J* 29:117, 1997.

51. Hunt LM, Valberg SJ, Steffenhagen K, et al: An epidemiological study of myopathies in Warmblood horses, *Equine Vet J* 40:171, 2008.

52. McCue ME, Valberg SJ: Estimated prevalence of polysaccharide storage myopathy among overtly healthy Quarter Horses in the United States, *Am J Vet Res* 231:746, 2007.

53. McCue ME, Ribeiro WP, Valberg SJ: Prevalence of polysaccharide storage myopathy in horses with neuromuscular disorders, *Equine Vet J* 36:340, 2006.

54. Firshman AM, Baird JD, Valberg SJ: Prevalences and clinical signs of polysaccharide storage myopathy and shivers in Belgian draft horses, *J Am Vet Med Assoc* 227:1958, 2005.

55. Valentine BA, Habecker PL, Patterson JS, et al: Incidence of polysaccharide storage myopathy in draft horse-related breeds: a necropsy study of 37 horses and a mule, *J Vet Diagn Invest* 13:63, 2001.

56. MacLeay JM, Sorum SA, Valberg SJ, et al: Epidemiologic analysis of factors influencing exertional rhabdomyolysis in Thoroughbreds, *Am J Vet Res* 60:1562, 1999.

57. McCue ME, Valberg SJ, Miller MB, et al: Glycogen synthase (GYS1) mutation causes a novel skeletal muscle glycogenosis, *Genomics* 91:458, 2008.

58. Valberg SJ, Cardinet GH III, Carlson GP, et al: Polysaccharide storage myopathy associated with recurrent exertional rhabdomyolysis in horses, *Neuromuscul Disord* 2:351, 1992.

59. McCue ME, Valberg SJ, Lucio M, et al: Glycogen synthase 1 (GYS1) mutation in diverse breeds with polysaccharide storage myopathy, *J Vet Intern Med* 22:1228, 2008.

60. MacLeay JM, Valberg SJ, Pagan JD, et al: Effect of ration and exercise on plasma creatine kinase activity and lactate concentration in Thoroughbred horses with

recurrent exertional rhabdomyolysis, *Am J Vet Res* 61:1390, 2000.

61. Harris P, Colles C: The use of creatinine clearance ratios in the prevention of equine rhabdomyolysis: a report of four cases, *Equine Vet J* 20:459, 1988.

62. Harris PA, Snow DH: Role of electrolyte imbalances in the pathophysiology of the equine rhabdomyolysis syndrome. In Persson S, Lindholm A, Jeffcott LB, eds: *Equine exercise physiology*, ed 3, Davis, CA, 1991, ICEEP Publications.

63. McKenzie EC, Valberg SJ, Godden SM, et al: Comparison of volumetric urine collection versus single-sample urine collection in horses consuming diets varying in cation-anion balance, *Am J Vet Res* 64:284, 2003.

64. Bain FT, Merritt AM: Decreased erythrocyte potassium concentration associated with exercise-related myopathy in horses, *J Am Vet Med Assoc* 196:1259, 1990.

65. Beech J, Lindborg S, Braund KG: Potassium concentrations in muscle, plasma and erythrocytes and urinary fractional excretion in normal horses and those with chronic intermittent exercise-associated rhabdomyolysis, *Res Vet Sci* 55:43, 1993.

66. Roneus B, Hakkarainen J: Vitamin E in serum and skeletal muscle tissue and blood glutathione peroxidase activity from horses with the azoturia-tying-up syndrome, *Acta Vet Scand* 26:425, 1985.

67. Hill H: Selenium-vitamin E treatment of tying-up in horses, *Mod Vet Pract* 43:66, 1962.

68. Upjohn MM, Archer RM, Christley RM, et al: Incidence and risk factors associated with exertional rhabdomyolysis syndrome in National Hunt racehorses in Great Britain, *Vet Rec* 156:763, 2005.

69. McGowan CM, Posner RE, Christley RM: Incidence of exertional rhabdomyolysis in polo horses in the USA and the United Kingdom in the 1999/2000 season, *Vet Rec* 150:535, 2002.

70. Dranchak PK, Valberg SJ, Onan GW, et al: Inheritance of recurrent exertional rhabdomyolysis in thoroughbreds, *J Am Vet Med Assoc* 227:762, 2005.

71. McGowan CM, Fordham T, Christley RM: Incidence and risk factors for exertional rhabdomyolysis in thoroughbred racehorses in the United Kingdom, *Vet Rec* 151:623, 2002.

72. McKenzie EC, Valberg SJ, Godden SM, et al: Effect of dietary starch, fat, and bicarbonate content on exercise responses and serum creatine kinase activity in equine recurrent exertional rhabdomyolysis, *J Vet Intern Med* 17:693, 2003.

73. Fraunfelder HC, Rossdale PD, Rickets SW: Changes in serum muscle enzyme levels in associated with training schedules and stages of oestrus cycle in thoroughbred racehorses, *Equine Vet J* 18:371, 1986.

74. Valberg S, Haggendal J, Lindholm A: Blood chemistry and skeletal muscle metabolic responses to exercise in horses with recurrent exertional rhabdomyolysis, *Equine Vet J* 25:17, 1993.

75. MacLeay JM, Valberg SJ, Pagan JD, et al: Effect of diet on thoroughbred horses with recurrent exertional rhabdomyolysis performing a standardised exercise test, *Equine Vet J Suppl* 30:458, 1999.

76. Waldron-Mease E: Hypothyroidism and myopathy in racing thoroughbreds and standardbreds, *J Equine Vet Sci* 3:124, 1979.

77. Lopez JR, Linares N, Cordovez G, et al: Elevated myoplasmic calcium in exercise-induced equine rhabdomyolysis, *Pflugers Arch* 430:293, 1995.

78. Ward TL, Valberg SJ, Gallant EM, et al: Calcium regulation by skeletal muscle membranes of horses with recurrent exertional rhabdomyolysis, *Am J Vet Res* 61:242, 2000.

79. Dranchak PK, Valberg SJ, Onan GW, et al: Exclusion of linkage of the RYR1, CACNA1S, and ATP2A1 genes to recurrent exertional rhabdomyolysis in Thoroughbreds, *Am J Vet Res* 67:1395, 2006.

80. Waldron-Mease E, Klein LV, Rosenberg H, et al: Malignant hyperthermia in a halothane-anesthetized horse, *J Am Vet Med Assoc* 179:896, 1981.

81. McKenzie EC, Valberg SJ, Godden SM, et al: Effect of oral administration of dantrolene sodium on serum creatine kinase activity after exercise in horses with recurrent exertional rhabdomyolysis, *Am J Vet Res* 65:74, 2004.

82. Edwards JG, Newtont JR, Ramzan PH, et al: The efficacy of dantrolene sodium in controlling exertional rhabdomyolysis in the Thoroughbred racehorse, *Equine Vet J* 35:707, 2003.

83. Beech J, Fletcher JE, Lizzo F, et al: Effect of phenytoin on the clinical signs and in vitro muscle twitch characteristics in horses with chronic intermittent rhabdomyolysis and myotonia, *Am J Vet Res* 49:2130, 1988.

84. McGowan CM, Menzies-Gow NJ, McDiarmid AM, et al: Four cases of equine polysaccharide storage myopathy in the United Kingdom, *Vet Rec* 152:109, 2003.

85. Valentine BA, Cooper BJ: Incidence of polysaccharide storage myopathy: necropsy study of 225 horses, *Vet Pathol* 42:823, 2005.

86. Valentine BA: Polysaccharide storage myopathy: a common metabolic disorder of horses, *Vet Pathol* 39:630, 2002.

87. Valberg SJ, MacLeay JM, Mickelson JR: Polysaccharide storage myopathy associated with exertional rhabdomyolysis in horses, *Comp Cont Educ Pract Vet* 19:1077, 1997.

88. Sprayberry KA, Madigan J, Lecouteur RA, et al: Renal failure, laminitis, and colitis following severe rhabdomyolysis in a draft horse-cross with polysaccharide storage myopathy, *Can Vet J* 39:500, 1998.

89. Valentine BA, de Lahunta A, Divers TJ, et al: Clinical and pathologic findings in two draft horses with progressive muscle atrophy, neuromuscular weakness, and abnormal gait characteristic of shivers syndrome, *J Am Vet Med Assoc* 215:1661, 1999.

90. Valentine BA, Credille KM, Lavoie JP, et al: Severe polysaccharide storage myopathy in Belgian and Percheron draught horses, *Equine Vet J* 29:220, 1997.

91. Valberg S: personal observation, 2009.

92. Annandale EJ, Valberg SJ, Mickelson JR, et al: Insulin sensitivity and skeletal muscle glucose transport in horses with equine polysaccharide storage myopathy, *Neuromuscul Disord* 14:666, 2004.

93. Annandale EJ, Valberg SJ, Essen-Gustavsson B: Effects of submaximal exercise on adenine nucleotide concentrations in skeletal muscle fibers of horses with polysaccharide storage myopathy, *Am J Vet Res* 66:839, 2005.

94. Ribeiro WP, Valberg SJ, Pagan JD, et al: The effect of varying dietary starch and fat content on serum creatine kinase activity and substrate availability in equine polysaccharide storage myopathy, *J Vet Intern Med* 18:887, 2004.

95. Valentine BA, Van Saun RJ, Thompson KN, et al: Role of dietary carbohydrate and fat in horses with equine polysaccharide storage myopathy, *J Am Vet Med Assoc* 219:1537, 2001.

96. Aleman M, Riehl J, Aldridge BM, et al: Association of a mutation in the ryanodine receptor 1 gene with equine malignant hyperthermia, *Muscle Nerve* 30:356, 2004.

97. McCue ME, Valberg SJ, Jackson M, et al: Polysaccharide storage myopathy phenotype in Quarter Horse-related breeds is modified by the presence of an *RYR1* mutation, *Neuromusc Disord* 19:37, 2009.

98. Aleman M, Brosnan RJ, Williams DC, et al: Malignant hyperthermia in a horse anesthetized with halothane, *J Vet Intern Med* 19:363, 2005.

99. Byrne E, Jones SL, Valberg SJ, et al: Rhabdomyolysis in two foals with polysaccharide storage myopathy and concurrent pneumonia, *Comp Cont Educ Pract Vet* 22:503, 2000.

100. Perkins G, Valberg SJ, Madigan JM, et al: Electrolyte disturbances in foals with severe rhabdomyolysis, *J Vet Intern Med* 12:173, 1998.

101. De La Corte FD, Valberg SJ, MacLeay JM, et al: Developmental onset of polysaccharide storage myopathy in 4 Quarter Horse foals, *J Vet Intern Med* 16:581, 2002.

102. Bernard W, Reimers JM, Cudd T, et al: Historical factors, clinicopathologic findings, clinical features and outcome of equine neonates presenting with or developing signs of central nervous system disease, *Proc Am Assoc Equine Pract* 41:222, 1995.

103. Dill SG, Rebhun WC: White muscle disease in foals, *Comp Cont Educ Pract Vet* 7:S627, 1985.

104. Sponseller BT, Valberg SJ, Tennent-Brown BS, et al: Severe acute rhabdomyolysis associated with Streptococcus equi infection in four horses, *J Am Vet Med Assoc* 227:1800, 2005.

105. Sponseller BT, Valberg SJ, Ward TL, et al: Muscular weakness and recumbency in a quarter horse colt due to glycogen branching enzyme deficiency, *Equine Vet Educ* 14:182, 2003.

106. Valberg SJ, Ward TL, Rush B, et al: Glycogen branching enzyme deficiency in quarter horse foals, *J Vet Intern Med* 15:572, 2001.

107. Ward TL, Valberg SJ, Adelson DL, et al: Glycogen branching enzyme (GBE1) mutation causing equine glycogen storage disease IV, *Mamm Genome* 15:570, 2004.

108. Wagner ML, Valberg SJ, Ames EG, et al: Allele frequency and likely impact of the glycogen branching enzyme deficiency

gene in Quarter Horse and Paint Horse populations, *J Vet Intern Med* 20:1207, 2006.

109. Tryon RC, Penedo MC, McCue ME, et al: Allele frequencies of inherited disease genes in subpopulations of American Quarter Horses, *J Am Vet Med Assoc* 234:120, 2009.

110. Kaese HJ, Valberg SJ, Hayden DW, et al: Infarctive purpura hemorrhagica in five horses, *J Am Vet Med Assoc* 226:1893, 2005.

111. Lewis SS, Valberg SJ, Nielsen IL: Suspected immune-mediated myositis in horses, *J Vet Intern Med* 21:495, 2007.

112. Barrott MJ, Brooks HW, McGowan CM: Suspected immune-mediated myositis in a pony, *Equine Vet Educ* April:80, 2004.

113. Traub-Dargatz JL, Schlipf JW Jr, Granstrom DE, et al: Multifocal myositis associated with Sarcocystis sp in a horse, *J Am Vet Med Assoc* 205:1574, 1994.

114. Hilton H, Madigan JE, Aleman M: Rhabdomyolysis associated with Anaplasma phagocytophilum infection in a horse, *J Vet Intern Med* 22:1061, 2008.

115. Peek SF, Semrad SD, Perkins GA: Clostridial myonecrosis in horses (37 cases 1985-2000), *Equine Vet J* 35:86, 2003.

116. Rebhun WC, Shin SJ, King JM, et al: Malignant edema in horses, *J Am Vet Med Assoc* 187:732, 1985.

117. Valberg SJ, Mckinnon AO: Clostridial cellulitis in the horse: a report of five cases, *Can Vet J* 25:67, 1984.

118. Vengust M, Arroyo LG, Weese JS, et al: Preliminary evidence for dormant clostridial spores in equine skeletal muscle, *Equine Vet J* 35:514, 2003.

119. Smith RK, Dyson SJ, Head MJ, et al: Ultrasonography of the equine triceps muscle before and after general anaesthesia and in postanaesthetic myopathy, *Equine Vet J* 28:311, 1996.

120. Hennig GE, Court MH: Equine postanesthetic myopathy: an update, *Compend Cont Educ* 13:1709, 1991.

121. Valverde A, Boyd CJ, Dyson DH, et al: Prophylactic use of dantrolene associated with prolonged postanesthetic recumbency in a horse, *J Am Vet Med Assoc* 197:1051, 1990.

122. Mubarek S, Hargens A: Acute compartment syndrome, *Surg Clin North Am* 63:539, 1983.

123. Hargens A, Akeson W: Pathophysiology of the compartment syndrome. In Mubarek S, Hargens A, eds: *Compartment syndromes and Volkmann's contracture*, Philadelphia, 1981, Saunders.

124. Sullins KE, Heath RB, Turner AS, et al: Possible antebrachial flexor compartment syndrome as a cause of lameness in two horses, *Equine Vet J* 19:147, 1987.

125. Maylin GA, Rubin DS, Lein DH: Selenium and vitamin E in horses, *Cornell Vet* 70:272, 1980.

126. McMurray CH, Rice DA: Vitamin E and selenium deficiency diseases, *Irish Vet J* 36:57, 1982.

127. Maas J, Galey FD, Peauroi JR, et al: The correlation between serum selenium and blood selenium in cattle, *J Vet Diagn Invest* 4:48, 1992.

128. Roneus B, Jonsson L: Muscular dystrophy in foals, *Zentralbl Veterinarmed A* 31:441, 1984.

129. Roneus BO, Hakkarainen RV, Lindholm CA, et al: Vitamin E requirements of adult Standardbred horses evaluated by tissue depletion and repletion, *Equine Vet J* 18:50, 1986.

130. Roneus B, Lindholm A: Glutathione peroxidase activity in the blood of healthy horses given different selenium supplementation, *Nord Vet Med* 35:337, 1983.

131. Roneus B: Glutathione peroxidase and selenium in the blood of healthy horses and foals affected by muscular dystrophy, *Nord Vet Med* 34:350, 1982.

132. Koller LD, Whitbeck GA, South PJ: Transplacental transfer and colostral concentrations of selenium in beef cattle, *Am J Vet Res* 45:2507, 1984.

133. Maas J, Peauroi JR, Tonjes T, et al: Intramuscular selenium administration in selenium-deficient cattle, *J Vet Intern Med* 7:342, 1993.

134. Ammend JF, Mallon FM, Wren WB: Equine monensin toxicosis: some experimental clinicopathological observations, *Comp Cont Educ Pract Vet* 2:S173, 1980.

135. Beier RC, Norman JO, Reagor JC, et al: Isolation of the major component in white snakeroot that is toxic after microsomal activation: possible explanation of sporadic toxicity of white snakeroot plants and extracts, *Nat Toxins* 1:286, 1993.

136. Olson CT, Keller WC, Gerken DF, et al: Suspected tremetol poisoning in horses, *J Am Vet Med Assoc* 185:1001, 1984.

137. Beier RC, Norman JO: The toxic factor in white snakeroot: identity, analysis and prevention, *Vet Hum Toxicol* 32 (Suppl): 81, 1990.

138. Martin BW, Terry MK, Bridges CH, et al: Toxicity of Cassia occidentalis in the horse, *Vet Hum Toxicol* 23:416, 1981.

139. Helman RG, Edwards WC: Clinical features of blister beetle poisoning in equids: 70 cases (1983-1996), *J Am Vet Med Assoc* 211:1018, 1997.

140. Whitwell KE, Harris P, Farrington PG: Atypical myoglobinuria: an acute myopathy in grazing horses, *Equine Vet J* 20:357, 1988.

141. Votion DM, Serteyn D: Equine atypical myopathy: a review, *Vet J* 178:185, 2008.

142. Finno CJ, Valberg SJ, Wunschmann A, et al: Seasonal pasture myopathy in horses in the midwestern United States: 14 cases (1998-2005), *J Am Vet Med Assoc* 229:1134, 2006.

143. Cassart D, Baise E, Cherel Y, et al: Morphological alterations in oxidative muscles and mitochondrial structure associated with equine atypical myopathy, *Equine Vet J* 39:26, 2007.

144. Westermann CM, Dorland L, Votion DM, et al: Acquired multiple Acyl-CoA dehydrogenase deficiency in 10 horses with atypical myopathy, *Neuromuscul Disord* 18:355, 2008.

145. Votion DM, Linden A, Delguste C, et al: Atypical myopathy in grazing horses: a first exploratory data analysis, *Vet J* 180:77, 2008.

146. Brewer BD: Disorders in calcium metabolism. In Robinson NE, ed: *Current therapy in equine medicine*, ed 2, Philadelphia, 1987, Saunders.

147. Baird JD: Lactation tetany (eclampsia) in a Shetland pony mare, *Aust Vet J* 47:402, 1971.

148. Blood DC, Radostis OM, Henderson JA: *Veterinary medicine*, ed 6, London, 1983, Baillière Tindall.

149. Day JW, Ranum LP: Genetics and molecular pathogenesis of the myotonic dystrophies, *Curr Neurol Neurosci Rep* 5:55, 2005.

150. Day JW, Ranum LP: RNA pathogenesis of the myotonic dystrophies, *Neuromuscul Disord* 15:5, 2005.

151. Roneus B, Lindholm A, Jonsson L: Myotonia in five horses, *Svensk Vet Tidning* 35:217, 1983.

152. Schooley EK, MacLeay JM, Cuddon P, et al: Myotonia congenita in a foal, *J Equine Vet Sci* 24:483, 2004.

153. Steinburg S, Bothelo S: Myotonia in a horse, *Science* 137:979, 1962.

154. Hegreberg GA, Reed SM: Skeletal muscle changes associated with equine myotonic dystrophy, *Acta Neuropathol (Berl)* 80:426, 1990.

155. Jamison JM, Baird JD, Smith-Maxie LL, et al: A congenital form of myotonia with dystrophic changes in a quarterhorse, *Equine Vet J* 19:353, 1987.

156. Montagna P, Liguori R, Monari L, et al: Equine muscular dystrophy with myotonia, *Clin Neurophysiol* 112:294, 2001.

157. Reed SM, Hegreberg GA, Bayly WM, et al: Progressive myotonia in foals resembling human dystrophia myotonica, *Muscle Nerve* 11:291, 1988.

158. Nollet H, Vanderstraeten G, Sustronck B, et al: Suspected case of stiff-horse syndrome, *Vet Rec* 146:282, 2000.

159. Dyson S: Unpublished data, 2000-2010.

160. Mayhew J: Personal communication, 2000.

161. Cox JH: An episodic weakness in four horses associated with intermittent serum hyperkalemia and the similarity of the disease to hyperkalemic periodic paralysis in man, *Proc Am Assoc Equine Pract* 383, 1985.

162. Spier SJ, Carlson GP, Holliday TA, et al: Hyperkalemic periodic paralysis in horses, *J Am Vet Med Assoc* 197:1009, 1990.

163. Rudolph JA, Spier SJ, Byrns G, et al: Periodic paralysis in quarter horses: a sodium channel mutation disseminated by selective breeding, *Nat Genet* 2:144, 1992.

164. Naylor JM: Selection of quarter horses affected with hyperkalemic periodic paralysis by show judges, *J Am Vet Med Assoc* 204:926, 1994.

165. Spier SJ, Carlson GP, Harrold D, et al: Genetic study of hyperkalemic periodic paralysis in horses, *J Am Vet Med Assoc* 202:933, 1993.

166. Naylor JM: Hyperkalemic periodic paralysis, *Vet Clin North Am Equine Pract* 13:129, 1997.

167. Reynolds AJ: Equine hyperkalemic periodic paralysis (HYPP): overview & management strategies. Available at: http://www.admani.com/AllianceEquine/TechBulletins/HYPP.htm. (Last accessed Jan. 5, 2008.)

168. Reynolds JA, Potter GD, Greene LW: Genetic-diet interactions in the hyperkalemic periodic paralysis syndrome in Quarter Horses fed varying amounts of potassium: III. The relationship between

plasma potassium concentration and HYPP symptoms, *J Equine Vet Sci* 18:731, 1998.

169. Carr EA, Spier SJ, Kortz GD, et al: Laryngeal and pharyngeal dysfunction in horses homozygous for hyperkalemic periodic paralysis, *J Am Vet Med Assoc* 209:798, 1996.

170. Traub-Dargatz JL, Ingram JT, Stashak TS, et al: Respiratory stridor associated with polymyopathy suspected to be hyperkalemic periodic paralysis in four quarter horse foals, *J Am Vet Med Assoc* 201:85, 1992.

171. Naylor JM, Robinson JA, Crichlow EC, et al: Inheritance of myotonic discharges in American quarter horses and the relationship to hyperkalemic periodic paralysis, *Can J Vet Res* 56:62, 1992.

CHAPTER 84   Principles and Practices of Joint Disease Treatment

1. Raker CW, Baker RH, Wheat JD: Patho-physiology of equine degenerative joint disease and lameness, *Proc Am Assoc Equine Pract* 12:229, 1966.

2. McIlwraith CW, Van Sickle DC: Experimentally induced arthritis of the equine carpus. Histologic and histochemical changes in the articular cartilage, *Am J Vet Res* 42:209, 1984.

3. Caron JP, Genovese RL: Principles and practices of joint disease treatment. In Ross MW, Dyson SJ, eds: *Diagnosis and management of lameness in the horse*, Philadelphia, 2003, Elsevier.

4. National Animal Health Monitoring Systems: *Lameness and laminitis in US horses*, Fort Collins, CO, 2000, USDA, APHIS, Veterinary Services—Centers for Epidemiology in Animal Health.

5. May SA, Lees P: Non-steroidal anti-inflammatory drugs. In McIlwraith CW, Trotter GW, eds: *Joint disease in the horse*, Philadelphia, 1996, Saunders.

6. Vane JR: Inhibition of prostaglandin synthesis as a mechanism of action for aspirin-like drugs, *Nature* 231:232, 1971.

7. Keegan KG, Messer NT, Reed SK, et al: Effectiveness of administration of phen-ylbutazone alone or concurrent administration of phenylbutazone and flunixin meglumine to eliminate lameness in horses, *Am J Vet Res* 69:167, 2008.

8. Frisbie DD, McIlwraith CW, Kawcak CE, et al: Evaluation of topically administered diclofenac liposomal crème for treatment of experimental osteoarthritis in horses, *Am J Vet Res* 70:210, 2009.

9. Frisbie DD: Current and future treatments of equine joint disease, *Proc Am Assoc Equinefocus meeting on Equine Joint Disease*, 2004.

10. Kunkel S, Chensue S: Arachidonic acid metabolites regulated interleukin-1 production, *BBRC* 128:892, 1985.

11. Dingle DJ: Prostaglandins in human articular cartilage metabolism, *J Lipid Med* 6:303, 1993.

12. Legendre LT, Tessmin RK, McClure SR, et al: Pharmacokinetics of firocoxib after administration of multiple consecutive daily doses to horses, *Am J Vet Res* 69:1399, 2008.

13. Jolly WT, Whittem T, Jolly AC, et al: The dose-related effects of phenylbutazone and methylprednisolone acetate formulation (Depo-Medrol®) on cultured explants of equine carpal articular cartilage, *J Vet Pharmacol Ther* 18:429, 1995.

14. Beluche LA, Bertone AL, Anderson DE, et al: Effects of oral administration of phenylbutazone to horses on in vitro articular cartilage metabolism, *Am J Vet Res* 62:1916, 2001.

15. Caldwell FJ, Mueller PO, Lynn RC, et al: Effect of topical application of diclopenac liposomal suspension on experimental induced subcutaneous inflammation in horses, *Am J Vet Res* 65:271, 2004.

16. Bertone JJ, Lynn RC, Vatistas NJ, et al: Clinical field trial to evaluate the efficacy of topically applied diclopenac liposomal cream for the relief of joint lameness in horses, *Proc Am Assoc Equine Pract* 48:190, 2002.

17. Trotter GW: Intra-articular corticosteroids. In McIlwraith CW, Trotter GW, eds: *Joint disease in the horse*, Philadelphia, 1996, Saunders.

18. Foland JW, McIlwraith CW, Trotter GW, et al: Effect of betamethasone and exercise on equine carpal joints with osteochondral fragments, *Vet Surg* 23:369, 1994.

19. Frisbie DD, Kawcak CE, Baxter GM, et al: Effects of 6α-methylprednisolone acetate on an in vivo equine osteochondral fragment exercise model, *Am J Vet Res* 59:1619, 1998.

20. Frisbie DD, Kawcak CE, Trotter GW, et al: Effects of triamcinolone acetonide on an in vivo osteochondral fragment exercise model, *Equine Vet J* 29:349, 1997.

21. Kawcak CE, Norrdin RW, Frisbie DD, et al: Effects of osteochondral fragmentation in intra-articular triamcinolone acetonide treatment on subchondral bone in the equine carpus, *Equine Vet J* 30:66, 1998.

22. Murray RC, DeBowes RM, Gaughn EM, et al: The effects of intra-articular methylprednisolone and exercise on the mechanical properties of articular cartilage in the horse, *Osteoarthritis Cartilage* 6:106, 1998.

23. Murray RC, Znaor N, Tanner KE, et al: The effect of intra-articular methylpred-nisolone acetate and energy on equine carpal subchondral and cancellous bone microhardness, *Equine Vet J* 34:306, 2002.

24. Bolt DM, Ishihara A, Weisbrode SE, et al: Effects of triamcinolone acetonide, sodium hyaluronate, amikacin sulfate and mipivican hydrochloride alone and in combination on morphology and matrix composition of lipopolysaccharide-challenged and unchallenged equine articular cartilage explants, *Am J Vet Res* 69:861, 2008.

25. Dechant JE, Baxter GM, Frisbie DD, et al: Effects of dosage titration of methyl-prednisolone acetate and triamcinolone acetonide on interleukin-l-conditioned equine articular cartilage explants in vitro, *Equine Vet J* 35:444, 2003.

26. Genovese RL: The use of corticosteroids in racetrack practice, *Proc Symp Effective Use Corticosteroids Vet Pract* 56, 1983.

27. McCluskey MJ, Kavenagh PD: Clinical use of triamcinolone acetonide in horses (205 cases) and the incidence of glucocorticoid-induced laminitis associated with its use, *Equine Vet Educ* 108, 2004.

28. Dutton H: The corticosteroid laminitis story: 1. Duty of care, *Equine Vet J* 39:5, 2007.

29. Bailey SR, Elliott J: The corticosteroid laminitis story: 2. Science of if, when and how, *Equine Vet J* 39:7, 2007.

30. Bathe AP: The corticosteroid laminitis story. 3. The clinician's viewpoint, *Equine Vet J* 39:12, 2007.

31. Labens R, Mellor DJ, Voute LC: Retrospective study of the effect of intra-articular treatment of osteoarthritis of the distal tarsal joints in 51 horses, *Vet Rec* 161:611, 2007.

32. Ozturk C, Athmaz F, Hepguler S, et al: The safety and efficacy of intra-articular hyaluronan with/without corticosteroid in knee osteoarthritis: 1 year, single-blind, randomized study, *Rheumatol Int* 26:314, 2006.

33. Doyle AJ, Stewart AA, Constable PD, et al: Effects of sodium hyaluronate and methylprednisolone acetate on proteo-glycan synthesis in equine articular cartilage explants, *Am J Vet Res* 66:48, 2006.

34. Yates AC, Stewart AA, Byron CR, et al: Effects of sodium hyaluronate and meth-ylprednisolone acetate on proteoglycan metabolism in equine articular chondro-cytes treated with interleukin-1, *Am J Vet Res* 67:1980, 2006.

35. McIlwraith CW, Frisbie DD, Kawcak CE: Current treatments for traumatic synovitis, capsulitis, and osteoarthritis, *Proc Am Assoc Equine Pract* 47:180, 2001.

36. Howard RD, McIlwraith CW: Hyaluronan and its use in the treatment of equine joint disease. In McIlwraith CW, Trotter GW, eds: *Joint disease in the horse*, Philadelphia, 1996, Saunders.

37. Gotoh S, Onya J, Abe M, et al: Effects of the molecular weight of hyaluronic acid and its action mechanisms on experimental joint pain in rats, *Ann Rheum Dis* 52:817, 1993.

38. Lynch TM, Caron JP, Arnoczky SP, et al: Influence of exogenous hyaluronan on synthesis of hyaluronan and collagenase by equine synoviocytes, *Am J Vet Res* 59:888, 1998.

39. Clegg PD, Jones MD, Carter SD: The effect of drugs commonly used in the treatment of equine articular disorders on the activity of equine matrix metal-loproteinases-2 and 9, *J Vet Pharmacol Ther* 21:406, 1998.

40. Goldberg VM, Buckwalter JA: Hyaluro-nans in the treatment of osteoarthritis in the knee: evidence for disease-modifying activity, *Osteoarthritis Cartilage* 13:216, 2005.

41. Aviad AD, Houpt JB: The molecular weight of therapeutic hyaluronan (sodium hyaluronate): how significant is it? *J Rheumatol* 21:297, 1994.

42. Smith MM, Ghosh P: The synthesis of hyaluronic acid by human synovial fibro-blasts is influenced by the extracellular environment, *Rheumatol Int* 7:113, 1987.

43. Gaustad G, Larsen S: Comparison of polysulfated glycosaminoglycan in sodium hyaluronate with placebo in treatment of traumatic arthritis in horses, *Equine Vet J* 27:356, 1995.

44. Gaustad G, Dolvik NI, Larsen S: Comparison of intra-articular injection of 2 mls of 0.9% NaCl solution with rest alone for treatment of horses with traumatic arthritis, *Am J Vet Res* 60:1117, 1999.

45. Frisbie DD, Kawcak CE, McIlwraith CW, et al: Evaluation of polysulfated glycosaminoglycan or sodium hyaluronan administered intra-articularly for treatment of experimental osteoarthritis in horses, *Am J Vet Res* 70:203, 2009.

46. Kawcak CE, Frisbie DD, McIlwraith CW, et al: Effects of intravenous administration of sodium hyaluronate on carpal joints in exercising horses after arthroscopic surgery and osteochondral fragmentation, *Am J Vet Res* 58:1132, 1997.

47. McIlwraith CW, Goodman NL, Frisbie DD: Prospective study on the prophylactic value of intravenous hyaluronan in 2-year old racing Quarter horses, *Proc Am Assoc Equine Pract* 44:271, 1998.

48. Trotter GW: Polysulfated glycosaminoglycan (Adequan®). In McIlwraith CW, Trotter GW, eds: *Joint disease in the horse*, Philadelphia, 1996, Saunders.

49. May SA, Hooke RE, Lees P: The effect of drugs used in the treatment of osteoarthritis on stromelysin (proteoglycanease) of equine synovial cell origin, *Equine Vet J* S6:28, 1988.

50. Glade MJ: Polysulfated glycosaminoglycan accelerates net synthesis of collagen in glycosaminoglycans by arthritic equine cartilage tissues in chondrocytes, *Am J Vet Res* 51:779, 1990.

51. Caron JP, Eberhart SW, Nachreiner R: Influence of polysulfated glycosaminoglycan on equine articular cartilage in explant culture, *Am J Vet Res* 52:1622, 1991.

52. Tew WP: Demonstration by synovial fluid analysis of the efficacy in horses of an investigational drug (L-1016), *J Equine Vet Sci* March/April:42, 1982.

53. White GW, Jones EW, Hamm J, et al: The efficacy of orally administered sulfated glycosaminoglycan in chemically-induced equine synovitis and degenerative joint disease, *J Equine Vet Sci* 14:350, 1994.

54. Trotter GW, Yovich J, McIlwraith CW, et al: Effects of intramuscular polysulfated glycosaminoglycan on chemical and physical defect in equine articular cartilage, *Can J Vet Res* 43:224, 1989.

55. Todhunter RJ, Minor RR, Wootton J, et al: Effects of exercise and polysulfated glycosaminoglycan on repair of articular cartilage defects in the equine carpus, *J Orthop Res* 11:782, 1993.

56. Yovich J, Trotter GW, McIlwraith CW, et al: Effects of polysulfated glycosaminoglycan upon chemical and physical defects in equine articular cartilage, *Am J Vet Res* 48:1407, 1987.

57. Frisbie DD, Kawcak CE, McIlwraith CW: Evaluation of the effect of extracorporeal shockwave treatment on experimentally induced e osteoarthritis in middle carpal joints of horses, *Am J Vet Res* 70:449, 2009.

58. Caron JP, Kaneene JB, Miller R: Results of a survey of equine practitioners on the use and efficacy of polysulfated glycosaminoglycan, *Am J Vet Res* 209:1564, 1996.

59. Burba DJ, Collier MA, Default LE, et al: In vivo kinetic study on uptake and distribution of intramuscular titanium-labeled polysulfated glycosaminoglycan in equine body fluid compartments and articular cartilage in an osteochondral defect model, *J Equine Vet Sci* 13:696, 1993.

60. Howell DS, Carreno MR, Palletta JP, et al: Articular cartilage breakdown in a lapine model of osteoarthritis: action of glycosaminoglycan polysulfate ester (GAGPS) on proteoglycan enzyme activity, hexuronate, and cell count, *Clin Orthop* 213:69, 1986.

61. Gustafson SB, McIlwraith CW, Jones RL: Comparison of the effect of polysulfated glycosaminoglycan, corticosteroids, and sodium hyaluronate in the potentiation of a sub infective dose of *Staphylococcus aureus* in the middle carpal joint of horses, *Am J Vet Res* 50:2014, 1989.

62. Gustafson DB, McIlwraith CW, Jones RL: Further investigations into the potentiation of infection by intra-articular injection of polysulfated glycosaminoglycan and the effect of filtration and intra-articular injection of Amikacin, *Am J Vet Res* 50:2018, 1989.

63. Kristiansen KK, Kold SE: Multi-variable analysis of factors influencing outcome of two treatment protocols in 128 cases of horses responding positively to intra-articular analgesia of the distal interphalangeal joint, *Equine Vet J* 39:150, 2007.

64. Little C, Ghosh P: Potential use of pentosan polysulfate for the treatment of equine joint disease, *Joint Dis Horse* 1:281, 1996.

65. Ghosh PM, Armstrong S, Read R, et al: Animal models of early osteoarthritis: their use for the evaluation of potential chondroprotective agents, *Joint Destruction Arthritis Osteoarthritis* 195, 1993.

66. Pagnano M, Westrich G: Successful non-operative management for chronic osteoarthritis pain of the knee: safety and efficacy of pre-treatment with intra-articular hyaluronans, *Osteoarthritis Cartilage* 13:751, 2005.

67. Raynauld JP, Goldsmith CH, Bellamy N, et al: Effectiveness and safety of repeat courses of hylan G-F 20 in patients with knee osteoarthritis, *Osteoarthritis Cartilage* 13:111, 2005.

68. Hamburger MI: Letter to the editor: Response to the article by Raynauld et al, *Osteoarthritis Cartilage* 13:1039, 2005.

69. Hamburger M, Settles M, Teutsch J: Identification of an immunogenic candidate for the elicitation of severe acute inflammatory reactions (SAIRs) to hylan G-F 20, *Osteoarthritis Cartilage* 13:266, 2005.

70. Frisbie DD, Sandler EA, Trotter GW, et al: Metabolic and mitogenic activities of insulin-like growth factors-1 and interleukin-1 conditioned equine cartilage, *Am J Vet Res* 62:436, 2000.

71. Duren S: Oral joint supplements: panacea or expensive fad? *Adv Equine Nutr* III:77, 2005.

72. Oke SL, McIlwraith CW: Review of the potential indications and contraindications for equine oral health supplements, *Proc Am Assoc Equine Pract* 54:261, 2008.

73. Setnikar I, Palumbo R, Canalis S, et al: Pharmacokinetics of glucosamine in man, *Arzneimittelforschung* 43:1109, 1993.

74. Adebowale AO, Cox DS, Linang I, et al: Analysis of glucosamine and chondroitin sulfate content in marketed products and CACO-2 permeability of chondroitin sulfate raw materials, *J Am Nutraceuticals Assoc* 3:37, 2003.

75. Adebowale AO, Du J, Liang I, et al: The bioavailability and pharmacokinetics of glucosamine hydrochloride and low molecular weight chondroitin sulfate after single and multiple doses to beagle dogs, *Biopharm Drug Dispos* 23:217, 2002.

76. Laverty S, Sandy JD, Celeste T, et al: Synovial fluid levels and serum pharmacokinetics in a large animal model following treatment with oral glycosaminoglycan at clinically relevant doses, *Arthritis Rheum* 52:181, 2005.

77. Du J, Liang I, Adebowale AO, et al: The bioavailability and pharmacokinetics of glucosamine hydrochloride and chondroitin sulfate after oral, intravenous single dose administration in the horse, *Biopharm Drug Dispos* 25:109, 2004.

78. Fenton JJ, Chlebek-Brown KA, Peters TL, et al: Glucosamine HCl reduces equine articular degeneration in explant cultures, *Osteoarthritis Cartilage* 6:258, 2000.

79. Dechant JE, Baxter GM, Frisbie DD, et al: Effects of glucosamine hydrochloride and chondroitin sulfate, alone and in combination, on normal and interleukin-1 conditioned equine articular cartilage explant metabolism, *Equine Vet J* 37:227, 2005.

80. Bergin BJ, Pierce SW, Bramlage LR, et al: Oral hyaluronan gel reduces post-operative tarsocrural effusion in the yearling Thoroughbred. Clinical evidence, *Equine Vet J* 38:375, 2005.

81. Kawcak CE, Frisbie DD, McIlwraith CW, et al: Evaluation of avocado and soybean unsaponifiable extracts for treatment of horses with experimentally induced osteoarthritis using an equine model, *Am J Vet Res* 68:598, 2007.

82. McCann MD, Moore IN, Carrick JB, et al: Effect of intravenous infusion of omega-3 and omega-6 lipid emulsions on equine monocyte fatty acid composition and inflammatory mediated production in vitro, *Shock* 14:222, 2000.

83. Henry MM, Moore IN, Feldman FB, et al: Effect of dietary alpha-linolenic acid on equine monocytes procoagulant activity and eichosanoid synthesis, *Circ Shock* 32:173, 1990.

84. Munsterman AS, Bertone AL, Zachosta, et al: Effect of the omega-3 fatty acid, alpha-linolenic acid, on lipopolysaccharide-challenged synovial explants from horses, *Am J Vet Res* 66:1503, 2005.

85. Billinghurst RC, O'Brien K, Poole AR, et al: Inhibition of articular cartilage degradation in culture by a non-peptidic matrix metalloproteinase inhibitor, *Ann N Y Acad Sci* 878:594, 1999.

86. Frisbie DD, McIlwraith CW, Kawcak CE: Unpublished data, 2005.

87. Frisbie DD: Future directions and treatment of joint disease in horses, *Vet Clin Equine* 21:713, 2005.

88. Frisbie DD, McIlwraith CW: Evaluation of gene therapy as a treatment for equine

traumatic arthritis and osteoarthritis, *Clin Orthop* 3795:S273, 2000.

89. Frisbie DD, Ghivizzani SC, Robbins PD, et al: Treatment of experimental equine osteoarthritis by in vivo delivery of the equine interleukin-1 receptor antagonist gene, *Gene Ther* 9:12, 2002.

90. Meijer H, Reinecke J, Becker C, et al: The production of anti-inflammatory cytokines in whole blood by physico-chemical induction, *Inflamm Res* 52:404, 2002.

91. Frisbie DD, Kawcak CE, Werpy NM, et al: Clinical, biochemical and histological effects of intra-articular administration of autologous conditioned serum in horses with experimentally induced osteoarthritis, *Am J Vet Res* 68:290, 2007.

92. Pittenger M, MacKay A, Beck S, et al: Multi-lineage potential of adult human mesenchymal stem cells, *Science* 284:143, 1999.

93. Frisbie DD, Kisiday JB, Kawcak CE, et al: Evaluation of adipose-derived stromal vascular fraction or bone marrow-derived mesenchymal stem cells for the treatment of osteoarthritis, *J Orthop Res* 27:1675,2009.

94. Murphy JM, Fink DJ, Hunziker EB, et al: Stem cell therapy in caprine model of osteoarthritis, *Arthritis Rheum* 48:3464, 2003.

95. Karsdel MA, Tanko LB, Riis BJ, et al: Calcitonin is involved in cartilage homeostasis: is calcitonin a treatment for OA? *Osteoarthritis Cartilage* 14:617, 2007.

96. Hajjaji HE, Williams JM, Devogelaer J-P, et al: Treatment with calcitonin prevents the net loss of collagen, hyaluronan and proteoglycan in aggregates from cartilage in the early stages of canine experimental osteoarthritis, *Osteoarthritis Cartilage* 12: 904, 2004.

97. Cranney A, Tugwell B, Zytaruk N, et al: Meta-analyses of therapies for post-menopausal osteoporosis. 6. Meta-analysis of calcitonin for the treatment of post-menopausal osteoporosis, *Endocr Rev* 23:540, 2002.

98. Hellio MP, Peschard MJ, Cohen C, et al: Calcitonin inhibits phospholipase A2 and collagenase activity of human osteoarthritic chondrocytes, *Osteoarthritis Cartilage* 5:121, 1997.

99. Yarborough TB, Lee MR, Hornof WJ, et al: Samarium 153-labelled hydroxyapatite microspheres for radiation synovectomy in the horse: a study of the biokinetics, dosimetry, clinical, and morphological response in normal metacarpophalangeal and metatarsophalangeal joints, *Vet Surg* 29:191, 2000.

100. Yarborough TB, Lee MR, Hornof WJ, et al: Evaluation of Samarium 153 for synovectomy in an osteochondral fragment-induced model of synovitis in horses, *Vet Surg* 29:252, 2000.

101. McIlwraith CW: *Diagnostic and surgical arthroscopy in the horse*, Philadelphia, 1990, Lea & Febiger.

102. McIlwraith CW, Bramlage LR: Surgical treatment of joint injuries. In McIlwraith CW, Trotter OW, eds: *Joint disease in the horse*, Philadelphia, 1996, Saunders.

103. McIlwraith CW, Fessler J: Arthroscopy in the diagnosis of equine joint disease, *J Am Vet Med Assoc* 172:263, 1978.

104. McIlwraith CW: *Diagnostic and surgical arthroscopy in the horse*, Lenexa, Kan., 1984, Veterinary Medicine Publishing Co.

105. McIlwraith CW, Yovich JV, Martin GS: Arthroscopic surgery for the treatment of osteochondral chip fractures in the equine carpus, *J Am Vet Med Assoc* 191:531, 1987.

106. Yovich JV, McIlwraith CW: Arthroscopic surgery for osteochondral fractures of the proximal phalanx of the metacarpophalangeal and metatarsophalangeal (fetlock) joints in horses, *J Am Vet Med Assoc* 188:243, 1986.

107. Richardson DW: Technique for arthroscopic repair of third carpal bone slab fractures in horses, *J Am Vet Med Assoc* 188:288, 1986.

108. Martin OS, McIlwraith CW: Arthroscopic anatomy of the equine femoropatellar joint and approaches for treatment of osteochondritis dissecans, *Vet Surg* 14:99, 1985.

109. McIlwraith CW, Martin GS: Arthroscopic surgery for the treatment of osteochondritis dissecans in the equine femoropatellar joint, *Vet Surg* 14:105, 1985.

110. Bertone AL, McIlwraith CW, Powers BE, et al: Arthroscopic surgery for the treatment of osteochondrosis in the equine shoulder joint, *Vet Surg* 16:303, 1987.

111. Lewis RB: Treatment of subchondral bone cysts of the medial condyle of the femur using arthroscopic surgery, *Proc Am Assoc Equine Pract* 33:887, 1987.

112. McIlwraith CW, Foerner JF, Davis DM: Osteochondritis dissecans of the tarsocrural joint: results of treatment with arthroscopic surgery, *Equine Vet J* 23:155, 1991.

113. McIlwraith CW: Arthroscopy—an update. In McIlwraith CW, ed: *Clinical techniques in equine practice*, Philadelphia, 2002, Saunders.

114. McIlwraith CW, Nixon AJ, Wright IM, et al, eds: *Diagnostic and surgical arthroscopy in the horse*, ed 3, Edinburgh, 2005, Mosby-Elsevier.

115. Kawcak CE, McIlwraith CW: Proximodorsal first phalanx osteochondral chip fragments in 320 horses, *Equine Vet J* 26:392, 1994.

116. Colon JL, Bramlage LR, Hance SR, et al: Qualitative and quantitative documentation of the racing performance of Thoroughbred racehorses after arthroscopic removal of dorsoproximal first phalanx osteochondral fractures (1986-1995), *Equine Vet J* 32:475, 2000.

117. Kawcak CE, McIlwraith CW, Norrdin RW, et al: Clinical effects of exercise on subchondral bone on carpometacarpophalangeal joints in horses, *Am J Vet Res* 61:1252, 2000.

118. Norrdin RW, Kawcak CE, Capwell BA, et al: Subchondral bone failure in an equine model of overload arthrosis, *Bone* 22:133, 1998.

119. Wilke M, Nixon AJ, Malark J: Fractures of the palmar aspect of carpal 7 bones in horses: 10 cases (1984-2000), *J Am Vet Med Assoc* 219:801, 2001.

120. Brommer H, Rijkenhuizen AM, van den Belt HAM, et al: Arthroscopic removal of an osteochondral fragment at the palmaroproximal aspect of the distal interphalangeal joint, *Equine Vet Educ* 13:294, 2001.

121. Vacek JR, Welch RD, Honnas CM: Arthroscopic approach and intra-articular anatomy of the palmaroproximal and plantaroproximal aspect of distal interphalangeal joints, *Vet Surg* 4:257, 1992.

122. McIlwraith CW: Tearing of the medial palmar intercarpal ligament in the equine mid-carpal joint, *Equine Vet J* 24:367, 1992.

123. Phillips TJ, Wright IM: Observations on the anatomy and pathology of the palmar intercarpal ligaments in the middle carpal joints of Thoroughbred racehorses, *Equine Vet J* 26:486, 1994.

124. Whitton RC, McCarthy Rose RJ: The intercarpal ligaments of equine mid-carpal joint. Part I: the anatomy of the palmar and dorsomedial intercarpal ligaments of the mid-carpal joint, *Vet Surg* 26:359, 1997.

125. Whitton RC, Rose RJ: The intercarpal ligaments of the equine mid-carpal joint. Part II: the role of the palmar intercarpal ligaments in the restraint of dorsal displacement of the proximal row of carpal bones, *Vet Surg* 26:367, 1997.

126. Whitton RC, Kannegieter NJ, Rose RJ: The intercarpal ligaments of the equine mid-carpal joint. Part III: clinical observations in 32 racing horses with mid-carpal joint disease, *Vet Surg* 26:374, 1997.

127. Foerner JJ, Barclay WP, Phillips TN, et al: Osteochondral fragments of the palmar/plantar aspect of the fetlock joint, *Proc Am Assoc Equine Pract* 33:739, 1987.

128. Fortier LA, Foerner JJ, Nixon AJ: Arthroscopic removal of axial osteochondral fragments of the plantar/palmar proximal aspect of the proximal phalanx in horses: 119 cases (1988-1992), *J Am Vet Med Assoc* 206:71, 1995.

129. McIlwraith CW, Vorhees SM: Management of osteochondritis dissecans of the dorsal aspect of the distal metacarpus and metatarsus, *Proc 36th Annual Meeting AAEP* 36:547, 1990.

130. Southwood LL, McIlwraith CW: Arthroscopic removal of fracture fragments involving a portion of the base of the sesamoid bone in horses, *J Am Vet Med Assoc* 217:236, 2000.

131. Southwood LL, Trotter GW, McIlwraith CW: Arthroscopic removal of abaxial fracture fragments of the proximal sesamoid bone in horses: 47 cases (1989-1997), *J Am Vet Med Assoc* 213: 1016, 1998.

132. Southwood LL, McIlwraith CW, Trotter GW, et al: Arthroscopic removal of apical fractures of the proximal sesamoid bone in horses: 98 cases (1989-1999), *Proc Am Assoc Equine Pract* 46:100, 2000.

133. Schnabel LV, Bramlage LR, Mohammed HO, et al: Racing performance after arthroscopic removal of sesamoid fracture fragments in Thoroughbred horses aged less than 2 years: 151 cases (1989-2002), *Equine Vet J* 39:64, 2007.

134. Schnabel LV, Bramlage LR, Mohammed HO, et al: Racing performance after arthroscopic removal of apical sesamoid fracture fragments in Thoroughbred horses aged >= 2 years: 84 cases (1989-2002), *Equine Vet J* 38:446, 2006.

135. Zamos DT, Honnas CM, Hoffman AG: Arthroscopic approach and intra-articular anatomy of the plantar pouch of the equine tarsocrural joint, *Vet Surg* 23:161, 1994.

136. Foland JW, McIlwraith CW, Trotter GW: Arthroscopic surgery for osteochondritis dissecans of the femoropatellar joint of the horse, *Equine Vet J* 24:419, 1992.

137. McIlwraith CW: Osteochondral fragmentation or the distal aspect or the patella in horses, *Equine Vet J* 22:157, 1990.

138. Marble GP, Sullins KE: Arthroscopic removal of patellar fracture fragments in horses: 5 cases (1989-1998), *J Am Vet Med Assoc* 216:1799, 2000.

139. Howard RD, McIlwraith CW, Trotter GW: Arthroscopic surgery for subchondral cystic lesions of the medial femoral condyle in horses: 41 cases (1988-1991), *J Am Vet Med Assoc* 206:846, 1995.

140. Textor JA, Nixon AJ, Lumsden J, et al: Subchondral cystic lesions of the proximal extremity or the tibia in horses: 12 cases (1983-2000), *J Am Vet Med Assoc* 218:408, 2001.

141. Ray CS, Baxter GM, McIlwraith CW, et al: Development of subchondral cystic lesions after articular cartilage and subchondral bone damage in young horses, *Equine Vet J* 28:225, 1996.

142. von Rechenberg B, Guenther H, McIlwraith CW, et al: Fibrous tissue of subchondral cystic lesions in horses produce local mediators in neutral metalloproteinases and cause bone resorption in vitro, *Vet Surg* 29:420, 2000.

143. von Rechenberg B, McIlwraith CW, Akens M: Spontaneous production of nitric oxide (NO) prostaglandins (PGE₂) in neutral metalloproteinases (MMPs) in media of explant cultures of equine synovial membrane and articular cartilage from normal and osteoarthritic joints, *Equine Vet J* 32:140, 2000.

144. Wallis TW, Goodrich LR, McIlwraith CW, et al: Arthroscopic injection of corticosteroid into the fibrous tissues of subchondral cystic lesions of the medial femoral condyles of horses: a retrospective study of 52 cases (2001-2006), *Equine Vet J* 40:461, 2007.

145. Schneider RK, Jenson P, Moore RM: Evaluation of cartilage lesions on the medial femoral condyle as a cause of lameness in horses: 11 cases (1988-1994), *J Am Vet Med Assoc* 210:1649, 1997.

146. Walmsley JP: Vertical tears in the cranial horn of the meniscus and its cranial ligament in the equine femorotibial joint: 7 cases and their treatment by arthroscopic surgery, *Equine Vet J* 27:20, 1997.

147. Walmsley JP: Arthroscopic surgery of the femorotibial joint, *Clin Tech Equine Pract* 1:226, 2002.

148. Walmsley JP, Philips TJ, Townsend HGG: Meniscal tears in horses: an evaluation of clinical signs and arthroscopic treatment of 80 cases, *Equine Vet J* 35:402, 2003.

149. Mueller POE, Allen D, Watson E, et al: Arthroscopic removal of a fragment from an intercondylar eminence fracture of the tibia in 2-year-old horse, *J Am Vet Med Assoc* 204:1793, 1994.

150. Walmsley JP: Fracture of the intercondylar eminence of the tibia treated by arthroscopic internal fixation, *Equine Vet J* 29:148, 1997.

151. Stick JA, Borg LA, Nickels FA, et al: Arthroscopic removal of osteochondral fragment from the caudal pouch of the lateral femorotibial joint in a colt, *J Am Vet Med Assoc* 200:1695, 1995.

152. Hance R, Schneider RK, Embertson RM, et al: Lesions of the caudal aspect of the femoral condyles in foals: 20 cases (1980-1990), *J Am Vet Med Assoc* 202:637, 1993.

153. Trumble TN, Stick AJ, Arnoczky SP, et al: Consideration of anatomic and radiographic features of the caudal pouches of the femorotibial joints of horses for the purpose of arthroscopy, *Am J Vet Res* 55:1682, 1994.

154. Watts AE, Nixon AJ: Comparison of arthroscopic approaches and accessible anatomic structures during arthroscopy of the caudal pouches of equine femorotibial joints, *Vet Surg* 35:219, 2006.

155. Honnas CM, Zamos DT, Ford TS: Arthroscopy of the coxofemoral joint of foals, *Vet Surg* 22:115, 1993.

156. Nixon AJ: Diagnostic and operative arthroscopy or the coxofemoral joint in horses, *Vet Surg* 23:377, 1994.

157. Weller RR, Maieler LJ, Bowen M, et al: The arthroscopic approach and intra-articular anatomy of the equine temporomandibular joint, *Equine Vet J* 34:421, 2002.

158. Richardson DW: Arthroscopically assisted repair of articular fractures, *Clin Equine Pract* 1:211, 2001.

159. Bassage LH II, Richardson DW: Longitudinal fractures of the condyles of the third metacarpal and metatarsal bones in racehorses: 224 cases (1986-1995), *J Am Vet Med Assoc* 212:1757, 1998.

160. Zekas LJ, Bramlage LR, Embertson RM, et al: Characterization of the type and location of fractures of the third metacarpal/metatarsal condyles in 135 horses in Central Kentucky (1986-1994), *Equine Vet J* 31:304, 1993.

161. Boening KJ: Arthroscopic surgery of the distal and proximal interphalangeal joints, *Clin Equine Pract* 1:218, 2002.

162. Boening KJ, Saldem FC, Leendertse I, et al: Diagnostic and surgical arthroscopy of equine coffin joints, *Proc Am Assoc Equine Pract* 36:331, 1990.

163. Vail TB, McIlwraith CW: Arthroscopic removal of an osteochondral fragment from the middle phalanx of a horse, *Vet Surg* 4:269, 1992.

164. Schneider RK, Ragle CA, Carter BG, et al: Arthroscopic removal of osteochondral fragments from the proximal interphalangeal joint of the pelvic limbs in three horses, *J Am Vet Med Assoc* 207:79, 1994.

165. Nixon AJ: Arthroscopic approaches and intra-articular anatomy of the equine elbow, *Vet Surg* 19:93, 1990.

166. McIlwraith CW, Nixon AJ: Joint resurfacing: attempts at repairing articular cartilage defects. In McIlwraith CW, Trotter GW, eds: *Joint disease in the horse*, Philadelphia, 1996, Saunders.

167. Nixon AJ: Arthroscopic techniques for cartilage repair, *Clin Tech Equine Pract* 1:257, 2002.

168. McIlwraith CW, Nixon AJ, Wright IM, et al: Arthroscopic methods for cartilage repair. In McIlwraith CW, Nixon AJ, Wright IM, et al, eds: *Diagnostic and surgical arthroscopy in the horse*, ed 3, Edinburgh, 2005, Mosby-Elsevier.

169. Frisbie DD, Trotter GW, Powers BE, et al: Arthroscopic subchondral bone plate microfracture technique augments healing of large chondral defects in the radial carpal bone and medial femoral condyle of horses, *Vet Surg* 28:242, 1999.

170. Vachon AM, McIlwraith CW, Powers BE, et al: Morphologic and biochemical study of sternal cartilage autografts for resurfacing induced osteochondral defects in horses, *Am J Vet Res* 53:1038, 1992.

171. Howard RD, McIlwraith CW, Powers BE, et al: Long term fate and effects of athletic exercise on sternal cartilage auto grafts used for repair of large osteochondral defects in horses, *Am J Vet Res* 55:1158, 1994.

172. Frisbie DD, Oxford JT, Southwood L, et al: Early events in cartilage repair after subchondral bone microfracture, *Clin Orthop Relat Res* 407:215, 2003.

173. Frisbie DD, Morisset S, Ho CB, et al: Effects of calcified cartilage on healing of chondral defects treated with micro fracture in horses, *Am J Sports Med* 11:1824, 2006.

174. Mitchell N, Shepherd N: Effects of patellar shaving in the rabbit, *J Orthop Res* 5:388, 1987.

175. Schmid A, Schmid F: Ultrastructural studies after arthroscopic cartilage shaving (abstract), *Arthroscopy* 3:137, 1987.

176. Johnson L: Arthroscopic abrasion arthroplasty: historical and pathologic perspective-present status, *Arthroscopy* 2:54, 1986.

177. Dandy DJ: Abrasion chondroplasty, *Arthroscopy* 2:51, 1986.

178. Bassett CA, Hermann I: Influence of oxygen concentrations and mechanical factors on differentiation of connective tissues in vitro, *Nature* 190:460, 1961.

179. Vachon A, Bramlage L, Gabel A, et al: Evaluation of the repair process of cartilage defects in the equine third carpal bone with and without subchondral bone perforation, *Am J Vet Res* 47:2637, 1986.

180. Rodrigo JJ, Steadman RJ, Silliman JF, et al: Improvement of full-thickness chondral defect in the human knee after debridement and microfracture using continuous passive motion, *Am J Knee Surg* 7:109, 1994.

181. Steadman JR, Rodkey WG, Briggs KK: Microfracture to treat full-thickness chondral defects: surgical technique, rehabilitation, and outcomes, *J Knee Surg* 15:170, 2002.

182. Knutsen G, Engebortsen L, Ludbigsen TC, et al: Autologous chondrocyte implantation compared with microfracture in the knee. A randomized trial, *J Bone Joint Surg* 86A:455, 2004.

183. Morales TI, Hascell VC: Factors involved in the regulation of proteoglycan metabolism in articular cartilage, *Arthritis Rheum* 32:1197, 1989.

184. Nixon AJ, Fortier LA: New horizons in articular cartilage repair, *Proc Am Assoc Equine Pract* 47:217, 2001.

185. Fortier LA, Nixon AJ, Mohammed HO, et al: Altered biological activity of equine chondrocytes cultured in a 3-D fibrin matrix and supplemented with transforming growth factor 1, *Am J Vet Res* 58:66, 1997.

186. Fortier LA, Lust TG, Mohammed HO, et al: Coordinated up-regulation of cartilage matrix synthesis in fibrin cultures supplemented with exogenous insulin-like growth factor-1, *J Orthop Res* 17:467, 1999.

187. Frisbie DD, Nixon AJ: Insulin-like growth factor and corticosteroid modulation of chondrocyte metabolic and mitogenic activities in interleukin-1 conditioned equine cartilage, *Am J Vet Res* 58:526, 1997.

188. Foley RL, Nixon AJ: Insulin-like growth factor-1 peptide elution profiles from fibrin polymers determined by high performance liquid chromatography, *Am J Vet Res* 58:1431, 1997.

189. Nixon AJ, Fortier LA, Williams J, et al: Enhanced repair of extensive articular defects by insulin-like growth factor-1 laden fibrin composites, *J Orthop Res* 17:475, 1999.

190. Hendrickson DA, Nixon AJ, Grande DA, et al: Chondrocyte-fibrin matrix transplants for resurfacing extensive articular cartilage defects, *J Orthop Res* 12:485, 1994.

191. Fortier LA, Lust G, Mohammad HO, et al: Insulin-like growth factor-1 enhances cell-based articular cartilage repair, *J Bone Joint Surg* 84B:276, 2002.

192. Nixon AJ, Brower-Toland BD, Bent SJ, et al: Insulin-like growth factor-1 gene therapy applications in cartilage repair and degenerative joint diseases, *Clin Orthop* 379S:S201, 2000.

193. Brower-Toland BD, Saxer RA, Goodrich LR, et al: Direct adenovirus-mediated insulin-like growth factor-1 gene transfer enhances transplant chondrocyte function, *Human Gene Therapy* 12:117, 2001.

194. Hidaka C, Goodrich LR, Chen CT et al: Acceleration of cartilage repair by genetically modified chondrocytes over expressing bone morphogenetic protein 7, *J Orthop Res* 4:573, 2003.

195. Houpt JL, Frisbie DD, McIlwraith CW, et al: Dual transduction of insulin-like growth factor-l in interleukin-l receptor antagonist protein controls cartilage degradation in an osteoarthritic culture model, *J Orthop Res* 23:118, 2005.

196. Nixon AJ, Houpt JL, Frisbie DD, et al: Gene mediated restoration of cartilage matrix by combination insulin-like growth factor-l/interleukin receptor-l antagonist, *Gene Ther* 12:177, 2005.

197. Morisset S, Frisbie DD, Robbins PD, et al: IL-IRa/IGF-l gene therapy modulates repair of microfractured chondral defects, *Clin Orthop Relat Res* 462:221, 2007.

198. Nixon AJ, Fortier LA, Goodrich LR, et al: Arthroscopic reattachment of osteochondritis dissecans lesion using resorbable polydioxanone pins, *Equine Vet J* 36:376, 2004.

199. Vachon AM, McIlwraith CW, Trotter GW: Morphologic study of induced osteochondral defects of the distal portion of the radial carpal bone in horses by use of glued periosteal autografts, *Am J Vet Res* 52:317, 1991.

200. Sams AE, Nixon AJ: Chondrocyte-laden collagen scaffolds for resurfacing extensive articular cartilage defects, *Osteoarthritis Cartilage* 3:47, 1995.

201. Nixon AJ, Sams AE, Lust G, et al: Temporal matrix synthesis and histologic features of a chondrocyte-laden porous collagen cartilage analog, *Am J Vet Res* 54:349, 1993.

202. Hendrickson DA, Nixon AJ, Herb HN: Phenotype and biological activity of neonatal equine chondrocytes cultured in a 3-dimensional fibrin matrix, *Am J Vet Res* 55:410, 1994.

203. Brittberg M, Lindahl A, Nilsson A, et al: Treatment of deep cartilage defects in the knee with autologous chondrocyte transplantation, *N Engl J Med* 331:889, 1994.

204. Peterson L, Minas T, Brittberg M, et al: Two- to 9-year outcome after autologous chondrocyte transplantation of the knee, *Clin Orthop* 374:212, 2003.

205. Peterson L, Minas T, Brittberg M, et al: Treatment of osteochondritis dissecans of the knee with autologous chondrocyte transplantation—results at two to ten years, *J Bone Joint Surg Am* 85A(Suppl 2):17, 2003.

206. Litzke L-F, Wagner E, Baumgartner, et al: Repair of extensive articular cartilage defects in horses by autologous chondrocyte transplantation, *Ann Biomed Eng* 32:57, 2004.

207. Frisbie DD, Bowman SM, Calhoun HA, et al: Evaluation of autologous chondrocyte transplantation via a collagen membrane in equine articular defects—results at 12 and 18 months, *Osteoarthritis Cartilage* 16:667, 2008.

208. Frisbie DD, Calhoun HA, Bowman S, et al: PDS/PGA staples compared to suture fixation of autologous chondrocyte constructs, *Proc 49th Annual Meeting Orthop Res Soc* 2003.

209. Kisiday JD, Kopesky PW, Evans CH, et al: Evaluation of adult equine bone marrow- and adipose-derived progenitor cell chondrogenesis in hydrogel cultures, *J Orthop Res* 26:322, 2008.

210. Wilke MM, Nydam DB, Nixon AJ: Enhanced early chondrogenesis in articular defects following arthroscopic mesenchymal stem cell implantation in an equine model, *J Orthop Res* 25:913, 2007.

211. Caplan AI, Dennis JE: Mesenchymal stem cells as trophic mediators, *J Cell Biochem* 98:1076, 2006.

212. Sullins KE, Veit HP, McIlwraith CW: Osteochondral grafts to fill large articular defects in horses, *Vet Surg* 18:77, 1989 (abstract).

213. Stover SM, Poole RR, Lloyd KCK: Repair of surgical created osteochondral defects with autogenous sternal osteochondral grafts in the horse, *Vet Surg* 18:76, 1989 (abstract).

214. Pearce SC, Hurtig MB, Calamette R, et al: An investigation of two techniques for optimizing joint surface congruency using multiple cylindrical osteochondral auto grafts, *Arthroscopy* 17:50, 2001.

215. Bodo G, Hangondy L, Modi S, et al: Autologous osteochondral grafting (mosaic) arthroplasty for treatment of subchondral cystic lesions in the equine stifle and fetlock joints, *Vet Surg* 33:588, 2004.

CHAPTER 85 Analgesia and Hindlimb Lameness

1. Kehlet H: Surgical stress: the role of pain and analgesia, *Br J Anaesth* 63:189, 1989.

2. Gourlay GK, Cherry DA, Plummer JL, et al: The influence of drug polarity on the absorption of opioid drugs into CSF and subsequent cephalad migration following lumbar epidural administration: application to morphine and pethidine, *Pain* 31:297, 1987.

3. Cousins MJ, Mather LE: Intrathecal and epidural administration of opioids, *Anesthesiology* 61:276, 1984.

4. Valverde A, Dyson DH, McDonell WN: Epidural morphine reduces halothane MAC in the dog, *Can J Anaesth* 36:629, 1989.

5. Doherty TJ, Geiser DR, Rohrbach BW: Effect of high volume epidural morphine, ketamine and butorphanol on halothane minimum alveolar concentration in ponies, *Equine Vet J* 29:370, 1997.

6. Robinson EP, Moncada-Suarez JR, Felice L: Dermatomal distribution of analgesia in horses after epidural morphine. Proceedings of the Fifth International Congress of Veterinary Anesthesia, Guelph, Ontario, Canada, 1994.

7. Robinson EP, Moncada-Suarez JR, Felice L: Epidural morphine analgesia in horses, *Vet Surg* 23:78, 1994 (abstract).

8. Skarda RT, Muir WW: Caudal analgesia induced by epidural or subarachnoid administration of detomidine hydrochloride solution in mares, *Am J Vet Res* 55:670, 1994.

9. Gomez DeSegura IA, DeRossi R, Santos M et al: Epidural injection of ketamine for perineal analgesia in the horse, *Vet Surg* 27:384, 1998.

10. Yaksh TL: Spinal opiate analgesia: characteristics and principles of action, *Pain* 11:293, 1981.

11. Bernards CM, Hill HF: Morphine and alfentanil permeability through the spinal dura, arachnoid, and pia mater of dogs and monkeys, *Anesthesiology* 73:1214, 1990.

12. Natalini CC, Robinson EP: Evaluation of the analgesic effects of epidurally administered morphine, alfentanil, butorphanol, tramadol, and U50488H in horses, *Am J Vet Res* 61:1579, 2000.

13. Valverde A, Little CB, Dyson DH, et al: Use of epidural morphine to relieve pain in a horse, *Can Vet J* 31:211, 1990.

14. Olbrich VH, Mosing M: A comparison of the analgesic effects of caudal epidural methadone and lidocaine in the horse, *Vet Anaes Analg* 30:156, 2003.

15. Natalini CC, Linardi RL: Analgesic effects of epidural administration of hydromorphone in horses, *Am J Vet Res* 67:11, 2006.

16. Sysel AM, Pleasant RS, Jacobson JD, et al: Efficacy of an epidural combination of morphine and detomidine in alleviating experimentally induced hindlimb lameness in horses, *Vet Surg* 25:511, 1996.

17. Sysel AM, Pleasant RS, Jacobson JD, et al: Systemic and local effects associated with long-term epidural catheterization and morphine-detomidine administration in horses, *Vet Surg* 26:141, 1997.

18. Burford JH, Corley KTT: Morphine-associated pruritus after single extradural administration in a horse, *Vet Anaes Analg* 33:193, 2006.
19. Yaksh TL: Pharmacology of spinal adrenergic systems which modulate spinal nociceptive processing, *Pharmacol Biochem Behav* 22:845, 1985.
20. Stamford JA: Descending control of pain, *Br J Anaesth* 75:217, 1995.
21. Howe JR, Yaksh TL, Go VLW: The effect of unilateral dorsal root ganglionectomies or ventral rhizotomies on alpha 2-adrenoceptor binding to, and the substance P, enkephalin, and neurotensin content of, the cat lumbar spinal cord, *Neuroscience* 21:385, 1987.
22. Osipov HM, Suarez LJ, Spoulding TC: Antinociceptive interactions between alpha-2 adrenergic and opiate agonists at the spinal level in rodents, *Anesth Analg* 68:194, 1989.
23. Skarda RT, Muir WW: Comparison of antinociceptive, cardiovascular, and respiratory effects, head ptosis, and position of pelvic limbs in mares after caudal epidural administration of xylazine and detomidine hydrochloride solution, *Am J Vet Res* 57:1338, 1996.
24. Redua MA, Valadao CAA, Duque JC, et al: The pre-emptive effect of epidural ketamine on wound sensitivity in horses tested by using von Frey filaments, *Vet Anaes Analg* 39:200, 2002.
25. Martin CA, Kerr CL, Pearce SG, et al: Outcome of epidural catheterization for delivery of analgesics in horses: 43 cases (1998-2001), *J Am Vet Med Assoc* 222:1394, 2003.
26. Maxwell LK, Thomasy SM, Slovis N, et al: Pharmacokinetics of fentanyl following intravenous and transdermal administration in horses, *Equine Vet J* 35:484, 2003.
27. Maxwell LK, Thomasy SM, Slovis N, et al: Transdermal fentanyl combined with nonsteroidal anti-inflammatory drugs for analgesia in horses, *J Vet Intern Med* 13:550, 2004.
28. Fielding CL, Brumbaugh GW, Matthews NS, et al: Pharmacokinetics and clinical effects of a subanesthetic continuous rate infusion of ketamine in awake horses, *Am J Vet Res* 67:1484, 2006.
29. Peterbauer C, Larenzaq PM, Knobloch M, et al: Effects of a low dose infusion of racemic and S-ketamine on the nociceptive withdrawal reflex in standing ponies, *Vet Anaesth Analg* 35:1467, 2008.
30. Field MJ, Cox PJ, Stott E, et al: Identification of the alpha2-delta-1 subunit of voltage-dependent calcium channels as a molecular target for pain mediation the analgesic actions of pregabalin, *Proc Natl Acad Sci U S A* 103:17537, 2006.
31. Dirikolu L, Dafalla A, Ely KJ, et al: Pharmacokinetics of gabapentin in horses, *J Vet Pharmacol Therap* 31:175, 2008.
32. Posner LP, Davis JL: Gabapentin for the treatment of neuropathic pain in a pregnant horse, *J Am Vet Med Assoc* 231:755, 2007.

CHAPTER 87 External Skeletal Fixation

1. Nemeth F, Black W: The use of the walking cast to repair fractures in horses and ponies, *Equine Vet J* 23:32, 1991.
2. McClure SR, Watkins JP, Bronson DG, et al: In vitro comparison of the standard short limb cast and three configurations of short limb transfixation casts in equine forelimbs, *Am J Vet Res* 55:1331, 1994.
3. McClure SR, Watkins JP, Ashman RB: In vitro comparison of the effect of parallel and divergent transfixation pins on breaking strength of equine third metacarpal bones, *Am J Vet Res* 55:1327, 1994.
4. Elce YA, Southwood LL, Nut JN, et al: Ex vivo comparison of a novel tapered-sleeve and traditional full-limb transfixation pin cast for distal radial fracture stabilization in the horse, *Vet Comp Orthop Traumatol* 19:93, 2006.
5. Nunamaker DM, Richardson DW, Butterweck DM, et al: A new external skeletal fixation device that allows immediate full weight bearing: application in the horse, *Vet Surg* 15:345, 1986.
6. Nunamaker DM, Richardson DW: External skeletal fixation in the horse, *Proc Am Assoc Equine Pract* 37:549, 1991.
7. Nash RA, Nunamaker DM, Baston R: Evaluation of a tapered-sleeve transcortical pin to reduce stress at the bone-pin interface in metacarpal bones obtained from horses, *Am J Vet Res* 62:955, 2001.
8. Kraus BM, Richardson DW, Nunamaker DM, et al: Management of comminuted fractures of the proximal phalanx in horses: 64 cases (1983-2001), *J Am Vet Med Assoc* 15:224, 2004.

CHAPTER 88 Counterirritation

1. Percivall W: *Lameness in the horse*, part 2, vol 4, London, 1871, Longmans, Green, Reader & Dyer.
2. Wooldridge GW: *Encyclopaedia of veterinary medicine, surgery and obstetrics*, London, 1921, Henry Frowde, Hodder & Stoughton.
3. Stashak TS, ed: *Adams' lameness in horses*, ed 4, Philadelphia, 1987, Lea & Febiger.
4. Silver I, Brown P, Goodship A, et al: A clinical and experimental study of tendon injury, healing and treatment in the horse, *Equine Vet J Suppl* 1:1, 1983.

CHAPTER 89 Cryotherapy

1. Hartwick RC: Review and update on 290 cases of bucked shins treated with cryosurgery. Proceedings of the Fourth Annual Meeting of the American College of Cryosurgery, Arlington, Virginia, 1981.
2. Montgomery TC: Cryotherapy of dorsal metacarpal disease, *Equine Pract* 3:219, 1981.
3. Wood WE: Treatment of tendonitis (bowed tendons) and bucked shins with cryosurgery. Proceedings of the Fourth Annual Meeting of the American College of Cryosurgery, Arlington, Virginia, 1981.
4. McKibbin LS, Paraschak DM: An investigation on the use of cryosurgery for treatment of bone spavin, splint, and fractured splint bone: injuries in standardbred horses, *Cryobiology* 22:468, 1985.
5. Schneider RK, Mayhew IG, Clarke GL: Effects of cryotherapy on the palmar and plantar digital nerves in the horse, *Am J Vet Res* 46:7, 1985.
6. Zhou L: Mechanism research of cryoanalgesia, *Neurol Res* 17:307, 1995.
7. Podkonjak KR: Veterinary cryotherapy. Part I. A comprehensive look at uses, principles, and successes, *Vet Med Small Anim Clin* 77:51, 1982.
8. Baxter JS: The machinery of veterinary cryosurgery, *J Small Anim Pract* 19:27, 1978.
9. Byrne MD: Cryosurgical instrumentation, *Vet Clin North Am* 10:771, 1980.
10. Tate LP, Evans LH: Cryoneurectomy in the horse, *J Am Vet Med Assoc* 177:423, 1980.

CHAPTER 90 Radiation Therapy

1. Desjardins AU: The analgesic property of roentgen rays, *Radiology* 17:317, 1927.
2. Mantell BS: The management of benign conditions In Hope-Stone HF, ed: *Radiotherapy in clinical practice*, Boston, 1986, Butterworths.
3. Pommer A: X-ray therapy in veterinary medicine, *J Am Vet Radiol Soc* 5:98, 1964.
4. Dixon RT, Gillette EL, Carlson WD: Some local effects of 60 cobalt gamma radiation on the equine carpus. 1. Effects on dermal blood flow and cutaneous temperature, *Aust Vet J* 49:130, 1973.
5. Adams OR, Stashak TS: *Adams' lameness in horses*, ed 4, Philadelphia, 1987, Lea & Febiger.
6. Silver IA, Rossdale PD, Brown PN, et al: A clinical and experimental study of tendon injury, healing and treatment in the horse, *Equine Vet J Suppl* 1:43, 1983.
7. Trott KR, Kamprad F: Radiobiological mechanisms of anti-inflammatory radiotherapy, *Radiother Oncology* 51:197, 1999.
8. Lowenthal JW, Harris AW: Activation of mouse lymphocytes inhibits induction of rapid cell death by x-irradiation, *J Immunol* 135:1119, 1985.
9. Hildebrandt G, Seed MP, Freemantle CN, et al: Effects of low dose ionizing radiation on murine chronic granulomatous tissue, *Strahlenther Onkol* 174:580-588, 1998.
10. Rodel F, Keilholz L, Herrmann M, et al: Radiobiological mechanisms in inflammatory diseases of low-dose radiation therapy, *Int J Radiat Biol* 83:357, 2007.
11. Hildebrandt G, Seed MP, Freemantle CN, et al: Mechanisms of the anti-inflammatory activity of low-dose radiation therapy, *Int J Radiat Biol* 74:367, 1998.
12. Rubin P, Soni A, Williams JP: The molecular and cellular biologic basis for the radiation treatment of benign proliferative diseases, *Semin Radiat Oncol* 9:203, 1999.
13. Dixon RT: Results of post-surgical radiation therapy, *J Am Vet Radiol Soc* 81, 1979.
14. Teskey GC, Kavaliers M: Ionizing radiation induces opioid-mediated analgesia in male mice, *Life Sci* 35:1547, 1984.
15. Holthusen H, Arndt JO: Nitric oxide evokes pain in humans on intracutaneous injection, *Neurosci Lett* 165:71, 1994.
16. Williams M, Kowaluk EA, Arneric SP: Emerging molecular approaches to pain therapy, *J Med Chem* 42:1481, 1999.
17. Kawabata A, Umeda N, Takagi H: L-Arginine exerts a dual role in nociceptive processing in the brain: involvement of the kyotorphin-Met-enkephalin pathway and NO-cyclic GMP pathway, *Br J Pharmacol* 109:73, 1993.

18. Chen X, Levine JD: NOS inhibitor antagonism of PGE2-induced mechanical sensitization of cutaneous C-fiber nociceptors in the rat, *J Neurophysiol* 81:963, 1999.

19. Levy D, Höke A, Zochodne DW: Local expression of inducible nitric oxide synthase in an animal model of neuropathic pain, *Neurosci Lett* 260:207, 1999.

20. Craven PL, Urist MR: Osteogenesis by radioisotope labelled cell populations in implants of bone matrix under the influence of ionizing radiation, *Clin Orthop Relat Res* 76:231, 1971.

21. Lo TC: Radiation therapy for heterotopic ossification, *Semin Radiat Oncology* 9:163, 1999.

22. Grant BD: Repair mechanisms of osteochondral defects in Equidae: a comparative study of untreated and x-irradiated defects, *Am Assoc Equine Pract* 95, 1975.

23. Dixon RT, Gillette EL, Carlson WD: Some local effects of 60 cobalt gamma radiation on the equine carpus. 2. Observed clinical effects and changes in estimated values of bone mineral content, *Aust Vet J* 49:135, 1973.

24. University of California, Davis, Veterinary Medical Teaching Hospital, unpublished data, 2001.

25. Alexander JE: The effects of therapeutic of therapeutic levels of x-irradiation on immature bone in horses, *Am Assoc Equine Pract* 221, 1967.

26. Clapp NK, Carlson WD, Morgan JP: Radiation therapy for lameness in horses, *J Am Vet Med Assoc* 145:277, 1963.

27. Meginnis PJ, Lutterbeck EF: Roentgen therapy of inflammatory conditions affecting the legs of Thoroughbred horses, *North Am Vet* 540, 1951.

28. Meginnis PJ, Lutterbeck EF: Further clinical experience with radiation therapy in race horses, *North Am Vet* 431, 1954.

29. Théon AP: Radiation therapy in the horse, *Vet Clin North Am Equine Pract* 14:673, 1998.

30. Franks PW: The use of ionising radiation for the treatment of injuries to flexor tendons and supporting ligaments in horses, *Equine Vet J* 11:106, 1979.

31. Burt JK, Johnson JH, Gillette EL: Preparing a radioisotope pack for plesiotherapy. A new technic, *Acta Radiol Suppl Stockh* 319:141, 1972.

32. Clunie G, Lovegrove FT: Radiation synovectomy. In Murray IPC, Ell PJ, Van der Wall H, eds: *Nuclear medicine in clinical diagnosis and treatment*, ed 2, New York, 1998, Churchill Livingstone.

33. Makela O, Sukura A, Penttila P, et al: Radiation synovectomy with holmium-166 ferric hydroxide macroaggregate in equine metacarpophalangeal and metatarsophalangeal joints, *Vet Surg* 32:402, 2003.

34. Yarbrough TB, Lee MR, Hornof WJ, et al: Samarium 153-labeled hydroxyapatite microspheres for radiation synovectomy in the horse: a study of the biokinetics, dosimetry, clinical, and morphologic response in normal metacarpophalangeal and metatarsophalangeal joints, *Vet Surg* 29:191, 2000.

35. Palmer JL, Bertone AL: Joint structure, biochemistry and biochemical disequilibrium in synovitis and equine joint disease, *Equine Vet J* 26:263, 1994.

36. Nickels FA, Grant BD, Lincoln SD: Villonodular synovitis of the equine metacarpophalangeal joint, *J Am Vet Med Assoc* 168:1043, 1976.

37. Barclay WP, White KK, Williams A: Equine villonodular synovitis: a case survey, *Cornell Vet* 70:72, 1980.

38. Yarbrough TB, Lee MR, Hornoff W, et al: Evaluation of Samarium-153 for synovectomy in an osteochondral fragment-induced model of synovitis in horses, *Vet Surg* 29:252, 2000.

39. Théon A: Radiation therapy. In Ross MW, Dyson SJ, eds: *Diagnosis and management of lameness in the horse*, Philadelphia, 2003, Saunders.

40. Silver IA: The treatment by radiotherapy of proliferative lesions in the horse, *Br Equine Vet Assoc* 49, 1963.

41. Dixon RT: A preliminary evaluation of Rn222 gamma radiation therapy in horses, *Aust Vet J* 45:389, 1969.

42. Dixon RT: The utilization of gamma radiation therapy as an integral part of equine practice, *J Am Vet Radiol Soc* 15:91, 1974.

CHAPTER 91   Rest and Rehabilitation

1. Richardson DW, Clark CC: Effects of short term cast immobilization on equine articular cartilage, *Am J Vet Res* 54:449, 1993.

2. French DA, Barber SM, Leach DH, et al: The effects of exercise on the healing of articular cartilage defects in the equine carpus, *Vet Surg* 18:312, 1989.

3. Todhunter RJ, Altman NS, Kallfelz FA, et al: Use of scintimetry to assess effects of exercise and polysulfated glycosaminoglycan on equine carpal joints with osteochondral defects, *Am J Vet Res* 54:997, 1993.

4. Foland JW, McIlwraith CW, Trotter GW, et al: The effect of betamethasone and exercise on equine carpal joints with osteochondral fragments, *Vet Surg* 23:369, 1994.

5. Grant BD: Repair mechanisms in osteochondral defects in the equine: a comparative study of untreated and x-irradiated defects, *Proc Am Assoc Equine Pract* 21:95, 1975.

6. Stover S: Personal communication, 2001.

7. Stover SM, Johnson BG, Daft BM, et al: An association between complete and incomplete stress fractures of the humerus in racehorses, *Equine Vet J* 24:260, 1992.

8. McCutcheon LJ, Bryd SK, Hodgson DR: Ultrastructural changes in fatigued equine muscles, *J Appl Physiol* 72:1111, 1992.

9. Nunamaker D: Personal communication, 2001.

10. Foss M: Personal communication, 2001.

11. Kawack C: Personal communication, 2001.

12. Grant BD, Smith LJ, Swenson K, et al: Hill training for high performance horses, *Equine Athlete* 1:6, 1988.

CHAPTER 92   Acupuncture

Equine Acupuncture for Lameness Diagnosis and Treatment

1. Jaggar D, Robinson N: History of veterinary acupuncture. In Schoen AM, ed: *Veterinary acupuncture: ancient art to modern medicine*, ed 2, St Louis, 2001, Mosby.

2. Cheng L: *China agricultural encyclopedia: traditional Chinese veterinary medicine*, Beijing, 1991, China Agriculture Press (in Chinese).

3. Guidelines for alternative and complementary veterinary medicine: In *AVMA Directory*, Schaumburg, Ill, 1996, American Veterinary Medical Association.

4. International Veterinary Acupuncture Society, Fort Collins, Colo.

5. Chi Institute of Traditional Chinese Medicine, Reddick, Fla.

6. Colorado State University, College of Veterinary Medicine, Department of Clinical Studies, Fort Collins, Colo.

7. Tufts University School of Veterinary Medicine, Continuing Education, North Grafton, Mass.

8. Veterinary Institute for Therapeutic Alternatives, Sherman, Conn.

9. Hwang Y, Egerbacher M: Anatomy and classification of acupoints. In Schoen AM, ed: *Veterinary acupuncture: ancient art to modern medicine*, St Louis, 2001, Mosby.

10. Steiss J: The neurophysiologic basis of acupuncture. In Schoen AM, ed: *Veterinary acupuncture: ancient art to modern medicine*, St Louis, 2001, Mosby.

11. Stux G, Pomeranz B: *Acupuncture: textbook and atlas*, New York, 1986, Springer-Verlag.

12. Chiu JH, Cheng HC, Tai CH, et al: Electroacupuncture-induced neural activation detected by use of manganese-enhanced functional magnetic resonance imaging in rabbits, *Am J Vet Res* 62:178, 2001.

13. Kendall DE: A scientific model for acupuncture. Part I, *Am J Acupunct* 17:251, 1989.

14. Luna SPL, Taylor PM: Effect of electroacupuncture on endogenous opioids, AVP, ACTH, cortisol and catecholamine concentrations measured in the cerebrospinal fluid (CSF), peripheral and pituitary effluent plasma of ponies. Proceedings of the Twenty-Fourth Annual International Congress on Veterinary Acupuncture, Chitou, Taiwan, 1998.

15. Bossut DFB, Leshin LS, Stromberg MW, et al: Plasma cortisol and beta-endorphin in horses subjected to electro-acupuncture for cutaneous analgesia, *Peptides* 4:501, 1983.

16. Shi FS, et al: Influence of EA on different acupoints on serum protein and its ingredients in donkey, *Chin J Vet Med* 24:31, 1998.

17. Shi FS, et al: Effect of EA on different acupoints on blood gas indicators in donkey, *Chin J Vet Med* 24:42, 1998.

18. Xie H, Ott EA, Harkins JD, et al: Influence of electro-acupuncture on pain threshold in horses and its mode of action, PhD dissertation, Gainesville, Fla, 1999, University of Gainesville.

19. Bossut DFB, Page EH, Stromberg MW: Production cutaneous analgesia by electro-acupuncture in horses: variations dependent on sex of subject and locus of stimulation, *Am J Vet Res* 45:620, 1984.

20. Farber PL, Tachibana A, Campiglia HM: Increased pain threshold following electro-acupuncture: analgesia is induced

mainly in meridian acupoints, *Acupunct Electrother Res* 22:109, 1997.

21. Xie HS: *Traditional Chinese veterinary medicine*, Beijing, 1994, Beijing Agricultural University Press.

22. Xie HS: Equine traditional Chinese medical diagnosis. In Schoen AM, ed: *Veterinary acupuncture: ancient art to modern medicine*, ed 2, St Louis, 2001, Mosby.

23. Fleming P: The location of equine back shu points: traditional Chinese versus transpositional. In Schoen AM, ed: *Veterinary acupuncture: ancient art to modern medicine*, St Louis, 2001, Mosby.

24. Xie H, Colahan PT, Ott EA: Electro-acupuncture for the treatment of chronic back pain in performance horses: a controlled clinical trial, PhD dissertation, Gainesville, Fla, 1999, University of Florida.

25. Altman S: Techniques and instrumentation. In Schoen AM, ed: *Veterinary acupuncture: ancient art to modern medicine*, St Louis, 2001, Mosby.

26. Fleming P: Diagnostic acupuncture palpation examination in the horse. In Schoen AM, ed: *Veterinary acupuncture: ancient art to modern medicine*, St Louis, 2001, Mosby.

27. Thoresen A: Equine *Ting* zone therapy. In Schoen AM, ed: *Veterinary acupuncture: ancient art to modern medicine*, St Louis, 2001, Mosby.

28. Gunn C: *Treating myofascial pain*, Seattle, 1989, University of Washington.

29. Seem M: *A new American acupuncture: acupuncture osteopathy*, Boulder, Colo, 1993, Blue Poppy Press.

30. Wang Z: Electro-acupuncture for treatment of 1 horse with cervical paralysis, *Chin J Tradit Vet Sci* 1:34, 1983 (in Chinese).

31. Gansu Institute of Veterinary Medicine: Aquapuncture on Bai-hui for equine sprain in lumbar region and hind limb. In *Scientific techniques of traditional Chinese veterinary medicine*, vol 1, Beijing, 1976, China Agriculture Press (in Chinese).

32. Klide A, Martin B: Acupuncture for treatment of chronic back pain in horses. In Schoen A, ed: *Veterinary acupuncture: ancient art to modern medicine*, St Louis, 2001, Mosby.

33. Fu LA: Treatment for back pain. In *Complete set of secret recipe of traditional Chinese veterinary medicine*, Shanxi, China, 1992, Shanxi Science and Technology Press (in Chinese).

34. Jeffcott LB: Back problems in the horse: a look at past, present and future progress, *Equine Vet J* 11:129, 1987.

35. Klide AM, Martin BB Jr: Methods of stimulating acupoints for treatment of chronic back pain in horses, *J Am Vet Med Assoc* 195:1375, 1989.

36. Martin BB Jr, Klide AM: Use of acupuncture for the treatment of chronic back pain in horses: stimulation of acupoints with saline solution injections, *J Am Vet Med Assoc* 190:1177, 1987.

37. Martin BB Jr, Klide AM: Treatment of chronic back pain in horses: stimulation of acupoints with a low powered infrared laser, *Vet Surg* 16:106, 1987.

38. Martin BB Jr, Klide AM: Acupuncture for the treatment of chronic back pain in 200 horses, *Proc Am Assoc Equine Pract* 593, 1991.

39. Martin BB Jr, Klide AM: Acupuncture for treatment of chronic back pain in horses. In Schoen AM, ed: *Veterinary acupuncture: ancient art to modern medicine*, ed 2, St Louis, 2001, Mosby.

40. Tang J: Aquapuncture in Bai-hui for back pain in horses and cattle, *J Tradit Chin Vet Med* 3:38, 1983 (in Chinese).

41. Tang ZY: Combination of acupuncture and herbal medicine for treatment of back pain in cattle, *Chin J Tradit Vet Sci* 1:30, 1991 (in Chinese).

42. Pei Y: Electro-acupuncture for treatment of back pain in horses, *Chin J Vet Sci Tech* 12:42, 1981 (in Chinese).

43. Bai AQ, Zhao XM, Zhang ZW, et al: Aquapuncture for treatment of lameness in horses and cattle, *Chin J Tradit Vet Sci* 2:22, 1989.

44. Bai ZR: Acupuncture for treatment of rheumatism in large animals, *Chin J Tradit Vet Sci* 3:39, 1988 (in Chinese).

45. Bao XM: Electro-acupuncture for treatment of stifle arthritis in cattle, *Chin J Tradit Vet Sci* 3:56, 1982.

46. Fleming P: Acupuncture for musculoskeletal and neurologic conditions in horses. In Schoen AM, ed: *Veterinary acupuncture: ancient art to modern medicine*, ed 2, St Louis, 2001, Mosby.

47. Gansu Institute of Veterinary Medicine: Pneumo-acupuncture treatment of 121 cases with equine lameness. In *Scientific techniques of traditional Chinese veterinary medicine*, vol 1, Beijing, 1976, China Agriculture Press (in Chinese).

48. Chen ZM: Aquapuncture in the Qiang-feng for treatment of equine contusion in the forelimbs, *Chin J Vet Sci Tech* 1:54, 1989 (in Chinese).

49. Guo L: Combination of Chinese and Western medicine for treatment of contusion in shoulder and hip, *J Tradit Chin Vet Med* 2:29, 1992 (in Chinese).

50. Guo SF, Li CY: Hemo-acupuncture and herbal medicine for treatment of equine cases with acute joint contusion, *Chin J Tradit Vet Sci* 3:6, 1983 (in Chinese).

51. He CM, Wang YM, Chen YD: A clinical trial on treatment of acute muscle rheumatism in mares, *Chin J Tradit Vet Sci Tech* 1:19, 1982 (in Chinese).

52. Li KC: Electro-acupuncture for treatment of lameness in horses, *Chin J Tradit Vet Sci* 1:13, 1993 (in Chinese).

53. Li SS: Hemo-acupuncture at Chan-wan for treatment of fetlock contusion in horses, *Chin J Tradit Vet Sci* 1:10, 1986 (in Chinese).

54. Tan ZH: Aquapuncture at Bai-hui for treatment of hindlimb rheumatism in cattle, *Chin J Tradit Vet Sci* 4:25, 1984 (in Chinese).

55. Ming SL, Gao XS: Combination of herbal medicine and aquapuncture for treatment of contusion in limbs in horses, *J Tradit Chin Vet Med* 4:47, 1989 (in Chinese).

56. Palmer SE: Lameness diagnosis and treatment in the standardbred racehorse, *Vet Clin North Am Equine Pract* 1:109, 1990.

57. Song ZD: Combination of herbal medicine and acupuncture for treatment of fetlock contusion in 128 cases, *Chin J Tradit Vet Sci* 2:26, 1982 (in Chinese).

58. Steiss JE, White NA, Bowen JM: Electro-acupuncture in the treatment of chronic lameness in horses and ponies: a controlled clinical trial, *Can J Vet Res* 53:239, 1989.

59. Sun TZ, Gao JH: Aquapuncture of vitamin B_{12} for treatment of forelimb contusion in horses, *J Tradit Chin Vet Med* 3:42, 1989 (in Chinese).

60. Tao BL, Wang GQ: The warm-needling acupuncture for treatment of 8 equine cases with rheumatism, *J Tradit Chin Vet Med* 2:15, 1984 (in Chinese).

61. Wang DG: Acupuncture in Qiang-feng and Zhou-shu for treatment of a donkey with shoulder contusion, *Chin J Tradit Vet Sci* 3:40, 1986 (in Chinese).

62. Wang H: An acupuncture method for Bi syndrome. In Yu C, ed: *Complete set of secret recipe of traditional Chinese veterinary medicine*, Shanxi, China, 1992, Shanxi Science & Technology Press (in Chinese).

63. Wang Y: Treatment of equine nerve peripheral paralysis, *Chin J Tradit Vet Sci* 4:36, 1991 (in Chinese).

64. Wang ZY: Aquapuncture for treatment of inflammation in brachialis and biceps brachii in horses, *Chin J Tradit Vet Sci* 2:47, 1991 (in Chinese).

65. Hackett G, Spitzfaden D, May K, et al: Acupuncture: is it effective for alleviating pain in the horse? *Proc Am Assoc Equine Pract* 43:333, 1997.

Acupuncture Channel Palpation and Equine Musculoskeletal Pain

1. Flaws B: *Sticking to the point*, Boulder, Colo, 1990, Blue Poppy Press.

2. Flaws B: *The secret of Chinese pulse diagnosis*, Boulder, Colo, 1995, Blue Poppy Press.

3. Xie H, Priest V: *Xie's veterinary acupuncture*, Ames, Iowa, 2007, Blackwell.

4. Urano K, Ogasawara A: Fundamental study on acupuncture point phenomena of dog body, *Kilsato Arch Exp Med* 51:95, 1978.

5. Yu C, Hwang Y-C, Liu Z, et al: *Handbook on Chinese veterinary acupuncture and moxibustion*, Bangkok, Thailand, 1990, FAO Regional Office for Asia and the Pacific.

6. Thoresen AS: *Alternative and complementary medicine*, Norway, 2001, Preutz Boktrykkeri.

7. Westermayer E: *Lehrbuch der Veterinarakupunktur, Band 2: Akupunktur des Pferdes*, Heidelberg, 1993, Karl F. Haug Verlag Gmb H & Co.

8. Cain M, Snader ML, Sutherland E, et al: Paper presented at International Veterinary Acupuncture Society Course, Santa Monica, California, 1987.

9. Snader ML: Transpositional equine acupuncture atlas. In Shoen A ed: *Veterinary acupuncture*, ed 1, Goleta, Calif, 1994, American Veterinary Publications.

10. Xie H: *Traditional Chinese veterinary medicine*, Beijing, China, 1994, Beijing Agricultural University Press.

11. Van Den Bosch E, Guray J-Y: *Acupuncture points and meridians in the horse*, Unpublished data, 1999.

12. McCormick WH: *The significance of ahshi points in shoulder lameness of the horse*. Proceedings of the Nineteenth International Congress in Veterinary Acupuncture. Thromso, Norway, 1993.

13. McCormick WH: Traditional Chinese channel diagnosis, myofascial pain syndrome and metacarpophalangeal joint trauma in the horse, *J Equine Vet Sci* 16:562, 1996.

14. McCormick WH: Oriental channel diagnosis in foot lameness of the equine forelimb *J Equine Vet Sci* 17:315, 1997.

15. McCormick WH: The origins of acupuncture channel imbalance in pain of the equine hindlimb, *Equine Vet Sci* 18:528, 1998.

16. McCormick WH: *The use of acupuncture channel imbalance in 350 sport horse purchase examinations, 1999-2007,* Proceedings of the American Academy of Veterinary Acupuncture Annual Meeting. Natick, Mass, 2008.

17. Cain M: *Acupuncture diagnosis and treatment of the equine,* Unpublished data, 1996.

18. Marks D: Personal communication, 2004.

19. Travell JG, Myofascial trigger points: a clinical view. In Bonica JJ, Albe-Fassard D, eds. Advances in pain research and therapy: proceedings of the First World Congress on Pain, vol 1, New York, 1976, Raven Press.

20. MacGregor J, Von Schweinitz DG: Needle electromyographic activity of myofascial trigger points and control sites in equine cleidobrachialis muscle, *Acupunct Med* 24:61, 2006.

21. Bowker RM, Abhold RH, Caron JP et al: Neuropeptidergic innervation of equine synovial joints, *Am J Vet Res* 54:1831, 1993.

22. Martin BB, Klide AM: Use of acupuncture for the treatment of chronic back pain in horses: stimulation of acupuncture points with saline solution injections, *J Am Vet Med Assoc* 190:1177, 1987.

23. Steiss JE: Electroacupuncture in the treatment of chronic lameness in horses and ponies: a controlled clinical trial, *Can J Vet Res* 53:239, 1998.

24. Hackett GE, Spitzfaden DM, May KJ: Acupuncture: is it effective for alleviating pain in the horse? *Proc Am Assoc Equine Pract* 43:333, 1997.

CHAPTER 93   Chiropractic Evaluation and Management of Musculoskeletal Disorders

1. Chapman-Smith DA: *The chiropractic profession,* West Des Moines, Iowa, 2000, NCMIC Group.

2. Leach RA: *The chiropractic theories: principles and clinical applications,* Baltimore, 1994, Williams & Wilkins.

3. Haldeman S: *Principles and practice of chiropractic,* New York, 2005, McGraw-Hill.

4. Wynn SG: Wherefore complementary medicine? *J Am Vet Med Assoc* 209:1228, 1996.

5. Haussler KK, Stover SM, Willits NH: Pathologic changes in the lumbosacral vertebrae and pelvis in Thoroughbred racehorses, *Am J Vet Res* 60:143, 1999.

6. Jeffcott LB: Disorders of the thoracolumbar spine of the horse—a survey of 443 cases, *Equine Vet J* 12:197, 1980.

7. Willoughby SL: *Equine chiropractic care,* Port Byron, Ill, 1991, Options for Animals Foundation.

8. Jeffcott LB: Guidelines for the diagnosis and treatment of back problems in horses, *Proc Am Assoc Equine Pract* 26:381, 1980.

9. Liebenson C: *Rehabilitation of the spine,* Baltimore, 1996, Williams & Wilkins.

10. Gatterman MI: *Foundations of chiropractic,* St Louis, 1995, Mosby.

11. Manga P, Angus DE, Papadopoulos C, et al: *The effectiveness and cost-effectiveness of chiropractic management of low-back pain,* Richmond Hill, Ontario, 1993, Kenilworth Publishing, Ontario Ministry of Health.

12. Cassidy JD, Lopes AA, Yong-Hing K: The immediate effect of manipulation versus mobilization on pain and range of motion in the cervical spine: a randomized controlled trial, *J Manipulative Physiol Ther* 15:570, 1992.

13. Brodeur R: The audible release associated with joint manipulation, *J Manipulative Physiol Ther* 18:155, 1995.

14. Reggars JW, Pollard HP: Analysis of zygapophyseal joint cracking during chiropractic manipulation, *J Manipulative Physiol Ther* 18:65, 1995.

15. Herzog W, Zhang YT, Conway PJW, et al: Cavitation sounds during spinal manipulative treatments, *J Manipulative Physiol Ther* 16:523, 1993.

16. Haussler KK, Bertram JEA, Gellman K: In-vivo segmental kinematics of the thoracolumbar spinal region in horses and effects of chiropractic manipulations, *Proc Am Assoc Equine Pract* 45:327, 1999.

17. Haussler KK, Erb HN: Pressure algometry: objective assessment of back pain and effects of chiropractic treatment, *Proc Am Assoc Equine Pract* 49:66, 2003.

18. Sullivan KA, Hill AE, Haussler KK: The effects of chiropractic, massage and phenylbutazone on spinal mechanical nociceptive thresholds in horses without clinical signs of back pain, *Equine Vet J* 40:14, 2008.

19. Haussler KK, Hill AE, Puttlitz CM, et al: Effects of vertebral mobilization and manipulation on kinematics of the thoracolumbar region, *Am J Vet Res* 68:508, 2007.

20. Wakeling JM, Barnett K, Price S, et al: Effects of manipulative therapy on the longissimus dorsi in the equine back, *Equine Comp Exerc Physiol* 3:153, 2006.

21. Faber MJ, van Weeren PR, Schepers M, et al: Long-term follow-up of manipulative treatment in a horse with back problems, *J Vet Med A Physiol Pathol Clin Med* 50:241, 2003.

22. Gómez Alvarez CB, L'Ami JJ, Moffat D, et al: Effect of chiropractic manipulations on the kinematics of back and limbs in horses with clinically diagnosed back problems, *Equine Vet J* 40:153, 2008.

23. Cauvin E: Assessment of back pain in horses, *In Pract* 19:522, 1997.

24. Steckel RR, Kraus-Hansen AE, Fackelman GE, et al: Scintigraphic diagnosis of thoracolumbar spinal disease in horses: a review of 50 cases, *Proc Am Assoc Equine Pract* 37:583, 1991.

25. Chaitow L: *Palpation skills,* New York, 1997, Churchill Livingston.

26. Van Schaik JPJ, Verbiest H, Van Schaik FDJ: Isolated spinous process deviation: a pitfall in the interpretation of AP radiographs of the lumbar spine, *Spine* 14:970, 1989.

27. Kessler RM, Hertling D: Assessment of musculoskeletal disorders. In Hertling D, Kessler RM, eds: *Management of common musculoskeletal disorders: physical therapy principles and methods,* ed 2, Philadelphia, 1990, Lippincott.

28. Gál JM, Herzog W, Kawchuk GN, et al: Movements of vertebrae during manipulative thrusts to unembalmed human cadavers, *J Manipulative Physiol Ther* 20:30, 1997.

29. Ahern TJ: Cervical vertebral mobilization under anesthetic (CVMUA): a physical therapy for the treatment of cervicospinal pain and stiffness, *J Equine Vet Sci* 14:540, 1994.

CHAPTER 94   Electrophysical Agents in Physiotherapy

1. Watson T: Ultrasound in contemporary physiotherapy practice, *Ultrasonics* 48:321, 2008.

2. Watson T: Masterclass. The role of electrotherapy in contemporary physiotherapy practice, *Manual Therapy* 5:132, 2000.

3. Grant BD: In McIlwraith CW, Trotter G, eds: *Joint disease in the horse,* Philadelphia, 1996, Saunders.

4. Steiss JE, Adams CC: Rate of temperature increase in canine muscle during 1 MHz ultrasound therapy: deleterious effect of hair coat, *Am J Vet Res* 60:76, 1999.

5. Schabrun S, Chipchase L, Rickard H: Are therapeutic ultrasound units a potential vector for nosocomial infection, *Physiother Res Int* 11:61, 2006.

6. Pye S: Ultrasound therapy equipment—does it perform, *Physiotherapy* 82:39, 1996.

7. ter Haar G: Therapeutic ultrasound, *Eur J Ultrasound* 9:3, 1999.

8. Watson T, Young S: Therapeutic ultrasound. In Watson T, ed: *Electrotherapy: evidence based practice,* New York, 2008, Churchill Livingstone-Elsevier.

9. Nussbaum EL: Ultrasound: to heat or not to heat—that is the question, *Phys Ther Rev* 2:59, 1997.

10. Lehmann J: *Therapeutic heat and cold,* Baltimore, 1992, Williams & Wilkins.

11. Dyson M, Suckling J: Stimulation of tissue repair by ultrasound: a survey of the mechanisms involved, *Physiotherapy* 64:105, 1978.

12. Baker KG, Robertson VJ, Duck FA: Review of therapeutic ultrasound: biophysical effects, *Phys Ther* 81:1351, 2001.

13. Leung MC, Ng GY, Yip KK: Effects of ultrasound on acute inflammation of transected medial collateral ligaments, *Arch Phys Med Rehabil* 85:963, 2004.

14. Hashish I, Harvey W, Harris M: Anti-inflammatory effects of ultrasound therapy: evidence for a major placebo effect, *Br J Rheumatol* 14:237, 1986.

15. Enwemeka CS, Rodriquez O, Mendosa S: The biomechanical effects of low intensity ultrasound on healing tendons, *Ultrasound Med Biol* 16:801, 1990.

16. Enwemeka CS: The effects of therapeutic ultrasound on tendon healing. A biomechanical study, *Am J Phys Med Rehabil* 68:283, 1989.

17. Ramirez A, Schwane JA, McFarland C, et al: The effects of ultrasound on collagen synthesis and fibroblast proliferation in vitro, *Med Sci Sports Exerc* 29:362, 1997.

18. Watson T: Soft tissue healing, *In Touch* 104:14, 2003.

19. Nussbaum E: The influence of ultrasound on healing tissues, *J Hand Ther Rev* 2:140, 1998.

20. Srbely JZ, Dickey JP: Randomized controlled study of the antinociceptive effects of ultrasound on trigger point sensitivity: novel applications in myofascial therapy, *Clin Rehabil* 21:411, 2007.

21. Watson T: Electrotherapy and tissue repair, *Sportex Med* 29:7, 2006.

22. Charman RA: In Forster A, Palastanga N, eds: *Clayton's electrotherapy theory and practice*, ed 10, London, 2002, Saunders.

23. Sanservino E: Membrane phenomena and cellular processes under action of pulsating magnetic fields. Lecture at the 2nd International Congress Magneto Medicine, Rome, November 1980.

24. Luben RA: Effects of microwave radiation on signal transduction processes of cells in vitro. In Bernhardt JH, Matthes R, Repacholi MH, eds: *Non-thermal effects of RF electromagnetic fields*, Munich, 1997, Maerkl-Druck Publishing.

25. Aronofsky DH: Reduction of dental post-surgical symptoms using non-thermal pulsed high-peak-power electromagnetic energy, *Oral Surg* 32:688, 1971.

26. Sanders-Shamis M, Bramlage LR, Weisbrode SE, et al: A preliminary investigation of the effect of selected electromagnetic field devices on healing of cannon bone osteotomies in horses, *Equine Vet J* 21:201, 1989.

27. Kold SE, Hickman J: Preliminary study of quantitative aspects and the effect of pulsed electromagnetic field treatment on the incorporation of equine cancellous bone grafts, *Equine Vet J* 19:120, 1987.

28. Goldin J: The effects of Diapulse on the healing of wounds: a double blind randomised controlled trial in man, *Br J Plast Surg* 34:267, 1981.

29. Robertson V, Ward A, Low J, et al: *Electrotherapy explained: principles and practice*, ed 4, Oxford, 2007, Butterworth Heinemann.

30. Baxter GD: *Therapeutic lasers, theory and practice*, ed 1, New York, 1994, Churchill Livingstone.

31. Baxter GD: Low-intensity laser therapy. In Watson T, ed: *Electrotherapy: evidence-based practice*, ed 12, London, 2008, Churchill Livingstone.

32. Kitchen SS, Partirdge CJ: A review of low level laser therapy, *Physiotherapy* 77:161, 1991.

33. King PR: Low level laser therapy: a review, *Physiother Theory Pract* 6:127, 1990.

34. Enwemeka CS: Attenuation and penetration of visible 632.8 nm and invisible infrared 904 nm light in soft tissues, *Laser Ther J* 13:16, 2003.

35. Ramey DW, Basford JR: Laser therapy in horses, *Comp Cont Educ* 22:263, 2000.

36. McNamara K, Macintosh S: Veterinary surgeons perceptions of animal physiotherapy, *Physiotherapy* 79:312, 1993.

37. Knowles D, Mackintosh S: A survey of animal physiotherapy practice in Britain, *Physiotherapy* 80:285, 1994.

38. Vasseljen O, Hoeg N, Kjeldstad B, et al: Low level laser versus placebo in the treatment of tennis elbow, *Scand J Rehab Med* 24:37, 1992.

39. Barclay J: As old as the hills—a historical review of treatment. In: *In good hands: the history of the Chartered Society of Physiotherapists*, Oxford, 1994, Butterworth Heinemann.

40. Del Mar CB, Glasziou PPI, Spinks AB: Is laser treatment effective and safe for musculoskeletal pain, *Med J Aust* 175:169, 2001.

41. Devor M: What's in a laser beam for pain therapy, *Pain* 43:139, 1990.

42. Goldman JA, Chiapella J, Bass N, et al: Laser therapy of rheumatoid arthritis, *Laser Surg Med* 1:93, 1980.

43. Bromiley M: *Equine injury, therapy and rehabilitation*, ed 2, Oxford, 1993, Blackwell Science.

44. Tunér J, Hode L: *Laser therapy: clinical practice & scientific background*, Grangesberg, Sweden, 2002, Prima Books AB.

45. Tunér J, Hode L: *The laser therapy handbook*, Grangesberg, Sweden, 2004, Prima Books AB.

46. Bayat M, Delbari A, Almaseyeh M, et al: Low-level laser therapy improves early healing of medial collateral ligament injuries in rats, *Photomed Laser Surg* 23:556, 2005.

47. Young S, Bolton P, Dyson M, et al: Macrophage responsiveness to laser light therapy, *Laser Surg Med* 9:497, 1989.

48. Honmura A, Yanase M, Obata J, et al: Therapeutic effects of Ga-Al-As diode laser irradiation on experimentally induced inflammation in rats, *Laser Surg Med* 12:411, 1992.

49. Bjordal JM, Demmink JH, Ljung AE: Low level laser therapy for tendinopathy. Evidence of a dose–response pattern, *Phys Ther Rev* 6:91, 2001.

50. Lucas C, Criens-Poublon LJ, Cockrell CT, et al: Wound healing in cell studies and animal model experiments of low level laser therapy: were clinical studies justified? A systematic review, *Lasers Med Sci* 17:110, 2002.

51. Brosseau L, Welch V, Wells G, et al: Low level laser therapy (classes I, II and III) for treating rheumatoid arthritis (Cochrane review). In *The Cochrane library*, issue 4, Chichester, UK, 2003, John Wiley and Sons.

52. Chow R: Dose dilemmas in low level laser therapy—the effects of different paradigms and historical perspectives, *Laser Ther J* 13:47, 2003.

53. Gur A, Cosut A, Sarac AJ, et al: Efficacy of different therapy regimes of low power laser in painful osteoarthritis of the knee: a double blind and randomised controlled trial, *Lasers Surg Med* 33:330, 2003.

54. Martin BJ, Kilde AM: Treatment of chronic back pain in horses—stimulation of acupuncture points with low powered infrared laser, *Vet Surg* 16:106, 1987.

55. Beckermann H, de Bie RA, Bouter LM, et al: The efficacy of laser therapy for musculoskeletal and skin disorders: a critical based meta-analysis of randomised clinical trials, *Phys Ther* 72:483, 1992.

56. De Bie R, Verhagen A, Lenssen T: Oral presentation: efficacy of 904 nm laser therapy in musculoskeletal disorders: a systematic review. In *The Cochrane library*, Chichester, UK, 1996, John Wiley and Sons.

57. Sharma R, Thukral A, Kumar S, et al: Effects of low level lasers in Quervains tenosynovitis, *Physiotherapy* 88:730, 2002.

58. Dyson M, Young S: Effects of laser therapy on wound contraction and cellularity in mice, *Laser Med Sci* 1:125, 1986.

59. McKibbin LS, Paraschak D: Use of laser light to treat certain lesions in Standardbreds, *Modern Vet Pract* 65:210, 1984.

60. McCaughan JS, Bethel BH, Jo T, et al: Effect of low dose argon irradiation on rate of wound closure, *Laser Surg Med* 5:607, 1985.

61. Lucroy MD, Edwards BF, Madwell BR: Low intensity laser light–inducted closure of chronic wound in dogs, *Vet Surg* 28:292, 1999.

62. Ghasmsari SM, Acorda JA, Taguchi K, et al: Evaluation of wound healing of the teat with and without low level laser therapy in dairy cattle by laser Doppler flowmetry in comparison with histopathology, tensiometry and hydroxyproline analysis, *Br Vet J* 152:583, 1996.

63. Fretz PB, Li Z: Low energy laser irradiation treatment for second intention wound healing in horses, *Can Vet J* 33:650, 1992.

64. Ng G, Fung D: Combining therapeutic laser and herbal remedy for treating ligament injury: an ultrastructural morphological study, *Photomed Laser Surg* 26:425, 2008.

65. Basford JR, Malanga, GA, Krause DA: A randomised controlled evaluation of low intensity laser therapy: plantar fasciitis, *Arch Phys Med Rehabil* 79:249, 1998.

66. Snyder-Mackler L, Ladin Z, Schepsis AA, et al: Electrical stimulation of the thigh muscle after reconstruction of the anterior cruciate ligament, *J Bone Joint Surg* 73A:1025, 1991.

67. Kanaya F, Tajima T: Effect of electro stimulation on denervated muscle, *Clin Orthop* 283:296, 1992.

68. Williams HB: The value of continuous electrical muscle stimulation using a completely implantable system in the preservation of muscle function following motor nerve injury and repair: an experimental study, *Microsurgery* 17:589, 1998.

69. Kernell D, Eerbeek O, Verhey BA, et al: Effects of physiological amounts of high- and low-rate chronic stimulation on fast-twitch muscle of the cat hindlimb. I. Speed- and force-related properties, *J Neurophysiol* 58:598, 1987.

70. Gorza L, Gundersen K, Lomo T, et al: Slow-to-fast transformation of denervated soleus muscles by chronic high-frequency stimulation in the rat, *J Physiol* 402:627, 1988.

71. Bigard A: Effects of surface electro stimulation on the structure and metabolic properties in monkey skeletal muscle, *Med Sci Sports Exer* 25:355, 1993.

72. Clemente FR, Barron KW: The influence of muscle contractions on the degree of microvascular perfusion in rat skeletal

muscle following transcutaneous neuro-muscular electrical stimulation, *J Orthop Sports Phys Ther* 17:177, 1993.

73. Millis DL, Levine D, Weigel JP: A preliminary study of early physical therapy following surgery for cranial cruciate ligament rupture in dogs, *Vet Surg* 26:254, 1997.

74. Millis DL, Levine D, Taylor RA: *Canine rehabilitation and physical therapy*, St. Louis, 2004, Saunders.

75. Watson T: www.electrotherapy.org. (Accessed March 21, 2009.)

76. Wolf SL, Gersh MR, Rao VR: Examination of electrode placements and stimulating parameters in treating chronic pain with conventional transcutaneous electrical nerve stimulation (TENS), *Pain* 11:37, 1981.

77. Baldry PE: *Acupuncture, trigger points and musculoskeletal pain*, Edinburgh, UK, 1989, Churchill Livingstone.

78. Zurgman C: Dermatitis from transcutaneous electrical nerve stimulation, *J Am Acad Derm* 6:936, 1982.

79. Binder-Macleod SA, Snyder-Mackler L: Muscle fatigue: clinical implications for fatigue assessment and neuromuscular electrical stimulation, *Phys Ther* 73:902, 1993.

80. Haker E, Lundeberg T: Laser treatment to acupuncture points in lateral humeral epicondylalgia—a double blind study, *Pain* 43:243, 1990.

CHAPTER 95   Osteopathic Treatment of the Axial Skeleton of the Horse

1. Williams N: Managing back pain in general practice: is osteopathy the new paradigm? *Br J Gen Pract* 47:653, 1997.

2. Pearson K, Gordon J: Locomotion. In Kendel E, Schwartz J, Jessel T, eds: *Principles of neuroscience*, New York, 2000, McGraw-Hill.

3. Hex X, Proske U, Schaible HG, et al: Acute inflammation of the knee joint in the cat alters responses of flexor motor neurons to leg movements, *J Neurophysiol* 59:326, 1988.

4. Sato A, Schmidt RF: Somatosympathetic reflexes: afferent fibres, central pathways, discharge characteristics, *Physiol Rev* 53:916, 1973.

5. Pernow B: Substance P, *Pharmacol Rev* 35:85, 1983.

6. Mantyh PW, DeMaster E, Malhotra A, et al: Receptor endocytosis and dendrite reshaping in spinal neurons after somatosensory reshaping, *Science* 268:1629, 1995.

7. Patterson MM, Worster RD: Neurophysiological system. In Ward RC, ed: *Foundations of osteopathic medicine*, Baltimore, 1997, Williams & Wilkins.

8. Sluka KA, Willis WD, Westlund KN: The role of dorsal root reflexes in neurogenic inflammation, *Pain Forum* 4:141, 1995.

9. Bakker DA, Richmond FJR: Muscle spindle complexes in muscles around upper cervical vertebra in the cat, *J Neurophysiol* 48:62, 1982.

10. Goldspink G, Williams F, Simpson H: Gene expression in response to muscle stretch, *Clin Orthop Related Res* 403(Suppl):S146, 2002.

11. Ward R: *Foundations of osteopathic medicine*, Baltimore, 1997, Williams & Wilkins.

12. Pusey A, Holah G, Colles C, et al: Detection of spinal dysfunction in horses using thermography, *Br Osteopath J* 20:27, 1997.

13. Colles C, Holah G, Pusey A: Thermal imaging as an aid to the diagnosis of back pain in the horse. In Ammer K, Ring E, eds: *Proceedings of the Sixth European Congress of Thermography*, Vienna, 1994, Uhlen Verlag.

14. Pusey A, Colles C, Brooks J: Osteopathic treatment of horses: a retrospective study, *Br Osteopath J* 16:30, 1995.

CHAPTER 96   Shock Wave Therapy

1. Graff J: Transmission of shock waves through bone: treatment of iliac ureteral stones in a supine position, *J Urol* 143:231, 1990.

2. Weinberger T: First Symposium of Extracorporeal Shock Wave Users in Veterinary Medicine, Pferdeklinik Burg Mueggenhausen, Weilerswist, Germany, 2000.

3. McCarroll GD, Hague B, Smitherman S, et al: The use of extracorporeal shock wave lithotripsy for treatment of distal tarsal arthropathies of the horse, *Proc Assoc Equine Sports Med* 18:40, 1999.

4. McCarroll GD, McClure SR: Initial experiences with extracorporeal shock wave therapy for treatment of bone spavin in horses, *Vet Comp Orthop Traumatol* 3:184, 2002.

5. McClure SR, Dorfmüller C: Extracorporeal shock wave therapy: theory and equipment, *Clin Tech Equine Pract* 2:348, 2003.

6. McClure SR: Extracorporeal shock-wave therapy and radial pressure-wave therapy: wave physics and equipment. In Robinson NE, Sprayberry K, eds: *Current therapy in equine medicine*, ed 6, St. Louis, 2009, Saunders.

7. Rompe JD, Kirkpatrick CJ, Kullmer K, et al: Dose-related effects of shock waves on rabbit tendo Achillis, *J Bone Joint Surg Br* 80:546, 1998.

8. Wang CJ, Huang HY, Pai CH: Shock wave-enhanced neovascularization at the tendon-bone junction: an experiment in dogs, *J Foot Ankle Surg* 41:16, 2002.

9. Chen YJ, Wang CJ, Yang KD, et al: Extracorporeal shock waves promote healing of collagenase-induced Achilles tendonitis and increased TGF-beta1 and IGF-1 expression, *J Orthop Res* 22:854, 2004.

10. Delius M, Draenert K, Diek YA, et al: Biological effects of shock waves: in vivo effect of high energy pulses on rabbit bone, *Ultrasound Med Biol* 21:1219, 1995.

11. Uslu MM, Bozdogan Ö, Güney S, et al: The effect of extracorporeal shock wave treatment (ESWT) on bone defects. An experimental study, *Bull Hosp Joint Dis* 58:114, 1999.

12. Johannes EJ, Dinesh MD, Daulesar Sukul DMKS, et al: High-energy shock waves for the treatment of nonunions: an experiment on dogs, *J Surg Res* 57:246, 1994.

13. Wang CJ, Chen HA, Chen CE, et al: Treatment of nonunions of long bone fractures with shock waves, *Clin Orthop Rel Res* 387:95, 2001.

14. Schaden W, Fischer A, Sailler A: Extracorporeal shockwave therapy for nonunion or delayed osseous union, *Clin Orthop Rel Res* 387:90, 2001.

15. Rompe JD, Rosendahy T, Schollner C, et al: High-energy extracorporeal shockwave treatment of nonunions, *Clin Orthop Rel Res* 387:102, 2001.

16. Da Costa Gomez TM, Radtke CL, Kalsherur VL, et al: Effect of focused and radial extracorporeal shockwave therapy on equine bone microdamage, *Vet Surg* 32:387, 2004.

17. Pauwels FE, McClure SR, Amin V, et al: Effects of extracorporeal shock wave therapy and radial pressure wave therapy on elasticity and microstructure of equine cortical bone, *Am J Vet Res* 65:207, 2004.

18. McClure SR, Van Sickle D, White MR: Effects of extracorporeal shock wave therapy on bone, *Vet Surg* 33:40, 2004.

19. Bischofberger AS, Ring SK, Geyer H, et al: Histomorphologic evaluation of extracorporeal shock wave therapy on the fourth metatarsal bone and the origin of the suspensory ligament in horses without lameness, *Am J Vet Res* 67:577, 2006.

20. Palmer SE: Treatment of dorsal metacarpal disease in the Thoroughbred racehorse with radial extracorporeal shock wave therapy, *Proc Am Assoc Equine Pract* 48:318, 2002.

21. Scheuch B, Whitcomb MB, Galuppo L, et al: Clinical evaluation of high-energy extracorporeal shock waves on equine orthopedic injuries, *Proc Assoc Equine Sports Med* 18:18, 1999.

22. McClure SR, Weinberger T: Extracorporeal shock wave therapy: clinical applications and regulation, *Clin Tech Equine Pract* 2:358, 2003.

23. Wang CJ, Huang HY, Chen HH, et al: Effect of shock wave therapy on acute factures of the tibia. A study in a dog model, *Clin Orthop Rel Res* 387:112, 2001.

24. Hus RW, Hsu WH, Tai Cl, et al: Effect of shock-wave therapy on patellar tendinopathy in a rabbit model, *J Orthop Res* 22:221, 2004.

25. Wang CJ, Wang FS, Yang KD, et al: The effect of shock wave treatment at the tendon-bone interface—a histomorphological and biomechanical study in rabbits, *J Orthop Res* 23:274, 2005.

26. Bosch G, Lin YL, van Schie HT, et al: Effect of extracorporeal shock wave therapy on the biochemical composition and metabolic activity of tenocytes in normal tendinous structures in ponies, *Equine Vet J* 39:226, 2007.

27. Bosch G, de Mos M, van Binsbergen R, et al: The effect of focused extracorporeal shock wave therapy on collagen matrix and gene expression in normal tendons and ligaments, *Equine Vet J* 41:335, 2009.

28. McClure SR, Van Sickle D, Evans R, et al: The effects of extracorporeal shock wave therapy on the ultrasonographic and histologic appearance of collagenase-induced equine forelimb suspensory ligament desmitis, *Ultrasound Med Biol* 30:461, 2004.

29. Caminoto EH, Alves ALG, Amorim RL, et al: Ultrastructural and immunocytochemical evaluation of the effects of extracorporeal shock wave treatment in

the hind limbs of horses with experimentally induces suspensory ligament desmitis, *Am J Vet Res* 66:892, 2005.

30. Lischer CJ, Ringer SK, Schnewlin M, et al: Treatment of chronic proximal suspensory desmitis in horses using focused electrohydraulic shockwave therapy, *Schweizer Archiv Tierheilkunde* 148:561, 2006.

31. Crowe O, Dyson S, Wright I, et al: Treatment of 45 cases of chronic hindlimb proximal suspensory desmitis by radial extracorporeal shockwave therapy, *Proc Am Assoc Equine Pract* 48:322, 2002.

32. Crowe O, Dyson S, Wright I, et al: Treatment of chronic or recurrent proximal suspensory desmitis using radial pressure wave therapy, *Equine Vet J* 36:313, 2004.

33. Kersh KD, McClure S, Evans RB, et al: Ultrasonographic evaluation of extracorporeal shock wave therapy on collagenase-induced superficial digital flexor tendonitis, *Proc Am Assoc Equine Pract* 50:257, 2004.

34. Alves ALG, da Fonseca BPA, Thomassian A, et al: Effects of extracorporeal shock wave treatment on equine tendon healing, *Int Soc Musculoskel Shockwave Ther Newslett* 1:12, 2006.

35. Revenaugh MS: Extracorporeal shock wave therapy for treatment of osteoarthritis in the horses: clinical applications, *Vet Clin North Am Equine Pract* 21:609, 2005.

36. McIlwraith CW, Frisbie DD, Park RD, et al: Evaluation of extracorporeal shockwave therapy for osteoarthritis using an equine model, *Proc Eur Coll Vet Surg* 13:257, 2004.

37. McClure SR, Evans RB, Miles KG, et al: Extracorporeal shock wave therapy for treatment of navicular syndrome, *Proc Am Assoc Equine Pract* 50:316, 2004.

38. Bär K, Mwiler M, Bodamer J, et al: Extrakorporale Stoßwellentherapie (ESWT)—eine Möglichkeit zur Therapie der Podotrochlose, *Tierärztl Prax* 29:163, 2001.

39. Dakin S, Dyson S, Murray R, Newton R: Osseous abnormalities associated with collateral desmopathy of the distal interphalangeal joint: Part 2: Treatment and outcome, *Equine Vet J* 41:794, 2009.

40. Weinberger T: The use of focused shock wave therapy in back problems of the horse. Symposium of Extracorporeal Shock Wave Users in Veterinary Medicine, Pferdeklinik Barkhof, Sottrum, Germany, 2002.

41. Cleveland RO, Chitnis PV, McClure SR: Acoustic field of a ballistic shock wave therapy device, *Ultrasound Med Biol* 33:1327, 2007.

42. Yeaman LD, Jerome CP, McCullough DL: Effects of shock waves on the structure and growth of the immature rat epiphysis, *J Urol* 141:670, 1989.

43. McClure SR, Sonea IM, Evans RB, et al: Evaluation of analgesia resulting from extracorporeal shockwave therapy and radial pressure wave therapy in the limbs of horses and sheep, *Am J Vet Res* 66:1702, 2005.

44. Dahlberg JA, McClure SR, Evans RB: Force platform evaluation of lameness severity following extracorporeal shock wave therapy in horses with unilateral forelimb lameness, *J Am Vet Med Assoc* 229:100, 2006.

45. Brown KE, Nickols FA, Leron JP, et al: Investigation of the immediate analgesic effects of extracorporeal shock wave therapy for treatment of navicular disease in horses, *Vet Surg* 34:554, 2005.

CHAPTER 97   Poor Performance and Lameness

1. Schamhardt H, Merkens H, Vogel V, et al: External loads on the limbs of jumping horses at take-off and landing, *Am J Vet Res* 54:675, 1993.

2. Merkens H, Schamhardt H, van Osch G, et al: Ground reaction force patterns of Dutch warmbloods at the canter, *Am J Vet Res* 54:670, 1993.

3. Clayton H: Performance in equestrian sports. In Back W, Clayton H, eds: *Equine locomotion*, London, 2001, Saunders.

CHAPTER 98   Experiences Using a High-Speed Treadmill to Evaluate Lameness

1. Morris EH, Seeherman HJ: Clinical evaluation of poor performance in the racehorse: the results of 275 evaluations, *Equine Vet J* 23:169, 1991.

2. Martin BB, Parente EJ, Maxson AD, et al: Clinical evaluation of poor performance in horses: the results of 693 examinations, *Proc Assoc Equine Sports Med* 16:17, 1997.

3. Martin BB, Reef VB, Parente EJ, et al: Causes of poor performance of horses during training, racing, or showing: 348 cases (1992-1996), *J Am Vet Med Assoc* 216:554, 2000.

4. King CM, Evans DL, Rose RJ: Cardiac, respiratory and metabolic responses to exercise in horses with various abnormalities of the upper respiratory tract, *Equine Vet J* 26:220, 1994.

5. Reef VB: Electrocardiography and echocardiography in the exercising horse. In Robinson NE, Wilson MR, eds: *Current therapy in equine medicine*, ed 4, Philadelphia, 1997, Saunders.

6. Foreman JH, Laurence LM: Lameness and heart rate elevation in the exercising horse, *J Equine Vet Sci* 11:353, 1991.

7. Foreman JH, Ferlazzo A: Physiological responses to stress in the horse, *Pferdeheilkunde* 12:401, 1996.

8. Parente EJ: Unpublished data, 2000.

9. Morris EA, Seeherman HJ: Redistribution of ground reaction forces in experimentally induced equine carpal lameness. In Robinson NE, Gillespie JR, eds: *Equine exercise physiology*, ed 2, Davis, Calif, 1987, ICEEP Publications.

10. Jeffcott LB, Dalin G, Drevmo S: Effect of induced back pain on gait and performance of trotting horses, *Equine Vet J* 14:129, 1980.

11. Nunamaker DM, Provost MW: Unpublished data, 1992.

12. Kobluk CN, Moncada-Suarez JR: Gait analysis. In Kobluk CN, Ames TR, Geor RJ, eds: *The horse: diseases and clinical management*, Philadelphia, 1995, Saunders.

13. Seeherman HJ: Lameness evaluation. In Auer JA, Stick JA, eds: *Equine surgery*, ed 2, Philadelphia, 1999, Saunders.

14. Schneider RK: Slow motion video gait analysis of gait abnormalities in horses, *Am Coll Vet Surg Ann Symp* 97, 1998.

15. Weishaupt MA, Weistner, Hermann PH, et al: Compensatory load redistribution of horses with weight-bearing forelimb lameness trotting on a treadmill, *Vet J* 171:135, 2004.

16. Keegan K, Yoshiharu Y, Pai PF, et al: Evaluation of a sensor based system of motion analysis for detection and quantification of forelimb and hindlimb lameness in horses, *Am J Vet Res* 65:665, 2004.

17. Martin BB: Complications of examination of horses for poor performance using a high-speed treadmill. Unpublished data 2000-2010.

18. Courouce A, Geffroy O, Barrey E, et al: Comparison of exercise tests in French trotters under training track, racetrack and treadmill conditions, *Equine Vet J Suppl* 30:528, 1999.

19. Galisteo AM, Cano MR, Morales JL, et al: Kinematics in horses at the trot before and after an induced forelimb supporting lameness, *Equine Vet J Suppl* 23:97, 1997.

20. McDonnell SM, Love CC, Reef VB, et al: Ejaculatory failure associated with aortic-iliac thrombosis in two stallions, *J Am Vet Med Assoc* 200:954, 1992.

21. Valberg SJ: Muscular causes of exercise intolerance in horses, *Vet Clin North Am Equine Pract* 12:495, 1996.

22. Waldron J: Personal communication, 2000.

23. Moyer W, Dabareiner R: Subjective evaluation of lameness and correlation with kinematic gait analysis, *Equine Med Rev* 9:4, 1999.

24. Keegan KG, Wilson DA, Wilson DJ: Evaluation of mild lameness in horses trotting on a treadmill by clinicians and interns or residents and correlation of their assessments with kinematic gait analysis, *Am J Vet Res* 59:1370, 1998.

CHAPTER 99   The Sales Yearling

Purchase Examination of a Thoroughbred Sales Yearling in North America

1. Reid CF: Radiographs and the purchase examination in the horse, *Vet Clin North Am Large Anim Pract* 2:151, 1980.

2. Teigland MB: Medical examination of horses at auction sales, *Vet Clin North Am Equine Pract* 8:413, 1992.

3. Ellis DR: Examinations at horse sales (Thoroughbreds). In Mabry T, ed: *The prepurchase examination*, Newmarket, 1998, Equine Veterinary Journal.

4. Hardy JA, Marcoux M, Breton L: Clinical relevance of radiographic findings in proximal sesamoid bones of two-year-old Standardbreds in their first year of race training, *J Am Vet Med Assoc* 198:2089, 1991.

5. Kane AJ, Park RD, McIlwraith CW, et al: Radiographic changes in Thoroughbred yearlings. Part 1: Prevalence at the time of the yearling sales, *Equine Vet J* 35:354, 2003.

6. Kane AJ, McIlwraith CW, Park RD, et al: Radiographic changes in Thoroughbred yearlings. Part 2: Associations with racing performance, *Equine Vet J* 35:366, 2003.

7. Park RD: Optimal views for evaluating Thoroughbred yearlings: quality control of the radiographic image, *Proc Am Assoc Equine Pract* 46:357, 2000.

8. Hance SR, Morehead JP: Radiographing Thoroughbred yearlings for the repository, *Proc Am Assoc Equine Pract* 46:359, 2000.
9. Marks D: Conformation and soundness, *Proc Am Assoc Equine Pract* 46:39, 2000.
10. Becht JB, Park RD: A review of selected normal radiographic variations of the equine fetlock, carpus, tarsus and stifle, *Proc Am Assoc Equine Pract* 46:362, 2000.
11. Martin BB: The pre-purchase examination and radiography in Thoroughbred yearlings. Proceeding of the Forty-Sixth Annual Meeting of the American College of Veterinary Surgeons, Chicago, 1998.
12. Maloney JW: Personal communication, 1976.
13. Freeman WC: Personal communication, 1993.
14. Bonnie ES: The legal aspects of pre-purchase examinations, *Vet Clin North Am Equine Pract* 8:273, 1992.
15. Reef VB: Personal communication, 1998.
16. Stashak TS: The relationship between conformation and lameness. In Stashak TS, ed: *Adams' lameness in horses*, ed 4, Philadelphia, 1987, Lea & Febiger.

CHAPTER 100 Pathophysiology and Clinical Diagnosis of Cortical and Subchondral Bone Injury

1. Frost HM: Structural adaptations to mechanical usage (SATMU): 1. redefining Wolff's Law: the bone modelling problem, *Anat Rec* 226:403, 1990.
2. Carrier TK, Estberg L, Stover SM, et al: Association between long periods without high-speed workouts and risk of complete humeral or pelvic fracture in Thoroughbred racehorses: 54 cases (1991-1994), *J Am Vet Med Assoc* 212:1582, 1998.
3. Nunamaker DM, Butterweck DM, Provost MT: Fatigue fractures in Thoroughbred racehorses: relationships with age, peak bone strain and training, *J Orthop Res* 8:604, 1990.
4. Stover SM: The epidemiology of the Thoroughbred racehorse injuries, *Clin Tech Equine Pract* 2:313, 2003.
5. Bennell KL, Malcolm SA, Brukner PD: Models for the pathogenesis of stress fracture in athletes, *Br J Sports Med* 30:200, 1996.
6. Stover SM, Johnson BJ, Daft BM, et al: An association between complete and incomplete stress fractures of the humerus in racehorses, *Equine Vet J* 24:260, 1992.
7. Norrdin RW, Kawcek CE, Capwell BA, et al: Subchondral bone failure in an equine model of overload arthrosis, *Bone* 22:133, 1998.
8. Riggs CM: Fractures—a preventable hazard of racing Thoroughbreds? *Vet J* 163:19, 2002.
9. Poole PR, Meagher DM: Pathological findings and pathogenesis of racetrack injuries, *Vet Clin North Am Equine Pract* 6:1, 1990.
10. Kaneko M, Oikawa M, Yoshihara T: Pathological analysis of bone fractures in race horses, *J Vet Med Sci* 55:181, 1993.
11. Haussler KK, Stover SM: Stress fractures of the vertebral lamina and pelvis in Thoroughbred racehorses, *Equine Vet J* 30:374, 1998.
12. Young DR, Richardson DW, Markel MD, et al: Mechanical and morphometric analysis of the third carpal bone of Thoroughbreds, *Am J Vet Res* 52:402, 1991.
13. Stover SM, Ardans AA, Read DH, et al: Patterns of stress fractures associated with complete bone fractures in racehorses, *Proc Am Assoc Equine Pract* 39:131, 1993.
14. Pilsworth RC: Incomplete fracture of the dorsal aspect of the proximal cortex of the third metatarsal bone as a cause of hind-limb lameness in the racing Thoroughbred: a review of three cases, *Equine Vet J* 24:147, 1992.
15. Shepherd MC, Pilsworth RC, Hopes R, et al: Clinical signs, diagnosis, management and outcome of complete and incomplete fracture to the ilium: a review of 20 cases, *Proc Am Assoc Equine Pract* 40:177, 1994.
16. Johnson PJ, Allhands RV, Baker GJ, et al: Incomplete linear tibial fractures in two horses, *J Am Vet Med Assoc* 192:522, 1988.
17. Bathe AP: 245 Fractures in Thoroughbred Racehorses: results of a 2-year prospective study in Newmarket, *Proc Am Assoc Equine Pract* 40:175, 1994.
18. Anastasiou A, Skioldebrand E, Ekman S, et al: Ex vivo magnetic resonance imaging of the distal row of equine carpal bones: assessment of bone sclerosis and cartilage damage, *Vet Radiol Ultrasound* 44:501, 2003.
19. Riggs CM, Boyde A: Effect of exercise on bone density in the distal regions of the equine third metacarpal bone in 2-year-old Thoroughbreds, *Equine Vet J Suppl* 30:555, 1999.
20. Norrdin RW, Stover SM: Subchondral bone failure in overload arthrosis: a scanning electron microscopic study in horses, *J Musculoskelet Neuronal Interact* 6:251, 2006.
21. Stover SM, Read DH, Johnson BJ, et al: Lateral condylar fracture histomorphology in racehorses, *Proc Am Assoc Equine Pract* 40:173, 1994.
22. Young AB, O'Brien TR, Pool RR: Exercise-related sclerosis in the third carpal bone of the racing Thoroughbred, *Proc Am Assoc Equine Pract* 34:333, 1988.
23. Lewis CW, Williamson AK, Chen AC, et al: Evaluation of subchondral bone mineral density associated with articular cartilage structure and integrity in healthy equine joints with different functional demands, *Am J Vet Res* 66:1823, 2005.
24. Murray RC, Whitton RC, Vedi S, et al: The effect of training on the calcified zone of middle carpal articular cartilage, *Equine Vet J Suppl* 30:274, 1999.
25. O'Sullivan CB, Lumsden JM: Stress fractures of the tibia and humerus in Thoroughbred racehorses: 99 cases (1992-2000), *J Am Vet Med Assoc* 222:491, 2003.
26. Mackey VS, Trout DR, Meagher DM, et al: Stress fractures of the humerus, radius, and tibia in horses, *Vet Radiol* 28:26, 1987.
27. Pleasant RS, Baker GJ, Muhlbauer MC, et al: Stress reactions and stress fractures of the proximal palmar aspect of the third metacarpal bone in horses: 58 cases (1980-1990), *J Am Med Assoc* 201:1918, 1992.
28. Ruggles AJ, Moore RM, Bertone AL, et al: Tibial stress fractures in racing Standardbreds: 13 cases (1989-1993), *J Am Vet Med Assoc* 209:634, 1996.
29. Koblik PD, Hornof WH, Seeherman HJ: Scintigraphic appearance of stress-induced trauma of the dorsal cortex of the third metacarpal bone in racing Thoroughbred horses: 121 cases (1978-1986), *J Am Vet Med Assoc* 192:390, 1988.
30. Pilsworth RC, Shepherd MC, Herinckx BMB, et al: A review of 10 horses with fracture of the wing of the ilium, *Equine Vet J* 26:94, 1994.
31. Peloso JG, Watkins JP, Keele SR, et al: Bilateral stress fractures of the tibia in a racing American quarter horse, *J Am Vet Med Assoc* 203:801, 1993.
32. Spike DL, Bramlage LR, Embertson RM, et al: Tibial stress fractures in 51 racehorses, *Proc Am Assoc Equine Pract* 42:280, 1996.
33. Verheyen KLP, Newton JR, Price JS, et al: A case-control study of factors associated with pelvic and tibial stress fractures in Thoroughbred racehorses in training in the UK, *Prev Vet Med* 74:21, 2006.
34. Kraus BM, Ross MW, Boswell RP: Stress remodeling and stress fracture of the humerus in four Standardbred racehorses, *Vet Radiol Ultrasound* 46:524, 2005.
35. Lloyd KC, Koblik P, Ragle C, et al: Incomplete palmar fracture of the proximal extremity of the third metacarpal bone in horses: ten cases (1981-1986), *J Am Vet Med Assoc* 192:798, 1988.
36. Ross MW: The metatarsophalangeal joint. In Ross MW, Dyson SJ, eds: *Lameness in the horse*, St Louis, 2003, Elsevier.
37. Davidson EJ, Ross MW, Parente EJ: Incomplete sagittal fractures of the talus in 11 racehorses, *Equine Vet J* 45:457, 2005.
38. Norwood GL: The bucked shin complex in Thoroughbreds, *Proc Am Assoc Equine Pract* 24:319, 1978.
39. Nunamaker DM, Butterweck DM, Black J: In vitro comparison of Thoroughbred and Standardbred racehorses with regard to local fatigue failure of the third metacarpal bone, *Am J Vet Res* 52:97, 1991.
40. Nunamaker DM: On bucked shins, *Proc Am Assoc Equine Pract* 48:76, 2002.
41. Edwards RB, Durcharme NG, Fubini SL, et al: Scintigraphy for diagnosis of avulsions of the origin of the suspensory ligament in horses: 51 cases (1980-1993), *J Am Vet Med Assoc* 207:608, 1995.
42. Ross MW, Ford TS, Orsini PG: Incomplete longitudinal fracture of the proximal palmar cortex on the third metacarpal bone in horses, *Vet Surg* 17:82, 1988.
43. Richardson DW: The metacarpophalangeal joint. In Ross MW, Dyson SJ, eds: *Lameness in the horse*, St Louis, 2003, Elsevier.
44. Arthur RM, Ross MW, Moloney PJ, et al: North American Thoroughbred. In Ross MW, Dyson SJ, eds: *Lameness in the horse*, St Louis, 2003, Elsevier.
45. Pilsworth RC: The European Thoroughbred. In Ross MW, Dyson SJ, eds: *Lameness in the horse*, St Louis, 2003, Elsevier.
46. Ross MW, Richardson DW, Beroza GA: Subchondral lucency of the third carpal bone in Standardbred racehorses: 13

cases (1982-1988), *J Am Vet Med Assoc* 195:789, 1989.

47. Steel CM, Hopper BJ, Richardson JL, et al: Clinical findings, diagnosis, prevalence and predisposing factors for lameness localized to the middle carpal joint in young Standardbred racehorses, *Equine Vet J* 38:152, 2006.

48. Davidson EJ, Martin BB: Stress fracture of the scapula in two horses, *Vet Radiol Ultrasound* 45:407, 2004.

49. Vallance SA, Lumsden JM, O'Sullivan CB: Scapula stress fractures in eight Thoroughbred racehorses, *Proc Am Assoc Equine Pract* 53:56, 2007.

50. Bramlage LR, Gabel AA, Hackett RP: Avulsion fractures of the origin of the suspensory ligament in the horse, *J Am Vet Med Assoc* 176:1004, 1980.

51. Davidson EJ, Ross MW: Clinical recognition of stress-related bone injury in racehorses, *Clin Tech Equine Pract* 2:296, 2003.

52. O'Callaghan MW: The integration of radiography and alternative imaging methods in the diagnosis of equine orthopedic disease, *Vet Clin North Am Equine Pract* 7:339, 1991.

53. Roub LW, Gumerman LW, Hanley EN, et al: Bone stress: a radionuclide imaging perspective, *Radiology* 132:431, 1979.

54. Wilcox JR, Moniot AL, Green JP: Bone scanning in the evaluation of exercise-related stress injuries, *Radiology* 123:699, 1977.

55. Ross MW: Scintigraphic and clinical findings in the Standardbred metatarsophalangeal joint: 114 cases (1993-1995), *Equine Vet J* 30:131, 1998.

56. Keegan KG, Twardock AR, Losonsky JM, et al: Scintigraphic evaluation of fractures of the distal phalanx in horses: 27 cases (1979-1988), *J Am Vet Med Assoc* 202:1993, 1993.

57. Rabuffo TS, Ross MW: Fractures of the distal phalanx in 72 racehorses: 1990-2001, *Proc Am Assoc Equine Pract* 48:375, 2002.

58. Dyson SJ: The distal phalanx and distal interphalangeal joint. In Ross MW, Dyson SJ, eds: *Lameness in the horse*, St Louis, 2003, Elsevier.

59. Kawcak CE, McIlwraith WC, Norrdin RW, et al: Clinical effects of exercise on subchondral bone of carpal and metacarpophalangeal joints in horses, *Am J Vet Res* 61:1252, 2000.

60. Foreman JH, Hungerford LL, Twardock AR, et al: Scintigraphic appearance of dorsal metacarpal and metatarsal stress changes in racing and nonracing horses, *Equine Exerc Physiol* 3:402, 1991.

61. Martinelli MJ, Chambers MD, Baker GJ, et al: A retrospective study of increased bone scintigraphic uptake in the palmarplantar fetlock and its relationship to performance: 50 horses (1989-1993), *Proc Am Assoc Equine Pract* 40:53, 1994.

62. Arthur RM and Constantinide D: Results of 428 nuclear scintigraphic examinations of the musculoskeletal system at a Thoroughbred racetrack, *Proc Am Assoc Equine Pract* 41:84, 1995.

63. Ehrlich PJ, Dohoo IR, O'Callaghan MW: Results of bone scintigraphy in racing Standardbred horses: 64 cases (1992-1994), *J Am Vet Med Assoc* 215:982, 1999.

64. Goltz KL, Bramlage LR: Retrospective analysis of nuclear scintigraphy using a radionuclide bone scanner: 191 cases, *Proc Am Assoc Equine Pract* 40:55, 1994.

65. Devous MD, Twardock AR: Techniques and applications of nuclear medicine in the diagnosis of equine lameness, *J Am Vet Med Assoc* 184:318, 1984.

66. Shepherd MC, Pilsworth RC: The use of ultrasound in the diagnosis of pelvic fractures, *Equine Vet Educ* 6:223, 1994.

67. Pilsworth RC: Diagnosis and management of pelvic fractures in the Thoroughbred racehorse. In Ross MW, Dyson SJ, eds: *Lameness in the horse*, St Louis, 2003, Elsevier.

68. Muir P, McCarthy J, Radtke CL, et al: Role of endochondral ossification of articular cartilage and functional adaptation of the subchondral plate in the development of fatigue microcracking of joints, *Bone* 38:342, 2006.

69. Morgan JW, Santschi EM, Zekas LJ, et al: Comparison of radiography and computed tomography to evaluate metacarpo/metatarsophalangeal joint pathology of paired limbs of Thoroughbred racehorses with severe condylar fracture, *Vet Surg* 35:611, 2006.

70. Radtke CL, Danova NA, Scollay MC, et al: Macroscopic changes in the distal ends of the third metacarpal and metatarsal bones of Thoroughbred racehorses with condylar fractures, *Am J Vet Res* 64:1110, 2003.

71. Riggs CM, Whitehouse GH, Boyde A: Pathology of the distal condyle of the third metacarpal and third metatarsal bones of the horse, *Equine Vet J* 31:140, 1999.

72. Zubrod CJ, Schneider RK, Tucker RL et al: Use of magnetic resonance imaging for identifying subchondral bone damage in horses: 11 cases (1999-2003), *J Am Vet Med Assoc* 223:411, 2004.

73. Nunamaker DM: Metacarpal stress fractures. In Nixon AJ, ed: *Equine fracture repair*, Philadelphia, 1996, Saunders.

74. Brokken MT, Schneider RK, Sampson SN, et al: Magnetic resonance imaging features of proximal metacarpal and metatarsal injuries in the horse, *Vet Radiol Ultrasound* 48:507, 2007.

75. Bischofberger AS, Konar M, Ohlerth S, et al: Magnetic resonance imaging, ultrasonography and histology of the suspensory ligament origin: a comparative study of normal anatomy of Warmblood horses, *Equine Vet J* 38:508, 2006.

76. Palmer JJ, Bertone JL, Litsky AS: Contact area and pressure distribution changes of the equine third carpal bone during loading, *Equine Vet J* 26:197, 1994.

77. Firth EC, Delahunt J, Wichel JW, et al: Galloping exercise induces regional changes in bone density within the third and radial carpal bones of Thoroughbred horses, *Equine Vet J* 31:111, 1999.

78. Young DR, Nunamaker DM, Markel MD: Quantitative evaluation of the remodeling response of the proximal sesamoid bone to training-related stimuli in Thoroughbreds, *Am J Vet Res* 52:1350, 1991.

79. Murray RC, Vedi S, Birch HL, et al: Subchondral bone thickness, hardness, and remodeling are influenced by short-term exercise in a site-specific manner, *J Orthop Res* 19:1035, 2001.

80. Firth EC, Rogers CW: Musculoskeletal responses of 2-year-old Thoroughbred horses to early training. 7. Bone and articular cartilage response in the carpus, *N Z Vet J* 53:113, 2005.

81. Radin EL, Rose RM: Role of subchondral bone in the initiation and progression of cartilage damage, *Clin Orthop Relat Research* 213:34, 1986.

82. Uhlhorn H, Ekman S, Haglund A, et al: The accuracy of the dorsoproximal-dorsodistal projection in assessing third carpal bone sclerosis in Standardbred trotters, *Vet Radiol Ultrasound* 39:412, 1998.

83. De Haan CE, O'Brien TR, Koblik PD: A radiographic investigation of third carpal bone injury in 42 racing Thoroughbreds, *Vet Radiol* 28:88, 1987.

84. Hooper BJ, Steel C, Richardson JL, et al: Radiographic evaluation of sclerosis of the third carpal bone associate with exercise and the development of lameness in Standardbred racehorses, *Equine Vet J* 36:441, 2004.

85. Uhlhorn H, Carlsten J: Retrospective study of subchondral sclerosis and lucency in the third carpal bone of Standardbred trotters, *Equine Vet J* 31:500, 1999.

86. O'Brien TR, deHann CE, Arthur R: Third carpal bone lesions of the racing Thoroughbred, *Proc Am Assoc Equine Pract* 31:515, 1985.

87. Bassage LH, Ross MW: Enostosis-like lesions in the long bones of 10 horses: scintigraphic and radiographic features, *Equine Vet J* 30:35, 1998.

88. Valdés-Martínez A, Seiler G, Mai G, et al: Quantitative analysis of scintigraphic findings in tibial stress fractures in Thoroughbred racehorses, *Am J Vet Res* 69:886, 2008.

89. Ross MW: The crus. In Ross MW, Dyson SJ, eds: *Lameness in the horse*, St Louis, 2003, Elsevier.

90. Ramzan PHL, Newton JR, Shepherd MC, et al: The application of a scintigraphic grading system to equine tibial stress fractures: 42 cases, *Equine Vet J* 35:382, 2003.

91. Hornof WJ, Stover SM, Koblik PD, et al: Oblique views of the ilium and the scintigraphic appearance of stress fractures of the ilium, *Equine Vet J* 28:355, 1996.

92. Steckel RR, Kraus-Hansen AE, Fackelman GE, et al: Scintigraphic diagnosis of thoracolumbar spinal disease in horses: a review of 50 cases, *Proc Am Assoc Equine Pract* 37:583, 1992.

CHAPTER 101   Bone Biomarkers

1. Marks CM, Hermey DC: The structure and development of bone. In Bilezikian JP, Raisz LG, Rodan G, eds: *Principles of bone biology*, London, 1996, Academic.

2. Martin TJ, Seeman E: Bone remodelling: its local regulation and the emergence of bone fragility, *Best Pract Res Clin Endocrinol Metab* 22:701, 2008.

3. Price JS, Russell RGG: Bone remodelling: regulation by systemic and local factors. In Whitehead CC, ed: *Bone biology and skeletal disorders in poultry*, Abingdon, UK, 1992, Carfax.

4. Evans RK, Antczak AJ, Lester M, et al: Effects of a 4-month recruit training program on markers of bone metabolism, *Med Sci Sports Exerc* 40:S660, 2008.

5. Parfitt AM: Bone remodelling, normal and abnormal: a biological basis for the understanding of cancer-related bone disease and its treatment, *Can J Oncol* 5:1, 1995.

6. Kaufman JM, Goemaere S: Osteoporosis in men, *Best Pract Res Clin Endocrinol Metab* 22:787, 2008.

7. Karsdal MA, Leeming DJ, Dam EB, et al: Should subchondral bone turnover be targeted when treating osteoarthritis? *Osteoarthritis Cartilage* 16:638, 2008.

8. Cruz AM, Hurtig MB: Multiple pathways to osteoarthritis and articular fractures: is subchondral bone the culprit? *Vet Clin North Am Equine Pract* 24:101, 2008.

9. Buckingham SHW, McCarthy RN, Anderson G, et al: Ultrasound speed in the metacarpal cortex—a survey of 347 Thoroughbreds in training, *Equine Vet J* 24:191, 1992.

10. Firth EC, Delahunt J, Wichtel JW, et al: Galloping exercise induces regional changes in bone density within the third and radial carpal bones of Thoroughbred horses, *Equine Vet J* 31:111, 1999.

11. Griffith JF, Genant HK: Bone mass and architecture determination: state of the art, *Best Pract Res Clin Endocrinol Metab* 22:737, 2008.

12. Haugeberg G: Imaging of metabolic bone diseases, *Best Pract Res Clin Rheumatol* 22:1127, 2008.

13. McIlwraith CW: Use of synovial fluid and serum biomarkers in equine bone and joint disease: a review, *Equine Vet J* 37:473, 2005.

14. Van Weeren PR, Firth EC: Future tools for early diagnosis and monitoring of musculoskeletal injury: biomarkers and CT, *Vet Clin North Am Equine Pract* 24:153, 2008.

15. Garnero P, Delmas PD: Non-invasive techniques for assessing skeletal changes in inflammatory arthritis: bone biomarkers, *Curr Opin Rheumatol* 16:428, 2004.

16. Seibel MJ: Clinical application of biochemical markers of bone turnover, *Arq Bras Endocrinol Metabol* 50:603, 2006.

17. Singer FR, Eyre DR: Using biochemical markers of bone turnover in clinical practice, *Cleve Clin J Med* 75:739, 2008.

18. Henthorn PS: Alkaline phosphatase. In Bilezikian JP, Raisz LG, Rodan G, eds: *Principles of bone biology*, London, 1996, Academic.

19. Jackson B, Eastell R, Russell RG, et al: The measurement of bone specific alkaline phosphatase in the horse: a comparison of two techniques, *Res Vet Sci* 61:160, 1996.

20. Rohde C, Anderson DE, Bertone AL: Effects of phenylbutazone on bone activity and formation in horses, *Am J Vet Res* 61:537, 2000.

21. Trumble TN, Brown MP, Merrit KA: Joint dependent concentrations of bone alkaline phosphatase in serum and synovial fluids of horses with osteochondral injury: an analytical and clinical validation, *Osteoarthritis Cartilage* 16:779, 2008.

22. Hank AM, Hoffmann WE, Saneki RK, et al: Quantitative determination of equine alkaline phosphatase isoenzymes in foal and adult serum, *J Vet Int Med* 7:20, 1993.

23. Van de Lest CH, Van den Hoogen BM, Van Weeren PR: Changes in bone morphogenic enzymes and lipid composition of equine osteochondrotic subchondral bone, *Equine Vet J Suppl* 31:31, 1999.

24. Lepage OM, Marcoux M, Tremblay A: Serum osteocalcin or bone Gla-protein, a biochemical marker for bone metabolism in horses: differences in serum levels with age, *Can J Vet Res* 54:223, 1990.

25. Lepage OM, DesCoteaux L, Marcoux M, et al: Circadian rhythms of osteocalcin in equine serum. Correlation with alkaline phosphatase, calcium, phosphate and total protein levels, *Can J Vet Res* 55:5, 1991.

26. Lepage OM, Eicher R, Ubelhart B, et al: Influence of type and breed of horses on serum osteocalcin concentration and evaluation of the applicability of a bovine RIA and human IRMA, *Am J Vet Res* 58:574, 1997.

27. Lepage OM, Hartmann DJ, Eicher R, et al: Biochemical markers of bone metabolism in draught and Warmblood horses, *Vet J* 156:169, 1988.

28. Hoyt S, Siciliano PD: A comparison of ELISA and RIA techniques for the detection of serum osteocalcin in horses. In *Proceedings of the 16th Equine Nutritional Physiology Society Symposium*, 351, 1999.

29. Hope E, Johnston SD, Hegstad RL, et al: Effects of sample collection on concentration of osteocalcin in equine serum, *Am J Vet Res* 54:1017, 1993.

30. Grafenau P, Eicher R, Ubelhart B, et al: General anaesthesia decreases osteocalcin plasma concentrations in horses, *Equine Vet J* 31:533, 1999.

31. Price JS, Jackson B, Eastell R, et al: Age related changes in biochemical markers of bone metabolism in horses, *Equine Vet J* 27:201, 1995.

32. Jackson BF, Smith RK, Price JS: A molecular marker of type I collagen metabolism reflects changes in connective tissue remodelling associated with injury to the superficial digital flexor tendon, *Equine Vet J* 35:211, 2003.

33. Price JS, Jackson B, Gray JA, et al: Biochemical markers of bone metabolism in growing Thoroughbreds, *Res Vet Sci* 71:1, 2001.

34. Jackson BF, Lonnell C, Verheyen K, et al: Gender differences in bone turnover in 2-year-old Thoroughbreds, *Equine Vet J* 35:702, 2003.

35. Jackson BF, Blumsohn A, Goodship AE, et al: Circadian variation in biochemical markers of bone cell activity and insulin-like growth factor-1 in two-year-old horses, *J Anim Sci* 81:2804, 2003.

36. Chapurlatt RD, Garnero P, Breart G, et al: Serum type I collagen breakdown product (serum CTX) predicts hip fracture risk in elderly women: the EPIDOS study, *Bone* 27:283, 2000.

37. Pastoret V, Carstanjen B, Lejeune F, et al: Evaluation of serum osteocalcin and CTX-I in Ardenner horses with special reference to juvenile interphalangeal joint disease, *J Vet Med A Physiol Pathol Clin Med* 54:458, 2007.

38. Donabadien M, Van Weeren PR, Perona G, et al: Early changes in biomarkers of skeletal metabolism and their association to the occurrence of osteochondrosis (OC) in the horse, *Equine Vet J* 40:253, 2008.

39. Schryver H, Millis DL, Soderholm LV et al: Metabolism of some essential minerals in ponies fed high aluminium, *Cornell Vet* 76:354, 1986.

40. Price JS, Colwell A, Eastell R, et al: Urinary excretion of deoxypyridinoline as a marker of bone resorption in the Thoroughbred racehorse, *Bone* 13:279, 1992.

41. Jackson BJ Eastell R, Russell RG, et al: The measurement of pyridinium crosslinks in serum as a biochemical marker of bone turnover in horses, *J Bone Miner Res* 10:S339, 1995.

42. Porr CA, Kronfeld DS, Lawrence LA, et al: Deconditioning reduces mineral content of the third metacarpal bone in horses, *J Anim Sci* 76:1875, 1998.

43. Robins SP: Fibrillogenesis and maturation of collagens. In Siebel MJ, Robins SP, Bilezikian JP, eds: *Dynamics of bone and cartilage metabolism*, 1999, Academic.

44. Black A, Schoknecht PA, Ralston, SL: Diurnal variation and age differences in the biochemical markers of bone turnover in horses, *J Anim Sci* 77:75, 1999.

45. Hoekstra KE, Nielsen BD, Orth MW, et al: Comparison of bone mineral content and biochemical markers of bone metabolism in stall-versus pasture-reared horses, *Equine Vet J* 30:601, 1999.

46. Kellerhouse PL, Brown C, Newall K, et al: Assessment of bone resorption marker assays in Thoroughbred horses, *J Bone Miner Res* 15:S526, 2000.

47. Billinghurst RC, Buxton EM, Edwards MG, et al: Use of an anti-neoepitope antibody for identification of type-II collagen degradation in equine articular cartilage, *Am J Vet Res* 62:1031, 2001.

48. Nelson F, Dahlberg L, Laverty S, et al: Evidence for altered synthesis of type II collagen in patients with osteoarthritis, *J Clin Invest* 102:2115, 1998.

49. Hannon R, Eastell R: Preanalytical variability of biochemical markers of bone turnover, *Osteoporosis Int* 11:30, 2000.

50. Jackson BF, Blumsohn A, Goodship AE, et al: Circadian variation in biochemical markers of bone cell activity and insulin-like growth factor-I in two-year-old horses, *J Animal Sci* 81:2804, 2003.

51. Carstanjen B, Hoyle NR, Gabriel A, et al: Evaluation of plasma carboxy terminal cross-linking telopeptides of type I collagen concentrations in horses, *Am J Vet Res* 64:104, 2004.

52. Christgau S, Bitsch-Jensen O, Hanover Bjarnason NH, et al: Serum crosslaps for monitoring the response in individuals using antiresorptive therapy, *Bone* 26:505, 2000.

53. Ginty F, Flynn A, Cashman KD: The effect of short-term calcium supplementation on biochemical markers of bone metabolism in healthy young adults, *Br J Nutr* 80:437, 1998.

54. Maenpaa PH, Pirskanen A, Koskinen E, et al: Biochemical indicators of bone formation in foals after transfer from pasture to stables for the winter months, *Am J Vet Res* 49:1990, 1988.

55. Chiappe A, Gonzalez G, Frandinger E, et al: The influence of age and sex in serum osteocalcin levels in Thoroughbred horses, *Arch Physiol Biochem* 107:50, 1999

56. Vervuert I, Winkelsett S, Christmann L, et al: Evaluation of the influences of exercise, birth date, and osteochondrosis on plasma bone marker concentrations in Hannovarian Warmblood foals, *Equine Vet J* 68:1319, 2007.

57. Billinghurst RC, Brama PAJ, van Weeren PR, et al: Significant exercise-related changes in serum levels of two biomarkers of collagen metabolism in young horses, *Osteoarthritis Cartilage* 11:760, 2003.

58. Naylor KE, Iqbal P, Ledius C, et al: The effect of pregnancy on bone density and bone turnover, *J Bone Miner Res* 15:129, 2000.

59. Davicco MJ, Faulconnier Y, Coxham V, et al: Systemic bone growth factors in light breed mares and their foals, *Arch Int Physiol Biochin Biophys* 102:115, 1994.

60. Venken K, Callewaert F, Boonen S, et al: Sex hormones their receptors and bone health, *Osteoporosis Int* 19:1517, 2008.

61. Jackson BF, Dyson PK, Hattersley RD, et al: Relationship between stages of the estrous cycle and bone cell activity in Thoroughbreds, *Am J Vet Res* 67:1527, 2006.

62. Garnero P: Markers of bone turnover for prediction of fracture risk, *Osteoporosis Int* 11:55, 2000.

63. Stepan JJ: Prediction of bone loss in menopausal women, *Osteoporosis Int* 11:45, 2000.

64. Delmas PD: Markers of bone turnover for monitoring treatment of osteoporosis with antiresorptive drugs, *Osteoporosis Int* 11:66, 2000.

65. Jackson BF, Dyson PK, Lonnell C, et al: Bone biomarkers and risk of fracture in two- and three-year-old Thoroughbreds, *Equine Vet J* 41:410, 2009.

66. Price J: Unpublished data, 2009.

67. McIlwraith CW: Personal communication, 2009.

68. Verheyen KL, Henley WE, Price JS, et al: Training-related factors associated with dorsometacarpal disease in young Thoroughbred racehorses in the UK, *Equine Vet J* 37:442, 2005.

69. Jackson BF, Lonnell C, Verheyen KL, et al: Biochemical markers of bone metabolism and risk of dorsal metacarpal disease in 2-year-old Thoroughbreds, *Equine Vet J* 37:87, 2005.

70. Ytrehus B, Carlson CS, Ekman S: Etiology and pathogenesis of osteochondrosis, *Vet Pathol* 44:429, 2007.

71. Price JS, Jackson B, Gray J, et al: Serum levels of molecular markers in growing horses: the effects of age, season, and orthopaedic disease, *Trans Orthop Res Soc* 22:587, 1997.

72. Billinghurst RC, Brama PAJ, van Weeren PR, et al: Evaluation of serum concentrations of biomarkers of skeletal metabolism and results of radiography as indicators of severity of osteochondrosis in foals, *Am J Vet Res* 65:143, 2004.

73. Dyson PK, Jackson BF, Pfeiffer DU, et al: Days lost from training in two and three year old Thoroughbreds: a survey of seven UK training yards, *Equine Vet J* 40:650, 2008.

74. Kawcak CE, McIlwraith CW, Norrdin RW, et al: The role of subchondral bone in joint disease: a review, *Equine Vet J* 33:120, 2001.

75. Fuller CJ, Barr AR, Sharif M, et al: Cross-sectional comparison of synovial fluid biochemical markers in equine osteoarthritis and the correlation of the markers with articular cartilage damage, *Osteoarthritis Cartilage* 9:49, 2001.

76. Kawcak CE: Effect of loading on subchondral bone of the equine carpal and metacarpophalangeal joints, PhD dissertation, Colorado, 1998, Colorado State University.

77. Frisbie DD, Al-Sobayil F, Billinghurst RC, et al: Serum fluid markers distinguish exercise from osteoarticular pathology, *Proc Am Assoc Equine Pract* 49:116, 2003.

78. Frisbie DD, Al-Sobayil F, Billinghurst RC, et al: Changes in synovial fluid and serum biomarkers with exercise and early osteoarthritis in horses, *Osteoarthritis Cartilage* 16:1196, 2008.

79. Lanyon LE: Functional strain in bone tissue, *J Biomech* 20:1083, 1997.

80. Price JS, Jackson B, Eastell R, et al: The response of the equine skeleton to physical training: a biochemical study in horses, *Bone* 17:221, 1995.

81. Jackson BF, Eastell R, Goodship AE, et al: Biochemical markers of bone metabolism reflect rapid adaptive responses in the skeleton of treadmill exercised two year old Thoroughbreds associated with changes in circulating insulin-like growth factor I, *Am J Vet Res* 64:1549. 2003.

82. Nielsen BD, Potter GD, Greene L, et al: Characterisation of changes related to mineral balance and bone metabolism in the young racing Quarter horse, *J Equine Vet Sci* 18:190, 1998.

83. Hiney KM, Potter GD, Gibbs PO, et al: Response of serum biochemical markers of bone metabolism to training in the juvenile racehorse, *J Equine Vet Sci* 20:851, 2000.

84. Vervuert I, Coenen M, Wedemeyer U, et al: Biochemical markers of bone activity in young Standardbred horses during different types of exercise and training, *J Vet Med A Physiol Pathol Clin Med* 49:396, 2002.

85. Caron JP, Peters TL, Hauptman JG, et al: Serum concentrations of keratan sulphate, osteocalcin, and pyridinoline crosslinks after oral administration of glucosamine to Standardbred horses during race training, *Am J Vet Res* 63:1106, 2002.

86. Fenton JI, Orth MW, Chelebek-Brown KA, et al: Effect of longeing and glucosamine supplementation on serum markers of bone and joint metabolism in yearling quarter horses, *Can J Vet Res* 63:288, 1999.

87. Geor R, Hope E, Lauper L, et al: Effect of glucocorticoids on serum osteocalcin concentration in horses, *Am J Vet Res* 56:1201, 1995.

88. Lepage OM, Laverty S, Marcoux M, et al: Serum osteocalcin concentration in horses treated with triamcinolone acetonide, *Am J Vet Res* 54:1209, 1993.

89. Fenton JI, Orth, MW, Chelebek-Brown KA, et al: Effect of longeing and glucosamine supplementation on serum markers of bone and joint metabolism in yearling quarter horses, *Can J Vet Res* 63:288, 1999.

90. Price JS, Jackson B, Noble GK, et al: Growth hormone administration increases bone turnover in horses, *J Endocrinol* 164:129, 2000.

91. Delguste C, Amory H, Doucet M, et al: Pharmacological effects of tiludronate in horses after long-term immobilization, *Bone* 41:414, 2007.

CHAPTER 102   The Bucked-Shin Complex

Etiology, Pathogenesis, and Conservative Management

1. Norwood GL: The bucked shin complex in Thoroughbreds, *Proc Am Assoc Equine Pract* 24:319, 1978.

2. Nunamaker DM, Provost MT: The bucked shin complex revisited, *Proc Am Assoc Equine Pract* 37:549, 1992.

3. Nunamaker DM: Bucked shins in horses in musculoskeletal fatigue and stress fractures. In Burr D, Milgrom C, eds: *Musculoskeletal fatigue and stress fractures*, Boca Raton, 2001, CRC Press.

4. Nunamaker DM, Butterweck CM, Provost MT: Some geometric properties of the third metacarpal bone: a comparison between the Standardbred and Thoroughbred racehorse, *J Biomech* 22:129, 1989.

5. Nunamaker DM, Butterweck DM, Black J: In vitro comparison of Thoroughbred and Standardbred racehorses with regard to local fatigue failure of the third metacarpal bone, *Am J Vet Res* 52:97, 1991.

6. Nunamaker DM, Provost MT, Bartel DL: Third metacarpal bone strain and stiffness measurements of Thoroughbred racehorses in training. Transactions of the Second Combined Meeting of the Orthopedic Research Societies of the United States, Japan, Canada, and Europe, San Diego, California, November 1995.

7. Nunamaker DM: The bucked shin complex, *Proc Am Assoc Equine Pract* 32:457, 1986.

8. Nunamaker DM, Butterweck DM, Provost MT: Fatigue fractures in Thoroughbred racehorses: relationship with age, peak bone strain and training, *J Orthop Res* 8:604, 1990.

9. Nunamaker DM, Butterweck DM: Bone modeling and remodeling in the Thoroughbred racehorse: relationships of exercise to bone morphometry. Transactions of the Thirty-Fifth Annual Meeting of the Orthopaedic Research Society, Las Vegas, Nevada, February 1989.

10. Boston RC, Nunamaker DM: Gait and speed as exercise components of risk factors associated with onset of fatigue injury of the third metacarpal bone in 2-year-old Thoroughbred racehorses, *Am J Vet Res* 61:602, 2000.

11. Nunamaker DM: Relationships of exercise regimen and racetrack surface to modeling/remodeling of the third metacarpal bone in two year-old thoroughbred racehorses, *Vet Comp Orthop Traumatol* 4:195, 2002.

12. Nunamaker DM: On bucked shins (Milne Lecture), *Proc Am Assoc Equine Pract* 48:76, 2002.

13. Estberg L, Stover S, Gardner IA, et al: High-speed exercise history and catastrophic racing fracture in Thoroughbreds, *Am J Vet Res* 57:1549, 1996.
14. Giladi M, Milgrom C, Simkin A, et al: Stress fractures and tibial bone width: a risk factor, *J Bone Joint Surg Br* 69:326, 1987.
15. Milgrom C, Giladi M, Simkin A, et al: The area moment of inertia of the tibia: a risk factor for stress fractures, *J Biomech* 22:1243, 1989.
16. Gibson VA, Stover SM, Martin RB, et al: Fatigue behavior of the equine third metacarpus: mechanical property analysis, *J Orthop Res* 13:861, 1995.
17. Rubin CT, Lanyon LE: Osteoregulatory nature of mechanical stimuli: function as a determinant for adaptive final, *J Orthop Res* 5:300, 1987.
18. Woo SLY, Kvei SC, Amiel D, et al: The effect of prolonged physical training on the properties of long bone: a study of Wolff's law, *J Bone Joint Surg Am* 63:780, 1981.
19. Milgrom C, Finestone A, Mendelson S, et al: The effect of pre-induction sport participation on the incidence of stress fractures in infantry recruits. Transactions of the Forty-Fourth Annual Meeting of the Orthopaedic Research Society, New Orleans, March, 1998.
20. Moyer W, Fisher JRS: Bucked shins: effects of differing track surfaces and proposed training regimens, *Proc Am Assoc Equine Pract* 37:541, 1992.

Stress Fractures of the Third Metacarpal Bone: Surgical Management
1. Specht TE, Miller GJ, Colahan PT: Effects of clustered drill holes on the breaking strength of the equine third metacarpal bone, *Am J Vet Res* 51:1242, 1990.
2. Dallap BL, Bramlage LR, Embertson RM: Results of screw fixation combined with cortical drilling for treatment of dorsal cortical stress fractures of the third metacarpal bone in 56 Thoroughbred racehorses, *Equine Vet J* 31:252, 1999.
3. Cervantes C, Madison JB, Ackerman N, et al: Surgical treatment of dorsal cortical fractures of the third metacarpal bone in Thoroughbred horses: 53 cases (1985-1989), *J Am Vet Med Assoc* 200:1997, 1992.

CHAPTER 103 On-the-Track Catastrophes in the Thoroughbred Racehorse
1. Mundy GD: Review of risk factors associated with racing injuries, *Proc Am Assoc Equine Pract* 43:204, 1997.
2. Verheyen K, Wood JLN, Lakhani KH: An epidemiological study to determine risk factors for fractures in British racehorses in training: a preliminary report. Proceedings of the Thirteenth International Conference of Racing Analysts and Veterinarians, Cambridge, UK, 2000.
3. Hill T: Track surfaces and factors associated with racing injuries, *World Veterinary Congress Abstracts* 54, 1995.
4. Peloso JG, Cohen ND, Mundy GD, et al: Epidemiological study of musculoskeletal injuries in racing thoroughbred horses in Kentucky, *Proc Am Assoc Equine Pract* 42:284, 1996.
5. New York Racing Association: Unpublished data, 1993-2000.
6. Hill T, Carmichael D, Maylin G, et al: Track condition and racing injuries in thoroughbred horses, *Cornell Vet* 76:361, 1986.
7. Mohammed HO, Hill T, Lowe J: Risk factors associated with injuries in thoroughbred horses, *Equine Vet J* 23:445, 1991.

CHAPTER 104 Catastrophic Injuries
1. Mudge MC, Bramlage LR: Field fracture management (trauma and emergency care), *Vet Clin North Am Equine Pract* 23:117, 2007.
2. Smith JJ: Emergency fracture stabilization, *Clin Tech Equine Pract* 5:154, 2006.
3. Bramlage LR: An initial report on a surgical technique for arthrodesis of the metacarpophalangeal joint in the horse, *Proc Am Assoc Equine Pract* 27:257, 1982.
4. Kraus BM, Richardson DW, Nunamaker DM, et al: Management of comminuted fractures of the proximal phalanx in horses: 64 cases (1983-2001), *J Am Vet Med Assoc* 224:254, 2004.
5. Lescun TB, McClure SR, Ward MP, et al: Evaluation of transfixation casting for treatment of third metacarpal, third metatarsal, and phalangeal fractures in horses: 37 cases (1994-2004), *J Am Vet Med Assoc* 230:1340, 2007.

CHAPTER 105 Track Surfaces and Lameness: Epidemiological Aspects of Racehorse Injury
1. Peters JE: Lameness incident to training and racing the Thoroughbred, *J Am Vet Med Assoc* 96:200, 1940.
2. Montgomery T: Leg problems in race horses, *Vet Med Small Anim Clin* 60:110, 1965.
3. Johnson BJ, Stover SM, Daft BM, et al: Causes of death in racehorses over a 2 year period, *Equine Vet J* 26:327, 1994.
4. McKee SL: An update on racing fatalities in the UK, *Equine Vet Educ* 7:202, 1995.
5. Bailey CJ, Reid SWJ, Hodgson DR, et al: Impact of injuries and disease on a cohort of two-and three-year old Thoroughbreds in training, *Vet Rec* 145:487, 1999.
6. Williams RB, Harkins LS, Hammond CJ, et al: Racehorse injuries, clinical problems and fatalities recorded on British racecourses from flat racing and National Hunt racing during 1996, 1997 and 1998, *Equine Vet J* 33:478, 2001.
7. Lam KH, Parkin TDH, Riggs CM, et al: Content analysis of free-text clinical records: their use in identifying syndromes and analysing health data, *Vet Rec* 161:547, 2007.
8. Parkin TDH, Clegg PD, French NP, et al: Risk of fatal distal limb fractures among Thoroughbreds involved in the five types of racing in the United Kingdom, *Vet Rec* 154:493, 2004.
9. Cruz AM, Poljak Z, Filejski C, et al: Epidemiologic characteristics of catastrophic musculoskeletal injuries in Thoroughbred racehorses, *Am J Vet Res* 68:1370, 2007.
10. Hill T, Carmichael D, Maylin G, et al: Track condition and racing injuries in Thoroughbred horses, *Cornell Vet J* 76:361, 1986.
11. Hernandez J, Hawkins DL, Scollay MC: Race-start characteristics and risk of catastrophic musculoskeletal injury in Thoroughbred racehorses, *J Am Vet Med Assoc* 218:83, 2001.
12. Rooney JR: The relationship of length of race to fatigue and lameness in Thoroughbred racehorses, *J Equine Vet Sci* 2:98, 1982.
13. Robinson RA, Kobluk CN, Clanton C: Epidemiological studies of musculoskeletal racing and training injuries in Thoroughbred horses, *Acta Vet Scand* 84(Suppl 1):340, 1988.
14. Peloso JG, Mundy GD, Cohen ND: Prevalence of and factors associated with musculoskeletal racing injuries of Thoroughbreds, *J Am Vet Med Assoc* 204:620, 1994.
15. Bailey CJ, Reid SWJ, Hodgson DR, et al: Risk factors associated with musculoskeletal injuries in Australian Thoroughbred racehorses, *Prev Vet Med* 32:47, 1997.
16. Wood JLN, Eastment J, Lakhani KH, et al: Modelling a retrospective study of death on racecourses. In Proceedings of the Society for Veterinary Epidemiology and Preventive Medicine, Noordwijkerhout, the Netherlands, 115, 2001.
17. Parkin TDH, Clegg PD, French NP, et al: Race and course level risk factors for fatal distal limb fracture in racing Thoroughbreds, *Equine Vet J* 36:521, 2004.
18. Estberg L, Stover SM, Gardner IA, et al: Fatal musculoskeletal injuries incurred during racing and training in Thoroughbreds, *J Am Vet Med Assoc* 208:92, 1996.
19. Cohen ND, Peloso JG, Mundy GD, et al: Racing-related factors and results of prerace physical inspection and their association with musculoskeletal injuries incurred in Thoroughbreds during races, *J Am Vet Med Assoc* 211:454, 1997.
20. Mohammed HO, Hill T, Lowe J: The risk of severity of limb injuries in racing Thoroughbred horses, *Cornell Vet* 82:331, 1992.
21. Wilson JH, Howe S, Jensen R, et al: Injuries sustained during racing at racetracks in the U.S. in 1992, *Proc Am Assoc Equine Pract* 39:267, 1993.
22. Ueda Y, Yoshida K, Oikawa M: Analyses of race accident conditions through use of patrol video, *J Equine Vet Sci* 13:707, 1993.
23. Boden LA, Charles JA, Slocombe RF, et al: Post-mortem study of Thoroughbred fatalities in Victoria, Australia between 2001 and 2004, *Proc Am Assoc Equine Pract* 51:303, 2005.
24. Kane AJ, Stover SM, Gardner IA, et al: Horseshoe characteristics as possible risk factors for fatal musculoskeletal injury of Thoroughbred racehorses, *Am J Vet Res* 57:1147, 1996.
25. Oikawa M, Ueda Y, Inada S, et al: Effect of restructuring a racetrack on the occurrence of racing injuries in Thoroughbred horses, *J Equine Vet Sci* 14:262, 1994.
26. Parkin TDH, Clegg PD, French NP, et al: Horse level risk factors for fatal distal limb fracture in racing Thoroughbreds in the UK, *Equine Vet J* 36:513, 2004.
27. Lam KH, Parkin TDH, Riggs CMR, et al: Evaluation of detailed training data

to identify risk factors for retirement because of tendon injuries in Thoroughbred racehorses, *Am J Vet Res* 68:1188, 2007.

28. Verheyen KLP, Newton JR, Price JS, et al: A case-control study of factors associated with pelvic and tibial stress fractures in Thoroughbred racehorses in training in the UK, *Prev Vet Med* 74:21, 2006.

29. Parkin TDH, Clegg PD, French NP, et al: Risk factors for fatal lateral condylar fracture of the third metacarpus/metatarsus in UK racing, *Equine Vet J* 37:192, 2005.

30. Boden LA, Anderson GA, Charles JA, et al: Risk factors for fatality in jump starts in Victoria (1989-2004), *Equine Vet J* 39:422, 2007.

31. Boden LA, Anderson GA, Charles JA, et al: Risk factors for Thoroughbred racehorse fatality in flat starts in Victoria (1989-2004), *Equine Vet J* 39:430, 2007.

32. Mohammed HO, Hill T, Lowe J: Risk factors associated with injuries in Thoroughbred horses, *Equine Vet J* 23:445, 1991.

33. Stirk AJ, Lifton P, Morris T: BHA Equine health and welfare data. Personal communication, 2008.

34. Bailey CJ, Reid SWJ, Hodgson DR, et al: Flat, hurdle and steeple racing: risk factors for musculoskeletal injury, *Equine Vet J* 30:498, 1998.

35. Cheney JA, Shen CK, Wheat JD: Relationship of racetrack surface to lameness in Thoroughbred racehorse, *Am J Vet Res* 34:1285, 1973.

36. Pratt GW: Racing surfaces—a survey of mechanical behaviour, *Proc Am Assoc Equine Pract* 321, 1984.

37. Zebarth BJ, Sheard RW: Impact and shear resistance of turf grass racing surfaces for Thoroughbreds, *Am J Vet Res* 46:778, 1985.

38. Riggs CM: Fractures—a preventable hazard of racing Thoroughbreds? *Vet J* 163:19, 2002.

39. Verheyen KLP, Wood JLN: Descriptive epidemiology of fractures occurring in British Thoroughbred racehorses in training, *Equine Vet J* 36:167, 2004.

40. Moyer W, Spencer PA, Kallish M: Relative incidence of dorsal metacarpal disease in young Thoroughbred racehorses training on two different surfaces, *Equine Vet J* 23:166, 1991.

41. Pickersgill CH, Reid SWJ, Marr CM: Musculoskeletal injuries and associated epidemiological risk factors among Thoroughbred flat racehorses, *Proc Br Equine Vet Assoc Congr* 39:208, 2000.

42. Clanton C, Kobluk C, Robinson RA, et al: Monitoring surface conditions of a Thoroughbred racetrack, *J Am Vet Med Assoc* 198:613, 1991.

43. Ratzlaff MH, Wilson PD, Hutton DV, et al: Relationships between hoof-acceleration patterns of galloping horses and dynamic properties of the track, *Am J Vet Res* 66:589, 2005.

44. Schaer BL, Ryan CT, Boston RC, et al: The horse-racetrack interface: a preliminary study on the effect of shoeing on impact trauma using a novel wireless data acquisition system, *Equine Vet J* 38:664, 2006.

45. Ryan CT, Schaer BL, Nunamaker DM: A novel wireless data acquisition system for the measurement of hoof accelerations in the exercising horse, *Equine Vet J* 38:671, 2006.

CHAPTER 107   The European Thoroughbred

1. Bathe AP: 245 fractures in Thoroughbred racehorses: results of a prospective study in Newmarket, *Proc Am Assoc Equine Pract* 40:175, 1994.

2. Stover SM, Johnson BJ, Daft BM, et al: An association between complete and incomplete stress fractures of the humerus in the racehorse, *Equine Vet J* 24:260, 1992.

3. Hornof W, O'Brien T: Radiographic evaluation of the palmar aspect of the equine metacarpal condyles: a new projection, *Vet Radiol* 21:161, 1980.

4. Pilsworth RC, Hopes R, Greet TR: A flexed dorsopalmar projection of the equine fetlock in demonstrating lesions of the distal third McIII, *Vet Rec* 122:332, 1988.

5. Ross MW: Scintigraphic and clinical findings in the Standardbred metatarsophalangeal joint: 114 cases (1993-1995), *Equine Vet J* 30:131, 1998.

6. Uhlhorn H, Eksell P: The dorsoproximal-dorsodistal projection of the distal carpal bones in horses: an evaluation of different beam-cassette angles, *Vet Radiol Ultrasound* 40:480, 1999.

7. Mackey VS, Trout DR, Meagher DM, et al: Stress fractures of the humerus, radius and tibia in horses, *Vet Radiol* 28:26, 1989.

8. Steckel RR: The role of scintigraphy in the lameness evaluation, *Vet Clin North Am Equine Pract* 7:207, 1991.

9. Dyson SJ, Martinelli MJ, Pilsworth RC, et al: *Equine scintigraphy*, Newmarket, UK, 2003, Equine Vet J Publications.

10. Gillis CL, Meagher DM, Pool RR, et al: Ultrasonographically detected changes in the superficial digital flexor tendons during the first months of race training, *Am J Vet Res* 54:1797, 1993.

11. Moyer W, Ford TS, Ross MW: Proximal suspensory desmitis, *Proc Am Assoc Equine Pract* 34:409, 1988.

12. Ford TS, Ross MW, Orsini PG: A comparison for methods for proximal palmar metacarpal analgesia in horses, *Vet Surg* 18:146, 1989.

13. Coudry V, Denoix J-M, Didierlaurent D, et al: Use of magnetic resonance imaging to diagnose the cause of proximal metacarpal pain in a Standardbred trotter, *Vet Rec* 162:790, 2008.

14. Shepherd MC, Pilsworth RC: Failure of intra-articular anaesthesia of the antebrachiocarpal joint to abolish lameness associated with chip fracture of the distal radius, *Equine Vet J* 25:458, 1993.

15. Shepherd MC, Pilsworth RC: Stress reactions to the plantarolateral condyles of Mt.III in UK thoroughbreds: 26 cases, *Proc Am Assoc Equine Pract* 43:128, 1997.

16. Pilsworth RC, Head MJ: A study of ten cases of focal peritarsal infection as a cause of severe lameness in the Thoroughbred racehorse: clinical signs, differential diagnosis, treatment and outcome, *Equine Vet J* 33:366, 2001.

17. Haussler KK, Stover SM: Stress fractures of the vertebral lamina and pelvis in thoroughbred racehorses, *Equine Vet J* 30:374, 1998.

CHAPTER 108   The North American Standardbred

1. Chateau H, Robin D, Falala S, et al: Effects of a synthetic all-weather waxed track versus a crushed sand track on 3D acceleration of the front hoof in three horses trotting at high speed, *Equine Vet J* 41:247, 2009.

2. Robin D, Chateau H, Pacquet L, et al: Use of a 3D dynamometric horseshoe to assess the effects of an all-weather waxed track and a crushed sand track at high speed trot: preliminary study, *Equine Vet J* 41:253, 2009.

3. Lucas JM, Ross MW, Richardson DW: Postoperative performance of racing standardbreds treated arthroscopically for carpal chip fracture: 176 cases, *Equine Vet J* 31:48, 1999.

4. Gill HE: Personal communication, 2001.

5. Ross MW: Unpublished data, 2009.

6. Ross MW, Nolan PM, Paimar JA, et al: The importance of the metatarsophalangeal joint in standardbred lameness, *Proc Am Assoc Equine Pract* 37:741, 1991.

7. Rabuffo TS, Ross MW: Fractures of the distal phalanx in 72 racehorses: 1990-2001, *Proc Am Assoc Equine Pract* 48:375, 2002.

8. Ross MW: Observations in horses with lameness abolished by palmar digital analgesia, *Proc Am Assoc Equine Pract* 44:230, 1998.

9. Hopper BJ, Steel C, Richardson JL, et al: Radiographic evaluation of sclerosis of the third carpal bone associated with exercise and the development of lameness in Standardbred racehorses, *Equine Vet J* 36:441, 2004.

10. Steel CM, Hopper BJ, Richardson JL, et al: Clinical findings, diagnosis, prevalence and predisposing factors for lameness localized to the middle carpal joint in young Standardbred racehorses, *Equine Vet J* 38:152, 2006.

11. Mitchell J: Unpublished data, 2001.

12. Ross MW: Scintigraphic and clinical findings in the standardbred metatarsophalangeal joint: 114 cases (1993-1995), *Equine Vet J* 30:131, 1998.

13. Gabel AA: Lameness caused by inflammation in the distal hock, *Vet Clin North Am* 2:101, 1980.

14. Woodie JB, Ruggles AJ, Bertone AL, et al: Apical fracture of the proximal sesamoid bone in Standardbred horses: 43 cases (1990-1996), *J Am Vet Med Assoc* 214:1653, 1999.

15. Bassage LH, Richardson DW: Longitudinal fractures of the condyles of the third metacarpal and metatarsal bones in racehorses: 224 cases (1986-1995), *J Am Vet Med Assoc* 212:1757, 1998.

16. Elce YA, Ross MW, Woodford AM: A review of central and third tarsal bone slab fractures in 57 horses, *Proc Am Assoc Equine Pract* 47:488, 2001.

17. Hammer EJ, Ross MW, Parente EJ: Incomplete sagittal fractures of the talus in 11 racehorses: outcome, *Equine Vet J* 37:457, 2005.

CHAPTER 109 The European and Australasian Standardbreds

The European Standardbred

1. Torre F, Motta M: Incidence and distribution of 369 proximal sesamoid bone fractures in 354 standardbred horses (1984-1995), *Equine Pract* 21:6, 1999.
2. Trotter GW: Aspects of palmar heel pain, *Proc Am Assoc Equine Pract* 45:195, 1999.
3. Buchner HHF: Gait adaptation in lameness. In Back W, Clayton H, eds: *Equine locomotion*, Philadelphia, 2001, Saunders.
4. Moyer W, O'Brien TR, Walker M: Nonseptic pedal osteitis: a cause of lameness and a diagnosis? *Proc Am Assoc Equine Pract* 45:178, 1999.
5. Ross MW, Richardson DW, Beroza GA: Subchondral lucency of the third carpal bone in standardbred racehorses: 13 cases (1982-1988), *J Am Vet Med Assoc* 195:789, 1989.
6. De Haan CE, O'Brien TR, Koblik PD: A radiographic investigation of third carpal bone injury in 42 racing thoroughbreds, *Vet Radiol* 28:88, 1987.
7. Pool RR, Meagher DM: Pathologic findings and pathogenesis of racetrack injuries, *Vet Clin North Am Equine Pract* 6:1, 1990.
8. Ehrlich PJ, Dohoo IR, O'Callaghan MW: Results of bone scintigraphy in racing standardbred horses: 64 cases (1992-1994), *J Am Vet Med Assoc* 215:982, 1999.
9. Trotter GW: Intra-articular corticosteroids. In McIlwraith CW, Trotter GW, eds: *Joint disease in the horse*, Philadelphia, 1996, Saunders.
10. Kawcak CE, Frisbie DD, Trotter GW, et al: Effects of intravenous administration of sodium hyaluronate on carpal joints in exercising horses after arthroscopic surgery and osteochondral fragmentation, *Am J Vet Res* 58:1132, 1997.
11. Schumacher J, Steiger R, Schumacher J, et al: Effects of analgesia of the distal interphalangeal joint or palmar digital nerves on lameness caused by solar pain in horses, *Vet Surg* 29:54, 2000.
12. Bramlage LR, Schneider RK, Gabel AA: A clinical perspective on the lameness originating in the carpus, *Equine Vet J Suppl* 6:12, 1988.
13. Palmer SE: Prevalence of carpal fractures in thoroughbred and standardbred racehorses, *J Am Vet Med Assoc* 188:1171, 1986.
14. Schneider RK, Bramlage LR, Gabel AA: The incidence and location of 371 third carpal bone fractures in 313 horses, *Equine Vet J Suppl* 6:33, 1988.
15. Lucas JM, Ross MW, Richardson DW: Postoperative performance of racing standardbreds treated arthroscopically for carpal chip fractures: 176 cases (1986-1993), *Equine Vet J* 31:48, 1999.
16. Torre F: A comparison of the radiographic and arthroscopic findings in the third carpal bone in the young standardbred horse, *Equine Pract* 19:14, 1997.
17. McIlwraith CW, Frisbie DD, Trotter GW, et al: Use of subchondral bone plate micropick technique to augment healing of articular cartilage defects, *Proc Am Assoc Equine Pract* 44:233, 1998.
18. McIlwraith CW: Tearing of the medial palmar intercarpal ligament in the equine midcarpal joint, *Equine Vet J* 24:367, 1992.
19. Palmer SE: Splints, fractures of the second and fourth metacarpal/metatarsal bones, and associated suspensory ligament desmitis. In Robinson N, Wilson MR, eds: *Current therapy in equine medicine*, ed 4, Philadelphia, 1997, Saunders.
20. Ross MW: Personal communication, 2001.
21. Hardy J, Marcoux M, Breton L: Clinical relevance of radiographic findings in proximal sesamoid bones of two-year-old standardbreds in their first year of race training, *J Am Vet Med Assoc* 198:2089, 1991.
22. Ross MW: Scintigraphic and clinical findings in the standardbred metatarsophalangeal joint: 114 cases (1993-1995), *Equine Vet J* 30:131, 1998.
23. Dyson SJ: Diagnosis and prognosis of suspensory desmitis. Proceedings of the Dubai International Equine Symposium, March 1996.
24. Ross MW, Nolan PM, Palmer JA, et al: The importance of the metatarsophalangeal joint in standardbred lameness, *Proc Am Assoc Equine Pract* 37:741, 1991.
25. Sandgren B: Bony fragments in the tarsocrural and metacarpo- or metatarsophalangeal joints in the standardbred horse: a radiographic survey, *Equine Vet J Suppl* 6:66, 1988.
26. Sandgren B, Dalin G, Carlsten J: Osteochondrosis in the tarsocrural joint and osteochondral fragments in the fetlock joints in standardbred trotters. I. Epidemiology, *Equine Vet J Suppl* 16:31, 1993.
27. Haakenstad LH, Birkeland R: Osteochondritis dissecans i haseleddet hos hest. Proceedings of the Twelfth Nordic Veterinary Congress, 1974.
28. Hartung K, Keller H, Munster B: Ein beitrag zur Roentgendiagnostik des Spat der Trabrennpferde, *Der Prakt Tierarzt* 59:177, 1978.
29. Alvarado AF, Marcoux M, Breton L: The incidence of osteochondrosis in a standardbred breeding farm in Quebec, *Proc Am Assoc Equine Pract* 35:293, 1989.
30. Schougaard H, Falk-Ronne J, Phillipson J: A radiographic survey of tibiotarsal osteochondrosis in a selected population of trotting horses in Denmark and its possible genetic significance, *Equine Vet J* 22:288, 1990.
31. Grondahl AM: The incidence of osteochondrosis in the tibiotarsal joint of Norwegian standardbred trotters: a radiographic study, *J Equine Vet Sci* 11:997, 1991.
32. Storgaard Jorgensen H, Proschowsky H, Falk-Ronne J, et al: The significance of routine radiographic findings with respect to subsequent racing performance and longevity in standardbred trotters, *Equine Vet J* 29:55, 1997.
33. Torre F, Motta M: Osteochondrosis of the tarsocrural joint and osteochondral fragments in the fetlock joints: incidence and influence on racing performance in a selected group of standardbred trotters, *Proc Am Assoc Equine Pract* 46:287, 2000.
34. Torre F, Toniato M: Osteochondral fragments from the medial malleolus in horses: a comparison between radiographic and arthroscopic findings, *Proc Am Assoc Equine Pract* 45:167, 1999.
35. Laws EG, Richardson DW, Ross MW, et al: Racing performance of standardbreds after conservative and surgical treatment for tarsocrural osteochondrosis, *Equine Vet J* 25:199, 1993.
36. McIlwraith CW, Foerner JJ, Davis DM: Osteochondritis dissecans of the tarsocrural joint: results of treatment with arthroscopic surgery, *Equine Vet J* 23:155, 1991.
37. Brehm W, Staecker W: Osteochondrosis (OCD) in the tarsocrural joint of standardbred trotters: correlation between radiographic findings and racing performance, *Proc Am Assoc Equine Pract* 45:164, 1999.

The Australasian Standardbred

1. Whitton RC, Kannegieter NJ: Osteochondral fragmentation of the plantar/palmar proximal aspect of the proximal phalanx in racing horses, *Aust Vet J* 71:318, 1994.
2. O'Sullivan CB, Dart AJ, Malikides N, et al: Nonsurgical management of type II fractures of the distal phalanx in 48 standardbred horses, *Aust Vet J* 77:501, 1999.
3. Steel CM, Hopper BJ, Richardson JL, et al: Clinical findings, diagnosis, prevalence and predisposing factors for lameness localised to the middle carpal joint in young Standardbred racehorses, *Equine Vet J* 38:152, 2006.

CHAPTER 110 The Racing Quarter Horse

1. http://www.aqharacing.com. (Last accessed, January 2009.)
2. *AQHA Handbook of Rules and Regulations*, 111:70, 2008.
3. Balch OK, Helman RG, Collier MA: Underrun heels and toe-grab length as possible risk factors for musculoskeletal injuries in Oklahoma racehorses, *Proc Am Assoc Equine Pract* 47:334, 2001.
4. McIlwraith CW, Goodman NL: Conditions of the interphalangeal joints, *Vet Clin North Am Equine Pract* 5:161, 1989.
5. Goodman NL: Lameness diagnosis and treatment in the Quarter Horse, *Vet Clin North Am Equine Pract* 6:85, 1990.
6. Nunamaker DM: The bucked shin complex, *Proc Am Assoc Equine Pract* 32:457, 1986.
7. McIlwraith CW, Yovich JB, Martin GS: Arthroscopic surgery for the treatment of osteochondral chip fractures in the equine carpus, *J Am Vet Med Assoc* 191:531, 1987.
8. Bramlage LR: A clinical perspective on lameness originating in the carpus, *Equine Vet J Suppl* 6:12, 1998.
9. McIlwraith CW: Tearing of the medial palmar intercarpal ligament in the equine mid-carpal joint, *Equine Vet J* 24:367, 1992.
10. Kawcak CE, McIlwraith CW: Proximal dorsal first phalanx osteochondral chip fragmentation in 336 horses, *Equine Vet J* 26:392, 1994.
11. Foerner JJ, McIlwraith CW: Orthopedic surgery in the racehorse, *Vet Clin North Am* 6:147, 1990.
12. Frisbie DD, Kawcak CE, Baxter GM, et al: Effects of 6α-methylprednisolone acetate on an in vivo equine osteochondral fragment exercise model, *Am J Vet Res* 59:1619, 1998.

13. Frisbie DD, Kawcak CE, Trotter GW, et al: Effects of triamcinolone acetonide on an in vivo equine osteochondral fragment exercise model, *Equine Vet J* 29:349, 1997.

14. Denoix J-M: Ultrasonographic examination in the diagnosis of joint disease. In McIlwraith CW, Trotter GW, eds: *Joint disease in the horse*, Philadelphia, 1996, Saunders.

15. Wallis TW, Goodrich LR, McIlwraith CW, et al: Arthroscopic injection of corticosteroids into the fibrous tissue of subchondral cystic lesions of the medial femoral condyle in horses: a retrospective study of 52 cases (2001-2006), *Equine Vet J* 40:461, 2008.

16. Saathoff B: Personal communication, 2008.

17. Johnson BJ, Stover SM, Daft BM: Causes of death in racehorses over a 2-year period, *Equine Vet J* 4:327, 1994.

CHAPTER 112   National Hunt Racehorse, Point to Point Horse, and Timber Racing Horse

1. Wood JLN, Harkins LS, Rogers K: A retrospective study of factors associated with racehorse fatality on British racecourses from 1990-1999. In Williams RB, Houghton E, Wade JF, eds: *Proceedings of the 13th International Conference of Racing Analysts and Veterinarians*, Newmarket, 2001, R&W Publications.

2. Parkin T, Clegg P, French N, et al: Risk of fatal distal limb fractures among Thoroughbreds involved in five types of racing in the United Kingdom, *Vet Rec* 154:493, 2004.

3. Pinchbeck G, Clegg PD, Proudman CJ, et al: Case-control study to investigate risk factors for hurdle racing in England and Wales, *Vet Rec* 152:582, 2003.

4. Stephen JO, White NA, McCormick WH, et al: Risk factors and prevalence of injuries in horses during various types of steeplechase races, *J Am Vet Med Assoc* 123:1788, 2003.

5. Pinchbeck G, Clegg P, Proudman C, et al: Horse injuries and racing practices in National Hunt racehorses in the UK: the results of a prospective cohort study, *Vet J* 167:45, 2004.

6. Boden L, Anderson G, Charles J, et al: Risk of fatality and causes of death of Thoroughbred horses associated with racing in Victoria, Australia, *Equine Vet J* 38:312, 2006.

7. Pickersgill C: Epidemiological studies into orthopedic conditions of the equine athlete, MVM thesis, Glasgow, Scotland, 2000, University of Glasgow.

8. Weller R, Pfau T, May SA, et al: Variation in conformation in a cohort of National Hunt horses, *Equine Vet J* 38:616, 2006.

9. Weller R, Pfau T, Verheyen K, et al: The effect of conformation on orthopaedic health in a cohort of National Hunt horses: preliminary results, *Equine Vet J* 38:622, 2006.

10. Avella C, Ely E, Verheyen K, et al: Ultrasonographic assessment of the superficial digital flexor tendons of National Hunt racehorses in training over two racing seasons, *Equine Vet J* 41:449, 2009.

11. Ely E, Avella C, Price J, et al: Descriptive epidemiology of fracture, tendon and suspensory ligament injuries in National Hunt racehorses in training, *Equine Vet J* 41:372, 2009.

12. Smith R: Personal communication, 2010.

13. Dyson SJ: Medical management of superficial digital flexor tendonitis: a comparative study in 219 horses, *Equine Vet J* 36:415, 2004.

14. Marr C, Love S, Boyd J, et al: Factors affecting the clinical outcome of injuries to the superficial digital flexor tendon in National Hunt and point to point racehorses, *Vet Rec* 132:476, 1993.

15. Ordidge R: Comparison of three methods of treating superficial digital flexor tendonitis in the racing Thoroughbred by transection of its accessory ligament alone (proximal check ligament desmotomy), or in combination with either intra-lesional injection of hyaluronidase or tendon splitting, *Proc Am Assoc Equine Pract* 42:164, 1996.

16. Bladon B: Pelvic fractures in Thoroughbred racehorses: plain bad news? *Proceedings of the 40th South African Equine Veterinary Association Annual Congress*, 2008, Kruger.

17. Hesse K, Verheyen K: Association between physiotherapy findings and subsequent diagnosis of pelvic or hindlimb fractures in racing Thoroughbreds, *Equine Vet J* 42:234, 2010.

CHAPTER 113   The Finnish Horse and Other Scandinavian Cold-Blooded Trotters

1. Ruohoniemi M, Ahtiainen H, Ojala M: Estimates of heritability for ossification of the cartilages of the front feet in the Finnhorse, *Equine Vet J* 35:55, 2003.

2. Ruohoniemi M, Mäkelä O, Eskonen T: Clinical significance of ossification of the cartilages of the front feet based on nuclear bone scintigraphy, radiography and lameness examinations in 21 Finnhorses, *Equine Vet J* 36:143, 2004.

CHAPTER 114   Prepurchase Examination of the Performance Horse

1. Dyson S: Evaluation of the musculoskeletal system. II. The limbs. In Mair T, ed: *British Equine Veterinary Association manual: the prepurchase examination*, Newmarket, 1998, Equine Veterinary Journal.

2. Dyson S: Evaluation of the musculoskeletal system. III. The feet and hooves. In Mair T, ed: *British Equine Veterinary Association manual: the prepurchase examination*, Newmarket, 1998, Equine Veterinary Journal.

3. Dyson S: Evaluation of the musculoskeletal system. IV. The use of flexion tests and small diameter lungeing. In Mair T, ed: *British Equine Veterinary Association manual: the prepurchase examination*, Newmarket, 1998, Equine Veterinary Journal.

4. Chandler N: Evaluation of the musculoskeletal system. V. The use of flexion tests and small diameter lungeing: an alternative view. In Mair T, ed: *British Equine Veterinary Association manual: the prepurchase examination*, Newmarket, 1998, Equine Veterinary Journal.

5. Cauvin E: Evaluation of the musculoskeletal system. I. The neck and back. In Mair T, ed: *British Equine Veterinary Association manual: the prepurchase examination*, Newmarket, 1998, Equine Veterinary Journal.

6. Dyson S: Evaluation of the musculoskeletal system. VI. The role of ridden exercise in identifying lameness. In Mair T, ed: *British Equine Veterinary Association manual: the prepurchase examination*, Newmarket, 1998, Equine Veterinary Journal.

7. Phillips T: The use of radiography in the prepurchase examination. In Mair T, ed: *British Equine Veterinary Association manual: the prepurchase examination*, Newmarket, 1998, Equine Veterinary Journal.

8. Fairburn A, Dyson S, Murray R: Osseous spurs on the dorsoproximal aspect of the third metatarsal bone, *Equine Vet J* (In press.)

CHAPTER 116   Lameness in the Dressage Horse

1. Holmström M: Quantitative studies on conformation and trotting traits in the Swedish warmblood riding horse, Dissertation, Uppsala, 1994, Swedish University of Agricultural Sciences.

2. Lundquist K: Kvalitetsbedömming av unge ridhäster, samband mellam bedönningsresultat och fremtida brukbarhet. Examensarbeta i husdjursförädling (in Swedish), Uppsala, 1983, Swedish University of Agricultural Sciences.

3. Murray R, Walters J, Snart H, et al: How do features of dressage arenas influence training surface properties which are potentially associated with lameness? *The Vet J* (In press.)

4. Murray R, Walters J, Snart H, et al: Identification of risk factors for lameness in dressage horses, *The Vet J* 184:27, 2010.

5. Butler J, Dyson SJ, Colles CM, et al: *Clinical radiology of the horse*, ed 3, Oxford, 2008, Wiley-Blackwell.

6. Denoix JM: Ultrasonographic evaluation of back lesions, *Vet Clin North Am Equine Pract* 15:131, 1999.

7. Murray R, Dyson S, Tranquille C, et al: Association of type of sport and performance level with anatomical site of orthopaedic injury diagnosis, *Equine Vet J Suppl* 36:411, 2006

8. Kristensen KK, Kold SE: Multivariable analysis of factors influencing outcome of two treatment protocols in 128 cases of horses responding positively to intra-articular analgesia of the distal interphalangeal joint, *Equine Vet J* 39:150, 2007.

9. Holmstrom M, Drevemo S: Effects of trot quality and collection on the angular velocity in the hindlimbs of riding horses, *Equine Vet Journal Supplt* 23:62, 1997.

10. Murray R, Branch M, Dyson S, et al: How does exercise intensity and type affect equine distal tarsal subchondral bone thickness? *J Appl Phys* 102:2194, 2007.

CHAPTER 117   Lameness in the Three Day Event Horse

1. Dyson SJ: Training the event horse. In Hodgson DR, Rose RJ, eds: *The athletic horse*, Philadelphia, 1994, Saunders.

2. Murray JK, Senior JM, Singer ER: A comparison of cross-country recovery rates at CCI 2* with and without steeplechase competitions, *Equine Vet J Suppl* 36:133, 2006.

3. Dyson SJ: Assessment of an acutely lame horse. In Dyson S, ed: *A guide to the management of emergencies at equine competitions*, Newmarket, England, 1996, Equine Veterinary Journal.

4. Dyson SJ, Pilsworth RC, Twardock AR, Martinelli MJ, eds: *Equine scintigraphy*, Newmarket, 2003, Equine Veterinary Journal.

5. Lambiase M, Henson FMD, Bathe AP: The use of scintigraphy as an indicator of osteoarthrosis of the distal tarsal bones of the hock. In British Equine Veterinary Association Congress Handbook, vol 38, London, 1999, British Equine Veterinary Association (abstract).

6. Lambiase M, Henson FMD, Jeffcott LB, et al: Use of dynamic force sensing array measurements to assess the benefits of various numnahs and therapeutic pads beneath the saddle. In *British Equine Veterinary Association Congress handbook*, vol 38, London, 1999, British Equine Veterinary Association (abstract).

7. Marks D: Back pain. In Robinson NE, Wilson MR, eds: *Current therapy in equine medicine*, ed 4, Philadelphia, 1997, Saunders.

8. Bathe AP, Humphrey DJ, Henson FMD: The oral bioavailability of chondroitin sulphate in horses: a pilot study. In Lindner A, ed: *The elite showjumper*. Proceedings of the Conference on Equine Sports Medicine and Science, Sicily, Italy, 2000.

9. Ramey R: Personal communication, 2001.

10. Du J, White N, Eddington ND: The bioavailability and pharmacokinetics of glucosamine hydrochloride and chondroitin sulfate after oral and intravenous single dose administration in the horse, *Biopharm Drug Dispos* 25:109, 2004.

11. Singer ER, Barnes J, Saxby F, et al: Injuries in the event horse: training versus competition, *Vet J* 175:76, 2008.

12. Murray JK, Singer ER, Saxby F, et al: Factors influencing risk of injury to horses falling during eventing, *Vet Rec* 154:207, 2004.

13. Bathe A, Bladon B, Smith R: Unpublished observations, 2006.

14. Bathe AP: Plantar metatarsal neurectomy and fasciotomy in the surgical treatment of hindlimb proximal suspensory desmitis: technique and preliminary results, *Vet Surg* 30:298, 2001 (abstract).

15. Dyson S, Wright I, Kold S, et al: Clinical and radiographic features, treatment and outcome in 15 horses with fracture of the medial pole of the patella, *Equine Vet J* 24:264, 1992.

16. Bathe AP: Resting haematological and biochemical parameters in a group of event horses, *Pferdeheilkunde* 12:712, 1996 (abstract).

17. Bathe A, Smith R: Unpublished observations, 1998.

CHAPTER 118 Lameness in Endurance Horses

1. Malton RJ: Personal communication, 2009.

2. Bryant JC: Personal communication, 2009.

3. Misheff MM: Unpublished data, 1996-2009.

4. Randall RW: Personal communication, 2000.

5. Castro VF, Schumacher J, Pauwels F, et al: A new approach to desensitizing the lateral palmar nerve of the horse, *Vet Surg* 34:539, 2005.

6. Rantanen NW: Personal communication, 2000.

7. Dyson SJ: Proximal palmar metacarpal pain: a diagnostic challenge, *Equine Vet Educ* 15:134, 2003.

8. Fortier, LA, Smith RK: Regenerative medicine for tendinous and ligamentous injuries of sport horses, *Vet Clin North Am Equine Pract* 24:191, 2008.

9. Launois MT, Vandeweerd JMEF, Perrin RAR, et al: Use of computed tomography to diagnose new bone formation associated with desmitis of the proximal aspect of the suspensory ligament in third metacarpal or third metatarsal bones of three horses, *J Am Vet Med Assoc* 234:514, 2009.

10. Alexander GR: Personal communication, 2009.

11. Powell SE: Personal communication, 2009.

12. Pollitt CC, Van Epps AW: Prolonged, continuous distal limb cryotherapy in the horse, *Equine Vet J* 36:216, 2004.

13. Van Epps AW, Pollitt CC: Equine laminitis model: cryotherapy reduces the severity of lesions evaluated seven days after the induction with oligofructose, *Equine Vet J* 41:741, 2009.

14. Misheff MM, Alexander GR, Hirst GR: Fractures in endurance horses, *Equine Vet Educ* (In press.)

15. Riggs CM: Aetiopathogenesis of parasagittal fractures of the distal condyles of the third metacarpal and third metatarsal bones—review of the literature, *Equine Vet J* 31:116, 1999.

16. Stover SM, Murray A: The California postmortem program: leading the way, *Vet Clin North Am Equine Pract* 24:21, 2008.

17. Muir P, McCarthy J, Radtke CL, et al: Role of endochondral ossification of articular cartilage and functional adaptation of the subchondral plate in the development of fatigue microcracking of joints, *Bone* 38:347, 2006.

18. Riggs CM, Whitehouse GH, Boyde A: Pathology of the distal condyles of the third metacarpal and third metatarsal bones of the horse, *Equine Vet J* 31:140, 1999.

19. Stepnik MW, Radke CL, Scollay MC, et al: Scanning electron microscopic examination of the third metacarpal/third metatarsal bone failure surfaces in Thoroughbred racehorses with condylar fracture, *Vet Surg* 33:2, 2004.

20. Zubrod CJ, Schneider RK, Tucker RL, et al: Use of magnetic resonance imaging for identifying subchondral bone damage in horses: 11 cases (1999-2003), *J Am Vet Med Assoc* 224:411, 2004.

21. Dyson SJ, Murray R: Osseous trauma in the fetlock region of mature sports horses, *AAEP Proc* 52:443, 2006.

22. Hill AE, Gardner IA, Carpenter TE, et al: Effects of injury to the suspensory apparatus, exercise, and horseshoe characteristics on the risk of lateral condylar fracture and suspensory apparatus failure in forelimbs of Thoroughbred racehorses, *Am J Vet Res* 65:1508, 2004.

23. Thomason JJ, Peterson ML: Biomechanical and mechanical investigations of the hoof-track interface in racing horses, *Vet Clin North Am Equine Pract* 24:53, 2008.

24. Mackay-Smith M, Cohen M: Exercise physiology and diseases of exertion. In: *Equine medicine and surgery*, Santa Barbara, Calif., 1983, American Vet Pub.

25. Whiting JM: The exhausted horse. In Robinson NE, Sprayberry KA, eds: *Current therapy in equine medicine*, ed 6, St. Louis, 2009, Saunders.

26. Carlson GP: Synchronous diaphragmatic flutter. In: *Current therapy in equine medicine*, ed 2, Philadelphia, 1987, Saunders.

CHAPTER 120 The Western Performance Horse

The Cutting Horse

1. Wallis TW, Goodrich LR, McIlwraith CW, et al: Arthroscopic injection of corticosteroids into the fibrous tissue of subchondral cystic lesions of the medial femoral condyle in horses: a retrospective study of 52 cases (2001-2006), *Equine Vet J* 40:461, 2008.

The Roping Horse

1. Dabareiner RM, Cohen ND, Carter GK, et al: Lameness and poor performance in horses used for team roping: 118 cases (2000-2003), *J Am Vet Med Assoc* 226:1694, 2005.

2. Dabareiner RM, Carter GK, Honnas CM: Injection of corticosteroids, hyaluronate, and amikacin into the navicular bursa in horses with signs of navicular area pain unresponsive to other treatments, *J Am Vet Med Assoc* 223:1469, 2003.

Barrel-Racing Horses

1. Stricklin JB: Barrel racing, *Proc Am Assoc Equine Pract* 43:37, 1997.

2. Cox J-B: Personal communication, 2002.

3. Galley RH: Personal communication, 2002.

4. Pearce G: Personal communication, 2002.

5. Women's Professional Rodeo Association, 1235 Lake Plaza Drive, Suite 13, Colorado Springs, Colo. At www.wpra.com.

6. Dabareiner RM, Cohen ND, Carter GK, et al: Musculoskeletal problems associated with lameness and poor performance among horses used for barrel racing: 118 cases (2000-2003), *J Am Vet Med Assoc* 227:1646, 2005.

CHAPTER 122 Lameness in the American Saddlebred and Other Trotting Breeds with Collection

1. Briggs HM: *Modern breeds of livestock*, ed 4, New York, 1980, MacMillan.

2. 2002 USA Equestrian rule book, Lexington, Ky, 2002, USA Equestrian.

CHAPTER 123 Lameness in the Arabian and Half-Arabian Show Horse

1. American Horse Shows Association: *General qualifications. 1998-1999 Arabian, Half-Arabian and Anglo Arabian division rule book*, New York, 1997, American Horse Shows Association.

2. Hahn CN, Mayhew IG, Mackay RJ, et al: Diseases of the spinal cord. In Colahan PT, Merritt AM, Moore JN, et al, eds:

Equine medicine and surgery, vol 1, ed 5, St Louis, 1999, Mosby.

3. Easter JL, Watkins J, Stephens S, et al: Effects of regional anesthesia on experimentally induced coffin joint synovitis, *Proc Am Assoc Equine Pract* 46:214, 2000.

CHAPTER 125   Lameness in Draft Horses

1. Stashak TS, ed: *Adams' lameness in horses*, ed 4, Philadelphia, 1987, Lea & Febiger.
2. Dyson SJ: Personal communication, 2001.

CHAPTER 126   Lameness in the Pony

1. Speed J: A cause of malformation of the limbs of Shetland ponies with a note on its phylogenic significance, *Br Vet J* 114:51, 1958.
2. Chan CC-H, Munroe GA: Congenital defects of the equine musculoskeletal system, *Equine Vet Educ* 8:157, 1996.
3. Voute LC, Henson FMD, Platt D, et al: Lesions of the lateral trochlear ridge of the distal femur in ponies with histological features of equine dyschondroplasia. Proceedings of the Thirty-Sixth British Equine Veterinary Association Congress, Harrogate, September 1997.
4. Voute L: Personal communication, 2001.
5. Clegg PD, Dyson SJ, Summerhays GES, et al: Scapulohumeral osteoarthritis in Shetland ponies, miniature horses and Falabella ponies (20 cases), *Vet Rec* 148:175, 2001.
6. Boswell JC, Schramme MC, Wilson AM, et al: Radiographic study to evaluate suspect scapulohumeral joint dysplasia in Shetland ponies, *Equine Vet J* 31:510, 1999.
7. Parth RA, Svalbe LS, Hazard GH, et al: Suspected primary scapulohumeral osteoarthritis in two miniature ponies, *Aust Vet J* 86:153, 2008.
8. Jones E, McDiarmid AM: Diagnosis of scapulohumeral joint arthritis in a Shetland pony by ultrasonography, *Vet Rec* 154:178, 2004.
9. Butler JA, Colles CM, Dyson SJ, et al: *Clinical radiology of the horse*, ed 3, Oxford, 2008, Wiley-Blackwell.
10. Jones E, McDiarmid AM: A retrospective study of 42 horses with pain originating from the stifle joint. Proceedings of the Thirty-Ninth British Equine Veterinary Association Congress, Birmingham, September 2000.
11. Schneider RK, Jenson P, Moore RM: Evaluation of cartilage lesions on the medial femoral condyle as a cause of lameness in horses: 11 cases (1988-1994), *J Am Vet Med Assoc* 210:1649, 1997.
12. Engelbert TA, Tate LP, Richardson DC, et al: Lateral patella luxation in miniature horses, *Vet Surg* 22:293, 1993.
13. Bjornsdottir S, Axelsson M, Eksell P, et al: Radiographic and clinical survey of degenerative joint disease in the distal tarsal joints in Icelandic horses, *Equine Vet J* 32:268, 2000.
14. Eksell P, Axelsson M, Brostrom H, et al: Prevalence and risk factors of bone spavin in Icelandic horses in Sweden, *Acta Vet Scand* 39:339, 1998.
15. Axelsson M, Bjornsdottir S, Eksell P, et al: Risk factors associated with hindlimb lameness and degenerative joint disease in the distal tarsus of Icelandic horses, *Equine Vet J* 33:84, 2001.
16. Smith RKW, Dyson SJ, Schramme MC, et al: Osteoarthritis of the talocalcaneal joint in 18 horses, *Equine Vet J* 37:166, 2005.
17. Malark JA, Nixon AJ, Haughland MA, et al: Equine coxofemoral luxations: 17 cases (1975-1990), *Cornell Vet* 82:79, 1992.
18. Stashak TS: Lameness. In Stashak TS, ed: *Adams' lameness in the horses*, ed 4, Philadelphia, 1987, Lea & Febiger.
19. Clegg PD, Comerford EJ: Coxofemoral luxation—how does our knowledge of treatment in other species help us in the horse? *Equine Vet Educ* 19:482, 2007.
20. Garcia-Lopez JM, Boudrieau RJ, Provost PJ: Surgical repair of a coxofemoral luxation in a horse, *J Am Vet Med Assoc* 219:1254, 2001.
21. Wright IM: Ligaments associated with joints, *Vet Clin North Am Equine Pract* 11:271, 1995.
22. McIlwraith CW: Diseases of joints, ligaments and related structures. In Stashak TS, ed: *Adams' lameness in the horse*, ed 4, Philadelphia, 1987, Lea & Febiger.
23. Hermans WA, Kersjes AW, van der Mey GJ, et al: Investigation into the heredity of congenital lateral patellar (sub)luxation in the Shetland pony, *Vet Q* 9:1, 1987.
24. Kobluk CN: Correction of patellar luxation by recession sulcoplasty in three foals, *Vet Surg* 22:298, 1993.
25. Knottenbelt D: Personal communication, 2001.
26. Shiroma JT, Engel HN, Wagner PC, et al: Dorsal subluxation of the proximal interphalangeal joint in the pelvic limb of three horses, *J Am Vet Med Assoc* 195:777, 1989.
27. McDiarmid A: Unpublished data, 1995.
28. Clark JO, Clark TP: Analgesia, *Vet Clin North Am Equine Pract* 15:712, 1999.
29. Eyre P, Elmes PJ, Strickland S: Corticosteroid-potentiated vascular responses of the equine digit: a possible pharmacological basis for laminitis, *Am J Vet Res* 40:135, 1979.
30. Scholes SF, Holliman A, May PD, et al: A syndrome of anaemia, immunodeficiency and peripheral ganglionopathy in Fell pony foals, *Vet Rec* 142:128, 1998.
31. Walmsley JP: First aid splinting for the equine fracture patient, *Equine Vet Educ* 5:61, 1993.
32. Auer JA: External coaptation and fixation. In Colahan PT, Mayhew IG, Merritt AM, et al, eds: *Equine medicine and surgery*, ed 5, St Louis, 1999, Mosby.
33. Nemeth F, Back W: The use of the walking cast to repair fractures in the horses and ponies, *Equine Vet J* 23:32, 1991.
34. Nunamaker DM, Richardson DW, Butterweck DM: A new external skeletal fixation devise in the horse, *Vet Surg* 15:345, 1986.
35. Baxter GM, Doran RE, Allen D: Complete excision of a fractured fourth metatarsal bone in eight horses, *Vet Surg* 21:273, 1992.
36. Barr ARS, Hillyer MH, Richardson JD: Partial carpal arthrodesis for multiple carpal fractures and subluxation in a pony, *Equine Vet Educ* 6:255, 1994.
37. Arighi M, Miller CR, Pennock PW: Arthrodesis of the scapulohumeral joint in a miniature horse, *J Am Vet Med Assoc* 191:713, 1987.
38. Pleasant RS, Baker GJ, Muhlbauer MC, et al: Stress reactions and stress fractures of the proximal palmar aspect of the third metacarpal bone in horse: 58 cases (1980-1990), *J Am Vet Med Assoc* 201:1918, 1992.
39. MacGregor CM: Studies of the pathology and treatment of equine navicular disease, PhD dissertation, Edinburgh, 1984, University of Edinburgh (Scotland).
40. Dyson SJ: Personal communication, 2008.
41. Aswad ASS: Ossification of the cartilages of the horse's foot (side bone), PhD dissertation, Edinburgh, 1971, University of Edinburgh (Scotland).
42. Field JR, Jeffcott LB: Equine laminitis: another hypothesis for pathogenesis, *Med Hypotheses* 30:203, 1989.
43. Durham AE, Rendle DI, Newton JE: The effect of metformin on measurements of insulin sensitivity and β cell response in 18 horses and ponies with insulin resistance, *Equine Vet J* 40:493, 2008.
44. Johnson PJ: The equine metabolic syndrome: peripheral Cushing's syndrome, *Vet Clin North Am Equine Pract* 18:271, 2002.
45. Freestone JF, Beadle R, Shoemaker K, et al: Improved insulin sensitivity in hyperinsulinaemic ponies through physical conditioning and controlled feed intake, *Equine Vet J* 24:187, 1992.
46. Ott EA, Kivipelto P: Influence of chromium tripicolinate on growth and glucose metabolism in growing horses, *J Anim Sci* 77:3022, 1999.
47. McGowan CM, Frost R, Pfeiffer DU, et al: Serum insulin concentrations in horses with equine Cushing's syndrome: response to a cortisol inhibitor and prognostic value, *Equine Vet J* 36:295, 2004.
48. Kuwano A, Yoshihara T, Takatori K, et al: Onychomycosis in white line disease in horses: pathology and clinical features, *Equine Vet J Suppl* 26:27, 1998.
49. Peremans K, Verschooten F, De Moor A, et al: Laminitis in the pony: conservative treatment vs dorsal wall hoof resection, *Equine Vet J* 23:243, 1991.
50. Curtis S, Ferguson DW, Luikart R, et al: Trimming of the chronically affected horse, *Vet Clin North Am Equine Pract* 15:463, 1995.
51. Cripps PJ, Eustace RA: Factors involved in the prognosis of equine laminitis in the UK, *Equine Vet J* 31:433, 1999.
52. Watson TD, Murphy D, Love S: Equine hyperlipaemia in the United Kingdom: clinical features and blood biochemistry of 18 cases, *Vet Rec* 131:48, 1992.
53. Love S: Personal communication, 2001.
54. Smith LJ, Mair TS: Rupture of the superficial flexor tendon in the forelimb in aged horses: a report of nine cases, *Equine Vet Educ* 19:183, 2007.
55. Palmer SE, Genovese R, Longo KL, et al: Practical management of superficial digital flexor tendonitis in the performance horse, *Vet Clin North Am Equine Pract* 10:468, 1994.
56. Dyson SJ: Superficial digital flexor tendon injuries in teenage and older horses, *Equine Vet Educ* 19:187, 2007.

57. Dyson SJ: Desmitis of the accessory ligament of the deep digital flexor tendon: 27 cases (1986-1990), *Equine Vet J* 23:438, 1991.

58. McDiarmid AM: Desmitis of the accessory ligament of the deep digital flexor tendon. In Robinson NE, Wilson MR, eds: *Current therapy in equine medicine*, ed 4, Philadelphia, 1997, Saunders.

59. Eliashar E, Dyson, SJ, Archer, RM, et al: Two clinical manifestations of desmopathy of the accessory ligament of the deep digital flexor tendon in the hindlimb of 23 horses, *Equine Vet J* 37:495, 2005.

60. Becker CK, Savelberg HHCM, Barneveld A: In vitro mechanical properties of the accessory ligaments of the deep digital flexor tendon in horses in relationship to age, *Equine Vet J* 26:454, 1994.

61. Dyson SJ, Dik KJ: Conditions of tendons, tendon sheaths and ligaments, *Vet Clin North Am Equine Pract* 11:315, 1995.

62. Barr ARS, Dyson SJ, Barr FJ, et al: Tendonitis of the deep digital flexor tendon in the distal metacarpal/metatarsal region associated with tenosynovitis of the digital sheath in the horse, *Equine Vet J* 27:348, 1995.

63. Smith MRW, Wright IM: Noninfected tenosynovitis of the digital flexor tendon sheath: a retrospective analysis of 76 cases, *Equine Vet J* 38:134, 2006.

64. Dyson SJ, Dik KJ: Tendon, tendon sheaths and ligament injuries in the Pastern, *Vet Clin North Am Equine Pract* 11:217, 1995.

65. Dik KJ, Dyson SJ, Vail TB: Aseptic tenosynovitis of the digital flexor tendon sheath, fetlock and pastern annular ligament constriction, *Vet Clin North Am Equine Pract* 11:151, 1995.

66. Owen R, Dyson S, Parkin T, et al: A retrospective study of palmar/plantar annular ligament injury in 71 horses: 2001-2006, *Equine Vet J* 40:237, 2008.

67. Wilmink JM, Stolk PWT, Van Weeren PR, et al: Differences in second intention wound healing between horses and ponies: macroscopic aspects, *Equine Vet J* 31:53, 1999.

68. Wilmink JM, Van Weeren PR: Second intention repair in the horse and pony and management of exuberant granulation tissue, *Vet Clin North Am Equine Pract* 21:15, 2005.

69. Miller CB, Wilson DA, Keegan KG: Growth characteristics of fibroblasts isolated from the trunk and distal aspect of the limb of horse and ponies, *Vet Surg* 29:1, 2000.

70. Ehrlich PJ, Seeherman HJ, O'Callaghan MW, et al: Results of bone scintigraphy in horse used for showjumping, hunting or eventing: 141 cases (1988-1994), *J Am Vet Med Assoc* 213:1460, 1998.

71. Jeffcott L: Personal communication, 2001.

72. Harris PA: The equine rhabdomyolysis syndrome in the United Kingdom: epidemiological and clinical descriptive information, *Br Vet J* 147:373, 1991.

73. Valentine BA, McDonough SP, Chang YF, et al: Polysaccharide storage myopathy in Morgan, Arabian and Standardbred related horses and Welsh-cross ponies, *Vet Pathol* 37:193, 2000.

74. Bjorck G, Everz KE, Hansen HJ, et al: Congenital cerebellar ataxia in the Gotland pony breed, *Zentralbl Veterinarmed A* 20:341, 1993.

75. Hahn CN, Mayhew IG, Mackay RJ: Diseases of vestibular and cerebellar structures. In Colahan PT, Mayhew IG, Merritt AM, et al, eds: *Equine medicine and surgery*, ed 5, St Louis, 1999, Mosby.

CHAPTER 127 Lameness in Breeding Stallions and Broodmares

1. McDonnell SM: Normal and abnormal sexual behavior, *Vet Clin North Am Equine Pract* 8:71, 1982.

2. Martin BB, McDonnell SM, Love CC: Effects of musculoskeletal and neurologic diseases on breeding performance in stallions, *Comp Clin Educ Pract Vet* 20:1159, 1998.

3. Varner DD, Schumacher J, Blanchard TL, et al: *Disease and management of breeding stallions*, Goleta, Calif, 1991, American Veterinary Publications.

4. Kenney RM, Hurtgen JP, Pierson R, et al: *Clinical fertility evaluation of the stallion*, Hastings, Neb, 1983, Society for Theriogenology.

5. Martin BB, Klide AM: Diagnosis and treatment of chronic back pain in horses, *Proc Am Assoc Equine Pract* 43:310, 1997.

6. Martin BB, Klide AM: Acupuncture for treatment of chronic back pain in horses. In Schoen AM, ed: *Veterinary acupuncture: ancient art to modern medicine*, Goleta, Calif, 1994, American Veterinary Publications.

7. Robinson NE: Appendix. In Robinson NE, ed: *Current therapy in equine medicine*, ed 3, Philadelphia, 1992, Saunders.

8. McDonnell SM, Love CC, Pozor MA, et al: Phenylbutazone treatment in breeding stallions: preliminary evidence for no effect on semen or testicular size, *Theriogenology* 37:1225, 1992.

9. Mitten LA, Hinchcliff KW: Nonsteroidal anti-inflammatory drugs. In Robinson N, ed: *Current therapy in equine medicine*, ed 4, Philadelphia, 1997, Saunders.

10. Oristaglio-Turner RM, McDonnell SM, Hawkins JF: Use of pharmacologically induced ejaculation to obtain semen in a stallion with fractured radius, *J Am Vet Med Assoc* 206:1906, 1995.

11. Wagner PC, Grant BD, Reed SN: Congenital vertebral malformation, *Vet Clin North Am* 3:385, 1987.

12. Fengar CK: Equine protozoal myeloencephalitis, *Comp Cont Educ Pract Vet* 19:513, 1997.

13. Bedford SJ, McDonnell SM: Measurements of reproductive function in stallions treated with trimethoprim-sulfamethoxazole and pyrimethamine, *J Am Vet Med Assoc* 215:1317, 1999.

14. Allen D: Acute laminitis: In White NA, Moore JN, eds: *Current techniques in equine surgery and lameness*, ed 2, Philadelphia, 1998, Saunders.

15. Hunt RJ: Chronic laminitis. In White NA, Moore JN, eds: *Current techniques in equine surgery and lameness*, ed 2, Philadelphia, 1998, Saunders.

16. Goetz TM: Treatment of chronic laminitis in horses, *Vet Clin North Am* 5:73, 1989.

17. Beech J: Rhabdomyolysis (tying up) in standardbred and thoroughbred racehorses. Proceedings of the International Equine Neurology Conference, Ithaca, NY, 1997.

18. McDonnell SM, Love CC, Martin BB, et al: Ejaculatory failure associated with aortic-iliac thrombosis in 2 stallions, *J Am Vet Med Assoc* 200:954, 1992.

19. Doucet MY, Bertone AL, Hendrickson D, et al: Comparison of efficacy and safety of paste formulations of firocoxib and phenylbutazone in horses with naturally occurring osteoarthritis, *J Am Vet Med Assoc* 232:91, 2008.

20. McConnell SM, Turner R: Unpublished observations, 2009.

21. Terry RL, McDonnell SM, Soma LS, et al: Pharmacokinetic profile, cardiovascular and behavioural changes following intravenous and oral gabapentin administration in the horse. Proceedings of the 48th British Equine Veterinary Association Congress, September 2009, Birmingham, UK, p 103.

22. McDonnell SM: Stallion behavior and endocrinology and behavior: what do we really know? *Proc Am Assoc Equine Pract* 41:18, 1995.

23. McDonnell SM: Ejaculation physiology and dysfunction, *Vet Clin North Am Equine Pract* 8:57, 1992.

24. McDonnell SM, Kenney RM, Meckley PE, et al: Conditioned suppression of sexual behavior in stallions and reversal with diazepam, *Physiol Behav* 34:951, 1985.

25. McDonnell SM, Kenney RM, Meckley PE, et al: Novel environment suppression of stallion sexual behavior and effects of diazepam, *Physiol Behav* 37:503, 1986.

26. McDonnell SM, Turner RM, Diehl NK: Modifying unruly breeding behavior in stallions, *Comp Cont Educ Pract Vet* 17:411, 1995.

27. Shideler RK: The mare examination: history. In McKinnon AO, Voss JL, eds: *Equine reproduction*, Philadelphia, 1993, Lea & Febiger.

28. Baird AN: Equine distal phalangeal sequestration, *Vet Radiol* 31:210, 1990.

29. Perkins NR, Frazer GS: Reproductive emergencies in the broodmare, *Vet Clin North Am Equine Pract* 10:643, 1994.

30. Brendemuehl JR, Waldridge BM, Bridges ER: Effects of sulfadiazine and pyrimethamine and concurrent folic acid supplementation on pregnancy and embryonic loss rates in broodmares, *Proc Am Assoc Equine Pract* 44:142, 1998.

31. McDonnell SM, Garcia MC, Kenney RM: Imipramine-induced erection, masturbation, and ejaculation in male horses, *Pharmacol Biochem Behav* 27:187, 1987.

32. Oristaglio-Turner RM, Love CC, McDonnell SM, et al: Use of imipramine hydrochloride for treatment of urospermia in a stallion with a dysfunctional bladder, *J Am Vet Med Assoc* 207:1602, 1995.

33. Johnston PF, DeLuca JL: Chemical ejaculation of stallions after the administration of oral imipramine followed by intravenous xylazine, *Proc Am Assoc Equine Pract* 44:12, 1998.

34. McDonnell SM: Pharmacologically induced ex-copula ejaculation in stallions using imipramine and xylazine, *Anim Reprod Sci* 68:153, 2001.

CHAPTER 128 Lameness in Foals

1. Stashak TS: Diagnosis of lameness. In Stashak TS, ed: *Adams' lameness in horses*, ed 4, Philadelphia, 1987, Lea & Febiger.
2. Bohanon TC: Developmental musculoskeletal disease. In Kobluk CN, Ames TR, Geor RJ, eds: The horse: diseases & clinical management, vol 2, Philadelphia, 1995, Saunders.
3. Douglas J: The pathogenesis and clinical manifestations of equine osteochondrosis, *Vet Med* 87:826, 1992.
4. Stashak TS: Diseases of joints, tendons, ligaments, and related structures. In Stashak TS, ed: *Adams' lameness in horses*, ed 4, Philadelphia, 1987, Lea & Febiger.
5. Dutton DM, Watkins JP, Honnas CM, et al: Treatment response and athletic outcome of foals with tarsal valgus deformities: 39 cases (1988-1997), *J Am Med Assoc* 215:1481, 1999.
6. Dutton DM, Watkins JP, Walker MA, et al: Incomplete ossification of the tarsal bones in foals: 22 cases (1988-1996), *J Am Vet Med Assoc* 213:1590, 1998.
7. Embertson RM, Bramlage LR, Herring DS, et al: Physeal fractures in the horse: classification and incidence, *Vet Surg* 15:223, 1986.
8. Pool R: Pathologic manifestations of osteochondrosis. Proceedings of the Developmental Orthopedic Disease Symposium, Dallas, April 1986.
9. Dik KJ, Enzerink E, van Weeren PR: Radiographic development of osteochondral abnormalities in the hock and stifle of Dutch Warmblood foals, from age 1 to 11 months, *Equine Vet J Suppl* 31:9, 1999.
10. Tull T, Woodie J, Ruggles A, et al: Management and assessment of prognosis after gastrocnemius disruption in Thoroughbred foals: 28 cases (1993-2007), *Equine Vet J* 41:541, 2009.
11. Madison JB: Infectious orthopedic disease in foals. In Robinson NE, ed: *Current therapy in equine medicine*, ed 4, Philadelphia, 1997, Saunders.
12. Vatistas NJ, Wilson WD, Pascoe JR, et al: Septic arthritis in foals: bacterial isolates, antimicrobial susceptibility, and factors influencing survival, *Proc Am Assoc Equine Pract* 39:259, 1993.
13. Firth EC: Infectious arthritis in foals. In White NA, Moore JN, eds: *Current practice of equine surgery*, Philadelphia, 1990, JB Lippincott.
14. Madison JB, Sommer M, Spencer PA: Relations among synovial membrane histopathologic findings, synovial fluid cytologic findings, and bacterial culture results in horses with suspected infectious arthritis: 64 cases (1979-1987), *J Am Vet Med Assoc* 198:1655, 1991.
15. Martens RJ, Auer JA: Haematogenous septic arthritis and osteomyelitis in the foal, *Proc Am Assoc Equine Pract* 26:47, 1980.
16. Schneider RK, Bramlage LR, Moore RM, et al: A retrospective study of 192 horses affected with septic arthritis/tenosynovitis, *Equine Vet J* 24:436, 1992.
17. McIlwraith CW: Treatment of septic arthritis. In Turner A, ed: *The veterinary clinics of North American large animal practice: equine orthopedic surgery*, Philadelphia, 1983, Saunders.
18. Bertone AL: Infectious arthritis in adult horses, *Proc Am Coll Vet Intern Med* 9:409, 1991.
19. Wagner PC, Watrous BJ, Darien BJ: Septic arthritis and osteomyelitis. In Robinson NE, ed: *Current therapy in equine medicine*, ed 3, Philadelphia, 1992, Saunders.
20. Steele CM, Hunt AR, Adams PLE, et al: Factors associated with prognosis for survival and athletic use in foals with septic arthritis (1987-1994), *J Am Vet Med Assoc* 215:973, 1999.
21. Madison JB, Scarratt WK: Immune-mediated polysynovitis in four foals, *J Am Vet Med Assoc* 192:1581, 1988.

Index

A

Abaxial extensions, usage, 296
Abaxial fractures, 405
  avulsion injuries, 405
Abaxial nonarticular fragments,
    493-494
  impact, 493-494
  lameness, mildness, 493
  occurrence, 493
  radiographs, 493
Abaxial sesamoid block,
    110-111
  performing, 111
  perineural analgesia, 125
Abdominal muscles, major
    hindlimb muscle rupture,
    162
Abductor digitus longus, 786
Abrasion arthroplasty, 850
  superficial intracortical
    debridement, 850
Abscesses, lameness, 985
Accessory carpal bone, 88
  fractures, 446
    occurrence, 446
    result, 780
  frontal slab fracture,
    lateromedial radiographic
    view, 446f
  horizontal/vertical fracture,
    1163
  nonarticular fractures,
    management, 446
  vertical slab fracture, 446
Accessory ligament, desmotomy,
    342
Accessory ligament of the DDFT
    (ALDDFT), 50
  anatomy, 734
  clinical signs, 735
  degenerative aging changes,
    734
  desmitis, 161-162, 422, 725
    incidence, 734
    occurrence, 734
    problem, 1111
    recurrence, deep digital flexor
      tendonitis (association),
      734
  desmopathy, 507
    observation, 734
  desmotomy, 342
    surgical intervention, 647
  force, decrease, 279
  history, 735
  injuries, exercise regimen,
    1174b
  insertion, 175
  occurrence, 161
  pathogenesis, 734
  treatment, 737-738
  ultrasonography, 735-737

Accessory ligament of the SDFT
    (ALSDFT), 263
  bilateral transection, 717-718
  desmitis, 778-779
    diagnosis, 778
    treatment, 778-779
  desmotomy, 264
  surgical procedure, 716
  transection, 715
    accomplishment, 716
    aftercare, 718
    function, explanation,
      716-717
    performing, timing, 717
Acetabulum fractures, 569-570
  clinical examination, 569
  scintigraphic examination, 569
  ultrasonographic examination,
    569-570
Acetylpromazine, administration,
    571
Acid firing, 868
Acoustic enhancement, 173
Acoustic shadowing, 174
Acoustic streaming, 902-903
Acquired flexural deformities,
    647-649
  causes, 647
  clinical signs, 647
  development, 647
  genetics, involvement, 647
  treatment, 647-649
Acrylic adhesives, 306-307
Acrylic-PVC copolymers, 307
Acrylonitrile butadrene styrene
    (ABS), 307
Action
  goose-step, treadmill (impact),
    931
  mechanism, 894, 906
  pathophysiology, 894
Active back movement, dynamic
    examination, 595f
Active training, 880
Acupoints, 888f, 889b
  palpation guidelines, 889-890
Acupuncture
  benefits, 886
  channel palpation, 887-892
  defining, 881
  diagnosis/therapy, basis,
    891-892
  diagnostic examination, 884
  history, 881
  interest, 881
  point, 882f
    selection, Western medical
      perspective, 884
    stimulation, 883
  scientific basis, 881-882
  techniques/instrumentation,
    883-884

Acupuncture (Continued)
  TENS, 906
  usage, 881-886
    evaluation, 887
    success, 886
Acute bone damage (assessment),
    scintigraphy (usage), 556
  physiological effects, 881-882
Acute carpal lameness, 428-429
Acute caudal antebrachial
    myositis, 454
  presumptive diagnosis, 454
  treatment, 454
Acute gluteal syndrome, 551
Acute hoof avulsions, 319
Acute infectious tenosynovitis,
    784-785
Acute lameness, racing/training
    (impact), 945
Acute laminitis
  grade 1 histopathology, 367-368
  grade 2 histopathology, 368
  grade 3 histopathology, 368-369
  histopathology, 367-369
  inflammation, 369
  leukocytes, 369
  shoe removal, 384-385
Acute left forelimb lameness,
    delayed-phase cranial image,
    451f
Acute medial collateral
    desmopathy, 211f
Acute noninfectious
    tenosynovitis, 766-767
Acu-TENS, 906
Acute-onset right hindlimb
    lameness, distal metatarsal
    region (transverse
    ultrasonographic images),
    730f
Acute-onset severe forelimb
    lameness, 156
Acute-onset severe lameness
    assessment, 159-163
  carpus examination, 161
  causes, 159
  chest examination, 160-161
  elbow examination, 161
  feet, examination, 162
  limb examination, 160
  medical history, 159-160
  shoulder examination, 160-161
  transportation, 163-164
Acute/repetitive overload injuries,
    395-399
Acute rhabdomyolysis
  clinical signs, 832
  treatment, 824-825
    intravenous/intragastric
      dimethyl sulfoxide,
      usage, 824
    objectives, 824

Acute sacroiliac joint injuries
    (identification), nuclear
    scintigraphy (usage), 590
Acute sacroiliac ligament injuries,
    585
Acute synovitis (flare), 101
Acute tenosynovitis
  characterization, 767
  treatment, 784
Acute traumatic tenosynovitis,
    789
  diagnosis, 789
Acute uncomplicated
    noninfectious tenosynovitis,
    prognosis, 769
Adaptive bony remodeling,
    exercise (usage), 957
Adaptive exercise, usage, 957
Adductor, major hindlimb muscle
    rupture, 162
Adequan, review, 843
Adhesives
  bonding ability, 306
  polymerization, speed
    (importance), 306
  types, 306-307
  use, 299, 306
Adipose-derived MSCs (A-MSCs),
    763
A disintegrin and
    metalloproteinase (ADAM),
    662
A disintegrin and metalloproteinase
    with thrombospondin type 1
    mofits (ADAMTS enzymes),
    662
Adjunctive therapies, 857-858
Adrenocorticotropic hormone
    (ACTH), impact, 370-371
Adult-derived mesenchymal stem
    cells, collection, 761
Adult equine tibia, lateromedial
    radiographic view, 528f
Adult horses
  acute onset lameness, 679
  distal phalanx, solar margin
    fracture, 360
    clinical signs/diagnosis,
      360
    treatment, 360
  femoral trochlear ridges/femoral
    condyles, fracture fragment
    origination, 546-547
  sedation, 678
  third metacarpal bone, dorsal
    sagittal ridge (fragments),
    409f
  tibial diaphyseal fractures,
    528-529
    dynamic compression plates/
      bone screws, usage,
      528-529

Page number followed by *f* indicate figures; *t,* tables; *b,* boxes.

1349

Adult jumper, hock (dorsomedial-plantarolateral oblique view), 637f
Advanced osteoarthritis, radiological changes (dorsopalmar radiographic projection), 667f
Age, clinical history, 9-11
Aged Thoroughbred broodmare, forelimb deformity, 10f
Aggrecan
　articular cartilage proteoglycan, 658
　monomer, schematic representation, 658f
Aggrecanase
　activation, 846-847
　interleukin-1 activation, 672f
Ah shi (tender points), 886
Albumin quotient (AQ), 138-139
Alkaline phosphatase (ALP), 948
All American Futurity, 1051-1052
Allodynia, development, 909
All-weather tracks, 976
　turf tracks, comparison, 974
Altered neurophysiology, clinical implications, 909
Aluminum rail shoes, 380-381
Ambulance
　design, improvements, 961
　operator training, 961
　supplies, 962
American Association of Equine Practitioners (AAEP)
　grading system framework, 71-72
　guidelines, 164
　information dissemination role, 2
　system, confusion, 72
American Endurance Ride Conference, 1137
American Quarter Horse Association (AQHA)
　formation, 1051-1052
　Racing Challenge, 1052
　stud book, 1052
American Quarter Horses, breaking, 1183
American Saddlebred, 1189
　back pain, 1191-1192
　breed, sport description, 1188-1189
　cervical myositis, 1195
　diagnostic analgesia, 1190
　distal hock joint pain, 1191
　distal phalanx
　　fractures, rarity, 1192
　　osteitis, 1192
　distal tarsitis, 1191
　fetlock joint, osteoarthritis/osteochondrosis, 1193
　frog pressure, maintenance, 1192
　gaits, 1189-1190
　　types, 1189-1190
　gluteal myositis, 1191-1192
　height, range, 1189
　hindlimb extensor tenosynovitis, 1195
　imaging considerations, 1190
　IRAP treatment, 1191
　lameness
　　conditions, 1191, 1194-1195
　　examination, 1190
　lateral gaits, ability, 1189
　navicular disease, 1192

American Saddlebred (Continued)
　palmar foot pain, 1192
　semimembranosus/semitendinosus myositis, 1194-1195
　shock wave therapy, 1191
　shoeing, 1190-1191
　soft tissue treatment, 1192
　stifle joint, osteoarthritis/osteochondrosis, 1193-1194
　stringhalt, 1194
　suspensory desmitis, 1194
　tarsocrural joint, osteoarthritis/osteochondrosis, 1192-1193
　tibial stress fractures, 1195
Amplitude, 905
Analgesia
　adjunctive therapies, 857-858
　benefits, 852
　characteristics, 856t
　SWT, impact, 919
Analog imaging, 218-219
Anamnesis, 9b
　clinical history, 9
Anaplasma-associated rhabdomyolysis, 832
Anatomy, language, 92
Anderson sling, 878
Anechoic, term (usage), 189t
Angiogram, three-dimensional volume-rendered images, 237f
Angiography, usage, 502-503
Angles, 20-21
Angular deformity, 33, 286-287
　compensation, 292
　objective assessment, radiology (usage), 641
Angular limb deformities
　congenital/developmental origin, 640-641
　diagnosis, 640-642
　growth rates, 641
　intervention, 642
　management, 640-642
　severity, 641
　subjective assessment, 641
　surgical management, 642-645
Animation, 300
Anlehnung (bit contract), 1112-1113
Anomalous first rib, postmortem specimen, 156f
Antebrachial region, lameness (association), 449
Antebrachiocarpal joints
　arthrocentesis, 120-121
　capsules, distention (detection), 999
　lameness, localization, 453
　osteoarthritis, 434
　pathological change, 1009
Antebrachium (forearm), 52
　anatomy, 449
　clinical diagnosis, 449-455
　compartment-like syndrome, 834
　digital palpation, 52
　distal aspect, analgesia, 114-115
　imaging, 449-455
　injuries, 1215
　puncture wounds, 454-455
　swelling, 455
　synovial cell sarcoma, identification, 693

Antibodies, serological testing, 137
Antidromic activity, development, 909
Antifungal drug administration regimens, 687t
Antiinflammatory drugs, usage, 142
Antimicrobial agents, bone concentration, 682
Antimicrobial drugs, constant rate infusion, 682
Antimicrobial-impregnated biodegradable drug delivery systems, 681
Antimicrobial susceptibility tests, 315
Aorta blood flow determination, first-pass radionuclide angiography (usage), 580
Aortoiliacofemoral thrombosis, 579-580
　clinical signs, 579-580
　rarity, 579
Apaloosa gelding, unbalance (weakness), 20f
Apical fractures, 404-405
Appendix QHs, 1182
Aquapuncture, 883-884
Aquatreds, 880
　usage, 880
Arabian Horse Registry of America, 1057, 1195
Arabian horses
　age, importance, 1198
　ALDDFT, desmitis, 1205
　conformation, lameness (relationship), 1197
　counterirritant therapy, 1203
　diagnostic analgesia, 1199
　distal hock joint pain, 1204
　distal interphalangeal joint, osteoarthritis, 1201-1202
　dynamic examination, 1198-1199
　feet, bruising/inflammation, 1200-1201
　flexion tests, 1198-1199
　gluteal pain (croup), 1203-1204
　history, 1195, 1197-1198
　hoof tester examination, 1198
　importation, 994
　lameness
　　conditions, 1200
　　diagnosis/management, 1200-1205
　　examination, 1197-1198
　　improvement, 1203
　metacarpophalangeal/metatarsophalangeal joints, osteoarthritis, 1204
　neurological examination, 1199-1200
　palmar foot pain, 1201-1202
　palpation, 1198
　performance classes, 1196, 1196b
　physical therapy, 1201
　proliferative periostitis, 1204
　proximal interphalangeal joint, osteoarthritis, 1205
　PSD, recurrence, 1202
　radiological abnormalities, 1201
　sacroiliac pain, 1203-1204
　saddle, examination, 1199
　shoeing, rules, 1197

Arabian horses (Continued)
　short-coupled lordotic back, 1089
　splint bone injuries, 1204-1205
　static examination, 1198
　stifle joints, osteoarthritis, 1202-1203
　suspensory desmitis, 1202
　thoracolumbar pain, 1203-1204
　training, impact, 1196-1197
　undiagnosed lameness, 1200
　visual examination, 1198
　work-related fractures, 1204-1205
Arabian international-level endurance horse, lateral radiographic view, 609f
Arabian mare, right carpus (dorsopalmar digital radiographic view), 10f
Arabian racehorses
　back pain, 1060-1061
　bones, fractures, 1061
　carpal osteochondral fragmentation, 1058
　diagnosis, absence, 1061
　distal hock joint pain, 1059-1060
　occurrence, 1060
　dorsal third metacarpal bone disease, 1061
　feet, lameness, 1060
　forelimb suspensory desmitis, 1059
　lineage, 1057
　metacarpophalangeal joint lameness, 1058
　myopathy, 1060
　origination, 1057
　primary hindlimb lameness, 1060-1061
　prognosis, 1059
　proliferative synovitis (villonodular synovitis), 1058
　proximal sesamoid bones, occurrence, 1061
　proximal suspensory desmitis, significance, 1059
　racing history, 1057
　racing-related lameness, 1057-1058
　recurrent exertional rhabdomyolysis, 1060
　stifle, carpal lameness (relationship), 1060
　stress fractures, 1061
　superficial digital flexor tendonitis, 1058-1059
　suspensory desmitis, 1059
　tarsocrural osteochondrosis, 1059-1060
　treatment, 1059
Arabian show horse, sporting event (history), 1195-1196
Arena maintenance, 1115
Arm, palpation, 53
Artemisia vulgaris, 883-884
Arthritis
　pain, 688-689
　pathological joint conditions, association, 688-689
Arthrocentesis
　approach, 117f
　performing, 119
Arthrodesis, indication, 445-446

Arthroscopic portals
  enlargement, 682
  open position, 255-257
Arthroscopic surgery
  advantages, 251-253
  aftercare instructions,
    differences, 259
  arthrotomy, comparison,
    251-253
  case selection, problems,
    252-253
  complications, 259
    reduction, 252
  disadvantages, 251-253
  fragment size, removal, 253
  functional capability, 252
  hyaluronan, intraarticular
    injections
    (recommendation), 438
  importance, 251
  instrumentation, 253-257
    expense, 252
  invasiveness, 258-259
  performing, 254-257
  postoperative care, 259
  principles, 253-257
  procedures, 258-259
  surgical experience, absence,
    252
  technique, 253-257
  usage, 439-440, 486-487
  versatility, increase, 252
  visibility, improvement, 251
Arthroscopy
  advantages, 260
  principles, 260
Articular cartilage, 244, 512-518,
    536-549
  biomechanical considerations,
    659-660
  changes, 255
  composition, 656
  defects, histology, 850f
  degradation
    occurrence, 661-662
    prevention, gene therapy
      (usage), 672-673
  dissecting flap, 618f
  extracellular matrix
    components, organization,
      657f
    presence, 668-669
  healing, models, 676
  lesions, healing (progress),
    849-852
  metabolism, skeletal
    biomarkers, 669-670
  MRI, usage, 244
  progressive loss, 849-850
  resurfacing treatments, 676
  structure/metabolism, 668-669
  traumatic damage, 353
Articular cartilage trauma,
    544-545
  prognosis, 545
  signs/diagnosis, 544
  treatment, 544-545
Articular chip fracture, 355
Articular contact, joint pressure
    (relationship), 279-280
Articular diseases, 536-549
Articular-epiphyseal cartilage
    complex (AECC), 617
  chondrocytes, impact, 617
  retained cartilage, thickening,
    618f
Articular fragments/lesions, 395

Articular grafting, 852
Articular margin, fractures, 175
Articular osteomyelitis, 683
Articular plantar process fractures,
    476-477
Articular processes
  abnormal findings, 601-602
  anatomy, 600-601
  synovial intervertebral
    articulations, 600-602
Articular soft tissue
  lubrication, requirement,
    659
  vascular supply, 1248f
Articular surface
  flattening, 465-466
  misalignment, mediolateral
    imbalance (impact),
      286f
Artifacts, 169, 229, 244-245
  impact, 169
  mirror image artifacts, 177
  MRI, usage, 244-245
  operator errors, 169-174
  urine contamination, 229
Artistic skills, development, 1
Aseptic preparation, performing,
    106
As low as reasonably achievable
    (ALARA), practice, 223
Aspartate aminotransferase (AST),
    136-137
Aspartate transaminase (AST)
  assessment usage, 818
  CK, serial activity comparison,
    818
  concentrations, impact, 1060
Association of Racing
    Commissioners International
    (ARCI) Class 4 drugs, 981
Asymmetrical physeal growth,
    641
Asymmetric hind torso
    movement, indicators, 249
Asymmetric vertical torso
    movement, expression, 249
Asymmetry, swelling (impact),
    33
Athletic function, return
    (prognosis), 357
Athletic injury, 282
Atypical equine rhabdomyolysis,
    157-158
Atypical myoglobinuria, 836-837
  occurrence, 836
  postmortem examination, 837
Australian Standardbred,
    1047-1051
  carpal joint disease, 1050
  diagnostic analgesia, 1048-1049
  distal phalanx, fracture, 1051
  distal tarsal joints,
    osteoarthritis, 1050
  fetlock joint, osteoarthritis,
    1049-1050
  flexion tests, 1048
  flexor tendons, ultrasonographic
    examination, 1049
  imaging considerations, 1049
  lameness
    conditions, 1049
    diagnosis/management,
      1049-1051
    examination, 1048
  nerve blocks, 1048
  pacers, involvement, 1047-1048
  proliferative synovitis, 1050

Australian Standardbred
    (Continued)
  proximal phalanx
    proximal plantar aspect,
      osteochondral fragments,
        1050
    sagittal fracture, 1051
  radiography, 1049
  rest, examination, 1048
  scintigraphy, 1049
  sport, description, 1047-1048
  stifle disease, 1051
  subsolar bruising, 1049
  superficial digital flexor
    tendonitis, 1050
  suspensory desmitis, 1050
  tarsocrural osteochondrosis,
    1051
  track surface, lameness
    (relationship), 1048
  training
    methods, 1048
    surface, lameness
      (relationship), 1048
  trotting, straight line, 1048
Autoimmune-mediated arthritis,
    689
Autologous chondrocytes,
    implantation, 852
Average fiber alignment score
    (A-FAS), 200
Avocado and soybean
    unsaponifiable (ASU) extracts,
    846
Avulsed fragment, detection, 404
Avulsion fractures, radiological
    detection, 404
Avulsion injuries, 405
Axial articular fragments, 492-493
  radiographic examination, 493
  removal, 493
Axial PSB fractures, 406
Axial skeleton, 86
  pelvis, attachment, 583
  racing injuries, 966
Axillary intertrigo infections, 1010
Azoturia, 1234-1235

B

Back
  caudodorsal views, 269f
  clinical examination, objective,
    593-594
  disorders, evaluation criteria,
    595t
  flexibility, 1090
  lesions, prognosis, 604
  problems, prevalence, 893-894
  thermographic evaluation, 924
Back-at-the-knee (calf knee), 15-16
  conformation, 25-26
  example, 26f
  impact, 434
Background radiation, 222
  impact, 222
Backing, 64
Back pain, 146f, 1161
  acupuncture, 605
    impact, 886
  alternative medicines, 605
  clinical assessment, difficulty,
    922
  diagnosis, 593-596
  inspection, 594
  local injections, 604-605
  management, 604-605
  mesotherapy, 605

Back pain (Continued)
  mobilization, 594-595
  movement, restriction
    (determination), 595
  palpation, 54, 594
  physical examination, 594-595
  presence/degree, 596
  pressure, 594
  prognosis, 604
  riding/harness, examination,
    596
  surgery, 605
  SWT application, 918
  systemic treatment, 604
  training management, 605
  in vivo kinematic studies,
    595-596
Backs
  problems, evaluation, 898
Bacterial infectious arthritis,
    fungal infectious arthritis
    (clinical manifestation
    comparison), 685
Badminton
  English event, 1123
  winner, 1124f
Balance, 18-19
  assessment, 18-19
    diagrammatic depiction, 19f
  dynamic balance, 285
  impact, 282
  optimum, 284-285
  radiological assessment, 290f
  static balance, 284-285
Balloon constant rate infusion
    systems, 682
Bandages
  application, 859f
  principles, 858
  stability/travel, 858
  usage, 426, 858
Bandaging, indications, 858
Bandy-legged conformation,
    22-23
Barefooted horse, natural balance
    trimming, 304-305
Bar firing, usage, 868
Barrel horses, turning, 1182f
Barrel racers, horse training,
    1181
Barrel racing, 1180-1181
  cloverleaf, diagram, 1180f
  discipline, 1181
  initiation, 1180
Barrel racing horses, 1180-1183
  conformation, 1181
  distal hock OA, 1182
  forelimbs, PSD (commonness),
    1182
  hindlimb proximal suspensory
    desmitis/suspensory branch
    desmitis, commonness,
    1182
  historical data, 1181
  lameness
    diagnosis/management,
      1182-1183
    examination, 1182
  medial femorotibial joint pain,
    occurrence, 1182-1183
  musculoskeletal problems, 1181
  performance problems, 1181
  shoeing considerations, 1183
  training, 1181
Barrel racing shoe, 295-296
Bars, 296-297, 303
  extension, 296-297

Baseline lameness, 3, 66, 80
  flexion tests, 80-86
  identification, 149
Base-narrow deformities, 30
Base-narrow forelimb
    conformation, 23f
Base-narrow travel, 30
Base-wide, toed-in conformation,
    22f
Base-wide, toed-out conformation,
    22f, 1024
Base-wide deformities, 30
Base-wide forelimb conformation,
    22f
Basillar fractures, 405
Basisesamoid block, perineural
    analgesia, 125
Basket weave, 309
Beat, term (usage), 64
Behavioral abnormalities, 11
Being broke in the middle, 1190
Belgian draft horse, shivers
    (raised tail/hindlimb
    overflexion characteristic),
    561f
Belgian gelding, right femoral
    head/neck fracture, 41f
Belgian Warmblood show
    jumper, left front pastern
    (lateromedial radiographic
    image), 1093f
Bench-knee conformation,
    171-172
Bench knee (offset knee), 15-16
Bending, 92
Beta-aminopropionitrile fumarate
    characteristics, 714
    treatment regimen, 868
Biceps brachii
  attachment, tearing, 462
  enthesopathy, 462
  humeral tubercles, transverse
    ultrasonographic image,
    464f
  lesions, 472
  tendonitis, 470, 806
    diagnosis, ultrasonographic
      examination, 470
    treatment, 470
Biceps brachii tendon
  lesions, 155
  mineralization/ossification,
    471
  rupture, 470
    rarity, 470
  transverse ultrasonographic
    image, 464f
Bicipital apparatus, congenital
    abnormalities, 470
Bicipital bursa, 456
  analgesia, 124
  diagnosis, 124
Bien jheng llun jhi, 887
Big lick, 1186-1187
Biglycan (proteoglycan), 700
Bilateral femoral nerve paralysis,
    occurrence, 562
Bilateral hindlimb suspensory
    desmitis, 39f
Bilateral ilial wing fractures, 555
Bilaterally symmetrical forelimb,
    71
Bilateral transection, 717-718
Biologically based therapies,
    846-848
Biological structures, breakage,
    270

Biomarkers
  circadian variability, impact,
    949
  diet, impact, 949-950
  measurability, 947
Biomechanical force, impact, 624
Biomechanics
  fundamentals, 90-91
  impact, 275-276
  terms, definition, 271b
Bipartite navicular bone, 343-344
Bisphosphonate drug, attention,
    490
Bisphosphonate treatment,
    impact, 952
Bi Syndrome, 889-891
Bit contact, 1113
Bitmap (BMP) formats, 170
Bladder
  meridian, acupuncture point,
    882f
  radioactive urine, 574
  superimposition, 228
Bleeding, blunt trauma/fractures
    (impact), 33
Blindfolding, 136
Blinding, 923
Blind spavin, 59-60
Blind splints, treatment, 1045
Blister beetles, 836
Blistering, 867-868
  process, 867
  usage, 867
Blocks, 297
Blood-brain barrier, compromise,
    139
Blood flow, increase, 688
  exercise/injury, impact, 697
Blood Stasis pattern, 887
Blunt trauma, impact, 33
Body length, importance, 20
Body lesions, 749-750
Body motion (measurement),
    kinematic technique (usage),
    246
Body-mounted inertial sensors,
    249
Body posture, clues, 39
Body segments, conformation
    (structural relationship),
    895-896
Body size, 621
Bog spavin, 517-518, 1225
  thoroughpin, differentiation, 59
Bone biomarkers, 947
  abbreviations, 947b
  age, relationship, 950
  classification, 947
  clinical applications, 950-951
  dorsal metacarpal disease,
    relationship, 951
  exercise, impact, 951-952
  fracture assessment, 951
  gender, impact, 950
  osteoarthritis, relationship, 951
  usage, 950-951
Bone bruising, 545
  prognosis, 546
  signs/diagnosis, 545
  treatment, 545-546
Bone curettes, usage, 254
Bone formation
  biomarkers, 948t
  changes, biomarker
    information, 948-949
Bone fragility disorder, 158
Bone glaprotein (BGP), 948

Bone islands (enostosis-like
    lesions), 464-465
Bone marrow
  aspirate, 762
  injection, 762
Bone marrow-derived MSCs
    (BM-MSCs), 761-762
  collection, 761-762
Bone-on-bone grating, 38
Bone-pin interface, total stress, 864
Bone resorption
  biomarkers, 948t, 949
  changes (measurement),
    biomarkers (usage), 949
Bones, 213-215, 243
  abscess, 214-215
    ultrasonographic imaging,
      214-215
  adaptation
    failure, 928
    jogging, usage, 957
  asymmetry, 35
  cell activity, biochemical
      markers (factors), 949-950
  density, localized increase, 942
  evaluation, care, 174
  fatigue, exercise (relationship),
      954-955
  fractures, 213-214
  geometric parameters (change),
      adaptive exercise (usage),
      957
  healing, gene therapy (usage),
      673
  locomotion, 278
  loss, 170
  modeling
    activity, 935
    existence, 225-226
    models, Wolff's law, 169
  MRI, usage, 243
  reduction, 271
  remodeling, 955
    activity, 935
    occurrence, 955
  repetitive overloading injury,
      1144-1145
  resorption
    osteolysis, 170
    Type I collagen
      C-telopeptides, marker
      (usefulness), 670
  scintigraphy, 215-216
    clinical tool, value, 229
    indications/case selection,
      229-230
  screws, usage, 390
  spavin, cryotherapy, 871
  spur, 171-172
  stimuli, reaction, 170
  stress, reduction, 489
  structure/metabolism, 668-669
  surfaces
    appearance, 213
    scanning, 169
  SWT application, 915-916
  tetracycline labeling, 326, 334
  trauma, 392
  turnover
    changes, 952
    ethic differences, 950
    seasonal changes, impact, 950
  uptake, problems, 222-223
  in vitro bone testing, 956
  in vivo strain measurements,
      954
  Wolff's law, application, 957

Bone scan phases, 223-224
Bone-seeking isotopes,
    accumulation, 667
Bone spavin
  fibrous/bony swelling, 60f
  term, usage, 59-60
Bone-specific alkaline phosphatase
    (BAP) (BALP), 670, 948
  isoform, 670
  usefulness, 951
Bony abnormalities, radiological
    evaluation, 941-942
Bony asymmetry, 37-39
Bony pelvis, position
    (assessment), 565f
Bony prominences, pressure
    (application), 572
Bony swelling, 33
Boots, usage, 426
Borrelia burgdoferi, 156, 690
  antibody titers, 137
Botulinum toxin type B, usage,
    560
Bowed tendon, 707
Bowlegged conformation, 22-23
Box rest, 357
  restriction, treatment, 574-575
Brachial plexus, 456
  damage, 473-474
Brachiocephalicus muscles
  lesions, 472
  palpation
    problems, 457
    resentment, 611-612
Brachium, 53
  anatomical considerations,
    456-457
  clinical signs, 457
  diagnosis, 457-458
  differential diagnosis, 460-474
  imaging, 458-460
  local analgesia, 457-458
  nuclear scintigraphy, 458-460
  radiography, 458
  ultrasonography, 458
Brachytherapy, 874
  treatment, 874
  involvement, 874
Braid, 309
Branch injury, PSB fracture
    (association), 754
Branch lesions, 751-754
Breakaway roping, calf roping
    (comparison), 1175
Breakaway roping horses,
    1175-1176
  conformation, 1175
  historical data, 1175
  lameness, diagnosis/
    management, 1175-1176
  performance problems, 1175
  shoeing considerations, 1176
  sport, description, 1175
Breakover
  calks, impact, 297
  modification, 299-300
  onset, 283
  phase, 284
  point, 299-300
    occurrence, 304
  position, sagittal plane, 287
  redirection, 300
Breed
  importance, 11
  pastern disorders, predilection,
    388
Breeders' Cup series, 978

Breeding stallions, 1235-1240
  aortoiliac thrombosis, 1238
  arthrodesis, 1236
  breeding
      management/schedule,
        1238-1240
    performance, monitoring,
        1240
  cervical vertebral malformation,
      treatment, 1236
  diagnostic considerations/
      therapy, 1236-1238
  distal phalanx, fractures, 1237
  ejaculation facilitation,
      management/
      pharmacological aids,
        1237b
  examination, 1235-1236
  fitness/weight management,
      1238
  ground semen collections,
      1240
  history, 1235
  injuries, 1237
  laminitis, 1237
  libido
    enhancement, management/
        pharmacological aids,
          1237b
    maintenance, 1238-1239
  management, 1238-1240
  mare, down grade position,
      1239f
  medications, usage, 1237t
  muscle disease, 1237
  musculoskeletal evaluation,
      1235
  neurological disease, 1236
  neurological examination,
      1235
  one mount rule, 1240
  osteoarthritis, 1236
  pain
    control, 1236
    management, 1238
  pharmacologically induced
      ex copula ejaculation,
      1240
  sheds
    flooring materials, 1239t
    handling considerations,
        1239-1240
  sore back, 1236
  sore feet, 1236-1237
  spotting, 1240f
  walk/trot, observation, 1235
Brief intense TENS, 906-907
Brisket
  injuries, 1215
  traumatic injury, 1215f
British Equine Veterinary
    Association (BEVA)
  establishment, 2
  guidelines, 164
  prepurchase examination
      worksheet, 1084f-1088f
British Horseracing Authority,
    Equine Welfare database,
    975
Broken-back foot-pastern,
    correction (complication),
    292-293
Broken-back hoof-pastern axis,
    treatment, 293
Broken-forward foot axis, DIP
    joint flexural deformity,
    291

Broken forward foot-pastern axis,
    31
Broodmare, 1240-1242
  breeding management
      considerations, 1242
  diagnostic considerations/
      therapy, 1241-1242
  foaling-related injuries, 1241
  husbandry, 1242
  laminitis, 1241
  limbs, enlargement/swelling,
      1241
  neurological disease, 1241-1242
  old injuries, 1242
  osteoarthritis, 1241
  prepubic tendon rrupture,
      1241
  rhabdomyolysis, 1241
  sore feet, 1241
  soundness, 1240
  ventral body wall hernias, 1241
Brucella abortus, 799
Brucella titers, measurement, 609
Bruise, 310-311
Bruised heels, lameness, 984-985
Bruising, diagnosis, 1005
Brushing, 74
  occurrence, 301
Bucked-knee, 39
Bucked-shin complex
  etiology/pathogenesis, 953-958
  exercise/bone fatigue,
      relationship, 954-955
  management, 953-958
  research findings, 953-956
  third metacarpal bone stiffness
      measurements, 954
  in vivo strain measurements,
      954
  Wolff's law, application, 957
Bucked shins, 502, 964, 1011
  commonness, 958
  cryotherapy, 871
  development, 940
  dorsal metacarpal disease,
      989-990
  likelihood, galloping (impact),
      956
  prevention, training
      program, principles, 957
    usage, 957-958
  rarity, 1018
  training schedule, interruption,
      958
Buckling, 136
Bull-noose foot conformation,
    32f
Bumpers, 1063
Burghley, English event, 1123
Bursae
  analgesia, 122
  flattening, 799
Bursa podotrochlearis, 316-317
Bursoscopy, 265-266
  equipment, 260
  infection, complications,
      265-266
  postoperative management/
      results, 265-266
  principles, 260
  reports, limitation, 265
  surgical principles, 260
  surgical technique, 260, 265
Bursoscopy, reports (limitation),
    265
Butter knife malleable retractors,
    384

Buttress foot, 32, 355
Byerley Turk, 1195

C

Cadence, 1112
Calcaneal bursa, 133, 799-800
  analgesia, indications, 133
  anatomical aspects, 509
  chronic distention, 799-800
  injuries, 799
Calcaneal osteitis
  prognosis, 525
  radiological signs, 524-525
Calcaneal tendonitis, 803
Calcanean fasciculus
  longitudinal ultrasound scan,
      211f
  proximal avulsion fracture,
      211
Calcaneus, 38-39
  dorsomedial-plantarolateral
      oblique radiographic view,
      782f
  flexed lateromedial/skyline
      views, 520
  flexed plantaroproximal-
      plantarodistal radiographic
      view, 524f
  infection (septic) osteitis,
      524-525
  IRU, lateral delayed phase
      scintigraphic image, 1031f
  proximal aspect
    swelling, 58f
    transverse anatomical section,
        93f
  skyline radiographic view,
      783f
Calcified cartilage
  debridement/removal
      requirement, 850
  microfracture, 438
Calcinosis circumscripta, 548-549,
    693
  examination, reason, 549
  lesions, 548-549
  prognosis, 549
  signs/diagnosis, 549
  treatment, 549
Calcitonin, 848
  direct chondroprotective effect,
      848
Calcium, deficiency, 625
Calf-knee (back-at-the-knee)
    conformation, conformation,
    26f
Calf-kneed conformation, 16
Calf-knee (sheep-knee)
    conformation, 25-26
Calf roping, breakaway roping
    (comparison), 1175
Calf roping horses, 1175-1176
  conformation, 1175
  historical data, 1175
  lameness, diagnosis/
      management, 1175-1176
  performance problem, 1175
  shoeing considerations, 1176
  sport, description, 1175
California Reined Cow Horse
    Association, 1176
Calks, 297
  forging, 297f
  impact, 297
  position, 297
Camera-based kinematic gait
    analysis, usage, 247

Camped-out in front, diagram,
    26f
Camped under, appearance, 41
Camped-under conformation, 29f
Camped under in front, 25
  diagram, 26f
Canadian National Horse Show,
    1195-1196
Cancellous bone plate, access,
    850
Canker, 319, 1221-1222
  occurrence, 319
Canter
  gait, 1190
  pirouette, 1113f
  three-beat gait, 4, 65
Cantharides (Spanish fly), impact,
    867
Capillary leakage, occurrence, 688
Capped elbow, 800
Capped hock, 58, 800
  swelling, 58f
Capsulitis, 1144
Capsulitis/synovitis, 395-396
  clinical signs, 395
  diagnosis, 395-396
  intraarticular hyaluronan, 396
  treatment, 396
Carboxyl propeptide, type II
    collagen concentrations, 669
Carpal arthrodesis, 445-446
Carpal bone
  attachment, 427
  distal row, dorsoproximal-
      dorsodistal (skyline)
      radiographic view, 430f,
        438f
  dorsal aspect, palpation, 52f
  incomplete ossification, 643f
  proximal row
    tangential view, 429
  proximal view
    transverse slices, 99f
  slab fractures, 443-444
Carpal canal
  anatomy, 777
  enclosure, 777
  SDF tendonitis, 779
Carpal chip fractures, 18
  development, 16
  osteochondral fragmentation,
      comparison, 434
Carpal flexion test, 83, 83f
  specificity, 429
Carpal flexor tendon sheath
    (carpal sheath, tenosynovitis,
    263
Carpal fractures, 988
Carpal hygroma, 448-449
Carpal joints, 120-121
  communications/boundaries,
      427-428
  flexural deformities, 645-646
  osteochondral fragmentation/
      chip fractures, 1058
Carpal lameness
  abduction, 73
  clinical characteristic/diagnosis,
      428-432
  pathognomonic facts, 428
  predisposition, 21-22
Carpal osteochondral fragments,
    434
  absence, 669
  occurrence, 434-435
Carpal palmar retinaculum,
    desmotomy, 264

Carpal region
  lameness, 1163
  soft tissue injuries, 447-448
Carpal retinacular release, 719
  accomplishment, 719
Carpal sheath (carpal flexor
      tendon sheath), 124, 263-264
  analgesia, 124
  anatomy, 263-264
  chronic enlargement, trauma
      (impact), 778
  deep digital flexor tendonitis,
      727
    unusualness, 779
  distal half, examination, 264
  distention, 423
  effusion, 777
  hemorrhage, 778
  postoperative care, 264
  solitary osteochondroma, 779
  surgical technique, 264
  synovitis, 777
  tenoscopy, 719
  tenosynovitis, 263, 709-710
Carpal synovial sheath
  extension, 777
  lameness, clinical signs, 777
Carpal tenosynovitis, 448
  differentiation, 51f
Carpometacarpal joints
  osteoarthritis, 401, 434
    clinical signs, 401
    diagnosis, 401
    treatment, 402
  positive contrast arthrogram,
      113f
Carpus, 51-52
  analgesic techniques,
      interpretation, 113-114
  anatomy, 426-428
  angulation, 290
  antebrachiocarpal joint,
      effusion (dorsal view),
      693f
  bilateral flexural deformity,
      646f
  catastrophic injury, rarity,
      964-965
  conditions, 432-449
  digit extensor tendon sheath,
      effusion (dorsal view),
      693f
  dorsal aspect
    aseptic preparation, 121
    chronic osteochondral
        fragments, 439
    warmth, detection, 51
  dorsal surface, temperature/heat
      (increase), 428
  dorsopalmar image, usage, 1041
  dorsopalmar radiographic view,
      643f
  effusion/heat, 435
  flexion, 52, 1052-1053
    ulnaris lateralis functions,
        462
  flexural deformity, 646f
  fractures, 447
  joint capsule, density, 427
  lameness, 964-965, 987-988
  lateral delayed scintigraphic
      image, 232f
  lateral views, 100f
  lateromedial radiographic view,
      789f
  osteoarthritis, 432-434
  osteochondrosis, rarity, 446

Carpus (Continued)
  palmar aspect, osteochondral
      fragments (occurrence),
      439
  racing injuries, 964-965
  radiological anatomy, 429-431
  sagittal T2 gradient echo image,
      243f
  soft tissue injuries, 447-448
  static flexion, response, 428-429
  synovitis, 1053
  valgus deformity, dorsopalmar
      radiographic view, 643f
Carpus valgus conformation,
      21-22
Carriage horses
  foot pain, 1211
Carriage horses
  tying up episodes, 1212
Cartilage
  abaxial surface, 321
  canals, involvement, 620-621
    mechanism, 621
  damage, 432, 435
  degeneration, subchondral
      bone plate thickening
      (cause-and-effect
      relationship), 660
  development, foot shape
      (impact), 322
  flaps, reattachment, 852
  healing (promotion), gene
      therapy (impact), 673
  ligamentous attachments, 321
  matrix degeneration
    MMPs, implication, 663t
    MMPs, role, 662
    pathological changes,
        photomicrograph, 661f
  metabolism, cytokines
      (classification/actions),
      663t
  necrosis, 1220-1221
  nutrition, 659
  proteins, presence, 658
  resurfacing, 259
    techniques, usage, 259, 438
  zones/layers, 656
Cartilage oligomeric matrix
      protein (COMP), 658,
      699-700
  abundance, 669
  levels
    elevation, 669-670
    variation, 700f
  molecule, cartoon, 700f
  subunits, 699-700
Cartilage-on-cartilage lubrication,
      mechanisms, 659
Cassia occidentalis, 836
Cast applications, 861-862
  indications, 858
  limitations, 862
Cast bandages, 861
  combination, 861
Cast removal, 787
Catastrophic distal limb fractures,
      972
Catastrophic forelimb distal
      limb fractures, distribution,
      973f
Catastrophic injuries
  defining, difficulty, 968
  McIII involvement, 963-964
  types, 969-972
Catastrophic musculoskeletal
      injuries, occurrence, 976

Catastrophic sinker foot,
      lateromedial radiograph,
      375f
Category IV T-lesions, 202t
Category VI T-lesions, 203t
Category V T-lesions, 202t
Cathepsins, 624
Catheters
  attachment, 855f
  placement, 855f
Caudal articular processes,
      synovial interverteral
      articulations, 592-593
Caudal cervical synovial
      articulations, muscle
      fasciculation (association),
      838
Caudal cervical vertebral articular
      processes, arthropathy, 650
Caudal cruciate ligament injuries,
      543-544
  prognosis, 544
  signs/diagnosis, 543
  treatment, 543-544
Caudal epidural drug
      administration, 853
Caudal margin, dorsal surface
      (evaluation), 589-590
Caudal neck
  nerve root impingement,
      613
  region, osteoarthritis, 613-614
Caudal PVC, full-limb forelimb
      bandage, 860f
Caudal radial osteochondroma/
      exotosis, impact, 162
Caudal thoracic vertebrae,
      vertebral bodies (lateral
      radiographic view), 603f
Cautery, 868-869
  performing, 868
Cell-based grafting, 676
Cellulitis, 33
  infection, impact, 166-167
  trauma, impact, 166
Center of balance (gravity), 4f
Central nervous system (CNS)
  disease, EHV-1 infection
      (impact), 139
Central pattern generators (CPGs),
      908
Central sensitization
  allodynia, development, 909
  antidromic activity,
      development, 909
  reduction, 910
Central tarsal bones
  fractures, 518-519
  incomplete ossification, 517
Centrodistal joint, 129
  arthrocentesis, difficulty, 129
  impact, 513
  osteoarthritis, 1120-1121
  synovial cavity separation,
      128-129
  tarsometatarsal joints,
      communication, 509
Cerebellar abiotrophy, 1235
Cerebrospinal fluid (CSF)
  albumin, predominance,
      138-139
  analysis, 137-139
  aspiration, 137-139
    performing, frequency
        (increase), 139
  cell count, values (usefulness),
      139

Cerebrospinal fluid (Continued)
  characteristics, 138
  CK concentrations, increase,
      138
  contamination, 139
  Western blot analysis,
      introduction, 139
Cervical cord compression,
      diagnosis, 143
Cervical myositis, 1195
Cervical osteoarthritis, pain,
      1111-1112
Cervical pain, cervical vertebral
      arthropathy (impact), 653
Cervical radiographs
  evaluation, semiquantitative
      scoring system (usage),
      140
  subjective/objective evaluation,
      651
Cervical spinal cord compression,
      142-143
  diagnosis, 143
Cervical spine
  anatomy, 606
  cervical vertebrae, cystlike
      lesions, 615
  cervical vertebral mobilization,
      general anesthesia, 616
  clinical conditions, 609-616
  clinical examination, 606-607
  clinical presentation, reasons,
      606
  computed tomography, 608
  congenital abnormalities, 609
  diagnostic tests, 609
  diskospondylitis, 614
  electromyography, 609
  first/second cervical vertebrae,
      subluxation, 609-610
  fracture, 614-615
  imaging considerations, 608-609
  jugular vein thrombophlebitis,
      615-616
  myeloma, 615
  neck, 53-54
    stiffness, 616
  neck musculature, disorders,
      611-612
  nuchal ligament, insertional
      desmopathy, 610-611
  nuclear scintigraphy, 608
  occipito-atlantoaxial
      malformation, 609
  osteoarthritis, 612-614
  palpation, 53-54
  radiography, 608
  semispinalis injury, 610-611
  sixth/seventh cervical vertebrae,
      subluxation, 610
  thermography, 609
  ultrasonography, 608
  vertebral osteomyelitis, 615
Cervical stenotic myelopathy
      (CSM)
  clinical signs, 649-650
    insidiousness, 649
  convalescence/rehabilitation,
      duration, 654
  diagnosis, 650-653
  fatal postoperative
      complications, 654
  grading scale, 649-650
  likelihood (prediction),
      radiography (usage), 652
  management, 653
  neurological deficits, 649

Cervical stenotic myelopathy
  (Continued)
  neurological status
      (improvement), cervical
      vertebral fusion (impact),
      654
  postoperative prognosis,
      determination, 654
  ratiometric measurements, use,
      652
  semiquantitative scoring
      system, 652
  surgical intervention, 653-654
  surgical treatment, 653-654
Cervical vertebrae
  components, 606
  cystlike lesions, 615
  fractures, 614
  lateral radiographic view, 651f
  myelographic examination,
      lateral radiographic view,
      650f
  plain radiography, usage, 651f
  radiological appearance,
      variations, 608
  ultrasonographic examination,
      653f
Cervical vertebral fusion, impact,
      654
Cervical vertebral malformation,
      631
  treatment, 1236
Cervical vertebral osteomyelitis,
      615
Channel pain
  diagnosis, acupoints, 888f
  mediation, 890f
Chemical neurectomy, 341-342
Chemical restraint, role, 106
Chemical synovectomy, 876
Chester bell, 1062
Chinese medical acupuncture
      diagnosis/treatment, 882-883
Chinese medical theories, 882-883
Chip fractures, 175
  occurrence, 1009
Chiropractic, 884, 892
  adverse effects, 900
  areas, clinical signs, 899
  care
      indications, 898-899
      response, 895-896
  clinical evaluation, 895-898
  complications, 900
  contraindications, 899
  diagnostic/therapeutic
      approaches, 898-899
  evaluation/treatment, clinical
      indications, 896b
  expertise, 894
  history, 893
  initiation, 895
  physical examination, 896
  posttreatment
      recommendations, 900
  practitioner qualifications,
      892-893
  prognosis, 900
  recommendations, 900
  research, 894-895
  techniques, 899-900
      effects, assessment, 895
      examination, 899-900
  treatment, 907
      goal, 894
  usage, success, 886
  usefulness, 893

Chiropractors
  animal treatment, 893
  training/experience, 899
Chondrocytes, 659
  clusters, 619f
  role, 661-664
Chondroitin sulfate (CS)
  components, 845
  glycosaminoglycan (GAG), 669
Chronic avulsion injury, repair,
      319
Chronic back pain, 886
Chronic canker, proliferative
      granulation tissue, 1222f
Chronic dietary imbalance,
      825-826
Chronic exertional
      rhabdomyolysis, 825-826
  chronic dietary imbalance,
      825-826
  storage disorder, 827-828
Chronic heel pain, distal phalanx,
      363f
Chronic infectious arthritis,
      678-679
Chronic infectious tenosynovitis,
      establishment, 790
Chronic lameness, front foot size
      (disparity), 34f
Chronic laminitic foot
  high-resolution sagittal 3D T1
      spoiled gradient-echo MRI
      image, 376f
  lateromedial venogram, 377f
Chronic laminitis, 374-377
  continuous supportive foot
      management, 374
  disease progression/
      exacerbation, 375
  toe modeling, association, 362
  treatment, 378
  venographic appearance,
      377-378
Chronic low-grade high-speed
      MTP joint lameness,
      occurrence, 493
Chronic osteochondral fragments,
      439
Chronic proliferative
      (villonodular) synovitis,
      396-397, 690
  clinical signs, 396
  diagnosis, 396
  treatment, 396-397
Chronic sacroiliac joint injuries,
      compensatory stiffness/pain,
      586-587
Chronic sacroiliac joint injuries
      (identification), nuclear
      scintigraphy (usage), 590
Chronic sacroiliac joint
      instability, acute sacroiliac
      ligament injuries (impact),
      585
Chronic sacroiliac joint
      subluxation, rectal
      examination, 586-587
Chronic synovitis
  radiation therapy, impact, 876
  treatment, 873
Chronic tarsal region pain, excess,
      510
Chronic tenosynovitis, 790-791
  diagnosis, 790
  origin, 790
  treatment, 790-791
Chronic traumatic synovitis, 690

Churchill hock test, 60-61
  demonstration, 61f
  development, 60
  performing, 61f
  usefulness, 60-61
Churchill test, 500, 513
Circadian variability, 949
Circle, lameness (worsening), 78
Circling, 77-79
  hindlimb lameness,
      relationship, 78-79
  lameness
      improvement, 78
      pronouncement, 77
Circumferential fibrocartilage, 94
Circumferential subcutaneous
      infiltration, 107
Claiming races, 979
Claudication, 3
Clinical examination, importance,
      147
Clinical history
  importance, 8-9
  information, 9-15
Clinical imaging, 267-269
Clinical physitis, recognition, 639
Clinical problems, types, 921b-922b
Clinical signs, confusion, 232-233
Clinical superficial digital flexor
      tendonopathy, 701
Clinical tendonitis, initiation,
      704
Clinical ultrasonography, 199-204
  quantitative analysis, 199-200
  quantitative terms, 200-203
Clips, 299
Closed suction drainage,
      management, 682
Close nail, 309
  placement, 310f
Clostridial myositis, 832-833
  clinical signs, 832
  diagnosis, 832
  treatment, 832-833
Clubfeet, 27f, 305
  conformation, presence, 33-34
  size, 305
  sole callus, difference, 305
Clydesdale yearling, calf-knee
      conformation, 27f
Cob gelding, feet (radiographic
      views), 365f
Coblation technology, usage, 260
Cob-type horses, movement
      (induction), 595
Coexistent lameness, 3-4
  assignation difficulty, 4
Cold-backed horse, 909
Cold-blooded trotters, training,
      1076
  duration, 1076
Cold edema, 164-165
Cold shoeing, hot shoeing
      (contrast), 298
Cold-water therapy, application,
      1033-1034
Colitis, 372
Collagenase-induced superficial
      digital flexor tendonitis, 917
Collagen fibril
  components, 696
  diameter, 696
      regional differences, 701-702
  organization, schematic
      representation, 657f
  populations, differences, 701f
  strength, 699

Collagens, 656-658
  fibers, location, 245
Collapsed heel conformation,
      324-325
Collateral blood supply,
      promotion, 580
Collateral desmitis, 498
Collateral ligament avulsions,
      410f
  injuries, 410
Collateral ligament injuries, 410,
      544
  cause, 691
  periarticular lesions, 148
  prognosis, 544
  signs/diagnosis, 544
  treatment, 410, 544
Collateral ligaments, 448, 812
  DIP/navicular bone,
      relationship, 329f
  disruption, 498
  luxation/subluxation, 498
  origination, 533
  tearing, 498
Collateral sesamoidean ligaments
      (CSLs), 324
  desmotomy, 342
  dorsal/palmar aspects, 116
  relationship, 89-90
  tension, increase, 324
Colt pacer, images, 1034f
Commercial breeders, public
      auction, 978
Commercial market, 978
Comminuted, term (usage), 445
Comminuted carpal fracture,
      443-444
Comminuted fractures, 361, 445
  occurrence, 445
  open reduction/reconstruction,
      bone screws (usage), 390
Common digital extensor (CDE),
      113-114
  muscle, compound muscle,
      785
  tendon, arthrocentesis, 119
Common digital extensor tendon
      (CDET)
  appearance, 785
  infection, 806
  location, 811
  rupture, 787-788
      diagnosis, 787
      occurrence, 787
Compartment syndrome,
      fasciotomy/relief, 506-507
Compensatory lameness, 3-4,
      66-67
  development, 67
  limbs, overloading, 66-67
  problem, 67
  three-dimensional
      reconstructions, voxel
      density value (usage), 235
Competitive driving, 1205
Complementary lameness, 66-67
Complete analgesia, goal, 102-103
Complete avulsion injuries,
      treatment, 319
Complete bar, 296-297
Complete ilial wing fracture, 557
Complete immobilization, 878
Complete radial fractures, open
      reduction/internal fixation
      (requirement), 452
Complete sacroiliac ligament
      disruption, 585

Composite materials, usage, 308-309
Compressed foam pad, trimming, 381f
Compression, 92
  force, clinical perspective, 77
Computed tomography (CT)
  advantages, 239
  angiogram, three-dimensional volume-rendered images, 237f
  availability, 431
  clinical applications, 236-238
  contrast media, 235-236
  diagnostic imaging modality, 234
  disadvantages, 239
  equine table, usage, 234f
  equipment, 234-235
  image
    display, 235-236
    processing, 235-236
    reconstruction, 235
  physics, 234
  tissues, density values, 235b
  transverse images, 237f
  usefulness, 237-238
Computer-image analysis, usage, 16-17
Computerized saddle pressure analysis images, 1131f
Concaved inner surface, 296
Concomitant bilateral forelimb/hindlimb lameness, 3-4
Concours Complet International (CCI), 1123
Condylar fractures, 408-409, 1029
  clinical signs, 408
  diagnosis, 408-409
  occurrence, 496
  prognosis, 408
  treatment, lag screws (usage), 408
Condyles, subchondral bone pain, 146-147
Cones (phase), 1206
Conformation, 282-293, 428
  balance, relationship, 18-19
  clinical outcomes, 17
  description, 282
  evaluation, 18-21
    relevance, 15
  fault, 434
  hereditary aspects, 15-16
  impact, 278-280, 282
  lameness, relationship, 6
  objective evaluation, possibility, 16-18
  optimum, 284-285
  problems, 285-288
    treatment, 291-293
  role, study, 17
  static conformation, 284-285
  structural relationship, 895-896
Congenital abnormalities, 609
Congenital bipartite navicular bone, history, 343
Congenital flexural deformities, 645-647
  distal interphalangeal (DIP) joints, involvement, 645
  prognosis, 647
  splint construction, 647
  treatment, 645
Connecting fibrocartilage, 94
Connective tissues, growth factors (impact), 699

Constant rate infusion (CRI), 682
Contact phase (stance phase), definition, 271b
Contact with the bit, 1113
Continuous linear echogenic structures, 169
Contralateral foot, shoe application, 866
Contralateral forelimb
  contact, 301
  front foot, hitting, 74
Contralateral hindlimb (diagonal hindlimb), front feet (hitting), 75
Contralateral limb, compensatory lameness, 67
Contrast radiography, usage, 388
Cooked linseed hoof packs, 1100-1101
Coon-footed axis, 31
Copper
  deficiency, 625
  dietary levels, studies, 623
  supplementation, impact, 630
  supplements, provision, 623
Cord, 133
Core injuries, 813
Core lesions, 814-815
  platelet-rich plasma, ultrasound-guided injection, 1118
Corium, progressive rotation/penetration, 381-382
Coronary band
  coronitis, inflammation, 1144
  palpation, 45
    dorsal joint pouch, assessment, 46f
  unevenness, 45f
  vasculature, 282
Coronary band lacerations, 318-319
  diagnosis, 319
  history/clinical signs, 318
  prognosis, 319
  treatment, 319
Corrective farriery, 930
Corrective shoeing, 289-290, 302
  diagnosis, usage, 302
Cortical bone
  changes (continuum), scintigraphic examination (usage), 230-231
  stress-related bone injury, 230-231
Cortical bone injury
  clinical examination, 936
  clinical signs, 936
  diagnostic analgesia, 936
  diagnostic imaging, 937-938
  locations, 938-946
  magnetic resonance imaging, 938
  nuclear scintigraphy, 937
  pathophysiology, 935-936
  radiography, 937
  ultrasonography, 937-938
Cortical stress-related bone injury, pathological continuum, 936
Cortical thickness, change, 170
Corticosteroids
  ARCI Class 4 drugs, 981
  HA, combination, 844-845
  injections, 439
  usage, policies/regulations, 981
Cortisone, presence, 370-371

Cosignors, contract separation, 933
Cosmetic results (improvement), arthroscopic surgery (usage), 252
Cotton wool, usage, 859
Counterirritation
  history, 867
  impact, 713-714
  techniques, outline, 867
Count numbers, 220-221
  usage, principles, 220-221
Country English Pleasure class, 1199
Count stealing, 220-221
Coupling media, 902
Cow-hocked conformation, 30f
  occurrence, 30
Cow sense, 1051-1052
Coxofemoral joint (hip joint), 131-133, 581-582
  dysplasia, 581
  fibrocartilaginous ring, 94
  injection site, blocking, 132-133
  lateral/dorsal view, 132f
  movement, degree, 564
  osseous cystlike lesions, 581
  osteoarthritis, 581
  radiographs, 573
  size/landmarks, 131-132
  trochanteric bursitis, 581
Coxofemoral region, pelvic fractures, 42-43
Crabbet Arabian Stud, 1195
Cranial articular processes, synovial interverteral articulations, 592-593
Cranial cruciate ligament, 1108
Cranial ligament injuries, 543-544
  prognosis, 544
  signs/diagnosis, 543
  treatment, 543-544
Cranial lumbar vertebrae, lateral radiographic view, 602f
Cranial thoracic dorsal spinous processes, fractures, 1161-1162
Cranial thoracic vertebrae, motion-corrected scintigraphic image, 598f
Cranial tibial cortex (lateral image), focal IRU (lateral/caudal delayed phase images), 229f
Creatine kinase (CK)
  assessment, usage, 818
  AST, serial activity comparison, 818
  concentrations, impact, 1060
Crepitus, 38
  presence, 522-523
  sound, 44
Crimp, 696
Cross-country fence, 1124f
Cross-country horses, bucked-knee conformation, 27-28
Cross-linked collagen telopeptides, 949
Cross-sectional area (CSA), 173, 178
  measurements, 173-174
Crossties, usage, 878
Croton oil, impact, 867
Croup, 1109-1110, 1203-1204
  height, 16-17
Cruciate distal sesamoidean desmitis, 816

Cruciate ligaments, injury, 691
Cruciate sesamoidean ligaments, 812
Crus, 57-58
  anatomy, 526
  conditions, 527-532
  injuries, 1215
  lameness
    clinical characteristics/diagnosis, 526-527
    degree, 526-527
    diagnostic analgesia, 527
    imaging considerations, 527
    tibial stress fractures, impact, 527
  muscles/tendons, locomotion importance, 526
  occurrence, 145
  palpation, 57-58
  soft tissue injuries, 532
  tumors, 532
Cryonecrosis, mechanisms, 869
Cryoneurectomy, 341-342, 871
Cryoprobes, usage, 870f
Cryotherapy, 373
  defense, 373-374
  efficacy, testing, 373
  instigation, 373
  metal probe tip, application, 870
  pain management usage, 870f
  popularity, 505
  technique, 869-870
  tolerance, 870
CS-846
  measurement, 669
  type II collagen concentrations, 669
C3 subchondral lucency, 942
CTX-1 concentrations, age (impact), 950
CTX decrease, 952
CTX-MMP immunoassay, development, 949
Cubital joint (elbow joint), 121
Culture-expanded BM-MSCs, 762-763
Cunean bursa, 133, 800
  injection, assessment, 133
Cunean tendonitis, cryotherapy, 871
Cunean tenectomy, 1226
Curb, 134, 1186
  clinical appearance, 792-793
  convex profile, 792
  cryotherapy, 871
  deep digital flexor tendonitis, impact, 798
  description, 796
  development, 29f
  examination, 794-795
  historical definition, 792
  lameness, relationship, 793
  osteoarthritis, 793
  peritendonous/periligamentous inflammation, 797
  racehorse injury, 796-797
  SDF tendonitis, 797
  soft tissue injuries, 794-798
  swelling, 60
  term, usage, 134
  treatment, 867
  ultrasonographic diagnosis, 795
  ultrasonographic examination, 798
Curby conformation, 29-30

Current lameness, 11-14
Cut out under the knee, 28
Cutting horse, 1165
  forelimb lameness, 1170
  skills, 1165
  training, 1165-1166
    initiation, 1165
Cyanoacrylate adhesive, usage, 307
Cyclohexyl methacrylate (CHMA), 306-307
Cyclooxygenase (COX) activity, NSAID inhibition, 840-841
Cytokines, 662-664
  classification/actions, 663t
  degradative effects, 664
  regulatory proteins, 662

D

Daily team roping, 1170
Dangerous horse, nerve blocks, 152
Darley Arabian, 1195
Dead-end host, 141
Decompression, usage, 342
Decorin (proteoglycan), 700
Deep digital flexor (DDF)
  tendonitis, 83, 422, 498
  pastern region impact, 731-732
Deep digital flexor (DDF)
  tenotomy
  performing, 383
    metacarpal region, 383f
    midpastern region, 384f
  usage, 382-384
Deep digital flexor tendon
  (DDFT), 48
  anastomosing vascular network, 696
  anatomy, 726-727
  blunt trauma, 732
  carpal sheath, organization, 263-264
  disruption, 161
  dorsal aspect, tenoscopic view, 262f
  dorsal surface, fibrillation, 326
  dorsomedial luxation, 733
  elasticity modulus, 727
  fibrosis, 729-730
  force, decrease, 279
  impact, 344
  infection, 733
  injuries, 479
  insertions, 98f
    strain, 301
  involvement, 315
  lateral border tear,
    oblique transverse
    ultrasonographic image,
    768f
  lateral margin, tenoscopic view, 731f
  lesions, description, 732
  marginal tears, 730-731
  mineralization, 729-730
  molding, 344
  palmar aspect, tenoscopic view, 262f
  primary lesions, tarsal region, 733
  puncture wounds, 732
  reciprocal apparatus, 95f
  rupture, 345
    impact, 732-733
  SDFT, blood flow differences, 697

Deep digital flexor tendon
  (Continued)
  shape, enlargement/change, 728-729
  tension, 283
    increase, 324
  transection, 382
  traumatic lacerations, 423
Deep digital flexor tendon (DDFT)
  primary lesions
  anatomy, 344-345
  computer tomography, 347
  history/clinical signs, 345
  local analgesia, 345-346
  magnetic resonance imaging, 347
    examination, results
    (correlation), 347
  nuclear scintigraphy, 346-347
  pathophysiology, 345
  radiography, 346
  surgical exploration, 348
  treatment, 348
  ultrasonography, 346
Deep digital flexor tenotomy, 382-384
Deep fibular nerve block, 127
Deep muscles, damage, 577
Deficiency pattern, 887-889
Degenerative joint disease, 177
Degenerative joint disorders, radiation therapy, 876
Degenerative musculoskeletal conditions, radiation therapy, 875t
Degenerative suspensory (ligament) desmitis (DSD), 10
Delamination injury, 398
Delayed images, osteochondrosis, 228-229
Delayed-onset muscular stiffness/soreness (DOMS), recognition, 821
Delayed patellar release, 538-539
  prognosis, 539
  signs/diagnosis, 538
  treatment, 538-539
Delayed phase images, 226f
Delayed phase scintigraphic images, 219f-220f
Delayed release of the patella, 556
Del Mar, 978
Deltoid tuberosity fracture, 462-463
  diagnosis, radiographic
  examination, 462-463
  healing, transverse/longitudinal
  ultrasonographic images, 214f
Dermis, cutaneous nerve entry, 882f
Desmitis, proximal interphalangeal
  joint (ultrasonographic
  images), 817f
Desmopathies, 599-600
Desmotomy, 261-262
Developmental orthopedic disease
  (DOD), 638, 1247
  dietary energy excesses, impact, 626
  early pregnancy, 629
  environmental contamination, 625-626
  evaluations, types, 627
  feeding practices, impact, 628-629

Developmental orthopedic disease
  (Continued)
  feeding program, goal, 630-631
  feedstuffs, intake determination, 627
  forage, provision, 628-629
  grain fortification, inadequacy, 629
  horses, description, 627
  lactation, 630
  late pregnancy, 629-630
  mineral excesses, 625-626
  mineral imbalances, 626
  nutrient requirements, defining, 627
  nutrition
    contributing factor, 626
    protocol, 627-628
  nutritional factors, 625-626
  nutritional management, 630-631
  osteochondrosis, relationship, 631
  overfeeding problem, 628
  physitis, 631
  prevention, feeding systems
  (usage), 629-630
  ration evaluations, 626-628
  sucklings, 630
  weanlings, 630
  yearlings, 630
Diagnostic acupoints, location, 884
Diagnostic acupuncture palpation
  points, 885f
Diagnostic analgesia, 429, 924
  complete analgesia, goal, 102-103
  false-negative responses, 145-148
  flexion tests, comparison, 87-88
  horse preparation, 106-107
  impact, 105-106
  injection techniques, 107
  intangible factors, 106
  perception, 106
  performing, 107
  principles, adherence, 101
  strategy/methodology/considerations, 101-106
  systemic side effects, 101
  value, 100
Diagnostic arthroscopy, 432
  indication, 486-487
  surgical arthroscopy, division, 254-255
Diagnostic medication, 924
Diagonal hindlimb, front feet
  (hitting), 75
Diaphyseal fractures, 464
Diaphysis, sagittal section, 618f
Diarthrosis, 93
Diclazuril, anti-*S. neurona* activity, 142
Diet, 13
  changes, 13
Dietary energy excesses, impact, 626
Dietary factors, changes, 13
Diffuse tendonitis/desmitis, 204
Digestible energy/protein, NRC
  values, 627
Digital annular ligaments, disease, 775-776
  diagnosis, 775-776
  etiopathogenesis, 775
  treatment, 776

Digital blood flow therapy, 373
Digital cushion, 321
  function, 321-322
  quality, impact, 304
Digital digital flexor tendon
  (DDFT), 48
  cross-sectional area,
  enlargement, 729
  medial/lateral palmar digital
  vein/artery/nerve, location, 50
Digital extensor attachment/pain,
  proliferative changes, 49f
Digital extensor tendon
  laceration, 786-787
  rupture, 648f
Digital flexor tendons
  absolute blood flow, 697f
  exercise, impact, 701t
  lacerations, convalescent period, 809-810
  racing injuries, 966-967
  strains, 695
  transection, 807
Digital flexor tendon sheath
  (DFTS)
  analgesia, 124
    alternatives, 124
  anatomical considerations, 764-765
  anatomy, 260-261
  deep digital flexor tendonitis,
  fetlock region, 727-731
  diagnostic ultrasonography, 765
  disease, diagnostic techniques, 765
  distal plantar outpouching fluid
  (isolation), pressure
  bandage (usage), 1213f
  distention, 33, 111
    needle insertion, 261
    plantar outline notch, 772f
  dorsal wall, formation, 764-765
  effusion, 49
  envelopment, 394
  extension, 49
  imaging, 765-766
  infection
    cause, 770
    surgical treatment, 770
  internal structures (evaluation),
  tenoscopy (usage), 766
  intrasynovial injection site, 124
  intrathecal analgesia, 396
    impact, 728
  proximal aspect, 61
  soft tissues, examination, 765-766
  stage 3 tenosynovitis, 767f
  surrounding, 811
  survey radiography, 766
  synovial fluid, characteristics, 765
  synovial ganglion (distal
  metatarsal region), lateral
  aspect (transverse
  ultrasonographic image),
  776f
  tenoscopy, 260-262, 719
  tenosynovitis, 498, 507,
  709-710, 816
    impact, 1121
    occurrence, 1111
  transverse ultrasonographic
  images, 729f
Digital flexor tenosynovitis, 1163

Digital nerves
dorsal branches, midpastern ring block (impact), 110
location, 812
Digital pulse
amplitudes
assessment, 90, 165
increase, 371
increase/elevation, 44, 48f
quality/strength, assessment, 44
Digital radiography, imaging plate usage, 182
Digital sheath tenoscopy, example, 261f
Digital synovial sheath, diseases, 766-771
diagnosis, 767-768
prognosis, 769
treatment, 768-769
unresponsiveness, 768-769
ultrasonographic examination, 767-768
Digital synovial sheath, synovial ganglion/hernia, 776
Digital vessels, enlargement, 328-329
Digits
arthrocentesis, dorsolateral view, 118f
conformation, 31-32
support structures, 304f
Direct digital palpation, impact, 708
Direct-glue shoes
techniques, 307
Direct local pressure, application, 86
Direct palpation, 86
Dirt compaction, 303
Dirt tracks, races, 1076
Diseases, examination, 141-145
Diskospondylitis, 144, 614
Displaced radial fractures, open reduction/internal fixation (requirement), 452
Distal border radiolucent zones, interpretation, 330
Distal caudal radial exostosis, lameness (association), 150
Distal crus, analgesia, 127
Distal digital annular desmitis, 816
Distal dorsal metacarpal region, transverse/longitudinal ultrasonographic images, 397f
Distal extremities
conformation, 6
edema, 33
external rotation, 24-25
internal rotation, 24
Distal forelimb, innervation, 323
Distal fragments, ostectomy, 870-871
Distal hock joint
fibrous/bony swelling, 60f
osteoarthritis, 512-516, 1146
impact, 281
Distal hock joint pain, 991-992, 1191
clinical signs, 513
commonness, 512-513
cryotherapy, 871
osteoarthritis, 512-516
PSD, coexistence, 745-746

Distal hock joint pain (Continued)
tarsal lameness, relationship, 1029-1032
Distal interphalangeal (DIP) joint, 322, 478-479
advanced flexural deformity, 648f
analgesia, 116
arthrocentesis, 117
articular surfaces (axial compression), DDFT (impact), 344
capsule, relationship, 89-90
collateral ligament injury, 918
collateral ligaments
DSIL, relationship, 329f
injuries, 356-357
diagnosis, 349-351
diagnostic arthroscopy, 351
dorsal aspect, osseous fragments, 355
dorsal joint pouch, assessment, 46f
effusion, 1020-1021
flexed dorsal 60° lateral-palmaromedial oblique view, 351f
flexion, heel elevation (impact), 287
flexural deformity
broken-forward foot axis, 291
self-limitation, 646-647
flexural deformity, surgical management, 11
functional anatomy, 349
history, 349
hoof, impact, 282
imaging techniques, 350-351
inflammation, 890
injection, care, 352
intraarticular analgesia, 116-117, 349-350
lateral approach, 117
lateral collateral ligament, transverse/longitudinal/ ultrasonographic images, 356f
lesions, 634
local analgesia, 349-350
magnetic resonance imaging, 351
movement, 349
nuclear scintigraphy, 351
osteoarthritis, 352-353, 985
pain
association, 355
presence, 349
palmar digital block, impact, 108
primary pain, association, 349-355
radiographic examination, 350
radiography, 350-351
synovial fluid, retrieval, 350
synovitis, 1053-1054
ultrasonography, 351
Distal limbs, 94
analgesia, 111
catastrophic fractures, 972
cryotherapy, 373
flexion, response (variation), 329
injuries, emergency first aid principles, 968-969
mechanics, conformation (impact), 278-280

Distal limbs (Continued)
palmarolateral view, 109f
passive stay apparatus, 94
reaction (change), shoe (impact), 280
swelling, 314
toe length/angle, impact, 278-279
Distal margin, progressive demineralization, 377
Distal metacarpal region
swelling, 709
transverse/longitudinal ultrasonographic images, 214f
transverse ultrasonographic image, 773f
Distal palmar metacarpal region, transverse ultrasonographic image, 1163f
Distal phalanx (distal phalanges) (DP)
anatomical dislocation, 375
articular fracture, 963
asymmetrical distal displacement, 375
body, fractures, 360-361
diagnosis, 360-361
treatment/prognosis, 361
chronic heel pain, 363f
comminuted fractures, 361
dislocation
anatomical variations, occurrence, 375
distal margin, progressive demineralization, 377
secondary changes, 376
vascular trauma, association, 376
distal displacement, 375
lateromedial radiograph, 375f
dorsoproximal-palmarodistal oblique radiographic view, 316f
extensor process, dorsoproximal aspect (osteochondral fragments), 634
focal IRU, 356-357
fracture, 146, 359-362, 476-477
occurrence, 476-477, 985
penetrating injury, association, 361
infectious osteitis, 315-316
prognosis, 316
IRU, association, 938-939
loading, 283-284
orientation, 363
osseous cystlike lesions, 357-358
dramatic lameness, association, 634
osseous trauma, 358
palmar processes, osteitis, 362-364
anatomy, 362
diagnosis, 363-364
history/clinical findings, 362-363
imaging techniques, 363-364
local analgesia, 363
magnetic resonance imaging, 364
nuclear scintigraphy, 364
radiography, 363-364
treatment/prognosis, 364
relationship, 89-90
solar angle, heel lowering, 384

Distal phalanx (Continued)
solar margin, fracture, 359-360
subchondral cyst, dorsal/sagittal plane magnetic resonance images, 636f
subchondral trauma, 361-362
suspension, 366-367
Distal phalanx (distal phalanges)
extensor process
clinical/imaging findings, 355
fracture, 355-356
fragmentation, 355-356
history, 355
lateromedial radiographic views, 350f
osteochondral fragments, 355
treatment/prognosis, 355-356
Distal radial physeal exostosis, 727, 779
Distal radial physis, closure, 450
radiographs, usage, 450
treatment, 450
Distal radius
nondisplaced fracture, craniocaudal radiographic view, 451f
osseous cystlike lesions, 453-454
management, 453-454
transverse ridge level, 765
Distal sagittal ridge
osteochondritis dissecans, 632f
Distal sesamoid bone, suspension, 322
Distal sesamoidean collateral ligaments (DSCL), transvere section, 97f
Distal sesamoidean desmitis, 814-816
Distal sesamoidean impar ligaments (DSILs), 324
injury, 355
insertion, endosteal irregularity, 327
relationship, 89-90
Distal sesamoidean ligaments
desmitis, 1163
injury, 498
palpation, 48
primary injury, 759
Distal tarsal bones, fractures, 518-520
Distal tarsal joints
communication, 128-129
intraarticular analgesia, performing, 511
Distal tarsal region, plantaromedial aspect (transverse ultrasonographic image), 733f
Distal tarsitis, 991, 1191
Distal third metacarpal disease, 986
Distal tibia
medial malleolus fractures, rarity, 522
physitis, 531
Disuse atrophy, 32
development, 32
Dog trotting, 552
Doppler ultrasonography, usage, 502-503
Dorsal chip fractures, 400
Dorsal 25° proximal
medial-plantarodistal lateral oblique digital radiographic view, 253f

Dorsal hoof wall
  angle, change, 278-279
  DIP joint center, dorsopalmar
    radiographic view, 285
  hoof capsule width/length,
    ground surface view, 285
  thickness, lateromedial
    radiographic view, 285
Dorsal metacarpal disease (DMD)
  bone biomarkers, relationship,
    951
  bucked shins, 989-990
  racehorse problem, 951
Dorsal osteochondral fragments,
  390
Dorsal pelvic images, 228
Dorsal periarticular proliferation,
  602
Dorsal pouch, prominence,
  118-119
Dorsal sacroiliac ligament,
  desmitis, 578
Dorsal spinous process
  impingement, 134-135,
    598-599
  summits, fracture, 155
Dorsal third metacarpal bone
  pain, signs, 940-941
Dorsolateral toe extension,
  placement, 642
Dorsomedial-plantarolateral
  oblique (DM-PILO)
  images, 1022-1023
  view, 519
Dorsopalmar balance (plantar
  balance), 282
Dorsopalmar digital radiographic
  view, 10f
Dorsopalmar foot balance,
  correction/preservation, 339
Dorsopalmar foot imbalance, 312
Dorsopalmar imbalance, 287-288,
  290-293
  effects, 288
  prolongation, delayed effects,
    287-288
  trimming response, 291
Dorsopalmar static balance,
  guidelines, 284f
Double plating techniques,
  522-523, 528-529
Down-angled oblique views,
  radiographic examination,
    493
Draft horses
  canker, 1221-1222
    treatment, 1222
  changes, 1216
  coronary band, defect, 476f
  cunean tenectomy, 1226
  developmental orthopedic
    disease, 1227-1228
  distal interphalangeal joints,
    osteoarthritis, 1222-1223
  distal phalanx, osteitis, 1221
  epiphysitis, 1227
  feet
    chronic scar/granulation
      tissue, 1221f
    lameness, 1217-1222
    thrush, 1221f
  flexural deformities, 1227
  foals, lameness, 1227-1228
  forelimb lameness, 1217-1227
  front foot, laminitis
    (lateromedial radiographic
    image), 1219f

Draft horses (Continued)
  hindlimb lameness, 5,
    1217-1227
  hock lameness, 1224
  hoof testers, 1217-1218
  hoof wall cracks, 1218-1219
  infectious arthritis, 1227
  lameness
    examination, 1216-1217
    management, 1223
    mange mites, impact, 1224
    problems, 1217
    sidebone, association, 1220
  laminitis, 1219-1220
    diagnosis, 1219
    management, 1219-1220
  medical management, 1226
  metacarpophalangeal joint
    lameness, 1223
  osteoarthritis, management,
    1225
  osteochondritis dissecans,
    1227-1228
  osteochondrosis, 1227-1228
  physitis, 1227
  proximal interphalangeal joint,
    osteoarthritis, 1222-1223
  quittor, 1220-1221
  radical hoof wall resection,
    avoidance, 1220
  ringbone, 1222-1223
  rubber inner tube, placement,
    1218f
  shivers, 1226-1227
  sidebone, 1220
  splint bones, fractures (rarity),
    1223
  splints, 1223
  stature, change, 1216
  status, 1216
  stifle joint, 1226
  subsolar abscess, 1217-1218
    location, 1218
  suspensory desmitis, 1223-1224
    management, 1224
  tarsocrural effusion (bog
    spavin), 1225
  tarsus, 1224-1226
  tendonitis, 1223-1224
    management, 1224
  upright pasterns, impact, 1222
  weanlings, lameness, 1227-1228
  yearling
    hock, dorsomedial-
      plantarolateral oblique
      radiographic image, 1225f
    lameness, 1227-1228
Draining tracts, 213
  cause, determination, 213
  scanning, 213
Dremel tool
  burr, usage, 313
  usage, 315-316
Dressage
  phase, 1206
  sport, 1112
Dressage horses, 1113-1114
  acute-onset moderately severe
    lameness, right shoulder
    (lateral scintigraphic
    image), 463f
  arena maintenance, 1115
  artificial surfaces, training,
    1114-1115
  back pain, causes, 1122
  balance, 1114
  bit, acceptance, 1115

Dressage horses (Continued)
  breaking, 1114
  caudal cervical vertebrae, lateral
    radiographic view, 614f
  centrodistal joint, osteoarthritis,
    1120-1121
  chronic left forelimb lameness,
    carpal sheath (transverse
    ultrasonographic image),
    778f
  clinical signs, correlation, 1120
  conformation/soundness, 1114
  description, terms, 1112
  diagnostic analgesia, 1116
  diagnostic nerve blocks,
    requirement, 1117-1118
  digital flexor tendon sheath,
    tenosynovitis, 1121-1122
  distal interphalangeal joint,
    synovitis/osteoarthritis,
    1119-1120
  examination, 1115
  forelimbs
    ALDDFT, desmitis, 1120
    proximal suspensory desmitis,
      1118-1119
    suspensory ligament
      branches, desmitis, 1119
  hindlimbs
    ALDDFT, desmitis, 1120
    proximal suspensory desmitis,
      1117-1118
    suspensory ligament
      branches, desmitis, 1119
  imaging considerations,
    1116-1117
  lameness, 472
    conditions, 1117
    examination, 1115-1116
  lateral movements, 1112
  management, success, 752-753
  medical therapy, response
    (failure), 1122
  metatarsophalangeal/
    metacarpophalangeal joints,
    synovitis/osteoarthritis,
    1121
  middle carpal joint, synovitis,
    1121
  nuclear scintigraphy, 1117
    usefulness, 1118
  palmar annular ligament
    desmitis, 1121
  plantar annular ligament
    desmitis, 1121
  proximal suspensory desmitis,
    1117-1119
  radial pressure wave treatment,
    1121
  radiography, value (absence),
    1119
  right hindlimb, chronic
    PSD (lateromedial
    radiographic view), 747f
  sacroiliac pain, 1122-1123
  sagittal short tau inversion
    recovery, MR image,
    335f
  sport, 1112-1113
  superficial digital flexor
    tendonitis, 721-726
  suspensory ligament
    desmitis, 1119
    ultrasonographic appearance,
      1118
  tarsometatarsal joints,
    osteoarthritis, 1120-1121

Dressage horses (Continued)
  third metacarpal bone,
    proximal palmar cortical
    stress fracture, 1122
  thoracolumbar pain, 1122-1123
  thoracolumbar/pelvic regions,
    diagnostic ultrasonography,
    1117
  training surfaces, 1114-1115
  ultrasonographic/radiological
    changes, 1118
  wear-and-tear lesions,
    occurrence, 1114
Drifting, 73
Driving horses
  ALDDFT, desmitis, 1215
  antebrachium, injuries, 1215
  arthrodesis, usage, 1212
  brisket, injuries, 1215
  bruises/corns, diagnosis, 1211
  conditioning, 1207
  conformation, 1208
  crus, injuries, 1215
  DFTS, tenosynovitis, 1213-1214
  diagnosis, difficulties, 1209
  diagnostic analgesia, 1208-1209
  direct trauma, 1214-1215
  distal hock joint pain,
    1211-1212
  distal interphalangeal joint,
    synovitis (occurrence),
    1211
  exertional rhabdomyolysis,
    1212-1213
  foot lameness, 1210-1211
  ground conditions, 1207-1208
  heel bulb laceration, 1214f
  hoof balance, assessment,
    1211
  imaging considerations, 1209
  interference injuries, 1214-1215
  joint capsule, distention,
    1208-1209
  lameness
    conditions, 1210
    diagnosis/management,
      1210-1215
    examination, 1208
    incidence, 1207
  lower limb joints, chronic
    osteoarthritis, 1214
  lower neck, injuries, 1215
  navicular syndrome, 1211
  osteoarthritis, treatment, 1214
  radiological examination, 1213
  rest, importance, 1210
  SDFT, 1215
  shoeing, 1209-1210
    assessment, 1211
  sport, description, 1205-1206
  stifle
    injuries, 1215
    lameness, 1214
  suspensory desmitis, 1210
    prevention, 1210
  training, 1207
  treatment, 1212
  trials, phases, 1206
  types, 1206-1207
    variation, 1206
  ultrasonography, 1209
  upper hindlimb, flexion tests,
    1211
Driving pony, left shoulder joint
  acute-onset instability
    (brachial plexus injury), 473f
Dropped elbow, 39

Dropped fetlock, 34f
Drugs
  administration, transdermal
    route, 857
  selection, 855-857
Dutch Warmblood
  dressage horses (third/fifth
    cervical vertebrae),
    neck pain/stiffness/
    incoordination (lateral
    radiographic view), 615f
  horse, right front foot
    (dorsoproximal-
    palmarodistal oblique
    image), 1093f
Duty cycle, 905
Duty factor, 274
  definition, 271b
Dynamic acquisition, 220
  composite image, 221f
Dynamic balance, 285
Dynamic Churchill test, 86
Dynamic examination, 1198-1199
Dynamic mediolateral balance,
  assessment, 289
Dynamic spinal cord compression,
  occurrence, 650
Dyschondroplasia, 617
Dysplasia, 468, 581
Dystrophic mineralization, 177,
  439

E

Early passive motion, 770-771
Early peritoneal new bone,
  hypertrophic osteopathy
  (association), 166
Early postinjury phase,
  antiinflammatory treatment,
  868
Early pregnancy, developmental
  orthopedic disease, 629
Ear tick-associated muscle
  cramping, 837
Echogenicity, 177-178
Edema, 88
Egg bar shoes, 1178
  fitting, 339
  impact, absence, 280
  lateral/palmar/solar views, 340f
EHV-1 infections, 139
Elastic modulus, 273
Elastic resilience, 273-274
Elbow, 52
  acute-onset severe left forelimb
    lameness, lateral
    scintigraphic images, 464f
  anatomical considerations,
    456-457
  clinical signs, 457
  collateral ligaments, injury, 461
    definitive diagnosis, 461
  diagnosis, 457-458
  differential diagnosis, 460-474
  ginglymus joint, 456
  imaging, 458-460
  inverse/simultaneous
    movement, 83-84
  lateral scintigraphic images,
    464f
  local analgesia, 457-458
  nuclear scintigraphy, 458-460
  osseous cystlike lesions, 460
  osteoarthritis, 460
    intraarticular analgesia,
      impact, 460
  osteochondrosis, 461

Elbow (Continued)
  radiographic examination,
    mediolateral/craniocaudal
    views (requirement), 458
  radiography, 458
  swelling/lameness, 52
  ultrasonography, 458
Elbow joint (cubital joint), 121
  components, 456
  luxation, 461-462
  mediolateral/craniocaudal
    radiographic views, 460f
  mediolateral radiographic view,
    458f
Electrical current/waveforms,
  905
Electrical stimulation, 905-907
Electrode placement, 907
Electrolyte depletion, 825
Electromyography (EMG), 140
  impact, 555
  performing, 820
Electrophysical agents
  contraindications, 902
  precautions, 902
  treatment record, 902
Electrotherapeutic windows, 901
Elevated wall, GRF shift, 286
Elite sport horses, conformation
  (evaluation), 16
Embryonic stem (ES) cells,
  definition, 761
Endochondral ossification, 617
  disorder, 174
  process, 617
Endogenous healing
  (manipulation), growth
  factors (usage), 851-852
Endogenous repair, stimulation,
  850-852
Endosteal new bone, 171
Endurance
  competition, evolution, 1139
  evolution, 1137
Endurance horses
  Arabian extraction, 1139
  bone injury, 1147
  capsulitis, 1144
  carpi, dorsal scintigraphic
    image, 150f
  chronic/recurrent lameness,
    1140-1141
  competition speeds, 1139
  coronary band (coronitis),
    inflammation, 1144
  course terrain, 1139
  diagnosis, absence, 1140
  distal hock joints, osteoarthritis,
    1146
  exertional myopathy, 1147
  feet, problems, 1143-1144
  full-body scintigraphy, 1140
  gluteal muscles, inflammation,
    1146
  gluteal myalgia, 1146
  handwalking, restriction, 1142
  high-volume fluid replacement,
    1148
  lameness
    categories, 1139-1140
    causes, 1140
    conformation, relationship,
      1139-1140
    examination, 1140
  laminitis, 1144
  metabolic problems, 1147-1149
    prevention, 1149

Endurance horses (Continued)
  metacarpal region, dorsopalmar
    radiographic image, 1143f
  metacarpophalangeal joint,
    dorsopalmar radiographic
    image, 1145f
  metacarpophalangeal/
    metatarsophalangeal
    osteoarthritis, 1144
  myositis, 1147
  national competitions, 1138
  palmar foot pain, 1143-1144
  palmar metacarpal soft
    tissues, longitudinal
    ultrasonographic images,
    1141f
  paravertebral myalgia, 1146
  periarticular pathology, 1144
  proximal palmar metacarpal
    pain, 1140-1143
    lameness cause, 1140
  proximal suspensory desmitis,
    1141-1142
  PSD management, 1141-1142
  rehabilitation program, 1142
  rhabdomyolysis, 1147
  second/fourth metacarpal
    bones, pathology,
    1142-1143
  sole bruises, occurrence, 1143
  sport, description, 1137-1138
  superficial digital flexor
    tendonitis, 1145-1146
  suspensory body/branches,
    desmitis, 1146-1147
  suspensory ligament, desmitis,
    1141
  synchronous diaphragmatic
    flutter (thumps),
    1148-1149
  synovitis, 1144
  tendon injuries, 1146
  third metacarpal bone
    bilateral fractures, diagnosis,
      1145
    condylar fractures, 1145
    distal aspect, stress pathology,
      1144-1145
    proximal palmar aspect, stress
      pathology, 1142
  third metatarsal bone
    bilateral fractures, diagnosis,
      1145
    condylar fractures, 1145
    distal aspect, stress pathology,
      1144-1145
  training methods, 1139
    differences, 1139
    types, 1139
  veterinary controls, 1138-1139
Endurance World Championships,
  1137
Energy density, skin surface
  measurement, 904
Energy dissipation, 321-322
Energy flux density (EFD), 915
English Pleasure horses, 1196,
  1199
English Show Hack, 1196
Enostosis-like lesions, 171, 424,
  452-453
  bone islands, 464-465
  intramedullary radiopaque
    lesions, comparison,
    943f
  term, usage, 450
  treatment, 453, 465

Enteritis, 372
Enterobacter cloacae, 524-525
Enthesophytes, 352-353
  formation, 172-173
Environmental contamination,
  625-626
Enzyme/cytokine ratios,
  identification, 679
Enzyme-linked immunosorbent
  assay (ELISA), 139
Enzymes, role, 624-625
Enzyme system, inhibition, 840
Eosinophilia, rarity, 138
Eosinophilic synovitis, 690
Epaxial structures, ultrasonographic
  examination, 596
Epaxial synovial intervertebral
  articulations, injections,
  596
Epidural α₂-adrenergic agonists,
  856
Epidural administration
  side effects, characteristics,
    856t
  technique, 853
Epidural analgesia, 852-853
  clinical applications, 857
  contraindications/
    complications, 857
  drugs, usage, 856-857
Epidural catheter
  insertion site, 853
  placement, 853-855
  threading, 855f
Epidural drug administration,
  853
Epidural injections, 853-855
Epidural opioids, 855-856
  action, onset/duration, 855-856
  side effects, 856
Epiphysis
  retained cartilage, thickening,
    618f
  sagittal section, 618f
  histological sections, 619f
Epoxy resins, environmental
  resistance, 307
Epson salt poultices, 1100-1101
Equimetrix, 250f, 251
Equine Cushing's dease (ECD),
  370-371
  development, 370
Equine degenerative
  myeloencephalopathy (EDM),
  143, 650
  misdiagnosis, 143
  vitamin E deficiency, 143
Equine digital flexor tendons,
  elasticity, 694
Equine Digital Support System
  (EDSS), 1100-1101
Equine distal limb, palmar/plantar
  supporting structures (in vitro
  biomechanical parameters),
  695t
Equine herpesvirus 1 infection,
  143-144
Equine joint disease model
  biomechanical models, 677
  instability models, 675-676
  types, 674-677
  usage, 673
  in vitro models, 674-675
  in vivo studies, 675-677
Equine joints, ultrasonographic
  examination (indications),
  206

Equine lameness
  interpretation, 69
  MRI indications, 245
  textbooks, 2
Equine limb, ultrasonographic
    evaluation
  equipment, 168-169
  indications, 169b
  sound, attenuation, 169
Equine lower motor neuron
    disease, 143
  clinical signs, 137
  diagnosis, 143
Equine metabolic syndrome,
    370
  term, usage, 370
Equine myelograms,
    interpretation, 652
Equine polysaccharide storage
    myopathy (EPSSM), 555,
    557
  changes, 562
Equine protozoal myelitis (EPM),
    7, 141-145
  Diclazuril, usage, 142
  evaluation, Western blot test,
    137
  forelimb/hindlimb gait
    abnormalities, 156
  motor neurons, involvement,
    555
  neurological signs, 1164
  prognosis accuracy, difficulty,
    142
  recognition, 141
  S. neurona, impact, 141
  Toltrazuril, usage, 142
  treatment, drugs (usage),
    141-142
Equine protozoal
    myeloencephalitis (EPM),
    650
Equine rhabdomyolysis (tying
    up), 575-576
  occurrence, 157-158
Equine scintigraphy, 215
Equine systemic proteoglycan
    accumulation, 10
Equine third metacarpal bone,
    distal aspect (post mortem
    specimen),
    661f
EquuSys, Inc., 250-251, 250f
Escherichia coli, 524-525, 677
E-series prostaglandins, regulation
    ability, 664
Estrogenic compounds,
    administration, 557
Estrous cycle, 950
  behavioral abnormalities, 11
Ether bandages, 859
  application, 859f
  usage, 859
Ethylenediamine tetraacetic
    acid (EDTA), usage, 677-678
Euglycemia, 370
Europe
  racetracks, 1036
    distribution, 1037t
  standardbreds, distribution,
    1037t
  training regimens, 996-997
European Standardbred,
    1036-1047
  centrodistal/tarsometatarsal
    joints, radiological
    appearance, 1041

European Standardbred
    (Continued)
  colt
    hock, dorsal 20°
      lateral-plantaromedial
      oblique radiographic
      image, 1042f
    metatarsophalangeal
      joint, dorsolateral-
      plantaromedial oblique
      radiographic image,
      1045f
  conformation, examination,
    1038
  corrective shoeing, 1042-1043
  crossbreeding, 1036
  curb, development, 1041
  diagnosis, absence, 1043
  diagnostic analgesia, 1040
    performing, 1040
    usefulness, 1040
  diagnostic imaging, 1040-1042
    inclusion, 1045
  dimensions/characteristics,
    1036-1037
  distal interphalangeal
    joint, osteoarthritis,
    1043-1044
  feet, examination, 1043
  fetlock joint, forelimb (effusion
    examination), 1039
  final diagnosis, 1042
  flexion tests, usage, 1040
  gait anomalies, 1038
  hind fetlock, dorsoproximal 45°
    medial-plantarodistolateral
    oblique radiographic image,
    1041f
  hindlimb, distal aspect
    (palpation), 1039
  hoof pain, 1043
  hoof tester examination,
    1039
  lameness
    conditions, 1043
    examination, 1038-1040
    problems, 1037-1038
  limbs, distal aspect
    (lateromedial radiographs),
    1044
  metacarpophalangeal joint,
    osteoarthritis, 1044
  metatarsophalangeal joint,
    hindlimb lameness source,
    1046
  middle carpal joint, lameness
    site, 1044-1045
  movement, examination,
    1039-1040
  palpation, 1038-1039
  prognosis, 1042
  proximal palmar metacarpal
    pain, 1045
  proximal suspensory desmitis,
    1045
  sesamoiditis, 1045-1046
  superficial digital flexor
    tendonitis, 1047
  suspensory branch desmitis,
    1046
  tarsocrural joint, osteoarthritis,
    1047
  training
    mechanical limitations,
      1037-1038
    programs, 1043
  treatment options, 1042

European Standardbred
    (Continued)
  trotters
    distal interphalangeal joint,
      lateromedial radiographic
      image, 1040f
    distal limb, pathological
      findings, 1040
    foot pain, flap/flip-flop shoe
      (usage), 1044f
    lameness, 1043-1047
    proximal metacarpal region,
      dorsopalmar radiographic
      image, 1041f
European Thoroughbreds
  clinical examination, 997-999
  clinical history, 997-1004
  diagnostic analgesia,
    1001-1003
  history, 994
  imaging considerations,
    999-1001
  racing, pattern, 994-995
  radiography, 999-1000
  scintigraphy, 1000-1001
  ultrasonography, 1001
European Western performance
    horses, 1183-1186
  carpus, lameness, 1186
  curb, 1186
  feet
    conformation, 1183
    lameness, 1183-1184
  fetlock joint, lameness,
    1185-1186
  hock
    dorsolateral aspect, long
      digital extensor tendon
      sheath (longitudinal
      ultrasonographic image),
      1184f
    lameness, 1184
    torsion test, usage, 1184
  lameness conditions, 1183
  long digital extensor tendon
    sheath, tenosynovitis,
    1184
  middle phalanx, plantar process
    (fracture), 1186
  osteoarthritis, treatment, 1184
  PSD, treatment, 1185
  second/fourth metacarpal/
    metatarsal bones, exostosis,
    1173
  stifle, lameness, 1185
  superficial digital flexor
    tendonitis, 1184-1185
  suspensory desmitis, 1185
  ultrasonographic examination,
    1185
Eventer gelding, right patella
    (cranioproximal-craniodistal
    radiographic view), 546f
Event horses
  acute-onset severe lameness
    history, left front foot
    (lateral pool phase
    scintigraphic image), 346f
  acute-onset severe left
    forelimb lameness,
    mediolateral radiographic
    view, 472f
  chronic right hindlimb
    lameness, distal metatarsal
    region (transverse
    ultrasonographic image),
    730f

Event horses *(Continued)*
  elbow joint, mediolateral/
    craniocaudal radiographic
    views, 460f
  forelimbs, carpal/proximal
    metacarpal regions (dorsal/
    lateral scintigraphic
    images), 396f
  lameness
    absence, 721
    left hindlimb (suspensory
      ligament), lateral
      branch (transverse
      ultrasonographic image),
      753f
    left elbow, mediolateral
      radiographic view, 161f
    left forelimb, metacarpal
      region (dorsomedial-
      palmarolateral oblique
      view), 158f
    left/right proximal pastern
      regions, right forelimb
      lameness (transverse
      ultrasonographic images),
      758f
    midcervical region, lateral
      radiographic view, 161f
    neck (base), forelimb gait
      restriction (longitudinal
      ultrasonographic images),
      822f
    neck stiffness, 611f
    palmar thermographic image,
      1130f
    pastern lesions, 723-724
    right forelimb
      midbody superficial digital
        flexor tendonitis, history,
        268f
      palmar aspect, transverse
        ultrasonographic image,
        722f
    right front fetlock,
      dorsolateral-palmaromedial
      oblique radiographic view,
      754f
    right front foot, sagittal spoiled
      gradient-echo MRI, 348f
    right hindlimb (lateral
      PSB), suspensory
      ligament (transverse
      ultrasonographic image),
      753f
    right stifle, cranioproximal-
      craniodistal oblique
      radiographic view, 163f
    subtle tendonitis, 722
      echogenicity, comparison,
        722
    superficial digital flexor
      tendonitis, 721-726
      clinical signs, 721-722
      diagnostic ultrasonography,
        722-723
      injury, occurrence, 722
      intralesional treatment,
        results, 723
      management, difficulty, 723
      treatment, 723
    tendon injury, severity
      (noncorrelation), 721-722
Eventing
  sport, 1123-1124
  stamp, 1124f
Excess, acupoint palpation,
    889-890

Excessive movement, reduction, 878
Excess pattern, 887-889
Exercise, 879-880
  bone fatigue, relationship, 954-955
  impact, 624
  intensity, approaches, 879
  levels, 168-169
    grading scale, 170b
  program, increase, 438
  rehabilitation component, 879
  response test, 819
  in vivo strain measurements, 954
Exercise-induced hindlimb lameness, aortoiliacofemoral thrombosis (impact), 579
Exercise-induced hyperthermia, 703
Exertional myopathy, 1147
Exertional rhabdomyolysis (ER), 824-829, 992
  cause, 825-826
  chronic dietary imbalance, 825-826
  impact, 825
Exhausted horse syndrome, 1147-1148
Exogenous corticosteroids, usage, 371
Exostoses, 419-421, 448
  axial impingement, 420-421
  presence, 62
Expected feed consumption, 629t
Experimental injections, credit, 2
Exposure
  factors, 168
  latitude, 168
Extension moment, 274-275
Extensions, 296
  shoe projections, 296
  usage, 296
Extensor carpi obliquus, 786
Extensor carpi radialis (ECR)
  muscle, 785
  tendon, portals (location), 120-121
  tendon sheath, chronic distention, 790f
  tenosynovitis, 52
Extensor carpi radialis tendon (ECRT)
  complete rupture, 788
  diagnosis, 788
  extension, 785
  insertion, enthesopathy, 788
  rupture, 788
  trauma, 788
Extensor moment, 274-275
Extensor process fragments/ fractures, rarity, 478-479
Extensor tendon, 448
  conditions, 786-788
  lacerations
    diagnosis, 786
    healing, 787
  sheaths, conditions, 788-791
  transection, 786, 807
    carpus, location, 807
    healing, 809
Extensor tendon injury
  anatomy, 785-786
  diagnostic techniques, 786
  graduated exercise, 809

External beam irradiation, 873-874
External blistering, 713-714
External coaptation, usage, 503
External genitalia, palpation, 54
External skeletal fixation
  history/development, 863-865
  mechanics, 863-865
  postoperative care, 866
External skeletal fixation device (ESFD), 863
  development, 863
  impact, 863
  removal, 866
  treatment, results, 866
External skeletal pin transfixation, usage (feasibility), 859
External trauma fractures, 422
  clinical signs, 422
  diagnosis, 422
  treatment, 422
Extraarticular fluid layer, detection, 214
Extracorporeal shock wave treatment, 744, 748
Ex vivo gene transfer, 671

F
Fabric cuff, 307
  PMMA/CHMA adhesive, usage, 307
Falabella ponies, sudden-onset severe lameness, 467
Fallen horse/jockey, 1067f
Falls, influence, 1067-1068
False-negative findings, 228
False-positive bone scans, occurrence, 227-228
False-positive findings, 227-228
False thoroughpin, 800-802
  diagnostic ultrasonography, 801
  longitudinal ultrasonographic image, 801f
Far gain, 170
Fasciotomy, accomplishment, 719
Fatigue failure
  decrease, exercise programs (usage), 955-956
  regression analysis, 956
  survival analysis, 956
Fatigue fractures
  radiologic detection, 175
  term, usage, 935
Fat-suppressed T2-weighted fast spin echo sequences, 938
Fédération Equestre Internationale (FEI), 1137
  dressage rules, 1112
  international rules, creation, 1205-1206
Feeding diets, effects (study), 623
Feedstuffs
  intake determination, 627
  nutrient determination, 627
Feet, 44-46, 63, 364-366
  abscesses, 985
  balance, 282-293
    assessment, 44-45
  balance, importance, 12
  built-in-protective mechanisms, 273
  cartilage disease
    anatomy, 364
    attachment, 364
    clinical signs/diagnosis, 365-366

Feet (Continued)
  cartilages
    ligamentous attachments, 321
    location, 320-321
    ossification, 365
    proximal aspect, 365
  chronic laminitis, sagittal section, 375f
  components, 321
  conformation, 1038
  derotating, 382f
  differential diagnostic analgesia, 110t
  dorsoproximal-palmaromedial oblique view, 364f
  elevation, palmar aspects, 46f
  exercise, 283-284
  finishing, 305
  forces, impact, 277
  function, 282-284
    shoeing, impact, 301-302
  ground interface, 272-273
  ground surface
    alteration, rotational deformities (impact), 287
    changes, 288-289
    elongation/narrowing, long toe (impact), 291
  horseshoes, preparation, 293-294
  imbalance, 1133
  importance, 44
  lameness, 1, 984-986
  lateral cartilage, extension, 320
  lateral placement, advancement/abduction, 75
  lateral view, arthrocentesis approach, 117f
  lateromedial venogram, 377f
  locomotion, 277-278
  long toes, 305
  medial cartilage, extension, 320
  navicular bursa, synoviocentesis (lateral view), 123f
  oblique dorsoproximal-palmarodistal oblique view, 359f
  oblique radiographic view, 315f
  pain, 1100-1103
  palmar portion, structures, 320
  palpation, 63
  penetrating injury, 361
  peptides, identification, 323
  placement, evaluation, 77
  poultice, 859-860
  racing injuries, 963
  rebalancing, 291
  rest, 282-283
  sagittal magnetic resonance imaging scan, 96f
  shape/balance/contour, assessment, 63
  shock-absorbing features, schematic drawing, 273f
  size, 33-34
  soreness, 1100, 1133
  strike, 69
  thrush, 1221f
  transverse sections, 97f
    chronic foot pain, appearance, 320f
  transverse T1-weighted gradient echo MRI, 1102f
  trimming, 279
    sequence, 304
  underrun heels, 305

Fell pony (left hind fetlock flexural deformity), ALDDFT (association), 736f
Femoral condyles, fracture
  fragment origination, 546-547
  prognosis, 547
  signs/diagnosis, 546-547
  treatment, 547
Femoral head, displacement, 582
Femoral nerve
  damage, 144-145
  paresis, 42
Femoral trochlear ridges, fracture
  fragment origination, 546-547
  prognosis, 547
  signs/diagnosis, 546-547
  treatment, 547
Femoropatellar compartments
  communication difficulty, 130
  lateral cul-de-sac, 130-131
Femoropatellar joint, 536-540
  arthrocentesis, 130-131
  osteoarthritis, 540
    prognosis, 540
    signs/diagnosis, 540
    treatment, 540
Femoropatellar OC, development, 621
Femorotibial joint, 541-545
  articular cartilage trauma, 544-545
  collateral ligament injuries, 544
  cranial/caudal cruciate ligament injuries, 543-544
  examination, 208
  medial collateral ligament, longitudinal ultrasound scan, 209f
  meniscal/meniscal ligament injuries, 542-543
  osteoarthritis, 545
  subchondral cystic lesions, 541-542
Femur
  greater trochanter, 575
  medial trochlear ridge, 533
  racing injuries, 965
  Salter-Harris fractures (types III/ IV), 547
    prognosis, 547
    signs/diagnosis, 547
    treatment, 547
  third trochanter, fracture/ enthesopathy, 582
Femur fractures, 552-554
  diagnosis, 553
  locking compression plate (LCP), 554
  occurrence, 552-553
  radiological evaluation, 553
  treatment/prognosis, case selection, 554
Fence-related injuries, 13
Feral foot, wall (wearing), 303f
Fetlock, 48-50, 206-208
  arthrodesis, 971
    infection, complication, 971
  dorsal aspect, 206-207
    sagittal ultrasound, 206f
  dorsomedial/dorsolateral aspects, 207
  drop, 72
    assessment, 72
    observation, 969

Fetlock (Continued)
evaluation, nuclear scintigraphy (usage), 395
flexion, 562
flexion test, 82-84
lower limb flexion test, comparison, 82
performing, 83f
height, 34, 39
hyperextension, 161
impact, 775
intersesamoidean ligament disease, 774-775
palmar/plantar ligament damage, 754-755
knuckling, 34
lameness, 1006-1008
offset knees, impact, 17
medial/lateral aspects, 207
palmar aspect, 207-208
scabs, 166
palmar ligament, focal tear (arthroscopic image), 756f
palmarolateral aspect, longitudinal ultrasound scan, 208f
position, assessment, 39
spherical masses, 802
valgus, 481
varus, impact, 641
Fetlock joint
anatomical constraints, 410
capsule distention/thickening, 1090
capsulitis, 1155
dorsal aspect, sagittal ultrasound scan, 207f
drop, 72
flexion, 62
imaging, ease, 395
intrasynovial analgesia, 394-395
lameness, 986-987
types, 395
Fetlock region
DDFT enlargement, 727
digital flexor tendon sheath, deep digital flexor tendonitis, 727-731
flexion test, 81
lateromedial radiographic view, 766f
Feustel, Louis, 977
Fiber alignment
pattern assessment, 178
scoring, 190b
Fiber alignment score (FAS), 173
usefulness, 173
Fibresand, Polytrack (change), 975
Fibrocartilage, degenerative changes, 326
Fibrocartilaginous structures, 93-94
Fibromas, occurrence, 693
Fibromodulin (proteoglycan), 700
Fibrosis, 33
Fibrotic myopathy, 56, 76, 554, 558-559
biomechanical basis, 559
cause, 559
clinical characteristics, 558-559
commonness, 559
medical therapy, 559
surgical therapy, 559
Fibrotic myopathy-type gait, 555
Fibrous ring, emanation, 765

Fibula fractures, 548
cause, 548
Fibular fractures, 531-532
occurrence, 531-532
Fibularis tertius
anatomy, 802
avulsion, 548
prognosis, 548
signs/diagnosis, 548
treatment, 548
clinical signs, 802-803
history, 802-803
peroneus tertius, disruption, 41
rupture, 163, 524, 802-803
cause, 802
diagnosis, 803
hock extension, 803f
treatment, 803
Fibular nerves
block, peroneal nerve block, 127
origination, 526
perineural analgesia, 511
Fibular tarsal bone, fractures, 520
trauma, impact, 520
Field hunters, bucked-knee conformation, 27-28
Field of view camera
recess/pit, construction, 218f
usage, 218f
Filled legs, 164-165
Filly, acute medial collateral desmopathy, 211f
Finnhorses
carpal canal syndrome, 1079
carpal synovitis, 1079
chronic suspensory desmitis, coping, 1079
curbs, 1080
diagnosis, radiological confirmation, 1080
diagnostic analgesia, 1079
lameness conditions, 1079-1081
original breed, 1076
SDF tendonitis, treatment, 1079-1080
second/fourth metacarpal bones, 1078
splints, 1080-1081
tarsal lameness, 1079
treatment options, limitation, 1080
trotters, radiological changes, 1079
Finnish horses
breed, history, 1076
conformation/lameness, 1077
flexion tests, 1078
imaging considerations, 1079
lameness
causes, 1079
diagnosis, absence, 1079
examination, 1077-1079
racetracks/weather conditions, 1077
shoeing considerations, 1077
tarsus, palpation, 1078
Firing, 868-869
performing, 868
usage, restrictions, 869
First cervical vertebrae, subluxation, 609-610
diagnosis, 609-610
First coccygeal interspace, identification, 853, 853f

First-opinion racehorse practice, 528
First rib, fracture, 474
First/second coccygeal vertebrae, first coccygeal interspace, 853f
Fistulous tracts (course determination), contrast radiography (usage), 388
Fistulous withers, 799
Five-gaited horses, examination, 1190
Five-gaited movements/transitions, complexity, 1189
Five-stage marathon, format, 1206t
Flare (acute synovitis), 101
Flat feet, 305
Flat racing, 995
popularity, 995
Flat shoe, 294
Flat shoe, usage, 301-302
Flat training, tendonitis (rarity), 996
Flat walk (gait), 1189
Flex-Free, 845
Flexion
duration, 81
exaggeration, gait abnormality, 156
paradoxical response, 83
tests
response, 573
usage, 1040
usefulness, 982
Flexion tests, 3, 80-86
diagnostic analgesia, relationship, 87-88
order/duration/force/venue, 81
results
evaluation, 81
pain, causes, 81
specificity, absence, 81
Flexor cortex (lateral aspect), palmar 45° proximal-palmarodistal oblique view, 338f
Flexor retinaculum, 779
Flexor tendonitis, 448
Flexor tendons
imaging, 170
lacerations, repairs, 809
loading, time-related pattern (relationship), 278
treatment, 809
Flexural limb deformity, 645
oxytetracycline, administration, 646
prognosis, 647
splint construction, 647
Flight phase, 283-284
Flip-flop shoe, 13
Flock-lined plastic cuff, 307
Fluid-filled osseous cystlike lesions, appearance, 327
Foals
acetabular fractures, prognosis, 571
angular limb deformity development, 642
examination, 641
persistence, 644-645
articular soft tissue, vascular supply, 1248f
articulating brace, carpus (flexural deformity), 646f

Foals (Continued)
carpus
dorsopalmar radiographic image, 1249f
fluctuant swelling, dorsolateral aspect, 787f
cervical stenotic myelopathy, management, 653
complex infection, diagnosis, 1250
conformation, correction, 291-292
crouched stance, 1243f
cuboidal bone injury, 1245
developmental orthopedic disease, 1247
digits, infection, 1251-1252
distal interphalangeal joint, advanced flexural deformity, 648f
distal phalanx
fractures, 1245-1246
solar margin, fracture, 359
clinical signs/diagnosis, 359
treatment/prognosis, 359
dorsopalmar/lateromedial/dorsoproximal-palmarodistal oblique radiographic views, 635f
epiphyseal-type infectious arthritis, 1249
examination, 641
external trauma, 1243
femur, oblique lateromedial radiographic image, 1244f
fetlock region, physitis, 639
flexural limb deformities, 645
treatment, 647-648
foot, dorsoproximal-palmarodistal oblique radiographic image, 1246f
gait deficits, 1243
hock
dorsoplantar radiographic image, 1250f
oblique lateromedial image, 1246f
immune-mediated synovitis, 1251
infectious arthritis, 683
treatment, 1250
infectious osteitis, 479
infectious osteomyelitis, 40f
infectious synovitis, 1249
joint/bone infections, treatments, 1250-1251
lameness
evaluation, 1242-1243
infectious causes, 1248-1252
noninfectious causes, 1243-1248
lateral recumbency, position, 644
left femur, transverse/longitudinal ultrasonographic images, 215f
long bones
fractures, 1243-1244
morphology, 1249f
vascular supply, 1248f
metacarpophalangeal joint, dorsolateral-palmaromedial oblique radiographic image, 1246f-1247f
myotonia congenita, 837

Foals (Continued)
odontoid peg fractures, 610
osteochondrosis, diagnosis, 1247
physeal type infection, 1249
physes, fractures, 1244-1245
categorization/definitions, Salter-Harris classification scheme, 1244
primary injuries, 787-788
proximal phalanx, Salter-Harris type II fractures (occurrence), 389
proximal sesamoid bones, fractures, 1246
proximal tibial physis, Salter-Harris type II fracture (caudocranial radiographic projection), 529f
PSB fractures, management problem, 407
radius, fractures, 1244
reactive arthritis, septicemia (impact), 677
right carpus valgus, frontal view, 642f
right forelimb, carpus valgus deformity, 1245f
soft tissue injury, 1248
stifle, lateromedial radiographic image, 1247f
stifle joint (medial tibial plateau), stifle joint (craniocaudal radiographic view), 683f
Sussmare-Raszynski intraosseous infusion needle, 1251f
third metacarpal bones (flexural deformity), distal aspect (dorsopalmar radiographic view), 639f
tibia
fractures, 1244
intermediate ridge, histological section, 619
tibial fractures, 529
toe extensions, application, 296
traumatic nerve injury, 1247-1248
ulna, fractures, 1244
vascular thrombosis, 1247
weanlings, dietary management, 830
Foam, precut block, 380f
Focal demineralization, 170
Focal hypoechoic lesions, 729
Focal IRU, 153-154
coxofemoral joint, association, 561
lateral/caudal delayed phase images, 229f
meaning, 225-226
scintigraphic evaluation, 946
Focal muscle soreness, 576-577
Focal peritarsal cellulitis, 1010
focal distention, 1010f
lymphatic damage architecture, relationship, 1010
Focal zone use, problem, 171-172
Foot-related lameness, 1005
Forage, inappropriate grain, 628-629
Forced exercise, 676
Forced flexion, 81
Forced tarsal flexion, racehorse objection, 999

Force-measuring equine treadmill, 246
Force (passive transfer), tendons (involvement), 694
Forces, 92
Forearm (antebrachium), 52
digital palpation, 52
Foreign bodies, 213
ultrasonographic appearance, 213
ultrasonographic examination, 213
Forelimb conformation, 21-28
lateral perspective, 25-28
Forelimb/hindlimb (F/H) weight distribution ratio, 4
Forelimb lameness, 19f, 78
cervical vertebral arthropathy, impact, 653
clinical determination, 69-70
correlation, 69-70
hindlimb lameness
concurrence, 160
confusion, 70-71
mimic, 70
neck lesions, relationship, 152
problems, occurrence, 4-5
recognition, 69-70
syndrome
appearance, 155
origin, 450
vagueness, 450
worsening, circle (impact), 78
Forelimb posture, 39-41
infectious osteomyelitis, 40f
radial nerve paresis/paralysis, 40f
Forelimbs
ALDDFT
desmitis, occurrence, 734
elasticity modulus, 734
anatomical drawing, 272f
bilateral branch desmitis, 1032
blocking strategy, 102f-103f
body desmitis, 1032
brushing interference, 1004
bursae, analgesia, 122-124
center of balance (gravity), 4f
conformation abnormalities, dorsal view, 1089f
distal aspect, 191-195
images, 267f
distal palmar outpouchings, 501
flexion tests, 82-84
fractures, 963-965
front perspective, 21-25
GRF vector/moment arms, schematic drawing, 275f
injury
ALDDFT enlargement, 737
ALDDFT treatment, 738
intraarticular analgesia, 116-122
limb flight abnormalities, 75
local infiltration, 133-135
mechanical/neurological lameness, considerations, 555-556
anatomical considerations, 556
metacarpal region, 50-51
palpation, 44-53
passive stay apparatus, 94, 94f
perineural analgesia, 108-116
proximal aspect, nuclear scintigraphic evaluation, 458-460

Forelimbs (Continued)
proximal suspensory desmitis (PSD), 739-744
commonness, 739
racing injuries, 963-965
SDFT injuries, occurrence, 707
soft tissue injuries, 161-162
stances, GRFs, 274f
stepping short, 155
suspensory ligament
injuries, exercise regimen, 1174b
transverse ultrasonographic image, 750f
total cross-sectional area (T-CSA), measurements, 200
unilateral branch desmitis, 1032
zone 0
longitudinal images, 192f
transverse images, 192f
zone 1A, transverse images, 193f
Forelimb symmetry, 32-35
Forging, 75, 1004
Four-beat gait (gallop), 4
4D competition, 1180
Fourth metacarpal bone (McIV)
cryotherapy, 870-871
distal fragments, ostectomy, 870-871
distal third fracture, suspensory desmitis (association), 751
exostosis, 1012
suspensory desmitis, association, 751
fractures, 505
healing, 505-506
SWT treatment, 916
palpation, 50
pathology, 1142-1143
proximal aspect, fracture, 447
second metacarpal bone
exostoses, 419-421
syndesmopathy, 419
Fourth metatarsal bone (MtIV)
cryotherapy, 870-871
distal fragments, ostectomy, 870-871
distal third fracture, suspensory desmitis (association), 751
exostoses, 1012
suspensory desmitis, association, 751
open comminuted fracture, dorsal 45° lateral-plantaromedial oblique digital radiographic view, 505f
Fourth metatarsal bone (MtIV), needle placement, 126
Fox hunting, 1062
Fractious horses, falling (traumatic injuries), 1199-1200
Fractures, 174-177, 213-214
aging, 176-177
assessment, CT (usage), 236
bone discontinuity, 174
detection, problem, 175
diagnosis, ultrasonography (usage), 213-214
evaluation, 175
fragments, impact, 401
healing process, 175
impact, 33

Fractures (Continued)
lateral-palmaromedial oblique radiographic view, 238f
nondisplacement, 496
occurrence, 981
repair, ultrasound, 903
risk (prediction), bone biomarkers (usage), 951
stability, 176
Fragment size, removal, 253
France, steeplechase race, 1064f
Free-legged, 64
Free radical scavengers, 373
Frequency transducer, problem, 172-173
Fresh bone marrow injection, 762
Frog
apex, 303
apex, spherical radiopaque markers, 379f
buttress, 303
central sulcus, cleft (trimming), 304-305
pressure, maintenance, 1192
proliferative pododermatitis, 319
puncture, 1210-1211
quality, impact, 304
sulci, 273
window, creation, 316-317
Frontal slab fracture
lameness, 441
management, 441-442
standing lateromedial digital radiographic view, 440f
Front feet
asymmetry, commonness, 932
hitting, 74-75
lameness, 1024-1026
lateral/solar scintigraphic images, 146f
size, disparity, 34f
symmetry, 13
ting points, 885f
Front shoes, fitting, 931
Fullering, 295
Full-limb forelimb bandage, 860f
Full-thickness cartilage damage, development, 488
Function, loss, 44
Functional neuroanatomy, knowledge, 90
Fungal infectious arthritis, 684-687
antifungal agents, local administration (intraarticular injection/regional limb perfusion), 685-687
antifungal drug administration regimens, 687t
bacterial infectious arthritis, clinical manifestation comparison, 685
clinical signs, 685
diagnosis, 685
literature review, 684-685
management, 685-687
medical therapy, 685
prognosis, 687
in vitro susceptibility testing, 686t
Fungal organisms, cytological observations, 685
Fusobacterium necrophorum, isolation, 311

G

GAG concentrations, 841-842
Gain settings, problem, 171
Gait, 64-66
  animation, 300
  anomalies, 1038
  clinical signs, 429
  contrast, 65
  deficits, 7
  distal hock joint pain, impact, 992
  evaluation, 807
  load, increase, 5f
  pathognomonic characteristics, 527
  stride cycle, 4
  walking manner, 64
Gait abnormalities, 3
  deficit, 562
  existence, 7
  trochanteric bursitis, impact, 552
Gait analysis, 79-80
  approaches, 246
  methodology, 246
Gaited horses
  fibrotic myopathy, 559
  lameness evaluation, 1187
  shoeing, 1190-1191
Gaited show horses, lameness, 1188
Gallop (four-beat gait), 4
  injuries, 962
Galloping horse, impact, 275-276
Galt trephine, usage, 315-316
Gambling, banning, 978
Gamma camera images, collection, 218
Gamma scintigraphy, 215-216
Ganglion, 692
  synovial hernia, contrast, 692
Gastrocnemius
  anatomical aspects, 509
  bursa, 800
  disruption, 805
  major hindlimb muscle rupture, 162
  muscle injury, 554-555, 834
  muscle/tendon, ultrasonographic examination, 527
  origin, injury, 549
  tendon, rupture, 41-42
Gastrocnemius tendonitis, 803-805
  anatomy, 803
  diagnosis, 804
  history/clinical signs, 803-804
  occurrence, 803
  treatment/prognosis, 804-805
Gelding
  aortoiliac thrombosis, clinical signs, 580f
  proximal metacarpal region, 399f
  riding horse, left carpus (non-weight-bearing dorsopalmar computed radiographic view), 445f
  Thoroughbred-cross Irish draft horse, 1124f
Generalized demineralization (osteopenia), 170
Generalized denervation atrophy, 560
General Stud Book, 1063-1064

Gene therapy, 851-852
  components, review, 671
  joint disease, relationship, 671-672
  therapeutic benefit, 673
  usage, 672-673
Gene transfer
  schematic drawing, 671f
  therapy, limitations, 847
Geometric balance, guidelines, 284f-285f
Geraderichten (straightness), 1112
Geriatric horse, lameness conditions (summary), 9b
Ginglymus joint, 456
Glucosamine hydrochloride, 845
  in vitro dose titration studies, 845-846
Glucose, presence, 370-371
Glue-on heart bar shoes, 384-385
Glue-on shoes, 306-309
  advantages, 307
  types, 307
Gluteal muscles, inflammation, 1146
Gluteal myalgia, 1146
Gluteal myositis, 1161
  occurrence, 992
Gluteal region, secondary muscle soreness, 1021
Gluteal syndrome, 550-552
  cadavers, dissection, 550
  cause, 551
  diagnosis, 550
    method, 550-551
  injury, treatment, 551
  management
    intramuscular injections, injection pattern, 551f
    shoeing, 552
  toe, dragging, 551
Glycogen branching enzyme deficiency (GBED), 830
  clinical signs, 830
    cause, 830
  diagnosis, 830
Glycogen synthase gene (GYS1), autosomal dominant gain-of-function mutation, 828
Glycosoaminoglycan chains, attachment, 658
Godolphin Barb, 1195
Grabs, 297
Gracilis
  major hindlimb muscle rupture, 162
  muscle injury, 554-555
  muscle tear, 1164
Grade 1 histological laminitis, 368f
Grade 3 histological laminitis, 368f
Grade 1 histopathology, 367-368
Grade 2 histopathology, 368
Grade 3 histopathology, 368-369
Gradient echo (GRE) image, 938
Graduated exercise, 809-810
Grain
  fortification, inadequacy, 629
  intake, restriction, 631
  overload, 372
Gram-negative bacteria, disappearance, 369
Grand National, 1062
  Chair, fall, 1069f

Grand Prix dressage horse
  action loss, thoracolumbar region (lateral nuclear scintigraphic image), 599f
  left forelimb
    lameness, left brachiocephalicus muscle (transverse ultrasonographic image), 823f
    palmar aspect, transverse ultrasonographic image, 725f-726f
  right forelimb (suspensory ligament), medial branch (transverse ultrasonographic image), 752f
Grand Prix show jumper
  dorsomedial-plantarolateral oblique radiographic images, 1092f
  left forelimb
    accessory carpal bone, proximal metacarpal region (transverse ultrasonographic image), 743f
    palmar aspect, transverse ultrasonographic image, 724f
  sagittal T1-weighted spoiled gradient-echo image, 336f
  Spruce Meadows jump, 1096f
  tubera ischii, 148f
Grasping forceps, usage, 254
Grass, training, 980
Gravel (subsolar abscess), 314
Greater trochanter, swelling, 38
Greater tubercles, fractures, 463-464
Ground reaction force (GRF), 65, 283
  definition, 271b
  experience, 274-275
  force (shift), mediolateral imbalance (impact), 288
  kinetic technique, usage, 246
  measurement, 71
    kinetic methods, usage, 246
  peak GRF, increase, 276
  quantification, 70
  representation, 274f
  result, 246
  shift, 286
  vertical GRF, schematic drawing, 275f
Growth
  management, 628
  rate, 641
    impact, 621
    measurement inability, 628
Growth factor-based biologics, 763-764
Growth factors
  intralesional injections, 1135
  study, 763
  usage, 851-852

H

Hackney Pony breed, 1188
Hair, clipping, 808
Hair coat, fineness, 169
Half-Arabian horses
  age, importance, 1198
  ALDDFT, desmitis, 1205

Half-Arabian horses (Continued)
  conformation, lameness (relationship), 1197
  counterirritant therapy, 1203
  diagnostic analgesia, 1199
  distal hock joint pain, 1204
  distal interphalangeal joint, osteoarthritis, 1201-1202
  dynamic examination, 1198-1199
  feet, bruising/inflammation, 1200-1201
  flexion tests, 1198-1199
  gluteal pain (croup), 1203-1204
  history, 1197-1198
  hoof tester examination, 1198
  lameness
    conditions, 1200
    diagnosis/management, 1200-1205
    examination, 1197-1198
    improvement, 1203
  medial-to-lateral hoof imbalances, 1198
  metacarpophalangeal/ metatarsophalangeal joints, osteoarthritis, 1204
  neurological examination, 1199-1200
  palmar foot pain, 1201-1202
  palpation, 1198
  performance classes, 1196, 1196b
  physical therapy, 1201
  proliferative periostitis, 1204
  proximal interphalangeal joint, osteoarthritis, 1205
  PSD, recurrence, 1202
  radiological abnormalities, detection, 1201
  sacroiliac pain, 1203-1204
  saddle examination, 1199
  shoeing, rules, 1197
  splint bone injuries, 1204-1205
  static examination, 1198
  stifle joints, osteoarthritis, 1202-1203
  suspensory desmitis, 1202
  thoracolumbar pain, 1203-1204
  toed-out carpus valgus back-at-the-knee conformation, 1197f
  training, impact, 1196-1197
  undiagnosed lameness, 1200
  visual examination, 1198
  work-related fractures, 1204-1205
Half-Arabian show horse
  metacarpophalangeal joint, lateromedial radiographic image, 1204f
  sporting event history, 1195-1196
Half-limb casts, usage, 390
Halicephalobrus (Micronema) deletrix, 144
Hallmarq 0.29-T MR system, 240f
Hand, displaced fractures, 561
Handle, 978-979
  emphasis, 979
Handler, safety, 65-66
Handwalking, 879-880
  exercise, 770-771
  restriction, 1142
Hanging-knee conformation, 27-28

Hard surfaces, 77
gait, 66
Harness, examination, 596
Haunch, downward settling, 70
Hay core, usage, 627
Head
conformation, 19
movement, asymmetric vertical
torso movement, 249
nod, 71
racing injuries, 966
Header, 1170-1171
Head horse
heeler, relationship, 1174f
right forelimb, transverse/
longitudinal
ultrasonographic images,
1174f
Heading horse, progressoin, 1171
Healing, turnout (contrast), 14
Healing deltoid tuberosity
fracture, transverse/
longitudinal ultrasonographic
images, 214f
Health, 13
Heart bar shoe, importance,
317-318
Heart deconditioning, 878
Heart Qi Vacuity, 887-889
Heat, loss, 266
Heel, 294
bruising, 310-311
bulb laceration, 1214f
elevation, impact, 287, 339
extensions, 296
impact, 296
usage, 296
height, impact, 279-280
hoof cracks, incompleteness,
318
loading, inability, 562
lowering/raising, impact, 287
rasping, 305
wedges, usage, 279
Heel-first landing, avoidance, 324
Heel horse, 1172f
Heeling horse, history, 1172
Heights, 20-21
Hemangiosarcoma, occurrence,
693
Hemarthrosis, 163, 690
result, 447
Hematology, 136-137
Hematoma resolution,
ultrasonography (usage), 212
Hematopoietic stem cells (HSCs),
761
Hemicircumferential periosteal
transection/elevation, 643
impact, 643-644
performing, 643
Hemorrhage, 423
Hemorrhagic synovitis,
postmortem examination,
678f
High-energy meal, ingestion,
622
Higher hyaluronan (HA)
concentrations, 841-842
corticosteroids, combination,
844-845
intraarticular corticosteroids,
combination, 842
tests, 843
usefulness, 842-843
High-motion joints, MPA usage
(avoidance), 842

High palmar analgesia,
comparison, 114
High palmar block, 112-114
importance, 125-126
modification, 114
High plantar block, performing,
126f
High plantar nerve block, 125-127
High-quality radiographic images,
168
High spavin, 59-60
High-speed lameness, history, 230
High-speed treadmills, 880
equipment, 925-926
history, collection, 925
horse preparation, 926-927
impact, 925
injury risk, minimization, 927
safety considerations, 926-927
systems, assembly, 926
Hill training, 880
Hind feet
anatomy, 475
arthroscopic examination,
486-487
chronic low-grade lameness,
482
clinical examination, 475-476
clinical signs, 475-476
computed tomography, 485-486
contralateral forelimb, contact,
301
diagnosis, 475-476
diagnostic analgesia, 482
dorsoplantar imbalance, 291
examination, 475-476
horizontal oblique views,
482-483
imaging considerations,
482-487
innervation, 475
interference, 75
keratoma, 478
laminitis, 477-478
magnetic resonance imaging,
484-485
radiographic examination,
482-483
scintigraphic examination,
483-484
ultrasonographic examination,
485
Hind fetlock, dorsal aspect
(acquired bursa), 800
Hind fetlock joint
evaluation, 62
physical appearance, 207f
Hindlimb conformation, 21f,
28-31
abnormalities, 30f
faults, 28
lateral perspective, 28-30
rear perspective, 30-31
Hindlimb extensor weakness, 562
Hindlimb flexion tests, 85
combination, 85f
specificity, absence, 84
usefulness, 81
Hindlimb lameness, 4-5, 71
back/muscle pain, relationship,
54
circling, relationship, 78-79
clinical recognition, 71
cranial phase reduction, 74
diagnosis, absence, 1012-1013
distal hock joint pain, 991
explanation, absence, 11

Hindlimb lameness (Continued)
forelimb lameness
concurrence, 160
confusion, 70-71
hind foot/pastern, contribution,
475
importance, 5
obscurity, 11
predisposition, 21f
recognition, 70
signs, appearance, 923
site distribution, consideration,
5
source, metatarsophalangeal
joint, 1046
Hindlimb proximal suspensory
desmitis, 744-749
computed tomography, 747
diagnostic analgesic techniques,
745
diagnostic ultrasonography,
745
differential diagnosis, 747
extracorporeal shock wave
therapy, 748
gross pathological/
histopathological findings,
749
high-quality ultrasonographic
images, importance, 745
magnetic resonance imaging,
747
nuclear scintigraphy, 746-747
postoperative management,
748
radial pressure wave therapy,
748
radiography/radiology, 745-746
treatment, 747-748
Hindlimbs
abduction
advancement phase, 76
problem, 563
activity, 1112
blocking strategy, 104f-105f
body desmitis, 506-507
bone/muscle mass, asymmetry,
35
broken-back hoof-pastern axis,
treatment, 293
brushing injuries, 1004
bursae, analgesia, 133
conformational faults,
diagrammatic
representation, 28f
DDFT, formation, 726-727
digital flexor tendonitis, 967
distal aspect, 195-198
perineural analgesia, 124-125
distal phalanx, inversion,
363-364
engagement, 18-19
extensor tenosynovitis, 1195
external rotation, 41
fetlock region, dorsal aspect
(soft tissue swelling), 791f
fractures, 965
gait
deficits, 76-77
stabbing, 75-76
injection, number (limitation),
125
injuries, 162-163
intraarticular analgesia, 128-133
investigation, 1003
limb flight, abnormalities, 75-76
local infiltration, 133-135

Hindlimbs (Continued)
lower limb flexion test,
performing, 84f
mechanical lameness, 76-77
mechanical/neurological
lameness, considerations,
555-556
anatomical considerations,
556
movement, abnormality, 77
muscle atrophy, 35-36
neurogenic muscle atrophy, 35
palpation, 56-60
passive stay apparatus, 94-95
pastern, scalping (impact), 1004
perineural analgesia, 124-127
pickup reluctance, 13
plaiting, commonness, 76
posture, 41-43
soft tissue injuries, impact,
41-42
protraction, 248
proximal desmitis, 506-507
proximal pastern, transverse
ultrasonographic image,
774f
resting, 41
rotational change, 30
selective atrophy, 36
stance phases, GRFs, 274f
stepping short, 563
swelling, 36-37
symmetry, 35-39
tail position, abnormality, 41
treading, 41
upper limb flexion tests,
demonstration, 85f
varus posture, 41
walk, stepping short, 563
Zone 1A, 195-196
Zone 2A, 196-197
Zone 3A, 197
Zone 1B, 196
Zone 2B, 197
Zone 3B, 197
Zone 4B, 198
Zone 4C, 198
zones, 195-198
Hindlimb sesamoiditis, 496-497
Hind pastern, 479-480
lameness, 479-480
Hind phalanges, fractures
(occurrence), 965
Hindquarters, muscle symmetry,
1090
Hind shoes, observation, 63f
Hip hike method centers, 249
Hip joint (coxofemoral joint),
131-133
injection site, blocking, 132-133
lateral/dorsal views, 132f
size/landmark, 131-132
Hip region pain, 1109-1110
History, 920-922
collection, 920
History, importance, 15, 135
Hi TENS, 906
Hobbles, impact, 927
Hock
acute injuries, 163
calcaneus, IRU (lateral delayed
phase scintigraphic image),
1031f
collateral ligaments, 211
dorsal 10° lateral-plantaromedial
oblique radiographic view,
636f

Hock (Continued)
dorsolateral-plantaromedial oblique radiographic views, 172f, 801f
dorsomedial-plantarolateral oblique view, 637f
dorsoplantar radiographic views, 636f
extension test, 85-86
usefulness, 85-86
flexed lateromedial view, 522f
flexion, 509
abduction, association, 508
reciprocal apparatus, impact, 95
flexion test, 84-85
lateromedial radiographic view, 172f
lateromedial view, 637f
ligaments, 509
plantar aspects, 29-30
transverse midline ultrasonographic image, 795f
plantar delayed phase scintigraphic image, 1030f
plantar distal aspect, transverse ultrasonographic image, 1080f
points, height (equivalence), 38
puncture wounds, 800
radiographic examination, 514-515
region
analgesia, 511
sagittal section, diagram, 799f
stressed dorsoplantar view, 522f-523f
torsion test, usage, 1184
transverse/longitudinal midline ultrasonographic images, 794f
transverse/longitudinal plantarolateral ultrasonographic images, 795f
transverse magnetic resonance image, 1147f
Hock-related lameness, 510
swelling, 510
Homeostatic pathways, diagram, 851f
Hoof capsule, 280
conformation/condition/ integrity, 45
deep digital flexor tendon, lesions, 733
DP dislocation, 376
grooving, 293
horn, arrangement, 280
load, impact, 277
resection, 293-294
soft tissue lesions, 148-149
strain patterns/peak strains, 278
Hoofs
avulsions, 318
balance
assessment, 44-45
characteristics, 489
role, 489
care, 379
goal, 380-381
cartilage (perforation), vascular foramina (impact), 321
cracks, 1025
dorsal aspect, lateromedial radiographic view, 379f

Hoofs (Continued)
examination, instruments (usage), 45f
flat shoe, nailing, 301-302
glue-on shoes, 306-309
growth, 282
imbalance, clinical identification, 288-291
keratomas, 358-359
lamellae, micrograph, 367f
lamellar tip, laminitis (development), 368f
lengths, 16-17
maladies, complication, 307-308
mechanism, 277
neoplastic space-occupying lesions, 358-359
nonneoplastic space-occupying lesions, 358-359
reconstruction materials, 306-309
repairs
composite materials, usage, 308-309
fabric characteristics, 308t
shoe attachment, 298-299
stiffness, 282
tester
examination, 1039
sensitivity, 1101
Hoof testers
adjustability, 48f
application, 47f
availability, 46f
examination, 46-47, 86-87
impact, 47
placement, 48f
Hoof wall
breakage, 304
reconstruction, 308-309
adhesives, usage, 309
fabric selection, 309
wire technique, limiting factor, 308
removal, 313f
stabilization, 317-318
thickness/strength, 318
thinning, shoeing (impact), 302
viscoelasticity, 282
Hoof wall cracks, 317-318
diagnosis, 317
hoof capsule, visual assessment, 317
history/clinical signs, 317
occurrence, 317
prognosis, 318
treatment, 317-318
variation, 317
Hoof wall lacerations, 318-319
diagnosis, 319
history/clinical signs, 318
prognosis, 319
treatment, 319
Hoof wall quality problem, 313-314
diagnosis, 313
impact, 313
prognosis, 314
treatment, 314
Hoof wall separation (white line disease) (seedy toe), 312-313
diagnosis, 312-313
history/clinical signs, 312
prognosis, 313
treatment, 313

Horse driving trials, 1205
Horse-produced artifacts (ultrasound tissue interaction artifacts), 173
Horses
age/sex/breed/use, facts, 9
confidence, 157
diagnostic analgesia preparation, 106-107
failure, complexity, 270
lateral perspective, 25-28
leading, lameness examination, 66
position, observation, 159-160
safety, 65-66
term, usage, 1205
toed in/toed out, 31
ultrasonographic preparation, 168
Horseshoes, 293-303
additives, 297
adhesives, usage, 299
application, 280, 306
attachment, 298-299
problem, 303
balance, 299
branch, cross-section profiles, 295f-296f
breakover modification, 299-300
closing, 297
eccentric setting, 303
edges, fullering/modifying, 295-296
foot preparation, 293-294
form, 294-298
functions, 299-301
glue, usage, 307-308
ground surface, devices (addition), 297
material, influence, 280
materials/size, 294
modification, 302
nails
placement, 310f
problems, 309-314
pads, insertion, 298f
placement, 306
protection, 299
quarter clips, usage, 280
removal, 310
selection, 303
importance, 306
solar surface, modification, 296
stock, cross-sectional profile, 294-296
support, 300-301
surface, projections, 297
toe clips, usage, 280
toe modification, 295f
traction, 299
increase, 299
requirement, 299
wear pattern/size, assessment, 45
web width, 294
weight, impact, 294
Horse-to-horse interactions, reduction, 13
Hospitalization, preference, 222-223
Hot shoeing, cold shoeing (contrast), 298
Hot water footbaths, 373
Household lameness names, 2
Housing, 13

Humeral head
caudal aspect, crushing, 469
radiological abnormalities, 465-466
Humeral tubercles
fracture, 470
osseous cystlike lesions, 467, 471
development, 471
osteitis, 470
Humeroradial joint, lateral collateral ligament, 456
Humerus, 462-465, 1012
cranial proximal aspect, transverse ultrasonographic image, 459f
deltoid tuberosity, fractures, 462-463
diaphyseal fractures, 464
distal aspect, osseous cystlike lesions, 460
enostosis-like lesions, 465
greater tubercle
cranial/caudal eminences, 456-457
fracture, 463-464
healing stress fracture, left elbow region (lateromedial radiographic image), 944f
lesser tubercle, fracture, 463-464
muscles, relationship, 456
proximal aspect, articular surface fracture, 469
stress fractures, 463
acute-onset forelimb lameness, 1012
commonness, 943-944
diagnosis, nuclear scintigraphy (usage), 944
SWT management, 916
Hunter
acute-onset lameness, antebrachium (longitudinal ultrasonographic image), 823f
scapulohumeral joint, mediolateral radiographic view, 467f
Hunter-bred horse, 1124f
Hunter Pleasure division, 1196
Hunters' Steeplechasers, 1063
Hurdle races, 1062
leading horse jump, 1063f
Hurdlers
lameness
causes, 1070
diagnosis/management, 1070-1075
superficial digital flexor tendonitis, 1070-1072
Hyaline cartilage, 321
Hyaluronan
injection, 433-434
intralesional/perilesional administration, 714-715
production, synovial cell (usage), 688
sodium hyaluronate, 842-843
synovial fluid lubrication, 688
systemic administration, 352
Hydrostatic mechanisms, function, 659
Hydroxylysyl pyridinoline (HP), presence, 949

Hygroma, 88, 691-692, 799
  spontaneous resolution, 692
  term, usage, 448-449
  treatment, 692
Hylan G-F 20, adverse reactions
    (risk), 844-845
Hypaxial muscles, location, 593
Hyperechoic, term (usage), 189t
Hyperinsulinemia, 370
  hormone imbalance, 370-371
Hyperkalemic periodic paralysis
    (HyPP), 838-839
  clinical episodes, 838
  clinical signs, 838
  control, 839
  diagnosis, 838-839
  etiology, 838
  prognosis, 839
  severity, 839
  treatment, 839
Hypertrophic osteopathy, 173,
    424-425, 449, 455
  clinical signs, 424-425
  diagnosis, 425
  early periosteal new bone,
      association, 166
  fibrous tissue/periosteal bone,
      bilaterally symmetrical
      proliferation (involvement),
      455
  treatment, 425
Hypocalcemia, 837
  treatment, 837
Hypochoeris radicata, 559-560
Hypoechoic, term (usage), 189t
Hysteresis, 273-274, 695

I

ICTP, effectiveness, 949
Idiopathic arthritis, 690
Idiopathic synovitis, 777
Idiopathic tenosynovitis, 783-784,
    788-789
  association, absence, 788-789
  defining, 788
  ultrasonographic examination,
      788
Idiopathic thoroughpin, 781
Iliac artery blood flow
    determination, first-pass
    radionuclide angiography
    (usage), 580
Iliac wing, dorsal surface
    (evaluation), 589-590
Ilial shaft examination, 559
Ilial shaft fractures, 568-569, 575
  clinical signs, 568
  pain, 568
  palpation/flexion, 568
  scintigraphic examination,
      568-569
  ultrasonographic examination,
      569
Ilial wing
  cranial/caudal margins, 555-556
  dorsal lateral oblique delayed
      phase scintigraphic image,
      568f
  focal IRU, scintigraphic
      evaluation, 946
  fractures, 567-568, 575
    clinical signs, 567
    scintigraphic examination, 568
    ultrasonographic detection,
        937-938
    ultrasonographic
        examination, 568

Ilial wing *(Continued)*
  stress fracture, 561f
    displacement, 562
    dorsal lateral oblique delayed
        phase scintigraphic
        image, 578f
Ilium
  sacral wing, fractures, 1012
  stress-related bone injury,
      945-946
IL-1ra gene
  benefits, 673
  direct transmission, 671
  sequence, transfer, 672
Image
  acquisition, 218-223, 266-267
  contrast, 168
  display, 235-236
  distance, 221
  dynamic acquisition, 221f
  findings, misinterpretation,
      152-154
  interpretation, principle, 219
  labeling, 168
  motion, 222
  obtaining, mode (usage), 219
  processing, 235-236
  reconstruction, 235
  resolution, 168-169
  sharpness, 168-169
  shielding, 221-222
Image quality, 220
  compromise, 222
  limitation, 556
  problems, 222
Imaging, 429-432
  equipment, 217-218
  modality, 216, 667-668
  performing, 266-267
  plates, usage, 182
Imbalance, 285-288
  forms, 288
  treatment, 291-293
Immature horses, subchondral
    bone cysts (enlargement),
    467
Immature periosteal new bone,
    overexposure, 177
Immobilization, 878
Immune-mediated arthritis, 689
Immune-mediated myopathies,
    831
Immune-mediated myositis
    (IMM), 831
  clinical signs, 831
  cryostate-cut sections, 831f
  diagnosis, 831
  treatment, 831
Immune-mediated polymyositis,
    occurrence, 831
Immune-mediated polysynovitis,
    156
Immune-related mechanisms,
    13
Immune stimulants, usage,
    142
Immunoglobulin G (IgG)
  complex deposition, presence,
      689
  index, 139
Immunohistochemistry, 141
Immunoradiometric (IRMA) assay,
    948
Impact, 275-276
  characteristics, 276
  resistance, importance, 306
  shock, 275-276

Implants, 215
  ultrasonographic examination,
      215
Impulse, 276
In-at-the-hock, angular deformity,
    31
In-at-the-knee conformation,
    21-22
  problem, 24f
Inclines, observation, 79
Incomplete bar, extension, 297
Incomplete fractures, occurrence,
    558
Incomplete lateral/medial
    condylar fractures,
    management, 496
Incomplete ossification, 517
Incomplete osteochondral
    fragments (diagnosis),
    scintigraphic examination
    (usage), 436-437
Increased radiopharmaceutical
    uptake (IRU), 67
  areas, identification, 228-229
  comparison, 170-171
  determination, 224
  focal areas, 431
    tibial stress fractures,
        relationship, 945
  gamma ray emission, 218-219
  increase, 216
  intensity, 224-225
  lateral delayed-phase
      scintigraphic view, 68f
  location, 224
  scintigraphic evidence, 432
Indian hedgehog (Ihh), role,
    624-625
Induced lameness, 3, 80
  concept, understanding, 80
  creation, tests (usage), 80
  flexion tests, 80-86
  hoof tester examination,
      impact, 86-87
Inertial sensor systems, examples,
    250f
Infarctive hemorrhagic purpura,
    831
Infected fracture, nonunion,
    503
Infection, 470-471
  cellulitis, association, 166-167
Infectious arthritis, 447, 526,
    677-684
  alternative therapy, 684
  antimicrobial agents, bone
      concentration, 682
  antimicrobial drugs
    direct local infusion, 680
    intraarticular injection/doses,
        680
    IV administration, 679
  antimicrobial-impregnated
      biodegradable drug delivery
      systems, usage, 681
  antimicrobial-impregnated
      biomaterials, usage,
      680-681
  antimicrobial therapy, 679-682
  bandaging, 684
  causes, 677
  clinical signs, 677
  criteria, requirements, 678
  diagnosis, 678-679
  diclofenac topical medications,
      684
  draft horses, 1227

Infectious arthritis *(Continued)*
  drugs, diffusion, 680
  epidural narcotics, 684
  examination, 677-678
  50:50 DL-lactide-glycolide
      copolymers, usage, 681
  infected bone (foci location),
      nuclear scintigraphy
      (usage), 679
  initial management, 677-678
  intravenous antimicrobial
      therapy, initiation, 679
  local therapy, 680-682
  models, 676-677
  NSAIDs, usage, 683-684
  pain management, 683-684
  PMMA
    biomechanics, 681
    usage, 680
  prognosis, 684
  rabbit model, 683
  regional perfusion, usage,
      681-682
  systemic therapy, 679-680
  topical treatment, 684
  treatment, 684
Infectious bursitis, 791
  occurrence, 791
Infectious injuries (evaluation),
    radiographs (usage),
    139
Infectious metritis, 372
Infectious myopathies, 831-833
Infectious myositis/cellulitis,
    454-455
  treatment, 455
Infectious navicular bursitis
    (septic navicular bursitis),
    316-317
  management, 317
Infectious osteitis/osteomyelitis,
    173
Infectious tenosynovitis, 770-771,
    782, 784-785, 789-790
  characterization, 789
  diagnosis, 770
  etiopathogenesis, 770
  prognosis, 771
  systemic antibiotic therapy,
      continuation, 790
  treatment, 770-771
    primary aim, 789
Inflamed joints, prostaglandins
    (elevated concentrations),
    664
Inflammation, 369
  sign, observation, 44
Inflammatory musculoskeletal
    conditions, radiation therapy,
    875t
Inflammatory myopathies,
    831-834
Infrared thermography, 266
  imaging, 911-913
Infraspinatus bursa, infection, 472
  occurrence, 472
Infraspinatus muscles, atrophy,
    53f, 473
Injured hind fetlock joint,
    physical appearance,
    207f
Injured horse
  field diagnosis, 159
  humane destruction, guidelines,
      164
  transportation, 861
Injured limb, transportation, 808

Injuries
  prevention, boots/bandages
      (usage), 425-426
  rate, comparisons, 974
  risk
      minimization, 927
      racing surface, impact, 972
  term, usage, 200
Innervation, 323
Inside rim shoes, 295-296
Instability models, 675-676
Instantaneous center of rotation
      (ICR), 16
Instrumented shoes
  customization, 246
  usage, 70
Insulin
  levels, osteochondral lesions
      (relationship), 622
  natural trigger factor, 370
  presence, 370-371
Insulin growth factor-I (IGF-I),
      851
Insulin-like growth factor I
      (IGF-I), in vitro evaluation,
      844-845
Interarticular fibrocartilage, 93
Intercalated bones, 93
Intercarpal ligament damage,
      988
Interference
  injury, 1004, 1018-1019
      decrease, 301
      prevention, 301
      occurrence, 301
      types, 74f
Interleukin-1 (IL-1)
  activation, diagram, 672f, 847f
  inhibition, 846-847
  receptor antagonist protein,
      synthesis (reduction),
      664
Interleukin-1 receptor antagonist
      (IL-1ra), 846-847
Interleukin-1 receptor antagonist
      protein (IRAP), 1155
  development, 847
  test, 847
Intermediate carpal bone,
      proximal aspect (dorsomedial-
      palmarolateral oblique
      radiographic view), 437f
Intermittent knuckling, 562
Intermittent upward fixation of
      the patella (IUFP), 56
Internal blistering, 713-714
Internal blisters, usage, 867-868
Internal fixation, usage, 503
Internal shielding, 221-222
Internal trauma fractures,
      421-422
  clinical signs, 421
  diagnosis, 421
  treatment, 421-422
International Federation of
      Arabian Horse Racing
      Authorities (IFAHR), 1057
International Federation of
      Horseracing Authorities
      (IFHA) rules, 980-981
International Veterinary
      Acupuncture Transpositional
      points, 889b
Interneuron pools, central
      sensitization, 909
Interosseous ligaments,
      attachment, 394

Interphalangeal joints
  flexion, 83
  tests, 84
Intersesamoidean ligament, 739
  body, focal tears, 754
  degeneration/partial rupture,
      754-755
  diseases, 774-775
      diagnosis, 775
      etiopathogenesis, 774-775
      treatment/prognosis, 775
  injury, 406-407
      diagnosis, 775
  insertion injury, 755
  perineural analgesia, four-point
      block (usage), 755
Interstitial brachytherapy, 874
Intersynovial fistulae, 791
  rarity, 791
Intertransverse joints,
      ultrasonographic evaluation,
      579, 604
Intertubercular bursa (bicipital
      bursa), 456, 470-471, 799
  bursoscopy, 265
  infection, 470
      treatment, 471
  intrathecal analgesia, 457
Interventional computed
      tomography, 238
Intervertebral disk, compression/
      traction forces, 571
Intraarticular analgesia
  impact, 394
  inconsistency, 105
  response, 387-388
Intraarticular blades, usage, 254
Intraarticular corticosteroids
  HA, combination, 842
  studies, 841-842
  usage, 841
Intraarticular fractures,
      occurrence, 175
Intraarticular fragmentation,
      suspensory branch injury
      (association), 406
Intraarticular HA, tests, 843
Intraarticular injections,
      nonracehorse response,
      492
Intraarticular plantar process
      osetochondritis dissecans
      fragments, 228-229
Intraarticular pressure, 659
  increase, 688
  variation, 659
Intraarticular PSGAG, usage
      (recommendation), 844
Intraarticular therapy, 844-845
Intraarticular volume, 659
  variation, 659
Intracavitary brachytherapy, 874
  development, 874
  formulations, development,
      874
Intralesional β-aminopropionitrile
      fumarate, usage, 714
Intralesional glycosaminoglycans,
      treatment regimen, 868
Intralimb compensatory lameness,
      482
Intrasynovial analgesia, false
      positive results, 149
Intrasynovial injections, 146
  performing, 107
Intrathecal hemorrhage, 778
Intravenous HA, usage, 843

Intravenous ketamine,
      subanesthetic doses, 857-858
Inversion, 363-364
In vitro bone testing, 956
In vivo strain measurements,
      954
Iodine-containing counterirritants,
      injection, 558
Ionizing radiation, administration,
      873
Ionophores, 836
Ipsilateral hindlimb, front foot
      (hitting), 74-75
Ipsilateral limbs, contact
      (occurrence), 301
Ipsilateral splint bone,
      radiographic examination,
      752
Irradiation
  clinical applications, 875-877
  recommendation, 876
  techniques, 873-874
Ischial tuberosity, laterally
      directed forces (application),
      589
Ischium fractures, 560
  scintigraphic examination,
      561-562
  ultrasonographic examination,
      561
Isoechoic, term (usage), 189t
Isoxsuprine, usage, 340-341

J
Jack spavin, cryotherapy, 871
Jack tendon, 133
Jockey Club, 1062
Jogging, increase, 1016
Joint-associated tumors, rarity,
      692-693
Joint capsule, 244
  dorsal aspects, large vessel
      (traversal), 517-518
  enthesophyte formation,
      172-173
  MRI, usage, 244
  palmar pouch distention,
      observation, 998
  trauma, 353-354
Joint disease
  anabolic processes, 670
  bone metabolism, skeletal
      biomarkers, 670
  catabolic processes, 670
  clinical evaluation, 664-668
  complexity, 674
  diagnosis/management,
      advances, 848
  factors, 674
  gene therapy, relationship,
      671-672
  intraarticular corticosteroids,
      841-842
  medical treatment, 840-846
  MRI role, 668
  NSAIDs, usage, 840-841
  surgical treatment, 848-852
  variables, 674
  in vitro study, tissues (usage),
      675
Joint disease model
  biomechanical models, 677
  instability models, 675-676
  types, 674-677
  usage, 673
  in vitro models, 674-675
  in vivo models, 675-677

Joint Photographic Experts Group
      (JPEG) formats, 170
Joints
  angles, impact, 279
  bleeding, 690
  debridement, 682-683
  disorders, radiation therapy,
      876
  dorsal aspect, evaluation, 268
  drainage, 682-683
      importance, 682
  effusion, viewing, 932
  environment (changes), forced
      exercise (usage), 676
  fluid, appearance, 678
  forced flexion, 81
  function, 92, 655-660
  infected tarsocrural joint,
      constant rate infusion
      balloon system, 682f
  internal architecture,
      importance, 92
  kinematics, 29-30
  lavage, importance, 682
  locomotion, 278
  lubrication, 659
  manipulation, 892
  mobilization, 892
  moment, reduction, 300
  motion
      active/passive ranges,
          assessment, 897
      articular zones, schematic
          representation, 892f
  movement, 272
  pain, 664-665
  pathophysiology (synovitis),
      687-688
  physiology, 687
  pressure, articular contact
      (relationship), 279-280
  range, patterns (diagram),
      894f
  sensory innervation, 103
  soft tissue diseases, 691-692
  structure, 92, 655-660
Jugular vein thrombophlebitis,
      615-616
Jumpers
  bucked-knee conformation,
      27-28
  forelimb, distal part (delayed
      image), 227f
Jumping pony,
      metacarpophalangeal joint
      (lateromedial radiographic
      image), 1230f
Jumping sports horses,
      characteristics, 1097

K
Kentucky Derby, 977
  initiation, 977
Keratan sulfate (KS), 669
  measurement, 669
Keratomas, 358-359
  clinical signs/diagnosis, 359
  history, 358
  treatment, 359
Ketamine, NMDA receptor
      antagonist, 856-857
Kick injury, 788
Kick wounds, 13
Kimzey Leg Saver Splint
  application, 968f
  usage, 861f
Kinematic analysis, 926

Kinematics, 247-251
  definition, 271b
  gait measurements, 510-511
  sensing element size, impact,
      249-250
  usage, 247
Kinetics, 246-247
  definition, 271b
  evaluation, 29-30
Kissing spines, 598-599
  presence, 599
  surgical treatment, 605
Knee, forward buckling, 39
Knee-sprung (over-at-the-knee,
    bucked-knee) conformation,
    27-28
Knocked-down hip, 37
Knock-kneed conformation,
    21-22

L

Lactate dehydrogenase (LDH),
    assessment usage, 818
Lactation, 630
  calcium requirements, 950
Lame foal, evaluation, 1242-1243
Lame horse, scintigraphic
    examination, 230-234
Lame limb, pain, 149
Lamellae, laminitis, 371
Lamellar anatomical
    characteristics, 367
Lamellar attachment, pathological
    deformation, 367
Lameness, 3, 282-293, 984-993
  acupuncture therapy, 884-886
  alleviation, intraarticular
      analgesia (usage), 82
  articular lesion, impact,
      103-105
  bacterial infection, 1009-1010
  categories, 67
  causes, 155-159
    correlation, 78
  characterization, 66-69
  clinical manifestations, 3
  clinical sign, 3
  comparison, 65
  compensation, understanding,
      67
  condition, 476-480
    initiation, 12
    list, 984
    worsening, 12
  conformation
    problem, impact, 288
    relationship, 6
  CT diagnosis, 236-238
  definition, 3
  degree, 428
    variation, 476, 513
  detection, 72-73
    inertial sensor systems,
        examples, 250f
    kinematic measures,
        248-249
  determination, 66-69
  diagnosis, 927-928
    acupuncture, usage, 881-886
    challenges, 149-152
    diagnostic analgesia, 982-983
    distal caudal radial exostosis,
        association, 150
    distribution, 4-5, 1018
    duration, 12
    elimination, 927-928
    etiquette, 7

Lameness (Continued)
  examination, 387-388, 981-983
    acupuncture, clinical
        applications, 884-886
    physical examination, role, 63
    shoes, wearing (requirement),
        927
    treadmill, usage, 927
  explanation, absence, 7,
      232-233
  grading, 66-69
  hard surfaces, impact, 13
  head conformation, irrelevance,
      19
  history, 54
    determination, questions,
        926b
    obtaining, 14-15
  imbalance, impact, 288
  importance, 6-7
  improvement, 12, 149, 771
    circling, impact, 78
    failure, 551-552
    intraarticular analgesia,
        administration, 394
  information/ideas, American
      Association of Equine
      Practitioners (dissemination
      role), 2
  intermittentness, 149
  investigation, principle, 89
  localization, 476
    preference, 220
  location, determination, 69-71
  management
    changes, 12-13
    information, 8
  medical conditions, association,
      13
  mediolateral imbalance, impact,
      290
  mimic, 63
  movement, 982
  muscle pain/injury, role, 821
  nuclear scintigraphic
      examination, 467
  observation, 54
  occurrence, 12-13
  osteochondrosis, impact, 1035
  pain, impact, 403
  palmar foot pain, impact, 1201
  past history, 14-15
  pattern, 997
  PIP lesions, impact, 633
  presence, 77-78, 156
  prognosis assessment, 7-8
  proliferative synovitis, impact,
      1050
  rectal examination, 55
  score, 71-72
  scoring, 72b
  severity
    observation, 969
    quantification, 71-72
    trauma, impact, 33
  shoeing, impact, 302-303
  slow-motion videotape,
      evaluation, 69
  strategy, components, 7-8
  treatment, acupuncture
    clinical applications, 884-886
    usage, 881-886
  variation, 151-152, 510, 517
  warming, 12
  worsening, 78
    diagnostic analgesia, impact,
        105-106

Lameness diagnosis
  change, 1
  critical issues, 2
  historical review, 2
Lameness evaluation, 87, 245
  inertial sensor systems,
      examples, 250f
  sound, usefulness, 72-73
  treadmill/gait analysis, usage,
      79-80
Lameness examination, 7, 65-66
  abbreviation, performing, 7
  components, 7-8, 7b
  horse, leading, 66
  movement, 77-79
  surface characteristics, 66
Lameness Locator, 250f, 251
Lameness problems
  determination, 11
  development, 11-12
  occurrence, 4-5
Laminar dermis, 321
Laminar ring, 371
Laminitic foot, lateromedial
    venogram, 378f
Laminitic horse, hoof care,
    379-382
Laminitis, 146, 369
  acute phase, 379-380
  characterization, 371
  chronic phase, hoof care goal,
      380-381
  clinical signs, 371
  cryotherapy, 373
  CT evaluation, 238
  development, 371-372, 374
  development, risk, 576
  developmental phase, 379
  diagnosis, 371-372
  digital blood therapy, 373
  exercise, impact, 373
  exogenous corticosteroids,
      usage, 371
  grade 1 histopathology, 367-368
  histopathology, descriptions,
      367
  hot water footbaths, 373
  hyperinsulinemia trigger, 370
  impact, 281
  lamellar disintegration
      (occurrence), 369
  management
    aspects, 384-386
    deep digital flexor tenotomy,
        usage, 382-384
  medical management, 384
  medical therapy, 372-374
  mineral oil, administration, 374
  NSAIDs, administration,
      372-373
  pathophysiology, 366-371
  pharmaceuticals,
      administration, 374
  phenylbutazone, usage, 372
  radiographic examination, 372
  risk, 370
  theories, 369
  treatment
    protocol/prognosis,
        radiographic
        examination, 372
    strategy, recommendation,
        373-374
  trigger factors, 369
  triggering, drug regimen, 372
  vasodilator therapy, 373
  venograms, usage, 377

Large breed horses, image quality,
    222
Large muscle masses, scanning,
    169
Large osteochondral fragments
    (slab fractures), 440-444
Laser
  animal studies, 905
  biophysics, 904
  therapy, 904-905
    human studies, 904
Lasing medium, 904
Late pregnancy, developmental
    orthopedic disease, 629-630
Lateral, term (usage), 429
Lateral carpal bones, impact,
    642
Lateral collateral cartilage, 320
Lateral collateral ligament, 456
  injury, 211
  transverse/longitudinal/
      ultrasonographic images,
      356f
Lateral condylar fracture,
    dorsopalmar projection,
    408f
Lateral condyle, displaced
    fracture (arthroscopic view),
    849f
Lateral delayed-phase
    scintigraphic view, 68f
Lateral digital extensor (LDE)
    muscle, 786
Lateral digital extensor tendon
    (LDET), 786
Lateral digital flexor tendon
    (LDFT), 262
  long digital extensor tendon,
      connection, 499
Lateral femorotibial (LFT) joint
  arthrocentesis, 130
  capsule, access, 56
  compartment challenge, 130
Lateral gaits, performing, 1189
Lateral malleolar fractures, trauma
    (origin), 521
Lateral malleolar fragments,
    trauma, 637
Lateral palmar block, 114
  performing, 114
Lateral palmar intercarpal
    ligaments, 447-448
  avulsion injury, 446-447
  description, 447-448
  displacement, resistance, 427
Lateral palmar nerves,
    desensitization, 110-111
Lateral patellar ligaments
  longitudinal ultrasound scan,
      208f
  palpation, 56
Lateral plantar metatarsal nerves,
    block, 126
Lateral plantar nerve
  block, 126
  dep branch, fasciotomy/
      neurectomy, 506-507
Lateral PVC, full-limb forelimb
    bandage, 860f
Lateral scintigraphic image, usage,
    228
Lateral splint bones, 499
Lateral thorax/abdomen,
    palpation, 54
Lateromedial foot balance,
    correction/preservation,
    339

Lathyrism, impact, 145
Lavage cannulae, usage, 254
Left antebrachium, craniocaudal
  radiograph, 14f
Left carpi (left carpus)
  dorsal 45° lateral-palmaromedial
    oblique radiographic view,
    431f
  dorsal 45° medial-palmarolateral
    digital radiographic view,
    439f
  flexed position
    diagram, 115f
    dorsal view, 120f
  joints, intraoperative
    arthroscopic images,
    256f
  lateromedial radiographs,
    26f
  non-weight-bearing
    dorsopalmar computed
    radiographic view, 445f
Left crus, lateral view, 127f
Left elbow region
  callus formation, lateromedial
    radiographic image,
    944f
Left elbow region, lateral view,
  122f
Left femur
  comminuted fracture, 38f
  lateromedial digital
    radiographic views, 553f
  transverse/longitudinal
    ultrasonographic images,
    215f
Left fore fetlock, dorsal 15°
  proximal-palmarodistal
  oblique/lateromedial images,
  1002f
Left fore (LF), dorsal 65°
  proximal-plantaro/palmaro
  distal digital radiographic
  views, 479f
Left fore (LF) SSL, ultrasonographic
  images, 816f
Left forelimb (LF), 64
  dorsal view, physitis, 640f
  lameness, head nod, 73
  lateral bone phase scintigraphic
    images, 1142f
  metacarpal region, dorsomedial-
    palmarolateral oblique
    view, 158f
Left front foot, sagittal short
  tau inversion recovery MRI,
  348f
Left front proximal
  interphalangeal joint,
  subluxation/osteoarthritis,
  49f
Left gastrocnemius, partial
  disruption, 38f
Left hind lateral OSL, origin
  (ultrasonographic images),
  814f
Left hind (LH)
  dorsal 65° proximal-plantaro/
    palmaro distal digital
    radiographic view,
    479f
  fetlock, flexural deformity,
    736f
  foot, dorsoproximal-
    plantarodistal oblique
    radiographic view,
    360f-361f

Left hindlimb (LH)
  abbreviation, 64
  lameness
    existence, 71
    midcrus, craniolateral
      aspect (transverse
      ultrasonographic images),
      802f
    transverse/longitudinal
      ultrasonographic images,
      728f
Left hind shoe, natural breakover
  indication, 1203f
Left hock, plantaromedial aspect
  (transverse/longitudinal
  ultrasonographic images),
  794f
Left humerus, lateral
  scintigraphic/mediolateral
  radiographic view, 465f
Left longissimus dorsi muscles,
  lactic acid (injection), 821
Left metacarpal region
  computer graphic, 203f
  transverse view, 114f
Left metacarpophalangeal
  (metatarsophalangeal)
  joint, dorsal 60° proximal-
  palmarodistal oblique image,
  1001f
Left metacarpophalangeal
  (metatarsophalangeal)
  joint/digit, palmarolateral
  (plantarolateral) view,
  119f
Left patella, arthroscopic view,
  546f
Left proximal metatarsal region
  left hand placement, 61f
  longitudinal image, 746f
Left-right asymmetry, problem,
  33
Left shoulder, mediolateral
  radiographic view, 160f
Left stifle, caudocranial view,
  147f
Left tarsus
  cross-section, 793f
  lateral view, 127f-128f
  plantar view, 128f
Left third carpal bone, flexed
  dorsal 60° proximal-
  dorsodistal oblique images,
  998f
Left third metacarpal bone,
  dorsopalmar radiographs,
  14f
Leg positions, 42
Lengths, 20-21
  measurements, 17f
Lesions
  age, determination, 178
  categories, 200-203
    exceptions, 204
  category I, 200
  category II, 200-201
  category II/category III injuries,
    201
  category III, 201
  category IV, 201-202
  category V, 202-203
  category VI, 203
  debridement, 261
  differentiation, 619
  hyperechoic/anechoic types,
    205
  identifiability, 155

Lesions (Continued)
  identification, nuclear
    scintigraphy (usage), 140
  suspicion, 178
  treatment, 870-872
Lesser tubercles, fractures,
  463-464
Leukocytes, 369
  counts, range (variation), 138
  detection, 369
Lexington (Kentucky), 977
Liautard's insistence,
  improvement, 64
Lidocaine, characteristics, 100-101
Ligament injury, 691, 812-816
  healing, slowness, 691
  localization, 587-588
  rehabilitation, 168
  in vivo studies, 916-917
Ligaments, 244
  cell population, elevation,
    698-699
  enthesophyte formation,
    172-173
  functional anatomy, 694
  histological features, 698f
  lesion characterization,
    parameters (usage), 189b
  MRI, usage, 244
  SW application, 916-917
  thermographic imaging,
    difficulty, 268
  transverse images, CSA
    measurements, 173-174
Limb flight
  abnormalities, 74-77
  evaluation, 73-74
  mechanical lameness, 76-77
  shoulder region lameness, 75
Limbs, 21
  abduction, 75
  blocking, 147
  bones, relationship, 271
  collapse, 135-136
  conformation, evaluation, 21
  diagonal pair, simultaneous
    lameness, 71
  direct trauma, 166
    boots/bandages, usage, 426
  distal aspect
    conformation problem/
      imbalance, 288
    fractures, 162
    imaging, 267
    lameness, pain (association),
      886
    rotational/angular
      conformation,
      examination, 289
    sagittal images, 242f
    tissues, function, 276
    transverse 3D T2 gradient
      echo image, 243f
  elevation, 62-63
  evolution, 279
  examination, 160
  flight arc, length/shape
    (perception), 248
  functional anatomy, 270-273
  immobilization, 861
  interference, 74
  manipulation, resentment, 572
  pain, multiple sources, 149
  passive movement, 823
  pogo sticks, comparison, 271
  proximal parts,
    ultrasonography, 199

Limbs (Continued)
  push-off, 249
  sinking, 135-136
  stiffness, 271
  swelling, local problem, 165
  weight-bearing position, 56-57
Linear array transducers, 169
Line firing, usage, 868
Listed and Group company, horse
  racing, 994
Liver Depression, 887
Load, bone adaptation rate
  (balance), 935
Load-deformation curves, 273-274
Loading, time-related pattern,
  278
Loading cycles, number, 276-277
Local analgesia
  incomplete response, 103
  response, 329-330
  techniques
    false-negative response,
      145-146
    responses, confusion, 148-149
Local anesthetics, 100-107
Local anesthetic solutions
  circumferential subcutaneous
    infiltration, 107
  effectiveness, time (allowance),
    146
  infiltration, 134
  injection, tissue damage
    occurrence, 101
  proximal diffusion, 101
  volume, variation, 107
Local area, blocking, 107
Local cold therapy, 505
Localized back muscle soreness,
  induction, 821-822
Localized muscle atrophy, 33
Localized muscle soreness, clinical
  significance, 611
Localized osteitis, small puncture
  wounds, 507-508
Local muscle soreness,
  observation, 612
Local myositis, 1169
Local palpation, 86
Locking compression plate (LCP),
  502-503
  impact, 554
Locking stifle, 556-558
Locomotion
  division, 274
  musculoskeletal element,
    277-278
Long bones
  enostosis-like lesions, 452
  fractures, emergency
    management, 451
  morphology, 1249f
  stress fractures, 1010-1012
  thermographic imaging,
    difficulty, 268
  vascular supply, 1248f
Long digital extensor (LoDE)
  muscle, situation, 786
Long digital extensor (LoDE)
  transection, 807
Long digital extensor tendon
  (LoDET)
  avulsion, 548
    prognosis, 548
    signs/diagnosis, 548
    treatment, 548
  LDET, connection, 786
Long hair coat, insulator, 267

Longitudinal image, obtaining, 173
Long lateral CLs, enthesopathy, 523-524
Long plantar desmitis, 798
  management, 798
Long radius (forearm), consideration, 20
Long-term lameness, 801-802
Long toes, 305
  impact, 291
Loose stifles, 562
Lope, three-beat gait, 65
Los Alamitos Racetrack, 1051-1052
Los Alamitos Two Million Futurity, 1051-1052
Lossgelassenheit (looseness/suppleness), 1112
Lo TENS, 906
Louisville Jockey Club, racetrack opening, 977
Low-dose radiation, antiinflammatory effects, 872-873
Lower hindlimb
  abnormal movement, 77
  lameness, clinical signs, 590-591
Lower limb flexion
  achievement, 82f
  positive response, 80
  test
    performing, 84
Lower limb flexion test, 81-82, 84
  fetlock flexion test, comparison, 82, 82f
  performing, 84f
  specificity, 82-83
Lower limb lameness, limb length (relationship), 18
Lower motor neuron diseases, 7, 136
Lower neck, injuries, 1215
Low-field magnets, developments, 668
Low four-point block, usage, 397
Low-grade equine rhabdomyolysis, occurrence, 923
Low-grade hindlimb stiffness, nuclear scintigraphy (usage), 576
Low-grade lameness, presence, 12, 355
Low-grade stifle lameness, positive diagnostic analgesia (usage), 534
Low-level laser therapy (LLLT), 904
  application, 904
  clinical applications, 904
  veterinary usage, 904-905
Low palmar analgesia, 111-112
Low palmar block, 111
  low plantar block, contrast, 125
Low palmar nerve block (plantar block), needle position (lateral view), 112f
Low plantar block, perineural analgesia, 125
Low plantar perineural technique, 482
Lumbar dorsal spinous process, prominence, 577
Lumbar regions
  muscles, assessment, 572
  myositis, impact, 992

Lumbar vertebrae, 946
  stress fractures, 946
Lumbosacral joint, 579
  abnormalities, clinical significance, 579
  lesions (treatment), deep paramedian injection (usage), 579
  ultrasonographic evaluation, 579, 604
Lumbosacral pathology, clinical signs, 579
Lumbosacral space, aspiration preparation, 137-138
Lumican (proteoglycan), 700
Luxation, 177, 468-469
  contact loss, 177
  patella, secondary upward fixation (impact), 581-582
Lyme disease, 156, 690
Lymphangitis, 33, 167
  occurrence, 167
Lysyl oxidase, copper (cofactor), 622

M

Magnetic field, homogeneity (disturbance), 245
Magnetic resonance imaging (MRI), 215
  acquisition, manipulation, 241
  advantages, 241
  disadvantages, 241
  equipment, 241
  Hallmarq 0.29-T MR system, 240f
  images
    contrast (determination), tissue proton density (usage), 241-242
  images, production, 240-241
  indications, 245
  interpretation, 241-244
  magnets, field strength, 240
  method, 239-240
  1.5-T GE Echospeed, 240f
  partial volume effects, 245
  pulse sequence, 240
  scan, 218
  slice-by-slice high-resolution images, 938
Major articular fractures, 395
Major vessel sites, knowledge, 90
Maladaptive/nonadaptive subchondral bone remodeling, lateral/plantar/flexed lateral delayed phase images, 233f
Malignant hyperthermia, 829
  clinical signs, 829
  diagnosis, 829
  etiology, 829
  treatment, 829
Mammaliam cartilage, regional organization (photomicrograph), 656f
Mange mites, impact, 1224
Manic flexoria tear, tenoscopic view, 769f
Man-made structures, safety factor, 270
Man o' War, 978
Manual therapies, 884, 892
  focus, 894-895
  hands, application, 892

Marathon phase, 1206
Mare, left hindlimb lameness crus (transverse ultrasonographic image), 804f
Marilyn Monroe trot, 998
Mast cells, degranulation, 903
Material properties, 273-274
  knowledge, 273
Matrix-degrading enzymes, 662
Matrix macromolecules, synthesis (decrease), 663-664
Matrix metalloproteinases (MMPs), 624, 661
  activation, 846-847
  expression, cytokine-mediated induction, 664
  inhibitors, 662
    BAY 12-9566, in vitro study assessment, 846
    inclusion, 846
    interleukin-1 activation, diagram, 672f
  role, 662
Matrix proteins, 658
Mature riding horse, foot (dorsoproximal-palmaromedial oblique view), 364f
Maximal zone cross-sectional area (MIZ-CSA), 200
Mean flexor tendon forces, calculation, 277f
Mechanical demands, structure coping, 273-278
Mechanical hindlimb gait abnormalities, diagrammatic representation, 557f
Mechanical lameness, 563
  biomechanical forces, 555
  pain, 555
Mechanical nociceptive thresholds (MNTs), 894-895
Mechanics
  alterations, 280-281
  changes
    laminitis, impact, 281
    osteoarthritis, impact, 281
    superficial digital flexor tendonitis, impact, 281
Medial collateral ligament
  calcanean fasciculus, longitudinal ultrasound scan, 211f
  deep palpation, 56-57
  desmopathy, 209
Medial cutaneous antebrachial block, 114-116
Medial cutaneous antebrachial nerve, cranial/caudal branches (block), 115-116
Medial femoral condyle, cartilage lesions (occurrence), 848
Medial femorotibial (MFT) compartments, communication inconsistency, 130
Medial femorotibial (MFT) joint
  arthrocentesis, 130
  cranial aspects, intraoperative arthroscopic images, 255f
  craniomedial aspect, proximodistal ultrasound scan, 210f
  effusion, 56
  medial aspect, proximodistal ultrasound scan, 210f

Medial femorotibial (MFT) joint (Continued)
  medial recess
    longitudinal ultrasound scan, 209f
    transverse ultrasound scan, 208f-209f
  pain, occurrence, 1182-1183
  site approach, cranial view, 131f
Medial femorotibial (MFT) osteoarthritis location, 57f
Medial lesion, lateral scintigraphic image (usage), 228
Medial malleolar fractures, rarity, 529
Medial meniscus, grade II tear, 849f
Medial nerve, block, 126
Medial oblique, term (usage), 429
Medial OSL, ultrasonographic images, 815f
Medial palmar intercarpal ligaments, 447
  displacement, resistance, 427
  tearing, observation, 447
  hemarthrosis, result, 447
Medial palmar nerves, desensitization, 110-111
Medial patellar desmotomy, 558
Medial patellar ligament
  deep palpation, 56-57
  location, 56
Medial recess, medial femorotibial joint, 208-209
Medial splint bones, 499
Medial-to-lateral hoof imbalances, 1198
Medial-to-lateral limb flight, 69
Medial trochlear ridge lesions, interpretation, 636
Median block, 114-116
Median nerve, block, 115
Medical injuries, categorization (attempts), 204
Medical records, 168
Medications
  changes/response, 13-14
  usage, 846
Mediolateral balance, 282
Mediolateral foot imbalance, 312
Mediolateral imbalance, 286-290, 292
  cause, 286
  dynamic effects, 286
  ensuring, 279
  flares/underrun walls, impact, 292
  impact, 279, 286f
  induction, 286
  prolongation, impact, 286
  trimming response, 291
  visual inspection, 288
Mediolateral static balance, guidelines, 285f
Medullary bone, trabecular structure (assessment), 177
Medullary cavity, radiopharmaceutical uptake increase (lateral/delayed bone phase scintigraphic view), 453f
Meniscal injuries, 1108
  observation, 209

Meniscal ligament injuries,
542-543
prognosis, 543
signs/diagnosis, 542-543
treatment, 543
Mepivacaine, characteristics,
100-101
Mesenchymal stem cells (MSCs),
847-848
intraarticular usage, 847-848
OA usage, 852
usage, 847
Mesenchymal stem cells (MSCs),
collection, 761
Mesotendon, 93
Mesotherapy, 605
usage, 605
Messenger (TB stallion), 1014
Metabolic myopathies, 829-830
Metacarpal region
analgesia
alternative, 114
provision, 112-113
anatomy, 394
border, 499
clinical examination, 395
diagnosis, 394-395
differential diagnosis, 396-397
diffuse filling, differential
diagnosis, 423-425, 423b
distal palmar aspects, transverse
ultrasonographic images,
171f
dorsomedial-palmarolateral
oblique view, 170f, 420f,
422f, 425f
dorsomedial-plantarolateral
oblique image, 1078f
imaging, 395-399
lameness, 78
lateral scintigraphic image, 90f
local analgesic techniques, 395
longitudinal image, 176f
MRI, 396
nuclear scintigraphy, 395-396
pain, elimination, 395
proximal palmar aspect, pain,
941-942
radiographic examination, 396
radiography, 395-396
SDFT, ultrasonographic images,
813f
swelling, 395
tendons/ligaments, palpation,
162
transverse images, 173f-174f,
176f
treatment, 397
ultrasonographic examination,
397
ultrasonography, 395
zone 3A, transverse/longitudinal
images, 190f-191f
Metacarpophalangeal (fetlock)
joint, 118-120
anatomical composition, 394
anatomical considerations, 394
arthrocentesis, 118-119
performing, 119-120
capsule, palpation, 48-49
catastrophic injury
involvement, 963-964
chronic proliferative synovitis,
396f
diagnosis, 394-395
dorsal osteochondral fragments,
390

Metacarpophalangeal (fetlock)
joint (Continued)
dorsolateral-palmaromedial
oblique radiographic view,
932f
dorsomedial-palmarolateral
radiographic view, 406f
dorsopalmar/flexed lateromedial
views, 409f
dorsopalmar radiographic
projection, 667f
dorsopalmar radiographic view,
633f
effusion, 398
examination, 998
extension, heel elevation
(impact), 287
flexed lateromedial radiographic
view, 405f
flexural deformities, 645-646
causes, 647
fractures, combinations, 964
high-motion joint, 394
imaging considerations, 395
intrasynovial analgesia, 394-395
lameness, test specificity, 82
lateromedial radiographic view,
398f, 405f-406f
lesions, 632-633
local anesthetic solution,
injection, 120
osteoarthritis, 397
osteochondral fragmentation/
chip fractures, 1058
palmar aspect, staphylococcal
abscesses, 1009-1010
palmar/plantar aspects, 939-940
palmar/plantar pouch,
arthroscopic examination,
753-754
physical examination, 394
positive contrast arthrogram,
118f
racing injuries, 963-964
region, analgesia, 111
sagittal fat-saturated T2 gradient
echo image, 243f
slightly flexed dorsopalmar
radiographic view, 399f
slightly oblique lateromedial
radiographic view, 406f
Metallic structures (imaging), CT
accuracy, 238
Metalloproteinase (MMP)
enzymes, 367
IL-1 activation, diagram, 847f
inhibition, therapeutic
approach, 846
inhibitors, 369
Metaphysis, sagittal section,
618f
Metastatic mineralization, 177
Metatarsal bones
disease, 986
orientation, 499
Metatarsal fascia, abaxial margins
(attachment), 499
Metatarsal region, 61
anatomy, 499-500
cellulitis, severity, 508
conditions, 502-508
diagnostic analgesia, 500-501
diffuse swelling, 508
high plantar perineural block,
500-501
imaging considerations,
501-502

Metatarsal region (Continued)
lameness
clinical characteristics/
diagnosis, 500-502
diagnosis, absence, 507
pain, pathognomonic historical
findings, absence, 500
pool/delayed phase
scintigraphic examination,
501-502
term, usage, 764
wounds, 507-508
Metatarsophalangeal (MTP) joint,
61-62
anatomy, 480-481
conditions, 488-498
conformation, 481
delayed phase lateral/plantar
scintigraphic images, 495f
dorsal osteochondral fragments,
390
dorsal subluxation, 497-498
dorsoplantar radiographic
views, 498f
evaluation, 62
flexor deformity, 497-498
flexural deformities, 645-646
fractures, 495
hindlimb lameness source, 1046
intermittent severe lameness,
481-482
lameness
clinical characteristics/
diagnosis, 481-482
clinical signs, 481
diagnosis, scintigraphic
examination, 483-484
occurrence, 481
lateral/plantar bone phase
scintigraphic images,
484f
lateral radiographic view, 776f
lesions, 632-633
longitudinal ultrasonographic
images, 767f
osteoarthritis, 63, 488-492
palmar/plantar aspects, 939-940
palmar/plantar pouch,
arthroscopic examination,
753-754
problems, 61-62
region
analgesia, 125
ignorance, 62f
ultrasonographic
examination, 485
scintigraphic images, 484f
Metatarsus, ultrasonographic zone
designations, 196f
Methylprednisolone acetate
(MPA), 841
intraarticular administration,
841-842
intraarticular injection, 992
Methylsulfonylmethane (MSM),
845
Microbial sensitivity testing,
315-316
Microconvex array transducers,
169
Microdamage, healing, 490
Microfracture, 259, 851
MicroSteed, components, 627
Midbody desmitis, 989
Midbody PSB fractures, 405-406
Midbody superficial digital flexor
tendonitis, history, 268f

Midcrus, craniolateral
aspect (transverse
ultrasonographic images),
802f
Middiaphyseal tibial fractures, 529
Middle-aged roping horses,
palmar foot pain (diagnosis),
1173
Middle carpal joints
arthrocentesis, 120-121
capsule, distention, 88
detection, 999
intraarticular analgesia, 740
intraoperative arthroscopic
images, 256f
lameness, association,
1008-1009
liquid acrylic injection, 113f
location, 426-427
palmar pouch, access, 121
positive contrast arthrogram,
113f
syndromes, 1008
synovitis, 1121
Middle East Arabian racehorse,
racing-related lameness,
1057-1058
Middle gluteal muscle
accessory head, lateral pelvic/
proximal thigh regions,
550f
pathological process, 550
Middle patellar ligaments,
palpation, 56
Middle phalanx (MP)
anatomical considerations, 387
articular chip fracture, 355
distal articular surface, 322
dorsal aspect, palisading new
bone, 355
fractures, 963
osseous trauma, 358
palmar/plantar eminence, 387
transverse contrast-enhanced
computed tomographic
image, 347f
transverse CT images, 238f
Midline-to-lateral pelvic width,
37
Midlumbar vertebrae, lateral
radiographic view, 602f
Midpastern region, deep digital
flexor tenotomy (performing),
384f
Midpastern ring block, 108-110
impact, 110
Midpastern tenotomy, 384
Mild carpal lameness, prodromal
clinical signs, 444
Mineralization, 471, 729-730
Minerals
excesses, 625-626
imbalances, 626
ratio, importance, 626
toxic levels, 626t
Miniature breeds, osteoarthritis,
467
Miniature horses, sudden-onset
severe lameness, 467
Miniature ponies, osteoarthritis,
1229-1230
Minimum sagittal diameter
(MSD), 140
Minor collagens, presence, 657-658
Mirror image artifacts, 177
Misdiagnosis, image findings
(misinterpretation), 152-154

Mixed lameness, 67-69
Mixed soft tissue injuries, 798
Mobilization techniques, 910
Modeling, 169
    term, usage, 935
Molybdenum-99, impact, 216
Moment arm, 274-275
    schematic drawing, 275f
Morgan breed, 1188
Morning workouts, injuries, 962
Morphine, selection, 856
Mosaic arthroplasty, 259
Mosaicplasty, 676
Motion, 222
    excess, sources, 222
    palpation, 897
        demonstration, 898f
    parameters, 247-248
        association, 248-249
Motion correction software, 668
Motor nerve conduction velocity,
    values, 140
Motor pattern, 908
Movement
    biomechanics, shoe weight
        (impact), 294
    determination, conformation
        (impact), 18
    excess, reduction, 878
Mucous membranes, examination,
    165-166
Mud fever, 166
Multiloculated abscess cavity,
    development, 612
Multiple frequency scanheads,
    availability, 169
Multivariable epidemiological
    studies, evidence, 975
Muscle atrophy, 32-33, 35-36
    assessment, 55
    detection, absence, 474
    localization, 33
Muscle disorders
    ancillary diagnostic tests,
        818-821
    clinical examination, 822-823
    diagnosis, 818-834
        scintigraphy usage,
            documentation (absence),
            819
    electromyography, 820-821
    history, 818, 822-823
    nuclear scintigraphy, 819, 823
    physical examination, 818
    prevention, 824
    thermography, 819, 823
    treatment, 823-824
    ultrasonography, 819-820, 823
Muscle Hill (trotting colt), 1014f
Muscles, 244, 472-473
    abscesses, 612, 821
        treatment/surgical drainage,
            612
    antebrachium (caudal aspect),
        myositis/traumatic injury
        (rarity), 454
    assessment, 458
    biopsy, 820
        collection, consideration,
            820
        histopathology samples,
            usage, 820
        impact, 555
        usage, 576
    cracking, 54
    damage, treatment, 823-824
    deconditioning, 878

Muscles (Continued)
    disease, rule-out reduction
        (classification system),
        820-821
    echogenicity (increase),
        postanesthetic myopathy
        (impact), 212
    electrical activity, recording,
        140
    enzymes
        concentrations,
            determination, 823
        examination, 818-819
    fasciculations
        caudal cervical synovial
            articulations, association,
            838
        disorders, 837-838
        knowledge, absence, 838
        osteoarthritis, association,
            838
    fiber tearing, 821
    fibrosis, documentation, 821
    groups, hypoperfusion, 833
    hemorrhage, 821
    inflammation, identification,
        268
    injuries, 148
        recognition problem, 824
    innervation patterns, 556
    knots, 822
    lesions, 472
    loss, 32
    mass
        asymmetry, 35
        infiltration, 212
    MDP absorption, 819
    mineralization, 821
    MRI, usage, 244
    pain, 821-824
        atrophy, assessment, 55
    pathological responses, 820
    soreness, 576
    stimulation, 823
    strain, 821-824
        diagnosis, thermography
            (usage), 590
    strength, increase, 906
    swelling, detection, 822
    tears, 821-824
    tumors, rarity, 212-213
Musculoskeletal disease,
    acupuncture diagnosis/
    therapy, 891-892
Musculoskeletal element,
    locomotion, 277-278
Musculoskeletal examination,
    897
Musculoskeletal extremity pain,
    889-891
Musculoskeletal injury
    elicitation, 275-276
    incidence, 960
Musculoskeletal pain, 887-892
    diagnosis/treatment, 887
Musculoskeletal problems
    (development), conformation
    (role), 17
Musculoskeletal structures, failure,
    270
Musculoskeletal system,
    requirements, 270
Musculoskeletal tissues,
    locomotion (impact), 274-275
Musculotendonous junction,
    transverse T2 gradient echo
    images, 244f

Myeloencephalitis, motor neurons
    (involvement), 555
Myelograms, interpretation, 652
Myelographic examination, usage,
    140
Myeloma, 615
    myeloproliferative disorder, 615
Myofascial pain, 891
Myoglobin, elevation, 819
Myositis, 212, 992, 1147
    impact, 992
    rarity, 454
Myotonia, 837
    clinical signs, 837
    diagnosis, 837
    disorders, 837-838
    treatment, 837

N

Nail bind, 309-310, 1133
    diagnosis, 309-310
        difficulty, 309-310
    history/clinical signs, 309
    term, usage, 309
    treatment/prognosis, 310
Nail prick, 303, 310
    diagnosis, 310
    discovery, 310
    history/clinical signs, 310
    prognosis, 310
    shoe removal, 310
    term, usage, 310
    treatment, 310
Nails
    driving, 298-299
    penetration, 316
Naive skeletal specimens, 571
National Cutting Horse
    Association, competition
    occurrence, 1165
National Hunt flat races, 1062
National hunt racehorse,
    1063-1065
    acute lesions, 1071
    back pain, 1074-1075
    carpus, lameness (association),
        1072
    chronic back pain, 1074-1075
    clinical examination, 1069
    conformation, lameness
        (relationship), 1068
    diagnosis, absence, 1070
    diagnostic analgesia, 1069-1070
    front feet, lameness
        (association), 1073
    hock, lameness (association),
        1072-1073
    imaging considerations, 1070
    injuries, 1075
    jump, teaching, 1065
    lameness, 1067-1068
        examination, 1068-1069
    metacarpophalangeal joint,
        lameness (association),
        1074
    neck lesions, 1074
    pelvis, lameness (association),
        1073
    racing, 1065-1067
    serial ultrasonographic
        examinations, 1071
    shoeing considerations,
        lameness (relationship),
        1070
    sport, description, 1062-1063
    structural damage, assessment,
        1072

National hunt racehorse
    (Continued)
    suspensory desmitis, 1072
        problems, 1072
    track surface, 1067-1068
    training, 1065, 1070
        surface, 1067-1068
National Hunt racing
    death rate, 1066-1067
    horses, sources, 1066
National hunt racing, categories,
    1062
National Hunt Steeplechase, 1062
National Reined Cow Horse
    Association, 1176
National Research Council (NRC),
    digestible energy/protein
    values, 627
National Show Horse, 1188
Natural Balance shoe
    design, 306f
    premade, usage, 306
Natural balance shoeing, 303-306
Natural balance trimming,
    303-306
Natural breakover, indication,
    1203f
Natural gait, 64
Natural trigger factors, 370-371
    bacterial origin, 370
Navicular apparatus, pain
    (factors), 324
Navicular bone
    aging changes, 325-326
    compressive forces/stress,
        comparison, 324
    computed tomography, 335-336
    cortices, thickness (variation),
        333
    decompression, surgical drilling
        (usage), 342
    distal aspect, gross post mortem
        specimen, 338f
    distal border, 322
        osseous fragments,
            occurrence, 330-332
    dorsoproximal-palmarodistal
        oblique radiographic views,
        325f, 327f, 343f
    dorsoproximal-palmarodistal
        oblique views, 332f
    evaluation, grading system, 330
    flexor aspect, distal/proximal
        borders (association), 326
    flexor border, new bone
        formation, 333
    IRU, 335
        lateral delayed-phase
            scintigraphic view, 68f
    lateral view, comparisons, 96f
    lateromedial view, 331f
    malformations, 478
    medulla, hyperintense signal,
        326-327
    MRI, 335-336
    nuclear scintigraphy, 334-335
    palmar aspect, fibrocartilage
        (degenerative changes), 326
    palmaroproximal-palmarodistal
        oblique view, 171f
    periarterial sympathectomy,
        342
    proximal border, margins, 330
    radiographic examination,
        330-334
    radiological appearance,
        interpretation, 1101

Navicular bone *(Continued)*
  radiological findings, 333b
  radiopharmaceutical uptake,
    lateral/plantar/solar delayed
    phase scintigraphic images,
    479f
  sagittal sections, 325f
  shape, determination, 325
    LM view, usage, 333
  spongiosa, trabecular
    architecture, 333
  transverse sections, 97f
Navicular bone fracture, 146
  clinical examination/diagnosis,
    343-344
  history, 343
  occurrence, 343
  treatment, 344
Navicular bursa (podotrochlear
    bursa), 122-124, 327-328, 799
  analgesia, 122-123
    palmar midline approach,
      usage, 123-124
    positive response, 330
  bursoscopy, 265-266
  compression, 123-124
  contrast radiography, 334
  endoscopic evaluation, 336-337
  endoscopic examination, 265
  infection, suspicion, 315
  penetrating wounds, 316-317
  postoperative management/
    results, 265-266
  primary bursitis, incidence/
    etiology, 327-328
  proximal, palmar injection
    technique, 124
  surgical access, 317
  surgical technique, 265
  synoviocentesis, lateral view,
    123f
Navicular bursoscopy, indication,
    265
Navicular disease
  biomechanical considerations,
    324-325
  chemical neurectomy/
    cryoneurectomy, 341-342
  chronic forelimb lameness, 324
  clinical presentations, 324
  clinical signs, 328-329
  development, risk factors, 324
  diagnostic considerations,
    328-337
  distal limb flexion, response
    (variation), 329
  entheseous changes, 327
  experimental reproduction,
    absence, 325
  histological sample, 330f
  histopathological studies,
    325-326
  history, 328
  injuries, association, 328
  intraarticular/intrathecal
    medication, 341
  isoxsuprine, usage, 340-341
  lameness, 329
  local analgesic techniques,
    response, 329-330
  management, shoes (usage),
    339
  management strategies,
    338-342
  NSAIDs, usage, 339-340
  nuclear scintigraphy/MRI
    observations, 326-327

Navicular disease *(Continued)*
  osteoarthritis, pathological
    similarities, 341
  pain, cause, 328
  palmar digital neurectomy, 342
  pathophysiology, 324-328
  shockwave therapy, 341
  therapy, 1101
  tiludronate, usage, 341
Navicular disease, default
    diagnosis, 231-232
Navicular force, 279
Navicular heel, pain (perception),
    281
Navicular position, location,
    123-124
Navicular suspensory apparatus,
    322
Navicular syndrome, 478, 985
  complexity, 918
  mechanics, 280-281
  SWT impact, 918
Near gain, 170
Neck
  base
    forelimb gait restriction,
      longitudinal
      ultrasonographic images,
      822f
    primary brachiocephalicus
      pain, 612
  bilateral symmetry,
    thermographic imaging,
    268-269
  bottom line, 16-17
  cervical spine, 53-54
  equidistant acupoints,
    existence, 607
  examination, 607
  flexibility, assessment, 607, 616,
    1090
  lateral scintigraphic image, 608
  lesions, 152
  mobility reduction, thermogram
    (lateral view), 912f
  movement, asymmetric vertical
    torso movement, 249
  muscle development, 53-54
  musculature, disorders, 611-612
  pain, 40-41
  palpation, limitation, 53-54
  passive movement, 823
  radiographic examination, 608
  reining, 1150
  stiffness, 616
    complaint, 606-607
  thermographic evaluation, 924
  topline, length, 16-17
  ventral scintigraphic image,
    608
Neck, soft tissues
  anatomy, 606
  cervical vertebrae, cystlike
    lesions, 615
  cervical vertebral mobilization,
    general anesthesia, 616
  clinical conditions, 609-616
  clinical examination, 606-607
  clinical presentation, reasons,
    606
  computed tomography, 608
  congenital abnormalities, 609
  diagnostic tests, 609
  diskospondylitis, 614
  electromyography, 609
  first/second cervical vertebrae,
    subluxation, 609-610

Neck, soft tissues *(Continued)*
  fracture, 614-615
  imaging considerations,
    608-609
  jugular vein thrombophlebitis,
    615-616
  myeloma, 615
  neck musculature, disorders,
    611-612
  neck stiffness, 616
  nuchal ligament, insertional
    desmopathy, 610-611
  nuclear scintigraphy, 608
  occipito-atlantoaxial
    malformation, 609
  osteoarthritis, 612-614
  radiography, 608
  semispinalis injury, 610-611
  sixth/seventh cervical vertebrae,
    subluxation, 610
  thermography, 609
  ultrasonography, 608
  vertebral osteomyelitis, 615
Necrosis of the cartilage,
    1220-1221
Negative bone scan results, 228
Negative responses, 152
Neonatal foals, gastrocnemius
    (disruption), 805
Neonatal tarsus, lateromedial
    radiographic view, 645f
Neoplasia, 144, 449, 692-693
Neoplastic space-occupying
    lesions, 358-359
  clinical signs/diagnosis, 359
  history, 358
  treatment, 359
Nerve blocks, 152, 229
  clinical clues, absence, 152
  negative responses, 152
  negative scintigraphic findings,
    152
  performing, failure, 147
Nerve impingement, space-
    occupying masses (impact),
    144-145
Nerve root impingement, 613
Nerves, 213, 473-474
  conduction studies, 140
  distinction, 213
  lesions, 144
Neuritis, 816-817
Neuroaxonal dystrophy, 143
Neurochemicals, presence, 323
Neurogenic atrophy, 32-33
Neurogenic muscle atrophy,
    occurrence, 35
Neurogenic pain, 891
Neurological deficit, detection,
    562
Neurological disease, suspicion,
    32
Neurological examination
  diagnosis, 135-141
  indication, 898
Neurological problems, 156
Neuroma, 816-817
  pain, association, 148
Neuromuscular electrical
    stimulation, parameters,
    905
Neuromuscular electrical
    stimulators (NMES), 905
  impact, 906
  machine parameters, 906
  treatment, indications, 906
  usage, 906

Neuromuscular system,
    functioning (importance),
    555
Neurons, categories, 908
Neurophysiology, 908
  alteration, 908-909
    clinical manifestations,
      909
Neurovascular bundle, schematic
    diagram, 882f
New bones
  formation, 333, 387
  growth, prevention, 877
  unknown origin, 173
Newmarket
  racing history, 994
  Rowley mile racetrack, 996f
New Zealand Thoroughbred
  gelding, 1124f
Nitazoxanide, impact, 142
Nitric oxide, 664
Nitric oxide synthases (NOSs),
    664
N-methyl-D-aspartate (NMDA)
    receptor antagonist,
    856-857
Nociceptor activity, 909
Nonarticular fragments, proximal
    sesamoid bones (impact),
    494
Noncollagenous glycoproteins,
    699-700
Noncovalent cross-links,
    provision, 699
Nondisplaced diaphyseal splint
    bone fractures, cryotherapy
    response, 1160
Nondisplaced incomplete
    fractures, usage, 667
Nonexertional rhabdomyolysis,
    829
Noninfectious arthritis
  blood flow, increase, 688
  capillary leakage, occurrence,
    688
  cellular influx, 688
  effusion, 688
  inflammation, impact, 688
  ischemia, 688
  joint pathophysiology
    (synovitis), 687-688
  joint physiology, 687
  neuropeptides, contribution,
    689
  pathological joint conditions,
    association, 688-689
Noninfectious bursitis, 471
  occurrence, 471
Noninfectious tenosynovitis,
    766-769
  etiopathogenesis, 766-767
Nonminiature breeds,
    osteoarthritis, 467-468
Nonneoplastic space-occupying
    lesions, 358-359
  clinical signs/diagnosis, 359
  history, 358
  treatment, 359
Nonracehorses
  dorsal chip fractures, 400
  intraarticular injection response,
    492
  osteoarthritis, insidiousness,
    488-489
  scintigraphic changes,
    483-484
Nonstakes races, categories, 979

Nonsteroidal antiinflammatory drugs (NSAIDs) prohibition, IFHA rules, 980-981
Non-weight-bearing state, 382-383
Nonwoven roving, 309
Normal TENS, 906
North American Arabian racehorse, racing-related lameness, 1058
North American racing, UK racing (comparison), 995-996
North American Standardbred
abscesses, 1024
base-wide toed-out conformation, 1024
blocking techniques, 1022
bruises, 1024
bucked shins, rarity, 1018
carpal lameness, 1018, 1026-1027
classes, 1015
clinical history, 1019-1020
colt pacer, images, 1034f
conformation, 1017-1018
contracted heel, 1025
corns, 1024
curb, 1036
diagnosis, absence, 1023
diagnostic analgesia, 1022
distal hock joint pain, 1018
tarsal lameness, relationship, 1029-1032
distal interphalangeal joint, osteoarthritis, 1026
distal phalanx, fractures, 1025-1026
exercise intensity, reduction, 1028
filly, carpal bones (dorsoproximal-dorsodistal digital radiographic image), 1027f
fourth metacarpal bones, exostoses/fractures, 1033-1034
fourth metatarsal bones, exostoses/fractures, 1034-1035
fractures, 1028-1029
front feet
IRU distribution, dorsal delayed scintigraphic image, 1026f
lameness, 1024-1026
gluteal region, secondary muscle soreness, 1021
hindlimb fault, 1018
hoof cracks, 1025
imaging considerations, 1022-1023
interference injuries, 1018-1019
jogging, increase, 1016
lameness, 1018-1019
diagnosis, clinical history (importance), 1019
distribution, 1018
examination, 1020-1022
overt signs, absence, 1020
low-heel underslung foot, rarity, 1024
low plantar block, usage, 1022
metacarpophalangeal joint lameness, 1033

North American Standardbred *(Continued)*
metatarsophalangeal joint lameness, 1027-1029
osteochondrosis, 1029
movement, examination, 1021-1022
muscle soreness, 1036
palpation, 1020-1021
proximal phalanx
dorsal frontal fractures, 1028-1029
midsagittal fractures, 1028
midsagittal fractures (dorsoplantar/flexed lateromedial xeroradiographic images), 1028f
quarter crack defect, 1024
race, initiation, 1015
racehorse
lameness conditions, 1024-1036
retraining, 1016-1017
right front foot, dorsomedial proximal-palmarolateral distal oblique xeroradiographic image, 1025f
racing performance, problem, 1017
radiography, 1022-1023
RER, occurrence, 1036
rest, impact, 1033
rhabdomyolysis, 1036
scintigraphic examination, 1023
second metacarpal bones, exostoses/fractures, 1033-1034
second metatarsal bones, exostoses/fractures, 1034-1035
sheared heel, 1024-1025
shoeing, lameness (relationship), 1023-1024
sidebone, 1025
splint bone disease, 1033-1035
sport, description, 1014-1016
stifle joint lameness, 1035
stress, maladaptive/nonadaptive remodeling (relationship), 1027-1028
superficial digital flexor tendonitis, 1036
suspensory desmitis, 1032-1033
talus, sagittal fracture (flexed lateral delayed phase scintigraphic image), 1031f
tarsocrural OA, occurrence, 1030
third metacarpal bone, condylar fractures, 1029
third metatarsal bone, condylar fractures, 1029
track size, lameness (relationship), 1017
training, 1016-1017
trotter, left stifle (caudocranial digital radiographic image), 1035f
ultrasonographic examination, 1023
underconditioning, fatigue, 1033
wall separation, gravel (relationship), 1025

North American Thoroughbred
abscesses, 985
conformation, 979
diagnosis, inability, 984
diagnostic analgesia, 982-983
requirement, 983
distal phalanx fractures, 985-986
drug testing considerations, 980-981
gluteal myositis, occurrence, 992
imaging considerations, 983
lameness conditions, 984
medication, 980-981
movement, consideration, 982
navicular syndrome, 985
NSAIDs, usage (IFHA prohibition), 980-981
osteoarthritis, 987
proximal suspensory desmitis, 988-989
quarter cracks, 985
scintigraphic examination, 983
shoeing, 983-984
sport, description, 977-979
stress fractures, 992-993
stress-related bone injuries, 992-993
suspensory desmitis, 988-989
unilateral hindlimb lameness, tibial stress fractures, 991
Norwegian horses, polyneuropathy, 42
Novel analgesic drugs, 857-858
Nuchal ligament, insertional desmopathy, 610-611
treatment, 611
Nuclear medicine
considerations, 215-216
diagnostic advancement, 215
facility, example, 218f
radioisotope involvement, 215-216
Nuclear scintigraphy, 140, 215-216
usage, 388
Nucleated cells, distribution, 679
Nutraceuticals, 845
license, 845
Nutrient intake
calculation, 627-628
comparison, 628
Nutrients
pharmaceuticals, combination, 845
requirements, defining, 627
Nutritional myodegeneration (NMD), 834-836
clinical pathology, 835
clinical signs, 834-835
diagnosis, 835
etiology, 834
pathology, 835
pathophysiology, 835
prevention/control, 836
treatment/prognosis, 835-836
Nutritional myopathies, 834-838

O

Objective information, subjective information (contrast), 8-9
Oblique distal sesamoidean ligaments, palpation, 48f

Oblique (middle) sesamoidean desmitis, 758-759
ultrasonographic abnormalities, 759
Oblique sesamoidean desmitis, 814-815
Oblique sesamoidean ligaments (OSLs)
acute injuries, 815
chronic injuries, 393
injury, 811-812
prognosis, 815
Occipito-atlantoaxial malformation (OAAM), 609
congenital abnormality, 609
diagnosis, confirmation, 609
Occult fissure lines/spiraling, 496
Occult osteochondral fragments (diagnosis), scintigraphic examination (usage), 436-437
Occult osteochondral fragments (identification), arthroscopic examination (usage), 254-255
Occult spavin, 59-60
Odd lameness, 155
Offset knee (bench knee), 15-16
conformation, 23-24
contribution, 17
Offset-knee conformation, 171-172
Offset ratios (determination), lines (usage), 18f
Older horses
long bone fractures, risk (increase), 10
problems, 9-10
Olecranon bursa, analgesia, 124
Olecranon fracture, 462
types, 462
Onchocerca cervicalis, 799
One Day Events, 1123
1.5-T GE Echospeed, 240f
On the bit, horse work, 19
Open gallop, 1139
Opposing articular surfaces, congruency, 660
Optimum balance/conformation, 284-285
Oral antioxidants, usage, 142
Oral HA product, efficacy (absence), 846
Oral joint supplements, 845-846
classification, 845
Oral supplements, license, 845
Oriental pattern-based therapy, Western disease-based approach (contrast), 887
Orthopedic disorders, mechanics (alterations), 280-281
Orthopedic implants, 135
Orthopedic laminitis, 477-478
Orthopedic surgery, 163-164
Osseous cystlike lesions, 173-174, 354, 446-447, 453-454
characteristics, 173
clinical/imaging findings, 357
detection, CT usage, 518
development, 174
full-thickness cartilage loss, association, 398
history, 357
identification, 405-406, 574, 930

Osseous cystlike lesions
(Continued)
occurrence, 354, 446-447,
466-467
result, 478-479
weight-bearing surface
occurrence, 632-633
Osseous fragments, 355
Ossification, impact, 620-621
Osteitis, 173, 214
clinical signs, 425
complicating factor (recognition),
radiography/
ultrasonography (usage),
770
diagnosis, 425
osteomyelitis, comparison,
524-525
term, usage, 524-525
treatment, 425
ultrasonography, 214
Osteoarthritis (OA), 177, 352-353,
397-398
abnormal findings, 601-602
anabolic processes, 669
articular cartilage
degradation (prevention),
gene therapy (usage),
672-673
articular cartilage metabolism,
skeletal biomarkers,
669-670
assessment, bone biomarkers
(value), 951
biomarkers, future, 670-671
catabolic processes, 669-670
clinical importance, 613
clinical signs, 397, 433
cytokines, degradative effects,
664
development, shoeing/hoof
balance role, 489
diagnosis, 397, 433
confirmation, 433
differentiation, difficulty,
215-216
direct/indirect molecular
markers, 669
early signs, 988
effusion, 665
etiopathogenesis, 660-661
identification, 668
imaging modalities, 667-668
indication, 177
joints
bone-seeking isotopes,
accumulation, 667
corticosteroids, direct
intraarticular injection
(assessment), 841f
trauma, 655
local signs, 665
magnetic resonance imaging
(MRI), usage, 665, 667-668
management, 433-434, 489-492
motion, limited range, 665
MSC usage, 852
muscle fasciculation,
association, 838
navicular disease, pathological
similarities, 341
nuclear scintigraphy, usage,
667
pathogenetic pathy, 660-661
pathophysiological events,
nitric oxide (mediator role),
664

Osteoarthritis (Continued)
presence, 349-350
prognosis, 545
radiography/radiology, role,
665-667
radiological abnormalities, 177,
352-353
absence, 352
inclusion, 613
radiological evidence, 433
radiological features, 667b
radiological findings, 665
scintigraphic evidence, 224
selective COX-2 inhibition,
beneficial effects, 841
signs/diagnosis, 545
SW application, 917
synovial fluid, changes, 665
synovium, role, 661
treatment, 397-398, 545
ultrasonography, 668
Osteoarthrosis, 177
indication, 177
Osteocalcin (OCa), 948
levels, measurement, 670
usage, 670
Osteochondral fracture fragment,
18
Osteochondral fragmentation,
434-445, 986-987
clinical signs, 435-437
management, 437-439
small fragments, 434-439
Osteochondral fragment-exercise
model, usage, 846
Osteochondral fragment model,
676
Osteochondral fragments, 176,
400-401, 494-495
arthroscopic removal, 1193
characterization, 400-401
clinical signs, 399-400
development, 434
predisposition, 434
diagnosis, 400
dorsomedial-palmarolateral
oblique radiographic view,
437f
identification, 494-495
intraoperative photograph,
494f
lameness, 435
location, 435
occurrence, 439
osteochondrosis, association,
391
presence, 482-483
proximal phalanx,
dorsoproximal aspect,
399-400
surgical removal, 439
prognosis, 438
treatment, 400
Osteochondral grafts, 852
Osteochondral lesions
insulin levels, relationship, 622
radiological identification, 618
size/location, impact, 676
toxic causes, 625
Osteochondral ossification,
overfeeding (impact), 622
Osteochondritis dissecans (OCD),
516-517, 1227-1228
lesion, 618f
Osteochondromata, removal, 264
Osteochondromatosis, 447, 693,
791

Osteochondrosis (OC), 27f, 174,
409-410, 446
articular disease, 536-538
biomechanical force, role, 624
body size, relationship, 621
calcium/phosphorus,
relationship, 622
cartilage canals, involvement,
620-621
causative factors, 620-625
characteristics, 617-619
clinical signs, 631
copper, relationship, 622-623
definitions/terminology, 617
delayed images, 228-229
delayed patellar release, 538-539
descriptions, variation, 619
digestible energy/protein,
impact, 621-622
endochondral ossification
disorder, 174
enzymes, role, 624-625
exercise, relationship, 624
flaps, osseous component,
631-632
gender, relationship, 624
genomic studies, 623
growth rate, relationship, 621
heredity, impact, 623-624
incidence, reduction (alternative
strategy), 623-624
lameness, association, 67-68
lesions, 537
arthroscopic removal, 637
features, 619
incidence/heritability, 623t
manifestation, 617-618
patella, upward fixation,
538-539
pathogenesis, 620-621, 631
exercise, role, 624
nutrition, impact, 621-623
peptide, involvement, 625
pathological condition, 623
pattern, 617
physeal dysplasia, relationship,
620
postmortem studies, 621
prognosis, 537-538
radiological changes, 537
recognition, 536-537
relationships, 620
signaling peptides, role,
624-625
signs/diagnosis, 537
subchondral bone cysts/osseous
cystlike lesions,
relationship, 620
trauma, role, 624
treatment, 537
Osteochondrositis dissecans
(OCD), 617
Osteolysis (bone resorption),
170
Osteomyelitis, 173, 214, 425
clinical signs, 425
complicating factor (recognition),
radiography/
ultrasonography (usage),
770
diagnosis, 425
osteitis, comparison, 524-525
term, usage, 173
treatment, 425
ultrasonography, 214
Osteopath, static/moving
examinations, 913-914

Osteopathic treatment
diagnosis/case selection,
910-911
Osteopathic treatment, effects,
909-910
Osteopathy, 884
approach, 907
autonomic component, 908
autonomic effects, 909
injury response, 908
motor component, 908
motor effects, 909
neurophysiological basis,
907-909
origination, 907
sensory component, 908
sensory effects, 908-909
treatment, 913-914
results, 914
Osteopenia (generalized
mineralization), 170
Osteophyte
bone spur, 171-172
development time, 171-172
formation, 171-172
Osteoprogenitor colony-forming
units, increase, 915-916
Out-at-the-knee conformation,
22-23
Outcome assessment, 8
Outdoor polo, 1150f
Outer hoof wall, curve (evenness),
305
Outside rim shoes, 295-296
Overall gain, 170
Over-at-the-fetlock, 28
Over-at-the-knee
bucked-knee (knee-sprung)
conformation, 27-28
conformation, 39
Overfeeding problem, 628
Overhead chains, usage, 878
Overreaching, 1004
Overriding spinous processes,
598-599
Ovnicek aluminum shoe, 381f

P

Pace, symmetrical lateral two-beat
gait, 64
Pacer
designation, 1019
third carpal bone (L-shaped
fracture), 442f
Pacing at the walk, 562
Pacing colt, left hindlimb
lameness (lateral/
plantar/flexed lateral
delayed-phase scintigraphic
images), 491f
Packed cell volume (PCV), 678
Paddock, horse introduction, 879
Paddock rest, 879
Pads, 297-298
design, 298
disadvantages, 298
insertion, 298f
Pain
abolishment
intraarticular analgesia, usage,
105
technique, alternative, 111
alleviation, alternative,
126-127
cause, 328
control, 385
elimination, 395

Pain (Continued)
gait control, 605
isolation, 148
localization, 3
management, LLLT (usage),
904
presence, 62
problem (determination),
phenylbutazone (usage),
923
reduction, 900
source, 91
desensitization, nerve blocks
(impact), 147-148
guess, 924
Painful area, digital compression,
86
Pain-related lameness, 562
Paint gelding
cervical pain/spinal ataxia,
caudal neck region (lateral
radiographic view), 650f
metatarsophalangeal joint,
medial aspect (acute
swelling), 691f
Paired gastrocnemius muscles,
origination, 526
PaL-DMO, 182
Palisading new bone, 355
Palmar annular desmitis, 422
Palmar annular desmotomy,
718-719
surgical approach, invasiveness
(reduction), 718
usage, 718
Palmar annular ligament (PAL)
desmitis, 1121, 1163
enlargement, 773
injury, impact, 771
insertion, PSB (avulsion
fracture), 754
intrasynovial injection site,
124
palmar annular ligament,
avulsion (attachment), 422
PSB palmar border insertion,
764
transection (desmotomy),
261-262
Palmar annular ligament (PAL)
syndrome, 771-774
diagnosis, 771-773
etiopathogenesis, 771
treatment, 774
Palmar carpal fragments, 439
Palmar carpal osteochondral
fragments, 439-440
lameness, occurrence, 439-440
Palmar digital analgesia, 108
clinical practice, 108
commonness, 108
concept, 108
contribution, quantification,
108
diagnostic blocks, performing,
108-110
ineffectiveness, 1003
radiograph, 111f
Palmar digital block, 108
phase image delay, 229
Palmar digital nerves, perineural
analgesia, 345-346
Palmar digital neurectomy, 342
Palmar foot pain, 1143-1144
definitive diagnosis, 337-338
mechanics, 280-281
soft tissue causes, 324-328

Palmar metacarpal nerve
analgesia, false-positive results,
134
subcarpal analgesia, 398
Palmar metacarpal region
longitudinal ultrasonographic
images, 172f
sagittal views, 89f
soft tissue structures, 50f
transverse sector scan image,
172f
transverse ultrasonographic
images, 170f
Palmar metacarpal soft tissues
longitudinal ultrasonographic
images, 1141f
structures, transverse
ultrasonographic image,
735f
transverse ultrasonographic
image, 150f, 420f
Palmar midline approach, usage,
123-124
Palmar nerves, perineural
analgesia, 395-396
Palmar osteochondral fragments,
removal, 439-440
Palmar pastern dermatitis, 66
Palmar pastern zones/descriptions,
198-199
Palpation
art, 43
importance, 43
physical examination, 981-982
Panosteitis-like lesions, 158-159
Paracentesis, performing, 315
Paralysis, signs, 145
Paratendon, absence, 706
Parathyroid hormone-related
protein (PTHrP), role,
624-625
Paravertebral myalgia, 1146
repetitive stress, relationship,
1146
Paresis, signs, 145
Partial bar, 296-297
Partial tendon lacerations, 809
Partial-thickness chondrectomy,
850
Passive exercise, 879
Passive stay apparatus, 94-95
Pastern, 48, 62-63
anatomical structure,
complexity, 198
anatomy, 475
angle, 31
arthroscopic examination,
486-487
chronic low-grade lameness,
482
clinical examination, 475-476
clinical signs, 475-476
computed tomography,
485-486
DDFT, 811
diagnosis, 475-476
diagnostic analgesic, 482
disorders, breed predilection,
388
dorsal ring block, 125
dorsolateral-palmaromedial
oblique radiographic view,
172f
examination, 475-476
fractures, 965
horizontal oblique views,
482-483

Pastern (Continued)
imaging considerations, 482-487
innervation, 475
joint, abnormalities, 816
keratoma, 478
laminitis, 477-478
length
impact, 287
importance, 31
lesions, 723-724
magnetic resonance imaging,
484-485
palmar aspect, transverse/
longitudinal
ultrasonographic image,
1110f
racing injuries, 963
radiographic examination,
482-483
sagittal anatomical section, 90f
scintigraphic examination,
483-484
SDFT, 811
soft tissue injuries, 810
anatomy, 810-811
SSL origin, 812
ultrasonographic anatomy,
811-812
tendon injury, 710
term, usage, 387
ultrasonographic examination,
485
ultrasonography, qualitative
assessments, 198
zone descriptions, 198-199
zone designations, 198-199,
198f
Zone P1A, 198
Zone P2A, 199
Zone P1B, 198-199
Zone P1C, 199
Pastern region
deep digital flexor injuries,
731-733
deep digital flexor tendon,
rupture, 732-733
deep digital flexor tendonitis,
731-732
ground, proximity, 387
infectious disorders, 393
injury, 1162
blunt trauma, impact, 732
lameness, 387
MRI, indication, 388
sepsis, 393
ultrasonographic evaluation,
388
wounds, 393
Past history, 11
Pasture-associated stringhalt, 560
Pasture intake
determination, 627-628
estimation method, usage, 628
Pasture myopathies, 836-837
Patella
delayed release, 556-558
biomechanical basis, 556
cause, 556
medical therapy, 556-558
surgical therapy, 558
distal luxation, 540
fragmentation, 539
complications, 538
prognosis, 539
sequela, 539
signs/diagnosis, 539
treatment, 539

Patella (Continued)
luxation, 539-540
signs/diagnosis, 539-540
treatment, 540
medial aspect, parapatellar
fibrocartilage, 94
secondary upward fixation,
impact, 581-582
upward fixation, 76, 538-539,
556-558
biomechanical basis, 556
cause, 556
clinical characteristics, 556
impact, 1168
medical therapy, 556-558
occurrence, 538
prognosis, 539
signs/diagnosis, 538
surgical therapy, 558
treatment, 538-539
Patellar ligaments
injuries, 540
prognosis, 540
signs/diagnosis, 540
treatment, 540
periarticular hemorrhage, 163
Patellar locking mechanism, 95f
Patellar manipulation, 87
performing, 57f
Patellar release, delay, 538-539
Pathological processes, 242-243
PDGF, 763
Peak force, 276
Peak GRF, increase, 276
Peak vertical GRFs, reduction,
246
Pectoral region, muscle soreness,
821
Pectorals, lesions, 472
Pedal osteitis, 362
inflammation, 362
term, inappropriateness, 362
Pelvic anatomy, 564
Pelvic asymmetry, 86
Pelvic canal region, examination,
572
Pelvic fractures, 42-43
acetylpromazine,
administration, 571
clinical examination, 564-565
diagnosis/management, 564
diagnostic techniques, 564-567
diagnostic ultrasonography,
565-566
impact, 570-571
occurrence, 567
radiography, 566
rectal examination, 565
scintigraphy, 566-567
surgical repair, 570-571
treatment, principles, 570-571
types, 570-571
ultrasonography, usefulness,
565-566
Pelvic heights/widths,
determination (perspective),
55f
Pelvic injury, 571
Pelvic regions
muscles, assessment, 572
nuclear scintigraphic
evaluation, 574
phase image problems, 224
structures, clinical assessment,
572
visual appraisal/palpation, 572
Pelvic rotation centers, 249

Pelvic stress fractures, 556
  catastrophic injuries, 993
  presumptive diagnosis, 587
  underestimation, 993
Pelvis
  anatomy, knowledge, 555
  asymmetrical movement, 70
  axial skeleton, attachment, 583
  bony elements, transcutaneous
    evaluation, 573-574
  diagram, 583f
  ilial wing, stress fracture (dorsal
    lateral oblique delayed
    phase scintigraphic image),
    568f
  ilium, stress-related bone injury,
    945-946
  lameness, relationship, 233
  palpation, 54-55
    performing, 54-55
    rectum, 55-56
  racing injuries, 965-966
  radiography, 556
    indications, 590
  right side, dorsal lateral oblique
    delayed phase scintigraphic
    image, 578f
  stress fractures, 1010-1012
  symmetrical halves, 555
Penetrating injuries, 213
  distal phalanx fractures,
    association, 361
  ultrasonographic examination,
    213
Penetrating wounds, 316-317
Penetration, wavelength
  dependence, 904
Pentosan Equine Injection, 844
Pentosan polysulfate (PPS), 844
  usage, review, 844
Peptides, presence, 323
Percutaneous cryotherapy, impact,
  869
Performance
  comparison, 923
  intensity, 13
  lameness, implication, 925
  shoeing, impact, 302
Performance horses
  blood tests, 1082-1083,
    1094-1095
    limitations, 1082-1083
  British Equine Veterinary
    Association prepurchase
    examination worksheet,
    1084f-1088f
  clinical findings
    (interpretation), nerve
    blocks (assistance), 1095
  conflicts of interest, 1083
  conformation, 1089-1090
  contract, 1082-1083
  distance examination, 1083
  examination, goals, 1081-1082
  flexion tests, 1091
  gait, assessment, 1090-1091
  insurance, 1082
  joints, assessment, 1090
  kissing spines, 599
  lunging, 1091
  magnetic resonance imaging,
    1094
  muscle symmetry, 1090
  nerve blocks, 1095
  nuclear scintigraphic
    examination, 1093
  observations, summary, 1095

Performance horses (Continued)
  prepurchase examination,
    1081
    reporting, guidelines,
      1095-1096
  problems, evaluation, 1091
  purchase
    client information, 1083
    examination, 1081
  purchaser reservations, 1082
  radiographic examination,
    1091-1093
  rectal examination, 1091
  regions, findings (examination/
    interpretation), 1092
  resale purchase, 1082
  ridden exercises, 1091
  tendons/ligaments, 1090
  thermographic examination,
    1094
  ultrasonographic examination,
    1094
  vendor communication, 1083
Performance problems, 6-7,
  924-925
  assessment, challenge, 920
  clinical assessment, 922-924
  list, 924b
  muscle pain/injury, role, 821
Periarticular cellulitis, 526
Periarticular edema, 88
Periarticular fibrosis, development,
  468-469
Periarticular laxity, 641
Periarticular lesions, 148
Periarticular osteophyte
  formation, development,
  172
Periarticular soft tissue, 655-656
  swelling, development, 469
Periarticular sympathectomy,
  342
Periarticular trauma, 469-470
Perineural analgesia, 108-116
  impact, 397
Perineural blocks
  assessment, 101
  efficacy, 101
  assessment process, 101
Perineural injections, performing,
  107
Periodic acid-Schiff (PAS) stain,
  367
Periosteal grafts, reattachment,
  852
Periosteal new bone, 170-171
  development, 171
Periosteal scratching, 990
Periosteal stripping, 643
Periostitis, 1011
Periovulatory discomfort, 157
Peripheral nerves
  deficits, 42
  distal axonopathy, 145
  distinction, 213
  injuries, 144-145
Peripheral sensory system, neuron
  categories, 908
Peritendonous-periligamentous
  (PT-PL) inflammation, 797
  clinical examination, 797
Peritendonous-periligamentous
  (PT-PL) swelling, 795
Peritendonous-periligamentous
  (PT-PL) tissue injury,
  797-798
Perna canaliculus, 845

Peroneal nerve block (fibular
  nerve block), 127
Peroneus tertius, 802-803
Personal Ensign, victory, 978
Phalangeal rotation, 375
Phalanges
  parasagittal fat suppressed STIR
    MRI, 1103f
  phalangeal axis, relationship,
    291
  rotation, mediolateral
    imbalance (impact), 286f
Pharmaceuticals, nutrients
  (combination), 845
Pharmacology, 100-107
Phase images
  delay, 229
  problems, 221
Phosphate-buffered saline (PBS)
  solution, 847
Phosphorus
  deficiency, 625
  overfeeding, effects, 622
Photo emission tomography
  (PET), 218
Photopenia, 226
Physeal dysplasia (physitis),
  relationship, 620
Physeal stimulation technique,
  644
Physeal uptake, delayed images,
  227f
Physical derangements, 387
Physical examination, usage,
  896
Physical limitation, 157
Physical restraint, usage, 106
Physis, IRU (presence), 450
Physitis, 449
  clinical signs, 639
  confinement, 638
  developmental orthopedic
    disease, 631
  observation, 639
  pathogenesis, 638-639
  physeal dysplasia, relationship,
    620
  treatment, 640
  type V Salter-Harris growth
    plate injury, relationship,
    638-639
Pick, 309
PICP, 949
Pin firing, 713-714
  usage, 868
PINP, 949
Pituitary pars intermedia
  dysfunction (PPID), 370
Plaiting, 75-76
  commonness, 76
Plantar annular ligament desmitis,
  1121
Plantar balance (dorsopalmar
  balance), 282
Plantar digital analgesia, 125
  perineural analgesia, 125
Plantar metatarsal nerves
  false-positive results, 134
  perineural analgesia, 745
Plantar metatarsal region,
  transverse ultrasonographic
  image, 424f
Plantar nerves, perineural
  analgesia, 745
Plantar pastern dermatitis, 66
Plantar pastern zones/
  descriptions, 198-199

Plantar pouches, arthrocentesis
  site (alternative), 130
Plantar process osteochondral
  fragments, 492-494
Plantar region, term (usage),
  764
Plantar soft tissue structures
  (evaluation), ultrasonographic
  evaluation (performing), 502
Plantar tarsus, transverse/
  longitudinal images, 196f
Plastic flock-line cuffs, 307
Platelet-rich plasma (PRP),
  763-764, 1118
  marketing, 763
Platinum Performance,
  components, 846
Pleasure horses
  DIP joint, lateromedial
    radiographic view, 353f
  superficial digital flexor tendon,
    rupture, 726
  superficial digital flexor
    tendonitis, 721-726
Pleasure horses, lumbosacral/
  pelvic injuries
  analgesic techniques, 573
  anatomical considerations,
    571
  aortoiliacofemoral thrombosis,
    579-580
  clinical examination, 572-573
  clinical signs, 571-573
  coxofemoral joint, 581-582
  diagnostic imaging, 573-574
  differential diagnosis, 574-582
  dorsal sacroiliac ligament,
    desmitis, 578
  equine rhabdomyolysis (tying
    up), 575-576
  femur, third trochanter (femur/
    enthesopathy), 582
  fractures, 574-575
  history, 571-572
  lumbosacral joint, 579
  muscle injury, 576-577
  nuclear scintigraphy, 574
  radiography, 573
  sacroiliac joint injury, 577-578
  sacrum wing, new bone (caudal
    aspect), 578-579
  serum muscle enzyme
    concentration, 573
  ultrasonography, 573-574
Pleasure riding horses
  cellulitis, impact, 1253
  drainage, creation, 1253
  foot, lateromedial radiographic
    image, 1253f
  lacerations/puncture wounds,
    risk, 1253
  lameness, causes, 1253
  laminitis, 1253
  left front foot, transverse T2
    gradient-echo MR image,
    336f
  local analgesic techniques,
    1252
  neurological problems, 1253
  right front pastern, longitudinal
    ultrasonographic image,
    759f
  tendon/ligament injuries,
    incidence, 1253
  uses, 1252
Plesiotherapy, 874
  efficacy, 876

Pleuropneumonia, 372
  onset, 561
Plexus, 321
Plumb line
  concept, 21
  usage, diagram, 22f
Pneumonia, onset, 561
Podotrochlear bursa (navicular
    bursa), 122-124
  analgesia, 122-123
    palmar midline approach,
      usage, 123-124
  compression, 123-124
  proximal, palmar injection
    technique, 124
  synoviocentesis, lateral view,
    123f
Pointing, 39
Point of zero moment (PZM),
    274-275, 283
Point to point horse
  acute lesions, 1071
  back pain, 1074-1075
  carpus, lameness (association),
    1072
  clinical examination, 1069
  conformation, lameness
    (relationship), 1068
  diagnosis, absence, 1070
  diagnostic analgesia, 1069-1070
  front feet, lameness
    (association), 1073
  hock, lameness (relationship),
    1072-1073
  imaging considerations, 1070
  injuries, 1075
  lameness, 1067-1068
    causes, 1070
    diagnosis/management,
      1070-1075
    examination, 1068-1069
  metacarpophalangeal joint,
    lameness (association),
    1074
  neck lesions, 1074
  pelvis, lameness (association),
    1073
  serial ultrasonographic
    examinations, 1071
  shoeing considerations,
    lameness (relationship),
    1070
  sport, description, 1062-1063
  structural damage, assessment,
    1072
  superficial digital flexor
    tendonitis, 1070-1072
  suspensory desmitis, 1072
    problem, 1072
  third metacarpal/metatarsal
    bones, fractures,
    1073-1074
  track surface, 1067-1068
  training surface, 1067-1068
Point to point races
  faller, 1066f
  nomenclature, 1063
  time, 1066
Polo
  industry, 1149-1151
  speed/stamina, 1150
  team, composition, 1149-1150
  types, 1149
Polo pony
  ALDDFT, desmitis, 1159
  ALSDFT, desmitis, 1164
  back pain, 1161

Polo pony (Continued)
  body suspensory desmitis, 1157
    career-ending injury, 1157
  carpal region lameness, 1163
  chronic proliferative synovitis
    (villonodular synovitis),
    1156
  chronic PSD, 1157
  conformation abnormalities,
    1151
  corticosteroids
    intramuscular injections,
      1161
    local infiltration, 1159
  cranial thoracic dorsal spinous
    processes, fractures,
    1161-1162
  diagnostic analgesia,
    performing, 1151
  diagnostic arthroscopy,
    1152-1153
  digital extensor tendon/
    metacarpophalangeal joint
    capsule, lateromedial
    radiographic image, 1155f
  digital flexor tenosynovitis,
    1163
  direct trauma, 1157-1158
  distal hock joint pain,
    1160-1161
  distal interphalangeal
    osteoarthritis, 1159
  distal phalanx
    fractures, 1158
    injury, 1157-1158
    pedal osteitis, osteitis, 1158
  distal sesamoidean ligaments,
    desmitis, 1163
  dorsal spinous process
    impingement, 1161
  drug testing, 1151
  equine protozoal myelitis,
    1164
  fetlock joint capsulitis, 1153
  forelimb, lateromedial
    radiographic image, 1156f
  gluteal myositis, 1161
  gracilis muscle tear, 1164
  hindlimb lameness, 1164
  hindlimb PSD, diagnosis, 1152
  hoof injury, 1157-1158
  imaging considerations,
    1152-1153
  intraarticular analgesia,
    1151-1152
  intralesional injections,
    1153-1154
  introduction, 1150
  lameness
    diagnosis, 1151
    examination, 1151-1152
    problems, 1153
    undiagnosed diagnosis, 1152
  left forelimb, distal aspect
    (dorsomedial-palmarolateral
    oblique radiographic
    image), 1162f
  left hock, dorsomedial-
    plantarolateral oblique
    radiographic image, 1160f
  magnetic resonance imaging,
    1152
  medical management,
    1153-1154
  metacarpal region, dorsolateral-
    palmaromedial oblique
    radiographic image, 1160f

Polo pony (Continued)
  metacarpophalangeal joint
    disease, pain sources, 1152
    dorsolateral-palmaromedial
      oblique radiographic
      image, 1157f
  metacarpophalangeal
    osteoarthritis, 1155-1156
  intraarticular injections,
    1155
  metatarsal region, dorsolateral-
    plantaromedial oblique
    radiographic image, 1159f
  navicular disease, 1158-1159
  neck reining, 1150
  nondisplaced diaphyseal splint
    bone fractures, cryotherapy
    response, 1160
  non-weight bearing, 1152
  osteitis, 1158
  osteoarthritis,
    metacarpophalangeal joint
    (dorsolateral-palmaromedial
    oblique radiographic
    image), 1155f
  palmar annular ligament,
    desmitis, 1163
  palmar foot pain, 1158-1159
  palmar metacarpal region,
    transverse ultrasonographic
    image, 1153f-1154f
  pastern region injuries, 1162
  peritendonous injections,
    1153-1154
  proximal interphalangeal
    osteoarthritis, 1162
  proximal suspensory desmitis,
    1156-1157
  proximity, 1150f
  PSBs, inflammation
    (sesamoiditis), 1162
  PSD, impact, 1156
  rhabdomyolysis, 1164
  rigid bars, attachment, 1162f
  rim shoes, 1150-1151
  SARAPIN, usage, 1159
  scintigraphic examination,
    1152
  sesamoiditis, 1162-1163
  shock wave therapy, 1157
  splint bone
    disease, 1159-1160
    injury, pain sources, 1152
  sport, history, 1149
  superficial digital flexor
    tendon, dislocation/
    luxation, 1161
  superficial digital flexor
    tendonitis, 1153-1155
  surgical management,
    1154-1155
  suspensory branch desmitis,
    1157
    commonness, 1157
  suspensory desmitis, 1156-1157
  tendons
    splitting, 1154
    ultrasonographic assessment,
      1154
  training, daily legging, 1150f
  traumatic exostoses, 1159
  ultrasonography, 1152
  upper forelimb lameness,
    1164
  withers, fracture, 1161-1162
Polydipsia, 370-371
Polyionic isotonic fluids, 784-785

Polymerase chain reaction (PCR)
  analysis, usage, 679
  testing, 139, 141
Polymerization
  reaction, 306
  speed, importance, 306
Polymethyl methacrylate (PMMA),
    306-307
  beads, usage, 680
Polysaccharide storage myopathy
    (PSSM), 827-829
  clinical signs, 828-829
  diagnosis, 828-830
  etiology, 828
  management, 828-829
  metabolic myopathies, 829-830
  semitendinosus biopsy,
    cryostat-cut sections, 830f
  treatment, 830
Polysulfated glycosaminoglycans
    (PSGAGs), 843-844
  effectiveness, HA effectiveness
    (comparison), 844
  intralesional/systemic
    administration, 715
  intramuscular administration,
    844
  usage, 396, 433-434
Polysynovitis, clinical syndrome,
    689
Polytrack, change, 975
Polyurethane adhesives, 307
Polyurethane tab type shoes,
    307
  cyanoacrylate adhesive, usage,
    307
Polyuria, 370-371
Polyvinyl chloride (PVC), 307
Pony
  ALDDFT, desmitis, 1233-1234
  antebrachiocarpal joint,
    osteoarthritis, 434
  back pain, 1234
  carpus, osteoarthritis, 1230
  cellulitis, antebrachium
    (transverse ultrasonographic
    image), 833f
  cerebellar abiotrophy, 1235
  characteristics, 1228
  coxofemoral joint
    dysplasia, 1230
    luxation, 1230
    luxation, appearance, 1231f
  DFTS, tendonitis, 1234
  diagnostic analgesia, 1228-1229
  digital flexor tendons, strains,
    695
  elbow, craniocaudal
    radiographic view, 461f
  foot, chronic laminitis, 1233f
  foot-related problems, 1233
  forelimb lameness, 149
  fractures, 1232
  gait assessment, 1228
  gelding
    acute-onset severe right
      forelimb lameness,
      shoulder region swelling,
      469f
    tibial tuberosity fracture,
      postoperative
      lateromedial radiographic
      view, 548f
  hemarthrosis, 1232
  hock, osteoarthritis, 1230
  imaging considerations, 1229
  joint conditions, 1230-1232

Pony (Continued)
joint disease, 1229-1232
treatment, 1232
lameness, 1228
conditions, 1229
examination, 1228
laminitis, 1233
risk, 370
limb deformities, 1229
muscular disorders, 1234-1235
patella
luxation, 1230-1231
upward fixation, 1231
proximal interphalangeal joint
bilateral nontraumatic dorsal
subluxation, 1232f
nontraumatic dorsal
subluxation, 1232
subluxation, 1232
right forelimb lameness, 156f
scapulohumeral joints,
osteoarthritis, 1229-1230
soft tissue injuries, 1233-1234
stifle, osteoarthritis, 1230
stringhalt, 560
subchondral bone, IRU (lateral/
solar delayed phase
images), 232f
superficial digital flexor
tendonitis, 1233
wounds, 1234
Poor-quality bone uptake,
222-223
Postanesthetic myopathy,
833-834
clinical signs, 833
diagnosis, 834
impact, 212
prevention, 834
treatment/prognosis, 834
Post-β peaks, decrease, 138
Postinjection muscle soreness/
abscessation, 833
Postmortem examination, 2
Post (posty) leg, 28
Posttraumatic exostosis,
occurrence, 877
Postulated radiolucent fracture
line, detection, 175
Posture, 39
Poultice, application, 1033-1034
Pregnancy, calcium requirements,
950
Preservative-free morphine, usage,
856
Pressage bandages, 859
production, 859
Pressure bandage, usage, 1213f
Pressure-measuring pads, force/
pressure distribution
measurement systems, 246
Pressure waves, schematic
demonstration, 915f
Pricked horseshoe nail placement,
310f
Primary brachiocephalicus pain,
612
Primary copper deficiency,
622-623
Primary deep digital flexor
tendonitis, 733
Primary DIP joint pain,
differential diagnosis,
351-355
Primary lameness, 66
Primary lateral digital flexor
tendon injuries, 781-782

Primary metatarsophalangeal joint
lameness, 67
Primary navicular disease
management strategies, 338-342
Primary navicular disease,
treatment, 338
Primary palmar annular ligament
thickening, 772-773
ultrasonographic evidence,
772-773
Primary tenosynovitis
secondary palmar annular
ligament thickening,
inclusion, 773
secondary tenosynovitis,
differentiation, 768
Primary traumatic synovitis, 690
Probes, usage, 254
Procel Cast Liner, application,
862f
Progressive lamellar separation,
376
Progressive osteoarthritis, 9
Proliferative synovitis, 48-49
diagnosis, 396
treatment, 396-397
villonodular synovitis, 690
Proliferative synovitis-like lesions,
260
Proprioception, mediation, 323
Prostagandin E$_2$
activation, 846-847
Prostagandin E$_2$ (PGE$_2$)
interleukin-1 activation, 672f
Prostagandins, 664
inhibition, 841
Protein administration, 851-852
Proteoglycan (PG), 658
composite molecules, 658
molecules, CS epitopes
(measurement), 669
Proteolytic enzymes, 704
Proton density (PD) image, 938
Proximal, dorsal metacarpal
region, palpation, 51f
Proximal check desmotomy, 715
Proximal digital annular desmitis,
816
Proximal dorsal articular fractures,
treatment, 389-390
Proximal dorsomedial
osteochondral fragments,
400f
Proximal humeral physis, injuries
(rarity), 464
Proximal interphalangeal (PIP)
joint, 117-118, 812
abaxial/axial palmar ligaments,
origination, 811
anatomical considerations, 387
arthrocentesis, 117
arthrodesis, 392
methods, 392
articular surfaces (axial
compression), DDFT
(impact), 344
capsule, assessment, 48
dorsal subluxation, 393
imaging considerations, 388
intraarticular analgesia,
response, 387-388
lateromedial/dorsopalmar
radiographic view, 634f
left abaxial plantar ligament,
ultrasonographic images,
817f
lesions, 633

Proximal interphalangeal (PIP)
joint (Continued)
osteoarthritis, 391-392
cryotherapy, 871
osteochondrosis, 391
palmar/plantar ligaments, 812
subluxation, 393
rarity/occurrence, 393
Proximal interphalangeal (PIP)
osteoarthritis, 1162
Proximal limb flexion tests, 513
Proximal metacarpal fasciotomy,
719
accomplishment, 719
Proximal metacarpal region
dorsolateral-palmaromedial
oblique radiographic, 425f
dorsopalmar radiographic views,
399
edema, occurrence, 740
longitudinal images, 171f,
741f
transverse computed
tomography images, 236f
transverse images, 172f
transverse sections, 89f
latex injection, 113f
Proximal metatarsal region
acute hindlimb injuries,
ALDDFT evaluation, 737
deep digital flexor tendon
lesions, 733
plantar scintigraphic images,
evaluation, 501-502
transverse anatomical section,
92f
transverse ultrasonographic
image, 746f
Proximal palmar metacarpal pain,
1032
Proximal palmar metacarpal
region
analgesic techniques,
interpretation, 113-114
longitudinal images, 188f
Proximal phalanx
anatomical considerations, 387
collateral ligament avulsions,
410f
comminuted fracture
lateromedial/dorsopalmar
radiographic views, 972f
radiographic views, 864f
dorsal frontal fractures, 402,
495-496, 1028-1029
occurrence, 495
result, 495-496
dorsal proximal aspect,
compression, 86
dorsoproximal aspect, osseous
opacities, 633
dorsoproximal aspect,
osteochondral fragments,
399-400, 494, 633
occurrence, 494
evaluation, radiographic
examination, 388
fractures, 388-390, 495-496
race occurrence, 963
types, 388
incomplete fractures
identification, nuclear
scintigraphy (usage), 388
occurrence, 389
injuries, 399-402
larger palmar fragments, 401
major fractures, 402

Proximal phalanx (Continued)
midsagittal fractures, 1028
dorsoplantar/flexed
lateromedial
xeroradiographic images,
1028f
palmar aspect
enthesophyte formation,
759
osteochondral fragments,
short sesamoidean
avulsions, 400-401
palmar fragments, 401
palmar/plantar avulsion
fractures, occurrence, 390
palmar/plantar osteochondral
fragments, 633
proximal aspect, dorsal frontal
fractures, 389-390
proximal-dorsal aspect,
horizontal oblique views
(usefulness), 482-483
proximal dorsal aspect,
palpation, 62f
proximal dorsomedial
osteochondral fragments,
400f
proximal palmar/plantar
margin, osteochondral
fragment, 401f
proximal physis, Salter-Harris
type II fracture
(lateromedial radiographic
image), 389f
proximodorsal aspect, chip
fractures, 400
sagittal fractures, 402
perineural analgesia, 402f
short incomplete sagittal
fractures, 1013
Proximal physeal injuries, 464
Proximal physeal tibial fractures,
529
Proximal plantar processes
acute fractures, 494
fragmentation, 492
Proximal pouch, bulge, 261
Proximal radius, cranial articular
margin, 458
Proximal sesamoid bones (PSBs),
44
abaxial aspect, fractures, 496
abaxial fractures, 405
abnormalities, 741
apical fractures, 404-405
aseptic necrosis, 755-756
avulsion fracture, 754
axial aspect
aseptic necrosis, 755
infection, 755-756
axial border, radiolucent
defects, 497
axial PSB fractures, 406
basilar fractures, 405
conditions, 402-407
desensitization, 395
distal metacarpal region,
transverse ultrasonographic
image, 773f
enlargement, 932
fractures, 404-407, 496
clinical signs, 404
diagnosis, 404-405
distribution, 496
importance, 402-403
intersesamoidean ligament
injury, 406-407

Proximal sesamoid bones
(Continued)
intraarticular fragmentation,
suspensory branch injury
(association), 406
midbody PSB fractures, 405-406
nonarticular fragments, impact,
494
nuclear scintigraphic
examination, 755
osteomyelitis, 755-756
palmar annular ligament,
avulsion (attachment), 422
palmar/plantar surface covering,
260-261
proximal aspect, 82
racing injuries, 964
radiographic examination, 752
training injury, 964
transverse lucencies, 404f
young foals, PSB fractures, 407
Proximal suspensory desmitis
(PSD), 50, 83, 422, 448
anatomy/cadaver specimen,
506f
differentiation, 740-741
importance, 988-989
management, 499-500
proximal metatarsal
region, transverse
ultrasonographic image,
745f
result, 739-740
Proximal tarsus, transverse
section, 781f
Proximal tibia
lateromedial view, 171f
nonossifying fibromas, 532
Proximopalmar metacarpal region,
palpation, 51f
Psoas minor/major muscles,
insertion, 593
Pubis fractures, 569
rarity, 569
scintigraphic examination, 569
ultrasonographic examination,
569
Pulse
duration, 905
elevation, 63
rate, 905
sequence, 240
Pulsed electromagnetic field
(PEMF)
contraindications, 904
emission, 903
therapy, 903-904
primary effects, 903-904
Punched shoe (stamped shoe),
294
Purpura hemorrhagica, 167
occurrence, 167
Pyramidal disease, 355
Pyridinoline (PYD), presence, 949

Q
Qi stagnation, 887
Quadriceps, major hindlimb
muscle rupture, 162
Quantitative analysis, 199-200
Quantitative measurements, 177
Quantitative terms, 200-203
Quarter, 294
Quarter cracks, 307-308
commonness, 985, 1024
debridement, 318f
incompleteness, 318

Quarter Horses (QHs)
barrel horses, 1182
colts (spinal ataxia), midneck
region (lateral radiographic
view), 651f
conformation, study, 18
distal foot, transverse section,
320f
distal metacarpal region,
transverse ultrasonographic
image, 1185f
evaluation, 16-17
right carpus, lateromedial
digital radiographic view,
433f
Quarter Milers, 1051
Quarter Pathers, 1051
Quarters, lameness, 984-985
Quickened horseshoe nail
placement, 310f
Quicken the Blood and Resolve
stasis, 887
Quicking, 310
Quittor, 1220-1221
definition, 1220-1221

R
Racecourse, studies, 975
Racehorses
advanced OA, 492
apical fractures, 404-405
arthroscopy, purpose, 432
athletic outcome, 710
injury assessment/goals, 710
carpal osteochondral fragments,
occurrence, 434-435
distal forelimbs, dorsal delayed
scintigraphic image,
231f
distal phalanx, fractures, 360
DMD problem, 951
early OA, diagnosis, 433
extensive osteoarthritis,
432-433
fetlock
evaluation, nuclear
scintigraphy (usage),
395
subchondral injury, locations,
398-399
forced tarsal flexion problem,
999
forelimbs, increase
radiopharmaceutical
uptake (site prevalence),
938t
gallop, 67
hindlimbs, increased
radiopharmaceutical uptake
(site prevalence), 938t
osteoarthritis
development, 432
subchondral bone,
maladaptive/nonadaptive
stress-related bone injury,
488
osteochondral fragmentation,
432-433
pain response, 998
prognosis, age (impact), 11
racing class, return, 8
radiological changes, absence,
433-434
retraining, 1016-1017
right forelimb, Kimzey Leg
Saver (application), 968f
sore shins, 1011

Racehorses (Continued)
superficial digital flexor
tendonitis, 706-715
clinical signs, 707-710
injuries, 707
surgical/conservative
management, prognosis
(evaluation), 8
symptomatic treatment, exercise
(continuation), 711-713
talus, incomplete sagittal
fractures, 520
tendon injury
acute phase, management,
710
long-term rehabilitation,
711-715
subacute phase treatment,
711-715
treatment, history, 711
Racehorses, performance problems
(cause), 6-7
Racetrack
comparisons, 974
configuration, variables, 974-975
injuries
correlation, 1068
location, 962-963
operators
change, 978-979
handle emphasis, 979
racing surface, quality, 975-976
type, multivariable
epidemiological studies,
975
variables, 974f
Racetrack surface
differences, 980
lameness, relationship, 980,
1052
speed, predisposition, 980
Racing
gambling, banning, 978
injuries, 963-967
pattern, 994-995
performance, evaluation, 8
Quarter Horse, training, 1052
return, chance (guidelines), 205
risk factors/interactions, 974f
sport, establishment, 977
turf tracks, 975-976
Racing Quarter Horse, 1186
antiinflammatory medications,
usage, 1054
carpal bones
dorsoproximal-dorsodistal
digital radiographic
image, 1056f
fractures, 1056
carpal joints, synovitis, 1053
carpus, osteochondral chip
fractures, 1054-1055
corrective shoeing, usage, 1054
distal hock joint pain, 1055
distal interphalangeal joint,
arthrosis, 1053-1054
feet, problems, 1053-1054
forelimb proximal suspensory
desmitis, 1055-1056
fractures, 1056
imaging considerations, 1053
intraarticular analgesia, 1054
lameness
conditions, 1053-1056
conformation, relationship,
1052
examination, 1052-1053

Racing Quarter Horse (Continued)
medial femoral condyle,
subchondral bone cysts,
1055
medial femorotibial joint, stifle
pain, 1055
metacarpophalangeal joints
lateromedial digital
radiographic image, 1055f
osteochondral chip fractures,
1055
synovitis, 1053
osteoarthritis, observation,
1055
osteochondral chip fractures,
incidence, 1054
pain relief, intraarticular
corticosteroids
(effectiveness), 1054
proximal phalanx, dorsal aspect
(intraarticular chip
fractures), 1055
proximal suspensory desmitis,
1055-1056
shoeing, 1053
problems, 1053
sport, history/description,
1051-1052
stifle problems, 1055
third carpal bone, frontal slab
fracture (lateromedial
digital radiographic image),
1056f
tibial stress fractures, 1056
track surface, lameness
(relationship), 1052
training, 1052
Racing surface
impact, 972
quality, 975-976
Racing TB (musculoskeletal
problem development),
conformation (role), 17
Rack (gait), 1190
Racking horses, 1186-1187
gait, 1187
confusion, 1187
Radial carpal bone
distal aspect, sclerosis,
1008-1009
distal dorsalarticular surface,
evaluation, 429-431
nonadaptive remodeling,
987-988
Radial fractures, 450-452
clinical signs, 450
rarity, 965
result, 450
Radial nerve
branch, damage, 156
injury, 144
paralysis, 474
paresis/paralysis, 40f, 144
Radial pressure wave (RPW),
914-915
shock waves, comparison, 915t
therapy, 744, 748
treatment, 916
Radial stress fractures,
management, 452
Radiation doses, expression, 873
Radiation-induced synovectomy,
876
Radiation safety, 169, 223
principles, 170b
rules/licenses, 223
Radiation synovectomy, 848

Radiation therapy
    analgesic effects, 873
    antiinflammatory effects,
        872-873
    antiproliferative effects, 873
    clinical applications, 875-877
    ionizing radiation, usage, 872
    prophylactic treatment, 877
    radiobiological aspects, 872-873
    treatment, 876
        side effects, 873
    usage, 876
        avoidance, 875
Radical hoof wall resection,
    avoidance, 1220
Radioactive gold, gamma ray
    emission, 874
Radioactive sources, radiation
    hazard, 876-877
Radiographic detail, 168-169
Radiographic examination,
    177-178
Radiographic images, factors,
    169b
Radiographic projections,
    178t-181t
Radiographic technique, 178-182
Radiographs
    evaluation, 178
    interpretation, 178
    permanent labeling, 182
    usage, 139
Radiography, 139-140, 168,
    429-431
    awareness, 91-92
    exposure factors, 168
    exposure latitude, 168
    film/screen factors, 169
    image
        contrast, 168
        resolution, 168-169
        sharpness, 168-169
    rare earth screens, usage, 458
Radioimmunoassay (RIA), 949
Radioisotopes, 216-217
    radiation, emission, 216
    in vivo/in vitro use, 215-216
Radiological abnormalities
    clinical significance, 154
    stall, confinement, 451-452
    variation, 174
Radiological changes, confusion/
    equivocation, 231-232
Radiolucent defect, dorsopalmar
    view, 407f
Radiopharmaceuticals, 216-217
    extravasation, 228
    perivascular injection, 228
Radiopharmaceutical uptake (RU),
    216-217
    decrease, 217
    increase, 608
        character, 225-227
    patterns, description/
        comparison, 597
Radiotherapy, clinical results,
    875-876
Radius
    craniodistal aspect, trauma, 434
    displaced (unstable) fractures,
        450-451
    distal aspect
        articular fracture, 447
        craniolateral-caudomedial
            oblique radiographic
            view, 791f
        lameness, localization, 453

Radius (Continued)
    osteochondroma, 449
    distal caudal aspect, exostoses,
        448
    enostosis-like lesions, 452-453
        radiological/scintigraphic
            finding, 452
        treatment, 453
    incomplete fractures, prognosis,
        452
    nondisplaced fractures,
        prognosis, 452
    osteitis/osteomyelitis, 455
        etiology, 455
        treatment, 455
    physitis, distal aspect (physeal
        dysplasia), 449
    proximal aspect, craniocaudal
        radiographic view, 461f
    racing injuries, 965
    stress fractures, rarity, 943
Radon gas, gamma ray emission,
    874
Ramp, 905
Rapid muscle atrophy,
    longissimus dorsi
    (cryostat-cut biopsy sections),
    831f
Ration evaluations, 626-628
    intention, 627
Reactive arthritis, septicemia
    (impact), 677
Reactive synovitis, 689-690
Reciprocal apparatus, 95f
    caudal component, disruption,
        41-42
    impact, 95
Rectal examination, 565
Recumbency, risk, 575-576
Recurrent exertional
    rhabdomyolysis (RER), 11,
    826-827
    acetylpromazine tranquilizers,
        usage, 827
    clinical signs, 826
    diagnosis, 826-827
    diet, adjustment, 827
    factors, 826
    incidence, 576
    management, 827
    muscle biopsies, histological
        appearance, 826-827
    prevention, 827
    restriction, 575
Red blood cell count, 678
Redden Ultimate, 381f
Redness, 44
Referred pain, 152
Refractive scattering, 173-174
Refractory exacerbative laminitis
    (RELs), 374
Regulatory veterinarian, 960-961
    duties, 960
Rehabilitation programs,
    principles, 877-878
Reined cow horse, 1176-1180
    centrodistal joint pain, 1179
    competition, 1176, 1178
    conformation
        lameness, relationship,
            1177
        problems, 1177
    corticosteroids, intraarticular
        injection, 1179
    diagnosis, absence, 1178
    distal interphalangeal joint
        pain, 1180

Reined cow horse (Continued)
    egg bar shoe, usage, 1178
    flexion tests, 1178
    imaging considerations, 1178
    lameness
        conditions, 1179
            prevention/detection, 1176
            shoeing considerations, 1178
            treatment, 1179-1180
    metatarsophalangeal joint pain,
        1180
    navicular syndrome, 1179
    sesamoiditis, 1180
    stifle pain, 1179-1180
    superficial digital flexor
        tendonitis, 1179
    suspensory desmitis, 1179
    tarsometatarsal joint pain,
        1179
    training, 1176
        lameness, relationship, 1177
        surfaces, 1176-1177
        surfaces, water content, 1177
        traumatic hoof injuries, 1179
Reining horses
    navicular syndrome, treatment,
        1184
    shoe, usage, 1184f
Renal dysfunction, diagnosis,
    228
Reparative healing, 707
Repetitive overload injuries,
    395-399
Repetitive stress injury,
    scintigraphic appearance,
    399f
Residual gait abnormality, 560
Respiratory disease, development,
    958
Respiratory rates, elevation, 63
Rest, 878-879
    amount, importance, 14
    programs, principles, 877-878
    quality, resistance, 14
Resurfacing joints, healing
    (progress), 849-852
Retained placenta, 372
Reverberation, 174-177
Rhabdomyolysis, 1147
    risk, reduction, 1137
Rheumatoid arthritis,
    steroid-responsive arthritis,
    689
Rhodococcus equi infection, 615
    impact, 677
Rib lesions, 155
Ridden exercise, importance,
    573
Ridden walking, 879
Riddle, Sam, 977
Rider, blinding, 923
Rider-induced problems, 157
Riding
    observation, 79
    odd lameness, 155
    performance, comparison, 923
Riding, examination, 596
Riding horse
    caudal cervical region, oblique
        lateral view, 613f
    left hind foot, dorsal
        three-dimensional T2
        gradient-echo MRI imaging,
        352f
    mineralized tissue, stifle
        (caudocranial radiographic
        view), 549f

Right carpus
    carpal bones, distal row
        (dorsoproximal-dorsodistal
        radiographic image),
        943f
    dorsal 45° medial-palmarolateral
        oblique radiographic view,
        437f
    dorsopalmar digital
        radiographic view, 10f
    joint, intraoperative
        arthroscopic images,
        256f
    lateral/dorsal delayed phase
        scintigraphic images,
        231f
    lateromedial digital
        radiographic view, 433f
    third carpal bone fractures,
        occurrence, 435
    unilateral flexural deformity,
        646f
Right coxofemoral joint,
    arthrocentesis, 132f
Right elbow
    mediolateral radiographic view,
        462f
    region, lateral scintigraphic
        image, 153f
Right fore lateral OSL,
    transverse/longitudinal
    ultrasonographic images,
    815f
Right forelimb (RL)
    abbreviation, 64
    deep digital flexor tendon
        rupture, distal aspect,
        732f
    lateral bone phase scintigraphic
        images, 1142f
    lateral/dorsal/flexed lateral/
        flexed dorsal delayed
        phase scintigraphic images,
        221f
    palmar metacarpal soft
        tissues, transverse
        ultrasonographic image,
        150f
    SDFT injury, computerized scan
        data, 712f-713f
Right fore medial palmar digital
    nerve, ultrasonographic
    images, 817f
Right front fetlock joint, forward
    knuckling (occurrence),
    35f
Right front foot, solar
    scintigraphic image, 153f
Right front metacarpal region,
    photograph, 709f
Right front proximal
    interphalangeal (PIP), flexed
    dorsolateral-palmaromedial
    oblique view, 154f
Right front SDFT, accessory carpal
    bone (transverse/longitudinal
    ultrasonographic images),
    717f
Right hind distal interphalangeal
    joint, intraoperative
    arthroscopic images, 256f
Right hindlimb (RH)
    abbreviation, 64
    proximal interphalangeal joint,
        lateral collateral ligament
        (ultrasonographic images),
        817f

Right hind metatarsophalangeal joint, dorsal 25° proximal medial-plantarodistal lateral oblique digital radiographic view, 253f
Right hind pastern, ultrasonographic images, 816f
Right ilial wing, ultrasonographic image, 566f
Right metacarpophalangeal joint, weight-bearing dorsal 20° proximal-palmarodistal oblique radiographic image, 1000f
Right radius
  distal aspect, craniocaudal digital radiographic view, 454f
  osteomyelitis, lateromedial radiographic view, 455f
Right stifle
  caudocranial radiographic view, 541f
  joint, lateromedial digital radiographic view, 558f
Rillito Park, 1051-1052
Rims, 294
Rim shoes, 295-296
Ring blocks, usage, 107
Ringbone, 1222-1223
Rives, Nathaniel, 977
Road nails/studs, usage, 1132
Robert Jones bandage, 522-523, 860, 1110-1111
  application, 1134
  usage, 860
ROI analysis, usage, 224-225
Roll cotton (cotton wool), usage, 859
Rollkur, 1112-1113
Rongeurs, usage, 254
Root signature, 40-41
Roping horses, 1170-1176
  management, 1173
Ross crossed-extensor phenomenon, 83
Rotation, severity, 381
Rotational deformities, 286-287
  compensation, 292
  impact, 287
Rowley mile racetrack, 996f
Royal Windsor International Driving Grand Prix, 1205-1206
Rump angle, factors, 21
Rump length, 20-21
  measurement, 20f
Run, four-beat gait, 64-65

S
Sacral fracture, 575f
Sacroiliac articulations
  bilateral osteoarthritis, 584f
  iliac wing/caudal margin, dorsal surface (evaluation), 589-590
  motion, limitation, 584
Sacroiliac desmitis, 585
Sacroiliac joint
  diagnostic analgesia, approaches, 589f
  disease
    diagnosis, 577
    occurrence, 578

Sacroiliac joint (Continued)
  dysfunction, clinical manifestations, 586
  intraarticular analgesia, 589
  intraarticular injection, 573
  needle placement, 589
  neurovascular structures, adjacency, 583-584
  osteoarthritis, 577
    bilateral condition, 584-585
    prevalence, 591
  pain, causes, 590-591
  pathological changes, 577
  provocation tests, dorsal view, 586f, 588f
  region, caudomedial approach, 589
  subluxation, 577
  synovial articulation, 583
Sacroiliac joint injuries, 577-578
  anatomical/functional features, 583-584
  antemortem diagnosis, 584
  clinical presentation, 585-586
    variation, 585
  clinical signs, 586
  diagnostic imaging, 589-590
  differential diagnosis, 590-591
  local analgesia, 589
  localization, 587-588
  long-term follow-up evaluation, 591
  pathological conditions, 584-585
  physical examination, 586-589
  presumptive diagnosis, 587
  prognosis, 591
  treatment, 591
Sacroiliac ligaments
  complete disruption, 585
  diagram, 583f
  injury, identification, 587
Sacroiliac region
  comparison, 55
  pain, 1136, 1169-1170
Sacroiliac strain, 1106-1107
Sacrum
  diagram, 583f
  fractures, 575
  ventral aspect, 55
  wing, new bone (caudal aspect), 578-579
Saddlebred gaits, 1189-1190
Saddle pressure analysis, 1129
Safety factor, definition, 271b
Safing, 294-295
Sagittal anatomical section, 88f
Sagittal slab fractures, 443
Sagittal T1-weighted magnetic resonance contrast venogram, 1192f
Salter-Harris type II fracture
  lateromedial radiographic image, 389f
  occurrence, 389, 529
Santa Anita Handicap, 978
Saphenous filling time, 61-63
Sarapin, 578-579
  usage, 1159
Sarcocystis neurona (S. neurona)
  antibodies, detection, 139
  impact, 141
  Nitazoxanide, impact, 142
  serological testing, 137
Sarcocystosis myositis, 831-832
Sawhorse stance, 1148

Scalping, 1004
  impact, 1004
Scandinavian cold-blooded trotters
  breed, history, 1076
  conformation/lameness, 1077
  diagnostic analgesia, 1079
  flexion tests, 1078
  imaging considerations, 1079
  lameness
    causes, 1079
    diagnosis, absence, 1079
    examination, 1077-1079
  racetracks/weather conditions, 1077
  shoeing considerations, 1077
  tarsus, palpation, 1078
  training, 1076
Scanning
  technique, 169
  timing, 204-205
Scans, interpretation, 224-229
Scapula, 471-472
  articular surface fracture, 469
  axial skeleton, attachment, 456
  body
    fracture, 472
    stress fractures, 471-472
  glenoid cavity
    postmortem appearance, 468f
    radiological abnormalities, 465-466
  neck, cranial aspect (suprascapular nerve relationship), 473
  ossification centers, 456, 471
  stress fractures
    postmortem examination, 944-945
    rarity, 993
Scapular height, 34-35
Scapular spine, fracture, 472
  result, 472
Scapulohumeral joint (shoulder joint), 121-122, 465-470
  capsule
    localized tearing, 468
    tearing, 468
  collateral ligaments, absence, 456
  dysplasia, 468
  lesions, 634-635
  luxation, 468
  mediolateral radiographic view, 458f
  osteochondrosis, 465-466
    clinical evidence, 465
Schwung (energy/swing), 1112
Sciatic nerve damage, 42
Scintigraphic examination
  impact, 230-231
  knowledge, 230-234
  usage, 431-432
Scintigraphy, 431-432
  diagnosis, 230
  examination, usage, 230
  images
    information, 226-227
    qualitative assessment, 224
  imaging modality, 216
  performing, methods, 217-218
  sensitivity, 937
  usefulness, 431
  value, 229, 937
Sclerosis, 171
  amount, consideration, 942-943

Screw-in calks, 297
Scrotal intertrigo infections, 1010
Scurry driving, 1205
Seating out, 296
Secondary copper deficiency, 622-623
Secondary lameness, 3-4, 66-67
Secondary palmar annular ligament constriction, 1050
Secondary shoulder region pain, 993
Secondary tenosynovitis, primary tenosynovitis (differentiation), 768
Second cervical vertebrae, subluxation, 609-610
  diagnosis, 609-610
Second metacarpal bone (McII)
  cryotherapy, 870-871
  distal fragments, ostectomy, 870-871
  distal third fracture, suspensory desmitis (association), 751
  dorsomedial-palmarolateral oblique radiographic view, 421f
  exostosis, 1012
    suspensory desmitis, association, 751
  fourth metacarpal bone, exostoses, 419-421
    clinical signs, 419
    diagnosis, 419-420
    treatment, 420-421
  fourth metacarpal bone, fractures, 421-422
  fractures, SWT treatment, 916
  head (plantar aspect), digital pressure (application), 60
  palpation, 50
  pathology, 1142-1143
  proximal aspect
    fracture, 447
    osseous cystlike lesions, 402
  stress fractures, SWT management, 916
  third metacarpal bone, syndesmopathy, 419
Second metatarsal bone (MtII)
  cryotherapy, 870-871
  distal fragments, ostectomy, 870-871
  distal third fracture, suspensory desmitis (association), 751
  exostoses, 504-505, 1012
    suspensory desmitis, association, 751
  fractures, 505
  interosseous ligaments, 504-505
  needle insertion, 126
Second sacral spinous process, apex, 587
Sector array transducers, 169
Seedy toe, 312-313
  term, usage, 312
Segmental vertebral contributions, diagram, 896f
Segmental vertebral motion
  diagram, 897f-898f
  increase, 900
Selective COX-2 inhibition, beneficial effects, 841
Selenium-responsive NMD, alleviation, 835

Self-maintained foot
  appearance, 303-304
  wall, wearing, 303
Selle Français breed, 1063-1064
Selle Français mare, lumbar region
    (transverse anatomical
    section), 593f
Semimembranosis muscle
    (tearing), longitudinal
    ultrasonographic image,
    212f
Semimembranosus, major
    hindlimb muscle rupture,
    162
Semimembranosus myositis,
    1194-1195
Semispinalis, injury, 610-611
  treatment, 611
Semitendinosus myositis,
    1194-1195
Sensations, mediation, 323
Sensing element size, impact,
    249-250
Sensory nerves
  conduction velocity, values,
    140
  functions, 323
Sepsis, 393
Septicemia, 677
Septic navicular bursitis,
    316-317
Serial ultrasonographic
    examinations, case
    management, 205
Serial venography, 378-379
Serology, 136-137
Seroma, inspissation, 376
Serratus ventralis, rupture,
    472-473
Serum amyloid protein A (SAA),
    561
Serum aspartate transminase
    (serum AST), 818
  activity, 818
Serum creatine kinase (serum CK),
    818
  concentration, measurement,
    162
  elevations, 826
  presence, 818
Serum lactate dehydrogenase
    (serum LDH), 819
Serum muscle enzyme
    concentration, 573
Sesamoiditis, 402-404, 496-497
  clinical signs, 402-403
  defining, 1045-1046
  diagnosis, 403
  lesions, radiological pathology,
    403f
  nuclear scintigraphy, 403
  radiological evidence, 403
  treatment, 404
Setaria species, 144
Setscrew model, usage, 116-117
Seventh cervical vertebrae,
    subluxation, 610
Severe acute inflammatory
    reactions (SAIRs), cross-linked
    HA products (association),
    844-845
Severe end-stage OS, intraarticular
    fractures, 481
Severe unrelenting lameness,
    481
Sex, importance, 11
Shear, 92

Sheared heel, 312, 1024-1025,
    1102
  diagnosis, 312
  history/clinical signs, 312
  presence, 312
  term, usage, 312
  treatment/prognosis, 312
Sheaths, swellings, 428-429
Sheep-knee (calf-knee)
    conformation, 25-26
Shetland ponies
  complete fibula, 525-526
  osteoarthritis, 1229-1230
  scapulohumeral joint,
      mediolateral radiographic
      view, 468f
  sudden-onset severe lameness,
    467
Shielding, 221-222
  importance, 221
Shin-hitting, 74-75
Shire riding horse, acute-onset left
    hindlimb lameness, caudal
    scintigraphic image, 574f
Shivers (shiverers) (shivering), 76,
    561-562, 1226-1227
  behavior, 156
  biomechanical basis, 561-562
  cause, 561
  clinical characteristic, 561
  clinical features, 561
  medical therapy, 562
  progressive disorder, 561
  stringhalt, comparison,
    145
  surgical therapy, 562
Shock, treatment, 808
Shock waves (SWs)
  application
    consideration, therapy
      planning, 918
    three-dimensional treatment
      plan, 918
  effect (evaluation) tissue
    explants (usage), 917
  radial pressure waves,
    comparison, 915t
  studies, 915
  SW-induced osteogenic
    stimulation, mechanisms,
    915-916
Shock wave (SW) generators,
    914-915
Shock wave therapy (shockwave
    therapy) (SWT), 341
  applications, 915-919
  complications, 918-919
  dose dependence, 915
  historical perspective, 914
Shoeing, 293-303, 338-339
  characteristics, 489
  convalescent therapy, 809
  deleterious effects, 302
  impact, 280, 301-302
  performance impact, 302
  practice, 301-303
  role, 489
  technique, 382f
Shoes
  wear, excess, 510
Shoe type
  impact, 280
  pattern/size, assessment, 45
Short format Three Day Event,
    1123
Short lateral CLs, enthesopathy,
    523-524

Short sesamoidean avulsions
    (osteochondral fragments),
    400-401
  clinical signs, 400-401
  diagnosis, 401
  treatment, 401
Short tau inversion recovery (STIR)
  image sequences, 484-485
  MR image, 335f
  sequences, 938
Shoulder, 53
  anatomical considerations,
    456-457
  clinical signs, 457
  diagnosis, 457-458
  differential diagnosis, 460-474
  fractures, rarity, 965
  imaging, 458-460
  instability, 473-474
    prognosis, 474
  intraarticular analgesia, 457
    false-negative results, 458
  lameness, 53
    diagnosis, 124
  local analgesia, 457-458
  nuclear scintigraphy, 458-460
  phase images, problems, 224
  racing injuries, 965
  radiography, 458
    importance, 458
  slip, 457, 473
  ultrasonography, 458
Shoulder angle
  factors, 21
  measurement, 20f
Shoulder joint (scapulohumeral
    joint), 121-122
  inverse/simultaneous
    movement, 83-84
Shoulder length, 20
  measurement, 20f
Shoulder region
  lameness, limb flight, 75
  lameness severity, 40
  lateral scintigraphic image, 147f
  lateral view, 122f
  lesions, 472
Show horses
  body weight, 1189
  fetlock joint conditions, 1193
  gaits, complexity, 1188-1189
  high heel, shodding, 1192
  longevity, 1189
  speed, performance, 1189
Show hunters
  ALDDFT, desmitis, 1111
  aseptic preparation, 1099
  back pain, 1106-1107
  cervical osteoarthritis, pain
    (relationship), 1111-1112
  clinical examination, 1103
  conformation, lameness
    (relationship), 1098
  cranial cruciate ligament, 1108
  croup, 1109-1110
  diagnosis, failure, 1099
  distal hock joint pain,
    1103-1104
    treatment, variation, 1104
  distal interphalangeal joint
    collateral ligament injury,
    1103
  synovitis, 1102-1103
  feet
    pain, 1100-1103
    soreness, 1100
  fetlock joint, 1107-1108

Show hunters (*Continued*)
  high level outdoor
    competitions, 1097
  hip region pain, 1109-1110
  imaging considerations, 1099
  lameness
    causes, diagnosis/
      management, 1100-1112
    examination, 1098-1099
    historical perspective, 1096
    problems, 1100
  management, therapeutic goals,
    1110-1111
  medical management, 1102
  meniscal injury, 1108
  muscle injury/pain, 1106
  navicular disease, 1101-1102
  nuclear scintigraphy, 1103
  osteoarthritis, 1102-1103,
    1107-1108
  over-at-the-knee conformation,
    1098
  pastern, 1109
  proximal/distal limb flexion
    tests, 1099
  radiographic examination, 1107
  SDFT, 1110-1111
    injury, 1110
  sesamoiditis, 1107-1108
  sheared heel, 1102
  shoeing considerations, 1098
  soft tissue injury, 1109
  spinous processes,
    impingement, 1106
  sport, structure, 1096-1097
  stifle joint pain, 1108-1109
  subchondral bone cysts, 1108
  subsolar bruising, 1100-1101
  suspensory desmitis, 1104-1106
  suspensory ligament
    injury, 1104-1105
    ultrasonographic
      examination, 1105
  synovitis, 1107
  third metacarpal/metatarsal
    bone, proximal aspect
    (radiographic examination),
    1105
  toe-in/toe-out forelimb
    conformation, 1098
  training, 1097
    competition surfaces,
      relationship, 1097-1098
  treatment, 1099-1100
  trimming/shoeing, 1101-1102
  withers fracture, 1106
Show jumpers
  acute-onset left forelimb
    lameness, images, 358f
  ALDDFT, desmitis, 1111
  aseptic preparation, 1099
  back pain, 1106-1107
  cervical osteoarthritis, pain
    (relationship), 1111-1112
  clinical examination, 1103
  conformation, lameness
    (relationship), 1098
  cranial cruciate ligament, 1108
  croup, 1109-1110
  diagnosis
    causes, diagnosis/
      management, 1100-1112
    failure, 1099
  DIP, lateral collateral ligament
    (transverse/longitudinal/
    ultrasonographic images),
    356f

Show jumpers (Continued)
distal hock joint pain,
1103-1104
treatment, variation, 1104
distal interphalangeal joint
collateral ligament injury,
1103
synovitis, 1102-1103
feet
pain, 1100-1103
soreness, 1100
fetlock joint, 1107-1108
flexed DIP, dorsolateral-
palmaromedial oblique
view, 353f
front feet, dorsal nuclear
scintigraphic image, 354f
high level outdoor
competitions, 1097
hip region pain, 1109-1110
imaging considerations, 1099
lameness
examination, 1098-1099
historical perspective, 1096
problems, 1100
left forelimb lameness,
midmetacarpal
region (transverse
ultrasonographic image),
751f
left front foot, solar/palmar
bone phase scintigraphic
image, 347f
management
success, 752-753
therapeutic goals, 1110-1111
mare (performance problem),
pelvic region (dorsal
scintigraphic image), 826f
medical management, 1102
meniscal injury, 1108
metacarpal region, proximal
injuries, 725
muscle injury/pain, 1106
navicular disease, 1101-1102
nuclear scintigraphy, 1103
origins, 1096
osteoarthritis, 1102-1103,
1107-1108
over-at-the-knee conformation,
1098
pastern, 1109
performance loss, lumbosacral
joint (ultrasonographic
image), 579f
proximal/distal limb flexion
tests, 1099
proximal metatarsal region,
transverse T2 gradient echo
low-field magnetic
resonance image, 748f
radiographic examination, 1107
right elbow, mediolateral
radiographic view, 462f
right hindlimb, proximal
suspensory desmitis, 744f
SDFT, 1110-1111
injury, 1110
sesamoiditis, 1107-1108
sheared heel, 1102
shoeing considerations, 1098
soft tissue injury, 1109
spinous processes,
impingement, 1106
sport, structure, 1096-1097
stifle joint pain, 1108-1109
subchondral bone cysts, 1108

Show jumpers (Continued)
subsolar bruising, 1100-1101
superficial digital flexor
tendonitis, 721-726
manifestations, 724-725
suspensory desmitis, 1104-1106
suspensory ligament
injury, 1104-1105
ultrasonographic
examination, 1105
synovitis, 1107
third metacarpal/metatarsal
bone, proximal aspect
(radiographic examination),
1105
toe-in/toe-out forelimb
conformation, 1098
training, 1097
competition surfaces,
relationship, 1097-1098
treatment, 1099-1100
trimming/shoeing, 1101-1102
withers fracture, 1106
Show pony, neck pain, 616f
Sickle-hock conformation, 507
Sickle-hocked conformation, 29f,
792, 979
commonness, 29-30
Sickle-hocked knee, 15-16
Sidebones, 1025
clinical relevance, 1080
Signaling peptides, role, 624-625
Signalment, 9-11
Simple acute luxation, 468-469
Simple base-wide conformation,
22f
Single abscess cavity,
development, 612
Single-foot gait, 1187
Single photon emission CT
(SPECT), 218
Single studs, palmar view, 1132f
Sinkers, 366-367
Sixth cervical vertebrae,
subluxation, 610
Skeletal muscle, 212-213
appearance, 212
damage, 233-234
necrosis, identification, 818
relaxants, systemic use, 1169
Skin
aseptic preparation, 605
markers, usage, 16-17
preparation, inadequacy,
170-171
schematic drawing, 882f
sensation, assessment, 607
surface contact, 173
Skyline view, 429
Slab fracture, 176, 440-444
term, usage, 440
Sleeves, concept, 860f
Sleipner Varg, 1076
Slings, improvement, 878
Slow gait, 1189-1190
Small-amplitude vibration, 276
Small fragments, 434-439
Small splits, observation, 815
Sodium technetium pertechnetate,
injection/mixing, 216
Soft surfaces, 77
gait, 66
Soft tissue
diseases, 691-692
injuries, 10, 161-162, 392
impact, 41-42
lesions, 148-149

Soft tissue (Continued)
racing injuries, 966
remodeling, 903
repair
inflammatory phase, 903
proliferation, 903
ultrasound application, 903
structures, injuries, 163
swelling, 816
cellulitis, impact, 37f
subcutaneous bleeding, 36f
thickening, 600
Solar bruising, 310-311
clinical signs, 311
history/etiology, 310-311
prognosis, 311
treatment, 311
Sole
bruises, occurrence, 1143
bruising, occurrence, 310-311
callus, difference, 305
pads, covering, 298
penetrating injuries, 314-316
surface, preparation, 305
Sole, deep penetrating injuries,
314-315
clinical signs, 314-315
diagnosis, 315
history, 314-315
treatment, 315
Solid brass cryoprobes, usage,
870f
Solitary bone islands, 464-465
Solitary osteochondroma, 727,
779
Solitary tibial nerve injury, rarity,
42
Somatic dysfunction
(confirmation),
thermographic examination
(usage), 911
Somatovisceral dysfunction,
890-891
Somebeachsomewhere (pacing
colt), 1014f
Sore hocks, commonness, 1013
Sore shins, 502
racehorse problem, 1011
Sound
attenuation, 169
usage, 72-73
waves, longitudinal waves, 901
Spavin
term, usage, 59
test, 84-85, 513
Specialized structures, 92-94
Speckle reduction software, 171
Speed, function, 276
Speedy cutting, 74-75
Spinal cord
diseases, 144
migrating parasites, impact,
144
dorsolateral compression,
asymmetrical ataxia/pain,
650
Spinal processes, ligaments
(association), 598-600
Spinal reflex, channel pain
mediation, 890f
Spinous processes
commonness, 896
contact/modeling
(demonstration),
ultrasonographic
examination (usage), 599
divergence, 592

Spinous processes (Continued)
fractures, 600
impingement
clinical significance
assessment, location
anesthetic solution
(diagnostic infiltration),
596
grading, 598
treatment, 1106
overriding, 599
Splint bones
disease, 1159-1160
proximal aspect, fractures, 1163
Splint exostoses (splints), 870
Splinting, 860-861
Splints, 134, 1012
analgesia, 134
availability, 861
exostoses, 504-505
lameness, association, 505
management, 505
removal, 787
usage, 860-861
Spondylosis, 173
Spongialization, 850
Spongiosa
flexor cortex, demarcation,
333
trabecular architecture, 333
Sporadic exertional
rhabdomyolysis, 824-825
clinical signs, 824
Sporadic lameness, 149-151
Sports horses
clinical assessment, 922-924
clinical problems, types,
921b-922b
questions, 920
Sports horses, lumbosacral/pelvic
injuries
analgesic techniques, 573
anatomical considerations, 571
aortoiliacofemoral thrombosis,
579-580
clinical examination, 572-573
clinical signs, 571-573
coxofemoral joint, 581-582
diagnostic imaging, 573-574
differential diagnosis, 574-582
dorsal sacroiliac ligament,
desmitis, 578
equine rhabdomyolysis (tying
up), 575-576
femur, third trochanter
(fracture/enthesopathy),
582
fractures, 574-575
history, 571-572
lumbosacral joint, 579
muscle injury, 576-577
nuclear scintigraphy, 574
radiography, 573
sacroiliac joint injury, 577-578
sacrum wing, new bone (caudal
aspect), 578-579
serum muscle enzyme
concentration, 573
ultrasonography, 573-574
Spruce Meadows, 1096f
Stabbing, 75-76
Stabby hindlimb gait, 75-76
Stable bandages, 858
application, 1134
usage, 858
Stable rest, 576
Stakes races, 979

Stall
confinement, 451-452
rest, 528, 878
Stamped shoe (punched shoe),
294
Stance phase (contact phase),
283
definition, 271b
Standardbred (STB)
abnormalities, detection,
435-436
carpal lameness development,
back-at-the-knee
conformation
(relationship), 434
curb, development, 1041
European racetracks, 1036
foals
osteochondrosis, 621
preoperative/postoperative
craniocaudal radiographic
views, 530f
hind fetlock, dorsoproximal 45°
medial-plantarodistolateral
oblique radiographic image,
1041f
hindlimb lameness (likelihood),
4
in-at-the-hock conformation,
30f
left gluteal atrophy, 35f
male, proximal metacarpal
region, dorsolateral-
palmaromedial oblique
xeroradiographic view,
397f
mare, right front SDFT
(transverse/longitudinal
ultrasonographic images),
717f
offset knees, 23-24
prominence, 24f
pacing filly, lateral/plantar
scintigraphic images, 512f
siblings, lameness conditions,
16
sickle-hocked conformation,
curb (development), 29f
stallion
left metatarsophalangeal
joint, plantar aspect
(intraoperative
arthroscopic images),
258f
pacer, lameness
(intraoperative
photograph), 720f
stress-related bone injury, right
carpus (lateral/dorsal
delayed phase scintigraphic
images), 231f
subchondral lucency, dorsal
30° proximal 45° lateral
plantar distal medial
oblique radiographic image,
937f
tarsocrural joint, OC
(radiological finding),
635
third carpal bone
frontal slab fracture,
442-443
subchondral lucency, 444
third carpal bones (focal intense
IRU), carpal region (dorsal
delayed scintigraphic
image), 943f

Standardbred (Continued)
third metacarpal bone,
geometric properties, 953
toe out behind, 30
in vitro fatigue data, 954f
weanling (right radius),
osseous cystlike lesion
(craniocaudal digital
radiographic view),
454f
Standardbred (STB) colt
carpal bones, dorsoproximal-
dorsodistal (skyline)
radiographic view, 438f
dorsopalmar xeroradiograph,
25f
hock, dorsal 20° lateral-
plantaromedial oblique
radiographic image,
1042f
left carpus, dorsal 45°
lateral-palmaromedial
oblique radiographic view,
431f
metatarsophalangeal joint,
dorsolateral-plantaromedial
oblique radiographic view,
391f, 1045f
pacer, images, 1034f
right middle carpal joint,
intraoperative arthroscopic
images, 257f
Standardbred (STB) filly
carpal bones, right distal row
(dorsoproximal-dorsodistal
digital radiographic image),
1027f
maladaptive subchondral bone
remodeling, dorsal 45°
lateral-plantaromedial
oblique digital radiographic
view, 483f
right tarsus, lateromedial
digital radiographic view,
519f
straight hindlimb
conformation/suspensory
desmitis, 29f
Standardbred (STB) gelding
hock, plantar aspect (transverse
midline ultrasonographic
image), 795f
left front SDFT (tendonitis), left
metacarpal region
(photograph), 709f
proximal lateral tibial epiphysis,
multioculated osseous
cystlike lesion/sclerosis
(lateromedial/caudocranial
digital radiographic view),
531f
Standardbred (STB) pacer
flow/pool phase images,
226f
left/right hindlimb, transverse
plantarolateral
ultrasonographic images,
796f
right hindlimb lameness, lateral
delayed phase scintigraphic
image, 477f
swelling, development,
202-203
walk/pace, 66
Standardbred (STB) racehorse
ALSDFT transection, 716
benefit, 716

Standardbred (STB) racehorse
(Continued)
carpus, dorsolateral-
palmaromedial radiographic
view, 683f
curb, appearance, 792f
hindlimb
load comparison, 6f
PSD, 744
hock, plantar aspect (transverse/
longitudinal midline
ultrasonographic images),
796f
hock/proximal metatarsal
region, dorsomedial-
plantarolateral
xeroradiographic view,
504f
interference, risk, 74
lateral/caudal delayed phase
scintigraphic images, 532f
lateral sesamoiditis, flexed
lateral delayed (bone)
phase scintigraphic image,
485f
metatarsophalangeal joint
lameness source, 5
scintigraphic images, 484f
middle carpal joint,
arthroscopic
endophotograph, 662f
pace, 64
right metatarsophalangeal joint,
dorsal T2-weighted gradient
echo magnetic resonance
image, 940f
SDF tendonitis, 767
management, 798
suspensory desmitis/dropped
fetlock, 34f
Standardbred (STB) sales yearling,
932-934
conformation, 934
lameness, development
(relationship), 934
disputes, resolution, 933-934
radiographic examination, 934
radiographs, collection, 934
sale conditions, 933
sales, location/time, 932
veterinarian, role, 934
videotapes, availability, 934
Standardbred (STB) trotters
lateral/caudal delayed phase
images, 225f
medial femorotibial joint,
caudocranial digital
radiographic image, 1035f
plantar/flexed lateral delayed
(bone) phase scintigraphic
images, 486f
third metatarsal bone,
stress-related bone injury
(intraoperative
photograph), 488f
toed-out conformation, 18
Standardbred (STB) yearling, neck
pain, 40f
Standing horse
abaxial sesamoid block, usage,
111
cast application, 862
deep digital flexor tenotomy,
performing, 383f
Standoff pads, 173
Staphylococcus aureus, 524-525
Staphylococcus species, 677

Static balance/conformation,
284-285
Static examination, 1198
Static manipulation, 47-48
Static palpation, 86
Stationary force plate, usage,
246-247
Steel shoes, usage, 1132
Steeplechasers
breeding, 1064
bucked-knee conformation,
27-28
lameness
causes, 1070
diagnosis/management,
1070-1075
osteoarthritis, left coxofemoral
joint (ventrodorsal
radiographic view), 582f
superficial digital flexor
tendonitis, 1070-1072
Steeplechases, distance, 1063
Steer, header roping, 1171f
Stem cells, 852
products, usage, 761-763
research, evolution, 761
therapies, 761-763
future, 763
popularity, 1135
Stenotic effect, cause, 774
Stent bandages, 859
towels/gauze rolls, 859
Stepping gaits, injury, 1192
Sternal bone marrow aspirate,
collection, 762f
Sternal cartilage grafts, 676
Sternal grafts, reattachment,
852
Sternal injury, 155
Sternum, sagittal section, 762f
Steward clog, 382f
Stickers, 297
Stiff horse syndrome (stiff-horse
syndrome), 156, 561, 838
Stiff joints, movement
(restoration), 910
Stiffness, 156
definition, 271b
Stifle, 56-57, 208-209
anatomy, 532-533
articular diseases, 536-549
caudal 30° lateral-craniomedial
oblique view, 535
caudocranial radiographic view,
549f
caudocranial view, 535
collateral ligaments
longitudinal imaging,
535-536
origination, 533
concurrent injury/infection,
absence, 549
considerations, 533-534
cranial aspect, soft tissue
coverage, 162
cranioproximal-craniodistal
oblique view, 535
developmental anatomy,
532-533
diagnosis, 533-534
diagnostic analgesia, 534
femoropatellar joint, 208, 533
femorotibial joints, 533
femur, medial trochlear ridge,
533
flexed lateromedial view, 535
flexion, 509

Stifle *(Continued)*
  flexion test, 86
    usage, 86f
  gait tests, 534
  hemorrhage, likeliness, 549
  history, 533-534
  imaging considerations,
    534-536
  injuries, 162-163, 1215
  joint pain, 1108-1109
  lameness, 993
    condition, 534
  lateromedial radiographic view,
    539f
  lateromedial view, 535
  lesions, 638
  manipulative tests, 534
  medial/lateral femorotibial
    joints, 208-209
  ossification centers, 532-533
  palpation, 56
  patellar ligaments, longitudinal
    imaging, 535-536
  racing injuries, 965
  radiography, 534-535
  radiological changes, 534-535
  reciprocal apparatus, 533
    impact, 533
  region, hematoma, 549
    prognosis, 549
    signs/diagnosis, 549
    treatment, 549
  scintigraphy, 536
  trauma, commonness, 162
  ultrasonography, 535-536
    value, 535
  valgus stress test, 57f
Stifle joint, 130-131
  arthroscopic surgery, advances,
    848
  compartments, 130
    blocking, 147
  dorsal turbo spin echo MRI,
    1194f
  independent injection, 130
  inflammation, 890
  pain, source, 1035
Still, Andrew Taylor, 907
Stimulation intensity, 907
Stimuli, bone response (Wolff's
  law), 169-174
Stocking-up, 33
Stovepipe swelling, 33
Straight behind, 28
Straight-behind condition, 15-16,
  28
Straight hocks, 28
Straight sesamoidean desmitis,
  756-758, 815
  treatment, 758
Straight sesamoidean ligaments
  (SSLs)
  chronic injuries, 393
  desmitis, treatment, 815
  dorsal-to-palmar thickness,
    812
  injuries, occurrence, 815
  origin, 812
  splits/lesions, observation,
    815
Strain, definition, 271b
Strangulating colic, 372
Stratiform fibrocartilage, 94
  occurrence, 94
Streetnail, 316-317
  term, usage, 316
Streptococcus equi infection, 615

Streptococcus equi rhabdomyolysis,
  832
  clinical signs, 832
  diagnosis, 832
  treatment, 832
Streptococcus lutetiensis, 370
Streptococcus zooepidemicus,
  524-525
Stress
  definition, 271b
  maladaptive/nonadaptive
    remodeling, impact,
    1027-1028
  mechanical measure, 274
  pathology, 1142, 1144-1145
  reactions, 396-397, 399-400
Stress fractures, 163, 463, 471-472
  radiologic detection, 175
  scintigraphic identification, 555
  SWT management, 916
  term, usage, 935
Stress-induced bone injuries, 997
Stress radiographs, usefulness, 33
Stress-related bone injury,
  230-231
  management, 489-492
  radiological diagnosis, 941
  RU decrease, 217
  suspicion, 230
Stress-related cortical bone injury,
  9
  term, reference, 935
Stress-related injury, 13
Stress-related subchondral bone
  injury, 9, 488-492
Stress-strain curve, regions, 694
Stride
  breakover phase, 284
  caudal phase, 73-74
    contrast, 73-74
    lengthening, 73
    severe lameness, 356
  characteristics, 284
  cranial phase, 68, 73-74
    contrast, 73-74
    reduction, 74
    shortening, 73-74
  cycle, weight bearing
    characteristic, 4
  flight phase, 283-284
  frequency, 276
    definition, 271b
  impact phase, 283
  initial contact, 283
  length, 276
  phases, 283-284
  SDFT, preferential loading, 704
  shortness, 19f
  stance phase, 283
  support phase, 283-284
  time, definition, 271b
Stringhalt, 144, 524, 559-560
  biomechanical basis, 560
  cause, 560
  clinical characteristics, 559-560
  gait abnormality, 156
  recognition, 145
  shivers, comparison, 145
  surgical therapy, 560
  upward flexion, exaggeration,
    559-560
Stringhalt-type gait, 555
Strong blisters, creation, 867
Structures
  deformation
    ability, 273-274
    response, 273

Structures *(Continued)*
  force, application, 273
  properties, 273-274
    changes, 274
Stud Book of the Finnhorse,
  1076
Studs, 297
Stumbling, 562
Subcarpal block, 134
  usage, 1003
Subchondral bone, 656
  change (continuum),
    scintigraphic examination
    (usage), 230-231
  cysts, 1108
  drilling, 850
  initial lesion, 489-490
  maladaptive/nonadaptive
    stress-related bone injury,
    488
  microcracks, propagation,
    490
  modeling, 942
  opaque band, radiolucent
    zones, 467
  plate thickening, cartilage
    degeneration (cause-
    and-effect relationship),
    660
  stress reactions, 461
  stress-related bone injury,
    230-231
Subchondral bone cysts, 173-174,
  466-467
  cause, 541
  enlargement, 467
  relationship, 620
  term, usage, 631
Subchondral bone injury,
  398-399
  clinical examination, 936
  clinical signs, 398, 936
  computed tomography, 938
  CT images, 239f
  diagnosis, 398-399
  diagnostic analgesia, 936
  diagnostic imaging, 937-938
  locations, 398-399, 938-946
  nuclear scintigraphy, 937
  pathophysiology, 935-936
  radiography, 937
  radiological identification,
    difficulty, 1007
  surgical management, 491-492
  treatment, 399
  ultrasonography, 937-938
Subchondral bone pain, 13-14
  bisphosphonate therapy,
    490-491
  importance, 148
  occurrence, 146-147
Subchondral bone trauma, 354,
  399-400, 518, 545
  prognosis, 546
  signs/diagnosis, 545
  treatment, 545-546
  unilateral lameness,
    characterization, 354
Subchondral cystic lesions,
  541-542
  prognosis, 542
  signs/diagnosis, 541
  treatment, 541-542
    stable/pasture rest, 541-542
  triamcinolone acetonide
    injection, arthroscopic
    view, 849f

Subchondral drilling, cancellous
  bone plate access, 850
Subchondral lucency, dorsal
  30° proximal 45° lateral
  plantar distal medial
  oblique radiographic image,
  937f
Subchondral micropicking, 676
  microfracture, 851
Subchondral plate
  microfracture, 259
  organization, 656
Subchondral stress-related bone
  injury, pathological
  continuum, 936
Subclinical pain, multipattern
  acupoint abnormality,
  891
Subcutaneous abscess, 800
Subcutaneous fibrosis, palmar
  annular ligament
  enlargement, 773
Subjective information, objective
  information (contrast), 8-9
Subluxation, 177
Submerged treadmills (aquatreds),
  usage, 880
Subsolar abscess (gravel), 314,
  1101
  diagnosis, 314
  history/clinical signs, 314
  prognosis, 314
  suspicion, 859-860
  treatment, 314
    goal, 314
Subsolar bruising, 1100-1101
Subtarsal block, 134
  importance, 125-126
Success criteria, 8
Sucklings
  developmental orthopedic
    disease, 630
  Salter-Harris type II fractures,
    occurrence, 529
Suckling Standardbred foal,
  digital dorsal 15°
  lateral-plantaromedial
  oblique radiographic view,
  521f
Superficial digital flexor (SDF)
  tendonitis, 31, 83, 423, 507
  advancement, 990
  career impact, 720
  cellulitis, 424
  commonness, 43-44
  development, complication,
    717-718
  impact, 281
  induction, 279
  management program, 721
  occurrence, 706-715
  recognition, 990
  rest, importance, 798
  risk, conformation (impact),
    704
  surgical management, 715-721
  SWT impact, 917
Superficial digital flexor tendon
  (SDFT), 43-44
  accessory ligament
    cutting, 90-91
  desmitis, 454
  transection, 715-718
  acute-onset lesions, 161
  anatomy, 802
  cellulitis, 424, 1071-1072
  clinical signs, 424

Superficial digital flexor tendon
   (Continued)
   characteristic, 175
   clinical signs, 707-710
   corticosteroids, usage, 715
   DDFT, blood flow differences,
      697
   displacement, 163
   heat, impact, 708
   history/clinical signs, 805
   laceration, 89
   lameness, result, 708
   lateral dislocation (luxation),
      59f
   left front lateral branch,
      ultrasonographic images,
      814f
   lesions (management), ALSDFT
      desmotomy (success), 723
   loading
      factors, 704
      ground surface, impact, 704
   muscles, characteristics, 694
   musculotendonous junction,
      transverse T2 gradient echo
      images, 244f
   necrosis, 424, 1071-1072
      clinical signs, 420-421
   preferential loading, 704
   right front medial branch,
      ultrasonographic images,
      813f
   rupture, 161
   skin necrosis, 424
      clinical signs, 424
   subluxaton/luxation, 805-806
      anatomy, 805
      diagnosis, 805
      history/clinical signs, 805
      treatment, 805-806
   support, 61
   swelling, 708
   swelling, right front metacarpal
      region (photograph), 709f
   tendonitis, 776
   thermographic imaging, 268
   thickening, indication, 708
   transforming growth factor-β3,
      immunohistolochemical
      staining, 699f
   traumatic lacerations, 423
   treatment, 424
Superficial digital flexor tendon
   (SDFT) injuries, 706-707,
   812-814
   baseline evaluation, 711
   initial evaluation, 710-711
   musculotendonous junction
      site, 779
   occurrence, 707
   treatment, beta-
      aminopropionitrile
      fumarate (usage), 714f
   ultrasonographic evaluation/
      categorization, 710-711
Superficial fibular/saphenous
   nerves, distal continuation,
   499-500
Superficial intracortical
   debridement, 850
Superior check desmotomy, 715
Support, 300-301
   bandages, 1134
   concept, application, 300
   term, usage, 300
Supporting lameness, 67-69
Supporting limb lameness, 67

Supporting limb laminitis, 371
Support phase, 283-284
   extension, 283
Supraglenoid tubercle fracture,
   471
   diagnosis, 471
   examination, 68
   prognosis, 471
Suprascapular nerve
   damage, 473
   injury, 11-12
Supraspinatus ligament
   injuries, 599-600
   thickening, impact, 600
Supraspinatus muscles, atrophy,
   53f, 473
Supraspinous bursa, 799
   clinical signs, 799
   treatment, 799
Supraspinous desmitis,
   impingement (treatment),
   1106
Supraspinous desmopathy,
   transverse/median ultrasound,
   600f
Supraspinous ligament (lumbar
   area), median/transverse
   ultrasound scans, 600f
Surface, 13
   characteristics, 66, 278
   impact, 13
   sensitivity, adhesive
      (interaction), 306
Surface brachytherapy
   (plesiotherapy), 874
   efficacy, 876
   surface applicator, usage, 874
Surgical arthroscopy, diagnostic
   arthroscopy (division),
   254-255
Surgical incisions (covering), ether
   bandages (usage), 859
Surgical synovectomy, 876
Surgical trauma, events sequence,
   873
Surgical wounds, creation,
   858-859
Survey radiography, 140
Suspensory apparatus
   anatomy, 738-739
   computed tomography, 743
   diagnostic analgesic techniques,
      740
   diagnostic ultrasonography,
      741
   differential diagnosis, 740-741
   distal sesamoidean ligaments,
      importance, 967
   extracorporeal shock wave
      treatment, 744
   magnetic resonance imaging,
      743
   nuclear scintigraphy, 742-743
   pathophysiology, 738-739
   radial pressure wave therapy,
      744
   radiography/radiology, 741-742
   traumatic disruption, 760,
      969-972
   complications, 971
   first aid, 970
   history/clinical presentation,
      969
   lateromedial radiographic
      view, 970f
   long-term complication, 971
   long-term splinting, 971

Suspensory apparatus *(Continued)*
   nonsurgical management,
      970-971
   nonsurgical management
      decisions, 971
   surgical management,
      971-972
   treatment, 743-744
   ultrasonographic abnormality,
      741
Suspensory apparatus of the distal
   phalanx (SADP), 374
Suspensory branches, appraisal,
   998
Suspensory desmitis, 29f, 498,
   506-507
   body lesions, 749-750
   branch lesions, 751-754
   clinical signs, 749, 751
   dependence, 751
   cryotherapy, 871
   diagnosis, 749-752
      basis, 749
   lameness observation,
      1005-1006
   management, 750, 752-754
   McII/McIV, radiographic
      examination, 750
   progress, monitoring, 750
   SWT, effects, 917
   treatment, 750, 752
   ultrasonographic abnormalities,
      749, 751-752
   ultrasonographic examination,
      1032
Suspensory ligament (SL)
   accessory ligament, extension,
      510
   branches, examination, 175
   distal sesamoidean ligaments,
      functional continuation,
      739
   front foot lameness, 67
   function, 739
   injury, predilection site, 1006
   medial/lateral branch, desmitis,
      422
   medial/lateral palmar digital
      vein/artery/nerve, location,
      50
   origin, 44, 134
      third metacarpal/metatarsal
         bone, avulsion fractures,
         749
   progressive atraumatic
      breakdown, 760
   proximal aspect, 82
      deep palpation, 62f
      examination, 998-999
      ultrasonographic appearance,
         987-988
   racing injuries, 967
   surgical splitting, usage, 744
   third interosseous muscle, term
      (usage), 738
   total collapse, 204
Suspensory ligament (SL) body
   desmitis, 422
   echogenicity, uniformity
      (absence), 749
   surgical splitting, 750
Sussmare-Raszynski intraosseous
   infusion needle, 1251f
Sustentaculum tali
   lesions, 525
   osteitis, 525
   plantaromedial aspect, 525

Swedging, 295-296
Sweeny nerve injury, 11-12
Swelling, 33
   clinical evidence, 204
   impact, 33
Swimming, 880
   pools, usage, 880
Swinging lameness, 67-69
Swinging limb lameness, 67-68
   comparison, 68
Swing phase
   parameters, association, 248
   protraction, definition, 271b
Swollen limbs
   clinical examination, 165-166
      results, 166
   diagnosis, 164-166
   history, 165
   management, 166-167
Sympathectomy, 342
Symphysis, 94
Synchronous diaphragmatic
   flutter (thumps), 1148-1149
Syndesmopathy, 419
Syndromes, examination, 141-145
Synovectomy, usage (recognition),
   848
Synovial bursae, 93
   function/structure, 92
Synovial cell sarcomas,
   identification, 693
Synovial chondromatosis, 693
Synovial facet joints, unilateral/
   bilateral modeling, 612
Synovial fistula, 692
   communication, 692
Synovial fluid, 244, 655
   bone formation biomarkers,
      948t
   changes, 665
   cytological studies, 315
   gross evaluation, 678
   laboratory analysis, 429
   lubrication, 688
   MRI, usage, 244
   nucleated cells, distribution,
      679
Synovial fluid cytology, clinical
   conditions/diagnostic/
   therapeutic manipulations,
   666t
Synovial ganglion, 448
Synovial hernia, 692
Synovial intervertebral
   articulations, 592-593,
   600-602
   anatomical specimen, 593f
   arthropathies (treatment),
      ultrasound-guided
      periarticular injection
      (transverse ultrasound
      scan), 604f
   lesions, 602
   radiological appearance,
      600f-601f
   transverse ultrasound scans,
      601f, 603f
Synovial intima, synoviocytes
   (presence), 655
Synovial joints, 271-272
Synovial pad, osteochondral
   fragments, 397
Synovial sheath, 93
Synovial structures, 92-93
Synovitis, 395-396
   occurrence, 690
   presence, 349-350, 689

Synovium, 244, 655
  gene transfer, schematic
    drawing, 671f
  MRI, usage, 244
  role, 661
  vascular connective tissue, 655
Synthetic all-weather track
    surface, differences, 995
Synthetic racing surfaces, shoeing
    (debate), 984
Syringe adapter attachment, 855f

T

Tack, 1115
  considerations, 1132
  observation, 982
Tack-induced pain, 156-157
Tail position, abnormality, 41
Takt (rhythm), 1112
Talocalcaneal-centroquartal joint
    (proximal intertarsal joint),
    fragments, 518
Talocalcaneal joint, osteoarthritis,
    516
  occurrence, 516
  tarsus, lateromedial
    radiographic view, 517f
Talus
  full-thickness cartilage erosion,
    638f
  incomplete sagittal fractures,
    520
  lateral trochlear ridge, distal
    aspect (lesions), 635
  medial trochlear ridge, surface
    depressions, 636-637
  sagittal fracture, 520
  rarity, 520, 1030
Tapered sleeve pin ESFD (TSP
    ESFD), 865f
  application, abbreviated
    instructions, 865-866
  availability, 865
  usage, 866f
Tarsal angles, evaluation, 29-30
Tarsal arthrocentesis, 128f
Tarsal bone fractures/luxations,
    518-523
  diagnosis, 519
  double plating techniques,
    522-523
  suspicion, 519
  treatment, 520
Tarsal bones
  incomplete ossification,
    lateromedial radiographic
    view, 645f
  osteitis, uncommonness,
    524-525
Tarsal groove, smoothing, 525
Tarsal injuries, 524-526
Tarsal joint capsule, fibrous part,
    509
Tarsal joint luxation, 522-523
Tarsal lameness, 1029-1032
Tarsal region, deep digital flexor
    tendon lesions, 733
Tarsal region pain
  passive flexion problem, 510
  upper limb flexion test
    response, 511
Tarsal sheath, 133, 262-265
  anatomy, 262-263
  characteristics, 780-781
  distention, 781f
  effusion, 59
  enclosure, 781

Tarsal sheath (Continued)
  functional anatomy, 780-781
  hemangiosarcoma, occurrence,
    693
  surgical technique, 262-263
  suspententaculum tali,
    tenoscopic views, 784f
  synovial sheath, similarity, 780
  tenoscopic views, 263f
  transverse ultrasonographic
    image, 783f
Tarsal sheath injuries
  clinical signs, 782
  diagnosis, 782-783
  radiographic examination, 782
  radiography, 782
  tenoscopy, 783
  tenovaginocentesis, 783
  ultrasonography, 783
Tarsal tenosynovitis
  causes, 781-782
  management, 783-785
  prognosis, 785
Tarsal valgus, angular deformity,
    31
Tarsocrural effusion, 59f, 1225
Tarsocrural joint, 129-130
  antimicrobial drug (delivery),
    regional limb perfusion
    (usage), 681f
  communication, 518
  lameness, 1192
    rarity, 1030
  lateral collateral ligaments,
    enthesopathy, 523-524
  long lateral collateral ligament,
    enthesitis, 1030-1031
  osteoarthritis, 516-517, 1047
    occurrence, 516-517
  osteochondrosis, 518, 635-638
    site, 1021
Tarsocrural joint capsule
  distention, 517-518
  treatment, 518
  ultrasonography, 518
Tarsocrural joint OCD, 846
Tarsocrural OA, occurrence, 1030
Tarsometatarsal (TMT) joint,
    128-129, 1134
  analgesia, 1003
  arthrocentesis, 128
  centrodistal joint,
    communication, 509
  complete luxation/subluxation,
    occurrence, 522-523
  impact, 513
  intraarticular analgesia, 745
  metatarsal region, border, 499
  osteoarthritis, 1120-1121
  pain, association, 1013
  positive contrast, 126f
  transverse ultrasonographic
    image, 746f
  value, 1191
Tarsus, 58-60, 128-130
  analgesia, 127
  anatomical considerations,
    508-511
  articular diseases, 512-518
    clinical signs, 513
    corticosteroid injections,
      repetition, 516
    diagnostic analgesia, 513-514
    history, 513
    nuclear scintigraphy, 515
    radiography/radiology,
      514-515

Tarsus (Continued)
  systemic medication, PSGAG
    (usage), 515
  treatment, 515-516
  treatment options, 515
  triamcinolone acetonide,
    usage, 515-516
  biomechanical studies, 508-509
  clinical signs, 510-511
  collateral ligament damage, 523
  components, 508
  congenital deformations,
    525-526
  corticosteroids (intraarticular
    medication), 515
  diagnosis, 510-511
  diagnostic analgesia, 511
  diagnostic imaging, 511-512
  dorsoplantar images, usage, 512
  dorsoplantar radiographic view,
    522f
  flexed lateromedial radiographic
    view, 521f
  intraarticular analgesia, 514
  lateral scintigraphic image,
    153f
  lateromedial radiographic view,
    517f
  lesions, absence, 512
  nuclear scintigraphy, 512
  palpation, 58
  periarticular osteophyte
    formation, dorsolateral-
    plantaromedial oblique
    radiographic view, 514f
  plantar aspect, 794f
    applied anatomy/
      ultrasonographic
      examination, 793-794
  plantar 25° lateral-dorsomedial
    oblique radiographic view,
    519f
  racing injuries, 965
  radiographic views, 511-512
  soft tissue injury, 523-524
  swelling, 510
  ultrasonographic zone
    designations, 196f
  valgus deformity, dorsoplantar
    radiographic view, 644f
Tarsus, lateral scintigraphic image,
    153f
Tarsus valgus
  conformation, 30f
  deformities, 645
Team roping
  categories, 1170
  conformation, 1171
  historical data, 1171
Team roping horses, 1170-1175
  lameness
    diagnosis/management,
      1172-1175
    examination, 1172
  ligament/tendon injury,
    occurrence, 1173
  musculoskeletal examination,
    1173
  palmar foot pain, 1172-1175
    diagnosis, 1173
  performance, decrease, 1171
  problems, 1172
  sport, description, 1170-1171
  training, 1171
Technetium hydroxymethylene
    diphosphonate (Tc-HDP), 216
  binding mechanism, 216

Technetium-99m
  half-life, shortness, 217
  usage, 216
Technetium methylene
    diphosphonate (Tc-MDP),
    216
  accumulation, 216-217
  binding
    importance, 217
    sites/stage, importance, 217
Technetium-99m-methylene
    diphosphonate (MDP),
    muscle absorption, 819
Teletherapy, 873-874
Temperament, 65-66, 157
Temporary lameness, occurrence,
    12-13
Temporomandibular joint pain,
    155
Tendon growth
  adaptive response/injury risk,
    schematic representation,
    703f
  cellular activity, confirmation,
    702-703
  loading/exercise sensitivity, 703
Tendon injury, 812-816
  acute phase, management, 710
  corticosteroids, usage, 715
  diagram, 806f
  exercise, control, 713-714
  graded exercise program, basis,
    713
  hyaluronan, intralesional/
    perilesional administration,
    714-715
  intralesional
    β-aminopropionitrile
    fumarate, 714
  limitation, 710
  long-term rehabilitation,
    713-714
  long-term treatment
    programs, 713-715
    proposal, 715
  mechanisms, 701-703
  physical therapies, 715
  polysulfated glycosaminoglycan
    (PSGAG), intralesional/
    systemic administration,
    715
  response, direct digital
    palpation, 708
  secondary palmar annular
    ligament thickening,
    inclusion, 773
    treatment/prognosis, 773-774
  severity (increase), racing return
    (difficulty), 711f
  surgical procedures,
    combination, 720-721
  training, absence, 713
  treatment, 721
  types, 700-701
  in vivo studies, 916-917
Tendonitis
  cryotherapy, 872
  prevention, strategies, 705f
  recurrence, severity, 966-967
Tendon lacerations
  convalescent therapy, 809-810
  diagnosis, 806-808
  emergency management, 808
  medical management, 808
  prognosis, 810
  shock, treatment, 808
  surgical treatment, 808-809

Tendon lacerations (Continued)
  systemic/local medications, usage, 808
  ultrasonographic evaluation, 807-808
Tendons, 243-244
  acute inflammatory phase, 705
  aging, effect, 701-703
  anatomical structure, 696-706
  associated structures, 696-699
  biomechanical parameters, 694
  biomechanical properties, 694-695
  blood flow, complexity, 703-704
  blood flow, increase
    exercise, induction, 697
    injury, impact, 697
  blood supply, 696-697
    laser Doppler flowmetry, usage, 704
    source, 696
  cells, reliance, 704
  cellular components, 697-699
  characterization, parameters (usage), 189b
  chronic remodeling phase, 706
  classification, 695-696
  clinical injury, risk factors, 705
  collagen, 699
  damage, 800
  degeneration, mechanisms, 703-704
  disease, prevention (strategies), 704-705
  dry weight, percentage, 699
  enthesophyte formation, 172-173
  exercise, effect, 701-703
  exercise-induced hyperthermia, 703
  force, palmar digital analgesia, 280-281
  function, relationship, 695-696
  functional anatomy, 694
  functional characteristics, 694-696
  healing, pathological conditions/phases, 705-706
  histological features, 698f
  hysteresis, 695
    loop, 696f
  infection, 423-424
    clinical signs, 423
    diagnosis, 423
    treatment, 424
  intrinsic/extrinsic injury, 700-701
  locomotion, 278
  material properties, 695
  matrix, molecular composition, 699-700
  mechanical influences, 703
  molecular composition, changes (occurrence), 702
  morphology, 696
  MRI, usage, 243-244
  nutrients, collection, 696
  pain, palpation, 990
  physical influence, 703
  profile, 708-709
  proteolytic enzymes, 704
  rehabilitation, 168
  reinjury, commonness, 706
  splitting, 720, 1154
  stability, ultrasonographic evaluation, 712-713
  stiffness, 694

Tendons (Continued)
  strain, 279
    measurement, 278
    stress-strain curve
      regions, 694
      simplification, 695f
    structural properties, 694
    subacute reparative phase, 705-706
    SW application, 916-917
    tensile strain, 695
    tensile stress, 695
    transverse images, CSA measurements, 173-174
    vascular theories, 703-704
Tendon sheaths, 265, 456
  analgesia, 122-124, 133
  function/structure, 92
  lacerations, 809
  wound debridement, 789-790
Tennessee Walking Horse, 1186
  stoicism, 1187
Tennessee Walking Horse Breeders' and Exhibitors' Association, 1186
Tenocyte metabolism, regulation, 699
Tenoplasty (tendon splitting), 720
Tenoscopy, 260-262
  advantages, 260
  equipment, 260
  postoperative care, 262
  principles, 260
  surgical principles, 260
  surgical techniques, 260-262
Tenosynovitis, 788-791
  induction, 781
  ultrasonographic examination, 767-768
Tenotomy
  rationale, 383
  repetition, 383
Tensile strain, 695
Tensile stress, 695
Tension, 92
Teres ligament, rupture, 582
Terminal aorta, longitudinal ultrasonographic images, 581f
Tetanus toxoid, administration, 808
Tevis Cup, 1137
Therapeutic ultrasound, 901-903
  applications, 903
  waves, 901
Therapy responses, monitoring, 952
Thermal imaging systems, availability, 266
Thermal print storage envelope, 168
Thermographic evaluation, helpfulness, 924
Thermographic examination, value, 911
Thermographic pattern, observation, 911
Thermographs, appearance, 912f
Thermography
  camera focus, 267
  clinical imaging, 267-269
  evaluation, usefulness, 268
  image acquisition, 266-267
  imaging, performing, 266-267
  sensitivity, 267-268
  usage, 90, 590
Thermoplastic adhesives, 307

Thickening, clinical evidence, 204
Thick-skinned cob-type horses, navicular bursa (surgical access), 317
Thigh, 56
  gluteal syndrome, 550-552
  injuries, 555
  swelling, assessment, 56
Third carpal bone
  avulsion fracture, 447
  frontal slab fractures, 440-443
    lameness, 441
    management, 441-442
  intermediate fossa, displaced frontal slab fracture (dorsal 45° medial-palmarolateral oblique digital radiographic view), 441f
  L-shaped fracture, 442f
  nonadaptive remodeling, 987-988
  radial facet, stress-related bone injury (lateral/dorsal delayed phase scintigraphic images), 231f
  radial fossa, displaced frontal slab fracture (standing lateromedial digital radiographic view), 440f
  sagittal slab fractures, 443
    management, 443
    radial fossa, medial aspect (involvement), 443
    skyline radiographic views, 443f
  sclerosis
    confinement, 1009
    development, 988
    severity, 1008-1009
  small osteochondral fragment, dorsolateral-palmaromedial oblique xeroradiographic/skyline radiographic views, 436f
  subchondral injury, 942-943
  subchondral lucency, 444-445
    carpal lameness, prodromal clinical signs, 444
    prognosis, 444-445
    surgical debridement, 444
Third interosseous muscle
  term, usage, 738
Third interosseous muscle, proximal aspect (attachment), 394
Third lumbar vertebra, caudal articular process (bone specimen), 602f
Third metacarpal bone (McIII)
  avulsion fracture, 83
  clinical signs, 400
  diagnosis, 400-401
  suspensory ligament, origin, 400
  treatment, 400-401
  bucked/sore shins, 396
  clinical signs, 397
  condylar fractures, 1029
  condyles
    stress reactions, 399-400
    subchondral bone pain, 146-147
    weight-bearing surface, osseous cystlike lesions (occurrence), 632-633

Third metacarpal bone (Continued)
  consideration, 20
  contrast, 65
  diagnosis, 397-398
  diagnostic ultrasonography, 399
  distal aspect, 48-49
    fetlock lameness, 1006-1008
    frontal plane microradiograph, 488f
    lateral condyle, displaced fracture (arthroscopic view), 849f
    subchondral bone changes, 939
    subchondral bone injuries, 1006-1008
  distal condyles, fractures, 1013
  distal palmar aspect repetitive stress injury (scintigraphic appearance), 399f
  distal plantarolateral aspect, intraoperative photograph, 488f
  distal sagittal ridge osteochondritis dissecans, 632f
  dorsal aspect
    assessment, 50
    fracture, 1011
    pressure, application, 44
  dorsal cortex, 86
    diffuse IRU, 941
    periostitis, 1011
    stress-related bone injury, 940
  dorsal cortical fracture, 964
  dorsolateral-palmaromedial oblique radiographic view, 953f
  dorsomedial articular fractures, 398
    clinical signs, 398-399
    diagnosis, 399
    treatment, 399-402
  fourth metacarpal bone, syndesmopathy, 419
  fractures, 83, 408-409
    management, 503
  geometric properties, 953
  incomplete longitudinal palmar cortical fatigue fractures, 396-397
  lateral condylar fractures, 396
  local fatigue failure, in vitro comparison, 953-954
  medial condylar fractures, 396
  microradiographs, fifty-percent length cross-sections, 955f
  nondisplaced axial fracture, displaced lateral condylar fracture, 407f
  osseous cystlike lesions, 409-410
  periostitis (bucked skins), 871
  plantarolateral focal increased radiopharmaceutical uptake, postmortem specimen, 1007f
  proximal aspect, dorsomedial articular fracture, 447
  proximal dorsal aspect, palpation, 50-51
  proximal palmar aspect, stress pathology, 1142
  proximal palmar cortex, incomplete longitudinal fracture, 447

Third metacarpal bone (Continued)
  proximal phalanx, fractures, 1013
  racing injuries, 964
  right distal aspect, physitis, 639f
  sagittal ridge
    osteochondritis dissecans, 632
    osteochondrosis, 409
  saucer (dorsal cortical) fractures, 396
  second metacarpal bone, syndesmopathy, 419
  shape/architecture, establishment, 958
  stiffness measurements, 954
  stress fractures
    postoperative treatment, 960
    prognosis, 960
    surgical management, 959-960
    surgical procedure, 959-960
  stress reactions, 396-397
  in vitro fatigue study, 957
Third metacarpal region, distal metaphyseal region (transverse stress fractures), 397
  clinical signs, 397-398
  diagnosis, 398
  nuclear scintigraphy, 401
  treatment, 398-399
Third metatarsal bone (MtIII)
  avulsion fractures
    focal triangular increased radiopharmaceutical uptake, delayed (bone) phase lateral scintigraphic image, 504f
    suspensory ligament origin, 503
  bucked/sore shins, 502
  comminuted fractures, 502-503
  condylar fractures, 1029
  condyles (weight-bearing surface), osseous cystlike lesions (occurrence), 632-633
  diaphyseal fractures, 502-503
  distal aspect
    fetlock lameness, 1006-1008
    fractures, 496
      condylar fractures, 496
    subchondral bone changes, 939
    subchondral bone injuries, 1006-1008
    transverse stress fractures, 503
  distal condyles, fractures, 1013
  distal plantarolateral aspect, radiolucent defect (dorsal 45° lateral 30° proximal-palmarodistal oblique radiographic image), 1047f
  dorsal cortical fractures, 502
  dorsoproximolateral aspect, articular fracture, 504
    occurrence, 504
  enostosis-like lesions, 506
  exostoses, 504-505
  lateral condyle
    bilateral stress injuries, plantar delayed phase scintigraphic image, 1008f
    subchondral bone injury, 1000

Third metatarsal bone (Continued)
  lesions, 632
  medial/lateral condylar fractures, 502
  midshaft fractures, 502-503
    management, 503f
  osteochondrosis, sagittal ridge, 494
  proximal aspect, coarse trabecular pattern (dorsoplantar radiographic view), 501f
  proximal phalanx, fractures, 1013
  racing injuries, 965
  sagittal ridge, osteochondritis dissecans, 632
  simple fractures, 502-503
  spiral fractures, 502
  subchondral stress remodeling, 1046
Third tarsal bones
  fractures, 518-519
  incomplete ossification, 517
  slab fracture, 519f
Third trochanters
  fracture/enthesopathy, 582
  palpation, 55f
Thoracic limbs, stumbling, 145
Thoracic vertebrae, spinous processes, 592
  lateral radiographic view, 599f
Thoracolumbar area
  dorsal profile, local deformation (supraspinous ligament thickening impact), 600
  thermograms, lateral views, 913f
Thoracolumbar injuries, 1169-1170
Thoracolumbar junction, lateral radiographic view, 602f
Thoracolumbar myositis, 1169
  clinical signs, 1169
Thoracolumbar region
  lateral nuclear scintigraphic image, 599f
  muscle tension/spasm, impact, 821
  passive movement, 823
  soft tissue injuries, 1169
Thoracolumbar region, phase image problems, 224
Thoracolumbar spine
  abnormal heat patterns, thermogram (dorsal view), 913f
  anatomy/function, 598
  back, 54
  blood vessels/nerves, 593
  bones, 592
  composition, 592
  exposure, technical parameters, 597t
  joints, 592-593
  lesions, 598-604
  ligaments, anatomical specimen, 592f
  local injections, 604-605
  movement
    examination, 595-596
    stimulation, 594
  muscles, 593
  palpation, 53-54
    performing, 54f
  phase images, problems, 221
  prognosis, 604

Thoracolumbar spine (Continued)
  radiographic examination, imaging plate position, 597f
Thoracolumbar spinous processes, radiology, 1106
Thoracolumbar synovial intervertebral articulations, radiographic lesions (types), 601t
Thoracolumbar synovial intervertebral joints, osteoarthritis, 1107
Thoracolumbar vertebrae, stability, 592
Thoracolumbar vertebral body, fracture/subluxation, 603
Thoracolumbar vertebral column
  induced extension, 898f
  induced left lateral flexion, motion palpation demonstration, 897f
Thoroughbred (TB)
  acute-onset lameness, left hock (medial view), 804f
  acute-onset severe left hindlimb lameness, ultrasonographic image, 576f
  bucked shins, development, 940
  carpal lameness development, back-at-the-knee conformation (relationship), 434
  caudal cervical vertebrae, lateral radiographic view, 608f
  cross-event horse
    acute-onset right hindlimb lameness, transverse ultrasonographic image, 737f
    right/left gracilis muscles, acute-onset right hindlimb lameness (transverse ultrasonographic images), 823f
  delayed images, 227f
  delayed phase scintigraphic images, 219f-220f
  digital flexor tendon injury (tendonitis), economic impact, 966
  distal forelimbs, delayed phase standing lateral scintigraphic images, 941f
  distal right forelimb, delayed phase lateral scintigraphic image, 941f
  dorsolateral-palmaromedial oblique image, 1093f
  event horse, left hock (lateromedial radiographic image), 1093f
  flat racehorse, fetlock region (dorsolateral-palmaromedial oblique radiographic views), 397f
  foals, angular limb deformitis (commonness), 644
  forelimb lameness, metacarpal region (transverse ultrasonographic image), 742f
  gelding, hind fetlock hyperextension, 760f

Thoroughbred (Continued)
  humerus (distal cranial aspect), focal intense IRU (lateral delayed phase scintigraphic image), 944f
  hurdler, right third metacarpal bone, dorsopalmar radiographic view, 396f
  jumper forelimb, distal part (delayed image), 227f
  left fore fetlock, dorsal 15° proximal-palmarodistal oblique/lateromedial images, 1002f
  left forelimb
    lameness, transverse ultrasonographic image, 759f
    lateromedial radiographic image, 1094f
  left hock, acute-onset lameness (medial view), 801f
  left metacarpal region (proximal aspect), acute-onset moderate left forelimb lameness (dorsopalmar radiographic view), 398f
  left third carpal bone, flexed dorsal 60° proximal-dorsodistal oblique images, 998f
  limbs, distal aspect (delayed phase lateral scintigraphic images), 939f
  lumbar stress fractures, identification, 946
  mare
    forelimb, proximal phalanx frontal plane fracture (lateromedial radiographic image), 390f
    pelvic region, dorsal bone phase scintigraphic view, 575f
  metacarpal region
    swelling, right metacarpophalangeal joint (dorsopalmar radiographic view), 757f
  midmetacarpal region, transverse/longitudinal ultrasonographic images, 933f
  proximal metacarpal region, dorsomedial-palmarolateral oblique radiographic view, 399f
  RER, semitendinosus muscle (biopsy cryostat-cut sections), 827f
  right hind fetlock, dorsoplantar radiographic image, 756f
  right ilium
    focal IRU (dorsal delayed phase pelvic scintigraphic image), 946f
    focal IRU (right oblique delayed phase scintigraphic image), 946f
  scapula, glenoid cavity (postmortem appearance), 468f
  scapulohumeral joint, craniomedial-caudolateral oblique view, 466f

Thoroughbred *(Continued)*
  third carpal bone
    fractures, occurrence, 435
    frontal slab fracture, 442-443
  third metacarpal bone
    geometric properties, 953
    lateromedial radiographic
      projection, 959f
    lateromedial radiographic
      view, 959f
  Thoroughbred-cross gelding
    (middle phalanx),
    comminuted articular
    fracture (lateromedial
    radiographic image), 392f
  tibial stress fractures,
    occurrence, 945
  in vitro fatigue data, 954f
  weanlings
    glycemic response test, 626
    Salter-Harris type II fracture,
      lateromedial radiographic
      image, 389f
Thoroughbred (TB) broodmare
  antibiotic/corticosteroid
    therapy, 167f
  lameness/swelling, 36f
Thoroughbred (TB) colt
  acute left forelimb lameness,
    delayed-phase cranial
    image, 451f
  cervical vertebrae, lateral
    radiographic view,
    650f-651f
  delayed-phase scintigraphic
    image, 254f, 448f
  lateral image, 226f
  lateral/solar delayed phase
    scintigraphic images,
    477f
  middle phalanx (proximal
    aspect), infectious arthritis/
    epiphysitis (dorsoplantar
    radiographic image),
    393f
  scapulohumeral joint,
    mediolateral radiographic
    view, 466f
  third metatarsal bone, midshaft
    fractures, 503f
Thoroughbred (TB) cross gelding
  left stifle
    lateral delayed phase
      scintigraphic image,
      536f
    lateromedial radiographic
      view, 542f
  stifle, lateromedial radiographic
    view, 539f
Thoroughbred (TB) filly
  asymmetrical shape/cranial
    neck region scoliosis,
    poll region (dorsal view),
    610f
  back pain/performance loss,
    thoracolumbar spine
    (lateral scintigraphic
    image), 603f
  left front foot, lateromedial
    radiographic view, 354f
  left humerus, lateral
    scintigraphic/mediolateral
    radiographic view, 465f
  metatarsophalangeal joints,
    delayed phase lateral/
    plantar scintigraphic
    images, 495f

Thoroughbred (TB) filly *(Continued)*
  neck pain/forelimb gait
    restriction, seventh cervical
    vertebra (displaced articular
    fracture), 607f
  proximal tibia, craniolateral-
    caudomedial oblique view,
    176f
  right metatarsophalangeal joint,
    dorosomedial aspect
    (intraoperative arthroscopic
    images), 257f
  stress-related bone injury,
    215-216
  third metatarsal bone,
    nondisplaced spiral fracture
    (digital radiographic
    images), 497f
  tubera sacrale height disparity,
    35f
Thoroughbred (TB) racehorse
  chronic synovitis/osteoarthritis,
    flexed lateromedial
    radiographic view, 397f
  collision injuries, 962
  computerized scan data, 712f
  desirability, consideration, 20
  distal radial carpal
    osteochondral fragment,
    dorsal 45° lateral-
    palmaromedial oblique
    radiographic projection,
    436f
  dorsal metacarpal disease, RPW
    treatment, 916
  elbows, lateral scintigraphic
    images, 464f
  euthanasia/insurance, 967-968
  fibularis terrius injury, 43f
  foal, external rotation, 25f
  front view, length/angle
    measurements, 17f
  gelding
    left fore SDFT, swelling
      (development), 203
    right fore SDFT injury,
      201-202
  hock, transverse/longitudinal
    midline ultrasonographic
    image, 795f
  horn quality/hoof conformation,
    problem, 1004
  humeral fractures, 942, 962
  injury, 481
  lameness, 2
    examination, 997
    sagittal low-field MRI, 487f
  lateral/caudal delayed phase
    images, 225f
  left carpi
    dorsoproximal-dorsodistal
      (skyline) digital
      radiographic view, 444f
    lateromedial radiographs,
      26f
  left forelimb lameness, 3-4
  left lateral view, angle
    measurements, 17f
  left tibia, lateral delayed phase
    scintigraphic image, 945f
  maladaptive/nonadaptive
    subchondral bone
    remodeling, lateral/plantar/
    flexed lateral delayed phase
    images, 233f
  metatarsophalangeal joint,
    lameness source, 5

Thoroughbred (TB) racehorse
  (Continued)
  on-the-track catastrophes
    emergency care, 961
    equipment, 961-962
    management considerations,
      961
    medication, 962
    public relations/media issues,
      963
    regulatory considerations,
      967
    track injury, location,
      962-963
  pelvic fractures, diagnosis/
    management, 564
  PSD, 1006
  racing performance, evaluation,
    8, 64-65
  radius, proximal aspect
    (craniocaudal radiographic
    view), 461f
  superficial digital flexor
    tendonitis, 43-44
  suspensory apparatus,
    traumatic disruption
    (lateromedial/dorsopalmar
    radiographic views),
    969f-970f
  training injuries, 962-963
  unilateral femoral nerve paresis,
    43f
  wastage, evaluation, 6-7
Thoroughbred (TB) sales yearling
  anabolic steroids, drug
    screening, 930
  clinical examination, 929
  endoscopy/echocardiography,
    929
  monitoring/sale selection,
    930
  ophthalmology, 929
  orthopedic conditions,
    931-932
  osseous cystlike lesion,
    identification, 930
  osteochondrosis, relevance,
    930
  preparation, 931
  presale injuries, 932
  presale/postsale examination,
    929
  purchase examination, 928-930
  purchase examination (Europe),
    930-932
  radiography, 929-930
  radiological findings, 929-930
  sale conditions, 928-929
  sale conditions (Europe), 931
  ultrasonographic examinations,
    932
  veterinary examination,
    conditions, 932
  views, 929
    Keeneland sales repository
      requirement, 929
Thoroughbred (TB) yearling
  back-at-the-knee (calf knee)
    conformation, 26f
  veterinary inspection, public
    auction, 928
Thoroughpin, 800-801
  bog spavin, differentiation,
    59
  swelling, 59f, 781f
Thread count, 309
Three-beat gait (canter), 4

Three Day Event horse, 1123
  clinical history, 1126
  coat, clipping, 1128
  conformation, lameness
    (relationship), 1126
  diagnosis, absence, 1129-1131
  diagnostic analgesia, 1127-1128
    importance, 1127
  emphasis, 1124
  examination, 1123-1124
  external trauma, 1136
  fence design, 1125
  fitness training, 1125
  flexion tests, 1127
  fractures, 1136
  growth factors, intralesional
    injections, 1135
  imaging considerations,
    1128-1129
  lameness
    conditions, 1132-1133
    diagnosis/management,
      1133-1137
    examination, 1126-1127
    prevention, 1137
    sport influence, 1125
  magnetic resonance imaging,
    1129
  pads, usage, 1131
  palpation, 1126
  prepurchase examination, 1126
  protective leg wear, 1132
  radiography, 1128
  rhabdomyolysis, 1137
    risk, reduction, 1137
  road nails/studs, usage, 1132
  sacroiliac region, pain, 1136
  saddle pressure analysis, 1129
  scintigraphy, 1128
  shoeing considerations,
    1131-1132
  soundness, determination,
    1127
  static examination, 1126-1127
  steel shoes, usage, 1132
  stem cell therapy, popularity,
    1135
  stifle fracture, 1136
  superficial digital flexor
    tendonitis, 1134-1135
  suspensory desmitis, 1135-1136
  tack considerations, 1132
  therapeutic shoe, 1131
  thermographic foot patterns,
    examples, 1129f
  thermography, 1128-1129
    usefulness, 1129
  thoracolumbar/cervical
    soreness/restriction, 1133
  training methods, 1125-1126
  types, 1124-1125
  ultrasonography, 1128
Three day event horse, sport,
  1123-1124
3D competition, 1180
Three-dimensional (3D) anatomy,
  95-100
Three-dimensional (3D) kinematic
  gait analysis, performing, 511
Three-dimensional (3D)
  reconstructions, voxel density
  value (usage), 235
Three-dimensional volume-
  rendered images, 237f
Three-gaited horses, examination,
  1190
Thrombosis, 423

Thrombus
formation, prevention, 580
palpation, 580
Thrush, 311-312
bacterial infection, 311
clinical signs/diagnosis, 311-312
prognosis, 312
treatment, 312
Tibia
circular path, 508
distal aspect
cranial intermediate ridge,
lesion site, 635
osseous cystlike lesions, 531
transverse anatomical section,
93f
distal physeal fractures, 529
occurrence, 529
enostosis-like lesions, 530
intercondylar eminence
fracture, 546
prognosis, 546
signs/diagnosis, 546
treatment, 546
intermediate ridge, histological
section, 621f
lateral malleolus, fracture,
521-522
ultrasonographic evaluation,
521-522
lateral scintigraphic image, 153f
medial aspect, palpation, 58f
medial malleolus, fractures, 522
osteochondroma, 530
proximal aspect, osseous
cystlike lesions, 530-531
racing injuries, 965
stress fractures
impact, 1011
occurrence, 945
SWT management, 916
stress-related bone injury, 527
torsion, application, 999f
Tibial malleolar fractures, 529
Tibial nerve block, 127
tuber calcanei proximal
location, 127
Tibial nerves
injury, 145
perineural analgesia, 511
Tibial stress fractures, 527-528, 991
diagnosis, 1011
IRU focal areas, 528
misdiagnosis, 991
occurrence, 527
treatment, 1011-1012
Tibial tuberosity, chronic
lameness/fracture
(lateromedial radiographic
view), 530f
Tibial tuberosity fractures, 530,
547-548
direct trauma, impact, 530
prognosis, 548
signs/diagnosis, 547
treatment, 547-548
Tied-in below the knee, 15-16
diagrammatic representation,
27f
notch description, 27-28
Tiludronate
attention, 490
usage, benefit, 490-491
Timber hurdles, 1062
Timber race, 1065f
Timber racing, 1067
popularity, 1067

Timber racing horse
acute lesions, 1071
back pain, 1074-1075
carpus, lameness (association),
1072
clinical examination, 1069
conformation, lameness
(relationship), 1068
diagnosis, absence, 1070
diagnosis/management, 1075
diagnostic analgesia, 1069-1070
front feet, lameness
(association), 1073
hock, lameness (association),
1072-1073
imaging considerations, 1070
injuries, 1075
lameness, 1067-1068
causes, 1075
examination, 1068-1069
metacarpophalangeal joint,
lameness (association),
1074
neck lesions, 1074
pelvis, lameness (association),
1073
serial ultrasonographic
examinations, 1071
shoeing considerations,
lameness (relationship),
1070
sport, description, 1062-1063
structural damage, assessment,
1072
suspensory desmitis, 1072
third metacarpal/metatarsal
bones, fractures,
1073-1074
track surface, 1067-1068
training surface, 1067-1068
Ting points, 885f
Tissue inhibitor of matrix
metalloproteinase-1 (TMP-1),
662
Tissues
damage (occurrence), local
anesthetic solution
(injection), 101
density values, 235b
destruction, cryotherapy
(impact), 869
explants, usage, 917
function, loss, 44
injury, stress relief, 300
interactions, 100-107
matrix, repair (improvement),
851
MR properties, 242
proton density, usage, 241-242
thermal injury, 868
ultrasound transmission, 902
TNF-α, proinflammatory cytokine,
664
Toe angle, impact, 278-279
Toe callus, wall (trimming), 304
Toed-in conformation, 23f
commonness, 24-25
existence, 24
Toed-out conformation, 18
Toe drag, 562
Toe extensions, application,
296
Toe first landing pattern, 562
Toe length
coronary band, proximal aspect,
290
impact, 278-279

Toe-out conformation, 979
Toe weights, usage, 25f
Tom Quality Gold Cup, 1137
T1-weighted spoiled gradient echo
sequence, 242f
Torsion, 92
Total cross-sectional area (T-CSA),
measurements, 200
Touch, mediation, 323
Toxemia, 372
Toxic mineral levels, 626t
Toxic myopathies, 836-838
Trabecular bone change
(detection), computed/
digital radiography (usage),
388
Trabecular pattern, radiolucent
changes (relationship), 403
Traction, 299
devices, usage (problem), 303
increase, 299
requirement, 299
Traditional Oriental Medicine
(TOM), 887
acupoints, 889b
examination, 887
Traditional TENS, 906
Trailers, 296
Training
history, 981
intensity, 13
decrease, 399
schedule, interruption, 958
stage, 997
surfaces, 976
Trakehner gelding, examination,
201
Tramadol, analgesic, 857
Transcutaneous electrical nerve
stimulation (TENS), 905
Hi TENS/Normal TENS, 906
Transducer, position, 209
Transection, horse selection,
717
Transfixation pins
casts, 862
loading regimen, 863
usage, 863
walking bar casts,
incorporation, 863
Transforming growth factor-β3,
immunohistochemical
staining, 699f
Transforming growth factor-B
(TGF-β), 763, 851
Transforming growth factor-β1
(TGF-β1), role, 625
Transphyseal bridging
performing, 644
surgical alternative, 644
Transplantation resurfacing
techniques, 259
Transportation, 163-164
Transverse 3D T2 gradient echo
image, 243f
Trauma
history, 11-12
impact, 624
reduction, arthroscopic surgery
(usage), 252
Trauma-related deformitis, 642
Traumatically induced cartilage,
398
Traumatic cervical vertebral
disorders, 650-651
Traumatic chip fractures,
occurrence, 409

Traumatic injuries (evaluation),
radiographs (usage), 139
Traumatic muscle injuries, 212
Traumatic myopathies, 833-834
Traumatic neuropathy, 560
Traumatic physitis, 450
treatment, 450
Traumatic synovitis, 690
Traumatic tenosynovitis,
783-784
Traumatic thoroughpin, 781
Traveling bandages, 858
Treading, 39, 41
Treadmill
lameness, case selection
criteria, 925
long-term training, 880
usage, 79-80, 880
Treadmill-integrated
force-measuring system,
247f
Tremetone, 836
pasture myopathy, 836
Triamcinolone acetonide (TA),
841
efficacy/chondroprotective
properties, 842
Triangulation
improvement, 264
techniques, application, 260
Triceps apparatus, failure, 39
Triceps myopathy, 472
Trigger factors, bacterial origin,
370
Trigger points, ultrasound, 903
Trimming, 338-339
sequence, 304
Tripartite navicular bone,
343-344
Triple Crown, stature (increase),
978
Triple plating technique,
528-529
Trochanteric bursa, 133, 799
Trochanteric bursitis, 552-555,
581
chronic condition, 552
impact, 552
injection pattern, diagrammatic
representation, 552f
pain, 552
positive diagnosis, achievement,
552
rest, 552
Trochanteric lameness, 552
Trot
comfort, 927
diagonal two-beat gait, 64
forelimb lameness, 70
gait, 1189
lameness
comparison, 65
relevance, 65
transition, 911
Trotter
designation, 1019
foot pain, flap/flip-flop shoe
(usage), 1044f
head, turning, 1015f
long toe, 46f
racing, 1015
right hock, zone 1B2
(transverse/longitudinal
ultrasonographic images),
795f
toed-out conformation, 25f
turns, negotiation, 1015f

Trotting, 79
  competitions, 1076
  observation, 136
Trotting breeds with collection, 1188
Trotting Finnhorses, examination, 1078
True stringhalt, 560
Tubera coxae, 37, 575
  determination, horse position, 37f
  evaluation technique, 567
  fractures, 567
    clinical signs, 567
    radiographic examination, 567
    scintigraphic examination, 567
    ultrasonographic examination, 567
  position, assessment, 555
Tubera ischii, dorsal oblique/caudal scintigraphic image, 148f
Tubera ischii, palpation, 55f
Tubera sacrale, 37
  asymmetry, 38f
  height
    asymmetry, phogoraph, 585f
    disparity, 35f
  prominence, 577
Tuber calcanei, 803-805
  osseous cystlike lesions, 524
    impact, identification, 524
  Zone 1B, transverse images, 196f
  Zone 2B, transverse images, 197f
Tuber coxae
  fracture, 54-55
  vertical displacement, 69-70
Tuber ischii, trauma/fractures, 574
Tuber ischium, fracture (diagnosis), 574
Tuber sacrale
  angle, change, 575f
  dorsal aspect, digital pressure (application), 587
  height, spontaneous/insidious differences (pathogenesis), 585
  tip, palpation, 567
  ventral displacement, 564-565
Tumors, 532
Tuohy needle
  curved point, 854f
  epidural catheter, 854f
Turf tracks, 975-976
  all-weather tracks, comparison, 974
Turnout, healing (contrast), 14
Tying up, 1060, 1234-1235
Type I collagen, carboxy-terminal propeptide, 949
Type I collagen C-telopeptides (CTX), usefulness, 670
Type I collagen N-terminal telopeptide (NTX), decrease, 952
Type II collagen, carboxyl propeptide, 669
Type 1 PSSM, diagnosis, 828
Type 1 sesamoiditis, treatment, 1046
Type 2 sesamoiditis, impact, 1046

Type V Salter-Harris growth plate injury, 638-639

U
Ulna
  olecranon, 456
    cranial aspect, 456
    fracture, 462
  osteitis/osteomyelitis, 455
    etiology, 455
    treatment, 455
Ulnar block, 114-116
Ulnar carpal bone
  lateral palmar intercarpal ligament, avulsion injury, 447-448
Ulnar carpal bone radiolucent defects, 446-447
Ulnaris lateralis, origin (avulsion), 462
Ulnar nerve, block, 115, 395-396
Ultrasonographic data, knowledge, 205
Ultrasonographic examinations
  indications, 206
  timing, 204-205
Ultrasonographic images, recording, 169
Ultrasonography, 141
  clinical findings, 168
  focal zone use, problem, 171-172
  frequency transducer, problem, 172-173
  future technology, 177
  gain settings, problem, 171
  images
    labeling, 168
    recording, 173
  importance, 206
  monitoring capability, 212
  operator errors, 169-174
  quantitative measurements, 177
  scanning technique, 169
  terminology, 177
Ultrasound (US)
  application, 903
  images, terms (usage), 173
  nonthermal effects, 902
  therapeutic effects, 902-903
  thermal effects, 902
  tissue interaction artifacts (horse-produced artifacts), 173
  transmission, 902
  waveform, 901-902
Ultrasound (US) beam
  angle, 171
  reflection, 169
Unbalanced Appaloosa gelding, weakness, 20f
Underrun heels, 305
Unexplained lameness, 7
Ungual cartilage, 320
Unilateral femoral nerve paralysis, occurrence, 562
Unilateral hindlimb lameness, 65, 491-492
  tibial stress fractures, 991
Unilateral hindlimb toe drag, 562
Unilateral lameness, 248
  pelvic fracture, impact, 570-571
  sudden onset, 353
Unilateral semitendinosus fibrotic myopathy, 68

United Kingdom (UK)
  flat racing, 995
    popularity, 995
  horse racing, history, 994
  races, catastrophic forelimb distal limb fractures (distribution), 973f
  racing, North American racing (comparison), 995-996
  training, 976
United States Arabian/Half-Arabian Show, 1195-1196
United States Army Remount Service, 1195
Unmyelinated fibers, characteristics, 323
Unroofing sole, 1210-1211
Unstable foot/feet, corium (progressive rotation/penetration), 381-382
Upper forelimb
  flexion, performing, 83f
  lameness, worsening, 78
  traumatic injury, 1215f
Upper hindlimb, lameness (worsening), 78
Upper limb extension test, performing, 84f
Upper limb flexion, 83-84
  test, 84-85
Upper limb manipulation, 53, 83-84
Upper thigh, caudal aspect (caved-in appearance), 559
Upright foot, size, 305
Urine contamination, 229
Urine dribbling, 575

V
Valgus deformity, dorsopalmar radiographic view, 643f
  transphyseal screw procedure, 644f
Valgus stress test, 57f, 87
Varus stress tests, 87
Vascular anatomy, importance, 90
Vascular channels, radiolucent changes (relationship), 403
Vascular foramina, impact, 321
Vascular leakage (vasculitis), 138
Vascular lesions, 158
Vascular thrombosis, 1247
Vascular trauma, DP dislocation (association), 376
Vasculitis, clinical syndrome, 689
Vasodilator therapy, 373
VEGF, 763
Venography, 377-379
  usefulness, 377
Ventral thorax/abdomen, palpation, 54
Versammlung (collection), 1112
Vertebral abnormalities, 142-143
Vertebral canal
  diameter, objective assessment, 651-652
  needle insertion, 854f
Vertebral column
  conformation, 895-896
  disorders, evaluation, 894
Vertebral laminar stress fractures, 603
Vertebral lesions, characterization, 894
Vertebral osteomyelitis, 144

Vertebral segments, evaluation, 897-898
Vertical GRF, schematic drawing, 275f
Vertical slab fracture, 446
Very intermittent lameness, 149-151
Very-low-grade lameness, 149
Vetalog, 841-842
Veterinary intervention, advantages, 205
Veterinary medicine, LLLT (usage), 904-905
Vet Gate, 1138
Vibration, magnitude, 276
Video camera, digital format, 926
Video-image analysis, usage, 16
Video technology, usage, 926
Villonodular synovitis, 48-49, 396-397
  traumatic injury, commonness, 693
Villonodular synovitis-like lesions, 260
Virus-associated myositis, 831
Virus isolation, 141
Vitamin E deficiency, 143
Voxel density value, usage, 235

W
Walk
  evaluation, 64
  four-beat gait, 562
  lameness, comparison, 65
  movement, information, 911
  pacing, 562
  trot, transition, 911
Walk (gait), 1189
Walking, 79
  bar cast, transfixation pins (incorporation), 863
  observation, 136
Walking horses
  gaits
    confusion, 1187
    types, 1186-1187
  lameness
    evaluation, 1187
    examination, 1187-1188
  sport, description, 1186-1187
Wall separation, gravel (relationship), 1025
War Admiral, 978
Warmblood (WBL)
  breeds, foot conformation, 1089-1090
  conformation, evaluation, 16
  foal, Salter-Harris type II fracture, dorsal 45° medial-plantarolateral obliqued digital radiographic views, 480f
  front foot, lateromedial radiographic view, 363f
  intermittent upward fixation, propensity, 1089
  left forelimb lameness, solar scintigraphic bone phase images, 334f
  mare, lameness (radiographic view), 366f
  metacarpal region, dorsomedial-palmarolateral radiographic view, 173f
  patella, upward fixation, 28
  right front foot, solar scintigraphic image, 153f

Warmblood (Continued)
  stifle, caudolateral-craniomedial oblique radiographic view, 174f
  toe out behind, 30
  trotters, toed-out conformation, 18
Warmblood (WBL) dressage horses
  chronic sacroiliac joint disease, dorsal delayed phase scintigraphic image, 578f
  left front foot, lateromedial radiographic view, 331f
  severe lameness, distal radius (lateromedial radiographic view), 780f
  severe right hindlimb lameness, right femur (lateral/caudal scintigraphic images), 582f
Warmblood (WBL) gelding
  bilateral hindlimb lameness, right stifle joint (lateromedial digital radiographic view), 558f
  bilateral hindlimb suspensory desmitis, 39f
  chronic recurrent proximal suspensory desmitis, interoperative photograph, 500f
  delayed phase image, 222f
  right femorotibial joint, arthroscopic view, 543f
Warmblood (WBL) show jumper
  PSD, left hindlimb (lateral scintigraphic image), 747f
  reluctance/stiffness, head (lateral view), 611f
  sagittal spoiled gradient-echo MR image, 337f
Warming into lameness, 12
Warming out of lameness, 12
Weakness, neurological problem (impact), 923-924
Weanlings
  developmental orthopedic disease, 630
  foals, dietary management, 830
  mineral requirements, 626t
  protein sweet feed, intention, 629
  proximal phalanx, Salter-Harris type II fractures (occurrence), 389
  Salter-Harris type II fractures, occurrence, 529
Wear-and-tear lesions, occurrence, 1114
Wedge test, 47-48, 87
  manipulation, 87
  usage, 47-48, 87f
Weight bearing, chronic reduction (impact), 33-34

Weight-bearing lameness, 248
Weight-bearing surface, osseous cystlike lesions (occurrence), 632-633
Welsh Cob gelding, right hindlimb patella (upward fixation), 538f
Western blot test, 137
Western performance horses
  clinical signs, 1166
  deep intramuscular injections, 1170
  diagnosis, basis, 1166
  distal hock joint pain, 1166-1167
  distal interphalangeal joint pain, 1180
  distal phalanx, osteitis, 1180
  distal tarsal joints, osteoarthritis, 1166-1167
  exploratory/diagnostic arthroscopy, 1167
  femorotibial joint pain, 1169
  fibrotic myopathy, 559
  handwalking, 1168
  hindlimb lameness, 1166
  intraarticular medication, usage, 1166-1167
  lameness
    diagnosis/management, 1166-1170
    examination, 1166
  NSAIDs, therapeutic levels, 1167
  osteochondrosis, 1167
  patella, upward fixatoin, 1168-1169
  sacroiliac region pain, 1169-1170
  shoeing considerations, 1175
  skeletal muscle relaxants, systemic use, 1169
  sport, description/history, 1165
  stifle, lameness, 1167-1169
  subchondral bone cysts, 1167-1168
    diagnosis, 1168
    surgery, adjunct, 1167
  tarsocrural joint
    arthrosis, 1167
    capsule, distention, 1167
  tarsus, lameness, 1166-1167
    therapy, variation, 1166
  thoracolumbar injuries, 1169-1170
  thoracolumbar myositis, 1169
    clinical signs, 1169
  thoracolumbar region, soft tissue injuries, 1169
  training, 1165-1166
Western Pleasure horses, 1196
Wet-to-dry bandages, 859
Wheat germ lectin (WGL), 948
White line disease, 312-313
  term, usage, 312

Whorl bone lameness, 552
Wickham, John, 977
Windgalls, 33
Wind puffs, 33
Wind puffs (windgalls), 49
Winging in/out, 75
Winn, Matt, 977
Winter racing, 1077f
Wire technique, limiting factor, 308
Withers
  fracture, 1106, 1161-1162
  height, 16-17
Wobbler syndrome, 649
Wolff's law, 169-174
  application, 957
Women's Professional Rodeo Association (WPRA), 1180
Wooden fabricated shoe, 382f
Working blisters, irritation, 867
World Equestrian Games, 1205-1206
Wounds, 393
  bandaging, 858-861
  cleansing/debridement, 808
  closure, surgery, 808
  digital palpation, 807
  existence, 263
  gross appearance, 806-807
  LLLT, usage, 905

X

X-ray beam, 177-178
Xylanzine, usage, 856

Y

Yan Chi, 890
Yao Zhong, 890
Yearlings
  collagen fibril populations, differences, 701f
  developmental orthopedic disease, 630
  dorsal chip fractures, 400
  draft horse, hock (dorsomedial-plantarolateral oblique radiographic image), 1225f
  feet, bilateral mediolateral static imbalance, 289f
  Salter-Harris type II fractures, occurrence, 529
  summer grazing, 931
  Thoroughbred colt
    caudocranial radiographic view, 541f
    femoropatellar joint, lateromedial radiographic view, 537f
Yearling Standardbred, neck pain, 40f
Young foals, PSB fractures, 407
Young growing animals, load (removal), 702

Young horses
  angular limb deformity, 644-645
  feeding program goal, 630-631
  lameness, improvement, 634-635
  osteoarthritis, radiological evidence, 433
  training, 65
Young's modulus, 273
Young Standardbred
  lameness, 1018-1019
  training, 1016
Youth National show, 1195-1196

Z

Zinc, deficiency, 625
Zone 0, 192
Zone 1A, 192-194
  distal extent, transverse images, 193f
  hindlimb zone, 195-196
  transverse/longitudinal images, 193f
Zone 1B, 194
  hindlimbs, 196
  transverse/longitudinal images, 194f
Zone 2A, 194
  hindlimbs, 196-197
  transverse images, 202f
Zone 2B, 194
  hindlimbs, 197
  transverse/longitudinal images, 191f, 197f, 201f
Zone 3A, 194
  hindlimbs, 197
  transverse/longitudinal images, 195f, 200f
Zone 3B, 194-195
  hindlimbs, 197
  transverse/longitudinal images, 202f
Zone 3C, 195
  transverse/longitudinal images, 195f
Zone 4A
  hindlimbs, 197
  transverse images, 197f
Zone 4B, hindlimbs, 198
Zone 4C, hindlimbs, 198
Zone P1A, pastern zone designations/descriptions, 198
Zone P2A, pastern zone designations/descriptions, 199
Zone P1B
  pastern zone designations/descriptions, 198-199
  transverse images, 198f
Zone P1C, transverse/longitudinal images, 199f
Zones
  definitions, 192-195
  designations, 191-199

ABBREVIATIONS

AAEP	American Association of Equine Practitioners
ACS	Autologous conditioned serum
ACTH	Adrenocorticotropic hormone
ADAMS	ADAM with thrombospondin type 1 motifs
A-MSCs	Adipose-derived mesenchymal stem cells
AECC	Articular epiphyseal cartilage complex
ALARA	As low as reasonably achievable
ALDDFT	Accessory ligament of the deep digital flexor tendon
ALSDFT	Accessory ligament of the superficial digital flexor tendon
ALP	Alkaline phosphatase
ANA	Antinuclear antibodies
AQ	Albumin quotient
AQHA	American Quarter Horse Association
ARCI	Association of Racing Commissioners International
AST	Aspartate aminotransferase, also known as aspartate transaminase
AVA	Arteriovenous anastomosis
BEVA	British Equine Veterinary Association
BGP	Bone gla-protein
BID	Twice daily
BLAP	Bone-specific alkaline phosphatase
BM-MSCs	Bone marrow–derived mesenchymal stem cells
BMD	Bone mineral density
BMP-2	Bone morphogenetic protein-2
bpm	Beats per minute
BSP	Bone sialoprotein
C1-C7	First to seventh cervical vertebrae
C3	Third carpal bone
$CaCO_3$	Calcium carbonate
CCI	Concours Complet International
CdCr	Caudocranial
CD joint	Centrodistal joint
CDE	Common digital extensor
CDET	Common digital extensor tendon
CdL-CrMO	Caudolateral-craniomedial oblique
CEI	Concours de Raid d'Endurance International
CHMA	Cyclohexyl methacrylate
Ci	Curie
CK	Creatine kinase
CL	Collateral ligament
CNS	Central nervous system
COMP	Cartilage oligomeric matrix protein
COX	Cyclooxygenase
CPG	Central pattern generator
CrCd	Craniocaudal
CRGP	Calcitonin gene–related peptide
CRL	Chronic remissive laminitic
CS	Chondroitin sulfate
CSA	Cross-sectional area
CSF	Cerebrospinal fluid
CSL	Collateral sesamoidean ligament
CSM	Cervical stenotic myelopathy
CSU	Colorado State University
CT	Computed tomography
CTX	Collagen C telopeptides
CVM	Cervical vertebral malformation
DDF	Deep digital flexor
DDFT	Deep digital flexor tendon
DE	Digestible energy
DEXA	Dual-energy x-ray absorbiometry
DFTS	Digital flexor tendon sheath
DIP joint	Distal interphalangeal joint
DL-PaMO	Dorsolateral-palmaromedial oblique
DL-PlMO	Dorsolateral-plantaromedial oblique
DM	Dry matter
DMD	Dorsal metacarpal disease
DMOAD	Disease-modifying osteoarthritic drug
DM-PaLO	Dorsomedial-palmarolateral oblique
DM-PlLO	Dorsomedial-plantarolateral oblique
DMSO	Dimethyl sulfoxide
DOD	Developmental orthopedic disease
DOMS	Delayed-onset muscular stiffness
DP	Distal phalanx
DPa	Dorsopalmar
DPD	Deoxypyridinoline
DPl	Dorsoplantar
DPr-PaDiO	Dorsoproximal-palmarodistal oblique
DSIL	Distal sesamoidean impar ligament
DSD	Degenerative suspensory desmitis
E	Modulus of elasticity
ECD	Equine Cushing's disease
ECR	Extensor carpi radialis
ECRT	Extensor carpi radialis tendon
EDM	Equine degenerative myeloencephalopathy
EDSS	Equine Digital Support System
EHVI	Equine herpesvirus I
EIPH	Exercise-induced pulmonary hemorrhage
EL	Exercise level
EM	Electron microscopy
EMG	Electromyography
EPM	Equine protozoal myelitis
EPSSM	Equine polysaccharide storage myopathy
ER	Exertional rhabdomyolysis
ES cells	Embryonic stem cells
ESFD	Equine skeletal fixation device
ESWT	Extracorporeal shockwave therapy
EVA	Equine viral arteritis
FAS	Fiber alignment score
FDA	(US) Food and Drug Administration
FEI	Fédération Équestre Internationale
FFD	Focus film distance
FSE	Fast spin echo
GAG	Glycosaminoglycan
GBE	Glycogen binding enzyme
GBED	Glycogen binding enzyme deficiency
GBq	Giga becquerel
GGHyl	Glucosylgalactosylhydroxylysine
Ghyl	Galactosylhydroxylysine
GRE	Gradient echo
GRF	Ground reaction force
GPS	Global positioning system
GSH-Px	Glutathione peroxidase
Gy	Gray
GYS1	Glycogen synthase gene
HA	Hyaluronan
HDP	Hydroxymethane diphosphonate
H & E	Hematoxylin and eosin
HPLC	High-performance liquid chromatography
HU	Hounsfield unit
Hyp	Hydroxyproline
HyPP	Hyperkalemic periodic paralysis
ICR	Instant center of rotation
ICTP/ CTX-MMP	Carboxy-terminal cross-linked telopeptide of type 1 collagen
IFAHR	International Federation of Arabian Horse Racing Authorities
IFHA	International Federation of Horseracing Authorities
IGF-I	Insulin-like growth factor I
IL1	Interleukin 1
IL-1ra	Interleukin-1 receptor antagonist
IM	Intramuscularly
IMM	Immune-mediated polymyositis
I_{min} and I_{max}	Minimum and maximum principal moments of inertia
IRMA	Immunoradiometric assay
iPS cells	Induced pluripotent stem cells
IRAP	Interleukin-1 receptor antagonist protein